Office
Practice
of Neurology

Office Practice of Neurology

Edited by

MARTIN A. SAMUELS, M.D.
Professor of Neurology
Harvard Medical School
Neurologist-in-Chief
Brigham and Women's Hospital
Co-Chair
Massachusetts General Hospital-Brigham and
Women's Hospital Partners Neurology Department
Boston, Massachusetts

STEVEN FESKE, M.D.
Instructor in Neurology
Harvard Medical School
Director
Ambulatory and Emergency Neurology
Department of Neurology
Brigham and Women's Hospital
Boston, Massachusetts

Section Editors
M.-Marsel Mesulam, M.D.
Michael S. Pessin, M.D.
David C. Preston, M.D.
Loren A. Rolak, M.D.
Egilius L. H. Spierings, M.D., Ph.D.
Lewis R. Sudarsky, M.D.
Patrick Y. Wen, M.D.

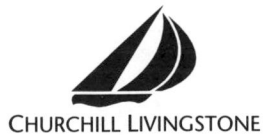

CHURCHILL LIVINGSTONE

New York, Edinburgh, London, Madrid, Melbourne, San Francisco, Tokyo

Library of Congress Cataloging-in-Publication Data

Office practice of neurology / edited by Martin A. Samuels ... [et
al.].
   p. cm.
  Includes bibliographical references and index.
  ISBN 0-443-08816-0
  1. Neurology.   2. Ambulatory medical care.   I. Samuels, Martin A.
  [DNLM: 1. Nervous System Diseases—diagnosis. 2. Nervous System
Diseases—therapy. WL 140 032 1996]
  RC346.034 1996
  616.8—dc20
  DNLM/DLC
  for Library of Congress   95-39775
                                       CIP

© Churchill Livingstone Inc. 1996

Distributed in the United Kingdom by Churchill Livingstone, Robert Stevenson House,
1–3 Baxter's Place, Leith Walk, Edinburgh EH1 3AF, and by associated companies,
branches, and representatives throughout the world.

Accurate indications, adverse reactions, and dosage schedules for drugs are provided in
this book, but it is possible that they may change. The reader is urged to review the
package information data of the manufacturers of the medications mentioned.

The Publishers have made every effort to trace the copyright holders for borrowed material. If they have inadvertently overlooked any, they will be pleased to make the necessary arrangements at the first opportunity.

Acquisitions Editor: *Kerry Willis*
Assistant Editor: *Marc Strauss*
Production Editor: *David Terry*
Production Supervisor: *Sharon Tuder*
Cover Design: *Paul Moran*

Printed in the United States of America

In memory of Eugene Rossitch, Jr., 1959–1994

CONTRIBUTORS

Robert J. Adams, M.S., M.D.
Professor, Department of Neurology, Medical College of Georgia, Augusta, Georgia

James W. Albers, M.D., Ph.D.
Professor, Department of Neurology, and Director, Neuromuscular Program, University of Michigan Medical School, Ann Arbor, Michigan

Lloyd M. Alderson, M.D., D.Sc.
Assistant Clinical Neurologist, Molecular Neuro-oncology Laboratory, Neurology Service, Massachusetts General Hospital, Boston, Massachusetts

Eben Alexander III, M.D.
Associate Professor of Neurosurgery and Radiation Oncology, Harvard Medical School; Co-Director, Stereotactic Radiosurgery/Radiotherapy Center, Brigham and Women's Hospital, Boston, Massachusetts

Michael P. Alexander, M.D.
Associate Professor, Department of Neurology, Boston University School of Medicine, Boston, Massachusetts; Director, Stroke Program, Braintree Hospital, Braintree, Massachusetts

Sepideh Amin-Hanjani, M.D.
Resident in Psychiatry, Harvard Medical School, Boston, Massachusetts

Richard M. Armstrong, M.D.
Associate Professor, Department of Neurology, Baylor College of Medicine; Neurologist, Department of Neurology, Methodist Hospital, Houston, Texas

Gerald M. Aronoff, M.D.
Assistant Clinical Professor, Department of Neurology, Tufts University School of Medicine, Boston, Massachusetts

Tetsuo Ashizawa, M.D.
Associate Professor, Department of Neurology, Baylor College of Medicine; Staff Physician, Department of Neurology, Veterans Affairs Medical Center and Methodist Hospital, Houston, Texas

Zahid H. Bajwa, M.D.
Instructor in Neurology, Harvard Medical School; Director of Education, Pain Management Center, Beth Israel Hospital, Boston, Massachusetts

Robert W. Baloh, M.D.
Professor, Department of Neurology, University of California, Los Angeles, UCLA School of Medicine, Los Angeles, California

Patrick D. Barnes, M.D.
Associate Professor of Radiology, Harvard Medical School; Chief, Section of Neuroradiology, Department of Radiology, Children's Hospital, Boston, Massachusetts

Richard J. Barohn, M.D.
Associate Professor, Department of Neurology, University of Texas Southwestern Medical Center at Dallas Southwestern Medical School, Dallas, Texas

Steven M. Baskin, M.D.
Director, New England Institute for Behavioral Medicine, Stamford, Connecticut; Program Director, New England Headache Treatment Program, Greenwich Hospital, Greenwich, Connecticut

Isabelita R. Bella, M.D.
Assistant Professor, Department of Neurology, University of Massachusetts Medical School; Neurologist, Department of Neurology, University of Massachusetts Medical Center, Worcester, Massachusetts

Susan R. Beluk, M.D.
Co-Director, Headache Management Program, Spaulding Rehabilitation Hospital, Boston, Massachusetts

Richard J. Benjamin, M.D.
Instructor in Pathology, Harvard Medical School; Associate Medical Director, Blood Bank, Department of Pathology, Brigham and Women's Hospital, Boston, Massachusetts

Alan R. Berger, M.D.
Professor, Department of Neurology, Albert Einstein College of Medicine of Yeshiva University; Vice-Chairman and Director of Clinical Electromyography Laboratory, Department of Neurology, Montefiore Hospital, Bronx, New York

Susan Biener Bergman, M.D.
Clinical Associate Professor, Department of Rehabilitation Medicine, Boston University School of Medicine; Clinical Director, New England Regional Spinal Cord Injury Center, Boston University Medical Center Hospital, Boston, Massachusetts

Peter McL. Black, M.D., Ph.D., F.A.C.S.
Frank D. Ingraham Professor of Neurosurgery, Harvard Medical School; Neurosurgeon-in-Chief, Children's Hospital and Brigham and Women's Hospital, Boston, Massachusetts

Charles F. Bolton, M.D.
Professor, Department of Clinical Neurological Sciences, University of Western Ontario Faculty of Medicine, London, Ontario, Canada

David Borsook, M.D., Ph.D.
Assistant Professor of Neurology, Harvard Medical School; Director, Massachusetts General Hospital Pain Center, Boston, Massachusetts

Lawrence M. Brass, M.D.
Associate Professor, Department of Neurology, Yale University School of Medicine; Chief, Neurology Service, Veterans Affairs Connecticut Healthcare System, New Haven, Connecticut

Jon Brillman, M.D.
Professor and Chairman, Department of Neurology, Hahnemann University School of Medicine (Allegheny), Pittsburgh, Pennsylvania

Edward B. Bromfield, M.D.
Assistant Professor of Neurology, Harvard Medical School; Director, Divisions of Electroencephalography and Epilepsy, Department of Neurology, Brigham and Women's Hospital, Boston, Massachusetts

Robert H. Brown, Jr., M.D.
Associate Professor of Neurology, Harvard Medical School; Director, Cecil B. Day Neuromuscular Research Laboratory, Neurology Service, Massachusetts General Hospital, Boston, Massachusetts

John C. M. Brust, M.D.
Professor, Department of Clinical Neurology, Columbia University College of Physicians and Surgeons; Director, Department of Neurology, Harlem Hospital Center, New York, New York

Wilson W. Bryan, M.D.
Assistant Professor, Department of Neurology, University of Texas Southwestern Medical Center at Dallas Southwestern Medical School, Dallas, Texas

Louis R. Caplan, M.D.
Professor and Chairman, Department of Neurology, Tufts University School of Medicine; Neurologist-in-Chief, Department of Neurology, New England Medical Center, Boston, Massachusetts

David A. Chad, M.D.
Professor, Department of Neurology, University of Massachusetts Medical School; Staff Neurologist, Department of Neurology, University of Massachusetts Medical Center, Worcester, Massachusetts

Michael E. Charness, M.D.
Associate Professor of Neurology, Harvard Medical School, Boston, Massachusetts; Chief, Neurology Service, Brockton/West Roxbury Veterans Affairs Medical Center, West Roxbury, Massachusetts; Director, Performing Artists Clinic, Department of Neurology, Brigham and Women's Hospital, Boston, Massachusetts

Marc I. Chimowitz, M.D.
Associate Professor, Department of Neurology, Emory University School of Medicine, Atlanta, Georgia

W. Hallowell Churchill, M.D.
Associate Professor of Hematology, Harvard Medical School; Medical Director, Blood Bank, Department of Clinical Pathology, Brigham and Women's Hospital, Boston, Massachusetts

Alan R. Cohen, M.D.
Associate Professor, Departments of Surgery and Pediatrics, Case Western Reserve University School of Medicine; Chief, Section of Pediatric Neurosurgery, Rainbow Babies and Children's Hospital, Cleveland, Ohio

Douglas G. Cole, M.D.

Instructor in Neurology, Harvard Medical School; Assistant Physician, Department of Neurology, Massachusetts General Hospital, Boston, Massachusetts

John P. Conomy, M.D.

Assistant Professor, Department of Neurology, Bowman Gray School of Medicine of Wake Forest University; Neurologist, Department of Neurology, North Carolina Baptist Hospital, Winston-Salem, North Carolina

Clifford C. Dacso, M.D.

Professor, Department of Medicine, Baylor College of Medicine, Houston, Texas

Kirk R. Daffner, M.D.

Assistant Professor of Neurology, Harvard Medical School; Director, Brigham Behavioral Neurology Group, Department of Neurology, Brigham and Women's Hospital, Boston, Massachusetts

Josep Dalmau, M.D., Ph.D.

Professor, Department of Neurology, Cornell University Medical College; Assistant Attending Physician, Department of Neurology, Memorial Sloan-Kettering Cancer Center, New York, New York

Basil T. Darras, M.D.

Associate Professor, Departments of Pediatrics and Neurology, Tufts University School of Medicine; Attending Physician, Division of Pediatric Neurology, Floating Hospital for Children at New England Medical Center, Boston, Massachusetts

Patricia H. Davis, M.D.

Assistant Professor, Department of Neurology, University of Iowa College of Medicine, Iowa City, Iowa

David M. Dawson, M.D.

Professor of Neurology, Harvard Medical School; Director, Massachusetts General Hospital-Brigham and Women's Hospital Partners Neurology Residency Training Program, Boston, Massachusetts

Lisa M. DeAngelis, M.D.

Associate Professor, Department of Neurology, Cornell University Medical College; Chief, Neurology Service, Memorial Sloan-Kettering Cancer Center, New York, New York

Umberto De Girolami, M.D.

Associate Professor of Pathology, Harvard Medical School; Neuropathologist, Department of Pathology, Brigham and Women's Hospital and Children's Hospital, Boston, Massachusetts

L. Dana DeWitt, M.D.

Assistant Professor, Department of Neurology, Tufts University School of Medicine; Staff Neurologist and Director, Transcranial Doppler Laboratory, Department of Neurology, New England Medical Center, Boston, Massachusetts

Luis D'Olhaberriague, M.D.

Neurologist, Department of Neurology, Henry Ford Hospital, Detroit, Michigan

James O. Donaldson, M.D

Professor, Department of Neurology, University of Connecticut School of Medicine, Farmington, Connecticut

Frank W. Drislane, M.D.

Assistant Professor of Neurology, Harvard Medical School; Neurologist, Department of Neurology, Beth Israel Hospital, and Division of Neurology, New England Deaconess Hospital, Boston, Massachusetts

Edward J. Dropcho, M.D.

Professor, Department of Neurology, Indiana University School of Medicine; Director, Department of Neurology, Indiana University Medical Center; Chief, Neurology Service, Richard Roudebush Veterans Affairs Medical Center, Indianapolis, Indiana

Bruce Ehrenberg, M.D.

Assistant Professor, Department of Neurology, Tufts University School of Medicine; Senior Neurologist, Department of Neurology, New England Medical Center, Boston, Massachusetts

Conrado J. Estol, M.D., Ph.D.

Chief, Stroke Section, Instituto Cardiovascular de Buenos Aires, Buenos Aires, Argentina

Bradley K. Evans, M.D.

Associate Professor, Department of Neurology, University of Alabama at Birmingham School of Medicine; Chief, Neurology Service, Department of Neurology, Birmingham Veterans Affairs Medical Center, Birmingham, Alabama

Gilbert J. Fanciullo, M.D., M.S.

Director, Pain Management Center, Holy Name Hospital, Teaneck, New Jersey

Robert G. Feldman, M.D.

Professor and Chairman, Department of Neurology, Boston University School of Medicine; Chief, Department of Neurology, Boston University Medical Center Hospital; Chief, Neurology Service, Veterans Affairs Medical Center, Boston, Massachusetts

Edward Feldmann, M.D.

Associate Professor, Department of Neurology, Brown University School of Medicine; Director, Cerebrovascular Laboratory, Rhode Island Hospital, Providence, Rhode Island

Steven Feske, M.D.

Instructor in Neurology, Harvard Medical School; Director, Ambulatory and Emergency Neurology, Department of Neurology, Brigham and Women's Hospital, Boston, Massachusetts

Howard A. Fine, M.D.

Assistant Professor of Medicine, Harvard Medical School; Director of Medical Neuro-oncology, Dana Farber Cancer Insititute, Boston, Massachusetts

Marvin A. Fishman, M.D.

Professor, Departments of Pediatrics and Neurology, Baylor College of Medicine; Chief, Neurology Service, Texas Children's Hospital, Houston, Texas

Scott M. Fishman, M.D.

Clinical and Research Fellow, Department of Neurology, Harvard Medical School, Boston, Massachusetts

Barry S. Fogel, M.D.

Associate Director, Center for Gerontology and Health Care Research, and Director, Division of Geriatric Psychology, Department of Psychiatry and Human Behavior, Brown University School of Medicine, Providence, Rhode Island; Medical Director of Psychiatric Services, Eileen Slater Hospital, Cranston, Rhode Island

Roy Freeman, M.D.

Assistant Professor of Neurology, Harvard Medical School; Neurologist, Division of Neurology, New England Deaconess Hospital, Boston, Massachusetts

Joseph H. Friedman, M.D.

Professor, Department of Clinical Neurosciences, Brown University School of Medicine; Chief, Division of Neurology, Roger Williams Medical Center, Providence, Rhode Island

Matthew P. Frosch, M.D., Ph.D.

Instructor in Pathology, Harvard Medical School; Associate Neuropathologist, Department of Pathology, Brigham and Women's Hospital, Boston, Massachusetts

Karen Furie, M.D.

Fellow, Division of Cerebrovascular Disease, Department of Medicine, Brown University School of Medicine, Providence, Rhode Island

Anthony J. Furlan, M.D.

Associate Professor, Department of Neurology, Ohio State University College of Medicine, Columbus, Ohio; Director, Department of Neurology, Cleveland Clinic Foundation; Head, Adult Neurology Section, Cerebrovascular Center, Cleveland, Ohio

George A. Gates, M.D., F.A.C.S.

Professor, Department of Otolaryngology, Head and Neck Surgery, University of Washington School of Medicine; Director, Virginia Merrill Brocdel Heming Research Center, Seattle, Washington

David S. Geckle, M.D.

Chief Resident, Department of Neurological Surgery, Case Western Reserve University School of Medicine, Cleveland, Ohio

Mel B. Glenn, M.D.

Professor and Chairman, Department of Rehabilitation Medicine, Boston University School of Medicine; Chief, Department of Rehabilitation Medicine, Boston University Medical Center Hospital; Director, Department of Rehabilitation Medicine, Boston City Hospital and Boston Specialty and Rehabilitation Hospital, Boston, Massachusetts

Clifton L. Gooch, M.D.

Assistant Professor, Department of Neurology, Baylor College of Medicine; Director, Electromyography Laboratory, Department of Neurology, Veterans Affairs Medical Center, Houston, Texas

C. David Gordon, M.D.

Attending Physician, Department of Head Pain Management, Michigan Head Pain and Neurological Institute, Ann Arbor, Michigan

Francesc Graus, M.D.

Assistant Professor, Department of Neurology, Barcelona University Faculty of Medicine; Attending Physician, Department of Neurology, Hospital Clinic, Barcelona, Spain

Harry S. Greenberg, M.D.

Professor, Departments of Neurology and Neurosurgery, University of Michigan School of Medicine, Ann Arbor, Michigan

Stephen B. Greenberg, M.D.

Professor and Vice-Chairman, Department of Medicine, Baylor College of Medicine; Chief, Medical Service and Infectious Diseases Section, Ben Taub Hospital, Houston, Texas

Melvin Greer, M.D.

Professor and Chairman, Department of Neurology, University of Florida College of Medicine, Gainesville, Florida

Robert C. Griggs, M.D.
Professor, Departments of Medicine, Pediatrics, Pathology, Laboratory Medicine, and Neurology, and Chair, Department of Neurology, University of Rochester School of Medicine and Dentistry, Rochester, New York

Stuart A. Grossman, M.D.
Associate Professor, Departments of Oncology, Medicine, and Neurosurgery, Johns Hopkins University School of Medicine; Director, Section of Neurology, Johns Hopkins Oncology Center, Baltimore, Maryland

Michael L. Gruber, M.D.
Clinical Associate Professor, Department of Neurology, and Associate Director, Division of Neuro-oncology, New York University School of Medicine, New York, New York

Ludwig Gutmann, M.D.
Professor and Chairman, Department of Neurology, West Virginia University School of Medicine, Morgantown, West Virginia

Walter A. Hall, M.D.
Associate Professor, Department of Neurosurgery, University of Minnesota Medical School—Minneapolis, Minneapolis, Minnesota

Julie E. Hammack, M.D.
Assistant Professor, Department of Neurology, Mayo Medical School, Rochester, Minnesota

Y. Harati, M.D.
Professor, Department of Neurology, and Medical Director, Muscle and Nerve Pathology Laboratory, Department of Neurology, Baylor College of Medicine; Chief, Neurology Service, Veterans Affairs Medical Center, Houston, Texas

Richard L. Harris, M.D.
Clinical Associate Professor, Department of Medicine, Baylor College of Medicine; Medical Epidemiologist, The Methodist Hospital, Houston, Texas

Michael T. Hayes, M.D.
Assistant Professor, Department of Neurology, Tufts University School of Medicine; Staff Neurologist and Co-Director, Electromyography Laboratory, Department of Neurology, St. Elizabeth's Hospital, Boston, Massachusetts

Simon M. Helfgott, M.D.
Assistant Professor of Medicine, Harvard Medical School, Boston, Massachusetts

John W. Henson, M.D.
Assistant Professor of Neurology, Harvard Medical School; Assistant Neurologist, Molecular Neurology Laboratory, Neurology Service, Massachusetts General Hospital, Boston, Massachusetts

Mary Louise Hlavin, M.D.
Assistant Professor, Department of Neurological Surgery, Case Western Reserve University, Cleveland, Ohio

Fred H. Hochberg, M.D.
Assistant Professor of Neurology, Harvard Medical School; Attending Neurologist, Section of Neuro-oncology, Neurology Service, Massachusetts General Hospital, Boston, Massachusetts

Dave Hollander, M.D. F.R.C.P.(C)
Assistant Professor, Department of Neurology, Tufts University School of Medicine; Associate Director, Neuromuscular Research Unit, New England Medical Center, Boston, Massachusetts

Gregory L. Holmes, M.D.
Associate Professor of Neurology, Harvard Medical School; Director, Division of Clinical Neurophysiology and Epilepsy, Department of Neurology, Children's Hospital, Boston, Massachusetts

Jennifer Horner, Ph.D.
Associate Professor of Speech-Language Pathology, Department of Surgery, Duke University Medical School; Director, Speech and Language Pathology Program, Department of Surgery, Duke University Medical Center, Durham, North Carolina

Liangge Hsu, M.D.
Instructor in Radiology, Harvard Medical School, Boston, Massachusetts

Steven B. Inbody, M.D.
Clinical Assistant Professor, Department of Neurology, Baylor College of Medicine, Houston, Texas

Robert N. Jamison, M.D.
Assistant Professor of Anaesthesia and Psychiatry, Harvard Medical School; Clinical Psychologist, Pain Management Center, Department of Anaesthesia, Brigham and Women's Hospital, Boston, Massachusetts

Joseph Jankovic, M.D.
Professor, Department of Neurology, Baylor College of Medicine, Houston, Texas

Gary W. Jay, M.D.
Medical Director, Headache and Neurorehabilitation Institute of Colorado, Northglenn, Colorado

Donald R. Johns, M.D.
Associate Professor of Neurology and Ophthalmology, Harvard Medical School; Neurologist, Department of Neurology, Beth Israel Hospital, Boston, Massachusetts

H. Royden Jones, Jr., M.D.

Associate Clinical Professor of Neurology, Harvard Medical School, Boston, Massachusetts; Chairman, Department of Neurology, Massachusetts Lahey Hitchcock Medical Center, Burlington, Massachusetts

Henry J. Kaminski, M.D.

Assistant Professor, Department of Neurology, Case Western Reserve University School of Medicine; Attending Physician, Department of Neurology, University Hospitals of Cleveland, Cleveland, Ohio

Percy N. Karanjia, M.D.

Associate Clinical Professor, Department of Neurology, University of Wisconsin Medical School, Madison, Wisconsin; Consulting Neurologist, Department of Neurology, The Marshfield Clinic, Marshfield, Wisconsin

Carlos S. Kase, M.D.

Professor, Department of Neurology, Boston University School of Medicine; Visiting Neurologist, Department of Neurology, University Hospital, Boston, Massachusetts

Bashar Katirji, M.D.

Associate Professor, Department of Neurology, Case Western Reserve University School of Medicine; Director, Electromyography Laboratory, and Chief, Division of Neuromuscular Diseases, University Hospitals of Cleveland, Cleveland, Ohio

Jonathan S. Katz, M.D.

Assistant Professor, Department of Neurology, University of Texas Southwestern Medical Center at Dallas Southwestern Medical School, Dallas, Texas

Nathaniel Katz, M.D.

Instructor in Anaesthesiology, Harvard Medical School; Interim Director, Pain Management Center, Brigham and Women's Hospital, Boston, Massachusetts

John J. Kelly, Jr., M.D.

Professor, Department of Neurology, George Washington University School of Medicine and Health Sciences; Chairman, Department of Neurology, George Washington Medical Center, Washington, D.C.

Shahram Khoshbin, M.D.

Associate Professor of Neurology, Harvard Medical School; Director, Teaching and Education Division, Department of Neurology, Brigham and Women's Hospital, Boston, Massachusetts

Howard S. Kirshner, M.D.

Professor and Vice Chairman, Department of Neurology, Vanderbilt University School of Medicine, Nashville, Tennessee

Edwin H. Kolodny, M.D.

Bernard A. and Charlotte Marden Professor and Chairman, Department of Neurology, New York University School of Medicine, New York, New York

Bruce R. Korf, M.D., Ph.D.

Associate Professor of Neurology, Harvard Medical School; Director, Clinical Genetics Program, Division of Genetics, Children's Hospital, Boston, Massachusetts

Walter J. Koroshetz, M.D.

Assistant Professor of Neurology and Medicine, Harvard Medical School; Associate Director, Clinical Neurology Service, Massachusetts General Hospital, Boston, Massachusetts

Kenneth Kraft, M.D.

Instructor in Psychology, Harvard Medical School; Consulting Psychologist, Pain Management Center, Division of Psychiatry, Brigham and Women's Hospital, Boston, Massachusetts

Lauren B. Krupp, M.D.

Associate Professor, Department of Neurology, State University of New York at Stony Brook School of Medicine, Stony Brook, New York

Lee Kudrow, M.D.

Co-Director, California Medical Clinic for Headache, Encino, California

Robert S. Kunkel, M.D., F.A.C.P.

Clinical Assistant Professor, Department of Medicine, Pennsylvania State University College of Medicine, Hershey, Pennsylvania; Staff Physician, Headache Center, Department of Internal Medicine, Cleveland Clinic Foundation, Cleveland, Ohio

Roger Kurlan, M.D.

Professor, Department of Neurology, and Chief, Movement and Inherited Disorders (MIND) Unit, University of Rochester School of Medicine and Dentistry; Attending Neurologist, Strong Memorial Hospital, Rochester, New York

David Lacomis, M.D.

Assistant Professor of Neurology and Pathology (Neuropathology), University of Pittsburgh School of Medicine; Staff Neurologist, Department of Neurology, University of Pittsburgh Medical Center, Pittsburgh, Pennsylvania

Eugene C. Lai, M.D., Ph.D.

Assistant Professor, Department of Neurology, Baylor College of Medicine, Houston, Texas

Robert Laureno, M.D.

Professor, Department of Neurology, George Washington University School of Medicine; Chairman, Department of Neurology, Washington Hospital Center, Washington, D.C.

Susan Laviolette, P.T.

Director, Lexington Physical Therapy Associates, Lexington, Massachusetts

Alyssa Lebel, M.D.

Instructor in Neurology, Harvard Medical School; Assistant Physician, Departments of Neurology and Anesthesia, Massachusetts General Hospital, Boston, Massachusetts

J. Douglas Lee, M.D.

Associate Clinical Professor, Department of Medicine, University of Wisconsin Medical School, Madison, Wisconsin; Infectious Diseases Consultant, Department of Infectious Diseases, The Marshfield Clinic, Marshfield, Wisconsin

Lance J. Lehmann, M.D.

Instructor in Anaesthesia, Harvard Medical School; Anaesthesiologist, Pain Management Center, Beth Israel Hospital, Boston, Massachusetts

Edward J. Levine, M.D.

Assistant Professor, Department of Medicine, Ohio State University College of Medicine, Columbus, Ohio

Steven R. Levine, M.D.

Clinical Instructor, Section of Otolaryngology, Department of Surgery, Yale University School of Medicine, New Haven, Connecticut

Peter LeWitt, M.D.

Professor, Departments of Neurology and Psychiatry, Wayne State University School of Medicine, Detroit, Michigan; Director, Clinical Neuroscience Center, Sinai Hospital, West Bloomfield, Michigan

Mark H. Libenson, M.D.

Assistant Professor, Departments of Neurology and Pediatrics, Tufts University School of Medicine; Attending Physician, Department of Neurology, New England Medical Center Hospitals, Boston, Massachusetts

Richard B. Lipton, M.D.

Associate Professor and Vice Chairman, Department of Neurology, Albert Einstein College of Medicine of Yeshiva University; Chief, Department of Neurology, and Director, Montefiore Manhattan Headache Unit, Montefiore Medical Center, Bronx, New York

Grant T. Liu, M.D.

Assistant Professor, Departments of Neurology and Ophthalmology, University of Pennsylvania School of Medicine, Philadelphia, Pennsylvania

Larry Z. Lockerman, D.D.S.

Active Medical Staff, Headache Center, Department of Neurology, Medical Center of Central Massachusetts, Worcester, Massachusetts

Elizabeth Loder, M.D.

Clinical Instructor in Medicine, Harvard Medical School; Director, Headache Management Program, Spaulding Rehabilitation Hospital, Boston, Massachusetts

Jay S. Loeffler, M.D.

Associate Professor of Radiation Therapy, Harvard Medical School; Director, The Brain Tumor Center, Brigham and Women's Hospital, Boston, Massachusetts

Eric L. Logigian, M.D.

Associate Professor of Neurology, Harvard Medical School; Director, Clinical Neurophysiology Laboratory, Department of Neurology, Brigham and Women's Hospital, Boston, Massachusetts

Jeffrey D. Macklis, M.D., D.Hst.

Associate Professor of Neurology and Program in Neuroscience, Harvard Medical School; Associate Physician, Deparment of Neurology, Brigham and Women's Hospital; Associate in Neurology, Division of Neuroscience, Department of Neurology, Children's Hospital, Boston, Massachusetts

Herbert G. Markley, M.D.

Associate Professor, Department of Neurology, University of Massachusetts School of Medicine; Associate Chief, Department of Neurology, The Medical Center of Central Massachusetts, Worcester, Massachusetts

Frederick J. Marshall, M.D.

Senior Instructor and Fellow in Experimental Therapeutics and Movement Disorders, Department of Neurology, University of Rochester School of Medicine and Dentistry; Attending Neurologist, Department of Neurology, Strong Memorial Hospital, Rochester, New York

R. S. Marshall, M.D.

Assistant Professor, Department of Neurology, Columbia University College of Physicians and Surgeons; Co-Director, Cerebral Localization Laboratory, Neurological Institute, Columbia-Presbyterian Hospital, New York, New York

E. Wayne Massey, M.D., F.A.C.P.

Director, Section of Neurorehabilitation, Duke University Medical Center, Durham, North Carolina

Jean K. Matheson, M.D.
Instructor in Neurology, Harvard Medical School; Co-Director, Sleep Center, Department of Neurology, Beth Israel Hospital, Boston, Massachusetts

Ninan T. Mathew, M.D., F.R.C.P.(C)
Clinical Professor, Department of Restorative Neurology and Human Neurobiology, Baylor College of Medicine; Director, Houston Headache Clinic, Houston, Texas

Kathleen McEvoy, M.D., Ph.D.
Assistant Professor, Department of Neurology, Mayo Medical School, Rochester, Minnesota

Robert R. McKendall, M.D.
Associate Professor, Departments of Neurology, Microbiology and Immunology, and Internal Medicine, University of Texas Medical School at Galveston, Galveston, Texas

M.-Marsel Mesulam, M.D.
Ruth and Evelyn Dunbar Professor, Departments of Neurology and Psychiatry and Behavioral Sciences, and Director, Center for Behavioral and Cognitive Neurology and The Alzheimer Program, Northwestern University Medical School, Evanston, Illinois

Edison Miyawaki, M.D.
Instructor in Neurology, Harvard Medical School; Staff Neurologist, Division of Neurology, New England Deaconess Hospital, Boston, Massachusetts

J. P. Mohr, M.S., M.D.
Sciarra Professor of Clinical Neurology, Department of Neurology, College of Physicians and Surgeons of Columbia University; Attending Neurologist, Neurological Institute, Columbia-Presbyterian Medical Center, New York, New York

Patricia M. Moore, M.D.
Associate Professor, Department of Neurology, Wayne State University School of Medicine; Neurologist, Department of Neurology, Harper Hospital and Detroit Receiving Hospital, Detroit, Michigan

Theodore L. Munsat, M.D.
Professor, Departments of Neurology and Pharmacology, Tufts University School of Medicine; Director, Neuromuscular Research Center, New England Medical Center, Boston, Massachusetts

Patrick E. Nolan, M.D.
Assistant Clinical Professor, Department of Internal Medicine, University of South Alabama College of Medicine; Attending Physician, Infections Limited, P.C., Mobile, Alabama

Thorkild Vad Norregaard, M.D.
Professor of Neuroimaging, Harvard Medical School; Neurosurgeon, Department of Surgery, New England Deaconess Hospital, New England Baptist Hospital, and Dana Farber Cancer Institute, Boston, Massachusetts

Kathryn N. North, M.D.
Fellow in Neurology, Harvard Medical School, Boston, Massachusetts

Cormac A. O'Donovan, M.D.
Assistant Professor, Department of Neurology, Bowman Gray School of Medicine of Wake Forest University, Winston-Salem, North Carolina

Richard K. Olney, M.D.
Professor, Department of Neurology, University of California, San Francisco, School of Medicine; Director, Electromyography Laboratory, Clinical Neurophysiology Laboratories, University of California Medical Center, San Francisco, California

Silvia Orengo-Nania, M.D.
Assistant Professor, Department of Ophthalmology, Baylor College of Medicine; Consultant, Departments of Glaucoma and Neuroophthalmology, Cullen Eye Institute, Houston Texas

Roy A. Patchell, M.D.
Associate Professor of Neurology and Neurosurgery and Chief, Department of Neurology, University of Kentucky College of Medicine, Lexington, Kentucky

Michael S. Pessin, M.D.
Professor, Department of Neurology, Tufts University School of Medicine; Director, Stroke Service, Department of Neurology, New England Medical Center, Boston, Massachusetts

John R. Peteet, M.D.
Assistant Professor of Psychiatry, Harvard Medical School; Physician, Division of Psychiatry, Brigham and Women's Hospital, Boston, Massachusetts

Ronald C. Petersen, Ph.D., M.D.
Associate Professor, Department of Neurology, Mayo Medical School; Director, Mayo Alzheimer's Disease Center, Rochester, Minnesota

Kendra Peterson, M.D.
Assistant Professor, Department of Neurology, University of Minnesota Medical School—Minneapolis, Minneapolis, Minnesota

Jackson Pickett, M.D.

Associate Professor, Department of Neurology, Medical University of South Carolina; Staff Neurologist, Department of Neurology, Ralph H. Johnson Veterans Administration Medical Center, Charlotte, South Carolina

William F. Pirl, M.D.

Clinical Instructor in Psychiatry, Harvard Medical School, Boston, Massachusetts

Joseph F. Polak, M.D., M.P.H.

Associate Professor of Radiology, Harvard Medical School; Staff Radiologist, Department of Radiology, Brigham and Women's Hospital, Boston, Massachusetts

Scott L. Pomeroy, M.D., Ph.D.

Assistant Professor of Neurology, Harvard Medical School; Director, Division of Neuro-oncology, Department of Neurology, Children's Hospital, Boston, Massachusetts

Frisso Potts, M.D.

Instructor in Neurology, Harvard Medical School, Boston, Massachusetts; Chief, Clinical Neurophysiology Service, Brockton/West Roxbury Veterans Affairs Medical Center, West Roxbury, Massachusetts

David C. Preston, M.D.

Assistant Professor of Neurology, Harvard Medical School; Director, Neuromuscular Service, Department of Neurology, Brigham and Women's Hospital, Boston, Massachusetts

Bruce H. Price, M.D.

Instructor in Neurology, Harvard Medical School; Neurologist, Neurology Service, Massachusetts General Hospital, Boston, Massachusetts; Chief, Department of Neurology, McLean Hospital, Belmont, Massachusetts

Amy Pruitt, M.D.

Assistant Professor, Department of Neurology, University of Pennsylvania School of Medicine, Philadelphia, Pennsylvania

Alan M. Rapoport, M.D.

Assistant Clinical Professor, Department of Neurology, Yale University School of Medicine, New Haven, Connecticut; Director, New England Center for Headache, Stamford, Connecticut; Medical Director, Inpatient Headache Unit, Greenwich Hospital, Greenwich, Connecticut

Paula Ravin, M.D.

Assistant Professor, Department of Neurology, University of Massachusetts Medical School, Worcester, Massachusetts

Elizabeth M. Raynor, M.D.

Clinical Instructor in Neurology, Harvard Medical School; Director, Electromyography Laboratory, Department of Neurology, Beth Israel Hospital, Boston, Massachusetts

Lawrence Recht, M.D.

Professor, Departments of Neurology and Surgery (Neurosurgery), University of Massachusetts Medical School, Worcester, Massachusetts

Kurt Reed, M.D.

Consultant, Department of Pathology, The Marshfield Clinic, Marshfield, Wisconsin

Gary S. Richardson, M.D.

Instructor in Medicine, Harvard Medical School; Director, Neuroendocrine Clinic, Brigham and Women's Hospital, Boston, Massachusetts

Ziad Rifai, M.D.

Assistant Professor, Department of Neurology, University of Rochester School of Medicine and Dentistry, Rochester, New York

Diana L. Rodriguez, M.D.

Assistant Professor, Departments of Pediatrics and Neurology, Baylor College of Medicine; Neurologist, Section of Child Neurology and Child Development, Child Neurology Clinical Care Center, Texas Children's Hospital, Houston, Texas

Loren A. Rolak, M.D.

Clinical Associate Professor, Department of Neurology, University of Wisconsin Medical School, Madison, Wisconsin; Director, Marshfield Multiple Sclerosis Center, The Marshfield Clinic, Marshfield, Wisconsin

Michael Ronthal, M.B., B.Ch., F.R.C.P.E.

Assistant Professor of Neurology, Harvard Medical School; Senior Neurologist, Department of Neurology, Beth Israel Hospital, Boston, Massachusetts

Marjorie H. Ross, M.D.

Instructor in Neurology, Harvard Medical School, Boston, Massachusetts

Eugene Rossitch, Jr., M.D.

Assistant Professor of Neurosurgery, Harvard Medical School, Boston, Massachusetts (deceased)

Patrick A. Roth, M.D.

Assistant Instructor, Department of Surgery, University of Medicine and Dentistry of New Jersey, Newark, New Jersey; Clinical Assistant Neurosurgeon, Department of Neurological Surgery, Hackensack Medical Center, Hackensack, New Jersey

Jeffrey D. Rothstein, M.D.

Associate Professor, Department of Neurology, Johns Hopkins University School of Medicine, Baltimore, Maryland

Jonathan P. Rozan, M.D.

Clinical and Research Fellow, Harvard Medical School; Physician, Pain Management Center, Beth Israel Hospital, Boston, Massachusetts

Robert L. Ruff, M.D.

Professor, Department of Neurology and Neurosciences, Case Western Reserve University School of Medicine; Chief, Neurology Service, Cleveland Veterans Affairs Medical Center, Cleveland, Ohio

James A. Russell, D.O.

Staff Neurologist and Director, Electromyography Laboratory, Department of Neurology, Lahey Clinic Medical Center, Burlington, Massachusetts

Thomas D. Sabin, M.D.

Professor, Departments of Neurology and Psychiatry, Boston University School of Medicine; Lecturer, Department of Neurology, Harvard Medical School; Lecturer, Department of Neurology, Tufts University School of Medicine; Director, Neurological Unit, Boston City Hospital, Boston, Massachusetts

Marie Saint-Hilaire, M.D.

Assistant Professor, Department of Neurology, Boston University School of Medicine; Attending Physician, Department of Neurology, Boston University Medical Center Hospital, Boston, Massachusetts

Nalini Samuel, M.D.

Fellow, Division of Clinical Neurophysiology and Epilepsy, Department of Neurology, University of Michigan Medical School, Ann Arbor, Michigan

Martin A. Samuels, M.D.

Professor of Neurology, Harvard Medical School; Neurologist-in-Chief, Brigham and Women's Hospital; Co-Chair, Massachusetts General Hospital-Brigham and Women's Hospital Partners Neurology Department, Boston, Massachusetts

Steven C. Schachter, M.D.

Assistant Professor of Neurology, Harvard Medical School; Director of Clinical Research, Comprehensive Epilepsy Center, Department of Neurology, Beth Israel Hospital, Boston, Massachusetts

David Schiff, M.D.

Instructor, Department of Neurology, Mayo Medical School; Senior Associate Consultant, Department of Neurology, Mayo Clinic and Mayo Foundation, Rochester, Minnesota

Donald L. Schomer, M.D.

Associate Professor of Neurology, Harvard Medical School; Director, Clinical Neurophysiology Laboratory, and Director, Comprehensive Epilepsy Program, Department of Neurology, Beth Israel Hospital, Boston, Massachusetts

R. Michael Scott, M.D.

Professor of Neurosurgery, Harvard Medical School; Director, Section of Pediatric Neurosurgery, Department of Surgery, Children's Hospital, Boston, Massachusetts

Allen M. Seiden, M.D., F.A.C.S.

Associate Professor, Department of Otolaryngology, University of Cincinnati College of Medicine, Cincinnati, Ohio

Elizabeth A. Sekul, M.D.

Assistant Professor, Departments of Neurology and Pediatrics, Medical College of Georgia, Augusta, Georgia

Barbara E. Shapiro, M.D., Ph.D.

Instructor in Neurology, Harvard Medical School; Director, Clinical Neuromuscular Unit, Neurology Service, Massachusetts General Hospital, Boston, Massachusetts

Jeremy M. Shefner, M.D., Ph.D.

Associate Professor of Neurology, Harvard Medical School; Co-Director, MDA Clinic, Department of Neurology, Brigham and Women's Hospital, Boston, Massachusetts

Fred D. Sheftell, M.D.

Assistant Professor, Department of Psychiatry, New York Medical College, Valhalla, New York; Director, New England Headache Treatment Program, New England Center for Headache, Stamford, Connecticut; Associate Medical Director, Headache Inpatient Unit, The Greenwich Hospital, Greenwich, Connecticut

Robert W. Shields, Jr., M.D.

Director, Quantitative Peripheral Nerve Laboratory, Department of Neurology, Cleveland Clinic Foundation, Cleveland, Ohio

Dennis C. Shrieve, M.D., Ph.D.

Assistant Professor of Radiation Oncology, Harvard Medical School; Radiation Oncologist, Department of Radiation Oncology, Brigham and Women's Hospital, Boston, Massachusetts

Joao O. Siffert, M.D.

Fellow, Division of Pediatric Neuro-oncology, Department of Neurology, New York University School of Medicine, New York, New York

Cathy A. Sila, M.D.

Assistant Clinical Professor, Department of Medicine, Pennsylvania State University College of Medicine, Hershey, Pennsylvania; Associate Medical Director, Cerebrovascular Center, Cleveland Clinic Foundation, Cleveland, Ohio

Linda A. Specht, M.D.

Director, Department of Neurology, Franciscan Children's Hospital, Boston, Massachusetts

William G. Speed, M.D.

Associate Professor, Department of Medicine, Johns Hopkins University School of Medicine; Director Emeritus, Speed Headache Associates, Baltimore, Maryland

Egilius L. H. Spierings, M.D., Ph.D.

Lecturer in Neurology, Harvard Medical School; Director of Headache Research, Department of Neurology, Brigham and Women's Hospital, Boston, Massachusetts

Steven J. Spindel, M.D.

Fellow, Division of Infectious Diseases, Department of Internal Medicine, Baylor College of Medicine, Houston, Texas

Barney J. Stern, M.D.

Professor, Department of Neurology, Emory University School of Medicine, Atlanta, Georgia

Guillermo A. Suarez, M.D.

Consultant, Department of Neurology, Mayo Clinic, Rochester, Minnesota

Lewis R. Sudarsky, M.D.

Assistant Professor of Neurology, Harvard Medical School; Associate Physician, Department of Neurology, Brigham and Women's Hospital, Boston, Massachusetts; Assistant Chief, Neurology Service, Brockton/West Roxbury Veterans Affairs Medical Center, West Roxbury, Massachusetts

Joshua J. Sunshine, M.D.

Fellow, Department of Neurology, Case Western Reserve University School of Medicine, Cleveland, Ohio

Katheryn Swoboda, M.D.

Fellow in Neurology, Harvard Medical School; Fellow in Neurology and Genetics, Children's Hospital, Boston, Massachusetts

William T. Talman, M.D.

Professor, Department of Neurology, University of Iowa College of Medicine; Chief, Neurology Service, Veterans Affairs Medical Center, Iowa City, Iowa

Nancy J. Tarbell, M.D.

Associate Professor of Radiation Oncology, Harvard Medical School; Chief, Joint Center for Radiation Therapy, Children's Hospital, Boston, Massachusetts

Daniel Tarsy, M.D.

Associate Professor of Neurology, Harvard Medical School; Chief, Division of Neurology, New England Deaconess Hospital, Boston, Massachusetts

Philip A. Teal, M.D.

Assistant Clinical Professor, Department of Neurology, University of British Columbia Faculty of Medicine; Director, Stroke Service, Department of Medicine, Vancouver Hospital and Health Sciences Centre, Vancouver, British Columbia, Canada

Daryl W. Thompson, M.D.

Director, Cerebrovascular Program, Department of Neurology, St. Louis University Health Science Center, St. Louis, Missouri

William R. Tyor, M.D.

Assistant Professor, Departments of Neurology and Microbiology and Immunology, Medical University of South Carolina College of Medicine, Charleston, South Carolina

David K. Urion, M.D.

Assistant Professor, Department of Neurology, Harvard Medical School; Assistant Neurologist, Department of Neurology; Director, Learning Disabilities and Behavioral Neurology Program; and Clinic Director, Neuromuscular Clinic, Children's Hospital, Boston, Massachusetts

Raul F. Valenzuela, M.D.

Neurologist, Department of Neurology, Catholic University of Chile, Santiago, Chile

David M. Vernick, M.D.

Assistant Professor of Otolaryngology, Harvard Medical School, Boston, Massachusetts

Thomas N. Ward, M.D.

Assistant Professor, Division of Neurology, Department of Medicine, Dartmouth Medical School, Hanover, New Hampshire; Director, Dartmouth—Mayday Regional Head-ache Program, Lahey—Hitchcock Clinic, Lebanon, New Hampshire

Carol A. Warfield, M.D.

Associate Professor of Anaesthesia, Harvard Medical School; Director, Pain Management Center, Beth Israel Hospital, Boston, Massachusetts

Lawrence R. Wechsler, M.D.

Associate Professor, Department of Neurology, University of Pittsburgh School of Medicine; Director, Noninvasive Cerebrovascular Laboratory, University of Pittsburgh Hospital, Pittsburgh, Pennsylvania

Randall E. Weeks, M.D.

Clinical Director, New England Headache Treatment Program, The Greenwich Hospital, Greenwich, Connecticut

David. H. Weinberg, M.D.

Assistant Professor, Department of Neurology, Tufts University School of Medicine; Director, Neurophysiology Laboratory, Department of Neurology, St. Elizabeth's Medical Center, Boston, Massachusetts

Sandra Weintraub, M.D.

Associate Professor, Departments of Psychiatry and Neurology, Northwestern University Medical School; Head, Neuropsychology, Neurobehavior—Alzheimer's Service, Northwestern Medical Faculty Foundation, Chicago, Illinois

Dennis Y. Wen, M.B.B.S.

Assistant Professor of Neurology, Harvard Medical School; Director, Division of Neuro-oncology, Department of Neurology, Brigham and Women's Hospital, Boston, Massachusetts

Patrick Y. Wen, M.D.

Assistant Professor of Neurology, Harvard Medical School; Director, Division of Neuro-oncology, Department of Neurology, Brigham and Women's Hospital, Boston, Massachusetts

Asa Wilbourn, M.D.

Associate Clinical Professor, Department of Neurology, Case Western Reserve University School of Medicine; Director, Electromyography Laboratory, Department of Neurology, Cleveland Clinic Foundation, Cleveland, Ohio

Dennis E. Wilkins, M.D.

Clinical Instructor in Neurology, Harvard Medical School; Staff Neurologist, Harvard Pilgrim Health Care, Boston, Massachusetts

Temple W. Williams, M.D.

Professor, Department of Medicine and Microbiology-Immunology, Baylor College of Medicine; Chief, Department of Infectious Diseases, The Methodist Hospital, Houston, Texas

Philip A. Wolf, M.D.

Professor, Department of Neurology; Research Professor of Medicine, Department of Preventive Medicine and Epidemiology; and Professor of Public Health (Epidemiology and Biostatistics), Boston University School of Medicine, Boston, Massachusetts

G. Bryan Young, M.D.

Associate Professor, Department of Clinical Neurological Sciences, University of Western Ontario Faculty of Medicine, London, Ontario, Canada

Amir A. Zamani, M.D.

Assistant Professor of Radiology, Harvard Medical School; Director, Neuroradiology Section, Department of Radiology, Brigham and Women's Hospital, Boston, Massachusetts

PREFACE

Somewhere deep in memory reverberates a saying to which we can supply no attribution, except to say that it is an ancient, and wry, curse: "May you live in interesting times." The past several years have been interesting times in the world of medicine, and the future promises to be more interesting still. For better and for worse, among the changes that we are living is a transportation of medical services from the inpatient to the outpatient setting and from the subspecialist to the generalist. Although a disease does not change its nature upon changing the location of the patient–doctor encounter, the outpatient style does limit the time for deliberation and access to the expertise of local colleagues, putting greater pressure on clinicians. We can no longer admit our difficult patient to the hospital to mull the problem over and see what everyone else thinks. And while time and assistance are becoming less available, advances in clinical science and technology continue to expand our understanding of the nature of diseases and to provide new tests to define them and new therapies to treat them. Keeping abreast of these changes and updating one's knowledge of and approach to illness places a high demand on the physician seeking to provide patients with the best care.

We have set out to create a practical book that serves the needs of clinicians seeing outpatients with neurologic problems. We have tried to provide the immediate handiness and explicitness of a manual in a book with a breadth that encompasses most of the neurologic problems that the practitioner of general neurology will confront. We have tried in this book to strike at the heart of the matter for neurologic clinicians. Section 2 of Part I is organized according to complaints, problems, and findings as they might present themselves prior to analysis, emphasizing the approach to the patient. Parts II through IX address problems gathered under traditional categories of disease. Where diagnosis is concerned, we have provided expanded differential diagnostic lists using tables while focusing the discussion on the most common, or otherwise most important, considerations. In Section 3 of Part I, we provide some basic information about commonly used diagnostic tests, and where appropriate throughout the book, we offer explicit suggestions about the use of diagnostic tests for specific problems. Where treatment is concerned, we have again discussed commonly used modalities in Part I, Section 4. Both

there and in later sections, we have included enough detail in selection and proper usage to provide a sound guide to practice. This commitment to explicitness makes the information here more prone to changes than a more general discussion would be and will thus make for a quicker dating of the text. We hope that in recompense our readers' approval of this format will demand that we correct this inherent fault with future updated editions. In the interest of focus, we have allowed the authors to suit their internal format to the topic at hand. Also, where different approaches represent different defensible interpretations of the literature and experience, we have let stand some competing recommendations within the text.

Several comprehensive texts of neurology provide extensive scientific background. We value these works and appreciate our dependence on basic and clinical research for the many advances currently moving neurology. However, here, we have chosen to devote our space to such background only enough to promote the discussion of clinical topics. Hence, the results of clinical science appear within the text where they enter into clinical decision making. Although it covers most of the field of neurology, the text is not comprehensive. We have chosen to omit many topics that we might have included. Some of these decisions were dictated by our focus on adults and on outpatient office practice. However, kids grow up sometimes bringing their neurologic diseases with them, and diseases do not respect hospital architecture—that is, our choice to see them as inpatient or outpatient problems—so we did cut some off here and add some there as we saw fit. For example, in Part I, coma is excluded as clearly an inpatient problem and beyond the scope of this book, and head injury is addressed as it confronts the outpatient physician after the acute issues have receded into the past. Yet in Section 2 of Part III on Infectious Diseases, we decided to include acute meningitis and other severe infections, and in Section 2 of Part VI on Epilepsy we include status epilepticus, because, although clearly inpatient problems, they represent important topics within their categories such that excluding them would have left conspicuous lacunae in our coverage. Within Part VIII on Neurology in General Medicine, we discuss some more common metabolic disorders, and Dr. Kolodny reviews the lysosomal storage diseases. However, many of the metabolic disorders that most commonly occur in children, we chose to exclude because of our adult focus and their rarity. To do them justice would have added greatly to the length of the book and altered its balance. This selectiveness has allowed us to broaden and deepen the discussions of those topics that we chose to include. We have not tried to provide comprehensive literature reviews of the topics covered. Instead, in the Suggested Readings at the end of each chapter, we have sought to supply useful references for more in-depth reading, to reference particular studies cited, and to support specific recommendations. Although this approach to the problem of selection leaves much unsaid, we feel that it has allowed us to create a book that discusses in explicit detail the great majority of problems that the adult neurologist or primary care physician will confront.

A project of this magnitude requires the work and cooperation of many people. We would like to express our sincere thanks to all of the contributors and section editors. Many of them are our colleagues in neurology. Others share their expertise from other fields: internal medicine, neuropsychology, neurosurgery, otolaryngology, pathology, psychiatry, radiology, radiation oncology, rehabilitation medicine, and speech and physical therapy. We appreciate the commitment and sacrifice of time and energy necessary to write these reviews and the care given to them. In a recent editorial in *The Boston Globe*, there appeared this quote attributed to Samuel Johnson: "Only a blockhead would write for any reason except money." We thank all of the blockheads who have given freely of themselves and trust that they have found their separate rewards.

We also wish to thank our editors at Churchill Livingstone who have urged us on to complete this awesome project in good time: Kerry Willis, Marc Strauss, and David Terry. Providing what little comic relief there is in Albert Camus' *La Peste*, there is a man, Grand, who sets out to write the perfect sentence. He imagines the scene on that day when his editors receive it: The chief editor rising after having silently read it and saying simply and solemnly to his colleagues around the table, "Gentlemen, hats off!" Need it be added that Grand never quite finishes his sentence. To those authors who had trouble putting that last period on their manuscript, we do understand. And although there are surely faults of haste and imperfections in this book, we hope that its merits overwhelm and, in part, excuse them.

Finally, the ultimate reason for this book is to give us a forum to provide our colleagues and students with a source that will, we hope, promote excellence in patient care for those who suffer with neurologic disease. We continue to learn from the integration of bookish study with close attention to our patients. Over the years, many of these patients have been generous enough to share their private medical problems with us in conference whereby we and our colleagues have broadened our experience far beyond what would have been possible in individual practices. To these patients, we express our deepest gratitude for having been among our teachers.

Martin A. Samuels, M.D.
Steven Feske, M.D.

CONTENTS

IX. Headache and Pain

Editor: Egilius L. H. Spierings

PRINCIPLES OF AMBULATORY NEUROLOGY AND THE APPROACH TO CLINICAL PROBLEMS

PART I

SECTION 1. PRINCIPLES OF DIAGNOSIS: THE GENERAL APPROACH TO NEUROLOGIC DIAGNOSIS

1. NEUROLOGIC HISTORY AND EXAMINATION

STEVEN FESKE

In every branch of medicine, the history and physical examinations are performed to answer several questions, including the following: In which parts of the body is there dysfunction? What is the underlying cause of the dysfunction? That is, from what disease is the patient suffering? Our goal in evaluating the patient with neurologic disease is to answer these same questions. We cannot answer them directly, however, but must do so by inference. The more immediate goal of the patient's history and physical examination, then, is to establish a firm basis from which we can make reliable inferences. In taking a history, we want to answer several more immediate questions: What happened? Which neurologic structures does this implicate? What was the context for the illness? Over what period of time did the illness develop? In performing our neurologic examination, we want to answer the following additional questions: What are the sites of neurologic dysfunction that might explain the neurologic signs that we can elicit? Do these signs fall into a known pattern of dysfunction or syndrome? What is the degree of dysfunction? In other words, our questions in the history and examination are directed to seek information about the localization, context, and timing of the disease process and, finally, the degree of disability.

By virtue of its intricate anatomic organization, the nervous system lends itself to a particularly fine analysis of localization. Because diseases tend to cause dysfunction in predictable sites, whether in certain tissue compartments (as in meningitis and subarachnoid hemorrhage), vascular territories (as in stroke), tissue types (as in multiple sclerosis), or in neuronal systems (as in amyotrophic lateral sclerosis), the neurologist's obsession with neurologic localization is critical to accurate diagnosis. The most informative examinations are those that are organized around working hypotheses about the possible localization of the lesion or lesions. Therefore, I strongly stress localization in this review of the techniques used in the clinical encounter.

The purpose of this chapter is to summarize an approach to the assessment of neurologic problems by the traditional patient history and physical examination. I point out useful ways to organize and develop the evaluation, but I do not describe the examination in detail. This is accomplished in various sections of the book where different anatomic sites and groups of disease are discussed: mental status examination (Ch. 131), cranial nerves (Chs. 7 to 12), motor and reflex examinations (Ch. 2), sensory examinations (Chs. 5 and 6), coordination (Ch. 120), and gait and station (Ch. 4).

PURPOSE OF EVALUATION

It is helpful to establish the purpose of a particular evaluation at the outset. This may be to diagnose an as yet unexplained problem; to follow the progression of a disease, either to make a diagnosis based on the course of the disease over time or to follow the progression or response to therapy in the case of an established diagnosis; or to assess the functional status of a patient with a disabling illness, such as stroke, multiple sclerosis, or Parkinson's disease. One's attention to certain details and recording methods may vary, depending on the purpose.

APPROACH TO THE PATIENT HISTORY AND PHYSICAL EXAMINATION

For the purpose of diagnosis, history is elicited to develop the nature of the complaints and the details of the events leading to them as well as to discover any medical, psychological, and social context that may offer epidemiologic clues to the cause. Both the patient history and physical examinations are used to identify the site or sites in the nervous system that have malfunctioned. Armed with this information and a solid foundation of medical and neurologic knowledge, one tries to identify the medical or neurologic syndrome into which the disease may fit. Often this will suggest an etiology or allow the examiner to generate a restricted list of possible etiologic diagnoses that can be further pruned by special tests. For the assessment of functional status and disease progression, details concerning the limitations of various functions must be explored along with the effects of these limitations on activities of daily living.

NEUROLOGIC HISTORY

Chief Complaint

It is helpful to physicians providing consultation to establish from the outset the reason for a visit, both as understood by the patient and as expressed by the consulting physician. This will allow the consultant to address specific questions posed by the patient and consulting physician and, in some cases, identify discrepancies of understanding and intent that may be important for diagnosis and management.

History of Present Illness

When possible, it is helpful to listen to the patient describe the problem in his or her own words, initially without much direction from the examiner. This allows the patient to present a story with emphasis on what has seemed most important for him or her and to bring in associated information that seems to be relevant. Many patients, given the floor, will focus on characteristic symptoms that will strongly suggest a diagnosis. Having heard this story, the examiner can begin to develop hypotheses about the possible causes of the problem and then direct the patient with specific questions that will help to distinguish among these possible causes. In some cases, such as transient events, it is important to develop the history of the onset of the event in second by second detail in an effort to distinguish such diagnoses as syncope, seizure, transient ischemic attack, migraine, and others. In cases where there has been an alteration in awareness, it is best to obtain the history from any available witnesses. Pain, weakness, numbness, paresthesias, other forms of dysfunction, and other related symptoms should be distinguished and characterized in detail, including sites, quality, temporal course, and modifiers.

The occurrence of similar or related symptoms in the past or the accumulation of symptoms over a long period of time may be important. In multiple sclerosis, a history of prior episodes suggestive of involvement of different anatomic sites is important. With transient ischemic attacks, very similar symptoms may recur many times. In epilepsy, recurrent seizures are typically stereotyped at onset. In chronic progressive illnesses, various symptoms may have emerged as subtle changes in the past and now become prominent symptoms, as is common in Parkinson's disease.

Precipitating factors may give clues to the cause. In cases of syncope, postural changes may prompt symptoms. In multiple sclerosis, immersion in warm water may provoke them. Many factors may trigger migraines. Emotional stimuli may trigger anxiety symptoms, but they also may exacerbate the manifestations of various neurologic diseases, including Parkinson's disease, other tremors, migraines, and others. The time of day at which symptoms occur may be the clue to the precipitating cause. Increased intracranial pressure will typically cause morning headaches, as will caffeine withdrawal. Tumor-related pain is often worse at night.

It is also helpful to ask about past evaluations and past treatments for the current problem or similar ones and the patient's responses to these. It is probably best to develop at this time other, earlier history that is directly relevant to the examiner's most favored hypotheses concerning the cause. This will include directly relevant epidemiologic information usually sought in the review of the past medical history as discussed below.

Past Medical History

It is helpful in most cases to review a list of major common medical and neurologic problems to fill in the patient's personal history. In my experience, a general question about past medical problems fails to elicit much relevant information, and a quick review of the following list will quickly bring out most past illnesses that have been established: diabetes mellitus, hypertension, heart disease, lung disease, gastrointestinal disease, renal disease, thyroid disease, arthritis, cancer, stroke, seizure, and migraine. A history of use of alcohol, other drugs, and cigarettes and other habits relevant to health should be sought in most cases. In many cases, it will be helpful to ask about risk factors for human immunodeficiency virus infection. Past trauma and surgery should be reviewed. In many cases when seeing adults, the early childhood history is not explored; however, it can be helpful in evaluating epilepsy and many chronic diseases with early onset. In patients with mild motor, cognitive, or behavioral abnormalities, movement disorders, or hydrocephalus, all having gone unnoticed, the explanation will sometimes be a mild static encephalopathy suggested by a history of prematurity or early childhood problems.

It is important to elicit a history of the medications that the patient is taking, since these will in some cases be the source of the problem, as is often so in cases of syncope, dizziness, and confusion. They will also give clues to otherwise unmentioned underlying problems. Knowing the current medications will also be important later when further evaluation and treatments are being planned.

Place of origin or travel may greatly color the assessment of a finding. Cerebral calcifications in a native of Central or South America or the Indian subcontinent or Southeast Asia all raise the likely possibility of cysticercosis, an unlikely explanation in patients from temperate climates. Various tropical diseases will be suggested by exposure. Lyme disease is endemic to certain areas and rare in others. Human immunodeficiency infection has become more widely disseminated but still has a higher incidence in sub-Saharan Africa, Haiti, and many urban areas. Human T cell leukemia virus type I infection is found mainly in the West Indies, parts of Africa, and Japan. Behçet's disease is more common in the Near East and the Pacific rim of eastern Asia, although many cases are now found in other areas. Several hereditary diseases also have been linked to restricted areas of the world. Machado-Joseph disease occurs in patients from Portugal, the Cape Verdean Islands, and areas populated by emigration from these sites, such as Brazil, Japan, and several areas in the United States. There are, of course, many other examples.

Exposure to animals is occasionally important. Mosquitos, ticks, and other insects bear many diseases, including encephalitis, Rocky Mountain spotted fever, Lyme disease, and others. Diseases associated with large animals include encephalitis borne by horses, Lyme disease borne by white-tailed deer, brucellosis borne by cattle, rabies borne by various small domestic and wild mammals, cat-scratch disease and toxoplasmosis borne by cats, and leptospirosis borne by rats. None of these are common. Unusual exposure may come from unusual work, such as laboratory technicians handling infectious pathogens.

Family History

Family history can provide important clues to diagnosis and, occasionally, incentive for screening and preventive treatment in several common diseases. Hypertension, diabetes, early atherosclerosis, migraine, epilepsy, and major depression all occur with a higher incidence in some families, although clear genetic causes have not been found. It is interesting to notice that many patients will report no family history of illnesses like migraine, but, when asked simply if anyone has frequent headaches, acknowledge that, in fact, a close family member has "routine headaches" all the time. For certain familial diseases, such as Huntington's disease, hereditary neuropathies, myotonic dystrophy, and many others, the family history is very important for diagnosis. Again, with diseases like the last two mentioned, it is common to be told initially that there is no family history of the disease, but to find on closer questioning for symptoms or on examination of family members that, in fact, there is. When familial diseases with established patterns of inheritance are being considered, it is important to construct a family tree with information as far back as possible.

Social History

When an illness has behavioral consequences, it is important to know the educational level, marital status and family situation, and occupation of the patient. Recent life events, new schools, new jobs, relocation, or the death of a close friend or relative can, of course, contribute to illnesses that have an emotional component. This information is also of great importance in planning for the chronic-care needs of patients with disabilities. Occupational risks are also important in many illnesses, such as carpal tunnel syndrome in patients who type or do other repetitive manual jobs.

Systems Review

After having extracted the apparently relevant information in the patient history, I use a quick systems review to ''cover all the bases'' when the diagnosis is still in question. This is intended to elicit symptoms that the patients may not spontaneously volunteer but that may be clues to unconsidered and contributory illnesses, as opposed to the questions concerning past diagnoses or symptoms of major concern that were sought earlier in the history of present illness and past medical history. Fever, chills, weight loss, and night sweats are important symptoms that suggest infectious or neoplastic disease. Surveying symptoms relevant to proper functioning of the head and neck, lungs, heart, digestive tract, urinary tract, endocrine system, and joints can be done quickly in most cases. Although one will usually have gotten most of the relevant information in earlier questioning, the unexpected history of major weight loss may turn one's thinking toward a malignancy. A history of lung disease and adenopathy in a patient with a facial palsy will make one think seriously of sarcoidosis, even though it is a rare cause. An unexpected history of diarrhea may make one seriously consider a rare case of Whipple's disease in a patient with spontaneous nystagmus and hypothalamic dysfunction. Although completeness in pursuing a review of systems will not often be rewarded by such rare diagnostic surprises, it is a good practice that sometimes will provide important clues.

NEUROLOGIC EXAMINATION

Many books are available describing the neurologic and medical physical examination in great detail, and the reader is referred to those mentioned at the end of this chapter for a detailed discussion of the neurologic examination. It is, of course, possible to carry out an exhaustive examination at great length. However, for a diagnostic examination, our goal is instead to apply a focused examination directed at the problem at hand, to apply a core screening examination to test the integrity of the nervous system as a whole, and to screen for significant medical illness. For an examination of functional status, our goal is to establish the level of function of a system in as objectifiable a manner as possible and to document it in a reproducible format for future comparison.

A complete neurologic examination should include the elements described below.

Mental Status

The mental status examination can be done, in large part, by observation during the course of history-taking. In patients with apparently normal mental function for whom the mental state is not brought into question by the complaints, the examiner can usually demonstrate a normal core of mental functions in this manner. When the mental state is in question, tests should address the level of consciousness, orientation, attention, moti-

vational tone, and affect/mood of the patient. These state functions provide the necessary substrate for normal interactions and the proper use of the more discrete mental functions. Language and memory should be tested and, when relevant, further mental status tests looking for evidence of focal disease should be done. Many of these are mentioned below in the discussion of localization.

Cranial Nerves

By testing smell and central and peripheral vision, visualizing the optic fundi, and testing pupils, lids, eye movements, hearing, facial sensation, facial movements, and oral, lingual, palatal, and sternocleidomastoid and trapezius movements, the examiner has screened for cranial nerve dysfunction. Each cranial nerve can be tested in further detail when its function is in question.

Motor Function

Muscles should be inspected for normal bulk, and abnormal postures and spontaneous movements of the muscles, body, and limbs should be noted. The muscle tone is noted to be decreased, normal, or increased. Hypertonicity should be characterized as spastic, paratonic (gegenhalten), or the lead pipe (often called cogwheel rigidity) of parkinsonism, or other types of rigidity, such as muscle spasm, myotonia, and voluntary rigidity. Power in the basic muscle groups should be assessed and recorded in a reproducible format. A common system is to record the power along a functional scale of five units, as follows: 5/5 = full power, 4/5 = movement against some resistance, 3/5 = movement against gravity, 2/5 = movement with gravity eliminated, 1/5 = a trace of movement, and 0/5 = no visible movement.

Sensory Function

The appreciation of light touch and deep pressure and pinprick, temperature, vibration, joint position, and cortical sensation should be tested. By strategically choosing the points to test, this screening can be completed quickly. I usually test light touch on the distal extremities, pinprick and temperature sensation at certain strategic sites on the dermatomal map (C3, supraclavicular fossa; C4, acromioclavicular joint; C5, lateral upper arm and lateral epicondyle; C6, thumb; C7, index and middle finger; C8, little finger; T1, medial epicondyle; T2, axilla; L1, inguinal crease; L2, anterior thigh; L3, medial knee; L4, medial malleolus; L5, dorsum of the foot between the great and second toes; S1, lateral heel; and S2, medial aspect of the popliteal fossa), and vibration and joint position in the fingers and toes. Cortical sensation is tested with graphesthesia, stereognosis, and two-point discrimination on the hands. This examination should be abnormal when there are deficits from peripheral neuropathies, various isolated neuropathies, the most common radiculopathies, myelopathies, and brain lesions; more detailed tests can be done, when indicated, to add precision and answer specific questions. For example, when a spinal cord lesion is in question, thoracic dermatomes should be tested and a sensory level sought.

Reflexes

The deep tendon reflexes are tested at the biceps (C5), brachioradialis (C6), triceps (C7), finger flexors (C8), knees (L2–L4), and ankles (S1). Additional ones can be added to answer localiz-

TABLE 1-1. Localization of Forebrain Lesions

Site	Finding
Left frontal lobe	"Anterior" aphasia (Broca's, transcortical motor), aphemia
	Ideomotor apraxia
	↓ Voluntary rightward saccades, left gaze preference
	Right hemiparesis, ↑ deep tendon reflex, and Babinski sign
Right frontal lobe	Motor neglect of left world
	Ideomotor apraxia
	↓ Voluntary leftward saccades, right gaze preference
	Left hemiparesis, ↑ deep tendon reflex, and Babinski sign
Bilateral frontal lobes	Perseveration, impersistence, stimulus-bound responses
	Impaired "executive functions"—planning, sequencing, judgment, insight, abstract reasoning
	Imparied motor (Luria) sequencing
	Snout, root, grasp, and palmomental reflexes
	Gegenhalten (paratonic rigidity)
Orbitofrontal	Dysinhibition, aggressive impulsivity
	Anosmia
	Memory disturbance
Frontal convexity	Abulia → akinetic mutism
	Incontinence
	"Magnetic" gait
Midline frontal	Bilateral leg weakness
	Behavioral changes (cingulate gyrus)
Left parietal lobe	Right cortical sensory loss (astereognosis, agraphesthesia, ↓ two-point discrimination)
	Anomic aphasia, transcortical sensory aphasia
	dysgraphia, dyscalculia, left-right disorientation, finger agnosia
	Right inferior quadrantanopsia
Right parietal lobe	Left cortical sensory loss (as above)
	Left-sided neglect, anisognosia
	Constructional apraxia, dressing apraxia
	Left inferior quadrantanopsia
Left temporal lobe	"Posterior" aphasia (Wernicke's, transcortical sensory)
	Conduction aphasia
	Amnesia for verbal material (usually bilateral lesions)
	Right superior quadrantanopsia
Right temporal lobe	Dysprosody, amusia, nonverbal auditory agnosia
	Amnesia for nonverbal material (usually bilateral lesions)
	Left superior quadrantanopsia
Bilateral temporal lobes	
Medial	Amnesia
Perisylvian	Coritcal deafness
	Auditory agnosia
Occipital lobe	Contralateral homonymous hemianopsia (macular sparing)
	Cortical bindness, Anton syndrome
Left	Alexia without agrahia (requires lesion of splenium of corpus callosum)
Parieto-occipital	Balint syndrome (simultanagnosia, optic ataxia, ocular apraxia)—impaired-visuospatial localization
Temporo-occipital	Visual agnosias (including prosopagnosia, color agnosia, achromatopsia)
	Visual amnesia
	Confusional state
Thalamus	Agitated confusional state
	Decreased level of consciousness
	Amnesia
	Aphasia (transcortical sensory)
	Hemisensory loss
	Cerebellar ataxia
Basal ganglia	Parkinsonism
	Aphasia (transcortical motor)
	Hyperkinetic syndromes (e.g., hemiballism with subthalamic nucleus infarction)

TABLE 1-2. Localization of Brainstem Lesions

Site	Finding
Midbrain	
Tectum and pretectum	Parinaud syndrome (large pupils with near-light dissociation, convergence-retraction nystagmus, impaired upgaze, eyelid retraction)
Tegmentum	Abnormal pupils—midrange, unequal, irregularly shaped
	Impaired vertical eye movements
	Anterior INO
	Skew deviation
	Decreased arousal
	Nuclear CN III lesions (including, bilateral ptosis and superior rectus deficits)
	Nuclear CN IV lesions (contralateral CN IV deficit)
Cerebral peduncles	Weber syndrome (ipsilateral CNIII, contralateral hemiparesis)
Red nucleus	Benedikt syndrome (ipsilateral CN III, contralateral tremor)
Ascending cerebellar fibers	Claude syndrome (ipsilateral CN III, contralateral cerebellar ataxia)
Pons	
Tegmentum	Ipsilateral gaze palsy ("wrong-way eyes")
	Intranuclear ophthalmoplegia
	One-and-a-half syndrome
	Skew deviation
	CN V, VI, VII, and VIII lesions
Basis pontis	Contralateral hemiparesis
	Contralateral ataxia
	Dysarthria
Medulla	
Lateral	Wallenberg syndrome (ipsilateral CN V, ipsilateral Horner syndrome, contralateral loss of pain and temperature below the neck [spinothalamic tract], vertigo and ipsilateral nystagmus, ipsilateral CN IX and X deficits, skew deviation)
Medial	Ipsilateral CN XII deficit, contralateral hemiparesis, contralateral medial lemniscus deficit (joint position and vibration)

Abbreviations: CN, cranial nerve; INO, internuclear ophthalmoplegia.

ing questions: jaw jerk (above the foramen magnum), hip adductors (L2–L4), tibialis posterior (L5). The degree of response, reproducibility, and symmetry of the reflexes are noted. Mass spread of the reflex to adjacent segments is noted. The main pathologic reflex that is included in the screening examination is a scratch to the lateral sole looking for the Babinski sign. The reflexes are usually recorded on a scale of 4 units, where 0/4 is absent, 1/4 and 2/4 are two degrees usually considered within normal limits when symmetric (although symmetrically 1/4 reflexes may be abnormal in certain contexts, such as a young person with early Guillain-Barré syndrome), 3/4 is hyperreflexic, and 4/4 is hyperreflexic with clonus. "Trace" and plus and minus signs are sometimes added to this scale to express intermediate degrees, but there is probably little reproducibility among examiners for these finer distinctions.

TABLE 1-3. Localization of Cerebellar Lesions

Site	Finding
Cerebellar hemisphere	Ipsilateral ataxia (intention temor, dysdiadochokinesia, dysmetria)
	Ipsilateral hypotonicity
Midline	Gait ataxia with widened base
	Truncal titubation
	Dysarthria (ataxic speech)
Vestibulocerebellum	Abnormal eye movements
	Skew deviation
	Hypo- and hypermetric saccades, micro- and macro-square-wave jerks, breakdown of smooth pursuit movements, opsoclonus
	Contralateral head tilt (cerebellopontine angle tumor)

Coordination

Tests of coordination, including rapid alternating movements and finger-to-nose and heel-to-shin maneuvers, are done. These can help to assess cerebellar as well as pyramidal and extrapyramidal motor function and sensory function.

Station and Gait

The patient should be observed to stand with the feet together and the eyes open and closed (Romberg sign) and to walk while balance, stride, arm swing, and posture are noted. Heel-to-toe (tandem) walking completes the screening neurologic examination per se.

Medical Status

A general medical examination should, of course, include as much detail as is necessary to address the problem. It is often important to know the vital signs, to examine head and neck structure and pulses and to listen for bruits, to listen to the heart for murmurs and abnormal rhythms, to palpate the abdomen for hepatosplenomegaly, to note the extremities for abnormalities of form (e.g., pes cavus), joint changes, or abnormal lymph nodes, and to inspect the skin for marks, such as café-au-lait spots, telangiectasias, petechiae, or other lesions.

NEUROLOGIC LOCALIZATION

The nervous system is organized in a way that lends itself to more or less precise localization of the anatomic site or sites of dysfunction. Since by identifying the part or subsystem of the nervous system affected by a disease (along with the context and timing of the illness), one can often accurately infer the nature of the disease process, localization is a major goal of the neurologic examination. Therefore, the rest of the discussion below of the diagnostic history and examination is organized around the knowledge used to localize the lesion.

The first question one asks is what is the gross location of the lesion? That is, is it in the muscle, neuromuscular junction, peripheral nerve, nerve plexus, nerve root, anterior horn cell, spinal cord, or brain? Is it on the left or right side of the brain, spinal cord, or body? If one can successfully make this determination, then one should try to make a more exact estimate of the precise localization within the nervous tissue. Information relevant to such localization is presented throughout the text. Tables 1-1 through 1-5 summarize some of the commonly used or classically described clues. As an example of this approach, clues that the brain is the site of concern include behavioral and cognitive symptoms; symptoms on one-half of the body, including more than one of the three possible locations—face, arm, and leg; a lack of peripheral pain, except headache; and features of an upper motor neuron or cortical sensory lesion. Having chosen to look closely at the brain for the lesion, one can ask if the lesion is diffuse or discrete and localized. Diffuse brain disease will usually cause impairment of the "state functions" mentioned above. Such lesions will underlie mainly cases of impaired level of consciousness (some of them) and impaired attention. Some cases of impaired motivation and altered mood will also be due to global disease. These will almost always include an impairment in attention. Many special

TABLE 1-4. Localization of Spinal Cord Lesions

Site	Finding

Spinal cord	Bilateral signs
	LMN signs at the level of the lesion
	UMN signs below the lesion
	  Marked spasticity with majestic Babinski signs
	  Absent jaw jerk
	  Sensory level at or below the level of the lesion

Craniocervical junction	Neck pain, head tilt Downbeating nystagmus UMN signs of all four extremities
Cervical spinal cord	Neck pain Root signs at the dermatomal level of the lesion in the neck, shoulders, or arms Long tract signs below the level of the lesion (usually bilateral) Sensory level at or below the level of the lesion Spastic bowel and bladder (later)
Thoracic spinal cord	Back pain Root signs at the level of the lesion Paraparesis—long tract signs below the level of involvement Sensory level below the level of involvement Spastic bowel and bladder
Conus medullaris (S3–Coc1)	Early bowel, bladder, and sexual dysfunction—usually areflexic (LMN) bladder Early perineal hypesthesia No motor signs in legs (if pure) Distal motor signs with loss of ankle jerks (if epiconus, L4–S2)
Cauda equina	See Table 1-5
Anterior cord syndrome	AHC (LMN) involvement at the level of the lesion Corticospinal tract involvement below the lesion Spinothalamic tract involvement below the lesion Sparing of the dorsal columns Spastic bowel and bladder
Central cord syndrome	Segmental loss of pain and temperature at the levels of the lesion UMN signs below the lesion Sparing of dorsal column modalities
Brown-Séquard (hemicord) syndrome	Ipsilateral corticospinal tract signs below the lesion Ipsilateral loss of vibration and joint position sense below the lesion Contralateral loss of pain and temperature below the lesion Band of ipsilateral hypesthesia to all modalities at the level of the lesion

Abbreviations: AHC, anterior horn cell; LMN, lower motor neuron; UMN, upper motor neuron.

TABLE 1-5. Localization of Lower Motor Neuron Lesions

Site	Finding
Anterior horn cells	Evolves to involve all four extremities (may not at first)—LMN involvement of the lower extremities may distinguish it from cervical spondylosis—in ALS Atrophy, fasciculations, and weakness Hypotonicity and loss of reflexes Tongue and other involvement above the neck (in ALS) Usually with associated UMN signs (in ALS)
Roots	Dermatomal pain and parasthesias Unilateral (unless multiple, as in GBS) Dermatomal sensory loss Myotomal weakness Isolated ↓ DTR
Caudal equina	Low back and perineal pain LMN deficits of the lower extremities (may be asymmetric) Early areflexic bladder and bowel
Nerve Mononeuropathy	Pain and parasthesias in sensory nerve distribution (light touch loss typically involves greater area than pinprick loss) Sensory and motor deficit characteristic of a peripheral nerve
Polyneuropathy	Usually distally predominant stocking glove distribution Deficit gradient from distal to proximal Symmetric deficits Loss of motor, sensory, or autonomic function, depending on the nerves involved Loss of ankle jerks in most

Abbreviations: ALS, amyotrophic lateral sclerosis; DTR, deep tendon reflex; GBS, Guillain-Barré syndrome; LMN, lower motor neuron; UMN, upper motor neuron.

TABLE 1-6. The Expanded Disability Status Scale

Score	Explanation
0	Normal neurologic exam (all grade 0 in FS; cerebral grade 1 acceptable).
1.0	No disability, minimal signs in one FS (i.e., grade 1 excluding cerebral grade 1).
1.5	No disability, minimal signs in more than one FS (more than one grade 1 excluding cerebral grade 1).
2.0	Minimal disability in one FS (one FS grade 2, others 0 or 1.)
2.5	Minimal disability in two FS (two FS grade 2, others 0 or 1).
3.0	Moderate disability in one FS (one FS grade 3, others 0 or 1), or mild disability in three or four FS (three/four FS grade 2, others 0 or 1) though fully ambulatory.
3.5	Fully ambulatory but with moderate disability in one FS (one grade 3) and one or two FS grade 2; or two FS grade 3; or five FS grade 2 (others 0 or 1.)
4.0	Fully ambulatory without aid, self-sufficient, up and about some 12 hours a day despite relatively severe disability consisting of one FS grade 4 (others 0 or 1), or combination of lesser grades exceeding limits of previous steps. Able to walk without aid or rest some 500 m.
4.5	Fully ambulatory without aid, up and about much of the day, able to work a full day—may otherwise have some limitation of full activity or require minimal assistance; characterized by relatively severe disability, usually consisting of one FS grade 4 (others 0 or 1) or combinations of lesser grades exceeding limits of previous steps. Able to walk without aid or rest for some 300 m.
5.0	Ambulatory without aid or rest for about 200 m; disability severe enough to impair full daily activities (e.g., to work full day without special provisions). (Usual FS equivalents are one grade 5 alone, others 0 or 1; or combinations of lesser grades usually exceeding specifications for step 4.0)
5.5	Ambulatory without aid or rest for about 100 m; disability severe enough to preclude full daily activities. (Usual FS equivalents are one grade 5 alone, others 0 or 1; or combinations of lesser grades usually exceeding those for step 4.0.)
6.0	Intermittent or unilateral constant assistance (cane, crutch, or brace) required to walk about 100 m with or without resting. (Usual FS equivalents are combinations with more than two FS grade 3 +.)
6.5	Constant bilateral assistance (canes, crutches, or braces) required to walk about 20 m without resting. (Usual FS equivalents are combinations with more than two FS grade 3 +.)
7.0	Unable to walk beyond about 5 m even with aid, essentially restricted to wheelchair; wheels self in standard wheelchair and transfers alone; up and about in wheelchair some 12 hours a day. (Usual FS equivalents are combinations with more than one FS grade 4 +; very rarely, pyramidal grade 5 alone.)
7.5	Unable to take more than a few steps; restricted to wheelchair; may need aid in transfer; wheels self but cannot carry on in standard wheelchair a full day; may require motorized wheelchair (Usual equivalents are combinations with more than one FS grade 4 +.)
8.0	Essentially restricted to bed or chair or perambulated in wheelchair, but may be out of bed much of the day; retains many self-care functions; generally has effective use of arms. (Usual FS equivalents are combinations, generally grade 4 + in several systems.)
8.5	Essentially restricted to bed much of the day; has some effective use of arm(s); retains some self-care functions. (Usual FS equivalents are combinations, generally 4 + in several systems.)
9.0	Helpless bed patient; unable to communicate effectively or eat/swallow. (Usual FS equivalents are combinations, almost all grade 4 +.)
9.5	Totally helpless bed patient; unable to communicate effectively or eat/swallow. (Usual FS equivalents are combinations, almost all grade 4 +.)
10	Death due to MS.

Abbreviations: FS, functional system; MS, multiple sclerosis.

(Adapted From Kurtzke JF; Rating neurologic impairment in multiple sclerosis: an expanded disability status scale (EDSS). Neurology 33: 1444–52, 1983, with permission.)

TABLE 1-7. Functional Systems Used in Expanded Disability Status Scale

Pyramidal functions
  0. Normal
  1. Abnormal signs without disability
  2. Minimal disability
  3. Mild or moderate paraparesis or hemiparesis; severe monoparesis
  4. Marked paraparesis or hemipareisis, quadriparesis, or monoplegia
  5. Paraplegia, hemiplegia, or marked quadriparesis
  6. Quadriplegia
  V. Unknown

Cerebellar functions
  0. Normal
  1. Abnormal signs without disability
  2. Mild ataxia
  3. Moderate truncal or limb ataxia
  4. Severe ataxia, all limbs
  5. Unable to perform coordinated movements due to ataxia
  V. Unknown
  X. Is used throughout after each number when weakness (grade 3 or more on pyramidal) interferes with testing

Brainstem functions
  0. Normal
  1. Signs only
  2. Moderate nystagmus or other mild disability
  3. Severe nystagmus, marked extraocular weakness, or moderate disability of other cranial nerves
  4. Marked dysarthria or other marked disability
  5. Inability to swallow or speak
  V. Unknown

Sensory functions
  0. Normal
  1. Vibration or figure-writing decrease only, in one or two limbs
  2. Mild decrease in touch or pain or position sense, and/or moderate decrease in vibration in one or two limbs; or vibratory (with or without figure writing) decrease alone in three or four limbs
  3. Moderate decrease in touch or pain or position sense, and/or essentially lost vibration in one or two limbs; or mild decrease in touch or pain and/or moderate decrease in all proprioceptive tests in three or four limbs
  4. Marked decrease in touch or pain or loss of proprioception, alone or combined, in one or two limbs; or moderate decrease in touch or pain and/or severe proprioceptive decrease in more than two limbs
  5. Loss (essentially) of sensation in one or two limbs; or moderate decrease in touch or pain and/or loss of proprioception for most of the body below the head
  6. Sensation essentially lost below the head
  V. Unknown

Bowel and bladder functions
  0. Normal
  1. Mild urinary hesitancy, urgency, or retention
  2. Moderate hesitancy, urgency, retention of bowel or bladder, or rare urinary incontinence
  3. Frequent urinary incontinence
  4. In need of almost constant catheterization
  5. Loss of bladder function
  6. Loss of bowel and bladder function
  V. Unknown

Visual (or optic) functions
  0. Normal
  1. Scotoma with visual acuity (corrected) better than 20/30
  2. Worse eye with scotoma with maximal visual acuity (corrected) of 20/30–20/59
  3. Worse eye with large scotoma, or moderate decrease in fields, but with maximal visual acuity (corrected) of 20/60–20/99
  4. Worse eye with marked decrease of fields and maximal visual acuity (corrected) of 20/100–20/200; grade 3 plus maximal acuity of better eye of 20/60 or less
  5. Worse eye with maximal visual acuity (corrected less than 20/200; grade 4 plus maximal acuity of better eye of 20/60 or less
  6. Grade 5 plus maximal visual acuity of better eye of 20/60 or less
  V. Unknown
  X. Is added to grades 0–6 for presence of temporal pallor

Cerebral (or mental) functions
  0. Normal
  1. Mood alteration only (does not affect score)
  2. Mild decrease in mentation
  3. Moderate decrease in mentation
  4. Marked decrease in mentation (chronic brain syndrome—moderate)
  5. Dementia or chronic brain syndrome—severe or incompetent
  V. Unknown

Other functions
  1. None
  2. Any other neurologic findings attributed to multiple sclerosis (specify)
  V. Unknown

(From Kurtzke JF: Rating neurolgic impairment in multiple sclerosis: an expanded disability status scale (EDSS). Neurology 33:1444–52, 1983, with permission.)

tests can be applied to probe for various focal brain lesions. It is helpful to organize the examination around the site one is testing and, when looking for evidence of disease at a locus, to test *multiple* functions governed by that locus. The outcome of the diagnostic assessment should be a formulation along the lines of the following scenario: An elderly man with a history of hypertension and atrial fibrillation presents with an acute right hemiparesis and Broca's aphasia. From this, one could infer that the most likely cause of such an illness is a stroke due to a cardiogenic embolus to the left middle cerebral

TABLE 1-8. Scripps Neurologic Rating Scale Worksheet[a]

System Examined	Maximum Points	Degree of Impairment			
		Normal	Mild	Moderate	Severe
Mentation and mood	10	10	7	4	0
Cranial nerves (eyes)	21				
Visual acuity		5	3	1	0
Fields, discs, pupils		6	4	2	0
Eye movements		5	3	1	0
Nystagmus		5	3	1	0
Lower cranial nerves	5	5	3	1	0
Motor	20				
RU		5	3	1	0
LU		5	3	1	0
RL		5	3	1	
LL		5	3	1	0
DTRs	8				
UE		4	3	1	0
LE		4	3	1	0
Babinski: R;L (2 each)	4	4	—	—	0
Sensory	12				
RU		3	2	1	0
LU		3	2	1	0
RL		3	2	1	0
LL		3	2	1	0
Cerebellar	10				
UE		5	3	1	0
LE		5	3	1	0
Gait, trunk, and balance	10	10	7	4	0
Special category: bladder bowel/sexual dysfunction	0	0	−3	−7	−10
Totals	100				

Abbreviations: DTR, deep tendon reflex; LU, left upper; RU, right upper; RL, right lower; LL, left lower; LE, lower extremity; UE, upper extremity.
[a] Points assigned for each component of the neurologic examination are subtotaled, and points for autonomic dysfunction are subtracted, leaving the final score.

(From Sipe JC, Knobler RL, Braheny SL, Rice GPA, Panitch HS, Oldstone MBA: A neurologic rating scale (NRS) for use in multiple sclerosis. Neurology 34:1368–72, 1984, with permission.)

artery and plan appropriate confirmatory evaluation and management.

FUNCTIONAL ASSESSMENT

When following the course of a chronic disease and when making recommendations concerning chronic-care needs, an assessment that answers questions about the degree of disability and provides a standard of comparison of patients and of a single patient over time is needed. A descriptive evaluation of function in the various areas—behavioral and cognitive, visual, auditory, motor, and sensory, ambulatory, and ability to perform activities of daily living, such as personal hygiene, bathroom activities, shopping, cooking, eating, and housekeeping—can be tailored to the situation at hand. For some diseases, standardized disability scales have been adopted by many practitioners. The Expanded Disability Status Scale is commonly used to follow the course of patients with multiple sclerosis and to define patient groups for clinical research. This is shown in Tables 1-6 and 1-7. Another instrument used for the rating of patients with multiple sclerosis, the Scripp's Neurologic Rating Scale, is more dependent on the neurologic examination alone than activities of daily living. It is shown in Table 1-8. The Intermediate Scale for Assessment of Parkinson's Disease is a simplified scale adapted for easy clinical use with patients who have Parkinson's disease. It is shown in Table 1-9.

TABLE 1-9 Intermediate Scale for Assessment of Parkinson's Disease

1. Self-care
   0 Normal.
   1 Independent, but some tasks require more time and effort than normal.
   2 Requires partial assistance to perform some activities (dressing, hygiene, standing up) or performance is achieved with considerable effort and slowness.
   3 Requires complete, or almost complete, assistance. Dependent.

2. Turning in bed
   0 Normal.
   1 Somewhat slow and clumsy. No help needed.
   2 Requires assistance but initiates and gives help to complete the movements, or performance is independent with considerable effort and slowness.
   3 Requires complete, or almost complete, assistance. Dependent.

3. Getting out of bed
   0 Normal.
   1 Somewhat slow and clumsy. No help needed.
   2 Initiates and gives help. The activity is performed with considerable slowness and effort or requires partial assistance.
   3 Dependent. Requires complete assistance.

4. Hygiene (washing, combing hair, shaving, brushing teeth, using toilet)
   0 Normal.
   1 Slight slowness, but independent.
   2 Requires partial assistance to perform some activities, or hygiene maintained independently with great effort and slowness.
   3 Requires complete assistance and/or special devices.

5. Bathing
   0 Normal.
   1 Slight slowness and effort, but independent.
   2 Requires partial assistance, but gives help and performs some activity with effort and slowness.
   3 Disabled and helpless.

6. Dressing.
   0 Normal.
   1 Slight slowness or effort. Independent.
   2 Moderate slowness and effort. Requires partial assistance (shoes, socks, tie, buttons).
   3 Even the simplest activities are performed with considerable effort. Requires complete assistance.

7. Speech
   0 Normal.
   1 Changes in voice or speech rhythm. Preserved volume of the voice. Clearly understood.
   2 Monotonous and/or dysarthric. Moderately difficult to understand.
   3 Very disturbed. Almost unintelligible, or speech not useful for communicative purposes.

8. Eating (chewing, swallowing)
   0 Normal.
   1 Normal diet. Chewing and swallowing are slow and labored.
   2 Ingests liquids and soft foods with ease. Requires time and effort to eat hard foods.
   3 Requires substitute methods (nasogastric tube or gastrostomy), or eats only liquids and soft foods with great effort.

9. Feeding (activities for nourishment)
   0 Normal.
   1 Slight to moderate slowness. Accidents are infrequent.
   2 Fully self-feeding with moderate slowness. Accidents are frequent and may require assistance with specific tasks (cutting meat, filling cup).
   3 Performs only a few feeding tasks with great slowness and effort, or requires complete assistance.

10. Walking
    0 Normal.
    1 Walks slowly; occasional instability. Does not require help.
    2 Moderately difficult, with considerable slowness and instability or freezing. Requires assistance.

11. Stairs
    0 Normal.

12. Arising from chair (straightback chair; arms folded across chest)
    0 Normal.

13. Gait
    0 Normal.
    1 Slow gait.

(From Martínez-Martín P: Intermediate Scale for Assessment of Parkinson's Disease and Assessment of Complications. p. 290–2. In Jankovic J, Tolosa E (eds): Parkinson's Disease and Movement Disorders. 2nd Ed. Williams & Wilkins, Baltimore, 1993, with permission.)

SUGGESTED READINGS

Brazis PW, Masdeu JC, Biller J: Localization in Clinical Neurology. 2nd Ed. Little, Brown, Boston, 1990

Haerer AF: DeJong's The Neurologic Examination. 5th Ed. JB Lippincott, Philadelphia, 1992.

Haymaker W: Bing's Local Diagnosis in Neurological Diseases. 15th Ed. CV Mosby, St. Louis, 1969

Hoehn MM, Yahr MD: Parkonsonism: onset, progression and mortality. Neurology 17:427–442, 1967

Kurtzke JF: Rating neurologic impairment in multiple sclerosis: an expanded disability status scale (EDSS). Neurology 33:1444–52, 1983

Martínez-Martín P: Intermediate Scale for Assessment of Parkinson's Disease and Assessment of Complications. pp. 290–2. In Jankovic J, Tolosa E (eds): Parkinson's Disease and Movement Disorders. 2nd Ed. Williams & Wilkins, Baltimore, 1993

Mesulam M-M: Principles of Behavioral Neurology. FA Davis, Philadelphia, 1985

Sipe JC, Knobler RL, Braheny SL et al: A neurologic rating scale (NRS) for use in multiple sclerosis. Neurology 34:1368–72, 1984

SECTION 2. PRINCIPLES OF DIAGNOSIS: COMMON PRESENTING SYMPTOMS AND FINDINGS

2. WEAKNESS

MICHAEL RONTHAL

Deficits in the motor system present primarily with weakness. This chapter is designed to help with the localization and diagnosis of weakness of somatic muscles.

The first step is to define broadly whether the deficit is due to a central lesion—that is, affecting upper motor neurons (UMN)—or to a peripheral process affecting the lower motor neuron (LMN). The UMN encompasses the central motor pathway from the cortex to, but not including, the anterior horn cell. The LMN includes the anterior horn cell, the motor nerves, endplates, and, for purposes of the localizing examination, the muscles. Careful examination of the patient will usually allow for differentiation between central and peripheral processes.

PATIENT HISTORY

As in all clinical diagnostic problems, data gathering begins with elicitation of the patient's history.

The patient complaint of "weakness," as with other primary complaints, may include a wide range of problems and hide a multitude of pathologies. For example, dyspnea of effort, rheumatologic pain produced by movement, ataxia, or even numbness may be meant. It is therefore important to probe into exactly what the patient means and to ask for localization of the symptoms.

If the complaint truly is weakness, it is often useful to ask the direct question, "In what daily life tasks does the weakness manifest?" Difficulty brushing hair and problems going up stairs may signify primarily a proximal distribution of weakness, suggestive of a myopathic process; difficulty with finger movements, a more distal distribution, suggestive of neuropathy; and weak legs, a myelopathy. Lateralized symptoms lead to the suspicion of a cranial process.

The evolution of the complaint over time may yield valuable clues as to the pathologic process. Sudden onset often implies a stroke; progressive lateralized weakness, an expanding mass lesion; and fluctuating weakness, particularly if related to repetitive effort, might suggest an endplate disorder. Sudden onset, short-lived episodes might suggest the diagnosis of transient ischemic attacks or even of atypical seizures.

Associated symptoms and events may be crucial to the diagnosis. The presence of palpitations at the onset of an episode of lateralized weakness supports the notion of cardiogenic emboli as the prime pathology. A vaccination or flulike illness 10 to 14 days prior to the onset may be the clue to a postinfectious syndrome at any level of the motor neuraxis. Inquiry as to the exact activity prior to onset will sometimes make the diagnosis, as in the so-called Saturday-night radial nerve palsy syndrome, a pressure palsy sustained at a time of drunken stupor. Muscular pain on exercise might suggest a metabolic myopathy.

The patient's occupational history may be of diagnostic importance. Exposure to lead might be the cause of a wrist drop, and pressure palsy or carpal tunnel syndrome may be suspected given the clue of specific work-related activities.

A history of urinary bladder dysfunction is of great importance. Frequency of micturition with urgency, urgency incontinence, and small quantities of urine voided each time implies a small, spastic irritable bladder, often seen in UMN syndromes. Cauda equina syndromes, too, may cause bladder dysfunction, frequently retention. In general, once neurogenic dysuria appears, the problem acquires a sense of urgency both in diagnosis and treatment. Abrupt neurogenic bladder dysfunction constitutes an emergency.

PHYSICAL SIGNS

The patient must be cooperative and pain-free for an accurate objective motor strength evaluation. The examiner attempts to resist or overcome the strength of the muscles. Muscle strength can be tested with the muscle at maximum contraction (having moved the joint it controls to its mechanical limit), as the joint begins to move, or at midposition. In the upper limbs, finger flexion is best tested starting with the fingers fully flexed over the examiner's fingers. Hand intrinsics, usually abductors, are tested in full abduction; extensors of fingers and wrists, in full extension; biceps and triceps, with the elbow joint held at a right angle; and the deltoid, with the arm abducted to shoulder height. In the lower limbs, hip flexion is best tested at midposition with the patient supine; quadriceps, foot and toe dorsiflexion, as well as toe plantar flexion are evaluated at maximum contraction. Plantar flexion is tested starting with the foot at midposition, hamstrings with the knee bent to a right angle, and thigh abductors with the patient lying on the side and abducting the uppermost thigh against the examiner's pressure.

If the patient is not cooperative, the power of the muscle being tested waxes briefly, and then strength falls away rapidly or else fluctuates. This is commonly referred to as "give-way" weakness. In order to test the power of the muscle in question, the examiner should resist the movement requested for only a brief second or two—during the short time span, normal or full power is likely to have been exerted before the give-way. Give-way implies either that there is a psychogenic component to the weakness or that pain associated with the movement inhibits the exertion of full strength.

Since various muscles vary in their strength, how can we be sure that there really is weakness and not just normal variability? How do we document and record weakness? If the examiner can overcome the power of a muscle, exerting resistance close to the joint that it moves and using an equivalent muscle of his or her own (e.g., fingers test finger strength), then that muscle is graded as "weak."

The most widely used grading system uses five grades: 5 is normal, 4 is "weak," 3 implies the ability to overcome gravity, 2 is movement with gravity eliminated, 1 is a flicker of movement, and 0 is paralysis. It will be readily apparent that within grade 4, there may be varying degrees of weakness. It is therefore common practice to expand grade 4 in some way. Various examiners use different systems. Provided that the system is constant and can be replicated by the examiner, any of these will do. A good system is simply to allow mild, moderate, and severe degrees of grade 4 weakness. Once accurately documented, the progress of the weakness, for better or for worse, can be followed.

ASSOCIATED PHYSICAL SIGNS

It is incumbent upon the examiner to differentiate weakness of central origin from that due to peripheral processes. The associated signs and the patterns of weakness help with this differentiation.

Upper Motor Neuron Lesions

Hypertonia and hyperreflexia, often combined with extensor plantar responses, are the clues to UMN localization.

Hypertonia or spasticity is evaluated by passively moving the limbs at the joints, commonly at the knees, wrists, and elbows. A catch of tone that rapidly settles—so-called clasp-knife rigidity—suggests an UMN lesion.

With the patient supine and relaxed, when the leg is passively rotated from side to side, the foot is normally "floppy" at the ankle and lags behind the rotatory movement. If the foot and leg move en bloc, hypertonia is present.

With the patient supine and relaxed, the examiner places hands under each popliteal fossa to gently support the legs. Quite abruptly the knees are jerked upward from this rest position. A normal response is for the heels to move proximally, scraping along the examining couch. If they jerk upward and then come to rest on the couch, spasticity is present.

Clonus at the ankles is tested for by abruptly passively dorsiflexing the foot on the ankle with the knee bent. Repetitive clonic jerking contractions of the calf muscles may fade after a few beats or be sustained.

Hyperreflexia refers to exaggerated tendon reflex responses. In extreme hyperreflexia, the reflex is repetitive or clonic. The limb to be tested should be supported so that it is perfectly relaxed, and the reflex hammer should be allowed to fall on the tendon close to the neighboring joint and more or less bounce off. The reflexes are commonly recorded in the chart on a stick figure using a "plus" grading system, which should be constant for any particular examiner. Thus, biceps, triceps, and brachioradialis reflexes are recorded in the upper limb, and knee and ankle reflexes are recorded in the lower limb.

Whereas hypertonia and hyperreflexia imply disinhibition of the final common pathway, a non- or extrapyramidal effect, the extensor plantar response implies a pyramidal tract lesion. The lateral aspect of the sole is scraped from heel to little toe with a somewhat sharp object. Often the end of a key will do. The full extensor response is extension of the great toe, fanning of the other toes, and contraction of the tensor fascia lata. This last sign can be extremely helpful if doubt exists as to the toe responses. Experimentally, a pure pyramidal tract lesion causes a flaccid paralysis or paresis with an extensor plantar response. On occasion, slowness of voluntary rapid alternating movements may be the only sign of pyramidal tract involvement.

In UMN lesions, the superficial or cutaneous reflexes are often suppressed or absent. The abdominal reflexes are elicited by gently scratching the abdominal wall in all four quadrants; the abdominal wall normally contracts spasmodically. This reflex may be absent unilaterally on the side of a hemiplegia. In males, the cremasteric reflex is elicited by gently scratching the upper inner aspect ot the thigh in broad sweeps. Normally the cremasteric muscle contracts and elevates the ipsilateral side of the scrotum.

Anatomic Substrate for Upper Motor Neuron Lesions

The Descending Corticospinal Tract. This is the major descending motor pathway. The tract is composed of axons of mainly cortical frontal cells, amongst them the pyramidal cells of Betz, of the contralateral hemisphere. This is therefore a crossed tract, the decussation occurring in the lower medulla as the pyramidal decussation. Seventy-five to 90 percent of fibers cross to become the lateral corticospinal tract. The remainder descend in the uncrossed ventral or direct pyramidal tract situated ventromedially in the anterior funiculus. The lateral corticospinal tract fibers terminate on the anterior horn of the central gray matter. Ten to 20 percent synapse directly with anterior horn cells. The rest terminate as arborizations around intercalated cells in the intermediate or ventral gray matter. This major motor tract shows a somatotopic arrangement of fibers in the cord such that those destined for sacral regions are laterally placed and those destined for cervical regions are medially situated with an orderly arrangement between.

Extrapyramidal Descending Tracts. The major nonpyramidal descending tracts originate in the brainstem. Their cells of origin receive connections from higher levels, and the tracts are named according to their brainstem level. They function in conjunction with the pyramidal tract to allow for smooth and coordinated movement and have excitatory and inhibitory effects on the motor neurons of the cord. The tectospinal, reticulospinal, and vestibulospinal tracts lie in the anterior funiculus, and the rubrospinal tract lies in the lateral funiculus just ventral to the corticospinal tract.

The more medially situated pathways—that is, those in the anterior funiculus as described above—are phylogenetically older and control axial and proximal muscles, those governing balance and posture. The rubrospinal tract is more concerned with distal muscles, those governing dexterity and fine movements. In humans, this latter function has largely been taken over by the corticospinal system, and the rubrospinal tract is vestigial.

Lower Motor Neuron Lesions

The hallmarks of LMN-associated signs are flaccidity, areflexia, and flexor plantar responses, provided that the foot flexor muscles retain the ability to contract. Testing is as described above for UMN lesions.

Fasciculations in the presence of weakness point to the anterior horn cell as the likely site of pathology.

The anatomic substrate is composed of the varied anatomy of the cranial nerves, anterior horn cells, spinal nerves, nerve plexuses, individual peripheral nerves, the neuromuscular junctions, and the muscles.

PATTERNS OF WEAKNESS

On occasion, the expected associated signs to support UMN versus LMN localization of a lesion are equivocal or absent. In that circumstance, the pattern of weakness in the limbs can be extremely useful in diagnosis.

Upper Motor Neuron Patterns

When the deficit is very severe, a paralysis is seen, and no pattern is evident. In more moderate and often subtle deficits, typical patterns of weakness are consistently present.

In the upper limb, the pattern of weakness in UMN lesions is that of weakness of extensor muscles. The muscles that are preferentially involved (i.e., the weaker muscles) are deltoid, triceps, wrist and finger extensors, and finger abductors. Conversely, biceps, shoulder adductor muscles, wrist and finger flexors, and finger adductors are mostly spared.

In the lower limb, hip flexors, foot and toe dorsiflexors, hamstrings, and thigh abductors are weaker than quadriceps and toe and foot plantar flexors.

Lower Motor Neuron Patterns

LMN patterns of weakness vary with the site of pathology, which may vary, ranging from dysfunction of anterior horn cell through spinal nerve root, plexus, nerve, endplate, and muscle itself.

Anterior Horn Cell. In degenerative diseases affecting the anterior horn cells, such as motor neuron disease (MND), there is no specific pattern. On occasion, the disease process may affect limbs sequentially but in a rather diffuse pattern.

The patient often presents with a combination of UMN and LMN signs. Thus whereas there may be atrophy with weakness predominantly in "LMN muscles," there is also hyperreflexia. Fasciculations may be prominent. If all the signs are localized

TABLE 2-1. Cervical Myotomes[a]

Segmental Level	Muscle(s)	Action
C5	Deltoid	Shoulder abduction
	Biceps/brachialis	Elbow flexion
C6, 7	Triceps	Elbow extension
	Brachioradialis	Elbow flexion in half supination
C6	Extensor carpi radialis	"Radial" wrist extension
C7	Extensor digitorum	Finger extension
C8	Flexor digitorum	Finger flexion
T1	Interossei	Finger abduction
	Abductor digiti V	Little-finger abduction

[a] Clinically useful main segmental innervation of muscle groups is shown. It should be appreciated that the nerve supply of all muscles is of multisegmental origin, and that this table is designed to help with clinical localization, rather than to present a complete anatomic guide.

to a midcervical level, cervical spondylosis is the likely diagnosis. If fasciculations are seen in noncervical myotomes or there are bulbar signs, MND is likely. The electromyogram (EMG) may be used as a diagnostic tool to study masseter and tongue muscles. EMG signs of diffuse and bulbar denervation strongly support the diagnosis of MND. At times cervical spondylosis and MND coexist in the same patient.

Spinal Nerve Root. Root involvement causes a "myotomal" pattern of weakness that varies with the root involved. Because of overlapping innevation, as described in anatomic texts, it may be quite bewildering to sort out involvement of one root from another. Experimentally, to produce segmental radicular paralysis, at least two roots need to be cut. In practice, we see weakness rather than paralysis, and it is usually possible to localize radicular weakness fairly accurately using a modified and simplified anatomy (Tables 2-1 and 2-2). The presence of a clearly defined root lesion, diagnosed by way of either myotomal weakness, dermatomal sensory loss, or a dropped reflex, is the only clear pointer to segmental localization within the spinal cord.

Nerve Plexus. The next level, moving distally, is the plexus—brachial in the upper limb and lumbosacral in the

TABLE 2-2. Lumbosacral Myotomes[a]

Segmental Level	Muscle(s)	Action
L1, L2	Iliopsoas	Hip flexion
L3	Adductor longus	
	Adductor brevs	
	Adductor magnus	Hip adduction
	Adductor minimus	
L3, L4	Quadriceps femoris	Knee extension
L4	Tibialis anterior	Ankle extension
L5	Extensor hallucis longus	
	Extensor hallucis brevis	
	Extensor digitorum longus	Toe extension
	Extensor digitorum brevis	
	Gluteus medius	Hip abduction
L5, S1	Semitendinosis	
	Semimembranosis	Knee flexion
	Biceps femoris	
S1	Gastrocnemius	
	Soleus	Ankle flexion
	Flexor digiti brevis	Toe flexion

[a] Clinically useful main segmental innervation of muscle groups is shown. It should be appreciated that the nerve supply of virtually all muscles is of multisegmental origin, and that this table is designed to help with clinical localization, rather than to present a complete anatomic guide.

lower limb. For plexus localization, the pattern of weakness fits neither a pure root distribution nor a single pure peripheral nerve distribution.

Peripheral Nerve. Although there is some variability, each single peripheral nerve consistently supplies specific muscles, which allows for localization based on the deficit found (Table 2-3).

Diffuse peripheral neuropathy causes a distal wasting and weakness syndrome. In severe cases, the weakness is so widespread as to cause total body paralysis with atonic muscles and areflexia. If of an acute or subacute onset, this suggests the diagnosis of Guillain-Barré syndrome.

Neuromuscular Junction. Variability in weakness over minutes or hours with waxing and waning suggests the diagnosis of myasthenia gravis. The diagnosis is established by demonstrating a myasthenic reaction or by reversing the signs with an injection of edrophonium. A myasthenic reaction is, by definition, increasing muscle weakness with exercise or weakness brought on by activity of the muscle being tested. It must be demonstrated that a muscle becomes weaker the more it is used. For eye muscles, prolonged lateral or vertical gaze results in progressive diplopia or observable progressive weakness of the extraocular muscles being exercised. In the limbs, one offers continual resistance to the muscle being exercised while evaluating its strength. Weakness ensues and becomes progressively worse. Pressure must be exerted continually and not intermittently, since even a brief rest can allow for restoration of power.

Muscle. Weakness localized to the pelvic and shoulder girdle muscles (i.e., proximal muscle weakness) supports the diagnosis of a myopathic disorder. Chronic spinal muscular atrophy, a neuropathic degenerative anterior horn cell syndrome, will often show the same distribution.

ADDITIONAL CLUES TO LOCALIZATION

The presence of cognitive deficits suggests that the lesion is in or undercuts the cortex.

Primarily proximal (i.e., limb girdle) weakness of an UMN type supports the notion of a high-convexity lesion. On the left side, this is often accompanied by a transcortical aphasia. This site of deficit is frequently due to an infarct in the watershed region and is seen primarily following an episode of acute circulatory failure with severe hypotension or after carotid occlusion with inadequate collateral perfusion.

A very dense hemiplegia without cognitive loss suggests that the lesion is in the deep white matter, often in the internal capsule.

A mild hemiparesis with prominent ataxia or dysarthria suggests a lacunar infarction either in the posterior limb of the internal capsule or in the pons. At times, lacunae in the corona radiata or larger lesions in the contralateral frontal lobe also cause an ataxic hemiparesis.

The finding of a cranial nerve deficit on one side with an UMN weakness on the contralateral side places the lesion in the brainstem precisely at the level of the cranial nerve involved. This is called an alternating hemiplegia or hemiparesis. Spinothalamic sensation may be affected in a similar fashion contralateral to a lateral medullary lesion, resulting in a so-called harlequin pattern of loss.

TABLE 2-3. Principle Motor Innervation of Peripheral Nerves[a]

Nerve	Muscle(s)	Action
Axillary	Deltoid	Shoulder abduction
Musculocutaneous	Biceps Brachialis	Flexion of elbow
Median	Flexor carpi radialis	Radial flexion of wrist
	Flexor digitorum sublimis	Flexion of middle phalanges (digiti II–V)
	Flexor digitorum profundus (lateral half)	Flexion of distal phalanges (digiti II and III)
	Pronator teres Pronator quadratus	Pronation of forearm
	Abductor pollicis brevis	Abduction of thumb
	Opponens pollicis brevis	Opposition of thumb
	Flexor pollicis longus	Flexion of distal phalanx of thumb
	Flexor pollicis brevis	Flexion of proximal phalanx of thumb
Ulnar	Flexor carpi ulnaris	Ulnar flexion of wrist
	Flexor digitorum profundus (medial half)	Flexion of distal phalanges (digiti IV and V)
	Abductor digiti minimi	Abduction digiti V
	All other intrinsics of hand	Finger abduction/adduction
Radial	Triceps	Extension at elbow
	Brachioradialis	Flexion of forearm
	Extensor carpi radialis/ulnaris	Extension at wrist with radial/ulnar deviation
	Supinator	Supination of forearm
	Extensor	
	Pollicis brevis	Extension of thumb—proximal
	Pollicis longus	Extension of thumb—distal
	Indicus proprius	Extension of index—proximal
	Digiti V proprius	Extension of little finger—proximal
	Digiti communis	Extension of digits II–V—proximal
Femoral	Iliopsoas	Flexion of thigh at hip
	Quadriceps	Extension of leg at knee
Obturator	Adductor longus Adductor brevis Adductor magnus	Adduction of thigh at hip
Superior gluteal	Gluteus medius Gluteus minimus	Abduction of thigh at hip
	Gluteus maximus	Extension of thigh at hip
Sciatic	Biceps femoris Semitendinosus Semimebranosus	Flexion of leg at knee
Sciatic branches Peroneal—deep	Tibialis anterior	Dorsiflexion of foot
	Extensor digitorum longus	Extension of toes
	Extensor hallucis longus	Extension of great toe
Peroneal—superficial	Peroneus	Pronation of foot
Tibial	Gastrocnemius Soleus	Plantar flexion of foot
	Flexor	
	Digitorum longus	Flexion of distal phalanges II–IV
	Hallucis longus	Flexion of distal phalanx 1
	Digitorum brevis	Flexion of middle phalanges II–V
	Hallucis brevis	Flexion of middle phalanx 1
Pudendal	Perineal and sphincters	Closure of sphincters Contraction of pelvic floor

[a] Clinically useful main segmental innervation of muscle groups is shown. It should be appreciated that this table is designed to help with clinical localization, rather than to present a complete anatomic guide.

Neck extensor muscles are normally very strong. Their power is tested by resting one's arms on the patient's shoulders and pushing forward with the fingers on the back of the head against maximal resistance. Weakness of the neck extensors has relatively few causes, which include myopathy, myasthenia, MND, and myotonic dystrophy.

Paraparesis suggests myelopathy. The long tract weakness will be in UMN distribution, often with other helpful signs, such as spasticity or hyperreflexia. Extensor plantar responses are hard signs to support the diagnosis of UMN dysfunction, but flexor responses in the presence of the other UMN cluster of signs do not negate the diagnosis. Just as in the sensory deficit of myelopathy, because of the so-called onion peeling somatotopic distribution of fibers within the major descending and ascending tracts, segmental localization based on UMN weakness can be difficult. The level of pathology is deduced by the finding of myotomal weakness, dermatomal sensory loss, or a dropped reflex (i.e., a root sign). Thus, the root signs of cord pathology are the counterpart of cranial nerve signs of brainstem pathology and allow for accurate segmental localization.

Bladder symptoms often help to raise the suspicion of myelopathy. The typical UMN bladder is of low capacity, hypertonic, and irritable. Thus urgency, frequency, and urgency incontinence are characteristic.

In brachial plexopathy, the combination of deltoid weakness (axillary nerve) with triceps weakness and wrist drop (radial nerve) localizes to the posterior cord of the plexus. The diagnosis of a more proximal brachial plexopathy may be strongly supported by the finding of a Horner syndrome.

Lateralized weakness of flexor hip girdle muscles may be of lumbosacral plexus origin. Here, diagnosis may be aided using the following paradigm: weakness of hip adductors, hip flexors, and quadriceps suggests high lumbar radiculopathy; weakness of adductors alone indicates an obturator nerve lesion, and weakness of quadriceps alone localizes to the femoral nerve; weakness of any two of the three groups supports the diagnosis of a plexus lesion. On occasion, a root lesion at L4 causes mild to moderate quadriceps weakness with an absent patellar reflex.

In wrist drop, there may be spurious weakness of the finger flexors. Since these can function at maximal power only if the wrist is in extension, when testing this movement the wrist should be held in passive forced extension. A proximal radial nerve palsy can be distinguished from cervical radiculopathy (C6–C7) by testing strength and bulk in the lower fibers of pectoralis major: if weakness is present here, the localization is likely to be fairly close to the root—the patient places hands on hips and forcefully adducts; the examiner places fingers posterior to the muscle in the anterior axillary fold and pushes forward.

In LMN foot drop, the common differential diagnosis is between a common peroneal palsy at the knee and a lumbar radiculopathy (L4–L5). In the former, foot inversion (posterior tibial nerve) is spared and is normal. In radiculopathy, both foot inversion and eversion are weak, as are knee flexion and hip abduction.

SUGGESTED READINGS

Berardelli A, Sabra AF, Hallett M et al: Stretch reflexes of triceps surae in patients with upper motor neuron syndromes. J Neurol Neurosurg Psychiatry 46:54–60, 1983

Bishop B: Spasticity: its physiology and management. Part 1. Neurophysiology of spasticity: classical concepts. Phys Ther 57:371–6, 1977

Davidoff RA: Skeletal muscle tone and the misunderstood stretch reflex. Neurology 42:951–63, 1992

Georgopoulos AP: Higher order motor control. Annu Rev Neurosci 14:361–77, 1991

Messina C: Pathophysiology of muscle tone. Funct Neurol 5:217–23, 1990

Young RR: Physiologic and pharmacologic approaches to spasticity. Neurol Clin 5:529–39, 1987

Younger DS: Differential diagnosis of progressive flaccid weakness. Semin Neurol 13:241–6, 1993

3. MOVEMENT DISORDERS

DANIEL TARSY

Movement disorders compose the neurologic conditions characterized by abnormalities of movement and posture. These are broadly and somewhat arbitrarily divided into akinetic and hyperkinetic or dyskinetic syndromes. Since akinesia is often accompanied by rigidity, the category of akinetic-rigid syndromes is used to designate what is usually referred to as parkinsonism. The hyperkinetic or dyskinetic syndromes comprise the disorders characterized by excessive or poorly regulated movements or postures and include tremor, chorea, ballismus, dystonia, dyskinesia, myoclonus, and tics. Most, but not all of these conditions, are attributable to disorders of the basal ganglia or extrapyramidal system, but it is important to realize that many have not been well localized in the nervous system. By tradition, motor disorders due to cerebellar, pyramidal tract, motor neuron, peripheral nerve, or muscle diseases are not included in this category and so are not discussed here.

AKINETIC-RIGID SYNDROMES

Akinetic-rigid syndromes are the most common movement disorders to require neurologic evaluation and include various combinations of akinesia, rigidity, and disturbed balance and posture. Tremor is commonly associated with akinesia and rigidity and is discussed separately below. The most common cause of these signs is idiopathic Parkinson's disease, but they also occur in other forms of parkinsonism, when they are commonly accompanied by other neurologic signs.

Idiopathic Parkinson's disease is the most common akinetic-rigid syndrome to present in middle to late life and is discussed in detail in Chapters 113 to 116. Major features are tremor, rigidity, akinesia, and postural abnormality. Patients typically present between ages 50 and 70 with complaints of tremor, usually accompanied by unilateral or asymmetric clumsiness of one hand and sometimes the leg on the same side. During initial evaluation, mild midline or contralateral symptoms or signs are often elicited from family members or observed on careful examination. These may include mildly reduced vocal or facial expression that is frequently mistaken for depression, a stare with reduced eyeblink frequency, slowing in routine activities of daily living, hesitation arising from deep chairs, flexed posture, and shuffling gait while turning. The characteristic rest tremor of Parkinson's disease is not always present and, when absent, often results in a delayed presentation with

TABLE 3-1. More Common Akinetic-Rigid Syndromes

Idiopathic Parkinson's disease
Postencephalitic parkinsonism
Parkinsonism due to drugs or toxins
Multiple system atrophy
    Striatonigral degeneration
    Shy-Drager syndrome
    Olivopontocerebellar degeneration (sporadic)
Other degenerative diseases
    Progressive supranuclear palsy
    Acquired hepatocerebral degeneration
    Corticobasal ganglionic degeneration
Genetically determined disorders
    Rigid Huntington's disease
    Wilson's disease
    Hallervorden-Spatz disease
    Pallidal degenerations
    Olivopontocerebellar degeneration (familial)
    Basal ganglia calcification
    Juvenile parkinsonism
    Dopa-responsive dystonia
    Metabolic disorders
Acquired secondary parkinsonism
    Multiple cerebral infarcts
    Postanoxic
    Hydrocephalus
    Punch-drunk syndrome
    Mass lesions (tumor, arterioventricular malformation)

(Modified from Weiner WJ, Lang AE: Movement Disorders: A Comprehensive Survey. Futura, Mt. Kisco, NY, 1989, with permission.)

midline akinetic signs. In more advanced cases, signs of akinesia and postural disturbance predominate. Progressive mutism, dysphagia, severe gait disturbance, freezing, and falls due to loss of postural reflexes may produce severe disability. The presence of such midline signs in advanced cases makes differentiation from other causes of parkinsonism more difficult than early in the disease.

A classification of the more common parkinsonian syndromes is listed in Table 3-1. Broad categories include primary idiopathic Parkinson's disease due to degeneration of substantia nigra; secondary forms of relatively pure parkinsonism such as neuroleptic induced, toxic, or postencephalitic parkinsonism; parkinsonism due to multiple system atrophy; parkinsonism associated with other degenerative or metabolic neurologic disorders, some of which are hereditary; and parkinsonism due to miscellaneous acquired structural or metabolic abnormalities. Any disorder that impairs nigral, striatal, or pallidal function may produce an akinetic-rigid syndrome. The term *parkinsonism-plus* is potentially confusing since it is often used to refer to both multiple sytematrophy as well as other less specific multisystem degenerations in which parkinsonism occurs in combination with other neurologic manifestations such as progressive supranuclear palsy.

The clinical characteristics and differential diagnosis of the akinetic-rigid syndromes will be discussed in greater detail in Part V of this book. It is sobering to note that, according to recent studies, 25 to 30 percent of patients diagnosed with idiopathic Parkinson's disease have been discovered to have other causes of parkinsonism at postmortem examination. The absence of resting tremor in a patient with akinesia, rigidity, and postural disturbance should serve as a clue that one is dealing with one of the other akinetic-rigid syndromes. This is particularly true if symmetric and midline motor manifestations appear early in the clinical course. Another useful clue to other forms of parkinsonism is the presence of pyramidal tract signs, cerebellar ataxia, nystagmus, oculomotor abnormalities, early and severe dementia, frontal release signs, sensory findings, or prominent autonomic disturbances early in the illness.

Parkinsonian syndromes due to multiple system atrophy are typically the most difficult to distinguish on clinical grounds from idiopathic Parkinson's disease. Multiple system atrophy is discussed in greater detail in Chapter 117. This specific group of three disorders comprises Shy-Drager syndrome, striatonigral degeneration, and the sporadic form of olivopontocerebellar atrophy. These are a heterogeneous group of disorders that share similar underlying neuropathology but exhibit a spectrum of variable and evolving neurologic findings that typically differ depending on when the patient is seen in the course of the disease. The presence of autonomic failure, such as orthostatic hypotension, bladder dysfunction, and impotence preceding the onset of significant motor disturbance is indicative of Shy-Drager syndrome. Predominant parkinsonism manifested by a rapidly progressive akinetic-rigid syndrome and relatively mild and variable tremor should suggest striatonigral degeneration. Cerebellar ataxia early in the course followed by parkinsonism and variable combinations of corticospinal tract deficits, oculomotor signs, pseudobulbar signs, dementia, lower cranial nerve palsies, optic atrophy and retinal degeneration, and muscle atrophy are the hallmarks of olivopontocerebellar atrophy. Other extrapyramidal features such as chorea and dystonia may also occur in olivopontocerebellar atrophy and complicate differential diagnosis.

Clinical differentiation among these three forms of multiple system atrophy is usually difficult and somewhat arbitrary. Since currently they are believed to be different clinical manifestations of a common distribution of neuropathology with a characteristic marker, the presence of oligodendroglial cytoplasmic inclusions, they are best grouped together under the diagnostic heading of multiple system atrophy. The most common clinical features of multiple system atrophy are parkinsonism with prominent akinesia, postural instability and falls; impotence, postural hypotension, and bladder dysfunction; relatively mild pyramidal signs without clinically important spasticity or weakness; and cerebellar ataxia. Less common but unique and helpful signs include respiratory stridor, myoclonic finger jerks, and antecollis. Mild tremor may be present but is more commonly an action than rest tremor. Dementia is notably absent in this group of disorders.

Progressive supranuclear palsy is sometimes included in the category of parkinson-plus syndromes but should be considered to be separate from multiple system atrophy because of its distinctive clinical presentation and neuropathology. The condition is best known for paralysis of voluntary vertical and horizontal gaze but produces a number of other highly characteristic motor manifestations that may precede the abnormal eye movements. Early symptoms include gait instability, sudden unexplained falls, generalized slowing, visual complaints, speech and swallowing difficulty, sleep disturbance, and personality change. By contrast with idiopathic Parkinson's disease, gait instability and falling are prominent early in the disease and are often the presenting manifestation. There are a number of characteristic neurologic findings in progressive supranuclear palsy. Supranuclear gaze palsy impairs downward more than upward gaze and also affects horizontal gaze. Initial eye findings may be subtle and limited to impaired saccadic movements. Progressive gaze difficulty and abnormalities of convergence and central fixation produce visual complaints such as difficulty reading and descending stairs, trouble focusing, and diplopia. Oculocephalic eye movements are disinhibited consistent with a supranuclear gaze paralysis. Other eye findings may include blepharospasm, levator inhibition with impaired voluntary eyelid opening, and square-wave jerks.

There is often a characteristic, sometimes astonished-appearing facial expression produced by the prominent stare, upper eyelid retraction, deep facial furrows, and impaired voluntary gaze that is considerably different from the facial masking of Parkinson's disease. Gait is lurching or stumbling, typically difficult to classify, and associated with impaired balance and tendency to fall easily. Rigidity is more marked in axial than limb muscles, but limb spasticity and dystonia may be prominent as late manifestations. Posture is relatively erect and there may be neck hyperextension. Tremor is uncommon but may occur. There is usually a pseudobulbar palsy with spastic dysarthria, dysphagia, and emotional release. Bilateral corticospinal tract findings are present, including hyperreflexia, spasticity, and extensor plantar responses. Dementia is usually not prominent early in the disease, although the abnormal facial expression and bradykinesia often convey a false impression of cognitive deficit. Cognitive function is typically difficult to evaluate late in the disease because of pseudobulbar anarthria, but may be impaired and is often associated with behavioral disturbance.

Parkinsonism may occur in association with a number of other primary degenerative neurologic disorders such as familial olivopontocerebellar atrophy, Huntington's disease, pallidal degenerations, corticobasal ganglionic degeneration, Alzheimer's and Pick's disease, basal ganglia calcification, Creutzfeldt-Jakob disease, Wilson's disease, and a number of metabolic and storage diseases of the nervous system. Differentiation of these disorders from idiopathic Parkinson's disease is usually assisted by the rest of the neurologic history and examination.

Acquired neurologic disorders that produce secondary parkinsonism can usually be differentiated clinically from idiopathic Parkinson's disease by history and examination and are described in Chapter 119. Neuroleptic- or metoclopramide-induced parkinsonism is relatively symmetric in distribution and more commonly associated with an action tremor than the typical resting tremor of idiopathic Parkinson's disease. However, asymmetry and rest tremor may also be observed. In such cases, often seen in older individuals, the possibility of underlying subclinical Parkinson's disease aggravated by dopamine-blocking medications should be considered. Parkinsonism due to toxin exposure is rare and is usually evident from the patient's medical history. Postencephalitic parkinsonism has disappeared as the population of patients who suffered encephalitis lethargica has declined. Occasional cases following viral encephalitis continue to occur but typically appear early without the prolonged latency characteristic of classic postencephalitic parkinsonism.

Other common causes of secondary parkinsonism include cerebrovascular disease with multiple small infarcts, anoxic encephalopathy, hydrocephalus, head trauma, brain tumor or arteriovenous malformation, and acquired hepatocerebral degeneration. Depending on the distribution of pathology, acquired brain disorders that cause parkinsonism are usually associated with dementia, corticospinal tract findings, pseudobulbar palsy, and gait ataxia. Severe dementia early in the clinical course can be a useful clue that one is dealing with secondary parkinsonism. Although multiple system atrophy also produces multisystem involvement, dementia is notably absent in multiple system atrophy, whereas autonomic manifestations are usually not present in the acquired disorders that produce parkinsonism.

A number of genetically mediated disorders may produce parkinsonism although usually in combination with other neurologic manifestations. The most important of these are the rigid form of Huntington's disease, Wilson's disease, familial olivopontocerebellar atrophy including Azorean disease, Hallervorden-Spatz disease, the pallidal degenerations, basal ganglia calcification, neuroacanthocytosis, dopa-responsive dystonia, juvenile parkinsonism, and rare metabolic and storage diseases usually seen in children or young adults such as GM_1 gangliosidosis and Gaucher's disease.

Approach to the Patient

Taking the medical history should be directed to eliciting symptoms of akinesia. *Akinesia* refers to impaired ability to move in the absence of paralysis and includes bradykinesia or slowness of movement and hypokinesia or reduced amplitude of movement. Akinesia is responsible for the vast majority of parkinsonian symptoms described by the patient and family, all of which relate to slowness and difficulty initiating, implementing, and maintaining motor movements. The pattern of akinetic symptoms will depend on whether there is unilateral, midline, or bilateral involvement. Idiopathic Parkinson's disease usually begins unilaterally or asymmetrically and typically presents with clumsiness and impaired dexterity in activities of daily living such as shaving, applying make-up, washing, dressing, using eating utensils, and handwriting. Shoulder or hip pain is an occasional early manifestation of limb akinesia. Midline involvement may produce facial masking with a staring and anxious expression, which may lead to a mistaken diagnosis of depression. Other midline symptoms may include soft and monotonic speech; stuttering; drooling; difficulty arising from a deep chair, turning in bed, or getting out of a car; and gait abnormality with short, shuffling steps and reduced armswing. More severe midline akinesia will cause impaired turning, propulsive and festinating gait, and episodes of freezing.

History related to cognitive, autonomic, and sensory function should be elicited from all patients. Dementia accompanies a number of the akinetic-rigid syndromes but is uncommon in multiple system atrophy. In parkinson's disease, dementia is a relatively late feature that occurs in approximately 25 to 30 percent of patients. When dementia is more severe and appears early, other akinetic-rigid syndromes such as multi-infarct dementia, normal pressure hydrocephalus, Creutzfeldt-Jakob disease, and progressive supranuclear palsy should be considered. Depression and passivity often characterize Parkinson's disease and may lead to a mistaken impression of dementia. In multiple system atrophy, autonomic symptoms typically precede motor symptoms, whereas they appear later in idiopathic Parkinson's disease. Constipation, urinary frequency, nocturia, and sexual dysfunction are particularly common in more advanced Parkinson's disease, whereas they appear earlier in multiple system atrophy. Orthostatic hypotension is a hallmark of multiple system atrophy but may also occur in milder form in Parkinson's disease with or without antiparkinson medications. Sensory symptoms such as pain or paresthesia occasionally occur in idiopathic Parkinson's disease and are of uncertain origin. Symptoms or signs of impaired cortical sensation are unique to corticobasal ganglionic degeneration.

Akinesia is readily evident throughout the neurologic examination during simple observation and when the patient is asked to carry out specific motor tasks. Facial expression and eyeblink frequency are reduced, and spontaneous gestures and repositioning movements may be lacking. Delay in initiating movements results in prolonged reaction time when a patient is asked to perform a movement. Slowness of movement is usually detectable by observation and confirmed by tests of distal and more proximal rapid alternating movements, including finger tapping, fist opening and closing, forearm pronation and supination, and foot tapping. In addition to being slow, there is a fatiguing of repetitive movements that produces a characteristic decremental pattern different from the more regular slowing produced by weakness and the poorly checked, ataxic movements produced by cerebellar dysfunction. In patients with tremor, repetitive movements may activate and assume the frequency of the associated tremor. Handwriting and drawing are slow and associated with fatiguing and micrographia.

Patients should be tested for ability to arise from a chair without use of the hands and should be observed walking back and forth in a long corridor. Postural abnormalities are frequent and may consist of postural deformity or postural instability. Examples of postural deformity include flexion of the neck, trunk, and joints of the extremities, which produces the characteristic simian posture of Parkinson's disease. Postural instability occurs late in the course of Parkinson's disease but may appear earlier in other akinetic-rigid syndromes such as progressive supranuclear palsy. Postural instability is manifested by impaired balance, unstable gait, retropulsion, and propulsive gait. There is a predisposition to sudden, unpredictable falls and failure of normal righting reflexes to prevent falls once they begin. The pull test or sternal shove are formal tests of righting responses in which the examiner either pulls back on the shoulders or shoves on the sternum. A mild deficit in postural righting reflexes is associated with several backward steps before balance is corrected. A more severe deficit produces falling backward en bloc without corrective movements of the arms or legs.

Rigidity is appreciated only during the formal examination and is an uncertain contributor to subjective motor symptoms. Many symptoms and signs that at one time were commonly attributed to muscle rigidity are actually due to akinesia and are known to remain after successful alleviation of rigidity with stereotactic thalamotomy. Rigidity is perceived as an increase in resistance to passive movement of the extremities or axial musculature. In the extremities, rigidity is equally distributed in flexors and extensors of the limb and may be associated with a cogwheel phenomenon if there is accompanying rest or action tremor. Mild rigidity may be elicited by reinforcement maneuvers such as having the patient perform repetitive movements of the contralateral limb.

TREMOR

Tremor is by far the most commonly observed movement disorder and, in fact, occurs from time to time in the vast majority of normal individuals, in whom it emerges as a result of exaggerated physiologic tremor. Tremor is defined as a rhythmic, oscillatory, and usually sinusoidal movement of a portion of the body with a relatively constant frequency and variable amplitude. Tremor occurs as a result of either alternating or relatively synchronous contractions of antagonistic muscles. Tremors may be broadly classified into static and action tremors. Static tremors have been broken down into tremors present at rest (rest tremor) and tremors present with the arms and hands held in a fixed posture (postural tremor). Action tremors may be divided into postural tremor and tremor that increases during goal-directed movement (intention tremor). In-

TABLE 3-2. Common Tremors

Rest tremor
  Parkinson's disease
  Parkinsonian syndromes
  Midbrain (rubral) tremor
  Wilson's disease
  Severe essential tremor
Postural-action tremor
  Enhanced physiologic tremor
  Essential tremor
  Primary writing tremor
  Other extrapyramidal disorders
    Parkinson's disease
    Wilson's disease
    Dystonia
  Cerebellar disease
  Peripheral neuropathy
Intention tremor (cerebellar outflow)
  Cerebellar disease
  Multiple sclerosis
  Midbrain stroke
  Midbrain trauma

(Modified from Weiner WJ, Lang AE: Movement Disorders: A Comprehensive Survey. Futura, Mt. Kisco, NY, 1989, with permission.)

tention tremor is sometimes also referred to as kinetic or terminal tremor. Since these categories are confusingly overlapping and inconsistently applied, tremors are classified here as resting, postural-action, and intention in type (Table 3-2). (More detailed discussions of tremor may be found in Ch. 121.)

Rest Tremor

The most common cause of rest tremor is Parkinson's disease. This is most evident when the affected body part is supported and completely at rest and temporarily dampens or disappears entirely during voluntary activity. Because of its suppression with activity, it usually produces less functional disability than postural-action or intention tremors. However, frequently, as soon as the body part assumes a new posture, the tremor reappears, thereby potentially interfering with use of eating utensils, handwriting, and similar motor activities. In most cases, rest tremor produces disability by its undesirable cosmetic effect and social embarrassment. Rest tremors characteristically fluctuate in amplitude and may appear and disappear depending on the degree of patient repose, if the patient feels he is under public observation, or related to other unidentifiable factors. In idiopathic Parkinson's disease, tremor usually appears first in one upper extremity and later spreads to involve the ipsilateral lower limb, followed by the contralateral side. Leg or foot tremor is more commonly due to Parkinson's disease than essential tremor. When the tremor is limited to distal muscles of the hand it often produces a characteristic ''pill rolling'' tremor. Tremor frequency is usually 4 to 6 Hz. When it increases in severity, it may become more continuous, larger in amplitude, and more proximal in distribution, but tremor frequency remains constant. The face, lips, and jaw may be involved, but unlike essential tremor or cerebellar disease, Parkinson's disease usually does not produce head tremor.

Rest tremor may also occur in isolation in other extrapyramidal disorders such as akinetic-rigid syndromes in which tremor is usually less prominent, Wilson's disease and non-Wilsonian hepatocerebral degeneration, and following midbrain injury due to stroke or trauma. An isolated low-amplitude rest tremor of the hand or jaw unaccompanied by other manifestations of parkinsonism sometimes occurs in elderly individuals in whom it usually does not progress to Parkinson's disease. This is to be distinguished from tremor-predominant Parkinson's disease, which occurs in younger patients who display other mild parkinsonian signs but often have a good prognosis for relatively slow progression. Rest tremor also occurs as a "spillover" phenomenon in a variety of disorders in which severe postural-action tremors predominate, such as Wilson's disease, severe forms of familial essential tremor, and other cerebellar or extrapyramidal syndromes. *Rubral tremor* refers to tremor that occurs following midbrain injury but that is due to lesions of superior cerebellar peduncle and possibly substantia nigra rather than red nucleus. This tremor is constant, occurs at rest, and either remains unchanged or more commonly increases with action and goal-directed activity.

Postural-Action Tremor

Postural and action tremors are the largest group of tremors and are elicited during examination under two circumstances: with the upper extremities suspended against gravity in a fixed posture and during the course of goal-directed activity.

Physiologic Tremor. All individuals have a very low amplitude, high-frequency tremor of about 10 to 12 Hz which is not visible under ordinary circumstances. Physiologic tremor results from a combination of mechanisms, including intrinsic motor neuron firing rates, suprasegmental influences on motor unit firing patterns, stretch reflex oscillations, and peripheral β-adrenergic mechanisms. Enhanced physiologic tremor is the most common cause of abnormal tremor. Many factors increase physiologic tremor, most by the common mechanism of increased sympathomimetic activity. Common drugs that increase adrenergic activity include β-adrenergic agonists such as terbutaline, isoproterenol, and epinephrine; amphetamines; tricyclic antidepressants; levodopa; nicotine; and xanthines such as theophylline and caffeine. Anxiety, excitement, fright, muscle fatigue, hypoglycemia, alcohol and narcotic withdrawal, thyrotoxicosis, fever, and pheochromocytoma also enhance physiologic tremor by adrenergic mechanisms. Miscellaneous toxic causes of increased physiologic tremor with unknown mechanisms include lithium, corticosteroids, sodium valproate, bromides, mercury, lead, and arsenic. Since enhanced physiologic tremor is the most common cause of postural-action tremor, it is apparent that a medical rather than primary neurologic cause for postural-action tremor will be found in most cases.

Essential Tremor. Essential tremor is a very common cause of postural-action tremor and is discussed in detail in Chapter 121. It is typically referred to as familial tremor when there is a family history, benign essential tremor when it is sporadic, and senile tremor when it appears for the first time after age 65. The use of *benign* as a modifier for essential tremor has historically been used to distinguish it from Parkinson's disease and other extrapyramidal disorders rather than as an indicator of its severity and is best omitted, since it is frequently associated with significant disability. Essential tremor often resembles enhanced physiologic tremor but results from abnormal central rather than peripheral nervous system mechanisms. However, in some cases, patients with essential tremor may develop superimposed enhanced physiologic tremor owing to anxiety or other adrenergic mechanisms, thereby increasing the severity of the tremor and potentially causing diagnostic confu-

sion. Subclasses of essential tremor based largely on the frequency and amplitude of the tremor have been suggested. These include benign essential tremor of relatively low amplitude and higher frequency; more severe essential tremor of higher amplitude and lower frequency often associated with rest tremor; postural-action tremor occurring with other neurologic disorders such as parkinsonism, dystonia, or peripheral neuropathy; and enhanced physiologic tremor.

Essential tremor most commonly affects the distal upper extremities but can also cause tremor of the head, voice, chin, trunk, and lower extremities. In the upper extremities, tremor becomes immediately apparent when the arms are held outstretched and typically increases at the very end of goal-directed movements such as drinking from a glass or finger-nose testing. If tremor oscillations increase steadily before arrival at the target rather than at the very termination of goal-directed activity, cerebellar outflow tremor should be considered, although a distinction between the two is often difficult. Lower extremity tremor rarely occurs in isolation and is usually associated with severe essential tremor. Head tremor may be vertical or horizontal and, although usually associated with upper extremity or voice tremor, is the predominant manifestation of essential tremor in some patients.

By definition, tremor should be the only manifestation of essential tremor. The most common differential diagnosis is with parkinsonian tremor. Although differentiation from classic rest tremor should be straightforward, some patients with Parkinson's disease have a postural-action tremor indistinguishable from essential tremor. In early cases of parkinsonian postural tremor, the presence of subtle bradykinesia or micrographia may assist in diagnosing Parkinson's disease, although these signs may not appear until later in the course. The presence of ataxia, dysmetria, proximal distribution of tremor, or gait disorder usually suggests a cerebellar disorder rather than essential tremor, although in some severe familial tremors, mild cerebellar signs appear to coexist with tremor. The presence of head tremor is particularly useful in separating essential tremor from parkinsonian tremor, in which head tremor is usually limited to the jaw or lips. Head tremor is also common in cervical dystonia, in which it may be due either to a coincidence of the two disorders or to a manifestation of dystonic spasm. Voice tremor rarely occurs in isolation and, when it does, should be differentiated from spasmodic dysphonia. Voice tremor produces a quavering voice unaccompanied by the straining and voice breaks characteristic of spasmodic dysphonia.

Essential Tremor Variants. Many postural-action tremors associated with essential or parkinsonian tremor are most severe during the act of writing. However, when tremor occurs exclusively while writing and not during other voluntary motor activities, it is referred to as *primary writing tremor*. This tremor is limited to the upper extremity while writing and causes relatively large amplitude supination-pronation movements at a frequency of 5 to 6 Hz. The low frequency and large amplitude of the tremor, its occasional association with writer's cramp, its relative resistance to propranolol, and its responsiveness to anticholinergic drugs suggest a closer relationship to dystonia than essential tremor.

Orthostatic tremor is limited to the legs and trunk and occurs exclusively while standing. Both high- and low-frequency tremors have been described; their relationship to essential tremor is uncertain. In cases of high-frequency tremor, the movements of the lower extremities may be so low in amplitude as to initially escape clinical detection.

Cerebellar Tremors.   Cerebellar tremors may be either postural-action or intention in type and, in severe cases, can spill over to occur at rest. They are relatively low in frequency at about 3 to 4 Hz and are associated with ataxia and dysmetria. *Rubral tremor* is due to disturbances of cerebellothalamic projections rather than the red nucleus itself, is characteristically present at rest, but increases during postural fixation and voluntary activity. Titubation of the head and neck may be associated with cerebellar tremor and is distinguished from essential head tremor by the presence of other cerebellar findings.

Other Extrapyramidal Disorders.   Postural-action tremor may occur in Parkinson's disease, other parkinsonian syndromes, Wilson's disease, and idiopathic torsion dystonia. Parkinsonian postural-action tremor is the most common of these and is discussed above. In Wilson's disease, postural-action tremor may be present in isolation or together with both rest and intention tremor. There is a high coincidence of postural-action tremor in dystonia, especially in cervical dystonia and writer's cramp.

Neuropathic Tremor.   Tremor is sometimes associated with large-fiber peripheral neuropathy. This association is most commonly observed in hereditary neuropathies, during the recovery phase of some cases of Guillain-Barré syndrome, and in chronic inflammatory demyelinating polyneuropathy. Muscle weakness and loss of proprioceptive or muscle spindle inputs have been offered as an explanation for this tremor. The type of tremor observed under these circumstances is variable and may be high-frequency and low-amplitude in type or low-frequency, high-amplitude and associated with proprioceptive or cerebellar ataxia.

Intention Tremor

Intention tremor is due to disturbances of the cerebellar outflow projection system mediated by the dentate nucleus and superior cerebellar peduncle. This large-amplitude tremor typically increases in severity as the body part moves closer to its target, in contrast to postural-action tremors, which either remain constant throughout the range of motion or increase at terminal fixation. These tremors are large in amplitude owing to involvement of proximal muscles and are sometimes difficult to distinguish from severe cerebellar ataxia and dysmetria. Nonetheless, the frequent association with ataxia, dysmetria, titubation, and other cerebellar signs is common and serves to identify the cerebellar origin of intention tremor. The most common causes are multiple sclerosis, midbrain trauma, and stroke. Degenerative diseases of the dentate nucleus and cerebellar outflow pathways, severe forms of essential tremor, Wilson's disease, hepatocerebral degeneration, and mercury poisoning may also produce intention tremor. Rubral tremor is due to lesions of the dentatothalamic projection system running through and near the red nucleus, which produce a combination of rest, postural-action, and intention tremor.

Approach to the Patient

Patient history concerning onset of tremor is usually straightforward, since this is a highly visible symptom readily evident to the patient and family members. Examination of old checkbook signatures may be useful in determining precise time of onset. Whether one is dealing with a rest, postural-action, or intention tremor is usually difficult to discern from patient history alone and is best left to the examination. Distribution of tremor and associated motor symptoms should be elicited, but here, too, it is usually more reliable to identify these by examination than through history. Precipitating, aggravating, or relieving factors, such as caffeine, alcohol, medications, exercise, fatigue, or stress, should be elicited. Family history is important in cases of essential or parkinsonian tremor.

Examination begins with observations of the tremor made during the interview. Many patients with tremor are more symptomatic early during the examination because of stress than after they become used to the situation. Patients should be observed while seated, lying down with the relevant body part fully supported, and while ambulating. Horizontal or vertical head tremor is usually associated with essential tremor but may also occur in cervical dystonia and midline cerebellar syndromes. Face, jaw, and lip tremors are more commonly a manifestation of parkinsonism, but palatal tremor should be sought as an indication of palatal myoclonus. Voice tremor is readily audible but may be enhanced by having the patient hold a prolonged note.

Extremity tremor is observed with the affected limb fully supported at rest, with the limb elevated against gravity, and during goal-directed movements. Most rest tremors cease with changes in limb posture but will quickly reappear following repositioning. Action-postural tremors are best elicited with the patient's arms held outstretched, with the patient's index fingers held an inch apart in front of the face, during patient finger–nose maneuvers, and while the patient drinks from a paper cup. Writing and drawing may demonstrate the large, tremulous, angulated loops of essential tremor or the micrographia of parkinsonism. Lower extremity tremor should be assessed at rest, during heel-shin testing, and while standing and walking. Leg tremor is more commonly due to parkinsonism than essential tremor. Frequency of tremor should be documented at rest and during postural and action maneuvers. Enhanced physiologic tremor is high in frequency at 10 to 12 Hz, essential tremor can be low- or high-frequency, and parkinsonian rest tremor is usually low in frequency at 4 to 6 Hz. Psychogenic tremors often vary in frequency from moment to moment and may subside when the patient is asked to carry out a repetitive motor task with the contralateral limb.

CHOREA

The term *chorea* means *dance* and is used to refer to an involuntary movement disorder characterized by a panoply of randomly appearing irregular, purposeless, jerky movements of various portions of the body, extremities, and face. The character, location, and duration of individual movements is unpredictable, although individual patients usually exhibit a certain repertoire of recurrent abnormal movements and postures that become stereotyped and characteristic for them. Involuntary movements are usually quick and jerky but may sometimes occur in the form of more prolonged alterations of posture. Quicker movements may resemble myoclonus or tics, whereas slower movements may appear dystonic. Early manifestations of chorea can be subtle and sometimes resemble fidgetiness more than a movement disorder. The patient and family are often unaware of abnormal movements at this stage and may report only motor restlessness. Early subjective complaints usually consist of clumsiness, dropping of objects, and loss of fine motor coordination of the extremities. Later in the course, unsteady gait, abnormal postures of the arms and hands while walking, and impaired balance may become prominent.

Examination may reveal a wide variety of involuntary movements of the face, extremities, and trunk. In mild chorea, involuntary movements may be infrequent, of small amplitude, and relatively isolated, giving an appearance difficult to distinguish from myoclonus or tics. Some choreic movements can be partly suppressed or successfully obscured by incorporation into semi-purposeful movements. In more advanced chorea, movements occur nearly continuously and appear to spread fluidly from site to site over the body. Abnormal facial expression is particularly prominent in chorea associated with Huntington's disease owing to a unique combination of reduced facial expression with superimposed involuntary facial movements such as elevation or frowning movements of the eyebrows, increased eye-blinking, pursing or puckering of the lips, blowing out of the cheeks, and various movements of the tongue and jaw. Abnormal movements and postures of the trunk may include arching of the back, flexion and extension of the trunk, stretching of the neck, shoulder shrugging, and rocking of the pelvis. Abnormal limb movements can be distributed proximally or distally and may include sudden and sustained twisting or extension postures of an arm or leg, distal twisting movements of the wrist or hands, small-amplitude, jerky movements of the hands or fingers, extensor posturing of the large toes, and piano-playing movements of individual fingers. The overall appearance often conveyed is that of a marionette being unpredictably jerked about by pulling on its strings. Respiratory dyskinesia may also be a manifestation of chorea and produce irregular breathing, grunting noises, and air gulping.

Depending on the etiology of the chorea, other motor abnormalities may coexist with the involuntary movements and may be a greater source of disability than the chorea itself. This is particularly true in Huntington's disease, in which dysarthria, gait disturbance, and eye movement abnormality may be prominent. Motor impersistence is particularly common in Huntington's disease and is manifest by inability to maintain a strong grip or keep the tongue protruded for more than several seconds. Oculomotor abnormalities in Huntington's disease may include impaired saccadic movements and saccadic pursuit. The gait is typically abnormal in Huntington's disease and is associated with more abnormal movements and postures than are evident when the patient is sitting down. This may produce a broad-based lurching and ataxic gait disorder over and above the effects of the chorea. In advanced cases, gait and balance become severely compromised, leading to multiple falls and wheelchair confinement.

The differential diagnosis of chorea in the adult is broad and includes a large number of hereditary, degenerative, and acquired disorders (Table 3-3). For practical purposes, the more common causes of chorea in adulthood other than Huntington's disease include tardive dyskinesia due to antipsychotic drugs; choreoathetosis due to stimulants, antiparkinson drugs, or anticonvulsants; cerebrovascular causes such as basal ganglia lacunar infarction and subthalamic hemorrhage; systemic diseases such as acquired hepatolenticular degeneration and systemic lupus erythematosis; metabolic disorders such as hyperthyroidism, hypoparathyroidism, and acute electrolyte imbalance; Sydenham's chorea; senile chorea; and hereditary disorders such as multiple system atrophy, Wilson's disease,

TABLE 3-3. Common Causes of Chorea

Hereditary disorders
  Neurometabolic disorders
    Wilson's disease
    Lesch-Nyhan disease
    Abnormal carbohydrate metabolism (e.g., galactosemia)
    Abnormal lipid metabolism (e.g., GM_1 and GM_2 gangliosidosis)
    Amino acidopathies (e.g., glutaric acidemia)
  Huntington's disease
  Hallervorden-Spatz disease
  Neuroacanthocytosis
  Sea-blue histiocytosis
  Ataxia telangiectasia
  Machado-Joseph disease
  Olivopontocerebellar atrophy
  Paroxysmal dystonic choreoathetosis
  Paroxysmal kinesigenic choreoathetosis
  Benign familial chorea
Drug-induced disorders
  Neuroleptics
  Stimulants
    Amphetamines
    Methyphenidate
    Pemoline
    Cocaine
    Caffeine
    Aminophylline
  Anti-parkinsonian agents
  Anticonvulsants
  Oral contraceptives
  Opiates
  Antihistamines
Systemic illnesses
  Systemic lupus erythematosus and the antiphospholipid antibody syndrome
  Acquired hepatolenticular degeneration
  Polycythemia rubra vera
  Vasculitis
  Behçet's disease
Toxins
  Carbon monoxide
  Alcohol
  Manganese
  Toluene
Metabolic disorders
  Hyperthyroidism
  Hypoparathyroidism
  Hyper- and hyponatremia
  Hyper- and hypoglycemia
  Hypocalcemia
  Hypomagnesemia
Infections and parainfectious disorders
  Sydenham's chorea
  Other post-infectious encephalitides
  Viral encephalitis
Neoplasia
  Primary and metastatic brain tumors
Cerebrovascular disorders
  Basal ganglion infarction
  Central nervous system hemorrhages
  Arteriovenous malformation
Others
  Pregnancy (chorea gravidarum)
  Senile chorea
  Cerebral palsy
  Kernicterus

(Modified from Weiner WJ, Lang AE: Movement Disorders: A Comprehensive Survey. Futura, Mt. Kisco, NY, 1989, with permission.)

benign familial chorea, neuroacanthocytosis, neurometabolic disorders, and paroxysmal choreoathetosis.

Huntington's disease is discussed in greater detail in Chapter 122. When there is a family history of chorea or other movement disorder, differentiation from benign familial chorea, multiple system atrophy, Wilson's disease, and paroxysmal dyskinesias is required. In benign familial chorea, onset occurs in very early childhood and is unassociated with akinetic-rigid features, cognitive changes, or progression, whereas multiple system atrophy and Wilson's disease rarely produce isolated chorea without other neurologic manifestations. The paroxysmal dyskinesias are discussed separately. The various causes of sporadic adult-onset chorea can usually be identified by history and appropriate laboratory tests. Huntington's disease may appear to be sporadic because of unavailability of accurate family history or genetic mutation. In such cases, the diagnosis may be established by DNA analysis for identification of excessive DNA triplet repeats. Senile chorea occurs after age 65, is unassociated with dementia, and is often limited to orofacial dyskinesia. Tardive dyskinesia (discussed in Chapter 123) may be differentiated from other choreiform disorders by the presence of more repetitive, stereotyped movements that predominantly but not exclusively involve muscles of the face, mouth, and tongue. Abnormal movements are often more dystonic than choreic, and the lack of progression, together with absence of other motor abnormalities such as motor impersistence, dysarthria, and gait ataxia, help to distinguish tardive dyskinesia from Huntington's disease. Chorea due to infarcts in basal ganglia is abrupt in onset and usually unilateral, although bilateral involvement occasionally occurs. Chorea may be the predominant manifestation of acquired hepatolenticular degeneration due to cirrhosis and portal hypertension. However, usually various combinations of tremor, akinesia, and rigidity are also present, together with asterixis and stigmata of chronic liver disease. Chorea due to drug intoxications or metabolic derangements is also abrupt in onset, usually associated with other acute neurologic manifestations, and identifiable by medical history and laboratory studies. Chorea due to streptococcal infection, systemic lupus erythematosis, pregnancy, or oral contraceptives is often relatively mild, is usually transient or fluctuating, and should be readily identifiable by history and appropriate laboratory studies.

Approach to the Patient

Taking a patient history must be directed at gathering possible clues to the large number of known medical and neurologic causes of chorea mentioned above. Family history, age of onset, progression, and associated cognitive or personality changes are particularly important with regard to Huntington's disease, benign hereditary chorea, degenerative diseases, and neurometabolic disorders. Acute onset in an adult should suggest drugs or drug withdrawal, systemic lupus, hyperthyroidism, recurrences of Sydenham's chorea due to oral contraceptives or pregnancy, or basal ganglia stroke.

Examination is observational in search of choreiform orofacial, extremity, or truncal movements. Subtle chorea may be difficult to distinguish from fidgety movements, some of which become incorporated into volitional movements. Dorsiflexion posturing of the large toe and piano-playing movements of the fingers while walking are characteristic of choreiform disorders. Involuntary respiratory movements and grunting noises are also frequently associated with chorea. Impersistence of tongue protrusion is typical of chorea but may be remarkably absent in severe orolingual dyskinesia due to neuroleptic drugs. Oculomotor abnormalities are present in Huntington's disease but also in other extrapyramidal disorders. Repetitive and goal-directed movements may appear awkward owing to either the chorea or other associated motor dysfunction. Gait may be ataxic in severe chorea, especially in Huntington's disease, in which motor abnormalities typically exceed the effects of cho-

rea. Dementia or other extrapyramidal signs, such as dystonia, akinesia, rigidity, tremor, myoclonus, or tics, should suggest a degenerative or neurometabolic disorder.

BALLISMUS

Ballismus refers to throwing or flinging movements of the limbs that are usually large in amplitude, of high velocity, and involve proximal more than distal musculature. Similar to chorea, movements are irregular and unpredictable but tend to be more continuous and higher in frequency than choreic movements. In most cases, ballismus is limited to one side of the body and is referred to as hemiballismus. The proximal distribution and rotatory character of the movements are often used to distinguish ballismus from chorea, but the distinction may be arbitrary, and there is much overlap in the characteristics of the two disorders and their pathologic substrate. Mild forms of hemiballismus sometimes present as a gait disorder due to proximal jerking movements of one leg. Hemiballismus is usually due to a focal destructive lesion of the contralateral subthalamic nucleus or its connections with globus pallidus, but has occasionally also been associated with lesions in the putamen, caudate nucleus, and thalamus. The most common cause is hemorrhage or infarction in the subthalamic nucleus. Although much less common, other focal processes, such as abscess, tumor, tuberculoma, toxoplasmosis, arteriovenous malformation, and multiple sclerosis, have also produced hemiballismus. The most common structural cause of bilateral ballismus is bilateral basal ganglia infarction, but it may also occur as a severe manifestation of degenerative disorders that produce chorea such as Huntington's disease. Toxic or metabolic abnormalities such as nonketotic hyperglycemia or intoxications with medications such as levodopa or anticonvulsants may also produce bilateral ballismus.

DYSTONIA

Dystonia is a disorder of abnormal posture and movement characterized by sustained muscle contraction that causes torsional and repetitive movements and abnormal postures. *Dystonia* is variously used to describe a specific type of focal or regional abnormal movement or posture, a syndrome that occurs secondary to a large number of specific nervous system diseases, or a primary disorder known as idiopathic torsion dystonia. Dystonic movements may be slow or rapid and are typically repetitive and patterned, by contrast with chorea, which is random and unpredictable, and myoclonus, which is rapid, rhythmic, and not associated with twisting changes in posture. Rapid dystonic movements are sometimes difficult to distinguish from myoclonus, and the term *myoclonic dystonia* is used. In some cases, rapid movements associated with dystonia are due to a patient's attempt to resist the abnormal posture, as in patients with cervical dystonia in whom as the head pulls to one side, it jerks intermittently in the opposite direction. The frequent association of postural-action tremor with focal dystonia also accounts for the presence of additional hyperkinetic movements in many cases.

Dystonic movements are characteristically more prominent during the execution of voluntary movements. *Action dystonia* refers to involuntary movements present only during voluntary use of a group of muscles and absent at rest. Some are task-specific and occur only with specific patterns of movement such as occupational cramp disorders; jaw, tongue, or vocal cord spasms while speaking; pharyngeal contractions while swallowing; and foot or toe dystonias while walking. As an action dystonia progresses, it may be precipitated by movements in body parts other than the involved area. In some cases, the dystonia progresses to produce a fixed posture at rest. Dystonia may be increased by fatigue or stress and improved or abolished by rest. Some patients discover sensory tricks that partially or completely suppress the abnormal movements or postures. These unusual characteristics of dystonia, together with otherwise normal neurologic examination results, sometimes lead to a mistaken diagnosis of conversion reaction.

Dystonia is classified in a number of ways, including age of onset, body distribution, and etiology. Age classification is broadly divided into childhood- and adult-onset dystonia. Distribution may be focal in one limb or body part; segmental in two or more adjacent body parts; multifocal in scattered body parts; generalized with face, limb, and axial involvement; or may have a hemidystonic distribution. Etiologic classification is divided into primary idiopathic and secondary symptomatic forms. Patients with idiopathic dystonia show no evidence for an identifiable cause of their symptoms and have normal neurologic examination results apart from dystonic manifestations. Childhood-onset dystonia is usually generalized and may be either idiopathic or due to underlying metabolic or structural disease. Idiopathic generalized dystonia in childhood typically begins focally, often in one lower extremity, and becomes generalized, whereas symptomatic forms are more likely to be generalized from onset. Adult-onset idiopathic dystonia usually remains focal or becomes segmental in distribution and only uncommonly becomes generalized. Hemidystonia is nearly always secondary to an identifiable structural abnormality in the contralateral putamen or thalamus. Common causes of dystonia are listed in Table 3-4.

Primary Dystonia

Primary dystonia is broadly divided into idiopathic generalized torsion dystonia and focal, segmental, and multifocal dystonia.

Generalized Dystonia. Generalized dystonia usually begins in childhood but may also appear in young adulthood. It typically has a focal onset involving the foot, hand, cranial, or axial muscles before spreading over months to years to involve adjacent and distant body regions. Childhood-onset torsion dystonia commonly begins in the lower extremity, whereas adult-onset torsion dystonia more commonly starts in the upper extremity, axial, or cranial musculature. Action dystonia is particularly common at the start but usually progresses to more constant dystonia and eventually to fixed dystonic postures. In children, inversion of one ankle and toe-walking are common presenting signs that initially may be alleviated by running, dancing, or walking backward. Later, dystonia spreads to other body regions and eventually causes major gait disturbance over a period of approximately 5 to 10 years. Childhood-onset idiopathic generalized torsional dystonia is usually genetically determined with an autosomal dominant pattern. Autosomal recessive and sex-linked recessive patterns of inheritance also occur.

Focal and segmental dystonias usually involve the upper extremity, cranial, and cervical musculature, do not progress after the first several months to years, and virtually always appear in adulthood. Most of these are sporadic, but a family history of focal dystonia has been observed in up to 25 percent of

TABLE 3-4. More Common Dystonias

Primary dystonia (idiopathic torsion dystonia)
  Hereditary
    Autosomal dominant
    Autosomal recessive
    X-linked recessive
    Paroxysmal dystonia
  Sporadic
    Childhood or adult-onset; generalized, segmental, or focal
Secondary dystonia
  Hereditary neurologic disorders due to identifiable metabolic defect
    Wilson's disease
    Dopa-responsive dystonia
    Gangliosidosis
    Metachromatic leukodystrophy
    Lesch-Nyhan syndrome
    Aminoacidurias
  Neurologic disorders (often hereditary) with undefined metabolic defect
    Leigh's disease
    Hallervorden-Spatz disease
    Neuronal ceroid-lipofuscinosis
    Dystonic lipidosis
    Basal ganglia calcification
    Ataxia-telangiectasis
    Neuroacanthocytosis
  Degenerative disorders
    Rigid Huntington's disease
    Parkinson's disease
    Pallidal degenerations
    Olivopontocerebellar degeneration
    Progressive supranuclear palsy
    Corticobasal ganglionic degeneration
  Acquired dystonia
    Perinatal brain injury, anoxia, kernicterus
    Anoxia, carbon monoxide
    Manganese toxicity
    Neuroleptic and antiparkinson drugs
    Stroke
    Head trauma
    Atrioventricular malformation
    Brain tumor
    Multiple sclerosis
    Peripheral trauma
  Psychogenic

(Modified from Weiner WJ, Lang AE: Movement Disorders: A Comprehensive Survey. Futura, Mt. Kisco, NY, 1989, with permission.)

cases. The clinical characteristics of these focal disorders are described in greater detail in Chapter 125, where their treatment with botulinum toxin is discussed.

Cervical Dystonia. Cervical dystonia or spasmodic torticollis is the most common focal dystonia that comes to medical attention. It usually begins in middle life when unlike in childhood, it is almost never due to a structural abnormality of the cervical spine. Several abnormal head positions occur, consisting of various combinations of torticollis (rotation), laterocollis (lateral tilt), retrocollis (head extension), and antecollis (head flexion). Unlike most other forms of dystonia, pain and discomfort are common and nearly always located in the posterior cervical region ipsilateral to the direction of head deviation. Sensory tricks that suppress the dystonia, such as placing a finger or hand on the chin or back of the neck, are more common than in other dystonias. Most patients exhibit tonic head deviation but clonic jerking or dystonic tremor is sometimes prominent and usually due to attempts to suppress the abnormal posture. Head tremor due to an associated essential tremor may also occur.

Cranial Dystonia. Cranial dystonia, also known as Meige's syndrome produces dystonic movements of the eyelids, face, tongue, and jaw. Blepharospasm is the most common manifestation and produces increased eyeblink frequency, forced closure of the eyelids, and apraxia of eyelid opening. Differential diagnosis includes secondary forms of blepharospasm due to neuroleptic drugs, Parkinson's disease, progressive supranuclear palsy, and rare brainstem lesions. Driving, bright lights, watching television and reading are common aggravating factors. There may be a variety of accompanying movements of the face, jaw, neck, or forehead that are secondary abortive attempts to control the blepharospasm and do not necessarily suggest a diagnosis of Meige syndrome. Oromandibular dystonia is the second most common manifestation of cranial dystonia. It may occur alone but usually accompanies other cranial dystonias such as blepharospasm, lingual, platysmal, or pharyngeal dystonia, and spasmodic dysphonia. Differential diagnosis includes tardive dystonia, edentulous jaw movements, and bruxism. Patterns of abnormal movements include jaw-opening, jaw-closing, and jaw deviation. The various movements typically occur synchronously in repetitive fashion. Oromandibular dystonia causes major disability, including pain, speech impairment, dysphagia, and oral trauma. Spasmodic dysphonia or laryngeal dystonia is an action dystonia in which involuntary adduction or abduction of the vocal cords is activated by speech. Adductor dysphonia is far more common and results from approximation of the vocal cords due to contraction or tensing of the thyroarytenoid muscles during speech. This causes a characteristic strained and staccato voice pattern with frequent voice breaks. In abductor dysphonia, there is involuntary separation of the vocal cords due to posterior cricoarytenoid contraction, which results in a breathy or whispered voice. Historically, spasmodic dysphonia was usually misdiagnosed as psychogenic in origin. Although this is usually not the case, it is sometimes appropriate to consider a psychological cause with the assistance of appropriate laryngologic evaluation and laboratory voice evaluation techniques. Differential diagnosis includes essential voice tremor, extrapyramidal dysarthria, and structural or inflammatory vocal cord abnormalities.

Limb Dystonia. Limb dystonia is discussed in detail in Chapter 124. Writer's cramp is the most common of the occupational cramp disorders but is not restricted to individuals who do a good deal of writing. Simple writer's cramp is a task-specific disorder in which other fine motor activities are unimpaired. In dystonic writer's cramp other manual activities of the hand become involved and there may eventually be progression to dystonia at rest and involvement of adjacent body parts. Patients present with complaints of slowness and deterioration of handwriting. Excessive squeezing of a pen by the index finger and thumb, involuntary extension movements of individual fingers away from the pen, and involuntary flexion or extension movements of the wrist occur individually or in various combinations. A variety of other cramps or craft palsies have been described affecting musicians, typists, tailors, and other occupations which are similar in their manifestations and are discussed in Chapter 126. Limb dystonia affecting the lower extremity is highly uncommon as a manifestation of primary dystonia and is more usually due to acquired injury of the central or peripheral nervous system.

Paroxysmal Dystonia. Paroxysmal dystonia is a rare disorder that may occur in primary idiopathic form or secondary to a variety of underlying neurologic disorders. Familial forms, as well as some sporadic cases, appear to be primary and associated with normal neurologic examination results. Paroxysmal dystonic choreoathetosis produces episodic dystonic movements that may occur several times daily and are often precipitated by alcohol, caffeine, or stress. Paroxysmal kinesogenic choreoathetosis typically produces more frequent episodes, is precipitated by sudden body or limb movements, and usually responds to treatment with anticonvulsant medications. Secondary forms of these disorders also occur, having a variety of causes, including multiple sclerosis, supplementary motor area seizures, endocrine or metabolic disorders, cerebral palsy, and psychogenic disorders.

Secondary Dystonia

The vast majority of dystonias are secondary and occur in the setting of underlying neurologic disorders. They are therefore nearly always associated with other neurologic findings in addition to dystonia. Dystonia may be associated with diseases with known metabolic defects, such as Wilson's disease, dopa-responsive dystonia, gangliosidosis, metachromatic leukodystrophy, and aminoacidurias. Dystonia may be prominent in disorders with suspected metabolic defects, such as dystonic lipidosis, ceroid lipofuscinosis, Leigh's disease, basal ganglia calcification, neuroacanthocytosis, and ataxia telangiectasia. A large number of degenerative diseases of the basal ganglia, such as Parkinson's disease, progressive supranuclear palsy, Huntington's disease, olivopontocerebellar atrophy, and pallidal degenerations, produce dystonia together with other extrapyramidal manifestations. Miscellaneous structural and toxic disorders that produce dystonia, many of which are associated with abnormal brain imaging, include perinatal anoxia or kernicterus, stroke, head trauma, multiple sclerosis, neoplasm, vascular malformations, neuroleptic and antiparkinson drugs, manganese toxicity, and peripheral trauma.

Approach to the Patient

It should be clear from the above that age of onset, distribution of dystonia, pattern of progression, and presence or absence of other neurologic findings will be particularly helpful in the evaluation of a dystonic syndrome. Childhood forms usually become generalized regardless of whether primary or secondary. Delayed onset of dystonia may occur following perinatal brain injury due to kernicterus, anoxia, or trauma. Adult forms of primary dystonia are usually nonprogressive and remain focal or segmental. Generalized or lower extremity dystonia in an adult should therefore raise the possibility of an identifiable underlying cause. Hemidystonia in a child or adult is strongly indicative of a contralateral basal ganglia abnormality. Action dystonia is more commonly a feature of primary dystonia, whereas the early appearance of a fixed dystonic posture is indicative of secondary dystonia. Diurnal variability should raise the possibility of dopa-responsive dystonia, which is remarkably sensitive to very small amounts of levodopa. Birth, developmental, medication, toxin, trauma, and family history are all important in identifying secondary dystonia.

Examination of patients with dystonia should emphasize careful observation under a variety of circumstances, especially as they carry out tasks that reportedly precipitate or aggravate their dystonia. Similar to tic disorders, some dystonias such as blepharospasm may be less evident in the office situation than suggested by the history. Variability of dystonia under different circumstances is often a hallmark of the disorder and should not necessarily imply a psychogenic cause. The presence of other abnormal central or peripheral neurologic findings should trigger a search for an underlying cause. In the absence of such findings, such a search is less likely to be fruitful. For example, the presence of tremor and akinesia should suggest Wilson's disease; cerebellar ataxia should suggest olivopontocerebellar atrophy, ataxia telangiectasia, or storage disorders; abnormal eye findings should suggest olivopontocerebellar atrophy, dystonic lipidosis, Huntington's disease, or Leigh's disease; and anterior horn cell or peripheral nerve findings should raise the question of metachromatic leukodystrophy, neuroacanthocytosis, ataxia telangiectasia, or olivopontocerebellar atrophy.

MYOCLONUS

The term *myoclonus* refers to quick, shocklike muscle contractions that produce brief and sudden movements of a limb or body part. Myoclonus presents in a number of patterns that should be carefully described in order to assist in its clinical classification. Frequency of muscle jerks may be individual and infrequent or constant and repetitive. Amplitude of movements may range from barely detectable movements within a limb to large jerks of the entire body. In most cases, the pattern of myoclonus is irregular, but it can be rhythmic. The distribution may be focal in one part of the body, segmental involving adjacent body regions, multifocal involving multiple body regions, or generalized involving the entire body. Myoclonus occurring in more than one body part may be asynchronous or synchronous. Muscle jerks may occur spontaneously, as a reflex response to inputs from sudden visual, auditory, or tactile stimuli, or as a result of active or passive voluntary movements.

Myoclonus occurs in a large variety of neurologic disorders (Table 3-5). The vast majority of these are central nervous system in origin but myoclonus occasionally occurs in peripheral neurologic disorders as well, such as hemifacial spasm, and rarely as an unusual manifestation of nerve or nerve root injuries. Unfortunately, the clinical features of myoclonus discussed above may not allow reliable classification of myoclonus by etiology or neuroanatomic origin. The various causes and clinical features of myoclonic syndromes are discussed in detail in Chapter 128. The more common etiologies include physiologic myoclonus, such as sleep startles, nocturnal myoclonus, and hiccough; epileptic myoclonus associated with idiopathic seizure disorders, benign or progressive myoclonic epilepsies of childhood, and epilepsy partialis continua; essential myoclonus, an early-onset hereditary or sporadic benign disorder that is usually action-induced and may overlap with essential tremor and myoclonic dystonia; and symptomatic myoclonus due to a wide variety of structural and metabolic disorders, such as storage diseases, cerebellar and basal ganglia degenerations, mitochondrial encephalopathies, dementias such as Alzheimer's disease and Creutzfeldt-Jakob disease, encephalitis, systemic metabolic disorders usually associated with asterixis, hypoxic and toxic encephalopathies, and focal damage to the brain or spinal cord from a variety of causes.

Approach to the Patient

A history of myoclonic jerks will usually be forthcoming from the patient or family, although small-amplitude myoclonus, especially in patients with other more serious neurologic manifestations, may be noticed only by the examiner. A history of toxin

TABLE 3-5. Common Causes of Myoclonus

Physiologic myoclonus (normal subjects)
  Nocturnal
  Anxiety
  Hiccough
Essential myoclonus (no known cause; no other manifestations)
  Hereditary
  Sporadic
  Benign neonatal sleep myoclonus
Epileptic myoclonus (seizures predominate; no encephalopathy)
  Fragments of epilepsy
    Isolated epileptic myoclonic jerks
    Epilepsia partialis continua
    Idiopathic stimulus-sensitive myoclonus
    Photosensitive myoclonus
    Myoclonic absences
  Childhood myoclonic epilepsies
    Infantile spasms
    Myoclonic astatic epilepsy
    Cryptogenic myoclonus epilepsy
    Juvenile myoclonus epilepsy
  Benign familial myoclonus epilepsy
  Baltic myoclonus
Symptomatic myoclonus (encephalopathy predominates)
  Storage disease
    Lafora body disease
    Lipidoses
    Ceroid-lipofuscinosis
    Sialidosis (cherry-red spot myoclonus)
  Spinocerebellar degeneration
    Ramsay Hunt syndrome
    Friedreich's ataxia
    Ataxia telangiectasia
  Basal ganglion degeneration
    Wilson's disease
    Torsion dystonia
    Hallervorden-Spatz disease
    Progressive supranuclear palsy
    Huntington's disease
    Corticobasal ganglionic degeneration
  Dementias
    Creutzfeldt-Jakob disease
    Alzheimer's disease
  Viral encephalopathies
    Subacute sclerosing panencephalitis
    Encephalitis lethargica
    Herpes simplex virus encephalitis
    Other viral encephalitides
    Postinfectious encephalitis
  Metabolic
    Hepatic failure
    Dialysis encephalopathy
    Hyponatremia
    Hyper- and hypoglycemia
    Infantile myoclonic encephalopathy with polymyoclonus
  Toxic encephalopathies
    Bismuth
    Heavy metals
    Methyl bromide
    DDT
    Drugs (e.g., levodopa, tricyclics)
  Physical encephalopathies
    Hypoxia
    Head trauma
    Heat stroke
    Electric shock
    Decompression injury
  Focal central nervous system
    Stroke
    Tumor
    Trauma
    Olivodentate lesions (palatal myoclonus)
    Spinal cord lesions (segmental myoclonus)
    Psychogenic

(Modified from Weiner WJ, Lang AE: Movement disorders: A Comprehensive Survey. Futura, Mt. Kisco, NY, 1989, with permission.)

exposure or drug use is important. Precipitants and circumstances under which the myoclonus appears should be elicited. Asterixis or negative myoclonus often presents as dropping of objects or sudden falls due to lapses in extensor muscle tone. Action myoclonus is characteristic of essential myoclonus, for which there may be a family history, but it is also the hallmark of postanoxic myoclonus, for which there should be an obvious history of acute cerebral anoxia. The most common forms of physiologic myoclonus occur only during sleep but are usually adequately described by the patient's spouse. In other cases, all night sleep recordings may be necessary for evaluation. Myoclonus not uncommonly accompanies idiopathic epilepsy. This myoclonus may be stimulus-sensitive in type and often occurs at times of reduced seizure control. The presence of myoclonus in a child either with or without epilepsy should prompt assessment of cognitive function and school performance. Symptomatic forms of myoclonus will usually be accompanied by other manifestations of what is usually a prominent underlying neurologic disorder.

In many patients, myoclonus may not be evident on routine neurologic examination. Efforts to elicit myoclonus by providing sudden auditory, tactile, or muscle stretch stimuli should be made. The muscle jerks should be characterized according to frequency, amplitude, rhythmicity, and distribution. Focal myoclonus limited to distal portions of one extremity suggests a cortical origin, whereas segmental involvement, especially if bilateral, may indicate a brainstem or spinal origin. Multifocal myoclonus is characteristic of systemic metabolic disorders, such as uremia or hepatic failure. When multiple body regions are involved, electromyographic study of synchrony and order of activation of muscle groups may be useful in identifying cortical and subcortical forms of myoclonus. Action myoclonus should be searched for in muscles of the limbs, face, and trunk. Action myoclonus of the upper extremities should be distinguished from severe postural-action or intention tremor, with which it sometimes coexists. Myoclonus is usually lower in frequency and more quick and jerky in its appearance than tremor. Myoclonus present at rest must be distinguished from chorea, which is usually more random, unpredictable, and multifocal in character. Tics usually produce more complex movements and postures, are more suppressible, and are often associated with inner tension and other subjective sensations. Since myoclonus is often accompanied by other manifestations of an underlying neurologic disorder, careful examination for associated cerebellar, extrapyramidal, and cognitive abnormalities is necessary for differential diagnosis.

TICS

Tics occur as a relatively common phenomenon at one time or another in a large number of neurologically normal individuals. Gilles de la Tourette syndrome is the best known neurologic condition characterized by the presence of motor and vocal tics and is discussed in detail in Chapter 127.

Motor tics most commonly appear as brief, high-velocity jerking movements of individual muscles, groups of muscles, or parts of the body. They are random and variable in pattern and frequency and usually can be voluntarily suppressed for limited periods of time. An infinite variety of motor tics may occur and may be classified as simple or complex and clonic or dystonic in type. Common examples of simple motor tics include eye blinking, blepharospasm, facial grimacing, platysma contractions, head jerking, shoulder shrugging, ab-

dominal or pelvic contractions, and arm or leg jerking. Complex motor tics produce patterned and coordinated movements that involve one or more regional groups of muscles and may appear purposeful, such as repetitive neck or limb shaking or stretching, hitting or touching movements, and whole-body movements such as turning, squatting, or jumping. Complex motor tics are often characterized by ritualistic, obsessive, and compulsive features, and in severe tic disorders such as Tourette syndrome, may include echopraxia and copropraxia. Clonic tics are brief, jerky, and characteristic of simple tics, Whereas dystonic tics are slower and more protracted movements that usually occur as part of complex tics.

Vocal tics are characteristic of Tourette syndrome and, similar to motor tics, may be simple or complex in type. Simple vocal tics include nonverbal noisemaking such as sniffing, coughing, throat clearing, humming, grunting, hooting, squealing, or barking. Complex vocal tics include verbal utterances, such as coprolalia, echolalia, cheers, and oaths, as well as nonverbal tics, such as belching, hiccoughing, and panting.

Motor tics are somewhat more common in the face, neck, and shoulders than in the trunk and extremities. Neither motor or vocal tics occur in response to external stimuli, but both are often increased during or following stressful situations. They often occur as an effort to relieve an internal urge and are at least temporarily suppressible. This is especially characteristic of dystonic tics in which uncomfortable internal sensations, sometimes referred to as "sensory" tics, are experienced in localized body regions, leading to repeated efforts at relief by movements or muscle contractions. A period of tic suppression is typically followed by a temporary flurry of increased tic frequency, which the individual will sometimes seek to carry out in private.

Approach to the Patient

The diagnosis of tic disorder should be readily apparent from the history provided by the patient and family members. Simple motor tics such as increased eye blinking are often mistakenly attributed to eye irritation, whereas simple vocal tics such as sniffing, throat clearing, or coughing are frequently blamed on nose or throat irritations. Many motor tics are initially thought to be normal phenomena and do not attract medical attention. It is typically when increasing numbers of more complex tics appear that patients present themselves or are brought by family members for neurologic evaluation. The description of an inner urge relieved by movement or muscle contraction is virtually pathognomonic of tics. However, this is mainly characteristic of dystonic tics and may not be prominent in patients with primarily simple tics. A history of fluctuating and changing tics over the course of months or years is particularly typical of Tourette syndrome but may be absent in patients with transient or chronic motor tic disorder.

Except for the presence of tics, neurologic examination results are normal in most patients who present for evaluation of tic disorder. Tourette syndrome may be accompanied by learning disabilities, attention deficit disorder, and obsessive-compulsive disorder, but not by abnormalities of the elementary neurologic examination. The presence of other neurologic findings should suggest a secondary tic disorder. Tics are best observed during the course of the interview rather than during the formal examination. In many patients, they are more prominent while sitting and quietly listening to the examiner than while actively engaged in relating the history. It is not unusual for patients with mild tics to exhibit little evidence of tics while in the presence of the examiner. In such cases, it is useful to observe the patient while he or she is in the waiting room, through a one-way mirror, or to listen for vocal tics through a closed examining room door. Mild choreic and dystonic manifestations may be present in patients with Tourette syndrome and difficult to separate from tics. Although ability to suppress movements is characteristic of tics, this feature may also be found in chorea, dystonia, or athetosis. Most dystonic and many simple tics are more reliably differentiated from dystonia or chorea by the inner urge and release that characterize tics and the historical features of the disorder.

Clinical criteria for the diagnosis of Tourette syndrome include childhood or adolescent onset, multiplicity of tics, presence of vocal tics, a historical pattern of variation in type and severity of tics over time, and suppressibility. Tourette syndrome must be differentiated from transient tic disorder and chronic motor tic disorder. Transient tics are common in children and may closely resemble Tourette syndrome but last less than a year and are usually unaccompanied by vocal tics. Chronic motor tic disorder appears in childhood or adult life but usually is limited to a single motor tic that remains constant in severity over an extended period of time. Both of these disorders may be present in family members of a patient with Tourette syndrome. Rare startle disorders characterized by sudden complex movements, such as hyperexplexia, jumping Frenchmen, latah, and myriachit, differ from tics in being triggered by external stimuli and unaccompanied by more usual tic manifestations. Secondary tic disorders may occur in a wide variety of neurologic disorders such as following chronic neuroleptic, amphetamine, or levodopa treatment; accompanying mental retardation; in postencephalitic syndromes; as sequelae of head trauma, stroke, and carbon monoxide poisoning; and in neuroacanthocytosis. In these cases, the history and presence of other neurologic findings will suggest a secondary tic disorder.

PSYCHOGENIC MOVEMENT DISORDERS

As in other categories of neurologic disease, psychogenic etiologies sometimes merit consideration in the evaluation of a movement disorder. Movement disorder specialty clinics are currently seeing increasing numbers of patients with movement disorders due to psychological causes. These include psychogenic dystonia, tremor, and gait disorder, which are the most common of the group, as well as psychogenic myoclonus, paroxysmal syndromes, and startle disorders. Unfortunately, the diagnosis of many movement disorders is based primarily on an observed pattern of symptoms and signs with few or no available methods of laboratory confirmation. This is especially true for hyperkinetic syndromes, in which the incidence of psychogenic disorders is higher than for hypokinetic disorders. Since the diagnosis commonly rests on clinical criteria, it is important to be particularly careful before attributing an unusual movement disorder to psychological causes. This is particularly important because historically a number of movement disorders, especially dystonias and tics, have been incorrectly attributed to psychological causes.

Criteria have been recommended for the likelihood that a psychogenic movement disorder is present. A documented psychogenic disorder is one in which the manifestations are rapidly and completely eliminated by psychological treatment such as psychotherapy, suggestion therapy, or placebo or the patient is documented to be free of signs when unknowingly observed. Since, with the exception of tics, acute drug-induced dyskinesias, and rare cases of cervical dystonia, organic movement disorders almost never remit suddenly and spontaneously, this serves to document psychogenic movement disorder. A clinically established psychogenic disorder is one in which the disorder is inconsistent over time or is incongruent with the known pattern of an established movement disorder and is accompanied by obvious psychiatric disturbance, other psychosomatic disorders, and other neurologic signs that are definitely psychogenic. A probable psychogenic disorder is one in which (1) the movements appear inconsistent or incongruent but there are no other findings to indicate a psychogenic cause or (2) the movements appear consistent and congruent but other psychogenic findings or somatizations are present. One may be suspicious of a possible psychogenic disorder in cases where the movement disorder appears consistent and congruent with an organic disorder but occurs in the setting of an obvious emotional disturbance.

Approach to the Patient

Certain clues in the history and examination may suggest the possibility of a psychogenic disorder. These include sudden onset, multiplicity of abnormal movements, inconsistency during the examination or from one examination to another, abnormal movements and postures that do not fit with recognized patterns, large-amplitude shaking movements, bizarre gait, excessive startle responses to a variety of stimuli, overly slow and deliberate voluntary movements, variable tremor frequency, marked relief of involuntary movements with distraction, a dystonia beginning as a fixed posture, and false weakness or sensory signs. Although these clues, together with an obvious psychiatric disorder, other somatizations, and identifiable secondary gain, may suggest a psychogenic etiology, it is important to view these signs in the context of the diagnostic criteria outlined above. This is especially true since one is sometimes dealing with rare, unique, or highly unusual movement disorders with variable manifestations that not uncommonly are also associated with psychiatric disturbance. Finally, as with any apparently psychogenic disorder, one has to be alert to the possibility that psychogenic abnormal movements may occur in patients with an underlying organic movement disorder. Inpatient or extended outpatient evaluation, reasonable and necessary laboratory tests, observed and unobserved video recording, psychiatric evaluation, and physical medicine evaluation and treatment should all be considered in the evaluation of such patients.

SUGGESTED READINGS

Dewey Jr. RB, Jankovic J: Hemiballism-hemichorea. Clinical and pharmacologic findings in 21 patients. Arch Neurol 46:862, 1989

Fahn S: Psychogenic movement disorders. p. 359. In Marsden CD, Fahn S (eds): Movement Disorders III. Butterworth-Heinemann, London, 1994

Fahn S, Marsden CD, Calne DB: Classification and investigation of dystonia. p. 332. In Marsden CD, Fahn S (eds): Movement Disorders II. Butterworth, London, 1987

Jankovic J, Stone L: Dystonic tics in patients with Tourette's syndrome. Mov Disord 6:248, 1991

Koller WC, Busenbark K, Gray C et al: Classification of essential tremor. Clin Neuropharm 15:81, 1992

Lang AE: Movement disorder symptomatology. p. 315. In Bradley WG, Daroff RB, Fenichel GM, Marsden CD (eds): Neurology in Clinical Practice. Butterworth-Heinemann, Boston, 1991

Marsden CD: The focal dystonias. Clin Neuropharm (suppl.) 9:S49, 1986

Marsden CD: Parkinson's disease. J Neurol Neurosurg Psychiatry 57:672, 1994

Marsden CD, Fahn S: Problems in the dyskinesias. In: Movement Disorders II. Butterworth, London, 1987

Obeso JA, Artieda J, Marsden CD: Different clinical presentations of myoclonus. p. 315. In Jankovic J, Tolosa E (eds): Parkinson's Disease and Movement Disorders. Williams & Wilkins, Baltimore, 1993

Quinn N: Multiple system atrophy—the nature of the beast. J Neurol Neurosurg Psychiatry (special suppl.) 52:78, 1989

The Tourette Syndrome Classification Study Group: Definitions and classification of tic disorders. Arch Neurol 50:1013, 1993

Weiner WJ, Lang AE: Movement Disorders: A Comprehensive Survey. Futura, Mt. Kisco, NY, 1989

TABLE 4-1. Classification of Gait Disorder by Etiology[a]

Etiology	1980–1982[b]	1990–1993	Total	%
Myelopathy	8	12	20	18.5
Parkinsonism	5	7	12	11.1
Hydrocephalus	2	4	6	5.6
Multiple infarcts	8	8	16	14.8
Cerebellar degeneration	4	4	8	7.4
Sensory deficits	9	11	20	18.5
Toxic/metabolic	3	0	3	2.8
Psychogenic causes	1	3	4	3.7
Other causes	3	2	5	4.6
Unknown causes	7	7	14	13.0

[a] n = 108 patients.

[b] Data from Sudarsky and Ronthal, Arch Neurol 40:740–3, 1983.

4. GAIT IMPAIRMENT AND FALLING

LEWIS R. SUDARSKY

Gait is a fundamental motor performance and a distinctive attribute of each individual. Walking undergoes characteristic changes over the life span. It is very sensitive to diseases of the nervous system, and the neurologic examination is not complete until the gait has been observed. Disorders of gait are particularly common among the very young and the very old. Delay in learning to walk can be the presenting manifestation of developmental or acquired neurologic disease in early childhood. Abnormalities of gait have been recorded in 15 percent of people over the age of 65. By age 80, 1 person in 4 will use mechanical aids to assist ambulation. Among persons 85 and older, the prevalence of gait disorder approaches 40 percent.

Falls are the main cause of accidental injury and sixth leading cause of death in the elderly, and gait disorders contribute measurably to the risk of falls and fall-related injury. In some instances, insecure ambulation and a history of falls are cause for nursing home admission. Nonambulatory nursing home patients have accelerated morbidity and mortality.

PRINCIPAL PATTERNS OF GAIT DISORDER AND THEIR CAUSE

To maintain a stable gait, the nervous system must simultaneously generate motor activity for locomotion and maintain balance. Locomotion involves phasic activity of trunk and limb muscles that coordinates the loading, unloading, and advance of the legs during the stance and swing phase. To prevent instability and falls, the nervous system also has to maintain a state of dynamic equilibrium, managing the center of mass in relation to the base of support.

The enormous heterogeneity of gait disorders observed clinically reflects the complexity of the anatomy involved in locomotion. A network of subcortical motor centers participate in the coordinated management of postural control and locomotion. The mesencephalic locomotor region, physiologically defined, lies in the region of the nucleus cuneiformis and (cholinergic) pedunculopontine nucleus. Locomotor synergies are executed through the reticular formation and reticulospinal pathway. Cortical modulation adapts the performance to suit a complex hierarchy of purposes and environmental needs. Bal-

ance is particularly dependent on sensory afferent systems that update the nervous system on the body's orientation with respect to the support surface and the vertical. Because of this anatomic complexity, there is a large potential for trouble, and walking is vulnerable to neurologic disease at every level.

Gait disorders have been classified descriptively, based on the abnormal physiology and biomechanics, and etiologically. In practice, many failing gaits look fundamentally similar. This overlap reflects common patterns of adaptation to declining performance. Gait disorder must be viewed as the product of a neurologic deficit and a functional adaptation. The unique features of the failing gait are often overwhelmed by the adaptive response. An example is the phenomenon of the cautious gait in the elderly. Many people with disorders of balance or locomotion adopt a timid or cautious style of walking, using short steps and a widened base of support like a person crossing a patch of ice. This pattern is entirely nonspecific; it is just a response to perceived imbalance.

A 1983 study conducted at our institution examined the common causes of gait disorder in a neurology office practice. Patients over 65 who were referred for an undiagnosed disorder of gait were examined. The study excluded patients with joint deformity and those on neuroleptic drugs. Older people frequently have comorbidity from arthritis, and minor orthopaedic deformity is a common source of gait abnormality. Table 4-1 includes our more recent experience with patients seen between 1990 and 1993.

In approximately 10 to 15 percent of older patients, no etiologic factors can be identified after a complete workup and lab studies. These cases are sometimes called essential senile gait, though it is unlikely that they represent a true morbid entity.

Spastic Gait

Spastic gait is characterized by stiffness and "bounce" in the legs, and a tendency to circumduct and scuff the feet. In extreme instances, the legs cross from increased tone in the adductors. Shoes often reflect an uneven pattern of wear across the outside.

Myelopathy from cervical spondylosis is a common cause of spastic or spastic-ataxic gait in the elderly. Spondylitic bars and ligamentous hypertrophy narrow the canal, causing mechanical compression and vascular compromise. Some degree of standing imbalance and bladder dysfunction (urgency, incontinence) accompany a mild spastic paresis of the legs. Magnetic resonance imaging (MRI) has improved the ease of diagnosis, though it sometimes demonstrates advanced pathology in the cervical spine in minimally symptomatic patients. Other causes of myelopathy in the elderly include vitamin B_{12} deficiency and degenerative disease (e.g., primary lateral sclerosis, hereditary spastic paraplegia).

Demyelinating disease and trauma are the leading causes of myelopathy in younger patients. In chronic progressive myelopathy of unknown cause, thorough workup with laboratory and imaging tests often establishes a diagnosis of multiple sclerosis. Myelopathy is sometimes due to a structural lesion, such as tumor or dural or spinal vascular malformation. Traumatic spinal injury may be incomplete or partial, such that the patient remains ambulatory. Motor vehicle and diving accidents, commonly alcohol-related, are the usual cause at our institution. Tropical spastic paraparesis related to human T cell virus type I is endemic in parts of the Caribbean and South America.

With cerebral spasticity, involvement of the upper extremities is sometimes observed, and dysarthria is usually an associated feature. Common causes include vascular disease (stroke) and multiple sclerosis. In the cerebral palsy population, a mild spastic diplegia is the most frequently observed syndrome.

Extrapyramidal Disorder

Parkinson's disease is common, affecting 1.5 percent of the population over 65. The flexed posture and shuffling gait are highly characteristic and distinctive. There may be difficulty with initiation and a tendency to turn en bloc. Patients sometimes accelerate (festinate) with progression or display retropulsion. Some patients with atypical parkinsonism present with axial stiffness, postural instability, and a shuffling gait (Ch 113). Drug-induced parkinsonism is increasingly recognized in ambulatory practice as a cause of impaired gait and balance. It is particularly common in a chronic care setting (chapter 119).

Hyperkinetic movement disorders also produce characteristic and recognizable disturbances in gait. Tardive dyskinesia is the cause of many odd, stereotypic gait disorders seen in chronic psychiatric patients. The gait in Huntington's disease is defined by the unpredictable occurrence of choreic movements which give a dancing quality. In generalized dystonia, muscular spasms produce a dysfunctional posture of the legs—typically adduction and inversion, sometimes with torsion of the trunk.

Frontal Gait Disorder ("Gait Apraxia")

Frontal gait disorder, sometimes known as gait apraxia, is more common in the elderly and has a variety of causes. Typical clinical features include a wide base of support, short stride, shuffling on the floor, and difficulty with starts and turns. Many exhibit a peculiar difficulty with gait initiation, descriptively characterized as the "slipping clutch" syndrome or gait ignition failure. The term *lower body Parkinsonism* is also used to describe this condition. In studies seeking clinicopathologic correlation, lesions are usually found in the deep frontal white matter.

Communicating hydrocephalus in the adult often presents with a gait disorder. Other features of the diagnostic triad (mental change, incontinence) may be absent in the initial stages. MRI demonstrates ventricular enlargement, an enlarged flow void about the aqueduct, and a variable degree of periventricular white matter change. A dynamic test is necessary to confirm the presence of hydrocephalus. The response to lumbar puncture, with removal of 30 to 50 ml of cerebrospinal fluid, has been used as a screening procedure (Ch. 16).

Another common cause of the frontal gait disorder is vascular disease, particularly subcortical small vessel disease. Of the patients in our series, 15 percent had multiple infarcts by computed tomography (CT) or MRI. Gait disorder is frequently seen in hypertensive patients with ischemic lesions of the deep hemisphere white matter (Binswanger's disease). The clinical syndrome includes mental change (variable in degree), dysarthria, pseudobulbar affect, increased tone, and hyperreflexia in the lower limbs.

Cerebellar Gait

Disorders of the cerebellum have a dramatic impact on gait and postural control. The ataxic gait is characterized by a wide base, lateral instability of the trunk, erratic foot placement, and decompensation of balance when attempting to walk tandem. Cerebellar patients have well-defined abnormalities of balance on platform posturography. They show considerable variation in their tendency to fall in the real world.

Posterior fossa tumors of childhood can present with an ataxic gait. Multiple sclerosis can produce ataxia and postural instability. Inherited and sporadic forms of cerebellar degeneration are described in Chapter 120. Other causes of cerebellar atrophy include toxins (alcohol, possibly phenytoin) and paraneoplastic cerebellar degeneration.

Sensory Ataxia and Disequilibrium

Patients with chronic imbalance due to a disorder of sensory afferent systems are now the largest single group, approaching 20 percent in our series. Balance depends on high-quality information from the visual system, the vestibular system, and proprioceptive afferents. When this information is degraded, standing balance is impaired and instability results. The sensory ataxia of tabetic neurosyphilis is a classic example. The contemporary equivalent is the patient with neuropathy affecting large-fiber afferents. The stance in such patients is destabilized by eye closure (Romberg's test). Patients have been described with imbalance from bilateral vestibular loss caused by disease or by exposure to ototoxic drugs.

Some older patients exhibit a syndrome of imbalance from the combined effect of multiple sensory deficits. Such patients, often elderly and diabetic, have disturbances in proprioception, vision, and vestibular sense that impair postural support. In the recent past, cataract surgery with external lenses has been a factor in the decompensation of some such patients.

Neuromuscular Disease

Patients with neuromuscular disease often have an abnormal gait, though it is not typically a presenting feature. With distal weakness (peripheral neuropathy), the step height is often increased to compensate for foot drop, and the sole of the foot may slap on the floor during weight acceptance. Neuropathy may be associated with a degree of sensory imbalance, as described above. Patients with myopathy or muscular dystrophy have primarily proximal weakness. Weakness of the hip girdle may produce a degree of excess pelvic rotation (waddle).

Toxic and Metabolic Disorders

Unquestionably the most common cause of difficulty walking is alcohol intoxication. Chronic toxicity from medications and metabolic disturbances can also impair motor function and gait. Static equilibrium is disturbed, and such patients are easily displaced backward. This is particularly dramatic in patients with chronic renal disease and those with hepatic failure in whom asterixis may impair postural support. Sedative drugs, especially neuroleptics and long-acting benzodiazepines, affect postural control and increase the risk for falls. These disorders are important to recognize because they are treatable.

Psychogenic Gait Disorder

Psychogenic disturbances of gait are among the most spectacular disorders encountered in neurology. Odd gyrations of posture (astasia-abasia) and dramatic fluctuations over time may be observed in the hysterical patient. Some patients with extreme anxiety walk with exaggerated caution, as if walking on a slippery surface. Depressed patients exhibit primarily slowness, a manifestation of psychomotor retardation, and lack of purpose in their stride.

Other Identifiable Causes

A few patients presenting with gait disorder have a mass lesion—primary central nervous system tumor or metastatic cancer. Lumbar spinal stenosis can severely limit ambulation and produce a flexed posture. Subdural hematoma should be ruled out in the patient with subacute evolution and a history of falls.

APPROACH TO THE PATIENT WITH A SLOWLY PROGRESSIVE DISORDER OF AMBULATION

In eliciting the patient's history, it is helpful to inquire about the pace of the illness. Stepwise evolution or sudden progression suggests vascular disease. Gait disorder may be associated with urinary urgency and incontinence, particularly in patients with subcortical frontal disease or spinal disease. Back pain or headache may be clues to a structural pathology, particularly in patients whose illness evolves over weeks to months. First awareness of a balance problem often follows a fall. It is always important to review the use of alcohol and medications that can affect gait and balance.

Because the list of possible diagnoses is lengthy, information on localization derived from the neurologic examination can be helpful in narrowing the search. This examination is often most informative, despite its focus on corticospinal systems, which play a minor role in locomotor control.

Gait observation provides an immediate sense of the patient's degree of disability. Cadence (steps per minute), velocity, and stride length can be recorded by timing a patient over a fixed distance. Watching the patient get out of a chair provides a good functional assessment of balance. Characteristic patterns of abnormality are sometimes observed, though failing gaits often look fundamentally similar as reviewed above.

Brain imaging studies (CT or MRI) are frequently informative in patients with an undiagnosed disorder of gait. MRI is sensitive for cerebral lesions of vascular or demyelinating disease and is a good screening test for occult hydrocephalus. Many elderly patients with gait and balance difficulty have lesions in the periventricular region and centrum semiovale. Although controversy persists about the clinical relevance of these lesions in the elderly, a substantial burden of white matter disease will inevitably affect cerebral control of locomotion.

EPIDEMIOLOGY OF FALLS

Prospective studies estimate that 20 to 30 percent of people over age 65 fall each year. The proportion is higher in hospital-ized elderly and nursing home residents. Roughly one of four falls results in serious injury, and 5 percent, in a fracture. Eight percent of persons over age 75 suffer a serious fall-related injury each year. By the age of 80, one in five women will have fractured a hip. For each person physically disabled, there are others whose functional independence is constrained by fear of falling. In a study conducted in New Haven, Connecticut, 18 percent of the elderly acknowledged that they voluntarily limited their activity (walking out of the home, shopping, bathing) because of fear of falling.

An epidemiologic, multiple risk factor model has been applied to study the problem of falls in the elderly. Independent risk factors for fall-related injury include cognitive impairment, decreased bone density, gait and balance impairment, and the presence of specific chronic illnesses, notably diabetes and stroke. In the prospective study of Tinetti et al. (1988) of people over age 75, cognitive impairment and the use of sedative medications substantially increased the risk of falling. A possible environmental factor was mentioned in 44 percent of the events. Tinetti and colleagues devised a functional assessment for gait and balance. They observed a direct correlation between number of gait and balance abnormalities recorded and risk of falling. A similar correlation was observed among inpatients in an intermediate-care facility.

In a more recent study, the same group looked at inability to get up after a fall. The phenomenon is rather more prevalent than generally thought. Thirty-nine percent of 660 fall events were associated with an inability to get up. Three percent of subjects were on the floor more than an hour. Such events were more likely to be associated with hospitalization. Absent evidence of serious cardiovascular disease, there was a marginally increased risk of death or functional decline over the next year.

APPROACH TO THE PATIENT WITH RECURRENT FALLS

Although falling is not a common cause for neurologic referral, there are some special circumstances, such as syncope and seizures, in which neurologic evaluation is sought. In epidemiologic surveys, 80 to 90 percent of fall events occur among 10 percent of patients, a group known as recurrent fallers. Some of these patients are frail older people with a large burden of chronic disease. Recurrent falls sometimes indicate a serious balance problem, a failure of postural control mechanisms.

A hierarchy of postural control systems can be demonstrated in humans. Static balance is examined by recording excursions of the center of pressure on a force platform. Sway can also be examined during eye closure and with other forms of sensory deprivation. Automatic postural adjustments maintain balance during quiet stance. Reactive postural adjustments can be recorded in the leg muscles beginning 110 msec after a perturbation. These are long-loop responses, not to be confused with the monosynaptic ankle stretch reflex. They are probably mediated at a brainstem level. As a last resort, rescue reactions protect against large displacements to prevent slipping and tripping falls. Anticipatory postural responses integrate balance control with other voluntary movement. The anatomic substrate for these systems has not been defined, but the cerebellum and vestibulospinal pathways are likely to be involved. All these physiologic adjustments depend on a redundancy of sensory information from vestibular, visual, and proprioceptive afferents. In the office, balance can be tested by simple functional measures such as one-limb stance, tandem stance, and response to posterior sternal displacement (pull test).

Relatively modest changes in balance function have been described in fit older subjects. Those who exhibit substantial imbalance are likely to have neurologic disorders affecting postural control. Parkinson's disease and other akinetic-rigid disorders can cause postural instability and falling. Patients with cerebellar degeneration likewise exhibit poorly coordinated postural synergies, and ataxic patients commonly present with falls. Sensory deficits involving proprioception, vestibular, or visual function can affect standing balance. Patients with bilateral vestibular deficits and those with severe sensory neuropathy are particularly unsteady in stance. Fife and Baloh (1993) have described a group of patients over age 75 with disequilibrium and a sense of imbalance in whom bilateral deficits can be demonstrated on sensitive laboratory tests of vestibular function. Vestibular testing may be appropriate for patients who exhibit balance difficulty that cannot be characterized using standard neurologic assessment.

Sheldon's classic study (1960) identified drop attacks and postural hypotension as the cause of a substantial number of falls. *Drop attacks* are defined as sudden lapse of postural tonus and collapse *without* loss of consciousness. In contemporary prospective studies of falls, drop attacks are an infrequent occurrence. They are probably a benign phenomenon, though some such cases are associated with serious cardiovascular disease. Orthostatic hypotension is identified as a factor in 5 to 10 percent of falls and should always be considered as a treatable cause. Postural hypotension is a common phenomenon in people over the age of 65, especially those on potent antihypertensive and vasodilator medications. Primary neurologic diseases, such as autonomic neuropathy or multiple system atrophy, are identified in occasional patients.

A correlation between cognitive impairment and falls is observed in community-based studies as well as in chronic-care facilities and nursing homes. The pathophysiology of falls in this context is not well understood. There may be a failure of attention or integrative control of posture at a high level. Sedative drugs are also associated with an increased risk of falls and fall-related injury. Neuroleptic drugs and benzodiazepines presumably compromise balance control systems at a brainstem or spinal level.

Subdural hematoma is always a concern in the patient with repeated falls. The significance of the cranial trauma may not emerge from the patient history. A low threshold for imaging studies is appropriate in this context, particularly if a disturbance in alertness or lateralized neurologic findings are apparent.

INTERVENTION TO REDUCE THE RISK OF FALL-RELATED INJURY

Therapeutic intervention is often recommended for the older person at substantial risk for falls, even if no neurologic disease is identified. Several intervention strategies have been examined since the 1970s. A home visit is frequently arranged to look for environmental hazards. Attention is focused on adequate lighting, installation of grab bars and nonslip surfaces in bathrooms, and elimination of slipping and tripping hazards from the floor. In some instances, the stairwells can be modified.

Rehabilitation techniques focus on the patient rather than the environment in an attempt to make the patient more resilient and less prone to injurious falls. High-intensity resistance strength training is now used to increase muscle mass in nursing home residents in their eighth and ninth decade. Improvements are realized in carriage and gait, which should translate to reduction in falls. Sensory balance training using a platform and visual feedback can enhance the stability of older subjects, and the benefits can be maintained over 6 months by a 10 to 20-min/d home program. This strategy is most successful in patients with vestibular and somatosensory balance disorders.

The NIA recently sponsored a multicenter study of intervention techniques to reduce the risk of fall-related injury (FICSIT trial). Two strategies emerged as having a measurable benefit in fall risk reduction. The Yale Health and Aging study employed a targeted, multiple risk factor abatement effort. Prescription medications were adjusted, and home-based exercise programs were tailored to the patients' needs. The targeted intervention was associated with a 44 percent reduction in the number of falls, compared with a control group of patients who had periodic social visits. The other strategy of proven success involves the use of Tai Chi exercises, which accomplish some of the same benefits as high-tech sensory-balance training.

SUGGESTED READINGS

Alexander NB: Postural control in older adults. J Am Geriatr Soc 42:93–108, 1994

Fife TD, Baloh RW: Disequilibrium of unknown cause in older people. Ann Neurology, 34:694–702, 1993

Masdeu J, Sudarsky L, Wolfson LI: Gait Disorders of Aging: With Special Reference to Falls. Little, Brown, Boston, 1995

Meisner I, Weibers DO, Swanson JH et al: The natural history of drop attacks. Neurology 36:1029–34, 1986

Nutt JG, Marsden CD, Thompson PD: Human walking and higher level gait disorders, particularly in the elderly. Neurology 43:268–79, 1993

Sheldon JH: On the natural history of falls in old age. Br Med J 2:1685–90, 1960

Sudarsky L: Gait disorders in the edlerly. N Engl J Med 322:1441–6, 1990

Tinetti ME, Speechley M, Ginter S: Risk factors for falls among elderly persons living in the community. N Engl J Med 319:1701–7, 1988

5. SENSORY LOSS AND PARESTHESIAS

THOMAS D. SABIN
DAVID M. DAWSON

PARESTHESIAS

Although many aspects of neurology increasingly depend upon neuroimaging, electrophysiologic data, and other laboratory data, the bedside sensory assessment remains a necessity for the clinician. During history taking the patient must be asked to use adjectives to describe abnormal sensory experiences. Burning, stinging, coldness, and heat suggest a problem in small-fiber systems; tingling, pins and needles, or "electricity" are more often features of malfunction in the large-fiber systems. Paresthesias are spontaneous abnormal sensations, whereas dysesthesias are usually unpleasant distortions of actual sensory stimuli in the patient's daily activities or during examination. The paresthesias of hyperventilation concentrate in the palms of the hands, around the mouth, and in the soles of the feet. The length of axons adds to the probability for tingling of hands and feet, but the richness of innervation accounts for the perioral symptoms. Lhermitte's phenomenon consists of an abnormal sensation that extends down the spine upon flexing the neck. Cervical cord lesions, particularly multiple sclerosis, are found in such patients; apparently neck movement stretches cord or dura. Vitamin B_{12} deficiency and cord compression may also cause Lhermitte's phenomenon. When both the centrally and peripherally directed axons of dorsal root ganglia are affected in sensory neuropathies (nitrous oxide, pyridoxine, cisplatin, carcinomatous), Lhermitte's sign is frequent. Some neurotic patients with nonanatomic paresthesias seem able to "tune into" the normal ongoing bombardment of afferent information that is ignored when attentional mechanisms are functioning normally. These patients have paresthesias every time they think about them and may develop a positive feedback system that causes increasing anxiety and more paresthesias. Strange sensations that ultimately come to focus on the genitalia are also often without a neurologic basis. A virtual symphony of paresthesias may be described by patients with panic disorders. When a sensory complaint is not accompanied by any abnormality in the sensory examination, the examiner must rely on a mastery of neuroanatomy because the distribution and quality of the paresthesias remain the only keys to a correct diagnosis.

TECHNIQUES OF SENSORY EXAMINATION

Elaborate quantification of sensory thresholds has only limited diagnostic use in daily practice, because these methods focus on a few sites and no overall pattern of sensory change is discerned. Since a complete sensory examination is infinite, the physician and the patient will be best served by one that is guided by a full patient history and done at the end of the neurologic examination. In this way, abnormalities already suspected can be rapidly documented. The patient's eyes usually should be closed for the sensory examination. When charting deficits, stimuli should always begin in the abnormal area and move toward the normal. The reverse technique will reveal quite a different sensory map. The experienced examiner is aware that the style of the examination may powerfully modify the results. An apparent difference in sensory thresholds between the two sides of the body can be induced commonly by suggestion and the mode of examination. With little effort, the examiner can sculpt a full-blown hemisensory loss in susceptible patients. If given the opportunity, patients with psychiatric disease will eventually use adjectives and describe anatomic distributions yielding important insights into the meaning of their complaints—and many a magnetic resonance imaging study or electromyelogram could be avoided. We urge that all sensory abnormalities be charted on a simple outline diagram. This discipline forces the examiner to commit to a localization and facilitates follow-up comparisons. Sensory deficits can be conveniently grouped into superficial, deep, and discriminative modalities.

Superficial Modalities

These cutaneous sensations are tested ordinarily as pain, temperature, and light touch. The bedside examination for *pain* sensibility is usually directed toward pinprick sensation. There are pain pathways that subserve a more primitive type of pain sensation which is less well localized and slower to appear in consciousness, sometimes called second pain, slow pain, or protopathic pain (see Ch. 6). The pain of pinprick that is local-

ized precisely and felt immediately is also known as first pain, fast pain, or epicritic pain. Cutaneous pain sense is tested by holding a sharp, sterile pin between the thumb and index finger with sufficient pressure so that it slides slightly on each contact with the patient. This causes no skin penetration and produces a constant stimulus. There are natural variations in thresholds over the surface of the body; increased sensitivity in the regions of the axillae, around the lips, and in the groin must be taken into account. Calluses can completely blunt the appreciation of pinprick. Comparison of one side of the body with a homologous area on the other side of the body is often useful. A rapid series of pinprick stimuli may cause temporal summation and give a false pattern of loss. This is particularly apt to occur at the fading border of peripheral neuropathies, the upper border of spinal cord lesions, or with lesions of the parietal operculum or thalamus. Temporal summation is a major reason why the "pinwheel" type of device for pinprick testing is discouraged. A second error occurs when the examiner does not appreciate the importance of skin temperature in the determination of sensory threshholds. Since the distal extremities tend to be cooler, a "pseudoneuropathy" to pin and temperature may be diagnosed by the overzealous examiner mapping out the normal increase in threshhold in the relatively cool parts distal of the body. When the patient is able to discern the sharpness of the pinpoint using preserved discriminative touch but is not actually reporting the painful qualities of the pin, another type of error may occur. Make sure the patient is reporting pain. Watching for a wince may help. Even in a confused patient, one can often rapidly map out an area of sensory loss to pinprick sensation simply by watching the patient's facial expressions with pinprick stimuli.

Areas of temperature loss often overlap with the areas of loss of sensitivity to pinprick. The most efficient way of confirming this pattern of loss is to use brief contact with a cool piece of metal such as the side of a tuning fork. This method will detect a subtler degree of sensory loss than comparing hot and cold. An ice cube in a thin plastic bag is useful for charting areas of complete loss of temperature sense. Since temperature is perceived on the basis of transfer of heat, skin temperatures may substanially alter thresholds. Uncomfortable distortion of cold stimuli is an early sign of small-fiber neuropathy.

Superficial touch stimuli can be graded satisfactorily if the examiner simply uses his or her own fingertip or a wisp of cotton fibers. (Caution—touching a hair results in a 100-fold amplification of signal.) Since patients often report qualitative alterations in touch perception within areas where pinprick and temperature sensation are reduced, the documentation of a true dissociated sensory loss relies upon the presence of normal touch thresholds. A set of graded nylon filaments as available in the Semmes-Weinstein Aesthesiometer (Research Media Inc., Hicksville, NY) helps solve this problem. The ticklish quality of a light stroking touch is absent in these areas of diminished pinprick and temperature sense.

Deep Sensory Modalities

Position sense is tested by inducing small-amplitude movements in the patient's distal digits. The digits should be grasped laterally to eliminate pressure cues. Some patients must be discouraged from using small palpatory movements of the digit to enhance position sense. One-degree displacements should be reported, but if a very slow drift is induced in the digit, more movement is required. Sensory ataxia and pseudochorea or pseudoathetosis in the outstretched hands appear when position sense loss is substantial. If there is distal position sense loss, then proximal joints should be assessed. The hip joints may be tested by having the blindfolded patient track the great toe with the opposite index finger. Romberg's sign is elicited by having the patient stand with the feet together and then close the eyes. The test is positive only if the posture is stable until the eyes are closed and then severe swaying or falling develops.

A 128-cycles per second tuning fork is used to assess vibration sense over the distal digits. The skeletal system transmits widely this modality and there is a normal falloff in vibration sense with aging. Demyelinating neuropathies cause elevated thresholds because of the demand for rapid conduction velocities required to transmit vibration sense. Corticosensory loss is suggested when position sense is absent but vibration sense is intact

PATTERNS OF SENSORY CHANGE

The remainder of this chapter is devoted to discussion of common patterns of sensory abnormalities and is arranged anatomically, beginning with intracutaneous nerve damage and following the pathways to the sensory cortex.

Intracutaneous Sensory Loss

Destruction of nerve endings and networks within the skin and superficial nerves is characteristic of the superficial neuropathy of leprosy. In high-resistance (tuberculoid) leprosy, there is a patch of sensory loss that does not obey the distribution of named peripheral nerves or roots; it is often associated with hypopigmented skin lesion, which has an elevated border. The loss is mostly to pinprick and temperature. Touch is sometimes sufficiently preserved so that the patient can tell the difference between the sharp and the blunt end of the pin using preserved discriminative sensation alone even though there is complete analgesia in the region. In low host resistance (lepromatous) forms of leprosy, the bacterial growth rate, which is greatest in the coolest tissues, determines the pattern (Fig. 5-1). The early involvement of the helices of the ears, the tip of the nose, malar areas, and the extensor surfaces (along with the preservation of reflexes) are important clues to this unique temperature-linked variety of sensory loss due to intracutaneous infection.

A pattern of pain and temperature loss somewhat resembling lepromatous leprosy occurs in tabes dorsalis (Fig. 5-2) Symmetric areas of pain and temperature loss known as Hitzig's zones develop on the abdominal protuberance around the breasts, the extensor surfaces of the forearms, and the anterior tibial region, as well as the tip of the nose and malar areas (the mask of Duchenne). This sensory loss is presumed to be due to the dorsal root lesions of tabes, but it is of interest that the treponeme of syphilis shares thermosensitivity with *Mycobacterium leprae* and is also capable of intracutaneous destruction of nerve endings as evidenced by the painless numb primary chancre. A point against a cutaneous origin for all of the disturbances of pain in tabes is the remarkable loss of deep pain sensation that occurs. Pressure applied to the Achilles tendons (Abadie sign), the testicles, or periosteum does not cause pain. Loss of deep pain sensation in the joints allows the accumulation of painless injuries resulting in Charcot joints. Delayed response to pinprick is another singular feature seen in some patients with tabes. Pinpricks given at too rapid a rate could confuse the examiner because the patient might be responding to a pinprick delivered several seconds before.

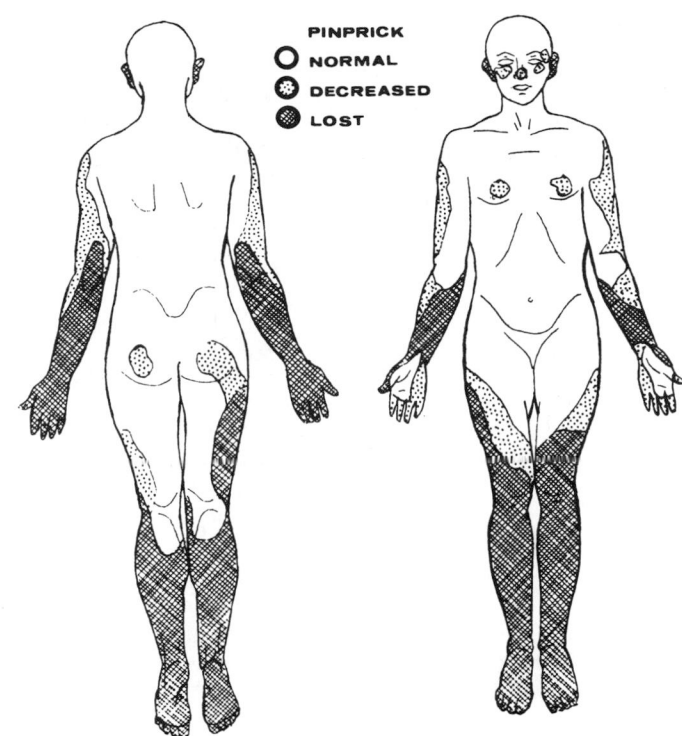

FIG. 5-1. Temperature-linked loss of pain sense in lepromatous leprosy. (From Sabin TD, Swift TR: Chapter 74. In Dyck RJ, Thomas PK (eds): Leprosy in Peripheral Neuropathy. 3rd Ed. WB Saunders, Philadelphia, 1993, with permission.)

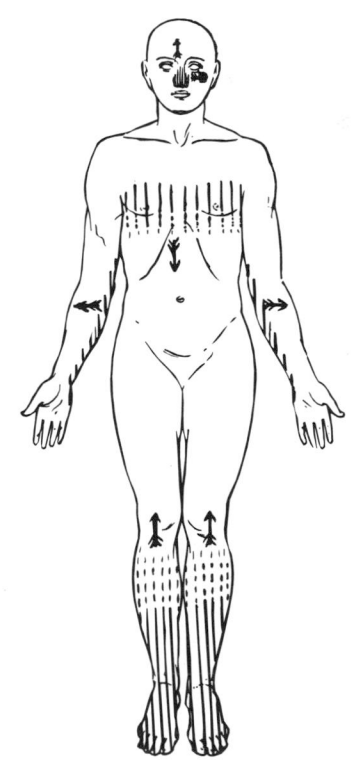

FIG. 5-2. Distribution of pain and temperature loss in Hitzig's zones of tabes dorsalis. The arrows indicate the manner of progression. (From Holmes G: Tabes dorsalis. p. 215. In: Nelson Loose-Leaf Medicine. Vol. 6. Thomas Nelson & Sons, New York, 1920, with permission.)

Functional Loss of Pinprick Sensation

Occasionally one will come across a patient with a nonanatomic patch of apparent total analgesia that may be related to hysteria, somatic delusions, or disability-seeking behavior. This can rapidly be sorted out by making a pinprick map on which the return from absent to normal sensation usually occurs across a distinct line, which should be inked in on the patient's skin. A similar absence of vibration sense across that same ink line, especially at a site where there is underlying bone to widely disperse the vibratory stimulation, reveals the nature of the apparent sensory loss. This testing should be done with the patient's eyes open so the ink line can be seen. When patients claims to suffer completely "numb" hands, they should have extreme difficulty in picking up a coin from a flat surface without bringing it to the edge. Naive patients with feigned sensory loss will respond with "yes" or "no" with each pinprick with the eyes closed. A rather sad commentary on our times is the patient who has been professionally trained to have "sensory loss" along a textbook nerve root distribution. Fortunately, this education is not usually adequate to dupe the sophisticated examiner.

Sensory and Mixed Nerves

Tingling paresthesias progressing to sensory loss with the greatest extent of loss affecting the modality of light touch is characteristic of a progressive mononeuropathy. Sensory complaints are common even with involvement of "pure" motor nerves. Such nerves do contain the sensory fibers subserving muscle pain and static and phasic stretch receptors. "Motor" nerve compression often causes "numbness" and "stiffness" as well as pain. If one nerve alone is involved, then a search for compression will usually yield the answer. When multiple named nerves are affected, then a mononeuritis multiplex such as that seen in certain collagen-vascular diseases, diabetes, and leprosy should be considered.

Polyneuropathy

The typical pattern of sensory loss in most sensory or sensori-motor polyneuropathies is distal and symmetric. A stocking-glove sensory loss that features abrupt loss of all modalities at sharply demarcated borders just above the ankles and the wrist is yet another variety of functional sensory loss. The loss of sensation in polyneuropathy is most often related to axonal length so that "knee socks" are present before the "gloves." Rather than an abrupt change to normal, there is a broad zone where the sensation on the limbs gradually returns. The greatest intensity of paresthesias and dysesthetic temporal summation is found where the sensory loss gradually shades off to normal. This distal loss can ultimately progress to affect proximal limbs and then the nerves traversing the body wall are involved. A "teardrop" plate of sensory loss appears over the anterior torso (Fig. 5-3). This loss is widest in the lower abdomen owing to the obliquity of the nerves and becomes narrower in the upper chest region, where the nerves follow the shorter ribs. This sensory loss may progress across the chest and be mistaken for a spinal sensory level. We have seen patients in whom there are just 10 or 12 cm of sensory sparing on either side of the midline of the back. In cases with dying-back type of neuropathy, sensory loss may be found in the distal branches of the first division of the trigeminal nerve in the posterior scalp. The distance from Gasser's ganglion out to the most distal reaches of this supply is about 28 cm. With a good sensory witness, the

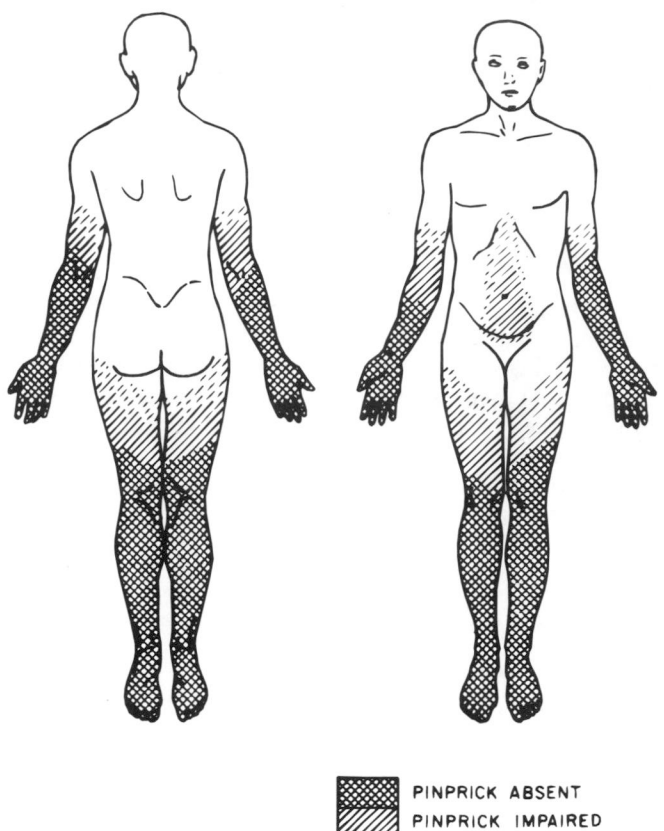

■ PINPRICK ABSENT
▨ PINPRICK IMPAIRED

FIG. 5-3. Advanced distal, symmetric sensory loss in sensory polyneuropathy with sensory loss over the anterior torso in a 43-year-old man with amyloid neuropathy. (From Sabin TD, Geschwind N, Waxman SG: Patterns of clinical deficits in peripheral nerve disease. p. 433. In Waxman SG (ed): Physiology and Pathobiology of Axons. Raven Press, New York, 1978, with permission.)

measurements from sensory ganglia to the border of abnormal sensation is constant over the head, torso, and on the four extremities. A distal symmetric pattern of deficits will also emerge with randomly scattered nerve lesions because of the statistical likelihood of accumulating more lesions in longer fibers.

Sensory Ganglionopathies

In sensory ganglionopathies, a clear distal-to-proximal pattern is not present because there is a direct toxic or immune attack on dorsal root ganglia. Large-fiber sensations are most affected, and the patients are often severely handicapped as a result of loss of proprioceptive and kinesthetic input from proximal as well as distal sources. The ataxia in these disorders is prominent. Widespread areflexia accompanies the loss of position and vibration sense. This constellation may be seen in an acute sensory ganglionopathy and the chronic ataxic neuropathy that may be associated with anti-myelin-associated glycoprotein antibodies, subacute carcinomatous sensory neuropathy associated with antibodies to dorsal root ganglia antigen, Sjögren syndrome, and pyridoxine toxicity. Pyridoxine toxicity illustrates the two possible variations in the basic patterns of sensory loss in the ganglionopathies. In experimental models, if the dose of pyridoxine is very large, early necrosis of the dorsal root ganglion cells with secondary degeneration of both the distally directed and centrally directed axons occurs immediately, whereas lower toxic doses allow survival of the dorsal root ganglia cells themselves but prevents them from maintaining axons, so that a distal-to-proximal degeneration of the centrally and peripherally directed axons occurs. The first symptoms in such ganglionopathies may begin in the face or over the torso and then spread distally, but sometimes the abnormalities appear in a widespread fashion simultaneously in both proximal and distal areas of the body.

Proximal Predilection Neuropathy

Porphyric neuropathy is an example of a acute process that may be associated with paralysis in the proximal musculature and a sensory loss over the torso and proximal limbs with sparing of the distal extremities. This is reflected by a loss of proximal deep tendon reflexes with a preservation of ankle jerks. One theory on the mechanism for this extraordinary pattern suggests that an endotoxin is brought back to the cell bodies by suicide retrograde transport, and the cells with shortest axons are injured first, resulting in a progressive proximal-to-distal sequence of deficits. Tangier disease may also spare distal sensation.

Nerve Roots

Individual Roots.   Nerve root impingement by a herniated disc in the lumbar or cervical spine may cause only tingling paresthesias within its distribution. If there is sensory loss, pinprick is most affected and usually only in a small portion of the dermatome because extensive overlap is a feature of root innervation. Tenderness of the nerve in which the entrapped root travels may indicate severe compression; tenderness along the course of nerves is otherwise a rare feature on physical examination.

Sensory Complaints in Guillain-Barré Syndrome.   In some cases of Guillain-Barré syndrome, sensory complaints are very prominent. The distribution of the deficits in this disease varies considerably, probably because individual differences in the blood–brain/root/nerve barrier. The distribution of "leakiness" to large immunologically active molecules that attack myelin determines the pattern of lesions. Some patients develop almost all their lesions in the nerve roots, so that proximal and distal sensory complaints (and paralysis) occur from the onset. The disturbance in 1A afferents with distortion of kinesthesia may be the cause of the ataxia in the Miller Fisher variant of Guillain-Barré syndrome.

Spinal Cord Syndromes

Sensory information undergoes both segregation by modalities and processing upon entering the cord. Substantial constriction or expansion on pinprick responsivity in experimentally isolated dorsal root receptive fields occurs with either selective ablation of the dorsal or ventral part of the Lissauer's tract or with application of various pharmacologic agents.

Once the sensory information is in the major sensory tracts, then compression by extrinsic lesions of the spinal cord causes clinical symptoms and deficits in the longest fiber systems first, so that paresthesias and sensory loss begin in the feet and gradually ascend to the level of the compressive lesion. A narrow segmental band of ipsilateral multimodal sensory loss due to involvement of roots or root entry zone may be the only sensory clue to the precise level of a compressive lesion.

The segregation of various sensory modalities accounts for several important clinical features in the bedside sensory examination. Since fibers carrying pinprick and temperature sensation decussate within a few segments of entering the spinal cord, the fibers subserving the lowest sacral segments are most superficial, so extrinsic compressive lesions produce early loss of pain and temperature in sacral segments. Intramedullary cord lesions tend to spare these superficial fibers and produce "sacral sparing." Since touch sensation is represented within the ipsilateral dorsal column system and in the crossed spinothalamic system, a careful search for the differential affection of pinprick and temperature versus position and vibration sense is often the key to unravelling spinal cord sensory syndromes.

Brown-Séquard Syndrome.   With hemisection of the cord, there is an ipsilateral band of loss of all modalities at the level of the lesion due to destruction of the fibers of all modalities at the root entry zone. Loss of position and vibration sense occurs below the level of the lesion on the same side, but on the opposite side of the body, there is only loss of pinprick and temperature sensation, whereas touch is preserved on both sides (Fig. 5-4). In the full-blown syndrome, ipsilateral upper motor neuron paralysis is present below the level of the lesion. The Brown-Séquard syndrome is nearly always present in the form fruste, but subtle variations on this pattern of sensory change are reliable indicators of lesion site. Certain monkey experiments indicate that the crossed pain and temperature loss are due to a physiologic state that can be abolished if there is complete section of the ventral funiculus on the side of the hemisection.

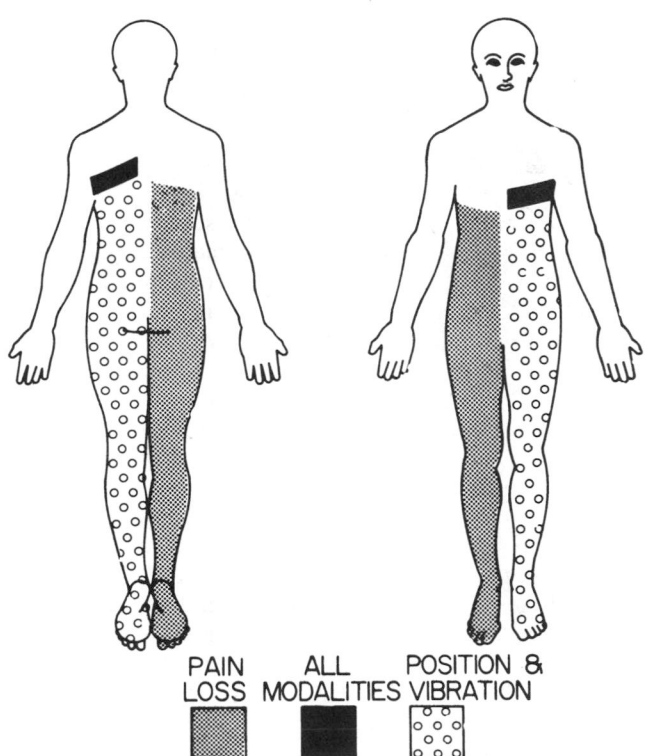

PAIN LOSS   ALL MODALITIES   POSITION & VIBRATION

FIG. 5-4.   The Brown-Séquard syndrome. Hemisection of the spinal cord showing ipsilateral loss of position and vibration sense and crossed loss of pinprick and temperature sensation below the lesion. (From Sabin TD, Geschwind N: The neurologic examination. p. 38. In Mark VH (ed): Tice's Practice of Surgery (Neurosurgery). Harper & Row, Hagerstown, PA, 1973, with permission.)

This lesion actually caused the pain and temperature loss to switch to the ipsilateral side, presumably owing to disinhibition of the systems serving these modalities. We have not seen an example of this phenomenon in human diseases; however, the fact that the loss of pin and temperature lasts only weeks or months after surgical tractotomy points to the physiologic state as a critical factor.

Dorsal Columns.   The information destined for the dorsal columns passes from the dorsal roots directly into these sensory tracts, resulting in lamination with the sacral areas and feet closest to the midline and the upper cervical segments most laterally. A demyelinating lesion in the center of the dorsal columns will therefore cause intense tingling of the feet, and as the lesion spreads laterally, tingling in the hands may develop. Such a patient is often misdiagnosed as having a neuropathy, but the preservation of ankle jerks rules this out. The diagnosis of peripheral neuropathy where large-fiber tingling is prominent should consistently be associated with loss of deep tendon reflexes, since the 1A fibers subserving the afferent loop of these reflexes are part of the heavily myelinated group and the ankle jerks rely on the function of only a few of the longest of them.

Suspended Sensory Loss.   The "suspended" sensory loss of central cord lesions is the most powerful diagnostic sensory syndrome of the spinal cord. The disruption of the pain and temperature pathways in the anterior white commissure as they cross the cord causes a profound loss of of these modalities in all segments so affected (Fig. 5-5). The sensory loss is dissociated

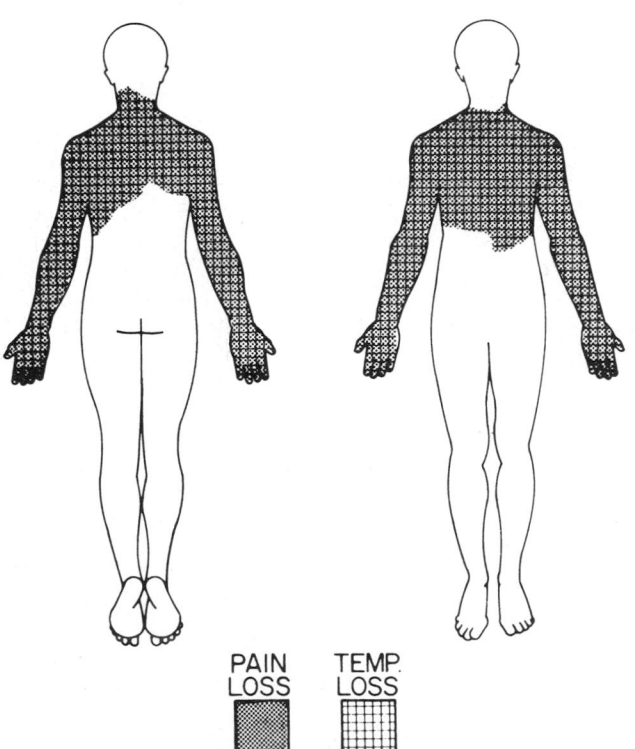

PAIN   TEMP.
LOSS   LOSS

FIG. 5-5.   Suspended sensory loss. A syrinx has interrupted crossing pain and temperature fibers from C3 to midthoracic levels, but the spinothalamic tracts themselves are spared. (From Sabin TD, Geschwind N: The neurologic examination. p. 39. In Mark VH (ed): Tice's Preactice of Surgery (Neurosurgery). Harper & Row, Hagerstown, PA, 1973, with permission.)

because there is excellent preservation of position, touch, and vibration in the areas devoid of pain and temperature sense. The patient will discriminate sharp from dull on the basis of well-preserved discriminative touch alone in the abnormal areas.

Craniocervical Junction.   "Reversed" dissociated sensory loss is one of the sensory syndromes that occurs with lesions at the junction between spinal cord and medulla. Basilar invagination, odontoid abnormalities, and foramen magnum meningioma are the most common causes. A loss of position and vibration limited to the upper extremities and upper torso is highly diagnostic of compression near the site of the decussation of the medial lemniscus. These patients have pseudochorea in the upper extremities and may demonstrate upper motor neuron findings that are also limited to the upper extremities. Loss of vibration sense over the clavicles is an unusual bedside finding in these patients.

Brainstem Syndromes

The dissociation of large- and small-fiber modalities continues in the lower brainstem, because the medial lemniscus remains distant from the spinothalamic system until the two converge in the rostral brainstem prior to entering the thalamus. The lateral medullary syndrome with ipsilateral loss of the pain and temperature in the face and crossed loss of these sensations over the rest of the body is the most common pattern seen in clinical practice. The medial medullary syndrome with loss of large-fiber modalities and upper motor neuron signs on the opposite side of the body and ipsilateral tongue paralysis is extremely rare. There has been one patient described with bilateral small lateral brainstem strokes with a universal loss of pinprick and temperature sensation but preserved deep pain to testicular, periosteal, and tendon pressure.

Thalamic Lesions

Lesions of the thalamus are capable of eliminating all modalities of sensation from the opposite side of the body. In this hemisensory loss, there is some sparing near the midline owing to bilateral representation of paramedian sites. In the thalamic Dejerine-Roussy syndrome there usually is a very small lesion; the patient may have minimal signs at time of onset, but over a period of a few weeks, severe spontaneous pain or stimulus-provoked, spreading, intense protopathic pain appears. The pain may be a dull, boring pressure that "explodes" over one-half of the body. The pain seems to resemble the normal experience of eating ice cream too rapidly and incurring intense pain in the forehead. This pain can also be imitated by plunging the hand and forearm into ice water. Within a few seconds after the stinging discomfort has disappeared, an extremely severe, boring ache in the shoulder and upper arm appears that rapidly becomes intolerable. One of our patients with a thalamic syndrome had his pain provoked by specific kinds of stimulation in all modalities except smell. The taste of salty foods or minimal tactile stimulation would provoke the pain. Specific sounds, such as his wife's ironing, could cause the pain, and each sweep of the iron would be associated with a wave of pain over the affected side of the body. This particular patient did not respond to medical treatment but improved following a stereotactic lesion placed in the centrum medianum.

Corticosensory Loss

Elementary sensory modalities are elaborated by the cerebral cortex into a much more complex sensory experience that has the qualities of space, weight, form, and texture. There is now experimental evidence to support the clinical observations that the regions of cortical sensory representation are not fixed anatomically or "hard wired" but may fluctuate according to the function of the innervated regions. Monkey experiments show a reallocation of up to 14 mm sensory cortex after prolonged peripheral deafferentation.

The power with which the cortex organizes body space is illustrated in the schoolboy trick of crossing the index finger over the middle finger and rubbing the point of intersection of the two fingers over the tip of the nose. This causes a powerful illusion that you have two noses. The cortical body map is obliged to account for the apparent palmar finger space of the unstimulated medial half of the index finger and lateral aspect of the middle finger by doubling the tip of the nose! Corticol sensory testing assesses this organization of sensory space. The ability to localize stimuli with the eyes closed using a single index finger or to discriminate between being touched with one or two close points are simple bedside tests for this function. Stimuli that are about 1 mm apart can be detected on the normal fingertips, whereas they may have to be as far as 7 cm apart in areas of the back. An unfolded paper clip is an adequate, inexpensive device for testing two-point discrimination.

Dissociation of position from vibration sense is a useful way to tell a cortical from a subcortical lesion. Vibration sense is present with cortical lesions but absent with subcortical/thalamic disorders. An excellent screening device for corticosensory disorder is graphesthesia. Some normal patients are unable to decipher numbers written on their skin; but if they can do this task, no other corticosensory disorder is likely.

Hemisensory extinction of bilateral touch or pinprick stimuli may be seen with large parietal lesions. The patient reports stimuli only on the side of the body opposite the intact hemisphere with stimultaneous stimuli but detects stimuli on each side when stimuli do not occur at the same time. Temporal and spatial summation overcome extinction, and the phenomenon can be tested in several modalities. Proximal over distal extinction also occurs on the same side of the body.

Patients with damage to the corticosensory systems rarely complain about any powerful paresthesias, unless these are part of a seizure or migraine. Large destructive hemispheric lesions cause the patient to say one side has "gone numb." Acutely, there is profound sensory loss to all modalities, most severe around the face and distal extremities, with relative preservation of the trunk and proximal limb girdles, roughly reflecting the proportions of sensory cortex subserving these areas. This sensory loss rapidly abates, flaccidity disappears, and spasticity appears. Motor disorders, even when they are "pure," often result in sensory complaints, and surely the limb without normal tone or movement must feel quite different, even though sensory pathways are apparently undisturbed according to the usual tests. The feeling that a limb is missing or gone from the body is often associated with anosognosia. This phenomenon can be viewed as the opposite of the phantom limb experience, for now the patient believes the limb does not exist, because brain awareness of it has been ablated. When the limb is amputated, the patient continues to sense its phantom existence, because its neural presence remains.

There is a paradox regarding pain perception and the sensory

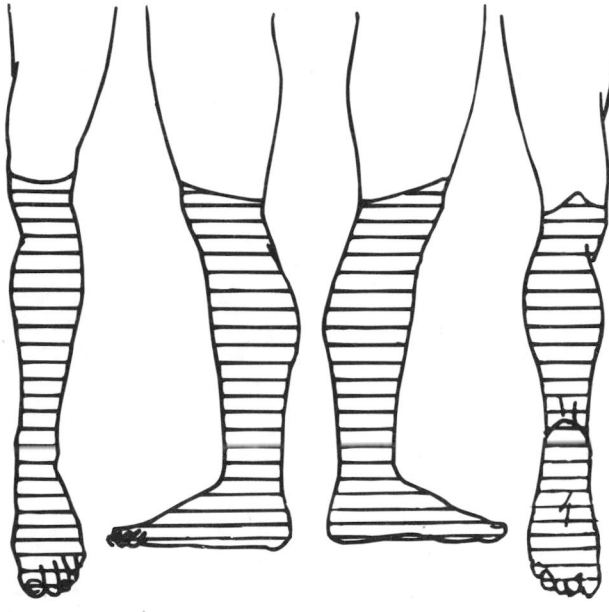

FIG. 5-6. Area of gross impairment of superficial and deep pain after a penetrating wound affecting the sensory cortex subserving this area. (From Marshall J: Sensory disturbances in cortical wounds with special reference to pain. J Neurol Neurosurg Psychiatry 14:187–204, 1957, with permission.)

cortex: pain sensation is intact with complete ablation of sensory cortex, but with focal lesions of the sensory cortex, pain loss appears on the opposite side of the body (Fig. 5-6). The muscles in the affected areas showed absent deep pain sensibility when injected with hypertonic saline. This suggests that widespread destruction of the sensory cortices may be necessary to disinhibit the thalamic mechanism required to bring pain to consciousness.

Focal lesions of the parietal operculum may produce a pseudothalamic syndrome with localized spontaneous pain that is more restricted and less severe than in the thalamic Dejerine-Roussy syndrome. Lesions undercutting the sensory association cortex may disconnect cortical pain representation from the limbic system and cause an asymbolia to pain. This seems to be a common but rarely described transient phenomenon in association with conduction aphasia.

SUGGESTED READINGS

Denny-Brown D: The enigma of crossed sensory loss with cord hemisection. pp. 889–95. In Bonica JJ, Chrubosik J, Cusins M (eds): Advances in Pain Research and Therapy. Vol. 3. Raven Press, New York, 1979

Denny-Brown D: The tract of lissauer in relation to sensory transmission in the dorsal horn of spinal cord in the Macaque monkey. J Comp Neurol 151:175–200, 1973

Marshall J: Sensory disturbances in cortical wounds with special reference to pain. J Neurol Neurosurg Psychiatry 14:187–204, 1951

Pons TB, Garraghty PE, Ommaya AK et al: Massive cortical reorganization after sensory deafferentiation in adult Macaques. Science 252:1857–60, 1991

Sabin TD: Classification of peripheral neuropathy: the long and the short of it. Muscle Nerve 8:711–9, 1986

Sabin TD: Temperature-linked sensory loss. A unique pattern in leprosy. Arch Neurol 3:257–62, 1969

Venna N, Sabin TD: Universal dissociated anesthesia due to bilateral brainstem infarcts. Arch Neurol 42:918–22, 1985

Waxman SG, Brill MHY, Geschwind N et al: Probability of conduction deficit as related to fiber length in random-distribution models of peripheral neuropathies. J Neurol Sci 1:39–53, 1976

Weiss JA, White JC: Correlation of IA afferent conduction with the ataxia of Fisher Syndrome. Muscle Nerve, 9:327, 1986

Xu Yue, Sladky JT, Brown MJ: Dose-dependent expression of neuronopathy after experimental pyridoxine intoxication. Neurology 39:1077–83, 1989

6. PAIN

DAVID M. DAWSON
THOMAS D. SABIN

The evaluation and treatment of specific categories of pain are discussed in detail in Part IX. This chapter discusses a general approach to the patient with pain.

Pain brings patients to medical care. Headache, visceral pain, pain in an extremity, long-term pain, and acute pain are all reasons for patients to go to their physicians. Neurologists deal with pain as do doctors in other specialties, but there are additional complexities when the nervous system is involved. Occasionally, the nervous system itself is the source of pain. At other times, the nervous system is damaged by the disease process, so that the reporting system for pain is inaccurate or misleading.

Many authors have commented on the importance of pain to the organism. Pain warns of damage or potential danger and serves a protective role; it is the most common symptom of disease and is often one of the earliest.

Throughout this discussion, the dual nature of pain is emphasized. It both alerts the patient and physician to the presence of disease and itself requires treatment. It is both an emotion and a perception, and as a perception has a dual nature: there is a fast-track system carrying one type of pain and a slow-track system carrying another. These interact, and both exist in most instances. Treatment of pain also is dual in nature, often focusing on the psychological and perceptual aspects and secondarily or when possible focusing on the cause and the removal of the cause.

The intensity of our reaction to pain is strongly controlled by the nervous system. Parts of the nervous system augment pain, and once in action, these systems can make pain intolerable. On the other hand, there are descending influences from higher centers that may inhibit our perception of pain and in some instances can obliterate it completely so that a sensation normally felt as painful is not even noticed.

There is one final way in which pain is dual: it has both an anatomic, hard-wired aspect and a biochemical aspect mediated by endorphins and chemical effectors, so that measurement and analysis of pain must deal with neuroanatomy on the one hand and with neurochemistry on the other.

CLINICAL ASSESSMENT

As neurologists, we are accustomed to investigating pain with patients via the history that they give. During history taking, reports of intensity of pain can be notoriously difficult to separate form the personal and psychological context of the patient's pain. Some authors draw a distinction between suffering and pain. Terror, depression, issues of financial compensation or disability payment, and simple concern that the physician will not be attentive can all play major roles in affecting the patient history. A terrible pain in the left shoulder will be much less intense, and the patient's suffering less, when the patient knows it represents bursitis and not a heart attack.

Patients are often asked to rate pain on a 1 to 10 scale. Sometimes that is useful; in acute settings, however, it is often not helpful. The patient's manner may help to indicate severity. Sweating, restlessness, cautious moving about, shallow breathing, and distractibility are often seen with severe pain. Yet lack of the appearance of pain does not indicate its absence.

Location

Neurologists deal mostly with face, head, and extremity pain. This reflects the fact that these are the common locations for nerve root pain, a common source of neurologic illness. More specifically, neurologists look for pain patterns that reflect a known anatomic pathway. For example, trigeminal pain affects the face, gums, eye, and forehead, but not the ear or neck. Pain from the fifth lumbar nerve root is located in the thigh, lateral calf, dorsum of the foot, and occasionally, down to the toes. Radicular pain in the chest tends to follow the distribution of an intercostal nerve. Location can be very helpful, even diagnostic in some instances. Often, however, pain is "nonanatomic." This does not mean that it is imaginary or that it has a psychologic basis. Central pain is often poorly localized. Patients with a cervical syringomyelia will have a dull aching pain over the entire shoulder, chest, and arm. Those with spinal cord infarctions may have pain that covers an entire extremity up to the abdomen. In diabetic amyotrophy due to vascular disease affecting nerve roots of the lumbar plexus, aching pain over the lower abdomen and upper leg occurs without good localization. The experienced observer will search for the anatomic pattern and hope that it can be discerned, but if it is absent, move on to other data.

Patterns of Diagnostic Value

Cutaneous Pain. A lesion of cutaneous branches of peripheral nerves has a very characteristic quality. It is prickling, tingling, and sensitive. The patient will avoid touching the area with clothing or with other objects. Tapping on the skin may produce intense burning or prickling sensations. When testing, one can usually find an elevation in threshold to pinprick, but more characteristic is the fact that threshold for light touch with a piece of cotton or thread is even more impaired than is cutaneous sensation for pinprick and cold. The border of the sensory loss on the skin is sharp and well defined. These kinds of cutaneous disorders are seen with lesions of the lateral femoral cutaneous nerve (meralgia paresthetica) or lesions of the sural nerve at the ankle or the radial nerve just above the wrist.

Cutaneous damage causing nerve damage is also seen following burns, closed trauma, crush injuries, or relatively deep lacerations. Sometimes in these conditions, one can find small areas—nowhere near as large as those of a peripheral nerve trunk—that are sensitive, prickling, and tingling in this same way. Every surgeon is aware of the patient with a painful scar over the abdomen following abdominal surgery, and hand surgeons know the pattern of nerve branching in the arms so as to avoid areas of skin incision that are most likely to produce these painful scars or lacerations. Again, tapping on the skin will often set off pain, paresthesias, and tingling, whereas areas of sensory loss, if present, are larger in size for light touch than they are for pinprick sensation.

Peripheral Nerve Pain.   Larger nerve trunks produce other kinds of pain. Many of us are aware of this from personal experience, since we have had sciatica or a contusion of the ulnar nerve at the elbow or other sources of large nerve trunk pain. Nerve pain is aching, widely radiating, and accompanied by paresthesias mostly in the distal territory of the nerve. A characteristic pattern with sciatica, for example, is a tingling, numb, paresthetic foot with loss of sensation in territories of several branches of that nerve accompanied by aching and severe pain all up and down the trunk of the nerve from top to bottom. Along these areas of pain, there will also be local tenderness. A person with sciatic pain will have tenderness to external pressure within the buttock, in the posterior thigh, and over the branches of the nerve around the fibular head.

One can recognize this as neuropathic pain because of its long extent up and down an extremity; by the characteristics of the pain, which include electric sensations, dysesthesias, and burning; and by the disturbance of sensory or motor function, which indicates nerve fiber loss. Other observations may clinch the conclusion that neuropathic pain is present. One of these observations is that of *allodynia,* a term implying that a sensation is altered in its character, most typically a cutaneous touch sensation becoming painful. Allodynia is very characteristic of partial peripheral nerve lesions, whether ischemic, metabolic, or compressive. Some authors assert that allodynia is especially seen after some reinnervation of a partially denervated area.

A second observation that may be clinically useful is that of recruitment with multiple stimuli. This is especially seen with axonal distal polyneuropathy, such as alcoholic neuropathy. A single pinprick is not felt over the foot, but multiple pinpricks produce sudden perception of pain, and then the pain will build up to a higher level with each successive pinprick. In alcoholic neuropathy, the build-up is seen commonly after one or two pinpricks; with other kinds of metabolic neuropathies, there may be more delay.

Allodynia has a particular feature that suggests a peripheral causation. Capsaicin extracts applied to the skin will often reduce pain and allodynia when used for a period of time as the content of substance P neurons within the skin diminishes. This observation indicates that a peripheral source for pain depends very specifically on the type of nerve ending that is damaged.

Nerve Root Pain.   One of the most common sources of pain is compression of a nerve root in the lumbar or cervical region by disk or bony spur. Pain due to lesions of nerve roots has many of the features of peripheral nerve pain, and testing for it is carried out in many of the same ways. However, several features of the pain and examination are characteristic of a root lesion:

1. Test for movement that will increase the pain, typically those that will stretch nerve roots as they pass out of the nerve foramina. The straight leg raising test for sciatic pain is the most common example. A positive straight leg raising test, whether done in the seated or prone position, is often seen when the fifth lumbar or first sacral nerve root is trapped at the foramen. In the cervical region, traction on the arm may produce pain or the patient may have noticed that certain neck movements, such as turning or lateral bending, can cause pain that radiates into the arm. These observations are very important diagnostically since they clearly localize the source of the pain. Pain with cough or sneeze, if present, is also a good indicator of nerve root compression.

2. Neurologic testing for monoradicular syndromes depends on detecting relatively minor findings. Nerve roots heavily overlap. Each muscle in the body receives primary nerve root innervation, but in only a few is the majority of the innervation from one nerve root. The deltoid muscle, for instance, receives much more than one-half of its innervation from the fifth cervical root, whereas the triceps muscle receives innervation from the sixth, seventh, and eighth cervical roots. All of the small muscles of the hand receive innervation from the eighth cervical and first thoracic roots. This kind of overlapping pattern is repeated in the lumbar and sacral roots. Therefore, one must discover weakness of a muscle group that is modest in degree in order to detect nerve root pathology.

3. The same goes for sensory examination: one is looking for minor differences. A fairly major loss of function in the sixth cervical nerve root on one side will cause numbness over the dorsal and palmar surfaces of the thumb and index finger, nearby portions of the wrist and dorsum of the hand, and possibly some loss in the forearm. All of this loss is modest in degree, incomplete, and certainly does not involve all of the territory to which the sixth cervical nerve fibers can be traced or that are shown on dermatome maps in textbooks. Allodynia and recruitment with repetitive stimulation are not commonly observed with root disorders. When found, these suggest peripheral nerve disease.

4. Pain is commonly out of proportion to the degree of sensory loss in nerve root disorders. This naturally brings to the forefront the question of malingering, hysteria, and psychologically enhanced pain. How is the examiner to distinguish the real from the false? Observation of the patient's behavior is useful. A person who makes exaggerated efforts to limp across the room, stands with severe grimacing yet arrives in the examining room fully dressed and has no trouble dressing after the examination is a patient of whom one is suspicious. In nerve root disorders, marked muscular weakness should be accompanied by loss of a corresponding tendon reflex and by muscular atrophy if of long standing. The sensory loss should bear some relationship to anatomic patterns, recognizing that these patterns are not invariable, and one must allow for this variation. The examiner needs to have experience, sympathy, anatomic knowledge, and a healthy skepticism when confronted with inconsistent patterns while maintaining an open mind for atypical presentations.

Plexus Disorders.   Diseases of the lumbosacral and brachial plexus are relatively uncommon compared to peripheral nerve or nerve root diseases. Nevertheless, they need to be carefully considered. In many instances, they cause serious problems with major loss of neurologic function. This applies especially to invasion by carcinoma, to radiation damage to the plexus, or to some of the inflammatory conditions, such as idiopathic brachial neuritis, in which the neurologic deficit can be quite marked.

Tricks that are useful in recognizing plexus disorders are to note that the pattern of deficit does not match that of a root or peripheral nerve, that proximal muscles such as the serratus anterior or pectoralis major are affected, or that the sensory loss seems very dense, and that in some instances sympathetic nervous system failure is evident by dryness of skin and lack of vasodilation. The electromyographic pattern may help by showing that the paraspinous muscles are spared, whereas all the distal muscles corresponding to a nerve root are affected.

The pain patterns produced by plexus disorders are not particularly typical. One exception is the lumbosacral plexus disorder seen in diabetic neuropathy. It is one of the few diseases in which pain and sensory loss occur over the lower abdomen in the T10–T12 dermatomes, and when this pattern is seen in a diabetic patient in the proper clinical setting, it is practically specific.

Pain with Spinal Cord Lesions.   The spinal cord is sometimes a source of pain, and examination of the pain-conducting pathways in patients with spinal cord disease is important. Several patterns are worth mentioning.

In patients with large central lesions of the spinal cord spanning a number of segments, the pain fibers are affected as they cross through the central gray matter. This is true of patients who have had contusions of the cord with central cord necrosis, of patients with primary tumors intrinsic to the cord, or of patients with cystic cavities, such as in syringomyelia. In these patients, a very dense ''dissociated'' sensory loss is found in which perception of pinprick, cold, and heat is absent over large areas of the torso and limbs, whereas perception of touch and posterior column function is preserved. The sensory deficit will be suspended (i.e., there will be normal sensation below the lowest level of the lesion) if the lesion includes the crossing spinothalamic fibers in the central gray while sparing the ascending spinothalamic tracts. True dissociated sensory loss of this type strongly implies disease of the spinal cord rather than disease of nerve roots or peripheral fibers.

It is characteristic of spinal cord lesions to produce a sensory level due to involvement of ascending sensory tracts. With cervical lesions, this level will be found around the neck; with thoracic lesions, over the trunk. It is an extremely important diagnostic test to look for this sensory level. One should start in a normal area of sensation, such as the face or upper neck, to give the patient a point of reference, then move from the distal parts of the body up the trunk toward the clavicles and ask the patient to compare stimuli, using no more than eight to ten stimuli to cover this whole area. If a sudden increase in sensitivity is found, one can go back and more precisely locate this level. The two sides should be compared, because often the level is lower on one side than it is on the other. A well-defined sensory level to cold, pinprick, and vibration is a strong indicator of spinal cord disease. Only very rarely will a higher lesion in the midbrain, pons, or medulla produce a level over the trunk when sensory tracts are affected, and even then it is accompanied by so many other signs that there should be no diagnostic confusion.

It has been known for nearly 100 years that the spinal level discovered by sensory testing may be removed by many segments from the associated lesion. If it is dense and well defined, as it is in traumatic paraplegia, the level accurately reflects the level of the lesion in the cord. In acute medical illness, in cord compression due to metastatic cancer, and in spinal cord infarction, among many other clinical settings, the level that is found by clinical examination is liable to be at least four or five segments below the actual anatomic level in the spinal cord itself. As noted above, with lesions involving the central gray matter, the level may be suspended.

In diseases with multiple lesions, such as multiple sclerosis, vitamin B_{12} deficiency with spinal cord involvement, or various hereditary degenerative diseases, the spinal tracts are damaged by means of accumulated lesions over a long area. Therefore, ''pseudolevels'' may be found. In multiple sclerosis, for instance, one can easily find that vibration sense over the sacrum is much less than it is over the spinous processes in the thoracic region. The level will be very much dependent upon the type of testing and the alertness of the patient. Pseudolevels of this type do indicate spinal cord disease but not segmental, localized, or transverse spinal disease.

Another pattern characteristic intrinsic spinal cord lesions is the Brown-Séquard syndrome. This is discussed along with sensory disorders in Chapter 5.

Pain with Brainstem Disorders.   With lesions in this area, again the pathologic change is in the pain-conducting sensory tracts. In lateral medullary stroke, for instance, the spinothalamic fibers that have crossed from the opposite side of the body are damaged in the lateral medulla. This produces a dissociated hemisensory loss below the neck, affecting primarily pinprick, cold, and heat sensation and sparing vibration and proprioception. There may be pain, usually a burning, poorly localized sensation.

The fibers of the fifth cranial nerve as they enter the pons mirror the pathways that are present in the spinal cord. Those fibers that subserve touch enter directly and pass upward, whereas those that subserve pain, cold, and heat sensation pursue a downward loop into the low medulla and then come back up again with the spinothalamic fibers. Theoretically, in lesions of the upper medulla and lower pons, one can find dissociated sensory loss affecting the face.

Disorders that affect the peripheral nerve fibers that directly enter the brainstem can be the cause of intense neuralgic pain. Trigeminal neuralgia is the most common example. In idiopathic cases, the patient is typically above the age of 60 and has intense unilateral lancinating pains in one or more divisions of the fifth cranial nerve. Usually these pains occur in the cheek, gum, or teeth. One should test for trigeminal sensation in such patients, but in idiopathic trigeminal neuralgia, there is typically no loss of function of any type. In patients with multiple sclerosis or pontine tumors, one can also find facial pain with either a neuralgic, sharp quality or burning dysesthesias with allodynia. In such settings it is more common to find loss of a corneal reflex or numbness over the face in the appropriate trigeminal distribution.

Thalamic Pain and Associated Syndromes.   By the time the sensory pathways reach the thalamus, they have been redistributed, and one is now dealing with hemisensory disturbances affecting the entire opposite side of the body, including the face. The peculiar crossed disorders seen with lateral medullary strokes and the dissociated loss seen with spinal cord lesions do not occur with thalamic lesions.

However, peculiar things can occur at this level. The thalamic syndrome, or Dejerine-Roussy syndrome, includes an *elevated* threshold to many sensory stimuli on the opposite side of the body that is, however, accompanied by intense burning pain in response to stimuli. Cold, touch, pinprick, or even psychological stimuli can produce this marked hemisensory pain. Most lesions producing the Dejerine-Roussy syndrome are not actually in the thalamus but slightly posterior to it, where they interrupt exiting and entering fibers.

A similar set of abnormalities can be found in other hemisphere diseases. Lesions that affect the deep part of the sylvian cortex, the so-called second sensory cortex located in the operculum, can produce painful sensory loss on the opposite side of the body. This is known as the pseudothalamic syndrome. It tends to be less severe and is, in fact, much more common than the true thalamic syndrome. A typical clinical picture is that of a patient who has had a cerebral embolus in the middle cerebral territory and months later has a hemiplegia accompanied by diffuse burning pain. Again, one can show elevated thresholds to many sensory stimuli and sometimes sensitivity to repeated pinprick.

Pain with Parietal Lobe Lesions. The parietal lobe is the final destination of the sensory pathways. It is at this level that judgments and comparisons are made so that the quality, intensity, and nature of stimuli can be finally analyzed. Lesions of this area are not ordinarily associated with pain, but they do produce loss of sensation of many types in the opposite limbs, trunk, and face. Patients with such lesions may have a universal disturbance of sensation that is quite difficult to analyze. In a number of patients, usually with right hemisphere damage, there is loss of awareness of a side of the body (neglect syndrome), which makes testing quite unpredictable. If there is a sensory loss, it will be maximal for such discriminative sensations as two-point discrimination, graphesthesia, judgments of textures and weights, and position sense, whereas it will be least apparent for more primary sensations as vibration sense, pinprick, and cold, which can be experienced using lower-level kinds of integrative activity.

Nonlocalized Pain Syndromes. A group of pain syndromes can occur following injury to tissues, including nerves, which do not follow the anatomic rules just reviewed above. Collectively, these syndromes are known as reflex sympathetic dystrophy. In spite of intense work by many authorities, they remain quite mysterious.

Pain experienced by these patients is typically present in one extremity, usually distally in the hand or foot. Evidence that reflex sympathetic dystrophy can affect the facial or trunk areas has been presented, but cases are rare and poorly documented. In the affected limb, diffuse dull pain occurs, following no neuroanatomic boundaries. For instance, after a crush injury of a hand, the hand may appear pale and sweaty or conversely reddish or dark purple in color with marked sensitivity to pressure or light tapping. All parts of the hand might be affected or several digits or one-half of the hand may be maximally affected. The hand is protected by the patient and will not be used. If the patient has reflex sympathetic dystrophy in the foot, he or she will arrive in the clinic on crutches. Sensitivity to touch or to light squeezing is one of the characteristic findings in these patients.

The term *sympathetic dystrophy* has been in use for many years but is gradually being replaced by the term *sympathetically maintained pain*. There are several reasons to invoke the sympathetic nervous system. First, the appearance of the hand

or foot suggests a disorder of sympathetic function with vasodilation, vasoconstriction, or an abnormality of sweating, and sympathetic block in the cervical or lumbar paraspinal region will often produce a dramatic response. That is not to say that these situations are easy to analyze. There is a very marked placebo response rate to sympathetic block for pain of any type. This may confuse the examiner and lead to an incorrect diagnosis of sympathetically mediated pain. Second, there are a number of patients with reflex sympathetic dystrophy or sympathetically maintained pain in whom sympathetic block is completely ineffective. Third, the exact nature of the involvement of the sympathetic nervous system has remained very controversial, and the literature remains specialized with little consensus. Majority opinion holds that trauma can produce changes within the spinal cord, based on the incoming traffic along sensory fibers, which lead to an alteration of adrenergic sensitivity of second- and third-order neurons within the dorsal horn. These changes can then affect the production of pain as well as sympathetic discharge.

Reflex sympathetic dystrophy or sympathetically maintained pain may occur in the presence of nerve injury. When there has been a nerve injury, most typically the sciatic or the median nerve, there will be deficit symptoms, and the pain will be maximally located in the area of the nerve supply. In other respects, the syndrome resembles reflex sympathetic dystrophy of non-neurologic origin. When a nerve trunk has been affected in this way, the diagnosis of causalgia is commonly applied. Even though the pain and sympathetic changes are distal, the injury to the nerve trunk is often proximal, as for instance, after a gunshot wound through the brachial plexus, a failed procedure for thoracic outlet syndrome, or trauma of the sciatic nerve in the upper buttock.

APPROACH TO THE PATIENT

The function of the examining physician in the assessment of pain is complex:

1. One must determine the importance of the pain as a symptom of disease. Diseases involving the viscera, such as cardiac disease, peritonitis, bone metastases from cancer, and deep infection may all have pain as their cardinal manifestation.
2. The examiner must decide about the psychological state of the patient, the accuracy of the report, the possibility of psychosis or severe depression as a source of pain, and other psychological issues. Every experienced physician is familiar with the patient with hysteria who has frequently reported pain before and has had many surgical procedures. Compensation or disability payments are common issues in pain management, as are complaints of fatigue, depression, anxiety, and resentment. There is a heavy overlap between pain and depression; each heightens the other.

A common problem in medicine in this era is that of chronic pain of undetermined cause in which psychological issues may play some role but do not seem to be primary. Such patients may move from one examiner to another and accumulate mountainous records of investigations.

When presented with a patient with pain, the examiner must make every effort to define his or her own concept of the neuroanatomy involved. Is it a nerve, a nerve root, many roots such as a plexus, or in the central nervous system? Is it a partial lesion? An irritative one? Are axons involved? Or is it more in the nature of a block in conduction? Too often, further testing is undertaken before these fundamental questions are thought through. Magnetic resonance imaging scans and electrophysiologic testing are nowadays extremely sensitive. Would minor slowing of median nerve velocity at the wrist have any meaning in this patient? Or would hypertrophic spurring at C5–C6 correlate? The thinking must precede the testing.

TREATMENT

In some instances, unfortunately not many, diagnosis leads directly to treatment and relief of pain. All too often, the clinician is faced with chronic pain for which no therapy will be directly successful, because a complex problem with a mixture of the physical and psychological is at work. Skillfully treading through these minefields is a mark of the expert clinician.

Responses to therapy should be carefully assessed. Did the patient initially respond to laminectomy only to have the pain recur 6 months later in a slightly different version of sciatica? If so, this suggests a recurrent disc. Did the patient have a prompt and complete response to carbamazepine and find that the stabbing facial pain was completely relieved? Trigeminal neuralgia will often respond in this way. Tricyclic antidepressants may help with pain of many types. The patient should be queried about this response. Was it immediate? The antidepressant effects of tricyclics often take weeks to build up; the analgesic effects are quicker.

In the past few years, treatment of pain has taken new directions. Pain treatment services have led the way in making changes. For postoperative pain and chronic pain of malignancy, the attitude is now widespread that severe or moderate pain should not be tolerated. Morphine intravenous pumps, intrathecal morphine, nerve blocks, and other new treatments are beginning to supplement or replace the older standbys. Fentanyl patches and long-acting oral morphine are better than standard oral narcotic agents with their peaks, valleys, and side effects.

Many patients do better on low-dose tricyclic antidepressants. Splinting, physiotherapy, and a host of nontraditional approaches all can make a difference. Recognizing that pain is a perception and an emotion, based in and arising from the brain, allows one to believe that these eclectic approaches all can play a valid role in patient care.

SUGGESTED READINGS

Alexander J, Black A: Pain mechanisms and the management of neuropathic pain. Curr Opin Neurol Neurosurg 5:228–34, 1992

Besson J-M, Chaouch A: Peripheral and spinal mechanisms of nociception. Physiol Rev 67:67–186, 1987

Fields HL, Heinricher MM, Mason P: Neurotransmmitters in nociceptive modulatory circuits. Annu Rev Neurosci 14:219, 1991

Kerr IG, Sone M, DeAngelis C et al: Continuous narcotic infusion with patient-controlled analgesia for chronic cancer pain in outpatients. Ann Intern Med 108:554–7, 1988

Krishnan KR, France RD: Antidepressants in chronic pain syndromes. Am Fam Physician 39:233–7, 1989

Levine JD, Gordon NC, Fields HL: The mechanism of placebo analgesia. Lancet 2:654, 1978

Payne R: Experience with transdermal fentanyl in advanced cancer pain. Eur J Pain 11:98–101, 1990

Richardson DE: Central stimulation-induced analgesia in humans—modulation by endogenous opioid peptides. Crit Rev Neurobiol 6:33–7, 1990

Watson CP, Evans RJ, Reed K et al: Amitriptyline versus placebo in postherpetic neuralgia. Neurol 32:671–3, 1982

Woolf CJ, Chong MS: Preemptive analgesia—treating postoperative pain by preventing establishment of central sensitization. Anesth Analg 77:362–9, 1993

7. DISORDERS OF THE EYES AND EYELIDS

GRANT T. LIU

Because a significant portion of the nervous system subserves vision, neurologic disorders frequently present with ophthalmic complaints. Lesions of the visual pathways can produce visual loss, whereas brainstem abnormalities or cranial neuropathies may result in ocular motility disturbances or abnormalities of the pupil or eyelid. The first section of this chapter reviews disorders of the afferent visual pathway, extending from the retina to occipital lobe; later sections deal with motility disturbances, disorders of the pupil, and disorders of the eyelids.

DISORDERS OF THE AFFERENT VISUAL PATHWAYS

The afferent visual pathways include those structures responsible for receiving, transmitting, and processing visual information: the eyes, optic nerves, chiasm, tracts and radiations, and the striate cortex. Higher-order processing occurs in visual association areas in extrastriate cortex. This chapter reviews the neuroanatomic features of these structures responsible for vision and describes a framework for the diagnosis of neurologic disorders affecting the visual pathways.

Neuroanatomy

The Eyes. The eyes are the primary sensory organs of the visual system. Before reaching the retina, light travels through the ocular media, consisting of the cornea, anterior chamber, lens, and vitreous. The size of the pupil, like the aperture of a camera, regulates the amount of light reaching the retina. The cornea and len focus light rays to produce a clear image on the retina, and the ciliary muscle can change the lens shape to adjust for objects at different distances (accommodation).

Retinal photoreceptors hyperpolarize in response to light. Cone photoreceptors are more sensitive to color and are concentrated in the middle of the retina, or macula, the center of which is the fovea. Rod photoreceptors, more important for night vision, predominate in the retinal periphery. Visual information is processed via horizontal, bipolar, and amacrine cells before reaching the ganglion cells, the axons of which make up the innermost portion of the retina and converge to form the optic disc and optic nerve (Fig. 7-1, Plate 7-1). The optic disc represents the intraocular portion of the optic nerve anterior to the lamina cribrosa. The retina is normally transparent, and the orange-red color visible on funduscopy is due to the pigment epithelium and choroidal circulation.

The retina nasal to the macula receives visual information from the temporal field, and the temporal retina, from the nasal field. The superior and inferior halves of the retina have a similar crossed relationship with respect to lower and upper fields of vision.

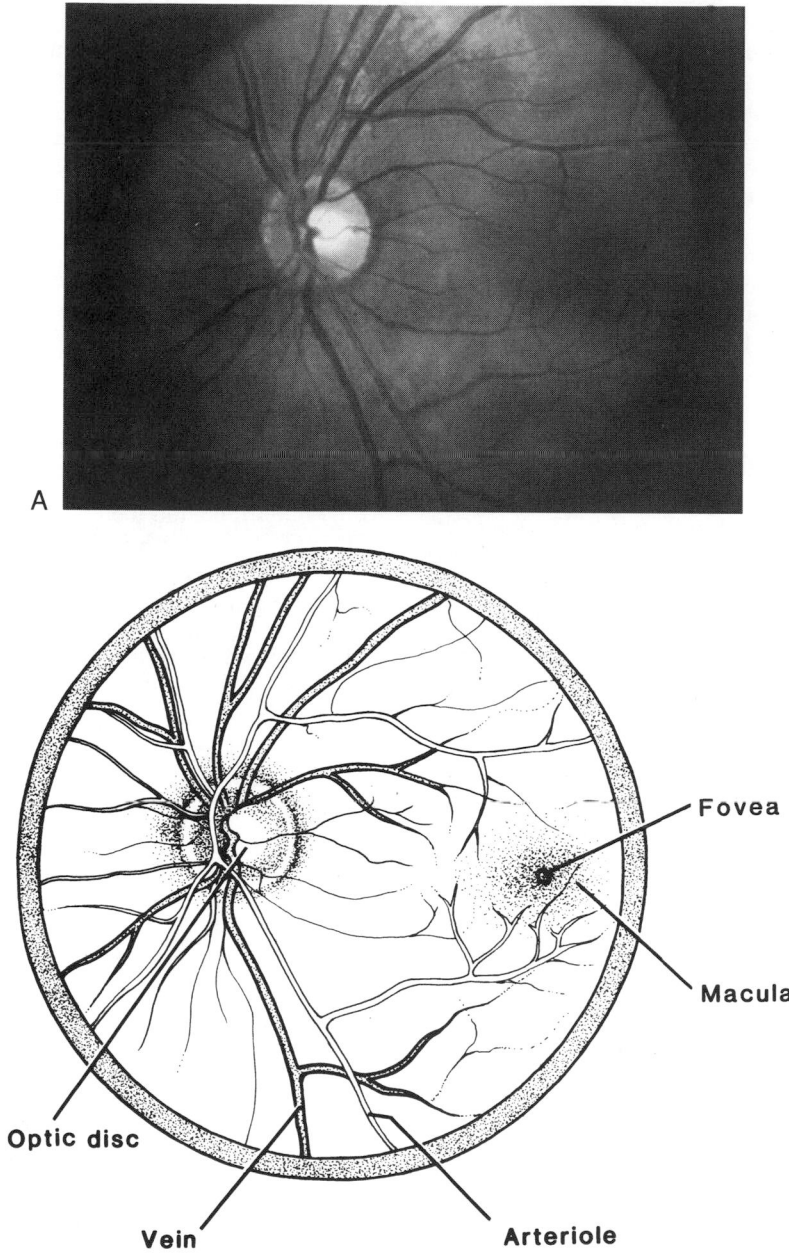

FIG. 7-1. **(A)** Normal left fundus. **(B)** Illustration identifying important structures.

The ophthalmic artery, a branch of the internal carotid, provides most of the blood supply to the eye, although there are external carotid anastomoses. The first major branch of the ophthalmic artery, the central retinal artery, pierces the dura of the optic nerve behind the globe, then travels within the nerve to emerge at the optic disc to supply the inner two-thirds of the retina. The ophthalmic artery also gives rise to the posterior ciliary arteries, which supply the optic nerve head, choroid, and outer one-third of the retina.

Optic Nerve, Chiasm, and Tract.   The optic nerve has four major portions: intraocular, intraorbital, intracanalicular, and intracranial. Posterior to the lamina cribrosa, optic nerve axons are myelinated by oligodendrocytes similar to those in white matter tracts in the brain and spinal cord.

The optic nerves join at the optic chiasm, which lies in the suprasellar region, superior to the diaphragma sella and inferior to the third ventricle and hypothalamus. At the chiasm, fibers from nasal retina cross, and the most ventral axons from the inferior nasal retina bend temporarily through the contralateral optic nerve (Wilbrand's knee), whereas the fibers from temporal retina remain ipsilateral (see Fig. 7-3). The ratio of crossed to uncrossed fibers is 53 percent to 47 percent. Ipsilateral temporal fibers and contralateral nasal fibers join to form the optic tracts.

Geniculocalcarine Pathway.   At the lateral geniculate nucleus, a part of the thalamus located above the ambient cistern, the ganglion cell axons in the optic tract synapse with neurons destined to become the optic radiations. This latter structure is divided functionally and anatomically. Fibers coursing through the temporal lobe, termed Meyer's loop, subserve visual information from the lower retina and connect to the inferior bank of the calcarine cortex. The parietal portion of the optic radiations relays information from upper retina to the superior bank of the calcarine cortex. Most of the optic radiations derive their blood supply from the middle cerebral artery. The mesial temporal section is supplied in part by branches of the posterior cerebral artery.

Striate Cortex.   Brodmann area 17 (or V1, primary or striate cortex) is the end organ of the afferent visual system and is located within the calcarine cortex in the occipital lobe. Most of the striate cortex, especially the portion situated posteriorly, is devoted to macular vision. Superior and inferior banks of calcarine cortex subserve contralateral inferior and superior quadrants, respectively. The majority of the occipital lobe is supplied by the posterior cerebral artery with a contribution from the middle cerebral artery in the occipital pole region.

Visual Association Areas.   Higher processing of visual information occurs, for example, in the lingual and fusiform gyri bordering the inferior calcarine bank in structures believed to be equivalent to monkey area V4, which is responsible for color vision. In an oversimplification, temporal lobe structures govern visual recognition and memory, whereas parietal lobe areas are responsible for spatial analysis.

Patient History

The temporal profile of the onset of visual loss might suggest an etiology, and its monocularity or binocularity will aid in localization. In general, acute visual deficits have ischemic or inflammatory etiologies, or may result from a vitreous hemorrhage or retinal detachment. Chronic or progressive visual loss may suggest a compressive, infiltrative, or degenerative process, but cataracts, refractive error, open-angle glaucoma, and retinal disorders such as age-related macular degeneration or diabetic retinopathy also should be considered. Monocular visual loss implies a lesion in one eye or optic nerve, whereas binocular visual loss usually results from involvement of both eyes or optic nerves or of the chiasm, tract, radiations, or occipital lobe.

Common complaints associated with visual loss include "blurry vision" or "gray vision." In addition to these negative symptoms, patients with lesions of the visual pathways may also complain of positive phenomena (e.g., flashing or colored lights [phosphenes], jagged lines, or formed hallucinations). The complexity of the visual images is nonlocalizing.

Examination

Patients with visual loss require an accurate assessment of acuity, color vision, visual fields, pupillary reactivity (see Relative Afferent Pupillary Defect, below), and funduscopic appearance. If possible, best corrected visual acuity should be tested for each eye—distance vision with a standard Snellen chart and near vision using a hand-held card. A pinhole can correct most refractive errors. Acuity can be recorded as 20/30, for instance, where the numerator refers to the distance (in feet) from which the patient sees the letters, and the denominator the distance from which a normal patient sees the same letters. Eyes unable to see the largest Snellen letters (20/200 or 20/400) should be graded according to their ability to count fingers (CF), see hand motions (HM), or have light perception (LP). Complete blind-

ness is termed *no light perception* (NLP). Color can be tested with standard pseudoisochromatic Ishihara, or Hardy-Rand-Ritter plates, pigment-based color vision tests in which the patient is asked to identify numbers or geometric shapes on pages of colored dots. Contrast sensitivity testing with sine-wave gratings is a useful adjunct, especially when results are abnormal despite other normal parameters.

Precise documentation of visual fields requires threshold perimetry or kinetic testing with a Goldmann perimeter or tangent screen. The kinetic technique, because it is shorter and allows interaction with the examiner, may be more appropriate for screening and for patients with significant neurologic impairment. Threshold computerized perimetry of the central 30 degrees of vision, although lengthy and tedious, is in many instances a better objective and more reproducible test for patients with optic neuropathies. At the bedside, visual fields can be documented carefully in all four quadrants of each eye using finger confrontation methods by asking the patient to "count fingers" or "tell me when you see the finger wiggling." In aphasic, intubated, uncooperative, stuporous, or very young patients, responses such as finger mimicry, pointing to targets presented, visually elicited eye movements, or reflex blink to visual threat can be gross indications of intact visual fields. Subjective hand or color comparison may elicit defects respecting vertical or horizontal meridians. The visual fields of each eye should be examined separately.

The posterior pole of the eye can be examined through an undilated pupil with a direct ophthalmoscope. Details of the optic nerve, retinal vasculature, macula, and peripapillary retina should be appreciated. A thorough examination of the retinal periphery requires a pharmacologically dilated pupil and indirect ophthalmoscopy.

Ocular causes of visual loss such as corneal or lens opacities, retinal detachments, or glaucoma should be excluded by an ophthalmologist. In general, patients with cataracts complain of blurry vision with glare, especially with automobile headlights, and those with glaucoma have peripheral visual field loss but preserved central acuity; the visual loss associated with both of these problems is insidious. Retinal detachments may present acutely with flashes of light, floaters, or peripheral field loss.

Ancillary Visual Testing.   Electrophysiologic testing such as a visual evoked potential (VEP) or electroretinogram (ERG) can confirm the localization to optic nerve or retina, but these tests should never replace the clinical examination. VEPs measure the cortical activity in response to flash or patterned stimuli and are abnormal in the presence of a lesion in the afferent visual pathway. ERGs, which measure rod and cone photoreceptor function, are particularly helpful in sorting out the retinal dystrophies and degenerations.

Topical Diagnosis

Figure 7-2 illustrates the visual field deficits characteristic of various lesions within the afferent visual pathway. Homonymous defects are those present in both eyes with the same laterality, whereas a hemianopia refers to loss of one-half of the visual field, respecting the vertical (usually) or horizontal meridian. Congruity refers to the symmetry of the field defect in both eyes.

Information garnered from the patient history and examination, in combination with the neuroanatomic principles outlined

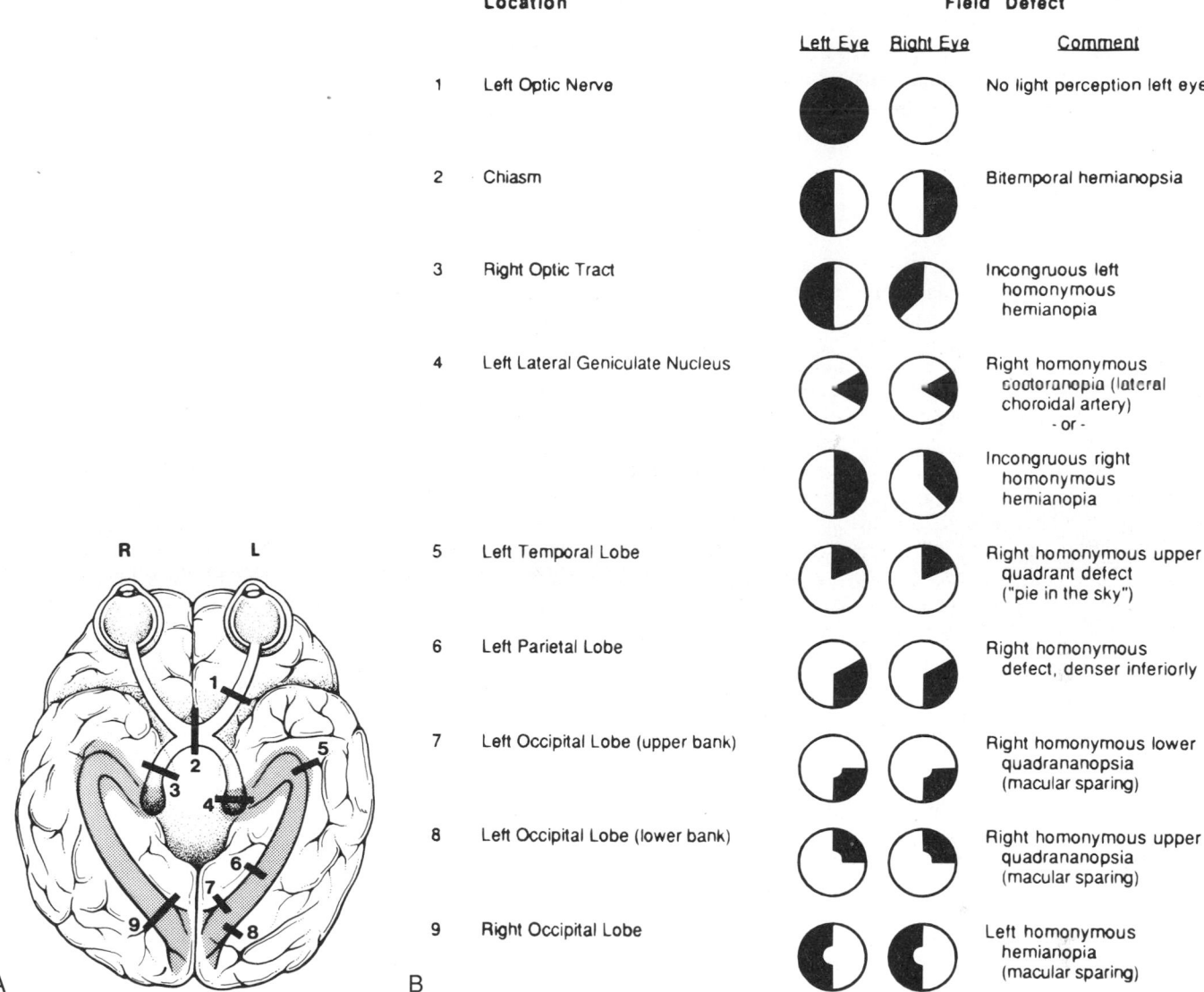

FIG. 7-2. **(A & B)** Visual pathways: correlation of lesion site and field defect, view of underside of the brain. Homonymous refers to a defect present in both eyes with the same laterality, whereas a hemianopia refers to visual loss that respects the vertical meridian. Congruous fields are symmetric in both eyes. Note that lesions of upper or lower occipital banks produce quadrantic defects, whereas lesions within temporal and parietal lobes cause field defects that tend not to respect the horizontal meridian. (Adapted from Mason C, Kandel ER: p. 437. In Kandel ER, Schwartz JH, Jessell T (eds): Principles of Neural Science. 3rd Ed. Appleton & Lange, Norwalk, CT, 1991, with permission.)

above, is usually sufficient for localization. The next step is identifying the pathologic process.

Clinical Diagnoses by Lesion Site

Retina.   The vascular and degenerative retinal disorders are important to neurologists because these problems may indicate underlying neurologic disease. Transient monocular blindness (amaurosis fugax) begins typically with a "gray shade" that encroaches on vision superiorly then resolves after seconds or minutes. This symptom is commonly the result of an atheromatous internal carotid lesion that embolizes to the retinal circulation, sometimes producing yellow cholesterol (Hollenhorst) plaques lodging at retinal vascular bifurcations (Plate 7-2). Emboli from calcific cardiac valves can cause similar symptoms but tend to be white. Other etiologies associated with amaurosis

fugax include giant cell arteritis (see below), retinal migraine, vasospasm, and cardiac thromboembolus.

Following more persistent interruption of blood supply, permanent visual loss may result from a branch or central retinal artery occlusion with a characteristic funduscopic appearance: a normal optic disc, vessel attenuation, segmentation of the blood column (termed "box-carring" of arterial blood flow), retinal edema (pale and opaque), and a macular cherry-red spot (Plate 7-3). The latter results from the visible perfused choroid in the macular region, surrounded by opaque, infarcted ganglion cell axons, which are absent in the macula. Central retinal artery occlusion requires urgent ophthalmic evaluation and consideration for ocular massage, anterior chamber paracentesis, acetazolamide, or carbon dioxide. Recently, thrombolytic therapy has been advocated for a subgroup of these patients.

Patients with retinal artery occlusion or amaurosis fugax

should undergo (1) evaluation of the carotid system first by auscultation to detect bruits, then by ultrasound or magnetic resonance imaging (MRI) to rule out stenoses; (2) echocardiography, transesophageal in some instances, to exclude a cardiac thrombus, myxoma, patent foramen ovale, or valvular lesion; (3) Holter monitoring in individuals with suspected cardiac arrhythmias such as atrial fibrillation, and (4) in elderly patients in whom giant cell arteritis should be considered, urgent measurement of the erythrocyte sedimentation rate.

The retinal examination can aid in the diagnosis of metabolic and energy disorders. A macular cherry-red spot can be seen in Tay-Sachs disease and sialidosis. Pigmentary disturbances are nonspecific but may be suggestive of Hallervorden-Spatz disease, abetalipoproteinemia, neuronal ceroid lipofucinosis, Refsum disease or a mucopolysaccharidosis. Patients with mitochondrial disorders such as Kearns-Sayre syndrome, chronic progressive external ophthalmoplegia, and MELAS syndrome (mitochondrial encephalomyopathy, lactic acidosis, and strokelike episodes) may develop a preferentially macular "salt and pepper" pigmentary retinopathy.

Retinal findings in neurocutaneous syndromes (phakomatoses) are frequently diagnostic. Examples include tapioca-like hamartomas in tuberous sclerosis, capillary angiomas in von Hippel-Lindau disease, retinal arteriovenous malformations in Wyburn-Mason syndrome, choroidal angiomas in Sturge-Weber syndrome, and choroidal hamartomas in neurofibromatosis type 1.

Optic Nerve. The hallmarks of an optic neuropathy are decreased visual acuity and color vision, unilateral visual field loss, and an afferent pupillary defect. Common field deficits include central, arcuate, and altitudinal scotomas, enlarged blind spots, and constriction. The most common optic neuropathy is glaucoma (elevated intraocular pressure), but the usual causes of optic neuropathies of neurologic importance are inflammation, vascular abnormalities, compression, infection, nutritional deficits, or elevated intracranial pressure.

The ophthalmoscopic appearance of the optic disc depends on the etiology and temporal profile of the optic neuropathy. Glaucomatous discs have enlarged cups, but the disc rim has normal color. Optic disc swelling, characterized by hyperemia, nerve fiber layer edema, obscuration of vessels, venous congestion, and peripapillary hemorrhages, usually indicates an acute or subacute process and is the result of axoplasmic stasis secondary to optic nerve injury, elevated intracranial pressure, compression or infiltration (Plate 7-4). Funduscopy is normal acutely in retrobulbar optic neuropathies, which by definition have no disc swelling, and the pathology presumably is more proximal, away from the optic nerve head. All optic neuropathies, once chronic, manifest with some degree of optic disc pallor, indicating atrophy (Plate 7-5).

Optic neuritis is the optic neuropathy most familiar to neurologists. Affected patients are typically young; many have multiple sclerosis. Visual loss results from inflammatory demyelination of the optic nerve. Although ocular involvement can be simultaneous, patients usually present with acute monocular visual loss with pain exacerbated by eye movements, and two-thirds of cases are retrobulbar. MRI may demonstrate optic nerve enhancement. By 1 year, 95 percent of patients will regain at least 20/40 acuity without treatment, though many will still have minor color, visual field, and pupillary abnormalities. Some will volunteer Uhthoff's symptom, a transient loss of vision in the previously affected eye during periods of elevated body temperature such as exercise or showering.

In previously healthy patients, the Optic Neuritis Treatment Trial demonstrated that pulse intravenous methylprednisolone hastens recovery, but the level of visual function is ultimately similar to that of patients given placebo. Patients given oral prednisone had a higher incidence of recurrent attacks. Forty-five to 80 percent of patients will eventually develop multiple sclerosis, but results of the 2-year follow-up of Optic Neuritis Treatment Trial patients suggest intravenous steroids may delay development of this disorder, especially in individuals with characteristic white matter lesions on MRI at presentation. The effect was transient, however. After a 3-year follow-up, there was no difference in the incidence of multiple sclerosis in the intravenous or placebo groups.

Nonarteritic anterior ischemic optic neuropathy, an idiopathic, presumed vascular insult to the optic nerve head, causes acute, painless loss of acuity, and a central scotoma or altitudinal field defect accompanied by disc swelling. In contrast to optic neuritis, the prognosis for visual recovery is poor, affected patients are usually in 50 or older, and a cupless optic disc, hypertension, and diabetes are apparent risk factors. Approximately one-third of patients will have subsequent involvement of the fellow eye. There is no effective medical or surgical treatment.

In all individuals with anterior ischemic optic neuropathy, symptoms of giant cell arteritis (jaw claudication, headache, scalp tenderness, weight loss, fatigue, and polymyalgia rheumatica) should be excluded through careful history taking, and an urgent erythrocyte sedimentation rate should be obtained (Plate 7-6). Most patients with arteritic visual loss are over 60 years old and have either systemic symptoms, an elevated sedimentation rate, or both. In my opinion, patients suspected of having visual loss due to giant cell arteritis should immediately receive high-dose intravenous methylprednisolone without waiting for temporal artery biopsy results. Intravenous corticosteroids may be more effective than oral prednisone in these patients by reducing the risk of fellow eye involvement and increasing the chances for some visual recovery. Histopathologic evidence of active arteritis may be present even up to 7 weeks after initiation of corticosteroids, but most biopsies should be performed within 1 week to ensure the greatest yield. Posterior (retrobulbar) ischemic optic neuropathy is rarely idiopathic, and suggests giant cell arteritis, systemic lupus erythematosis, or a compressive lesion.

Pseudotumor cerebri (idiopathic intracranial hypertension) should be mentioned here because its major morbidity is visual loss related to optic nerve dysfunction. Patients should satisfy the following (modified Dandy) criteria (see Smith, 1985): (1) signs and symptoms due to elevated intracranial pressure, (2) normal neurologic examination results except for an abducens palsy, (3) modern neuroimaging excluding a mass lesion or other cause of elevated intracranial pressure, and (4) normal cerebrospinal fluid parameters, except an elevated opening pressure (> 250 mmH$_2$O). Patients are usually young obese females and may complain of headache, transient visual obscurations (seconds), pulsatile intracranial noises, or double vision. Almost uniformly, patients have papilledema (Plates 7-4 and 7-7), and other causes of disc elevation, such as pseudopapilledema (optic nerve drusen) (Plate 7-8) or congenital nerve head elevation), should be excluded. Typically, visual acuity and color are preserved, but optic nerve-related visual field defects, best detected with threshold perimetry, are present in over 90 percent of patients and include enlarged blind spots, generalized constriction, and inferior nasal field loss. The modern management of pseudotumor cerebri is based upon the severity and progression of visual deficits. Patients with no or mild visual loss should be treated with weight reduction, symptomatic headache therapy, and acetazolamide, whereas those failing medical therapy with severe or progressive visual loss are candidates for optic nerve sheath decompression. Serial lumbar punctures probably have no role in the management of this disorder. Lumboperitoneal shunting, because of significant failure and complication rates, is more appropriate for individuals with headache as their primary symptom and for those who fail sheath decompression. In rare malignant cases, patients may be refractory to all therapies and develop chronic atrophic papilledema with debilitating visual loss.

A detailed review of all optic neuropathies is beyond the scope of this chapter; however, Table 7-1 lists several etiologies according to pathogenesis and frequency. The list can be overwhelming, but the cause of most optic neuropathies is apparent after eliciting a careful patient history and conducting a thorough examination. Glaucoma, optic neuritis, and ischemic optic neuropathy are the most commonly encountered and have characteristic presentations as described, but several other optic neu-

TABLE 7-1. Optic Neuropathies According to Etiology and Frequency

Etiology	More Common	Less Common	Etiology	More Common	Less Common

Compressive	Carotid-ophthalmic aneurysm
	Metastases
	  Canalicular
	  Intraorbital
	Orbital pseudotumor
	Sellar mass lesions (see Table 7-2)
	Spheno-orbital meningioma
	Thyroid eye (Grave's) disease
		Bone dysplasias
		Ectatic carotid artery
		Orbital mass lesion
		Arteriovenous malformation
		Dermoid
		Hemangioma
		Lymphangioma
		Mucocele
		Venous varix
		Nasopharyngeal tumor
		Sinus disease
		Paranasal tumor
					Neuroretinitis
					Neuromyelitis optica
					Optochiasmatic arachnoiditis
					Vaccination
					Sarcoidosis
					Steroid-responsive perineuritis (pseudotumor variant)
					Systemic lupus erythematosus
					Wegener's granulomatosis

Congenital disc anomalies	Disc hypoplasia Congenital disc elevation Optic nerve head drusen	Coloboma de Morsier syndrome Disc aplasia Megalopapilla Morning glory syndrome Myelinated nerve fibers Optic nerve pit	Neoplastic (primary)	Childhood optic nerve glioma Malignant optic nerve glioma Perioptic meningioma	Hemangioma Melanocytoma

Heredodegenerative	Leber's hereditary optic neuropathy	Behr's complicated optic atrophy
		Charcot-Marie-Tooth disease
		Diabetes and deafness
		Friedreich's ataxia
		Infantile recessive optic atrophy
		Kjer's dominant optic atrophy
		Marie's ataxia
		Mucopolysaccaridoses
		Polyneuropathy and deafness
		Sphingolipidoses
		  Adrenoleukodystrophy
		  Alexander's disease
		  Krabbe's disease
		  Metachromatic leukodystrophy
		  Niemann-Pick disease type A
		  Pelizaus-Merzbacher disease
		  Tay-Sachs disease
			Nutritional (deficiency)	Cobalamin (B_{12})
				Thiamine (B_1)
				Tobacco/alcohol amblyopia
					Niacin
					Jamaican

			Toxic	Ethambutol Methanol	Amantadine Amiodarone Arsenic Bischloroethyl nitrosourea (BCNU) (intracarotid) Carbon tetrachloride Chloramphenicol Chlorpropamide Cisplatin Ciprofloxacin Digitalis Disulfiram Ethchlorvinol Ethylene glycol 5-Fluorouracil Hexachlorophene Hydroquinolines Isoniazid Lead Penicillamine Quinine Thallium Toluene Vincristine
Infectious	Syphilis	Cat-scratch disease Cryptococcus infection Cytomegalovirus infection Herpes zoster Human immunodeficiency virus infection Intraocular nematode infection Orbital cellulitis Lyme disease Toxoplasmosis Tuberculosis	Vascular	Ischemic optic neuropathy Nonarteritic Giant cell arteritis Blood loss Hypotension Papillophlebitis	Carotid-cavernous sinus fistula Cataract extraction Diabetic papillopathy Hypotony Migraine Ophthalmic artery occlusion Radiation-induced (delayed) Systemic lupus erythematosus
Infiltrative	Carcinomatous meningitis Leukemia Lymphoma	Gliomatosis cerebri Optic nerve metastases	Other	Glaucoma Papilledema Pseudotumor cerebri Trauma	Big blind spot syndrome Uremia
Inflammatory	Optic neuritis Acute disseminated encephalomyelitis	Guillain-Barré syndrome Histiocytosis Inflammatory bowel disease			

ropathies also have telltale features. Tobacco/alcoholic ambly-opia is associated with cecocentral scotomas; Leber's hereditary optic neuropathy follows a maternal inheritance pattern, usually presents in young males with profound, sometimes sequential, visual loss, has a typical fundus picture with pseudo-disc edema and peripapillary telangiectasias, and is associated with specific mitochondrial DNA mutations. Optic nerve gliomas are associated with neurofibromatosis type 1. Hereditary, nutrition, or toxic factors are usually evident in the patient history. Progressive visual loss accompanied by optic atrophy implies a compressive lesion, such an aneurysm or tumor.

Thin-section MRI of the orbits with fat suppression and gadolinium can confirm optic nerve inflammation or establish the etiology of a mass lesion. Lumbar puncture with cytology may be necessary in instances of suspected neoplastic infiltration.

Optic Chiasm.   Temporal field defects respecting the vertical meridian, in either or both eyes, suggest a chiasmal process.

Although a bitemporal hemianopsia is classic, the actual pattern of field loss depends on the chiasm's position and the exact location of the culprit lesion (Fig. 7-3). If the chiasm is post-fixed, or if the lesion affects the anterior portion of the chiasm, patients may present with an optic neuropathy or a junctional scotoma resulting from involvement of the ipsilateral optic nerve and Wilbrand's knee. Central hemianopic scotomas or optic tract syndromes may be the product of prefixed chiasms or more posteriorly situated lesions.

Patients with chiasmal field loss are often without visual complaints unless acuity is abnormal, and a temporal field defect may not be apparent until the patient reads only the nasal half of the acuity chart. Rarely, others may complain of double vision caused by an inability to align the noncorresponding nasal visual fields of each eye (hemifield slide phenomenon). Color vision may be altered only in defective fields, and asymmetric lesions may produce an afferent pupillary defect. Lesions solely of the chiasm rarely cause optic disc swelling without third ventricular compression, but chronic processes may lead

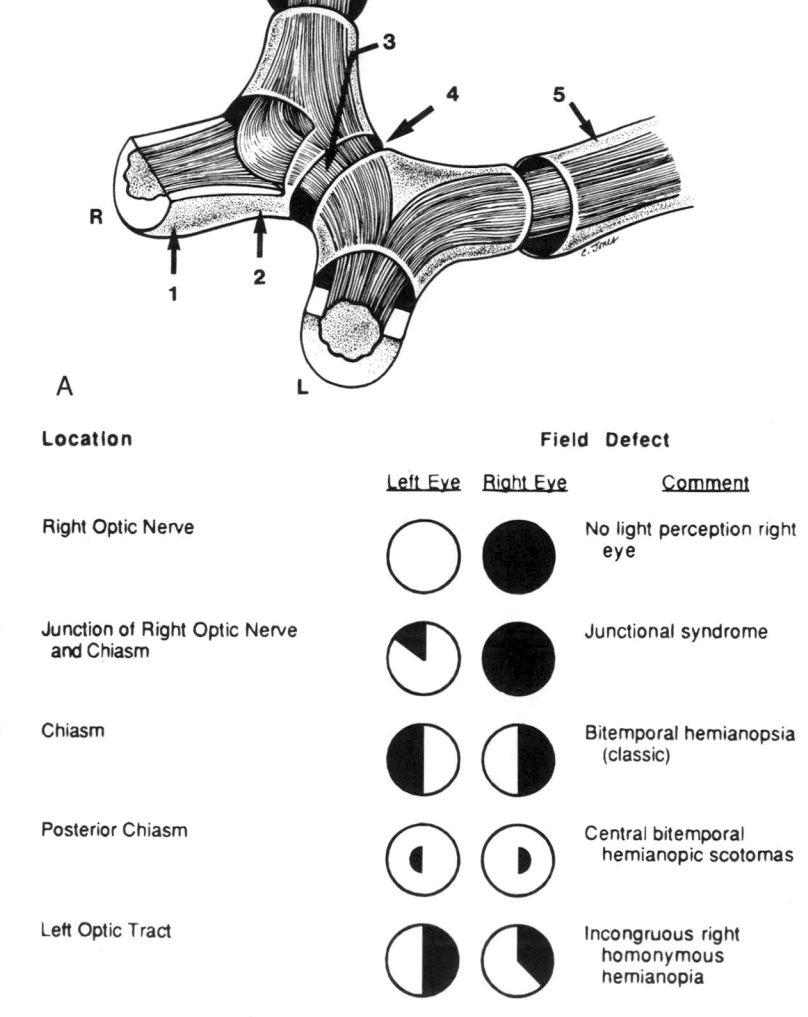

FIG. 7-3.   (A & B) Optic chiasm: correlation of lesion site and field defect. Note the most ventral nasal fibers (mostly from inferior nasal retina) temporarily travel within the fellow optic nerve in Wilbrand's knee. (Adapted from Hoyt WF, Luis O: Arch Ophthalmol 70:69–85, 1963, with permission.)

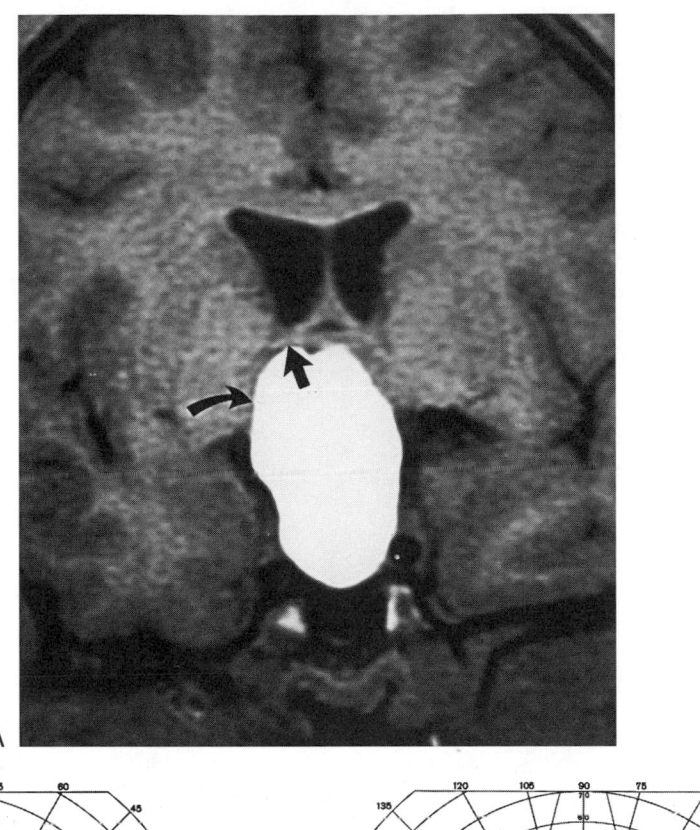

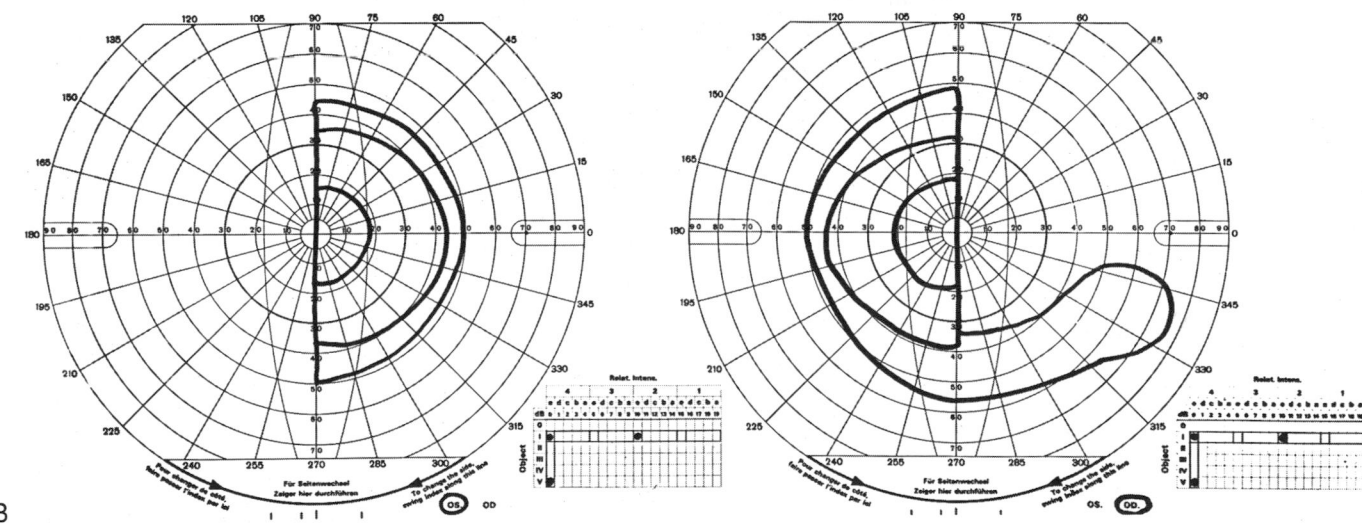

FIG. 7-4. **(A)** T1-weighted magnetic resonance image, coronal view, demonstrating a craniopharyngioma (*curved arrow*), with homogeneous high-signal characteristics, compressing the optic chiasm (*straight arrow*). **(B)** Goldmann visual fields of the same patient, demonstrating a bitemporal hemianopsia resulting from chiasmal compression.

to optic atrophy. Seesaw nystagmus can occur in association with parasellar lesions, and the presence of ocular motor palsies suggests cavernous sinus involvement (see Disorders of Eye Movements, below).

Chiasmal syndromes are usually caused by sellar and suprasellar compressive masses (Fig. 7-4), and this differential diagnosis is best considered according to the patient's age, since many lesions are congenital (Table 7-2). Historical evidence of pituitary dysfunction, such as galactorrhea, hypothyroidism, amenorrhea, decreased libido, hypogonadism, hypoadrenalism, hypercortisolism (Cushing syndrome), or acromegaly, should be investigated. Hypothalamic involvement may manifest with diabetes insipidus, feeding disorders, temperature dysregula-

tion, precocious puberty, or Russell diencephalic syndrome (hyperkinesis, euphoria, and emaciation). Visual loss in these instances is insidious, and medical or surgical decompression may result in partial or complete visual recovery, especially in patients without optic atrophy.

Most processes that cause optic neuropathies, especially the infectious, infiltrative, and inflammatory ones (Table 7-1), can also affect the chiasm. Congenital malformation and vascular infarction of the chiasm are rare.

MRI of the sellar region, especially with coronal and sagittal thin sections, is the neuroimaging procedure of choice in this setting. Computed tomographic (CT) scanning, by demonstrating calcification associated with craniopharyngiomas or bony

TABLE 7-2. Sellar and Suprasellar Compressive Lesions According to Age Group, Etiology, and Frequency

Age Group	More Common	Less Common

Pediatric–young adult	Chiasmal-hypothalmic glioma
	Craniopharyngioma
		Arachnoid cyst
		Arteriovenous malformation
		Choristomas
		Dermoid
		Empty sella syndrome
		Epidermoid
		Ganglioglioma
		Germ cell tumors
		  Choriocarcinoma
		  Endodermal sinus tumor
		  Germinoma
		  Embryonal carcinoma
		  Teratoma
		Pituitary adenoma
		Rathke's pouch cyst

Middle age–elderly	Aneurysm (internal carotid) Craniopharyngioma Meningioma Pituitary adenoma Pituitary apoplexy	Malignant optic glioma Metastases to chiasm, sella, or suprasellar region Sphenoethmoidal mucocele

No particular age predilection		Histiocytosis
		Lymphocytic hypophysitis
		Meningitis
		  Bacterial
		  Tuberculous
		  Sarcoidosis

erosion due to a meningioma, may be complementary. Mass lesions in this region will obviously necessitate endocrine and neurosurgical evaluation.

Optic Tract/Lateral Geniculate Body. Isolated syndromes of the optic tract and lateral geniculate body, both characterized in most cases by incongruous homonymous hemianopias, are uncommon. Optic tract lesions may be associated with asymmetrically impaired visual acuity (usually worse in the eye ipsilateral to the lesion), and a contralateral afferent pupillary defect. Extremely rare pupillary findings include contralateral mydriasis (Behr's pupil), and hemianopic pupillary reactivity (Wernicke's pupil—see Disorders of the Pupils, below). Because of presynaptic interruption, patients may have bilateral optic atrophy with ipsilateral temporal pallor and contralateral "bow tie" or "band" atrophy. As stated previously, sellar and parasellar masses, especially craniopharyngiomas and aneurysms, may involve the tract. Isolated tract syndromes may also result from demyelination.

Clinically, lateral geniculate and tract syndromes may be difficult to distinguish. The unique exceptions are related to the geniculate's dual vascular supply. A lateral choroidal artery infarction causes a congruous homonymous horizontal wedge-shaped sectoranopia, and an anterior choroidal artery syndrome leads to upper and lower homonymous sectoranopias. There should be no afferent pupillary defect with a pure geniculate lesion (see Disorders of the Pupils, below).

Optic Radiations. Interruption of Meyer's loop classically causes congruous or incongruous contralateral homonymous field defects denser superiorly ("pie in the sky"), whereas high parietal lesions are associated with deficits more prominent inferiorly. In reality, there is considerable variation, and complete disruption of the optic radiations leads to a dense homonymous hemianopia (Fig. 7-5). Visual acuity is normal in unilateral cases, but may be abnormal with bilateral lesions. The pupils always react normally in lesions posterior to the optic tract.

Hemianopias due to lesions of the radiations usually have additional lateralizing and localizing signs. Temporal lobe lesions may lead to personality changes and complex partial seizures, or fluent aphasias if the left side is involved, and the usual cause is neoplastic, such as a low-grade glioma. Left neglect (see below) accompanying a left hemianopia implies a right parietal lesion, whereas conduction aphasias or Gerstmann syndrome suggests a left-sided process. A homonymous field defect accompanied by ipsilateral sensory loss, astereognosis, or graphesthesia implies a parietal localization, whereas one associated with a dense ipsilateral hemiparesis involving face, arm, and leg might suggest a more deep-seated lesion with involvement of the internal capsule. Patients with hemianopias due to parietal lesions have abnormal pursuit and optokinetic responses when stripes or objects are drawn toward the side of the lesion, indicating concurrent involvement of deep, descending parieto-occipital pursuit fibers. Parietal mass lesions can be distinguished from middle cerebral artery occlusion by a more insidious course, history of headache, and papilledema.

Occipital Lobe. Unilateral striate cortex lesions, most commonly due to vascular insult or mass lesion, produce congruous homonymous hemianopias respecting the vertical meridian, and processes preferentially affecting upper or lower banks of calcarine cortex lead to quadrantic field defects. Altitudinal hemianopias with respect to the horizontal meridian are the result of bilateral upper or lower bank disturbances. Patients may complain of blurry vision in the defective field as if they were looking through water or smoked glass. Others may be unaware of their deficit until they have a car accident or family members notice the patient bumping into household objects.

Posterior cerebral artery occlusions may not involve the occipital pole, which also receives distal branches from the middle cerebral artery, thereby sparing macular vision. Bilateral cortical representation of the macula may also account for some instances of sparing. Acuity and color vision are unaffected with unilateral occipital injury and are diminished only following bilateral geniculocalcarine lesions. A variable but characteristic temporal crescent in the unpaired 60- to 90-degree field of the eye ipsilateral to the hemianopia results from preservation of the rostral portion of the striate cortex, supplied by end branches of the anterior cerebral artery. Homonymous hemianopic central scotomas also localize exclusively to a unilateral occipital lobe lesion.

Patients may have a gaze preference away from the hemianopia, and the optokinetic response (see next section) is normal in the setting of occipital lobe infarction and abnormal with occipital mass lesions with edema extending into the parietal lobe (Cogan's rule). Stroke-related hemianopias are usually isolated, unless proximal posterior cerebral artery occlusion causes an ipsilateral hemiparesis, third-nerve palsy, or ataxia from mesencephalic infarction, and memory or personality changes from mesial-temporal or thalamic involvement.

Bilateral posterior cerebral artery occlusion may result in tunnel fields with preservation of central vision only, but oftentimes bilateral processes lead to cortical blindness. These patients have no reflex blink to threat or optokinetic response, and their intact pupillary light responses distinguish them from those with bilateral optic nerve involvement. Cortically blind individuals with Anton syndrome confabulate and deny their blindness, in some instances because additional cerebral lesions have altered memory, recognition, and behavior.

Positive visual phenomena, such as colored shapes, people, or objects, may occur within the blind field, or visual images

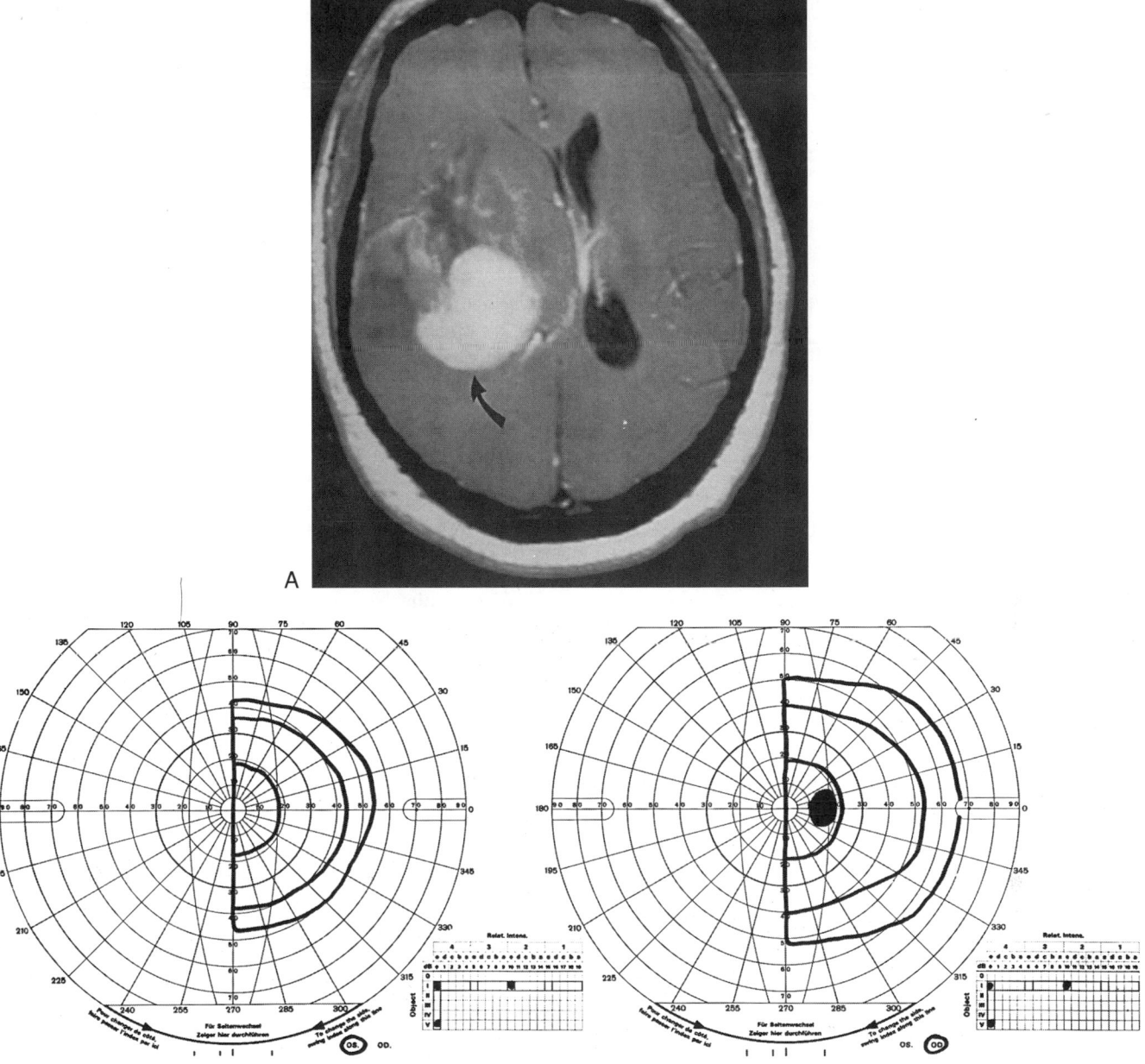

FIG. 7-5. **(A)** T1-weighted magnetic resonance image with gadolinium, axial view, demonstrating a contrast-enhancing parietal lobe anaplastic glioma (*arrow*) with mass effect and surrounding edema. **(B)** Goldmann visual fields of the same patient, demonstrating a left homonymous hemianopia due to interruption of the optic radiations.

may persist (palinopsia). Constant visual hallucinations are typically ''release'' phenomena, whereas those that are episodic usually represent irritative (convulsive) foci.

Other unique and unusual features following occipital lobe injury include the recovery of motion perception, called the Riddoch phenomenon, and blindsight, which is unconscious vision in the blind hemifield. Both of these may in part represent the residual capacities of the ''second'' more primitive retinal-tectal-pulvinar subcortical, extrastriate visual pathway.

Headaches preceded by transient hemianopic phenomena, with or without scintillations or phosphenes, are usually indicative of migraine. Some patients may present only with the visual prodrome, without the headache, in so-called acephalgic mi-

graine. Rarely, patients with complicated migraine may develop occipital lobe infarction and fixed hemianopic defects.

Other etiologies should be entertained in the differential diagnosis of occipital lobe dysfunction. Posterior cerebral artery infarction may occur in the setting of transtentorial herniation. Hypertensive encephalopathy or ecclampsia may cause transient hemianopias or cortical blindness. In elderly patients, Alzheimer's disease should be considered, and in this age group, posteriorly situated hemorrhages are uncommon secondary to long-standing hypertension and instead should suggest amyloid angiopathy. Infectious causes include abscesses, progressive multifocal leukoencephalopathy, and Creutzfeld-Jakob disease. In children, meningoencephalitis, MELAS, and adrenal leukodystrophy should be considered. Postictal hemianopias are uncommon.

In patients with permanent, dense hemianopias as their only neurologic deficit, I have attempted adaptive hemianopic Fresnel paste-on prisms with varied success.

Higher Cortical Lesions.   With involvement of visual association areas, individuals may have additional visual symptoms unexplained by field deficits. Although subjective complaints are usually vague (''blurry'' or ''I'm having trouble seeing''), many are easily characterized after further investigation.

Inferior occipital lobe injury involving lingual and fusiform gyri may result in a contralateral homonymous upper quadrantanopsia and defective color vision in the inferior quadrant (cerebral hemiachromatopsia). Patients with a left-sided lesion and coinvolvement of the splenium of the corpus callosum or adjacent periventricular white matter may develop alexia without agraphia (or pure alexia or ''word blindness''), a disconnection syndrome characterized by a right homonymous field deficit and an inability to access lexical visual information processed in the right occipital lobe.

Inability to recognize visualized objects (''visual agnosia'') despite a normal afferent pathway often suggests bilateral medial occipitotemporal lesions disrupting the inferior longitudinal fasciculus, a white matter pathway connecting striate cortex with visual association areas in temporal lobe. Prosopagnosia, resulting from similar lesions, is a dramatic visual agnosia for faces only.

Recent evidence has demonstrated that lateral occipitotemporal lesions affecting Brodmann area 39, believed to be analogous to monkey area MT, may result in defective motion perception.

Right hemispheric lesions, especially those involving the inferior parietal lobule, may result in neglect or inattention to visual, tactile, and auditory stimuli in left hemispace, dressing and constructional apraxia, or spatial disorientation. Hemineglect can be present even without visual field deficits. The degree of visual inattention varies from dense neglect of all stimuli on one side to subtle instances in which the patient is able to detect objects in left and right fields if shown separately, but ignores the ones on the left when presented bilaterally (double simultaneous stimulation).

Balint syndrome consists of ocular apraxia (a deficit in shifting gaze), optic ataxia (a defect in reaching under visual guidance), and simultanagnosia (an inability to perceive a whole scene in its entirety, or visual disorientation). The deficits, which sometimes include absent blink to threat, may reflect bilaterally defective visual attention, as the culprit lesions are typically bilateral occipitoparietal in the areas important for visual attention and foveal refixation. The accompanying visual field defect is usually inferior and altitudinal but sometimes the fields are normal. The usual etiology is watershed infarction in the setting of hypoperfusion following cardiac or respiratory arrest, but patients with Alzheimer's disease may also present with complex visual disturbances resembling any or all of the elements of Balint syndrome.

Functional Visual Loss.   Clinicians should always be wary about functional (hysterical) visual loss when there is a mismatch between the patient's complaints and the examination results, or when the visual loss is nonphysiologic. Examples of the latter include monocular temporal field loss that persists binocularly or constricted visual fields on tangent screen testing that fail to expand physiologically when the patient is moved

from 1 to 2 m away from the screen (tubular fields). Mismatches include complaints of no light perception in one eye and normal vision in the other with normal stereo vision or without an afferent pupillary defect in the supposed defective eye. An optokinetic response in a patient claiming blindness is also evidence of a functional disorder.

DISORDERS OF EYE MOVEMENTS

Eye movements facilitate refoveation and maintenance of visual fixation. Diagnostically, it is easiest to consider ocular motility disorders in two major groups: those that are primarily ophthalmoparetic, with impairment of eye movements, versus those that are characterized by nystagmus or inappropriate saccades (''too little versus too much''). With this framework in mind, this section reviews history-taking, examination techniques, and the diagnosis of important eye movement abnormalities encountered in neurologic practice.

Patient History

Patients with ophthalmoparesis usually have double vision (diplopia), but other common complaints include blurry vision, dizziness (dysequilibrium), or an inability to focus. Those with chronic and symmetric processes, and others with dysconjugate eye movements but poor vision, complete unilateral ptosis, or long-standing suppression of one eye (amblyopia), may not have any visual complaints.

Individuals should be asked if the the diplopia is binocular, since monocular double vision usually suggests refractive error, conversion disorder, or in rare instances, cerebral dysfunction. Two other questions will help isolate the involved muscle: is the diplopia (1) vertical, often implying a vertical rectus or oblique dysfunction, or horizontal, usually suggesting medial or lateral rectus impairment; or (2) worse in any cardinal position of gaze, since the double vision should be maximal in the direction of action of the paretic muscle. For instance, horizontal binocular diplopia that is worse in left gaze and at distance suggests left lateral rectus dysfunction.

The temporal profile and accompanying symptoms often suggest etiology and localization. A history of acute, painful diplopia can be consistent with a vasculopathic cranial mononeuropathy, orbital process, or cavernous sinus lesion. Insidious painless diplopia in association with other bulbar signs such as hoarseness or dysphagia may indicate a chronic meningitis or myasthenia gravis. The latter, however, often produces ptosis and fluctuating symptoms with diurnal variation. Sudden diplopia with ataxia, dysarthria, dysphagia, or vertigo usually indicates a brainstem process such as demyelination or vascular infarction; posterior fossa masses with similar symptoms are usually accompanied by headache, nausea and vomiting, and papilledema due to fourth ventricular compression and noncommunicating hydrocephalus.

Patients with nystagmus or inappropriate saccades often complain of dizziness (vertigo) or may experience the illusion of environmental motion (oscillopsia).

Examination

The ocular motility examination consists of observation in primary gaze, evaluation of ductions and vergences, then detection of misalignment.

The presence of any obvious ocular misalignment or abnormal, spontaneous eye movements should be assessed first in primary gaze while the patient fixates on a distant target. An esotropia means one eye is deviated inward relative to the other, whereas an exotropia describes one eye deviated outward relative to the other. Any vertical misalignment is described by the laterality of the higher eye (e.g., a left hypertropia indicates the left eye is higher than the right). Adjunctive observations should include the presence or absence of head turn or tilt, pupillary reactivity (see next section), examination of the eyelids, palpebral fissures, and orbicularis oculi (see next section), and relative proptosis either by inspection or quantitatively by Hertel exophthalmometry.

Ductions refer to monocular eye movements, and rotations laterally are termed abduction, medial adduction, upward elevation, and downward depression. Ductions can be tested by having the patient voluntarily direct gaze in the cardinal fields (up and right, up, up and left, right, left, down and right, down, and down and left). Limitation of eye movement despite pushing on the globe with a cotton-tipped swab (at the limbus following instillation of a topical anesthetic agent) suggests mechanical restriction (''positive forced duction test''). An intact Bell's phenomenon, the upward rotation of the globe elicited by having patients try to close their eyes while the examiner holds the lids open, indicates intact nuclear and infranuclear oculomotor nerve function for upgaze.

Vergences are binocular eye movements. Convergence can be evaluated by having patients look at their thumb or other accommodative target as it approaches their nose, and both eyes should adduct with pupillary constriction. Pursuit movements should then be tested by having the patients keep the head still and visually track a target moved horizontally or vertically. The speed and accuracy of saccades, which are high-velocity conjugate eye movements, should be examined by asking the patient to look eccentrically then quickly refixate on a target in primary gaze (the examiner's nose, for instance). Optokinetic nystagmus can be elicited by rotating a striped drum or moving a striped tape horizontally and vertically and asking the patient to ''count the stripes as they go by.'' The slow phases of optokinetic nystagmus are generated as the patient follows a target; the optokinetic nystagmus fast phase is a corrective saccade to view the next target. Oculocephalic responses can be evaluated by having the patient fix on a stationary target while the examiner gently rotates the head and extends and flexes the neck. The stimulus is either from proprioceptive afferents in the neck or the vestibular system, or both. In addition, with an arm extended and their chair rotated, most patients should be able to

maintain visual fixation on their thumb; difficulty with this task suggests an inability to suppress the vestibulo-ocular response. When rotated around the examiner, infants, normally with poor fixation, manifest a vestibulo-ocular response with tonic eye deviation toward the direction of rotation followed by quick corrective jerks. The vestibulo-ocular response can be tested in comatose patients by cold caloric stimulation with ice water injected into the ear.

Ophthalmoparesis often will be evident on evaluation of ductions alone; however, more subtle instances of misalignment may require cover or Maddox-rod testing. While the patient fixates on a target in distance, any refixation movement of the fellow eye after monocular occlusion confirms a tropia (Fig. 7-6). An outward movement of the uncovered eye signifies an esotropia, an inward movement implies an exotropia, and a downward movement indicates a hypertropia. In the absence of a tropia, alternately covering each eye breaks binocular fusion and can reveal a latent phoria.

The Maddox rod (Fig. 7-7), containing parallel half-cylinders, can help detect small deviations, but by itself does not identify the paretic eye. If misalignment is detected, the direction of gaze that produces the greatest separation between images should be determined by moving the fixation light in the cardinal positions. Vertical deviations should also be evaluated with the head tilted toward the right and left shoulders.

Ophthalmoparesis

In a logical, hierarchic control of eye movements, the supranuclear centers in the cortex and brainstem (see Fig. 7-14) direct the three ocular motor cranial nerves (III, IV, and VI), which in turn innervate the six extraocular muscles of each eye (Fig. 7-8). Supranuclear and nuclear structures have additional vestibular, cerebellar, and basal ganglia input.

The oculomotor nerve (III) activates the medial rectus (adduction), inferior rectus (depression), and superior rectus and inferior oblique (elevation) muscles, as well as the pupillary sphincter muscle (constriction) and levator palpebrae of the upper lid (Fig. 7-8). A complete, isolated infranuclear third-nerve palsy causes ipsilateral elevation, adduction, and depression weakness, accompanied by abduction, hypodeviation, pupillary mydriasis, and ptosis (Fig. 7-9).

The trochlear nerve (IV) supplies the superior oblique muscle, which intorts the eye and and depresses it in adduction.

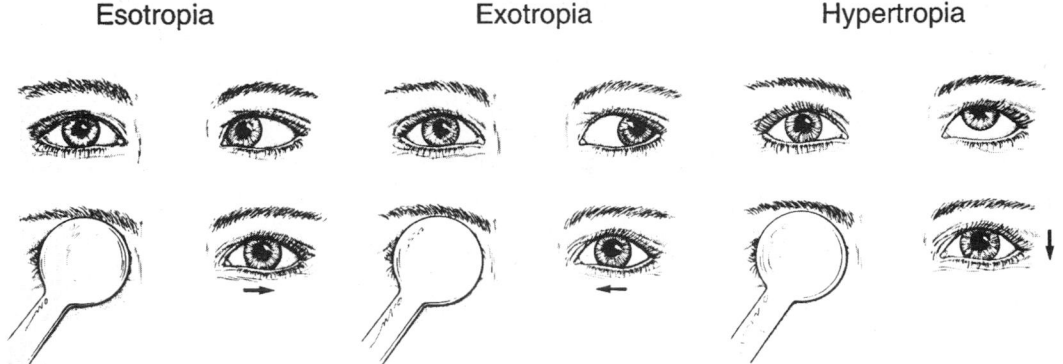

FIG. 7-6. Cover testing for ocular misalignment. In each case, the patient is fixing with the nonparetic right eye. Upon occlusion of the right eye, the misaligned left eye is forced to fixate. Esotropic eyes move laterally to fixate, whereas exotropic eyes move medially and hypertropic eyes move downward to fixate. Thus, ocular deviations can be determined by the direction of the fixation movements.

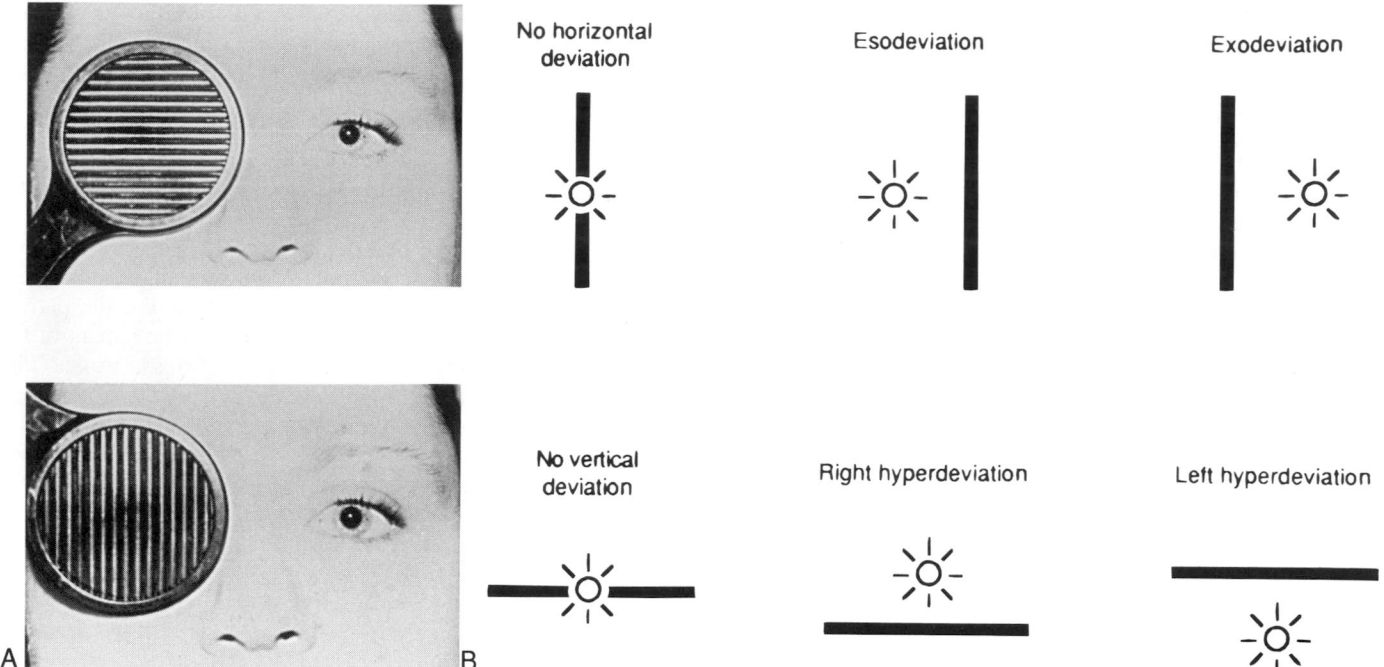

FIG. 7-7. (A & B) Maddox-rod testing for ocular misalignment. By convention, the Maddox rod is always placed over the right eye, and the patient is asked to fixate on a distant, bright white light. A binocular patient's right eye sees a red line, whereas the uncovered left eye sees the white light. The illustrations on the right are drawn from the patient's perspective. *Top row:* To evaluate horizontal ocular deviations, the bars on the Maddox rod are aligned horizontally, so the patient sees a vertical red line with the right eye. If there is no horizontal deviation, the patient perceives the red line passing through the white light. If the eyes are esodeviated, the red line, whose image would abnormally fall on the nasal retina, appears to the right of the white light ("uncrossed diplopia"). Exodeviated eyes would result in the red line appearing to the left of the light ("crossed diplopia") because the red image would abnormally fall on temporal retina. *Bottom row:* To evaluate vertical deviations, the bars on the Maddox rod should be oriented vertically, so the patient will see a horizontal red line with the right eye. The red line passes through the white light when there is no vertical deviation, whereas a red line perceived below the light implies a right hyperdeviation, and a white light perceived below the red line indicates a left hyperdeviation (i.e., the lower image corresponds to the hyperdeviated eye). Note: this test will characterize the ocular misalignment, but by itself it does not indicate which eye has the abnormal motility.

Patients with superior oblique paresis complain of vertical diplopia, often with a torsional component, and they have an ipsilateral hypertropia worse on contraversive (contralateral conjugate) horizontal gaze and ipsilateral head tilt (Parks' three-step test, best demonstrated with alternate cover or Maddox-rod testing) (Fig. 7-10).

The abducens nerve (VI) innervates the lateral rectus muscle, which abducts the eye. Patients with a lateral rectus palsy complain of binocular horizontal double vision worse on ipsiversive gaze and at a distance. In many cases, the limitation of abduction is evident (Fig. 7-11), but in more subtle instances, alternate cover or Maddox-rod testing would confirm an esotropia largest on ipsiversive gaze.

In adults, the most common identifiable cause of acquired third- and sixth-nerve palsies is vascular insufficiency due to diabetes, hypertension, or atherosclerosis. The most common identifiable cause of a fourth-nerve palsy is head trauma. However, most frequently, the cause of an isolated single ocular motor palsy is undetermined. In children, the most common cause of acquired third-, fourth-, and sixth-nerve palsies is trauma (Table 7-3). In all age groups, when the ocular motor palsies occur in combination, an etiology is almost always identified.

Often, the ophthalmoparesis and abnormal motility pattern is characteristic, but historical features or accompanying neurologic findings frequently aid in localization and diagnosis.

Nuclear and Infranuclear Disorders in the Brainstem. The oculomotor complex lies within the mesencephalic periaqueductal gray matter, and unique features include the central caudal subnucleus, which subserves bilateral levator function, and the superior rectus subnuclei, which each innervate the contralateral superior rectus muscle (Fig. 7-8). A unilateral lesion of the third-nerve nucleus therefore results in bilateral ptosis, worse ipsilaterally, ipsilateral mydriasis, ipsilateral palsy of the medial rectus, inferior rectus and inferior oblique muscles, and bilateral superior rectus palsies.

Lesions of the midbrain tegmentum can affect the oculomotor nerve fascicles as they travel ventrally, often with "crossed" neurologic signs. Involvement of the fascicle as it passes through the crossing dentatorubrothalamic fibers produces an ipsilateral oculomotor palsy and contralateral ataxia (Claude syndrome). A lesion of the cerebral peduncle results in ipsilateral oculomotor palsy and contralateral hemiparesis (Weber syndrome), and a larger process also involving the red nucleus can cause the same findings plus contralateral involuntary limb movements or tremor (Benedikt syndrome). The usual cause of a nuclear or fascicular oculomotor palsy is infarction in the territory of a mesencephalic paramedian penetrating vessel arising from the proximal posterior cerebral artery, but other etiologies include metastatic tumors and abscesses.

The trochlear nucleus lies ventral to the aqueduct in the pontomesencephalic junction, caudal to the oculomotor complex.

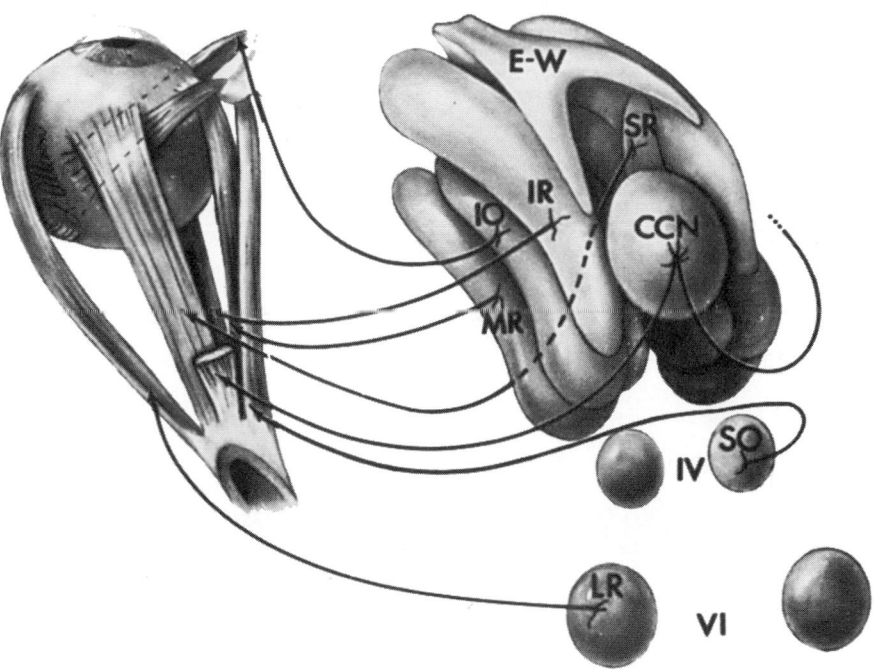

FIG. 7-8. Oculomotor nuclear complex and innervation of the extraocular muscles. Note that the central caudal nucleus (CCN) supplies both lid levators, and the superior rectus subnucleus (SR) and superior oblique nucleus (SO) innervate the contralateral muscle. Other oculomotor subnuclei: E-W, Edinger-Westphal; IR, inferior rectus; IO, inferior oblique; and MR, medial rectus. LR, lateral rectus nucleus. (From Glaser JS, Bachynski B: Infranuclear disorders of eye movement. p. 363. In Glaser JS: Neuro-ophthalmology. 2nd Ed. JP Lippincott, Philadelphia, 1990; adapted from Warnick R: Representation of the extra-ocular muscles in the oculomotor nuclei of the monkey. J Comp Neurol 98:449–95, 1953, with permission.)

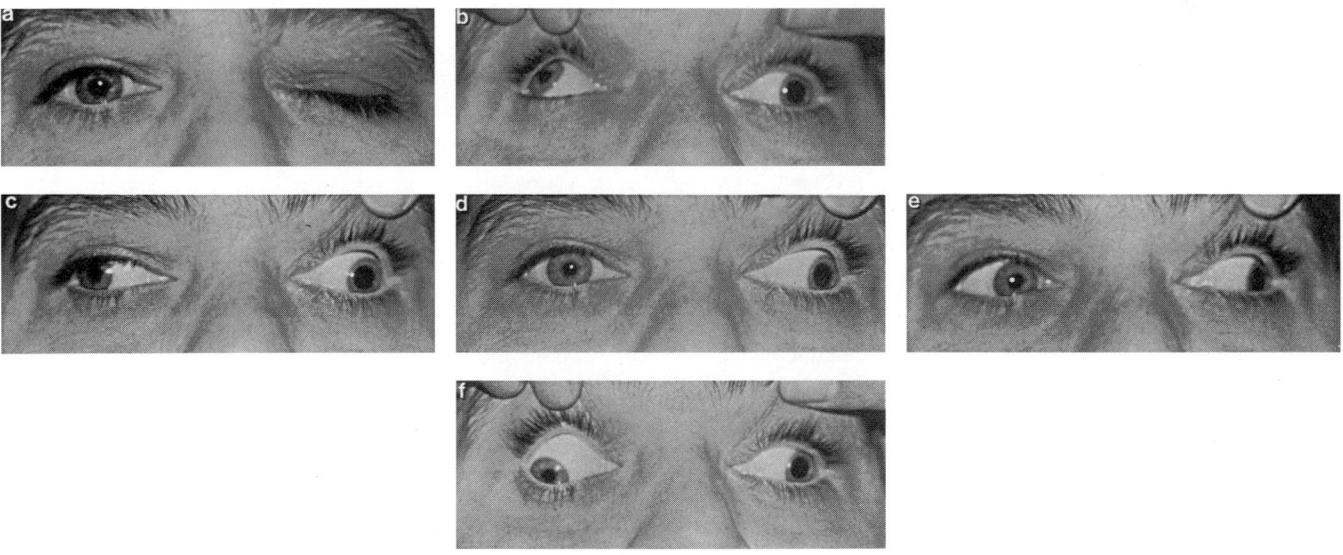

FIG. 7-9. Complete left fascicular third-nerve palsy due to mesencephalic infarction. The left eye has **(A)** complete ptosis, **(B)** defective upgaze, **(C)** absent adduction, **(D)** a down and out position in primary gaze with a large, unreactive pupil, **(E)** intact abduction, and **(F)** deficient downgaze.

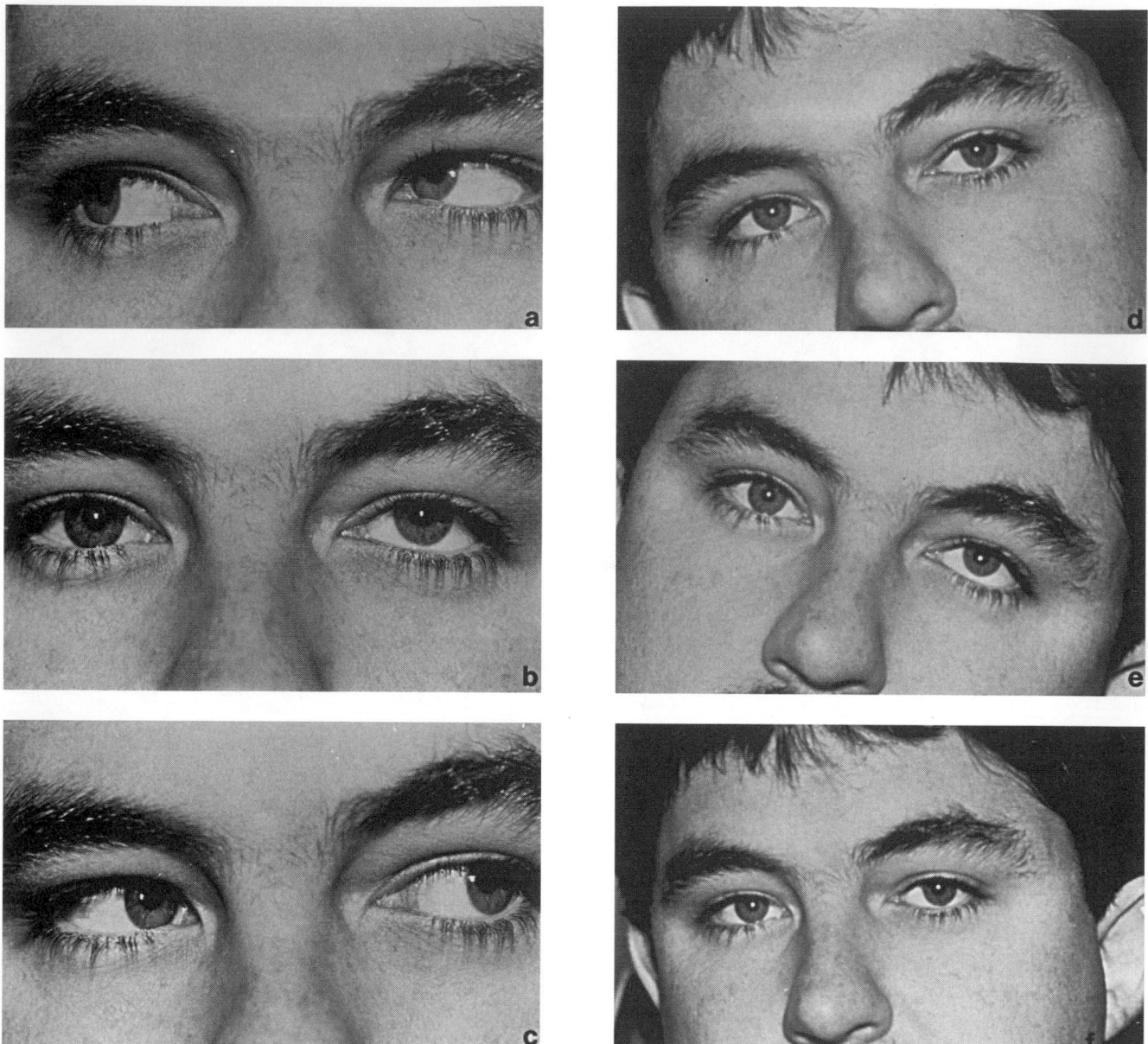

FIG. 7-10. Traumatic left fourth-nerve palsy, three-step test: **(A)** right gaze, **(B)** primary gaze, **(C)** left gaze, **(D)** Right head tilt, **(E)** left head tilt, and **(F)** preference for a right head turn (left gaze) and right head tilt, which minimizes the patient's vertical diplopia. Step 1: Which eye is hypertropic? (Left—see Fig. B); Step 2: Is hypertropia worse in left or right gaze? (Right—see Fig. A versus Fig. C); Step 3: Is hypertropia worse in left or right head tilt? (Left— see Fig. E versus Fig. D). The left hypertropia, which is worse in right gaze and left head tilt, is consistent with weakness of the left superior oblique muscle.

Fourth-nerve axons decussate near the roof of the aqueduct and exit the brainstem dorsally just beneath the inferior colliculi to innervate the contralateral superior oblique muscle. Lesions involving the decussation (anterior medullary vellum), usually the result of trauma, characteristically cause bilateral fourth nerve palsies.

The abducens nucleus lies immediately ventral to the genu of the facial nerve (facial colliculus in dorsal pons), and the fascicles travel ventrally before exiting the pons. The nucleus also gives rise to fibers that ascend within the medial longitudinal fasciculus to reach the contralateral medial rectus subnucleus in the mesencephalon. Thus, a lesion in the region of the sixth-nerve nucleus would result in an ipsiversive conjugate gaze palsy and ipsilateral facial weakness. A lesion of the caudal ventral pons involving the abducens fascicle and corticospinal tract would result in a lateral rectus palsy and a contralateral hemiparesis (Raymond syndrome). Embolic or thrombotic occlusion of paramedian penetrating branches of the basilar artery is the usual cause for disturbances in these areas, but demyelination, vascular malformations, and metastases should also be considered

Möbius syndrome is characterized by a congenital disturbance of horizontal eye movements and bifacial paresis due in part to malformation or injury to brainstem nuclei. In Duane's retraction syndrome, an abduction deficit is accompanied by ipsilateral globe retraction and narrowing of the palpebral fissure during adduction, and in one autopsy case, the oculomotor nerve anomalously innervated the lateral rectus muscle.

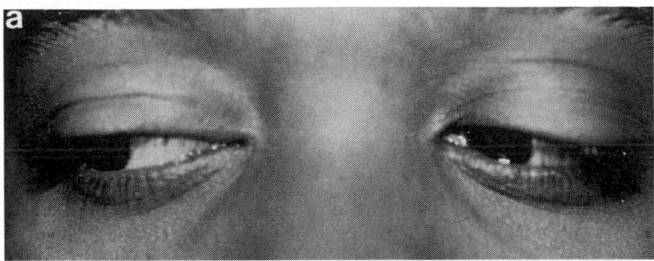
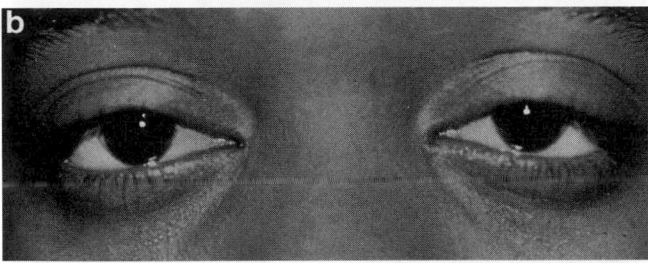
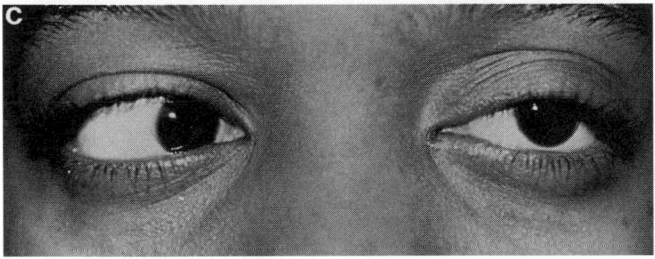

FIG. 7-11. Left sixth nerve palsy due to obstructive hydrocephalus with intracranial hypertension: **(A)** normal right gaze, **(B)** normal primary gaze, **(C)** defective abduction of the left eye.

TABLE 7-3. Causes of Acquired Third-, Fourth, and Sixth-Nerve Palsies According to Frquency and Age Group[a]

Nerve Palsy	Adult[b]		Childhood[c]	
	Etiology	%	Etiology	%
Cranial nerve III	Undetermined	23.1	Trauma	40.0
	Vascular	20.7	Undetermined	17.1
	Head trauma	16.2	Neoplasm	14.3
	Aneurysm	13.8	Ophthalmoplegic migraine	8.6
	Neoplasm	11.7	Surgical	8.6
	Other	14.5	Meningitis	2.9
			Other	8.6
Cranial nerve IV	Undetermined	36.0	Trauma	36.8
	Head trauma	32.0	Undetermined	21.1
	Vascular	18.6	Hydrocephalus	10.5
	Neoplasm	4.1	Meningitis	5.3
	Aneurysm	1.7	Neoplasm	5.3
	Other	7.6	Surgical	5.3
			Other	15.8
Cranial nerve VI	Undetermined	29.6	Trauma	42.0
	Vascular	17.7	Neoplasm	20.5
	Head trauma	16.7	Undetermined	14.8
	Neoplasm	14.6	Viral infection	3.4
	Aneurysm	3.6	Hydrocephalus	2.3
	Other	17.9	Meningitis	2.3
			Surgical	1.1
			Other	13.6
Multiple (any combination of cranial nerve III, IV, or VI)	Neoplasm	34.4	Trauma	55.6
	Head trauma	21.0	Neoplasm	16.7
	Aneurysm	10.9	Aneurysm	11.1
	Undetermined	8.4	Surgical	5.6
	Vascular	5.0	Meningitis	5.6
	Other	20.2	Other	5.6

[a] *Vascular* refers to associated diabetes mellitus, hypertension, or atherosclerosis.
[b] (Data from Rush JA, Younge BR: Paralysis of cranial nerves III, IV, and VI. Arch Ophthalmol 99:76–9, 1981.)
[c] (Data from Kodsi SR, Younge BR: Acquired oculomotor, trochlear, and abducent cranial nerve palsies in pediatric patients. Am J Ophthalmol 114:568–74, 1992.)

In amyotropic lateral sclerosis and the spinal muscle atrophies, the nuclei of the ocular motor nerves are usually spared.

Infranuclear Disorders: Subarachnoid Space, Cavernous Sinus, and Orbital Apex. The three ocular motor nerves traverse the subarachnoid space at the skull base before reaching the cavernous sinus, then ultimately they pass through the superior orbital fissure to innervate the extraocular muscles just distal to the orbital apex.

Acute bacterial and chronic fungal, tuberculous, spirochetal (syphilitic and Lyme borrelia), and inflammatory (sarcoid) meningitic processes may affect the ocular motor nerves within the subarachnoid space, and other cranial nerves may be involved. Carcinomatous or lymphomatous meningitis may produce a similar clinical picture, sometimes accompanied by radicular signs and symptoms indicating more widespread meningeal involvement. The ocular motor nerves can be involved in Guillain-Barré syndrome, the Miller Fisher variant (ophthalmoparesis, ataxia, and areflexia), and chronic inflammatory demyelinating polyneuropathy, usually in the setting of systemic weakness. Cerebrospinal fluid examination is essential for diagnosing and sorting out these infectious, neoplastic, and inflammatory disorders.

Within the subarachnoid space, posterior communicating aneurysms may compress the third nerve, almost always with pupillary dilatation. A third-nerve palsy accompanied by altered mental status and ipsilateral hemiparesis should suggest uncal herniation, causing third-nerve compression and contralateral impingement of the cerebral peduncle along the tentorial edge (Kernohan's notch).

The sixth nerve, as it climbs along the clivus and then over the petrous apex, is vulnerable to injury during downward brainstem shifts resulting from supratentorial masses (''false localizing sign''). Changes in intracranial pressure that occur in pseudotumor cerebri (intracranial hypertension) or after lumbar puncture (intracranial hypotension) may also cause sixth-nerve palsies. Injury to the ocular motor nerves in this area may be due to trauma and skull-base tumors such as chordomas, clivus meningiomas, and chondrosarcomas.

The three ocular motor nerves and the first and second divisions of the trigeminal nerve (V_1 and V_2) lie along the lateral wall of the cavernous sinus, whereas the internal carotid artery and third-order oculosympathetic fibers from the superior cervical ganglion lie more medially (Fig. 7-12). Cavernous sinus involvement would be suggested by any combination of unilateral third-, fourth-, or sixth-nerve dysfunction accompanied by hypesthesia of the forehead, cornea, or cheek, or by a Horner syndrome. Complete interruption of all three ocular motor nerves would result in total ophthalmoplegia, ptosis, and mydriasis.

Idiopathic granulomatous inflammation of the cavernous sinus (Tolosa-Hunt) is characterized by painful ophthalmoplegia, and affected patients have a rapid response to corticosteroids. Sellar masses (Table 7-2), if large enough, may compress cavernous sinus structures, and the clinical scenario of acute headache, visual loss, and ophthalmoplegia should suggest pituitary apoplexy. The differential diagnosis of cavernous sinus lesions also includes metastases, infection (mucormycosis in an immunocompromised individual), septic cavernous sinus thrombosis, carotid-cavernous sinus fistulas and intracavernous aneurysms. Thin-section MRI through the sellar region with

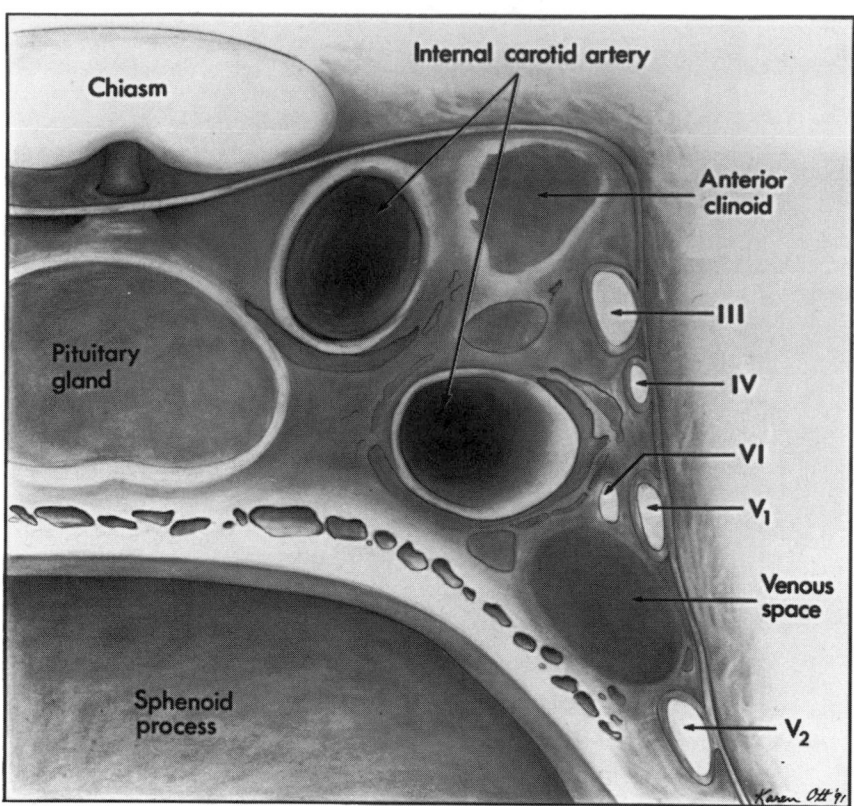

FIG. 7-12. Cavernous sinus, coronal view. Note that the third and fourth cranial nerves are located in the wall of the cavernous sinus, whereas the sixth nerve lies freely next to the carotid artery. Because the carotid siphon is cut in cross section, two arterial lumens are seen; the sympathetic plexus surrounds the more caudal portion of cavernous carotid artery. The sphenoid sinus is medial and inferior to this region, whereas the optic chiasm lies directly above the pituitary gland. III, ocular motor nerve; IV trochlear nerve; VI, abducens nerve; V_1, ophthalmic division of the trigeminal nerve; V_2, maxillary division of the trigeminal nerve. (From Galetta SL: Cavernous sinus syndromes. p. 610. In Margo CE, Hamed LM, Mames RN (eds): Diagnostic Problems in Clinical Ophthalmology. WB Saunders Philadelphia, 1994, with permission.)

coronal views and gadolinium are optimal for detecting and discerning cavernous sinus pathology.

Ischemic ocular motor palsies, associated with hypertension or diabetes, are often preceded by orbital ache or pain. The ischemic third-nerve palsies, characterized by pupillary sparing, may be due to infarction of the nerve in the intracavernous or subarachnoid portions, or within the mesencephalon. Most patients with vasculopathic ocular motor palsies recover spontaneously within 8 to 12 weeks.

Except for sparing of V_2, lesions of the superior orbital fissure are clinically difficult to distinguish from those of the cavernous sinus, and the differential diagnosis is similar. The orbital apex syndrome consists of third-, fourth- and sixth-nerve paresis, V_1 distribution sensory loss, oculosympathetic paresis, and visual loss due to optic nerve involvement.

Patients with traumatic or chronic compressive third-nerve palsies (but not diabetes- or hypertension-related ones) may develop aberrant regeneration, or synkinesis. Common abnormal motility patterns include lid elevation during adduction or depression and miosis during adduction.

Infranuclear Disorders: Neuromuscular Junction. The extraocular muscles are involved in over 90 percent of patients with myasthenia gravis. Fifty percent present with motility abnormalities or ptosis only, and of this group, one-half will remain ''ocular myasthenics,'' whereas the other one-half will develop generalized symptoms, usually within 2 years. The diagnosis is supported by painlessness, diurnal variation, fatigability, and eyelid signs such as ptosis or Cogan's lid twitch (see Disorders of the Eyelids, below). Any eye muscle can be affected, and the motility pattern may mimic a pupil-sparing third-, fourth-, or sixth-nerve palsy, as well as supranuclear disturbances (see below) such as a conjugate gaze palsy, internuclear ophthalmoplegia, or one-and-a-half syndrome. As a rule, the pupil is uninvolved. Resolution of appreciable ptosis or motility deficits following administration of intravenous edrophonium (Tensilon test) helps establish the diagnosis, but interpretation is more difficult with subtle ocular abnormalities. Acetylcholine receptor antibody levels, abnormal in one-half of patients with solely ocular myasthenia, and electromyography with repetitive stimulation and single-fiber studies are important complementary tests. Acetylcholinesterases usually fail to control the diplopia, which often requires additional corticosteroids.

Eye muscle involvement is unusual in Lambert-Eaton myasthenic syndrome, although rare patients may develop ptosis or minor motility disturbances. Ocular motility and pupillary reactivity may be affected in botulism.

Infranuclear Disorders: Ocular Myopathies. Restrictive thyroid myopathy is the most common cause of diplopia in middle-aged patients. The double vision is typically insidious and painless, often accompanied by complaints of dry eye due to re-

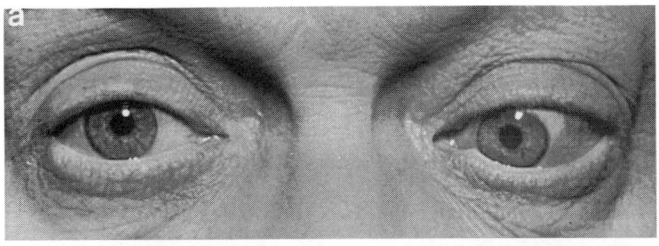
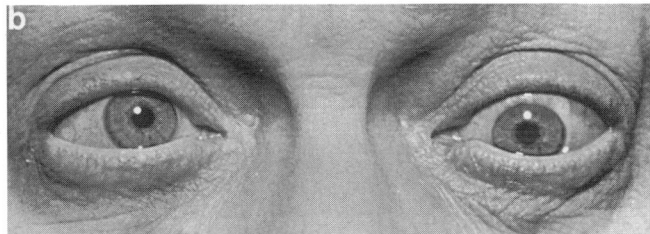
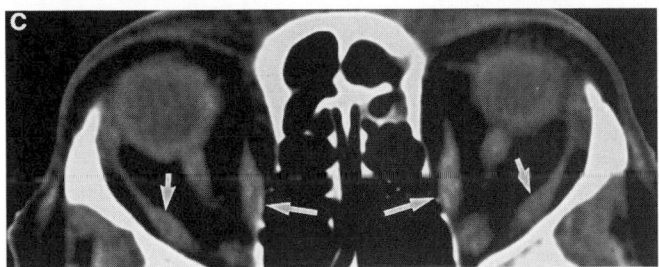
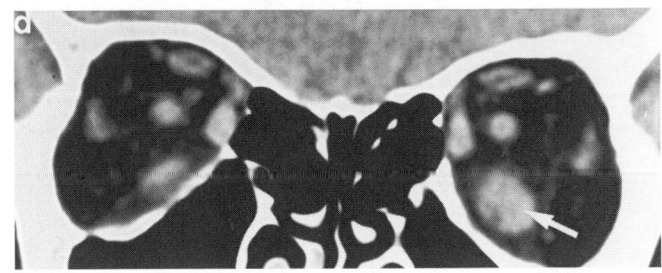

FIG. 7-13.   Thyroid eye (Grave's) disease causing left elevation deficit. **(A)** In primary gaze, there is a right hypertropia and mild left proptosis. **(B)** On attempted upgaze, the left eye has no elevation; forced duction test was positive. **(C)** Computed tomographic scan of the orbits, axial view, demonstrating bilaterally enlarged medial rectus (*larger arrows*) and lateral rectus muscles (*smaller arrows*). **(D)** Computed tomographic scan, coronal view of the orbits, showing diffusely enlarged extraocular muscles; the inferior rectus on the left (*arrow*) is especially large, and accounts for the tethering of the left eye in attempted upgaze and the positive forced duction test.

duced tear film and decreased blink rate. One or both eyes may be proptotic with eyelid edema, lid retraction, and lagophthalmos (see Disorders of the Eyelids, below). Restriction of elevation with a positive forced duction test is characteristic of the disorder (Fig. 7-13), but any muscle or combination may be involved. Affected patients have either primary hyperthyroidism (Grave's disease), primary hypothyroidism (Hashimoto's thyroiditis), or hypothyroidism due to treated hyperthyroidism. For unknown reasons, the extraocular muscles develop lymphocytic and plasmacytic infiltration with secondary production of acid mucopolysaccharides and fibrosis. CT and MRI scanning of the orbits may demonstrate thickening of the extraocular muscles (Fig. 7-13). Thyroxine (T_4), free T_4 index, triiodothyronine (T_3), and thyroid-stimulating hormone (TSH) should all be evaluated if dysthyroid myopathy is suspected, although many patients will be clinically euthyroid. The disorder is often self-limited, but treatment modalities include head elevation during sleep, corticosteroids, radiation, and surgical orbital decompression. Optic nerve compression due to expansion of orbital contents requires urgent surgery or radiation.

Insidious, symmetric loss of eye movements, lack of diplopia, bilateral ptosis, and weakness of orbicularis oculi characterize chronic progressive external ophthalmoplegia due to mitochondrial dysfunction (*external* refers to extraocular muscles; *internal* refers to the pupillary sphincter). The Kearns-Sayre syndrome, typified by chronic progressive external ophthalmoplegia, pigmentary retinopathy, and cardiac conduction defects, is associated with mitochondrial DNA deletions. Patients with oculopharyngeal dystrophy, myotonic dystrophy, myotubular myopathy, congenital fiber-type disproportion, Bassen-Kornzweig syndrome (abetalipoproteinemia), and Refsum's disease may also develop slowly progressive ptosis and ophthalmoparesis. Congenital fibrosis syndrome is a rare familial disorder in which patients are born with bilateral ptosis and ophthalmoparesis due to fibrosis of the extraocular muscles.

Orbital myositis, with inflammation of muscles only, and orbital pseudotumor, with involvement of muscles and other contiguous structures, are characterized by painful double vision and restrictive ophthalmoplegia. Usually idiopathic but sometimes associated with systemic lupus erythematosus or Crohn's disease, they probably represent the orbital versions of the Tolosa-Hunt syndrome. The pain and diplopia are usually responsive to oral corticosteroids.

Isolated metastases to extraocular muscles are uncommon, but orbital metastasis from lung or breast carcinoma or lymphoma can involve the extraocular muscles. CT or MRI usually reveals an orbital soft-tissue mass.

Although uncommon, extraocular muscle ischemia due to giant cell arteritis should be considered in any patient over 60 years of age with diplopia.

Supranuclear Disorders: Cortical Lesions.   The frontal eye fields (FEFs), located in premotor cortex area 8, initiate contraversive horizontal eye deviation. Thus, patients with a frontal lobe tumor or stroke will have a voluntary contraversive horizontal gaze deficit and an ipsiversive gaze preference. Epileptogenic frontal foci may result in contraversive gaze deviation and nystagmus. Patients with hemianopias or visual neglect may have a gaze preference away from the defective hemifield and into their good field.

Deep parietal lesions may cause a homonymous hemianopia and poor tracking of objects (optokinetic stimuli are best) moving ipsilaterally owing to interruption of the optic radiations and adjacent descending corticobulbar fibers from the parieto-occipitotemporal pursuit area (Fig. 7-14). This combination is highly localizing, since patients with lesions restricted to the occipital lobe have hemianopias but normal optokinetic responses.

Bilateral parietal lesions, usually due to watershed infarction, can lead to deficient initiation of voluntary eye movements but preservation of reflex saccades and pursuit (ocular motor apraxia). This abnormality also can be congenital or part of Balint syndrome (see Disorders of the Afferent Visual Pathways, above).

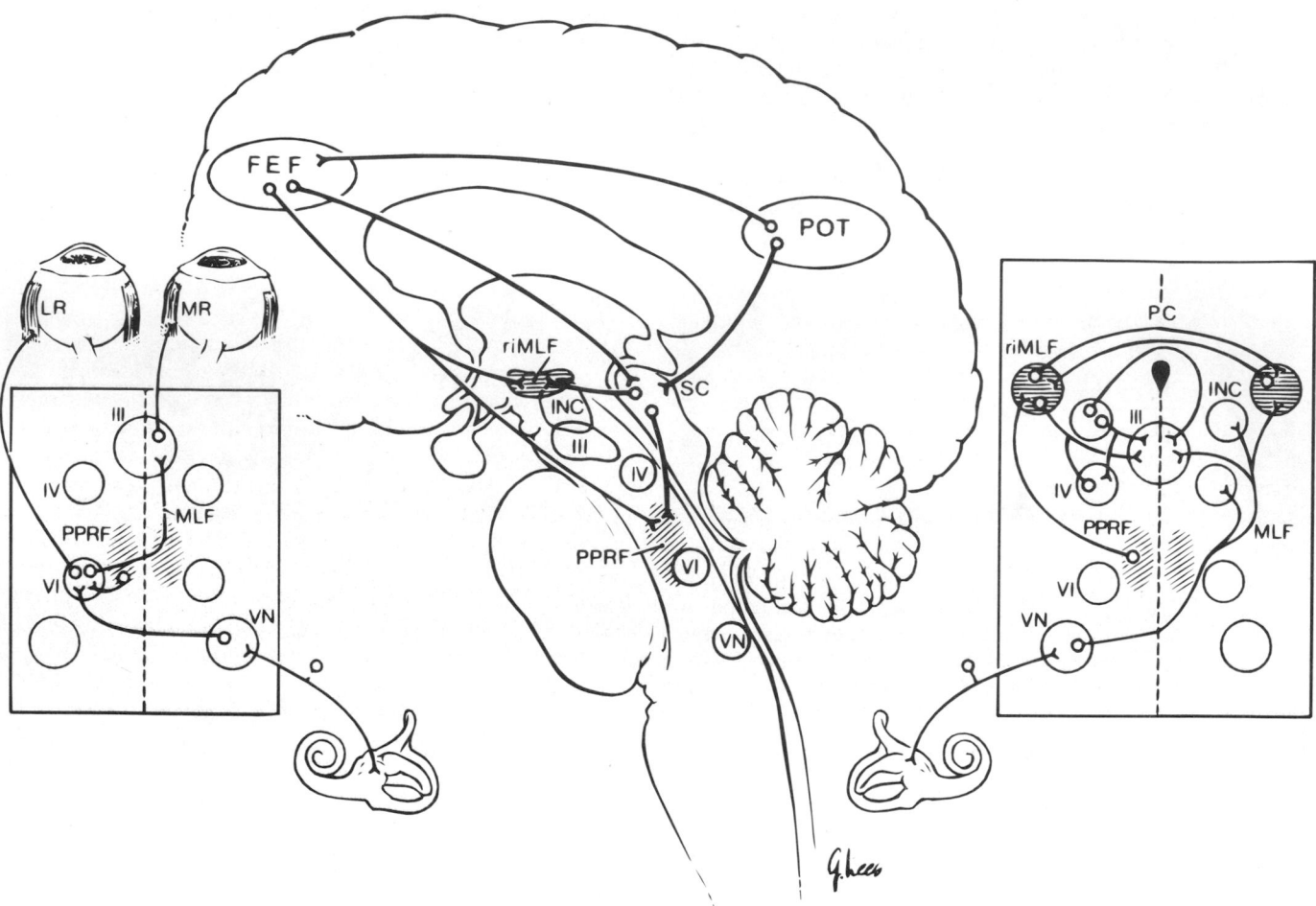

FIG. 7-14.   Summary of eye movement control. Center: The supranuclear connections from the frontal eye fields (FEF) and the parieto-occipito-temporal junction region (POT) to the superior colliculus (SC), rostral interstitial nucleus of the medial longitudinal fasciculus (riMLF), and the paramedian pontine reticular formation (PPRF). The FEF and SC are involved in the production of saccades, whereas the POT is thought to be important in the production of pursuit. Left: Schematic drawing shows the brainstem pathways for horizontal gaze. Axons from the cell bodies located in the PPRF travel to the ipsilateral abducens nucleus (VI), where they synapse with abducens motoneurons whose axons travel to the ipsilateral lateral rectus muscle (LR) and with abducens internuclear neurons whose axons cross the midline and travel in the medial longitudinal fasciculus (MLF) to the portion(s) of the oculomotor nucleus (III) concerned with medial rectus (MR) function (in the contralateral eye). Right: Schematic drawing shows the brainstem pathways for vertical gaze. Important structures include the riMLF, PPRF, the interstitial nucleus of Cajal (INC), and the posterior commissure (PC). Note that axons from cell bodies located in the vestibular nuclei (VN) travel directly to the abducens nuclei and, mostly via the MLF, to the oculomotor nuclei. IV, trochlear nucleus. (From Miller NR: Neural control of eye movements. p. 627. In: Walsh and Hoyt's Clinical Neuro-ophthalmology, Vol. 2. 4th Ed. Williams & Wilkins, Baltimore, 1985, with permission.)

Supranuclear Disorders: Brainstem Lesions.   Each frontal eye field activates the contralateral paramedian pontine reticular formation (PPRF). Neurons of the paramedian pontine reticular formation in turn excite the adjacent sixth-nerve nucleus, which, via the medial longitudinal fasciculus (MLF), innervates the contralateral medial rectus subnucleus (Fig. 7-14, left). Upgaze and downgaze, also under voluntary control by the frontal eye fields, are initiated by neurons in the mesencephalic rostral interstitial nucleus of the medial longitudinal fasciculus (riMLF) and regulated by cells in the interstitial nucleus of Cajal (INC), areas that exert supranuclear control over the third- and fourth-nerve nuclei (Fig. 7-14, right). The vestibular nuclei have direct and indirect connections with the third- and fourth-nerve nuclei, via the medial longitudinal fasciculus (Fig. 7-14, left and right).

MESENCEPHALON.   The dorsal midbrain (Parinaud) syndrome is characterized by a supranuclear vertical gaze paresis

(upward > downward), lid retraction, convergence-retraction nystagmus, pupillary light-near dissociation, and pseudoabduction deficits due to excessive convergence tone. Affected patients have difficulty with voluntary vertical gaze, but oculocephalic and pursuit eye movements are normal. Hydrocephalus, compression of the pretectum by pineal region or thalamic masses, or infarction are the usual causes. The abnormality of vertical gaze results from involvement of supranuclear fibers for upgaze, which originate from the rostral interstitial nucleus of the medial longitudinal fasciculus and interstitial nucleus of Cajal, and cross dorsally within the posterior commissure (Fig. 7-14, right). Skew deviation, a supranuclear vertical ocular misalignment secondary to disruption of vestibular influences, can occur after midbrain injury with the hypertropic eye ipsilateral to the lesion.

PONS.   Disruption of the medial longitudinal fasciculus in the pons results in an internuclear ophthalmoplegia typified by an ipsilateral adduction deficit, contralateral abducting nystagmus, and preservation of convergence. The side of the adduction deficit determines the side of the internuclear ophthalmoplegia. In a young individual, an internuclear ophthalmoplegia is suggestive of demyelination, but bilateral internuclear ophthalmoplegias are virtually diagnostic. Other etiologies include tumor or vascular infarction or malformation. Damage to the paramedian pontine reticular formation results in an ipsilateral conjugate gaze palsy. The combination of an internuclear ophthalmoplegia with a ipsiversive conjugate palsy is a pontine "one-and-a-half" syndrome due to simultaneous ipsilateral involvement of the paramedian pontine reticular formation and median longitudinal fasciculus. Damage to either of these structures in addition to the corticospinal tracts results in Foville syndrome, consisting of a facial palsy, conjugate gaze paresis, and contralateral hemiparesis, and the Raymond-Cestan syndrome, characterized by an internuclear ophthalmoplegia and contralateral hemiparesis.

MEDULLA.   Both skew deviation, with the hypertropic eye contralateral to the lesion, and ipsilateral conjugate gaze deviation may be associated with lateral medullary infarcts (Wallenberg syndrome).

Basal Ganglia Disorders.   In progressive supranuclear palsy, a supranuclear deficit in downward eye movements may be an early and prominent finding. Patients may complain of blurry vision, trouble going down stairs, or difficulty focusing. As the disease progresses, first upward, then horizontal eye movements may be affected, and in the late stages, there may be complete ophthalmoplegia. Patients with Parkinson's disease may have hypometric saccades and pursuit, and individuals with Huntington's disease may have defective initiation of saccades, but these are inconsistent findings and unhelpful in diagnosing the two disorders.

Treatment.   The ophthalmoparesis in some of the disorders described, such as ischemic and traumatic ocular motor palsies, will usually resolve spontaneously. Other cases, such as those due to myasthenia gravis or bacterial meningitis, will improve as the underlying cause is treated. In the meantime, patients with diplopia can wear an eyepatch over one eye to resolve the double vision, or one lens of a pair of eyeglasses can be taped over. The eye being patched should be alternated daily in children to prevent amblyopia. Some authors have advocated botulinum toxin injections into the antagonist muscle of a paretic one. For instance, in a left lateral rectus palsy, the left medial rectus palsy is injected with botulinum to decrease the likelihood of medial rectus contraction and facilitate recovery of binocularity when the lateral rectus palsy recovers.

Individuals with ophthalmoparesis who do not improve spontaneously, and whose examination results remain stable for 6 months, may be candidates for eye muscle surgery. Surgical correction of palsies of single muscles, such as a lateral rectus and superior oblique palsy, is more straightforward than cases where multiple muscles may be involved, as in thyroid eye disease.

Nystagmus and Inappropriate Saccades

Nystagmus.   Nystagmus is a to-and-fro rhythmic oscillation of the eyes. Most types of nystagmus fall in two groups: pendular nystagmus, with symmetric oscillations, and jerk nystagmus, which has slow and fast phases—the latter determines the direc-

tion (as in "leftward-beating nystagmus"). Pathologic nystagmus usually results from posterior fossa or peripheral vestibular abnormalities, but some subtypes are unique and highly localizable.

Pendular eye movements in infancy usually indicate congenital nystagmus, whose other characteristic features include binocularity, appearance at age 2 to 4 months during development of visual fixation, superimposition of jerk nystagmus, lack of oscillopsia, and dampening by convergence. Patients with a null point, where the amplitude of the nystagmus is smallest, may adopt a head turn to achieve this position. The nystagmus wave forms do not distinguish the patients with congenital nystagmus due to abnormal visual pathways (e.g., retinopathies, optic nerve hypoplasia, periventricular leukomalacia) versus those with normal vision. Acquired forms of pendular nystagmus in childhood include the Heimann-Bielchowsky phenonemon, a slow monocular vertical oscillation associated with unilateral visual loss (e.g., due to an optic nerve glioma), and spasmus nutans, a benign, self-limited disorder typified by the triad of asymmetric nystagmus, head bobbing, and torticollis. In rare instances, patients with chiasmal gliomas or other suprasellar tumors may develop a spasmus nutans-like syndrome, but visual loss, optic atrophy, or endocrine abnormalities are also usually evident.

Acquired pendular nystagmus in adults may result from lesions in the cerebellar pathways, usually following demyelination or infarction. In oculopalatal myoclonus, 3-Hz pendular ocular oscillations are accompanied by synchronous movements of the palate and sometimes face and pharynx. The disorder is a delayed complication of injury to the central tegmental tract or dentatorubral pathway (Mollaret's triangle) and is associated with olivary hypertrophy. Trihexyphenidyl may be effective in this disorder.

Horizontal jerk nystagmus usually signifies an abnormality in the vestibulocerebellar pathways. As a general rule, nystagmus that is right-beating in right gaze and left-beating in left gaze (bidirectional, direction-changing, or gaze-evoked nystagmus) reflects a posterior fossa process disrupting the neural integrator, a network responsible for gaze holding. Structures comprising the neural integrator include the cerebellar flocculus and paraflocculus, the nucleus prepositus hypoglossi, and the adjacent medial vestibular nucleus. Symmetric gaze-evoked nystagmus may result from sedatives or anticonvulsants, whereas cerebellar lesions may produce an asymmetric bidirectional nystagmus greater in amplitude ipsilaterally. Physiologic end-gaze nystagmus, usually present only in extremes of gaze, has a smaller amplitude and higher frequency than pathologic nystagmus.

Jerk nystagmus that is horizontal and unidirectional or has a torsional component usually indicates a vestibular abnormality. Purely vertical, horizontal, or torsional nystagmus suggests a nuclear (central) vestibular lesion such as a lateral medullary infarction. Cold-water irrigation of the tympanic membrane mimics a destructive lesion of the vestibular end organ (peripheral) by producing nystagmus with an ipsilateral slow phase and contralateral fast phase; warm-water irrigation mimics an irritative lesion and produces an ipsilateral fast phase (the mnemonic COWS: cold, opposite; warm, same). Peripheral vestibular abnormalities include labyrinthitis, Menière's disease, benign positional vertigo, or neuronitis (see Ch. 9). Bilateral cold-water irrigation produces conjugate downgaze, whereas warm-water irrigation elicits upgaze.

Downbeat nystagmus is very suggestive of a cervicomedullary junction disturbance, such as an Arnold-Chiari malformation, foramen magnum meningioma, or drug toxicity. Periodic alternating nystagmus, which can be congenital or acquired, has the same localization and is characterized by repetitive cycles of horizontal nystagmus beating in one direction for 90 seconds, then 10 seconds in a neutral phase, followed by 90 seconds of nystagmus beating in the opposite direction. Most patients respond to baclofen. Asymmetry of optokinetic nystagmus has localizing value with regard to parietal lesions as discussed in Disorders of the Afferent Visual Pathways, above. Convergence-retraction nystagmus, a dramatic condition in which the globes turn inward and retract into the orbit, occurs in association with dorsal midbrain lesions (Parinaud syndrome) and is elicited during attempted upward saccades. Seesaw nystagmus, in which alternately one eye elevates and intorts while the other depresses and extorts, is associated with large parasellar tumors and mesencephalic lesions.

Saccadic Abnormalities. Hypermetric saccades overshoot the target, whereas hypometric saccades undershoot. Saccadic dysmetria, a sign of vestibulocerebellar dysfunction, is often accompanied by gaze-evoked nystagmus and appendicular and gait ataxia. Often, the direction of the hypermetria lateralizes to the side of a cerebellar hemispheric lesion.

Inappropriate Saccades. Square-wave jerks are characterized by small-amplitude back-to-back horizontal saccades away from fixation, with an intersaccadic interval. They may occur in progressive supranuclear palsy or schizophrenia and represent the subtle end of the spectrum of eye-movement abnormalities grouped under saccadic intrusions. Saccadic oscillations occur around fixation, usually following a saccade and in the setting of cerebellar disease. Ocular flutter, typified by back-to-back bursts of horizontal saccades without an intersaccadic interval, and opsoclonus, in which the eyes conjugately saccade in random, chaotic directions ("saccadomania") are the dramatic saccadic intrusions. Both occur in association with meningoencephalitis and drug toxicity and as a paraneoplastic phenomenon in children harboring occult neuroblastoma or in adults with breast cancer.

Miscellaneous Conditions. Superior oblique myokymia is an intermittent rapid contraction of the superior oblique muscle and causes diplopia and monocular oscillopsia. Carbamazepine is the treatment of choice.

Treatment. As indicated above, some forms of nystagmus respond to pharmacologic treatments. Congenital nystagmus can be treated with base-out prisms in both eyes to induce convergence, or other prism strategies to help move the eyes into the null position. Another alternative is the Anderson-Kestenbaum surgical procedure, in which the attachments of the extraocular muscles are relocated to shift the null position to primary gaze, thereby eliminating the head turn.

Recent reports have suggested using retrobulbar injections of botulinum toxin to treat patients with acquired pendular nystagmus associated with oscillopsia and visual acuity loss. Injections into specific muscles has also been advocated. Although successful in decreasing the amplitude of the nystagmus and improving visual acuity in some instances, many patients develop ptosis or diplopia.

Eye Movements in Coma

In comatose patients, the positions of the eyes and any spontaneous movements should be observed first. Conjugate lateral eye deviation may indicate a destructive lesion in the ipsilateral frontal lobe or contralateral pons, or a seizure focus in the contralateral cerebral hemisphere. Rarely, a thalamic lesion causes "wrong-way eyes," with contraversive horizontal eye deviation. Conjugate downward eye deviation implies a dorsal midbrain lesion or hydrocephalus.

Dysconjugate eyes might suggest an extraocular muscle palsy, although depressed mentation often uncovers a latent eso- or exophoria. A pupil involving third-nerve palsy might indicate uncal herniation or posterior communicating artery aneurysm.

If ocular motor function in the brainstem is intact, there may be roving eye movements, characterized by conjugate or dysconjugate slow ocular deviations in random directions. *Periodic alternating or "ping-pong" gaze* refers to slow, repetitive, back and forth, horizontal conjugate eye movements. Spontaneous nystagmus is unusual in coma except in dorsal midbrain lesions associated with convergence-retraction nystagmus. Patients with ocular bobbing, usually comatose due to severely distructive pontine lesions, have a fast conjugate downward deviation followed by a slow upward correction to midposition. Ocular dipping, with a quick upward deviation followed by a slow downward movement, has the same neuroanatomic localization.

Comatose patients exhibiting spontaneous full, conjugate eye movements, as well as normal pupillary reactivity and eyelids, can be considered to have intact third-, fourth-, and sixth-nerve function, as well as preserved internuclear connections. Individuals having absent or abnormal spontaneous eye movements should be tested using oculocephalic (head turning or doll's head) or oculovestibular (ice-water caloric) maneuvers. Cervical spine trauma and a perforated tympanic membrane should be excluded before performing these tests. The normal oculocephalic response is conjugate eye deviation away from the head turn. In comatose patients with intact brainstem function but abnormal cortical influences, the oculocephalic response may be overly brisk (disinhibited), and ice-water stimulation in one ear may result in ipsiversive eye deviation without the contraversive corrective phase. These maneuvers may uncover a vertical gaze paresis, skew deviation, sixth-nerve palsy, or internuclear ophthalmoplegia useful for brainstem localization. In early metabolic coma, the oculocephalic and oculovestibular reflexes are usually preserved. Absent oculocephalic and oculovestibular reflexes may indicate diffuse brainstem dysfunction, and is seen in late transtentorial (rostral-caudal) herniation and brain death.

DISORDERS OF THE PUPILS

The pupil has three major functions: to vary the quantity of light reaching the retina, to minimize the spherical aberrations of the peripheral cornea and lens, and to increase depth of field. This section reviews pupillary abnormalities encountered in neurologic settings.

Neuroanatomy

The pupillary light reflex is mediated by a parasympathetic pathway (Fig. 7-15), and light directed in either eye leads to bilateral pupillary constriction (miosis). Light is transmitted via the anterior visual pathway and reaches parasympathic structures in the midbrain; parasympathic fibers to the eye exit within the third nerve before synapsing at the ciliary ganglion.

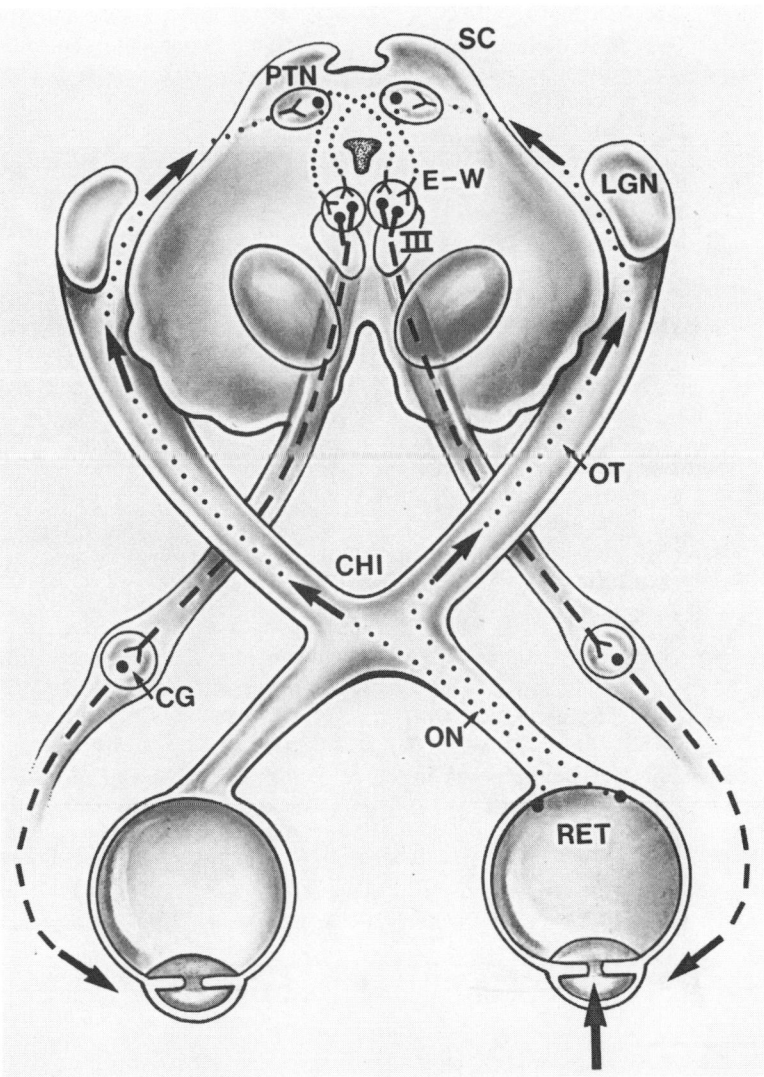

FIG. 7-15. Pupillary light reflex—parasympathetic pathway. Light entering one eye (*straight black arrow, bottom right*) stimulates the retinal photoreceptors (RET), resulting in excitation of ganglion cells, whose axons travel within the optic nerve (ON), partially decussate in the chiasm (CHI), then leave the optic tract (OT) (before the lateral geniculate nucleus [LGN]) and pass through the brachium of the superior colliculus (SC) before synapsing at the mesencephalic pretectal nucleus (PTN). This structure connects bilaterally within the oculomotor nuclear complex at the Edinger-Westphal (E-W) nuclei, which issue parasympathetic fibers that travel within the third nerve (inferior division) and terminate at the ciliary ganglion (CG) in the orbit. Postsynaptic cells innervate the pupillary sphincter, resulting in miosis. Note that light in one eye causes bilaterally pupillary constriction. (Adapted from Slamovits TL, Glaser JS: The pupils and accommodation. p. 460. In Glaser JS (ed): Neuro-ophthalmology. 2nd Ed. JP Lippincott, Philadelphia, 1990, with permission.)

Pupillary dilation (mydriasis) is the function of the oculo-sympathetic system, which contains three neurons beginning in the hypothalmus and ending at the iris and eyelids (Fig. 7-16).

Examination

Pupillary size can be measured in light and dark using the pupil scale available on most near acuity cards. Transient fluctuations in pupillary diameter are normal and are termed hippus. Pupillary light reactivity should be tested with a bright light, such as a halogen transilluminator or indirect ophthalmoscope, while the patient views a distant target (to prevent accomodation). With the light shined in one eye, the ipsilateral pupillary light reflex is the direct response, whereas the contralateral is the consensual response. In the swinging flashlight test, the light is alternately directed at each eye (without too much hesitation between eyes and with equal exposure to light in both eyes) to compare each pupil's constriction to light (Fig. 7-17). Pupillary miosis can also be elicited during accommodation to a near target (thumb, pen, or written material). The examiner should also screen for afferent visual pathway, ocular motility, and eyelid abnormalities.

Pupillary Abnormalities Due to Lesions of the Afferent Visual Pathways

In a subtotal unilateral optic neuropathy or severe retinal or macular abnormality, both pupils have the same size, but the direct and consensual pupillary light responses may be diminished when light is directed in the involved eye. In unilateral blindness (no light perception) due to complete optic nerve or retinal injury, the pupillary light reflex is absent (amaurotic).

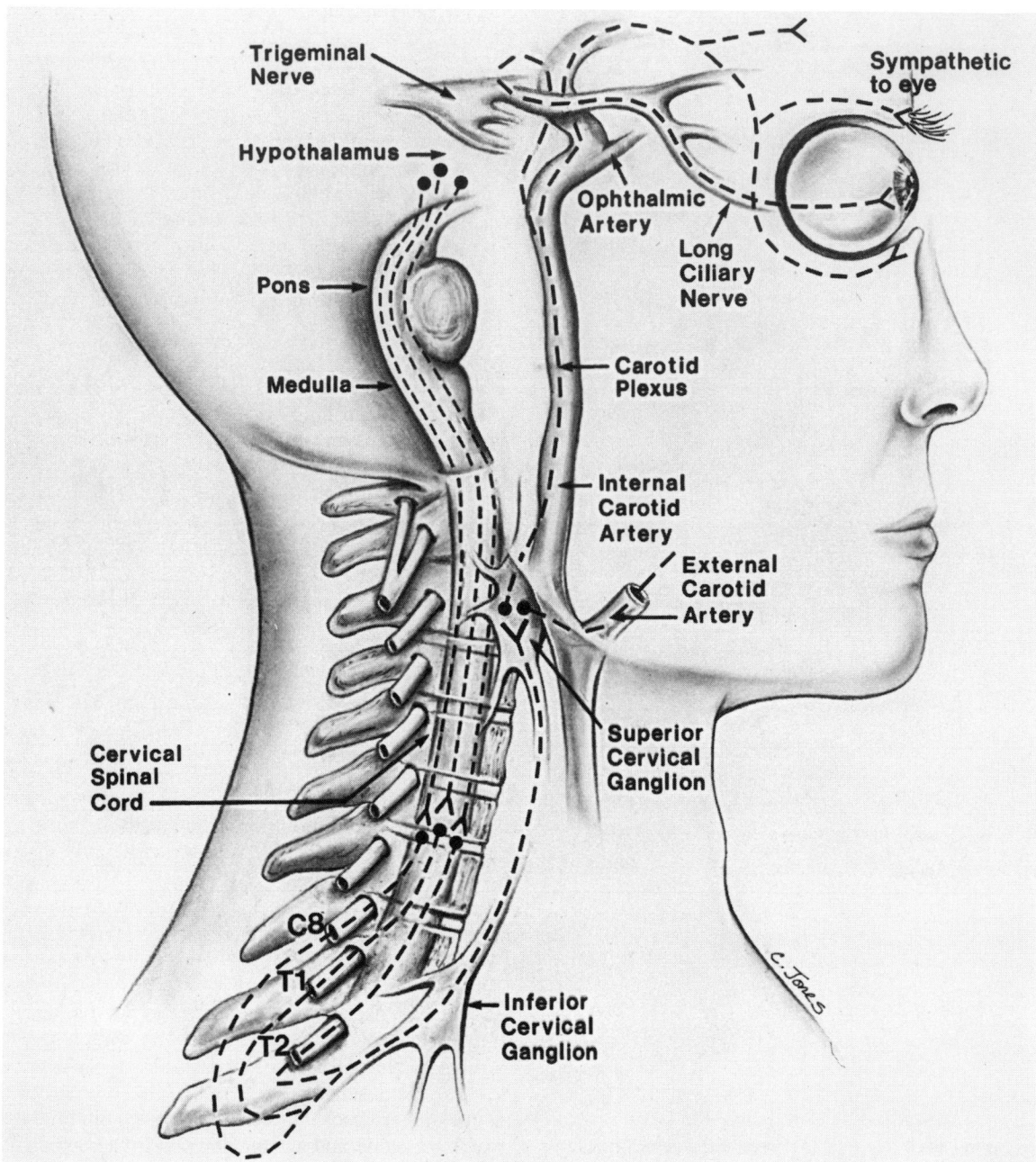

FIG. 7-16. Sympathetic innervation of the pupil and eyelids. First-order hypothalamic (central) neurons descend through the brainstem (midbrain, pons, medulla) and cervical spinal cord. These fibers then synapse with preganglionic neurons, whose cell bodies lie in the intermediolateral gray column and whose axons exit the cord ipsilaterally at C8, T1, and T2. These second-order fibers then travel rostrally via the sympathetic chain and terminate in the superior cervical ganglion. The postganglionic axons ascend within the carotid plexus, which surrounds the internal carotid artery, to reach the cavernous sinus and arrive at the iris via branches of the first division of the trigeminal nerve and then the long ciliary nerve. Sudomotor fibers to the lower face follow the external carotid then facial arteries. Sympathetic fibers to Müller's muscles also travel within the carotid plexus into the cavernous sinus, then may join branches of the third nerve before reaching the upper and lower eyelids.

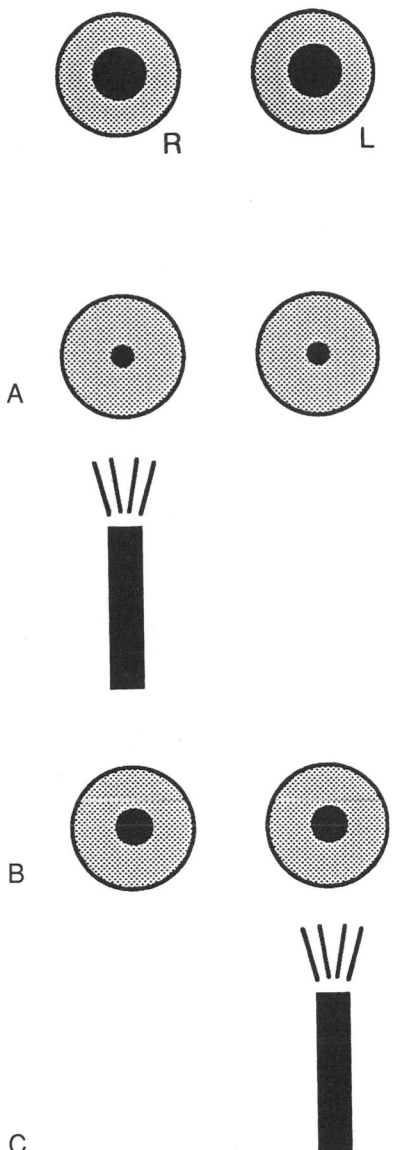

FIG. 7-17. Swinging flashlight test revealing a left relative afferent pupillary defect (L RAPD) in the hypothetical setting of visual loss in the left eye due to an optic neuropathy. **(A)** Pupillary sizes are equal at rest in ambient lighting. **(B)** Light stimulation of the good right eye results in brisk bilateral pupillary constriction. **(C)** Light stimulation of the defective left eye produces comparatively weaker pupillary constriction, and the pupils dilate.

During the swinging flashlight test, when light is directed in the unaffected eye, both pupils will react normally. When the light is returned to the abnormal eye, both pupils will dilate because of the comparatively weaker pupillary constriction (relative afferent pupillary defect) (Fig. 7-17). Even if each pupil constricts to light, but a secondary redilation (pupillary escape) occurs in one eye, the interpretation is the same; this is what Marcus Gunn originally described.

Abnormal visual acuity and color vision, a central scotoma, and a relative afferent pupillary defect collectively are highly suggestive of an optic neuropathy, although a large macular lesion could produce similar findings. In bilateral optic nerve disease, a relative afferent pupillary defect may not be present unless the visual loss is highly asymmetric. A severe unilateral visual loss without a relative afferent pupillary defect may be

functional. Visual loss due to corneal, lens, and vitreous opacities and refractive errors does not produce a relative afferent pupillary defect, but rarely, an amblyopic eye may have a relative afferent pupillary defect.

Asymmetric chiasmal syndromes may be associated with a relative afferent pupillary defect, especially if an eye has subnormal visual acuity. Isolated optic tract lesions may have a contralateral relative afferent pupillary defect, despite normal visual acuities, because the defective temporal field in the contralateral eye is larger than the nasal field of the ipsilateral eye. Behr's pupil (a large contralateral pupil) and Wernicke's hemianopic pupil, one which reacts more briskly to light projected from within the intact hemifield than to light within the abnormal field, are associated with optic tract syndromes, but in clinical practice are rare. As a rule, isolated lesions of the geniculate, optic radiations, and visual cortex do not affect pupillary size or reactivity.

Anisocoria

Asymmetric pupillary sizes is termed anisocoria. Pupillary inequality greater in light suggests the larger pupil is abnormal, owing to a parasympathetic defect, pharmacologic blockade, or iris damage. A greater difference in darkness implies either oculosympathetic paresis or, less commonly, nonpathologic simple (essential) anisocoria. The latter occurs in 15 to 30 percent of the normal population, is characterized by normal pupillary constriction and dilation, and may be less evident in light, owing to mechanical limitations of the iris. More often in clinical practice, simple anisocoria is characterized by a difference in pupillary sizes that is unchanged in light and dark. Often, the simple anisocoria will be evident on old photographs or a driver's license.

Figure 7-18 is an algorithm for evaluating anisocoria when only one pupil is abnormal.

Parasympathetic Disruption—Disorders of Pupillary Constriction. Lesions affecting the dorsal midbrain, causing Parinaud syndrome, may interfere with pupillary reactivity by disrupting ganglion cell axons entering the brachium of the superior colliculus. Bilaterally, the pupils may be midposition to large, poorly reactive to light, but briskly reactive to near stimuli owing to intact supranuclear influences upon midbrain accommodative centers (pupillary light-near dissociation). Ectopic pupils (corectopia) may occur in patients with severe midbrain damage.

In a complete third-nerve palsy (see previous section), the pupil is large and unreactive to light or near stimuli, either directly or consensually (internal ophthalmoplegia) (Fig. 7-9). A nuclear or fascicular lesion in the midbrain rarely causes mydriasis alone and is almost always accompanied by ptosis or ophthalmoparesis. On the other hand, processes in the subarachnoid space such as meningitis, aneurysmal compression (posterior communicating or internal carotid), and uncal herniation (Hutchinson's pupil) may present with a dilated pupil with minimal other indications of a third-nerve palsy. Pupil-sparing third-nerve palsies in middle-aged to elderly patients are usually related to diabetes or hypertension. An aneurysm that presents initially with external ophthalmoparesis or ptosis typically will involve the pupil within several days. Abnormal miosis during ocular adduction or depression may be a sign of aberrantregeneration following a third-nerve palsy associated with head trauma or compression.

Pupils dilated surreptitiously, or as part of an ophthalmic evaluation with tropicamide or cyclopentolate (both anticholin-

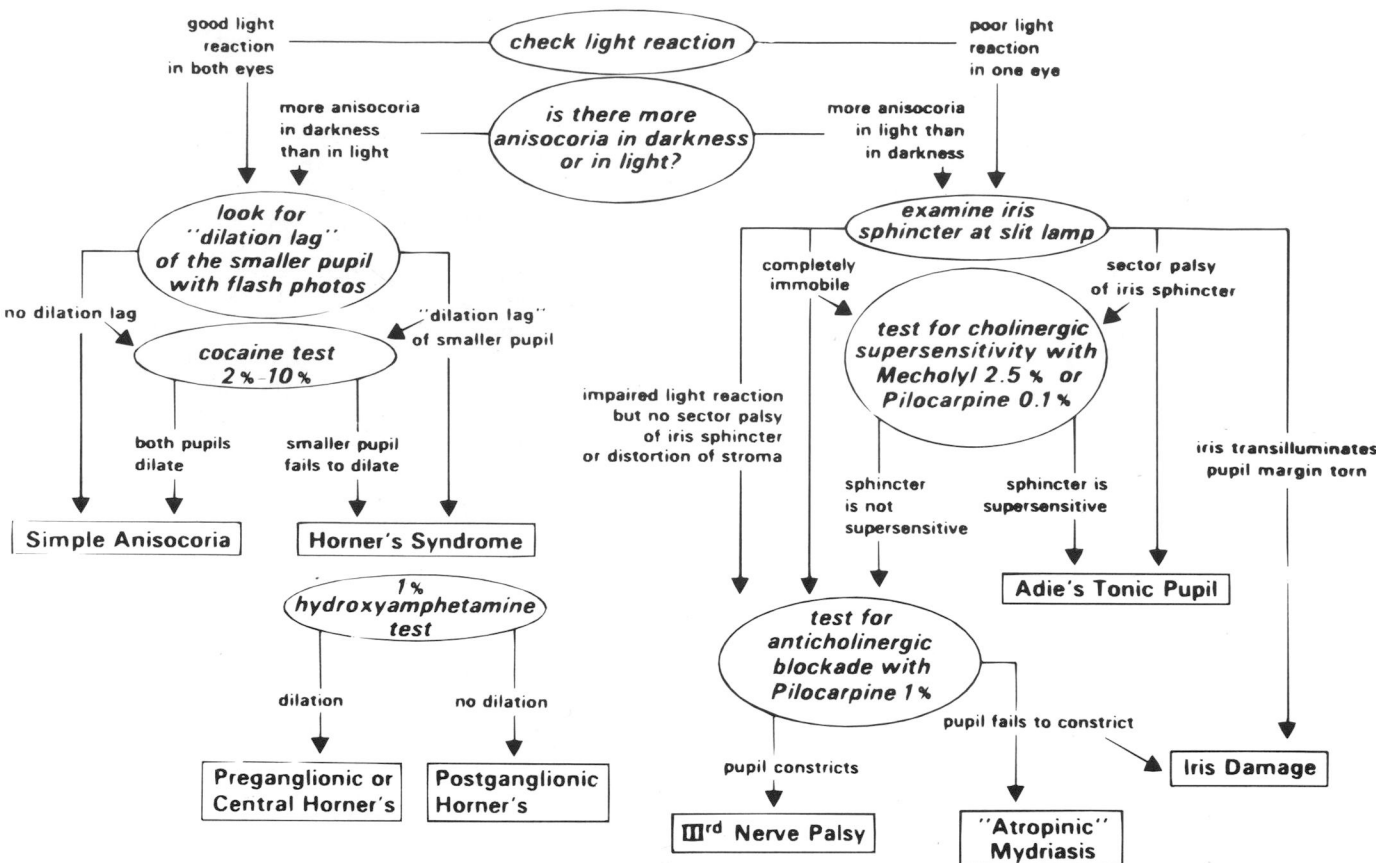

FIG. 7-18. Flow chart for evaluating anisocoria. The chart guides the workup of an abnormal pupil and assumes the other pupil is normal. (From Thompson HS, Pilley SFJ: Unequal pupils. A flow chart for sorting out the anisocorias. Surv Ophthalmol 21:45–8, 1976, with permission.)

ergic agents), or accidentally by an individual who has contact with atropine or a scopolamine patch who then touches his eye, are generally large (>7 to 8 mm) and unreactive. One percent pilocarpine drops would fail to constrict these pharmacologically dilated pupils, but would be effective in third-nerve palsy-related mydriasis.

Tonic pupils result from damage to the ciliary ganglion or the postganglionic short ciliary nerves that innervate the pupillary sphincter and ciliary muscles. Characteristically, they are large, have light-near dissociation (Fig. 7-19), and redilate slowly after constriction. In some instances, the near response may also be defective. Patients may have accommodation paresis, resulting in difficulty with near vision. On slit-lamp examination, the pupils may be irregular, with sectoral paralysis or vermiform movements. After 1 or 2 months, a tonic pupil may become miotic and smaller than the fellow pupil. Tonic pupils may be isolated following viral illnesses or eye or orbital trauma, or part of Adie syndrome, which also includes absent deep tendon reflexes. They may also occur in association with dysautonomias, diabetes mellitus, Guillain-Barré syndrome, or Miller Fisher syndrome. Because of iris sphincter denervation hypersensitivity, tonic pupils will constrict following administration of dilute (0.125 percent) pilocarpine (Fig. 7-19), which does not affect most normal pupils. Tonic pupils usually have a benign etiology, necessitating only symptomatic treatment, such as refractive correction for reading or dilute pilocarpine for photophobia.

Argyll Robertson pupils also exhibit light-near dissociation with a brisk near response, but are typically miotic with poor dilation in the dark (Fig. 7-20). Although nonspecific, they are highly suggestive of syphilis and should therefore prompt serologic testing. The lesion responsible for the pupillary abnormality is uncertain but may result from a disturbance in the midbrain light-reflex pathway between the pretectal nucleus (Fig. 7-15) and Edinger-Westphal nuclei.

Ocular causes of unreactive pupils, including direct eye trauma, angle closure glaucoma, or iritis should be addressed by an ophthalmologist with a slit-lamp examination.

In spasm of the near reflex, miosis is associated with convergence and accomodation. Usually indicative of a functional disorder, this symptom rarely may be associated with brainstem lesions.

Sympathetic Disruption—Disorders of Pupillary Dilation. Interruption of any of the three oculosympathetic neurons may result in Horner syndrome, characterized by unilateral miosis, facial anhidrosis, and upper and lower eyelid ptosis (Fig. 7-21). Usually, the patient will have no ocular complaints. The miotic pupil dilates slowly in the dark (dilation lag), so the anisocoria is accentuated in darkness. The eyelid abnormality may give the false impression that the eye is set back in the orbit (pseudo-enophthalmos). Lesions of the third-order neuron distal to the carotid bifurcation result in loss of sweating on the medial aspect of the forehead and side of the nose, whereas more proxi-

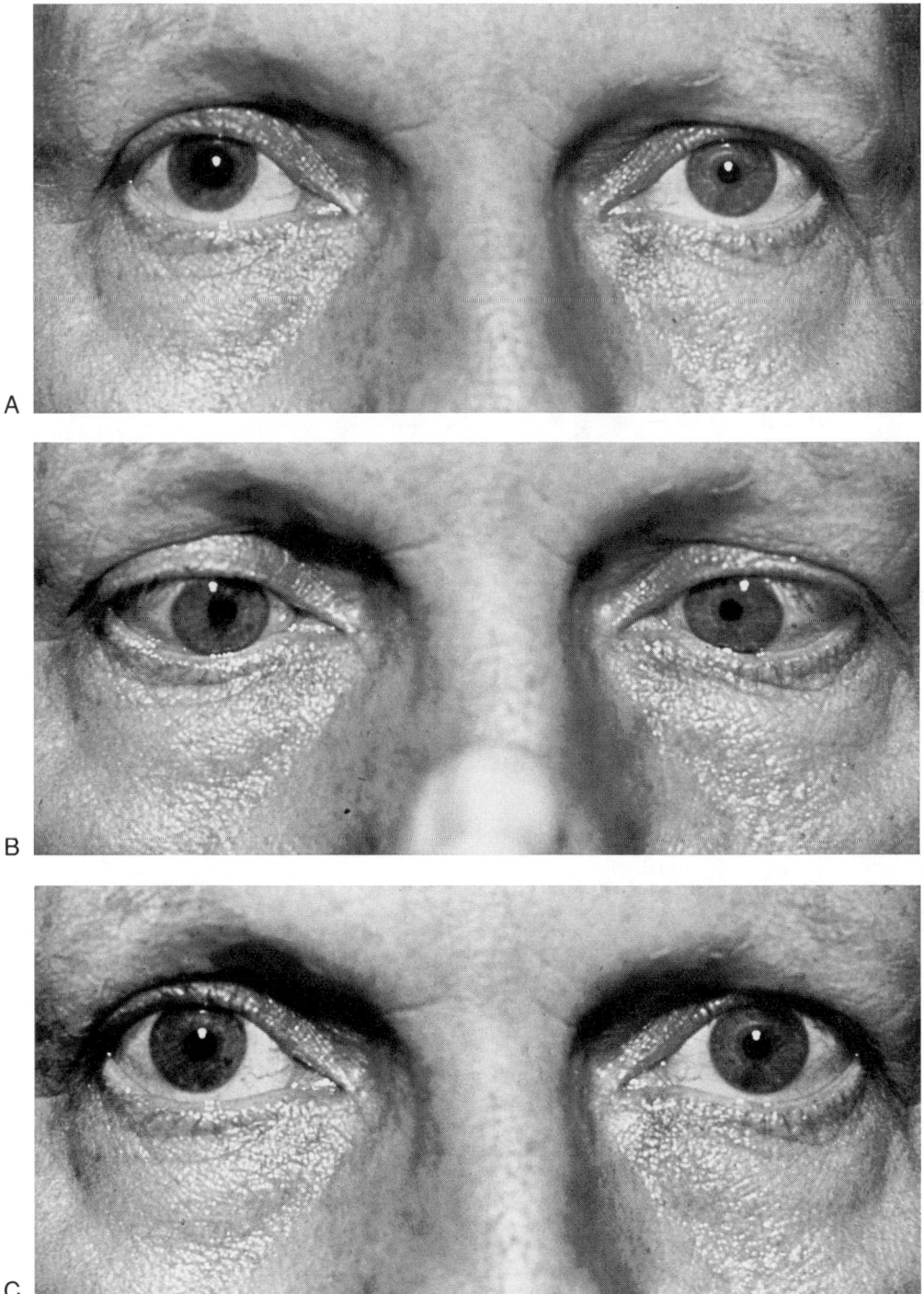

FIG. 7-19. Idiopathic right tonic pupil. **(A)** The right pupil is midposition and larger than the left, poorly reactive to light, but **(B)** reactive to near stimulus (the examiner's thumb). The patient complained of blurry vision in the right eye while attempting to read, consistent with accommodation paresis. **(C)** After instillation of 0.125 percent pilocarpine eye drops at 0 and 5 minutes into both eyes, which were checked 30 minutes later, the right pupil had constricted, whereas the left was relatively unchanged when compared with Fig. A, indicating denervation hypersensitivity on the right.

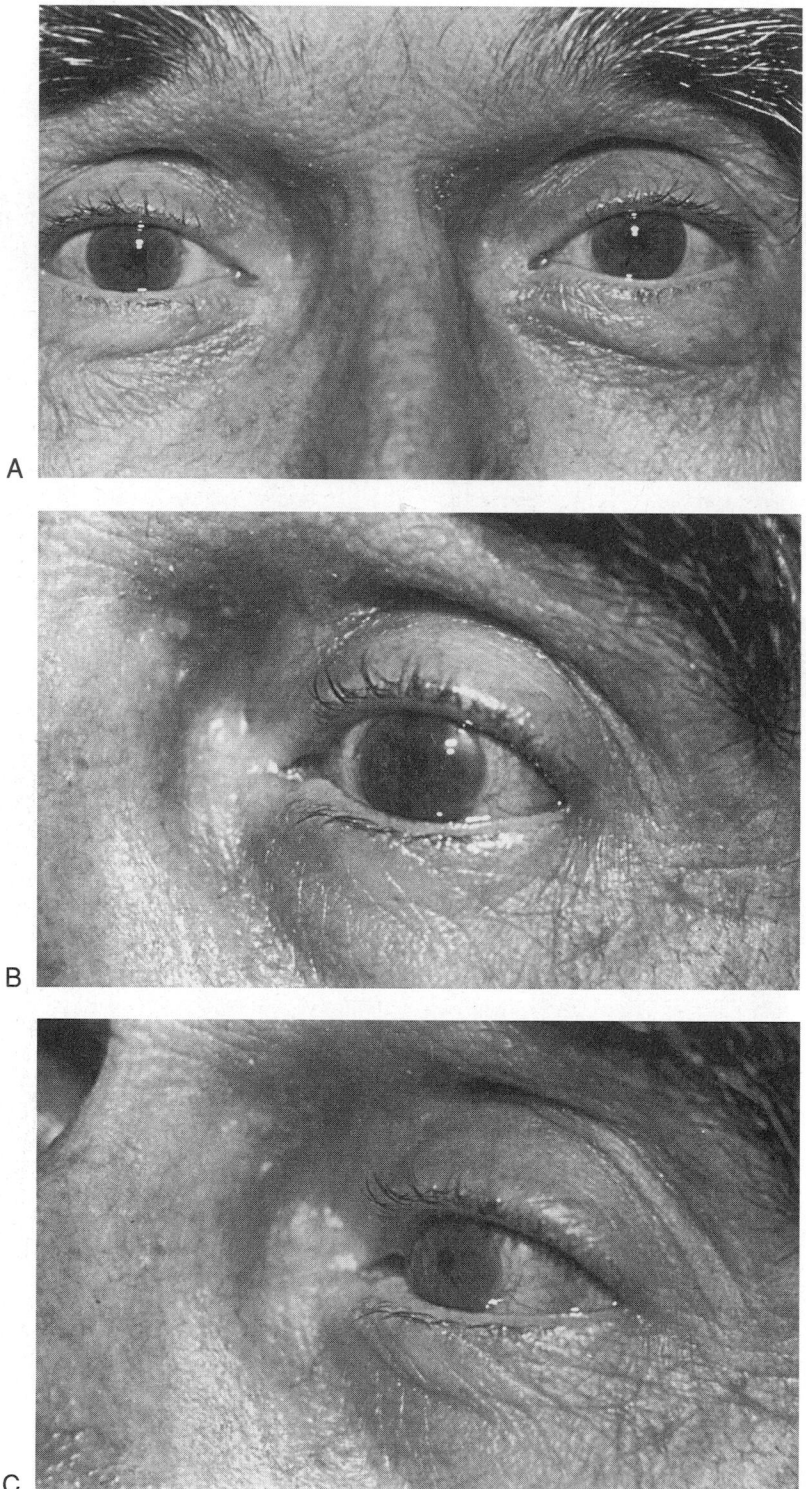

FIG. 7-20.   Argyll Robertson pupils in tabes dorsalis (absent deep tendon reflexes, loss of vibratory sense and proprioception in the lower extremities, and Charcot joints). The pupils are **(A)** small and **(B)** poorly reactive to light, but **(C)** constrict to near stimuli. (The patient was seen courtesy of J. Lawton Smith, M.D.)

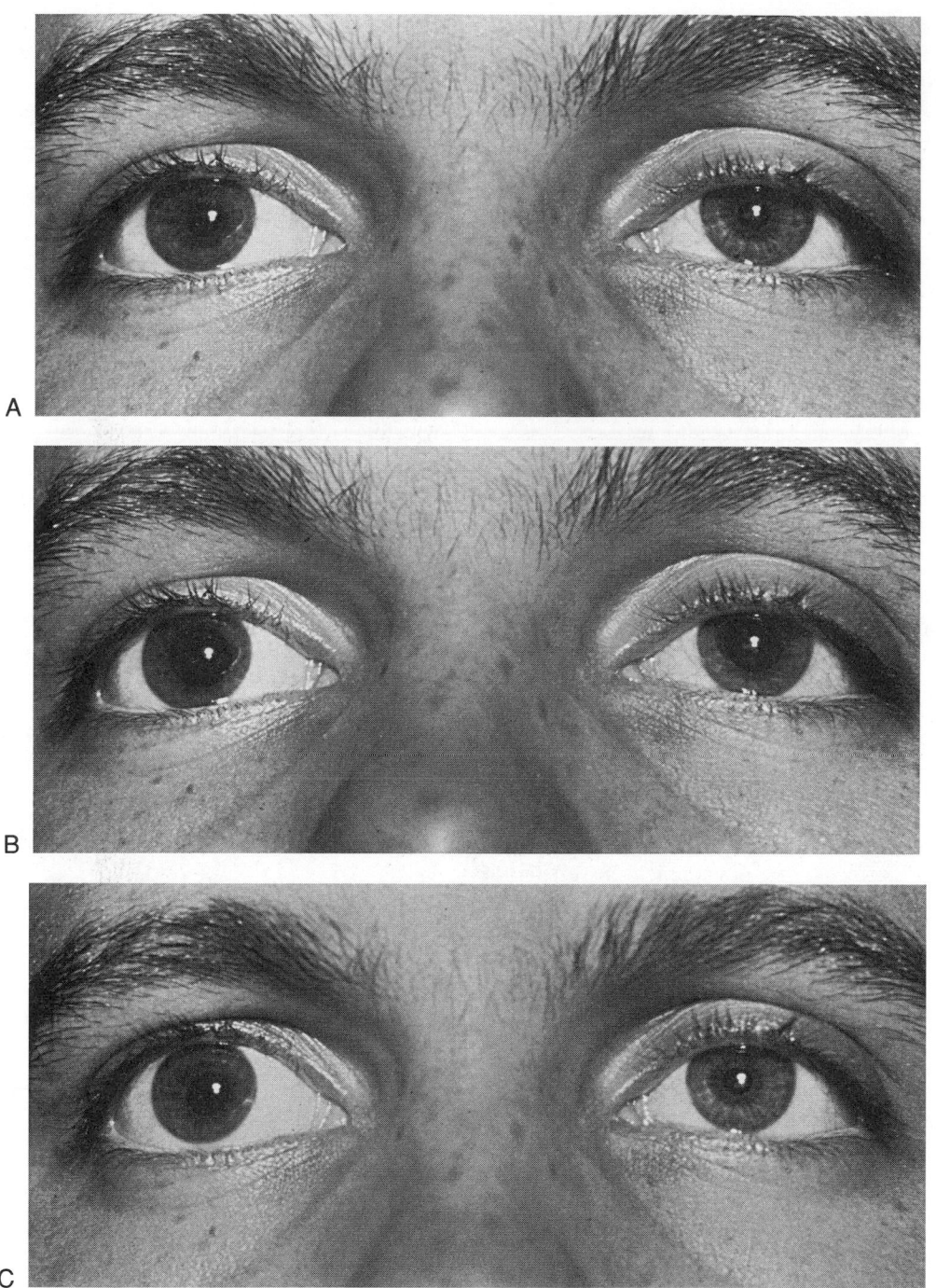

FIG. 7-21. Left Horner syndrome due to cervical spinal cord trauma. **(A)** In room light, the left pupil is miotic, and there is left upper lid ptosis. **(B)** The anisocoria is greater in the dark. **(C)** After instillation of 10 percent cocaine at 0 and 1 minutes into both eyes, which were then checked 45 minutes later, the normal right pupil dilated, whereas the left pupil remained the same, confirming oculosympathetic paresis on the left.

mal lesions, including those of the first- and second-order neurons, involve the whole one-half of the face.

In a study of inpatients with acquired oculosympathetic palsy (Keane, 1979), 63 percent had involvement of the first-order neuron, usually due to lateral medullary or other brainstem stroke. Cerebral infarction or hemorrhage and intracranial tumor, presumably involving the hypothalamus, and syrinx and transverse myelopathy were other central etiologies. Twenty-one percent were due to disruption of the preganglionic, or

second-order neuron (the ganglion referred to is the superior cervical ganglion; thus, *preganglionic* refers to the second-order neuron, and *postganglionic* to the third-order neuron), in most instances resulting from thoracic (e.g., Pancoast's tumors) and neck tumors, but also from surgical and nonsurgical trauma such as attempted direct carotid artery puncture. Third-order neuron (postganglionic) injury was least common (13 percent, with cavernous sinus tumors, trauma, and vascular (cluster) headache as listed etiologies. Carotid dissection should always be considered in the setting of ipsilateral Horner syndrome, carotidynia, dysgeusia, and neurologic symptoms consistent with ipsilateral cerebral ischemia. Carotid thrombosis, by interrupting the blood supply to the superior cervical ganglion or carotid plexus, can cause oculosympathetic paresis. A Horner syndrome and ipsilateral third-, fourth-, V_1, V_2, or sixth-nerve involvement indicates a cavernous sinus process. In two outpatient series, the central neuron was implicated in only 9 and 15 percent of the patients. The second-order neuron was the most common lesion site in one study (Maloney et al., 1980), whereas the third-order neuron was most frequent in another (Grimson and Thompson, 1975).

Etiologies in children include occult neuroblastoma in the upper thorax or cervical sympathetic chain and birth-related brachial plexus trauma. Because iris melanocytes require oculosympathetic input, congenital Horner syndromes can be associated with an ipsilateral lighter colored iris (iris heterochromia).

The diagnosis of a Horner syndrome associated with a lateral medullary stroke, brachial plexus injury, or spinal cord trauma, for instance, is often straightforward. However, the distinction between ipsilateral ptosis and miosis due to oculosympathetic paresis and other causes, such as physiologic anisocoria combined with levator dehiscence-disinsertion on the side of the miotic pupil (so-called pseudo-Horner syndrome), may require pharmacologic testing. Cocaine, which blocks reuptake of norepinephrine at the sympathetic nerve terminal in the iris dilator muscle, allows a relative increase of neurotransmitter available for the postsynaptic receptors. Iris dilator tone depends on the intactness of each neuron in the oculosympathetic pathway; interruption of any one of the three neurons results in decreased norepinephrine release by the third-order neuron, and cocaine will have no or little effect. Thus, after topical instillation of 10 percent cocaine into the eyes (the corneas have to be pristine without previous intraocular pressure measurements or corneal reflex testing during that office visit—disturbances of the corneal epithelium will alter the absorption of the cocaine), repeated 1 minute later, then checked after 45 minutes, a Horner's pupil will either remain miotic or dilate poorly, and an unaffected one will dilate normally (Fig. 7-21). In simple anisocoria, both pupils will dilate with cocaine.

If the cocaine test indicates oculosympathetic paresis (i.e., a positive cocaine test), 24 to 48 hours later 1 percent hydroxyamphetamine drops can be applied (and repeated after 5 minutes, and then examined 30 minutes later) topically to both eyes to test whether the lesion is pre- or postganglionic. The ability of the third-order neuron to synthesize norepinephrine is independent of the other two neurons. Hydroxyamphetamine, which enhances release of presynaptic norepinephrine, will dilate a Horner's pupil only if the third-order neuron is intact. Thus, in a third-order Horner syndrome, the involved pupil will not dilate with hydroxyamphetamine, but in first- or second-order sympathetic interruption, both pupils will dilate.

Oculosympathetic spasm refers to irritation of the oculosympathetic pathway, resulting in unilateral pupillary mydriasis, occasionally accompanied by ipsilateral facial flushing and hyperhydrosis. Cervical cord lesions, thoracic tumors, and carotid artery puncture have been reported causes.

Pupils in Neuromuscular Disease

In general, the pupils are unaffected in myasthenia gravis. Patients with botulism who develop defective release of acetylcho-

line can have bilaterally dilated pupils and accomodative paresis with varying degrees of ptosis and ophthalmoparesis.

Pupils in Coma

Pupillary signs may be extremely important in the evaluation of comatose patients, especially with regard to localization. As stated above, hypothalamic lesions may cause small but reactive pupils owing to oculosympathetic paresis, whereas thalamic and mesencephalic lesions may result in third-nerve palsies, midposition or large pupils with light-near dissociation, or, less likely, pupillary corectopia. Destructive lesions of the pons may disrupt the descending oculosympathetic pathways and result in bilateral pinpoint pupils. Pupillary dilation may be the first sign of uncal herniation before other signs of third-nerve paresis develop.

In metabolic encephalopathies, the pupils may be small but remain reactive to light until midbrain dysfunction ensues. Opiate intoxication causes pinpoint pupils resembling those seen with large pontine lesions. Atropine poisoning causes dilated and fixed pupils.

DISORDERS OF THE EYELIDS

The upper and lower eyelids protect the eye. Aside from insufficient eyelid closure, which is discussed with facial palsy in Chapter 8, ptosis (drooping), retraction (abnormal elevation),

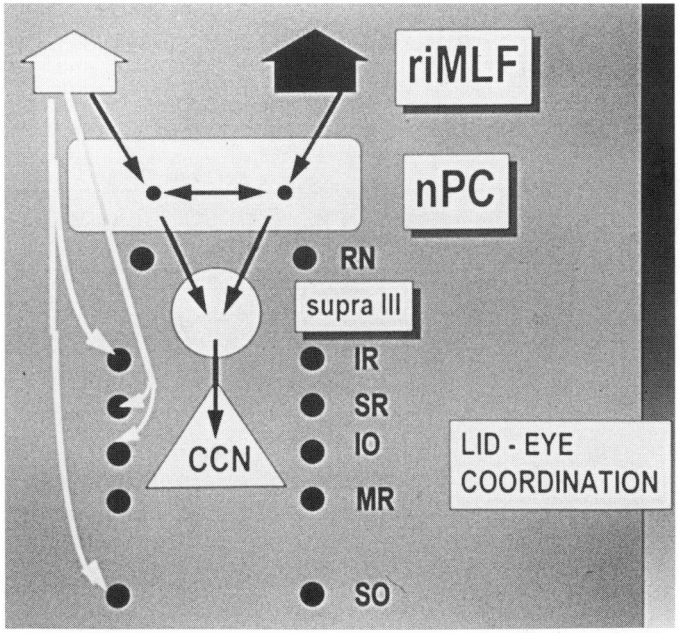

FIG. 7-22. Theoretic scheme of lid-eye coordination based on data from Schmidtke and Büttner-Ennever (1992). The rostral interstitial nucleus of the medial longitudinal fasciculus (riMLF) is interconnected to the nucleus of the posterior commissure (nPC) (*black arrows*) to coordinate lid and vertical eye movements. The inhibitory pathway from the nucleus of the posterior commissure may pass through an intermediary region called the supraoculomotor area (supra III) to influence the central caudal nucleus (CCN). The rostral interstitial nucleus of the medial longitudinal fasciculus also projects to the subnuclei of the third nerve to mediate up and downgaze. IR, inferior rectus; SR, superior rectus; IO, inferior oblique (*white arrows*); MR, medial rectus; SO, superior oblique; RN, red nucleus. (From Galetta SL, Gray LG, Raps EC et al: Unilateral ptosis and contralateral eyelid retraction from a thalamic-midbrain infarction. J Clin Neuro-ophthalmol 13:221–4, 1993, with permission.)

and abnormal blinking are the most important neurologic eyelid disorders. This section reviews the differential diagnosis of these and other eyelid abnormalities encountered by neurologists.

Neuroanatomy

The levator palpebrae superioris muscle, with minor contributions from Müller's and the frontalis muscles, maintains the normal position of the upper eyelid. Both levator muscles are supplied by the central caudal nucleus of the oculomotor complex (Fig. 7-8), Müller's muscle is innervated by oculosympathetic neurons (Fig. 7-16), whereas the frontalis receives fibers from the facial nerve. Eyelid position depends mainly on the resting tone of the levator muscles, which varies according to the patient's state of arousal, with alert individuals having wider palpebral fissures than drowsy ones. Experimental lesions of the frontal lobes, angular gyrus, and temporal lobes may produce ptosis, and experimental stimulation of areas within frontal, temporal, and occipital lobes may produce eyelid opening, but the exact nature of the cortical control of the eyelids is unclear.

Recent evidence suggests that vertical eye movements and lid position are coordinated in the midbrain by the nucleus of the posterior commissure, whose neurons pass through the supraoculomotor area (supra III) to inhibit the central caudal nucleus (Fig. 7-22). Thus, in upgaze, the levator muscles contract and the eyelids open, whereas during downgaze, nucleus of the posterior commissure neurons of the fire, allowing eyelid relaxation. Each nucleus of the posterior commissure lies dorsolateral to the third-nerve nucleus, and interconnecting neurons between the nucleus of the posterior commissure on each side travel through the posterior commissure in the dorsal midbrain (Fig. 7-23).

Hering's law of equal innervation, which refers to the yoking of agonist muscles, applies to both levator muscles. Thus, ptosis on one side may be accompanied by lid retraction on the other, owing to the excess tonus required to keep the ptotic lid open.

Examination

First, the eyelids and their position should be observed at rest with the eyes straight ahead. The palpebral fissure, the opening between the upper and lower eyelids, usually measures between 9 and 15 mm in height (in the middle) when the lids are open. In an adult, normally the upper eyelid covers the top of the cornea (Fig. 7-24), whereas the lower eyelid lies at or just below the limbus (junction of cornea and sclera). In a neonate, the upper eyelid may be above the cornea, and the lower lid just above the limbus. Any obvious abnormalities in the shape or size of the lid also should be noted. An upper eyelid above the limbus ("scleral show") implies that the palpebral fissure is widened, and disorders causing lid retraction or poor eyelid closure should be considered. Fissure narrowing suggests either excessive orbicularis contraction or ptosis due to a neurogenic, myogenic, or mechanical problem.

Next, the lids should be examined during eye movements. During horizontal conjugate gaze, the palpebral fissure widens in the abducting eye in approximately one-half of normal individuals, and in about 15 percent, the lid elevates in the adducting eye as well. During upgaze, levator tone increases to lift the upper eyelid, whereas in downgaze, the eyelids should relax and follow the eyes smoothly. If when the patient looks at a target moved downward, the eyelids lag behind (lid lag or lagophthalmos), thyroid eye disease should be suspected (see below).

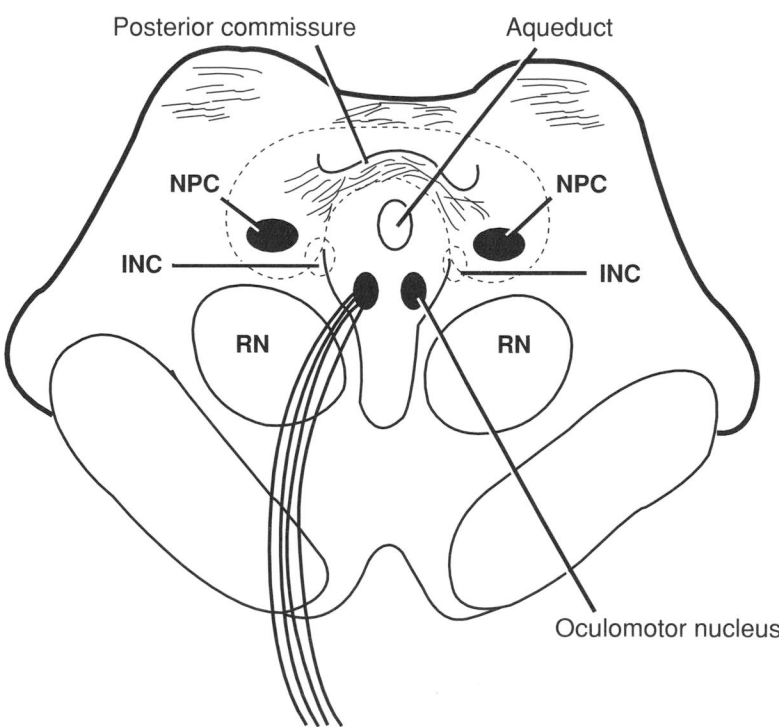

FIG. 7-23. Diagram of the mesencephalon at the level of the superior colliculus demonstrating the connection between each nucleus of the posterior commissure (NPC) through the posterior commissure, which lies dorsal to the aqueduct. Each NPC lies dorsolateral to the oculomotor (III) nuclei. INC, interstitial nucleus of Cajal; RN, red nucleus. (Courtesy of Steven L. Galetta, M.D.)

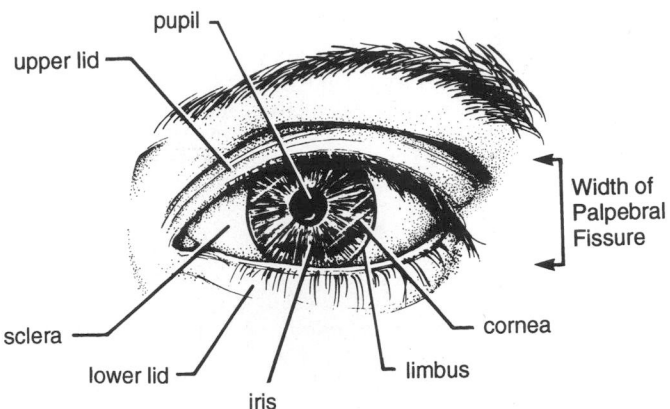

FIG. 7-24.   Normal eye and eyelids. The palpebral fissure is the opening between the upper and lower lids, and its width should be measured along the 12-o'clock meridian of the cornea (at the pupil). Normally, the upper lid covers the limbus (junction of cornea and sclera), whereas the lower lid usually lies at or just below it.

In any patient with a suspected eyelid abnormality, ocular motility and the pupils also should be evaluated carefully.

Ptosis

A detailed differential diagnosis of ptosis is outlined in Table 7-4, but the text here concentrates on the most common causes. Etiologies should be considered according to age (congenital versus acquired in adulthood), acuity of onset, the appearance of the eyelid, and accompanying neurologic signs.

Isolated ptosis in the neonate is usually due to congenital maldevelopment of the levator palpebrae or its tendon, which also causes incomplete lowering of the eyelid in downgaze. Commonly, the involved eye has deficient elevation (double elevator palsy), and if both eyes are ptotic, neither eye may have normal upgaze. Patients with Marcus Gunn jaw-winking have a ptotic eyelid that retracts during contraction of the external pterygoid muscle (e.g., nursing, chewing, mouth opening, or moving jaw forward or side to side) (Fig. 7-25), presumably from anomolous innervation of the levator by the trigeminal nucleus (trigemino-oculomotor synkinesis). Neurofibromas and lid tumors such as hemangiomas should also be suspected in children with ptosis. Oculomotor palsies and Horner syndrome (see below) related to birth trauma should also be considered in this age group.

Acquired painless ptosis of gradual onset is usually due to levator-dehiscence-disinsertion (see below), but neurologic causes include disorders of neuromuscular transmission or myogenic etiologies. In myasthenia gravis, the ptosis may fluctuate, with a tendency to worsen at the end of the day, and the lids are usually affected bilaterally and asymmetrically. Ptosis may be the only manifestation of myasthenia gravis, or there may be varying degrees of accompanying orbicularis oculi weakness, ophthalmoparesis, or generalized weakness, and the pupils are normal. Fatigue, Cogan's lid twitch, and curtaining are other important eyelid signs in myasthenia, although they are nonspecific and may be seen with ptosis due to other etiologies. In sustained upgaze, a myasthenic eyelid may fatigue and droop. Cogan's lid twitch is a "jump" in eyelid position elicited by having the patient look down for several seconds then back up to primary gaze, during which the upper eyelid may overshoot, then fall back down, due to rapid recovery and then

TABLE 7-4.   Causes of Ptosis

Congenital
  Isolated
  With double-elevator palsy
  Anomalous synkineses (including Marcus Gunn jaw-winking)
  Lid or orbital tumors (hemangioma, dermoid)
  Birth trauma (third-nerve palsy, Horner syndrome)
  Neurofibromatosis (neurofibroma)
  Neonatal myasthenia (transient)
  Congenital fibrosis syndrome

Acquired
  Myogenic
    Chronic progressive external ophthalmoplegia (CPEO)
    Kearns-Sayre syndrome ("CPEO-plus")
    Myotonic dystrophy
    Oculopharyngeal dystrophy
    Topical steroid eyedrops
  Disorder of neuromuscular transmission
    Myasthenia gravis
    Eaton-Lambert syndrome
    Botulism
  Neurogenic
    Horner syndrome
    Oculomotor nerve palsy
    "Cortical" ptosis
    Obtundation, drowsiness, coma
    Apraxia of eyelid opening
  Mechanical
    Inflammatory (edema, allergy, chalazion, hordeolum, blepharitis, conjunctivitis)
    Cicatricial
    Tumor (lid, orbit)
  Blepharochalasis
  Levator dehiscence-disinsertion syndrome
    Aging
    Inflammation (ocular, lids, orbit)
    Surgery (ocular, orbital, postcataract)
    Trauma
  Pseudoptosis
    Dermatochalasis
    Duane retraction syndrome
    Microphthalmos/phthisis bulbi
    Enophthalmos
    Pathologic lid retraction of the opposite eye
    Chronic (old) Bell's palsy
    Voluntary blepharospasm
    Hypotropia
    Hysteria

(Adapted from Thompson BM, Corbett JJ, Kline LB, Thompson HS: Pseudo-Horner's syndrome. Arch Neurol 39:108–11, 1982, and pp. 37–60. Glaser JS, (ed): Neuro-ophthalmology. 2nd Ed. JB Lippincott, Philadelphia, 1990, with permission.)

fatigability of the levator muscle. With unilateral ptosis (the abnormal one) and contralateral lid retraction (the normal one—obeying Hering's law), manual elevation of the ptotic lid may allow the retracted one to fall slowly—so-called curtaining. Myasthenic lids may also flutter near the lash margin. Edrophonium may dramatically elevate a ptotic lid in myasthenia (Fig. 7-26), thereby establishing the diagnosis, and acetylcholine receptor antibodies and electromyography may also be helpful. Patients with Lambert-Eaton syndrome may have bilateral ptosis, usually without ophthalmoparesis. In chronic progressive external ophthalmoplegia, the ptosis is usually symmetric and accompanied by bilateral ophthalmoparesis and orbicularis oculi weakness. In myotonic dystrophy, bilateral ptosis is associated with bifacial weakness, "hatchet facies," temporal balding, and myotonia.

Acquired painless ptosis of sudden onset strongly suggests a neurologic cause, especially in unilateral cases with pupillary involvement. Mild unilateral ptosis accompanied by miosis and pupillary dilation lag in the dark implies Horner syndrome (see Disorders of the Pupils, above), whereas more prominent unilateral ptosis with adduction, elevation, and depression deficits, with or without pupillary mydriasis, suggests an infranuclear third-nerve palsy (see Disorders of Eye Movements, above). A unilateral nuclear oculomotor lesion causes bilateral ptosis

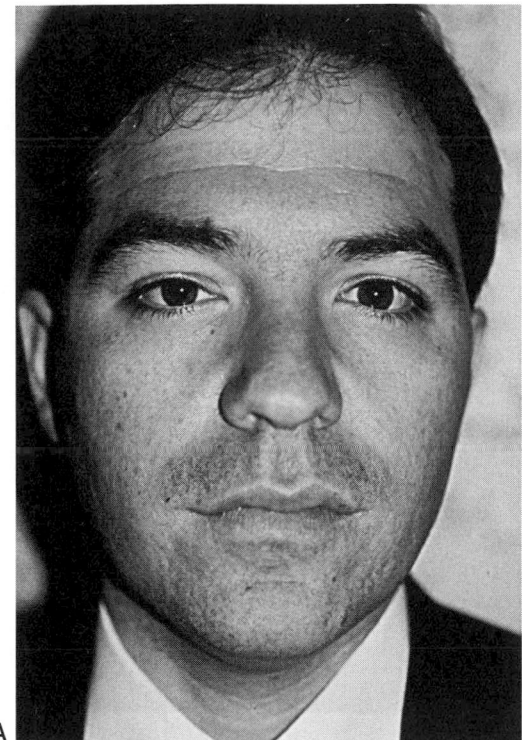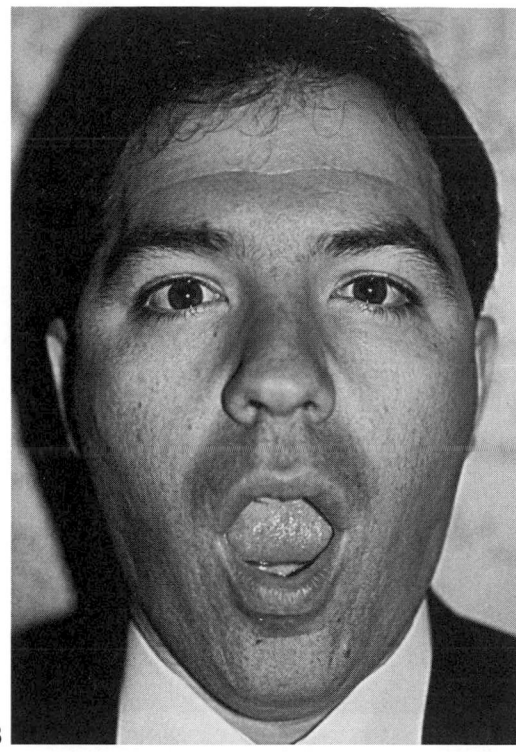

FIG. 7-25. Marcus Gunn jaw-wink phenomenon. **(A)** This man has had ptosis of the right upper eyelid since birth (congenital ptosis). **(B)** Upon opening his mouth, the right upper eyelid elevates, presumably due to congenital aberrant innervation of the levator palpebrae muscle (normally third nerve) by the motor nucleus of the trigeminal nerve (V). Chewing, sucking, and moving the jaw from side to side also elicit right upper eyelid elevation. (Courtesy of Brian R. Watts, M.D.)

(nuclear ptosis), worse ipsilaterally, ipsilateral third-nerve dysfunction, and contralateral superior rectus weakness (see Disorders of Eye Movements). A unilateral cerebral hemispheric lesion may in rare instances cause contralateral or bilateral ptosis (cortical ptosis) without third nerve or sympathetic involvement. Deficient voluntary lid elevation (apraxia of eyelid opening) can mimic levator paralysis until the patient opens the eyes without ptosis after a sudden command or stimulation. This disorder occurs insidiously in association with extrapyramidal disorders such as Parkinson's disease, Huntington's disease, and progressive supranuclear palsy, and, rarely, acutely with hemispheric lesions.

Non-neurologic causes of ptosis are probably more common in the general population than the etiologies discussed above, and these disorders should be suspected in isolated cases. In particular, in many elderly patients the aponeurosis of the levator muscle may dehisce or disinsert from the tarsal plate of the upper eyelid. The eyelids are usually affected bilaterally, but levator function is still relatively preserved. Dermatochalasis, the hanging of skin over the eyelid due to loss of skin elasticity, may mimic ptosis (pseudoptosis). In addition, ptosis may be suspected incorrectly when in fact the upper eyelid of the other eye is pathologically retracted.

Other than treating the primary cause, ptosis can be managed by taping the eyelids open or with eyelid "crutches" attached to eyeglasses. Surgical management of ptosis is more effective in chronic cases, and popular procedures include shortening of the levator muscle or aponeurosis and Müller's muscle resection.

Eyelid Retraction

The two most common causes of eyelid retraction are thyroid eye disease and dorsal midbrain lesions. Thyroid lid retraction, sometimes the only ocular abnormality in these patients, is either uni- or bilateral and is often accompanied by lid lag (Fig. 7-27). The exact mechanism is unclear. Exposure keratopathy and dry eye can complicate the lid retraction and lid lag, especially in individuals with infrequent blinking. Artificial tears are usually sufficient, but some thyroid patients with lid retraction require surgical levator lengthening or excision of Müller's muscle.

Supranuclear eyelid retraction due to dorsal midbrain dysfunction (Collier sign) is usually bilateral and often associated with the supranuclear vertical gaze paresis characteristic of Parinaud syndrome (Fig. 7-28). Pupillary light-near dissociation and convergence-retraction nystagmus may also be observed. The eyelid retraction is exacerbated on attempted upgaze, but normally, the lids relax on downgaze. Children with hydrocephalus may develop bilateral lid retraction and tonic downward eye deviation ("setting sun sign") due to periaqueductal involvement. Schmidtke and Büttner-Ennever (1992) postulated that neurogenic lid retraction can result from either a unilateral nucleus of the posterior commissure lesion or interruption of the posterior commissure, both of which would result in decreased inhibition of levator neurons in the central caudal nucleus (Fig. 7-22). A unilateral lesion involving the nucleus of the posterior commissure and the oculomotor fascicle would produce an ipsilateral third-nerve palsy with ptosis and contralateral lid retraction (plus-minus lid syndrome). Rarely, lid lag can accompany lid retraction in individuals with these dorsal midbrain disturbances.

Lid retraction may also be associated with parkinsonism, myotonia, myositis, sympathetic overexcitation, Marcus Gunn jaw-winking, pseudoretraction due to contralateral ptosis, and oculomotor synkinesis (eyelid elevation during adduction).

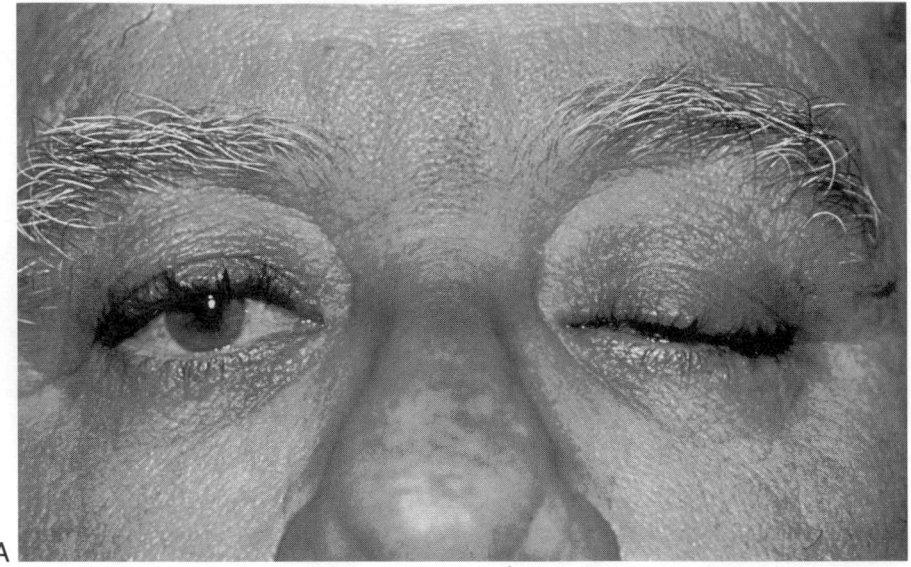

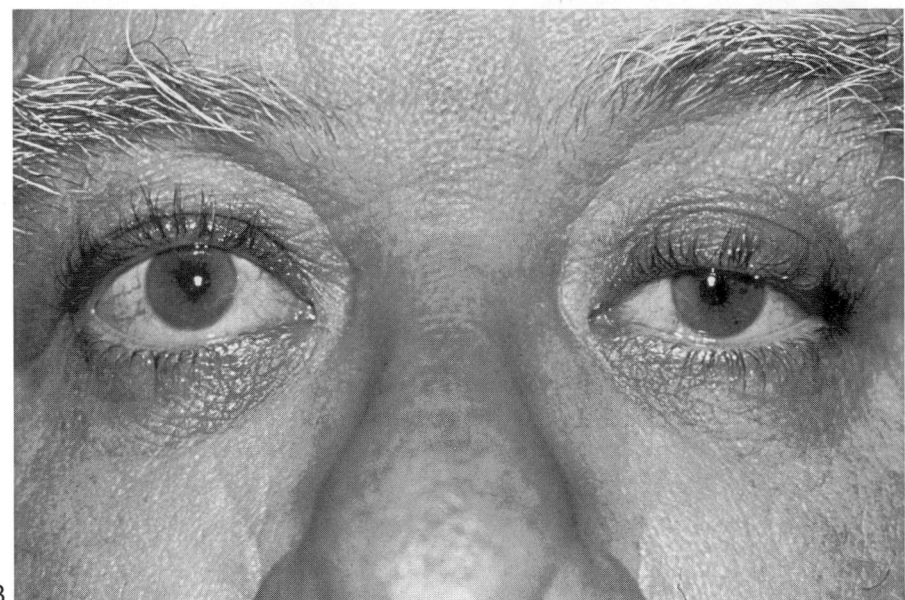

FIG. 7-26. **(A)** Bilateral ptosis in ocular myasthenia gravis (left eyelid much worse than right eyelid). The patient also had bilateral ophthalmoparesis and orbicularis weakness. **(B)** Both eyelids elevated after intravenous administration of 10 mg of edrophonium.

Abnormal Blinking

A blink is a temporary closure of both eyelids and normally does not interfere with the continuity of vision. The mean spontaneous blink rate is 16 ± 9 blinks per minute. Stimulation of the cornea or eyelashes normally produces a blink, and this reflex, mediated by the trigeminal and facial nerves, can be abnormal if corneal sensation or eyelid closure is defective. Other normal blink reflexes include blinking to bright light or dazzle (brainstem mediated) and to a threatening gesture such as a menacing hand. There is evidence to suggest that this blink to visual threat is cortically mediated, since patients with hemianopias from occipital and parietal lesions as well as those with visual neglect from right parietal lesions may not blink when menaced from within the defective field.

Decreased spontaneous blink rates may be characteristic of thyroid eye disease or parkinsonism, although reflex blinking can be increased in the latter (Myerson sign—the patient persis-

tently blinks with each tap by the examiner on the forehead). Increased blink rates are associated with schizophrenia and Tourette syndrome.

Essential blepharospasm is an idiopathic disorder characterized by involuntary bilateral eyelid closure ranging from increased blink frequency to severe, sustained spasms of the orbicularis oculi. The treatment of choice is localized injections of botulinum toxin around the eyelids. Blepharospasm accompanied by dystonic movements of the lower face or neck is termed Meige syndrome.

In hemifacial spasm, the whole face on one side contracts with eyelid closure and elevation of the corner of the mouth. This disorder may be idiopathic or may indicate vascular compression of the facial nerve, and it should be distinguished from facial tics that begin in childhood and from focal seizures, which should correlate with an abnormal electroencephalogram. Botulinum injections as well as neurosurgical de-

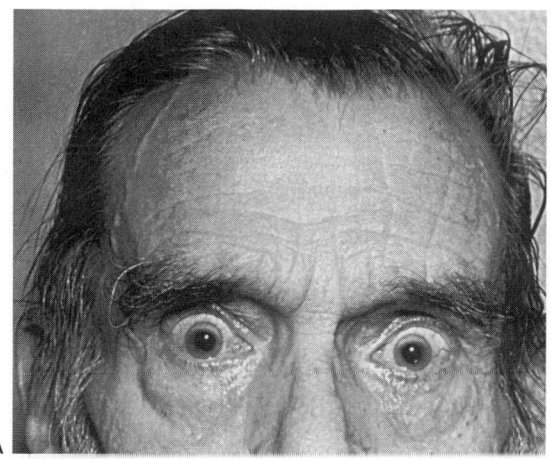 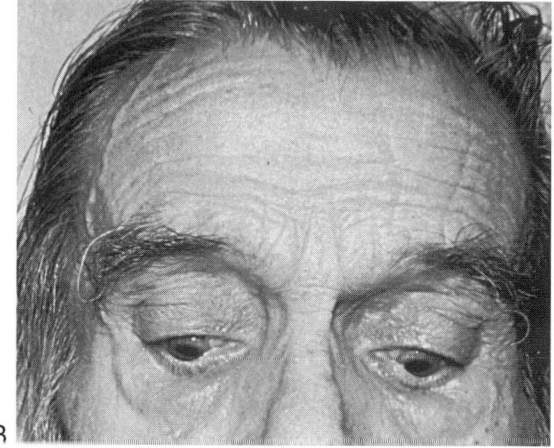

A   B

FIG. 7-27. **(A)** Eyelid retraction and **(B)** lid lag (the lids fail to relax in downgaze) related to hyperthyroidism (Grave's disease). This 80-year-old man presented with 2 months of horizontal double vision and a 30-pound weight loss over 1 year. He had partially restricted eye movements in all directions of gaze, and magnetic resonance imaging revealed enlargement of several extraocular muscles. The patient was emaciated and in atrial fibrillation. The pupils were partially dilated owing to mydriatic drops.

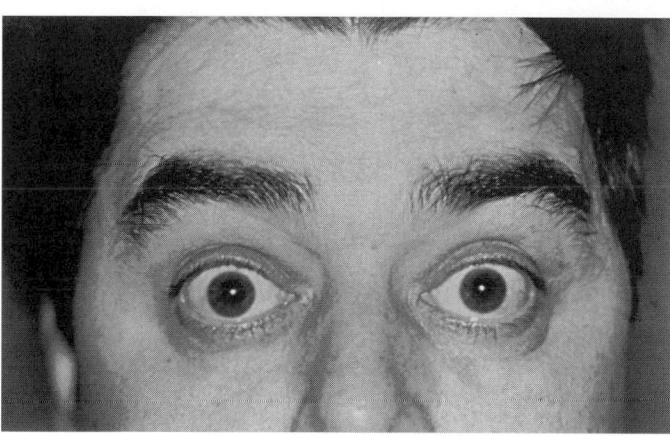

FIG. 7-28. Eyelid retraction due to dorsal midbrain infarction (Collier sign). The patient also had a mild supranuclear upgaze paresis as part of Parinaud syndrome. (Courtesy of Steven L. Galetta M.D.)

compression of the facial nerve trunk near a tortuous or dolichoectatic artery of the posterior circulation have both been advocated as effective therapies.

Small unilateral contractions of the facial muscles characterize facial myokymia, which, when associated with ipsilateral facial contracture and weakness (spastic-paretic facial contracture), suggests a pontine lesion rostral to the seventh nerve nucleus. Eyelid myokymia, small annoying twitches of the upper or lower eyelids, is usually benign and may be due to stress, fatigue, nicotine, or caffeine.

SUGGESTED READINGS

Disorders of the Afferent Visual Pathways

Albert DM, Jakobiec FA: Principles and Practice of Ophthalmology. WB Saunders, Philadelphia, 1994

Beck RW, Cleary PA, Trobe JD et al: The effect of corticosteroids for acute optic neuritis on the subsequent development of multiple sclerosis. N Engl J Med 329:1764–9, 1993

Beck RW, Cleary PA, the Optic Neuritis Study Group: Optic neuritis treatment trial. One year follow-up results. Arch Ophthalmol 111:773–5, 1993

Beck RW: The optic neuritis treatment trial: three-year follow-up results. Arch Ophthalmol 113:136, 1995

Damasio AR: Disorders of complex visual processing: agnosias, achromatopsia, Balint's syndrome, and related difficulties of orientation and construction. pp. 259–88. In Mesulam M-M (ed): Principles of Behavioral Neurology. FA Davis, Philadelphia, 1985

Frisen L: Clinical Tests of Vision. Raven Press, New York, 1990

Gautier J-C: Amaurosis fugax [editorial]. N Engl J Med 329:426–8, 1993

Glaser JS: Neuro-ophthalmology. 2nd Ed. JP Lippincott, Philadelphia, 1990

Liu GT, Glaser JS, Schatz NJ, Smith JL: Visual morbidity in giant cell arteritis: clinical characteristics and prognosis for vision. Ophthalmology 101: 1779–85, 1994

Miller NR: The visual sensory system, the optic nerve. In Walsh and Hoyt's Clinical Neuro-ophthalmology. Vol. 1. 4th Ed. Williams & Wilkins, Baltimore, 1982

Smith JL: Whence pseudotumor cerebri? [editorial] J Clin Neuroophthalmol 5:55–6, 1985

Wall M: Idiopathic intracranial hypertension. Neurol Clin 9:73–95, 1991

Disorders of Eye Movements

Caplan LR: "Top of the basilar" syndrome. Neurology 30:72–9, 1980

Galetta SL: Cavernous sinus syndromes. pp. 609–15. In Margo CE, Hamed LM, Mames RN (eds): Diagnostic Problems in Clinical Ophthalmology. WB Saunders, Philadelphia, 1994

Glaser JS: Neuro-ophthalmology. 2nd Ed. JP Lippincott, Philadelphia, 1990

Kodsi SR, Younge BR: Acquired oculomotor, trochlear, and abducent cranial nerve palsies in pediatric patients. Am J Ophthalmol 114:568–74, 1992

Leigh RJ, Averbuch-Heller L, Tomsak RL et al: Treatment of abnormal eye movements that impair vision: strategies based on current concepts of physiology and pharmacology. Ann Neurol 36:129–41, 1994

Leigh RJ, Zee DS: The Neurology of Eye Movements. 2nd Ed. FA Davis, Philadelphia, 1991

Liu GT, Crenner CW, Logigian EL et al: Midbrain syndromes of Benedikt, Claude, and Nothnagel: setting the record straight. Neurology 42:1820–2, 1992

Miller NR: Walsh and Hoyt's Clinical Neuro-ophthalmology. Vol. 2. 4th Ed. pp. 559–998. The Ocular Motor System: Embryology, Anatomy, Physiology, and Topographic Diagnosis. Williams & Wilkins, Baltimore, 1985

Plum F, Posner JB: The Diagnosis of Stupor and Coma. 3rd Ed. FA Davis, Philadelphia, 1980

Rush JA, Younge BR: Paralysis of cranial nerves III, IV, and VI Arch Ophthalmol 99:76–9, 1981

Silverman IE, Liu GT, Volpe NJ, Galetta SL: The crossed paralyses: the original brainstem syndromes of Millard-Gubler, Foville, Weber, and Raymond-Cestan. Arch Neurol 52:635–38, 1995

Spector RH: Vertical diplopia. Surv Ophthalmol 38:31–62, 1993

Disorders of the Pupils

Burde RM, Landau WM: Clinical neuromythology XII. Shooting backward with Marcus Gunn: a circular exercise in paralogic. Neurology 43:2444–7, 1993

Grimson BS, Thompson HS: Drug testing in Horner's syndrome. pp. 265–70. In Glaser JS, Smith JL (eds): Neuro-ophthalmology. Symposium of the University of Miami and the Bascom Palmer Eye Institute. Vol. VIII. CV Mosby, St. Louis, 1975

Keane JR: Oculosympathetic paresis. Analysis of 100 hospitalized patients. Arch Neurol 36:13–16, 1979

Loewenfeld IE: The Pupil. Anatomy, Physiology, and Clinical Applications. Vol 1. Wayne State University Press, Detroit, 1993

Maloney WF, Younge BR, Moyer NJ: Evaluation of the causes and accuracy of pharmacologic localization in Horner's syndrome. Am J Ophthalmol 90:394–402, 1980

Miller NR: The autonomic nervous system: pupillary function, accomodation and lacrimation. pp. 385–86. In Walsh and Hoyt's Clinical Neuro-ophthalmology. pp. 385–556. Vol. 2. 4th Ed. Williams & Wilkins, Baltimore, 1985

Morris JGL, Lee J, Lim CL: Facial sweating in Horner's syndrome. Brain 107: 751–8, 1984

Plum F, Posner JB: The Diagnosis of Stupor and Coma. 3rd Ed. pp. 44–7. FA Davis, Philadelphia, 1980

Slamovits TL, Glaser JS: The pupils and accommodation. pp. 459–86. In Glaser JS (ed): Neuro-ophthalmology. 2nd Ed. JP Lippincott, Philadelphia, 1990

Thompson HS, Pilley SFJ: Unequal pupils. A flow chart for sorting out the anisocorias. Surv Ophthalmol 21:45–8, 1976

Thompson BM, Corbett JJ, Kline LB, Thompson HS: Pseudo-Horner's syndrome. Arch Neurol 39:108–11, 1982

Disorders of the Eyelids

Caplan LR: Ptosis. J Neurol Neurosurg Psychiat 37:1–7, 1974

Galetta SL, Gray LG, Raps EC et al: Unilateral ptosis and contralateral eyelid retraction from a thalamic-midbrain infarction. J Clin Neuroophthalmol 13:221–4, 1993

Glaser JS: Neuro-ophthalmology. 2nd Ed. pp. 46–51. Philadelphia, JP Lippincott, 1990

Karson CN, LeWitt PA, Calne DB, Wyatt RJ: Blink rates in parkinsonism. Ann Neurol 12:580–3, 1982

Lepore FE: Bilateral cerebral ptosis. Neurology 37:1043–6, 1987

Liu GT, Ronthal M: Reflex blink to visual threat. J Clin Neuroophthalmol 12: 47–56, 1992

May M, Galetta S: The facial nerve and related disorders of the face. pp. 239–78. In Glaser JS (ed): Neuro-ophthalmology. 2nd Ed. JP Lippincott, Philadelphia, 1990

Miller NR: Anatomy and physiology of normal abnormal eyelid position and movement. pp. 932–95. In Walsh and Hoyt's Clinical Neuro-ophthalmology. Vol. 2. 4th Ed. Williams & Wilkins, Baltimore, 1985

Schmidtke K, Büttner-Ennever JA: Nervous control of eyelid function. A review of clinical, experimental and pathological data. Brain 115:227–47, 1992

Thompson BM, Corbett JJ, Kline LB, Thompson HS: Pseudo-Horner's syndrome. Arch Neurol 39:108–11, 1982

8. FACIAL PALSY

GEORGE A. GATES

Facial palsy (FP), the most common of the cranial neuropathies, results in a distorted and dysfunctional face that may affect a patient's social and employment status. It affects speech, eating, and other activities that use the lip musculature (such as playing a wind instrument), and it places the eye at risk for ulceration caused by inadequate lid function. Patients with FP are often afraid they have had a stroke (or worse), are dismayed about their prognosis and the risks and complications of treatment, and are confused about the choice of therapy because of contradictory evidence. Most cases of FP represent idiopathic FP (IFP), formerly called Bell's palsy. This disorder occurs suddenly in otherwise healthy people and has few symptoms besides pain and the inability to move one side of the face. The

palsy is nearly always unilateral and is demonstrably peripheral in localization. In 85 percent of patients with IFP, spontaneous satisfactory recovery occurs over several weeks. However, this fairly benign scenario does not apply to the appreciable number of cases of FP that are due to other etiologies, such as systemic infection, invasive infection of the middle ear cleft and skull base, neoplasm, or trauma.

Because most patients with FP will recover spontaneously but a minority require prompt intervention, the physician is placed in somewhat of a dilemma. On the one hand, it is important not to assume that all cases of FP represent IFP. On the other hand, for reasons of cost it is advisable to follow a logical, stepwise approach to the management of these patients and to be prudent in ordering tests. One should not behave from the start as though an unusual etiology is present unless there are indications that it is. Unfortunately, society does not tolerate delayed or inaccurate diagnosis well, and many physicians opt to order a large battery of initial studies to reduce the risk of later legal action.

This chapter reviews the types of peripheral FP that the neurologist is likely to see in a consultative office practice. A brief review of the pertinent anatomy and physiology is given, followed by a synopsis of etiologic considerations and a discussion of current therapies. The term *palsy* is used to indicate any weakness of the facial muscles upon voluntary effort. *Paresis* implies present but diminished movement, and *paralysis* indicates absence of volitional movement.

ANATOMIC CONSIDERATIONS
Description

The facial nerve arises from the facial nucleus and loops around the abducens nucleus and exits the pons just anterior to the root entry zone of cranial nerve VIII (Fig. 8-1). It crosses the cerebellopontine angle slightly anterior to the cochleovestibular nerve, from which it picks up the nervus intermedius. In the fundus of the internal auditory canal, the facial nerve exits through a separate foramen superior to the transverse crest and anterior to the vertical crest. Within the temporal bone, the nerve has four segments with differing susceptibility to disease or injury. Each segment is separated from the next by a bend or genu, in which the direction of the nerve changes markedly.

Labyrinthine Segment.   The first part of the fallopian canal is the short, narrow labyrinthine segment that passes in immediate proximity to the basilar turn of the cochlea anteriorly and the anterior (superior) semicircular canal posteriorly. Here the nerve is tightly encased in bone with little soft-tissue support.

Geniculate Segment.   The nerve then widens markedly because of the geniculate ganglion, which houses the cell bodies of the special sensory fibers that supply taste sense to the anterior two-thirds of the tongue. The greater superficial petrosal nerve arises anteriorly at the geniculum to exit via the hiatus of the facial canal, traverses the middle cranial fossa, and synapses in the sphenopalatine ganglion. It carries secretomotor fibers from the salivatory nucleus in the pons to the sphenopalatine ganglion, from which postganglionic fibers pass to the lacrimal gland. Interruption of the facial nerve at or proximal to the level of the geniculate ganglion results in a marked decrease of lacrimation on the ipsilateral side.

Tympanic Segment.   The nerve then turns posteriorly to cross the middle ear in the tympanic segment of the fallopian canal.

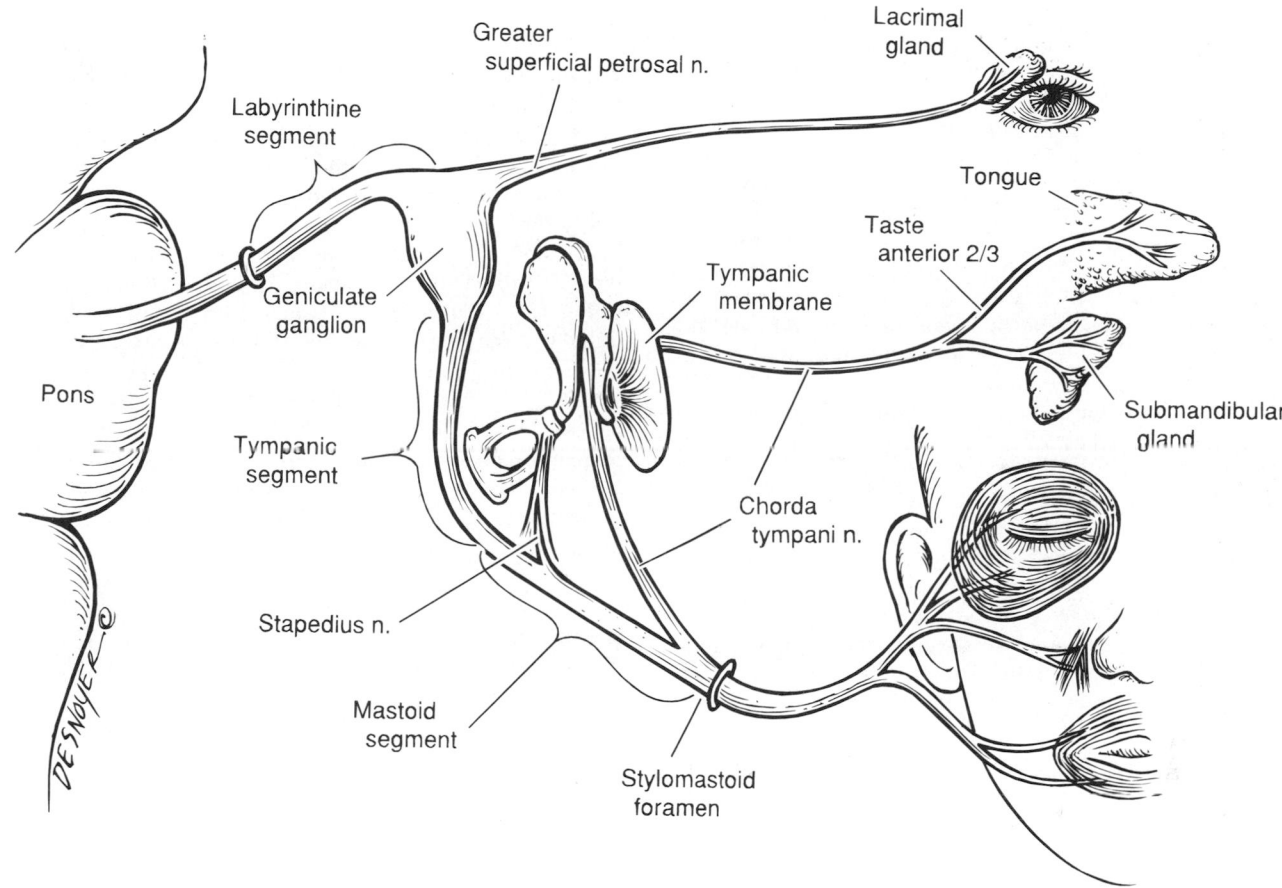

FIG. 8-1. The anatomy of the facial nerve and related structures.

This segment lies adjacent to the oval window, and in 15 percent of people, the nerve is exposed to the middle ear mucosa, owing to incomplete bony closure of the canal. At the external genu, the next bend of the facial nerve, it turns inferiorly beneath the ledge of the lateral semicircular canal to enter the vertical mastoid segment. There may be great variability in this segment, with the nerve passing beneath the oval window or even splitting in two to surround the oval window.

Mastoid Segment. The greatest frequency of positional variation occurs in the mastoid segment. The external genu may be at the level of the inferior end of the lateral semicircular canal or several millimeters posterior to it. This is the segment most often injured in mastoid surgery. The very short motor branch to the stapedius muscle exits in the upper part of this segment. Lesions of the facial nerve above this level are associated with loss of the stapedius (acoustic) reflex. Below this, the chorda tympani nerve exits the main trunk just 4 mm above the stylomastoid foramen, passing antegrade to cross the middle ear between incus and malleus. The chorda tympani can often be seen otoscopically at this point. It carries taste fibers to the anterior two-thirds of the tongue and secretomotor parasympathetic fibers to the submandibular and sublingual salivary glands. Loss of taste sensation and decreased salivation from these two glands are characteristic of lesions above the takeoff of the chorda tympani nerve.

After exiting the temporal bone at the stylomastoid foramen, the nerve takes its fourth bend as it turns in an anterosuperior direction to pass through the parotid gland on its way to the facial muscles. The nerves to the postauricular muscles and to the posterior belly of the digastric muscle arise at the stylomastoid foramen level. From the stylomastoid foramen to the motor endplates, the nerve length varies from 8 to 12 cm in the adult, depending on patient's size and the muscle group in question.

The soft-tissue structures that surround the facial nerve in the fallopian canal form a multilayered sheath consisting of (1) the periosteum lining the inside of the fallopian canal; (2) the layer of vessels, primarily veins, that surround and cushion the nerve proper (the fallopian canal is the primary vascular channel for the temporal bone); and (3) the epineurium, which, in a single fascicular nerve such as the facial, is contiguous with the perineurium. The perineurium is a thin, epithelioid layer of cells and connective tissue that surrounds the entire monofascicular intratemporal facial nerve. It acts as a diffusion barrier to prevent extracellular fluid from entering or leaving the endoneurium. It has radial fibrous connections that segregate the fasicle into compartments.

Clinical Implications

The long intraosseous course (33 mm) of the fallopian canal through the temporal bone renders the facial nerve vulnerable to trauma at the skull base. In addition, because of its intimate proximity to the middle ear cleft, the nerve is frequently involved by inflammatory processes arising therein. The narrowness of the intralabyrinthine segment of the proximal fallopian canal appears to be an important factor in poor recovery from lesions affecting the proximal portion of the nerve. With the exception of this short segment, the nerve is surrounded by a cushion; here, the nerve literally is encased in a bony sleeve. This leaves little room for expansion when the nerve is injured or infiltrated by disease.

The unique sheath surrounding the facial nerve is thought to contribute to IFP. The sheath limits the inflammatory swelling of the nerve and probably contributes to the increase in pressure that occurs in IFP and trauma. Cutting the sheath is essential in decompression. The perineurium limits the egress of inflammatory endoneurial fluid, which probably delays recovery from inflammatory lesions.

The facial nerve carries motor, secretomotor, pain, and special sense (taste) fibers. Throughout its intratemporal course, the facial nerve is a single fasicle and the axonal fibers are distributed randomly across its cross-sectional area. Thus, it is unusual to develop a weakness of a single part of the face (e.g., the forehead) from a discrete injury, such as a partial section of the nerve; rather, there is weakness of all parts of the face. Because of this admixture of fibers, faulty reinnervation (synkinesis) is a common sequel of facial neuropathy, even in the absence of measurable degeneration of the nerve.

Testing of the functions subserved by the fibers carried in these branches of the facial nerve should permit a judgment to be made about the level of the lesion. Clinical applications of the topographic anatomy of the facial nerve are discussed below.

CLASSIFICATION

In 1943, Seddon created a classification of nerve injuries that serves as a convenient conceptual framework for describing degrees of injury. In neurapraxia (conduction block), the axon is anatomically normal and full recovery is expected. The majority of patients with IFP have a neurapraxic lesion. In axonotmesis, Wallerian degeneration of some axons occurs and good but not perfect recovery results from regeneration of these axons through intact nerve sheaths. The degree of recovery is proportional to the number of degenerating axons and the number that reinnervate the appropriate motor endplates. The major sequel of axonotmesis is synkinesis, which is thought to occur from misdirection of regenerating axons. Patients with complete paralysis due to IFP usually have an axonotmetic lesion. Neurotmesis refers to interruption of both the axon and the sheath, and recovery in this instance is much poorer. Here, the loss of axons and the potential for misdirected regeneration is greater. Trauma is the prototypical cause of neurotmesis.

Sunderland's five-degree classification system expands Seddon's neurotmesis into three levels of injury. First and second degrees of injury correspond to Seddon's neurapraxia and axonotmesis, respectively. Third degree implies loss of endoneural tubes; fourth degree, the interruption of the perineurium; and fifth degree, complete physical transsection of the nerve. Spontaneous recovery predictions are based on the degree of damage: (1) complete, (2) synkinesis, (3) incomplete with synkinesis, (4) poor, and (5) minimal or none. First-degree injury is seen in mild cases of IFP with paresis; second-degree, with paralysis due to IFP or herpes zoster oticus; third-degree, with more invasive inflammatory lesions; fourth-degree, from contusion associated with blunt trauma; and fifth-degree, from penetrating trauma (e.g., knife wound).

CLINICAL SYNDROMES

Idiopathic Facial Palsy

Most cases of FP have no obvious cause and thus represent IFP. The older term *Bell's palsy,* given in honor of the great British neurologist Sir Charles Bell, is best avoided becuase it is often used as a generic term for FP of any type. IFP usually afflicts adults and generally resoves without sequelae.

Etiology. Theories of causation abound. Autonomic dysfunction, allergy, and reactivation of latent herpes simplex virus infection have been proposed over the years; the latter is currently the most favored theory. Evidence of viral etiology is indirect but appears plausible. Mori and colleagues (1982) studied 299 patients over the age of 10 with a clinical diagnosis of Bell's palsy during the 15-year period ending in 1981. They found that the yearly incidence of a significant rise in the serum complement-fixing antibody to the following viruses varied from 25 to 37 percent of cases; herpes simplex was noted in 35 cases, varicella-zoster in 21, influenza virus (A and B) in 39, and mumps virus and adenovirus in 11 cases, respectively. Because increases in serum antibodies to these viruses also occur in the general population without FP, meaningful interpretation of these uncontrolled data is difficult.

Histopathology. The known histologic changes occurring in IFP are the result of chance examinations and are all at the light microscopic level and consist of intraneural hemorrhages, edema, and cellular infiltration, and perivascular lymphocytic infiltrates in the fallopian canal. The spectrum of pathology in the average case is unknown, and attempts to develop an animal model have not been successful. It seems clear that the cases associated with severe degeneration and poor outcome have involvement of the nerve proximally in the intralabyrinthine segment. Evidence from intraoperative electric stimulation suggests that the level of distal extension varies and that many sites within the fallopian canal are affected. However, these observations can be made only in cases undergoing surgical decompression because of severe degeneration of the nerve, and they may not apply to all cases of IFP.

Natural History. Most cases are of rapid onset, generally within a few hours. In 40 percent, the patient is able to move the face, though weakly (paresis). In the rest, the face is totally paralyzed. Even within the latter group, degeneration of the nerve is not the rule; neurapraxia (conduction block) is. Recovery from neurapraxia is prompt and complete. Incomplete recovery rates varied from 15 to 43 percent of cases in a series spanning 15 years. Incomplete recovery may be due to another etiology indistinguishable clinically (except for the poor recovery) from IFP, such as a form fruste of the Ramsay Hunt syndrome. Recovery of some degree of facial motion is the rule and absence of any return by 3 months after onset raises the possibility that the presumptive diagnosis of IFP is incorrect.

Facial Palsy Due to Systemic Infection

Viral. FP is known to occur in infections due to the varicella-zoster virus, Epstein-Barr virus (infectious mononucleosis), measles, rubella, rabies, mumps, cytomegalovirus, infectious hepatitis, and human immunodeficiency virus. Herpes zoster oticus, described by J. Ramsay Hunt and also known as the cephalic zoster syndrome, is characterized by severe retroauricular pain; vesicles in the tympanic membrane, external auditory canal, and pinna as well as the base of the tongue; redness of the chorda tympani nerve; complete facial paralysis; hyperacusis with dysacusis; and vertigo. It is more prevalent in older patients, and the outlook for complete recovery is poor, although most are not left with a disabling defect.

Bacterial. Numerous bacterial disorders cause systemic neuropathy, which may include FP. Well-known but rare examples in North America are tetanus, brucellosis, typhoid fever, leptospirosis, and diphtheria. In general, it is unlikely that FP would be the sole manifestation of the underlying disorder. Approximately 10 percent of patients with Lyme disease, a systemic spirochetal infection with *Borrelia burgdorferi* that follows the bite of the deer tick, *Ixodes dammini,* develop FP, and in one-quarter of these cases, the palsy is bilateral. Of note, full recovery of facial function occurred in 86 percent of a study group of patients with Lyme disease, with or without treatment, in an average of 30 days. Chronic granulomatous disorders known to be associated with facial paralysis are sarcoidosis (in which bilateral palsy is not uncommon), leprosy, and syphilis.

Facial Palsy Associated with Middle Ear Disease

FP was a common complication of middle ear and mastoid disease in the preantibiotic era. Acute otitis media is still an occasional cause of FP in children. Children experience FP infrequently, and seldom is the cause idiopathic. However, most cases of FP secondary to middle ear disease are due to cholesteatoma or chronic otitis media. It is generally assumed that FP occurring in the course of acute otitis media is due to congenital dehiscences in the fallopian canal, which permit diffusion of inflammatory mediators onto the exposed nerve. In this instance, the FP remits as the otitis media subsides. Subacute otitis media with masked infection of the mastoid (so-called masked mastoiditis) is an occasional cause of FP in children. Clinically, the patient's tympanic membrane and middle ear may have recovered from the acute inflammation and are normal upon examination. Persistent pain over the mastoid and subtle radiographic evidence of clouding and demineralization are the chief clinical manifestations. Prompt facial nerve decompression is indicated. In chronic otitis media, the facial nerve may be involved at any point within the temporal bone, but most often in the mastoid segment. Cholesteatomatous or osteitic erosion of bone is the pathologic mechanism. Prompt surgical intervention is essential to prevent irreversible paralysis.

Immunocompromised patients, notably elderly diabetics, may develop a progressive infection of the external ear canal known as necrotizing or malignant otitis externa. The facial nerve is the most common of the posterior cranial nerves to be involved in necrotizing otitis externa. The site of lesion is nearly always extratemporal, and the mechanism of palsy is a neurotoxin elaborated by the causative organism, *Pseudomonas aeruginosa.* Except for local debridement, surgical therapy is contraindicated.

Facial Palsy Due to Neoplasm

Primary neoplasms of the facial nerve are rare and generally suspected clinically only when the presumed diagnosis of IFP is proved erroneous by the absence of any signs of recovery by 3 months. Schwannomas of the facial nerve usually grow to substantial size before weakness of the face occurs, and only about one-quarter of cases present with FP. Neoplasms involving the facial nerve secondarily are more common. Among these, the acoustic neuroma (vestibular schwannoma) and other cerebellopontine angle tumors are important but infrequent causes. Patients with neoplasms of the temporal bone, such as the glomus jugulare tumor, may present with FP.

Facial Palsy Due to Trauma

The second most common cause of FP is trauma, which includes penetrating as well as closed head injury. External injury is far more common than are iatrogenic lesions. Birth trauma, secondary to forceps application or extension of the head during version, is infrequent; excellent recovery is the rule. Patients with delayed-onset FP following blunt head trauma are treated expectantly as for IFP. If the paralysis is of immediate onset, there is no recovery of motion in 25 percent or more of cases. Therefore, surgical decompression is usually recommended in traumatic facial paralysis of immediate onset.

Facial Palsy in Primary Neurologic Disorders

Guillain Barré Syndrome. FP of more proximal origin is generally related to infection, most often the postinfectious polyneuritis syndrome of Guillain-Barré. FP is common in the Guillain-Barré but rarely the sole manifestation of it. Bilateral FP (facial diplegia) is often seen in this syndrome. Other causes of facial diplegia are sarcoidosis and Lyme disease. Infectious polyneuritis is a self-limited disorder, and therapy is directed toward general support of the patient.

Melkersson Syndrome. A familial disorder, Melkersson (or Melkersson-Rosenthal) syndrome is characterized by recurrent, sometimes alternating, FP associated with facial edema and fissured tongue. The pathogenic mechanisms triggering this enigmatic disorder are unknown. Spontaneous but incomplete recovery is the rule, but recurrence is common. Because repeated episodes result in progressively poorer recovery, surgical decompression should be considered after two episodes.

DIAGNOSTIC EVALUATION

Patient History and Physical Examination

Important aspects of the patient history are the rapidity of progression and any related events at the time of onset. Pain is common, more so in older patients, and provides little help in differential diagnosis. A history of chronic otorrhea should be sought. Intermittent spasm or facial tic and a palsy that progresses slowly suggest a slow-growing neoplasm as the cause. In most cases of IFP, the onset is fairly rapid—over a few hours to 1 or 2 days—and no other symptoms except for pain are present. The physical examination should establish first that all branches of the facial nerve are affected (upper motor lesions spare the forehead and orbicularis oculi), and second, the extent of the palsy. Is tone present? Is any movement possible? Examination of the cornea for abrasion or ulceration should be routine, as should testing for absence of the corneal reflex that might be seen with a large cerebellopontine angle lesion.

Special attention must be paid to the tympanic membrane and external auditory canal, looking for even subtle signs of inflammation, especially if there has been a recent history of otalgia, ear pressure, or otorrhea. Any patient with abnormalities of the tympanic membrane should be referred to an otologist for otomicroscopic evaluation. A crust on the drumhead, for example, might be the only sign of a cholesteatoma. Occasionally, the chorda tympani nerve appears red as it passes across the underside of the posterosuperior aspect of the tympanic membrane. This is a subtle sign of the Ramsay Hunt syndrome. Be careful to examine behind the pinna: Battle sign (postauricular ecchymosis) is a subtle clue to recent trauma.

Physical Examination of Facial Motor Function.   Three degrees of motor impairment are seen in lower motor nerve lesions: paresis, paralysis with tone, and flaccid paralysis. *Paresis* describes weakness of voluntary motion; *paralysis* indicates absence of motion. Paralysis with preservation of muscle tone is typical in most cases of IFP. Flaccid paralysis (i.e., with sagging of the face) occurs infrequently (and generally in older patients) and indicates a severe loss of neuronal input to the facial muscles, and thus the extent of nerve dysfunction is judged to be maximal. There are also three clinical phases of palsy. The first is loss of emotional expression: the patient is not able to smile at a joke, for example, but can smile voluntarily. The second phase is loss of voluntary motion. The third is loss of resting tone. Recovery from paralysis follows the reverse order: for example, recovery of facial tone precedes restoration of voluntary motion. This progression of clinical findings applies to all peripheral lesions regardless of the specific etiology.

Upper motor neuron facial palsy involves only the lower part of the face, owing to bilateral innervation of the neurons supplying the upper face and eyelids.

Hearing Testing.   Tuning-fork tests are useful to search for hearing loss on the side of the palsy. Placing a stethoscope in the patient's ears and sounding a tuning fork softly and again loudly at the bell may reveal unequal suprathreshold hearing. In the Ramsay Hunt syndrome, the patient may experience the sound louder and often distorted on the affected side, especially with the louder stimulus. Clinical hearing tests such as the finger-rub or whispered-voice testing are commonly used by neurologists for screening purposes. However, these clinical tests are imprecise and little weight should be placed on them for diagnosis. Any complaint of hearing loss or asymmetry of these screening tests should be followed by standard audiometric testing.

Head and Neck Examination.   Careful palpation of the parotid gland and upper neck should always be done. FP occurs often in cases of parotid malignancy. The onset is slow and begins in one branch, as a rule. It may be the presenting symptom in deeply seated tumors. Metastatic squamous cell carcinoma and lymphoma are other invasive lesions that may cause FP.

Staging of Palsy

Staging is a dynamic process and may change over the first 3 weeks of the disorder. Therefore, patients should be observed closely during this time before a final staging and prognosis is offered.

The most useful clinical staging system is the simplest—the House-Brackmann scale, shown in Table 8-1. This has been widely used by otologic surgeons and has shown great merit because it is applicable to all types of facial nerve disorders and is easily learned and used. Stage I indicates normal voluntary facial function, and stage VI, complete absence of motor function. Stage II patients have very mild weakness detectable by close inspection, and stage V patients have only slight volitional motion that also requires close inspection to detect. Stage

TABLE 8-1. House-Brackmann Facial Paralysis Rating Scale[a]

Stage	Description
I	Normal facial motion
II	Slight weakness
III	Mild to moderate weakness
IV	Moderate to severe weakness
V	Minimal motion
VI	Complete paralysis

[a] As modified to apply to the acute stage of paralysis. Additional descriptors for synkinesis, tic, contracture may be used to describe the recovery stage of facial paralysis. Interpretation of this scale varies, but in general, stages I and VI correspond to 100% and 0% motion; stages II and V correspond to 10–25% loss or persistence of motion, respectively; and stages III and IV correspond to 25–50% loss and 50–75% loss of motion, respectively. The scale implies assessment of voluntary motion, but may be applied to loss of involuntary motion, such as seen in central lesions; however, this should be noted separately.

III and IV cases have obvious decrements, with stage III being slightly better than a theoretic 50 percent decrease in motion and stage IV being slightly worse. The classification applies only to an overall assessment of voluntary movement, which, in fact, encompasses the parameters of strength, range, and speed of motion. In practical terms, however, one compares the magnitude of maximum displacement of distinct structures (e.g., oral commissure, brow elevation, eye closure) from their resting position on the opposite sides of the face.

Patients with IFP who have residual facial motion (paresis) should be considered a distinct group because they will recover satisfactorily without treatment and do not need additional testing after the history has been elicited and the physical examination conducted. These patients would be staged II to IV, depending on the degree of paresis. Patients with grade V to VI IFP should undergo electrical testing and basic topognostic testing (Schirmer's) in anticipation of delayed recovery.

Topognosis

It is useful in prognosis and therapy for patients with complete paralysis to study the various branches of the facial nerve in an attempt to localize the site or level of the lesion. Most important are the status of ipsilateral lacrimal function and acoustic reflex. Patients with a poor prognosis are potential candidates for surgical decompression. The site of lesion materially affects the surgical approach.

Schirmer's II Test.   Lesions at or proximal to the geniculate ganglion usually affect lacrimal function to a noticeable degree. Tests of resting lacrimal activity (Schirmer's I) are less sensitive than stimulated function tests (Schirmer's II). Absence or severe diminution of lacrimation generally indicates a poor prognosis because of both the nature of the lesion and its proximal site. Proximal lesions recover slowly and incompletely as a rule because of the long distance over which regenerated axons must pass and because the etiology, which is often the varicella-zoster virus, is usually associated with severe neural degeneration.

The stimulated Schirmer's test is done with porous paper strips placed over the lower lid into the conjunctival sac, and after a short wait, both nasal cavities are touched briefly with cotton applicators to stimulate reflex lacrimation. The reason for waiting is to let the tears pooled in the lower fornix to wet the paper to achieve a starting point from which to note further wetting due to stimulated lacrimation. Generally, the degree of wetting is measured after 1 or 2 minutes and the two sides are compared. A reduction to 25 percent of the normal side indicates a significant impairment. Usually, there is little if any flow on the abnormal side when the lesion is at the geniculate ganglion. The test may be falsely positive in trauma cases in which the greater superficial petrosal nerve is injured independent of the facial nerve.

Stapedius Reflex. Both stapedius muscles contract reflexly in response to the loudness of a sound presented to either ear. Also known as the acoustic reflex, it is best measured with an electroacoustic imittance audiometer that has the capability of testing the reflex ipsilaterally and contralaterally. Loss of the efferent limb of the reflex is seen in most cases of facial paralysis, and recovery of the reflex occurs before facial motion returns. The reflex may be normal in patients with paretic lesions and has no localizing value in that instance. Absence of the stapedius reflex is expected in all cases of intratemporal facial paralysis arising proximal to the stapedius muscle, and its return is an early sign of recovery that usually preceeds recovery of facial motion. The test takes only 1 to 2 minutes per ear and is widely available in otologists' offices. The chief value of the test is to exclude the uncommon case of FP due to occult extracranial etiologies, such as neoplasm in the parotid gland.

Taste and Salivation. Loss of taste and stimulated submandibular salivation are to be expected in most cases of FP. Because of the variability in taste testing in normal people, taste testing has little value for either localization or prognosis in routine cases. Similarly, saliva flow measurements are no longer used in clinical practice.

Electrical Studies

Assessment of neural status by electrical tests is useful only for patients with complete paralysis. The tests are virtually always normal in paretic patients.

Threshold of Stimulability. The normal facial nerve can be stimulated using a square-wave pulse with an active electrode on the overlying skin and an indifferent electrode at a distance. By varying the current intensity, one can determine the electrical threshold of the nerve (i.e., that amount of current flow necessary to produce a just visible twitching of the face). The test is most reproducible when the thin skin over the branch to the eyelid is selected and the skin is thoroughly cleaned. Avoid electrode paste: it promotes lateral spread of the current and artifactually raises the observed threshold. The average threshold for the nerve to the orbicularis in my hands is 0.75 mA, and for the marginal mandibular branch, it is 1.0 mA. I use as abnormal a threshold of greater than 2.0 mA. There appears to be little justification to use the old criterion of abnormality (a 3-mA difference between the two sides of the face) that was advocated in Europe in the 1960s. I use the Hilger facial nerve stimulator and stimulate over the nerve to the orbicularis oculi and over the marginal mandibular nerve. The normal nerve and the neurapraxic nerve distal to the lesion have identical thresholds; rising thresholds indicate degeneration. Given that axonal degeneration proceeds distally at a slow rate, it may take

72 hours or more for the electrical thresholds on the face to become abnormal. Retention of normal thresholds after 72 hours in the presence of a complete facial paralysis suggests that the lesion is neurapraxic and that recovery will be complete. However, thresholds may worsen over the first week or two, so it is advisable to retest during the first 3 weeks. Absence of stimulability indicates severe degeneration and indicates a poorer prognosis. Elevated thresholds would suggest partial degeneration, but the correlation of abnormal thresholds with outcome is too variable to use for clinical decision making. Thresholds of the regenerated nerve remain elevated, although at levels lower than during the acute episode.

Maximal Nerve Stimulation. Advocates of this test suggest that it becomes abnormal sooner than threshold tests and provides better clinical evidence of nerve degeneration. It is done with the facial nerve stimulator turned to a suprathreshold level. The examiner visually compares the strength of the response on the two sides using a scale of 0 to 4. A score of 4 is assigned if the two sides have equal contraction and a score of 2 is given when the palsied side contracts only 50 percent of the normal side. The test is more painful than the threshold test and is subject to interpretation by the examiner. In my experience, the maximal stimulation test results parallel the nerve excitablility threshold test results. Others rely heavily on the maximal stimulation test results to indicate neural degeneration, which corresponds to a score of 0 to 1 (25 percent or less of the normal side).

Nerve Conduction. Nerve conduction studies also employ percutaneous stimulation, and in general the results parallel those of threshold testing. Needle electrodes placed within the muscle record the response and the internal circuitry of the stimulator-recorder calculates the conduction velocity.

Electromyography. The electromyogram (EMG) is most useful to verify that degeneration has occurred and is also employed on occasion to determine if regeneration is underway. Unfortunately, the EMG cannot detect fibrillations, the EMG hallmark of degeneration, until nearly 3 weeks after the onset of the paralysis, too late to make any useful treatment decision. On the other side of the coin, voluntary motor units are noticeable on the EMG weeks before any return of visible facial motion. Such information may be of interest and reassurance to concerned patients.

Electroneuronography. Electroneurography (ENOG) compares the amplitude of the compound muscular action potential evoked by percutaneous stimulation over the main trunk of the nerve and recorded via skin electrodes on the two sides of the face. It presumes that the number of functioning axons is proportional to the height of the evoked electric potential. Test results may vary with the positioning of the electrodes and the skill of the examiner; variations of up to 20 percent between sides of normal subjects have been noted. ENOG is used by some as an indicator of the need for facial nerve decompression in IFP, herpes zosteroticus and trauma. A compound muscular action potential decrease on the affected side to less than 10 percent of that on the normal side is good evidence of substantial degeneration of the nerve, which warrants consideration of decompression (see Surgical Treatment, below, for a full discussion). Correspondingly, when the ENOG on the affected side is greater than that amount, the spontaneous outcome is likely to be favorable.

Laboratory Tests

Hematologic.   If systemic infection is suspected, the peripheral blood should be studied to determine the hemaglobin, hematocrit, white blood cell count, and sedimentation rate. Antibodies to specific disorders may be ordered at the discretion of the physcian. The value of the routine blood studies is marginal in young patients with facial paresis due to IFP. However, in older patients with IFP, the prevalence of diabetes mellitus is higher than in the general population and screening for systemic metabolic disorders is appropriate. A fasting blood sugar and urinalysis should be done in older patients who have not had periodic assessment of their health status. Routine tests for systemic disease are generally not warranted in cases of IFP in the absence of some indication in the patient history and physical examination of an underlying process.

Radiologic.   Routine imaging of the temporal bone or posterior cranial fossa is not indicated in patients with paresis due to suspected IFP who have a normal otologic examination. It is highly unusual to discover occult mastoid disease in patients with no prior history and normal physical examination results Magnetic resonance imaging (MRI) studies have shown transient increases in gadolinium uptake in some cases of acute FP, but this finding has no value in treatment decisions. In patients with recurrent FP, slowly progressive palsy, or an abnormal physical examination, computed tomography (CT) and MRI images of the temporal bone and posterior fossa are vital. Suspected causes would be temporal bone pathology, including facial nerve schwannoma. Patients with a presumptive diagnosis of IFP who fail to show any evidence of recovery by 3 months, and certainly by 6 months, should have a complete neuroradiographic examination to evaluate the possibility of an occult etiology. CT scans are very helpful in assessing the status of the fallopian canal with the possibility of facial neuroma in mind.

MANAGEMENT OF IDIOPATHIC FACIAL PARALYSIS

The principal treatment decision—to use corticosteroid or not—is based upon degree of paralysis, presence of pain, and indicators of poor prognosis. Patients with paresis recover fully and therefore do not need therapy. However, pain relief is notable following the administration of a corticosteroid agent. Corticosteroid is given to prevent worsening of the process causing the paralysis. Therefore, the earlier the onset of therapy, the better. Although the evidence for a better outcome in patients with IFP treated with corticosteroid is not consistent, it is generally persuasive. In cases of suspected herpes zoster oticus, acyclovir therapy is warranted. For patients with suspected Lyme disease, a course of antimicrobial agent should be considered.

Corticosteroid Treatment

The chief pharmacologic agent used for IFP is one of the oral glucocorticoids, most often prednisone or methylprednisolone. Corticosteroid therapy is controversial in terms of proven efficacy but widely used because of relief of pain. Three randomized double-blinded studies have been reported. The first (May et al., 1976) had insufficient numbers of cases to justify its negative conclusions; the second (Wolf et al., 1978) showed improved outcomes in the corticosteroid-treated patients in all categories, but none of the differences were statistically significant, except for the prevention of crocodile tears. The third (Austin et al., 1993) compared the status of patients with IFP treated with 60 mg/d prednisone ($n = 35$) versus placebo ($n = 41$), using a prospective randomized double-blind design. There was a fourfold reduction in ENOG evidence of degeneration in the prednisone group ($P = .06$) and a significant difference ($P = .03$) in the number of subjects having a poor result (grade III: 0 percent treatment versus 17 percent control). These results support the use of prednisone in cases of grade V to VI IFP to reduce the incidence of poor results in those at greatest risk. Interestingly, the incidence of autonomic synkinesis was about 11 percent in both groups, which is in contrast to the results of Wolf and colleagues.

Stennert in West Germany used a intensive in-hospital multiple-drug regimen in a nonrandomized uncontrolled study (Stennert, 1981). The agents used were large doses of corticosteroid (200 to 250 mg of prednisone daily), intravenous rheomacrodex (Dextran), and oral pentoxifylline. Ninety-four percent of the patients had complete recovery, often before discharge from the hospital, which is in contrast to the untreated spontaneous complete recovery rate of 71 percent noted by Pieterson (1982). Whether this high recovery rate is due to timing of treatment, the duration of treatment, a single agent, or the combination is not known. Such a regimen, which involved hospitalization for 2 weeks, would not be considered cost-effective in the United States. Currently, some neurologists in Europe advocate massive short-term doses of prednisone (1 to 2 g daily for 3 to 5 days) and report a very high rate of success (Stennert, personal communication, 1994). The anecdotal success of this approach invites a systematic study with appropriate controls and outcome measures.

Oral prednisone is used in my institution for patients with pain and with complete paralysis, beginning with 60 to 80 mg/d for 6 days, with a progressive taper over the next 4 days. There appears to be little justification for treating patients with paresis. The use of corticosteroid in patients with palsy (i.e., House-Brackmann grade II to IV) to prevent degeneration is controversial, but may be used if no contraindications exist when the physician's judgment leads to suspicion of impending degeneration. The patients are examined weekly during the first 3 weeks to monitor their palsy, nerve excitability thresholds, and corneal integrity. Patients with incomplete paralysis who show worsening of their palsy or rising thresholds are started on prednisone. Should the paralysis be complete and electrical thresholds rise progressively during the first 3 weeks, the patient is sent for ENOG testing and counseled in regard to the usefulness of surgical decompression its complications and the controversy surrounding its indications (see Surgical Treatment, below).

Acyclovir

Acyclovir is a virostatic drug that is effective against replicating viruses. It has been used for herpes zoster oticus and for IFP. Reports of administration to patients with herpes zoster oticus have been uncontrolled; intravenous dosing (5mg/kg every 8 hours for 3 to 8 days) followed by oral administration of 400 mg five times daily for 2 weeks was the most common regimen. Resolution was faster and better than with historical controls

(Uri et al., 1992). Adour (1994) randomly assigned 94 patients with IFP to receive acyclovir 200 mg orally five times a day plus prednisone (1 mg/kg orally) or placebo/prednisone and found significantly better outcomes in the group taking acyclovir.

Lyme Disease

The diagnosis of Lyme disease in a patient with apparent IFP should be sought through a history of tick bites, arthralgias, and erythema migrans. Serologic confirmation of *B. burgdoferi* should be sought. Antimicrobial therapy is the primary treatment. Amoxicillin (500 mg three or four times daily), tetracycline (500 mg four times daily), or doxycycline (100 mg twice daily) given orally as an outpatient for 3 to 4 weeks is the recommended initial therapy.

Counseling and Reassurance

Patients often assume that their facial paralysis is due to a stroke, and many are distraught because of the facial deformity as well as the fear that it may progress. It is important to specifically reassure the patient in this regard when the diagnosis is IFP.

Eye Protection

Corneal exposure and drying are common sequelae of facial paralysis, particularly when tone is lost and ectropion results. The normal pump action of the orbicularis oculi, which holds the lid against the globe, is lost, and the tears accumulate in the lower conjunctival sac rather than spreading out across the surface of the globe. Blinking ceases with facial paralysis, and thus an important mechanism for preserving corneal humidification is lost. Two aspects of eye treatment should be noted. First is the use of artificial tears; the second relates to taping the eyelids at night. Patients should be advised about the risks of corneal exposure and instructed to instill methylcellulose solution into the affected eye regularly during the day. This will help keep the cornea moist. Ointments may provide slightly better protection, but they keep the patient from seeing clearly. A commercially available moisture chamber is helpful for patients who work outdoors to keep wind and particles out of the eye while keeping vision near normal.

At night, the upper lid should be taped closed by a strip of quarter-inch paper tape placed obliquely from the middle of the upper lid down to the malar eminence (not straight down across the cornea). This will ensure eye protection during sleep. Patients who are young and have adequate eye protection because of good lid tone and an active Bell's phenomenon (upward rolling of the globe during lid closure) do not need taping, but older patients usually do. I recommend it to all both for safety's sake and to call attention to the risk of eye damage as a result of the facial paralysis. Should the patient develop eye pain, a slit-lamp examination after fluorescein staining of the cornea is mandatory. I inspect the stained cornea with an ophthalmoscope routinely during follow-up care. Consultation with an ophthalmologist is requested if the paralysis is prolonged, the lagophthalmos severe, or if corneal abrasion or ulceration occurs.

Physical Therapy

Unfortunately, no amount of physical maneuvering will affect the rate of recovery of the affected nerve. Some have employed massage, external straps, and electric stimulation in the management of patients with idiopathic facial paralysis. They are not needed.

Prosthetics

In cases in which recovery is incomplete, lower lip weakness and asymmetry is common. A modified denture or dental appliance can be made by a prosthodontist to push out the lower lip and restore facial symmetry at rest.

Surgical Treatment

Decompression. Surgical decompression of the facial nerve has been the main treatment of traumatic paralysis and has been applied in severe cases of IFP for over 40 years. Surgical treatment consists of removing one-half the circumference of the bony fallopian canal at the site of the lesion and incising the tripartite nerve sheath. It is advocated as a means of halting the progression of neural degeneration in those cases with clear-cut evidence of degeneration. Once the degeneration is complete, surgical decompression has little value. It is also advocated for patients with apparent idiopathic facial paralysis in whom there is no evidence of recovery after 3 months. In this situation, decompression is used as a means of surgical exploration of the nerve to rule out a nerve tumor or occult invasive infection.

Although evidence of efficacy of decompression for IFP is anecdotal and controversial, the procedure is still advocated by some neurotologists in highly selected cases. Given that less than 5 percent of cases of IFP have a sufficiently poor prognosis to warrant consideration of an operation and that these patients cannot be identified without electrical testing during the 21-day window when decompression is most effective, it is highly unlikely that a sufficient number of cases could ever be found to conduct a randomized clinical trial. Moreover, the variability in surgical skill and experience among the large number of otologists who would of necessity have to participate in such a study would be likely to seriously bias the outcome of the study. Therefore, the isolated reports from experienced clinical investigators remains the best evidence of efficacy to date.

To be effective, surgical decompression should encompass the involved segments of the nerve. Early techniques focused on the vertical segment of the nerve, which is accessible with minimal morbidity. However, later research has indicated that it is the intralabyrinthine segment that is involved in the severe cases, which requires decompression via a middle fossa mini-craniotomy. Gantz et al (1982) found that the block is proximal to the geniculate ganglion in the majority of cases and that the Schirmer's I test was misleading in 39 percent of cases. Therefore, in IFP, the operation must begin in the intralabyrinthine segment and extend distally until a normal nerve is encountered. As such, the surgical approach involves both the middle cranial fossa and mastoid—rather extensive surgery for the group of older patients most likely to need it.

An extensive anecdotal literature has developed on the subject. Many, like May, who once advocated surgical decompression have stopped decompressing patients with IFP. Fisch (1982) studied 14 patients with severe facial paralysis due to IFP and showed a difference of only 15 percentage points in outcome (78.8 percent recovery versus 63.9 percent) between the 7 patients who chose decompression and the 7 who did not. All 14 patients had 95 to 100 percent degeneration within 1 to

14 days after onset. For patients with herpes zoster oticus, the difference was 22 points (70.2 percent—5 patients versus 48.3 percent—2 patients).

Clearly, surgical decompression for patients with severe IFP is controversial. In defense of surgical decompression to treat IFP, the procedure is logical within the current theoretic understanding of the disorder and is used only for that small select group of informed patients whose outcome is predicted to be poor by ENOG. It is also used for patients with traumatic lesions of the facial nerve of immediate onset in whom laceration is suspected and in those with delayed onset in whom severe degeneration occurs. For informed patients who are willing to accept the risk of auditory complications in order to achieve the greatest chance of minimizing undesirable sequelae of their paralysis, early surgical intervention by a skilled, experienced neurotologic surgeon is an option.

PROGNOSIS

The outlook for complete recovery in IFP is good as long as some motion persists. Once the paresis progresses to paralysis, the prognosis depends on the degree of degeneration, which is estimated by electrical tests. A rising threshold suggests axonal degeneration and signals the need for ENOG, which gives a more precise estimate of the degree of degeneration. If the ENOG falls to over 90 percent of the normal side within 21 days after the onset of paralysis, the outlook for normal recovery is poor.

SEQUELAE

Most cases of idiopathic facial paralysis are neurapraxic in type and recovery is rapid and complete. Pieterson (1982) reported that 71 percent of 1,100 cases of IFP occurring in a Danish county over a 15-year period had perfect recovery, usually within a 6-week period. This time course is compatible with the Gates-Mikiten hypothesis of endoneurial fluid formation as the cause of neurapraxia and its gradual resorption through the perineurial sheath as the mechanism for recovery.

In approximately 30 percent of cases, recovery is not complete and various stigmata of axonal degeneration appear: persistent weakness, motor synkinesis, spasm, contracture, crocodile tears. Regeneration is a slow and usually incomplete process. Regenerating axons elongate at the rate of 1 mm/d. Thus, after degeneration of the nerve within the proximal labyrinthine segment, it would take 400 days for the new axons to reach the motor endplates.

Weakness

During regeneration, axons sprout and proliferate and push forward to the motor endplates. Even under ideal circumstances, return of muscle strength to normal is unusual. The extent of return is proportional to the number, size, and degree of myelination of the fibers that return to their original motor endplate. Some fibers may not regenerate, and others may be diverted to other muscle groups. Thus, the number of axons reaching the muscle is reduced. In addition, the regenerated axons that do reach the appropriate muscles are smaller and less well myelinated than the original fibers. Thus, impulses are transmitted more slowly and with greater variation in speed. Since motor strength depends on coordinated impulse transmission, a regenerated nerve is nearly always an impaired one.

Synkinesis

Axons regenerate by first forming multiple buds, which, as alluded to above, may become diverted from their original axon sheaths and end in other muscle fibers. When this happens, the patient has great difficulty in moving each muscle group independently; the resultant mass action of muscle is termed synkinesis. A typical example is eye closure (or blinking) when, for example, one tries to smile. In this case it is apparent that some fibers of nerve branch to the orbicularis oris had found their way into the orbicularis oculi. Synkinesis is the clinical hallmark of axonal degeneration.

Spasm and Contracture

Involuntary muscle spasms are common sequelae of severe degeneration. In addition, contracture and permanent distortion of the face are also noted. Prevention of these complications is an important goal of therapy.

Crocodile Tears

The facial nerve carries two groups of sympathomimetic fibers—those to the nose and lacrimal gland (via the greater superficial petrosal nerve) and those to the submandibular gland (via the chorda tympani). Faulty regeneration when the lesion is quite proximal may result in autonomic synkinesis. Thus, during mealtime, discharges of the salivary fibers, which have been rerouted to the lacrimal gland, result in diffuse tearing instead of salivation.

SUMMARY

FP is a common problem due to epidemics of IPF, which is probably due to viral infection. A patient history and physical examination are adequate evaluation for paretic patients who fit the diagnostic criteria of IFP. Most cases resolve satisfactorily without therapy. Extensive evaluation is reserved for those who have complete paralysis and electrical test evidence of degeneration. These cases should receive corticosteroid therapy. Diabetics appear to have a higher prevalence of IFP than the general population, and older patients should be screened for glucose intolerance. Patients with complete paralysis and ENOG evidence of severe degeneration while receiving corticosteroid are at risk of an unsatisfactory outcome and should be counseled about surgical decompression.

SUGGESTED READINGS

Adour KK: Bell's palsy: Results of a double-blind, placebo-controlled acyclovir-prednisone and placebo-prednisone treatment study. Br Med J (in press), 1995

Austin JR, Peskind SP, Austin SG, Rice DH: Idiopathic facial nerve paralysis: a randomized double blind controlled study of placebo versus prednisone. Laryngoscope 103:1326–33, 1993

Clark JR, Carlson RD, Sasaki CT et al: Facial paralysis in Lyme disease. Laryngoscope 95:1341–5, 1985

Fisch U: Results of surgery versus conservative treatment in Bell's palsy and herpes zoster oticus. pp. 273–8. In Graham MD, House WF (eds): Disorders of the Facial Nerve. Raven Press, New York, 1982

Gantz BJ, Gmur A, Fisch U: Intraoperative evoked electromyography in Bell's palsy. Am J Otolaryngol 3:273–8, 1982

Gates GA: Nerve excitability testing: technical pitfalls and threshold norms using absolute values. Laryngoscope 103:379–85, 1993

Gates GA, Mikiten TM: The idiopathic facial paralyses (Bell's palsies). pp. 279–86. In Graham MD, House WF (eds): Disorders of the Facial Nerve. Raven Press, New York, 1982

House JW, Brackmann DE: Facial nerve grading system. Otolaryngol Head Neck Surg 93:146–7, 1985

May M, Klein SR, Taylor FH: Idiopathic (Bell's) facial palsy: natural history defies steroid or surgical treatment. Laryngoscope 95:406–9, 1985

May M, Wette R, Hardin WB, Sullivan J: The use of steroids in Bell's palsy: a prospective controlled study. Laryngoscope 86:1111–22, 1976

Morgan M, Nathwani D: Facial palsy and infection: the unfolding story. Clin Infect Dis 2:263–71, 1992

Mori H, Kita M, Takahashi H et al: Bell's palsy and virus—analysis of 299 cases for six years. Facial N Res 2:83–6, 1982

Pietersen E: Natural history of Bell's palsy. In Graham MD, House WF (eds): Disorders of the Facial Nerve. Raven Press, New York, 1982

Seddon HJ: Three types of nerve injury. Brain 66:237–88, 1943

Sigal LH: Current recommendations for the treatment of Lyme disease. Drugs 43:683–99, 1992

Stennert E: Pathomechanisms in cell metabolism: a key to treatment of Bell's palsy. Ann Otol Rhinol Laryngol 190:577–83, 1981

Sunderland S: The peripheral nerve trunk in relation to injury. A classification of nerve injury. pp. 133–41 In: Nerves and Nerve Injury. Churchill Livingstone, Edinburgh, 1978

Uri N, Greenberg E, Meyer W, Kitzes-Cohen R: Herpes zoster oticus: treatment with acyclovir. Ann Otol Rhinol Laryngol 101:161–2, 1992

Wolf SM, Wagner JH, Davidson S, Forsyth A: Treatment of Bell's palsy with prednisone: a propspective randomized study. Neurology 28:158–61, 1978

9. DIZZINESS AND VERTIGO

ROBERT W. BALOH

HISTORY OF THE DIZZY PATIENT

Dizziness is a common symptom; it can be caused by many different pathophysiologic mechanisms and is associated with a variety of diagnoses (Table 9-1). Since the evaluation and management of the different general types of dizziness differ markedly, it is critical that the examining physician first determine the type of dizziness before proceeding with diagnostic studies. The history usually provides the key information.

A sensation of spinning nearly always indicates a vestibular disorder. Patients with nonvestibular dizziness occasionally report a sensation of spinning inside the head, but the environment seems still and they do not have nystagmus. Patients with vestibular lesions often liken the sensation to that of being drunk or motion sick; they feel off balance and may tilt or fall to one side. Patients with presyncopal or hypoglycemic dizziness typically use terms such as lightheaded, floating, feeling giddy, or swimming. The sensation that one has left one's own body is characteristic of psychophysiologic dizziness. Drugs can produce several different types of dizziness. Most sedating drugs cause a nonspecific dizziness described as a fogginess, cloudiness, or giddiness that is presumably due to diffuse depression of the central nervous system. Alcohol can cause this nonspecific dizziness but can also produce a positional vertigo and nystagmus as a result of differential changes in specific gravity of the endolymph and cupula. The common anticonvulsants phenytoin and carbamazepine cause disequilibrium and ataxia as a result of both acute and chronic cerebellar dysfunction. Most of the commonly used antihypertensive drugs predispose patients to orthostatic hypotension and presyncopal dizziness.

Patients often use the term dizziness to describe a sensation of imbalance or disequilibrium that occurs only when they are standing or walking and is unrelated to an abnormal head sensation. Such imbalance is common with acute unilateral peripheral vestibular lesions, but it is transient and invariably associated with subjective vertigo. Both the vertigo and imbalance are compensated within a few days. Patients who slowly lose vestibular function, either on one side or both sides, typically do not experience vertigo but describe a vague feeling of imbalance and unsteadiness on their feet. Bilateral vestibular loss can cause persistent unsteadiness that may be incapacitating, particularly in older patients. Ototoxic drugs, such as the aminoglycosides, produce a characteristic combination of gait unsteadiness and oscillopsia caused by loss of vestibulospinal and vestibulo-ocular reflex function, respectively. Imbalance associated with loss of proprioceptive function is nearly always associated with other findings of peripheral neuropathy. When imbalance is due to loss of vestibulospinal or proprioceptive function, it is typically more pronounced in the dark when the patient is unable to use vision to compensate for the loss. On the other hand, patients with cerebellar lesions have severe imbalance even with vision.

Vertigo is an episodic phenomenon, whereas other types of dizziness are usually more persistent. Exceptions would be presyncopal dizziness caused by postural hypotension or cardiac arrhythmias or hypoglycemic dizziness caused by excessive insulin or lack of food intake. Patients with psychophysiologic dizziness often report being dizzy from morning to night without change for months to years at a time. Vertigo is invariably aggravated by head movements, whereas other types of dizziness may even improve with head or body movements. Episodes of dizziness induced by position change suggest a vestibular cause if postural hypotension has been ruled out. Although stress can aggravate both vestibular and nonvestibular dizziness, dizziness that is reliably precipitated by stress suggests a nonvestibular cause. Episodes of dizziness occurring only in specific situations such as when the patient is driving on a freeway or shopping in a busy supermarket suggest a psychophysiologic cause. Nausea and vomiting are usual with vertigo but uncommon with other types of dizziness. Associated auditory or neurologic symptoms suggest a vestibular disorder; presyncopal symptoms and syncope suggest a nonvestibular disorder.

TABLE 9-1. Mechanisms and Common Causes of Dizziness

Type	Mechanism	Common Causes
Vertigo	Imbalance of tonic vestibular signals	Benign positional vertigo, viral neurolabyrinthitis, Menière's disease, migraine, vertebrobasilar insufficiency
Presyncopal dizziness	Pancerebral ischemia	Hyperventilation, orthostatic hypotension, vasovagal, cardiac arrhythmia
Hypoglycemic dizziness	Inadequate brain glucose level; increased circulating catecholamine levels	Insulin treatment of diabetes mellitus; alcoholism, insulin-secreting tumors
Psychophysiologic dizziness	Impaired central integration of sensory signals	Anxiety, phobias, panic syndrome
Drug intoxication	Depression of central nervous function	Alcohol, tranquilizers, anticonvulsants
Disequilibrium	Loss of vestibulospinal, proprioceptive, or cerebellar function	Ototoxicity, peripheral neuropathy, stroke, cerebellar degeneration

EXAMINATION

Evaluation of the dizzy patient should include a general medical examination as well as a complete otologic and neurologic examination. Whenever possible, the examining physician should attempt to reproduce the patient's dizziness. Bedside provocative tests can assist in making a pathophysiologic diagnosis.

Rapid head movements commonly induce vertigo because they accentuate an imbalance within the vestibular pathways. Even after compensation has occurred, head movements or change in position can lead to episodes of vertigo. Patients with perilymph fistula develop brief episodes of vertigo precipitated by changes in middle ear pressure commonly associated with coughing or sneezing. A bedside fistula test can be performed by pressing the tragus into the ear canal or by changing the pressure in the canal with a pneumatoscope. A brief spell of vertigo and nystagmus indicates a positive test.

Presyncopal dizziness as a result of orthostatic hypotension can develop immediately on standing or insidiously after several minutes of standing. The diagnosis is made by documenting an acute or progressive decline in mean blood pressure of more than 15 mmHg while the patient is in the erect position. In patients with autonomic insufficiency, the pulse rate may remain unchanged despite the hypotension. In patients suspected of hyperventilating, it is helpful to have the patient voluntarily overbreathe to reproduce symptoms and provide insight into the mechanism.

Examination of a patient complaining of disequilibrium should focus on assessment of gait. Patients are encouraged to walk as they normally do and to narrow their base by walking in tandem. Acute unilateral peripheral vestibular lesions cause falling toward the side of the lesion, but within a few days balance returns to normal. Patients with bilateral peripheral vestibular loss have more difficulty compensating and usually show persistent imbalance on tandem walking tests, particularly with eyes closed. The broad-based ataxic gait of cerebellar disorders is usually easily distinguished from the milder gait disorders associated with vestibular or sensory loss.

Bedside Tests of Vestibular Function

In an alert person, rotating the head back and forth in the horizontal plane (the doll's eye test) induces compensatory horizontal eye movements that are dependent on both the visual and vestibular systems. Because of the combined visual and vestibular input, a patient with complete loss of vestibular function and normal visual pursuit may have normal-appearing compensatory eye movements on this test. The doll's eye test is a useful bedside test of vestibular function in a comatose patient, however, because such patients cannot generate visual tracking eye movements. In this setting, slow conjugate compensatory eye movements indicate normally functioning vestibulo-ocular pathways. Because the vestibulo-ocular reflex has a much

higher frequency range than the smooth pursuit system, a semiquantitative bedside test of vestibular function can be made by having patients shake their head back and forth at frequencies above 1 cycle/s while reading a standard visual acuity chart. A decrease in visual acuity of more than one line compared with testing with the head still suggests an abnormal vestibulo-ocular reflex. A complete unilateral or bilateral vestibular loss can also be identified by rapidly moving the head to the side while the patient fixates on the examiner's nose. Normally, the eyes move smoothly in the orbit to maintain fixation. In patients with vestibular loss, the eyes deviate from the target, and catch-up saccades are required. Patients with compensated vestibular lesions (peripheral or central) may develop a transient spontaneous nystagmus after vigorous head shaking (so-called head-shaking nystagmus). With unilateral peripheral vestibular lesions, the nystagmus beats toward the intact side.

The caloric test uses a nonphysiologic stimulus to induce endolymphatic flow in the horizontal semicircular canal and horizontal nystagmus by creating a temperature gradient from one side of the canal to the other. With a cold caloric stimulus, the column of endolymph nearest the middle ear falls because of its increased density. This causes the cupula to deviate away from the utricle and produces horizontal nystagmus with the fast phase directed away from the stimulated ear. A warm stimulus produces the opposite effect, causing ampullopetal endolymph flow and nystagmus directed toward the stimulated ear (mnemonic: COWS for cold opposite, warm same). Because of its ready availability, ice water is usually used for bedside caloric testing. To bring the horizontal canal into the vertical plane, the patient lies in the supine position with head tilted 30° forward. Infusion of a few milliliters of ice water induces a burst of nystagmus usually lasting 1 minute or so. A comatose patient shows only a slow tonic deviation toward the side of stimulation. Greater than a 20 percent asymmetry in nystagmus duration suggests a lesion on the side of decreased response. This should always be confirmed, however, with standard bithermal caloric testing (see below).

Tests for Pathologic Nystagmus

Nystagmus by definition is a nonvoluntary rhythmic oscillation of the eyes. It usually has a clearly defined slow and fast component, alternating in directions. By convention, the direction of the fast component defines the direction of nystagmus. Physiologic nystagmus refers to nystagmus that occurs in normal subjects (e.g., caloric-induced nystagmus), whereas pathologic nystagmus implies an underlying abnormality. Spontaneous nystagmus refers to nystagmus that occurs with the patient seated, eyes in the primary position, without external stimulation. Gaze-evoked nystagmus is induced by changes in gaze position. Nystagmus that is not present in the sitting position but is present in some other head and body position is called positional nystagmus.

TABLE 9-2. Differentiating Between Spontaneous Nystagmus of Peripheral and Central Origin

	Appearance	Fixation	Gaze	Mechanism	Localization
Peripheral	Combined torsional, horizontal	Inhibited	Unidirectional (Alexander's law)	Asymmetric loss of peripheral vestibular tone	Labyrinthine or vestibular nerve
Central	Often pure vertical, horizontal, or torsional	Usually little effect	Usually changes direction	Imbalance in central oculomotor tone; usually, central vestibular; may be visual	Central nervous system, usually brainstem or cerebellum

Examination for pathologic nystagmus should include a careful search for spontaneous, gaze-evoked, and positional nystagmus. Spontaneous nystagmus may be present with fixation, or it may occur only when fixation is inhibited. There are several simple methods for inhibiting fixation at the bedside. Frenzel glasses consist of +30 lenses mounted in a frame that contains a light source on the inside so that the patient's eyes are easily visualized. An ophthalmoscope can also be used to block fixation and bring out a spontaneous nystagmus. While the fundus of one eye is being viewed, the patient is asked to cover the other eye lightly. Features that distinguish between spontaneous nystagmus of peripheral and central origin are summarized in Table 9-2. Spontaneous nystagmus of peripheral vestibular origin is typically inhibited with fixation and does not change direction with gaze, whereas that of central origin is usually prominent with fixation and often changes direction with change in the direction of gaze. Several varieties of central nystagmus have localizing value (Table 9-3).

Patients with gaze-evoked nystagmus are unable to maintain stable conjugate eye deviation away from the primary position. The eyes drift back toward the center, and corrective saccades (fast components) are needed to reset the desired gaze position. Gaze-evoked nystagmus is therefore always in the direction of gaze. The site of abnormality can be anywhere from the neuromuscular junction to the multiple brain centers controlling conjugate gaze. Dysfunction of the so-called oculomotor integrator may be a common mechanism for several types of gaze-evoked nystagmus.

Two general types of positional nystagmus can be identified on the basis of nystagmus duration: static and paroxysmal (also known as positional and positioning nystagmus). One induces static positional nystagmus by slowly placing the patient into the supine and right lateral and then left lateral positions. This type of positional nystagmus persists as long as the position is held. Because direction-changing and direction-fixed static positional nystagmus occur with both peripheral and central vestibular lesions, their presence indicates only a dysfunction somewhere in the vestibular system. As with spontaneous nystagmus, however, lack of suppression with fixation and signs of associated brainstem dysfunction suggest a central lesion. Positioning nystagmus is induced, after a brief delay, by a rapid change from erect sitting to supine head-hanging left or head-hanging right (the so-called Hallpike maneuver). It is initially high in frequency but dissipates rapidly (within 30 seconds to 1 minute). The most common variety of positioning nystagmus, so-called benign positional nystagmus, usually has a 3- to 10-second latency before onset and rarely lasts longer than 30 seconds. The nystagmus is usually torsional with fast phase directed upward (i.e., toward the forehead). It is usually only prominent in one head-hanging position, and a burst of nystagmus in the reverse direction occurs when the patient resumes the sitting position. Another key feature is that the vertigo and nystagmus that the patient experiences with the initial positioning rapidly decreases with repeated positioning (fatigability).

LABORATORY EVALUATION

Electronystagmography

Electronystagmography is a technique for recording eye movements that allows precise quantification of both physiologic and pathologic nystagmus. A standard electronystagmography test battery includes (1) tests of visual ocular control (saccades, smooth pursuit, and optokinetic nystagmus); (2) a careful search for pathologic nystagmus with fixation and with eyes open in darkness; and (3) a bithermal caloric test. An electronystagmography test is helpful in identifying a vestibular lesion and localizing it within the peripheral and central pathways.

With the bithermal caloric test, each ear is irrigated for a fixed duration (30 to 40 seconds) with a constant flow rate of water that is 7° below body temperature (30°C) and 7° above body temperature (44°C). The main advantages of this test method are (1) both ampullopetal and ampullofugal endolymph flow are serially induced in each horizontal semicircular canal, (2) the caloric stimulus is highly reproducible from patient to patient, and (3) the test is well tolerated by most patients. The major limitation is the need for constant temperature baths and plumbing to maintain continuous circulation of water through the infusion hose. The response to caloric stimulation can be assessed in several ways. The simplest method is to measure the duration of nystagmus after each infusion using a stopwatch. Prior to the development of electronystagmography, this was the only practical way to quantify the bithermal caloric test. With electronystagmography, one can measure the velocity profile of the slow phases and calculate the maximum slow phase velocity after each stimulus. The vestibular paresis formula

$$\frac{(R30° + R44°) - (L30° + L44°)}{R30° + R44° + L30° + L44°} \times 100$$

compares the maximum slow phase velocity of right-sided responses with that of left-sided responses, and the directional preponderance formula

$$\frac{(L30° + R44°) - (L44° + R30°)}{L30° + R44° + L44° + R30°} \times 100$$

compares the maximum slow phase velocity of nystagmus to the right with that of nystagmus to the left in the same subject. Dividing by the total response normalizes the measurements to remove the large variability in absolute magnitude of normal caloric responses.

The finding of a significant vestibular paresis (greater than 25 percent) with bithermal caloric stimulation suggests a lesion in the vestibular system that is located anywhere from the end organ to the vestibular nerve root entry zone in the brainstem. It is a reliable sign of unilateral peripheral vestibular disease. A significant directional preponderance on caloric testing (greater than 30 percent) indicates an imbalance in the vestibular system

TABLE 9-3. Localizing Value and Common Causes of Different Types of Central Nystagmus

Type	Localization	Common Causes
Downbeat	Cervical-medullary junction (flocculus?)	Chiari malformation, cerebellar atrophy, multiple sclerosis
Upbeat	Caudal midline brainstem	Infarction, tumor, multiple sclerosis
Periodic alternating	Cerebellovestibular pathways	Infarction, multiple sclerosis, syrinx
Rebound	Cerebellum	Cerebellar atrophy, infarction
Dissociated	Medial longitudinal fasciculus	Multiple sclerosis, infarction
Convergence retraction	Pretectum	Pineal tumors, infarction
Palato-ocular myoclonus	Mollaret triangle, olivodentatorubral pathways	Infarction, degenerative disease

but is nonlocalizing, occurring with both peripheral and central vestibular lesions.

Rotational Testing

Electronystagmography can also be used with rotational testing, but such tests are not generally available because expensive equipment is required to generate precise rotational stimuli. Rotational tests do have several advantages over caloric tests, however. Multiple graded stimuli can be applied in a relatively short period, and rotational testing is usually less bothersome to some patients than caloric testing. Unlike caloric testing, a rotational stimulus to the semicircular canals is unrelated to physical features of the external ear or temporal bone; therefore, a more exact relationship between stimulus and response is possible.

Rotational testing is most useful for evaluating patients with presumed bilateral peripheral vestibular loss (e.g., as a result of ototoxic drug exposure) because both labyrinths are stimulated simultaneously and the degree of remaining function is accurately quantified. Because the variance associated with normal rotational responses is less than that associated with caloric responses, diminished function is identified earlier. Artifactually diminished caloric responses occasionally occur in patients with angular narrow external canals or with thickened temporal bones. Because a rotational stimulus is unrelated to these factors, rotationally induced nystagmus is normal in such patients. Furthermore, patients with absent caloric responses may have decreased but measurable rotationally induced nystagmus, particularly at higher stimulus velocities. The ability to identify remaining vestibular function, even when it is small, is an important advantage of rotational testing, particularly when the physician is contemplating ablative surgery or monitoring the effects of ototoxic drugs.

Posturography

Body sway is a normal phenomenon that occurs in everyone. Sway increases in older people and in patients with balance problems. Because sway tends to be slight when subjects stand on a stable platform, moving platforms have been developed in an attempt to increase test sensitivity (dynamic posturography). The platform can either be tilted or linearly displaced, and the sway can be measured immediately after the movement or during the movement. Furthermore, in an effort to dissect the different sensory contributions to the maintenance of balance, systems have been developed to manipulate somatosensation and vision selectively. With these devices, the angle of sway is fed back to a dynamic posture platform or to a movable visual surround so that movement about the ankle joint or movement of the visual surround is sway referenced.

Posturography is a method for quantifying balance. It is not a diagnostic test and is of little use for localizing a lesion. It can be helpful for following the course of a patient and may serve as a quantitative measure of the response to therapy. As noted above, sway increases in older people, and several studies have shown that the frequency of falls increases as sway increases, suggesting that posturography may be a useful clinical tool for identifying older people at risk for falling.

Neuroimaging

Computed tomography (CT) and magnetic resonance imaging (MRI) have revolutionized the diagnosis of lesions involving the temporal bone and posterior fossa. The relative merit of these two imaging techniques is still being defined, although MRI is clearly superior to CT for imaging soft tissue lesions. MRI can identify small acoustic neuromas confined to the internal auditory canal, tumors that are missed with CT. Infusion of contrast further increases the sensitivity of MRI for identifying small tumors. MRI can also reliably identify gliomas of the brainstem and cerebellum, tumors that may be isodense on CT. CT is useful for identifying bony erosion, hemorrhage, and/or calcification within tumors. The decision on whether to order neuroimaging studies is easy in patients with dizziness and associated neurologic symptoms and signs but is difficult in patients with isolated dizziness. Acoustic neuromas and other cerebellopontine angle tumors rarely present with vertigo because they slowly compress the vestibular nerve and the brain compensates. Rarely, cerebellar infarcts can present with just vertigo and imbalance (see below), but as a general rule isolated attacks of vertigo indicate a peripheral vestibular lesions (i.e. neuroimaging will not be helpful).

DIAGNOSIS AND TREATMENT OF COMMON NEUROTOLOGIC SYNDROMES

Table 9-4 summarizes the diagnosis and management of common neurotologic conditions.

Benign Positional Vertigo

Benign positional vertigo is by far the most common cause of vertigo. It is not a disease but rather a syndrome that can be the sequela of several different inner ear diseases; in about one-half of cases, no cause can be found. Patients with this condition develop brief episodes of vertigo with position change, typically when turning over in bed, getting in and out of bed, bending over and straightening up, or extending the neck to look up.

TABLE 9-4. Diagnosis and Management of Common Neurotologic Syndromes

	Diagnosis	Management
Benign positional vertigo	Brief (<1 min), positioning-induced vertigo and nystagmus	Maneuver to remove debris from semicircular canal
Acute unilateral vestibulopathy	Prolonged (days) vertigo, spontaneous nystagmus, unilateral reduced caloric response	Antivertiginous drugs first few days; begin vestibular rehabilitation as soon as possible
Chronic bilateral vestibulopathy	Vertigo infrequent, disequilibrium and oscillopsia, bilateral reduced caloric response	Stop ototoxin, vestibular rehabilitation
Ménière's disease	Vertigo (hours), tinnitus, hearing loss, ear fullness, spontaneous nystagmus, fluctuating hearing levels	Low salt diet (1 g of Na^+/day), ± diuretic, antivertiginous drugs during attack, surgery for intractable cases (<5%)
Migraine	Recurrent vertigo (variable duration), headache, visual aura, motion sensitivity, family history	Control potential triggers (foods, stress); antimigraine drugs (β blockers, calcium channel blockers, acetazolamide)
Vertebrobasilar insufficiency	Abrupt vertigo (minutes), disequilibrium and oscillopsia, other neurologic symptoms and signs, risk factors for vascular disease	Antiplatelet drugs (aspirin or ticlopidine); if spells continue, anticoagulation (heparin or warfarin)

So-called top-shelf vertigo is nearly always due to benign positional vertigo. The diagnosis rests on finding the characteristic fatigable positioning nystagmus after a rapid change from the sitting to the head-hanging position (see above). There is now convincing evidence that benign positional vertigo results from free-floating debris (probably calcium carbonate crystals) within the posterior semicircular canal that moves under the influence of gravity. The debris forms a clot within the canal; when it moves, it displaces the cupula, resulting in a burst of nystagmus and vertigo. Dispersion of the debris with repeated movements accounts for fatigability of the vertigo and nystagmus. This so-called canalithiasis theory has led to a simple bedside treatment of benign positional vertigo that cures the vast majority of patients. If the history and physical findings are typical, no further evaluation is necessary. If the history or findings are atypical, however, the condition must be distinguished from other causes of positional vertigo that may occur with tumors or infarcts in the posterior fossa.

Management.   Once the diagnosis of benign positional vertigo is made, a simple explanation of the nature of the disorder and its favorable prognosis can help relieve the patient's anxiety. Because of the dramatic nature of the episodes of vertigo, many patients believe they have a life-threatening disorder such as a tumor or stroke, and they are reassured to learn that there is simply a mechanical problem in their inner ear. Once the diagnosis is confirmed with the Hallpike positional test, a positioning maneuver is performed to liberate the clot of debris from the posterior semicircular canal. We use a modified Epley maneuver as shown in Figure 9-1, but other maneuvers may be equally effective. The key feature of these maneuvers is to move the patient from one head-hanging position to the other so that the clot rotates around the posterior semicircular canal. Once the clot enters the utricle, it presumably becomes attached to the membrane or is cleared through the endolymphatic duct and sac so it can no longer interfere with semicircular canal dynamics. The patient is instructed to avoid lying flat for at least 2 days after the maneuver is performed to prevent the clot from re-entering the posterior canal orifice. Cure rates of 70 to 90 percent have been consistently reported after a single session with these liberatory maneuvers. The maneuver should be repeated if the patient continues to be symptomatic after the initial maneuver. Between 10 and 20 percent of patients will have an exacerbation within 1 to 2 weeks after performing the maneuver, and as many as 50 percent will have an exacerbation at some time. Other similar maneuvers have been developed to remove debris from the anterior and horizontal semicircular canals when the direction of nystagmus indicates that these canals are involved.

Acute Peripheral Vestibulopathy

One of the most common clinical neurologic syndromes at any age is the acute onset of vertigo, nausea, and vomiting lasting for several days and not associated with auditory or neurologic symptoms. Most affected patients gradually improve over a few weeks, but some, particularly older patients, can have persistent symptoms for months. About 50 percent of such patients report an upper respiratory tract illness within a few weeks prior to the onset of vertigo. This syndrome occasionally occurs in epidemics, may affect several members of the same family, and may often erupt in the spring and early summer. All of these facts suggest a viral origin, but attempts to isolate an agent have

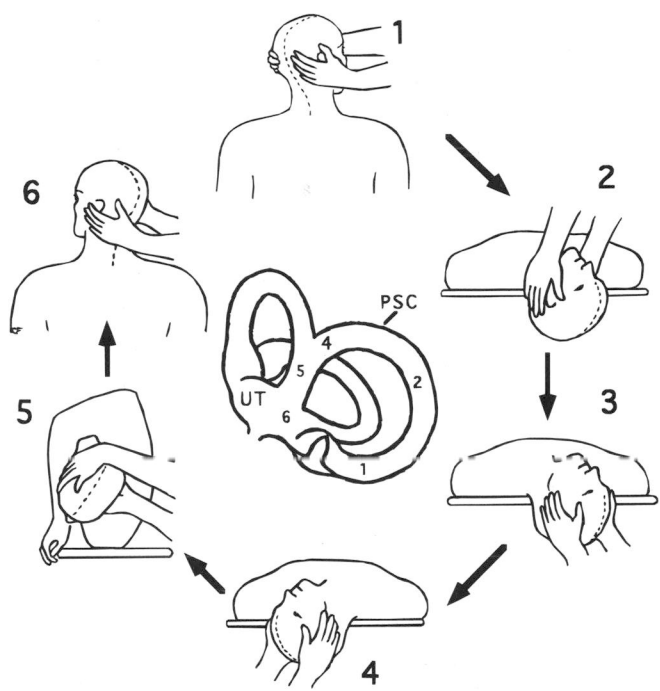

FIG. 9-1.   Method for treating benign positional vertigo affecting the right ear. The procedure is reversed for treating the left ear. The drawing of the labyrinth illustrates the position of the debris as it moves around the posterior semicircular canal (PSC) and into the utricle (UT). (*1*) Patient in upright position. (*2*) Patient is moved rapidly to head-hanging right (Hallpike test). (*3*) Operator moves to head of bed, repositioning hands. (*4*) Head is rotated quickly to the left with right ear upward. Position maintained for 30 seconds. (*5*) Patient rolls onto the left side while operator rapidly rotates head leftward until the nose is toward ground. Position maintained for 30 seconds. (*6*) Patient is rapidly lifted into the sitting position, now facing left. The sequence is repeated until no nystagmus can be elicited. The patient is instructed to avoid lying flat for 2 days to prevent the debris from re-entering the posterior canal.

been unsuccessful, except for occasional findings of a herpes zoster infection. Pathologic studies showing atrophy of one or more vestibular nerve trunks, with or without atrophy of their associated sense organs, are evidence of vestibular nerve site and probably viral etiology in many patients with this syndrome. In some patients, attacks of acute vestibulopathy, usually less severe, recur months or years after the initial attack. Whether this represents reactivation of a latent virus or some other pathophysiologic mechanism is unknown.

Vertigo often follows a blow to the head that does not result in temporal bone fracture, so-called labyrinthine concussion. Although they are protected by a bony capsule, the delicate labyrinthine membranes are susceptible to blunt trauma. Blows to the occipital or mastoid region are particularly likely to produce labyrinthine damage. Transverse fractures of the temporal bone typically pass through the vestibule of the inner ear, tearing the membranous labyrinth and lacerating the vestibular and cochlear nerves. Complete loss of vestibular and cochlear function is the usual sequela, and the facial nerve is damaged in approximately 50 percent of cases. Fistulae of the oval and round windows can result from impact noise, deep water diving, severe physical exertion, or blunt head injury without skull fracture. The mechanism of the rupture is a sudden negative or positive pressure change in the middle ear or a sudden increase in cerebrospinal fluid pressure transmitted to the inner ear via the cochlear aqueduct or the internal auditory canal. Clinically, the rupture leads to the onset of vertigo or hearing loss or both. A perilymph fistula should be seriously considered when there is clear relationship between the onset of vertigo and the onset of severe exertion, barometric change, head injury, or impact noise.

Occlusion of the internal auditory artery leads to a sudden profound loss of both auditory and vestibular function. However, ischemia confined to the anterior vestibular artery distribution can result in isolated vertigo caused by infarction of only the vestibular labyrinth. This diagnosis should usually only be considered in older patients, particularly those with a history of transient ischemic attacks, stroke, or known atherosclerotic vascular disease. It can be seen in association with hyperviscosity syndromes such as hyperlipidemia, polycythemia, macroglobulinemia, and sickle cell anemia. After recovering from the acute manifestations, patients may develop episodes of typical benign positional vertigo either months or years later. The positional vertigo presumably results from an ischemic necrosis of the utricular macula, causing a release of otoconia that make their way into the long arm of the posterior semicircular canal (see above).

Management. Treatment of patients who present with isolated episodes of auditory and/or vestibular loss is controversial because the pathophysiology is often uncertain. As suggested above, unless there is convincing evidence to support a vascular or nonviral infectious cause, the patient should be managed as a presumed case of viral neurolabyrinthitis, that is, with symptomatic treatment. Although steroids have been recommended for their anti-inflammatory effect, there have been no controlled studies to assess the risk-benefit ratio for these drugs. About one-half of the patients with vestibular neurolabyrinthitis are left with permanent loss of vestibular function (as documented by serial caloric examinations), but the central nervous system is able to adapt to the vestibular loss, and residual symptoms are usually minimal once the compensation has occurred. Vestibular rehabilitation should be started immediately after the acute nausea and vomiting symptoms subside and should be continued until the dizziness and imbalance are minimal. Although antiviral agents such as cytarabine and acyclovir have been used for treating systemic viral illnesses in children, it is unclear whether the hearing loss that is often associated with disorders such as cytomegalovirus and rubella infections is altered by such treatment. There have been no reports on the efficacy of antiviral agents in adults with viral neurolabyrinthitis.

Patients who lose vestibular function on one side owing to trauma or vascular occlusion recover through central compensation despite the continued loss of function. As with viral neurolabyrinthitis, management consists of early symptomatic treatment to relieve nausea and vomiting followed immediately by vestibular rehabilitation to accelerate the compensation process. Patients with suspected perilymph fistulae are typically put at bed rest for several days to allow the fistula to close spontaneously. A small percentage of patients require exploration of the middle ear and surgical repair of the fistula.

Chronic Bilateral Vestibulopathy

Unlike patients with an acute imbalance in vestibular tone, patients with bilateral vestibulopathy often present with subtle symptoms of nonspecific dizziness and disequilibrium that may be difficult to separate from other neurologic causes of disequilibrium. The associated oscillopsia may be incorrectly interpreted as a problem with vision, leading to an ophthalmologic evaluation. By far, the most common cause of bilateral vestibulopathy is ototoxic drug damage from aminoglycosides. Such patients may experience vertigo during the acute phase if the toxic effect is asymmetric. More often, there is a gradual progressive symmetric loss of vestibular function, leading to imbalance but not vertigo. Unfortunately, many patients being treated with ototoxic drugs are initially bedridden and unaware of the vestibular impairment until they recover from the acute illness and try to walk. Then they discover that they are unsteady on their feet and that the environment tends to jiggle in front of their eyes (oscillopsia). Although the aminoglycosides usually produce auditory and vestibular damage, some such as streptomycin and gentamicin are relatively specific for the vestibular system, whereas others such as kanamycin, tobramycin, and amikacin cause more damage to the auditory system. The ototoxicity of aminoglycosides is due to hair cell damage in the inner ear. Because they are excreted almost exclusively by glomerular filtration, patients with renal impairment are at high risk for developing ototoxicity.

Management. The clinician must be constantly on the alert for early symptoms of damage from ototoxic drugs. This is particularly important in the patient who is seriously ill and confined to bed or in a patient who has renal impairment. Younger patients usually adapt to bilateral vestibular loss by using other sensory signals to replace the lost vestibular signals. Older patients, on the other hand, may be left permanently disabled. Vestibular rehabilitation can help patients learn to substitute other sensory signals for the vestibular loss. The best treatment is prevention. If the drug is discontinued early during the course of symptoms, the disorder may stabilize or improve.

Menière's Disease

Menière's disease typically develops with a sensation of fullness and pressure along with tinnitus and decreased hearing in one ear. Vertigo rapidly follows, reaching a maximum intensity within minutes and then slowly subsiding over several hours. The patient is usually left with a sense of unsteadiness and dizziness for days after the acute vertiginous episode. In the early stages, the hearing loss is completely reversible but in later stages a residual hearing loss remains. Tinnitus may persist between episodes but usually increases in intensity immediately before or during the acute episode. It is typically described as a roaring sound like the sound of the ocean or a hollow seashell. Such episodes occur in irregular intervals for years, with periods of remissions unpredictably intermixed. Eventually severe permanent hearing loss develops, and the episodic nature spontaneously disappears (burnt-out phase). About one-third of patients will develop bilateral Menière's disease.

Variations from this classic picture occur, particularly in the early stages of the disease process, but the diagnosis remains uncertain until the combination of fluctuating hearing loss and vertigo occurs. Some patients experience abrupt episodes of falling to the ground without loss of consciousness or associated neurologic symptoms. These episodes have been called otolithic catastrophes based on the presumed sudden stimulation of an otolith organ by the increased inner ear pressure. So-called delayed Menière's disease develops in an ear that has been damaged years before, usually by a viral or bacterial infection. When the hearing loss is profound, as it often is, the episodic vertigo will not be accompanied by fluctuating hearing levels and tinnitus.

Management. Medical management of Menière's disease consists of symptomatic treatment of the acute spells of vertigo and long-term prophylaxis with salt restriction and diuretics. The mechanism by which a low salt diet decreases the frequency and severity of attacks with Menière's disease is unclear, but there is strong empiric evidence for its efficacy. We recommend salt restriction in the range of 1 g of sodium per day, with a minimum therapeutic trial of 6 months to 1 year. Food intake should be regularly distributed throughout the day. Binges (particularly food with high sugar or salt content) should be avoided. Occasionally, patients will notice that certain foods (e.g., alcohol, coffee, or chocolate) may precipitate attacks. Diuretics (acetazolamide 250 mg bid or hydrochlorothiazide 50 mg bid) provide additional benefit in some patients, although they cannot replace a salt restriction diet.

Migraine

Vertigo is a common symptom with migraine, occurring either with the headaches or in separate isolated episodes. Furthermore, vertigo attacks can predate the onset of headaches, and in some cases vertigo is the only manifestation of migraine (a so-called migraine equivalent). The diagnosis of migraine should be entertained in any patient with chronic recurrent attacks of vertigo of unknown cause. The duration of attacks is variable, and therefore migraine can mimic several other common neurotologic vertigo syndromes. The magnitude of the problem is apparent when one considers that migraine may affect as many as 25 percent of women and 15 percent of men and that vertigo attacks occur in at least one-quarter of these.

The diagnosis of migraine-associated vertigo is straightforward when the vertigo is part of an aura that is followed by typical unilateral throbbing headache. The diagnosis becomes more problematic when the vertigo attacks and headache occur independently or the vertigo attacks occur without headaches. Long-standing motion sensitivity, including carsickness and a clear family history of migraine, help support the diagnosis. Also some patients have typical migraine visual aura or other focal neurologic symptoms unassociated with headache. Bickerstaff described a type of migraine in which the aura consisted of posterior fossa symptoms such as vertigo, ataxia, dysarthria, and tinnitus along with visual phenomena consistent with ischemia in the distribution of the posterior cerebral arteries. He emphasized that the symptoms were particularly common in adolescent girls and commonly in association with their menstrual period. Others have subsequently described a more widespread age distribution. One must be alert to the possibility of posterior fossa migraine in any patient presenting with transient vertigo and other posterior fossa symptoms. In some individuals, the headache is not severe and is adequately managed by aspirin, sleep, or mild analgesics and sedatives. Many of these patients are much more concerned about the aura phenomena than their headaches.

Management. If infrequent, vertigo attacks associated with migraine can be treated with symptomatic medications that produce sedation and relieve nausea. As with the headache, if the patients can fall asleep, the symptom is often gone when they awaken. Migraine prophylactic medications can be useful in patients with frequent recurrent attacks of vertigo or in patients with a persistent motion sick sensation that can go on for days or weeks at a time. We have found that acetazolamide (250 mg bid) is particularly effective for preventing vestibular symptoms associated with migraine. Propranolol (80 to 160 mg/day) and amitriptyline (75 to 150 mg/day) are also effective for relieving both headache and vertigo associated with migraine.

Acoustic Neuroma

Acoustic neuromas (vestibular schwannoma) usually begin in the internal auditory canal, producing symptoms by compressing the nerves in the narrow confines of the canal. As the tumor enlarges, it protrudes through the internal auditory meatus, producing a funnel-shaped erosion of the bone surrounding the canal, stretching adjacent nerves over the surface of the mass, and deforming the brainstem and cerebellum. Acoustic neuromas account for about 5 percent of intracranial tumors and over 90 percent of cerebellar-pontine angle tumors. By far, the most common symptoms associated with acoustic neuromas are slowly progressive unilateral hearing loss and tinnitus from compression of the cochlear nerve. Rarely, acute hearing loss occurs, apparently from compression of the labyrinthine vasculature. Vertigo occurs in fewer than 20 percent of patients, but approximately 50 percent complain of mild imbalance or disequilibrium.

Management. With few exceptions, the management of tumors in the internal auditory canal and cerebellopontine angle is surgical. Occasionally, one might follow the course of a patient with a small acoustic neuroma, particularly if the patient is elderly or has underlying medical problems. These tumors can remain confined to the internal auditory canal for years; symptoms may be restricted to those of the eighth cranial nerve.

Vertebrobasilar Insufficiency

Vertebrobasilar insufficiency is a common cause of vertigo in older people. Whether the vertigo originates from ischemia of the labyrinth, brainstem, or both structures is not always clear because the blood supply to the labyrinth, eighth cranial nerve, and vestibular nuclei originates from the same source, the vertebrobasilar circulation. Vertigo with vertebrobasilar insufficiency is abrupt in onset, usually lasts minutes, and is frequently associated with nausea, vomiting, and severe imbalance. Associated symptoms resulting from ischemia in the remaining territories supplied by the posterior circulation include visual blurring or blacking out, diplopia, drop attacks, weakness and numbness of the extremities, and headache. These symptoms occur in episodes, either in combination with the vertigo or separately. Vertigo may be an isolated initial symptom of vertebrobasilar insufficiency, but repeated episodes of vertigo without other symptoms should suggest another diagnosis. Vertebrobasilar insufficiency is usually caused by atherosclerosis of the subclavian, vertebral, and basilar arteries. Emboli in the posterior circulation are probably more common than has been generally appreciated. About one in five posterior circulation infarcts is cardioembolic, and another one in five is due to interarterial embolism arising most often from occlusive lesions of the extracranial and intracranial vertebral arteries. Other less common causes of arterial occlusion include dissection, arteritis, polycythemia, and hypercoagulation syndromes. Occasionally episodes of vertebrobasilar insufficiency are precipitated by postural hypotension, Stokes-Adams attacks, or mechanical compression from cervical spondylosis. Regarding the latter, cervical spondylosis is extremely common in older people, but documented cases of mechanical compression of vertebral arteries or extension are rare.

Occasionally, cerebellar infarction presents with severe vertigo, vomiting, and ataxia without associated brainstem symptoms and signs that might suggest the erroneous diagnosis of an acute peripheral vestibular disorder. The key differential point is the finding of cerebellar signs (gait ataxia and gaze-evoked nystagmus). Such patients must be watched carefully for several days because they may develop progressive brainstem dysfunction owing to compression by a swollen cerebellum. The diagnosis of vertebrobasilar insufficiency or stroke within the posterior circulation can usually be made at the bedside based on the characteristic combination of symptoms and signs. One should focus on risk factors for atherosclerosis, including history of coronary artery disease, hypertension, diabetes mellitus, and hyperlipidemia. In younger subjects without obvious risk factors for atherosclerosis, one should consider the possibility of trauma and other systemic illnesses that might predispose to hypercoagulation syndrome.

Specific stroke syndromes in the distribution of a single vessel are now easily identified with MRI. The decision on whether to perform angiography with suspected vertebrobasilar insufficiency can be difficult. In an older patient with multiple risk factors for atherosclerosis and infrequent transient ischemic attacks, one might reasonably choose to treat with antiplatelet drugs without performing angiography. However, in patients without obvious risk factors for atherosclerosis, for those with severe incapacitating attacks or rapidly increasing frequency of transient ischemic attacks, angiography is nearly always required.

Management. Treatment of vertebrobasilar insufficiency usually consists of controlling risk factors (diabetes, hypertension, or hyperlipidemia) and the use of antiplatelet drugs (aspirin and ticlopidine). Anticoagulation (heparin and warfarin) is reserved for patients with frequent incapacitating episodes or for patients with symptoms and signs suggesting a stroke in evolution, particularly basilar artery thrombosis.

Other Central Causes of Vertigo

Familial Ataxia Syndromes.   Vestibular symptoms and signs are common with several of the hereditary ataxia syndromes, including Friedreich's ataxia, olivopontocerebellar atrophy, Refsum's disease, late-onset cerebellar atrophy, and familial periodic ataxia. In most of these syndromes, the symptoms are slowly progressive, with the cerebellar ataxia and incoordination overshadowing loss of vestibular function. Head movement-induced oscillopsia and dizziness commonly occur because the patient is unable to suppress the vestibulo-ocular reflex with fixation. Vertigo is usually not present because the vestibular loss occurs gradually in a bilateral symmetric fashion. However, patients with familial periodic ataxia often have episodes of vertigo, nausea, and vomiting, which may be misinterpreted as a peripheral vestibular disorder such as Menière's disease. The key to the diagnosis in all of these syndromes is the finding of ataxia of the trunk and extremities and the characteristic oculomotor signs, including several varieties of central nystagmus.

Chiari Malformation.   With the Chiari congenital malformation, the brainstem and cerebellum are elongated downward into the cervical canal, causing pressure on both the caudal midline cerebellum and the cervical-medullary junction. Symptoms and signs can be delayed until adult life; in which case, they are usually unassociated with any other developmental defects. The most common neurologic symptom is a slowly progressive unsteadiness of gait, which patients often describe as dizziness. Vertigo and hearing loss are infrequent, occurring in about 10 percent of patients. Spontaneous downbeat nystagmus is particularly common with Chiari malformation, but other forms of central nystagmus also occur. Dysphagia, hoarseness, and dysarthria can result from stretching of the lower cranial nerves, and obstructive hydrocephalus can result from occlusion of the basilar cisterns. MRI is the procedure of choice for identifying Chiari malformations; midline sagittal sections clearly show the level of the cerebellar tonsils.

Multiple Sclerosis.   Vertigo is the initial symptom in about 5 percent of patients with multiple sclerosis and is reported sometime during the disease in as many of 50 percent. The typical bout of vertigo associated with multiple sclerosis lasts from hours to days, although positional vertigo lasting seconds is also a common feature. The key to the diagnosis is to find disseminated lesions within the nervous system occurring with a remitting and exacerbating course. Nearly all varieties of central spontaneous and positional nystagmus occur with multiple sclerosis, and occasionally patients show typical peripheral vestibular nystagmus when the lesion affects the root entry zone of the vestibular nerve. MRI of the brain will identify white matter lesions in about 95 percent of patients with multiple sclerosis, although similar lesions are sometimes seen in patients without the clinical criteria for the diagnosis of multiple sclerosis.

Vertigo and Focal Seizures.   Vestibular symptoms are common with focal seizures, particularly those originating in the temporal and parietal lobes. Common associated symptoms include an abnormal epigastric sensation, nausea, mastication, and salivation. Visual illusions and hallucinations are also commonly associated, suggesting a close functional relationship between cortical visual and vestibular projections. The key to differentiating vertigo with seizures from other causes of vertigo is that seizures are invariably associated with an altered level of consciousness. There are usually associated stereotyped motor phenomena, and the patient is usually unresponsive for part of the seizure. Episodic vertigo as an isolated manifestation of a focal seizure disorder is a rarity, if it occurs at all. The diagnosis rests on finding characteristic electroencephalographic changes and focal structural lesions on neuroimaging.

Management.   Because the specific enzymatic defect is unknown in most of the degenerative cerebellar disorders, treatment is symptomatic. Regular physical therapy to maintain range of motion about all joints is critical to avoid painful contractions. A special diet low in long chain fatty acids can be effective in controlling the progressive symptoms and signs with Refsum's disease. Acetazolamide is effective for relieving the episodic symptoms in patients with familial periodic ataxia. The usual dosage is 250 mg bid or tid. How acetazolamide affects this disorder is unknown, but a therapeutic trial of acetazolamide should be undertaken in any patient with recurrent episodes of vertigo and/or ataxia who has a family history of similar episodes. In patients with Chiari type I malformations, suboccipital decompression of the foramen magnum region can stop the progression and occasionally lead to improvement in neurologic symptoms and signs. Management of multiple sclerosis and focal seizure disorders is discussed in detail in other sections of this book.

TABLE 9-5. Dosage and Effects of Commonly Used Antivertiginous Medications

Class	Drug	Dosage	Sedation	Antiemetic Actions	Dryness of Mucous Membranes	Precautions
Anticholinergic agent	Scopolamine	0.6 mg PO q4–6h or 0.5 mg transdermally q3d	+	+	+ + +	Asthma, prostate enlargement, older people
Antihistamine	Meclizine (Antivert)	25 mg PO q4–6h	+	+	+	Asthma, glaucoma
	Dimenhydrinate (Dramamine)	50 mg PO or IM q4–6h or 100 mg suppository q8h	+	+	+	
	Promethazine (Phenergan)	25 or 50 mg PO or IM or as suppository q4–6h	+ +	+ +	+	
Benzodiazepine	Diazepam (Valium)	5 or 10 mg PO, IM, or IV q4–6h	+ + +	+	−	Pregnancy, prior drug addiction
Phenothiazine	Prochlorperazine (Compazine)	5 or 10 mg PO or IM q6h or 25 mg suppository q12h	+	+ + +	+	Liver disease, extrapyramidal reactions
Benzamide	Metoclopramide (Reglan)	5 or 50 mg PO, IM, or IV q4–6h	+	+ + +	+	Bowel obstruction, liver or renal disease

SYMPTOMATIC TREATMENT OF VERTIGO

Treatment of vertigo can be divided into three general categories: specific, symptomatic, and rehabilitative. Whenever a specific therapy, such as those discussed in the prior section, exists, obviously, it is the treatment of choice. However, in many cases, there is no specific therapy, or symptomatic treatment is combined with specific therapy. A major change in treatment strategy that has evolved over the past several years is that vestibular rehabilitation therapy should be begun as soon as possible after an acute vestibular lesion. Prolonged use of sedating, symptomatic medications is contraindicated because this can slow down the vestibular compensation process.

The commonly used antivertiginous drugs and their dosages are listed in Table 9-5. It is often difficult to predict which drug or combinations of drugs will be most effective in a given patient; some respond to one drug but not to others in the same class. The mechanism of action of these drugs is not completely known, although most have been shown either to decrease the efficacy of transmission from primary to secondary vestibular neurons or to decrease the overall excitability of neurons in the vestibular nucleus.

The choice of a drug or combination of drugs is based on the known effects of each drug (Table 9-5) and on the severity and time course of symptoms. In patients with acute severe vertigo, sedation is desirable, and drugs such as promethazine and diazepam are particularly useful. If nausea and vomiting are severe, the antiemetics prochlorperazine and metoclopramide can be combined with another antivertiginous medication. The patient with chronic recurrent vertigo usually is attempting to carry on normal activities, and therefore sedation is undesirable. In this setting, meclizine, dimenhydrinate, and scopolamine are often useful.

Vestibular rehabilitation exercises are designed to retrain the eye and body musculature gradually to use visual and somatosensory signals to compensate for loss of vestibular signals. Eye and head movements are performed in bed as soon as possible after acute vertigo, nausea, and vomiting have subsided. More vigorous exercises while standing and moving about are then gradually introduced as the patient recovers. For example, walking across a room, up and down a slope, and up and down steps with eyes open and closed can be introduced within the first few days. Games that require eye-hand coordination are ideal as the patient progresses with recovery. The patient should be encouraged to seek out the head positions and movements that cause dizziness as far as can be tolerated because the more frequently dizziness is induced the more quickly compensation occurs. Grouping patients together for vestibular exercises is often ideal because they can encourage each other and beginners can witness the progress of long-term members. The purpose of the exercises should be explained to each patient, and each should receive written instructions outlining an exercise regimen. The exercises are usually continued for 1 to 3 months. During this time, the patient is encouraged to return to a normal schedule of work and leisure activity as soon as possible.

SUGGESTED READINGS

Baloh RW, Honrubia V: Clinical Neurophysiology of the Vestibular System. 2nd Ed. FA Davis, Philadelphia, 1990
Baloh RW, Honrubia V, Jacobson K: Benign positional vertigo: clinical and oculographic features in 240 cases. Neurology 17:173, 1987
Brandt T: Vertigo. Its Multisensory Syndromes. Springer-Verlag, London, 1991
Epley JM: The canalith repositioning procedure: for treatment of benign paroxysmal positional vertigo. Otolaryngol Head Neck Surg 107:399, 1992
Grad A, Baloh RW: Vertigo of vascular origin: clinical and ENG features in 84 cases. Arch Neurol 46:281, 1989
Huang CY, Yu YL: Small cerebellar strokes may mimic labyrinthine lesions. J Neurol Neurosurg Psychiatry 48:263, 1985
Kayan A, Hood JD: Neuro-otological manifestations of migraine. Brain 107:1123, 1984
Rybak LP, Matz GJ: Auditory and vestibular effects of toxins. p. 3161. In Cummings CW, Fredrickson JM, Harker LA et al (eds): Otolaryngology—Head and Neck Surgery. CV Mosby, St. Louis, 1986
Schuknecht HF: Delayed endolymphatic hydrops. Ann Otol 87:743, 1978
Schuknecht HF: Neurolabyrinthitis. Viral infections of the peripheral auditory and vestibular systems. p. 1. In Nomura Y (ed): Hearing Loss and Dizziness. Igaku-Shoin, Tokyo, 1985

10. HEARING LOSS AND TINNITUS

DAVID M. VERNICK

Hearing loss and tinnitus affect over 20 percent of the United States population. Whether the cause is congenital, aging, trauma, loud noise exposure, drugs, infection, foreign body, cerumen, or less common causes, the physician needs first to recognize and then to diagnose the problem before anything can be done to help alleviate the patient's suffering. As the average age of the population increases, the number of people with hearing losses increases. (About 30 percent of people over age 65 and 35 percent over age 75 have a significant loss.) Similar numbers can be found for tinnitus. The impact of hearing loss and tinnitus on our society continues to grow, making their recognition and treatment more critical.

AUDITORY ANATOMY

The auditory system can be divided into several segments for purposes of localizing impairments. The auricle, the external auditory canal, and middle ear make up the conductive sound-transmission component; the inner ear, auditory nerve, and brain make up the sensorineural sound-transmission component.

Conductive System

Sound is funneled into the external auditory canal via the auricle. The sound strikes the eardrum, causing it to vibrate at a frequency-specific rate. This vibration is transmitted through the ossicles (malleus, incus, and stapes) into the inner ear to the perilymph. The usual loss of energy when sounds goes from air to fluid is made up by the mechanical advantage of the middle ear ossicles and the size ratio of the eardrum to the stapes footplate. Any interference with this sequential process, like cerumen, infection, tympanic membrane perforation, or middle ear fluid can lead to a conductive hearing loss.

Sensorineural System

Fluid vibrations in the inner ear are converted into electrical impulses at the hair cell level in a tonotopic distribution. High frequencies stimulate the cochlear base, and low frequencies stimulate the apex. Humans have about 15,000 hair cells, which synapse with and send their signals to about 30,000 first-order neurons. Although outer hair cells outnumber inner hair cells three to one, 90 percent of the neurons synapse with the inner hair cells. These first-order neurons have their cell bodies located in the spiral ganglion in the cochlea and synapse at the cochlear nucleus of the pollens. Sound then ascends through the brainstem in bilateral pathways to the auditory cortex. This information continues to be relayed in a frequency-specific tonotopic pattern.

Injury to the inner ear, either the auditory nerve or the hair cells, usually causes a unilateral sensorineural hearing loss that is frequency specific to the area of injury. Because of the bilateral distribution of information, injuries to the auditory neurons, brainstem, and cortex usually cause a more subtle processing type of problem not recorded on routine audiometry, such as the inability to localize sounds seen in multiple sclerosis. Bilateral sensorineural hearing loss from a brainstem lesion is rare and usually overshadowed by concomitant neural deficits.

HEARING LOSS

Conductive Versus Sensorineural

Alteration of the auditory process can occur at any step of sound transmission from the auricle to the auditory cortex (Figs. 10-1 and 10-2). When this alteration occurs at any step up to the transmission of sound energy to the perilymph by the stapes, the type of hearing loss produced is called conductive. This means that any process that affects the outer or middle ear sound transmission causes a conductive hearing loss. When the alteration occurs at any step after the sound has entered the inner ear (from the cochlea to the cortex), it is called sensorineural. Table 10-1 lists common causes of conductive and sensorineural hearing loss and tinnitus.

Conductive hearing loss can occur from any process that occludes the ear canal. Wax, water, or a foreign body can all block sound transmission. Alteration of the eardrum, either from injury or infection, can limit its vibratory ability. A perforation, especially when it is located posterosuperiorly over the ossicles, can be particularly severe. A floppy, redundant eardrum can produce the same effect. (Interestingly, a very stiff eardrum from tympanosclerosis usually does not cause hearing loss.) Erosion of the ossicles from infection or cholesteatoma, limitation of their motion by scarring or otosclerosis, tumors in the middle ear, and fluid in the middle ear all create a conductive hearing loss by interfering with tympanic membrane and ossicular mobility.

Sensorineural hearing loss occurs from a problem in the inner ear, along the auditory nerve, or in the central nervous system. Fluid balance problems in the inner ear such as Menière's disease or perilymphatic fistulae can cause hearing to fluctuate or deteriorate. Inner ear infections from bacteria and viruses can cause sudden hearing loss with or without vertigo. Tumors along the auditory nerves in the posterior fossa, such as acoustic neuromas, can cause a progressive or sudden sensorineural hearing loss (see Ch. 158). Autoimmune diseases, such as Cogan syndrome and lupus, can have a rapidly progressive inner ear component to them, causing hearing loss. Brainstem and cortical lesions can cause hearing loss or lead to problems in processing the auditory information once it is received.

HISTORY AND PHYSICAL EXAMINATION

The diagnosis of many causes of hearing loss comes from taking a careful history. The time of onset of the loss, whether gradual or sudden; the severity of the loss; the presence or absence of fluctuation of the hearing; and the presence of other illnesses all can help limit the differential diagnosis. Associated symptoms such as pain, vertigo, tinnitus, and otorrhea can also help. Activities around the time of onset such as flying and diving can lead to the etiology. A family history of hearing loss can alert one to the possibility of otosclerosis, early presbycusis, or genetic causes of hearing loss.

Physical examination of the ear can further differentiate most causes of hearing loss. Cerumen, foreign bodies, outer and middle ear infections, fluid in the middle ear, perforations, cholesteatomas, and glomus tumors can all be distinguished by a careful ear examination. Wax in the ear canal needs to be removed

TABLE 10-1. Causes of Hearing Loss and Tinnitus

Conductive	Sensorineural
Cerumen	Presbycusis
Foreign body	Menière's disease
External otitis	Labyrinthitis
Acute otitis media	Autoimmune hearing loss
Serous otitis media	Acoustic neuroma
Cholesteatoma	Noise
Otosclerosis	Drugs
Glomus tympanicum and jugulare tumors	Congenital
Perforations of the tympanic membrane	Strokes
Ossicular discontinuity	
Congenital	

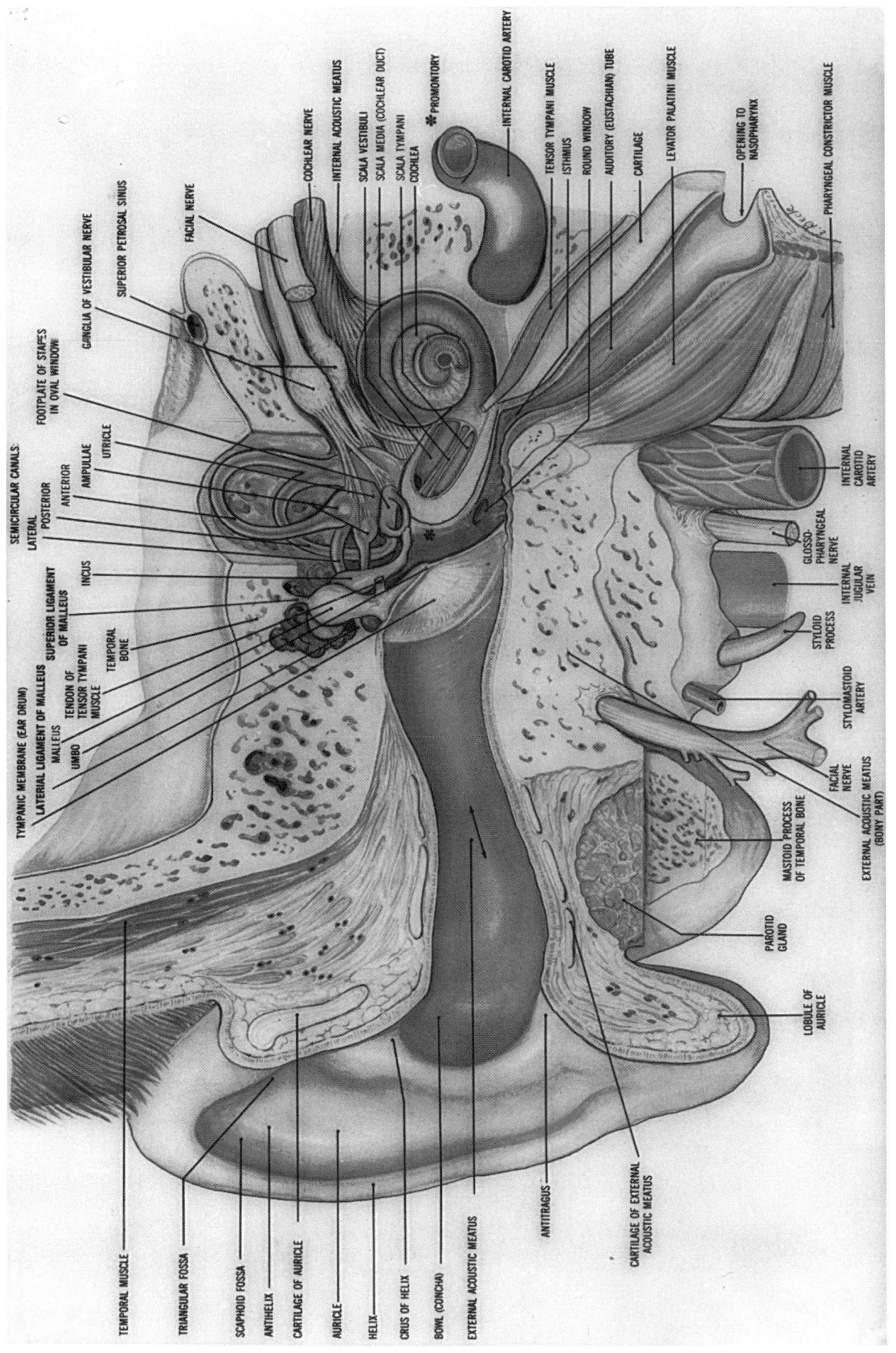

FIG. 10-1. The anatomy of the ear.

TEMPORAL MUSCLE

TRIANGULAR FOSSA

SCAPHOID FOSSA

ANTIHELIX

CARTILAGE OF AURICLE

AURICLE

HELIX

CRUS OF HELIX

BOWL (CONCHA)

EXTERNAL ACOUSTIC MEATUS

ANTITRAGUS

CARTILAGE OF EXTERNAL ACOUSTIC MEATUS

LOBULE OF AURICLE

PAROTID GLAND

MASTOID PROCESS OF TEMPORAL BONE

EXTERNAL ACOUSTIC MEATUS (BONY PART)

FACIAL NERVE

STYLOMASTOID ARTERY

STYLOID PROCESS

INTERNAL JUGULAR VEIN

GLOSSO-PHARYNGEAL NERVE

INTERNAL CAROTID ARTERY

PHARYNGEAL CONSTRICTOR MUSCLE

OPENING TO NASOPHARYNX

LEVATOR PALATINI MUSCLE

CARTILAGE

AUDITORY (EUSTACHIAN) TUBE

ROUND WINDOW

ISTHMUS

TENSOR TYMPANI MUSCLE

INTERNAL CAROTID ARTERY

* PROMONTORY

COCHLEA

SCALA TYMPANI

SCALA MEDIA (COCHLEAR DUCT)

SCALA VESTIBULI

INTERNAL ACOUSTIC MEATUS

COCHLEAR NERVE

SUPERIOR PETROSAL SINUS

GANGLIA OF VESTIBULAR NERVE

FACIAL NERVE

FOOTPLATE OF STAPES IN OVAL WINDOW

SEMICIRCULAR CANALS:
LATERAL
POSTERIOR
ANTERIOR

AMPULLAE

UTRICLE

INCUS

SUPERIOR LIGAMENT OF MALLEUS

MALLEUS

TENDON OF TENSOR TYMPANI MUSCLE

UMBO

TEMPORAL BONE

LATERAL LIGAMENT OF MALLEUS

TYMPANIC MEMBRANE (EAR DRUM)

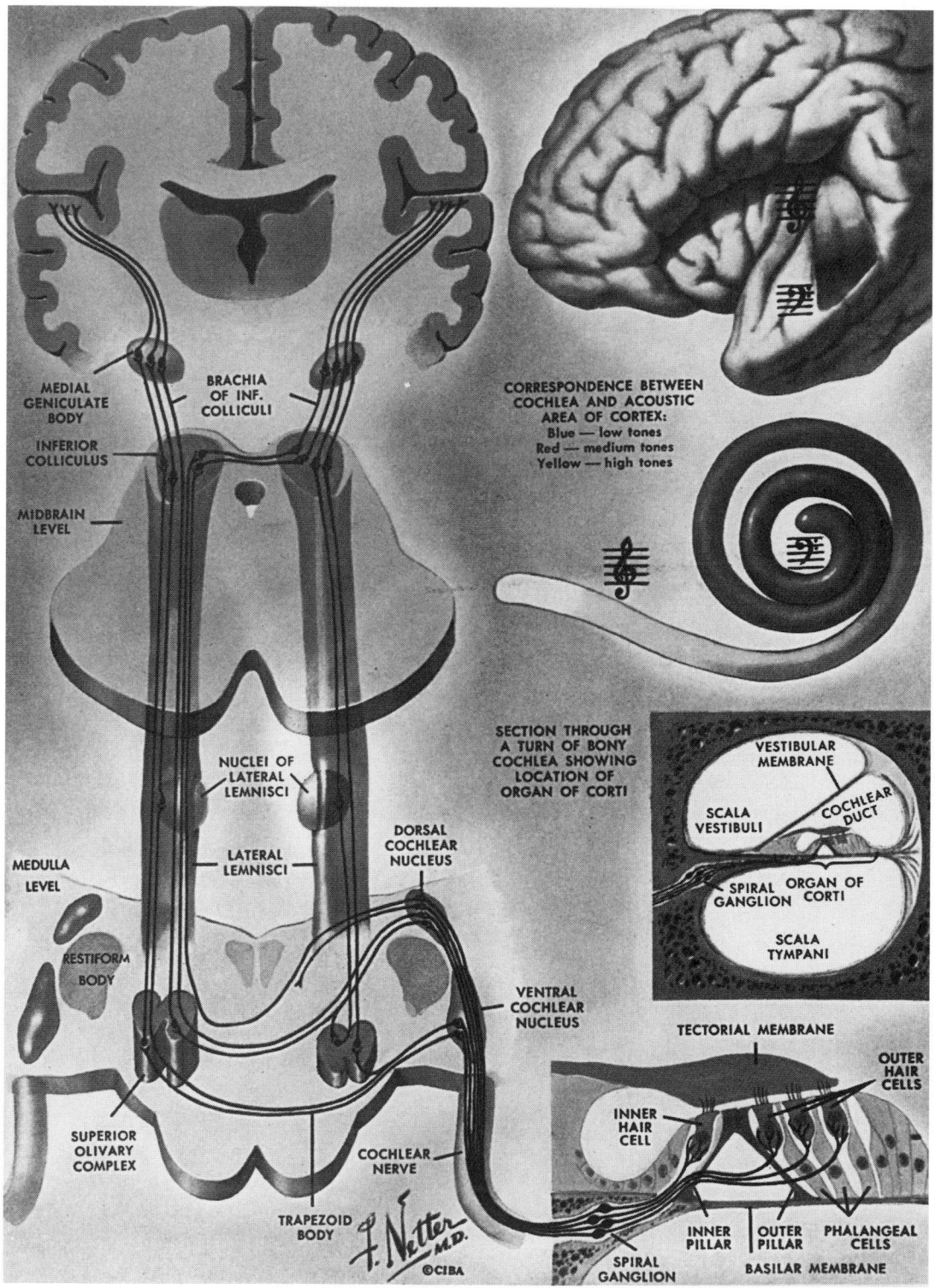

FIG. 10-2.   The cochlea and the central anatomy of hearing.

even if it is not the cause of the hearing loss, so that it does not obscure another cause. Balance function should be assessed because the vestibular system is connected to the auditory system in the inner ear. Facial nerve function should also be checked because the facial nerve traverses the ear. Although lower cranial nerves can be involved in some skull-based tumors, hearing loss is usually not the presenting feature.

TESTING

When hearing loss is suspected, a hearing test should be performed. Auditory testing can be done crudely in the office using a whisper in the ear, a rubbing of fingers next to the ear, or the tick of a watch. Background noises around the office can make such testing inaccurate.

Use of a tuning fork can determine whether a hearing loss is conductive or sensorineural. A 512-Hz tuning fork should be used because lower frequencies give too much vibrational sensation, many times interfering with the auditory testing. Two common tests with the tuning fork should be performed. The first test, the Rinne test, involves testing air conduction versus bone conduction in each ear. Care should be taken to ensure that the tuning fork is placed firmly against the mastoid bone when testing the bone level of hearing. Normally, air conduction is greater than bone conduction. When bone conduction is greater than air conduction, a conductive hearing loss is present in the ear. The second test, the Weber test, is designed to determine whether hearing is equal in the two ears. The vibrating tuning fork is placed in the midline, either on the forehead or base of the nose. The tone should not lateralize to either side. If it does, the hearing is asymmetric. If it lateralizes to the side where air conduction is greater than bone conduction on Rinne testing, then the person has a sensorineural hearing loss in the opposite ear. If it lateralizes to the side where bone conduction is greater than air conduction, than it confirms the presence of a conductive hearing loss in the lateralized side. If it stays in the midline, hearing may still not be normal. A person could still have a significant hearing loss that is bilaterally symmetric.

Multiple tests of auditory function have been developed to try to determine the site of the hearing loss, whether cochlear or retrocochlear. Bekesy audiometry, impedance audiometry, short increment sensitivity index testing, and acoustic reflex decay are but a few. Historically, they are interesting, but because these tests are all fraught with inaccuracy they have been replaced with auditory-evoked response testing. Auditory-evoked response testing is discussed in detail in Chapter 19. Of importance here is that it can help determine whether the lesion is cochlear or retrocochlear in location. It is quick, painless, noninvasive, accurate, reproducible, and requires minimal, if any, patient cooperation.

When structural evaluation of the mastoid, inner ear, or intracranial cavity is necessary, computed tomography (CT) or magnetic resonance imaging (MRI) is required. Bony detail of the temporal bone is best delineated by the CT scan. Soft tissue details of the internal auditory canal, posterior fossa, and brain are best shown by MRI, usually with gadolinium contrast. Magnetic resonance angiography can be helpful for evaluating vascular lesions, such as glomus tumors and aneurysms, that might impinge on auditory function.

TREATMENT

The successful treatment of hearing loss depends on an accurate diagnosis. Wax should be removed, and infection should be treated with antibiotics. Tympanic membrane perforations and ossicular problems can be corrected surgically. Tumors should be treated with radiation or surgery or both. Steroid therapy may promote recovery from sudden hearing loss. Hearing aids can be used whenever surgery is not desired or when the loss is sensorineural. Dispensing of the hearing aid should be done by a trained professional to ensure optimal fit. Cochlear implants can be placed in those who are deaf.

Hearing loss has many etiologies. The assessment of these is essential to proper treatment. Hearing loss that is new in onset, unilateral, or rapidly changing should alert the physician that full evaluation is necessary, and referral to a specialist should be considered.

COMMON CAUSES OF HEARING LOSS

Presbycusis

The most common cause of hearing loss is presbycusis, hearing loss secondary to aging. It is a high-frequency loss that is bilaterally symmetric and gradual in onset. Treatment is with hearing aids.

Cerumen

Cerumen can cause a gradual or sudden hearing loss. Treatment is removal.

Foreign Body

Obstruction of the ear canal by a foreign body can cause a conductive hearing loss. Treatment is removal.

Infection

Otitis Externa.   Infections in the external ear canal can cause hearing loss late in their course. Typically, the canal has to swell practically shut before there is significant hearing loss. Most patients have such severe pain at that point that hearing loss is a minor issue. Treatment is with ear drops and sometimes oral antibiotics.

Acute Otitis Media.   This middle ear infection causes hearing loss because fluid builds up in the middle ear and the eardrum becomes inflamed. Treatment involves the use of oral antibiotics. If the eardrum is ruptured from the ear infection, then ear drops may be used to prevent an external ear infection. Resolution of the hearing usually follows days to weeks after the infection has cleared. A serous effusion often remains until all the swelling has resolved.

Labrynthitis.   A viral or bacterial infection in the inner ear can cause severe vertigo (see Ch. 9). Often, it also involves the auditory system, resulting in hearing loss. There is usually a sudden onset of severe vertigo associated with nausea and vomiting. Nystagmus is present early in the infection. Mild cases can resolve within days to weeks. More severe cases can require 3 to 6 months for recovery. Treatment includes antiemetics and supportive measures. Vestibular suppressant drugs, such as meclizine, may be helpful initially but probably retard long-term recovery. Vestibular physical therapy can hasten recovery in severe cases.

Serous Otitis Media.   Fluid in the middle ear can cause mild to moderate hearing loss. The fluid can be thin, causing a mild hearing loss, or thicker, causing increasing hearing loss. There are multiple causes for serous otitis media, and treatment depends on the cause. In children, the most common cause is eustachian tube dysfunction. Treatment involves the use of antibiotics and ventilation tubes in the ears. In adults, especially if the serous otitis media is unilateral, one must rule out a nasopharyngeal tumor if no other etiology is obvious.

Tympanic Membrane Perforations

Perforations in the eardrum can cause hearing loss, depending on the size and location of the perforation. Total eardrum perforations cause approximately 40 dB of hearing loss. Treatment involves repair of the perforation. If the cause is traumatic, most perforations heal spontaneously.

Cholesteatomas

Cholesteatomas are skin cysts that grow in the middle ear. These can cause destruction of bone, including the ossicles. Treatment involves surgical removal of the cholesteatoma and, if necessary, ossicular reconstruction.

Trauma

Blows to the head can cause a high-frequency sensorineural hearing loss. They can also cause a conductive hearing loss by disrupting the ossicular chain. Temporal bone fractures can do either or both as well as tear the eardrum. A bleeding ear or blood behind the eardrum after injury is a classic sign of a temporal bone fracture. Bruising of the skull base in the mastoid region (Battle's sign) also identifies the injury. The diagnosis is best made on clinical grounds because skull radiographs and even CT scanning may miss up to one-half of temporal bone fractures. Treatment is usually observation during the healing phase and surgery only if the cerebrospinal fluid leak or conductive hearing loss persists. If the patient has acute vertigo or immediate facial nerve palsy, a special evaluation needs to be done for possible surgical exploration of the ear. Antibiotics are contraindicated, unless the fracture is from a penetrating injury. The prophylactic use of antibiotics usually leads to emergence of resistant organisms if later infection occurs.

Noise

Noises louder then 80 dB can cause damage to the inner ear hair cells. This damage can occur over years of exposure, as in construction work, or suddenly, as from an explosion. The typical loss will center at 4,000 Hz, where the inner ear is most sensitive. Wearing ear plugs or earmuffs is the best way to avoid injury.

Tumors

Acoustic neuromas are tumors that grow on the vestibular nerve in the internal auditory canal (see Ch. 158). They cause unilateral hearing loss by compressing the auditory nerve. A hallmark of an acoustic neuroma is decrease discrimination greater than expected given the level of hearing loss. Neurofibromatosis type II is a genetic disorder that causes bilateral acoustic neuromas (see Ch. 159). These, however, are rare. Other tumors, such as glomus jugulare tumors, squamous cell carcinomas, and metastatic tumors of the ear are unusual. Glomus tumors usually present with pulsatile tinnitus. Squamous cell carcinoma and metastatic tumors very often present with a nonhealing lesion or severe pain in the ear. Treatment depends on the extent of the disease. Surgery, radiation, or both are the usual options.

Drugs

Multiple drugs can cause hearing loss. Aminoglycosides, such as gentamicin, and chemotherapeutic drugs, such as cisplatin, are the usual drugs implicated. Other drugs, such as aspirin, can cause reversible hearing loss and tinnitus.

Menière's Disease

Fluctuating low-frequency hearing loss, tinnitus, and episodic vertigo are the classic triad of Menière's disease (see Ch. 9). Hearing usually decreases and tinnitus increases prior to the onset of the vertigo. Episodes of vertigo usually last from 0.5 to 4 hours. Between episodes, balance is usually normal. Hearing loss and tinnitus, however, persist. The etiology of Menière's disease is, in most cases, unclear. The pathophysiology is a relative overproduction of endolymph, leading to ballooning of the inner ear membranes. The eventual rupture of these membranes leads to the severe vertiginous attacks. Treatment to date varies from dietary restrictions, such as salt restrictions, to diuretic therapy. Surgery can be performed in refractory cases. Because of the unpredictable nature of the illness, the efficacy of most therapies is not well documented.

Otosclerosis

Otosclerosis is an inherited enchondral bone disorder that causes conductive hearing loss by fixing the stapes in the oval window. The onset is usually in the third or fourth decade of life. Stapedectomy or hearing aids are the usual treatment options available.

Autoimmune Hearing Loss

A rapidly progressive sensorineural hearing loss has been seen in many autoimmune diseases, such as Cogan syndrome, systemic lupus erythematosus, and Behçet's disease. A similar bilateral rapidly progressive sensorineural hearing loss without associated systemic illness has been recently described. Diagnosis to date is based on clinical features. Western blot immunoassay for the inner ear 68-kd protein may serve as a diagnostic marker.

Treatment consists of immunosuppressive doses of steroids (prednisone 60 mg per day) usually for 4 to 8 weeks with a gradual taper if the patient responds and a quick taper if not. Methotrexate has been used in some instances where steroids either lose their effectiveness or are initially ineffective.

Congenital

Hearing loss can be present at birth. Infections in utero, such as rubella, syphilis, and cytomegalovirus, can cause congenital hearing loss. Multiple genetic syndromes can also cause maldevelopment of the inner ear and hearing loss. Treatment is with hearing aids to amplify the sounds.

Strokes

Brainstem strokes are a rare cause of sensorineural hearing loss. Because of the bilateral innervation of the cochlear nucleus to the cortex, strokes are much more likely to cause problems with sound interpretation rather than actual sound perception. An argument is always made that sudden hearing loss may be a stroke phenomenon, especially in the elderly patient. Differentiation of such an isolated stroke from a viral infection is difficult at best.

TINNITUS

Noises in our heads that are not the result of outside stimuli are called tinnitus. Seventeen percent of the United States population, or over 40 million people, hear such noises. These noises can be anything from a constant hum to music to pulsatile beats. The noise and its intensity can vary from moment to moment, many times without obvious explanation. Its effects on the person can vary from an inconsequential annoyance to a major life crisis. Many times, the initial onset leads directly to an emergency room visit to rule out a brain tumor or stroke. Although usually benign in nature, tinnitus can be a major problem for many.

Types

Tinnitus is classified as either objective or subjective. Objective tinnitus can be heard by people other than those afflicted. Subjective tinnitus can be heard only by those afflicted. Much more is known about objective tinnitus because it lends itself more readily to investigation. The vast majority of patients with tinnitus, however, have the subjective type.

Objective tinnitus is usually pulsatile. Vascular causes include carotid artery aneurysms, vascular tumors such as glomus jugulare and glomus tympanicum tumors, arteriovenous malformations, and flow noises, such as a venous hum or carotid artery turbulence secondary to atherosclerosis. Spasms of muscles, such as the tensor tympani, the stapedius muscle, the palatal muscles, or the tensor and levator veli palatini can give intermittent runs of tinnitus. Spontaneously generated inner ear noises (otoacoustic emissions) are rarely loud enough to be heard.

Subjective tinnitus is more often constant or intermittent (not pulsatile). Cerumen, acute otis media, trauma to the temporal bone, and loud noise exposure are but a few of the causes. Any process that affects the hearing can lead to tinnitus. Processes that affect the central auditory system can also lead to tinnitus. The noise that is heard bears no relationship to its cause. The intensity of the tinnitus also seems to be independent of the cause. Although tinnitus can often go away, most times, when it is present for over 1 year, it is permanent.

Evaluation of Patients With Tinnitus

Evaluation of a patient with tinnitus starts out as any other evaluation should, that is, with a thorough history. Questions should be directed at determining the characteristics of the noise, such as pulsatile versus constant, unilateral versus bilateral, and intermittent versus continuous. The time of and activities surrounding the onset of the noise may also help. A history of loud noise exposure, head injury, upper respiratory infection, or change in medication may give a clue to the cause. The presence of medical problems, such as hypertension, hyperlipidemia, and hyperthyroidism, may also help pinpoint the cause.

A history of associated change in hearing or of dizziness can also be helpful.

Once the historical background is known, a physical examination should follow. The presence of wax, infection, or foreign body in the ear can lead to easily corrected causes. More often, however, the ears look normal. A thorough cranial nerve examination and cardiovascular check should follow. When the tinnitus is pulsatile, auscultation of the neck is needed to rule out a bruit.

Testing

Laboratory testing depends on what is found in the history and physical examination. When no obvious cause, such as cerumen or infection, is apparent, an audiogram should be obtained. This should include tests of air and bone conduction and speech discrimination. If the tinnitus is bilateral and a symmetric hearing loss is found, no further testing need be done. If the tinnitus is unilateral or the hearing loss is asymmetric, further testing is needed.

Brainstem auditory-evoked responses are good screening tests for retrocochlear lesions. Imaging studies, such as CT and MRI, can show up the temporal bones, skull base, and brain in great detail. Lesions such as cerebellopontine angle tumors, multiple sclerosis, infarcts, and vascular lesions can be identified. Magnetic resonance angiograms can help distinguish vascular tumors, aneurysms, arteriovenous malformations, and severe atherosclerosis.

Blood work can occasionally help pinpoint the etiology of tinnitus. Hematocrit, erythrocyte sedimentation rate, lipid studies, thyroid function tests, syphilis screening, and autoimmune evaluation can all be done. Usually, the history dictates whether these tests are indicated.

A whole battery of tests exists to characterize tinnitus and attempt to quantify it. When a person has objective tinnitus, this can be very helpful in determining the etiology. Tympanometry can show muscle myoclonus. Spontaneous otoacoustic emissions can be recorded. When a person has subjective tinnitus, however, the testing is more appropriate for a research laboratory because benefit has yet to be shown for this further type of characterization.

Treatment

Treatment for tinnitus depends on the etiology. Pulsatile tinnitus secondary to vascular tumors such as glomus jugulare and glomus tympanicum tumors can be treated with surgery or radiation. Pulsatile tinnitus secondary to hypertension can be treated medically. A venous hum can be eliminated by ligation of the jugular vein.

Audible tinnitus secondary to spontaneous acoustic emissions can be treated with salicylates. Tinnitus from muscle spasms can be controlled either surgically, by cutting the stapedius muscle or tensor tympani muscle, or with medications, such as phenytoin or carbamazepine in the case of palatal myoclonus.

Response to therapy in subjective tinnitus depends on the etiology. When a treatable cause is present, such as fluid, wax, or infection, appropriate therapy for the underlying problem usually eliminates the tinnitus. When a drug, such as a salicylate, causes the tinnitus, a change in medication eliminates the noise. When exposure to loud noise is producing the problem, ear noise protection or a change of environment may alleviate the problem.

For most people with tinnitus, none of the above situations exist. Instead the tinnitus is due to an uncorrectable cause, such as sensorineural hearing loss. For most of these patients, a knowledge of the nature of tinnitus and its benign course is satisfying. Because of the prevalence of the disorder, multiple therapeutic regimens have been devised and touted as the ultimate cure. Although a comprehensive review would not be worthwhile, a few highlights should be known.

Electrical stimulation of the ear has been tried to override the tinnitus. Alternating and direct currents have been applied to multiple different sites. Cochlear implants have been placed in the inner ear. For all of these therapies, the results thus far are not encouraging.

Tinnitus maskers are devices that replace the perceived noise with an applied noise. Some people find the applied noise more pleasant. Occasionally, the external noise causes the internal noise to go away for a short period of time after the external noise is stopped. This result, known as postmasking suppression, is however unpredictable and short-lived.

Multiple medications have been tried to block the tinnitus. Phenytoin, primidone, tocainide, niacin, vitamin A, histamine, and carbogen have all met with limited success. Many of these medications have had great initial results with minimal long-term lasting effects.

Multiple diets and alternative medicine therapies have been tried. Because stress, fatigue, and anxiety are major factors in the perception of tinnitus, therapy designed at reducing them is usually helpful, although seldom curative. Yoga, biofeedback, hypnosis, and relaxation training all help through the mechanism of stress reduction.

Most people with tinnitus learn to live with the noise. About 1 percent of patients, however, do not. These people can become severely depressed and suicidal. Appropriate psychological referral and counseling is necessary in this group to help them adjust to their illness.

For all tinnitus sufferers, a little knowledge can go a long way in alleviating anxiety. Patients need to know that tinnitus will not cause hearing loss or make them deaf. It only interferes with concentration. They need to know that tinnitus can fluctuate in tone and intensity, depending on the patient's state of mind. They need to know that the noise may be permanent but usually fades into the background. They need some reassurance that they can continue with their lives despite the presence of the noise. Fortunately, in most cases, the advice works.

SUGGESTED READINGS

Alberti PW, Ruben RJ: Otologic Medicine and Surgery. New York: Churchill Livingstone, 1988

Kitahara M: Tinnitus Pathophysiology and Management. New York: Igoku-Shoin, 1988

Konigamark BW, Godin RJ: Genetic and Metabolic Deafness. WB Saunders, Philadelphia, 1976

Mattox DE, Richtsmeier WJ: Tinnitus—the initial evaluation. Otolaryngol Head Neck Surg 96:172–4, 1987

Nadol JB Jr: Hearing loss. N Engl J Med 329:1092–102, 1993

Paparella MM, Shumrick DA: Otolaryngology. Vol. 2. WB Saunders, Philadelphia,

Puckert LG, Rees TS: Placebo effect in tinnitus management. Otolaryngol Head Neck Surg. 92:697–9, 1984

Strome M, Kelly JH, Fried MP: Manual of Otolaryngology. Little, Brown, Boston, 1992

Vernick DM: Tinnitus. pp. 1397–9. In May HL (ed): Emergency Medicine. 2nd Ed. Vol. 2. Little Brown & Company, Boston, 1992

Vernick DM, Branch WT: The painful or discharging ear. pp. 203–10. In Branch, WT, Jr (ed): Office Practice of Medicine. 3rd Ed. WB Saunders, Philadelphia, 1994

11. DISORDERS OF TASTE AND SMELL

ALLEN M. SEIDEN

The prevalence of taste and smell disorders is difficult to determine, although it has been estimated that as many as 1 to 2 percent of Americans develop chemosensory complaints. Traditionally, these patients have been difficult to diagnose and treat, owing to a general lack of knowledge about the chemical senses, as well as to the lack of clinically accessible testing methods. Although many physicians consider such a complaint a potential harbinger of intracranial pathology, little is known about the frequency with which such lesions will actually present with a chemosensory loss or when radiographs are actually indicated. In addition, the relative importance of a chemosensory problem continues to be underestimated because most clinicians fail to appreciate the devastating effect it can have on a patient's quality of life.

Typically, these patients have been to a number of health professionals in an unsuccessful attempt to get help. It is likely that they will see an internist or neurologist. If the specialist is not able to verify their disorder objectively, their complaint begins to be questioned by family, friends, and even health care providers. This lack of support only worsens their sense of isolation and despair, while at the same time increasing the likelihood that an important diagnosis may be missed.

Fortunately, chemosensory disorders have been receiving increasing attention and are currently the focus of a number of clinical taste and smell research centers that have developed around the United States. There are now well-established and proven methods for evaluating both taste and smell loss and, with these, has come an appreciation for the common causes of such dysfunction. It is important that neurologists be familiar with the current knowledge regarding chemosensory assessment and diagnosis.

ANATOMY AND PHYSIOLOGY

Three anatomically and physiologically distinct chemosensory systems interact extensively to determine our overall chemosensory experience: olfaction, gustation, and irritation (also known as the common chemical sense). The sense of smell is mediated through olfactory receptors located high in the nasal vault along the upper septum, the cribriform plate, and the medial wall of the superior turbinate. These receptors are bipolar sensory neurons the cell bodies of which lie in the basal two-thirds of the epithelium. An apical dendrite extends to the surface where it forms the olfactory knob from which several immotile cilia extend into the overlying mucous layer. Proximal to the cell body, an unmyelinated axon passes through the basal lamina where it joins other axons to form bundles now ensheathed by Schwann cells. These ultimately make up the 15 to 20 fascicles of the olfactory nerve that pass through perforations in the cribriform plate to synapse in the olfactory bulb.

To stimulate odorant perception, airborne molecules must reach the olfactory cleft and then pass through the layer of mucus that covers the epithelium. The site of chemosensory transduction is believed to be the olfactory cilia, from which the information is transmitted along the first cranial nerve to the glomerular layer of the olfactory bulb. Here a considerable convergence of information occurs, after which second-order neurons project to the olfactory cortex. The olfactory cortex, in turn, maintains widespread interconnections with other areas of the brain, including the mediodorsal thalamus, hippocampus, hypothalamus, and other areas of the limbic system. The complexity of the olfactory system is clear from the fact that we can readily identify thousands of different odorants. The method of coding this diverse information is not known. Individual receptors generally respond to several different odorants, and attempts to classify them based on their patterns of sensitivity have been unsuccessful. Studies suggest, however, that different odorants produce different sorption patterns across the olfactory mucosa, which thus functions almost like a chromatograph, and this may be instrumental in coding for different odors.

Olfactory receptor neurons undergo constant turnover. Therefore, while cutting the olfactory nerve causes retrograde degeneration of the olfactory neuroepithelium, it later regenerates from basal cells located near the lamina propria and, in animal experiments, has demonstrated reconnection to the olfactory bulb. This regenerative capacity provides, at least in theory, for the possibility of recovery following environmental insult.

The innervation for taste is more complex; as a result, true taste loss less commonly occurs. Taste buds are found in the fungiform papillae on the anterior two-thirds of the tongue, innervated by the chorda tympani nerve (cranial nerve VII); on the posterior third of the tongue within the circumvallate and foliate papillae, innervated by the glossopharyngeal nerve (cranial nerve IX); on the soft palate, innervated by the greater superficial petrosal nerve (cranial nerve VII); and within the pharynx, epiglottis, and upper esophagus, innervated by the vagus nerve (cranial nerve X).

Primary taste afferents synapse in the nucleus of the solitary tract in the medulla. Information is then transmitted via the parabrachial nuclei of the pons to the thalamus and insular cortex and to the lateral hypothalamus, stria terminalis, and amygdala. An alternative pathway connects via the reticular formation to cranial motor nuclei that control muscles involved in facial expression, licking, chewing, and swallowing.

Taste buds are modified epithelial cells containing taste receptors arranged in a columnar pattern, each projecting microvilli into a taste pore that opens into the oral cavity. This appears to be the site of transduction. A given taste receptor is responsive to more than one taste quality. In fact, contrary to popular opinion, different areas of the oral cavity do not selectively discriminate between salty, sour, sweet, and bitter; rather, all four taste qualities can be perceived throughout, although some regional differences in sensitivity are present. Precisely how this correlates with the coding of sensory information remains unknown.

Owing to their superficial location, taste buds are susceptible to injury. However, similar to the olfactory system, taste-receptor cells undergo constant regeneration from an underlying layer of basal cells. This too, then, should allow for some recovery following environmental insult.

The third chemosensory system is that of irritation, otherwise known as the common chemical sense, mediated primarily by the trigeminal nerve. The ophthalmic and maxillary divisions of the trigeminal nerve distribute free nerve endings throughout the nasal and oral mucosa. Stimulation of these receptors is perceived as burning or irritation and usually precipitates nasal and oral reflexes meant to eradicate the noxious stimulus.

Hot peppers, mustards, and similar spices add to olfactory and gustatory information by stimulating these free nerve endings. One does not ordinarily distinguish among these chemosensory systems, so that the entire sensory experience is perceived as flavor. It is important to recognize that patients sometimes confuse the ability to detect irritation as an intact sense of taste or smell. By the same token, because the common chemical sense usually remains intact in patients with taste or smell dysfunction, it can be useful in the assessment of the malingering patient.

DIFFERENTIAL DIAGNOSIS

Numerous terms have been used to describe the various manifestations of taste and smell dysfunction; however, it is important that terminology be standardized (Table 11-1). It is worth noting that anosmia, hyposmia, ageusia, and hypogeusia are readily detected by current testing methods. Hyperosmia and hypergeusia, while occasionally reported by patients, are difficult to measure objectively.

By the same token, dysosmia and dysgeusia are frequent complaints but are not measurable by current methods. Dysosmia usually occurs in association with an olfactory loss that may be from any number of etiologies, although in our experience it seems to occur more commonly with viral-induced loss. In addition, phantosmias have been described in association with seizure activity, psychiatric illness, and Alzheimer's disease.

In contrast, dysgeusia tends to occur without a complaint of taste loss, although thorough testing often reveals an associated spatial ageusia. Dysgeusia is often caused by dental disease and the use of certain medications, but it may also occur in association with gastroesophageal reflux and postnasal drip or be caused by peripheral nerve injury, exposure to toxins, or stroke.

More than 200 conditions and 40 medications have been reported to cause taste and smell disorders, although much of this information remains anecdotal. However, as the various clinical taste and smell research centers continue to gather data, more is learned about the common causes of taste and smell problems. Table 11-2 lists the etiology of dysfunction in 307 consecutive patients seen at the University of Cincinnati Taste and Smell Center. The majority of these patients were found to have an olfactory loss, whereas only a very small minority in fact had a measurable taste loss (see below).

TABLE 11-1. Definitions of Chemosensory Dysfunction

Anosmia: complete loss of smell
Hyposmia: diminished smell sensitivity
Partial anosmia: inability to detect certain odorants
Partial hyposmia: diminished sensitivity to some odorants
Hyprosmia: increased odorant sensitivity
Dysosmia: distortion in odorant perception
  Parosmia: in response to a specific stimulus
  Phantosmia: no external stimulus present
Ageusia: complete loss of taste
Hypogeusia: diminished taste sensitivity
Hypergeusia: increased taste sensitivity
Dysgeusia: distortion in taste perception

TABLE 11-2. Etiologies of Taste and Smell Dysfunction at the University of Cincinnati Taste and Smell Center

Category	No.	%
Nasal/sinus disease	55	18
Head trauma	56	18
Prior upper respiratory infection	56	18
Idiopathic	67	22
Multiple	17	6
Toxic exposure	18	6
Congenital	8	3
Miscellaneous	26	8
Age	4	1
Total	307	100

Olfactory Loss

It has been our experience that the most common causes of smell loss clearly relate to nasal or sinus disease, a prior viral infection, or an episode of head trauma. These categories account for 54 percent of our patients, and other centers have reported similar results.

In the case of nasal and sinus disease, secondary inflammatory changes in the nose obstruct the nasal vault and, therefore, the olfactory receptors. It is a conductive loss rather than a neurosensory loss and, as such, is usually amenable to therapy. For this reason, it is important to make the appropriate diagnosis and not to mistake these patients for those with a viral-induced loss.

It is obvious that patients with severe nasal obstruction secondary to diffuse nasal polyps also have an olfactory impairment. However, in many cases, the nasal airway may be preserved while the olfactory vault is obstructed by polyps located high in the nose or by mucosal edema secondary to chronic underlying sinus obstruction. Such findings are not readily apparent on a routine nasal examination, and such patients may be lacking in other nasal symptoms.

There are a number of clues that suggest a conductive loss. The degree of smell loss is usually severe, with most patients found to be anosmic or severely hyposmic. However, this loss usually fluctuates with the degree of nasal congestion. Activities that are associated with nasal decongestion, such as exercise, heavy lifting, or showering, sometimes produce a temporary improvement in smell sensitivity. Administration of systemic corticosteroid and, less often, topical steroids will also improve olfactory function in these patients and can be used diagnostically because they should have no effect on olfactory loss secondary to other causes. Ultimately, a thorough nasal examination, which is best done endoscopically with a fiberoptic telescope, is necessary. This usually requires referral to an otolaryngologist, which is recommended in any patient with a history suggesting nasal or sinus pathology.

The diagnosis of viral-induced anosmia or hyposmia is based primarily on the occurrence of a viral illness or cold just prior to the onset of olfactory loss in the absence of any other clear etiology. These patients often describe an upper respiratory infection that was more severe than usual. As the symptoms of congestion resolved, however, their sense of smell never returned. Exactly what predisposes some cases of viral illness to result in olfactory loss is as yet unknown; however, the pathophysiologic mechanism seems to involve a direct insult to the olfactory epithelium. On the other hand, the olfactory epithelium has been demonstrated to be a possible route of viral invasion to the central nervous system, and therefore central olfactory pathways may also be involved.

There are no confirmatory physical findings to help diagnose postviral olfactory loss. However, in contrast to patients with nasal and sinus disease, these patients tend more often to be hyposmic rather than anosmic, and symptoms do not fluctuate. In addition, they frequently complain of dysosmia, tend to be older, and tend to be female.

Prognosis in this group has been uncertain. In theory, the possibility of recovery exists because of the capacity of the olfactory epithelium to regenerate, but this has never been systematically studied. Recently, however, we reviewed this group of patients and found that, in fact, almost all of them demonstrate some improvement over a 3 to 5-year period. This occurs spontaneously, with no specific effective therapy having been found.

Post-traumatic olfactory loss is also commonly seen in our clinic and is also diagnosed largely by history; it occurs in approximately 5 percent of patients with head trauma. The loss is immediate, although depending on the severity of injury, it may not be immediately recognized by the patient. The presumed mechanism is shearing of the olfactory fila as they pass through the cribriform plate as a result of coup-contrecoup forces, and it is, therefore, more likely to occur with a frontal or occipital blow. However, smell loss may also occur following intracranial hemorrhage and cerebral ischemia without disruption of the olfactory nerve.

These patients typically present with anosmia or severe hyposmia. Again, there is a potential for regeneration and recovery, but in our experience this seems unlikely. Reports generally indicate that one-third of patients demonstrate some improvement; however, whether this is due to actual neural regeneration or simply to resolution of the contusion has not been determined.

The next and largest category in Table 11-2 encompasses idiopathic cases, those patients for whom a specific cause for their taste or smell complaint was not determined. This simply points out that there is still a great deal about chemosensory disorders that remains unclear. It is expected that, as our experience increases, so will our ability to identify cause and effect.

In a number of patients, multiple potential causes appeared to exist; a single specific cause could not be identified. For example, a patient may have described having an upper respiratory infection at the same time as being exposed to toxic inhalants at work.

We have, in fact, seen 18 patients in whom a measurable olfactory loss could be traced to a toxic exposure, usually experienced at the workplace. Unfortunately, the diagnosis is based solely on the coincidence of exposure just prior to the onset of loss, and histologic correlation is lacking. A number of environmental and industrial agents have been linked to anosmia or hyposmia, such as benzene, formaldehyde, paint solvents, and cadmium and nickel dusts, but reports remain largely anecdotal. The exposure in such cases is usually excessive, and the prognosis for recovery remains uncertain.

We have seen eight patients with congenital olfactory loss, all of whom were found to be anosmic. The literature describes a number of endocrine disorders associated with congenital anosmia, such as Kallmann syndrome (hypogonadotropic hypogonadism) and Turner syndrome, but our patients had no such abnormalities. A preliminary biopsy study has shown the presence of an incompletely developed olfactory neuroepithelium in these patients.

The category of miscellaneous in Table 11-2 refers to a variety of clearly definable etiologies that perhaps are not unusual causes of olfactory loss but are uncommon in patients presenting to a taste and smell clinic. As such, they are grouped together, but include, for example, prior craniofacial surgery, stroke, seizure disorder, and radiation therapy. Potential neurologic causes of olfactory loss are discussed further below.

Although olfactory loss may frequently be attributed to age, in reality, there appears to be little effect until the age of 65, after which there is generally a gradual decline in identification ability and elevation in threshold. This seems to be related to a progressive but patchy replacement of the olfactory epithelium with respiratory epithelium. Whether this occurs secondary to the aging process or to repeated environmental insult is unclear. In any event, it is important to compare olfactory testing in the older age group with age-matched controls.

Olfactory Loss Related to Systemic Neurologic Diseases

As alluded to earlier, our taste and smell clinic is an ambulatory center to which patients generally are referred with a primary chemosensory complaint. In that respect, this may be a somewhat skewed population, such that we do not often see patients with a variety of systemic or metabolic disorders that frequently may be associated with taste or smell dysfunction. Nevertheless, there are reports that have explored olfactory loss as an associated symptom of neurodegenerative disease.

Smell function may be impaired when disease involves central or peripheral olfactory pathways. For example, the demyelinating effects of multiple sclerosis have been found to be associated with smell loss, although the pattern varies depending on the distribution of disease. Patients with temporal lobe epilepsy have diminished odor identification but maintain normal thresholds; it is thought that this may relate more to defective odor memory processing rather than a true sensory impairment.

A great deal of research has focused on the neuropathology of the olfactory pathways in Alzheimer's disease. Damage has been demonstrated in the olfactory epithelium, and characteristic neuritic plaques and neurofibrillary tangles seem to involve the olfactory bulb, tract, and olfactory cortex preferentially. As stated above, there is evidence that environmental toxins or infectious agents may gain access to the central nervous system through the olfactory neuroepithelium. Therefore, it has been theorized that the olfactory system may provide a route of entry to the central nervous system for some neurotoxic agent that may well be responsible for the development of Alzheimer's disease and perhaps other neurodegenerative diseases.

Olfactory loss is present early in the development of Alzheimer's disease and, in time, may serve as a useful clinical marker for the illness. However, the degree of dysfunction is clearly related to the severity of the dementia. This was verified in patients who were able to demonstrate the cognitive ability to perform olfactory testing correctly, as determined by their performance on picture identification testing.

Significant olfactory dysfunction has also been demonstrated in Parkinson's disease with elevated thresholds and impaired identification ability. The degree of loss in these cases does not seem to correlate with patient age, the duration of symptoms, or the severity of disease. In addition, pharmacologic manipulation with various antiparkinsonian medications has not been found to alter the olfactory loss.

Other disorders associated with dementia that have also been found to involve olfactory loss include Huntington's chorea and Korsakoff's psychosis.

As previously stated, most of these patients will likely develop other neurologic signs that prompt presentation to a physician. Nevertheless, olfactory loss is one manifestation that can be measured and, ultimately, may prove useful in the early detection of some of these disorders as well as in their differential diagnosis.

Gustatory Loss

Although complaints of taste loss are common, such complaints are, in fact, usually the result of an olfactory loss (see below). A true measurable taste loss is distinctly uncommon, and this is due to the wider distribution of gustatory receptors that are innervated by several different cranial nerves as compared to the olfactory system (see Anatomy and Physiology above).

Both a prior viral respiratory infection and head injury have been related to subsequent taste loss. Bilateral traumatically induced taste loss is seen in 0.5 percent of head-injured patients and in 5 to 6 percent of patients with post-traumatic anosmia. However, it is more likely that a localized or spatial ageusia will occur from injury to specific cranial nerves. For example, a temporal bone fracture may injure the chorda tympani nerve, depleting taste to the anterior two-thirds of the tongue, while the remainder of gustatory innervation remains intact.

Such spatial ageusia is usually asymptomatic in that the patient rarely recognizes a taste loss. This may be related to a release-of-inhibition phenomenon. In other words, it has been suggested that, under ordinary circumstances, each of the gustatory nerves produces a reciprocal inhibition of the other, influencing the overall taste sensation. When injury occurs to one of these nerves, this in essence releases its inhibitory effect, with the result being that overall taste perception remains the same. On the other hand, many of these patients seem to experience dysgeusia, which may also be related to this release-of-inhibition phenomenon.

Dysgeusia is a particularly troubling problem because it is essentially always unpleasant and often interferes with the enjoyment of eating. It is often described as a persistent salty, bitter, or rancid taste that may or may not be masked by food. Although, in many cases, an etiology remains obscure, it is important to rule out any oral or dental pathology. For example, older, debilitated, or immunocompromised patients are prone to oral thrush or xerostomia, both of which may cause dysgeusia. A listing of medications is important because a number of medications may yield detectable levels in saliva, resulting in secondary dysgeusia.

EVALUATION

History

When taking a history with regard to olfactory or taste loss, it is important to try to assess the degree of loss and its duration. It may take some time for patients to recognize the presence of such a loss; so the loss is usually of fairly long standing when they present for medical evaluation. Particular attention should be paid to any antecedent event that may be related to symptom onset, such as a prior upper respiratory infection, traumatic incident, or toxic exposure. One should focus initially on ruling out the three most common causes of chemosensory loss (see above), unless other specific symptoms direct otherwise.

It is also important to question associated complaints, including dysosmia and dysgeusia. If the patient admits to a fluctuation in smell sensitivity, this would suggest that the problem is conductive and likely related to nasal or sinus pathology. Any associated systemic symptoms or medical conditions that might be contributory need to be evaluated, as does the list of medications that can often be associated with chemosensory disorders.

An important point needs to be emphasized. It is very unusual for a patient to present with complaints of smell loss and not have that loss borne out by olfactory testing. On the other hand, many of these patients also complain of taste loss and, in fact, may even present for that reason, unaware that an associated olfactory deficit exists. On actual testing, however, most of these patients have a normal sense of taste.

Of 750 patients presenting to the University of Pennsylvania Smell and Taste Center, 78.1 percent complained of a reduced ability to smell and 66.4 percent of a reduced ability to taste. Measurement of taste and smell function in these patients revealed that 70.9 percent did, in fact, have an olfactory deficit; however, less than 3 percent had a measurable taste deficit.

The point is that there is a common confusion among patients regarding taste and flavor. The appreciation of flavor involves olfactory, tactile, and thermal qualities as well as taste, so that a loss of any of these modalities might be interpreted as a diminution in ''taste.'' Olfactory input is perhaps the most important contribution to flavor perception. Therefore, when taking a history, it is much more predictive if the clinician asks specifically whether the patient can distinguish the four taste qualities (i.e. salty, sour, sweet, and bitter).

A true taste loss is distinctly uncommon and, as mentioned earlier, may go unnoticed if confined to localized areas. When a measurable taste loss is present, the history needs to focus on any possible illness or procedure that may have resulted in neurologic injury. These may include neurologic and otologic procedures and also tonsillectomy and recent dental surgery. Because of the extensive neural input responsible for taste, complete ageusia is uncommon and has been detected by us in only one patient in over 300. The etiology in this patient remains obscure but presumably reflects some sort of central neurologic pathology.

Physical Examination

A complete head and neck examination is essential; the remainder of the examination is largely directed by the history. In the case of prior head injury, few other findings may be present. On the other hand, it may not always be possible to distinguish a viral-induced loss from a conductive loss simply based on the history. The former group may continue to have symptoms of rhinitis. The latter may describe recurrent bouts of infection that clearly may have been viral in origin, and they will not always experience a fluctuation in their olfactory sensitivity. Therefore, a thorough nasal examination is very important.

As alluded to earlier, if patients complain of other nasal symptoms or if the etiology of their loss remains unknown, then referral to an otolaryngologist is warranted. A thorough endoscopic examination of the nose is necessary to rule out underlying infection, polyps, neoplasia, or other inflammatory conditions that may sufficiently obstruct the olfactory vault.

If the patient's loss cannot be related to nasal or viral pathology, trauma, or some sort of toxic exposure, then a search must

be made for another less common etiology. In this case, a full neurologic examination is important. Although it is unlikely that a patient who has had a stroke, for example, would present initially with only a chemosensory complaint, there are a number of neurologic disorders for which olfactory loss may be an early symptom (see above).

When patients present with hypogeusia or dysgeusia, a thorough oral examination is imperative. This includes an assessment of oral hygiene and the condition of the teeth, restorations, prostheses, gingivitis, halitosis, and the presence of any mucosal lesions. Common underlying maladies include candidiasis, xerostomia, chronic sialadenitis, and cryptic tonsillitis. A referral to a dentist or otolaryngologist should again be considered. A further delineation of dysgeusia as a manifestation of central or peripheral origin can be made by the application of a mild topical anesthetic.

Olfactory Testing

A number of well-established, standardized tests are now available for measuring an olfactory loss. Perhaps the most popular is the University of Pennsylvania Smell Identification Test, developed at the University of Pennsylvania and available from Sensonics (Haddonfield, NJ). This test consists of four booklets, each with 10 microencapsulated odorants on a small scratch and sniff pad (Fig. 11-1). The patient must scratch the pad, sniff the odorant, and select one of four possible odorant choices for each question.

Extensive normative data for both sex and age exists for this test, allowing for accurate interpretation (Doty et al., 1984). In addition, it has demonstrated excellent test-retest reliability. Normal subjects in general should be able to identify 35 to 40 of the odorants correctly. A score of 20 to 34 is considered representative of hyposmia, and a score below 20 is consistent with anosmia. Because this is a forced-choice test, a score of approximately 10 would be expected based simply on chance. Therefore, a score much below this suggests malingering.

A significant advantage of this test is that it is simple and inexpensive to administer, requiring no trained personnel, and

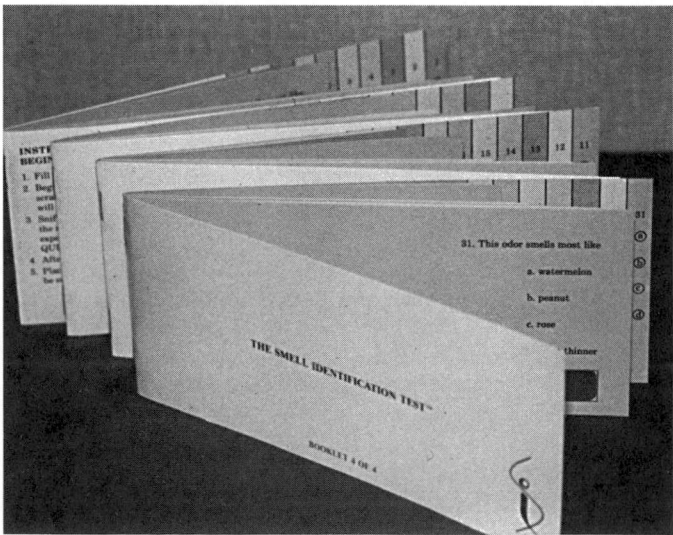

FIG. 11-1. University of Pennsylvania Smell Identification Test, which consists of four booklets. Each booklet contains 10 microencapsulated odorants on a scratch and sniff pad, available through Sensonics (Haddenfield, NJ).

therefore probably makes the most sense in a clinical setting that is not specialized to evaluate chemosensory disorders.

In our clinic, we also administer two tests that were developed at the Connecticut Chemosensory Clinical Research Center (Cain et al., 1988). The first is a threshold test, utilizing butanol as a reference odorant. The patient is presented with a series of dilutions in opaque squeeze bottles, alternating with bottles containing only water. The threshold is that dilution that the patient correctly selects on five consecutive trials, and this is determined for each nostril.

The second test is another odor identification test, in which the patient is presented with seven different odorants each wrapped in gauze and placed in a glass jar. The test items are commonly found food and household products. The patient holds one nostril closed and then, after sniffing the jar, must identify the name of the odorant from a list of 20 choices. An eighth jar contains a trigeminal stimulant, usually Vicks VapoRub, that serves as a useful control for malingering.

Typically, the threshold and identification test scores are combined into a composite score for each nostril. This result then indicates the level of olfactory loss. The advantage of this battery is the ability to detect unilateral differences.

Currently, there is no method of testing for dysosmia. However, dysosmia is usually associated with some degree of olfactory loss, more commonly seen in cases of mild to moderate hyposmia. Therefore, olfactory testing is important in these patients. The abnormal smell should be characterized by history as to its quality, frequency, intensity, and relationship to any particular environmental exposure.

Taste Testing

Taste testing is not performed in every patient who presents with a taste complaint because, as mentioned earlier, most of these patients actually have an olfactory loss. Such testing is indicated if (1) by history, the patient cannot distinguish the four basic taste qualities, (2) the patient complains of a taste loss despite normal olfactory test results, (3) the patient complains of dysgeusia, or (4) the patient with an olfactory loss is not convinced that this loss accounts for the perceived decreased appreciation of food but also feels that a true taste loss has been suffered.

Stock solutions of the four taste qualities are used (i.e., sweet [1 M sucrose], salty [1 M sodium chloride], sour [0.032 M citric acid], and bitter [0.001 M quinine hydrochloride]). Four serial dilutions are made for each, all of which are both colorless and odorless.

A simple screen for taste loss is to ask the patient to identify 5 ml of each of the four strongest solutions. The patient is given the sample in a medicine cup, swishes it around the mouth, and then spits it out. Between samples, the mouth is rinsed with distilled water.

A more thorough assessment involves a taste scaling procedure in which the patient is given various dilutions, and is asked to identify both its quality and intensity. To try to standardize intensity ratings, a method of magnitude matching is used. Patients are asked to equate a very strong taste stimulus with a very loud sound, and a very weak taste stimulus with a barely audible sound. A rating scale of 1 to 9 is used.

Someone with a focal taste deficit would nevertheless tend to perform normally on the taste scaling test, which involves whole-mouth testing. Spatial testing allows an evaluation of each of the cranial nerves involved in gustation and should

therefore detect such a loss. A cotton-tipped applicator is used to apply a sample of the strongest concentration of each of the four taste solutions. Application is made to the four quadrants of the tongue and to the left and right soft palate, and the patient must again identify the quality and rate the intensity of the solution. If necessary, the lingual nerve can also be tested by applying cold or hot distilled water.

Radiologic Evaluation

In the evaluation of olfactory loss, it must be remembered that the most common causes are diagnosed by history and physical examination. Therefore, radiologic studies are not ordered routinely. For example, if the patient's history clearly indicates that an upper respiratory infection preceded the loss and there are no associated neurologic signs or symptoms, we do not obtain radiologic studies.

On the other hand, in the absence of a clear etiology, the possibility of intracranial pathology becomes more relevant, albeit remote. An enlarging olfactory groove meningioma, pituitary tumors with suprasellar extension, frontal lobe gliomas, and large aneurysms of the anterior cerebral or anterior communicating arteries may produce a gradual onset of anosmia. Most of these patients will, of course, not likely present with olfactory loss as their only complaint. However, when a measurable olfactory loss is present and its cause is not apparent, then we usually obtain a magnetic resonance imaging scan.

If the clinician suspects underlying inflammatory sinus disease, then radiographs are helpful to delineate the extent of disease. In these cases, computed tomographic scans are usually more valuable than plain radiographs because the bony anatomy is more apparent. The coronal plane is preferred because the olfactory cleft, nasal vault, and ostiomeatal complex are more clearly displayed. If neoplasia of the nose or sinuses is suspected, then a magnetic resonance imaging scan should also be considered to delineate any intracranial extension more clearly.

THERAPY

In most patients presenting with a chemosensory loss, the etiology will be definable. However, at our current level of understanding, only those with a conductive olfactory loss or an inflammatory oral condition producing hypogeusia or dysgeusia will be amenable to treatment.

Clearly, patients with nasal or sinus disease should be referred to an otolaryngologist for aggressive medical and, in some cases, surgical therapy. In general, these patients should expect improvement in their conductive smell loss, although this may require ongoing therapy, depending on the underlying condition. In the case of postviral smell or taste loss, no specific therapy has been found to be effective, including topical or systemic steroids.

Although the diagnosis of traumatically induced olfactory loss is fairly straightforward, there is again no specific therapy. Recovery in this group seems less likely to occur, indicating that the injury suffered is more difficult for the system to repair. This would coincide with a more proximal site of injury (i.e., the cribriform plate and olfactory nerve) rather than the peripheral neuroepithelium.

Based on studies done in the 1960s, there is a widespread misconception that zinc therapy is helpful in patients with chemosensory dysfunction. However, more recent data refute this notion, and clearly there is no basis for zinc supplementation unless the patient has a zinc deficiency. This is a rare occurrence but has been reported to be associated with hypogeusia. This is the only established indication for zinc.

Unfortunately, for most patients who present with chemosensory loss, no specific therapy is currently available. Nevertheless, it is important to document the degree of loss and try to determine its etiology. This not only facilitates the diagnosis of any associated pathology but also allows counseling of the patient about the prognosis. In addition, patients generally describe a certain sense of relief that their loss is real and that their complaint is taken seriously. Therefore, it is important that any patient presenting with a complaint of taste or smell loss be appropriately and thoroughly evaluated.

SUGGESTED READINGS

Amoore JE: Effects of chemical exposure on olfaction in humans. pp. 155–90. In Barrow CS (ed): Toxicology of the Nasal Passages. Hemisphere Publishing, Washington, DC, 1986

Bartoshuk LM: Taste: robust across the age span? Ann N Y Acad Sci 561: 65–75, 1989

Bartoshuk LM, Gent J, Catalanotto FA et al: Clinical evaluation of taste. Am J Otolaryngol 4:257–60, 1983

Cain WS, Gent J, Goodspeed RB et al: Evaluation of olfactory dysfunction in the Connecticut Chemosensory Clinical Research Center. Laryngoscope 98:83–8, 1988

Costanzo RM, Becker DP: Smell and taste disorders in head injury and neurosurgery patients. p. 565. In Meiselman HL, Rivlin RS (eds): Clinical Measurement of Taste and Smell. MacMillan, New York, 1986

Deems DA, Doty RL, Settle G et al: Smell and taste disorders, a study of 750 patients from the University of Pennsylvania Smell and Taste Center. Arch Otolaryngol Head Neck Surg 117:519, 1991

Doty RL: Olfactory dysfunction in neurodegenerative disorders. pp. 735–51. In Getchell TV, Doty RL, Bartoshuk LM, Snow JB (eds): Smell and Taste in Health and Disease. Raven Press, New York, 1991

Doty RL, Reyes PF, Gregor T: Presence of both odor identification and detection deficits in Alzheimer's disease. Brain Res Bull 18:597–600, 1987

Doty RL, Shaman P, Dann M: Development of the University of Pennsylvania Identification Test: a standardized microencapsulated test of olfactory function. Physiol Behav 32:489–502, 1984

Duncan HJ, Seiden AM, Smith DV: Long term follow-up of olfactory loss secondary to head trauma and upper respiratory infections. Arch Otolaryngol Head Neck Surg (accepted for publication)

Goodspeed RB, Gent JF, Catalanotto FA: Chemosensory dysfunction: clinical evaluation results from a taste and smell clinic. Postgrad Med 81:251–60, 1987

Graziadei PPC, Monti-Graziadei GA: Regeneration in the olfactory system of vertebrates. Am J Otolaryngol 4:228–33, 1983

Henkin RI, Schecter PJ, Friedewald WT et al: A double blind study of the effects of zinc sulfate on taste and smell dysfunction. Am J Med Sci 272: 285, 1976

Hornung DE, Mozell MM: Factors influencing the differential sorption of odorant molecules across the olfactory mucosa. J Gen Physiol 69:343–61, 1977

Jafek BW: Ultrastructure of human nasal mucosa. Laryngoscope 93:1576–99, 1983

Jafek BW, Hartmen D, Eller PM et al: Postviral olfactory dysfunction. Am J Rhinol 4:91–100, 1990

Monath TP, Cropp CB, Harrison AK: Mode of entry of a neurotropic arbovirus into the central nervous system: reinvestigation of an old controversy. Lab Invest 48:399–410, 1983

Nakashima T, Kimmelman CP, Snow JB: Progressive olfactory degeneration due to ischemia. Surg Forum 34:566–68, 1983

Paik SI, Lehman MN, Seiden AM et al: Human olfactory biopsy: the influence of age and receptor distribution. Arch Otolaryngol Head Neck Surg 118: 731–8, 1992

Paik SI, Seiden AM, Duncan HJ, Smith DV: Olfactory mucosal biopsy in patients with congenital anosmia. Chem Senses 16:566, 1991

Pryse-Phillips W: Disturbance in the sense of smell in psychiatric patients. Proc R Soc Med 68:472, 1975

Report of the Panel on Communicative Disorders to the National Advisory Neurological and Communicative Disorders and Stroke Council. Public Health Service, Washington, DC, 1979

Rollin H: Drug-related gustatory disorders. Ann Otol 87:37, 1978

Schecter PJ, Friedewald WT, Bronzert OA et al: Idiopathic hypogeusia: a description of the syndrome and a single-blind study with zinc sulfate. Int Rev Neurobiol, suppl. 1:125, 1972

Seiden AM, Duncan HJ, Smith DV: Office management of taste and smell disorders. Otolaryngol Clin North Am 25:817–35, 1992

Smith DV: Taste and smell dysfunction. pp. 1911–34. In Paparella MM, Shumrick DA, Gluckman JL et al (eds): Otolaryngology-Head and Neck. 3rd Ed. Vol. 3. WB Saunders, Philadelphia, 1990

Smith DV, Shipley MT: Anatomy and physiology of taste and smell. J Head Trauma Rehabil 7:1–14, 1992

Talamo BR, Rudel RA, Kosik KS et al: Pathologic changes in olfactory neurons in patients with Alzheimer's disease. Nature 337:736–9, 1989

12. DYSARTHRIA AND DYSPHAGIA

JENNIFER HORNER
E. WAYNE MASSEY

Acquired neurogenic speech and oropharyngeal swallowing disorders are both fascinating and useful to the neurology clinician. They are useful because they may herald the onset of a neurologic disease, reflect its pathophysiology, correlate with its progression, or mark its regression as a result of either natural history or treatment. Dysarthria and dysphagia can be acute, paroxysmal, or insidious and slowly progressive, and they can occur in isolation or as part of a multifaceted neurologic syndrome. Despite their frequent concurrence, dysarthria and dysphagia are dissociable, a phenomenon that speaks to the specificity of the disease process. Although the various manifestations or "types" of dysarthria typically signal the location of the neurologic disease, oropharyngeal dysphagia is usually more general in its presentation and therefore less localizable. Disease processes associated with these disorders include vascular disease (e.g., infarction, hemorrhage, and malformations), neoplasms (intra- and extracranial), inflammations (central or peripheral), demyelinating disease (e.g., multiple sclerosis), immunologic disorders (e.g., myasthenia gravis), infections (e.g., Lyme disease, herpes, rabies, and leprosy), toxins (e.g., drugs, arsenic, lead, and mercury), immunodeficiency diseases (e.g., acquired immunodeficiency syndrome), and extrinsic compression (e.g., cervical spondylosis and lymphadenopathy). Neurologic syndromes associated with dysarthria and/or oropharyngeal dysphagia are summarized in Table 12-1.

DYSARTHRIA

Characterization

Acquired dysarthria is not attributable to a speech delay or learning disorder, aphasia, delirium, dementia, anatomic anomaly, or psychiatric illness, though these disorders may at times concur with, mask, or mimic a dysarthria. *Dysarthria is caused by, and attributable to, motor and/or sensory impairments of the neural control mechanisms subserving respiration, phonation, resonance, articulation, and/or prosody.* Dysarthria may result from central or peripheral nervous system compromise, be it unilateral or bilateral in character. Dysarthria reflects neurologic abnormalities in many muscle groups (e.g., spastic dysarthria in pseudobulbar palsy) or single muscles (e.g., dysphonia secondary to unilateral vocal fold paralysis). Dysarthria is com-

TABLE 12-1. Some Syndromes Associated With Dysarthria and Oropharyngeal Dysphagia

Anatomic Level	Syndrome
Cortex	Stroke syndromes (e.g., opercular syndrome, akinetic mutism)
	Dementia (e.g., Alzheimer's disease)
	Phakomatosis (e.g., Sturge-Weber)
Subcortex	Unilateral and bilateral upper motor neuron stroke
	Pseudobulbar palsy
	Multi-infarct syndrome and small vessel disease
	Progressive supranuclear palsy
	Capsular syndrome
	Hypophonia (thalamus, caudate)
	Mutism (bilateral thalamus)
	Tabes dorsalis
Extrapyramidal	Parkinsonism
	Parkinson's disease
	Tardive dyskinesia
	Huntington's disease
	Sydenham's chorea
	Choreoacanthocytosis
	Perivenous encephalomyelitis
	Hepatolenticular degeneration (Wilson's disease)
	Tourette's syndrome
	Orofacial dyskinesia (Meige)
	Spasmodic torticollis
	Paraneoplastic disorders
Cerebellum	Cerebellar degeneration (toxic, paraneoplastic)
	Spinocerebellar degeneration (e.g., Friedreich's ataxia)
	Stroke
	Paroxysmal dysarthria
	Developmental malformations (e.g., Chiari)
Brainstem	Stroke syndromes (e.g., dysarthria-clumsy hand syndrome, lateral medullary syndrome)
	Jugular foramen syndrome
	Central pontine myelinolysis
	Locked-in syndrome
	Akinetic mutism (reticular activating system)
	Palatopharyngolaryngeal myoclonus
	Essential (familial) tremor
	Syringobulbia
	Chiari malformation
Motor neuron	Motor neuron disease (amyotrophic lateral sclerosis)
	Poliomyelitis
	Postpolio syndrome
Myoneural junction	Myasthenia gravis
	Lambert-Eaton myasthenic syndrome
	Botulism, reaction to botulinum toxin
Peripheral nerves and muscles	Muscular dystrophies
	Myotonic disorders
	Metabolic myopathies
	Polymyositis/dermatomyositis
	Polyarteritis nodosa
	Collagen vascular diseases (e.g., systemic lupus erythematosis)
	Reaction to botulinum toxin
	Polyneuroradiculopathies (e.g., Guillain-Barré syndrome)
	Idiopathic seventh cranial nerve palsy (Bell's palsy)
	Amyloidosis
	Glosopharyngeal neuralgia
	Hereditary neuropathies (e.g., Charcot-Marie-Tooth disease)
Multiple anatomic sites	Demyelinating disease (e.g., multiple sclerosis)
	Acquired immunodeficiency syndome
	Creutzfeldt-Jakob disease
	Multisystem atrophy (e.g., Shy-Drager)
	Tetanus
	Hyperparathyroidism
	Paraneoplastic syndromes
	Encephalomyelitis (e.g., Rocky Mountain spotted fever, Lyme disease)
	Sarcoidosis

mon in neurologic disease and may manifest as subtle alterations in speech quality or as a severe limitation of speech production to the point of mutism. In this chapter, the singular term "dysarthria" will be used to refer to this heterogeneous group of neurologic speech disorders. Table 12-2 defines the basic subsystems of speech and associated deviant speech dimensions; Table 12-3 shows the recognized neural substrates of major types of dysarthria.

History and Examination

A neurologic examination should look for findings associated with the diseases mentioned in Table 12-1. A more detailed examination of speech should seek to characterize the dysarthria to provide clues to the neurologic localization of dysfunction (Table 12-3) and the subsystems of speech involved (Table 12-2). This last goal especially is greatly facilitated by consultation with a speech-language pathologist with specialized training and experience in neurologic disorders. Other specialty consultations and referrals are helpful once the diagnostic questions are defined (e.g., otolaryngology and pulmonary medicine).

Special Tests

The sole instrument for detecting the presence of dysarthria is the ear of the examiner. If the trained listener does not hear dysarthria, it does not exist. Modalities helpful for determining the underlying physiologic deficits are familiar to the neurologist and include visual observation (e.g., of abnormal range, dysmetria, or dystonia), and tactile assessment (e.g., of posture, strength, reflexes, and tone). Clinical and instrumental evaluation approaches are summarized in Table 12-4.

Differential Diagnosis

Broadly defined, the term dysarthria properly includes all aberrations of speech attributable to neurologic impairment, including acquired fluency disorders (e.g., palilalia) and voice disorders (e.g., spasmodic dysphonia). For the sake of clarity, and out of respect for traditional taxonomies, these disorders have been included among the differential diagnoses (Table 12-5).

Management

Management is directed to the underlying causes, as discussed in other sections of this text. In addition, the dysarthria per se may be amenable to several general approaches to therapy (Table 12-6). The management of dysarthria requires a shared emphasis on the physiologic deficits underlying the dysarthria and the perceptual end product, speech intelligibility. The therapies for dysarthria are directed to the remediation or amelioration of the physiologic impairments, as manifested in abnormal speech quality. General management considerations include the acuity or chronicity of the disease, the cognitive status of the patient (including learning ability, motivation, and compliance), the presence of coexisting diseases, the overall severity of dysarthria, as well as the effectiveness of concurrent medical treatment. A multitude of individualized therapy techniques usually involve some combination of preventive, compensatory, restorative, augmented, and prosthetic therapy approaches.

DYSPHAGIA

Characterization

Disorders of the oropharyngeal or esophageal swallowing mechanism often reflect an underlying structural or neurologic abnormality. When caused by either congenital or acquired neurologic disease, the term neurogenic dysphagia is commonly used, and the term neurogenic oropharyngeal dysphagia specifically refers to oropharyngeal dysfunction, as distinct from esophageal dysfunction. Although many non-neurologic organic etiologies can account for dysphagia, and psychological factors may aggravate the condition, our discussion is limited

TABLE 12-2. Basic Subsystems of Speech and Associated Deviant Speech Dimensions

Speech Subsystem	Definition	Neurologic Substrates	Deviant Speech Dimensions[a]
Respiration	The pulmonary foundation of speech: expiratory air drives vocal fold abduction and adduction and effects the production of sound throughout the upper respiratory tract; intricately related to phonation.	Subserved for inspiration by spinal nerves at levels C2–C8, T1–T12, the phrenic nerve, and CN XI spinal accessory and for expiration, spinal nerves T1–T12.	Short phrases Monoloudness Loudness decay; decrescendo Excessively elevated or low loudness Excess loudness variation; alternating loudness Forced inspiration-expiration Grunt at end of expiration
Phonation	The production of voice as a by-product of respiratory air flow, contraction-relaxation of intrinsic laryngeal muscles, passive and active movement of the vocal folds, and elevation-depression of the larynx by virtue of the activity of extrinsic laryngeal muscles.	Intrinsic laryngeal muscles, subserved by CN X; extrinsic laryngeal muscles, by CN V, VII, XI, and XII, and C1–C3 via ansa cervicalis.	Audible inspiration; inspiratory stridor Excessively low or high pitch Monopitch Pitch breaks Diplophonia Voice tremor Voice stoppages Continuous voicing, mistiming of voice on-offset Hoarse voice (aperiodic roughness) Harsh voice (periodic roughness) Strain-strangled voice Continuous or transient breathiness
Resonance	The product of complex aerodynamic and vibratory forces and dependent on alterations in the size and shape of the upper respiratory tract during speech. Narrowly defined, resonance is the by-product of opening and closing of the velopharynx in coordination with respiration, phonation, and articulation.	Velopharynx subserved by CN V (tensor veli palatini) and X; pharynx subserved by CN IX and X.	Hypernasality Hyponasality Nasal air emission (audible)
Articulation	Broadly defined, articulation is the product of the juxtaposition of muscles that cause alterations in air flow and, therefore, differentiated sound qualities. In English, the major distinctions among speech sounds are (1) vowel vs. consonant, (2) place of articulation, (3) manner of articulation (sonorant [nasal vs. oral] vs. obstruent [stop vs. fricative]), and (4) voice-voiceless.	Broadly defined, articulation is subserved by all the respiratory, laryngeal, velopharyngeal, and oral musculature and their respective central and peripheral sources of innervation, including CN V, VII, IX, X, XI, and XII and C1–C3 via ansa cervicalis.	Imprecise consonants Distorted vowels Irregular articulatory breakdown Prolonged speech sounds
Prosody	Refers to the melody of speech, defined as rate, rhythm (stress variation and pause), and intonation or inflection (rising and falling pitch).	All speech subsystems and their neural substrates participate in the production of prosody, as well as the speaker's whole body posture, emotional state, and affective drive.	Repeated segments Abnormally slow or fast rate (overall) Increasing rate overall Increased rate in segments Prolonged intervals Inappropriate silences Reduced or diminished stress Excess and equal stress Reduced stress variation

Abbreviations: CN, cranial nerve.
[a] Data from Darley FL, Aronson AE, Brown JR. Motor Speech Disorders. WB Saunders, Philadelphia, 1975.

to neurogenic dysphagia. Neurogenic oropharyngeal dysphagia in adults has been estimated to occur in 12 percent of the generally ill hospitalized population, in up to 30 percent in poststroke patients, and in as many as 50 percent of nursing home residents.

Acquired neurogenic oropharyngeal dysphagia is not attributable to dysarthria, aphasia, dementia, psychiatric illness, or gastroenterologic disorder, but, because of overlapping neural substrates and coexisting disease, dysphagia often concurs with, or is exacerbated by, these entities. *Neurologic oropharyngeal dysphagia is caused by, and attributable to, motor and/or sensory impairments subserving oral function and the complex pharyngeal reflex.* Although robust in the face of acute and rigorously managed neurologic illnesses (e.g., stroke), swallowing often appears to be fragile in the context of chronic or multiple disease states. Dysphagia may manifest as subtle alterations in the efficiency or comfort of prandial swallowing or as a severe limitation in the quantity of nutritional intake to the extent that nonoral means of nutrition must be instituted.

Swallowing dysfunction of any type places the patient at risk for aspiration pneumonia, malnutrition, and dehydration with subsequent morbidity and mortality. Prandial aspiration is the spilling of food or liquid below the level of the true vocal cords.

When audible, aspiration elicits a reflexive laryngeal cough; when silent, it elicits no cough. Silent aspiration is elusive during bedside evaluation, and diagnostic tests such as videofluoroscopy are necessary to identify it.

Though the swallowing mechanism may change in subtle ways as a function of normal aging, no study has revealed aspiration of food or liquid into the lungs during swallowing by healthy, elderly patients except during sleep. However, the threshold for a cough reflex is known to increase during aging. Decreased sensitivity of the cough may explain silent aspiration in elderly patients with neurologic impairment, especially when sedation is involved.

Swallowing requires an intricate interplay of cortical-subcortical and brainstem neuronal systems. These include voluntary bolus control in the oral-preparatory phase, the swallowing reflex threshold (which depends on the stimulus and oral-pharyngeal "awareness"), cortical-subcortical descending pathways, the brainstem swallowing centers located in the reticular formation bilaterally, and the lower cranial nerves. Coordination of these neural systems allows the oral preparatory phase, the reflex initiation phase, the pharyngeal phase, and the upper esophageal phase to proceed in a normal way. The neural substrates of oropharyngeal swallowing are described in Table 12-7; general

TABLE 12-3. Anatomic Substrates of the Dysarthrias

Anatomic Substrate	Typical Perceptual Hallmarks	Dysarthria Type
Cortex	Slow, labored speech with exaggerated prosody (dysprosody), articulatory prolongation and syllable segregation	Aphemia (or cortical dysarthria, compare with apraxia of speech)
	Fast rate with attenuated prosody (aprosody), monotone quality, and indistinct articulation	Aprosody
Subcortex	Imprecise consonants, short phrases, slow rate, monoloudness, monopitch	Unilateral upper motor neuron dysarthria
	Slow rate is prominent, hypernasality, articulatory distortions (consonants and vowels), short phrases, harsh or strain-strangled voice	Bilateral upper motor neuron dysarthria or spastic dysarthria
Extrapyramidal	Increased rate, decreased articulatory range and precision, hypophonia (low volume); voice tremor may be present	Hypokinetic dysarthria (e.g., in Parkinson's disease)
	Unsteady rate and loudness; sound prolongations; irregular articulatory breakdown	Slow hyperkinetic dysarthria (e.g., in dyskinesia, dystonia)
	Variability in precision of speech sounds, variable loudness (at times excessive), and hypernasality	Quick hyperkinetic dysarthria (e.g., in chorea, myoclonus)
Cerebellum	Excess and equal stress, articulatory imprecision prolonged phonemes, harsh voice; voice tremor may be present	Ataxic dysarthria (type I[a])
	Reduced stress variation with articulatory imprecision ("slurring"), prolonged phonemes, harsh voice; voice tremor may be present	Ataxic dysarthria (type II[a])
Brainstem	Hypernasality, dysphonia (hoarse-breathy), articulatory imprecision; if severe, rate is slow, voice is aphonic, and inspiratory stridor may be present	Flaccid dysarthria, bilateral
	Flaccid weakness and associated perceptual speech deviance dependent on which peripheral nerves are involved	Flaccid dysarthria, discrete (e.g., dysphonia secondary to unilateral vocal fold paralysis)
Mixed anatomic substrates	Cerebellum, subcortex (e.g., multiple sclerosis)	Mixed ataxic-spastic dysarthria
	Upper motor and lower motor neuron (e.g., amyotrophic lateral sclerosis)	Mixed flaccid-spastic dysarthria
	Cerebellum, subcortex, basal ganglia (e.g., hepatolenticular degeneration, Wilson's disease)	Mixed ataxic-spastic-hypokinetic dysarthria

[a] Personal observation.

TABLE 12-4. Special Tests for Dysarthria[a]

Test	Purpose
Perceptual evaluation	Descriptive analysis of spontaneous speech using operationalized terms, such as Mayo's deviant speech dimensions (see Table 12-2); rating of overall intelligibility.
Oral motor-sensory examination	Examination of cranial nerves V, VII, IX, X, XI, and XII, using isolated voluntary oral movements (e.g., protrusion, retraction, lateralization, elevation) and sensory testing (including bilateral face, lips, tongue, velum, and pharyngeal gag).
Discrete speech subsystems examination	Oral production of discrete tasks by speech subsystem (e.g., *respiration*: sigh, pant, hold breath, cough, loudness range and control tasks); *phonation*: vowels and diphthongs, vowel prolongation, pitch range and control tasks; *resonance*: nasal oral contrasts (e.g., hamper), oral syllables with nares open and occluded (e.g., beat, bat, boat, boot); *articulation*: oral word and sentence repetition, and standard articulation inventories; *rate and coordination*: diadochokinesis for isolated syllables /pˆ/, tˆ/, kˆ/ and syllable sequences /pˆtˆkˆ/; *prosody*: contrastive stress, intonation, and speech rhythm assessed in spontaneous speech and oral paragraph reading.
Spirometry	Quantification of forced vital capacity, phonation volume, phonation time, mean air flow rate (for a sustained vowel).
Air flow and air pressure	Quantification of oral pressrue, laryngeal air flow, laryngeal airway resistance, nasal air flow, and differential oral-nasal pressure.
Vocal tract visualization and imaging	Rigid oral endoscopy with stroboscopy is ideal for observing vocal fold adduction, asymmetry, and aperiodicity.
Oscillographic analysis	A two-dimensional (amplitude, time) waveform display of acoustic events, allowing visualization and measurement of fundamental frequency, pitch range, pitch perturbation, and oral diadochokinetic rates.
Spectrographic analysis	A three-dimensional (amplitude, frequency, time) display of acoustic events, providing a graphic display of energy regions ("formants") corresponding to resonant frequencies of the vocal tract during speech.
Nasalence measures	The ratio of acoustic energy output from the nasal and oral cavities, yielding an objective correlate of nasality.
Electroglottography (electrolaryngography)	By placing electrodes on the thyroid cartilage, the electrical impedance across the larynx is measured, and a waveform representing vocal fold adduction and abduction is obtained as well as the percentage of open versus closed phases.

[a] For a review and critique of comprehensive acoustic speech analysis systems, see Read, Buder, and Kent (1992).

subtypes of oropharyngeal dysphagia are shown in Table 12-8.

History and Examination

As for dysarthria, the history and and examination for dysphagia should be directed to seek out evidence for the underlying cause (Table 12-1) and a more detailed characterization of the dyspha-gia, which will help to establish the neurologic localization (Table 12-8). History should include neurologic, gastrointestinal, pulmonary, and nutritional areas as well as current feeding status, including oral diet, caloric needs, weight, and status of dentition. A complete neurologic examination should include a detailed cranial nerve evaluation. Specialty consultations are often essential (e.g., speech-language pathology, gastroenterology, pulmonary medicine, and radiology).

TABLE 12-5. Differential Diagnosis of Dysarthria

Diagnosis	Definition
Dysarthria	"A speech disorder resulting from damage to neural mechanisms that regulate speech movements" (Netsell, 1984)
Apraxia of speech	A neurologic disorder of articulation and prosody characterized by an inability to achieve spatial and temporal speech targets in a smooth and coordinated fashion; frequently coexists with but is not attributable to aphasia. Variability of articulation and prosody, a hallmark of this disorder, suggests that it is due neither to linguistic (phonologic) knowledge nor to elementary motor-sensory impairment, but rather to an intermediate (perhaps programming) stage of speech production (compare with aphemia, cortical dysarthria).
Cortical stuttering	A form of acquired neurogenic dysfluency characterized by speech initiation difficulty and repetition of sounds and syllables at the beginning of utterances.
Palilalia	A form of acquired neurogenic dysfluency characterized by compulsive reiteration of words and phrases, usually at the latter part of the utterance, often accompanied by decreasing loudness and increasing rate of speech.
Foreign accent syndrome	An acquired speech disorder in which speech assumes phonetic characteristics consistent with a foreign language caused by abnormalities in the production of vowels and consonants and to alterations in stress and intonation patterns.
Spasmodic dysphonia	A voice disorder characterized by an intermittently "strained-strangled" voice quality, including adductor, abductor, and mixed adductor-abductor types, attributed to neurologic, psychogenic, or idiopathic causes.
Structurally based speech disorders	Speech disorders resulting from structural changes caused by a birth defect (e.g., cleft palate), injury (e.g., gunshot wound), or surgery for malignant tumor (e.g., glossectomy, pharyngectomy, laryngectomy, mandibulectomy, etc.). Surgical interventions may lead to compromise of peripheral nerves, such that the resultant speech disorder is properly diagnosed as both neurologic and structural in origin.
Non-neurologic speech disorders	Nonmalignant lesions and growths (e.g., vocal fold polyp, contact ulcer, or nodule; pharyngeal abscess; enlarged adenoids); nasal congestion from viral illness or allergies; polypoid degeneration or leukoplakia associated with a smoking history; voice disorders secondary to endocrine disorders, etc.
Developmental speech disorders	Speech articulation disorders resulting from delayed or disordered learning; may coexist with a language disorder, learning disability, or mental retardation.
Psychogenic speech disorders	Disorders of articulation, fluency, or voice that mimic neurologic or other organic articulation, fluency, or voice disorders but are caused by neurosis, anxiety, conversion disorder, or other psychopathology.
Dialectal variation	A rule-based variation in speech articulation and prosody that is normal in the context of a given sociolinguistic community.
Aging	Speech changes associated with normal aging include breathy-weak voice quality (e.g., from vocal fold bowing and thinning or mucosal edema and dehydration) and normal geriatric changes in pitch (lower in females, higher in males).
Iatrogenic speech disorders	Changes in voice from postintubation trauma (e.g., laryngeal edema), prolonged intubation (e.g., vocal fold web), presence of tracheostomy, or xerostomia caused by radiation therapy or pharmacologic agents.

TABLE 12-6. Management Approaches for Dysarthria

Approach	Definition and Examples
Distinguish primary from secondary features	Diagnostic evaluation should determine which dysarthric features are intrinsic to the disorder and which are premorbid (e.g., smoking history); coexisting (e.g., pulmonary disease); or secondary, compensatory features of the speech disorder. Secondary features should be distinguished as adaptive (e.g., slower rate in compensation for articulatory impreciseon) or maladaptive (e.g., hyperfunctional, strained voice in compensation for reduced respiratory support).
Preventive approaches	Through direct instruction and clinician modeling, these techniques are used to prevent the habituation of maladaptive behaviors (e.g., vocal strain, excessive loudness, excessive mandibular excursion). On a speech subsystem basis, the clinician adjusts speech stimuli to the appropriate level of difficulty in order to re-establish and reinforce normal range and effort parameters to provide optimal conditions for speech production.
Compensatory techniques	Through direct therapy, patients are taught to compensate for reduced speech intelligibility using individualized strategies (e.g., intersyllabic, interword, or interphrase pause) to regulate nonoptimal speech rate, prolonging speech sounds to compensate for reduced stress variation, strategic placement of pause before complex speech sounds, use of intrusive "schwa" for complex sound blends, speaking in short phrases to compensate for reduced respiratory support, etc.
Restorative treatments	The clinician introduces restorative techniques on an individualized basis and with reference to the relatively spared or impaired speech subsystems. For *respiration*, incentive inspiratory training; for *phonation* from flaccid weakness, adduction exercises; for *resonance*, biofeedback regarding nasalence; for *articulation and prosody*, traditional auditory verbal training (structured and hierarchical repetitive speech exercises, supplemented with audio- and videotape feedback), as well as oscillogrpahic biofeedback regarding oral plosion, speech rate, pitch inflection, loudness modulation, contrastive stress, etc. Other forms of biofeedback potentially useful in dysarthria therapy include delayed auditory feedback, electromyography, and electroglottography. Behavioral modification techniques (e.g, modeling, evaluative feedback, and reinforcement) in addition to more current biofeedback approaches are standard speech-language pathology approaches in the treatment of the dysarthric individual.
Augmented approaches	Depending on the patients, motor abilities, cognitive status, literacy, and motivation, speech may be simulated or augmented by communication boards (pictures, alphabet cards, word grids, sentence construction notebooks), hand-held typewriters, synthesized voice devices, and adapted computers.
Prosthetic approaches	In select patients, prostheses might include palatal lift or obturator, chin strap or cervical collar for head and neck stabilization, or a bite block for jaw stabilization. In hypophonic patients, a voice amplifier is often helpful; in tracheostomized patients, a "communication valve" is essential for speech/voice restoration.

Special Tests

Abnormal findings on the examination or evidence of aspiration may guide the clinician's decision to request a videofluoroscopic examination. Evidence of aspiration or increased risk of aspiration includes diminished or absent pharyngeal sensation, dysphonia (e.g., wet, forced, harsh, breathy, or strained voice), reduced laryngeal excursion during swallowing, cough after a trial of ice chips, weak voluntary or reflexive cough, upper airway congestion, abnormal chest examination, or noncardiac chest pain. Aspiration pneumonia, current or past, would also alert the clinician. If bilateral neurologic (including cranial nerve) signs are found or the patient is somnolent, the risk of

TABLE 12-7. Phrases of Oropharyngeal Swallowing and Common Clinical and Videofluoroscopic Abnormalities

Phase	Definition	Neurologic Substrates	Common Abnormalities
Oral-preparatory phase	The lips close to retain food and liquid boluses; the buccal cavities and tongue, in concert with jaw movement, hold, manipulate and masticate boluses; peristaltic motion of the tongue against the palate moves boluses to the posterior oral cavity; boluses are retained in the oral cavity posteriorly by virtue of posterior tongue to velar contact.	Motor and sensory aspects of CN V, VII, X, and XII	Lip incompetency (with drooling) Retention of food in the buccal cavities Inefficient bolus formation Incomplete mastication Slow anterior-posterior transport of boluses Residue along the tongue Premature leakage of material into the pharynx
Reflex initiation phase	The reflex is initiated by virtue of tactile, taste, temperature, and/or kinesthetic stimulation of the tongue base, anterior faucial pillars, velum, and oropharynx. The anatomic and temporal aspects of reflex initiation are modulated, in part, by bolus size and texture. Typically, the reflex initiates as the bolus passes over the base of the tongue (just above the mandibular ramus). Reflex initiation marks the onset of the pharyngeal phase and the onset of an apneic interval that is sustained through the duration of the swallow.	The lower portion of the motor strip is considered to be the substrate for voluntary swallowing; the medullary "swallowing centers," for the reflexive aspect of swallowing (i.e., nucleus tractus solitarius [sensory] and nucleus ambiguus [motor] situated in the dorsal medulla bilaterally)	*Delayed swallow reflex* characterized by passage of the bolus below the ramus of the mandible prior to laryngeal closure, hesitation of the bolus during its oral-to-pharyngeal transit, preswallow "pooling" of the bolus in the midpharynx (vallecular spaces) or in the lower pharynx (pyriform sinuses), and/or poor coordination between the swallow reflex and the mandatory apneic interval.
Pharyngeal phase	The pharyngeal phase entails laryngeal closure and elevation and pharyngeal clearance. Three major physiologic events are responsible for pharyngeal clearance: (1) the propulsion force of the tongue *pushing* the bolus downward; (2) the upward and forward movement of the larynx *pulling* the larynx out of the bolus path and *pulling* the pharyngeal esophageal segment open; and (3) the rapid peristaltic contractions of the pharyngeal constrictor muscles, *clearing* the bolus through the lower pharynx.	CN IX, X, XI, and XII and innervation to extrinsic neck and laryngeal muscles to sustain head posture during swallowing and effect laryngeal excursion, with input from C1–C3 via ansa cervicalis.	*Posterior tongue weakness,* undermining the force of bolus propulsion into the pharynx. *Incomplete laryngeal closure,* effectively lowering pressure in the parhyngeal cavity and allowing spillage of food into the airway. *Incomplete laryngeal excursion,* undermining opening of the pharyngeal-esophageal segment. *Weak contraction* of the pharyngeal constrictors, causing residue in the pharynx after the swallow and undermining complementary relaxation of the pharyngeal-esophageal segment. *Aspiration* (i.e., passage of material below the level of the true vocal folds); audible (with a cough) or silent (no cough).
PES phase	Opening of the pharyngeal-esophageal segment (upper esophageal sphincter) entails a complementary interaction of mechanical forces (increased pressure in the closed pharyngeal cavity, and upward pulling on the PES secondary to laryngeal movement) as well as muscular forces (pharyngeal constrictor contraction, which effects PES relaxation).	CN IX, X, XI, and XII and innervation to extrinsic neck and laryngeal muscles to sustain head posture during swallowing and effect laryngeal excursion, with input from C1–C3 via ansa cervicalis.	Premature or delayed PES opening (relative to bolus position) or reduced duration of PES opening (relative to bolus size) can lead to residue in the lower pharynx and potential spillover of residue into the larynx.

Abbreviations: PES, pharyngeal-esophageal segment; CN, cranial nerve.

TABLE 12-8. Anatomic Substrates of Neurogenic Oropharyngeal Dysphagias

Anatomic Substrate	Typical Oropharyngeal Manifestation	Dysphagia Type
Hemispheric, unilateral	Mildly delayed reflex Trace liquid aspiration Mild pharyngeal residue Contralateral pyriform sinus "droop" Thicker substances usually swallowed with greater ease than liquids	"Hemispheric dysphagia" 20–30% aspiration incidence 2–6-week recovery 90%⁺ favorable outcome[a]
Hemispheric, bilateral (cortical, subcortical, and extrapyramidal neural systems)	Markedly delayed reflex Greater-than-trace liquid aspiration Thicker substances swallowed without aspiration but often characterized by significant pharyngeal residue	"Bihemispheric dysphagia" 40–50% aspiration incidence 4–12-week recovery 90%⁺ favorable outcome[a]
Brainstem	Absent swallow reflex likely in acute medullary lesions Incomplete laryngeal excursion Impaired pharyngeal function (unilaterally or bilaterally depending on the extent of lesions) Aspiration, often significant Liquids usually swallowed with greater ease than thicker substances and solids	"Bulbar dysphagia" 60–70% aspiration incidence 8–24-week recovery 80%⁺ favorable outcome[a]
Myoneural junction	Similar to bulbar dysphagia Notable for deterioration with fatigue Nasal regurgitation and pharyngeal residue common	"Myoneural dysphagia" Function varies with effectiveness of medical therapy
Peripheral nerves and muscles	Mandibular: reduced mastication Lingual: inefficient bolus formation and slow oral motility Facial: poor bolus retention in buccal cavity, lip incompetency (with drooling) Velar: nasal regurgitation Pharyngeal: pharyngeal residue Laryngeal, intrinsic: aspiration risk (very high with bilateral vocal fold paralysis) Laryngeal, extrinsic: reduced laryngeal excursion, diminished pharyngeal-esophageal segment opening	"Myodysphagia" The degree of oropharyngeal dysphagia is greater in the context of multiple muscle group involvement (e.g., polymyositis) than in isolated muscle group involvement (e.g., unilateral recurrent laryngeal nerve paralysis). Recovery depends on the underlying etiology and the efficacy of treatment.

[a] Favorable outcome defined as resumption of oral feeding with few to no restrictions.

TABLE 12-9. Special Tests for Dysphagia

Test	Purpose
Focused clinical examination	Bedside examination of the lower cranial nerves and assessment of the pharyngeal gag reflex bilaterally, glottal coup, laryngeal excursion during dry and bolus swallows, and speech quality (notably phonation).
Videofluoroscopy (oropharynx)	Dynamic, videotaped image of the oral cavity, pharynx, larynx, and proxmial esophagus in lateral and anterior-posterior projections, allowing observation of temporal and spatial characteristics of swallowing, the presence and degree of aspiration, the presence and degree of oropharyngeal residue, and on-line observation of the benefits of postural or bolus modifications.
Vocal tract visualization and imaging	Indirect laryngoscopy (mirror imaging) and rigid oral endoscopy allow observation of the oropharynx, epiglottis, and aryepiglottic folds, true vocal folds (especially helpful for detecting vocal fold lesions). Rigid scope or fiberoptic imaging with stroboscopy is ideal for observing vocal fold adduction, asymmetry, and aperiodicity.
Fiberoptic endoscopic evaluation of swallowing	Dynamic nasal endoscopic image of the oropharynx, epiglottis, and supraglottic region during swallowing of foods and liquids; postswallow observation of aspiration and pharyngeal residue.
Skull radiography	Observation of skeletal and cartilagenous structures (e.g., spinal vertebrae, palate, mandible, thyroid cartilage, hyoid bone).
Manofluorography	Simultaneous manometric recording of oropharyngeal pressure changes and videofluoroscopic images of oropharyngeal bolus swallows.
Ultrasonography	Dynamic images of soft tissue well suited for observation of oral structures and suprahyoid swallowing function.
Head computed tomography or magnetic resonance imaging	Observation of brain, brainstem, and cervical spine (for hemorrhage, neoplasm, and skeletal abnormalities).
Scintigraphy	Quantification of a tracer present in the lungs, pharynx, or esophagus using radionuclide scanning.
Electromyography	Record electrical activity from muscles to measure motor neuron activity; used selectively to assess pharyngeal and laryngeal function; may be helpful to evaluate systemic disease when suspected.

aspiration is increased. Special tests used in the evaluation of dysphagia are described in Table 12-9.

Differential Diagnosis

Dysphagia varies depending on the type of neurologic disorder and the extent of the disease. Other causes of oropharyngeal dysphagia often coexist with, exacerbate, or mimic neurogenic dysphagia and should be considered in the differential diagnosis (Table 12-10).

Management

As with dysarthria, therapy is directed to the underlying cause and to the dysphagia itself. The management approaches to dysphagia are multifaceted and individualized. General management considerations include the acuity or chronicity of the disease; the cognitive status of the patient (including learning ability, motivation, and compliance); the presence of coexisting diseases that affects overall posture, strength, endurance; as well as the effectiveness of concurrent medical treatment. As summarized in Table 12-11, there are several principles that guide our management of swallowing disorders, including the importance of distinguishing primary from coexisting or confounding secondary features, followed by the clinician's judi-

TABLE 12-10. Differential Diagnosis of Dysphagia

Diagnosis	Definition
Neurogenic dysphagia	A swallowing disorder resulting from damage to neural mechanisms that regulate oropharyngeal movements, both reflexive and voluntary.
Apraxia of swallowing	An oral phase dysfunction resulting from an inability to control voluntary movement of the lips and tongue, usually characterized by stasis of food or liquid in the oral cavity.
Mechanical (structural) dysphagia	Swallowing difficulty attributable to structural abnormalities caused by congenital abnormalities (e.g., cleft palate), trauma, or surgical ablation of tissue (e.g., glossectomy, mandibulectory, laryngectomy) and associated sequelae. Surgical interventions may lead to compromise of peripheral nerves, such that the resultant swallowing disorder is properly diagnosed as both neurologic and structural in origin. Mechanical dysphagia is frequently exacerbated (temporarily or permanently) by postsurgical treatments.
Developmental dysphagia	In infants, a failure to develop and thrive often results in poor feeding ability; often associated with medical illness and long-term hospitalization during which normal developmental milestones are not achieved; often coexist with gastroenterologic disease.
Postural dysphagia	Alterations in posture of the head and neck (e.g., spasmodic torticollis, tardive dyskinesia) causing abnormalities of bolus control, motility, or clearance with actual aspiration or an increased risk for aspiration. Postural and neurogenic dysphagia frequently coexist.
Pulmonary-related dysphagia	Altered respiratory patterns (e.g., chronic obstructive pulmonary disease) may interfere with the normal swallowing-respiration interface.
Esophageal dysphagia	A host of esophageal disorders, both anatomic and physiologic in etiology, may coexist with and potentially exacerbate oropharyngeal dysphagia (e.g., gastroesophageal reflux disease; Zenker's diverticulum; and esophageal spasms, strictures, infections).
Skeletal dysphagia	Spinal abnormalities, when severe, may impinge on the pharyngeal cavity and proximal esophagus and thereby interfere with swallowing (e.g., osteophytes, diffuse interstitial sclerotic hyperostosis, spinal curvature, etc.).
Functional swallowing disorders	The so-called globus syndrome or hypopharyngeal syndrome is characterized by discomfort and strain during pharyngeal swallowing often subsequent to pharyngeal infection or irritation. Because true psychogenic dysphagia is rare, rigorous evaluation is necessary to rule out structural or physiological etiologies (e.g., cricopharyngeal spasm secondary to reflux disease).
Aging and disease with dysphagia	Normal, healthy elderly persons experience developmental changes in oropharyngeal function (e.g., diminished taste and smell, slower oropharyngeal motility, altered dentition) but are able to swallow efficiently and without prandial aspiration. In the context of acute and chronic illnesses, dementia, polypharmacy, reduced mobility and reduced alertness, elderly patients are vulnerable to anorexia, dehydration, malnutrition, and aspiration. The heightened threshold for the cough reflex increases the likelihood of silent aspiration in elderly patients.
Iatrogenic swallowing disorders	Changes in swallowing caused by postintubation trauma (e.g., laryngeal and pharyngeal edema), prolonged intubation with cuffed tracheostomy (e.g., alteration of the respiratory-swallowing interface, mechanical obstruction of the proximal esophagus), presence of tracheostomy (potentially restricting laryngeal excursion and disallowing closure of the larynx during swallowing), sequelae of botulinum toxin therapy, and xerostomia as a result of radiation therapy and pharmacologic agents.

TABLE 12-11. Management Approaches for Oropharyngeal Dysphagia

Approach	Definition and Examples
Distinguish primary from secondary features	Diagnostic evaluation should determine which dysphagic features are intrinsic to the neurologic deficit, which are premorbid (e.g., cervical spine degenerative changes), coexisting (e.g., reflux disease), or compensatory features of the disorder. During clinical observation, secondary features should be distinguished as adaptive (e.g., avoidance of problematic food textures), or maladaptive (e.g., abnormal, nonfacilitative head positioning).
Preventive approaches	Prevention of aspiration is vital in acute and chronic phases of illness and entails using optimal torso and head postures during meals (usually fully upright), restriction of oral intake to safe textures (using specially designed "dysphagia diets," as indicated), restriction of bolus size, restriction of utensil choice (e.g., avoiding use of a straw), and close monitoring of vital signs and nutritional values.
Compensatory techniques	Compensatory approaches are conscious maneuvers used by the patient and caregiver and are essential to aspiration prevention and optimal nutritional intake. For example, postural modifications (forward neck flexion, or lateral rotation), in combination with management of bolus size can minimize aspiration risk. Videofluoroscopy is typically used as a brief therapeutic trial to confirm the benefit of postural compensations.
Restorative treatments	Numerous restorative approaches are described in the literature, but anecdotal evidence only is available regarding efficacy in most instances.[a]
Augmented approaches	For patients at risk for aspiration and/or nutritional compromise, enteral nutritional methods (nasogastric, nasoduodenal, gastrostomy, and jejunostomy tubes) and parenteral (intravenous) fluids, feedings, or supplements are indicated. These may be either temporary or permanent, depending on patients' swallowing and nutritional limitations and requirements.
Prosthetic approaches	Motorically limited patients may benefit from adaptive equipment (dishes and utensils) alone or in combination with arm slings, orthoses, and postural supports. When functional self-feeding is a goal for the dysphagic patient, the integration of swallowing techniques and adaptive feeding goals is essential.

[a] For a summary of current dysphagia treatments, see Alberts MJ, Horner J: Dysphagia and aspiration syndromes. In Bogousslevsky J, Caplan LR (eds): Stroke Syndromes. Cambridge University Press, Cambridge, 1995 (in press).

cious selection and combination of preventive, compensatory, restorative, augmented, or prosthetic therapy approaches. Baseline and periodic evaluations by the speech-language pathologist are advisable and, ideally, should be done in concert with clinic visits to the neurologist.

SUGGESTED READINGS

Alberts MJ, Horner J: Dysphagia and aspiration syndromes. In Bogousslevsky J, Caplan LR (eds): Stroke Syndromes. Cambridge University Press, 1995 (in press)

American Speech-Language-Hearing Association: Instrumental diagnostic procedures for swallowing ASHA 34, suppl. 7, 25, 1992

Aronson AE: Clinical Voice Disorders. 3rd Ed. Thieme, New York, 1990

Blumstein SE, Alexander MP, Ryalls RH, Katz W, Dworetzky B: On the nature of the foreign accent syndrome: a case study. Brain Lang 31:215, 1987

Castell DO, Donner MW: Evaluation of dysphagia: a careful history is crucial. Dysphagia 2:65, 1987

Darley FL, Aronson AE, Brown JR: Motor Speech Disorders. WB Saunders, Philadelphia, 1975

DePippo KL, Holas MA, Reding MJ et al: Dysphagia therapy following stroke: a controlled trial. Neurology 44:1655, 1994

Duffy JR, Folger WN: Dysarthria in Unilateral Central Nervous System Lesions. Presented to the American Speech-Language-Hearing Association, Detroit, 1986

Gray LP: The relationship of "inferior constrictor swallow" and "globus hystericus" or the hypopharyngeal syndrome. J Laryngol Otol 97:607, 1983

Hartman DE, Abbs JA: Perceptual and physiologic characteristics of unilateral upper motor neuron (UUMN) dysarthria. Presented to the American Speech-Language-Hearing Association, St. Louis, 1992

Horner J, Alberts MJ, Dawson DV, Cook GM: Swallowing in Alzheimer's disease. Alzheimer Dis Assoc Dis 8:177, 1994

Horner J, Buoyer FG, Alberts MJ, Helms MJ: Dysphagia following brainstem stroke: clinical correlates and outcome. Arch Neurol 48:1170, 1991

Horner J, Massey EW: Managing dysphagia: special problems in patients with neurologic disease. Postgraduate Med 89:203, 1991

Horner J, Massey EW, Riski JE et al: Aspiration following stroke: clinical correlates and outcome. Neurology 38:1359, 1988

Kahrilas PJ: The anatomy and physiology of dysphagia. p. 11. In Gelfand DW, Richter JE (eds): Dysphagia: Diagnosis and treatment. Igaku-Shoin, New York, 1989

Kent RD, Rosenbek JC: Prosodic disturbance and neurologic lesion. Brain Lang 15:259, 1982

Kent RD, Rosenbek JC: Acoustic patterns of apraxia of speech. J Speech Hear Res 26:231, 1983

Logemann JA: Swallowing physiology and pathophysiology. Otolaryngol Clin North Am 21:613, 1988

McConnel FMS: Analysis of pressure generation and bolus transit during pharyngeal swallowing. Laryngoscope 98:71, 1988

Netsell R: A neurobiologic view of the dysarthrias. p. 1. In McNeil MR, Rosenbek JC, Aronson AE (eds): The Dysarthrias: Physiology, Acoustics, Perception, Management. College-Hill, San Diego, 1984

Pontoppidan H, Beecher HK: Progressive loss of protective reflexes in the airway with the advance of age. JAMA 174:2209, 1960

Read C, Buder EH, Kent RD: Speech analysis systems: an evaluation. J Speech Hear Res 35:314, 1992

Rosenbek JC: Treating the dysarthric talker. p. 359. In Rosenbek JC (ed): Current Views of Dysarthria. Seminars in Speech and Language 5(4), 1984

Rosenbek JC, Robbins J, Fishback B, Levine RL: Effects of thermal application on dysphagia after stroke. J Speech Hear Res 34:1257, 1991

Schiff HP, Alexander MP, Naeser MA, Galaburda AM: Aphemia: clinical-anatomic correlations. Arch Neurol 40:720, 1983

Sonies BC: Oropharyngeal dysphagia in the elderly. Clin Geriatr Med 8:569, 1992

Sonies BC, Baum BJ: Evaluation of swallowing pathophysiology. Otolaryngol Clin North Am 21:701, 1988

Wertz RT, Rosenbek JC: Where the ear fits: a perceptual evaluation of motor speech disorders. p. 39. In Webb WG (ed): Oral Motor Dysfunction in Children and Adults. Sem Speech Lang 13(1), 1992

Yorkston KM, Beukelman DR, Bell KR: Clinical Management of Dysarthric Speakers. Little, Brown/College-Hill, Boston, 1988

13. TRANSIENT EVENTS

FRANK W. DRISLANE

Transient neurologic symptoms come in a tremendous variety and can be particularly vexing because the symptoms have usually resolved by the time of evaluation and patients often have a difficult time describing them. The history usually contains most of the diagnostic information, but the neurologic examination remains important.

As elsewhere in neurology, localization assists diagnosis. Consideration of the neural structures or functions affected during a spell helps to organize the many possibilities and guide investigations. Transient events may affect the whole brain (usually leading to loss of consciousness), may affect particular functions that are not precisely localized, or may have a localizable focal onset. With this perspective on localization, one considers the epidemiology or risk factors of an individual patient; associated earlier symptoms; and the onset, progression, and nature of the event. This is usually sufficient to bring one diagnosis to the fore, though many transient events remain unexplained. The variety of pathophysiologic processes that produce transient symptoms is great, and this chapter concentrates on the differentiation of one syndrome from another rather than on the management of individual diseases.

SYNCOPE AND NEAR-SYNCOPE

Syncope, a relatively sudden nonepileptic loss of consciousness, is due to a global diminution in brain metabolism. Most episodes are due to a generalized decrease in brain perfusion and oxygen delivery. Often, perfusion declines over seconds, and the patient has premonitory symptoms, such as lightheadedness, gradually dimming vision, generalized weakness, occasional tinnitus or vertigo, nausea, or peripheral paresthesias. Observers may note pallor or sweating. Respiration continues, but blood pressure usually declines. The pulse, often weak, may be faster or slower, depending on the mechanism of syncope. Muscle tone is diminished. A few brief clonic jerks of the limbs are common accompaniments, but jerking may be more prolonged ("convulsive syncope") if the head remains elevated. Incontinence is rare. With a gradual onset, falls are also more gradual, and patients may be able to protect themselves to some degree. Injuries are less common than with the more sudden epileptic falls. Most syncope is strongly related to body position, occurring with the subject upright and usually relieved quickly on reclining. When the patient is lying down, perfusion improves, and most recover quickly, often within seconds and much faster than with seizures. Rarely does unconsciousness last for minutes. Subsequently, brief confusion is common, but a long "postictal" confusion is not.

Causes of Syncope

Most causes of syncope can be kept in mind by considering mechanisms of diminished cerebral perfusion (Table 13-1), including insufficient blood volume, inadequate or malfunctioning peripheral vasoconstrictive reflexes necessary for the maintenance of blood pressure, and cardiac disease.

Decreased Perfusion. VOLUME LOSS. Volume loss, as in hemorrhage, is a primary consideration. Adrenal failure may also diminish blood volume. A drop in blood pressure of more than 15 mmHg or a pulse increase of greater than 20 beats/min on rising from lying to standing suggests hypovolemia or inadequate postural reflexes. Volume-dependent syncope is exacerbated by starvation, inadequate fluid intake, diuretics, and deconditioning and prompted by prolonged standing, especially in a warm environment, which promotes peripheral vasodilation.

LOSS OF POSTURAL REFLEXES. Even with an adequate intravascular volume, syncope occurs when postural reflexes fail. Baroreceptors in the carotid sinus, aortic arch, and elsewhere in thoracic structures prompt a reflex diminution in vagal tone and a sympathetic response, increasing heart rate and peripheral vasoconstriction when effective intravascular volume diminishes. Interruption of this reflex can occur in the afferent or efferent limb, either centrally or in the peripheral autonomic nervous system. Central causes of autonomic failure include Parkinson's disease, the Shy-Drager syndrome, striatonigral de-

TABLE 13-1. Causes of Transient Global Dysfunction/Syncope

Hypoperfusion
  Volume loss
    Acute hemorrhage
    Diuretics, starvation
    Hypoadrenalism (Addison's disease)
  Inadequate postural reflexes
    Autonomic dysfunction
    Central   Parkinson's disease
              Striatonigral degeneration
              Multiple system atrophy
              Pure autonomic failure
    Peripheral Baroreceptor dysfunction
              Familial dysautonomia
              Pure autonomic failure
              Spinal cord disease
              Sympathectomy
              Guillain-Barré syndrome
              Neuropathies (e.g., diabetes, amyloidosis, rarely porphyria)
    Antihypertensive medications and others, including phenothiazines, tricyclics, levodopa
  Increased vagal tone
    Emotional stimulus (e.g., pain, fear, unpleasant sight)
    Carotid sinus hypersensitivity
    Glossopharyngeal neuralgia
    Valsalva maneuver
    Micturition syncope
  Cardiac
    Electrical
      Conduction
        Sinoatrial (sick sinus syndrome)
        Atrioventricular, including complete heart block
      Atrial arrhythmias (e.g., atrial fibrillation, supraventricular tachycardias)
      Ventricular arrhythmias (e.g., ventricular tachycardia, associated with long QT syndrome)
    Valvular, especially aortic stenosis, prosthetic valve malfunction
      Other obstructions
        Hypertrophic cardiomyopathies
        Congenital heart disease
        Atrial myxomas
        Pericardial tamponade
        Chest masses
        Impaired venous return
          Cough (tussive) syncope
          Pericardial tamponade
          Abdominal and thoracic masses
    Pulmonary hypertension
    Low output cardiac failure
      Myocardial infarction
      Cardiomegalies
      Some congenital diseases
  Situational (combination of mechanisms)
    Micturition
    Cough
    Breath-holding
    Hyperventilation or hypercarbia
    Valsalva maneuver
  Acute intracranial hypertension
    Cerebrospinal fluid obstruction, third ventricular tumors and cysts
    Masses
    Hemorrhage
Metabolic impairment with adequate perfusion
  Inadequate oxygen delivery
    Hypoxia
    Carbon monoxide and other poisonings
    Anemia, hemoglobinopathies
  Impaired metabolism
    Hypoglycemia
    Poisons

generation, and other multisystem atrophies (see Ch. 117). These diseases often include degeneration of brainstem nuclei that serve as essential relay stations in effecting postural reflexes. Pure autonomic failure includes both central and peripheral autonomic nervous system pathology. Spinal cord injuries above the upper thoracic sympathetic outflow may also impair postural reflexes. Surgical sympathectomy may have the logical side effect of syncope as a result of interruption of a needed postural reflex. Peripherally, Guillain-Barré syndrome (which may affect autonomic nerves with or without others) and autonomic neuropathies (see Ch. 15) may cause severe postural hypotension. Autonomic neuropathies cause syncope primarily through blood pressure changes rather than by their effects on the heart rate, which may be abnormally regular. The most important cause is diabetes, with amyloidosis and porphyria as rarer causes. Alcohol may lead to other causes of syncope but generally causes a sensory neuropathy with less autonomic nerve damage. Other symptoms of autonomic dysfunction include abnormalities in temperature and sweating regulation, gastrointestinal dysmotility, and sphincter and sexual dysfunction. Antihypertensive medications often interfere with vasoconstriction, and phenothiazines, tricyclic antidepressants, and levodopa can contribute to syncope.

INCREASED VAGAL TONE. Even if peripheral vasoconstriction functions properly most of the time, syncope may be caused by the opposition of excessive vagal stimulation. Vasovagal (vasodepressor) syncope is especially common in adolescents and young adults, frequently with an emotional precipitant, such as pain, fear, or an unpleasant sight, such as blood, blood drawing, or another's injury. It usually provides seconds of premonitory warning symptoms, such as nausea, gastrointestinal distress, sweating, and pupillary dilation. The primary vagal response is bradycardia, but this may lead to more serious arrhythmias, such as conduction block or sinus arrest. The loss of consciousness is usually brief, and recovery is rapid.

Carotid sinus hypersensitivity can cause excessive vagal function. Carotid sinus massage usually leads to a reflex bradycardia in normal subjects, but an excessive reaction can cause syncope. There is usually an identifiable precipitant such as a tight collar or turning the head. The bradycardia, rather than vasodilation, then leads to syncope. Glossopharyngeal neuralgia may also lead to bradycardic syncope, more commonly in older patients. There should usually be a history of pain in the throat before the syncope, sometimes precipitated by speaking, swallowing, or other oral movements.

CARDIAC DISEASE. Although not the most frequent, the most important and serious cause of syncope is cardiac disease. In contrast to most other forms of syncope, cardiac syncope need not occur in the upright position and may be much more rapid and lead to injury.

Cardiac arrhythmias are particularly important, especially in older patients, and may be the sign of serious ischemic or other cardiac disease. Complete or third-degree heart block may cause a very rapid loss of consciousness with no evident cardiac pulse and a long period of electrocardiographic silence; ventricular arrhythmias may supervene. Sick sinus syndrome and sinus node disease may lead to severe bradycardias and syncope. Sinoatrial node block often leads to a ventricular escape rhythm and less severe symptoms than with complete heart block. Paroxysmal supraventricular tachycardias are less life threatening than heart block and ventricular arrhythmias. They more often lead to palpitations or presyncope than to complete loss of consciousness. Ventricular tachycardias are more dangerous, and therapy remains controversial and difficult. The long QT syndrome is a marker for risk of ventricular arrhythmias.

Valvular disease, especially aortic stenosis, can lead to life-threatening syncope. Left ventricular outflow obstructions (as in hypertrophic cardiomyopathies) may be detected by a careful cardiac examination and, certainly, by echocardiography. Rare myxomas can cause sudden cardiac obstruction. Other mechanisms of syncope include prosthetic valve malfunction, pulmonary hypertension, and pulmonary embolism. Low-output cardiac failure following a myocardial infarction or in congenital heart disease, sometimes worsened by hypoxia, may also lead to syncope. Pericardial tamponade and chest tumors can also cause mechanical obstruction to cardiac output. Cardiac syncope is more likely to be manifested during exertion, including competitive sports, when cardiac output cannot meet demand; exertional vasodilation in large muscles may help precipitate the syncope.

SITUATIONAL SYNCOPE. Some syncopal episodes have a characteristic precipitant. Micturition syncope typically occurs in older men when they arise to urinate at night. There is a postural component of arising to a standing position, and mechanical effects alone can decrease venous return to the heart. Cutaneous vasodilation from a warm sleeping environment may contribute. Urination may diminish the sympathetic stimulus of a full bladder, and vagal input may also be important. Many of the same factors allow a vigorous Valsalva maneuver to lead to syncope.

Cough syncope occurs in patients with severe chronic obstructive pulmonary disease during paroxysms of prolonged coughing rather than from a single or simple cough alone. The buildup of intrathoracic pressure and diminished venous return are likely to be the main contributors. Treatment is aimed at the pulmonary disease. Breath-holding spells may cause syncope in the same way, particularly after hyperventilation and a Valsalva maneuver, as practiced in adolescent pranks. Breath-holding spells also occur in children under the age of 5, often triggered by crying or emotional stimuli, and can lead to loss of consciousness, with some clonic jerking limb movements suggesting epilepsy. Interictally, however, the neurologic examination and electroencephalogram (EEG) remain normal. Both cyanotic and pallid forms have been described. The latter appears to involve increased vagal tone and bradycardia.

INCREASED INTRACRANIAL PRESSURE. A sudden increase in intracranial pressure with acute or intermittent hydrocephalus may decrease perfusion. Colloid cysts may obstruct cerebrospinal fluid outflow; these attacks are rare and should be positional. Other mass lesions such as tumors or the effects of a sudden hemorrhage may decrease perfusion through pressure effects.

Metabolic Causes. Although most cases of syncope can be attributed to diminished brain perfusion, cerebral metabolism may be interrupted in other ways. Acute hypoxia or diminution of oxygen-carrying capacity through anemias, hemoglobinopathies, or poisoning by toxins, such as carbon monoxide, can also cause syncope. Finally, cerebral metabolism requires glucose, and hypoglycemia may cause syncope, typically in diabetic patients after an excess of insulin, sometimes precipitated by exertion. Usually, there is a prodrome of hunger, altered behavior, and agitation with sympathetic activation, including tachycardia, before a gradual loss of consciousness.

Near-Syncope

Some spells are difficult to distinguish from syncope. Near-syncope or presyncope often includes lightheadedness and the same premonitory symptoms as early syncope, and it may have the same causes. The evaluation is similar to that for syncope though the symptoms are of an even less certain nature. Hypovolemia may lead to a feeling of generalized weakness and presyncope rather than to actual syncope. Hyperventilation and hypocarbia diminish cerebral blood flow through vasoconstriction and are a relatively common cause of near-syncope in young people, often associated with anxiety. Perioral and acral paresthesias are common; reproduction of symptoms by hyperventilation is confirmatory. Psychiatric problems such as anxiety and panic attacks may present similarly.

Mimickers of Syncope

Epilepsy, transient ischemic attacks (TIAs), and migraine cause many transient symptoms, but rarely syncope alone. Seizures can cause a sudden loss of consciousness, but there is almost always a history of seizures and other current signs of a seizure. Seizures more often cause an immediate loss of consciousness rather than a prolonged prodrome and are more likely to lead to physical injury, incontinence, and a prolonged postictal confusional state. A few brief clonic jerks may accompany syncope and do not implicate seizures. Although globally diminished brain perfusion may be considered a TIA in the broadest sense, the usual carotid or vertebrobasilar TIAs have symptoms and signs of focal ischemia and rarely cause syncope. Vertebrobasilar ischemia and migraine can impair consciousness, but almost always with other posterior circulation deficits, including cranial nerve abnormalities, and the onset of symptoms is generally slow.

Evaluation of Syncope

The evaluation of a patient with syncope begins with a second-by-second history of the episode's very beginning, including the patient's position, activities such as exertion or change in posture, and precipitating events such as urination or an unpleasant sight. Premonitory symptoms and whether a subject falls or is injured help to narrow the possible causes. Witnesses are crucial in describing the onset of syncope and the patient's appearance (e.g., agitation or pallor). The suddenness and duration of loss of consciousness are important, as is the speed of recovery. Staring, automatisms, or stereotyped motor activity are important if seizures are suspected. A history of cardiac disease is important, particularly in older patients. In younger patients, hyperventilation and vagally mediated syncope are more common. Impaired venous return and baseline low blood pressures in pregnancy may predispose to syncope.

Medication history is always important. As noted, medications with potentially adverse effects on autonomic function include antihypertensives, calcium channel blockers, diuretics, phenothiazines, levodopa, and tricyclic antidepressants. Alcohol can contribute to syncope in many ways.

Physical examination during the episode, including blood pressure and cardiac rhythm, can make the diagnosis. Subsequently, the evaluation includes orthostatic vital signs and a cardiac examination. The neurologic examination looks for persistent signs of prior focal disease such as strokes; a peripheral neuropathy may be related to many possible diagnoses. Basal ganglia disorders with autonomic failure should be recognizable from the associated motor abnormalities, which are not transient. Reproduction of symptoms through hyperventilation or carotid sinus massage can be very helpful, but the latter has risks and must be performed in a setting with the capacity for resuscitation.

Testing generally includes a cardiogram and, with any serious concern for a cardiac cause, echocardiography and monitoring for arrhythmias. Exercise tolerance testing is considered with a high suspicion of ischemic cardiac disease and after a cardiologist's evaluation. Patients with dangerous arrhythmias may need invasive electrophysiologic cardiac testing to define

the arrhythmia and its possible source or medications that might ameliorate it. The EEG may show flattening during an episode of syncope, but this is seldom available. Subsequently, nonepileptic EEG abnormalities tend to confuse the diagnosis. Seizures are a rare cause of syncope alone; EEGs are generally unnecessary without a clinical suspicion of seizures. Some patients with syncope prove to have epilepsy eventually, but the diagnosis is usually made through observation of subsequent events. Without suspicion of focal lesions or raised intracranial pressure, computed tomographic and magnetic resonance imaging scans are usually unnecessary.

Not rarely, the cause of syncope remains undetermined, even after a thorough investigation. Fortunately, the prognosis is generally excellent if serious cardiac disease has been excluded. Accordingly, the search for cardiac causes of syncope is the most important part of the investigation. Seizures and TIAs are unlikely causes of most cases of pure syncope, and presumptive treatment with anticonvulsants or anticoagulation is ill advised without a secure diagnosis. The diagnosis may emerge with follow-up and continued observation.

SPELLS WITHOUT SYNCOPE OR CLEAR FOCAL ONSET

Spells that provide neither the consideration of cerebral perfusion nor precise neurologic localization to aid in diagnosis can be among the most difficult to evaluate (Table 13-2). Still, the

TABLE 13-2. Causes of Spells Without Syncope or Clear Focal Signs

Confusional states
  Complex partial seizures, complex partial status epilepticus
  Absence seizures, absence status
  Migraine
  Dialysis dysequilibrium
  Porphyria
  Psychiatric disease
  Fluctuating encephaopathies (e.g., medication, metabolic, toxic, infectious)
Memory loss
  Transient global amnesia
  Benzodiazepines, anticholinergics
  Alcoholic blackouts
  Fugue states
  Less transient, including head injury, Wernicke's disease, postictal state, electroconvulsive therapy, dementia
Drop attacks
  Vertebrobasilar ischemia
  Anterior cerebral ischemia
  Foramen magnum and upper cord lesions
  Acute vestibulopathies, Menière's disease
  Raised intracranial pressure
  Severe asterixis, myoclonus
  Cataplexy
  Imbalance, including cerebral and cerebellar lesions, basal ganglia disorders, myelopathy, myopathy, peripheral neuropathies, sensory deprivation. (Exclude impaired consciousness with syncope, presyncope, or drop seizures)
Sleep disorders
  Narcolepsy, cataplexy
  Parasomnias, including somnambulism, night terrors, paroxysmal dystonias, rapid eye movement sleep/behavior disorder
  Base of the brain masses
Dizziness (including presyncope, imbalance, above)
  Vertigo (e.g., benign positional vertigo, Menière's disease eighth cranial nerve lesions)
  Temporal lobe seizures
  Posterior fossa lesions, multiple sclerosis, head injury, ear pathology
Hallucinations
  Visual, including withdrawal states, occipital lesions, occasional seizures, migraine, midbrain lesions, ocular deafferentation
  Auditory, including temporal lobe seizures, schizophrenia
Psychiatric episodes
  Panic attacks, anxiety disorders
  Episodic dyscontrol
Pseudoseizures

epidemiologic background, time course, and nature of the spell can narrow the possibilities and guide testing.

Confusional Spells

Confusional spells are particularly difficult because neither the patient nor observers may be able to recall details of the spell well. Confusional states are characterized by a marked diminution in attention, with a patient shifting sets too frequently and too widely to focus on any task. This usually implies bilateral brain dysfunction, particularly in the limbic system. Thinking may be very disorganized. Delirium implies some agitation amid the confusion.

Complex partial seizures are one of the most important of the many causes of confusional spells. The onset is focal ("partial"), and confusion or other alterations in consciousness occur when seizures spread to involve limbic structures bilaterally. Complex partial seizures typically have neither the focal motor onset of a simple partial seizure nor the convulsions of a generalized seizure. Often, there are prolonged periods of uninterruptible staring or automatisms, such as blinking, chewing, smacking, licking, or other orobuccal movements, or repetitive, stereotyped behavior, such as picking at clothing. Psychiatrically based spells are more likely to have a clear precipitant and no automatisms. Complex partial seizures seldom have a clear precipitant, though sleep deprivation, infection, toxic and metabolic factors, head injury, endocrinologic changes such as pregnancy, and lowered anticonvulsant levels can contribute.

Many different abnormal behaviors are possible in complex partial seizures, but an individual patient usually has stereotyped spells. The greater the number of symptoms and the more varied behavior, the less likely is the diagnosis of epilepsy. Complex partial seizures usually last no more than a few minutes but may be difficult to distinguish from prolonged postictal confusional states. The strangest behavior may occur postictally, and witnesses may be injured when trying to restrain a confused patient postictally; this is not "ictal violence."

In the evaluation of complex partial seizures, the history of the earliest onset of symptoms is crucial. Unless specifically asked, patients do not necessarily remember such symptoms as olfactory hallucinations before subsequent aspects of a spell. Staring spells and automatisms are seldom noticed by patients but are very important observations of witnesses.

Complex partial status epilepticus is far less common and may involve frequent complex partial seizures or a prolonged recovery between recurrent seizures. The EEG is crucial in diagnosis.

Prolonged absence seizures may also produce confusional episodes. Patients often display blinking or simple automatisms. They can generally continue walking, without falling or hurting themselves. Absence status may continue for days. A history of seizures increases clinical suspicion, but the patient may have been off medications and seizure-free for years. Absence status may recur after years in older patients or may arise anew, particularly after benzodiazepine withdrawal. A characteristic EEG confirms the diagnosis. Intravenous benzodiazepines may interrupt nonconvulsive status quickly.

Dialysis dysequilibrium is characterized by hours of confusion during or just after hemodialysis. It may also include seizures and headaches. The setting provides the diagnosis.

TIAs rarely cause confusion alone without focal neurologic signs. Strokes, especially right parietal, can cause confusion and occasionally resolve quickly. Confusional migraine is uncommon but may lead to several hours of confusion or even stupor, especially in adolescents with a history of migraine. Porphyria may produce episodic confusion and altered behavior.

Most confused behavior is not so transient. Among the most common causes are metabolic abnormalities, infection, and medications; steroids, sedatives, anticonvulsants, and medications for Parkinson's disease are frequent offenders. Medication withdrawal can cause similar confusion, and all of these causes are more likely to affect older patients or those already impaired through strokes, dementia, or other illnesses. These episodes rarely abate within hours but may fluctuate a good deal. Confusion may be precipitated by trauma and sensory or sleep deprivation. Wernicke's encephalopathy can occur suddenly; often attention is normal, and there are oculomotor signs as well as ataxia and confusion. Psychiatric illnesses that cause confusion rarely fluctuate so quickly.

The evaluation of patients with transient confusion relies heavily on the earlier history, which emphasizes seizure disorders, medication use, psychiatric illness, or other chronic illnesses that make a patient more vulnerable. Witnesses may observe helpful signs such as blinking or abnormal movements, possibly suggesting seizures. Because of fluctuations in metabolic encephalopathies, blood testing for such abnormalities is important. With a suspicion of seizures, and occasionally without, the EEG can be informative, not only for epilepsy but also for corroboration of a diffuse encephalopathy if this is not already clear clinically. Thiamine and glucose treatment are usually appropriate.

Transient Memory Loss

Sudden, transient, and isolated memory loss is relatively uncommon but can be dramatic. Transient global amnesia is a well-recognized syndrome, including the sudden onset of anterograde amnesia lasting several hours. Many authors exclude cases attributable to head injury, epilepsy, or migraine, but these diagnoses are not always obvious at presentation. Transient global amnesia generally occurs in subjects over 50 years old. About one-third have some intense emotional experience as a precipitant. A minority have recurrences. Immediate recall and long-present memory are preserved, but memory for the recent past and for new information is severely impaired. There may also be minimal retrograde amnesia. Most patients are slightly agitated and characteristically repeat over and over the same questions about what is happening to them. Patients are usually attentive, and semantic memory, language function, personal identity, visuospatial capabilities, and social interactions are preserved. Newly presented information must be tested to demonstrate the amnesia. Patients may be labeled as having acute confusional episodes, but most can focus on a task and reason effectively. The amnesia usually resolves within 8 hours, though mild symptoms may linger for days, and events during the episode are lost permanently.

The cause is a subject of much debate, but several different processes can produce the same result. Brief and recurrent episodes, especially without the repetitive questioning behavior, suggest the possibility of epilepsy. Particularly in these cases, an EEG is appropriate, but the structures serving memory are deep, and abnormalities may be missed. Vascular disease in older patients may also produce EEG abnormalities not diagnostic of seizures. The low recurrence rate lessens the likelihood of seizures. Relatively few cases of transient global amnesia appear to be epileptic, but memory can be altered in a postical state. Several reported cases have occurred in clear migraine attacks. Other characteristic symptoms such as visual auras, subsequent headache, and a positive family history are strongly suggestive. The common precipitants and benign course are also suggestive of migraine.

Most cases have no obvious cause. Some authors find a correlation with vascular risk factors and postulate simultaneous bilateral hippocampal ischemia as a result of posterior circulation vascular disease. Vertebral angiography has led to transient global amnesia, and thalamic lesions, including masses, have been found. Most memory loss is presumed to involve bilateral structures that subtend memory function in the medial temporal lobes (particularly hippocampus) or in the thalamus, but in a few cases left-sided mesial temporal or thalamic lesions have produced an indistinguishable syndrome, probably caused in part by the dependence of testing on verbal function.

The benign course, otherwise normal neurologic examination, and low recurrence rate argue that most patients with transient global amnesia need minimal investigation and no treatment, particularly in younger patients with a suggestion of migraine. A history of headache, seizures, head injury, and recent medication are pertinent, but a patient may not remember them, and witnesses are valuable. Visual field testing can indicate a posterior circulation stroke or other lesion. Older patients with cardiovascular risk factors should be investigated as for TIAs (below). Patients with histories suggestive of seizures merit an EEG, preferably after sleep deprivation, and an examination for focal lesions.

Benzodiazepines produce an occasional isolated amnesia, even without sedation; their widespread use produces many episodes. Amnesia occurs with all different benzodiazepines and is dose related. As in transient global amnesia, semantic memory and reasoning are usually preserved, and subjects may function normally in complex tasks, only to realize a large gap in memory subsequently. The amnesia is usually inapparent to observers, as behavior and performance remain normal. There appears to be a disruption in new learning and consolidation rather than in retrieval. The effect may last a few hours. Indeed, midazolam is often used by anesthesiologists, in part for its amnestic effects during medical procedures. Anticholinergics may produce both anterograde and retrograde amnesia. Older patients and those receiving other psychotropic medications, including alcohol, are more susceptible.

Alcoholic ''blackouts'' are hours to days of amnesia for performed activities during heavy alcohol use rather than a loss of consciousness. Performance is more likely to decline during alcoholic amnesia than with benzodiazepines. Chronic alcoholism and prior head injury may contribute.

The term *fugue state* refers to more prolonged episodes of apparently purposeful behavior, including driving long distances, with preservation of performance but with amnesia for actions and their rationale. Many are associated with depression or other psychiatric illness, and this history should be sought. Head injury and medication use are also pertinent. Briefer episodes can represent a seizure or postical state. An EEG is often warranted, but most fugue states are more prolonged than typical seizures.

Often, an isolated memory loss is suspected, but a more extensive examination shows a confusional state. These are often due to acute metabolic derangements, medications, other toxins, or infections. Episodes are usually more prolonged. Right hemisphere strokes or mass lesions may produce a confusional state,

also of longer duration, and not memory loss per se. Seizures and postictal states usually produce prominent confusion rather than pure amnesia, although memory loss alone may be reported subsequently. Dementias produce nontransient memory loss as part of more extensive cognitive dysfunction.

Head trauma, especially with bitemporal injury, is one of the most common causes of memory loss, but the amnesia is seldom brief. Acutely, an injury may be forgotten, and memory loss may be brief. The history or examination for trauma may make the diagnosis clear. Wernicke's disease, the residua of herpes encephalitis, and electroconvulsive therapy for depression can also produce more prolonged memory deficits. Psychiatric disease or factitious memory loss must be suspected when patients appear to have forgotten overlearned materials such as their own names and have preservation of language function with apparent loss of reasoning.

The evaluation of patients with isolated amnesia includes a history that looks for similar prior episodes, migraine, head injury, epilepsy, or psychiatric illness. History and laboratory studies look for benzodiazepine, alcohol, or other medication use. The examination should exclude a confusional state and check for visual field loss and other neurologic deficits. Treatment can only be aimed at a specific diagnosis rather than at memory loss per se.

Drop Attacks

The term *drop attack* should generally be restricted to a sudden fall without impairment of consciousness. It implies a sudden dysfunction of truncal and leg muscle tone or sudden leg weakness. Without affecting consciousness, such attacks implicate lower brainstem or spinal cord structures where postural maintenance reflexes and control of the trunk and both legs are governed in a region compact enough to be affected by a single process.

In older patients, hypoperfusion and syncope or near-syncope are always important considerations when it is uncertain that consciousness has been maintained. Cardiac syncope can occur suddenly, with rapid recovery, and the loss of consciousness may be forgotten. Because of the high morbidity rate, it is very important not to mistake cardiac syncope for drop attacks.

With truly maintained consciousness, brainstem ischemia is a major consideration. Pontine ischemia that affects the corticospinal tracts bilaterally can cause a loss of tone with preserved consciousness. Compression of ventral brainstem structures by a mass or ectatic basilar artery can do the same. With severe vertebrobasilar or cervical spine disease, compression of one vertebral artery by head turning can be sufficient. Brainstem ischemia is more common in older patients, usually includes other signs of cranial nerve dysfunction or ataxia, and usually comes on gradually. Much more rarely, transient anterior cerebral ischemia can lead to bilateral leg weakness.

Just a bit caudally, foramen magnum mass lesions can compress the brainstem or upper spinal cord. Especially with preexisting rheumatoid arthritis or severe cervical spondylosis, neck movement may cause transient compression. This can be exacerbated by trauma. Often, the examination shows signs of a myelopathy. Rarely, mass lesions or midline, third ventricular cysts cause sudden obstruction of cerebrospinal fluid pathways and acute hydrocephalus, leading to drop attacks. Usually, headaches are suggestive.

Atonic seizures may be called drop attacks but include a loss of consciousness. They can be rapid and dangerous. Most are generalized or generalize rapidly from a frontal or other focus. More violent myoclonic seizures explain some falls. Most patients with atonic seizures also have other seizures, and many suffer from Lennox-Gastaut syndrome or other childhood epilepsies with several seizure types. Tonic seizures, often part of Lennox-Gastaut syndrome also, may cause falls by sudden rigid extension of the legs and trunk. Some seizures remain focal but include enough weakness or limb malfunction to cause falls. Seizures tend to be stereotyped, and most cause falls with a longer loss of consciousness. They are an unlikely explanation for isolated drop attacks without other clear seizure types, especially in adults. Occasionally, myoclonus or asterixis in the legs or trunk can be severe enough to cause drops.

Other than simply tripping, patients may fall because of imbalance. This may be due to cerebral, cerebellar, vestibular, spinal cord, or peripheral nerve dysfunction. Weakness, as a result of myopathy, infarcts, or other deficits, and spasticity are possible causes, as is impaired sensation (particularly somesthetic, though impaired vision and hearing can contribute). Parkinson's disease and other basal ganglia disorders often impair postural reflexes. The falls may be transient, but basal ganglia disease, myelopathy, and peripheral neuropathy should be evident on neurologic examination. Patients with vestibular disease severe enough to cause imbalance and falls often have vertigo. Sudden, nearly violent vestibular dysfunction and imbalance may occur in Menière's disease; this should include sensorineural hearing loss and tinnitus along with the vertigo and generally occurs in older patients. Medications are always a concern and may exacerbate prior neurologic illness. Nonneurologic disease such as arthritis and orthopaedic problems can also prompt falls.

A few authors have described a curious entity of isolated falls occurring during walking in women over the age of 40, often recurring a few times a year, with no leg weakness, myelopathy, basal ganglia disorder, or other identifiable cause. The legs seem to give out suddenly. Some events are prompted by pregnancy, suggesting a hormonal influence, though the etiology is entirely unclear.

Finally, cataplexy may be the purest form of drop attack, with a perfectly maintained consciousness and sudden atonia, often precipitated by a sudden emotional stimulus such as fear or laughter. Respiration is maintained. Patients may remain atonic for several minutes. Cataplexy appears to represent the atonia of rapid eye movement (REM) sleep occurring in waking. The abnormalities in tone at inappropriate times with regard to sleep, as well as the abnormal dreaming or hallucinations in wakefulness, indicate abnormalities in upper brainstem structures that control the onset of dreaming and atonia. At least some cataplexy is found in most patients with narcolepsy, and almost all cataplexy is part of narcolepsy. Less frequently, it may occur with other brainstem lesions or masses at the base of the skull.

Evaluation of drop attacks begins with a history, which seeks to determine whether syncope, especially cardiac, or seizures were actually involved. Prior cardiac disease, palpitations, TIAs, headache, hearing loss, vertigo, any sensory loss (including visual and auditory), or symptoms of narcolepsy are of interest. Medication history is always pertinent. The exact onset of the fall and the progression are important, and witnesses are valuable. The examination looks for raised intracranial pressure; evidence of old cerebrovascular disease; basal ganglia disorders with alterations in tone or movement; signs of a my-

elopathy, including spasticity; ataxia; and a search for weakness, especially in the legs.

With such varied causes, drop attacks can have no single therapy. One must treat the underlying cause, and anticoagulation for presumed TIAs or anticonvulsants for possible seizures are inappropriate without a reasonable diagnosis.

Sleep Disorders

Sleep disorders can produce transient or paroxysmal symptoms in addition to cataplexy. Narcoleptic sleep attacks can be relatively sudden, and patients can have lapses in attention or fall asleep at inappropriate times, suggesting syncope. The history may suggest narcolepsy, especially if associated with cataplexy, sleep paralysis, or hallucinations at the onset or end of sleep. The EEG can help differentiate sudden attacks of sleepiness from seizures, showing drowsiness and sleep in the former; postictal slowing is not the same as a sleepy record.

Other paroxysms of abnormal movement or behavior may occur during sleep. Parasomnias, including sleepwalking and night terrors, occur in slow wave sleep rather than in REM; patients are amnestic for the attacks. Similar episodes can be epileptic. REM sleep behavior disorder can lead to very disruptive activities during dreaming without the usual atonia. The restless legs syndrome may respond to levodopa, and nocturnal dystonias can be responsive to anticonvulsants (see Ch. 162). Polysomnography with EEG can help distinguish parasomnias and movement disorders of sleep from nocturnal seizures.

Dizziness

Dizziness is a relatively useless term clinically and must be further differentiated. Three categories encompass much of dizziness. Lightheadedness is often presyncope, and investigations follow the same rationale. Imbalance or unsteadiness suggests incoordination, weakness, or disturbances in tone or sensation, as discussed earlier regarding falling spells. Finally, "dizziness" can mean vertigo or the perception of movement in the absence of true movement; most is rotational. Vertigo is often associated with unilateral vestibular system dysfunction, but the laterality is not always clear at the time of presentation, especially with transient symptoms (see Ch. 9).

Brief episodes of severe rotational vertigo with nausea and gait instability and a definite relationship to head position are strongly suggestive of benign positional vertigo. Episodes often last less than 1 minute but may recur months after apparent resolution. Often, the neurologic examination is normal, and no treatment is required. Attacks of vertigo with nausea and vomiting along with hearing loss and tinnitus suggest Menière's disease; its acute vestibular dysfunction can even lead to falls without loss of consciousness. Both of these conditions involve extra-axial vestibular dysfunction (i.e., in inner ear structures or in the eighth cranial nerve). Rarely, abnormal input to the vestibular system caused by cervical spine or other neck disease can lead to vertigo.

Vertigo from brainstem disease is often less severe and may be associated with diplopia, facial numbness, absent corneal reflexes, dysarthria, dysphagia, or abnormal visual fields or acuity. Less dramatic vertigo (often translational rather than rotational) can occur with temporal lobe seizures. Occasionally, vertigo, tinnitus, and hearing loss can be part of presyncope. Strokes can produce more lasting vertigo, but TIAs involving the basilar and internal auditory artery supplying the eighth cranial nerve can also include vertigo.

Less transient vertigo can occur with chronic ear disease such as infections, skull fractures or other head injury, barotrauma, and aminoglycoside toxicity. Cerebellopontine angle tumors more often present with hearing loss than with vertigo. Posterior fossa tumors and multiple sclerosis produce less transient symptoms and signs.

The examination focuses on peripheral ear and eighth cranial nerve dysfunction, including signs of infection, hearing loss, and associated cranial nerve and brainstem signs. Hearing loss on audiometry can help diagnose Menière's disease. Provocative maneuvers involving head turning and vestibular apparatus positioning, such as the Hallpike maneuver, attempt to elicit the patient's typical symptoms and concomitant nystagmus.

Hallucinations

Hallucinations often localize to a sensory region. Visual hallucinations are common in migraine and occipital seizures. They may also occur along with delirium in encephalopathies, including those caused by metabolic derangements, medications, and medication withdrawal, particularly from alcohol. Poor visual acuity predisposes to visual hallucinations. Raised intracranial pressure can lead to fleeting bilateral visual loss; visual loss is discussed more extensively in Chapter 7. Auditory hallucinations may occur with temporal lobe dysfunction, including seizures. Epileptic auditory hallucinations are generally less well formed, varied, and directive than those in schizophrenia.

Psychiatric Conditions

Psychiatric diseases can also produce paroxysmal symptoms. Panic attacks can come on abruptly and include autonomic symptoms such as palpitations, nausea, sweating, and flushing, along with feelings of shortness of breath, choking, vertigo, lightheadedness, tremor, chest pain, depression, fear, and a feeling of impending doom. Paresthesias can follow hyperventilation. A sense of depersonalization is less common, and very rare attacks may lead to a loss of consciousness, possibly through hyperventilation.

Many panic attacks can be diagnosed on the basis of the autonomic and respiratory symptoms, along with fear or dread. Alteration in consciousness raises the question of complex partial seizures. Panic attacks often occur in patients with related psychiatric problems, and many have an emotional precipitant. Lateralized symptoms are unlikely, and loss of consciousness or injury are rare. More than with seizures, there is variability in symptoms from episode to episode, and EEGs should remain normal. EEG monitoring during the episodes can be very helpful in distinguishing the two.

Episodic dyscontrol with angry or even "directed" and violent reactions to seemingly minor, though identifiable, stimuli is generally considered a psychiatric problem. Episodes last for minutes, usually followed by profuse apologies. Between episodes, patients have relatively normal behavior and are not psychotic. Head injury, encephalitis, and mild or moderate mental retardation are common settings. With a well-identified precipitant and no other clear signs of seizures, these episodes are rarely epileptic.

Nonepileptic seizures or *pseudoseizures* may produce bizarre spells. Unfortunately, for diagnostic simplicity, perhaps one-half of patients with nonepileptic seizures also have true epilepsy. Often, patients have severe psychiatric problems and have a model for seizure manifestations. Epileptic seizures are more often stereotyped; pseudoseizures last longer and tend to have more variety. They may be provoked by suggestion or stress, include poorly coordinated movements and more complex vocalizations, and usually do not respond to anticonvulsants. Pseudoseizures more often occur with an audience and less often during sleep. Injuries are rare. Actions or violence may appear more directed, and patients may resist examination during the event.

EEG monitoring can help, but many seizures, including frontal seizures, can have unusual manifestations and be difficult to record. Interictal EEGs are of less value because epileptic patients may have normal EEGs, and pseudoseizures occur in patients with epilepsy. Thus, a diagnosis of epilepsy cannot be absolutely "ruled out" but can be rendered less likely, provided that the typical spells are recorded and the EEG shows a normal background without epileptic changes or postictal slowing. A diagnosis of nonepileptic seizures helps to minimize medication toxicity and points the way to psychiatric therapy, though this is not always curative.

FOCAL OR LOCALIZED SYMPTOMS

Transient symptoms with clear focal features help make the neurologic diagnosis in the traditional way, through localization (Table 13-3). The "big three" diagnostic entities are TIAs, epileptic seizures, and migraine. They can cause very similar spells, but several features may help to distinguish one from the other (Table 13-4).

Transient Ischemic Attacks

TIAs are temporary dysfunction of brain tissue caused by inadequate blood flow. Vague spells and "dizziness" unaccompanied by localizable symptoms do not constitute TIAs; symptoms must correspond to dysfunction of an identifiable vascular territory.

Carotid artery territory TIAs often produce contralateral hand and arm weakness and sensory loss. Face and leg symptoms are often less severe, particularly with primary involvement of the middle cerebral artery, but the signs and symptoms change depending on the vascular territory involved (e.g., leg weakness is more likely with anterior cerebral artery ischemia). Carotid TIAs can be limited to ipsilateral visual symptoms with involvement of the ophthalmic artery. In the hemisphere dominant for language they can produce aphasia; less frequently, language disturbances occur in isolation.

TIAs, without completed strokes, may be more common in the vertebrobasilar territory and often include combinations of diplopia, ataxia, vertigo, dysarthria, unilateral or bilateral visual symptoms, and weakness on one or both sides, especially in the legs. Although isolated vertigo or imbalance can be a posterior circulation TIA, there are usually other associated symptoms

TABLE 13-3. Causes of Transient Events With Focal Onset

Common
Transient ischemic attacks
Epilepsy with partial onset
Migraine
Less Common
Overlap syndromes (migraine ± seizure ± ischemia)
Mass lesions
Multiple sclerosis
Movement disorders

TABLE 13-4. Differentiating Features of Common Spells With Focal Symptoms

	Seizure	Transient Ischemic Attack	Migraine
Epidemiology, risks	Any age; different age-related syndromes Birth, childhood injury, head injury, encephalitis	Older patient Risks for vascular disease	Younger Female:male 3:1
Family history	+	−	+ +
Precipitants	Infection, sleep disturbance, head injury, medication change, stress, hormonal change; not postural	Activity (embolic) Upright posture; poor perfusion	Foods, medication Stress Hormonal change
Localization; clinical features	Several foci, including motor Positive symptoms (e.g., motor and hallucinations)	Must correspond to a vascular territory: Carotid: unilateral, especially in limbs Vertebrobasilar: brainstem, occipital, can be unilateral or bilateral in legs Negative symptoms (e.g., paralysis)	Posterior cerebrum common Visual symptoms, including positive hallucinations; some negative
Time course	March over seconds May progress to complex partial, generalized seizures	Lasts minutes usually Often maximal at onset but may stutter	March over minutes, can be 20 minutes Often precedes headache by 20–30 minutes
Altered consciousness	With progression to complex partial and generalized seizures	Rare	Rare May occur in adolescents with basilar migraine, but with slow onset and incomplete
Appearance to observers	Motor abnormalities, jerking common Staring, automatisms, incontinence, falls in some with progression	Sudden loss of function, weakness, clumsiness, dysarthria, aphasia	Often appears normal Occasional slurring, clumsiness
Examination	Focal at the onset Postictal focal deficits May have old focal lesions	Evidence of vascular disease May have focal or multifocal deficits, some old	Usually normal during and between episodes
Imaging studies	Usually normal except for prior and predisposing lesions	New (and old) vascular lesions	Usually normal
Electroencephalogram	May have epileptiform abnormalities, depending on type and localization of seizures	Frequently with focal or multifocal slowing Epileptiform abnormalities not rare	Often normal Prominent focal slowing may long outlast the episode

and signs. TIAs should have the same manifestations as strokes, if only briefly; these syndromes are further elaborated in the chapters on vascular disease.

TIAs usually present suddenly, often in older patients with a history or risks for vascular disease. Symptoms are almost always ''negative'' (i.e., a loss of function) rather than ''positive'' phenomena, such as involuntary movements or visual sensations or hallucinations. Alteration in consciousness or confusion are rare, but an aphasia may be mistaken for confusion. The definition of TIAs as lasting less than 24 hours is somewhat misleading because most last just minutes, and events of over 1 hour are much less common.

The history of a patient with TIAs should include a search for risk factors and a history of similar or related events, including transient monocular blindness when carotid disease is suspected. TIAs tend to be stereotyped, though emboli may recur in different vascular territories. Cardiogenic emboli often occur during activity. New headaches may follow cerebral ischemia. Cocaine use may cause transient or more permanent ischemia, and medication history is important in evaluating any transient event.

Neurologists rarely have the opportunity to examine a patient during a TIA, but the examination is still important afterward; the event is not transient if signs persist. Funduscopic examination can show vascular disease or even emboli themselves. Cardiac examination for arrhythmias and murmurs is important. Rarely, a blood pressure difference between the two arms signifies subclavian stenosis causing vertebrobasilar ischemia, exacerbated by arm use in a ''steal'' syndrome. The neurologic examination (including testing of cognition, visual fields, cranial nerves, and more distal motor and sensory function) may

show that an event is not transient or may show evidence of prior strokes.

By definition, TIAs resolve. Investigation is directed at preventing recurrences or strokes by looking for causes of strokes. Focal symptoms warrant a search for focal lesions, and the magnetic resonance imaging scan is the most sensitive and useful test. Cardiac and hematologic evaluations (including for coagulopathies and dysproteinemias) are usually appropriate. Direct evaluation of individual vessels depends on the clinical localization. In older patients, temporal arteritis and erythrocyte sedimentation rates are too often overlooked. More extensive evaluations are appropriate in younger patients and in those with new symptoms rather than recurrences of the same symptom.

Seizures

In addition to the falls, loss of consciousness, and confusional spells described earlier, seizures produce focal or ''partial'' symptoms. Seizures often occur in patients with risk factors such as congenital, birth, or other early injuries; prior meningitis or encephalitis; strokes; tumors; or head injury. They are precipitated by irregular sleep, medications, infection, head injury, stress, or hormonal flux. Certain seizure syndromes are age related, and a substantial minority of patients have family histories of epilepsy.

When seizure symptoms spread over the body, the progression is rapid, usually within seconds. The resolution of seizures is slower and may require hours. Some lead to a confusional state or prolonged focal deficits (motor, sensory, or cognitive) postictally (e.g., a ''Todd's'' paralysis) for up to hours. Seizures have a great variety, but repeated episodes tend to be stereo-typed in the same patient. Accordingly, a tremendous variety of paroxysmal symptoms is unlikely to be epileptic.

Simple partial or focal seizures leave consciousness unaffected, and patients can report focal symptoms. With a progression to complex partial seizures, however, there is an impairment of consciousness, and amnesia for the event may occur. The observations of patients and witnesses are crucial. Family members may report many more spells than the patients themselves. The exact onset of symptoms is important; uninterruptible staring spells and orobuccal automatisms are important clues. Jerking motor activity, the character of hallucinations, and the time course of spells all help to characterize a seizure. Patients usually refer to focal seizure onsets as "auras." Some begin with olfactory or other hallucinations, and patients will not necessarily report these symptoms without being asked. Some features of an episode may suggest or discourage a diagnosis of epilepsy (Table 13-5).

The history should include a family history and that of gestation, delivery, and early development, as well as prior illnesses or injuries that predispose to seizures. The general examination searches for related findings (e.g., the skin lesions in tuberous sclerosis or other neurocutaneous syndromes) and neurologic deficits that indicate a greater risk of seizures.

As with TIAs, focal seizures mandate a search for focal lesions, including a magnetic resonance imaging or computed tomographic scan. Interictal EEG epileptiform abnormalities increase the likelihood of seizures, but discharges can occur without epilepsy, and EEG abnormalities are also found in vascular disease, migraine, and other illnesses. Abnormalities such as focal slowing are insufficient to diagnose seizures, and there are artifacts and normal variants with sharp features on EEG. EEGs may remain normal in patients with seizures, especially with a frontal focus. When symptoms are frequent enough, long-term EEG monitoring can be diagnostic if electrographic seizure activity is recorded at the time of symptoms. Postictal

slowing can also be a useful finding. Seizure diagnosis is detailed further in the chapters on epilepsy.

Migraine

Migraine is extremely common, affecting approximately 18 percent of the female and 6 percent of the male population of the United States (see Ch. 205). Many have headaches alone, but migraine often includes unilateral or bilateral "positive" visual symptoms, visual loss, or unilateral sensory and motor symptoms. Its pathophysiology is poorly understood, but cerebral vasculature and trigeminal nerve nociceptive afferents are involved; the progressive cortical dysfunction of spells, however, does not respect vascular boundaries. Focal symptoms typically occur in patients with known migraine and in patients much younger than those with TIAs. Spells usually precede a typical headache but can occur without headache. A family history of migraine is very common. New symptoms may occur with new stresses, including hormonal (e.g., a woman with no prior migraine but with a significant family history may have new migrainous visual symptoms, without headache, during pregnancy).

A gradual onset of symptoms is typical. With limb involvement, numbness may "march" over a period of up to 30 minutes compared to the spread of seizures over seconds. The neurologic deficit tends to precede the headache by 20 minutes and may last 20 to 30 minutes, resolving during the headache; some are more prolonged. "Positive" visual symptoms are more suggestive of migraine or seizure than of TIAs. Jagged bright lines in a "fortification spectrum" are strongly suggestive of migraine. Marked focal EEG slowing in migraine may outlast the neurologic deficit or headache by many hours.

Basilar artery migraine usually occurs in younger subjects, typically adolescents with a history of migraine, and often includes brainstem dysfunction such as vertigo, diplopia, bilateral visual field loss, ataxia, and dysarthria. In more severe episodes, loss of consciousness occurs over minutes but is less severe than with seizures, typically with ready rousability. Confusion may last hours. Visual symptoms are often first. Motor symptoms are generally clumsiness and weakness, not positive signs such as limb jerking. Recovery is usually rapid. Benefit from typical migraine medication can be a diagnostic aid. Paroxysmal vertebrobasilar symptoms in children rarely represent ischemia and are more likely to be migraine.

Overlap Syndromes

Among migraine, seizures, and ischemia, there are many complicated overlapping syndromes. Rarely, migraine can lead to focal ischemia and a stroke. Vascular disease is probably the most common cause of focal seizures in older adults. Focal lesions may lead to "symptomatic" migraine headaches. Headaches can occur postictally.

In some syndromes, such as benign occipital epilepsy of childhood, it may be impossible to separate migraine from epilepsy. These patients have prominent focal occipital spike wave discharges and a very high incidence of migraine. Seizures typically occur during the migraine aura but may follow attacks of migraine. Clonic movements, complex partial seizures, and generalized convulsions may follow typical migrainous visual phenomena. Negative phenomena such as blindness may occur with occipital seizures. The family history is often positive, but manifestations are uncommon in adults. The prognosis is

TABLE 13-5. Myths About Spells and Seizures

"I don't have seizures any more, just frequent auras."
  The "aura" is the partial onset of the seizure (though auras may also be part of migraine); it may progress to a convulsion.
"Incontinence and tongue-biting are reliable signs of convulsions."
  These symptoms occur more often with seizures than with other paroxysmal attacks, but their absence does not argue strongly against epilepsy; even with convulsions, they are found in a minority of patients.
"Bilateral motor activity without loss of consciousness indicates pseudoseizure."
  Some bilateral jerking activity, especially when prolonged and somewhat irregular, along with apparently purposeful behavior, is suggestive of pseudoseizure. Nevertheless, complex partial seizures of frontal origin may include bilateral leg activity such as "bicycling" or running with a preserved consciousness and even memory for the event.
"The patient has several bizarre symptoms. It must be temporal lobe epilepsy."
  Seizures tend to be stereotyped from episode to episode with an individual. An individual seizure may progress from an olfactory hallucination to a staring spell and on to a generalized convulsion; in addition, some patients have a few types of seizures. Nevertheless, a wide variety of symptoms is unlikely to be attributable to epilepsy.
"Drop attacks are commonly caused by seizures."
  Atonic seizures are relatively rare and generally found in patients with refractory seizure disorders, including several types of seizures. These drop attacks tend to occur with loss of consciousness.
"An EEG will diagnose epilepsy ("rule out" seizures)."
  EEG findings aid in the diagnosis of seizures and may help to indicate an individual type of epilepsy, but up to one-half of patients wtih epilepsy have a normal EEG at a given time. Also, there are many EEG abnormalities not diagnostic of epilepsy, and epileptiform discharges occur occasionally without clinical epilepsy. The EEG must be used with the clinical history and observations.

Abbreviations: EEG, electroencephalogram.

usually excellent. Concurrent migraine and epilepsy can also be traced to mitochondrial encephalopathies.

Other Causes of Focal Symptoms

Less often, transient focal symptoms arise from causes other than epilepsy, ischemia, or migraine. *Mass lesions* may present with transient focal symptoms, possibly caused by venous insufficiency or focal seizures. The neurologic examination may show less transient signs. *Multiple sclerosis* can produce focal weakness, sensory changes, or incoordination lasting minutes or hours, but there is almost always other, nontransient evidence of the disease such as optic nerve or eye movement dysfunction, spasticity, or ataxia. Transient multiple sclerosis symptoms usually last much longer. They may occur with an increase in body temperature.

Occasionally, *movement disorders* can present paroxysmally. Paroxysmal dystonias may last minutes, hours, or days. Some such movement disorders occur in the context of multiple sclerosis, cerebral palsy, or hypoparathyroidism. Though the events do not appear to be epileptic and the EEG is usually normal, anticonvulsants help in some cases, as they can for paroxysmal nocturnal dystonias.

Gilles de la Tourette syndrome or other tic disorders are occasionally mistaken for seizures. The grunting, barking, or forced and occasionally obscene vocalizations may be difficult to manage. Tics often respond to neuroleptic medications but with potential complications. Tardive dyskinesias occur after antipsychotic medication use but may be inconstant in appearance (see Ch. 123). Often, basal ganglia dysfunction is evident such as in Parkinson's disease, and this is not intermittent. In a startle syndrome called hyperekplexia, a sudden stimulus (usually noise) leads to violent body stiffening and falls. The syndrome is familial but not epileptic. Sudden movement disorders such as chorea, athetosis, and hemiballismus occur in basal ganglia disorders, including those caused by strokes. Usually, the neurologic examination is abnormal, and scans may show lesions, especially in vascular cases.

Transient neurologic symptoms challenge the neurologist with a bewildering array of diagnostic possibilities. The events have usually resolved before one has a chance to observe them, and witnesses must always be sought. Nevertheless, a reasonable diagnosis can usually be reached within the framework of considering which part of the brain is involved, along with epidemiologic factors, the time course and character of events, and some characteristic features of certain syndromes. Foremost consideration is given to the more threatening diagnoses such as cardiac disease, epilepsy, and cerebrovascular disease, although many conditions are relatively benign. Often, it is more prudent to wait for recurrence of events for additional data rather than to jump to prescribe therapy without a clear diagnosis.

SUGGESTED READINGS

Andermann F, Lugaresi E: Migraine and Epilepsy. Butterworth, Boston, 1987
Camfield PR, Metrakos K, Andermann F: Basilar migraine, seizures, and severe epileptiform EEG abnormalities. Neurology 28:584–8, 1978
Engel J Jr: Seizures and Epilepsy. FA Davis, Philadelphia, 1989
Kapoor WN, Karpf M, Wieand S et al: A prospective evaluation and follow-up of patients with syncope. N Engl J Med 309:197–204, 1983
Kushner MJ, Hauser WA: Transient global amnesia: a case-control study. Ann Neurol 18:684–91, 1985
Luders H, Lesser RP: Epilepsy: Electroclinical Syndromes. Springer-Verlag, London, 1987
McLeod JG, Tuck RR: Disorders of the autonomic nervous system. Ann Neurol 21:419–30, 519–29, 1987
Meissner I, Wiebers DO, Swanson JW, O'Fallon WM: The natural history of drop attacks. Neurology 36:1029–34, 1986
Morrell MJ: Differential diagnosis of seizures. Neurol Clin 11:737–54, 1993
Thorpy MJ: Handbook of Sleep Disorders. Marcel Dekker, New York, 1990

14. RESPIRATORY DYSFUNCTION

DAVID LACOMIS

Respiratory dysfunction is usually caused by cardiopulmonary disorders or by upper airway obstruction; however, neurologic diseases may also impair respiration. Such nervous system disorders may present with acute respiratory dysfunction and require emergency assessment, or they may progress more insidiously and so come to the attention of the neurologist or primary care physician in ambulatory practice. In many of these patients, associated clinical features reveal the cause of the respiratory disorder, such as Guillain-Barré syndrome. In others, such as some patients with amyotrophic lateral sclerosis, respiratory dysfunction may appear alone. As with all nervous system diseases, clinical diagnosis is founded on an understanding of the neuroanatomy and of the pathologic processes that may occur in the relevant structures.

NEUROANATOMY OF RESPIRATION

Muscles of Respiration

A respiratory bellows mechanism moves air repetitively into and out of the lung alveoli, allowing gas exchange to occur. The inspiratory phase of this biphasic process is active; the expiratory phase is predominantly passive. During quiet inspiration, the diaphragm, which is attached to the xiphoid process, the lower six ribs, and the upper lumbar vertebrae, performs most of the work. When this dome-shaped circumferential muscle group contracts, its central tendon is pulled down and forward, causing the abdominal viscera to descend and the abdomen to protrude. The central tendon then becomes fixed. Further expansion of the chest cavity is accomplished by elevation of the lower ribs and forward displacement of the sternum and upper ribs. The resultant increase in intrathoracic volume lowers intrapleural and intrapulmonary pressures, causing air to rush into the lungs from the upper air passages. Intercostal and scalene as well as paraspinal and sternocleidomastoid muscles serve as accessory muscles of respiration to increase the thoracic volume further during deep respiration or when there is respiratory compromise. Muscles of the upper airway (genioglossus, pharyngeal constrictors, and the laryngeal and neck strap muscles) work to keep the airway open. During normal expiration, there is passive recoil of the thoracic cage and lungs along with abdominal and intercostal muscle contraction, causing an elevation in intrathoracic pressure and the expulsion of air from the lungs.

Peripheral Nerve Supply of the Respiratory Muscles and Lung

The diaphragm is innervated bilaterally by the phrenic nerves, which are derived from the third, fourth, and fifth cervical segments and their respective anterior horn cells and motor roots. The phrenic nerves descend across the scalene muscles, diving deep to the internal jugular veins, and enter the thorax in front of the internal thoracic artery. In the thorax, the nerves then descend anterior to the roots of the lungs, traverse the fibrous pericardium and mediastinal pleura, and, finally, innervate the diaphragm. The left phrenic nerve also passes anterior to the arch of the aorta. Thus, the phrenic nerves are vulnerable to injury at multiple sites from the neck to the lower thorax.

Intercostal and respiratory paraspinal muscles are supplied by thoracic spinal roots. Abdominal muscles receive their innervation from lower thoracic and upper lumbar segments. The strap muscles of the neck (sternohyoideus, sternothyroideus, thyrohyoideus, and omohyoideus) are supplied by the upper cervical roots; the sternocleidomastoid muscles, by the spinal accessory nerves predominantly; and the nasopharyngeal muscles, by the ninth, tenth, and twelfth cranial nerves. Pulmonary innervation to bronchial muscles, glands, blood vessels, and mucous membranes is both sympathetic and parasympathetic. The parasympathetic supply is from the vagal nerve and mediates bronchconstriction by stimulating muscle contraction; the sympathetic influence is inhibitory and facilitates relaxation of bronchial smooth muscles and, hence, bronchodilation.

Central Control of Respiration

The upper motor neuron pathways governing respiratory control are complex and have been reviewed in detail by Kelly and Luce (1991) (Fig. 14-1). Both automatic and voluntary control mechanisms orchestrate the complex movements of respiration. The afferent limb of the automatic component begins with pulmonary and respiratory muscle stretch mechanoreceptors and with blood oxygen and CO_2 chemoreceptors located on the floor of the fourth ventricle and in the aortic and carotid bodies. These receptors provide sensory input to specialized neurons in the medulla, the central respiratory pattern generator. The dorsal respiratory group is adjacent to the tractus solitarius and contains ''inspiratory'' neurons; the ventral group is associated with the nucleus ambiguus and retroambiguus and contains ''inspiratory'' and ''expiratory'' neurons. Centers in the pons, including the so-called pneumotaxic center, and in the pontomedullary junction modulate respiratory control.

Efferent fibers travel to the contralateral lungs and pharyngeal and laryngeal muscles via the vagus nerve and to the respiratory muscles via the phrenic and intercostal nerves and their spinal roots. The associated spinal cord pathways are located ventrolaterally. Voluntary overdrive mechanisms, such as those governing breath-holding and voluntary hyperventilation, have not been fully characterized, but the motor cortex, reticular activating system, cerebellum, midbrain, and forebrain all have postulated roles.

Much of the pathway that mediates respiration is also involved in the production of hiccups or singultus. This phenomenon results from repetitive contraction of the diaphragm while the glottis is closed. Phrenic, vagal, and sympathetic afferents are involved in addition to phrenic efferents. These nerves are controlled by the central respiratory structures in the brainstem. Therefore, a lesion along this exended pathway may cause hiccups with or without respiratory dysfunction.

SYMPTOMS AND SIGNS OF NEUROGENIC RESPIRATORY DYSFUNCTION

Dyspnea is usually the first symptom of respiratory dysfunction from any cause. In addition to the well-known features from the

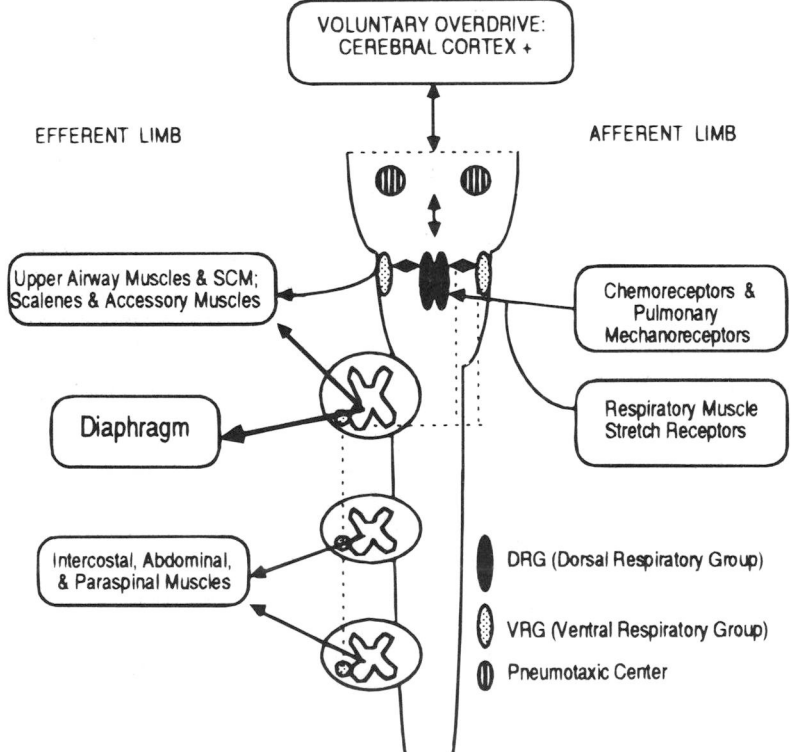

FIG. 14-1. The neuroanatomic pathways of respiration are outlined. See text for description. SCM, sternocleidomastoid muscle. (Adapted from Kelly BJ, Luce JM: The diagnosis and management of neuromuscular diseases causing respiratory failure. Chest 99:1485–94, 1991, with permission.)

history and neurologic examination that may suggest nervous system disease, certain nonspecific and respiratory symptoms and signs should lead to consideration of neurogenic respiratory dysfunction. Lethargy, morning headache, anxiety, fatigue, hypersomnolence, and confusion may be reported. Dyspnea may worsen with exertion and when the patient is supine, as the diaphragm then works against gravity. The resting respiratory rate may be increased, and accessory muscles of respiration may be called into action at rest. Neurogenic respiratory dysfunction may also worsen during sleep, especially rapid eye movement sleep, when there is atonia of all respiratory muscles, except the diaphragm, and when central control mechanisms are less responsive to afferent input.

Patients with isolated neurogenic respiratory dysfunction usually have normal breath sounds. Percussion may reveal evidence of decreased diaphragmatic excursion. The overall pattern of respiration can be evaluated by observing the rhythmicity of breathing (or of diaphragmatic contraction by electromyography [EMG]). The chest radiograph may be clear or reveal plate-like atelectasis or elevated hemidiaphragms. Fluoroscopy, especially in conjunction with the ''sniff test,'' may confirm abnormal diaphragmatic movements. Recognizing the phenomenon of *alveolar hypoventilation,* however, is perhaps the most important clue that a neurogenic process is causing respiratory compromise.

ALVEOLAR HYPOVENTILATION

Alveolar hypoventilation occurs when ventilation of the alveoli is low in relation to O_2 consumption and CO_2 production such that the partial oxygen tension (PO_2) falls and the partial carbon dioxide tension (PCO_2) rises. The hypoxemia may improve after administering supplemental O_2, but hypercapnia can only improve after increasing the ventilatory rate when respiratory muscle weakness precludes an increase in the tidal volume. Both central and peripheral nervous system diseases may cause alveolar hypoventilation. This is characterized by arterial blood gas measurements that demonstrate hypoxemia and hypercapnia with a normal alveolar-arterial oxygen gradient (A-a gradient).* Although hypercapnia and hypoventilation may also occur with pulmonary diseases, many lung diseases also produce hypoxemia by causing ventilation to perfusion inequalities rather than hypoventilation. This results in an elevation of the A-a O_2 gradient.

Fortunately, alveolar hypoventilation does not occur until the advanced stages of neurogenic respiratory failure. Therefore, in the early stages, clinicians must rely on other measures, including pulmonary function tests, to determine whether or not the respiratory dysfunction is due to a neurologic disorder.

PULMONARY FUNCTION TESTS

The mechanical and metabolic aspects of respiration that are most useful in evaluating patients with suspected neurogenic

respiratory dysfunction are those that can be readily measured, followed over time, and utilized in separating pulmonary from neurologic causes of respiratory compromise. Static and dynamic lung volumes and expiratory and inspiratory pressures meet these criteria

Static Lung Volumes

Total lung capacity (TLC) is the volume of air present in the chest after full inspiration (Fig. 14-2). During quiet ventilation, the volume of air inspired and expired in one breath is the tidal volume (TV), normally 500 to 750 ml. The vital capacitiy (VC) is, perhaps, the most commonly measured bedside volume. It is the amount of air that can be moved into or out of the lungs on a single breath, normally about 65 mg/kg. The forced vital capacity (FVC) is the volume of air that can be forcefully exhaled after a maximal inspiration. The volume of air left in the lungs at the end of quiet expiration is the functional residual capacity (FRC), and the amount remaining at the end of maximal expiration is the residual volume (RV). Unlike the other lungs volumes defined above, RV and FRC cannot be measured by spirometry. Gas dilution techniques or body plethysmography are required. RV, but not FRC, is dependent on expiratory muscle strength in addition to the elastic recoil of the chest wall and airway closure.

Lung volumes, especially the FVC, are useful to follow in patients with neuromuscular diseases that may affect respiration because improvement in the FVC may parallel clinical improvement and reflect successful therapy; a falling FVC can warn the clinician of impending respiratory failure.

Time-Volume Curves and Flow-Volume Loops

Lung volumes may also be measured against time. For example, the forced expiratory volume in 1 second (FEV_1) is the volume of air expired in 1 second after a maximal inspiration. The midmaximal forced expiratory flow (FEF_{25-75}) measures the flow during the middle half of the VC (i.e., from 75 to 25 percent of VC). The FEV_1 and the FEF_{25-75} are not generally dependent on respiratory muscle strength. In addition to effort, they are dependent on the elastic recoil of the lungs and airway resistence and compliance. These measures can be plotted as time-volume curves (Fig. 14-3).

A forced expiration can also be plotted as a flow-volume tracing comparing expiratory flow from TLC to RV with inspiratory flow back to TLC. On flow volume tracings, the midpoints of expiration ($V_{50}E$) and inspiration ($V_{50}I$) can be determined. These points should be about equal for both phases of the respiratory cycle creating a $V_{50}E$ to $V_{50}I$ ratio of 1. If there is an alteration in the expiratory or inspiratory phase of respiration, this ratio will readily reflect it.

The flow-volume loop is useful in evaluating possible upper airway obstruction, which may be caused by bulbar weakness as well as other extra- or intrathoracic processes. Flow-volume loops from patients with bulbar or upper airway muscle weakness may reveal oscillations in inspiratory or expiratory flow or both. Flow plateaus in either phase of respiration may also be demonstrated (Fig. 14-4).

Restrictive Versus Obstructive Patterns and Disorders

The FEV_1 to FVC ratio is particularly useful in separating so-called restrictive from obstructive patterns on pulmonary func-

---

*If you know the FIO_2, PCO_2, and PO_2, the A-a gradient can be calculated as follows:

A-a gradient = PAO_2 − PaO_2 < 15 to 30 mmHg, depending on the age

If PAO_2 = FIO_2 (PB − P_{H_2O}) − PCO_2/ 0.8

PAO_2 = 0.21 (760-47) − 1.25 (PCO_2)

hence, PAO_2 = 150 − 1.25 (PCO_2)

PaO_2 is measured directly. In these equations, PAO_2 = alveolar PO_2; PaO_2 = arterial PO_2; FIO_2 = fractional O_2 inspired (FIO_2 of room air is 0.21); PB = barometric pressure; P_{H_2O} = partial pressure of H_2O; (47 mmHg when saturated); and 0.8 is the respiratory quotient.

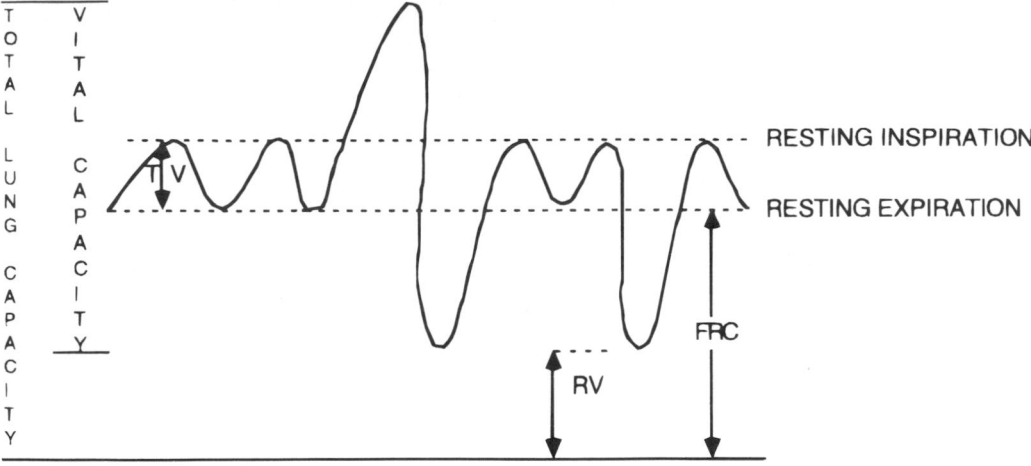

FIG. 14-2. Lung volumes at rest and after forced inspiration and expiration. See text for description. TV, tidal volume; RV, residual volume; FRC, functional residual capacity

tion tests (Table 14-1). These patterns correlate with primary pulmonary obstructive and restrictive diseases, but restrictive patterns may also point toward other extrapulmonary processes, such as respiratory muscle weakness or kyphoscoliosis.

Normal patients usually have an FEV_1 and FVC that are at least 80 percent of the predicted values obtained from a normal population, and normals can usually expire 80 percent of their FVC in 1 second. The FEV_1 to FVC ratio is normally 0.70 or greater. With restrictive disorders, there is a decrease in both the VC and air flow because of limitations in lung and chest wall expansion, for example, from pulmonary fibrosis, vascular disease, mass lesions compressing the pulmonary space, kyphoscoliosis, or ankylosing spondylitis. Moderate to severe *respiratory muscle weakness* is another important cause of a restrictive

pattern. In restrictive disorders, the FVC and FEV_1 are symmetrically reduced (Fig. 14-3). In some primary restrictive pulmonary diseases associated with increased lung recoil, the FEV_1 may actually be elevated. Thus, the FEV_1 to FVC ratio generally remains greater than 0.70 in all restrictive disorders. In addition, other lung volumes, including TLC, RV, and FRC, are reduced in most restrictive disorders. Descending to the RV is dependent on expiratory muscle strength, so that it may be increased in some patients with neuromuscular disease in contrast to the usual restrictive pattern.

In obstructive disorders in which there is an impediment to

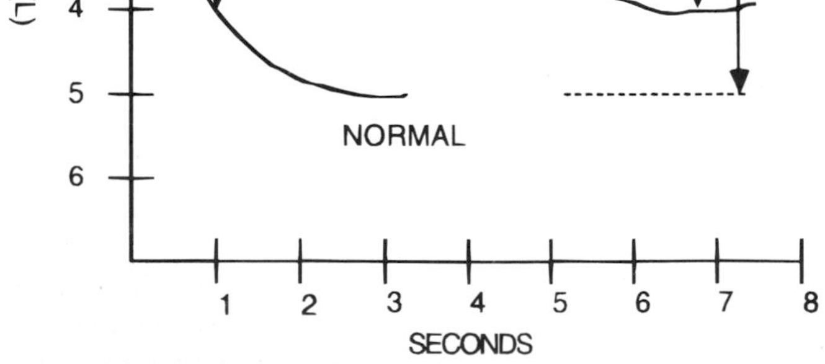

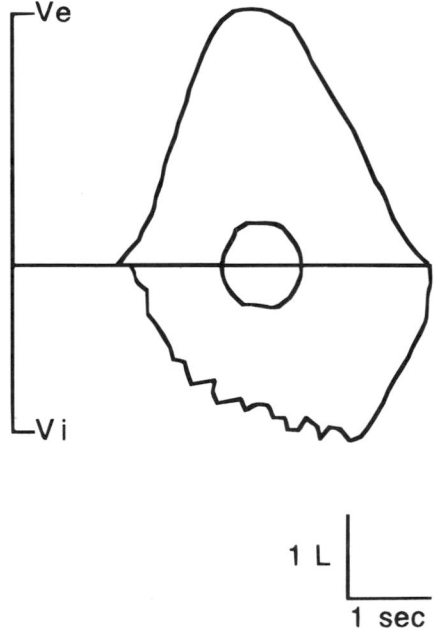

FIG. 14-4. Example of a flow-volume loop from a patient with amyotrophic lateral sclerosis. There are inspiratory flow oscillations and a reduced inspiratory flow volume (Vi). Ve, expiratory flow volume. (The inner circle represents tidal volume. The inspiratory phase of respiration is depicted below the horizontal meridian, and the expiratory phase is above the horizontal meridian). (Modified from Vincken W, Elleker G, Cosio MG: Detection of upper airway muscle involvement in neuromuscular disorders using the flow-volume loop. Chest 90:52–7, 1986, with permission.)

FIG. 14-3. Representative time-volume curves from a normal patient (bottom curve), a patient with an obstructive pulmonary disorder (top curve), and a patient with restrictive "pulmonary" disorder (middle curve) are superimposed. FVC, forced vital capacity; FEV_1, forced expiratory volume in the first second of expiration. In the obstructive disorder, the FEV_1 is markedly reduced while the FVC is mildly reduced. In the restrictive disorder, the FEV_1 and FVC are symmetrically reduced.

TABLE 14-1. Classic Findings on Pulmonary Function Testing in Restrictive and Obstructive Disorders[a]

	Measures of Pulmonary Function						
	FEB_1	VC	FEV_1/FVC	MVV	FEF_{25-75}	RV	FRC
Restrictive pattern							
Neuromuscular disease	DEC	DEC	>70%	DEC[b]	DEC	INC	DEC
Primary lung disease	DEC-INC	DEC	>70%	N/DEC	DEC	DEC	DEC
Obstructive pattern	DEC	N/DEC	<70%	DEC	DEC	INC	INC

Abbreviations: DEC, decreased; N, normal; INC, increased; FEV_1, forced expiratory volume in 1 second; VC, vital capacity; FVC, forced vital capacity; MVV, maximal voluntary ventilation; FEF_{25-75}, midmaximal forced expiratory flow; RV, residual volume; FRC, functional residual capacity.
[a] Some variability in these patterns is expected among individuals.
[b] May be decreased out of proportion to the FEV_1.

air expulsion, the FEV_1 is significantly reduced while the FVC is preserved or mildly reduced (Fig. 14-3). Therefore, the FEV_1 to FVC ratio is less than 70 percent. In addition, obstructive diseases of pulmonary origin, (e.g., chronic bronchitis) are usually associated with a high RV or FRC. Patients with neuromuscular diseases usually do not manifest this obstructive pattern unless there is an associated pulmonary disease.

Assessment of Respiratory Muscle Fatigue

Most lung volumes, including expiratory flows, are not affected by mild losses in respiratory muscle strength. One exception may be the *maximal voluntary ventilation* (MVV), which is measured as the amount of air exchanged during 12 to 15 seconds of maximal effort with the reported value extrapolated to 1 minute. Because the maximum number of breaths that one can take in 1 minute is about 35 to 40, the MVV is usually about 35 to 40 times greater than the FEV_1. Like the FEV_1, the MVV is dependent on the effort and pulmonary mechanics, but it is also a measure of endurance and *is* affected by respiratory muscle power and fatigue. Disorders that cause a decrease in FEV_1 also affect MVV, but a reduction in MVV out of proportion to a reduction in FEV_1 should raise suspicion that a neuromuscular disorder is affecting respiration, if the patient has given a full effort.

Inspiratory and Expiratory Pressures

When lung volumes are still normal in the early stages of neurogenic respiratory dysfunction, maximum inspiratory and expiratory forces may be reduced. These forces can be measured as pressures at the mouth by a manometer and are also dependent on effort, lung volume, mouth seal, age, and sex. The maximum expiratory pressure (PEmax) is normally $100 \, cmH_2O$, while the maximum inspiratory pressure (PImax), also called the negative inspiratory force, is usually $-70 \, cmH_2O$ or more (i.e., more negative). In theory, because the PImax parallels diaphragm function, it should be the more sensitive indicator of respiratory muscle weakness. In practice, PEmax may be more sensitive. In one study, it was abnormal in 87 percent of patients with respiratory dysfunction of neuromuscular origin.

Many of these tests are best suited to the study of the lower motor neuron limb of the neurologic pathways of respiratory control. Clinical assessment of the upper motor neuron pathway is more difficult. The overall pattern of respiration can be evaluated by observing the rhythmicity of respiration or of the contractions of the diaphragm by EMG. Minute ventilation, the product of the TV and the respiratory rate, also gives a measure of the overall integrity of breathing. The mouth occlusion pressure, the mouth pressure response to random occlusion of the airway during inspiration, is determined by an involuntary reaction and may also be decreased in lesions of central control.

Central chemical drive can be assessed by CO_2 inhalation techniques and by the response to hypoxia.

Once the presence of a neurogenic cause of respiratory dysfunction has been confirmed using the measures of respiratory physiology outlined above, one's knowledge of general and respiratory neuroanatomy can be directed toward determining the anatomic localization of the lesion.

LOCALIZATION AND CAUSES OF NEUROGENIC RESPIRATORY DYSFUNCTION

Upper Motor Neuron Disorders

Upper motor neuron disorders that affect automatic respiration usually produce *central (primary) alveolar hypoventilation*. Although these patients exhibit resting hypoxemia and hypercapnia, they can normalize their blood gases with increased respiratory effort because of intact voluntary overdrive mechanisms. They are most vulnerable to hypoxia and hypercapnia while asleep, when voluntary mechanisms are inactive, and while the central automatic driving mechanisms are inadequate (Ondine's curse). Lung volumes and inspiratory and expiratory pressures are usually not reduced.

The most common site of a lesion that affects central respiratory control is the medulla oblongata. Usually, other brainstem signs accompany such a lesion. Imaging studies, especially magnetic resonance imaging, may be helpful in identifying a structural abnormality. Upper cervical spinal cord lesions can also produce this syndrome. A wide variety of pathologic processes, listed below and discussed later in the text, may cause central alveolar hypoventilation.

Disorders of the brainstem or high cervical spinal cord
    Tumor
    Encephalitis and polio
    Infarction or hemorrhage
    Trauma
    Demyelination
    Chiari malformations
    Degenerative diseases, e.g., Leigh's disease
    Association with Hirschsprung's disease
    Drugs
    Idiopathic

A unique association occurs with Hirschsprung's disease. In these rare patients, the combination of congenital brainstem and neural intestinal lesions raises the possibility that a developmental abnormality in serotonergic neurons in both the intestine and brainstem may lead to gut atonia and Ondine's curse. In addition to structural lesions, drugs such as sedatives and narcotics can impair central respiratory control, especially in patients harboring underlying central nervous system or pulmonary disorders.

Many brainstem lesions that cause coma can lead to central neurogenic *hyper*ventilation (midbrain), apneustic (pontine), or ataxic (medullary) breathing. This subject has been reviewed by Plum and Posner (1982). More subtle dysfunction of the central sleep generator can cause central sleep apnea.

High cervical spinal cord lesions (C4 and above), usually traumatic, produce a variety of respiratory abnormalities, from Ondine's curse to persistent apnea, as a result of bilateral hemidiaphragm paralysis. Lower cervical and thoracic lesions may affect upper airway, paraspinal, intercostal, and abdominal muscle innervation and lead to decreased expiratory and inspiratory pressures and a restriction in lung and chest wall expansion. Hypoventilation and atelectasis may then become chronic problems.

Pathologic processes above the brainstem may also affect respiration in more subtle fashion, but their mechanisms and clinical significance are not clear. The cerebral cortex, for example, innervates the contralateral hemidiaphragm. Thus, a cortical lesion, such as a stroke, may weaken the diaphragm, but such unilateral lesions do not appear to produce respiratory dysfunction. Cerebellar atrophy has occasionally been associated with a disordered rhythm of breathing. Disorders of the basal ganglia, especially Parkinson's disease, may cause dyspnea. Respiratory muscle rigidity with associated shallow breathing, impaired laryngeal and respiratory muscle coordination, and airway obstruction are proposed causes. Other movement disorders, such as tardive dyskinesia, may occasionally interfere with the rhythm of respiration.

Lower Motor Neuron Disorders

Lower motor neuron disorders (Table 14-2) account for the majority of neurologic diseases that affect respiration and ultimately result in alveolar hypoventilation. These disorders may cause diaphragmatic dysfunction and present with dyspnea, especially on exertion and when supine. Other signs of lower motor neuron disease, including limb and sometimes extraocular and oropharyngeal (bulbar) muscle weakness, frequently accompany the respiratory dysfunction. The degree of limb and bulbar weakness does not correlate well with the degree of respiratory muscle weakness. However, in some neuromuscular diseases, significant proximal limb weakness is more likely to accompany respiratory muscle weakness than is isolated distal limb weakness. Serious underlying diaphragm weakness is asymptomatic in many patients predisposed by their underlying

TABLE 14-2. Peripheral Nervous System Disorders Associated With Respiratory Dysfunction

Anatomic Localization	Disease
Anterior horn cell	Amyotrophic lateral sclerosis Polio/postpolio syndrome Tetanus[a]
Peripheral nerve	Guillain-Barré syndrome Charcot-Marie-Tooth disease Critical illness polyneuropathy
Neuromuscular junction	Myasthenia gravis Botulism Lambert-Eaton myasthenic syndrome
Muscle	Dystrophies Inflammatory myopathies Acid maltase deficiency Toxic myopathies Hypokalemia and rhabdomyolysis Hypophosphatemia

[a] Predominantly affects spinal cord interneurons.

disease to have eventual respiratory decompensation; therefore, the physician should routinely assess the respiratory function in everyone presenting with one of the disorders in Table 14-2.

CLINICAL AND LABORATORY ASSESSMENT IN PATIENTS WITH LOWER MOTOR NEURON RESPIRATORY DYSFUNCTION

When respiratory muscle weakness of lower motor neuron origin is identified, the physician should try to determine the precise anatomic localization (i.e., anterior horn cell, motor root, peripheral nerve, neuromuscular junction, or muscle) and the cause of the neurologic lesion. The detailed neurologic history and examination help to localize the process, unless it is isolated to respiratory muscles, a rare occurrence. A pertinent laboratory screen should then be undertaken. In addition to routine serologic studies, measurements of the level of serum creatine kinase and antibody titers to the acetylcholine receptor may be especially useful in suspected muscle diseases and myasthenia gravis. In the latter case, an edrophonium test may also be helpful (see Ch. 103). EMG helps to identify the level of the motor unit affected in patients with respiratory muscle weakness. In addition to routine nerve conduction studies and needle examination of the limbs and paraspinal muscles, repetitive nerve stimulation is done to assess the function of the neuromuscular junction. If myasthenia gravis is highly suspected and repetitive stimulation of a distal and proximal nerve is normal, single-fiber EMG, although nonspecific, increases the sensitivity of diagnosis of a generalized neuromuscular junction disorder to nearly 100 percent if two muscles are studied. Unfortunately, some patients are unable to cooperate with this demanding examination (see Ch. 103).

Electrophysiologic evaluation of the phrenic nerves is now being performed more commonly in many centers and may be useful for anatomic localization of the lesion causing respiratory dysfunction, especially with lesions producing axonal loss. The phrenic nerves can be stimulated percutaneously at the posterior border of the sternocleidomastoid muscles. EMG of the diaphragm can also be performed with minimal risk of pneumothorax. One technique has been reviewed by Bolton (1993). Evidence of denervation may be seen with anterior horn cell diseases, upper cervical root degeneration, or other lesions of the phrenic nerves producing axonal loss. Myotonic discharges may be recorded from the diaphragm and suggest a myotonic disorder, but typical motor unit potential changes of myopathy are difficult to separate from normal diaphragmatic motor unit potentials. Therefore, the EMG of the diaphragm does not sensitively identify myopathy. Repetitive stimulation of the phrenic nerve for evaluation of neuromuscular junction transmission is also technically difficult.

SPECIFIC LOWER MOTOR NEURON DISEASES

Anterior Horn Cell Diseases

Amyotrophic lateral sclerosis is currently the most common disorder of the anterior horn cells (and upper motor neurons) that affects respiration, and it does so often. Such patients frequently have bulbar and limb weakness and fasciculations in addition to upper motor neuron signs. In the early stages of their illness, however, rare patients may have only subtle limb weakness, fasciculations, or both, and exertional dyspnea or hypoventilation may be the presenting manifestation of their disease. Preferential phrenic nerve-associated motor neuron loss may cause such a presentation. Treatment is supportive, and long-term management of respiratory failure is based on ethical and medical factors. Some patients do well with intermittent noninvasive positive airway pressure ventilation via the nasal or oral route, and some benefit from continuous home mechanical ventilation via tracheostomy.

Poliomyelitis

Poliomyelitis, now rare, was once a common cause of respiratory failure. Lower brainstem or cervical segment involvement leads to respiratory paralysis. Cerebrospinal fluid pleocytosis and an associated viral syndrome are important diagnostic clues. Rarely, patients with a remote history of polio develop hypoventilation as a component of the postpolio syndrome, especially if the VC falls below 40 to 50 percent of the predicted value. These patients usually have residual respiratory weakness caused by their initial bout with poliomyelitis.

Tetanus

Tetanus affects spinal cord inhibitory interneurons rather than anterior horn cells and may cause respiratory dysfunction by impairing diaphragm relaxation. Recognition of a recent wound and associated clinical features, such as muscle rigidity, are helpful in making the diagnosis.

Peripheral Neuropathies

The Guillain-Barré syndrome, an acute inflammatory demyelinating polyneuropathy, is the most common cause of acute neurogenic respiratory failure. Approximately 20 to 33 percent of patients with Guillain-Barré syndrome require ventilatory assistance. Respiratory failure, if it occurs, usually does so in the first 2 weeks of the illness. Patients with respiratory failure also tend to have the greatest generalized weakness, but again, there is no reliable correlation between limb and respiratory muscle weakness. Fortunately, most recover with good supportive care, and plasma exchange shortens the duration of mechanical ventilation.

Rarely, porphyria, vasculitis, paralytic shellfish poisons, and other toxins, including organophosphates, produce a neuropathic syndrome associated with respiratory failure. Intensive care unit patients may also develop phrenic nerve axonal loss and polyneuropathy in association with sepsis and multiorgan failure, termed critical illness polyneuropathy. Some patients with the demyelinating form of Charcot-Marie-Tooth disease (hereditary motor and sensory neuropathy type I) may develop mild respiratory dysfunction, although this clinical observation has not been frequently made. These patients with Charcot-Marie-Tooth disease and those without respiratory symptoms have normal lung volumes but may have decreased inspiratory and expiratory pressures.

Unilateral phrenic nerve injury or compression does not usually cause respiratory failure, unless it is associated with a pulmonary disorder or another cause of respiratory muscle weakness. Bilateral phrenic nerve injury, which may rarely occur intraoperatively, does cause respiratory failure.

Neuromuscular Junction Disorders

Approximately 30 percent of patients with myasthenia gravis have respiratory muscle weakness, and 10 to 15 percent may develop respiratory failure as a major component of "myasthenic crisis." Most of these patients have already been diagnosed with myasthenia gravis, but some present with respiratory distress as their initial complaint, often after a precipitating illness or after administration of drugs, such as neuromuscular junction blocking agents.

Botulism, a presynaptic neuromuscular junction disorder in which acetylcholine release is blocked by an ingested neurotoxin, may cause respiratory failure along with gastrointestinal symptoms, pupillary paralysis, and extraocular and bulbar weakness.

Respiratory dysfunction occurs in about 6 percent of patients with another rare presynaptic disorder, Lambert-Eaton myastenic syndrome. The respiratory dysfunction may develop spontaneously, or it may be precipitated by anesthesia. The diagnosis is often confused with myasthenia gravis, but the presence of low-amplitude motor responses that markedly increase in amplitude after a brief period of exercise should help to distinguish Lambert-Eaton myasthenic syndrome from myasthenia gravis.

Tick paralysis is caused by the bite and persistent attachment of *Dermacentor andersoni,* usually along the hairline. It may cause respiratory and limb paralysis as a result of neuromuscular junction blockade. Removal of the tick completely cures this illness.

Drugs, such a magnesium in antacids, aminoglycosides, lithium, and acetylcholinesterase inhibitors may potentiate or cause defects in neuromuscular transmission.

Myopathic Disorders

Long-standing severe dystrophies, especially Duchenne muscular dystrophy, produce respiratory muscle weakness that causes a restrictive disorder, atelectasis, and hypoventilation. Superimposed scoliosis in many patients exacerbates the restrictive limitation. Thus, surgery for scoliosis is often performed early after boys with Duchenne muscular dystrophy become wheelchair-bound and before pulmonary function deteriortates further.

Rare patients with myotonic dystrophy develop alveolar hypoventilation with a restrictive spirometric pattern, probably as a result of respiratory muscle weakness. Myotonic discharges may be identified by EMG of the diaphragm. Some patients with myotonic dystrophy may also develop hypersomnolence of central origin.

Acid maltase deficiency is a rare glycogen storage disease that occurs in infantile, childhood, and adult forms. In the adult form, up to one-third of the patients present with respiratory failure. Most patients also have proximal weakness, an elevation in creatine kinase levels, and increased insertional activity with complex repetitive discharges and even myotonic discharges in affected muscles, especially the paraspinals. Muscle pathology and biochemical studies reveal a vacuolar myopathy with low or absent acid maltase activity.

Acquired myopathies, especially the inflammatory disorders polymyositis and dermatomyositis, are frequently associated with respiratory muscle weakness of varying degrees, as identified by pulmonary function studies. Overt respiratory failure is less common. Respiratory muscle weakness may be the presenting feature in up to 4 percent of patients with polymyositis.

Myopathies caused by toxins, such as alcohol, may also involve respiratory muscles. In particular, the combination of high-dose intravenous corticosteroids and neuromuscular blocking agents administered to some critically ill patients, especially those in status asthmaticus, can cause a myopathy that frequently affects respiratory muscles.

Hypophosphatemia can cause rapidly reversible respiratory weakness, probably on the basis of muscle dysfunction, but the anatomic localization of the abnormality is uncertain. Severe hypokalemia with or without rhabdomyolysis can cause limb and respiratory muscle weakness. Other electrolyte disturbances, such as hyponatremia, hyperkalemia, hypercalcemia, and hypermagnesemia, may also result in generalized weakness without preferential diaphragm involvement.

MANAGEMENT OF NEUROGENIC RESPIRATORY DYSFUNCTION

Treatments for the specific disorders mentioned in this chapter are discussed in later chapters that address these diseases in greater detail. Here follow some general guidelines for the management of neurogenic respiratory failure. To handle this problem expertly, it is often helpful to enlist the assistance of colleagues in critical care and pulmonary medicine.

Acute Management

As with all causes of respiratory distress, assessment of airway, respiration, and vital signs are the first steps. Patients must be individually evaluated regarding the need for acute intervention (hospitalization, intensive care unit management, endotracheal intubation, etc.) based on the clinician's judgment and laboratory assessment. Evidence of intercurrent illnesses, especially pulmonary infections, should be sought. Abnormalities of electrolytes and other metabolic disturbances can also worsen respiratory weakness. A chest radiograph, arterial blood gas measurement, and bedside FVC, PEmax, or PImax should be obtained on all patients.

There is usually a correlation between the clinical state and inspiratory and expiratory pressures. A PEmax of less than 40 cmH_2O may be associated with the inability to clear secretions, and a PImax of less than -20 cmH_2O (absolute value) may indicate imminent progression to hypoventilation with hypercapnia. With progression of diaphragm weakness to the point that the VC is less than 10 to 15 ml/kg, respiratory failure with hypoxemia and hypercapnia often occurs and may culminate in stupor and coma if untreated. With such a decline in the VC, paradoxic respirations may develop such that the abdomen moves inward instead of outward as the rib cage expands. If intercostal (expiratory) muscle weakness is also present, the rib cage may move inward instead of outward as the abdomen expands.

Based on the VC and associated respiratory pathophysiology, Ropper (1993) has devised an approach to respiratory management that applies to all patients with neurogenic respiratory dysfunction (Fig. 14-5). In general, tracheal intubation is undertaken when mechanical ventilation is required or if airway protection is desired to prevent aspiration. In patients with worsening neuromuscular respiratory muscle weakness, tracheal intubation should usually be performed before significant hypercapnia occurs. In addition, use of paralytic agents should be minimized; if anesthetics are used in patients with certain

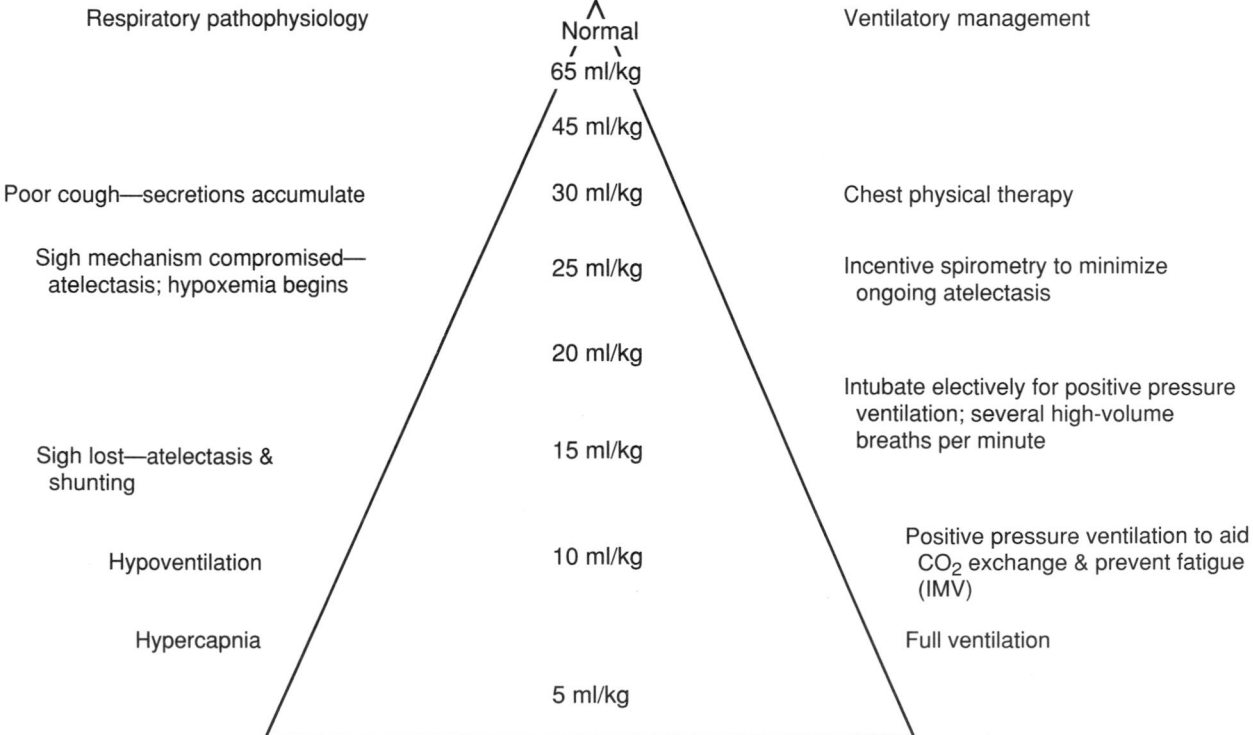

FIG. 14-5. Relationship between vital capacity, pathophysiology of lung function, and suggested therapy in respiratory failure. (From Ropper AH: Neurological and Neurosurgical Intensive Care. 3rd Ed. Raven Press, New York, 1993, with permission.)

myopathies, such as myotonic dystrophy, one should be vigilant for the possible development of malignant hyperthermia.

Chronic Management

Patients with chronic neurologic disorders that cause respiratory muscle weakness require good pulmonary toilet with postural drainage and chest physiotherapy. They may benefit from incentive inspiratory spirometry. Preventative care is also paramount. If they are bed-bound, patients should be turned frequently and have pressure points padded, and they should receive prophylaxis for venous thrombosis. Good nutrition and mobilization with physical and occupational therapy are important. Patients should receive influenza and pneumococcal vaccinations. Underlying pulmonary and neurologic diseases and intercurrent illnesses should be treated aggressively.

Alveolar hypoventilation may be treated with supplemental oxygen, but positive-pressure mechanical ventilation via tracheostomy may be necessary to prevent hypercapnia. Some patients may require only intermittent ventilation. In lieu of tracheostomy, this subset of patients who require only intermittent ventilation may benefit from intermittent positive-pressure ventilation delivered by nasal or oral mask, especially at night. This technique allows respiratory muscles to rest and improves ventilatory performance in some patients. Oxygen saturation, hypercapnia, and symptoms of hypoventilation may all improve. This group of patients may also benefit from negative-pressure (cuirass) ventilation. Finally, in some patients with chronic central neurogenic hypoventilation, phrenic nerve pacing may be considered.

ACKNOWLEDGMENTS

I appreciate the careful and thoughtful reviews of the manuscript by Drs. David Chad (Neurology Department, University of Massachusetts Medical Center) and Ronald Stiller (Pulmonary and Critical Care Medicine, University of Pittsburgh Medical Center).

SUGGESTED READINGS

Bach JR, Alba AS: Management of chronic alveolar hypoventilation by nasal ventilation. Chest 97:53–7, 1990

Bolton CF: AAEM minimonograph #40: clinical neurophysiology of the respiratory system. Muscle Nerve 16:809–18, 1993

Burki N: Measurements of ventilatory regulation. Clin Chest Med 10:215–26, 1989

Demedts M, Beckers J, Rochette F, Bulcke J: Pulmonary function in moderate neuromuscular disease without respiratory complaints. Eur J Respir Dis 63:62–7, 1982

Eichacker PQ, Spiro A, Sherman M et al: Respiratory muscle dysfunction in hereditary motor sensory neuropathy, type I. Arch Intern Med 148:1739–40, 1988

Fostad H, Nilsson S: Intractable singultus: a diagnostic and therapeutic challenge. Br J Neurosurg 7:255–62, 1993

Griggs RC, Donohoe KM, Utell MJ et al: Evaluation of pulmonary function in neuromuscular disease. Arch Neurol 38:9–12, 1981

Haddad GG, Mazza NM, Defendini R et al: Congenital failure of autonomic control of ventilation, gastrointestinal motility and heart rate. Medicine (Baltimore) 57:517–24, 1978

Kelly BJ, Luce JM: The diagnosis and management of neuromuscular diseases causing respiratory failure. Chest 99:1485–94, 1991

Plum F, Posner JB: The Diagnosis of Stupor and Coma. 3rd Ed. FA Davis, Philadelphia, 1982

Ropper AH: Neurological and Neurosurgical Intensive Care. 3rd Ed. Raven Press, New York, 1993

Vincken W, Elleker G, Cosio MG: Detection of upper airway muscle involvement in neuromuscular disorders using the flow-volume loop. Chest 90:52–7, 1986

Vincken W, Elleker G, Cosio MG: Determinants of respiratory muscle weakness in stable chronic neuromuscular disease. Am J Med 82:53–58, 1987

15. AUTONOMIC DYSFUNCTION

ROY FREEMAN

The extensive afferent and efferent connections of the autonomic nervous system provide the anatomic basis for the diverse constellation of symptoms that accompany the autonomic degenerative diseases. The symptoms of dysautonomia, however, are not only found in the rare primary autonomic nervous system diseases but are also responsible for much of the morbidity associated with frequently encountered neurologic disorders such as multiple sclerosis, cerebrovascular disease, Parkinson's disease, and peripheral neuropathies. Recognition of the signs and symptoms of autonomic dysfunction and knowledge of its pathophysiology and treatment is thus of obvious importance to the clinical neurologist. This chapter covers the common diseases of the autonomic nervous system, the pathophysiology of dysautonomia, and the treatment of those features of autonomic dysfunction that are most frequently encountered by the practicing neurologist, that is, orthostatic hypotension, bladder dysfunction, and the disorders of gastrointestinal motility.

DISEASES OF THE AUTONOMIC NERVOUS SYSTEM

A wide variety of disorders may produce the signs and symptoms of autonomic dysfunction. Careful history taking and physical examination with appropriate use of special investigations usually permits an accurate clinical diagnosis of these diseases to be made. A useful practical approach is to classify the disorders associated with autonomic failure into those diseases accompanied by predominantly central nervous system features, those diseases accompanied by predominantly peripheral nervous system features, and those diseases without neurologic features (Tables 15-1 to 15-3).

TABLE 15-1. Autonomic Dysfunction With Central Nervous System Manifestations

Multiple system atrophy with autonomic failure (Shy-Drager syndrome)
Olivopontocerebellar atrophy
Striatonigral degeneration
Parkinson's disease
Brain tumors (brainstem, cerebellum, diencephalon)
Wernicke's encephalopathy
Multiple infarcts
Syringomyelia and syringobulbia
Hydrocephalus
Multiple sclerosis
Myelopathies
Traumatic
Inflammatory
Pernicious anemia
System degenerative
Tabes dorsalis
Progressive supranuclear palsy
Huntington's disease
Amyotrophic lateral sclerosis

TABLE 15-2. Autonomic Dysfunction With Peripheral
Nervous System Manifestations

Diabetes
Amyloidosis
Guillain-Barré syndrome
Acute and subacute autonomic neuropathies
Chronic inflammatory polyneuropathy
Hereditary neuropathies
  Hereditary sensory and autonomic neuropathies
  Fabry's disease
  Navajo Indian neuropathy
  Hereditary motor and sensory neuropathy
  Tangier disease
Infectious diseases
  Chagas disease
  Human immunodeficiency virus neuropathy
  Botulism
  Diphtheria
  Leprosy
Toxic neuropathies
  Vacor
  Vincristine
  Perhexilene maleate
  Cisplatin
  Taxol
  Organic solvents
  Acrylamide
  Heavy metals
Connective tissue diseases
  Sjögren's syndrome
  Systemic lupus erythematosus
  Rheumatoid arthritis
Pernicious anemia
Porphyria
Uremia
Alcoholic neuropathy
Hepatic disease
Paraneoplastic neuropathies
Eaton-Lambert syndrome
Dopamine β-hydroxylase deficiency
Adie syndrome

Autonomic Dysfunction With Central Nervous System Features

There are numerous disorders with autonomic manifestations and central nervous system signs. Of these diseases, multiple system atrophy with autonomic failure (MSA) and idiopathic Parkinson's disease most frequently produce clinically significant autonomic dysfunction. Patients with MSA or Shy-Drager syndrome typically present with autonomic symptoms such as orthostatic hypotension, bowel and bladder dysfunction, anhidrosis, and impotence, together with motor dysfunction that can involve the extrapyramidal, cerebellar, and pyramidal systems. Impotence in males is characteristically the first autonomic symptom of this disease, although usually the symptoms of orthostatic hypotension lead patients to seek medical attention. In contrast to idiopathic Parkinson's disease, MSA is more

TABLE 15-3. Isolated Autonomic Dysfunction

Pure autonomic failure
Medications
  Antihypertensive agents
  Tricyclic agents
  Monoamine oxidase inhibitors
  Dopamine blocking agents
Aging
Endocrine diseases
  Adrenocortical deficiencies
  Pheochromocytoma
Surgical sympathectomy
Mitral valve prolapse
Hypovolemia
Electrolyte disturbance
Hyperbradykinism
Postural orthostatic tachycardia

likely to have a symmetric onset and is less responsive to levodopa and dopamine agonists. The resting parkinsonian tremor is rarely present in MSA, but inspiratory stridor, vocal cord paralysis, and antecollis commonly occur. The median survival of MSA is usually less than 10 years. Pathologic studies have demonstrated cell loss and gliosis that involves the striatonigral, olivopontocerebellar, and autonomic systems. An argyrophilic, intracytoplasmic oligodendroglial inclusion may be a specific pathologic hallmark of multiple system atrophy.

In contrast, the autonomic symptoms accompanying Parkinson's disease are usually not as severe as those seen in patients with MSA. They characteristically occur late in the course of the illness and are often associated with levodopa and dopamine agonist therapy. Nevertheless, autonomic dysfunction is frequently the source of significant morbidity for the parkinsonian patient. There are many other disorders with autonomic dysfunction and central nervous system signs; however, the autonomic symptoms are usually of secondary importance. These disorders are also unlikely to be confused with MSA or Parkinson's disease (Table 15-1).

Autonomic Dysfunction With Peripheral Nervous System Features

Autonomic dysfunction occurs with most peripheral neuropathies, particularly those that predominantly involve the small or unmyelinated fibers. This review covers those peripheral neuropathies in which autonomic dysfunction is a clinically significant manifestation. A complete list of peripheral neuropathies with autonomic manifestations is found in Table 15-2.

Diabetes Mellitus. Diabetes mellitus is the most common cause of autonomic neuropathy in the developed world. A constellation of signs and symptoms occurs that affects cardiovascular, gastrointestinal, urogenital, thermoregulatory, sudomotor, and pupillomotor function. An increased resting heart rate is frequently observed in diabetic patients. With progression of the autonomic neuropathy, some patients display a fixed heart rate that responds only minimally to physiologic stimuli. The initial tachycardia is due to a vagal cardiac neuropathy that may be followed by a decrease in heart rate and, ultimately, a fixed heart rate caused by progressive cardiac sympathetic nervous system dysfunction. Orthostatic hypotension occurs in diabetes as a consequence of efferent sympathetic vasomotor denervation, causing reduced vasoconstriction of the splanchnic and other peripheral vascular beds. There is an increased frequency of sudden death in patients with autonomic neuropathy. Proposed etiologies for sudden unexplained death in diabetic patients include cardiorespiratory arrest as a result of cardiac arrhythmias, silent cardiac ischemia, and sleep apnea.

Bladder symptoms associated with autonomic neuropathy include hesitancy, poor stream, increased intervals between micturition, and a sense of inadequate bladder emptying. These symptoms may be followed by urinary retention and overflow incontinence. Detrusor muscle sensory abnormalities are the earliest bladder autonomic manifestation. These sensory abnormalities impair bladder sensation and increase the threshold for initiating the micturition reflex. A decrease in detrusor activity (detrusor areflexia) follows that leads to incomplete bladder emptying, an increased postvoid residual, decreased peak urinary flow rate, bladder overdistention, and ultimately urinary retention.

Impotence is a frequent and disturbing symptom in male diabetic patients. Reported incidence has ranged from 30 to

75 percent of diabetic males. Impotence may be the earliest symptom of diabetic autonomic neuropathy, although sensory, vascular, and psychogenic etiologies, alone or in varying combinations may also be responsible for this symptom. Sympathetically mediated ejaculatory failure may precede the appearance of impotence, although impotence can occur with retained ability to ejaculate and experience orgasm.

Autonomic dysfunction occurs throughout the gastrointestinal tract, producing several specific clinical syndromes. Diabetic gastroparesis may manifest as nausea, postprandial vomiting, bloating, belching, loss of appetite, and early satiety. Food residue is retained in the stomach as a result of impaired gastric peristalsis compounded by lower intestinal dysmotility. Gastroparesis often impairs the establishment of adequate glycemic control. Denervation of the vagus nerve may be play a role in this disorder.

Constipation is the most frequently reported gastrointestinal autonomic symptom and is found in up to 60 percent of diabetic patients. The pathophysiology of diabetic constipation is poorly understood but may reflect loss of the postprandial gastrocolic reflex. Diarrhea and other lower gastrointestinal tract symptoms may also occur. Diabetic diarrhea is profuse, watery, and typically occurs at night. The diarrhea can last for hours or days and frequently alternates with constipation. Fecal incontinence, as a result of anal sphincter incompetence or reduced rectal sensation, is another manifestation of diabetic autonomic neuropathy. The pathogenesis of diabetic diarrhea includes abnormalities in gastrointestinal motility, decreased gut transit time, reduced α_2-adrenergic receptor-mediated fluid absorption, bacterial overgrowth, pancreatic insufficiency, coexistent celiac disease, and abnormalities in bile salt metabolism.

Diabetic autonomic neuropathy initially results in a loss of thermoregulatory sweating in a glove-and-stocking distribution that can extend to the upper aspects of the limbs and anterior abdomen, conforming to the well-recognized length dependence of diabetic neuropathy. This process ultimately results in global anhidrosis that usually accompanies a profound generalized autonomic neuropathy. Hyperhidrosis may also accompany diabetic autonomic neuropathy. Excessive sweating may occur as a compensatory phenomenon, involving proximal regions such as the head and trunk that are spared in a dying-back neuropathy. Gustatory sweating, an abnormal production of sweating that appears over the face, head, neck, shoulders, and chest after eating even nonspicy foods, is occasionally observed.

Amyloid Neuropathy. Autonomic dysfunction frequently accompanies the polyneuropathy of both primary and familial amyloidosis. Patients with amyloid neuropathy typically present with distal sensory symptoms such as numbness, paresthesias, and dysesthesias, although the autonomic manifestations may occasionally be the presenting feature of amyloid neuropathy. On examination, there are signs of a sensorimotor polyneuropathy that predominantly involves the small fibers that mediate pain and temperature sensation. Characteristic autonomic signs and symptoms include postural hypotension, diarrhea, constipation, fecal incontinence, disturbances in bladder function, pupillary abnormalities, and erectile failure. These autonomic manifestations are similar to those described with diabetic autonomic neuropathy.

The variant transthyretin, in which methionine substitutes for valine at position 30, is the point mutation that is the most common cause of familial amyloid polyneuropathy in the United States. Other transthyretin mutations also give rise to familial amyloid polyneuropathy. Proposed mechanisms of injury include pressure exerted by amyloid deposits on peripheral nerves, dorsal nerve root ganglia, or autonomic ganglia and ischemic damage caused by amyloid infiltration of epineural and intraneural blood vessel walls.

Acute and Subacute Autonomic Neuropathies. Autonomic manifestations usually accompany the Guillain-Barré syndrome, although they are usually overshadowed by motor features of that disorder. Autonomic manifestations may, however, be the sole or predominant feature of an acute or subacute peripheral neuropathy. The hallmark of these autonomic neuropathies is the acute or subacute presentation of varying combinations of orthostatic hypotension, constipation, bladder atony, impotence, secretomotor paralysis, and blurring of vision associated with tonic pupils. Sensorimotor manifestations may accompany the autonomic manifestations but are not the predominant aspect of the presentation. The autonomic manifestations of this disorder may involve both the sympathetic and parasympathetic divisions of the autonomic nervous system (pandysautonomia) or the parasympathetic nervous system alone (cholinergic dysautonomia).

Only 40 percent of cases recover fully to premorbid status. For an estimated 12 percent, symptoms persist to a significant degree. Full or partial recovery, when reported, occurred over the course of months to years. Autonomic testing in the recovery phase of illness in these patients often showed evidence of persistent subclinical autonomic dysfunction. Acute dysautonomia has been described in relationship to the Epstein-Barr virus, streptococcal infection, and herpes simplex infection, in addition to other nondiagnosed viral syndromes. Associations with malignancies and connective tissue diseases have been described in other cases.

Hereditary Autonomic Neuropathies. The hereditary neuropathies are a heterogeneous group of disorders, some of which have significant involvement of autonomic fibers. The hereditary sensory and autonomic neuropathies (HSAN) are characterized by prominent sensory loss without motor involvement and by often striking dysautonomia. Autonomic manifestations are modest in autosomal-dominant sensory neuropathy (HSAN type I) and autosomal-recessive sensory neuropathy (HSAN type II) with the possible exception of bladder dysfunction. These disorders are associated with severe sensory loss with acral injuries.

HSAN type III, or Riley-Day syndrome (familial dysautonomia), is an autosomal recessive disorder seen primarily in Ashkenazi Jewish children. The clinical features of this disease include insensitivity to pain and temperature but sparing visceral pain, absence of tears, hypoactive corneal and tendon reflexes, and absence of fungiform papillae. Poor suck and feeding, esophageal reflux with vomiting and aspiration, and an uncoordinated swallow may be the first clinical manifestations. Later in the course of the illness, vibratory sensory loss and impaired appendicular coordination manifest. Autonomic disturbances may be prominent at any point in the disease course. Autonomic manifestations include episodic hyperhidrosis, vasomotor instability with defective temperature homeostasis, postural hypotension, hypertensive crises, and supersensitivity to cholinergic and adrenergic agents. A decline in blood pressure on standing without compensatory tachycardia is characteristic of the disorder.

Anhidrotic sensory neuropathy, a disorder with autosomal recessive inheritance (HSAN type IV), manifests in the first months of life with insensitivity to pain, anhidrosis, episodes of unexplained fever, and retardation of motor development. Virtual absence of unmyelinated fibers has been described in peripheral nerves.

Anhidrosis is also prominent in an autosomal recessive disorder observed among Navajo Indians, first described by Johnsen et al. (1985). These patients exhibit relatively little sensory loss except for deep pain sensibility. Of the hereditary motor and sensory neuropathies, peroneal muscular atrophy or Charcot-Marie-Tooth disease has been most clearly associated with autonomic disturbances.

Fabry's disease or angiokeratoma corporis diffusum is an X-linked, recessively inherited disorder that is associated with deficiency of the enzyme α-galactosidase A (ceramide trihexosidase). The enzyme deficiency results in the accumulation of ceramide trihexoside in various tissues that include the skin, nervous system, kidney, cardiovascular system, and eye. The neurologic manifestations of this disorder are secondary to the deposition of glycolipid in autonomic and dorsal root ganglia, in perineurial cells, and in unmyelinated and myelinated axons. Young males with this disorder typically present with severe distal extremity paroxysmal pains and tenderness; a truncal reddish-purple maculopapular rash; and angiectases of the skin, conjunctiva, nail bed, and oral mucosa. These corpora angiokeratoma that result from deposition of the glycolipid in skin together with the painful distal peripheral neuropathy, progressive renal disease, corneal opacities, and cerebrovascular accidents in adult life constitute the typical clinical manifestations of this disorder. The autonomic manifestations include hypo- or anhidrosis, reduced saliva and tear formation, impaired cutaneous flare response to scratch and histamine, and disordered intestinal motility. Patients' gastrointestinal symptoms may be as severe as their sensory complaints. Pupillary constriction to dilute pilocarpine has been documented, suggesting denervation supersensitivity, although cardiovascular autonomic reflexes in one series were normal. The generalized presentation of the anhidrosis has suggested sweat gland dysfunction that may be due to intracytoplasmic inclusions in the eccrine glands rather than autonomic neuropathy. Neuropathologic studies have demonstrated degeneration and loss of unmyelinated fibers. Fabry's disease can be diagnosed by assaying the enzyme α-galactosidase A in leukocytes or skin fibroblasts.

Paraneoplastic Autonomic Neuropathy.   Dysautonomia may be an isolated manifestation of a paraneoplastic disorder or part of a generalized paraneoplastic syndrome. Autonomic neuropathies have been documented in case reports in association with carcinoma of the lung, pancreatic carcinoma, Hodgkin's disease, and testicular cancer. Paraneoplastic constipation and intestinal pseudo-obstruction have been associated with small cell carcinoma of the lung. Such patients have inflammatory infiltrates of the myenteric plexus of the stomach and antineuronal antibodies.

Paraneoplastic dysautonomia has been associated with anti-Hu antibodies directed against neuronal nuclear antigen. These antibodies are also found in patients with a paraneoplastic sensory neuronopathy and encephalomyelitis. The autonomic features that accompany this paraneoplastic syndrome include orthostatic hypotension, pupillomotor dysfunction, sudomotor dysfunction, constipation, urinary retention, impotence, and xerophthalmia. In one large series, the autonomic nervous system was involved in 28 percent of patients with anti-Hu antibodies and was the predominant symptom in one-third of these patients.

Dysautonomia is a common manifestation of the Lambert-Eaton syndrome in patients with and without malignancies. Symptoms suggesting cholinergic dysfunction such as dry mouth, erectile and ejaculatory failure, constipation, blurred vision, and impaired sweating occur most frequently. Autonomic tests, however, have demonstrated both cholinergic and adrenergic abnormalities.

Infectious Diseases.   The peripheral neuropathies associated with a number of infectious diseases have accompanying autonomic manifestations. Autonomic dysfunction may occur in patients with human immunodeficiency virus infection. The symptoms of dysautonomia have included orthostatic hypotension, syncope, presyncope, sweating disturbances, bladder and bowel dysfunction, and impotence.

There is an increasing incidence of Chagas disease in the United States, and the autonomic manifestations of this disease should be considered in the differential diagnosis of dysautonomia. Chagas disease, which is due to a parasitic infection by *Trypanosoma cruzi,* is associated in the late stages of illness with severe cardiovascular and gastrointestinal dysautonomia. The pathogenesis of the autonomic dysfunction is unresolved and may be due to direct neural injury during the acute illness or to a persistent immune-mediated response. Reduced bowel motility, sialorrhea, megaesophagus, and megacolon are the most frequent gastrointestinal manifestations. Cardiovascular manifestations include impairment in the blood pressure response to standing, resting bradycardia, anhidrosis, conduction abnormalities, arrhythmias, cardiac failure, and cardiomegaly.

Isolated Autonomic Nervous System Dysfunction

Pure autonomic failure is an idiopathic peripheral autonomic nervous system degeneration that, in contrast to the Shy-Drager syndrome, has no motor manifestations. There are also no signs or minimal signs of a somatic peripheral neuropathy. Because this disorder is slowly progressive and has a significantly better prognosis than the Shy-Drager syndrome, it is important to differentiate between these two disorders. The autonomic features of the Shy-Drager syndrome may, however, precede the other neurologic signs by several years, preventing an early definitive diagnosis. Patients with pure autonomic failure typically have a low resting plasma norepinephrine level caused by degeneration or dysfunction of the postganglionic sympathetic neuron. The plasma norepinephrine level, which in normal subjects increases by 100 to 200 percent when the subject moves from the supine to the upright position, does not change significantly in patients with pure autonomic failure. There is, however, a wide scatter of results within the group of patients with pure autonomic failure that often makes it difficult to classify individual patients. Other conditions with isolated autonomic manifestations are listed in Table 15-3.

SIGNS, SYMPTOMS, AND TREATMENT OF AUTONOMIC FAILURE

Orthostatic Hypotension

The assumption of the upright posture results in a complex sequence of physiologic reactions in response to the pooling of approximately 500 ml of blood in the lower extremities and splanchnic circulation. There is a decrease in venous return to the heart, and the reduced ventricular filling results in diminished cardiac output and blood pressure. The hemodynamic changes provoke a baroreceptor-initiated compensatory reflex mediated via the central nervous system and effected by the peripheral efferent autonomic outflow. These compensatory mechanisms increase the peripheral resistance, venous return, and cardiac output and thus limit the fall in blood pressure. The normal response to the assumption of the erect posture is a fall in systolic blood pressure (5 to 10 mmHg), an increase in diastolic blood pressure (5 to 10 mmHg), and an increase in the pulse rate (10 to 25 beats/min). Should these mechanisms fail, the symptoms of cerebral hypoperfusion will ensue. The hallmark of both central and peripheral causes of neurogenic orthostatic hypotension is the failure to release norepinephrine levels appropriately on standing. Normally, norepinephrine is released into the synaptic cleft in response to standing, resulting in an increase in plasma norepinephrine concentration.

Treatment. Patient education is the cornerstone of the management of orthostatic hypotension. Patients with orthostatic hypotension should move from a supine to standing position in gradual stages, particularly in the morning when orthostatic tolerance is lowest. Maneuvers such as straining, coughing, and raising the arms above the head should be avoided. The removal of potential reversible causes of orthostatic hypotension is the first and most important management step. Medications such as diuretics, antihypertensive agents, antianginal agents, and antidepressants are the most common offending agents. The excessive natriuresis and reduction in central blood volume can be attenuated or minimized by increasing sodium intake with high sodium-containing foods or salt tablets. Raising the head of the bed 10 to 20 degrees activates the renin-angiotensin-aldosterone system and decreases the nocturnal diuresis. Raising the head of the bed may also reduce the supine hypertension that is prevalent in these patients, either as a consequence of baroreceptor denervation or as a side effect of treatment. Severe supine hypertension often limits therapeutic intervention, although surprisingly, most patients tolerate sustained supine blood pressures without untoward effect. The use of custom-fitted elastic stockings permits the application of graded pressure to the lower extremities and abdomen. These stockings minimize peripheral blood pooling in the lower extremities and splanchnic circulation.

These nonpharmacologic measures, unfortunately, help only the mildly afflicted, and pharmacologic intervention is usually required. Numerous agents from diverse pharmacologic groups have been implemented in the treatment of orthostatic hypotension (Table 15-4). The therapeutic goal is merely to ameliorate all symptoms while minimizing side effects. There is rarely the need to restore normotension. The most effective pharmacologic measures include mineralocorticoids, direct and indirect sympathomimetic agents, and other pressors, prostaglandin synthesis inhibitors, and recently reported erythropoietin.

Fludrocortisone acetate, a synthetic mineralocorticoid, is the medication of first choice for most patients with orthostatic hypotension. This agent has a long duration of action and may be taken once or twice daily. Fludrocortisone increases the blood volume and enhances the sensitivity of blood vessels to circulating catecholamines. Other potential modes of action include enhancing norepinephrine release from sympathetic neurons and increasing vascular fluid content. Treatment is initiated with a 0.1-mg tablet and can be increased to 1 mg daily,

TABLE 15-4. Pharmacologic Agents to Treat Orthostatic Hypotension

Mineralocorticoids
  Fludrocortisone
Sympathomimetic agents
  Ephedrine
  Pseudoephedrine
  Phenylpropanolamine
  Phenylephrine
  Methylphenidate
  Dextroamphetamine
  Tyramine (with monamine oxidase inhibition)
  Midodrine
  Clonidine
  Yohimbine
  DL- and L-dihydroxyphenylserine
Nonspecific pressor agents
  Ergot derivatives
  Caffeine
  Somatostatin analogues
β-Adrenergic blocking agents
  Propranolol
  Pindolol
  Xamoterol
  Prenalterol
Prostaglandin synthetase inhibitors
  Indomethacin
  Flurbiprofen
  Ibuprofen
  Naproxen
Dopamine blocking agents
  Metoclopramide
  Domperidone
V1 and V2 receptor agonists
  Desmopressin acetate
  Lysine-vasopressin
Erythropoietin

although little benefit is obtained by increasing beyond 0.5 mg. Treatment may unfortunately be limited by supine hypertension caused by an increase in the peripheral vascular resistance. Other side effects include ankle edema, hypokalemia, and rarely congestive heart failure. Potassium supplementation is usually required, particularly when higher doses are used.

Direct and indirect sympathomimetic agents have a long history of use in the treatment of orthostatic hypotension. Commonly used α_1-adrenoreceptor agonists include those with direct and indirect effects (ephedrine, pseudoephedrine, and phenylpropanolamine), those with direct effects (phenylephrine), and those with only indirect effects (methylphenidate and dextroamphetamine sulfate). The use of all these medications is complicated by tachyphylaxis, although efficacy may be regained after a short drug holiday. The sympathomimetic side effects, such as anxiety, tremulousness, tachycardia, and supine hypertension that inevitably accompany the use of these agents are frequently intolerable to patients. The peripheral selective α-agonist, midodrine, shows some promise in the treatment of orthostatic hypotension. The efficacy of this agent has been demonstrated in small open-label and double-blind studies. Potential side effects of this agent include pilomotor reactions, pruritus, supine hypertension, gastrointestinal complaints, and urinary urgency. Tachyphylaxis may occur less frequently with this agent.

The prostaglandin synthesis inhibitors, such as indomethacin, naproxen, and flurbiprofen, have been used to treat orthostatic hypotension. The probable mode of action of these agents is to limit the vasodilating effects of circulating prostaglandins and arachidonic acid derivatives. Erythropoietin has recently been shown to improve orthostatic tolerance in patients with orthostatic hypotension.

Most patients respond to the interventions described above. A complete list of medications used to treat orthostatic hypotension is present in Table 15-4.

Autonomic Dysfunction of the Urinary Bladder

The bladder wall is composed of three layers of interdigitating smooth muscle and serves as a receptacle for the storage and appropriate evacuation of urine. This smooth muscle (the detrusor muscle) forms the internal sphincter at the junction of the bladder neck and urethra. The internal sphincter is not anatomically discrete and functions as a physiologic sphincter. In contrast, the external sphincter is formed from the striated muscle of the urogenital diaphragm and is a true anatomic sphincter. Higher centers involved in bladder control include the anterior and medial frontal lobes, limbic regions, basal ganglia, thalamus, hypothalamus, and brainstem. These regions receive afferent fibers from and send efferent fibers to "micturition centers" in the lower spinal cord.

The bladder has parasympathetic, sympathetic, and somatic innervation. The parasympathetic nerves originate in the intermediolateral column of the second, third, and fourth sacral segments of the spinal cord and provide the major excitatory input to the urinary bladder. The nerve fibers from these segment pass through the ventral nerve roots of the spinal cord and form pelvic nerves that synapse with postganglionic neurons on the surface of the bladder. Activation of these muscarinic, cholinergic, postganglionic nerves produces detrusor muscle contraction.

The sympathetic nerve supply to the bladder originates in the intermediolateral column of spinal segments T10–L2 and passes through the sympathetic ganglia to reach the hypogastric plexus via the splanchnic nerves. Postganglionic sympathetic neurons then innervate the dome of the bladder, producing inhibition via the β-adrenergic receptors of the detrusor muscle and excitation at the α-adrenergic receptors of the internal sphincter, bladder base, and urethra via the hypogastric nerves.

The striated muscle of the external urethral sphincter is innervated by the pudendal nerves, which originate from the lateral anterior horn cells of the second, third, and fourth sacral segments, a region known as the sphincter motor nucleus or Onuf's nucleus. This sphincter is under voluntary control but undergoes reflex relaxation during micturition. Afferent fibers mediating bladder sensation and reflex bladder contraction are carried by sympathetic, parasympathetic, and somatic nerves to the spinal cord.

Treatment. The innervation of the bladder described above provides the basis for understanding bladder autonomic dysfunction. There are several different schemas classifying voiding dysfunction. The classification of Krane and Siroky (Table 15-5) incorporates a functional description of detrusor muscle

and sphincter function and provides a logical basis for instituting therapy. Therapies directed at reducing bladder hyperreflexia and maintaining urinary continence may decrease bladder contractility, enhance bladder outlet resistance, or employ other means to bypass vesicular or sphincteric abnormalities. Therapies for bladder hypomotility, conversely, attempt either to increase bladder contractility, to decrease outlet resistance, or to achieve both.

The nonpharmacologic interventions that include toileting regimens, Credé's maneuver, intermittent catheterization, indwelling Foley catheterization, palliative or definitive surgical interventions, and biofeedback are often used in concert with medications. The patient's customized therapy is best pursued with the aid of urologic consultation. Individualized treatment regimens should be guided by the history, examination, urodynamic studies, and measurement of the postvoid residual volume.

PHARMACOTHERAPY FOR BLADDER HYPERREFLEXIA. The pharmacotherapy for urinary incontinence caused by detrusor hyperreflexia attempts either to decrease bladder contractility or to increase outlet resistance (Table 15-6). Atropine and associated antimuscarinic substances depress involuntary bladder contractions. Propantheline bromide is the oral antimuscarinic agent most commonly used; its usual dose is 15 to 30 mg every 4 to 6 hours. Higher doses may be of benefit, but such trials are often limited by anticholinergic side effects. Direct-acting, smooth muscle relaxants constitute the other major category of inhibitors of bladder contractility. The suggested mechanism of action of such agents involves papaverine-like "antispasmodic" action, although their anticholinergic and local anesthetic properties may contribute to clinical efficacy. Oxybutynin (5 mg three or four times per day), dicyclomine hydrochloride (20 mg three times per day), and flavoxate hydrochloride (100 to 200 mg three or four times per day) are other commonly used agents. Anticholinergic side effects of these

TABLE 15-5. Classification of Bladder Dysfunction

Detrusor hyperreflexia (or normoreflexia)
   Coordinated sphincters
   Striated sphincter dyssynergia
   Smooth muscle sphincter dyssynergia
   Nonrelaxing smooth muscle sphincter
Detrusor areflexia
   Coordinated sphincter
   Nonrelaxing striated sphincter
   Denervated striated sphincter
   Nonrelaxing smooth muscle sphincter

TABLE 15-6. Therapy of Bladder Hypermotility

Behavioral therapy
   Timed bladder emptying
   Biofeedback
Catheterization and collecting devices
   Clean intermittent self-catheterization
   Urine collection devices
      Condom catheters
      Indwelling catheters
      Diapers and pads
Pharmacotherapy to inhibit bladder contractility
   Anticholinergic agents
   Smooth muscle relaxants
   Polysynaptic inhibitors
   Calcium channel antagonists
   β-Adrenergic agonists
   α-Adrenergic antagonists
   Prostaglandin synthetase inhibitors
   Tricyclic antidepressants
Pharmacotherapy to increase outlet resistance
   β-Adrenergic antagonists
   α-Adrenergic agonists
   Tricyclic antidepressants
   Estrogen
Surgical therapy
   Denervation procedures
   Augmentation cystoplasty
   Vesicourethral suspension
   Bladder outlet reconstruction
Treatment of urinary tract infection
Treatment of autonomic dysreflexia

medications, though clinically encountered, are reported to be less common than with atropine.

The tricyclic antidepressants are effective in the management of incontinence, probably by a combination of mechanisms. Both decreased bladder contractility and increased outlet resistance are the proposed mechanisms of action. Doses used in the management of incontinence are typically less than those used in depression. Among the various agents, the greatest experience has been reported with the tertiary amine imipramine. Small initial doses at bedtime (10 to 25 mg) are often effective, although a slow increment of dosage to 150 mg or more per day in single or divided doses may be needed. Orthostatic hypotension, sedation (most likely an antihistaminic effect), as well as anticholinergic side effects may limit trials with this medication. Other agents used to decrease bladder contractility include β_2-agonists, calcium channel antagonists, prostaglandin-synthetase inhibitors and polysynaptic inhibitors such as baclofen.

The medications that decrease bladder contractility are often used in conjunction with therapy that increases bladder outlet resistance, although the use of these agents would depend on the sphincter characteristics noted on urodynamic studies. The bladder neck and proximal urethra are richly populated by α-adrenergic receptors, which, when stimulated, result in smooth muscle contraction. α-Adrenergic agonists are the principal agents used to increase bladder outlet resistance; ephedrine (25 to 50 mg four times per day), pseudoephedrine (30 to 60 mg four times per day), phenylpropanolamine hydrochloride (25 to 50 mg three times per day), and others have been studied. Elevated blood pressure, anxiety, insomnia, and significant neurologic sequelae (headache, seizures) may limit dosage, and, as is the case with amphetamine-like substances, tachyphylaxis may develop.

PHARMACOTHERAPY FOR BLADDER HYPOMOTILITY. Stimulation of muscarinic, postganglionic receptors results in enhanced bladder contractility. Bethanechol chloride is a parasympathomimetic drug with relatively selective action at the urinary bladder. It is effective in chronic states of detrusor atony or hypotonicity, although it has also been used to facilitate reflex bladder contraction in patients with suprasacral cord injury. The dosing and route of administration of bethanechol vary with the clinical indications for its use. Typical oral doses range from 25 to 100 mg four times daily. The cholinergic agonist carbachol chloride, which may have additional ganglion-stimulating properties, also may enhance bladder motility.

Other agents used to enhance detrusor contractility include methyldopa, phenoxybenzamine, prostaglandins, and narcotic antagonists. Striated sphincter tone may also be attenuated by α-adrenergic blockade. Other agents that reduce striated muscle tone, such as baclofen, dantrolene, and the benzodiazepines, may also be of benefit. The high doses necessary frequently result in excessive central nervous system effects or generalized weakness (Table 15-7).

Autonomic Dysfunction of the Gastrointestinal Tract

The myoelectrical activity of gastrointestinal smooth muscle may be influenced by neural input intrinsic to the gut (the enteric nervous system), by extrinsic parasympathetic and sympathetic pathways, and by gastrointestinal neuropeptides acting either as neurotransmitters or as circulating hormones. Variation in smooth muscle activity has been described in the gut

TABLE 15-7. Therapy of Bladder Hypomotility

Catheterization and collecting devices
  See Table 15-6
Compressive and reflex maneuvers
  Credé's maneuver
  Valsalva maneuver
  Trigger zone stimulation
Pharmacotherapy to enhance bladder contractility
  Parasympathomimetic agents
  Prostaglandins
  α-Adrenergic antagonists
  Opioid antagonists
  Metoclopramide
Pharmacotherapy to relax the smooth muscle sphincter
  α-Adrenergic antagonists
  β-Adrenergic agonists
Pharmacotherapy to relax the striated muscle sphincter
  Centrally acting muscle relaxants
  Baclofen
  Dantrolene
Electrical stimulation of the paralyzed bladder
  Direct stimulation
  Stimulation of the spinal bladder innervation
    Conus medulloaris
    Pelvic nerve
    Anterior roots
Surgery
  Reduction cystoplasty
  Bladder neck and sphincter surgery

that appears to be a function of regional differences in the generation of transmembrane potentials.

Superimposed on the inherent differences in smooth muscle activity is the enteric nervous system, which consists of a myenteric plexus located between the inner-circular and outer-longitudinal smooth muscle layers (Auerbach's plexus) and a submucosal plexus (Meissner's plexus). A number of different intrinsic enteric neurons have been identified, and any individual neuron may contain multiple neuropeptides. For example, cholinergic-substance P neurons probably mediate motor excitation; motor inhibition is a function of dynorphin-vasoactive intestinal polypeptide neurons. Even in the absence of extrinsic autonomic nervous system influences, the enteric nervous system governs basic gut functions.

The "extrinsic" autonomic nervous system appears to integrate functions in anatomically separate areas of the gastrointestinal tract. Autonomic nervous system regulation of sphincteric function is of particular importance. The internal anal sphincter, consisting of a circumferential layer of smooth muscle, is responsible for 80 percent of resting sphincter tone and is under autonomic control, particularly tonic sympathetic excitation. Striated muscle sphincters, both at the anus (external anal sphincter) and at the level of the esophagus, are also subject to extrinsic autonomic nervous system influences. Parasympathetic efferents in the vagus nerve and second, third, and fourth sacral segments synapse with both myenteric cholinergic neurons, which mediate excitation of smooth muscle, as well as with myenteric inhibitory neurons. Extrinsic sympathetic efferents arising in the intermediolateral gray column synapse in the celiac and superior and inferior mesenteric ganglia and ramify throughout the gastrointestinal tract in the distribution of their respective arterial trunks. Histochemical studies have discriminated subpopulations of sympathetic postganglionic fibers on the basis of immunoreactive neuropeptides that colocalize in norepinephrine-containing cells.

Treatment. BOWEL HYPOMOTILITY. An increase in dietary fiber (up to 25 g/day) with water (10 ounces four times per day) and exercise is the first line of therapy for bowel hypomotility in most patients. The use of psyllium (up to 30 g/day) or methylcellulose (up to 6 g/day) with a concomitant increase in fluid intake further increases stool bulk. Appropriate caution must be exercised with these agents; for example, high fiber may be disadvantageous in diabetic gastroparesis because of distention and cramping pain that can be associated with its use or because of the potential of bezoar formation.

Stool softeners (e.g., docusate sodium 100 to 500 mg/day) or lubricants (e.g., mineral oil) together with an osmotic laxative (e.g., lactulose 15 to 60 ml/day) may be used if the above measures are ineffective. Glycerin suppositories or sodium phosphate enemas stimulate evacuation by promoting fluid retention in the rectum. (Table 15-8)

The contact cathartics such as the diphenylmethane derivatives (phenolphthalein and bisacodyl) and the anthraquinones (senna and cascara) should be used sparingly, although the use of these agents cannot be avoided in patients with constipation caused by autonomic failure. Extensive use of these agents may damage the myenteric plexus, producing cathartic bowel.

One or more of three general mechanisms of action have been described for the laxatives as a group. A given drug may increase intestinal bulk because of its hydrophilic or osmotic properties, it may decrease the net absorption of electrolytes and water by the intestinal mucosa by damaging the enterocytes or weakening intercellular junctions, or it may have its effects by enhancing intestinal motility and thus reducing fluid and electrolyte absorption.

The individual agents may be classified by their response latency and clinical effects. Softening of feces over 1 to 3 days occurs with the bulk-forming preparations and docusates, a semifluid stool may be induced over 6 to 8 hours by diphenylmethane and anthraquinone laxatives, and a watery evacuation in 1 to 3 hours occurs with the saline cathartics, such as magnesium citrate and milk of magnesia.

The benzamide, metoclopramide (5 to 20 mg orally 30 min-

TABLE 15-8. Pharmacotherapy of Bowel Hypomotility

Bulk agents
  Bran
  Psyllium
  Methylcellulose
Laxatives and cathartics
  Osmotic laxatives and cathartics
  Lactulose
  Sorbitol
  Magnesium salts
  Sodium phosphate
  Polyethylene glycol-saline solutions
  Glycerin suppositories
  Contact cathartics
    Diphenylmethane derivatives
     Phenolphthalein
     Bisacodyl tablets or suppositories
    Anthraquinone derivatives
     Senna
     Cascara
    Ricinoleic acid (castor oil)
Stool softeners and lubricants
  Mineral oil
  Docusates
Prokinetic agents
  Metoclopramide
  Cisapride
  Domperidone
  Erythromycin
  Cholinomimetics
    Bethanechol
    Acetylcholinesterase inhibitors
  Opioid antagonists
  Misoprostol

utes before meals and at bedtime), accelerates gastric emptying and has a central antiemetic action. Metoclopramide action is inhibited by atropine and is not affected by vagotomy, suggesting that its mode of action, which is primarily on antral motor activity, involves release of acetylcholine from intramural cholinergic neurons or direct stimulation of antral muscle by intact postganglionic cholinergic neurons. A dopaminergic mechanism has been inferred from studies demonstrating that levodopa-related inhibition of gastric emptying is reversed by metoclopromide.

In diabetic patients with concurrent gastroparesis and constipation, metoclopramide therapy may improve both symptoms, although its effect on colonic motility is controversial. Tolerance to metoclopramide therapy has been described. Patients maintained long term on metoclopramide theoretically may be at risk for the development of tardive dyskinesia and other side effects related to the antagonism of dopamine. Concurrent renal failure may increase the risk for acute toxicity. The cholinomimetic agent, bethanechol chloride, may be used in combination with metoclopramide and in cases of metoclopramide resistance. Domperidone, a peripheral antidopaminergic agent, may provide symptomatic relief in patients with gastroparesis, although it is not clear that the medication improves objective measures of gastric emptying.

Erythromycin and related macrolide compounds exhibit strong in vitro affinity for motilin receptors and have agonist properties that mimic the prokinetic action of exogenous motilin, a gastrointestinal polypeptide. Infusions of motilin in diabetic patients with gastroparesis result in accelerated gastric emptying, but therapeutic use of the agent is limited by its need for intravenous administration and by its short half-life. Single intravenous doses of erythromycin shorten postprandial, gastric emptying time to normal levels in diabetic patients with gastroparesis. Oral erythromycin (250 mg three times per day), also improves gastric emptying, although not to the degree noted after a single parenteral administration.

Cisapride is a benzamide cholinomimetic agent that increases motility in the esophagus, stomach, and bowel by enhancing release of acetylcholine from neurons of the myenteric plexus. In contrast to metoclopramide, cisapride lacks dopamine-blocking activity. This agent has been used with some success in several clinical conditions, including idiopathic gastric stasis, intestinal pseudo-obstruction, chronic constipation associated with laxative use, diabetic constipation, and diabetic gastroparesis. In a comparison of intravenously administered doses of cisapride and metoclopromide, cisapride may accelerate postprandial emptying to a slightly greater degree. Its effect on colonic motility is superior to that of metoclopramide.

The somatostatin analogue octreotide may stimulate intestinal motor complexes, and this agent has been used to treat sclerodermatous pseudo-obstruction. Somatostatin, however, is known to impair motor responses to feeding, and treatment with octreotide in other conditions has been associated with hypomotility and bacterial overgrowth. Clinical experience to date with octreotide suggests that its various side effects may potentially limit therapeutic use. Nausea and abdominal cramping pain occur with administration of the medication. Fat malabsorption and cholelithiasis have been described with chronic use.

The synthetic prostaglandin E_1 analogue misoprostol enhances intestinal motility and affects intestinal fluid and electrolyte secretion. Preliminary studies suggest that this agent may be of benefit in refractory constipation. Rare patients who do not respond to medical therapy may require colonic surgery. Such patients should have documented slow colonic transit time and intact rectal sphincter function.

BOWEL HYPERMOTILITY. Diabetic diarrhea best exemplifies the diagnostic complexity involved in the evaluation and treatment of neurogenic diarrheal conditions. Prior to the diagnosis of neurogenic diarrhea, other causes must systematically be excluded. Diarrhea as a result of bacterial overgrowth has been a subject of some controversy. One theory regarding the pathogenesis of diabetic diarrhea holds that gastric and small bowel hypomotility may predispose to the proliferation of bacteria that deconjugate bile salts and thus inhibit micelle formation. Steatorrhea and diarrhea thus result indirectly as a consequence of neurogenic dysmotility.

A trial of tetracycline (500 to 1,000 mg per day) is therefore conducted in most patients with unexplained chronic diarrhea, especially when steatorrhea is present. Treatment with prokinetic agents (see above) may also improve diarrhea. Should these measures fail, opioid agonists should be used. These agents decrease peristalsis and increase rectal sphincter tone. The synthetic opioids (diphenoxylate and loperamide) are preferable to alcohol solutions of opium. In the individual case, empiric management with tetracycline, opiates, prokinetic agents, psyllium, anticholinergics, and other agents is often required.

An alternative theory implicates a dysregulation of α_2-adrenoreceptor-mediated intestinal ion transport in diabetic diarrhea. Clonidine, a specific α_2-adrenergic receptor agonist, may be used to treat diarrhea in doses of up to 1.2 mg per day. The somatostatin analogue octreotide has been studied as a potential antidiarrheal agent in small numbers of patients with various conditions. As noted above, it may have a prokinetic action, but somatostatin has also been shown to inhibit stimulated water secretion in gut.

FECAL INCONTINENCE. Studies of idiopathic fecal incontinence have found delayed conduction in pudendal nerves supplying the external sphincter and denervation changes in pelvic muscles. Impaired rectal sensation may be responsible for incontinence in such cases because detecting the presence of stool in the anal canal is essential to normal continence. Other authors have argued that the neuropathy is secondary to prolonged straining at stool and traction on pudendal nerves.

Medical treatments generally attempt to rectify conditions that are either associated with or predispose to fecal incontinence. Use of high-fiber diets and bulking agents may be beneficial because a semiformed stool is more easily controlled than liquid feces. Fecal disimpaction is indicated in some cases. Daily tap water enemas aid in clearing residua in the rectum between evacuations and may allow for functional continence. Antidiarrheal agents may benefit patients for whom incontinence and diarrhea coexist. Biofeedback based on the patient's perception of a distensible balloon in the rectum and training to increase external sphincter pressure has met with success in some reports, although the response to biofeedback is likely to be dependent on the state of afferent pathways from the rectum.

Most patients who undergo surgical sphincter repair regain continence for solid stool, although the presence of pelvic floor neuropathy is associated with poorer outcome. Other surgical interventions, including colostomy, artificial anal sphincters, and creation of a reconstructed sphincter with muscle grafts, may be necessary in treatment-resistant cases.

SUGGESTED READINGS

Bannister R, Mathias CJ: Clinical features and investigations of the primary autonomic failure syndromes. p. 531. In Bannister R, Mathias CJ (eds): Autonomic Failure. Oxford University Press, Oxford, 1992

Bannister R, Oppenheimer DR: Degenerative diseases of the nervous system associated with autonomic failure. Brain 95:457, 1972

Blaivas JG: The neurophysiology of micturition: a clinical study of 550 patients. J Urol 127:958, 1982

Brunton LL: Agents affecting gastrointestinal water flux and motility, digestants, and bile acids. p. 914. In Gilman AG, Rall TW, Nies AS, Taylor P (eds): The Pharmacological Basis of Therapeutics. Pergamon Press, New York, 1990

Cable WJ, Kolodny EH, Adams RD: Fabry disease: impaired autonomic function. Neurology 32:498, 1982

Camilleri M: Disorders of gastrointestinal motility in neurologic diseases. Mayo Clin Proc 65:825, 1990

Camilleri M, Thompson WG, Fleshman JW, Pemberton JH: Clinical management of intractable constipation. Ann Intern Med 121:520, 1994

Cohen J, Low P, Fealey R et al: Somatic and autonomic function in progressive autonomic failure and multiple system atrophy. Ann Neurol 22:692, 1987

Dalmau J, Graus F, Rosenblum MK, Posner JB: Anti-Hu–associated paraneoplastic encephalomyelitis/sensory neuronopathy. A clinical study of 71 patients. Medicine (Baltimore) 71:59, 1992

Dyck PJ: Neuronal atrophy and degeneration predominantly affecting peripheral sensory and autonomic neurons. p. 1065. In Dyck PJ, Thomas PK, Griffin JW (eds): Peripheral Neuropathy. Vol. 2. WB Saunders, Philadelphia, 1993

Fedorak RN, Field M, Chang EB: Treatment of diabetic diarrhea with clonidine. Ann Intern Med 102:197, 1985

Feldman M, Schiller LR: Disorders of gastrointestinal motility associated with diabetes mellitus. Ann Intern Med 98:378, 1983

Freeman R, Miyawaki E: The treatment of autonomic dysfunction (review). J Clin Neurophysiol 10:61, 1993

Freeman R, Roberts MS, Friedman LS, Broadbridge C: Autonomic function and human immunodeficiency virus infection. Neurology 40:575, 1990

Hart RG, Kanter MC: Acute autonomic neuropathy. Two cases and a clinical review. Arch Intern Med 150:2373, 1990

Hilsted J, Low PA: Diabetic autonomic neuropathy. p. 423. In Low PA (ed): Clinical Autonomic Disorders. Little, Brown, Boston, 1993

Ingall TJ, McLeod JG: Autonomic function in hereditary motor and sensory neuropathy (Charcot-Marie-Tooth disease). Muscle Nerve 14:1080, 1991

Iosa D, Dequattro V, De-Ping Lee D et al: Pathogenesis of cardiac neuromyopathy in Chagas' disease and the role of the autonomic nervous system. J Auton Nerv Syst 30:S83, 1990

Johnsen SD, Johnsen P, Stein SC: A new hereditary sensory autonomic neuropathy in a Navajo population. Ann Neurol 18:400, 1985

Khurana RK: Paraneoplastic autonomic dysfunction. p. 505. In Low PA (ed): Clinical Autonomic Disorders. Little, Brown, Boston, 1993

Kyle RA, Dyck PJ: Amyloidosis and neuropathy. p. 1294. In Dyck PJ, Thomas PK, Griffin JW et al (eds): Peripheral Neuropathy. WB Saunders, Philadelphia, 1993

Lennon VA, Sas DF, Busk MF et al: Enteric neuronal autoantibodies in pseudoobstruction with small cell lung carcinoma. Gastroenterology 100:137, 1991

Madoff RD, Williams JG, Caushaj PF: Fecal incontinence. N Engl J Med 326:1002, 1992

Mamdani MB, Walsh RL, Rubino FA et al: Autonomic dysfunction and Eaton Lambert syndrome. J Auton Nerv Syst 12:315, 1985

Miyawaki E, Freeman R: Peripheral autonomic neuropathies. p. 253. In Korczyn A (ed): Handbook of Autonomic Nervous System Dysfunction. Marcel Dekker, New York, 1994

Papp MI, Lantos PL: The distribution of oligodendroglial inclusions in multiple system atrophy and its relevance to clinical symptomatology. Brain 117:235, 1994

Saraiva MJM, Costa PP, Goodman DS: Biochemical marker in familial amyloidotic polyneuropathy, Portuguese type: family studies of transthyretin (prealbumin)-methionine-30 variant. J Clin Invest 76:2171, 1985

Staskin DR: Classification of voiding dysfunction. p. 411. In Krane RJ, Siroky MB (eds): Clinical Neuro-Urology. Little, Brown, Boston, 1992

Tarsy D, Freeman R: The nervous system and diabetes. p. 794. In Weir G, Kahn R (eds): Joslin's Diabetes Mellitus. Lea & Febiger, Philadelphia, 1994

Thomas PK: Autonomic involvement in inherited neuropathies. Clin Auton Res 2:51, 1992

Tuck RR, McLeod JG: Autonomic dysfunction in Guillain-Barré syndrome. J Neurol Neurosurg Psychiatry 44:983, 1981

Wein AJ: Evaluation and treatment of urinary incontinence: practical uropharmacology. Urol Clin North Am 18:269, 1991

Wein AJ, Van Arsdalen K, Levin RM: Pharmacologic therapy. p. 523. In Krane RJ, Siroky MB (eds): Clinical Neuro-Urology. Little, Brown, Boston, 1992

Wingate DL: Autonomic dysfunction and the gut. p. 510. In Bannister R, Mathias CJ (eds): Autonomic Failure. Oxford University Press, Oxford, 1992

Wood JD: Physiology of the enteric nervous system. p. 67. In Johnson LR, Christensen J, Jackson MJ et al (eds): Physiology of the Gastrointestinal Tract. Raven Press, New York, 1987

Ziegler MG, Lake CR, Kopin IJ: The sympathetic-nervous-system defect in primary orthostatic hypotension. N Engl J Med 296:293, 1977

16. HYDROCEPHALUS AND DISORDERS OF CEREBROSPINAL FLUID FLOW

SEPIDEH AMIN-HANJANI
WILLIAM F. PIRL
PETER McL. BLACK

Hydrocephalus is ventricular dilation caused by a disturbance in cerebrospinal fluid (CSF) circulation. This disturbance can occur anywhere in the CSF system. It is important to recognize hydrocephalus in the office practice of neurology and internal medicine because it can be associated with common complaints such as headache, gait disturbance, and memory difficulty, and should be recognized as it can be successfully treated.

Several terms are used to describe the anatomy of the particular hydrocephalic problem. *Communicating hydrocephalus* is characterized by continuity of the CSF in the ventricular system with the subarachnoid space of the brain and spinal cord. *Noncommunicating hydrocephalus* occurs when there is a blockage in the ventricular system or its outlets so that the ventricles and the subarachnoid space are not in continuity. It is important to recognize this distinction because a lumbar puncture is unsafe in the noncommunicating form. *Hydrocephalus ex vacuo* is not actually a form of hydrocephalus, but rather is a state of increased ventricular size resulting from cortical atrophy. Although hydrocephalus has many different manifestations, it is instructive to group cases into two clinical syndromes: high-pressure hydrocephalus and normal-pressure hydrocephalus (NPH), with gradations between them.

This chapter describes the clinical presentations, diagnosis, and management of hydrocephalus in adults. Similar principles, however, apply to hydrocephalus in children.

CLINICAL PRESENTATIONS

High-Pressure Hydrocephalus

The onset of high-pressure hydrocephalus can be acute, over hours to days, or chronic, over weeks to months. High-pressure hydrocephalus can be life-threatening, causing obtundation, coma, and death. Its symptoms are related to increased intracranial pressure (ICP).

Headache is the most frequent complaint. The headache, usually bifrontal, is most severe in the morning; it tends to be worse when the patient lies flat and to be relieved by sitting, and it can be exacerbated by coughing. It can progress to a generalized headache and may even wake up the patient at night. Nausea and vomiting commonly occur in association with the headache and are also most severe in the morning. The nausea is not associated with head movements or any abdominal discomfort. The patient may also complain of visual changes, including decreased visual acuity, diplopia, and an inability to look up. "Graying-out" of vision may occur if a pressure wave causes serious optic nerve compression.

The gait disorder is typically an unsteady, broad-based gait, which may first appear as slow and uncertain and then develop into short, staggering steps.

Changes in mental status can range from impairment of recent memory to confusion. Signs of frontal lobe disorder with slowness of response, inattentiveness, distractibility, inability to plan or sustain complex actions, and perseveration may be present. However, in contrast to primary cortical dementias, such as Alzheimer's disease, there is no aphasia, agnosia, or apraxia.

Physical examination may reveal papilledema from increased ICP, but it is not invariably present. Testing extraocular movements may indicate lateral rectus weakness caused by compression of abducens nerve fibers. This is a sign of generalized increased ICP; it is not a localizing sign even when it is unilateral. Paralysis of upward gaze and of accommodation result from pressure on the tectal plate. Truncal ataxia may be present.

Almost all cases of high-pressure hydrocephalus in adults are caused by an obstruction of flow through the ventricular system and subarachnoid pathways. This results in increased mean pulsatile pressures in the ventricular system and a consequent increase in ventricular size. The ventricles will continue to expand until the pressure can no longer be compensated, eventually leading to central herniation and death.

An obstruction can occur anywhere along the CSF pathway. The etiologies are the same as those listed in Table 16-1 for NPH. Even with a specific cause, there may be no localizing signs to help the examiner discern the underlying etiology. Subarachnoid hemorrhage is the most common cause of obstruction, with hydrocephalus occurring in as many as 67 percent of cases of subarachnoid hemorrhage. Because of this frequency, patients with a subarachnoid hemorrhage should be monitored for symptoms of hydrocephalus for up to 3 weeks after the event. Tumors causing obstruction of the ventricles or their

TABLE 16-1. Some Causes of Adult Normal-Pressure Hydrocephalus

Cause	Percentage
Subarachnoid hemorrhage	34
Idiopathic	34
Head injury	11
Tumors	6
Prior surgery	5
Aqueduct stenosis	3
Meningitis	3
Others	4

(Modified from Katzman R: Low pressure hydrocephalus. p. 29. In Wells CE (ed): Dementia. FA Davis, Philadelphia, 1977, with permission.)

outflow are another important cause of high-pressure hydrocephalus. In addition to intraventricular tumors, tumors may also obstruct the ventricular system extrinsically. Compression of the third ventricle can occur posteriorly by a pineal tumor or inferiorly by a craniopharyngioma or pituitary adenoma. Similarly, the fourth ventricle can be compressed by posterior fossa tumors. Aqueduct stenosis, a congenital disorder that may present in adulthood, should also be seriously considered in the differential diagnosis.

Normal-Pressure Hydrocephalus

NPH is characterized by enlargement of the ventricles and normal CSF pressure. It is best diagnosed by its clinical presentation: the classic triad of gait disturbance, disturbances in mentation (usually slowing of thought and action), and urinary incontinence. Symptoms of high-pressure hydrocephalus such as headache, nausea and vomiting, and visual changes are not seen.

Gait Disorder. Gait disturbance is the most prominent symptom in NPH and is usually the earliest in onset. It has been described as unsteady or uneven, and patients often complain of falling. The gait is characterized by its wide base, slow speed, short steps, and vertical ataxia. (Patients place their feet on the ground with variable forces.) Patients sometimes describe feelings of weakness in their legs, and they may actually be consuming more energy in walking than is normal. The problems with walking can progress to complete inability to walk and even inability to stand or sit because of unsteadiness. However, the gait disorder appears to be more of a frontal "gait apraxia," which poses difficulties in organizing a smooth gait, rather than an actual ataxia. The same NPH patients who are unable to walk demonstrate unimpaired functioning of the legs when lying on their back. There may also be some upper extremity involvement with tremor and deterioration of handwriting.

Gait disorders are regularly encountered in the elderly, and NPH may account for only 4 percent of these cases. Some features of the disordered gait of NPH may help to distinguish it from other causes of gait disorder, although this may often be difficult. Patients with Alzheimer's disease may have a gait disorder but, compared to NPH, the gait tends to be shuffling and scuffing with increased double-support stride. It occurs late in disease Alzheimers, after cognitive deterioration. Cerebellar ataxia must also be considered in the differential diagnosis. In contrast to the vertical ataxia of NPH, in cerebellar ataxia movements of the legs are more variable in the transverse and sagittal planes. Other evidence of cerebellar incoordination, such as dysmetria and terminal tremor, is not present in NPH. Parkinson's disease is also characterized by a gait disorder and may be confused with NPH because both can display bradykinesia, increased tone, and dysarthria. However, the parkinsonian gait is described as hesitant with festination, en bloc turning, flexed posture, and lack of accessory movements such as arm swinging. In addition, cogwheel rigidity and masked facies are distinguishing features of Parkinson's disease. Patients with Binswanger's disease or multi-infarct dementia may also present with a gait disorder that is difficult to distinguish from NPH, although patients with NPH tend to present at a later age and more frequently have gait disturbance at onset.

Disturbance of Mentation. A variety of mental changes have been described in NPH, ranging from mild memory loss to severe dementia. Impairment of recent memory is the most frequent complaint. A loss of initiative, spontaneity, and interest may progress to apathy and abulia, that is, a slowing of thought and action. Responses and voluntary movements are slow and delayed. Abulia is so characteristic of NPH that it may even be considered separately from the dementia as a fourth component of the syndrome. Some cognitive impairment may be present with verbal abilities unaffected, while nonverbal tasks such as copying, drawing, and arranging objects become difficult. Changes in mood, behavior, and personality may also be evident.

This clinical picture represents a subcortical type of dementia—frequently encountered in the elderly—which may be very difficult to distinguish from other subcortical dementias like Binswanger's disease and multi-infarct dementia, from depression, and, at times, from cortical dementias like Alzheimer's disease. When they are present, Alzheimer's disease can be distinguished by aphasia, agnosia, and apraxia, which are not components of the dementia of NPH. The changes in mentation seen in Alzheimer's disease occur much earlier than the gait disturbance, which is usually a late symptom. In NPH, gait disorder usually precedes or occurs concurrently with changes in mentation. Major depression may present as a pseudodementia with memory loss and psychomotor retardation; however, neurovegetative symptoms and depressed mood should be present. Incontinence is generally not seen in depression. Binswanger's disease and the multi-infarct state may cause a dementia very similar to that of NPH and pose a diagnostic difficulty that can only be resolved by other tests, for example, magnetic resonance imaging (MRI).

Incontinence. Urinary incontinence is the third part of the NPH triad, and, although it occurs commonly in NPH, it is not seen with the same frequency as gait disorder and changes in mentation. It may occur as a late symptom. The incontinence ranges from a sense of urgency to a frontal lobe type of incontinence in which the appropriate awareness of the need to urinate is lost, leading to a loss of sphincter control. Fecal incontinence is rare. Urinary incontinence can also be seen in atrophic processes such as Alzheimer's disease.

Physical Examination. The physical examination reveals no focal signs, unless there is a specific cause for the NPH, such as tumor. Papilledema is absent and extraocular movements and upward gaze are intact. Increased tone may or may not be present. Weakness is not present, but limb movement may be slow. Increased tendon reflexes may be observed, and a positive Babinski sign may be present in one or both feet. Sucking or grasping reflexes may appear in later stages. No sensory loss is seen. Cerebellar ataxia is not present. Patients are unable to achieve tandem walking, and they have positive Romberg signs. Gait difficulties are described above.

Etiology. NPH can be caused by anything that results in low-grade scarring or obstruction of the ventricular system or subarachnoid pathways. The etiologies are listed in Table 16-1. Subarachnoid hemorrhage is the most common cause of NPH with a known etiology. Other causes include meningitis, partial obstruction of the CSF pathways by tumor, cranial radiation, and neurosurgery, particularly following a posterior fossa operation. NPH may follow trauma that causes a subarachnoid hemorrhage that subsequently obstructs the basal cisterns. Less commonly, it may follow an obstruction of a major venous sinus or the third ventricle and its outflow. Aqueduct stenosis more frequently leads to high-pressure hydrocephalus, but may cause NPH as well. Idiopathic NPH, seen in a large number of cases, is more common in patients who are over 60.

Pathogenesis.   In the pathogenesis of NPH, Hakim and Adams have suggested that there is an initial rise in CSF pressure that leads to ventricular enlargement. This enlargement is maintained despite normal pressure because of the relationship of pressure and area described by LaPlace's law, pressure = force/area. The increased force on the ventricular wall is distributed at a lower pressure over the greater area of the enlarged ventricular wall. Even though the pressure appears normal most of the day, continuous intracranial pressure monitoring in some patients also shows periods of increased intracranial pressure waves at night.

INVESTIGATIONAL STUDIES

The purpose of ancillary testing in patients with hydrocephalus is twofold: to establish a reliable diagnosis, and to predict the utility of CSF diversion in the treatment of the disorder. Once a patient has presented with a clinical picture suggestive of hydrocephalus, the initial diagnostic test of choice is the computed tomographic (CT) scan. This should be performed both with and without contrast; an unenhanced scan will visualize the ventricular contours, while contrast enhancement may reveal otherwise indistinguishable underlying lesions. The cardinal CT features of hydrocephalus include (1) enlargement of ventricles, with rounding of the ventricular contour; (2) the presence of periventricular lucencies, especially around the frontal horns; and (3) normal-sized subarachnoid spaces. Enlargement of the subarachnoid spaces and prominent cortical sulci suggest atrophy with ex vacuo ventricular enlargement, but these conditions may also be present with hydrocephalus.

If CT scanning reveals ventricular enlargement characteristic of hydrocephalus and a clear etiologic lesion, further imaging is costly and of no additional benefit. MRI is an important adjunctive test if CT scanning fails to establish a reliable diagnosis. It is better than CT in identifying underlying lesions, such as small periaqueductal or posterior fossa tumors. MRI is also the modality best equipped to assess parenchymal disease seen with Binswanger's disease or multi-infarct dementia, which may be difficult to distinguish from NPH on clinical grounds alone. Furthermore, sagittal imaging with MRI helps to distinguish hydrocephalus from atrophy by showing distinctive features of the former, such as thinning and bowing of the corpus callosum. Periventricular hypointensity on T1-weighted MRI is, however, less specific and can be seen in the setting of edema, ischemia, demyelination, and other disorders. Measurement of proton relaxation times of periventricular abnormalities may prove to be a useful technique for distinguishing these processes.

MRI also allows measurement of intracranial CSF volume, which may provide a sensitive volumetric index of ventricular size. Quantification of the volumes of various intracranial compartments may prove beneficial in the differentiation of hydrocephalus from other causes of ventriculomegaly.

In addition to volumetric determinations, MRI can show CSF flow patterns through the aqueduct of Sylvius. A variety of MRI techniques have been applied to establish flow and pulsatility patterns through the Sylvian aqueduct in patients with hydrocephalus. Recent reports suggest that these techniques may have value in differentiating the various types of hydrocephalus, although they are not yet clinically applicable.

Cisternography has been widely used in evaluating CSF dynamics in patients with ventricular enlargement and suspected NPH. It is performed by intrathecal injection of a radioactive isotope (isotope cisternography) or contrast material and serial CT scanning (CT cisternography). The passage of the isotope or contrast into the ventricles and subarachnoid space is visualized. A normal pattern shows flow over the convexities and not into the ventricles. The typical pattern of NPH is ventricular entry and stasis without ascent over the convexities. Most patients show a "mixed" pattern. The value of cisternography in diagnosis and prediction of shunt responsiveness has been brought into question. Recent reports indicate that cisternography provides no additional diagnostic accuracy over the combination of clinical and CT criteria.

Determination of CSF pressure by lumbar puncture is an important component of diagnosis in some patients. Those individuals who do not have findings of high-pressure hydrocephalus and are suspected clinically to have NPH without an identifiable etiology should undergo lumbar puncture. An opening pressure less than 180 mmH$_2$O in this group of patients is consistent with a diagnosis of idiopathic NPH. The value of shunting in such patients may be further elucidated by a CSF-tap test, which involves removal of 50 ml fluid. Alternatively, serial lumbar punctures, which presumably create an ongoing dural leak acting as a temporary shunt, can be performed. Clinical improvement, especially of gait, predicts a good response to shunting. Temporary lumbar drainage has been suggested as a further maneuver for prediction of shunt responsiveness.

Continuous ICP monitoring can also help to identify those patients with idiopathic NPH who are likely to benefit from CSF diversion. Monitoring can be performed using a frontal ventricular catheter, lumbar catheter, or epidural transducer, all of which allow prolonged pressure recording over at least 24 hours. Increased baseline CSF pressure or pressure waves (A or B waves) can be used as criteria for shunt responsiveness. A more quantitative analysis of ICP waves may allow greater accuracy in these determinations.

An adjunct to prolonged pressure recording is the use of infusion tests to assess resistance to CSF absorption. Lumbar infusion of normal saline has been shown to detect prolonged increases in ICP, indicating deficits in CSF absorptive capacity. A similar technique measuring the resistance to ventricular infusion may be useful in patients with noncommunicating hydrocephalus. A well-proven technique involves measurement of CSF conductance by lumboventricular perfusion. Outflow resistance greater than 12.5 ml/min/mmHg has been correlated with improvement after shunting. The disadvantages of these testing modalities are their invasiveness and potential for equivocal measurements of CSF outflow resistance. They may offer prognostic information for shunting in a selected group of patients with idiopathic NPH in whom other less invasive testing has been unhelpful.

There is some evidence that functional tests such as single photon emission computed tomography (SPECT), which shows patterns of cerebral blood flow, positron emission tomography (PET), which demonstrates brain metabolism, and magnetic resonance spectroscopy, which measures ratios of chemical markers in the brain, may help to differentiate NPH from other causes of dementia and may also be of some predictive value in determining shunt responsiveness. However, these tests are still under investigation and need further validation before they enter mainstream clinical practice. Electroencephalography and evoked responses have no utility in the diagnosis of hydrocephalus.

DECISION MAKING AND MANAGEMENT

The optimal management of a patient with suspected hydrocephalus relies on the strength of the clinical diagnosis and the validity of ancillary tests aimed at prognostication. When making management decisions, it is useful to consider separately the clinical entities that result from high- and normal-pressure hydrocephalus.

The patient with symptoms of increased ICP and ventriculomegaly, who is acutely deteriorating as indicated by a worsening level of conciousness or loss of vision, requires emergent neurosurgical consultation for placement of ventriculostomy.

In less acute situations involving high-pressure hydrocephalus, CSF diversion by operative placement of a shunt is indicated. In cases of hydrocephalus secondary to an obstructive mass, however, primary management that includes removal of the mass may relieve the hydrocephalus. Operative removal is increasingly the treatment of choice, given recent improvements in microsurgical technique, although there may be a need for CSF diversion at a later date. Preoperative shunting carries the risk of upward tentorial herniation with large midline cerebellar masses, as well as the potential for spreading malignant cells to the peritoneum via the shunt.

The definitive treatment for NPH is shunting, but poor responses in some groups and the potential for serious complications must be considered in the decision to proceed with shunt placement. Patients with the diagnosis of NPH as supported by the clinical syndrome and CT findings should undergo careful evaluation for an underlying cause. When a clear etiology is present, such as recent subarachnoid hemorrhage, meningitis, evidence of aqueduct stenosis, or obstructive tumor, shunting is the treatment of choice and is associated with good outcome. As with high-pressure hydrocephalus due to a mass, it is reasonable to remove an obstructive lesion as primary management for NPH.

For cases of idiopathic NPH the decision is more complex. Numerous clinical findings and tests have been advocated as predictors of shunt responsiveness, some of which are discussed above. Many studies have addressed this issue. The following parameters have consistently proven to be good prognosticators for shunt response:

1. NPH of known etiology
2. Shorter duration of symptoms (although long duration is not a contraindication)
3. Prominent gait disturbance
4. Improvement after serial lumbar punctures
5. Altered CSF dynamics as demonstrated by long-term monitoring or infusion testing, especially lumboventricular perfusion
6. A CT scan showing periventricular lucency

Studies of shunt responsiveness report response rates in the range of 30 to 80 percent. In our experience about two-thirds of patients improve and perhaps 5 percent may worsen in some way with shunt placement. Differences in outcome may be due to differential selection for shunting and analysis of outcomes. Standardized preshunting selection criteria may increase the likelihood of improvement.

Of special interest are patients with ventricular enlargement who are free of symptoms related to hydrocephalus. The incidental finding of ventriculomegaly on imaging in such patients should prompt careful evaluation for subtle symptoms or signs of hydrocephalus. If the patient is truly asymptomatic, no further investigation or intervention is indicated; however, interval follow-up to assess the possible development of symptoms is warranted.

SHUNTS

Shunt Systems

Currently the commonly employed systems for CSF diversion are ventriculoperitoneal, ventriculoatrial, ventriculopleural, and lumboperitoneal shunts. The most widely used is the ventriculoperitoneal shunt.

The components of a typical CSF diversion system include the following:

1. *Proximal catheter: ventricular or lumbar catheter*. A ventricular catheter is inserted into the right frontal horn via a right frontal or right parieto-occipital burr hole. A lumbar catheter for lumbar CSF diversion is an option in communicating hydrocephalus and carries the advantage of avoiding ventricular puncture and general anesthesia. However, lumbar shunts have a much greater tendency for obstruction and have generally fallen out of favor.
2. *Distal tubing*. Silastic tubing is attached to the proximal catheter and tunneled subcutaneously to the distal site of drainage, that is, the peritoneal cavity (ventriculo- and lumboperitoneal shunts), the right atrium via the common facial vein (ventriculoatrial shunt), or the pleural cavity (ventriculopleural shunt).
3. *Valve*. A valve is interposed between the proximal and distal shunt components, usually near the site of the ventricular catheter. It regulates the pressure and prevents retrograde flow of shunted CSF. Several valve designs exist, including spring-loaded, slit, or resistance valves, which vary by their mechanism of outflow regulation. These are fixed-pressure valves functioning at high, medium, or low settings. More recently, variable-pressure valves, which allow percutaneous adjustment of pressure settings, have become available. These valves allow the surgeon to fine-tune ICP in shunted patients without the need for reoperation. The ideal opening pressure of the valve for hydrocephalic patients is controversial. Low- and medium-pressure valves have been advocated in the past; others have indicated the effectiveness of high-pressure systems. The utility of variable-pressure valves is under investigation.
4. *Ancillary components: ventricular reservoir and antisiphon device*. Ventricular reservoirs are commonly placed proximal to the valve system in ventricular shunts and are generally palpable. They serve as an access for extracranial measurement of the ICP, CSF removal, and testing of the shunt system. When shunted patients are in an upright position, the ICP may become subatmospheric, leading to overdrainage. Antisiphon devices are designed to prevent intraventricular pressure from falling below atmospheric pressure at the level of the antisiphon device, thus preventing overdrainage.

Shunt-Related Complications

The most important shunt-related complications are discussed in the following sections.

Obstruction.   Shunt obstruction can be of insidious, intermittent, or sudden onset and presents with clinical deterioration indicative of shunt malfunction. The ventricular catheter may become obstructed by debris, coagulum, or contact with choroid plexus or brain secondary to decreased size of the ventricles. Proximal catheter obstruction is the most common cause of shunt malfunction. The distal end may become blocked in ventriculoperitoneal shunts by omentum or peritoneal adhesions. Shunt blockage requires surgical exploration and revision.

Infection.   The rate of shunt infections in adults is less than 5 percent, which is lower than the rate in the pediatric population. Infection can manifest in several ways: wound infection at the site of shunt insertion, ventriculitis and meningitis, or secondary infection of the vascular system, including endocarditis (ventriculoatrial shunts) and peritoneal infection (ventriculoperitoneal shunts). However, most commonly, shunt infection presents insidiously as shunt malfunction, and typical findings of meningitis are generally not present. Most infections occur immediately or within a few months of shunt insertion and are generally attributed to bacterial contamination during surgery. Shunt infection may also occur in the setting of systemic infection, such as pneumonia or urinary tract infection. The most common pathogens are *Staphylococcus epidermidis* and, less frequently, *S. aureus, Pseudomonas aeruginosa,* and *Escherichia coli.* The general approach to shunt infection is removal of the entire shunt system and external ventricular drainage until the infection has cleared following a full course of intravenous antibiotics.

Subdural Collections.   Subdural hematomas may form after the shunting of hydrocephalus as a result of tears in the cortical bridging veins when the brain matter has not yet adequately expanded to fully occupy the increased cranial space caused by the drainage of fluid. Even minor head trauma can increase the risk of subdural hematoma. Collections of low protein fluid, called subdural hygromas, may also develop. These likely represent effusions that develop in response to the excess space within the cranial vault unoccupied by brain matter. Subdural collections of blood or fluid are generally a complication of overdrainage after too-rapid ventricular decompression. Use of the higher pressure valves or variable-pressure valves that allow graded ventricular decompression may decrease the incidence of this complication. For symptomatic collections, burr hole drainage is initially attempted. It may be necessary to temporarily clamp off the shunt so that the brain can expand and occlude the subdural space.

Overdrainage.   Symptoms of overdrainage often mimic those of underdrainage; they include headache, nausea and vomiting, lethargy, diplopia, impaired upgaze, and visual impairment. However, unlike those of increased ICP, the symptoms of overdrainage are typically worse when the patient is upright and are relieved when lying down. Overdrainage can give rise to two distinct syndromes: the low ICP syndrome, which can be distinguished by positional measurement of ICP, and the slit ventricle syndrome, which is apparent on CT or MRI as reduction of the ventricles to subnormal size. The latter syndrome is more prominent in the pediatric population but may be seen in adults who were initially shunted at a young age. Encroachment of the ventricular walls onto the draining catheter leads to intermittent or complete CSF obstruction with accompanying signs and symptoms of suddenly increased ICP.

For unclear reasons that may relate to decreased compliance of the system, the ventricles do not enlarge despite shunt obstruction. Both of these syndromes require shunt revision with substitution of a new system, perhaps incorporating an antisiphon device or a valve with higher opening pressure.

Mechanical Failure.   Disconnection of shunt components or fracture of the Silastic tubing at stress points may occur, especially with head trauma. Palpation of the subcutaneous shunt tubing throughout its length may reveal a gap or bulge at the site of disconnection. A radiographic shunt series, comprising a selection of films showing anteroposterior and lateral views of the skull and chest or KUB and lateral views of the abdomen, depending on shunt type, can be helpful in determining the site of disconnection. Surgical exploration and revision will be necessary in cases of mechanical failure.

Shunt Type-Specific Complications.   Ventricular shunts carry a small risk (approximately 5 percent) of seizures; the incidence of this may be decreased with the use of an occipital rather than a frontal catheter. Prophylactic anticonvulsant medication is not indicated in routine management. Ventriculoatrial shunts carry the unique risk of thromboembolic episodes such as pulmonary embolism; with the shunt materials currently in use, these risks are small. Lumboperitoneal shunts are often obstructive and have been associated with acquired tonsillar herniation.

Evaluation of a Patient With Suspected Shunt Malfunction

Shunt malfunction must be suspected in patients presenting with headache, nausea and vomiting, lethargy, or visual changes. These patients should be evaluated for signs of increased ICP, including papilledema and abducens or upward gaze palsy. Alternatively, shunt malfunction may manifest as a recurrence of prior hydrocephalic symptoms, such as worsening of gait, memory, or incontinence. In fact, regression of clinical improvements at any time after shunt placement should raise the question of shunt malfunction. The clinical deterioration is often stereotyped in any one patient. Malfunction is most frequently a consequence of obstruction, infection, or malposition of the shunt system.

On physical examination, palpation of the shunt tubing may reveal disconnection. Palpation and compression of the valve suggest blockage of the ventricular catheter if the valve can be compressed but refills very slowly. Blockage within the valve or distally is likely if the valve is incompressible. A normally working shunt should allow easy valve emptying and refill within 5 to 30 seconds. Valve pumping, however, is not considered to be a reliable indicator of shunt function, and some shunt systems have no palpable valve.

A shunt series is of variable benefit, since disconnection is a relatively uncommon cause of shunt malfunction. It is indicated if there is clear suspicion of disconnection on examination. To determine the CSF pressure, lumbar puncture or tapping of the shunt reservoir can be performed. Lumbar puncture is preferable if it can be performed safely, because shunt tapping carries a 1 percent risk of infection. A shunt tap should be considered an invasive procedure requiring meticulous attention to sterile technique. Neurosurgical consultation before the procedure is warranted.

An attempt to withdraw CSF after puncture of the reservoir may help to localize the site of malfunction. Inability to withdraw suggests proximal obstruction at the level of the ventricular catheter. Easy withdrawal suggests distal obstruction. It is important to note that flushing of the system via shunt tap is unwise, since it may further increase an already decompensating ICP. A shuntogram can be performed by injecting water-soluble iodine contrast dye into the reservoir, followed by serial radiographs over 30 minutes. The test is aimed at defining a site of obstruction and indicating the rate of dye clearance from the system. However, results are often inconclusive, and shuntograms are not commonly used. Ultimately, surgical exploration can identify the source of malfunction. It is important to exclude infection in any malfunction, therefore CSF should be analyzed at the time of lumbar puncture, shunt tap, or operative revision.

SUGGESTED READINGS

Adams RD, Victor M: Principles of Neurology, 5th Ed. McGraw-Hill, New York, 1993

Benzel EC, Pelletier AL, Levy PG: Communicating hydrocephalus in adults: prediction of outcome after ventricular shunting procedures. Neurosurgery 26:655, 1990

Black PM: Hydrocephalus and vasospasm following subarachnoid hemorrhage from ruptured intracranial aneurysm. Neurosurgery 18:12, 1986

Black PM, Hakim R, Olsen Bailey N: The use of the Codman-Medos programmable Hakim valve in the management of patients with hydrocephalus: illustrative cases. Neurosurgery 34:1110, 1994

Black PM, Ojemann RG, Tzouras A: CSF shunts for dementia, incontinence and gait disturbances. Clin Neurosurg 32:632, 1985

Borgesen SE, Gjerris F: The predictive value of conductance to outflow of CSF in normal pressure hydrocephalus. Brain 105:65, 1982

Condon B, Patterson J, Wyper D et al: Use of magnetic resonance imaging to measure intracranial cerebrospinal fluid volume. Lancet 1:1355, 1986

Crockard HA, Hanlon K, Duda EE, Mullan JF: Hydrocephalus as a cause of dementia: evaluation by computerized tomography and intracranial pressure monitoring. J Neurol Neurosurg Psychiatry 40:736, 1977

Fisher CM: Hydrocephalus as a cause of disturbances of gait in the elderly. Neurology 32:1358, 1982

Gallassi R, Morreale A, Montagna P et al: Binswanger's disease and normal-pressure hydrocephalus: a clinical and neuropsychological comparison. Arch Neurol 48:1156, 1991

Haan J, Thomeer RTWM: Predictive value of temporary external lumbar drainage in normal pressure hydrocephalus. Neurosurgery 22:388, 1988

Hakim S, Adams RD: The special clinical problem of symptomatic hydrocephalus with normal cerebrospinal fluid pressure: observations on cerebrospinal fluid hydrodynamics. J Neurol Sci 2:307, 1965

Hussey F, Schanzer B, Katzman R: A simple constant-infusion manometric test for measurement of CSF absorption. II. Clinical studies. Neurology 20:665, 1970

Jagust WJ, Friedland RP, Budinger TF: Positron emission tomography with [^{18}F] fluorodeoxyglucose differentiates normal pressure hydrocephalus from Alzheimer-type dementia. J Neurol Neurosurg Psychiatry 48:1091, 1985

Kamiya K, Yamashita N, Nagai H, Mizawa I: Investigation of normal pressure hydrocephalus by 123I-IMP SPECT. Neurol Med Chir 31:503, 1991

Katayama S, Asari S, Ohmoto T: Quantitative measurement of normal and hydrocephalic cerebrospinal fluid flow using phase contrast cine MR imaging. Acta Med Okayama 47:157, 1993

Katzman R: Low pressure hydrocephalus. In Wells CD (ed): Dementia. FA Davis, Philadelphia, 1977

Larsson A, Jensen C, Bilting M et al: Does the shunt opening pressure influence the effect of shunt surgery in normal pressure hydrocephalus? Acta Neurochir (Wien) 117:15, 1992

Larsson A, Wikkelso C, Bilting M, Stephensen H: Clinical parameters in 74 consecutive patients shunt operated for normal pressure hydrocephalus. Acta Neurol Scand 84:475, 1991

Mascalchi M, Ciraolo L, Bucciolini M et al: Fast multiphase MR imaging of aqueductal CSF flow: 2. Study in patients with hydrocephalus. AJNR 11:597, 1990

Matsumae M, Kikinis R, Lorenzo AV et al: Intracranial compartments in patients with enlarged ventricles assessed by MRI based image processing. (submitted)

McQuarrie IG, Saint-Louis L, Scherer PB: Treatment of normal pressure hydrocephalus with low versus medium pressure cerebrospinal fluid shunts. Neurosurgery 15:484, 1984

Morgan MK, Johnston IH, Spittaler PJ: A ventricular infusion technique for the evaluation of treated and untreated hydrocephalus. Neurosurgery 29:832, 1991

Nitz WR, Bradley WG, Watanabe AS et al: Flow dynamics of cerebrospinal fluid: assessment with phase-contrast velocity MR imaging performed with retrospective cardiac gating. Radiology 183:395, 1992

Puca A, Anile C, Maira G, Rossi G: Cerebrospinal fluid shunting for hydrocephalus in the adult: factors related to shunt revision. Neurosurgery 29:822, 1991

Pudenz RH, Foltz EL: Hydrocephalus: overdrainage by ventricular shunts: a review and recommendations. Surg Neurol 35:200, 1991

Raftopoulos C, Chaskis C, Delecluse F et al: Morphological quantitative analysis of intracranial pressure waves in normal pressure hydrocephalus. Neurol Res 14:389, 1992

Roman GC: White matter lesions and normal-pressure hydrocephalus: Binswanger's disease or Hakim syndrome? AJNR 12:40, 1991

Shiino A, Matsuda M, Morikawa S et al: Proton magnetic resonance spectroscopy with dementia. Surg Neurol 39:143, 1993

Sindou M, Guyotat-Pelissou, Chidiac A, Goutelle A: Transcutaneous pressure adjustable valve for the treatment of hydrocephalus and arachnoid cysts in adults: experience with 75 cases. Acta Neurochir (Wien) 121:135, 1993

Sorensen PS, Jansen EC, Gjerris F: Motor disturbance in normal-pressure hydrocephalus: special reference to stance and gait. Arch Neurol 43:34, 1986

Sudarsky L, Ronthal M: Gait disorders among elderly patients: a survey study of fifty patients. Arch Neurol 40:740, 1983

Symon L, Dorsch NWC: Use of long-term intracranial pressure measurement to assess hydrocephalic patients prior to shunt surgery. J Neurosurg 42:258, 1975

Tamaki N, Nagashima T, Ehara K et al: Hydrocephalic oedema in normal-pressure hydrocephalus. Acta Neurochir Suppl 51:348, 1990

Vanneste J, Augustin P, Davies GAG et al: Normal-pressure hydrocephalus: is cisternography still useful in selecting patients for a shunt? Arch Neurol 49:366, 1992

Vanneste J, Augutijn P, Dirven et al: Shunting normal-pressure hydrocephalus: do the benefits outweigh the risks? A multicenter study and literature review. Neurology 42:54, 1992

Waldemar G, Schmidt JF, Delecluse F, Andersen AR et al: High resolution SPECT with 99MTc-d,l-HMPAO in normal pressure hydrocephalus before and after shunt operation. J Neurol Neurosurg Psychiatry 56:655, 1993

Welch K, Shillito JS, Strand R et al: Chiari I malformation: an acquired disorder? J Neurosurg 55:604, 1981

Wikkelso C, Andersson H, Bloomstrand C, Lindqvist G: The clinical effect of lumbar puncture in normal pressure hydrocephalus. J Neurol Neurosurg Psychiatry 45:64, 1982

Wood JH, Bartlet D, James AE, Udvarhelyi GB: Normal-pressure hydrocephalus: diagnosis and patient selection for shunt surgery. Neurology 24:517, 1974

17. TRAUMATIC BRAIN INJURY

MICHAEL P. ALEXANDER

This chapter covers three aspects of traumatic brain injury (TBI) that may involve neurologists: the mild injury in the emergency room, the spectrum of problems of severe TBI, and the office management of mild TBI, including the patient who never recovers.

ACUTE MANAGEMENT OF TRAUMATIC BRAIN INJURY

In the United Kingdom 10 percent of all emergency room visits are for TBI—mostly minor. Of the minor TBI patients, the overwhelming majority will have no neurologic deterioration and will not require hospital care. Approximately 2 percent will deteriorate and potentially require neurosurgical management. As summarized by Vollmer and coworkers (1991), "the major practical problem in [minor TBI] involves developing a management scheme that prevents delay in treatment of the small number of intracranial complications without causing excessive rates of hospitalization, inconvenience, and cost to the vast majority of patients." In the mid-1980's in both the United Kingdom and the United States, multidisciplinary groups proposed management schemes. During the same decade, prospective studies from Scotland provided data sufficient to stratify overall risk for different segments of the minor TBI population. This stratification of risk has been supported by several additional investigations.

The large prospective series carried out by Teasdale and colleagues (1990) in Glasgow illuminates the real locus of risk. A Glasgow Coma Scale (GCS) score of 15 with no skull fracture carries a 1/6,000 risk of deterioration. A GCS score of 15 with a skull fracture carries a risk of 1/32, a 188-fold increase. A GCS score of 13–14 without skull fracture, has a risk of 1/21, but with skull fracture, a risk of 1/4. In the entire group, a skull fracture alone raises the risk of deterioration 400-fold. Studies from the United States also demonstrate the substantially lower risk of deterioration in the GCS 15 group (approximately 2 percent overall in several studies) compared to the GCS 13–14 group. Most investigators now do not consider a patient with a GCS score of 13–14, that is, with any impairment of consciousness in the emergency room, as a minor, low-risk case. The Glasgow Coma Scale is given in Table 17-1.

In the United Kingdom, Shackford and colleagues (1992) have identified several criteria as the indicators of increased risk, and it has been recommended that any patient with even one criterion should be admitted for observation and computed tomography (CT) scanning as clinically indicated. These criteria are as follows:

1. Confusion or altered level of consciousness in the emergency room (i.e., GCS 13 to 14)
2. Skull fracture
3. Neurologic signs or severe headache or vomiting
4. Difficult assessment (young age, intoxication, etc.)
5. Other high-risk medical conditions (e.g., use of anticoagulants)
6. No reliable home observer

In the United States, Masters and colleagues (1987) have proposed a three-tiered strategy. For the mildest cases with no loss of consciousness, a normal neurologic examination, and no clinical signs of basilar skull fracture, discharge to home is appropriate. For patients with a history of loss of consciousness and amnesia but with normal examination results, "extended observation" and "consideration of CT" are recommended. For patients with GCS scores of 13 to 14 or with focal signs, immediate CT is indicated. There are problems with both sets of recommendations. The UK criteria generate a large number of admissions. The patients are probably not closely observed, given the low risk of clinical problems, and the high number of admissions are costly. Recent analysis suggests also that the criteria are too easily ignored, often just to avoid the paperwork of admissions in a low-risk group. The US criteria probably underestimate the value of skull radiographs in narrowing the population at risk. The US criteria for moderate cases ignore the large number of likely missed skull fractures with the markedly increased risk of possible deterioration. It has also been difficult to implement the use of these criteria.

Recent studies clarify how these apparently different approaches, employing observation, skull radiographs, and CT scans, result in fairly similar outcomes. Taheri and coworkers (1993) in the United States report 310 consecutive admissions with a GCS score of 15, five (1.7 percent) deteriorated, that is, required neurosurgery. All 5 patients who deteriorated were among the 10 patients with skull fracture. Of the 273 patients who had skull radiographs but no fracture, there were no delayed deteriorations. Using the UK criteria, all five patients would have been admitted for observation or CT scanning—four for focal signs and one for intoxication. (Recall that *all* 310 were actually admitted.) Using the US criteria, four would have had immediate CT scan (focal signs), and one would have been observed. It is impossible to reconstruct how many others would have been observed. Servadei and associates (1993) reported 113 patients with a GCS score of 15 who were referred to a neurosurgical center because of a positive CT scan; 95 percent also had a skull fracture on radiograph. The five patients without fracture included four cases with "small" hemorrhages not requiring surgery and one child who would have been observed or had a CT scan by both US and UK criteria.

This is a clinical management problem that every hospital with an emergency room should probably resolve through a quality improvement project. The current literature supports the following scheme (Fig. 17-1):

1. Any minor TBI patient with focal signs or GCS scores of 13 to 14 (i.e., altered mental state) in the emergency room should have a head CT scan.
2. Patients with GCS 15 and no focal signs should be sent home if there was no loss of consciousness or amnesia, there are no worrisome medical issues, there is no intoxication, they are older than 14 years of age, and the home setting is reasonable.

TABLE 17-1. The Glasgow Coma Scale

Eye Opening		
None	1	Not attributable to ocular swelling
To pain	2	Pain stimulus is applied to chest or limbs
To speech	3	Nonspecific response to speech or shout, does not imply the patient obeys command to open eyes
Spontaneous	4	Eyes are open, but this does not imply intact awareness
Motor Response		
No response	1	Flaccid
Extension	2	"Decerebrate." Adduction, internal rotation of shoulder, and pronation of the forearm
Abnormal flexion	3	"Decorticate." Abnormal flexion, adduction of the shoulder
Withdrawal	4	Normal flexor response; withdraws from pain stimulus with abduction of the shoulder
Localized pain	5	Pain stimulus applied to supraocular region or fingertip causes limb to move so as to attempt to remove it
Obeys commands	6	Follows simple commands
Verbal Response		
No response	1	(Self-explanatory)
Incomprehensible	2	Moaning and groaning, but no recognizable words
Inappropriate	3	Intelligible speech (e.g., shouting or swearing), but no sustained or coherent conversation
Confused	4	Patient responds to questions in a conversational manner, but the responses indicate varying degrees of disorientation and confusion
Oriented	5	Normal orientation to time, place, and person

Summed Glasgow Coma Scale Score = E + M + V (3 to 15).

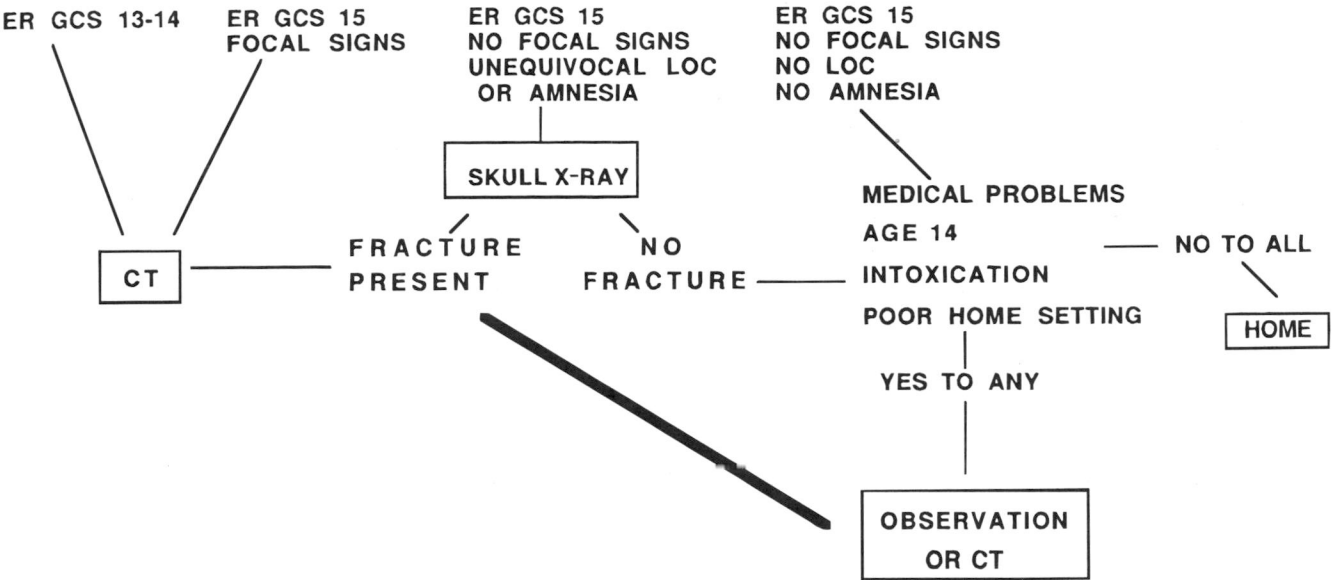

FIG. 17-1. Suggested emergency room (ER) management of mild TBI. GCS, Glasgow Coma Scale; LOC, loss of consciousness; CT, computed tomography.

3. Patients with a GCS score of 15 and no focal signs but who have had unequivocal loss of consciousness and amnesia should be given skull radiography and, if these radiographs are negative for fracture and if there are no medical issues, they should be sent home.

4. Patients listed under item 3 *with* skull fracture should either be kept for observation or have a CT scan, depending on relative costs, time of day, and local preferences.

Shackford's group, in their major multicenter US study, used a retrospective analysis of the role of CT in minor TBI assessment and came to similar conclusions, although the nature of the study limits its utility for prospective management decisions. A more important discovery was the frighteningly high number of admitted patients (30.2 percent) who had no documentation of any follow-up neurologic examination. Admit for "observation" at your peril! I recommend CT scanning for any patient who is admitted, but local preferences should be spelled out as *specific* practice guidelines, and a quality improvement committee should follow compliance for risk management purposes.

THE BEHAVIORAL NEUROLOGY OF SEVERE TRAUMATIC BRAIN INJURY

Patients with severe TBI are usually managed by neurosurgeons, often in the intensive care unit when their care requires respiratory assistance. There are only a few points to note regarding acute care:

1. There is no definite role for prophylactic anticonvulsants after the first week following the injury.
2. The value of dexamethasone is unknown.
3. Even hyperventilation is of uncertain overall value, balancing reduced edema against vasoconstriction with possible ischemia, although it is always reasonable management.
4. New classes of agents that may reduce or block cell death in the acute period are under study, and these may be added to the therapeutic armamentarium in the near future.

The neurologic management of severe TBI survivors at the rehabilitation center requires a specific diagnosis of the injury type.

Diffuse Axonal Injury

Sudden acceleration-deceleration is the most important physical agent of TBI. Powerful inertial forces are generated. The microscopic structure of the brain leaves it most susceptible to inertial shear injury. Shearing disrupts axons and small blood vessels. Axonal disruptions lead to eventual cell death and, perhaps, to downstream neuronal injury from release of excitatory neurotransmitters. The small blood vessel injury can produce simple petechial hemorrhages, which are maximal in parasagittal white matter—increasing centripetally from the cortex to deep white matter—or focal or diffuse edema. This entire neuropathologic picture is called diffuse axonal injury, and clinical severity is directly related to the extent of neuronal and vascular damage. Recovery from diffuse axonal injury is highly correlated with several measures of injury severity, including GCS, duration of coma, and duration of post-traumatic amnesia.

The clinical evolution of diffuse axonal injury from coma follows characteristic stages:

1. Coma: no eye opening, no verbalization, no meaningful response
2. Unresponsive wakefulness: eye opening (vegetative state)
3. Mute vigilance: watchful, irregular direct responsiveness
4. Responsive confusional state: severe impairment in attention and memory, which may be quiet, agitated, or fluctuating
5. Oriented cognitive impairment: recovered day-to-day memory and usually independent basic self-care (physical limitations allowing)
6. Supervised functional independence
7. Independent functional competence

Note that even at stage 7, there may be residual cognitive impairments. Although many patients with diffuse axonal injury have no motor impairments, severe cases may have a variety of motor deficits reflecting parasagittal, deep white matter lesions, superior cerebellar outflow and midbrain tegmental lesions, and, in the most severe cases, deeper brainstem lesions.

As a rule, patients should receive inpatient rehabilitation until the transition from stage 5 to stage 6 from which point they can be managed at home. The transition from coma to functional competence depends on the severity of diffuse axonal injury. The mildest possible diffuse axonal injuries probably are "ding" injuries in sports. Careful assessment of a well-motivated patient with "ding" demonstrates recovery over 7 to 10 days. For injuries with brief loss of consciousness and 20 to 60 minutes of post-traumatic amnesia, the common concussion, the recovery period is probably 1 1/2 to 6 months. For more "severe" mild TBI with post-traumatic amnesia lasting longer than 60 to 90 minutes (GCS 13–14), recovery might require 4 to 12 months. As severity measures increase, the duration of recovery gets longer. These times are *much* longer than most neurologists realize. Only the most severe cases stall at stages 2 through 5.

Focal Cerebral Contusions

In addition to diffuse axonal injury, TBI can cause focal cerebral contusions, which may occur directly at a point of contact, but most are caused by inertial forces driving the basal frontal and temporal cortex into rough adjacent bony surfaces. Focal cerebral contusions are abrasions that originate in cortex, include disruption of vascular structures, and may cause physical disruption, ischemic injury, or hemorrhagic injury of adjacent white matter. These abrasions may be seen anywhere, but the inferior and anterior temporal and orbital and polar frontal regions are most common. Focal cerebral contusions have very poor correlation with the markers for severity of diffuse axonal injury, that is, the initial GCS score and loss of consciousness. In fact, patients with focal cerebral contusions may never, or only transiently, have been unconscious, that is, have had apparently "minor" TBI. Patients with multiple focal cerebral contusions, especially those with accompanying subdural hematomas, have a very high mortality rate.

The clinical profile of focal cerebral contusions depends upon location, number, and size. In the most common locations, behavioral problems predominate. Damage to orbital frontal cortex produces poor regulation of emotions with overreactivity, irritability, social disruptiveness, and lability. Damage to the polar frontal cortex produces impaired complex, motivated behaviors with shallow and distractible problem-solving and disorganized complex social behaviors. Recovery depends on size, depth, and number of these contusions; they are often bilateral and symmetrical. The timing of recovery is similar to other focal destructive lesions, such as infarcts and hemorrhages. Recovery is potentially rapid for 2 to 4 months and then is relatively flat. It is important to note the similarity between the cognitive clinical profiles of *late* severe diffuse axonal injury and frontal focal cerebral contusions and also to note the markedly different probabilities of late recovery between severe diffuse axonal injury (good) and focal cerebral contusions (poor).

Hypoxic-Ischemic Injury

Although diffuse axonal injury and focal cerebral contusions are the defining injuries of TBI, hypoxic-ischemic injury is also common in more severe cases and in certain cases of herniation, often from epidural hematomas. Diffuse hypoxic-ischemic injury is due to a mixture of factors, including edema, increased intracranial pressure, local vascular damage, and systemic shock or chest or airway injury impairing ventilation; there may be no specific clinical markers beyond clinical suspicion. Diffuse hypoxic-ischemic injury has a dramatically worse prognosis for recovery for any given duration of loss of consciousness, falling to essentially zero when the loss of consciousness associated with this injury lasts for 7 days. Focal hypoxic-ischemic injury is usually caused by posterior cerebral artery entrapment lesions due to herniation. Clinical consequences are the same as those predicted for more common posterior cerebral artery infarctions and depend on whether it is temporal or occipital and whether it is left, right, or bilateral. Recovery patterns mimic infarctions of more common origins.

Mixed Pathologies

Many patients have a mixture of pathologies, with GCS scores determined by either severity of diffuse axonal injury or by severity of early herniation. Duration of coma is determined by severity of diffuse axonal injury or hypoxic-ischemic injury. Post-traumatic amnesia is determined by severity of diffuse axonal injury, severity of diffuse hypoxic-ischemic injury, or location of focal cerebral contusions. Long-term outcome is determined by severity of diffuse axonal injury and diffuse hypoxic-ischemic injury and by location, size, and number of focal cerebral contusions and focal hypoxic-ischemic injury. The long-term prospects of patients over 40 years old are delayed and constrained.

Patients with severe TBI seen months to years after injury and after acute rehabilitation may present because of seizures or some other neuromedical problem, such as headaches or spasticity, because of behavioral or cognitive problems, or for advice about the next stages in rehabilitation. Behavioral and cognitive diagnoses require competence at detailed mental status assessment and absolute clarity about the relative role of diffuse axonal injury and focal cerebral contusions in the clinical profile because of their differing prognoses. If not previously performed, magnetic resonance imaging (MRI) is essential. It has advantages in revealing old focal cerebral contusions, particularly for demonstrating basal focal cerebral contusions without bone artifact, and for demonstrating petechial hemorrhages from diffuse axonal injury (paramagnetic foci). Neuropsychological assessment is essential in characterizing cognitive limits and strengths.

Treatment

Treatment issues that arise in the late assessment of patients with severe TBI are of two types: retraining/remediation and behavioral. The late rehabilitation recommendations are determined by three factors: (1) the patient's profile of deficits, (2) the probable prognosis for improvement and learning as determined by the neuropathology, and (3) financial, personal, and social resources. Rehabilitation of severe TBI is emotionally draining for patients and families. It is expensive and may take a long time and enormous patience.

As noted above, the deficits are usually predominantly cognitive and behavioral. Neuropsychological and neuropsychiatric assessment are essential to proper characterization. Postacute rehabilitation of cognitive deficits takes several possible forms. There are programs that attempt to combine direct treatment of cognitive deficits with compensatory strategies for the patient, family, and workplace or school. The claims for direct treatment of attentional, memory, or other cognitive deficits are controversial for three reasons. First, it has been hard to demonstrate efficacy beyond natural recovery. Second, it has been difficult to demonstrate generalization of any recovered process for tasks beyond those trained. Third, the treatment tasks often lack common sense. If you want a patient to be able to work as a receptionist again, why have that patient do computer vigilance tasks? Why not do simplified ''receptionist vigilance'' tasks? Programs of direct treatment are often called ''cognitive rehabilitation,'' and they demand skepticism.

A second type of program emphasizes the compensation strategies and directly treats only tasks of functional relevance, such as budgeting, check handling, riding public transportation, and filling out applications. These programs do not suffer from the three weaknesses of direct treatment programs, but they must be judged by how they match treatment goals with reasonable neurologic prognoses. These programs may also be called ''cognitive rehabilitation,'' but the two types of programs differ in a critical dimension of treatment. Physicians should know the structure of the programs to which they refer patients.

For some patients behavioral disorders are a primary obstacle to functional recovery. Behavioral management also depends on precise diagnosis. Only a taste of the diagnostic dilemmas can be presented here. For instance, does a patient with a unilateral frontal polar contusion have low motivation because of limitations in higher order mental processes like goal setting, setting mental representation of strategies to goals, or organizing complex activities? Or is the patient depressed? Or both? Does a patient with disinhibition and intrusive behavior have an attentional problem related to severe diffuse axonal injury, to orbitofrontal injury, to anxiety, or to a combination of these? Neuropsychiatric assessment may clarify these questions.

Treatment may involve behavioral treatment, perhaps ''cognitively based,'' as in the second program type described above, or, perhaps, ''behaviorally based.'' Treatment may also be pharmacologic. There are two overriding lessons about drug treatment: First, there are no magic potions for the TBI patient. For every patient with periodic agitation who responds to haloperidol, there is another who does not, but who responds to benzodiazepines. There are concrete reasons *not* to use all known drugs in the TBI patients, for example, motor side effects or worsened alertness. Claims for several generations of ''mood regulators'' in TBI, such as carbamazepine, propanolol, lithium, and others, are only weakly supported. Second, when a clear psychiatric disorder is established, even if it is believed to be neurogenic, treatment should start with the same agents that have been efficacious in the purely psychiatric form of the disorder.

Patients with severe diffuse axonal injury can often make good functional recovery even if their basic neurologic deficits and limitations do not change. Careful use of progressively more demanding rehabilitation programs leading to vocational and educational programs is always justified. Patients with substantial frontal focal cerebral contusions do not typically benefit greatly, but behavioral and compensatory strategies may improve their function within a particular setting, if realistic goals are set.

BEHAVIORAL NEUROLOGY OF MINOR TRAUMATIC BRAIN INJURY

As reviewed above, minor TBI is defined by injury characteristics, not, in some circular manner, by outcome characteristics.

Some minor TBI patients have a bad functional outcome, and some severe TBI cases have an excellent outcome. The outcome does not define the injury! As mentioned above, there is no reliable biologic marker for severity, although functional imaging or cognitive evoked potentials may yet provide such a marker. At present, minor TBI is defined by a melange of clinical measures: (1) GCS at first examination, (2) duration of loss of consciousness, and (3) duration of post-traumatic amnesia. There are patients with minor TBI by those measures who have intracerebral hemorrhages, so-called ''complicated minor TBI.'' ''Complicated'' cases should be set aside from this discussion and considered as the mild end of the spectrum of severe TBI.

As outlined above, it is currently believed that diffuse axonal injury underlies all of these injuries, minor TBI cases simply having less injury than severe ones. There may be crucial idiosyncratic differences in the *location* of diffuse axonal injury between cases that account for differences in outcome, but at present, these potential differences cannot be detected clinically or with imaging. This uncertainty should induce humility in clinicians willing to write off deficits as ''psychogenic.''

Although it is customary to view GCS scores 13 to 15 as minor, both in the emergency room and in outcome, there are probably differences between patients who have a GCS score of 15 and those who have GCS scores of 13 to 14. The mildest TBIs are the ''ding'' injuries and, perhaps, the pure inertial injuries from whiplash without loss of consciousness. In the ''modal'' mild TBI, there is brief loss of consciousness (less than 1 to 2 minutes), post-traumatic amnesia, including much of the accident scene or even transport to the emergency room (20 to 60 minutes), and a GCS score of 15 in the emergency room. Retrograde amnesia is often remarkably brief if inquired about after post-traumatic amnesia has cleared. In ''more severe'' mild TBI, loss of consciousness may be up to 1 hour, post-traumatic amnesia up to 24 hours, and GCS scores of 13–14 in the emergency room. These cases clearly shade into severe TBI with GCS scores of 11 to 12 and post-traumatic amnesia of 1 to 2 days. The more prolonged the injury measures, the more severe the injury.

This discussion briefly covers four topics: (1) the natural history of neurologic recovery, (2) the other injuries associated with brain injury, such as head and neck, vestibular, and psychological injuries, that together produce the postconcussive syndrome, (3) the natural history of postconcussive syndrome and (4) the persistent postconcussive syndrome.

Neurologic Recovery

The primary neurologic deficits of minor TBI are in attention and memory. It is arguable that other deficits—complex mental operations, often called ''executive functions,'' and behavioral regulation—are due to these two primary deficits. Many patients also complain of sleep disorders. This may represent primary damage to sleep structures, or it may be due to superimposed pain states, medications, enforced inactivity, or attentional deficits. Numerous studies have demonstrated that recovery of attention and memory requires a considerable time even in the mildest cases. ''Ding'' injuries seem to take 7 to 10 days to recover. The ''modal'' cases may require 1 1/2 to 6 months. Increasing age above 40 years may prolong these times. In the later stages of recovery, deficits may be subtle, and well-designed tasks, such as information processing, choice reaction times, and stressed recall tasks, may be required to demonstrate them. Some patients may even have effectively recovered and still show subtle deficits. The more subtle the deficits, the more they are affected by situational, psychological, comorbid medical, and premorbid personal factors. The same mild deficit in sustained attention may be much more symptomatic in a 46-year-old police officer with daily headaches and a sick spouse than in a 19-year-old part-time student who is otherwise asymptomatic and living with parents. There is no formula that maps neuropsychological deficits (at least mild ones) directly onto functional status. There are no known treatments that accelerate recovery. Note that the times to recover are *much longer* than the ''few days rest'' often prescribed. The key management action is to arrange sufficient time for recovery, allowing for comorbid injuries, age, and employment status.

Injuries Associated With Postconcussive Syndrome

When heads hit windshields, more than the brain may be injured. The head may be injured causing lacerations, abrasions, fractures, and other injuries. The peripheral vestibular system may be disrupted. The neck may be strained. For that matter, systemic injuries may be severe enough to cause the minor TBI to be totally overlooked as care is directed to other life-threatening injuries. Finally, patients with mild TBI may have an experience that patients with severe TBI never have. They may remember the injury circumstances if not the actual point of injury. The psychological traumas—anxiety, fear, guilt—are accessible to many mild TBI patients.

Headache, cervical strain, and peripheral vestibular disorders are dealt with elsewhere in this text, but a few points relevant to TBI should be mentioned here. Patients with evidence of cervical soft tissue injury require early appropriate symptomatic treatment: limited immobilization, including cervical pillows, physical therapy, and analgesics. The emergence of headaches unrelated to simple local trauma is essentially universal after minor TBI. Most of these will clear in days to weeks, and simple analgesics are sufficient. Acute peripheral vestibular injury can be treated with rest and vestibular suppressants, such as clonazepam, although sedation may be an unacceptable side effect in these patients.

Patients with severe psychological trauma—feelings of responsibility for a fatality, nightmares, avoidance behaviors, sadness over a death, etc.—should receive early counseling. The likely time course of recovery needs to be established early. Patients should understand the high probability of recovery, but they should receive assistance during the time this takes.

Natural History of Postconcussive Syndrome

The interaction of neurologic deficits, pain, vestibular injury, psychological trauma, other systemic injuries, and psychosocial disruptions, such as financial loss, temporary unemployment, and increased time at home, is the postconcussive syndrome. The most common symptoms are headache, poor memory, poor sleep, poor concentration, dizziness, anxiety, depression, and a variety of sensory sensitivities (photophobia, positional vertigo, hyperacusis, etc.). Most are multifactorial. Symptomatology declines after the first few weeks to 40 to 50 percent, after a few months to 30 percent, and by 1 year to 15 to 20 percent. Treatment has been discussed above. The neurologic injury requires time. Symptomatic treatment of other injuries is essential. Psychological counseling may be needed. A plan for gradual resti-

tution of preinjury activities will prevent patients from returning too quickly and failing or from struggling in their routine activities and thus increasing psychological stress.

Persistent Postconcussive Syndrome

Postconcussive syndrome is considered persistent when it is present for 1 year; in many patients, symptoms, in fact, *increase* over time. Several studies have shown that symptoms in patients with persistent postconcussive syndrome undergo a shift from purely somatic initially to increasingly psychological-vegetative symptoms. A number of factors are said to be associated with an increased risk of persistent postconcussive syndrome: female sex, ongoing litigation, low socioeconomic status, prior mild TBI, severity of initial neck pain, and preinjury emotional state. Note that differences in ''mildness'' from ''dings'' to a GCS score of 13 have not been implicated. No one factor is, however, a very potent predictor.

Dickmen and colleagues (1986) have eloquently described the role of postinjury ''psychological factors'' in persistent postconcussive syndrome while observing that these factors have largely eluded prospective definition. Lishman (1988) has provided an elegant description of how physiogenesis is transformed to psychogenesis. In recent years, some prospective analyses have yielded insights into persistent postconcussive syndrome, for example, these patients have more significant head and neck pain than their recovered counterparts. That chronic pain alone can produce symptoms of cognitive impairment is well known.

Patients with persistent postconcussive syndrome are much more likely to have reached diagnostic criteria for specific psychiatric disorders by 6 months after the injury. Depression is most common. Global anxiety, at times with features of post-traumatic stress disorder, is also common. Memory for the injury scene may be a factor in the qualities of post-traumatic stress disorder. Peripheral vestibular disorder is a potent contributor to the anxiety that develops in a large number of patients with acute vestibular disease within 6 months of onset. Even frank phobic disorder can develop. That depression or anxiety can produce symptoms, and even signs, of cognitive dysfunction is also well known. Depressed patients with cognitive impairment even have a consistent pattern of frontal hypoperfusion in positron emission tomography (PET) studies.

Finally, patients with persistent postconcussive syndrome have a larger number of chronic social problems than their recovered counterparts. As patients remain symptomatic, and perhaps even worsen, families become transformed. The families of patients with persistent postconcussive syndrome have a different belief structure: the patient *is* disabled; the doctors *can't or aren't trying* to find the cause; the family's role is to take over and support the now disabled patient. Arguments about injury characteristics, negative CT scans, and depression fall flat against this belief structure. Very few patients are frankly malingering.

Treatment of persistent postconcussive syndrome is often unrewarding. Few approaches are open. First, symptomatic treatment should be offered where appropriate. This might include analgesia, vestibular suppressants, counseling, physical therapy. Antidepressants can be used as headache treatment or sleeping aids. Antianxiety agents can be used as vestibular suppressants. Physical therapy for neck pain can be used to mobilize the patient into a schedule, a home program, and some fitness activities. Because these patients actually have trivial neurologic impairments, they are often, if ironically, ideal for cognitive rehabilitation programs designed for the late severe TBI patient. Only programs of the second type described above are appropriate. Because of their good neurologic recovery, programs to reenter community activities and to practice interviews and time management can be quite successful. Treatment of basic psychiatric symptoms is an essential part of this plan. Depressed TBI patients are no more swayed by cajoling and encouragement than functionally depressed patients.

Treatment of these patients is quite difficult and requires simultaneous attention to somatic symptoms and to psychological processes. Two mistakes to avoid are attributing persistent postconcussive syndrome to malingering or to pending litigation without further neuropsychiatric assessment and endlessly pursuing symptomatic treatment of one somatic complaint without attempting to place the treatment in a broader medical, rehabilitative, and psychological context.

SUGGESTED READINGS

Alexander MP: Neuropsychiatric correlates of persistent postconcussive syndrome. J Head Trauma Rehabil 7:60, 1992

Dikmen S, McLean A, Temkin N, Wyler A: Neuropsychological and psychosocial consequences of minor head injury. J Neurol Neurosurg Psychiatry 49:1227, 1986

Eagger S, Luxon LM, Davies RA, Coelho A, Ron MA: Psychiatric morbidity in patients with peripheral vestibular disorder: a clinical and neuro-otological study. J Neurol Neurosurg Psychiatry 55:383, 1992

Katz DI, Alexander MP: Predicting outcome and course of recovery in patients admitted to rehabilitation. Arch Neurol 51:661, 1994

Lishman WA: Physiogenesis and psychogenesis in the 'post-concussional syndrome.' Br J Psychiatry 153:460, 1988

Masters SJ, McClean PM, Arcarese JS: Skull x-ray examinations after head trauma: recommendations by a multidisciplinary panel and validation study. N Engl J Med 316:84, 1987

Servadei F, Vergoni G, Nasi MT et al: Management of low-risk head injuries in an entire area: results of an 18 month survey. Surg Neurol 39:269, 1993

Shackford SR, Ward SI, Ross SE et al: The clinical utility of computed tomographic scanning and neurologic examination in the management of patients with minor head injuries. J Trauma 33:385, 1992

Taheri PA, Karamanoukian H, Gibbons K et al: Can patients with minor head injuries be safely discharged home? Arch Surg 128:289, 1993

Teasdale GM, Murray G, Anderson E et al: Risks of acute traumatic intracranial haematoma in children and adults: implications for managing head injuries. Br Med J 300:363, 1990

Vollmer DG, Dacey RG, Jane JA: Craniocerebral trauma. p. 63. In Joynt R (ed): Clinical Neurology. Lea & Febiger, Philadelphia, 1991

Williams DH, Levin HS, Eisenberg HM: Mild head injury classification. Neurosurgery 27:422, 1990

SECTION 3. PRINCIPLES OF DIAGNOSIS: SPECIAL TESTS

18. LABORATORY EVALUATION

STEVEN FESKE

The neurologic history and examination will allow the physician to make an anatomic or syndromic diagnosis. Additional studies, including laboratory tests, electrophysiology, and neuroimaging, can add precision to this diagnosis and often support an etiologic diagnosis. The chapters in this section describe the use of many of the ancillary tests that are helpful in neurologic diagnosis. The goal of these chapters is to provide a brief general description of the nature and interpretation of commonly used tests. More specific information about the indications and interpretations of certain tests can be found in the discussions of particular diseases. This chapter addresses selected general laboratory tests significant in neurologic diagnosis.

TESTS OF COAGULATION

Stroke is the most common life-threatening neurologic disease and among the most common causes of death. The neurologist must understand the laboratory tests that contribute to the proper evaluation and management of vascular disease. The coagulation system is shown in Figure 18-1. The cascade of reactions following from the activation of factor X constitutes the common pathway. The cascade of reactions beginning with the activation of factor XII and including the reactions of the common pathway constitutes the intrinsic pathway. Activation of factor X via factor VII and tissue factor and the resultant cascade of reactions through the common pathway constitute the extrinsic pathway.

Normal coagulation depends on the interaction of the coagulant proteins that exist in blood as proenzymes and three anticoagulant systems, the protein C-protein S system, the antithrombin III system, and the newly recognized tissue factor pathway inhibitor system, along with a fourth plasmin fibrinolytic system. Many functional and antigenic tests have been devised to assess the state of the coagulant systems. The sites of entry of the anticoagulant inhibitory systems and the fibrinolytic system and the sites of reagent activation or sampled products of many of the assays of coagulation are also shown in Figure 18-1; the descriptions of the tests of coagulation that follow refer to this figure.

Prothrombin Time

The prothrombin time is the time in seconds that it takes plasma to clot after the addition of thromboplastin (tissue factor). Therefore, it depends on the normal function of factor VII of the extrinsic pathway and the common pathway downstream to it. The prothrombin time can be prolonged by any disease

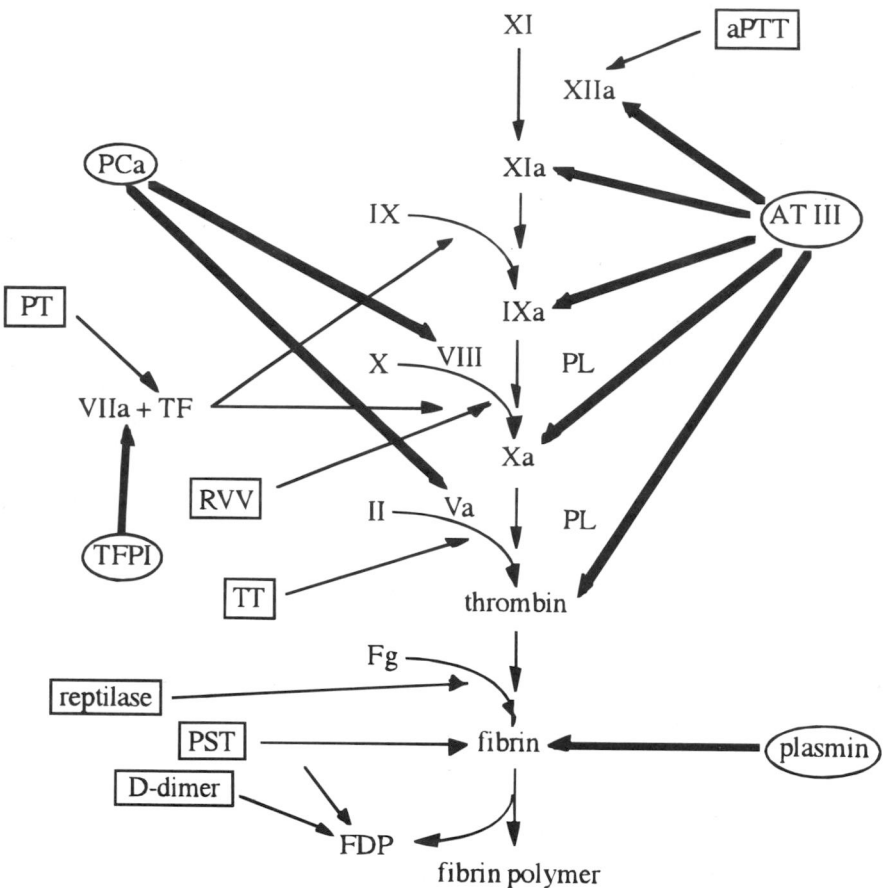

FIG. 18-1. The coagulation cascade, anticoagulant inhibitory systems, and tests of coagulation function. The interaction of the four anticoagulant systems are shown in ovals: antithrombin III (AT III), protein C and S system (PCa), tissue factor pathway inhibitor (TFPI), and plasmin. Some of the functional tests of coagulation are shown in rectangles: activated partial thromboplastin time (aPTT), prothrombin time (PT), thrombin time (TT), Russell's viper venom test (RVV), protamine sulfate test (PST), and D-dimer. PL, cellular phospholipid surface; II, prothrombin; Fg, fibrinogen; FDP, fibrin degradation products. (Modified from Nachman RL, Silverstein R: Hypercoagulable states. Ann Intern Med 120:520, 1994, with permission.)

or medication affecting these factors. Warfarin inhibits synthesis of the vitamin K-dependent factors II, VII, IX, and X. Three of these are necessary for proper function of the extrinsic and common pathways, and the prothrombin time is a sensitive assay of the intensity of anticoagulation by warfarin. Until recently, it had been customary to report the prothrombin time as a ratio of the patient's value and a control value: PT_p/PT_c. Recommendations for the desirable intensity of anticoagulation were published as prothrombin time ratios. In recent years, it has been suggested that the prothrombin time value be reported as a standardized ratio, that is, the international normalized ratio (INR). This value normalizes differences based on the variable sensitivities of lots of reagent thromboplastin. The INR is defined as

$$INR = (PT_p/PT_c)^{ISI}$$

where PT_p is the patient's prothrombin time in seconds, PT_c is the mean of a series of control values, and ISI is the international sensitivity index, a measure of the sensitivity (reactivity) of the thromboplastin used. The ISI is calculated by the manufacturer of the thromboplastin or the laboratory and is a property of the particular lot of thromboplastin. A thromboplastin with a sensitivity equal to that of the World Health Organization standard will have an ISI of 1 and hence will yield an INR equal to the prothrombin time ratio. With less sensitive thromboplastins

(higher ISI) the prothrombin time value for a given INR is lower, and the range of values is narrower; for more sensitive thromboplastins, the range of values for prothrombin time is wider, and subtler abnormalities of coagulation can be detected. An INR ≤ 1.4 suggests hemodynamically adequate levels of coagulation factors. Recent recommendations for the desirable intensity of anticoagulation in various clinical situations are discussed in Chapter 25 and in Part II.

Activated Partial Thromboplastin Time

The activated partial thromboplastin time (aPTT), usually called simply PTT, is the time in seconds that it takes plasma to clot after the addition of a contact agent that fully activates factors XII and XI along with calcium and phospholipid. These reagents activate factors XII and XI, and therefore the PTT depends on the normal function of these factors and the other factors of the intrinsic pathway. It can be prolonged by any disease or medication affecting these factors. It is more sensitive than the prothrombin time for the detection of acquired circulating anticoagulants, often called lupus anticoagulants (see below). It is also sensitive to the multiple level effects of heparin, and therefore is used as the functional assay of adequate heparinization. For most indications for which full heparinization is desirable, a PTT of 1.5 to 2.5 times the normal value is the therapeutic goal. Heparin therapy is discussed in Chapter 25.

It is widely accepted that hereditary and acquired dysfunction of these coagulation systems can cause thromboembolic disease, including strokes. Tests for the presence of hypercoagulability are now a part of the evaluation of stroke and other thrombotic events when the more common risk factors are absent. Abnormalities of two of the three anticoagulant systems, the protein C-protein S and antithrombin III systems, have been associated with thrombosis. The tissue factor pathway inhibitor system has not yet been reported to cause disease. Also, abnormalities of fibrinogen and the plasmin fibrinolytic system can rarely cause clinical thrombosis.

Protein C and Protein S

Protein C is a vitamin K-dependent serine protease, that is, one of a family of proteolytic enzymes with serine in the active site. Protein S is its vitamin K-dependent cofactor. The protein C-protein S complex inactivates factors Va and VIIIa. This probably prevents thrombus formation at the capillary level. Decreased levels or dysfunctional molecules with low enzymatic activity can cause hereditary hypercoagulable states. Also, many conditions can cause acquired deficiencies. Assays for antigenic levels and enzymatic activity exist for both proteins. Protein S can be measured in the free (active) and bound states. Because they are vitamin K-dependent, these proteins are depleted by warfarin. It is best to wait 1 to 2 weeks after warfarin therapy has been discontinued to measure them. If warfarin therapy cannot be stopped, the ratio of protein C antigen:prothrombin antigen can estimate the effective level.

Antithrombin III

Antithrombin III is a vitamin K-dependent serine protease inhibitor that irreversibly inactivates factors XIIa, XIa, IXa, Xa, and IIa (thrombin), all serine proteases. Heparin binds to antithrombin III, enhancing its natural anticoagulant effects. As with proteins C and S, decreased activity can result from hereditary decreased synthesis with low levels of a normal molecule or synthesis of a dysfunctional molecule, or it can be acquired due to loss of hepatic synthetic function. Antigenic and functional activity assays are available.

Fibrinogen

Elevated fibrinogen has been identified in the Framingham study as a risk factor for stroke in men, although because no treatment has yet been recommended in its presence, it has not been useful to measure fibrinogen levels routinely. Dysfibrinogenemia, synthesis of an abnormal fibrinogen molecule, is usually associated with pathologic hemorrhage; however, thrombosis rarely occurs. Fibrinogen function can be assayed with tests of the final steps of the coagulation cascade, the thrombin time and the reptilase clotting time. The thrombin time is the time in seconds that it takes for plasma to clot after the addition of thrombin. This tests the generation of a fibrin clot from the existing fibrinogen. Reptilase hydrolyzes fibrinogen to promote clotting directly. Both of these clotting times are prolonged in the presence of an abnormal fibrinogen. An antigenic assay for the fibrinogen level is also available.

The Plasmin Fibrinolytic System

Abnormal plasmin generation is a rare cause of hypercoagulability. These disorders can also be hereditary or acquired. Antigenic and functional assays are available in special circumstances; however, because these disorders are rare, screening is not routine.

The Antiphospholipid Antibody Syndrome

The presence of circulating antibodies to negatively charged phospholipids has been associated with pathologic thrombosis. The mechanism of thrombogenesis is unknown but probably a result of a reaction of the antibody with phospholipid of the endothelial cell or platelet membrane. Several tests are available to look for the presence of such antibodies. So far, their optimal use and interpretation have not been clarified. These antibodies were originally identified in patients with systemic lupus erythematosus and named lupus anticoagulants because of their effect in prolonging phospholipid-dependent coagulation times. Binding to phospholipid inhibits the generation of the thrombin activator complex, which is produced by the interaction of factors Xa and Va and phospholipid (Fig. 18-1). This may prolong the PTT and, less commonly, the prothrombin time. This prolongation is not corrected by the addition of normal plasma in mixing studies when a circulating anticoagulant is present. However, these routine tests are not sensitive indicators of a lupus anticoagulant. Russell's viper venom test and the kaolin clotting time depend on the direct activation of factor X. These are more sensitive screening tests for a lupus anticoagulant. Using these tests to define the lupus anticoagulant, the false-negative rate of the PTT is 22 to 33 percent. Therefore, one of these two tests is recommended to screen for lupus anticoagulants. Russell's viper venom test has been favored because it is simple, easy to perform, not influenced by inhibitors of factors VIII and IX, which can confound the interpretation of the kaolin clotting time, and does not require a confirmatory test (as does the kaolin clotting time). (The kaolin clotting time corrects with the addition of phospholipid but not normal plasma.) Refinements of the PTT and Russell's viper venom test that are more sensitive to the presence of lupus anticoagulants have been developed, and these have become the favored screening tests in many laboratories.

Antigenic tests for the presence of antibodies to cardiolipin are more sensitive and reproducible than tests for a lupus anticoagulant, and they allow for a quantitative assessment. An enzyme-linked immunosorbent assay (ELISA) for IgG (GPL) and IgM (MPL) anticardiolipin antibodies is available. Specificity for clinical disease, such as thrombosis, fetal loss, and thrombocytopenia, correlates with higher titers and with the presence of anticardiolipin of the IgG class. Harris and colleagues (1987) have recommended cutoff values for the interpretation of the clinical significance of anticardiolipin antibodies (Table 18-1). Most laboratories report this test as positive if values are at the lower end of the moderate positive range seen in Table 18-1. Harris and colleagues (1986) reported that predictive values for disease increase with increasing titers.

The tests for lupus anticoagulant and anticardiolipin are dis-

TABLE 18-1. The Clinical Significance of Anticardiolipin Titers

Antibody Class	Normal	Low Positive	Moderate Positive	High Positive
IgG (μg/ml)	≤5	6–14	15–80	>80
IgM (μg/ml), MPL (U/ml)	≤3	4–5	6–50	>50

(Adapted from Harris EN et al: Evaluation of the anticardiolipin antibody test: report of an international workshop held 4 April 1986. Clin Exp Immunol 68:215, 1987, with permission.)

cordant. Depending on the method used to test for the lupus anticoagulant, it detects 50 to 94 percent of those with anticardiolipin by ELISA. A positive anticardiolipin test detects 70 to 80 percent of those with a lupus anticoagulant by a sensitive assay. Because of this discordance, and because it remains unclear which test best correlates with disease, it is recommended that in the appropriate clinical setting, screening be done with both the ELISA for anticardiolipin and a sensitive test for lupus anticoagulants, such as the Russell viper venom test. A positive anticardiolipin value can then be quantitated to estimate the risk of thrombosis (Table 18-1).

Disseminated Intravascular Coagulation

Disseminated intravascular coagulation (DIC) can be an acute and fulminant process, usually accompanied by hemorrhage or a subtle subacute or chronic process that can lead to hemorrhage or pathologic thrombosis. Therefore, screening tests for DIC are sometimes an appropriate part of the evaluation of thromboembolic disease. A battery of tests is available to assay the several steps in this coagulopathy. Consumption of fibrinogen, thrombin, and coagulation factors higher up in the clotting cascade leads to a fall in the fibrinogen level and a prolongation of the clotting times—partial thromboplastin, prothrombin, and thrombin times. If the fibrinogen was high at the start, it may remain in the normal range. Consumption of platelets results in a fall in the platelet count and prolongation of the bleeding time. Intravascular fibrin deposition in the small vessels causes a microangiopathic hemolytic anemia, which is detected by a fall in the hemoglobin and hematocrit and schizocytes on a peripheral blood smear. If thrombosis and fibrinolysis are activated, fibrin monomer and fibrin degradation products are formed. Fibrin degradation products can be quantitated and are usually greater than 40 µg/ml in DIC. The serial dilution protamine sulfate test detects fibrin monomer and fibrin degradation products. Protamine sulfate causes the dissociation of soluble complexes of fibrin monomer and fibrin degradation products. Since these complexes prevent polymerization, this dissociation by protamine sulfate allows polymerization to proceed. A positive test means that fibrin monomer and fibrin degradation products are present and that fibrinogen and fibrinolysis have been activated. The protamine sulfate test is a sensitive, though nonspecific, test of DIC.

IMMUNOLOGIC MARKERS OF DISEASE

Many neurologic diseases have an established or presumed autoimmune etiology. These include many inflammatory medical diseases with neurologic complications, many neuropathies, myasthenia gravis, and many paraneoplastic syndromes. Many of these autoantibodies are useful in clinical diagnosis. Further discussions of most of the tests described in this section are found in later chapters discussing the diseases with which they are associated.

Autoantibodies in Rheumatic Disease

Rheumatic disease enters into the differential diagnosis of several neurologic disorders, including neuropathies, sensory neuronopathy, myositis, aseptic meningitis, and stroke. Autoantibodies are never diagnostic; however, in the appropriate clinical

TABLE 18-2. Some Autoantibodies in Immunologically Mediated Diseases With Neurologic Complications

Antigen	Clinical Significance
Rheumatoid factors	Nonspecific, sensitive for RA and Sjögren syndrome
ANA	Nonspecific
ds DNA, peripheral pattern	Specific for SLE, active renal disease
ss DNA, peripheral pattern	Nonspecific, very sensitive for SLE
Antihistone, homogeneous	In SLE and drug-induced LE; if present alone, suggestive of drug-induced LE
Sm, speckled	Specific for SLE, renal and CNS disease
RNP, speckled	Nonspecific: PM with MCTD, SLE, Sjögren syndrome, scleroderma
Jo-1	PM with interstitial lung disease
PM-Scl	PM with scleroderma
Ro (SSA)	SLE, Sjögren syndrome
La (SSB)	Primary Sjögren syndrome, if no other autoantibodies are present
cANCA	Vasculitis from Wegener's granulomatosis or microscopic periarteritis
pANCA	Glomerulonephritis; also classic PAN and other vasculitides and rheumatic diseases

Abbreviations: RA, rheumatoid arthritis; ANA, antinuclear antibodies; SLE, systemic lupus erythematosus; LE, lupus erythematosus; CNS, central nervous system; RNP, ribonuclear protein; PM, polymyositis; MCTD, mixed connective tissue disease; cANCA, antineutrophilic cytoplasmic antibodies, cytoplasmic pattern; pANCA, perinuclear pattern; PAN, polyarteritis nodosa.

(Adapted from Condemi JJ: Autoimmune diseases. JAMA 268:2883, 1992, with permission.)

context, they can support the diagnosis of an underlying rheumatic disease (Table 18-2).

Rheumatoid Factors.   The routinely used rheumatoid factor tests for the presence of IgM antibodies to certain immunoglobulins. This test is about 90 percent sensitive for typical rheumatoid arthritis. It is, however, nonspecific and can be positive in many other rheumatic and nonrheumatic diseases, many of which cause neurologic disease, including systemic lupus erythematosus (SLE), dermatomyositis, Sjögren syndrome, sarcoidosis, and endocarditis. Ninety percent of patients with Sjögren syndrome have rheumatoid factors.

Antinuclear Antibodies.   Over 90 percent of patients with SLE will have high titers of antinuclear antibodies (ANA). These, too, are nonspecific. The pattern of nuclear immunofluorescent staining can add specificity. A peripheral staining pattern is specific for active SLE. Diffuse and speckled patterns are nonspecific. Antibodies to certain nuclear antigens are more specific for SLE. These include antibodies to double-stranded DNA and anti-Sm. Antibodies to the antigens Ro (also called SSA) and La (also called SSB) and single-stranded DNA are nonspecific; they are present in most patients with clinical SLE and a negative ANA screen. Antihistone antibodies also appear in lupus and, when found alone, suggest that it is drug-induced.

A positive ANA is found in about 70 percent of patients with Sjögren syndrome. The staining pattern is usually diffuse or speckled. Antibodies to the small nuclear ribonuclear proteins Ro and La are often seen as well, although they are nonspecific as noted above. The presence of isolated anti-La antibodies suggests primary Sjögren syndrome.

Mixed connective tissue disease enters into the diagnosis of neuropathies, myositis, and aseptic meningitis. High titers of antibodies to ribonuclear protein (also called extractable nuclear antigens because they are soluble in aqueous buffers) are characteristic of this disease, although they too are nonspecific.

Polymyositis can occur in association with various rheumatic diseases. Characteristic antinuclear antibodies may accompany these different syndromes. As noted above, ribonuclear protein is found in polymyositis with mixed connective tissue disease. Autoantibodies to Jo-1 accompany polymyositis in interstitial lung disease. Autoantibodies to PM-Scl, a nucleolar antigen, accompany polymyositis in scleroderma.

Autoantibodies in Systemic Vasculitis: Antineutrophilic Cytoplasmic Antibodies

Antineutrophilic cytoplasmic antibodies (ANCA) bind with enzymes within granules of polymorphonuclear leukocytes. Two patterns can be detected by immunofluorescent staining; a cytoplasmic pattern detected by ELISA and a perinuclear pattern detected by indirect immnofluorescence. The cytoplasmic pattern has a high sensitivity and specificity for certain types of systemic vasculitis, Wegener's granulomatosis, and microscopic periarteritis. The perinuclear pattern is most commonly found in crescentic necrotizing glomerulonephritis, but it can be seen with low sensitivity and specificity in other inflammatory diseases, such as classic periarteritis nodosa and other systemic vasculitides, rheumatoid arthritis, SLE, inflammatory bowel disease, and chronic liver disease.

Autoantibodies in Myasthenia Gravis

Acetylcholine Receptor Antibodies. Antibodies to the nicotinic acetylcholine (ACh) receptor are detected by Western blot analysis. They are found on the order of 75 to 95 percent of the time in patients with acquired generalized myasthenia gravis with only rare false positives reported. The sensitivity is reduced to about 50 to 70 percent in myasthenia gravis limited to the ocular muscles. These antibodies have been implicated in the pathogenesis of myasthenia gravis to establish it convincingly as an autoimmune disease. In the appropriate clinical setting, a positive test can corroborate the diagnosis of adult and neonatal myasthenia gravis. The levels of these autoantibodies do not, however, correlate with disease activity in populations, although there may be a correlation in a given case. These autoantibodies are also found in cases of drug-induced myasthenia. They are not present in congenital myasthenia.

Antistriated Muscle Antibodies. In patients with myasthenia gravis, the presence of antibodies to striated muscle suggests that the patient harbors a thymoma.

Autoantibodies in Paraneoplastic Syndromes

Several paraneoplastic neurologic syndromes have been associated with specific autoantibodies (Table 18.3). Although these

TABLE 18-3. Autoantibodies in Paraneoplastic Neurologic Syndromes

Antigen	Clinical Syndrome	Tumor Types
Yo	Subacute cerebellar degeneration	Ovarian, breast, other gynecologic cancers
Hu	Subacute sensory neuronopathy, limbic and brainstem encephalitis, subacute cerebellar degeneration	Small cell lung cancer
Ri	Opsoclonus in adults	Breast cancer
CAR	Retinal degeneration	Small cell lung cancer
VGCC	Lambert-Eaton myasthenic syndrome	Small cell lung cancer
MAG	Paraproteinemia with indolent sensory-motor neuropathy	MGUS

Abbreviations: CAR, cancer-associated retinopathy; VGCC, voltage-gated calcium channels; MAG, myelin-associated glycoprotein; MGUS, monoclonal gammopathy of undetermined significance.

autoantibodies have not been as clearly implicated in the pathogenesis of the neurologic syndrome as have ACh receptor antibodies in myasthenia gravis, when present they can help to direct the physician to the appropriate search for underlying tumors, and they can provide evidence that a given syndrome is, in fact, a remote effect of cancer.

Anti-Yo Antibodies. Anti-Yo antibodies react with an antigen found in the cytoplasm of cerebellar Purkinje cells. A subset of patients with paraneoplastic subacute cerebellar degeneration have these antibodies in the serum and cerebrospinal fluid (CSF). Almost all patients with subacute cerebellar degeneration and a high titer of anti-Yo antibodies have been women with ovarian, breast, or other gynecologic malignancies. Only rare cases of other malignancies have been reported, including a lung cancer and a lymphoma. Patients with the syndrome of subacute cerebellar degeneration without anti-Yo antibodies are most likely to have lung cancer, especially small cell cancer, or Hodgkin's disease. Rarely, other cancers, such as lymphomas, have been identified, or no tumor has been found. Therefore, the presence of these antibodies should prompt a careful search for an underlying gynecologic malignancy. Tumor diagnosis may be delayed until long after the onset of the neurologic syndrome.

Anti-Hu Antibodies. Anti-Hu antibodies react with an antigen found in neuronal nuclei. Most patients with these antibodies in serum or CSF have been found to harbor a small cell cancer. Rarely other tumors have been found: prostate carcinoma, neuroblastoma, and chondromyxosarcoma. Tumor diagnosis may be delayed, and, rarely, no tumor has been found. Several neurologic syndromes may accompany these antibodies. The major associated syndromes include subacute sensory neuronopathy; paraneoplastic encephalomyelitis, including limbic encephalitis, brainstem encephalitis, and myelitis; and cerebellar degeneration with loss of Purkinje cells (anti-Yo negative). The presence of these antibodies in the context of these neurologic syndromes should prompt a careful search for a small cell carcinoma or other less common tumor. High titers of them in a patient with known small cell carcinoma support the paraneoplastic etiology of the neurologic findings. Low titers are found in about 16 percent of all patients with small cell carcinoma.

Anti-Ri Antibodies. Anti-Ri antibodies also react with a neuronal nuclear antigen. These antibodies are found in high titers in the serum and CSF of patients with paraneoplastic opsoclonus associated with breast cancer. They have not been found in childhood opsoclonus-myoclonus with or without neuroblastoma nor in breast cancer without opsoclonus. Their presence should stimulate a search for an underlying breast tumor. The clinical usefulness of this autoantibody is less well established than that of anti-Yo and anti-Hu.

Cancer-Associated Retinopathy Antibodies. The cancer-associated retinopathy antigen and possibly other ocular antigens are the target of autoantibodies of cancer-associated retinopathy. High titers of these antibodies have been associated with paraneoplastic retinal degeneration. This syndrome is rare. Most patients have had small cell lung cancer. Other associated cancers include those of the breast, prostate, colon, and cervix.

Anti-Voltage-Gated Calcium Channels. Autoantibodies to voltage-gated calcium channels at nerve terminals have been found in some patients with small cell lung cancer, some of whom had the Lambert-Eaton myasthenic syndrome. About 50 to 60 percent of patients with Lambert-Eaton myasthenic syndrome whether with or without cancer, have been found to have such antibodies in their serum. This strongly suggests an autoimmune etiology for this syndrome, however, the clinical significance of these antibodies has not yet been defined, and no commercially available test for them exists.

Antibodies to Myelin-Associated Glycoprotein. Several different syndromes of neuroradiculopathy accompany monoclonal paraproteinemias. About one-fourth to one-half of the patients with an IgM monoclonal spike on serum protein electrophoresis have serum antibodies to myelin-associated glycoprotein (MAG), a glycoprotein that participates in myelin interactions with the axon. Usually these monoclonal IgM proteins have kappa light chains; however, occasionally IgM-lambda immunoglobulins are found with similar anti-MAG activity. These patients typically have a demyelinating sensorimotor neuropathy with indolent progression and elevated CSF protein. Although it has not been shown that these antibodies are responsible for the neuropathy, treatment that lowers the M protein may be effective.

Autoantibodies in Other Diseases

Anti-GM₁ Ganglioside Antibodies. Gangliosides are macromolecules made up of an oligosaccharide with at least one acid sugar associated with the lipid ceramide. They are widely distributed in the membranes of the central and peripheral nervous system tissues. Anti-GM_1 ganglioside antibodies have been found in the serum of some patients with a lower motor neuron syndrome that resembles amyotrophic lateral sclerosis (ALS). This syndrome is more common in males and is characterized by lower motor neuron dysfunction, typically without upper motor neuron signs, with less atrophy than in anterior horn cell disease, and with a more prolonged course, multifocal motor conduction block, and high titers of anti-GM_1 ganglioside antibodies. It has been called multifocal motor neuropathy with conduction block. An ELISA is available, and serum titers above 1:350 are considered specific for the syndrome. Typically they are much higher. Low titers, 1:300 or less, are nonspecific and may be found with central nervous system (CNS) damage from, for instance, multiple sclerosis and ALS. Multifocal motor neuropathy with conduction block has been successfully treated with cyclophosphamide. Since it cannot be reliably distinguished by the clinical examination from lower motor neuron forms of motor system disease, nerve conduction studies and assays of GM_1 ganglioside antibodies have been useful to define it. Successful treatment usually results in a fall in antibody titers, so the antibody test has also been used to follow the response to treatment. Other anti-ganglioside antibodies have been identified, but their assays have not yet found clinical use.

Antibodies to Glutamic Acid Decarboxylase. Glutamic acid decarboxylase is the enzyme that catalyzes the formation of gamma-aminobutyric acid (GABA) from glutamic acid. GABA is a major inhibitory neurotransmitter in the CNS, and glutamic acid decarboxylase is present in high concentrations in the terminals of GABAergic neurons. Antibodies to glutamic acid decarboxylase have been found in the serum and CSF of about 60 percent of patients with the stiff-man syndrome. They have also been found in some patients with insulin-dependent diabetes, a disease with a probable autoimmune mechanism that may co-occur with it. It has been hypothesized that an autoimmune attack on GABAergic neurons causes the stiff-man syndrome. Although this hypothesis remains to be proven, these autoantibodies have been used along with clinical and electrophysiologic findings as a possible marker for the syndrome.

TESTS OF INFECTION

Bacterial cultures and viral isolation from CSF, blood, and other tissues and fluids will be used to diagnose many infectious neurologic diseases. Titers of specific antiviral immunoglobulins can also be used to indicate past infection (IgG) or recent infection (IgM or four fold or higher rise of IgG titers from acute to convalescent specimens drawn 4 to 6 weeks apart). In many cases, however, the diagnosis is not easily made by culture or viral isolation. This section discusses some of the other tests used to diagnose neurologic infections.

Antigen Detection

Bacterial meningitis can usually be diagnosed by Gram stain and culture of CSF and blood. At times, especially when patients present having already received antibiotics, all stains and cultures will be negative. Latex agglutination has largely replaced counterimmunoelectrophoresis to identify the antigens of many of the more common organisms that cause meningitis. Tests are available for *Haemophilus influenzae, Streptococcus pneumoniae, Neisseria meningitidis,* group B streptococci, and *Cryptococcus neoformans*. These tests have sensitivities in the 80 to 100 percent range, although reports vary, and one study of the meningococcal latex agglutination test found it to be only 33 percent sensitive. The cryptococcal antigen is widely used for diagnosis and to follow the response to treatment. It is about 95 percent sensitive. False positives occur rarely.

Polymerase Chain Reaction

With the proper primers, a heat-resistant DNA polymerase, and a process of repeated heating and cooling to denature and rehybridize DNA, minute quantities of DNA can be amplified and detected in tissues. RNA can be similarly detected after synthesis of a complementary DNA (cDNA) using reverse transcriptase. This technique has been developed into a sensitive and specific clinical test for a few pathogens, including herpes simplex virus, *Mycobacterium tuberculosis,* cytomegalovirus, and *Borrelia burgdorferi*. Other viral assays are being developed: enteroviruses, varicella-zoster virus, Epstein-Barr virus, JC virus, HIV. Polymerase chain reaction for herpes simplex virus is very sensitive when specimens are collected early in the infection; however, the sensitivity falls off significantly in the days after presentation. Specificity for active CNS disease is good. Herpes simplex virus DNA is not found in the CSF of patients with latent herpes simplex virus infection but no CNS disease or non-herpes simplex virus neurologic disease.

Serology for Syphilis

The VDRL (Venereal Disease Research Laboratories) test is a flocculation test that detects antibodies produced by treponemal infection. These antibodies, called reagins, are produced upon the invasion of host tissues. The rapid plasma reagin (RPR) test is a refinement of the VDRL. It uses purified cardiolipin-lecithin-cholesterol antigen to detect the anticardiolipin antibodies produced by treponemal infection. It is more sensitive than the VDRL. The advantage of the VDRL is that it can be quantitated and its titer reflects disease activity. After treatment, the titer usually falls, and the test becomes nonreactive over 6 to 12 months. Occasionally, a positive serum reaction of low titer (1:1, 1:2, or slightly greater) persists after successful treatment. The VDRL can also be used to assay CSF. The CSF VDRL is very specific. Although false positive tests can occur with contamination of the CSF with reactive blood or with CSF paraproteinemias and autoimmune disease, such false positives are rare. The sensitivity of the CSF VDRL is, however, reported to be low. False-negative rates of up to 60 to 63 percent have been reported. Although this estimate may be too high, and false-negative rates as low as 6 percent have been reported, with current data it remains unreliable as a final criterion for the diagnosis of neurosyphilis.

All positive nontreponemal tests should be confirmed by a serum treponemal test to eliminate false positive serologies. Treponemal tests assay directly for antibodies to treponemal antigens. The two most commonly used tests are the fluorescent treponemal antibody-absorption (FTA-ABS) and the microhemagglutination assay for *Treponema pallidum* (MHA-TP). These tests use antigens to nonpathogenic treponemes to "absorb" the nonspecific treponemal group antigens. With the serum free of these antigens, the tests detect the presence of specific serum antibodies by their reaction with *T. pallidum*. These tests are more sensitive and specific for syphilis than the nontreponemal tests. The reaction does not vary with treatment and once reactive will remain so indefinitely. To increase its postive predictive value, it is best used as a confirmatory test when the reagin test is reactive. Most authors do not recommend the use of the treponemal tests on CSF because they are so sensitive that the passive diffusion of tiny amounts of blood into the CSF will cause a false-positive reaction.

There is no clear consensus for the best approach to the diagnosis of neurosyphilis. Minimal findings should probably include (1) a reactive serum treponemal test and (2) an abnormal CSF (>5 WBC/mm^3 or protein >45). Yet with neither a positive CSF VDRL nor clinical disease consistent with neurosyphilis, the diagnosis must be questioned.

Serologic Tests for Lyme Disease

Culture of *B. burgdorferi* is difficult and not useful for routine diagnosis of Lyme disease. Diagnosis has therefore depended on the presence of positive serologic tests in the appropriate clinical setting. Screening is usually done with ELISA for IgG, but the humoral response is delayed, so that the sensitivity is poor in the first few weeks of infection. EIA antibody capture assays are also available for IgM (and IgA), which may increase the sensitivity in early disease. Because of cross-reactivity with other antigens, the false-positive rate for these serolgic tests is high in the presence of many other inflammatory diseases. Western blotting has been used to confirm the diagnosis of Lyme disease in indeterminate cases. Dressler and associates (1993) have proposed criteria for positive Western blots based on the presence of characteristic bands: two of the common IgM bands in early Lyme disease and five of the common IgG bands after the first few weeks. Their sensitivity and specificity data are shown in Table 18-4. Polymerase chain reaction for *B. burgdorferi* has been introduced as a test with high sensitivity and specificity; however, its use with the other diagnostic tests for Lyme disease has not yet been well defined. For all of the

TABLE 18-4. Sensitivity and Specificity of Serologic Tests for Lyme Disease

	Sensitivity (%)	Specificity (%)
Early Lyme disease		
IgM ELISA	40	94
IgM Western blot	32	100
Lyme disease after first weeks		
IgG ELISA	89	72
IgG Western blot	83	95

Positive ELISA results include "indeterminate" cases (1:200 to 1:400).

(Adapted from Dressler F, Whalen JA, Reinhardt BN, Steere AC: Western blotting in the serodiagnosis of Lyme disease. J Infect Dis 167:398, 1993, with permission.)

serologic tests and for polymerase chain reaction, it is important to remember that positive tests may persist long after successful treatment, and they alone are not indications of active infection.

CEREBROSPINAL FLUID ANALYSIS

CSF analysis provides important information for diagnosis in many neurologic diseases. The lumbar puncture is safe and quickly and easily performed in most patients. The exceptions to this constitute the absolute or relative contraindications to lumbar puncture: patients with local infection at the puncture site, those with brain masses or masses involving the spinal cord above the puncture site, and those with bleeding diatheses or on anticoagulant therapy. When the physician cannot successfully reach the subarachnoid space using the usual technique, fluoroscopy can visually guide the insertion of the spinal needle. In cases where CSF must be obtained above a spinal mass or infection, the neurosurgeon or neurologist can achieve this by lateral C1-C2 puncture. In many cases of bleeding diatheses, an infusion of coagulation factors, such as fresh frozen plasma, cryoprecipitate, platelets, or a specific factor can precede the procedure to allow sampling. In some cases, CSF is obtained upon the placement of an intracranial pressure monitor or ventricular catheter for monitoring or therapy.

Normal CSF is clear and colorless. The normal pressure in the lumbar subarachnoid space with the patient relaxed in the decubitus position is 50 to 200 mm CSF (4 to 15 mmHg). With normal CSF flow, the pressure decreases with inspiration and increases with expiration and jugular compression (Queckenstedt test).

Pigments

The CSF can be colored by pigments that are the products of hemoglobin breakdown after its release from lysed erythrocytes (RBCs). Initially, oxyhemoglobin can be detected as a pink or orange pigment. Bilirubin stains the CSF yellow. It may not be detectable for up to 12 hours after the release of RBCs into the CSF. Eventually, methemoglobin may stain the fluid dark yellow or brown. The presence of such pigments is one cause of xanthochromia. Xanthochromia can be detected by visual inspection or, with greater sensitivity, by spectrophotometry. Clinically, xanthochromia is primarily of interest in distinguishing subarachnoid hemorrhage from blood introduced into the CSF by minor trauma during the lumbar puncture (traumatic tap). In a study of serial samples of CSF in patients with well-established diagnoses of subarachnoid hemorrhage, Vermeulen and coworkers (1989) found that with spectrophotometric analysis, all of these patients had xanthochromia after 12 hours, which persisted for 2 weeks. Many, and perhaps most, patients will have xanthochromia before 12 hours have elapsed, however, earlier samples have not been reported in systematic studies. Based on these data, the authors recommend that lumbar puncture be delayed for 12 hours after subarachnoid hemorrhage to avoid the scenario of the uninterpretable tap without xanthochromia. Although the spectrophotometric analysis of xanthochromia is very sensitive under these conditions of delay, it is less specific, and traumatic puncture can be accompanied by xanthochromia. The issue is important because other techniques traditionally used to differentiate these two diagnoses are known to be unreliable:

1. *Declining RBC counts.* It is customary to establish the RBC count in an early and a late collection tube. If this results in a normal later tube, then it reliably indicates a traumatic tap. However, a fall to a significant, though smaller, number of RBCs is not reliable and can occur in subarachnoid hemorrhage.
2. *Clotting of CSF blood.* Blood introduced by a traumatic tap may clot within minutes, unlike the defibrinogenated blood after subarachnoid hemorrhage. However, this test is reliable only when large numbers of RBCs are present.
3. *Crenation of RBCs.* Crenation of normal RBCs occurs by an osmotic loss of water. Although the presence of crenated RBCs has been suggested as an indication of true subarachnoid hemorrhage, crenation can occur early, and this test is not reliable.
4. *Erythrophages.* Erythrophages, which are macrophages that have engulfed RBCs, reliably attest to the presence of blood that has been in the CSF too long to be compatible with a traumatic tap unless an earlier lumbar puncture was performed, introducing RBCs. However, their detection requires cytology, and they are rarely seen. Therefore, this test is too slow and insensitive to be of practical use.

A newer test, the D-dimer assay, may prove to be both sensitive and specific for old blood in the CSF. In a small study by Lang and colleagues (1990) 6/6 patients with subarachnoid hemor-

rhage had positive tests, and there were no false positives among 14 traumatic taps and 20 normal controls. Further study of this test will decide its clinical reliability. Causes of xanthochromia other than pigments include the following:

1. Jaundice
2. CSF protein greater than 150 mg/dl
3. Certain drugs, such as rifampin
4. Carotenoids in food faddists taking large doses
5. Melanin in meningeal melanomatosis
6. Contamination with the cleansing iodine solution

Cell Counts

CSF samples should be refrigerated and promptly analyzed to avoid systematic errors in cell counts. This is a real problem that must be circumvented in large hospitals where specimens are transported by messengers and often sit for long periods before analysis. Leukocytes (WBCs) begin to lyse within 1 hour of collection at room temperature. Most authors consider 5 or less mononuclear cells/mm^3 to be normal. In adults, more than 10 cells is clearly abnormal. In the case of a traumatic tap, the WBC differential count should be approximately proportional to the peripheral WBC differential count. A rough calculation will allow for one WBC per 500 to 1,500 RBCs; however, this calculation is very error-prone, and clinical judgment must enter into it. In normal CSF, virtually all WBCs are mononuclear, mostly T lymphocytes. In inflammatory diseases, polymorphonuclear leukocytes and lymphocytes (again mainly T cells) will rise. A predominance of polymorphonuclear cells suggests bacterial infection, early viral infection, or occasionally other infections, chemical meningitis, tumor, or infarction. Chronic infections, viral infections after the early phase, and noninfectious inflammatory disorders usually cause a rise in T lymphocytes. In leptomeningeal lymphoma, the lymphocytes are typically monoclonal B cells. Therefore monoclonal antibody staining can help to differentiate lymphoma from inflammation. The

TABLE 18-5. Cerebrospinal Fluid Findings in Meningitis

Etiology	Cell Counts (cells/mm^3)	Glucose (mg/dl)	Protein (mg/dl)	Comments
Normal	≤5	45–80	20–45	
Bacterial	>200 cells (most >1,000); PMN predominance	Low	>100	Gram stain; latex agglutination; culture
Viral	Fewer; usually 5 to several hundred; lymph predominance	Normal	<100	May have PMNs early, esp. HSV, mumps, LCM; these organisms may also cause low glucose and protein up to about 200; PCR for HSV and CMV
Tuberculosis	<500; lymphs	Low	100–500	Glucose is almost always low; AFB; PCR
Fungal	Increased	Low	>100	May have PMN predominance; glucose is almost always low; with immune compromise as in AIDS, the formula may be normal; cryptococcal Ag
Syphilis	Increased	Normal or low	Normal or mildly high	About ¼ have low glucose when active
Parameningeal	Increased	Normal or low	Variable	About 10% have low glucose
Neoplastic	Lymphocytes; neoplastic cells	Low	High	Cytology; monoclonal antibodies typing
SAH	RBCs; may have increased WBCs	Low	Varies with RBC count	Early WBC proportional to blood count; later WBC proportion rises with meningeal inflammation
Sarcoidosis	<100	Normal or low	High	About ½ have low glucose; ACE has low sensitivity and specificity

Abbreviations: PMN, polymorphonuclear leukocytes; HSV, herpes simplex virus; LCM, lymphocytic choriomeningitis; PCR, polymerase chain reaction; CMV, cytomegalovirus; AFB, acid fast bacillus stain; SAH, subarachnoid hemorrhage; RBCs, red blood cells; WBCs, white blood cells; ACE, angiotensin-converting enzyme activity.

numbers of cells can vary greatly, so only rough guidelines can be suggested for differential diagnosis based on cell counts (Table 18-5).

Cytopathology

Cytopathologic evaluation is useful to diagnose leptomeningeal or ependymal malignancy, usually carcinoma or lymphoma. This test is specific but insensitive. To optimize the sensitivity, a large volume of fluid should be sent, and it should be processed immediately to avoid cell lysis or loss of characteristic morphologic features. In suspected cases, sometimes multiple samples must be analyzed before a diagnosis is confirmed. As noted above, because lymphomas usually produce monoclonal B cells, monoclonal antibody staining can help differentiate malignant from inflammatory lymphocytes when morphology does not.

Glucose

Glucose enters the CSF by facilitated diffusion across endothelial cells mediated by a specific transporter. The CSF level depends on the serum level during the prior 4 hours or so and the rate of metabolism of glucose within the CSF. Therefore, a serum glucose level drawn within a few hours before the lumbar puncture should accompany any CSF sampling. When taken from the lumbar subarachnoid space, the normal CSF glucose is about 65 percent of the serum level. This ratio increases as sampling moves rostrally. When the serum glucose rises in diabetes mellitus, the CSF to serum ratio of glucose can fall to as low as 31 percent. In disease, the CSF glucose can be low as a result of increased metabolism by WBCs or brain or as a result of decreased entry of glucose following from transporter inhibition. A low value always indicates some diffuse meningeal process. With a normal serum glucose, a CSF value of less than 50 percent of the serum value or less than 45 mg/dl usually indicates disease. Many infections, subarachnoid hemorrhage, chemical meningitis, noninfectious inflammatory diseases, and leptomeningeal malignancy can all lower the glucose level. Typically, the level is normal in viral infections, except herpes simplex virus, varicella-zoster virus, and mumps. Therefore, the glucose value is used clinically to help to differentiate viral and bacterial meningitis (Table 18-5). Certain diseases characteristically cause a low CSF glucose. These include tuberculosis, fungal meningitis, carcinomatous meningitis, and

TABLE 18-6. Some Causes of Elevated Cerebrospinal Fluid Protein

Infections
　　meningitis, tuberculosis, syphilis, HIV, abscess of brain and epidural space.
Tumor
　　brain tumor, meningeal carcinoma or leukemia, neurofibroma, paraneoplastic syndromes of the nervous system
Central demyelination
　　multiple sclerosis, acute demyelinating encephalomyelitis
Polyneuropathy
　　Guillain-Barré syndrome, chronic inflammatory demyelinating neuropathy, diabetic polyneuropathy
Cerebrovascular disease
　　infarction, hemorrhage
Metabolic disease
　　hypothyroidism, uremia, diabetes mellitus with polyneuropathy
Degenerative diseases of the nervous system
Miscellaneous
　　CNS trauma, spinal subarachnoid block, arachnoiditis, noninfectious inflammatory disorders of the brain and meninges

(Data from Fishman RA: Cerebrospinal Fluid in Diseases of the Nervous System. 2nd Ed. p. 199. WP Saunders, Philadelphia, 1992.)

TABLE 18-7. Some Causes of Low Cerebrospinal Fluid Protein

Children less than 2 years
After removal of large volumes of lumbar cerebrospinal fluid
Cerebrospinal fluid leak
Benign intracranial hypertension
Water intoxication with increased intracranial pressure
Hyperthyroidism
Leukemia

(Data from Fishman RA: Cerebrospinal Fluid in Diseases of the Nervous System. 2nd Ed. p. 201. WP Saunders, Philadelphia, 1992.)

subarachnoid hemorrhage. In a significant proportion of cases of active neurosyphilis and parameningeal infection, the glucose will also be low.

Protein

Most CSF proteins are derived from the serum. A small fraction of them are synthesized in the CNS. Proteins exit by passing into the venous sinuses via the arachnoid villi. There is a rostral-caudal gradient of CSF protein concentration. In adults, approximate normal levels are 20 to 45 mg/dl in the lumbar subarachnoid space, 15 to 25 mg/dl in the cisterna magna, and 6 to 15 mg/dl in the ventricles. The total protein level is elevated in many diseases. Bacterial meningitis typically elevates the protein significantly, while viral meningitis usually does not; therefore this also is used to differentiate these two diseases before culture information is available (Table 18-5). Mild to moderate elevations are common and nonspecific (Table 18-6). Great elevations (above 500 mg/dl) usually indicate spinal subarachnoid block, meningitis, arachnoiditis, or subarachnoid hemorrhage. The Froin syndrome is a coagulation of CSF that occurs with elevations usually greater than 1,000 mg/dl as is seen in spinal subarachnoid block. Low CSF protein values may be seen in a few diseases (Table 18-7).

Diseases that cause intrathecal synthesis of gamma-globulin may cause an elevation of gamma-globulin, IgG index, and oligoclonal bands. Normal CSF IgG is 5 to 12 percent of the total CSF protein. The IgG index can be used to identify intrathecal synthesis:

$$\text{IgG index} = \frac{\text{IgG}_{CSF}/\text{IgG}_{serum}}{\text{alb}_{CSF}/\text{alb}_{serum}}$$

The normal IgG index is 0.85 or less. A small volume of contaminating serum, as in a traumatic tap, can falsely elevate the IgG index. This requires about 0.2 percent serum or enough to allow 5,000 to 10,000 RBCs/mm^3. Oligoclonal bands are spikes of two or more clonal expansions of immunoglobulin found on CSF protein electrophoresis. Their presence suggests an immune-mediated CNS process. They are most commonly sought to give laboratory support to a diagnosis of multiple sclerosis. In definite multiple sclerosis, they are said to be present 83 to 94 percent of the time. The sensitivity is much lower when patients with probable and possible multiple sclerosis are included. Other diseases that result in intrathecal synthesis of immunoglobulin can cause oligoclonal bands. Almost all patients with SSPE have them. Many other CNS infections can cause them, including progressive rubella encephalitis, herpes simplex virus and other encephalitides, neurosyphilis, Lyme disease, and bacterial and viral meningitis.

SUGGESTED READINGS

Condemi JJ: Autoimmune diseases. JAMA 268:2883, 1992
Coull BM, Levine SR, Brey RL: The role of antiphospholipid antibodies in stroke. Neurol Clin 10:125, 1992

Dalman J, Graus F, Rosenblum MK et al: Anti-Hu-associated paraneoplastic encephalomyelitis/sensory neuronopathy: a clinical study of 71 patients. Medicine 71:59, 1992

Dressler F, Whalen JA, Reinhardt BN, Steere AC: Western blotting in the serodiagnosis of Lyme disease. J Infect Dis 167:392, 1993

Fishman RA: Cerebrospinal Fluid in Diseases of the Nervous System. 2nd Ed. WS Saunders, Philadelphia, 1992

Hagen EC, Ballieux BEPB, van Es LA et al: Antineutrophilic cytoplasmic autoantibodies: a review of the antigens involved, the assays, and the clinical and possible pathogenetic consequences. Blood 81:1996, 1993

Harris EN, Chan JKH, Asherson RA: Thrombosis, recurrent fetal loss, and thrombocytopenia: predictive value of the anticardiolipin antibody test. Arch Intern Med 146:2153, 1986

Harris EN, Gharavi AE, Patel SP, Hughes GRV: Evaluation of the anticardiolipin antibody test: report of an international workshop held 4 April 1986. Clin Exp Immunol 68:215, 1987

Herndon RM, Brumback RA: The Cerebrospinal Fluid. Kluwer Academic, Boston, 1989

Jordan KG: Modern neurosyphilis: a critical analysis. West J Med 149:47, 1988

Lang DT, Berberian LB, Lee S et al: Rapid differentiation of subarachnoid hemorrhage from traumatic lumbar puncture using the D-dimer assay. Am J Clin Pathol 93:403, 1990

Nachman RL, Silverstein R: Hypercoagulable states. Ann Intern Med 119:819, 1993

Posner JB: Paraneoplastic syndromes. Neurol Clin 9:919, 1991

Sigal LH: The polymerase chain reaction assay for *Borrelia burgdorferi* in the diagnosis of Lyme disease. Ann Intern Med 120:520, 1994

Simon RP: Neurosyphilis. Arch Neurol 42:606, 1985

Vermeulen M: Xanthochromia after subarachnoid haemorrhage needs no revisitation. J Neurol Neurosurg Psychiatry 52:826, 1989

19. ELECTROPHYSIOLOGY: ELECTROENCEPHALOGRAPHY AND EVOKED POTENTIALS

EDWARD B. BROMFIELD

Even in the present age of sophisticated neuroimaging, the neurophysiologic techniques of electroencephalography (EEG) and evoked potentials (EP) can provide the clinician with noninvasive and relatively inexpensive means of obtaining information about neurologic function that is not otherwise available. Despite major advances in molecular biology and neurochemistry, the nervous system is still best considered as an electrical system; electrodiagnostic techniques are in this sense fundamental to an understanding of its function and dysfunction. From a clinical point of view, it is necessary to appreciate how these techniques complement the information obtained from history, physical examination, and other diagnostic studies.

ELECTROENCEPHALOGRAPHY

Physiology and Anatomic Correlations

Routine EEG recordings summarize the electrical fields generated by large neuronal populations behaving in a synchronous manner; the physiologic correlates of the scalp EEG are thought to be excitatory and inhibitory postsynaptic potentials generated at the apical dendrites of cortical pyramidal cells. A single standard scalp electrode records activity from approximately 6 cm² of gyral surface. Cortical activity at the sides and depths of

sulci, as well as at deeply located cortex such as the medial temporal or orbitofrontal regions, is less well represented. Nevertheless, a sufficiently large area of cortex is sampled to reflect many aspects of focal and global function. Furthermore, because cortical activity is affected in somewhat predictable ways by changes in other regions that are not directly accessed, including white matter, deep gray structures, and the brainstem, EEG can provide information about a wide variety of conditions. Its utility is greatest, however, for diseases that primarily affect cortical function, such as epilepsy.

Technique and Analysis

Scalp EEG is generally recorded using metal cup electrodes filled with conducting gel or paste. Placement of electrodes on the head was standardized in 1958 with the adoption of the International 10–20 System, which uses percentage measurements of distances between skull landmarks (Fig. 19-1). Newer nomenclature has been proposed mainly to include intermediate placements which allow many more than the 21 standard positions shown in Figure 19-1. The number of channels used for recording and display is, in theory, unlimited; in practice, paper tracings are made on machines with 16 to 21 channels, while digital systems often record 32 or more channels.

Because of the low amplitude of scalp-recorded signals relative to electrical noise in the laboratory environment, a *differential amplifier,* which amplifies the difference between two inputs, is used. Each channel, therefore, records the time-varying difference in electrical potential between two points. The arrangement on the page of the specific electrode pairs whose potential difference is displayed in each channel is called a *montage.* Although this arrangement is arbitrary, montages are devised to reflect a logical spatial approach that facilitates analysis. There are two main types of montages: referential and bipolar. In referential recording, the second input is the same for all channels. This arrangement is useful for certain types of analysis, but technical factors, particularly the impossibility of designating a truly inactive, artifact-free reference, limit its usefulness. In the other type of montage, termed *bipolar,* a common reference electrode is not used; typically, pairs of adjacent electrodes are connected in chains such that the second input of one channel becomes the first input of the next (see Figs. 19-2 to 19-6). Some montages are better than others for displaying various normal and abnormal phenomena, and routine 20- to 30-minute studies usually make use of three to six different ones, including both the referential and bipolar types.

Analysis of EEG depends on identifying the dominant frequencies and important transient electrical events over different regions during waking, drowsy, and sleeping states. Wave-frequency is classified as α (8 to less than 14 Hz), β (14 Hz and greater), θ (4 to less than 8 Hz), and δ (less than 4 Hz). The normal adult waking EEG is characterized by posterior α-wave activity that attenuates on eye opening (Fig. 19-2). Lower amplitude β-waves usually predominate anteriorly, intermixed with small amounts of slower frequency waves. β-Waves may be increased by certain drugs, especially sedatives (Fig. 19-3). Prominent θ and δ waves during the waking state in adults, particularly if asymmetric (Fig. 19-4), are abnormal. Normal stage 1 sleep is characterized by attenuation of α-wave and increased prominence of θ-wave frequencies. Characteristic sharp transients over the vertex are seen in late stage 1; stage 2 sleep is characterized by lower voltage, rhythmic sleep spindles (Fig. 19-5), as well as K complexes, which resemble combina-

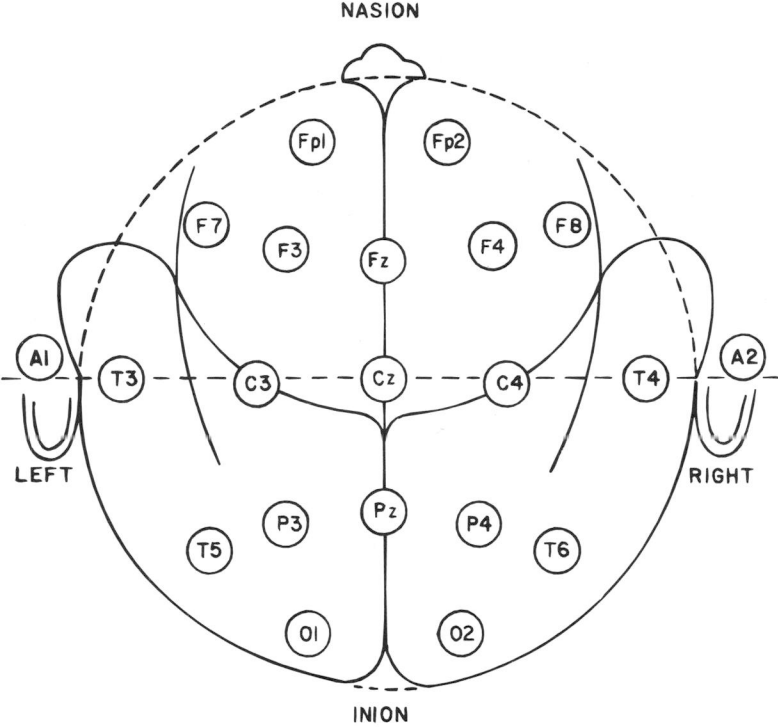

FIG. 19-1. The International 10–20 System of electrode placement. Fp, frontopolar; F, frontal; C, central (near the central sulcus); P, parietal; T, temporal; O, occipital; A, earlobe or mastoid. The numerical designation indicates left (odd), right (even), or midline (Z for zero) location, with higher numbers indicating distance from the midline. (From Aminoff MJ: Electroencephalography: General Principles and Clinical Applications. p. 41. In: Electrodiagnosis in Clinical Neurology. 3rd Ed. Churchill Livingstone, New York, 1995, with permission.)

tions of vertex waves and spindles. Stage 3 is defined by high-voltage δ-waves occurring during 20 to 50 percent of the analyzed segment, and stage 4 by the presence of δ-waves more than 50 percent of the time. EEG during rapid eye movement (REM) sleep resembles that of stage 1, but rapid horizontal eye movements and attenuation of muscle activity are also present. Neither slow wave sleep (stage 3 or 4) nor REM is typically recorded during a routine daytime study.

Interpretation of an EEG requires knowledge of the age as well as the state of consciousness of the patient. Prenatal development, as manifested in the EEG of premature infants, is characterized by differentiation of the states of waking, active sleep, and quiet sleep (the latter two analogous to REM and non-REM sleep), and synchronization of the two hemispheres. Spindles first occur about 2 months after term, and a posterior waking rhythm of about 4 Hz after approximately 3 months; frequency gradually increases to the alpha range by 3 years and reaches adult frequencies at about 10 years. During childhood, slow waves in the waking state become less prominent, with δ-waves disappearing and θ-waves diminishing. EEG is rather stable through adolescence and maturity. In later adulthood, slower waves may again be normally present, with even a small amount of δ-waves allowable in elderly individuals, and the α-wave rhythm may also slow slightly.

Characterization of normal and abnormal waveforms includes description of frequency, amplitude, contour (e.g., sharpness), rhythmicity, topographic distribution, polarity (surface positive vs surface negative), persistence, and reactivity. Some patterns are sufficiently distinct to have their own, often acronymic, names (see below and Table 19-1).

Indicators of cerebral dysfunction include a posterior rhythm that is too slow (relative to age-matched controls or a previous study) or marked left-right asymmetries of frequency or reactivity; amplitude is commonly higher over the right hemisphere, and right:left ratio can normally be as high as 2:1 or as low as 2:3. β-wave asymmetries, however, should not exceed 2:3 in either direction, lower amplitude being an indicator of lateralized or localized cortical dysfunction. In the presence of a cranial defect, however, the high-frequency filtering effect of the skull is diminished, resulting in improved transmission and therefore higher amplitude of β-waves under the skull breach.

The most common indicators of abnormal cerebral function are slow waves, with the degree of slowing being proportional to the severity of dysfunction, δ-waves signifying more severe dysfunction than θ-waves. Generalized slowing is the most common correlate of a diffuse encephalopathy, although a multifocal process can at times be indistinguishable. Localized slowing is of particular importance as it may in some circumstances be the only indication of a focal neurologic process. Structural lesions involving white matter typically correspond to areas of irregular slowing, while rhythmic slowing more often reflects involvement of deep midline structures or of both cortical and deep gray matter, as in metabolic processes.

The interictal EEG correlate of a seizure tendency is the epileptiform discharge (Figs. 19-6 and 19-7), which may take the form of spikes, sharp waves, and spike-wave complexes. A spike is a transient electrical event that stands out from the background, has a sharp peak at the conventional paper speed of 30 mm/s, and has a duration at its base of 20 to just under 70 ms. Because of the organization of cortical pyramidal cells, polarity as recorded at the cortical surface or scalp is usually negative. A sharp wave is similar but has a duration of 70 to

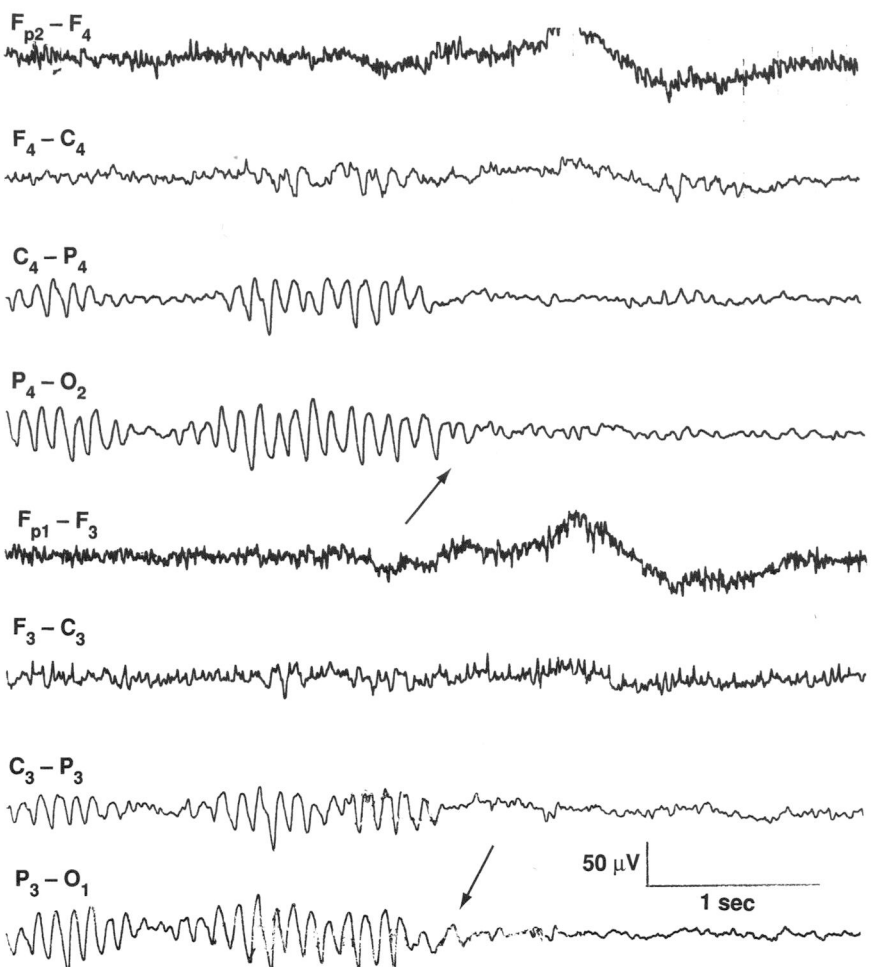

FIG. 19-2.   Normal adult α-rhythm. Note attenuation with eye opening (*arrow*), as well as muscle (fast) and eye opening (slow) artifact in frontopolar derivations.

200 ms. A spike-wave complex is a spike immediately followed by a distinct θ-wave or, more commonly, δ-wave; these often occur in rhythmic bursts. Variants include sharp-slow complexes and polyspike-wave or multiple-spike and slow-wave complexes. Distinguishing these interictal epileptiform discharges from normal or nonspecific phenomena is not always straightforward, however, and may depend on such characteristics as age and state of the patient as well as morphology, location, polarity, reactivity, amplitude, and context of the waveform. There are also distinct patterns, discussed in several of the Suggested Readings, that resemble single or repetitive discharges but in fact correlate weakly, if at all, with a seizure tendency or other aspects of brain dysfunction. These include benign epileptiform transients of sleep (BETS or small sharp spikes), rhythmic midtemporal θ-waves of drowsiness (also called *psychomotor variant*), 14- and 6-Hz positive spikes, 6 per second phantom spike-waves, and subclinical rhythmic EEG discharge of adults (SREDA).

Finally, there are several distinctly abnormal patterns, often of a repetitive, periodic, or rhythmic nature. Periodic lateralized epileptiform discharges (PLEDs) are commonly seen in the setting of acute or subacute disturbances, such as strokes and inflammations and, like sporadic localized sharp waves, are strongly associated with partial seizures. Bilateral insults may be manifested as bilateral independent or bisynchronous peri-

odic discharges, with morphology and rate providing some information about etiology (see below). Triphasic waves are a characteristic repetitive waveform that can resemble generalized sharp-slow complexes but occur in the context of metabolic encephalopathy rather than seizures. The *burst-suppression* pattern, where periods of electrical silence alternate with bursts of mixed frequency activity, indicates severe underlying dysfunction. Transient rhythmic abnormal activity may represent an actual seizure, although an ictal recording during a routine study is unusual except in cases of status epilepticus.

Clinical Uses

In contemporary practice, EEG is used primarily in cases of known or suspected epilepsy, more prolonged states of altered consciousness, or other instances of focally or globally impaired cerebral function. The most common scenario is that of an adult or child seen after a transient event that may have represented a seizure. The EEG result can contribute to clinical decision-making in several ways: first, it can help to assess the probability that the event represented a seizure; second, it can in some instances indicate the relative susceptibility of this individual to another seizure in the future. These probabilities are critical in deciding whether or not to treat the patient for presumed epilepsy. Furthermore, the type of interictal epileptiform activ-

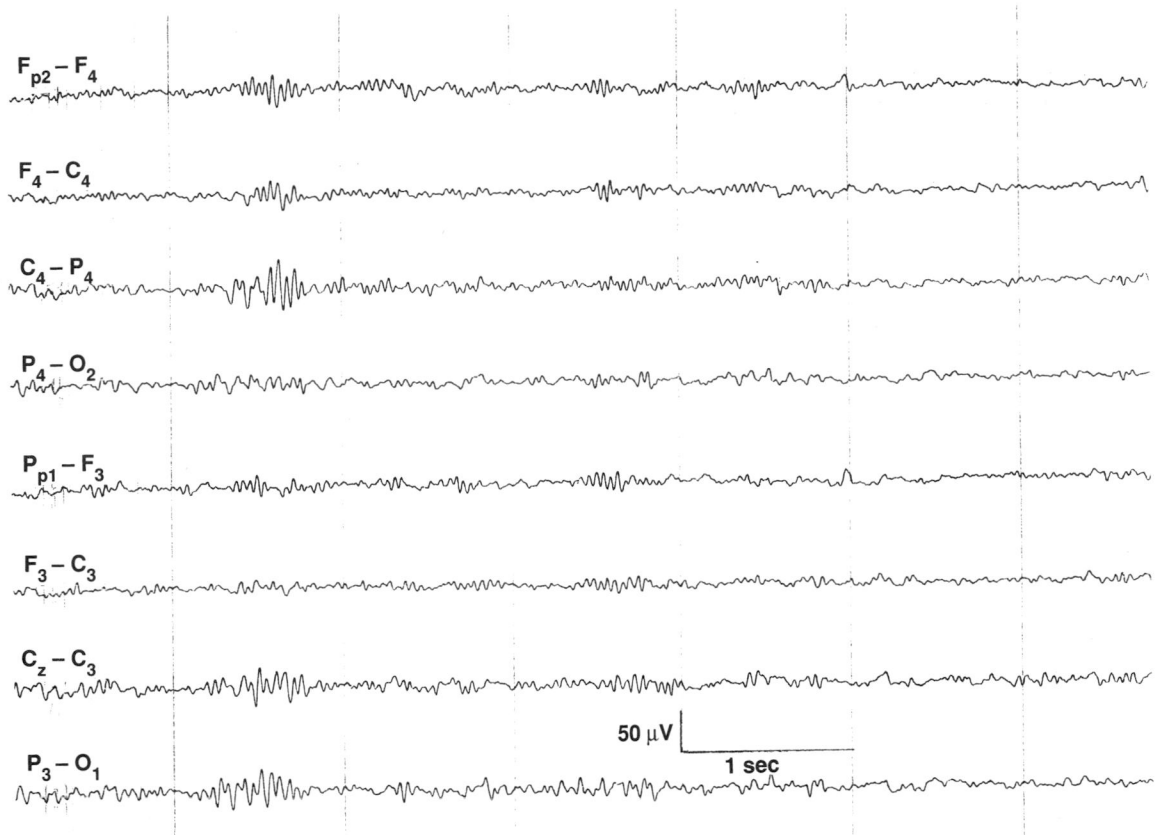

FIG. 19-3. Excessive β-waves seen diffusely in patient on sedative medications.

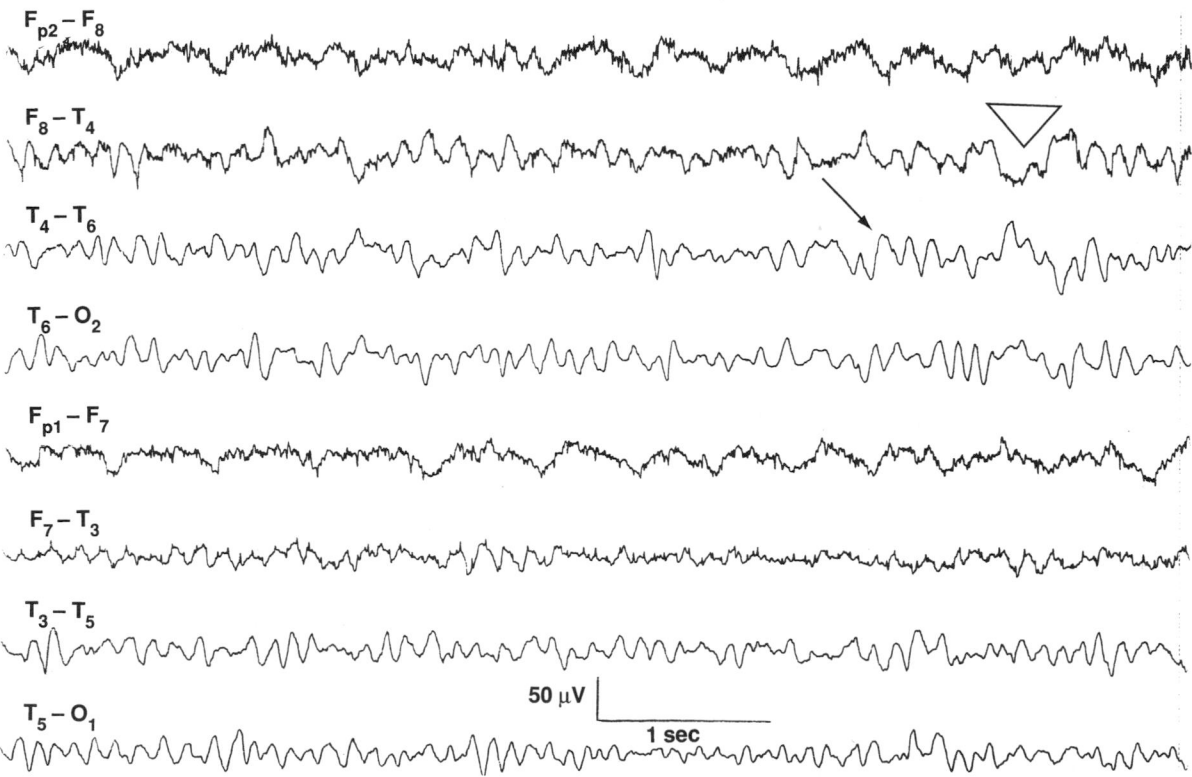

FIG. 19-4. Right temporal θ-waves (*arrow*) and δ-waves (*arrowhead*) in patient with history of stroke. Bilateral anterior δ-frequency waveforms are contaminated by eye movement artifact as well as high-frequency muscle artifact.

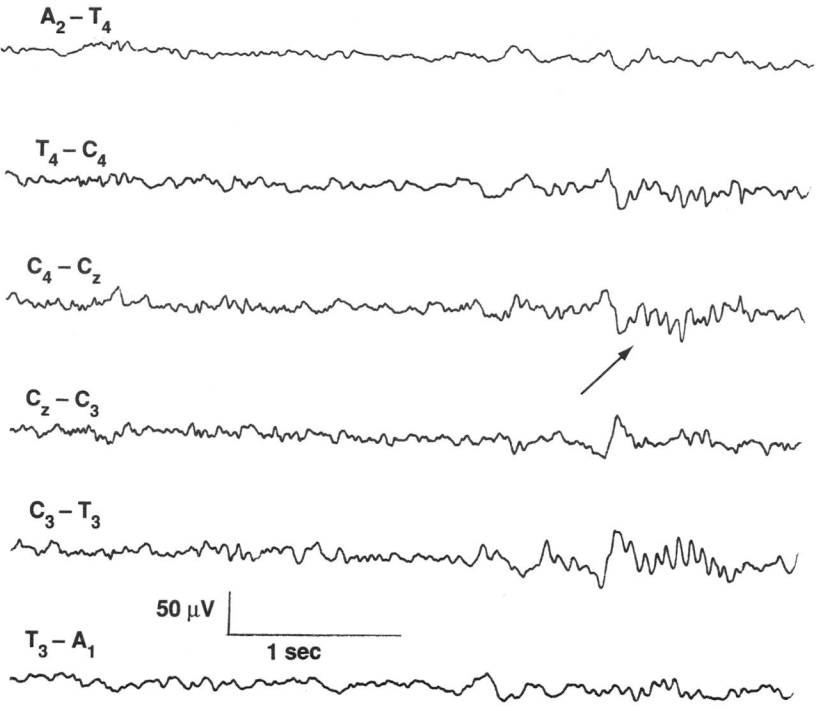

FIG. 19-5.   Vertex wave and sleep spindle (*arrow*) during stage 2 sleep.

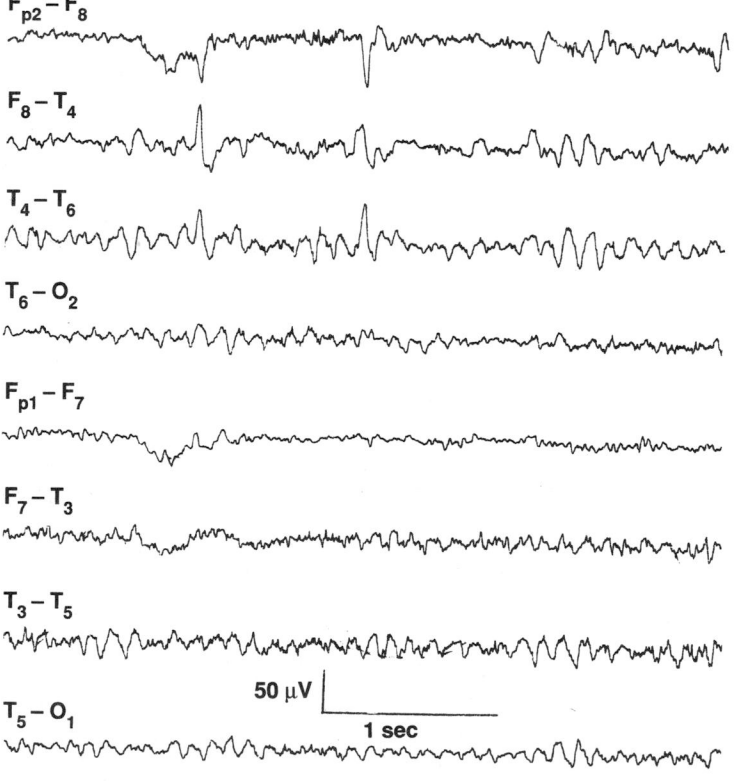

FIG. 19-6.   Repetitive sharp waves over right frontotemporal region.

TABLE 19-1. Anatomic and Clinical Correlates of Common EEG Findings

Finding	Anatomic	Clinical
Slow background (bilateral)	Diffuse/thalamocortical dysfunction	Encephalopathy (acute or chronic)
Asymmetric/unilateral slow background	Ipsilateral diffuse or posterior dysfunction	Probable structural lesion
Widespread intermittent rhythmic δ-wave activity (IRDA; usually anterior in adults, posterior in children)	Deep and cortical gray matter	Toxic-metabolic encephalopathy; midline lesion; hydrocephalus; if unilateral, migraine, postictal state, structural lesion
Persistent bilateral irregular slowing (especially delta)	Diffuse, bihemispheric, and/or upper brainstem reticular dysfunction	More severe encephalopathy; bihemispheric or brainstem lesions
Irregular slowing, unilateral or focal	Focal subcortical dysfunction (slower and more persistent with increased dysfunction)	Underlying structural lesion
Consistently asymmetric beta and/or sleep spindles	Cortical dysfunction on side of lower amplitude, or skull/dural defect on opposite side	Structural lesion or subdural collection on lower side; skull defect on higher side
Sharp waves/spikes/spike-wave complexes, focal or multifocal	Localized cortical irritability	Partial epilepsy; focal or multifocal disturbance with seizure tendency
Spike-wave complexes, generalized	Diffuse cortical irritability	Probable generalized epilepsy, either idiopathic (3 Hz or faster complexes, normal background), or symptomatic (slow rate, abnormal background)
Periodic lateralized epileptiform discharges	Localized or hemispheric dysfunction with cortical irritability	Acute or subacute process, often vascular or inflammatory (e.g., encephalitis), with seizure tendency; postictal or interictal in relation to serial seizures/status epilepticus
Triphasic waves	Diffuse cortical and subcortical dysfunction	Encephalopathy, especially hepatic, less commonly uremic or postanoxic

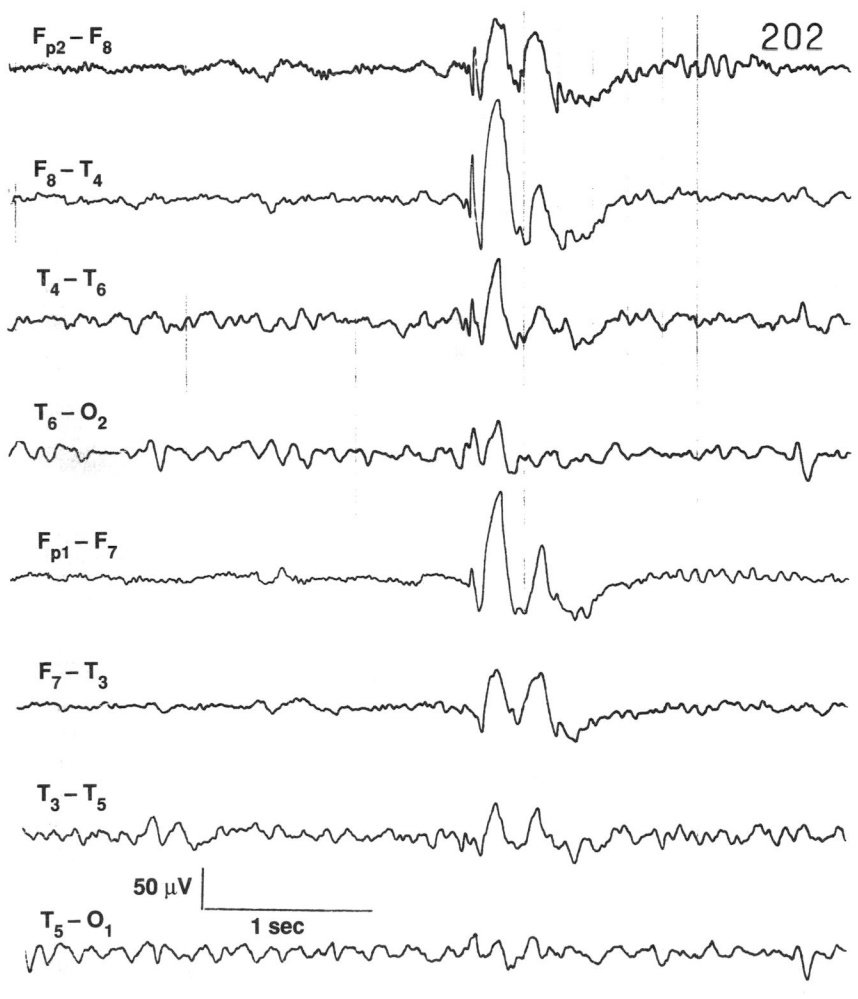

FIG. 19-7.   Generalized spike-wave complex with anterior predominance and slight right greater than left asymmetry.

ity present is important in identifying the underlying epilepsy syndrome (see Chapter 139), which can influence the choice of treatment. A staring spell, for example, can be the manifestation of either a partial seizure of temporal lobe origin or an inherited tendency toward generalized absence seizures; in the first case, one would likely find temporal sharp waves or spikes, and in the second, 3-Hz generalized spike-wave complexes. When there are repeated or prolonged seizures, constituting status epilepticus, EEG is needed to guide therapy if motor manifestations are absent. In many cases of nonconvulsive status (see Chapter 141), diagnosis would be impossible without EEG confirmation.

The EEG can help in assessing severity, localization, and, in some cases, etiology and prognosis of a wide variety of other conditions that affect cerebral function. In toxic or metabolic encephalopathies, the characteristic finding is diffuse slowing. Clues to etiology include excess fast activity in the case of sedative toxicity and triphasic waves in the case of hepatic encephalopathy. (If there is no evidence of the latter, uremia or hypoxia-ischemia should be considered.) More severe abnormalities, from burst-suppression to continuously low voltage to electrocerebral inactivity, are most commonly seen after anoxia, although severe toxic or metabolic disturbances can also be the cause. The nonreactive "α-coma" pattern, in the most common setting of postanoxia, indicates a dismal prognosis but, like other patterns, may be less ominous if resulting from another etiology. True electrocerebral inactivity, for which specific technical criteria have been adopted, can be a useful adjunct in the diagnosis of brain death as long as drug intoxication and hypothermia have been ruled out. In encephalopathy and coma, serial studies are often useful, since EEG deterioration or improvement may precede clinical changes. Also worth noting is the use of EEG in suspected psychogenic coma, where a normal waking pattern with reactive posterior alpha rules out a cerebral cause. Alternatively, a normal background may be present in the locked-in syndrome due to pontine pathology.

EEG can also be very useful in diagnosis of inflammatory and dementing conditions. While findings in meningitis are similar to those of metabolic encephalopathies, encephalitis may be associated with focal or multifocal slowing as well as sharp waves or spikes. Herpes simplex encephalitis, in particular, is characteristically associated with unilateral or bilateral frontotemporal slowing, often with sharp waves or periodic complexes that may be synchronous or asynchronous between the hemispheres and recur at 1- to 5-second intervals; these changes may precede neuroimaging abnormalities. In the rare pediatric disease of subacute sclerosing panencephalitis, the EEG finding of slowly periodic (every 5 to 10 seconds) bursts of very high voltage, bilateral slow and sharp waves is virtually pathognomonic. Creutzfeldt-Jakob disease in its middle and later phases typically shows simpler diphasic or triphasic, more rapidly repeated (every 0.5 to 1.5 second) periodic complexes. Senile dementia of the Alzheimer type, by contrast, is usually associated with background disorganization, showing increasing amounts of theta and delta as the condition progresses. Early in the disease, EEG may be normal, but a marked dissociation between clinical and electrographic findings may also suggest the diagnosis of pseudodementia secondary to depression.

Vascular disease, including multi-infarct dementia, characteristically is associated with focal or multifocal slowing (Fig. 19-4), with or without loss of faster frequencies, depending on extent of cortical involvement. Localized sharp waves may be present and may be periodic in the acute or subacute stroke phase. An EEG performed during a hemispheric transient ischemic attack, when imaging may be negative, typically shows slowing over the involved area. Resolution on follow-up study can confirm the vascular nature of the process, although this does not rule out the possibility of a postictal deficit with associated slowing. Complicated migraine can show EEG findings identical to those of a stroke or transient ischemic attack, although rhythmic rather than irregular slowing may be more common in migraine. Between attacks, patients with migraine may have a variety of nonspecific abnormalities, including temporal theta and sharp transients, that can be confused with those seen in patients with epilepsy.

Use of EEG in patients with progressive focal lesions, such as tumors or abscesses, has been largely overtaken by neuroimaging, but EEG may still be useful in following more widespread changes that can result from radiation or medications, in assessing the role of seizures in causing ictal or interictal functional impairment, or in showing progression of the underlying condition.

The utility of EEG in psychiatric disorders, especially of computerized methods of display (see below), remains controversial, but EEG is clearly helpful in ruling out neurologic causes of abnormal behavior. When combined with recording of other physiologic variables, EEG plays an integral role in the study of sleep disorders via polysomnography (see Chapter 144).

The EEG Report: Contents and Terminology

Many physicians, including some neurologists, view the EEG report as an arcane, jargon-laden document not worthy of detailed perusal and skip as quickly as possible to the "bottom line." As with any laboratory test, the ordering clinician should specify the reason for the study, and the report should answer insofar as possible the specific question or questions asked. The accompanying detailed description is also important, however, and can provide clues about the usefulness of a particular study. The report should mention any special preparation or recording methods (see below) and then describe the dominant or important electrical activity noted in each of the waking, drowsy, and sleeping states, if represented. Description of the waking EEG usually uses the term "background" to refer to the dominant posterior rhythm, specifying the frequency and approximate amplitude range. Description of the waking record may also include reference to beta frequencies, particularly as regards amount, amplitude, and symmetry.

The description should next include any slower waves that are consistently seen, especially if abnormal based on age and state of the patient. Finally, any significant transient waveforms, specifically epileptiform discharges, should be described. If these are difficult to distinguish from normal or nonspecific phenomena alluded to earlier, the description should reflect this uncertainty.

Description of the EEG recorded in drowsiness and sleep is similar, but the concept of a "background" is more nebulous. At the least, the report should note how any abnormal findings seen in the waking state evolve during subsequent states. Finally, activation procedures are described. In most cases these include hyperventilation for 3 to 4 minutes, which normally causes diffuse slowing but may bring out focal or epileptiform abnormalities, and intermittent photic (strobe light) stimulation, which is a general indicator of visual system function and which in occasional patients precipitates epileptiform activity not noted under other conditions or even a clinical seizure. Additional activation procedures may be tailored to the individual patient, particularly if clinical events are known to be precipitated by, for example, auditory stimuli, cognitive tasks, position changes, or anxiety.

Each report should follow with a section summarizing the study. This begins with a global statement of whether it is normal or abnormal, perhaps including a modifier concerning degree of abnormality, and a listing of the abnormal features. Most electroencephalographers prefer to call questionable findings normal rather than abnormal. This propensity makes clinical sense in the case of suspected epilepsy, since a single EEG may be normal in approximately 50 percent of individuals with the condition, whereas a frankly abnormal EEG with definite epileptiform discharges may have a specificity in excess of 95 percent. Finally, there should be an interpretation regarding the clinical implications of the findings, specifically in relation to the reason that the EEG was requested. Comparisons to previous studies of the same patient and suggestions for future EEG studies can be useful. In the case of suspected epilepsy, although a single study is only about 50 percent sensitive, two more repeat recordings up to a total of three can increase the yield to approximately 90 percent.

An important part of the electroencephalographer's art is wording the conclusion so as to answer the clinical question with the appropriate degree of confidence, neither too much nor too little. Phrases such as ''consistent with'' or ''suggestive of'' may be frustrating for the clinician but do accurately represent the uncertainty of many clinical correlations. While the evidence for dysfunction may be unequivocal, the cause of that dysfunction is rarely clear from the EEG alone.

Table 19-1 shows the main types of EEG abnormalities with their anatomic and, where possible, etiologic correlates. More complete listings and discussions may be found in several excellent texts of electroencephalography.

Special Studies

This category includes both special patient preparation and special recording techniques, including electrode placements beyond those of the standard ''10–20'' system. The most important patient preparation techniques include sedation and sleep deprivation. These are particularly useful in the evaluation of seizures or suspected seizures, especially if the waking record shows no epileptiform discharges. Numerous studies have documented increased sensitivity of recordings that include drowsiness and stage 2 sleep, and some suggest an additional ''activating'' effect of sleep deprivation itself. It is unclear whether or not complete sleep deprivation is required. In children or uncooperative adults, sedation may be needed not just to record sleep but also to obtain a record sufficiently free of artifact to allow interpretation. It should be emphasized that neither sleep deprivation nor sedation is indicated when the purpose of the study is to evaluate encephalopathy, for which a fully awake recording provides the most reliable data.

Special electrode placements are most often used to help detect or localize a seizure focus, especially when the mesial temporal lobe, not well sampled by standard electrodes, is suspected. Useful information is provided by ''anterior temporal'' or ''T1/T2'' electrodes, standard disc electrodes placed anteriorly and inferiorly to the standard midtemporal placements. Sphenoidal electrodes are thin wires introduced by means of a needle approximately 3 to 5 cm medial to the mandibular notch,

with the tips located near the foramen ovale. These must be inserted by a physician and are generally used only in long-term recordings (see below). A simpler variant of these is the so-called ''minisphenoidal'' electrode, which is a standard 1-cm needle electrode bent at the hub inserted at the same infrazygomatic location; surface electrodes at this site are also useful. Nasopharyngeal electrodes are uncomfortable, prone to artifact, and not clearly more sensitive than supplementary surface electrodes and so are now rarely used.

Additional techniques of EEG study include prolonged recordings with or without simultaneous video recording; these are especially useful in correlating specific clinical behaviors with EEG, thus demonstrating whether or not the behaviors have an epileptic basis. This is generally a reliable test for complex partial seizures, which are nearly always accompanied by some ictal or postictal EEG change. However, simple partial seizures, that is, with preserved consciousness, are often not detected on surface EEG recording. Also, artifacts produced by movement of the head and eyes can interfere with interpretation. Ambulatory studies, which generally are not accompanied by video recording, are particularly problematic in this regard. These long-term studies, therefore, must be interpreted by an experienced electroencephalographer.

Computerized methods of EEG analysis or ''brain mapping'' have been used increasingly over the past decade. Most commonly, spectral analysis of waveforms recorded over several seconds is converted to a gray-scale or color map based on the amount of activity in various frequency bands at different sites. While this method of data display can convey useful information, the information is usually apparent to an experienced reader on routine EEG and may be misleading if artifacts are not carefully screened out. Also, complex statistical issues render controversial the mapping profiles of various patient groups; though some of these distinctions may be valid on a population basis, their usefulness in diagnosis of individual patients is debated.

EVOKED POTENTIALS

Evoked potentials used in clinical practice measure conduction along visual, auditory, or somatosensory pathways from the periphery to the central nervous system. Since the amplitude of these responses is small, generally less than that of the background EEG noise, routine use of these studies did not become possible until the advent of computer averaging techniques. Averaging results in a marked increase in signal-to-noise ratio because the evoked response is time-locked to the stimulus, while background noise occurs randomly. The smaller the evoked potential in relation to ongoing EEG activity, the greater the number of repetitions needed to visualize the signal.

Clinically useful conclusions can be drawn from evoked potential studies even though the exact generators are not known in many instances. Electrodes placed close to the relevant nerve, tract, or cortical region can reveal the timing of impulse conduction in a relatively straightforward manner. Because of specific characteristics of electrical fields generated by various sensory nuclei, however, even potentials generated by deep structures in the brainstem and elsewhere can be recorded by appropriately placed surface electrodes.

In general, latency determinations are more reliable than amplitude changes; a readily identifiable but delayed peak is a strong indicator of slowed conduction, usually a consequence of demyelination; although a reliably decreased amplitude can

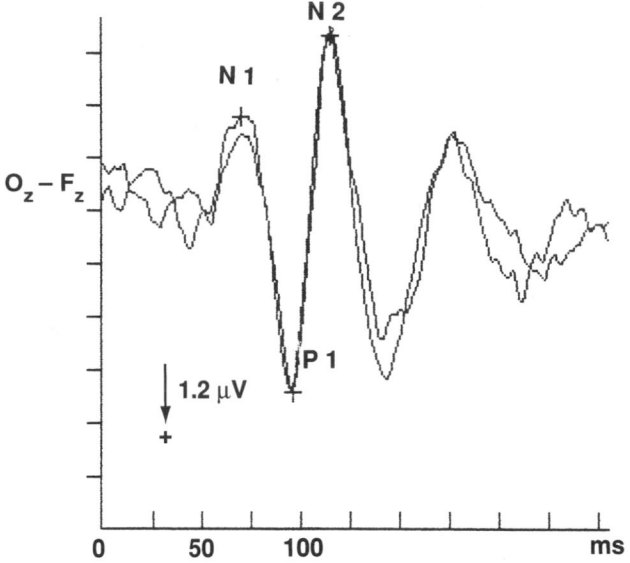

FIG. 19-8.   Normal pattern-shift visual evoked potential. The major positive peak, also called P100, is labeled P1.

reflect fewer involved axons producing the response, it is often difficult to exclude technical factors as an explanation for small or even absent peaks. For all evoked potential peaks, latencies are normally distributed in the general population. "Abnormal" prolongation of latencies, therefore, must be statistically determined; in most laboratories, a cutoff of 2.5 or 3 standard deviations is used. By the stricter criterion, false positives would tend to occur less than 1 percent of the time; this degree of specificity is gained at the expense of some increase in the incidence of false negatives.

Visual Evoked Potentials

Electrical responses to visual stimulation may be produced by neural elements in the retina (electroretinogram), but for neurologists the cortically generated visual evoked potentials (VEP),

recorded at the occiput, are of greatest use. These may be produced by a simple flash of light, but latency and waveform are highly dependent on patient and stimulus characteristics. In infants or other individuals who cannot be instructed to attend to a specific stimulus, flash-induced VEPs can verify that the visual pathway from eye to brain is at least functioning but are insensitive to subtotal dysfunction. By far the most widely used method of visual testing is pattern-shift VEP, recorded in relation to abrupt reversal of the light and dark squares of a checkerboard pattern, usually displayed on a video terminal. Generally, a rate of approximately two reversals per second is used for 100 to 200 stimuli. The normal response as recorded from the midoccipital region is a positive deflection approximately 100 ms after the stimulus, sometimes called the P100, or P1 (Fig. 19-8). At the usual check sizes, field sizes, and distances used, macular vision is important in generating this potential, and visual acuity must be at least 20/100 for a valid test. Since response can also be affected by such variables as ambient light, total luminance of the display, and degree of contrast between light and dark squares, it is important that each laboratory determine its own normal values.

If ophthalmic pathology can be ruled out, a prolonged latency of the major positive peak, either absolutely or in relation to the contralateral eye, is highly specific for optic nerve or chiasmal pathology. This is the basis for the most common clinical uses of pattern-shift VEP, particularly in documenting optic nerve impairment in suspected multiple sclerosis. This study is nearly 100 percent sensitive in known optic neuritis, even after clinical recovery. Perhaps more importantly, more than 50 percent of multiple sclerosis patients without clinical optic nerve involvement have abnormal pattern-shift VEP, although the percentage is probably lower in those without a firm diagnosis. Another major use of pattern-shift VEP is in confirming psychogenic visual loss; this presupposes some patient cooperation, however, in that the patient must visually focus on the center of the checkerboard pattern during a sufficient number of stimuli. Unless fixation can be verified, therefore, an abnormal study is inconclusive in this context; a normal study, by contrast,

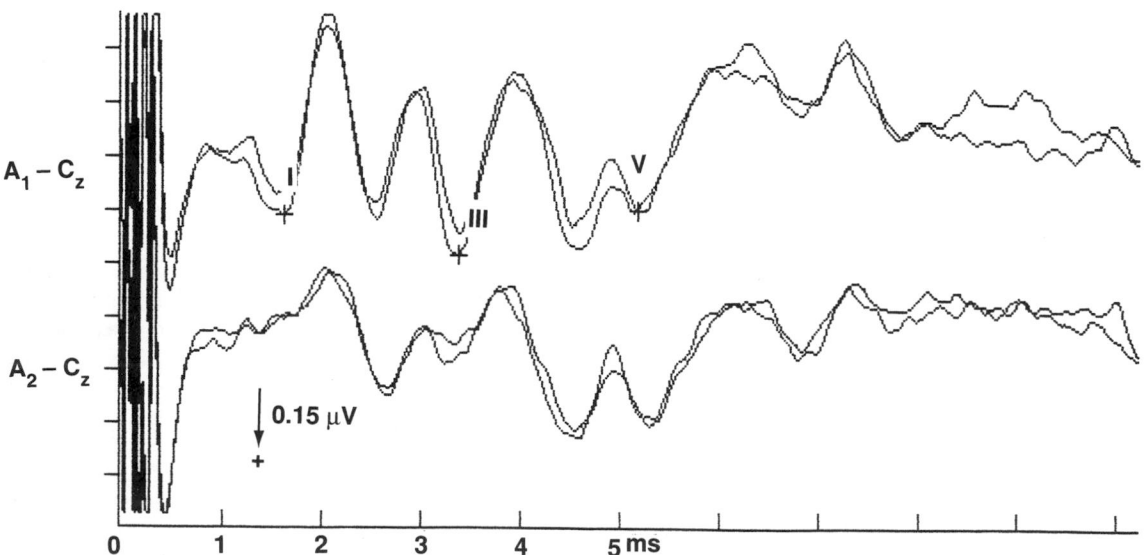

FIG. 19-9.   Normal left ear brainstem auditory evoked potential. Peaks I, III, and V are labeled. (Downward deflection to represent positive polarity is in keeping with EEG convention, but many laboratories reverse this for BAER studies.) Note stimulus artifact at onset of tracing.

argues strongly against an organic basis for major visual impairment, especially if monocular. Pattern-shift VEP may be normal with postchiasmal abnormalities, rarely even in the case of cortical blindness. Hemifield pattern reversal stimulation may be used to investigate hemianopias, but is more difficult than full-field studies and less often used.

Auditory Evoked Responses

Clinically used auditory evoked potentials are those generated by brainstem structures, and are therefore often called brainstem auditory evoked responses (AER). In contrast to the VEP, which is recorded immediately over its generator in the visual cortex, the brainstem AER is a series of ''far-field'' potentials recorded at the earlobe or mastoid linked to a vertex electrode. Using a broadband click stimulus, one can generally record at least five successive peaks, designated I to V (Fig. 19-9). Wave

I, generated by the acoustic nerve, occurs approximately 2 ms after the stimulus, and the succeeding four peaks are approximately 1 ms apart; wave III is thought to be generated by the cochlear nucleus, and wave V is considered to reflect arrival of the signal at the inferior colliculus. Diencephalic and cortical auditory evoked potentials can also be recorded, but these are generally used only for research purposes. Because the latencies are so short, stimuli can be given rapidly, approximately 9 to 12 per second, but because the amplitudes are so small, 1,000 to 4,000 stimuli must be given. As with VEP, latency of peaks is more informative than amplitude; absolute and especially interpeak latencies can generally distinguish between lesions affecting the acoustic nerve or cochlear apparatus and those affecting either the lower or upper brainstem. Audiography and other otolaryngologic studies can be helpful in more fully characterizing peripheral abnormalities suggested by brainstem AER.

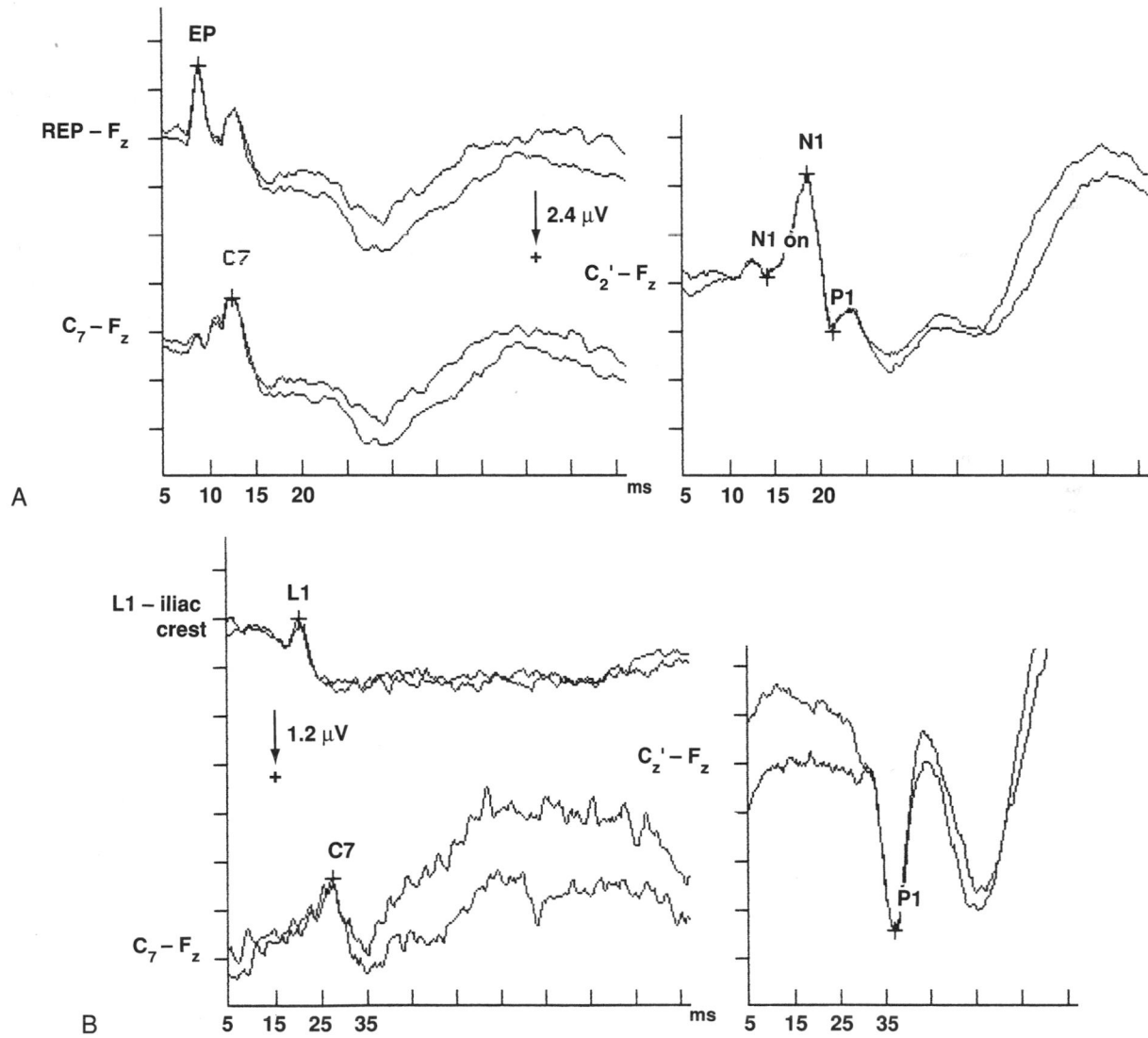

FIG. 19-10. Normal somatosensory evoked potentials elicited by stimulation of **(A)** right median and **(B)** left posterior tibial nerves. To eliminate stimulus artifact horizontal axis of display starts after time zero of stimulus presentation. Reference (second input to amplifier) is Fz unless otherwise noted. REP, right Erb's point; EP (also called N9), Erb's point potential; C7 (also called N13), potential at seventh cervical spinous process; N1 (also called N20), major cortical negative peak recorded over C3', 2 cm posterior to C3 of 10–20 system; N1 on, onset of N1 peak; P1 (also called P23), cortical positive peak; L1, peak recorded at first lumbar spinous process (iliac crest reference); C7, peak recorded at seventh cervical spinous process; P1 (also called P37), major cortical peak recorded at Cz', 2 cm posterior to Cz of 10–20 system.

Because of the proximity of both peripheral and central structures subserving vestibular and auditory function, brainstem AERs may be helpful in assessing complaints of vertigo as well as of diminished hearing and tinnitus. Brainstem AERs remain a highly sensitive means of screening for acoustic neuromas and other infratentorial tumors, although this function has been largely overtaken by advances in magnetic resonance imaging (MRI). Regarding the evaluation for possible multiple sclerosis, brainstem AER is less likely to reveal an asymptomatic (brainstem) lesion than VEP or somatosensory evoked potential. An abnormal brainstem AER in a patient with clinical involvement at a single site outside the brainstem, however, can be highly suggestive of the diagnosis. Other uses of brainstem AERs include any condition where brainstem involvement, especially of the white matter, is suspected clinically, such as in the leukodystrophies.

An advantage of brainstem AER is that this test does not require patient cooperation, as does pattern-shift VEP, and is generally resistant to the effects of anesthesia (unless hypothermia is produced). Reliable information can be obtained, therefore, in unresponsive patients and in infants. In the latter case, age-matched controls must be used, as adult values are not reached until approximately age 2. A further use in infants is estimation of auditory threshold in those unable to cooperate with audiography.

Somatosensory Evoked Potentials

Stimulation of a peripheral nerve allows measurement of peak latencies at various sites between that stimulated and the sensory cortex. Use of mixed motor and sensory nerves, such as the median in the upper extremity (Fig. 19-10A) and the posterior tibial (Fig. 19-10B) or peroneal in the lower extremity, produces a twitch response of the muscle innervated by the stimulated nerve, demonstrating adequacy of the stimulus; intensity does not have to be submaximal as with compound muscle action potential testing. Recording sites generally include peripheral nerve or plexus, site of entrance into the spinal cord, one or more rostral spinal and/or brainstem locations, and the corresponding sensory cortex. Stimulus frequency is generally 4 to 7 Hz, with 500 to 2,000 repetitions needed per trial.

Somatosensory evoked potentials (SSEPs) are produced by the fastest conducting fibers, that is, those traveling in the posterior columns, and therefore may be insensitive to lesions affecting only spinothalamic or motor tracts in the spinal cord or brainstem. On the other hand, SSEPs test large areas of the nervous system; lower extremity studies in particular can screen for dysfunction along the entire length of the neuraxis. Approximately 80 percent of patients with multiple sclerosis have abnormal SSEP, even if there is no clinical sensory loss, but the percentage is less than 50 percent among those in whom the diagnosis is not yet established. Lower extremity studies may be more sensitive than upper extremity but are more difficult to perform satisfactorily. SSEP can be helpful in confirming an organic basis for otherwise unclear sensory complaints, and can often help to localize the site of the abnormality to peripheral nerve or plexus, spinal cord (cervical vs thoracolumbar), or brainstem-cerebral hemisphere. Although interpeak latencies can be helpful, detection of a superimposed central abnormality in those with significant peripheral delay can be difficult. Finally, SSEP can be useful in prognosis of nontraumatic coma, with several studies suggesting that preservation of unilateral and especially bilateral cortical responses to median nerve stimulation implies a more favorable prognosis.

SUMMARY

EEG and evoked potential studies provide noninvasive, relatively inexpensive means of assessing physiologic function, thus complementing structural information obtained from neuroradiologic and other investigations. While degree and location of abnormalities can often be assessed, specific etiology cannot be determined by these tests alone, and results must be integrated with history, physical examination, and other laboratory studies.

SUGGESTED READINGS

Aminoff MJ: Electrodiagnosis in Clinical Neurology. 3rd Ed. Churchill Livingstone, New York, 1992

Chiappa KH: Evoked Potentials in Clinical Medicine. 2nd Ed. Raven Press, New York, 1990

Daly DD, Pedley TA: Current Practice of Clinical Electroencephalography. 2nd Ed. Raven Press, New York, 1990

Misulis KE: Spehlmann's Evoked Potential Primer. 2nd Ed. Butterworth-Heinemann, Boston, 1994

Niedermeyer E, Lopes da Silva F: Electroencephalography: Basic Principles, Clinical Applications, and Related Fields. 3rd Ed. Williams & Wilkins, Baltimore, 1993

20. ELECTROPHYSIOLOGY: NERVE CONDUCTION STUDIES AND ELECTROMYOGRAPHY

ELIZABETH M. RAYNOR
DAVID C. PRESTON

GENERAL PRINCIPLES OF ELECTRODIAGNOSIS

The term electromyography (EMG) is commonly used inclusively to refer to electrodiagnostic testing, which involves nerve conduction studies in addition to the needle electrode examination of muscle. These studies are used primarily in the evaluation of the peripheral nervous system, including both motor and sensory nerves as well as muscle and neuromuscular junction. When correlated with the clinical examination, they provide a powerful tool for localizing and determining the extent, severity, approximate time course, and pathophysiology of a lesion. The importance of clinical correlation for planning the appropriate study and interpreting the results cannot be overemphasized. Thus, every electrophysiologic evaluation should be preceded by an appropriately tailored history and neurologic examination, and the results of the study should be viewed in light of the clinical picture.

PHYSIOLOGIC VARIABLES

There are several physiologic variables that may significantly influence the results of nerve conduction studies as well as needle electromyography. Correct interpretation of electrophysiologic data is dependent on a full understanding of these and other external factors that affect the results.

Age

Normal values for nerve conduction studies are age-dependent. Nerve conduction velocities, in particular, are related to the maturational stage of myelin. Conduction velocity for a motor nerve of a normal infant is approximately half that of a normal adult and increases gradually to reach adult values by the age of 4 years.

Temperature

Nerve conduction studies are most significantly influenced by temperature. Nerve conduction velocity slows in direct proportion to a fall in temperature, at a rate of 1.5 to 2.0 m/s for each degree centigrade below 34°. Similarly, distal latencies increase by approximately 0.3 ms per degree fall in temperature.

Height

Nerve conduction studies, particularly late responses, are influenced by the height of the patient, which dictates the length of the nerves. This translates into different normal values for conduction velocity in the upper and lower extremity, the latter being about 10 m/s slower. Also, normal values for F responses and H reflexes are based on height.

ANATOMY, PHYSIOLOGY, AND PATHOPHYSIOLOGY

Anatomy and Physiology of Nerve and Muscle

The peripheral nervous system includes the motor and sensory neurons (i.e., anterior horn cells and dorsal root ganglia), motor, sensory, and autonomic nerve fibers, neuromuscular junction, and muscle. The term *motor unit* refers to an anterior horn cell, its accompanying motor axon, and all the muscle fibers it innervates. The concept of the motor unit has great clinical importance.

Nerve fibers are composed of axons of varying diameter, both myelinated and unmyelinated. In the sensory system, large diameter myelinated fibers are responsible for transmitting vibration and proprioceptive information, while small unmyelinated fibers transmit pain and temperature sense. Motor axons are myelinated fibers of mostly intermediate and large diameters. Myelinated fibers are unique in their ability to rapidly transmit neural impulses via saltatory conduction, while along unmyelinated fibers, impulses travel slowly by continuous propogation. Nerve conduction studies, both motor and sensory, provide information about myelinated axons of large and intermediate diameter. It is not possible to routinely measure the function of small unmyelinated fibers using current methods.

Individual motor nerve fibers terminate via smaller twigs to multiple neuromuscular junctions, each of which is in direct contact with a single muscle fiber. Normally, when a motor neuron or its axon is activated (i.e., threshold for depolarization is reached), all the muscle fibers it innervates contract in a synchronous, all-or-none fashion.

Pathologic Processes Affecting Peripheral Nerves

A number of different pathologic processes affect peripheral nerves, and the distribution of the lesions they produce may be generalized, focal, or multifocal, depending on the underlying etiology. All neuropathic processes ultimately produce characteristic histologic and electrophysiologic abnormalities, which fall into three distinct categories, discussed below. In many instances, these abnormalities coexist in some combination;

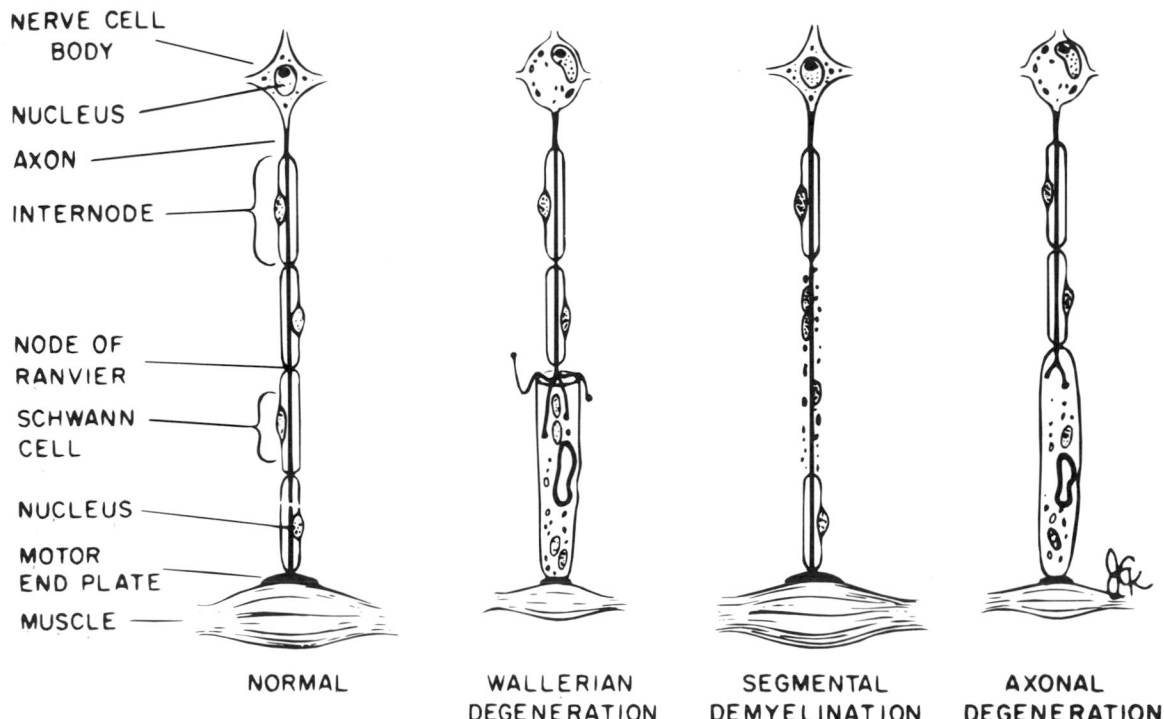

NERVE CELL BODY
NUCLEUS
AXON
INTERNODE
NODE OF RANVIER
SCHWANN CELL
NUCLEUS
MOTOR END PLATE
MUSCLE

NORMAL   WALLERIAN DEGENERATION   SEGMENTAL DEMYELINATION   AXONAL DEGENERATION

FIG. 20-1.   Normal and pathologic processes affecting peripheral nerve. (From Asbury AK, Johnson PC: Pathology of peripheral nerve. p. 5. In Bennington JL (ed): Major Problems in Pathology. Vol. 9. WB Saunders, Philadelphia, 1978, with permission.)

however, one pathologic change is usually primary or predominant (Fig. 20-1).

Axonal Degeneration.   Often described as ''dying-back,'' degeneration of the axon begins distally and proceeds proximally in the setting of toxic or other metabolic injury to the nerve. Mechanical injury to nerve or death of the parent neuron will also result in axonal degeneration. Degeneration ultimately leads to denervation of muscle fibers associated with the motor unit. Examples include axonal polyneuropathies and most toxic and metabolic neuropathies.

Wallerian Degeneration.   When a nerve is physically interrupted, the stump distal to the point of trauma will degenerate. It usually takes 3 to 5 days to complete this process, after which the nerve is inexcitable. The nerve can be stimulated proximally, but the impulse will not be conducted across the interrupted segment. Regeneration of the nerve must occur from the proximal stump at the site of the injury. Examples include focal trauma to the nerve and ischemic injury to the nerve.

Segmental Demyelination.   Focal disruption in the myelin sheath often leads to denuded segments of nerve. Marked slowing of conduction velocity across these sites ensues, since impulses must travel along demyelinated segments in a continuous fashion. Conduction failure or block along a particular nerve fiber may occur if impulses cannot traverse the demyelinated segment. The important clinical consequence of conduction block is weakness. Examples include the inflammatory demyelinating neuropathies, Guillain-Barré syndrome, and chronic inflammatory demyelinating polyneuropathy.

Pathologic Processes Affecting Muscle

The pathologic changes that affect muscle may be separated into two broad categories: neurogenic and myopathic. In general, these are accompanied by characteristic electromyographic abnormalities which allow fairly reliable distinction between them (Fig. 20-2).

Neurogenic Processes.   When any portion of the motor unit proximal to the muscle fiber degenerates, the muscle fiber will ultimately become denervated. Following such injury, denervation changes develop in muscles according to their physical proximity to the site of the lesion, earliest in those muscles nearest the lesion. Subsequent reinnervation of these muscle fibers occurs by collateral sprouting from the distal terminals of nearby healthy motor units. Following reinnervation, there are fewer motor units than normal, each of which now carries a larger burden of muscle fibers than before.

Myopathic Processes.   In primary disorders of muscle, motor neurons and their axons are intact, but the individual muscle fibers contributing to the motor unit degenerate. Consequently, each motor unit now has a much smaller number of muscle fibers than previously. As opposed to the situation in neurogenic disorders, there is a normal complement of motor units with an abnormally reduced number of muscle fibers in each individual motor unit.

NERVE CONDUCTION STUDIES

Motor Nerve Conduction Studies

To perform motor conduction studies, recording electrodes are placed on the skin overlying the belly of a muscle, and an

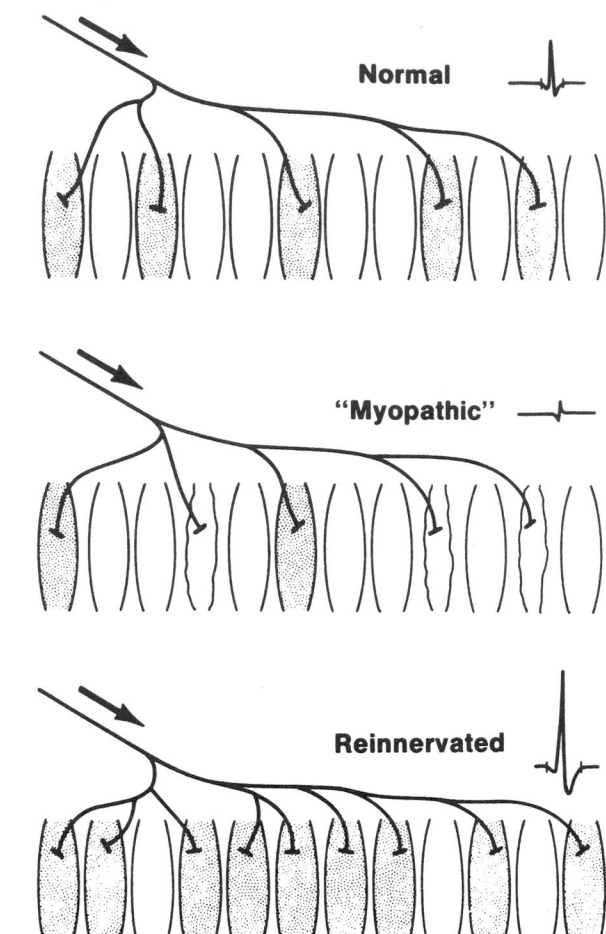

FIG. 20-2.   Normal, myopathic, and neuropathic motor units. Changes in motor unit size and shape are accompanied by similar electromyographic changes. (From Young RR, Jarcho LW, Petajan JH: Laboratory aids in the diagnosis of neuromuscular disease. In Wintrobe MM (ed): Harrison's Principles of Internal Medicine. 7th Ed. McGraw-Hill, New York, 1974, with permission.)

inactive reference electrode is placed on a nearby tendon. The motor nerve innervating this muscle is stimulated with electrical current at low levels, increasing incrementally until the recorded response no longer gains amplitude. This *supramaximal* stimulation ensures that all the motor fibers belonging to the particular muscle have been depolarized. The recorded response is called a compound muscle action potential (CMAP) or M wave. It represents the summation of all muscle fiber action potentials activated by the stimulation of a motor nerve at a given site. Typical motor recordings from a normal subject are shown in Figure 20-3. There are several parameters of importance, which are discussed in the following subsections.

Latency.   The latency is the time, in milliseconds, from stimulation to the onset of the CMAP. The latency reflects the time required for conduction of the stimulus along the length of a nerve, transmission of the neurotransmitter-mediated signal across the neuromuscular junction, and depolarization of the muscle fiber membrane. It is a measure of the conduction time of the fastest conducting fibers only. Distal latency is measured from the stimulation site closest to the muscle. Abnormal prolongation of distal latency reflects focal slowing across the segment, as in compressive neuropathies (e.g., carpal tunnel

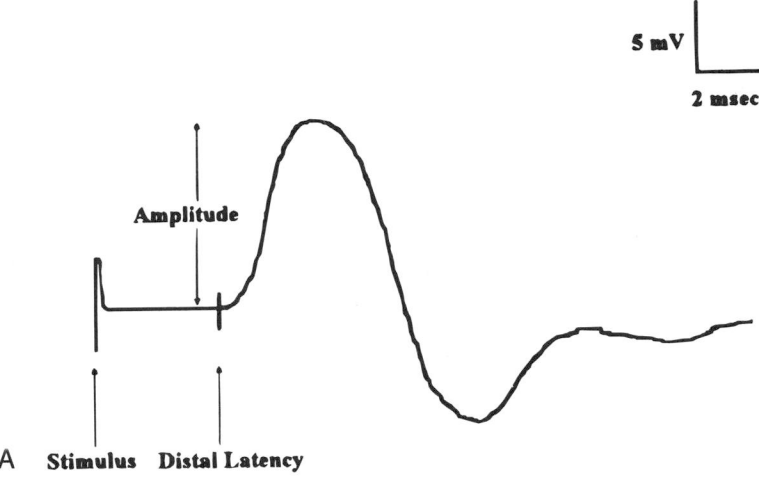

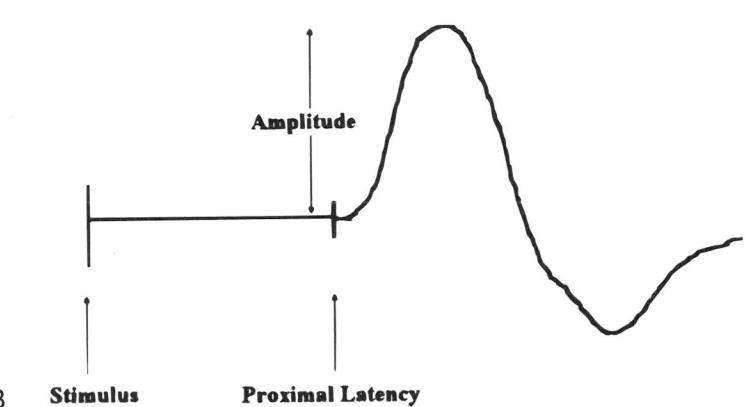

FIG. 20-3. Motor nerve conduction study. Recording of **(A)** the abductor pollicis brevis muscle and stimulating the median nerve at the wrist and **(B)** at the antecubital fossa. The compound muscle action potential (CMAP) represents the summation of individual muscle fiber action potentials stimulated at each site. Amplitude is measured from baseline to peak. Latencies are measured from the stimulus to the onset of the potential and represent the fastest conducting fibers. By stimulating distal and proximal sites, conduction velocity between the two sites can be determined.

syndrome) or demyelinating neuropathies. Less significant prolongation occurs with axonal neuropathies.

Amplitude. The amplitude is the height, in millivolts, of the potential measured from baseline to peak. The CMAP amplitude is a reflection of the number of muscle fibers activated by the stimulus at a particular site. Any disease process that reduces the number of axons or the number of muscle fibers that can be brought to action potential will reduce the CMAP amplitude. Examples include axonal neuropathies, nerve trauma, motor neuron disease, and severe myopathy.

Conduction Velocity. The conduction velocity is the speed, in meters per second, of nerve impulse conduction. For motor studies, a direct measure of conduction velocity along a nerve segment cannot be obtained simply by dividing the distance between stimulation site and recording site by the onset latency, since the time for neuromuscular transmission and muscle membrane depolarization is included in the latency measurement. Therefore two stimulation sites are used, and the distance between proximal and distal stimulation sites divided by the

difference in latencies for the two sites gives a measure of conduction velocity along the nerve segment between them. Again, this value represents the conduction speed of the fastest conducting fibers only. Minimal slowing can occur in the setting of severe axonal loss with dropout of the fastest conducting fibers. Abnormal slowing of conduction velocity, out of proportion to that expected from axonal loss, indicates segmental demyelination.

Sensory Nerve Conduction Studies

In antidromic recordings, the recording electrodes are placed on the skin in an area of innervation of a single sensory nerve, and the nerve is stimulated supramaximally at a site proximal to the recording electrode. The recorded sensory nerve action potential (SNAP) is a summation of the individual action potentials of all the fibers activated. Since sensory nerves normally carry information from the periphery toward the sensory neuron, this setup is in the direction opposite to the natural movement of impulses along a sensory nerve. However, stimulation of a nerve creates a wave of depolarization that travels bidirec-

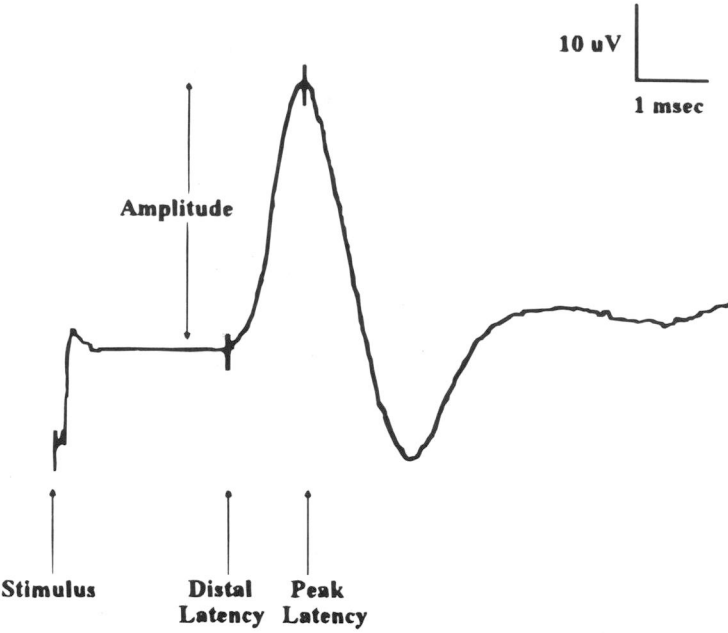

FIG. 20-4. Sensory nerve action potential (SNAP). Recording over the second digit of the hand and stimulating the median nerve at the wrist (antidromic recording). The SNAP represents the summation of all individual sensory fiber action potentials. Amplitude is measured from baseline to peak. Latencies are measured from the stimulus to onset (representing the fastest fibers) and to peak. Conduction velocity can be determined by dividing the distance between the stimulus and recording electrodes by the onset latency.

tionally, allowing recording of sensory impulses distal or proximal to the stimulation site. In the latter situation, the recording technique is called orthodromic. An example of an antidromically recorded potential is shown in Figure 20-4.

The parameters examined are as for motor nerves; however, several important differences should be noted. First, the latency measurement for sensory nerves is a direct reflection of conduction time of the fastest conducting fibers along a given segment, since there is no neuromuscular transmission or muscle fiber activation time. Second, these potentials are considerably smaller, with the amplitude measured in microvolts. This is partly due to the natural amplification of motor signals which results from the innervation of several hundred muscle fibers by one motor nerve fiber. Third, abnormalities in amplitude, latency, and velocity mirror those seen in motor fibers, given similar pathophysiology, with one important caveat: *SNAP amplitudes are not affected by axonal or neuronal lesions proximal to the dorsal root ganglion.* Axonal lesions proximal to the dorsal root ganglion will cause degeneration up to the dorsal root ganglion cell, leaving the dorsal root ganglion and its peripheral axon intact and effectively disconnected from the spinal cord. Thus, if sensory loss is due to a radiculopathy, the recorded SNAP will be normal, no matter how severe the clinical deficit.

Late Responses

F Wave. With supramaximal stimulation of a motor nerve, the depolarizing wave is propagated bidirectionally, and the impulse traveling proximally will reach and activate a small number of anterior horn cells. The resulting action potential is propagated down the motor nerve and creates a small potential of variable configuration occurring many milliseconds after the CMAP. The exact latency and configuration vary as the anterior

horn cells involved in each F response vary from stimulation to stimulation. Figure 20-5 illustrates normal F-wave recordings. The latency of this response measures conduction up and back down the length of the motor nerve from the point of stimulation to the recording site. It indirectly provides a measure of conduction along the proximal portion of the motor nerve. The most commonly measured parameter is the minimum F-wave latency. F waves are most widely used in evaluating patients with demyelinating neuropathies in whom F-wave latencies are prolonged due to demyelination in proximal nerve and root segments.

H Reflex. Another late response, the H reflex, is actually otherwise unrelated to the F response. The H reflex is analogous to the ankle deep tendon reflex and is similarly mediated by the S1 root. Rather than a stretch stimulus, the stimulus is a submaximal electrical current that selectively activates IA afferent sensory fibers. The depolarizing wave travels up the sensory nerve, which activates a motor neuron, creating a reflex contraction of the muscle. The H reflex is measured from the soleus muscle following stimulation of the tibial nerve at the knee. It is not readily obtainable from other sites in normal adults. Unilateral abnormalities are indicative of an S1 radiculopathy. Bilateral abnormalities may represent bilateral S1 radiculopathies or, more commonly, peripheral neuropathy.

ELECTROMYOGRAPHY

Recording Methods and Normal Findings

The EMG (electromyogram) is a recording of the electrical activity in muscle fiber membranes which provides information about the muscle and related nerves. In a routine examination, a small needle electrode is inserted into various muscles, and activity is observed in a number of sites within each muscle.

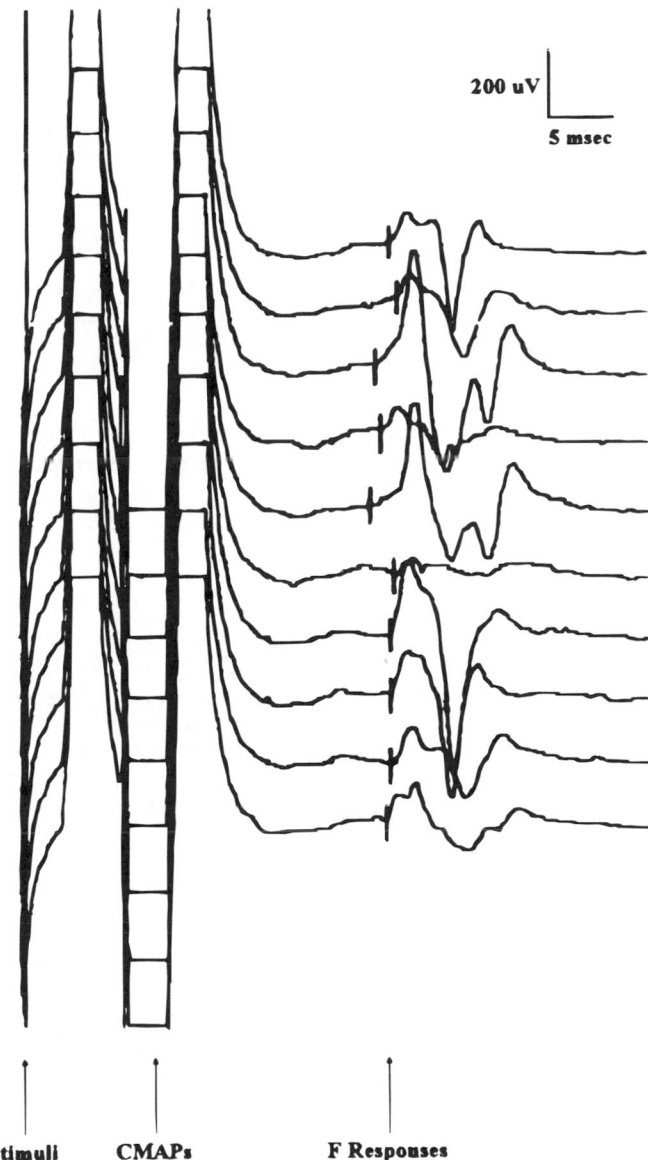

Spontaneous Activity. Normal muscle is silent at rest except when the needle is in the vicinity of the neuromuscular junction. Here, endplate activity may normally be recorded. This physiologic spontaneous activity is of little importance except that it may be mistaken for abnormal spontaneous activity.

Motor Unit Potentials and Firing Pattern

With minimal voluntary contraction of the muscle, motor unit action potentials (MUAPs) are recorded. MUAPs are the summated action potentials of 10 to 20 muscle fibers derived from a single motor unit near the needle electrode. These complex potentials have a definable duration, amplitude, and number of phases. Normal values for MUAP parameters vary from one muscle to another and with different age groups. In addition to their configuration, MUAPs are characterized by their firing pattern. Although no pattern of abnormalities is pathognomonic of a specific disease process, it is usually possible to define MUAP abnormalities as neurogenic or myopathic (see below). Figure 20-6 shows a normal MUAP and its parameters. Table 20-1 outlines changes in these parameters in neurogenic and myopathic lesions. The individual parameters of a MUAP are discussed in the following subsections.

Amplitude. The amplitude is highly variable and dependent primarily on the distance between the recording electrode and the actively firing muscle fibers. Only a small percentage of fibers in a given motor unit contribute to the MUAP amplitude. Those not within the immediate vicinity of the tip of the recording electrode are not recorded. Amplitude increases with proximity to the electrode and with increasing number or diameter of muscle fibers (as in neurogenic disorders). Amplitude decreases with decreasing number of muscle fibers (as in myopathies) and with increasing distance from the electrode.

Duration. The parameter of duration probably best reflects the size of the motor unit territory, that is, the number of muscle fibers innervated by a single motor unit. Duration is increased in neurogenic disorders in which healthy motor units reinnervate

FIG. 20-5. F Responses (10 rastered traces). Recording the abductor pollicis brevis muscle and stimulating the median nerve at the wrist. The F responses are late potentials which occur after the compound muscle action potential (CMAP) resulting from antidromic travel to the anterior horn cell in the spinal cord and back again. (Note the gain and sweep speed required to measure the F responses and the resulting distortion of the CMAP potentials.) Each F response varies slightly in configuration and latency, representing a different population of motor fibers.

Findings are observed during needle insertion, with the muscle at rest, and during voluntary contraction. The selection of muscles for study is usually made by the electromyographer based on the clinical question and the prior nerve conduction and EMG findings.

Insertional Activity. Mechanical deformation of the muscle membrane by the needle causes brief discharge of the muscle fiber, normally lasting less than 500 ms after needle movement ceases. Insertional activity is increased in disorders that cause abnormal excitability of muscle membrane, most commonly in neurogenic disorders. Decreased insertional activity results from muscle fibrosis or fatty replacement, which may be present in long-standing muscle disorders, such as dystrophies.

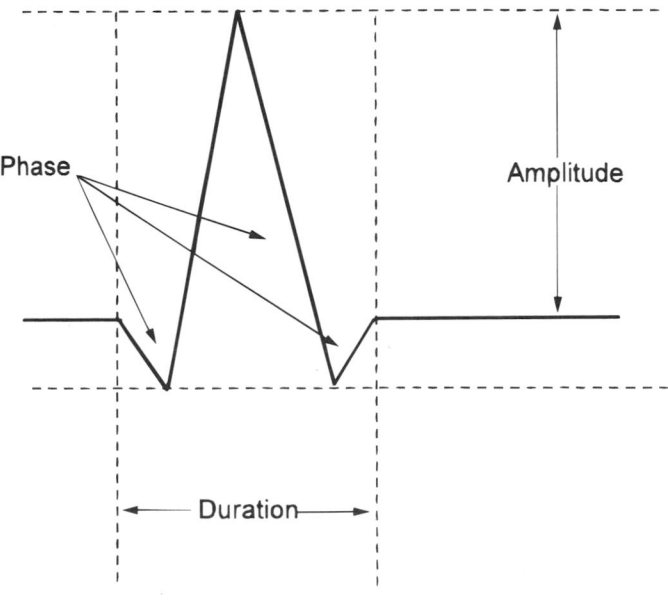

FIG. 20-6. Motor unit action potential parameters.

TABLE 20-1. EMG Features of Neurogenic and Myopathic Disorders

Lesion	Insertional Activity	Spontaneous Activity	MUAP Amplitude	MUAP Duration	MUAP Phases	Activation	Recruitment
Neurogenic							
Denervation							
Acute (<3 wk)	NL	None	NL	NL	NL	NL	Reduced
Subacute (3 wk–3 mo)	Increased	Fibs, PSW	NL	NL	NL	NL	Reduced
Chronic reinnervation (3–6 mo)	NL or increased	None[a]	High	Increased	Polyphasic	NL	Reduced
Myopathic							
Inflammatory	Increased	Fibs, PSW, CRDs	Low	Short	Polyphasic	NL	Early
Noninflammatory	Normal	None	Low	Short	Polyphasic	NL	Early

Abbreviations: MUAP, motor unit action potential; NL, normal; Fibs, fibrillations; PSW, positive sharp waves; CRDS, complex repetitive discharges.
[a] May see Fibs and PSW if ongoing denervation is occurring.

denervated muscle fibers, consequently increasing their motor unit territories. Duration is shortened in myopathic disorders, since the number of muscle fibers per motor unit is less than normal. This parameter is more reliable than amplitude as a measure of abnormality, since it is less dependent on needle placement.

Phases. The number of phases is equal to the number of baseline crossings plus one (see Fig. 20-6). This parameter is a measure of the synchronicity of firing of the muscle fibers contributing to the CMAP. Normally, the number of phases equals four or less; anything greater is considered polyphasic. Polyphasic potentials may occur normally in up to approximately 10 percent of motor units. Increased polyphasia occurs commonly in both neurogenic disorders with reinnervation and myopathic disorders.

Firing Pattern. With voluntary contraction, force increases in two ways. First, the motor unit that initially fires increases its *firing rate* to about 10 to 15 per second (Hz). Second, at that point the firing frequency stabilizes, and force is increased further by the *recruitment* of another motor unit that fires at a rate similar to the first. Motor units are recruited in an orderly arrangement according to their size, with the smaller motor units being recruited first. Another term related to firing rate is *activation*. Activation requires voluntary effort and depends on the central control of movement. Thus, activation may be abnormal in upper motor neuron lesions or with poor effort. If activation is poor enough, the firing rate will remain below that required to recruit second and third motor units. In such cases, determination of the recruitment pattern becomes extremely dif-

ficult. Abnormal recruitment is distinct from abnormal activation and is an important hallmark of neurogenic lesions. Characteristic changes in recruitment actually help differentiate neurogenic from myopathic lesions, as discussed in the following section.

EMG Abnormalities

Abnormal Spontaneous Discharges. Except for endplate activity, all spontaneous activity occurring with the muscle at rest is abnormal. A variety of different discharge patterns are described. Table 20-2 outlines common abnormal EMG activity observed during rest. Figure 20-7 illustrates denervation potentials in the form of fibrillation potentials and positive sharp waves.

Abnormal Motor Units (Neurogenic Versus Myopathic Lesions). Individual characteristics of the MUAP may be affected similarly by these two types of lesions; however, the overall picture often defines an EMG abnormality as either neurogenic or myopathic. When the distinction is unclear, usually the recruitment pattern is of greatest relevance. Table 20-1 outlines the characteristic EMG features of neurogenic and myopathic lesions. Figure 20-8 compares normal, neurogenic, and myopathic MUAPs.

MYOPATHIC LESIONS. Myopathic MUAPs have a small amplitude and short duration and are highly polyphasic. Each motor unit has lost individual muscle fibers so that increasing force requires activation of more motor units than previously. There is no shortage of motor units so that *recruitment* occurs *earlier* than normal.

TABLE 20-2. Characteristics of EMG Activity Recorded at Rest (Spontaneous Activity)

Activity	Normal/Abnormal	Source	Associations
End plate Activity	Normal	Miniature endplate potentials (neuromuscular junction)	Normal finding
Fibrillations and positive sharp waves	Abnormal	Spontaneous discharge of individual muscle fibers	Neurogenic lesions with denervation Inflammatory myopathies
Complex repetitive discharges ("CRDs")	Abnormal	Spontaneous repetitive discharge of grouped muscle fibers	Neurogenic lesions with denervation Inflammatory myopathies (usually in chronic lesions)
Fasciculations	Abnormal	Spontaneous discharge of motor unit	Lower motor neuron lesions, particularly of anterior horn cell Radiculopathies
Myotonia	Abnormal	Spontaneous repetitive discharge of muscle fiber	Myotonic dystrophy Myotonia congenita, paramyotonia Inflammatory myopathies Acid maltase deficiency
Myokymia	Abnormal	Repetitive grouped discharge of motor units	Radiation plexopathy Demyelinating neuropathy Compressive neuropathy

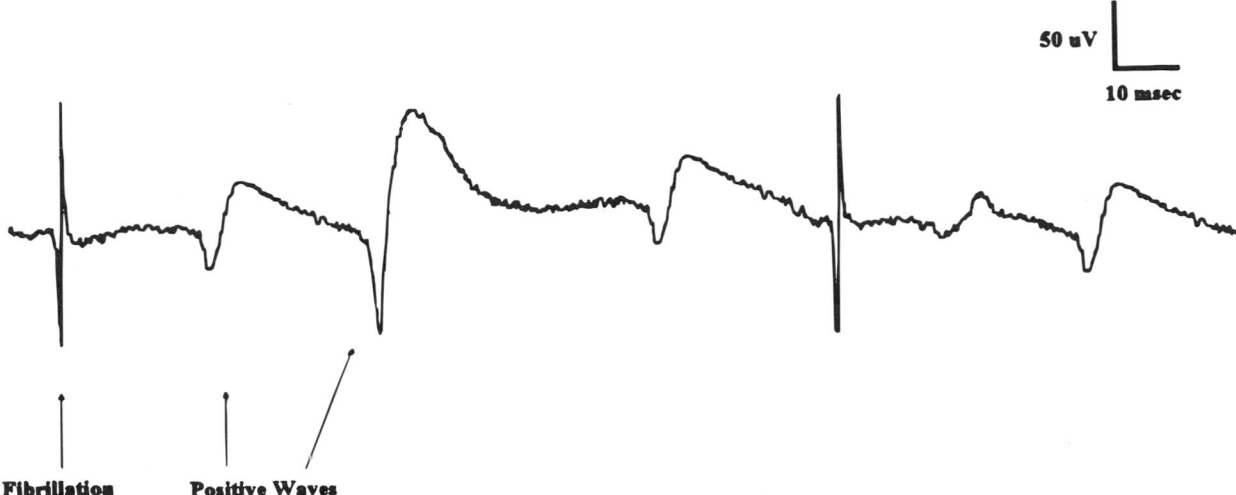

50 uV

10 msec

Fibrillation   Positive Waves

FIG. 20-7. Denervating potentials on EMG. When denervated, individual muscle fibers spontaneously depolarize. They may take the form of either fibrillation potentials (spike waveform) or positive waves (abrupt positive downward deflection followed by a slow negative phase). Although classically associated with neuropathic disease, they may also be seen in myopathies, especially inflammatory myopathies.

NEUROGENIC LESIONS. The hallmark of neurogenic lesions is *reduced* recruitment. Since motor units have been lost, there are fewer available for recruitment. The remaining motor units fire at an abnormally rapid rate in an effort to increase force. In severe lesions a single motor unit may fire at rates of 40 to 50 Hz. Changes associated with denervation and subsequent reinnervation occur over a predictable time course, thus EMG findings are dependent on timing of the study in relationship to the lesion. Reduced recruitment is the only feature that is present acutely. *Denervation* is characterized by abnormal spontaneous activity. Following *reinnervation,* motor units have high amplitude and long duration and are polyphasic.

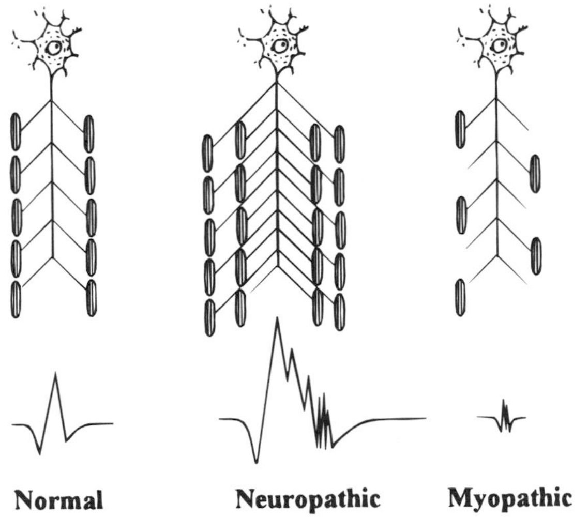

Time Course of Denervation-Reinnervation. Following axonal injury, muscles will become denervated according to their proximity to the injury. In a nerve root lesion, denervation will be present (in the form of fibrillation potentials and positive sharp waves) in the related paraspinal muscles within 7 to 10 days; in the proximal limb muscles in 2 weeks, and in the distal limb muscles in 3 weeks. Reinnervation changes require approximately 3 to 6 months to develop. The presence of abundant fibrillation potentials in a muscle indicates ongoing axonal loss. One exception occurs following spinal surgical procedures in which the paraspinal examination may continue to show denervation changes for years, which are nonspecific and do not necessarily imply ongoing root involvement.

ELECTRODIAGNOSIS OF COMMON NEUROMUSCULAR DISORDERS

Compressive Neuropathies

Carpal Tunnel Syndrome. When questioning carpal tunnel syndrome, the goals are to localize the median neuropathy to the wrist and to rule out other diagnostic possibilities. The differential diagnosis includes more proximal median nerve compression, upper trunk brachial plexopathy, and C6 radiculopathy. The latter may co-occur with the carpal tunnel syndrome, creating a "double crush." Characteristic findings from nerve conduction studies (NCS) and EMG include

NCS: There is focal slowing of median motor conduction across the carpal tunnel (i.e., wrist) segment. Distal motor latency may be prolonged. Sensory conduction velocity may be slowed across the wrist. Reduction in median SNAP or CMAP amplitudes implies axonal loss.

EMG: Ongoing denervation in the abductor pollicis brevis indicates significant, progressive axonal loss. Median innervated C6 muscles should be screened to eliminate the diagnosis of a double crush.

Normal   Neuropathic   Myopathic

FIG. 20-8. Motor unit action potentials (MUAP) on EMG. A MUAP represents the depolarization of all muscle fibers within one motor unit (i.e., one anterior horn cell, its axon, and all muscle fibers connected to it). Most normal MUAPs are within 5 to 15 ms in duration and have three phases. In neuropathic disease, MUAPs become large, long, and polyphasic, representing reinnervation. In myopathic disease, the MUAP becomes smaller, briefer, and polyphasic as individual muscle fibers die out or become dysfunctional.

Ulnar Neuropathy at the Elbow. When ulnar neuropathy at the elbow is suspected, the goals are to localize the ulnar lesion to the elbow. The differential diagnosis includes lower trunk brachial plexopathy (i.e., neurogenic thoracic outlet syndrome) and C8-T1 radiculopathy. Characteristic findings include

NCS: There is focal slowing of conduction velocity across the elbow segment with or without conduction block. With the elbow flexed to 90 degrees, a dropoff in conduction velocity of more than 10 m/s is abnormal. The amplitude of the ulnar SNAP is frequently reduced.

EMG: There are signs of denervation and reinnervation in ulnar-innervated hand and forearm muscles. Median and radial innervated C8-T1 muscles are screened to rule out a C8 radiculopathy.

Peroneal Neuropathy at the Knee. When evaluating suspected peroneal neuropathy at the knee, the goals are to localize the lesion to the peroneal nerve segment at the level of the fibular neck. The differential diagnosis includes sciatic nerve lesions, lumbosacral plexopathy, and L5 radiculopathy. Characteristic findings include

NCS: There is reduced peroneal CMAP amplitude associated with abnormal slowing of motor conduction velocity across the fibular neck segment (dropoff of greater than 10m/s). If the superficial peroneal division is involved, SNAP amplitude will be reduced. Tibial motor NCS are normal.

EMG: Denervation and reinnervation changes are present in peroneal innervated muscles of the lower leg. L5 muscles innervated by nerves other than the peroneal are screened to rule out a more proximal lesion.

Polyneuropathy

In evaluating polyneuropathies by EMG, the goals are primarily to determine whether the neuropathy is axonal or demyelinating in nature.

Axonal Neuropathies. Axonal neuropathies are characterized by a distal predominance of axonal loss. The electrophysiologic findings in generalized sensorimotor neuropathy include

NCS: There are reductions of SNAP and CMAP amplitudes distally (i.e., lower extremity greater than upper) with relative preservation of the conduction velocities such that values below 75 percent lower limit of normal are rare, even with marked reduction in amplitude. F responses are normal or mildly prolonged, as are distal motor latencies. H reflexes are symmetrically prolonged or absent, corresponding to the severity of the neuropathy.

EMG: There are EMG signs of reinnervation which demonstrate a distal-to-proximal gradient of severity. Ongoing denervation with a similar distal predominance is present in more severe cases.

Demyelinating Neuropathies. Demyelinating neuropathies are characterized by segmental demyelination, which is best reflected in the nerve conduction studies:

NCS: There is marked slowing of the conduction velocity to less than 75 percent of the lower limit of normal, which may be accompanied by prolongation of distal motor laten-

cies, dispersion of the CMAP, and conduction block. SNAP amplitudes are usually reduced and slowed. Marked reduction in CMAP amplitude indicates significant axonal loss or conduction block and implies a worse prognosis. F wave latencies are markedly prolonged or unobtainable.

EMG: Recruitment is reduced in proportion to the severity of weakness. Denervation may be present in severely affected nerves, if there is secondary axonal degeneration.

Radiculopathy

When considering a possible radiculopathy, the goals are to localize the lesion to the nerve root (versus the plexus or nerve) and to determine its distribution (e.g., L4-L5, L5-S1). Characteristically:

NCS: The CMAP amplitudes may be reduced, if recorded from the appropriate myotomal territory. However SNAPs recorded from an area of sensory loss will always be *normal* in a lesion proximal to the dorsal root ganglion.

EMG: There are denervation and reinnervation signs in the limb in the appropriate myotomal distribution. Additionally, paraspinal muscles show ongoing denervation (fibrillations) at the appropriate root level.

Myopathy

In myopathies, the nerve conduction studies are usually normal, although CMAP amplitudes may be reduced if there is significant distal involvement. The EMG is characteristic and shows small-amplitude, short-duration MUAPs that are highly polyphasic and recruited early with minimal voluntary contraction. The interference pattern is full but of low amplitude. Ongoing denervation (fibrillations, positive sharp waves, and complex repetitive discharges) is often present in inflammatory myopathies.

Motor Neuron Disease

In motor neuron disease, the anterior horn cell is the primary site of pathology. As with all lesions proximal to the dorsal root ganglion, the sensory system is normal on electrophysiologic testing, as it is clinically in this case. The findings include

NCS: Sensory nerve conduction studies are normal. CMAP amplitudes may be reduced or normal with no significant slowing of conduction velocity.

EMG: Ongoing denervation and reinnervation in multiple root distributions must be present in at least three limbs to diagnose a generalized motor neuron disorder.

TESTS OF NEUROMUSCULAR TRANSMISSION

Repetitive Stimulation Studies

Repetitive stimulation studies are the most common electrodiagnostic technique for evaluation of neuromuscular transmission disorders. When testing for postsynaptic disorders (e.g., myasthenia gravis), the technique is similar to motor nerve conduction studies. Rather than a single supramaximal stimulus, trains of repetitive stimuli are delivered at a rate of 3 stimuli per second with 6 to 10 stimuli in a train. For each train of stimuli, the CMAP amplitude of the first response is compared

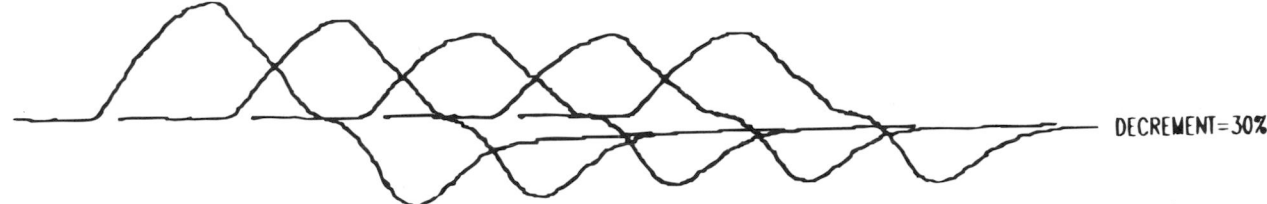

DECREMENT=30%

FIG. 20-9. Repetitive nerve stimulation. In normal subjects, repetitive motor nerve stimulation at 3 Hz results in no decrement of the compound muscle action potential. In disorders of neuromuscular transmission, decrements greater than 10 percent are typically seen. The figure shows abnormal decrement stimulating the ulnar nerve in a patient with myasthenia gravis.

to that of the fifth response and the percent decrement is measured. Decrements of *greater than 10 percent* are abnormal and are characteristic of postsynaptic transmission disorders of which myasthenia gravis is the prototype (Fig. 20-9). The sensitivity of the test is increased if performed after 1 minute of exercise with the maximal decrement usually seen at 3 to 4 minutes after exercise. The greatest diagnostic yield is obtained if a weak muscle is examined. The trapezius is often chosen for this reason.

Single-Fiber Electromyography

The specialized technique of single-fiber electromyography is highly sensitive for detecting neuromuscular transmission defects. Special expertise and equipment are required, and the study may not be available at all centers. The electrode records simultaneously from a pair of single muscle fibers belonging to the same motor unit and measures the amount of variability between discharges, or *jitter*. Jitter is a reflection of neuromuscular transmission time and is abnormally increased in disorders of neuromuscular transmission. While highly sensitive, it is nonspecific and may be abnormal in neurogenic lesions.

Electrodiagnosis of Common Disorders

The electrodiagnostic approach varies considerably, depending on whether one is looking for a postsynaptic neuromuscular transmission disorder, as in myasthenia gravis, or a presynaptic disorder, as in the Lambert-Eaton myasthenic syndrome (LEMS).

Myasthenia Gravis.   In generalized myasthenia gravis, motor nerve conduction studies and EMG are usually normal, although CMAP amplitudes may rarely be reduced, and EMG may have a myopathic appearance. Repetitive stimulation studies will usually show an abnormal decremental response to 3 Hz stimulation. The diagnostic yield is greater in those with obvious weakness; therefore, it may be helpful to withhold anticholinesterase medications prior to testing. Single-fiber EMG studies show abnormally increased jitter.

Lambert-Eaton Myasthenic Syndrome.   When testing for LEMS, one can usually find abnormalities in any muscle examined. Routine motor nerve conduction studies are often suggestive of the diagnosis, since CMAP amplitudes are universally low. EMG may show myopathic changes or may be normal. Repetitive stimulation studies are not routinely used for diagnosis, unless a patient is unable to cooperate. If necessary, the stimulation is carried out at rapid rates of 30 to 50 Hz, looking

for an abnormal increment or post-tetanic facilitation in the CMAP amplitude of greater than 100 percent. The preferred method of electrodiagnosis involves recording a single CMAP before and after 10 seconds of maximal voluntary contraction. A dramatic increase in the recorded CMAP amplitude of 100 percent or more is diagnostic. Single-fiber EMG studies are usually not necessary for diagnosis. *Botulism*, another common presynaptic neuromuscular transmission disorder, has an electrophysiologic picture similar to LEMS.

UTILITY AND LIMITATIONS OF ELECTRODIAGNOSTIC STUDIES

There are several ways that a referring physician can improve the results obtained from electrodiagnostic testing. First, it is important to carefully select patients who are appropriately diagnosed by the tests performed in the EMG laboratory. Central or upper motor neuron disorders are not usually diagnosed by nerve conduction or EMG studies. Timing of the study in relationship to injury is also important. Localization of nerve injuries may be quite difficult if studies are done before wallerian degeneration is complete (5 to 7 days) and the full extent of the lesion may still not be appreciated until denervation develops on EMG (3 to 6 weeks). The appropriate study is best determined by a clear clinical question, as in "question right carpal tunnel syndrome versus C6 radiculopathy," as opposed to something vague, such as "arm pain." Often, a brief capsule of the history and examination are all that is needed, as in "proximal weakness, arms and legs." Finally, it is best to prepare patients for the study by letting them know what is involved and that it may be moderately uncomfortable.

While electrodiagnostic testing is very valuable to the clinician and in some cases is diagnostic, there are frequently situations in which studies are abnormal but not clearly localizing. In those cases, the electromyographer reports the physiologic findings, and it is up to the clinician to interpret the results in light of the clinical picture. The EMG should always be considered an extension of, not a substitute for, the clinical evaluation.

SUGGESTED READINGS

Brown WF: The Physiological and Technical Basis of Electromyography. Boston: Butterworth-Heinemann Publishers, 1984
Brown WF, Bolton CF: Clinical Electromyography. 2nd Ed. Butterworth-Heinemann, Boston, 1993
Keesey JC: AAEE Minimonograph #33: Electrodiagnostic approach to defects of neuromuscular transmission. Muscle Nerve 12:613, 1989
Kimura J: Electrodiagnosis in Diseases of Nerve and Muscle. 2nd Ed. FA Davis, Philadelphia, 1989

Oh SJ: Clinical Electromyography: Nerve Conduction Studies. 2nd Ed. Williams & Wilkins, Baltimore, 1993

Sethi RK, Thompson LL: The Electromyographer's Handbook. 2nd Ed. Little, Brown, Boston, 1989

21. NEUROIMAGING: RADIOLOGY, MAGNETIC RESONANCE IMAGING, POSITRON EMISSION TOMOGRAPHY, AND SINGLE-PHOTON EMISSION COMPUTED TOMOGRAPHY

AMIR A. ZAMANI

Radiologic methods of investigating neurologic disease have improved significantly over the past two decades. Invasive procedures have been replaced with less invasive and more accurate diagnostic tests. These better and safer techniques and equipment permit faster and more accurate diagnosis and therapy.

COMPUTED TOMOGRAPHY

Background and Technique

The technology of computed tomography (CT) is the result of ingenious work by Hounsfield in the EMI laboratory in England. The equipment became available for diagnostic testing in 1973, a year after Hounsfield announced his invention of "computerized axial transverse scanning" at the meeting of the British Institute of Radiology. CT has had an enormous effect on the radiologic evaluation of neurologic disease. Before CT, the only radiologic tests for the brain were pneumoencephalography, angiography, and radionuclide brain scanning, which had the disadvantages of being invasive, insensitive, or nonspecific. For the first time a diagnostic test provided direct images of brain pathology in a noninvasive way. Within a few years, CT scanning of the head and body would become routine in many hospitals around the globe.

A simplified explanation of CT scanning is as follows: A collimated beam of x-ray photons enter the body and are attenuated by being absorbed as photons interact with the matter. A detector on the opposite side of the body receives the attenuated beam. The x-ray source and the detector are coupled together and rotate about the body. Therefore a thin cross section of the body is exposed to the x-ray beam from different "vantage points," and with each exposure the detectors receive the attenuated beam. Powerful computers attached to the detectors calculate the attenuation at different points on this section and display these as a two-dimensional picture. On this picture, contrast between adjacent tissues represents their relative attenuation properties. Intravenous contrast injection enhances the

inherent absorptive differences. At the same time, it adds a small risk to an otherwise relatively safe procedure. Minor reactions include nausea and hives. More severe reactions include asthma, laryngeal edema, and anaphylaxis. Death is very rare (1 in 60,000 injections). Deterioration of renal function may be seen in patients with preexisting renal disease, especially in those with diabetes. Radiation dose received by the part being examined is usually quite small.

Clinical Applications

Despite its power, cranial CT has limitations, including poor visualization of the posterior cranial fossa, poor sensitivity to demyelating processes, and nonspecificity of many CT findings. Obtaining images in coronal and sagittal planes is difficult.

In patients with head trauma, brain contusions and extra- and intracerebral hematomas are easily identified. Fractures of the calvarium may be visible. Midline shifts and subfalcine herniations can be measured, and findings may suggest transtentorial herniation. The fear that an isodense subdural collection may be missed is exaggerated. The diagnosis of diffuse axonal injury is difficult from CT scans, however, and in patients with sustained mental status change after head trauma, magnetic resonance imaging (MRI) of the brain is indicated.

CT is usually the first radiologic test employed in patients who have had a cerebrovascular events. The method is very sensitive to subarachnoid hemorrhage (90 percent are detected in the first 24 hours) and intracerebral hemorrhage (Fig. 21-1). About 40 percent of bland infarctions may not be seen in the first 24 hours. A brainstem or small cortical infarct may not be detected at all. Hemorrhagic conversion of a bland infarct is believed to occur in 20 to 25 percent of infarcts followed by CT scan.

CT scanning and MRI are the two competing tests for patients suspected of harboring a brain tumor. The overall sensitivity of MRI is probably higher, although CT scanning is cheaper, more easily available, and more sensitive to calcification. At times, detection of calcification has significant diagnostic value (in craniopharyngiomas, meningiomas, dermoids, and in nonneoplastic conditions, such as aneurysms and cysticercosis). Small posterior fossa tumors (e.g., small intracanalicular acoustic schwannomas and small cerebellar metastases) may be missed on a CT scan.

In patients with infection, most intracranial parenchymal loci are detected. The appearance of the CT scan is not diagnostic in many cases, however. Meningeal infection, with few exceptions (tuberculosis, syphilis), is poorly detected. Detection of lesions in herpes simplex encephalitis may lag up to 5 days behind the onset of symptoms.

In patients with dementia, CT scanning is able to rule out hydrocephalus and to detect infarctions, intracranial collections, and mass lesions. In patients with brain atrophy, the pattern of brain shrinkage may allow a more specific diagnosis.

Abdominal and pelvic CT scans are useful tests in patients presenting with plexopathy: Psoas abscess, retroperitoneal hemorrhage, and abdominal and pelvic masses may be detected. Radiologic tests do not reveal any specific findings in many patients with plexopathy.

CT scanning of the lumbar spine is a useful diagnostic test in patients with herniated lumbar disks or lumbar stenosis. Disk hernations, symptomatic or asymptomatic, can be easily detected. However, questions regarding the metastatic involvement of the spine are best answered by MRI.

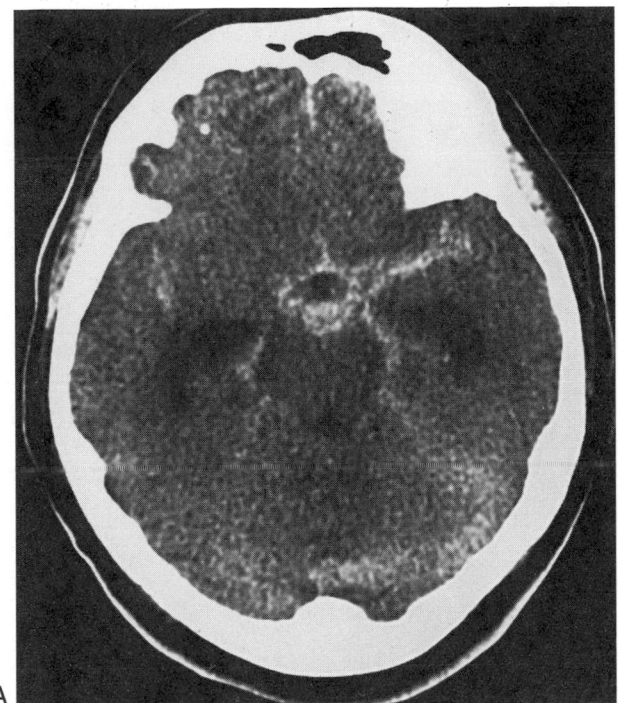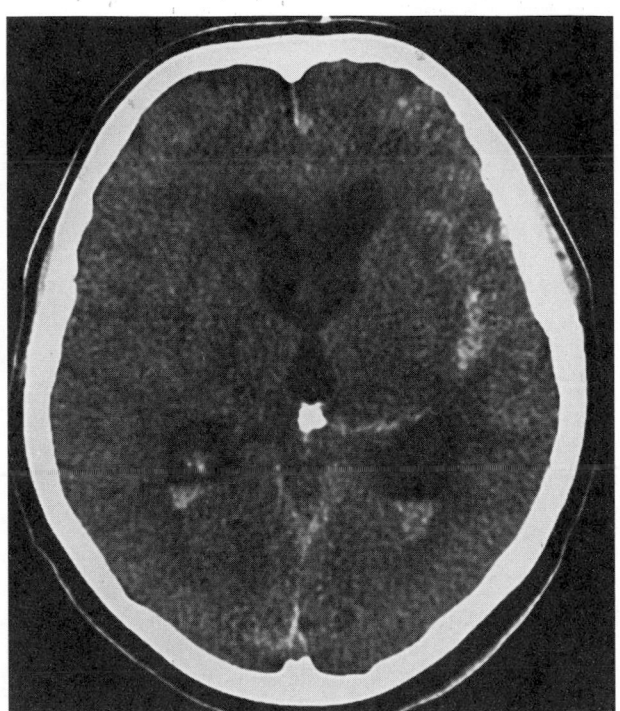

FIG. 21-1.   **(A & B)** CT scan of subarachnoid hemorrhage. Blood is seen in basal cisterns and ventricles. There is moderate hydrocephalus.

MAGNETIC RESONANCE IMAGING

Background and Technique

The phenomenon of nuclear magnetic resonance (NMR) was discovered by Block and Purcell in 1946 and earned them the Nobel Prize in 1951. For years, the technique was used in spectral analysis of small samples. Medical MRI is fairly new, and owes its status today to the pioneering work of Damadian and Lauterbur. Widespread use of MRI would not have been possible if the medical profession had not had the CT experience earlier.

The MRI technique uses a strong magnetic field (0.25 to 1.5 T) with which a small number of protons (being small magnets themselves) become aligned. Then external energy is added to the system in the form of radiowaves and imparts a higher (and unstable) energy status to the protons. As the protons return to their more stable energy level, the surplus energy is dispersed as radiowave signals. The location of the protons in the body is encoded in the wavelength of the emitted signal. By adding three different magnetic gradients (in three different directions) to the main magnetic field, this location can be exactly determined. Using the Fourier transform technique, an image is then produced.

The speed with which a sample becomes magnetized and the signal decays are related to T1 and T2 relaxation times of the sample. Every magnetic resonance image has T1 and T2 information; by changing imaging parameters, one can produce predominantly T1, predominantly T2, and intermediate (spin density) images. Cerebrospinal fluid is dark on T1 and bright on T2 images. Fat is bright on T1-weighted images but becomes darker with increasing T2 weighting. Most brain lesions are low intensity on T1 and high intensity (bright) on T2 images.

Clinical Applications

MRI is not subject to many of the limitations of CT. Images of the posterior fossa are very clear and artifact-free. Obtaining images in coronal or sagittal planes is difficult with CT; MRI can be obtained effortlessly in any plane.

One of the greatest advantages of MRI is its ability to provide images of flowing blood. Magnetic resonance angiography (MRA), developed in the past few years, is now able to provide diagnostic quality images in many patients. In addition to narrowing at the carotid bifurcation (and the rare tandem lesion in the siphon), MRA can demonstrate aneurysms larger than 3 to 4 mm and different components of arteriovenous malformations.

The disadvantages of MRI include its relative insensitivity to small calcification, poor delineation of bony structure, and expense. CT imaging and interpretation are relatively easy to learn, but MRI interpretation is considerably more complex and requires more in-depth knowledge and effort.

MRI is very sensitive to changes seen in multiple sclerosis. In one study, 95 to 99 percent of patients had positive brain MRI scans (Fig. 21-2). A negative study of brains, however, does not exclude this diagnosis. Gadolinium-enhanced study reveals enhancement in the more active lesions.

About 80 percent of acute infarctions can be detected on the first day. Lesions can be detected earlier by MRI than by CT scans, but it still takes a few hours for the lesions to be seen. Perfusion-diffusion MRI may allow earlier detection of an infarct and assessment of its size. Brainstem infarcts are shown with relative ease. Concomitant MRA delineates carotid bifurcation, siphon, basilar artery, or middle cerebral artery narrowing. The most commonly used MRA technique (time-of-flight) frequently overestimates and, less frequently, underestimates narrowing at the bifurcation. If MRA and Doppler ultrasonography results concur, many centers will not need additional conventional angiography.

Very early cerebral hemorrhage is hard to differentiate from other lesions on MRI and is much easier to detect on CT scans. The best detection rate of early subarachnoid hemorrhage by

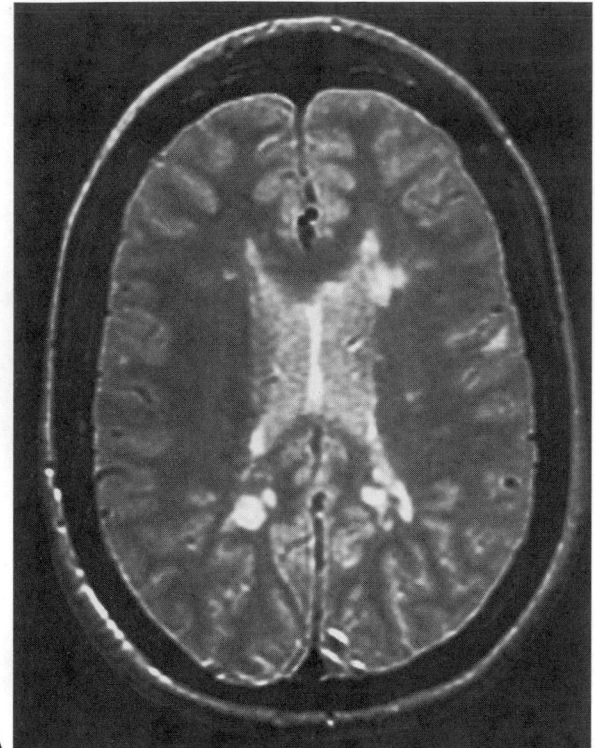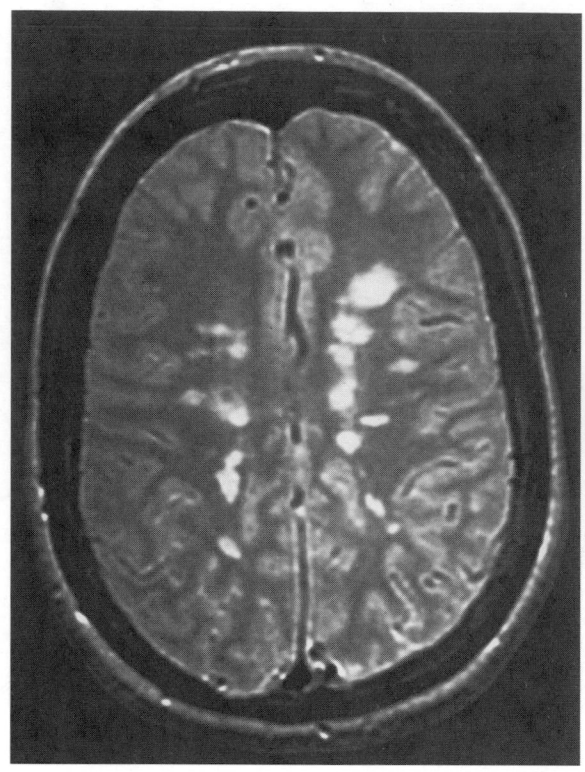

A

B

FIG. 21-2.   (A or B) MRI in multiple sclerosis. Numerous discrete foci of increased signal intensity are seen on these intermediate images in periventricular and subcortical regions.

MRI is 50 percent—far below the performance of CT. Conversely, MRI detects later products of hemorrhage (deoxyhemoglobin, methemoglobin, and hemosiderin) without difficulty (Fig. 21-3). Subacute intracerebral hemorrhage can present with a confusing CT picture, difficult to differentiate from abscess and tumor. Diagnosis of subacute hemorrhages with MRI is relatively easy. The angiographically occult cerebrovascular malformation (OCVM) is usually a cavernous angioma; these lesions have characteristic MRI features (Fig. 21-4).

After acute head trauma, a patient is usually studied by CT scanning. MRI examination may not be possible, since patients are frequently unstable or uncooperative. CT scans are also more sensitive in the detection of early products of hemorrhage. MRI is able to detect all lesions secondary to trauma (with the exception of skull fractures) and definitely is more sensitive than CT scans in the detection of diffuse axonal injury.

In patients with brain tumors, gadolinium-enhanced MRI is superior to contrast-enhanced CT in demonstrating small extra-axial posterior fossa tumors and meningeal carcinomatosis. By obtaining three-dimensional reconstructions and images in three orthogonal planes, the spatial relations of a tumor are well demonstrated. This information may be helpful to a neurosurgeon in choosing the best possible approach to a deep lesion.

Intracranial infection can be studied successfully with MRI, but a specific diagnosis may not be possible in many cases. For example, secure differentiation of lesions due to toxoplasmosis from those due to other infections and lymphoma in patients with AIDS may not be possible from MRI findings alone. Meningeal involvement is easier to detect on MRI than on CT scans. In herpes simplex encephalitis, the MRI changes (foci of increased intensity in temporal and inferior frontal lobes) appear earlier (2 days vs 3 to 5 days) than the changes on CT scans. In addition, MRI is more sensitive and more accurate in demonstrating the extent of the lesions.

MRI abnormalities (increased T2 intensity in basal ganglia and thalami) have been reported in Creutzfeldt-Jakob disease. Hydrocephalus, multiple infarcts, and intracranial fluid collections and mass lesions can be seen or ruled out in patients presenting with dementia. Abnormalities of iron deposition have been described in patients with Parkinson's disease (excessive iron accumulation in the putamen) and Parkinson-like syndromes.

In few other areas has MRI had more impact than in the spinal cord. Areas of demyelination, myelitis, traumatic cord lesions, syrinx, and tumors can be successfully demonstrated. By judicious use of the imaging sequences, location of an extramedullary (extradural vs intradural) lesion can be correctly appreciated (Fig. 21-5). Cord compression is no longer an indication for emergency myelography; this can be assessed satisfactorily with MRI.

Patients with cardiac pacemakers, metal workers who may have tiny ferromagnetic fragments in their eyes, and pregnant women in their first trimester are usually excluded from MRI examinations. Extreme care must be exercised to avoid subjecting a patient with an unknown intracranial aneurysm clip to a strong magnetic field. A few instances of fatal outcome have already been reported. Gadolinium enhancement is comparatively safer than contrast enhancement on CT scans. The most common adverse reactions are headaches, coldness at the injection site, and nausea. Anaphylactoid reactions are extremely rare. Caution should be exercised in administering gadolinium in patients with hemolytic anemia, pregnant women, and children less than 2 years old, since the safety of this drug has not been established in these patients.

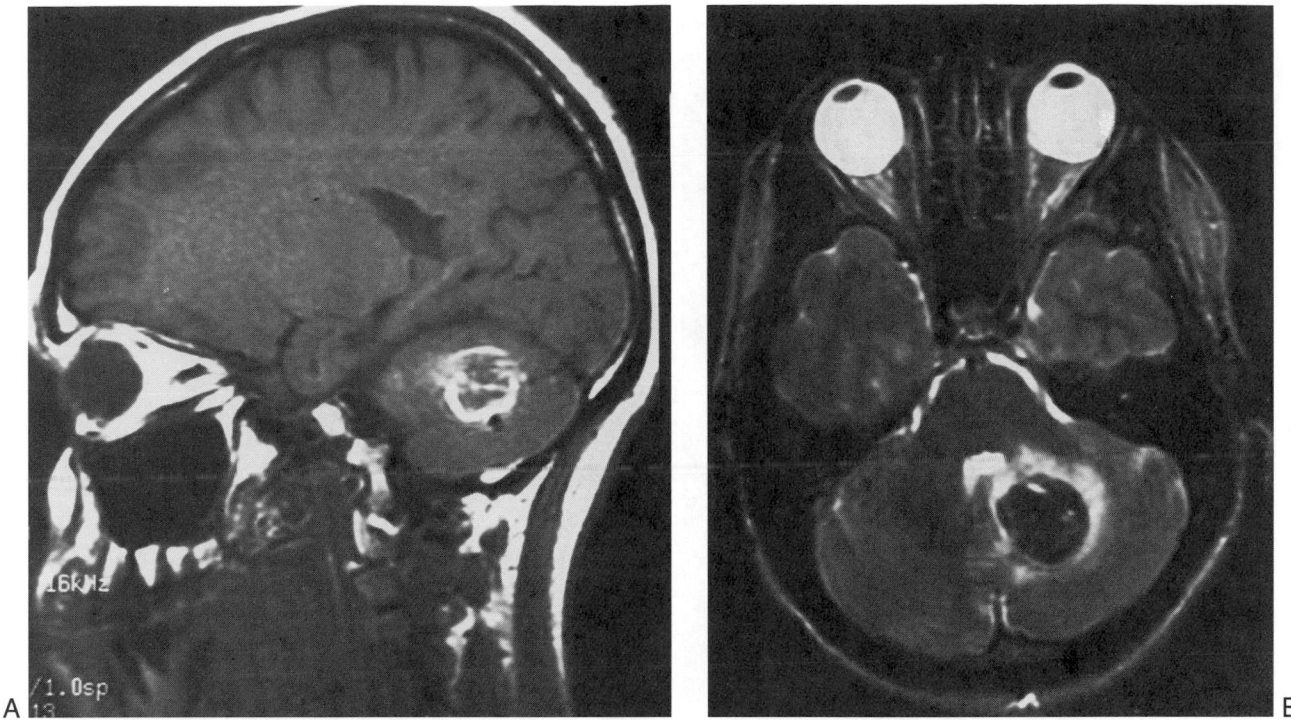

FIG. 21-3. MRI of acute cerebellar hemorrhage. **(A)** A lesion with increased intensity in the periphery is seen on this T1-weighted image in left cerebellar hemisphere. **(B)** Significant hypointensity on T2-weighted images is typical for acute hemorrhage.

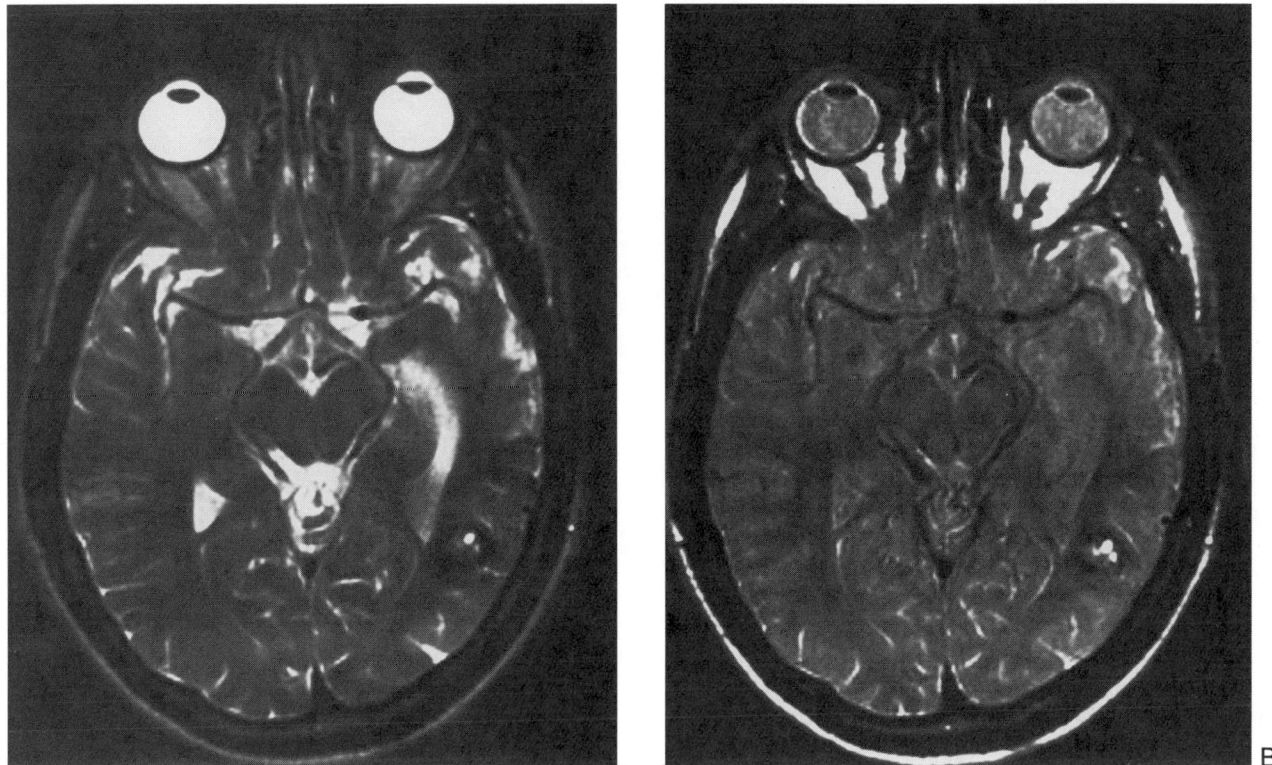

FIG. 21-4. MRI of cavernous angioma. **(A)** On T2-weighted and **(B)** intermediate images, the lesion has an irregular hyperintense center surrounded by a hypointense ring of hemosiderin.

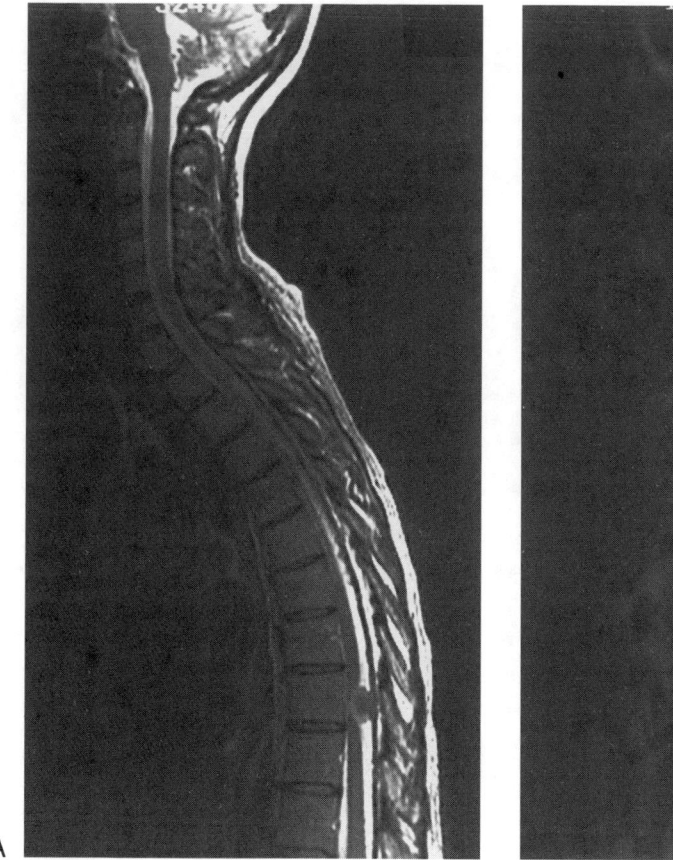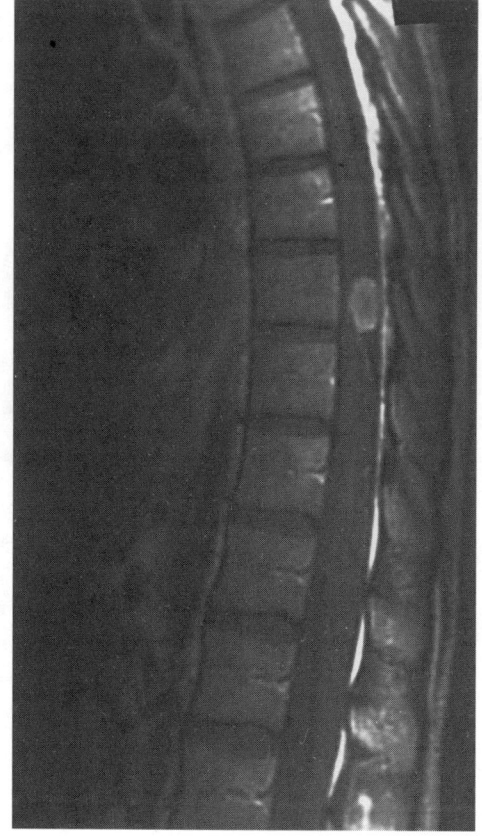

FIG. 21-5. Thoracic meningioma in spine MRI. **(A)** A survey of cervical and thoracic canal demonstrates an extramedullary, intradural lesion posterior to the cord. **(B)** Injection of contrast enhances the lesion on this T1-weighted image.

PET AND SPECT

Positron emission tomography (PET) and single-photon emission computed tomography (SPECT) provide important functional and metabolic information, including regional cerebral blood flow and normal brain response to a variety of sensory stimuli. These techniques also have been used to study stroke, epilepsy, brain tumors, radiation necrosis, and a variety of psychiatric illnesses.

Soon after a positron is emitted it collides with an electron. The two particles are lost in this encounter and two photons are produced. PET is based on the detection of annihilation photons thus produced. This detection requires strong cameras with exquisite spatial resolution. Positron-emitting isotopes are produced in a nearby cyclotron and incorporated into physiologic tracers to monitor a variety of processes. The high cost of cyclotron and special cameras limits the availability of PET to selected research centers.

SPECT uses readily available pharmaceuticals and modified conventional nuclear medicine cameras. These advantages have facilitated widespread use of SPECT across the country. Nowadays, SPECT is commonly used to differentiate radiation necrosis from recurrent tumor and to evaluate dementias and epilepsy.[^{99m} T$_c$] HMPAO SPECT can be used to give a semiquantative measure of regional cerebral blood flow. Perfusion defects can be seen in acute stroke long before changes on CT scans are appreciated. The spatial resolution of SPECT is, however, far below that of CT scans and MRI.

CEREBRAL ANGIOGRAPHY

Transfemoral cerebral angiography has become a much faster and safer test, mainly due to digital imaging systems, safer radiographic agents, and smaller catheters. Most centers now perform this procedure on an outpatient basis with a short stay in a recovery room after the procedure.

The major indication for cerebral angiography is vascular disease. Angiography remains the gold standard in evaluating atherosclerotic bifurcation disease; cerebral aneurysms, vascular malformations, and vasculitides are other indications. Better techniques, safer catheters, and faster imaging equipment have led to successful transcatheter endovascular therapy of a variety of cerebrovascular conditions, such as thrombolytic therapy of stroke and treatment of arteriovenous malformations and aneurysms. Angiography is now rarely used to study brain tumors, since CT scans and MRI can provide more information with less risk.

The incidence of complications has diminished with the newer techniques. Still, permanent neurologic deficits, although rare, can occur. Stroke as a result of angiography should occur at a rate of 0.5 percent or less in good hands. The most common local complication is groin hematoma.

MYELOGRAPHY

With widespread use of CT scans and MRI, the number of myelograms performed in the United States has diminished. In patients suspected of harboring a cord tumor, myelography is now rarely used. Cord tumors, whether extramedullary or intramedullary, are now studied with MRI. The great majority of patients with lumbar or cervical disk disease and stenosis are studied with CT scanning and MRI. In fact, CT scanning may be the most convenient radiologic method in patients suspected of having a lumbar disk herniation. In complicated cases, including some postoperative backs, in patients with possible arachnoiditis, and in selected cervical disk disease cases with equivocal MRI findings, myelography and postmyelography CT scans may be indicated.

Safer aqueous contrast agents (iohexol and iopamidol) have replaced older aqueous (metrizamide) and oily (pantopaque) agents. The most common adverse reactions are headache (20 percent), nausea, and vomiting. Back pain and leg pain may occur during or after the procedure. With these new agents, more significant neuropsychiatric side effects (confusion, restlessness, nightmares) are very rare. Universal employment of smaller lumbar puncture needles (25G) and decreased dose of contrast offer hope for further reduction in the incidence of these complications.

Contraindications to myelography are the same as those to lumbar puncture (e.g., increased intracranial pressure, especially with posterior fossa mass lesions, and severe thrombocytopenia) and a history of reactions to contrast material.

SUGGESTED READINGS

Atlas SW: Magnetic Resonance Imaging of the Brain and Spine. Raven Press, New York, 1991

Bradley WG: MR appearance of hemorrhage in the brain. Radiology 189:15, 1993

Bryan RN et al: Diagnosis of acute cerebral infarction: comparison of CT and MR imaging. Radiology 180:541, 1991

Edelmann RR, Warach S: Magnetic resonance imaging. N Engl J Med 328: 708, 1993

Edelmann RR, Warach S: Magnetic resonance imaging. N Engl J Med 328: 785, 1993

Gentry LR: Imaging of closed head injury. Radiology 191:1, 1994

Latchaw RE: MR and CT Imaging of the Head, Neck, and Spine. 2nd Ed. Mosby Year Book, St. Louis, 1991

Osborn A: Diagnostic Neuroradiology. 1st Ed. CV Mosby, St. Louis, 1994

Stark DD, Bradley WG: Magnetic Resonance Imaging. 2nd Ed. Mosby Year Book, St. Louis, 1992

Schwartz RB, Mantello MT: Primary brain tumors in adults. Semin Ultrasound CT MRI 13:449, 1992

22. NEUROIMAGING: SONOGRAPHIC APPROACHES

JOSEPH F. POLAK

Sonography can be used to evaluate both the extracranial and intracranial arteries. Sonographic imaging of extracranial arteries concentrates on the carotid bifurcation. Since most carotid lesions occur there, sonography serves as a very cost-effective screen for the common atherosclerotic lesions of the extracranial carotids. It can reliably image neither the origin of the major arteries from the aorta nor the proximal intracranial portions of

TABLE 22-1. Use of Sonography for Intra-Cranial Artery Evaluation

Type of Imaging	Advantage	Disadvantage
Pulsed-Doppler evaluation	Inexpensive	Large operator experience necessary; time consuming
Duplex imaging	Angle correction possible	Difficulties in identifying middle cerebral artery not alleviated
Color-flow imaging	Rapid vessel identification; angle correction facilitated	Additional expense

the internal carotid artery. The evaluation of the intracranial circulation by transcranial Doppler sonography is limited by the need to penetrate the cranium with sound waves, which greatly reduces its resolution. Although its value as a clinical test is less well established, it is used to evaluate patterns of blood flow in the cerebral vessels and, on occasion, to detect focal lesions. Tables 22-1 and 22-2 summarize the uses of sonography for extracranial and intracranial artery evaluation.

GENERAL PRINCIPLES

As the ultrasound beam penetrates the soft tissues of the body, three interactions can be defined: scattering, attenuation, and reflection. These interactions occur simultaneously and are responsible for the formation of the final image. *Scattering* is the basic interaction between the ultrasound beam and the soft tissues of the body. It occurs when the sound waves encounter heterogeneous media, such as particles in suspension and irregular surfaces. The intensity of the echo measured by the transducer is proportional to the degree of scattering. The amount of energy scattered and its direction depend on the relative orientations of the tissues of interest, their density, and the size of the cells that make up the tissues. The plasma does not cause significant scattering but allows almost all the energy of the sound waves to travel through it. The cellular elements of blood, the red cells and, to a lesser extent, the white cells and platelets, cause much less scattering than the normal surrounding tissues, typically one-ten thousandth that of surrounding soft tissues. Hence one-ten thousandth the intensity of the echogenic signal is detected from blood as compared to its surrounding tissues (Fig. 22-1). Scattering (as well as absorption and reflection) causes the energy of the ultrasound beam to dissipate as the depth of the tissue increases. This dissipation of energy with tissue penetration is called *attenuation*. The attenuation is more pronounced at high frequencies, so that the ultrasound beam loses the ability to penetrate tissues as the carrier frequency increases. Attenuation is dependent on scatter and, therefore, on tissue type; it is more pronounced in muscle than it is in the soft tissues of the brain, and it is lower in structures containing blood or clear fluid. When tissues of greatly different acoustic characteristics (*acoustic impedance*) have interfaces that are relatively large and smooth (i.e., when scatterers are aligned), the ultrasound wavefront is reflected almost perfectly. This *reflection* causes a sharp increase in signal strength. The transition between the lumen and the intima of the arterial wall is a smooth interface with a great difference in impedence. *Spatial resolution* is a measure of the ability of the image to distinguish two structures lying beside each other; it improves as the frequency of the sound waves increases.

TABLE 22-2. Use of Sonography for Carotid Artery Evaluation

Type of Imaging	Advantage	Disadvantage
Gray-scale imaging	Atherosclerotic plaque evaluation with high resolution (0.2 mm)	Less reliable with more severe stenoses
Periorbital Doppler evaluation	Determines presence of high-grade lesions of the internal carotid by changes in blood flow direction	Sensitive only to very high-grade stenoses of at least 80 to 90% diameter narrowing
Doppler waveform analysis with continuous-wave probe	Accurate for detection of 50% diameter stenosis or more	Operator expertise required; lesion characteristics cannot be evaluated by this nonimaging approach
Duplex imaging	Accuracy of 90% for detecting stenoses of 50% diameter narrowing or more	May fail to detect or differentiate total from subtotal occlusions
Color-flow imaging	Accuracy of 90% for detecting stenoses of 50% diameter narrowing or more; decreases time of examination	Cannot be reliably used to measure the residual flow lumen of the artery

TYPES OF SONOGRAPHIC IMAGES

Gray Scale Image

Gray scale imaging, or B-mode ultrasound, is accomplished with a device consisting of an electronic array of piezoelectric crystals. The crystals generate sound waves that are transmitted within the soft tissues of the body. The returning echoes are detected, amplified, processed, and displayed as a two-dimensional image (Fig. 22-1). The physical properties discussed above explain the appearance of carotid and intracranial sonograms. Blood does not produce much signal, therefore the arterial lumen is black. Thrombus or atherosclerotic plaque in the artery lumen constrasts with the blood. Superficially located carotid arteries can be readily imaged with a high-frequency transducer and show exquisite resolution of detail. Deeper lying arteries are more difficult to image, since the ultrasound beam is attenuated. Adopting a lower frequency transducer improves penetration, but the lower frequencies entail a loss in the resolution of detail. Calcification hinders penetration of the ultrasound

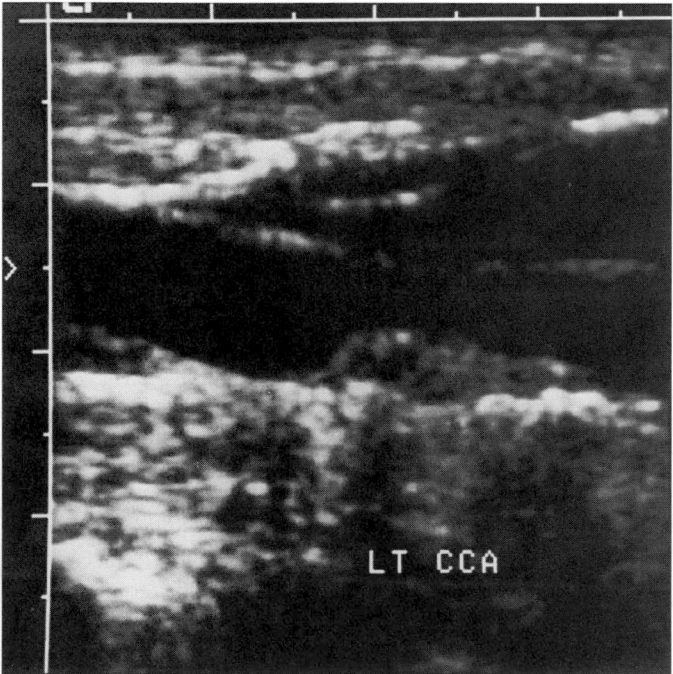

FIG. 22-1. Gray scale (B-mode) image showing a plaque in the common carotid. Plaque structure is defined by the strength of the echoes within the lesion. Here, a mixture of dense and less dense elements are seen. The focal area of decreased signals on the left of the plaque likely represents a hemorrhage within the plaque. The lumen of the artery is dark since the signal intensity of blood is much lower than that of the surrounding soft tissues.

beam, obscuring the sonographic image of the underlying lesion.

Doppler Ultrasound

Doppler ultrasound provides additional information about the velocity and direction of blood flow within vessels. This allows ultrasound to identify and quantitate arterial stenoses and to identify other types of lesions.

Transcranial Doppler ultrasound

Attenuation is enhanced at higher frequencies, and penetration is enhanced at lower frequencies. Intracranial sonography necessitates the use of frequencies of 2 MHz or less (compared with 5 MHz or greater for extracranial sonography) to penetrate the thinnest portion of the temporal bone. As a result, resolution of detail is very poor.

FLOW INFORMATION: DOPPLER ULTRASOUND

The major indication for cerebrovascular sonography is the detection of arterial stenosis or abnormalities of flow dynamics within vessels. For this, Doppler ultrasound plays a critical role. The basic principle underlying the use of Doppler ultrasound is as follows. A sound beam emitted or deflected from a moving object undergoes a frequency shift, the magnitude and valence of which depend on the speed and direction of the movement, respectively, with respect to the transducer. Motion toward the transducer increases the frequency of the returning sound waves, and motion away from the transducer decreases their frequency. The magnitude of the frequency shift is determined by the speed of the object and the angle between the direction of motion and the "line-of-sight." This principle is exploited to measure the *velocity* of arterial blood. It can be summarized by the Doppler equation, which relates the measured frequency shift to the relative motion between two objects: the ultrasound carrier frequency and the angle created between the moving body and the direction of the ultrasound beam. If the ultrasound beam and motion are in the same direction ($\theta = 0$), the frequency shift is maximal. The frequency shift decreases as this angle increases toward 90 degrees. The Doppler equation is given by

$$\Delta V = 2(V_0/c)V \cos \theta$$

where Δv is the frequency change, v_0 is the original frequency, c is the velocity of sound in the body, V is the blood velocity, and θ is the angle between the direction of blood flow and the direction of the sound beam. This equation relates the frequency shift to the velocity of blood flow and the Doppler angle. Note again that to measure the velocity, the direction of flow must be known, since it enters into the equation as the angle (cos θ) between the ultrasound beam and the object in motion (the flowing blood).

Continuous-Wave Doppler Ultrasound

Continuous-wave Doppler ultrasound employs a nonimaging probe that continuously transmits and receives sound waves along its line of sight. Motion of blood in the beam causes frequency shifts in the returning echoes. Since the actual depth of the returning echoes cannot be determined, there is ambiguity as to the location and orientation of the vessel being imaged. The signal from the moving blood can be displayed as an auditory output tone, as a digital output that represents the average velocity, or, most commonly, as a visual output—the Doppler spectral waveform. An experienced ear is needed to interpret the frequency shifts that occur in the auditory signals when blood flow velocity increases at stenotic lesions. A display of the average velocity of blood and its direction is normally used to verify the direction of blood flow in the periorbital branches of the carotid system. The Doppler spectral waveform—the preferred method of display of frequency shift to detect stenotic lesions—is an instantaneous display of the frequency shifts in the returning ultrasound echoes. The intensity of the display is roughly proportional to the number of red cells while the height is that of the fastest moving red cells (Fig. 22-2).

Pulsed Doppler Ultrasound

Pulsed Doppler ultrasound is used to send a pulse of a finite duration into the soft tissues. The ultrasound device then waits for a finite amount of time before detecting the returning echoes. The delay between transmission and return of the echoes measures the depth of the source of these echoes. By selecting a particular time delay, the operator can listen to signals from a specific chosen depth. The returning frequency shift information can be displayed as a Doppler spectral waveform and used to determine the velocity of blood. This can be done without the aid of an image, as in traditional transcranial Doppler sonography. If both pulsed Doppler and real-time gray-scale imaging are done simultaneously, then the direction of the sound beam can be depicted on a two-dimensional image. This imaging approach, called *duplex sonography* (Fig. 22-3), is very useful in the evaluation of the extracranial carotid vessels but may be less important for the intracranial circulation, since the vessels of interest tend to be located at a fixed depth from the temporal bone. Duplex sonography remains the only way to achieve appropriate angle correction and subsequent accurate velocity estimation because it allows accurate determination of the direction of flow (see equation above).

Color-Flow Imaging

Color-flow imaging is a modification of the pulsed Doppler ultrasound principle. In this technique, the equivalent of multi-

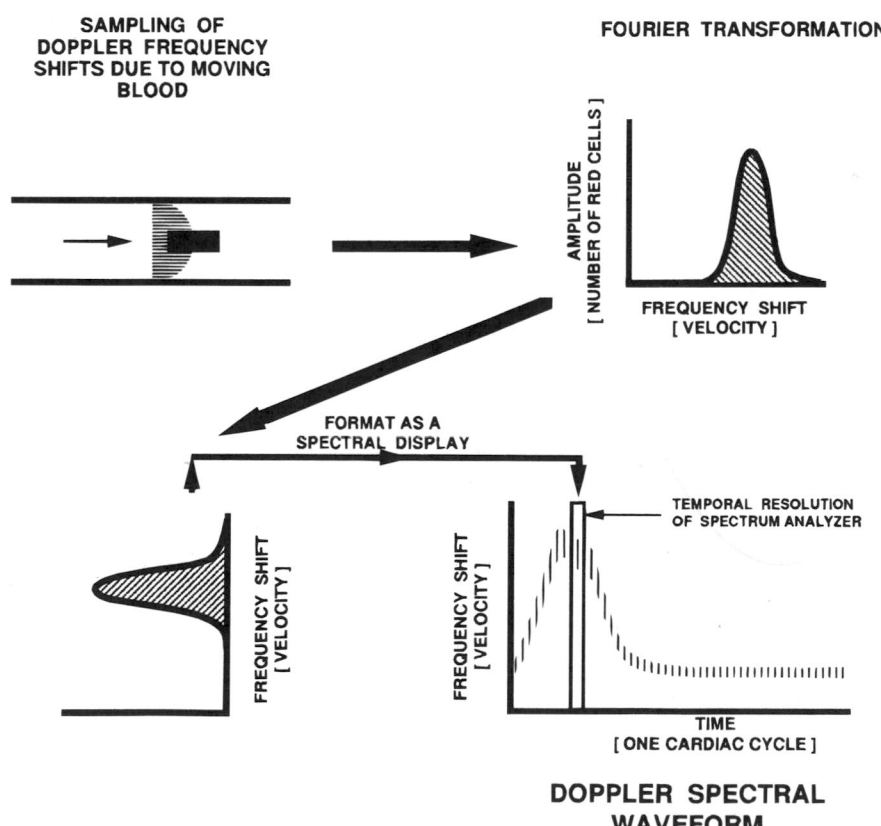

FIG. 22-2. Diagram showing the steps taken to create a Doppler spectral waveform. Frequency shift information is extracted from the echoes generated by moving blood and presented in the form of a frequency shift histogram (often with the aid of a Fourier transformation). This histogram is created at time increments of 1 to 10 ms. The histograms are processed and rendered as a waveform where intensity of the trace is roughly proportional to the number of red cells and the *y* axis is a reflection of the Doppler peak frequency shifts (velocities).

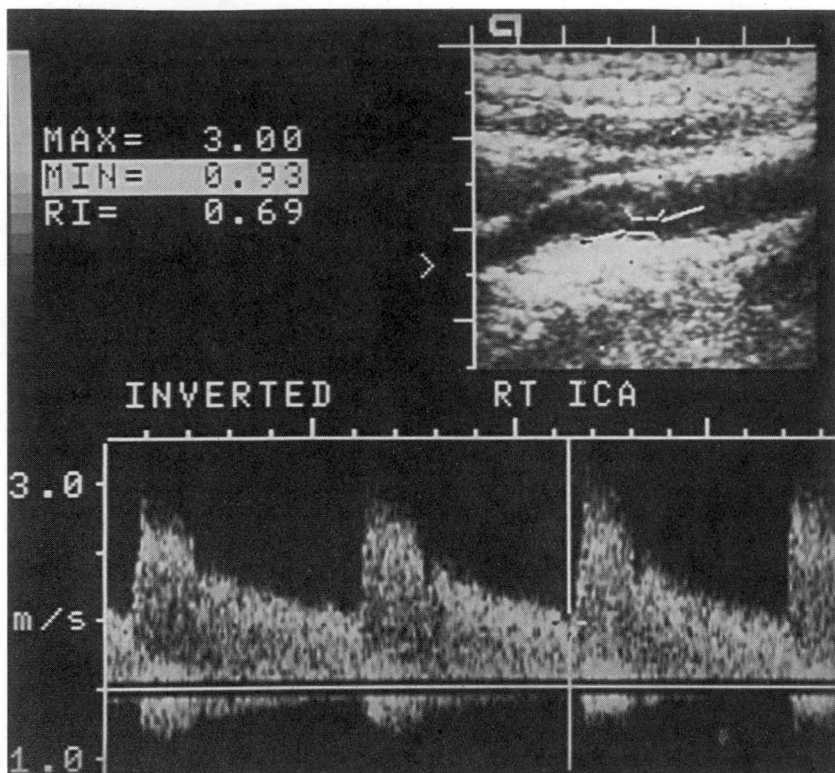

FIG. 22-3.   Doppler waveform sampled at a site of increased velocity. The waveform has a peak systolic velocity of 3.0 m/s, corresponding to a diameter stenosis of 80 percent. A lesion is not clearly shown on the gray scale image. This is a common limitation of gray scale imaging since it tends to be less reliable when stenosis of more than 50 percent diameter narrowing is present.

ple Doppler gates are positioned throughout the imaging field and used to sample the relative magnitude and direction of moving blood. This information is then processed, and the frequency shift information is encoded as a color overlay to the gray-scale image. While the velocity information obtained with pulsed Doppler sonography is traditionally displayed as a spectrum, the color image does not have such a level of discrimination. Instead, it maps the average velocity in a volume element as a color. Such a display is useful in identifying arteries and veins that have flowing blood within them. It is more often used as a guide for imaging, for selective pulsed Doppler sonography, and for subsequent waveform analysis.

USES OF GRAY-SCALE IMAGING OF CAROTID ATHEROSCLEROTIC LESIONS

Early Lesions

The atherosclerotic changes detectable by gray-scale imaging of the extracranial carotid arteries include focal lesions, preferentially located at the origin of the internal carotid artery, and a diffuse thickening of the common carotid wall. Much interest is now being paid to measurements of diffuse wall thickness changes or of focal areas of thickening in the arterial wall early in the development of atherosclerotic lesions. These changes are of submillimeter magnitudes and may be useful for monitoring the effects of medical interventions on early atherosclerosis. Their measurement requires specialized protocols and computer software.

Plaque Deposition

The sonographic characterization and classification of atherosclerotic plaques depend on the ability to detect the presence

of hemorrhage within a plaque. Plaques having zones of hemorrhage within them are thought to be more active or unstable. The detection of these plaques may identify those prone to repeated episodes of rupture and hence those conveying risk for embolic strokes. Yet, while it is true that most carotid endarterectomy samples show zones of recent hemorrhage within the excised plaque, not all episodes of hemorrhage are associated with symptoms. In fact, such intraplaque hemorrhage is probably most often asymptomatic.

Plaque density correlates with the constituents of the plaque. Material that is isodense or hypodense to normal vessel wall causes low- or very low-intensity echoes within the plaque. These areas of low echogenicity may represent smooth muscle cells, hematoma, or lipid. Fibrous tissue causes hyperdense signals on the B-mode image. The structure of the plaque is described as homogeneous or heterogeneous. Homogeneous plaque contains material of similar echo intensity and can be isodense, hypodense, or, occasionally, hyperdense. Hyperdense plaques tend to have areas of strong echogenic signals intermixed with areas of weaker echogenic signals and therefore are called heterogeneous; these plaques have probably undergone previous episodes of hemorrhage. The likelihood that a plaque will produce heterogeneous signals increases as the severity of the stenosis increases.

The surface characteristics of a plaque are normally described as the relative smoothness or irregularity of its contour. Ulceration is defined sonographically as an excavation of 2 mm or more in the plaque surface. Detecting and documenting the presence of ulceration is, however, difficult by sonography. Accuracy is often quoted to be above 80 to 85 percent; however, in some studies the accuracy is much lower. A major problem in determining the accuracy of sonography for lesions not removed at surgery is the variable accuracy of arteriography as a ''gold standard.'' This may be as low as 60 to 70 percent. Irregularities in the plaque contour by arteriography are known to correlate with a high rate of transient ischemic attacks and stroke. This presumably results from the thrombogencity of the internal portions of the plaque in contact with the blood.

USES OF DOPPLER WAVEFORM ANALYSIS FOR STENOSIS DETECTION AND GRADING

Hemodynamically significant stenoses are defined as those stenoses causing a pressure gradient. In general, this occurs for stenoses that cause 50 percent or greater narrowing of the lumen. The velocity of blood increases as the lumen narrows and is typically highest at the point of maximal stenosis. The zone of increased velocity established at the stenosis continues downstream as a jet. The jet will typically extend from 1 to 2 cm distal to the stenosis. The velocity can be measured by the Doppler ultrasound, and the correlation of blood flow velocity changes with degrees of stenosis is the basis for Doppler sonography of the carotid system. Blood, as it decelerates quickly at the boundary of the jet, will typically develop turbulent flow. This causes a spread in the measured velocities of moving blood and is detected as a broadening of the Doppler spectrum. This broadening is difficult to measure, and because nonlaminar flow is also seen in lesions that do not cause a hemodynamically significant narrowing, it has limited value as a diagnostic measure of the severity of stenosis.

Elevation of the peak systolic velocity above 125 cm/s is an accepted diagnostic criterion for the presence of more than 50 percent stenosis in the internal carotid artery. This correlation assumes a cardiac output within the normal range and average common carotid velocity values of 80 cm/s. In one series, 130 cm/s was used as the cutoff for 60 percent stenosis. It is also possible to use the peak systolic frequency shift to grade the severity of a stenotic lesion. A carotid stenosis will also cause an increase in the velocity of blood during diastole, but this effect may be more variable. One hemodynamic effect of a high-grade lesion in the internal carotid artery is to decrease the common carotid systolic and diastolic velocities. This fact can be used to make velocity ratios that compensate for the effect of decreased blood flow. The following velocity ratios have been, at one time or another, proposed as parameters for grading the severity of internal carotid artery stenosis:

1. The ratio of the peak systolic velocity within the internal carotid artery divided by that in the common carotid artery
2. The ratio of internal carotid artery peak end-diastolic velocity to the common carotid artery peak end-diastolic velocity
3. The ratio of the peak systolic velocity within the internal carotid artery divided by the peak end-diastolic velocity within the common carotid artery

These different ways of grading the severity of carotid artery stenosis were compared in a large series that concluded that the end-diastolic velocity ratio was a better parameter for grading the presence of significant stenosis of 80 percent or more. Other authors report that the peak systolic velocity is the more robust parameter. A velocity ratio such as the internal carotid artery to the common carotid artery peak systolic velocity does offer a simple means of correcting for changes in cardiac output in patients with heart disease.

Tandem Lesions

The velocity ratio is useful because the increasingly narrowed internal carotid artery is likely to depress flow velocities within the common carotid artery. A mean peak systolic velocity below 25 cm/s in the common carotid artery indicates the presence of significant downstream internal carotid artery stenosis. This parameter has low sensitivity, since many high-grade internal carotid artery stenoses will not significantly affect the common carotid artery velocity waveforms. Presumably, this is due to the development of collateral flow either through the circle of Willis or through the ipsilateral external carotid artery.

Ipsilateral stenosis at sites removed from the accessible cervical carotid artery bifurcation may, however, be so severe that it affects the waveform sampled downstream or upstream to the lesion. A lesion located downstream, for example, an intracranial stenosis or occlusion, will cause a relatively greater effect on the diastolic flow, decreasing it to the point that it may be absent. Systolic flow velocity also tends to decrease. These effects can be taken as indicators of a downstream lesion. In the case of an upstream lesion, relative vasodilation causes diastolic flow to be preserved while systolic flow is depressed, and the time to reach peak systolic velocity is delayed. This situation can arise in the case of an origin stenosis of the left common carotid artery or the innominate artery. These effects on the Doppler spectrum are only seen with very high-grade stenoses, that is, at least 80 percent diameter narrowing.

Limitations

The presence of calcification hampers the penetration of the ultrasound beam and may mask the presence of stenotic lesions. In general, calcified lesions of 1 cm or less in length can be reliably evaluated.

Doppler sonography remains limited in its ability to distinguish total from subtotal internal carotid artery occlusions. The high-grade lesion above 95 percent diameter stenosis is often called a pseudo-occlusion. Velocities and the intensity of the returning echoes sampled in the artery are severely depressed. Echo detection may be almost impossible when the diseased artery is located deep in the neck where the ultrasound signals cannot reliably penetrate. Color-flow imaging may help achieve some improvement in distinguishing total from subtotal occlusions. Currently, the accurate diagnosis of such lesions requires a long-injection arteriogram.

SPECIFIC CLINICAL USES OF DOPPLER SONOGRAPHY

Carotid Artery Stenosis

It is possible to conduct a simple survey of the carotid arteries and to detect the presence of atherosclerotic lesions using gray-scale imaging alone. However, this has been shown to be unreliable, especially when higher grade lesions are present. Duplex sonography is sufficient to achieve accurate detection and grading of carotid artery stenoses. The addition of color-flow imaging facilitates and shortens the examination. In general, the accuracy of Doppler sonography for detecting carotid artery stenoses of 50 percent or more is estimated at 90 percent.

The identification of patients that have clinically significant stenoses now relies on data from two studies, the North American Symptomatic Carotid Endarterectomy Trial (NASCET 1991) and the European Carotid Surgery Trialists' Collaborative Group study (ECST 1991), that suggest carotid endarterectomy is beneficial in selected symptomatic patients with stenosis of 70 percent or greater. Recall that the cutoff for hemodynamically significant (above 50 percent) internal carotid artery stenosis has been established to be 125 cm/s. Moneta and colleagues (1993) observe that the threshold of 250 cm/s or a peak systolic velocity ratio of 4 can identify patients with a 70 percent diameter stenosis with high accuracy. Hunink and colleagues (1993) suggest that a threshold of 230 cm/s peak systolic velocity is sufficient to identify these patients. A regression equation that permits the actual measurement of the percentage of stenosis from peak systolic velocity and adjusts for common carotid artery velocity can also be used. Peak systolic velocity is a robust parameter that offers a sensitivity and specificity in the range of 90 percent. In addition, it seems to be less affected by selection bias than other velocity parameters. This bias is introduced because the population examined by sonography is selected for arteriography based on the results of sonography. This selection bias may affect the overall performance of the diagnostic test. Although accurate estimates of the degree of stenosis by ultrasound are now possible with certain limitations, it must be remembered that ultrasound usually cannot adequately distinguish stenoses of 95 percent or more from total occlusions.

Other Lesions of the Carotid Arteries and Great Vessels

Subclavian Steal Syndrome. The subclavian steal syndrome is due to the presence of a high-grade stenosis in the proximal subclavian artery. The vertebral arteries, occasionally excepting the left vertebral, originate from the subclavian artery. In this syndrome, blood flow in the ipsilateral vertebral artery is reversed, and blood originally destined for the brain is shunted to supply the arm through the subclavian artery distal to the stenosis. Flow within the vertebral artery may also be partly reversed. In less severe subclavian artery stenosis, the application of a blood pressure cuff or use of another method, such as exercise, to induce vasodilation of the arteries of the arm can increase demand and cause orthograde flow to reverse in the vertebral artery. By detecting this flow reversal, sonography can help to diagnose this syndrome.

Vasculitis. Takayasu's arteritis causes a diffuse inflammatory reaction of the media and adventitia of large arterial branches of the aorta. Additional involvement of the subclavian artery and axillary arteries is often seen. Carotid sonography can help to distinguish between atherosclerosis and diffuse vasculitis. Atherosclerosis preferentially affects the region of the carotid bifurcation, and focal lesions are common, while diffuse thickening of the arterial wall is common in vasculitis.

Radiation Arteropathy. Accelerated atherosclerosis can occur following irradiation. Patients having had head and neck surgery and subsequent irradiation develop a diffuse thickening of the common carotid artery wall with relative sparing of the internal carotid artery bifurcation. Pathologically, this process resembles atherosclerosis. It typically becomes apparent within 10 years following radiation treatment.

Arterial Dissection. One type of carotid artery dissection is an extension of an aortic dissection. This is seen by sonography to extend proximally from the internal carotid artery into the common carotid artery and to end at variable levels along the more distal internal carotid artery. The dissection is best visualized on a longitudinal image.

The second type of dissection is localized to the internal carotid artery. It is post-traumatic or idiopathic and affects young patients. Permanent stroke is the exception rather than the rule. The lesion typically develops in the high portion of the internal carotid artery as it enters the bony canal. Because of this, the lesion is often not visualized directly. However, flow profiles in the more proximal internal carotid artery show the effect of the more distal flow obstruction. The waveform will tend to be blunted—with signals above and below baseline—or almost absent.

Pseudoaneurysms and Aneurysms. Aneurysms or pseudoaneurysms of the vertebral and extracranial carotid arteries are rare. Pseudoaneurysm formation may follow trauma due to penetrating injuries. Aneurysms may arise spontaneously at the bifurcation. Patients typically present with a pulsatile mass in the neck. Carotid sonography can identify the presence of these lesions and determine the level of involvement. Most pulsatile masses referred for sonographic studies are shown to be ectatic carotid arteries or slightly enlarged segments of the carotid arteries. True aneurysms are quite rare.

Neoplasms. Neoplastic lesions involving the carotid artery bifurcation are rare. Carotid body tumors are extremely hypervascular masses growing in the carotid artery bifurcation. Other neoplastic masses, such as enlarged lymph nodes, may involve the carotid artery and the nearby structures. Neoplastic involvement of the wall of the carotid artery causes the loss of the interface normally seen between the adventitia and periadventitia of the arterial wall. This loss of interface can be demonstrated by sonography as evidence of neoplastic invasion.

Vertebral Arteries

The vertebral artery Doppler waveform resembles that of the internal carotid artery. The Doppler evaluation is limited to sampling the waveforms in the accessible portions of the vertebral artery that are found between the transverse processes of the cervical vertebrae. This is mainly used to confirm the presence of antegrade flow and to characterize the overall appearance of the spectral waveform. Color-flow imaging can help identify high-grade stenoses, since it can detect zones of flow disturbance projected beyond the areas obscured by the transverse processes of the cervical vertebrae. Less severe lesions may be missed, since the short systolic jet may be masked by bone. The reported accuracy of sonography for stenosis detection varies between 38 and 83 percent. Accuracy at the higher end of this range can be achieved when the origin of the vertebral artery is visualized. Increased peak systolic velocity may also suggest that the vertebral artery serves as the important collateral pathway to the circle of Willis when the carotid arteries are severely diseased.

Vertebrobasilar Arterial Insufficiency. High-grade stenosis or occlusion of the vertebral or basilar arteries or the subclavian steal phenomenon may result in compromise of blood flow to the brainstem, cerebellum, and occipital lobes. Patients may complain of dizziness, vertigo, unsteady gait, diplopia, drop attacks, and other symptoms referable to this territory. Such patients are difficult to evaluate. Not uncommonly, posterior circulation symptoms will be incorrectly attributed to carotid artery system atherosclerotic lesions simply because the carotid artery system is more accessible to evaluation. Evaluation of flow patterns in the vertebral arteries by Doppler sonography may contribute to the assessment of patients when symptoms point to the posterior circulation.

INTRACEREBRAL SONOGRAPHY (TRANSCRANIAL DOPPLER)

The bone of the cranium acts as an obstacle to the penetration of ultrasound energy. The evaluation of the intracerebral vessels is, however, possible with low-frequency ultrasound that can penetrate the thin layer of bone in the temporal region to evaluate the anterior circulation or pass through the foramen magnum to evaluate the posterior circulation. Most transcranial sonography has been performed using nonimaging probes equipped with range-gated pulsed Doppler. Evaluation for the presence and direction of blood flow is achieved with the knowledge of the relative location and depth of the different intracranial arteries. This type of examination can be quite time-consuming. The use of duplex sonography and color flow imaging facilitate the examination.

The traditional velocity parameter is the mean velocity, and values are not angle-corrected, since a nonimaging approach is used. Angle-corrected peak velocities can be measured with duplex sonography. Two parameters derived from the Doppler waveform can be used with both approaches: the pulsatility index and the resistive index. Both are angle independent. Pulsatility indices range from 0.6 to 0.8 in the middle cerebral artery. They may be reduced on the side of high-grade internal carotid artery stenosis.[55] Assessment for reversal of the direction of flow within the different branches of the circle of Willis when the internal carotid artery is totally or subtotally occluded can be done subjectively. Subtle changes in intracerebral velocities are difficult to interpret because stenosis cannot reliably be distinguished from autoregulatory constriction of the cerebral vessels. There are, therefore, no specific findings in the intracranial branches that can be used to predict the presence of a significant stenosis of the proximal internal carotid artery.

Cerebrovascular Spasm. Cerebral artery spasm tends to develop approximately 2 to 14 days following an episode of subarachnoid hemorrhage. This is most often associated with rupture of an aneurysm. Symptoms suggesting the presence of spasm can be quite vague. Increases in mean velocities above 200 cm/s in the middle cerebral artery are suggestive of arterial spasm in the appropriate context. Increased peak velocities also correlate with an arteriographic finding of narrowed vessels in spasm.

Intracerebral Lesions. There are no large series giving the overall accuracy of transcranial Doppler sonography for detecting the presence of tandem lesions in the intracranial internal carotid artery or of isolated focal lesions in the middle cerebral branches. The presence of high-grade velocity signal within the middle cerebral branches in patients with sickle cell disease is indicative of arterial stenosis. The findings for focal atherosclerotic lesions of the intracranial arteries are variable and include increases in velocity as well as decreases. The clinical reliability of this technology to confirm brain death is based on the presence of a high-resistance Doppler waveform pattern. Accuracy

is heavily dependent on the operator and on the adjustment of velocity scales and sensitivity of the imaging device.

Collateral Pathway Assessment. The collateral pathway assessment is often recognized as the major strength of transcranial Doppler sonography. The presence of high-grade lesions in arteries may be accompanied by marked collateralization. Absence of significant collaterals may affect the surgical approach to carotid endarterectomy and lead to the use of a shunt. Conversely, well-developed collaterals, despite the presence of a high-grade stenosis in a patient who is a high-risk surgical candidate, may suggest that repair of the lesion is not warranted. To aid in this assessement, a provocative test, such as a common carotid artery compression, can be performed to see if the intracranial flow patterns are affected.

Effect of High-Grade Internal Carotid Artery Stenosis. In asymptomatic patients, a high-grade lesion of 80 to 90 percent diameter stenosis may affect flow dynamics within the intracerebral vasculature. A potential use of transcranial Doppler sonography is the study of this effect of extracranial stenosis on intracranial flow dynamics. Ultimately, such an evaluation may help identify patients who would benefit from surgical revision. There are, as yet, no large series evaluating this hypothesis.

SUGGESTED READINGS

Aaslid R, Huber P, Nornes H: Evaluation of cerebrovascular spasm with transcranial Doppler ultrasound. J Neurosurg 60:37, 1984

Adams R, McKie V, Nichols F et al: The use of ultrasonography to predict stroke in sickle cell disease. N Engl J Med 326:605, 1992

Becker G, Lindner A, Bigdahn U: Imaging of the vertebrobasilar system by transcranial color-coded real-time sonography. J Ultrasound Med 12:395, 1993

Bluth EI, McVay LV, Merritt CRB et al: The identification of ulcerative plaque with high-resolution duplex carotid scanning. J Ultrasound Med 7:73, 1988

Bluth EI, Stavros AT, Marich KW et al: Carotid duplex sonography: a multicenter recommendation for standardized imaging and Doppler criteria. RadioGraphics 8:487, 1988

Bogdahn U, Becker G, Winkler J et al: Transcranial color-coded real-time sonography in adults. Stroke 21:1680, 1990

Buckley A, Southwood T, Culham G et al: The role of ultrasound in evaluation of Takayasu's arteritis. J Rheumatol 18:1073, 1991

Chuang VP: Radiation-induced arteritis. Semin Roentgenol 29:64, 1994

Davis PC, Nilsen B, Braun IF et al: A prospective comparison of duplex sonography vs angiography of the vertebral arteries. AJNR 7:1059, 1986

deBray J-M, Joseph P-A, Jeanvoine H et al: Transcranial Doppler evaluation of middle cerebral artery stenosis. J Ultrasound Med 7:611, 1988

European Carotid Surgery Trialists' Collaborative Group. MRC European Carotid Surgery Trial: interim results for symptomatic patients with severe (70–99%) or with mild (0–29%) carotid stenosis. Lancet 337:1235, 1991

Glasier CM, Seibert JJ, Chadduck WM et al: Brain death in infants: evaluation with Doppler US. Radiology 172:377, 1989

Gooding GAW, Langman AW, Dillon WP et al: Malignant carotid artery invasion: sonographic detection. Radiology 171:435, 1989

Hunink MGM, Polak JF, Barlan MM et al: Detection and quantification of carotid artery stenosis: efficacy of various Doppler velocity parameters. AJR 160:619, 1993

Imparato AM, Riles TS, Mintzer R et al: The importance of hemorrhage in the relationship between gross morphologic characteristics and cerebral symptoms in 376 carotid artery plaques. Ann Surg 197:195, 1983

Kotval PS, Babu SC, Shah PM: Doppler diagnosis of partial vertebral/subclavian steals convertible to full steals with physiologic maneuvers. J Ultrasound Med 9:207, 1990

Lennihan L, Kupsky WJ, Mohr JP et al: Lack of association between carotid plaque hematoma and ischemic cerebral symptoms. Stroke 18:879, 1987

Lindegaard K-F, Bakke SJ, Grolimund P et al: Assessment of intracranial hemodynamics in carotid artery disease by transcranial Doppler ultrasound. J Neurosurg 63:890, 1985

Moneta GL, Edwards JM, Chitwood RW et al: Correlation of North American Symptomatic Carotid Endarterectomy Trial (NASCET) angiographic definition of 70% to 99% internal carotid stenosis with duplex scanning. J Vasc Surg 17:152, 1993

North American Carotid Endarterectomy Trial Collaborators. Beneficial effect of carotid endarterectomy in symptomatic patients with high-grade stenosis. N Engl J Med 325:445, 1991

O'Donnell TF, Erdoes L, Mackey WC et al: Correlation of B-mode ultrasound imaging and arteriography with pathologic findings at carotid endarterectomy. Arch Surg 120:443, 1985

O'Leary DH, Polak JF, Kronmal RA et al: Distribution and correlates of sonographically detected carotid artery disease in the Cardiovascular Health Study: the Cardiovascular Health Study group. Stroke 23:1752, 1992

Polak JF, Dobkin GR, O'Leary DH et al: Internal carotid artery stenosis: accuracy and reproducibility of color-Doppler-assisted duplex imaging. Radiology 173:793, 1989

Ricotta JJ, Bryan FA, Bond MG et al: Multicenter validation study of real-time (B-mode) ultrasound, arteriography, and pathologic examination. Vasc Surg 6:512, 1987

Robinson ML, Sacks D, Perlmutter GS et al: Diagnostic criteria for carotid duplex sonography. AJR 151:1045, 1988

Spencer MP, Reid JM: Quantitation of carotid stenosis with continuous-wave (C-W) Doppler ultrasound. Stroke 10:326, 1979

Steinke W, Hennerici M, Anlick A: Doppler color flow imaging of carotid body tumors. Stroke 20:1574, 1989

Steinke W, Rautenberg W, Schwartz A et al: Noninvasive monitoring of internal carotid artery dissection. Stroke 25:998, 1994

Visona A, Lusiana L, Castellani V et al: The echo-Doppler (duplex) system for the detection of vertebral artery occlusive disease: comparison with angiography. J Ultrasound Med 5:247, 1986

Walker DW, Acker JD, Cole CA: Subclavian steal syndrome detected with duplex pulsed Doppler sonography. AJNR 3:615, 1982

Wang A-M, O'Leary DH: Common carotid aneurysm: ultrasonic diagnosis. JCU 16:262, 1988

Wilkinson DL, Polak JF, Grassi CJ et al: Pseudoaneurysm of the vertebral artery: appearance on color-flow Doppler sonography. AJR 151:1051, 1988

Zurbrugg HR, Leupi F, Schupbach P et al: Duplex scanner study of carotid artery dissection following surgical treatment of aortic dissection type A. Stroke 19:970, 1988

23. BIOPSY OF THE BRAIN

MATTHEW P. FROSCH
UMBERTO DE GIROLAMI

A brain biopsy is an important procedure that can contribute to neurologic diagnosis and influence therapy. This benefit needs to be balanced against the fact that sampling of brain tissue carries with it the risk of neurologic disability. The clinical course, location, and type of lesion, and the information desired from the biopsy are all determinants that help shape the decision to perform a biopsy. These factors will also influence the manner with which the biopsy is handled. Once the decision to perform a brain biopsy has been reached, the interaction between the neurologist, neurosurgeons, neuroradiologists, and neuropathologists should continue. The pathologic interpretation of brain biopsies is beyond the scope of this chapter and is covered in detail in standard textbooks. This brief review is intended to offer some guidance regarding the general approach and evaluation of brain biopsies.

TYPES OF BIOPSY

The clinical setting, the medical condition of the patient, and the nature of the anticipated pathologic process contribute to the selection of the biopsy method. Brain biopsies can be performed as open neurosurgical procedures with direct visualization of the tissue to be sampled or by stereotactic procedures. An open biopsy can allow for additional resection, drainage, or other manipulation based on findings at the time of intraoperative pathologic consultation. Thus, for metastatic lesions it is possible to resect the tumor nodule, while for abscesses effective drainage of the lesion can be achieved. Open biopsies are limited by the anatomic site of the lesion (for example, intrinsic brainstem lesions) and the underlying medical condition of the patient. In contrast, stereotactic biopsies do not require an extensive surgical procedure and can reach areas of the brain that are inaccessible to open biopsies. Recent advances in stereotactic neurosurgical techniques and more precise localization of lesions by computed tomography and magnetic resonance imaging have resulted in more widespread use of this method for brain biopsy.

Although it may seem self-evident, it is worth stating that when a patient with a focal lesion requires a brain biopsy, the biopsy should be taken from the region of lesion so as to maximize the likelihood of reaching a diagnosis. Stereotactic biopsies are often used for focal lesions that are defined by imaging studies; they are less useful in the context of diffuse or multifocal processes where the larger sampling area afforded by open biopsy increases the likelihood of obtaining a diagnostic specimen.

SAMPLING

A major issue in the interpretation of brain biopsies is the adequacy of sampling. In any context, the biopsy must include the site of the suspected disease process. Thus, when attempting to provide histologic evidence of vasculitis, it is important that the biopsy sample include adequate representation of meningeal and cortical vessels. Similarly, when a demyelinating process is suspected, as with progressive multifocal leukoencephalopathy, the specimen needs to contain white matter from the area of radiologic abnormality. At least as important as providing pathologic support for a suspected diagnosis, a brain biopsy provides the opportunity to exclude disease processes under consideration in the clinical differential diagnosis. Furthermore, in a patient with multiple lesions, a biopsy of a single lesion provides information only about that lesion and may not be representative of the others, that is, different disease processes may be active in a given patient. This is an important issue in immunosuppressed patients who may be affected simultaneously by multiple opportunistic infections.

An erroneous diagnosis of a discrete mass lesion can be reached if tissue sampling is inadequate. For example, if necrotic tissue is obtained from the center of a ring-enhancing lesion, it will be impossible to distinguish between an associated high-grade neoplasm (either primary or metastatic) or an infectious process. Similarly, within glial tumors, the histologic grade can vary greatly from one area of the lesion to another.

INTRAOPERATIVE PATHOLOGIC INTERPRETATIONS

Examination of brain biopsy tissue by neuropathologists during the course of the neurosurgical procedure is carried out routinely. The aims of this consultation include (1) the confirmation that lesional tissue has been obtained, (2) an attempt to make an intraoperative diagnosis, and (3) proper triage of specimen handling for special studies. Gross and microscopic examination of the tissue as well as examination of radiologic studies and discussions with the neurosurgeon are necessary to achieve these aims.

The intraoperative histopathologic examination of tissue is most commonly performed by "frozen sections." For this procedure, a portion of tissue—chosen to adequately represent the biopsy—is rapidly frozen in a mounting medium that solidifies in the cold. Sections are then cut on a cryostat at approximately 8 to 12 mm thickness, picked up on glass slides, rapidly fixed in alcohol, and stained with a rapid hematoxylin and eosin procedure. They may also be stained with an aniline dye and mounted in an aqueous medium. Frozen sections are also useful for detection of compounds that are partially soluble in the media used for preparation of standard histologic sections, such as lipid (with Oil red O or Sudan black) and glycogen (PAS).

The frozen section method has certain advantages over other methods as well as drawbacks. This method of diagnosis is well established around the world because the histopathologic changes and artifacts are similar to those of conventional tissue sections. Frozen sections, thus, provide information regarding the histologic architecture of the lesion similar to that seen with permanent sections (Plate 23-1). Because the tissue used for frozen section analysis is at a later time routinely processed for permanent sections, confirmation of the intraoperative diagnosis is possible on the exact piece of tissue to be used for these sections.

On the other hand, frozen sections of brain are technically more difficult to perform than comparable sections on tissues from other regions of the body. The freezing process introduces artifacts; there is often poor nuclear detail on frozen sections, and permanent sections prepared from tissue that was frozen will usually show artifacts (clefts in the tissue, hyperchromatic and/or atypical nuclei).

An important complement to frozen sections are the smear and touch preparations. These methods do not subject tissue to the trauma of freezing. Although these preparations do not yield significant information regarding the architecture of the lesion, they allow excellent demonstration of nuclear detail (Plate 23-2). The methods also have the advantage of requiring extremely small amounts of tissue.

Touch preparations are performed by applying a glass slide to the surface of the biopsy with a small amount of pressure, then rapidly fixing the slide and staining it in the usual manner. This method is extremely helpful in poorly cohesive lesions, such as lymphomas, some carcinomas, and inflammatory lesions with areas of necrosis.

For the preparation of smears, a small fragment of tissue is placed on the surface of the slide and then smeared rapidly against another slide, in a manner similar to that used for preparation of a thick blood smear. The slide is stained with hematoxylin and eosin after rapid alcohol fixation. In addition to providing excellent nuclear detail, smear and touch preparations also show individual cell morphology. Delicate processes of tumor cells, as seen in pilocytic astrocytomas, can be well visualized (Plate 23-3A), as can the perivascular arrangement of processes in ependymomas (Plate 23-3B). Similarly, the syncytial knots of cells from meningiomas (Plate 23-3C) and the cytologic features of medullolblastoma can be well seen (Plate 23-3D). Smear preparations, because of their excellent preservation of nuclei, can also be used for analysis of DNA content (ploidy).

SPECIAL STUDIES

At the time of intraoperative consultation, a number of decisions are made by the neuropathologist and neurosurgeon based on examination of the specimens. A most critical decision regards the adequacy of the tissue sample. If the material provided is inadequate to allow for a definitive diagnosis, this information must be conveyed to the neurosurgeon.

Given the histologic appearance of the sampled tissue, the pathologist will need to initiate a variety of procedures. In general, biopsy tissue is fixed in 10 percent buffered formalin and processed by routine procedures. A variety of alternative or supplementary procedures can be followed, based on preliminary diagnoses from intraoperative consultation. These so-called "special studies" are intended to provide additional information and aid the pathologist in rendering a diagnosis. Some of the methods are considered here briefly.

For the diagnosis of processes involving lymphoid cells (either neoplastic or reactive) it is often useful to have access to the wide range of immunohistochemical procedures used by the hematopathologist, many of which work best on either frozen tissue or material fixed with fixatives other than formalin (Plate 23-4A,B). Thus, if such studies are considered, a portion of the specimen may be handled in this manner. When indicated, tissue should be frozen rapidly in liquid nitrogen or a cooled dry ice/isopentane bath. Material prepared in this fashion can also be used for immunofluorescence studies in the evaluation of vasculitides.

Similarly, special fixation is required if it is intended that tissue will be used for electron microscopy, which may be helpful in cases of poorly differentiated neoplasms, viral infections, and storage diseases. Additional special handling may be necessary in storage diseases since the "stored" material might be dissolved out of tissue during standard processing. Preparation of additional frozen sections as well as nonaqueous fixation and processing can preserve intracellular storage material.

When either preoperative considerations or intraoperative consultation has raised the possibility of an infectious process, microbiologic cultures (including viral, bacterial, and fungal cultures) are indicated. These may be complemented by stains for specific classes of organisms (Plate 23-4C), although some organisms can be seen with standard hematoxylin and eosin staining (Plate 23-4D).

The past twenty years have seen the expansion of the role of immunohistochemical stains, especially in the study of tumors. This method can provide various types of information. It can, for example, confirm the glial nature of a lesion through immunoreactivity for the glial intermediate filament protein GFAP (Plate 23-4E) or reveal the nature of germ cells within a germinoma through immunoreactivity for placental alkaline phosphatase. With appropriate reagents, this method can also be useful in the diagnosis of infectious diseases (Plate 23-4F).

Recent developments in the understanding of the molecular genetics of neoplasia, and, in particular, of the genetic alterations found in primary central nervous system tumors has generated interest in additional studies of tumors. Specifically, samples of fresh sterile tumors can be submitted in some institutions for cytogenetic analysis. These can be performed either on direct preparations of cells (useful in highly proliferative neoplasms) or after short-term culture of tumor cells. The presence of certain chromosomal alterations can be characteristic of specific lesions (e.g., monosomy 22 in meningiomas) or predictive of natural history (e.g., role of aneuploidy in medulloblastomas). There has also been a recent expansion in the use of direct molecular methods based on PCR determinations of allelic loss or specific classes of mutations. While these studies can be performed on fixed archival material, they are greatly facilitated by taking representative samples of lesional and nonlesional tissue for rapid freezing. In the absence of nonlesional material at the time of surgery, DNA prepared from the patient's blood can be used for comparison purposes.

SPECIAL CONSIDERATIONS

Unfixed biopsy tissue from all patients needs to be treated with universal precautions. However, in patients with known or highly suspected infection by certain pathogens, some additional considerations may be relevant. In many institutions, cryostats require decontamination following introduction of tissue from patients infected with hepatitis B virus, *Mycobacterium tuberculosis,* or HIV, in addition to regularly scheduled decontamination. For this reason, specimens from patients known to be infected by these agents are rarely processed for frozen section; they are either fixed promptly or, if necessary, are evaluated by smear and touch preparations.

When brain biopsies are performed for the purpose of confirmation or exclusion of a spongiform encephalopathy, including Creutzfeldt-Jakob disease, certain additional precautions are observed because of the special nature of the infectious prion agent. Since this diagnosis requires excellent, artifact-free histologic preparation, no frozen sections or smear preparations are performed. The biopsy is placed directly into formalin by the surgeon and allowed to fix. It is then fixed briefly in formic acid, followed by additional formalin fixation. This procedure provides for adequate histologic detail (Plate 23-5), while resulting in near complete inactivation of the infectious agent.

DIAGNOSTIC ISSUES

The consideration of neuropathologic interpretation of brain biopsies falls outside the scope of this chapter; however, a few general comments are appropriate regarding the major categories of disease that are encountered (Table 23-1). Consideration of the individual entities appears elsewhere in this text. A large proportion of brain biopsies are performed to determine if a neoplasm is present. Depending on the institution involved and the pattern of neurosurgical referrals, there can be a wide range of ratios between primary and metastatic tumors. The neuropathologist frequently provides the essential information regarding the nature of a tumor and its histologic grade—information critical for the subsequent therapy and care of the patient. Similarly, in cases of infectious diseases, the choice of antimicrobial therapy depends on the combination of microbiologic results and histologic interpretations. Under some circumstances, diseases that are ordinarily diagnosed without resort to brain biopsy may present in an atypical manner and lead to such a procedure. An example of this would be the infrequent presentation of multiple sclerosis as a single lesion with moderate mass effect.

AREAS OF DIFFICULTY

Although neuropathologic examination of biopsied brain tissue can be extremely important in guiding patient care, it is not an infallible technique and has several areas of intrinsic difficulty. Some of these have been considered above in the discussion of sampling effects. Apart from this and other technical issues, some histopathologic patterns, while distinctive, are not diagnostic. Thus, a biopsy may show a pattern of reactive gliosis with increased numbers of astrocytes, many of which have well-

TABLE 23-1. Entities Diagnosed by Brain Biopsy

Focal lesions (mass lesions; some may be multifocal)
  Tumors
    Primary brain tumors
    Metastatic tumors
    Lymphoma
    Germ cell tumors
    Pituitary lesions
  Infections
    Bacterial abscesses
    Fungal infections (aspergillosis, candida, mucormycosis)
    Parasitic infections (toxoplasmosis)
    Viral infections with focal findings
      Herpes encephalitis
      Progressive multifocal leukoencephalopathy
  Other focal processes
    Multiple sclerosis (may rarely present as a mass lesion)
    Strokes with atypical features
    Vascular malformations
    Seizure foci
  Cysts
    Colloid cysts
    Arachnoid cysts
    Pineal region cysts
  Effects of prior treatment (radionecrosis)
Diffuse processes
  Meningitic processes
    Meningeal carcinomatosis
    Vasculitis
    Infections
    Sarcoidosis
  Infections
    Viral encephalitis
  Demyelinating diseases
    ADEM
    AHL
  Inflammatory, autoimmune processes (including paraneoplastic)
  Dementia
    Alzheimer disease
    Other neurodegenerative diseases (e.g., Pick's disease, Lewy body disease)
    Creutzfeldt-Jakob disease
    Storage diseases (e.g., neuronal ceroid lipofuscinosis)
  Metabolic disorders

Abbreviations: ADEM, acute disseminated encephalomyelitis; AHL, acute hemorrhagic leukoencephalitis.

defined cytoplasm but do not give evidence of what has evoked the reaction. Similarly, the biopsy may demonstrate destructive lesions with evidence of tissue necrosis and inflammation and yet be nondiagnostic.

SUGGESTED READINGS

Adams JH, Duchen LW: Greenfield's Neuropathology. 5th Ed., Oxford University Press, New York, 1992

Brown P, Wolff A, Gajdusek DC: A simple and effective method for inactivating virus infectivity in formalin-fixed tissue samples from patients with Creutzfeldt-Jakob disease. Neurology 40:887, 1990

Burger PC, Scheithauer BW, Vogel FS: Surgical Pathology of the Nervous System and its Coverings. 3rd Ed., Churchill Livingstone, New York, 1991

Burger PC, Scheithauer BW: Tumors of the Central Nervous System. 3rd Ser., Fasc. 10. Armed Forces Institute of Pathology, Washington, DC, 1994

Chandrasoma PT, Apuzzo MLJ: Stereotactic Brain Biopsy. Igaku-Shoin, New York, 199???

Fletcher JA, Kozakewich HP, Hoffer FA et al: Diagnostic relevance of clonal cytogenetic aberrations in malignant soft-tissue tumors. N Engl J Med 324:436, 1989

Folkerth RD: Smears and frozen sections in the intraoperative diagnosis of central nervous system lesions. Neurosurg Clin 5:1, 1994

Ganju V, Jenkins RB, O'Fallon JR et al: Prognostic factors in gliomas: a multivariate analysis of clinical, pathologic, flow cytometric, cytogenetic and molecular markers. Cancer 74:920, 1994

Hu DJ, Kane MA, Heymann DL: Transmission of HIV, hepatitis B virus, and other bloodborne pathogens in health care settings: a review of risk factors and guidelines for prevention. Bull WHO 69:623, 1991

Louis DN: The p53 gene and protein in human brain tumors. J Neuropathol Exp Neurol 53:11, 1994

Russell DS, Rubinstein LJ: Pathology of Tumors of the Nervous System. 5th Ed., Williams & Wilkins, Baltimore 1989

24. BIOPSY OF NERVE AND MUSCLE

UMBERTO DE GIROLAMI
MATTHEW P. FROSCH

BIOPSY OF NERVE

The comprehensive treatise on peripheral nerve diseases by Dyck and collaborators (1993), the textbook on neurology by Adams and Victor (1993), and *Greenfield's Neuropathology* (1992) give excellent accounts of nerve biopsy techniques and interpretation. The monographs by Ouvrier and colleagues (1990) and Bouche and Vallat (1992) are especially noteworthy; we have also written on the subject (Richardson and De Girolami, 1995). The simple classification scheme that we follow for purposes of neuropathologic assessment of a peripheral nerve biopsy combines the following attributes:

1. Etiologic basis of the disorder: Is the process acquired or hereditary?
2. Topography of the injury: Is the peripheral nervous system diffusely (polyneuropathy) or focally involved (mononeuropathy, single or multiple)?
3. Chronology of pathologic process: Does the disease follow an acute, subacute, or chronic course?
4. Underlying pathologic process: What pattern of injury is present (axonal degeneration vs segmental demyelination vs infection vs vascular injury vs other)?

As is clear from this list, interpretation of a nerve biopsy requires the correlation of histologic changes with clinical information and electrophysiologic investigations.

INDICATIONS AND TECHNIQUES

Nerve biopsy is sometimes necessary to establish a diagnosis of a peripheral neuropathy and, when so, it is most often needed to tailor specific treatment or to better define a hereditary disorder. The most common indications are

1. Evaluation of pathologic process in multifocal asymmetric mononeuropathies: commonly found processes include vasculitis, amyloidosis, infectious disease (leprosy, acquired immunodeficiency syndrome).
2. Evaluation of hereditary polyneuropathies of childhood and young adulthood: these biopsies often reveal inborn errors of metabolism or HMSN/HSAN variants.
3. Evaluation of the severity of a neuropathy and underlying pathologic process in acquired polyneuropathies of adulthood: these biopsies may provide evidence of demyelination or axonal degeneration, of remyelination or axonal regeneration (clusters), as well as show changes of toxic polyneuropathies.

The nerve chosen for biopsy is generally the sural nerve, a sensory nerve. Biopsy of this nerve leads only to a restricted area of sensory loss on the lateral aspect of the ankle and foot; however, it must be remembered that sampling of a single distal sensory nerve may not be representative of focal disease processes elsewhere in the peripheral nervous system (especially in processes with predominant motor involvement).

Nerve biopsies are performed under local anesthesia in adults; general anesthesia is often required to obtain an adequate specimen from children. The laboratory should be contacted in advance of the surgery so that the tissue can be picked up directly from the operating room and processed immediately. A 2- to 3-cm-long section is removed just above the lateral malleolus. It is important not to flood the nerve itself with anesthetic and to handle it very gently in transit and maintain it wrapped in a saline-moistened gauze, rather than immersed in fluid. A frozen section can be required to ascertain that peripheral nervous tissue is present since the macroscopic appearance of sclerotic veins at surgery may resemble nervous tissue.

The biopsy is divided into several portions so that different types of studies can be performed. A portion is rapidly frozen in a histology-mounting medium and stored for possible immunofluorescence studies; these studies can reveal the deposition of immunoglobulins or other inflammatory markers such as complement or fibrinogen. A second small fragment is snap-frozen in liquid nitrogen for potential biochemical studies, when a metabolic disorder is suspected.

The remainder of the tissue (the bulk of it) is stretched delicately on a cardboard strip or kept isometric with staples (or needles) or on a muscle biopsy clamp and fixed in glutaraldehyde. From this tissue, material will be embedded in plastic (resin) and processed for semithin (1-μm sections) and thin sections for electron microscopy. The semithin sections yield the most important morphologic information regarding the integrity of axons and myelin sheaths. Quantitative morphometric methods (comparing the patient's sample with age-matched controls) can be extremely useful to detect variations in the range of fiber diameters, the thickness of the myelin sheath in proportion to the diameter of the axon, and the internodal length. Other portions of this fixed material may be used for nerve teasing. With this method, individual myelinated fibers are separated from the nerve fascicles and stained, allowing examination of the integrity and thickness of the myelin sheath as well as revealing alterations in internodal length. Finally, routine formalin fixation and paraffin embedding is performed on a portion of the biopsy. These preparations are most often contributory in the setting of inflammatory, neoplastic, or infectious diseases.

Structure of Normal Nerve

The principal structural component of peripheral nerve is the *nerve fiber,* an axon with its Schwann cells and myelin sheath (Fig. 24-1). A nerve consists of numerous fibers grouped into fascicles by connective tissue sheaths. *Myelinated* and *unmyelinated* nerve fibers are intermingled across the fascicle. In sural nerve, myelinated fibers range between 2 and 15 μm in diameter and have a bimodal distribution. Small myelinated axons, which average 4 μm, are about twice as numerous as the larger size population, which average 11 μm. Axons are myelinated in segments (internodes) separated by *nodes of Ranvier.* A single Schwann cell supplies the myelin sheath for each internode. The thickness of the myelin sheath is directly propor-

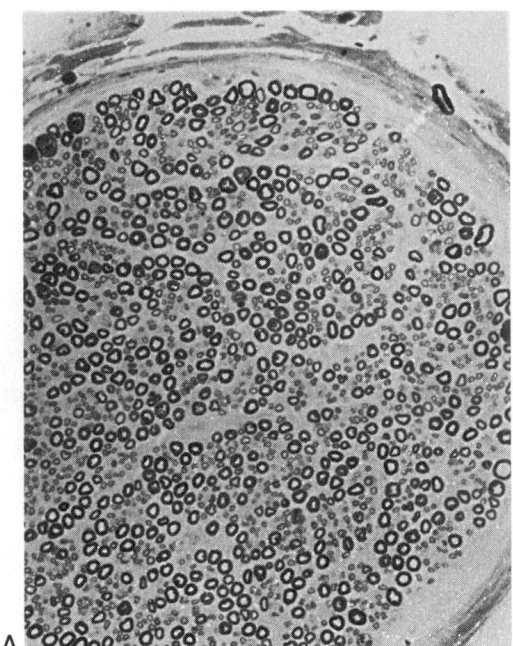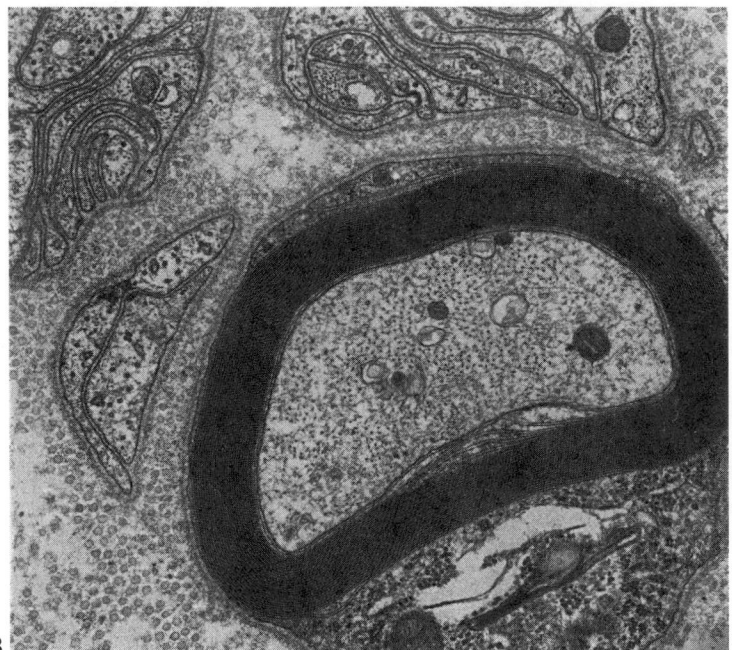

FIG. 24-1. (A) Transverse section of normal sural nerve showing densely packed myelinated fibers of varying sizes and a rim of perineurial layers. (Plastic-embedded 1-μm-thick section stained with toluidine blue). (B)—Electron micrograph of a transverse section through the internodal region of a single normal myelinated fiber with surrounding Schwann cell (*bottom right*) and several unmyelinated fibers (*top left*).

tional to the diameter of the axon, and the larger the axon diameter, the longer the internodal distance.

Unmyelinated axons are more numerous than myelinated axons and range in size from 0.2 to 3 μm. They occur in groups of 5 to 20, each group enveloped by a single Schwann cell. Each axon is invested by a region of Schwann cell membrane but without the specialized differentiation to form myelin.

Schwann cells, regardless of their association with myelinated or unmyelinated fibers, have pale oval nuclei with an even chromatin distribution and an elongated bipolar cell body. Electron microscopy shows that Schwann cells, unlike fibroblasts, have a basement membrane. Peripheral axons contain organelles and cytoskeletal structures, including microfilaments, neurofilaments, microtubules, mitochondria, vesicles, smooth endoplasmic reticulum, and lysosomes. Dense-cored and coated vesicles are located in the nerve terminals. Protein synthesis does not occur in the axon, and axoplasmic flow delivers proteins and other substances synthesized in the perikaryon down the axon. A retrograde transport system serves as a feedback to the cell body.

The connective tissue sheaths of peripheral nerve include the *epineurium,* which encloses the entire nerve, the *perineurium,* a multilayered concentric connective tissue sheath that encloses each fascicle, and the *endoneurium,* which surrounds individual nerve fibers. The nerve microenvironment is regulated by the *perineurial barrier* (formed by the tight junctions between the perineurial cells), the *blood-nerve barrier,* and the *nerve-cerebrospinal fluid (CSF) barrier.* Endoneurial capillaries derived from the vasa nervorum form tight junctions and establish the blood-nerve barrier. The blood-nerve barrier has been found to be relatively less competent within nerve roots, dorsal root ganglia, and autonomic ganglia. The nerve-CSF barrier is formed by the tight junctions between the cells that form the outer layer of the arachnoid membrane. These cells fuse with

the perineurium of the roots and cranial nerves as they leave the subarachnoid space, and the motor and sensory fibers, which are separated within anterior and posterior roots intermingle within the mixed sensorimotor nerves that exit the spinal canal.

Reactions to Injury

Although disease processes of many kinds with differing pathogenic mechanisms may affect the peripheral nervous system, there are essentially two principal reactions to injury: segmental demyelination and axonal degeneration. These pathologic processes can also occur in combination.

Segmental demyelination is the morphologic expression of dysfunction of the Schwann cell or damage to the myelin sheath. The process characteristically is "segmental" along the length of the nerve fiber in that it affects some Schwann cells and their corresponding internodes while sparing others. The disintegrating myelin is phagocytosed by Schwann cells and macrophages. The denuded axon segment provides a stimulus for remyelination, and cells within the endoneurium remyelinate it forming new myelinated internodes that are shorter and thinner than normal (features that are best seen with teased nerve preparations). With sequential episodes of demyelination and remyelination, there is an accumulation of tiers of Schwann cell processes, which, on transverse section, appear as concentric skeins of cell cytoplasm surrounding the axon (onion bulbs) (Fig. 24-2).

Axonal degeneration is characterized by primary destruction of the axon, with secondary disintegration of its myelin sheath (Fig. 24-3). The damage to the axon may either be due to a discrete, localized event (trauma, ischemia) or to an underlying abnormality of the neuron (*neuronopathy*) or its axon (*axonopathy*). When axonal degeneration occurs as the result of transection, the distal portion of the fiber undergoes an acute process

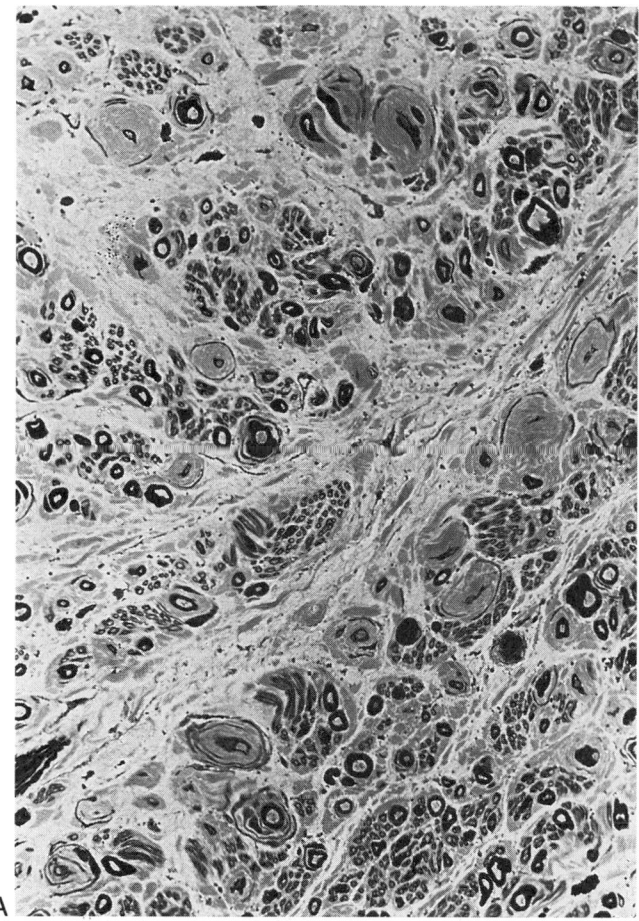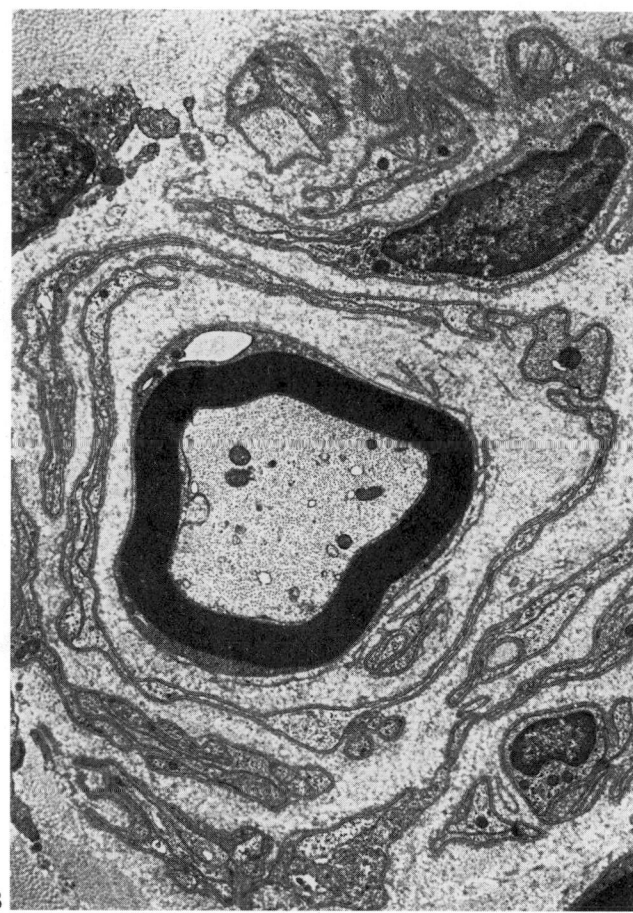

FIG. 24-2. **(A)** Chronic and repeated segmental demyelination and remyelination in hereditary onion bulb neuropathy (Charcot-Marie-Tooth). Note decrease in the number of myelinated fibers, increase in endoneurial connective tissue, and numerous onion bulbs. **(B)** Electron micrograph of onion bulb showing myelinated axon surrounded by overlapping Schwann cell processes alternating with collagen fibers.

of disintegration (termed *wallerian degeneration*) characterized by breakdown and phagocytosis of the axon and its myelin sheath into fragments forming small oval compartments (*myelin ovoids*). In the slowly evolving neuronopathies or axonopathies, evidence of myelin breakdown is scant because only a few fibers are degenerating at any given time.

The proximal stumps of axons that have degenerated may develop new growth cones, which extend along the course of the degenerated axon. The presence of multiple, closely aggregated, thinly myelinated, small-caliber axons can be recognized as evidence of regeneration (regenerating cluster). This regrowth of axons is a slow process, on the order of 2 mm/day. In spite of its slow pace, axonal regeneration accounts for some of the potential for functional recovery following peripheral axonal injury.

In addition to these pathologic reactions affecting the nerve fiber, examination of the supporting tissues of the nerve can reveal evidence of inflammatory/infectious, vascular, connective tissue, and neoplastic disease processes similar to those found in other organ systems.

BIOPSY OF SKELETAL MUSCLE

Over the past thirty years there has been a growing recognition of the value of the muscle biopsy as a diagnostic tool in the evaluation of patients with muscle disease. The single standard treatise available on the topic in 1962, *Diseases of Muscle* by Adams and colleagues, was followed by a number of excellent monographs, which included the newer techniques of enzyme histochemistry, electron microscopy, and molecular biology. In spite of (or because of) the advances in the laboratory, the necessity to correlate the information obtained from the muscle biopsy with the clinical neurologic assessment and the electromyographic (EMG) and nerve conduction velocity studies remains all the more essential today.

Muscle diseases are classified on histopathologic/etiologic grounds into three major categories:

1. Neurogenic atrophy or denervation atrophy: the pathologic changes found in muscle reflect alterations in its innervation
2. Myopathies: a large category of diseases, including inherited, congenital, acquired, metabolic, and toxic disorders with abnormalities in the muscle fibers
3. Disorders of the neuromuscular junction: a small group of disorders where the abnormalities are restricted to the neuromuscular junction; patients with these disorders have minimal structural alterations and are rarely biopsied

Indications and Techniques

The evaluation of a skeletal muscle biopsy specimen is dependent on careful selection of the site of the biopsy based on

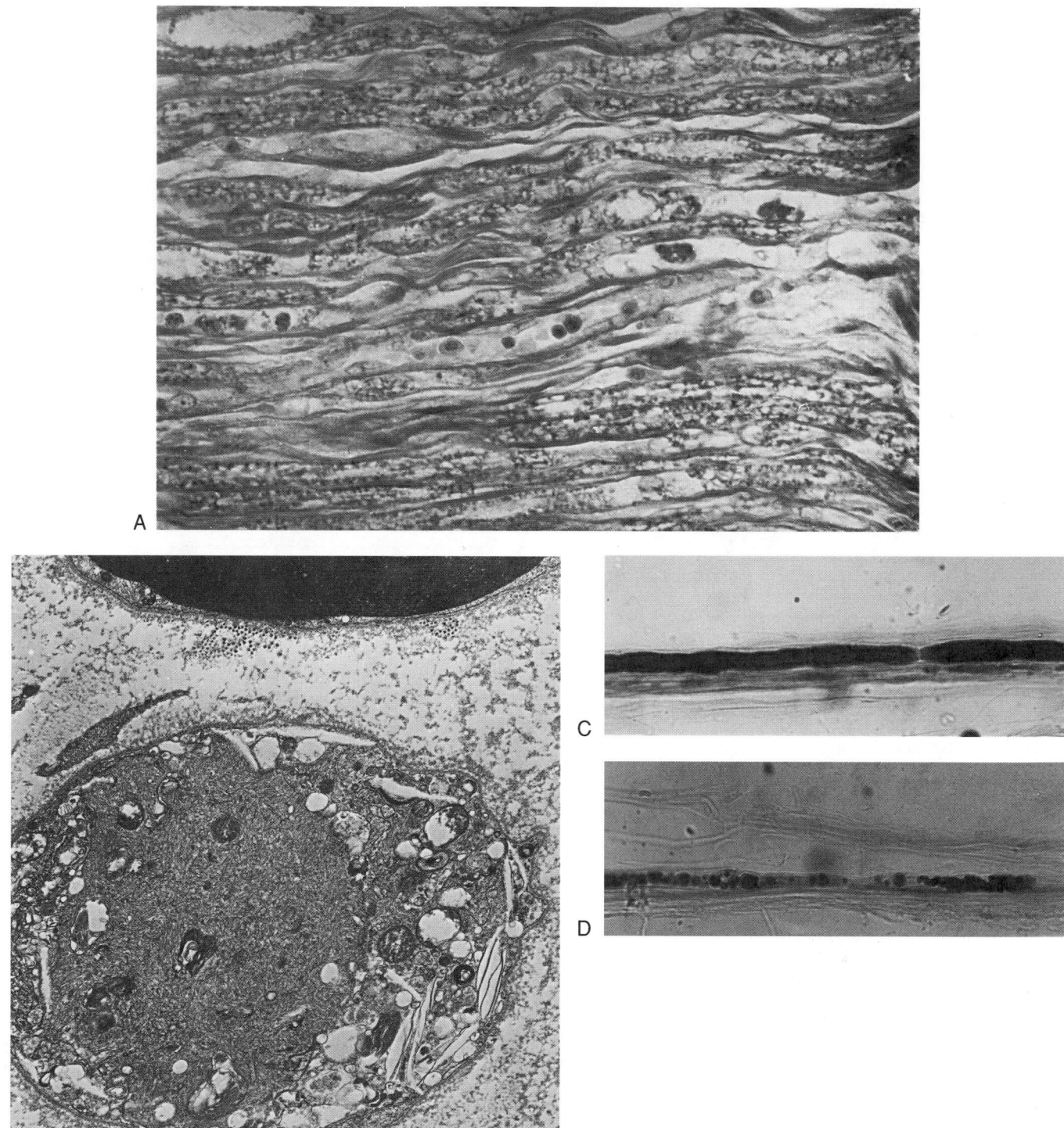

FIG. 24-3. **(A)** Longitudinal section of paraffin-embedded nerve showing breakdown of myelinated fiber. (Woelke's stain for myelin.) **(B)** Electron micrograph of axonal degeneration. Note disappearance of myelin and accumulation of filaments and organelles in the axon. Normal myelin sheath is shown at top. **(C)** Nerve teasing: normal fiber stains intensely black at the internode; node of Ranvier is located at the clear zone between the two internodes. **(D)** Nerve teasing: axonal degeneration is characterized by irregular beading and fragmentation of the myelin sheath and axon.

clinical and neurophysiologic data. Since the physician who requests the biopsy is often not the person who performs the surgery, communication between the two is essential to ensure that the proper site is chosen. The muscle chosen should be easily accessible and should be involved by the disease process to a moderate degree. Severely weak or atrophic muscles should not be biopsied nor should the biopsy be taken from the sites of prior EMG needle examinations or areas of previous trauma, since the ensuing tissue reaction to injury response may confuse the interpretation of the biopsy. The biopsy should be taken with as little trauma as possible from the belly of the muscle—never from the tendinous insertion. The specimen should be brought to the neuropathology laboratory *immediately* after removal. Biopsy specimens should be transported from the operating room wrapped in a saline-moistened gauze to prevent drying en route.

Specimens should include "clamped" biopsies, which are prevented from contracting by the use of a muscle biopsy clamp or stretched out by suturing the muscle over a tongue blade. Each specimen should be about 1 cm in length and 0.5 cm in width. These specimens are intended for (1) formalin fixation and paraffin-embedding for light microscopic examination and (2) fixation with glutaraldehyde/paraformaldehyde and plastic embedding for electron microscopy. In addition, a comparable fragment of tissue should be provided; the majority of this tissue is rapidly frozen in liquid nitrogen-cooled isopentane and carefully oriented to obtain transverse sections (or, if sufficient, both transverse and longitudinal sections) and is sectioned on a cryostat for a battery of histochemical reactions (ATPase at alkaline and acid pHs, oxidative enzyme reactions), hematoxylin and eosin, Trichrome, PAS + diastase, and lipids. Appreciation of individual myocyte size and shape can best be made from this material, which is comparably free of the shrinkage and preparation artifacts. Morphometric evaluation of the size and number of muscle fibers of each histochemical type can be performed on these sections. The frozen sections and the

TABLE 24-1. Muscle Fiber Types

Characteristic	Type 1	Type 2
Action:	Sustained force Weightbearing	Sudden movements Purposeful motion
Enzyme content:	NADH: dark staining ATPase pH 4.2: dark staining ATPase pH 9.4: light staining	NADH: light staining ATPase pH 4.2: dark staining ATPase pH 9.4: dark staining
Lipids:	Abundant	Scant
Glycogen:	Scant	Abundant
Ultrastructure:	Many mitochondria Wide Z band	Few mitochondria Narrow Z band
Physiology:	Slow twitch	Fast twitch
Color:	Red	White

histochemical reactions performed on them thus form a very important basis for the interpretation of muscle biopsies. A small portion is also stored frozen for subsequent biochemical studies. Similar to the handling of a nerve biopsy, the apportioning of the biopsy specimen for a variety of studies allows for a wide range of studies to be performed from a single biopsy procedure.

Structure of Normal Skeletal Muscle

Skeletal muscles are composed of individual muscle fibers, which are multinucleated syncytia derived from numerous cells. The nuclei are normally located just beneath the plasma membrane (sarcolemma); they are slender, oval, and oriented parallel to the length of the fiber with evenly distributed chromatin and inconspicuous nucleoli. Internal nuclei, best seen in transverse section, are estimated to be found in no more than about 3 percent of normal adult fibers; they occur in higher frequency in some pathologic conditions. Satellite cells, a reserve cell population, are located adjacent to the sarcolemma and are covered by basement membrane which encircles the entire muscle fiber. Almost the entire cytoplasm of the muscle fiber is filled with myofilaments which form the contractile apparatus. A my-

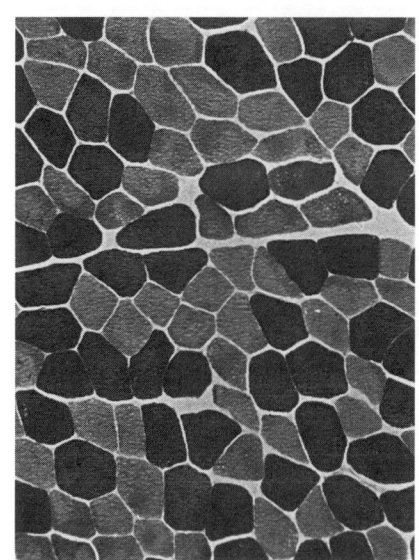 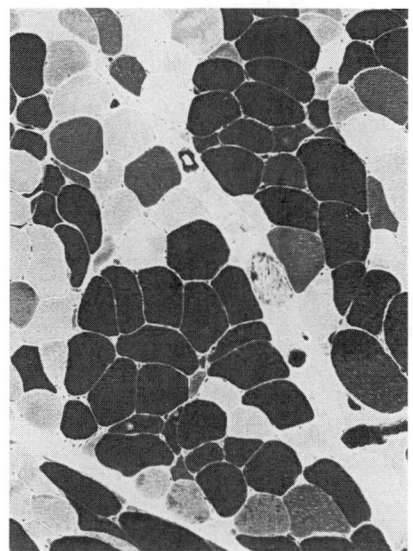 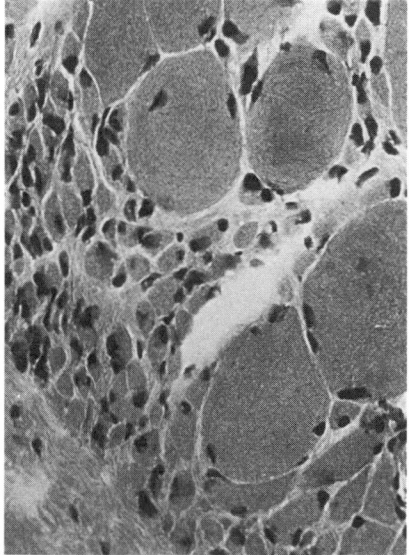

FIG. 24-4. **(A)** Normal muscle showing a checkerboard pattern of type 1 and type 2 fibers. (ATPase enzyme histochemistry on frozen sections.) **(B)** Denervation and reinnervation showing clustering of fibers of the same histochemical type and loss of the checkerboard pattern. (ATPase enzyme histochemistry on frozen sections.) **(C)** End-stage denervation showing grouping of atrophic fibers. (Hematoxylin and eosin.)

ofibril is composed of identical repeating units (sarcomeres) of interlaced, longitudinally directed thin filaments and thick filaments and perpendicularly disposed Z bands. The T-tubule system, involved in calcium release during excitation, is an invagination of the sarcolemmal membrane into the interior of the cell which courses parallel to the Z bands accompanied on each side by smooth endoplasmic reticulum.

The adult muscle fiber is polygonal on transverse section; in infancy, fibers tend to be round, as are those of the extrinsic eye muscles and some facial and pharyngeal muscles in adults. The cross-sectional diameter of individual fibers varies, depending on the specific muscle and its functional status. The functional unit of a muscle is a motor unit, which consists of multiple muscle fibers innervated by a single motor neuron. The size of motor units depends on the particular muscle being studied as well as on any pathologic process present. The individual muscle fibers of a motor unit are randomly distributed throughout the cross section of a normal muscle, although this may be altered in some disease states.

In diagnostic muscle biopsy histochemistry, two major types of fibers (type 1 and type 2) are recognized, and these correspond to some extent to the general physiologic subclassifications of skeletal muscle cells (Fig. 24-4A and Table 24-1). Type 1 fibers are high in myoglobin and oxidative enzymes and have many mitochondria; these features are in keeping with their ability to perform tonic contraction. They stain dark with ATPase at pH 4.2 and light at pH 9.4. Type 2 fibers are rich in glycolytic enzymes and are involved in rapid phasic contractions; they stain dark with ATPase at pH 9.4 and light at pH 4.2.

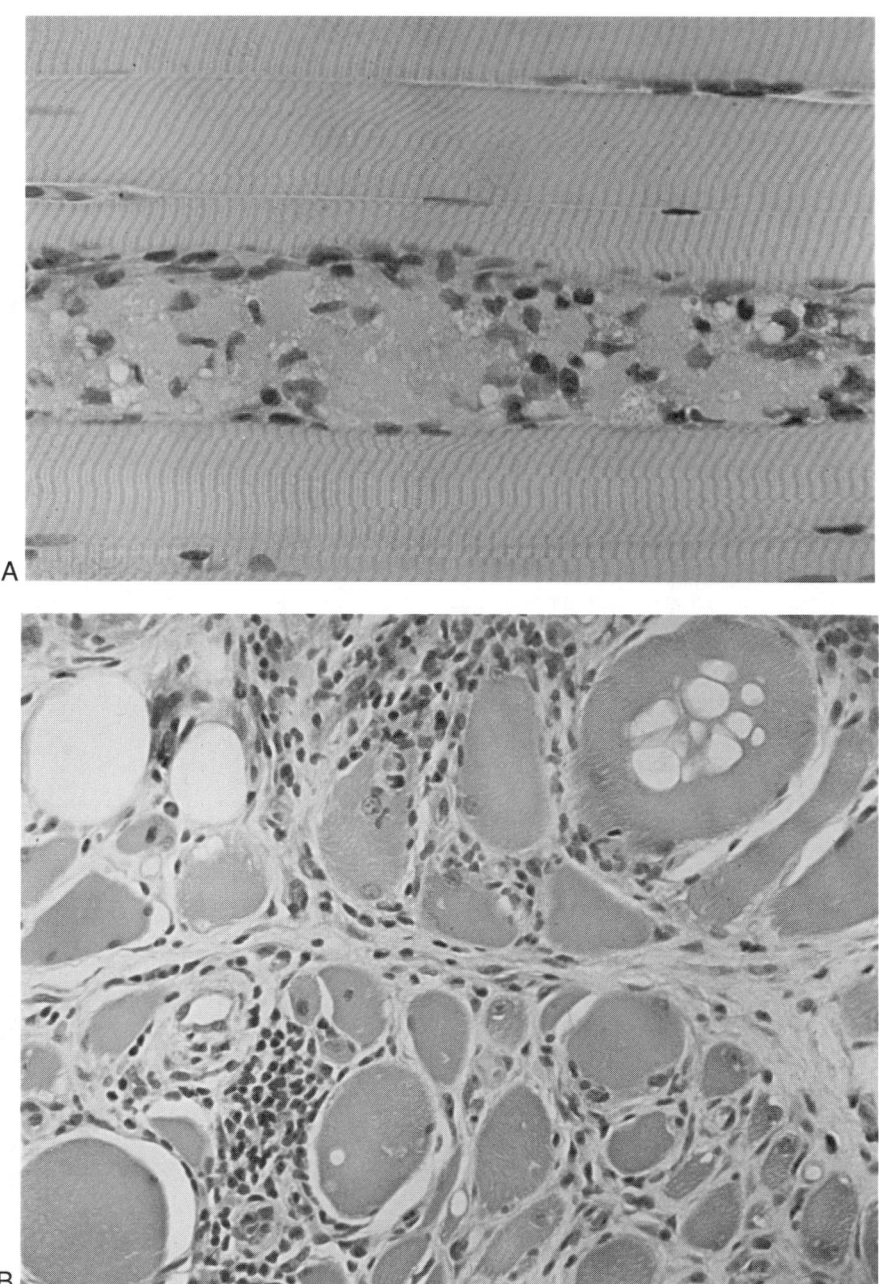

FIG. 24-5. **(A)** Longitudinal section of paraffin-embedded muscle showing muscle fiber necrosis. (Hematoxylin and eosin.) **(B)** Transverse section of paraffin-embedded muscle showing inflammatory infiltrates.

The innervating motor neuron determines the type of an individual fiber; therefore, all fibers of a single motor unit are of the same type. Since these fibers are distributed randomly across the muscle, normal muscle shows a "checkerboard" pattern of alternating light and dark fibers as demonstrated with ATPase or other of histochemical reactions. There is variability in the relative abundance of fiber types among muscles.

Muscle spindles are fusiform structures that respond to stretch in muscles and thus have a role in maintaining tone. They consist of specialized muscle and nerve fibers delimited by a connective tissue capsule. The connective tissue sheath of muscles include the endomysium, which surrounds individual muscle fibers, the perimysium, which groups muscle fibers into primary and secondary bundles (fasciculi), and the epimysium, which envelops single muscles or large groups of fibers.

Reactions to Injury

The two principal pathologic processes seen in skeletal muscle are those consequent to interruption of innervation (*denervation atrophy*) and those due to a primary abnormality of the muscle fiber itself (*myopathic change*). When axonal degeneration occurs, the muscle fibers within that motor unit lose their neural input and undergo denervation atrophy. Denervation of muscle leads to downregulation of myosin and actin synthesis, a resorption of myofibrils, and a decrease in the cell size while allowing the cell to survive. In cross section, the atrophic fibers are smaller than normal and have a roughly triangular shape ("angulated"). There is also cytoskeletal reorganization of some muscle cells, which results in a rounded central zone of disorganized filaments (target fiber).

Reinnervation of muscle fibers may precede the regeneration of motor axons. Surviving axons from intact motor units can extend sprouts, which will reinnervate the neighboring denervated muscle fibers. These newly incorporated muscle fibers now will assume the fiber type of their new parent motor unit. A patch of 15 to 30 adjoining fibers of the same histochemical type will form ("fiber type grouping") (Fig. 24-4B), and the normal checkerboard pattern of alternating light and dark fibers is lost. In chronic denervation, over time, there is atrophy of the fibers of the "type group" ("group atrophy") (Fig. 24-4C).

Myopathic changes comprise those abnormalities of the muscle fibers found in primary disorders of the muscle cell itself and represent a wide spectrum of histopathologic alterations. They include those changes that result in destruction of the fiber with consequent regeneration and those structural changes not leading directly to cell death but associated with fiber dysfunction. *Segmental necrosis,* destruction of a portion of a myocyte (Fig. 24-5A), may be followed by *myophagocytosis* as macrophages infiltrate the region. *Regeneration* occurs as the peripherally located satellite cells proliferate and reconstitute the destroyed portion of the fiber. The regenerating cell has large internalized nuclei with prominent nucleoli, and the cytoplasm, laden with RNA, becomes basophilic. Other characteristics of myopathic injury include vacuolation, inflammation, alterations in structural proteins or organelles, and accumulation of intracytoplasmic deposits (Fig. 24-5B). Whatever the cause, the loss of fibers is associated with extensive deposition of collagen and fatty infiltration.

Individual myofiber *hypertrophy* occurs in response to increased load, either in the setting of exercise or in pathologic conditions where other muscle fibers are injured. Large fibers may divide along a segment (*muscle fiber splitting*) so that, in cross section, a single large fiber contains a cell membrane traversing its diameter, often with adjacent nuclei.

Other types of structural alterations in the muscle fibers are seen in various disorders. These include those seen in the congenital myopathies where a variety of abnormalities in myofilament or organelle structure are evident, particularly by electron microscopy. In the so-called mitochondrial myopathies, there are alterations in mitochondrial organization and number. Among the metabolic myopathies, lipid-storage myopathies demonstrate abnormally numerous and misshapen lipid droplets, and certain metabolic myopathies show subsarcolemmal and intracytoplasmic vacuoles.

One last pattern of injury which requires comment is type 2 atrophy in which this fiber type shows relatively selective atrophy. This pattern may occur in association with inactivity or disuse in a variety of clinical settings as a well as with steroid treatment. It may be a superimposed process in cases where muscle pain or other problems have resulted in decreased activity.

SUGGESTED READINGS

Adams RD, Denny-Brown D, Pearson CM: Diseases of Muscle: A Study in Pathology. 2nd Ed Harper & Row, New York, 1962

Adams JH, Duchen LW: Greenfield's Neuropathology. 5th Ed. Oxford University Press, New York, 1992

Adams RD, Victor M: Principles of Neurology. 5th Ed. McGraw-Hill, New York, 1993

Bouche P, Vallat J-M: Neuropathies Périphériques. Doin, Paris, 1992

Carpenter S, Karpati G: Pathology of Skeletal Muscle. Churchill Livingstone, New York, 1984

Dubowitz V, Brooke MH: Muscle Biopsy: A Modern Approach. WB Saunders, Philadelphia, 1973

Dyck PJ, Thomas PK, Griffin JW, Low PA, Poduslo JF: Peripheral Neuropathy. 3rd Ed, WB Saunders, Philadelphia, 1993

Engel AG, Franzini-Armstrong C: Myology: Basic and Clinical. WB Saunders, Philadelphia, 1994

Ferreire G, Denef J-F, Rodriguez J, Guzzetta F: Morphometric studies of normal sural nerves in children. Muscle Nerve 8:697, 1985

Ouvrier RA, McLeod JG, Pollard JD: Peripheral Neuropathy in Childhood. Raven Press, New York, 1990

Richardson EP Jr, De Girolami U: Pathology of the Peripheral Nerve, WB Saunders, Philadelphia, 1995

SECTION 4. PRINCIPLES OF TREATMENT

25. PHARMACOLOGY OF COMMONLY USED DRUGS

STEVEN FESKE

This chapter provides some basic information about some of the drugs that are commonly used in the therapy of neurologic diseases. The discussions here are general and selective in an attempt to target certain issues that repeatedly arise in the use of the drugs chosen for mention. Indications and further information about the use of a drug in a specific disease can be found in the discussion of that disease in later chapters.

THROMBOEMBOLIC DISEASE

Antiplatelet Agents

Aspirin.   Acetylsalicylic acid is the ester of acetic and salicylic acids. It irreversibly inhibits cyclo-oxygenase, which is the enzyme that catalyzes the conversion of arachidonic acid to prostaglandins and thromboxanes. The major product of this metabolic pathway in platelets is thromboxane, which promotes platelet adhesion. Because the platelet does not have the machinery to resynthesize cyclo-oxygenase, aspirin renders a platelet permanently deficient in thromboxane, and hence poorly adherent, for its lifetime. The major product of this metabolic pathway in endothelial cells is prostacyclin, which inhibits platelet adhesion. After irreversible inhibition of its cyclo-oxygenase by aspirin, an endothelial cell can replenish it, if left unexposed to further aspirin. Aspirin is readily absorbed by the gastrointestinal (GI) tract; biotransformation occurs mainly in the liver. Aspirin and its inactive metabolites are excreted in the urine; alkaline pH promotes excretion of free salicylate by ''trapping'' the ionized form in the urine. Initial studies on the effect of aspirin in transient ischemic attacks used 1,300 mg/day. Because low doses offer a possible theoretical advantage—irreversibly inhibiting platelet adhesion while allowing a return of prostacyclin production by the endothelium—and surely lower side effects, later studies have tested smaller doses. It is now most common to use 325 mg/day for antiplatelet therapy, and even lower doses have been shown to have clinical antithrombotic effects. Some patients may derive benefit from higher doses. Details concerning its use in the prevention of thromboembolic disease are discussed in Chapter 44. The major side effects are GI symptoms and erosion with bleeding and other abnormal bleeding secondary to platelet dysfunction. The former can be minimized by the use of enteric-coated preparations. The antithrombotic effect can be assayed by the bleeding time, which is prolonged by aspirin.

Ticlopidine.   Ticlopidine hydrochloride inhibits adenosine diphosphate-induced platelet aggregation. Unlike aspirin, it does not inhibit cyclo-oxygenase, and it has no effect on platelet thromboxane or endothelial cell prostacyclin. Like aspirin, its effect lasts for the life of the platelet. It is readily absorbed by the gastrointestinal tract, and is highly, about 98 percent, protein bound. It is metabolized by the liver to inactive compounds that are excreted in the urine and feces and small amounts are excreted unchanged. The plasma half-life is 4 to 5 days. The dosage and use have been established primarily by two large studies, the Canadian American Ticlopidine Study (CATS) and the Ticlopidine Aspirin Stroke Study (TASS), reported in 1989. At 250 mg twice a day, ticlopidine was superior to placebo and slightly superior to aspirin for secondary prevention of stroke and other vascular events. These issues are discussed in detail in Chapter 44. Ticlopidine caused significantly more side effects than aspirin. Its serious side effect is neutropenia, which can result from arrest of granulocyte maturation. Severe neutropenia has occurred in about 1 percent of patients, generally within the first 3 months of ticlopidine use and is reversible upon discontinuation of the drug. Other significant side effects are diarrhea (about 20 percent), rash, bleeding disorders, elevated values of liver function tests, and a slight elevation of serum lipoproteins. All are dose-dependent and reversible. Because of these side effects, the manufacturer recommends that monitoring include a baseline complete blood count (CBC) and differential count and repeated CBCs and differential counts every 2 weeks for 3 months or for 2 weeks after therapy has been discontinued. If the absolute neutrophil count (white blood cell count [WBC] × fractional neutrophil count) falls to ≤ 1,200/mm^3, ticlopidine should be stopped and the patient closely monitored until the neutrophil count returns to normal. This recovery is usually complete within 3 weeks. Liver function tests should also be monitored during the first 3 months of treatment.

Anticoagulants

Heparin.   Heparin is a large mucopolysaccharide polymer of repeating D-glucosamine-L-iduronic acid and D-glucosamine-D-glucuronic acid disaccharide units. Commercially available heparin contains varying proportions of these disaccharides in polymers of various lengths. Heparin works through its interaction with the naturally occurring anticoagulants antithrombin III (AT III) and heparin cofactor II. AT III is a serine protease inhibitor (see Chapter 18 and Fig. 18-1) that irreversibly binds to the activated clotting factors XIIa, XIa, IXa, Xa, IIa (thrombin), and XIIIa. This complex formation inactivates these factors, especially factors Xa and thrombin, and inhibits thrombus formation. Heparin greatly accelerates the reaction of AT III with these factors. Because of its large molecular size and polarity, it is poorly absorbed through the gastrointestinal tract, and it does not readily cross the placenta. It must be given intravenously or subcutaneously. Heparin is transformed by the liver into inactive metabolites, which are eliminated in the urine. The half-life increases with increasing doses, and during continuous infusion, a steady state may not be reached for more than 48 hours. Large thrombi, as in pulmonary embolism, increase the clearance, decrease the half-life, and increase the doses needed to achieve a given degree of anticoagulation. Low-dose heparin for prophylaxis against deep-vein thrombosis is usually given subcutaneously at 5,000 U twice daily, and this dose usually has little, if any, effect on the partial thromboplastin time (PTT). For prophylaxis after a stroke or transient ischemic attack, full heparin anticoagulation is usually given by an infusion at approximately 1,000 U/h. No loading or a low-loading dose of 500–1,000 U probably decreases the risk of reperfusion hemorrhage (see Ch. 44). The PTT is checked in 6 to 8 hours, and the infusion is adjusted to maintain a PTT of 1.5 to 2.5 times the control value (about 45 to 60). Daily PTT values are measured to maintain the desired degree of anticoagulation. The use of heparin for stroke prevention is discussed in Chapter 44. The most common adverse effect is hemorrhage. Higher PTT values and large loading doses have been associated with an increased risk of intracerebral hemorrhage after ischemic stroke. Other side effects include hypersensitivity and thrombocytopenia; the latter is generally caused by heparin-induced platelet aggregation. A more severe thrombocytopenia can result from the formation of antiplatelet antibodies, which can occasionally cause heparin-induced thrombosis. Therefore, all patients receiving full- or low-dose heparin should have serial platelet counts. Low molecular weight heparinoids cause fewer side effects and are under study for the treatment of stroke.

Warfarin. Warfarin sodium is a congener of dicumerol, which acts by interfering with post-translational modification in the liver of the vitamin K-dependent clotting factors, II (prothrombin), VII, IX, and X. It also decreases the activity of the vitamin K-dependent proteins C and S, which interact to inhibit thrombosis (Fig. 18-1). Warfarin is well absorbed after an oral dose. It is almost totally bound to albumin. It is metabolized by the hepatic microsomal enzymes to inactive products and excreted in urine and stool. The degradation half-lives of the affected clotting factors differ. They are approximately 6, 24, 40, and 60 hours for factors VII, IX, X, and II, respectively. The earliest anticoagulant effect in 8 to 12 hours is due to depletion of factor VII. The peak effect is delayed by 2 to 4 days after the peak serum concentration and is due to the depletion of factors X and II. Usual practice is to start with the expected maintenance dose of 2 to 5 mg/day or to give a loading dose of 10 mg/day for 2 to 3 days and then lower the dose to 5 mg/day when the international normalized ratio (INR; prothrombin) begins to rise. The dose can then be adjusted, usually to 2 to 10 mg/day to achieve the desired INR (see Chapter 18). Recent recommendations have simplified the therapeutic goals for INR prolongation to 2 to 3 for all indications, except embolic prophylaxis in patients with a mechanical heart valve. These issues are discussed in Chapter 44. Because of the delay of peak effect, a dose should be expected to prolong the INR maximally in 2 to 3 days. Prothrombin checks and dose adjustments should take this delay into account. Approximately weekly checks of the prothrombin should be followed until a stable dose is found. Thereafter, periodic checking, approximately monthly, must continue as long as the patient is taking the drug, since various drugs and conditions can alter the effect of a given dose. The major side effect is hemorrhage. Higher prothrombin values, the addition of aspirin, and a tendency to fall correlate with an increased risk. A transient procoagulant effect with resultant thrombosis can occur early in therapy. This is because protein C, like factor VII, has a short half-life and is depleted before factors X and II. This relatively uncompensated early depletion of protein C may also be responsible for the skin necrosis that

TABLE 25-1. Warfarin Drug Interactions

Drugs that may enhance the anticoagulant effect	
Alcohol	Metronidazole
Allopurinol	Paroxetine
Cephalosporins	Pentoxifylline
Cimetidine	Phenytoin
Clofibrate	Quinidine, quinine
Disulfiram	Salicylates
Ethycrinic acid	Sertraline
Fluoxetine	Tamoxifen
Heparin	Thyroid supplements
Lovastatin	TMP-SMZ
MAOIs	
Drugs that may inhibit the anticoagulant effect	
Antacids	Haloperidol
Antihistamines	Nafcillin
Barbiturates	Oral contraceptives
Carbamazepine	Paraldehyde
Cholestyramine	Primidone
Corticosteroids	Rifampin
Glutethimide	Trazodone
Griseofulvin	Vitamin C

Abbreviations: MAOIs, monoamine oxidase inhibitors; TMP-SMZ, trimethoprim-sulfamethoxazole.

can rarely follow warfarin use. To prevent these potential early complications, many authors recommend overlapping the heparin with warfarin for 2 to 3 days after a therapeutic INR is achieved in cases requiring acute anticoagulation. Vitamin K deficiency, alcoholism, hepatic disease, and hypermetabolic states increase the anticoagulant response to warfarin. A high intake of vitamin K-rich vegetables like broccoli and spinach, pregnancy, nephrotic syndrome, hypometabolic states, and hereditary resistence decrease the anticoagulant response. Warfarin has important interactions with many other commonly used drugs (Table 25-1).

IMMUNE FUNCTION

Corticosteroids

Several corticosteroids are used for different indications in many neurologic diseases. Dexamethasone, methylprednisolone, and prednisone, the most common choices, are congeners of cortisol, the primary endogenous glucocorticoid. Dexamethasone is fluorinated, which increases its potency. Corticosteroids act by forming a complex with an intracytoplasmic receptor. This complex enters the nucleus where it binds to chromatin and alters RNA transcription and, ultimately, protein synthesis. This general basic mechanism is responsible for the many effects of corticosteroids on function. These effects include the stabilization of the blood-brain barrier and a decrease in the production of vasogenic edema, an inhibition of the inflammatory and immune responses by multiple effects on lymphocytes, macrophages, and immunoglobulins, and a lytic effect on neoplasms, especially lymphomas and myelomas. Dexamethasone and methylprednisolone are available in oral and injectable forms, and prednisone is given orally. They are protein-bound by a specific binding protein, transcortin, and, at pharmacologic doses, more importantly by albumin. Prednisone is inactive and must be converted to prednisolone to have its effect; this conversion occurs rapidly in the liver. The corticosteroids are further metabolized in the liver and other tissues and excreted primarily in the urine. The doses vary greatly with the indication and response. Potency equivalencies are shown in Table 25-2. Recommended doses of dexamethasone for brain edema are given in Chapter 149 and for spinal cord compression in Chapter 167. For acute spinal cord trauma, an infusion of methylprednisolone has been recommended (Bracken 1990). For mul-

TABLE 25-2. Relative Potencies and Equivalent Doses of Corticosteroids

Drug	Relative Anti-inflammatory Potency	Equivalent Dose (mg)
Cortisol	1	20
Prednisone	4	5
Methylprednisolone	5	4
Dexamethasone	25	0.75

(Adapted from Haynes RC, Murad F: Adrenocorticotropic hormone. p. 1475. In Gilman AG, Goodman LS, Rall TW: Goodman and Gilman's The Pharmacological Basis of Therapeutics. Macmillan, New York, 1985, with permission.)

tiple sclerosis, methylprednisolone is often used, as discussed in Chapter 45. Various regimens and doses are used for steroid-responsive neuromuscular diseases. Although it is not possible to recommend a single regimen for all indications, it is perhaps helpful to emphasize some of the general principles of the proper use of chronic corticosteroids and to give an example of a reasonable tapering schedule that can be used as a model from which to deviate based on the clinical circumstances. Table 25-3 gives a conservative schedule for the slow tapering of high-dose prednisone. Many patients may tolerate a more rapid taper, and some will not require a maintenance dose. When relapses occur on such a tapering schedule, it is usually necessary to raise the dose to a level higher than the prior one on which the patient was stable and to slowly work back to the lower dose. Therefore, it behooves the physician to remain cautious during prednisone tapering to avoid such setbacks that may significantly increase the time spent on high doses of medication. The many side effects of corticosteroids are well known. Acutely in large doses, they may cause sodium and water retention, elevated blood pressure, glucose intolerance, gastrointestinal bleeding, and an agitated confusional state. Chronically, they cause all of these problems and more, including a cushingoid appearance, osteoporosis, avascular necrosis, acneform and atrophic skin changes, cataracts, type II muscle fiber atrophy, potassium depletion, and susceptibility to opportunistic infections. In general, prednisone is safe for short-term use in pregnancy, such as in Bell's palsy. By accelerating hepatic metabolism of the corticosteriods, the anticonvulsants phenobarbital, phenytoin, and carbamazepine may increase the doses necessary to achieve a given effect. To minimize the side effects and possibly to increase the therapeutic effect, the entire daily dose of corticosteroid should be given in the morning, and alternate-day regimens should be used when possible. All patients on chronic doses should be counseled to follow a low-sodium, low-carbohydrate, high-protein diet and to avoid weight gain. Potassium should be supplemented by food choices or KCl

supplements. H-2 blockers or antacids are often helpful to prevent gastrointestinal side effects. Monitoring for the treatable side effects should be done with periodic urine or serum glucose measurements, serum K^+, blood pressure, and stool hematests. When patients receiving chronic steroids become acutely ill, it is important to give them stress doses of replacement corticosteroids (about 300 mg/day of cortisol or its equivalent), since the exogenous corticosteroids inhibit the hypothalamic-pituitary-adrenal axis. Patients with a history of tuberculosis or a positive PPD should receive isoniazid to prevent reactivation of TB. Pyridoxine 50 to 100 mg/day is given with isoniazid to prevent neuropathy.

Azathioprine

Azathioprine is a purine analogue, a derivative of mercaptopurine, that functions as an antimetabolite by virtue of its structural relationship to endogenous purines. Thus it decreases synthesis of adenine and guanine and, hence, of DNA. It impairs lymphocyte function and decreases the numbers of lymphocytes to cause its immunosuppressive effects. It is well absorbed orally and is also available for intravenous use. It is converted to 6-mercaptopurine and then to ribonucleotide thioinosinic acid, which is the active metabolite. This active metabolite and the unconverted azathioprine are converted to inactive metabolites in the liver and erythrocytes. Conversion by xanthine oxidase constitutes one important pathway of inactivation. It is eliminated in the urine to an extent adequate to cause accumulation in patients with renal insufficiency so that dosage reduction is necessary. In neuromuscular disease, it has been used largely for its steroid-sparing effects, that is, in patients requiring large doses of corticosteroids, its use may allow a reduction in the dose of the steroids and thus in their side effects. The usual doses are 1 to 3 mg/kg daily on a once or twice a day schedule. Onset of its therapeutic effect is typically delayed by 2 to 3 months. The major side effects are bone marrow suppression with leukopenia, macrocytosis, and toxic hepatitis. Anemia, thrombocytopenia, and opportunistic infections are rare. Myelosuppression is dose-dependent and will often reverse after reduction or temporary withdrawal of the dose. Other drugs that cause myelosuppression can potentiate this effect. Skin rash, gastrointestinal complaints, and fever can also occur. Because it is metabolized by xanthine oxidase, the dose must be markedly reduced (by about one-fourth) when allopurinol is used at the same time. Periodic monitoring of CBC and liver function tests is necessary throughout therapy.

TABLE 25-3. Slow Tapering Schedule for Alternate-Day Prednisone Treatment of Neuromuscular Disease[a]

High Day (mg)	Low Day (mg)	Duration	Taper Method
100	100	3–4 wk	Approximately 1 mg/kg daily starting dose
100	100–10	9 wk	After 3–4 weeks, taper the alternate day dose by 10 mg/wk
100	10–0	2 wk	Slow the taper to 5 mg/wk for the last 2 weeks before stopping the alternate day's dose
100	0	2–4 wk	If no benefit by this time, consider alternative treatment
100–70	0	18–24 wk	Taper by 5 mg every 3–4 weeks
70–40	0	36–48 wk	Taper by 2.5 mg every 3–4 weeks
40–20	0	8–16 mo	Taper by 2.5 mg every 1–2 months
15–10	0	Maintenance	Taper by 2.5 mg every 3–4 months to 10–15 mg on alternate days

[a] Each day's dose is given as a single morning dose. The starting dose may be higher or lower, depending on the patient's weight. This schedule tapers slowly, and a more rapid taper may be tolerated in many patients. Although many patients require a low maintenance dose, some will be able to discontinue the medication.

(Adapted from Dalakas M: Pharmacologic concerns of corticosteroids in the treatment of patients with immune-related neuromuscular disorders. Neurol Clin 8:100, 1990, with permission.)

Cyclophosphamide

Cyclophosphamide is a nitrogen mustard alkylating agent. It binds to DNA causing cross-linking. This disrupts cell division and other cell functions and is responsible for its cytotoxic effect. It decreases the production of anti-GM_1 antibodies in patients with multifocal motor neuropathy. It is well absorbed orally and is also available for intravenous use. It undergoes metabolic activation by hepatic microsomal enzymes. Inactivation also occurs in the liver. Inactive metabolites and unchanged drug are excreted by the kidney. It has found several uses in neurologic patients, including some cases of chronic inflammatory demyelinating polyneuropathy, multifocal motor neuropathy, and isolated angiitis of the central nervous system. Some practitioners use it in the treatment of multiple sclerosis. Many approaches to intravenous and oral treatment are taken. Several of these are discussed in the following chapters on specific diseases. For daily oral dosing, the usual starting dose is a single 50-mg pill daily. This dose can be increased by 50 mg/day every 3 to 4 weeks, if side effects allow, to the usual maintenance dose of 100 to 150 mg daily (2 to 3 mg/kg/day). The dose must be adjusted based on the WBC count. A usual approach is to follow the CBC weekly and maintain the WBC count between 3,000 and $4,000/mm^3$ and the ANC $> 1,500/mm^3$. (Occasionally, the desired therapeutic effect will be achieved without leukopenia.) When counts fall below these levels, the medication should be held until the counts rise and then restarted at a lower dose. The major side effects result from its cytotoxicity. Myelosuppression always occurs and must be closely followed as noted above. Nausea, vomiting, and alopecia may occur. The nausea and vomiting can be assuaged by taking the medication with meals or cold foods, although this may decrease absorption. Hemorrhagic cystitis results from contact of the toxic metabolite acrolein with the bladder mucosa. This risk can be diminished by maintaining increased urine flow with adequate fluid intake, but care must be taken to avoid water intoxication, since cyclophosphamide can also promote renal water retention. If evidence of cystitis is found the drug should be immediately discontinued. Infertility occurs in both men and women after exposure. Men may wish to arrange for cryopreservation of sperm before treatment. Cyclophosphamide induces the potential to develop later malignancies, especially leukemia, lymphoma, and urologic carcinomas. This risk is thought to be significant after cumulative doses exceeding 85 g, therefore it is important to maintain cumulative dose records. Uncommon sides effects include hepatotoxicity, pulmonary fibrosis, and opportunistic infections. In addition to the monitoring of CBCs mentioned above, urine analysis for evidence of hemorrhagic cystitis, urine cytologies for evidence of malignancy, and liver function tests should be followed periodically while the medication is in use.

Intravenous Immunoglobulin

Human immunoglobulin is a pooled product of plasma containing a high concentration of gamma globulins. Plasma is screened for ALT elevation and reactivity to HBsAg, anti-HBc, HCV, anti-HCV, HIV, and HTLV I before pooling. The product undergoes a fractionation process that decreases the viral burden. Some manufacturers have introduced an additional solvent detergent step to ensure further viral inactivation. The mechanism of action in autoimmune disease is not known. Possible mechanisms include downregulation of autoantibody production and the introduction of anti-idiotype antibodies in the foreign immunoglobulin. These large proteins must be administered intravenously. During the first week the levels fall as the immunoglobulins are redistributed between the intra- and extravascular compartments. The elimination half-life is about 3 weeks but varies significantly among individuals. It has been given for various neuromuscular diseases with a proven or presumed immune pathogenesis, especially the Guillain-Barré syndrome and myasthenia gravis. The dose used by the Dutch Guillain-Barré Study Group was 0.4 g/kg daily for 5 days. The past experience and indications for it in neurologic disease are discussed in Chapters 93, 103, and 199. Fever, chills, headache, urticaria, flushing, nausea, vomiting, chest tightness, shortness of breath, abdominal pain, arthralgias, and myalgias may be related to the infusion rate. If the side effects are mild, the infusion can be temporarily halted and resumed after symptoms subside. Prophylaxis with aspirin, acetaminophen, and diphenhydramine may also be given. Those with IgA deficiency and known antibodies to IgA and those with a history of anaphylaxis or other severe reactions to intravenous immunoglobulins should not receive them. No cases of immunoglobulin-associated HBV or HIV infection have been reported after widespread use. There have recently been some reported cases of associated HCV infection, although this risk is very low.

Interferon-β_{1b}

Interferon-β_{1b} is a form of recombinant interferon beta, an immunoregulatory cytokine. Its precise mechanism of action is not known; however, it seems to stimulate T-suppressor cell function, which is decreased in patients with progressive multiple sclerosis, to decrease T-helper activation, to inhibit the interferon-γ (IFNG)-induced expression of class II major histocompatibility complex antigens on antigen-presenting cells, and to decrease production of IFNG, which increases the T-cell mediated inflammatory response in multiple sclerosis and promotes exacerbations. The Multiple Sclerosis Study Group compared placebo to 1.6 million international units (MIU) and 8 MIU every other day and found that interferon-β_{1b} decreased exacerbation rates in relapsing-remitting multiple sclerosis in a dose-dependent manner at 2 and 3 years. At higher doses it increased the number of patients who remained exacerbation-free for 2 years. The study showed no effect on disability scores in the 3 years of follow-up. MRIs also showed fewer active scans, fewer new lesions, and a reduced burden of disease in the group receiving the higher dose. The Food and Drug Administration has approved the use of interferon-β_{1b} for the treatment of ambulatory patients with relapsing-remitting multiple sclerosis. The drug is given at a dose of 8 MIU subcutaneously every other day. The major side effects include flulike symptoms, such as fever, chills, sweating, and myalgias, and inflammatory reactions at the injection site. Depression and suicidal ideation are possible side effects. One suicide and four suicide attempts occurred in the treatment groups (249 patients). It may have an abortifacient effect, and patients should be warned of this. Rarely there may be a reversible decrease in blood counts or an increase in liver function tests results. It is recommended that the CBC, platelets, and liver functions be monitored periodically.

ACETYLCHOLINESTERASE INHIBITORS

Table 25-4 summarizes information on acetylcholinesterase inhibitors.

Edrophonium (Tensilon)

Edrophonium is a rapid-onset, short-acting acetylcholinesterase inhibitor because of its reversible binding to acetylcholinester-

TABLE 25-4. Acetylcholinesterase Inhibitors

Drug	Route of Administration	Onset of Action / Duration of Action	Dose	Equivalence to Oral Pyridostigmine
Edrophonium (Tensilon)	IV	20–30 s / 2–4 min	2–10 mg	
Neostigmine methylsulfate (Prostigmin)	IV SQ IM	20–30 min (IM) / 2.5–4 h	0.5 mg	120
Pyridostigmine bromide (Mestinon)	IV SQ IM	Rapid (minutes) / 2–3 h	2.0 mg	30
Pyridostigmine bromide (Mestinon)	PO	10–30 min / 3.5–4.5 h	30–120 mg	1
Neostigmine bromide (Prostigmin)	PO	10–20 min / 3–4 h	7.5–30 mg	4

(Adapted from Johns TR: Summing up: The use of cholinesterase inhibitors. Semin Neurol 2:299, 1982, with permission.)

ase and its rapid elimination by the kidney. Its onset of action is usually within 30 seconds to 1 minute, and the effect lasts less than 10 minutes. It comes in vials of 1 ml containing 10 mg of medication. A test dose of 1 to 2 mg (0.1 to 0.2 ml) is given over about 30 seconds. If no adverse reaction occurs, the remaining 8 mg can be injected. Seybold (1986) and Daroff (1986) suggest a modified test with smaller incremental increases in the dose. It is helpful to pretreat with 0.5 to 1.0 mg of intravenous atropine to prevent the muscarinic side effects. In addition to relieving discomfort, this helps to preserve patient blinding. The most important side effects are bradycardia and bronchospasm, and the testing physician must be prepared to respond with atropine and resuscitative measures to these problems should they arise. Caution should be taken in elderly patients. Patients with heart disease who might be expected to be sensitive to the cholinergic effects on the heart and patients with bronchospastic lung disease should not be tested with edrophonium.

Pyridostigmine (Mestinon)

Pyridostigmine is a competitive inhibitor of acetylcholinesterase. It is a close congener of neostigmine, with fewer side effects, and has become the major anticholinesterase used for therapy in myasthenia gravis. It is available for oral and parenteral use. The usual starting dose is 30 mg every 4 to 6 hours with doses timed to achieve the greatest benefit at times of greatest need, for example, 30 minutes before meals in patients with oropharyngeal weakness. The dose is adjusted according to the symptoms. Most patients achieve maximum benefit at a dose of 30 to 120 mg every 4 hours. Occasionally lower or higher doses are necessary. To achieve the maximum benefit while minimizing the risk of overdose, it is best to keep the dose low enough so that a definite improvement is detectable 30 to 45 minutes after a dose and there is some wearing-off effect before the next dose. Many patients can tolerate daytime-only dosing. For patients who have respiratory symptoms in the morning extended-release tablets are available (Mestinon Timespan 180 mg). These tablets can be broken into halves or fourths to titrate the dose without sacrificing the delayed absorption. Absorption is erratic, however, and these are usually not recommended for daytime use. Most side effects occur from the increased effect at cholinergic receptors in the central nervous system, (CNS), at smooth muscle, and at autonomic glands. Abdominal cramps, nausea, vomiting, and diarrhea are most common. Increased bronchial and oral secretions and wheezing occur less commonly and should warn the physician of possible cholinergic overdose. Loperimide, propantheline, glycopyrrolate, or diphenoxylate with atropine can be used to minimize these side effects, but if the side effects are severe enough to necessitate their frequent use, treatments other than cholinesterase inhibitors may be preferable. Enhanced vagal effects on the heart are uncommon, except with intravenous acetylcholinesterase inhibitors.

Neostigmine (Prostigmin)

Like pyridostigmine, neostigmine is a competitive inhibitor of acetylcholinesterase. It is also available for oral and parenteral use. It has therapeutic and side effects similar to pyridostigmine, and, because it may have a slightly higher incidence of side effects, its use has been largely replaced by pyridostigmine. An intramuscular injection of neostigmine has also been used as a diagnostic test. Neostigmine 0.04 mg/kg is given intramuscularly. The effect begins in 20 to 30 minutes, peaks in about 1 hour, and lasts for 3 to 4 hours. This provides a more prolonged period for diagnostic testing than does edrophonium.

ANTIPARKINSON AGENTS

Levodopa/carbidopa (Sinemet)

Levodopa, an aromatic amino acid, is the metabolic precursor of dopamine. Carbidopa is an inhibitor of aromatic amino acid decarboxylase, the enzyme that converts L-dopa to dopamine. Dopamine does not cross the blood-brain barrier, therefore it is ineffective when given to patients with Parkinson's disease. Levodopa does cross the blood-brain barrier and can be converted to dopamine in the striatum. Levodopa, however, is converted rapidly to dopamine by extracerebral tissues when given orally, requiring large doses and their attendant side effects to achieve significant CNS effects. Since carbidopa does not cross the blood-brain barrier, it serves to prevent peripheral conversion to dopamine and, thus, to allow more levodopa to enter the CNS at lower doses and with fewer side effects. In the striatum levodopa must be taken up into the terminals of nigrostriatal neurons and decarboxylated to dopamine, which is then stored and released. Levodopa competes with other amino acids for absorption in the GI tract. Therefore, a high protein diet may significantly impair its absorption. It is excreted in the urine as dopamine and unconverted levodopa. The clinical use of levodopa-carbidopa is complex; this is discussed in Chapters 113 and 115. The major side effects are abnormal involuntary movements, confusion and other mental changes, and nausea and other GI symptoms. Early in Parkinson's disease, the involuntary movements usually occur only at supratherapeutic doses, while late in the disease, the abnormal movement may occur at the doses needed for the therapeutic effect. Abrupt discontinuance of levodopa can result in a syndrome of severe muscle rigidity, fever, and elevated CPK (creatine kinase) that resembles the neuroleptic malignant syndrome. The major drug interaction is with nonselective monamine oxidase inhibitors, and these drugs should not be given together. It is, however, often given safely with the selective MAO-B inhibitor selegiline (see below).

Selegiline (Eldepryl)

Selegiline, L-deprenyl, is an irreversible inhibitor of monamine oxidase (MAO). When given at the low doses typically used for Parkinson's disease, it is relatively selective for MAO type B, which is the primary MAO in the brain that catalyzes the breakdown of catecholamine neurotransmitters. Selegiline may ameliorate symptoms of Parkinson's disease by inhibiting the catabolism of striatal dopamine and therefore increasing the dopamine available to postsynaptic receptors. It may also have a protective effect. By decreasing oxidative catabolic reactions in the striatum, it may inhibit the generation of neurotoxic free radicals. This pathogenetic hypothesis for Parkinson's disease has not been proven. The clinical effectiveness of selegiline for neuroprotection has been addressed by the Deprenyl and Tocopherol Antioxidative Therapy of Parkinsonism (DATA-TOP) study (Parkinson Study Group 1989); however, the results were not conclusive. After absorption in the gastrointestinal tract, selegiline is rapidly converted to the active metabolites *N*-desmethyldeprenyl, amphetamine, and methamphetamine. These metabolites have different half-lives and are excreted in the urine over several days. The usual dose is 5 mg twice daily. The major side effects are the potential drug interactions. Since MAO type A is the subtype primarily responsible for detoxification of exogenous vasoactive amines as they enter the system through the gastrointestinal tract, low doses of selegiline usually do not lead to a hypertensive reaction to amine-containing foods, and therefore, at these doses, it is not necessary to enforce dietary restrictions as with nonselective MAO inhibitors (MAOIs). However, at higher doses the selectivity can be lost, and hypertensive crises can occur as with other MAOIs. Severe toxicity with stupor or agititation, fever, and rigidity have been reported when selegiline has been given with meperidine, as with meperidine and other MAOIs. Similar reactions may also occur when used in combination with fluoxetine and other serotonin reuptake inhibitors.

Dopamine Agonists

Bromocriptine. Bromocriptine is an ergot alkaloid derivative. It is a relatively selective D-2 dopamine receptor agonist with mild D-1 antagonist effects. These effects confer symptomatic relief in some patients with parkinsonism. It is rapidly absorbed in the GI tract. It undergoes extensive first-pass conversion in the liver and is excreted largely in the bile and stool. It is about 90 to 95 percent protein-bound. The doses are based on the clinical response. It should be started at low doses of about 1.25 to 2.5 mg daily. The dose is raised slowly, by about 1.25 mg each week, until the desired effect is achieved or side effects emerge. The usual doses are in the range of 2.5 to 25 mg daily in divided doses. Higher doses are sometimes used. The major side effects are orthostatic hypotension, nausea, vomiting, hepatitis, dyskinesias, dizziness, and various behavioral problems, including agitation, confusion, hallucinations, and psychosis. Distal paresthesias, livedo reticularis, and angina

pectoris may occur as a result of the ergot properties. The effect of dopamine agonists may be inhibited by dopamine blockers, such as neuroleptics. Their effect may be enhanced by MAOIs and monamine reuptake inhibitors.

Pergolide. Pergolide, also an ergot derivative, is a D-2 dopamine receptor agonist and a weak D-1 agonist. Its indications are similar to those of bromocriptine. It is well aborbed by the GI tract. Multiple metabolites, some active, are excreted in the urine. It is 10 to 20 times more potent than bromocriptine and has a longer half-life. It should be started at low doses, about 0.05 mg daily. Because of the prolonged half-life, the dose should be raised slowly, and as with bromocriptine, small (about 0.1–0.15 mg) dose increases should be made at intervals of about a week or more. Usual doses are 1 to 5 mg daily divided into three doses. The side effects and drug interactions are similar to those of bromocriptine. Hepatotoxicity and pleural thickening can occur but are rare.

BEHAVIORAL NEUROLOGY AND PSYCHIATRY

Tacrine

Tacrine is a centrally active, reversible inhibitor of cholinesterase. It presumably acts by increasing the pool of acetylcholine available to postsynaptic receptors in the cerebral cortex and hippocampus. It is well absorbed in the GI tract. Absorption is significantly reduced by food. It is metabolized by hepatic microsomal enzymes. It is inactivated mainly by transformation in the liver. The half-life is about 2 to 4 hours. The recommended starting dose is 40 mg/day (10 mg qid). If it is tolerated, this dose can be increased by 40 mg/day every 6 weeks until a dose of 160 mg/day is reached. The most common side effect is hepatotoxicity. Elevations of the ALT of greater than three times normal occur in about 25% of patients. This elevation may not respond to a dose reduction. It usually occurs within the first 12 weeks and is initially asymptomatic. It reverses after the tacrine is discontinued, and about three quarters of patients will tolerate the dose on rechallenge, although those who again develop ALT elevations will tend to do so more rapidly than on first exposure. Because of this common asymptomatic side effect, it is currently recommended that patients have weekly tests of ALT for the first 18 to 24 weeks of therapy and then every 3 months. It is also recommended that weekly monitoring be resumed for at least 6 weeks after any dose increase. Other side effects include anorexia, nausea, vomiting, diarrhea, abdominal pain, headache, dizziness, and confusion. Drug interactions are related to competition for the hepatic P450 enzyme system. Theophylline levels will increase. Anticholinergic agents may be inhibited and cholinomimetic ones potentiated by tacrine.

Antidepressants

Monamine reuptake inhibitors are most often used in psychiatric practice for the treatment of affective disorders. However, it behooves the physician treating patients with neurologic disease to be familiar with these medications because they are useful in the treatment of neurologic diseases such as neuropathic pain syndromes and headache; they are used as therapeutic trials in patients with possible depression presenting as pseudodementia; and many patients with neurologic complaints may be receiving these drugs for primary psychiatric illness. I will not try to discuss these agents here; however, they are compared

TABLE 25-5. Adverse Effects of Commonly Used Antidepressants

Drug	Sedation	Anticholinergic	Orthostatic Hypotension	Cardiac Conduction Effects
Heterocyclics				
Amitriptyline	H	H	M	H
Imipramine	M	M	H	H
Doxepin	H	M	M	M
Desipramine	L	L	L	M
Nortriptyline	M	M	L	M
Clomipramine	H	H	L	M
Serotonin reuptake inhibitors				
Fluoxetine	VL	N	VL	VL
Sertraline	L	N	N	VL
Paroxetine	L	N	N	VL
Triazolopyridines				
Trazodone	H	VL	M	L
Amino ketones				
Bupropion	L	VL	VL	N
Triazolobenzodiazepines				
Alprazolam	H	VL	VL	N

Abbreviations: H, high; M, moderate, L, low; VL, very low; N, none.

(Adapted from Janicak PG, Davis JM, Preskorn SK, Ayd FJ: Principles and Practice of Psychopharmacotherapy. p. 272. Williams & Wilkins, Baltimore, 1993, with permission.)

according to several clinically relevant parameters in Table 25-5. Janicak and colleagues have published (1993) an excellent discussion of the use of these drugs in psychiatric illness.

ANTIEPILEPTIC DRUGS

Information on antiepileptic drugs is summarized in Table 25-6.

Phenytoin

Phenytoin decreases ion flux through voltage-sensitive sodium channels in the resting state and during action potential generation. It also decreases calcium and potassium flux. This reduces the spread of excitation from epileptogenic foci. It is slowly and variably absorbed in the GI tract. It precipitates at the site of intramuscular injection and is slowly absorbed, so that this route of administration is not recommended. It can be given intravenously. Phenytoin will preciptitate in glucose solutions, therefore it must be given in saline without glucose. After absorption or intravenous injection, it rapidly enters the brain. It is approximately 90 percent protein bound, mainly to albumin. Renal failure, liver disease, old age, pregnancy, and other conditions that lower the serum albumin decrease the ratio of bound to total phenytoin. It is transformed to inactive metabolites primarily by the hepatic microsomal enzymes. At low concentrations the inactivation is linear (first order), however, at higher doses the half-life increases with increasing dose (zero order),

probably due to saturation of the hepatic enzymes or inhibition of them by metabolites. This effect is often clinically relevant with disproportionately great increases in the serum level after dose increases in the higher dose ranges. The inactive metabolites are eliminated in the stool and urine. At usual doses, the half-life is about 22 hours. The doses do not usually require adjustment for renal insufficiency, although the total level will be lower for a given free level due to changes in protein binding ratio as noted above. The usual adult starting dose is 300 mg daily. This can be given in a single daily dose or divided into two or three doses if gastrointestinal upset is a problem. Dose adjustments can then be based on the clinical response and serum levels. Intravenous phenytoin can be given in a loading dose of about 18 mg/kg (about 1,200 mg in a 70-kg patient) given no faster than 50 mg/min with close monitoring of the cardiac rhythm and vital signs. Phenytoin has many side effects, although these usually do not prevent its use. Hirsutism can be a bothersome side effect, especially in women. Gingival hyperplasia is common and can be minimized by good dental hygiene. Hypersensitivity is not uncommon and can manifest as a mild pruritic rash or bullus eruptions (Stevens-Johnson syndrome), eosinophilia, hepatitis, interstitial nephritis, and fever. Lymphadenopathy resembling Hodgkin's disease, pseudolymphoma, can occur. Altered folate absorption and probably metabolism can cause folate depletion and megaloblastic anemia. Increased catabolism of vitamin K reduces the concentrations of vitamin K-dependent clotting factors. This can cause neonatal hemorrhage in the infant of a mother taking phenytoin.

TABLE 25-6. Antiepileptic Drugs

Drug	Half-life (hours)	Usual Dose[a] (mg/24 hours)	Therapeutic Level[a] (µg/ml)	Available Preparations (mg)
Phenobarbital	100	60–240	15–40	30, 60, 100 syrup
Phenytoin	22	300	10–20	30, 50, 100 syrup
Primidone	7–14	750–1,500	5–12	50, 250 syrup
Carbamazepine	10–20	600–1,200 (begin 100 bid)	6–12	100, 200 suspension 100 mg/5 ml
Ethosuximide	50–60	500–1,500	40–100	250 syrup
Valproic acid (divalproex)	6–16	1,000–4,000 (begin 15 mg/kg)	50–100	250, 500 sprinkles
Clonazepam	18–50	0.5 mg tid increase to 20 mg/d	5–70 (rarely used)	0.5, 1.0, 2.0
Felbamate	15–23	1,800–3,600	20–80 (not used)	400, 600 oral suspension
Gabapentin	5–7	900–2,400	Not used	100, 300, 400
Lamotrigine	22 (monotherapy)	50–100	0.5–3	25, 100, 150, 200

[a] Optimal doses and therapeutic levels may vary from the typical recommendations in some patients.

TABLE 25-7. Phenytoin Drug Interactions

Drugs that increase phenytoin levels
  Dicumarol
  Chloramphenicol
  Disulfuram
  Isoniazid
  Cimetidine
  Sulfonamides

Drugs that lower the total and free phenytoin levels
  Carbamazepine
  Theophylline
  Phenobarbital (may occasionally raise level)
  Alcohol (may occasionally raise level)

Drugs that lower the total level and increase the free fraction
  Valproate
  Phenylbutazone
  Sulfisoxazole
  Salicylates

Drugs whose levels are lowered by phenytoin
  Carbamazepine
  Theophylline
  Oral contraceptives
  Corticosteroids

It can be prevented by the oral replacement of vitamin K in the last 2 weeks of pregnancy and by the administration of parenteral vitamin K to these newborns. Alteration of vitamin D metabolism and impairment of calcium absorption can cause osteopenia. Gastrointestinal symptoms are rarely limiting and can be lessened by dividing the dose and giving the medicine with food. With long-term use cerebellar degeneration and peripheral neuropathy may develop; however, these problems are usually not severe enough to be clinically significant. With overdoses and rapid intravenous use cardiac arrhythmias can be serious side effects. Toxic levels are initally accompanied by high-amplitude gaze-evoked nystagmus (roughly higher than 20 μg/ml), by ataxia at higher levels (roughly 30 μg/ml), and finally by CNS depression (40 μg/ml). Cardiac toxicity can emerge in susceptible patients. Erythromycin and propoxyphene can elevate levels of phenytoin by inhibiting hepatic microsomal enzymes. Some of the many drug interactions are displayed in Table 25-7. Total, free, and salivary levels of phenytoin have been used to monitor therapy. In most cases, optimal total levels are 10 to 20 μg/ml. When the protein binding is altered, as in renal failure and valproate therapy, so that the binding ratio is significantly less than 90 percent, lower total levels should be maintained. Free levels are not routinely measured, but they may help when problems arise. Therapeutic free levels are about 0.8 to 2.5 μg/ml. Salivary levels of phenytoin correlate well with free levels.

Phenobarbital

Phenobarbital is a barbiturate sedative. It facilitates the inhibitory neurotransmitter action of γ-aminobutyric acid (GABA) by allosteric modulation of its receptor. It is well absorbed orally and can also be given intravenously. It is 40 to 60 percent bound by plasma protein. It is largely transformed to inactive metabolites by hepatic microsomal enzymes. About 25 percent is excreted unchanged in the urine. The elimination half-life is about 100 hours. The typical adult maintenance dose is about 1 to 4 mg/kg or 60 to 240 mg/day. Despite its long half-life, it is usually given on a twice daily schedule to minimize sedation caused by large single doses. Intravenous loading with 10 to 20 mg/kg can be administered at a rate of up to 100 mg/min with careful monitoring of the vital signs. Slow oral loading can be achieved by giving double the expected maintenance

dose over the first 4 to 5 days of use. The major side effect is sedation. Usually tolerance develops to this side effect. Behavioral changes, especially irritability, hyperactivity in children, and agitation and confusion in the elderly may occur. Like phenytoin it can impair vitamin K metabolism, causing neonatal hemorrhage, folate metabolism, causing megaloblastic anemia, and vitamin D metabolism, causing osteomalacia or osteoporosis. When given rapidly intravenously, it can cause hypotension, sedation, and respiratory depression necessitating ventilatory assistance. This effect is greatly potentiated by the simultaneous use of benzodiazepines. It decreases the half-life of many drugs by inducing hepatic microsomal enzymes. Valproic acid raises the phenobarbital level by up to 40 percent by decreasing its inactivation. Therapeutic levels vary. Typical effective ranges are 15 to 40 μg/ml.

Primidone

Primidone is a congener of phenobarbital. Its mechanism is thought to be similar to that of phenobarbital. It is rapidly absorbed from the gastrointestinal tract. It is metabolized by the liver to two active metabolites: phenobarbital and phenylethylmalonamide (PEMA). About 40 percent of the primidone is excreted unchanged in the urine. The half-life of primidone is about 7 to 14 hours; that of PEMA is about 16 hours. Phenobarbital's half-life is about 100 hours as noted above. The active metabolites, especially phenobarbital, can accumulate with chronic use. The dose is usually begun at 100 mg/day and increased to 750 to 1500 mg/day. The daily dose is divided to provide twice or thrice daily dosing. Many patients will not tolerate primidone because of its frequent side effects. These include sedation, dizziness, nausea, and vomiting. As with phenytoin and phenobarbital it can impair metabolism of vitamins K and D and folate. Its use carries with it the same potential drug interactions as does phenobarbital. Phenytoin increases the conversion to phenobarbital. Isoniazid decreases this conversion. When monitoring of levels is indicated, both phenobarbital and primidone levels should be measured. The typical therapeutic levels of primidone are 5 to 12 μg/ml.

Carbamazepine

Carbamazepine has a tricyclic structure related to the tricyclic antidepressants. Like phenytoin it inhibits neuronal firing by blocking voltage-sensitive sodium channels. It is absorbed slowly and erratically by the gastrointestinal tract. It is about 75 percent bound to plasma proteins. It is transformed by hepatic microsomal enzymes to an active epoxide metabolite whose serum concentration can reach 50 percent of the carbamazepine level and have significant anticonvulsant effect. The epoxide is further transformed to inactive metabolites that are excreted in the urine. The elimination half-life is about 10 to 20 hours during long-term therapy. At the onset of therapy the half-life is much longer; however, carbamazepine induces the hepatic microsomal enzymes that metabolize it (autoinduction), thereby shortening its own half-life with chronic use. The epoxide has a shorter half-life. Because of the long early half-life and the frequency of toxic symptoms even at low doses at the beginning of treatment, it is best to start at a low dose of about 100 mg twice a day. This dose can be raised by 200 mg every 5 to 7 days to the desired maintenance dose. This is usually in the range of 600 to 1,200 mg daily given in three to four divided doses. The most common side effects are dose-related vertigo, ataxia, nystagmus, nausea, and vomiting. It can cause an elevation in liver enzymes and the syndrome of inappropriate antidiuretic hormone (SIADH) with hyponatremia. The most serious side effects are agranulocytosis and aplastic anemia, but these are very rare. More commonly, mild leukopenia will occur. This may be transient, static, or progressive and typically responds to discontinuation of the drug. It is recommended that the medication be discontinued if the total WBC count falls below 3,000 cells/mm^3 or the granulocyte count falls below 1,500 cell/mm^3. Most of its drug interactions result from induction of hepatic microsomal enzymes by carbamazepine and other drugs. Phenytoin, phenobarbital, and primidone decrease carbamazepine levels. Carbamazepine decreases phenytoin and valproate levels and increases the conversion of primidone to phenobarbital. Erythromycin and propoxyphene inhibit the microsomal enzymes causing a rise in carbamazepine levels. Therapeutic levels are usually 6 to 12 μg/ml. Periodic monitoring of the Na, CBC, and transaminases is recommended during chronic therapy.

Valproic Acid

Valproic acid (VPA) (Depakene) is a simple branched-chain carboxylic acid. Sodium divalproex (Depakote) is a 1:1 mixture of the acid and its sodium salt. VPA probably potentiates GABAergic inhibition, and it may have effects on both GABAergic systems and excitatory neurotransmitters. VPA is absorbed well by the gastrointestinal tract, although absorption varies slightly with the formulation and is delayed by food. It is highly (90 percent) protein bound and displaces many other drugs from albumin binding sites. It is metabolized by the liver to inactive products. The half-life is from 6 to 16 hours. It is pushed to the lower end of this range by drugs, such as other antiepileptic drugs, that induce hepatic microsomal enzymes. The initial dose is 15 mg/kg/day, that is, about 1,000 mg/day in the average adult, usually divided into three or four daily doses. Doses are then increased by 5 to 10 mg/kg/day (about 500 mg/day) at intervals of about a week to the effective dose. The maximal dose is about 60 mg/kg/day (about 4,000 mg/day). The major adverse effects are hepatic dysfunction and thrombocytopenia. Severe hepatic dysfunction with liver failure is uncommon; it usually occurs within the first 6 months of therapy and is more likely in younger children. Acute pancreatitis has also occurred. A dose-related and reversible elevation in the liver function tests is more common. When mild this may be addressed by lowering the dose with close follow-up. Thrombocytopenia can occur as a result of decreased platelet production by the marrow or increased platelet destruction with antiplatelet antibodies. Impaired function of platelets in normal numbers may also occur, and depending on the cause, may respond to dose reduction. More common but less severe side effects include nausea, vomiting, indigestion, and weight gain due to increased appetite. An action tremor is common and may respond to dose reduction. VPA decreases levels of carnitine and has many drug interactions. Because it is highly protein-bound, it displaces many other drugs from plasma albumin, in most cases, reducing the total level without significantly changing the free (active) level. The clinician must be aware of this effect when adjusting other agents, most importantly, phenytoin. VPA inhibits the inactivation of phenobarbital and raises its level by about 40 percent. Phenobarbital doses should be lowered accordingly when VPA is added. Other agents that induce hepatic microsomal enzymes will shorten the half-life and lower the levels of VPA. The published therapeutic range is 50 to 100 μg/ml. Levels significantly above this may be used in many patients. Liver function tests and CBC with platelets must be closely monitored in the first 6 months of therapy and periodically thereafter. When trying to achieve optimal dosing of phenytoin in combination with VPA, free drug levels may be helpful.

Clonazepam

Clonazepam is a long-acting benzodiazepine, which, like phenobarbital, acts by facilitating the action of GABA with its receptor. It is well absorbed by the gastrointestinal tract and metabolized by the liver to other active and inactive metabolites. The half-life of the parent clonazepam is 18 to 50 hours. Elimination is by metabolism to inactive compounds and urinary excretion. The usual initial dose is 0.5 mg two or three times a day. This dose can be slowly increased to achieve the desired effect. Maximum recommended doses are about 20 mg/day, although doses much lower than this are usually used. The major adverse effect is CNS depression, which may lead to confusion, depression, and pseudodementia; it should be used with caution in the elderly. Tolerance develops, and withdrawal can be difficult, causing CNS irritability. Rapid withdrawal can precipitate an acute withdrawal syndrome with seizures similar to that caused by withdrawal from alcohol and other benzodiazepines. The major drug interactions are a potentiation of the CNS depressant effects of other agents. Usual levels are 5 to 70 μg/ml; however, these are rarely used clinically, and the dose is adjusted based on the therapeutic and adverse effects.

Ethosuximide

Ethosuximide is a succinimide. Although many physiologic and molecular effects of ethosuximide have been described, its mechanism of action as an antiepileptic agent remains unknown. It is well absorbed after an oral dose and is not significantly bound by plasma proteins. It is metabolized by hepatic microsomal enzymes to inactive metabolites; about 25 percent of the drug is excreted unchanged in the urine along with these metabolites. The half-life in adults is about 40 to 50 hours. In adults, the initial dose is usually 250 mg twice a day. This may be increased by 250-mg increments weekly until the desired effect is achieved without excessive side effects. In adults, usual maintenance doses range from 500 to 1,500 mg/day given in three or four doses. Gastrointestinal symptoms occur commonly: anorexia, nausea, vomiting, cramps, and diarrhea. CNS side effects may include drowsiness, irritability, and sleep disturbances. Bone marrow suppression may occur. Phenytoin levels may increase when ethosuximide is added. The therapeutic range is 40 to 100 μg/ml. Sore throat or fever should prompt an examination and check of the CBC and platelets.

Felbamate

Felbamate has a structure unrelated to other antiepileptic agents. Its mechanism of action is unknown; however, it has been shown both to inhibit NMDA receptor excitatory responses and to potentiate GABA receptor inhibitory responses by modulating their respective ion channel functions for calcium and chloride. It is well absorbed in the gastrointestinal tract without inhibition by food. About half of it is eliminated unchanged in the urine, and half is transformed by the liver to inactive metabolites. It is not highly protein bound. Its elimination follows first-order kinetics in the usual therapeutic doses. The half-life is about 15 to 23 hours. When first released in September

1993, the dosing recommendations were as follows: The recommended starting dose was 1,200 mg daily in three or four divided doses. Typical maintenance doses were 2,400 to 3,600 mg daily. For initial anticonvulsant therapy, the manufacturers recommended a slow dose increase (by 600 mg every 2 weeks) to 2,400 mg/day, continuing up to 3,600 mg/day, if clinically indicated. Most patients can tolerate a much more rapid titration to the full dose. For conversion to felbamate and for adjunctive therapy, the manufacturers recommended increasing by 1,200 mg/day weekly from the starting dose of 1,200 mg/day. Because it causes a rise in the levels of phenytoin, valproic acid, and the active epoxide metabolite of carbamazepine, concurrent dose reductions of up to one-third the prior dose of these drugs are recommended with the initial dose and the first increase in dose, with further adjustments based on the clinical response. In the summer of 1994, it was recommended that the routine use of felbamate be suspended because of 10 reported cases of aplastic anemia with two deaths. Reports of serious hepatic failure followed shortly thereafter. Prior to these reports, the most common known side effects were CNS effects (insomnia, somnolence, headache, dizziness, and diplopia) and gastrointestinal effects (anorexia, nausea, and vomiting), all of which were usually mild. It does have significant interactions with other antiepileptic drugs. It increases plasma concentrations of phenytoin and VPA by 20 to 40 percent and reduces plasma concentrations of carbamazepine by about one-third. The level of the active epoxide metabolite of carbamazepine increases by about 50 percent as the carbamazepine level falls. Phenytoin and carbamazepine lower the concentration of felbamate. Valproic acid does not affect felbamate levels. It is not known if felbamate interferes with the metabolism of warfarin, oral contraceptives, corticosteroids, or cyclosporin. The therapeutic range in most studies has been about 20 to 80 μg/ml; however, serum levels are a poor indication of the concentration in the brain, and monitoring of felbamate levels is not recommended. Because of the newly reported serious side effects, it now appears that the use of felbamate will be strictly limited to special cases of refractory epilepsy.

Gabapentin

Gabapentin became available for use in the United States in 1993. It is structurally related to GABA but, unlike GABA, readily crosses the blood-brain barrier. However, it does not seem to be an agonist of GABA receptors, and its mechanism is not known. It binds to a neuronal protein found only in the brain, and its antiepilepic efficacy is proportional to this binding. It is well absorbed by the gastrointestinal tract and is not affected by food. It is not protein bound. It is not metabolized. Elimination follows linear kinetics at therapeutic doses. It is eliminated by the kidney with a half-life of about 5 to 7 hours. Dosage adjustment is necessary with renal insufficiency. On the first day of the regimen 300 mg is administered, and on each of the next 2 days 300 mg is added until a starting dose of 300 mg three times a day is reached. The usual therapeutic dose is 900 to 1,800 mg daily, although higher doses, up to 3,600 mg daily, have been well tolerated in clinical studies. The dose should be raised above 900 to 1,200 mg/day based on the clinical response. Rapid titration in 2 to 3 days has been well tolerated. The side effects have been mild in clinical studies: somnolence, dizziness, ataxia, fatigue, and headache have been the most prominent ones. No long-term data are available. It has no known significant interactions with other drugs and probably does not inhibit the effectiveness of contraceptives.

No drug concentration, hematologic, or liver function monitoring is necessary, although there is so far little clinical experience with this new drug.

Lamotrigine

Lamotrigine is a phenyltriazine unrelated to other antiepileptic agents. Like phenytoin and carbamazepine, it acts on voltage-sensitive sodium channels to inhibit neuronal firing. It also may reduce the release of the excitatory neurotransmitters, glutamate and aspartate. By virtue of complementary mechanisms, lamotrigine and VPA may have a synergistic effect that benefits patients with intractable seizures. It is rapidly absorbed by the gastrointestinal tract. It is about 55 percent bound to plasma proteins. It is metabolized by hepatic microsomal enzymes to inactive compounds. During monotherapy, the half-life is about 22 hours. In combination with phenytoin, carbamazepine, and phenobarbital, the half-life falls to 15 hours. With VPA the half-life of lamotrigine is prolonged to 59 hours, necessitating a downward adjustment in the dose. The usual dose is 50 to 100 mg daily, but daily doses as high as 600 mg have been used. It is recommended that it be started with 25 mg at night and raised by 25 mg every 2 weeks to the effective dose. It has a low toxicity. Side effects include diplopia, drowsiness, dizziness, ataxia, headache, nausea, and vomiting. These are all dose-related and common with doses greater than 100 mg/day. The main drug interactions are with other antiepileptic drugs. A severe disabling tremor has been reported in patients treated with a combination of lamotrigine and VPA. As noted above, VPA increases its half-life significantly, and drugs that induce hepatic microsomal enzymes shorten its half-life. It does not alter the metabolism of other antiepileptic drugs, except by raising the carbamazepine epoxide level by about 10 percent. Therapeutic trough levels are 0.5 to 3 μg/ml in most studies. No laboratory monitoring is necessary during maintenance, but, clinical experience is still limited.

SUGGESTED READINGS

American Academy of Neurology Quality Standards Subcommittee: Practice advisory on selection of patients with multiple sclerosis for treatment with Betaseron. Report of the Quality Standards Subcommittee of the American Academy of Neurology. Neurology 44:1537, 1994

Bracken MB, Shepard MJ, Collins WF et al: A randomised, controlled trial of methylprednisolone or naloxone in the treatment of acute spinal-cord injury. N Engl J Med 322:1405, 1990

Brodie MJ: Felbamate: a new antiepileptic drug. Lancet 341:1445, 1993

Chadwick D: Gabapentin. Lancet 343:89, 1994

Dalakas M: Pharmacologic concerns of corticosteroids in the treatment of patients with immune-related neuromuscular disorders. Neurol Clin 8:93, 1990

Daroff RB: The office Tensilon test for ocular myasthenia gravis. Arch Neurol 43:843, 1986

Davis KL, Thal LJ, Gamzu ER et al: A double-blind, placebo-controlled multicenter study of tacrine for Alzheimer's disease. N Engl J Med 327:1253, 1992

Farlow M, Gracon SI, Hershey LA et al: A controlled trial of tacrine in Alzheimer's disease. JAMA 268:2523, 1992

Gent M, Easton JD, Hachinski VC et al: The Canadian American Ticlopidine Study (CATS) in thromboembolic stroke. Lancet 1:1215, 1989

Gilman AG, Goodman LS, Rall TW et al: Goodman and Gilman's The Pharmacological Basis of Therapeutics. Macmillan, New York, 1985

Hass WK, Easton JD, Adams HP et al: A randomized trial comparing ticlopidine hydrochloride with aspirin for the prevention of stroke in high-risk patients. N Engl J Med 321:501, 1989

The INFB Multiple Sclerosis Study Group: Interferon beta-1b is effective in relapsing-remitting multiple sclerosis. I. Clinical results of a multicenter, randomized, double-blind, placebo-controlled trial. Neurology 43:655, 1993

Janicak PG, Davis JM, Preskorn SH, Ayd FJ: Principles and Practice of Psychopharmacotherapy. Williams & Wilkins, Baltimore, 1993

Leppik IE: Antiepileptic drugs in development: prospects for the near future. Epilepsia 35(Suppl 4):S29, 1994

Parkinson Study Group: DATATOP: a multicenter controlled clinical trial in early Parkinson's disease. Arch Neurol 46:1052, 1989

The Parkinson Study Group: Effect of deprenyl on the progression of disability in early Parkinson's disease. N Engl J Med 321:1364, 1989

Sanders DB, Scoppetta C: The treatment of patients with myasthenia gravis. Neurol Clin 12:343, 1994

Seybold ME: The office Tensilon test for ocular myasthenia gravis. Arch Neurol 43:842, 1986

Watkins PB, Zimmerman HJ, Knapp MJ et al: Hepatotoxic effects of tacrine administration in patients with Alzheimer's disease. JAMA 271:992, 1994

26. THERAPEUTIC PLASMA EXCHANGE

RICHARD J. BENJAMIN
W. HALLOWELL CHURCHILL

RATIONALE

Therapeutic plasma exchange (TPE) is a dramatic procedure with an intuitively simple rationale: if a plasma factor is the cause of disease, then its removal should be the cure. Evolving from the dubious historical practice of bloodletting, the removal of blood, separation of its formed elements, and their reinfusion with plasma replacement was suggested as a treatment for hyperviscosity as early as 1914 and accepted as standard therapy in 1960. However, it was only with the availability of modern apheresis machines, initially developed to facilitate the selective donation of blood components, that widespread therapeutic trials of plasma exchange have become feasible.

Plasma exchange with either allogeneic plasma or, more commonly, human serum albumin in saline, is by its very nature a nonspecific therapy. Specificity, however, may be derived from the relative delay with which a particular noxious agent is regenerated. In particular, antibodies, with their relatively long half-lives (about 21 days), may remain depleted for prolonged periods following a short course of TPE. By this rationale, any autoimmune diseases with demonstrable autoantibodies became a legitimate subject for clinical trials, and just as bloodletting was advocated for a multitude of mysterious maladies, the availability of plasma exchange by apheresis rapidly found favor as the intervention of last resort in a variety of serious immune-mediated diseases.

Several decades have passed, and plasma exchange has begun to find its proper niche in the medical armamentarium (Table 26-1). This process of validation has been instructive in itself. In practically every disease for which TPE has been advocated, initial case reports of dramatic efficacy in a small number of patients spurred interest and excitement. Thereafter,

validation has been accomplished by several mechanisms. In some diseases, most notably myasthenia gravis, TPE became accepted medical practice by consensus without formal trial. In the 1986 Consensus Development Conference, TPE was endorsed as therapy for the short-term reduction of symptoms in myasthenia gravis based on the rationale that autoantibodies play a major etiologic role and on several uncontrolled, open clinical trials. For other diseases, a more conventional path was followed. In Guillain Barré syndrome benefit was demonstrated in a number of formal controlled trials. In thrombotic thrombocytopenic purpura, therapeutic efficacy was already assumed on the basis of a decade of uncontrolled studies and then confirmed by controlled comparison of plasma infusion versus plasma replacement. In diseases such as polymyositis, dermatomyositis, and lupus nephritis, efficacy assumed on the basis of case studies was not confirmed by properly controlled clinical trials. The importance of properly designed studies is best illustrated by the use of plasma exchange in rheumatoid arthritis. Initial reports of effectiveness were popularized in the lay media and appeared to be confirmed by trials that did not include sham pheresis and blinded observation of outcome. When these controls were included, no clinical benefit was demonstrated despite significant differences in laboratory indices. The precedent has now been set: whereas anecdotal reports are useful in directing attention to the potential of TPE in various diseases, full controlled trials, including sham TPE, are necessary before employing this relatively expensive, potentially harmful procedure as accepted practice in new applications.

With these caveats, this chapter discusses the use of TPE in a limited number of neurologic diseases to illustrate the technical principles and potential complications inherent in this therapy. This serves as a basis for evaluating its role, potential or proven, in the many other neurologic conditions discussed in this book.

INDICATIONS

The clinical impact of TPE can be summarized as relatively fast, temporary, and expensive. TPE seldom induces disease remission by itself, and the ideal applications are therefore acute, self-limited disorders such as Guillain-Barré syndrome, or chronic disorders, such as myasthenia gravis, in which rapid short-term therapeutic effects are needed. To be considered in chronic diseases, TPE must be compared to less invasive and less expensive procedures. Nevertheless, neurologic diseases are now the most common indications for TPE, constituting 89 percent of procedures in the recent report of Couriel and Weinstein (1994). Furthermore, the total number of TPE procedures and the proportion performed for neurologic indications appear to be increasing. The list of neurologic conditions for which TPE has shown benefit on occasion is long and will be discussed in detail in the chapters concerning specific diseases; however, a few well-documented indications are illustrative.

The benefit of TPE in the Guillain-Barré syndrome has been established in three large randomized trials that included more

TABLE 26-1. Indications for Therapeutic Plasma Exchange and Their Basis

Randomized Trial	Consensus/Case Report	Possible But Not Proven
Guillain-Barré syndrome	Myasthenia gravis	Pemphegus
Chronic inflammatory polyradiculopathy	Hyperviscosity	Goodpasture syndrome
Peripheral neuropathy with monoclonal gammopathy of undetermined significance	Hemolytic uremic syndrome	Autoimmune hemolytic anemia
Thrombotic thrombocytopenic purpura	Cryoglobulinemia	Cold agglutinin disease
	Familial hypercholesterolemia	Antibody to coagulation factors
	Post-transfusion purpura	Idiopathic thrombocytopenic purpura

than 500 patients. Based on the rationale that humoral immunity may play an etiologic role in Guillain-Barré syndrome, these studies show that TPE, begun early in the course of the disease, results in a decreased need for ventilatory assistance and more rapid improvement in muscular strength when compared to conservative therapy. Improvement was more marked in patients randomized to TPE within 1 week of clinical onset, although these patients may be more liable to relapse once TPE is stopped, presumably owing to the regeneration of the putative toxic etiologic plasma factor. For this reason, it has been suggested that if TPE is initiated in the first week of disease, it should be continued through the third week in order to decrease the likelihood of relapse. Recently, a randomized trial compared the use of intravenous immunoglobulin G (IVIG) and TPE in the treatment of Guillain-Barré syndrome. This study claimed to show a significantly better rate and degree of response in IVIG-treated patients. A number of observers have noted that the TPE-treated patients in this trial fared no better that the controls (non-TPE) in the prior North American trial that demonstrated the efficacy of TPE in Guillain-Barré syndrome and have therefore expressed some reservations about these findings.

In myasthenia gravis, an autoimmune disease usually associated with circulating antinicotinic acetylcholine receptor antibodies and muscular weakness, there is a clear theoretic basis for trial of TPE, and there are many anecdotal reports of its efficacy. TPE generally effects a rapid (2 to 4 days) improvement in muscular strength, although maximal improvement may be delayed for several weeks. These effects are short-lived, and long-term remissions are not seen. Despite the fact that TPE has never been subjected to formal trial, the 1986 National Institute of Health (NIH) Consensus Conference recommended that TPE has a role in acute exacerbations of myasthenia gravis ("myasthenic crises"), pre- and post-thymectomy, in which TPE may reduce the need for postoperative ventilation, and during the introduction of more conventional anticholinergic and immunosuppressive therapy, when many patients experience a clinical deterioration. Although not a recommendation of the consensus conference, there are isolated reports of response to chronic TPE therapy in a minority of patients unresponsive to conventional therapy.

Chronic inflammatory demyelinating polyradiculopathy (CIDP) and disease-associated polyradiculopathies, both thought to be due to poorly defined autoimmune processes, are ameliorated by TPE regimens. In particular, Dyck et al. (1986) showed in a sham TPE controlled formal trial that a 3-week course of TPE led to significant improvement in nerve conduction studies, neurologic disability score, and motor function. These authors concluded that in some patients with CIDP, TPE has a clear ameliorating effect, but in others, no improvement is observed. Although TPE alone may benefit CIDP patients, its role compared to, or in combination with, IVIG and immunosuppressive drugs has not been established. Published results have employed schedules of 1 to 3 single-volume plasma exchange procedures per week for at least a month or until a clear plateau phase has been reached. Periodic retreatments have then been tailored to the individual patient's symptoms.

TPE has been attempted in paraproteinemic peripheral neuropathy, including paraproteinemias associated with myeloma, lymphoma, amyloidosis, Waldenström's macroglobulinemia, and monoclonal gammopathy of undetermined significance (MGUS). In these conditions, peripheral neuropathy may be due to a variety of pathologic mechanisms, including ischemia, cryoglobulinemia, hyperviscosity, or direct attack on the myelin sheath by specific antibodies. Whatever the mechanism, the rationale for removal of the paraprotein is strong; however, only limited trial results are available, and no clear recommendation on efficacy of TPE versus conventional cytotoxic therapy can be made, with the notable exception of the neuropathy associated with MGUS. Dyck et al. 1991 published results of a controlled trial of TPE versus sham TPE in patients with stable or worsening polyneuropathy with MGUS. A short course of TPE (six procedures over 3 weeks) produced a significant improvement in the neuropathy disability score, the weakness score, and the summed compound muscle action potential. On completion of the double-blind study, the sham-treated patients were crossed over to TPE and again showed significant improvement. In both arms of the study, patients with IgG or IgA gammopathy fared better than those with IgM gammopathy, and improvement was limited to 7 to 20 days. These findings support the use of TPE, with concomitant immunosuppressive therapy, in patients with debilitating neuropathy.

By contrast with the above studies in which TPE therapy is based on controlled trials or consensus, there are a number of conditions in which its use remains controversial. A good example is multiple sclerosis, for which large double-blind trials in both chronic progressive and acute relapsing multiple sclerosis both support and fail to support the use of TPE in conjunction with immunosuppressive agents. These studies place multiple sclerosis onto the long list of diseases for which anecdotal reports of improvement induced by TPE will continue to justify therapeutic trials when no other alternative is available or situations are particularly desperate.

TECHNICAL ASPECTS

Whatever the indication, once the decision to treat a patient by TPE has been made, a series of further choices are necessary with respect to (1) the site of venous access to be employed, (2) the type of plasmapheresis equipment needed, (3) the nature of the anticoagulant and replacement fluid to be used, and finally, (4) the level of monitoring required during the process.

Excellent venous access is essential—inadequate access is a major barrier to TPE. Modern plasmapheresis equipment requires relatively high blood flow rates of 40 to 100 ml/min, usually through two venous sites. Whereas peripheral veins may be most suited for short courses of therapy, especially in the outpatient setting, adequate peripheral access is often not available in obese patients or those with sclerosed peripheral veins. Furthermore, use of peripheral veins requires patient cooperation because hand squeezing is often required to ensure adequate flow from antecubital veins. The alternative, a centrally placed large-bore multilumen venous catheter, offers high flow rates and convenience but exposes the patient to the risks inherent in placing and maintaining these lines. These risks include potentially life-threatening problems, such as catheter infection, hemorrhage, air embolism, and pneumothorax, as well as loss of access due to thrombosis. Central pheresis catheters require meticulous toilet to prevent infection. Patency may be maintained by filling with a small volume of heparin solution (e.g., 1.2 ml saline with 1,000 IU heparin) at the end of each procedure. Heparin in the lines, if accidently flushed into the patient rather than being withdrawn, can cause abnormal laboratory tests, heparin-induced thrombocytopenia, and occasionally in patients with underlying coagulopathy, significant bleeding. Notwithstanding these risks, central lines are more convenient for repeated procedures and are most suited to prolonged courses of TPE, especially in severely compromised patients in intensive care units.

The choice of plasmapheresis equipment to be used is usually determined by availability. Modern machines all operate on one of three basic principles: continuous- or discontinuous-flow centrifugation or membrane filtration. Centrifugation methods offer the advantage that the same equipment may be used by the hematology services for white blood cell and platelet collection. Discontinuous centrifugation machines (e.g., Haemonetics 30, 30s, and V50, Haemonetics Inc., Braintree, MA) withdraw up to 350 ml blood per cycle, separate the cellular elements from plasma, and then return the former to the patient prior to starting the next cycle. Although this method has the advantage that a single venous access site may be used, it involves large changes in extracorporeal volume, which may not be tolerated in compromised patients. This problem can be minimized by using two vascular sites and infusing replacement fluid simultaneously with blood removal. Nevertheless, the high extracorporeal volume required may still be a problem in severely anemic patients or those with cardiovascular instability, and such patients may need to be treated with repeated cycles of lower volume.

By contrast, with continuous flow machines (e.g., Cobe Spectra, Cobe Laboratories Inc., Lakewood, CO; Fenwal CS3000, Baxter Health Care Corp., Deerfield, IL), blood flows at a constant rate from one venous site and is separated into components that are selectively recombined and reinfused via a second venous access site. These systems generally require lower extracorporeal volumes of 220 to 350 ml and are more efficient; indeed, there is suggestive evidence that continuous-flow machines may offer marginally better clinical outcomes than discontinuous machines in Guillain-Barré syndrome and multiple sclerosis, although the scientific basis for this observation is not clear.

The third principle, plasma filtration, uses pressure over a selective membrane to separate plasma from cells and platelets. This process uses small extracorporeal volumes (< 100 ml) and may be run on standard hemodialysis equipment; however, it requires high blood flow rates (approximately 100 ml/min) via excellent venous access. Furthermore, separation may become less than optimal because of changes in the selective properties of the membrane due to adsorption of proteins, clotting, and the accumulation of partially rejected solutes adjacent to the membrane surface. This is particularly likely to be a problem in patients with polyclonal or monoclonal gammopathies.

The filtration and continuous-flow centrifugation machines have been further adapted to allow the selective removal of solutes by in-line affinity columns or specific precipitation. In this manner, immune complexes, antibodies, bile acids, or lipoproteins may be selectively removed with reinfusion of the cleared plasma. These systems allow major savings on the costs of replacement fluids, and preliminary evidence, such as the increased levels of high-density lipoprotein found after selective removal of low-density lipoprotein, may suggest the possibility of benefit; however, they have yet to justify their use with evidence of significant direct clinical improvement.

Whichever type of plasmapheresis equipment is used, blood must be anticoagulated in the extracorporeal circulation, either by heparinization of the entire patient, or more commonly by the addition of acid citrate dextrose at the proximal venous site. The amount of acid citrate dextrose added is usually specified by the plasmapheresis equipment manufacturer. In both cases, most of the anticoagulant is removed with the plasma; however, problems with residual anticoagulant are a common cause of complications in TPE (see below) and may necessitate reversal of anticoagulation.

The volume and type of replacement fluid used may also affect the clinical outcome. Since the constant withdrawal and reinfusion of blood involves the dilution of the native plasma by the replacement fluid in vivo, total replacement is not feasible. A single exchange of one plasma volume theoretically removes 60 to 70 percent of native plasma, with larger proportional exchange requiring exponentially increasing exchange volumes. Most programs therefore adopt strategies of 1 to 1.5 times plasma volume exchanges repeated regularly, thereby achieving over 90 percent depletion of proteins such as immunoglobulins. This translates into a 2- to 3-L plasma exchange in an adult, using the empiric estimate of plasma volume in women at 40 ml/kg and in men at 45 ml/kg. Whereas tables are available to determine plasma volume, most modern plasmapheresis machines are programmed to compute the optimum volume automatically based on the patient's weight and hematocrit. Clinical allowance, however, must still be made for preexisting fluid shifts caused by the patient's underlying condition.

Plasma must be replaced by a similar colloid solution. Historically, fresh frozen plasma was the natural choice; however, a high incidence of allergic reactions and the risk of viral infections have now restricted its use to diseases (e.g., thrombotic thrombocytopenic pupura) in which plasma has a direct beneficial effect. Synthetic plasma expanders have yet to gain popularity in this application, as their short plasma half-life renders them unsuitable for sick patients undergoing repeated procedures. For these reasons, pasteurized human albumin diluted in saline is now commonly used, providing maintenance of oncotic pressure, a minimal risk of infection, and a low incidence of side effects. Albumin in saline, however, does not replace coagulation factors and leads to a dilution coagulopathy, including hypofibrinogenemia, which persists for 24 to 48 hours after TPE. Consequently, TPE is usually scheduled every second day to minimize the effects of this acquired coagulopathy and to avoid the need for supplementary fresh frozen plasma, with its attendant risks of infection and allergy.

The level of monitoring patients require when undergoing regular TPE varies according to the clinical situation. In all cases, a supervising physician must make the initial therapeutic plan and be readily available to manage any complications that may emerge. At one extreme, severely compromised patients (e.g., severe Guillain-Barré syndrome) may require the cardiovascular and respiratory care of an intensive care unit, whereas multiple sclerosis patients in remission may be treated as outpatients. At a minimum, a trained operator must be present throughout the procedure to carry out regular monitoring of the patient's vital signs and the plasmapheresis equipment's operational status. A constant record of the fluid balance, anticoagulant use, and flow rates should be available to allow rapid interpretation of adverse reactions. Routine assessments over a course of exchanges should include platelet counts, fibrinogen levels, and immunoglobulin levels, since these are factors that are known to be depleted by TPE. Ultimately, the care of TPE patients requires a thorough familiarity with the complications commonly encountered during TPE and a sound knowledge of their management.

COMPLICATIONS

Like any major medical procedure, the potential benefits of TPE must be weighed against the risks to the patient. These may vary from life-threatening, requiring immediate termination of the procedure, to mild, causing minimal interference. Indeed, recent surveys suggest that almost one-half (40 to 49 percent) of all patients treated may demonstrate untoward effects at some point during their course of therapy, although these occur during a minority (12 to 17 percent) of individual exchange procedures. Most complications are mild to moderately severe and do not prevent the successful completion of a procedure; however, serious complications and even deaths have been reported.

In general, TPE complications may be divided into common problems usually related to the nature of the replacement fluid or the anticoagulant and less common complications related to vascular access, hemostasis, cardiovascular stability, or the underlying disease process.

Historically, the most frequent life-threatening reactions were due to anaphylaxis in response to fresh frozen plasma, especially in IgA-deficient patients. Moreover, mild allergic reactions, including fever, chills, and urticarial rashes, were the most common mild complications (Table 26-2). These problems are dramatically reduced by the use of albumin in saline as replacement. In recent surveys, life-threatening or fatal reactions have usually related to the use of vascular access catheters. Whereas these are clearly necessary to allow repeated procedures with minimal discomfort to the patient, the threat of catheter-related bacteremia, hemo- and pneumothorax, and hematomata is ever present. Indeed, anecdotal reports of venous catheters mistakenly placed in major arteries and at least one report of death relating to subclavian artery laceration during catheter placement demand consideration.

Less severe complications that require medical intervention but do not result in termination of the procedure include nausea, vomiting, vasovagal reactions, and hypotension. In these cases, positioning of the patient, infusion of 0.9 percent saline, and the treatment of citrate toxicity usually allow the procedure to continue after a suitable delay. Reactions to citrate, the calcium-chelating anticoagulant used in most plasmapheresis machines, are now the single most common type of complication related to TPE (Table 26-2). This requires routine patient counseling about hypocalcemia and its common sequelae, including paraesthesias and muscle cramps. When symptoms occur, slowing

the whole blood flow rate, adjustment of the anticoagulant ratio and oral calcium supplementation are often all that are required; however, intravenous calcium supplementation administered in 5 percent dextrose water may be used. A less common reaction to citrate is metabolic alkalosis, especially in renal failure patients unable to excrete the excess bicarbonate load generated by the hepatic metabolism of citrate. Such alkalosis may require treatment with acetazolamide or, in severe cases, by infusion of diluted hydrochloric acid through a dedicated central line.

Hypofibrinogenemia due to dilution by replacement fluid is another common finding after plasma exchange, although bleeding complications are relatively rare. Nevertheless, it is important to monitor serum fibrinogen levels and to consider replacement therapy should concentrations fall below 50 mg/dl. This is especially true in patients with an underlying hemostasis problems, including thrombocytopenia or after major surgery. Rarer mild complications related to the replacement fluid include metabolic defects such as hypomagnesemia, hypophosphatemia, and urticarial rashes due to minor components of purified human serum albumin.

Finally, one has to consider the spectrum of complications related to the underlying disease process. For example, patients with Guillain-Barré syndrome may be more prone to hypotensive episodes, or those with thrombotic microangiopathies, to bleeding problems.

CONCLUSION

Plasma exchange is sometimes a startlingly effective and dramatic procedure in selected patients with otherwise untreatable disease. Whereas the "nontrivial" rate of complications in TPE demands intensive screening of patients before commiting them to this hazardous and relatively expensive therapy, the rarity of life-threatening complications and the potential benefits in suitably selected patients argue strongly that it is a worthwhile procedure if performed by experienced personnel with appropriate monitoring.

SUGGESTED READINGS

Abel JJ, Rowntree LG, Turner BB: Plasma removal with return of corpuscles (plasma pheresis). J Pharmacol Exp Ther 5:625–34, 1914

Burgstaler EA, Pineda AA: Plasma exchange versus affinity column for cholesterol reduction. J Clin Apheresis 7:69–74, 1992

Campion EW: Desperate diseases and plasmapheresis. N Engl J Med 326:1425–7, 1992

Ciavarella D, Wuest D, Strauss RG et al: Management of neurological disorders. J Clin Apheresis 8:242–57, 1993

Consensus Conference: The utility of therapeutic plasmapheresis for neurological disorders. JAMA 256:1333–7, 1986

Couriel DC, Weinstein R: Complications of therapeutic plasma exchange: a recent assessment. J Clin Apheresis 9:1–5, 1994

Domen RE, Kennedy MS, Jones LL, Senhauser DA: Hemostatic imbalances produced by plasma exchange. Transfusion 24:336–9, 1984

Dwosh IL, Giles AR, Ford PM et al and the Queens University plasmapheresis study group: Plasmapheresis therapy in rheumatoid arthritis: a control double blinded cross over trial. N Engl J Med 308:1124–9, 1983

Dyck PJ, Daube J, O'Brien P et al: Plasma exchange in chronic demyelinating polyradiculoneuropathy. N Engl J Med 314:461–5, 1986

Dyck PJ, Low PA, Windebank AJ et al: Plasma exchange in polyneuropathy associated with monoclonal gammopathy of undetermined significance. N Engl J Med 325:1482–6, 1991

French cooperative group on plasma exchange in Guillain-Barré syndrome: Plasma exchange in Guillain-Barré syndrome: one year followup. Ann Neurol 32:94–7, 1992

Grishaber JE, Cunningham MC, Rohret PA, Strauss RG: Analysis of venous access for therapeutic plasma exchange in patients with neurological disease. J Clin Apheresis 7:119–23, 1992

TABLE 26-2. Incidence of Adverse Reactions with Therapeutc Plasma Exchange

Complication	Sutton et al. (1989) (%)	Couriel and Weinstein (1994) (%)
Fever, chills, urticaria	3.7	0.3
Muscle cramps, paresthesias	2.5	5.5
Hypotension	2.3	2.1
Nausea, vomiting, abdominal pain	1.5	3.9
Headache	1.2	—
Chest pain	0.2	—
Cardiac arrythmia	0.1	—
Dyspnea, bronchospasm	0.1	—
Convulsions	0.04	—
Respiratory arrest	0.04	—
Other	0.8	1.0
Hypofibrinogenemia	—	3.7
Percentage incidence	12.5	16.5
Total number of procedures	5,235	381

Guillain-Barré study group: Plasmapheresis and acute Guillain-Barré syndrome. Neurol 85:1096–104, 1985

Huestis DW: Mortality in therapeutic hemapheresis. Lancet 1:1043, 1983

Kornfeld P, Fox S, Maier K, Mahjoub M: Ten years experience with therapeutic apheresis in a community hospital. J Clin Apheresis 7:63–8, 1992

Lewis EJ, Hunsicker LS, Lan S-P et al: A controlled trial of plasmapheresis therapy in severe lupus nephritis. N Engl J Med 326:1373–9, 1992

Mckhann G, Griffen J, Cornblath D et al: Plasmapheresis and Guillain-Barré syndrome: analysis of prognostic factors and the effect of plasmapheresis. Ann Neurol 23:347–53, 1988

Miller FW, Leitman SF, Cronin ME et al: Controlled trial of plasma exchange and leukapheresis in polymyositis and dermatomyositis. N Engl J Med 326:1380–4, 1992

Moake JL: TTP—desperation, empiricism, progress. N Engl J Med 325:426–8, 1992

Noseworthy JH, Vandervoort MK, Penman M et al: Cyclophosphamide and plasma exchange in multiple sclerosis. Lancet 337(i):1540–1, 1991

Osterman PO, Fagius J, Lundemo G et al: Beneficial effects of plasma exchange in acute inflammatory polyradiculoneuropathy. Lancet (ii) 1296–8, 1984

Parker TS, Gordon BR, Saal SD et al: Plasma high density lipoprotein is increased in man when low density lipoprotein (LDL) is lowered by LDL-pheresis. Proc Natl Acad Sci USA 83:777–81, 1986

Pearl RG, Rosenthal MM: Metabolic alkaosis due to plasmapheresis. Am J Med 79:391–3, 1985

Reimann PM, Mason PD: Plasmapheresis: technique and complications. Int Care Med 16:3–10, 1990

Rock GA, Shumak KH, Buskard NA et al: Comparison of plasma exchange with plasma infusion in the treatment of thrombotic thrombocytopenic purpura. Canadian apheresis study group. N Engl J Med 325:393–7, 1991

Ropper AH, Albers JW, Addison R: Limited relapse in Guillain-Barré syndrome after plasma exchange. Arch Neurol 45:314–5, 1988

Samtleben W, Randerson DH, Blumenstein M et al: Membrane plasma exchange: principles and application techniques. J Clin Apheresis 2:163–9, 1984

Schwab PJ, Fahey JL: Treatment of Waldenström's macroglobulinemia by plasmapheresis. N Engl J Med 263:574–9, 1960

Strauss RG: Current status of hemapheresis in the United States. J Clin Apheresis 6:95–8, 1991

Sutton DMC, Nair RC, Rock G and the Canadian apheresis study group: Complications of plasma exchange. Transfusion 29:124–7, 1989

Thornton CA, Griggs RC: Plasma exchange and intravenous immunoglobulin treatment of neurological disease. Ann Neurol 85:260–8, 1994

van der Meche FGA, Schmitz PIM and the Dutch Guillain-Barré study group: A randomized trial comparing intravenous immune globulin and plasma exchange in Guillain-Barré syndrome. N Engl J Med 326:1123–9, 1992

Wood L, Jacobs P: The effect of serial therapeutic plasmapheresis on platelet count, coagulation factors, plasma immunoglobulin, and complement levels. J Clin Apheresis 3:124–8, 1986

Ziselman EW, Bongiovanni MB, Wurzel HA: The complications of therapeutic plasma exchange. Vox Sang 46:270–6, 1984 1984

27. REHABILITATION OF NEUROLOGIC DISABILITY

MEL B. GLENN
SUSAN BIENER BERGMAN

The development of a disabling neurologic condition can affect the medical health, mobility, self-care and independent living skills, vocational and recreational abilities, social roles, and psychological health of the individual. Each of these areas must be evaluated and then addressed in a coordinated team approach. The physician leading the rehabilitation effort must be trained to work as part of the team, tackling not only the medical aspects of neurologic disease but also treating the impairments, disabilities, and handicaps, as well as the psychosocial concerns

that have resulted. Residency training in physical medicine and rehabilitation specifically addresses these issues. However, some neurologists have spent much of their careers in a rehabilitation setting, and there has been a growing awareness among neurologists of rehabilitation issues. In recognition of the link between the two specialties, the American Board of Physical Medicine and Rehabilitation and the American Board of Psychiatry and Neurology have approved 5-year joint training that can lead to board certification in both specialties.

Although traditionally the bulk of the initial rehabilitation after the onset of severe neurologic disability has been attended to in an inpatient hospital setting, as health care changes, rehabilitation too is moving to a greater extent to the home, skilled nursing facility, and outpatient setting. The physician is therefore more likely to see a more disabled outpatient than in the past and must be prepared to address the more acute rehabilitation needs with a team-oriented outpatient approach. This chapter addresses some of the more common issues facing the clinician working with the neurologically disabled outpatient.

MOTOR CONTROL

Central Nervous System Disorders

Spasticity is common with central nervous system (CNS) disease, and other motor problems may coexist with it, depending on the locus of injury. Spasticity is often prominent with spinal cord disease, stroke, cerebral palsy, traumatic brain injury, and hypoxic and other encephalopathies. With it are often seen weakness; primitive motor behaviors, such as the synergies, postural and labyrinthine reflexes, and prominent nociceptive reflexes (e.g., flexor spasms); and at times rigidity, dystonia, ataxia, and tremors. Proper treatment is dependent upon a thorough inventory of the motor disturbances as well as an evaluation of their relative contribution to disability. What may be a problem at one time may be an asset at another, as in the use of spastic knee extensor muscles to aid in weight bearing or the use of spastic finger flexors to assist in grasping.

A search for nociceptive influences is called for when spasticity or flexor spasms are severe or increased from baseline. Problems with the urinary tract, bowel, or skin are the most common contributors. Treating these exacerbating factors may result in a reduction of spasticity or spasms.

Physical and occupational therapy play a primary role in the treatment of many of the motor disorders seen with CNS disease. Range-of-motion (ROM) exercises with slow, sustained stretch of muscle are pivotal in the treatment of spasticity and other hypertonias. Patients and their caregivers should be taught to perform these exercises on a regular basis to aid in the inhibition of increased muscle tone and to prevent contractures from developing or worsening. Therapists use a variety of other techniques to inhibit problematic hypertonia or reflex movements and to facilitate isolation of the controlled active movement when patterned movements tend to predominate. Proper positioning in bed or chairs is essential to this process. When these abnormal movements cannot be inhibited, therapists can assist the patient in learning to use them functionally. Strengthening exercises can be included when weakness is contributing to loss of motor control. Strengthening can also be used to decrease spasticity in the antagonist muscles.

A variety of physical modalities are frequently useful as well. These include heat, cold, vibration at lower frequencies, electric stimulation of antagonists, high-frequency electrical stimulation of the hypertonic muscle, electromyographic biofeedback, and ultrasound. Casts or carefully fitted orthotic devices can assist in the normalization of muscle tone and control of movement. They are most commonly employed at the foot and ankle or the hand and wrist. Ankle-foot orthoses (AFOs) can assist in restoring a heel-toe gait by preventing excessive plantar flexion and inversion. Plastic orthoses can be made more restrictive to control more severe problems with hypertonia. Alternatively, they can be extensively customized to support critical areas of the foot, with customized footplates if necessary. Metal AFOs can be made with double-action ankle joints that allow for adjustment of ankle position and its secondary effect on knee and hip positioning, which can then be titrated and changed as the patient's motor control evolves. Medial or lateral straps can be used to control eversion and inversion. Children with spasticity and weakness at the knees and hips will at times require long-leg braces and pelvic bands, with the more proximal components gradually weaned as control improves.

Patients and their assistants can be taught to use other equipment such as reachers, adapted splints, canes, crutches, walkers, wheelchairs, hospital beds, lifts, and other devices to improve activity of daily living (ADL) and mobility skills. Electronically based environmental control units can be used for more remote tasks, such as turning on radios and televisions or opening doors. Speaker phones can now follow voice commands, and voice-operated computers have evolved to become a practical alternative for some individuals. For those with impairments of speech, a variety of augmentative communication devices are available.

Medications can be useful when more conservative approaches are not adequately addressing the problem or are not practical. Muscle tone can be assessed using a scale such as the Ashworth Scale, although such scales may not be sensitive or reliable enough to pick up the changes seen with medications. Response is best gauged by targeting specific functional or prefunctional goals and observing and discussing the response with the patient and therapists. Diazepam and other benzodiazepines are useful for spasticity, flexor spasms, and dystonic posturing. The usual dose range of diazepam is from 4 to 60 mg/d. The proclivity of the benzodiazepines to cause sedation and impairment of attention and memory often precludes their use in those with supraspinal disease and the elderly, who are most susceptible to these effects. Benzodiazepines should not be discontinued abruptly, since withdrawal symptoms may occur. Baclofen tends to be somewhat less problematic with regard to cognitive side effects, but often causes similar problems. Baclofen is probably more effective at addressing problematic flexor spasms than in decreasing hypertonia. It is generally started at 5 mg three times daily and increased gradually to 20 mg four times daily or the lowest dose providing maximal benefit. Considerably higher doses are sometimes used without adverse effect. It should not be discontinued abruptly, since hallucinations can occur. Although it can be sedating, dantrolene sodium is the least likely to be so, and in this respect is the best of the three commonly used agents for spasticity in patients with cerebral disorders. Dantrolene is generally started at 25 mg once or twice daily and gradually increased to as much as 100 mg four times daily. It occasionally causes hepatotoxicity and should be used only in situations in which liver function tests can be monitored. Because it affects hypertonia by inhibiting the release of calcium from the sarcoplasmic reticulum, it has a propensity to weaken muscles as well. This does not usually affect function except in areas where already weak muscles are strong enough to be useful, but where the balance can easily be tipped. Clono-

dine has been used to treat spasticity and flexor spasms, though it has not been studied as well as the other medications described above. The treatment of parkinsonian rigidity is described in Chapter 113.

Side effects and lack of the desired efficacy often limit the usefulness of medications in the treatment of hypertonia, and more invasive approaches may be necessary. Chemical neurolysis with phenol or alcohol is an effective means of addressing spasticity and targets a specific muscle or muscle group. The duration of effect ranges from days to years but generally can be expected to be 6 months or more. Blocks can be performed at the level of the nerve root or plexus, the mixed sensorimotor peripheral nerve, or the motor nerve or branch. Although active function can be diminished in weak muscles or those in which hypertonia is being used to the patient's advantage, with proper assessment prior to the block, this is not usually a problem. Only a small percentage of axons are usually affected by the block. When mixed sensorimotor nerves are lysed, dysesthesias can develop in the sensory distribution, but this typically lasts only a few weeks, and the level of pain is generally manageable. Rarely, the pain is severe or unremitting, in which case low-dose tricyclic antidepressants, a course of systemic corticosteroids, or ultimately a reblock at the same site will usually relieve the pain. This issue can be avoided entirely by blocking motor branches only. Sensory loss is rare with chemical neurolysis of mixed sensorimotor nerves. Chemical neurolysis is most effective for spasticity but can have a modest effect on dystonia, rigidity, and the hypertonia associated with primitive motor behaviors. Injection of botulinum toxin into the muscle can achieve a similar effect, but lasts for only 2 to 4 months. This can be an advantage or disadvantage, depending upon the situation. Botulinum toxin may be more effective than chemical neurolysis for dystonias.

Baclofen can also be delivered via an intrathecal pump with greater effect and avoidance of systemic side effects. The effectiveness of intrathecal baclofen has been demonstrated largely in patients with spinal cord injury and multiple sclerosis, although there is evidence that it can be useful for spasticity caused by supraspinal lesions as well. The dose can be titrated and programmed for the individual's needs.

Spasticity can also be diminished with radiofrequency dorsal rhizotomy. The procedure is quite effective for spasticity and usually lasts longer than chemical neurolysis. However, it can permanently impair sensation. Therefore, it is best reserved for those with complete sensory loss due to spinal cord injury or for those with brain injury who are so physically incapacitated that they rely on others for ADLs, mobility, and skin care. It is not indicated for those whose major dysfunction or problem with care is being caused by dystonic posturing. Selective surgical dorsal rhizotomy does not generally cause impaired sensation and has been effectively employed to diminish spasticity in children with cerebral palsy. It is a significantly more invasive procedure than radiofrequency rhizotomy. Dorsal column stimulation is used in some centers with reports of successful reduction of spasticity. It is rarely necessary to resort to other procedures with greater associated risks, such as myelotomy and intrathecal phenol injection, since the development of this greater armamentarium of approaches to problems with muscle tone.

Orthopaedic procedures can also contribute to the control of hypertonia. Musculotendinous transfers can be used to balance the tone about a joint but must be approached with great care, owing to the possibility of creating an imbalance on the antagonist side. Musculotendinous lengthening allows for greater stretch of muscle, particularly when contracture has developed in the context of spasticity. Lengthenings may need to be combined with other approaches so that the neurologic component is controlled as well.

Ataxia can be an extremely disabling condition and is difficult to address. Occupational and physical therapists can help a patient to learn to stabilize an upper extremity proximally for more effective use of the distal extremity. Stabilizing devices can assist walking. Functional motor control, however, will have a chance of improving only with numerous repetitions of the skill to be learned over weeks, months, and years. A variety of medications (e.g., β-adrenergic blockers, clonazepam, isoniazid) have been reported to improve ataxia, though none has been proven to be consistently effective. The pharmacologic management of other tremors and dyskinesias associated with CNS disorders is discussed in Chapter 121.

Motor Unit Disorders

Muscle weakness is the sine qua non of the muscular dystrophies and is often a major issue in the rehabilitation of persons with motor neuron disease, peripheral neuropathy, or radiculopathy. The role of strengthening exercises in motor unit disorders has been controversial. In the early 1970s, the observation that some individuals with muscular dystrophy developed overwork weakness contributed to concern about the safety of active exercise. Indeed, overwork weakness may be the basis of postpolio syndrome. Numerous studies have demonstrated both the potential for the development of overwork weakness following heavy exercise and the safety and efficacy of submaximal resistance exercise, stopping well short of muscle fatigue. The latter can strengthen muscles in those with static disorders and retard the progression of weakness and maximize function in those with progressive disorders.

Exercise plays a crucial role in the treatment of radiculopathy. Pain can be reduced and further injury prevented by optimizing posture, flexibility, and strength in key areas. For example, when lumbosacral radiculopathy causes low back pain, strengthening exercises to the abdominals, paraspinals, and hip and knee extensors are usually prescribed as well as stretching exercises for the hamstrings, paraspinals, and other hip and pelvic muscles. Proper body mechanics during basic and more strenuous ADLs help to prevent further injury.

In entrapment neuropathies and cumulative trauma disorders, proper positioning, ergonomically optimal work stations and tools, and strengthening of supporting musculature are most useful. Judicious use of nonsteroidal anti-inflammatory drugs (NSAIDs) (e.g., ibuprofen, 600 mg four times daily) can help relieve pain so that exercise is better tolerated. Chronic pain can be treated effectively with low-dose tricyclic antidepressants (e.g., amitriptyline, starting at 10 mg QHS). Transcutaneous electrical nerve stimulation (TENS) may help control localized discomfort. Pain management is discussed in greater depth in Chapters 228 through 230.

Progressive disorders, especially those that present in childhood, offer special challenges. Therapeutic goals include postponing loss of ambulation and enhancing independence in activities of daily living. ROM exercises help to retard the development of contractures. Normal ADLs or play should not be overlooked as a therapeutic regimen. They can provide submaximal active exercise, will be easier to comply with than formal exercise sessions, and can have psychological benefit. Avoiding obesity will also help to maintain mobility.

In the progressive disorders of childhood, as muscle weakness progresses, compensatory postures will develop facilitating the development of joint contractures (see Contracture, below). Together, weakness and contractures severely threaten mobility. Certain signs and symptoms herald the loss of ambulation, including falls, decreased active hip and knee extension, loss of stair climbing, decreased ROM in hips, knees, and ankles, and decreased cumulative standing and walking time per day. Hip and knee flexion contractures and ankle plantar flexion contractures should be monitored.

Once these signs are noted, bracing should be initiated. Selection of the proper type of braces depends on the degree of weakness present. AFOs can relieve foot drop and reduce the stress on weakened hip girdle musculature. In patients with more severe hip weakness, lightweight knee-ankle-foot orthoses (KAFOs) can be beneficial. Bracing can also be used to enhance safety and reduce pain and fatigue in neuropathies and radiculopathies. By normalizing gait patterns, energy consumption drops and injury to supporting muscles is minimized.

Night splints to hold the neutral position can be used to reduce contractures and maintain ROM at the ankle in severe neuromuscular diseases. They can also reduce pain in entrapment neuropathies while facilitating resolution. Care must be taken to assure proper fit and adequate padding to prevent skin breakdown.

Contracture prevention is also important in the upper extremities. Wrist and finger deformities in progressive neuromuscular diseases can accelerate the loss of hand strength and function in the progressive neuromuscular diseases or severe neuropathies.

For individuals who can not ambulate safely, care must be taken in selecting the proper wheelchair. Instead of representing a loss, the right wheelchair can herald increased freedom and a new opportunity to keep up with peers. In progressive disorders, moving to full-time wheelchair use can hasten the progression of scoliosis and respiratory muscle weakness, particularly in children. Thus, proper positioning is vital. The patient should be comfortable and sit squarely on a firm but not rigid surface to prevent pelvic obliquity. A seat belt will prevent loss of positioning. Lateral supports and hip pads may help to maintain proper alignment of the trunk. Cushions and back supports can be adjusted to accommodate individual structural deformities and provide a stable seating surface. Custom-molded systems can be useful for those with deformities that are difficult to correct or accommodate. Overly rigid systems should be avoided—more compliant materials are better tolerated by fully sensate individuals. Specific prescription considerations are well outlined by Brammel and Maloney. The choice of power chair-control mechanisms will depend on the degree of residual hand function.

Adaptive equipment, ranging from the high-tech to the low-tech, can be very useful in prolonging independence with ADLs. Such equipment includes long-handled combs, brushes, and sponges; toilet paper holders, shoehorns, flexible shower hoses, tub transfer seats, elastic shoelaces, reaches, plate guards, built-up utensils, sandwich holders, and the like. Electronic equipment such as environmental control units and robotic devices may be helpful to augment function. Home modifications such as installment of ramps, widening of doorways, and elimination of architectural barriers can enhance independence.

Contracture

Contracture of joints is caused by shortening of muscles, tendons, ligaments, and joint capsules or by heterotopic ossification. Contractures are a common consequence of weakness, hypertonia, or hypotonia, and disuse. Passive, active, or active-assisted ROM exercises should be started as soon as possible after the onset of a disorder that results in one or more of these abnormalities to prevent contractures. And such exercises should be started as soon as possible to promote remediation, if therapy begins after contractures have developed. Orthotics and other devices to control positioning are often also essential to prevention. Hypertonia must often be addressed to prevent or remediate contractures. Serial casting or splinting is an effective method for regaining ROM once it has been lost. Traction is occasionally employed but is often not practical. Surgical release or lengthening is often necessary when other approaches have failed. Contracture of nervous and vascular structures may limit the ability to lengthen soft tissues after long-standing contracture. Contractures are most easily reversed when they have recently developed but can usually be substantially corrected after months, and sometimes even after years.

Shoulder stiffness often develops in the hemiplegic patient after stroke, and this is frequently followed by shoulder-hand syndrome, which is believed to be a variant of reflex sympathetic dystrophy. The joints of the hand become stiff and flexion contractures begin to develop. Pain, edema, and vasomotor changes are prominent. The patient vigilantly protects the hand and may resist ROM exercises. The key to remediating this problem is to reduce edema and stiffness of the hand and stiffness of the shoulder. Edema is best controlled by elevation, edema-reducing gloves, or graded wrapping of the fingers and hand, ROM exercises, and massage. Warm or cold packs to the hand and shoulder can make ROM movements less painful. A course of an NSAID may reduce pain and inflammation, though a short course of a corticosteroid is more likely to be effective for more severe shoulder-hand syndrome. A low dose of a tricyclic antidepressant may also help to reduce pain. Stellate ganglion blocks may be necessary when other interventions have failed. If spasticity is causing pain and limiting ROM at the shoulder, nerve blocks to affect the shoulder adductors and internal rotators can be helpful.

Neurogenic heterotopic ossification commonly occurs after a traumatic spinal cord injury (SCI) or severe traumatic brain injury (TBI) and occasionally can be seen with nontraumatic lesions of the CNS or peripheral nervous system. Often heralded by signs of a local inflammatory response, it occasionally causes significant disability in the individual with SCI, but more commonly results in disability in the patient with severe TBI by causing pain and contracture at the shoulders, elbows, hips, and knees. The etiology is uncertain, but an unknown neurologic factor combined with trauma to the joint during ROM exercises or assisted transfers may be the essential ingredients that lead to an interaction between undifferentiated mesenchymal cells and endogenous chemical mediators. Avoiding ROM exercises is not a satisfactory preventive measure in most instances, since contracture will almost certainly develop if they are not done. Therapists must walk a fine line marking the unseen boundary between contracture formation and the possibility of the development of heterotopic ossification. Once ossification starts to form, ROM exercises are generally necessary to prevent the possibility of ankylosis, although the severe pain caused by the presence of the heterotopic bone can be a limiting factor in the patient whose sensation is intact. The administration of disodium etidronate can effectively prevent the deposition of hydroxyapatite crystals on the bony matrix but does not prevent the development of the osteoid. Once the medication is stopped, mineralization is likely to proceed. Although it is possible that there is some long-term benefit to using etidronate prophylactically for a period of 3 to 6 months, this issue has not yet been studied sufficiently. NSAIDs have been studied for the prevention of postsurgical recurrence of heterotopic ossification but not as a prophylactic measure shortly following an injury. Ultimately, if heterotopic ossification results in limitation of ROM with functional consequences, surgical excision can be considered. However, recurrence is a common problem. To minimize this, the surgery is usually delayed until more than a year after the injury to allow the bone to mature. NSAIDs and radiotherapy appear to be promising approaches to prevent recurrence, although further studies are needed. In those with heterotopic ossification following TBI, the better the cognitive and motor function of the patient, the less likely recurrence seems to be. Participation in postoperative therapy will be better as well.

Scoliosis

Rapidly progressive spinal curvature represents a significant source of morbidity in pediatric neuromuscular disease and is not uncommon in children with upper motor neuron dysfunction. If left untreated, curve progression can result in incapacitating deformities that can interfere with seating, worsen restrictive lung disease, and wreak havoc on body image. Until fairly recently, scoliosis had been treated with various types of orthoses. Some may slow the course of progression, but none has effectively prevented progression. As survival has increased with mechanical ventilation, more aggressive surgical approaches have been tried. Timing of surgical intervention is critical in order to avoid both rapid increase in the magnitude of the curve and pulmonary complications. Laprade advocates offering surgery to patients whose curves approach 30 degrees and who have vital capacities of at least 30 percent the predicted value. Early surgical techniques such as Harrington rod instrumentation have given way to segmental spinal stabilization, which does not require postoperative external immobilization.

RESPIRATORY INSUFFICIENCY

In the late stages of progressive neuromuscular disorders and motor neuron disease, detection and treatment of respiratory insufficiency become the most pressing issues. Careful history taking may reveal symptoms of mild hypercarbia or hypoxemia, including anxiety, insomnia, morning headaches, somnolence, and nightmares. Pulmonary function testing in both sitting and supine positions may be helpful. Appropriate preventive measures include annual influenza vaccines and aggressive chest physical therapy for respiratory infections. Individuals with high cervical SCI should receive these prophylactic therapies as well. Sleep apnea is common in persons with cervical SCI.

Splaingard et al. offer criteria for beginning mechanical ventilation in neuromuscular disease, including vital capacity below 25 percent predicted along with at least one of the following:

1. PCO_2 greater than 55 mmHg
2. Recurrent atelectasis or pneumonia
3. Moderate dyspnea at rest
4. Congestive heart failure

They further suggest instituting nighttime ventilation on a semi-elective basis after careful discussion. Negative-pressure devices may be helpful at this stage. As the disease progresses further, daytime ventilation will eventually be required. Tracheostomy may be necessary in the presence of upper airway obstruction.

Technologic advances have allowed us to offer patients the opportunity to extend their lives significantly. However, before such treatment is started, some ethical issues must be addressed. Some argue that the quality of life once the patient becomes ventilator-dependent is unacceptable. This argument is inconsistent with recent studies. Despite the fact that in Muscular Dystrophy Association clinics only one-third of practioners routinely prescribe respirators for patients developing respiratory failure, most respirator-dependent patients scored similarly to healthy controls in a recent life satisfaction survey. Despite decreased activity, patients can maintain their satisfaction with life. However, patients and families deserve to be fully informed about all aspects of living with a ventilator. Discussions with peers who have been through a similar experience may be helpful.

The most beneficial approach to this problem is to discuss the options with the patient and family before respiratory failure becomes evident. This information should be repeated to be sure it is understood. The impact on family life, the ethical and legal difficulties involved in withdrawing support, and the fact that mechanical ventilation is not a cure should be emphasized. Ultimately, the decision belongs to the patient and family. The health-care team can facilitate discussion of these issues. Counseling for the patient and the family can also help them to sort out their feelings about death and dying.

As society becomes more accepting of those with disabilities and as technology affords more effective devices, not only the length but also the pleasure in life for such patients will continue to improve. A well-managed patient can live significantly longer. With appropriate concern for psychological issues, this extended life can be satisfying.

URINARY TRACT DYSFUNCTION

Upper motor neuron disease can cause impairment of the urinary tract, resulting in incontinence, infection, stone formation, and the potential for renal insufficiency. Spinal cord lesions cause a hyperreflexic detrusor and the potential for detrusor-sphincter dyssynergia (simultaneous contraction of the detrusor and external or internal sphincters) and increased intravesical pressure. Increased intravesical presure can result in bladder trabeculation and diverticulae, vesicoureteral reflux, pyelonephritis, and hydronephrosis. When the bladder is not emptying properly, intermittent catheterization, aided by anticholinergic drugs if necessary, is generally the best approach but may not be practical, owing to motor impairment of the upper extremities, lack of availability of others to do catheterization, work schedules, or compliance problems. Indwelling catheters tend to encourage infection, stone formation, urethral erosion, and may be associated with an increased risk of carcinoma of the bladder. Suprapubic catheters avoid urethral problems and may be an acceptable choice. Surgical sphincterotomy or periodic application of phenol or botulinum toxin to the external urethral sphincter are other options that allow the use of an external drainage system without catheterization in the male. Some male patients will be able to empty their bladders reasonably well and safely to use an external drainage system without the need

for any procedures. Absorbent diapers may be necessary in some females. Diversion and bladder augmentation procedures are other alternatives for providing continence and greater ease of catheterization.

Measurement of voided volume plus postvoid residual volume is a simple method for determining bladder capacity and assessing whether the patient with a neurologic disorder has a problem with storage or emptying. Urodynamic studies determine the dynamics of the detrusor and sphincters and measure the intravesical pressure. In individuals with SCI, they should be obtained when increased voiding between intermittent catheterizations and lower postvoid volumes indicate that the transition from a hypo- to hyperreflexic bladder is occurring. A cystometrogram is useful when reflux is suspected. Those patients with potential for upper tract problems due to increased intravesical pressure or reflux should have their upper tracts examined periodically with, for example, renal ultrasound and renal scan.

Because detrusor-sphincter coordination is controlled at the pontine level patients with intracranial lesions rarely develop detrusor-sphincter dyssynergia and therefore do not tend to have problems with increased intravesical pressure, reflux, and hydronephrosis. In such patients, the urodynamic study will generally indicate that there is a hyperreflexic bladder that empties at low volumes without undue reflexive sphincter contraction. Urodynamic and upper tract studies are necessary only when repeated urinary tract infections occur or outlet obstruction is suspected.

Lower motor neuron lesions result in a hyporeflexic detrusor with difficulty voiding and leakage due to overflow. This situation is best managed with intermittent catheterization, but if this is not practical, suprapubic catheters can be a reasonable alternative. If incontinence is primarily the result of inability to toilet oneself, then condom catheters and leg bags can be useful in males. Although indwelling urethral catheters may be a viable alternative for some females, they too often result in urethral dilation or breakdown. In addition, they promote urinary tract infection and stone formation. In males, indwelling urethral catheters often cause penile-scrotal fistulae and abscesses. Adult diapers may be a necessary alternative if assistance is not available on a frequent enough basis.

Symptomatic infections should be treated with antibiotics, but it is futile to attempt to treat persistent asymptomatic bacteriuria with course after course of antibiotics. Many patients with neurogenic bladders adapt to ongoing colonization with only occasional problems. Those who have vesicoureteral reflux, hydronephrosis, or urea-splitting organisms are at greater risk, and eradication of asymptomatic bacteriuria should at least be attempted. The value of continuous prophylactic antibiotic treatment is controversial.

BOWEL DYSFUNCTION

Patients with lower and upper motor neuron lesions may experience constipation and incontinence of bowel. A regular bowel program can usually minimize these problems. After adequately emptying a constipated gastrointestinal tract with laxatives and enemas if necessary, a regular daily or every-other-day suppository or digital stimulation combined with a fiber-rich diet and plenty of fluids is a good starting point. If this is unsuccessful, a stool softener—or, if the stool needs added bulk, psyllium hydrophilic mucilloid—can be added. A laxative such as senna can be given, timed so that its action coincides with the administration of the suppository or digital stimulation. Glycerin suppositories may suffice for some, whereas bisacodyl suppositories or minienemas may be needed for others. If treatment proves difficult, rectodynamic studies, if available, can be used to identify anorectal dyssynergia, which can be treated with topical viscous lidocaine or prolonged anal stretch. If megarectum is diagnosed, high-volume enemas may be necessary. Colostomy should be reserved for those for whom all other approaches have failed.

SEXUAL FUNCTION

All too frequently, health-care professionals do not address, and may even avoid, discussion of sexuality with disabled individuals. By taking a sexual history, the physician validates the legitimacy of the patient's often unspoken concerns. Significant others should be brought into the discussion whenever possible. Although sexual dysfunction should be fully discussed, ultimately, emphasis should also be placed on the individual's abilities, whether physical or psychological in nature. In a sexual relationship, ownership of the problems should be placed on the couple as a unit and not solely upon the person with the disability. Physicians can play an important role as counselors, providing correct information about neurogenic sexual dysfunction and the effects of motor, sensory, language, cognitive, and behavioral impairment on sexuality, while offering approaches to address each of these areas. Avoidance of sexually transmitted diseases as well as contraceptive needs and child care should be discussed. Psychological etiologies (e.g., depression, anxiety) for sexual dysfunction should be explored as should the possibility of drug-induced, vascular, or endocrine causes. When needed, the patient should be referred for counseling by professionals experienced in working with the sexual concerns of people with disabilities.

When nongenital sensorimotor dysfunction is affecting sexuality, these problems should be specifically addressed through physical and occupational therapy as well as the other approaches discussed above under Motor Unit Disorders. Speech and language issues should be treated by a speech and language pathologist who is aware of the sexual issues involved. Cognitive and behavioral issues can be explored with the assistance of a neuropsychologist who can work with the patient and significant other to develop strategies that will reduce the impact of these problems on the sexual relationship. The use of sexual aides such as vibrators should be discussed when relevant.

Erectile dysfunction can be addressed with medications, including the intracavernosal injection of vasoactive substances (e.g., papaverine, phentolamine). Externally applied vacuum or entrapment devices or penile orthoses can be tried. A variety of surgically implanted penile prostheses are available. Higher erosion and infection rates must be considered in the population with SCI. These complications may be less of a problem with the inflatable prostheses than with the rigid type. Problems with vaginal lubrication can be treated with artificial lubricants.

Conception is generally normal in women with SCI. Men with SCI usually cannot conceive, in part due to ejaculatory dysfunction and in part due to spermatozoal dysfunction. However, electroejaculation and electrovibration techniques are improving, making conception more likely. Pregnancy, labor, and delivery can usually be carried to a good outcome in women with SCI, although further loss of mobility, skin breakdown, inability to detect labor, and autonomic dysreflexia are potential problems.

AUTONOMIC DYSREFLEXIA

In addition to the hyperreflexia of the somatic and parasympathetically innervated systems noted above, individuals with SCI above the level of the major sympathetic splanchnic outflow (T6 and above) commonly have hyperactive sympathetic reflexes. A noxious stimulus, usually from the bladder, bowel, or skin, will initiate a sympathetic nervous system response that includes increased blood pressure, sweating, and piloerection. The spinal cord is isolated from the usual supraspinal control mechanisms, and so the response goes unchecked. Vasodilation results in flushing of the face and neck and nasal and conjunctival congestion. Blood pressure can reach dangerous levels, resulting in intracerebral hemorrhage or seizures, if the noxious stimulus is not removed. The patient will usually experience a pounding headache and, at times, chest pain. Most SCI patients will have been educated about this condition during their inpatient rehabilitation stay and will alert uninformed caregivers or manage the problem themselves. The treatment is to identify the cause and eliminate it, if possible. Some of the common etiologies include a distended bladder, blocked catheter, urinary tract infection, urinary tract stones, constipation, pressure ulcer, ingrown toenail, tight clothing, and need for a change in position. Intra-abdominal pathology may occasionally be the culprit.

While waiting for an infection to respond to treatment, intravesical lidocaine or pyridium may help to control blood pressure by decreasing bladder irritation and spasm and so decreasing afferent input into the reflex arc. Anticholinergic medications can similarly diminish nociceptive input by decreasing bladder irritability. If necessary, antihypertensives such as topical nitroglycerin or nifedipine can be used when the etiology is elusive or temporarily unresolvable. Care must be taken to avoid hypotension when the condition resolves. Patients going for urinary tract or other procedures may need prophylactic medication or at least frequent monitoring of their blood pressure. Similar precautions must be taken for women anticipating labor and delivery. Autonomic dysreflexia must be distinguished from preeclampsia/eclampsia to prevent serious maternal morbidity.

COGNITIVE, PERCEPTUAL, AND BEHAVIORAL DYSFUNCTION

Supraspinal disorders frequently result in cognitive, language, perceptual, and behavioral impairment with adverse consequences on ADLs, other independent living skills and community skills, and social interactions. These problems may reflect relatively focal lesions, as seen after stroke, or diffuse injuries with superimposed focal lesions, such as those after TBI or anoxic encephalopathy. Those working with such patients must address these issues as well as any physical impairment that might be present. Neuropsychological evaluation can help to identify the core components of the cognitive disability so that strategies can be based on a thorough understanding of the deficits and the residual strengths of the individual. Language and cognitive treatments are generally designed to challenge the patient at a level at which success can be achieved with the support and structure provided by the therapist. Instruction and cues are intended to assist the patient to incorporate consistent strategies for overcoming or compensating for the deficit in question. It may be necessary to address core language and cognitive and perceptual impairment as a starting point, but therapists should move toward working with the patient in a functional context as soon as is practical. It is important to address any sleep disturbances that may be exacerbating cognitive impairment. Psychostimulant (e.g., methylphenidate) and dopaminergic (e.g., amantadine) drugs can also be useful to address problems with arousal, initiation, and attention, as can also the more adrenergic antidepressants (e.g., protriptyline). However, first any medical issues, such as infection or hydrocephalus, should be addressed. Medications that might be exacerbating these problems should be withdrawn, if possible.

The treatment of behavioral disorders (e.g., disruptive and combative behaviors) should also be based on an evaluation of the underlying impairments contributing to the problem at hand. Premorbid conditions, frustration, depression, and anxiety in reaction to the disability or environment, and neuropsychological conditions can all contribute and must be addressed. Complex partial seizures may occasionally play a role. Planned behavioral interventions must be consistently employed by those working with the patient. Underlying arousal, initiation, and attentional problems are common contributors to aggressive behavior and should be dealt with as noted above. If other approaches are not adequately effective, a wide variety of pharmacologic interventions can be used to assist in the treatment of aggressive and disruptive behaviors. Sedating or otherwise cognition-impairing drugs such as neuroleptics and benzodiazepines should be avoided when possible, unless they are necessary to control dangerous situations or there are specific indications for their use (e.g., psychosis, anxiety).

Depression is common after the onset of severe disability. The support of family, peers, and staff, success during rehabilitation, and individual counseling can all be helpful. Cognitively impaired individuals may be less able to benefit from these interventions. Medications should be used when depression interferes with the patient's ability to participate in rehabilitation and other activities or when it is causing considerable pain for extended periods of time.

PSYCHOLOGICAL ADJUSTMENT FOLLOWING NEUROLOGIC DISABILITY

The development of a disability has a profound effect not only on the person with the disability but on the family and significant others as well. The disability may of necessity alter well-established roles. For example, the provider or nurturer must suddenly rely on others to a much greater extent or the developing adolescent or young adult is suddenly thrust into a state of greater dependency than that from which he or she was struggling to emerge. Festering or latent interpersonal conflict may flare up. Even the most well-adjusted patient or family member will be placed under severe stress.

The physician treating a patient with a neurologic disability should question the patient and family regarding adjustment issues, then counsel or refer for counseling if necessary. The stress felt by the patient and family may manifest itself as anger toward the physician or other rehabilitation team members. Despite the personal feelings that this may arouse in the treatment team, such a response should be approached sympathetically as a rehabilitation issue. At times, the patient or family may split the team into "allies" and "enemies." As team leader, the physician must be aware of such dynamics in order to prevent discord among the team members. Other patients and family members may not outwardly express any signs of stress or may deal with stress by avoiding difficult situations as much as possible. These responses should be explored by the physician or other team members, such as the social worker or psychologist.

Psychological adjustment after the disability is affected by society's response to people with disabilities. The constant reminders of the limited access to services readily available to others can be daunting. The individual with a disability should be encouraged to seek out peer support, if possible in the context of constructive political action. Consumer advocacy groups have had a substantial impact on legislation and funding for the needs of people with disabilities, and the process can be empowering to those involved.

SUGGESTED READINGS

Ashworth B: Preliminary trial of carisoprodol in multiple sclerosis. Practioner 162:540, 1964

Bach JR: Rehabilitation of the patient with respiratory dysfunction. In DeLisa JA (ed): Rehabilitation Medicine: Principles and Practice. 2nd Ed. JB Lippincott, Philadelphia, 1993

Bach JR, Campagnolo DI, Hoeman S: Life satisfaction of individuals with Duchenne muscular dystrophy using long term mechanical ventilatory support. Am J Phys Med Rehabil 70:129, 1991

Bach JR, Lieberman JS: Rehabilitation of the patient with disease affecting the motor unit. In DeLisa JA (ed): Rehabilitation Medicine: Principles and Practice. 2nd Ed. JB Lippincott, Philadelphia, 1993

Bach JR, Zedenberg A, Winter C: Wheelchair mounted robot manipulators: long term use by patients with Duchenne muscular dystrophy. Arch Phys Med Rehabil 69:59, 1990

Brooke MH: A Clinician's View of Neuromuscular Diseases. 2nd Ed. Williams & Wilkins, Baltimore, 1986

Brammell CA, Maloney FP: Wheelchair prescriptions. In Maloney FP, Burks JS, Ringel SP (eds): Interdisciplinary Rehabilitation of Multiple Sclerosis and Neuromuscular Disorders. JB Lippincott, Philadelphia, 1985

Craig C, Zimbler S: Orthopaedic procedures. In Glenn MB, Whyte J (eds): The Practical Management of Spasticity in Children and Adults. Lea & Febiger, Philadelphia, 1990

Cole TM: Gathering a sex history from a physically disabled adult. Sex Disability 9:29–37, 1991

Fowler WM: Rehabilitation management of muscular dystrophy and related disorders: I. the role of exercise. Arch Phys Med Rehabil 63:31, 1982

Gans BM, Glenn MB: Introduction. In Glenn MB, Whyte J (eds): The Practical Management and Spasticity in Children and Adults. Lea & Febiger, Philadelphia, 1990

Garrison SJ, Rolak LA: Rehabilitation of the stroke patient. p. 801. In DeLisa JA (ed): Rehabilitation Medicine: Principles and Practice. 2nd Ed. JB Lippincott, Philadelphia, 1993

Giebler K: Physical modalities. In Glenn MB, Whyte J (eds): The Practical Management of Spasticity in Children and Adults. Lea & Febiger, Philadelphia, 1990

Glenn MB: Nerve blocks for the treatment of spasticity. p. 481. In Katz R (ed): Spasticity. Physical Medicine and Rehabilitation State of the Art Reviews. Vol. 3. Hanley and Belfus, Philadelphia, 1994

Glenn MB: Nerve blocks. In Glenn MB, Whyte J (eds): The Practical Management of Spasticity in Children in Adults. Lea & Febiger, Philadelphia, 1990

Glenn MB: Update on pharmacology: a pharmacological approach to aggressive and disruptive behaviors after traumatic brain injury (Part 1). J Head Trauma Rehabil 2:71–3, 1987

Glenn MB: Update on pharmacology: a pharmacological approach to aggressive and disruptive behaviors after traumatic brain injury (Part 2). J Head Trauma Rehabil 2:80–1, 1987

Glenn MB: Update on pharmacology: a pharmacological approach to aggressive and disruptive behaviors after traumatic brain injury (Part 3). J Head Trauma Rehabil 2:85–7, 1987

Halar EM, Bell KR: Contracture and other deleterious effects of immobility. p. 681. In DeLisa. JA (ed): Rehabilitation Medicine: Principles and Practice. 2nd Ed. JB Lippincott, Philadelphia, 1993

Hylton N: Dynamic casting and orthotics. In Glenn MB, Whyte J (eds): The Practical Management of Spasticity in Children and Adults. Lea & Febiger, Philadelphia, 1990

Kasdon D: Neurosurgical approaches. In Glenn MB, Whyte J (eds): The Practical Management of Spasticity in Children and Adults. Lea & Febiger, Philadelphia, 1990

Katz D: Update on pharmacology: movement disorders following traumatic head injury. J Head Trauma Rehabil 5:86–90, 1990

Krane RJ, Siroky MB: Neuro-Urology. 2nd Ed. Little, Brown, Boston, 1991

LaPrade RF, Rowe DE: The operative treatment of scoliosis in Duchenne muscular dystrophy. Orth Rev 21:39, 1992

Linsenmeyer TA, Stone JM: Neurogenic bladder and bowel dysfunction. p. 733. In DeLisa JA (ed): Rehabilitation Medicine. Principles and Practice. 2nd. Ed. JB Lippincott, Philadelphia, 1993

Little JW, Massagli TL: Spasticity and associated abnormalities of muscle tone. p. 666. In DeLisa JA (ed): Rehabilitation Medicine: Principles and Practice. 2nd Ed. JB Lippincott, Philadelphia, 1993

Splaingard ML, Frates RC, Harrison GM: Respiratory function in hereditary neuromuscular diseases: pathophysiology and management. Curr Concepts Rehabil Med 2:3, 1985

Staas Jr WE, Formal CS, Gershkoff AM et al: Rehabilitation of the spinal cord-injured patient. p. 886. In DeLisa JA (ed): Rehabilitation Medicine: Principles and Practice. 2nd Ed. JB Lippincott, Philadelphia, 1993

Varghese G: Heterotopic ossification, p. 407. In Berrol S (ed): Traumatic Brain Injury. In Kraft GH (ed): Physical Medicine and Rehabilitation Clinics of North America. Vol. 3. WB Saunders, Philadelphia, 1992

Whyte J, Morrissey J: Motor learning and relearning. In Glenn MB, Whyte J: The Practical Management of Spasticity in Children and Adults. Lea & Febiger, Philadelphia, 1990

Whyte J, Rosenthal M: Rehabilitation of the patient with traumatic brain injury. p. 825, In DeLisa. JA (ed): Rehabilitation Medicine: Principles and Practice. 2nd Ed. JB Lippincott, Philadelphia, 1993

Whyte J, Robinson K: Pharmacologic management. In Glenn MB, Whyte J (ed): The Practical Management of Spasticity in Children and Adults. Lea & Febiger, Philadelphia, 1990

Zasler ND: Sexuality in neurologic disability: an overview. Sex Disability 9: 11–27, 1991.

CEREBROVASCULAR
DISEASE

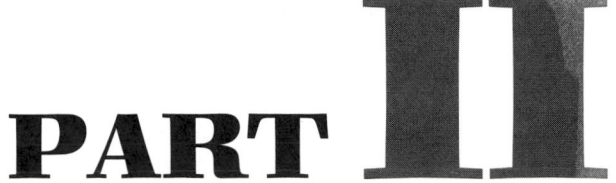

SECTION 1. GENERAL ASPECTS OF CEREBROVASCULAR DISEASE

28. EPIDEMIOLOGY AND STROKE RISK FACTORS

PHILIP A. WOLF

Cerebrovascular diseases leading to stroke are among the most common neurologic problems encountered by the physician. Each year in the United States alone there are 500,000 new strokes, which are accompanied by significant disability, lost productivity, and enormous health-care costs, currently estimated at $18 billion per year. Physician awareness of the recognized stroke risk factors, early symptoms and signs, and reversible phases of the condition may afford the opportunity to prevent more serious, recurrent, and costly consequences. Even after stroke has occurred, the physician who has an understanding of the underlying pathophysiology may provide helpful common-sense measures to prevent further neurologic deterioration and to promote early, effective rehabilitation.

Stroke is a condition that leads to hospitalization, but many of its early manifestations are encountered in everyday office practice in patients with or without other medical conditions. The chapters in this section of the book try to balance the office approach to cerebrovascular disease with the basic pathophysiology and the medical demands of caring for stroke patients during hospitalization. This chapter deals with epidemiology of stroke and its risk factors; subsequent chapters deal with basic pathogenetic mechanisms and with the cardinal clinical symptoms of the most common forms of cerebrovascular disease leading to stroke. Less common forms of stroke are also presented, since they are encountered in any busy medical practice. Chapter 29 provides a discussion of the ever-expanding field of neurodiagnostic testing. An approach to patient evaluation that is based on the usual clinical features of the major pathogeneses of stroke and builds on the information from diagnostic tests is presented, followed by a chapter on current treatment strategies.

MORTALITY AND INCIDENCE OF STROKE

Stroke is the most frequent life-threatening disease of the nervous system, accounting for 20 percent of all cardiovascular disease deaths and ranking third as a leading cause of death in the United States, after heart disease and cancer. Whereas stroke is four times more likely to lead to disability than death, the American Heart Association estimates that in 1991 there were 144,070 deaths from stroke in the United States. Mortality data provide rates of stroke deaths according to age, gender, race, and geographic area and supply information on mortality trends over time. Although these death certificate data are crude, the large numbers of uniformly coded events provide a broad picture of stroke mortality (Table 28-1).

Variation by Age, Gender, and Race

Stroke mortality in the United States increased exponentially with age, approximately tripling in successive decades of life (Table 28-1). Rates were approximately 50 percent higher overall in blacks than whites, and the greatest differences were seen in the younger ages, particularly below the age of 65 years (Fig. 28-1).

In the National Health and Nutrition Examination Survey I Epidemiologic Follow-up Study (NHEFS), age-adjusted mortality for blacks from stroke was 1.98 times that of whites. Of interest, 31 percent of excess mortality could be accounted for by six key risk factors for cardiovascular disease. A further 38 percent of the excess deaths could be accounted for by family income. However, nearly one-third (31 percent) of the excess black total mortality remained unexplained. When compared to whites, blacks had increased prevalence rates of hypertension and diabetes. They also had more intracerebral hemorrhage and less extracranial and large artery atherosclerotic disease than whites. The epidemiology of stroke in blacks and hispanics is being investigated with increased intensity in a number of multiracial populations in the United States.

Orientals have been known to have a low rate of coronary heart disease and a high prevalence of stroke. A high incidence and prevalence of stroke in Chinese was found in a survey of six mainland cities with rates that were comparable to those of native Japanese in Japan. The disparity between the stroke and

TABLE 28-1. Stroke Mortality Rates per 100,000 and Change in Stroke Mortality, by Sociodemographic Group, Ages 35 and Older, in the United States, 1980–1989

Group	Stroke Mortality Rates		Average Annual Percent Change in Stroke Mortality Rates 1980–1989
	1980	1989	
Age			
35–44	8.5	6.5	−2.6
45–54	25.4	18.6	−3.4
55–64	65.2	49.3	−2.9
65–74	218.8	145.8	−4.1
75–84	783.9	523.4	−4.0
85 +	2,260.0	1,640.8	−3.2
Race and sex[a]			
Black men	276.5	193.2	−3.5
Black women	228.3	169.5	−3.1
White men	181.8	123.3	−3.9
White women	159.4	111.2	−3.6
Region[a]			
South	196.6	134.8	−3.9
North Central	173.9	122.3	−3.6
West	169.2	121.9	−3.3
Northeast	154.0	104.2	−3.7
United States	175.7	122.3	−3.6

[a] Age-adjusted rates, ages 35 +.

(From Centers for Disease Control and Prevention: Cardiovascular Disease Surveillance, Stroke, 1980–1989; issued 1994.)

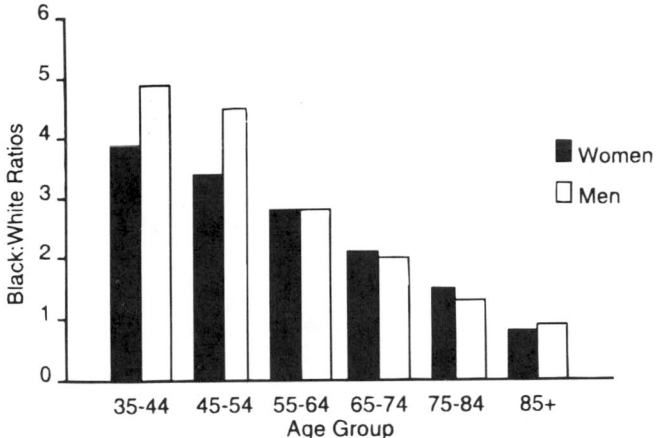

FIG. 28-1. Black to white ratios of stroke mortality rates by age group and sex, 1989. (From Centers for Disease Control and Prevention: Cardiovascular Disease Surveillance, Stroke, 1980–1989. p. 8. 1994.)

Variation by Geographic Region

In the 1980s, the highest age-adjusted stroke mortality rates occurred in the South and the lowest rates in the Northeast and the West (Table 28-1, Fig. 28-2). The map of state-specific mortality rates in 1990 indicates the highest rates were concentrated in the southeastern states—the "stroke belt." These regional differences are apparent for each gender and racial group. The existence of these regional variations suggest an environmental basis for the variation in stroke mortality (and perhaps in stroke incidence). Mortality rates from stroke vary widely between countries (Fig. 28-3). Among 33 industrial countries, the United States had one of the lowest stroke death rates, whereas Eastern European countries and Portugal had substantially higher rates.

Secular Trends in Stroke Mortality

Death rates for stroke in the United States have declined consistently since 1915. This decline has occurred in all age groups, in both races and sexes, and in all regions. The rate of decline up to 1968 averages 1 percent per year. From 1972 to 1992, mortality rates for stroke decreased more than 60 percent in the United States. As seen in Table 28-1, stroke mortality rates declined between 1980 and 1989, as they had in the previous decade. Death rates fell in all age groups, in men and women, in blacks and whites, and in all regions of the United States. This remarkable recent decline was real and not an artifact of coding or death certification practices. Similar declines have also occurred in most other westernized industrial nations. This decline in death rates is due to a decrease in stroke severity and perhaps to a falling stroke incidence.

Incidence of Stroke

Mortality statistics, however, fail to convey the degree of distress of stroke survivors and their families, whose lives are irrevocably altered by this catastrophe. Cerebrovascular disease is a major problem; approximately 500,000 persons sustained a new or recurrent stroke, and there were 3,060,000 survivors

coronary heart disease death rates, and presumably a similar disparity in incidence rates, is attributed to the high prevalence of hypertension and the low levels of blood lipids in Orientals. Cerebrovascular disease was the most frequently certified cause of death in Japan during the three decades following World War II, and the mechanism of stroke was most frequently thought to be intracerebral hemorrhage. In Japanese men in Hawaii and San Francisco, deaths attributed to stroke also fell relative to those from coronary heart disease and cancer.

It is now well established that infarction, not hemorrhage, is the most frequent stroke mechanism and accounts for two-thirds of stroke events in Japanese, be they residents of Japan or Hawaii. However, hemorrhage does occur several times more frequently in Japanese than in U.S. whites or blacks. There is also a difference in the site of the atherosclerotic arterial pathology, with a predominance of intracranial disease in Japanese, in contrast to the pattern in white Americans, in whom the extracranial arteries are the focus of the atherosclerotic process.

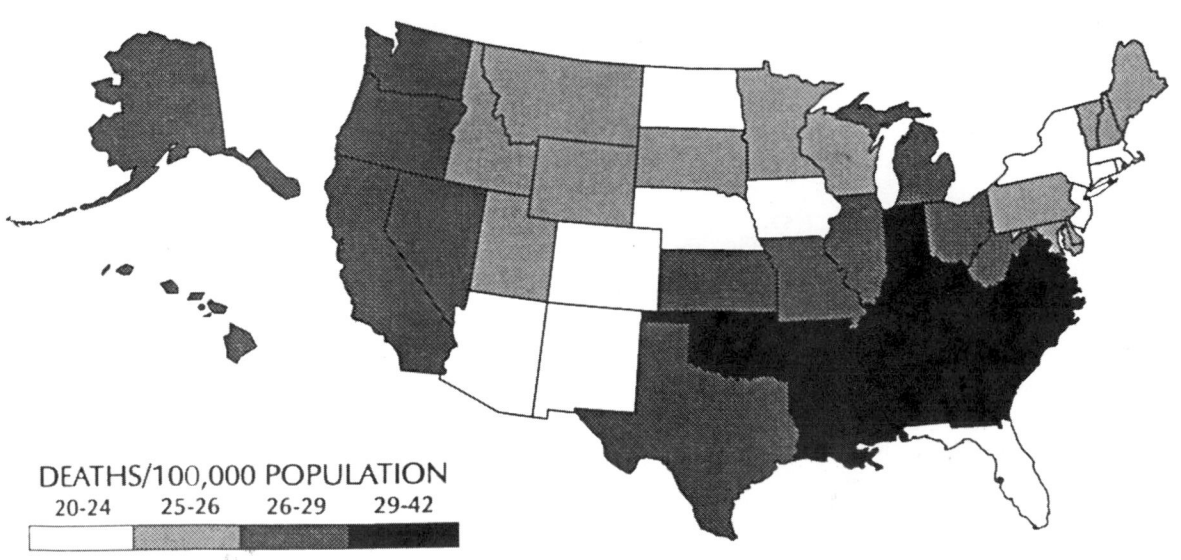

DEATHS/100,000 POPULATION
20-24   25-26   26-29   29-42

FIG. 28-2. Age-adjusted death rates for stroke by state in the United States, 1990. (From Morbidity and Mortality, Chartbook on Cardiovascular, Lung and Blood Diseases. U.S. Department of Health and Human Services, Washington, D.C., May, 1994.)

AGE-ADJUSTED RATE/100,000 POPULATION

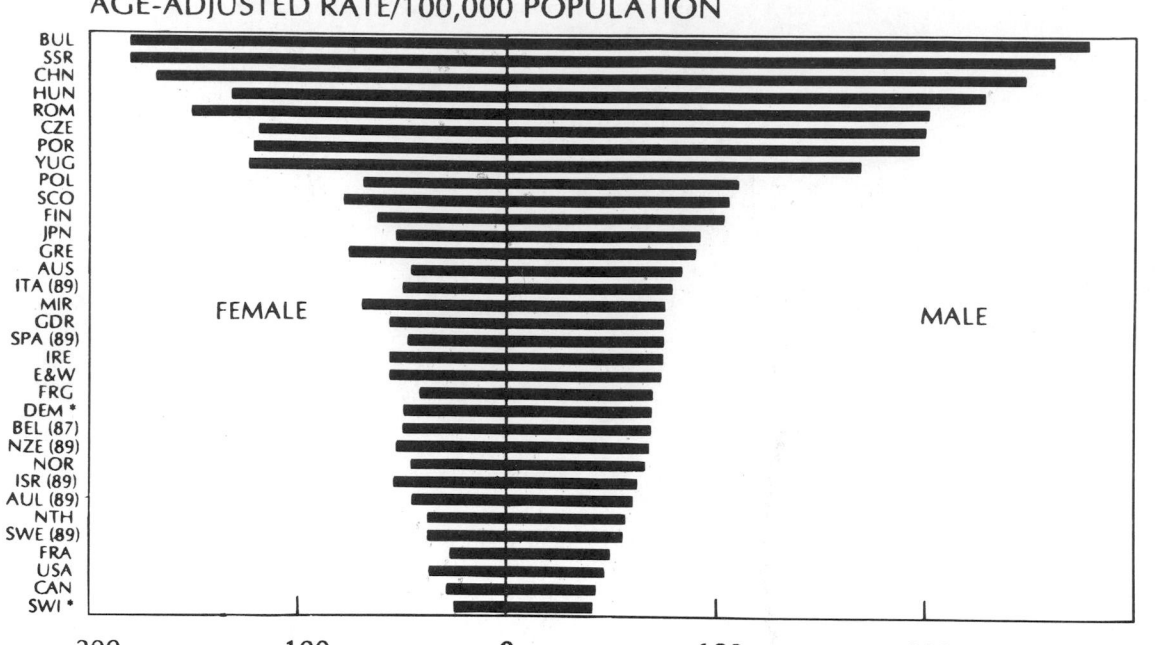

FIG. 28-3. Death rates for stroke, ages 35 to 74, by country and sex, 1990. (From Morbidity and Mortality, Chartbook on Cardiovascular, Lung and Blood Diseases. U.S. Department of Health and Human Services, Washington, D.C., May, 1994.)

of stroke alive in the United States in 1991, many of whom required chronic care. In the elderly, the segment of the population in which most stroke occurs, it is a major source of disability leading to institutionalization.

Incidence of stroke was determined over 36 years of follow-up of 5,070 men and women, aged 30 to 62, who were free of cardiovascular disease at entry in the study in 1950. The population was examined every 2 years and follow-up was quite satisfactory. After 36 years of follow-up in the Framingham Study, there were 693 cases of stroke and transient ischemic attack. The average annual incidence of all strokes combined increased with age and doubled in successive decades. Unlike myocardial infarction, which predominates in men, particularly below age 65, an age group for which myocardial infarction rates are more than three times higher in men, stroke incidence is only 30 percent greater in men than women. Incidence of stroke has been reported in a number of other populations, and the same age/gender trends were seen.

RISK FACTORS FOR STROKE

The term *risk factor* was coined by William B. Kannel in one of the early Framingham Study publications. That report identified, for the first time in prospective epidemiologic study, certain "factors of risk" predisposing to the development of coronary heart disease. Risk factors have now been identified for stroke and the relative magnitude of each has been determined. Since the pathologic processes underlying the various stroke types differ, it is reasonable to expect that risk factors for infarction differ from risk factors for hemorrhage. Furthermore, precursors of parenchymatous bleeding need not be identical to those for subarachnoid hemorrhage. There is also reason to believe that risk factors for stroke due to atherosclerosis of the carotid and vertebral arteries differ in their impact when compared to lacunar stroke. It is likely that the risk factor profile

for embolic stroke will also be different. Nevertheless, certain predisposing factors, particularly elevated blood pressure, appear to be common to most stroke types.

Whereas innovations in medical and surgical therapies to reduce the damage from stroke offer promise, it seems likely that prevention will continue to be the most effective strategy in reducing the impact of cerebrovascular disease. Prevention is facilitated by an understanding of predisposing risk factors and diseases identified chiefly through prospective epidemiologic study. The relative impact of each of these risk factors has become clearer and controlled clinical trials have demonstrated the effectiveness of modification of a number of these risk factors for stroke prevention.

Atherogenic Host Factors

Assessment of the importance of each of the major atherogenic risk factors was made specifically in that stroke type resulting most directly from the atherosclerotic process, atherothrombotic brain infarction. This category includes all ischemic stroke: large-artery atherothrombosis, lacunar infarction, and infarct of undetermined cause, excluding cardiogenic embolism. The major host factors to consider are hypertension; systolic and diastolic blood pressure levels; blood lipids, including serum cholesterol; diabetes; and fibrinogen. Hematocrit and obesity as well as serum proteins have also been implicated.

Hypertension. Hypertension is the chief risk factor for stroke. The age-adjusted relative risk of stroke among definite hypertensives ($\geq 160/\geq 95$ mmHg), compared to normotensives ($\leq 140/\leq 90$ mmHg), is 3.1 in men and 2.9 in women, and even borderline levels (levels between definite hypertension and normotension) carry a 50 percent increased stroke risk (Fig. 28-4). The impact of hypertension was seen in men and women and at all ages up to age 84 years. Whereas brain infarction

COLOR PLATES

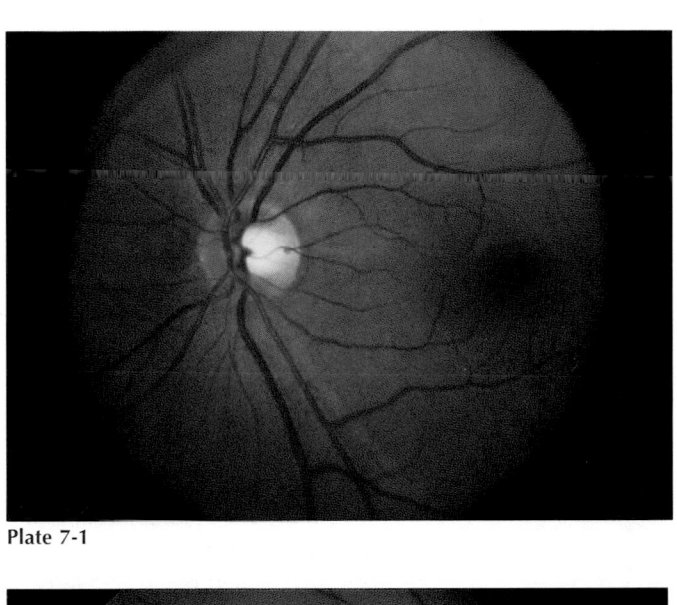

Plate 7-1

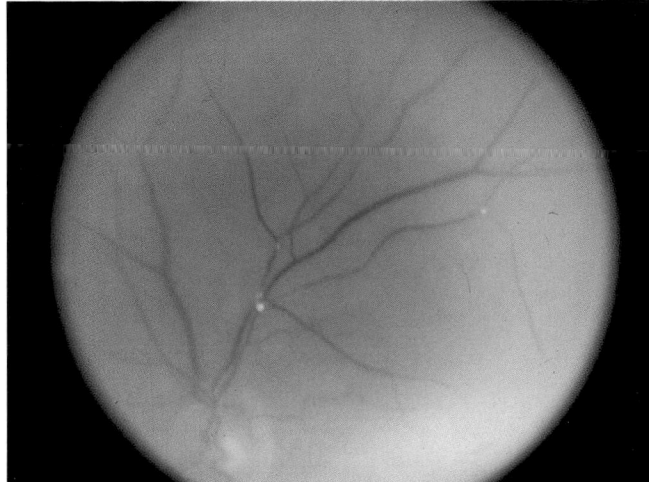

Plate 7-2

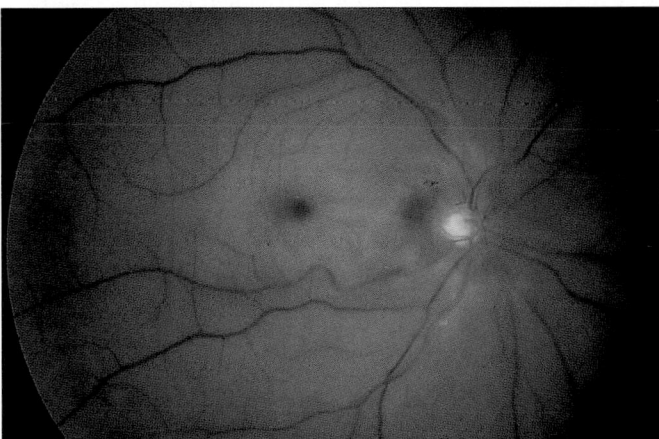

Plate 7-3

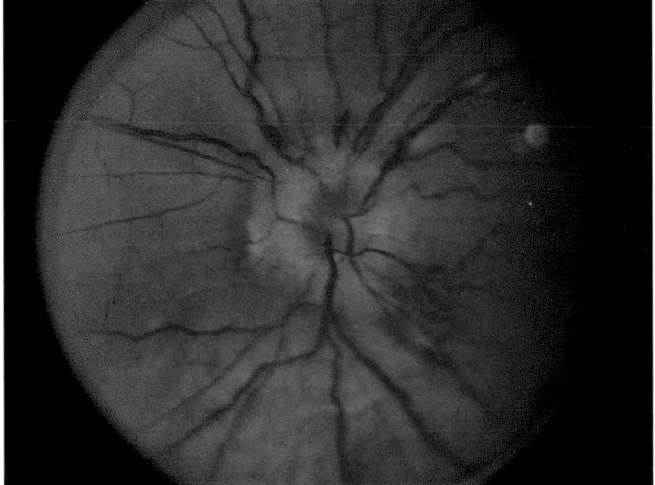

Plate 7-4

PLATE 7-1. Normal left fundus (see Fig. 7-1).

PLATE 7-2. View of the retina and retinal vessels in the left eye supratemporal to the optic disc. Four Hollenhorst plaques, seen as shiny yellow lesions at arterial bifurcations, can be seen. This patient had a left internal carotid artery occlusion.

PLATE 7-3. Central retinal artery occlusion with opaque retinal edema, macular cherry-red spot, and arteriolar attenuation. (Courtesy of Steven L. Galetta, M.D.)

PLATE 7-4. Acute papilledema due to pseudotumor cerebri (left eye). Note peripapillary hemorrhages superiorly and infratemporally, disc hyperemia, venous tortuosity, and obscuration of vessels at the disc margin owing to nerve fiber layer elevation. The round light area in the upper right of the plate is a photographic artifact.

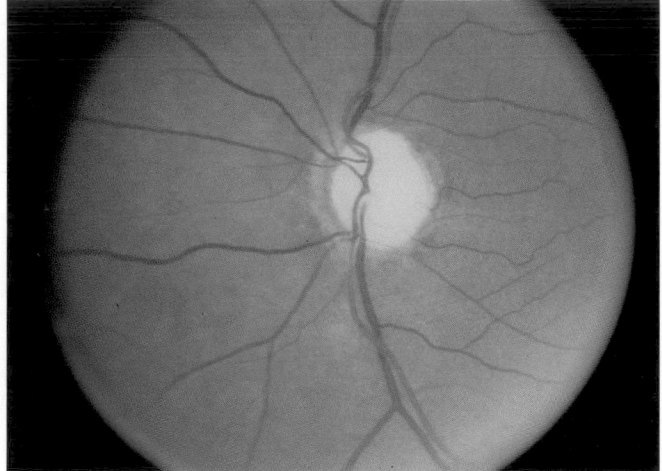

Plate 7-5

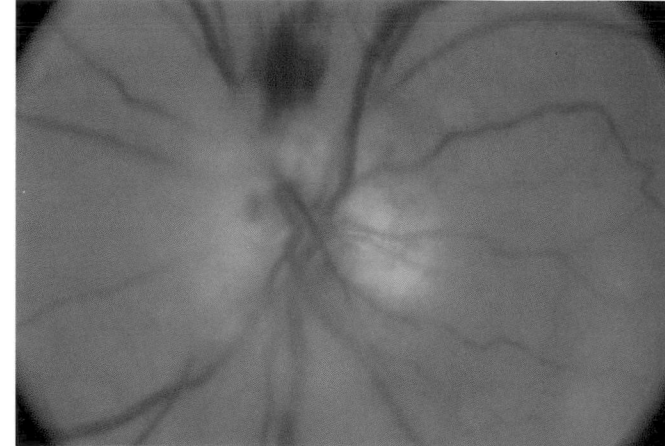

Plate 7-6

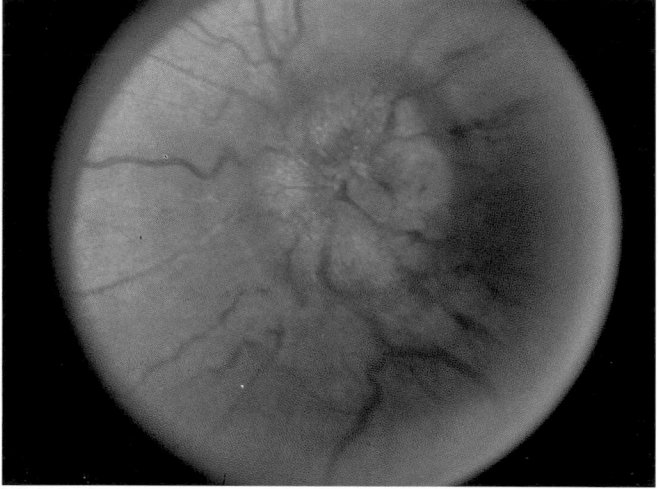

Plate 7-7

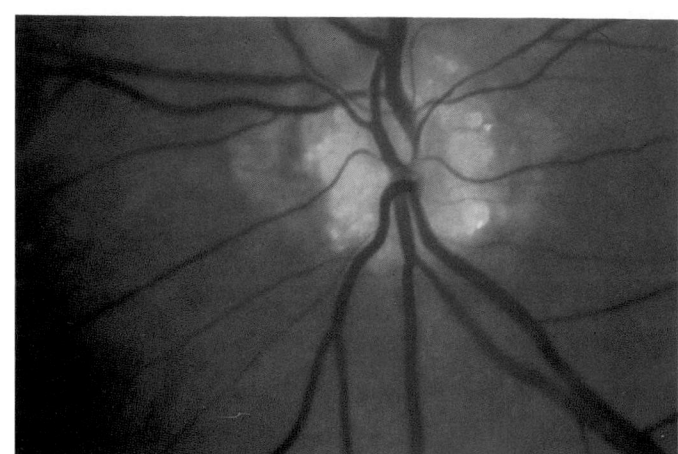

Plate 7-8

PLATE 7-5. Optic disc pallor several months after nonarteritic ischemic optic neuropathy.

PLATE 7-6. Pallid disc swelling of anterior ischemic optic neuropathy owing to giant cell arteritis (20/200 vision). Note the peripapillary hemorrhage superiorly.

PLATE 7-7. Chronic papilledema ("champagne cork" appearance) owing to pseudotumor cerebri. Note whitish exudate overlying the disc as well as venous dilation and tortuosity.

PLATE 7-8. Pseudopapilledema caused by optic nerve head drusen.

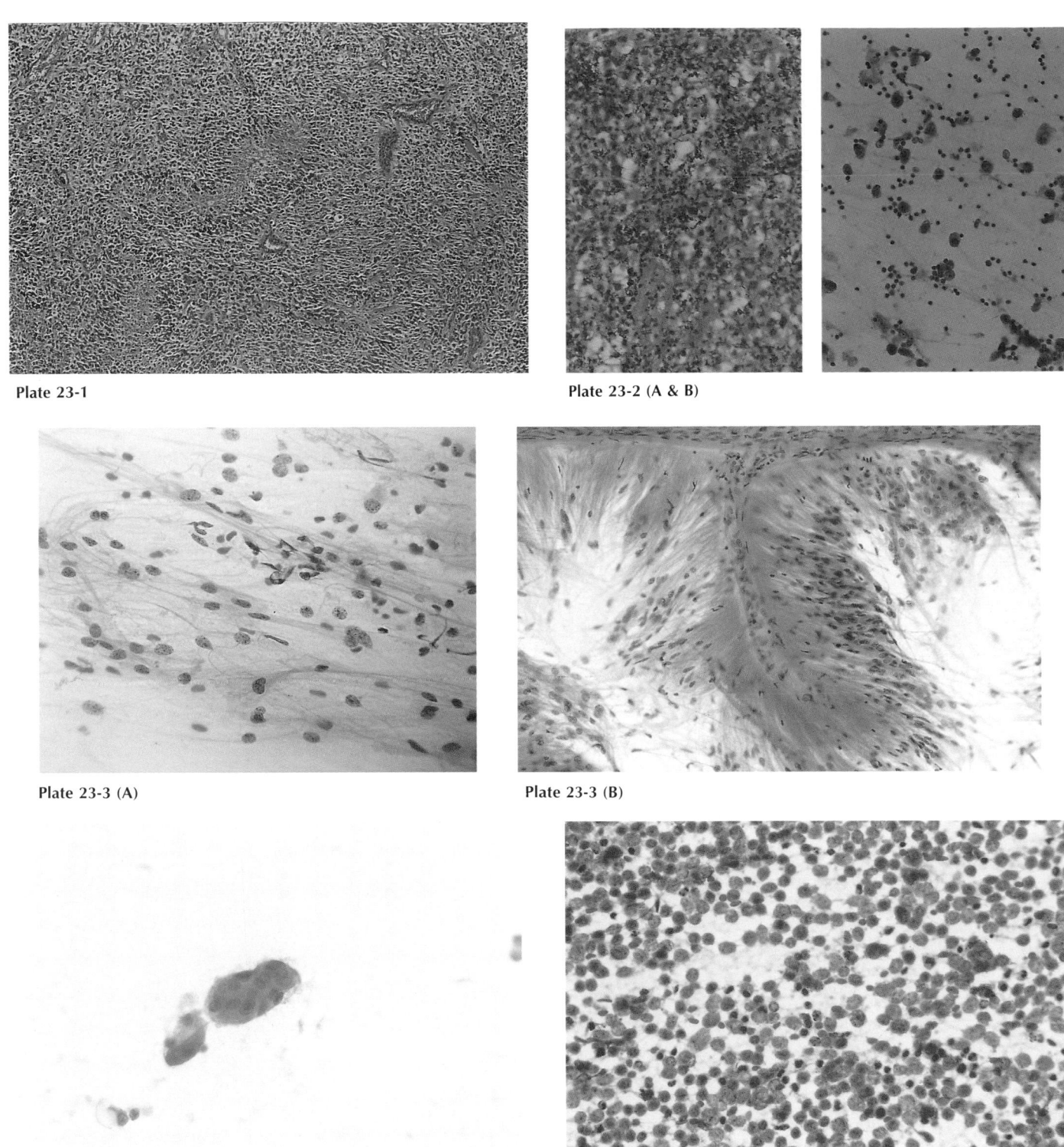

Plate 23-1

Plate 23-2 (A & B)

Plate 23-3 (A)

Plate 23-3 (B)

Plate 23-3 (C)

Plate 23-3 (D)

PLATE 23-1. Glioblastoma multiforme showing a densely cellular tumor with extensive pleomorphism and two of the architectural features characteristic of this high grade glioma: the presence of areas of necrosis surrounded by pseudopalisading of tumor cells and vascular cell proliferation. (H&E)

PLATE 23-2. Comparison of nuclear detail as seen with **(A)** frozen section and **(B)** smear prep. Both slides come from a suprasellar region tumor and contain two populations of cells: a small, benign-appearing lymphoid population and a larger, more pleomorphic population of germ cells. These findings, which are strikingly revealed on the smear preparation, are those of a germinoma. (H&E)

PLATE 23-3. Examples of smear preparations. **(A)** Elongated nuclei, delicate hairlike processes, and Rosenthal fibers are seen in a pilocytic astrocytoma. **(B)** Perivascular arrangement of processes (''perivascular pseudorosettes'') are found in an ependymoma. **(C)** A well-defined syncytial cluster of cells is present in a meningioma. **(D)** An abundant sheet of small, poorly differentiated cells characterize a medulloblastoma. (H&E)

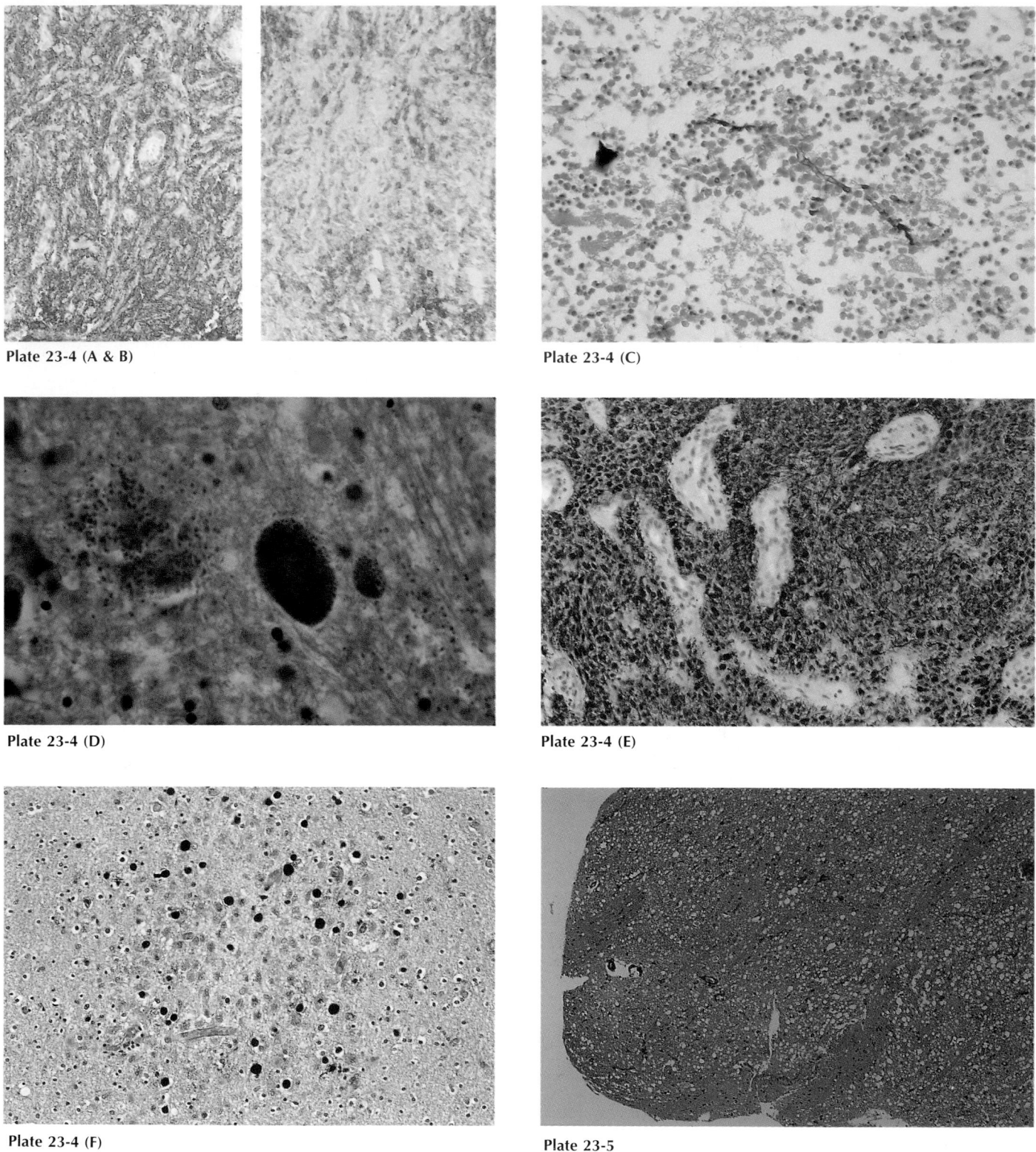

Plate 23-4 (A & B)

Plate 23-4 (C)

Plate 23-4 (D)

Plate 23-4 (E)

Plate 23-4 (F)

Plate 23-5

PLATE 23-4. Examples of special studies. **(A & B)** Immunohistochemical marking of a lymphoma reveals that the tumor cells stain for a pan B-cell marker (Plate A) but not for a pan T-cell marker (Plate B). **(C)** Methenamine silver stain reveals the presence of fungal forms within the debris of an abscess. **(D)** *Toxoplasma* organisms can be seen as both free tachyzoites and as bradyzoites within a pseudocyst (H&E). **(E)** Immunohistochemistry for intermediate filament protein GFAP in a high-grade glioma shows staining of the tumor cells (the pale unstained islands of cells represent areas of vascular cell proliferation). **(F)** Immunohistochemistry for JC virus antigen in a small lesion of progressive multifocal leukoencephalopathy shows the presence of numerous infected oligodendrocytes (counterstained with Luxol Fast Blue/PAS).

PLATE 23-5. Stereotactic biopsy of the putamen from a patient with a rapidly progressive dementing illness. The biopsy shows the vacuolar change in the grey matter characteristic of Creutzfeldt-Jakob disease, with no changes present in the adjacent white matter. (H&E)

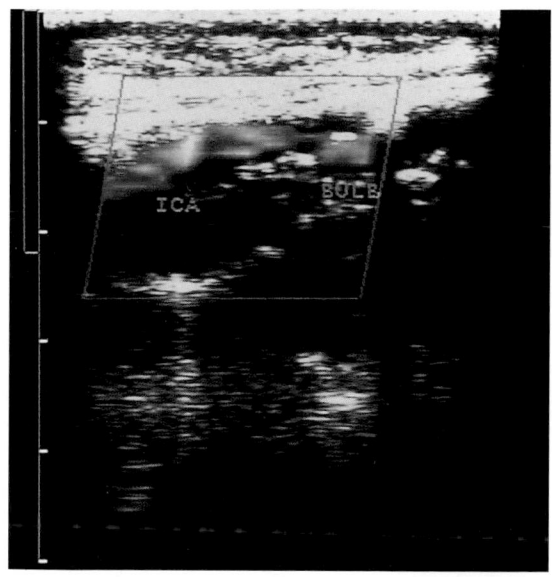

Plate 29-1

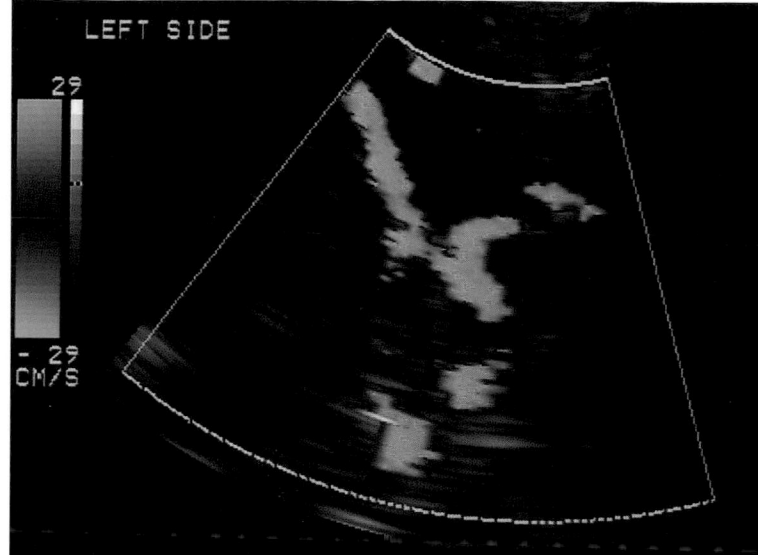

Plate 29-2

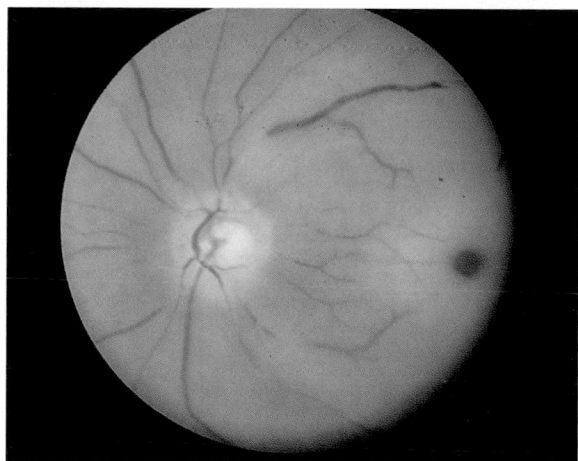

Plate 43-1 (A)

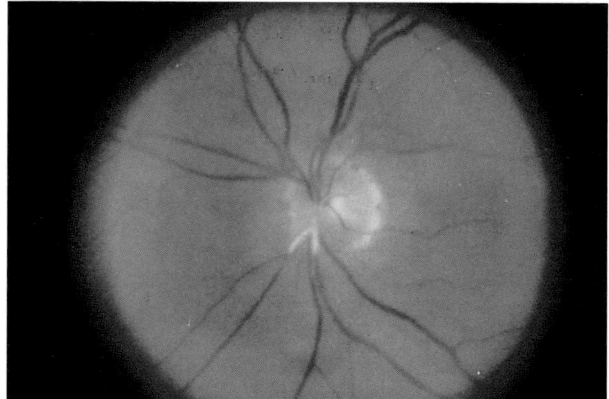

Plate 43-1 (B)

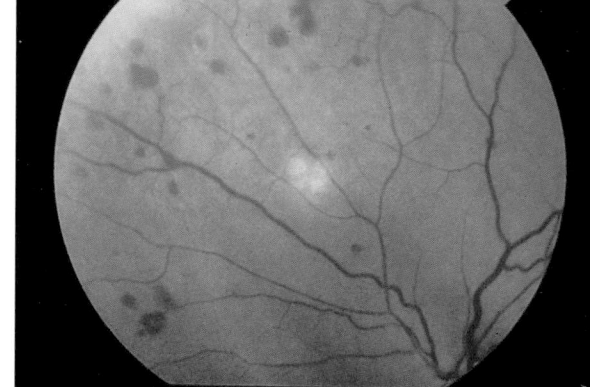

Plate 43-1 (C)

PLATE 29-1. Color duplex image of the left carotid bifurcation in a patient with asymptomatic carotid artery stenosis.

PLATE 29-2. Transcranial color image of the intracranial circulation demonstrating middle cerebral artery, posterior communicating artery, distal internal carotid artery, and origin of posterior cerebral artery. (Courtesy of V. L. Babikian, M.D.)

PLATE 43-1. Retinal manifestations of carotid disease. **(A)** Central retinal artery occlusion with ischemic retinal pallor, narrowing of the arterioles, and a cherry-red macula. **(B)** Branch retinal artery occlusion owing to a saddle embolus of platelet-fibrin material in the inferior retinal artery. **(C)** Venous stasis retinopathy with dot and blot hemorrhages in the midretinal periphery, and attenuation of arterioles owing to low retinal perfusion in a patient with a high-grade carotid stenosis.

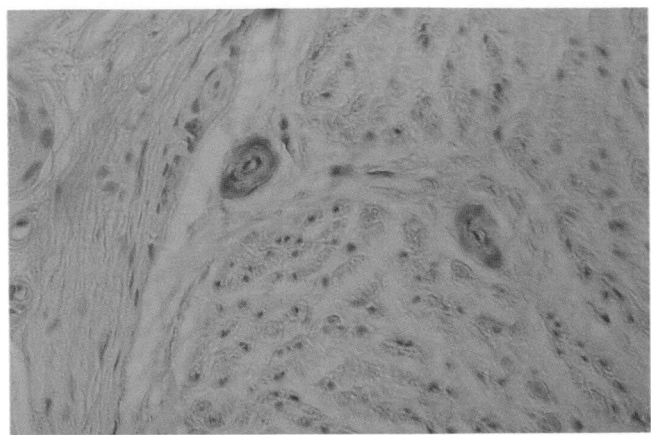

Plate 100-1

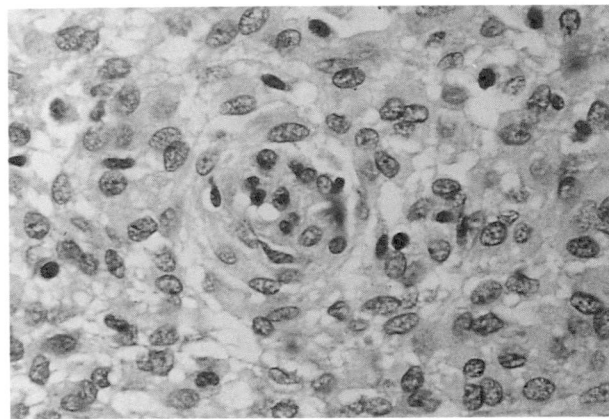

Plate 155-1 (A)

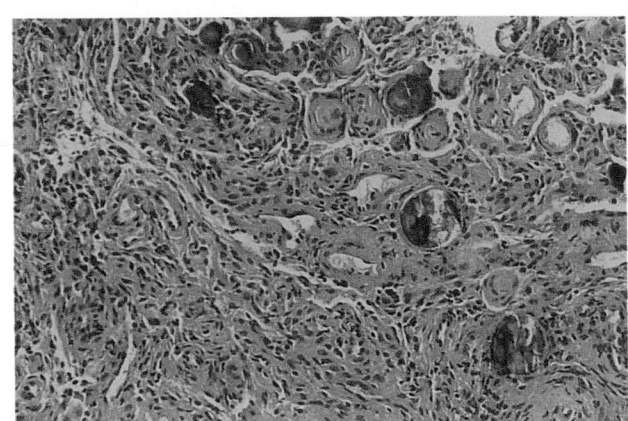

Plate 155-1 (B)

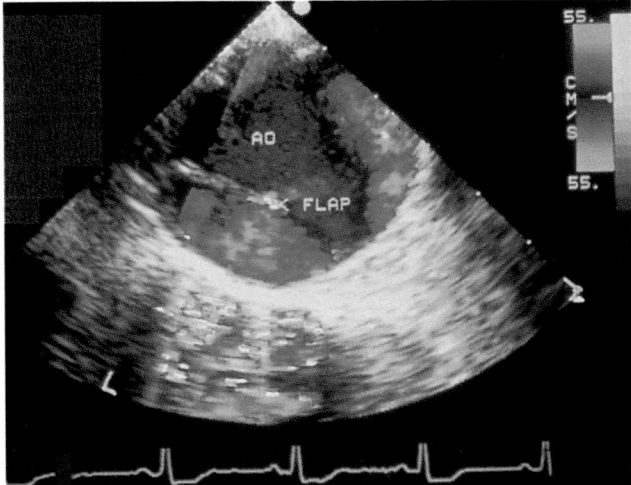

Plate 183-1

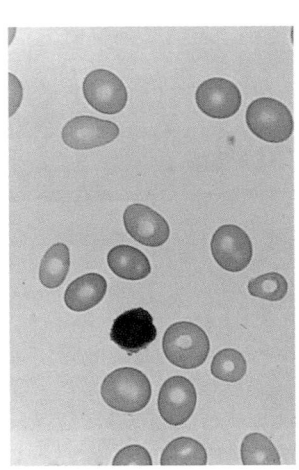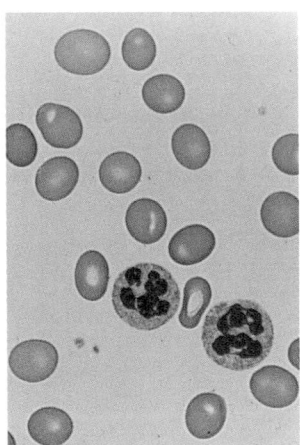

Plate 187-1 (A & B)

PLATE 100-1. Sural nerve biopsy of a patient with familial amyloidosis. Transverse section embedded in paraffin and stained with monoclonal antibodies to transthyretin (TTR). Note amyloid deposits showing a positive reaction with a monoclonal antibody to TTR.

PLATE 155-1. Typical histology of meningiomas (H&E). **(A)** Whorl formation. **(B)** Psammoma bodes. (From Al-Mefty O, Origitano TC: Meningiomas. pp. 28.1–28.12. In Rengachary SS, Wilkins RH (eds): Principles of Neurosurgery. Wolfe Publishing, London, 1994, with permission.)

PLATE 183-1. Transesophageal echocardiogram showing intimal flap entry site is marked by blood flow into false channel (yellow). (Courtesy of T. Marwick, M.D., Cleveland Clinic Foundation, Cleveland, OH.)

PLATE 187-1. Peripheral blood smears of patients with megaloblastic anemia. **(A)** Macrocytosis. **(B)** Hypersegmented neutrophils. (Courtesy of Jackie Mitus, M.D., Brigham and Women's Hospital, Boston, MA.)

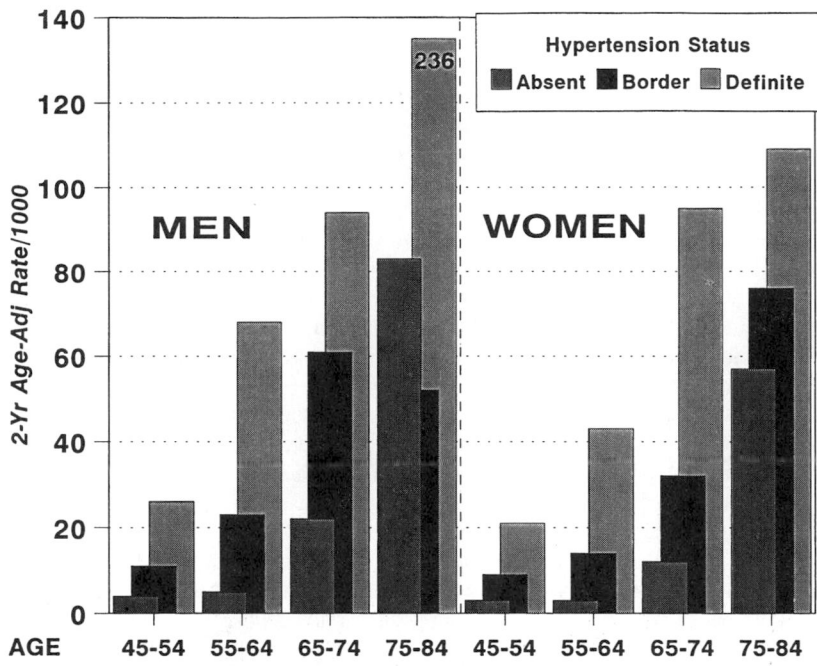

FIG. 28-4. Incidence of atherothrombotic brain infarction and hypertensive status, 36-year follow-up, the Framingham Study. (From Wolf PA: Cerebrovascular disease in the elderly. p. 130. In Tresch DD, Aronow WS, (eds): Cardiovascular Disease in the Elderly Patient, Marcel Dekker, New York, 1987 with permission.)

incidence is increased in hypertensives, this categoric classification does not portray the strong relationship to the level of the blood pressure. Risk of stroke generally, and brain infarction specifically, is directly related to the level of the blood pressure throughout its range, with no critical value of pressure, systolic or diastolic, below which stroke does not occur.

A substantial portion of stroke incidence is directly attributable to hypertension, and a portion of stroke in the population would be eliminated if hypertension were effectively treated. This portion, the population attributable fraction, was estimated to be 56.4 percent of strokes in men and 66.1 percent in women, based on an analysis of 26-year follow-up of Framingham Heart Study data.

Systolic Versus Diastolic Pressure Level. Both systolic and diastolic blood pressure level are strongly and independently related to atherothrombotic brain infarction incidence, although the diastolic component has been thought to be of primary importance. Clinical trials of antihypertensive treatment and disease prevention, principally stroke, have used diastolic blood pressure as the basis for categorization of subjects. However, evidence for the ascendancy of diastolic blood pressure over systolic is lacking. Diastolic blood pressure, which is more difficult to measure accurately and varies within a narrower range than the systolic component, seems to provide no advantage in predicting the cardiovascular complications of hypertension. To further emphasize the ascendancy of systolic over diastolic blood pressure level, Fisher reports that he determines only the systolic pressure and no longer routinely measures the diastolic pressure (once aortic valvular disease has been excluded). Data from the Framingham Study support this contention. Among persons with systolic blood pressures of 160 mmHg or higher, stroke risk does not increase with increasing levels of diastolic blood pressure. On the other hand, among persons with diastolic hypertension, incidence of stroke increases steadily with level of systolic blood pressure.

Isolated Systolic Hypertension. With advancing age, there is a disproportionate rise in systolic blood pressure, whereas the diastolic pressure levels off and then begins to decline. In the elderly, this isolated elevation of systolic pressure becomes highly prevalent. Isolated systolic hypertension (i.e., systolic pressure of 160 mmHg or higher and diastolic pressure less than 90 mmHg) occurs in 20 percent of men and 30 percent of women age 80 years and older. Increased systolic blood pressure in the presence of normal diastolic levels in the elderly resulted from decreased elasticity of the walls of the great arteries. As such, these isolated systolic pressure elevations were considered to be the consequence rather than a risk factor for cardiovascular disease. However, it has been demonstrated in the Framingham Heart Study and in other epidemiologic studies that stroke and cardiovascular disease incidence was significantly increased in persons with isolated systolic hypertension. Risk was proportional to the level of systolic pressure even after diastolic pressure, age, and digital pulse-wave configuration (an index of arterial rigidity) were taken into account. The Systolic Hypertension in the Elderly Program (SHEP Trial) found a clear beneficial effect of systolic blood pressure reduction in elderly with isolated systolic hypertension and is discussed below.

It is now apparent that even borderline isolated systolic hypertension (systolic blood pressure level of 140 to 160 mmHg with a diastolic pressure of less than 90 mmHg) was associated with an increased risk of developing definite hypertension and had a 42 percent greater risk of developing a stroke or transient ischemic attack, even after other pertinent risk factors were taken into account.

Blood Lipids. The positive relationship between total serum cholesterol and incidence of coronary heart disease in men and women is well established. High-density lipoprotein (HDL) cholesterol has an inverse association and low-density lipoprotein (LDL) cholesterol and a direct relationship to incidence of coronary heart disease. A significant impact on coronary heart disease incidence can be shown by blood lipids using the total serum cholesterol HDL cholesterol ratio up to age 80. These relationships do not apply to stroke generally or to brain infarction in particular, and a low total cholesterol level seems to predispose to parenchymatous hemorrhage.

A recent meta-analysis consisting of 460,000 subjects with 46,000 strokes showed no significant association between total serum cholesterol and total stroke incidence. However, a relationship was found in the Honolulu Heart Study of Japanese men and in the Multiple Risk Factor Intervention Trial (MRFIT) screenees. In Honolulu, the level of total cholesterol measured years before was directly related to the incidence of thromboembolism. No such relationship existed, long or short term, between ischemic stroke and total or LDL cholesterol in Framingham and no protective effect of HDL cholesterol. In MRFIT, the incidence of death certificate–diagnosed ischemic stroke was greater in those with the highest levels of serum total cholesterol obtained 6 years before. Furthermore, in a meta-analysis of cholesterol-lowering trials, the rate of myocardial infarction was decreased but there was no significant benefit in stroke prevention in the treated groups.

A surprisingly consistent finding has been the relationship between low total serum cholesterol and increased incidence of intracerebral hemorrhage. This finding was first noted among rural Japanese following World War II Serum cholesterol levels were, by Western standards, quite low—frequently below 160 mg/dl. An etiologic link has been suggested by the recent confirmation of this relationship in other Oriental populations, in Ha-

waiian Japanese, as well as in white men in the United States. In 350,977 men aged 35 to 57 years were screened for entry into the MRFIT; after 6 years of follow-up, there were 83 deaths from intracerebral hemorrhage and 55 deaths from subarachnoid hemorrhage. In the lowest serum cholesterol category, less than 160 mg/dl, the risk factor–adjusted relative risk of intracranial hemorrhage was 1.0 and relative risk at all higher levels of serum cholesterol was approximately 0.32 (Fig. 28-5). When deaths from intracranial hemorrhage were examined by entry diastolic blood pressure, the age-adjusted rate of death was significant only in persons with pressures of 90 mmHg or higher. Death rates per 10,000 were 23.07 in the lowest serum cholesterol category, less than 160 mg/dl, and ranged from 3.09 to 4.83 in the four higher categories. The interaction of high diastolic blood pressure and low serum cholesterol in promoting intracerebral hemorrhage suggested to some investigators "that very low serum cholesterol levels weaken the endothelium of intracerebral arteries, resulting in hemorrhagic stroke in the presence of hypertension." Other factors predisposing to intracerebral hemorrhage are increased alcohol consumption, dietary protein deficiency, and a high intake of polyunsaturated fatty acids. These polyunsaturated fatty acids, both linoleic acid derived from vegetable oils and eicosapentanoic acid from fish oil, act to reduce platelet aggregability and may thereby promote hemorrhage.

Although the relationship between blood lipids and stroke is unclear, serum lipid levels have been directly related to extracranial carotid artery atherosclerosis and to extracranial carotid artery wall thickness. Atherosclerosis of the carotid artery, and the circle of Willis in autopsy studies, is directly related to levels of blood lipids. On the other hand, the relationship to stroke generally may be obscured by the differing influence of

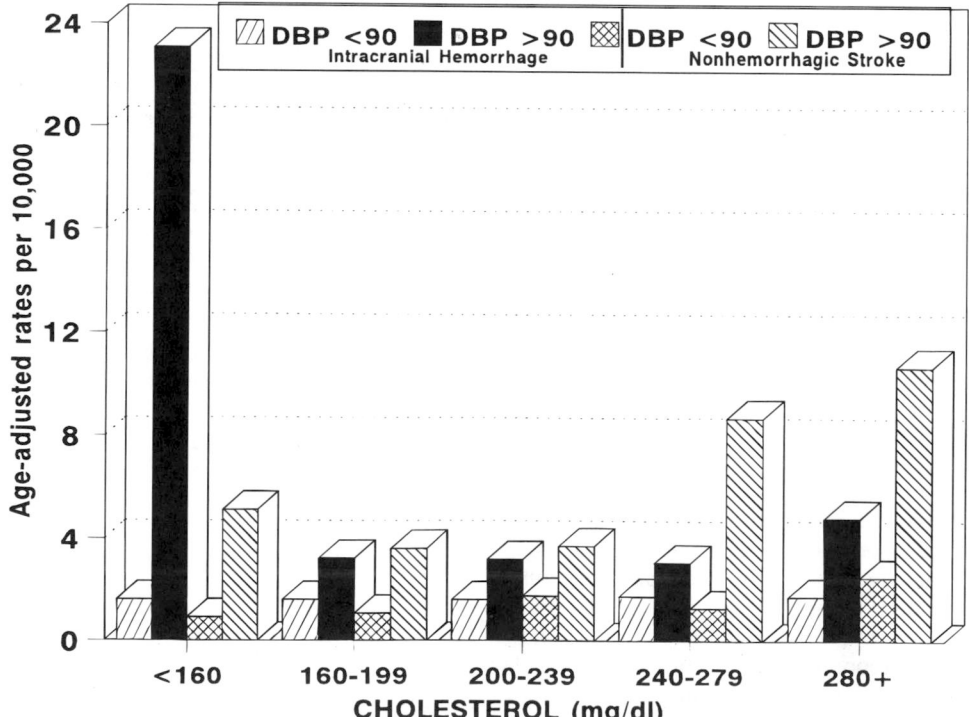

FIG. 28-5. Ischemic stroke and intracerebral hemorrhage death rates in men with normal and elevated diastolic blood pressure (DBP) according to screening serum cholesterol level. Multiple Risk Factor Intervention Trial screenees, 6-year follow-up. (From Wolf PA, Cobb JL, D'Agostino RB: Epidemiology of stroke. p. 16. In Barnett HJM, Mohr JP, Stein BM, Yatsu FM: Pathophysiology, Diagnosis, and Management. 2nd Ed. Churchill Livingstone, New York, 1992, with permission.)

lipids on the varying vascular pathologies underlying stroke. There is no apparent influence of lipids on lacunar infarcts or on strokes secondary to cerebral embolism.

Diabetes.   Diabetic patients have an increased susceptibility to atherosclerosis. Case-control studies of stroke patients and prospective epidemiologic study have confirmed the increased risk of ischemic stroke in diabetic patients, ranging from 1.8 to 3-fold. In the United States, in the period 1976 to 1980, a medical history of stroke was 2.5 to four times more common in diabetic patients than in persons with normal glucose tolerance. In the Honolulu Heart Program, Japanese men living in Hawaii with diabetes had double the risk of thromboembolic stroke of nondiabetic patients that was independent of other risk factors. In a population-based cohort in Rancho Bernardo, diabetic patients had a relative risk of stroke that was 1.8 in men and 2.2 in women, after adjusting for the effect of other pertinent risk factors.

In the Framingham Study, peripheral arterial disease with intermittent claudication occurred more than four times as often in diabetic patients. The coronary and cerebral arteries were also affected, but to a lesser extent. For brain infarction, the impact of glucose intolerance (i.e., physician-diagnosed diabetes, glycosuria, or a blood sugar $\geq$150 mg/100 ml) is greater in women than men and was significant as an independent contributor to incidence only in older women. Overall, persons with glucose intolerance have double the risk of brain infarction as nondiabetics.

Obesity.   Obesity is associated with higher levels of blood pressure, blood glucose, and atherogenic serum lipids, and on that account alone could be expected to increase stroke incidence. Obesity, as expressed as a Metropolitan Relative Weight that is more than 30 percent above average, is a significant independent contributor to brain infarction incidence in men aged 35 to 64 and women aged 65 to 94 years. However, even in the other two age/sex groups, obesity exerts an adverse influence on health status that is probably mediated through elevated blood pressure, impaired glucose tolerance, and other mechanisms. In the Honolulu Heart Study, obesity has been recently identified as an independent factor related to stroke incidence. The pattern of obesity has also been identified to be important. Persons with central obesity manifested by abdominal deposition of fat, rather than obesity involving the hips and thighs, has been related to the occurrence of atherosclerotic disease.

Family History of Stroke.   Although family history of stroke is perceived to be an important marker of increased stroke risk, definitive confirmation by epidemiologic study has been lacking. Maternal history of death from stroke, but not paternal, was recently found to be significantly related to stroke incidence in a cohort of Swedish men born in 1913. Other significant risk factors included hypertension, abdominal pattern of obesity, and fibrinogen level. Maternal history of fatal stroke was independently related to stroke even after these variables were taken into account.

In the Framingham Study, no relationship was found between a history of stroke death in parents and documented stroke in subjects. Verified stroke cases, nonfatal and fatal, in these cohort members were then related to the occurrence of stroke in their children (members of the Framingham Offspring Study cohort). In these analyses, both maternal and paternal stroke was associated with an approximately 1.5-fold increased risk of stroke even after other risk factors were taken into account.

Thus, family history of stroke, so frequently mentioned and nearly universally acknowledged as risk factor for stroke, has been only recently identified and documented by epidemiologic study.

Fibrinogen.   Elevated serum fibrinogen has been implicated in atherogenesis and in arterial thrombus formation. In prospective epidemiologic study, there was a substantial and significant independent impact of fibrinogen on cardiovascular disease incidence including stroke. In a prospective study of 54-year-old Swedish men, fibrinogen in combination with elevated systolic blood pressure, was found to be a potent risk factor for stroke. Level of fibrinogen, measured on the tenth biennial examination in the Framingham Study, was also significantly related to incidence of cardiovascular disease, including stroke. However, fibrinogen was also positively associated with most of the major risk factors for stroke, including age, hypertension, hematocrit level, obesity, and diabetes.

Hematocrit.   Some studies, including the Framingham Study, have demonstrated a relationship between high normal hematocrit level and incidence of cerebral infarction. Confirmation of this relationship has come from an autopsy study of Japanese stroke patients and from several clinical and radiologic studies of patients with stroke. In these 36-year follow-up data, elevated blood hematocrit, within the normal range, and generally not pathologically elevated red blood cell mass, is significantly and independently associated with brain infarction only in men aged 35 to 64, but not in women or in older men. This significant relationship persisted even after the impact of cigarette smoking and hypertension were taken into account. Increased concentration of red blood cells in combination with high blood fibrinogen levels raises blood viscosity. This interaction may become significant in narrowed small penetrating arteries and in high-grade stenosis of a major cerebral artery.

Heart Disease and Impaired Cardiac Function

Cardiac disease and impaired cardiac function are frequent accompaniments and precursors of stroke. These cardiac contributors are disease states or organ dysfunctions and not risk factors. Although hypertension is the preeminent risk factor for stroke of all types, at each blood pressure level, persons with impaired cardiac function have a significantly increased stroke risk. Cardiovascular disease is highly prevalent among stroke cases. In the Framingham Study, after 36 years of follow-up of more than 600 stroke and transient ischemic attack cases, 80.8 percent were hypertensive, 32.7 percent had prior coronary heart disease, 14.5 percent had congestive heart failure, 14.5 percent had atrial fibrillation, and only 13.6 percent had none of these.

Coronary Heart Disease.   In the Framingham Study, coronary heart disease was ascertained prospectively on biennial examination as well as by monitoring hospitalizations over 36 years of follow-up. Acute myocardial infarction predisposes to stroke, particularly in the days and weeks following the event. Stroke incidence has been clearly demonstrated to be reduced by aspirin or warfarin administered after an acute myocardial infarction. Among Q-wave myocardial infarctions, anterior wall infarcts are more likely to lead to stroke than infarcts at other sites. The mechanism is presumed to be cerebral embolism from an intracardiac mural thrombus. Often, however, the mechanism of stroke in persons with coronary heart disease is less apparent. Persons with uncomplicated angina pectoris, non-

Q-wave infarction, and clinically silent myocardial infarction also have an increased incidence of ischemic stroke. Recent data from the Framingham Study suggest that silent, or unrecognized, myocardial infarction survivors had a 10-year incidence of stroke of 17.8 percent in men and 17.3 percent in women, an incidence not that much less than the 19.5 percent and 29.3 percent in men and women, respectively, that is seen following recognized myocardial infarction.

Congestive Heart Failure. Congestive heart failure prevalence increases with age, from a low of 0.8 percent at ages 50 to 59 to 9.1 percent at 80 to 89 years, usually as a consequence of hypertension and coronary heart disease. It predisposes to atrial fibrillation, which may precipitate or exacerbate congestive heart failure. However, even after the impact of atrial fibrillation, hypertension, and coronary heart disease are taken into account, congestive heart failure increases the risk of stroke more than fourfold. The hazard posed by congestive heart failure persists, despite the availability of many new drugs, with no good evidence of improved survival over the past 20 years in the Framingham Study. Congestive heart failure is a serious and highly lethal condition with survival following onset that is similar to that of lung cancer.

Atrial Fibrillation. In association with rheumatic heart disease and mitral stenosis, atrial fibrillation has long been believed to predispose to stroke. In the recent years, atrial fibrillation without valvular heart disease, previously considered to be innocuous, has been associated with more than a fivefold increased incidence of stroke. Atrial fibrillation is also a fairly common cardiac arrhythmia in the elderly. In the Framingham Study, atrial fibrillation prevalence more than doubled in successive decades to 8 percent at ages 80 to 89 years. Although 15 percent of stroke occurred in persons with atrial fibrillation, the proportion of strokes associated with this arrhythmia increased steadily with age, reaching 36.2 percent for ages 80 to 89 years. There is clearly a powerful impact of atrial fibrillation on stroke incidence in the elderly that is independent of cardiac disease and hypertension. The success of a series of clinical trials using warfarin to prevent stroke in atrial fibrillation has validated the independent importance of atrial fibrillation, since nearly 70 percent risk reduction occurred without any specific measures to improve the associated cardiac conditions.

Left Ventricular Hypertrophy by Electrocardiogram. Left ventricular hypertrophy (LVH) by electrocardiogram (ECG) increases in prevalence with age and blood pressure. Risk of brain infarction increased by more than fourfold in men and sixfold in women with this abnormal ECG pattern. The increased risk persisted even after the influence of age and other pertinent risk factors were accounted for.

Echocardiographic Factors. Using ECG, a number of structural changes that predispose to stroke have been identified. Although none are routinely available in the office practice of neurology, several sources of emboli, aortic arch thrombi, and patent foramen ovale have been identified and are discussed elsewhere in this section. ECG has also identified structural changes that make an independent contribution to stroke incidence. These include mitral annular calcification, increased left atrial size, and increased left ventricular mass (LVM). Mitral annular calcification and increased left atrial size serve to predispose to atrial fibrillation. However, each exerts an impact on stroke incidence that is independent of atrial fibrillation by mechanisms that are not entirely clear. Mitral valve prolapse, often cited in the past as a risk factor for stroke, has not held up as an important abnormality despite the relatively high prevalence in the population.

LVM-to-height ratio determined by echocardiography offers a more sensitive and quantitative assessment of cardiac muscle hypertrophy than LVH by ECG. Recently, LVM as determined on M-mode echocardiography has been shown to be directly related to incidence of stroke. The hazard ratio for stroke and transient ischemic attack, comparing the uppermost quartile to the lowest, was 2.72 after adjusting for age, gender, and cardiovascular risk factors. There was a graded response with a hazard ratio of 1.45 for each quartile increment of LVM-to-height ratio. Thus, echocardiography offers prognostic information beyond that provided by traditional risk factors.

Environmental Factors

Cigarette Smoking. Cigarette smoking, a powerful risk factor for myocardial infarction and sudden death, has been clearly linked to brain infarction, as well as to subarachnoid hemorrhage (Table 28-2). A similar relationship between cigarette smoking and stroke has been seen in Hawaiian Japanese men after 10 years of follow-up in the Honolulu Heart Study, in which cigarette smoking made a significant independent contribution to cerebral infarction and intracranial hemorrhage risk. In the late 1970s, several studies of oral contraceptives and stroke in young women identified cigarette smoking as an important risk factor. Surprisingly, the association between cigarette smoking, oral contraceptives, and stroke was primarily related to subarachnoid hemorrhage. In the Nurses' Health Study, a cohort of nearly 120,000 women followed prospectively for 8 years for the development of stroke, there was an increased risk of subarachnoid hemorrhage as well as thrombotic stroke in cigarette smokers. Relative risk of subarachnoid hemorrhage showed a dose–response relationship of from fourfold in light smokers to 9.8-fold in smokers of 25 or more cigarettes daily. Of note, in each smoking category, the relative risk of subarachnoid hemorrhage, whether or not other associated risk factors were taken into account, was twice as great as for thromboembolic stroke (Table 28-2).

The association between cigarette smoking and subarachnoid hemorrhage from aneurysm was also found in men (as well as women) in Framingham and in New Zealand in case-control analyses. In a case-control study of 114 patients with subarachnoid hemorrhage in a defined region in Finland, cigarette smokers were significantly more prevalent among cases than matched controls. Relative risk of subarachnoid hemorrhage in smokers, as compared with nonsmokers, was 2.7 in men and 3.0 in women. The authors suggested that smoking promoted a temporary increase in blood pressure, which, acting in concert with the "metastatic emphysema effect," was responsible for subarachnoid hemorrhage from cerebral aneurysm. No more reasonable hypothesis has been promulgated to explain this powerful relationship. In a population-based case-control study in several counties in the Seattle, Washington, area, cigarette smoking was found to increase risk of subarachnoid hemorrhage from aneurysm ninefold. The relationship of cigarette smoking to intracerebral hemorrhage is currently unclear.

In a meta-analysis of 32 separate studies, including those cited above, cigarette smoking was a significant independent contributor to stroke incidence in both sexes and at all ages,

TABLE 28-2. Age-Adjusted Relative Risks[a] of Stroke (Fatal and Nonfatal Combined), by Daily Number of Cigarettes Consumed Among Current Smokers

Event	Never Smoked	Former Smoker	Current Smoker	No. Cigarettes Smoked per Day Among Current Smokers			
				1–14	15–24	25–34	≥35
Total Stroke[b]	1.00	1.35 (0.98–1.85)	2.73 (2.18–3.41)	2.02 (1.29–3.14)	3.34 (2.38–4.70)	3.08 (1.94–4.87)	4.48 (2.78–7.23)
Subarachnoid hemorrhage[b]	1.00	2.26 (1.16–4.42)	4.85 (2.90–8.11)	4.28 (1.88–9.77)	4.02 (1.90–8.54)	7.95 (3.50–18.07)	10.22 (4.03–25.94)
Ischemic stroke[b]	1.00	1.27 (0.85–1.89)	2.53 (1.91–3.35)	1.83 (1.04–3.23)	3.57 (2.36–5.42)	2.73 (1.49–5.03)	3.97 (2.09–7.53)
Cerebral hemorrhage[b]	1.00	1.24 (0.64–2.42)	1.24 (0.64–2.42)	1.68 (0.34–5.28)	2.53 (0.71–6.05)	1.41 (0.39–5.05)	1.41 (0.39–5.05)

[a] Relative risks adjusted for age in 5-year intervals, follow-up period (1976–78, 1978–80, 1980–82, 1982–84, 1984–86, or 1986–88), history of hypertension, diabetes, high cholesterol levels, body mass index, past use of oral contraceptives, postmenopausal estrogen therapy, and age at starting smoking.
[b] Numbers in parentheses are 95% confidence intervals.

(Adapted from Kawachi I, Colditz GA, Stampfer MJ: Smoking cessation and decreased risk of stroke in women. JAMA 269:233, 1993, with permission.)

and was associated with an approximately 50 percent increased risk overall when compared with nonsmokers. The risk of stroke generally, and of ischemic stroke specifically, rose as number of cigarettes smoked per day increased, in both men and women.

Smoking Cessation. Observational studies have demonstrated a decrease in stroke incidence following smoking cessation. In the Framingham Heart Study, risk of stroke in former cigarette smokers fell within 1 or 2 years following cessation. Within 5 years of smoking cessation, risk of stroke in former smokers was no greater than in persons who had never smoked. This seemed true even in the elderly and in persons who had been heavy smokers for many years. In the Nurses' Health Study, relative risk of stroke in former smokers fell to 0.4 within 5 years following cessation (Fig. 28-6). This is the same risk, relative to current smokers, as subjects who had never smoked. Clearly, the axiom "It's never too late to quit" holds true for stroke as it does for coronary heart disease. However, the impact of cigarette smoking is more long-lasting for other diseases with risk of peripheral arterial disease and certain cancers, particularly carcinoma of the lung, persisting beyond 10 years following cessation.

The rapid reduction of the effect of cigarette smoking on coronary heart disease and stroke strongly suggests a precipitating effect of smoking on disease rather than an influence of promoting atherogenesis. An effect on endothelium and blood clotting might be the mechanism. In any case, it is certain that smoking cessation has been accepted as a proven way to reduce stroke risk and to do so quite promptly.

Oral Contraceptives. An increased risk of stroke was reported in users of oral contraceptives, particularly in older women (i.e., above age 35), and predominantly in those with other cardiovascular risk factors, particularly hypertension and cigarette smoking. The relative risk of stroke was estimated to be increased fivefold in oral contraceptive users and former users, with risk concentrated in cigarette smokers above age 35. However, the mechanism of stroke in oral contraceptive users is unclear. Cerebral infarction is more likely to be due to thrombotic disease than to atherosclerosis; it is known that clotting is enhanced by the oral contraceptive-induced increased platelet aggregability and by its alteration of clotting factors to favor thrombogenesis. In young women with unexplained ischemic stroke, use of oral contraceptives is presumed to be the "cause" of the infarct; however, the stroke was attributed to oral contraceptive use in no more than 10 percent of a series of carefully studied patients. Although there have been few systematic investigations of oral contraceptives and stroke in the 1980s, among case-control studies of stroke in oral contraceptive users conducted in the 1970s, "thromboembolism" was the type of stroke said to occur most frequently in oral contraceptive users. However, women in the case group often experienced transient episodes of neurologic dysfunction, transient ischemic attacks, or stroke events categorized as being due to "ill-defined and uncertain" causes. Risk of stroke was highest in women who took oral contraceptives containing higher levels of estrogen; the lower levels of estrogen in the newer oral contraceptive formulations seem to have substantially reduced the hazard, and former users seem to be at no increased risk of stroke.

Of particular interest is the interaction between oral contraceptives, cigarette smoking, and subarachnoid hemorrhage. Prospective observation of over 40,000 women, one-half of whom were taking oral contraceptives, showed an increased risk of fatal subarachnoid hemorrhage (not cerebral infarction) in women taking oral contraceptives. Risk was increased fourfold in cigarette smokers above age 35, with most cases confined to this group.

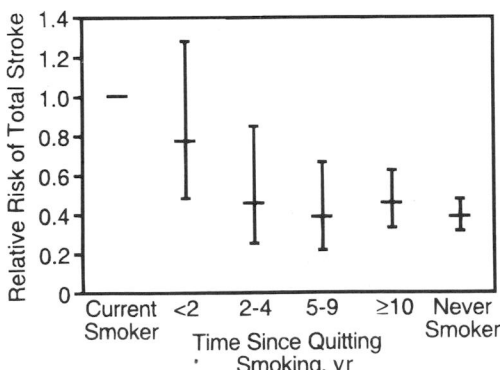

FIG. 28-6. Smoking cessation and risk of stroke in women. Age-adjusted relative risks of total stroke in relation to time since stopping smoking. Current smoker was the reference category. Error bars represent 95 percent confidence intervals. (From Kawachi I, Colditz GA, Stampfer MJ et al: Smoking cessation and decreased risk of stroke in women. JAMA 269:234, 1993, with permission.)

Alcohol Consumption. As in myocardial infarction, impact of alcohol consumption on stroke risk is related to the amount of alcohol consumed. Heavy alcohol use, either habitual daily heavy alcohol consumption or binge drinking, seems to be related to an excess of stroke and stroke deaths. Light or moderate alcohol consumption, on the other hand, is convincingly associated with a reduced incidence of coronary heart disease, and recent evidence suggests moderate alcohol consumption may reduce the risk of stroke as well. Light and moderate alcohol use tends to raise the HDL cholesterol and may be associated with a reduction in coronary heart disease incidence, whereas high levels of alcohol intake are linked to hypertension and hypertriglyceridemia and may in this way be associated with an increased rate of coronary heart disease.

Heavy alcohol consumption seems to increase the incidence of stroke, particularly parenchymatous hemorrhage. In a prospective study in Yugoslavia, heavy alcohol consumption was associated with increased stroke incidence, though the stroke subtype was not clearly determined. Increased incidence of intracerebral hemorrhage has been related to alcohol consumption in the Honolulu Heart Program, with a strong dose–response relationship. Increases in alcohol consumption were related to increasing levels of blood pressure, cigarette smoking, and to lower serum cholesterol levels, all risk factors for intracerebral hemorrhage. However, even after taking these factors into account, heavy alcohol consumption was independently related to incidence of intracranial hemorrhage, both subarachnoid and intracerebral; no significant relationship was found between alcohol and thromboembolic stroke. Age-adjusted estimated relative risk of intracerebral hemorrhage for light drinkers (1 to 14 oz per month), as compared to nondrinkers, was 2.1; for moderate drinkers (15 to 39 oz per month), 2.4; and for heavy drinkers, (40+ oz per month), 4.0. After adjustment was made for other associated risk factors, intracerebral hemorrhage was 2.0, 2.0, and 2.4 times more frequent, respectively, in these alcohol consumption categories. Data from the Framingham Study also suggest an increased incidence of brain infarction and stroke with increased levels of alcohol use, but only in men.

There are a number of mechanisms by which heavy alcohol consumption may predispose to and moderate alcohol consumption protect from stroke. Cigarette smoking is more frequent in heavy drinkers, and there is attendant hemoconcentra-

tion. Alcohol drinking and cigarette smoking have been shown to increase both blood hematocrit and viscosity, and rebound thrombocytosis during abstinence has been observed. Cardiac rhythm disturbances, particularly atrial fibrillation, occur with alcohol intoxication, producing what has been termed ''holiday heart.'' Acute alcohol intoxication has been named as a precipitating factor in stroke in young people, both in thrombotic stroke and in subarachnoid hemorrhage.

Physical Activity. Leisure time- and work-associated vigorous physical activity has been linked to lower coronary heart disease incidence. More physically active longshoremen had lower rates of myocardial infarction but had no reduction in stroke incidence. In a study of 17,000 former Harvard students, those who were more physically active had about one-half the risk of fatal coronary heart disease and one-third the mortality rate of their least active fellow alumni. In recent years, there is evidence supporting a protective effect of moderate physical activity on stroke incidence that is independent of other risk factors. In the Framingham Study, physical activity determined in older individuals, mean age 65 years, was associated with a reduced stroke incidence when compared with the least active group in a gender-specific Cox proportional hazards model. For men, the relative risk was 0.41 (95 percent confidence interval, 0.24 to 0.69; $P = .0007$) after taking into account the effects of potential confounders, which included age, systolic blood pressure, serum cholesterol, glucose intolerance, vital capacity, body mass index, LVH by ECG; atrial fibrillation, valvular heart disease, congestive heart failure, coronary heart disease, and occupation. However, there was no evidence of a protective effect of physical activity on risk of stroke in women. Furthermore, as is the case in coronary heart disease, there was no evidence that heavy levels of physical activity conferred any greater benefit than moderate levels. In a number of other population studies and in a series of case-control studies, low levels of physical activity were associated with increased incidence of stroke. In 7,735 men aged 40 to 59, there was a protective

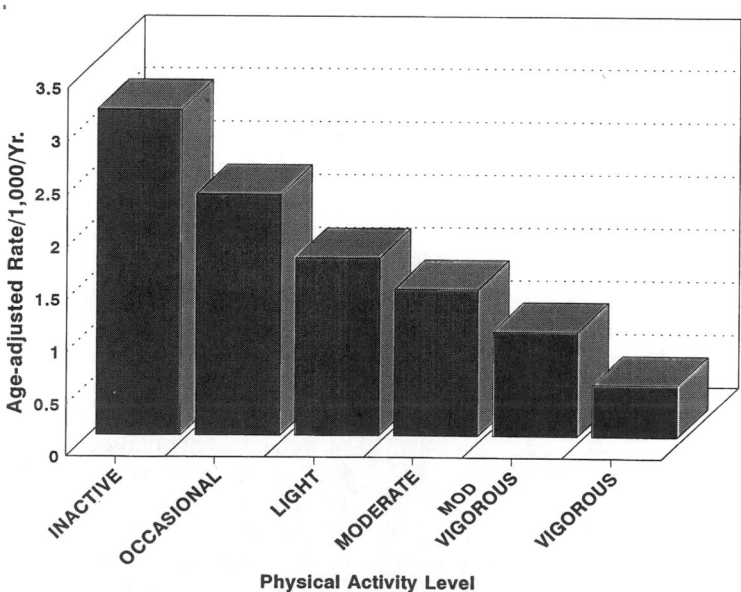

FIG. 28-7. Physical activity and stroke, men 40 to 59 years of age. Age-adjusted rates of stroke according to physical activity. (Adapted from Wannamethee G, Shaper AG: Physical activity and stroke in British middle aged men. Br Med J 304:598, 1992, with permission.)

effect of high levels of physical activity on stroke incidence (Fig. 28-7). In this latter study, there was a clear graded inverse relationship between physical activity level and stroke incidence. Why no such beneficial effect has not been demonstrated in women is unclear. It is possible that the measures of physical activity in older women whose workplace is the home do not adequately measure different levels of activity. A preliminary analysis disclosed an inverse relationship between physical "fitness," not activity, in women and incidence of stroke. This suggests women who have higher vital capacities, slower pulse rates, and less obesity have lower stroke incidence on the basis of increased physical activity. The increased physical activity, however, was not reflected in their responses to the questionnaire used in the Framingham Study.

Physical activity exerts a beneficial influence on risk factors for atherosclerotic disease by reducing blood pressure and weight, by reducing the pulse rate, raising the HDL cholesterol and lowering the LDL cholesterol, improving glucose tolerance, and by promoting a life style conducive to changing diet and promoting cessation of cigarette smoking. Physical activity level may now be added to the list of modifiable risk factors that can reduce stroke incidence.

STROKE PREVENTION THROUGH RISK FACTOR MANAGEMENT

There has been rapid decline in death rates from stroke in the United States and in most other industrialized nations since 1968. In the United States, this decline of more than 50 percent in mortality rates in a 20-year span supports the notion that modifiable environmental influences are operating in stroke and cardiovascular disease occurrence. At least part of the decline results from a reduction in the severity of stroke, which most attribute to improved detection and treatment of hypertension. Prevention of stroke, and perhaps stroke recurrence, has been shown to occur by reduction of elevated blood pressure, by cigarette smoking cessation, and by warfarin anticoagulation in the presence of atrial fibrillation. It seems likely that prevention and treatment of predisposing cardiac diseases would help. There is little evidence that cholesterol reduction per se would reduce stroke directly. Of course, coronary heart disease is a major precursor of stroke and is the principal cause of death of stroke and transient ischemic attack survivors, and on that account, coronary heart disease prevention is certainly worthwhile.

Control of Hypertension and Stroke Prevention

Based on a combined analysis of nine major prospective studies involving 420,000 individuals with a mean 10-year follow-up, there was clear evidence of a graded relationship between diastolic pressure and stroke and coronary heart disease incidence. There was no threshold level below which risk gradients were flat. For every 7.5-mmHg diastolic pressure increase, there was a 46 percent increase in stroke incidence and a 29 percent increase in coronary heart disease.

Relating these findings from prospective observational study to randomized trials of blood pressure reduction demonstrated that treatment prevented stroke. The findings should put to rest the concern that reduction of blood pressure in hypertensives serves to precipitate stroke. From a statistical analysis of fourteen treatment trials with a total of 37,000 hypertensive sub-

jects, it was clear that reduction of blood pressure in hypertensives reduced stroke incidence. There was an average blood pressure reduction of 5.8 mmHg and a corresponding reduction in stroke incidence of 42 percent. This observed reduction in stroke closely approximated that expected on the basis of prospective observational studies. In these studies, the duration of blood pressure reduction was brief—from 2 to 5 years—suggesting interruption of a precipitating factor rather than interfering with atherogenesis. Presumably, more prolonged blood pressure control would have both effects.

Emphasis has been placed on the diastolic component in virtually all treatment trials, although stroke risk is clearly no less directly related to systolic pressure levels. In the elderly, in whom isolated elevation of the systolic pressure is common, treatment was thought to be ineffective in reducing pressure, hazardous in terms of side effects, and unwarranted on the basis of availability epidemiologic data. In the SHEP Trial, 4,736 persons above age 60, with systolic blood pressure levels above 160 mmHg and diastolic pressures below 90 mmHg, blood pressure reduction was associated with a 36 percent reduction in stroke and a 27 percent reduction in myocardial infarction and coronary death after 4.5 years of follow-up (Fig. 28-8). These findings have enormous importance, since two-thirds of all individuals with hypertension between the ages of 65 and 89 years have isolated systolic hypertension. The bulk of strokes occur in this age group.

It is clear from the SHEP Trial and from the European Working Party on Hypertension in the Elderly (EWPHE) study that antihypertensive medication was well tolerated by the elderly. SHEP demonstrated that reduction of pressure was accomplished with relative ease, was controlled in approximately one-half with chlorthalidone alone, and was well tolerated as evidenced by a 90 percent compliance rates in the active treatment group at 5 years. Since increased blood pressure is the most powerful risk factor for stroke, and since the benefits of treatment occur so promptly, control of increased blood pressure, systolic as well as diastolic levels, is the cornerstone of stroke prevention.

Treatment of Nonvalvular Atrial Fibrillation with Warfarin

It has been estimated that approximately 25 percent of persons with nonrheumatic atrial fibrillation will sustain a stroke within 10 years. It was suspected on the basis of clinical experience that chronic warfarin anticoagulation could prevent stroke recurrence in atrial fibrillation. However, warfarin anticoagulation carries a risk of hemorrhage, particularly intracranial hemorrhage. For this reason, clinicians were reluctant to prescribe warfarin, particularly in elderly patients with atrial fibrillation. However, since 1990, the benefit and safety of low-intensity Coumadin anticoagulation for stroke prevention in atrial fibrillation has been demonstrated by a series of randomized clinical trials. These trials have also validated the concept that it is the atrial fibrillation and not the associated cardiac conditions that is responsible for the increased stroke incidence in the presence of atrial fibrillation. Since treatment with warfarin has no effect on hypertension, coronary heart disease, or congestive heart failure, the anticoagulant action must be responsible for the benefit seen.

When the data from the five primary prevention trials were pooled, there was a remarkable 68 percent reduction in the rate

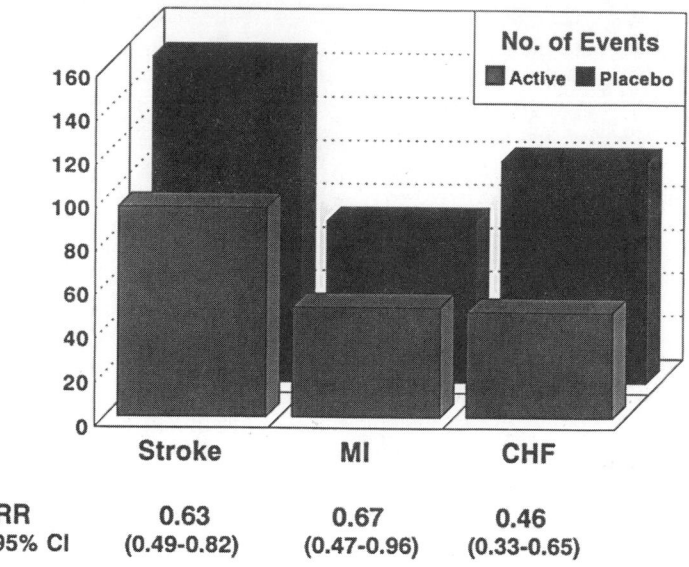

FIG. 28-8. Results of the Systolic Hypertension in the Elderly Trial: nonfatal events (From Wolf PA: Lewis A. Conner lecture. Contributions of epidemiology to the prevention of stroke. Circulation 88:2474, 1993, with permission.)

of stroke by warfarin anticoagulation. A more modest benefit of aspirin in stroke prevention was seen. In the Stroke Prevention in Atrial Fibrillation Study (SPAF II trial), a 44 percent reduction was achieved with 325 mg/d of aspirin. The benefit of aspirin is not entirely clear, and there was no benefit for the prevention of ''cardioembolic'' stroke in SPAF II Most of the effect was seen in the prevention of transient ischemic attacks and mild ischemic events; there was no benefit in those above

age 75, in whom atrial fibrillation has its greatest impact. No benefit of aspirin was seen in the European Atrial Fibrillation Trial (EAFT), as described below.

Factors that predisposed to stroke were identified from the pooled analysis by testing previously identified factors for the individual trials. The independent risk factors for stroke were found to include increasing age, previous stroke or transient ischemic attack, history of hypertension, and diabetes (Fig. 28-

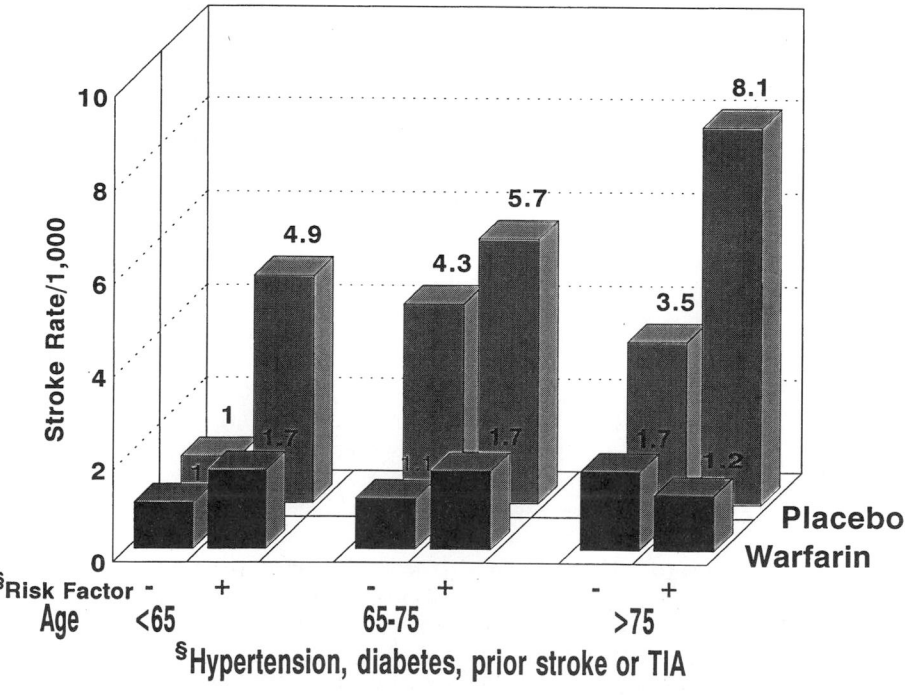

FIG. 28-9. Efficacy of warfarin by risk category—pooled analysis of atrial fibrillation trials. (Adapted from Risk factors for stroke and efficacy of antithrombotic therapy in atrial fibrillation, analysis of pooled data from five randomized controlled trials. Arch Intern Med 154:1454, 1994, with permission.)

9). The presence of one of these risk factors was associated with an increased incidence of stroke in each of the three age groups: under 65, 65 to 74, and 75+ years. In all but one of the categories, persons with atrial fibrillation with or without associated risk factors warranted treatment with low-intensity warfarin anticoagulation. Subjects with atrial fibrillation who were under 65 years of age and had no risk factors had a stroke risk of approximately 1 percent per year. These individuals, the data for whom have been extrapolated to include that of younger individuals with lone atrial fibrillation, would appear to have such a low stroke risk that warfarin can be withheld (and 325 mg/d of aspirin given).

This dramatic reduction in stroke incidence by low-intensity warfarin anticoagulation was achieved with a 0.3 percent rate of intracranial hemorrhage and an overall major hemorrhage rate of 1.3 percent. Recurrent stroke in patients with atrial fibrillation was also strikingly reduced by warfarin. In the EAFT, the 12 percent per year stroke rate in the placebo group was reduced to 4 percent in an intention-to-treat analysis, and there were no intracerebral hemorrhages in the warfarin group of 225 patients, followed for 2.3 years. Of interest, there was no significant risk reduction from aspirin in this secondary prevention trial.

Thus, with the exception of SPAF II, in which a higher intensity of warfarin anticoagulation occurred and was associated with an intracranial hemorrhage rate of 1.8 percent per year in persons 75 years of age or older, the other five trials achieved a remarkably low rate of major hemorrhage. Risk of bleeding with warfarin was significantly outweighed by the benefits of stroke prevention. Taken together, the five primary prevention trials of warfarin therapy resulted in rates of intracranial hemorrhage lower than 0.3 percent per year.

Cessation of Cigarette Smoking

Based on data from the Nurses' Health Study and from the Framingham Study, it seems clear that stopping smoking is followed by a reduction in stroke risk in a remarkably short time. Risk of coronary heart disease decreases by approximately 50 percent within 1 year of smoking cessation and reaches the level of those who never smoked within 5 years. In the Framingham Heart Study, in both men and women, risk of stroke in former cigarette smokers did not differ from that of persons who never smoked by the end of 5 years. Since smoking confers an increase in stroke risk of 40 percent in men and 60 percent in women, after all other pertinent risk factors have been taken into account, cessation may be expected to significantly reduce risk of stroke.

Physical Activity Promotion

As with cigarette smoking, data from observational studies strongly suggest a beneficial role of moderate sustained physical activity in cardiovascular disease prevention. No randomized clinical trial data are likely to appear that will bolster these data. The beneficial effects of vigor and a feeling of well-being, as well as the salutary effects on cardiovascular risk factors, are compelling. Taken together, it is clear that regular moderate physical activity should be an integral part of a life style that will help to reduce the risk of stroke and other cardiovascular diseases.

Prevention and Treatment of Heart Disease, Including Atrial Fibrillation

Since coronary heart disease, cardiac failure, and atrial fibrillation predispose to stroke, prevention of these cardiovascular contributors can be anticipated to reduce incidence of stroke. On the basis of current knowledge of the epidemiology of cardiac failure, prevention of obesity and treatment of hypertension may be beneficial. Reduction of coronary heart disease risk requires, in addition to hypertension control and smoking cessation, dietary or pharmacologic treatment to reduce elevated total and LDL cholesterol and to increase the HDL cholesterol fraction. Prevention of atrial fibrillation might best be accomplished

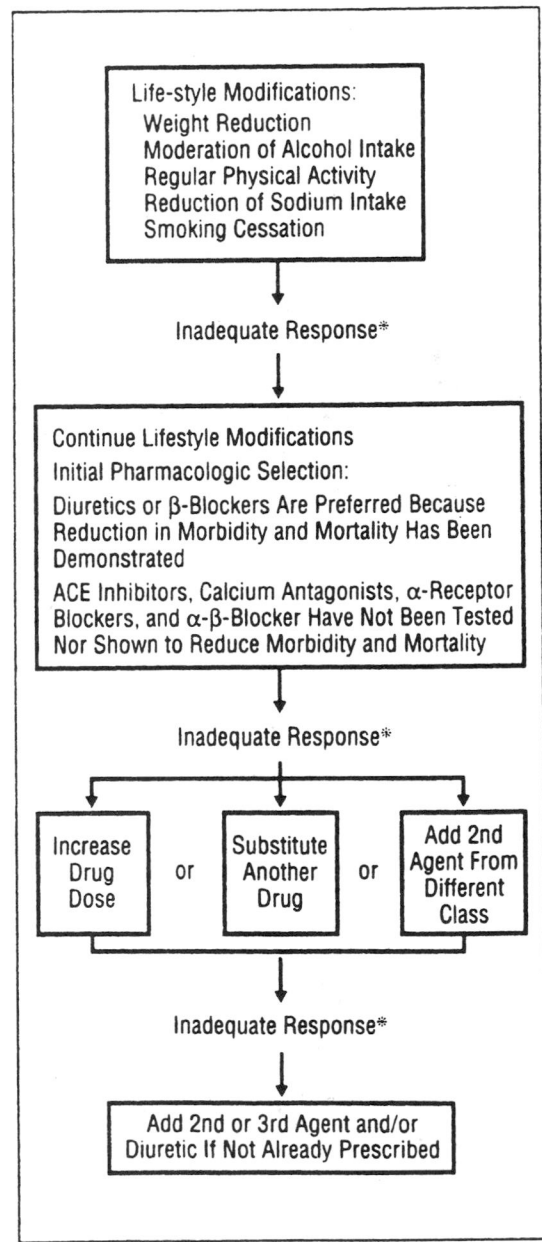

FIG. 28-10. Treatment algorithm. Asterisk response means the patient achieved goal blood pressure or is making considerable progress toward this goal; ACE, angiotensin-converting enzyme. (From Joint National Committee: The fifth report of the Joint National Committee on Detection, Evaluation, and Treatment of High Blood Pressure (JNC V). Arch Intern Med 153:164, 1993, with permission.)

by preventing the appearance of the major precursor of atrial fibrillation, which is heart disease.

Identification of High-Risk Candidates for Stroke Prevention

Each physician can identify "prime" candidates for stroke among asymptomatic patients. Control of elevated blood pressure, including isolated systolic hypertension, will definitely prevent stroke. Among asymptomatic persons with borderline elevations of blood pressure it would be helpful to ascertain which are at increased risk of developing a stroke. Primary prevention of hypertension and control of mild blood pressure elevations, particularly in persons at low risk of cardiovascular disease, may be accomplished with hygienic measures. These include weight loss by restriction of calories, increase in dietary potassium intake, reduction in dietary sodium intake, moderation in alcohol consumption, and moderate physical activity. These measures can also be advocated for most people (Fig. 28-10). Persons with higher blood pressure levels or those with a less benign risk factor profile will probably warrant pharmacologic intervention for blood pressure control.

In order to select those persons at greatest risk of developing cardiovascular disease and stroke, a risk profile has been developed based on 36 years of follow-up data from the Framingham Study. Using information collected during the course of taking a comprehensive medical history and conducting a physical examination, plus obtaining an ECG, a patient's probability of stroke may be determined. Using a separate table for men and women, stroke probability is determined by a point system

based on age, systolic blood pressure, antihypertensive therapy use, presence of diabetes, cigarette smoking, history of cardiovascular disease (coronary heart disease or congestive heart failure), and ECG abnormalities (LVH or atrial fibrillation). It is apparent that in persons at varying levels of blood pressure, probability of stroke varies across a wide range. Probability rises with increased systolic blood pressure (120 mmHg and 180 mmHg are shown), depending on the presence of other abnormalities in the risk profile (Fig. 28-11). Probability of stroke in the hypothetical 70-year-old woman depicted in Figure 28-11 may be higher in the presence of multiple risk factor abnormalities at a systolic blood pressure of 120 mmHg than at 180 mm Hg in the absence of such abnormalities. This quantitative determination of the probability of stroke, relative to what is average for a woman of this age, may help the patient (and the physician) more fully appreciate the patient's increased level of risk.

The stroke risk profile will help the physician identify those borderline hypertensives warranting pharmacologic treatment by virtue of an increased probability of stroke. Clearly, there are other situations—not considered here—in which a patient can also be noted to be at substantially increased risk of stroke, such as recent transient ischemic attack, recent-onset atrial fibrillation, recent myocardial infarction, during and immediately following cardiac surgery, and others that are dealt with elsewhere in Part II of this book.

ACKNOWLEDGMENTS

This chapter was supported in part by grants 2-RO1-NS-17950-13 (National Institute of Neurological Disorders and Stroke),

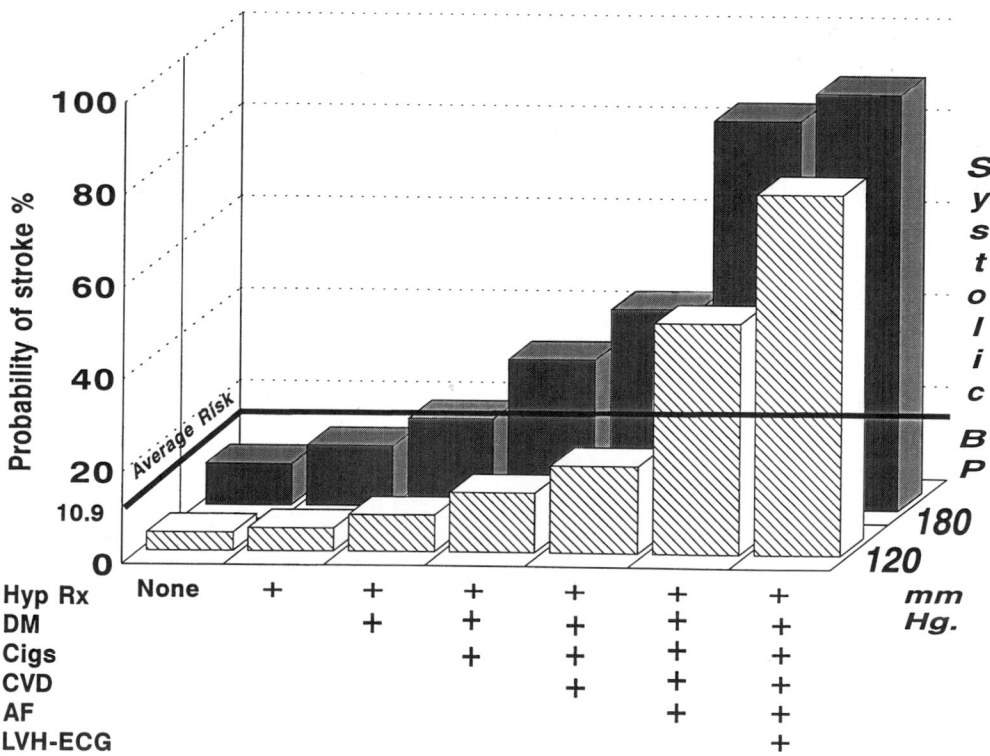

FIG. 28-11. Probability of stroke during 10 years in women aged 70 years at two systolic blood pressure levels: impact of other risk factors. Hyp Rx, antihypertensive therapy; DM, diabetes mellitus; CIGS, cigarette smoking; CVD, previously diagnosed coronary heart disease, cardiac failure, or intermittent claudication; AF, atrial fibrillation; LVH-ECG, left ventricular hypertrophy by electrocardiogram. (From Wolf PA, D'Agostino RB: Hypertension and risk of stroke: the influence of associated risk factors in the Framingham Study. Hypertens Res 17 (Suppl I): S85, 1994, with permission.)

RO1-HL40423 (National Institute on Aging, National Heart, Lung, and Blood Institute), and Contract NIH-NO1-HC-38038 (National Heart, Lung, and Blood Institute).

SUGGESTED READINGS

Collins R, Peto R, MacMahon S et al: Blood Pressure, stroke, and coronary heart disease. Part 2. Short-term reductions in blood pressure: overview of randomised drug trials in their epidemiological context. Lancet 335: 827–38, 1990

Fisher CM: The ascendancy of diastolic blood pressure over systolic. Lancet: 1349–1350, 1985

Fletcher AE, Bulpitt CJ: How far should blood pressure be lowered? N Engl J Med 326:251–254, 1992

Joint National Committee: The Fifth Report of the Joint National Committee on Detection, Evaluation, and Treatment of High Blood Pressure [JNC V]. Arch Intern Med 153:154–83, 1993

Kawachi I, Colditz GA, Stampfer MJ et al: Smoking cessation and decreased risk of stroke in women. JAMA 269:232–6, 1993

Laupacis A: Anticoagulants for atrial fibrillation. Lancet 342:1251–2, 1993

Morbidity and Mortality, Chartbook on Cardiovascular, Lung, and Blood Diseases. U.S. Department of Health and Human Services, Washington, D.C., May, 1994

SHEP Cooperative Research Group: Prevention of stroke by antihypertensive drug treatment in older persons with isolated systolic hypertension. Final results of the Systolic Hypertension in the Elderly Program (SHEP). JAMA 265:3255–64, 1991

Wolf PA: Lewis A. Conner lecture. Contributions of epidemiology to the prevention of stroke. Circulation 88:2471–8, 1993

Wolf PA, D'Agostino RB, Belanger AJ, Kannel WB: Probability of stroke: a risk profile from the Framingham Study. Stroke 22:312–8, 1991

29. NEURODIAGNOSTIC TESTING

LAWRENCE R. WECHSLER
L. DANA DeWITT

Evaluation of a patient with stroke begins with gathering a thorough medical history and conducting a detailed physical examination. From this information, the astute clinician attempts to decide upon localization of the ischemic insult and the mechanism of the event. Once these initial impressions are formulated, further evaluation using appropriate neurodiagnostic tests is planned to confirm or alter the original diagnosis. Ultimately, treatment decisions are based upon knowledge of the pathophysiology and location of the stroke. Neurodiagnostic testing helps clarify each of these components.

Many procedures have been developed or improved to aid in the clinical evaluation of cerebrovascular disease. For many years, angiography was performed by direct carotid puncture, but was used sparingly until the transfemoral approach reduced complications. The use of ultrasound for evaluation of the carotid arteries by Doppler, B-mode imaging, and recently duplex Doppler has steadily grown and its efficacy has improved. Transcranial Doppler (TCD) and magnetic resonance angiography (MRA) now provide a noninvasive evaluation of the intracranial circulation. Computed tomography (CT) and magnetic resonance imaging (MRI) techniques add a further dimension available for patients with stroke.

The challenge for the clinician is to select the appropriate tests and sequence to clarify each clinical situation while minimizing time, cost, and risk to the patient. This requires the physician to have a basic understanding of the results generated by a test, its strengths and weaknesses, and any pitfalls in interpretation. This chapter briefly describes each of the tests commonly used for the evaluation of patients with cerebrovascular disease and helps the clinician to apply these tests intelligently to clinical vascular problems.

NONINVASIVE CAROTID ARTERY EVALUATION

In patients with stroke in the anterior circulation (carotid artery, middle cerebral artery, and anterior cerebral artery), evaluation focuses on possible sources of ischemia, including the carotid arteries and heart. Evaluation for carotid disease usually begins with a noninvasive vascular evaluation. Occasional patients with fluctuating signs or a crescendo pattern of transient ischemic attacks (TIAs) may warrant immediate angiography because significant carotid stenosis is almost certain, and rapid diagnosis is essential to prevent progression to stroke. However, most others with a single ischemic event or stable neurologic symptoms undergo noninvasive evaluation of the carotids as the initial test. Several different methods for ultrasound evaluation of the carotid arteries are available (Table 29-1).

Continuous-Wave Doppler

Doppler evaluation of the carotid arteries is based upon the reflection of ultrasound from red blood cells traveling through the carotid bifurcation. An ultrasound probe emits a signal that penetrates the skin and reflects from the flowing blood back to the probe. A receiving crystal within the probe then converts the signal into electric impulses. The frequency of the reflected signal is changed slightly from the emitted signal and that change is directly proportional to the velocity at which the red blood cells are traveling. The faster the velocity, the greater the frequency shift. This relationship is known as the Doppler principal. The formula that describes the relationship between velocity and frequency shift is as follows:

$$V = \frac{cf}{2 \cos \phi \, f_0}$$

where V = velocity; f_0 = emitted frequency, f = received frequency shift, c = constant, and ϕ = angle of insonation.

Continuous-wave (CW) Doppler transducers include a separate transmitting and receiving crystal from which signals are continuously both sent and received. Any reflectors in the path of the emitted signal are included in the received signal; thus, two vessels in the same path cannot be distinguished. This method has an advantage, however, when the depth of a vessel in the neck is unknown, since it is unlikely a very deep artery or a small focal area of stenosis will be missed by CW Doppler. When an artery becomes narrowed, red blood cell velocity increases, allowing the same volume of blood to pass through the stenosis per unit of time. Thus, increased velocity, reflected in increased frequency shift recorded by CW Doppler, indicates stenosis. The more severe the stenosis, the greater the velocity and therefore the frequency shift recorded by CW Doppler.

Probe frequencies of 5 to 10 mHz are most commonly used for CW Doppler. Higher frequencies provide greater resolution but less penetration. The amount of frequency shift expected for any given velocity is greater the higher the probe frequency. Thus, minor differences in degree of stenosis are distinguished more easily with a higher frequency Doppler probe. Since the angle of insonation between the ultrasound beam and the artery is not known with CW Doppler, velocity cannot be directly calculated from frequency shift (see equation above). However, assuming a constant angle, greater frequency shifts reflect

TABLE 29-1. Comparison of Various Modes of Carotid Imaging

Mode	Doppler	Image	Expense	Accuracy	Advantage	Disadvantage
Continuous-wave Doppler	+	−	+	+	No aliasing	No depth information
B-mode ultrasound imaging	−	+	+ +	+	Identifies nonstenotic plaque	Velocity change not detected
Duplex Doppler	+	+	+ + +	+ + +	Corrects for angle of insonation	Small jet of high velocity may be missed
Color-flow imaging	+	+	+ + + +	+ + + +	Site of maximal velocity easily found	Insonation angle alters reliability of color analysis

higher velocities. The degree of stenosis indicated by a given frequency shift depends upon the frequency of the probe. To properly interpret CW Doppler, the frequency of the probe must be known.

B-Mode Ultrasound Imaging

Ultrasound imaging uses frequencies similar to CW Doppler but depends upon signals reflected from interfaces between two structures of different acoustic impedance. An emitted ultrasound signal travels unimpeded through tissue until it reaches an interface between two acoustically dissimilar media. Some of the signal passes through the interface, but a component is reflected and detected by the original transducer. The strength of the reflected signal is proportional to the difference in acoustic impedance at the interface. Knowing the speed ultrasound travels in the tissue, and time from emitted signal to reception of the reflected signal, the distance to the interface can be calculated. Each reflection is represented by a dot on a screen at the appropriate distance, and the intensity of the dot is proportional to the strength of the reflected signal. From information obtained by scanning a large area or sector an image is reconstructed. Modern probes include an array of transducers that allow real-time imaging by updating the image at a frequency fast enough to view continuous motion. Like CW Doppler, the resolution increases with higher transducer frequency, but tissue penetration is sacrificed. Thus, a high-frequency imaging probe improves resolution, but is often unable to provide adequate images of deep arteries.

Duplex Doppler

The combination of B-mode imaging and Doppler evaluation is referred to as duplex Doppler. In most cases, pulsed Doppler (PD) is used instead of CW Doppler. PD uses the same transducer to both emit and receive. A brief ultrasound signal is transmitted into the tissue. The transmitter is then turned off and the receiver opened for a short time. The timing of the receive cycle can be varied so that only signals reflected from a particular depth are received. Signals traveling shorter or longer distances reach the transducer but do not register since the receiver is not active at that time. The depth can be varied simply by changing the interval during which signals are received. Imaging and PD cycles alternate very rapidly, allowing simultaneous real-time imaging and Doppler analysis of a selected portion of the artery.

Duplex Doppler provides several advantages over either B-mode imaging or PD alone. Since the artery from which the Doppler signals are derived can be seen, the angle of insonation is measurable and therefore velocity can be calculated directly from the PD information without making assumptions about the relationship between the probe and the artery. In addition, the Doppler window can be steered directly into the area that appears stenotic on the image. This assures that areas of dense plaque will be thoroughly investigated by PD.

B-mode imaging provides excellent definition of the size, location, composition, and surface characteristics of plaque.

However, it is difficult to accurately image a three-dimensional object in two dimensions. Multiple views through the area help reconstruct a three-dimensional picture, but a very small eccentric lumen is often difficult to assess even by the best ultrasonographers. Velocity does not generally increase until lumen diameter is narrowed by approximately 60 percent; thus, no Doppler velocity changes are seen with minor stenoses. Spectral broadening, an increase in the number of different velocities present in the Doppler signal, sometimes reflects lesser degrees of stenosis, but B-mode imaging should be more accurate in estimating minor degrees of luminal narrowing. Beyond 60 percent stenosis, velocity increases rapidly with decreasing lumen size. This relationship is predictable (Fig. 29-1) and allows estimation of severe degrees of stenosis more accurately than by B-mode alone. The combination of the two in the form of duplex Doppler maximizes the definition of both the plaque and the degree of stenosis. Since the same transducer is alternately used for imaging and PD, there is a limit to the frequency that can be detected by these instruments. No such limit exists for CW Doppler. In addition, if the Doppler window is not placed in the critical area because of operator error, or because the plaque causing stenosis is not well seen by imaging, the maximal stenosis may not be detected.

Color-Flow Imaging

Some Duplex instruments provide an additional modality, color-flow imaging. The velocity of blood flow recorded by Doppler is translated into a color scale, with red and blue indicating flow in one direction or the other and brightness of the color proportional to velocity. This is then superimposed on the B-mode image (Plate 29-1). Color-flow imaging improves detection of short segments of high-grade stenosis or stenosis within hypoechoic plaque that may not be easily identified by B-mode imaging. The high-velocity flow is seen as a bright jet of bright color within the lumen. PD can then by directed to the area of maximal stenosis to record the highest velocity.

Indirect Tests of the Carotid Circulation

In some noninvasive laboratories indirect tests of the carotid circulation are added to carotid duplex or color-flow imaging to enhance the accuracy of the overall test battery for detecting carotid stenosis. These tests include oculoplethysmography (OPG-Gee or Kartchner type), and supraorbital Doppler. In contrast to the direct examination of the carotid bifurcation, these studies detect flow abnormalities in the orbital circulation and reflect reduced perfusion distal to a hemodynamically significant stenosis at the carotid bifurcation. OPG is performed with a small cup applied to the eye through which negative pressure is applied until intraocular pressure exceeds ophthalmic systolic pressure. When the vacuum is released, return of pulsations marks systolic pressure (Fig. 29-2). A difference of 6 mm or greater between the two eyes is considered abnormal and suggests a high-grade stenosis on the side of the lower pressure. Bilateral abnormalities are detected by comparison with the brachial arterial pressure.

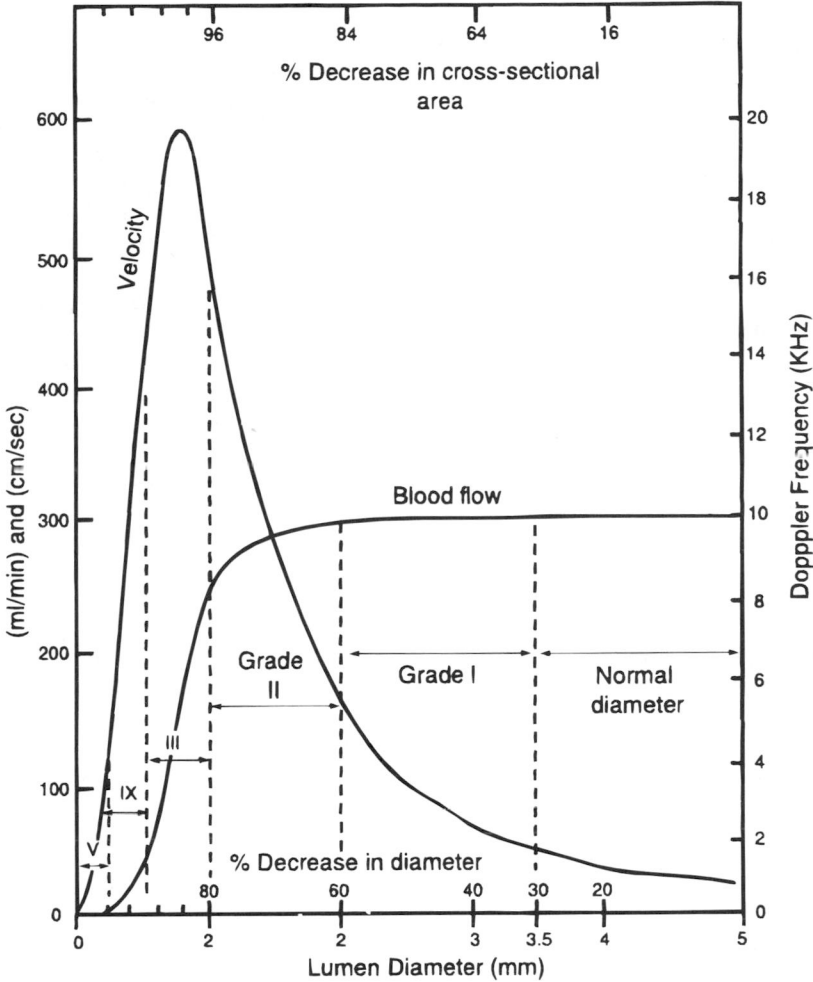

FIG. 29-1.   Relationship between residual lumen diameter or percent stenosis and frequency shift measured by Doppler. (From Spencer MP, Reid JM: Quantitation of carotid stenosis with continuous-wave (C-W) Doppler ultrasound. Stroke 10:326, 1979, with permission.)

Supraorbital Doppler measures direction of flow in the supraorbital and supratrochlear arteries, branches of the ophthalmic artery. Normally, flow is outward from the orbit to the supraorbital area, but when the external carotid artery supplies collateral to the internal carotid artery circulation through the ophthalmic artery, flow in these branches becomes reversed. The reversed direction of flow is detected with a high-frequency Doppler probe positioned over the superior rim of the orbit. Reversal of both arteries usually indicates a more severe stenosis than reversal of only the supraorbital artery.

When used alone, the indirect tests are not highly accurate. However, in combination with carotid duplex or color-flow imaging, they add to the sensitivity and specificity of noninvasive evaluation. If the carotid bifurcation is deep in the neck and suboptimally visualized, or if it is difficult to be certain whether a stenosis is in the internal or external carotid artery, abnormalities of the indirect tests may help avoid misinterpretations. In addition, stenosis above the bifurcation, such as distal stenosis due to dissection or carotid siphon stenosis may be missed by duplex examination but detected by these indirect tests. Although some experts argue the additional yield does not justify the added cost, even a few patients with stenosis correctly classified because of indirect tests improves overall accuracy and thus makes noninvasive testing more clinically useful.

Interpretation of Noninvasive Carotid Studies

An experienced examiner with the highest quality equipment can achieve higher than 90 percent sensitivity and specificity for detecting more than 50 percent stenosis at the carotid bifurcation and accurately estimate the degree of stenosis within 10 to 20 percent. A typical report includes the peak systolic velocity recorded in the common internal and external carotid arteries on both sides, description of the amount of plaque, and the maximal stenosis observed by B-mode examination, usually based upon an image obtained in the transverse plane. Some laboratories also report the ratio of internal carotid to common carotid artery velocity. Values greater than 2 are considered abnormal. Information is obtained regarding the irregularity of the plaque surface and the characteristics of the plaque, such as homogeneous, nonhomogeneous, hypoechoic, or calcified (Fig. 29-3). It remains unclear whether these features of the plaque correlate with embolic potential or stroke risk. Highly stenotic plaques with ulceration are associated with a greater subsequent stroke risk than nonulcerated plaques, but it may be difficult to accurately identify ulceration by ultrasound. A smooth depression in a plaque or normal area of artery between two plaques sometimes mimics the appearance of an ulceration. Most clinicians rely upon the degree of stenosis reported by carotid noninvasive testing for clinical decision making but

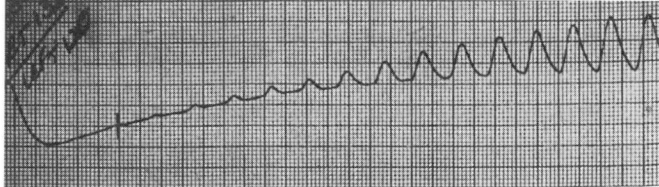

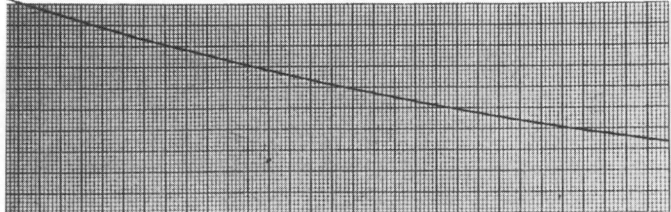

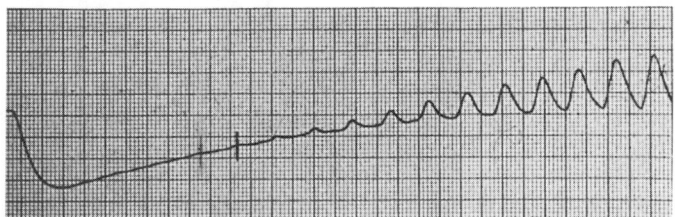

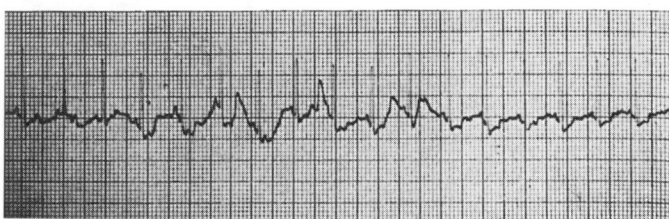

FIG. 29-2. Normal oculoplethysmographic Gee recording from a patient with no significant carotid artery disease.

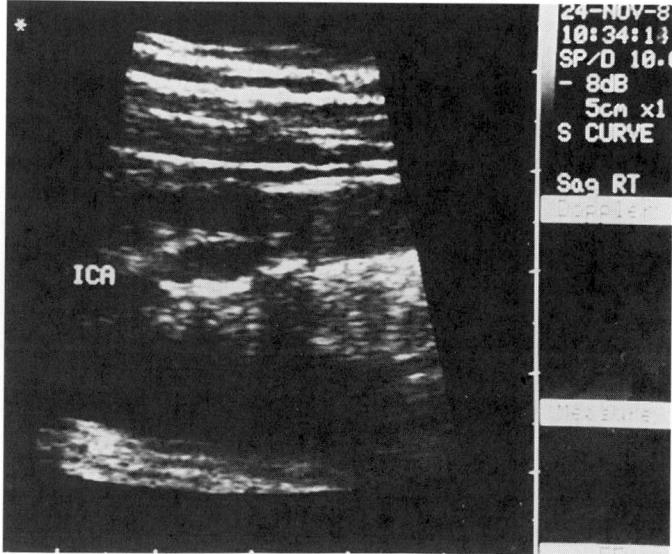

FIG. 29-3. B-mode ultrasound image of the carotid bifurcation demonstrating plaque in the internal carotid artery. ICA, Internal carotid artery.

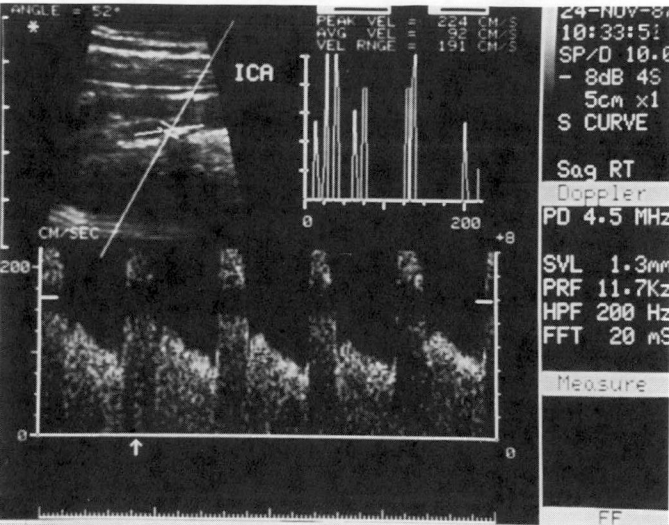

FIG. 29-4. Duplex Doppler examination of the same patient shown in Figure 29-3. The Doppler probe is directed to the area of stenosis and the Doppler spectra recorded from this area is displayed below the image. Velocity is increased, with spectral broadening indicating a severe hemodynamic change. ICA, Internal carotid artery.

apply information regarding irregularity or plaque characteristics with great caution. Peak velocities in the internal carotid artery (ICA) greater than 140 cm/sec using a 5-mHz Doppler probe are associated with diameter stenosis of at least 60 percent. Velocity continues to increase as the degree of stenosis increases. With severe stenosis (>75 percent diameter), end-diastolic velocity begins to rise (>125 cm/sec) (Fig. 29-4). Most reports classify diameter stenosis as less than 50%, 50 to 75 percent, 75 to 95 percent, over 95 percent, or occluded. This is usually based upon the Doppler results, but may be supported by the degree of stenosis seen on B-mode imaging. When there is a discrepancy-between the B-mode and Doppler estimates of stenosis, the Doppler is usually more accurate for high degrees of stenosis, and the B-mode image for minor degrees of narrowing.

False negative results occasionally occur with carotid duplex, and the clinician should be aware of the possibility that a significant stenosis or occlusion may not be detected. If the report seems inconsistent with the clinical syndrome and there is a high index of suspicion of carotid disease, the quality of the ultrasound examination should be evaluated. In some patients, very deep arteries; short, thick necks; or heavily calcified arteries limit the ability to visualize the vessel and detect a stenotic signal by Doppler. Angiography should be considered when there is doubt about the reliability of the ultrasound results. The ICA may be very tortuous and turn abruptly downward after takeoff from the common carotid artery. If the aberrant position is not identified, no ICA Doppler signal is detected and the examiner may mistakenly diagnose carotid occlusion. Stenosis may be overlooked because of a short area of sudden narrowing with incomplete examination of this area by Doppler. However, when a high-velocity signal is found, signifying stenosis, this is rarely a false positive. Normal arteries should not produce high velocities in a focal segment. If angiography fails to confirm a stenosis in such cases, a web or kink may cause stenosis but not be seen on the views obtained by angiography. The angiogram is more likely to be falsely negative than the ultrasound falsely positive.

False negative studies also occur when the stenosis is beyond the first few centimeters of the ICA. This is seen with dissection, or when plaque begins high in the neck. False positive results may occur when an external carotid stenosis is mistaken for the ICA, or due to incorrect setting of the angle of insonation, falsely increasing the velocity calculation based upon the frequency shift. If one of the arteries at the carotid bifurcation is occluded, it may be difficult to determine whether the remaining artery is the internal or external carotid artery. A well-trained examiner improves the overall accuracy of the test by knowing these pitfalls and avoiding errors in those few cases where questions arise. In any noninvasive laboratory, quality assurance and ongoing correlations with angiographic results strengthens the ability of the physicians interpreting the study and establishes the reliability of the laboratory upon which other clinicians depend for proper evaluation of their patients.

Applications of Carotid Noninvasive Testing

Stroke and Transient Ischemic Attack. When a patient presents with a TIA or stroke, the major clinical concern is the mechanism of the ischemic event and institution of appropriate therapy to prevent recurrence or progression of neurologic deficits. Severe carotid stenosis or recent carotid occlusion are associated with a substantial short-term stroke risk, and anticoagulation and/or carotid endarterectomy are treatment options. Because of the high sensitivity and specificity of carotid noninvasive testing, this is an excellent screening test for significant carotid stenosis. If the study reveals more 70 percent diameter stenosis and symptoms are clearly attributable to the carotid circulation on the side of stenosis, carotid endarterectomy should be strongly considered. The risk of stroke in symptomatic patients reported in the North American Symptomatic Carotid Endarterectomy Trial (NASCET) applies to a specific measurement of residual lumen diameter defined angiographically; at present, a similar threshold for carotid noninvasive studies has not been identified. Therefore, patients with stenosis by noninvasive testing in the 50 to 70 percent range should be considered for angiography to be certain they do not reach the 70 percent diameter stenosis threshold for consideration of carotid endarterectomy. Seventy percent diameter stenosis equates with 95 percent area stenosis; thus, it is important to determine whether the results of carotid studies are reported as diameter or area stenosis. If this information is not included in the report, the ultrasonographer should be called to clarify this issue in order to properly assess the significance of the test results.

Despite improvement in detection of very tight stenosis by color-flow imaging, carotid noninvasive testing in any form cannot distinguish a near-occlusion from complete occlusion with certainty. For this reason, when no Doppler signal is obtained from the internal carotid artery, most ultrasonographers report a virtual or complete carotid occlusion. Since patients are still at risk for stroke and carotid endarterectomy can be performed if a small residual lumen remains, patients with this pattern should undergo angiography if they are candidates for carotid endarterectomy. At present, only angiography reliably differentiates complete occlusion from pseudo-occlusion.

Patients with multiple TIAs in the same vascular territory have an arterial lesion until proven otherwise. Although carotid noninvasive tests remain a good screen for the presence of significant carotid bifurcation disease, it is likely angiography will be necessary regardless of the results to exclude tandem intracranial disease. Although the carotid studies may provide clues as to what to expect on angiography, in some cases, noninvasive testing can be deferred and angiography performed as the initial test.

Vertebrobasilar Ischemia. Vertebrobasilar TIAs are typically not related to carotid disease, and carotid noninvasive testing is not always necessary. Carotid disease, even when significant, is incidental except for rare patients with unusual anomalies of the circle of Willis. Similarly, a typical lacunar stroke syndrome in a patient with appropriate risk factors for small-vessel vascular disease need not always undergo noninvasive carotid testing. However, if there are any atypical features suggesting cortical involvement or the typical risk factors are absent, carotid noninvasives should be included in the stroke assessment.

Syncope. Syncope has been reported in association with bilateral severe carotid stenosis or occlusion, but in most cases the carotid disease is known or previously suspected. Even when bilateral severe carotid disease is present, other etiologies for syncope, particularly cardiac causes, should be vigorously pursued. Mild or moderate degrees of carotid stenosis do not predispose to syncope. In the typical patient with syncope and no clear indication of carotid disease, the yield of carotid noninvasive testing is low and should not be considered an essential component of the evaluation.

Asymptomatic Stenosis. There has been considerable debate about whether patients with asymptomatic carotid bruits should have carotid noninvasive testing. In some cases, finding stenosis by noninvasives leads to angiography and then carotid endarterectomy despite the asymptomatic state. Recent results from the Asymptomatic Carotid Atherosclerosis Study (ACAS) indicate a 55 percent reduction in ipsilateral stroke in asymptomatic patients with 60 percent or greater stenosis treated with carotid endarterectomy. These results apply to patients with reasonable surgical risks operated on by highly skilled surgeons demonstrating a low surgical morbidity. Carotid bruits may not be a reliable indicator of significant carotid stenosis; thus, carotid noninvasive testing may become a screening test for individuals with risk factors for atherosclerotic carotid artery disease. Assessment of the degree of carotid stenosis in asymptomatic individuals is helpful in long-term management even if immediate carotid endarterectomy is not considered. Rather than explaining TIAs to all patients with bruits and alarming many of them with little or no stenosis, noninvasive testing identifies those with high degrees of carotid stenosis who are at highest risk for stroke should a TIA occur. Since TIAs may not be recognized, it is useful to review with patients the possible symptoms of carotid TIAs and ask them to call or go to an emergency room if these symptoms occur. In some patients, carotid stenosis may be stable in serial studies performed over several years. In others, the degree of stenosis progresses between studies. When stenosis progresses to high levels (e.g., > 60 percent diameter stenosis), prophylactic carotid endarterectomy might be more seriously considered, particularly in relatively young patients who are excellent surgical candidates.

TRANSCRANIAL DOPPLER

Until the development of TCD, evaluation of the intracranial circulation required cerebral angiography. TCD takes advantage of relative areas of thinning of the skull or natural "windows" that allow penetration of ultrasound (Table 29-2). A

TABLE 29-2. Comparison of Transcranial Doppler Techniques

	Doppler	Image	Expense	Accuracy	Advantage	Disadvantage
Transcranial Doppler	+	−	+	+ +	Rapid bedside examination	No angle correction
Transcranial color imaging	+	+	+ + +	+ + +	Arteries more easily identified	Equipment not as portable; need good window

transducer is positioned in these windows and directed toward the arteries at the base of the brain. The middle cerebral artery (MCA), anterior cerebral artery (ACA), posterior cerebral artery (PCA), and terminal ICA are insonated from a temporal window located above the zygomatic arch and anterior to the pinna. The vertebral arteries and basilar artery are approached from the occipital window along the midline below the occipital protuberance. The orbital window is accessed by placing the probe over the eye and pointing directly posterior to insonate the ICA siphon and ophthalmic artery. TCD uses a 2-mHz probe, in contrast to 5- to 10-mHz probes typically used for extracranial Doppler applications. The lower frequency allows a greater percent of emitted ultrasound to pass through bone and reflect from moving red blood cells in the intracranial arteries. At higher transducer frequencies, the bone would absorb nearly all the ultrasound and no reflected signal could be obtained. The velocity of blood flow is then determined from the frequency shift of the received signal according to the Doppler equation above. Like carotid duplex, the velocity calculation depends upon knowledge of the angle of insonation between the probe and the artery. Since velocity is proportional to cosine ϕ (angle of insonation), the calculated velocity would be within 15 percent of the true value, assuming the angle remains less than 30 degrees. For most of the intracranial arteries, the angle of insonation is small, although it may occasionally exceed 30 degrees when the artery is tortuous or displaced from its usual position due to mass effect or edema.

Arteries are identified from each window based upon the position of the probe, the depth at which the signal is obtained, and the direction of blood flow. TCD instruments use a pulsed Doppler so that signals from varying depth can be discerned without overlap. The direction of blood flow is also distinguished so that two signals with flow in different directions can be displayed simultaneously. For example, from the temporal window, with the probe directed anteriorly and superiorly at a depth of 50 to 65 mm, flow toward the probe in the MCA is found. Increasing the depth to 70 to 75 mm places the focus of the ultrasound beam in the ACA with blood flow away from the probe. Directing the transducer more posteriorly, flow toward the probe appears in the proximal PCA at depths of 60 to 70 mm, and away from the probe as the signal centers on the P2 segment of the PCA. Similar alterations in direction and depth differentiate the vertebral arteries from the basilar artery, and the ICA siphon from the ophthalmic artery.

Interpretation of Transcranial Doppler

A typical TCD report includes peak and mean velocities recorded from the MCAs, ACAs, PCAs, ICA siphons, ophthalmic arteries, vertebral arteries, and basilar artery. In some cases, pulsatility is also reported. Pulsatility index (peak end-diastolic velocity/mean velocity) provides a measure of resistance in the distal arterial bed. Vasodilation due to ischemia reduces pulsatility in the basal cerebral arteries. Increased pulsatility is occasionally seen with multiple distal emboli or raised intracranial pressure. Pulsatility is more variable than velocity, and is used

for interpretation only when clearly different in one arterial territory compared with all others. Stenosis of the intracranial arteries increases peak and/or mean velocity above the normal range. This is determined by laboratory normals or published values for each artery. Abnormality is usually defined as velocities beyond 2.5 or 3 standard deviations from the mean. Stenosis often produces an increased velocity in a focal segment of the artery with a sudden decrement in velocity beyond the stenosis (Fig. 29-5). Elevated velocities are not always due to stenosis. Vasospasm increases velocity and cannot be reliably distinguished from stenosis due to atherosclerosis. Increased velocities also occur when an artery supplies collateral blood flow. For example, ACA velocity may be increased when the contralateral carotid artery is occluded and there is collateral blood flow to the hemisphere on the side of the occlusion across the anterior communicating artery (Fig. 29-6). The increased velocity occurs in a more diffuse pattern throughout the course of the artery rather than the focal pattern characteristic of stenosis. In addition, other abnormalities such as reversed direction of blood flow in the ipsilateral ACA or asymmetric MCA velocities support collateral blood flow as the cause of increased velocity. Decreased velocity may occur in the MCA on the side of an extracranial carotid artery stenosis or occlusion, but is rarely a significant finding when present in multiple intracranial arteries. The inability to find a signal from an artery suggests occlusion, but only if other arteries are easily found from the same window, assuring that the absent signal is not due to inadequate penetration of ultrasound through bone. Five to 10 percent of individuals do not have an adequate temporal window, and a complete study cannot be obtained.

Transcranial Color Imaging

Although the angle of insonation for most intracranial arteries is less than 30 degrees, direct determination of the position of the artery by B-mode ultrasound increases the reliability of this measurement and more precisely determines velocity. Transcranial color imaging (TCI) combines a B-mode image of the intracranial compartment with color-flow imaging of the basal cerebral arteries (Plate 29-2). Since a low transducer frequency is used for TCI (2 to 3 mHz), resolution is not optimal, but in many cases the major cerebral arteries can be identified. The Doppler is focused on the artery of interest, and velocities can be measured accurately after correction for the observed angle of insonation. Using this technique, preliminary studies indicate velocities may be as much as 30 percent higher than those recorded with TCD alone. In addition to greater accuracy, TCI shortens examination time and enhances test reproducibility. However, the failure rate is higher with TCI owing to the need for greater reflected signal, and it is technically a more difficult study. In addition, it may be difficult to image a sufficiently long segment of artery to obtain adequate Doppler recordings.

Applications of Transcranial Doppler

Intracranial Stenosis. Intracranial atherosclerotic disease is an uncommon cause of ischemia, although it is more frequent

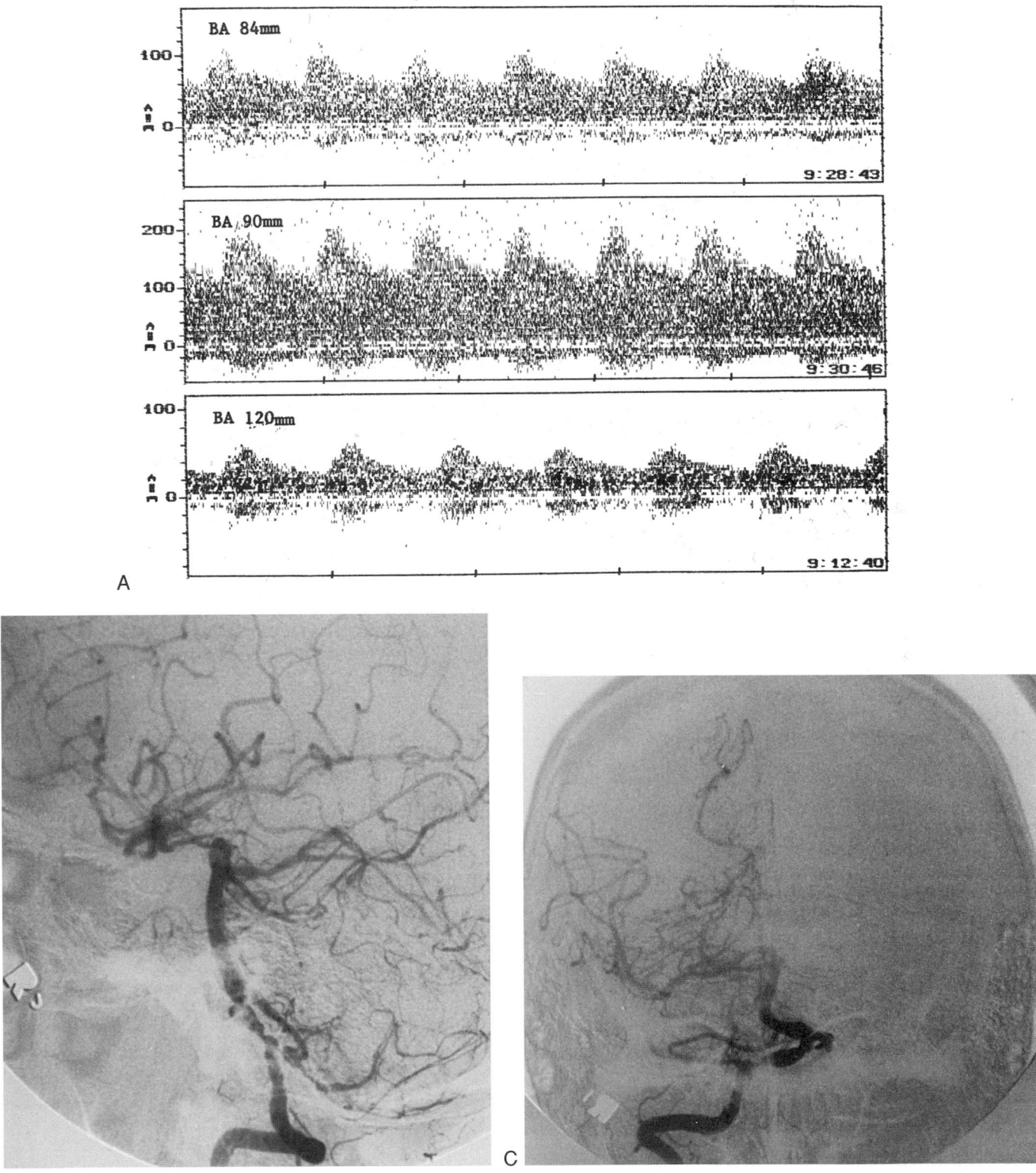

FIG. 29-5. **(A)** Transcranial Doppler from a patient with episodic dizziness and visual blurring demonstrating a focal increase in velocity in the middle panel with a decrease in velocity beyond this area (*lower panel*) **(B)** Corresponding lateral and **(C)** anteroposterior angiogram from the same patient showing stenosis in the distal vertebral or proximal basilar artery.

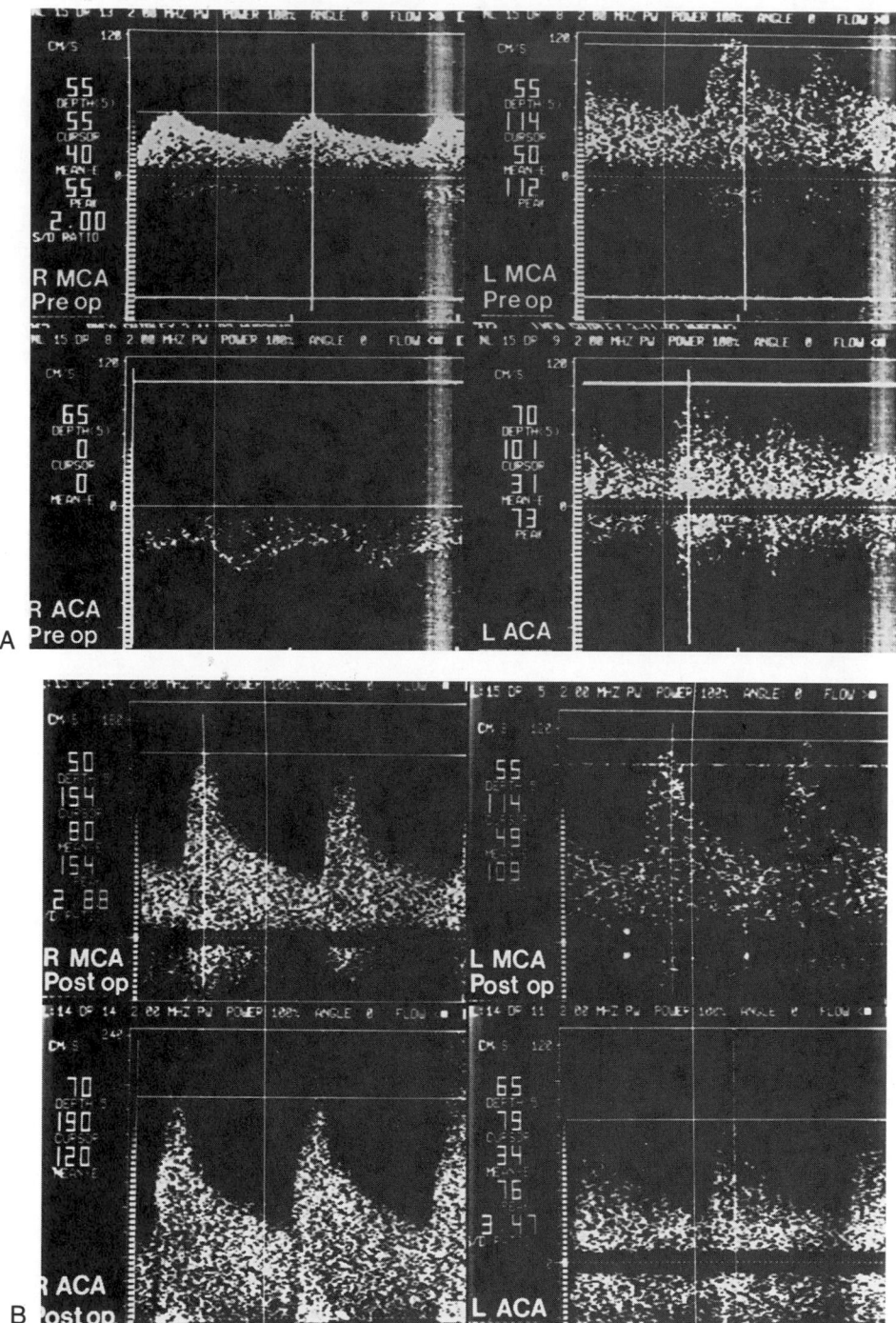

FIG. 29-6. **(A)** Transcranial Doppler recordings from both middle cerebral arteries (MCAs) and anterior cerebral arteries (ACAs) in a patient with severe extracranial carotid artery stenosis on the right. MCA velocity is reduced with blunting of the waveform on the side of the stenosis (*top left*). ACA velocity is increased contralateral to the extracranial stenosis (*bottom right*) with reversal of the normal direction of flow in the ACA ipsilateral to the stenosis (*bottom left*). **(B)** Recordings from the same patient following carotid endarterectomy. MCA velocity has increased with loss of the blunting on the operated side. ACA flow is now anterograde bilaterally with elevated velocities on the operated side.

in the African-American and Asian population. However, the risk of recurrent stroke after an ischemic event related to ICA siphon or MCA stenosis is substantial, and detection of lesions facilitates treatment that may prevent further ischemic injury. Basilar artery and vertebral artery stenosis or occlusion can also be detected by TCD. In such cases, anticoagulation may be indicated.

Velocity elevation beyond the normal range in a segment of the intracranial artery with an abrupt decrement in velocity beyond the stenosis is the characteristic TCD pattern of stenosis (Fig. 29-5). The extent of velocity elevation correlates with the degree of stenosis in the MCA, but this correlation is less precise for the basilar, vertebral arteries, and particularly the ACA. Sensitivity and specificity of TCD for detection of MCA stenosis is 80 to 90 percent or greater in most studies. Limited data is available for other intracranial arteries, including the vertebrals and basilar artery, but sensitivity and specificities of over 80 percent have been documented in a few small studies published to date. In the posterior circulation, a very short segment of stenosis in the vertebral or proximal basilar artery may be overlooked, owing to the relatively large sample volume used by most TCD instruments. In addition, the distal basilar is difficult to consistently insonate, and stenosis in this segment may not be detected.

Despite these drawbacks, TCD provides an excellent screening tool for intracranial disease in patients with TIA or stroke. In the anterior circulation, intracranial stenosis can be detected without the need for angiography. Multiple ischemic events or stereotyped TIAs with normal extracranial carotid duplex studies should prompt a search for intracranial stenosis. Patients with TIAs or stroke attributable to the posterior circulation can be screened for significant large vessel stenosis with TCD. Many elderly patients present with vague symptoms of dizziness or visual disturbances for which vertebrobasilar ischemia is considered a possible etiology. Rather than resorting to angiography, TCD evaluation identifies the few individuals with significant stenosis who may benefit from medical treatment for stroke prevention. If basilar or vertebral artery stenosis is highly suspected based upon the clinical presentation, angiography should be performed because of the possibility of a false negative TCD.

The absence of a signal from one of the intracranial arteries is not always due to occlusion. Technical factors such as a poor window or a tortuous artery may explain the inability to insonate an artery. Anomalies of the circle of Willis, such as an atretic A1 segment of the ACA or an atretic vertebral artery, may also mimic occlusion.

MRA combined with TCD often provides more information about the intracranial circulation than either test alone. MRA suffers from artifacts due to turbulent flow and overestimates the degree of stenosis. Movement degrades the images and claustrophobic reactions excludes some individuals from completing the procedure. However, high-quality images identify arterial lesions accurately, whereas TCD provides velocity information to assess the hemodynamic significance of the stenosis. An absent signal by TCD or nonvisualization of an artery by MRA may be due to technical artifacts, but when both tests are abnormal, occlusion is likely. In a patient with stroke or TIA, conventional angiography may be avoided if both studies are normal or both confirm an intracranial arterial stenosis or occlusion.

Extracranial Carotid Artery Disease. TCD findings in patients with extracranial carotid artery disease reflect distal hemodynamic effects of the carotid lesion. Thus, changes do not usually occur until stenosis becomes severe or the artery is occluded. Velocity in the MCA ipsilateral to the stenosis may be reduced in comparison to the contralateral MCA, and ipsilateral MCA pulsatility may be decreased (Fig. 29-6). A side-to-side difference of at least 30 cm/sec peak velocity must be present to suggest an abnormality. In addition, contralateral ACA velocity may be increased and ipsilateral ACA flow direction reversed when there is collateral from the contralateral carotid across the anterior communicating artery. Proximal PCA and basilar artery velocities increase when collateral arises from the posterior communicating artery. Ophthalmic artery flow is reversed in some cases, or this artery may be absent on the side of the extracranial lesion. If only one of these findings is present, the diagnosis is uncertain, but two or more abnormalities increase the likelihood of an extracranial carotid lesion.

In most cases, however, extracranial stenosis or occlusion is identified by carotid noninvasive testing. TCD adds additional information that may be important in deciding on treatment. If severe stenosis is found by carotid noninvasive procedures in a patient with minor stroke or TIA, carotid endarterectomy should be considered. Angiography is necessary to confirm the degree of stenosis and exclude tandem lesions in the carotid siphon or MCA. With high-quality carotid duplex studies indicating more than 90 percent diameter stenosis, it is unlikely that angiography will demonstrate less than 70 percent diameter stenosis, the current threshold for carotid endarterectomy in symptomatic individuals. A normal TCD study excludes tandem lesions, and in appropriate cases surgery can be performed without the need for angiography. Information obtained by TCD may help manage an individual patient by assessing adequacy of collateral blood flow. Collateral flow in the anterior and posterior communicating arteries can be detected, or TCD examination may indicate the absence of collateral. Carbon dioxide reactivity can be assessed by monitoring TCD velocity with varying carbon dioxide concentrations or after Diamox administration. Reduced reactivity implies vasodilation of the distal vascular bed due to reduced cerebral perfusion. A few small studies suggest such individuals are at higher risk for subsequent stroke, but larger studies are needed to confirm these results. Whether collateral patterns and reactivity are useful in deciding on treatment of patients is unknown, but this information contributes to the overall picture of patients with cerebrovascular disease. If collateralization is limited and reactivity reduced, blood pressure management might be less aggressive to help maintain cerebral perfusion. In contrast, concern about hypotension during surgery or hypertensive therapy would be less in a patient with normal reactivity and excellent collaterals.

Vasospasm. Despite treatment with calcium channel-blockers, symptomatic vasospasm occurs in 10 to 20 percent of patients with subarachnoid hemorrhage from ruptured aneurysms. Vasospasm causes increased velocities in the basal cerebral vessels similar to stenosis due to atherosclerosis. As vasospasm worsens, velocity increases. Thus, TCD can be used to detect vasospasm before symptoms occur, and to follow the progression of vasospasm over time. Selection of patients at risk for ischemia based upon steadily increasing velocities allows early institution of treatment to prevent progression to infarction. Once therapy such as induced hypertension is started, vasospasm may be monitored by daily TCD studies. When velocities begin to decline, therapy may be discontinued (Fig. 29-7). TCD

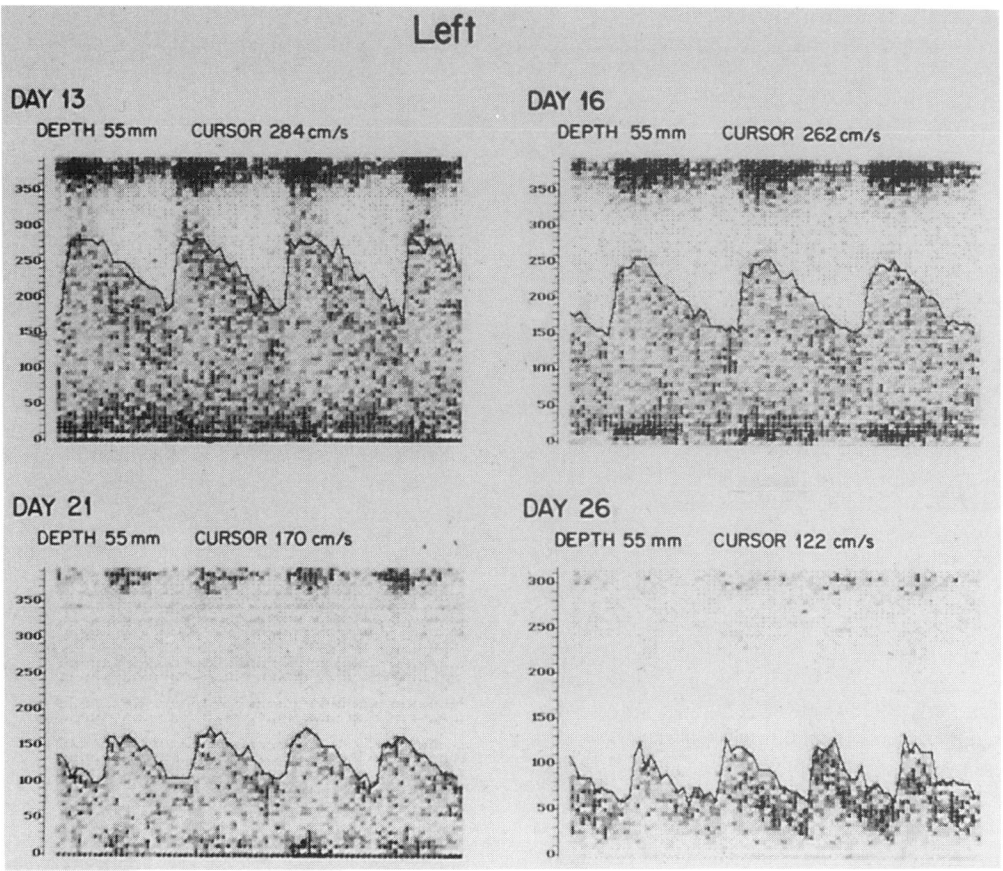

FIG. 29-7.   Transcranial Doppler recording from the left middle cerebral artery (MCA) in patient with symptomatic vasospasm following subarachnoid hemorrhage. Aphasia and right-hand weakness developed 10 days postoperatively and 13 days after the hemorrhage. Her symptoms resolved when blood pressure was raised. On day 16, MCA velocities remained elevated and symptoms recurred when pressor therapy was tapered. Twenty-one days after the hemorrhage, velocities by transcranial Doppler had decreased, indicating less severe vasospasm. Her blood pressure was reduced without return of neurologic symptoms. On day 26, velocities in the MCA had returned to normal and she remained asymptomatic. (From Wechsler LR, Ropper AH, Kistler JP: Transcranial Doppler in cerebrovascular disease. Stroke 17:905–12, 1986, with permission.)

offers the advantage of convenient bedside testing that can be repeated at frequent intervals without risk to the patient.

TCD detects MCA vasospasm with a sensitivity of 70 to 90 percent and specificity of 90 to 100 percent, but similar to atherosclerotic disease, corresponding figures are lower for other intracranial arteries. Elevated velocities may also occur with hyperemia, although this is much less common than vasospasm. Increased velocity in the submandibular ICA sometimes reflects hyperemia. The ratio of the MCA to submandibular ICA velocities is used as an index of hyperemia. Ratios greater than 3 usually indicate vasospasm. In rare cases, diffuse vasospasm in distal arteries beyond the basal cerebral vessels leads to infarction and clinical deterioration. This is not detected by TCD, since only the proximal arteries are insonated. When available, cerebral blood flow (CBF) studies compliment TCD information. TCD only reflects changes in the basal cerebral vessels, whereas CBF measures tissue perfusion. Distal vasospasm would be detected by reduced CBF despite relatively normal TCD velocities. In asymptomatic patients with rapidly rising velocities, CBF may remain normal until vasospasm becomes severe. Once perfusion falls, ischemia is probably imminent. Measurement of CBF when velocities reach high levels (> 300 cm/sec systolic or 200 cm/sec mean) may better select those at high risk who would benefit from aggressive hypertension therapy.

Systemic factors that alter TCD velocity must be considered when comparing serial studies in the same patient. Velocity varies with hematocrit. As hematocrit decreases, velocity increases in all arteries. Carbon dioxide changes also alter velocity; decreasing carbon dioxide reduces velocity and increases pulsatility. Increasing carbon dioxide has the opposite effect. Medications may also directly modify velocity by changing the caliber of the basal cerebral arteries. Vasodilators decrease velocity, assuming blood flow remains constant. In most ambulatory patients, these factors are not operative, but in critically ill patients with subarachnoid hemorrhage, systemic factors must be monitored and considered in interpreting daily fluctuations in velocity.

Embolus Detection.   High-intensity transient signals within the TCD recording signify small emboli traveling through the intracranial circulation. This may be particulate (e.g., fibrin platelet) or gaseous (e.g., air) or represent cavitation due to a mechanical disturbance such as from a prosthetic valve. An audible "thud" is detected and a characteristic high-intensity signal is superimposed upon the normal TCD pattern (Figure 29-8). High-intensity transient signals have been recorded during carotid surgery, coronary bypass surgery, and in patients with atrial fibrillation or carotid stenosis. High-intensity transient signals in the MCA are more common ipsilateral to severe

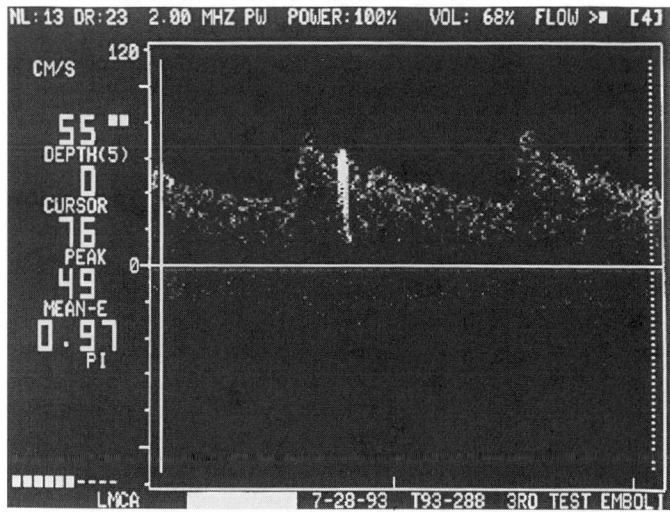

FIG. 29-8. Transcranial Doppler recording from a patient with a prosthetic valve demonstrating a high-intensity transient signal indicating embolic material in the middle cerebral artery.

carotid stenosis. There is typically no clinical correlate to high-intensity transient signals, and the clinical significance of these abnormalities has yet to be defined. However, preliminary studies indicate high-intensity transient signals are more common with symptomatic carotid stenosis than asymptomatic stenosis, and occur with large-vessel strokes more frequently than lacunes. Embolus monitoring in patients with carotid stenosis may eventually be helpful in predicting stroke risk or in determining and monitoring medical therapy.

COMPUTED TOMOGRAPHY

Creation of an image of the brain by CT scanning represented a major breakthrough in evaluation of neurologic disorders. It allowed examination of intracranial contents without the risks and discomfort inherent in pneumoplethysmography or angiography. CT constructs an image from passage of x-rays through a thin section of the brain. A detector on the opposite side measures the number of emitted x-rays that are not scattered or absorbed by the tissue. Beams of x-rays pass through each area of the tissue slice from many different angles to create a map of tissue density. The brightness of each point in the tissue is mathematically represented by fast Fourier transformation, and the summed value from multiple projections is displayed on a cathode ray tube as relative brightness. Many advances in technology and design have resulted in improved resolution without excessive x-ray exposure. Scanning time continues to decrease, while image quality and information increases.

Applications of Computed Tomography

The use of CT in the evaluation of stroke dates back to 1974, when the first units were installed in the United States at Massachusetts General Hospital and the Mayo Clinic. It remains widely used for this purpose. With the development of MRI and the age of the cost-effective practice of medicine, it is important to recognize the advantages and disadvantages of CT compared to other modalities.

In patients with stroke, CT is often the first study performed because it is likely to be the most readily available imaging procedure. It is rapid, requiring the patient to be still for only a short period of time, and provides information quickly. CT is the most important early imaging procedure when brain hemorrhage is highly suspected or must be ruled out prior to administration of anticoagulant therapy. In the evaluation of acute stroke, CT tends to be abnormal early only if the stroke is quite large and there is accompanying edema. CT is limited in the evaluation of lacunar strokes, which may not be evident on CT. In addition, CT does not visualize infarction well in the posterior fossa due to artifacts produced by the temporal bones. Arteriovenous malformations (AVMs) can be observed with CT if contrast if given, but small arterial malformations and cavernous angiomas may be missed.

If contrast is necessary during CT evaluation, allergic reactions as well as renal disease can be limitations. Patients with iodine allergy should be premedicated if contrast CT must be performed, although MRI might be a safer alternative in such situations. Patients with renal compromise should be well hydrated prior to contrast administration. Again, if renal disease is severe, it might be advisable to perform MRI rather than contrast CT. The CT gantry is quite narrow and limited to the head; thus, claustrophobic reactions are far less problematic, compared to MRI. CT scanning with modern scanners is accomplished in much less time than MRI, minimizing movement artifacts in agitated patients.

Ischemic Stroke. Ischemic stroke appears as an area of hypodensity on CT. The shape and location of the region of hypodensity can help delineate the vascular territory involved and aid in the formulation of pathophysiology. Small, deep lesions suggest a lacunar stroke due to small-vessel vascular disease. A wedge-shaped abnormality involving the cortex is characteristic of an embolic mechanism. Edema also appears as a region of hypointensity; therefore, early on, the area of infarction may appear larger than the actual territory of infarcted brain. However, CT is excellent for detecting changes due to mass effect, with ventricular or cisternal compression, shift, or obliteration and displacement of midline structures.

CT is more often readily available than newer modalities, and in the acute evaluation of the stroke patient, this is an important factor. However, CT in acute ischemic stroke is often normal, and detection of ischemic tissue can take at least 48 hours to become visible.

Ischemic stroke will enhance from a few days to a few weeks after infarction. However, under most circumstances, performing enhanced CT on ischemic stroke is unnecessary and tends only to confuse things; ischemic stroke may enhance irregularly or along the borders and give the appearance of abscess or tumor.

The appearance of vessels on unenhanced and enhanced CT can sometimes be helpful in determining pathophysiology in ischemic stroke. Acute occlusive emboli can appear as cylindric hyperdensities in the basal cisterns and subarachnoid spaces. This has been noted most often in the MCA and has been described as the "hyperdense MCA sign" (Figure 29-9).

Hemorrhagic Stroke. Intracerebral hemorrhage on CT is seen as a region of high density, either parenchymal, subarachnoid, intraventricular, subdural, or a combination of these. Unlike ischemic stroke, acute hemorrhage appears immediately and is very well delineated by CT and should be the first imaging evaluation when acute hemorrhage is suspected. Parenchymal hemorrhage can occur secondary to a variety of causes,

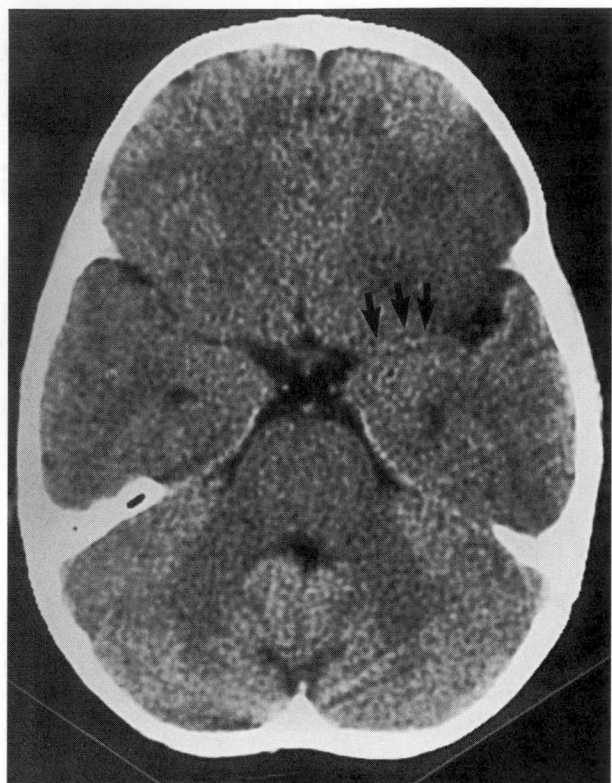

FIG. 29-9. Embolic occlusion of the middle cerebral artery following an internal carotid artery dissection. Thrombus is seen in the middle cerebral artery as a region of increased density in the stem of the artery (*arrows*).

such as hypertension, amyloid angiopathy, rupture of an AVM, cavernous angioma or aneurysm, hemorrhage into tumor, coagulopathy, and hemorrhagic conversion of ischemic stroke. The location and appearance of the hemorrhage on CT can sometimes help to determine the etiology. A well-circumscribed ball-shaped lobar hemorrhage or hemorrhage into the basal ganglia or cerebellum in a hypertensive patient is most likely secondary to rupture of small penetrating vessels secondary to hypertensive damage. In a young, nonhypertensive person hemorrhage into a tumor or a vascular malformation must be considered. Sometimes in the latter instance, the hemorrhage borders will be somewhat irregular, though this is not always the case. Occasionally, performing contrast CT in addition to plain CT may help to demonstrate tumor or vascular malformation; however, if the lesion is small, it may be engulfed by the hemorrhage and not be visible until a few months later when the blood resolves. Hemorrhagic infarction can often be differentiated from other causes of parenchymal hemorrhage owing to its inhomogeneous appearance and high density within a low-density, wedge-shaped vascular lesion.

Mass effect from hemorrhage as well as surrounding edema can be well delineated by CT. In addition, extension into the ventricles can be identified by CT. Although this allows for some spontaneous drainage of blood out of the brain substance and with it some lessening of mass effect, extension of parenchymal blood into the ventricles is usually associated with a poorer prognosis.

CT is the study of choice when acute subarachnoid hemorrhage is suspected. The distribution of blood in the basal cisterns or fissures is often helpful in discerning the location of the aneurysm. Anterior communicating artery aneurysms often rupture into the interhemispheric fissure with blood near the anterior perforated substance and occasionally into the basal frontal lobe. MCA aneurysms often rupture primarily into the sylvian cisterns and sylvian fissure on the side of the aneurysm. Patients with hemorrhage from posterior communicating artery aneurysms have more blood posteriorly, near the posterior perforating substance, and the ICA on the side of the aneurysm. Hemorrhage from aneurysm rupture in the posterior fossa is primarily into the posterior fossa cisterns. The thickness of blood and persistence of clot has also been noted to correlate in many instances with the development of vasospasm.

Subdural hematomas (SDH) in the acute and subacute stages are well visualized on CT. However, in the later stages, a chronic SDH may be isointense to brain and be missed except for its mass effect. Bilateral SDH may also be difficult to identify, particularly in the isodense stage, because the mass effect from one side offsets the other. Absence of sulcal markings and inappropriately small ventricles may provide the only clues to the correct diagnosis.

Spiral Computed Tomography

Spiral CT is a new approach to CT that allows continuous data collection while a subject is advanced through the CT gantry. An uninterrupted volume of data can then be reconstructed to produce a three-dimension representation of CT information. Contrast material is injected intravenously, and after an appropriate delay, vascular structures are visualized.

Evaluation of the common carotid artery bifurcation by spiral CT has been compared with images obtained with conventional angiography, ultrasound, and MRA. The degree of carotid stenosis determined with spiral CT correlated with angiography in 92 percent of cases, with that determined with ultrasound in 97 percent of cases, and with that determined with MRA in 100 percent of cases. Calcifications and large ulcers were well seen.

This suggests that spiral CT may be an excellent noninvasive technique for evaluation of carotid artery disease. Whether this can be extended to evaluation of disease intracranially remains to be seen. In addition, more work is necessary to assess the advantages and disadvantages of spiral CT over the presently used noninvasive techniques of ultrasound and MRA.

MAGNETIC RESONANCE IMAGING

MRI utilizes a magnetic field and radio waves to produce brain images. Rather than being an x-ray picture, MRI is based upon different tissue responses to magnetic resonance. Magnetic resonance is defined as the enhanced absorption of energy occurring when the nuclei of atoms or molecules within an external magnetic field are exposed to radiofrequency energy at a specific frequency, called the Larmour or resonance frequency. In the production of an MRI, randomly oriented tissue nuclei are aligned by a powerful, uniform magnetic field. This alignment is then disrupted by properly tuned radiofrequency pulses. The nuclei recover their alignment by relaxation processes; tissue contrast develops as a result of the different rates at which nuclei realign with the magnetic field. The positions of nuclei are localized by the application of spatially dependent magnetic fields, called gradients. The signals are measured after a user-determined time has elapsed from the initial radiofrequency excitation. The signal is then transformed into an image by the computer using a mathematic process called Fourier transformation.

Several tissue-related factors affect the strength of the MR signal, including proton density, relaxation times, magnetic susceptibility, chemical shift, flow, and contrast agents. The most important factors are the relaxation times, T1 and T2. Relaxation represents the process by which the spins respond to the perturbing effects of the radiofrequency pulse. The duration of these processes, expressed by the T1 and T2 relaxation times, is dependent on certain physical and chemical characteristics of the tissues being imaged.

Interpretation of Magnetic Resonance Imaging

Knowledge of the appearance of both normal brain elements and pathologic lesions on various scanning sequences is necessary to properly interpret MRI. Scanning sequences are designed to emphasize T1 or T2 characteristics of tissue. This depends upon parameters called TE (echo time), and TR (repetition time). Short TE and TR enhance T1, whereas long TE and TR enhance T2. Gray and white matter, cerebrospinal fluid and fat all have characteristic T1 and T2 appearances that help identify normal structures. Differential diagnosis of abnormalities depends upon the T1 and T2 appearance in relation to known structures such as brain and cerebrospinal fluid. A typical MRI report usually includes a list of the scanning sequences performed as well as a description of any abnormalities in terms of hyperintensity or hypointensity on T1- and T2-weighted images. In some cases, injection of gadolinium shortens T1 in abnormal tissue and produces increased brightness on T1-weighted images.

In addition to scanning sequences, magnet field strength also may alter the appearance of normal and abnormal brain tissues. High field strength (1.5 Tesla) magnets provide faster scanning times and improved signal to noise ratios. Lower field strengths (0.1 to 0.3 Tesla) allow mobile operation and reduce costs. Unfortunately, techniques such as MRA are often not possible with low field strength, limiting these instruments to routine scanning of the brain and spine.

Applications of Magnetic Resonance Imaging

MRI is completely noninvasive, providing brain images without exposing the patient to x-radiation. It does require that the patient lie very still for a longer period of time than for CT, though with newer developments, the time required for acquiring data is becoming shorter. MRI cannot be performed on all patients. Pacemakers, metal implants, some mechanical valves, and aneurysm clips preclude MRI scanning. Claustrophobic reactions are common, although some low-field-strength magnets have open gantries that are more easily tolerated. Movement degrades MRI images, and renders the test less useful in agitated or poorly cooperative patients unless sedated. Gadolinium reactions occur but are rare.

Ischemic Stroke. Because of the sensitivity of MRI for detecting early changes in brain water content, MRI is the most sensitive method for imaging the early infarction; ischemic changes are seen early because of water changes within cells that are usually the earliest morphologic signs of cell death. An increase in the bulk water content of tissue causes prolongation of both T1 and T2 relaxation times. Infarction is therefore visualized as an area of hypointensity on T1- and hyperintensity

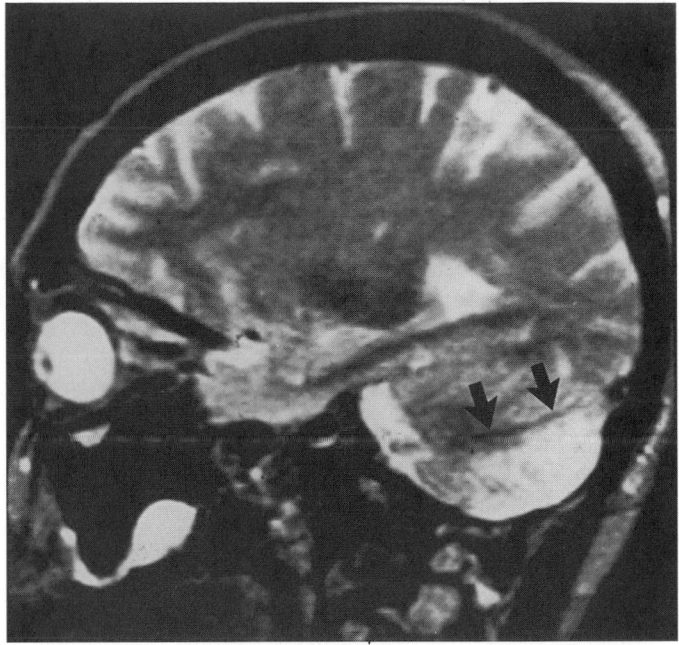

FIG. 29-10. Sagittal T2-weighted magnetic resonance imaging study showing posterior inferior cerebellar artery distribution infarction (*arrows*).

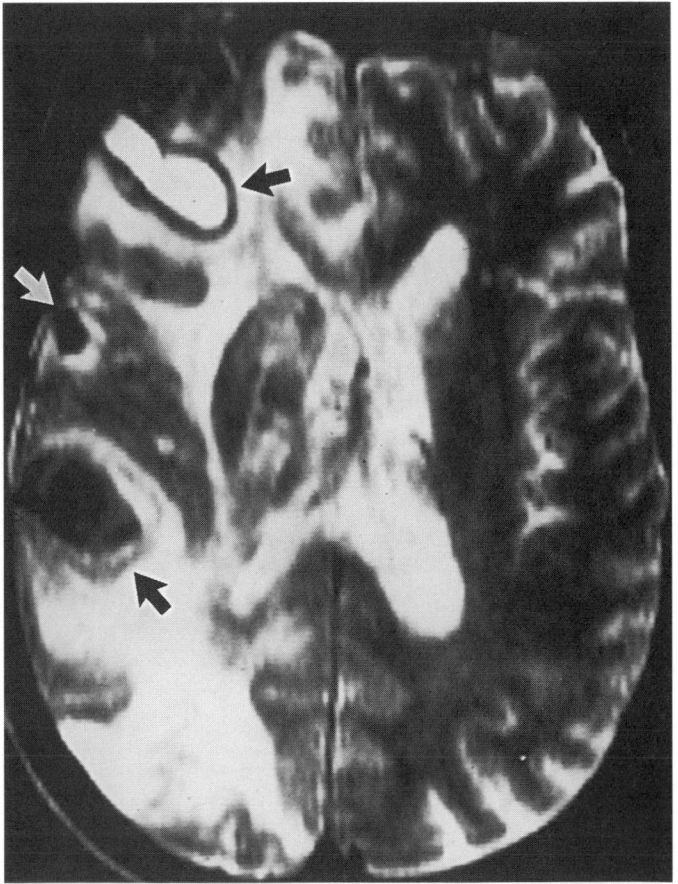

FIG. 29-11. Magnetic resonance image showing three intracerebral hemorrhages of different ages (*arrows*).

on T2-weighted studies, with T2-weighted images being more sensitive.

There is rarely a need for gadolinium when performing MRI in the evaluation of ischemic infarction. When used, gadolinium enhances a rim of tissue surrounding the infarction on the T1 study. This is usually seen with infarction in the subacute stage. Similar to iodinated contrast and CT, this pattern of enhancement tends to confuse the evaluation rather than clarify because of the overlap in appearance with tumors and abcess.

Small lesions such as lacunes are visualized better with MRI than with CT. In addition, because MR images are not degraded by bone artifact, MRI is superior to CT in the evaluation of lesions in the posterior fossa. Also, different image orientation (i.e., sagittal views for evaluation of cerebellar infarction) (Fig. 29-10) can be an extremely helpful aid in lesion localization. When an MRA is planned in addition to an image of the brain, MRI is preferred to CT, since the vascular and imaging studies can be completed sequentially.

The newer technique of diffusion-weighted MRI appears to provide a much earlier detection of ischemia than does conventional MRI. It is likely to become the favored method for testing various stroke therapies, and when it becomes more universally available, may become the test of choice for evaluating acute stroke.

Hemorrhagic Stroke. MRI characteristics of hemorrhage are determined primarily by the densities and paramagnetic qualities of hemoglobin and its breakdown products. For this reason, a hemorrhage changes its MRI characteristics as it undergoes degradation. MRI is excellent for staging the time of hemor-

rhage as well as for detecting old hemorrhage (Fig. 29-11) however, for the same reason, it is not good for evaluating acute hemorrhage.

Hyperacute hemorrhages, those less than 24 hours old, consist primarily of intracellular oxyhemoglobin that is isointense on both T1- and T2-weighted images. These hemorrhages are therefore difficult to detect. Sometimes they are slightly bright on T2-weighted images because of the similar intensities of intracellular oxyhemoglobin and water. Twenty-four to 48 hours after the hemorrhage, referred to as acute hemorrhage, intracellular oxyhemoglobin has broken down into intracellular deoxyhemoglobin. This is nearly isointense on T1-weighted images, or it may have a slightly prolonged T1. Intracellular deoxyhemoglobin has a very short T2 relaxation time and appears black on T2-weighted images. There may be a rim of brightness on T2-weighted images due to the surrounding edema. This is also not an optimal time for MR detection of hemorrhage. CT is clearly better at this stage.

From day 2 or 3 to weeks after the hemorrhage, intracellular deoxyhemoglobin is oxidized to intracellular methemoglobin, which has a short T1 phase and is therefore bright on T1-weighted images. This process begins at the periphery of a hematoma and gradually moves toward the center (Fig. 29-12A). With further degradation and lysis of red blood cells, methemoglobin is released into the extracellular space. Intracellular and extracellular methemoglobin are bright on T1-weighted images, though intracellular methemoglobin remains dark on T2-weighted images and becomes bright when it is released extracellularly. Thus, in early subacute hemorrhages, intracellular methemoglobin will appear bright on T1 and dark

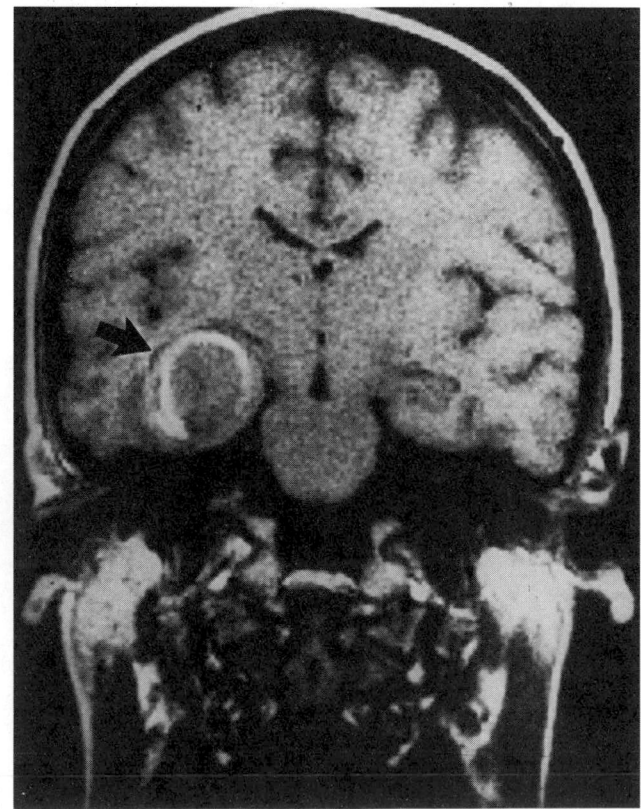
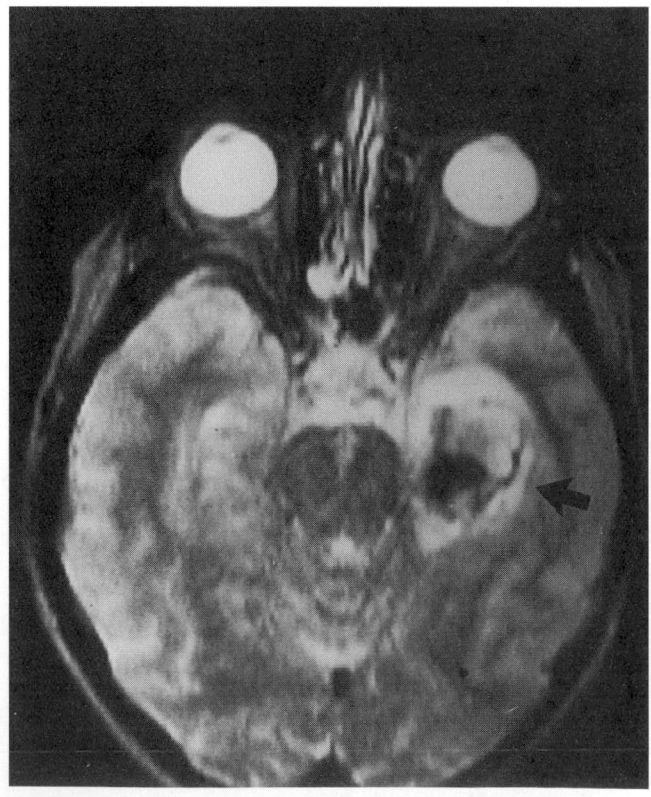

A   B

FIG. 29-12. **(A)** T1-weighted and **(B)** T2-weighted magnetic resonance image of a subacute intracerebral hemorrhage (*arrows*).

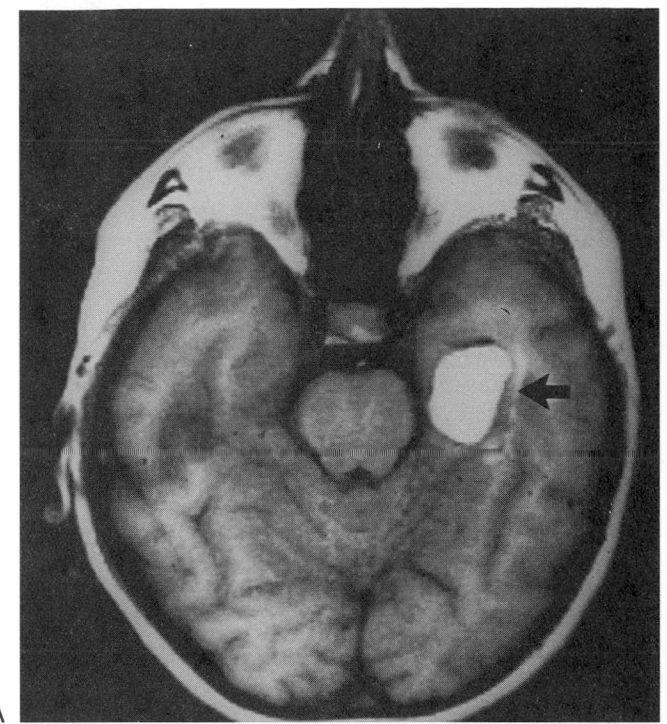 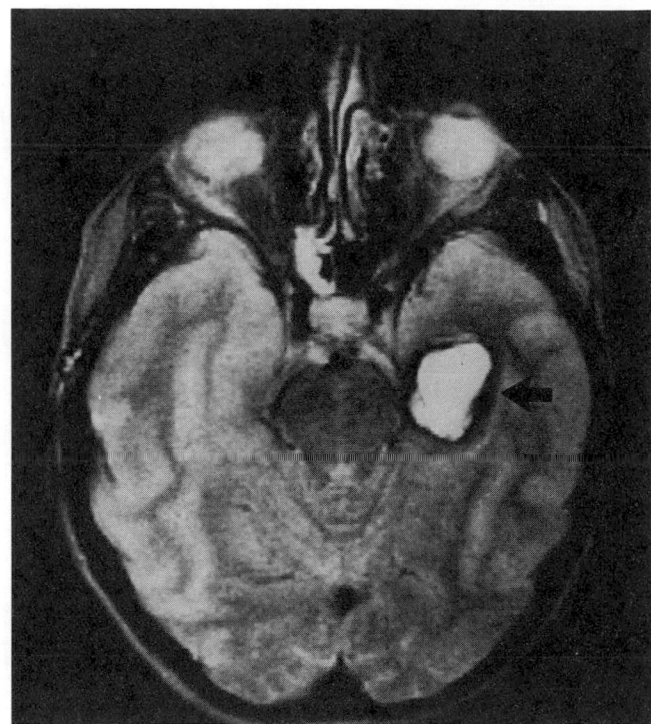

FIG. 29-13. **(A)** T1-weighted and **(B)** T2-weighted magnetic resonance image of an intracerebral hemorrhage (*arrows*) age 3 months.

on T2. As time progresses, the hemorrhage will appear bright on T1 and become bright on T2. Again, this process progresses from the periphery of the hematoma inward; therefore, at this stage, on T2 images one could see a bright periphery surrounding a dark center (Fig. 29-12B). Eventually, the hemorrhage will appear bright on both T1- and T2-weighted images (Fig. 29-13A). Later, the blood products are further broken down into hemosiderin, which appears hypodense on both T1- and T2-weighted images. This is initially seen as a dark rim surrounding a bright center on T2-weighted studies (Fig. 29-13B). MRI is far superior to CT for identifying the site of old hemorrhage. Some hemosiderin remains even after all the hematoma has been resorbed, leaving a black slit on T2-weighted images.

The basic appearance of hemorrhagic infarction on MRI is the same as previously described with CT (i.e., a lesion in a vascular distribution with inhomogeneous blood). The MRI characteristics of the blood are the same as previously outlined in MRI features of hematoma. Again, hyperacute and acute lesions are better imaged by CT. In addition, if hemorrhagic infarction is comprised of petechial blood rather than clot, it may not be imaged by MRI.

For the reasons previously outlined, CT is better than MRI for the evaluation of presumed subdural hematoma in the hyperacute and acute stages. In ruling out subacute and more chronic SDHs, MRI may show clot that appears white on both T1- and T2-weighted studies. MRI is less sensitive than CT for detecting acute subarachnoid hemorrhage. This is partially secondary to the inability of MRI to detect oxyhemoglobin, and high oxygen tension in the cerebrospinal fluid favors a higher concentration of oxyhemoglobin over deoxyhemoglobin. Also, subtle signal changes in the hemorrhage average with the long T1 and T2 values of cerebrospinal fluid, causing it to be difficult to detect.

However, in the subacute stage, when the CT attenuation of cisterns have returned to near normal, small remnants of subarachnoid clot might appear as bright signals on T1-weighted images.

Vascular Malformations.   Flowing blood causes a loss of signal on MRI; therefore, vessels appear as dark voids on T1- and T2-weighted studies. These flow voids can be used to assess patency of a vessel on MRI (e.g., in looking for basilar occlusion). In AVMs, a serpiginous tangle of vessels can be seen well on non-contrast-enhanced MRI (Fig. 29-14). With contrast, this becomes hyperintense, although contrast is usually not necessary when screening for the presence of AVMs. Increased signal in the cerebral veins or sinuses on routine MRI suggests sinus thrombosis (Fig. 29-15) and may be confirmed with magnetic resonance venography (MRV). MRI has been found to be much better than CT for detecting cryptic AVMs. Cavernous angiomas have a distinct appearance on MRI. Because they have a tendency to hemorrhage repetitively under low pressure, sometimes asymptomatically, they appear as a round, encapsulated-looking lesion, dark on T1- and T2-weighted images, and filled with hemosiderin (Fig. 29-16 and 29-17).

Arterial Dissection.   Dissection can sometimes be detected on plain MRI without conventional angiography or MRA. Clot can be seen in the vessel wall and has the characteristics of hematoma as outlined previously. Typically, the intramural thrombus shows high intensity on axial T1-weighted images and remains white on T2-weighted images. This can be seen with axial sections through the head with intracranial dissection (Fig. 29-18) and axial cuts through the neck with extracranial dissection.

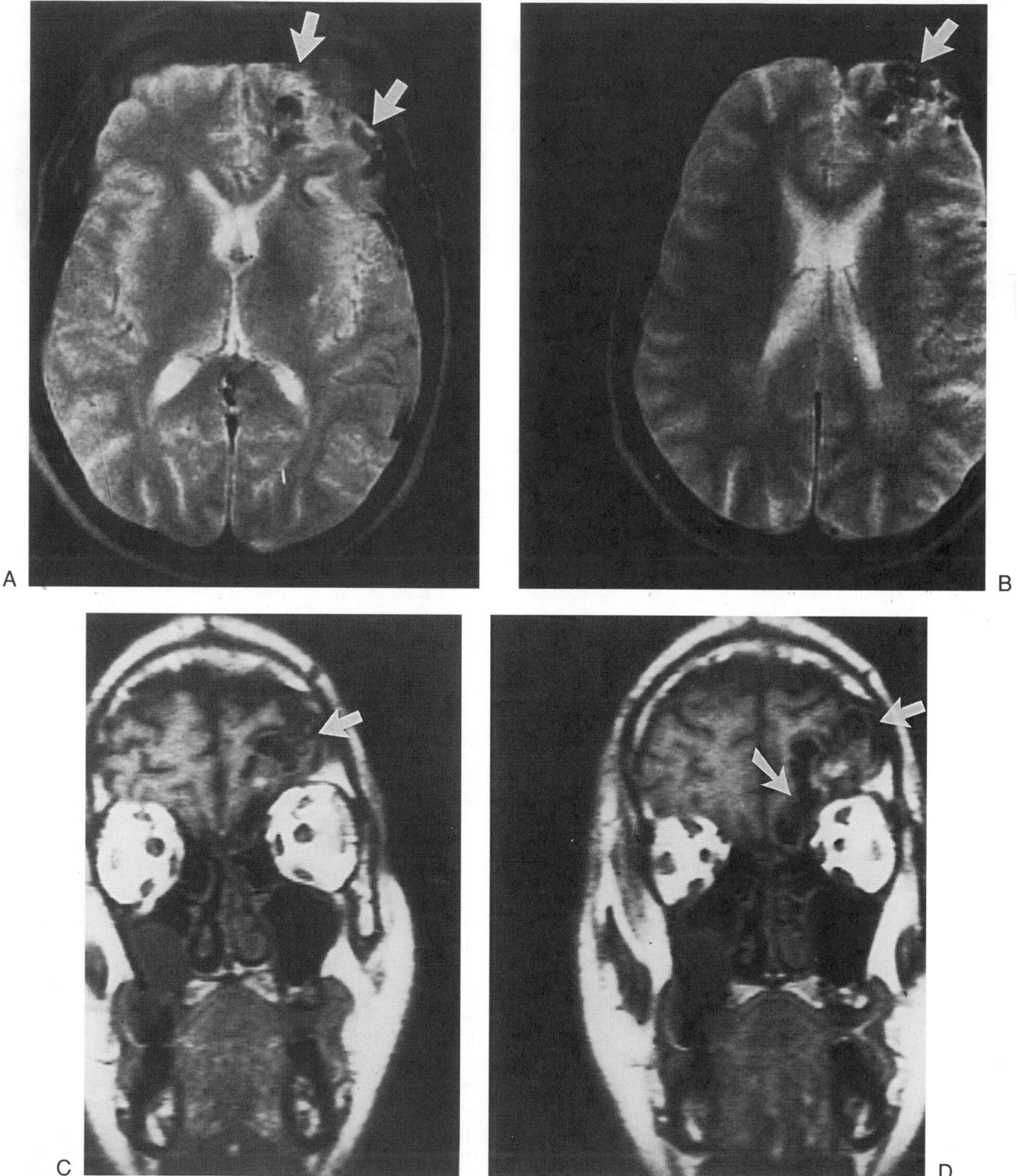

FIG. 29-14. **(A & B)** Axial T2-weighted and **(C & D)** coronal T1-weighted magnetic resonance image showing flow voids in vessels of a frontal arteriovenous malformation (*arrows*).

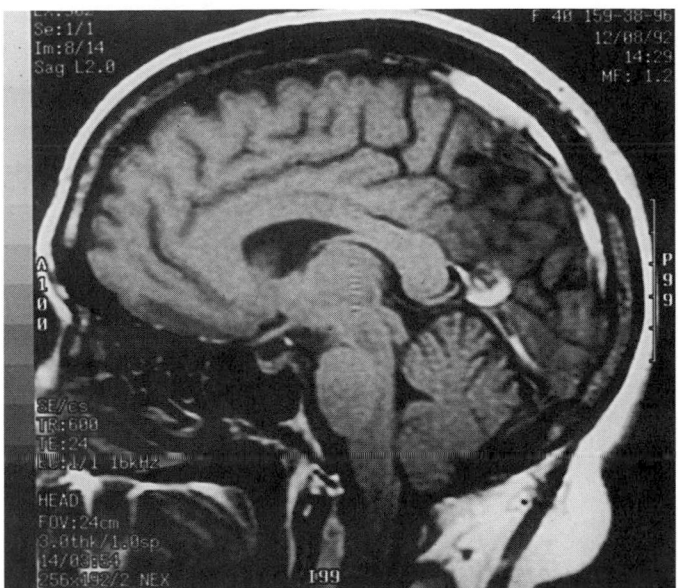

FIG. 29-15. T1-weighted magnetic resonance image showing bright signal in venous sinuses in patient with sinus thrombosis.

MAGNETIC RESONANCE ANGIOGRAPHY

MRA is a relatively new means of visualizing arteries in the head and neck. The study can be performed noninvasively at the same time that MRI is done. Unlike conventional angiography, the images are reflective of flow within the vessel, not anatomy; this always needs to be kept in mind when viewing and interpreting MRA.

MRA includes different evolving MRI techniques that can be used to directly image flow in arteries, veins, and cerebrospinal fluid. The imaging techniques presently used, two-dimensional time-of-flight (2D-TOF), three-dimensional time-of-flight (3D-

TOF), two-dimensional phase contrast (2D-PC), and three-dimensional phase contrast (3D-PC), each have their advantages and disadvantages. A consensus has not been entirely reached as to which technique should be used in a given application. In addition, it is very important that the one choosing the technique be completely aware of the clinical information and the purpose of the study.

TOF techniques exploit the contrast between the high signal intensity of inflowing, fully magnetized blood and the low signal intensity of saturated stationary tissue. During acquisitions, the imaging volume repeatedly experiences radiofrequency pulses that result in saturation of nonmoving spins. As fully magnetized flowing spins enter the imaging section or volume, there is greater signal intensity from the unsaturated spins than from the surrounding tissue, resulting in a difference in signal intensity between flowing blood and stationary tissue. The advantages of 2D-TOF is sensitivity to slow flow, making it ideal for venography, to image the patency of dural venous sinuses or venous outflow from an AVM. 3D-TOF has the advantages of short scan times and high spatial resolution. A disadvantage and pitfall to the TOF technique is that thrombus or other short T1 substances may be confused with flow.

PC MRA detects and images flow on the basis of the shift in the phase of magnetization that occurs when material moves in the presence of a magnetic field gradient. Recent advances have reduced the total imaging time for 3D-PC sequences by one-third, which has resulted in imaging times that are more acceptable for clinical conditions. 2D-PC is a fast sequence with excellent background suppression that can enable assessment of the patency of major vascular structures. This technique is frequently used as a scout view for other MRA images.

MRA shows drop-out of signal within a vessel when turbulence is present, either secondary to a stenosis or tortuosity in a vessel. MRA is excellent for visualizing the carotid bifurcation in the neck and demonstrating ICA stenotic disease. How-

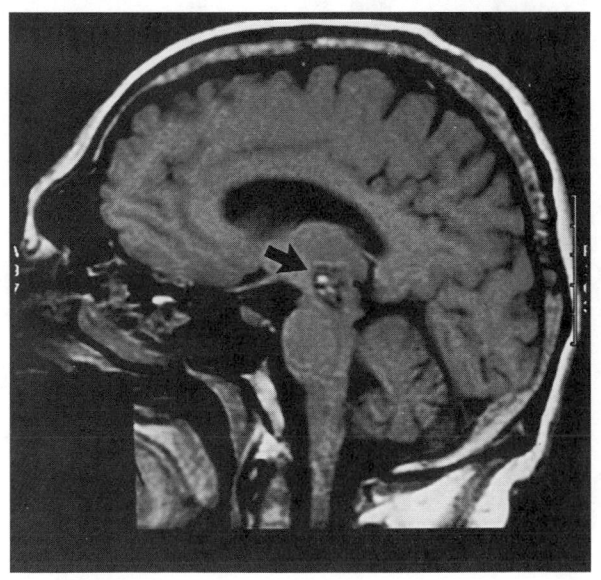 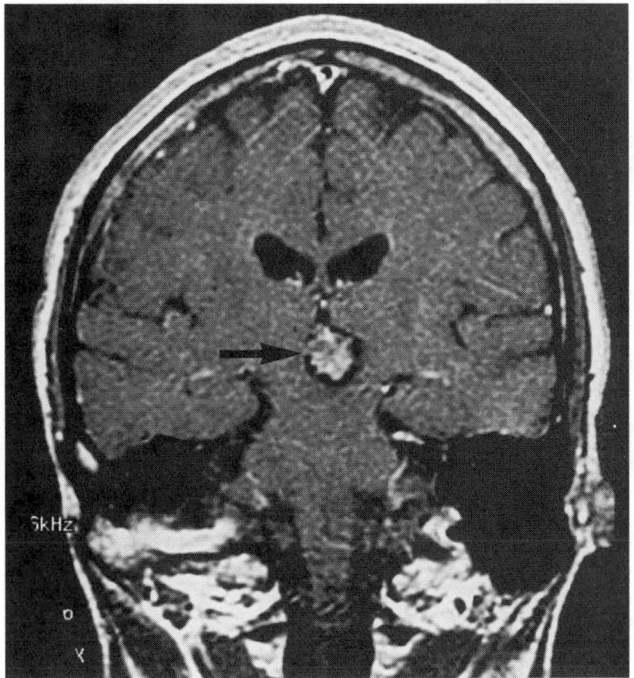

FIG. 29-16. **(A)** T1-weighted sagittal and **(B)** coronal magnetic resonance image of an upper midbrain cavernous angioma (*arrows*).

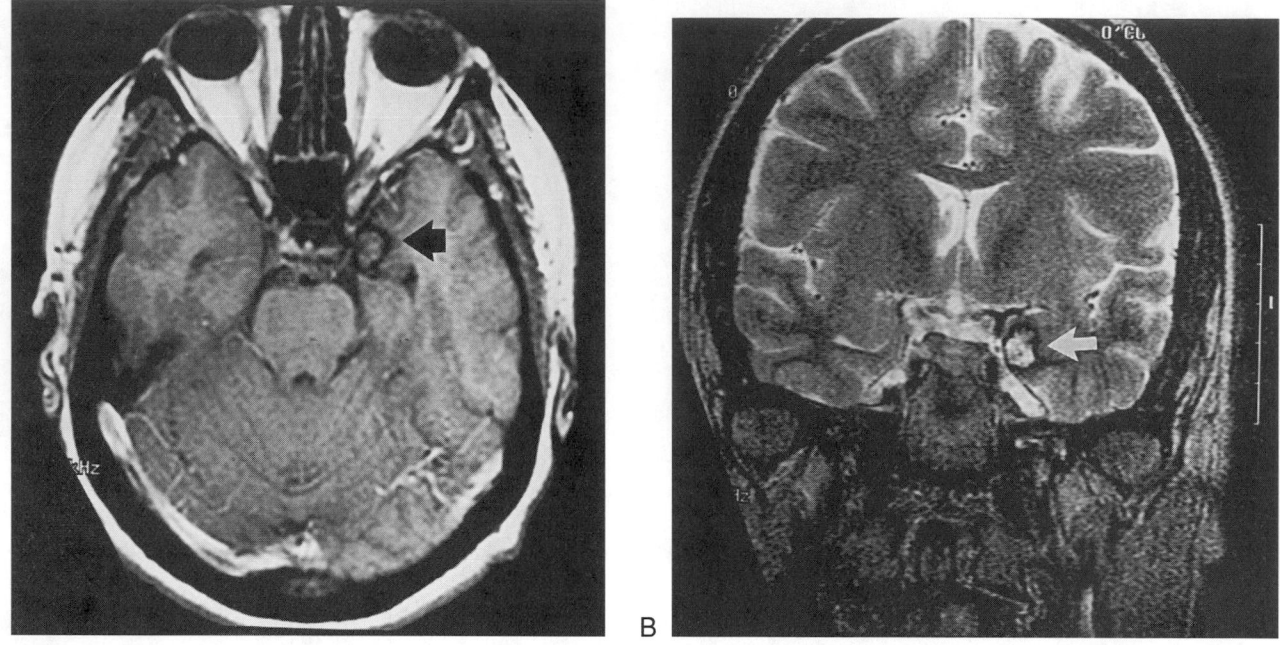

FIG. 29-17. **(A)** T1-weighted axial and **(B)** T2-weighted coronal magnetic resonance image of a cavernous angioma in the medial left temporal lobe (*arrows*).

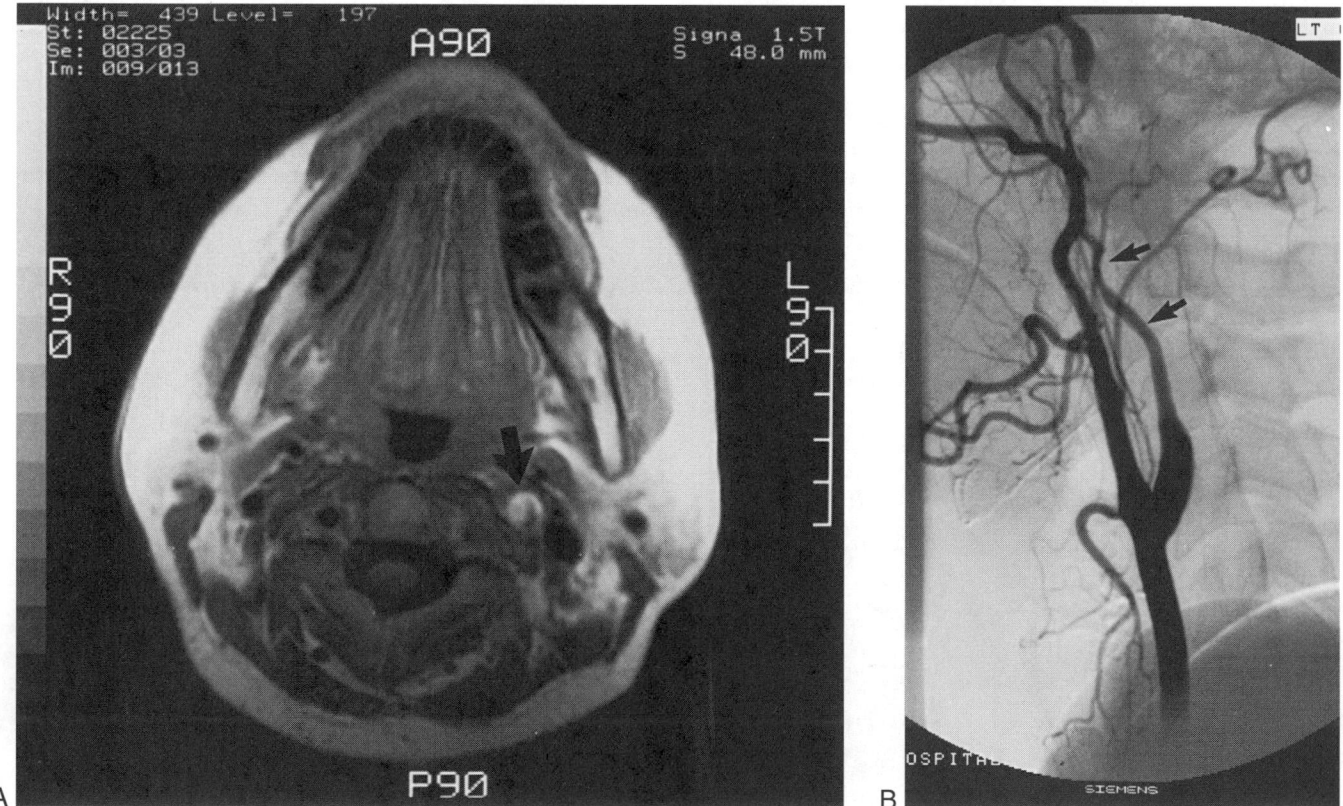

FIG. 29-18. **(A)** Magnetic resonance image showing clot in the wall of the left internal carotid artery (ICA) caused by dissection. **(B)** Corresponding angiogram of the left ICA showing tapered narrowing characteristic of dissection.

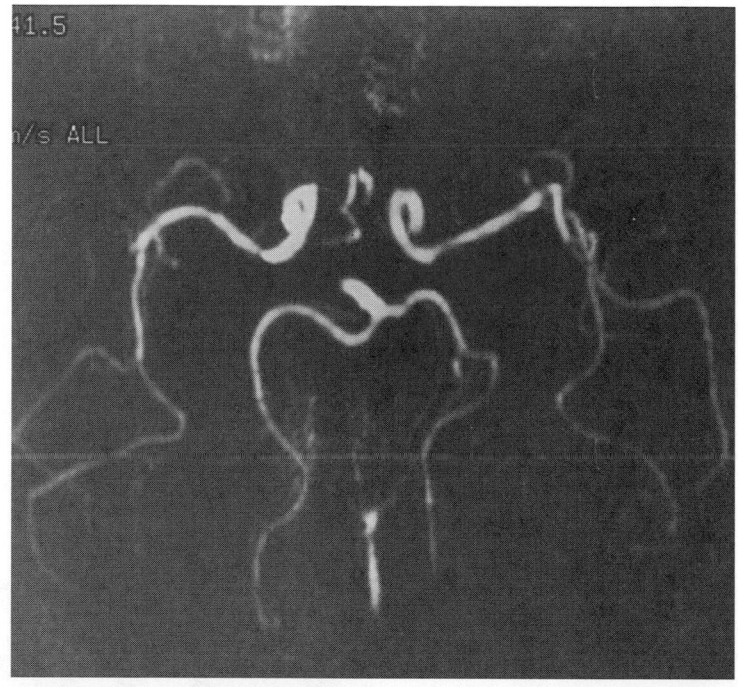

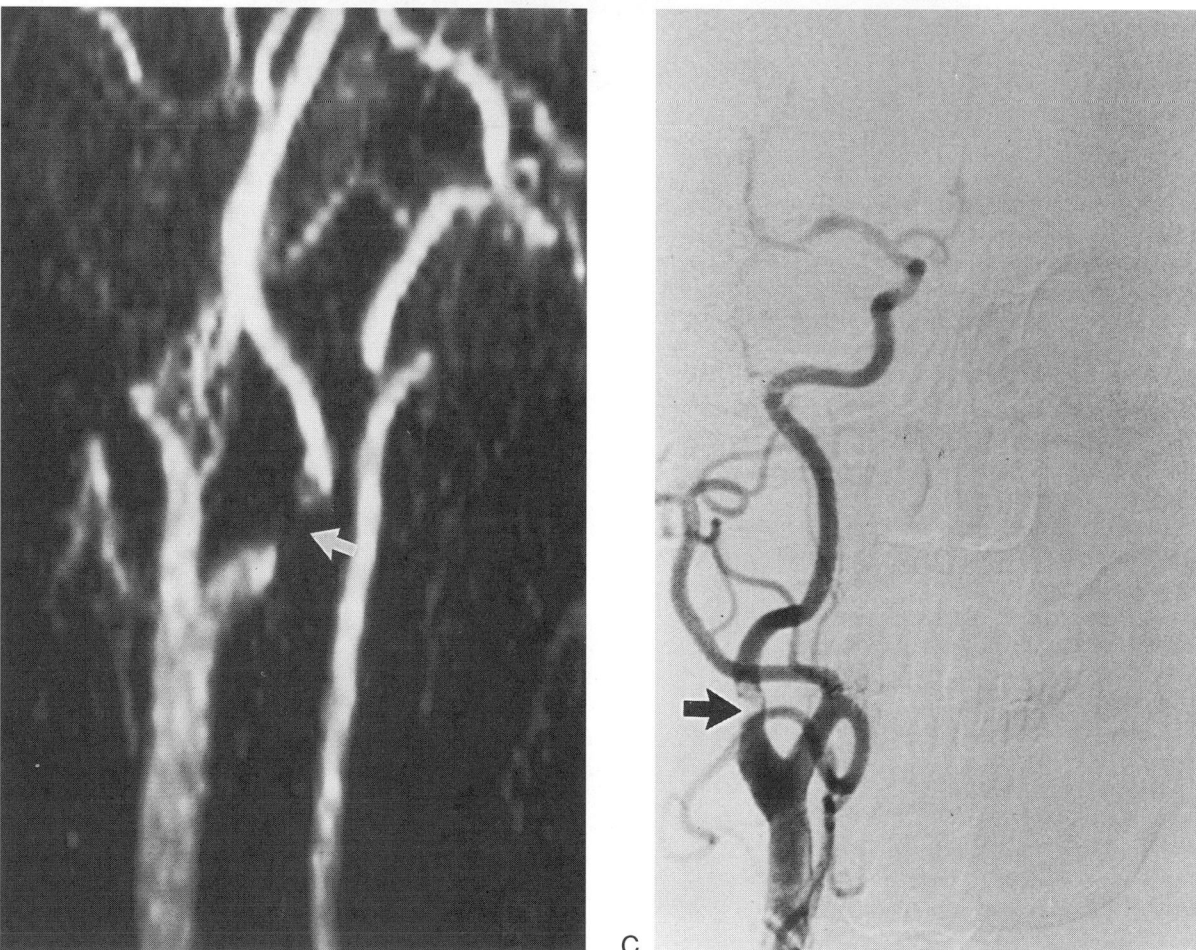

FIG. 29-19. **(A)** Magnetic resonance angiogram (MRA) showing skip area in region of very tight internal carotid artery (ICA) bifurcation stenosis (*arrow*) with reconstitution above. **(B)** MRA showing signal of flowing blood in carotid siphon above a tight ICA stenosis. **(C)** Angiogram corresponding to MRA in Fig. A.

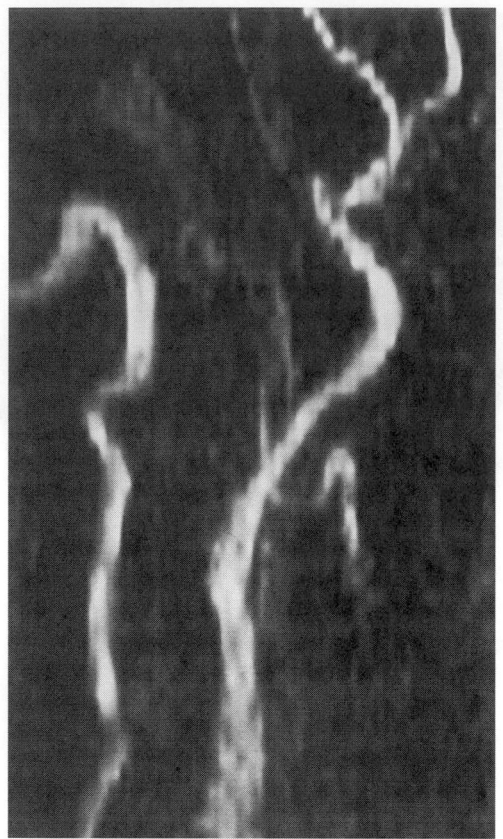
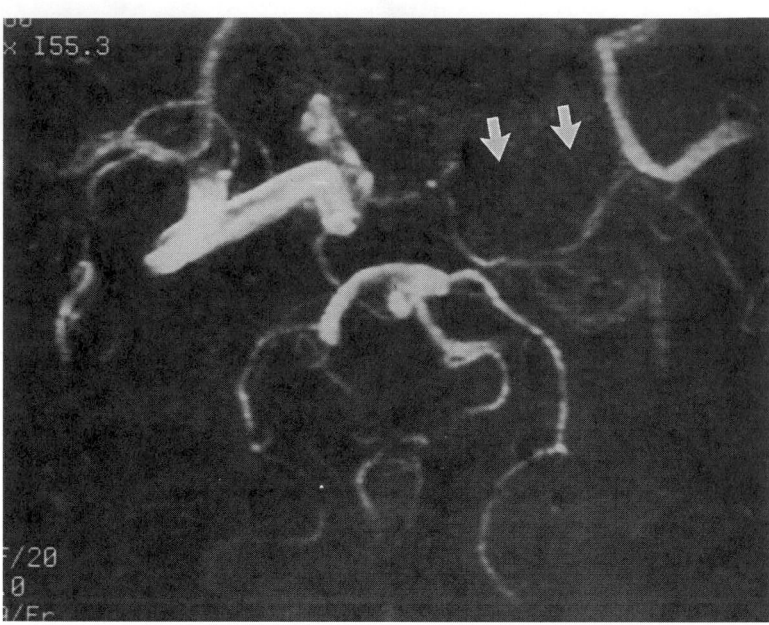

FIG. 29-20. **(A)** Magnetic resonance angiogram (MRA) in internal carotid artery (ICA) occlusion. **(B)** MRA showing absence of signal indicating lack of flowing blood in carotid siphon above a complete ICA occlusion (*arrow*).

ever, because of turbulence caused by stenosis, MRA tends to overestimate the degree of narrowing of the vessels. Extracranially, with a very tight, critical ICA stenosis, a region of total drop-out of signal may be seen, with reconstitution of flow above (Fig. 29-19). With complete occlusion, there is complete loss of signal from the occluded region extending caudally (Fig. 29-20A) and intracranially. This can be visualized as loss of signal in the carotid siphon (Fig. 29-20B). Critical ICA stenosis in the neck resulting in very slow flow past the stenosis can appear as an occlusion. Though MRA can actually be better

than angiography for detecting slow flow above a critical stenosis, this can still be missed with MRA. Therefore, if carotid endarterectomy is considered, angiography with a trickle study should be performed.

Carotid siphons are well-visualized by MRA; however, because of the bends in the vessel, there may be drop-out of signal that can be confusing when evaluating this region. The intracranial anterior circulation vessels are well seen when evaluating for regions of proximal stenosis. Tight MCA stenosis is seen as a narrowed vessel or region of signal drop-out (Fig. 29-21).

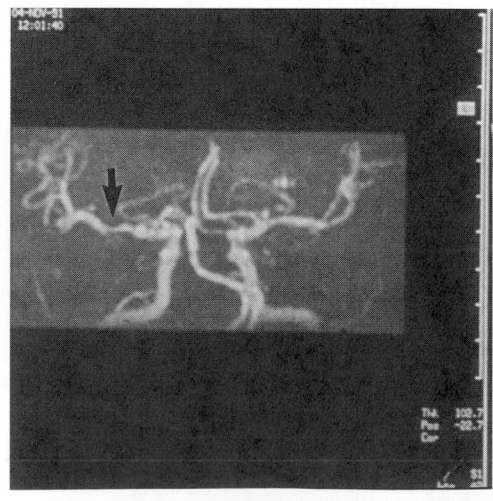
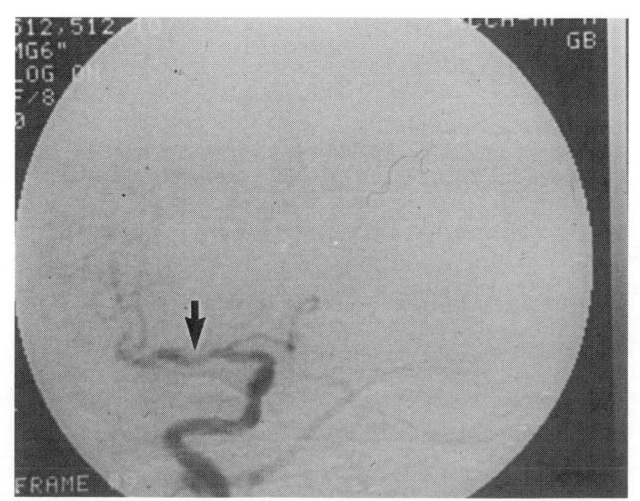

FIG. 29-21. **(A)** Magnetic resonance angiogram and **(B)** conventional angiogram of middle cerebral artery stenosis (*arrow*).

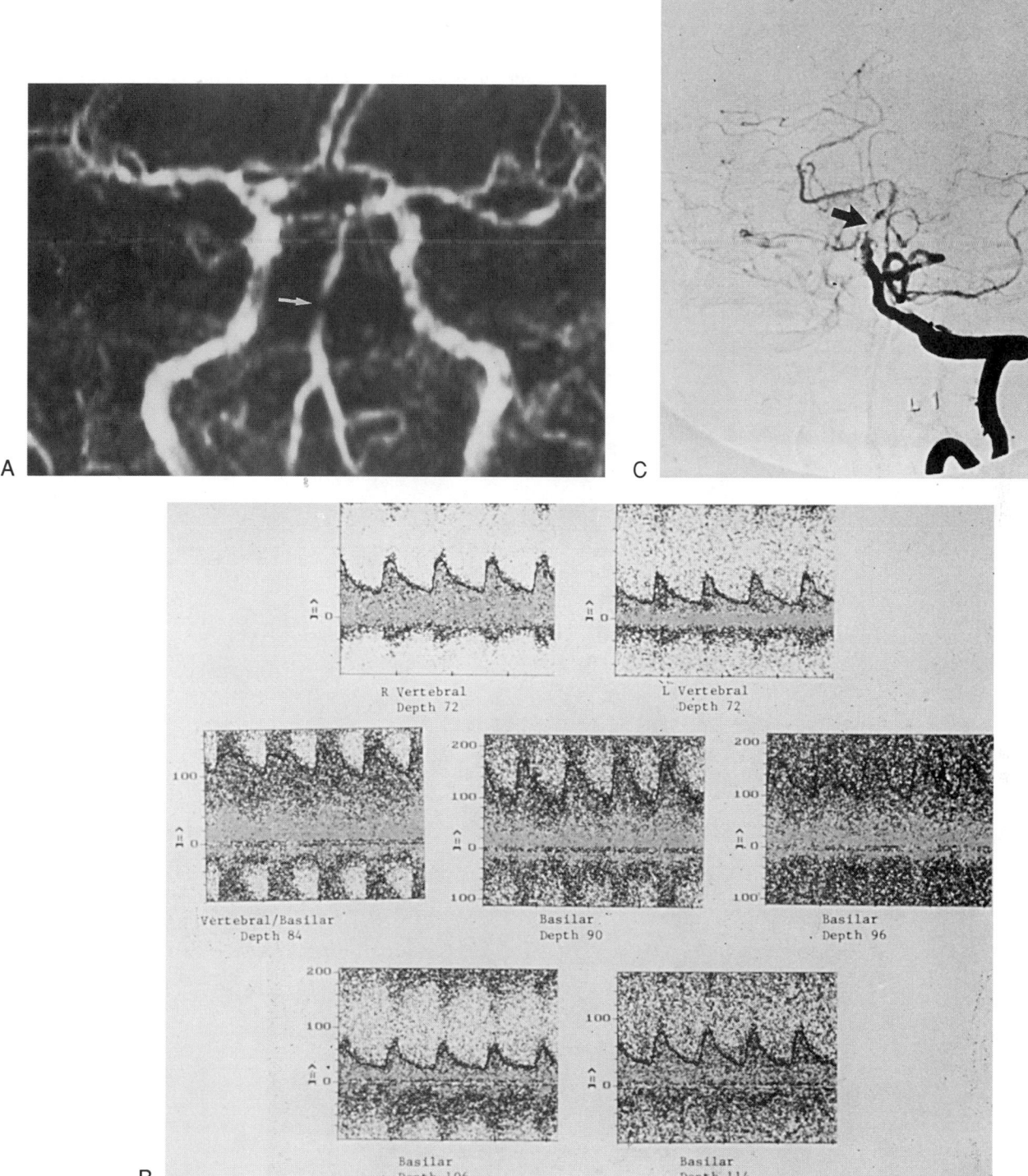

FIG. 29-22. **(A)** Magnetic resonance angiogram in basilar stenosis showing region of complete drop-out of signal (*arrow*). **(B)** Transcranial Doppler recording from the same patient showing elevated velocities in the midbasilar artery consistent with a region of stenosis. **(C)** Angiogram from the same patient showing basilar stenosis (*arrow*).

In the posterior circulation, the extracranial vertebral arteries are well visualized in the neck in the region between the origin and the bony portion and in that portion of the vessel going through the bony vertebral foramina. MRA of the vertebral artery origins off the subclavian arteries is usually not adequate because of artifact from cardiac movement. Newer techniques are attempting to place receiving coils over this region to selectively image it, though this is not done routinely. The portion of the vertebral artery that bends around the rostral cervical vertebrae can again be a problematic region for evaluation because of the sharp angulation and curvature of the artery. The intracranial vertebral arteries and the basilar artery are well visualized by MRA. Basilar stenosis appears as a region of signal drop-out (Fig. 29-22A), which without specialized flow studies, can be difficult to differentiate from occlusion. TCD

ultrasound (Fig. 29-22B) or angiography (Fig. 29-22C) may be necessary for further clarification.

Depending on the MRA technique, flow In the posterior circulation, may be shown as an open vessel, no matter what the direction. Figure 29-23 outlines a major pitfall with MRA. This patient had severe bilateral intracranial vertebral disease with reversed flow in the basilar artery. The regions of vertebral disease were lost in the images between the extracranial study, which showed a very small right vertebral artery and a normal left vertebral artery, and the intracranial study, which did not demonstrate a right vertebral artery, but the left vertebral artery again appeared normal. On angiography, the right vertebral artery was occluded, the left was tightly stenotic in the intracranial portion, and the basilar artery filled retrograde via the carotids. Transcranial Doppler ultrasound also demonstrated the reversal

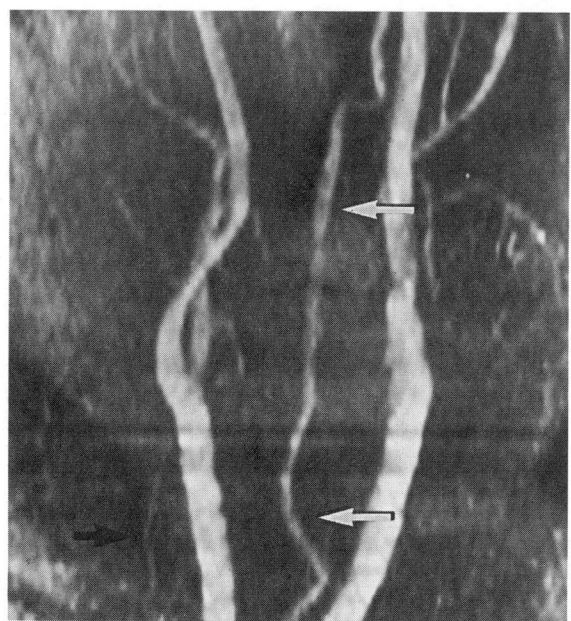

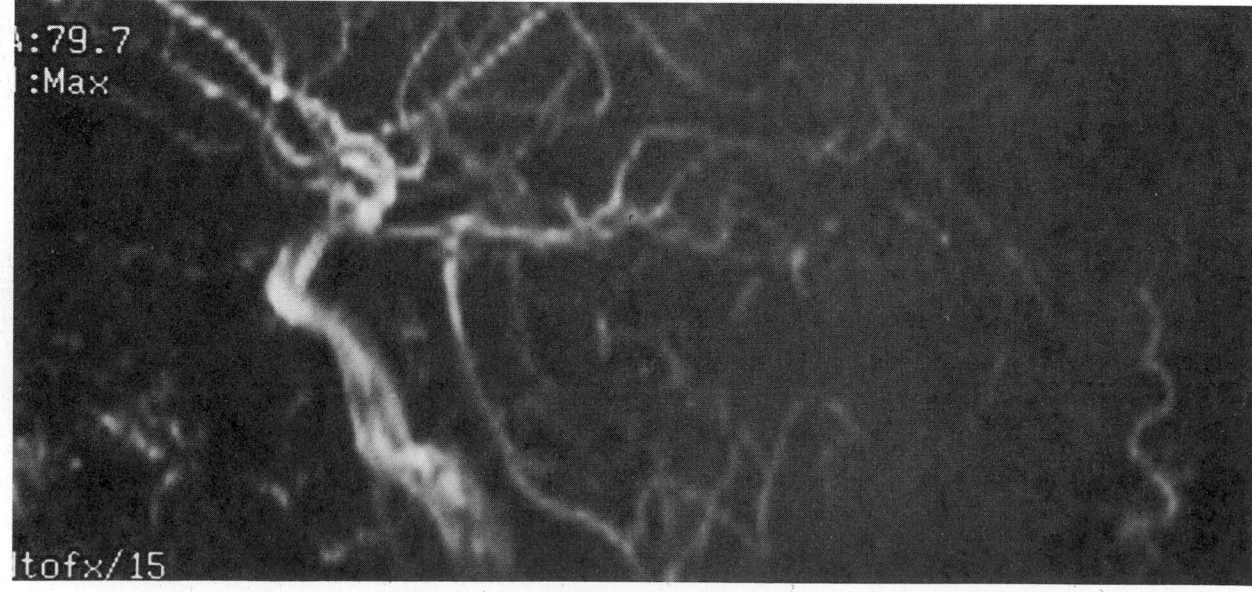

FIG. 29-23.   **(A)** Magnetic resonance angiogram of extracranial vessels showing normal flow in the left vertebral (*arrows*) and small right vertebral arteries. (*Figure continues.*) **(B)** Magnetic resonance image of the head showing normal-appearing flow in the left vertebral and basilar arteries.

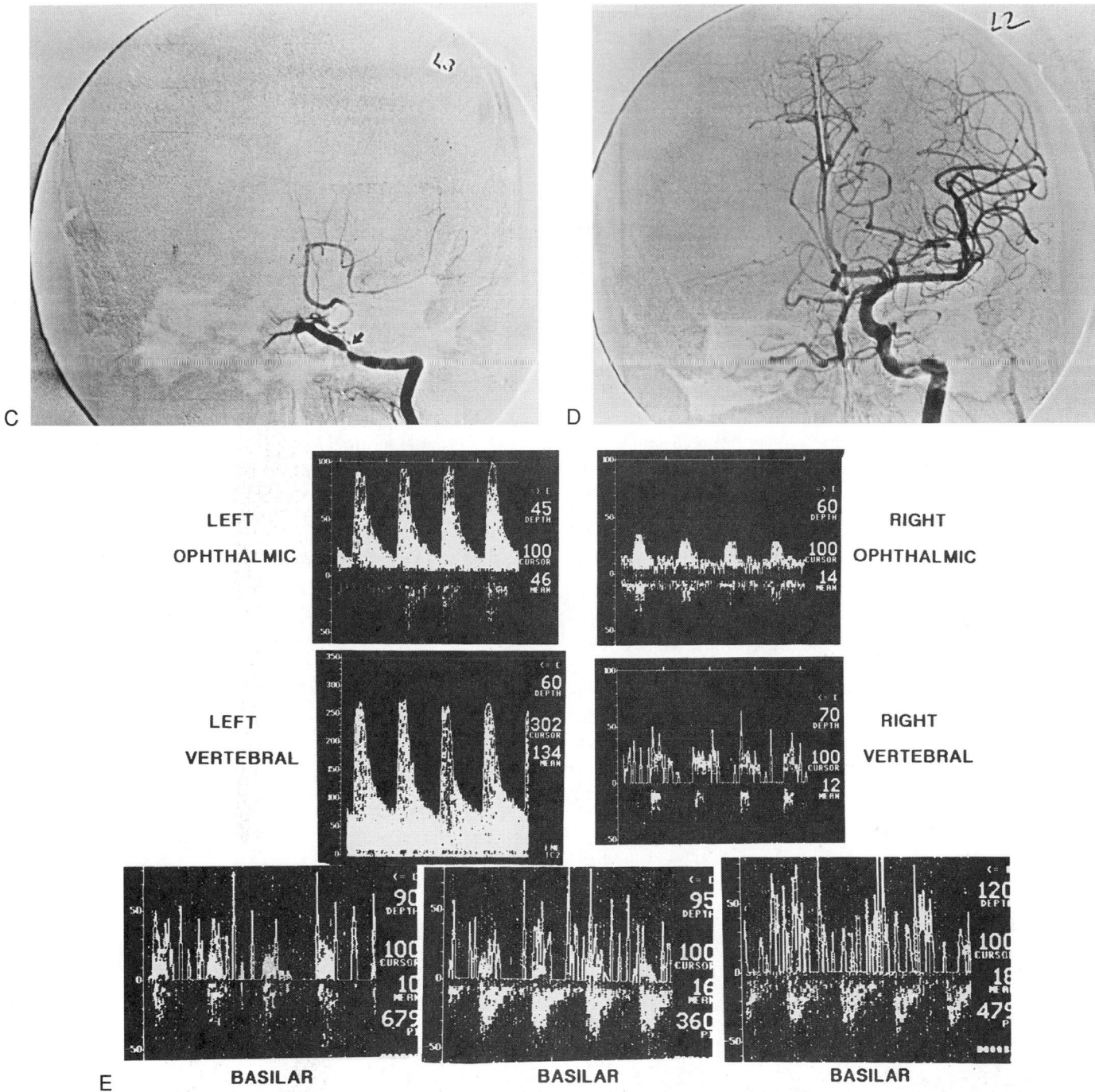

FIG. 29-23. *(Continued).* **(C)** Angiogram showing tight left intracranial vertebral stenosis and **(D)** basilar artery filling retrograde from the carotid artery injection. **(E)** Transcranial Doppler recording showing elevated velocities in the left vertebral artery consistent with stenosis, and reversed flow in the basilar artery (this patient also had a tight left ophthalmic artery stenosis).

of flow in the basilar artery. MRA techniques can be adapted to record the direction of flow in the vessels and eliminate these pitfalls. In addition, the extracranial and intracranial vessels can be viewed together or images can be overlapped to avoid this problem.

Branch vessels such as the posteroinferior cerebellar arteries, anteroinferior cerebellar arteries and superior cerebellar arteries are often well demonstrated on MRA. However, the smaller the vessel, the more likely that MRA will not detect it. MRA is not as good as angiography for evaluating small vessel occlusions or patterns of vasculitis.

Applications of Magnetic Resonance Angiography

Ischemic Stroke. In a patient with TIA or stroke attributable to ischemia in the distribution of the MCA or ACA, MRA may provide important information. It is probably not the optimal test for evaluation of the carotid bifurcation because of the tendency to overestimate the degree of stenosis. Since recommendations regarding carotid endarterectomy in both symptomatic and asymptomatic patients depends upon percent stenosis, the most accurate measurement of lumen diameter should be obtained. Conventional angiography is preferred by most clinicians, although at some centers the combination of carotid duplex and MRA has replaced angiography if both studies indicate very severe stenosis. In a patient with TIA or stroke and no significant carotid disease by noninvasive carotid testing, intracranial disease should be suspected. This is particularly true when repeated stereotyped attacks occur in the absence of carotid bifurcation disease. MRA, similar to TCD, provides a noninvasive examination of the intracranial circulation. Narrowing of the carotid siphon or MCA can be identified, then further defined by TCD or conventional angiography. Negative study results should obviate the need for conventional angiography in most cases.

Evaluation of vertebrobasilar TIAs or stroke may also include MRA. Similar to the anterior circulation, MRA provides a noninvasive screening test for stenosis in the vertebral and basilar arteries. Multiple stereotyped events or a stepwise progression of neurologic deficits not clearly attributable to a single branch of the basilar artery suggests large-vessel disease in the posterior circulation. MRA allows rapid identification of stenosis (although the severity of stenosis may not be accurate) and may obviate the need for conventional angiography or at least delay angiography until the patient's clinical status stabilizes. Although the use of heparin is controversial, knowledge of the vascular anatomy early on facilitates decisions regarding management of blood pressure, anticoagulants, and activity.

Aneurysms and Arteriovenous Malformations. With a sensitivity of 95 percent, MRA may be a useful screening test for intracranial aneurysms, if one is willing to accept some false negative studies for lesions less than 5 mm in diameter. In the setting of subarachnoid hemorrhage, angiography is necessary since even small aneurysms must be detected. AVMs that are seen as serpiginous flow voids on standard spin-echo MRI can be better delineated by MRA, though conventional angiography remains the method of choice for definitive evaluation of intracranial aneurysms and AVMs.

Magnetic Resonance Venography

MRV is a new technique that is excellent for visualization of the intracerebral veins and sinuses. It is particularly good when suspecting venous sinus thrombosis, in that it is noninvasive, can be performed at the same time as the MRI, and can demonstrate the open vessels well. The occluded vessels are seen as absence of flow. MRV is very helpful in identifying sagittal sinus thrombosis as the etiology of chronic headaches and increased cerebrospinal fluid pressure (Fig. 29-24). Venous infarction appears on CT or MRI as a superficial cortical wedged-shaped abnormality, often with a prominent hemorrhagic component. When such lesions are seen, MRV is helpful to identify occlusion of a cortical vein or sinus without the need for conventional arteriography with venous imaging.

CONVENTIONAL ANGIOGRAPHY

Conventional angiography remains the "gold standard" for optimally visualizing the cerebral and neck vessels. However, it is an invasive procedure with complications of stroke and bleeding as well as limitations such as dye allergy. In some situations,

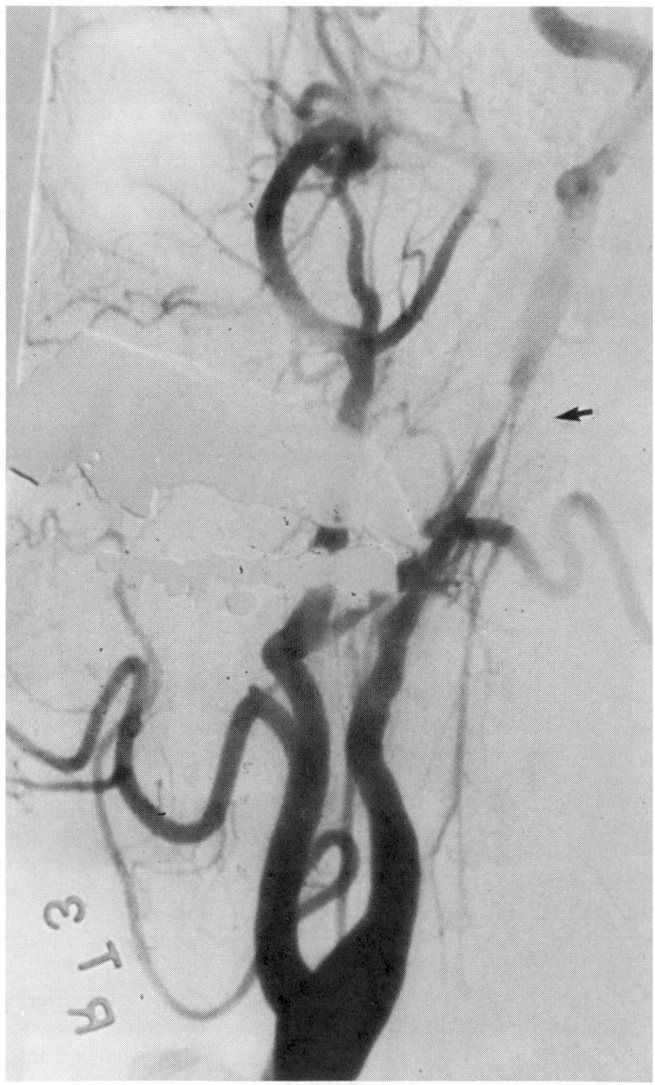

FIG. 29-25. Long, tapered narrowing of the extracranial internal carotid artery in a dissection (*arrow*).

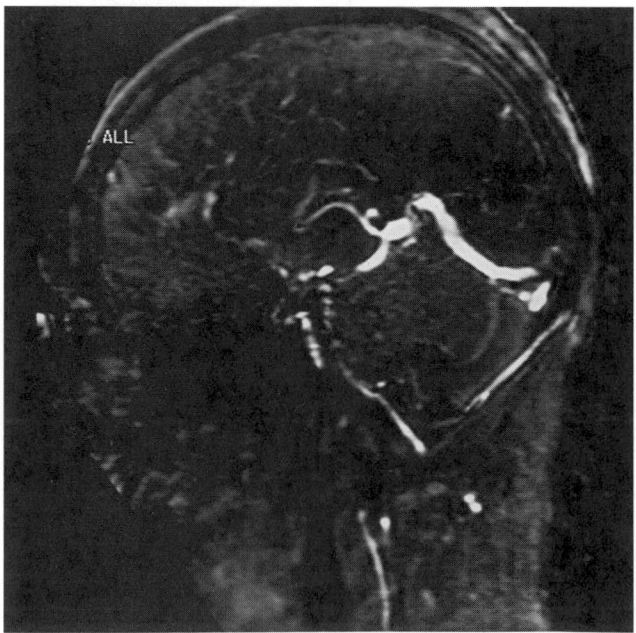

FIG. 29-24. Magnetic resonance venography showing absence of flow in the superior and inferior sagittal sinuses.

MRA may replace conventional angiography. Angiography carries a complication rate of 0.5 to 1 percent, whereas MRA presents virtually no risk. Three-dimensional acquisitions by MRA allow multiple views of vascular anatomy. Conventional angiography typically obtains only two or three views, which may not optimally visualize the pathology. Angiography takes time and may delay appropriate therapy. However, when definitive information is needed regarding the status of the cerebral circulation, conventional angiography remains the test of choice.

Applications of Conventional Angiography

Cerebrovascular Disease. Standard catheter angiography remains the optimal method for evaluation of arterial lesions. Unlike MRA, conventional angiography is an actual anatomic diagram of the vessels and their pathology. In the evaluation of extracranial vascular disease, angiography can differentiate between mild, moderate, or severe occlusive disease and shows regions of irregularity. It remains the method of choice for evaluating the aortic arch and the origins of the great vessels. In extracranial carotid dissection, angiography shows the well-described tapered stenosis or string sign (Fig. 29-25) and "tell-tale pouch."

Angiography performed acutely following large-vessel territory strokes can often be helpful in defining the pathophysiology of the stroke. It is excellent for identifying intracranial stenotic lesions as well as showing abrupt cut-off of vessels with embolic occlusion. If angiography is being performed to document embolic occlusion of a vessel, it is best performed within 48 hours of the ischemic event because emboli often break up via the body's own thrombolytic mechanisms.

Differentiating near occlusion of the carotid artery from total occlusion in symptomatic patients is important, since those with near occlusion may be amenable to carotid endarterectomy. At present, neither MRA or ultrasound reliably diagnoses total carotid occlusion. When either study suggests occlusion, conventional angiography should be pursued to definitively exclude a small residual lumen. The standard filming sequence should be extended to detect very slow antegrade flow. Technical improvements may eventually document the reliability of other techniques; however, until that time, conventional angiography should be performed unless other factors preclude the possibility of carotid surgery.

Aneurysm and Arteriovenous Malformations. Angiography remains the evaluation of choice for imaging aneurysms and outlining AVMs with detail, showing feeding and draining vessels. For patients in whom surgery is being considered for either of these entities, angiography is essential. Angiography is often performed prior to evacuation of an intracerebral hematoma, in an attempt to demonstrate an aneurysm or AVM before surgery. If nothing is found and surgery is not performed, angiography should be repeated in a few months once the blood has resorbed.

Angiography demonstrates small vessels well and is the best imaging method available for outlining the "beading" of vessels seen with vasculitis. However, vasculitis affecting only the very small penetrating vessels can be missed with angiography and can be seen only on brain biopsy. Regions of segmental

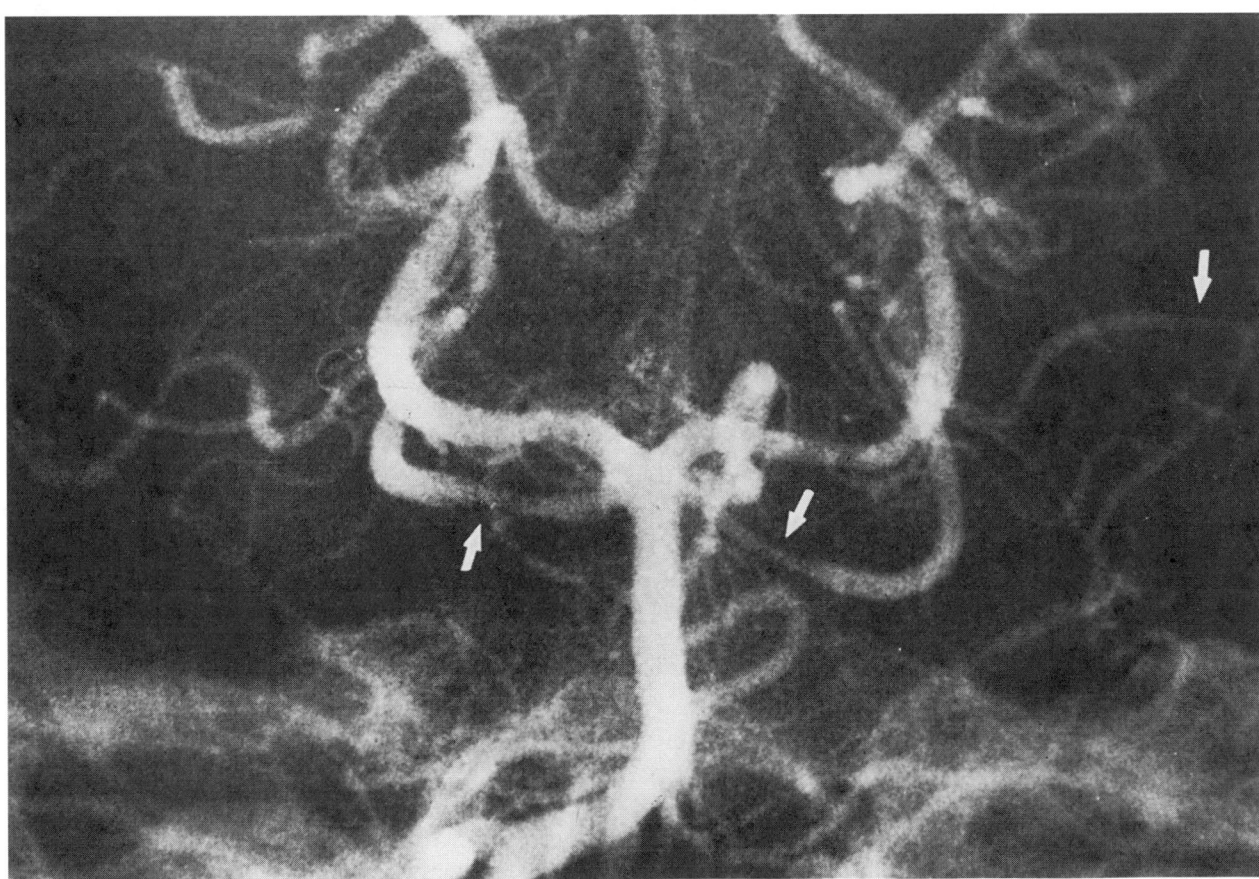

FIG. 29-26. Regions of segmental narrowing presumed due to vasospasm (*arrows*).

narrowing also occur in the absence of vasculitis and may be due to reversible vasospasm (Fig. 29-26).

Interventional Angiography

Angiography has become a method for performing interventional techniques to treat various conditions. In the case of an acute vessel occlusion, a catheter can be placed directly into the clot for delivery of thrombolytic agents. Occluding balloons or embolic materials can be placed via catheter into large aneurysms or into feeding vessels to an AVM either to occlude them completely or shrink them prior to surgical removal. Angioplasty is a technique now being performed on both extracranial as well as intracranial stenotic vessels; a catheter is placed through the region of stenosis and a balloon is expanded, ''cracking'' the plaque and widening the vessel.

SUGGESTED READINGS

Aaslid R, Markwalder T-M, Nornes H: Noninvasive transcranial Doppler ultrasound recording of flow velocity in basal cerebral arteries. J Neurosurg 57:769, 1982

Ackerman RH, Candia MR: Assessment of the vascular substrate of ischemic brain disease. pp. 138–46. In Fisher M, Bogousslavsky J (eds): Current Review of Cerebrovascular Disease. Current Medicine, Philadelphia, 1993

Babikian VL, Hyde C, Pochay V, Winter MR: Clinical correlates of high-intensity transient signals detected on transcranial Doppler sonography in patients with cerebrovascular disease. Stroke 25:1570, 1994

Babikian VL, Wechsler LR: Transcranial Doppler Ultrasonography. CV Mosby, St. Louis, 1993

Bartels E, Flugel KA: Quantitative measurements of blood flow velocity in basal cerebral arteries with transcranial duplex color-flow imaging. J Neuroimag 4:77, 1994

Call GK, Fleming MC, Sealfon S et al: Reversible cerebral segmental vasoconstriction. Stroke 19:1159, 1988

DeWitt LD, Wechsler LR: Transcranial Doppler. Stroke 19:915, 1988

Eliasziw M, Streifler JY, Fox AJ et al: Significance of plaque ulceration in symptomatic patients with high-grade carotid stenosis. Stroke 25:304, 1994

Estol CJ, DeWitt LD, Tettenborn B et al: Accuracy of transcranial Doppler in the vertebrobasilar circulation. Ann Neurol 28:225, 1990

Goldberg HI, Grossman RI, Gomori JM et al: Cervical internal carotid artery dissecting hemorrhage: diagnosis using MR. Radiology 158:157, 1986

Gracs G, Fox A, Barnett HJM, Vinuela F: CT visualization of intracranial arterial thromboembolism. Stroke 14:756, 1983

Hennerici MG, Daffertshofer M: Noninvasive vascular testing. pp. 121–37. In Fisher M, Bogousslavsky J (eds): Current Review of Cerebrovascular Disease. Current Medicine, Philadelphia, 1993

Huston III J, Ehman RL: Comparison of time-of-flight and phase contrast MR neuroangiographic techniques. Radiographics 13:5, 1993

Ley-Pozo J, Ringelstein EB: Noninvasive detection of occlusive disease of the carotid siphon and middle cerebral artery. Ann Neurol 28:640, 1990

Mattle HP, Kent KC, Edelman RR et al: Evaluation of the extracranial carotid arteries: correlation of magnetic resonance angiography, duplex ultrasonography, and conventional angiography. J Vasc Surg 13:838, 1991

Minematsu K, Fisher M, Li L et al: Diffusion-weighted magnetic resonance imaging: rapid quantitative detection of focal brain ischemia. Neurology 42:235, 1992

North American Symptomatic Carotid Endarterectomy Trial (NASCET) collaborators: Beneficial effect of carotid endarterectomy in symptomatic patients with high-grade carotid stenosis. N Engl J Med 325:445, 1991

Ruggieri PM, Masaryk T, Ross JS: Magnetic resonance angiography: cerebrovascular applications. Stroke 23:774, 1992

Schwartz RB, Jones KM, Chernoff DM et al: Common carotid artery bifurcation: evaluation with spiral CT. Radiology 185:513, 1992

Sloan MA: Detection of vasospasm following subarachnoid hemorrhage. p. 105. In Babikian VL, Wechsler LR (eds): Transcranial Doppler Ultrasonography. CV Mosby, St. Louis, 1993

SECTION 2.   COMMON PATHOGENESES OF STROKE

30. ATHEROTHROMBOTIC CEREBRAL INFARCTION

CARLOS S. KASE
CONRADO J. ESTOL

The mechanisms of ischemic and hemorrhagic stroke are multiple, in part reflecting the variability in size and location of the arteries involved. The chapters in this section present the pathogenetic mechanisms that underlie most cases of stroke. The frequency of these pathogeneses reflects the prevalence in the population of stroke risk factors, as discussed in Chapter 28, and is in turn reflected by the frequency of the different types of stroke. Table 30-1 lists the stroke subtypes and their frequencies as determined in the hospital-based Harvard Stroke Registry.

ATHEROGENESIS

Atherothrombotic occlusion of cerebral arteries, also referred to as large vessel disease, is most commonly the result of atheroma deposition in the vessel wall, frequently complicated by formation of fresh clot in an area of intimal disruption. The process of atheroma formation, which typically affects large and medium muscular arteries at branching points, involves the progressive deposition of fatty materials along with fibrous tissue in the subintimal region. Through a complex interaction of presumably injured endothelial cells with macrophages, smooth muscle cells, and platelets, the arterial wall becomes the site where lipids, especially cholesterol, become deposited, at the same time triggering major changes in the smooth muscle cells in

TABLE 30-1. Stroke Subtypes, Hospital-Based Series ($n = 694$)

Subtype	No. Patients	%
Large artery thrombosis	233	34
Lacunar infarction	131	19
Embolism	215	31
Intracerebral hemorrhage	70	10
Subarachnoid hemorrhage	45	6

(From Mohr JP, Caplan LR, Melski JW et al: The Harvard Cooperative Stroke Registry: a prospective registry. Neurology 28:754, 1978, with permission.)

the arterial media. This results in progressive focal changes in the artery, with encroachment of the lumen.

The development of luminal stenosis secondary to enlargement of the atheromatous plaque is subject to individual variability, and is thought to be accelerated by atherogenic risk factors such as hypertension, diabetes, hypercholesterolemia, and smoking, as well as by poorly understood local changes in the atheromatous plaque such as ulceration and subplaque hemorrhage. The resulting focal stenosis is the first event that eventually leads to symptoms in large-vessel atheromatosis, either transient ischemic attacks (TIAs), or ischemic stroke.

ATHEROMA DISTRIBUTION AND MECHANISM OF SYMPTOMS

The distribution of atherothrombosis in cerebral arteries favors the large proximal trunks at sites of bifurcation (Fig. 30-1). These proximally located lesions can become symptomatic by

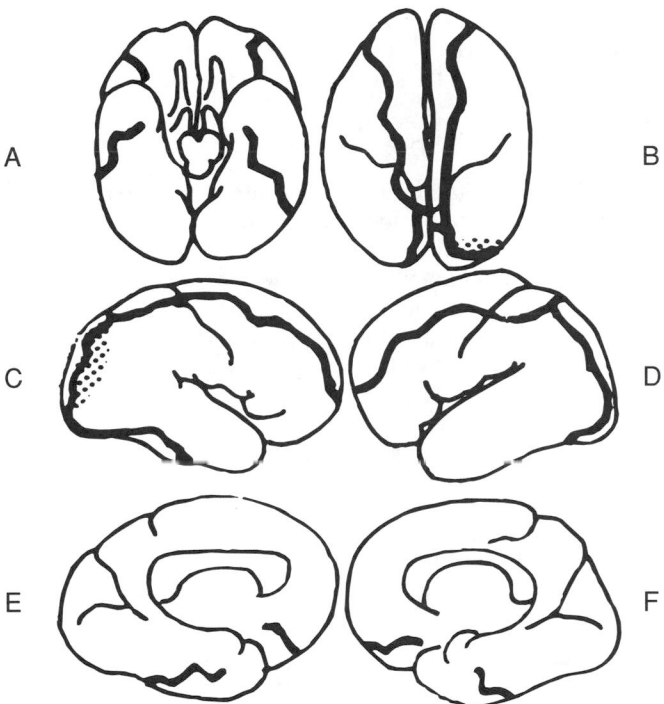

FIG. 30-2. Arterial borderzones between anterior, middle, and posterior cerebral arteries. **(A)** Base of brain; **(B)** upper surface of hemispheres; **(C)** right lateral convexity; **(D)** left lateral convexity; **(E)** left medial view; **(F)** right medial view. (From Mohr JP: Neurological complications of cardiac valvular disease and cardiac surgery including systemic hypotension. p. 143. In Vinken PJ, Bruyn GW (eds): Handbook of Clinical Neurology. North Holland Publishing, Amsterdam, 1979, with permission.)

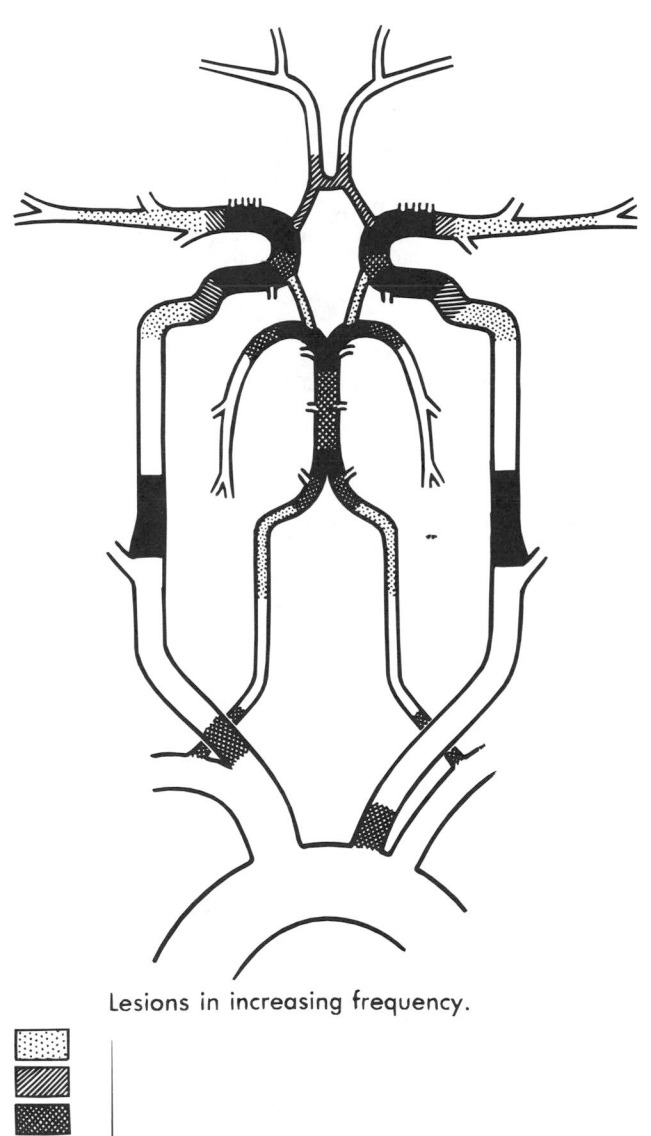

Lesions in increasing frequency.

FIG. 30-1. Frequency and severity of atherosclerotic lesions in the arterial cervicocerebral tree. (From Poirier J, Gray F, Escourolle R: Manual of Basic Neuropathology. pp. 65–102. WB Saunders, Philadelphia, 1990, with permission.)

several mechanisms: (1) progressive lumen reduction to the point of compromising the distal cerebral flow, generally producing TIAs; (2) disruption of thrombus on the plaque with embolization of thrombus fragments, resulting in the so-called artery-to-artery emboli that lodge in a distal branch of the affected artery; or (3) in situ clot formation on an atheromatous plaque with total occlusion of the affected artery. The artery-to-artery embolic occlusions resulting from extracranial internal carotid artery (ICA) atheroma involve the main trunk or the divisions of the middle cerebral artery (MCA) more commonly than the anterior cerebral artery (ACA), whereas those of proximal vertebral artery or basilar artery origin affect the cerebellum, brainstem, or posterior cerebral artery (PCA) territory. Complete arterial occlusion by fresh thrombus superimposed on atheroma, on the other hand, can result in either cerebral infarction or TIAs, but this event can be fully asymptomatic, the latter being for the most part due to the availability of collateral blood flow that results in sparing of ischemic brain tissue.

In the event of cerebral infarction occurring at the time of acute atherothrombosis, the stroke mechanism can be either distal embolization by clot (generally thought to occur at the time of the acute thrombotic occlusion) or, less commonly, distal hemodynamic insufficiency resulting in infarction along the borderzones of the major intracranial arteries that are branches of the involved proximal artery. For the ICA, these infarcts generally involve the MCA/ACA borderzone along the upper hemispheric convexity and the MCA/PCA borderzone in the posterior parietal-superior-temporal convexity (Fig. 30-2); for the vertebral artery, the infarcts occur along the posterior edge of the cerebellar hemisphere, in the posterior-inferior cerebellar artery to superior cerebellar artery borderzone; for the proximal basilar artery, such infarcts can involve the PCA/MCA border-zone and, less commonly, the thalami, bilaterally.

CLINICAL PRESENTATION

The clinical presentation in cerebral atherothrombosis varies depending on multiple factors, such as the location of the artery involved, the degree and speed of arterial stenosis or occlusion, the availability of collateral blood flow, and probably the level and variations of systemic blood pressure. The latter three factors relate to the severity of the initial clinical deficit, whereas the location of the involved artery determines the specific stroke syndrome. Since the latter are presented in detail in Chapter 41, the discussion here is limited to the general clinical features of cerebral atherothrombosis that apply to this condition regardless of the location of the affected artery.

Transient Ischemic Attacks

TIAs—brief episodes of fully reversible focal neurologic deficits—can occur in instances of atheromatosis of extracranial or intracranial arteries such as the ICA, vertebral artery, basilar artery, MCA, and PCA. The mechanism is thought to be either transient hemodynamic failure of hypoperfused distal branches of the affected artery, or distal embolization of particulate material (thrombus) that after producing symptoms by blocking an intracranial artery is rapidly fragmented and pushed distally into the circulation, to account for the rapid resolution of symptoms. The duration of TIAs is more often on the order of minutes than hours, and this factor relates to some extent to the mechanism of the TIAs; those lasting minutes are more commonly due to hemodynamic factors, whereas those that last longer (hours) have features that favor an embolic mechanism.

Unusual Clinical Presentations.   Although TIAs are by definition characterized by transient focal deficits or "negative" phenomena, an exception to the rule may be the occasional observation of transient "positive" phenomena in the setting of tight stenosis or occlusion of the appropriate artery. This includes the observation of transient repetitive clonic jerking of the contralateral arm or leg (limb shaking), without electroencephalographic changes or response to antiepileptic drugs to suggest a partial motor seizure, in instances of ICA stenosis or occlusion, and the occasional report of visual phenomena ("flashing lights") in the hemifield contralateral to a stenotic or occluded PCA or in the eye ipsilateral to a stenotic or occluded ICA, in an elderly person without history of migraine headaches or previous episodes of hemianopsia or transient monocular blindness. These rare events probably correspond to cortical ischemia with "irritative, positive" phenomena rather than the more common transient deficits of focal neurologic function that define TIAs. In the proper setting, which generally includes negative electroencephalographic examination results for a seizure phenomenon and imaging procedures such as computed tomography (CT) and magnetic resonance (MRI) that rule out a focal mass lesion or scar, TIAs should be considered in the differential diagnosis of these phenomena, and appropriate vascular studies aimed at detecting focal atherostenotic disease should follow.

Clinical Significance.   TIAs correlate with atheromatosis of the corresponding artery in from 50 percent to close to 90 percent of cases, with some variability that depends on the clinical characteristics and vascular territory involved. As a result of this correlation, they are helpful in detecting symptomatic arterial stenosis and, most importantly, in preventing cerebral infarction, the most serious neurologic event that may follow the onset of TIAs. It has been estimated that as many as 20 to 35 percent of patients with symptomatic ICA stenosis in the 70 to 79 percent through 90 to 99 percent range, respectively, will develop ipsilateral hemispheric infarction within 24 months from TIA onset. This relatively early occurrence of stroke events after TIA onset determines the recommendations for management of the patient with recent onset of TIAs.

Patient Management.   The need for hospital admission is most critical for patients with onset of TIAs within days, for those who have had repeated episodes over periods of days, and for patients who evidence appropriate focal neurologic deficits on examination despite reporting full subjective resolution of symptoms. The latter situation is indicative of the development of cerebral infarction, an event that may be documented in as many as 30 to 40 percent of patients when they are assessed with CT or MRI, respectively, after TIA symptoms with full clinical resolution.

We recommend the use of continuous intravenous heparin infusion after recent onset of TIAs, while further evaluation continues, on the unproven assumption that cerebral infarction can be averted by short-term in-hospital use of this medication during the period of highest stroke risk after TIA onset. Heparin is used without an initial bolus, at a rate of 1,000 U/h, adjusting the infusion rate to maintain an activated partial thromboplastin time of 1.5 times control, while monitoring hematocrit and stool guaiac for blood loss and platelet counts for heparin-induced thrombocytopenia.

Ischemic Stroke

Stroke as a result of atherothrombosis of a major arterial trunk can be due to either distal embolization of thrombus (artery-to-artery mechanism) or local thrombus formation with distal hemodynamic consequences. In the first instance, the clinical presentation will be indistinguishable from that of intracranial embolism of other types, such as cardiogenic embolism, in which the type of onset and course reflects the sudden occlusion of a previously healthy intracranial artery by unstable particulate materials. The clinical features of cerebral embolism are discussed in Chapter 31.

Atherothrombosis with "hemodynamic" ischemic stroke often presents as stroke during sleep, the patient waking with the neurologic deficit. This type of onset is thought to relate to a propensity for clot formation during sleep as a result of changes in blood viscosity/coagulability, perhaps also facilitated by relatively low blood pressure during sleep. In those instances in which the onset of atherothrombotic stroke is during activity, a gradual progression of neurologic deficits is characteristic. Gradual, smooth progression or more commonly a "stepwise" course over minutes to hours is the rule. In the latter situation, a minimal focal neurologic deficit at onset, with initial stabilization, is followed by subsequent worsening and stabilization, until a final, persistent level of dysfunction is reached. These "steps" in the early progression of atherothrombotic brain infarction can at times be related to lowering of blood pressure (including attempts at tightly controlling hypertension present on admission with a mild neurologic deficit), but in most instances they are unrelated to a detectable event, most likely representing the gradual build-up of thrombus at the occlusion site. Another feature of the presentation of atherothrombotic stroke is the relative paucity of associated clinical findings at onset. These include a low figure of around 10 percent of headache and vomiting and a virtual absence of seizures at onset, features that distinguish this stroke subtype from cerebral embolism and especially the hemorrhagic stroke varieties. Seizures at onset are so rare that their presence in the setting of a progressive focal neurologic deficit (otherwise suggestive of atherothrombotic infarction) should raise the alternative diagnosis of brain tumor or abscess, rather than cerebral infarction.

It should be stressed that the effects of large-vessel atherothrombosis include presentations with TIAs and ischemic stroke, as well as its potential for being a fully asymptomatic event. In the event of ICA occlusion, either stroke, TIA, or an asymptomatic presentation occur with similar frequencies of 37 percent, 30 percent, and 33 percent, respectively.

LABORATORY DIAGNOSIS

The diagnosis of stenosis or occlusion of large extracerebral and intracerebral arteries relies on a number of techniques that are being increasingly used in the management of patients with TIAs or stroke and, to a lesser extent, in asymptomatic individuals with suspected atherostenosis of those arteries. These tests are labeled as noninvasive when they rely on pulse, pressure measurements, neuroimaging (magnetic resonance angiography), or ultrasound techniques, in contradistinction to the invasive technique of contrast cerebral angiography. They are discussed in detail in Chapter 29.

Our policy in the use of noninvasive diagnostic techniques is to obtain duplex ultrasound in all patients with suspected extracranial ICA disease, along with transcranial Doppler for the evaluation of intracranial arteries in those suspected of having atherostenosis or occlusion in the carotid or vertebrobasilar system.

TREATMENT

A number of treatments for cerebral atherothrombosis have been added in recent years to the available therapeutic options, largely as a result of the conduction of multicenter clinical trials. Among these, two major clinical trials (the North American Symptomatic Carotid Endarterectomy Trial [NASCET] and the European Carotid Surgery Trial [ECST]) have definitely established carotid endarterectomy as the treatment of choice for stroke prevention in patients with symptomatic (TIA or minor stroke) extracranial atherosclerosis of the ICA with stenosis of 70 percent or more. In both studies, the comparison between the randomized groups of medical and surgical therapy conclusively demonstrated a significantly lower frequency of stroke events in patients in the surgical group: in NASCET, after 24 months of follow-up, 26 percent of the medical group patients had a stroke ipsilaterally to the symptomatic ICA, whereas only 9 percent in the surgical group experienced this endpoint (Fig. 30-3). In the ECST trial, these figures were 16.8 percent for the medical group and 10.3 percent for the surgical group, after a follow-up of 33 months. The difference between the groups was statistically significant in both trials. In the ECST, patients with symptomatic ICA stenosis of 30 percent or less were also included, and there was no demonstrated superiority of surgery

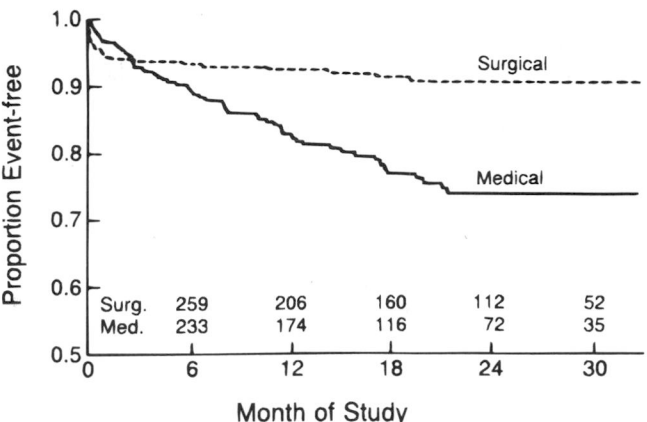

FIG. 30-3. Survival curves of patients free of ipsilateral stroke in the surgical and medical groups. Difference significant ($P < .001$) at 18 months of followup. (From North American Symptomatic Carotid Endarterectomy Trial Collaborators: Beneficial effect of carotid endarterectomy in symptomatic patients with high-grade carotid stenosis. N Engl J Med 325:445, 1991, with permission.)

over medical management. In the intermediate group of moderately severe ICA stenosis (between 30 and 69 percent), both studies still are continuing patient recruitment, since no difference between the surgical and medical group has been detected in interim analysis of the data.

In patients with carotid TIAs without a surgical lesion in the appropriate ICA, and in those with vertebrobasilar TIAs, the currently recommended treatment for stroke prevention is with antiplatelet agents. The most commonly used agent is aspirin (acetylsalicylic acid [ASA]) since it has been shown to be superior to placebo in a number of clinical trials involving over 9,000 patients. Its ideal dose has not been determined yet, and the controversy over the use of high (975 to 1,300 mg/d) or low (80 to 300 mg/d) doses of ASA still continues. In instances of ASA intolerance or failure of ASA to prevent stroke in TIA patients, a commonly used drug is ticlopidine, which has been shown to be superior to placebo and ASA, in secondary and primary stroke prevention studies, respectively. Its mechanism of action differs from that of ASA (a cyclo-oxygenase inhibitor) and other antiplatelet agents such as dipyridamole (a phosphodiasterase inhibitor), as it acts by inhibiting the binding of fibrinogen to the platelet wall, as a first step leading to platelet aggregation. Given in a dose of 250 mg twice a day, ticlopidine decreased by 13 percent the rate of stroke events in TIA patients in comparison with ASA. Its main side effects are gastrointestinal intolerance, primarily diarrhea, and a low-frequency but potentially life-threatening risk of neutropenia. The latter requires close monitoring of the neutrophil counts every 2 weeks, for a period of 3 months, since all reported instances of severe ticlopidine-related neutropenia (absolute neutrophil count $\leq$ $450/mm^3$) have occurred within 90 days from treatment onset—none beyond that period of time. A secondary inconvenience with the use of ticlopidine is its higher price, estimated in 1995 at approximately $85 per month for a dose of 250 mg twice a day, as opposed to $1.33 to $6 per month with enteric-coated ASA treatment at a dose of 325 mg/day or 650 mg twice a day, respectively.

The role of warfarin in the treatment of TIAs is still unclear. In most situations in which surgical treatment is not an option, failure to prevent stroke with ASA or ticlopidine is followed by treatment with warfarin. However, the value of warfarin in this setting has not been properly evaluated in comparison with antiplatelet agents or in relationship to its significant potential for producing life-threatening hemorrhagic complications. In agreement with old opinion and practice, recent data have suggested a benefit of warfarin over ASA for stroke prevention in patients with TIAs due to intracranial atherosclerotic disease in the carotid circulation. By extrapolating these data to the vertebrobasilar circulation, warfarin is generally favored over the antiplatelet agents for stroke prevention in patients with posterior circulation TIAs and documented (by magnetic resonance angiography or contrast angiography) atherosclerotic disease in that territory.

SUGGESTED READINGS

Castaigne P, Lhermitte F, Gautier JC et al: Internal carotid artery occlusion: a study of 61 instances in 50 patients with post-mortem data. Brain 93: 231, 1970

European Carotid Surgery Trialists' Collaborative Group: MRC European Carotid Surgery Trial: interim results for symptomatic patients with severe (70–99%) or with mild (0–29%) carotid stenosis. Lancet 337:1235, 1991

Fisher CM, Ojemann RG: A clinico-pathologic study of carotid endarterectomy plaques. Rev Neurol 142:573, 1986

Hass WK, Easton JD, Adams HP et al: A randomized trial comparing ticlopidine hydrochloride with aspirin for the prevention of stroke in high risk patients. N Engl J Med 321:501, 1989

Jonas S: Anticoagulant therapy in cerebrovascular disease: review and meta-analysis. Stroke 19:1043, 1988

Mohr JP, Caplan LR, Melski JW et al: The Harvard cooperative stroke registry: a prospective registry. Neurology 28:754, 1978

North American Symptomatic Carotid Endarterectomy Trial Collaborators (NASCET): Beneficial effect of carotid endarterectomy in symptomatic patients with high-grade carotid stenosis. N Engl J Med 325:445, 1991

Patrono C: Aspirin as an antiplatelet drug. N Engl J Med 330:1287, 1994

Pessin MS, Hinton RC, Davis KR et al: Mechanisms of acute carotid stroke. Ann Neurol 6:245, 1979

Tatemichi TK, Young WL, Prohovnik I et al: Perfusion insufficiency in limb shaking transient ischemic attacks. Stroke 21:341, 1990

31. CEREBRAL EMBOLISM

CARLOS S. KASE
CONRADO J. ESTOL

Stroke due to embolism is common and results from the sudden obstruction of a cerebral artery by particulate material that originates proximal to the occlusion site and has been carried to it by the circulation. The sources of such material are usually located in the heart and the large vessels (aorta, carotid artery, vertebral artery) (Table 31-1). This mechanism of ischemic stroke is characterized by a number of distinctive clinical and anatomic features that separate it from the atherothrombotic variety of brain infarction.

SOURCES OF EMBOLIC MATERIAL

Embolic material may differ in type, size, and mechanical characteristics that in turn determine to some extent its behavior in the cerebral circulation.

Embolic material of cardiac origin is often composed of fragments of thrombus that originate from either the left atrium or atrial appendage in instances of chronic atrial fibrillation with

TABLE 31-1. Sources of Cerebral Embolism

High-risk sources
  Mechanical prosthetic valve
  Mitral stenosis with atrial fibrillation
  Atrial fibrillation (other than lone atrial fibrillation)
  Left atrial/atrial appendage thrombus
  Sick sinus syndrome
  Recent myocardial infarction (<4 weeks)
  Left ventricular thrombus
  Dilated cardiomyopathy
  Akinetic left ventricular segment
  Atrial myxoma
  Infective endocarditis

Medium-risk sources
  Mitral valve prolapse
  Mitral annulus calcification
  Mitral stenosis without atrial fibrillation
  Left atrial turbulence (smoke)
  Atrial septal aneurysm
  Patent foramen ovale
  Atrial flutter
  Lone atrial fibrillation
  Bioprosthetic cardiac valve
  Nonbacterial thrombotic endocarditis
  Congestive heart failure
  Hypokinetic left ventricular segment
  Myocardial infarction (>4 weeks, <6 months)

(From Adams HP, Bendixen BH, Kappelle LJ et al: Classification of subtype of acute ischemic stroke: definitions for use in a multicenter clinical trial. Stroke 24:35, 1993, with permission.)

or without associated rheumatic valvular disease, or the left ventricle as a result of mural thrombus formation after recent or remote myocardial infarction. In each instance, the embolic material is mechanically unstable at the site of final occlusion, and is prone to spontaneous fragmentation or dissolution by the body's fibrinolytic system, with eventual partial or complete reestablishment of the circulation at the site of the occlusion. Other forms of unstable particulate material of cardiac origin include air bubbles or platelet aggregates formed during open-heart surgery under cardiopulmonary bypass. Embolic fragments that are mechanically more stable include septic emboli originating in infected valvular vegetations in bacterial endocarditis, fibrocalcific materials from degenerated mitral or aortic valves, and cholesterol-fibrin emboli from denuded (ulcerated) aortic, carotid, or vertebral atheromatous plaques.

Cardiac Sources

Atrial Fibrillation. Chronic and, to a lesser extent, paroxysmal atrial fibrillation in the setting of rheumatic heart disease increases the risk of cerebral embolism 17-fold in comparison with control populations. Even nonrheumatic atrial fibrillation carries a five- to six-fold increase in the risk of cerebral embolism, making atrial fibrillation the single most important cardiac risk factor for cerebral embolism. The prevalence of atrial fibrillation increases steadily with age, to approximately 15 percent in individuals older than 75 years of age, and it carries a risk of stroke of at least 5 percent per year in the absence of oral anticoagulant treatment. Factors that increase the risk of systemic (including cerebral) embolism in patients with atrial fibrillation include recent conversion from paroxysmal to chronic atrial fibrillation, congestive heart failure, "spontaneous echo contrast" on transesophageal echocardiogram (TEE), and changes between atrial fibrillation and sinus rhythm as a result of electric or pharmacologic cardioversion.

Myocardial Infarction. Recent myocardial infarction, especially of the anterior wall, carries a 2 to 3 percent risk of cerebral embolism within the first 30 days, largely as a result of fresh mural thrombus formation. Factors that increase the embolic risk in this setting include concomitant atrial arrhythmias and congestive heart failure. In the chronic state of a healed myocardial infarction, a persistent risk of cerebral embolic events in the order of 5 percent per year results from residual ventricular aneurysms or akinetic segments of the left ventricle, within which clot can occasionally be documented by TEE.

Bacterial Endocarditis.   The presence of infected mitral or aortic valvular vegetations in bacterial endocarditis constitutes a major source of cerebral embolism. Among the neurologic complications of bacterial endocarditis, cerebral embolism accounts for as many as 29 percent, a frequency that surpasses that of hemorrhagic stroke related to septic arteritis or mycotic aneurysm rupture. In the modern era of decreasing rheumatic heart disease but increasing use of intravascular manipulations, illicit intravenous drugs, and immunosuppression, the most common responsible organisms in bacterial endocarditis have shifted from the low-virulence *Streptococcus viridans* to the more virulent *Staphylococcus aureus* and fungi. The general resistance of these more virulent organisms to antibiotic and antifungal agents results in an increased frequency of cerebral septic emboli and mortality, in comparison with infection with the *Streptococcus* species.

Prosthetic Heart Valves.   Mechanical heart valves carry a substantial risk of cerebral embolism of about 3 percent per year, even in the presence of chronic oral anticoagulation. The embolic risk is higher with mitral than with aortic valves, and it is potentiated by the concomitant occurrence of atrial fibrillation. The introduction of bioprosthetic valves with lower potential for clot formation, along with the routine use of anticoagulants (at times in association with antiplatelet agents) has dramatically reduced the frequency of this complication.

Mitral Valve Prolapse.   The high frequency of mitral valve prolapse in the general, asymptomatic population (2 to 6 percent), especially in women, makes the interpretation of its association with ischemic stroke difficult. However, instances of embolic stroke in young patients with mitral valve prolapse and no other identifiable cause of stroke has been reported, especially in the setting of myxomatous degeneration of the mitral valve with resulting insufficiency. Additional factors such as atrial fibrillation or infectious endocarditis may be necessary for cerebral embolism to occur in some patients with mitral valve prolapse.

Patent Foramen Ovale and Interatrial Septal Aneurysm.   An abnormal communication between the right and left atria via a patent foramen ovale is found in about 10 percent of the general asymptomatic population in those younger than 45 years of age. In patients with an otherwise unexplained ischemic stroke in the same age group, the prevalence of patent foramen ovale as detected by "air contrast" echocardiography with Valsalva maneuver rises significantly to 40 to 50 percent, suggesting that paradoxic embolism (of venous origin) through an abnormal right-to-left shunt is a potential source of embolic cerebral infarction. In addition, interatrial septal aneurysms, at times associated with a patent foramen ovale, also carry a risk of cerebral embolism.

Atrial Myxoma.   Atrial myxoma, a rare tumor of the left atrium and mitral valve, can be a source of multiple cerebral emboli, generally in the setting of systemic symptoms of malaise, fever, weight loss. The tumor emboli may be associated with the development of cerebral aneurysms that in their multiplicity and peripheral location in the cerebral circulation resemble the "mycotic" aneurysms of infectious endocarditis.

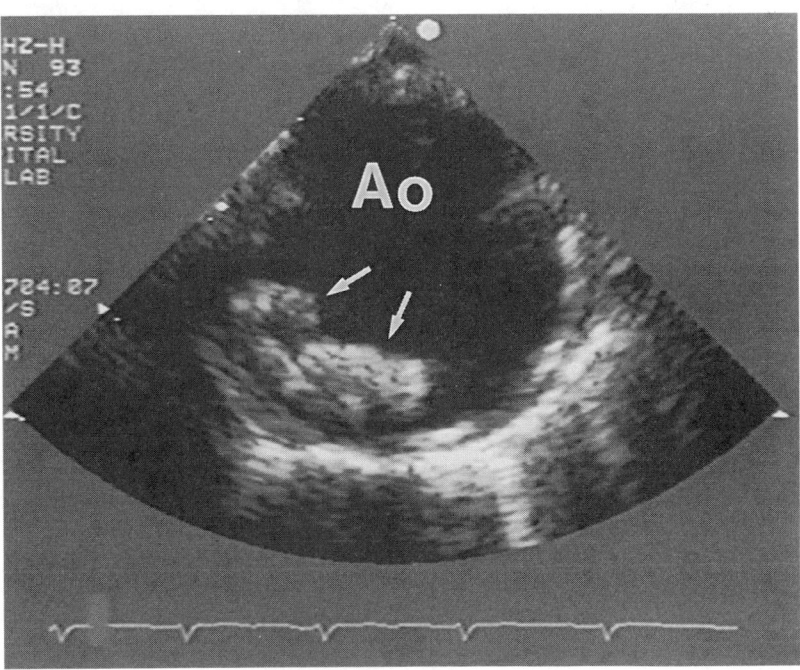

FIG. 31-1.   Transesophageal echocardiogram of descending aorta (Ao), with ulcerated atheromatous plaque and atheromatous debris and thrombus protruding into the aortic lumen (*arrows*). (Courtesy of Lisa A. Mendes, M.D., Department of Cardiology, Boston University Medical Center, Boston, MA.)

Arterial Sources

Arterial embolic sources lead to cerebral embolism by releasing particulate materials (generally thrombus, platelet-fibrin aggregates, or cholesterol-calcium particles) into distal arterial branches, generally intracranial, corresponding to the so-called artery-to-artery mechanism of embolism.

Ulcerated Aortic Atheroma.

As a mechanism of cerebral embolism, ulcerated aortic atheroma has been recently recognized in autopsy material. The transesophageal technique of echocardiography has allowed the visualization of extensive mobile thrombi protruding into the aortic lumen (Fig. 31-1). In patients without other detected embolic sources, this finding on TEE is considered the putative mechanism of cerebral embolism.

Carotid Artery Atheroma.

Cerebral embolism is assumed to be the stroke mechanism in instances of tight stenosis and acute occlusion of the extracranial internal carotid artery (ICA). The actual occurrence of distal embolism in patients with ulcerated carotid atheroma in the absence of significant stenosis is unclear. In the setting of acute ICA occlusion, the stroke mechanism has been inferred to be distal intracranial embolization in as many as two-thirds of the cases, the remaining one-third being on the basis of "distal insufficiency" with resulting borderzone infarcts. A similar mechanism of distal embolization of fresh clot is thought to be the main cause of stroke in acute carotid artery dissection. In yet another situation, that of long-standing extracranial ICA occlusion with formation of a "stump," presumed cerebral embolization has occurred as clot from the "stump" has traveled intracranially via the external carotid artery-to-ophthalmic artery collaterals to the intracranial ICA.

Vertebral Artery.

The extracranial vertebral artery is prone to trauma in the area of the C1–C2 junction, where extreme head rotation and hyperextension, after chiropractic neck manipulations, car and skiing accidents, voluntary neck "cracking" movements, and sneezing, can lead to dissection. This in turn can produce occlusion of the vertebral artery and distal embolization, generally into the ipsilateral posterior-inferior cerebellar artery (PICA), but also into the basilar artery and its distal branches (superior cerebellar artery [SCA] and posterior cerebral artery [PCA]).

CONSEQUENCES OF EMBOLIZATION OF INTRACRANIAL ARTERIES

Depending on their size, embolic particles can obstruct intracranial arteries either proximally or at distal branch sites, thus leading to great variability in infarct size, as well as location. In addition, the absence of local disease of the obstructed artery may result in only transient occlusion. Even with established infarction, autopsy studies of cerebral embolism performed days after stroke onset may fail to disclose the arterial obstruction. This is further confirmed by angiography, which documents the appropriate occlusion in up to 75 percent of the cases if the study is performed within 48 hours from onset, but in only 11 percent of patients if the study is delayed beyond that time.

The transient character of some cerebral embolic occlusions

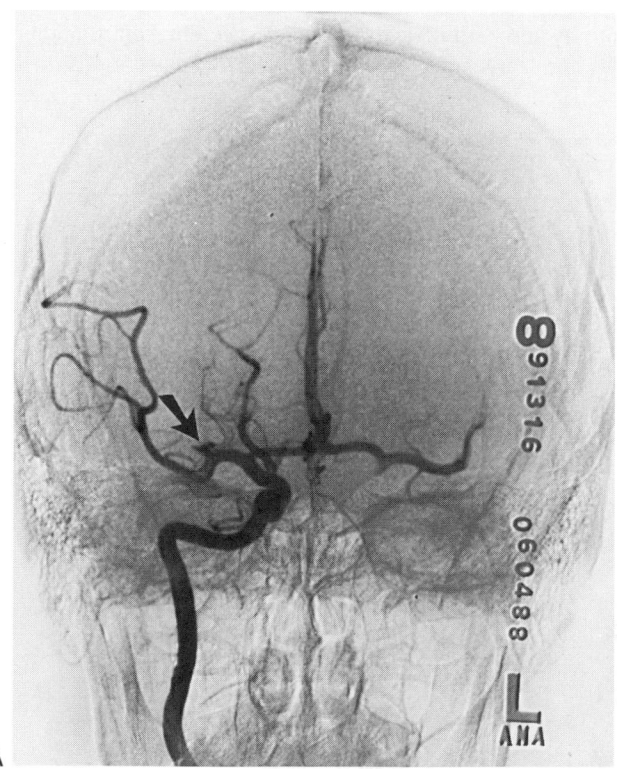
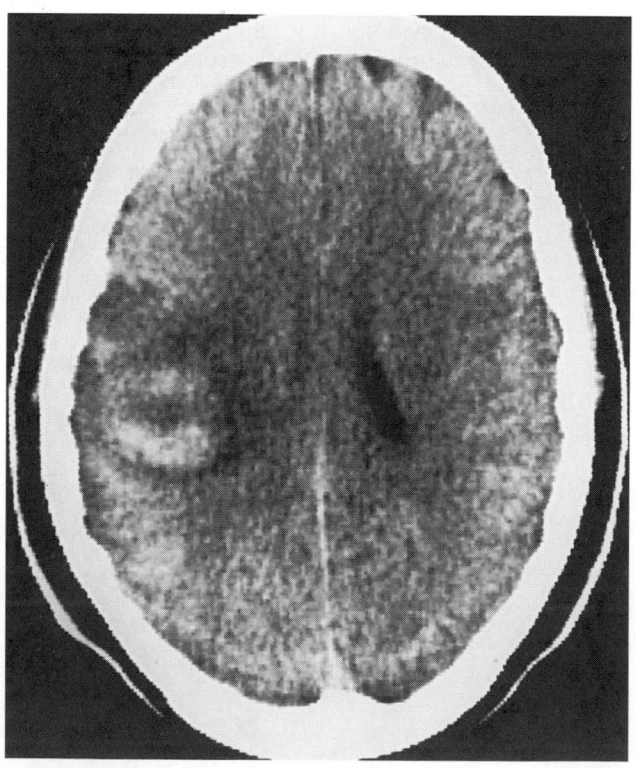

A   B

FIG. 31-2. **(A)** Embolic occlusion of the upper division of the middle cerebral artery (*arrow*), which did not reopen after treatment with rt-PA. **(B)** CT showing hemorrhagic infarction in the distal middle cerebral artery territory in the same patient. (From García JH, Ho K-L, Caccamo DV: Intracerebral hemorrhage: pathology of selected topics. pp. 49–72. In Kase CS, Caplan LR (eds): Intracerebral Hemorrhage. Butterworth-Heinemann, Boston, 1994, with permission.)

is also responsible for another characteristic feature, hemorrhagic infarction, in contrast to the "pale" or "bland" infarct that characterizes atherothrombotic infarcts. Hemorrhagic infarction results from spontaneous fragmentation and lysis of the embolus and reperfusion bleeding of vessels in the area of ischemia. Abnormal permeability of hypoxically injured capillaries results in leakage of red blood cells into the infarcted parenchyma by diapedesis (rather than actual rupture of the vascular wall as in parenchymal hemorrhage), with petechial hemorrhagic staining of the necrotic brain. Additionally, hemorrhagic infarction may in some instances result when bleeding occurs from collateral channels supplying the infarct, despite persistence of the embolic occlusion (Fig. 31-2). In both settings, the petechial staining of the already necrotic tissue usually has no clinical consequences, as there is no added tissue damage or mass effect as a result of the hemorrhagic transformation. Hemorrhagic infarction is more often seen pathologically (in 50 to 70 percent of cases) than by computed tomographic (CT) scan (in 5 to 43 percent of cases), suggesting the relative insensitivity of CT. Hemorrhagic infarct occurs after variable periods from the onset of the stroke, generally starting after at least 6

hours, reaching its peak by day 3 to 4, but may occur as late as 2 to 4 weeks after stroke onset if serial CT scanning is performed. The occurrence of hemorrhagic infarction after cerebral embolism may affect management decisions (see below).

SITES OF OCCLUSION

Cerebral embolism typically affects intracranial arteries. The larger extracranial ICA and vertebral artery are most susceptible to atherothrombotic occlusions (Fig. 31-3). Depending on the size of the embolus, the occlusion may affect a proximal artery at the circle of Willis, or a more distal vessel, such as a division or a cortical branch. Intracranial branch occlusions are virtually diagnostic of embolism, as atherothrombotic occlusions at these sites are rare.

Embolic particles have a predilection for certain intracranial vessels (Table 31-2), presumably reflecting the hemodynamics of the cerebral circulation and the patterns of angulation of the various branches off the main arterial trunks. The predominance of middle cerebral artery (MCA) embolic occlusions has been documented pathologically and angiographically, as well as by

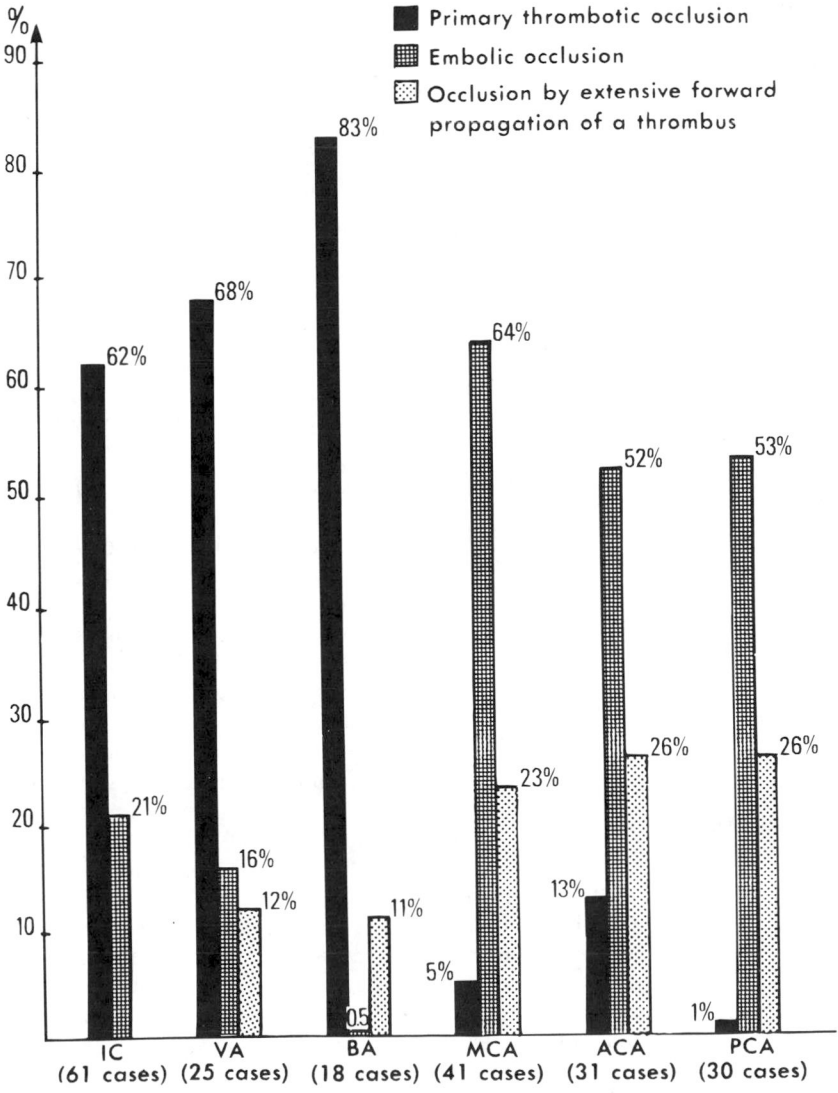

FIG. 31-3. Autopsy data of causes of cerebral infarction in the various vascular territories. (From Poirier J, Gray F, Escourolle R: Manual of Basic Neuropathology. pp. 65–102. WB Saunders, Philadelphia, 1990, with permission.)

TABLE 31-2. Intracranial Arteries Affected in Cerebral Embolism (*n* = 148)

MCA				PCA		
Stem	*UD*	*LD*	*ACA*	*Stem*	*Branch*	*Basilar*
55 (37%)	48 (32%)	20 (13%)	1 (0.6%)	10 (7%)	3 (2%)	11 (7%)

Abbreviations: MCA, middle cerebral artery; ACA, anterior cerebral artery; PCA, posterior cerebral artery; UD, upper division; LD, lower division.

(From Kunitz SC, Gross CR, Heyman A et al: The pilot Stroke Data Bank: definition, design, and data. Stroke 15:740, 1984, with permission.)

the observed destination of particles released in the proximal circulation in the process of performing therapeutic embolization of arteriovenous malformations.

CLINICAL FEATURES

Embolic occlusion typically produces a sudden focal neurologic deficit that is of maximal severity at its onset. The almost instantaneous character of a motor deficit often leads the patient to fall to the ground, not allowing time to sit down or hold onto a nearby source of support. The same features occur with the onset of aphasia or hemianopia, resulting in sudden speech dysfunction or ''jargon'' during conversation, or inability to see to one side. This contrasts with the more gradual and progressive onset of the neurologic deficits in atherothrombotic and lacunar infarction and, to a lesser extent, in intracerebral hemorrhage.

The focal deficits in cerebral embolism characteristically occur during activity, in the awake state, and the presence of a deficit on awakening is distinctly unusual. Other clinical features that may accompany cerebral embolism include the presence of headache, seizures, and loss of consciousness. Although infrequent, these manifestations occur in embolism more often than in atherothrombotic infarction, with figures in the order of 10 percent for headache and 5 to 7 percent for seizures and loss of consciousness. The latter are thought to be due to the sudden interruption of blood flow to a segment of the cerebral cortex, as a result of the embolic cortical branch occlusion. The mechanism of the headache is less clear, but possible contributors are distention of the pain-sensitive artery by the impacted embolus and possibly vasodilation of arteries adjacent to the occlusion as potential sources of collateral flow. The latter mechanism is favored by reported instances of headache onset occurring at the time of resolution, rather than at the onset, of a focal neurologic deficit. The location of the headache is at times correlated with the site of arterial embolic occlusion: the temporal area in MCA stem occlusion, lateral retro-ocular in PCA occlusion, occipitocervical in vertebral artery (VA) occlusion or dissection, and cervical and/or hemifacial in extracranial ICA occlusion or dissection.

Patterns of Evolution of Neurologic Deficits Due to Cerebral Embolism

The course that follows in the first hours after the ''maximal from the onset'' deficit is quite variable, with either stability, fluctuation, dramatic improvement, or, rarely, worsening. A fluctuating course after onset, the ''nonsudden onset of cerebral embolism,'' refers to deficits that occur suddenly, then improve rapidly, to be followed by recurrence of the same initial deficits or, more commonly, one that additionally reflects occlusion of a more distal branch in the same territory of the vessel involved initially. An example of this course occurs from embolic occlusion of the intracranial ICA with sudden onset of a large hemi-

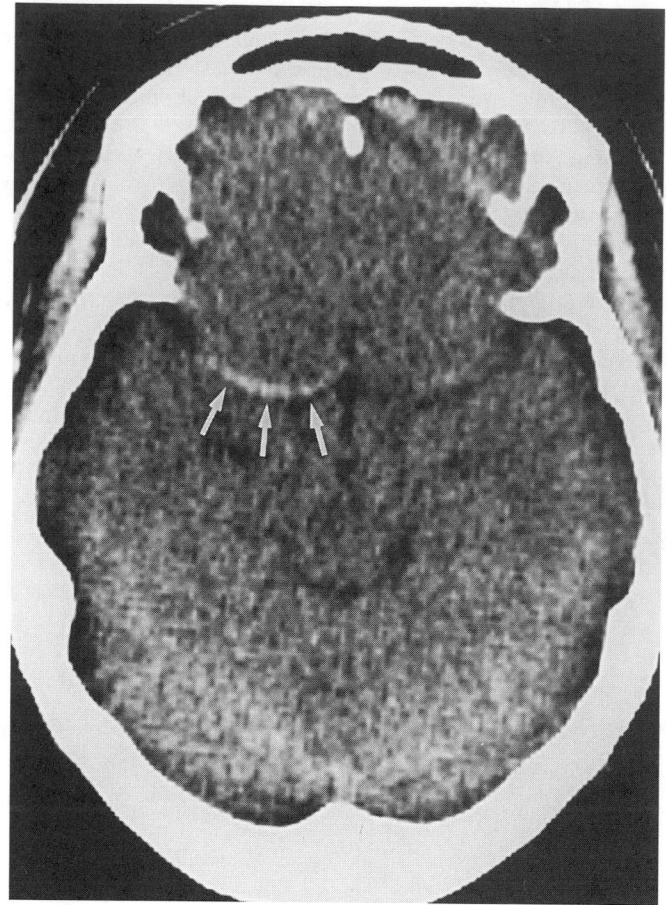

FIG. 31-4. Noncontrast CT scan with hyperdense MCA sign, representing clot within the middle cerebral artery trunk (*arrows*).

spheric syndrome, with rapid improvement (presumably due to effective distal collateral flow), followed by recurrence of a deficit indicative of distal MCA branch occlusion (such as aphasia). The latter is thought to result from migration of fragments of the original embolus into more distal branches in the MCA territory.

A similar mechanism accounts for instances of sudden onset of a major hemispheric deficit that is followed by a dramatic improvement within hours from onset. This course, referred to as ''the spectacular shrinking deficit'' syndrome, is often caused by embolic occlusion of the MCA stem with later spontaneous recanalization that may at times be suggested by the initial CT scan (Fig. 31-4). After a few hours from onset, the patient shows a remarkable improvement in neurologic function, with total or partial resolution of the hemiplegia, hemisensory defect, hemianopia, and aphasia. Subsequent CT scans often show signs of infarction in the deep MCA (lenticulostriate) territory, at times along with a second, separate focus of infarction in one of the divisional territories of the MCA.

A deteriorating course after a cerebral embolism is uncommon and may reflect antegrade or retrograde clot extension from the initial site, or massive hemorrhagic transformation of the infarct. Further clot extension at the site of the initial embolic occlusion can at times be demonstrated angiographically; its clinical manifestations are those of a gradual worsening of neurologic deficits, reflecting an enlarging area of ischemia, superimposed on the abrupt, and more restricted, initial deficit. Instances of neurologic deterioration subsequent to hemorrhagic transformation of the infarct are uncommon, since most hemorrhagic infarctions do not add further to the initial neurologic deficits. However, on occasion a massive hemorrhage within the infarcts (unlike a hemorrhagic infarction) may follow in the course of an otherwise uncomplicated embolic stroke and is most often associated with institution of anticoagulant and/or fibrinolytic treatment in the first few hours after stroke onset. Although such complications can also occur in the absence of treatments for unclear reasons, as part of the natural history of cerebral embolism, its frequency appears to be enhanced by the use of these agents, especially when used in combination. This suggests that a likely mechanism of this complication may be early reperfusion of the affected artery (generally the MCA stem) by the effect of the fibrinolytic agent, followed by massive hemorrhagic infarction/intracerebral hemorrhage due to reflow of blood into an ischemic vascular bed with abnormally increased permeability. The severity of the latter process of extravasation may be enhanced by the concomitant use of anticoagulation at the time of the reperfusion.

The clinical syndromes of cerebral embolism are varied, reflecting different sites of intracranial occlusions. They are discussed in detail in Chapter 41.

LABORATORY DIAGNOSIS

The laboratory diagnosis of cerebral embolism is divided into (1) the imaging documentation of the embolic occlusion and infarct topography by CT, magnetic resonance imaging (MRI), and angiography; and (2) the documentation of a cardiac or vascular embolic source by ultrasound and angiographic techniques.

Imaging

In the first hours after embolic infarction, both CT and MRI are usually negative for attenuation or signal changes in the parenchyma. However, noncontrast CT scan can document a hyperdensity consistent with clot in the area of the MCA stem in embolic occlusions (the hyperdense MCA sign) (Fig. 31-4); the MRI correlate is absence of a flow void in the artery occluded by an embolus.

CT scan shows the early signs of hypodensity in the parenchyma after about 6 to 12 hours from onset, and a well-established low-density area does not occur before 24 hours. In instances of early hemorrhagic transformation, the hyperdensity of hemorrhagic infarction may be documented earlier, but not usually before 6 hours from stroke onset. Other more subtle signs of early cerebral infarction can be detected after about 6 hours from onset. These include suggestions of obliteration of cortical sulci in massive MCA infarcts, representing early cerebral edema, and blurring of the gray/white matter distinction in the insular cortex area in MCA infarcts.

MRI shows the parenchymal changes of infarction earlier than CT, generally after about 8 hours from onset. The changes occur first in T2-weighted images as a ''bright signal'' in the area of infarction, followed by subsequent demonstration of infarction as ''low signal'' changes in T1-weighted sequences. This test is also sensitive in showing the early changes of cerebral edema as mass effect causing obliteration of sulci and cisterns, and as hyperintensity of the white more than the gray matter in the area of infarction. It is also accurate in the detection of subtle hemorrhagic changes within the infarct.

Contrast cerebral angiography has the ability to document embolic occlusions dependent on the time elapsed between stroke onset and the performance of the test. Its yield decreases dramatically (to about 17 percent) if the test is performed beyond 48 hours from onset, whereas it is high (about 75 percent) if performed within that period of time. This reflects the natural instability of embolic particles. The role of magnetic resonance angiography in the detection of intracranial embolic occlusions is still evolving. This technique still has poor resolution for demonstrating occlusion of branches of intracranial arteries, although missing groups of branches may be apparent. Furthermore, the degree of larger extracranial artery luminal stenosis/occlusion may be overestimated. It is expected that further refinements in technique will make it an alternative to conventional contrast angiography in the future.

Detection of Cardiac and Vascular Sources

Many of the common cardiac sources of systemic embolism can be suspected or confirmed with clinical examination (cardiac auscultation) and routine laboratory data such as chest x-rays and electrocardiogram. Such studies will uncover instances of atrial fibrillation, sick sinus syndrome, valvular disease, recent or remote myocardial infarction, and cardiomyopathy. The additional use of transthoracic echocardiography and especially TEE is indicated for confirmation of valvular disease (including mitral or aortic stenosis or insufficiency, mitral valve prolapse, vegetations in bacterial endocarditis or nonbacterial thrombotic endocarditis), atrial myxoma, documentation of post-myocardial infarction akinetic ventricular segments, ventricular aneurysms, mural thrombus, dilated cardiomyopathy with reduced ejection fraction, atrial septal aneurysm, and patent foramen ovale. The identification of ''spontaneous echo contrast'' in the dilated atria in atrial fibrillation correlates with embolic potential. The value of additional techniques, such as continuous (Holter) electrocardiographic monitoring, is low but helpful for the occasional detection of intermittent atrial arrhythmias (mainly atrial fibrillation). Only patients who have been symptomatic with lightheadedness or presyncope/syncope should be further investigated for intermittent arrhythmias with potential for cerebral embolization.

Although the finding of one of the above sources of cardiac embolism is an important element in assigning a presumptive embolic cause to a stroke in the proper clinical setting, it does not always prove a cause and effect relationship. In approximately 17 percent of patients with a high-risk cardioembolic source such as atrial fibrillation, noninvasive techniques document a concomitant stenosis of more than 50 percent in the extracranial carotid artery appropriate to the location of the ischemic stroke.

The investigation of vascular sources of systemic embolism (artery-to-artery) involves the study of extracranial arteries such as the carotid and VAs with ultrasound and angiography. In addition, the role of ulcerated atheroma with clot formation in the thoracic aorta can be effectively investigated with TEE. The techniques of vascular imaging are described in Chapter 30. Their application to the diagnostic evaluation of patients with suspected cerebral embolism aims at documenting a tightly stenotic proximal arterial lesion, with or without ulceration, appropriate to the intracranial occlusion. In the absence of a documented cardiac embolic source, such ultrasound findings should be considered the putative explanation for the embolic intracranial occlusion, and managed accordingly. If management involves plans for treating a surgically correctable lesion, most surgeons require the confirmatory use of contrast angiography prior to performing surgery. The alternative of substituting contrast angiography with the combined information of Doppler ultrasound and magnetic resonance angiography of the extracranial circulation in the presurgical assessment of these patients is currently being evaluated.

TREATMENT AND PREVENTION

Acute Treatment

The treatment of patients with an acute embolic stroke involves the principal issue of whether to use intravenous heparin anticoagulation for prevention of recurrent embolism. In patients with a high-risk embolic source such as atrial fibrillation or rheumatic heart disease, the risk of reembolization is thought to be in the order of 1 percent per day, for a cumulative rate of about 10 percent in the first 2 weeks after stroke onset. This high risk of stroke recurrence is the basis for the recommendation of early institution of heparin anticoagulation as a continuous intravenous infusion. Heparin is generally given without an initial bolus (because it often causes excessive prolongation of the activated partial thromboplastin time [aPTT] within the first 1 to 2 hours after administration), at a rate of 1,000 U/h, adjusting it to maintain an aPTT of 1.5 times control, generally corresponding to a value between 45 and 55 seconds. This treatment is maintained for several days, while the evaluation of the stroke mechanism proceeds. If the decision is made to treat the patient with long-term oral anticoagulants (warfarin), this is started, and upon reaching the dose necessary to maintain a prothrombin time (PT) of 1.5 times control (generally 16 to 20 seconds) and an international normalized ratio (INR) of 2 to 3, heparin is discontinued.

Treatment with heparin has to be closely monitored in order to avoid intracranial or systemic bleeding and drug-induced thrombocytopenia. Intracranial hemorrhage is a potential but low-risk complication of continuous intravenous heparin infusion in patients with an acute embolic infarct. Heparin is contraindicated in patients with septic cerebral embolism, because of the high propensity of septic emboli to produce necrosis of the arterial wall with potentially massive hemorrhage. In the setting of nonseptic emboli, early heparin anticoagulation to prevent recurrent embolism is a safe treatment, provided the level of anticoagulation is not excessive and the patient does not have a massive infarct or uncontrolled hypertension (i.e., a blood pressure more than 180/100 mmHg). The presence of a CT-detected hemorrhagic infarction has been considered a contraindication to the use of anticoagulation because of the fear of promoting further hemorrhagic transformation or even intracerebral hemorrhage by the anticoagulant effect. However, in instances in which the risk of recurrent embolism is great, as in patients with mechanical prosthetic heart valves or atrial fibrillation, heparin may be used safely if excessive anticoagulation is avoided and blood pressure is monitored closely.

Heparin-induced thrombocytopenia occurs in approximately 10 percent of patients treated. This complication takes two forms. Early thrombocytopenia (type I) occurs within the first 4 or 5 days of treatment, and is generally of mild character (not reaching platelet counts below 50,000/mm^3) and rarely associated with bleeding phenomena or thromboembolism. The platelet count usually recovers on its own, even without drug discontinuation. The cause is thought to be direct heparin-induced platelet aggregation. Late thrombocytopenia (type II) occurs toward the end of the first or second week of treatment and is serious (generally producing platelet counts below 50,000/ mm^3—often below 10,000/mm^3). It can be associated with hemorrhagic and especially thrombotic phenomena that can lead to stroke, myocardial infarction, or limb loss secondary to gangrene. These vascular complications result from massive intravascular aggregates of platelets (the "white clot" syndrome). The mechanism of this serious form of heparin-induced thrombocytopenia is thought to be a IgG- and IgM-induced immune response. The identification of this potentially serious complication requires routine monitoring of platelet counts in patients treated with intravenous heparin.

Other therapeutic modalities for acute cerebral embolism, such as thrombolytic and neuroprotector agents, are being actively evaluated, but currently these are still investigational strategies (see Ch. 44). Thrombolytic agents have the potential to lyse embolic occlusions and restore critical cerebral perfusion. Thrombolysis can be achieved by systemic (intravenous) or intra-arterial administration, but as yet, no direct comparison of these delivery modes has been studied. Preliminary evidence suggests that intra-arterial delivery is more effective than intravenous delivery in producing recanalization, but this technique requires sophisticated facilities and trained personnel, which may limit accessibility to treatment and exceed the narrow time frame before ischemic tissue becomes irreversibly injured. The critical issue of improved clinical outcome related to recanalization has not been unequivocally established.

Another group of agents, so-called neuroprotectors, have properties designed to limit the cascading toxic effects of the initial ischemic injury on the neuronal population at risk. These include calcium channel-blockers, n-methyl-D-aspartate (NMDA) receptor antagonists, and free-radical scavengers. Neuroprotective agents may limit the ischemic damage and, importantly, may provide additional time for the initiation of other treatments to restore arrested circulation, such as thrombolysis.

Primary Prevention

Primary prevention is most effective in patients with cardiac conditions with high potential for embolization, such as mechanical prosthetic heart valves and atrial fibrillation. In patients with mechanical prosthetic heart valves, the rate of systemic embolization is dramatically reduced by the use of chronic oral (warfarin) anticoagulation. The protection conferred by this agent can be further enhanced by the addition of antiplatelet agents, such as dipyridamole and especially aspirin (acetylsalicylic acid [ASA]). The recommended PT is 2 to 2.5 times control, with an INR of 2.5 to 3.5, values that are higher than those used for other indications for warfarin use. The dose of combined ASA treatment is 325 mg/day.

In patients with chronic atrial fibrillation, who are neurologically intact at the onset of the prophylactic treatment, the use of chronic warfarin anticoagulation results in a dramatic overall reduction of 86 percent in the risk of cerebral embolic events. Such effect has been documented in five consecutive clinical trials (see Section I). These studies have shown (1) a consistent beneficial effect of warfarin over placebo; (2) a smaller benefit from ASA over placebo in some studies (SPAF) but not in others (AFASAK, BAATAF); (3) a low rate of hemorrhagic complications when the PT and INR are tightly controlled, with PT values in the range of 1.25 times control; and (4) a benefit of warfarin that applies to secondary stroke prevention as well. These data have clearly established the value of warfarin anticoagulation for primary and secondary stroke prevention in patients with chronic atrial fibrillation. The value of ASA as a single agent is less impressive than that of warfarin, but its role in certain subgroups of patients, especially those over 75 years of age, will be further defined after the completion of ongoing clinical trials.

SUGGESTED READINGS

Amarenco P, Cohen A, Tzourio C et al: Atherosclerotic disease of the aortic arch and the risk of ischemic stroke. N Engl J Med 331:1474, 1994

Bogousslavsky J, Cachin D, Regli F et al: Cardiac sources of embolism and cerebral infarction: clinical consequences and vascular concomitants: the Lausanne Stroke Registry. Neurology 41:855, 1991

Caplan LR: Brain embolism, revisited. Neurology 43:1281, 1993

Caplan LR, Hier DB, D'Cruz I: Cerebral embolism in the Michael Reese Stroke Registry. Stroke 14:530, 1983

Cerebral Embolism Task Force: Cardiogenic brain embolism. Arch Neurol 43: 71, 1986

Fisher CM, Adams RD: Observations on brain embolism with special reference to the mechanism of hemorrhagic infarction. J Neuropathol Exp Neurol 10:92, 1951

Gács G, Merei FT, Bodosi M: Balloon catheter as a model of cerebral emboli in humans. Stroke 13:39, 1982

Hacke W, Zeumer H, Ferbert A et al: Intra-arterial thrombolytic therapy improves outcome in patients with acute vertebrobasilar occlusive disease. Stroke 19:1216, 1988

Hart RG, Easton JD: Hemorrhagic infarcts. Stroke 17:586, 1986

Yatsu FM, Hart RG, Mohr JP, Grotta JC: Anticoagulation of embolic strokes of cardiac origin: an update. Neurology 38:314, 1988

32. LACUNAR INFARCTION

CARLOS S. KASE
CONRADO J. ESTOL

Twenty percent of strokes are classified as lacunar infarctions (see Table 30-1). They represent areas of cerebral infarction measuring between a few millimeters and 1.5 cm, and they are also referred to as penetrating artery disease or small-vessel disease because affected vessels are the perforating branches of the main cerebral arteries—middle cerebral artery (MCA), anterior cerebral artery (ACA), posterior cerebral artery (PCA), basilar artery. These vessels measure between 40 and 400 μm (less than 0.5 mm) in diameter, and they supply deep hemispheric structures such as the basal ganglia, internal capsule, and thalamus, as well as portions of the brainstem, such as the basis pontis. As a result of the small size and parenchymal location of the affected vessels, lacunar infarcts are, by definition, small and deep infarcts. Their common sites are (1) the internal capsule (the posterior limb, genu, or less commonly, the anterior limb); (2) the caudate nucleus; (3) the basal ganglia (putamen, globus pallidus); (4) the thalamus (rarely in combination with the internal capsule); (5) the centrum semiovale and corona radiata; (6) the basis pontis; and (7) the cerebellum.

PATHOGENESIS

Lipohyalinosis

In a number of landmark neuropathologic studies, Fisher defined the arterial abnormalities related to lacunar infarctions. Affected vessels were found to have an abnormality referred to as lipohyalinosis, a process different from large-vessel ather-

oma. This is a degenerative change due to hypertension, which results in the deposit of a hyaline, amorphous substance within the arterial wall, at times progressing to occlusion of the lumen, causing a small ischemic infarct (lacune) (Fig. 32-1). Usually the obstructing lesion is along the course of the small vessel some distance from its origin. Hypertension was found in as many as 75 percent of patients with lacunar infarcts documented in the Harvard Stroke Registry. However, lacunar infarcts can also be the result of other mechanisms described in this chapter.

In some patients the lipohyalinotic changes in the arterial wall progressively weaken the wall, leading to dilation and microaneurysm formation. This lesion may express itself by either a small lacunar infarct, or it may rupture and cause a hypertensive intracerebral hemorrhage.

Embolism

Both the classic small lacunes and larger deep infarcts of greater than 2 cm in diameter can be the result of small cardiac or artery-to-artery (from the carotid, aorta) embolism. This notion is supported by the demonstration of lacunar infarcts at autopsy, in which the perforating artery leading to the lacune is free of disease in its wall, a finding highly suggestive of an embolic mechanism of occlusion, assuming disappearance of the original occluding embolus. However, the mere coexistence of a lacunar infarct with a proximal cardiac or vascular source of embolism does not necessarily establish a cause and effect relationship. Other clinical criteria, in particular the mode of onset and the course and clinical features of the neurologic deficit, need to be considered in the diagnosis of the mechanism of a lacunar infarct.

Branch Artery Disease (Junctional Plaque and Microatheroma Mechanism)

Mechanisms that affect the entire territory of a branch produce an infarct larger than the typical lacune, and result from junctional plaques or microatheroma involving the penetrator at its origin. Caplan and Fisher called attention to lacunar infarcts, generally larger than the classical small lacunes, that were caused by occlusion of penetrating branches at their origin from the parent vessels, producing a large swath of infarction. A plaque of atheroma in the MCA or the basilar artery could grow to involve the emerging penetrating artery, leading to its occlusion. Because these plaques affect the parent vessel and a penetrating artery simultaneously, they are also known as junctional plaques. Other possible mechanisms of occlusion involve the growth of microatheroma within the very origin of the penetrating vessel.

CLINICAL FEATURES

The mode of onset and course of lacunar infarcts differ from those of large-vessel disease. Lacunar infarcts are preceded by transient ischemic attacks (TIAs) in 15 to 20 percent of cases, whereas at least 50 percent of atherothrombotic infarcts are preceded by TIAs. Some features characterize the TIAs of lacunar mechanism:

(1) They generally occur over shorter periods of time (2 to 5 days) before the onset of infarction, in comparison with weeks to months in cases of large artery atherothrombosis.

(2) TIAs from small-vessel disease tend to occur in clusters,

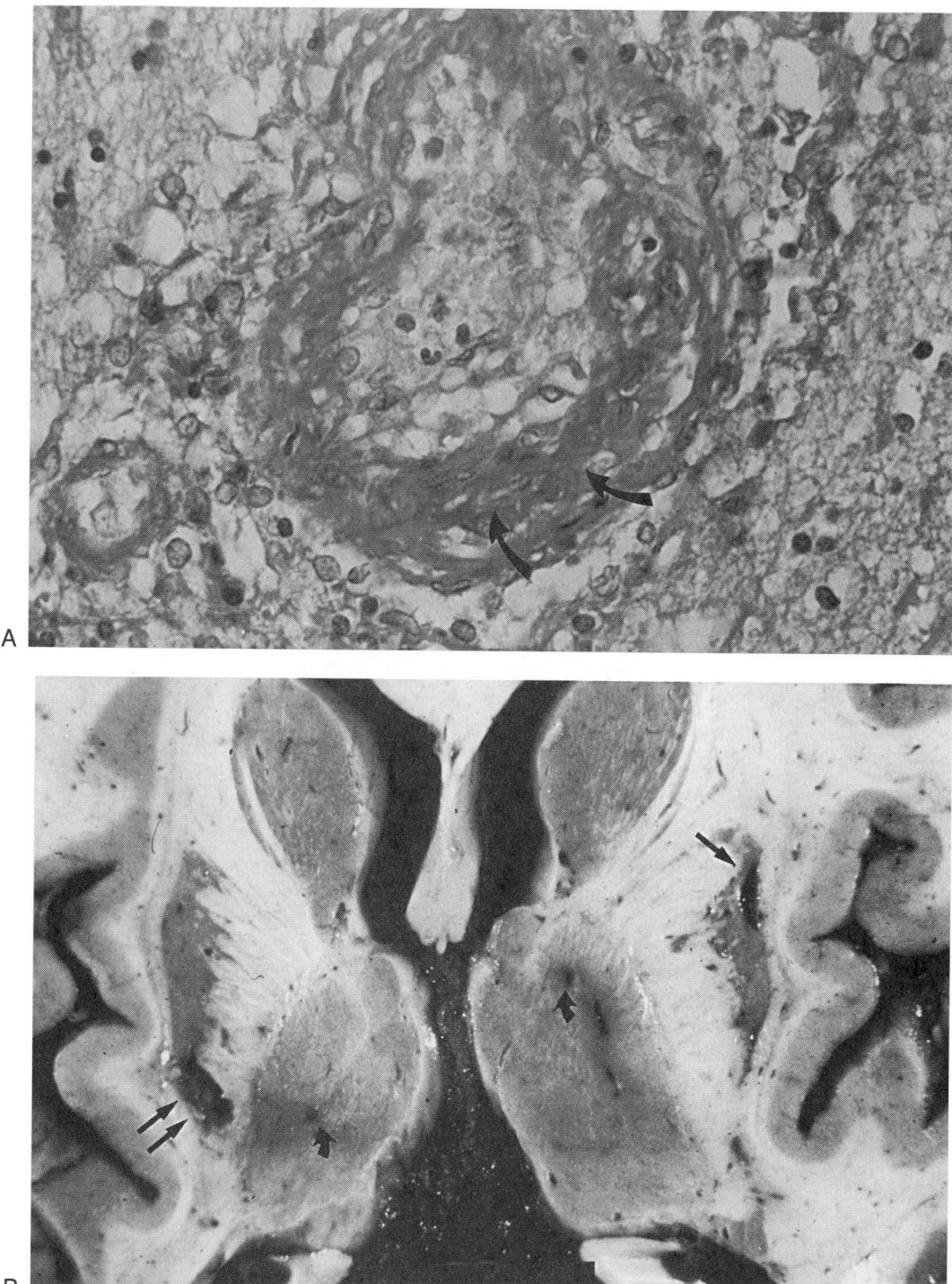

FIG. 32-1. **(A)** Small parenchymal artery with lipohyalinosis (*curved arrows*). (H&E, × 45.) **(B)** Multiple lacunar infarcts in the putamen (*arrow*), posterior limb of the internal capsule (*double arrows*), and thalami (*curved arrows*). (Courtesy of Michael S. Pessin, M.D., Department of Neurology, New England Medical Center, Boston, MA.)

occasionally even several times a day (a so-called flurry of TIAs), whereas large-vessel TIAs usually present as recurrent isolated episodes

(3) TIAs from small-vessel ischemia are more stereotyped (e.g., weakness of the entire hemibody) as compared to the more variable features of large vessel TIAs (transient monocular blindness, monoparesis, or dysphasia in the case of internal carotid artery [ICA] stenosis).

The time of onset in lacunar infarcts (and atherothrombotic strokes) is equally distributed during sleep and activity, as opposed to embolism and intracranial hemorrhage, which virtually always occur during the waking hours. The deficits caused by lacunar infarcts often have an insidious onset and a progressive course, in contrast with the sudden onset that characterizes embolism. Lacunar infarcts are the most commonly observed ischemic strokes that feature a gradually progressive course after onset.

Headache, seizures and mental status changes, which are frequent findings in cerebral embolism and intracranial hemorrhage, do not occur with lacunar infarcts. The absence of cognitive changes and seizures reflects the subcortical nature of lacunes, and the lack of headache presumably is due to the absence of pain fibers in small parenchymal penetrating arteries.

Lacunar Syndromes

The clinical syndromes related to lacunar infarcts have been described in detail since 1965 by Fisher, and they are discussed in detail in Chapter 42. There are approximately 50 possible lacunar syndromes, but the most frequently encountered include pure motor hemiparesis, pure sensory stroke, sensorimotor stroke, ataxic hemiparesis, and the dysarthria-clumsy hand syndrome. Multiple lacunar infarctions in the deep portions of the cerebral hemispheres cause the ''lacunar state'' (''état lacunaire''), characterized by a pseudobulbar syndrome with dysarthria, dysphagia, emotional lability, and a small-stepped gait (''marche à petits pas'').

Binswanger's Disease and Related Subcortical Degenerations

The relationship between small-vessel vasculopathy causing discrete lacunes and the more widespread cerebral white matter degeneration associated with progressive cognitive impairment and focal neurologic deficits (Binswanger's encephalopathy) is unsettled. The ready identification of white-matter hypodensities on computed tomography (CT), or high-signal lesions on T2-weighted magnetic resonance imaging (MRI) have led to correlation studies in both nondemented older patients and those with progressive dementia. Limited CT-neuropathologic observations in nondemented and demented patients with periventricular white-matter hypodensities and presumed Binswanger's encephalopathy have shown the triad of demyelination, axonal loss, and thickening of arteriolar walls. General cerebral atrophy, with ventricular enlargement, and multiple lacunes are frequently present. However, the CT findings alone do not reliably predict the presence of dementia since they are frequently seen in older patients with or without dementia who have hypertension and other vascular risk factors.

Patients with multiple lacunes may develop a pseudobulbar state characterized by progressive bulbar dysfunction and, rarely, cognitive impairment, resulting from the cumulative effects of discrete lacunes from small penetrating arterial disease. The occurrence of progressive cognitive impairment in association with multiple white-matter lesions on neuroimaging has led to a broader differential diagnosis that includes Binswanger's encephalopathy, congophilic angiopathy, normal pressure hydrocephalus, and other leukoencephalopathies. Often, the diagnosis of Binswanger's disease is raised because of the neuroimaging findings in patients with progressive dementia. Whether this reflects chronic white-matter ischemia from small penetrating arterial disease related to hypertension or other pathogenetic factors is unclear. At least one genetic variant, cerebral autosomal dominant arteriopathy with subcortical infarcts and leukoencephalopathy (CADASIL), has been identified in some familial clusterings. The diagnosis of Binswanger's encephalopathy and related subcortical white-matter conditions reflects our sharpened clinical observations and improved neuroimaging techniques, but their exact pathogenesis awaits further clarification from cliniconeuropathologic studies.

DIFFERENTIAL DIAGNOSIS

The presence of a pure motor hemiparesis may at times be associated with isolated signs of either visual neglect, dysphasia, or other cognitive deficits. This combination generally results from embolism to the MCA stem leading to a deep, large striatocapsular and cortical infarct as shown by MRI or CT. These features reinforce the important clinical dictum that pure motor hemiparesis secondary to lacunar infarction should be diagnosed only in the presence of a deficit limited to the motor system. In addition, the presence of headache, seizures, mental status changes, an unusual distribution of weakness, and an absent history of hypertension should all raise the suspicion that the syndrome is not lacunar, prompting the use of further diagnostic testing. Rarely, a subdural hematoma, small parenchymal hemorrhage, tumor, or limited large-artery cortical infarction may explain these imitators of pure motor hemiparesis.

Since large- and small-artery disease share common risk factors, large-vessel atherosclerosis of varying degrees can exist coincidentally in some patients with lacunar infarcts. This could potentially lead to an unnecessary carotid endarterectomy if the physician is not familiar with the presentation of lacunar disease. On the other hand, patients with typical lacunar syndromes may have a small hemorrhage or cortical infarct resulting in a limited deficit unrelated to penetrating artery disease.

Hypertensive hemorrhages and lacunar infarcts have the common neuropathologic substrate of lipohyalinosis affecting small penetrating arteries, and occasionally may result in similar clinical signs such as pure motor hemiparesis or pure sensory stroke from a small capsular or thalamic hemorrhage, respectively. However, clinical differentiation is relatively simple since the CT or MRI will readily document the hemorrhage.

A severe stenosis of the ICA may cause hemodynamic insufficiency and ischemia in the MCA penetrator territory (the lenticulostriate arteries), with resulting internal capsule infarction and pure motor hemiparesis. Extracranial ICA disease may be suspected if there is a history of carotid TIAs, or a carotid bruit. A duplex Doppler scan of the carotids, a contrast angiogram, or magnetic resonance angiography (MRA) should be obtained to confirm the diagnosis and consider carotid endarterectomy.

DIAGNOSIS

The clinical history and findings on examination in most cases will strongly suggest the diagnosis of a lacunar syndrome. Neu-

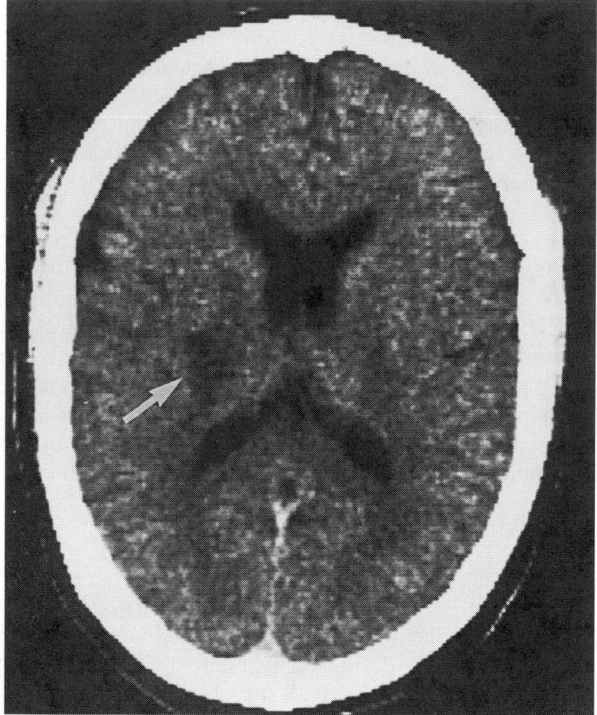

FIG. 32-2. CT showing lacunar infarction in the posterior limb of the right internal capsule (*arrows*) 5 days after onset of left pure motor hemiparesis, following a normal CT scan on the day of onset. (Courtesy of Michael S. Pessin, M.D., Department of Neurology, New England Medical Center, Boston, MA.)

roimaging will usually provide confirmation of the clinical suspicion; if the initial scan is negative, a later scan at 2 to 5 days may show the infarct (Fig. 32-2). MRI is superior to CT in the detection of lacunar infarctions, especially in the brainstem, cerebellum, and thalamus (Fig. 32-3). In most patients with lacunar syndromes, especially pure motor hemiparesis, the lacune will be documented by CT or MRI.

The use of diagnostic techniques for documentation of cardiac or vascular embolic sources is necessary only in patients who present with an unclear history and clinical and imaging evidence of a lacunar infarction appropriate to the neurologic findings. Evaluation should include a search for both cardiac and vascular embolic sources, especially intracranial atherosclerotic disease. The latter is important in the documentation of "branch syndromes" (in the basilar artery, MCA) due to atherosclerotic disease of the parent artery that gives rise to the involved perforator(s). This is currently being increasingly investigated with MRA instead of contrast cerebral angiography in order to minimize the potential risks of cerebral angiography.

TREATMENT

Inadvertent or purposeful excessive lowering of blood pressure in patients with lacunar infarction is a common mistake that can at times result in marked neurologic worsening. The blood pressure should be lowered only if it is consistently higher than 220 mmHg systolic and 120 mmHg diastolic on three successive measurements every 15 minutes. It is preferable not to decrease the blood pressure below 170/90 during the first few days after stroke onset, and it should subsequently be slowly lowered to normal or near normotensive values over the following 2 to 4 weeks. Aspirin (acetylsalicylic acid [ASA]), 325 mg/d, is often given, more for reducing general cardiovascular effects than as a proven agent in the prevention of stroke progression or recurrence. Anticoagulation should be considered in branch artery disease when the parent vessel (large artery) shows significant narrowing and is not accessible to surgical correction. The potential value of ASA or warfarin for secondary prevention of recurrent lacunar (and other) infarcts is currently being investigated in the multicenter Warfarin-Aspirin Recurrent Stroke Study (WARSS). Results from this trial should be available sometime after 1998.

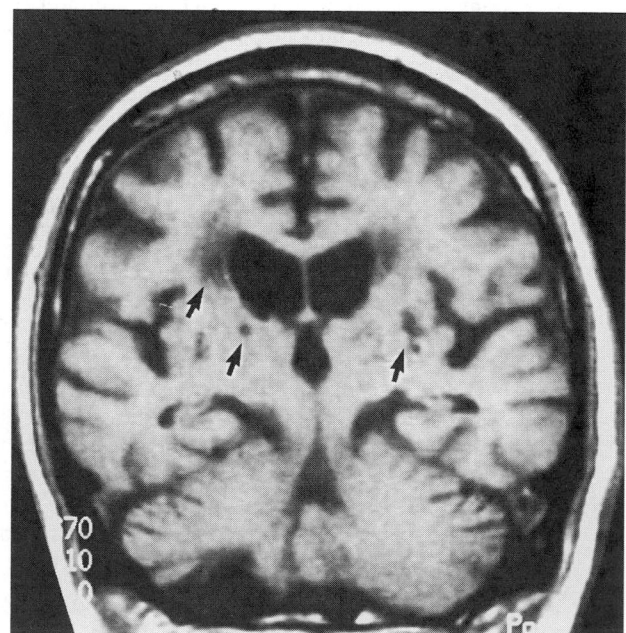
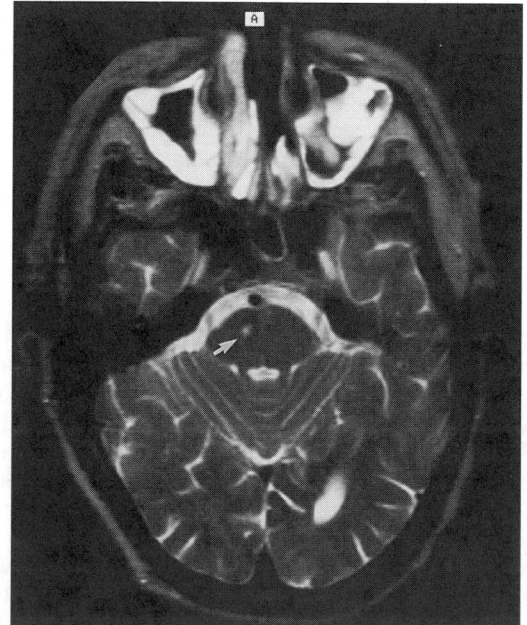

FIG. 32-3. **(A)** T1-weighted MRI showing old lacunes in right thalamus, right caudate, and left putamen (*arrows*). **(B)** T2-weighted MRI showing lacune in right basis pontis (*arrow*). (Courtesy of Rita Bhatia, M.D., Department of Radiology, Boston University Medical Center, Boston, MA.)

SUGGESTED READINGS

Fisher CM: Lacunar infarcts: a review. Cerebrovasc Dis 1:311, 1991

Fisher CM: Pure sensory stroke and allied conditions. Stroke 13:434, 1982

Fisher CM: Ataxic hemiparesis. Arch Neurol 35:126, 1978

Fisher CM: The arterial lesions underlying lacunes. Acta Neuropathol 12:1, 1969

Fisher CM: A lacunar stroke, the dysarthria-clumsy hand syndrome. Neurology 17:614, 1967

Fisher CM: Lacunes, small deep cerebral infarcts. Neurology 15:774, 1965

Fisher CM: Pure motor hemiplegia of vascular origin. Arch Neurol 13:30, 1965

Fisher CM, Caplan LR: Basilar artery branch occlusion: a cause of pontine infarction. Neurology 21:900, 1971

Miller V: Lacunar stroke: a reassessment. Arch Neurol 40:129, 1983

Mohr JP: Lacunes. Stroke 13:3, 1982

Mohr JP, Kase CS, Meckler R et al: Sensorimotor stroke. Arch Neurol 34:734, 1977

33. INTRACEREBRAL HEMORRHAGE

CARLOS S. KASE
CONRADO J. ESTOL

Intracerebral hemorrhage (ICH) results from direct bleeding into the substance of the brain, with local accumulation of blood and formation of a hematoma. Intracranial hemorrhage constitutes approximately 15 percent of all strokes, and its cause is hypertension in 50 to 70 percent of the cases. The majority of these hemorrhages are located in the depth of the cerebral hemispheres (Table 33-1).

PATHOGENESIS

Hypertension

The pathogenesis of hypertensive ICH involves the rupture of small (50 to 200 μm in diameter) parenchymal perforating arteries, as a result of hypertension-induced degenerative changes in their walls. These include the focal degenerative change of the vessel wall labeled lipohyalinosis, and the formation of local outpouchings of the arterial wall, the so-called microaneurysms described by Charcot and Bouchard. There is still controversy as to which of these lesions causes the rupture of the arterial wall. Their pathogenic role in ICH is favored by their higher frequency in hypertensives in comparison with normotensives, as well as their preferential location to the areas of the brain in which ICH occurs most frequently (deep gray nuclei and

TABLE 33-1. Locations of Intracerebral Hemorrhage

Location	%
Putamen	33
Cerebral lobes	23
Thalamus	20
Cerebellum	8
Pons	7
Miscellaneous	9

(From Kase CS, Williams JP, Wyatt DA et al: Lobar intracerebral hematomas: clinical and CT analysis of 22 cases. Neurology 32:1146, 1982, with permission.)

TABLE 33-2. Nonhypertensive Causes of Intracerebral Hemorrhage

Cerebral amyloid angiopathy
Vascular malformations
Anticoagulants
Thrombolytic agents
Brain tumors
Sympathomimetic drugs
Vasculitis

subcortical white matter of the cerebral hemispheres). Once the arterial rupture has occurred, the period of actual bleeding into the brain parenchyma is thought to be relatively brief, in the order of 30 minutes or so. However, recent data derived from use of serial computed tomographic (CT) scanning after onset of ICH suggest that bleeding can actually proceed over periods of several hours. This results in the frequent observation of substantial increases in hematoma size after hours from onset. Hemorrhage eventually stops due to formation of a platelet plug that blocks the rupture site in the arterial wall, outside of which fibrin and red blood cells accumulate.

Nonhypertensive Mechanisms

A number of nonhypertensive mechanisms play a role in ICH (Table 33-2).

Cerebral Amyloid Angiopathy. Cerebral amyloid angiopathy is a unique form of cerebral angiopathy with deposits of amyloid in the media and adventitia of small and medium arteries of the cerebral hemispheres. The affected arteries are those located in the superficial layers of the cerebral cortex and the leptomeninges. Cerebral amyloid angiopathy typically affects elderly individuals, in whom histopathologic features of Alzheimer's disease are often found. Pathologically, it is characterized by deposits of Congo-red positive material in the media and adventitia of cortical and leptomeningeal arteries, which show birrefringence under polarized light. The ICHs occur in superficial, subcortical, or lobar locations since the angiopathy selectively affects arteries of the cortical surface and leptomeninges. An additional feature of cerebral amyloid angiopathy is a tendency to produce recurrent ICHs over periods of months or years, occasionally even leading to simultaneous acute hematomas in different brain locations.

Vascular Malformations. Previously unsuspected small vascular malformations, including arteriovenous malformations (AVMs), cavernous angiomas, and venous angiomas, can present as spontaneous ICH in adults. Their frequency in series of ICH varies between 4 and 8 percent of the cases. They are being increasingly diagnosed with the advent of CT scanning and magnetic resonance imaging (MRI). AVMs appear as multiple vascular channels, often accompanied by calcification; cavernous angiomas have a characteristic aspect on the T2-weighted MRI sequences, with a mixed-signal central core surrounded by a low-signal hemosiderin ring (Fig. 33-1); venous angiomas appear as a large, dilated venous channel that is connected to a series of smaller veins, the so-called caput medusae (Fig. 33-2). The risk of bleeding is highest in AVMs, lowest in venous angiomas, and intermediate in cavernous angiomas. Recent data suggest that venous angiomas have a negligible tendency to bleed, and when that occurs it is the result of rupture of an associated cavernous angioma. The hemorrhages produced by

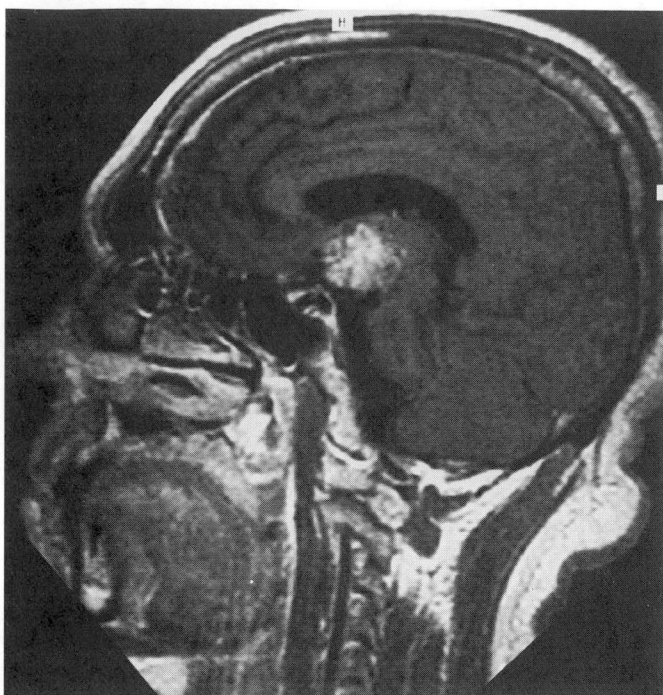

FIG. 33-1. T2-weighted sagittal MRI of cavernous angioma of the basal ganglia, showing mixed-signal central core with peripheral hypodense areas of hemosiderin deposition. (Courtesy of Rita Bhatia, M.D., Department of Radiology, Boston University Medical Center, Boston, MA.)

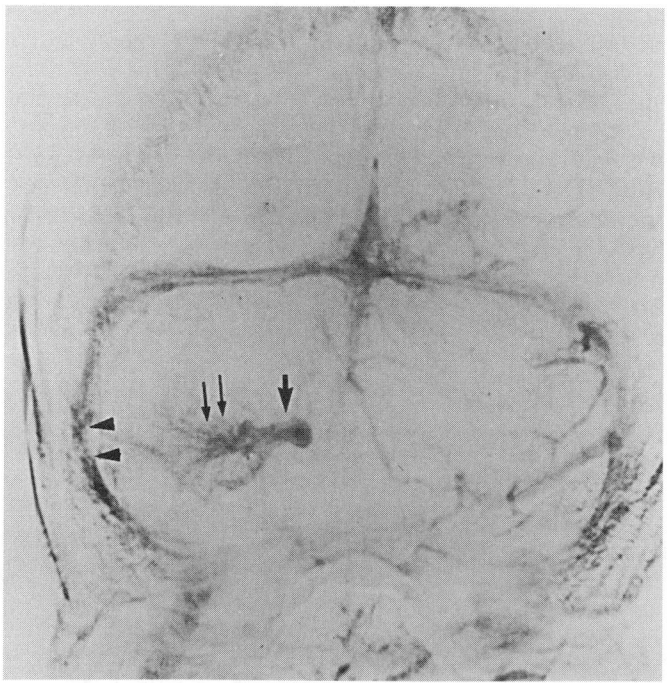

FIG. 33-2. Vertebral angiogram, venous phase, showing venous angioma as the "caput medusae" medullary veins (*double small arrows*) that drain into a large medially placed vein (*large arrow*), which in turn drains into the transverse sinus (*arrowheads*). (From Kase CS: Aneurysms and vascular malformations. pp. 153–78. In Kase CS, Caplan LR (eds): Intracerebral Hemorrhage. Butterworth-Heinemann, Boston, 1994, with permission.)

these lesions, especially those due to AVMs, tend to be more often in the subcortical white matter (rather than in the deep portions of the hemisphere), reflecting their usually more superficial location.

Oral Anticoagulants. Oral anticoagulants (warfarin sodium) increase the risk of ICH between 8- and 11-fold. These ICHs have been linked by some authors to the coexistence of hypertension, but a more consistent risk factor is an excessive prolongation of the prothrombin time (PT) beyond the "therapeutic" range. Clinically, these hemorrhages have some distinct features. A gradual and slow progression of the neurologic deficit occurs in as many as 50 percent of the cases, suggesting a process of slow bleeding into the parenchyma (as opposed to the usually faster course of hypertensive ICH), possibly resulting from rupture of different type or size vessels than those affected in hypertensive ICH.

Thrombolytic Agents. Thrombolytic agents, which are extensively used in the treatment of patients with acute myocardial infarction, have been associated with intracranial hemorrhage in approximately 0.5 percent of patients treated. Intracerebral hemorrhage in this setting is often of lobar location and large size, the latter leading to high mortality rates (44 percent). Among the potential risk factors for this complication of thrombolysis, an excessive prolongation of the activated partial thromboplastin time (aPTT) from the concomitant use of intravenous heparin has been suggested. In other instances, a preexistent angiopathy with bleeding potential, such as cerebral amyloid angiopathy, has been identified at autopsy examination. This suggests that the choice of this form of therapy should be properly assessed in the elderly presenting with acute myocardial infarction, to exclude those who may be at substantially increased risk of bleeding intracranially.

Brain Tumors. Brain tumors are found in 2 to 10 percent of cases of ICH. Those likely to present as ICH are largely malignant, either primary (glioblastoma multiforme) or metastatic, the latter most commonly corresponding to bronchogenic carcinoma, melanoma, choriocarcinoma, or renal-cell carcinoma. The sites of hemorrhage relate to the type of underlying tumor: deep-seated white-matter tumors such as glioblastoma multiforme produce deep hemispheric hemorrhages, whereas hemorrhages into metastatic tumors are more often corticosubcortical, reflecting the predilection of secondary tumors for the superficial portions of the cerebral hemispheres.

Sympathomimetic Drugs. A number of sympathomimetic drugs have been implicated in causing ICH. These include the amphetamines, phenylpropanolamine, and cocaine. Hemorrhage has generally occurred shortly after use of the drug, within minutes to a few hours after exposure. The majority of the hematomas are lobar, with only occasional ones in the basal ganglia or thalamus. Transiently elevated blood pressure has been noted in approximately 50 percent of the reported cases, and angiographic changes of multifocal areas of arterial constriction and dilation ("beading") have been documented, raising the possibility of a drug-induced angiopathy as their cause. On rare occasions, this angiographic pattern has been shown histologically to correspond to a true drug-induced vasculitis, after use of either phenylpropanolamine or cocaine.

Vasculitis. Vasculitis affecting cerebral vessels is rare, in particular in the systemic vasculitides. A primary cerebral form, isolated (or granulomatous) angiitis of the nervous system, which often leads to repeated episodes of ischemic infarction, can, on rare occasions, be the cause of episodes of ICH. In some instances, the ICH has been the first manifestation of the vasculitis.

CLINICAL FEATURES

The onset of ICH occurs virtually always in the awake period, with a focal deficit that develops smoothly and steadily over seconds or minutes. The syndrome may cease further development at any stage or continue to death in a few hours, the latter being occasionally associated with CT scan documentation of progressive enlargement of the hematoma. This type of smooth onset is seen in approximately two-thirds of the cases, whereas in the remainder it develops so rapidly that the deficit seems maximal at onset. None experience fluctuation or early resolution of the deficit.

Putaminal Hemorrhage

The bleeding site in the putaminal hemorrhagic variety of ICH is most commonly in the posterior half of the putamen (Fig. 33-3). From that area, the hemorrhage can spread into the centrum semiovale, the isthmus of the temporal lobe (along the course of the arcuate fasciculus), or across the internal capsule (frequently reaching the ventricular system). These patterns of extension of the hemorrhage result in further neurologic signs, and the larger hematomas will be eventually accompanied by signs of intracranial hypertension. The rare instances in which the bleeding is small and remains confined to the posterior putamen can result in a surprisingly mild motor deficit, at times conforming to a ''pure motor hemiparesis'' syndrome.

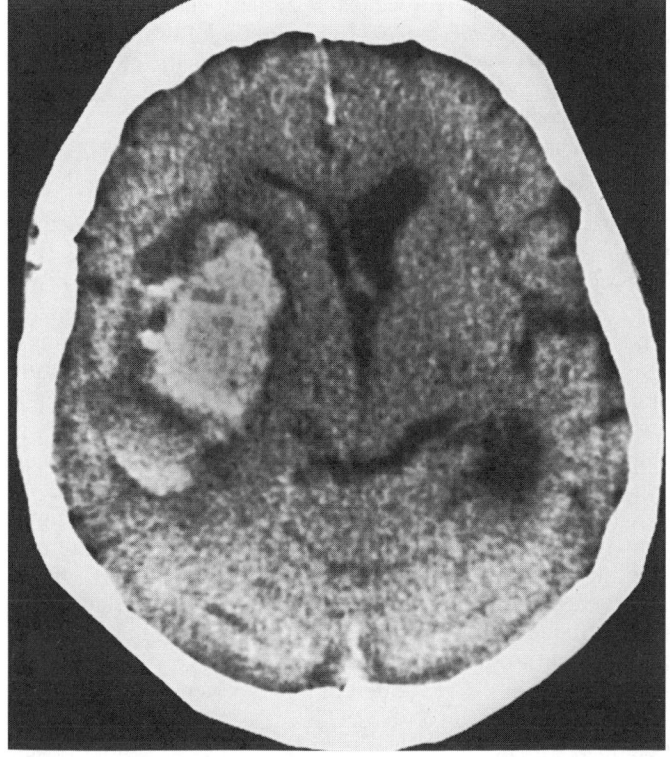

FIG. 33-3. CT of large right putaminal hemorrhage with moderate mass effect.

In the typical example of putaminal hemorrhage of moderate or large size, the patient develops a usually severe hemiparesis or hemiplegia affecting arm, face, and leg, reflecting bleeding into the area of the internal capsule. This is accompanied by a hemisensory syndrome, hemianopia, and aphasia if the dominant hemisphere is affected. Unawareness of the deficit develops when the nondominant hemisphere is involved. The aphasia encountered has generally been either slight or of the global variety; conduction aphasia is rare to nonexistent in this setting. Eye movement disorders feature conjugate horizontal gaze deviation toward the hematoma side when the hemiplegia is well developed, but eye movements are frequently normal when the hematoma is smaller, and the resulting hemiparesis is mild. More complex disorders of eye movements occur in the event of uncal herniation and midbrain compression. Pupillary size and reactivity to light are usually normal unless uncal herniation with resultant third-nerve palsy has occurred. Functional recovery can be predicted often by the degree of deficit present on examination. Patients with a dense hemiplegia show very little functional recovery, whereas those with only milder weakness may show complete resolution. Surgery to evacuate the hematoma is generally not done, except in some patients with larger hematomas. Surgical intervention can lessen mortality, but functional prognosis remains poor.

Caudate Hemorrhage

Hemorrhage into the head of the caudate nucleus is characterized by abrupt onset of headache and vomiting, frequently accompanied by decreased level of consciousness and neck stiffness, in a manner similar to subarachnoid hemorrhage from ruptured aneurysm. Focal neurologic deficits such as hemiparesis or gaze palsy occur infrequently and are of transient nature. Occasional patients develop signs of Horner syndrome ipsilateral to the hemorrhage.

CT scan shows a hematoma in the head of the caudate nucleus, with extension into the adjacent lateral ventricle (Fig. 33-4), frequently associated with hydrocephalus. In cases with transient focal motor deficits, the hemorrhages tend to be larger, extending into the internal capsule and along the body of the caudate nucleus. Their outcome is in general benign, with progressive resolution of the clinical deficits and gradual reduction of ventricular size. Although it is frequently present at onset, hydrocephalus rarely requires surgical shunting. The main mechanism in primary caudate hemorrhage is hypertension, but ruptured anterior communicating aneurysm or parenchymal AVM need to be ruled out by angiographic studies.

Thalamic Hemorrhage

The hemorrhage that arises in the thalamus frequently enlarges and tracks laterally to involve the internal capsule, in addition extending posterolaterally into the parietotemporal region, or downward into the midbrain (Fig. 33-5). Its location in the vicinities of the third ventricle frequently results in ventricular extension, at times with early obstructive hydrocephalus.

The initial contralateral complete hemisensory syndrome and capsular hemiparesis/hemiplegia occur immediately. If the hemorrhage enlarges laterally, conjugate horizontal gaze deviation toward the lesion occurs, but in rare instances a contralateral conjugate eye deviation (''wrong-way eyes'') is seen. As the hemorrhage spreads inferiorly and compresses the dorsal midbrain, ocular findings characteristically feature upward gaze

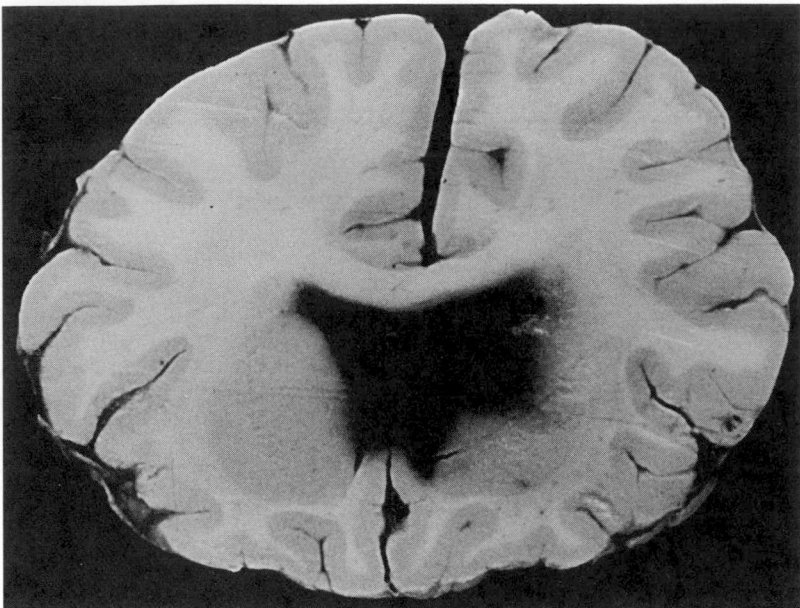

FIG. 33-4.   Left caudate nucleus hemorrhage with extension into the lateral ventricles.

palsy with miotic unreactive pupils. Because of the upward gaze palsy, the ocular position at rest is one of conjugate downward deviation, sometimes associated with convergence. The sensory deficit is often of striking severity and widely distributed over the contralateral limbs and face, including the scalp, neck, and trunk. A thalamic pain syndrome can be the permanent sequela of the destructive lesion affecting the thalamus. An aphasia

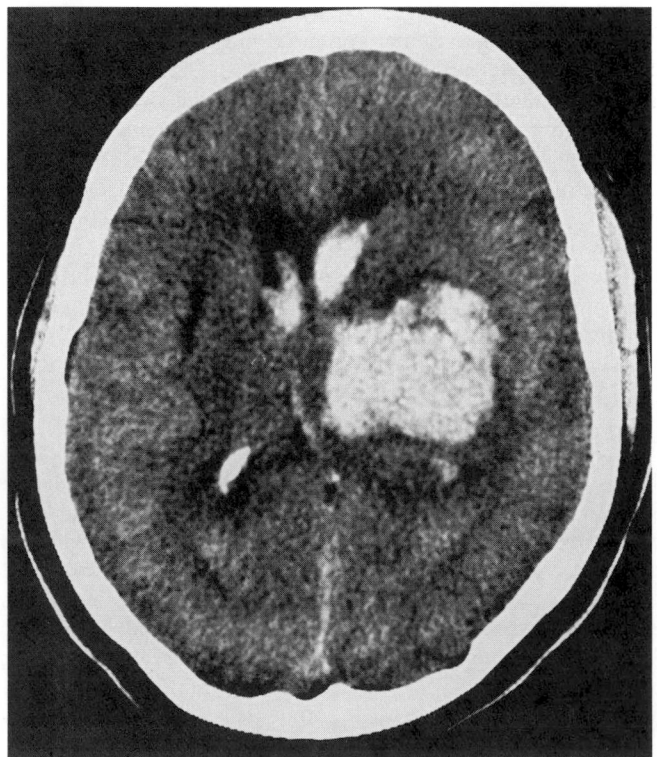

FIG. 33-5.   CT of left thalamic hemorrhage with extension into the third and lateral ventricles.

lasting several days is encountered in the smaller dominant hemisphere cases. It has been described as a fluctuating delirium-like state with disproportionate literal paraphasias.

CT scan information on the size of the hematoma has useful prognostic significance: hematomas larger than 3.3 cm are often fatal, whereas patients with hematomas smaller than 2.7 cm show significantly better survival rates. Owing to the inaccessibility of these hematomas, direct surgical evacuation is attempted rarely. It is possible that patients presenting with marked obstructive hydrocephalus at onset can benefit by ventriculostomy or cerebrospinal fluid shunting. In some instances, these surgical procedures have produced dramatic improvement in the clinical picture, and they may represent a useful therapy for selected cases of thalamic ICH.

Lobar Hemorrhage

Approximately one-fourth of the spontaneous ICHs occur in the subcortical white matter of the cerebral hemispheres (Fig. 33-6), predominantly in the parietooccipital region. The hematoma develops at the junction of the gray and white matter, producing a globular mass that separates the two. At autopsy years later, the remnant of the hemorrhage appears as a shallow orange-stained cavity, given the name ''slit hemorrhage.''

The clinical manifestations depend on the location of the hematoma: hemiparesis predominating in the arm in frontal hemorrhages, sensorimotor deficit with visual field defect in parietal hematomas, homonymous hemianopsia in occipital hemorrhages, Wernicke-type aphasia in dominant temporal lobe hematomas. The latter speech deficit is at times surprisingly evanescent. Seizures occur in lobar hemorrhage with higher frequency than in other forms, reflecting the proximity of the lesion to the cerebral cortex.

This variety of ICH is often of nonhypertensive mechanism, suggesting that other causes such as ''occult'' vascular malformations, cerebral amyloid angiopathy, underlying tumors, and angiopathies related to drug use or abuse need to be investigated once the lobar location of the ICH has been determined.

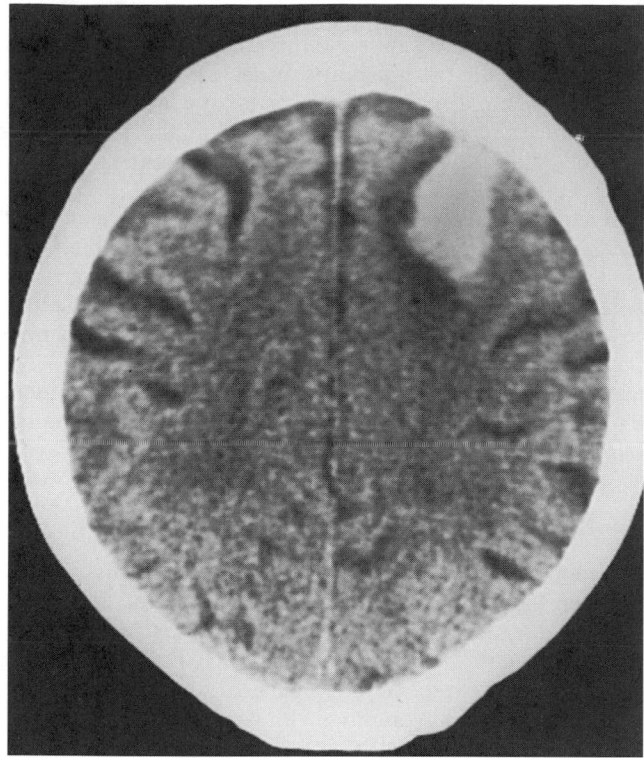

FIG. 33-6. Right frontal lobar hemorrhage.

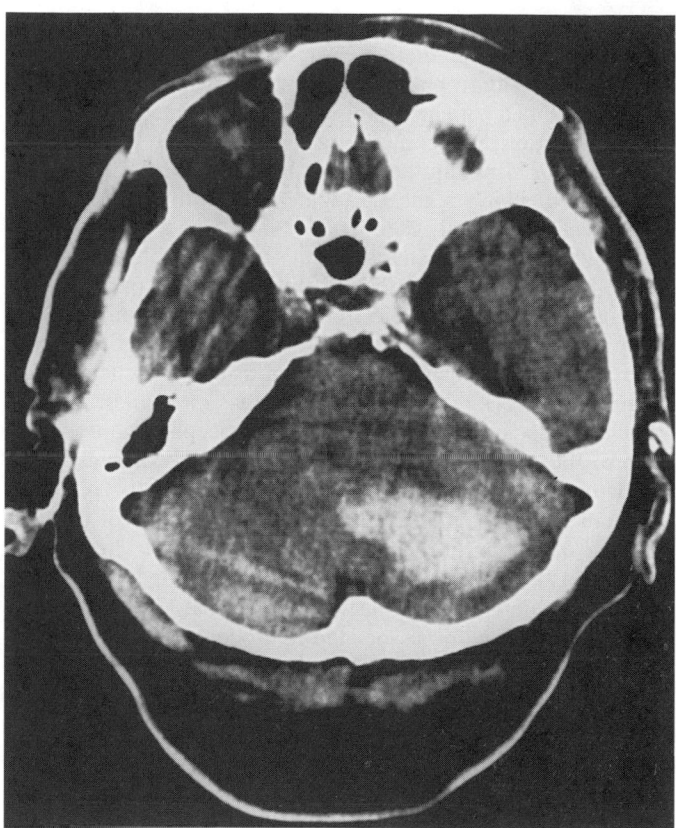

FIG. 33-7. Left hemispheric cerebellar hemorrhage with compression of the fourth ventricle.

Lobar ICHs generally show a less severe degree of disability in survivors, as well as lower mortality as compared with other supratentorial sites of ICH. Furthermore, they are accessible to surgical drainage and, if untreated, they may be fatal as a result of prominent pressure effects. If the CT scan shows that the hemorrhage is near the cortical surface, and if there is significant mass effect, consideration should be given to its surgical evacuation.

Cerebellar Hemorrhage

Hemorrhage in the cerebellum represents 10 to 15 percent of intracerebral hematomas. The majority of the hemorrhages develop in the area of the dentate nucleus, spreading laterally into one hemisphere (Fig. 33-7) or superomedially to the midline of the superior vermis.

The onset is sudden in 95 percent of cases, with prominent nausea, vomiting, dizziness, and inability to stand and walk. Headache occurs in 74 percent, but loss of consciousness at onset is rare (14 percent). Clinical examination shows limb or gait ataxia, peripheral facial palsy, and ipsilateral gaze palsy, a useful diagnostic triad. Hemiplegia and subhyaloid hemorrhages are extremely rare. Occasionally, small cerebellar hemorrhages present with pure vertigo, nausea and vomiting sometimes misdiagnosed as Menière's disease, acute labyrinthitis, or vestibular neuronitis. For this reason, one should maintain a high index of suspicion and perform a CT scan early in the course of the illness to evaluate the possibility of cerebellar hemorrhage.

Cerebellar hemorrhage has a notorious tendency to produce sudden worsening in the patient's condition after an initial benign course: 50 percent of patients presenting in an alert state on admission went on to develop sudden coma within 48 hours

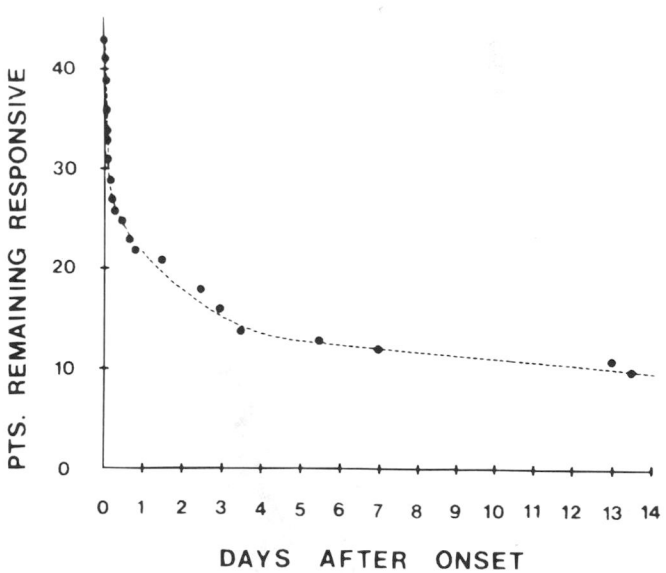

FIG. 33-8. Development of coma in 43 patients with cerebellar hemorrhage as a function of time from onset of symptoms. (From Ott KH, Kase CS, Ojemann RG et al: Cerebellar hemorrhage: diagnosis and treatment: a review of 56 cases. Arch Neurol 31:160, 1974, with permission.)

from onset in one series (Fig. 33-8). This course could not be related to reliable predictors on admission evaluation. Since surgical intervention has a low morbidity when performed in alert or obtunded patients, and is usually associated with a satisfactory functional outcome, surgery is generally planned for cases diagnosed within the first 48 hours, particularly in those instances in which signs of tegmental pontine involvement (ipsilateral horizontal gaze palsy, sixth-nerve palsy, facial palsy) are present. The characteristics of the hematomas on CT can be useful early predictors of clinical course: patients with a benign, stable course tend to have hematomas smaller than 3 cm in diameter. Those patients with abrupt onset and more severely depressed level of consciousness and tendency toward progressive deterioration show hematomas of 3 cm or more in diameter, associated with obstructive hydrocephalus and effacement of the quadrigeminal cistern. Surgical decompression is mandatory in the larger hemorrhages, but the results are generally poor if the patient has already reached a state of coma at the time of surgery. Consequently, it is important to operate early in instances of large cerebellar hemorrhages to prevent progressive brainstem dysfunction and coma. The smaller hematomas that show no associated hydrocephalus can be managed medically, but at the earliest indication of signs of brainstem dysfunction, surgery should be undertaken promptly.

Pontine Hemorrhage

The most dramatic and least treatable of the hypertensive hemorrhages, pontine hemorrhage, produces the more uncommon syndromes. They usually affect the ventral pons, arising from bleeding from the paramedian penetrators, then extending into the rest of the basis pontis and tegmentum (Fig. 33-9). The larger hemorrhages can lead to deep coma within minutes of onset, usually in association with quadriplegia and decerebrate rigidity. In addition, reactive, small (''pinpoint'') pupils occur, along with a variety of ocular motility disorders, including ocular ''bobbing,'' uni- or bilateral internuclear ophthalmoplegia, and uni- or bilateral sixth-nerve palsy, all of which are replaced by bilateral horizontal ophthalmoplegia in the most severe cases. In addition, abnormal respiratory rhythms and hyperthermia are commonly seen.

Large pontine hemorrhages are almost invariably fatal. Small laterally placed hemorrhages in the pontine or midbrain tegmentum usually spare consciousness and produce an array of cranial nerve findings and lateralized weakness and ataxia. These smaller hematomas mimic syndromes of partial pontine ischemia to a degree that CT scanning is necessary to separate hemorrhage from infarction. Prognosis is better in the unilateral than in the bilateral variety of pontine hemorrhage. Surgical intervention is not generally attempted.

Mesencephalic Hemorrhage

The midbrain is a rare location for primary ICH; only 12 cases have been reported over the past 10 years. Six of these cases have been due to hypertension or AVMs, the rest being normotensive and without other risk factors for ICH.

Their clinical presentation frequently involves the abrupt onset of headache and vomiting, with variable motor signs. The latter have been described in primarily unilateral hematomas, and have corresponded to either contralateral hemiparesis or ipsilateral cerebellar ataxia, with a corresponding gait disturbance. The most common physical findings have reflected the tectal-tegmental location of the hemorrhages, leading to ocular signs that include paralysis of upward gaze, small unreactive pupils with preserved near reflex (i.e., light-near dissociation), and palpebral ptosis. One instance of a caudally placed tectal hemorrhage presented with bilateral fourth-nerve palsies and

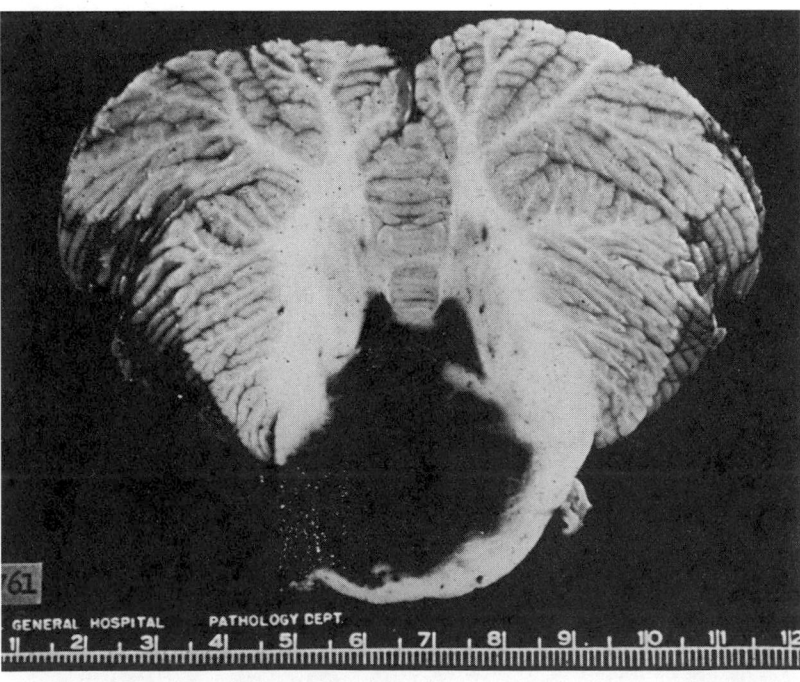

FIG. 33-9.   Massive bilateral pontine hemorrhage with involvement of most of the basis and tegmentum, with extension into the fourth ventricle. (Courtesy of Michael S. Pessin, M.D., Department of Neurology, New England Medical Center, Boston, MA.)

TABLE 33-3. Hemoglobin and MRI Evolution in Hematoma

Stage	Time	Hb Form	Magnetic Property	Hematoma SI, T1	Hematoma SI, T2	Hemosiderin Rim (SI, T2)	Edema (SI, T2)
Hyperacute	Hours	Oxyhemoglobin	Diamagnetic	= or ↓	↑	—	↑↑
Acute	Days	Deoxyhemoglobin	Paramagnetic	= or ↓	↓↓	—	↑↑
Early subacute	Weeks	Methemoglobin (intracellular)	Paramagnetic	↑	↓	↓↓	↑↑
Late subacute	Weeks-months	Methemoglobin (extracellular)	Paramagnetic	↑↑	↑↑	↓↓	—
Chronic	Months-years	Hemosiderin	Paramagnetic	= or ↓	↓↓	↓↓	—

Abbreviations: Hb, hemoglobin; SI, signal intensity relative to normal gray matter; T1, T1-weighted sequences; T2, T2-weighted sequences.

(From Dul K, Drayer BP: CT and MR imaging of intracerebral hemorrhage. pp. 73–93. In Kase CS, Caplan LR (eds): Intracerebral Hemorrhage. Butterworth-Heinemann, Boston, 1994, with permission.)

unilateral Horner syndrome. Hydrocephalus from aqueductal compression has been frequently reported, in some instances requiring ventricular shunting. In general, the prognosis has been good, most patients surviving with persistent ocular and pupillary changes.

Medullary Hemorrhage

Hemorrhage into the substance of the medulla oblongata is the least common form of ICH. It is at times seen as part of the caudal extension of a pontine hemorrhage, but in its primary medullary form has been reported in only 12 cases in the last 30 years. Its clinical presentation is highlighted by the sudden onset of features indicative of largely unilateral tegmental or basal medullary involvement, with vertigo, vomiting, gait imbalance, limb ataxia, and paresis of lower cranial nerves. Its findings on neurologic examination can be similar to those of Wallenberg's lateral medullary syndrome, with the exception that medullary hemorrhage often presents with hemiparesis and hypoglossal nerve palsy, reflecting extension of the ICH ventrally and medially, respectively, away from the dorsolateral area.

DIAGNOSIS

The diagnosis of ICH relies heavily on the imaging techniques of CT and MRI, since they can essentially diagnose the condition with a 100 percent reliability. CT is particularly useful in establishing the diagnosis of ICH, as opposed to ischemic stroke, a distinction that is not always possible on clinical grounds alone, especially in instances of small hemorrhages that produce minimal signs of increased intracranial pressure (ICP). The advent of MRI has added to the diagnostic precision of brain imaging by providing useful data on the evolution of the ICH. These data derive from the paramagnetic properties of the hemoglobin contained in the hematoma, which undergoes predictable biochemical changes that are time-dependent, thus allowing precise timing of the duration of the ICH (Table 33-3).

MANAGEMENT

Management of patients with ICH should be directed toward preserving remaining neurologic function and preventing deterioration due to elevated ICP with resultant coma or death. A CT scan of the brain should follow promptly the initial clinical evaluation. These patients should be managed in a neurologic/neurosurgical intensive care unit whether they are to be managed conservatively or are to receive pre- or postoperative care.

The patients should be kept at bed rest with the head elevated 30 degrees to reduce ICP by facilitating venous drainage.

In patients with ICH who present with lethargy or in coma, or who were initially alert and then deteriorated, an airway should be established, preferably with endotracheal intubation, and oxygenation to PO₂ of 100 to 150 mmHg should be maintained. The management of increased ICP includes the use of hyperventilation (to produce hypocarbia of PCO₂ of 25 to 30 mmHg, which effectively reduces ICP by producing cerebral vasoconstriction), and osmotic diuretics (mannitol) that reduce cerebral volume (and ICP) by causing a shift in water from the cerebral to the intravascular space. The value of corticosteroids (dexamethasone) in improving outcome by reducing ICP has not been proven, since their potential beneficial effects are often offset by their systemic complications.

Many patients with ICH may present with markedly elevated blood pressure. It is often impossible to determine whether this represents an exacerbation of previously long-standing hypertension or is a reflex response to increased ICP. In the presence of increased ICP, excessive reductions of blood pressure in the setting of impaired cerebral autoregulation may substantially reduce cerebral blood flow and cause further deterioration owing to added cerebral ischemia.

Another important therapeutic issue in ICH relates to the choice of surgical or nonsurgical management. In most instances of supratentorial ICH, in particular in thalamic and putaminal locations, there is no evidence that surgical intervention has an impact on outcome. The same is true for the primary brainstem (midbrain, pontine, and medullary) hemorrhages, despite the anecdotal reporting of successful surgical treatment in selected instances. The varieties of ICH that are often benefited by surgical intervention are the lobar and, especially, cerebellar locations.

SUGGESTED READINGS

Barinagarrementeria F, Cantú C: Primary medullary hemorrhage: report of four cases and review of the literature. Stroke 25:1684, 1994

Broderick JP, Brott TG, Tomsick T et al: Ultra-early evaluation of intracerebral hemorrhage. J Neurosurg 72:195, 1990

Caplan LR: Intracerebral hemorrhage revisited. Neurology 38:624, 1988

Kase CS: Intracerebral hemorrhage: non-hypertensive causes. Stroke 17:590, 1986

Kase CS, Pessin MS, Zivin JA et al: Intracranial hemorrhage after coronary thrombolysis with tissue plasminogen activator. Am J Med 92:384, 1992

Levine SR, Brust JCM, Futrell N et al: Cerebrovascular complications of the use of the ''crack'' form of alkaloidal cocaine. N Engl J Med 323:699, 1990

Rådberg JA, Olsson JE, Rådberg CT: Prognostic parameters in spontaneous intracerebral hematomas with special reference to anticoagulant treatment. Stroke 22:571, 1991

Simard JM, Garcia-Bengochea F, Ballinger WE et al: Cavernous angioma: a review of 126 collected and 12 new clinical cases. Neurosurgery 18:162, 1986

Schütz H, Bödeker R-H, Damian M et al: Age-related spontaneous intracerebral hematoma in a German community. Stroke 21:1412, 1990

Wijdicks EFM, Jack CR: Intracerebral hemorrhage after fibrinolytic therapy for acute myocardial infarction. Stroke 24:554, 1993

34. SUBARACHNOID HEMORRHAGE

CARLOS S. KASE
CONRADO J. ESTOL

The greatest fear of many people is to "have an aneurysm in the brain." The fear is justified considering the devastating effects of subarachnoid hemorrhage (SAH) secondary to aneurysmal rupture. Prevention of SAH is difficult because of the lack of symptoms prior to aneurysmal rupture, and its treatment is associated with many obstacles related to the complications of SAH and the need and timing of neurosurgical management.

MECHANISMS

SAH is the result of bleeding from arteries and veins that are located close to the brain surface, with accumulation of blood in the basal cisterns and surrounding subarachnoid space. The vast majority (80 percent) of nontraumatic SAHs are caused by rupture of "congenital" or "berry" aneurysms, which result from the effects of blood pressure on areas of congenitally mal-formed and weakened arterial walls, usually at bifurcation sites. Eighty-five percent of aneurysms are distributed in the carotid circulation (35 percent in the anterior communicating and anterior cerebral arteries, 30 percent in the internal carotid artery at the origin of the posterior communicating artery, and 20 percent in the middle cerebral artery [MCA]). The posterior circulation accounts for 15 percent of aneurysms, and the distribution is 10 percent at the top of the basilar artery and basilar-superior cerebellar artery junction and 5 percent in the VA at the origin of the posterior inferior communicating artery (Fig. 34-1).

Miscellaneous Causes of Aneurysmal Subarachnoid Hemorrhage

Mycotic Aneurysms.   These aneurysms are more appropriately called "infectious" or "bacterial." Infected embolic material from cardiac valves with bacterial endocarditis causes an inflammation in the arterial wall with formation of a focal aneurysmal dilation of the vessel wall. The arteries affected are usually peripheral MCA branches. Mycotic aneurysms occur in 2 to 12 percent of patients with bacterial endocarditis. Therefore, angiography to rule out aneurysms is mandatory in the event of symptoms of SAH or intracranial hemorrhage, and, if an aneurysm is diagnosed, follow-up angiography is essential in planning management. The treatment is intravenous antibiotics to promote vessel wall healing, and surgery is not encouraged because of vessel wall friability. However, there is controversy as to which of these treatment options is preferable. It is generally agreed that patients who have a mycotic aneurysm, which either did not disappear or became larger after an appropriate course of intravenous antibiotics, should be treated by surgical clipping of the aneurysm.

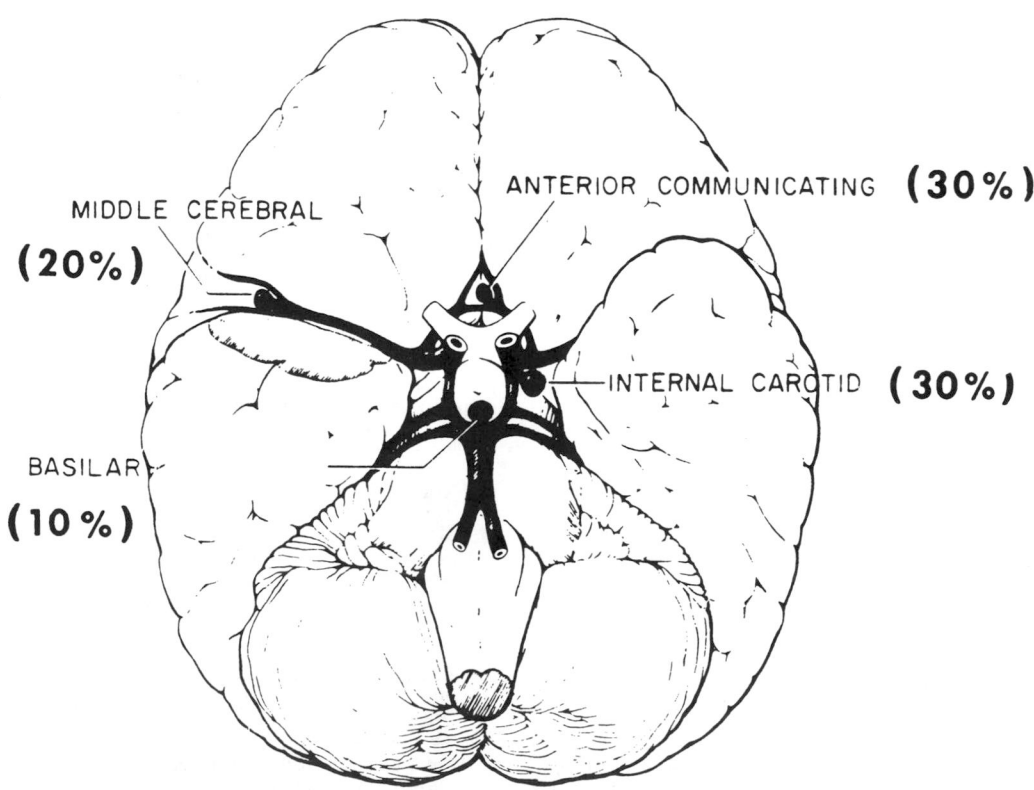

FIG. 34-1.   Frequency of aneurysms of the arteries of the circle of Willis. (From Crowell RM, Zervas NT: Management of intracranial aneurysm. Med Clin North Am 63:695–713, 1979, with permission.)

Aneurysms may also result from embolization to distal MCA branches from *atrial myxoma* or from *choriocarcinoma*. They are similar to infectious aneurysms in their peripheral location in the cerebral circulation.

Nonaneurysmal Subarachnoid Hemorrhage

Not all SAHs are secondary to ruptured aneurysms. Perimesencephalic hemorrhage is a condition with a good prognosis in which the SAH is almost exclusively limited to the perimesencephalic cisterns. The hemorrhage probably arises from capillary or venous bleeding in the pontomesencephalic region. The rule is an uncomplicated clinical course with no risk of rebleeding and virtually no incidence of vasospasm. It is reasonable to obtain an angiogram as part of the initial workup in order to rule out the unlikely alternative diagnosis of ruptured aneurysm of the top of the basilar artery. However, if the study is negative for aneurysm, a second angiogram is usually not necessary.

EPIDEMIOLOGY

Intracranial hemorrhages account for approximately 15 percent of all strokes. SAH represents approximately one-third of these hemorrhages. In the United States, 28,000 aneurysmal hemorrhages occur each year. According to autopsy data, approximately 5 percent of the population harbor intracranial aneurysms. The mortality rate of SAH is 10 percent in the first few days and 50 percent during the first month. The main causes of mortality during the first 2 weeks are, in order of frequency, the direct effects of the initial hemorrhage, rebleeding, and vasospasm. Among the patients who survive, 50 percent are left with neurologic sequelae that prevent them from regaining employment.

PATHOGENESIS

Aneurysm refers to the abnormal dilation of an arterial segment. Since the tension in the wall increases proportionally to the vessel's radius, the risk of arterial rupture is greater with increasing diameter of the aneurysm. This observation refutes the old notion that giant aneurysms are less likely to rupture than small ones; recent data suggest that giant aneurysms (greater than 2.5 cm; Fig. 34-2) have a high risk of rupture. They represent 3 to 5 percent of all intracranial aneurysms and are more frequent in women. They also carry a risk of ischemic infarction that results from embolization of intra-aneurysmal thrombus into arteries distal to the aneurysm.

The most common aneurysms are the so-called congenital, berry, or saccular aneurysms. Although their exact mechanism of origin has not been clearly defined, they probably develop during life in areas of congenitally malformed arteries. Others have proposed that aneurysms are lesions acquired during life that form in areas where the internal elastic lamina has suffered degenerative changes secondary to atherosclerosis. This theory also implies that coexisting medial defects, acquired or congenital, are necessary for aneurysm formation. Chronic hypertension is thought to be a predisposing factor for aneurysmal growth.

Fusiform or dolichoectatic aneurysms are elongated, tortuous, and dilated segments of arteries. These abnormal vessels are often associated with atherosclerotic changes in elderly patients with hypertension. In some patients, especially the young, these aneurysms may result from structural abnormalities in the

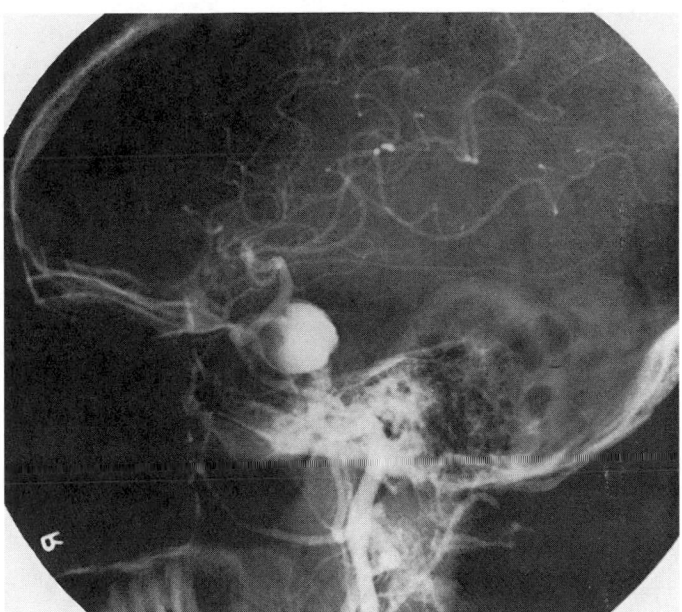

FIG. 34-2. Arteriogram with giant aneurysm of the left internal carotid artery. (Courtesy of Shripad Tilak, M.D., Department of Radiology, Boston University Medical Center, Boston, MA.)

vessel wall in the absence of atherosclerosis. Fusiform aneurysms can affect any of the main intracerebral vessels. These aneurysms (especially those in the posterior circulation) frequently cause symptoms through either mass effect on adjacent structures or ischemia from embolic material dislodged from the wall, causing occlusion of distal branches.

CLINICAL FEATURES

Few symptoms in neurology have received as much attention as the *headache* of SAH. The most typical is that described as "the worst headache in the patient's life," but less severe headaches may represent slight "leaking" from aneurysms (which could even occur within the wall of the aneurysm without blood entering the subarachnoid space). The so-called sentinel headache, which is of sudden onset but often transient in duration, is frequently the prologue to the major episode of SAH, and occurs in 50 percent of patients during the 3 weeks preceding the SAH. In one-third of patients, the site of the headache may help localize the aneurysm. There are conditions, however, with severe headache that are not related to SAH, such as the "thunderclap headache," the headache associated with arterial dissection, and coital headache. Even in these latter situations, one cannot overemphasize the importance of obtaining a cerebrospinal fluid (CSF) sample and computed tomographic scan (CT) to rule out SAH in questionable cases.

In about 30 percent of cases, the patient *loses consciousness* at the time of onset of SAH, as a result of the sudden increase in intracranial pressure. Many patients regain consciousness after a few minutes or hours and remain obtunded.

Neurologic examination may reveal a wide spectrum of signs, varying from normal to a deeply comatose patient with no brainstem function. Certain findings help localize the aneurysm, such as a *third nerve palsy* caused by an internal carotid artery aneurysm at the junction with the posterior communicating artery. *Neck stiffness* has also been considered a cardinal sign in SAH. However, it is important to know that irritation of cervical roots by the subarachnoid blood can take a few hours

TABLE 34-1. The Hunt-Hess Classification of Subarachnoid Hemorrhage

Grade	Description
0	Unruptured aneurysm
1	Asymptomatic or mild headache and slight nuchal rigidity
2	Cranial nerve palsy (i.e., third nerve palsy), moderate to severe headache, and nuchal rigidity
3	Mild focal deficit and lethargy or confusion
4	Stupor, moderate to severe hemiparesis, and early decerebrate rigidity
5	Deep coma, decerebrate rigidity, and moribund appearance

to develop and that a supple neck on early examination does not exclude SAH. On funduscopic examination, *subhyaloid hemorrhages* are seen in 25 percent of patients. They are located in proximity to the optic disc and are caused by increased intracranial pressure interfering with the venous outflow from the eye. These hemorrhages appear to have a fluid level and result from accumulation of blood anterior to the retina. Subhyaloid hemorrhages may extend into the vitreous humor (Terson syndrome), and their presence is associated with a poor outcome from the SAH.

Systemic Diseases and Intracranial Aneurysms

Some systemic disorders are associated with an increased incidence of intracranial aneurysms. These include coarctation of the aorta, polycystic kidney disease, Marfan syndrome, fibromuscular dysplasia (with greater incidence of cerebral aneurysms in aortic, cervical, and intracranial locations than in the kidney), arteriovenous malformations, moyamoya disease, Ehlers-Danlos syndrome (type IV), and Rendu-Osler-Weber syndrome. The recognition of these disorders and their association with cerebral aneurysms may help in diagnosis at the asymptomatic, prerupture stage, allowing for treatment prior to the potentially devastating SAH.

Grading Scales

In dealing with a disease such as SAH, which has a varied prognosis and several serious complications, it is useful to classify patients in clinical subgroups that predict outcomes. This has led to the creation of several clinical scales. An additional value of these scales is for comparison of patients from different series to assess treatment strategies. The most widely used scale is that of Hunt and Hess, which grades the patient's condition based on the presence of headache and other meningeal signs, mental status, and focal neurologic deficits (Table 34-1).

The following are treatment strategies based on this scale: patients in grades 0 and 1 are candidates for early aneurysmal clipping (within the first 72 hours); grade 2 patients may also be considered for early surgery. Grade 3 patients should be managed medically until an improvement to grade 1 or 2 occurs, making them candidates for surgery; patients in grades 4 and 5 have a poor prognosis, and they are not candidates for surgical treatment.

DIAGNOSIS

The single most important issue in the diagnosis of SAH is a high index of suspicion for the condition. Studies have shown that up to 25 percent of patients with SAH have been discharged home from emergency rooms with a diagnosis of benign headache. In patients presenting with a sudden, severe headache

(even if it is *not* the "worst headache of their lives"), a CT and/or lumbar puncture should be done.

Computed Tomography

The first diagnostic step should be to obtain a noncontrast CT. Subarachnoid blood is seen in the majority of cases on the day of SAH (Fig. 34-3), but 4 percent of scans may show no blood in the subarachnoid spaces when bleeding has been slight. Also, the positivity of CT declines with time, to 90 percent after day 1, 80 percent after day 5, 50 percent after week 1, and 30 percent at week 2, most CTs showing no subarachnoid blood after week 3. Contrast administration may show the aneurysm (especially if its diameter is greater than 10 mm), as well as most arteriovenous malformations. The CT distribution of the SAH can predict the location of the aneurysm in approximately 70 percent of cases: greater accumulation of blood in the interhemispheric fissure suggests an anterior communicating artery aneurysm, blood in the sylvian fissure correlates with MCA aneurysm, and a lateralized SAH at the chiasmatic cistern suggests a posterior communicating artery aneurysm. Basilar artery aneurysms and the benign form of perimesencephalic SAH result in accumulation of blood in the entire suprasellar cistern, mimicking the distribution of blood from anterior circulation aneurysms.

CT also shows parenchymal blood, which is frequently (in 20 to 40 percent of cases) associated with certain aneurysm sites; temporal lobe hemorrhage suggests a posterior communicating artery or MCA aneurysm rupture, and frontal lobe hemorrhage is associated with anterior cerebral artery or anterior

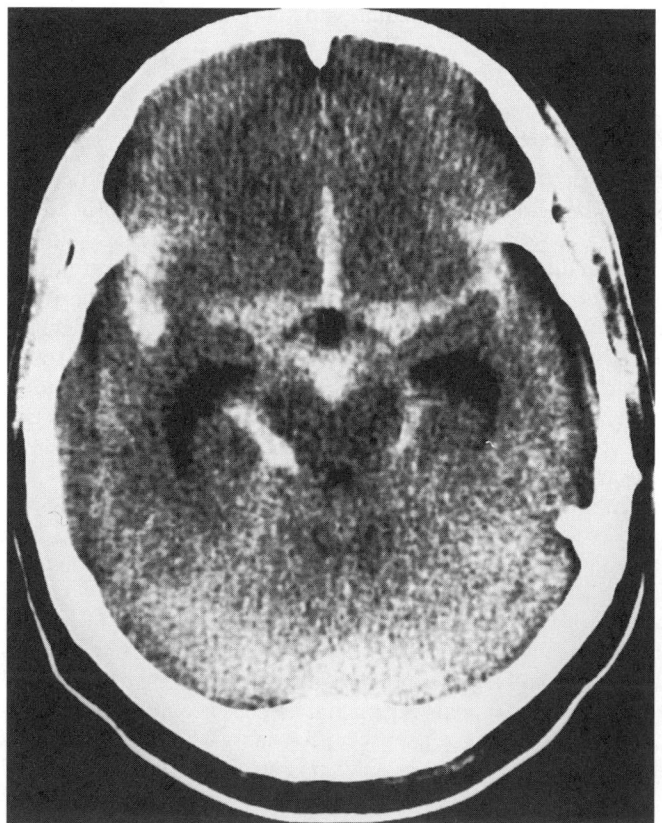

FIG. 34-3. CT of acute subarachnoid hemorrhage showing diffuse distribution of blood in the basal cisterns and sylvian fissures. (Courtesy of Shripad Tilak, M.D., Department of Radiology, Boston University Medical Center, Boston, MA.)

communicating artery aneurysms. Intraventricular extension of blood (seen in 20 percent of patients) is associated with obstructive hydrocephalus if the third ventricle is involved; on the other hand, the pooling of blood in the occipital horns may only reflect the effect of gravity, with no prognostic value.

An important nonhemorrhagic finding in CT is hydrocephalus. A baseline CT with normal ventricular size can be followed for changes of hydrocephalus, which at times may explain the onset of clinical deterioration in the absence of rebleeding.

Lumbar Puncture

Lumbar puncture can be of significant help in the diagnosis and follow-up of patients with SAH. Serial lumbar punctures may confirm improvement with progressive reabsorption of the blood in the subarachnoid space. In addition, if rebleeding is suspected, an increase in the amount of red blood cells may help confirm the diagnosis in the presence of equivocal CT results.

When Is a Tap Traumatic?   The notion that a decreasing number of red blood cells in successive tubes supports the diagnosis of a traumatic puncture is correct but has too many exceptions to be a useful rule. The only reliable method to confirm SAH is to spin the tube with bloody CSF and examine the supernatant with a spectrophotometer to search for xanthochromia (dark yellow color), which reflects the presence of bilirubin and other pigments released by the prior occurrence of bleeding. When a spectrophotometer is not available, a less reliable method of assessing xanthochromia of the CSF supernatant is to compare it visually with a tube containing water or saline against a white background under good illumination.

Timing of the Lumbar Puncture.   A false-negative result for CSF xanthochromia is possible if the CSF is analyzed too early after SAH. Pigments are released from the red blood cells no earlier than 2 to 4 hours after the bleeding; to be certain about absence of xanthochromia, it is recommended to delay the lumbar puncture for 6 to 12 hours after the hemorrhage. In the event of a negative CT in a patient suspected of having a SAH, the lumbar puncture should be performed after at least 6 hours have elapsed from headache onset.

Magnetic Resonance Imaging

Magnetic resonance imaging (MRI) is not a useful diagnostic tool in the first few hours after SAH since hemorrhages are isointense (i.e., not visible) because of the presence of deoxyhemoglobin and the absence of methemoglobin in the CSF. After the first few days, the presence of methemoglobin in the subarachnoid blood will turn the subarachnoid space hyperintense on T1-weighted sequences. In the chronic stage, the accumulation of hemosiderin gives a hypointense signal to the subarachnoid space on both MRI sequences. MRI is also useful for the detection of aneurysms and arteriovenous malformations, and it is the ideal imaging technique to visualize the "true" size of giant aneurysms, which is often underestimated in angiography because of partial intraluminal filling with thrombus.

Angiography

In most cases, cerebral angiography provides information about the location and size of an aneurysm and the presence of vaso-spasm. In up to 15 percent of cases, the angiogram may appear negative, but this may be due to an inadequate study without the special (oblique) views needed to locate an aneurysm. If an aneurysm is identified after first injecting the suspected artery, the other arteries should be surveyed to rule out multiple aneurysms, which are present in 20 to 25 percent of patients presenting with aneurysmal SAH. When multiple aneurysms are found on angiography, helpful hints that point to the one that bled include the largest aneurysm, the one closest to the greatest amount of subarachnoid blood, and the one in relation to vessels that may be affected by vasospasm.

Aneurysmal SAH With Negative Angiography.   Angiography may be negative in cases of aneurysmal SAH for different reasons: the aneurysm may decrease in size or may be accompanied by spasm of its parent artery, resulting in poor filling and visualization; surrounding blood clots may exert mass effect that obliterates the aneurysm; blood in the neck of the aneurysm may clot, preventing dye from entering the aneurysmal sac; and bleeding may be secondary to an aneurysm that is too small to be visualized by angiography. Most studies suggest that if aneurysms are not found after properly performed panangiography, the risk of recurrent bleeding is very low. If the initial angiogram is negative, we recommend repeat angiography after 7 to 10 days and even consider a third study a few weeks later if the index of suspicion remains high after two negative studies.

COMPLICATIONS

Rebleeding

The risk of rebleeding is greatest during the first few hours after the initial hemorrhage, and its actual frequency may be underestimated because of the difficulty in separating early rebleeding from the effects of the initial hemorrhage, especially in patients who are stuporous or have a high Hunt and Hess grade. The risk of rebleeding approaches 4 percent during the first day, decreasing to 1.5 percent per day during the following 2 weeks (20 percent in the first 2 weeks), reaching 50 percent in the first 6 months, and maintaining a plateau of 3 percent per year thereafter. Patients with a high Hunt and Hess grade on admission have higher rebleeding rates. The mortality rate from rebleeding can be as high as 70 to 90 percent.

Vasospasm

Vasospasm refers to sustained constriction of basal cerebral arteries, generally in the vicinities of the ruptured aneurysm, but sometimes it is widespread. Its main effect is ischemic cerebral infarction. Vasospasm uncommonly occurs earlier than the third day after SAH, has its peak frequency on day 7, and rarely occurs after day 17. This complication carries a 7 percent mortality rate and an even higher rate of permanent neurologic disability.

The pathogenesis of vasospasm remains unsettled. It is, in part, the result of the vasoactive effects of various substances released into the subarachnoid space as a consequence of the SAH. These include prostaglandins, free radicals, epinephrine, and oxyhemoglobin. Although vasospasm is usually reversible, some of the vascular changes may be permanent, resulting in structural changes in the arterial wall. Neuropathologic studies during the first few days of vasospasm have shown an inflammatory reaction in the adventitia, smooth muscle necrosis in the media with involvement of the elastic lamina, and swelling

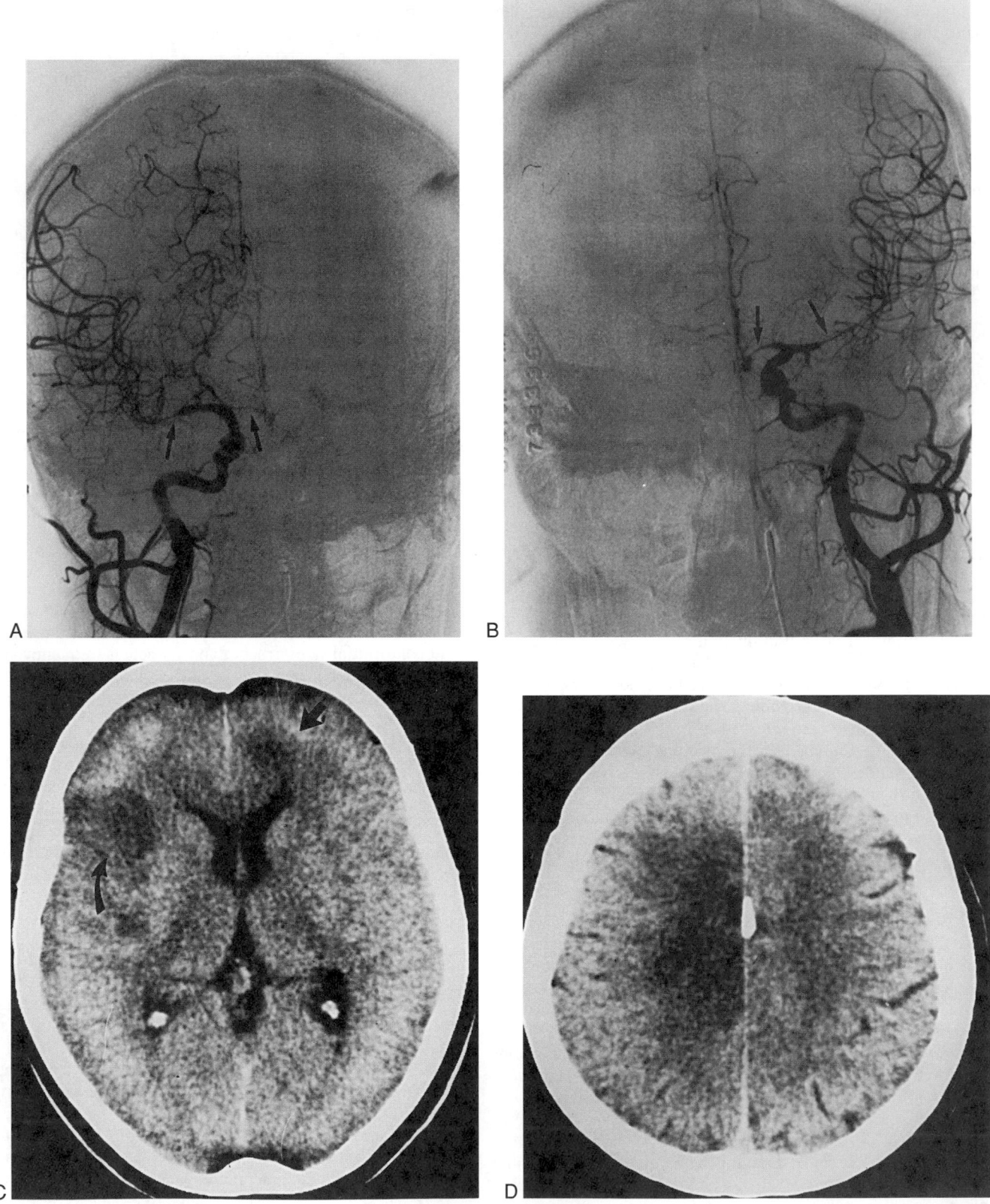

FIG. 34-4. **(A)** Right carotid angiogram with marked spasm of the proximal anterior and middle cerebral arteries (*arrows*); note paucity of flow in the distal anterior cerebral artery branches. **(B)** Marked spasm in left anterior and middle cerebral arteries (*arrows*). **(C)** CT with infarction in the right middle cerebral artery *(curved arrow)* and left anterior cerebral artery *(arrow)* territories. **(D)** Large infarct in the left anterior cerebral artery territory.

of intimal cells with an increase in the intercellular distance and loss of endothelial tight junctions. These changes are caused by a combination of stimuli that include the vasoactive substances, alteration of the ''endothelium-derived relaxing factor,'' and immunologically mediated phenomena.

Vasospasm usually affects the vessels in closest proximity to the area of bleeding and is most severe in the presence of large clots in the subarachnoid space. It is present on angiography in 50 to 70 percent of patients during the first 2 weeks after SAH (Fig. 34-4), subsiding after about 3 to 4 weeks. However, angiographically identified vasospasm is clinically symptomatic in only 20 to 30 percent of patients. The use of transcranial Doppler has greatly facilitated the diagnosis and follow-up of vasospasm. This noninvasive technique can be repeated often and is easily performed at the bedside. Important limitations of this technique are that it is highly operator dependent and that the transcranial windows may not be permeable to the ultrasound in 15 percent of the elderly population.

The clinical presentation of vasospasm is usually marked by a decrease in the level of consciousness and focal neurologic signs. Since ischemia is the clinical hallmark, patients may have any of the ischemic syndromes that relate to the arterial territory affected.

Hydrocephalus

Hydrocephalus can be found in the first few hours after SAH, and its presence correlates with increasing age, hypertension, a large accumulation of subarachnoid blood, or aneurysms located in the posterior circulation. Subacute hydrocephalus occurs after the first week and chronic hydrocephalus, after a few weeks or months. In the acute cases, CSF drainage can be life saving, and shunt placement should be considered.

Seizures

Seizures occur in 25 percent of patients with SAH and usually complicate the early stages of the hemorrhage. In the absence of seizures acutely, less than 5 percent of patients develop them later. There is no consensus on whether to give prophylactic anticonvulsants to patients with SAH, but, based on the potential for catastrophic aneurysmal rebleeding in the event of a seizure, their use is favored. An intravenous loading dose of phenytoin (17 mg/kg administered not faster than 50 mg/min) followed by 300 mg/day is recommended. Phenobarbital, at a dose of 90 to 120 mg/day, is also an effective anticonvulsant and may also be useful as a mild sedative.

Hyponatremia

Hyponatremia may produce an encephalopathy and can precipitate seizures, complicating the course of SAH. Determining the cause of hyponatremia in SAH may be difficult and presents a treatment dilemma. On the one hand, it can be due to the syndrome of inappropriate secretion of antidiuretic hormone, which improves with water restriction. On the other hand, hyponatremia can be caused by sodium loss with hypovolemia (cerebral salt wasting syndrome), and treatment with water restriction may cause dehydration and worsening of the ischemic effects of vasospasm. The distinction between these two conditions can be made with clinical (presence of dehydration or hypovolemia) and laboratory (serum and urinary sodium levels and osmolality) information. Depending on the degree of hyponatremia, treatment requires intravenous normal saline or, rarely, hypertonic saline. Usually, the establishment of normo-

volemia corrects the hyponatremia. A circulating digoxin-like substance or the atrial natriuretic factor may be related to the occurrence of hyponatremia in patients with SAH.

Cardiac Complications

A number of electrocardiogram changes can occur as a result of SAH. Changes in the ST segment and T wave (''waterfall Ts''), Q waves, sinus arrhythmia, and prolongation of the QT segment are frequently found. Life-threatening *torsade de pointes,* ventricular tachycardia, and ventricular fibrillation can also occur. Most arrhythmias are reversible, although myocardial ischemia from massive hypersympathetic discharge can result in necrosis of myocardial fibers. The cause of this abnormal autonomic response is thought to be hypothalamic injury from the acute SAH.

TREATMENT

General Medical Treatment

The patient with SAH should always be admitted to an intensive care unit bed. The environment should be quiet, and absolute bed rest is essential. After 5 days, the patient is allowed to use a bedside commode. Stool softeners are prescribed routinely to prevent constipation and straining.

Most management strategies depend on the patient's initial condition. The most frequently used measures are regular recording of vital signs, neurologic checks, intake and output monitoring, daily laboratory (arterial blood gases and serum sodium level), intravenous fluids (0.45 percent saline and 5 percent dextrose in water at 100 ml/h), nasal oxygen (some patients will be intubated), cardiac monitoring, arterial and central lines, prophylactic anticonvulsants, antiemetics, dexamethasone, and analgesics (codeine) as needed.

Antifibrinolytic Therapy

Although antifibrinolytic therapy is effective in decreasing the risk of rebleeding, its use is not recommended because of several serious complications. Aminocaproic acid and tranexamic acid are associated with an increased incidence of vasospasm and ischemic infarction, hydrocephalus, and other complications presumably related to a hypercoagulable state.

Vasospasm

Treatment of vasospasm is directed at augmenting blood flow in the affected areas. This goal can be achieved in several ways, but some carry a high risk of aneurysmal rupture if surgical clipping has not been performed during the first few days after the hemorrhage. The treatment modalities used to counteract the effects of vasospasm include

1. *Pharmacologic Agents.* The partially cerebral-selective vasodilator calcium channel blocker, nimodipine, in an oral dose of 60 mg every 4 hours (started within 4 days of onset of SAH and continued for 21 days) has been effective in improving neurologic outcome. Although it has not been shown to reverse angiographic vasospasm, it may produce its beneficial effects through improvement in leptomeningeal collateral circulation, decreased platelet aggregation, increased red cell deformability, and a neuroprotective effect mediated by limitation of entry of calcium into neurons. Potential side effects include hypotension, renal failure, and pulmonary edema.

2. *Induced Hypertension.* The first step should be to produce volume expansion with colloids. Then, medications to increase blood pressure, such as dopamine in a 4-μg/kg/h dose, can be administered. The aim is to reach a mean blood pressure of 140 mmHg. This therapy carries the potential risk of aneurysmal rupture in nonoperated patients, in whom maximal systolic pressure should not exceed 160 mmHg.

3. *Hemodilution.* Using albumin or other colloids may improve circulation through the narrowed vessels. A hematocrit around 33 ± 3 percent is ideal, since it improves blood flow (via a decrease in blood viscosity) without compromising the oxygen-carrying capacity of the blood.

4. *Mechanical Measures.* In recent years, interventional neuroradiologic techniques have offered new treatments. Vasospasm may be mechanically reversed by introducing a balloon in the artery (in a similar way to the procedure of coronary angioplasty) and then inflating it until vessel dilation is achieved.

Surgery

The controversy has revolved around the issue of performing early (first 3 days) or late (after the tenth day) surgery. The principal advantage for early clipping of the aneurysm is the prevention of rebleeding. The disadvantages include the surgical difficulties of operating on an acutely injured brain with the risk of rupturing the aneurysm or inducing vasospasm from surgical manipulation. However, advances in neuroanesthesia have improved the local surgical field, and the possibility of washing the subarachnoid space free of clot or even using thrombolytic agents to achieve this may reduce later vasospasm.

Delayed surgery allows time for the patient to stabilize clinically and for the brain to recover partially from the initial hemorrhage, but disastrous rebleeding may occur in the interim. Surgery is technically easier in the nonacute SAH, as there is better definition of anatomic landmarks and the aneurysm is less susceptible to rupture during the surgery.

This controversy was partially resolved by the results of the Cooperative Study on the Timing of Aneurysm Surgery (Haley et al., 1992), which showed that early and delayed surgery are associated with similar mortality rate at 6 months. However, functional outcome was significantly better for the early surgery group. Other findings of this trial included poor results that occurred when surgery was performed between days 5 and 10 because of an increased frequency of vasospasm and cerebral infarction; delayed surgery is indicated in patients with a poor clinical status (Hunt and Hess grade 4 or more), evidence of vasospasm on admission, active medical complications, giant aneurysms, or aneurysms of the top of the basilar artery; and early surgery with clipping of the aneurysm allows safe, aggressive treatment of vasospasm with induced hypertension and volume expansion. We favor early surgery in patients who present with a Hunt and Hess grade 1 or 2 and who have none of the contraindications described above.

UNRUPTURED ANEURYSM DETECTED INCIDENTALLY OR DURING EVALUATION OF A HIGH-RISK PATIENT

A decision to treat an incidental, unruptured aneurysm surgically must weigh the natural history of the risk of rupture (and its consequences) against the surgical morbidity and mortality rates. For aneurysms less than 10 mm, the annual risk of rupture is 0 to 4 percent, and it is greater if the aneurysm is larger. Surgical treatment by experienced surgeons has been accomplished with a low mortality rate of 0 to 1 percent, and a morbidity rate of 14.5 percent. The surgical risks are greater with larger aneurysms and those located at the carotid bifurcation, with intermediate risks for MCA, ophthalmic artery, and anterior communicating artery aneurysms and the lowest risk for internal carotid artery-posterior communicating aneurysms.

We recommend surgery for unruptured aneurysms in healthy patients who have a life expectancy greater than 5 years. In the case of very small aneurysms in elderly patients with chronic but not necessarily fatal associated diseases, follow-up of the aneurysm, if possible with magnetic resonance angiography, will help decide whether surgical treatment is indicated in the event of documented enlargement of the aneurysm.

SUBARACHNOID HEMORRHAGE AND PREGNANCY

Although previous opinions suggested an increased frequency of aneurysmal rupture in the third trimester, the rate is probably similar throughout the various stages of pregnancy. Rupture occurs more frequently in multiparous women. The hypervolemia of pregnancy and the stress of delivery increase the risk of aneurysmal rupture. Decisions about treatment are made as in any other patient with SAH. CT and angiography should be performed using abdominal shielding to protect the fetus. If the patient is in favorable neurologic and general clinical condition, early surgery should be performed. Fetal maturation should be initiated on admission, especially if the episode occurs early in the third trimester. Cesarean section is performed with epidural anesthesia followed immediately by general anesthesia for aneurysm clipping. Earlier pregnancy with a nonviable fetus should not delay surgery, and clipping of the aneurysm should be done under general anesthesia, avoiding hypotension, with the mother in the lateral decubitus position to minimize the compromise of fetal circulation. There are no contraindications to the use of nimodipine to prevent vasospasm, although cautious fetal monitoring is advised to detect the fetal acidosis syndrome and myocardial depression. The physiologic volume expansion of pregnancy may help in limiting the ischemic effects of vasospasm. Unruptured aneurysms should be treated surgically if they are larger than 10 mm in diameter; otherwise, surgical clipping should take place after delivery.

SUGGESTED READINGS

Adams HP: Calcium antagonists in the management of patients with aneurysmal subarachnoid hemorrhage: a review. Angiology 41:1010, 1990

Dias MS, Sekhar LN: Intracranial hemorrhage from aneurysms and arteriovenous malformations during pregnancy and the puerperium. Neurosurgery 27:855, 1990

Fisher CM, Kistler JP, Davis JM: Relation of cerebral vasospasm to subarachnoid hemorrhage visualized by computed tomographic scanning. Neurosurgery 6:1, 1980

Haley EC, Kassell NF, Torner JC: The International Cooperative Study on the Timing of Aneurysm Surgery: the North American experience. Stroke 23: 205, 1992

Hijdra A, van Gijn J, Nagelkerke NJD et al: Prediction of delayed cerebral ischemia, rebleeding and outcome after aneurysmal subarachnoid hemorrhage. Stroke 19:1250, 1988

Lindegaard KF, Nornes H, Bakke SJ et al: Cerebral vasospasm after subarachnoid hemorrhage investigated by means of transcranial Doppler ultrasound. Acta Neurochir 42:81, 1988

Rinkel GJE, Wijdicks EFM, Vermeulen M et al: Outcome in perimesencephalic (nonaneurysmal) subarachnoid hemorrhage: a follow up study in 37 patients. Neurology 40:1130, 1990 van Crevel H, Habbema JDF, Braakman R: Decision analysis of the management of incidental intracranial saccular aneurysms. Neurology 36:1335, 1986

Vermeulen M, van Gijn J: The diagnosis of subarachnoid hemorrhage. J Neurol Neurosurg Psychiatry 53:365, 1990

Wiebers DO, Whisnant JP, O'Fallon WM: The natural history of unruptured intracranial aneurysms. N Engl J Med 304:696, 1981

Wijdicks EFM, Ropper AH, Hunnicutt EJ et al: Atrial natriuretic factor and salt wasting after aneurysmal subarachnoid hemorrhage. Stroke 22:1519, 1991

Wilkins RH: Attempts at prevention or treatment of intracranial arterial spasm: an update. Neurosurgery 18:808, 1986

35. VASCULAR MALFORMATIONS

CARLOS S. KASE
CONRADO J. ESTOL

Vascular malformations correspond to developmentally abnormal vessels that can be of different types, depending on their histologic configuration. The four main types of vascular malformations are arteriovenous malformations (AVMs), cavernous angiomas, venous angiomas, and telangiectasias.

ARTERIOVENOUS MALFORMATIONS

AVMs are abnormal "tangles" of arteries and veins, with one or a group of feeding arteries that end in a central nidus, which drains, without interposed capillaries, into enlarged veins (that receive arterialized blood; Fig. 35-1). They are the second most common cause of subarachnoid hemorrhage and occur in a ratio of 1:10 with aneurysms. The mortality rate from the first hemorrhage is lower (10 percent) than that of aneurysmal subarachnoid hemorrhage, as is also its morbidity rate (30 to 50 percent); vasospasm does not occur after hemorrhages secondary to AVMs, and rebleeding rates are lower than those for aneurysmal rupture. Affected patients are usually younger (15 to 20 years) than those with aneurysms. Seven percent of patients with AVMs have coexisting cerebral aneurysms, which are located in the feeding artery in two-thirds of the patients.

Clinical Findings

Hemorrhage is the most common presentation (50 percent) of AVMs, followed by seizures and focal neurologic signs secondary to mass effect. Seizures are more frequent in patients diagnosed at a younger age and can also occur at the time of presentation of hemorrhage. However, the risk of hemorrhage in patients with seizures as the initial symptom is low. Seizures are thought to result in part from electrical neuronal instability caused by partial focal ischemia, resulting from a "steal" phenomenon caused by blood shunting in the malformation. This same mechanism explains the occasional observation of ischemia leading to infarction in areas adjacent to an AVM.

Headache is a frequent symptom but does not generally have the intensity described with aneurysmal rupture. It can be chronic and at times difficult to differentiate from "migraine with aura," especially in patients with occipital AVMs and accompanying transient visual phenomena, in particular homonymous hemianopia. The prevailing dogma is to suspect an AVM in young patients with hemicranial (migraine) headaches that are always located on the same side of the head, never on the opposite side. A bruit is often heard over the scalp with dural AVMs and occasionally with large superficial parenchymal malformations.

Their diagnosis is greatly facilitated by the use of imaging techniques that depict not only the meningocerebral hemorrhage in instances of acute bleeding but also the malformation itself. Computed tomographic (CT) scan often shows calcification in the area of the AVM, along with a serpiginous pattern of blood vessels, both arterial and venous, which is best depicted after intravenous contrast infusion. An even better definition of the AVM can be obtained with magnetic resonance imaging (MRI), which often shows the arterial and venous portions of the malformation as "flow voids" seen in T1-weighted images (Fig. 35-2). The more specific characteristics of the malformation, in terms of the anatomy of feeding arteries and draining veins that is essential to the surgical planning, still requires the use of contrast angiography.

Treatment

The conventional treatment for AVMs has been surgical resection. Ligation of feeding arteries, which carries the risk of brain infarction from ischemia, is limited to major arteries, followed by ligation of the draining veins. The nidus is then isolated from the brain parenchyma and excised using microsurgical techniques. In the perioperative period, β-blockers are administered to decrease the risk of "breakthrough" bleeding when the small vessels left at the surgical site cannot handle the large volumes of blood previously flowing into the malformation.

Embolization techniques are rapidly evolving in the aneurysm and AVM field, although they have not yet replaced conventional surgery. In this technique, microcatheters are advanced to the feeding arteries and nidus to deliver in situ different types of embolic materials. In various series, the mortality rate ranges from 2 to 4 percent. In some AVMs, embolization alone can completely obliterate the malformation; in others, embolization is used to decrease flow into the AVM prior to microsurgical resection or radiosurgical obliteration.

Stereotactic radiosurgery (γ knife), developed over the last decade, is an effective method for treatment of AVMs less than 4 cm in size. Larger AVMs can also be treated with this technique, but the degree of obliteration decreases with increasing lesion size. It should be kept in mind that the obliterating process depends on proliferative endothelial changes, collagen deposition, and vascular wall fibrosis, which are progressive, and usually takes a few years to be completed (100 percent occlusion in 3 years for AVMs less than 4 cm^3, 95 percent between 4 and 25 cm^3, and 70 percent for those more than 25 cm^3). Because of this, patients continue to be at risk of rebleeding during that period of time. In addition, radionecrosis of brain tissue adjacent to the AVM can result in cognitive deficits that are yet to be defined fully.

Although different combinations of microsurgery, embolization techniques, and radiosurgery are indicated, depending on the lesion's size and location, some general treatment guidelines are followed. Since most patients are previously healthy young individuals, we favor an aggressive approach with the goal of total resection of the AVM once the patient has recovered from

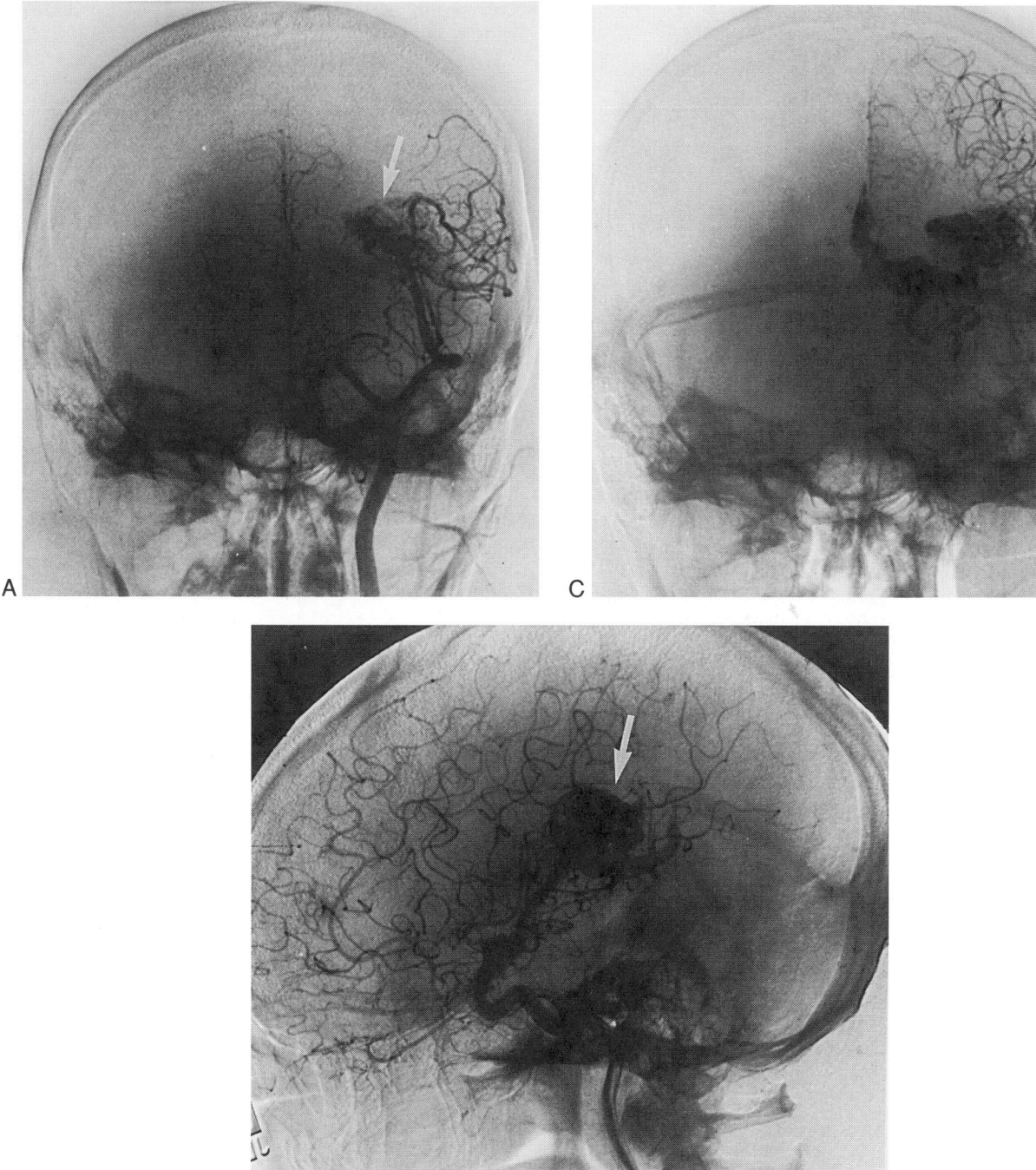

FIG. 35-1. **(A)** Anteroposterior carotid angiogram showing AVM (*arrow*) fed by distal middle cerebral artery branches. **(B)** Lateral angiogram of large parietal AVM (*arrow*) fed by the middle cerebral artery. **(C)** Arterial phase angiogram with early draining of parietal AVM into the deep venous system and the transverse sinuses. (Courtesy of Shripad Tilak, M.D., Department of Radiology, Boston University Medical Center, Boston, MA.)

the initial effects of acute hemorrhage. In older patients and in those with severe deficits from the initial bleeding episode, conservative treatment is favored, with either radiotherapy or embolization techniques. Patients with seizures as the only manifestation of the AVM and those who are fully asymptomatic need to be individualized in terms of the need for treatment, based on the location, size, and anatomy of the AVM. If seizures are intractable, surgery should be considered, although AVM resection may not alter an established brain injury that is likely to remain as a seizure focus.

Dural Arteriovenous Malformations

These lesions are located in close proximity to the venous sinuses, especially the transverse and sigmoid sinuses. The feeding vessel is most commonly the occipital artery, although branches from the vertebral or carotid arteries can also be feeders. In contrast to parenchymal AVMs, the dural types usually become symptomatic after age 40. Because of their location, they often present with an occipital bruit, pulsatile tinnitus, headache, and visual disturbances. As with any other posterior fossa mass, they can cause papilledema. Their surgical treat-

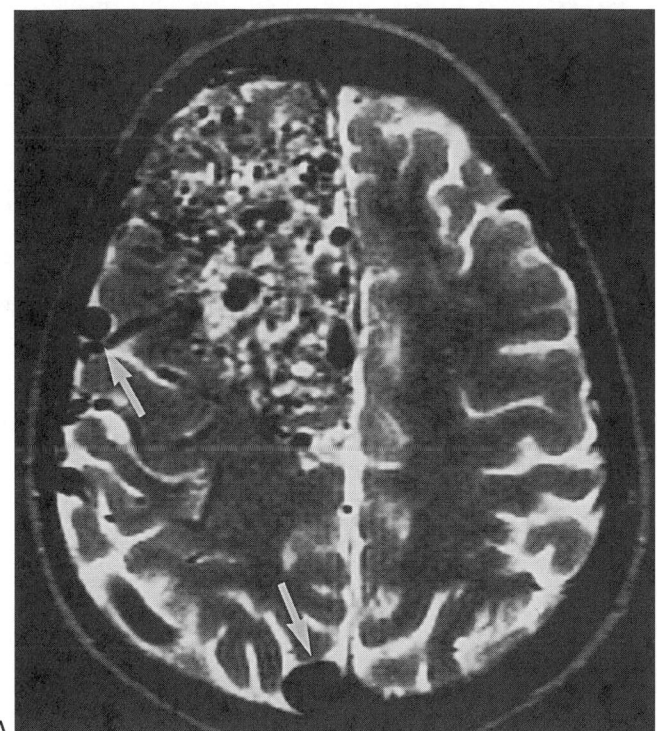
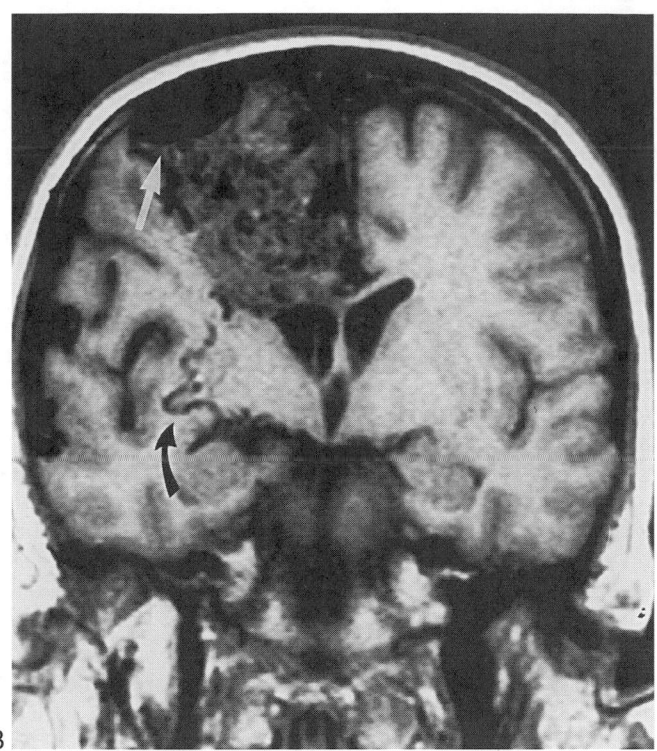

FIG. 35-2. **(A)** T1-weighted MRI showing large AVM as multiple "flow voids" in the left frontal lobe, along with prominent superficial venous channels (*arrows*). **(B)** T1-weighted MRI of same AVM in the coronal plane, showing markedly enlarged venous drainage channel in the cerebral surface (*arrow*) and an arterial feeder originating from the MCA trunk (*curved arrow*). (Courtesy of Rita Bhatia, M.D., Department of Radiology, Boston University Medical Center, Boston, MA.)

ment is difficult because of their tendency to bleed profusely. To limit this problem, embolization previous to surgery is often performed.

Spinal Arteriovenous Malformations

These malformations merit separate mention because of the importance of their consideration in the differential diagnosis of subarachnoid hemorrhage. In the event of subarachnoid hemorrhage followed by negative angiography for cerebral aneurysm or AVM, a spinal AVM should be considered. Its typical presentation includes abrupt onset of severe back pain and myelopathy (may also cause radiculopathy), but they can also cause headache and other focal neurologic phenomena such as visual changes, ocular nerve palsies, seizures, and loss of consciousness. A slowly progressive spinal cord compression syndrome has also been recognized.

Arteriovenous Malformations and Pregnancy

The popular notion that pregnancy increases the risk of bleeding from an AVM is probably incorrect and derives from the fact that most AVMs bleed by age 40, thus including women in their early, reproductive years. However, the increased volemia of pregnancy, especially during the third trimester, and the increase in blood and intracranial pressure of the peripartum period may increase the risk of AVM rupture.

As is recommended for aneurysms, management should be undertaken if AVMs present with bleeding during pregnancy. Depending on the anatomic characteristics of the lesion, the most appropriate treatment is selected. Partial treatments with embolization or radiosurgery started during pregnancy can be completed after delivery, since no differences in maternal mortality rate have been documented between surgical and nonsurgical treatment. Vaginal delivery is acceptable using epidural anesthesia.

CAVERNOUS ANGIOMAS ("CAVERNOMAS")

This lesion is characterized by groups of malformed vascular channels without arterial or venous structure, surrounded by connective tissue, without neural tissue in between them. Cavernous angiomas are generally single but, occasionally, are multiple, in which case familial incidence is highly likely. They can occur in any area of the brain, although they have a certain predilection for the pons. Their diagnosis is currently made routinely with MRI, owing to their highly characteristic pattern of a mixed-signal central core surrounded by a low-density hemosiderin ring in T2-weighted sequences (see Fig. 33-1).

Clinically, cavernous angiomas present similarly to AVMs, causing bleeding, but with lower rebleeding and mortality rates. Seizures and slowly progressive neurologic deficits can also occur, with the latter being a result of repeated episodes of small bleeding, often leading to a misdiagnosis of brain tumor or multiple sclerosis. Cavernous angiomas are often incidental findings after contrast CT or MRI; they are not detectable on angiography because of their small size and slow flow.

Treatment is often surgical, with the malformation generally being removed at the time of drainage of an intracerebral hematoma. Modern microsurgical techniques are allowing the removal of cavernous angiomas in areas of difficult surgical access, such as the pons, where these lesions were deemed inoperable in the past.

VENOUS ANGIOMAS

These lesions are formed by one or more enlarged veins that are most commonly an incidental CT or MRI finding. Angiography shows no abnormal vessels in the arterial and capillary phases, but a characteristic pattern of a cluster of abnormal veins (''caput medusae'') draining into a larger one in the venous phase of the angiogram is diagnostic of venous angioma (see Fig. 33-2).

Since they carry essentially no bleeding risk, they should not be treated. In the rare instances of bleeding associated with venous angiomas, it is now apparent that the cause is an associated cavernous angioma, not the venous angioma itself. In these instances, surgical therapy should be directed only at the cavernous angioma, since removal or ligation of the venous angioma is contraindicated, as it carries a high risk of postoperative venous hemorrhagic infarction. This is due to the fact that venous angiomas, despite being malformed vessels, effectively perform the venous drainage in the area of the brain where they are located.

TELANGIECTASIAS

These malformations are made of multiple enlarged blood vessels of capillary structure. They rarely cause neurologic deficits of brainstem origin, but their bleeding tendency is nil. They cannot be diagnosed with angiography on account of their small size and slow flow, but they can be detected by MRI. Occasionally, they are associated with cavernous angiomas in the same area of the brain, generally in the brainstem.

SUGGESTED READINGS

Caroscio JT, Brannan T, Budabin M et al: Subarachnoid hemorrhage secondary to spinal arteriovenous malformation and aneurysm. Arch Neurol 37:101, 1980

Drake CG: Arteriovenous malformations of the brain: the options for management. N Engl J Med 309:308, 1983

Gomori JM, Grossman RI, Goldberg HI et al: Occult cerebral vascular malformations: high-field MR imaging. Radiology 158:707, 1986

Horton JC, Chambers WA, Lyons SL et al: Pregnancy and the risk of hemorrhage from cerebral arteriovenous malformations. Neurosurgery 27:867, 1990

Malik GM, Pearce JE, Ausman JI: Dural arteriovenous malformations and intracranial hemorrhage. Neurosurgery 15:332, 1984

Rigamonti D, Hadley MN, Drayer BP et al: Cerebral cavernous malformations: incidence and familial occurrence. N Engl J Med 319:343, 1988

Stahl SM, Johnson KP, Malamud N: The clinical and pathological spectrum of brainstem vascular malformations. Arch Neurol 37:25, 1980

Stein BM, Wolpert SM: Arteriovenous malformations of the brain: current concepts and treatment. Arch Neurol 37:1, 1980

Steinberg GK, Fabrikant JI, Marks MP et al: Stereotactic heavy charged particle Bragg-peak radiation for intracranial arteriovenous malformations. N Engl J Med 323:96, 1990

Viñuela F, Fox AJ: Interventional neuroradiology and the management of arteriovenous malformations and fistulas. p. 131. In Barnett HJM (ed): Neurologic Clinics: Cerebrovascular Disease. WB Saunders, Philadelphia, 1983

SECTION 3. LESS COMMON CAUSES OF STROKE

36. LESS COMMON VASCULAR CAUSES OF STROKE

NALINI SAMUEL
LUIS D'OLHABERRIAGUE
STEVEN R. LEVINE
LAWRENCE M. BRASS

Stroke results from a variety of diseases that affect the vascular supply of the brain. Although classified into half a dozen major mechanisms, many different underlying etiologies can contribute to, or may directly result in, a stroke. Even an abridged listing of the diseases associated with stroke can be daunting (Tables 36-1 and 36-2). In this and the following four chapters, some of the less common causes of stroke are selected for detailed discussion, others are covered elsewhere in this volume. The topics reviewed are included because of their importance in helping the clinician better understand, and manage, patients with stroke.

Although the diseases discussed in these chapters are generally considered uncommon causes for stroke as a whole, in clinically important subgroups, they may predominate. For example, in younger patients, dissection and fibromuscular dysplasia are among the most common causes of nonatherosclerotic carotid narrowing. Other diseases, although uncommon, were selected because they may illustrate an important mechanism of stroke, such as the venous-to-arterial shunts associated with pulmonary arteriovenous malformations or vasospasm in migraine.

DISSECTION

Arterial dissection occurs when a tear in the intima or injury in the media allows blood to accumulate within the potential space between the layers of the arterial wall, usually within the medial layer. In about one-half of the cases, an obvious traumatic injury can be identified. This is often attributed to an abrupt or extreme extension of the neck. Reported associations include chiropractic manipulation, sports injuries, whiplash injury, and endotracheal intubation. The other half are often referred to as ''spontaneous dissection.'' In many cases of spontaneous dissection, subtle or minor activities have been

TABLE 36-1. Causes of Ischemic Stroke

Arteropathy
  Noninflammatory
    Atherosclerosis
    Sneddon syndrome
    Homocystinemia
    Rendu-Osler disease
    Moyamoya disease
    Hereditary hyperlipidemia
    Pseudoxanthoma elasticum
    Marfan syndrome
    Fabry's disease
    Neurofibromatosis
    Arterial dissection
    Trauma to the cervical arteries
    Fibromuscular dysplasia
    Basilar artery ectasia
    Arteriovenous malformations
    Arterial spasm (subarachnoid hemorrhage, migraine, neurosurgery, hypercalcemia)
    Arteral kinking
    Cervico-occipital and cervical abnormalities (Arnold-Chiari syndrome, basilar impression, cleidocranial dysostosis, atlantoaxial subluxation, odontoid dislocation, cervical spine subluxation, chiropractic maneuvers)
    Cervical rib
    Scalenus syndrome
    Cervical spondylosis
    Steal syndromes
    Cocaine
  Inflammatory
    Periarteritis nodosa
    Systemic lupus erythematosus
    Wegener's arteritis
    Systemic sclerosis
    Giant cell arteritis
    Rheumatoid arthritis
    Mixed connective tissue disease
    Granulomatous angiitis of central nervous system
    Sjögren syndrome
    Takayasu disease
    Inflammatory bowel disease
    Köhlmeier-Degos disease
    Lymphomatoid granulomatosis
    Aortoarteritis
    Infectious arteritis (tuberculosis, brucellosis, syphilis, fungal, viral, endocarditis, malaria, *haemophilus influenzae* infection, pneumococcosis, mycoplasmosis)
    Drugs (amphetamines)
    Acquired immunodeficiency syndrome
    Fibrinoid hypertensive arteritis
    Cysticerosis
    Neoplastic angioendotheliosis
    Intravascular malignant histiocytosis
    Radiation arteritis
    Angiography
Blood (coagulation)
  Polycythemia vera
  Hypereosinophilic syndrome
  Secondary polycythemia (lung disease, cyanotic heart disease, high altitude, high oxygen-affinity hemoglobins, hypernephroma, hemangioblastoma)
  Stress polycythemia
  Hyperfibrinogenemia
  Antiphospholipid antibodies
  Ferropenic anemia
  Macrolobulinemia
  Myeloma
  Leukemia
  Thrombocythemia
  Thrombotic thrombocytopenic purpura
  Sickle cell disease
  Paroxysmal nocturnal hemoglobinuria
  Nephrotic syndrome
  Antithrombin III deficiency
  Amniotic fluid embolism
  Fat embolism
  Foreign body embolism
  Cartilagenous embolism
Unusual cardiac embolic disorders
  Atrial septal aneurysms
  Fibroelastoma of cardiac valve
  Postpartum cardiomyopathy
  Libman-Sacks endocarditis (verrucous endocarditis)
  Cardiac tumors

Acute hypotension (bleeding, myocardial infarction, surgery, anesthesia, pulmonary embolism)

TABLE 36-2. Causes of Hemorrhagic Stroke

Noninflammatory arterial disease
  Amyloidosis
  Rendu-Osler disease
  Moyamoya disease
  Ehlers-Danlos disease
  Arterial dissection
  Arteriovenous malformations
  Cocaine
Inflammatory arterial disease
  Periarteritis nodosa
  Systemic lupus erythematosus
  Wegener's arteritis
  Systemic sclerosis
  Mixed connective tissue disease
  Granulomatous angiitis of central nervous system
  Infectious arteritis (tuberculosis, brucellosis, syphilis, fungal, viral, endocarditis, malaria, *Haemophilus influenzae* infection, pneumococcosis, mycoplasmosis)
  Drugs (amphetamines, phenypropanolamine)
  Acquired immunodeficiency syndrome
  Fibrinoid hypertensive arteritis
  Familial cortical arteritis
Mass lesions
  Cerebral tumors (astrocytoma, meningioma, pituitary adenoma, subependymoma, hemangioma, metastases)
Blood dyscrasias
  Macroglobulinemia
  Myeloma
  Leukemia
  Thrombotic thrombocytopenic purpura
  Thrombocytopenia (acute leukemia, aplastic anemia, chronic lymphoid leukemia, dysmyelopoietic syndromes, septicemia, angioimmunoblastic lymphadenopathy, post-transfusional purpura)
  Acquired qualitative platelet defects (uremia, surgery, paraproteinemia, polycythemia, myelofibrosis, drugs)
  Sickle cell disease
  Scurvy
  Coagulation factors diseases (hemophilia, Christmas disease, von Willebrand disease, deficiency of factors V, VII, XII, or XIII)
  Vitamin K disorders (liver diseases, anticoagulation)
  Intravascular disseminated coagulation (septicemia, viral diseases, heat stroke, giant hemangioma, shock, cancer, leukemia, snake bite, acute intravascular hemolysis)

implicated in causing arterial injury such as sneezing and coughing bouts, vomiting, or turning the head while backing an automobile. The etiologic role of these minor ''traumas'' remains speculative; however, they may be important for those with structural abnormalities of the vessel wall (e.g., Ehlers-Danlos syndrome).

As the false lumen accumulates blood within the vessel wall, the lumen of the artery narrows. Stroke may be caused by hemodynamic compromise secondary to vessel narrowing or the formation of thrombus with secondary embolization.

The characteristic clinical presentation of dissection is a focal neurologic syndrome with unilateral headache or neck pain following a neck injury. With dissection of the carotid artery, the pain is often referred to the eye, temple, or forehead. Because the sympathetic nerves that surround the carotid artery may also be injured, there is often an accompanying Horner syndrome. With a vertebral artery dissection, the pain is often referred to the neck or back of the head, and a lateral medullary syndrome often occurs. With either location of dissection, patients may describe pulsatile tinnitus, and an arterial bruit may be heard on auscultation.

The most common sites for dissection are within the proximal internal carotid artery, usually 2 cm or more beyond the bifurcation, or the distal extracranial vertebral artery. Cerebral angiography is usually required for the diagnosis. The classic angiographic finding is a smooth, long, tapered narrowing of the arterial lumen (Fig. 36-1). Pseudoaneurysm formation or intraluminal thrombus may also been seen. Dissections may involve

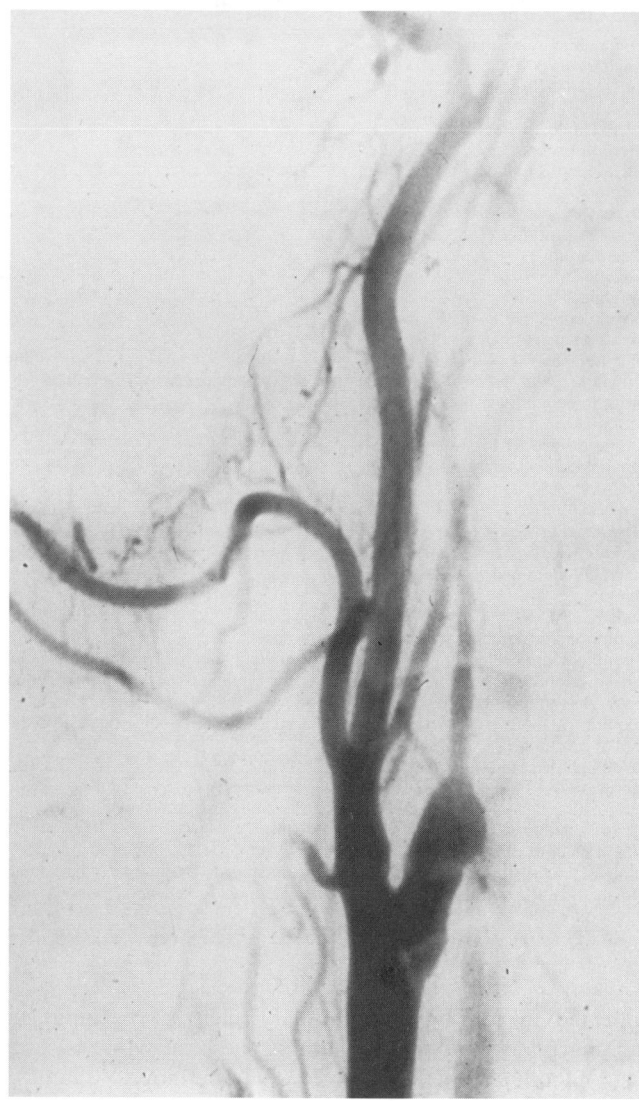

FIG. 36-1. Carotid dissection.

There should be an aggressive consideration of diseases affecting the arterial wall for patients with a family or personal history of dissection or more than one vessel affected. The diseases associated with cervical dissection include fibromuscular dysplasia, Marfan syndrome, cystic medial degeneration, atherosclerosis, luetic arthritis, and Ehlers-Danlos syndrome. In addition, for all patients with dissection, the clinician should review the medical history and physical examination for clues to suggest one of these diagnoses.

FIBROMUSCULAR DYSPLASIA

Fibromuscular dysplasia is a nonatherosclerotic and noninflammatory vasculopathy. It affects small and medium sized arteries. The most commonly affected vessels are the renal arteries (75 percent of cases) and the carotid arteries (25 percent). The disease is commonly multifocal and affects other vascular beds such as the visceral arteries, iliac and femoral arteries, axillary and subclavian arteries, as well as the intracranial vessels.

Pathologically, any of the layers of the arterial wall (intima, media, or adventitia) may be involved. Typically, there is hypertrophy of fibrous tissue or proliferation of smooth muscle with irregular narrowing of the vessel lumen. Angiographically, this typically appears as a segmental narrowing of the artery, which may look similar to a "string of beads" (Fig. 36-2).

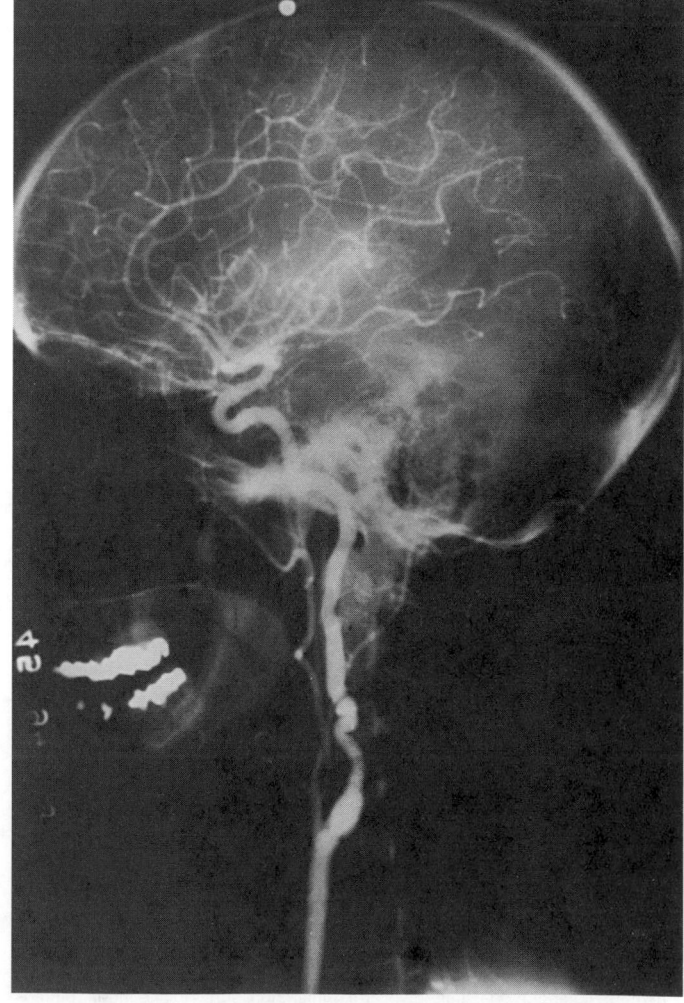

FIG. 36-2. Carotid fibromuscular dysplasia.

more than one vessel. This is more commonly seen in patients with widespread abnormalities of the vessel wall.

Other techniques for the diagnosis of dissection are less reliable. Duplex ultrasound often misses a dissection. The head of the duplex imaging device is usually too large to examine the internal carotid artery much beyond the bifurcation in the neck; so the more distal dissections are easily missed. The vertebral arteries are difficult to image because of their path through the transverse processes of the vertebral bodies. Magnetic resonance imaging (MRI) has a high enough resolution, and is able to demonstrate the extraluminal blood directly within the media of the arterial wall. The reliability of this finding, and of detecting dissection with magnetic resonance angiography, is unknown.

Opinions concerning therapy vary, and no studies to date have documented an unequivocal beneficial treatment. Anticoagulation is often used because of the potential for embolization from the region of the narrowed lumen. Many authorities recommend acute anticoagulation followed by 6 to 12 months of warfarin therapy. Others authorities cite the low rate of recurrent stroke in untreated patients and advocate antiplatelet therapy.

The etiology is unknown, but women are affected about twice as often as men. The condition is uncommon, and the reported rate in clinical stroke series is about 0.5 percent. Fibromuscular dysplasia is noted incidentally (in any arterial bed) in about 1 percent of autopsy cases, which illustrates that most patients are asymptomatic. Fibromuscular dysplasia has been associated with a variety of stroke mechanisms, including carotid dissection, embolization, and aneurysm formation, but its role as a causative factor remains unclear.

Angioplasty has emerged as a treatment for those patients with renal artery stenosis and secondary hypertension, but its role in carotid fibromuscular dysplasia is uncertain except perhaps for the exceptional patient with high-grade stenosis and symptoms related to low perfusion. The reported low rate of stroke in patients with fibromuscular dysplasia favors a conservative approach using antiplatelet agents. If the disease is discovered incidentally, specific therapy is not indicated.

MIGRAINE

Migraine is a common neurologic disorder, which is diagnosed primarily by clinical history. This creates a challenge to the clinician who must rely heavily on the patient's account of what is typical or atypical about a particular migraine attack. Migraines are frequently associated with other neurologic accompaniments. The definition of a migrainous infarction requires a positive brain imaging study and the persistence of symptoms for more than 1 week, following an otherwise typical migraine attack. Patients with migraine and persisting aura should be evaluated fully for stroke.

The pathophysiology of migraine is not completely understood, but several mechanisms have been proposed, including hormone-induced vasospasm, spreading depression, and platelet aggregation. The overall effect on cerebral blood flow parameters and cerebrovascular patency can contribute to the evolution of a stroke.

Estimates of the quantitative importance of migraine as a cause of (ischemic) stroke are at best uncertain. From our meta-analysis of 2,168 cases of stroke in the young, published in the literature, there were 77 (3.5 percent) migraine-related strokes. However, the diagnostic criteria were so different from study to study that these figures can only be taken as a crude approximation. The new definition of migraine-related stroke is from the International Headache Society Classification of Head Pain (Table 36-3).

There are four main subtypes of migraine-related strokes (Table 36-4). The first subtype (coexisting migraine and stroke) refers to a stroke that occurs remotely in time from a migraine attack in a migraineur. The second subtype (stroke with clinical features of migraine) describes migrainous syndromes caused by an established structural cause such as arteriovenous malformation (AVM) or an old infarct or migrainous symptoms related to a new cause such as an acute stroke. The third subtype

TABLE 36-3. Criteria for the Diagnosis of Migrainous Stroke

One or more migrainous aura symptoms that are not fully reversible within 7 days and/or are associated with neuroimaging confirmation of ischemic infarction
Patient has previously fulfilled criteria for migraine with neurologic aura

The present attack is typical of previous attacks, but neurologic deficits are not completely reversible within 7 days and/or neuroimaging demonstrates ischemic infarction in the relevant area

Other cases of infarction ruled out by appropriate investigations

TABLE 36-4. Classification of Migraine-Related Strokes

I	Coexisting migraine and stroke
II	Stroke with clinical features of migraine
	IIa Established (symptomatic migraine): arteriovenous malformation, old infarct, brain tumor
	IIb New-onset (migraine mimic): arterial dissection, stroke
III	Migraine-induced stroke
	IIIa Without risk factors
	IIIb With risk factors: oral contraceptives, smoking
IV	Uncertain: mitral valve prolapse, antiphospholipid antibodies

(migraine-induced stroke (MIS) refers to stroke in a person with a history of migraine with aura, whose symptoms are similar to the previous migraine attacks, and in whom other causes of stroke are absent. Finally, the fourth subtype (uncertain group) includes cases that do not fit in any of the other categories.

In conclusion, migraine and stroke can be casually linked (MIS). In people younger than 45, this association is easier to demonstrate than in older patients, in which multiple risk factors and causes of stroke are likely to coexist. The diagnosis of MIS must be limited to migraineurs who suffer a stroke during a typical attack after a complete etiologic investigation has ruled out cardiac, arterial, and hematologic causes of stroke. Although angiography can sometimes induce migraine attacks, transient global amnesia, and infarcts, there were no complications of angiography in MIS in the largest of the referred series. Other studies found an equally low rate of complications of angiography in a migraine group compared to control patients. It can be argued, on the other hand, that the yield of angiography in MIS is low, although this could reflect the well known loss of sensibility of angiography, with time after ictus. Further progress in ultrasound techniques and magnetic resonance angiography may soon resolve the dilemma of angiography in migraine. Most migraine-related infarcts occur in the posterior circulation and are associated with migraine attacks of long duration and with a history of migraine with aura. These data support the view that there is a continuum between migraine with aura and MIS. Once computed tomography (CT) or MRI have excluded structural lesions that can cause symptomatic migraine (especially an AVM) and migraine mimics, arterial dissection is the most common condition to be considered when migraine-related stroke is investigated (see next section).

Arterial hypertension, diabetes, cardiac diseases, hypercholesterolemia, smoking, and other risk factors for stroke clearly operate also in migraineurs. However, there are three conditions that merit special consideration in the context of migraine-related stroke: mitral valve prolapse (MVP), antiphospholipid antibodies (aPL), and oral contraceptives. MVP is present in up to 5 percent of the general population and, similar to migraine, is more common in women. The prevalence of MVP in migraineurs ranges between 20 and 30 percent. Aged males with MVP, redundant, thickened valve leaflets and other valve-associated anomalies represent a high-risk group for stroke. Strokes associated with MVP and migraine may not be cardioembolic. One reported case of a migraineur who took oral contraceptives and had a stroke also had associated patent foramen ovale and MVP. Protein C or S deficiencies, aPL, and platelet disorders have also been reported in MVP.

Clearly, there exists a link, causal or more complex, between migraine, MVP, and stroke. The importance of aPL—anticardiolipin antibodies (aCL) and lupus anticoagulant—in migraine-related strokes might be twofold. First, there is now clear evidence that aCL are present in at least 10 percent of all stroke patients and aCL are an independent risk factor for stroke. Second, aPL have been related to migraine and other neurologic nonischemic conditions. However, two recent studies failed to associate migraine and aPL reactivity. To complicate the issue further, aPL have also been associated with mitral valve lesions. Although the issue is still unsettled, it seems currently reasonable to look for aPL in migraine patients and in all stroke patients. The use of oral contraceptives, especially early preparations with high doses of estrogen, have been associated with an increased risk of ischemic stroke. Although in one study there was no difference in oral contraceptive use between migraineurs with and without stroke, most evidences suggests that migraineurs who use oral contraceptives have a 2.5 to 6 increased relative risk of stroke than migraineurs who do not, particularly if they also smoke. Other conditions that have occasionally been associated with migraine-related stroke are MELAS syndrome, migraine with cerebrospinal fluid pleocytosis, overuse of ergotamine, and sickle cell trait.

The general principles of migraine management include the avoidance of known triggers of migraine attacks and the use of drugs. Drug therapy is directed, first, to abort the migraine attack and, second, to prevent the frequency of attacks. Migraine prophylaxis, in general, should be limited to patients who suffer more than two or three disabling attacks per month, in whom symptomatic therapies have failed or caused severe side effects, and in whom nonpharmacologic treatment has also failed. The treatment of migraine-related stroke depends on the assumed stroke mechanism. The first steps in the management of migraine-related stroke are directed toward identifying risk factors for thromboembolic stroke (arterial [carotid dissection], cardiac [MVP], or hematologic [aPL]) and treating them accordingly. The management of MIS should stress control of precipitating factors, such as avoiding tobacco and oral contraceptive use. Antimigraine drugs with vasoconstrictor effects (such as ergotamine and methysergide) must be stopped. Antiplatelet drugs to be used in the prophylaxis of stroke are aspirin or ticlopidine. No study has addressed the need for primary prophylaxis of stroke in migraine. However, clinical judgment suggests the use of aspirin, which is useful both for migraine treatment and stroke prevention, in patients with severe, frequent (two or three per month) attacks of migraine with aura, especially when there are clear deficits such as aphasia or hemiparesis.

MOYAMOYA SYNDROME

Moyamoya syndrome refers to a group of diseases resulting in intracranial arterial occlusions. The name moyamoya (Japanese for a puff of smoke) refers to the angiographic blush of fine collateral vessels that form around the arterial occlusions. The arterial occlusion is the disease. The appearance of moyamoya is a secondary reaction (Fig. 36-3).

This syndrome is most common during the first three decades of life. After this age, the ability to form these collaterals is markedly diminished. The initial cerebrovascular syndrome is usually ischemic, secondary to hypoperfusion. In later life (third to fifth decades), there is an increased risk of intracerebral hemorrhagic from rupture of these small, fragile collateral vessels. These collateral vessels may bleed from the long-term effects of stress, fibrinoid necrosis, or microaneurysm formation. Many of the cases in later life present with a parenchymal hemorrhage.

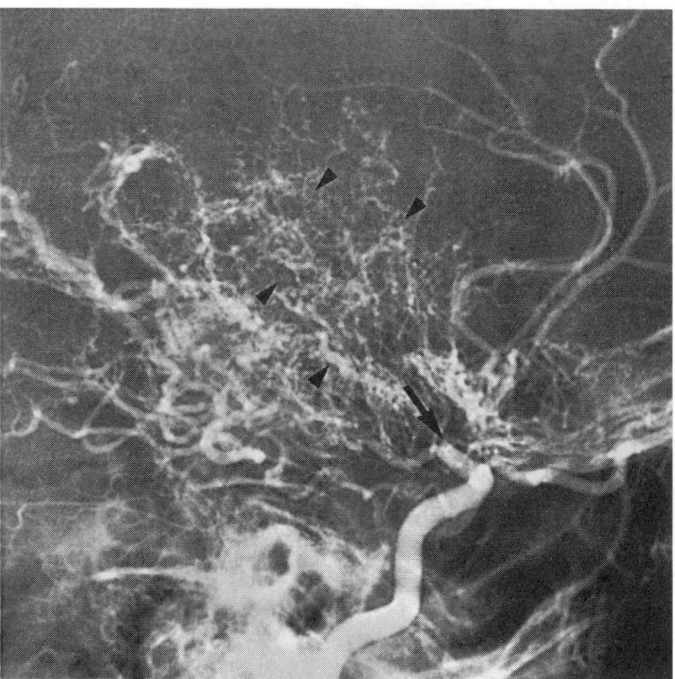

FIG. 36-3. Moyamoya (*arrowheads*). The large arrow indicates high-grade stenosis of the intracranial internal carotid artery.

In both age groups, the syndrome is about twice as common in girls and women.

The term *moyamoya disease* is often used to refer to idiopathic intracranial carotid occlusion in young children, usually younger than 4 years old. The carotid occlusive disease is often bilateral. The prognosis for this group is poor; seizures, hemiparesis, and encephalopathy are common. As the name suggests, the syndrome was initially described in Japan, where the estimated incidence is 1 per 1,000,000 per year. It is now being recognized in the Western nations, but the incidence appear to be lower in whites.

The etiology of moyamoya disease is unclear, but a limited number of autopsy examinations suggest that the occlusive process is an intimal hyperplasia. Numerous theories to account for the condition have been proposed, including genetic transmission, congenital anomaly, acquired infectious agent, autoimmune process, hyperactivity of cervical sympathetic nerves, and abnormal thrombogenesis. Between 7 and 12 percent of cases are familial, and the syndrome has been associated with genetic diseases such as neurofibromatosis, sickle cell disease, Marfan syndrome, radiation therapy, type I glycogenesis, pseudoxanthoma elasticum, and Down syndrome.

The diagnostic evaluation is dependent on the angiographic demonstration of intracranial large artery occlusions at the skull base and the moyamoya vessels. The infarcts are usually readily demonstrated by CT or MRI and are usually bihemispheric. The hemorrhages are deep in the distribution of the fine collaterals. The abnormal collateral vessels, however, are below the resolution of magnetic resonance angiography. The presence of moyamoya may be suggested on MRI, magnetic resonance angiography, or CT when there is stenosis or occlusion of the intracranial internal carotid artery or the proximal middle cerebral artery (MCA).

Other testing often done as part of the early evaluation of a patient with moyamoya includes duplex carotid ultrasound, which may demonstrate a high-resistance velocity waveform in the internal carotid artery, suggesting distal occlusive disease. Transcranial Doppler ultrasound shows low velocity in the distal internal carotid artery and proximal MCA with impaired cerebral reactivity. If the stenosis is not complete, there may be a focal increase in blood velocity in the region of the stenosis. Laboratory studies are usually not helpful but may be indicated to exclude other disease processes that may be associated with the moyamoya syndrome (see above).

A variety of medical and surgical management strategies have been used. Medical management includes antiplatelet agents, anticoagulants, steroids, and vasodilators. Most commonly, aspirin is used. Other symptomatic medical treatment addresses the common problems of epilepsy and headache. Surgical management has focused on procedures that aim to bypass the occlusion by creating an anastomotic connection between the intracranial and extracranial circulation. The goal is to improve the circulation beyond the occlusive area and relieve the strong pressure gradient across the fine collateral vessels to minimize the secondary bleeding complications. The procedure most often performed is the superficial temporal artery-MCA bypass, which connects a branch of the superficial temporal artery (from the extracranial circulation) to a branch of the MCA (in the intracranial circulation).

FUSIFORM (DOLICHOECTATIC) ANEURYSMS

Fusiform aneurysms are tortuous, ectatic, elongated variations of the normal arterial anatomy, which have also been called dolichoectatic (dolicho = long, ectatic = distended) arteries. The condition may affect any of the major cerebral arteries but is most commonly seen in the vertebrobasilar vessels (Figs. 36-4 and 36-5). They were thought to be an uncommon vascular anomaly, but, with the increasing use of high-resolution CT, MRI, and magnetic resonance angiography, they are being found more frequently. Depending on the definition, their prevalence ranges between 0.06 and 6 percent.

On neuroimaging, the vertebrobasilar aneurysms appear as

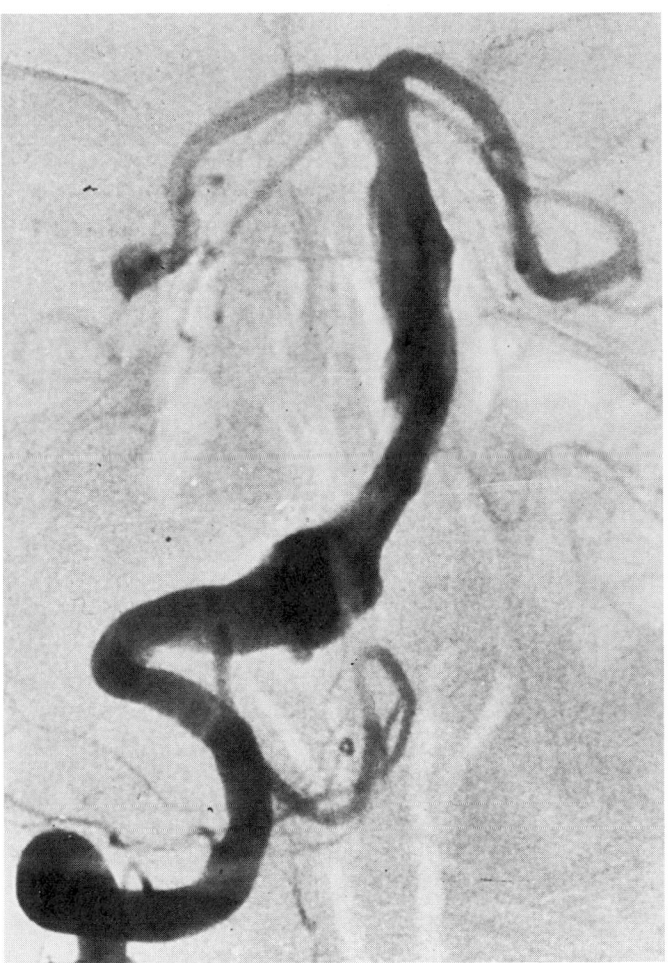

FIG. 36-5. Dolichoectatic basilar artery.

curvilinear, enhancing channels crossing the cerebellopontine angle (Figs. 36-6 and 36-7). These enlarged arteries can cause cranial nerve and brainstem compression or hydrocephalus. The most frequently affected cranial nerves are the trigeminal nerve (with associated facial pain) and the facial nerve (causing hemifacial spasm). Tinnitus, cerebellar or vestibular ataxia, and gaze abnormalities are frequently associated with brainstem compression.

Fusiform aneurysms of the vertebrobasilar arteries have also been implicated as a cause of stroke. Several mechanism have been proposed. Clinically, the causes may be multiple and difficult to determine in an individual case (Table 36-5). Complete or partial thrombosis of the aneurysm can cause ischemic stroke in different ways. The enlarged, tortuous artery may have areas of stasis, which harbor clots. An intraluminal clot may be the origin of emboli to the distal basilar or posterior cerebral arteries. Thrombosis may also occur and have local effects in occluding the parent vessel or compressing the origin of small penetrating vessels at the base of the brainstem. In addition, a thrombosed aneurysm may also contribute to local neural compression. Although fusiform aneurysms have a wider caliber than the normal artery, they may be compromised by atherosclerosis. Stroke syndromes associated with localized atheroocclusive disease may also occur.

Subarachnoid hemorrhage from fusiform aneurysm rupture, although rare, has been reported. Rupture is thought to be re-

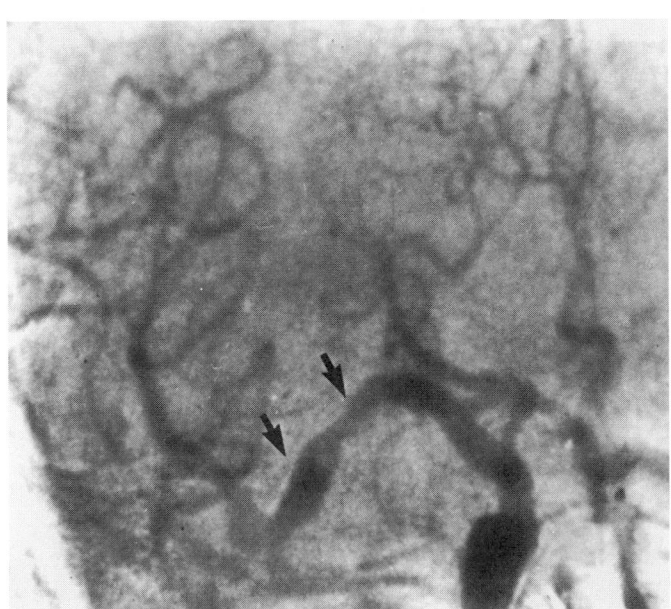

FIG. 36-4. Dolichoectasia of middle cerebral artery (*arrows*).

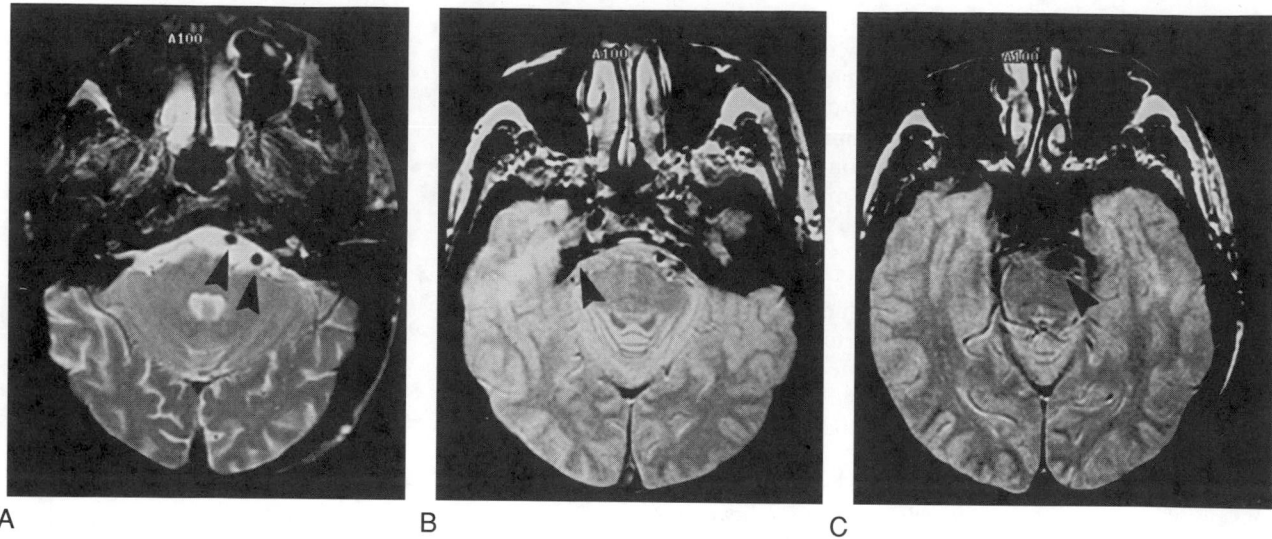

FIG. 36-6. **(A)** T2-weighted image showing both vertebral arteries (*arrowheads*) on the right. **(B & C)** Dolichoectatic basilar artery.

lated to structural defects in the vessel wall, such as a deficiency in elastin or fibrous dysplasia of the intima. These structural anomalies may occur as part of a systemic arteriopathy reported to affect the pancreas, spleen, and other organs. It has also been associated with α-glucosidase deficiency. Saccular aneurysms, more commonly associated with subarachnoid hemorrhage, also occur in association with fusiform aneurysms. Finally, hemorrhage may occur through minor trauma in these abnormally weak arteries with rupture or dissection.

Diagnostic tests that can be useful to study fusiform aneurysms include ultrasonography, CT scan, MRI, magnetic resonance angiography, and conventional angiography. Doppler studies, although the reliability is unknown, may show low blood velocities in dilated arteries. On a CT scan, vertebrobasilar ectatic arteries appear as tortuous, dilated vascular channels crossing the brainstem from one cerebellopontine angle to the other side. MRI and magnetic resonance angiography have better resolution and often demonstrate that the vertebral arteries are also distorted or displaced. Angiography is still necessary, however, to demonstrate the aneurysms clearly and to help differentiate among the possible mechanisms for stroke (arteriosclerosis, intraluminal thrombus, dissection, and so forth).

The best management for these fusiform aneurysms, especially when found incidentally, is unknown. When compression is present and symptomatic, success with surgical therapy has been reported in a few small series of cases. The use of surgery for secondary prevention of stroke is not known.

HEREDITARY HEMORRHAGIC TELANGIECTASIA

Hereditary hemorrhagic telangiectasia (HHT) is a familial disorder of systemic angiomatosis. Vascular malformations may occur in nearly any organ system but typically involve the skin, central nervous system, lungs, and mucosal membranes.

Although the disease is characterized by telangiectasia, other vascular malformations, including AVMs may occur. The most common neurologic syndromes are caused by central nervous system and pulmonary AVMs. About 10 percent of patients with HHT have vascular malformations of the central nervous system. These are most often detected only after patients present with intracranial hemorrhage, seizures, headaches, or focal neurologic symptoms. Pulmonary AVMs occur in about one-quarter of cases. When large and multiple, they may impair pulmonary function by allowing mixing of venous and arterial

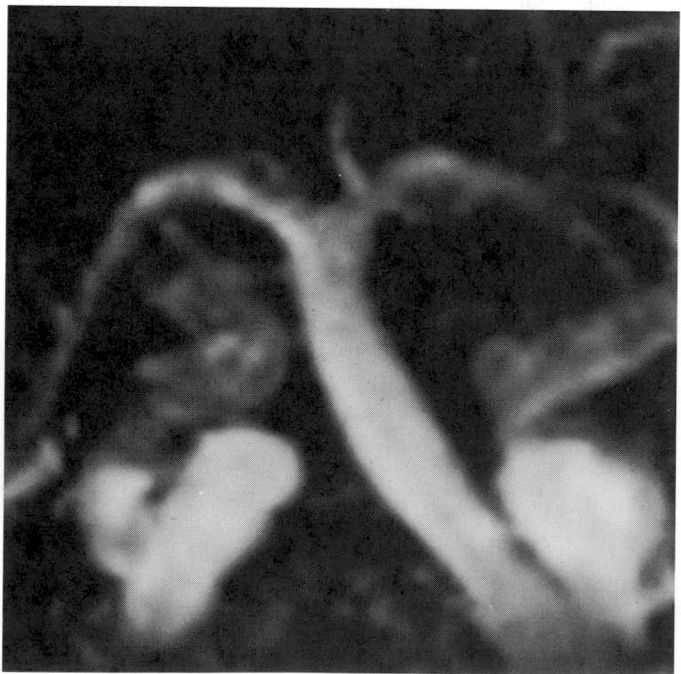

FIG. 36-7. Magnetic resonance angiography showing a dilated, ectatic basilar artery of the same patient as in Figure 36-6.

TABLE 36-5. Mechanisms of Stroke Related to Fusiform Aneurysms

Thrombosis of the aneurysm or parent artery
Intraluminal clot
Artery-to-artery embolism
Distortion/occlusion of the origin of penetrating branch arteries
Dissection
Subarachnoid hemorrhage

blood. This may result in oxygen desaturation and secondary polycythemia. Pulmonary AVMs may also act as a shunt from the venous circulation to the arterial circulation, without blood passing through the pulmonary capillary bed.

Much of our current understanding of right-to-left (venous-to-arterial) shunts is derived from diseases that affect the cardiac septa (e.g., patent foramen ovale). Strokes in those with intracardiac shunts have been attributed to direct effects of the shunt, but the cardiac abnormality is also a marker for an associated risk for stroke. Pulmonary AVMs serve as a second model for understanding right-to-left shunts and their role in stroke.

Patients with pulmonary AVMs have an increased risk of cerebral embolism and cerebral abscess, each arising from the loss of the filtering effect of the capillary bed of the lungs. About 5 percent of patients with pulmonary AVMs develop a brain abscess. One-third of all patients have MRI evidence of an ischemic stroke. The associated ischemic cerebral syndromes range from transient ischemic attacks to massive hemispheric infarction. Still unexplained is an increased frequency of migraine with aura. This may occur in up to one-half of patients with pulmonary AVM and HHT.

The diagnosis of HHT is made if two of the three main criteria are met: (1) presence of telangiectasias, (2) recurrent episodes of bleeding, and (3) family history of HHT. Bleeding is the most common symptom, with 95 percent of patients reporting recurrent epistaxis, usually by the age of 20. Bleeding may also occur within the gastrointestinal tract and may be severe enough to require blood transfusion.

Telangiectasias can be seen in 75 percent of patients. They evolve over time, however, and one-half of those affected do not develop visible external telangiectasia until after age 30. They are most commonly found on the mucosal membranes of the lips, tongue, and eyes. They are also frequently seen on the face and finger tips.

Although HHT is believed to be autosomal dominant, there is a high rate of spontaneous mutations. The disease may also be asymptomatic or may skip a generation, making the initial diagnosis difficult. Because of the difficulty of presymptomatic diagnosis and the variable penetrance, the estimated prevalence varies from 1 in 100,000 to as high as 20 in 100,000.

The treatment is directed at minimizing bleeding from the telangiectasias and obliterating AVMs that are responsible for bleeding or venous-arterial shunting. Long-term therapy may be problematic as the vascular malformations tend to be multiple and frequently recur. Screening in family members, and early therapy, may help lower the risk for first and recurrent strokes.

VENOUS INFARCTS

Cerebral venous and dural sinus thrombosis (CVT) is an uncommon cause of stroke, although it is probably underdiagnosed. The physician should be suspicious of its occurrence in the setting of a young stroke patient without obvious risk factors and a CT or MRI showing an atypical distribution of one or more infarcts with a hemorrhagic component. Its manifestations are protean. Typically, patients present with headache or seizures with focal deficits, encephalopathy, or progressive deterioration in level of consciousness. The temporal evolution of symptoms and signs can be acute, subacute, or chronic.

The typical settings include the postpartum period, known or discovered hypercoagulable states, post-traumatic status, dehydration, malignancy, oral contraceptives, or connective tissue disease.

Headache is common (75 percent of patients) and is often worse with bending over, Valsalva maneuver, or head turning. The pain may have a throbbing vascular quality. Nausea, photophobia, phonophobia, or vomiting may be due to increased intracranial pressure, tissue ischemia, or hemorrhage into the parenchyma. Seizures are often focal but may be generalized and are associated with hemorrhagic changes.

Papilledema is not a reliable sign of CVT, being present in only about 50 percent of patients with proved CVT. Focal signs may fluctuate and refer to the area of parenchymal ischemia, hemorrhage, or mass effect. Papilledema, hemiparesis, sixth cranial nerve palsies, and parietal dysfunction may be present. The most common venous structure involved is the superior sagittal sinus.

Diagnosis can be suggested on CT scan when either bland or hemorrhagic infarcts are present in adjacent regions or when the low attenuation is not in a typical arterial distribution. A delta sign (filling defect in the torcular herophili on contrast CT, representing clot in the sinus) may be present but is not specific or sensitive. Further evidence for CVT can be obtained by MRI, especially midsagittal views for imaging the full extent of the superior sagittal sinus. Magnetic resonance angiography of the venous phase can aid in the diagnosis and has replaced conventional angiography in some centers as the study of choice. Catheter angiography of the venous phase may still be necessary in some patients.

In pursuit of an underlying cause, a careful history should be obtained for pregnancy, head or neck trauma, prior or current malignancy, diabetes, dehydration, infectious/inflammatory conditions, prior miscarriages, prior clotting problems, and a family history of clotting problems. Laboratory studies should be obtained when the cause is not certain and include complete blood count, platelet count, renal function, erythrocyte sedimentation rate, antinuclear antibody, serum protein electrophoresis, prothrombin time, activated partial thromboplastin time, aCL, lupus anticoagulant, proteins S and C, antithrombin III, dysfunctional activated protein C complex, fibrinogen, and evaluation for occult malignancy.

Treatment includes management of headache and seizures, avoiding dehydration, administering intravenous heparin (maintaining the partial thromboplastin time at 2 to 2.5 times control) when no significant hemorrhagic component is present, and administering corticosteroids if a disease amenable to steroids is found. The use of warfarin for several months is common based on the underlying cause. Acute thrombolysis of CVT has been tried in a few cases with reasonable success but carries increased risk of hemorrhage.

Prognosis is related to age and level of consciousness, although even comatose patients can make remarkable recoveries. The mortality rate from CVT has been declining, and recurrence is rare.

SUGGESTED READINGS

Ameri A, Bousser MG: Cerebral venous thrombosis. Neurol Clin 10:87–111, 1992

Barnett H, Mohr JP, Stein BM, Yatsu FM: Stroke: Pathophysiology, Diagnosis and Management. 2nd Ed. Churchill Livingstone, New York, 1992

Bousser M-G, Barnett HJM: Cerebral venous thrombosis. p. 517. In Barnett HJM, Stein BM, Mohr JP, Yatsu FM (eds): Stroke: Pathophysiology, Diagnosis and Management. 2nd Ed. Churchill Livingstone, New York, 1992

Brass LM: Stroke in younger patients. In Fisher M (ed): Clinical Atlas of Cerebrovascular Diseases. Wolfe, Boston, 1994
Caplan LR: Stroke: A Clinical Approach. 2nd Ed. Butterworths, Boston, 1993

TABLE 37-1. Medications Most Frequently Associated With Drug-Induced Antiphospholipid Antibodies

Phenothiazines (chlorpromazine)
Hydralazine
Procainamide
Quinidine
Phenytoin
Valproic acid

37. COAGULATION-RELATED CAUSES OF STROKE

NALINI SAMUEL
LUIS D'OLHABERRIAGUE
STEVEN R. LEVINE
LAWRENCE M. BRASS

COAGULOPATHIES

A wide variety of hematologic disorders can produce stroke. They have been implicated in about 5 percent of all strokes, but there is a higher portion in younger patients (approximately 10 percent). Most disorders are associated with an increased thrombotic tendency and an increased risk of ischemic stroke. Less commonly, a bleeding diathesis may predispose a patient to hemorrhage.

Hemostasis is a delicate interplay between a large number of checks and balances in the coagulation pathway. The abnormalities implicated include deficiencies of factors inhibiting coagulation (antithrombin III, protein S, and protein C), increased levels of factors promoting coagulation (factors V and VII), and decreased activity in the fibrinolytic pathway (plasminogen or plasminogen activator deficiencies). More recently, increased levels of fibrinogen have been implicated as a risk factor for ischemic stroke.

The most commonly investigated coagulopathies in the clinical evaluation of patients with stroke are deficiencies of protein C, protein S, and antithrombin III. As with most coagulopathies, the factor deficiencies may be either hereditary or acquired. Protein C and protein S are both vitamin K-dependent cofactors. Protein C is activated by thrombin. It has lytic effects on activated factor VIII. A deficiency results in an enhanced tendency to thrombosis. The hereditary form has been reported in association with recurrent venous thrombosis, usually in children or young adults. An acquired reduction in the levels of protein C is seen with liver disease, leukemia, and disseminated intravascular coagulation. Protein S is required for protein C to have its full effect. Venous infarction is commonly reported in protein S deficiency, similar to protein C. Reported cases include older patients, including middle-aged adults. Antithrombin III deficiency is believed to be among the most common of the coagulopathies with a reported incidence of 1 in 2,000 people. Acquired deficiency has been reported with severe liver disease, disseminated intravascular coagulation, nephrotic syndrome, and the use of birth control medication.

For all of these coagulopathies, venous disease has been reported more frequently than arterial disease. Patients typically present with headache, nuchal rigidity, papilledema, focal neurologic deficits, seizures, fever, and an altered mental status. Normal contrast enhancement within the venous sinuses will not occur in the presence of thrombosis. On computed tomographic scan, the superior sagittal sinus is normally seen near the occipital pole in cross-section (where it appears as a radiodense triangle). For those with superior sagittal thrombosis, an "empty delta" sign may be noted (because of the lack of contrast enhancement in the sinus).

The trigger for an individual stroke, associated with a coagulopathy, is usually unknown, but surgery, trauma, pregnancy, hormone use, and systemic illness have been postulated. When a coagulation abnormality is detected, therapy should be tailored to the individual case. For those with an acquired coagulopathy, treatment of the underlying condition may reverse the risk. In hereditary deficiencies, especially with recurrent ischemic episodes, warfarin is often recommended. Well-designed clinical trials, however, are lacking.

Increased blood viscosity has been associated with decreased blood flow and a higher risk of ischemic stroke. This may occur as a result of diseases of red blood cell morphology or quantity. Macroglobulinemia (Waldenström's disease) may produce a hyperviscosity state or a bleeding diathesis, leading to either an ischemic or hemorrhagic infarction. The recommended management is usually with plasmapheresis. In addition, multiple myeloma, particularly IgA myeloma, predisposes to a hyperviscosity state. Other causes of hyperviscosity syndrome are polycythemia vera, cryoglobulinemia, and collagen vascular disorders. Treatment is usually directed at the underlying disorder. Phlebotomy may be useful if the hematocrit is extremely elevated.

A large number of other hematologic disorders have been associated with stroke (see Tables 36-1 and 36-2). Some of the diagnostic assays are difficult to perform. For example, although antiplatelet medication reduces the risk of stroke, the

TABLE 37-2. Features Associated With Antiphospholipid Antibodies and the Antiphospholipid Antibody Syndrome

Clinical	Laboratory
Arterial thrombosis	Prolonged activated partial thromboplastin time
Cerebral	
Ocular	False-positive VDRL syphilis test
Peripheral	Thrombocytopenia
Myocardial	Hemolytic anemia
Dermal/digital	Positive antinuclear antibody test
Pulmonary	Reduced C4
Mesenteric	
Venous thrombosis	
Deep leg	
Hepatic (Budd-Chiari syndrome)	
Retinal	
Cerebral	
Adrenal	
Miscarriages	
Livedo reticularis	
Pulmonary hypertension	
Left-sided cardiac valvular lesions	
Verrucous endocarditis (Libman-Sacks endocarditis)	
Myxomatous mitral valve degeneration	
Intracardiac thrombi	
Chorea	

role of platelet abnormalities has been difficult to demonstrate in clinical studies. Platelet function testing is technically difficult to perform, and even the process of venipuncture can activate platelets.

In spite of the difficulties in diagnosing disorders of platelets and coagulation, the importance of this group of disorders is likely to increase in the future. An example of just one of the coagulation-related abnormalities gaining in recognition is antiphospholipid antibodies (aPL).

ANTIPHOSPHOLIPID SYNDROME

The aPL are circulating immunoglobulins (IgG, IgM, and IgA isotypes) that bind anionic and neutral phospholipid-containing moieties. The two most clinically studied and relevant aPL are the lupus anticoagulant and anticardiolipin antibodies. They are primarily acquired but can be inherited. Several medications may be associated with drug-induced aPL (Table 37-1).

While aPL have been recognized since 1906 with the discovery of the Wassermann test for syphilis (syphilitic sera contains aPL), it has only been 10 years since the coining of a syndrome associated with these antibodies. This syndrome, the antiphospholipid antibody syndrome, has distinct clinical and laboratory features.

The principal clinical features include thrombotic events, both venous (most commonly deep vein thrombosis) and arterial (most commonly ischemic stroke), and left-sided cardiac valve lesions akin to verrucous or Libman-Sacks endocarditis with fibrin-platelet deposits on the valvular surface. Other neurologic disturbances include migrainelike events and less commonly chorea, myelopathy, miscarriages, adrenal thrombosis with orthostatic hypotension, pulmonary hypertension, and livedo reticularis (Table 37-2). Age at onset is generally younger than 50 years.

Laboratory features include prolonged phospholipid-dependent coagulation tests (activated partial thromboplastin time) as a sign of lupus anticoagulant, thrombocytopenia, false-positive VDRL syphilis test result, IgG anticardiolipin antibodies, reduced complement C_4 positive antinuclear antibody (usually low titer) test, and occasionally hemolytic anemia (Table 37-3).

Antiphospholipid antibodies are linked to a prothrombic state, are seen in approximately 10 percent of first ischemic stroke patients, and are an independent risk marker for first ischemic stroke. The aPL are more common in younger stroke patients, and only the IgG isotype has been statistically linked to stroke in case-control studies. The IgM isotype may represent an acute-phase reaction and can be seen following a variety of infections. IgA isotype has been the least studied and has only anecdotal associations with stroke, Guillain-Barré syndrome,

TABLE 37-3. Laboratory Diagnosis of Lupus Anticoagulant

Prolonged phospholipid-dependent coagulation screening test
Failure to correct with mixing studies
Demonstration of phospholipid specificity

Studies:
Prothrombin time
Activated partial thromboplastin time
Tissue thromboplastin inhibition
Platelet neutralization procedure
Dilute phospholipid activated partial thromboplastin time
Kaolin clotting time
Russell viper venom time
Dilute Russell viper venom time
STACLOT LA

TABLE 37-4. Screening for Antiphospholipid Antibodies (Anticardiolipin Antibodies and Lupus Anticoagulant)

Any patient with ischemic symptoms in the brain or eye without a clear cause
If one or more of the clinical or laboratory features are present to suggest antiphospholipid syndrome, even in the presence of known vascular risk factors
Any patient with recurrent thrombosis

and myelopathy. The reasons for the non-neurologist to screen patients for aPL include ischemic brain, eye, or spinal cord events or chorea without clear cause in a patient with recurrent thrombolic events and one or more clinical (systemic or neurologic) or laboratory features of antiphospholipid syndrome (Table 37-4).

Mechanisms of the most common neurologic manifestations of antiphospholipid syndrome and transient ischemic attacks (stroke) are probably heterogeneous and include embolism from cardiac valve lesions (verrucous endocarditis, left-sided valve thickening and myxomatous degeneration, and intracardiac clot), a hypercoagulable state with in situ thrombosis, and a cerebral vascular endotheliopathy (Fig. 37-1). The aPL within the antiphospholipid syndrome, as opposed to aPL not associated with the syndrome, appear to require a cofactor for binding. This cofactor is β_2-glucoprotein-1, also called apolipoprotein H. This cofactor is a naturally occurring anticoagulant that inhibits the intrinsic coagulation pathway and the prothrombinase activity of platelets. Binding and subsequent alteration of the function of the cofactor could therefore lead to a prothrombotic state. Preliminary evidence suggests that aPL are directed at the fifth repeating domain (C terminal) of the cofactor molecule and can inhibit prostaglandins I_2, reduce protein C and protein S levels, and alter thrombomodulin binding. Also, aPL bind to activated platelets (not normally inactivated platelets). The ability of aPL to bind activated platelets appears to be directly related to the amount of phosphatidylserine exposure on the platelet membrane. Sera from patients with aPL and stroke have significantly higher IgG binding to human brain microvascular endothelium compared to stroke patients' sera without aPL and sera from healthy controls. However, there is a poor correlation between binding to brain endothelium and binding to anticardiolipin antibodies. The binding is also nonspecific, as similar binding to human umbilical vein cells has been demonstrated. There is no evidence for complement-mediated brain endothelium cytotoxicity.

The treatment of antiphospholipid syndrome remains empiric. The optimal therapy is unknown. Rational therapy has been hampered by the lack of precise understanding (probably multiple mechanisms) of how aPL leads to thrombosis. There have been no rigorous treatment studies nor any controlled trials for neurologic disease within the antiphospholipid syndrome. Most treatment data come from studies of recurrent aborters with systemic lupus erythematosus. The Antiphospholipid Antibodies and Stroke Study Group initiated plans for pilot treatment studies to prevent recurrent thrombotic events, including stroke in patients with stroke and antiphospholipid syndrome. Therapeutic options in these patients include antithrombotics and immune-based treatment. Antithrombotics include anticoagulants (warfarin [low-versus high International Normalized Ratio, INR], subcutaneous heparin, or low molecular weight heparin [oid]) and antiplatelet agents (aspirin, ticlopidine, and dipyridamole). Immune-based therapies include corticosteroids, immunosuppressants (azathioprine, cyclophosphamide, and cyclosporine), (intravenous immune globulin), plasmapheresis, ''binding'' paresis, and anti-idiotype antibodies.

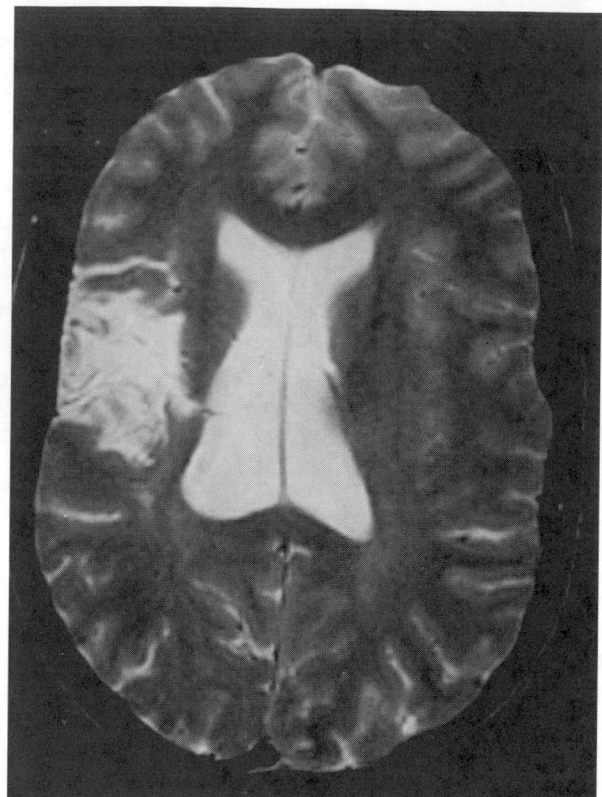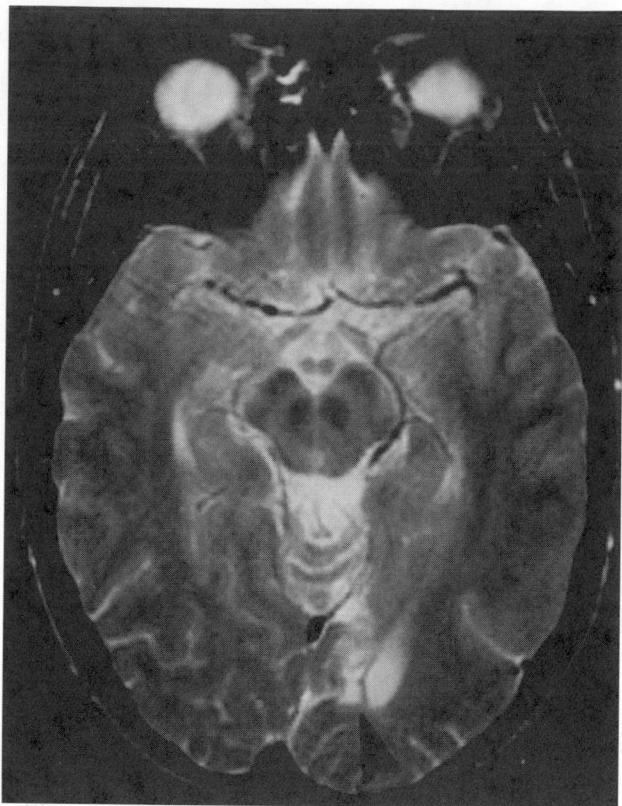

FIG. 37-1. **(A)** T2-weighted magnetic resonance image showing a perisylvian, chronic infarct (note lack of mass effect) in a young woman with antiphospholipid antibody syndrome. At the time, echocardiography did not reveal any specific abnormality. **(B)** Contralateral subcortical posterior communicating artery infarct (arrowhead) in the same woman whose echocardiography now showed a noninfective vegetation of the mitral valve.

HOMOCYSTINEMIA

Homocyst(e)inemia refers to the sum of free and protein-bound homocysteine and homocysteinyl derivatives. In plasma, free homocysteine, and cysteine-homocysteine mixed disulfide account for about 20 percent of the total. The remainder is protein-bound homocysteine. Homocystinuria is used to designate a group of biochemical abnormalities, not a single disease entity. Several autosomal recessive enzyme deficiencies are associated with homocystinuria and an increased risk for cardiovascular disease and stroke.

Homocysteine is at an important metabolic branch point. It is synthesized from methionine and metabolized via transulfuration to cystathionine or methylated to form methionine (as part of the sulfur conservation cycle). Methylation can occur via several pathways that are dependent on folate and vitamin B_{12} containing enzymes.

Cystathionine β-synthase deficiency is the most common enzymatic deficiency causing homocystinuria and increased plasma levels of homocysteine (because of impaired conversion of homocysteine to cystathionine). The homozygous state has been associated with vascular disease and variable degrees of marfanoid (tall and thin) body type, lens dislocation, and mental retardation. Nearly every syndrome associated with atherosclerosis—including ischemic stroke—can be seen by early childhood, sometimes during the first year of life. The mechanism for stroke is thought to be secondary abnormalities in the vascular endothelium with an increased tendency for thrombosis. There may be a direct toxic effect of homocysteine on the vascular endothelium, stimulating proliferation of vascular smooth mus-

cle, an impairment of endothelium-derived relaxation factor, or a thrombogenic effect via expression of thrombomodulin and activation of protein C. Although cystathione β-synthase deficiency is inherited as an autosomal-dominant trait, there appears to be considerable genetic heterogeneity. This may account for the wide variation in the age of onset and severity of the clinical syndrome.

Recently, the heterozygous state and a variety of acquired disorders of methionine metabolism have been associated with an increased risk of stroke (and cardiovascular disease). A gene for homocystinuria may be present in as many as 1 in 70 people.

Over the last few years, more than 20 case-control and cross-sectional studies, which together included more than 2,000 patients, have consistently reported an association between higher blood levels of homocysteine and an increased risk for vascular disease. For example, in the physician's health study, a plasma homocysteine level of just 12 percent over the upper limit of the normal range was associated with a 3.4-fold increase in the risk of myocardial infarction. The true upper limit of "normal" is not clear. Homocysteine levels above 14 μmol/L has been used as an upper limit of normal, yet patients from the Framingham Study with homocysteine levels between 11 and 14 μmol/L were at increased risk for carotid stenosis. The importance of homocyst(e)ienemia as a risk factor, and those groups of stroke patients in which it should be considered, however, is still unclear.

In younger patients, elevated plasma homocysteine appears to be an independent risk factor for vascular disease. At least for cardiovascular disease, it appears to be associated with premature (age less than 55 years) atherosclerosis. Modest elevations of homocystine levels may also occur in up to a quarter of young patients with stroke.

There is also evidence that elevated plasma homocysteine may be a risk factor for vascular disease in elderly patients. Increased levels of homocysteine have also been associated with an increased likelihood of carotid atherosclerosis and greater degrees of carotid stenosis in elderly patients. This may be related to modest decreases in enzyme cofactors. One-third to one-half of those with low to normal serum vitamin B_{12} levels also have increased levels of homocysteine. How this combination of low B_{12} and increased homocysteine might contribute to vascular disease is still being evaluated. In pilot studies of elderly patients, 20 to 40 percent of those with cardiovascular disease also had increased levels of homocysteine and decreased levels of vitamin B_{12}. Deficiencies of vitamin B_6 and folic acid may also result in an elevation in homocysteine levels.

Measuring serum homocysteine levels is likely to become much more common in the near future; however, the availability is currently limited. Testing patients for the heterozygote state is currently even more difficult to perform, expensive, and not widely available. The most commonly performed screen involves measuring homocyst(e)inemia in response to methionine loading. At the present time, testing is recommended only for those who have a normal vascular risk factor profile by routine testing, especially in younger patients or those with a strong family history of premature atherosclerosis.

In the mid-1960s it was shown that treating patients with cystathionine β-synthase deficiency using pyridoxine could reduce plasma levels of methionine to normal and dramatically reduce homocystine levels in the plasma and urine. Not all of those with this enzyme deficiency responded. Responsiveness may be linked to the presence of residual activity of the mutant enzyme.

It also appears as if other forms of both inherited and acquired homocystinuria (and the elevated levels of homocystine) may respond to dietary manipulation and treatment with folic acid, vitamin B_6 or vitamin B_{12}. Clinical trials for dietary supplementation are already underway for cardiovascular disease and are being planned for prevention of stroke.

SUGGESTED READINGS

Ameri A, Bousser MG: Cerebral venous thrombosis. Neurol Clin 10:87–111, 1992

Barnett H, Mohr JP, Stein BM, Yatsu FM: Stroke: Pathophysiology, Diagnosis and Management. 2nd Ed. Churchill Livingstone, New York, 1992

Brass LM: Stroke in Younger Patients. In Fisher M (ed): Clinical Atlas of Cerebrovascular Diseases. Wolfe, Boston, 1994

Bousser M-G, Barnett HJM: Cerebral venous thrombosis. p. 517. In Barnett HJM, Stein BM, Mohr JP, Yatsu FM (eds): Stroke: Pathophysiology, Diagnosis and Management. 2nd Ed. Churchill Livingstone, New York, 1992

Caplan LR: Stroke: A Clinical Approach. 2nd Ed. Butterworths, Boston, 1993

Coull BM, Levine SR, Brey RL: The role of antiphospholipid antibodies in stroke. Neurol Clin 10:125–143, 1992

Feldmann E, Levine SR: Cerebrovascular disease with antiphospholipid antibodies: immune mechanisms, significance, and therapeutic options. Ann Neurol (Suppl): in press, 1994

Feldmann E: Intracerebral Hemorrhage. Futura Publishing, Mt. Kisco, NY, 1994

Levine SR, Welch KMA: The spectrum of neurologic disorders associated with antiphospholipid antibodies: lupus anticoagulants and anticardiolipin antibodies. Arch Neurol 44:876–83, 1987

Levine SR, Deegan MJ, Futrell N, Welch KMA: Cerebrovascular and neurological disease associated with antiphospholipid antibodies: 48 cases. Neurology 40:1181–9, 1990

Levine SR, Brey RL: Antiphospholipid antibodies and ischemic cerebrovascular disease. Semin Neurol 11:329–38, 1991

Selhub J, Jacques PF et al: Association between plasma homocysteine concentrations and extracranial carotid-artery stenosis. N Engl J Med 322:286, 1995

Selhub J, Jacques PF et al: Vitamin status and intake as primary determinants of homocysteinemia in an elderly population. JAMA 270:2693, 1993

Stampfer MJ, Malinow MR: Can lowering homocysteine levels reduce cardiovascular risk? N Engl J Med 332:328, 1995

38. ILLICIT DRUGS AND STROKE

NALINI SAMUEL
LUIS D'OLHABERRIAGUE
STEVEN R. LEVINE
LAWRENCE M. BRASS

ILLICIT DRUGS

It is important to consider the use of illicit drugs as an unusual cause of stroke, particularly in the young. Various drugs (see Tables 36-1 and 36-2) can produce immediate and long-term effects on the vascular network that may predispose the patient to stroke. Besides, drug users commonly develop an addictive lifestyle that includes the simultaneous use of different drugs and lack of hygienic habits, resulting in multiple infections. Parenteral drug users have an increased risk of blood-borne and other infections (infectious endocarditis, hepatitis, syphilis, and acquired immunodeficiency syndrome [AIDS]) that also cause stroke.

Cocaine

Cocaine, a local anesthetic, may be used as a recreational, stimulant drug in the form of powder of cocaine hydrochloride for intranasal administration (''snorting''). Rectal, oral, vaginal, or sublingual administration are also employed. Alkaloidal free base of cocaine, or ''crack,'' is inhaled or smoked. Crack has become the most popular form of cocaine since it has a higher power of addiction and is cheaper and easier to handle than cocaine hydrochloride. Since the introduction of crack in 1983, its use and the number of its medical and neurologic complications have become epidemic. By 1982, 28 percent of people between 18 and 25 years had used cocaine, whereas, in 1990, 34 percent of people between ages 15 and 44 years had used drugs, with cocaine being the predominant one. Since 1977, when Brust and Richter reported the first case of cocaine-related stroke, the number of reported cases remained below 10 per year until 1987, jumping from zero in 1985 and three in 1986 to 29 in 1987. Since then, the number of cocaine-related strokes has increased ceaselessly. It is likely that the increasing number of reported cases reflects not only the spreading crack epidemic but also the greater cerebrovascular specificity and higher potency of this drug.

The effects of cocaine include hypertension, central nervous system stimulation, and local anesthesia. Cocaine blocks reuptake of dopamine, serotonin, and norepinephrine and binds to dopamine transport protein at nerve terminals, thus blocking its presynaptic reuptake and increasing dopamine levels. It also blocks serotonin and norepinephrine reuptake. Dopaminergic effects include hypertension, tachycardia, and vasoconstriction. Cocaine intake results in marked increases in blood pressure, myocardial oxygen demand, and heart rate. Coronary blood flow, which increases in response to exercise, is decreased by cocaine intake. Therefore, cocaine simultaneously increases myocardial oxygen demand and decreases myocardial oxygen supply. These latter two effects of cocaine are potentiated by simultaneous tobacco smoking. In the cerebral arteries, enhanced sympathetic activity accompanied by hypertension could be a major factor for stroke via vasoconstriction and vasospasm. Increased perfusion pressure can give rise to hypertensive opening of the blood-brain barrier, which facilitates the entry of circulating catecholamines into the brain. Finally, cocaine has been shown to decrease acutely, and on a long-term basis, cerebral metabolism, cerebral blood flow (CBF), and brain glucose metabolism. Single photon-emission computed tomographic studies in former cocaine users found regions of hypoperfusion in frontal, periventricular, and/or temporal-parietal areas. Serotonergic effects include vasoconstriction on large and medium-sized cerebral arteries, and increased platelet response to arachidonic acid with increased thromboxane production and platelet aggregation. A possible noradrenergic effect is a lack of increase in CBF in response to hypertension, since norepinephrine increases cerebrovascular resistance. A direct inhibitory effect of cocaine in platelet aggregation has also been described.

The mechanisms of cocaine-related stroke are multiple. Cocaine users often employ simultaneously other potentially stroke-inducing drugs, either voluntarily or because they are adulterants of cocaine. Cocaine-induced hemorrhagic strokes are associated in more than 50 percent of cases with arteriovenous malformations (AVMs) and aneurysms. Cocaine causes severe hypertension, which, together with increased cardiac output, can promote aneurysm or AVM rupture, thus causing hemorrhages (intracranial [ICH] and subarachnoid hemorrhages [SAH]). Extreme hypertension may also cause primary ICH. After vasoconstriction, rapid reperfusion of previously ischemic brain tissue can also cause ICH. Vasoconstriction induced by increased monoamine activity, together with increased thrombotic activity as a result of a serotonin-induced rise in synthesis of thromboxane, may underlie some ischemic strokes. Vasospasm, either as a result of severe hypertension or related to SAH, is another possible cause of ischemic stroke (Fig. 38-1). Vasculitis has rarely, if ever, caused cocaine-related ischemic stroke, which contrasts with amphetamine-induced ICH. Cocaine causes cardiac arrhythmia, cardiomyopathy, and myocardial infarction, with a potential risk of cardioembolic stroke. Parenteral cocaine users are at increased risk of infectious endocarditis.

Cocaine-related stroke is an ailment of drug users, fetuses and newborns whose mothers employ the drug, and pregnant women. Cocaine-related strokes affect mainly young people with a male preponderance. Ischemic—including transient ischemic attacks and cerebral, retinal, and spinal cord infarcts—and hemorrhagic strokes occur with approximately equal frequency. There are, however, clinically important differences, depending on the type of cocaine used. In cocaine hydrochloride users, hemorrhagic strokes are twice as common as ischemic strokes, whereas, in alkaloidal cocaine users, ischemic and hemorrhagic strokes are equally likely. Aneurysms and AVMs are twice as frequent with cocaine hydrochloride stroke than with alkaloidal cocaine stroke. Concomitant alcohol use is more frequent in cocaine hydrochloride users than in alkaloidal cocaine users. Alcohol depresses the degradation of cocaine, and alcoholism is a risk factor for all types of stroke, but especially for hemorrhagic stroke. Finally, alkaloidal cocaine is related to a more rapid absorption of the drug and higher cocaine blood levels than cocaine hydrochloride. Crack

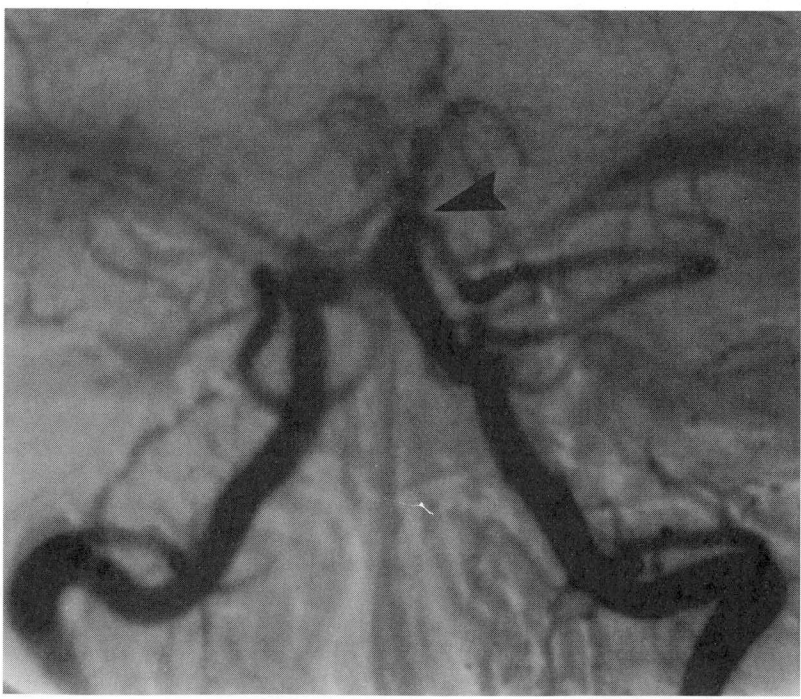

FIG. 38-1. • Basilar artery narrowing (*arrowhead*) in a chronic intranasal cocaine user.

cocaine smokers are also more likely than cocaine hydrochloride intranasal users to escalate dosage. A proof of cocaine use can be obtained either by history taking or toxicologic screening. Cocaine, or its metabolite benzoylecgonine, can be detected from the urine of a novice user for up to 48 hours after intranasal use and for up to 3 weeks following chronic use.

Anterior circulation ischemic strokes predominate over posterior circulation strokes. Small deep infarcts and specific brainstem syndromes also occur. Hemorrhagic strokes are more often hemispheric, deep basal-ganglionic, or lobar and sometimes multiple. Angiographic findings include aneurysms, AVMs, branch stenosis or occlusions, beading, spasm, and very rarely vasculitis. Emboli rising from cardiomyopathies are probably an underrated cause of stroke in cocaine users who are prone to infectious endocarditis. Infectious endocarditis causes ischemic and hemorrhagic strokes, multiple microemboli presenting as toxic encephalopathy, meningitis, pyogenic arteritis, mycotic aneurysms, and SAH. Headache is the most common associated complaint in cocaine-related strokes and is more common than among unselected stroke patients. Serotonergic effect of cocaine on platelets may be related to these headaches. The prognosis for patients suffering from cocaine stroke is poor; one-third of patients will die, and another one-third will remain severely handicapped. Treatment does not differ from stroke from other etiologies, although there is some evidence that magnesium could ameliorate cocaine-induced cerebral vasospasm. Aneurysms and AVMs should be treated as required. Mycotic aneurysms do not usually disappear after antimicrobial therapy, and their bleeding is associated with a high mortality rate; so surgical removal should be performed. Prevention of cocaine strokes depends on discontinuation of drug use.

In cocaine-induced central nervous system disorders other than stroke, seizures and status epilepticus may occur with or without associated stroke as a result of a decrease in seizure threshold. Drug intoxication is commonly a cause of status epilepticus. Animal studies demonstrated increased glucose metabolism in dopaminergic pathways after cocaine administration, and cocaine binding in humans is the highest in the corpus striatum. Movement disorders related to cocaine include tremor, dystonia, myoclonus, chorea, tics, parkinsonism, akathisia, and neuroleptic malignant syndrome. Positron emission tomographic studies found CBF decreasing, especially in frontal areas, in chronic users, even after detoxication, and computed tomographic studies demonstrated brain atrophy. Cognitive and behavioral deficits found in chronic users include impaired attention, concentration, new leaning, memory, word production and visuomotor integration, euphoria, and psychotic behavior, especially paranoia.

Amphetamine and Psychostimulant Drugs

Amphetamine, methamphetamine, and dextroamphetamine are powerful analeptics that are used because of their psychostimulant and appetite depressant effects. Two patterns of abuse exist. Truck drivers, housewives, and students employ oral preparations; intravenous administration is used by drug addicts. Nasal administration and concurrent intake of alcohol or other drugs is also common. Cerebrovascular complications of amphetamine use are worldwide.

Amphetamine and methamphetamine release cytoplasmic dopamine from the nerve terminals with general dopaminergic stimulation. There are also noradrenergic and serotonergic effects. Amphetamine induces tachycardia, hypertension, and increased respiratory rate, which can result in hypocapnia. Acute effects of amphetamine overdose include extreme hypertension, hyperpyrexia, coma, vascular collapse, and death. In extreme cases, neuropathologic examination shows diffuse brain edema without large infarctions or hemorrhages.

Mechanisms underlying ICH include extreme hypertension, AVM rupture, and vasculitis. When these mechanisms are compared with those of cocaine-related hemorrhages, there are two main differences. AVMs in amphetamine users are uncommon, and amphetamine-induced vasculitis is frequently inferred radiologically or found at autopsy. Two different types of vasculitis have been described, one that resembles polyarteritis nodosa and one that affects small arterioles and resembles "hypersensitivity" vasculitis. Ischemic strokes have also been related to vasospasm or endocarditis.

Ischemic strokes and transient ischemic attacks are less common than hemorrhagic strokes after amphetamine use. The mean age of patients with ICHs was 25 years, and oral use of amphetamine followed by intravenous use was the most common route of administration. Lobar hemorrhages predominate over basal-ganglionic hemorrhages. Angiography may be negative or show AVMs or a pattern of segmental areas of constriction, irregularity, and occasional fusiform dilation and beading suggestive of vasculitis. At times, angiographic abnormalities are transient and disappear on a second examination. The clinical picture is often characterized by a paucity of focal signs in spite of large focal lesions. Oddly enough, signs of sympathetic overactivity are generally absent, but headache is common. Prognosis is poor, with the mortality rate ranging up to 20 percent. Amphetamine-induced central nervous system disorders other than stroke include restlessness, talkativeness, tremor, insomnia, psychomotor hyperactivity, psychotic behavior of paranoid schizophrenic type, seizures, and rhabdomyolysis.

Phenylpropanolamine

Phenylpropanolamine is a drug structurally related to amphetamine, though less potent. Its use is not under the Food and Drug Administration restrictions that apply to amphetamine, and it is found in more than 70 over-the-counter medications, including nasal decongestants, cough and cold remedies, and appetite suppressants. Reported associations include hypertension, headache, seizures, psychiatric reactions, and ICH. Most of the reported hemorrhages are parenchymal, although SAH secondary to aneurysm rupture has also been described. Potential stroke mechanisms of hypertension and vasculitis have been reported. Some cases have been related to concomitant use of alcohol, caffeine, monoamine oxidase inhibitors, or cocaine. Cases have also been reported in the puerperium.

Making a causal association between stroke and a common drug or risk factor is difficult. There are only a few dozen reported cases of stroke, but billions of doses of phenylpropanolamine are ingested each year in the United States. In a review of the existing literature, there are many reporting biases, which makes it impossible to implicate phenylpropanolamine as a causal agent. The issue can best be resolved with a well-designed case-control study.

Ephedrine and pseudoephedrine have been related to ICHs; phentermine and probably phendimetrazine, to ischemic strokes; and methylphenidate, to ischemic and hemorrhagic strokes.

Phencyclidine and Lysergic Acid Diethylamide

Phencyclidine (PCP) ("angel dust") was used legally as an animal immobilizing agent and illegally as an hallucinogen. PCP became very popular during the 1970s and was smoked, eaten, or injected. The mechanisms of action of PCP are not clear, although PCP enhances catecholamine and serotonin transmission and is a noncompetitive N-methyl-D-aspartic acid antagonist. One to 5 mg of PCP induces euphoria, emotional lability, and a feeling of numbness; 5 to 15 mg causes confusion, decreased sensory perception, and body distortions; higher doses produce psychosis, myoclonus, nystagmus, seizures, coma, and respiratory collapse. Hypertension, leading to hypertensive encephalopathy, can occur. A few cases of ICHs and SAH, occasionally associated with aneurysms, and a single case of brainstem ischemia, have been related to PCP use.

Lysergic acid diethylamide (LSD) has occasionally been related to ischemic strokes, sometimes with angiographic findings suggestive of vasculitis.

Opiates and Barbiturates

There are about half a million heroin abusers in the United States. Heroin is usually taken parenterally, so addicts have an increased risk of blood-borne and other infections (infectious endocarditis, hepatitis, syphilis and AIDS). Violence, drug overdose, and AIDS are the most common causes of death in heroin addicts. Among the other medical complications of heroin users are ischemic and hemorrhagic strokes.

Heroin overdose develops as a result of miscalculation of the dose, suicide attempts, and circumstances that decrease drug tolerance (Addison's disease, myxedema, liver disease, or pneumonia) and upon resuming the habit after a long period of withdrawal. Depressed consciousness with small, pinpoint pupils and respiratory depression are the hallmarks of heroin overdose. Patients surviving cardiorespiratory arrest are sometimes left with residual anoxic encephalopathy.

There are multiple mechanisms of strokes in heroin addicts. ICH and SAH are most often the result of mycotic aneurysm rupture in the setting of infectious endocarditis. Altered clotting caused by liver failure in the setting of hepatitis or malignant hypertension from heroin nephropathy are other causes of hemorrhagic strokes. Infectious endocarditis is the main cause of ischemic stroke in heroin addicts. *Candida albicans* and *Staphylococcus aureus* are the most common pathogens, with the latter leading to underlying microbia in endocarditis with neurologic complications. Infectious endocarditis causes ischemic and hemorrhagic strokes, multiple microemboli presenting as toxic encephalopathy, meningitis, pyogenic arteritis, mycotic aneurysms, and SAH. A cerebral vasculitis has been described in some heroin-related infarcts. Increased erythrocyte sedimentation rate, positive latex test, eosinophilia, and hypergammaglobulinemia suggest a possible immunologic mechanism. Delayed anoxic encephalopathy and bilateral globus pallidus infarction have been described in heroin addicts after cardiorespiratory arrest. An acute or subacute myelopathy has been reported in heroin users. Its pathogenesis is unknown, although some cases presented an anterior spinal artery syndrome.

Pentazocine and tripelennamine ("T's and blues") caused stroke in three of 13 patients with neurologic symptoms. The most likely mechanism was foreign body embolization.

Barbiturates and other sedative drugs cause stroke as a result of overdose and decreased brain perfusion. Rarely, barbiturate abuse has been related to vasculitis or moyamoya.

Alcohol

Alcohol affects 10.6 million adults in the United States, and about 20 percent of adolescents are problem drinkers. Alcohol intoxication is one of the two leading causes of status epilepticus. However, the relationships between alcohol and stroke are not clear. Coronary artery disease may be more prevalent in abstainers than in moderate drinkers, and some evidence suggests that internal carotid artery stenosis is related inversely with light to moderate alcohol intake. Light to moderate alcohol intake decreases low-density lipoprotein (LDL) cholesterol and increases high-density lipoprotein (HDL) cholesterol, whereas heavy alcohol consumption increases triglyceride levels and blood pressure. The pattern of increased HDL and decreased LDL seems to protect from coronary artery arteriosclerosis; increased LDL (and intermediate-density lipoprotein) with decreased HDL are commonly found in patients with cerebral infarction.

The impact of alcohol consumption on stroke risk depends on the study population, sex, race, alcohol dose, alcoholism definition, presence of confounding factors (age, diabetes, and arterial hypertension), concomitant use of other drugs (tobacco and cocaine), and type of stroke (ischemic or hemorrhagic). Low to moderate alcohol consumption (5 to 25 g/day) is associated with a decreased relative risk of both myocardial and cerebral infarction and increased the risk of SAH in women. Lifelong abstainers of both sexes appear to bear an increased risk of stroke. The likelihood of hospitalization for ischemic stroke, in both sexes and in whites as well as in blacks, was decreased in people who drank. People who consumed three or more drinks a day had an increased risk of hospitalization for ICH. Aging, hypertension, and black race are associated with a further increase in risk. Among men, the relative risk of stroke is greater in abstainers than in light drinkers (10 to 90 g of alcohol weekly), but heavy drinkers (300 g of alcohol or more weekly) have a four times greater increase in relative risk of stroke as compared with abstainers.

Several mechanisms might explain the different effects of different doses of alcohol as well as differences in the risks of ischemic versus hemorrhagic strokes. In humans, ethanol in small doses produces cerebral vasodilatation, and higher doses induce cerebral vasoconstriction. Acute ethanol intoxication reduces the difference between carotid artery and jugular vein oxygen concentration, reflecting a reduced cerebral oxygen metabolism. Cardiac arrhythmias, especially atrial fibrillation, can result from underlying alcoholic cardiomyopathy or directly from alcohol-induced sympathetic stimulation in acute intoxication ("holiday heart"). Arterial hypertension results both from acute and chronic use. Acutely, alcohol decreases fibrinolytic activity, increases factor VIII and platelet activity, and shortens bleeding time. Ethanol consumption can also cause stroke by vasospasm and increased blood viscosity. Chronic alcoholic patients present with decreased levels of vitamin K-dependent clotting factors, increased fibrinolysis, and platelet abnormalities that are secondary to hepatic disease. Alcohol withdrawal has been related to both increased and decreased CBF.

In conclusion, moderate alcohol may decrease the risk of cerebral infarction, but the stroke risk is higher in heavy drinkers than in abstainers. Acute intoxication is related to an increased risk of both ischemic and hemorrhagic strokes. Chronic alcoholic patients have an increased risk of all types of stroke, especially hemorrhagic stroke.

Tobacco

Tobacco smoking is an important risk factor for coronary artery disease. Although a few studies failed to prove such a relationship between smoking and stroke, there is overwhelming evidence linking smoking with increased risk of stroke. In the Nurses' Health Study, smokers had a dose-dependent increased risk for both ischemic stroke and SAH. Cessation of smoking appears to decrease the previously increased risk, and, in a Finnish study, the observed declining incidence of stroke was attributed to the declining prevalence of smoking. There is an especially high risk of ischemic stroke and SAH in young women who smoke and use oral contraceptives. Oral contraceptives and smoking further potentiate each other in migraineurs. Among ischemic stroke subtypes, smoking is more common among noncardioembolic than cardioembolic stroke victims.

Tobacco can induce stroke by multiple mechanisms. Tobacco smoking increases the risk of myocardial infarction, increases myocardial oxygen demand, and decreases myocardial oxygen supply. Concurrent use of cocaine potentiates the latter two effects of smoking. Smoking aggravates coronary artery disease, constricts coronary arteries, decreases HDL levels, raises systolic and diastolic blood pressure, increases heart rate, and can precipitate atrial fibrillation. Although smoking is not by itself a risk factor for arterial hypertension, it accelerates its progression. Extracranial internal carotid artery stenosis seems to correlate in a dose-dependent fashion with smoking. CBF is decreased in smokers, and ex-smokers show CBF values between those of smokers and nonsmokers. Tobacco smoking increases platelet reactivity and fibrinogen concentration and decreases prostacyclin formation. Chronic obstructive pulmonary disease is associated with increased hematocrit, which could further decrease CBF. Finally, lung cancer causes ICH as a result of bleeding into metastases and ischemic stroke from nonbacterial thrombotic endocarditis, tumor embolism, and disseminated intravascular coagulation.

SUGGESTED READINGS

Ameri A, Bousser MG: Cerebral venous thrombosis. Neurol Clin 10:87–111, 1992

Barnett H, Mohr JP, Stein BM, Yatsu FM (eds): Stroke: Pathophysiology, Diagnosis and Management. 2nd Ed. Churchill Livingstone, New York, 1992

Brass LM: Stroke in Younger Patients. In Fisher M (ed): Clinical Atlas of Cerebrovascular Diseases. Wolfe, Boston, 1994

Bousser M-G, Barnett HJM: Cerebral venous thrombosis. p. 517. In Barnett HJM, Stein BM, Mohr JP, Yatsu FM (eds): Stroke: Pathophysiology, Diagnosis and Management. 2nd Ed. Churchill Livingstone, New York, 1992

Caplan LR: Stroke: A Clinical Approach. 2nd Ed. Butterworths, Boston, 1993

39. INFLAMMATORY DISORDERS CAUSING STROKE

NALINI SAMUEL
LUIS D'OLHABERRIAGUE
STEVEN R. LEVINE
LAWRENCE M. BRASS

Vasculitis refers to any inflammation of blood vessels. Arteritis and angiitis are often used interchangeably with vasculitis because, in most conditions, arteries, capillaries, and veins are all affected. The clinical features of cerebral vasculitis are usually nonspecific and diverse. The most common feature, especially early in the course, is encephalopathy (fluctuating confusion and memory changes, along with personality changes—sometimes with paranoid or psychotic reactions). Often, headache, seizures, and focal signs (including hemiparesis and cranial nerve palsies) occur. Hypothalamic disturbances, involuntary movements, and spinal paraplegia may also be seen.

Many types of vasculitis can affect the intracranial blood vessels and have been associated with stroke, usually as part of a larger, systemic process (Table 39-1). The most common processes are herpes zoster infection, lymphoma, and sarcoidosis. Also important are systemic lupus erythematosus, polyarteritis nodosa, Wegener's granulomatosis, and Takayasu's disease. Inflammatory changes in cerebral vessels have also been reported with drug use (heroin, cocaine, lysergic acid diethylamide, and amphetamines). Infectious processes (bacterial, viral, or fungal) can, but rarely do, cause cerebral vasculitis. For the infectious processes, the vasculitis usually arises from direct extension from an adjacent inflammatory process. With

TABLE 39-1. Defined Causes of Central Nervous System Vasculitis

Processes	Etiology
Systemic necrotizing arteritis	Systemic necrotizing arteritis (including polyarteritis nodosa)
	Wegener's granulomatosis
	Lymphomatoid granulomatosis
	Sarcoidosis
Autoimmune diseases	Rheumatoid arthritis
	Systemic lupus erythematosus
	Scleroderma
	Sjögren's syndrome
	Ulcerative colitis
	Celiac disease
Infectious disease	Herpes zoster
	Cytomegalovirus
	Human immunodeficiency virus
	Fungal infection
	Syphilis
	Borrelia burgdorferi infection
	Tuberculosis
	Bacterial meningitis
	Strongyloides stercoralis infestation
	Relapsing polychondritis
Neoplasm	Hodgkin's and non-Hodgkin's lymphoma
	Neoplastic angioendotheliosis
	Malignant histiocytosis
	Hairy cell leukemia
Toxic	Drugs
	Sympathomimetic agents
	Irradiation

(Modified from Hankey GJ: Isolated angiitis/angiopathy of the central nervous system. Cerebrovasc Dis 1:2, 1991, with permission.)

any of these etiologies, stroke rarely occurs as an isolated syndrome.

ISOLATED ANGIITIS

In this chapter, we focus on isolated angiitis of the central nervous system. For a more detailed and comprehensive discussion of central nervous system vasculitis, consult Chapter 49. As the name suggests, it is restricted to the cranial vessels, and central nervous system symptoms predominate. Isolated (granulomatous) angiitis of the central nervous system is a rare condition. Younger patients are most often affected. It is a segmental inflammatory disease of the small and medium sized vessels with infiltration by monocytes, plasma cells, and giant cells. Small granulomata are often present histologically. Although restricted to the central nervous system, the disease is often multifocal within it. The absence of systemic inflammation is a key point in the diagnosis. It is the absence of systemic symptoms that also makes the condition difficult to diagnose.

Diagnosis and Treatment

Early symptoms may be subtle and include headache, confusion, intellectual decline, changes in memory, and malaise. As the disease progresses, focal signs are typically seen. These include focal deficits (stroke), seizures, and myelopathies. Angiographic findings of multiple areas of segmental narrowing and occlusion or delayed emptying of vessels suggest the diagnosis, but the angiogram may appear normal when the disease affects vessels too small to be visualized. Since the angiographic changes are not specific, a biopsy may be necessary. False-negative biopsy findings are common because of the segmental nature of the disease.

The following criteria have been proposed for the diagnosis: (1) headache and multifocal neurologic deficits present for at least 6 months, unless the deficits are severe at onset or rapidly progressive; (2) angiographic demonstration of segmental arterial narrowing; (3) exclusion of systemic inflammation or infection; and (4) leptomeningeal biopsy demonstrating inflammation or excluding alternative diagnoses.

The etiology is unknown. The presence of granulomata, and the absence of antibodies or immune complex deposition within the vessel walls, suggests a disorder of cell-mediated immunity. Viral and neoplastic triggers have been suggested but remain highly speculative.

An aggressive treatment approach appears indicated because the disease is often progressive (with recurrent stroke leading to death). Although not tested in randomized trials, immunotherapy with prednisone and cyclophosphamide has been recommended. It is not clear whether immunosuppression results in prolonged remission or cure.

GIANT CELL ARTERITIS

Another type of vasculitis restricted to the head is giant cell arteritis (also known as temporal arteritis or cranial arteritis). It predominantly involves medium and large arteries, but only rarely extends beyond the dura (i.e., rarely involves the intracranial vessels). It occurs in older patients and is rare before age 50. Systemic signs and symptoms are present in the majority of patients and should lead the clinician to suspect the diagnosis. In addition to symptoms directly related to cranial arteritis (headache, temporal tenderness, decreased temporal artery pulse, and jaw claudication), there are nearly always systemic signs (including sedimentation rate greater than 50 mm/h, poly-

myalgia rheumatica, malaise, fever, and weight loss). The diagnosis is most often made on biopsy of extracranial vessels (usually the temporal artery). Treatment includes corticosteroids and may be required for 1 year or longer.

SUGGESTED READINGS

Hankey GJ: Isolated angiitis/angiopathy of the central nervous system. Cerebrovasc Dis 1:2, 1991

40. STROKE RELATED TO PREGNANCY AND THE PUERPERIUM

NALINI SAMUEL
LUIS D'OLHABERRIAGUE
STEVEN R. LEVINE
LAWRENCE M. BRASS

Pregnancy and the puerperium carries an increased risk for both ischemic and hemorrhagic stroke. Approximately one pregnant woman per 1,000 to 2,500 will have a stroke, and treatment is aimed at the underlying cause. Women with eclampsia may have nonfatal or fatal intracranial hemorrhage or ischemic stroke during the peak of eclampsia, pre-eclampsia, or shortly following resolution of eclampsia (Fig. 40-1). Clues to this

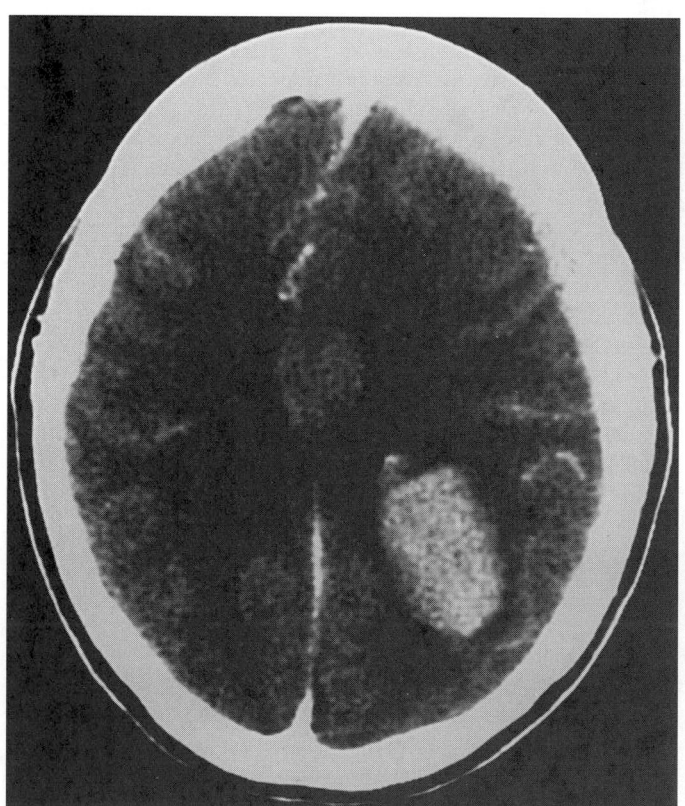

FIG. 40-1. Parietal hemorrhage surrounded by a rim of edema in a young woman with postpartum eclampsia. Note collapse of the ipsilateral ventricle and midline shift.

cause include hypertension, proteinuria, papilledema, hyperreflexia, and pitting edema.

The clinical neurologic manifestations of pre-eclampsia/eclampsia include headache, change in vision (including cortical blindness), seizures (often generalized), and depressed level of consciousness (including coma). Focal neurologic signs are rare, and, in the absence of parenchymal hemorrhage, their mechanism is unclear but may be related to cerebral vasospasm (based on angiographic data in several cases).

Brain imaging studies demonstrate areas of ischemia/edema in regions of the cortex, basal ganglia, and white matter. Lesions may disappear with resolution of the eclamptic process.

Speculation concerning the mechanism of cerebral vasoconstriction has included increased levels of endothelin, a highly potent vasoconstrictive peptide that is released from the uterus postpartum.

Cerebral venous thrombosis may complicate pregnancy and the puerperium and is discussed above. Other factors that contribute to puerperal stroke include postpartum cardiomyopathy (rare cause of cardioembolic stroke) and hypercoagulable states (antithrombin III deficiency, protein S and protein C deficiency, antiphospholipid antibodies, elevated levels of factors V and VIII and fibrinogen, polycythemia, and thrombocytosis).

SUGGESTED READINGS

Ameri A, Bousser MG: Cerebral venous thrombosis. Neurol Clin 10:87–111, 1992

Barnett H, Mohr JP, Stein BM, Yatsu FM: Stroke: Pathophysiology, Diagnosis and Management. 2nd Ed. Churchill Livingstone, New York, 1992

Bousser M-G, Barnett HJM: Cerebral venous thrombosis. p. 517. In Barnett HJM, Stein BM, Mohr JP, Yatsu FM (eds): Stroke: Pathophysiology, Diagnosis and Management. 2nd Ed. Churchill Livingstone, New York, 1992

Caplan LR: Stroke: A Clinical Approach. 2nd Ed. Butterworths, Boston, 1993

SECTION 4. CLINICAL FEATURES AND MANAGEMENT OF CEREBROVASCULAR DISEASE

---

41. CARDINAL CLINICAL FEATURES OF ISCHEMIC CEREBROVASCULAR DISEASE IN RELATION TO VASCULAR TERRITORIES

MICHAEL S. PESSIN
PHILIP A. TEAL

The clinical symptoms and signs of cerebrovascular disease are varied and, at first impression, may seem too heterogeneous and complex to classify by vascular territory. However, the goal of identifying which artery(ies) is responsible for the patient's symptoms is the very cornerstone of vascular diagnosis. Careful assessment of the clinical features can often aid the physician in clarifying the affected vascular territory and even the specific artery. Differentiation of large artery from small penetrating artery disease may help elucidate the underlying pathogenesis and guide diagnostic and management efforts. This chapter describes the common clinical vascular syndromes.

CAROTID TERRITORY

Anatomy

Figure 41-1 illustrates the anatomy of the internal carotid artery (ICA) and its principal branches. Each ICA arises from the bifurcation of the common carotid artery and has a cervical (extracranial) and intracranial course. The right common carotid artery takes origin from the innominate artery, and the left common carotid artery usually arises directly from the aortic arch, although variations are common. The bifurcation of the common carotid artery into the external carotid artery and ICA occurs in the cervical region at approximately the level of the superior thyroid cartilage (C4 to C5), although individual variations proximal or distal are common. The location of the carotid bifurcation makes auscultation of bruits readily accessible.

The external carotid artery is recognized by its several facial branches, which form important collateral channels when the circulation is compromised by occlusive lesions of the ICA or vertebral artery (VA). Anastomotic channels around and in the orbit may establish blood flow via the ophthalmic artery to the intracranial portion of the ICA when occlusion is at or just beyond the cervical bifurcation. The external carotid artery and the VA provide important reciprocal collaterals to each other in the presence of occlusive disease. The external carotid artery supplies branches that anastomose with the distal extracranial VA when the proximal, extracranial VA is occluded. Also, muscular branches of the VA may reconstitute the external carotid artery in the presence of common carotid artery occlusion.

The extracranial ICA, free of branches, extends from the bifurcation into the entrance of the petrous bone at the skull base. The intracranial ICA has three distinct segments: the petrosal, cavernous, and supraclinoid. The supraclinoid segment is the most important because of its several major branches. The first is the ophthalmic artery, which enters the orbit through

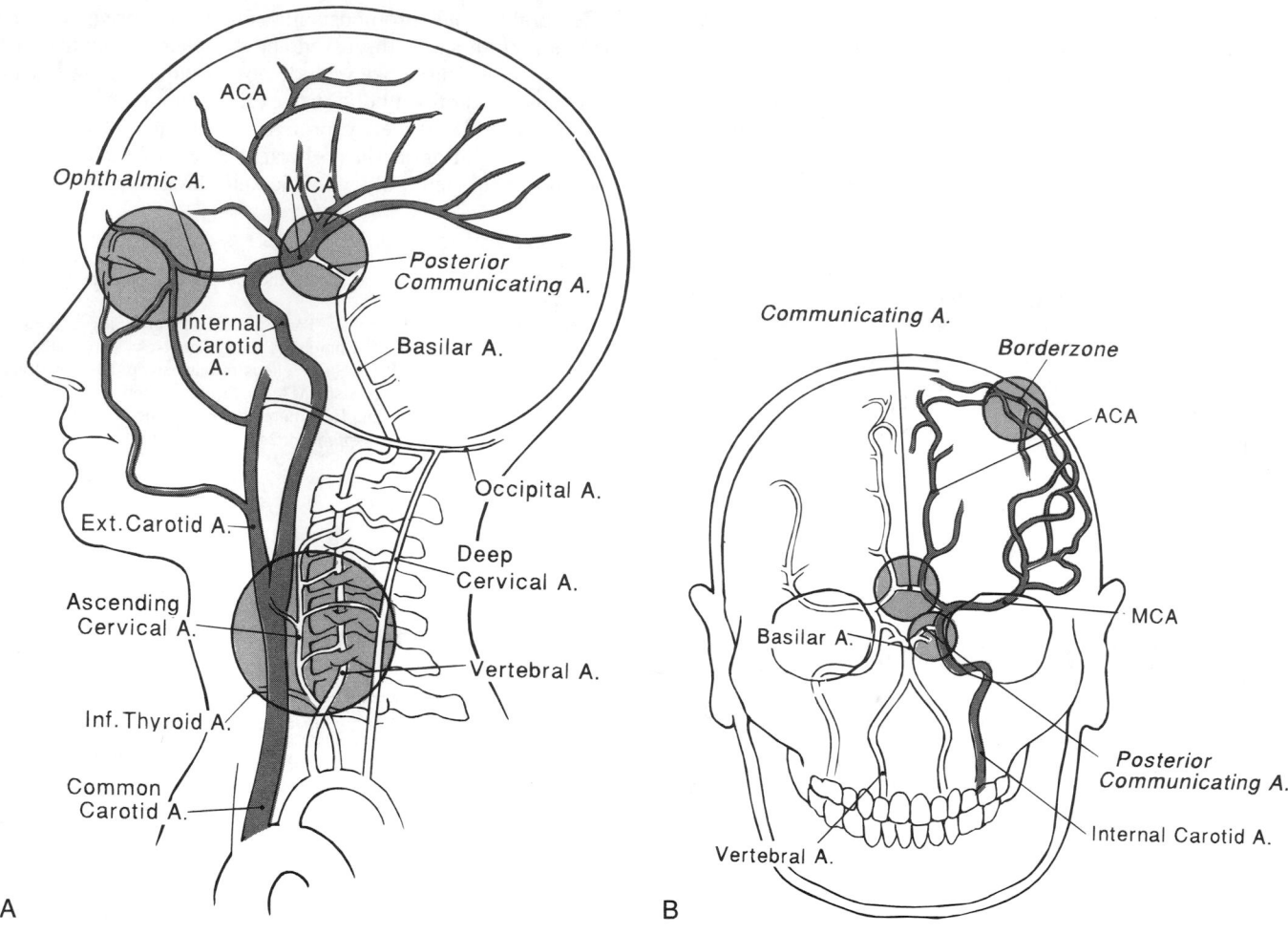

FIG. 41-1. Cerebral circulation showing the extra- and intracranial course of the carotid artery and its principal intracranial branches. Encircled areas highlight important collateral pathways. **(A)** Lateral view. Transorbital anastomoses via the ophthalmic artery link the external and internal carotid arteries. The posterior communicating arteries connect the carotid and vertebrobasilar circulation. Muscular branches of the cervical arteries from extracranial anastomoses between the vertebral artery and the external carotid artery. **(B)** Anteroposterior view. The anterior communicating artery connects the right and left carotid circulations. Leptomeningeal anastomoses form important collateral pathways in the borderzones between major arterial territories. ACA, anterior cerebral artery; MCA, middle cerebral artery.

the optic foramen and gives rise to several branches, including the important central retinal artery, which supplies the retina. The next branch is the posterior communicating artery, which joins the posterior cerebral artery (PCA) and, when fully developed, serves as an important conduit between the carotid (anterior) and vertebrobasilar (posterior) circulations. The anterior choroidal artery arises from the ICA just distal to the posterior communicating artery. The ICA then divides into its terminal branches, the anterior cerebral artery (ACA) and middle cerebral artery (MCA). The ACA supplies the upper medial surface of the hemisphere from the frontal pole to the posterior parietal area, extending over the convexity of the hemisphere to form an important anastomotic network with the distal branches of the MCA. The MCA supplies the entire lateral aspect of the hemisphere through several branches and is the largest extension of the terminating ICA.

Collateral Circulation

Several of the important collateral channels have already been described. These include connections between the external carotid artery and ICA via the orbital vessels; connections be-

tween the external carotid artery and VA; the circle of Willis, which connects the two intracranial carotid circulations via the anterior communicating artery; and the important carotid to vertebrobasilar connection through the posterior communicating artery. In addition, important leptomeningeal networks exist between the small terminal branches of the ACA and MCA and PCA and MCA, providing so-called borderzone collaterals. All of these collateral channels provide critical safeguards to compensate for various extra- and intracranial occlusive lesions (Fig. 41-1).

MANIFESTATIONS (PRESTROKE) OF INTERNAL CAROTID ARTERY DISEASE

Two important prestroke manifestations of ICA disease are bruits and transient ischemic attacks (TIAs). The presence of a carotid bruit heard on auscultation may be an important sign of silent carotid artery disease or a reassuring corroboration of an occlusive lesion in the presence of symptoms. The carotid bruit, the sound of turbulent blood flow, suggesting an underlying stenosis, is best heard at the bifurcation area in the region of the superior thyroid cartilage to the angle of the mandible.

Careful auscultation can almost always identify a bruit when severe stenosis is present. The quality of the bruit may vary and is not as predictive of underlying stenosis as the location at the bifurcation area. The bruit may be soft or loud with a harsh or high pitched quality. When the stenosis becomes critical or the artery occludes, the bruit may disappear or be absent from the start because of the reduced blood flow.

A carotid bruit must be distinguished from other sounds that may reflect conditions other than carotid stenosis, such as a radiated cardiac murmur, external carotid stenosis, nonstenosing lesions of the ICA, and venous sounds. Cardiac murmurs that radiate to the neck usually diminish in intensity the greater the distance they are from the heart in contrast to bifurcation bruits, which are localized and remain constant or increase in intensity. Noncritical stenoses of the ICA may produce sounds of turbulent flow and may be difficult to differentiate from more severe stenosis, without noninvasive testing. External carotid stenosis alone might produce a bifurcation area bruit. Its differentiation from ICA stenosis may be possible by detecting a diminished preauricular pulse from reduced flow in the ipsilateral superficial temporal artery compared to the normal side. Finally, venous sounds may confuse interpretation of neck bruits. Venous sounds, however, are usually heard low in the neck in the supraclavicular area. They may be obliterated by light compression of the external jugular vein or disappear in the supine position. All neck bruits, especially those suspected of reflecting ICA stenosis, should be investigated further with noninvasive carotid testing.

In the presence of carotid occlusion, an ocular bruit may be heard with a stethoscope over the contralateral orbit in up to 25 percent of patients, at least during the early phase following occlusion. The ocular bruit is thought to reflect increased blood flow in the contralateral ICA. Sometimes an ocular bruit may be present with severe ipsilateral carotid siphon stenosis.

Carotid Territory Transient Ischemic Attacks

TIAs are an important symptom of carotid artery disease and occur in 50 to 75 percent of patients with proven carotid stroke in retrospective series. TIAs refer to brief, reversible focal neurologic deficits that reflect temporary ischemia in a specific arterial territory. They last only minutes and must be differentiated from other common transient focal neurologic symptoms that reflect other mechanisms such as migraine, seizures, and isolated dizziness (vestibulopathy) (see Ch. 43). TIAs may occur in any vascular territory but are broadly classified into carotid (anterior) and vertebrobasilar (posterior) circulation events. Carotid territory TIAs include transient monocular blindness (TMB) and transient hemispheric attacks (THAs), reflecting the principal target areas of the retina and hemisphere.

Transient Monocular Blindness

TMB refers to the occurrence of temporary monocular visual obscuration. It may take several forms in which the patients describe a ''blur,'' ''fog,'' ''mist,'' ''cloud,'' or ''like Saran wrap,'' affecting visual clarity in one eye. The classic form of a shade or curtain effect of visual loss, descending or ascending to obscure all or part of monocular vision, occurs in only a minority of patients. Positive visual phenomena such as sparkles, lights, or colors, are uncommon and help to distinguish TMB from a migrainous event.

TMB is brief in duration, lasting 1 to 5 minutes, usually less than 15 minutes. Patients may have a few episodes or hundreds over many months or even years before seeking medical evaluation. TMB occurs without other symptoms and, together with its brief duration, is often perceived by patient and physician as a benign, inconsequential event. Although TMB usually occurs without any obvious inciting stimulus, occasionally occurrence after standing up or after other position changes or reduction in blood pressure related to antihypertensive medications may precipitate the visual obscuration. Exposure to bright sunlight may provoke an episode of TMB in patients with severe carotid stenosis by the mechanism of retinal hypoperfusion with reduced resynthesis of visual pigments, stressed by the bright stimulus. The pathogenesis of TMB, when related to carotid disease, may reflect embolism into the retinal circulation from platelet-fibrin thrombi superimposed on extracranial ICA atheromatous disease or a hemodynamic effect from severe stenosis or occlusion.

Chance observations of the ocular fundus during an attack of TMB in a small number of dramatic instances have documented embolic material traversing the retinal circulation. Usually, the embolus is grayish-white in appearance, reflecting platelet-fibrin material. Cholesterol emboli, also known as Hollenhorst plaques, named for the ophthalmologist who described them, are characterized by bright orange-gold birefringent crystals, but their relationship to TMB is unclear. Hollenhorst described these cholesterol crystals in patients with generalized cerebrovascular disease but found no association in a separate group of patients with TMB. They are often an incidental finding on funduscopic examination in patients with systemic atherosclerotic disease, and their principal importance is as a marker for generalized atherosclerosis. A poor prognosis related to a high mortality rate from cardiac death is associated with their discovery. The source of cholesterol emboli observed in the retinal circulation may arise from debris on a carotid atherosclerotic plaque or a more proximal atheroma from the aortic arch. Usually, no fundic abnormalities are seen during or after an attack of TMB, leading some to infer that embolic material has already passed from the retinal circulation. Undoubtedly, some attacks of TMB are caused by embolic material circulating through the retinal vasculature. Single or only a few attacks of TMB may be accounted for by this mechanism, but multiple, recurrent similar episodes of TMB over an extended period probably reflect retinal hypoperfusion from hemodynamic insufficiency related to carotid occlusive disease. Since the retinal circulation, like the hemisphere beyond, is a distal field of the carotid artery circulation, it is subject to hemodynamic effects in the presence of severe extracranial ICA stenosis or occlusion. A symptomatic low-perfusion state implies intermittent failure of collateral circulation. Conditions known to stress the delicate balance between adequate retinal perfusion and insufficiency include orthostatic blood pressure changes, hypotension induced by excessive antihypertensive medications, and exposure to bright light. Typically, patients with a hemodynamic mechanism may have many attacks over long periods without visual sequelae. The clinical features of such attacks are often similar or even identical (stereotyped) each time.

The occurrence of TMB in an adult with known vascular risk factors carries a strong relationship to carotid artery occlusive disease in as many as 30 to 50 percent of patients. As expected, TMB also has a strong relationship to other manifestations of carotid occlusive disease. Patients may have a history of THAs, but, interestingly, these attacks do not occur simultaneously with TMB. The mechanisms for both types of attacks are similar, but factors sufficient to produce retinal ischemia seem to have little effect on the hemispheric circulation. A rare exception has been the report of simultaneous ocular and hemisphere infarction in a few patients with carotid disease, but this exception reinforces the general principle of nonsimultaneity. Patients with both eye and hemisphere attacks have a higher incidence of carotid disease than do patients with TMB alone. Patients with only TMB at the time of presentation have a lower 2-year stroke risk than do those patients presenting with THAs. This conforms to clinical experience, which suggests that stroke seldom follows an attack of TMB alone, until THAs occur.

Benign Variants of Transient Monocular Blindness

Young women and otherwise healthy adults younger than 45 years of age may have attacks of TMB with a benign course. These patients have no tendency toward generalized atherosclerosis, and carotid occlusive disease is not the underlying mechanism. Until recently, the actual mechanism was uncertain, but vasospasm of the retinal circulation, perhaps similar to a migrainous mechanism, has now been documented. Recognition of this benign variant is important in order to avoid unnecessary, costly, and potentially risky diagnostic procedures in search of the more common atherosclerotic causes of TMB.

Transient Hemispheric Attacks

Transient ischemia that affects hemispheric function is the other common and important carotid TIA, referred to as a THA. In general, hemispheric dysfunction is reflected by weakness and/or numbness of part or all of the opposite side from the affected carotid artery. Speech may be involved when the dominant hemisphere is the target, and a behavioral alteration characterized by poor awareness of the deficit is common in nondominant hemispheric dysfunction. The latter affliction makes patients unreliable reporters of their own disability and often leads physicians astray in attempting to interpret their patients' concocted symptoms.

The most common symptoms experienced by the patient with carotid THAs are motor and sensory impairment of the contralateral limbs, followed by pure motor dysfunction, then pure sensory symptoms, and finally isolated dysphasia. Brachial paresis is the most consistent effect and may be the only symptom. It is common, as the sole manifestation of carotid occlusive disease, for the patient to describe suddenly dropping a utensil because of unexpected weakness. This specific deficit occurs presumably because of ischemia in the distal field of the carotid serving the suprasylvian motor area of arm function.

THAs are brief in duration, usually lasting less than 15 minutes, with many only 1 to 10 minutes. Patients may have only one or many THAs, spanning weeks to months, but rarely for more than 1 year, before coming to medical attention.

An unusual form of carotid THA referred to as limb shaking involves movements of the contralateral limbs. The limb shaking tends to be recurrent, involuntary, irregular movements described as "shaking," "trembling," "twitching," and "flapping." When limb shaking is the initial manifestation of carotid insufficiency, its differentiation from focal epilepsy may be difficult. Epilepsy, however, is more stereotyped and rhythmic than typical limb shaking. When other types of carotid TIA are part of the patient's history, then limb shaking may be more easily recognized as another ischemic manifestation.

Limb-shaking TIAs are regularly associated with hemodynamically significant ICA stenosis or occlusion, presumably reflecting a motor instability. A few patients have been reported with bilateral carotid occlusive disease with limb shaking on both sides of the body, on different occasions. Carotid endarterectomy, in a limited number of patients, has abolished these limb-shaking spells.

The pathogenesis of carotid THAs involves hemodynamic and embolic factors. Usually, patients with recurrent similar attacks have significant flow impairment from ICA stenosis or occlusion. In contrast, patients with only one or a few hemispheric attacks of different features may have an embolic mechanism affecting different MCA branches. Of course, both mechanisms and their effects may express themselves at different times in a patient.

THAs associated with carotid stenosis of 70 percent or more carry a significant risk of subsequent stroke over a 2-year period, estimated to be approximately 26 percent, higher than TMB alone based on data from the North American Symptomatic Carotid Endarterectomy Trial.

OCULAR STROKE

Extracranial carotid artery occlusive disease may present as ocular ischemia in the form of central retinal artery occlusion, retinal artery branch occlusion, or venous stasis retinopathy. These and other ocular ischemic syndromes are discussed in Chapter 43.

CEREBRAL INFARCTION IN THE CAROTID TERRITORY

Internal Carotid Artery

Occlusive disease of the ICA may be asymptomatic or cause stroke of varying severity from mild to devastating, depending on the mechanism(s) of ischemia (whether hemodynamic or embolic), availability of collateral blood flow, and size/location of the resulting infarct. The evolution or tempo of the fixed neurologic deficit may take one of several forms. Transient ischemic attacks (ocular or hemispheric) may precede the stroke by days, weeks, or months. With this background, the patient may awaken one morning with minor arm-hand weakness and speech difficulty. This persists for several hours and may improve, only to worsen later the same day or over the next few days to a major hemisphere disturbance with aphasia and hemiplegia. This classic "stepwise onset" marks the process as atherothrombotic and implies a worsening hemodynamic condition with a final arterial-to-arterial embolic occlusion of the MCA stem or its branches. A stepwise onset with a less severe outcome may occur from pure hemodynamic insufficiency and watershed infarction without intracranial embolism. Another scenario involves TIAs followed by a sudden, severe major hemispheric stroke, implying direct embolism to the MCA. Sometimes, with no history of preceding TIAs, the patient presents with a sudden partial or even complete MCA territory infarct as the first and only expression of their ICA disease, mimicking cardiac embolism. The absence of TIAs with a sudden, isolated embolic-type stroke may be questioned, but many patients do not report previous TIAs to the physician or family, and when the stroke occurs they are either unaware (nondominant hemisphere syndrome) or severely aphasic (dominant hemisphere) and unable to provide this history.

The impact of the infarct usually involves the MCA territory, less commonly the ACA territory. One angiographic study of patients with symptomatic ICA occlusive disease found intra-

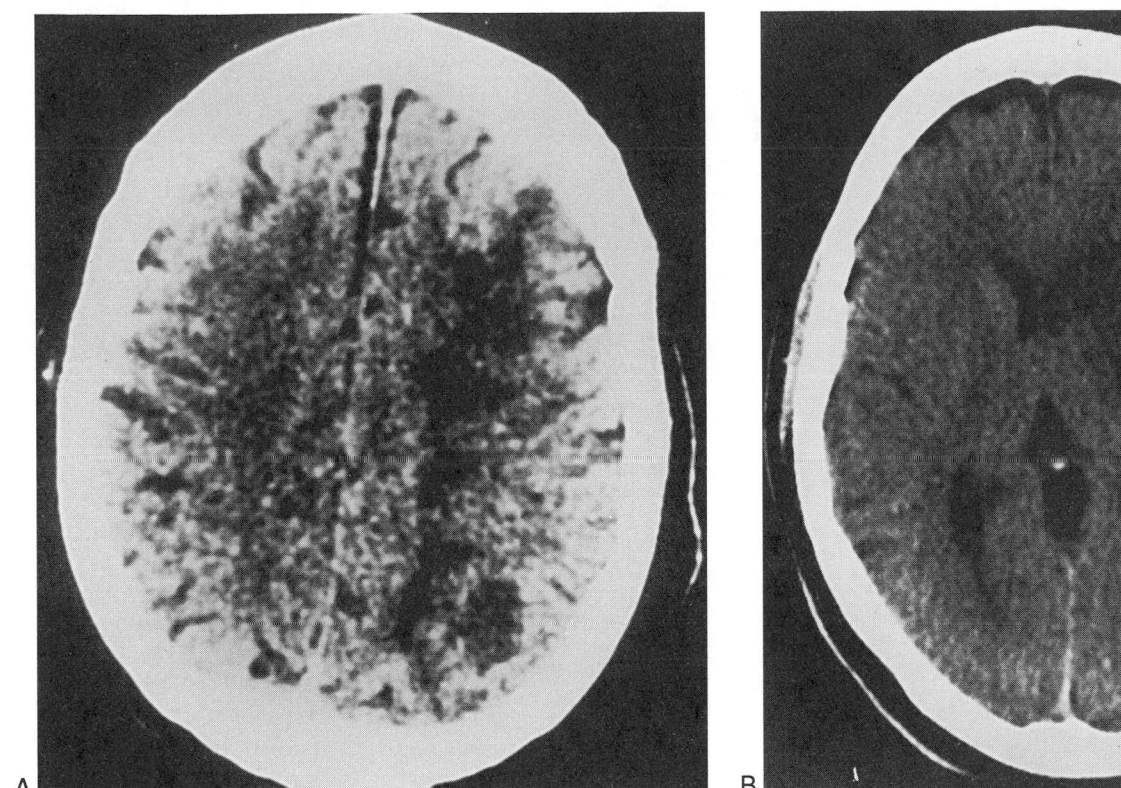

FIG. 41-2. **(A)** Computed tomographic scan of a patient with a watershed infarction, showing low attenuation along the anterior and posterior borderzones caused by low perfusion, resulting from a carotid artery occlusion. **(B)** Computed tomographic scan of a patient with an embolic infarction shows a discrete area of low attenuation in the territory of the superior division of the middle cerebral artery.

cranial embolism to be the predominant mechanism for infarction in two-thirds of patients studied with a nonembolic, presumed low-perfusion, state in one-third. These two groups were further characterized by a high frequency of preceding TIAs and a milder clinical deficit in patients with a nonembolic mechanism. Infarctions resulting from these two mechanisms have a different hemisphere topography (Fig. 41-2A). The impact of the hemodynamic mechanism affects the suprasylvian area of the frontal-parietal cortical convexity in the distal field of the carotid (MCA) supply. The resulting infarct lies high on the convexity and disproportionately affects motor function of the arm and hand, less so for the leg, with relatively sparing of the face, which is situated lower in the sylvian area. Language abnormalities associated with these suprasylvian infarcts are generally not as severe as those with sylvian localizations and take the form of the transcortical aphasias characterized by the relative preservation of repetition. The embolic infarct pattern is a discrete hypodensity involving the cortex and underlying white matter, usually in the sylvian region (Fig. 41-2B).

Embolism from the occlusive ICA atheroma often blocks the MCA stem or branches, but the ACA may also be involved, especially if the embolus occludes the top of the carotid where both major arterial supplies arise. Since ICA territory strokes most often affect the MCA territory, the distinction from primary athero-occlusive disease of the MCA stem or cardiogenic embolism may not be possible on clinical grounds alone unless markers of previous carotid disease exist in the form of TMB. The majority of MCA occlusions result from embolism, either carotid or cardiac source. This fact makes it important to investigate for a carotid source when MCA territory infarction is present, even if obvious cardiac embologenic disease is present, since both mechanisms may coexist.

MIDDLE CEREBRAL ARTERY TERRITORY

The MCA and its branches supply the largest portion of the cerebral hemisphere, including the deep basal ganglia-internal capsular area and lateral surface of the hemisphere. The MCA territory accounts for the most common stroke syndromes because of its large blood supply and susceptibility to occlusion.

Anatomy

The most common anatomic pattern is the MCA originating as a stem from the terminal ICA, which then divides into a superior and inferior division, from which approximately 12 branches arise to supply the lateral aspect of each hemisphere. The lenticulostriate arteries (LSAs), small vessels that originate from the MCA stem, or less often the superior division, are endarteries supplying the putamen, part of the internal capsule, and caudate nucleus (Fig. 41-3).

Either the superior or inferior divisions may be individually blocked by embolism, resulting in a restricted cortical territory infarct. The superior division territory supplies the lateral frontal and anterior parietal regions in a sylvian-suprasylvian distribution; the inferior division supplies the temporal-posterior parietal region. The functional anatomy underlying these vascular territories leads to specific neurologic deficits. Occlusion of individual branches of the superior and inferior division are usually caused by embolism and result in partial clinical syndromes, depending on the vessel and brain location affected.

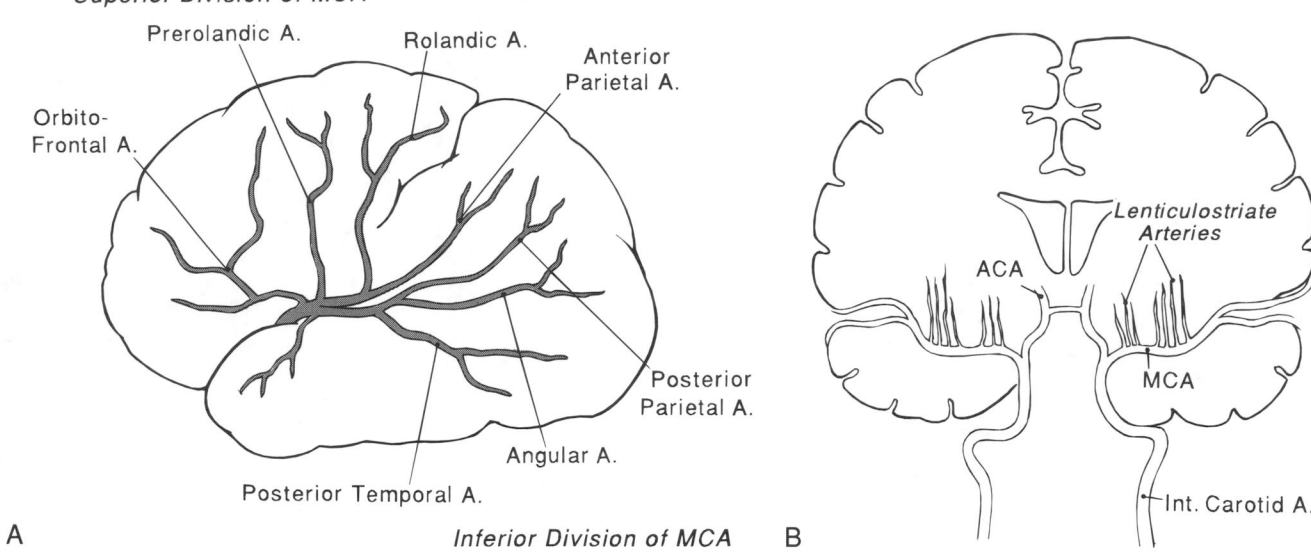

FIG. 41-3. Anatomy of the middle cerebral artery. **(A)** Lateral view showing the most common vascular pattern with cortical branches arising from superior and inferior divisions. **(B)** Anteroposterior view showing the lenticulostriate arteries originating from the stem of the middle cerebral artery (MCA). ACA, anterior cerebral artery.

Pathogenesis of Middle Cerebral Artery Territory Stroke

The most common cause of MCA occlusion is embolism, either from a cardiac or artery-to-artery source from extracranial ICA atherosclerosis. Primary atherosclerosis may produce a focal stenosis or occlusion of the MCA stem, but overall it is a relatively uncommon cause of occlusion compared to embolism.

Clinical Features

Middle Cerebral Artery Stem.   Table 41-1 illustrates the computed tomographic (CT) patterns and attendant clinical deficits for MCA territory infarcts. The maximal neurologic syndrome, well known to the clinician, results from a large infarct involv-

ing the deep territory and cortical surface produced by occlusion of the MCA stem proximal to the take-off of the LSAs. The principal clinical signs include hemiplegia of face, arm, and leg; head and eye deviation to the affected hemisphere; hemisensory loss; homonymous hemianopsia; and global aphasia (dominant hemisphere) or neglect (nondominant hemisphere). The neurologic outcome associated with MCA stem occlusion produces an unacceptably severe deficit, although, rarely, a benign outcome has been noted in patients with effective collaterals who have had a progressive occlusive lesion, allowing time for compensatory collaterals to develop.

Middle Cerebral Artery Penetrator Territory.   The LSAs arise from the MCA stem and consist of a medial and lateral group

TABLE 41-1. Middle Cerebral Artery Territory Infarct Patterns and Clinical Features

Arterial Territory	CT	Motor	Sensory	Visual	Language	Behavior
MCA stem complete territory		Hemiplegia; F-A-L Head and eye deviation	Hemianesthesia	Homonymous hemianopsia	Global aphasia	Neglect (ND > D)
MCA superior division		Hemiparesis; F-A > L Head and eye deviation	Hemianesthesia; F + A > L	—	Expressive aphasia (Broca's) (D)	Neglect (ND)
MCA inferior division		Minimal weakness	Rapidly resolving hemisensory	Homonymous hemianopsia or upper quadrant anopsia	Receptive aphasia (Wernicke's) (D)	Behavioral disturbances Constructional apraxia, delirium (ND)

Abbreviations: F, face; A, arm; L, leg; D, dominant hemisphere; ND, nondominant hemisphere; CT, computed tomography; MCA, middle cerebral artery.

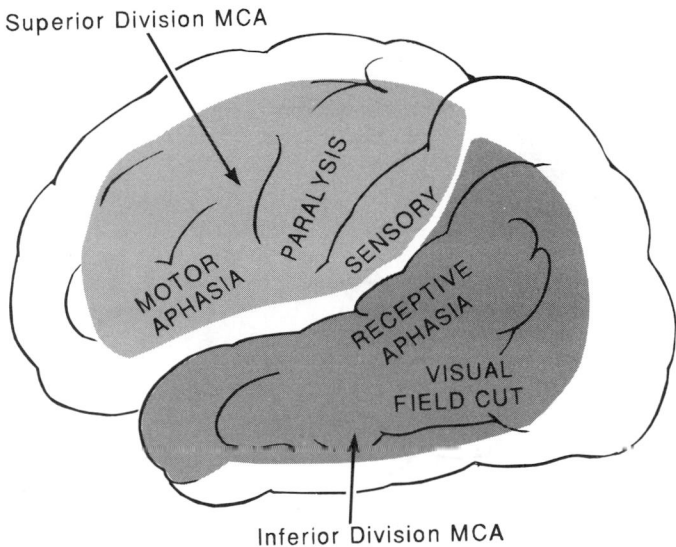

FIG. 41-4. Surface anatomy and functional correlates of territorial infarctions of superior and inferior divisions of the middle cerebral artery (MCA).

of vessels. Occlusion of one or more of these penetrators results in a small deep infarct in the striatocapsular area. The resulting neurologic deficit is usually a pure motor hemiparesis from the capsular infarct. The prognosis for functional recovery is excellent.

Middle Cerebral Artery Divisions. The clinical syndrome associated with superior division occlusion results from infarction of the anterior sylvian and suprasylvian part of the hemisphere involving the frontal-parietal region (Fig. 41-4). The deep penetrating territory of the LSAs is spared since the superior division originates distal to their origin. Motor deficits predominate in superior division territory infarction. Hemiparesis follows the distribution of face and arm, which are more affected than the leg. Head and eye deviation is common. The hemisensory loss follows the pattern of the motor deficit with the face and arm more affected than the leg. An expressive-type (Broca's) aphasia results in the dominant hemisphere and neglect, in the non-dominant hemisphere. The inferior division clinical syndrome results from infarction in the temporal-parietal area and is usually below the sylvian fissure (Fig. 41-4). Here, motor deficits are overshadowed by a predominantly fading hemisensory loss and either homonymous hemianopsia or inferior quadrantanopsia related to injury of the optic radiation deep to this region. A receptive-type (Wernicke's) aphasia occurs in the dominant hemisphere, and behavioral disturbances of agitation and constructional apraxia result from the nondominant hemisphere.

Middle Cerebral Artery Branches. Individual branches or combinations of two or more branch occlusions of either the superior or inferior division result in restrictive clinical signs referable to the focal brain region and its functional anatomy (Fig. 41-3).

ANTERIOR CEREBRAL ARTERY

Anatomy

The ACA and its cortical branches supply the anterior and medial aspects of each cerebral hemisphere except for the most posterior portion supplied by the PCA (Fig. 41-5). Deep branches, including Heubner's artery, supply the anterior limb of the internal capsule and part of the head of the caudate nucleus. The anterior communicating artery, which is a critical conduit of the circle of Willis, joins both ACAs in the midline. The cortical branches of the ACA supply the medial orbital surface of the frontal lobe, the frontal pole, the supplementary motor area, and the motor-sensory cortex supplying the foot, leg, and urinary bladder. Branches also supply the corpus callosum. The leptomeningeal branches of the ACA course over the convexity of the hemisphere to form the important borderzone anastomoses with the distal branches of the MCA from the lateral surface of the hemisphere. Variations of ACA anatomy are common, and frequently both ACAs are supplied from one carotid circulation because of an atretic or absent proximal (A-1) segment.

Pathogenesis of Anterior Cerebral Artery Territory Stroke

Occlusive disease of the ACA usually results from embolism either from a carotid or cardiac origin. Intrinsic athero-occlusive disease of the ACA, like the MCA, is uncommon. Bilateral ACA territory infarcts are usually caused by vasospasm following rupture of a saccular aneurysm of the anterior communicating artery. Ischemic stroke in the territory of an ACA is relatively uncommon, accounting for approximately 5 percent of all anterior circulation infarcts, compared to stroke in the MCA territory.

Clinical Features

The principal clinical features of ACA territory infarction include motor and sensory dysfunction of the contralateral foot and leg. The proximal arm may also be weak, but the face and hand are usually spared. Sensory loss, confined to the foot and leg, is mild and involves two-point discrimination, localization, stereognosis, and position sense. Pain and temperature are less affected. The distribution of the weakness and sensory loss, which disproportionately affects the leg and proximal rather than distal arm, with the face spared, stamps the process as ACA territory in contrast to MCA distribution deficits, which heavily affect the lower face, arm, and hand but less often the leg. This distribution presumably reflects the cortical localization of foot and leg, located superiorly and medially in the hemisphere. With bilateral ACA territory infarcts, the patient may have a paraparesis mimicking a spinal cord syndrome. Another feature is abulia, a behavioral alteration characterized by lack of volition and spontaneity. Abulia is a profound state of reduced responsiveness to verbal and environmental stimuli in an otherwise alert patient. Soft, whispering speech and delayed and laconic responses to questions are common. Abulia reflects injury to the anterior and medial frontal cortex. It may result from only unilateral ACA territory infarction or from bilateral infarcts that produce a more profound state of unresponsiveness. Aphasia does not occur but can be mistakenly suggested by the behavioral alterations and tendency for echolalia. Dyspraxia of the left limbs for verbal and tactile stimuli may be present from a presumed disconnection syndrome when the corpus callosum is involved in the infarct. Urinary incontinence may occur, with unilateral or bilateral lesions reflecting involvement of the paracentral lobule.

Heubner's artery(ies) includes two to four arteries that arise

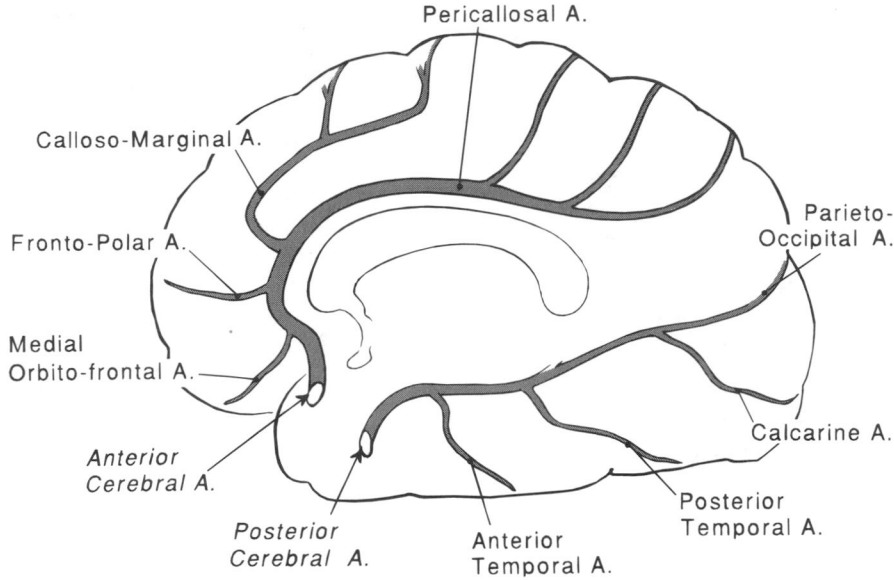

FIG. 41-5.   Cortical branches of the anterior and posterior cerebral arteries on the medial surface of the cerebral hemisphere.

from the proximal ACA and supply part of the caudate nucleus, anterior limb of the internal capsule, and anterior part of the putamen. The clinical features resulting from Heubner arterial territory infarction include dysarthria and behavioral-cognitive deficits such as abulia, neglect, or aphasia.

ANTERIOR CHOROIDAL ARTERY

Anatomy and Pathogenesis

The anterior choroidal artery is a small vessel that originates from the internal carotid artery a few millimeters distal to the origin of the posterior communicating artery. It supplies branches to the optic tract. As it courses posteriorly, it gives off branches to the medial aspect of the temporal lobe, cerebral peduncle, and thalamus. Branches supply the lateral geniculate body and posterior half of the posterior limb of the internal capsule. The vessel terminates in the choroid plexus. Stroke in the territory of anterior choroidal artery is uncommon but can be recognized by the topography of the CT infarct encompassing the deeper territories of the hemisphere (Fig. 41-6). The most common stroke mechanism is small vessel disease in patients with hypertension and diabetes. Cardiac embolism may also account for some cases of infarction.

Clinical Features

The most consistent clinical features are hemiparesis and hemisensory loss from infarction of the posterior limb of the internal capsule and homonymous visual field defects from ischemia to the optic radiations or lateral geniculate body. The absence of higher cortical dysfunction in a patient with hemiparesis, hemisensory loss, and hemianopsia reflects the large subcortical extent of the infarct and helps differentiate anterior choroidal artery territory stroke from large infarcts in the MCA territory.

VERTEBROBASILAR TERRITORY

The vertebrobasilar (VB) circulation supplies the brainstem; cerebellum; and, through the PCA, the medial temporal lobe,

thalamus, and visual centers, including the primary visual (calcarine) cortex. Physicians have traditionally viewed the VB circulation as somehow uniquely different from the carotid or anterior circulation. The clinical symptoms are often confusing to the physician, and the stroke mechanisms are thought to be mysterious. Often, the patient's symptoms, which are not readily consistent with carotid ischemia, are casually labeled ''VB insufficiency,'' and, without further diagnostic effort, anticoagulants are prescribed. This attitude, in contrast to the efforts made to clarify carotid territory ischemia, reflects in part the perceived absence of surgical treatment such as carotid endar-

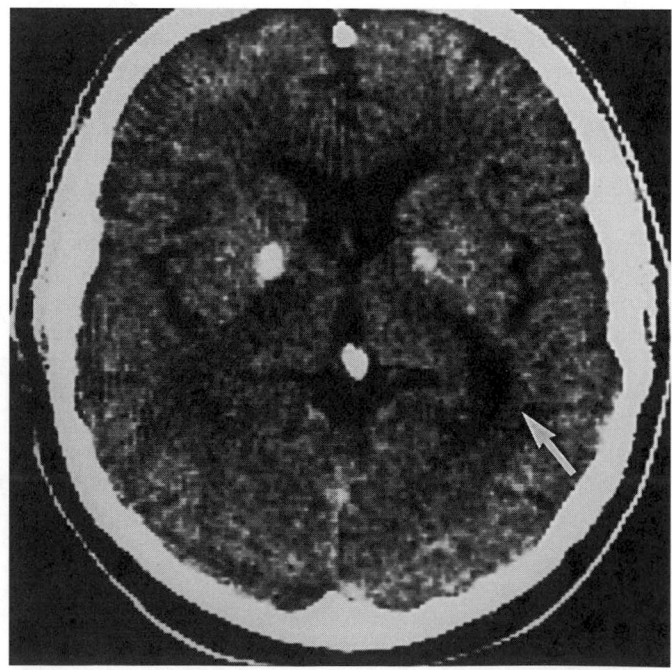

FIG. 41-6.   Computed tomographic appearance of an anterior choroidal artery infarction showing an area of low attenuation in the posterior limb of the internal capsule and lateral geniculate body (*arrow*).

terectomy, the puzzling array of symptoms and signs, and a poor understanding of the pathophysiology of VB stroke. Earlier attempts at understanding VB ischemia by Mayo Clinic clinicians lead to the term ''VB insufficiency'' and treatment with warfarin anticoagulation, based on favorable results in small uncontrolled studies that lacked angiographic clarification of the underlying vascular disease. This approach has unfortunately persisted despite new information that has emerged from neurodiagnostic techniques and detailed clinical studies of various VB syndromes. As Caplan et al. (1992) pointed out in comparing the VB to the carotid circulation, ''Consider two arterial systems. They are located only a few inches apart, have the same anatomic constitutions, and, except for size, cannot be easily distinguished from each other grossly or under a microscope. They are exposed to the same blood, the same cardiac output, and the same blood pressure. Would you expect that diseases of the two systems would be very different? The answer is a resounding no.'' We now know that the two circulations are more similar than different in terms of stroke risk factors, mechanisms of ischemia (primary atherosclerosis, artery-to-artery embolism, cardiac origin embolism, and all other common mechanisms of VB territory ischemia), and potential

treatments. Even the unusual conditions of dissection, vasculitis, and fibromuscular hyperplasia occur in the VB circulation. An understanding of the clinicopathologic features of the VB circulation should help eliminate the double standard in our approach to these problems and enable the clinician to approach VB vascular disease with the same confidence as in the carotid territory.

Anatomy

Figure 41-7 illustrates the anatomy of the VB circulation. The two VAs arise extracranially from the subclavian arteries and join at the pontomedullary junction to form the single basilar artery. The basilar artery lies on the ventral surface of the pons and, at the pontomesencephalic junction, divides into the two PCAs.

The two VAs are not usually equal in size. The dominant, larger VA is often the left one. One VA may be absent, atretic, or terminate at the posterior inferior cerebellar artery (PICA) without joining to form the basilar artery. The VAs have four segments; the first segment includes the origin of the VA from the subclavian artery to its entrance in the transverse foramen

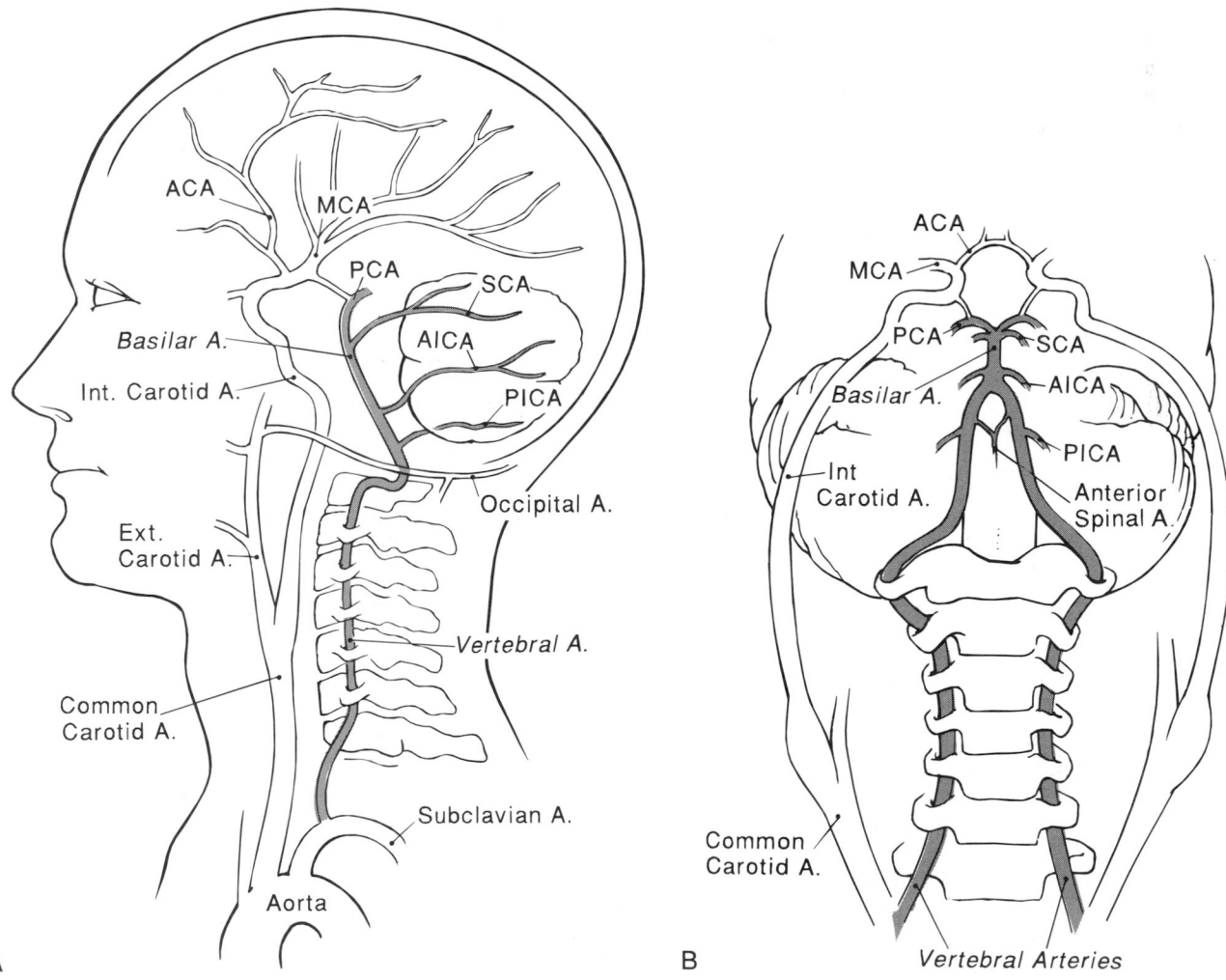

FIG. 41-7. Anatomy of the vertebrobasilar circulation. **(A)** Lateral view showing the origin and extracranial course of the left vertebral artery, the basilar artery, and its major branches. **(B)** Anteroposterior view showing the merging of the vertebral arteries to form the basilar artery and their principal branches. ACA, anterior cerebral artery; MCA, middle cerebral artery; PCA, posterior cerebral artery; SCA, superior cerebellar artery; AICA, anterior inferior cerebellar artery; PICA, posterior inferior cerebellar artery.

of the cervical vertebra at the level of C6 or C5. The second segment is entirely within the bony canal of the transverse foramina from its entrance to C2. The third segment is that portion with a tortuous route emerging from C2 and coursing posteriorly and laterally, circling the posterior arch of C1, and passing between the atlas and occiput. The fourth segment is the intracranial portion that pierces the dura mater to enter the foramen magnum. Its long extracranial course, bony encasement, and tortuous exit make the VA susceptible to traumatic injury, a common cause of stroke.

The PICA is the largest branch of the VA, originating a few millimeters above the foramen magnum, approximately 1.5 cm below the origin of the basilar artery. The PICA supplies the posterior inferior cerebellar hemispheres and provides a branch to the dorsal medullary area. Direct branches from the VA, just distal to the origin of PICA, are the major supply to the lateral medullary region. Near the confluence of the two VAs that form the basilar artery, small branches form the anterior spinal artery, which courses caudally to supply a major portion of the anterior spinal cord.

The largest branches of the basilar artery are the paired cerebellar arteries, the anterior inferior cerebellar artery (AICA), and superior cerebellar artery (SCA). The AICA originates at approximately the midbasilar level and supplies the anterior inferior aspect of each cerebellar hemisphere. The AICA and PICA may provide important anastomotic pathways to compensate for occlusive disease in the proximal basilar artery. The internal auditory artery is usually a branch of AICA but may arise directly from the basilar artery.

The SCA takes origin from the rostral basilar just proximal to its bifurcation into the PCAs. The SCA supplies the superior surface of the cerebellum and part of the rostral lateral pontine tegmentum. The basilar artery then usually bifurcates into the two PCAs unless one, or uncommonly both PCAs, arise directly from the ICA.

The other group of vessels arising from the basilar are the penetrating arteries, which supply the medial and lateral pons and part of the midbrain. This paramedium group consists of seven to 10 vessels arising from the posterior wall of the basilar artery and supplies the basal and tegmental pons on either side of the midline. Another group, the short lateral circumferential arteries, numbering five to seven arteries, supplys the more lateral pontine base and lateral tegmentum.

VERTEBRAL ARTERY

Pathogenesis of Vertebral Artery Territory Stroke

Disease of the VA is a common cause of brainstem and cerebellar stroke. The consequences of VA occlusion are variable and, like other vascular territories, depend on the pathogenesis, occurrence of local embolism to distal sites, and availability of effective collateral channels. Unilateral VA occlusion, especially in its extracranial segments, may be well tolerated without symptoms because of effective collaterals and patency of the other VA. On the other hand, distal embolism to the basilar artery or its branches can lead to disastrous consequences. One reason why extracranial disease is so well tolerated is the abundance of collateral circulation, leading to reconstitution of the more distal VA (Fig. 41-1A). The external carotid artery may effectively re-establish antegrade VA flow via the occipital branch to the VA. Also, muscular branches of the deep cervical and ascending cervical arteries and thyrocervical trunk may reconstitute the distal VA when proximal VA occlusion is present. Increasingly, it has been recognized that extracranial VA occlusive disease, like the carotid, can serve as a source for distal embolism into the basilar artery or its branches and lead to stroke.

The extracranial VA is also susceptible to traumatic injury because of its encasement in the bony part of the cervical canal. Either spontaneously or after minor trauma from neck manipulation, the VA may be injured, and dissection with luminal compromise and clot embolization may occur. This is a common cause of stroke, especially in young patients without other vascular risk factors.

Intracranial VA occlusive disease results from atheromatous disease and is a frequent cause of stroke. It is the usual cause of lateral medullary and cerebellar infarction. When occlusion is associated with thrombus propagation or local embolism, the basilar artery may be swept into the occlusive process, leading to a major pontine infarct.

Clinical

Extracranial VA occlusive disease is usually well tolerated unless distal embolism occurs. These effects are discussed with the specific arterial syndromes that follow. The most well known extracranial VA vascular problem is the "subclavian steal" syndrome. This results from subclavian atherostenosis but affects the VB circulation (Fig. 41-8). Subclavian stenosis just proximal to the origin of the left VA impairs antegrade flow and creates a low-pressure system in the VA. Since the subclavian also supplies the arm circulation, the pulse is reduced or absent, and exercise of the limb may precipitate the diversion of blood out of the intracranial circulation from the right VA and basilar artery into the low pressure left VA system. With angiographic visualization, the contrast is seen filling the right VA antegrade and then flows retrograde down into the left VA instead of continuing into the intracranial basilar circulation. In effect, blood is diverted from the basilar circulation by the pressure differential in the left VA as a result of the subclavian occlusive lesion. The clinical effects of subclavian steal are inversely related to the prominent acclaim associated with this vascular condition. That is, it is a benign syndrome in relationship to brainstem ischemic effects. Neurologic symptoms are usually transient and may include episodic posterior headache, dizziness, loss of balance, and double vision. Stroke is rare. Symptoms in the ischemic arm are common, and patients complain of fatigue, tiredness, cramping, or coldness. The left subclavian artery is more often affected than the right subclavian, and a bruit caused by the stenosis may be heard along the subclavian artery.

Intracranial Vertebral Artery

The lateral medullary syndrome is the most common stroke associated with intracranial VA occlusive disease. In approximately 20 percent of patients, associated cerebellar infarcts are present as a result of compromise of the PICA circulation, which is in close proximity to the VA occlusive process. More often, the infarct is restricted to a small wedge of tissue in the dorsal lateral medulla, resulting from occlusion of direct VA branches that supply this area (Fig. 41-9). Table 41-2 shows the typical symptoms and signs of lateral medullary infarction. While initial disability may be severe, by 6 months, recovery is excellent. Magnetic resonance imaging (MRI) may show the infarct, but CT rarely delineates this small area of the medulla

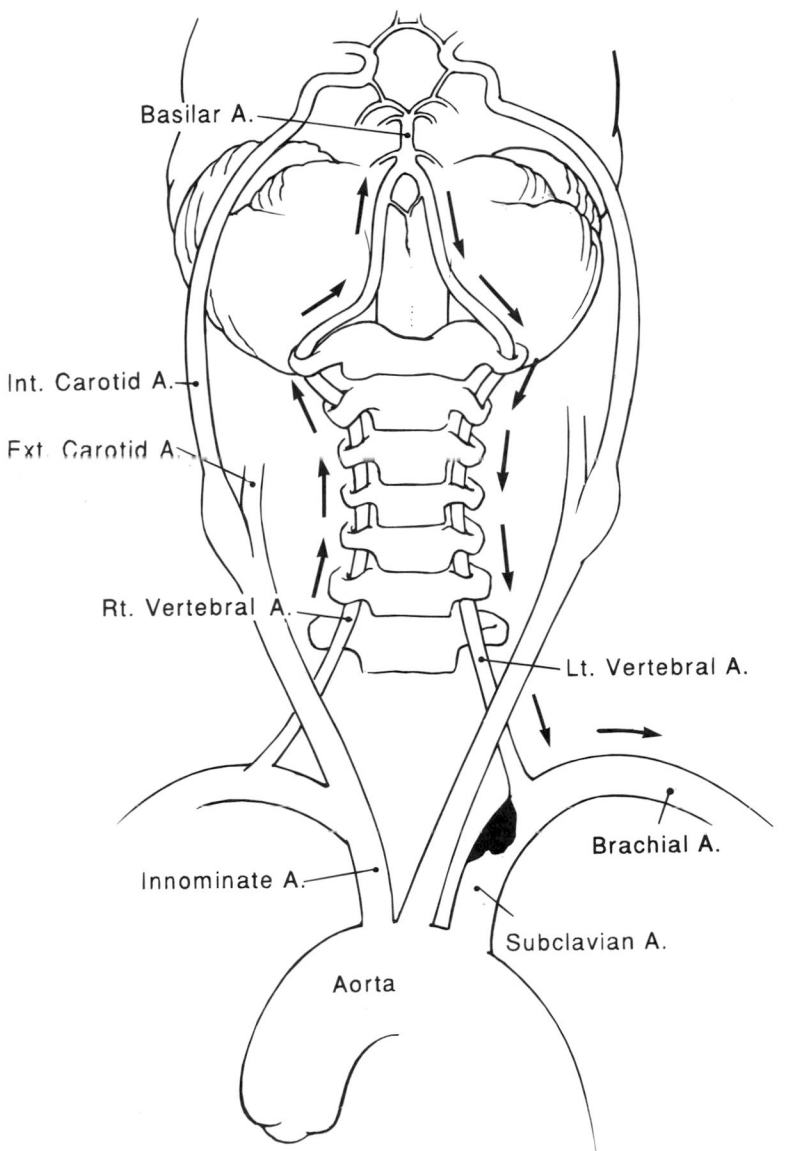

FIG. 41-8. Subclavian steal with right-to-left vertebrovertebral crossover flow caused by a proximal stenosis of the left subclavian artery.

because of reduced sensitivity and artifacts from adjacent bony structures.

CEREBELLAR INFARCTION

Cerebellar infarction is usually caused by atheromatous disease of the parent VA or basilar artery or embolism to one of the long circumferential cerebellar arteries (PICA, AICA, or SCA). The cerebellar infarct may be restricted to only the cerebellum or may be part of a larger syndrome that includes other brainstem structures, as in the lateral medullary syndrome. The clinical diagnosis of cerebellar infarct is often confused with the more benign medical condition of peripheral vestibulopathy because dizziness and vertigo, with accompanying vomiting, are a prominent part of the cerebellar syndromes, mimicking an isolated vestibular dysfunction. Differentiation is critical since the pathogenesis, treatment, and prognosis are different. Often, neuroimaging (CT/MRI) may be necessary to differentiate and clarify the clinical picture. The clinical features may help differentiate the cerebellar vascular territory (Table 41-3).

Posterior Inferior Cerebellar Artery

PICA territory infarcts are the most common of the cerebellar strokes and generally produce the largest infarcts. The pathogeneses of PICA territory infarcts are equally divided between intracranial VA athero-occlusive disease and embolism from either a cardiac or proximal arterial source. The most common clinical features include sudden spinning dizziness, gait ataxia, and posterior headache. Nausea and vomiting are a regular accompaniment. Appendicular dysfunction on the side of the infarct is usually present. If only the medial PICA branch is involved, the midline vermis may be most affected, producing gait ataxia. If the lateral PICA branch is affected, then the infarct lies laterally in the cerebellar hemisphere, and lateropulsion, veering to the side of the infarct when walking or standing, is common. In larger PICA territory infarcts, mass effect compromising brainstem structures, obstructive hydrocephalus from compression of the fourth ventricle, and herniation through the foramen magnum may jeopardize life. Other signs accompanying these seriously ill patients include reduced level of con-

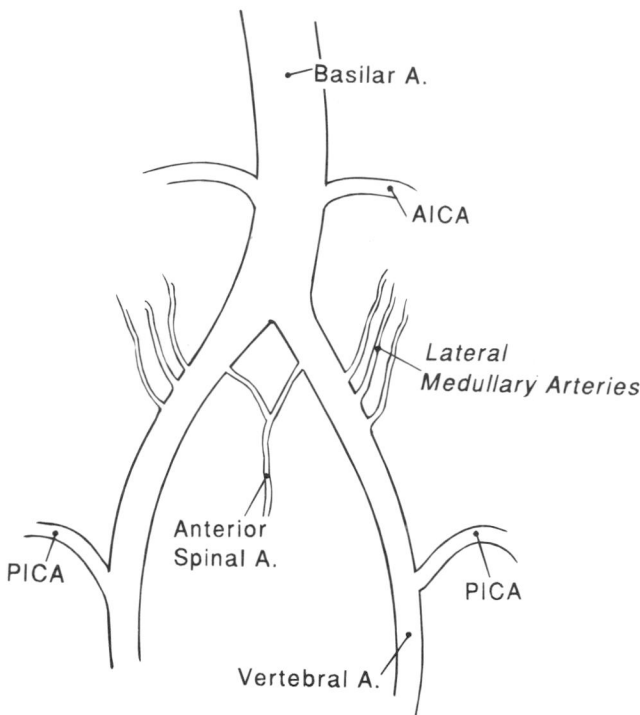

FIG. 41-9. Vascular anatomy of the vertebrobasilar junction. Small branches arising directly from the distal vertebral artery supply the lateral medulla. AICA, anterior inferior cerebellar artery; PICA, posterior inferior cerebellar artery.

TABLE 41-2. Lateral Medullary Syndrome

Ipsilateral to the lesion
  Facial pain
  Decreased facial pain and temperature sensation
  Decreased corneal sensation
  Horner syndrome
  Dysphagia, hoarseness, and decreased gag reflex caused by paralysis of palate, pharynx, and larynx (nucleus ambiguus)
  Ipsilateral cerebellar signs
Contralateral to the lesion
  Decreased pain and temperature on trunk and extremities
Nonlateralized features
  Vertigo, nausea, and vomiting (caused by involvement of vestibular nuclei)
  Nystagmus, usually greatest to side of lesion; gait ataxia

TABLE 41-3. Cerebellar Infarction: Vascular Territory and Clinical Features

Vascular Territory	Clinical Features	Associated Infarcts
PICA	Vertigo, ataxia, vomiting, lateropulsion, headache, delayed coma (large infarction)	± Lateral medulla syndrome
AICA	Dysmetria (ipsilateral), crossed syndrome-ipsilateral Horner, facial palsy, deafness, lateral gaze palsy, contralateral temperature and pain loss	Lateral pons, middle cerebellar peduncle
SCA	Ataxia, unilateral limb dysmetria, dysarthria, nystagmus; headache and vertigo less common; Horner syndrome, contralateral pain and temperature loss, and fourth nerve palsy may be seen; rostral basilar artery syndrome or coma, often with tetraplegia, may occur	± Midbrain, thalamic, occipitotemporal lobes

Abbreviations: PICA, posterior inferior cerebellar artery; AICA, anterior inferior cerebellar artery; SCA, superior cerebellar artery

sciousness, ipsilateral face paresis, decreased corneal response, and a Babinski sign, indicating a progressive mass effect. If medical measures fail to reverse the process, urgent ventricular drainage and surgical evacuation of the necrotic cerebellar tissue may be life-saving measures. Once the acute phase has passed, functional recovery is generally good with some rehabilitation effort.

Anterior Inferior Cerebellar Artery

AICA territory infarcts are commonly accompanied by other brainstem signs from involvement of nearby structures in the pons. The reason is that the offending obstructive lesion usually originated in the adjacent basilar artery and affected the AICA circulation in the limited number of patients studied. The cerebellar component of the infarct is usually smaller than those caused by PICA and SCA occlusion and, by itself, has a favorable course. The brainstem signs usually produce maximal involvement at the midpontine level, extending from the midline to the lateral margin. The signs are similar to the lateral medullary syndrome with the addition of peripheral involvement of the seventh (facial) cranial nerve and eighth cranial nerve (ipsilateral hearing impairment) but sparing of cranial nerves IX and X.

Superior Cerebellar Artery

Occlusion of the SCA is often due to embolism, which blocks the rostral basilar artery and includes the SCA territory; occasionally, isolated SCA embolic occlusion occurs, as seen in Figure 41-10 in a patient with mitral stenosis. Gait and limb ataxia and dysarthria are the most prominent signs; vertigo and headache are less common than in PICA territory infarcts. Since the penetrating short circumferential branches of the SCA supply the upper pontine and midbrain tegmentum, other signs are frequently present. Horner syndrome, contralateral pain, and

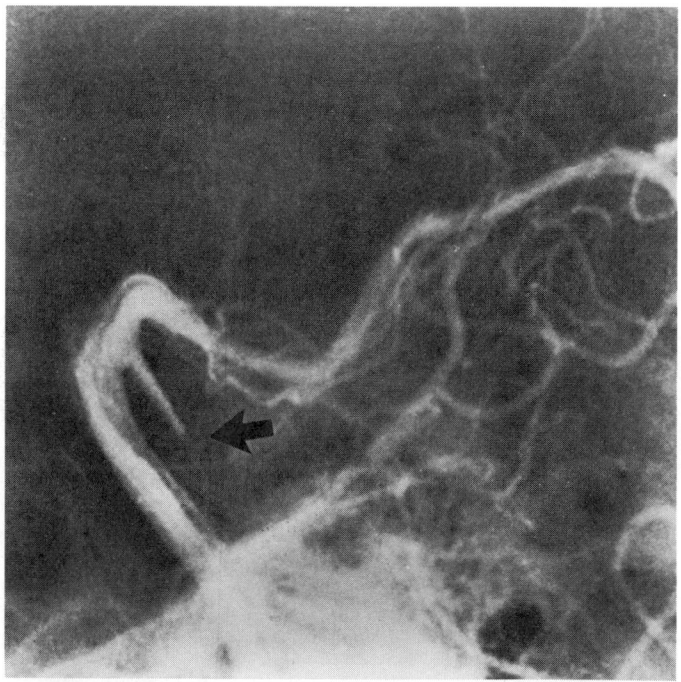

FIG. 41-10. Angiogram showing an abrupt occlusion of the superior cerebellar artery (*arrow*) caused by a cardiac embolus.

temperature impairment of the face and limbs, contralateral fourth cranial nerve paresis, and ipsilateral involuntary movements have all been recorded.

BASILAR ARTERY

The early reports of basilar artery occlusive disease were based on autopsy material and naturally portrayed a dismal outcome. In fact, the deficits associated with basilar artery occlusion were viewed as incompatible with life or as so devastating as to be unacceptable for functional recovery. We now know that basilar artery occlusion can encompass a spectrum of neurologic dysfunction, which is relatively minor in some patients and life threatening in others. In between these extremes, a variety of disability may occur. This is similar to the effects of large artery disease in the anterior carotid arterial territory.

The critical factors influencing outcome relate to the mechanism(s) of the vascular disease, the availability of effective collaterals, and the size and distribution of the resulting infarct. In a survey of the New England Medical Center stroke registry, all 20 patients with angiographically proven basilar artery occlusion collected over a 5-year period survived with varying disability, many with a surprisingly good functional outcome. The diagnosis of basilar artery occlusion has been enhanced by modern neurovascular techniques such as angiography, MRI and magnetic resonance angiography, and transcranial Doppler ultrasound so that an accurate and more representative population of patients can be assessed.

Pathogenesis of Basilar Artery Territory Stroke

Occlusive lesions of the basilar artery usually affect the proximal, middle, or distal segments of the artery, although the mechanisms differ for each site; the proximal and midportions are susceptible to atherothrombosis, and the more distal basilar artery is most often affected by embolism. Basilar artery stenosis, from atherosclerosis, usually precedes the occluding atherothrombotic lesion and may involve any segment of the artery in approximately equal frequency (Fig. 41-11). The common belief that the proximal basilar is most susceptible to focal stenosis is not borne out by a review of available reports based on autopsy and angiographic series.

Early recognition of basilar artery disease at the stage of TIAs may allow treatment to prevent the full-blown deficits

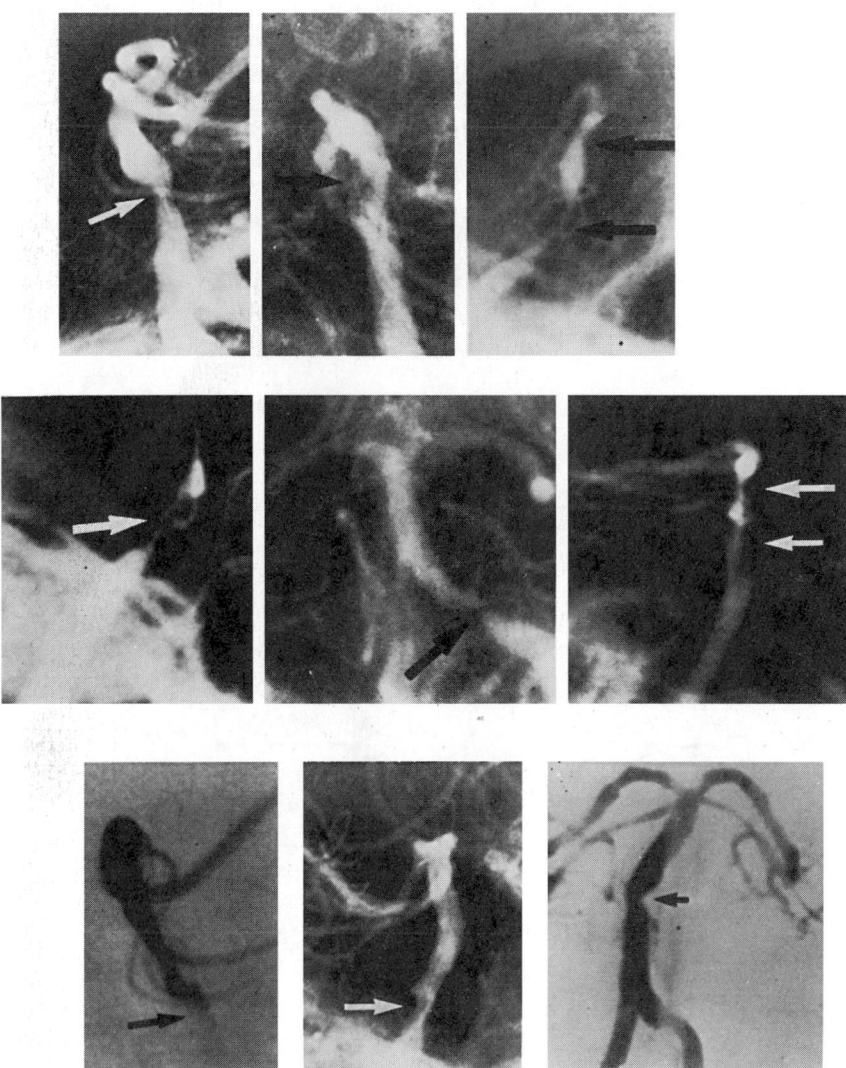

FIG. 41-11. Angiograms showing focal atherostenosis occurring in the proximal, middle, and distal segments of the basilar artery (*arrows*).

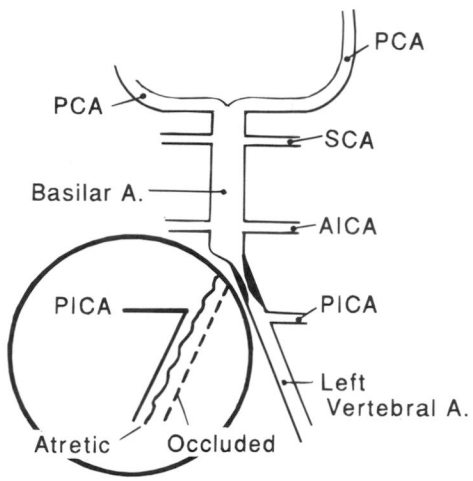

FIG. 41-12. The basilar artery may be supplied by a single vertebral artery as a result of congenital or acquired vascular anomalies, as shown in the circle. Stenosis of the dominant or solitary vertebral artery may result in severe compromise of basilar artery perfusion. PCA, posterior cerebral artery; SCA, superior cerebellar artery; AICA, anterior inferior cerebellar artery; PICA, posterior inferior cerebellar artery.

that may be associated with complete occlusion. In our own series of nine patients with basilar artery stenosis, TIAs were the common initial presentation, occurring in six patients. The TIAs preceded stroke except in two patients whose only clinical manifestation was TIAs. Seven patients had brainstem stroke; in four, it was preceded by TIAs. The TIA features included two or more of the following symptoms: dizziness, diplopia, perioral numbness, dysphagia, weakness, or loss of consciousness.

The complete clinical picture of basilar artery occlusion depends on the distribution and extent of brainstem infarction.

Several variations in VB anatomy may complicate the final result. For example, if only one VA supplies the basilar artery because the other is hypoplastic, occluded, or ends as a PICA, then occlusion of the dominant VA may act as a primary basilar occlusion (so-called basilarization of the VA; Fig. 41-12). Bilateral intracranial VA occlusions may produce an effect similar to isolated proximal or middle basilar artery occlusion.

TIAs frequently precede basilar artery occlusion in up to 50 percent of patients. The tempo of the onset of stroke is variable and depends on the mechanism. In embolism to the basilar apex, the onset is abrupt with a maximal deficit, as in other embolic syndromes. If atherothrombosis is the mechanism, a subacute and stepwise onset is typical, as in carotid occlusive disease. For example, a patient may have TIAs over days to weeks followed by a partial deficit involving slurred speech, gaze paresis, and hemiparesis. This may stabilize or even improve for hours, up to a few days, only to be followed by progression to include bilateral weakness, ophthalmoplegia, hemianopsia, and impaired consciousness. Often, the process may abate at any point in the course. The full picture usually evolves over 2 to 5 days.

The distribution of brainstem infarction is variable. The pons is the principal target area of maximal injury with proximal and middle basilar artery segmental occlusion (Fig. 41-13). The infarct is often bilateral but asymmetric and usually affects the basis pontis and medial tegmentum, producing bilateral weakness or paralysis. With extension to the tegmentum, cranial nerve palsies and pseudobulbar effects such as dysarthria and dysphagia may be present. If the infarct involves part of the midbrain tegmentum, an array of oculomotor abnormalities is common, including bilaterally ptosis and partial or complete ophthalmoplegia. When the infarct is extensive and involves the pontine base and tegmentum bilaterally, limb weakness, bulbar paralysis, and extraocular palsies occur. The patient may

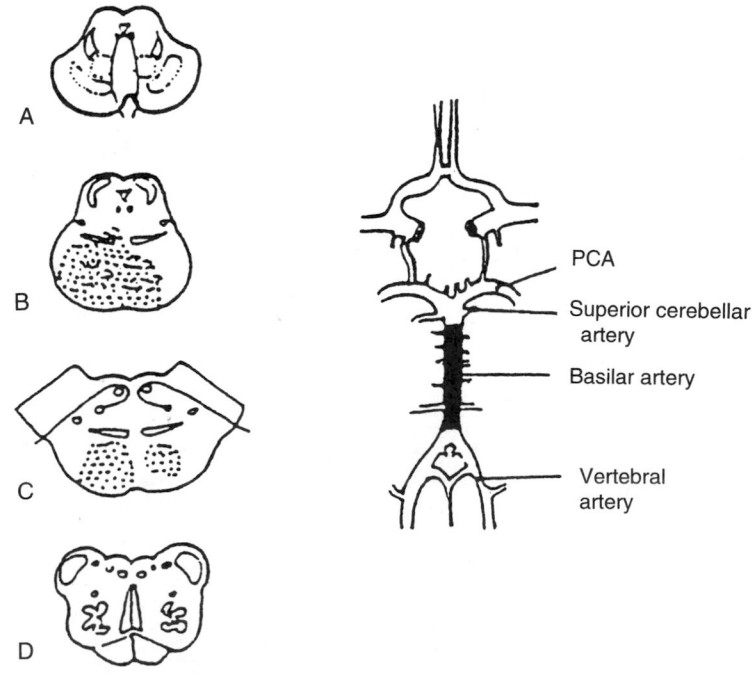

FIG. 41-13. Bilateral infarction of the pons (shaded areas) caused by basilar artery occlusion. **(A)** midbrain; **(B)** upper pons; **(C)** lower pons; **(D)** medulla.

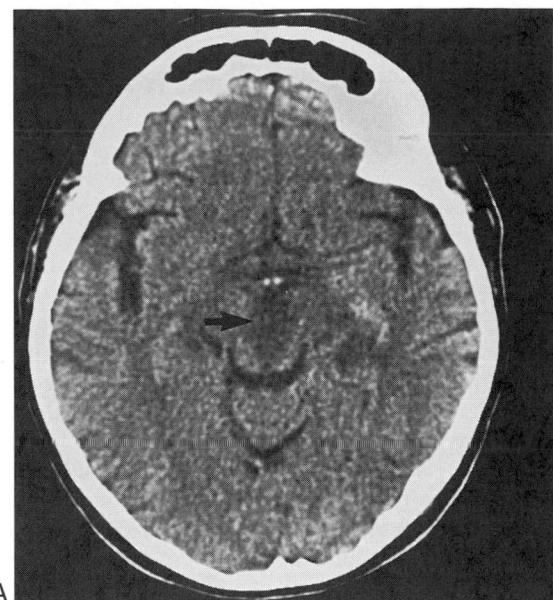 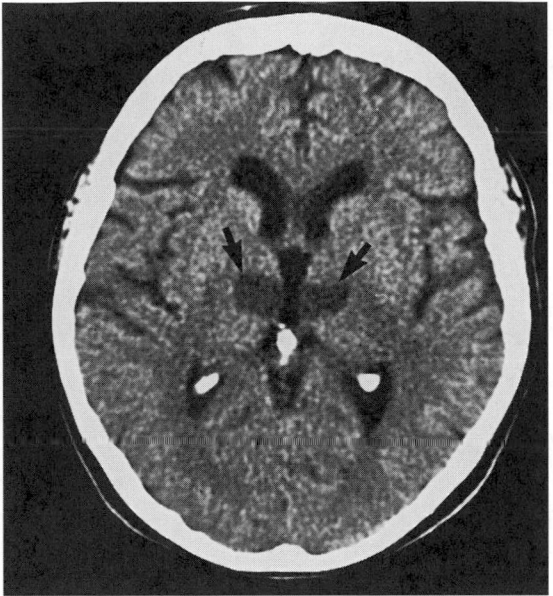

FIG. 41-14. Computed tomographic scans showing low-density areas of infarction in the midbrain and both medial thalami in a patient with an embolic stroke resulting in a "top of the basilar syndrome" (*arrows*).

be alert but unable to move except for eye blinking. This alert but immobile state is called the "locked-in syndrome."

Top of the Basilar Syndrome

When embolism blocks the rostral basilar artery, the resulting infarct involves penetrating branches from the basilar apex, posterior communicating artery, and PCA and may include the SCA territory in the infarct as well. The infarct is usually bilateral but asymmetric, involving midbrain, thalamus, medial temporal lobe, as well as the occipital territory of the cortical branches of the PCA (Fig. 41-14). Behavioral and visual and oculomotor disturbances predominant, with weakness absent or minor. Abnormalities in alertness with excessive sleep-like behavior are common from bilateral medial thalamic involvement. If awake, the patient may be abulic, lacking in spontaneity. Depending on the extent of midbrain infarction, paralysis of voluntary vertical and downgaze may be impaired, with relative sparing of vertical movements with reflex maneuvers. Conversion nystagmus, bilateral ptosis, and lid retraction also occur if the medial midbrain tegmentum is affected. If the occlusive process extends into one or both PCAs, then unilateral or bilateral hemianopic defects that produce cortical blindness occur. Cortical visual disturbances include Balint syndrome (absence of voluntary eye movements, optic ataxia in coordinating visual-motor function, and asimultagnosia). Sometimes patients are poorly aware of their blindness or actively refute its existence (Anton syndrome), attempting to perform as a normally sighted person with disastrous consequences.

Basilar Artery Penetrator Territory

Small paramedian and short circumferential arteries arise from the posterior wall of the basilar artery and supply the paramedian and lateral pontine regions. A variety of clinical signs may occur, depending on the extent and exact location of the infarct. Pure motor hemiparesis with dysarthria and ataxia are the most common features associated with occlusive disease of these

small vessels. Despite the common occurrence of these small pontine infarcts, the spectrum of clinical features has not been fully defined to date. Although the basis pontis is a favorite site for these infarcts, the pontine tegmentum is also often involved, producing various cranial nerve dysfunction, especially involving eye movements. Double vision, unilateral or bilateral internuclear ophthalmoplegia, paresthesias, and other cranial nerve abnormalities occur.

POSTERIOR CEREBRAL ARTERY

Anatomy

The PCAs arise at the pontomesencephalic junction from the termination of the basilar artery in 70 percent of patients; of the remainder, one or sometimes both PCAs may originate from the ICA from a large posterior communicating artery. The PCAs course around the cerebral peduncles and give off penetrating branches to the midbrain and thalamus. The branches to the thalamus include the thalmoperferants, thalmogeniculates, and posterior choroidal arteries. After circling the peduncle in the ambient cistern, the artery divides into its cortical-supplying branches; these include the anterior and posterior temporal branches, which supply the medial and lateral surfaces of the temporal lobe, respectively; the parietal-occipital artery, which supplies the deep white matter of the occipital lobe; and the medial placed calcarine artery, which supplies the primary visual cortex (Fig. 41-15).

Pathogenesis of Posterior Cerebral Artery Stroke

Occlusion of the cortical branches of the PCA is usually caused by embolism, either cardiac in origin or from a more proximal VB source. Intrinsic atheromatous disease of the PCA stem, similar to its MCA stem counterpart, is not as common as embolism. The rarity of PCA stem stenosis was documented in our identification of only six symptomatic patients in a 7-year review of angiographic records at New England Medical Center (Fig. 41-16). The stenosis occurs at the more proximal (perime-

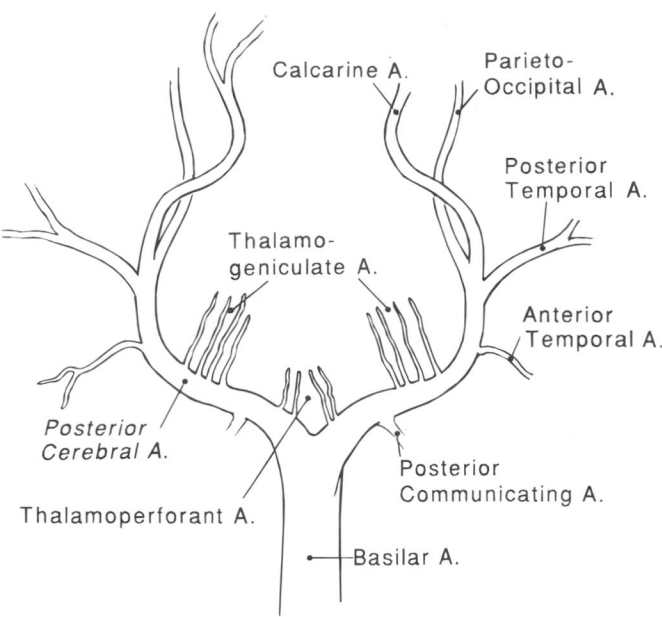

FIG. 41-15.   Anatomy of the posterior cerebral artery. Small penetrating branches arise from the proximal segments to supply the thalamus and deep structures, and the cortical branches arise more distally.

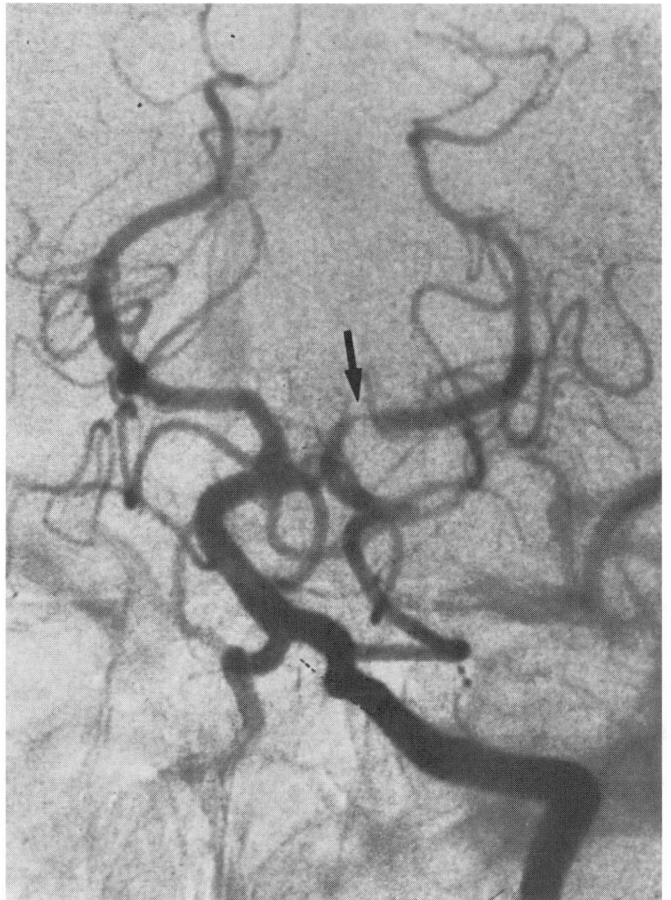

FIG. 41-16.   Angiogram showing a stenosis of the proximal stem of the left posterior cerebral artery (*arrow*).

sencephalic) segment of the artery as it courses around the midbrain.

Clinical

TIAs may be associated with PCA disease if the primary lesion is atherostenosis. In our series of PCA stenosis, transient hemianoptic visual disturbances and paresthetic sensory symptoms were common and contrasted with MCA stem stenosis in which motor and speech TIAs predominate.

The most common and consistent feature of PCA territory infarction is a hemianopsia. It is usually congruous, spares macular (central) vision, and reflects unilateral infarction of the calcarine visual cortex. The visual defect may be limited to a superior quadrantanopsia if the fusiform and lingual gyri below the calcarine fissure are the principal target of infarction or an inferior quandrantanopsia if the upper bank (cuneus) of the calcarine cortex is primarily affected. Superior quadrantanopsia is more common than inferior visual field defects. Hemianopsia may be the only clinical sign. Approximately three-fourths of patients are aware of their hemivisual field defect but may not recognize that it involves both eyes. They quickly adjust by turning their head or adjusting visual materials to compensate for their awareness of unilateral visual impairment. This clear awareness by the patient helps distinguish visual fields loss in the PCA territory from loss in the MCA territory in which infarction of the parietal lobe leaves the patient invariably unaware.

Sensory abnormalities are also part of PCA territory infarction, and together with hemianopsia stamp the localization as PCA territory. Sensory symptoms result from ventral posterolateral thalamic infarction supplied by the small branches of the thalamogeniculate pedicle. The patient complains of a dysesthetic feeling involving all or part of the contralateral face, limbs, and body, described as a prickly, cold, warm, or tingling sensation. Usually, the complaints exceed any abnormalities found on examination, which tends to be negative. This pure sensory stroke, when it occurs in isolation, reflects a small infarct in the distribution of the thalamic penetrating branches. If the infarct is larger, as a result of multiple branch occlusions, then objective findings on examination are usually present.

Other interesting cognitive abnormalities may occur with large-territory PCA infarcts. If the medial temporal lobe in the dominant hemisphere is affected, a severe but temporary amnestic syndrome may occur. Rarely does memory impairment last longer than a few months, if that long. Recent and immediate memory functions are most affected, and patients may attempt to ''fill-in'' for their absent memories with fabrications (confabulation). With large infarcts involving the visual cortex and surrounding deep visual association territory, several classic syndromes may result:

1. *Alexia without agraphia.* In this striking syndrome, patients are able to write correctly and legibly but cannot read their own production or other lexical material. Sometimes, individual words may be read, but sentence material is impaired. Visual color naming may be abnormal in the presence of intact color matching and the ability to recite color names for familiar objects.
2. *Amnestic dysnomia.* Patients are unable to name common objects and have difficulty producing proper names in spontaneous speech but can describe the function and nature of objects.
3. *Visual agnosia.* Patients are unable to name objects at sight

but may copy objects correctly and name them when presented by other input modalities such as touch, sound, or description. Bilateral lesions in the parietal-occipital territory produce even more spectacular behavior abnormalities.

4. *Prosopagnosia.* When lesions involve the temporal occipital areas (lower banks of the calcarine fissure) bilaterally, patients may be unable to recognize and name familiar faces.

5. *Balint syndrome.* In bilateral parietal-occipital lesions, patients may be unable to move their eyes voluntarily, although reflex eye movements are normal (psychic paralysis of gaze); to coordinate visual-motor performance, so it appears the patient is ataxic in reaching for objects (optic ataxia); and to assess a picture in its totality instead focusing on detailed aspects without ''seeing'' the meaning of the picture (asimultagnosia).

6. *Anton syndrome.* Cortical blindness from bilateral occipital lesions leaves patients with poor awareness or active denial of their blindness. In this extraordinary syndrome, patients deny their blindness and attempt to perform as a sighted person, walking into objects, and then making lame excuses for their clumsiness.

Usually, motor function is preserved in PCA territory infarcts except for the uncommon occurrence of midbrain peduncular lesions that may produce a hemiparesis. The predominance of visual and sensory symptoms, including higher cortical behavioral abnormalities, is the hallmark of PCA territory infarction. This helps distinguish PCA territory infarcts from those in the MCA territory in which motor and speech disturbances predominate.

PENETRATOR ARTERIAL DISEASE—LACUNAR AND BRANCH ARTERY INFARCTS

Small infarcts in the deep parts of the brain have been called lacunes, describing the small residual fluid-filled cavity of infarcted tissue. They range in size from 2 to 3 mm up to 15 mm and result from occlusion of a *single,* small penetrating artery along its course after arising from the larger parent intracranial vessels, the MCA, anterior choroidal artery, ACA, PCA, posterior communicate artery, VA, basilar artery, and cerebellar arteries. Branch artery infarcts differ from lacunes in that they are larger and tend to represent infarction in the distribution of more than one penetrator. There are three principal vascular processes associated with lacunes and branch artery disease: (1) lipohyalinosis, a vasculopathy associated with hypertension that leads to occlusion of tiny arteries 40 to 200 μm in diameter along their course some distance from the origin; (2) atherosclerosis; and (3) embolism. The latter two processes involve larger

arteries, 200 to 800 μm in diameter. Atherosclerosis operates in two ways to affect small penetrating arteries. A mural plaque, with or without superimposed thrombus, may develop in the parent large artery lumen and block the orifice of one or more branch penetrators, or a tiny bead of atheroma may develop just inside the orifice of the branch and compromise blood flow (Fig. 41-17). Embolic occlusion of the branch is a presumptive mechanism based on the finding of a normal branch supplying an area of infarct after presumed spontaneous lysis of an embolic plug has occurred.

Branch orifice disease usually produces larger infarcts than lacunes and is usually associated with symptoms. The smallest lacunae resulting from occlusion of tiny penetrators are often asymptomatic and detected only with neuroimaging techniques. This probably accounts for the unexpected discovery of one or more small lacunes on imaging studies performed for reasons other than vascular symptoms. Hypertension plays a role in both the development of lipohyalinosis and atheroma, but diabetes is a less certain risk factor for lipohyalinosis, although it is associated with large artery atherosclerosis. The distinction between small lacunes and branch artery infarcts is important because the mechanism(s), diagnostic evaluation, and treatment may differ.

Both types of small, deep infarcts may develop in one of three characteristic ways: quickly over a few hours; subacute evolution over 2 to 3 days, up to 6 days; or preceded by TIAs that may be multiple and hectic in the 24-hour period before stroke.

PENETRATING ARTERY TERRITORIES

Middle Cerebral Artery

The most common presentation of a symptomatic lacune in the LSA territory of the MCA is pure motor hemiparesis. The clinical syndrome results from a strategically placed small infarct in the posterior limb of the internal capsule from occlusion of a penetrating LSA. Originally, it was thought that pure motor hemiparesis equally involved the face, arm, and leg on the opposite side, but, as further cases were documented, unequal permutations affecting the face, arm, and leg were found to occur. Vision, speech, language, behavior, and sensation are spared, reinforcing the apparently redundant designation as pure motor hemiparesis. Fisher (1991) described other concomitants of pure motor hemiparesis under the general classification of pure motor hemiparesis *plus,* but these additional features are uncommon compared to the usual pure motor stroke and often result from extension of the infarct to adjacent structures in the internal capsule or pons. Pure motor hemiparesis has also been

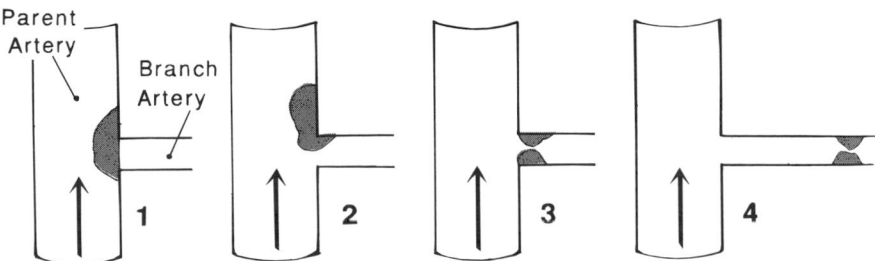

FIG. 41-17. Pathogenesis of lacunar and branch artery infarcts. (*1*) Mural plaque in the parent artery occluding the branch orifice. (*2*) Mural plaque with partial obstruction of the branch orifice. (*3*) Microatheroma caused by atherosclerosis. (*4*) Lipohyalinosis resulting from hypertension.

reported in infarcts in the corona radiata, pons, and even the medullary pyramid. Larger striatocapsular infarcts may more accurately reflect branch occlusive disease, affecting several LSA penetrators and producing an infarct that involves part of the internal capsule, head of the caudate, and putamen. Technically, this is not a lacunar infarction since it involves more than one penetrating vessel and likely reflects embolism or primary atherosclerosis of the MCA stem occluding several LSA branches, despite the apparent absence of significant cortical MCA territory infarction.

Ataxic hemiparesis is another common lacunar syndrome that occurs in the LSA territory as well as in the pons. The infarct lies in the anterior limb of the internal capsule or adjacent corona radiata. The clinical features include the unusual combination of cerebellar and pyramidal dysfunction on the same side, with the leg and ankle disproportionately weak and little or no weakness of face and upper extremity. Attempts to distinguish the location of the infarct on clinical grounds alone are generally unsuccessful, although dysarthria may be more prominent with pontine lacunes.

Dysarthria, clumsy hand syndrome, describes the principal clinical deficits in this uncommon lacune. The syndrome may involve additional features of facial weakness, mild degrees of hand or even leg weakness, and dysphagia. The most consistent localization has the been the anterior limb or genu of the internal capsule; a few reports have identified lesions in the basis pontis.

Anterior Cerebral Artery

The recurrent artery(ies) of Heubner arise as a single or multiple branches from the proximal ACA and supply part of the head of the caudate nucleus, anterior limb of the internal capsule, and frontal lobe. Occlusion of Heubner's artery may produce an infarct in the caudate and anterior limb of the internal capsule. The clinical syndrome from the caudate portion of the infarct includes dysarthria and behavioral-cognitive abnormalities such as abulia, neglect, and aphasia. Unilateral weakness may result from the capsular infarct.

Posterior Communicating and Posterior Cerebral Artery

Thalamoperferating branches arise from the posterior communicating artery and proximal PCA to supply the anteriomedial thalamus and ventral posterolateral thalamic nuclei, respectively. The polar artery (also called the tuberothalamic artery) arises from the posterior communicating artery and supplies the anteriomedial and anterolateral thalamic nuclei in the midline. Infarction causes abulia and transient cognitive abnormalities such as aphasia and visual neglect. The thalamic-subthalamic artery arises from the proximal PCA. One common anatomic variation involves a single unilateral artery branching to supply both thalamic areas, which may produce a butterfly-shaped paramedian thalamic infarct. The clinical syndromes include an amnestic disorder, sleepiness, and abnormalities of upward gaze. With bilateral infarcts, disturbances in alertness with hypersomnolence may result. The thalamogeniculate arteries arise from the ambient segment of the PCA and supply the ventral posterolateral thalamic nuclei. They are the counterpart of the LSA arteries arising from the MCA stem (Fig. 41-18). Infarction in this area produces the classic pure sensory stroke syndrome. The patient's sensory complaints exceed objective findings, which in small infarcts are absent. Patients describe tingling, numbness, warmth, cold, tightness, a swollen feeling, and hypersensitivity. The distribution of sensory symptoms usually involve parts of face, trunk, and one or both limbs. In

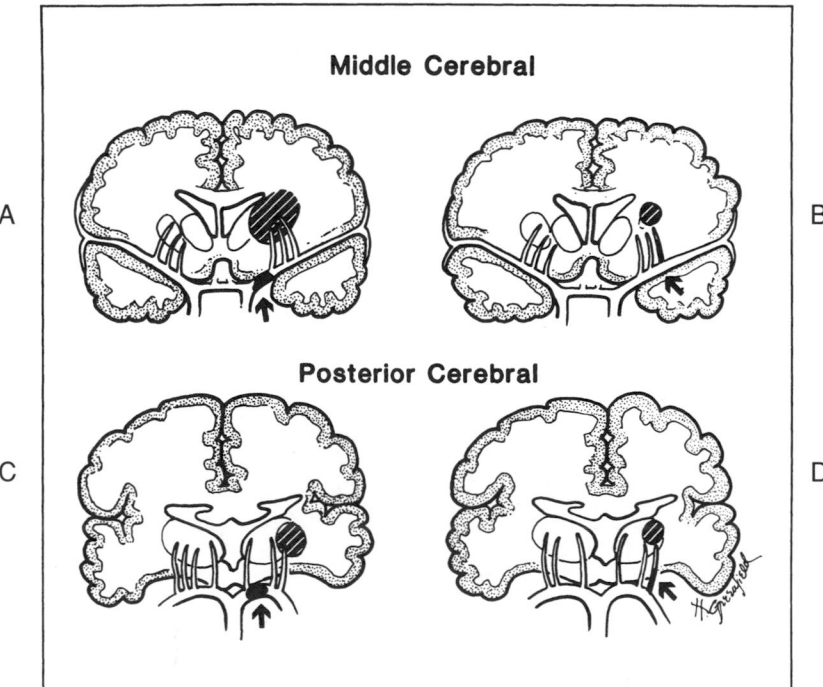

FIG. 41-18. Mechanisms of deep infarction. **(A)** Large striatocapsular infarction caused by middle cerebral artery stem occlusion (arrow). **(B)** Small deep capsular infarction resulting from occlusion of a lenticulostriate artery from lipohyalinosis. **(C)** Large lateral thalamic infarction caused by embolic occlusion of the parent posterior cerebral artery. **(D)** Small lateral thalamic infarction resulting from occlusion of a small thalamogeniculate artery.

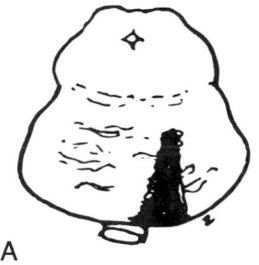 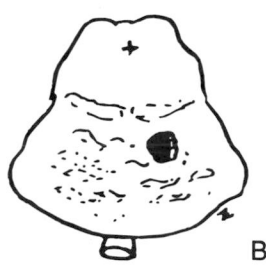

A   B

FIG. 41-19. (A) Wedge-shaped pontine infarct extending to basal surface caused by an atherosclerotic branch occlusion. (B) Small, deep lacunar infarct in pons resulting from lipohyalinosis.

the extreme example, a complete hemisensory deficit may split the midline from face to trunk, including the genitalia. Usually, the sensory symptoms involve tactile, temperature, and pain sensitivity, less often vibratory and joint position sense. Sensory complaints may wax and wane over many months, serving as a frustrating and fearful annoyance to the patient. Rarely, painful hyperpathic sensory syndrome may follow the acute stroke and persist (Dejerine-Roussy syndrome).

Basilar Artery Penetrators

A spectrum of clinical brainstem syndromes may result from occlusion of basilar artery paramedian and short circumferential branches. The pons is the principal focus of these lacunes and larger branch territory infarcts. CT or MRI can help distinguish between a lacune and branch artery disease based on the topography of the infarct. Lacunes occur in the basis pontis and tegmentum, are irregular in shape, and generally are smaller than branch infarcts, which abut the basal surface (Fig. 41-19).

Pure motor hemiparesis is the most frequent clinical syndrome plus additional abnormalities the spectrum of which continues to evolve with clinical-imaging case correlations. Other accompaniments to pontine pure motor hemiparesis include dysarthria, sixth nerve palsy, internuclear ophthalmoplegia, one-and-a-half syndrome, and conjugate gaze paresis. The clinical features of the larger branch territory infarcts are yet to be defined. Other pontine lacunar syndromes related to penetrator disease have been mentioned and include ataxic hemiparesis and dysarthria-clumsy hand.

SUGGESTED READINGS

Amarenco P: The spectrum of cerebellar infarctions. Neurology 41:973, 1991

Brust JCM: Anterior cerebral artery disease. p. 337. In Barnett HJM, Stein BM, Mohr JP, Yatsu FM (eds): Stroke: Pathophysiology, Diagnosis, and Management. 2nd Ed. Churchill Livingstone, New York, 1992

Caplan LR: Intracranial branch atheromatous disease: a neglected, understudied, and underused concept. Neurology 39:1246, 1989

Caplan LR, Pessin MS, Mohr JP: Vertebrobasilar occlusive disease. p. 443. In Barnett HJM, Stein BM, Mohr JP, Yatsu FM (eds): Stroke: Pathophysiology, Diagnosis, and Management. 2nd Ed. Churchill Livingstone, New York, 1992

Fisher CM: Occlusion of the internal carotid artery. Arch Neurol Psychiatry 69:346, 1951

Fisher CM: Occlusion of the carotid arteries: further experiences. Arch Neurol Psychiatry 72:187, 1954

Fisher CM: Observations of the fundus oculi in transient monocular blindness. Neurology 9:333, 1959

Fisher CM: Concerning recurrent transient cerebral ischemic attacks. Can Med Assoc J 86:1091, 1962

Fisher CM: Lacunar infarcts—a review. Cerebrovasc Dis 1:311, 1991

Helgason C, Caplan LR, Goodwin J, Hedges T: Anterior choroidal artery-territory infarction. Arch Neurol 43:681, 1986

Kase CS, Norrving B, Levine SR et al: Cerebellar infarction. Clinical and anatomic observations in 66 cases. Stroke 24:76, 1993

Mohr JP, Gautier JC, Hier DB: Middle cerebral artery disease. p. 361. In Barnett HJM, Stein BM, Mohr JP, Yatsu FM (eds): Stroke: Pathophysiology, Diagnosis, and Management. 2nd Ed. Churchill Livingstone, New York, 1992

Mohr JP, Gautier JC, Pessin MS: Internal carotid artery disease. p. 285. In Barnett HJM, Stein BM, Mohr JP, Yatsu FM (eds): Stroke: Pathophysiology, Diagnosis, and Management. 2nd Ed. Churchill Livingstone, New York, 1992

Mohr JP, Pessin MS: Posterior cerebral artery disease. p. 419. In Barnett HJM, Stein BM, Mohr JP, Yatsu FM (eds): Stroke: Pathophysiology, Diagnosis, and Management. 2nd Ed. Churchill Livingstone, New York, 1992

North American Symptomatic Carotid Endarterectomy Trial Collaborators: Beneficial effect of carotid endarterectomy in symptomatic patients with high-grade carotid stenosis. N Engl J Med 325:445, 1991

Pessin MS, Duncan GW, Mohr JP, Poskanzer DC: Clinical and angiographic features of carotid transient ischemic attacks. N Engl J Med 296:358, 1977

Pessin MS, Hinton RC, Davis KR et al: Mechanisms of acute carotid stroke. Ann Neurol 6:245, 1979

42. DIFFERENTIAL DIAGNOSIS OF THE MAJOR STROKE SUBTYPES

LOUIS R. CAPLAN

Effective management of patients with cerebrovascular disease depends on accurate diagnosis. An outpatient ambulatory setting offers the physician advantages and disadvantages over an inpatient encounter in caring for patients with cerebrovascular disease, and different issues may sometimes arise. The office usually allows more privacy, room, time, and relative freedom from distractions. The patient and any accompanying friends or family can be interviewed behind closed doors and at more leisure than in the usual hospital room. Somehow, seeing the patient and significant others in their usual attire adds an insight into their character that is not gotten from seeing the patient in hospital uniform.

The hospital environment is more anxiety producing; the decision to place the patient in the hospital itself implies grave illness. Hospital routines and the many personnel are hard to adapt to, and patients lose their autonomy. The physician can, however, return to see the hospitalized patient as often as feasible and has several opportunities to ask questions of the patient, and examine, instruct, and interact with the patient. In the outpatient setting, the doctor has a finite time to arrive at a diagnosis and plan. A revisit may be needed to get another shot at the diagnosis and management plan. In the outpatient setting, the decision of whether to hospitalize a patient with cerebrovascular disease is often central; in hospitalized patients, that decision has already been made.

In ambulatory patients, the key questions are as follows. What is the diagnosis (what and where are the vascular and brain lesions)? What tests should be ordered, and how soon? What treatment should be prescribed? What instructions and explanations should be given to the patient? These decisions must be made quickly, directly after the outpatient encounter.

This section concentrates on the first two issues—making the diagnosis and planning the evaluation of a patient suspected of having cerebrovascular disease.

GENERAL STRATEGIES, RULES, AND AIMS OF DIAGNOSIS

A few general strategies help the physician arrive at an accurate stroke diagnosis. In order to manage a stroke patient effectively, the physician would like optimally to know the following.

1. The stroke mechanism, ischemic or hemorrhagic and their subtypes. Figure 42-1 shows a diagnostic tree that lists the major differential diagnostic considerations.
2. The nature, location, and severity of the causative cerebrovascular lesions.
3. The pathophysiology of the vascular lesion that caused the brain injury.
4. The nature and function of the key cellular and serologic blood components and any disorder of coagulation.
5. The state of the brain, whether normal, infarcted, or injured but recoverable.

Modern diagnostic methods can yield the bulk of this information. In most circumstances, the testing can be performed safely and quickly on an ambulatory basis, provided that the pace and severity of the symptoms and signs permit.

Rule 1. The diagnostic encounter should be hypothesis based. The physician aims to know *what* disease process is occurring and *where* the lesion is, both in the *nervous system* and in the *cardiovascular bed.* Initially, it is important to let the patient tell the story uninterrupted. This offers great insight into patients, intelligence, language, and organizing skills as well as their concerns. As they tell their story, aided by any accompanying family or significant others, the physician should begin to generate what and where hypotheses and to test them actively as the history is taken. Tables 42-1 and 42-2 contain lists of the types of information used to arrive at what and where diagnoses.

The patient's sex, age, and past illnesses are known and can give the first clues. For example, suppose the patient is an elderly hypertensive man who developed a slight left hemiplegia 4 days ago. Hypertension raises the possibility of intracerebral hemorrhage (ICH). His age also favors some types of hemorrhage (e.g., amyloid angiopathy or minor trauma). Alternatively, the hypertension might have caused penetrating artery disease (the cause of lacunar infarcts) on accelerated the development of large artery extracranial and intracranial atherosclerosis. Already there are three hypotheses about the stroke type. Then, as the course of development of the deficit is pursued, the physician mentally decides whether the patient's and family's account of the early symptoms and their subsequent course favors one of these hypotheses or suggests a different possibil-

ity. This process of generating and testing what hypotheses should continue throughout the entire patient encounter.

At the same time, the physician also pursues the thinking about where diagnosis, the localization of the lesion in the nervous system and the arteries that supply these regions. The patient's description of what is or was wrong should generate anatomic hypotheses. Full awareness of a left hemiparesis by the patient makes a subcortical or brainstem locus more likely than a frontal or parietal lobe cortical lesion. If a homonymous visual field defect is present, the lesion must be supratentorial and posteriorly located in the contralateral cerebral hemisphere. An arm monoparesis or a great discrepancy in the degree of weakness in the patient's face, arm, hand, and leg suggests a more cortical, paracentral localization. As the history taking proceeds, physicians should construct a picture in their mind's eye of the location of the lesion.

Rule 2. The diagnoses should be attacked vigorously and sequentially during each part of the encounter. Much hinges on the completeness and accuracy of the diagnoses. Go after the diagnosis tenaciously, first during the history, then during the general and neurologic examinations, and then during each step of the laboratory and imaging evaluations.

Rule 3. The diagnoses should be considered using probabilities. The likelihood of a given diagnosis affects the evaluation. After the history, it is useful to list possible what and where diagnoses with their likely probabilities. Table 42-3 is an example of such a list in a patient with a left hemiparesis.

The general and neurologic examinations should be planned ahead of time. What features could be found during the examination that would clarify the stroke mechanism and the pathologic anatomy? For example, in a patient with left hemiparesis, visual field testing, tests for neglect, drawing, and copying, somatosensory testing, and careful cranial nerve examination should allow more precise localization. Clearly, the neck should be auscultated with a stethoscope for carotid and vertebral artery bruits, and a careful cardiac and peripheral vascular examination is warranted. Are there any signs of systemic bleeding or head injury? At times, the examination uncovers findings completely unsuspected from the history. For example, the pa-

TABLE 42-1. Data Used for the *"What"* Diagnosis

Ecology
  Demography and medical conditions known in the past and/or recognized now (age, race, sex, hypertension, angina pectoris, diabetes, hypercholesterolemia, rheumatic heart disease, etc.)
Past cerebrovascular events
  Transient ischemic attacks and past strokes: distribution, nature, and cause
Activity at onset of cerebrovascular event
Course
  Maximal at outset, fluctuating from normal to abnormal, stepwise, gradually progressive, or rapid improvement
Associated symptoms
  Headache, vomiting, loss of consciousness, or seizures
Neuroimaging
  Computed tomography or magnetic resonance imaging

TABLE 42-2. Data Used for *"Where"* Diagnosis

Neurologic symptoms described by patient
Neurologic signs found on neurologic examination
Vascular examination
Brain neuroimaging
  CT and MRI
Vascular diagnostic tests
  Ultrasound (extracranial and intracranial), MRA, spiral CT, standard angiography

Abbreviations: CT, computed tomography; MRI, magnetic resonance imaging; MRA, magnetic resonance angiography.

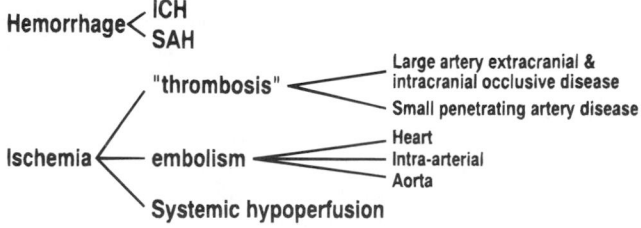

FIG. 42-1. Differential diagnostic considerations in major stroke. ICH, internal cerebral hemorrhage; SAH, subarachnoid hemorrhage.

TABLE 42-3. Weighting of Risk Factors

	Thrombosis	Lacunae	Embolism	Intercerebral Hemorrhage	Subarachnoid Hemorrhage
Hypertension	+ +	+ + +		+ +	+
Severe hypertension	+ + +	+	+ +	+ + + +	+ +
Coronary artery disease	+ + +		+ +		
Claudication	+ + +		+		
Atrial fibrillation			+ + + +		
Sick sinus syndrome			+ +		
Valvular heart disease			+ + +		
Diabetes	+ + +	+	+		
Bleeding diathesis				+ + + +	+
Hyperlipidemia	+ + +	+	+		
Cancer			+ +	+	+
Old age	+ + +	+ +		+	−
Black or Japanese origin	+	+		+ +	

tient with left hemiparesis might have additional right-sided weakness and a bilateral Babinski sign or nystagmus suggesting a brainstem (pontine) localization or an enlarged nodular liver that may indicate metastatic disease. As the examination proceeds, the physician should continue to weigh hypotheses and their probabilities.

Now, the laboratory and imaging evaluation should be planned to test the existing hypotheses. Ordinarily a neuroimaging test, either computed tomography (CT) or magnetic resonance imaging (MRI), is the first test in a patient who has had a stroke or has neurologic signs. The presence of a hemorrhage dictates a battery of tests that are different than if the process were ischemic. Most patients require some blood testing, including hemoglobin, hematocrit, white blood count, platelet count, prothrombin time, and activated partial thromboplastin time (aPTT). Vascular diagnostic tests and cardiac testing usually are planned after the results of imaging and blood tests are known.

DEMOGRAPHICS AND PAST ILLNESSES

Age, sex, race, family history, and the patient's medical history strongly affect the probability of the various stroke mechanisms. Some illnesses heavily favor only one mechanism (e.g., rheumatic mitral stenosis with atrial fibrillation strongly suggests cardiac origin embolism). Others, such as hypertension, can predispose to a number of possibilities. Factors such as race and sex affect the likelihood of particular vascular occlusive lesions. In general, white men have more extracranial occlusive disease of the internal carotid (ICA) and vertebral artery origins in the neck; women, blacks, and Asians have more intracranial large artery occlusive disease. Blacks and Asians have a higher frequency of ICH. Table 42-3 estimates the relative weights attributable to the various risk factors.

TABLE 42-4. Modifiable Stroke Risk Factors

Smoking
Hypertension
Diabetes
Polycythemia
Thrombocytosis
Obesity
Physical inactivity
Excess alcohol use
Use of high-dose estrogen oral contraceptives
Use of amphetamines, cocaine, and other sympathomimetic drugs

Risk factors also help the physician assess the chances of future vascular disease—stroke, coronary artery disease, and peripheral vascular occlusive disease. These risk factors should be identified and discussed with the patient and family before they leave the office. Table 42-4 lists the key modifiable risk factors.

PAST AND RECENT CEREBROVASCULAR EVENTS

A history of a stroke or transient ischemic attack (TIA) can yield important clues to the present cerebrovascular event. As arteries gradually occlude, there are often brief periods of intermittent reduced distal blood flow and embolization of white platelet-fibrin aggregates, red fibrin-dependent clots, and plaque material into the intracranial branches supplied by that artery. In the Harvard stroke registry, about 50 percent of patients with large artery occlusive lesions and one-fourth of patients with penetrating artery disease had preceding TIAs in the same vascular territory as their stroke. In large artery lesions (e.g., the ICA in the neck), the attacks are spread over a long interval and are often heterogeneous, with, for example, transient monocular blindness in one attack, hand and face numbness in a second attack, and aphasia with hand weakness in a third spell. In penetrating artery disease, attacks usually, but not always, occur during a shorter time span and closer to the time of the stroke. Attacks are often similar in their features and reflect the subcortical blood supply (e.g., tingling on the left side of the body in each attack is most often due to disease of a thalamogeniculate branch artery supplying the lateral thalamus).

Patients whose present stroke is a small deep infarction caused by penetrating artery or branch atheromatous disease have often had past lacunar strokes in different regions. Similarly, patients with emboli originating from the heart have often also had prior embolic strokes or unrecognized brain infarcts in other vascular territories. These past lacunae and embolic brain infarcts may be detectable clinically but sometimes are evident only on CT and MRI images.

The nature of the prior attacks or recent TIAs as revealed by history, examination, or imaging provides a clue to the nature of the present event. Unfortunately, most individuals are naive about the workings of their bodies, especially their nervous systems. A patient may attribute temporary hand numbness and weakness to a local lesion in the limb and may not think of reporting it. Similarly, most patients would be unlikely to report having white sparkles in the left visual field 10 days ago. Thinking it a symptom for the eye doctor. To elicit the history of prior TIAs or strokes, the physician must doggedly and tenaciously ask and reask about specific functions. Did you ever have your foot or leg go temporarily limp. . . . your vision fade temporarily in one eye. . . . your speech fail you or come out garbled, slurred, or wrong . . . and so forth? Family members may remember such spells that the patient did not recognize or recall. The patient may not recall symptoms the first time the questions are asked but may recall the events later. For example, a patient with transient monocular blindness when questioned about loss of vision on at least three occasions always gave a negative response. The day after he said no for the third time, he spontaneously said, "Doc, now I remember. About a week ago I was in line at the food store, and my left eye went gray for about a minute. The clerk said that I must have gotten a speck of dirt in the eye. Because it went away, I didn't make much of it."

COURSE OF DEVELOPMENT OF A STROKE

Each stroke subtype has its usual common signature of development. Emboli most often (more than 80 percent) occur suddenly and create deficits that are maximal immediately. Patients suddenly slump in their chair with a hemiplegia. In contrast, ICHs grow gradually over minutes, and the signs gradually increase. If the hematoma becomes large, then headache, vomiting, and decreased consciousness ensue, after the initial signs of focal brain dysfunction. Subarachnoid hemorrhages (SAH) also begin suddenly, but the blood released into the cerebrospinal fluid under arterial pressure causes severe headache, vomiting, and transient interuption in posture or activities. Unlike ICH, focal symptoms of brain dysfunction are not usually present at outset. In patients with large artery occlusive disease, fluctuations in the symptoms and signs are characteristic, with stepwise increases in deficits, temporary improvements or return to normal function, and the gradual but erratic progression of symptoms and signs during a few days. These fluctuations and changes are presumed to be due to changes in the systemic circulation affecting collateral blood flow and propagation and embolization of thrombi distally into downstream branches.

Few patients can give an accurate account of the development of symptoms. Those with right hemisphere frontal and parietal lobe strokes may not recognize any deficit. Again, family and friends can supply useful data. Have the patient *walk through* the events before and after the stroke began. A patient reported that she gradually developed a left-sided paralysis that morning. When she described the events in more detail she said, "At the breakfast table, my left hand and arm went weak and clumsy, and I dropped the coffee cup from my hand. I went upstairs to my bedroom, and I walked OK on the stairs. I rested for a half hour, and then when I came downstairs my hand was all right. I cleaned the room without trouble. An hour later, my hand and arm went weak again. This time I stumbled on the steps and had to limp with my left leg. When I called my daughter, my words were slurred. I lay down again, but this time, when I tried to get up, I couldn't use my left side at all." This fluctuating pattern of the development of the deficit are characteristic of a so-called thrombotic stroke in which the deficit is due to occlusion of a feeding artery with distal hypoperfusion. In her case, the symptoms fit the pattern of a pure motor hemiparesis most likely caused by penetrating artery or branch atheromatous disease.

ACTIVITY AT ONSET OF THE STROKE OR TRANSIENT ISCHEMIC ATTACK

Most strokes and TIAs occur during activities of daily living. Emboli can be precipitated by a cough, sneeze, suddenly rising from bed during the night to go to the bathroom, or sexual intercourse (especially paradoxic emboli). SAH and ICH can be precipitated by intercourse or emotional stress. In patients with large artery occlusive disease, standing or rising after bending can precipitate brief ischemic attacks. Vigorous turning or stretching of the neck can cause extracranial arterial dissections. Always inquire what the patient was doing before and during the attack. Was there any unusual or vigorous physical activity or emotional duress in the minutes, hours, or days before the attack?

ACCOMPANYING SYMPTOMS

Headache, loss of consciousness, vomiting, and seizures all provide clues to the stroke's etiology. Headaches, unusual for the patient prior to the stroke, may signify large artery occlusive disease or recent elevation in blood pressure. Headache at stroke onset is invariable in SAH and sometimes occurs in brain embolism. In ICH, headache usually follows the onset of other symptoms and signs. Figure 42-2 shows the relationship of headache and vomiting to types of stroke in the Michael Reese and University of Illinois stroke registries. Vomiting is very frequent near the onset of SAH and is common in large supratentorial and infratentorial ICHs. Vomiting is also frequent in patients with cerebellar and medullary infarcts. Seizures are slightly more common in patients with embolic infarcts and lobar ICHs than in patients with other stroke subtypes. Loss of consciousness is common in patients with SAH, large ICHs, and brainstem infarcts that affect the tegmentum bilaterally.

LABORATORY AND IMAGING EVALUATION

After completing the history and examination and constructing a list of *what* and *where* differential diagnoses, the physician is ready to plan the investigations. In some cases, the patient has already had some investigations. It is best to obtain the history and examine the patient before reviewing such accompanying information. Clearly, the nature and speed of the evaluation depend on the circumstances.

Acute Stroke

In the case of acute stroke, nearly always, a hospital admission is in order. CT or MRI and blood screening tests should be ordered as the patient is admitted. Subsequent testing depends on the results of imaging and blood tests. The exception might be a patient with a clear cut lacunar stroke who prefers to stay at home and can be managed by the family there. Such a patient would have (1) risk factors for a lacune, especially hypertension and or diabetes, and (2) a typical clinical picture of a lacunar syndrome with nondisabling signs, such as pure sensory stroke, dysarthria with minor arm clumsiness, pure dysarthria, and so forth. In that patient, an MRI before sending the patient home would help confirm the diagnosis and eliminate the presence of any unexpected lesions. If the scan shows a small deep infarct that explains the clinical findings, then the diagnosis is clear. If the MRI, or CT, scan shows old lacunes and no cortical infarct, then the diagnosis of lacunar infarction is still highly

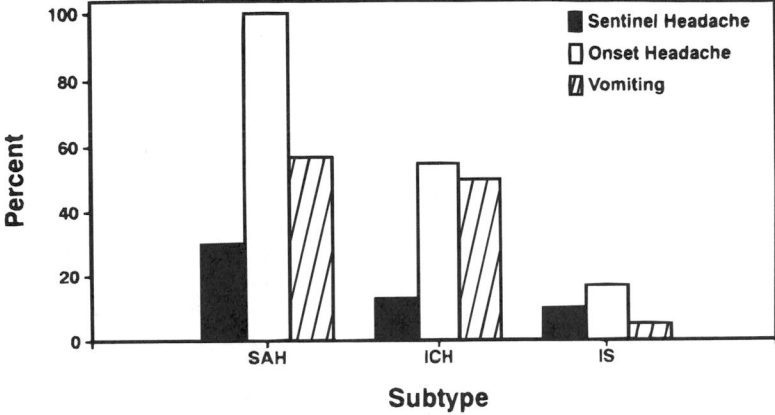

FIG. 42-2. Headache and vomiting frequencies by stroke subtypes. SAH, subarachnoid hemorrhage; IPH, intraparenchymal hemorrhage; IS, ischemic stroke (embolic and thrombotic). (From Gorelick PB, Hier DB, Caplan LR, Langenberg P: Headache in acute cerebrovascular disease. Neurology 36:1445, 1986, with permission.)

probable. If a cortical infarct or small hemorrhage is found, then further diagnostic testing, usually in the hospital, is warranted.

Remote Stroke

If the patient has a remote stroke (i.e., a stroke more than one week old), a scan brought with the patient (or a reliable description of the films) should suffice to tell whether the lesion was a hemorrhage or an infarct. If it was a hemorrhage, the site, size, and pattern of spread should be evident. If the problem was ischemic, the scan might show the infarct or have only slight or nondiagnostic abnormalities. If the studies are old, inadequate, or nondiagnostic, then a new scan (optimally an MRI) should be ordered.

Hemorrhage

An angioma or arteriovenous malformation may be evident from the films. If such a lesion is present and potentially resectable, then angiography may be in order. If the patient is hypertensive and the ICH is in a typical locale for a hypertensive hematoma (putamen, caudate, thalamus, cerebellum, or pons), then antihypertensive therapy is indicated without the need for other workup except blood screening. Ordinarily, all patients should have a platelet count, prothrombin time, and aPTT. An inquiry about the use of drugs (cocaine, diet pills, or methamphetamine) and medicines (especially warfarin derivatives) is important. The location of the hemorrhage might suggest a contusion caused by trauma. If the scan suggests SAH or an aneurysm is seen, then admission for angiography is warranted.

Infarction

If the lesion is a small deep infarct and the patient has hypertension or diabetes and compatible clinical findings, then blood testing is usually sufficient (complete blood count, platelet count, and fibrinogen level). If the scan shows a cortical lesion or, in fact, any lesion unlikely to represent a lacune, then usually a triad of *blood screening tests* (complete blood count, platelet count, prothrombin time, aPTT, and serum calcium), *cardiac tests* (electrocardiography and echocardiography), and *noninvasive vascular tests* (extracranial and intracranial ultrasound) and/or magnetic resonance angiography (MRA) should be ordered. The localization of the ischemia, of course, determines the main vessels to be studied. If the lesion is in the right cerebral hemisphere, then a carotid duplex and color-flow Doppler of the ICA in the neck and transcranial Doppler of the anterior circulation arteries would be indicated. Alternatively, an MRA or spiral CT examination of the ICA and its tributaries could be performed. If the lesion is in the posterior circulation, then a duplex and color-flow Doppler examination of the vertebral arteries in the neck, a continuous-wave Doppler insonation of the upper neck in the region of the atlas loop (V_3) portion of the vertebral artery to determine the direction of flow in this area, and transcranial Doppler using a suboccipital window to insonate the intracranial vertebral arteries and basilar artery should be performed. Alternatively, head and neck MRA or spiral CT angiography could be done with attention to the vertebrobasilar arteries. In patients who will undergo MRI, an accompanying MRA can be done while the patient is still in the magnet *after* reviewing the preliminary results of the MRI so that the vascular study can be adequately planned.

Transient Ischemic Attacks in the Absence of a Stroke

What if the patient had one or more TIAs and not a stroke? If the evaluation can be performed urgently (that day), then outpatient preliminary testing is an option. If the nature or frequency of the attacks is very worrisome, then hospital admission is prudent. Usually, a scan (CT or MRI) and ultrasound and/or MRA are scheduled concurrently. Blood screening, as described above, is also done. If the pattern of the clinical findings or the scan suggests large artery occlusive disease (TIAs in the same vascular territory), then cardiac testing can be postponed until the results of ultrasound and/or MRA are available. If there is only one attack or there were attacks in a number of vascular territories, cardiac testing is scheduled first or concurrently with noninvasive vascular testing. When the clinical localization is unclear, then a review of the scan is necessary before deciding on the order and nature of the cardiac and vascular testing.

SUGGESTED READINGS

Caplan LR: Intracranial branch atheromatous disease: a neglected, under-studied, and under-used concept. Neurology 39:1246, 1989

Caplan LR: Cerebrovascular disease (stroke). p. 1957. In Stein J (ed): Internal Medicine. 3rd Ed. Little, Brown, Boston, 1990

Caplan LR: The Effective Clinical Neurologist. Blackwell, Boston, 1990

Caplan LR: Diagnosis and treatment of ischemic stroke. JAMA 266:2413, 1991

Caplan LR: Stroke neuroimaging: evaluation of a recent stroke patient. J Neuroimaging 3:48, 1993

Caplan LR: Stroke: a Clinical Approach. 2nd Ed. Butterworth-Heinemann Boston, 1993

Caplan LR, Gorelick PB, Hier DB: Race, sex, and occlusive cerebrovascular disease: a review. Stroke 17:649, 1986

Chimowitz MI, Logigian EL, Caplan LR: The accuracy of bedside neurological diagnosis. Ann Neurol 28:78, 1990

Gorelick PB, Hier DB, Caplan LR, Langenberg P: Headache in acute cerebrovascular disease. *Neurology* 36:1445, 1986

Kase CS, Caplan LR: Intracerebral Hemorrhage, Butterworth-Heinemann, Boston, 1994

43. COMMON VASCULAR PROBLEMS IN OFFICE PRACTICE

MARC I. CHIMOWITZ
DARYL W. THOMPSON
ANTHONY J. FURLAN

Internists and neurologists frequently evaluate patients with a wide variety of cerebrovascular problems. In this chapter, we discuss some of the more common cerebrovascular problems seen in office practice and focus on the diagnosis and management of these problems.

CAROTID BRUITS AND ASYMPTOMATIC CAROTID STENOSIS

Clinical Detection and Prognosis

Carotid bruits are detected in 4 to 5 percent of the population aged 45 to 80 years and are associated with internal carotid artery stenosis in 50 percent of cases. Other causes of neck bruits include increased venous flow, external carotid stenosis, or a transmitted cardiac murmur. Localized bruits just below the jaw angle correlate best with underlying internal carotid artery stenosis, especially those with a diastolic component ("the longer the bruit, the tighter the stenosis"). Bruit loudness does not reliably predict the presence or severity of internal carotid stenosis; loud bruits may be heard with increased venous flow, whereas preocclusive internal carotid stenosis may produce a very soft bruit. Venous noises are usually a low-pitched rumble that are continuous through diastole and often change with body position or Valsalva maneuver. Cardiac murmurs are loudest below the clavicle and fade away as one auscultates up the neck. Subclavian bruits are loudest in the supraclavicular fossa or base of the neck and may disappear with light supraclavicular compression. Bruits from cervical vertebral artery stenosis are uncommon but can occasionally be heard in the posterior neck triangle. The absence of a carotid bruit does not rule out the diagnosis of carotid occlusive disease (e.g., a bruit may not be heard if there is low flow through a severe stenosis or if the internal carotid artery is occluded). In the latter case, a contralateral orbital bruit may be heard because of increased flow through the contralateral internal carotid artery.

Patients with asymptomatic carotid bruits have an increased risk of stroke. The annual risk of unheralded stroke (i.e., stroke without a preceding transient ischemic attack [TIA]) in these patients is 1.5 to 4 percent; however, many of these strokes occur contralateral to the side of the bruit and are related to other mechanisms of stroke (e.g., penetrating artery disease or cardioembolism).

A carotid bruit is a strong indicator of systemic atherosclerosis, in particular, coronary artery disease. Several studies have shown that the annual risk of myocardial infarction in patients with asymptomatic carotid bruits or stenosis is approximately 5 percent per year, which exceeds the 1.5 to 4 percent rate of stroke. Moreover, this high rate of myocardial infarction occurs in patients with or without previous symptoms of coronary artery disease.

Evaluation and Treatment of Patients With Asymptomatic Carotid Bruit

Until very recently, there was little consensus on whether patients with a carotid bruit should undergo testing to determine the presence of carotid stenosis. The lack of consensus was based on uncertainty regarding the best therapy for asymptomatic carotid stenosis. Within the past year, however, the results of the Asymptomatic Carotid Atherosclerosis Study have established that carotid endarterectomy, in addition to medical therapy (aspirin and aggressive management of modifiable risk factors), is superior to medical therapy alone for the prevention of unheralded stroke in patients with asymptomatic carotid stenosis greater than 60 percent. In that study, Kaplan-Meier projections showed that the risk of stroke over 5 years was 4.8 percent for patients treated surgically compared with 10.6 percent for patients treated medically. This represents a relative risk reduction of 55 percent in patients undergoing endarterectomy. Of note, however, is that the success of the operation is dependent on surgeons performing the procedure with perioperative morbidity and mortality rates less than 3 percent.

Based on the results of the above study, patients with an asymptomatic carotid bruit should undergo a noninvasive diagnostic study to determine whether they have carotid stenosis that is a greater than 60 percent reduction in diameter. Most centers employ duplex (Doppler and B mode) carotid ultrasound as the initial screening test. In laboratories with good quality assurance, carotid ultrasound has a sensitivity of 85 percent and a specificity of 90 percent for detecting carotid occlusive disease. An emerging alternative to duplex ultrasound is magnetic resonance angiography (MRA), which is easier to read than ultrasound and provides a "picture" of the carotid artery based on blood flow characteristics. The sensitivity and specificity of MRA is equal to or superior to ultrasound but less than angiography for detecting high-grade carotid stenosis. MRA and ultrasound tend to overestimate the degree of stenosis and frequently cannot distinguish subtotal from complete carotid artery occlusion.

Some surgeons perform endarterectomy based solely on noninvasive testing. While this approach avoids the risk and expense of angiography, it may result in at least a 5 percent false-postive rate of severe stenosis and lead to unnecessary surgery. With refinement in MRA technology, however, noninvasive evaluation is expected to replace angiography eventually except in disputed cases.

BRAIN SPELLS

Internists and neurologists frequently encounter patients with recurrent episodic neurologic symptoms (brain spells). The differential diagnosis of brain spells includes isolated dizziness, TIAs, migraine, seizure, metabolic derangements (e.g., hypoglycemia), presyncope, and a functional disorder. To determine the cause of the patient's spells, it is useful to separate nonfocal from focal spells; the former are rarely due to cerebrovascular occlusive disease, whereas the latter may be. Excluded from this discussion are functional spells, the manifestations of which are myriad.

Nonfocal Spells

Isolated Dizziness. "Dizziness" is a nonspecific term used by patients to describe a variety of different sensory symptoms. A detailed history usually enables the physician to ascertain whether the patient is referring to lightheadedness/faintness, unsteadiness/imbalance, or true vertigo (subjective sense of self or environmental rotatory motion).

Faintness or lightheadedness is rarely neurologic in origin. The causes are varied and include anemia, volume depletion, postural hypotension, vasovagal disorders, dysautonomia, arrhythmias, hyperventilation, panic attacks, and other anxiety disorders. Unsteadiness or imbalance also has many possible causes (disease of cerebellum and its connections, vestibular disease, posterior column dysfunction, and peripheral neuropathy). From a cerebrovascular point of view, the most common cause of acute isolated unsteadiness or imbalance (ataxia) is cerebellar infarction or hemorrhage.

Vertigo can be caused by peripheral or central vestibular dysfunction. Postural aggravation suggests a peripheral cause. Other associated features help distinguish peripheral from central vertigo. For example, the coexistence of deafness or tinnitus suggests that the vertigo is of peripheral origin. The presence of diplopia, dysarthria, or sensory or motor dysfunction indicates a central origin. Both peripheral and central vertigo can be associated with nausea, vomiting, and gait ataxia. Vertebrobasilar occlusive disease should always be considered in the differential diagnosis of vertigo. Patients with vertebrobasilar disease often present with recurrent stereotypical spells of vertigo, diplopia, dysarthria, perioral numbness, and ataxia. Episodes of isolated vertigo that occur over several months are virtually never caused by vertebrobasilar disease and usually are the result of a peripheral vestibular disorder.

Syncope. Syncope is the loss of consciousness and postural tone as a result of globally diminished blood flow to the brain. It is invariably caused by disorders that cause low cardiac output (e.g., aortic stenosis, heart block, ventricular arrhythmia, vasovagal syncope, and so forth). Occasionally, patients with vertebrobasilar occlusive disease may lose consciousness because of ischemia to the reticular activating system in the brainstem; however, these patients invariably have associated brainstem symptoms and signs prior to losing or on regaining consciousness.

The diagnostic evaluation of syncope should focus on the cardiovascular system. The workup should include an electrocardiogram, Holter monitoring (though it has a low diagnostic yield) and occasionally electrophysiologic studies, a tilt table test, and autonomic testing. Neurologic testing should be restricted to an electroencephalogram (EEG) if a generalized seizure cannot be ruled out by the history. Carotid imaging is not indicated unless the patient has associated slurred speech, monocular visual loss, or hemiparesis prior to losing or on regaining consciousness.

The prognosis of patients with syncope depends on the results of the cardiac evaluation. Patients with a serious cardiac cause of syncope (e.g., ventricular arrhythmia) have a 20 percent annual mortality rate, whereas patients without a cardiac or other identifiable cause have a substantially more benign outcome.

Focal Brain Spells

The differential diagnosis of transient, focal neurologic spells includes seizures, migraine, transient global amnesia, and TIAs. The latter refer to acute focal neurologic deficits caused by cerebral ischemia that, by definition, clear within 24 hours. Most TIAs, however, last only a few minutes. Typically, with TIAs, the deficit is maximal at onset, and there is no "march" of symptoms, altered awareness, or clonic motor activity. TIAs associated with carotid occlusive disease usually consist of episodes of transient monocular blindness (amaurosis fugax), dysarthria or dysphasia, and contralateral hemiparesis involving the hand and face predominantly. Rare TIAs in patients with high-grade carotid occlusive disease include transient monocular blindness precipitated by bright light and focal clonic limb shaking ("limb-shaking TIAs") that may mimic focal seizures. Transient ischemic attacks associated with vertebrobasilar occlusive disease consist of episodes of visual loss of both eyes, diplopia, dysarthria, vertigo, ataxia, perioral numbness, hemiparesis, and quadraparesis.

Focal seizures (partial simple seizures) that manifest as motor, sensory, or speech disturbances may be difficult to distinguish from TIAs. Motor or sensory symptoms that "march" over seconds up or down one side of the body suggest a focal seizure rather than a TIA. Clonic limb shaking is usually caused by a seizure but may also be a manifestation of a carotid TIA. The cause of the limb shaking in this setting is hypoperfusion of the cerebral cortex caused by a high-grade carotid stenosis or occlusion.

TIAs may also be difficult to distinguish from migraine. Headache is not always a distinguishing feature since TIAs may be associated with head pain in up to 40 percent of patients and migrainous neurologic symptoms may be unaccompanied by headache ("acephalgic migraine"). Carotid distribution ischemia typically causes frontotemporal head pain, whereas vertebrobasilar ischemia causes occipital head pain. The mechanism is probably related to collateral arteries dilating in response to ischemia. Visual symptoms may be a prominent feature of both disorders. Whereas a scintillating scotoma is highly suggestive of a migrainous event, a retinal or occipital embolus may cause a similar phenomenon. Similarly, transient monocular blindness points to ischemia in the carotid distribution, but migraine may produce retinal dysfunction that mimics amaurosis fugax. The visual aura of a migraine tends to spread across the visual field over the course of a few minutes, usually has positive features such as motion or color, and is generally followed by a headache. The headache of cerebral ischemia has a more variable time relationship to the neurologic symptoms.

Rarely, weakness of the limbs or facial muscles on one side of the body occurs as a migrainous aura. Migraine weakness generally lasts 20 to 30 minutes and, again, often has a spreading evolution over minutes. Attacks of migraine with hemiparesis are sometimes familial (hemiplegic migraine). Aphasia can also occur as the aura of migraine, further complicating the distinction from TIA. The syndrome of basilar artery migraine has many features in common with vertebrobasilar ischemia. Each may manifest as disturbances of consciousness, vision, equilibrium, or motor and sensory function.

Occasionally, migraine disappears for years only to re-emerge in later life to be easily confused with TIAs. The 70-year-old patient may have completely forgotten the menstrual headaches she had at age 20, with identical visual scintillations now mimicking vertebrobasilar insufficiency. Fisher termed such attacks "transient migrainous accompaniments," and they are common in any large office practice!

Distinguishing TIA from migrainous events should not be made based on a single feature of either disorder. They are clinical diagnoses requiring several features to be present to suggest one or the other. Features suggestive of cerebral ischemia include multiple risk factors for vascular disease, age greater than 60 years, and previous ischemic events. Features suggestive of migraine include recurrent attacks of headache, a family history of migraine, onset of headaches prior to 40 years of age, scintillating scotoma, and the marching onset of neurologic symptoms.

Transient global amnesia is characterized by the abrupt onset of severe anterograde amnesia without disturbance of consciousness, focal neurologic symptoms, or epileptic features, which resolves within 24 hours. Most patients are middle-aged or elderly. The etiology is uncertain, but growing evidence suggests that it is most often related to migraine. In some cases, transient global amnesia may be due to thromboembolic vertebrobasilar occlusive disease or complex partial seizures.

Patients usually only have a single attack, but occasionally the attacks may be multiple and occur over several years. If the clinical presentation is typical, expensive and invasive tests (e.g., brain magnetic resonance imaging or angiography) should be avoided because they are invariably normal and may pose a risk to the patient.

OCULAR STROKE

The retina and optic nerve may be the primary targets for certain cerebrovascular disorders. Branches of the ophthalmic artery supply both these ocular structures; the central retinal artery supplies the retina, and the posterior ciliary artery supplies the optic nerve. These two branches of the ophthalmic artery are affected by different vascular disorders.

Retinal Ischemia

The most common cause of retinal ischemia is carotid occlusive disease followed by other sources of embolism (e.g., the heart or aortic arch) and some hyperviscosity states (e.g., polycythemia vera). The mechanism of retinal ischemia in patients with carotid disease is either embolism to the central retinal artery or its branches or hypoperfusion of the retina caused by high-grade carotid stenosis or carotid occlusion. Transient retinal ischemia is manifested by transient monocular blindness (amaurosis fugax), which is classically, but uncommonly, described by patients as a "shade being pulled down" over the eye. It is more common for patients to describe fuzzy, blurred, or cloudy vision in the eye. When evaluating patients with a complaint of transient monocular visual loss, it is important to ask if they covered one eye and then the other eye to verify that the visual

loss was monocular. Patients with homonymous hemianopsia (e.g., from occipital ischemia), who do not cover one eye at a time to test their vision, often complain of monocular visual loss in the eye corresponding to the side of the hemianopsia.

Clues to the mechanism of transient retinal ischemia may be obtained from the history. Sector or altitudinal visual field defects with a horizontal meridian suggest embolism to the retina, whereas slow monocular dimming of vision, like a camera shutter, suggests hypoperfusion. A variant of this symptom is monocular visual dimming in bright light related to retinal hypoperfusion from ipsilateral carotid artery occlusion or critical stenosis.

The ophthalmoscopic examination may reveal other clues to the mechanism of ischemia. Hollenhorst plaques, which are yellowish, refractile retinal emboli composed of cholesterol flakes, suggest an arterial source of embolism. Platelet-fibrin emboli, which are grayish-white and lodge in peripheral vessel bifurcations, also suggest an arterial source of embolism. Calcific emboli, which are large and chalk white and lodge in the central retinal artery over the disc head, may arise from a heart valve or complex carotid plaque. Septic emboli (Roth spots), which appear as whitish cores surrounded by hemorrhage, suggest endocarditis.

Central Retinal Artery and Retinal Branch Artery Occlusion

Prolonged occlusion of the central retinal artery causes permanent damage to the retina. Central retinal artery occlusion typically causes total blindness of the eye that is usually painless. The pupil may fail to react because of diffuse retinal ischemia. The retina becomes pale and edematous, and the retinal vessels narrow. The optic disc becomes pale but the fovea retains its color and stands out as a cherry red spot (Plate 43-1A). Occasionally, the actual embolus may be seen, but usually no obstruction is visualized since the occlusion is proximal to the emergence of the retinal vessels from the disc. Obstruction of a retinal artery branch results in a focal retinal infarct and restricted visual loss, reflecting the local area supplied by the branch. Usually, embolism is the cause, and the source may be the ipsilateral carotid artery or the heart. When visualized funduscopically, the embolic material is often grayish-white (platelet-fibrin) and not cholesterol (Plate 43-1B). While some studies suggest a low correlation between central retinal artery occlusion or retinal artery branch occlusion and ipsilateral carotid occlusive disease, more recent studies show a much higher correlation. We suggest that all patients with central retinal artery occlusion or retinal artery branch occlusion undergo duplex carotid ultrasound to rule out carotid occlusive disease. If the carotid ultrasound is unrevealing, echocardiography should be performed to rule out a cardiac source of embolism.

Venous Stasis Retinopathy

A less recognized cause of retinal ischemia is venous stasis retinopathy (VSR), which is caused by chronic retinal hypoperfusion, usually from internal carotid artery occlusion. VSR appears similar to diabetic retinopathy with dot and blot hemorrhages and cotton wool patches (Plate 43-1C); the distinction is that VSR is usually unilateral. Eventually VSR may lead to neovascular glaucoma and blindness unless the hypoperfusion is reversed. In this setting, if a stenotic external carotid artery is supplying blood flow to the orbit, external carotid endarterectomy should be considered. On the other hand, if blood flow to the eye is largely from limited collateral flow from the contralateral hemisphere through the anterior communicating artery, ipsilateral extracranial-intracranial bypass surgery should be considered.

Optic Nerve Ischemia

Anterior ischemic optic neuropathy (AION) is usually caused by diseases that involve the posterior ciliary arteries. The most common of these diseases are intrinsic atherosclerosis and temporal arteritis. Rarely, optic nerve ischemia may be caused by sudden, severe hypotension. Carotid stenosis is rarely associated with AION. Patients with AION present with unilateral visual loss that is maximal in the temporal field. An afferent pupillary defect is invariably present, and ophthalmoscopy shows a pale, swollen disc that is frequently associated with flame hemorrhages around the disc. Ischemia of the optic nerve may rarely involve the posterior portion of the optic nerve. We have seen a few patients who, on awaking from major surgery that is associated with severe blood loss, complain of monocular blindness. The examination initially shows an afferent pupillary defect but no abnormality of the disc. In time, optic atrophy develops.

INOBVIOUS STROKE

Acute onset of hemiparesis is the archetypal presentation of stroke. The diagnostic challenge in patients with this presentation is not to recognize that the cause is vascular but rather to establish the specific cause of stroke (e.g., large artery occlusive disease, penetrating artery disease, or cardioembolism). In patients with stroke that is not manifested by hemiparesis ("stroke without paralysis"), it may be difficult to recognize that the cause of the patient's neurologic presentation is vascular. This is particularly true when the cardinal feature of the patient's presentation is a behavioral abnormality. Awareness of the stroke syndromes described below should prevent physicians from attributing these presentations to nonvascular causes.

Nondominant Temporoparietal Infarction

Occlusion of the inferior division of the middle cerebral artery (MCA) causes infarction of the temporal and parietal lobes in the region of the sylvian fissure. Involvement of the dominant hemisphere produces the neurologic syndrome of Wernicke's aphasia, hemianopsia, and agitation, which is more readily recognized as having a vascular etiology. The mirror image infarct in the nondominant hemisphere produces the syndrome of confusion, agitation, hemianopsia, and poor drawing and copying, which may be misinterpreted as having a psychiatric cause because of the prominent behavioral abnormalities. We have seen a few patients with nondominant inferior division MCA territory infarction who were admitted to the psychiatry service with a diagnosis of delirium (Fig. 43-1). Recognition of the hemianopsia is critical to prevent this error.

Dominant Hemisphere Infarction

Occlusion of the superior division of the MCA in the dominant hemisphere produces Broca's aphasia, which is usually associated with hemiparesis. This syndrome is readily recognized as having a vascular etiology. Occasionally, a Broca's type of aphasia may be the only manifestation of an infarct in this

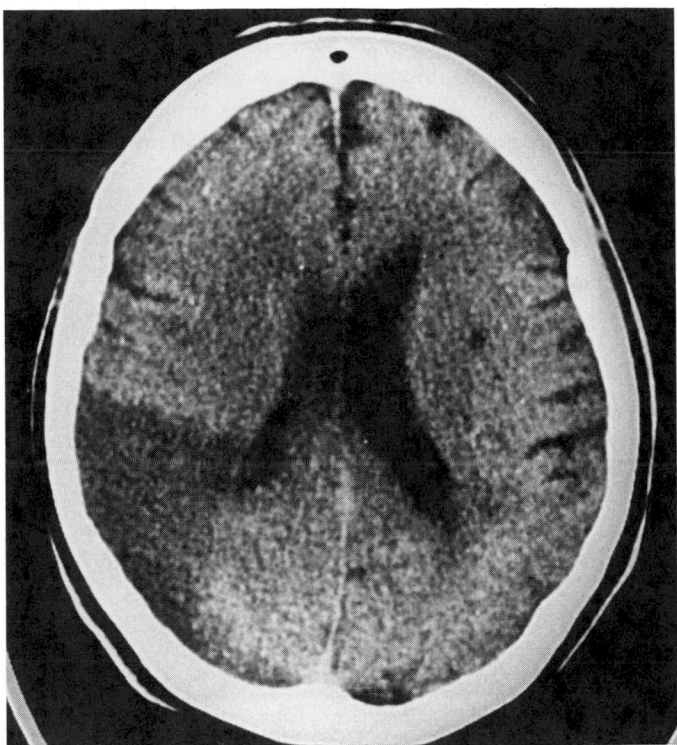

FIG. 43-1. A 67-year-old man admitted to psychiatry service with delirium. Computed tomography showed a wedge-shaped cortical infarct in the territory supplied by the inferior division of the right middle cerebral artery.

territory, but a vascular etiology should be suspected because of the sudden onset of the aphasia.

Infarction of the entire territory supplied by the inferior division of the MCA in the dominant hemisphere produces Wernicke's aphasia, hemianopsia, and agitation. This syndrome can also be seen with lobar hemorrhages in the temporal lobe and after traumatic brain injury. Smaller, discrete cortical infarcts in the territory supplied by the inferior division of the MCA produce subtypes of receptive aphasia that are not associated with visual or behavioral abnormalities. These subtypes include conduction aphasia, pure word deafness, and alexia with agraphia. These presentations are usually recognized as having a vascular etiology because of the sudden onset of the deficit. Occasionally, Alzheimer's disease may present with a receptive-type aphasia, but the onset is always more gradual if an accurate history is obtained. Patients with pure word deafness, a rare aphasic syndrome characterized by impaired auditory comprehension with normal reading comprehension, usually report that they cannot hear, which may lead to the incorrect diagnosis of an otologic problem. This error can be avoided by showing that the patient hears auditory stimuli (e.g., able to count the number of times hands are clapped or a bell rings) but has impaired auditory comprehension.

Most occlusions of the superior or inferior divisions of the MCA or their branches are caused by an embolus from the heart or carotid artery and less commonly by intrinsic atherosclerosis.

Occipital Infarction

The cardinal sign in patients with an occipital infarct caused by occlusion of the posterior cerebral artery is a contralateral, congruous, homonymous hemianopsia or quadrantanopsia. Visual loss is usually recognized immediately by the patient when the lesion involves the dominant hemisphere; however, the patient often reports that the visual loss involves the contralateral eye only. This may lead the unsuspecting physician to a diagnosis of ocular pathology rather than occipital infarction. Careful visual field testing of each eye separately uncovers the homonymous hemianopsia and leads to the correct diagnosis. Patients with infarction of the dominant occipital lobe may have other signs such as alexia without agraphia, hemiachromatopsia, dysnomia, and memory loss (the latter two signs imply associated medial temporal lobe involvement) that help to clarify the diagnosis.

When the nondominant occipital lobe is infarcted, patients may not recognize their visual loss because of inattention to the contralateral hemifield. This type of infarction is sometimes only recognized when these patients undergo a routine examination by an ophthalmologist. In some cases of nondominant occipital infarction, agitation may be a prominent feature that brings the patient to medical attention. Detection of the homonymous hemianopsia leads to the correct diagnosis. As with MCA division territory infarcts, most posterior cerebral artery territory infarcts are caused by an embolus from the heart or vertebral or basilar arteries.

Bilateral occipital infarction causes cortical blindness, which is often denied by the patient (Anton syndrome). This usually occurs in the setting of a hypotensive event (e.g., cardiac arrest) or occlusion of the top of the basilar artery. Associated signs may include agitation, confusion, and memory disturbance (from associated bilateral medial temporal infarctions).

Caudate and Medial Thalamic Infarcts

Infarction of the caudate nucleus without extension into the adjacent anterior limb of the internal capsule often causes isolated cognitive and behavioral abnormalities. These abnormalities may include abulia, agitation and hyperactivity, contralateral neglect (right caudate), and language abnormalities (left caudate). Lipohyalinotic or atherosclerotic occlusion of Heubner's artery, a branch of the anterior cerebral artery, or a medial striate artery that arises from the proximal anterior cerebral artery or MCA is the usual cause of infarction. The acute onset of these neurobehavioral abnormalities should suggest the possibility of a vascular etiology, especially in a patient with risk factors for penetrating artery disease.

Thalamic infarction is readily recognized when a patient presents with acute hemisensory loss involving the face, arm, leg, and torso. An infarct in the ventroposterolateral thalamic nucleus caused by occlusion of a thalamogeniculate artery is responsible for this syndrome. Less commonly, thalamic infarction may involve the paramedian thalamic nuclei (intralaminar nuclei and dorsomedial nuclei) that are supplied by the thalamoperforating arteries. Patients with these infarcts usually present with cognitive and behavioral abnormalities such as confusion, memory disturbance, hemineglect (nondominant), aphasia (dominant), and somnolence (Fig. 43-2).

SEIZURES AFTER STROKE

Seizures have been recognized as a complication of stroke since 1864 when Hughlings Jackson described a patient with partial seizures following cerebral infarction. Subsequently, studies have clarified the frequency of seizures after stroke and the risk factors for developing seizures.

The percentage of patients who have at least one seizure within 2 years of stroke is 4.4 to 8.4 percent. The onset of the initial seizure is within the first week of stroke in 33 to 65 percent patients and within 1 year in 73 to 90 percent. Only 2 percent of initial seizures occur more than 2 years after stroke. Lobar hemorrhages are associated with the highest rate of early seizures (12 to 15 percent), followed by subarachnoid hemorrhage (8.5 percent), and cortical infarction (6.5 to 8 percent). Small subcortical infarcts are rarely associated with seizures. In patients with ischemic stroke, early studies suggested that cardioembolism was particularly associated with a high rate of seizures; however, more recent studies have shown that other mechanisms of ischemic stroke (e.g., artery-to-artery embolism and low flow from high-grade stenosis) are associated with similar rates of seizures.

Partial simple (56 percent) or partial complex (24 percent) seizures account for 80 percent of seizures after stroke. The epileptic phenomenology typically reflects the site of cerebral injury (e.g., focal motor seizure with infarction of the precentral gyrus or partial complex seizures with medial temporal infarction). Status epilepticus occurs in only 8 percent of initial seizures after stroke and usually involves focal seizures only (epilepsia partialis continua).

Most studies have shown that initial seizures occurring more than 2 weeks after stroke are associated with a high rate of multiple, recurrent seizures (i.e., epilepsy); however, the risk of epilepsy after early poststroke seizures (i.e., seizures within 2

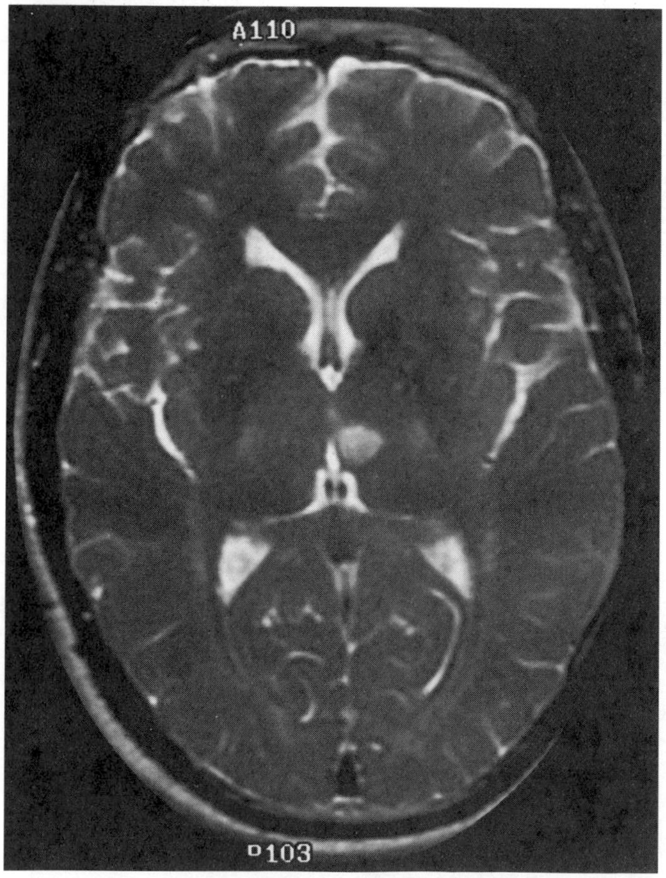

FIG. 43-2. A 47-year-old man presented with acute confusion and memory disturbance. Magnetic resonance imaging showed a left medial thalamic infarct.

weeks of stroke) has long been debated. Whereas initial studies suggested that the long-term risk of epilepsy was only 6 percent after early poststroke seizures, more recent studies have shown epilepsy rates of 22 to 32 percent during a mean follow-up of 26 to 30 months. In one study by Kilpatrick et al. (1992) of consecutive patients with ischemic or hemorrhagic stroke, epilepsy rates were compared in 31 patients with early poststroke seizures versus 31 patients without early seizures who were matched for age and stroke mechanism. The epilepsy rate over 26 months in the group with early seizures was 32 percent compared with 10 percent in patients without early seizures ($P < 0.05$). Risk factors that have predicted multiple, recurrent seizures after an initial poststroke seizure are hemorrhagic stroke (superficial or deep), large cortical infarcts, and periodic lateralized epileptiform discharges (PLEDS) or diffuse slowing on EEG.

Anticonvulsant therapy is usually very successful in controlling poststroke epilepsy. Since most of these seizures are partial simple or partial complex seizures with occasional secondary generalization, monotherapy with either phenytoin or carbamazepine is sufficient to control seizures in 90 percent of these patients. In a few intractable cases, polytherapy (using combinations of phenytoin, carbamazepine, and valproic acid) is sometimes necessary.

While some physicians use anticonvulsants routinely in all patients with acute hemorrhagic or ischemic stroke, the low overall rate of seizures after stroke (4.4 to 8.4 percent) argues against this approach. Our current practice is to initiate phenytoin or carbamazepine once a seizure occurs because of the high rate of recurrence. A baseline EEG is useful to determine whether PLEDS or diffuse slowing is present since these findings may influence a later decision to continue or discontinue anticonvulsant therapy. We prescribe a sufficient dose of anticonvulsant monotherapy to control the seizures without causing drug toxicity, and, once the patient has been seizure free for at least 18 to 24 months, we discuss the option of discontinuing the anticonvulsant. A repeat EEG is helpful in making that decision. Factors that would argue against discontinuing the anticonvulsants are the presence of PLEDS or diffuse slowing on the baseline EEG, persistent spikes on a recent EEG, hemorrhagic stroke, a large cortical infarct, or when the patient's occupation involves driving or working with moving machinery.

Seizures After Carotid Endarterectomy

Seizures occur in approximately 1 percent of patients within 2 to 13 days of carotid endarterectomy. The seizures invariably are focal motor seizures contralateral to the side of the endarterectomy that occasionally generalize. These seizures are usually caused by hyperperfusion injury following endarterectomy or an infarct occurring during endarterectomy.

In the former case, postoperative hypertension and failure of autoregulation ipsilateral to carotid endarterectomy results in hyperperfusion of the ipsilateral hemisphere. This may manifest as ipsilateral headache, contralateral motor seizures, and occasionally intracerebral hemorrhage. Brain imaging usually shows patchy cerebral edema and occasionally hemorrhage ipsilateral to the side of the carotid endarterectomy. Transcranial Doppler ultrasound shows markedly elevated ipsilateral MCA blood flow velocities. With judicious management of blood pressure, the headache and focal brain edema usually resolves within 1 to 2 weeks. Anecdotal data suggests that the

long-term risk of recurrent seizures in patients who have an initial seizure related to postendarterectomy hyperperfusion is low. These patients typically have not required long-term anticonvulsants, whereas patients with seizures related to stroke during endarterectomy have a higher rate of recurrent seizures and therefore require anticonvulsant therapy.

ISCHEMIC STROKE IN YOUNG PATIENTS

Although the risk of stroke is much lower in the population aged 15 to 50 years than in the population older than 50 years, it is relatively common for neurologists to encounter stroke in the young, particularly at a tertiary referral center. Establishing the cause of stroke in the young is often a challenging process. While some causes of stroke in the young are similar to causes of stroke in the elderly (e.g., carotid atherosclerosis or cardiac embolism), the list of diseases that need to be considered as a potential cause of stroke in the young is longer than it is in the elderly. Furthermore, the cause of stroke remains uncertain in a substantially higher percentage of younger patients (up to 40 percent) than in older patients despite a thorough diagnostic evaluation.

It is useful to categorize causes of stroke in the young into the following major groups: (1) atherosclerotic large artery occlusive disease of the carotid or vertebrobasilar circulation, (2) nonatherosclerotic large artery occlusive disease (e.g., dissection or moyamoya disease), (3) occlusive disease of small penetrating arteries that arise from the major intracranial arteries (also termed small vessel disease), (4) cardioembolism, (5) prothrombotic states, (6) miscellaneous causes (e.g., migraine, oral contraceptives, or substance abuse), and (7) stroke of undetermined cause. A detailed list of specific diseases in approximate order of frequency within each of these major groups is shown in Table 43-1.

Data from several studies indicate that 21 to 48 percent of strokes in the young are caused by atherosclerotic large artery occlusive disease, 10 to 33 percent by nonatherosclerotic large artery occlusive disease (dissections constituted 10 to 20 percent in some studies), 13 to 35 percent by cardioembolism, 3 to 18 percent by penetrating artery disease, 8 to 15 percent by prothrombotic states, and 4 to 15 percent from miscellaneous causes. Stroke of undetermined causes include 7 to 40 percent of cases.

Although many heterogeneous disorders need to be considered when attempting to establish the cause of stroke in the young, a detailed history and bedside examination are useful for narrowing the diagnostic possibilities. Atherosclerotic large artery occlusive disease should be strongly considered in patients with atherosclerotic risk factors; coronary or peripheral vascular disease; a family history of premature atherosclerosis; a history of multiple, stereotypical TIAs; and the presence of a carotid bruit. Prominent facial pain (usually periorbital) preceding or accompanying the stroke, head or neck trauma preceding the stroke, and the presence of an ipsilateral Horner syndrome should suggest carotid dissection. Prominent posterior neck pain should suggest a vertebral artery dissection. A history of atrial fibrillation, cardiac valve replacement, cardiomyopathy, recent myocardial infarction, or rheumatic mitral stenosis suggests cardioembolism. Stroke occurring during a Valsalva maneuver (e.g., while defecating) should suggest the possibility of paradoxic embolism through an interatrial septal defect.

Lipohyalinotic or atherosclerotic penetrating artery disease

TABLE 43-1. Potential Causes of Ischemic Stroke in the Young

Atherosclerotic large artery disease
  Predisposition to early atherosclerosis in patients with familial hyperlipidemia, onset of diabetes in childhood or adolescence, severe hypertension, homocysteinuria (especially homozygote state), pseudoxanthoma elasticum, radiation therapy to neck or cranium
Nonatherosclerotic large or medium-sized artery disease
  Carotid or vertebral artery dissection
  Fibromuscular dysplasia
  Idiopathic moyamoya disease
  Moyamoya pattern from sickle cell disease or neurofibromatosis
  Sarcoid vasculopathy
  Infectious (e.g., mucormycosis and other fungal infections, tuberculosis, cysticercosis)
  Herpes zoster vasculopathy
  Angiitis associated with polyarteritis nodosa, Wegener's granulomatosis, Churg-Strauss syndrome, Takayasu's disease, lupus erythematosus, lymphomatoid granulomatosis, giant cell arteritis (rare in young patients)
  Primary angiitis of the nervous system
Penetrating artery disease
  Lipohyalinotic
  Atherosclerotic
  Infectious causes (usually associated with meningeal infection) (e.g., syphilis, cryptococcus, tuberculosis)
  Small vessel vasculitis (e.g., Behçet's, primary angiitis of central nervous system, Wegener's, hypersensitivity vasculitis)
Cardioembolism
  Probable association
    Bacterial endocarditis
    Prosthetic valve
    Acute myocardial infarction
    Cardiomyopathy
    Right-to-left interatrial shunt with associated deep vein thrombosis or pulmonary embolus
    Atrial fibrillation
    Mitral stenosis (higher on the list in developing countries)
    Left atrial thrombus or spontaneous contrast (invariably associated with cardiomyopathy, atrial fibrillation, or mitral stenosis)
    Left atrial myxoma or other tumor
  Possible association
    Right-to-left interatrial shunt without associated deep vein thrombosis or pulmonary embolus
    Mitral valve prolapse
    Interatrial septal aneurysm, especially the types associated with an interatrial shunt
    Akinetic or hypokinetic ventricular segment without associated thrombus
    Mitral annular calcification
    Bicuspid aortic valve, especially if calcified
Prothrombotic states
  Probable association with stroke
    Antiphospholipid antibody syndrome
    Sickle cell disease
    Cancer-related thrombosis
    Polycythemia vera
    Essential thrombocytosis
    Thrombotic thrombocytopenic purpura
    Disseminated intravascular coagulation
  Possible association with stroke
    Markedly elevated factor VIII level
    Protein C deficiency
    Protein S deficiency
    Antithrombin III deficiency
    Dysfibrinogenemia
    Disorders of fibrinolysis (e.g., dysplasminogenemia, elevated plasminogen activator inhibitor)
Miscellaneous associations with increased stroke risk
  Substance abuse (especially with cocaine and amphetamines)
  Migraine
  Oral contraception
  Pregnancy and postpartum period
  MELAS syndrome (mitochondrial encephalopathy, lactic acidosis, and stroke-like episodes)
Stroke of undetermined cause

should only be considered in patients with an established history of hypertension or diabetes, pure motor hemiparesis or pure sensory stroke, a subcortical infarct 1.5 cm or less in size that correlates with the neurologic deficit, and no evidence of large artery disease or a cardioembolic source. Prothrombotic states should be considered in patients with a personal or family history of recurrent venous or arterial thromboses (especially if the thromboses affected unusual sites such as the arm), those with cancer, and those with an intraluminal carotid or vertebrobasilar clot on vascular imaging. The presence of antiphospholipid antibodies contributing to the cause of stroke should be considered in patients with recurrent fetal loss or thrombocytopenia (the antiphospholipid antibody syndrome) or in those with lupus erythematosus. Other mechanisms of ischemic stroke in patients with lupus erythematosus are large artery atherosclerosis from lupus-related hypertension, Libman-Sacks endocarditis, thrombotic thrombocytopenic purpura, and rarely cerebral vasculitis. The presence of systemic cancer raises the possibility of a prothrombotic state or nonbacterial thrombotic (marantic) endocarditis.

Substance abuse raises the possibility of stroke related to vasospasm, vasculitis, or bacterial endocarditis (if intravenous drugs are used). Cocaine and amphetamines are associated with the highest risk of stroke. Although the use of oral contraceptives has been associated with an increased risk of stroke in large epidemiologic studies, the overall risk to an individual patient remains very low. Therefore, an extensive diagnostic evaluation should be performed in all young stroke patients who are receiving oral contraceptives to rule out the possibility of another cause of stroke. While migraine has been reported to cause stroke, it has been our experience that the diagnosis of migraine-related stroke is usually incorrect. The presence of headache after stroke is common regardless of the cause of stroke. Migraine-related stroke should only be diagnosed in patients with a history of migraine with aura who have a persistent neurologic deficit after a typical migraine attack for which *no other cause can be found.* Primary angiitis of the central nervous system is another disorder that, in our opinion, is overdiagnosed in young patients with stroke. Typically, patients with primary angiitis present with chronic headaches, seizures, or encephalopathy rather than a single stroke. They usually have inflammatory cerebrospinal fluid, and angiography may show multiple areas of segmental narrowing of small and medium sized arteries, though larger arteries may occasionally be involved. Since the angiographic findings are not specific for vasculitis (seen also with reversible segmental vasospasm as in migraine, diffuse intracranial atherosclerosis, and lymphomatous or infectious infiltration of arteries), a brain biopsy is usually necessary to establish the diagnosis.

An Approach to Diagnostic Testing in Young Stroke Patients

The following tests are recommended routinely in all young (15 to 50 years) stroke patients: complete blood count, platelet count, prothrombin time, partial thromboplastin time, cholesterol, high-density lipoproteins, low-density lipoproteins, triglycerides, fluorescent treponemal antibody, IgG and IgM anticardiolipin antibodies, electrocardiography, brain imaging (magnetic resonance imaging is preferable to computed tomography CT), and cerebrovascular imaging. One approach to cerebrovascular imaging is to begin noninvasively with carotid and transcranial Doppler ultrasound and MRA. If intracranial occlusive disease (e.g., moyamoya disease or vasculitis) is a strong consideration, based on the clinical and brain imaging findings, or if the results of transcranial Doppler ultrasound and MRA are discordant, conventional angiography is required to clarify the diagnosis. In patients with fever, blood cultures, transesophageal echocardiography, and a lumbar puncture are also recommended. In black patients, a sickle cell preparation (followed by hemoglobin electrophoresis if the preparation is positive) should also be included in the routine studies to rule out sickle cell disease.

If the diagnosis is established by these routine tests (e.g., angiography shows atherosclerotic carotid occlusive or a dissection), the diagnostic evaluation is terminated. In patients with normal routine blood tests and vascular imaging or in patients with an occluded intracranial artery without a proximal large artery source of embolus, echocardiography is recommended. Transesophageal rather than transthoracic echocardiography is the preferred procedure because of its higher sensitivity and specificity for detecting cardiac abnormalities such as an interatrial septal aneurysm, atrial septal defect, left atrial spontaneous contrast (''smoke''), and small vegetations. Bubble contrast echocardiography is routinely performed in this setting to rule out a right-to-left shunt through an interatrial septal defect. If a right-to-left shunt is found, venous ultrasound of the lower extremities is performed to evaluate for deep venous thrombosis.

If the diagnostic evaluation remains negative, the following assays are usually performed: antithrombin III, protein C antigen and activity, protein S antigen and activity, factor VIII, D-dimer, fibrin split products, fibrinogen, plasminogen activator inhibitor-1, and serum homocysteine. Since low levels of protein C and protein S and high levels of factor VIII, fibrinogen, and plasminogen activator inhibitor-1 may be acute-phase responses to stroke, it is advisable to repeat these tests at least 3 months after stroke to determine whether the abnormalities persist. Since anticoagulation influences the results of some of these tests (e.g., protein C and protein S), these tests need to be modified to take this into account. Consultation with a hematologist is important in the evaluation and treatment of a suspected prothrombotic state in patients with stroke.

Prevention of Recurrent Stroke in the Young Patient

Therapeutic strategies to prevent recurrent stroke are similar in young and old patients. Regardless of the cause of stroke, vascu-

TABLE 43-2. Some Cause-Specific Treatments to Prevent Recurrent Stroke

Cause of Stroke	Treatment[a]
≥70% internal carotid stenosis	Carotid endarterectomy[a] followed by aspirin therapy
Atherosclerotic occlusive disease of a major intracranial artery	Warfarin, aspirin, or ticlopidine
Carotid or vertebral dissection	Warfarin or antiplatelet therapy
Moyamoya disease	Antiplatelet agents, consider warfarin or surgical therapy (extracranial-intracranial bypass, encephalomyosynangiosis)
Prosthetic valve	Change to warfarin if stroke occurred while patient receiving aspirin; add antiplatelet agent if stroke occurred while patient receiving warfarin; consider replacing valve if recurrent strokes
Bacterial endocarditis	Antibiotics; consider valve replacement
Atrial fibrillation or mitral stenosis	Warfarin more efficacious than aspirin for secondary stroke prevention[a]
Right-to-left interatrial shunt with associated deep vein thrombosis	Warfarin or Greenfield filter
Right-to-left interatrial shunt without associated deep vein thrombosis	Antiplatelet agents, warfarin, or closure of interatrial defect
Interatrial septal aneurysm	Antiplatelet agents, warfarin
Antiphospholipid antibody syndrome	Antiplatelet agent or warfarin, questionable role for immunotherapy
Prothrombotic states associated with deficiency of natural anticoagulants (e.g., protein C or S deficiency)	Warfarin

[a] Proved in randomized prospective trials.

lar risk factors such as hypertension, diabetes, hyperlipidemia, and smoking need to be treated aggressively. Specific stroke preventive therapy such as antiplatelet agents, anticoagulation, and carotid endarterectomy is recommended based on the cause of the stroke (Table 43-2). Patients should be told to report recurrent symptoms suggestive of TIAs after discharge from the hospital, and return visits should be scheduled periodically (e.g., every 3 to 6 months initially and then annually). In our experience, the rate of recurrent stroke in young patients is approximately 2 to 4 percent per year depending on the cause of stroke, which is substantially lower than the rate of recurrent stroke in elderly patients (approximately 5 to 10 percent per year).

SELECTED READINGS

Abi-Samra FM, Fouad FM, Sweeney PJ, Maloney JD: Syncope: a practical diagnostic approach. pp. 249–83. In Furlan AJ (ed): The Heart and Stroke. Springer-Verlag, Berlin, 1987

Bogousslavsky J, Regli F, Uske A: Thalamic infarcts: clinical syndromes, etiology, and prognosis. Neurology 38:837, 1988

Caplan LR, Kelly CS, Kase CS et al: Infarcts of the inferior division of the right middle cerebral artery: mirror image of Wernicke's aphasia. Neurology 36:1015, 1986

Chimowitz MI, Weiss DG, Cohen SL et al: Cardiac prognosis of patients with carotid stenosis and no history of coronary artery disease. Veterans Affairs Cooperative Study Group 167. Stroke 25:759, 1994

Fisher CM: Late-life migraine accompaniments as a cause of unexplained transient ischemic attacks. Can J Neurol Sci 7:9, 1980

Hoyt WF: Retinal ischemic symptoms in cardiovascular diagnosis. Postgrad Med 52:85, 1972

Kilpatrick CJ, Davis SM, Hopper JL, Rossiter SC: Early seizures after acute stroke. Risk of late seizures. Arch Neurol 49:509, 1992

Sandok BA, Whisnant JP, Furlan AJ, Mickell JL: Carotid artery bruits—prevalence survey and differential diagnosis. Mayo Clin Proc 57:227, 1982

Stern BJ, Kittner S, Sloan M et al: Stroke in the young: part I. MMJ 40:453, 1991

Stern BJ, Kittner S, Sloan M et al: Stroke in the young: part II. MMJ 40:565, 1991

The Asymptomatic Carotid Atherosclerosis Study Group: Study design for randomized prospective trial of carotid endarterectomy for asymptomatic atherosclerosis. Stroke 20:844, 1989

Wolf PA, Kannel WB, Sorlie P et al: Asymptomatic carotid bruit and risk of stroke: the Framingham Study. JAMA 245:1442, 1981

44. CURRENT TREATMENT STRATEGIES FOR CEREBROVASCULAR DISEASES

R. S. MARSHALL
J. P. MOHR

Few therapies for stroke have met the demands of well-designed clinical trials. Antiplatelet therapy, warfarin anticoagulation for prevention of cardioembolic stroke, and carotid endarterectomy for high-grade carotid stenosis have become standard fare for internists and neurologists familiar with the current literature. Stroke diagnosis in the modern age has focused on defining cardiac pathology or carotid disease that would warrant anticoagulation or surgical referral; however, most patients with cerebrovascular disease fit imperfectly into categories that offer standard therapeutic responses. Conflicting data from the diagnostic workup, identification of stroke mechanisms with putative, but unproven, significance, and the presentation of strokes in the hyperacute phase confront the responsible physician with difficult clinical decisions that could mean the difference between a benign course and major disability. In addition, a growing armamentarium of diagnostic tools, burgeoning preclinical evidence that ischemia may be a modifiable process, and an increasingly well-informed public have increased the options for treating patients with transient ischemic attacks (TIAs) and stroke. We present here the evidence for the established therapies as well as a survey of recent avenues of research that will likely form the basis for stroke treatment in the future.

ANTIPLATELET THERAPY

Aspirin therapy in primary and secondary stroke prevention has been widely employed because of its ease of administration, its documented prophylactic effect in coronary artery disease, and its perception by physicians and the public as a benign treatment. This last point is not entirely to its advantage: many patients (and some physicians) continue to think of aspirin as adjunct therapy and often fail to mention its use when answering inquiries about medications being taken. Other antiplatelet drugs, such as sulfinpyrazone and dipyridamole used alone, have not proved beneficial in clinical testing.

More than 10 randomized placebo-controlled trials of aspirin following TIAs or minor stroke have been completed. Most showed a significant risk reduction with aspirin. The results of the aspirin trials, combined with the decline in stroke incidence over the past few decades has led statisticians to calculate that modern clinical trials of stroke prevention may require approximately 1,000 patients enrolled and followed for an average of 5 years to detect a 50 percent difference at a significance level of $p < .05$. Smaller studies may conclude benefit when none exists or overlook a true benefit.

All of the four largest clinical trials—the British, European, French, and Canadian—found some degree of benefit, ranging from 20 percent reduction in stroke and vascular death in the British trial to 50 percent reduction in stroke and stroke-death in the French trial. Two slightly smaller trials—the Danish and the Swedish—found no benefit. The Danish study used an acetylsalicylic acid (ASA) dose of 50 to 75 mg/day, and the Swedish study entered only patients who had suffered major strokes. Differences found in other studies are of uncertain significance. A lack of benefit in women, reported in the British and Canadian studies, may have been due to a lack of statistical power, as the risk of stroke and stroke recurrence is lower for women. The optimum dose of aspirin remains controversial. The Dutch trial for stroke prevention after TIA, using calcium salicylates, showed no difference between 30 mg/day and 283 mg/day. The British trial found no difference between 300 mg/day and 1,300 mg/day but the meaning of the data has been disputed. Patients in the Stroke Prevention in Atrial Fibrillation were benefitted by ASA 325 mg/day in a setting of atrial fibrillation only, not TIA or prior stroke. Consequently, it remains unsettled whether ultra-low-dose aspirin or aspirin in doses as high as 1,300 mg/day offers slight, wide, or no major differences in rates of first or recurrent stroke. The only source of agreement is that the higher doses produce more disagreeable gastrointestinal side effects.

Ticlopidine, a novel platelet antiaggregant newly available in North America, has been in use in Europe and the rest of the world for over 15 years. Its maximum antiplatelet action is at a dose of 500 mg/day, it reaches maximum effect at 3 to 5 days, and its effects last the lifetime of the platelets. Adverse side effects include gastrointestinal disturbance in 20 percent of patients, which may resolve with temporary dose reduction, rash in 10 percent, neutropenia in 2.4 percent, and severe neutropenia in 0.8 percent, which is seen in the first few months and is reversible. Significant hemorrhage occurs in less than 1 percent of patients and gastrointestinal bleeding is three times less likely in patients taking 500 mg of ticlopidine than 1,300 mg of ASA. Two large clinical trials found a benefit in ticlopidine over ASA and placebo.

The Canadian-American Ticlopidine Study randomized 1,053 patients with recent noncardioembolic stroke to receive ticlopidine 250 mg bid or placebo. The study excluded patients who had significant comorbidity and those with TIA alone. The incidence of primary endpoints (ischemic stroke, myocardial infarction, and vascular death) was 10.8 percent in the ticlopidine group versus 15.3 percent in the placebo group for a relative risk reduction of 30.2 percent by "on-treatment" analysis. Intention-to-treat analysis concluded a 23 percent risk reduction for the treatment group. Treatment was discontinued by 52 percent of patients in the ticlopidine group and 40 percent of those in the placebo group. Relative reduction in stroke or stroke-death was found on secondary analysis to be 33.5 percent. Ticlopidine proved equally effective in men and women.

The Ticlopidine-Aspirin Stroke Study randomized 3,069 patients to ticlopidine 250 mg bid or ASA 650 mg bid. The study consisted of patients with TIAs, transient monocular blindness, or minor stroke; the average follow-up period was 2.3 years. In their intention-to-treat analysis, these investigators showed a 12 percent reduction in stroke or stroke-death. In a 3-year follow-up, the incidence of fatal or nonfatal stroke was reduced 21 percent. The drug was discontinued by 21 percent of the ticlopidine group and 14.5 percent of the ASA group.

For those who can tolerate the medicine, ticlopidine appears to have a slight advantage over aspirin and a definite advantage over placebo in secondary stroke prevention. In a subsequent subgroup analysis of the two studies, women and those for whom aspirin therapy had failed appeared to benefit more from ticlopidine than aspirin. Patients with diabetes mellitus requiring treatment, those on antihypertensives, and those with elevated creatinine levels also showed greater treatment effects versus aspirin. It remains to be determined in patterns of practice whether the slight improvement in stroke-event rates that results from ticlopidine therapy, compared with slightly less improvement under aspirin therapy, will offset the side effects and annoyances in monitoring to permit ticlopidine to become popular.

ANTICOAGULATION

Although the evidence for the use of intravenous heparin in acute stroke is scanty, most physicians heparinize acute stroke patients when (1) there is a proven cardioembolic source, (2) TIAs are increasing in frequency or severity, or (3) a patient is awaiting imminent carotid endarterectomy. Long-term anticoagulation with warfarin is better established, but no less controversial.

Heparin

Anticoagulation with intravenous heparin is not intended to dissolve a thrombus, but to impair the thrombogenesis created by the "clotting cascade." Considering that experience with warfarin and heparin is decades long, one might be forgiven in thinking their utility had been settled, but such is not the case. The debate on heparin use has continued undiminished, and only lately have major trials been mounted to settle its utility. Only two clinical trials in the computed tomography (CT) era evaluated the effect of heparin anticoagulation in acute stroke treatment. One study treated patients with cardioembolic stroke and demonstrated probable benefit. The other study failed to show a treatment effect in noncardioembolic stroke.

The first study reported 45 patients with presumed cardioembolic stroke randomized into two groups: immediate anticoagulation with intravenous heparin versus delayed anticoagulation with warfarin after 14 days. The intravenous heparin group received a bolus of 5,000 to 10,000 units of heparin within 48 hours of stroke onset, followed by a maintenance infusion to keep the partial thromboplastin time (PTT) at 1.5 to 2.5 times the patient's baseline. After at least 96 hours of heparin the study group was switched to long-term anticoagulation with warfarin. Patients younger than 18 or older than 78 were excluded, as were those with persistent, severe hypertension. Of the 24 patients randomized to receive early anticoagulation there were no recurrences and no hemorrhages during the 2-week study period. Of the 21 patients randomized to receive delayed anticoagulation, two had early recurrent embolism, one had a deep-vein thrombosis, two had hemorrhagic conversions, and two died. The study was terminated early because of the strong trend toward benefit in the immediate anticoagulation group, despite the small sample size.

The second study randomized 225 patients to receive either intravenous placebo or heparin within 48 hours of stroke onset, with a target PTT of 50 to 70 seconds. The study period was 7 days, and no long-term anticoagulation was given. Patients were excluded from the study if they had a possible cardioembolic source, if their deficit was too severe or resolved prior to the initiation of therapy, if previous deficits existed, or if stroke progression was noted within 1 hour of study onset. No significant differences in stroke progression or death was seen at 7 days. No difference in functional level was seen at 1 year. There were significantly more deaths in the heparin group at 1 year, although most of these deaths occurred 3 to 12 months after the initial stroke and "appeared unrelated to treatment."

Both studies suffered from a small sample size. They established that early recurrence was not so common as to make estimation of any therapeutic effect an easy task. Because the first study focused on cardioembolic stroke and the second excluded such patients, the conflicting conclusions cannot be directly compared. A subsequent meta-analysis was unable to show a benefit of anticoagulation, although most trials were surveyed before CT was devised. The findings were of sufficient interest that a multicenter trial is under way in the United States to compare a synthetic heparin with placebo in acute stroke. No heparin studies have thus far determined whether there are differences in benefit for stroke patients according to the route of administration (intravenous or subcutaneous), or, if intravenous, the form of administration to continuous or bolus, or the exact dose and duration of therapy. The matter is not trivial, since evidence favoring similar effects for intermittent subcutaneous heparin could easily allow treatment at home. Similarly, if continuous intravenous administration is needed, it could be given by a subcutaneous pump, thereby sparing hospital expense in ambulatory patients.

Warfarin

Warfarin anticoagulation was brought early into clinical practice and has long been standard treatment of patients with rheumatic mitral stenosis and prosthetic valves; it has never been subjected to the kinds of trials demanded nowadays, and is not likely soon to undergo any such trial. Large epidemiologic studies, for which the Framingham study is a model, have established high risk for stroke in patients with cardiac disease. The highest risk was seen in patients with atrial fibrillation in combination with valvular disease. The overall risk of stroke in patients with chronic atrial fibrillation is 5 percent per year. With the decline in incidence of rheumatic heart disease and rising uncertainty of the best management for nonvalvular atrial fibrillation, such patients have been considered suitable for such trials. Six prospective, randomized trials have now proved there is a benefit in long-term anticoagulation and a low risk of serious complications.

The six studies are the Copenhagen Atrial Fibrillation, Aspirin, Anticoagulation Study (AFASAK), SPAF, Boston Area Anticoagulation Trial for Atrial Fibrillation (BAATAF), Canadian Atrial Fibrillation Anticoagulation (CAFA) trial, Veterans' Administration Stroke Prevention in Nonrheumatic Atrial Fibrillation (SPINAF) trial, and European Atrial Fibrillation Trial (EAFT). Overall, patients on warfarin had a 64 percent reduction in stroke risk in an "intention-to-treat" analysis and an 83 percent reduction in an "on-treatment" analysis. Patients with strokes in the warfarin groups were no more likely to have hemorrhagic than ischemic strokes. The rate of major bleeding was nearly identical for the warfarin and control groups at about 2 percent; minor bleeding was three times more likely in the warfarin group.

The design of the studies varied slightly. All six studies excluded highest-risk cardiac patients; those with recent embolic events, recent myocardial infarction and significant congestive heart failure, or cardiomyopathy were not enrolled. SPAF excluded patients with lone atrial fibrillation, randomizing them to aspirin or placebo groups only because of a low stroke risk of less than 0.5 percent per year. AFASAK excluded patients with paroxysmal atrial fibrillation for the same reason. The level of anticoagulation differed slightly. AFASAK and EAFT used a prothrombin time of 1.5 to 2.0 times control, SPAF a prothrombin time of 1.3 to 1.8 times control, and CAFA, SPINAF, and BATAAF a prothrombin time of approximately 1.2 to 1.5 times control. For the control groups AFASAK used ASA 75 mg/day or placebo, SPAF and EAFT used 325 mg/day or placebo, and BATAAF allowed ASA or no treatment to be used, at the discretion of the investigators.

The AFASAK study randomized 1,007 patients over a 2-year period. The unblinded warfarin group showed an incidence rate of 2 percent per year for TIA, stroke, or systemic thromboembolism, percent compared with a 5.5 percent incidence rate in the ASA and placebo arms. Three of the five stroke patients in the warfarin group had strokes when they were off warfarin. Nonfatal bleeding occurred in 6 percent of the warfarin group (43 percent of these patients were found to have inflammatory or malignant disease) as compared with 1 percent in the control groups. A drawback to this study was that 38 percent of patients in the warfarin group dropped out, mostly because of the inconvenience of frequent blood draws.

The SPAF study randomized 1,330 patients and was terminated early at a mean follow-up period of 1.3 years. The incidence of stroke or systemic embolism was 2.3 percent in the warfarin group, 3.6 percent in the ASA group, and 7.4 percent in the placebo group. In this study as well, four of six patients with ischemic stroke in the warfarin group had strokes off therapy. Major bleeding complications were comparable in the warfarin, ASA, and placebo groups at 1.5, 1.4, and 1.6 percent respectively.

Of the 420 patients randomized in the BAATAF study, who

were followed for an average of 2.2 years, ischemic stroke occurred in the warfarin group at a rate of 0.41 percent per year and in the control group at 2.98 percent per year for a risk reduction of 86 percent. The two strokes in the warfarin group occurred at prothrombin times of less than 1.2. Among the strokes in the control group, 8 of 13 occurred in patients taking aspirin. The death rate in the warfarin group was 2.25 percent and in the control group, 5.97 percent. Two fatal hemorrhages occurred, one presumed intracerebral hematoma (ICH) in the warfarin group and a pulmonary hemorrhage in the control group. Minor bleeding occurred in 38 patients in the warfarin group and in 21 patients in the control group.

The CAFA trial was altered midway because of the superior benefit conferred by warfarin in the AFASAK and SPAF trials. Patients were then allowed open-label access to warfarin. The results from the study were then reported in an "efficacy analysis" in which endpoint events occurring more than 28 days after stopping therapy were not counted. A risk reduction of 52 percent was counted among the 378 patients randomized in the trial.

The SPINAF trial randomized 525 men to receive warfarin or placebo. This trial was the only one among the five to fully blind the warfarin assessment. A 12-hour cutoff was used to distinguish TIA from stroke. A 79 percent risk reduction was found for the warfarin group before the trial was terminated.

Only the EAFT, of the six trials discussed here, addressed secondary stroke prevention. In this study, 1,007 patients with TIA or minor ischemic stroke were randomized to receive open-label warfarin, aspirin 300 mg/day, or placebo. During the mean follow-up period of 2.3 years, 8 percent in the anticoagulation group reached an endpoint of stroke, myocardial infarction, systemic embolism, or death related to any vascular disease. By contrast, 17 percent in the placebo group reached these endpoints. The relative risk reduction for stroke alone was 66 percent. Warfarin was also found to be much more effective when compared with the aspirin group (relative risk [R] = .60; 95 percent confidence interval [95% CI] = 0.41 to 0.87).

With regular monitoring and the international normalized ratio (INR), now widely available to ascertain anticoagulation levels, warfarin has become much safer than in the early trials. The current consensus on anticoagulation, as approved by the National Heart, Lung and Blood Institute, recommends an INR range of 2.0 to 3.0 for cerebrovascular disease in the absence of cardiac valvular disease. Recent trials, including the Warfarin Aspirin Recurrent Stroke Study, are using lower INRs (1.4 to 2.8). Further testing of the efficacy of very low levels of anticoagulation is in progress.

SURGICAL INTERVENTION

Carotid endarterectomy was introduced in 1954. Although efficacy was unproven in the early years, the operation grew in popularity from 15,000 in 1971 to 105,000 in 1985. Following the 1985 trial that suggested extracranial-intracranial bypass procedure was ineffective therapy, a series of randomized clinical trials was initiated to assess the efficacy of endarterectomy. Three large multicenter trials addressed the question of operating in the setting of symptomatic carotid artery disease. Results from these trials demonstrate a 10 to 18 percent absolute reduction in stroke risk for endarterectomy in high-grade (greater than 70 percent) stenosis. Mild-to-moderate disease remains under investigation, and despite the completion of two recent randomized trials, the issue of asymptomatic carotid stenosis has not been fully resolved.

The North American Symptomatic Carotid Endarterectomy Trial drew data from 50 centers in the United States and Canada, randomizing patients to surgery and best medical therapy (mostly ASA 1,300 mg/day) or medical therapy alone. The patients were stratified to 30 to 69 percent stenosis or 70 to 99 percent stenosis documented by angiogram. After 659 patients had been randomized in the high-grade stenosis group—half the number projected as necessary to prove a 10 percent risk reduction—the study was terminated because of a dramatic therapeutic benefit favoring surgery. The cumulative risk of ipsilateral stroke at 2 years was found to be 9 percent in the surgical group and 26 percent in the medical group for a risk reduction of 17 percent. The cumulative risk of major or fatal ipsilateral stroke was 2.5 percent in the surgical group and 13.1 percent in the medical group. The risk of all strokes was 12.6 percent versus 27.6 percent, and the risk of death or major stroke was 8 percent versus 18.1 percent, for the surgical and medical groups, respectively. Average perioperative morbidity and mortality for all involved centers was 5.8 percent. Perioperative incidence of major stroke or death was 2.1 percent. The group with 30 to 69 percent stenosis is still under investigation.

Another multicenter trial, the Veterans Administration study, randomized 189 patients with greater than 50 percent internal carotid artery (ICA) stenosis to surgical plus medical therapy (ASA 325 mg) versus medical therapy alone and found similar results. At a mean follow-up of 11.9 months, crescendo TIAs and stroke were found in 7.7 percent of patients in the surgical group versus 19.4 percent in the medical group for a risk reduction of 11.7 percent. Patients with greater than 70 percent stenosis showed a risk reduction of 17.7 percent. Perioperative morbidity and mortality in this study was 5.5 percent.

The largest, longest running trial is the European Carotid Surgery Trial, which also found a striking benefit of surgical intervention for high-grade carotid stenosis among the 2,518 patients they recruited. Their comparison groups were surgery plus aspirin versus aspirin alone. The high-grade stenosis (greater than 70 percent) portion was terminated for this trial after a 9.3 percent risk reduction was noted for stroke or death in less than 30 days and a 9.6 percent reduction in stroke or death at 3 years. Recruitment continues in this study for patients with 30 to 69 percent stenosis.

The challenge of what to do with asymptomatic carotid artery disease has been addressed by three randomized trials. Overall, the evidence favors surgery; however, gender and severity of stenosis remain contentious issues. Asymptomatic bruits are present in 4 to 5 percent of the general population aged 45 to 80, but the reported risk of carotid stenosis without symptoms has varied widely in the literature. Often quoted is a relatively small study of 50 patients with greater than 50 percent stenosis: stroke occurred in 4.5 percent and TIAs in 16.5 percent. At the other extreme is a study of patients with asymptomatic stenotic carotid arteries contralateral to operated symptomatic arteries, and no strokes occurred in a 20-year follow-up period. Nonuniformity of definitions and follow-up contributes to the problem in defining risk. Radiographic evidence of prior strokes may be found in 15 to 20 percent of all stroke patients presenting with their "first" acute stroke.

An older multicenter trial of asymptomatic carotid stenosis, Carotid Artery Stenosis with Asymptomatic Narrowing: Operation Versus Aspirin (CASANOVA), randomized 410 patients to surgery and medical therapy (ASA 330 mg, dipyridamole 75 mg) versus surgery alone. Those with more than 90 percent stenosis were excluded. Their end points were stroke or death. Patients were removed from the study and operated on if a TIA occurred in the ipsilateral territory, if more than 90 percent stenosis developed, or if there was more than 50 percent bilateral disease. These investigators observed no difference between the two groups; however, the exclusion of patients with more severe arterial disease and the small number of participants left the issue unresolved.

A Veterans Administration trial of patients with greater than 50 percent carotid stenosis randomized 444 men to receive either 1,300 mg of aspirin daily or aspirin therapy plus carotid endarterectomy. Perioperative stroke or death, including angiographic complications, was 4.7 percent in the surgical group. Neurologic endpoints, which included fatal and nonfatal stroke, TIAs, and transient monocular blindness, were found in 12.8 percent of patients in the surgical group and in 24.5 percent in the medical group for a relative risk reduction of 51 percent, favoring surgery. Elimination of transient neurologic events from the analysis, however, made the differences between the two groups nonsignificant. Furthermore, when only ipsilateral events were considered, the difference between surgery and medical therapy disappeared as well.

The Asymptomatic Carotid Artery Study (ACAS) fared slightly better in defining a benefit for surgery, at least for men. In this study, 40 U.S. centers randomized 1,644 patients with greater than 60 percent ICA stenosis to receive either "best medical therapy" (usually an antiplatelet agent and agressive management of modifiable risk factors) versus best medical therapy plus endarterectomy. The aggregate risk of any stroke or death in the perioperative period was 2.3 percent. After a mean follow-up period of 2.7 years, the Kaplan-Meier projections from an intention-to-treat analysis showed the incidence of any stroke or death over 5 years to be 5.1 percent for the endarterectomy group versus 11.0 percent for patients treated with medical therapy alone over the same period. The relative risk reduction conferred by surgery was therefore 55 percent (95% CI = 23 to 73). Explanations for a fourfold difference in the relative risk reduction for men versus women in this study (69 percent versus 16 percent) awaits further analysis.

Although the two asymptomatic carotid stenosis studies appear to support a more widespread use of surgical intervention, it will remain up to the individual clinician to assess the risk versus benefit in a given individual. Supplementary laboratory data may help assess the significance of a carotid stenosis. Positive-emission tomography may identify areas of "misery perfusion" in the borderzone regions representing tissue at risk that could be better perfused after operation. Regional cerebral blood flow (rCBF) measurements may show low flow areas as well as areas of decreased vasoreactivity following CO_2 inhalation. The existence of adequate collaterals may be inferred by the reestablishment of low resistance flow in the common carotid artery on duplex Doppler (external carotid artery to ophthalmic to ICA collateral) or a reversal of flow in the anterior cerebral artery on transcranial Doppler (collateral via the anterior communicating artery).

HYPERACUTE TREATMENT OF STROKE

A major thrust of current research in stroke therapy is the treatment of the ischemic process within the first few hours after ictus. In the interval between the termination of substrate delivery to brain tissue and irreversible cell death, there may be a window of opportunity to modify what was once considered to be an inevitable pathophysiologic progression. Systemic or intra-arterial thrombolysis and hyperacute neronal protection are two lines of research that have begun to address the issue.

Although most of the therapies that follow are still in safety and dosing phases of clinical trial, such treatment modalities are likely to become standard treatment in the future.

THROMBOLYTIC THERAPY

Increasing experience with thrombolytic agents, including urokinase, streptokinase, and, more recently, recombinant tissue plasminogen activator (rtPA), has demonstrated instances of significant and sustained neurologic improvement when thrombolytic treatment is initiated within the first few hours. Better outcomes are generally associated with documented recanalization of the artery feeding the symptomatic region. What remains uncertain is whether the timing of therapy is more important than specific dose and whether delays increase the risk of complications, negating any benefits. Depleted plasminogen in the aging thrombus may reduce the thrombolytic potential of these agents after a few hours. A multicenter Phase I trial evaluated the safety and efficacy of intravenous administration of (rtPA) in the treatment of acute ischemic stroke. Patients were stratified and evaluated separately for those treated within 90 minutes and between 91 and 180 minutes of stroke onset. An open-label, dose escalation study design was used; 94 consecutive patients were treated with intravenous rtPA at one of seven doses, over 60 or 90 minutes. Subsequent use of anticoagulation was at the discretion of the investigators. Endpoints included ICH, hemorrhagic transformation without ICH, systemic hemorrhagic complication, death, major neurologic improvement at 2 and 24 hours, and neurologic deterioration. Of the 74 patients treated within 90 minutes, 32 percent had decreased level of consciousness, 37 percent had gaze deviation, and 40 percent had hemiparesis. Major neurologic improvement at 2 hours occurred in 30 percent of patients, correlating with smaller infarct size, but not with patient age, race, gender, infarct location, severity of initial deficit, or presence of edema. In 46 percent of patients there was improvement at 24 hours. Neurologic deterioration occurred in 11 percent of patients at 24 hours (two cases of ICH), and in 8 percent at 7 to 10 days. Six patients had died at 30 days and six more by 3 months. Asymptomatic bleeding occurred in 4 percent and was not dose related. Symptomatic bleeding correlated only with total dose. The three patients (4 percent) who developed ICH within 24 hours had all received doses greater than 0.85 mg/kg. Of the 20 patients treated at 91 to 180 minutes under the same study design, 2 had fatal ICH and 3 had major neurologic improvement after 24 hours. Those who died had received higher doses (0.85 or 0.95 mg/kg).

Three other studies, based on angiographic criteria for the diagnosis of arterial occlusion, used intravenous rtPA within 6 to 8 hours of onset of stroke. Recanalization was demonstrated angiographically in 20 to 50 percent of patients, asymptomatic hemorrhagic conversion in 30 to 40 percent, hemorrhage causing deterioration or death occurred in 10 percent, and good outcome clinically at 24 hours in 40 percent.

Improved neuroradiologic techniques, using urokinase or streptokinase to perform intra-arterial thrombolysis, have produced some beneficial results in a small series, renewing an interest in the use of these agents. A multicenter trial of prourokinase in acute middle cerebral artery occlusion is now underway in the United States.

Early encouraging results of thrombolytic therapy have thus far been in open-label studies and leave unsettled how well they compare with the natural history. In a recent study assessing

29 strokes within 12 hours of onset, 24 percent showed spontaneous improvement within the first hour after baseline examination, and 52 percent had improved by 18 hours after stroke onset. Spontaneous recanalization has been documented in individual cases by angiogram or by Doppler in the same time frame as that from rtPA, so eventually studies will have to involve a placebo arm. For now, the main issues of safety are being worked out in the hope that justification for placebo studies will eventually be demonstrated.

NEURONAL RESCUE

Calcium Channel Antagonists

In vitro studies and animal models have indicated a pathologic role of calcium entry in neuronal injury. Ischemia induces the release of excitatory amino acid neurotransmitters, such as glutamate and glycine, which promote calcium entry into neurons via such receptor-mediated membrane channels as the kainate, the α-amino-3-hydroxy-5-methyl-4-isoxazolepropionic acid (AMPA), and the N-methyl-D-aspartate (NMDA) channels. A variety of enzymatic reactions follows, including those mediated by calmodulin. Destruction of neurofilaments, disruption of cell membrane integrity and consequent cell death most likely result from the production of nitric oxide and the subsequent formation of other free radicals. The NMDA channel has at least six sites that may be susceptible to pharmacologic blockade. The glutamate recognition site has been blocked experimentally by the compound CGS-19755, the glycine site by HA-966, the "upper competitive site" by MK-801, NS-1102, and d-Methorphan, the polyamine site by Ifenprofil, and another competitive site by Mg^{2+}. At a sixth site—a site of phosphorylation—no antagonist has yet been identified. Enzymatic inhibition of nitric oxide synthetase by N-nitro-L-arginine also appears to protect against glutamate neurotoxicity. The efficacy of these agents in humans awaits clinical trials.

Voltage-dependent calcium channel antagonists are the only agents that, thus far, have reached the stage of clinical trials. Verapamil, diltiazem, and nifedipine have poor brain penetration and were never considered viable candidates for cerebral protection. Nicardipine was evaluated in a small Phase I trial: 35 patients were randomized to receive 3 to 7 mg/kg/h IV infusion versus placebo. All patients showed improvement, with a slight difference favoring nicardipine. No further studies have been performed.

The greatest experience to date has been with nimodipine, which has fewer systemic effects than the other calcium channel blockers and penetrates the blood-brain barrier well. In a large multicenter trial of subarachnoid hemorrhage, infarction was reduced by 34 percent and poor outcome by 40 percent. Early trials for ischemic stroke, using nimodipine 120 mg/day, showed decreased mortality when treatment was administered within 24 hours of stroke onset, but no significant difference in long-term functional recovery. The largest trial, conducted by the Nimodipine Study Group, enrolled 1,064 patients for 21 days in doses of 60 mg, 120 mg, or 240 mg/day compared to placebo. Heparin was allowed in cases of suspected cardioembolic stroke. Exclusion criteria included intracranial hemorrhage and significant comorbidity. Although no significant differences in mortality or neurologic function were seen across the groups for the overall cohort treated within 48 hours of stroke, subgroup analysis of those patients treated with 120 mg/day within 18 hours of stroke onset showed significantly better outcome scores and a 30 percent reduction in worsening frequency. Benefit also correlated with negative initial brain computed tomography (CT) scan.

Although only this trial among nine double-blind, placebo-controlled studies showed such significant benefit, the numbers of those treated early in the other trials was too small for individual analysis. A meta-analysis of all nine trials, totaling 3,714 patients, indicated a benefit for those receiving early therapy: the 616 patients treated within 12 hours showed a pooled odds ratio of 0.62 favoring nimodipine (95% CI, 0.44 to 0.87). No effect on outcome was seen for age, sex, hypertension, diabetes, or cardiac disease. There was no drug effect for those treated 13 to 24 hours, and a slightly worse outcome for those treated after 24 hours. Further studies appear to be in order, but at the least, useful therapy seems in the offing. Of especial note is that the human studies corroborate the animal models, which emphasize the importance of early intervention.

Other Neuroprotective Agents

Currently, clinical trials around the world have begun to test the potential benefits of a variety of other neuroprotective agents. Table 44-1 lists some agents currently under investigation. Most will fail to prove efficacious; others will produce unmanageable side-effect profiles. At this time, the appearance of white matter vacuolar changes, apparently produced by the NMDA antagonists, has halted some of the clinical trials. Enthusiasm for the development of new agents is unlikely to wane in the near future, however, since the weight of preclinical evidence suggests that neuroprotection is possible, and the therapeutic implications that such evidence brings to the clinical arena is monumental.

INTERVENTIONAL NEUROVASCULAR PROCEDURES

Interventional neurovascular techniques have evolved rapidly in recent years to allow superselective arterial catheterization into previously inaccessible sites. The success of balloon angioplasty in the treatment of coronary and peripheral vascular disease has stimulated interest in the treatment of cerebrovascular conditions and stroke. Increasing experience with superselective catheterization procedures in the treatment of surgically inaccessible aneurysms and arteriovenous malformations has been extended to the investigational use of endovascular procedures for ischemic cerebrovascular disease in the treatment of acute stroke. Three areas currently under investigation include (1) the treatment of cerebral vasospasm secondary to subarachnoid hemorrhage with balloon angioplasty and pharmacologic antispasmodic agents, (2) percutaneous transluminal angioplasty for extracranial and intracranial stenoses, and (3) the local intra-arterial delivery of thrombolytic agents for acute stroke. The safety and effectiveness of these procedures has not been established in scientifically designed studies, but growing experience with these techniques suggest their potential benefits. Clinical trials will undoubtedly soon be organized to assess the clinical indications, safety, and potential benefits of these procedures.

RECOMMENDATIONS FOR MANAGEMENT

From the outset of the encounter with an acute stroke patient, the conscientious clinician must accrue sufficient data to make informed and timely management decisions. Settling the diagnosis of stroke subtype is no longer pro forma but can help predict likely outcome and direct therapy. From the history, TIAs, hypertension, glucose level, cardiac disease, and stroke subtype predict recurrence. Particular attention should be paid

TABLE 44-1. Investigational Neuroprotective Agents for Acute Stroke

Agent	Putative Mechanism	Status
Ramacemide (Fisons)	NMDA antagonist-noncompetitive	Phase II
Dextromethorphan	NMDA antagonist-noncompetitive	Phase I
Dizoclipine (MK-801)	NMDA antagonist-noncompetitive	Canceled
CNS 1102 (Cambridge Neuroscience)	NMDA antagonist-noncompetitive	Phase II
Eliprodil (Lorex)	NMDA antagonist-noncompetitive	Planned phase II
CGS 19755 (Ciba-Geigy)	NMDA and glutamate antagonist	Planned phase III
Lubeluzole (Janssen)	Inhibitor of glutamate-activated NOS pathway	Planned phase I
Tiralazide (Upjohn)	Free radical scavenger	Phase II
Nimodipine (Bayer)	Voltage-dependent calcium channel antagonist	Phase III completed
Nicardipine	Voltage-dependent calcium channel antagonist	Canceled
PY 108-068	Voltage-dependent calcium channel antagonist	Canceled
Pertussis toxin	Voltage-dependent calcium channel antagonist	Preclinical
γ-Conopeptide GVIA (Zeneca)	Presynaptic calcium antagonist	Preclinical

Abbreviations: NMDA, *N*-methyl-D-aspartate; NOS, nitric oxide synthetase.

to indicators of cardioembolic sources, such as recent myocardial infarction, arrhythmias, or congestive heart failure. Headache suggests subarachnoid bleeding in the absence of focal signs, while in the latter setting lobar hemorrhage is more common than ischemic stroke. Pain in the neck, side of face, teeth or jaw, or retro-orbital area may indicate vertebral or carotid artery dissection, even without a history of neck trauma.

The physical examination can give an impression of the size and and a fair estimate of the location of the infarct, and thus guide the urgency of subsequent management steps. Hemiparesis and forced gaze deviation suggests a large hemispheral or critical brainstem lesion, particularly if accompanied by decreased level of consciousness, whereas hemiparesis involving face, arm, and leg in an alert patient suggests a small, deep lesion involving a confluence of motor fibers. When isolated, behavioral abnormalities such as aphasia or hemineglect without a gaze preference suggest smaller hemispheral lesions. General examination may reveal a carotid bruit, and physical examination and an electrocardiogram may reveal an arrhythmia or signs of cardiomyopathy or congestive heart failure.

Magnetic resonance imaging (MRI) should identify all but the smallest lesions and is superior to the CT for brainstem and small, deep, so-called lacunar infarcts. CT scans are the equal of MRI in documenting an infarct within the first hours and are better for a diagnosis of acute hemorrhage or bony abnormalities. Either technology may miss an infarct within the first several hours of onset. Data collected should suggest stroke etiology. From 15 to 30 percent of strokes are embolic from a cardiac source such as atrial fibrillation or valvular disease. Although 5 to 6 percent of patients may have a fluctuating course, the classical clinical presentation of cardioembolic stroke is of sudden deficit, maximal at onset. Syndromes more likely to be embolic include hemianopia without hemiparesis, pure Wernicke aphasia, and ideomotor apraxia. CT and MRI that show a single cortical branch territory infarct also are consistent with an embolic source because atheroma rarely extends out onto the surface vessels, although the source of the inferred embolus may not be readily apparent even after full evaluation. Mainstem branch occlusions are also often embolic, but local atherostenosis is a possibility in such a setting as well. One difficult pitfall on initial CT is the deep-lying lucency involving the internal capsule and basal ganglia of some 2 to 3 cm in size, apparently sparing cortex, which can be labeled as a large lacune. Often such instances are also of embolic origin, involving several lenticulostriate branches of the middle cerebral artery from temporary occlusion of the middle cerebral stem,

followed by rapid collateralization from anterior or posterior cerebral branches or recanalization of the occlusion with distal migration of the embolus. A right-to-left shunt, usually a patent cardiac foramen ovale, can be inferred when transcranial Doppler shows microbubbles in the intracranial vessels after injection of 10 ml of agitated saline in the antecubital vein and contrast transesophageal or standard transthoracic echocardiography usually can find the defect in the cardiac atrial wall or mitral valve prolapse. Holter monitoring may infer a cardiac emboligenic source by documenting atrial fibrillation.

In 15 percent of cases, severe large vessel atherosclerosis is present and seems to be responsible for the stroke. It is best appreciated when there is severe extracranial internal carotid stenosis or occlusion and the "distal field" lesion is imaged on CT scan or MRI as an infarct high over the convexity, spreading caudally from the borderzone between arterial territories. The most common clinical profile of this type of infarct is fractional arm weakness (shoulder different from hand). Male gender, hypertension, and diabetes mellitus appear significantly more often in this group than in patients with cardioembolic stroke. Although the standard angiogram most reliably demonstrates large vessel stenosis, when it is severe enough to be of hemodynamic significance, duplex Doppler usually readily delineates the severity of the internal carotid stenosis and shows high-velocity, turbulent flow. Intracranial ICA stenosis may produce detectable high resistance flow on Doppler examinations of the extracranial carotid. Transcranial Doppler often shows dampened pulsatility in the ipsilateral middle cerebral artery. Duplex Doppler, in combination with magnetic resonance angiography, is rapidly becoming a reliable alternative to the more invasive traditional angiogram. Cerebral blood flow measurements with xenon CT, single-photon emission computed tomography, and rCBF techniques are also being used to evaluate regional hypoperfusion.

In perhaps 15 percent of all stroke, large vessel atherosclerosis with less than hemodynamic stenosis (less than 80 percent occluded or with an ulcerated plaque) occurs in the absence of a cardioembolic source, and the etiology of artery-to-artery embolus is inferred. Embolic fragments may arise from atherosclerotic lesions in the ICA, the basilar artery, intracranial large vessels, the proximal stump of an occluded carotid, or the distal tail of a thrombus in an occluded ICA. Distinguishing intra-arterial embolism from possible cardioembolic etiology may be difficult; however, the former usually produces a smaller cortical infarct, and the latter is more often associated with a decreased level of consciousness and an abnormal initial CT scan.

Small deep lesions in the subcortical white matter, the thalamus, the basal ganglia, or the pons accompanied by an appropriate clinical syndrome suggest lacunar disease, accounting for 15 to 20 percent of all stroke. Arteriolar wall lipohyalinosis, microatheroma, or even microembli may produce the pathology. Early studies described only a handful of classic syndromes, but case reports have expanded the number to more than 70. Positive scans in the capsule, adjacent corona radiata, thalamus or pons have been reported for clumsy hand-dysarthria, ataxic hemiparesis, and hemiballism; pure sensory syndromes have been associated with small thalamic lesions. CT scanning is positive in only half of lacunar strokes, with MRI increasing the yield somewhat. Larger lacunes are more often symptomatic. Hypertension is the risk factor most associated with lacunar infarction.

Despite efforts to arrive at a diagnosis, the cause of infarction in up to 40 percent of cases remains undetermined. This may result from an inability to perform appropriate laboratory studies because of the patient's advanced age or comorbidity, or because of unwillingness on the part of the physician or patient. It may also result from improper timing of tests, such as an angiogram performed after an embolus has cleared, or a CT scan or MRI performed before the infarction appears. In a majority of these cases, however, appropriate testing done at the proper time produces normal or ambiguous findings. Evaluation of patients classified as infarct of undetermined cause in the Stroke Data Bank revealed certain common features. They tended not to have prior TIAs, infarcts, carotid bruits, or cardiac risk factors; 57 percent had clinically relevant CT images; surface infarcts were found in 40 percent; hemispheral syndromes predominated in 66 percent, and basilar syndromes occurred in 15 percent; 27 percent worsened in the hospital, and 41 percent had moderate to severe weakness. Some of these cases may be explained by hypercoagulable states from protein C, free protein S, fibrinogen, lupus anticoagulant, or anticardiolipin antibody abnormalities. Paradoxical emboli through a patent foramen ovale may explain other cases. Migraine, meningitis, dissection, arteritis, or inherited metabolic abnormality may explain rare cases. Rather than force a classification into one of the four established categories, we recommend maintaining the classification of infarct of undetermined cause (or "cryptogenic infarction") until a definite cause can be established.

SUMMARY OF PRESENT PRACTICE

1. All patients with suspected stroke in which a deficit persists for more than 1 hour should undergo a CT or MRI head scan. Subsequent investigation is directed toward identifying stroke etiology.
2. If the clinical picture and CT scan/MRI appearances are consistent with a small or moderate-sized ischemic stroke, heparin should be administered by intravenous infusion until the stroke subtype is determined, maintaining an INR of 1.4 to 2.8. This treatment may also be given if there is minor, but only minor, hemorrhagic infarction on brain imaging.
3. If the stroke is large and disabling, there is greater risk of hemorrhagic transformation; brain imaging should be repeated 48 to 72 hours after stroke onset and anticoagulation started only if hemorrhagic conversion has not occurred. If the clinical and imaging diagnosis is intracranial hemorrhage, anticoagulants and antiplatelet agents should not be given.

4. Investigation of stroke etiology should focus first on cardioembolic sources and large vessel atherothrombosis. Transthoracic echogardiography, carotid duplex Doppler, and transcranial Doppler should be performed in nearly all cases. Magnetic resonance angiography and transesophageal echocardiography may deliver a diagnosis when the aforementioned studies are inconclusive.
5. Patients with recent myocardial infarction, atrial fibrillation, valvular disease, or intracardiac thrombus should be orally anticoagulated for at least 1 year. The prothrombin time should be kept at 1.2 to 2.5 times control (INR = 2.0 to 3.0). If there is atrial fibrillation, warfarin should be continued indefinitely, provided that reliable monitoring is available.
6. If the stroke is small, the heart is normal, and a duplex Doppler sonogram shows significant carotid stenosis (greater than 70 percent), intravenous heparin should be continued until the exact degree of stenosis has been determined by digital subtraction angiography or magnetic resonance angiography (if available). Prophylactic endarterectomy for patients with greater than 70 percent stenosis should be undertaken as soon as possible. For patients with lesser degrees of stenosis, Doppler monitoring should be undertaken at intervals of 3, 6, or 12 months to document those whose stenosis increases to more than 70 percent, which qualifies them for surgery. Patients in whom asymptomatic carotid stenosis greater than 60 percent is identified should be considered for endarterectomy, provided the operation is performed at a center where the perioperative morbidity and mortality is less than 3 percent.
7. If no cardioembolic source or operable carotid stenosis in identified, and the patient is not considered at risk for hemorrhage, antiplatelet treatment with aspirin 325 mg daily should be prescribed as chronic outpatient therapy. Ticlopidine may also be considered, particularly if the patient is female or has failed aspirin therapy. Close attention to the neutrophil count is essential when using ticlopidine.

SUGGESTED READINGS

Alberts GW: Role of ticlopidine for prevention of stroke. Stroke 23:912, 1992

The American Nimodipine Study Group: Clinical trial of nimodipine in acute ischemic stroke. Stroke 23:3, 1992

Barnett HJM: Aspirin in stroke prevention: an overview. Stroke 21(suppl. IV): IV40, 1990

Boysen G: Anticoagulation for atrial fibrillation and stroke prevention. Neuroepidemiology 12:280, 1993

Endarterectomy for Asymptomatic Carotid Artery Stenosis: Executive Committee for the Asymptomatic Carotid Atherosclerosis Study. JAMA 273:1421, 1995

Choi DW: Cerebral hypoxia: some new approaches and unanswered questions. J Neurosci 10:2493, 1990

Easton JD, Wilterdink JL: Carotid endarterectomy trials and tribulations. Ann Neurol 35:5, 1994

European Atrial Fibrillation Trial (EAFT) Study Group: Secondary prevention in non-rheumatic atrial fibrillation after transient ischaemic attack or minor stroke. Lancet 342:1251, 1993

Higashida RT, Halbach VV, Tsai FY, Dowd CF, Hieshima GB. Interventional neurovascular techniques for cerebral revascularization in the treatment of stroke. AJR 163:793, 1994

North American Symptomatic Carotid Endarterectomy Trial Collaborators: Beneficial effect of carotid endarterectomy in symptomatic patients with high-grade carotid stenosis. N Engl J Med 325:452, 1991

Rothman SM, Olney JW: Glutamate and the pathophysiology of hypoxic-ischemic brain damage. Ann Neurol 19:105, 1986

Sherman DG, Dyken ML, Fisher M et al: Antithrombotic therapy for cerebrovascular disorders. Chest 102:529S, 1992

von Kummer R, Hacke W: Safety and efficacy of intravenous tissue plasminogen activator and heparin in acute middle cerebral artery stroke. Stroke 23:646, 1992

IMMUNE AND INFECTIOUS DISEASE

PART III

SECTION 1. IMMUNE-MEDIATED DISEASES

45. MULTIPLE SCLEROSIS

LOREN A. ROLAK

Multiple sclerosis (MS) is the most common disabling neurologic disease of young people, afflicting at least a quarter of a million Americans. The symptoms of MS result from recurrent attacks of inflammation in the central nervous system (CNS), and there is very strong, although circumstantial, evidence that it is an autoimmune disorder. The target of the immune attack is myelin, the lipoprotein sheath that surrounds the axons and provides extremely efficient insulation, which enhances nerve conduction. The white matter of the brain takes its name from the glistening white appearance of this lipid wrapping and contains most of the tracts, pathways, and axonal projections of the CNS; the gray matter contains primarily the cell bodies of the neurons themselves. Inflammation and damage to the myelin (which is made by cells called oligodendrocytes) interrupts nerve conduction and thus nerve function, thereby producing the symptoms of MS.

EPIDEMIOLOGY

Multiple sclerosis favors women over men by a ratio of nearly 2 to 1, and strikes most often between the ages of 20 and 40, with a peak at age 30. Caucasians are especially vulnerable, particularly those of northern European extraction and those living in northern latitudes, where the incidence of the disease is highest, but the "melting pot" of America is so intermixed and geographically mobile that these epidemiologic features provide little useful information to the clinician. While clearly not inherited in any direct fashion, it tends to cluster slightly within families—there is a 1 to 3 percent risk of developing MS if a parent or sibling has the disease, and a 25 percent concordance among monozygotic twins.

CLINICAL FEATURES

Variability and diversity characterize the symptoms and presentation of MS. There is virtually no neurologic complaint that has not been traced to MS at one time or another, and a comprehensive account of its clinical features can become nothing more than a mere recitation of a positive neurologic review of systems. The most common symptoms are as follows:

Weakness or numbness in one or more limbs
Optic neuritis: painful loss of vision in one eye
Tremor and incoordination, especially of gait, from cerebellar dysfunction
Double vision, dysarthria, or vertigo, from brainstem dysfunction
Bowel or bladder dysfunction
Fatigue

Some symptoms, however, reflecting primarily gray matter damage, occur so rarely that their appearance casts doubt on the diagnosis of MS, for example:

Dementia, lethargy, or other altered mental status
Aphasia
Seizures, syncope, or loss of consciousness
Pain
Dystonia, chorea, or other involuntary movements
Muscle atrophy or fasciculations

Most symptoms of MS are focal, representing the inflammation of a specific tract or pathway within the CNS, such as monocular visual loss from optic neuritis, weakness or numbness in one or more limbs from damage to the spinal cord, or ataxia and tremors from lesions in the cerebellar pathways. Diffuse, nonfocal symptoms occur less commonly, for example, dementia, confusion, syncope, and vague dizziness. An exception to this rule is fatigue—an overwhelming sense of exhaustion and lassitude that often accompanies focal symptoms of MS.

Most symptoms develop abruptly, within minutes or hours. These exacerbations or "attacks" of MS typically last 6 to 8 weeks from onset to recovery and involve multiple areas of the CNS simultaneously, producing a polysymptomatic presentation. Resolution is often complete. However, the pattern of presentation, like so many features of MS, is highly variable, and symptoms may fluctuate considerably or even progress with little resolution. Attacks strike approximately every 14 to 16 months (or about 0.7 attacks per year). In many patients, over a span of 5 to 10 years, the attacks begin more indolently, persist more chronically, and remit less completely, transforming into a pattern of steady deterioration rather than episodic flares. The temporal profile of symptoms is so unpredictable, however, and patients may fluctuate so readily from a progressive course to a recovering one and back again, that traditional labels such as "exacerbating-remitting" and "chronic-progressive" are not very useful.

PROGNOSIS

MS is seldom fatal, and the life expectancy is shortened only by months; concerns about prognosis center primarily on the quality of life and prospects for disability. Most patients and clinicians harbor an unfounded view of MS as a relentlessly progressive, inevitably disabling disease. In fact, 15 years after the onset of MS, 20 percent of patients may be bedridden or institutionalized, another 20 percent may require a wheelchair, crutches, or a cane to ambulate, but 60 percent will be ambulatory without assistance and may have little deficit at all. Probably one-third of all MS victims go through life without any persistent disability and with only intermittent, transient episodes of symptoms. The following factors predict a good prognosis in MS:

Young age at onset
Sensory symptoms at onset (numbness, paresthesias, visual loss)
Rapid resolution of initial symptoms
Benign course during the first 5 years

A patient who has accumulated little disability after 5 to 7 years is unlikely ever to do so.

DIAGNOSIS

MS is among the most difficult of all diseases to diagnose because of the bewildering number of symptoms it causes and the multiple ways they can present. The "typical" MS patient is a young woman with abrupt, focal neurologic symptoms occurring discretely or in combinations, lasting weeks to months and then resolving, with new or recurrent symptoms developing months to years later. A definite diagnosis may be difficult or indeed impossible when the situation is not "typical," that is, when the patient is older, when symptoms are strictly progressive, or when there has been only one episode of neurologic dysfunction. Tests can buttress the clinical diagnosis of MS, but no laboratory findings are specific for MS, and all have pitfalls that limit their usefulness.

Magnetic resonance imaging (MRI) is a highly sensitive but disappointingly nonspecific technique for visualizing the inflammatory lesions of MS, which appear as multiple, irregular, confluent areas of increased signal intensity, ranging in size from 0.5 to 3.0 cm, scattered deep within the brain, especially around the ventricles (Fig. 45-1). Nearly 90 percent of patients with definite MS have abnormal MRI scans, and various analyses have shown that MRI of the head should be the first test performed to evaluate suspected MS patients. A major disadvantage of MRI remains it lack of specificity, since many conditions mimic MS on MRI. While it is a sensitive, noninvasive technique, it is also nonspecific and frequently detects "abnormalities" in patients without clear pathology, thus inappropriately labeling many patients with the diagnosis of MS. The use of MRI requires considerable expertise, and overdiagnosis of MS based on MRI changes occurs too frequently.

Abnormalities in the cerebrospinal fluid (CSF) are sufficiently common and characteristic to make CSF analysis accurate for the diagnosis of MS. Spinal fluid protein and white blood cell counts are occasionally mildly elevated, but the most useful findings are immunologic changes, including an increase in the immunoglobulin G (IgG) level and synthesis rate. Immunoglobulins in the spinal fluid, presumably reflecting an underlying autoimmune activation, appear as distinct oligoclonal bands when electrophoresed. The pattern formed by these bands varies from patient to patient, but they are present in some form in nearly 90 percent of all MS patients, and other diseases that produce similar banding are seldom mistaken for MS. The major obstacle to the use of CSF for the diagnosis of MS is the reluctance of patients to undergo lumbar puncture.

Evoked potentials play a limited, but occasionally useful, role in the diagnosis of MS. Evoked potentials measure conduction along specific CNS pathways by recording the electroencephalographic response to visual, auditory, or sensory (electrical) stimulation; a slowing in conduction is presumed to reflect inflammation and demyelination in that pathway, thus detecting an asymptomatic or subclinical MS lesion. The sensitivity and specificity of these techniques do not approach those of the MRI or cerebrospinal fluid (CSF), but they can often reveal unsuspected lesions or confirm an organic basis for vague complaints, and thereby heighten the probability of MS.

The following is a nonexhaustive list of diseases that often mimic MS:

1. Hysteria and somatization disorders
2. Postviral demyelination (acute disseminated encephalomyelitis)
3. Vasculitis affecting the central nervous system (either primarily or secondary to other conditions, such as lupus erythematosus, Sjögren syndrome, or polyarteritis nodosa)
4. Spinocerebellar degenerations
5. Spirochetal infections: Lyme disease or syphilis
6. Sarcoidosis
7. Retroviral infections: acquired immune deficiency syndrome, human T-cell lymphotrophic virus-1
8. Stroke in the young
9. Inherited white matter diseases (leukodystrophies)
10. Tumors: metastases, lymphoma
11. Syringomyelia

A diagnosis of definite MS can be made by fulfilling six clinical criteria:

1. The patient must have two separate central nervous system lesions.
2. The symptoms must have occurred in two or more separate episodes.
3. The symptoms must involve the white matter, not the gray matter.
4. The neurologic examination must show objective abnormalities.
5. The patient must be between ages 10 and 50, but preferably between 20 and 40.
6. The patient must have no other disease accounting for the symptoms.

If all clinical criteria are not met, a diagnosis of definite MS can still be made using laboratory support:

1. Two attacks with only one lesion, plus abnormal spinal fluid oligoclonal bands
2. One attack with two lesions, plus abnormal spinal fluid

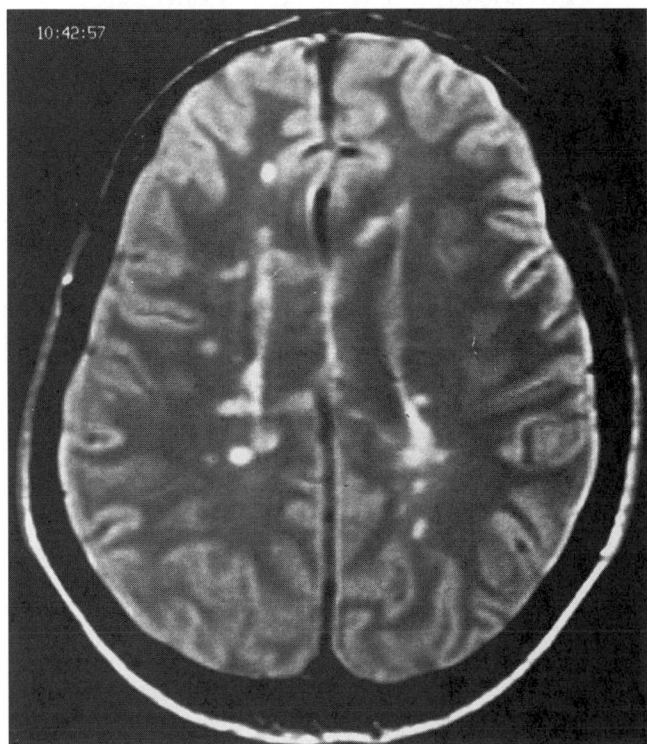

FIG. 45-1. MRI of the brain (using a T2-weighted technique) showing the typical multiple, scattered, and periventricular signal abnormalities of multiple sclerosis.

3. One attack with one lesion, plus abnormal spinal fluid and abnormal MRI

Because of the many pitfalls and nuances in diagnosing MS, and the implications of this diagnosis for future disability, employability, insurance, and lifestyle planning for the patient, most patients suspected of having MS should be referred to a neurologist for confirmation of that diagnosis.

TREATMENT

Multiple sclerosis should be attacked on two fronts: treatment to suppress the disease itself and alter its natural history, and treatment to improve the symptoms of MS and mask the deficits it causes.

Steroid therapy suppresses MS by inhibiting the immune system and reducing inflammation. Despite a solid scientific rationale for its use, steroid therapy remains empirical, with considerable controversy as to the most effective type of steroids, route of administration, and duration of therapy. For mild attacks of MS, oral steroids may be given as prednisone 60 mg PO qd for 7 to 10 days or, more commonly, as a Medrol dosepak in a preplanned tapered regimen. For more severe MS attacks, or chronically progressing symptoms, standard treatment employs high doses of methylprednisolone (Solu-Medrol) 500 to 1,000 mg IV drip (such as with 500 ml D_5W) for several consecutive days (usually 3 to 5 days), often followed by an oral taper. Despite several properties that might benefit MS patients, steroids probably do not in fact alter the fundamental pathology of MS to any great degree, and, although they often rapidly improve attacks, they seem ineffective in changing the natural history of the disease or preventing ultimate disability.

β-Interferon has received provisional approval from the Food and Drug Administration for use in ambulatory patients with frequent attacks of MS, based on positive results from a large controlled trial (and in spite of negative results from several smaller ones) that indicated the drug can affect the underlying pathophysiology of MS and alter its natural history by minimizing the frequency and severity of attacks. Although it is not clear which of the complex immunoregulatory actions of β-interferon produces therapeutic effects in MS patients, it may provide benefits by stimulating the function of suppressor T cells, thus enhancing immune suppression. The drug is self-administered in subcutaneous injections every other day (although other forms of β-interferon are being developed using different regimens). Patients do not improve while on the drug, but therapy seems to reduce the rate of attacks and the volume of MRI lesions. These benefits are modest, however, and there is no major effect on disability within the first few years of treatment. Initially, the scarce availability of β-interferon, which is produced by recombinant DNA technology, slowed its introduction, and the high incidence of side effects (nausea, fevers, myalgias, and debilitating malaise) has further limited its usefulness. At this time, β-interferon therapy not a practical option for many patients with MS, although its ultimate role awaits the introduction of additional, modified β-interferons and further testing on other groups of MS patients.

Other immunologically based treatments for MS are under investigation at a variety of centers throughout the country, including promising studies on copolymer-I, a myelinlike peptide also capable of delaying or preventing MS attacks. The

TABLE 45-1. Commonly Used Treatments for the Symptoms of Multiple Sclerosis

Spasticity	Baclofen (Lioresal) 10 to 40 mg tid
Tremor/ataxia	Clonazepam (Klonopin) 0.5 to 2.0 mg bid
Paresthesias	Amitriptyline (Elavil, Endep) 75 to 150 mg qhs
Fatigue	Amantadine (Symmetrel) 100 mg bid
Spastic bladder	Oxybutynin (Ditropan) 5 mg qd to qid

National Multiple Sclerosis Society maintains a registry of research protocols to which patients may be referred.

In the absence of a cure for MS, patient management often emphasizes symptomatic treatment, usually with considerable improvement in the quality of life. Table 45-1 summarizes the most useful treatments for the major symptoms of MS.

Spasticity refers to the tightness, muscle spasms, and increased tone commonly seen, especially in the legs, as a disabling symptom in MS victims with spinal cord damage. Although the stiffness often impairs ambulation, alleviation of spasticity seldom results in a dramatic improvement in walking, but rather is most helpful for patients with flexor spasm and pain, to improve transfers, minimize decubiti, and enhance self-care. Therapeutic expectations should be modest. Baclofen (Lioresal), diazepam (Valium), and dantrolene (Dantrium), all effectively reduce spasticity, but, primarily for reasons of toxicity, baclofen is the preferred drug. Treatment can start as 10 mg tid and increase up to 40 mg tid or qid. Sedation is the main limiting side effect.

The tremor caused from cerebellar damage produces major disability and stubbornly resists any therapy. Drugs that enhance γ-aminobutyric acid (GABA), the primary inhibitory neurotransmitter of the cerebellum, have produced sporadic successes and warrant a therapeutic trial. Clonazepam (Klonopin) is the most useful agent, starting in doses of 0.5 mg bid and increasing gradually as permitted by the sedative side effects. Isoniazid (INH) in doses of 900 to 1,200 mg daily has shown benefit in several studies, but the hepatic and peripheral nerve toxicity, and the need to closely monitor laboratory abnormalities, diminish the enthusiasm for this drug. Modest improvement can occasionally result from the use of more nonspecific CNS depressants, such as propranolol (80 mg or more daily, in a long-acting format), or primidone (Mysoline, in doses of 250 mg bid or more).

The neurogenic bladder, which commonly accompanies MS, usually causes considerable distress and embarrassment for patients, and restoration of normal continence provides welcome improvement in their quality of life. Urologic symptoms should be specifically inquired about, to penetrate patients' natural reticence about the subject, but, because of the complexities of neurologic bladder control, specific testing and management is best left to a knowledgeable urologist. The same advice applies to sexual dysfunction, another frequent problem.

The fatigue of MS produces considerable disability and is the primary reason why most patients quit their jobs. This malaise and lack of energy can usually be differentiated from the depression commonly seen in MS patients by its characteristic dramatic worsening with heat, and its description as an overwhelming exhaustion that actually prevents any sustained physical activity. Commonsense measures help allay this fatigue, such as daytime naps, and it also responds, for completely mysterious reasons, to amantadine (Symmetrel) 100 mg PO bid.

Finally, psychological support and patient rapport are crucial to the management of MS. Careful studies suggest that most patients wish to be told their diagnosis as soon as it is suspected. Most patients also, understandably, want to participate in their own treatment and to do anything they can to help themselves. In this regard, it is frustrating that the two areas of greatest concern to most patients have little effect on MS, namely, diet and exercise. Nutritionally, there are no foods or supplements to be enhanced or avoided, despite a proliferation of "MS diets" in the lay literature. Similarly, a good general exercise regimen is as desirable for MS patients as for any other person, but, beyond a general maintenance of fitness, exercise has no effect on MS itself. In fact, the increased body heat often produces at least transient worsening of symptoms.

SUGGESTED READINGS

Ebers GC: Treatment of multiple sclerosis. Lancet 343:275, 1994

ffrench-Constant C: Pathogenesis of multiple sclerosis. Lancet 343:271, 1994

Reingold SC: Advances in the understanding and treatment of multiple sclerosis. J Neuroimmunol 44:221, 1993

Rolak L: Prognosis of multiple sclerosis. In Evans R, Yatsu F, Baskin D (eds): Prognosis of Neurologic Disease. Oxford University Press, Oxford, UK, 1992

Weinstock-Guttman B, Ransohoff RM, Kinkel RP, Rudick RA: The interferons: biological effects, mechanisms of action, and use in multiple sclerosis. Ann Neurol 37:7, 1995

46. OPTIC NEURITIS

SILVIA ORENGO-NANIA

Optic neuritis, which is a syndrome rather than a primary disease, results from inflammation of the optic nerve and leads to sudden, painful loss of vision in one eye. A variety of disorders can cause optic neuritis, usually demyelinating disease such as multiple sclerosis. However, in most cases optic neuritis is a monosymptomatic event without any identifiable underlying etiology. Optic neuritis is the most common cause of neurogenic vision loss in patients under the age of 50 (Table 46-1).

CLINICAL PRESENTATION

Optic neuritis attacks women nearly twice as often as men. It involves young adults most frequently; the average age of onset is 30, and it is rarely seen in patients over 50. Caucasians are

TABLE 46-1. Differential Diagnosis of Sudden Vision Loss

Painful causes
  Optic neuritis
  Trauma
  Migraine
  Angle closure glaucoma
  Giant cell arteritis
Nonpainful causes
  Central retinal artery occlusion
  Central retinal vein occlusion
  Retinal detachment
  Optic nerve tumor
  Anterior ischemic optic neuropathy
  Vitreous hemorrhage
  Toxin (quinine, methanol, ethambutol)
  Hysteria
  Ophthalmic artery occlusion
  Occipital lobe stroke

affected eight times more often than any other racial group, while African-Americans are rarely afflicted.

The inflammation of the optic nerve destroys many aspects of visual function in patients with optic neuritis. At presentation, the visual acuity may range from normal to complete blindness, but usually the visual loss begins slowly, followed by a precipitous drop. It remains poor for days to weeks and then begins to improve steadily over weeks to months. During the attack, approximately one-third of patients maintain good vision (20/40 vision or better), one-third develop moderate visual impairment (20/50 to 20/190), and one-third suffer severe loss of vision (worse than 20/200). However, vision ultimately recovers to 20/50 or better in almost 95 percent of patients regardless of the extent of visual loss or type of treatment administered. Contrast sensitivity and color vision are also impaired in almost all patients, and usually remain at least somewhat abnormal following resolution of the visual acuity. Patients may complain of other associated visual aberrations, including the Riddoch phenomenon (the ability to see moving objects better than static objects), and Uhthoff's phenomenon (the worsening of visual function with increased body temperature, for example, during exercise).

Pain accompanies optic neuritis in over 90 percent of patients and may precede or occur simultaneously with the loss of vision. As the vision worsens, the pain tends to abate. Characteristically, eye movements aggravate the pain.

Pupillary involvement is inevitable and takes the form of an afferent pupillary defect (also called a Marcus-Gunn pupil). This is best demonstrated with a bright light source in a dim room. The light is shown in the normal eye first and then quickly flashed to the affected eye. In a normal patient, the pupil constricts in the normal eye with exposure to the light and a consensual constriction is seen in the opposite eye. When the light is then quickly shifted to the opposite eye, it will constrict in a normal patient but will appear to dilate in a patient with optic neuritis. This dilation occurs because the inflamed optic nerve cannot respond to light, and the pupil passively enlarges, consensually with the opposite, normal pupil. An afferent pupillary defect is seen in essentially all cases of optic neuritis.

The appearance of the optic nerve at the onset of the disease can vary from completely normal to papillitis (disc edema with surrounding hemorrhage and cotton wool patches). Most patients develop inflammation in the retrobulbar portion of the optic nerve so the disc appears normal; only one-third of patients will show classic disc edema. In all cases of optic neuritis, whether bulbar or retrobulbar, the late optic nerve findings include generalized or temporal optic nerve pallor, which persists permanently despite visual recovery.

Visual field abnormalities take many forms. The classic visual field defect is a central scotoma. However, altitudinal, nasal step, paracentral, enlarged blind spot, hemianopic, and arcuate defects may appear.

Interestingly, the opposite eye may also show some decrease in visual function on formal ophthalmologic testing, but patients usually complain of only unilateral symptoms. Most fellow eye abnormalities resolve quickly. Significant bilateral optic neuritis is unusual in adults, but is seen more commonly in children, especially when secondary to a viral infection. However, new attacks of optic neuritis, in the affected eye or the opposite eye, can occur in up to 30 percent of patients within 2 years.

ETIOLOGY

Demyelination is the most common identifiable cause of optic neuritis, and multiple sclerosis (MS) is the most frequent cause

TABLE 46-2. Common Causes of Optic Neuritis

Idiopathic
Demyelination
  Multiple sclerosis
  Acute disseminated encephalomyelitis (postinfectious and
    postvaccinal disease)
Viral infection
Bacterial infection
  Syphilis
  Lyme disease
  Tuberculosis
Fungal infection
  Cryptococcus
  Histoplasmosis
Systemic inflammation
  Sarcoidosis
  Systemic lupus erythematosus
  Reiter syndrome
  Crohn's disease
  Behçet's disease

of demyelination. Because of this intimate association, some experts feel that idiopathic optic neuritis is merely a forme fruste or variant of MS. It is the first symptom in 20 percent of MS patients and occurs in 70 percent of all MS patients at some point. The percentage of patients presenting with isolated optic neuritis who will subsequently develop full-blown clinical MS varies among studies from 17 to 90 percent, with an average of approximately 50 percent. Other infectious and inflammatory diseases that cause optic neuritis are listed in Table 46-2.

DIAGNOSIS

Despite the lengthy differential diagnosis of sudden monocular visual loss, research protocols have shown a negligible yield for any laboratory tests in a patient with typical clinical features of optic neuritis. Routine blood work or imaging studies are seldom helpful in the patient with classic signs and symptoms of this disease. However, any patient with an unusual course may require further diagnostic testing. A lumbar puncture may show evidence of a specific infection. (In patients with idiopathic optic neuritis or secondary to MS, the immunoglobulin G (IgG) level may be elevated, often with oligoclonal bands.) In the patient with symptoms suggestive of collagen vascular disease, an antinuclear antibody test should be considered. A fluorescent treponemal antibody/absorption (FTA-ABS) titer may help diagnose syphilitic vasculitis, and a chest radiograph may help diagnose sarcoidosis.

Although controversial, some authorities advocate performing magnetic resonance imaging (MRI) on all patients for the detection of white matter changes characteristic of demyelination. If the findings are consistent with MS, more aggressive treatment may be indicated.

TREATMENT

Many patients with optic neuritis require no treatment. Most recover good visual function within several weeks or months, regardless of therapy.

The recent Optic Neuritis Treatment Trial studied patients between the ages of 18 and 45 who were randomized to one of three treatment arms: (1) oral prednisone (1 mg/kg/day) for 14 days, (2) intravenous methylprednisolone sodium succinate (1,000 mg/day) for 3 days followed by oral prednisone (1 mg/kg/day) for 11 days, or (3) oral placebo for 14 days. Visual recovery was more rapid among patients who received steroids administered intravenously, but there was no long-term benefit

when compared to the placebo or oral regimens. There was no difference between the groups at 1 year with respect to visual acuity, contrast sensitivity, color vision, or visual fields. The oral regimen was associated, however, with a higher recurrence rate of new attacks of optic neuritis in both the initially affected and the fellow eye. The recurrence rate, defined as a new attack either in the affected eye or the opposite eye within 2 years of follow-up, was 27 percent in the group that received steroids orally, compared to 13 percent in the group on the intravenous regimen, and 15 percent in the group on placebos.

A controversial finding was the reduction of the 2-year incidence of definite MS in patients with isolated optic neuritis in the group receiving intravenous treatment. Overall, 7.5 percent of patients developed MS in the group that received intravenous steroid treatment, compared to 14.7 percent in the group on oral steroids, and 16.7 percent in the group on placebos at 2 years. Regardless of treatment, most MRI findings were consistent with demyelination, suggesting that MRI is useful for prognosis and for guiding therapy, since patients with abnormal scans (and thus a high risk for MS) could be strongly considered for intravenous steroid treatment to delay the development of any MS symptoms.

Side effects of glucocorticoid treatment of patients with optic neuritis are minimal. Minor symptoms such as restlessness, insomnia, tremor, mood change, weight gain, and stomach upset are the most common. Serious side effects may be rare because the patient population is young and relatively healthy.

SUMMARY

In a young (especially female) patient who presents with unilateral progressive loss of vision and pain with eye movement, and with an afferent pupillary defect, optic neuritis is the most likely diagnosis. Extensive testing is not required, but MRI may be useful. If MRI shows lesions consistent with demyelination, the clinician should consider treatment with intravenous methylprednisolone 1,000 mg/day for 3 days followed by oral prednisone 1 mg/kg/day for 11 days. If there is no visual recovery, other etiologies should be considered.

SUGGESTED READINGS

Beck RW, Cleary PA, Anderson MA et al: A randomized controlled trial of corticosteroids in the treatment of acute optic neuritis. N Engl J Med 326: 581, 1992
Beck RW, Cleary PA, Trobe JD et al: The effect of corticosteroids for acute optic neuritis on the subsequent development of multiple sclerosis. N Engl J Med 329:1764, 1993
Beck RW, The Optic Neuritis Study Group: Corticosteroid treatment of optic neuritis: a need to change treatment practices. Neurology 42:1133, 1992
Ebers GC: Optic neuritis and multiple sclerosis. Arch Neurol 42:702, 1985
Kurtzke JF: Optic neuritis or multiple sclerosis. Arch Neurol 42:705, 1985
Optic Neuritis Study Group: The clinical profile of optic neuritis. Arch Ophthalmol 109:1673, 1991

47. TRANSVERSE MYELITIS
LOREN A. ROLAK

Transverse myelitis is a syndrome of acute inflammation cutting across the entire spinal cord, producing weakness, numbness, and bowel and bladder dysfunction. It afflicts all ages in

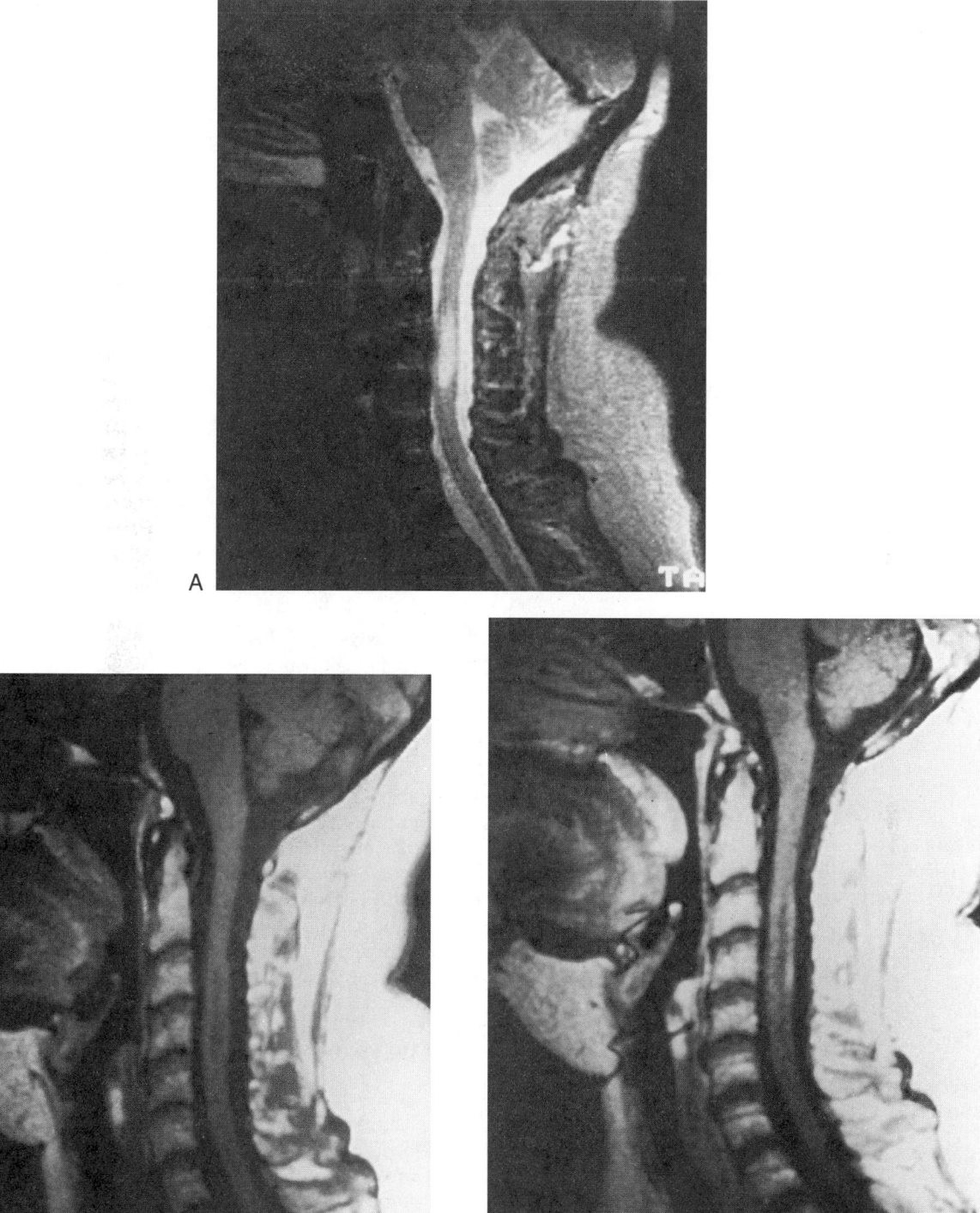

FIG. 47-1. Magnetic resonance imaging of a patient with transverse myelitis, showing inflammation in the cervical spinal cord. **(A)** T2-weighted image. **(B)** T1-weighted image. **(C)** T1-weighted image with gadolinium enhancement.

all parts of the world, affecting males and females equally. Nearly one-third of patients, especially those in the younger age groups, report a preceding viral illness, often a nonspecific upper respiratory infection. Most cases presumably represent an idiopathic, autoimmune inflammation and demyelination of the spinal cord, similar to an attack of multiple sclerosis (MS) or acute disseminated encephalomyelitis, but the syndrome can be produced by a direct viral infection of the cord, as a paraneoplastic remote effect of cancer, or other etiology.

CLINICAL FEATURES

Transverse myelitis has a dramatic presentation, with the rapid onset of symptoms over several hours to a few days. As is typical of most spinal cord lesions, patients develop a sensory level that is almost always in the midthoracic region, below which they lose all sensation. Muscular strength is lost, often to the point of paraplegia. Patients will have increased reflexes, spasticity, and Babinski signs, but in approximately 30 percent of patients the inflammation is so severe and abrupt as to produce "spinal shock" with flaccid hyporeflexia at onset. Because the myelitis usually involves the midthoracic region, the weakness and numbness spare the arms, but in the 20 percent of patients whose myelitis is cervical, the arms are affected. Bowel and bladder control are lost, however. Sharp, gnawing back pain develops in over half the patients.

DIAGNOSIS

The urgent goal in a patient with acute development of a spinal cord syndrome is to exclude a mechanical, compressive lesion. A diagnostic evaluation of suspected transverse myelitis is as follows:

1. MRI of the spinal cord may visualize the myelitis, and exclude other processes, especially compression.
2. MRI of the head is particularly useful to exclude multiple sclerosis.
3. Lumbar puncture assesses inflammation and excludes infections (such as syphilis) and multiple sclerosis.
4. Laboratory screening: vitamin B_{12}, folate, sedimentation rate, antinuclear antibodies, VDRL test, human immunodeficiency virus.

Compression from cervical spondylosis or metastatic cancer frequently mimics transverse myelitis, so immediate imaging of the spinal cord takes highest priority. Magnetic resonance imaging (MRI) is preferred over conventional contrast myelography because of its noninvasive nature, detailed anatomic resolution, and ability to detect intrinsic lesions within the spinal cord (Fig. 46-1). The cord should be scanned through the patient's sensory level, and carried up to the level of the brainstem to ascertain any high lesions. The purpose of cord imaging is not so much to detect the inflammation of transverse myelitis, which is visible in less than 50 percent of cases, but rather to exclude other processes in the differential diagnosis, particularly compressive lesions.

The spinal fluid generally reflects nonspecific inflammation, with a mildly elevated protein and modest lymphocytic pleocytosis. Some patients have immunologic abnormalities as well, with elevated immunoglobulin levels or oligoclonal immunoglobulin G (IgG) bands on electrophoresis.

Transverse myelitis is a syndrome, and may be caused by many diseases, for example:

1. Idiopathic autoimmune transverse myelitis
2. Acute disseminated encephalomyelitis (postinfectious or postvaccinal inflammation)
3. Multiple sclerosis
4. Viral myelitis
5. Vasculitis, from lupus or other vasculitides
6. Spinal cord infarction
7. Paraneoplastic myelopathy
8. Human immunodeficiency virus vacuolar myelopathy
9. Subacute combined degeneration (vitamin B_{12} deficiency)
10. Spirochetal infections, such as syphilis or Lyme disease
11. Intrinsic, intraspinal tumor

A specific etiology is seldom found, and most patients with an acute, noncompressive cord lesion have "idiopathic" inflammatory transverse myelitis. Because it is an abrupt, inflammatory lesion of the central nervous system, transverse myelitis in a young patient raises the specter of MS. However, unlike optic neuritis, which is a similar monophasic idiopathic inflammatory attack, transverse myelitis seldom heralds the development of MS, and no more than 20 percent of transverse myelitis victims will ultimately develop further lesions and proceed onto MS. Nevertheless, MRI scanning of the brain, to search for disseminated inflammatory lesions, is routinely performed in most patients with transverse myelitis.

PROGNOSIS

Transverse myelitis runs a variable course: one-third of patients develop only mild weakness and numbness and little disability, one-third are moderately disabled, and one-third suffer devastating paralysis, anesthesia, and loss of sphincter control. Surprisingly, the degree of initial deficit correlates poorly with the degree of recovery. Prognosis cannot be predicted based on age, sex, preceding illnesses, MRI findings, or spinal fluid abnormalities, and the only useful forecaster is rapidity of onset; patients whose symptoms strike very abruptly, especially with spinal shock, are unlikely to recover. Overall, approximately one-fourth of patients recover nearly to normal, half persist with moderate disability, and one-fourth remain severely affected. Symptoms that have not abated within 3 to 6 months are unlikely ever to do so.

TREATMENT

Transverse myelitis is best treated with high-dose intravenous steroids, such as the common regimen of methylprednisolone (Solu-Medrol) 1 g IV daily for 3 to 5 days, often followed by an oral steroid taper. Steroids suppress the immune system, reduce inflammation, stabilize the blood-brain barrier, interfere with inflammatory proteolytic enzymes, and enhance nerve conduction, so the rationale for their use is sound. Nevertheless, most reviews and analyses have not been able to show that they ultimately affect outcome, or that treated patients have a better prognosis than the natural history of the disease. Because no careful studies have ever been done, the true value of steroids remains uncertain. They continue to be routinely employed, but it is disconcerting that their benefits are not more obvious.

Treatment otherwise centers on management appropriate to any patient with an acute spinal cord injury, such as attention to bowel and bladder dysfunction, decubiti and skin care, pulmonary embolus from immobility, and muscle contractures from spasticity. Once the acute phase has passed, severely impaired patients should be referred to spinal cord injury units, rehabilitation facilities, or other specialized centers.

SUGGESTED READINGS

Ford B, Tampieri D, Francis G: Long-term follow-up of acute partial transverse myelopathy. Neurology 42:250, 1992

Jeffery DR, Mandler RN, Davis LE: Transverse myelitis. Arch Neurol 50:532, 1993

Tyler KL, Gross RA, Cascino GD: Unusual viral causes of transverse myelitis. Neurology 36:855, 1986

48. ACUTE DISSEMINATED ENCEPHALOMYELITIS

WILLIAM R. TYOR

Acute disseminated encephalomyelitis (ADEM) is a demyelinating disease. It is also called parainfectious, postinfectious, or postvaccinial encephalomyelitis because of its association with infectious illnesses and vaccines (Table 48-1), and, in its most aggressive form, it is called acute hemorrhagic leukoencephalitis. The best-characterized relationship of ADEM with infectious disease is with measles infection; before the introduction of measles vaccine, this was a relatively common association, occurring in 1:400 to 1:1,000 measles cases. Development of ADEM following other infections, including rubella, mumps, herpes viruses, influenza, Lyme disease, and mycoplasma, has also been described (Table 48-1). ADEM associated with rabies vaccines prepared from animal brain is well known, and early studies involving the injection of rabbit brain into monkeys led to our current concept of the autoimmune nature of this disease

TABLE 48-1. Some Parainfectious and Postvaccinal Agents Associated With Acute Disseminated Encephalomyelitis

Infections
  Viral
    Coxsackie
    Epstein-Barr
    Herpes zoster
    Herpes simplex
    Influenza
    Measles
    Mumps
    Rubella
  Bacterial
    Borrelia burgdorferi
    Legionella pneumophila
    Leptospira
Vaccinations
  Diphtheria
  Influenza
  Measles
  Pertussis
  Rabies
  Rubella
  Vaccinia

TABLE 48-2. Clinical Features of Acute Disseminated Encephalomyelitis

Demographics and initial symptoms
  Any age, but unusual before 10 years
  Usually follows infection or vaccination by 1 to 3 weeks
  May be several days of fever, chills, and malaise
Possible neurologic manifestations (uniphasic)
  Abrupt onset of seizures with rapid progression to coma
  Subacute onset evolving over days
    Headache, fever, nausea, vomiting, meningismus
    Progression to delirium
    Sensory abnormalities, hemiparesis, paraparesis
    Ataxia, visual disturbances, cranial nerve signs
    Bladder and/or bowel dysfunction
    Involuntary movements, myoclonus
    Behavioral and cognitive disturbances
    Increased intracranial pressure
  More chronic course developing over weeks

and the development of the first animal model of experimental allergic encephalomyelitis. Other vaccines that have been linked with occasional cases of ADEM include smallpox, pertussis, influenza, rubella, diphtheria, and measles. However, in many cases, the relationship between ADEM and infectious disease or vaccination is not clear, and therefore these represent idiopathic events.

CLINICAL PRESENTATION

Typically, the onset of ADEM begins 1 to 3 weeks after an infection or immunization and may affect all ages, although it is uncommon in children under 10 years old. In some patients, a prodrome of fever, malaise, and myalgia occurs for several days prior to the onset of focal or multifocal neurologic deficits (Table 48-2).

Symptoms may develop abruptly, with seizures and rapid deterioration to coma, or they may evolve over a period of days involving primarily white matter in the cerebral hemispheres, optic nerves, brainstem, cerebellum, and spinal cord. Signs include encephalopathy, hemiparesis, cranial nerve palsies, visual dysfunction, ataxia, and myelopathy (i.e., paraparesis and sphincter dysfunction). However, signs referable to gray matter involvement are not uncommon and consist of movement disorders such as choreoathetosis, seizures, and myoclonus. There also may be signs of increased intracranial pressure.

PROGNOSIS

Generally, deficits peak within several days and begin to resolve, but occasionally a protracted course lasting weeks and, rarely, months is observed. It should be emphasized that ADEM is a uniphasic disease, and this important feature helps to distinguish it from multiple sclerosis, which can also cause abrupt, multifocal neurologic deficits. Relapses that can be considered manifestations of ADEM and not of multiple sclerosis are rare. The mortality rate for ADEM has been estimated as high as 30 percent, but complete recovery occurs in at least half of the patients. Rapid onset with severe manifestations portends a poor prognosis.

DIAGNOSIS

No laboratory abnormality is pathognomonic for ADEM, but there are common findings (Table 48-3). Cerebrospinal fluid (CSF) pressure may be increased, and the CSF may demonstrate moderate leukocytosis (fewer than 100 cells/μl, usually mono-

IMMUNE AND INFECTIOUS DISEASE • IMMUNE-MEDIATED DISEASES

TABLE 48-3. Magnetic Resonance Imaging and Cerebrospinal Fluid Findings in Acute Disseminated Encephalomyelitis

Cerebrospinal fluid
  Pressure
    May be elevated
  Cell count
    Usually between 5 and 100 white cells/ml
    Predominantly polymorphonuclear early and mononuclear later
  Chemistries
    Glucose normal
    Protein usually between 45 and 100 mg/dl
  Other
    Myelin basic protein may be elevated
    Immunoglobulin G index may be elevated
    Oligoclonal bands may be present
Magnetic resonance imaging
  Multifocal areas of increased T2-weighted intensity, usually in the white matter

TABLE 48-4. General Guidelines for Therapy of Acute Disseminated Encephalomyelitis

Immunosuppression
  Intravenous methylprednisolone 1 g/day for 3 days
  If no response, consider prolonged IV steroids or other immunosuppressive therapy
  Then prednisone 60 mg/day for 1 week followed by a rapid taper
Supportive care
  Prevention of complications in bedridden patients
    Decubitus ulcers
    Thrombophlebitis
    Contractures
    Bowel dysfunction
    Atelectasis
  Symptomatic therapy
    Seizures
    Bladder dysfunction
    Dysphagia
    Pain
    Spasticity
    Depression
  Physical and occupational therapy

nuclear cells) and a modest increase in protein (less than 100 mg/dl). However, infrequently the CSF is normal. Occasionally the CSF shows an increased IgG index and oligoclonal bands, although increased myelin basic protein occurs in a larger proportion of patients, especially in ADEM after measles infection or Semple vaccination (inactivated rabies prepared from sheep brain). Computed tomography (CT) scans reveal multifocal hypodense lesions, usually in the white matter, which may enhance with contrast. MRI is more sensitive and demonstrates areas of increased intensity on T2-weighted scan, mainly in the white matter. The electroencephalogram is frequently abnormal but nonspecific, displaying generalized, multifocal, or focal slowing. Systemic findings can include an increased erythrocyte sedimentation rate and mild proteinuria.

The most important differential diagnosis of ADEM is multiple sclerosis, and the clinical, laboratory, and pathologic similarities of these two diseases have long been appreciated. It is often impossible, using any criteria, to separate ADEM from a single, first attack of multiple sclerosis. The diagnosis of multiple sclerosis is clear when multifocal neurologic signs relapse and remit, but the discrimination between ADEM and multiple sclerosis is difficult when neurologic deficits do not relapse, remain static, or slowly progress over months. Distinguishing between these diseases must often await the passage of time, even years.

Other diagnostic considerations include viral encephalitis, tumor, meningitis, cerebrovascular disease, endocarditis with cerebral embolization, intracranial abscess, intracranial hemorrhage, central nervous system vasculitis, and central nervous system sarcoidosis.

TREATMENT

There are no controlled trials of corticosteroids in ADEM. Based on the similarities of ADEM with multiple sclerosis, and the likelihood that they are autoimmune diseases, as well as numerous anecdotal reports of the beneficial effects of steroids, intravenous methylprednisolone followed by prednisone is recommended (Table 48-4). Normally, 1 g methylprednisolone administered intravenously in 500 ml of normal saline over 2 hours is given for 3 days, followed by prednisone, 60 to 80 mg (1 mg/kg) taken orally for 7 days and then tapered rapidly over the next 10 days. In severe or refractory cases, intravenous steroids may be given for longer periods or more vigorous immunosuppression such as with cyclophosphamide or azathioprine should be considered. However, data on these types of

prolonged or intense immunotherapy are deficient. Information regarding the efficacy of other treatments, such as plasmapheresis and γ-globulin, is also lacking. In cases where there is significant increased intracranial pressure, it may be necessary to administer mannitol, reverse Trendelenburg position, hyperventilation, and even surgical placement of intracranial pressure monitoring and decompression.

Some complications of ADEM can be ameliorated (Table 48-4). Seizures are usually well controlled with the standard recommended doses of phenytoin, carbamazepine, or phenobarbital. Cognizance of bladder dysfunction and its treatment are important to help prevent further complications of urinary tract infection and potential sepsis. Bowel dysfunction, usually manifest by constipation, is also a frequent complication, especially in patients who are bedridden. Decubitus ulcers, thrombophlebitis, contractures, and peripheral nerve compression often afflict bedridden patients. Atelectasis and pneumonia may develop, so respiratory care is important.

Occasionally, patients with ADEM become dysphagic and require special diets or tube feeding. Dysesthetic pain may develop and can be improved with nonsteroidal anti-inflammatory drugs, tricyclic agents such as amitriptyline, or anticonvulsants like carbamazepine. Spasticity is a frequent complication and may require treatment with baclofen, diazepam, and physical therapy. Physical therapy is useful early for passive range of motion, and later for more active exercises. Occupational therapy is also an important adjunct, especially in patients with persistent deficits requiring special needs for daily living. Utilization of social services and vocational rehabilitation may ultimately be necessary. Most patients with ADEM recover significantly, but many have residual deficits that often require continued care and support. Mild depression is to be expected and occasionally requires treatment with antidepressants or mental health referral.

SUGGESTED READINGS

Johnson RT: Viral infections of the nervous system. Raven Press, New York, 1982
Miller HG, Gibbons JL: Acute disseminated encephalomyelitis and acute disseminated sclerosis: results of treatment with ACTH. Br Med J 2:1345, 1953
Sriram S, Steinman L: Postinfectious and postvaccinal encephalomyelitis. Neurol Clin North Am 2:341, 1984

Tyor WR: Postinfectious encephalomyelitis and transverse myelitis. p. 155. In Johnson RT, Griffin JW (eds): Current Therapy in Neurologic Disease. 4th Ed. Mosby, St. Louis, 1993

Ziegler DK: Acute disseminated encephalitis: some therapeutic and diagnostic considerations. Arch Neurol 23:476, 1966

49. CENTRAL NERVOUS SYSTEM VASCULITIS

STEVEN B. INBODY

Although primary angiitis of the central nervous system (PACNS) is often discussed in the context of disorders of the cerebral vasculature, its clinical manifestations seldom mimic stroke, but rather more closely resemble those observed in inflammatory and immune-mediated disorders of the central nervous system (CNS). Most patients present with the subacute onset of a diffuse encephalopathy without focal neurologic symptoms. Further diagnostic confusion can arise from reliance on laboratory screening tests such as the erythrocyte sedimentation rate (ESR), antinuclear antibody (ANA), and rheumatoid factor (RF), which are frequently normal, leading to the mistaken exclusion of PACNS. These potential diagnostic pitfalls have undoubtedly delayed the early diagnosis of suspected CNS vasculitis in many cases. However, if diagnosed early and treated aggressively, PACNS can be controlled with little neurologic morbidity.

CLINICAL FEATURES

Patients with PACNS usually present with a subacute encephalopathy, or occasionally with a focal or multifocal disturbance in brain or spinal cord function (Table 49-1). Generalized features may include headache, stiff neck, confusion, psychosis, disorientation, dementia, emotional disturbances including depression, anxiety, or apathy, and alterations of consciousness ranging from lethargy to coma. The gradual onset of headache and altered mental status is by far the most common presenting picture. Focal features often appear gradually, rather than abruptly or "strokelike," and include hemiparesis, paresthesias, hemianopsia, disorders of gait (ataxic or apractic), seizures, aphasia, and extrapyramidal symptoms ranging from chorea and tremor to parkinsonism.

TABLE 49-1. Clinical Features at Time of Diagnosis in 40 Cases of Histologically Confirmed PACNS

Clinical Finding	No. (%) of Patients
Diffuse cortical dysfunction	38 (95)
Headache	27 (68)
Focal cerebral dysfunction	20 (50)
Evidence of increased intracranial pressure	17 (43)
Brainstem or cranial nerve disease	16 (40)
Seizures	10 (25)
Spinal cord disease	9 (23)
Fever/sweats	8 (20)
Anorexia/weight loss	8 (20)
History, physical examination inadequate for assessment	2 (5)

(Modified from Vollmer TL, Guarnaccia J, Harrington W et al: Idiopathic granulomatous angiitis of the central nervous system. Arch Neurol 50:92, 1993, with permission.)

Cranial mononeuropathies, either singularly or multiply, may also be seen. Cranial nerves II through VIII appear to be most commonly involved, causing monocular visual loss, diplopia, facial paresthesias and paresis, deafness, tinnitus, and vertigo.

Generalized symptoms, sometimes very suspicious for a systemic vasculitis or collagen vascular disease, may develop in up to 20 percent of patients. These complaints include fevers, night sweats, anorexia, weight loss, and malaise.

Patients with histologically proven PACNS have ranged in age from 3 to 78, with most cases occurring between 35 and 65, and with a slight male predominance. The mean duration of symptoms prior to diagnosis is approximately 6 months, although some patients have had complaints as long as 5 years before confirmation of their disease.

DIAGNOSIS

Since its original description by Cravioto and Feigin in 1959, granulomatosis angiitis restricted to the CNS has been reported under a wide variety of names and associated with multiple causes, including Hodgkin's disease, Varicella zoster, and herpes ophthalmicus. The descriptive term "granulomatosis angiitis" has remained a popular synonym even though less than 50 percent of PACNS cases are granulomatous histologically. Primary angiitis of the CNS is now used to refer to a vasculitis, causally unrelated to any systemic disorder, confined to the brain and spinal cord. Definitive diagnosis often depends exclusively on histopathologic confirmation.

Primary angiitis of the CNS characteristically involves the small to medium-sized leptomeningeal and intracerebral blood vessels, although occurrence in large arteries has been reported (Fig. 49-1). The angiitis is typically focal and segmental, with regions of normal vasculature often occurring between lesions (Fig. 49-2). Thus, an isolated negative biopsy would not necessarily exclude the diagnosis of PACNS. The histologic changes may be granulomatous or nongranulomatous (Fig. 49-3). Thrombosis may occur in blood vessels of different sizes, with or without involvement by the angiitis.

The differential diagnosis of vasculitis confined to the CNS would, of course, include systemic vasculitides that involve other organs as well (Table 49-2). While the history and physical examination are often adequate to confirm (or exclude) these generalized inflammations, Table 49-3 lists some studies that may be helpful for diagnosing specific causes of vasculitis.

No characteristic abnormalities on blood analysis have been reported in cases of PACNS. Of particular importance has been the consistent finding of normal (or only mildly elevated) laboratory values for ESR, ANA, RF, and complement levels. This observation has prompted several investigators to strongly recommend searching for alternative diagnoses if in fact these laboratory values are abnormal.

Nonspecific changes appear in the cerebrospinal fluid (CSF) of many patients (Table 49-4) and represent the findings expected in an inflammatory process. The CSF exhibits a primarily mononuclear pleocytosis in more than 50 percent of patients. CSF protein levels are elevated, sometimes markedly, in more than 80 percent of the patients tested. To date, only limited information is available concerning elevations in the CSF immunoglobulin G (IgG) synthesis rate or IgG index, which may be abnormal due to impairment of the blood-brain barrier. Oligoclonal bands are usually not present. These CSF findings represent a frequent laboratory abnormality in PACNS, although they are nonspecific. However, some patients, perhaps

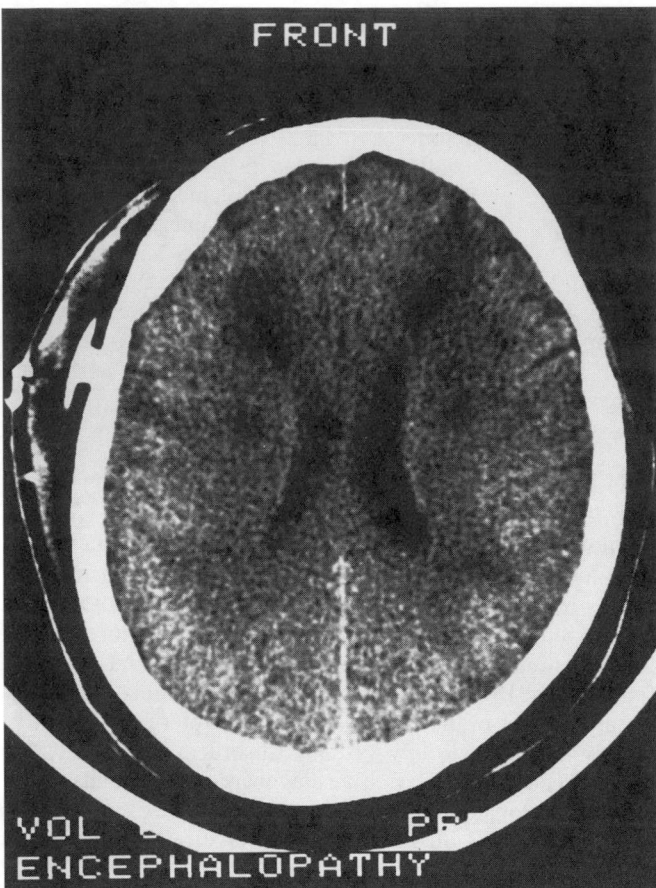

FIG. 49-1. Contrast-enhanced CT scan of the brain of a 54-year-old man with primary angiitis of the central nervous system, showing multifocal, hypodense ischemic lesions.

as many as 20 percent, will have completely normal CSF, and unfortunately, this does not exclude the diagnosis of PACNS.

Most large studies of histologically proven PACNS have utilized computed tomography scans for (CT) evaluation of the brain, and two-thirds of patients have shown focal, hypodense lesions, consistent with ischemia, especially involving the cortex, and with a predilection for the temporal lobes (Fig. 49-1). The advent of magnetic resonance imaging (MRI) with infusion of gadolinium has shown even greater sensitivity in demonstrating small, multifocal parenchymal lesions involving both gray and white matter, with many more exhibiting enhancement by MRI as compared to conventional CT scanning. Meningeal enhancement is also common (Fig. 49-2).

Electroencephalography (EEG) is abnormal in up to 90 percent of cases, and frequently shows diffuse slowing early in the clinical course of PACNS, often providing the first objective evidence of an organic basis for the patient presenting with a subacute confusional state. The EEG shows generalized, nonspecific slowing and only rarely demonstrates focal defects. Epileptiform activity is uncommon.

Although angiography is often advocated as a screening (or even definitive) test for PACNS, it shows changes diagnostic of vasculitis in fewer than half of all patients. This disappointingly low yield may reflect the fact that the pathology in PACNS prefers small blood vessels, below the resolution of conventional angiograms.

It is apparent, then, that patients may present with a picture consistent with PACNS, but with entirely normal laboratory studies, or only nondiagnostic changes, such as a few punctate signal changes on an MRI, nonspecific inflammation in the CSF, or generalized slowing on an EEG. In this setting, brain biopsy is indicated to establish a definitive diagnosis. The biopsy is usually taken from the nondominant hemisphere, often in the temporal lobe, and includes tissue from meninges and from a core of underlying brain. This procedure is relatively

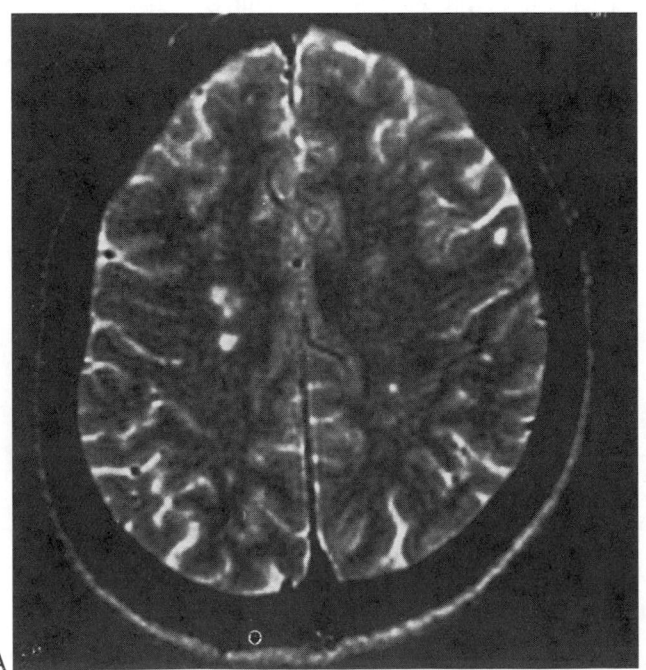
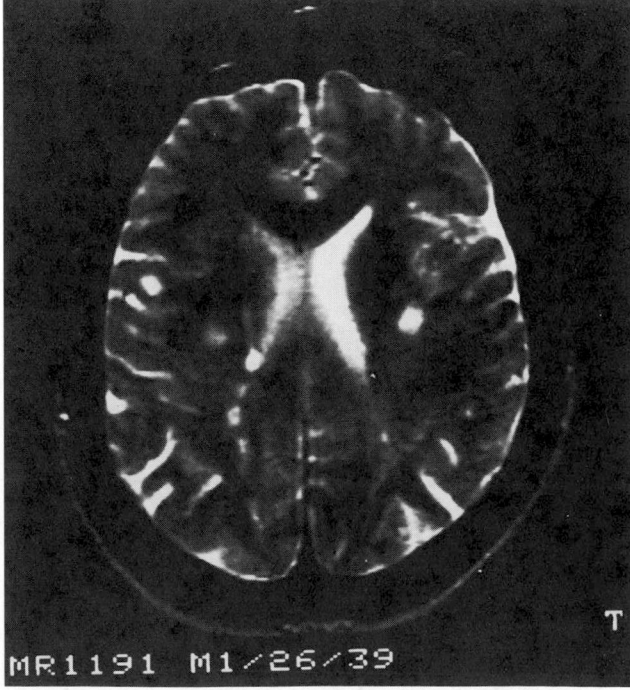

FIG. 49-2. **(A & B)** T2-weighted MRI scans of the same patient as in Fig. 49-1, showing multifocal scattered ischemic lesions. (Courtesy of Kenneth Madden, M.D., and Lawrence Hutchins, M.D., The Marshfield Clinic, Marshfield, WI.)

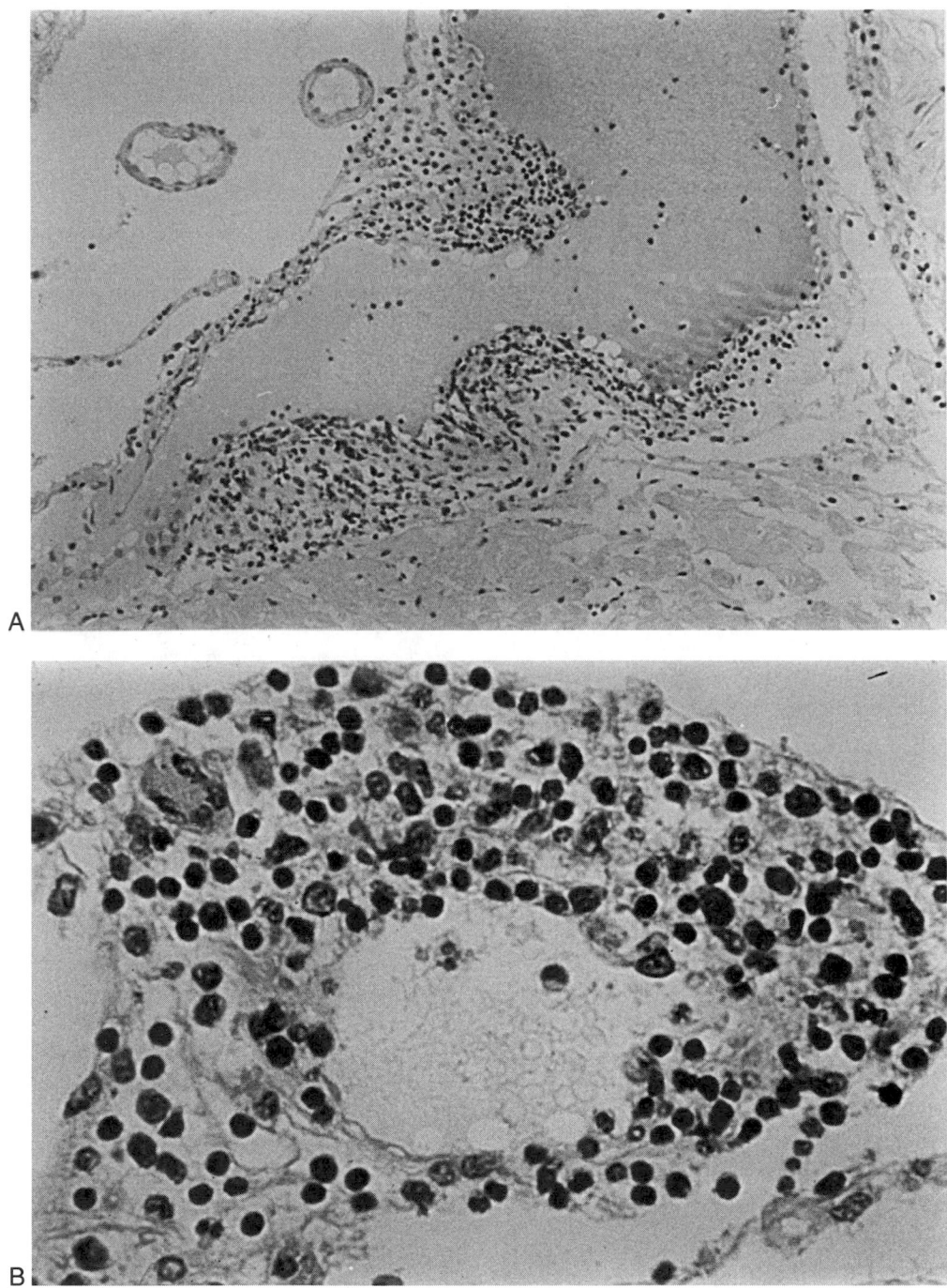

FIG. 49-3. **(A)** Biopsy showing intense vasculitis in a patient with primary angiitis of the central nervous system. **(B)** High-power magnification demonstrates the characteristic granulomatous inflammation of the vessel wall. (Courtesy of Bruce Krawisz, M.D., The Marshfield Clinic, Marshfield, WI.)

TABLE 49-2. Classification of Central Nervous System Vasculitis

Nonsystemic (Localized) Vasculitis

Idiopathic	Secondary Causes
Primary (granulomatous) angiitis	Malignancy
	Hodgkin's disease
Isolated benign cerebral vasculitis	Non-Hodgkin's lymphoma
(without biopsy confirmation)	
	Infection-related vasculitis
	Herpes zoster
	Cytomegalovirus
	Human immunodeficiency virus

Systemic Vasculitis

Idiopathic	Secondary Causes
Systemic necrotizing vasculitis	Connective tissue disease
Polyarteritis nodosa	Systemic lupus erythematous
Polyangiitis overlap syndrome	Rheumatoid arthritis
Microscopic polyangiitis	Sjögren syndrome
Wegener's granulomatosis	Mixed connective tissue disease
Churg-Strauss syndrome	Scleroderma
Kawasaki's disease	
	Miscellaneous Systemic Disease
Hypersensitivity vasculitis	Sarcoidosis
Henoch-Schonlein purpura	Behçet's disease
Systemic leukocytoclastic vasculitis	Cogan syndrome
(idiopathic)	Hypersensitivity angiitis
	Drug-induced angiitis
Giant cell arteritis	Serum sickness
Temporal arteritis	Cryoglobulinemia
Takayasu's arteritis	Infection-related vasculitis
	Bacterial
Miscellaneous vasculitides	Fungal
Eales' disease	Viral
Optic disc vasculitis	Protozoal
Buerger's disease	Mycoplasma
	Rickettsial
	Hepatitis B
	Tuberculosis
	Syphilis
	Malignancy-related
	Lymphoma
	Leukemia
	Paraneoplastic
	Vasculitis in substance abuse
	Amphetamines, cocaine, heroin

TABLE 49-3. Diagnostic Studies Recommended in Suspected Vasculitis

Nonspecific studies consistent with possible vasculitis
  ESR
  CBC
  C-reactive protein
  EEG
  CSF cell count and protein
  MRI of the cervical or thoracic spinal cord
  MRI/CT of brain
  EMG/NCV

Specific studies supportive of secondary causes of vasculitis
  Hepatitis B
  HIV
  Cryoglobulins
  Serum complement
  Angiotensin-converting enzyme
  ANA
  Rheumatoid factor
  ANCA
  VDRL (FTA-ABS)
  CSF fungal serology
  Blood cultures
  CSF fungal and AFB cultures and stains
  Anti-double-stranded DNA
  Anti-Ro
  Anti-La

Specific studies consistent with other organ involvement in systemic vasculitis
  Transaminases
  Creatinine
  Urinalysis
  CPK
  CXR
  Sinus x-rays

Specific studies supportive of probable vasculitis
  Cerebral angiography
  Selective organ-specific (noncerebral) angiography

Specific studies suggestive of an alternative diagnosis simulating vasculitis
  Lyme disease serology
  CSF oligoclonal bands
  Antiphospholipid antibodies
  Echocardiogram
  CSF cytology and lymphocyte cell surface markers

Diagnostic studies of definite vasculitis
  Brain biopsy
  Nerve and muscle biopsy
  Other organ biopsy (i.e., skin, kidney)

Abbreviations: ESR, erythrocyte sedimentation rate; CBC, complete blood count; EEG, electroencephalogram; CSF, cerebrospinal fluid; MRI, magnetic resonance imaging; CT, computed tomography; EMG, electromyogram; NCV, nerve conduction velocity; HIV, human immunodeficiency virus; ANA, antinuclear antibody; ANCA, antineutrophilic cytoplasmic antibodies; VDRL, Venereal Disease Research Laboratory; FTA-ABS, fluorescent treponemal antibody-absorption; AFB, acid-fast bacilli; CPK, creatine phosphokinase; CXR, chest x-ray.

benign and has a very high yield, and should not cause hesitancy or reluctance when necessary to establish a diagnosis in this often fatal disease.

TREATMENT

Although immunotherapy for PACNS has been successful, the infrequent occurrence and variable clinical course of this disorder has limited the necessary prospective controlled trials needed to determine the most efficacious and least toxic regimens. The current mainstay of PACNS therapy is combination cyclophosphamide/glucocorticoid treatment, which has dramatically reduced the morbidity and mortality of the disease. The complimentary immunosuppressant actions of these two drugs, however, must be weighted against the additive risk of infection and side effects when used in combination.

The appropriate starting dose of glucocorticoids is chosen to rapidly suppress disease activity, and typically requires prednisone .5 to 1 mg/kg daily. The alternate use of high-dose, pulsed intravenous glucocorticoid therapy (i.e., methylprednisolone 1 mg/day) has not yet been proven justified for extended use. Cyclophosphamide can be administered orally at a dose of 1.5 to 2.5 mg/kg daily. Intravenous pulsed therapy with doses between 500 mg and 1,000 mg/m^2 body surface each month are less toxic, but potentially less efficacious.

TABLE 49-4. Cerebrospinal Fluid Findings in Patients with Histologically Confirmed PACNS

CSF Findings	No. (%) of Patients
WBC count, $\times 10^6$/L	
0–9	8 (20)
10–99	8 (20)
100–250	12 (30)
>250	1 (3)
Not recorded	11 (27)
Protein, g/L	
<0.50	3 (8)
0.50–0.99	8 (20)
1.00–2.00	16 (40)
>2.00	5 (12)
Not recorded	8 (20)
Opening pressure, mmH$_2$O	
<200	7 (18)
>200	13 (32)
Not recorded	20 (50)

(Modified from Vollmer TL, Guarnaccia J, Harrington W et al: Idiopathic granulomatous angiitis of the central nervous system. Arch Neurol 50:92, 1993.)

Clinical assessment of the patient at regular intervals and serial monitoring of laboratory parameters of inflammation, such as an elevated CSF protein, will allow the rate of glucocorticoid and cyclophosphamide reduction to be adjusted for each individual patient. Immunosuppression with this regimen should be maintained until patients are symptom-free for 1 year, after which the prednisone and cyclophosphamide can be tapered over 3 to 6 months.

Any immunosuppressant therapy has the potential for complications. The patient and physician should be aware of the potential complications of both medications prior to initiating therapy. Blood counts must be monitored to maintain white blood cells at rates greater than 3,000 to 4,000 mm³, and urinalysis should be checked to detect hemorrhagic cystitis.

CONCLUSION

The diagnosis of PACNS remains difficult in the absence of specific laboratory tests. Timely diagnosis depends on the physician maintaining a high index of suspicion and a vigilance for alternate disease processes. Until the immunopathologic mechanisms underlying PACNS are identified, the necessary early diagnosis of this potentially treatable syndrome will depend on clinical judgement and careful, but aggressive pursuit of the diagnosis.

SUGGESTED READINGS

Kissel JT, Rammohan KW: Pathogenesis and therapy of nervous system vasculitis. Clin Neuropharmacol 14:28, 1991
Lie JT: Primary (granulomatous) angiitis of the central nervous system: a clinicopathologic analysis of 15 new cases and a review of the literature. Hum Pathol 23:164, 1992
Nadeau SE, Watson RT: Neurologic manifestations of vasculitis and collagen vascular syndromes. Clin Neurol 59:1, 1990
Tarvaert JWC, Kallenberg C: Neurologic manifestations of systemic vasculitides. Rheumatic Dis Clin North Am 4:913, 1993
Vollmer TL, Guarnaccia J, Harrington W et al: Idiopathic granulomatous angiitis of the central nervous system. Arch Neurol 50:925, 1993

SECTION 2. INFECTIOUS DISEASES

50. APPROACH TO THE PATIENT WITH A CENTRAL NERVOUS SYSTEM INFECTION

J. DOUGLAS LEE
KURT REED

When presented with a patient thought to have an infection of the central nervous system (CNS), consideration of the disease features in a sequential manner can allow considerable limiting of the differential diagnosis and thus earlier specific diagnosis and treatment. The steps, in order of use, consist of defining the clinical syndrome being evaluated, the characteristics of the affected patient, the circumstances in which the disease was contracted, and the laboratory and imaging data.

DELINEATION OF THE CLINICAL SYNDROME

The primary CNS infections include meningitis, encephalitis, myelitis, abscess, radiculopathy, and combinations of these. Each of these in turn can be defined as acute or chronic. Acute disease is usually due to viral or bacterial infections, and chronic disease to syphilis, or granulomatous disease, or other less common infections.

Meningitis in the acute form presents with an altered level of consciousness and fever or hypothermia as the most consistent features. Headache is combined in many cases with evidence of meningeal irritation (stiff neck), and the diagnosis of menin-gitis is confirmed by finding significant cerebrospinal fluid (CSF) pleocytosis. The duration of illness spans hours to days before presentation. The cause is usually viral or readily culturable bacterial infections, although rickettsial disease, syphilis, Lyme borreliosis, Listeria monocytogenes, and leptospirosis can cause this syndrome.

Chronic meningitis usually causes a degree of encephalitis as well, producing cortical dysfunction, at times fluctuating and often combined with cranial nerve palsies, and mononuclear CSF pleocytosis. Common etiologies include granulomatous diseases, tumor, or syphilis, but many cases are idiopathic.

Encephalitis of the acute type presents with the rapid onset of cortical dysfunction and fever, with a relatively modest CSF pleocytosis. Common etiologies include viruses, especially herpes viruses, enteroviruses, human immunodeficiency virus (HIV), and mumps. Chronic encephalitis presenting as dementia is usually not of infectious origin, but syphilis or HIV should be excluded, as should the same conditions responsible for chronic meningitis.

Myelitis is often associated with encephalitis, and has a similar differential diagnosis. It may present as transverse myelitis or as ascending disease with motor (poliomyelitis syndrome) or mixed sensory and motor findings. More diffuse cord involvement produces cord dysfunction combining motor and sensory deficits in a bilateral distribution at multiple cord levels. Mechanical cord compression, including that caused by abscesses, must be excluded as a first priority in cases consistent with a single level of cord dysfunction.

Space-occupying lesions, such as brain abscesses or the lesions of toxoplasmosis in acquired immune deficiency syndrome (AIDS), are accompanied by headache, altered mental status, and focal or lateralized signs indicating an intracranial site of involvement. Seizures are common. In the spinal canal the presentation is one of transverse myelitis.

Radiculopathy, with evidence of sensory and motor dysfunction in a radicular distribution, is usually mechanical, but Lyme disease is the most common local infectious process.

Involvement of multiple sites (e.g., meningitis with radiculopathy, or cranial neuritis and encephalopathy, or myelopathy with chronic encephalitis) in the acute state suggests syphilitic disease, Lyme borreliosis, or postinfectious phenomena and in the chronic state suggests syphilis, granulomatous disease, neoplastic meningitis, or other noninfectious etiologies.

CHARACTERISTICS OF THE AFFECTED PATIENT

Immune Status

The immune status of the patient can be the most important piece of epidemiologic information the physician possesses. Patients with antibody deficiency or dysfunction are predisposed to infections with encapsulated bacteria such as *Neisseria meningitidis, Streptococcus pneumoniae,* and *Haemophilus influenzae,* which are major causes of meningitis. Deficiencies of the terminal components of the complement pathway predispose to *Neisseria,* and patients with a family history of these infections or a recurrent history of *Neisseria* infections should be evaluated for these deficiencies. Patients with impaired inflammatory responses (e.g., chronic steroid use) or deficient cell-mediated immunity are particularly prone to intracellular infections such as fungal infections, *Listeria,* and herpetic infection. In the presence of advanced HIV disease all of the above are considered, but reactivation toxoplasmosis, tuberculosis, progressive multifocal leukoencephalopathy, cryptococcosis, syphilis, HIV dementia, and fungal infections are common.

Associated Diseases

There are a number of medical conditions that predispose to specific neurologic infections. Patients with chronic sinus or mastoid infection are predisposed to brain abscess, as are patients with chronic suppurative pulmonary infections (bronchiectasis and lung abscess), dental sepsis, endocarditis, or intracardiac or intrapulmonary right-to-left shunts. Chest radiographic evidence of pulmonary disease should raise the question of nocardiosis, tuberculosis, histoplasmosis, blastomycosis, or coccidioidomycosis in patients with CNS disease. Chronic or recurrent uveitis may indicate the existence of systemic lupus erythematosus (SLE), toxoplasmosis, Behçet syndrome, sarcoidosis, leprosy, or Vogt-Koyanaga-Harada (VKH) syndrome. Skin depigmentation is also seen in VKH, as well as in other autoimmune diseases. Neoplastic disease may cause carcinomatous meningitis or space-occupying lesions, mimicking meningitis or abscess, respectively. Certain drugs are known to cause sterile meningitis (sulfa-trimethoprim, nonsteroidal anti-inflammatory drugs [NSAIDs], and azathioprine), as can connective tissue diseases (SLE, Behçet syndrome, vasculitis, and sarcoidosis). Surgical or traumatic damage to the meninges predisposes to skin flora, gram-negative rod and staphylococcal infections, and, if associated with mucosal surfaces, pneumococcal meningitis.

CIRCUMSTANCES OF THE INFECTION

Epidemic or Sporadic

When other individuals appear to have the same condition during the same time period (an epidemic), a viral etiology is the

TABLE 50-1. Geographic Aspects of CNS Infections

Location	Agent	Disease
Africa	Malaria	Cerebral malaria
	Trypanosome	Sleeping sickness
Southwest United States	Coccidioidomyces	Chronic meningitis
Rocky Mountains	Coltivirus	Colorado tick fever
Third world	Rabies	Rabies encephalitis
	Taenia	Cysticercosis
	Tuberculosis	Chronic meningitis
Most continents	Various viruses	Encephalitis

usual cause. With the exception of meningococcal disease in closed populations, secondary cases of bacterial infection of the CNS are rare. The distribution of cases in time and place (family, work, school, or community at large), and history of animal or insect exposure, may indicate the nature of transmission (airborne, arthropod vector) and thus the etiology. Although an individual who is the first in a viral epidemic is often treated for bacterial disease, after the first few cases information from the laboratory will allow presumptive diagnosis of subsequent cases.

Travel and Geography

The CNS infections with strong geographic aspects are outlined in Table 50-1. The various insectborne encephalitis viruses have specific primary hosts, ranges, and vectors. When patients are seen with encephalitis after returning from travel, consideration of a viral encephalitis is recommended.

Insect and Animal Exposure

Animal, mosquito, mite, and tick exposure histories may also suggest diagnostic possibilities (Table 50-2).

Vocational and Avocational Exposures

Vocational and avocational exposures mainly relate to zoonotic diseases. Individuals who work or recreate in the outdoors are at particular risk of Lyme disease (borreliosis), rickettsial diseases, and other arthropodborne illnesses. Animal handlers are at risk for the zoonoses described above. On occasion living or working in crowded, poorly ventilated areas has resulted in epidemics, particularly of *Neisseria meningitidis* in military recruits.

LABORATORY DATA

Blood Tests

Of the routine available laboratory tests, the complete blood count may indicate chronicity of disease or underlying disease (anemia). Leukopenia or absence of leukocytosis may speak for severe sepsis, viral etiology, connective tissue disease, or a noninfectious etiology. Lymphocytosis and particularly atypical lymphocytosis is suggestive of a viral etiology, but may be present in toxoplasmosis and other intracellular infections. Thrombocytopenia may indicate sepsis, disseminated intravascular coagulation underlying marrow disease or an autoimmune disease.

Hyperglobulinemia suggests either a chronic inflammatory disorder (HIV, chronic infection, or connective tissue disease) or a plasma cell or lymphocytic disorder. Abnormalities of liver or renal function imply a multisystem disease and indicate the

TABLE 50-2. Exposure Histories and CNS Infections

Exposure	Agent	Disease
Mosquito	Arboviruses (worldwide)	Encephalitis
Tick	Arboviruses	Encephalitis
	Rickettsia	Rocky Mountain spotted fever; typhus
	Borrelia burgdorferi	Lyme disease
Fleas and lice	Rickettsia	Scrub typhus
Mites	Rickettsia	Scrub typhus
Monkeys	Herpes B virus	Encephalitis
Cats	Toxoplasma	Toxoplasmosis
	Rabies virus	Rabies
	Coxiella burnettii	Q fever
Mice	Hantaan virus	Multisystem failure
	Lymphocytic choriomeningitis virus	Meningoencephalitis
Cattle	Brucella	Chronic meningitis
	Rabies virus	Rabies
	C. burnettii	Q fever
Rodents	Leptospira	Meningoencephalitis
	Rabies virus	Rabies
Horses	Rabies virus	Rabies
	Brucella	Chronic meningitis
	Leptospira	Encephalitis
Swine	Rabies virus	Rabies
	Brucella	Chronic meningitis
	Leptospira	Encephalitis
Goats and sheep	Rabies virus	Rabies
	C. burnettii	Q fever
	Brucella	Chronic meningitis
	Leptospira	Encephalitis
Skunks	Rabies virus	Rabies
Dogs	Rabies virus	Rabies
	Toxocara canis	Meningoencephalitis
Bats	Rabies virus	Rabies

need to look for disseminated infections (viral, spirochetal, rickettsial, or granulomatous infections), as well as noninfectious etiologies.

Spinal Fluid Tests

Examination of the CSF is usually the single most valuable laboratory test available. In all diseases the range of values for any CSF test is very large and much overlap exists, but some guidelines are useful.

The CSF white blood cell counts and differential must be interpreted with caution. In general, infections of the parenchyma and parameningeal foci of infection show less intense pleocytosis, a tendency toward mononuclear pleocytosis, and lower protein levels than those seen in meningeal inflammation. Cell counts in bacterial infection are higher (1,000 to 5,000/mm^3) than in viral infection (100 to 1,000/mm^3), but there are many exceptions. Although bacterial meningitis usually has a neutrophilic pleocytosis (above 85 percent), in partially treated bacterial infections the differential may shift toward the right. Viral meningitis (especially mumps) may also present with a neutrophilic pleocytosis before changing to a lymphocytosis after a day or so. The presence of eosinophils (rare) suggests allergic or parasitic disease but may be seen with tuberculosis, fungal infections, and lymphoma. Large numbers of red blood cells in the CSF, if not due to a traumatic tap, suggest subarachnoid bleed, herpes encephalitis, or another necrotizing process.

The presence of elevated protein is expected in all CNS infections, but very high levels (more than 400 mg/dl) with few cells suggest neoplasm. Proteins of 100 to 400 mg/dl are typical of bacterial meningitis, while levels are lower in viral meningitis. In chronic infections or inflammation the CSF γ-globulin levels may be high relative to albumin, suggesting intracompartmental antibody production.

Glucose in bacterial meningitis is usually less than 35 mg/dl but normal in viral infections and parenchymal infections. Numerous exceptions to this rule will be seen.

Microbiologic Tests

Recovery of the etiologic agent in culture provides a definitive diagnosis and should always be attempted when infection is a consideration and CSF has been obtained. Since some fungal and bacterial pathogens may be present in low concentrations (e.g., Cryptococcus and Mycobacterium tuberculosis), it is important to provide at least several milliliters of CSF to the laboratory. If unusual pathogens (e.g., Leptospira or Borrelia) are a consideration, consultation with the laboratory will allow the most appropriate culture methods to be used.

During community outbreaks of viral meningitis, the agent should be fully identified from at least several patients and the results forwarded to public health officials for epidemiologic purposes.

Serologic Tests

Serologic studies to detect organism-specific antibodies may complement microbiologic results. For fastidious organisms or those that are not cultivable in most laboratories, diagnosis may depend on serologic testing (such as syphilis, borreliosis, many viruses, rickettsia, mycoplasma, protozoa, and parasites). A few diseases may be diagnosed using a single serum specimen (syphilis, brucellosis, HIV, human T-cell leukemia/lymphoma virus-1); but when these or any serology is negative, paired serum samples drawn 2 or more weeks apart, in the acute and convalescent stages of illness, are more sensitive and specific. In advanced HIV disease or comparable states of immunosuppression, negative serologies may remain negative because of the patient's inability to produce antibody.

Detection of localized antibody production in the CNS (CNS antibody index) is possible for many organisms but is not well standardized, and interpretive criteria originate in the laboratory that performs the test. It is essential that these tests be performed after consultation with the reference laboratory to ensure that the data obtained will be useful.

Antigen Tests

Antigen detection in the CSF is the rapid diagnostic method of choice for cryptococcal infection. Patients with HIV disease and cryptococcal infection have positive serum cryptococcal antigen more frequently than do non-HIV patients. Detection of bacterial antigens in CSF, serum, or urine is not cost effective, and should not be used routinely, but this test plays a role in making a diagnosis in the patient with partially treated meningitis.

Imaging Tests

Imaging studies (CT scan or MRI) are indicated if space-occupying lesions or hydrocephalus are suspected. If imaging is needed in a setting that is compatible with acute meningitis and a lumbar puncture is deemed inadvisable, then empirical therapy must be used, pending imaging and lumbar puncture. If images cannot be obtained immediately, empirical therapy is unlikely to obscure the diagnosis, since blood cultures are often positive, the CSF will not be sterilized immediately, and CSF antigen tests are often positive.

SUGGESTED READING

Naber SP: Molecular pathology: diagnosis of infectious disease. N Engl J Med 331:1212, 1994

BACTERIAL INFECTIONS

51. BACTERIAL MENINGITIS

STEVEN J. SPINDEL
RICHARD L. HARRIS

Bacterial meningitis is a serious and potentially overwhelming infection that results in severe morbidity and mortality. The annual incidence of bacterial meningitis in the United States is 3 per 100,000 people, which is approximately 25,000 cases. In spite of recent medical advances, the mortality from bacterial meningitis has not improved in the past three decades and neurologic sequelae remain a significant complication.

EPIDEMIOLOGY

Etiologies of acute bacterial meningitis can be divided into community and nosocomial acquired. One-half of community-acquired infections are caused by *Streptococcus pneumoniae* and *Neisseria meningitidis* (Table 51-1). Other organisms causing meningitis are *Listeria monocytogenes,* streptococci, *Staphylococcus aureus* and *Haemophilus influenzae* type B. Until recently, *H. influenzae* contributed a significant portion of community-acquired meningitis, especially in younger age groups. However, the incidence of *H. influenzae* invasive disease has declined dramatically since the advent of conjugated *H. influenzae* type B vaccine in 1988.

Nosocomial episodes of meningitis are defined as those that occur while hospitalized (typically more than 48 hours after

TABLE 51-1. Causative Organisms in All Cases of Adult Bacterial Meningitis

Organism	Community-acquired (%)	Nosocomial (%)
Streptococcus pneumoniae	37	5
Neisseria meningitidis	13	<1
Haemophilus influenzae	4	3
Listeria monocytogenes	10	3
Streptococci	7	7
Gram-negative bacilli (not *H. influenzae*)	3	39
Staphylococcus aureus	5	10
Coagulase-negative staphylococci	0	8
Anaerobes	1	1

(Data from Durand ML, Calderwood SB, Weber DJ et al: Acute bacterial meningitis in adults. N Engl J Med 328:21, 1993, with permission.)

admission) or within 1 week after discharge. The proportion of meningitis that is nosocomially acquired has risen significantly over the past three decades, increasing from 28 percent in the 1960s to 48 percent in the 1980s, because of advancing medical technology in neurosurgical techniques and the care of trauma patients. Most cases of nosocomial meningitis occur in patients after recent neurosurgery, placement of a neurosurgical device, or head trauma. Nosocomial meningitis without antecedent neurosurgical procedures or trauma is unusual, but occurs in patients who have contiguous or extracranial sites of infection and are otherwise debilitated. The incidence and proportion of meningitis due to gram-negative bacilli (other than *H. influenzae*) and staphylococci has increased primarily due to these factors. The incidence of infection of ventricular shunts, ventriculostomies, intracranial pressure (ICP) monitors, or cerebrospinal fluid (CSF) reservoirs varies, but averages 5 to 15 percent. The risk of infection is proportional to the amount of time the device is externalized and, with ICP monitors, increases when in place for 72 hours or more. CSF reservoirs and shunts usually become infected within 1 to 2 months of placement. Staphylococci and gram-negative bacilli account for up to 50 percent and 25 percent of these infections, respectively. Nosocomial meningitis can occur in almost one-fifth of patients suffering head trauma and can increase up to 50 percent if a CSF leak is present. CSF leaks are most frequently associated with patients who have a basilar skull fracture. Pathogens associated with meningitis due to basilar skull fractures frequently reflect nasopharyngeal colonization that are similar to those in community-acquired infection (*S. pneumoniae, N. meningitidis, H. influenzae*), rather than staphylococci and gram-negative bacilli which account for only 5 percent of infections.

PATHOPHYSIOLOGY

Bacteria that invade the CSF and cause meningitis have several virulence factors. They must be able to colonize the nasopharynx, penetrate into and survive in the bloodstream, and breach the blood-brain barrier to enter the CSF. Once in the CSF, there are few if any host immune defenses. The lack of complement-mediated or humoral immunity enables the bacteria to replicate with ease. Resultant damage within the central nervous system (CNS) is most likely due to the local production of cytokines such as interleukin-1, interleukin-6, and tumor necrosis factor. Cytokines are stimulated by bacterial cell wall components such as lipoteichoic acid of *S. pneumoniae* and lipopolysaccharide of gram-negative bacteria. These cytokines directly and indirectly initiate a cascade of immune responses that allow leukocytes to adhere to endothelial cells in the cerebral vasculature and migrate into the CSF. Intercellular junctions become leaky and albumin is able to exude into the CSF. The resultant brain edema, increased intracranial pressure, and altered cerebral blood flow results in severe consequences such as ischemic brain damage, seizures, cranial nerve injuries, and herniation.

Meningitis after head trauma is initiated when organisms colonizing the nasopharynx and/or the skin are directly introduced into the CSF. Basilar skull fractures allow organisms from the sinuses, ear canal, and mastoid air cells to enter the CSF. Meningitis due to ventricular shunts and ventriculostomies most commonly occurs as infection progresses in a retrograde fashion from the distal end. Other routes of infection for shunts include skin or wound breakdown, hematogenous seeding and contamination of the surgical device at the time of placement.

COMMUNITY-ACQUIRED PATHOGENS

Pneumococcal meningitis is the most frequent etiology of bacterial meningitis in adults, accounting for one-third to one-half of all cases. Pneumococcal meningitis occurs in the late fall and winter, and outbreaks are associated with overcrowded conditions. *S. pneumoniae* is the most common organism associated with CSF leaks and also represents the most common cause of recurrent episodes of bacterial meningitis. Pneumonia is seen in one-quarter of cases, and, frequently, concomitant disease such as sinusitis, mastoiditis, or otitis is present. Pneumococcal meningitis is seen in all age groups, but has an increased incidence at the extremes of age, and in patients with underlying medical disorders. Predisposing factors include alcoholism, cirrhosis, sickle cell anemia, asplenia, thalassemia, multiple myeloma, chronic lymphocytic leukemia, and immunoglobulin deficiencies.

Meningococcal meningitis is caused by serogroups A, B, C, Y, and W135 of *N. meningitidis*. Group B accounts for approximately half and group C for 22 to 45 percent of the sporadic cases of meningitis. The overwhelming majority of cases of meningococcal meningitis in the United States are sporadic and epidemic outbreaks are very rare, though such outbreaks remain common in developing areas of the world. This disease follows seasonal trends, occurring in the winter and early spring. It afflicts mostly children and young adults. Its peak incidence occurs in infants less than 4 months of age, with half of the cases occurring in infants less than 2 years old. Only 10 percent of cases occur in patients over 45 years old, unless an epidemic is in progress. Nasopharyngeal carriage of virulent strains is found in 20 to 40 percent of young adults and contacts, although in epidemic situations this can approach 90 percent. Predisposing factors for the development of disease consist of primary complement deficiencies (deficiency of terminal complement C5–C9), and diseases that impair humoral immunity or complement function. These include nephrotic syndrome, multiple myeloma, systemic lupus erythematosus, and hepatic failure.

Meningitis due to *H. influenzae* is usually caused by serotype B, with less than 15 percent being non-type B. In the northern United States there is a biphasic incidence pattern peaking in the spring and in the fall. There has been a dramatic change in the epidemiology of all *H. influenzae* disease since the introduction of conjugated vaccines and earlier vaccination schedules since 1988. *H. influenzae* once represented the most common cause of meningitis in children between the neonatal period and age 6, and 80 percent of these cases occurred in children less than 2 years old. Only 5 percent of cases occurred in adolescents between the ages of 10 and 18. Since the use of the new vaccines, the incidence of *H. influenzae* disease has decreased remarkably by almost 95 percent in children under the age of 5, and has now become an uncommon cause of meningitis. *H. influenzae* meningitis is an even rarer pathogen in adults, but when present, more than half of these patients will have a significant risk factor. Major predispositions to *H. influenzae* meningitis include a CSF leak, head trauma, or contiguous infections such as otitis or sinusitis. Additional risk factors include immunodeficiencies such as hypogammaglobulinemia, diabetes mellitus, alcoholism, asplenia, and HIV infection.

L. monocytogenes causes meningitis primarily in neonates, and occasionally in adults. It can occur in otherwise healthy patients, but remains the leading cause of bacterial meningitis in immunocompromised hosts. Patients at risk include alcoholics, renal transplant recipients, and neutropenic patients. Cases have also been reported in HIV-infected patients. Infections usually occur in the summer and early fall. Meningitis results from bacteremia, the source of which is presumed to be the gastrointestinal tract. *L. monocytogenes* is a beta-hemolytic gram-positive bacillus, and therefore, a laboratory report of diphtheroids or beta-hemolytic streptococci would prompt suspicion of possible *Listeria* meningitis. The physician must work closely with the microbiology laboratory to assist in the diagnosis of this disease.

Various streptococci can cause meningitis in the elderly, and are associated with pneumonia, endocarditis, or brain abscess. Underlying diseases in susceptible patients include diabetes mellitus, cancer, alcohol abuse, hepatic failure, renal failure, and corticosteroid use.

NOSOCOMIAL PATHOGENS

The frequency of meningitis due to gram-negative bacilli other than *H. influenzae* has increased from 11 to 24 percent between 1962 and 1988. Gram-negative bacilli are an uncommon cause of community acquired meningitis (3 percent); however, they are a constant and significant source of nosocomial meningitis (40 percent). Half of the cases occur in postneurosurgical patients, and one-third will occur following head trauma. The remainder occur in neutropenic patients, and other immunocompromised hosts such as those with acquired immune deficiency syndrome (AIDS), cirrhosis, and diabetes mellitus. Gram-negative bacillary meningitis occurs primarily in patients over the age of 60. *Escherichia coli* and *Klebsiella pneumoniae* are the most common etiologies, accounting for three-quarters of meningitis due to gram-negative organisms. Other pathogens include *Pseudomonas aeruginosa*, *Proteus*, *Enterobacter*, and *Serratia*.

Staphylococci account for the majority of ventricular shunt infections, and also cause meningitis in patients who have suffered head trauma and required invasive neurosurgical procedures. Community-acquired cases of staphylococcal meningitis are uncommon (5 percent). Most of these patients have extracranial sources of infection such as endocarditis or skin and soft tissue infections that seed the meninges hematogenously. One-half the patients have underlying diabetes mellitus, cancer, renal failure, alcoholism or other immunodeficiencies.

CLINICAL MANIFESTATIONS

The classic symptoms of meningitis which include fever, headache, and cognitive dysfunction occur in over 75 percent of cases. Other common symptoms are nausea, vomiting, rigors, sweats, weakness, myalgias, and photophobia. Confusion, lethargy, obtundation, and coma represent the range of mental status changes that can occur. Seizures are seen in up to one-third of cases. Focal neurologic deficits such as cranial nerve palsies, hemiparesis, aphasia, or visual field defects can occur in 10 to 20 percent of cases. However, papilledema is a rare finding and, if present, raises the suspicion of an intracranial mass or abscess. Nuchal rigidity is very common (88 percent). Pneumococcal meningitis is more likely to cause altered mental status and focal neurologic defects than meningitis due to other pathogens. A petechial rash is classically associated with meningococcemia, but can be seen with other infections, such as pneumococci or *H. influenzae,* especially in asplenic patients. Echovirus, rickettsiae, and *S. aureus* also cause similar rashes. Atypical skin rashes such as purpuric changes and maculopapular lesions can also be seen. Elderly patients may present with very subtle signs and symptoms, and confusion is the most common presenting symptom. Nuchal rigidity is less common in the elderly, appearing in only about one-half of the cases. However, these patients may have neck stiffness due to other diseases, and frequently a lumbar puncture must be performed in a febrile elderly patient with neck stiffness and altered mental status to rule out meningitis. Neutropenic patients can also present with mild and nonspecific signs and symptoms because of their inability to mount an inflammatory response.

The clinical manifestations of meningitis in patients who have suffered head trauma or have undergone neurosurgery are similar to those with community-acquired meningitis. However, because the patient's underlying condition can mimic or obscure meningeal symptoms, the diagnosis can be difficult. Rhinorrhea or otorrhea may be indicative of a CSF leak, which can occur in patients with basilar skull fractures. Patients with intraventricular shunt infections may exhibit fewer meningeal signs because infection is primarily limited to the ventricles. Signs and symptoms such as headache, nausea, vomiting, and mental status changes probably result from shunt malfunction rather than infection itself. There may be associated clinical findings from bacteremia or peritonitis because of infection at the distal end of the ventricular shunt.

OUTCOME

Bacterial meningitis was associated with a 25 percent case-fatality rate in a large series of adult bacterial meningitis at Massachusetts General Hospital during a 27-year period (1962–1988). Mortality associated with meningitis due to *S. pneumoniae, N. meningitidis,* and *H. influenzae* was 28 percent, 10 percent, and 11 percent, respectively. Mortality due to gram-negative bacteria was markedly higher (36 percent). Risk factors found to increase mortality were age—older than 60—obtunded mental status upon admission, and onset of seizures within 24 hours of admission. Morbidity from bacterial meningitis is significant, with 10 percent of children suffering sensorineural hearing loss and 30 to 50 percent having residual neurologic deficits such as seizures, hydrocephalus, and physical and developmental disabilities. More than 50 percent of adults suffering from meningitis due to *S. pneumoniae* will have long-term neurologic sequelae.

DIAGNOSIS

The suspicion of bacterial meningitis is a medical emergency, and it is critical that the diagnosis be made urgently, since infection can be rapidly progressive and fatal. Empirical antimicrobial therapy should be initiated as soon as possible, preferably once CSF and blood cultures have been obtained. As long as focal neurologic findings and papilledema are absent, a lumbar puncture should be performed immediately. If papilledema or focal neurologic deficits are present, an intracranial mass or abscess should be excluded by a computed tomography (CT) scan. Before performing an imaging study, the clinician should obtain blood cultures from these patients and administer antibiotics. Further management and refinement of antibiotics can be performed after the Gram stain of the CSF and other laboratory data become available. A difficult and often controversial situa-

TABLE 51-2. Typical Findings in Normal and Infected Cerebrospinal Fluid

	Normal	Bacterial meningitis
White blood cells (per mm^3)	<5	>1,000
Pleocytosis	>85% lymphocytes	Average 85% neutrophils
Glucose (mg/dl)	45–60	<40
CSF:serum glucose ratio	0.6	<0.5
Protein (mg/dl)	10–60	>150

tion arises when lumbar puncture has not been, or cannot be, performed for various reasons, but meningitis is highly suspected. We recommend obtaining blood cultures immediately and initiating empirical therapy. Remember, the etiologic agent is still likely to be identified via the blood cultures (positive in 50 percent), cultures of CSF obtained after antibiotics are given, or by latex agglutination tests.

It is important to evaluate the results of the CSF cell count and differential, and glucose and protein levels. The CSF studies in bacterial meningitis typically reveal a white blood cell (WBC) count greater than 1,000/mm^3, neutrophil predominance, glucose less than 40 mg/dl or less than 50 percent of the serum glucose, and protein greater than 100 mg/dl (Table 51-2). It is important to remember that any or all of the CSF studies may be normal in up to 30 percent of cases of bacterial meningitis. The differential on the white blood cells will have a predominance of neutrophils, although lymphocytosis occurs in 14 percent of cases (especially in meningitis due to *L. monocytogenes* or in patients with partially treated meningitis caused by any etiology). Hypoglycorrhachia will occur in 50 to 70 percent of patients, and almost all have elevated protein levels. Normal ventricular fluid has slightly higher glucose and lower protein concentrations than lumbar CSF, which should be taken into account when evaluating ventricular CSF. Organisms will be seen on Gram stain in 60 to 90 percent of culture-positive cases, and the yield can be improved with cytospin preparations of the CSF. (The most frequent error on CSF analysis is the misidentification of *L. monocytogenes* as pneumococci.) Cultures will be positive in at least 70 percent of patients with bacterial meningitis. Prior antibiotics usually have little effect on initial CSF findings, however, they can convert the pleocytosis to a lymphocytic predominance, decrease the yield of CSF Gram stains to 40 to 60 percent, and also decrease the yield of CSF cultures by one-third. The opening pressure is elevated in 75 percent or more patients (above 140 to 200 mmH$_2$O), although extremely high values (e.g., higher than 600 mmH$_2$O) should suggest an intracranial mass or communicating hydrocephalus.

Rapid diagnostic tests such as counterimmunoelectrophoresis (CIE) and latex agglutination are available for most bacterial pathogens. They have good specificity, but sensitivities are highly variable and dependent on the methods employed. It is important to realize that the diagnosis of meningitis should not be excluded by a negative test. Rapid tests can detect nonviable bacteria and can be helpful, especially in those patients who receive antibiotics prior to obtaining CSF for cultures. CIE and latex agglutination tests can be obtained for *H. influenzae* type B, *S. pneumoniae,* group B streptococci, and *N. meningitidis* groups A, C, Y, and W135.

It may be more difficult to diagnose meningitis in patients after trauma or neurosurgery because of the underlying CSF changes and pleocytosis that occur in these conditions. However, a neutrophilic pleocytosis usually is present, and the WBC to red blood cell ratio in the CSF should be elevated when compared to CSF values after trauma or neurosurgery. Nevertheless, the diagnosis of meningitis may ultimately be based on culture results. In meningitis due to CSF leaks, radiographic imaging can detect clues such as basilar skull fractures or opacification of sinuses. Nuclear medicine tests such a radionuclide cisternography are sensitive but nonspecific for the site of CSF leaks. The best test to detect the site of CSF leakage is a CT scan with CSF contrast enhancement with metrizamide. These tests should not be performed acutely but rather after the infection has been cooled down. When a ventricular shunt infection or ventriculitis is suspected, the CSF should be sampled from the ventricle, since CSF obtained from the lumbar area may not accurately reflect the presence of infection. CSF glucose is frequently normal, and the WBC count may be normal or increased in these cases.

CT scans may demonstrate the route by which meningeal infection has been introduced, such as erosive lesions, septic emboli, or abscesses. Other findings may include meningeal enhancement, ventriculomegaly, hydrocephalus, infarcts, cavernous sinus thrombosis, and subdural effusions or empyemas.

TREATMENT

Antimicrobial agents for the treatment of bacterial meningitis must be able to penetrate the blood-brain barrier into the CSF and attain high bactericidal concentrations in the CSF. Empirical therapy can be based on the age, clinical syndrome, and the risk factors of the host.

The necessity for urgent treatment often dictates that an antibiotic be started before the causative agent can be identified definitively. A reasonable empirical therapeutic regimen for community-acquired meningitis consists of ampicillin 2 g IV q4h plus ceftriaxone 2 to 3 g IV q12h (or cefotaxime). Nosocomial meningitis should initially be treated with vancomycin 1 g IV q12h and ceftazidime 2 g IV q8h. (Recommended dosages for these antimicrobials are listed in Table 51-3.) Once the identification and susceptibility of the organism is confirmed, antibiotic treatment can be tailored for the specific etiology (Table

TABLE 51-3. Dosages of Antibiotics Used for Bacterial Meningitis in Adults

Antibiotic	Dosage & Interval
Penicillin G	4 million units IV q4h
Ceftriaxone	2–3 g IV q12h
Cefotaxime	2 g IV q4h
Vancomycin	1 g IV q12h[a]
	± 5–20 mg IT q24–48h to keep CSF levels >10 μg/ml
Ampicillin	2 g IV q4h
Chloramphenicol	1.5–2 g IV q6h
Trimethoprim/sulfamethoxazole	10 mg/kg IV q8h[b]
Piperacillin	3–4 g IV q4–6h
Ceftazidime	2 g IV q8h
Nafcillin or oxacillin	2–3 g IV q4h
Gentamicin or tobramycin	5 mg/kg/day IV in 2 or 3 divided doses
	± 4 mg IT q12–24h to keep CSF levels 2–10 μg/ml
Amikacin	15 mg/kg/day IV in 2 or 3 divided doses
	± 5–10 mg IT q12–24h to keep CSF levels 2–10 μg/ml
Rifampin	300 mg PO or IV q6h

Abbreviations: IT, intrathecal (or intraventricular).
[a] Higher dosages may be required to give adequate CSF levels.
[b] Dosage based on trimethoprim component.

51-4). Duration of therapy is traditionally 10 to 14 days for most organisms.

Gram-negative meningitis should be treated for at least 21 days or until 10 days after a negative CSF culture. Third-generation cephalosporins are the treatment of choice, and systemic aminoglycosides can also be added (amikacin has better CSF penetration than gentamicin or tobramycin). Piperacillin, imipenem, or trimethoprim/sulfamethoxazole can be substituted for cephalosporins if resistant organisms are suspected. Intraventricular or intrathecal aminoglycosides may be added in these cases or when the patient is not responding, especially if concentrations of antibiotics in the CSF are low. Treatment of infections associated with neurosurgical devices may be difficult. The use of intravenous antibiotics alone is successful in only one-quarter of patients, and the addition of intrathecal or intraventricular antibiotics increases the success rate to 40 percent. This outcome can be improved further to 75 percent by the immediate replacement of the shunt, which is acting as a nidus of persistent infection. CSF leaks should be repaired if recurrent infection occurs or the leak does not spontaneously cease within 1 month.

Antibiotic-resistant organisms are an emerging problem. Penicillin-resistant pneumococci were reported initially in Europe and represent a growing percentage of strains (5 to 15 percent) in the United States. (These are screened for by the use of an oxacillin disk diffusion method, and a zone less than 20 mm around the oxacillin disk represents penicillin resistance. Pneumococcal strains can possess either relative [minimum inhibitory concentration [(MIC) = 0.1 to 1.0 μg/ml] or absolute penicillin resistance [MIC greater than 1.0 μg/ml].) Strains that are relatively resistant to penicillin may also be cephalosporin-resistant. Therefore, MICs for cefotaxime and ceftriaxone should be checked (by standard broth dilution methods) so that the utility of these cephalosporins can be determined. Vancomycin with or without rifampin should be used for cephalosporin-resistant cases (MIC levels of 2 μg/ml or greater), and strains of pneumococci that are absolutely resistant to penicillin. Some experts have begun to recommend the addition of vancomycin as empirical therapy for community-acquired meningitis because of the growing problem of cephalosporin resistance; however, individual treatment decisions should be based upon the knowledge of local resistance patterns. The penetration of vancomycin into the CSF is very unpredictable and high doses of vancomycin are required for treatment. CSF levels of vancomycin should be monitored, and, if low, the dosage of vancomycin can be adjusted. Intrathecal administration of vancomycin can also be used to achieve bactericidal CSF concentrations. Resistance to ampicillin by *H. influenzae* has been increasing, with beta-lactamase producing strains responsible for up to one-third of all cases of *H. influenzae* meningitis. There are also penicillin-resistant strains of *N. meningitidis* with low-affinity penicillin-binding proteins that have been reported, predominantly in Europe. Therefore, extended spectrum cephalosporins are the drugs of choice for both of these organisms until the susceptibility patterns of the strain can be established.

Therapeutic choices can be confusing in the patient claiming an allergy to penicillin. Many people carry the label of penicillin allergy, but only a small minority have life-threatening reactions. A careful history should be obtained of the allergic reaction, and if not consistent with an anaphylactic or immediate type I (immunoglobulin E [IgE]-mediated) allergy, penicillin or a cephalosporin can be used. If no history can be obtained, we recommend the use of cephalosporins, given the low risk:

TABLE 51-4. Antimicrobial Therapy for Adult Bacterial Meningitis

Organism	Risk Factors and Clinical Syndrome	Therapy
S. pneumoniae	Community-acquired, CSF leak, recurrent meningitis	PCN-sensitive: penicillin G PCN-relative resistance: ceftriaxone or cefotaxime PCN-absolute resistance: vancomycin ± IT vancomycin[a] PCN allergy: vancomycin[b]
N. meningitidis	Community-acquired, contact to meningitis	PCN-sensitive: penicillin G or ampicillin PCN-resistant: ceftriaxone or cefotaxime PCN allergy: chloramphenicol
H. influenzae	Community-acquired, basilar skull fracture, daycare exposure, sinusitis, otitis	β-Lactamase-negative: ampicillin β-Lactamase positive: ceftriaxone or cefotaxime PCN allergy: chloramphenicol
L. monocytogenes	Community-acquired, age >50 years, immunocompromised	Penicillin G or ampicillin PCN allergy; Trimethoprim-sulfamethoxazole
Gram-negative bacilli	Age >50 years, nosocomial infection, postneurosurgery	Ceftriaxone or cefotaxime or piperacillin If *Pseudomonas aeruginosa*, use ceftazidime + IV aminoglycosides ± IT or intraventricular aminoglycosides
Streptococci	Endocarditis	Penicillin G or ampicillin + IV aminoglycosides
S. aureus	Post-trauma, neurosurgery, shunt placement, endocarditis, other site of infection	MSSA: nafcillin or oxacillin MRSA: vancomycin ± IT vancomycin
Coagulase-negative staphylococci	Shunt placement, ventriculostomy, post-trauma, neurosurgery	Vancomycin ± IT vancomycin + rifampin

Abbreviations: IV, intravenous; PCN, penicillin; MSSA, methicillin sensitive *S. aureus*; MRSA, methicillin resistant *S. aureus*.
[a] IT, intrathecal administration if CSF concentrations are persistently low, or patient is not clinically responding.
[b] PCN-Allergy: Vancomycin as an alternative only in the setting of a history of anaphylaxis (see text).

benefit ratio of using these antibiotics for a life-threatening meningitis. Skin testing may be performed; however, antibiotics should not be delayed while this is done.

There has been intensive investigation into the use of adjunctive anti-inflammatory measures to prevent much of the sequelae of meningitis. Antibiotics cause rapid bacterial killing, cell lysis and the release of cell wall components that have inflammatory properties. There is speculation that antibiotics with less bacteriolytic properties may decrease these severe effects (e.g., new carbapenems). In children with *H. influenzae* meningitis, corticosteroids have been determined to decrease morbidity such as sensorineural hearing loss, ataxia, and hemiparesis. However, there are no good studies of the adjunctive use of corticosteroids in adults, and it is debated whether steroids should be used routinely in all cases of meningitis. Controlled studies are ongoing, but many experts currently recommend the use of corticosteroids in adults with meningitis when bacterial loads are high (e.g., when the Gram stain is positive), or with an elevated opening pressure or other evidence of cerebral edema and increased intracranial pressure.

PROPHYLAXIS

Close family, household, and intimate contacts, classmates, and day care attendees of documented cases of *N. meningitidis* should be treated with rifampin immediately after exposure to prevent infection (Table 51-5). Transmission to health care workers is very rare and occurs via direct contact with respiratory secretions. The risk of transmission is very low with meningococcal meningitis or meningococcemia. Treatment is indicated only for health care workers with intensive close contact (e.g., cardiopulmonary resuscitation or exposure to respiratory secretions). Rifampin prophylaxis should be prescribed when there are susceptible children who have had contact with the index case in the prior week. Rifampin should be given to children of all ages and adults in the household or day care setting because immunized individuals can serve as a reservoir for infection of susceptible children. Studies of the efficacy of prophylactic antibiotics in patients with CSF leaks have yielded conflicting results. None of these were well-controlled prospective trials, and therefore no clear-cut current recommendations can be given.

SUGGESTED READINGS

CDC: Progress toward elimination of *Haemophilus influenzae* type B disease among infants and children—United States, 1987–1993. MMWR 43:144, 1994

Durand ML, Calderwood SB, Weber DJ et al: Acute bacterial meningitis is adults. N Engl J Med 328:21, 1993

Geiseler PJ, Nelson KE, Levin S et al: Community-acquired purulent meningitis: a review of 1,316 cases during the antibiotic era, 1954–1976. Rev Infect Dis 2:725, 1980

McGee ZA, Baringer JR: Acute Meningitis. p. 741. In Mandell GL, Douglas RG Jr, Bennett JE (eds): Principles and Practices of Infectious Diseases. 3rd Ed. Churchill Livingstone, New York, 1990

Moellering RC, Scheld WM, Wispelwey B: Meningitis. Infect Dis Clin North Am 4: 1990

Quagliarello VJ, Scheld WM: New perspectives on bacterial meningitis. Clin Infect Dis 17:603, 1993

Schlech WF III, Ward JI, Band JD et al: Bacterial meningitis in the United States, 1978 through 1981. JAMA 253:1749, 1985

Schlesinger LS, Ross SC, Schaber DR: *Staphylococcus aureus* meningitis: a broad-based epidemiologic study. Medicine 66:148, 1987

Wenger JD, Hightower AW, Facklam PR et al: Bacterial meningitis in the United States, 1986: report of a multistate surveillance study. J Infect Dis 162:1316, 1990

TABLE 51-5. Recommendations for Prophylaxis of Meningitis

Organism	Prophylaxis	Comments
Neisseria meningitidis	Rifampin 600 mg PO bid for 2 days Rifampin 10 mg/kg dose (up to 600 mg) for children	Minocycline is an alternative Ciprofloxacin is effective as a one time dose Ceftriaxone for pregnant contacts
Haemophilus influenzae	Rifampin 600 mg PO qd for 4 days Rifampin 20 mg/kg dose (up to 600 mg) for children	Day care prophylaxis if children <1 year old with ≥25 contact hours per week, or ≥2 cases in 60 days

52. BRAIN AND SPINAL ABSCESSES

LOREN A. ROLAK

Bacteria seldom cause abscesses within the parenchyma of the brain, and when they do it is usually as a complication of an infection elsewhere in the body. Although rare, brain abscesses produce devastating consequences, so their detection and treatment are urgent medical matters.

EPIDEMIOLOGY

Although a quarter of all brain abscesses occur in previously healthy patients, with no predisposing infections or medical complications, most arise as the result of either local extension or hematogenous spread of infection by pyogenic bacteria in other locations. Table 52-1 shows the most frequent sites of underlying infections and the organisms most likely to cause brain abscesses in each setting. Within the brain, at least half of abscesses contain two or even more pathogenic bacteria, which often complicates both diagnosis and treatment. Around 75 percent of patients have only a solitary abscess, especially those patients in whom the abscess arises from a perimeningeal infection, or other contiguous site. Most patients with multiple abscesses have a hematogenous source of infection, such as endocarditis, or have an underlying immune deficiency, including acquired immune deficiency syndrome (AIDS).

CLINICAL FEATURES

Although brain abscesses obviously represent a pyogenic infection, most do not present with the features of an infection—fever, nuchal rigidity, and elevated peripheral white blood cell (WBC) count are rare. Even the spinal fluid is usually normal. Instead, the usual presentation is of a mass lesion, with clinical features reflecting the subacute onset of a progressively enlarging space-occupying lesion. Table 52-2 shows the most com-

TABLE 52-1. Causes of Brain Abscesses

Underlying Infection (%)	Common Pathogens
Otitis or mastoiditis (15)	Gram-negative bacilli Streptococcus Bacteroides
Dental infections (15)	Streptococcus Bacteroides
Sinusitis (20)	Staphylococcus aureus Streptococcus Bacteroides Haemophilus influenzae
Head wound or neurosurgery (5)	S. aureus Gram-negative bacilli Streptococcus
Pulmonary infection (15)	Streptococcus Mixed flora Nocardia
Endocarditis (5)	Streptococcus S. aureus
Idiopathic or unknown (25)	S. aureus Streptococcus Bacteroides
Acquired immune deficiency syndrome (or other immune deficiency)	Toxoplasma gondii Nocardia Aspergillus Candida

TABLE 52-2. Most Common Presenting Symptoms of a Brain Abscess

Symptom	Frequency (%)
Headache	75
Focal deficit	65
Altered mental status	60
Seizures	40
Fever	30
Increased intracranial pressure (vomiting, papilledema)	20
Nuchal rigidity	20

mon presenting symptoms of a brain abscess, with focal deficits, seizures (often focal) and increased intracranial pressure dominating the picture. The onset of symptoms is generally subacute and gradual, evolving over 2 weeks or more, as the infection progresses from a localized cerebritis to a focal, well-encapsulated abscess, with a necrotic center and well-defined capsule (Table 52-3).

DIAGNOSIS

Imaging of the brain, with either magnetic resonance imaging (MRI) or computed tomography (CT) scanning, provides the key to the diagnosis of abscesses. Surgical biopsy, guided by the imaging, is usually required for a definitive diagnosis. Paradoxically, many standard tests for infections provide little useful information in patients with brain abscesses. Cultures of the blood and the spinal fluid seldom yield the causative organisms. For this reason, as well as the fact that lumbar punctures may carry a risk of neurologic deterioration in patients with increased intracranial pressure from a brain abscess, a spinal tap is seldom indicated for the diagnosis of brain abscesses. Very little information exists regarding the value of serologic or immunologic methods of identifying the pathogens responsible for the abscess, such as counterimmunoelectrophoresis and other techniques, but their utility is most likely limited.

Both CT and MRI are quite accurate for detecting abscesses, showing a focal lesion with a necrotic center and an enhancing ring (the collagen capsule) surrounding it, generating considerable edema and mass effect (Fig. 52-1). This appearance can be definitive in the proper clinical setting, but an identical radiographic appearance may be produced by certain tumors (especially metastases) and even occasional ischemic infarctions, resolving hematomas, and radiation necrosis. Therefore, to provide greater diagnostic certainty as well as to obtain exact identification of the causative organisms, a biopsy is usually required.

When brain imaging shows changes compatible with an abscess, further diagnostic testing should often include a chest radiograph, blood cultures, electrocardiogram, and echocardiography. The physical examination should focus particular attention on the sinuses, teeth, and ears, and all patients should have their human immunodeficiency virus (HIV) status determined.

Brain abscesses can seldom be diagnosed or treated successfully without surgical intervention. In most cases, a stereotactic CT-guided needle aspiration should be performed for confirma-

TABLE 52-3. Formation of a Brain Abscess

Stage	Time (days)	Process
Early cerebritis	1–3	Acute inflammation Polymorphonuclear infiltration
Late cerebritis	4–9	Necrotic center Fibroblast activity Edema New vessel formation
Capsule formation	10–14	Mature collagen capsule

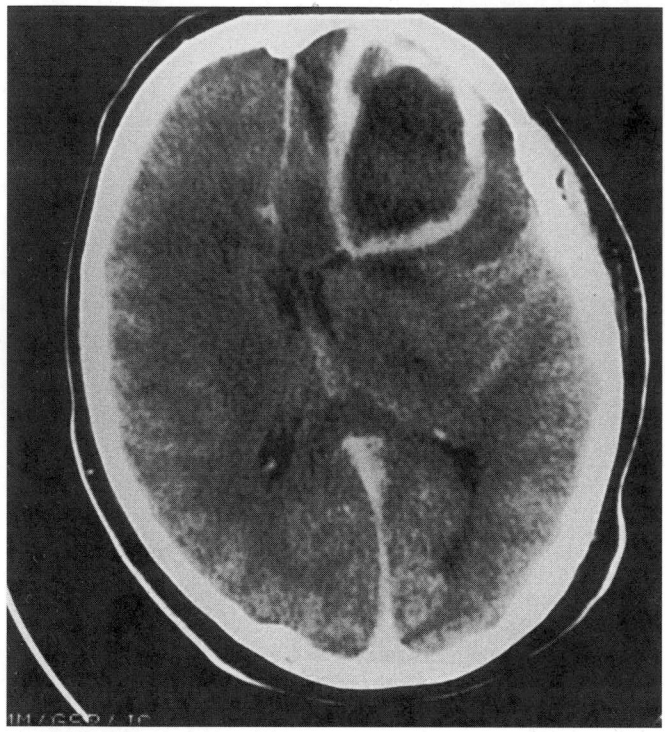

FIG. 52-1. CT scan with contrast enhancement from a 68-year-old man with a bacterial abscess (of unknown cause) in the left frontal lobe. The scan shows the necrotic abscess surrounded by an enhancing capsule, with edema and mass effect.

tion of the diagnosis and culturing of the responsible bacteria. Over 90 percent of patients have positive bacterial cultures in this setting.

TREATMENT

Ideal treatment consists of specific antibiotics tailored to the specific culture and sensitivity results for the individual organisms obtained from the abscess. In most cases, such specific cultures can in fact be obtained through surgical intervention. However, if surgery is not possible, or the surgical specimen proves sterile (which occurs in up to 20 percent of cases in some series, although the yield is generally excellent), or if empirical therapy must be started prior to a definitive diagnosis because of the seriousness of the patient's medical condition or because of anticipated delays in further management, then the initial antibiotic regimen will necessarily be less precise. Many abscesses contain multiple organisms, and therefore empirical therapy must include broad-spectrum coverage. Streptococci, common organisms in many abscesses, respond well to penicillin, which is also an effective agent against most gram-positive organisms and many anaerobes. Metronidazole has an excellent action against bacteroids, and penetrates abscess walls well. The third-generation cephalosporins provide good coverage against gram-negative bacteria and so should also be included in an empirical regimen for brain abscesses. A suggested empirical therapy for brain abscesses is as follows:

1. Penicillin G 4 million units IV q4h
   plus
2. Ceftriaxone 4 g IV q12h
   plus
3. Metronidazole 500 mg IV q6h

Surgery greatly facilitates the management of brain abscesses. In addition to biopsy and culture for diagnosis, drainage of the abscess almost always accelerates healing and recovery. This can generally be accomplished stereotactically, and repeated drainage can be performed if necessary. Definitive surgical excision of an abscess is seldom necessary: it is a major surgical procedure with significant morbidity and mortality, abscesses are not always localized in easily resected areas, and drainage alone usually leads to adequate clinical recovery. Complete excision is thus generally reserved for those lesions that do not respond to stereotactic drainage plus antibiotic treatment.

Nonsurgical management of brain abscesses has been effective in some cases. However, such treatment is seldom successful for large abscesses—larger than 3 cm—and certainly is much more difficult than treatment that is aided by surgical drainage. Therapy with antibiotics alone is usually recommended only if multiple abscesses are present, making surgical drainage too difficult, or if the patient is otherwise an unacceptable surgical candidate because of underlying medical complications or other factors.

Even with surgical drainage, antibiotic therapy must generally continue for at least 6 to 8 weeks. Repeated MRI or CT scan can effectively document the response to treatment, but therapy need not continue until the scans are entirely normal, since complete radiographic resolution always lags behind successful treatment, often by many months. Despite the frequent presence of edema and mass effect, often to a considerable extent, the concomitant use of steroids is not advised for abscesses. Steroids often delay healing and impair antibiotic effectiveness by solidifying the abscess capsule and inhibiting drug penetration across the blood-brain barrier.

In the modern era of neuroimaging and sophisticated antibiotics, the mortality from brain abscesses has declined to approximately 20 percent, from a greater than 80 percent mortality in the preantibiotic era. Nevertheless, as many as 50 percent of survivors will suffer permanent neurologic sequelae from the abscess. Focal neurologic findings may persist, depending on the location of the abscess. Permanent seizures frequently complicate brain abscesses, and as many as 30 to 50 percent of patients experience seizures following successful treatment of their infection. Fortunately, conventional anticonvulsant therapy, such as with phenytoin or carbamazepine, generally successfully suppresses these seizures.

SPINAL EPIDURAL ABSCESS

In the spine, bacterial abscesses seldom involve the substance of the cord itself, but rather tend to arise in the epidural space, between the dura that surrounds the spinal cord and the bony vertebral bodies themselves. Similar to brain abscesses, these lesions often arise in patients with underlying infections, especially osteomyelitis of the vertebral bodies; intravenous drug abuse is also a particular risk factor for the development of spinal epidural abscesses. Also analogously with brain abscesses, these lesions seldom present as an infection, and fever or elevated peripheral WBC counts seldom appear. Rather, the presentation usually takes the form of an acute spinal cord compression from the mass effect, resembling cord compression from a metastatic neoplasm. Pain at the level of the abscess is almost always present, followed by signs of spinal cord compression, including paralysis, a sensory level, and loss of bowel and bladder function. Most abscesses arise in the thoracic or lumbar region, and develop subacutely, over days or even weeks.

Diagnostically, lumbar puncture and examination of the CSF almost never yields a specific diagnosis, and may dangerously spread the infection. Instead, diagnostic testing should begin with imaging of the spine, by MRI if possible. MRI accurately detects the abscess, which then guides the surgeons for definitive decompression and drainage of the abscess. Urgent surgical decompression is almost always indicated.

Culture of surgical specimens will provide a definitive diagnosis and accurate identification of the causative organisms in almost all cases. Empirical antibiotic therapy, pending the final culture results, should be directed at coverage for *Staphylococcus aureus* and streptococci, which account for 75 to 90 percent of all cases. Gram-negative aerobes cause almost all other cases (especially in intravenous drug users) and thus an appropriate regimen would be vancomycin 1 g q8h or nafcillin 2 g q4h plus a third-generation cephalosporin such as ceftriaxone 4 g q12h. Intravenous antibiotics must be continued for 4 to 8 weeks. Neurologic recovery is excellent if spinal cord damage is minimal at the time of presentation and decompression, but is very poor if paraparesis or paralysis has been present longer than 48 to 72 hours.

SUGGESTED READINGS

Chun CH, Johnson JD, Hofstetter M, Raf MJ: Brain abscess: a study of 45 consecutive cases. Medicine (Baltimore) 65:414, 1986

Mampalam TJ, Rosenblum ML: Trends in the management of bacterial brain abscesses: a review of 102 cases over 17 years. Neurosurgery 23:451, 1988

Sandhu FS, Dillon WP: Spinal epidural abscess: evaluation with contrast-enhanced MR imaging. AJR 158:45, 1992

Wheeler D, Keiser P, Rigamonti D, Keay S: Medical management of spinal epidural abscesses: case report and review. Clin Infect Dis 15:22, 1992

53. TUBERCULOSIS

CLIFFORD C. DACSO

Mycobacteria cause a broad repertoire of human disease. In the nervous system, the most important of the mycobacteria are *Mycobacterium tuberculosis* and *M. leprae*. Nontuberculous mycobacteria, historically known as ''atypical mycobacteria,'' have also been implicated in nervous system disease, but only rarely. Mycobacteria share the characteristic of producing surface lipids that render them acid-fast, meaning that they cannot be decolorized by acid-alcohol after staining. Although some other organisms (such as *Nocardia*) are sometimes acid-fast, the vast majority of organisms with this staining characteristic are mycobacteria. Mycobacteria are generally slow-growing, and in the laboratory they require supplemented media and 5 to 10 percent CO_2.

EPIDEMIOLOGY

Tuberculosis syndromes are caused either by *M. tuberculosis* or *M. bovis,* but since the latter has virtually been eradicated in cattle in the United States, domestic tuberculosis is virtually always *M. tuberculosis*. The incidence of tuberculosis infection in the United States is approximately 9 cases per 100,000. Developing countries have an incidence approximately 15 times the rate in the United States. Nationally, tuberculosis showed a progressive decline since systematic surveil-

lance was introduced in 1953, but this decline has halted and even reversed. The causes for this resurgence are believed to be the epidemic of acquired immune deficiency syndrome (AIDS), increased immigration from the Pacific rim, and higher levels of poverty and homelessness. Despite the changes in pulmonary tuberculosis, extrapulmonary and nervous system tuberculosis rates have remained constant.

CLINICAL FEATURES

Tuberculosis infection usually begins as a respiratory infection, after which the bacilli are ingested by macrophages and carried to lymph nodes and then are disseminated hematogenously throughout the body. In 90 percent or more of patients, the primary pulmonary focus heals, as do the disseminated lesions, forming granulomas and often later calcifying. These sites may serve as foci for later reactivation, however. Tuberculous infection of the central nervous system may develop following reactivation from such a distant site, although the most common pathogenesis is not from direct hematogenous seeding, but rather from rupture of an adjacent focus of tuberculosis, called a tubercle.

Organisms are widely disseminated throughout the central nervous system and, under the appropriate host conditions, may proliferate. Conditions of immunosuppression, such as waning cellular immunity of age, corticosteroids or other immunosuppressing drugs, or trauma, promote the reactivation of tuberculosis.

Tuberculous meningitis has a broad and protean range of presentations. It is best thought of as a chronic meningitis with gradual onset, although it may present abruptly, mimicking acute bacterial meningitis. An acute onset of symptoms cannot rule out tuberculosis as the etiology of meningitis. Nevertheless, the most typical picture is a gradual headache and confusion, often with little or no fever. Personality changes also occur frequently as the disease progresses. A more insidious form of tuberculosis of the central nervous system (CNS) is even more chronic, with personality changes occurring over months to years.

Tuberculous meningitis generally also causes signs and symptoms characteristic of a chronic basilar meningitis. As a consequence, cranial nerve abnormalities are common. The inflammation frequently begins to involve blood vessels as well, producing a secondary vasculitis and subsequent strokes. These are often major infarcts, resulting in severe hemiparesis. The inflammation and exudate at the base of the brain may lead to another major complication, hydrocephalus. This can be sufficiently severe to cause increased intracranial pressure and herniation.

Table 53-1 shows the staging of tuberculous meningitis. A patient's recovery depends upon the stage at which therapy is instituted. Untreated, tuberculous meningitis is usually fatal within weeks.

DIAGNOSIS

Although most patients have extrameningeal tuberculosis, and a chest radiograph can be diagnostically useful, failure to find other organs involved with the disease cannot exclude tuberculosis as the etiology of meningitis. In the urban setting, social ills, alcoholism, AIDS, and drug use are frequent concomitants, and diagnostic suspicion should be higher in these patients. The diagnosis of tuberculous meningitis often rests on finding compatible signs and symptoms in a suitable clinical situation. These signs and symptoms are listed on p. 374.

TABLE 53-1. Staging of Tuberculous Meningitis

Stage	Mental Status	Signs
1	Conscious, alert	Meningismus, nonfocal examination
2	Confused	Cranial nerve involvement, hemiparesis
3	Comatose	Dense hemiplegia or paraplegia

1. Fungal meningitis
2. Sarcoidosis
3. Lyme disease
4. Borreliosis
5. Syphilis
6. Parameningeal focus of infection
7. Brain abscess
8. Toxoplasmosis
9. Carcinomatous meningitis
10. Partially treated pyogenic meningitis

Peripheral blood tests are often normal, including the complete blood count. Hyponatremia may be seen as a result of the syndrome of inappropriate secretion of antidiuretic hormone (SIADH) that develops in as many as 30 percent of patients with tuberculous meningitis. A positive PPD (purified protein derivative [tuberculin]) test is useful, although a negative one will occur in as many as one-third of cases.

The imaging modalities of magnetic resonance imaging (MRI) or computed tomography (CT) scanning can be extremely helpful in the diagnosis and management of patients with tuberculous meningitis. The CT scan can usually demonstrate (and follow) the major features of tuberculous meningitis, including basilar inflammation, cerebral infarction and edema, tuberculomas, and hydrocephalus.

Spinal fluid examination is the cornerstone of the diagnosis of tuberculous meningitis. Almost all patients have a substantial lymphocytic pleocytosis. Hypoglycorrhachia is seen in the majority of cases and can be useful in distinguishing tuberculosis from other causes of chronic basilar meningitis. Although the protein is usually elevated in the spinal fluid, a normal protein does not rule out the disease. The key to the diagnosis of tuberculous meningitis is the demonstration of acid-fast bacilli. In order to find the organisms, the importance of large-volume taps done repeatedly cannot be overemphasized.

Culture of these slow-growing bacilli is not useful because of the length of time a culture result may require. Recent reports of enzyme-linked immunosorbent assay (ELISA) for mycobacterial antigens and the use of polymerase chain reaction offer hope of a more accurate and rapid diagnosis.

TREATMENT

Therapy for tuberculous meningitis should consist of three drugs, although resistant organisms require more, as shown in Table 53-2. Corticosteroids are generally added when there are focal neurologic signs (stages 2 and 3), cerebral edema, elevated intracranial pressure, spinal fluid block, or deteriorating mental

TABLE 53-2. Therapy for Tuberculous Meningitis[a]

Antituberculous therapy should consist of three drugs given once daily for 9 months
  Isoniazid (INH) 10 mg/kg
  Rifampin 600 mg
  Pyrazinamide 25 to 35 mg/kg

Prednisone 60 to 80 mg daily for 1 to 2 weeks should be added in severe cases.

[a] When resistant organisms are suspected, multidrug regimens are required.

status. Some authors have also recommended steroids when there is involvement of the optic nerve. Surgery is reserved for those patients with hydrocephalus or whose increased intracranial pressure has not responded to corticosteroids and repeated lumbar puncture.

Success of treatment is related to the clinical stage at which treatment is begun (Table 53-1). Patients in stage 1 have virtually no mortality, while 40 to 60 percent of patients in stage 3 die despite aggressive treatment.

TUBERCULOMA

Tuberculomas are space-occupying lesions resulting from the containment of the inflammatory process in metastatic tuberculosis. Tuberculomas are more common in developing countries, particularly in children. In the United States, tuberculomas are seen most frequently in the setting of AIDS.

Presenting signs of tuberculomas are dependent on the site of the lesion. When adjacent to the arachnoid they may rupture, causing arachnoiditis. In the brain, tuberculomas present as mass lesions, often with seizures. In the spinal cord, tuberculomas may cause cord compression and spinal fluid block; combined surgery and chemotherapy should be instituted for these cases.

Fewer than one-third of patients have signs of tuberculosis elsewhere, as contrasted with tuberculous meningitis. CT scans are very useful in the diagnosis. Early tuberculomas show edema and low-density or isodense lesions. As the lesions progress, they become hyperdense, with ring enhancement.

Medical treatment is preferable to surgery, which is reserved for lesions in critical locations or for diagnosis. Steroids are useful if cerebral edema causes symptoms.

SUGGESTED READINGS

Davis LE, Rastogi KR, Lambert LC et al: Tuberculous meningitis in the southwest United States: a community based study. Neurology 43:1775, 1993
Kaneko K, Onodera O, Miyatake T et al: Rapid diagnosis of tuberculous meningitis by polymerase chain reaction (PCR). Neurology 40:1617, 1990
Kennedy DH, Fallon RJ: Tuberculous meningitis. JAMA 241:64, 1979
Leonard JM, Des Prez RM: Tuberculous meningitis. Infect Dis Clin North Am 4:769, 1990

54. LEPROSY

Y. HARATI

Leprosy (Hansen's disease) is a chronic, infectious, granulomatous disease caused by the intracellular acid-fast bacillus *Mycobacterium leprae*. It is considered to be primarily a disease of peripheral nerves, but the skin, eyes, mucosa of the upper respiratory tract, muscles, bones, and testes may also be affected. The spectrum of clinical and pathologic manifestations depends on the immune status of the infected individual.

Only a small portion of any given population is susceptible to *M. leprae*. Despite a very low transmission rate, and available medical treatment, a significant stigma is still associated with the disease. Until recently, the estimated number of patients with leprosy around the world was about 10 to 12 million, but the most recent estimates by the World Health Organization (WHO) in 1987, 1992, and 1994 have reduced this number to

5.1, 3.1, and 2.4 million, respectively. This steady decline is credited to the introduction of multidrug therapy against leprosy in 1982 by the WHO. The infection occurs in nearly all countries, but it is found primarily in the Indian subcontinent, sub-Saharan Africa, and Southeast Asia. Six countries alone account for more than 85 percent of the estimated cases; these are, in order of frequency, India, Brazil, Bangladesh, Indonesia, Myanmar and Nigeria.

In the United States there have been up to 350 new cases reported every year for the past 20 years, most of which have been acquired in other countries. There are about 6,000 active cases in the United States, mostly in the states bordering the Gulf of Mexico (Louisiana, Florida, and Texas) but also in Hawaii. Because of the fact that almost all states in the United States have reported at least a few cases of leprosy, there are 10 Hansen's disease clinics around the country funded by the U.S. Public Health Services. The Hansen's Disease Center in Carville, Louisiana is the sole focus of centralized care for leprosy in the United States. When a patient with leprosy is encountered it is advisable to contact the experienced staff of this center for information on the latest therapeutic regimen and advise. Their telephone number is (504)642-4700.

EPIDEMIOLOGY

Although close human contact has been traditionally accepted as the mode of infection with *M. leprae,* the precise modes of transmission have not been established. A major portal of entry may be the respiratory tract, as the nasal secretions of those with lepromatous leprosy may contain up to 2×10^8 *M. leprae* in a single nose blow. Other possibilities such as inoculation via the skin, gastrointestinal transmission, or insect bite have been considered but not proven. As many as 70 percent, and no fewer than 50 percent, of patients with leprosy have no history whatsoever of contact with another known leprosy patient. Nonhuman sources of infection, such as infected wild armadillos (*Dasypus novemcinctus*), have been suggested as the source of leprosy in these patients. Approximately 5 to 10 percent of wild armadillos in Louisiana and eastern Texas have leprosy. Leprosy has also been discovered in the sooty mangabey, a New World monkey. The reason for the greater susceptibility of some individuals to the disease is not known; there is no strong support for genetic, racial, ethnic, or nutritional factors.

CLINICAL FEATURES

Few diseases present as wide a spectrum of clinical and pathologic forms as leprosy. It exists in three major forms: tuberculoid (TT), borderline (BB), and lepromatous (LL) (Table 54-1). The borderline type may be further divided into borderline-tuberculoid (BT), midborderline (BB), and borderline lepromatous (BL). A minor form, called indeterminate leprosy, is a nascent stage of the disease in which the clinical and histopathologic destiny of the disease is uncertain.

A practicing physician may encounter a patient with leprosy when there is evidence of peripheral nerve lesions affecting cutaneous nerves, single or multiple motor-sensory nerves or nerves of distal lower limbs. Because of the proclivity of *M. leprae* to grow in cooler areas of the body (i.e., pinnae of the ears, the extensor surfaces of the limbs, the face or the buttock), the patchy cutaneous sensory deficits are more commonly seen in these areas. They do not usually involve the palms of the

TABLE 54-1. Classification and Clinical Characteristics of Leprosy

Tuberculoid leprosy (TT)
 Few well-defined anesthetic macules or papules
 Nerve involvement is common

Borderline forms
 Borderline tuberculoid (BT)
  More skin lesions with less distinct borders
  Nerve involvement
 Midborderline (BB)
  More skin lesions than BT with vague borders
  Nerve involvement is common
 Borderline lepromatous (BL)
  Numerous skin lesions with vague borders
  Nerve involvement is less than BB

Lepromatous leprosy (LL)
 Multiple skin lesions (macules, nodules or diffuse infiltration) with systemic distribution
 Late nerve involvement

Indeterminate
 Vaguely defined, hypopigmented or erythematous macules

hands and soles of feet, inguinal areas, intergluteal fold, perineum, axillae or scalp, the warmer areas of the skin. Sensory loss, patchy or diffuse, precedes paralysis in all types of leprosy. The involved areas have decreased temperature and pain sensation, but position and vibration sensations are normal. The pattern of sensory loss, being caused by the intracutaneous nerve involvement, does not follow the pattern of any peripheral nerve or nerve root distribution. This, along with the intact tendon reflexes due to preservation of deep and warmer intramuscular nerves, should raise the possibility of leprosy. The preservation of reflexes remains the most helpful sign in differentiating all forms of leprosy with nerve involvement from other polyneuropathies. The evolution, pattern, and extent of the sensory involvement and subsequent motor weakness are determined by the type of leprosy.

Tuberculoid leprosy is the most common and localized form of the disease, associated with delayed-type hypersensitivity and limited spread and proliferation of bacilli. Patients with this form of leprosy are likely to seek medical attention early in the disease process and be seen by a neurologist. Characteristically, there are only a single or several asymmetrically distributed hypopigmented and hypoesthetic and analgesic skin lesions, with firmly papulated borders. The involved areas are also anhidrotic and eventually lose hairs. Cutaneous nerves adjacent to lesions are frequently enlarged and nearby peripheral nerves are frequently palpable. The most frequently enlarged nerves are the greater auricular, the ulnar above the elbow, the peroneal at the fibular bone head, and the posterior tibial nerve. The involved nerves usually display slowed nerve conduction from the earliest stage. The enlarged ulnar nerve extends 10 to 12 cm proximal to the olecranon groove area. In other neuropathies with enlarged nerves (e.g., amyloidosis, hypertrophic neuropathies, Refsum's disease) there are typically widespread areflexia and distal symmetric deficits allowing the differentiation from leprosy. Patients with tuberculoid leprosy are immunocompetent and mount an intense tissue reaction at the site of entry into nerve of *M. leprae,* preventing the bacilli from multiplying. However, the vigorous immune response against the microorganism results in the nerve damage at the outset. Nerve biopsy shows only a few organisms, even in the face of complete nerve destruction by profound tissue proliferation.

In contrast to tuberculoid leprosy, the poor specific cellular immune response of patients with *lepromatous leprosy* permits unchecked bacillary proliferation and hematogenous dissemination. These patients do not present to the physician early in their disease process because there are no early signs of nerve involvement and early dermal lesions are not likely to be noticed by the patient. The patients are highly infectious, however. The two symptoms that usually cause the patient to seek medical attention are nasal stuffiness and pedal edema. Because of the absence of tissue reaction, including little intraneural macrophage invasion, there is minimal early nerve damage despite massive bacillary invasion of Schwann cells. The loss of nerve function is gradual, as opposed to the rapid nerve destruction seen in tuberculoid leprosy and many borderline forms. Loss of sensation in limbs in advanced neuropathies leads to repeated injuries and ulcerations of the feet and hands. Nerves of the cooler parts of the body are more prominently involved and a pattern of multiple mononeuropathies emerges in the early stages of nerve involvement. Because of the deeper and warmer location of autonomic nerves and ganglia, prominent clinical autonomic dysfunction is not seen in leprosy. Biopsy or smear of skin, cutaneous nerves, and nasal mucosa reveals rampant acid-fast bacilli infiltrations.

Borderline cases have a variable combination of clinical, bacteriologic, histologic and immunologic abnormalities of the two polar types. They usually ''downgrade'' toward lepromatous leprosy if not treated. Nerve involvement is variable with either asymmetric nerve enlargement in ''downgrading'' disease or symmetric neuropathy when disease is ''upgrading'' from the lepromatous pole. In certain borderline cases, a prolonged mononeuropathy multiplex phase may occur before the appearance of skin lesions, leading to misdiagnosis if peripheral nerve enlargement is not detected by palpation.

It should be remembered that, in the absence of sensory loss, leprosy should not be diagnosed. In leprosy, deep tendon reflexes and position and vibration sense are usually preserved, proximal muscle wasting and weakness are uncommon and pyramidal tract signs are not observed.

LEPROSY REACTIONS

Aside from the slow progressive illness, there are several specific reactions that may be associated with sudden deterioration of neurologic functions. The first type of reaction, known as reversal reaction (type 1 reaction), occurs in tuberculoid leprosy, causing a sudden exacerbation of the existing lesions. Acute neurologic deficit and severe pain may occur following the treatment with chemotherapy, and is thought to be caused by the sudden change in the cell-mediated immunity response to *M. leprae.*

The second type, known as erythema nodosum leprosum (ENL), or type 2 reaction, occurs in about 50 percent of patients with lepromatous leprosy after several months of therapy and is characterized by fever, malaise, generalized lymphadenopathy, hepatosplenomegaly and arthritis. Acute painful neuritis may also develop. The reaction is presumably due to an acute hypersensitivity reaction precipitated by the release of antigens from dead mycobacteria.

Leprosy reactions and the acute neuritis must be recognized early and treated immediately. If untreated the neurologic deficits may remain permanent.

DIAGNOSIS

A definitive diagnosis is best made by the demonstration of acid-fast bacilli in skin or peripheral nerve biopsies, although organisms may be difficult to detect in tuberculoid disease.

TABLE 54-2. Recommendations for the Treatment of Hansen's Disease in the United States

Disease Type	Initial Therapy	Maintenance Therapy
Paucibacillary	Dapsone 100 mg/day plus rifampin 600 mg/mo for 6 mo	Dapsone monotherapy for 3 yr (indeterminate and TT), or 5 yr (BT)
Multibacillary	Dapsone 100 mg/d plus rifampin 600 mg/day for 3 y	Dapsone monotherapy for 10 yr (BB) or life (BL and LL)
Multibacillary with questionable resistance	Clofazimine 50 mg/day be added to the multibacillary regimen and should be used if any uncertainty exists whether the patient's bacilli are fully dapsone-sensitive	
Multibacillary with resistant *Mycobacterium leprae*	Dapsone-clofazimine 50 mg/day plus rifampin 600 mg/ day for 3 yr	Indefinite clofazimine monotherapy

Abbreviations: BB, mid borderline; BL, borderline lepromatous; BT, borderline tuberculoid; LL, lepromatous; TT, tubculoid.

Detection of antibody against leprosy (phenolic glycolipid I) is extremely specific, but again insensitive in polar tuberculoid disease.

TREATMENT

The treatment of leprosy should be conducted under the auspices of an infectious disease specialist. State and local health departments should be notified for the purpose of locating and evaluating contacts as well as assisting with the treatment. It is important that family members and other intimate contacts be examined both clinically and electrophysiologically.

The recommended chemotherapy for different forms of leprosy in the United States is outlined in Table 54-2. The World Health Organization recommendation is somewhat different but contains the main therapeutic agents: dapson, rifampin, and clofazimine. Recent clinical trials with sparfloxacin and ofloxacin in the treatment of lepromatous leprosy have reported encouraging results.

Treatment of leprosy reactions must be initiated promptly. Corticosteroids (60 to 80 mg prednisone/day), thalidomide (an investigational drug, but may be obtained from Hansen's Disease Center, in Carville, Louisiana), and clofazimine are the major drugs used. The effect of thalidomide is rapid (2 to 3 days) and impressive. Its mechanism of action, however, is unknown.

Surgical intervention when nerve compression is present is of significant value. Due to the complexity and chronicity of the disease the optimum management of patients requires the cooperation and skills of many health providers including internist, neurologist, orthopedic surgeon, neurosurgeon, ophthalmologist, rehabilitation specialist, occupational therapist, and social worker.

SUGGESTED READINGS

Black LA, West BC, Lary CH, Todd IV Jr: Environmental nonhuman sources of leprosy. Rev Infect Dis 9:562, 1987

Chan PG, Garcia-Ignacio BY, Chavez VE et al: Clinical trial of sparfloxacin for lepromatous leprosy. Antimicrob Agents Chemother 38:61, 1994

Harati Y, Kolimas R: Infectious peripheral neuropathies. Curr Neurol 8:37, 1988

Jakeman P, Smith WCS: Thalidomide in leprosy reaction. Lancet 343:432, 1994

Koch HP: Thalidomide and congeners as anti-inflammatory agents. Prog Med Chem 22:165, 1985

Meyer WM, Marty AM: Current concepts in the pathogenesis of leprosy. Drugs 41:832, 1991

Sabin TD, Swift TR, Jacobson RR: Leprosy. p. 1354. In Dyck PJ, Thomas PK (eds): Peripheral Neuropathy. WB Saunders, Philadelphia, 1993

Waters MFR: Leprosy 1962–1993. Trans R Soc Trop Med Hygiene 87:500, 1993

55. BRUCELLOSIS

CLIFFORD C. DACSO

Brucellosis is a zoonosis caused by *Brucella* species. Brucellosis is sometimes called undulant fever because of the waxing and waning course of the chronic disease. David Bruce identified the causative organism, a small gram-negative coccobacillus, from the spleen of a patient in 1886. Traditionally, there are six species of brucellae: *abortus, suis, melitensis, canis, ovis,* and *neotomae,* but recent genetic studies show that all brucellae are probably from a single species, *Brucella melitensis.* Because of the variety of the clinical presentation, however, the older names have been retained and continue to be used in the literature.

EPIDEMIOLOGY

Brucellae exist in nature in a broad variety of animals and locations. Humans usually become ill when they ingest milk or milk products contaminated with brucellae. Mucosal and respiratory inoculation are other important routes of acquisition, as is direct contact through breaks in the integument. Laboratory exposures have also been reported, and occupations where animal contact is frequent such as slaughterhouse (*abattoir*) workers and veterinarians have an increased risk of brucellosis.

CLINICAL FEATURES

Brucellosis has a broad repertoire of clinical manifestations by virtue of its chronicity and its ability to infect a large number of organ systems. The onset of illness usually is within weeks of exposure and is often insidious, with headache, backache, myalgias, malaise, and low-grade fever. There are few physical findings, however. If left untreated, brucellosis often becomes chronic with multiple areas of focal infection. Organs involved include the heart, liver, lungs, musculoskeletal system, skin, and other reticuloendothelial tissue-bearing organs. Brucellosis is considered in the differential diagnosis of conditions that are difficult to diagnose, such as fever of unknown origin, suppurative arthritis, osteomyelitis, and ''culture-negative endocarditis.'' Descriptions of clinical brucellosis frequently use the words ''protean manifestations.''

NEUROLOGIC MANIFESTATIONS

Brucellosis affects the central nervous system (CNS) in 2 to 6 percent of reported cases, but because the symptoms of neurobrucellosis are as nonspecific as headache and depression, the actual incidence is probably higher. Neurobrucellosis can be the presenting symptom of systemic brucella infection or it can occur later in the disease. Although data are not specific on psychiatric complications, depression is said to be more common with brucellosis than with other chronic infections. Headache is another common symptom, although meningismus is seen in only one-half of the patients. Cerebrovascular complications, including mycotic aneurysms and strokes, have been reported in rare cases, as have optic neuritis and cranial neuropathy.

DIAGNOSIS

The diagnosis of neurobrucellosis requires a high degree of clinical suspicion. Although culture and serology may each be diagnostic, neither alone is usually sufficient. The complete evaluation of suspected neurobrucellosis should include lumbar puncture with culture, serum and cerebrospinal fluid brucella serology and blood culture. Neurobrucellosis usually presents with a CSF mononuclear pleocytosis, hypoglycorrachia, and increased protein. Bone marrow culture can be useful, particularly in chronic cases. Because of the predilection of the organism for blood vessels and the incidence of mycotic aneurysm, thrombosis, and hemorrhage, CNS imaging may be useful in the evaluation of selected cases, particularly in patients presenting with a focal neurologic examination.

TREATMENT

Treatment of neurobrucellosis involves first the treatment of the systemic disease with doxycycline (100 mg bid) and either oral rifampin (900 mg qd) or parenteral streptomycin (15 mg/kg IM). The combination with streptomycin is thought to be better when spondylitis is present, but there are no prospective studies comparing regimens for neurobrucellosis. Many authorities feel that additional drugs should be added to the regimen if there is neurologic involvement, and thus a combination of doxycycline, streptomycin, rifampin, and trimethoprim-sulfamethoxazole (480/2,400 mg qd) for 2 to 4 months has been suggested. (Streptomycin is usually only given for the first 2 or 3 weeks because of toxicity.) Although third-generation cephalosporins achieve good CNS penetration, their efficacy versus brucellae is variable and in vitro susceptibilities should be confirmed before their use.

Corticosteroids have been used in neurobrucellosis based on the advice of ''most authorities,'' although their efficacy has not been demonstrated by trials. Dexamethasone is speculated to be beneficial in neurobrucellosis, particularly if initiated prior to antimicrobial chemotherapy.

When treatment is initiated early in the course of neurobrucellosis, the outcome is generally good.

SUGGESTED READINGS

McClean DR, Russell N, Khan MY: Neurobrucellosis: clinical and therapeutic features. Clin Infect Dis 15:582, 1992

Mousa AM, Bahar RH, Araj GF et al: Neurological complications of brucella spondylitis. Acta Neurol Scand 81:16, 1990

Mousa AM, Koshy TS, Araj GF et al: Brucella meningitis: presentation, diagnosis, and treatment. J Med 60:873, 1986

56. LEGIONELLOSIS

CLIFFORD C. DACSO

Legionellosis is the collective name of clinical syndromes produced by the family Legionellaceae, a group of gram-negative intracellular bacilli. Although there are more than 30 species in this family, most of the clinical illness is produced by *Legionella pneumophila.*

EPIDEMIOLOGY

Legionellae are ubiquitous aquatic organisms that thrive in artificial reservoirs such as air conditioning cooling towers and water distribution systems. Aerosolization and inhalation of contaminated water is a major mode of transmission. Patients with chronic lung disease, airway compromise, and immunosuppression are more likely to develop clinical manifestations of *Legionella* infection. The preponderance of clinical disease caused by legionellae occurs in the lung.

CLINICAL MANIFESTATIONS

Clinical legionellosis can present in two ways: Legionnaire's disease and Pontiac fever. Pontiac fever is a self-limited illness characterized by flulike symptoms, cough, and headache. Although seroconversion to legionellae occurs, there is no pulmonary parenchymal disease and complete recovery occurs without any more than supportive treatment.

Legionnaire's disease is the name given to pulmonary and multisystem disease. Onset of the disease usually follows inoculation by 2 days to 2 weeks. Flulike symptoms are prominent early, followed by pulmonary symptoms of nonproductive cough and chest pain. Gastrointestinal symptoms of diarrhea, nausea, and abdominal pain are common, as are constitutional symptoms of fever, headache, malaise, and myalgias.

NEUROLOGIC MANIFESTATIONS

Neurologic manifestations are common concomitants of Legionnaire's disease. Headache is very frequent. Abnormal mentation occurs in up to 30 percent of infected patients, including lethargy, confusion, delirium, and hallucinations, and is out of proportion to any hypoxia present. This has no prognostic significance and tends to resolve with the illness. Other neurologic conditions such as peripheral neuropathy (primarily motor), chorea, seizures, sixth nerve palsies, and brain abscess have been reported, but their incidence is unknown. Cerebellar dysfunction, including ataxia and dysarthria, is a particularly prominent complication, and may persist as a permanent residual.

DIAGNOSIS

Legionellosis should be suspected clinically in patients with an acute febrile pneumonia with a nonproductive cough, diarrhea, and altered mental status. The EEG is abnormal (diffusely slow) in 40 percent of patients, and the cerebrospinal fluid is abnormal (mildly elevated protein and pleocytosis) in 20 percent.

Despite its ubiquity in nature, legionellae are difficult to cultivate in vitro. Using special media, legionellae have been recovered from respiratory secretions, pleural fluid, abscesses, blood, and wounds. Direct fluorescent antibody tests can give a rapid diagnosis and should be performed on the appropriate specimen when legionellosis is suspected, but tests are positive in only 50 percent of cases. Although serodiagnosis is possible, its use requires the demonstration of an antibody rise, which may take months. A combination of all these test methods gives the best yield.

TREATMENT

Erythromycin has been the cornerstone of treatment of legionellosis. Controlled studies evaluating the newer macrolide antibiotics have yet to be performed; however, they may well be superior because of their pharmacokinetics. Quinolone antibiotics, and rifampin have in vitro activity versus legionellae. Although there are no clinical trials, it is reasonable to combine erythromycin 4/day IV with rifampin 600 mg bid when central nervous system disease is suspected. Similarly, quinolones have been used successfully in Legionnaire's disease unresponsive to erythromycin.

Legionella pneumonia is fatal in 15 percent of those who are infected, but the rate is 25 to 80 percent if the patient is immunosuppressed. Recovery when it occurs, however, is usually complete.

SUGGESTED READINGS

Johnson JD, Raff MJ, Van Arsdall JA: Neurologic manifestations of Legionnaire's disease. Medicine (Baltimore) 63:303, 1984

Nguyen MN: Legionellosis. Infect Dis Clin North Am 5:561, 1991

57. TETANUS

CLIFTON L. GOOCH

The fearsome effects of tetanus were well known long before contemporary immunization programs. Despite widespread immunization in the United States, however, cases of tetanus continue to appear and, for the unfortunate patient, the well-described hazards of this condition remain considerable. Approximately 100 cases are reported nationwide each year, with mortality rates of 30 percent despite aggressive therapy. Inadequately immunized individuals (up to 10 percent of the U.S. population) constitute the vast majority of cases. High-risk groups include those over 50 years old, African-Americans from the rural South, and intravenous drug abusers, especially heroin addicts. In developing countries lacking adequate immunization programs, tetanus is a common cause of death, with an estimated 500,000 cases per year internationally and a mortality rate of 45 percent.

EPIDEMIOLOGY

The causative bacteria, *Clostridium tetani,* may exist as a spore in topsoil, clothing, and dust for long periods. It is strictly anaerobic, and must enter its host through a contaminated wound for successful infection and subsequent production of its pathogenic toxin, tetanospasmin. Approximately 70 percent of cases are associated with acute trauma, and, although puncture wounds are classically associated with tetanus, lacerations are an equally likely cause. Potential causes of tetanus are as follows:

1. Puncture wound
2. Laceration
3. Otitis media
4. Corneal abrasion
5. Intramuscular injection
6. Foreign body injuries

7. Dental manipulation
8. Cutaneous ulcerations
9. Burns
10. Abortions
11. Pregnancy and delivery
12. Gastrointestinal or genitourinary surgery

Neonatal tetanus may also be caused by infection of the umbilical stump. From 5 to 10 percent of cases have no identifiable antecedents.

Following contamination, germination and local infection cause clinical disease in an average of 3 to 21 days, although the incubation period ranges from 1 day to several months. Once established, the organisms begin to produce tetanospasmin, an extremely powerful toxin. Tetanospasmin then undergoes retrograde axonal transport via local nerves to the central nervous system where it interferes with the release of inhibitory neurotransmitters such as GABA (gamma-aminobutyric acid), diversely affecting the spinal cord, brainstem, cerebral cortex, and hypothalamus. Resultant disinhibition of motor systems and altered sympathetic nervous system function ultimately result in increased muscle contraction, rigidity, reflex spasms and autonomic dysfunction. Restricted local symptoms may be the first manifestation, but if the toxin disseminates by hematogenous, lymphatic, and intra-axonal spread, generalized symptoms may appear.

CLINICAL FEATURES

Tetanus may be classified clinically as generalized, local, cephalic, and neonatal (Table 57-1). Unfortunately, generalized tetanus is the most common form of the disease. Some patients report headache, low-grade fever, and irritability early, but jaw stiffness with subsequent difficulty opening the mouth (trismus or ''lockjaw'') is usually the presenting symptom. Sequential spread to other facial, bulbar, neck, axial, and limb muscles then ensues, culminating in generalized rigidity. The patient's extremities may be firmly extended with persistent contraction of the facial muscles and lip retraction, producing *risus sardonicus* (a sardonic smile).

With further progression, torturing generalized tonic spasms begin. These consist of severely painful episodes of arching of the back with extension of the legs (opisthotonus), adduction and flexion of the arms, and flexion of the fists over the chest. These spasms may occur in response to minor emotional or visual stimuli and can be violent enough to cause tendon detachments as well as long-bone and vertebral fractures. Consciousness is not impaired. In addition to the excruciating pain of these tetanic spasms, involvement of the pharyngeal, laryngeal, and diaphragm musculature may precipitate aspiration or death by suffocation. Further dangers appear with sympathetic nervous system involvement. Tachycardia may herald this complication, which can include arrhythmias, bradycardia, and sinus arrest. Labile hypertension, refractory hypotension, excessive sweating, and fever may also be encountered.

If the patient survives the initial phase of the illness, recovery may be quite prolonged. Spasms typically improve after 2 weeks and slowly resolve over 3 to 4 weeks, with resolution of all symptoms over 1 to 2 months, provided secondary complications do not occur. Rehabilitation may require several more months.

Local tetanus appears as progressively increasing muscular stiffness (eventually becoming continuous) in the vicinity of a local trauma or surgical site, with intermittent superimposed spasms which, like generalized tetanic spasms, may be induced by a number of different stimuli. It is more common in the extremities, and may cause significant rigidity of the affected limb. Typically it persists for weeks to months, then gradually resolves without sequela. Patients in this category have a good prognosis with less than 1 percent mortality, and usually recover completely if they do not progress to the generalized form.

Cephalic tetanus typically follows injury of the face and head and may appear after otitis media. Symptoms may occur after as few as 1 to 2 days, most often as weakness of the facial and ocular muscles with later localized tetanic spasm. Trismus may also be an early sign. This variety is more likely to progress to generalized disease, although a nonprogressive cephalic form may occur.

Neonatal tetanus usually appears after umbilical cord contamination in the first 7 to 10 days following delivery, most commonly in underdeveloped regions with poor maternal immunization and unsterile delivery environments. Poor feeding and irritability quickly give way to diffuse rigidity, opisthotonus, and intermittent generalized spasms with minimal stimulation. The prognosis for recovery is very poor.

DIAGNOSIS

The diagnosis of tetanus is a clinical one, based on those features just described. Serum antibody levels greater than 0.01 IU/ml make the diagnosis less probable, but do not exclude it. Wound cultures may be negative. The differential diagnosis includes other conditions, most of them noninfectious, which produce severe muscle spasms, such as strychnine poisoning, black widow spider bite, dystonia associated with neuroleptic use, rabies, hysteria, and the stiff-person syndrome.

TREATMENT

Prevention

The most effective and simple way to eliminate tetanus is through appropriate immunization. Primary immunization (Table 57-2) can be achieved in infancy with DTP (diphtheria, tetanus, and pertussis) vaccines administered at 2, 4, 6, and 15 months of age, with a booster at 4 to 6 years of age, and every 10 years thereafter. If immunization is not achieved in infancy,

TABLE 57-1. Clinical Types of Tetanus

Clinical Type	Symptoms	Prognosis
Generalized	Trismus, generalized rigidity, risus sardonicus, painful tetanic spasms, opisthotonus, dysphagia, laryngeal and pharyngeal spasm, autonomic dysfunction (labile hypertension, arrhythmias, etc.)	30% mortality, significant secondary morbidity
Local	Localized muscular stiffness, superimposed localized spasm, isolated limb rigidity	Good, <1% mortality, but may generalize
Cephalic	Facial and ocular muscle weakness, localized spasm, early trismus	Guarded, more likely to generalize
Neonatal	Follows umbilical cord contamination by 7 to 10 days, poor feeding, irritability, then opisthotonus and generalized tetanic spasms	Very poor

TABLE 57-2. Primary Tetanus Immunization

Patient	Vaccine	Schedule
Infant	DTP	Four doses 2 months of age, 4 months of age, 6 months of age, and 15 months of age Booster 4 to 6 years, every 10 years thereafter
Under 7 years	DTP	Four doses Primary vaccination Second dose 6 to 12 weeks after the first Third dose 6 to 12 weeks after the second Fourth dose 6 to 12 weeks after the third Booster 4 to 6 years old Every 10 years thereafter
Over 7 years	Td	Three doses Primary vaccination Second dose 4 weeks after the first Third dose 6 months after the second Booster Every 10 years thereafter
Pregnant	Td	Two doses During second and third trimester only, at least 4 months apart Booster Every 10 years thereafter

Abbreviations: DTP, diphtheria, tetanus, and pertussis; Td, tetanus and diphtheria. (Data from Groleau, G: Tetanus. Emergency Med Clin North Am 10:351, 1992.)

patients under 7 years old may receive DTP vaccination on the following schedule: initial dose; second dose 4 to 8 weeks after the first; third dose 4 to 8 weeks after the second; fourth dose 6 to 12 weeks after the third; booster dose at 4 to 6 years old; and every 10 years thereafter. Unimmunized patients older than 7 years should receive three injections of Td (tetanus and diphtheria) on the following schedule: initial dose; second dose 4 weeks after the first; third dose 6 months after the second; and every 10 years thereafter. Unimmunized pregnant patients should receive two injections of Td during the last two trimesters, at least 1 month apart, and every 10 years thereafter. Vaccination should not be attempted during the first trimester. Tetanus vaccination is well tolerated and is contraindicated only by a history of anaphylaxis or other adverse reaction following vaccination, although these are rarely encountered.

After acute injury, appropriate wound care, including debridement, irrigation, and indicated antibiotics, are paramount. Further treatment depends upon the nature of the wound. In "tetanus-prone" wounds (older than 6 hours, infected, contaminated, or ischemic) in patients with an incomplete or unclear immunization history, human tetanus immune globulin (HTIG) 250 units should be administered intramuscularly, followed by completion of the primary immunization schedule described above. Patients with such wounds and a clear history of complete immunization with adsorbed tetanus vaccine do not require HTIG, but should receive a booster (Td in patients older than 7 years, DTP in patients younger than 7 years) if their last booster was more than 5 years ago. Pregnant patients in the first trimester, with a history of full immunization, may receive HTIG without risk to the fetus. Second- and third-trimester patients may receive routine boosters as indicated. For more minor clean wounds, nonimmunized patients do not require HTIG, but should begin the appropriate vaccination schedule immediately. Immunized patients without a booster in the last 10 years should receive a booster vaccination.

Acute Treatment

Patients diagnosed with tetanus should be admitted to the intensive care unit for close observation. A one-time dose of HTIG, 3,000 to 10,000 units should be given intramuscularly in an attempt to neutralize the toxin. Appropriate wound care, followed by antibiotic administration to eradicate the infection is the next step, and procaine penicillin, 10 to 12 million units IV or IM daily in divided doses for 10 days is the therapy of choice. For the penicillin-allergic patient, clindamycin 150 to 300 mg q6h, erythromycin 500 mg PO q6h, or tetracycline 500 mg PO or IV q6h for 10 days are acceptable alternatives.

The patient should be maintained in as dark and quiet an environment as possible. Mild tetanus without tetanic spasms may be treated with diazepam 2 to 10 mg IV q4–12h, or phenobarbital 50 to 100 mg q3–6h, titrated to response. Dantrolene may also be effective. More severe tetanus with tetanic spasms necessitates tracheostomy because of the danger of associated laryngospasm, and mechanical ventilation is needed prior to the institution of more intensive pharmacotherapy as all recommended therapies may cause significant respiratory depression. Benzodiazepines are the most effective agents for the treatment of tetanic spasms, and diazepam, in high doses of 40 to 120 mg IV per day in divided doses every 2 to 8 hours is recommended. Alternatively, phenobarbital or short acting barbiturates such as pentobarbital (initially given in doses of 50 to 200 mg IM q2–8h, titrated to response) in combination with chlorpromazine, 200 to 300 mg/day may be used. Tachyphylaxis from chlorpromazine and worsening muscle spasm may limit this approach, however. Barbiturates and diazepam in combination may cause cardiac arrest and should be used with great care.

Severe rigidity and spasms refractory to the above therapy should be treated with neuromuscular blockade, which can be instituted with succinylcholine and maintained with pancuronium with continuation of heavy sedation to minimize patient discomfort. Alternative use of higher dose intravenous dantrolene (140 mg bolus, followed by 1 mg/kg IV q4h, with ultimate conversion to 100 mg PO q4h) has been reported to be an effective substitute for neuromuscular paralysis in a few severe cases.

Autonomic dysfunction does not reliably respond to medical therapy, but treatment of labile hypertension may be attempted with intravenous morphine in 5- to 30-mg infusions over 30 minutes repeated every 2 to 8 hours. General principles regarding care of the debilitated critically ill patient should be closely observed, with particular attention to nutritional needs and the prevention of decubitus ulcers, gastric ulcers, and deep-vein thrombosis.

Tetanus is a horrible affliction and, once contracted, carries a high risk of death. It is preventable, however, and physicians should be attentive to the immunization status of their patients and take every opportunity to provide them with the protection our modern era has made available.

SUGGESTED READINGS

Groleau G: Tetanus. Emergency Med Clin North Am 10:351, 1992
Kefer M: Tetanus. Am J Emergency Med 10:445, 1992
Tidyman M, Prichard JG, Deamer RL, Mac N: Adjunctive use of dantrolene in severe tetanus. Anesth Analg 64:538, 1985
Walsh TM: Diseases of nerve and muscle. p. 358. In Samuels MA (ed): Manual of Neurology. 4th Ed. Little, Brown, Boston, 1991
Weinstein L: Current concepts: tetanus. N Engl J Med 289:1293, 1973

Wright DK, Lalloo UG, Nayiager S, Govender P: Autonomic nervous system dysfunction in severe tetanus: current perspectives. Crit Care Med 17:371, 1989

SPIROCHETAL INFECTIONS

58. NEUROSYPHILIS

J. DOUGLAS LEE

Syphilis is a sexually transmitted disease caused by the spirochete *Treponema pallidum*. At the time of primary infection, the spirochetes replicate at the site of inoculation and within 3 weeks create a painless chancre. This chancre may last 2 to 8 weeks, or longer in human immunodeficiency virus (HIV) infected patients. Within several weeks of the primary chancre, a spirochetemia produces the second stage of syphilis, and it is at this stage that spirochetes invade the central nervous system in one-third of patients. Although acute syphilitic meningitis may occur (1 to 3 percent of patients), neurologic symptoms are usually absent at this stage. Secondary syphilis is self-limited and is followed by a latent period of chronic infection that may last months, years, or a lifetime (Table 58-1). In 30 percent of untreated patients, tertiary syphilis will subsequently appear, and it is these tertiary manifestations that are of major concern to the neurologist (Table 58-2).

CLINICAL FEATURES OF NEUROSYPHILIS

In the secondary stage, 1 to 2 percent of all syphilis patients will show evidence of acute aseptic meningitis or meningoencephalitis. Clinical manifestations may also include cranial neuropathies of nerves II to XII, particularly cranial nerve VIII.

Tertiary syphilis generally produces three patterns of neurologic involvement, all based on obliterative endarteritis. It is important to remember, however, that there are few neurologic entities that syphilis cannot mimic. The typical syndromes are as follows:

1. *Meningovascular syphilis.* This is a chronic syphilitic meningitis associated with arteritis with occlusion of blood vessels producing cerebral infarctions. The clinical picture may be that of a chronic meningitis, or a dementia, but most patients present with a stroke syndrome.
2. *General paresis.* Invasion of the brain by spirochetes causes a chronic low-grade encephalitis producing neuropsychiatric abnormalities and dementia. Pupillary changes are also common.
3. *Tabes dorsalis.* In this syndrome, the dorsal columns of the spinal cord and the proprioceptive pathways are preferentially involved, creating a sensory ataxia with painful paresthesias, loss of deep sensation in the legs, and, in the end stage, Charcot joints. Optic atrophy and Argyll-Robertson pupils may also occur.

Neurosyphilis, therefore, must be suspected in a wide variety of both peripheral and central nervous system disease, as well as any patient with a positive syphilis serology. Diagnostic considerations are as follows:

1. Dementia
2. Chronic meningitis
3. Stroke in the young (under age 45)
4. Visual loss (retinitis, optic atrophy)
5. Acoustic and vestibular (cranial nerve VIII) dysfunction
6. Peripheral neuropathy (lower extremity numbness)
7. HIV infection with neurologic symptoms
8. Patients with a positive syphilis serology

DIAGNOSIS OF NEUROSYPHILIS

Patients with any clinical problem typical of syphilis, and that includes a large number of patients, should be tested for neurosyphilis. To confirm the clinical suspicion of neurosyphilis, a patient should have both serologic abnormalities and characteristic spinal fluid changes. A definite case of neurosyphilis will be one who has a typical syndrome, positive treponemal serology, and abnormal spinal fluid with a positive spinal fluid VDRL. Confirmation of neurosyphilis requires three criteria:

1. Appropriate clinical signs and symptoms
plus
2. Reactive specific treponemal serology in the serum (FTA or MHA-TP)
plus
3. At least one abnormal spinal fluid parameter
   a. Pleocytosis
   b. Increased protein
   c. Reactive CSF-VDRL test

There are other patients who will have lesser degrees of certainty of diagnosis, but because of the treatable nature of this disease, many patients will require treatment when the diagno-

TABLE 58-2. Neurologic Manifestations of Tertiary Syphilis

Meningovascular
  Strokes
  Chronic meningitis
General paresis
  Dementia
  Personality change
  Irregular (Argyll-Robertson) pupils
Tabes dorsalis
  Numbness in feet and legs
  Lightening pains in legs
Other
  Optic neuritis or atrophy
  Hearing loss or dizziness

TABLE 58-1. Stages of Syphilis

Stage	Time From Infection	Neurologic Manifestations
Primary	0–4 weeks	None
Secondary	4–8 weeks	Acute syphilitic meningitis or asymptomatic meningitis
Latent	8 weeks-lifetime	None
Tertiary	1–30 years	Meningovasculitis General paresis Tabes dorsalis Gummas Optic atrophy, otitis Cardiovascular

sis is not definite. It is very important that patients in these situations understand the uncertainty of the diagnosis.

Serologic Testing

There are two types of serologic tests for syphilis: treponemal and nontreponemal. The nontreponemal tests quantitatively measure a patient's antibody response to cardiolipin-lecithin-cholesterol antigens. These tests included the Venereal Disease Research Laboratory (VDRL) serology and the rapid plasma reagin (RPR) serology. These antibodies are reliably produced during infection with *Treponema pallidum,* making these tests very sensitive, but because they are also present in other diseases, false positives are common. A false-positive result is defined as a positive reagin nontreponemal serology and a negative treponemal antibody test. Reagin tests may be done in spinal fluid and in serum.

The treponemal tests detect antibodies specifically directed toward treponemal antigens. These include the fluorescent treponema antibody (FTA) and the microhemagglutinin assay for antibodies to *T. pallidum* (MHA-TP). Although lacking some sensitivity, they are very specific, with few false positives. These tests are standardized in serum only, not in cerebrospinal fluid (CSF). Neurosyphilis is unlikely with a negative serum treponemal antibody test.

Both types of tests are useful for the diagnosis of neurosyphilis. The nontreponemal tests are used as screening tests, and the specific treponemal tests are used to confirm syphilitic infection and exclude false positives.

In addition to their diagnostic usefulness, the nontreponemal tests provide a measure of disease activity, with titers proportionate to the activity of disease. Serial measurements after treatment provide a reliable monitor of therapeutic efficacy. The specific treponemal tests (FTA, MHA-TP) remain positive even after the disease has been successfully treated, and are not useful for the determining the effectiveness of therapy.

Cerebrospinal Fluid Analysis

In patients with suggestive symptoms and positive serum serologies, the diagnosis of neurosyphilis can be confirmed by spinal fluid analysis. The CSF must be examined in all patients with suspected neurosyphilis who have a positive serum FTA or MHA-TP, unless their spinal fluid is known to be negative and they have received treatment adequate for their stage of syphilis. If adequacy of treatment is uncertain or if the CSF has not been evaluated, lumbar puncture is necessary. CSF examination is mandatory before beginning antibiotic therapy for secondary latent or tertiary syphilis. Although active neurosyphilis can probably occur with normal spinal fluid, a diagnosis of neurosyphilis usually requires an abnormality of at least one of the following spinal fluid studies:

1. *Protein:* The CSF protein is usually elevated. Levels greater than 200 mg percent are rare.
2. *Pleocytosis:* The increased white blood cells in the spinal fluid are predominantly lymphocytes and may number up to 200 white blood cells (WBCs)/mm^3.
3. *Reactive CSF syphilis tests:* A positive VDRL test in the spinal fluid is an extremely specific test for neurosyphilis and is considered diagnostic. It is, however, not sensitive, and the test may be normal in half of all patients with active disease.

Although not part of the diagnostic criteria for syphilis, most patients will have elevated immunoglobulin G (IgG) levels in the spinal fluid, with oligoclonal bands.

Patients, therefore, should be treated for neurosyphilis specifically if they have a positive serum FTA (or equivalent test), and any abnormality of the spinal fluid (including increased protein, pleocytosis, or a positive CSF VDRL test).

NEUROSYPHILIS WITH HIV INFECTION

In patients with acquired immune deficiency syndrome (AIDS), neurosyphilis is usually more virulent, because of the impaired immune response. This allows the disease in all stages to progress more rapidly and particularly alters the secondary stage of syphilis, when the central nervous system (CNS) is invaded by the spirochete. This usually subclinical infection often produces significant symptoms in the HIV-infected patient. Acute syphilitic meningitis is especially common at this stage. Because of impaired immune response, atypical manifestations may appear, including severe necrotizing brain and spinal cord lesions.

The diagnosis of neurosyphilis is often more difficult because serum and CSF serologic tests may be nonreactive. HIV infection itself often produces spinal fluid changes of pleocytosis and elevated protein, which can mimic changes seen in syphilis. HIV may also cause dementia, myelopathy, and other symptoms and signs consistent with neurosyphilis. Thus, the clinical, serologic, and CSF values required to diagnose syphilis may be altered. Patients with AIDS, who are suspected of having neurosyphilis, should nevertheless have their blood and spinal fluid examined, and treatment is recommended for HIV-positive patients in whom there is any reasonable suspicion of neurosyphilis.

THERAPY

Any patient who has definite or possible neurosyphilis should be treated. Particularly in low prevalence areas, patients will be seen who have minimal CNS disease (e.g., unilateral cranial nerve VIII disease), normal CSF, and a positive serum FTA only. Another problem is the patient with a positive VDRL test and an FTA test that is positive weakly and intermittently. These patients should be treated, recognizing the limitations of biologic tests in producing a definite diagnosis and recognizing the potential harm in missing a diagnosis. The patient should be informed of the uncertainty of the diagnosis and the rationale for treatment to minimize legal, social, and emotional consequences. All follow-up should be undertaken for these patients as for definite cases.

High-dose intravenous penicillin is the drug of choice for treatment of neurosyphilis. Patients should receive intravenous aqueous crystalline penicillin G in a dose of 4 million units every 4 hours for 10 days. Traditional intramuscular therapy of 2.4 million units of benzathine penicillin a week does not achieve reliably bacteriocidal concentrations of penicillin in the nervous system.

Patients who claim to be "allergic to penicillin" often are not, and should be evaluated with skin testing and chart reviews to confirm the existence of the allergic response, since penicillin is considered to be the best therapy. A variety of other antibiotic regimens are recommended, but there are not good studies to prove equivalency. Antibiotic regimens for tertiary syphilis are as follows:

1. Penicillin G 4 million units q4h 10 days or
2. Amoxicillin 3 g plus probenecid 1 g bid 15 days or
3. Doxycycline 200 mg PO bid 21 days or
4. Ceftriaxone 1 g IM qd 14 days.

Adequate antibiotic therapy for neurosyphilis should arrest the progression of clinical signs and symptoms, but may not restore existing neurologic damage nor improve baseline CSF abnormalities. However, the spinal fluid usually returns toward normal and should be reexamined at 3- to 6-month intervals after treatment to verify a decline in cell count and protein. In secondary syphilis, the CSF cell count, protein, and VDRL test are usually negative by 6 months and the VDRL test is virtually always negative at 2 years. In tertiary syphilis, most patients have normal CSF within 2 years, but it may require as long as 5 years for the CSF VDRL test to become nonreactive. After adequate therapy, the VDRL test should be followed until it is negative, and further treatment is not necessary as long as it continues to decline in titer. A rebound in any parameter suggests recurrence and necessitates an additional full course of antibiotic therapy. This is particularly a problem in HIV patients where treatment failures have been shown to occur much more frequently.

SUGGESTED READINGS

Davis LE, Schmitt JW: Clinical significance of cerebrospinal fluid tests for neurosyphilis. Ann Neurol 25:50, 1989

Hart G: Syphilis tests in diagnostic and therapeutic decision making. Ann Intern Med 104:368, 1986

Hook EW, Marra CM: Acquired syphilis in adults. N Engl J Med 326:1060, 1992

Musher DM, Hamill RJ, Baughn RE: Effect of human immunodeficiency virus (HIV) infection on the course of syphilis and on the response to treatment. Ann Intern Med 113:872, 1990

Simon RP: Neurosyphilis. Neurology 44:2228, 1994

Wolters EC: Treatment of neurosyphilis. Clin Neuropharmacol 10:143, 1987

59. LYME DISEASE

LAUREN B. KRUPP

Lyme disease results from a bacterial infection caused by the tick-transmitted spirochete, *Borrelia burgdorferi*. The disease involves multiple systems, and clinical features range in severity from a mild transient flulike illness to a more severe and chronic condition with rheumatologic, neurologic, and cardiac complications. Major target organs of the infection are the skin, joints, heart, eye, and nervous system. The neurologic consequences of this infection are varied and multiple. Some are certainly a direct consequence of nervous system infection, while others may be secondary to the host's immune reaction.

The classic description of neuralgia, neuritis, and chronic lymphocytic meningitis associated with this disorder occurred in 1941 when Bannwarth reported on a series of patients with radicular pain, aseptic meningitis, and involvement of the peripheral and cranial nerves. In subsequent decades, European authors recognized that this syndrome consisted of dermatologic features and symptoms of meningoradiculoneuritis. Often a preceding tick bite was recalled. Wider recognition of the disorder came later in the mid-1970s when Steere and colleagues described an unusual outbreak of arthritis among children in Lyme, Connecticut. This outbreak was associated with a skin rash in 25 percent of patients, and in 21 percent it was preceded by a tick bite. By the end of the decade, the illness was termed Lyme disease. In 1982, a unique spirochete was recovered from a deer tick and named *Borrelia burgdorferi* after its discoverer. This spirochete was subsequently identified as the etiologic agent for Lyme disease.

The term Lyme disease replaces former labels of ''Bannwarth syndrome,'' ''Garin-Bujadoux disease,'' and ''tickborne meningoencephalitis.'' In Europe, neurologic Lyme disease is still often referred to as neuroborreliosis.

EPIDEMIOLOGY

Lyme disease is now the leading tickborne disease in Europe and the United States. Over 50,000 cases have been reported to the Centers for Disease Control and Prevention (CDC) since the establishment of national surveillance for the infection in 1982. Epidemiologic surveys document spread of the tick vector and increased tick infection rates within endemic areas. States with the highest incidence are New York, Connecticut, New Jersey, Pennsylvania, Rhode Island, Massachusetts, Maryland, Minnesota, and California. New York alone accounts for 40 percent of the cases, with most clustering in Suffolk and Westchester Counties, where the tick vector is most abundant.

B. burgdorferi, the spirochete responsible for Lyme disease, shares some features common to other spirochetal agents, such as those that produce syphilis, leptospirosis, and relapsing fever. Spirochetes first infect locally and involve the skin or entry site, then produce a spirochetmia, and disseminate throughout the body. Later, chronic organ infection can occur. As is true for several other spirochetes, *B. burgdorferi* is very difficult to grow in culture, making the laboratory diagnosis of the infection often problematic.

B. burgdorferi infects several different species of tick, each unique to a specific geographic area of the United States. Ticks commonly feed on wildlife such as deer or field mice. When a human, serving as an incidental host, is bitten by an infected tick, the disease may be transmitted.

CLINICAL FEATURES

The CDC has specific guidelines for the diagnosis of Lyme disease that are useful clinically. A case is defined by the CDC as a person with the erythema migrans rash or a person with at least one late objective manifestation and laboratory confirmation of infection. Erythema migrans is a pathognomonic marker that appears 1 to 30 days after infection as a patch that expands centrifugally from 5 to 42 cm. It may be multiple, has central clearing, and is absent from soles and palms. The rash lasts for days to weeks. Histologic tests show a superficial and deep perivascular interstitial plasma cell infiltrate; spirochetes may be present at the periphery. Objective late systemic manifestations of Lyme disease include any of the following when an alternative explanation is not found: musculoskeletal (recurrent brief attacks of objective joint swelling in one or a few joints, sometimes followed by chronic arthritis), cardiac (acute onset high-grade atrioventricular conduction defect that resolves in days to weeks and is sometimes associated with myocarditis), or neurologic (cranial neuritis, particularly unilateral or bilateral facial palsy, radiculoneuropathy, or, rarely, encephalomyelitis

TABLE 59-1. Lyme Disease Stages

Acute
  Localized
    Unifocal erythema migrans
    Flulike illness
  Disseminated
    Multifocal erythema migrans
    Cardiac conduction abnormalities
    Hepatitis
    Arthritis
    Lymphocytic meningitis
    Headache without meningitis
    Cranial neuropathy
    Radiculitis
Chronic
  Arthritis and arthralgia
  Encephalomyelitis
  Encephalopathy
  Chronic neuropathy
  Entrapment neuropathies
Post-treatment/remote effects
  Fatigue
  Cognitive difficulty
  Fibromyalgia
  Sleep disturbance
  Headache
  Arthralgia

if associated with intrathecal *B. burgdorferi* antibody production). Although the CDC criteria are helpful, rigid adherence to the case definition is likely to exclude some true Lyme disease patients.

Lyme disease has been divided into early (acute localized and disseminated) and later (chronic) stages (Table 59-1). Although specific syndromes are most common to particular stages of the infection, a great deal of overlap exists in the time course of clinical manifestations. In general, lymphocytic meningitis, facial nerve palsy, severe encephalitides, and painful radiculitis occur soon, within weeks to months of infection. Patients with long-standing disease commonly have encephalopathy of mild to moderate severity, peripheral neuropathy, or both. Following resolution of the infection, many patients suffer from persistent remote effects such as fatigue and headache.

NEUROLOGIC CLINICAL SYNDROMES

Both the central nervous system (CNS) and peripheral nervous system (PNS) can be involved in Lyme disease.

Peripheral Nerve and Muscle

The specific PNS disorders of Lyme disease are listed in Table 59-2. Paresthesias and radiculopathy, of varying severity, are often associated with Lyme disease. An intense radicular pain may develop in the dermatologic distribution of either the arthropod bite or the rash. The peripheral neuropathy is usually milder, of the axonal type (causing atrophy and denervation

TABLE 59-2. Peripheral Nervous System Manifestations

Multifocal axonal neuropathy
  Painful radiculitis
  Guillain Barré-like
  Mononeuritis multiplex
  Chronic mild sensorimotor neuropathy
  Facial nerve palsy
Entrapment neuropathy
  Carpal tunnel syndrome
Myositis

but without much slowing of nerve conduction velocities), and usually affects the lower extremities.

Frequently patients with PNS involvement also experience meningeal symptoms and cerebrospinal fluid (CSF) abnormalities. Thoracic sensory radiculitis, mononeuritis multiplex, and brachial plexitis associated with meningeal involvement are well documented.

Another neuropathy common to Lyme disease is entrapment neuropathy, particularly carpal tunnel syndrome. Much rarer are cases of polyradicular motor neuropathy suggestive of Guillain-Barré syndrome (GBS). The presence of CSF pleocytosis distinguishes these cases from classic GBS, and frequently the neuropathy is axonal as opposed to the demyelinating radiculopathy with slowed conduction times in GBS. Myositis and polymyositis have also been noted in Lyme disease, but are uncommon.

Cranial Nerve

The seventh (facial) nerve is commonly affected in Lyme disease, with an incidence as high as 10 percent of patients with disseminated infection. Bilateral facial nerve palsy may occur. Damage may develop as part of a peripheral nerve process, or as part of a basal meningitis.

Cranial nerves III, IV, V, VI, and VIII can be affected in Lyme disease, and Lyme disease has also occasionly been associated with optic neuritis. A few cases of recurrent laryngeal nerve abnormalities have occurred, but the lowest cranial nerves otherwise seem to be spared.

Central Nervous System

A large number of different CNS syndromes have been associated with Lyme disease, but in only a few is the evidence for a causal relationship compelling. The main syndromes are shown in Table 59-3 and include meningitis, encephalitis, encephalomyelitis, and encephalopathy.

The hallmark of neurologic Lyme disease is meningitis. This occurs during the early disseminated phase and may vary from a mild illness to, less frequently, a severe meningoencephalitis. Headache is common in 50 to 89 percent of cases, and sometimes persists post-treatment. Fever may occur but frequently is absent. Many (20 to 50 percent) patients with meningeal symptoms experience memory and concentration difficulty, mood disturbance, disrupted sleep, and, in more severe cases, obtundation and stupor. Approximately half of patients with meningitis have cranial neuropathy, and a third have radiculoneuropathy. Systemic symptoms include weight loss, profound fatigue, and myalgia. The CSF generally reveals pleocytosis, elevated immunoglobulin G (IgG), and intrathecal antibody production to B. burgdorferi, or other evidence of *B. burgdorferi* CNS invasion such as borrelial antigens or DNA.

Encephalomyelitis and encephalitis can occur in Lyme disease but are much less common than meningitis. The clinical

TABLE 59-3. Central Nervous System Manifestations

Lymphocytic meningitis
  With secondary cranial neuropathies
Focal encephalitis/encephalomyelitis
  Severe, with focal findings
  Mild, with encephalopathy
Encephalopathy
  Usually mild, occasionally moderate to severe, associated headache, fatigue, and
    malaise frequent

presentations occasionally mimic mass lesions. These include progressive spastic paraparesis, hemiparesis, ataxia, stupor, aphasia, apraxia, psychosis, or dementia. Hearing loss and headache are frequent milder accompanying problems. Seizures are rare. Varying degrees of cognitive impairment may be present. An acute or subacute monophasic illness is the usual time course. In patients who remain untreated, a relapsing-remitting or progressive course spanning months to years is possible. Although symptoms can be alarming, most patients with Lyme disease encephalomyelitis are only mildly affected. Mild confusion, irritability, and lethargy are by far the most frequently encountered clinical syndromes.

A syndrome common to late infection is a mild to moderate encephalopathy with noninflammatory CSF. The most frequent complaints are memory difficulties, mild confusion, and word-finding difficulty. Several studies using neuropsychological testing have confirmed cognitive deficits, which frequently improve following antibiotic therapy. In a subset of patients, however, complaints of cognitive dysfunction may persist. In the seropositive Lyme cases with encephalopathy and normal CSF it is difficult to know whether active persistent infection is etiologically responsible. In most cases the electroencephalogram (EEG) or magnetic resonance imaging (MRI) is not helpful. Borrelial antigen and DNA have been recovered from the CSF of a few of these patients, which suggest that active infection is present. However, it is also possible that immune mechanisms contribute to this syndrome.

Other neurologic manifestations of Lyme disease have been reported, including vasculitis, movement disorders, and dementia. Many of these syndromes were in patients lacking CSF abnormalities or measurement of anti-*B. burgdorferi* antibody in the CSF, and hence their relationship to the disease requires further study.

Post-treatment Lyme Manifestations and Remote Effects

Remote effects of Lyme disease include those symptoms that persist months after vigorous antibiotic therapy (Table 59-1). The most common persistent symptoms are fatigue, confusion, cognitive loss, and headache. Many Lyme patients experience mild to moderate depressive symptoms, as occurs with other chronic medical disorders. Psychosis and severe anxiety disorder have been observed in rare cases of Lyme disease. In some instances, inadequate initial treatment leads to continued symptoms. For other cases, the initial therapy may have been adequate, and the recovery period takes longer than expected. The relationship between remote effects or post-treatment syndromes to continued infection is still under investigation. Eventually, most patients make excellent recoveries.

DIAGNOSIS

As a result of the clinical diversity of Lyme disease presentations, and the fact that many patients may have no recollection of the tick bite or may lack the pathognomonic erythema migrans rash, the diagnosis has become increasingly dependent on laboratory testing. The laboratory may be a great aid in the evaluation of a suspected case, but the diagnosis remains a clinical one. Furthermore, laboratory diagnosis is not infallible and has three major areas of difficulty:

1. The diagnostic methods that are most accurate and specific (either culture or visualization of *B. burgdorferi*) are too insensitive and too slow for practical application. Thus, diagnosis relies upon indirect means, such as detection of an antibody response. However, due to the nature of the immunologic response, early in the illness (within the first few weeks after exposure), many infected patients will not be seropositive in even the best of clinical laboratories.
2. There is a plethora of different commercial diagnostic assays for detecting antibodies to *B. burgdorferi*. Most have failed the standards established by the CDC because of lack of standardization, reliability, and sensitivity.
3. Some cross-reactivity develops between autoantibodies or antibodies to other inflammatory conditions and those directed against *B. burgdorferi*. Also, persons exposed to the organism may remain asymptomatic and never develop a clinical infection. Hence, in areas where Lyme is endemic, physicians may inappropriately use a low or borderline Lyme test as a basis for treatment while ignoring the absence of a supporting clinical history.

To effectively deal with each of these problems the strengths and limitations of the different diagnostic methods available for this infection must be understood.

Culture

Successful growth of *B. burgdorferi* has been achieved using special media, but in only 10 percent of meningitis cases is the organism recovered from CSF. In most reports, the yield for recovering the organism from blood is even lower, ranging from 1.3 to 5 percent. Similarly, identification of *B. burgdorferi* in tissue has a very low yield, since the organisms are very sparse.

Antibody Assay

Measurement of anti-*B. burgdorferi* antibodies is currently the most useful diagnostic test for Lyme disease. The preferable technique is the enzyme-linked immunosorbent assay (ELISA). In reliable experienced laboratories, up to 93 percent of infected patients are seropositive. The incidence of false positives is less than 2 percent.

The problem of false-negative results is particular to the early phase of the infection. In suspected seronegative Lyme cases the antibody test should be repeated in 4 weeks. Occasionally, antibiotics may abrogate the antibody response in an infected patient so that the ELISA will be falsely negative.

To determine whether there is CNS infection, both serum and CSF analyses must be obtained, and antibody from both compartments measured and compared. A CSF:serum antibody titer ratio of greater than 1 indicates intrathecal synthesis. The presence of intrathecal antibody synthesis is the only laboratory marker currently recognized by the CDC for diagnosing active CNS infection. In cases of meningitis, the relationship between the organism that has invaded the CNS and the resultant neurologic syndrome is straightforward. On the other hand, the relationship of some of the neurologic complaints in Lyme disease is still not as well understood. For example, encephalopathy associated with Lyme disease may be due to active infection, but in some cases it may result from immunologic or other indirect effects of the illness. Intrathecal antibody synthesis is often absent in such patients.

Several experimental tests that look promising for diagnosis of CNS infection are borrelial-specific antigen detection in CSF, polymerase chain reaction (PCR), and borrelial-specific immune complexes. Unfortunately these tests are not yet available outside of research centers.

Ancillary Tests

The CSF may be abnormal in patients with radicular syndromes, facial palsy, or CNS disorders, and often shows a lymphocytic pleocytosis. Oligoclonal bands in the CSF are rare, but may be present. Protein elevation may occur but is usually mild. Patients with meningitis and radiculitis often have intrathecal production of specific antibodies to *B. burgdorferi*. In contrast, patients with mild axonal neuropathy or entrapment neuropathy generally lack a CSF pleocytosis or evidence of intrathecal antibody synthesis.

Electrophysiologic studies in patients with PNS syndromes are either normal or show an axonal neuropathy. In some patients with encephalitis, the EEG reveals focal or generalized slowing, but more often the EEG is normal.

In cases where the MRI is abnormal, the findings are typical of an inflammatory process. Singular or multiple punctate lesions on T2-weighted images involving the subcortical white matter are most often seen. Lesions may also appear in the brainstem, thalamus, or periventricular areas.

In summary, most patients suspected of neurologic Lyme disease will need the CSF examination and blood work. Diseases to exclude in the blood include other spirochetal infections, collagen vascular diseases, and disorders that might lead to a false-positive serology. In special cases additional studies, including EEG, electromyography, MRI, and neuropsychological testing, will be helpful.

TREATMENT

Choosing the appropriate antibiotic therapy for patients with Lyme disease depends on correctly identifying their clinical syndromes (Table 59-4). Choosing antibiotics with good CSF penetration is important.

Patients with early localized disease, such as erythema migrans and flulike symptoms respond well to oral antibiotics, which shorten the course of the skin infection and reduce the frequency of later syndromes. Although no longer widely used, oral penicillin was also a successful treatment.

Certain neurologic complications respond well to oral therapy. For patients with mild symptoms of peripheral neuropathy or entrapment neuropathy, oral antibiotic therapy is quite effective. Some patients treated for symptoms of radicular pain, vertigo, or leg weakness improve with high-dose oral doxycycline. On the other hand, many patients require parenteral treatment for these syndromes. If there is evidence of CNS involvement, such as CSF pleocytosis, protein elevation, intrathecal antibody synthesis, or signs of meningitis, parenteral therapy is indicated.

Patients with meningitis, meningoencephalitis, encephalitis, or severe encephalopathy require parenteral therapy. Currently, the preferred parenteral antibiotic for neurologic Lyme disease is ceftriaxone or cefotaxime, which cross the blood-brain barrier readily and yield CSF levels that exceed the mean inhibitory concentration for the spirochete. A practical advantage of ceftriaxone is that is has a long half-life, allowing for once-daily administration. In many circumstances this can be done in the home with a visiting nurse. A problem with ceftriaxone is the possibility of developing pseudomembranous colitis and gallbladder disease. Pseudomembranous colitis can be avoided with a diet supplement of active yogurt or acidophilus. However, patients with gastrointestinal histories need to be closely followed.

A Jarisch-Herxheimer reaction occurs in 10 to 20 percent of parenteral antibiotic-treated cases, usually within the first 24 hours of treatment. It is best managed with anti-inflammatory agents. In most cases steroids are best avoided; they may interfere with therapy and increase treatment failures. Patients who are allergic to penicillin can still often be treated with ceftriaxone or cefotaxime; however, the clinician should proceed cautiously. An alternative is high-dose oral doxycycline (200 mg bid).

Occasionally patients given oral therapy progress to develop late neurologic syndromes. Parenteral treatment is also indicated in these cases. Most patients do respond to these regimens. In rare instances, relapse may occur. In such cases reevaluation is appropriate, and it is imperative to distinguish persistent symptoms that are not antibiotic-responsive from genuine treatment failure, in which case additional antibiotic therapy is appropriate. Finally, reinfection can occur and requires retreatment. In highly endemic areas or in persons with occupations that place them at high risk (landscaper, park ranger), reinfection is not unusual.

Prophylactic treatment of deer tick bites depends on whether the potential exposure occurred in an highly endemic area, but in general prophylaxis is not recommended.

Treatment response should be determined by the clinical response and not by serum serology. Many patients adequately treated will have persistently elevated serum Lyme titers for

TABLE 59-4. Antibiotic Therapy for Lyme Disease

Route	Indications	Antibiotic
Oral	Early localized infection: erythema migrans rash & flulike symptoms such as fatigue, malaise, mild concentration difficulty	Amoxicillin, 500 mg qid × 3–4 weeks *or* Doxycycline, 100 mg bid or tid × 3–4 weeks
	Early disseminated infection without CSF abnormalities, i.e., facial nerve palsy	
	Late infection: mild neuropathy, axonal or entrapment neuropathy, radiculitis (mild) without CSF abnormalities	
Intravenous	Meningitis	Ceftriazone, 2 g daily × 3–4 weeks *or* Cefotaxime, 2 g tid × 3–4 weeks *or* Penicillin G, 24 mU × 3–4 weeks
	Encephalitis, encephalomyelitis, cranial neuritis, facial nerve palsy, or radiculitis with CSF abnormalities	
	Severe encephalopathy, or documented progressive cognitive loss and evidence of systemic Lyme borreliosis	In cases of cephalosporin or penicillin allergy, an alternative is high-dose doxycycline, 200 mg bid
	Systemic disseminated late disease: cardiac-pericarditis or conduction block, arthritis, multifocal erythema migrans, acrodermatitis chronica atropicans	

months and, rarely, years after treatment. Hence following the Lyme titer alone is not a reliable treatment guide. On the other hand, patients with severe CNS syndromes, who are not responding after several weeks of parenteral therapy, should have repeat CSF examinations. If the CSF shows persistent pleocytosis or elevated protein then an additional 2 or 3 weeks of parenteral therapy is advised.

New medications such as azithromycin for Lyme disease are being compared to more established therapies. Until additional studies are available to definitively establish relative efficacy and side-effect profiles, it is unclear whether the disadvantages of higher cost will be offset by the benefits of azithromycin or other new antibiotic medications.

SUGGESTED READINGS

Coyle PK: Neurologic complications of Lyme disease. Rheum Dis Clin North Am 19:993, 1993

Pfister HW, Wilske B, Weber K: Lyme borreliosis: basic science and clinical aspects. Lancet 393:1013, 1994

Reik LR: Lyme disease and the nervous system. Thieme, New York, 1991

Weber K, Pfister HW: Clinical management of lyme borreliosis. Lancet 393: 1017, 1994

60. LEPTOSPIROSIS

PATRICK E. NOLAN

Leptospirosis is an uncommon systemic infectious disease in which meningitis is a common feature, caused by a spirochete of the genus *Leptospira*. A worldwide zoonotic disease, leptospirosis is transmitted and propagated among wild and domestic animals, with humans considered accidental, "dead-end" hosts. *L. interrogans* is the only species that causes disease in humans. There are over 170 serotypes of *L. interrogans*, which is a finely coiled, motile spirochete, 0.1 μm in width by 6 to 20 μm in length, with a characteristic bent, hooked end.

EPIDEMIOLOGY

Leptospirosis is reported about 100 times per year in the United States, with a seasonal predilection for the summer and early fall. It has most often affected males with occupational or recreational exposure to animals. Traditionally, sewermen, miners, and fish workers, work characterized by exposure to rats, represented most cases. Now more cases are seen in farmers, veterinarians, abattoir workers, campers, swimmers, canoeists, and kayakers. In the United States, dogs, livestock, rodents, wild mammals, and cats are the most prevalent animal exposures.

Rats are the "classic" enzootic reservoir and are the most common disease source worldwide. Poor sanitary conditions such as rat-infested urban dwellings, homes where pet dogs share close proximity to humans and exhibit urinary incontinence, or recreational activities in inland, stagnant waters where infected animals have urinated, are frequent epidemiologic associations. Part of the difficulty in the control of this zoonosis lies in the fact that a symbiotic relationship can occur in the animal host whereby a healthy-appearing animal can harbor the spirochete in the renal tubules and excrete live and contagious microorganisms in the urine for prolonged periods. Even fully vaccinated pet dogs have been known to transmit disease in this fashion.

CLINICAL FEATURES

The coiled spirochete is able to penetrate intact mucous membranes and abraded skin. Cuts or abrasions of the skin or a history of immersion or splash that may contaminate the mucous membranes of the eyes or nasopharynx are pertinent historical findings. From the mucocutaneous site of infection, the spirochete enters the bloodstream and disseminates to every organ system, including the central nervous system, eye, liver, and kidney. Tissue injury occurs by an unknown mechanism, but vasculitis is usually a prominent feature; nonspecific inflammatory changes occur most commonly in the liver and kidney, but can be widespread. Most cases are subclinical, and because of this the disease is felt to be largely underreported. Infections associated with clinical disease sometimes follow a biphasic course. Although most often a monophasic illness, this biphasic paradigm is helpful in thinking about the pathogenesis of the disease.

After an incubation period of 7 to 12 days, a flulike illness ensues associated with fever, headache, and myalgia. Often this has an abrupt onset. The headache is intense and may be associated with photophobia. A relative bradycardia has been described. During this phase, spirochetes can be found circulating in the blood, cerebrospinal fluid, and most tissues. Myofibrils with cytoplasmic vacuoles and a mild polymorphonuclear infiltration can be demonstrated histologically in the muscles during this period of often intense myalgia. Toward the end of the first week, there may be improvement, and the patient may actually become afebrile for a few days.

The second phase is characterized by the disappearance of spirochetes from the bloodstream, cerebrospinal fluid, and organs, and the presence of circulating antibody. Culture of the blood and cerebrospinal fluid (CSF) are usually negative, and cultivation of leptospires can usually be made only from the urine. This second "immune" or "leptospiruric" phase is thought to be mediated by circulating immune complexes and is manifested clinically by lymphadenopathy, a skin rash, meningitis, hepatitis, nephritis, and uveitis. Conjunctival suffusion is particularly characteristic and can be a clue to this disease. This may be associated with photophobia, ocular pain, and a conjunctival hemorrhage.

About 90 percent of cases are mild and without jaundice—"anicteric leptospirosis." About 10 percent of the time a severe course with jaundice and renal failure unfolds in a syndrome known as Weil's disease. This was first described by Weil in 1886 and was referred to as "acute febrile icterus" in Osler's textbook. Fever, severe headache often uncontrolled by analgesics, and a mild delirium are characteristic. Nausea, vomiting, and abdominal pain are common and splenomegaly occurs in 15 to 25 percent of patients. Abnormal urinalysis is described in 70 percent of cases. Myocarditis can be one feature of the immune phase inflammatory process and a fatal hemorrhagic myocarditis with cardiogenic shock has been described. The full-blown syndrome of renal and hepatic failure, bleeding diathesis, vascular collapse, and coma, has a 5 to 10 percent mortality rate.

During the second, leptospiruric phase, an aseptic meningitis can be demonstrated on cerebrospinal fluid examination in 50 to 90 percent of patients, usually with a mononuclear pleocytosis of less than 500 cells. Typically, the CSF protein is moderately elevated and the glucose normal, in a picture resembling viral meningitis. There have been reports of both neutrophilic pleocytosis and hypoglycorrhachia, however. Leptospires can no longer be isolated, and the meningitis may be caused by secondary immune reactions. The meningitis seldom persists more than a few days, and is never fatal.

Although aseptic meningitis is the most common neurologic manifestation, peripheral neuropathy, flaccid paraplegia, and mononeuritis multiplex have been reported in the medical literature.

DIAGNOSIS

The differential diagnosis includes the causes of fever associated with a multisystem disease, or, in severe cases, icteric multisystem disease. *Staphylococcus aureus,* group A streptococci, and *Neisseria meningitidis* can mimic the acute, undifferentiated fever. Viral aseptic meningitis or toxin exposure could also be considered in the differential diagnosis. With a history of zoonotic exposure, *Brucella,* tularemia, plaque, and rickettsial infections such as Q fever and Rocky Mountain spotted fever could all reasonably be considered with leptospirosis. The severe icteric form can mimic obstructive jaundice or viral hepatitis. The presence of fever, zoonotic exposure, the conjunction of hepatic and renal abnormalities, and elevated creatine kinase (reflecting the prominence of muscle involvement), can be good clinical clues to the diagnosis.

Culture requires a special semisolid medium and it may take up to 8 weeks, although growth usually appears 6 to 10 days after inoculation. Diagnosis is most frequently confirmed serologically. Agglutinins begin to appear during the second week of the illness and generally peak during the third or fourth week. A microscopic slide agglutination method uses killed antigen pooled from the most common serotypes, and is often employed as a screening test. A fourfold rise in titer in an appropriate clinical setting is diagnostic. The microscopic agglutination test uses live antigen and is more specific, although cross-reactions still make serotyping problematic. Culture is the only reliable way to identify the infecting serotype, but is most useful for epidemiologic purposes.

TREATMENT

Treatment with tetracycline or doxycycline instituted within the first 2 to 4 days of anicteric disease has been shown to shorten the course of illness. Because of the inherent delay in diagnosis, an early index of suspicion for leptospirosis and empirical treatment are most appropriate. Doxycycline 100 mg PO or IV bid is the recommended dose. Penicillin G, even when given late in severe icteric disease, can also attenuate the severity and shorten the course. Penicillin G 1.5 million units IV q6h should be given in these cases. Cefotaxime and erythromycin have experimental support for use in situations such as allergy to penicillin or tetracycline. The duration of treatment is 5 to 7 days. Despite early use of appropriate antibiotics, some patients have died nevertheless. Early suspicion, appropriate antibiotic therapy, and meticulous intensive care offer the best chance to lessen the 5 to 10 percent mortality rate in severe disease.

SUGGESTED READINGS

Edwards GA, Domm BM: Human leptospirosis. Medicine 39:117, 1960
Kreisberg RA: An abundance of options. N Engl J Med 329:413, 1993
Sperber SJ, Schleupner CJ: Leptospirosis: a forgotten cause of aseptic meningitis and multisystem febrile illness. South Med J 82:1285, 1989
Westblom TU, Everett ED, Satalowich M: Leptospirosis: a 10-year experience. Missouri Med 83:744, 1986

61. FUNGAL INFECTIONS

TEMPLE W. WILLIAMS

Fungi are nonphotosynthetic eukaryotic microorganisms that typically grow as a mass of branching filaments (''hyphae'') known as a mycelium. Some fungi grow only in the yeast form. Most pathogenic fungi are dimorphic: the mycelial phase occurs in nature and conversion to the yeast phase occurs at body temperature. Unlike the vast armies of bacterial and viral pathogens, only a few fungi cause human disease, and often only in immune-compromised patients. However, most fungi that cause systemic disease can also affect the central nervous system (CNS). The incidence of fungal infections of the CNS has dramatically increased because of the ever-increasing number of immunosuppressed patients with cancer, transplanted organs, or acquired immunodeficiency syndrome (AIDS). The clinical manifestations of fungal CNS infection vary widely and include meningitis, meningoencephalitis, and abscesses of the brain and spinal cord.

The clinical presentation of fungal meningitis or encephalitis in non-AIDS patients is typically subacute to chronic and includes symptoms and signs suggestive of meningeal inflammation and, eventually, basilar meningitis with cranial nerve abnormalities. Symptoms and signs include headache, fever, malaise, nausea, vomiting, mental status changes, signs of meningeal inflammation (nuchal rigidity, Kernig and Brudzinski signs), visual changes or photophobia, or seizures.

In contrast, AIDS patients with fungal meningitis frequently present with a new headache or fever as their only clue to the etiology of a nonspecific deterioration. Other physical findings are also frequently absent—meningismus occurs in less than one-third of patients. As many as 15 percent of AIDS patients with fungal meningitis may have no CNS symptoms or signs, and therefore a high degree of suspicion must be maintained in these patients, and the threshold for diagnostic lumbar punctures must be much lower than in patients with normal immune systems.

The most common fungal pathogens that cause CNS infection are *Cryptococcus neoformans* and *Coccidioides immitis.* Many other fungi are less frequent but potential CNS pathogens, including *Histoplasma capsulatum, Blastomyces dermatitidis, Candida* species, *Sporothrix schenckii,* the *Mucoraceae,* and some exotic molds (Table 61-1).

Successful treatment of fungal infections of the CNS depends on early diagnosis and early institution of appropriate therapy. Also important to a successful outcome is the underlying immune status of the patient—AIDS patients pose the most difficult challenge therapeutically.

CRYPTOCOCCOSIS

Cryptococcus neoformans has always been the most common cause of fungal meningitis. Before the AIDS epidemic, over 50

TABLE 61-1. Diagnosis of Fungal Meningitis

Organism	Initial Infection	Distribution in America	India Ink	Antigen/Antibody Tests in CSF	Antigen/Antibody Tests in Serum	CSF Cultures
Cryptococcosis	Pulmonary	Widespread	+	Yes	Yes	+, often within 1 week
Coccidiodomycosis	Pulmonary	Southwest	−	Yes	Yes	+, but may take weeks
Histoplasmosis	Pulmonary	Ohio and Mississippi river valleys	−	Yes, occasionally	Yes	+, but may take weeks
Blastomycosis	Pulmonary	Southeastern and Great Lakes	−	No	Yes	+, but difficult
Candidosis	Commensals, normal flora	Widespread	−	No	Yes	+, often high colony count
Sporotrichosis	Skin wound, pulmonary	Widespread	−	Yes	?	+, but difficult

Symbols: +, positive; −, negative.

percent of patients with cryptococcal meningitis had a serious underlying disease, often with altered cell-mediated immunity. Some underlying conditions predisposing to the development of fungal meningitis are as follows:

1. AIDS
2. Lymphoproliferative malignancies
3. Organ transplant recipients
4. Corticosteroid therapy
5. Diabetes mellitus
6. Sarcoidosis

In recent years, most cases of cryptococcosis occur in AIDS patients—10 to 15 percent are eventually infected.

C. neoformans is linked to pigeons and pigeon droppings, which form a fertile medium for growth of the fungus, which is found worldwide. The route of infection is pulmonary, but the primary infection frequently is asymptomatic or passed off as a cold or flulike illness. There is invasion of the lung, however, and hematogenous spread of the yeast to the brain as well as to other organs, including the kidney and the prostate gland. The neurotropism of this organism is an essential feature of the infection and accounts for its preeminence as the leading cause of fungal CNS infection. The CNS infection usually manifests as meningitis or meningoencephalitis, but rarely as an isolated granulomatous lesion (cryptococcoma).

The pathogenic strains of *C. neoformans* typically have a large polysaccharide capsule surrounding the yeast. This capsule is antiphagocytic and accounts for the very minimal inflammatory response in infected tissues. This polysaccharide is shed into CSF and body tissues, and its detection forms the basis for the cryptococcal antigen test. The capsule also is the basis for the India ink preparation, in which the carbon black particles of the ink are displaced away from the red, cell-sized yeast by the large polysaccharide capsule (Fig. 61-1).

Cryptococcal meningitis is typically a subacute to chronic illness except in AIDS patients, where it may present as an acute fulminant infection. Most patients appear after days to weeks of headache; fever is not constant, but often present. Other manifestations include nausea, vomiting, altered mental status, malaise, meningeal signs, papilledema, visual changes, photophobia, and seizures or focal neurologic deficits. As many as 10 percent of patients with cryptococcal meningitis will have no neurologic symptoms or signs and will be discovered by serologic tests and/or lumbar puncture performed as a part of an evaluation for fever.

Specific diagnosis should depend upon a positive culture from CSF. The CSF in patients with fungal meningitis, including cryptococcal meningitis, is usually grossly clear but has a lymphocytic pleocytosis, low glucose (frequently very low; range: 5 to 10 mg/dl) and an elevated protein level. These CSF

parameters may be normal, however, in AIDS patients, although they will more often have an elevated opening pressure. India ink preparations of spun CSF sediment should be positive in half the non-AIDS patients and in three-fourths of the AIDS patients. In AIDS patients, the large number of organisms frequently allows a positive India ink preparation using unspun CSF, and allows a presumptive diagnosis pending culture results. *C. neoformans* is relatively easy to grow and frequently can be grown and identified on culture within the first week.

In patients with a negative India ink preparation, a presumptive diagnosis can be made by detection of cryptococcal antigen by latex agglutination in CSF and/or serum. This is a highly sensitive and specific test, and is readily available. The antigen is positive in CSF in 95 to 99 percent of infected AIDS patients and in serum in 90 to 95 percent. The very rare negative CSF antigen tests in patients with subsequently positive CSF cultures are attributed to infection with a rare nonencapsulated strain of *C. neoformans*. False-positive tests in the CSF are most frequently caused by a positive rheumatoid factor, chronic lymphocytic leukemia with cerebral involvement, or disseminated *Trichosporon beigelii* infection, but such false-positive titers are rarely higher than a 1:4 dilution.

Although a positive culture of CSF provides the definitive diagnosis, the organism can also be grown from urine, bone marrow, and from blood when cultured using the lysis-centrifugation method. Therefore, the initial clue to the possibility of

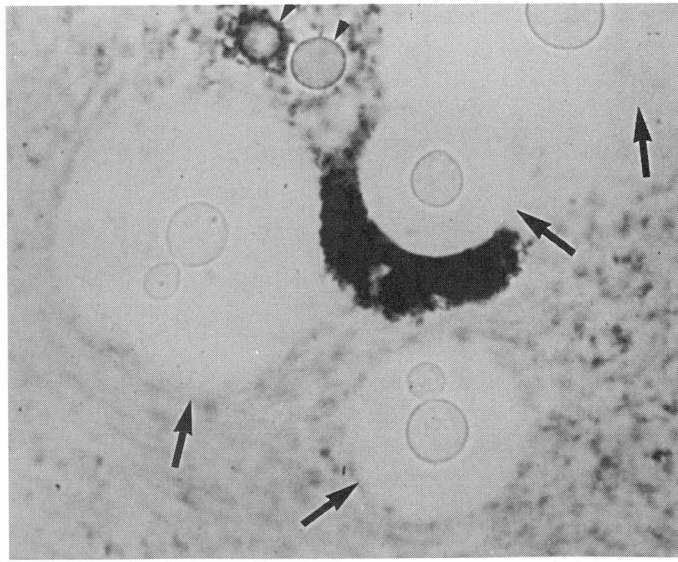

FIG. 61-1. India ink preparation in the CSF, showing the cryptococcal organism. Arrowheads indicate red blood cells; arrows, *C. neoformans*.

cryptococcal meningitis may come from a positive urine or blood culture obtained during a fever evaluation.

Treatment for cryptococcal meningitis has traditionally been systemic amphotericin B, with or without 5-fluorocytosine (5FC), used early in the course in acutely ill patients. In the non-AIDS patient with chronic meningitis who is not moribund or acutely and fulminantly ill, the practical approach is still the regimen for administration of intravenous amphotericin B: On day 1, the patient receives a test dose of 5 mg amphotericin B in 50 ml D_5W infused over 1 hour, with vital signs checked every 15 minutes; 4 hours later, the dose is increased to 10 mg in 100 ml D_5W over 1 hour, with 15-minute vital signs recorded; and 4 hours later, the dose is further increased to 25 mg in 250 ml D_5W over 2 hours; on day 2, the maximum dose is given as 50 mg in 500 ml D_5W over 2 hours. This dose is repeated 50 mg/dl daily until creatinine = 3.0 mg/dl or blood urea nitrogen (BUN) = 50 mg/dl; then the same dose is given every other day. Treatment should be continued a minimum of 6 weeks or until 1 g amphotericin B has been given after the first negative CSF culture was obtained. The CSF should be recultured at 0.5 g, 1.0 g, 2.0 g, and 3.0 g of amphotericin B administration. The most common side effects of amphotericin B are as follows, in order of frequency:

1. Increased blood urea nitrogen and creatinine
2. Fever and chills
3. Nausea, vomiting, and anorexia
4. Local phlebitis
5. Hypokalemia and hypomagnesemia
6. Anemia
7. Headache
8. Bronchospasm
9. Hypotension
10. Anaphylaxis

Treatment of these side effects may include an antiemetic and meperidine (Demerol) 25 to 50 mg IV slowly for severe chills. A central line may be quite useful in the patient with poor peripheral venous access and in the patient who may elect to complete treatment at home. In most patients, the symptomatic reactions will actually decrease as the daily dose is increased. If the reactions persist with each dose, pretreatment may be necessary with a nonsteroidal anti-inflammatory agent orally or parenterally, or a small dose of hydrocortisone (25 to 50 mg) IV just before the start of the daily amphotericin B infusion. Another major toxic effect of amphotericin B treatment is a usually reversible rise in BUN and serum creatinine. The dosage regimen should be modified based on this side effect, and BUN, and serum creatinine must be monitored twice weekly until stable, and then once weekly during the course of treatment. The BUN and creatinine should return to the pretreatment level if the total dose of amphotericin B does not exceed 3.5 g in a lifetime.

Additional toxic effects include a drop in serum potassium and magnesium and a drop in hemoglobin and hematocrit. The serum potassium and magnesium may drop precipitously and should be monitored along with the BUN and serum creatinine, and replacements should be given as indicated. The drop in hemoglobin and hematocrit will probably be much slower and does not require treatment unless the patient becomes symptomatic or has a coexisting medical condition that would be made critically worse by the anemia, in which case treatment consists of blood transfusions. Once the amphotericin is discontinued, the hemoglobin and hematocrit will return to the pretreatment levels without specific iron or vitamin therapy. Iron and B_{12} or folate treatment is not effective, since this is a direct toxic effect of the amphotericin B on the bone marrow.

Intrathecal administration of amphotericin B is probably not useful in the treatment of cryptococcal meningitis.

Other ancillary treatment measures in the non-AIDS patient include the addition of 5FC given orally or by nasogastric tube in a dose of 150 mg/kg/day in the patient who is moribund or critically ill when the diagnosis is established. The 5FC can be initiated in full dosage while simultaneously building up to the full daily dose of amphotericin B. This combination may lead to more rapid sterilization of the CSF and is believed by some to be superior to amphotericin B alone in the treatment of non-AIDS patients. However, once the BUN and serum creatinine start to rise, the serum levels of 5FC rise and bone marrow and/or hepatic toxicity may occur. It is necessary to stop the 5FC at this point, or monitor levels and keep them under 100 μg/ml (draw levels 2 hours after dose) if it is essential to continue the drug because of the severity of the illness. Liver functions as well as complete blood counts should be checked weekly during the course of treatment.

In AIDS patients with cryptococcal meningitis, no therapeutic regimen is curative. The best method for initial treatment, and then long-term suppression to prevent relapse, is currently being investigated. To date the usual treatment in AIDS patients has consisted of 6 weeks of amphotericin B treatment (with or without 5FC initially, in a dose of 100 mg/kg/day) followed by long-term suppression with either weekly infusion of intravenous amphotericin B (1 mg/kg/week) or daily oral fluconazole (200 mg/day). A critical point is that the CSF culture must be negative before switching to the long-term suppressive or maintenance therapy in AIDS patients. In this patient population, repeat lumbar puncture should probably be performed at 2 and 4 weeks of treatment, then monthly until cultures are negative and the patient can be switched to maintenance therapy.

Many other treatment and maintenance regimens are currently under investigation with the hope that an effective oral treatment regimen can be established with a higher dose of fluconazole or with itraconazole, another new triazole antifungal agent, or some combination of these agents. New recommendations concerning treatment and maintenance regimens in AIDS patients may emerge as these trials are completed and published.

COCCIDIOIDOMYCOSIS

Coccidioides immitis is the etiologic agent of coccidioidomycosis and is the second most common pathogen in fungal meningitis. In contrast to *C. neoformans,* which exists only in the yeast form, *C. immitis* is a dimorphic fungus, growing as a mold in nature and converting to a pathogenic yeast when inhaled into the lung at body temperature. This fungus is limited in its geographic distribution to the semiarid regions of the southwestern United States, Mexico, and areas of Central and South America between latitudes 40 degrees north and 40 degrees south. This endemic region is marked by the growth of the creosote bush.

Infection with this fungus occurs when a susceptible person inhales the mold (arthroconidia) form of the fungus while traveling in or residing in the endemic area. A primary pulmonary infection occurs when the mold phase converts to the yeast phase at body temperature. There is then invasion of the lung by the yeast phase with spread to the hilar nodes as well as systemic hematogenous spread throughout the body, including the brain and meninges. In hosts with normal immune systems, this primary pulmonary illness with hematogenous dissemination may manifest as a cold or flulike illness and is usually self-limited without specific treatment. Once infected, blacks, Filipinos, Native Americans, AIDS victims, and pregnant women have an increased risk of progressive disseminated disease and a higher mortality.

Coccidioidal meningitis is the most severe form of disseminated disease and is probably incurable even in patients with normal immune systems. In blacks, Filipinos, Native American Indians, and AIDS patients, the presentation is often that of an acute meningitis occurring within 3 months of the primary infection, with multiple other organs involved as well. In non-AIDS whites, the presentation is more often that of chronic meningitis occurring long after the primary infection, with a protracted course and periods of spontaneous remission of symptoms. This is particularly common in nonpregnant white women, in whom the CNS alone is infected and there is a predilection for the meninges, in contrast to cryptococcal meningitis where involvement of the brain is extensive. The clinical presentation of either the acute or chronic meningitis may include headache, varying degrees of fever, altered mental status, nausea, vomiting, and seizures. Signs of meningeal irritation are usually absent in the chronic form, but hydrocephalus or focal neurologic deficits may be found.

The diagnosis is established by growth of the organism from CSF. This is much more difficult in coccidioidomycosis than in cryptococcosis because the colony count of yeast in the CSF is much lower. The diagnosis should be considered in any patient with a lymphocytic pleocytosis in the CSF and a very low CSF glucose level, with or without an elevated CSF protein level. Once cryptococcus has been excluded by a negative India ink preparation and a negative cryptococcal antigen in the CSF and serum, the differential diagnosis should turn to coccidioidomycosis and tuberculosis. A careful travel history as well as history of exposure to tuberculosis becomes very helpful at this point.

A presumptive diagnosis can be established by a positive test for complement-fixing antibodies in the CSF for coccidioidomycosis. This is a very sensitive (75 to 95 percent) and specific test in patients with CNS coccidioidomycosis. To corroborate this etiologic diagnosis a repeat lumbar puncture with removal of a large volume (50 to 60 ml) of CSF for culture may be necessary. Cultures of C. immitis may take several weeks, so treatment can be started based on the presumptive diagnosis established by the positive complement fixation test on CSF. Serum antibody titers are useful in the immunocompetent patient in establishing an early diagnosis of disseminated disease, but it is important to establish the presence or absence of CNS infection by specific serologic tests and cultures of CSF because the treatment of meningitis and disseminated coccidioidomycosis without meningitis are different. Patients with immunodeficiency states, including AIDS, may fail to develop complement-fixing antibodies in either serum or CSF, but their CSF cultures are more likely to be positive because of more aggressive infection.

Therapy for coccidioidal meningitis requires prolonged treatment with both intravenous and intrathecal amphotericin B. The intravenous administration of amphotericin B is as discussed earlier in this chapter in the section "Cryptococcosis." Intrathecal amphotericin B can be administered by cisternal tap or via an Ommaya reservoir, which can be inserted surgically with direct access to a lateral ventricle. If the patient has noncom-

municating hydrocephalus and needs a shunt, a combination apparatus with Ommaya reservoir and shunt can be inserted.

Intrathecal amphotericin B is quite irritating, so the doses must be very low. Therapy should begin with 0.01 mg given into the cisternal CSF or lateral ventricle via an Ommaya reservoir. If this is tolerated, increase the dose to 0.05 mg, then 0.1 mg, then 0.2 mg, working up by 0.1 mg per dose until the side effects are intolerable, and then reduce the dose to the maximum tolerable level. This tolerable dose will probably be in the 0.5 to 1.5 mg range, although some patients may tolerate as much as 3 to 5 mg per dose. Once the maintenance dose has been reached, therapy can continue with alternate days of intravenous and intrathecal amphotericin B, giving 50 mg of amphotericin B intravenously on the days between the intrathecal doses, provided the BUN remains below 50 mg/dl and the serum creatinine below 3.0 mg/dl. The total dose of intravenous amphotericin B for treatment of coccidioidal meningitis is often 3.0 to 3.5 g and this dose should be continued until the CSF culture and complement-fixation titer are negative or until the latter levels off at 1:2 or 1:4. At that point, intrathecal maintenance therapy alone can be continued and the interval of treatments reduced over time to the minimum dose required to keep the CSF complement-fixation titer negative or stable at its low level, which may require one to three intrathecal doses per week. This suppressive maintenance therapy must be continued indefinitely to prevent relapse.

The new triazoles, fluconazole and itraconazole, show promise in treating coccidioidal meningitis. Both are given in a dose of 400 mg/day orally and show benefits in non-AIDS patients. Clinical trials are underway to better define an alternative to intravenous and intrathecal amphotericin B in the treatment of coccidioidal meningitis in both AIDS and non-AIDS patients.

HISTOPLASMOSIS

Histoplasma capsulatum is the etiologic agent of histoplasmosis. It is a thermal dimorphic fungus found commonly in the Ohio and Mississippi river valleys. Like C. immitis, H. capsulatum grows as a mold in nature, and the primary infection results from inhalation of the mold. Once in the lung, the mold converts to the yeast phase, which invades the lung and spreads hematogenously. Most patients with progressive histoplasmosis have widespread infection of the reticuloendothelial system. Central nervous system involvement is quite rare in the non-AIDS patient. When it does occur, it usually presents as chronic meningitis, and the cerebrospinal fluid reveals a lymphocytic pleocytosis (with or without elevated CSF protein) and low CSF glucose, sometimes very low (in the 5 to 10 mg/dl range). In AIDS patients, disseminated disease and meningitis are more frequent and can result from primary exposure or reactivation of a quiescent focus. Therefore, a history of recent travel in the endemic area is not critical in suspecting the diagnosis if the patient has ever lived in the endemic regions.

In AIDS patients, CNS manifestations may be subclinical, or can range from frank acute meningitis to acute confusional states to a picture of single or multiple space-occupying lesions. The diagnosis is established by a positive culture of CSF. As in coccidioidal meningitis, the colony count of fungi in CSF may be very low. To compensate for this, large volumes of CSF should be cultured if initial cultures are negative. H. capsulatum can be very slow-growing, and the cultures must be held for a full 6 to 8 weeks before being reported as negative. A presumptive diagnosis can be established by positive complement-fixation antibody titers to yeast-phase and mycelial-phase antigens in CSF. Unfortunately, these are not so sensitive nor specific as the similar serologic tests in the CSF in coccidioidal meningitis. AIDS patients frequently fail to demonstrate an antibody response.

There is a new radioimmunoassay for *H. capsulatum* polysaccharide antigen (HPA), which seems more specific but still not very sensitive, being present in only a quarter of non-AIDS patients with culture-proven meningitis. This test is being evaluated at present.

Treatment of histoplasma meningitis in the non-AIDS patient is parenteral amphotericin B in a total dose of 2.0 to 2.5 g. In AIDS patients, the initial intensive course of amphotericin B can be stopped at 1.0 to 1.5 g if the clinical response is adequate. Relapse will occur, however, and maintenance therapy must be continued with parenteral amphotericin B 50 mg once or twice weekly or itraconazole 400 mg/day given orally. If successful, this maintenance therapy should be continued indefinitely in the AIDS patient.

BLASTOMYCOSIS

Blastomyces dermatitidis is the etiologic agent in North American blastomycosis. This is another thermal dimorphic fungus found principally in North America, particularly in the southeastern United States and in the Mississippi, Ohio, and St. Lawrence river areas as well as around the Great Lakes. It grows as a mold in nature and the primary infection is in the lungs. There is conversion of the mold to the yeast phase at body temperature and then invasion of the lung and hematogenous seeding. CNS infection can occur from this seeding, or by direct extension, as from osteomyelitis of the spine.

CNS blastomycosis is extremely rare and is usually a late manifestation of disseminated disease. It can present in three clinical patterns: focal pyogranulomas, spinal abscess secondary to extension of an epidural abscess, or as an exudative or chronic meningitis. Focal neurologic deficits may be present if the presentation is with a mass lesion of a pyogranuloma. The patient with meningitis may present with headache, fever, lethargy, or altered mental status and a stiff neck. Back pain and signs of cord compression accompany the epidural abscess form. In any case, the CSF will reveal an elevated cell count, but this fungus can elicit a pyogenic response so the differential count can be mixed rather than the lymphocytic pleocytosis typical of most fungal infections. The CSF protein is usually elevated and the glucose level is low. Serologic tests for blastomycosis are notoriously poor, so they cannot be relied upon to help make a presumptive diagnosis. The diagnosis is established by culture of the spinal fluid and, again, large volumes should be cultured to compensate for the low colony count of the yeast in the CSF if initial fungal cultures are negative in routine small volume samples of CSF.

Treatment in the non-AIDS patient consists of parenteral amphotericin B in a total dose of 2.0 to 2.5 g. The role of azoles is currently being investigated. Blastomycosis is rare in AIDS patients and meningitis is rare in patients with disseminated blastomycosis. Therefore, there is no proven treatment regimen to recommend in this situation. The treatment regimen recommended for AIDS patients with histoplasma meningitis should be effective.

CANDIDOSIS

Candida species number more than 80, but only 10 or so species are proven pathogens. Most are commensals and part of the normal flora of the gastrointestinal tract. Tissue invasion is associated with altered host defenses. The organism can reach the bloodstream from the gut, the urinary tract, or by infection of a venous or arterial line. Dissemination is hematogenous, and CNS infection is usually part of widespread disseminated disease. The clinical picture mirrors the disseminated nature of the infection, with fever and headache being common complaints and meningismus being a common sign. The CSF reveals a lymphocytic pleocytosis, elevated protein level, and normal to decreased glucose levels. The colony count of yeast is frequently high so that a Gram stain of CSF sediment is positive in half the patients, and the cultures rapidly become positive. Diagnosis is established by a positive culture. Serologic tests are currently being evaluated.

Treatment for candidal meningitis is parenteral amphotericin B in a total dose of 2.0 to 2.5 g in the non-AIDS patient. In AIDS patients, the regimen used for cryptococcal meningitis should be adequate.

SPOROTRICHOSIS

Sporothrix schenckii is the etiologic agent of sporotrichosis. This is another thermal dimorphic fungus. It grows in nature as a mold, frequently in association with sphagnum moss. Its usual presentation is as a cutaneous or subcutaneous infection following a puncture wound or abrasion of the skin. Spread is via lymphatics. If not recognized and treated, the lymphatic drainage can lead to hematogenous dissemination to the CNS. CNS involvement is very rare and usually presents as a chronic meningitis: headache is the most common symptom, followed by altered mental status and fever. The CSF reveals a lymphocytic pleocytosis with elevated protein level and normal to low glucose levels. The colony count is low, so culture of a large volume of CSF may be necessary to establish the diagnosis. A presumptive diagnosis can be established by detecting antibody to *S. schenckii* in the CSF by latex agglutination or enzyme immunoassay.

Treatment in the non-AIDS patient is parenteral amphotericin B in a total dose of 2.0 to 2.5 g. In AIDS patients a regimen of parenteral amphotericin B followed by suppressive itraconazole would seem appropriate, but data are lacking at present because of the paucity of cases.

OTHER FUNGAL INFECTIONS

Other fungi cause CNS infections, but the clinical picture is more often that of a mass lesion with blood vessel invasion and infarction, or focal parenchymal lesions, rather than meningitis. The common pathogens producing this form of CNS disease include the molds, *Aspergillus* species, and the zygomycetes which cause mucormycosis.

Mucormycosis is usually caused by *Rhizopus arrhizus* or *R. oryzae* molds in the zygomycete class. It is ubiquitous and usually incapable of infection except in patients with serious underlying diseases, including diabetes mellitus. Unlike yeasts, molds may grow fulminantly, as a mass lesion, or produce a cerebritis that involves arteries and leads to infarctions. Rhinocerebral mucormycosis often presents with diplopia, face pain, and nasal stuffiness arising from inflammation and necrosis of the nose and orbit. The mass erodes the skull and sinuses, picking off cranial nerves, and then invades intracranially, causing coma and death within days or weeks. Fever and headache are common, as is an abnormal CSF, showing mild pleocytosis and elevated protein. Computed tomography scans or magnetic resonance imaging shows characteristic sinus opacification and bony erosion, and cerebral involvement is seen as a nonspecific mass lesion. Confirmation of the diagnosis usually requires biopsy.

Treatment for these pathogens frequently requires extensive surgical debridement of the craniofacial lesions or the brain masses, plus appropriate chemotherapy of intravenous amphotericin B. A team approach utilizing neurosurgical and infection disease consultation is recommended, since survival rates are only 50 percent or less.

SUGGESTED READINGS

Bennett JE: Current therapy of deep mycoses. Update 11 to Mandell GL, Douglas RG, Jr, and Bennett JE (eds): Principles and Practice of Infectious Diseases. Churchill Livingstone, New York, 1991

Katzman M, Ellner JJ: Chronic meningitis. p. 755. In Mandell GL, Douglas RG, Jr, and Bennett JE (eds): Principles and Practice of Infectious Diseases. 3rd Ed. Churchill Livingstone, New York, 1990

Pietroski NA, Safir E, Stern JJ: Neurology: CNS fungal infections in AIDS patients. p. 194. The AIDS Reader, 1992

Treseler CB, Sugar AM: Fungal meningitis. Infect Dis Clin North Am 4:755, 1990

62. CYSTICERCOSIS

RICHARD M. ARMSTRONG

Neurocysticercosis is one of the most common parasitic infections affecting the nervous system. It results from the encystation of the larval form of the pork tapeworm *Taenia solium* in the brain parenchyma, the ventricular system, or the meninges.

EPIDEMIOLOGY

Tapeworms, or cestodes, are segmented worms that attach to the intestinal mucosa with their head, or scolex, which contains sucking disks and hooks. Behind the scolex form the ribbonlike segments, or proglottids, each of which contains several thousand eggs. The pork tapeworm generally has 1,000 proglottids and extends up to 3 m in length. When the proglottids are shed into the feces, the eggs are infective and, if ingested by a human, will develop into larval oncospheres that penetrate the gut wall, enter the bloodstream, and disseminate throughout the body, with a predilection for the central nervous system (CNS). The larvae may then develop into a cyst containing a scolex, which is known as a cysticercus. In this sequence of events, the infected person is acting as an intermediate host for the parasite. The pig also functions as an intermediate host for *T. solium* and is crucial to the continued presence of the disease in endemic areas.

Humans can also function as the primary or definitive host when they harbor the adult *T. solium* worm in the small intestine. Ingestion of cysts, usually in infected pork, results in colonization of the small intestine when the scolex, released from the ingested cyst, affixes to the gut wall and proceeds to mature into an adult worm with numerous proglottid segments. Usually only a single worm is present in the lumen of the small bowel, and the host is asymptomatic, possibly harboring a worm for many years. Fecally contaminated foodstuffs are then ingested by humans (autoinfection) or other intermediate hosts, usually the pig.

Neurocysticercosis is endemic in many regions of the world and is most common where there is a high rate of infestation in pigs. It is a significant problem among immigrants to the United States. The actual prevalence is not known, but autopsy series in Mexico indicate that up to 3.6 percent of the population may be infected.

CLINICAL FEATURES

Humans, the primary hosts of *T. solium,* are usually asymptomatic when infected. However, when infected by the larval stage they function as intermediate hosts and may be symptomatic with fever and headache as the larvae invade the tissues. Once the cysts are established in the tissues they may remain viable for many years, be well tolerated by the host, and persist without clinical manifestations. Neurocysticercosis may become symptomatic up to 30 years after infection. Neurologic symptoms usually result either from the local inflammatory response induced by the parasite, or from the mass effect of the space-occupying lesion.

Following implantation, the cyst consists of a thin-walled sac that contains the scolex attached to the cyst wall. In this vesicular stage the parasite elicits little response from the host. If they remain small and few in number, they may persist in the brain parenchyma through a long asymptomatic phase. Computed tomography (CT) scans and magnetic resonance imaging (MRI) show circumscribed hypodense lesions without associated enhancement or edema.

Eventually, the cyst begins to undergo degenerative changes and enters into a colloidal phase. The vesicular liquid takes on a gelatinous-colloidal character, and the cyst wall thickens. This change elicits an inflammatory host response, and radiologically the cyst and surrounding edema are enhanced by contrast media.

The degenerating cyst then enters a nodular granular phase in which the vesicle shrinks and its contents become semisolid. It is progressively replaced by granulomatous tissue, and on CT scan it appears as a hypodense area with irregular borders and surrounding edema. With contrast media enhancement, small, rounded hyperdensities are seen.

Finally, the lesion retracts further and becomes a calcified, inactive mass.

Small parenchymal cysts may remain asymptomatic until they begin to degenerate and the host mounts an inflammatory response. This inflammation, with edema, may then act as an irritative focus, and seizures may develop. If the cyst size or number is large, there may be mass effect with resulting headache and focal neurologic signs. If there is diffuse involvement with multiple reacting lesions, the clinical picture may be that of an acute encephalitis.

Seizures and headaches are the most frequent presenting clinical features. The seizures are often focal in onset. Less commonly, there may be nausea, vomiting, papilledema, meningeal irritation, altered mental status, and other signs of increased intracranial pressure. Cranial nerve palsies, focal neurologic deficits from cerebral lesions, ataxia, and signs of cord compression may also present or occur during the course of the disease. Meningeal inflammation, in reaction to neurocysticercosis, may result in vascular occlusion and infarction.

Cysts may develop within the ventricles and cause obstruc-

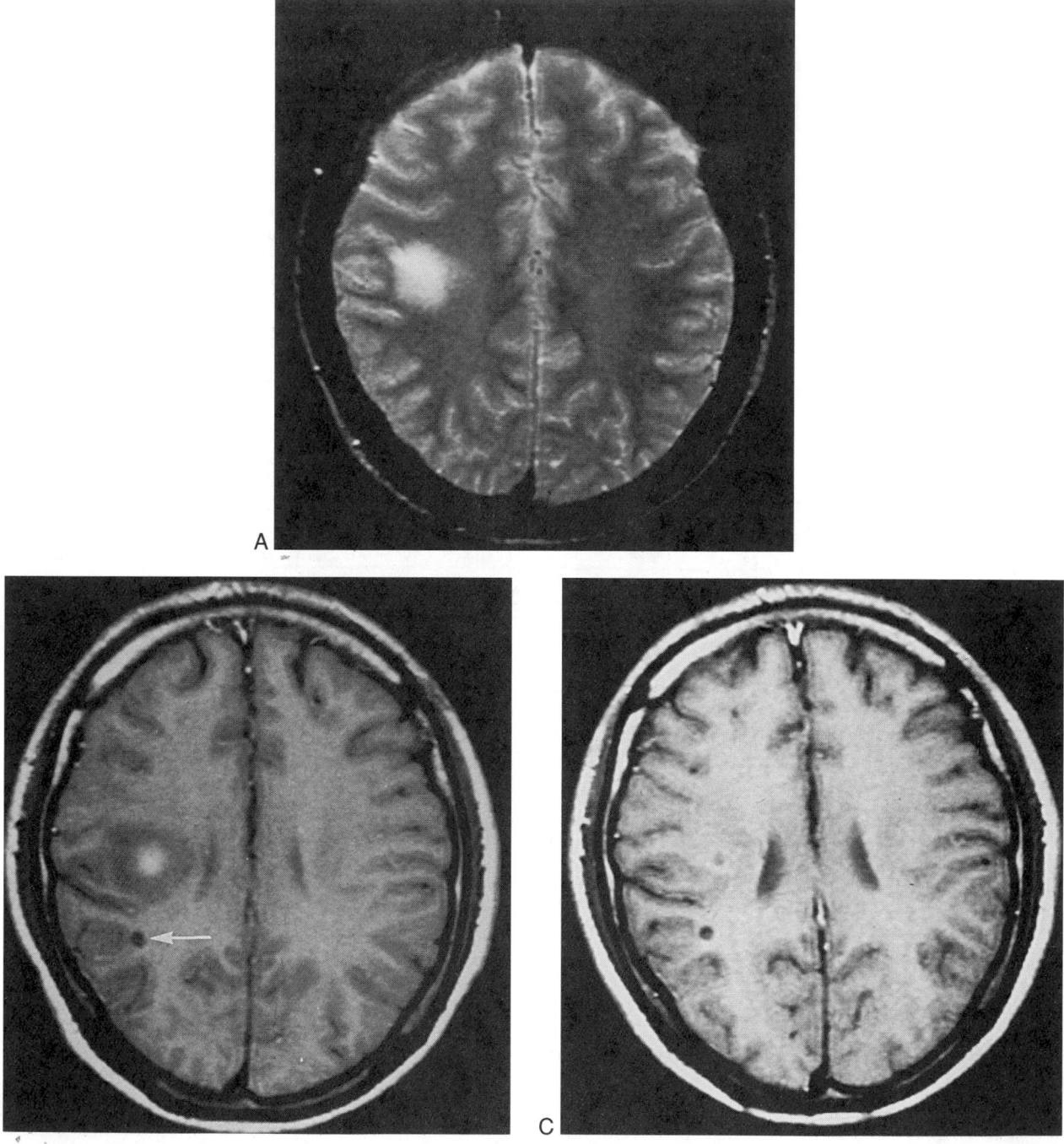

FIG. 62-1. **(A)** T2-weighted MRI scan showing an active cyst at the gray-white matter junction in the right cerebral hemisphere. **(B)** The same lesion on gadolinium-enhanced T1 imaging, showing the characteristic enhancement and surrounding edema. This T1 technique also shows a small, nonenhancing punctate lesion (*arrow*), which is an old, degenerated, inactive cyst. **(C)** Contrast-enhanced T1-weighted MRI 7 weeks after adequate therapy with praziquantel, showing shrinkage, resolution of edema, and loss of enhancement. The old, inactive lesion is unchanged. (Courtesy of J. Douglas Lee, M.D., and Lawrence Hutchins, M.D., The Marshfield Clinic, Marshfield, WI.)

tive hydrocephalus as a result of their anatomic location, and not because of degenerative changes or host reactions. However, these latter may occur, and the resulting inflammatory response may also produce an obstructive hydrocephalus and signs of meningeal irritation.

In the spinal canal, meningeal lesions can produce cord compression. The cervical region is most commonly involved. Meningeal cysts may have a mass effect by themselves or by the inflammatory response they elicit in the meninges, which may result in vessel occlusion and infarction of the cord. Intramedullary cysts also occur within the spinal cord.

Ocular cysticercosis is rare but can occur. Extraocular, intraorbital, subretinal, conjunctival, and palpebral lesions have all been reported.

Many patients will have involvement of multiple anatomic sites and present with various combinations of symptoms and syndromes. The clinical manifestations will reflect the number, size, viability or biologic status of the parasite, and the host response to the parasite. MRI and CT studies are informative in defining location and the biologic status of the cysts.

DIAGNOSIS

Headaches and seizures are the primary presenting features, and neurocysticercosis should be considered in the differential diagnosis of any patient who has a history of exposure in an endemic area. Neurocysticercosis is the most common identified cause of adult seizures in Mexico, and also accounts for a

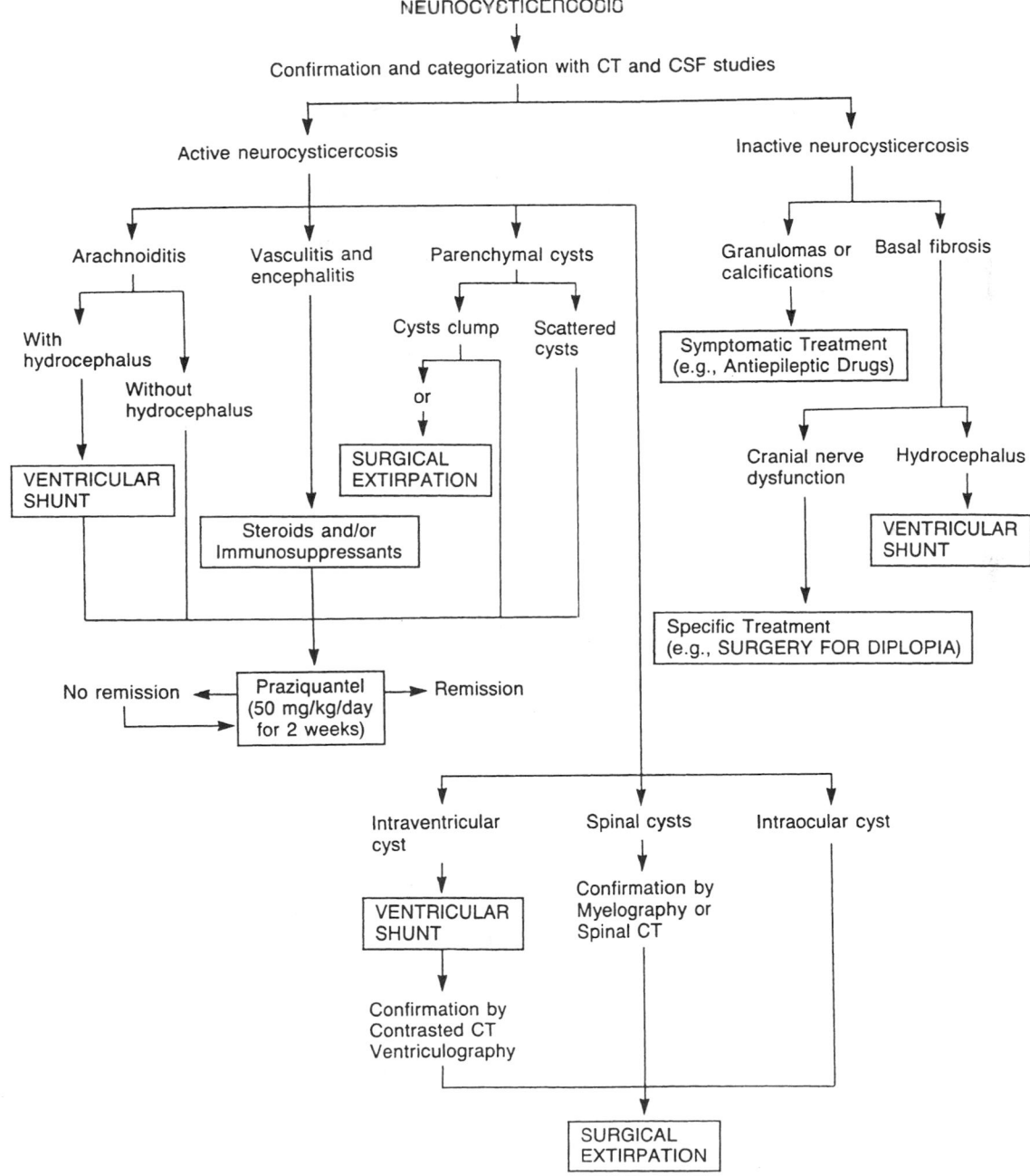

FIG. 62-2.   Algorithm for the treatment of neurocysticercosis. (From Johnson RT: Neurocysticercosis in Current Therapy in Neurologic Disease. 2nd Ed. Mosby-Year Book, St. Louis, MO, 1992, with permission.)

significant proportion of cases of hydrocephalus or intracranial masses.

Calcified, palpable subcutaneous or intramuscular nodules are found in fewer than 5 percent of patients in modern series. Peripheral blood eosinophilia is inconstant. CSF analysis is normal in approximately two-thirds of cases, but in one-third there may be a pleocytosis of polymorphonuclear or lymphocytic cells and an associated increase of protein. Occasionally, eosinophils may be seen in the cerebrospinal fluid (CSF).

Serologic and CSF tests to detect antibodies are available. The enzyme-linked immunoabsorbent assay (ELISA) or enzyme-linked immunoelectrotransfer blot (EITB) can be useful in confirming the diagnosis. The EITB has a specificity of 100 percent and a sensitivity greater than 93 percent in the serum and approximately 80 percent in the CSF. The ELISA is less sensitive in the serum and CSF. These tests are not readily available in all areas, and for the present they are used as confirmatory, rather than diagnostic, tests. ELISA and EITB are more sensitive and specific than the earlier techniques of complement fixation, immunoprecipitation, and other tests to detect antibody and antigen.

CT and MRI studies are informative in diagnosing neurocysticercosis (Fig. 62-1). The appearance of typical lesions, combined with a history and physical examination that are consistent with cysticercosis, allows the diagnosis to be made with a high degree of confidence. Cysts in the vesicular stage will be seen as low-density rounded lesions without associated contrast media enhancement or edema. Once degeneration begins, the cysts appear as hypodense or isodense rounded lesions with ring or nodular enhancement and adjacent edema. End-stage neurocysticercosis may appear as small calcifications at multiple sites, but predominantly at the gray-white junction. These are best seen by CT examination. CT scanning and MRI also allows definition of cysts in the ventricular and arachnoid spaces. It is not uncommon for the CT or MRI studies to show multiple lesions in various phases of evolution.

TREATMENT

Figure 62-2 shows an algorithm for the treatment of neurocysticercosis. Praziquantel and albendazole are the most commonly used anticysticercal drugs, with albendazole probably superior in reducing the total number of cysts. Praziquantel is usually given in a dose of 50 mg/kg/day in three divided doses for 12 to 14 days. The regimen for albendazole is 15 mg/kg/day in three doses for 8 days.

If only calcified lesions are seen on CT and the spinal fluid is normal, then no anticysticercal treatment is required. Active cysts in a symptomatic patient should be treated with either praziquantel or, preferably, albendazole, both of which are effective against viable and degenerating cysts.

During treatment, parenchymal lesions that have been tolerated asymptomatically may begin to undergo degeneration and activate an inflammatory host response, which results in associated edema. If the lesion is large, there may be mass effect and compromise of adjacent neurons, producing neurologic deficits. The lesion may also act as an irritative focus, which produces seizures. Drug-induced death of cysticerci may thus result in an increased inflammatory response analogous to the Herxheimer response. Clinically, this may be manifest as increased intracranial pressure, meningeal irritation, or general malaise. Some authorities recommend the concomitant administration of corticosteroids (prednisone or dexamethasone), but this may decrease, significantly, the bioavailability of praziquantel. If the lesion load is not great and there is little or no meningeal involvement, then it is appropriate to treat without corticosteroids and to monitor the patient for the first few days of treatment, adding corticosteroids if there is a significant reaction. Nonsteroidal anti-inflammatory drugs may be used as an alternative to steroids.

If recurrent seizures occur, they can usually be effectively managed with phenytoin or carbamazepine in the usual therapeutic doses. There is some suggestion that anticonvulsants may decrease the bioavailability of the anticysticercal agents, but this is probably not significant in most cases.

Imaging studies should be repeated 3 months after treatment to assess the efficacy of the treatment by documenting a decrease in size and number of cysts.

Occasionally, complications mandate surgical treatment of neurocysticercosis. Intraventricular cysts may cause obstructive hydrocephalus, for which early surgical intervention is indicated. Shunting may be required acutely to treat the hydrocephalus, and, if possible, the cyst should be removed. Ventricular shunting and brain decompression may also be required to manage cases of acute fulminant cysticercosis encephalitis. Cysts may develop in the meninges around the spinal cord or within the cord, and these, too, should be treated surgically. Anticysticercal agents, anticonvulsants, and corticosteroids, when appropriate, should be used concomitantly.

Neurocysticercosis can be prevented with proper cooking of pork and by the implementation of appropriate sanitary practices. Carriers of the adult worm should be treated. Handwashing by food handlers and the elimination of contaminated foods for pigs have been effective in developed countries.

SUGGESTED READINGS

Alarcon F, Hidalgo F, Moncayo J et al: Cerebral cysticercosis and stroke. Stroke 23:224, 1992

DelBrutto OH: Medical treatment of cysticercosis: effective. Arch Neurol 52: 102, 1995

Del Brutto OH, Santibanez R, Noboa CA et al: Epilepsy due to neurocysticercosis: analysis of 203 patients. Neurology 42:389, 1992

Kramer LD: Medical treatment of cysticercosis: ineffective. Arch Neurol 52: 101, 1995

Scharf D: Neurocysticercosis: 238 cases from a California hospital. Arch Neurol 45:777, 1988

Takayanagui OM, Jardim E: Therapy for neurocysticercosis: comparison between albendazole and praziquantel. Arch Neurol 49:290, 1992

Teitelbaum GP: MR imaging of neurocysticercosis. Am J Radiol 153:857, 1989

63. TRICHINOSIS

Y. HARATI

Human trichinosis, the best-known parasitic infection of muscles, is caused by nematodes of the species *Trichinella spiralis*. It develops after the ingestion of raw of incompletely cooked infected pork, bear, horse, or walrus meat containing viable cysts of the parasite. Trichinosis has been documented in 39 countries of North and South America, Europe, and Africa. Its prevalence is increased in ethnic groups with a culinary preference for raw or inadequately cooked pork products including individuals of Laotian, Cambodian, German, Italian, and Polish descent—several recent outbreaks of trichinosis among Southeast Asian refugees in the United States have also been reported. With the ease of world travel, and heightened immigration, the likelihood of a practicing physician in the United States to encounter patients with trichinosis has significantly increased, and the diagnosis should be considered in any patient presenting with fever, myalgias, periorbital edema, and eosinophilia.

EPIDEMIOLOGY

Approximately 28 million people worldwide are infected with this parasite, but most are asymptomatic or minimally symptomatic and thus do not come to medical attention. The annual incidence of trichinosis in the United States has steadily declined; only 206 cases were reported to the Centers for Disease Control and Prevention from 1987 to 1990. There is no gender difference in reported cases; about 60 percent of patients are between the ages of 20 and 50. The highest number of cases come from the northeastern and mid-Atlantic states, which reflects both higher rates of infection among swine in these areas and a higher concentration of ethnic groups with culinary preference for raw or lightly cooked pork. Pork and pork products, especially sausages, account for 75 percent of all human *Trichinella* infection; nonpork products including game animals, bear, and walrus meat account for 13 percent, and in 12 percent of patients the source is undetermined. Ground beef contaminated by pork (e.g., in a meat grinder) is a common source of nonpork-induced disease.

Although in suspected cases of trichinosis a detailed dietary and travel history is important, failure to elicit a history of raw pork consumption does not exclude the diagnosis. Travelers to Mexico, Asia, and Africa make up 65 percent of reported cases of travel-associated trichinosis in the United States; this percentage appears to be increasing in parallel with an increase in the total number of travelers to high-risk countries. Trichinosis should be suspected in any individual with eosinophilia returning from abroad.

Enactment of several federal and state laws prohibiting the feeding of non-heat-treated garbage to swine has all but eliminated commercial pork products as a cause of trichinosis. However, the noncommercial sources of pork, as from wild animals and small farms not using modern hog management and slaughter practices, are emerging as an important remaining source of human trichinosis in the United States. Case reporting of trichinosis consistently increases from December through March, probably as a result of homemade pork products eaten during the holiday season.

CLINICAL FEATURES

Following the ingestion of contaminated meat, the encysted larva is digested by stomach and proximal intestinal enzymes, leading to liberation of the organism in the upper small bowel. The released larvae burrow into the mucosa of the small intestine, and after 24 to 36 hours develop into mating male and female adult worms. Each female worm then produces up to 1,500 new larva during her lifetime of 2 to 5 weeks. The progeny larva penetrate through the mucosa of the small intestine, gaining access to the lymphatic and venous circulation, and disseminate widely, especially to striated muscles. The muscles most commonly invaded are, in order of frequency, as follows:

diaphragm, extraocular, tongue, pharyngeal, jaw, intercostal, neck, back, abdominal, and limb muscles. Immature larva reaching striated muscles will encyst, but larva reaching nonstriated muscles or other tissues do not encyst and may continue to migrate, resulting in marked inflammation and tissue necrosis. This process is usually self-limited but may result in severe multiorgan pathology, chronic sequela, or even death. The muscle cystic structures may begin to calcify as early as 6 months following the initial infection. However, as in animals, the larva may remain viable within cysts for several years.

The clinical symptoms of trichinosis arise from successive phases of parasitic enteric invasion, larval migration, and tissue encystment. When muscle invasion involves less than 10 larvae per gram of muscle no symptoms may arise, but infection of 50 to 100 larvae per gram can produce severe symptoms. Most infections are asymptomatic and are not recognized clinically. During the first week of infection, when larval invasion of the gut occurs, transient diarrhea, abdominal pain, nausea, or vomiting may occur. During the second week after infection, when larval migration and muscle invasion begin, local and systemic hypersensitivity reactions occur. Fever, chills, headache, periorbital and facial edema, subconjunctival, retinal, and nailbed hemorrhage, macular, petechial or urticarial skin rash, hoarseness, cough and dyspnea, dysphagia, and hypereosinophilia develop. When infection is severe and hypereosinophilia exceeds $4,000/mm^3$, a cardioneurologic syndrome consisting of diffuse and focal encephalopathy (microinfarcts or focal cerebritis), hypodensities on brain computed tomography (CT) scan, diffuse ischemic or focal myocarditis with tachyarrhythmia, heart failure, and creatine kinase-(CK-MB) isoenzyme elevation may occur. The myocarditis may initially manifest as tachycardia or chest pain and may mimic acute myocardial infarction. Electrocardiographic evidence of myocardial involvement may be found in up to 75 percent of patients with trichinosis. Most fatalities of trichinosis are due to myocarditis, pneumonitis, or encephalitis and occur in the third to ninth week of the disease.

Upon larval invasion and encystment of muscles at the end of the first week, pain and tenderness develops, particularly of proximal muscles. This symptom, along with generalized weakness, malaise, and elevated serum CK levels, may result in considerable diagnostic confusion with polymyositis (or dermatomyositis if skin rash is also present). However, in trichinosis the pain is more severe than polymyositis, and pain in the jaws, neck, and back may be prominent. Involvement of extraocular muscles, intercostal muscles, and the diaphragm are also more common in trichinosis. Electromyography in both conditions demonstrates myopathic features and fibrillation potentials. Only eosinophilia, other systemic symptoms, and the travel and culinary history may permit the correct diagnosis.

DIAGNOSIS

Confirmation of the diagnosis is often accomplished by serologic testing and/or muscle biopsy. Serologic testing is simple, highly sensitive, and specific. Antibodies to *T. spiralis,* however, are not detected until 3 weeks or more after the onset of infection, although ultimately significant antibody titers develop in about 95 percent of individuals. Available serologic tests include rapid screening counterimmunoelectrophoresis, enzyme-linked immunosorbent assay (ELISA), passive hemagglutination, and indirect immunofluorescence. The bentonite flocculation test is most widely used; a titer of 1:5 or greater is considered positive, although a fourfold risk in the titer is more convincing. The test may be repeated in 4 to 6 weeks to determine a rise in the titer. An elevated titer may persist for many months.

The quickest way to establish the diagnosis during the muscle phase of the illness is to find *Trichinella* larva within the striated muscles. An open muscle biopsy to obtain at least 1 g of muscle is required. The highest yield of larvae is near the tendon insertion of the muscle. An inflammatory infiltrate—mainly eosinophils and neutrophils, with fewer lymphocytes, plasma cells, and other mononuclear cells—is seen around parasite-containing muscle fibers and in the interstitium. When larvae are not observed because of a sampling error, such an inflammatory reaction to larvae may be the only pathologic abnormality present. If the biopsy is obtained 3 or 4 weeks after the infection, encapsulation or even calcification of the capsule may be seen.

The differential diagnosis of trichinosis, which is a disease with multisystem involvement, is extensive:

Polymyositis
Dermatomyositis
Viral syndromes: influenza, gastroenteritis, exanthems
Periarteritis
Sepsis: pneumonitis, meningitis, typhoid
Allergic phenomena
Encephalitis

Trichinosis should be considered in patients who present with fever and myalgias, especially if they show allergic phenomena such as periorbital edema and eosinophilia. Patients should be thoroughly questioned regarding their consumption of pork and wild animal meat, and whether other individuals became ill after a common meal.

PROGNOSIS

Most lightly infected patients recover uneventfully with supportive care consisting of bed rest, analgesics, and antipyretics. In prospective studies of patients who had severe acute trichinosis 10 years earlier, 60 percent have shown lingering symptoms of muscle pain, burning eyes, and decreased tolerance for stress; 56 percent had impaired muscle strength; 55 percent had conjunctivitis; and 32 percent had impaired coordination. More than one-third of patients continued to have detectable immunoglobulin G antibodies to *T. spiralis* 10 years later. However, soft tissue radiographs, brain MRI, or muscle biopsy failed to show calcified residual larva. The cause of these persistent symptoms remains unknown but may suggest ''chronic trichinosis'' or persevering immune reaction.

TREATMENT

As soon as the disease is suspected, it is advisable to treat the patient with menzimidazole compounds such as thiabendazole (Mintezol) 25 mg/kg bid (maximum 3.0 g/day) for 5 to 7 days to remove intestinal larva and worms. The drug is ineffective against *Trichinella* in the muscle. However, mebendazole, a carbamate derivative of thiabendazole, has been shown to be active against both the invasive phase and the encystment of infection at a dose of 400 mg PO tid for 10 days. The drug is better tolerated than thiabendazole. (Another effective drug, albendazole, is not currently licensed by the Food and Drug Administration for use in the United States.) Because a Herxheimer-like reaction may result from the simultaneous disintegration of many larvae following antihelminthic therapy, corticosteroids (prednisone 40 to 60 mg PO for 5 to 10 days) are usually given. Severe trichinosis should be treated with antihelminthic drugs as well as high-dose corticosteroids orally or intravenously (methylprednisolone 250 to 500 mg/day).

PREVENTION

Prevention of trichinosis is possible by thorough cooking of infected meat; a temperature of 58.3°C throughout the meat is adequate. The pork should be cooked until it is no longer pink. Freezing at −15°C (home freezers) for 3 weeks or at −32°C for 24 hours is also effective in larval elimination. Smoking, salting, or drying of meat does not exclude *Trichinella* infection. *Trichinella* of arctic meat (walrus or bear) are most resistant and may remain viable despite freezing.

SUGGESTED READINGS

McAuley JB, Michelson MK, Hightower AW et al: A trichinosis outbreak among southeast Asian refugees. Am J Epidemiol 135:1404, 1992

McAuley JB, Michelson MK, Schantz PM: *Trichinella* infection in travelers. J Infect Dis 164:1013, 1991

Bailey TM, Schantz PM: Trends in the incidence and transmission patterns of human trichinellosis in the United States, 1982–1986. Rev Infect Dis 12: 5, 1990

Compton JS, Celum CL, Lee C et al: Trichinosis with ventilatory failure and persistent myocarditis. Clin Infect Dis 16:500, 1993

Fourstie V, Douceron H, Brugieres P et al: Neurotrichinosis. Brain 116:603, 1993

Harms G, Binz P, Feldmeier H et al: Trichinosis: a prospective controlled study of patients ten years after acute infection. Clin Infect Dis 17:637, 1993

Herrera R, Varela E, Morales G et al: Dermatomyositis-like syndrome caused by trichinosis: report of two cases. J Rheumatol 12:782, 1985

Landry SM et al: Trichinosis: common source outbreak related to commercial pork. South Med J 85:428, 1992

64. TOXOPLASMOSIS

BRADLEY K. EVANS

Toxoplasma gondii is an obligate intracellular parasite. Although cats are the definitive hosts for this organism, it can infect a wide variety of animals, with preferential invasion of intestinal, muscle, brain, and eye tissue. In humans, the central nervous system (CNS) is especially vulnerable, and infection with this organism can cause three neurologic syndromes: congenital toxoplasmosis, meningoencephalitis associated with a mononucleosislike syndrome, and CNS toxoplasmosis in patients with acquired immunodeficiency syndrome (AIDS).

EPIDEMIOLOGY

The *T. gondii* organism may pass through several forms and infect a variety of hosts in its complex life cycle. The primary source of transmission to humans is controversial, but probably comes from ingesting contaminated soil (such as by cat or other animal feces) or, more commonly, from eating undercooked meat (particularly pork or lamb). Digestion releases the cysts, which multiply in the gastrointestinal tract and become invasive. The parasite can penetrate any mammalian cell, divide, then rupture the cell as new organisms are released. The CNS is most frequently affected, and muscle is another preferential tissue.

Serologic surveys document from 25 to 75 percent of adult humans as having been exposed to toxoplasmosis; seropositivity is more common in people who eat undercooked meat and in those from poverty-stricken areas. This is true as well in HIV-infected patients, where Europeans and Haitians are the most commonly seropositive (50 to 75 percent) for toxoplasmosis.

CLINICAL FEATURES

Toxoplasmosis acquired after birth rarely produces symptoms in immunocompetent patients. In the unusual case where infection produces clinical illness, it generally takes the form of a picture resembling mononucleosis, with cervical lymphadenopathy, malaise, fatigue, fever, myalgia, pharyngitis, and, rarely, a maculopapular rash. Around 20 percent of such patients may have meningitis, with headache and abnormal cerebrospinal fluid (CSF) showing mild elevations in protein and white blood cell count (less than 50 WBC/mm^3).

The primary importance of *T. gondii* as a human pathogen arises from its prominence as a cause of disease, especially encephalitis, in immunosuppressed patients. It is the major opportunistic infection of the CNS. Although deficits may appear insidiously, over several weeks, AIDS patients with CNS toxoplasmosis usually have a rapid onset of neurologic symptoms and signs, evolving within a few days. Sometimes the onset is rapid enough to mimic a stroke. Common symptomatic findings are headache (70 percent), altered mental status (60 percent), fever (50 percent), seizures (33 percent), and focal neurologic deficits (60 percent). Although patients may present with diffuse symptoms, such as confusion or headache, focal signs and symptoms ultimately develop in most of them, including hemiparesis, visual field defects, and aphasia.

Nearly all patients with CNS toxoplasmosis have immunoglobulin G (IgG) antibodies to *T. gondii*, indicating previous exposure to the organism. This implies that CNS toxoplasmosis in AIDS patients almost always represents reactivation of a latent toxoplasmal infection, rather than a primary infection. Encephalitis can develop when CD4 counts fall below 200/mm^3.

In the patient with AIDS, CNS toxoplasmosis is the most common cause of a focal brain lesion. At least 10 percent of HIV-infected patients will have CNS toxoplasmosis during the course of their illness. This risk increases in patients known to be seropositive to *T. gondii*, of whom about one-third will later develop CNS toxoplasmosis. The risk for CNS toxoplasmosis is markedly reduced in patients who are known to be seronegative.

DIAGNOSIS

The diagnosis of CNS toxoplasmosis is usually made presumptively, without tissue confirmation. The diagnosis can be assumed in an AIDS patient known to have measurable antitoxoplasmal antibodies, with a typical clinical syndrome, and with typical findings on neuroimaging studies. In these patients, antitoxoplasmal therapy is begun (see below). Improvement—within 2 weeks clinically and within 4 weeks by neuroimaging studies—then confirms the diagnosis.

Blood tests are not of much help. If the CD4 count is known, it is almost always below 200/mm^3 (it is below 100/mm^3 in 80 percent of patients). Approximately 97 to 100 percent of patients have a measurable IgG antibody titer to *T. gondii*, but this only indicates past exposure. Current serologic tests to confirm an active infection (positive IgM titer, high IgG titer, or rising IgG titer) are of little practical diagnostic use in AIDS patients.

When the patient has a headache, altered mental status, seizures, or focal neurologic deficits, head computed tomography (CT) or head magnetic resonance imaging (MRI) is the key test leading to the diagnosis of CNS toxoplasmosis. Both neuroimaging tests are valuable, but MRI is more sensitive than CT in showing the lesions. Most clinicians first perform the head MRI, without and with contrast, reserving the CT for those patients who are too critically ill to have an MRI or who have another contraindication to MRI.

In CNS toxoplasmosis, there are four cardinal findings on neuroimaging studies. First, there are usually multiple lesions, particularly if an MRI is done. In fact, if the MRI shows only a single lesion, this should alert the clinician to consider alternative diagnoses. Second, the lesions are preferentially located in the basal ganglia and gray-white junction of the cerebrum. Third, the lesions have a mass effect, and fourth, they enhance (Fig. 64-1). These four findings are not diagnostic of CNS toxoplasmosis; similar findings can be seen in primary CNS lymphoma.

Patients who are known to be seronegative or who have atypical findings on neuroimaging studies should be considered for early brain biopsy for a definitive diagnosis. Other indications for brain biopsy include worsening after 1 week of antitoxoplasmal treatment, failure to improve 14 days after initiating treatment, and worsening of an individual lesion by neuroimaging studies.

Even a brain biopsy may not provide a definitive diagnosis, since the toxoplasmal cysts and individual organisms (tachyzoites) can be difficult to identify amid the intense inflammation. The highest yield is obtained with an open rather than a stereotactic biopsy, if immunostaining for tachyzoites is performed, and if mouse inoculation with brain tissue is done. Despite these precautions, it is still possible that the organisms will not be identified, and that the inflammation will be misidentified as CNS lymphoma or a viral encephalitis.

In considering the differential diagnosis, one should remember that a patient may have multiple concurrent intracranial disease processes. The following list gives the differential diagnosis of CNS toxoplasmosis in AIDS patients:

Primary CNS lymphoma
Progressive multifocal leukoencephalopathy
Multiple bacterial abscesses
Tuberculous abscesses
Fungal abscesses
Brain metastases
Herpes simplex encephalitis
HIV encephalitis

CNS lymphoma is the main alternative diagnosis, since it can present with a fairly rapid onset over 1 or 2 weeks, and can be associated with an identical clinical picture and identical neuroimaging findings, and is common in AIDS patients (about 2 percent of AIDS patients develop CNS lymphoma). The diagnosis of CNS lymphoma is usually made by stereotactic biopsy (since patients with this tumor do worse after open biopsy with resection). The diagnosis of CNS lymphoma can be rendered much more difficult if the patient has been treated with corticosteroids, which should therefore be avoided if possible in pa-

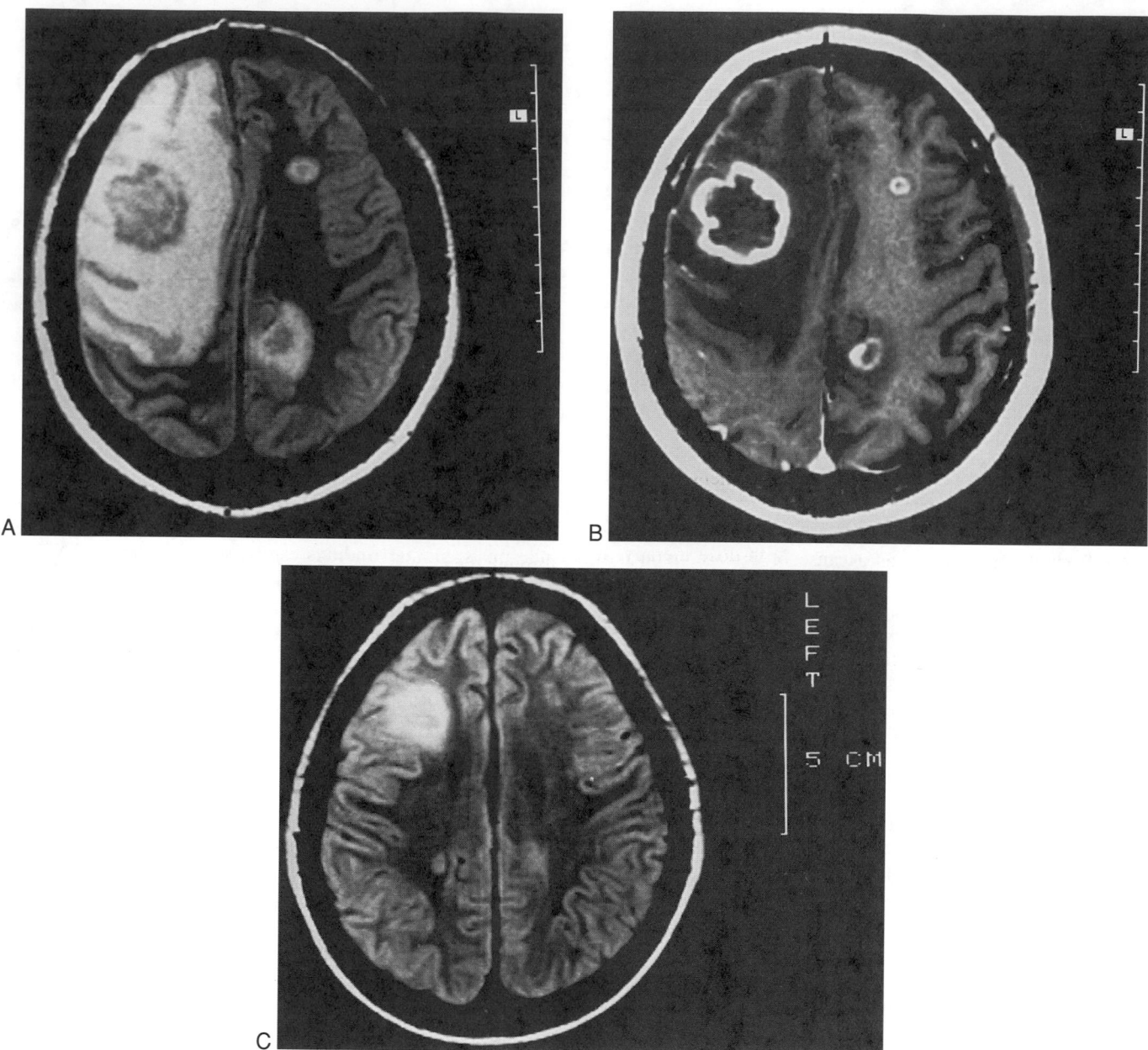

FIG. 64-1. An immunocompromised patient with toxoplasmosis. **(A)** T2-weighted MRI of the brain showing a large lesion at the gray-white junction of the cerebrum of the right frontal lobe, with a mass effect. Two smaller lesions are seen in the left hemisphere. **(B)** T1-weighted MRI of the same patient after infusion of gadolinium, showing the characteristic enhancement of toxoplasmosis. **(C)** T2-weighted MRI of the same patient 4 weeks after treatment with high-dose pyrimethamine, sulfadiazine, and leucovorin, showing substantial resolution of the lesions. (Courtesy of J. Douglas Lee, M.D. and Lawrence Hutchins, M.D., The Marshfield Clinic.)

tients thought to have CNS toxoplasmosis: CNS lymphoma may temporarily "melt away" after corticosteroid therapy, which leads to mistaken attribution of improvement to antitoxoplasmal therapy and to later difficulties in proper diagnosis. Brain metastases, fungal or tuberculous abscesses, and multiple bacterial abscesses associated with acute endocarditis can also mimic CNS toxoplasmosis. These diagnoses are often initially considered if the patient is not known to be HIV-infected. Viral encephalitis, HIV encephalitis, and progressive multifocal leukoencephalopathy can also produce abnormalities on neuroimaging studies in AIDS patients, but do not usually produce the combination of acute onset, focal neurologic findings, and multiple mass lesions on neuroimaging studies seen with CNS toxo-

plasmosis. Finally, in AIDS patients about 20 percent of brain biopsies performed to evaluate focal brain lesions are nondiagnostic.

PREVENTION AND TREATMENT

Although CNS toxoplasmosis represents reactivation of a latent infection, it is still important to advise HIV-infected patients to avoid primary infection by handling raw meat carefully, eating only well-cooked meat, and minimizing contact with cats.

To date, there is no proven prophylactic treatment for patients who have a positive toxoplasmal serology, although trimethoprim-sulfamethoxazole (often used to prevent *Pneumocystis* pneumonia) may have some effect in primary prevention of CNS toxoplasmosis.

After a presumptive diagnosis of CNS toxoplasmosis, primary treatment with high-dose pyrimethamine (200 mg initially, then 50 to 100 mg/day), sulfadiazine (4 to 6 g/day), and folinic acid (leucovorin, 10 to 50 mg/day) is begun. Pyrimethamine is associated with bone marrow toxicity and sulfadiazine with sensitivity reactions, and up to 40 percent of patients therefore will not tolerate the high-dose pyrimethamine-sulfadiazine combination. As an alternative to sulfadiazine, clindamycin can be used. Clinical improvement should occur within 10 to 14 days, and radiologic improvement should be seen within 2 to 4 weeks. Corticosteroids are best avoided if possible (see above).

After 4 to 6 weeks of primary treatment with high-dose pyrimethamine, sulfadiazine, and leucovorin, patients must be on lifelong daily maintenance therapy with the same drugs, but at about half the dose of primary treatment. Without maintenance therapy, nearly all patients will relapse. Even with maintenance therapy, perhaps as many as 25 percent of patients will relapse; of these, about 80 percent will respond to retreatment with high-dose therapy. Therefore, a patient with acute clinical deterioration and worsened abnormalities on neuroimaging is probably in relapse, and should be retreated with high-dose therapy. It is not clear whether patients with new seizures, or new headaches, but without worsening on neuroimaging studies, should be considered to be in relapse, but empirical retreatment is often advised.

SUGGESTED READINGS

Israelski DM, Remington JS: AIDS-associated toxoplasmosis. p. 319. In Sande MA, Volberding PA (eds): The Medical Management of AIDS. 3rd Ed. WB Saunders, Philadelphia, 1992

Navia BA, Petito CK, Gold JWM et al: Cerebral toxoplasmosis complicating the acquired immune deficiency syndrome: clinical and neuropathological findings in 27 patients. Ann Neurol 19:224, 1986

Wijdicks EFM, Borlefffs JCC, Hoepelman AIM, Jansen GH: Fatal disseminated hemorrhagic toxoplasmic encephalitis as the initial manifestation of AIDS. Ann Neurol 29:683, 1991

VIRAL INFECTIONS

65. VIRAL MENINGITIS AND ENCEPHALITIS

STEPHEN B. GREENBERG

Many viruses can invade the central nervous system (CNS). Viral CNS infections (often referred to as aseptic meningitis) may be asymptomatic or associated with only mild symptoms, but they can occasionally cause severe meningitis or encephalitis. The criteria for diagnosis of the acute aseptic meningitis syndrome are as follows:

1. Signs and symptoms of acute meningeal irritation
2. Mononuclear cell predominance in cerebrospinal fluid (CSF)
3. Absence of detectable bacteria in the CSF
4. Absence of parameningeal or systemic illness
5. Brief and benign illness

The criterion for diagnosis of encephalitis is alteration of consciousness or focal neurologic findings with evidence of meningeal inflammation. Thus, the term "meningoencephalitis" may be appropriate in many cases.

An estimated 8,000 to 20,000 cases of acute aseptic meningitis occur annually in the United States. Approximately 1,000 to 2,000 cases of encephalitis are reported annually to the Centers for Disease Control. Viral causes of meningoencephalitis are numerous, but clinical signs and symptoms alone usually cannot establish a specific diagnosis. However, new laboratory methods are becoming available that will aid in rapid and specific identification of viral agents and will lead to new knowledge of the epidemiology of these viral infections.

PATHOGENESIS

Entry and replication of the viruses that cause meningitis and encephalitis occur extraneurally. Most viruses reach the CNS by the hematogenous route. Viruses may invade the CNS through the choroid plexus or by direct penetration of the endothelium of cerebral blood vessels. Nonhematogenous routes of transmission also exist; these routes may be important in the pathogenesis of rabies or adult-onset herpes simplex encephalitis (HSE). In these cases, the virus may infect the brain by retrograde travel along axons in the spinal cord and/or the brain. With viral replication in neural cells, cell death or dysfunction results. The extent of neuronal damage may contribute to the clinical severity of viral meningoencephalitis.

EPIDEMIOLOGY

When the viral etiologies of acute aseptic meningitis syndrome were first reported in the 1960s, most infections were caused by enteroviruses or mumps, with a few cases secondary to lymphocytic choriomeningitis (LCM), herpes simplex virus (HSV), or arboviruses. Although the spread of human immuno-

TABLE 65-1. Viruses Causing Aseptic Meningitis Syndrome and/or Encephalitis

Virus	Meningitis	Encephalitis
Adenoviruses	—	—
Arboviruses	+ + +	+ + +
Coronaviruses	—	—
Cytomegalovirus (CMV)	—	+
Enteroviruses	+ + +	+ + +
Epstein-Barr virus (EBV)	—	+
Herpes simplex type 1 (HSV type 1)	+	+ +
Human immunodeficiency virus (HIV)	+	—
Influenza	—	—
Lymphocytic choriomeningitis (LCM)	+	—
Measles	—	+
Mumps	+	+
Parainfluenza	+	—
Rabies	—	+
Rotavirus	—	—
Rubella	—	—
Varicella zoster virus (VZV)	—	+

Symbols: + + +, common/sporadic or epidemic; + +, common/sporadic; +, uncommon; —, rarely reported cases.

TABLE 65-2. Classification of the Most Common Viruses Causing Epidemic Aseptic Meningitis or Encephalitis

Enterovirus (gastrointestinal spread)
  Poliovirus
  Coxsackievirus
  Echovirus

Arbovirus (arthropodborne [insect] spread)
  Eastern equine encephalitis
  Western equine encephalitis
  Venezuelan equine encephalitis
  St. Louis encephalitis
  California encephalitis

deficiency virus (HIV) and increased vaccine usage has led to a change in common etiologies, enteroviruses and arboviruses still account for the majority of viral aseptic meningitis and encephalitis (Tables 65-1 and 65-2).

Viral meningitis or encephalitis can occur either sporadically or epidemically. Enteroviruses and arboviruses are most often the agents in epidemics, while HSV type 1 is the most common cause of sporadic cases of encephalitis in the United States. Less common causes of encephalitis are the herpes viruses (Epstein-Barr virus [EBV], cytomegalovirus [CMV], varicella-zoster virus [VZV]), measles, and rabies (Table 65-1).

Of the many factors influencing the epidemiology of acute aseptic meningitis syndrome or viral encephalitis, the most important for determining etiology are the patient's age, status of immunocompetence, and geographic location, and the season. Certain viral infections occur worldwide, infect humans of all ages, and display little or no seasonal variation; others are specific to season and geographic area, especially those caused by insectborne viruses (Table 65-3). Typical clinical findings with enteroviral infections are myocarditis and pleurodynia, which can cause epidemics, especially in the summer and fall. HIV should be considered in high-risk populations and will often present with a mononucleosis syndrome. Contact with rodents is often an indication of possible infection with LCM, and patients with HSV type 2 will often have primary genital lesions. Mumps, although less frequently seen since the widespread use of vaccines, can have associated parotitis. Focal neurologic deficits are seen with HSE, although there is no seasonality. The characteristic rash of VZV is seen with this infection, and encephalitis in children is often manifested by cerebellar ataxia. The mononucleosis syndrome will be seen in patients with EBV- or CMV-associated encephalitis. A history of mosquito bite may be helpful for detecting the common arbovirus-associated encephalitides. Adenovirus may have preceding respiratory symptoms. Rabies, characteristically, will be associated with an animal bite, although cases have occurred where this history is lacking.

CLINICAL FEATURES AND DIAGNOSIS

The clinical features of meningitis or encephalitis range from mild febrile illnesses associated with headache to severe illnesses associated with convulsions, coma, and death. Usual signs and symptoms of aseptic meningitis are fever, headache, vomiting, photophobia, and stiff neck. Usual signs and symptoms of encephalitis include altered consciousness, seizures, and focal deficits. These clinical features are so universal, and so nonspecific, that diagnosis of the precise virus causing the infection is seldom possible.

There are also few diagnostically specific laboratory tests. In most cases, a complete blood count is normal. Opening pressure of the CSF is usually elevated. The CSF white blood cell counts range from a few cells to more than 1,000 cells/ml. Early on, neutrophils may be present, but after 48 hours, lymphocytes predominate. A moderately elevated protein level is often found. Glucose concentration is usually normal, but cases of mumps or HSV have been associated with hypoglycorrhachia. Gram stain is negative.

All patients with presumed viral meningitis or encephalitis should have an acute serum obtained for serologic studies, as well as CSF sent for virus culture. Isolation of virus from the CSF may be possible in many viral infections (Table 65-4), especially the enteroviruses. Throat washings and stool specimens may be positive in some viral infections, but one should be cautious in interpreting positive cultures outside of the CNS, since these may reflect chronic or previous infection rather than relate to the acute episode. In the case of serum, whether the patient recovers or continues to be ill over several weeks, if virus cultures are negative, a convalescent serum should be obtained and both the acute and convalescent sample tested for antibody titers. An exception is arbovirus encephalitis, where a single high titer in an acute phase serum may be diagnostic. Newer techniques are available for the detection of many viruses using immunofluorescence, polymerase chain reaction (PCR), and EIA. These newer techniques, although not readily available, will soon provide the clinician with more rapid and specific diagnosis of viral meningitis and encephalitis.

TABLE 65-3. Epidemiology of Viral Meningoencephalitis

Agent	Typical Clinical Findings or History	Season/Epidemiology
Enteroviruses	Myocarditis/pleurodynia	Summer/fall; epidemic and sporadic
Human immunodeficiency virus	High-risk populations, mononucleosis symptoms	No seasonality; sporadic
Lymphocytic choriomeningitis	Contact with rodents	Winter; sporadic
Herpes simplex type 2	Primary genital lesions	No seasonality; sporadic
Mumps	Parotitis	Spring/summer; sporadic
Herpes simplex type 1	Focal neurologic deficits	No seasonality; sporadic
Varicella-zoster	Characteristic rash, cerebellar ataxia	No seasonality; sporadic
Epstein-Barr virus/cytomegalovirus	Mononucleosis syndrome, immunosuppressed	No seasonality; sporadic
Togaviridae (eastern/western equine)	Mosquitoborne	Summer; epidemic
Flaviviridae (St. Louis)	Mosquitoborne	Summer; epidemic
Bunyaviridae (California)	North Central states	Summer; epidemic
Adenovirus	Prior respiratory symptoms	No seasonality; sporadic
Rabies	History of animal bite, hydrophobia	No seasonality; sporadic

(From Greenberg S: Viral infections. In Kelley WN (ed): Textbook of Internal Medicine. 2nd JB Lippincott, Philadelphia, 1992, with permission.)

TABLE 65-4. Viral Diagnosis of Aseptic Meningitis Syndrome and Encephalitis

Virus	Tissue Culture	Antigen Detection	Serology
Adenovirus	+ + +	+	+ + +
Arboviruses	+ +	+	+ + +
Coronaviruses	+	+	+
Cytomegalovirus (CMV)	+ + +	+ + +	+ + +
Enteroviruses	+ + +	+	+ +
Epstein-Barr virus (EBV)	+	+	+ + +
Herpes simplex type 1 (HSV type 1)	+ + +	+ +	+ + +
Herpes simplex type 2 (HSV type 2)	+ + +	+ +	+ + +
Human immunodeficiency virus	+ +	+ + +	+ + +
Influenza	+ +	+ +	+ + +
Lymphocytic choriomeningitis (LCM)	+	+	+ +
Measles	+ +	+	+ + +
Mumps	+	+	+ +
Parainfluenza	+ + +	+ +	+
Rabies	+	+ +	+ +
Rotavirus	+	+ + +	+ + +
Rubella	+ +	+	+ + +
Varicella zoster virus (VZV)	+ + +	+ +	+ + +

Symbols: +, method not available or research laboratory only; + +, method available in specialized references laboratories; + + +, method used in most virology laboratories.

SPECIFIC VIRUSES THAT CAUSE MENINGITIS OR ENCEPHALITIS

Enteroviruses

Enteroviruses cause more than 80 percent of identified cases of the aseptic meningitis syndrome. These viruses appear to be transmitted by the fecal-oral route. Infections occur worldwide and year-round, but peak during the summer, are more common in young infants and children than in adults, and may occur sporadically or epidemically. Only a few types are common, although many serotypes may cause aseptic meningitis or encephalitis. The clinical presentation of the infections includes fever, malaise, nausea, vomiting, pharyngitis, signs of meningeal irritation, and occasionally a maculopapular rash. Infants may not present with these typical signs and symptoms, often showing only irritability or a change in behavior.

Clues to identifying an enterovirus meningitis or encephalitis are time of year (summer), presence of other cases in the community, presence of exanthems, mild pericarditis or conjunctivitis, or pleurodynia. Most laboratory tests are not helpful. Initially, the CSF may show a polymorphonuclear predominance, but in approximately 66 percent of cases there is a shift to lymphocytes in the CSF during the first 6 to 48 hours. In approximately 15 percent of cases the CSF shows low glucose levels. Diagnosis can be most readily made by culturing the CSF for virus. In initial studies, newer tests of the CSF for PCR detection of viral RNA appear to be exquisitely sensitive and specific. Treatment is supportive and, although late sequelae have been reported, most patients recover uneventfully. However, significant sequelae have been reported in agammaglobulinemic patients with enteroviruses. In a few of these cases, treatment by intravenous and intrathecal immunoglobulin has been beneficial.

Arboviruses

The arboviruses that infect humans in the United States include western equine encephalomyelitis (WEE), eastern equine en-cephalomyelitis (EEE), Venezuelan equine encephalomyelitis (VEE), St. Louis encephalitis (SLE), and California encephalitis (CE). There are marked geographic differences among each of these agents: WEE extends from the west coast to the midwestern and southern United States; EEE extends from the Atlantic coast to the gulf coast; VEE is found in the southern states; SLE is widely distributed among many states; and CE is found in the eastern and north central United States. Deaths have been reported for all the arboviruses, especially in very young and elderly patients. Mosquitos and birds serve as the animal hosts for WEE, EEE, and SLE.

Clinically, there are few clues to identifying an arbovirus encephalitis. Diagnosis of these infections requires serologic tests, since these viruses are not easily cultured. A presumptive diagnosis may be made with a high titer in an acute-phase serum sample. Treatment is supportive, since no specific antiviral agent is effective. Severe neurologic sequelae have been reported in many patients with SLE and EEE, but are rare in patients with VEE and CE.

Herpes Simplex Type 1 and Type 2

Herpes simplex encephalitis (HSE) presents with altered levels of consciousness and either focal or diffuse neurologic signs and symptoms, especially hallucinations, personality change, and headache. Focal or generalized seizures occur in approximately 50 percent of all cases. Electroencephalography (EEG) may show a periodic spike/slow wave activity in the temporal lobe, and computed tomography (CT) scans or magnetic resonance imaging (MRI) may show contrast enhancement and mass effect, especially in the frontotemporal areas of the brain. In many patients, CSF shows a lymphocytic pleocytosis and red blood cells. Rarely is HSV-1 cultured from CSF in patients with HSE, and diagnosis requires detection of the virus by brain biopsy or, more recently, by amplification of HSV-DNA is the CSF of patients by PCR. Acyclovir, when added to basic supportive management and treatment of increased intracranial pressure, has been shown to be of benefit in reducing the morbidity and mortality of severe cases of HSE. Acyclovir 10 mg/kg should be given every 8 hours for a 2-week course. It is most effective in patients begun on therapy before coma.

Herpes simplex type 2 (HSV-2) can cause aseptic meningitis. Evidence of acute genital tract infection with HSV-2 is frequently found at the time of the neurologic infection. Although the genital disease tends to recur, the meningitis seldom relapses.

Other Viruses

Acute HIV infection has been associated with the aseptic meningitis syndrome. Often, the diagnosis can only be made by detection of p24 antigen in the CSF, since late conversion of ELISA and Western blot serologic tests only occurs several weeks later. Patients with high-risk behavior should be suspected of having acute HIV meningitis.

Less common causes of meningoencephalitis include LCM, and the group of other herpesviruses such as CMV, EBV, and VZV. Each of these viruses can be diagnosed using a combination of serologies and/or virus cultures. No specific epidemiology is associated with these viruses, except for the exposure to animals in LCM, and the appearance of the typical chicken pox or shingles lesions in patients with VZV meningoencephalitis.

DIFFERENTIAL DIAGNOSIS

There are many nonviral causes of meningitis and encephalitis, which can be confused clinically with viral infections. Such nonviral causes include the following:

Leptospirosis (Weil's disease)
Tuberculosis
Toxoplasmosis
Rocky Mountain spotted fever
Mycoplasma infection
Lyme disease
Syphilis
Cryptococcosis
Histoplasmosis
Cysticercosis
Systemic lupus erythematosus
Granulomatous angiitis
Uveomeningoencephalitis (Vogt-Koyanagi-Harada syndrome)
Behçet's disease
Whipple's disease
Sarcoidosis
Mollaret's disease

The differentiation of viral from nonviral causes of meningitis and encephalitis is important, because there is effective treatment for bacteria, spirochetes, *Rickettsia, Mycoplasma,* fungi, and protozoa. In addition, noninfectious causes, such as collagen vascular disease, sarcoidosis, and tumor have also been reported to give a similar picture.

Tuberculous meningitis is one of the most serious mimics of viral meningitis or encephalitis. The incidence of tuberculous meningitis has increased in adults in recent years, and it may occur as an isolated finding separate from pulmonary or disseminated infection. A lymphocyte predominance appears in the spinal fluid, and the protein levels will range from 100 to 500 mg/dl. The CSF glucose level is often below mg/dl in half the patients, and only in 10 to 40 percent of patients will there be acid-fast bacilli on microscopic examination of the CSF. Although ring-enhancing or other inflammatory lesions may be demonstrated on CT or MRI scans, these are not always present and not specific to tuberculosis. Thus, in some cases it may be necessary to initiate empirical therapy when clinical suspicion and laboratory data suggest possible tuberculous meningitis.

TREATMENT

If the initial CSF findings are compatible with viral meningitis or encephalitis, treatment consists of close observation and supportive therapy. There is no specific antiviral therapy for the patient with aseptic meningitis.

SUGGESTED READINGS

Bale JF: Viral encephalitis. Med Clin North Am 77:25, 1993

Connolly KJ, Hammer SM: The acute septic meningitis syndrome. Infect Dis Clin North Am 4:599, 1990

Feigin RD, Shackelford PG: Value of repeat lumbar puncture in the differential diagnosis of meningitis. N Engl J Med 1973, 289:571

Johnson RT: Viral Infections of the Nervous System. Rowan, New York, 1982

McKinney WP, Hendebert GR, Harper SA et al: Validation of a clinical prediction rule for the differential diagnosis of acute meningitis. J Gen Intern Med 9:8, 1994

Rotbart HA: Viral meningitis and the aseptic meningitis syndrome. In Scheld WM, Whitley RJ, Durack DT (eds): Infections of the Central Nervous System. Raven Press, New York, 1991

Rotbart HA: Diagnosis of enteroviral meningitis with the polymerase chain reaction. J Pediatr 117:85, 1990

Spanos A, Harrell FE Jr, Durack DT: Differential diagnosis of acute meningitis: an analysis of the predictive value of initial observations. JAMA 262: 2700, 1989

Tsai TF: Arboviral infections in the United States. Infect Dis Clin North Am 5:73, 1991

66. HERPES SIMPLEX ENCEPHALITIS

PERCY N. KARANJIA

The herpes simplex family of viruses is a group of ubiquitous, complex, double-stranded DNA viruses that are responsible for a variety of acute infections of the central nervous system (CNS). These include herpes simplex encephalitis (HSE), meningitis, myelitis, and radiculitis. Herpes simplex type I (HSV-1) is responsible for most cases of HSE, and herpes simplex type II (HSV-2) is the usual agent for herpetic myelitis and radiculitis in adults and for neonatal HSE. Both agents have been implicated in aseptic meningitis.

Primary infection with HSV-1 is presumed to occur in childhood or early adulthood, resulting in gingivostomatitis and, uncommonly, keratitis or skin lesions. Antibodies to HSV-1 are detectable in at least 75 percent of the world's population by adolescence. HSV-1 is transmitted most commonly in saliva, and HSV-2 is transmitted by genital contact. Primary involvement of the CNS is uncommon.

After replication in epithelial tissue, HSV is believed to be transported to neurons by retrograde axoplasmic transport, where it remains latent. At autopsy, HSV has been detected in trigeminal, dorsal root, and autonomic ganglia. Host factors for reactivation of the virus have not been identified—the disease has been described in those with AIDS, but it is not common in this population. On reactivation, the virus may be transmitted to the periphery by orthograde axoplasmic transport, resulting in common herpes labialis. In rare instances, HSV may be transported to the orbitofrontal and temporal lobes of the brain by the olfactory nerves or dural branches of the trigeminal nerves; the result is a severe, necrotizing, hemorrhagic encephalitis, which is often fatal.

EPIDEMIOLOGY

Herpes simplex encephalitis constitutes approximately 10 to 20 percent of all cases of acute encephalitis. It shows no seasonal or geographical preference and is equally prevalent in both men and women. The disease occurs at all ages, although most adult cases are seen in patients who are over 50.

CLINICAL FEATURES

There are no clinical features that are pathognomonic for HSE (Table 66-1). However, the virus shows a predilection for the temporal and orbitofrontal lobes, resulting in a characteristic clinical picture that should alert the clinician to the diagnosis. Headaches and fever (101° to 104°F), evolving over a few days,

TABLE 66-1. Clinical Features of HSE

Symptoms	Percent of Patients
Change in consciousness	95
Fever	90
Change in personality	85
Headache	80
Seizures	65
Autonomic changes	60
Aphasia	50
Amnesia	25
Hallucinations	20

TABLE 66-2. Initial CSF Findings in HSE

	Typical	Atypical
Opening pressure	Elevated	Normal
White blood cells	Lymphocytes 50–100 WBC/mm³	Neutrophils Acellular
Red blood cells	Present	Absent
Protein	50–100 mg%	>100 mg%
Glucose	Normal	Low

are the usual initial symptoms, sometimes preceded by a mild flulike illness. Occasionally, the onset of the disease may be subacute or even chronic. There is nothing about the headache that differentiates it from other less severe illnesses. Alteration of consciousness occurs invariably, ranging from a minor clouding of consciousness to coma. Subtle changes in personality, agitation, or frank psychosis are common. Partial or generalized seizures are frequent and may be difficult to control; status epilepticus may occur. Focal neurologic signs evolve over the next few days in approximately 50 percent of patients, of which language disorders and hemiparesis are the most common. Hallucinations of an olfactory and gustatory type or autonomic dysfunction due to orbitofrontal involvement, and memory loss due to temporal lobe involvement are characteristic, the latter usually being a striking late feature. On rare occasions a brainstem encephalitis occurs. The course of the untreated illness is progressive over several days or weeks in the majority of patients, with severe cerebral edema leading to brain herniation and death.

DIAGNOSIS

The diagnosis of HSE is urgent because the virus multiplies rapidly, and the prognosis is dependent on the stage of the patient when a treatment is begun. Although focal findings re-

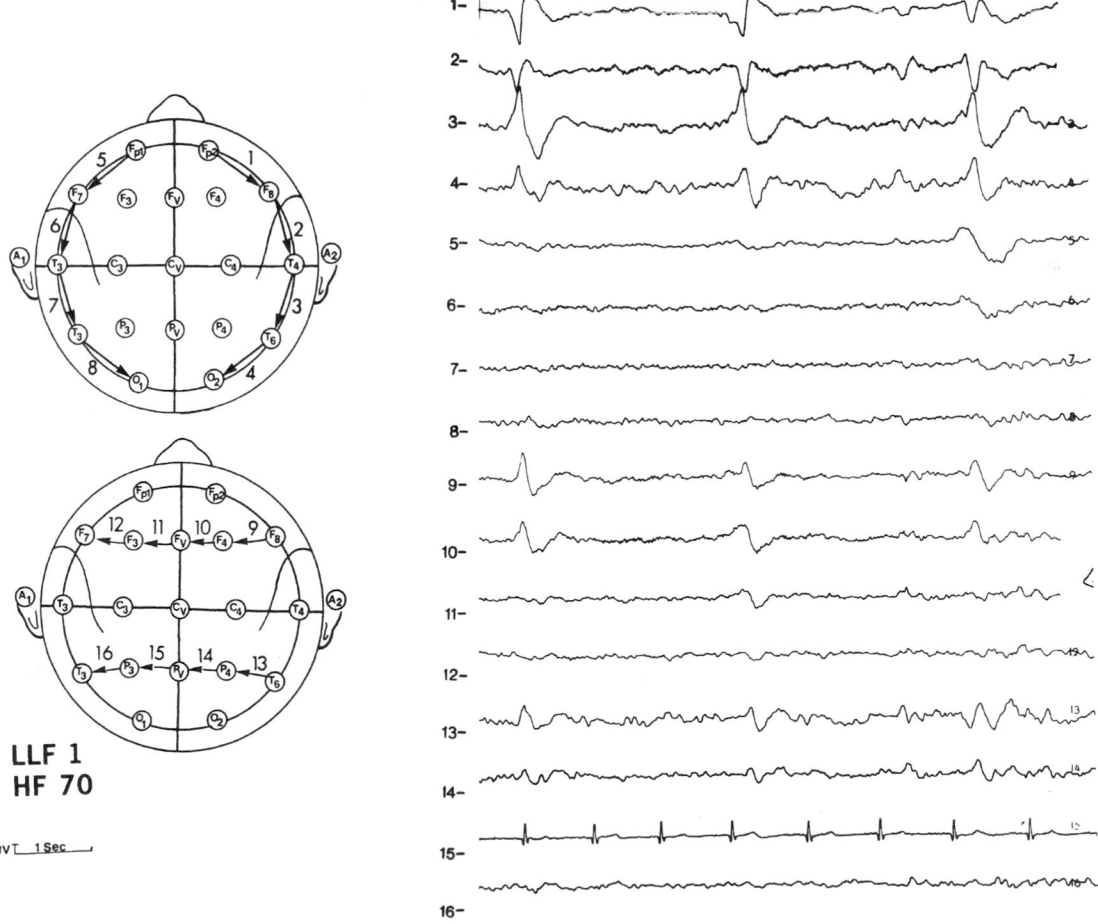

FIG. 66-1. EEG showing PLEDs over the right temporal area (especially in leads 1–4, and 9 + 10) in a 26-year-old woman with HSE, seizures, and confusion. The background is slow and disorganized.

flecting frontal and temporal lobe damage are characteristic, there are no clinical features that reliably differentiate HSE from other forms of encephalitis. Laboratory tests that are useful in the diagnosis include examination of the CSF, electroencephalography (EEG), computed tomography (CT) scanning, and magnetic resonance imaging (MRI). These tests are not specific for HSE but can be obtained readily in most community settings and, when taken in the context of an appropriate clinical picture, are highly suggestive of the diagnosis. Firm confirmation of the diagnosis requires brain biopsy or serologic evidence in the cerebrospinal fluid (CSF).

In most cases the CSF is abnormal (Table 66-2). The opening pressure is often raised. The leukocyte count is 50 to 100 cells/mm^3 with lymphocytes generally predominant, although neutrophils may sometimes dominate early in the illness. Red blood cells are frequently present (40 percent or more), and some xanthochromia may be seen, which substantiates the necrotic nature of the virus and helps distinguish HSE from most other viral encephalitides. The protein level is moderately elevated—50 to 100 mg/dl early in the illness—but may be very high as the disease progresses and may remain elevated for several months. The glucose level is usually normal but is moderately depressed in 25 percent of cases. Mumps and varicella are other encephalitides that may show a low CSF glucose.

Immunodiagnostic techniques using the polymerase chain reaction (PCR) to amplify viral DNA are highly sensitive and specific for HSV and should be obtained whenever possible, although presently the test is only available in selected centers. About 95 percent of spinal taps performed within 1 to 2 days of onset of symptoms will demonstrate a positive PCR. Serial examinations are therefore only suggested if the diagnosis is strongly suspected and the initial PCR is negative. Preliminary results are available in about 8 hours, but confirmation takes longer. The PCR may remain positive in the CSF for up to 5 days after acyclovir treatment is instituted. Tests for the detection of viral antigen in the CSF and the detection of intrathecal synthesis of HSV immunoglobulin G are also used in the diagnosis.

Serum antibody analysis is of little use in the diagnosis since the general population has a very high prevalence of HSV antibodies and a rise in titer may occur with a variety of non-HSV illnesses.

If the patient fails to improve clinically, or if the initial CSF shows a predominance of neutrophils with a low glucose level, a repeat lumbar puncture must be performed to exclude bacterial infection. If there are no atypical features, the lumbar puncture should not be repeated, since the CSF takes several weeks to normalize and a worsening CSF profile with a rise in white blood cell (WBC) count, and protein may be seen despite clinical improvement, which may be misleading.

The EEG is abnormal in about 85 percent of patients, with periodic, predominantly lateralized sharp or spike activity known as periodic lateralized epileptiform discharges (PLEDs) superimposed on a disorganized slow background localized over one or both temporal or frontal areas (Fig. 66-1). This EEG picture in a patient with encephalitis is very suggestive of the diagnosis.

The CT scan may be normal early in the illness, but 5 or 6 days later shows low attenuation lesions in one or both anterior and mesial temporal lobes or orbitofrontal lobes in 60 percent of patients. Areas of patchy hemorrhage are frequently seen; mass effect is common. The lesions show contrast enhance-

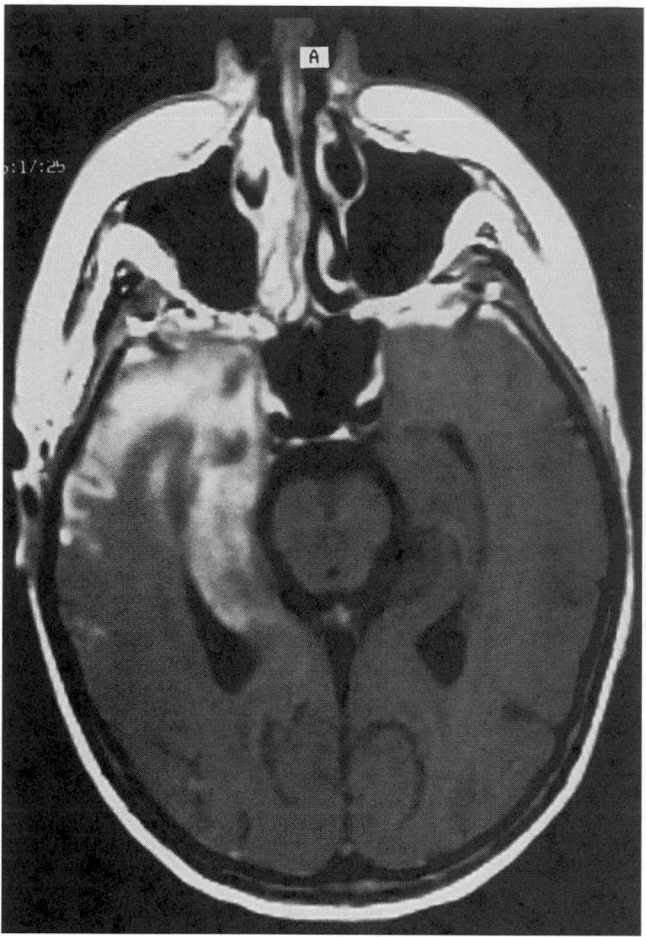

FIG. 66-2. Postcontrast T1-weighted MRI scan showing typical enhancement of the parenchyma and cortical ribbon in the right temporal lobe in a 70-year-old woman with HSE.

ment due to disruption of the blood-brain barrier after the first week.

MRI is the imaging procedure of choice in HSE. It is more sensitive than CT in the early detection of HSE because it is more sensitive to small quantities of edema, shows axial and coronal views, and is less susceptible to artifacts. MRI may show unilateral or bilateral abnormalities of the mesial temporal and orbitofrontal cortices even when the CT scan is normal. The T2-weighted images show signal hyperintensity in the temporal or orbitofrontal lobes (Fig. 66-2). Contrast enhancement of the parenchyma and cortical ribbon are frequently seen. Methemoglobin, as evidence of hemorrhage, is also common.

Radionuclide scans show increased uptake of the tracer over the temporal and frontal lobes, but are rarely performed today, since they give no useful additional information. The value of single-photon-emission tomography (SPECT) in HSE is unclear.

Brain biopsy provides a definitive diagnosis in most cases, provided it is taken from an affected area. Since the disease is often asymmetric, stereotactic biopsy under radiologic control is desirable. The material should be sent for histopathology, electron microscopy, immunologic studies, and cultures for viruses, bacteria, and fungi. Microscopically, areas of necrosis, hemorrhage, and polymorphonuclear infiltrates are seen in the more severely affected areas. Eosinophilic intranuclear inclusions (Cowdry A bodies) are seen in neurons and glial cells and are characteristic, but are also seen with varicella-zoster, cytomegalovirus, and measles.

Unfortunately, there is considerable controversy regarding who should have a brain biopsy. The fear is that other treatable diseases masquerading as HSE may be missed, since only 40 percent of patients undergoing a biopsy for HSE in early studies actually had the disease. However, with the availability of MRI, and the polymerase chain reaction in CSF, the likelihood of diagnostic errors has greatly diminished. Brain biopsy is not a benign procedure, despite the reported low complication rates (0 to 3 percent). Serious complications include hemorrhage and increased brain swelling leading to herniation. Valuable time may also be lost before treatment is begun if one awaits a biopsy. Therefore, a biopsy should be reserved for the patient who has an atypical clinical, radiologic, or laboratory picture, who cannot undergo further testing, or who has not shown the anticipated clinical response to treatment. Immunosuppressed

patients pose a different problem, as they are known to harbor unusual illnesses; in this group, early biopsy is generally favored.

The differential diagnosis of HSE includes other viral encephalitides, bacterial infections including tuberculosis, fungal infections, and brain abscess. Cerebral infarction, tumors, and acute disseminated encephalomyelitis (ADEM) are other conditions that need to be considered.

Diagnostically, once HSE is clinically suspected, the following things need to be done (Fig. 66-3):

1. Obtain an imaging procedure of the head emergently, preferably MRI. If this shows the typical temporofrontal lesion and no mass effect, proceed with lumbar puncture and send CSF for cell count, protein, glucose, cultures for bacteria, mycobacteria, cryptococcal antigen, and fungi. If mass effect is demonstrated on brain imaging, do not perform a lumbar puncture. Instead, reduce intracranial pressure with a 20-mg bolus of dexamethasone administered intravenously, fol-

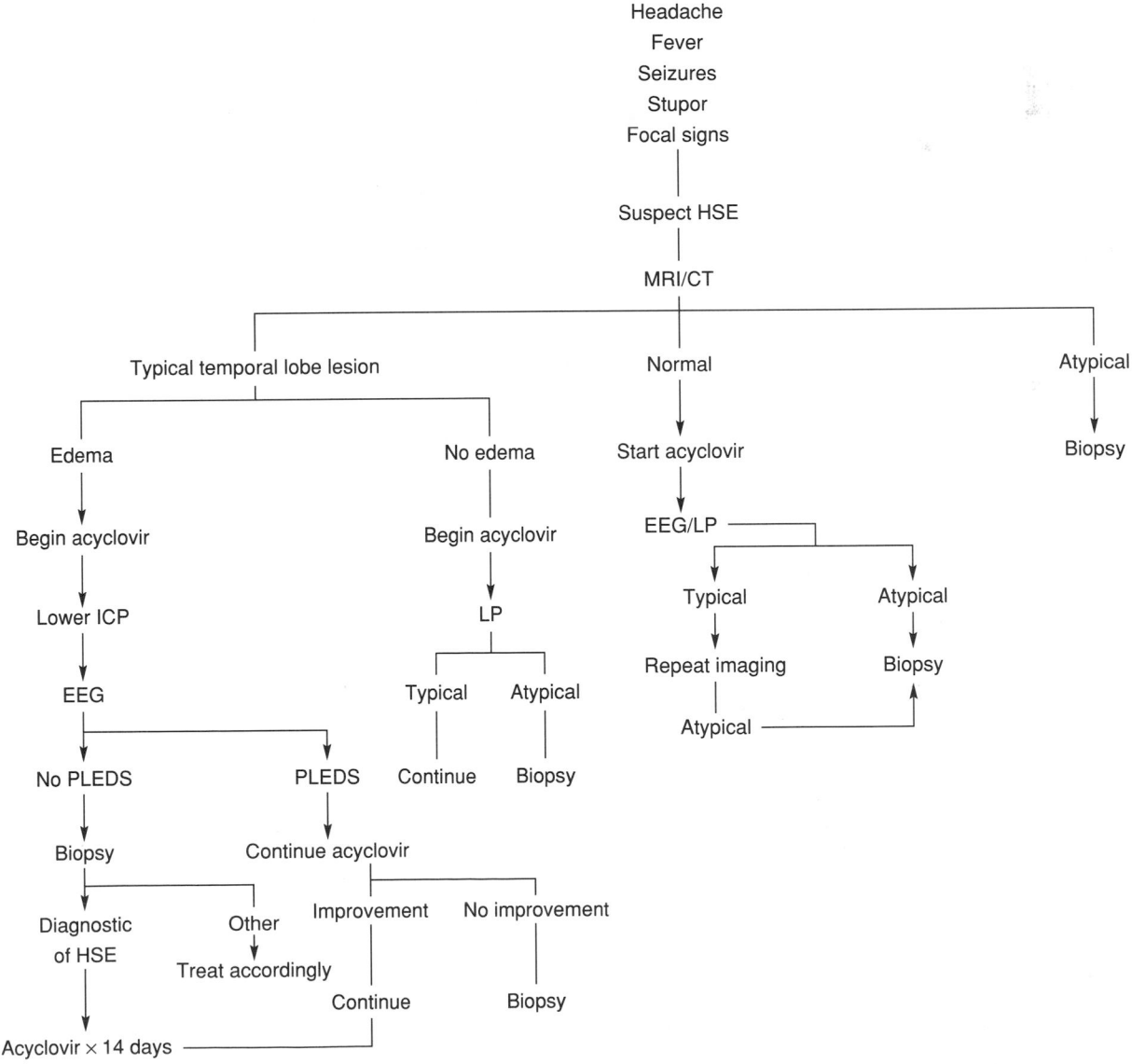

FIG. 66-3. Algorithm for management of suspected HSE.

lowed by 4 mg every 4 hours. If the mass effect produces a midline shift of greater than 3 mm, or if the patient continues to deteriorate or is comatose, admit the patient to the intensive care unit, intubate, and hyperventilate (to a P_{CO_2} of 28 to 30 mmHg). Use a bolus of intravenous mannitol (50 to 100 g) if the imaging suggests incipient herniation, and alert the neurosurgeon. Obtain an open biopsy with brain decompression at the earliest possibility.
2. If the CSF results are atypical, repeat the lumbar puncture and proceed with a brain biopsy.
3. Obtain an EEG. If the EEG is characteristic, proceed with acyclovir therapy and wait to see if a clinical response occurs within the next 72 to 96 hours.

TREATMENT

As soon as the diagnosis is suspected, even while definitive test results are pending, start acyclovir, 10 mg/kg IV q8h. After confirmation of HSE, acyclovir therapy should be continued for 2 weeks. Use vidarabine (encephalomyelitis/kg/day) intravenously if acyclovir cannot be used for any reason. Unfortunately, it is neither as effective an agent as acyclovir nor as safe because it is insoluble and requires large volumes of fluid to be administered.

Start anticonvulsants if seizures occur. Because seizures are frequently multiple, intravenous loading with phenytoin, 18 mg/kg given slowly over 30 minutes, followed the next day by 5 mg/kg/day, is the fastest way of attaining adequate anticonvulsant coverage. Status epilepticus, when it occurs, needs to be aggressively treated.

General management includes close attention to details of fluid and electrolyte balance, as well as renal function. Frequent checks of neurologic function looking for signs of raised intracranial pressure, such as yawning, progressive drowsiness, pupillary asymmetry, and rise in blood pressure while pulse rate decreases, must be obtained. A neurologist or neurosurgeon must be informed immediately if there is any clinical deterioration.

PROGNOSIS

HSE carries a mortality rate of 70 percent if untreated. Therapy with acyclovir decreases the mortality rate to 15 to 20 percent, but with vidarabine the mortality rate is 50 percent. Memory disturbance, altered personality, hemiparesis, and seizures are frequent sequelae, occurring in as many as 50 percent of acyclovir-treated survivors. Despite the disability, many are able to return to ''near-normal'' lives. The prognosis is worse in the elderly, in the immunocompromised, and in the patient who is comatose upon presentation.

Relapse rarely occurs in the adequately treated patient. Should this happen, restart acyclovir in a higher dose (15 mg/kg q8h) for a longer duration of time (3 weeks).

SUGGESTED READINGS

Aurelius E: Herpes simplex encephalitis: early diagnosis and immune activation in the acute stage and during long-term follow-up. Scand J Infect Dis [Suppl] 89:3, 1993
Demaerel P, Wilms G, Robberecht W et al: MRI of herpes simplex encephalitis. Neuroradiology 34:490, 1992
Skoldenberg B: Herpes simplex encephalitis. Scand J Infect Dis [Suppl] 80: 40, 1991
Whitley RJ: Herpes simplex virus infections of the central nervous system. Drugs 42:406, 1991
Whitley RJ, Cobbs CJ, Alford CA Jr et al: Diseases that mimic herpes simplex encephalitis: diagnosis, presentation and outcome. NIAID Collaborative Antiviral Study Group. JAMA 262:234, 1989

67. VARICELLA-ZOSTER VIRUS INFECTION

Y. HARATI

Primary infection by the highly contagious varicella-zoster virus (VZV), a DNA virus, produces chicken pox (varicella) described first in the ninth century a.d. by the Persian physician, Rhazes. Following the initial infection, the virus, in keeping with its nature as a herpes virus, becomes latent in multiple sensory ganglia for decades. (It appears that VZV ascends to sensory ganglia from the skin lesions of varicella.) The subsequent and delayed reactivation of VZV may cause many neurologic manifestations, for example:

Herpes zoster (shingles)
Postherpetic neuralgia
Postherpetic dermatomal anesthesia
Cranial neuropathies: cranial nerves VII, VIII (Ramsay-Hunt syndrome); III, IX, VI (ophthalmoplegia); II, V, IX, X
Motor neuropathies
Radiculopathies
Diaphragmatic paralysis
Myelitis
Meningoencephalitis
Cerebral vasculopathy
Myositis
Cystitis and urinary retention
Colonic pseudo-obstruction (Ogilvie syndrome)

Herpes zoster (shingles), the most common neurologic complication, has been recognized from antiquity as a creeping eruption (*herpes,* Greek: to creep) that girdles the body (*zoster,* Greek: girdle, belt); from this characteristic feature the common name shingles is derived (*cingulum,* Latin: a girdle). Exactly why and by what mechanism the virus remains latent for so long, what reawakens it from latency, and why such reactivation occurs infrequently when compared to herpes virus infection, is not clear.

EPIDEMIOLOGY

Unlike varicella, herpes zoster is a sporadic disease occurring at all ages, but mainly among the elderly. The disease is uncommon in children, relatively constant in frequency between 20 and 50 years of age (2.5 cases per 1,000 annually), and thereafter doubles its incidence each decade. The cumulative risk of zoster, if one lives to age 80, is about 15 percent.

The recurrence of herpes zoster infection, unlike herpes simplex, is uncommon and only about 2 percent of patients experience a second episode. There is often no apparent provoking factor, but the well-known predisposing factors include immunosuppression by cytotoxic drugs, corticosteroid treatment, radiation therapy, acquired immunodeficiency syndrome (AIDS), organ transplantation, systemic disorders such as systemic lupus erythematosus (SLE), and, in particular, malignancies. The association with lymphomas and leukemia is very close. In one series, 7.9 percent of 303 patients with lymphoma and leukemia developed zoster, and of these 40 percent had Hodgkin's disease. The association between malignancy and the risk for developing zoster should not lead to the converse notion that patients with zoster are more likely to have underlying malignancy. Population-based studies have disapproved this assumption, thereby obviating the need for thorough evaluation of otherwise healthy individuals with zoster to search for an underlying malignancy.

Immunosuppression predisposes the patient to spread of the virus beyond the dermatome and sensory ganglia and into the central nervous system or systemically. In HIV infection, one of the most common causes of immunodeficiency in recent years, the incidence of herpes virus is seven times greater than that of the general population. Diagnosis of disseminated zoster in a young, previously healthy patient should be an indication for HIV testing.

CLINICAL FEATURES

The first sign of herpes zoster is often a gradual onset of unilateral hyperesthesia or paresthesia of the affected dermatome. This is soon followed by dermatomal pain of variable intensity. During this phase, which usually lasts about 1 or 2 days but may be prolonged up to 21 days, the pain may be misdiagnosed as myocardial infarction, pleurisy, appendicitis, ovarian cyst, herniated intervertebral disk, thrombophlebitis, duodenal ulcer, cholecystitis, or thoracoabdominal diabetic neuropathy, depending on the dermatome involved. The zoster pain, however, is usually associated with pruritus and hypersensitivity of the involved dermatome to touch. The dermatomes frequently involved are T3 to L3, with T5 and T6 having the highest affliction (about 60 percent). The ophthalmic division of the trigeminal nerve is the most frequently affected cranial nerve (about 15 percent). In approximately 5 percent of patients fever, headache, mild stiff neck, regional adenopathy, and nausea may coincide with the painful phase and precede the development of rash, but these symptoms do not seem to be correlated with the likelihood of any complications, including postherpetic neuralgia.

The rash usually appears as erythematous macules, papules, and then vesicular eruptions in a beltlike distribution following one or, rarely, two or more sensory dermatomes. They become turbid and begin to crust within 5 to 10 days and occasionally become pustular or hemorrhagic, often with superficial necrosis. The crusts usually fall off in 2 to 3 weeks, commonly leaving scars and increased or decreased pigmentation with or without skin anesthesia. Weakness and denervation of intercostal and abdominal muscles, which may pass unnoticed, sometimes develops. In the immunocompromised host, especially patients with AIDS, this time course may become protracted, and a picture of chronic zoster emerges.

Dissemination reflects a viremia and can be defined, arbitrarily, as the appearance of more than 20 lesions outside the primary and adjacent dermatomes. In about one-half of patients with disseminated lesions, other neurologic complications (see the list in the first section of this chapter) visceral involvement (particularly pneumonitis) and ocular involvement, contribute to the morbidity and mortality. Even with aggressive antiviral therapy, the mortality rate in such patients is in the range of 4 to 15 percent.

Involvement of the ophthalmic branch of the trigeminal nerve may be complicated by local spread, causing eye damage, cranial nerve palsies, meningoencephalitis, postherpetic neuralgia, and delayed cerebral angitis and cerebral infarction. Ocular damage occurs in nearly 50 percent of such patients, especially when it affects the nasociliary nerve branch (supplying sensation to the eyeball and the tip of the nose), resulting in corneal scarring and inflammation. The presence of the vesicles at the end of the nose (Hutchinson sign) indicates involvement of this branch and should prompt ophthalmologic consultation. In addition to retinal vasculitis, necrotizing retinitis, and arterial sheathing, optic neuritis and retrobulbar neuritis may also be present. Untreated patients have an extremely poor outcome, and retinal detachment resulting from retinal holes may subsequently develop. About 64 percent of patients with retinal necrosis become legally blind.

The clinical triad of eruption on the ear and within the ear canal, hearing impairment, and ipsilateral facial paralysis, described by J. Ramsay Hunt, may extend to other areas, including the 2nd and 3rd cervical root, oral and nasopharyngeal region. The earliest otologic symptom is usually unilateral pain in the ear, and before the development of any objective finding, the diagnosis may be difficult to secure. Tinnitus, vertigo, nausea, often incapacitating gait unsteadiness, and occasionally a Menière-like syndrome may develop. With the appearance of the rash and facial palsy the diagnosis will become clear. The facial weakness in Ramsay Hunt syndrome is more severe than Bell's palsy and when complete, recovers less frequently. Hearing deficit may be partial or total, and often there is reduced speech discrimination. The Ramsay Hunt syndrome is believed to result from a herpetic inflammation of the geniculate ganglion, the somatic sensory locus of the facial nerve.

Involvement of peripheral motor nerves or nerve roots resulting in paralysis varies from 0.5 to 31 percent and is more common in the elderly and in association with malignancies. Motor weakness nearly always follows the cutaneous lesions, the time interval between the two commonly being no more than 2 to 3 weeks. Within hours or days the weakness reaches its peak level with no further progression or spread to other muscles. Involvement of upper extremities, especially C5–C6 segments, occurs twice as often as lower extremities. In patients with a motor neuropathy of the limbs, about 50 to 70 percent have complete functional recovery. When the phrenic nerve is involved with herpes zoster, paralysis of the hemidiaphragm will occur. A neurogenic bladder due to involvement of motor or sensory nerves innervating the bladder or sacral segments of the spinal cord can develop following cutaneus eruption in sacral dermatomes. Gastrointestinal visceral motor complications manifesting as paralytic ileus, colonic pseudo-obstruction (Ogilvie syndrome) or localized colonic spasm may occur following lumbar and sacral segment involvement. Although the prognosis of this manifestation of herpes zoster is generally good, its recognition may be difficult when the preceding cutaneus eruptions are not reported or not noticed.

Myelitis, of variable extent, occurs in less than 1 percent of herpes zoster and results from direct viral invasion of the spinal cord from dorsal root ganglia. It usually follows the rash of thoracic dermatomes by a few days or up to 10 weeks. It can, however, precede the rash and cause diagnostic difficulties, requiring imaging and myelographic studies to exclude other causes. Prominent weakness and back pain may be present, but a sensory level occurs in less than half of patients. The CSF examination usually discloses mononuclear pleocytosis, increased protein and normal glucose levels.

At least three types of brain involvement may complicate herpes zoster: diffuse encephalitis, focal parenchymal infection, and vasculitis. Older patients and immunodeficient individuals may present with acute encephalitis a few days following the cutaneus rash. The clinical picture is that of an acute or subacute delirium accompanied by CSF pleocytosis, with few focal features. Here, again, the encephalitis may precede the skin eruption, creating diagnostic difficulties. At the onset of encephalitis, fever is common, and headache, nuchal rigidity, and ataxia are also frequent. The electroencephalogram shows diffuse slow-wave activity, and about 10 percent of patients have seizures. In 94 percent of patients with clinical encephalitis, VZV antibody, measured by indirect membrane immunofluorescence, is present in the CSF at a titer of 1:2 or more. Most patients with encephalitis recover if other complications of the disease do not intervene.

Focal encephalitis is seen in immunosuppressed patients and resembles progressive multifocal leukoencephalopathy, with cerebral lesions mainly involving the white matter. Its onset may be temporally remote from the cutaneus rash or occur without the presence of skin eruption. It may be associated with vasculopathy and focal infarction. Brain biopsy may be required for accurate diagnosis. Cowdry type A intranuclear inclusions on microscopic examination, and visualization of herpes virus nucleocapsids by electron microscopy, confirm the diagnosis.

Delayed cerebral vasculitis involving the internal carotid artery or its major branches, resulting in a catastrophic onset of hemiplegia, is observed following the ophthalmic-division zoster. The delay between the rash and onset of cerebral dysfunction varies from none to as long as 6 months, with a mean interval of 7 weeks. The syndrome results from direct viral invasion of the arterial wall by viral spread from the infected ganglion or a delayed granulomatous reaction.

POSTHERPETIC NEURALGIA

The syndrome of postherpetic neuralgia (PHN) is defined solely by the persistence of pain after herpes zoster. A conservative definition is when pain in the affected region lasts longer than 3 months after crusting of the skin lesions. PHN occurs in about 10 to 15 percent of all herpes zoster patients and is the most feared complication of this condition. The incidence of PHN progressively increases to more than 60 percent in patients over age 60, but gradually disappears in most, and is still present at 6 months in only 13 percent of those older than 60. In some patients, however, PHN persists for years or even a lifetime. PHN is more common after ophthalmic herpes zoster than it is after spinal segment involvement. The more severe the initial herpes zoster involvement, the greater the likelihood of the pain becoming chronic

Pain is usually described as a constant nagging, burning, aching, tearing, and itching, upon which may be superimposed shocks and jabs. Many patients describe "tenderness" (allodynia) even with light contact with clothing or hyperpathia superimposed on the continuous component of the pain. The misery of patients is such that PHN is known in Danish as *Helvedesild,* meaning "hell-fire"

The differential diagnosis of PHN should not be difficult. Virtually all patients will describe the acute episode of herpes zoster and will manifest pigmentary changes in the skin. However, the diagnosis of PHN following herpes zoster in the ab-

sence of skin rash, known as *zoster sine herpete,* is difficult to establish. The existence of this form of herpes zoster has been questioned, but recent studies demonstrating VZV DNA in the CSF of several patients tends to support this syndrome as a clinical variant of PHN. The diagnosis, however, must be made only after excluding other causes of radiculopathy, such as nerve compression and diabetic thoracoabdominal neuropathy.

TREATMENT

Treatment of individual patients must take into account their background risk for particular complications (Table 67-1). In some young immunocompetent patients with uncomplicated truncal or limb herpes zoster, the usual analgesics such as aspirin, local compresses such as Calamine lotion, or local anesthetic-containing creams may be sufficient to reduce the intensity of pain. In older patients, amitriptyline and fluphenazine, alone or in combination, are useful. When the zoster appears to be complicated, or herpes ophthalmicus or Ramsay Hunt syndrome has developed, it is prudent to start early treatment with oral antiviral agents such as acyclovir, 600 to 800 mg five times per day for 10 days, or the newer agent famciclovir 500 to 750 mg tid. Although there is no controlled clinical trial of antiviral therapy in cases of myelitis, encephalitis, or cerebrovascular diseases, in such cases it is best to administer acyclovir intravenously due to its superior bioavailability to the oral form. In herpes ophthalmicus, when acyclovir is started within 7 days after the rash, the incidence of corneal ulceration and uveitis is diminished, but that of PHN is not altered. Similar treatments, when given to immunocompetent and immunocompromised patients with truncal zoster, results in a slightly faster relief from pain, and reduced healing time of lesions, but has no significant effect on PHN.

Of the newer antiviral agents, valaciclovir and famciclovir have been shown to be equally or more effective than acyclovir in treatment of acute herpes zoster, and have a more convenient

TABLE 67-1. Treatment of Acute Herpes Zoster

Young, immunocompetent, uncomplicated zoster
  Nonopioid analgesics
  Local anesthetic creams
  Supportive care
Young, immunocompetent, with cephalic zoster
  Analgesics
  Local anesthetic creams
  Antidepressants
  Oral antiviral (famciclovir or acyclovir)
Young, immunocompetent, complicated zoster (encephalitis, myelitis, vasculitis)
  Analgesics
  Local anesthetic creams
  Antidepressants
  Intravenous acyclovir
  Corticosteroids
Elderly, immunocompetent, spinal or limb zoster
  Analgesics
  Local anesthetic creams
  Antidepressants with or without carbamazepine
  Short-course oral corticosteroid for very severe pain
Elderly, immunocompetent, cephalic zoster
  Analgesics
  Local anesthetic creams
  Antidepressants with or without carbamazepine
  Oral antivirals (famciclovir or acyclovir)
  Corticosteroids
Any age, immunocompromised, with or without complications
  Analgesics
  Topical anesthetics
  Antidepressants with or without carbamazepine
  Intravenous acyclovir

dosing schedule. They also have a modest effect on shortening the duration of PHN.

Famciclovir, a prodrug of penciclovir, is readily absorbed following oral administration. Penciclovir is similar to acyclovir in terms of structure, spectrum of activity, and mechanism of action. Famciclovir, when given at a dose of 500 mg or 750 mg three times daily to immunocompetent zoster patients, results in a modest improvement in cutaneus healing and shortens the duration of PHN to nearly half if no treatment was given. In comparison to acyclovir, the primary advantages of famciclovir are the more convenient dosing schedule and perhaps shortening the duration of PHN. Neither drug effectively prevents the development of PHN.

Valaciclovir, the ʟ-valin ester of acyclovir, is converted rapidly to acyclovir after oral administration. Like famciclovir it is absorbed significantly better than acyclovir when taken orally and requires fewer daily doses. When compared with acyclovir, immunocompetent patients over 50 years old have 1 or 2 weeks less herpetic pain. The dose of valaciclovir is 1 g orally three times per day for 7 days.

Patients of any age who are immunocompromised, including those with cancer, cephalic zoster, or who have any complications of zoster, should be treated promptly, preferably within 24 hours of onset, with intravenous acyclovir to prevent systemic spread. The recommended intravenous dose is 5 to 10 mg/kg infused every 8 hours for 5 days. It is not known, however, that such a regimen will in fact reduce the outcome of motor weakness or zoster-associated cerebral vasculitis. In acyclovir-resistant patients with VZV infection, foscarnet, 40 mg/kg intravenously every 8 hours for 7 to 14 days is recommended. The drug is more expensive and generally less well tolerated than acyclovir and requires controlled rates of infusion in large volumes of fluid.

The place of corticosteroids in the treatment of acute herpes zoster remains unanswered. Randomized, double-blind trials of acyclovir for 7 or 21 days, with or without prednisone 40 mg/day, showed no additional benefit from steroid therapy in the rate of PHN, although steroids did seem to reduce the pain during the first 3 days of therapy when the inflammation was at its maximum. Until the results of ongoing studies on the use of steroids in herpes zoster become available, the use of systemic steroids should be reserved for older immunocompetent patients with severe herpes zoster pain, or for complicated zoster (e.g., encephalitis, myelitis, or vasculitis) in combination with antiviral drugs. Although dissemination after steroid use in immunocompetent patients has been observed anecdotally, it has not been observed in several controlled studies, suggesting that the therapy is safe in otherwise healthy patients.

Treatments such as subcutaneous injections of local anesthetics, peripheral nerve block, paravertebral or epidural block, and sympathetic block, although anecdotally and empirically effective, cannot be recommended for routine use.

TREATMENT OF POSTHERPETIC NEURALGIA

Treatment of PHN is a formidable task (Table 67-2). Amitriptyline or nortriptyline are effective in pain relief in 44 to 67 percent of patients with PHN, an effect that is independent of the antidepressant properties of the drugs. The dose can be gradually increased (10 mg/day at bedtime) until pain relief or a maximum dose of 150 mg/day is reached. Specific 5-hydroxytryptamine (5HT) reuptake blockers (e.g., fluoxetine, paroxetine, and citalopram), which are safer in the elderly and lack

TABLE 67-2. Treatments Employed for Postherapeutic Neuralgia

Nonpharmacologic
  Support and education
  Physical therapy
  Transcutaneous electrical nerve stimulation
  Cognitive and behavioral therapy
Pharmacologic
  Topical anesthetics
  Antidepressants
  Anticonvulsants (carbamazepine, phenytoins)
  Topical capsaicin
  Lidocaine analogues (mexiletine)
  Intravenous lidocaine
  Opioids
Surgical (see text)
  Sympathectomy
  Dorsal root entry zone lesions
  Dorsal column and brainstem stimulation
  Various nerve blocks
  Cryoanalgesia

cardiovascular toxicity, may prove effective and should be tried if amitriptyline or nortriptyline are of no benefit or cause side effects. The addition of carbamazepine may alleviate shooting and jabbing pains.

If these treatments are not successful or pain relief is only partial, a transcutaneous electrical nerve stimulation (TENS) unit along with physical therapy may prove helpful. However, in most patients the beneficial effect of TENS will decline with time. Infiltration of lidocaine into painfully sensitive skin may result in temporary (a few hours to days) but significant improvement. Local applications of topical lidocaine (5 or 10 percent in cream, ointment, gel, or patches) have been effective when used in combination with other therapies. Capsaicin cream, a substance P depletor, applied three times per day, results in modest pain relief after several days of application. Patients who do not respond to these therapeutic modalities may be given an oral lidocaine analogue, mexiletine, at a dose of 150 mg bid or tid to be increased to a total of 600 mg daily. Gastrointestinal and central nervous system side effects of mexiletine may prohibit its use. Those with more severe and long-term PHN may benefit from intravenous lidocaine (5 mg/kg) resulting in pain relief comparable to intravenous morphine. The beneficial effect, however, is usually short lasting.

Opioids, used intravenously or orally, may result in substantial relief and should not be withheld from patients with severe PHN for fear of addiction liability, tolerance, or safety. Clinical experience in the management of cancer pain as well as chronic nonmalignant pain indicates that addiction and tolerance to opioid analgesics do not constitute relevant treatment complications. Upward titration of slow-release oral morphine or oxycodone results in good to excellent pain control without significant effects on cognition. This treatment, however, should be reserved for those patients proven refractory to all other pharmacologic therapies.

There have been several invasive and surgical treatments employed in the therapy of PHN. Acupuncture, nerve block, dorsal column and brain stimulation, dorsal root entry zone operation, ganglionectomy, sympathetic block, and cryoanalgesia are either entirely ineffective or provide only transient relief at much greater risk of morbidity. Only patients who are truly refractory to all other treatment modalities should be considered for ablative surgeries.

SUGGESTED READINGS

Anon: Varicella-zoster virus infection: new insights into pathogenesis and postherpetic neuralgia. Ann Neurol 35:S1, 1994

Gilden DH, Wright RR, Schneck SA et al: Zoster sine herpete, a clinical variant. Ann Neurol 35:530, 1994

Hirschmann JV: Herpes zoster. Semin Neurol 12:322, 1992

Rowbotham M: Treatment of postherpetic neuralgia. Semin Dermatol 11:218, 1992

Straus SE, Ostrove JM, Inchauspé G et al: Varicella-zoster infection. Ann Intern Med 108:221, 1988

Watson CPN: Postherpetic neuralgia. Neurol Clin 7:231, 1989

68. CYTOMEGALOVIRUS INFECTION

DIANA L. RODRIGUEZ
MARVIN A. FISHMAN

Cytomegalovirus (CMV) is a prevalent agent that commonly infects persons of all ages, geographic locations, and socioeconomic and cultural backgrounds. Human CMV is a species-specific, double-stranded DNA herpesvirus that is widely disseminated in nature and is capable of remaining latent in the host. Most CMV infections are inapparent; however, clinical illness may range from mild to fatal.

EPIDEMIOLOGY

CMV infections occur worldwide and are influenced by many factors, including age, geographic location, cultural and socioeconomic status, and child-rearing practices. CMV is the most common cause of congenital and perinatal viral infections throughout the world. The incidence is not seasonal, and there is no sexual predilection. CMV may be acquired congenitally, perinatally, or postnatally, with postnatal acquisition being highest in early childhood, adolescence, and during the childbearing years.

Approximately 1 percent of all newborns are congenitally infected with CMV; the incidence is highest in populations with low standards of living. Infection of the fetus may occur via primary (newly acquired) or recurrent (reactivated) maternal CMV infection. Although most newborns congenitally infected with CMV are likely to be asymptomatic, symptoms and sequelae are much more common in those infants whose mothers experienced a primary, rather than a recurrent, CMV infection during pregnancy.

Perinatal infections are much more prevalent than congenital infections because of more potential exposure via the mother's cervicovaginal secretions, urine, saliva, and breast milk. The usual incubation period for perinatal infection is 5 to 6 weeks.

Children not congenitally or perinatally infected with CMV may be infected during toddler or preschool years. Infection is influenced by day-care attendance and low socioeconomic status of the family. In developing countries and in lower socioeconomic populations, over 80 percent of children acquire CMV infection by age 3 years, and almost all persons have been infected by adulthood.

CMV infection in adolescents and adults also varies according to geographic location and socioeconomic status. CMV infection increases in adolescence, presumably due to the more intimate physical contact that occurs in that age group; it appears to be more prevalent in nonwhite races.

CMV infection may be conferred via other routes, such as bone marrow and organ transplantation, blood transfusion, and very rarely by nonintimate person-to-person contact. It is the most frequent debilitating and dangerous viral infection in immunosuppressed bone marrow and organ transplantation recipients and in patients with acquired immunodeficiency syndrome (AIDS). An active infection with CMV occurs in almost all such patients and usually becomes apparent clinically and virologically about 30 to 90 days after transplantation. Although reactivation, reinfection, and primary CMV infections all can produce symptoms in immunosuppressed transplant recipients, primary CMV infections are much more likely to be severe.

CLINICAL FEATURES

Although most CMV infections are asymptomatic, they can range from minor to severe, or even fatal. Common manifestations of CMV infection may include a mononucleosis syndrome, or an interstitial pneumonitis, and less commonly the virus may cause congenital or acquired chorioretinitis, hepatitis, various gastrointestinal illnesses, myocarditis, endocrinopathies, genitourinary system infections, and several neurologic illnesses, especially in immunosuppressed patients.

CMV-induced mononucleosis can occur as a primary infection in both immunocompetent and immunocompromised individuals, as well as a reactivation infection in immunocompromised patients. Although it may be seen at any age, it most commonly occurs in young adults between 20 and 40 years old. It is characterized by very pronounced malaise and fever that may last 1 to 4 weeks, peripheral lymphocytosis with atypical lymphocytes, and mild elevation of liver enzymes. Pharyngitis, splenomegaly, and the production of heterophil antibodies are not as common in the CMV-induced infectious mononucleosis as it is in the Epstein-Barr virus (EBV)-induced mononucleosis syndrome. Complications are rare, but may include Guillain-Barré syndrome, and meningoencephalitis.

Interstitial pneumonitis caused by CMV is a frequent and serious infection in immunosuppressed children and adults, especially in organ transplantation patients and those with AIDS. It is characterized by fever and dry, nonproductive cough, which then progresses to respiratory distress with dyspnea, retractions, wheezing, and hypoxia. Its mortality rate in transplant patients is close to 90 percent. Radiographically, it is a diffuse, interstitial infiltrate.

NEUROLOGIC MANIFESTATIONS

The most significant neurologic illnesses caused by CMV are listed below:

Congenital CMV infection
Meningoencephalitis
Retinitis pigmentosa/chorioretinitis
Transverse myelitis
Polyneuritis
Illnesses in immunosuppressed patients
    Encephalitis
    Myeloradiculitis
    Mononeuritis multiplex
    Peripheral neuropathy

TABLE 68-1. Clinical Manifestations of Congenital Cytomegalic Inclusion Disease

Symptom	Percent of Patients
Deafness	90
Hepatomegaly	70
Splenomegaly	70
Jaundice	64
Intrauterine growth retardation	63
Petechiae, purpura	57
Cataracts	50
Microcephaly	40
Microphthalmia	18
Retinopathy	18
Cerebral calcifications	17
Congenital heart disease	5
Glaucoma	3
Pneumonia	3

(Modified from Feigin RD, Cherry JD (eds): Textbook of Pediatric Infectious Diseases. p. 931. WB Saunders, Philadelphia, 1991, with permission.)

Prenatal transmission of CMV to the fetus occurs by way of maternal viremia and transplacental passage of the virus, perhaps within virus-infected leukocytes. Symptomatic patients are infected during the second or third trimester of pregnancy, in contrast to rubella infections, which are felt to occur during the first trimester. Each year, approximately 30,000 to 40,000 babies are born with congenital CMV infection. Of these, 5 to 10 percent will have typical cytomegalic inclusion disease (CID) (Table 68-1), another 5 percent will have atypical involvement, and 90 percent will have no clinical manifestations at birth. Neurologic sequelae or deafness occur in up to 90 percent of infants who are symptomatic at birth.

Involvement of the central nervous system (CNS) produces the most severe sequelae of the disease. The most common ophthalmologic findings include optic atrophy, strabismus, and chorioretinitis. The chorioretinitis cannot be differentiated from that due to congenital toxoplasmosis, either in appearance or location in the retina (Fig. 68-1).

Microcephaly is another common CNS manifestation. It may not be present at birth, but may become apparent at 1 year of age or later. When associated with cerebral calcifications, microcephaly carries a high probability of psychomotor retardation. The cerebral calcifications are typically periventricular in distribution, a pattern that may also be observed in congenital toxoplasmosis (Fig. 68-2). Other cerebral lesions include microgyria and other cortical malformations, cerebellar aplasia, subdural effusions, polycystic encephalomalacia, porencephaly, and calcifications of cerebral arteries. Hydrocephalus, which may be progressive, may also rarely be seen.

Meningoencephalitis caused by CMV is rare. It may occur as a complication of CMV mononucleosis, secondary to a primary infection in an immunocompetent individual, or as a primary or recurrent infection in an immunosuppressed patient. Symptoms include headache, photophobia, nuchal rigidity, memory deficits, and inability to concentrate. The cerebrospinal fluid (CSF) reveals a mild mononuclear pleocytosis and slightly elevated protein content. Although CMV is rarely isolated from the CSF or brain parenchyma, neuropathologic findings of intranuclear inclusions and microglial nodules are characteristic.

CMV may also cause an acquired chorioretinitis, especially in immunosuppressed individuals such as bone marrow transplant recipients and in patients with AIDS. It probably occurs secondary to hematogenous spread of the virus to the retina. The appearance of the funduscopic and congenital CMV chorioretinitis is similar. Because CMV retinitis can progress to complete blindness if the macula is involved, immunosuppressed patients should receive regular ophthalmologic evaluations for early diagnosis and therapy.

The other important CNS disease produced by CMV is transverse myelitis. Although this syndrome of acute spinal cord

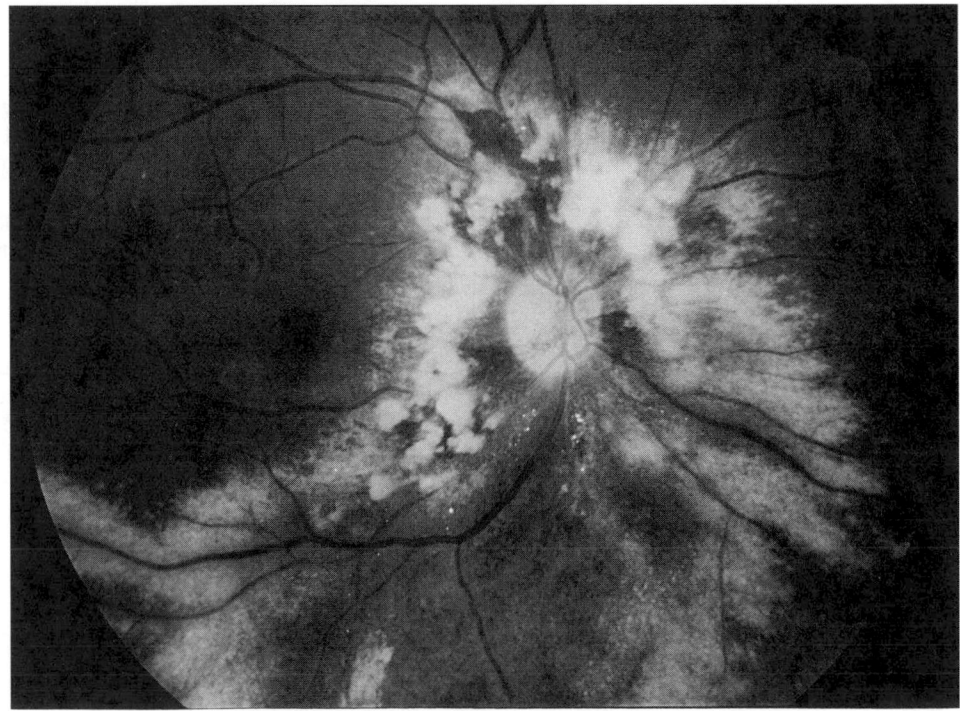

FIG. 68-1.   CMV chorioretinitis. (Courtesy of Richard A. Lewis, M.D., Baylor College of Medicine, Houston, Texas.)

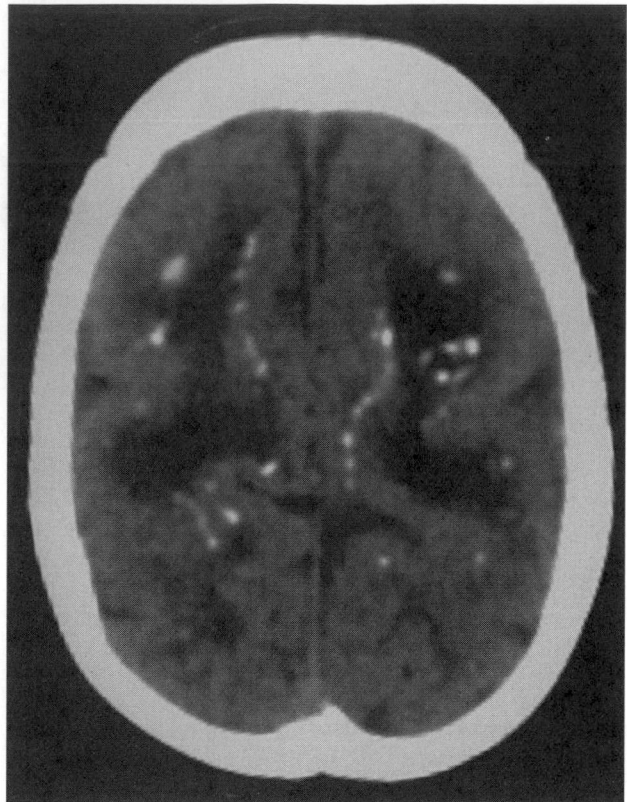

FIG. 68-2. CT scan showing periventricular calcifications in a patient with congenital CMV infection. (Courtesy of Gail Demmler, M.D., Baylor College of Medicine, Houston, Texas.)

inflammation results in most cases from demyelination and autoimmune phenomena, it can arise from viral infections including, albeit rarely, CMV.

The virus can also invade the peripheral nervous system. It is associated with a polyradiculopathy and a painful peripheral neuropathy in AIDS patients, and with the Guillain-Barré syndrome in immunocompetent patients. Bell's palsy has been noted in a pregnant woman during a primary CMV infection.

There is a growing recognition of CMV infections in AIDS patients; 50 percent may show evidence of CMV infection of the CNS at postmortem examination. It is one of the most common opportunistic infections in patients with AIDS, and has been reported to cause encephalitis, myeloradiculitis or polyradiculomyelopathy, mononeuritis multiplex, and polyneuropathy. A peculiar polyradiculomyelopathy, especially lumbosacral, has been associated with CMV infection. It is a rapidly progressing syndrome occurring in about 1 percent of AIDS patients, characterized by low back pain, subacute ascending motor weakness, areflexia, sphincter disturbance, progressive flaccid paraparesis, and a neutrophilic cerebrospinal fluid pleocytosis. Electrophysiologic studies typically demonstrate features of axonal neuropathy associated with varying degrees of demyelination.

There have been several reports of patients with AIDS who have developed a mononeuritis multiplex comprised of multifocal subacute sensorimotor neuropathy in whom CMV has been found in the peripheral nerve. Involvement has been patchy and symmetrical, as confirmed by electrophysiology. Cranial nerves occasionally have been affected, notably the recurrent laryngeal nerve. The CSF is usually normal, although polymorphonuclear

pleocytosis may occur. Peripheral nerve biopsy demonstrates multiple foci of endoneurial necrosis with CMV inclusions in Schwann cells.

DIAGNOSIS

Infection with CMV, whether congenital or acquired in adulthood, can only absolutely be established by isolation of the virus from urine, saliva, CSF, or blood, together with a fourfold or greater antibody rise. Techniques for detecting antibody to make the diagnosis include immunofluorescence, demonstration of complement-fixing or neutralizing antibody, or enzyme-linked immunosorbent assay (ELISA). Unfortunately, these serologic techniques are difficult to interpret, since antibody elevations may not be detectable for up to 4 weeks after the primary infection, and titers often remain high for years afterward.

TREATMENT

Ganciclovir, previously called 9-(1,3-dihydroxy-2-propoxymethyl)guanine, or DHPG, was the first antiviral compound licensed specifically for the treatment of life-threatening and sight-threatening infections with CMV. This agent acts by inhibiting replication of viral DNA polymerase; ganciclovir must be metabolized to the triphosphate form intracellularly to effect this inhibition. Ganciclovir is virostatic and therefore suppresses active infection, but does not produce a cure. CSF concentration of the drug is usually 25 to 70 percent of the plasma concentration. Ganciclovir is indicated for the treatment of CMV retinitis in immunocompromised patients, and may also be effective in CMV meningoencephalitis. Therapeutic trials of ganciclovir in newborns with evidence of CNS involvement are in progress.

Ganciclovir treatment is usually given in two phases: induction and maintenance. The usual dosage for induction is 5 mg/kg IV bid for 2 to 3 weeks. Following induction, a maintenance treatment of 5 mg/kg/day given 5 to 7 days of the week is necessary for many patients who remain immunosuppressed, especially patients with AIDS. If the disease progresses on maintenance therapy, then another course of the induction treatment should be considered. Important side effects include bone marrow suppression with neutropenia, anemia, and thrombocytopenia.

Foscarnet (trisodium phosphonoformate) is a compound which inhibits the DNA polymerase of human herpes viruses, including CMV. It is also active against human immunodeficiency virus (HIV). It has been used in AIDS patients who have CMV retinitis and polyradiculomyelopathy. As with ganciclovir, foscarnet treatment is given as induction and then maintenance therapy. Induction therapy is administered intravenously as 60 mg/kg q8h for 2 to 3 weeks, depending on the patient's response. Following induction, maintenance therapy of 90 to 120 mg/kg/day intravenously is administered. If progression of the disease occurs, the patient may be retreated with the induction and maintenance phases again. Foscarnet is very nephrotoxic; the majority of patients will experience some decrease in renal function in response to its administration. It also may cause electrolyte abnormalities as well as anemia and leukopenia. Therefore, these parameters should be closely monitored during administration.

SUGGESTED READINGS

Alford CA, Stagno S, Pass RF, Britt WJ: Congenital and perinatal cytomegalovirus infections. Rev Infect Dis 12:745, 1990

Bale JF Jr: Human cytomegalovirus infection and disorders of the nervous system. Arch Neurol 41:310, 1984

Drew WL: Cytomegalovirus infection in patients with AIDS. J Infect Dis 158: 449, 1988

Swaiman KF: Pediatric Neurology, Principles and Practice. 2nd Ed. CV Mosby, St. Louis, 1993

Menkes JH: Textbook of Child Neurology. 4th Ed. Lea & Febiger, Philadelphia, 1990

69. EPSTEIN-BARR VIRUS INFECTION

CLIFFORD C. DACSO

The Epstein-Barr virus (EBV) is one of the herpes viruses that infect humans. Other members of this group include herpes simplex types I and II, varicella-zoster virus, cytomegalovirus, human herpes virus type 6, and simian herpes B virus. (The latter is primarily an infection of nonhuman primates, with humans as accidental hosts.) Herpes viruses all share some common characteristics. They all produce viral latency, meaning that the viral genetic material is integrated into that of the host. However, this does not mean that the virus is completely dormant, as there is production and display of virus antigens of EBV on host cell surfaces. EBV is different from other human herpes viruses in that it possesses several distinct antigens that do not cross-react. These antigens provide unique serologic markers for EBV activity.

Herpes viruses contain double-stranded DNA. EBV DNA can exist in a circular form called the EBV episome, and replication of this form by host DNA polymerase plays a role in the persistence of EBV infections. Viral transmission is usually either by direct transfusion of infected material, or by mucosal exposure.

EPIDEMIOLOGY

EBV is a ubiquitous infector of humans. Initially described as a virus associated with Burkitt's lymphoma, its etiologic role in the pathogenesis of infectious mononucleosis has since become clear. Much like the other herpes viruses, EBV persists in human tissues and is shed for long periods after the acute infection. Since the major mode of transmission of EBV is salivary and respiratory secretions, the prolonged shedding of the virus provides ample opportunity for transmission. Although EBV can be transmitted by blood transfusion, the oropharyngeal route is the major one.

As with cytomegalovirus, the acquisition of the infection occurs at a younger age in lower socioeconomic groups. The incidence of primary infection with EBV coincides with the beginning of social activity in adolescents, during which there is exposure to oropharyngeal secretions. About 90 percent of adults have serologic evidence of exposure to the virus.

CLINICAL FEATURES

Following an incubation period of 4 to 8 weeks, the illness usually begins insidiously. Infectious mononucleosis has a fairly stereotyped repertoire of signs and symptoms. Fever, pharyngitis, and anterior or posterior cervical lymphadenopathy are almost universal findings. Splenomegaly and hepatomegaly are frequently found. These features of the acute infection resolve within 5 to 14 days, but the malaise of mononucleosis may persist for months, and delay the return to school or work.

Although neurologic manifestations of EBV infection occur in only 1 percent of patients, they can be the presenting signs and symptoms and can be quite severe. Neurologic manifestations of infectious mononucleosis have been recognized for many years, well before the identification of the etiologic agent.

Infectious mononucleosis may present as meningitis or encephalitis. When this occurs, examination of the CSF will show a lymphocytic pleocytosis, sometimes even with atypical lymphocytes seen in the smear. Symptoms often develop abruptly and become quite severe, but recovery without complications is the most common outcome of EBV meningitis in the immunocompetent host. EBV meningoencephalitis usually is indistinguishable from other diffuse viral encephalitides; however, involvement of the cerebellum seems to be more prominent. Because of the rarity of this condition, the incidence of cerebellitis is difficult to ascertain, but it can be a striking, albeit transient, complication.

Other neurologic conditions that have been associated with EBV infection are listed below:

Encephalitis
Meningitis
Meningoencephalitis
Bell's palsy
Other cranial nerve palsies
Transverse myelitis
Brachial plexopathy
Mononeuritis multiplex
Seizures
Demyelinating disease
Optic neuritis
Guillain-Barré syndrome
B-cell lymphoma
Transient global amnesia

Again, because of the rarity of neurologic complications of EBV, most of the data about these conditions exist in case report form, often as a serologic finding of acute infection in patients presenting with a neurologic symptom. However, at least two conditions, Guillain-Barré syndrome and central nervous system demyelination, can apparently occur as a result of EBV infection directly, without signs of infectious mononucleosis and often without positive antibodies.

Although the rare deaths that occur with infectious mononucleosis usually result from neurologic complications, most damage to the nervous system resolves completely, leaving no sequelae. Persistent deficits are rare.

In the setting of the acquired immunodeficiency syndrome (AIDS), EBV is a very common infecting agent. B-cell lymphomas in the central nervous system have been associated with EBV infection in patients with AIDS, and in those receiving immunosuppressive agents over a long period of time, such as after organ transplantation. This malignancy is relatively resistant to therapy.

DIAGNOSIS

Nonspecific laboratory abnormalities abound in EBV infection. Mild transaminase elevation is very common, and cryoglobulinemia to a greater or lesser extent is virtually universal. Circulating atypical lymphocytes are seen in almost all cases but are not pathognomonic, since other virus infections, hematologic malignancies, and toxoplasmosis can also produce atypical lymphocytes in the peripheral blood smear.

The laboratory diagnosis of EBV infection rests on the demonstration of the serologic response. Antibodies reactive with sheep red blood cells (heterophil) are manifestations of the polyclonal immunoglobulin production that occur during EBV infection, and may even mediate some of the complications of infectious mononucleosis. The heterophil antibody test is positive in more than 90 percent of patients. These antibodies are checked by using the highly accurate and reproducible Monospot test. Although the Monospot test is positive in the preponderance of cases and false positives are rare, the appearance of heterophil antibodies in the course of the disease is variable. Therefore, EBV infection should not be ruled out on the basis of a single negative Monospot.

Antibodies to the viral capsid antigen (VCA) can be demonstrated and immunoglobulin G (IgG) differentiated from IgM. IgG antibody rises early in clinical disease and persists for life, but IgM antibody does not persist. For this reason, IgM VCA antibody is diagnostic of acute disease.

Although the data are preliminary, the polymerase chain reaction (PCR) holds out hope for rapid diagnosis of EBV disease in the central nervous system.

A syndrome consisting of usually abrupt onset fatigue and lassitude, variously coupled with low-grade fever, myalgias, arthralgias, lymphadenopathy, and evanescent rashes, has been reported sporadically for at least the last 100 years. At one time this "chronic fatigue syndrome" was thought to represent chronic infection with the EBV, based on rising antibody titers to the EBV early antigens. When examined closely, it became evident that there is no consistent association, either virologically or epidemiologically, between chronic fatigue syndrome and EBV. There still remains, however, a large number of clinicians and patients who insist on this association. Despite the lack of correlation with EBV, chronic fatigue syndrome is quite debilitating and responds poorly to therapy. It appears, however, to be self-limited.

TREATMENT

Specific antiviral treatment effective in vivo is not yet available; however, many agents can be shown to decrease viral replication in vitro. For the rare severe manifestations of EBV, including impending airway closure, some have recommended a rapidly tapering course of corticosteroids. Since most of the EBV complications are self-limited, including the neurologic manifestations, this intervention is seldom required.

SUGGESTED READINGS

Bray PF, Culp KW, McFarlin DE et al: Demyelinating disease after neurologically complicated primary Epstein-Barr virus infection. Neurology 42: 278, 1992

Grose C, Henle W, Henle G et al: Epstein-Barr virus infections in acute neurological disease. N Engl J Med 292:392, 1975

Holmes GP, Kaplan JE, Gantz NM et al: Chronic fatigue syndrome: a working case definition. Ann Intern Med 108:387, 1988

Ito H, Sayama S, Irie S et al: Antineuronal antibodies in acute cerebellar ataxia following Epstein-Barr virus infection. Neurology 44:1506, 1994

Silverstein A, Steinberg G, Nathanson M: Nervous system involvement in infectious mononucleosis. Arch Neurol 6:353, 1972

Tsutsumi H: Epstein-Barr virus infection and neurological disorders in children: detection of Epstein-Barr virus genomes in the cerebrospinal fluid by polymerase chain reaction technique, abstracted in English. No To Hattatsu 25:135, 1993

70. POLIOMYELITIS

CLIFTON L. GOOCH

Although the dread inspired by the polio epidemics of the 1950s, which left an estimated 250,000 to 300,000 survivors with paralysis, has been largely forgotten by recent generations, poliomyelitis remains a significant threat in underdeveloped countries with inadequate immunization programs. Because of immigration, imported cases continue to appear in the United States and vaccine-associated paralytic polio, though rare, is a well-documented risk. Recurrent weakness in polio survivors (the postpolio syndrome) is a late complication in approximately 25 percent of cases, and has been reported with increasing frequency over the last decade. Although considered eradicated for the present in many developed countries, polio epidemics recur when vaccination standards fall. Even in the United States, despite aggressive vaccination, some communities are poorly immunized (with survey documentation of inadequate immunization in 50 percent of children younger than 2 years), providing unprotected populations for the reappearance of polio.

The polioviruses are single-stranded RNA viruses belonging to the enterovirus subgroup of the picornaviruses. They are spread by fecal-oral contamination, surviving in sewage or contaminated water for prolonged periods. Once ingested, the virus enters the lymphatic tissue in the ileum and pharynx and disseminates locally by lymphatic, followed by hematogenous, spread. The infection may then enter the central nervous system (CNS), possibly through defects in the blood-brain barrier, where it prominently affects the motor nerves (anterior horn cells) and/or brainstem motor nuclei. These lesions are responsible for the areflexic weakness that is the hallmark of the disease, as well as the bulbar weakness and, depending on distribution, may impair respiratory muscle function. Thalamic and reticular formation involvement may rarely precipitate autonomic instability.

EPIDEMIOLOGY

Prior to the development of effective immunization, polio epidemics occurred primarily in northern, temperate countries with excellent sanitation. Populations living under less sanitary conditions are more likely to be exposed to endemic polio in early infancy, usually while still protected from severe disease by maternal antibodies, and thus may develop lifelong immunity. In the absence of immunization, more sanitary conditions prevent such early exposure, creating large groups highly susceptible to the virus and setting the stage for recurrent epidemics. These typically occur in late summer and affect predominately children older than 6 months, adolescents, and young adults.

TABLE 70-1. Clinical Types of Poliovirus Infection

Clinical Type	% of Total	Features	Prognosis
Subclinical	90	No symptoms	Excellent
Abortive (4 days–5 weeks postexposure)	8	Malaise, fever, headache, sore throat, cough, diarrhea, nausea and vomiting	Excellent
Nonparalytic with "aseptic" meningitis (2–10 days after above illness)	1.98	Malaise, fever, sore throat, cough, diarrhea, nausea and vomiting, severe headache, meningismus, CSF pleocytosis, elevated protein	Good, with small chance of progression
Paralytic (3–5 days after onset of CNS symptoms)	0.02	Muscular stiffness, spasm (early), resolution of fever, coarse fasciculations, focal weakness, urinary bladder dysfunction, respiratory failure, rare bulbar weakness (pharyngeal, facial), rare autonomic dysfunction	15–30% mortality; 33% of survivors with permanent weakness

Older patients, when affected, are more likely to have severe disease.

CLINICAL FEATURES

Clinically, poliovirus infection can be divided into four types: subclinical infection, abortive poliomyelitis, nonparalytic poliomyelitis with "aseptic" meningitis, and paralytic poliomyelitis (Table 70-1). The incubation period following ingestion of the virus is typically 1 to 2 weeks, but may range from 4 days to 5 weeks. Dissemination and viremia cause no symptoms in 90 percent of cases (*subclinical infection*). Malaise, fever, headaches, sore throat, cough, diarrhea, nausea, and vomiting are prominent in the remaining 10 percent. In this group with clinically apparent infections most patient have self-limited symptoms that resolve after 2 to 3 days, without recurrence (*abortive poliomyelitis*). Only 2 percent of infections progress to the central nervous system. These patients report persistence of their systemic symptoms, or recurrence 2 to 10 days after apparent recovery, accompanied by constant headache and painful neck stiffness due to meningeal irritation. Cerebrospinal fluid analysis demonstrates an early leukocytosis (25 to 500 cells/mm^3) with neutrophilic predominance in the first few days, superseded by lymphocytic predominance. Normal glucose and mildly to moderately elevated protein (usually less than 150 mg/dl) are also present. These symptoms usually resolve without sequela in 7 to 14 days (*nonparalytic poliomyelitis with "aseptic" meningitis*).

Unfortunately, 0.1 to 1 percent of infections invade the motor system after CNS penetration, resulting in *paralytic poliomyelitis*. These patients complain of back and hamstring stiffness, spasm and muscle tenderness, in addition to the above symptoms. The onset of weakness and paralysis follows closely, occurring during or after resolution of the fever and 3 to 5 days after the onset of CNS symptoms (although it may range from a presenting symptom of nervous system involvement to late appearance 2 or 3 weeks into the illness). Weakness progresses rapidly over hours to days, with coarse fasciculations early and atrophy starting in 1 to 3 weeks. Asymmetric onset is common, and the lower extremities are more often affected, especially in young children under 5 years. Associated arm weakness and bilateral lower extremity weakness is more common in older children and adolescents, while young adults are most at risk for quadriplegia. Although hyperreflexia may be present in some cases initially, diminution and loss of deep-tendon reflexes ultimately occurs, often as an early finding. Muscles of the trunk and thorax, including the muscles of respiration, may also be affected.

Bulbar involvement complicates 10 to 15 percent of cases, most commonly affecting the tenth cranial nerve and causing paralysis of the pharyngeal musculature. Laryngeal weakness may also develop. Facial palsies are less likely, although facial diplegia may sometimes appear. Urinary bladder muscle dysfunction is a common complication in adults. Myocarditis, autonomic dysfunction with hypertension, acute cerebellar ataxia and transverse myelitis are less often accompaniments. Approximately 15 to 30 percent of adults and 2 to 5 percent of children with paralytic disease die, and patients with bulbar disease and respiratory involvement are at the greatest risk. Mortality peaks in the first week of paralysis, chiefly from respiratory failure due to depression of the respiratory centers and from destruction of the motor neurons supplying the intercostal and diaphragm muscles. Other causes of death include aspiration due to bulbar weakness and disturbed control of vascular tone.

Strength may begin to recover within the first month after onset, and maximal recovery usually occurs by 6 to 9 months. Approximately one-third of patients will have significant permanent weakness. Appropriate care is essential to minimize musculoskeletal deformities such as scoliosis, subluxations, and joint dislocations, and equinovarus deformities.

Weakness typically remains stable after infection, but 25 to 30 percent of paretic patients will develop a progressive weakness, sometimes involving previously asymptomatic muscles, approximately 25 to 35 years after infection. This condition, termed the *postpolio syndrome*, advances extremely slowly, with an average decline in strength of 1 percent per year. Its etiology remains controversial, but it does not appear to cause significant additional paralysis in most cases.

DIAGNOSIS

The diagnosis of polio is made in the appropriate clinical setting and can be supported by the isolation of viruses from the throat, stool, and cerebrospinal fluid (CSF). Virus grown in tissue culture systems should enable identification of enterovirus in 3 to 4 days, with specification of poliovirus in 10 to 11 days. Submission of all the above specimens is highly important, as CSF cultures alone are rarely positive. Acute and convalescent serum antibody titers to the three pathogenic types of poliovirus can also be measured, with a fourfold increase considered diagnostic of acute infection.

Because neurologic symptoms often develop after (or in the absence of) systemic symptoms, paralytic polio seldom presents with clinical features of an infection. Instead, the differential diagnosis of polio includes other conditions that cause rapid, flaccid paralysis:

Guillain-Barré syndrome
Transverse myelitis
Botulism
Heavy metal poisoning
Tick paralysis

TREATMENT

Therapy is supportive. Patients should be hospitalized when they manifest signs of nervous system infection. Early muscle and meningeal pain may respond to hot packs and analgesics. Close attention to early signs of respiratory insufficiency such as increasing restlessness and anxiety is critical, and serial vital capacities should be monitored and mechanical ventilation instituted when measurements fall below 30 to 50 percent of predicted values. Tracheostomy may be necessary due to excessive secretions in bulbar and spinal disease. Bladder paralysis is typically transient, lasting only a few days, and may be treated with bethanechol, 5 to 10 mg PO or 2.5 to 5 mg SQ as needed to induce voiding, although some patients may nevertheless require catheterization. Constipation, secondary to abdominal muscle weakness, should be treated with enemas. Appropriate positioning of weak limbs with splints, boards, and sandbags, as well as early physical therapy is critical to minimize deformity, but surgical correction of specific abnormalities may be required in some cases and should be performed by an experienced orthopedic surgeon.

Two vaccines are currently available for polio, each of which offers protection against all three antigenic types of the virus: the live oral polio vaccine (OPV) and the formalin-inactivated polio vaccine (IPV). OPV is the currently recommended regimen in the United States because of increased intestinal immunity and because of transfer of the virus, and hence immunity, to close contacts of the recipient. Four doses are given: one each at 2, 4, and 15 to 18 months, and at 4 to 6 years of age. Fecal viral shedding continues for 6 to 8 weeks following inoculation. Unfortunately, rare cases of paralytic disease following this vaccination are reported (1 per 550,000 first doses, 1 per 12.3 million subsequent doses) and adults are at increased risk. This vaccine should not be given to immunodeficient patients or their contacts.

IPV is administered in four doses with a 4- to 8-week interval between the first and second doses, followed in 6 to 12 months by the third dose, and a booster at 4 to 6 years. Further adult boosters may be needed to maintain immunity with IPV. Immunocompromised patients and their contacts may receive this vaccine without any risk of infection, but it is contraindicated in patients with a history of neomycin or streptomycin allergy requiring medical treatment. Some investigators recommend IPV for the primary vaccination of unimmunized adults as well.

With the announcement by the Pan American Health Organization of a 2-year interval free of wild-type poliovirus infection in the Americas following an aggressive immunization campaign, the potential eradication of polio seems one step closer. The practitioner must remain vigilant, however, in our increasingly mobile international community, and must realize that a future polio outbreak remains possible until the last patient is immunized and the last host clear of disease.

SUGGESTED READINGS

Agree JC, Rodriguez AA, Tafel JA: Late effects of polio: critical review of the literature on neuromuscular function. Arch Phys Med Rehabil 72:923, 1991

Centers for Disease Control: Polio: what you need to know. U.S. Department of Health and Human Services, Public Health Service, Atlanta, 1992

Foege WH: Eradication of polio in the Americas. JAMA 270:1857, 1993

Munsat TM: Poliomyelitis: new problems with an old disease. N Engl J Med 324:1206, 1991

Nkowane BM, Wassilak SGF, Orenstein WA et al: Vaccine-associated paralytic poliomyelitis: United States: 1973 through 1984. JAMA 257:1335, 1987

Patriarca PA, Foege WH, Swartz TA: Progress in polio eradication. Lancet 342:1461, 1993

Patriarca PA: Polio outbreaks: a tale of torment. Lancet 344:630, 1994

Ramlow J, Alexander M, LaPorte R et al: Epidemiology of the post-polio syndrome. Am J Epidemiol 136:769, 1992

71. MEASLES AND SUBACUTE SCLEROSING PANENCEPHALITIS

DIANA L. RODRIGUEZ
MARVIN A. FISHMAN

Measles, or rubeola, is caused by an RNA virus that produces a fever, cough, coryza, conjunctivitis, and an erythematous maculopapular confluent rash. There is a pathognomonic enanthem called Koplik spots located on the buccal surface of the cheeks. Complications due to measles infection are numerous and affect many organ systems, including the central nervous system (CNS). Fortunately, in 1963, measles vaccines became available and their administration led to a dramatic reduction in epidemic measles as well as its complications.

EPIDEMIOLOGY

Measles is primarily a disease of children. In the prevaccine era, the highest rate of occurrence was in children 5 to 10 years old, but since the introduction of the vaccine, half of all cases now occur in adolescents and young adults. In many developing countries, measles is the most important cause of death from ages 1 through 5 years, and accounts for 1 to 2 million deaths per year worldwide.

CLINICAL FEATURES

Measles is a highly contagious disease characterized by three stages:

1. An incubation stage of approximately 10 to 14 days with few, if any, symptoms
2. A prodromal or catarrhal stage of approximately 3 to 5 days with Koplik spots, mild to moderate fever, mild conjunctivitis, coryza, and progressively worsening, brassy cough
3. A final or exanthem stage with a maculopapular rash erupting from head to toe, accompanied by high fever

Measles is spread via the respiratory route and is most contagious during the prodromal period, or catarrhal stage of illness. Patients should be considered contagious from 1 to 2 days before the onset of symptoms (3 to 5 days before the rash) to at least 7 days after the onset of the rash. Patients with subacute sclerosing panencephalitis (SSPE), a complication of measles, are not infectious.

In typical measles, the exanthem occurs at about the peak of the respiratory symptoms. The duration of the rash is usually 6 to 7 days. During the exanthem phase, the fever usually peaks on the second or third day and then declines over a 24-hour period. Fever that persists after the third or fourth day of exanthem is usually an indication of a complication. Other manifestations during this period may include pharyngitis, localized or generalized lymphadenopathy, diarrhea, vomiting, laryngitis, croup, and abdominal pain.

NEUROLOGIC COMPLICATIONS

The neurologic complications and sequelae are not rare. Neurologic manifestations of a primary measles infection most frequently include a parainfectious encephalitis/encephalomyelitis, acute measles encephalitis of the delayed type, and SSPE.

Parainfectious Encephalomyelitis

Parainfectious encephalomyelitis (a type of acute disseminated encephalomyelitis) is a demyelinating illness that occurs more often in association with measles infection than with other exanthematous illnesses, complicating approximately 1 in 800 to 2,000 measles cases. Although the encephalitis may be relatively mild, the mortality rate is 10 to 20 percent, and a similar percentage suffer persistent neurologic sequelae. Prevention of this neurologic complication of measles alone provides sufficient justification for immunization against the disease.

The encephalomyelitic syndrome may precede the rash, but, characteristically, the rash is fading and other symptoms are improving when the patient suddenly experiences a recrudescence of fever, convulsions, stupor, and deepening coma. Other less common manifestations include hemiplegia, cerebellar disease, and occasionally a transverse myelitis or other signs of spinal cord involvement. Choreoathetotic movements occur infrequently. In many cases the syndrome is much less severe and the patient suffers a transient encephalitic illness with abrupt recurrence of fever, headaches, irritability, listlessness, lethargy, confusion, and signs of meningeal irritation.

Long-term sequelae of parainfectious measles encephalitis may include various degrees of retardation, epilepsy, deafness, a syndrome of postencephalitic hyperkinesia, and hemiplegia or paraplegia. The occurrence of neurologic sequelae does not correlate with the severity of the initial symptoms.

The CNS complications may occur after measles immunization, but only with an incidence of approximately 1.68/1,000,000 vaccine doses. Fever and rash develop 7 to 12 days after immunization, followed by lethargy, irritability, and possibly seizures.

Considerable controversy relates to the mechanisms responsible for the neurologic syndromes. Recent investigations have failed to isolate measles virus or to demonstrate measles virus RNA or other viral antigens in the brains of most affected patients. These findings have led to the hypothesis that the illness may be autoimmune and that viral invasion of the CNS is unnecessary.

Acute Measles Encephalitis of the Delayed Type

A unique measles encephalitis that occurs in immunosuppressed patients is sometimes referred to as acute measles encephalitis of the delayed type. Although the symptoms vary, the illness appears to be different from either the acute encephalitis that occurs in patients without known immunodeficiencies or the chronic picture of SSPE. The incubation period has varied between 5 weeks and 6 months. Convulsions are frequently the initial symptom, and they are a prominent aspect of the illness. The seizures may be focal, unilateral, or continuous localized clonic activity (epilepsia partialis continua). Other findings include hemiplegia, stupor, coma, hypertonia, and slurred speech. Most cases have been fatal, and the duration of illness has been from 1 week to 2 months. Investigators have isolated measles virus from the brain of a patient with this illness. The lesions are similar to those of SSPE except that the inflammatory changes are lacking. In a sense, this subacute measles encephalitis is an opportunistic infection of the brain in an immunodeficient patient. The interval between exposure and onset of neurologic disease, the rapid subsequent course, and lack of antibodies, distinguish this subacute measles encephalitis from both postmeasles encephalitis and SSPE.

SUBACUTE SCLEROSING PANENCEPHALITIS

A more delayed form of measles encephalitis is SSPE, a progressive inflammatory disease of the CNS caused by a persistent, aberrant measles virus infection. The risk of SSPE in children who previously had natural measles is between 0.6 and 2.2 per 100,000 infections, with a mean latency to onset of SSPE of 7 to 12 years. In contrast to natural measles, the risk of SSPE after measles immunization is about 1 per 1 million. In vaccinees who develop SSPE, the mean incubation period is approximately 3 to 7 years.

SSPE affects mainly children and adolescents and rarely occurs beyond the age of 18 years, with a usual age of onset between 5 and 15 years of age. Typically, there is a history of primary measles infection at a very early age, often prior to age 2 years. It is more common in rural than urban populations, and it appears to be five times more common in males than in females. The National SSPE Registry, which was established to monitor cases after the introduction of the measles vaccine in 1964, continues to record 10 to 20 new cases each year (some of which may be vaccine-induced).

SSPE has been divided into four clinical stages. Stage I (0 to 30 percent disability) involves impairment of intellectual functions, especially behavior and learning. There is slowing of mental processes and behavioral reactions. This stage may be missed, because of its insidious onset and progression. It may last a few weeks to a few years. Stage II (30 to 55 percent disability) is marked by seizure activity and progression of the dementia. Rhythmic myoclonic jerks are the characteristic finding, occurring at 5- to 15-second intervals, initially involving the head and then the trunk and limbs. These rhythmic myoclonic jerks are the unique hallmark of SSPE. They do not occur in sleep nor do they impair consciousness. Also seen in Stage II is a decrease in spontaneous movement and speech, though comprehension remains intact. Stage II lasts approximately 1 month to 1 year. Stage III (55 to 80 percent disability) is marked by further loss of cortical function, hyperthermia, difficulty swallowing, drooling, choreoathetoid movements, decorticate or decerebrate posturing, more extrapyramidal and pyramidal symptoms, disappearance of the characteristic involuntary movements, and alteration of consciousness. Half of these patients have ophthalmologic abnormalities such as optic atrophy, papilledema, or a focal chorioretinitis which can affect the periphery or the macula with subsequent visual loss. Stage III lasts approximately 3 to 18 months. The patient with stage IV disease (end stage and 80 percent disability to death) is mute and quadriplegic. This stage may last from 1 to 6 years.

Remissions in SSPE have been described, but the patients ultimately succumb to the illness. The length of survival seems to depend on the age of onset; younger patients tend to survive longer than older patients. Most patients die 1 to 3 years after the onset of the illness, although survival for as long as 16 years has been described. There are no reliable clinical or laboratory indicators to predict length of survival. Death is usually a result of loss of central control mechanisms for temperature, respiratory and cardiac functions, or from secondary infection.

The pathogenesis of SSPE is not entirely understood but seems to involve an alteration of the virus as it infects the CNS, allowing it to escape immune surveillance. There appears to be an abnormality in the synthesis of the matrix (M) protein, a polypeptide, which is important in the assembly of the viral nucleocapsid; however, the full complement of genetic material needed to code for all proteins, including the M protein, is present and functional. Patients with SSPE therefore lack antibody to the M protein even though they have high titers of antibody to other measles-virus polypeptides. In addition, most patients who develop SSPE had their acute measles infection at a very young age, which suggests that immature or altered immunity may play a role.

DIAGNOSIS

The diagnosis of measles is usually made from the typical clinical picture; laboratory confirmation is rarely needed. During the prodromal stage, multinucleated giant cells can be demonstrated in smears of the nasal mucosa. Virus can be isolated if necessary in tissue culture. Finally, diagnostic rises in antibody titer can be demonstrated between acute and convalescent sera.

Interestingly, Gibbs and associates noted that 51 percent of 680 measles patients without clinical evidence of encephalitis had abnormal EEGs during acute or immediate postacute illness.

The diagnosis of measles postinfectious encephalomyelitis is usually suggested by the history of preceding measles infection and the ensuing encephalomyelitic picture. The cerebrospinal fluid (CSF) usually shows a lymphocytic pleocytosis and increased protein content. Magnetic resonance imaging (MRI) may reveal areas of demyelination.

Measles encephalitis of the delayed type, compared to SSPE, has a relatively short interval between exposure and onset of neurologic disease, and a subsequent rapid course. The CSF may be normal, and there may not be any increase in measles antibody titers. Pathologically, brain lesions are similar to those of SSPE except that the inflammatory changes are lacking.

The characteristic clinical and laboratory features of SSPE are progressive dementia, myoclonic movements, a typical EEG pattern, elevated immunoglobulin G (IgG) and oligoclonal bands in the CSF, and very high titers of anti-measles antibody in the serum and CSF. Characteristic, although not pathognomonic, of SSPE is an EEG pattern of periodic paroxysmal bursts seen in stage II disease (Fig. 71-1). These consist of 2- to 3-second high-voltage diphasic activity occurring at 5- to 8-second intervals, often associated with spike discharges. They occur in approximately 80 percent of SSPE patients, sometimes several years prior to the clinical onset of myoclonus.

The CSF in SSPE is often abnormal. The CSF IgG, most of which is directed against the measles virus, rises to levels greater than 20 percent of the total protein. Oligoclonal banding is observed, and an excessive number of plasmacytes are found in the CSF.

High anti-measles antibody titers in serum and CSF confirm the diagnosis of SSPE. Other tests that help corroborate the diagnosis are MRI and brain biopsy. Imaging studies obtained during early stages of SSPE demonstrate small ventricles with obliteration of hemispheric sulci and fissures. With a prolonged course, they reflect changes consistent with demyelination and atrophy of gray and white matter.

A brain biopsy may be performed if the diagnosis is uncertain. In SSPE, the pathologic process represents a subacute encephalitis accompanied by demyelination. Light microscopy reveals inflammatory lesions of the gray and white matter, including demyelination, intranuclear and intracytoplasmic inclusion bodies of neurons and glial cells (Cowdry A and Cowdry B bodies), inflammatory cells, and gliosis (Fig. 71-2). Electron microscopy reveals intracellular inclusions that can be shown to contain measles virus nucleocapsids.

TREATMENT

Treatment of the typical case of self-limited measles is supportive. Likewise, the treatment of measles encephalomyelitis and acute measles encephalitis of the delayed type is also symptomatic and supportive. Neither γ-globulins nor corticosteroids offer benefit or prevent the development of sequelae. Seizures should be aggressively controlled.

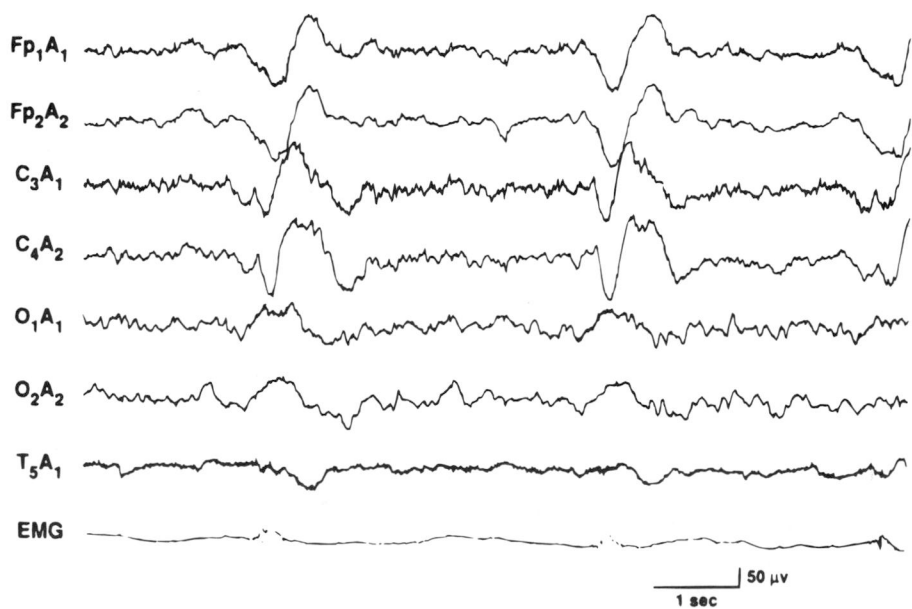

FIG. 71-1. EEG showing the periodic paroxysmal bursts with accompanying myoclonus seen in SSPE.

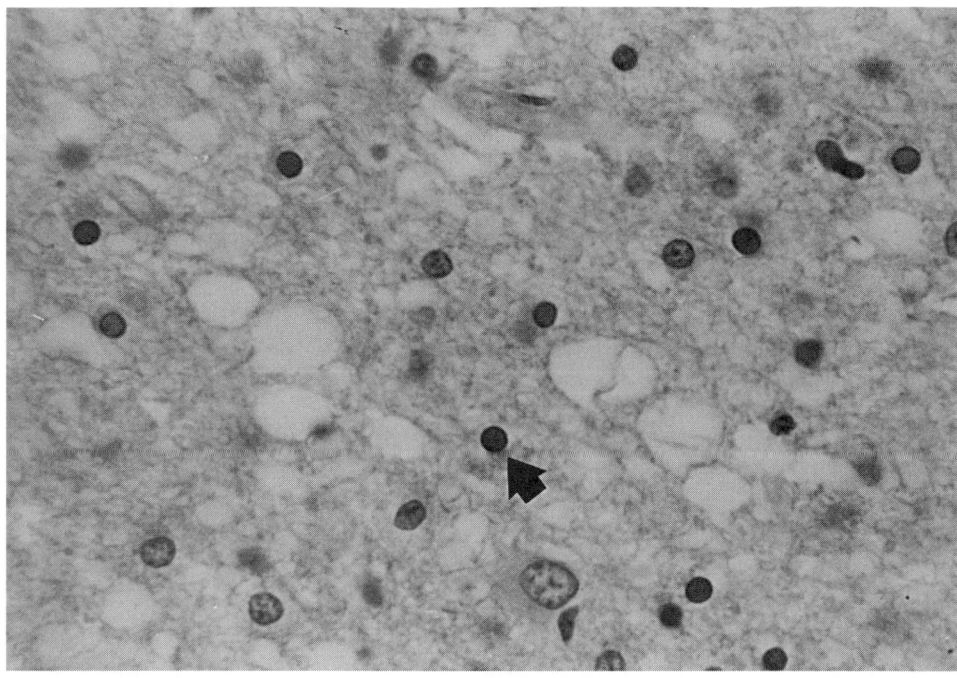

FIG. 71-2. Light microscopy demonstration of an eosinophilic intranuclear inclusion (*arrow*) and reactive gliosis in SSPE. (Courtesy of Marvin A. Fishman, M.D., Baylor College of Medicine, Houston, Texas.)

There is no proven effective treatment for SSPE, although case reports of the use of inosiplex and intrathecal α-interferon have suggested a possible beneficial effect. Despite these hopeful treatments, the cornerstone of care is still supportive: airway protection, nutrition, prevention of contractures and decubiti, monitoring for and treating secondary infections. Seizures are difficult to control in these patients but carbamazepine, valproic acid, diazepam, and primidone may be useful in controlling myoclonic, generalized, and psychomotor seizures.

SUGGESTED READINGS

Aarli JA: Nervous complications of measles. Eur Neurol 12:79, 1974

Grattan-Smith PJ, Procopis PG, Wise A, Grigor WG: Serious neurological complications of measles: a continuing preventable problem. Med J Aust 143:385, 1985

Lyon G, Ponsot G, Lebon P: Acute measles encephalitis of the delayed type. Ann Neurol 2:322, 1977

Menkes JH: Textbook of Child Neurology. 4th Ed. Lea & Febiger, Philadelphia, 1990

Swaiman KF: Pediatric Neurology, Principles and Practice. 2nd Ed. CV Mosby, St. Louis, 1993

72. PROGRESSIVE MULTIFOCAL LEUKOENCEPHALOPATHY

BRADLEY K. EVANS

Progressive multifocal leukoencephalopathy (PML), a rare disease of brain white matter, occurs exclusively in immunosuppressed patients, particularly those with acquired immunodeficiency syndrome (AIDS). The disease is caused by JC virus, a small, circular, double-stranded DNA virus in the papovavirus family. PML results from JC virus infection of oligodendrogliocytes, the cells that produce the myelin (white matter) of the brain. Dysfunction and death of these cells, with demyelination secondary to oligodendrogliocyte damage, causes the symptoms of PML.

EPIDEMIOLOGY

Seroepidemilogic studies confirm that most people have been exposed in childhood (asymptomatically) to the JC virus. Because some normal individuals intermittently excrete the virus in urine, it is assumed that JC virus can establish a latent infection in kidney and perhaps in other tissues as well. JC virus may cause PML either by reactivation of a latent infection in the brain or by reactivation in another organ, leading subsequently to brain infection. (AIDS patients may have intermittent JC viremia, for which they are asymptomatic, which probably represents a reactivation.) Compared to JC virus in kidney, however, the JC virus in PML lesions has multiple mutations, and these may be important for conferring the qualities needed to produce clinical disease.

Currently, over half of patients with PML have AIDS. Because of this association, human immunodeficiency virus (HIV) testing is indicated in all patients diagnosed with PML. In HIV-infected patients, the risk for developing PML during the course of their illness is approximately 2 to 5 percent. Even though PML may be the first manifestation of HIV infection, the CD4 count in AIDS patients with PML is very low, typically less than $50/\text{mm}^3$. Other causes of immunosuppression associated with PML are lymphocytic malignancies (e.g., chronic lymphocytic leukemia and Hodgkin's disease), organ transplantations, corticosteroid therapy, and cancer chemotherapy.

CLINICAL FEATURES

PML usually progresses indolently, over several weeks. Sometimes the onset seems to be more precipitous, particularly if the lesion is in a relatively clinically vital area of the brain. Typically, PML causes one or more focal brain lesions, usually arising at the gray-white junction, and later spreading into adjacent white matter. Lesions can affect the cerebral hemispheres, the cerebellum, or the brainstem, and they produce symptoms depending upon their location. Typical early symptoms are hemiparesis, hemianopsia, and ataxia. Besides these signs of a focal brain lesion, which are present in approximately 75 percent of patients, PML may produce altered mental status (about 50 percent of patients), particularly late in the illness, when the lesions are multiple and large. Fever and headache are infrequent, probably no more common than in other AIDS patients. Seizures are slightly more frequent in AIDS patients with PML (10 to 20 percent of patients).

DIAGNOSIS

Blood and spinal fluid tests seldom aid in the diagnosis. Some patients with PML may have a high CSF myelin basic protein level, reflecting intense myelin breakdown, but this is a nonspecific finding.

Neuroimaging, particularly head MRI, is the key test in this disorder. The MRI shows one or more hyperintense lesions on T2-weighted imaging, which do not have mass effect and do not enhance. The lesions are focal, in contrast to AIDS-dementia complex, in which the MRI shows diffuse changes in both cerebral hemispheres. The head CT in patients with PML typically shows one or more hypolucent lesions, without mass effect and without enhancement, but the CT is less sensitive than the MRI (Fig. 72-1). These neuroimaging findings, although highly suggestive of PML, are not diagnostic: focal virus encephalitis due to cytomegalovirus (CMV) infection or to Herpes zoster can produce an identical radiologic picture.

Thus, the keys to the diagnosis are recognition of the patient's immunosuppressed state and proper interpretation of the MRI. In an immunosuppressed patient with a typical clinical picture and neuroimaging findings, the diagnosis may be made presumptively, without tissue confirmation. This occurs particularly if the patient is too ill to undergo a biopsy, if lesions are in areas difficult to biopsy, or if vigorous treatment is not contemplated.

Definitive diagnosis is by brain biopsy, usually done stereotactically. Because biopsies from patients with PML can be misread as a demyelinating plaque, an astrocytoma, or viral encephalitis, tissue from these biopsies must be stained and examined carefully. By light microscopy, PML produces demyelination, giant astrocytes that have bizarre nuclei or are multinucleate (mimicking cell changes seen in astrocytomas), and oligodendroglial cells with intranuclear inclusions that can be eosinophilic or basophilic. These inclusions are crystalline masses of viral particles, which immunostain for JC virus. Immunostaining will definitely identify the inclusions as JC virus, and not cytomegalovirus (CMV) or the varicella-zoster virus.

In HIV-infected patients, the differential diagnosis of PML is CNS toxoplasmosis, CNS lymphoma, AIDS-dementia complex, and focal viral encephalitis. CNS toxoplasmosis and CNS lymphoma are more rapid illnesses, often progressing over a few days to weeks. Seizures, altered mental status, and headache are more common in these two illnesses than in PML, and neuroimaging in these conditions shows lesions with mass effect and enhancement. AIDS-dementia complex presents with altered mental status and no focal findings. CMV and herpes zoster can cause a focal encephalitis that can mimic PML clinically, radiologically, and pathologically. Finally, it is important to remember that 20 percent of AIDS patients with focal lesions by head CT or MRI have nondiagnostic brain biopsies. Note that if the patient is not recognized as being immunosuppressed, PML may be mistaken for ischemic stroke, multiple sclerosis, a leukodystrophy, or a low-grade glioma.

TREATMENT

PML progresses inexorably to death in nearly all patients. In possibly 2 to 5 percent of patients, the disease will "burn out." The chances this will happen are probably greater in patients

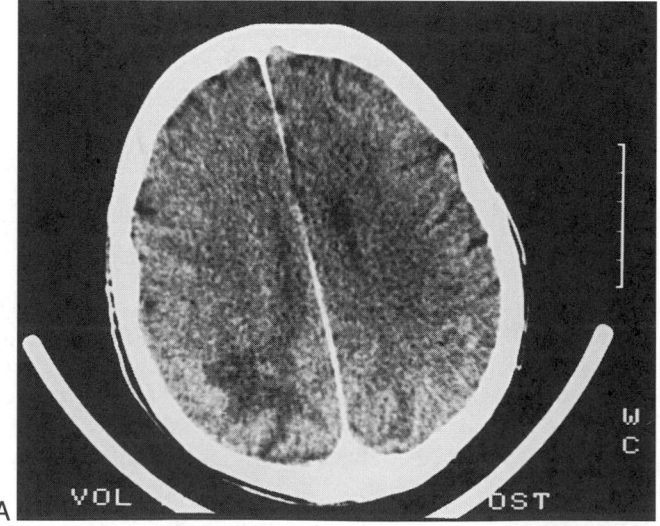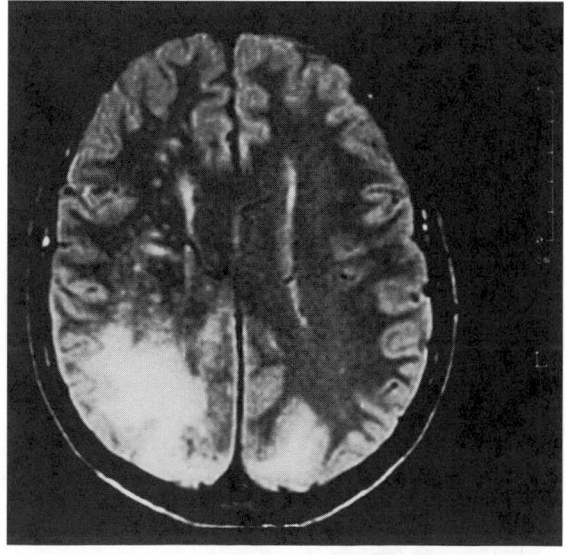

FIG. 72-1.   **(A)** Contrast-enhanced CT scan of the head of an immunocompromised patient with PML. In both occipital lobes there are patchy hypolucent lesions, without mass effect and without enhancement. **(B)** T2-weighted MRI scan of the same patient showing the characteristic findings in PML of focal, hyperintense lesions without mass effect.

who have inflammatory changes on brain biopsy (reflecting an active immune response) and in patients whose immune suppression can be reversed.

No effective treatment for PML is known. Since JC virus can be grown in cell culture, possible treatments for PML can first be tested in the laboratory. Cytosine arabinoside, in cell culture at doses achievable therapeutically, successfully inhibits JC virus replication. Case reports suggest that cytosine arabinoside may be an effective treatment in some patients, and there is an ongoing trial in AIDS patients with PML using cytosine arabinoside given either intravenously or intrathecally.

SUGGESTED READINGS

Berger JR: AIDS and the nervous system. p. 757. In Aminoff M (ed). Neurology and General Medicine. Churchill Livingstone, New York, 1995

Berger JR, Mucke L: Prolonged survival and partial recovery in AIDS-associated progressive multifocal leukoencephalopathy. Neurology 38:1060, 1988

Krupp LB, Lipton RB, Swerdlow ML et al: Progressive multifocal leukoencephalopathy: clinical and radiographic features. Ann Neurol 17:107, 1985

Tornatore C, Berger JR, Houff SA et al: Detection of JC virus DNA in peripheral lymphocytes from patients with and without progressive multifocal leukoencephalopathy. Ann Neurol 31:454, 1992

Walker DL: Progressive multifocal leukoencephalopathy. p. 503. In Vinken PJ, Bruyn GW, Klawans HL (eds): Handbook of Clinical Neurology: Demyelinating Diseases. Vol. 47. Elsevier, Amsterdam, 1985.

73. RABIES

PATRICK E. NOLAN

Rabies is an ancient, almost uniformly fatal infectious disease in which the clinical manifestations are distinctly neurologic, most often causing an encephalitis. It is caused by an RNA virus of the rhabdovirus family and is primarily a disease of animals, with most human infections developing after an animal bite. Although rabies claims fewer than a dozen victims in America each year, over one million Americans are bitten by animals annually, making at least the specter of infection a common health problem.

EPIDEMIOLOGY

Because it is a zoonotic disease, the frequency of occurrence is directly related to the animal reservoir in a given locale. In developing countries, the primary reservoir is domestic dogs and cats. Except on the Texas/Mexico border, there is essentially no endemic domestic rabies in the United States, and most cases of human rabies are imported by patients exposed to dogs or cats in foreign countries. The few exposures occurring within the United States usually involve wild carnivores, with only 10 percent traced to domestic animals infected by the endemic wildlife reservoir. The main responsible species is the skunk, and less common sources are racoons, foxes, wolves, and bats. Bats are a somewhat insidious source in that most infections retrospectively identified by isolation of bat-associated strains occur in patients who cannot recall any exposure to bats. An important rule regarding the implicated species is that an "un-provoked" attack by any animal is cause for concern. (Bites or scratches that occur while petting or feeding animals are considered "provoked" in most circumstances.) Among domestic animals, cats are more often implicated than dogs, because of the tighter controls and regulations of rabies vaccination in dogs, and the more independent and predatory nature of cats.

Animal saliva and central nervous system tissue are considered the only infectious material when determining what constitutes an exposure. Dried secretions and blood, feces, and urine are not considered contagious. An animal bite with a break in the skin and contamination of the wound with rabid saliva is the most efficient route of transmission. Nonbite exposures rarely transmit infection, but "high-risk" animal contamination of an open wound or mucous membrane does warrant intervention. Aerosolization of virus in bat-infested caves and transplantation of infected human tissue, especially corneas, have been the most efficient nonbite exposures. Simple contact such as petting a rabid animal does not constitute a significant exposure. The risk of infections to humans after significant exposure to a rabid animal is variable; from 5 to 80 percent after a bite and from 0.1 to 1 percent after a scratch.

CLINICAL FEATURES

After infection, the rabies virus is sequestered at the local site of the bite or wound, and probably replicates as an intracellular infection of local skeletal muscle cells. This partially explains the long incubation period of 30 to 90 days (and occasionally over a year) in humans. (The incubation period in domestic animals is only 3 to 5 days and is the basis for holding animals for observation in questionable cases of transmission.) Spread occurs out of the muscles by way of peripheral nerves back to the spinal ganglia and central nervous system, where the virus appears most concentrated in the gray matter of the limbic system and lower brain. Subsequently, the virus may spread outward via autonomic nerves to almost every organ system, including the salivary glands, which can transmit the virus through infected saliva.

The clinical manifestations of rabies include the prodrome, the acute neurologic period or second phase, and the final phase of coma and death. The prodrome lasts 1 to 4 days and is very nonspecific, with low-grade fever, malaise, gastrointestinal upset, cough, and headache. In 50 to 80 percent of patients, pain, paresthesias, and/or pruritus develop at the site of the bite.

Subtle neurologic changes herald the second phase with confusion and anxiety progressing to agitation, combativeness, and excessive motor activity. Aggressive behavior with a waxing and waning pattern may occur with intervals of relatively normal mental status. Hallucinations are frequent. Vocal paralysis, hyperreflexia, and ataxia paint a rather distinctive picture of the acute neurologic phase. Muscle contractions with jerking movements and facial grimacing are characteristic, with contractures of the pharynx and larynx occurring with attempts to swallow liquids. "Hydrophobia" refers to episodes of uncontrolled muscle spasm, lasting 1 to 5 minutes, precipitated by attempts to drink water. Choking, gagging, hypersalivation, diplopia, optic neuritis, and facial palsies are further evidence of brainstem and cranial nerve dysfunction. Such brainstem involvement helps distinguish rabies from other viral encephalitides, and accounts for its fulminantly fatal course. This presentation characterizes approximately 80 percent of cases and is called "classic" or "furious" rabies.

The remaining 20 percent of cases may manifest so-called "paralytic" rabies. In this presentation, an ascending paralysis, either symmetric or asymmetric, is the predominant presentation. This may mimic Guillain-Barré syndrome. For unclear reasons, "paralytic" rabies occurs more commonly after exposure to bats. It may also complicate the more primitive neural tissue-derived rabies vaccines still used in some developing countries.

The final phase is characterized by autonomic instability, dysrhythmias, coma, and death from a brainstem respiratory center damage. Survival after the onset of neurologic symptoms is only 4 to 20 days. There have been only three survivors reported from clinical human rabies, and these patients received partial passive and active immunization prior to onset of symptoms.

DIAGNOSIS

The differential diagnosis includes the spectrum of unexplained encephalitis. Botulism, cerebral malaria, epilepsy, metabolic encephalopathy, illicit drug effect, rabies hysteria, rickettsial disease, stroke, tetanus, or arboviral encephalitis might all be considered, depending upon the clinical presentation.

The diagnosis can be confirmed by viral isolation from the saliva or cerebrospinal fluid, (CSF), but this requires a minimum of 6 days. Rabies antibody levels can be detected in the serum or CSF, but occasionally are negative early in the illness. Direct fluorescent antibody staining for antigen detection on saliva, a corneal impression, or a skin biopsy from the nape of the neck, has a diagnostic sensitivity of 50 to 90 percent and a diagnostic specificity of close to 100 percent. This test is usually positive before antibody formation and is probably the best test available. Brain biopsy specimens demonstrating the characteristic cytoplasmic inclusion bodies known as Negri bodies may help confirm the diagnosis.

TREATMENT

Determining when to treat after a possible exposure can pose a considerable dilemma, and the algorithm in Figure 73-1 may provide some broad guidance.

Treatment consists of a triadic approach with local wound care, passive immunoglobulin administration, and active immunization with rabies vaccine—all vitally important. The only clinical failures have been related to failure to properly perform all three steps in this approach:

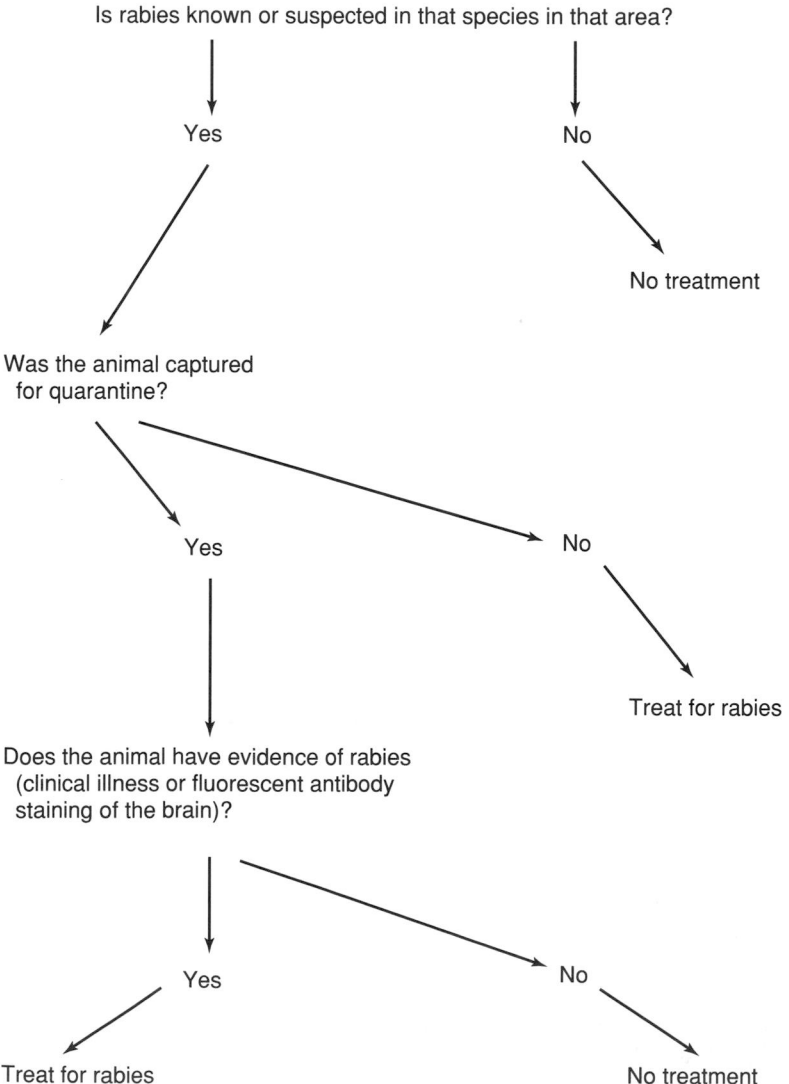

FIG. 73-1. Treatment algorithm for a person bitten or licked on an open wound by a possibly rabid animal.

1. *Local wound care* consists of a thorough and vigorous cleaning of the wound with soap and water. This can significantly reduce the risk in superficial wounds, as has been appreciated since the time of Celsius in a.d. 100 when he recommended excising and cauterizing the wound. Quaternary ammonium compounds such as benzalkonium chloride may also be used as cleansers. Tetanus toxoid is often used as well.
2. *Passive immunization* is accomplished using human rabies immunoglobulin (HRIG). Administration of 200 IU/kg of HRIG at the time of exposure offers antibody protection during the initial 2-week period before the active vaccine has elicited an antibody response. One-half of this dose is infiltrated into the wound, and the other half is injected intramuscularly at a site different from the vaccine and with a syringe that is not used for the vaccine.
3. *Active immunization* is provided by the human diploid cell vaccine (HDCV), administered in five 1-ml intramuscular doses on days 1, 3, 7, 14, and 28. These doses should always be injected in the deltoid muscle, as failures have occurred with gluteal injections.

Note that veterinarians and others with a high risk of exposure to the rabies virus may consider preexposure prophylaxis. The preferred regimen uses three intramuscular injections of HDCV on days 1, 7, and 28. A neutralizing antibody titer should be checked after vaccination.

Local and state health departments are good resources when a question arises regarding decisions of pre- or postexposure prophylaxis. The Division of Viral and Rickettsial Diseases at the Center for Disease Control and Prevention in Atlanta is also available for rabies advice, at (404)639-1075 during working hours or (404)639-2888 after hours.

SUGGESTED READINGS

Baer GM, Fishbein DB: Rabies postexposure prophylaxis. N Engl J Med 316: 1270, 1987
Fishbein DB, Robinson LE: Rabies. N Engl J Med 329:1632, 1993
Hoff GL, Mellon GF, Thomas MC, Geidinghagen DH: Bats, cats and rabies in an urban community. South Med J 86:1115, 1993
Rosenthal KE, Thornton GF: The ten most common questions about rabies. Infect Dis in Clin Pract 3:44, 1993

74. LYMPHOCYTIC CHORIOMENINGITIS

CLIFFORD C. DACSO

Lymphocytic choriomeningitis (LCM) virus is a member of the *Arenavirus* family of pleomorphic single-stranded RNA viruses. All arenaviruses exist in a rodent reservoir, and humans are accidental hosts. Other members of the group include the Old World species such as Lassa virus and the Tacaribe virus complex. Like the others in its class, LCM virus produces asymptomatic infections in rodents but can be devastating in humans.

EPIDEMIOLOGY

LCM virus is ubiquitous in European and American mice. There is no reason to suspect that the virus is not present in other parts of the world, although it has not been definitively identified. Infection is sporadic and appears to be related to contact with infected mouse urine. Laboratory workers who handle hamsters and mice are particularly at risk. Transmission is by direct inoculation or aerosol, although the route of transmission is not clear in many cases. Infections are isolated, not epidemic, and human-to-human transmission has not been reported.

CLINICAL FEATURES

Following infection, two separate syndromes of LCM may appear (Table 74-1). The first is an influenzalike syndrome, with arthralgias, pharyngitis, and orchitis beginning a few days after infection and lasting 3 to 10 days. Liver enzymes may rise slightly, and a chest radiograph may show basilar pneumonitis.

Meningitis usually appears 2 to 3 weeks following inoculation. Typically, the acute viral illness appears first, followed by meningitis in 2 weeks. Fever, headache, and pharyngitis are prominent signs. Relapse is common within a few days or weeks after apparent recovery. In mice, the meningitis, when it occurs, is attributed not to the direct infection but rather to a cell-mediated immune reaction. This reaction may contribute to the pathogenesis of the disease in humans also, although virus has been recovered from the spinal fluid of infected individuals.

DIAGNOSIS

The peripheral blood usually shows mildly elevated liver enzymes, neutropenia, and thrombocytopenia. The cerebrospinal fluid (CSF) has a lymphocytic pleocytosis with a few hundred cells per microliter. As opposed to other viral meningitides, LCM infection shows hypoglycorrhachia in a quarter of cases.

Although the virus can be isolated from the spinal fluid, it is a dangerous procedure and should only be performed in laboratories equipped to handle arenaviruses. The diagnosis is commonly made by direct immunofluorescence of cells in the CSF, or by serologic response using enzyme-linked immunosorbent assay or radioimmunoassay. With the exception of specific serology, the disease is often indistinguishable from other viral encephalitides.

TREATMENT

There is no effective treatment for LCM, although recovery from meningitis is almost universal. On the rare occasions when encephalitis supervenes, residual neurologic deficits can be seen in a quarter of the patients.

TABLE 74-1. Signs and Symptoms of Lymphocytic Choriomeningitis Infection

Sign/Symptom	Frequency (%)
Fever and chills	75–100
Malaise, weakness	50–75
Retro-orbital headache	50–75
Photophobia	50–75
Anorexia, nausea	50–75
Pharyngitis	25–50
Vomiting	25–50
Dysesthesia	25–50

SUGGESTED READINGS

Borrow P, Oldstone MB: Mechanism of lymphocytic choriomeningitis virus entry into cells. Virology 198:1, 1994

Hammer SM, Connolly KJ: Viral aseptic meningitis in the United States: clinical features, viral etiologies, and differential diagnosis. Curr Clin Top Infect Dis 12:1, 1992

Jahrling PB, Peters CJ: Lymphocytic choriomeningitis virus: a neglected pathogen of man. Arch Pathol Lab Med 116:486, 1992

Stephensen CB, Blount SR, Lanford RE et al: Prevalence of serum antibodies against lymphocytic choriomeningitis virus in selected populations from two U.S. cities. J Med Virol 38:27, 1992

Turkovic B, Ljubicic M: ELISA and indirect immunofluorescence in the diagnosis of LCM virus infections. Acta Virol 36:576, 1992

75. RUBELLA

DIANA L. RODRIGUEZ
MARVIN A. FISHMAN

Rubella is caused by an RNA virus. Except in cases of congenital infection, the virus usually causes a mild exanthematous, infectious illness with low morbidity and mortality rates. Prior to the introduction of the rubella vaccine in 1969, children were the most frequently affected, but now most cases appear in adolescents and young adults. In 1941, the Australian ophthalmologist Gregg reported congenital defects in babies of mothers who had rubella during early pregnancy. This led to the recognition of the congenital rubella syndrome (CRS), a postnatal manifestation of a prenatally acquired infection. Neurologic damage may complicate either CRS or adult acquired disease.

EPIDEMIOLOGY

Rubella occurs worldwide. Epidemics occur every 6 to 9 years and pandemics every 10 to 30 years. The last worldwide pandemic occurred from 1962 to 1964. During this time in the United States, there were 12.5 million cases of acquired rubella. There were also 11,000 fetal deaths, and 20,000 infants were born with defects consistent with CRS, 2,100 of whom died. After the introduction of routine vaccination during infancy, rubella activity has decreased by 99 percent. In recent years, however, rubella outbreaks have occurred in prisons, colleges and universities, hospitals, and among office workers. In community epidemics, attack rates in susceptible persons are estimated to range from 50 to 90 percent.

Humans are the only natural host for rubella. It is spread by the respiratory route, and infected persons shed large concentrations of the virus from the nose and throat. Rubella occurs seasonally, mostly in the winter and spring months. In adults, more cases of rubella are reported in women than in men, but this finding may be more related to the concern for CRS than a true difference on the basis of sex.

CLINICAL FEATURES

Postnatally acquired rubella infection is generally a very benign, exanthemous infection, and symptoms are typically more pronounced in adults than in children. The incubation period is usually from 14 to 21 days. In children, there are typically no prodromal symptoms; the first symptom is usually the rash.

In older persons, however, the rash is usually preceded by 1 to 5 days of prodromal symptoms, which may include low-grade fever, headache, malaise, anorexia, mild conjunctivitis and eye pain, coryza, pharyngitis, cough, and tender lymphadenopathy (suboccipital, postauricular, or cervical nodes). An enanthem (Forchheimer spots), consisting of small, red macules on the soft palate, occasionally precedes or accompanies the rash.

Once the exanthem becomes apparent, the prodromal symptoms subside. The characteristic rash is pruritic, appears erythematous and maculopapular, and lasts 1 to 5 days or longer. In contrast to the measles exanthem, the rash is usually less coppery and pinker in appearance and heals with desquamation or brownish discoloration.

The duration of illness in uncomplicated rubella is variable. Most patients would continue normal activity if the rash were not present. In general, full return to normal activity occurs within 3 days. Treatment is symptomatic.

NEUROLOGIC COMPLICATIONS

Neurologic sequelae of rubella infection are uncommon; a conservative estimate of the complication rate is approximately 1 in 5,000 to 6,000 cases. These usually take the form of CRS in children or an encephalitis or encephalomyelitis in acquired infections of both children and adults.

Congenital Rubella Syndrome

CRS is a multisystem disease characterized by intrauterine growth retardation, cataracts, chorioretinitis, congenital heart disease, sensorineural deafness, hepatosplenomegaly, jaundice, anemia, thrombocytopenia, and rash.

Approximately 5 to 25 percent of women of childbearing age do not have rubella antibodies and therefore are at risk for primary infection. Transplacental transmission of the infection occurs via maternal viremia.

Although as many as two-thirds of proven congenitally infected infants may be asymptomatic at birth, almost 75 percent of these will develop long-term sequelae within the first 5 years of life. However, clinical manifestations, when present, are often very apparent (Table 75-1). Growth retardation is apparent at birth. Eye findings are frequent and include cataracts (usually present at birth), pigmentary or "salt-and-pepper" retinopathy (Fig. 75-1), microphthalmia (usually unilateral), and congenital glaucoma. Sensorineural hearing loss, which is most often bilateral, is another very frequent finding; some degree of hearing loss is noted in almost all patients. Cardiac findings may be a cause of early infant morbidity and mortality and include myocarditis and a variety of structural anomalies.

TABLE 75-1. Manifestations of Congenital Rubella Syndrome

Manifestation	Percent
Deafness	67
Heart disease	48
Psychomotor retardation	45
Chorioretinitis	39
Thrombocytopenia	22
Bilateral cataracts	15
Unilateral cataracts	13
Spasticity	12
Glaucoma	3

(Modified from Cooper LZ, Ziring PR, Ockerse AB et al: Rubella: clinical manifestations and management. Am J Dis Child 118:18, 1969, with permission.)

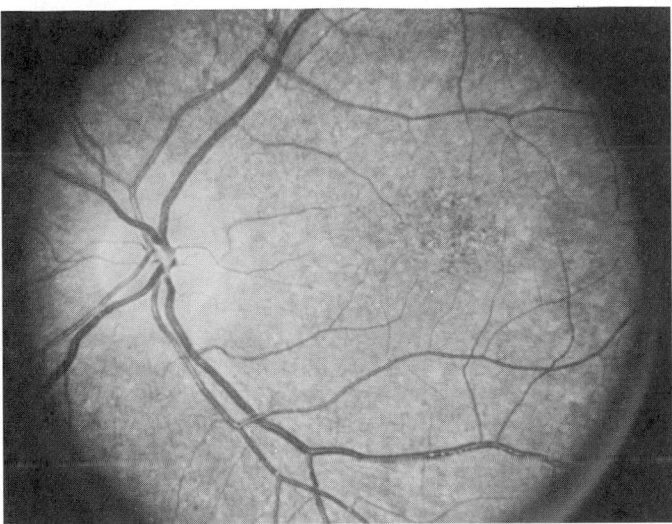

FIG. 75-1. Rubella "salt-and-pepper" retinopathy. (Courtesy of Dr. Richard A. Lewis, Baylor College of Medicine, Houston, Texas.)

Central nervous system manifestations in congenitally infected infants are pervasive. Signs and symptoms may occur at birth or become apparent as the child grows and matures. Ten to 20 percent of congenitally infected infants have active meningoencephalitis at birth. Findings may include a large, full, or bulging anterior fontanel, irritability, hypotonia, seizures (usually not observed until after the neonatal period), lethargy, disturbances of tone, and head retraction with arching of the back. The seizures, which may occur in 25 percent of infected infants, are most commonly minor motor seizures or abrupt vasomotor changes. Cerebrospinal fluid (CSF) examination reveals an elevated protein content and a mild pleocytosis; rubella virus can often be isolated from the CSF.

By 1 to 4 months of age, affected children may demonstrate irritability, restlessness, vasomotor instability, photophobia, opisthotonic posturing, and developmental delay. Remarkably, however, between 6 and 12 months of age, approximately one-half of these infants appear to improve and acquire developmental milestones.

Later neurologic disease, such as mental and motor retardation, can be related to the severity and persistence of the initial meningoencephalitis. Active central nervous system infection has been demonstrated for 1 year of more, and rubella virus has been isolated from the CSF as long as 18 months after birth.

Behavior disorders frequently are seen in children with deafness but often cannot always be associated with a preceding meningoencephalitis. Reactive behavior disorders and infantile autism may occur. Children with CRS and generalized growth retardation, but a proportionally small head size, often have normal intelligence. In contrast, the prognosis for mental development in a child with true microcephaly is poor.

Acquired Adult Rubella

Rubella can be associated with postinfectious encephalitis and/or myelitis. Postrubella encephalomyelitis tends to be a more severe but shorter illness than measles postinfectious encephalitides. This entity is an acute demyelinating, possibly autoimmune, disease, with numerous foci of demyelination (surrounding small- and medium-sized vessels) throughout the brain and spinal cord.

The onset of the encephalomyelitic syndrome most often occurs 2 to 4 days after the appearance of rash, but occasionally rash and neurologic symptoms occur at the same time; in other instances, the appearance of encephalitis is delayed as much as 1 week after the onset of illness. Typically, the rash is fading and other symptoms are improving when the patient suddenly develops a recrudescence of fever, headache, neck stiffness, convulsions, stupor, and deepening coma. Coma and seizures are more frequent than in measles encephalitis and carry a poor prognosis. Other less common manifestations include hemiplegia and evidence of cerebellar disease (such as ataxia) and occasionally spinal cord disease. With spinal cord involvement, there may be partial or complete paraplegia or quadriplegia, diminution or loss of reflexes, sensory impairment, and varying degrees of paralysis of bladder and bowel. Myoclonic movements or choreoathetosis may be observed.

The mortality rate for rubella encephalomyelitis is approximately 20 percent, and most patients die early in the course of the illness, usually in the first 3 days. Despite the gravity of the illness, recovery is usually complete, with most cases returning to baseline neurologic function is approximately 2 weeks.

Another grave illness associated with rubella is a progressive rubella panencephalitis syndrome, which is now rare; no new cases have been reported in the last decade. Four to 14 years after either a congenital or acquired rubella infection, patients developed a progressive, insidious dementia, often associated with seizures. Clumsiness of gait was an early symptom, followed by a frank ataxia of gait and then of the limbs. Death usually occurred 3 to 8 years after the onset of new neurologic symptoms.

Thus, it appears that rubella virus infection, acquired in utero or in the postnatal period, may persist in the nervous system for years before rekindling into a chronic active infection. Finally, there are other less common entities previously associated with rubella infection that bear mentioning. These include transverse myelitis, carotid artery thrombosis, optic neuritis, polyradiculopathy, polyneuropathy (such as carpal tunnel syndrome), and Guillain-Barré syndrome. Most of these manifestations occur within 1 to 2 weeks after rubella infection. Rubella vaccine has also been associated with a polyneuropathy and a myeloradiculoneuritis.

DIAGNOSIS

Diagnosis of congenital rubella infection at birth can be accomplished by isolation of the virus from nasopharynx, urine, stool, buffy coat of the blood, or CSF or by demonstration of an elevated IgM level at birth identified as specific rubella antibody. Retrospective diagnosis of congenital rubella infection in older children may be suggested by administering rubella vaccine. In seronegative children with congenital rubella, only 10 percent respond with a rise in titer of hemagglutination-inhibition antibodies, as opposed to 98 percent of nonimmune normal children.

Postnatally acquired disease can be diagnosed by viral isolation from nasal or throat specimens, by a significant change in hemagglutination-inhibition antibodies (classically, the most standard diagnostic test), by enzyme-linked immunosorbent assay values or neutralizing antibody titers, or by the demonstration of specific IgM rubella antibody in a single serum sample.

Examination of the CSF in rubella encephalomyelitis usually reveals a mild pleocytosis (20 to 100 cells/mm), with most cells being lymphocytes. The protein content is normal or slightly elevated, and the sugar concentration is normal.

In rubella panencephalitis, the CSF shows a mild increase in cells (lymphocytes), a modest elevation of protein, and a marked increase in the proportion of gamma globulin (35 to 52 percent of total protein), which assumes an oligoclonal pattern when analyzed by agarose gel electrophoresis. The CSF and serum rubella antibody titers are elevated. Electroencephalograms have shown consistent abnormalities consisting of high-voltage slow-wave activity without the periodicity characteristic of subacute sclerosing panencephalitis. Pathologic examination of the brain has shown a widespread, progressive subacute panencephalitis, mainly affecting the white matter. No inclusion-bearing cells have been seen.

TREATMENT

Unfortunately, no specific treatment exists for either CRS or progressive rubella panencephalitis syndrome. Steroids have sometimes been tried for postrubella encephalomyelitis, as with other forms of postinfectious immune-mediated inflammatory syndromes, but their value is unclear. Care is primarily supportive in these cases. Isoprinosine (Inosiplex) and other antiviral agents have not been found to be effective.

SUGGESTED READINGS

Connolly JH, Hutchinson WM, Allen IV et al: Carotid artery thrombosis, encephalitis, myelitis and optic neuritis associated with rubella virus infections. Brain 98:583, 1975

Menkes JH: Textbook of Child Neurology. 4th Ed. Lea & Febiger, Philadelphia, 1990

Swaiman KF: Pediatric Neurology, Principles and Practice. 2nd Ed. CV Mosby, St. Louis, 1993

Townsend JJ, Baringer JR, Wolinsky JS et al: Progressive rubella panencephalitis. N Engl J Med 292:990, 1975

Wolinsky JS, Berg BO, Maitland CJ: Progressive rubella panencephalitis. Arch Neurol 33:722, 1976

76. HIV INFECTION AND DISEASES OF THE BRAIN

BRADLEY K. EVANS

Human immunodeficiency virus (HIV) is an RNA virus. When it infects a cell, its RNA enters the cell and is reverse transcribed to DNA. Reverse transcription is the step of infection affected by the Therapeutic agents zidovudine (AZT), zalcitabine (dideoxycytosine), didanosine (dideoxyinosine) and most other drugs currently available for the treatment of HIV infection.

After HIV RNA is reverse transcribed to DNA, some of this DNA is inserted into the cell's genome. From the safety of the cell's nucleus, the DNA can produce viruses and virus-related material until the cell dies. The strategy of the HIV virus is to control the production of viruses very carefully so that the cell survives for a long time. This is a "slow virus" infection.

One important viral protein made by an infected cell is gp160, a large protein that extends through the cell's plasma membrane. In the course of normal processing, gp160 is cleaved to gp120 and gp41. These two proteins provide a way for HIV to infect cells and thus represent a key step in the pathogenesis of infection. The larger protein, gp120, binds to a helper T lymphocyte and monocyte cell surface protein called CD4; the smaller one, gp41, is responsible for the fusion of lipid membranes that allows the viral RNA to enter cells. Many HIV vaccine candidates are variants of the gp160 or gp120 proteins.

HIV TESTING

Common diagnostic tests for HIV infection are the HIV antibody test and the p24 antigen test. The HIV antibody test is sensitive and specific for HIV infection. It actually refers to two tests: an enzyme-linked immunosorbent assay (ELISA), which, if positive, is followed by a Western blot. The ELISA alone has many false-positive results. The western blot is technically difficult to perform, making it unfeasible to do routinely. In the Western blot, many problems of interpretation can arise. If the patient's serum contains antibodies to normal cell proteins, the Western blot may show abnormal bands that can be mistaken for bands caused by anti-HIV antibodies.

A major problem with all HIV antibody tests is that anti-HIV antibodies may not appear in the serum for a highly variable period of time after the initial infection, typically weeks to a few months. This period of HIV infection, in which a patient is infected but anti-HIV antibodies cannot be detected, is popularly called the "window." Diagnosis during the window period may require repeating the HIV antibody test a few months later, or using a diagnostic test that relies upon detection of HIV antigens, instead of antibody. The common HIV antigen tested for is p24. This is a viral protein contained within infected cells, within viral particles, and, sometimes, free in serum. The p24 antigen is detectable only in very early or very late infections, when antigen is in excess compared to antibody. Most of the time, in HIV-infected patients, p24 antigen is negative because antibody is in excess. The p24 antigen test's practical usefulness is limited to diagnosis of HIV infection during the window period.

The "CD4 count" refers to an enumeration of peripherally circulating lymphocytes that express the CD4 antigen on their surface. Functionally, these are T-helper cells. In normal, uninfected people, the CD4 count is usually 500 to 1,600 cells/mm^3. Early in HIV infection, the CD4 count often transiently drops, and then, late in infection, the CD4 count reliably decreases, reflecting the inexorable depletion of T-helper lymphocytes by HIV infection. A low CD4 count correlates highly with impaired immune function, that is, patients with opportunistic infections almost always have a CD4 count less than 200/mm^3. Recently, the CD4 count has become accepted as a "surrogate marker" for gauging the severity of HIV infection. In an HIV-infected patient, a CD4 count less than 200/mm^3, by itself, indicates full-blown acquired immunodeficiency syndrome (AIDS). Serial CD4 counts are used to monitor the success of treatment with antiretroviral drugs; a sudden decrease in the CD4 count may prompt a change in antiretroviral therapy. However, the CD4 count can fluctuate in response to factors other than HIV infection. For example, other viral infections can result in fewer circulating CD4 cells. Comparing the CD4 count to the "CD4/CD8 ratio" (the ratio of T-helper cells to T-suppressor and T-cytotoxic cells) is often helpful in interpreting a low CD4 count. With HIV infection, the CD4 count and the CD4/CD8 ratio decrease in tandem (in AIDS, typically less than 200/mm^3 and less than 0.2, respectively); other causes of

TABLE 76-1. Human Immunodeficiency Virus Infection and Diseases of the Central Nervous System

HIV meningoencephalitis
AIDS-dementia complex
Parenchymal infections
    Toxoplasmosis
    Progressive multifocal leukoencephalopathy
    Focal encephalitis
    Syphilitic gumma
    Tuberculoma
    Cryptococcoma
    Nocardial abscess
Central nervous system lymphoma
Ischemic stroke
Meningeal infections
    Acute meningitis
    Chronic meningitis

Abbreviations: HIV, human immunodeficiency virus; AIDS, acquired immunodeficiency syndrome.

a low CD4 count usually are also associated with a decreased number of CD8-positive lymphocytes, leaving the CD4/CD8 ratio in its normal range (0.5 to 2.0).

Other tests, such as viral culture, virus quantitation in plasma, acidified p24 antigen test, polyethylene glycol precipitation, and various polymerase chain reaction techniques are, at the moment, research tools only. One or more of these tests, or variations of them, may eventually replace either the HIV antibody test or the CD4 count because of the problems discussed above.

Table 76-1 lists the central nervous system diseases that are commonly associated with HIV infection and AIDS.

HIV MENINGOENCEPHALITIS

Even at the time of primary infection, HIV is present in the brain of most patients. By the time of AIDS, the virus titer in the brain is higher than in any other organ. However, most patients with HIV infection have no neurologic complaints, and most have a normal neurologic examination and unremarkable neuroimaging. Even when the patient is asymptomatic, however, the cerebrospinal fluid (CSF) may show a range of abnormalities: a pleocytosis of up to 50 mononuclear cells/mm^3, a protein level up to 100 mg/ml, oligoclonal bands, and, sometimes, hypoglycorrhachia. These CSF abnormalities may be present at any time during infection. In fact, CSF pleocytosis becomes less common as the illness progresses.

Any time during the illness, but particularly at 1 month after primary infection, patients may have a mononucleosis-like illness that may present with any combination of headache, meningismus, fever, altered mental status, and isolated cranial nerve palsies. Investigation shows only a CSF lymphocytic pleocytosis. The diagnosis may be complicated since the HIV antibody test may not become positive for weeks or a few months after this illness. Treatment is symptomatic.

AIDS-DEMENTIA COMPLEX

This illness is also called HIV encephalitis, HIV dementia, and HIV-associated cognitive/motor complex. The diagnosis of AIDS-dementia complex (ADC) is an AIDS-defining illness. Although sometimes the patient's CD4 count is as high as 500/mm^3, ADC is more common the lower the CD4 count is. ADC is the most frequent neurologic diagnosis in AIDS patients.

The pathophysiology of ADC is not known, but some pathologic and laboratory data, and a complicated chain of reasoning,

implicate excitotoxicity as a possible mechanism. In the white matter of the cerebral hemispheres of patients with ADC, there are "microglial nodules." These are collections of microglial cells and monocytes, both cell types infected with HIV. Multinucleated giant cells may also be seen in the white matter of patients with severe ADC. These cells are thought to be the result of fusion of infected cells with adjacent cells, perhaps mediated by gp41 on the surface of the infected cells. The severity of dementia correlates with the number of microglial nodules and the presence of multinucleated giant cells, and these are the only brain cells definitely known to be infected with HIV. These infected cells release gp120 and cytokines, which can induce an astroglial enzyme, indoleamine-2, 3-dioxygenase. This is the key enzyme in the synthesis of an N-methyl-D-aspartic acid (NMDA) receptor agonist, quinolinic acid. Quinolinic acid is increased in the CSF of patients with ADC. In certain neurons, excessive NMDA agonist activity causes intracellular calcium to rise and the neurons to die (excitotoxicity). In fact, there are fewer neurons in the cerebral cortices of AIDS patients than in uninfected controls, supporting the idea that excitotoxicity may play a role in the pathophysiology of ADC.

Clinical Manifestations

Common early complaints are memory problems, slowed thinking, and apathy. The usual memory tasks (three-object recall, serial sevens, and spelling words backward) are usually performed accurately. Patients have difficulty with verbal fluency tests (e.g., name as many fruits as possible in 30 seconds; as a general rule, the ability to name 10 or more fruits in 30 seconds is normal, 5 to 9 is mildly impaired, and 0 to 4 is consistent with moderate or severe dementia). Complex motor tasks (grooved pegboard, trailmaking, and timed walking) are performed slowly, too. Patients may have an unsteady gait, sometimes severe enough to suggest that the patient has vacuolar myelopathy.

Besides this common presentation of mental slowness, patients may present with fulminant psychosis. These patients have grossly disturbed thinking, often with extreme agitation, sexual impulsivity, and violence. In the late stages of ADC, patients become apathetic, withdrawn, and eventually quadriparetic and bedridden.

Patients do not necessarily progress inexorably to the late stage. A patient's clinical condition can fluctuate remarkably over weeks or months, sometimes because of changes in treatment, but sometimes for no apparent reason.

In ADC, head magnetic resonance imaging shows cerebral atrophy and deep white matter hyperintensities on T2-weighted images. The hyperintensities are "fluffy" and symmetric in the cerebral hemispheres. There is no mass effect and no enhancement. These white matter changes are characteristic, but not diagnostic, of ADC. Head computed tomography may be normal or show faint white matter abnormalities and may also reveal striking atrophy (Fig. 76-1).

A lumbar puncture is often performed, primarily to exclude other conditions. In patients with ADC, as with all HIV-infected patients, the CSF may show pleocytosis, increased protein, or hypoglycorrhachia. The CSF also shows increased amounts of β-microglobulin and neopterin, which correlate with the severity of ADC. Neopterin and β-microglobulin are proteins released by activated immune cells. CSF quinolinic acid is also increased in ADC.

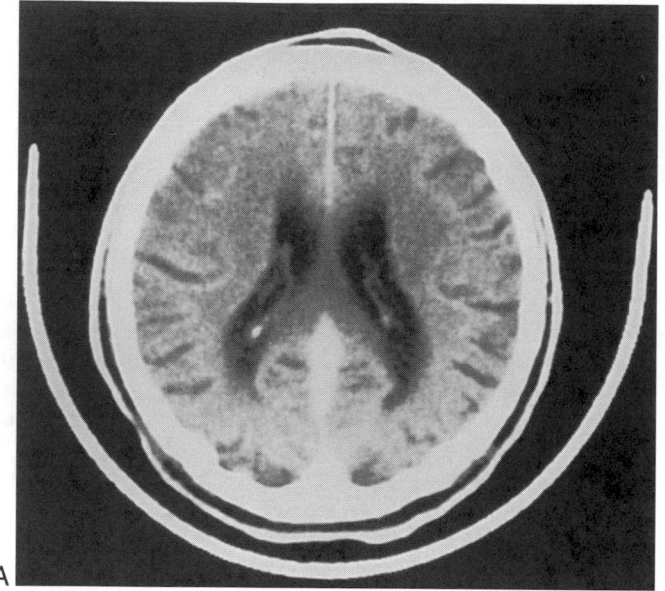 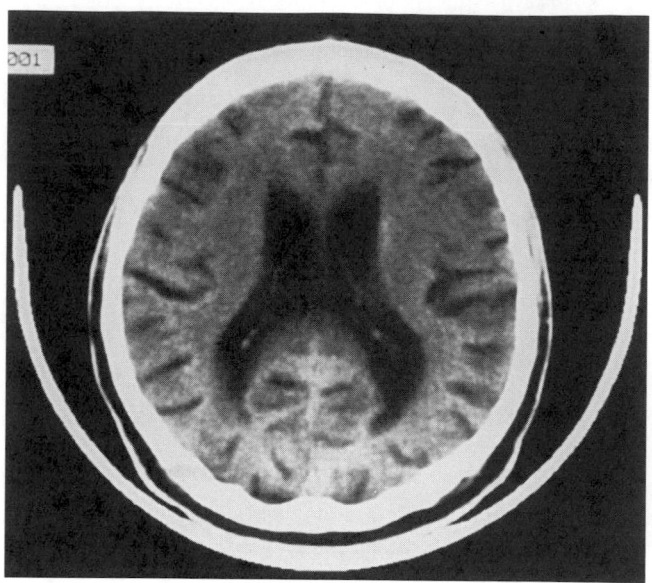

FIG. 76-1. **(A)** CT scan of a 31-year-old man with AIDS-dementia complex, showing mild diffuse atrophy. **(B)** CT scan done only 6 weeks later, showing a marked increase in the amount of atrophy. (Courtesy of Susan Weathers, M.D., Baylor College of Medicine, Houston, Texas.)

Diagnosis and Differential Diagnosis

ADC is considered a diagnosis of exclusion. The differential diagnosis of ADC is psychiatric illness (e.g., depression and mania), systemic illness, a side effect of a medication, disease of the brain parenchyma other than ADC, chronic meningitis, malnutrition, and vitamin deficiencies. Two vitamin deficiencies, thiamine deficiency and cyanocobalamin deficiency, are important to consider.

Thiamine deficiency is a treatable cause of altered mental status. AIDS patients may develop thiamine deficiency if they are alcoholic or if they have esophagitis, pancreatitis, or other gastrointestinal disease. Patients who do not eat may become thiamine deficient within a couple of weeks. These patients develop ''quiet'' confusion and motor incoordination that may be mistaken for ADC. Nystagmus and poor short-term memory are important neurologic signs of possible thiamine deficiency, but thiamine should be given to any malnourished patient thought to have ADC, whether these neurologic signs are present or not.

Vitamin B_{12} deficiency may also cause mild mental confusion and gait abnormalities similar to those seen in ADC. Patients with subacute combined degeneration have impaired vibration sensation in the lower extremities and a Romberg sign. A low serum cyanocobalamin level confirms the diagnosis.

Treatment

Treatment of ADC is with AZT. The current recommendation is that high doses—at least 1,000 mg/day—be used. Improvement may be delayed for weeks to a few months after starting treatment. AZT not only treats ADC but also prevents its development. Other antiretroviral agents have not been well studied, but they seem to be less effective than AZT.

Other possible treatments of ADC—memantine (an NMDA receptor antagonist) and nimodipine (a calcium channel blocker)—are now in clinical trials. They are based on the idea that excitotoxicity is involved in the pathophysiology of ADC.

OTHER PARENCHYMAL BRAIN DISEASES

The three most common diseases affecting the brain parenchyma are central nervous system (CNS) toxoplasmosis (see Ch. 64), CNS lymphoma, and progressive multifocal leukoencephalopathy (PML) (see Ch. 72). Other parenchymal brain diseases are neurosyphilitic gummas, tuberculomas, cryptococcomas, nocardial brain abscesses, or focal encephalitides caused by cytomegalovirus, varicella-zoster virus, or Herpes simplex virus type 1. This category also includes ischemic and embolic strokes. Ischemic strokes may be caused by vasculitis due to *Treponema pallidum,* varicella-zoster virus, hepatitis B virus, or HIV.

Any of these diseases might present primarily with altered mental status and mimic ADC. Seizures, headaches, papilledema, and focal or lateralizing findings on neurologic examination are indications that the patient may have a parenchymal brain disease.

Neuroimaging studies are usually abnormal, showing focal or multifocal disease, sometimes with mass effect and enhancement. CNS toxoplasmosis and CNS lymphoma cause multifocal lesions with mass effect and enhancement; these are not seen with PML. The other parenchymal diseases cause variable amounts of mass effect and enhancement. Cryptococcomas usually are multiple, cystic, and located in the basal ganglia (Fig. 76-2). Lumbar puncture is contraindicated when the neuroimaging studies show a large mass effect.

Diagnosis may require brain biopsy, but brain biopsy is nondiagnostic in at least 20 percent of patients. In addition, brain biopsy itself involves risk to the patient. It is sometimes better to treat mass lesions of the brain presumptively, without tissue confirmation of the diagnosis, and follow the success of treatment by clinical examination and serial neuroimaging studies. This approach is now widely accepted for CNS toxoplasmosis, when the patient has positive serologic findings and multiple mass lesions in the brain.

Treatment of CNS toxoplasmosis and PML are considered in separate chapters. CNS lymphoma is treated with chemotherapy

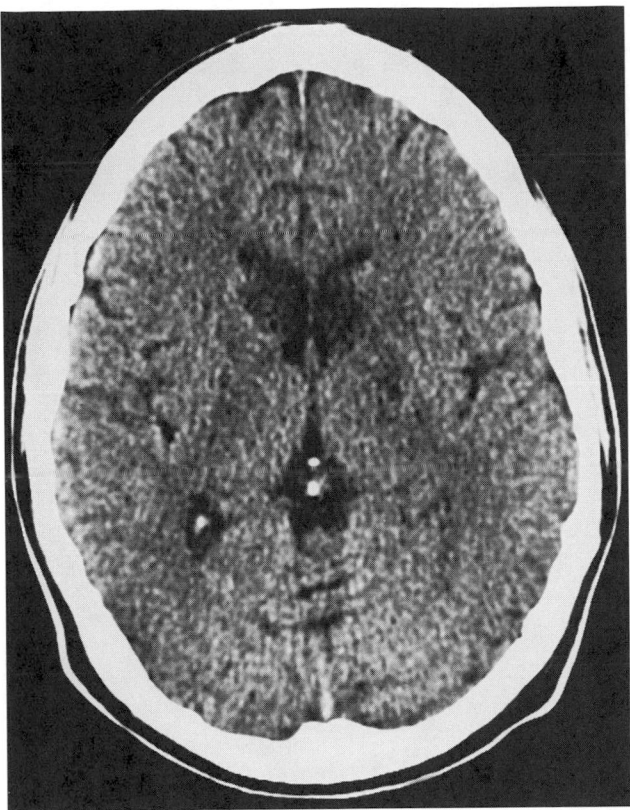

FIG. 76-2. CT scan of a patient with AIDS, showing multiple, cystic cryptococcomas located primarily in the basal ganglia. (Courtesy of Michael Hillman, M.D., and Lawrence Hutchins, M.D., The Marshfield Clinic.)

and cranial irradiation. The other diseases are treated as they are in patients who are not HIV infected, except one has to remember that higher doses and more prolonged courses of acute treatment may be needed and that maintenance therapy may be necessary.

MENINGITIS IN HIV-INFECTED PATIENTS

Among diseases that primarily affect the meninges, common presenting signs are fever, cranial nerve palsies, seizures, strokes due to vasculitis or venous thrombosis, and increased intracranial pressure (caused by obstructive hydrocephalus, nonobstructive hydrocephalus, or diffuse cerebral edema).

Acute meningitis is not common in AIDS patients, surprisingly. The most common causative organisms are *Streptococcus pneumoniae, Salmonella,* and *Listeria monocytogenes. Listeria* causes more of a subacute meningitis, with a lymphocytic pleocytosis. By Gram stain, *Listeria* organisms may be mistaken for diphtheroids. *T. pallidum* may occasionally cause acute meningitis and a polymorphonuclear pleocytosis. Patients with a gram-negative meningitis may have disseminated strongyloidiasis; fresh feces, sputum, and CSF should be specifically examined for the motile larvae of *Strongyloides stercoralis.* Treatment of these infections is the same as for patients who are not HIV infected.

Chronic meningitis is most commonly due to *Cryptococcus neoformans,* but *Mycobacterium tuberculosis, T. pallidum,* lymphoma, *Histoplasma capsulatum, Coccidioides immitis, L. monocytogenes,* cytomegalovirus, herpes zoster, and herpes simplex type 2 can also cause CSF lymphocytic pleocytosis.

Only 25 percent of AIDS patients with cryptococcal meningitis have meningeal signs. Some patients have normal CSF cell counts, protein, and glucose. Diagnostic tests are serum cryptococcal antigen (positive in 90 to 99 percent of AIDS patients with cryptococcal meningitis), blood fungal culture, CSF cryptococcal antigen, India ink examination of CSF, and CSF fungal culture. Rheumatoid factor can cause a false-positive cryptococcal antigen test result unless the CSF or serum is specifically pretreated to eliminate this possibility. Cryptococcal antigen tests can also be falsely negative in the presence of extremely high titers of antigen (prozone phenomenon). Serial dilutions should be done to show positivity at higher titers. Treatment of cryptococcal meningitis in AIDS patients requires acute treatment and maintenance therapy. In patients treated with fluconazole as maintenance therapy, there is a 3 percent relapse rate within the first 3 months.

Neurosyphilis in HIV-infected patients presents special problems in diagnosis and treatment. Neurosyphilis may present at any stage of HIV infection. Interpretation of CSF studies in HIV-infected patients is complicated by the fact that many of these patients have a CSF pleocytosis due to the HIV infection. Serologic tests for syphilis and the specific antitreponemal tests (such as FTA-Abs) rely upon the patient producing antibody, but antibody production may be impaired in patients with AIDS. These serologic tests also may show a prozone phenomenon, that is, a positive test is only seen at high titers, when serial dilutions are done. The polymerase chain reaction test for syphilis is, so far, experimental. Early versions of this test show a lack of sensitivity for detection of syphilis.

The usual treatment of early syphilis is associated with a high rate of failure in HIV-infected patients. Failure is often manifest as neurosyphilis, particularly meningitis and strokes. High-dose intravenous penicillin G treatment for neurosyphilis may also be associated with a high rate of treatment failure.

Because of these diagnostic and treatment problems in HIV-infected patients, because syphilis can be clinically evident at any stage of HIV infection, and because HIV and syphilis are sexually transmitted diseases, it is recommended that all patients diagnosed with syphilis have HIV testing, and all patients with HIV have testing for syphilis.

PROBLEMS IN DIAGNOSIS

Mental confusion and headaches in an HIV-infected patient can be due to a bewildering variety of diseases. By the history and examination alone, it is often not possible to reach a definite diagnosis. For the most common diseases, that is, ADC, CNS toxoplasmosis, CNS lymphoma, PML, and cryptococcal meningitis, there is great overlap in their clinical features (Table 76-2).

"HIBGIA"—Sometimes Useful in Diagnosis

One principle sometimes helpful in diagnosis is called "HIBGIA" ("Had it before, got it again"). This refers to the fact that disease recurrence is common in AIDS patients because of failure of acute therapy, failure of maintenance therapy, or failure to take maintenance therapy. By this principle, if a patient had a disease, particularly an infectious disease, and now has new neurologic complaints, then it is likely that the patient has recurrence of the disease. As an example, if a patient was previously treated for syphilis and now has neurologic complaints, then neurosyphilis is a primary consideration as a diagnosis.

TABLE 76-2. Human Immunodeficiency Virus Infection and the Central Nervous System[a]

Disease	Percent[b]	Onset	Altered Mental Status (%)	Headache (%)	Focal Signs (%)	Seizures (%)	Other (%)
None	—	—	0	20	0	2	—
ADC	33	Varies	100	20	0	2	—
CNS toxo	10	Days	75	50	75	25	Fever 50%, (+) serology >95
CNS lymph	2	Days-weeks	75	50	75	25	—
PML	2	Wks-months	50	20	95	10	—
Cryptomeningitis	10	Weeks	25	75	10	10	Fever 75, (+) serum CRAG

Abbreviations: ADC = acquired immunodeficiency syndrome-dementia complex; CNS toxo = CNS toxoplasmosis; CNS lymph = CNS lymphoma; PML = progressive multifocal leukoencephalopathy; CRAG = cryptococcal antigen.
[a] Percentages are approximate.
[b] Percentage of patients who will develop the disease.

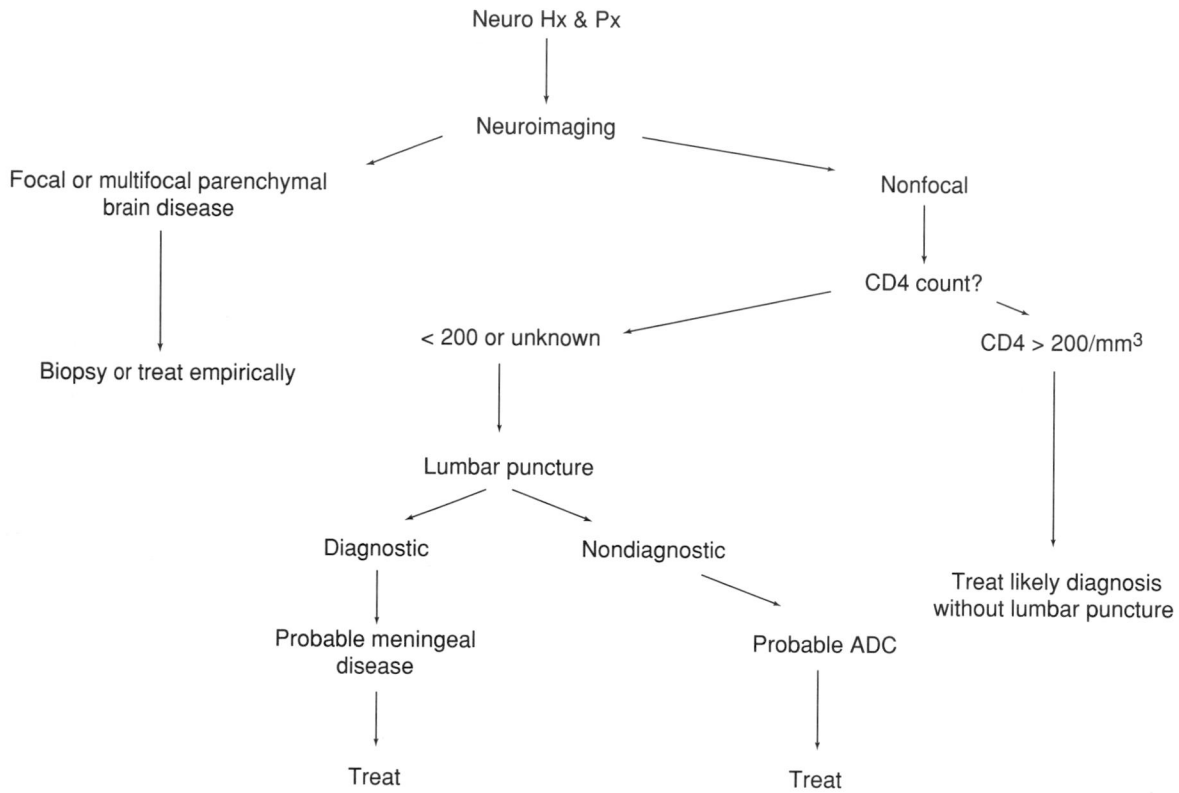

FIG. 76-3. Approach to the diagnosis of patients with HIV infection and central nervous system symptoms.

Lumbar Puncture in AIDS Patients

The lumbar puncture can be hazardous in HIV-infected patients. Such patients may have parenchymal brain disease with mass effect and be asymptomatic or relatively asymptomatic. For that reason, neuroimaging should be done first, before the lumbar puncture, in all HIV-infected patients. For patients with a large amount of mass effect, lumbar puncture is contraindicated.

The CSF can be difficult to interpret in HIV-infected patients, and careful thought should be given to what information is needed from the lumbar puncture. An opening pressure should be obtained every time, since many CNS diseases in AIDS patients are complicated by increased intracranial pressure. An increased CSF white cell count (more than 5/mm³) is seen in 25 percent of HIV-infected patients undergoing a diagnostic lumbar puncture, an increased CSF protein level (more than 50 mg/dl) in 50 percent, and hypoglycorrhachia in 10 percent. Since hypoglycorrhachia is so common, a concomitant blood glucose level should be obtained with every lumbar puncture

to be able to evaluate a low CSF glucose level. Even when one or more of these abnormalities are present, it still may not be possible to reach a definite diagnosis.

An Approach To Clinical Diagnosis

Based on the above information, the diagnostic strategy shown in Figure 76-3 is suggested. The neuroimaging study itself, and not just the report of the study, should be reviewed by the clinician.

SUGGESTED READINGS

Gordon SM, Eaton ME, George R et al: The response of symptomatic neuro-syphilis to high-dose intravenous penicillin G in patients with human immunodeficiency virus infection. N Engl J Med 331:1469–73, 1994
Hollander H, McGuire D, Burack JH: Diagnostic lumbar puncture in HIV-infected patients: analysis of 138 cases. Am J Med 96:223–8, 1994
Sidtis JJ, Gatsonis, Price RW et al: Zidovudine treatment of the AIDS dementia complex: results of a placebo-controlled trial. Ann Neurol 33:343–9, 1993
Simpson DM, Tagliati M: Neurologic manifestations of HIV infection (Review). Ann Intern Med 121:769–85, 1994

Worley JM, Price RW: Management of neurologic complications of HIV-1 infection and AIDS. pp. 193–217. In Sande MA, Volberding PA (eds): The Medical Management of AIDS. 3rd Ed. WB Saunders, Philadelphia, 1992

77. HIV INFECTION AND DISEASES OF THE SPINAL CORD, NERVE ROOTS, PERIPHERAL NERVES, AND MUSCLE

BRADLEY K. EVANS

In patients with acquired immunodeficiency syndrome (AIDS), three common reasons for neurologic consultation are gait instability, painful feet, and urinary retention with inability to walk. These are usually due to disease of the spinal cord (vacuolar myelopathy), peripheral nerves (distal sensory polyneuropathy), and nerve roots (cytomegalovirus [CMV] polyradiculitis), respectively. In addition to these common syndromes, human immunodeficiency virus (HIV)-infected patients can also develop other neuropathies and myopathies.

VACUOLAR MYELOPATHY

Vacuolar myelopathy is the most common cause of walking problems in HIV-infected patients. Patients tend to have a CD4 count less than 200/mm^3, but the CD4 count may occasionally be as high as 500/mm^3. Vacuolar myelopathy is a unique spinal cord syndrome, seen only in HIV-infected patients. Despite this strong association with HIV infection, the exact pathophysiology is not known. There is no effective treatment. Over several months, walking deteriorates, and patients eventually need gait assistance and sometimes a wheelchair.

Clinical Manifestations

Symptoms begin with gait instability, which is slowly progressive over several weeks. The upper extremities are not affected. Some patients notice proximal weakness, but there is no urinary incontinence, except perhaps in the latest stages of the illness.

Neurologic abnormalities are confined to the lower extremities and are symmetric. The gait is wide based and unsteady. Patients are unable to tandem walk, but they do not have a Romberg sign. Patients have proximal weakness, brisk reflexes, and bilateral Babinski toe signs. Sensation, including vibration sensation, is normal or nearly normal.

Neuroimaging is unremarkable. The cerebrospinal fluid (CSF) may show mild pleocytosis, slightly increased protein level, and, sometimes, a slight hypoglycorrhachia, but these CSF findings are nonspecific and usually are not helpful in the diagnosis.

Diagnosis and Differential Diagnosis

This clinical pattern is sufficiently distinctive to be virtually diagnostic, and any patient with these clinical findings should be suspected of being HIV infected. Somewhat similar clinical pictures can be seen in spinal cord compression, subacute combined degeneration, and cervical stenosis.

Patients with spinal cord compression usually present more acutely with walking problems. They may have back pain and tenderness, urinary incontinence, or asymmetric findings suggesting a partial Brown-Séquard syndrome. A patient with any one of these findings should have neuroimaging of the spinal canal. Lymphoma is the most common cause of spinal cord compression in AIDS patients, and neuroimaging may also be indicated in patients with lymphoma who have typical findings of vacuolar myelopathy.

HIV-infected patients have an increased risk of developing vitamin B$_{12}$ deficiency. Macrocytosis and pancytopenia, typical clues to this diagnosis, may either be absent or wrongly attributed to HIV infection or its treatment. Because vitamin B$_{12}$ deficiency is treatable, a serum vitamin B$_{12}$ level should be done in all patients suspected of having vacuolar myelopathy. Although patients with subacute combined degeneration have a similar gait instability, they also have marked loss of vibration sensation and the Romberg sign, which are not seen in vacuolar myelopathy.

Subacute combined degeneration and vacuolar myelopathy are very similar pathologically. Because of this, it seemed that vacuolar myelopathy might be the result of abnormal vitamin B$_{12}$ metabolism in these patients (despite their normal serum vitamin B$_{12}$ levels). Further study has shown that plasma and urinary homocysteine and methylmalonic acid values are normal in these patients, and that cyanocobalamin, l-methionine, or a combination of the two are not effective treatments for vacuolar myelopathy. Some HIV-infected patients, who were already receiving adequate cyanocobalamin treatment for vitamin B$_{12}$ deficiency, have developed vacuolar myelopathy. The pathogenesis of vacuolar myelopathy thus remains unknown.

Cervical stenosis may also mimic vacuolar myelopathy. Patients with cervical stenosis tend to have distal, not proximal, lower extremity weakness. Neuroimaging tests establish the diagnosis of cervical stenosis.

Because most patients with vacuolar myelopathy have proximal weakness, physicians may diagnostically consider a treatable myopathy or neuropathy. Sometimes, a patient has an elevated serum creatine kinase level or other evidence of a myopathy or has electrodiagnostic findings suggesting a concomitant neuropathy, but, even in these patients, treatment of the myopathy or neuropathy does not usually improve walking.

DISTAL SENSORY, SYMMETRIC POLYNEUROPATHY

Distal sensory, symmetric polyneuropathy (DSP) is common in patients with AIDS, particularly in those with very low CD4 counts. DSP is an axonal, "dying-back" polyneuropathy, with pathologic changes not only in the distal peripheral nerve but also in the fasciculus gracilis in the cervical spinal cord. It is assumed that HIV itself causes DSP, but how it does is not known. Why some AIDS patients—about 30 percent—have DSP, but others do not, also is unknown.

Clinical Manifestations

Patients with DSP have dysesthesias in their feet. They may suffer pain, burning, coldness, aching, or just uncomfortable feelings, and walking is painful. They may present in a wheelchair with a primary complaint of "inability to walk."

There may be no neurologic abnormalities, or patients may have a "stocking" loss of light touch and pinprick sensations. Pain sensation remains intact. If there is sensory loss, it does not extend much above the ankles. Ankle jerks often are lost. Clinical abnormalities progress either very slowly or not at all. Patients developing signs of a more severe neuropathy (such as weakness in the lower extremities or any neurologic abnormality in the upper extremities) do not have DSP, but another type of peripheral neuropathy.

In DSP, electrodiagnostic tests, if they are done, are normal or show only mild distal denervation changes.

Diagnosis and Differential Diagnosis

Any mild peripheral neuropathy can cause complaints and neurologic findings similar to DSP. For instance, diabetes mellitus and alcoholism, the most common causes of peripheral neuropathies, frequently produce neuropathies in HIV-infected patients, too.

Medications can cause a peripheral neuropathy, which, in its early stages, can mimic DSP. In HIV-infected patients, the most commonly implicated drugs are zalcitabine (dideoxycytosine or ddC) vincristine, and isoniazid. The neuropathy due to ddC is not only dose related but also dependent upon individual susceptibility. However, it is not possible to predict who will develop a neuropathy from ddC. Treatment consists of stopping the drug, but the neuropathy may continue to worsen (or "coast") for up to 8 weeks after ddC is stopped. The neuropathy of vincristine is also related both to dose and to individual susceptibility. For some of these patients, vincristine neuropathy may be extremely severe, resembling Guillain-Barré syndrome. Isoniazid neuropathy can vary from a mild peripheral neuropathy to a fulminant syndrome of encephalopathy and diffuse weakness. Patients with a pre-existing neuropathy, and who are malnourished and alcoholic, are particularly susceptible. Pyridoxine (vitamin B_6) 100 mg/day, given with isoniazid, helps prevent neuropathy and does not diminish isoniazid's antimycobacterial actions. Preventative treatment with pyridoxine is important, since, for serious tuberculous infections, there may be no practical alternative to isoniazid, even when a patient develops a neuropathy.

Treatment

In general, treatment of DSP is symptomatic; however, there is an ongoing clinical trial of nerve growth factor treatment to see if this will directly improve the neuropathy. As far as symptomatic treatment for DSP is concerned, amitriptyline is most commonly prescribed, usually beginning at 25 mg at bedtime and increasing to 100 to 150 mg at bedtime. Its side effects are mental confusion, orthostatic hypotension, and urinary retention. Mexiletine, clonazepam, and capsaicin cream are useful alternatives to amitriptyline for some patients. Opiates are also effective.

CYTOMEGALOVIRUS POLYRADICULITIS

This syndrome occurs exclusively in patients with AIDS, usually when the CD4 count is less than 50/mm³. In fact, many patients are being treated for a CMV infection elsewhere in the body at the time this illness begins.

Clinical Manifestations

The first complaint is either inability to walk or urinary retention. Symptoms progress over a few days to a couple of weeks; so patients may develop both problems. In addition to these primary complaints, about one-half of patients have superficial pain and dysesthesias in the pelvic girdle area. In the full-blown syndrome, patients have severe proximal weakness, loss of sensation in a bathing-trunk distribution, loss of knee jerks, and a large, flaccid urinary bladder.

Diagnosis and Differential Diagnosis

If diagnosed early, this is a treatable condition. Suspicion of CMV polyradiculitis should arise if the patient has an extremely low CD4 count, known CMV infection elsewhere in the body, rapid onset of proximal weakness, urinary retention, pain and dysesthesias of the proximal lower extremities, or any combination of these findings.

The diagnostic test is a lumbar puncture. The CSF shows a polymorphonuclear pleocytosis (usually more than 100/mm³) and hypoglycorrhachia. About one-half of the time, CMV can be cultured from the CSF. Since neurosyphilis, human T-cell lymphotrophic virus type I, and lymphomatous meningitis can rarely cause a similar polyradiculitis, it is important to do diagnostic tests for these conditions. Other neurodiagnostic tests are only inconsistently helpful. Lumbar magnetic resonance imaging may, or may not, show contrast enhancement, suggesting inflammation of the meninges and nerve roots. Electromyogram may show denervation changes proximally, but it may not because of the acuteness of the illness.

Treatment

Untreated, a patient with CMV polyradiculitis becomes bedridden, with urinary retention. With early treatment, urinary bladder function and ability to walk can return. Treatment is high-dose ganciclovir. Patients with negative CSF culture for CMV are just as likely to respond as are those with positive cultures. If the patient is already receiving high-dose ganciclovir, foscarnet is added. Whether glucocorticoids are beneficial is not known.

INFLAMMATORY DEMYELINATING POLYNEUROPATHIES

The inflammatory demyelinating polyneuropathies include Guillain-Barré syndrome (or acute inflammatory demyelinating polyneuropathy) and chronic inflammatory demyelinating polyneuropathy (CIDP). These neuropathies tend to occur in the early or middle stages of the illness, often when the patient is not known to be HIV-infected. The neuropathy is identical to Guillain-Barré syndrome and CIDP occurring in patients who are not HIV infected. In HIV-infected patients, the CSF may show a pleocytosis; CSF pleocytosis is unusual in patients who are not HIV infected and thus is a valuable clue that the patient might have an HIV infection.

Diagnosis of HIV infection in inflammatory demyelinating neuropathies requires specific HIV testing. The HIV antibody test may be falsely normal early in the infection, when inflammatory demyelinating neuropathies often occur. Either a p24 antigen test or repeat HIV antibody test in 2 to 6 months is required for diagnosis in this situation.

Whether or not the neuropathy is associated with HIV infection, treatment options are the same: glucocorticoids (for CIDP), plasmapheresis, and gammaglobulin.

MONONEURITIS MULTIPLEX

This is a poorly understood condition, which is rare. Patients notice localized pain or sensory loss and focal weakness. If symptoms begin in a single nerve distribution, the condition may initially be misdiagnosed as a compression neuropathy. Later, neurologic deficits indicate involvement of multiple, individual nerves. Sometimes localization points to brachial or lumbar plexus lesions. Although this syndrome is vasculitic, the cause or causes are not known, but HIV, CMV, and hepatitis B virus have been implicated. Reportedly, mononeuritis multiplex early in the course of HIV infection may spontaneously remit, while mononeuritis multiplex in patients with low CD4 counts tends to progress. With progression, mononeuritis multiplex becomes symmetric and clinically resembles a generalized polyneuropathy. There is no recognized treatment for mononeuritis multiplex in HIV-infected patients. Case reports suggest that ganciclovir may be effective treatment for some patients with mononeuritis multiplex and low CD4 counts.

MYOPATHIES

In AIDS patients, weakness is most commonly due to malnutrition and concurrent illness. Proximal weakness is more commonly seen with vacuolar myelopathy than with myopathy. Although patients with vacuolar myelopathy and CMV polyradiculitis have proximal weakness, the upper extremities are spared, and there are other neurologic findings in the lower extremities that point to the correct diagnosis. In patients with a clinically important myopathy, the serum creatine kinase level is nearly always elevated. Therefore, this test is useful as a simple screening test for AIDS patients with unexplained proximal weakness. Serum creatine kinase elevations occur in AIDS patients who do not have a myopathy; so a high creatine kinase value alone, even in a patient with proximal weakness, is not diagnostic of a myopathy. In AIDS patients with myopathy, electromyography shows brief, low-amplitude muscle potentials and helps confirm the diagnosis.

There are three myopathic syndromes in HIV-infected patients: HIV wasting syndrome, inflammatory myopathy, and mitochondrial myopathy.

Patients with the HIV wasting syndrome, which is common, have loss of gluteal mass (''saggy butt syndrome''). This may be due to a myopathy, but it is usually unaccompanied by any weakness that the patient notices.

Inflammatory myopathy can occur anytime during the course of HIV infection, but it is rare. Patients complain of proximal weakness involving the upper and lower extremities. There are no sensory abnormalities. Muscle stretch reflexes are usually diminished in proportion to the weakness. The immune pathophysiology of this inflammatory myopathy is not known; HIV is not found in muscle fibers. Treatment is administration of glucocorticoids (e.g., prednisone 60 mg/day).

HIV-infected patients may also have changes in their muscle biopsies consistent with a mitochondrial myopathy (''ragged-red fibers''). The mitochondrial changes presumably reflect direct muscle toxicity of zidovudine, which inhibits mitochondrial DNA polymerase in vitro. This myopathy is more common in patients who have taken high doses (e.g., more than 1,000 mg/day) of zidovudine for more than 6 months. Now that lower daily doses of zidovudine are commonly used, this myopathy is rarely a clinical problem. The treatment is to decrease or eliminate zidovudine.

On muscle biopsy, an AIDS patient with a myopathy may have multiple abnormalities: inflammation, ragged-red fibers, and rod (or ''nemaline'') bodies. The presence of all these changes makes it difficult to know what therapy to recommend for the patient. Either glucocorticoid treatment or decreasing zidovudine can be tried first.

SUGGESTED READINGS

Dalakas M, Illa I, Pezeshkpour GH et al: Mitochondrial myopathy caused by long-term zidovudine therapy. N Engl J Med 322:1098–105, 1990

Simpson DM, Tagliati M: Neurologic manifestations of HIV infection. Ann Intern Med 121:769–85, 1994

So YT, Olney RK: Acute lumbosacral polyradiculopathy in acquired immunodeficiency syndrome: experience in 23 patients. Ann Neurol 35:53–8, 1994

Worley JM, Price RW: Management of neurologic complications of HIV-1 infection and AIDS. pp. 193–217. In Sande MA, Volberding PA (eds): The Medical Management of AIDS. 3rd Ed. WB Saunders, Philadelphia, 1992

78. HTLV-I INFECTION

ROBERT R. McKENDALL

The discovery of human T-cell lymphotrophic virus type I (HTLV-I) and its linkage to an unusual leukemia and chronic myelopathy is an extraordinary story of modern day medical scientific investigation. In 1980, Poeisz and his collaborators isolated a retrovirus from fresh lymphocytes of an American patient with cutaneous T-cell lymphoma. This was the first human retrovirus isolated, and it was called HTLV-I. A worldwide search for links between hematologic malignancies and human retroviruses ensued. In Martinique, neurologist Jean Claude Vernant noted a patient with tropical spastic paraparesis (TSP) who had serum antibodies to HTLV-I. He had a group of 25 TSP patients tested for serum HTLV-I antibodies, and 78 percent were positive. This was the first link of TSP with HTLV-I.

Independently, Mitsuhiro Osame observed multilobulated ''flower'' lymphocytes in the blood and cerebrospinal fluid CSF of some Japanese patients with spastic paraparesis. These cells were similar to the leukemic cells of adult T-cell lymphoma. Osame's patients were shown to have serum and CSF antibodies to HTLV-I, and he reported on a new clinical entity, which he named HTLV-I-associated myelopathy (HAM). Soon, the DNA from HAM cell lines was shown to be identical to DNA from adult T-cell leukemia cell lines. Finally, based on seroepidemiologic, clinical, pathologic, and viral isolation similarities, HAM and TSP were shown to be the same disease, caused by the retrovirus responsible for adult T-cell lymphoma (HTLV-I).

EPIDEMIOLOGY

Seroepidemiologic studies have expanded the known HTLV-I endemic areas far beyond the original descriptions in Japan and the Caribbean. Endemic regions exist in Central America, South America (Columbia, Venezuela, Peru, Bolivia, and Brazil), and Africa (Uganda, Ivory Coast, Tanzania, and Zaire). The virus remains rare in Europe and Australia.

In North America, seropositive individuals have been found in Canada, the United States, and Mexico. The prevalence rate in United States volunteer blood donors is 0.025 percent. Most cases of HAM/TSP in the United States have occurred in immigrants, patients who had sexual partners from endemic areas, recipients of blood transfusions, or in association with intravenous drug abuse. Endemic infection in the United States has been well documented or is highly likely in Texas, North Carolina, Alabama, South Carolina, New York, Alaska, and Florida. Overall epidemiologic studies of HAM frequency and seropositivity rates have estimated that seropositive individuals have a 1 percent risk of developing adult T-cell lymphoma or HAM/TSP.

CLINICAL FEATURES

Progressive leg weakness, spasticity, and urinary symptoms are the hallmarks of this disease. Back pain is less consistent. Patients frequently complain of difficulty walking rather than leg weakness; stiffness is the most common complaint. Foot dragging, falling, and difficulty running are other symptoms, and some impairment of ambulation is present in 60 to 80 percent of patients. Urinary retention, urgency, or incontinence are commonly present, though not as primary presenting complaints. Impotence and constipation occur less often. Sensory disturbances are occasional and usually mild. Paresthesias occur in 25 to 33 percent of cases, and sensory cord levels are present in only 10 to 25 percent of cases. Cranial nerves are usually not impaired, though nystagmus and diplopia occur in 8 percent, and transient seventh nerve paralysis has been reported. Intention tremor, dysmetria, deafness, and retrobulbar neuropathy are other rare features, seen in occasional patients.

On neurologic examination, the findings primarily reflect involvement of the pyramidal tracts (motor), with lesser involvement of the posterior columns (proprioception). Weakness is primarily proximal, in the iliopsoas and gluteus medius. The legs are uniformly involved, and the arms are weak in up to 33 percent of patients. Hyperreflexia with or without clonus is present in 100 percent of patients, and upgoing Babinski signs are present in over 90 percent of patients. A jaw jerk is present in 12 to 33 percent of patients in the larger series. The gait exhibits mild scissoring and an awkward stiffness. About 50 percent require a cane or other gait appliance. The diminished vibration and proprioception in the feet and toes is mild. Involvement of touch and pain fibers is uncommon (6 to 10 percent). By brain magnetic resonance imaging (MRI), electroencephalography (EEG), and pathologic evaluation, the disease clearly involves widespread areas of the nervous system; however, clinical symptoms of involvement outside the spinal cord are not often prominent.

The onset and course is highly variable; most (75 percent) patients have an insidious course progressing over months to years. About 10 to 20 percent of cases progress to severe gait impairment over 1 to 3 months. Rarely, a more acute onset simulating a transverse myelopathy or even a vascular event has been observed.

The disease usually begins with asymmetric leg weakness and stiffness. Over months, the other leg becomes involved. Mild paresthesias may develop, and the patient may begin to notice jumping or jerking of one or both legs due to spasticity. Backachea may then develop as the spasticity becomes more pronounced. Occasional urinary incontinence or difficulty starting the urine stream develops. When the patient notes interfer-

ence with ambulation or athletic activities, medical attention is sought.

DIAGNOSIS

Laboratory Studies

Table 78-1 summarizes the laboratory findings in HAM/TSP. The leukocyte count is normal, but blood smears may show flower lymphocytes, named for their multilobulated nuclei, which are morphologically similar to adult T-cell lymphoma cells. These cells are 1 percent of the leukocytes and must be searched for carefully. They may also be present in the CSF, and they are pathognomonic of HTLV-I infection. Flower lymphocytes are $CD4^+$ $CD10^+$, indicating activated T-helper cells. Hypergammaglobulinemia (IgG and IgA) or serum oligoclonal bands may be important diagnostic clues. Most patients are seropositive for HTLV-I by enzyme-linked immunosorbent assay and Western blot. Interestingly, abnormal tests for syphilis and Lyme disease are common in both serum and CSF.

Cerebrospinal Fluid Abnormalities

Routine CSF analysis may be normal or may show various abnormalities. The glucose level is uniformly normal. Protein is elevated in up to 40 percent of patients, ranging from 50 to 210 mg/dl. Cell counts are elevated in up to 57 percent of patients, consisting of all mononuclear cells. Flower lymphocytes appear in 12 to 100 percent of cases. Elevated intrathecal production of IgG, as measured by oligoclonal IgG bands, IgG index, or CSF IgG synthesis rate, occurs in 21 to 85 percent of patients. The specificity of most of the antibody is unknown, but some of the IgG bands contain antibody to the viral gag protein p24.

Imaging

The imaging study of choice for both spinal cord and brain evaluation is MRI. The spinal cord frequently shows atrophy and high-intensity T2-weighted lesions, which are diffuse in

TABLE 78-1. Laboratory Features in Human T-Cell Lymphotrophic Virus-Associated Myelopathy and Tropical Spastic Paraparesis

Serum
  Flower lymphocytes
  Hypergammaglobulinemia, IgG and IgA
  Oligoclonal bands
  Antibodies to gag, env, and tax viral proteins
  VDRL positive
  Increased $CD4^+4B4^+$ (helper/inducer) T cells
  Normal $CD4^+2H2^+$ (suppressor/inducer) T cells
  Elevation of circulating adhesion glycoprotein cICAM-1
Cerebrospinal fluid
  Glucose level normal
  Protein variably elevated
  Mononuclear pleocytosis
  Flower lymphocytes
  Oligoclonal bands
  Elevated IgG synthesis rate
  Anti-HTLV-I–specific antibodies by ELISA and Western blot
  Elevated neopterin level
  Tumor necrosis factor-α detectable in mononuclear cells
  Elevated interferon-γ

Abbreviations: HTLV-I, human T-cell lymphotrophic virus type I; ELISA, enzyme-linked immunosorbent assay.

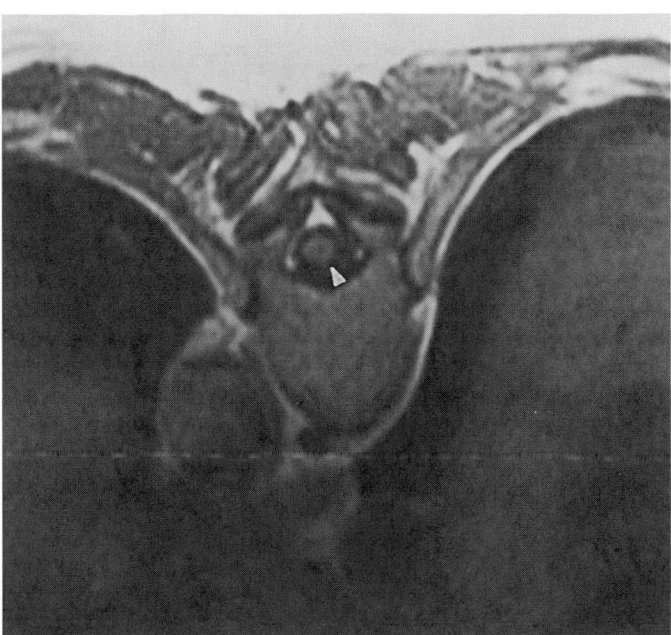

FIG. 78-1. Spinal cord MRI in a 64-year-old woman with myelopathy and HTLV-I virologically proved to be in cerebrospinal fluid cells. Transverse cut at T8 shows a small spinal cord in a spinal canal that appears large owing to the loss in diameter of the spinal cord.

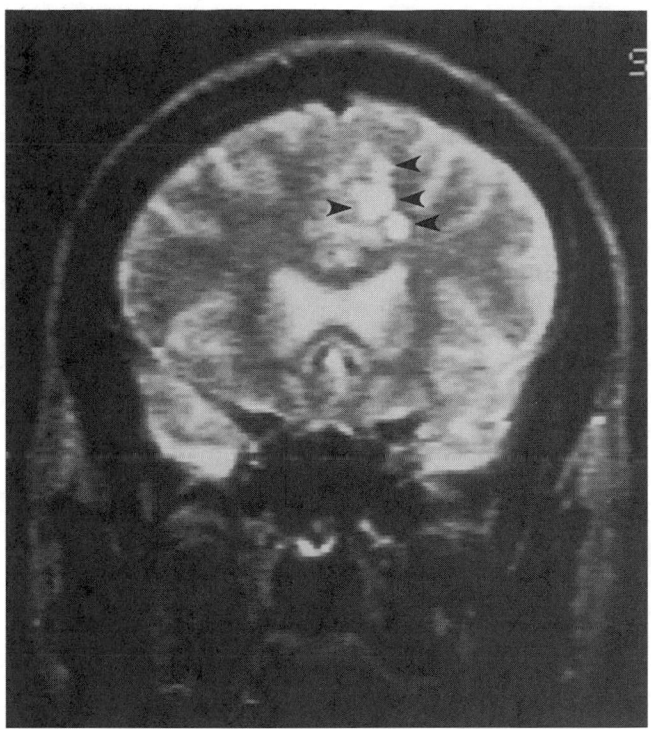

FIG. 78-2. Brain MRI abnormalities in a 53-year-old black man with virologically proved HTLV-I–associated myelopathy and with bilateral lower extremity weakness and urinary hesitation. Multiple areas of high signal intensity clustered in the left medial cerebrum on a T2-weighted scan.

the cervical and thoracic cord (Fig. 78-1). The incidence of MRI abnormalities in the brain ranges between 25 and 80 percent. Lesions appear in subcortical, deep cerebral, and periventricular areas (Fig. 78-2). The periventricular lesions are usually contiguous with the lateral ventricles, often near the posterior horn, and usually appear as large confluent areas. The subcortical and deep lesions are usually small and multifocal.

Electroencephalography and Evoked Potentials

Diffuse EEG abnormalities occur in 64 percent of patients, and delays in visual, brainstem auditory, and somatosensory-evoked potentials have been described. However, these studies are nonspecific and not particularly useful diagnostically.

Differential Diagnosis

To make a presumptive diagnosis of HTLV-I myelopathy requires a compatible clinical presentation of progressive or mildly relapsing and remitting myelopathy, a CSF with a low-grade inflammatory and immunoglobulin profile, MRI showing spinal cord atrophy or diffuse T2-weighted bright abnormalities, presence of Western blot confirmed HTLV-I specific antibodies in the serum and/or CSF, and exclusion of other causes, including cord compression, multiple sclerosis, vitamin B^{12} deficiency, human immunodeficiency virus disease, and Lyme disease. The presumptive diagnosis is strengthened by residence in a high-seroprevalence endemic area, by transfusion exposure, and by a history of intravenous drug abuse. Finding one of the associated systemic diseases commonly accompanying HTLV-I may also be helpful, including pulmonary alveolitis, arthritis not attributable to other causes, uveitis, persistent prostatitis, cystitis, infective dermatitis, or polymyositis. Pulmonary bronchoalveolitis may be detected as a persistent or fluctuating infiltrate on chest radiography.

To make a definitive diagnosis requires demonstration of

virus or viral genes in CSF cells by isolation or polymerase chain reaction, evidence of intrathecal synthesis of specific HTLV-I antibody by comparison of Western blots run with serum and CSF at equal IgG concentrations (this is easy to do; just ask your laboratory), or presence of unexplained serum hypergammaglobulinemia or serum oligoclonal bands. Without at least one of the latter three findings, a diagnosis of HTLV-I myelopathy is only presumptive and is especially likely to be wrong in patients from areas of low seroprevalence. Multiple sclerosis would be more likely in those instances.

PREVENTION AND TREATMENT

Prevention involves four major areas: blood transfusions, sexual transmission, breast feeding, and vaccine development. The rare instances of seronegative HAM/TSP indicate that transmission by blood cannot be completely eliminated. Strong public health educational programs and marital counseling are needed to promote condom use and to warn seropositive mothers of the risk of transmission by breast feeding. Vaccines would be cost effective, at least in high-prevalence endemic areas, but currently no vaccines are in trials.

Several treatment approaches are in development, but most have not been subjected to placebo-controlled, blinded trials, and therefore the results must be interpreted cautiously. Oral prednisolone has been the most extensively tried treatment. It was reported to induce improvement over 6 months in the first Japanese reports, but improvement was not maintained after a 2-year follow-up period. There are other reports of continued improvement in a few patients treated with prednisone.

Systemic interferon-α has been reported to be effective in two uncontrolled open trials. Heparin has also been used based on its ability to inhibit migration of activated T-cells into the central nervous system and to inhibit induction of autoimmune diseases such as experimental allergic encephalomyelitis. Danazol has been used in two open trials, also with modest success. Plasmapheresis has been used in small trials, usually with other immunologic therapies, and it should be tried in the patient who does not respond to steroids or interferon-α; however, the improvement seen with plasmapheresis may not be maintained.

HTLV-I reverse transcriptase is an essential enzyme for viral replication. Some reverse transcriptase–inhibiting drugs used to treat human immunodeficiency virus are also active against HTLV-I virus. However, results of treatment with azidovudine at doses of 0.5 to 1 g/d have been decidedly mixed and largely disappointing.

Supportive therapy of spasticity and urinary sphincter disturbances can be very helpful. Administration of baclofen, α-adrenergic medications, and anticholinergic medications is similar to that of myelopathies of other causes.

SUGGESTED READINGS

McKendall RR: HTLV-I diseases. pp. 737–72. In McKendall RR, Stroop WG (eds): Handbook of Neurovirology. Marcel Dekker, New York, 1994

Roman GC: Tropical spastic paraparesis and HTLV-I myelitis. pp. 525–42. In McKendall RR (ed): Handbook of Clinical Neurology. Vol. 56. Elsevier, Amsterdam, 1989

Roman GC, Vernant JC, Osame M (eds): HTLV-I and the Nervous System. Alan R Liss, New York, 1989

79. CHRONIC AND RECURRENT NONINFECTIOUS MENINGITIS

ELIZABETH A. SEKUL
TETSUO ASHIZAWA

Chronic or recurrent lymphocytic meningitis can present a diagnostic challenge, particularly when it is the initial manifestation of a multisystem disease. Chronic meningitis is defined as cerebrospinal fluid (CSF) pleocytosis for greater than 4 weeks in association with clinical signs of meningitis such as headache, fever, and neck stiffness. Recurrent meningitis implies cellular clearing from the CSF between episodes. The underlying disease processes that can present with these meningitides are varied, but they can be classified into several categories. Infectious etiologies, particularly viral, fungal, rickettsial, tubercular, and syphilitic, are probably the most common cause and should be aggressively sought via direct culture, antibody titers, and antigen presence (such as VDRL). Parameningeal foci of infection such as mastoiditis can also produce a picture of chronic CSF pleocytosis. Noninfectious causes of chronic or recurrent meningitis include a group of rarer disorders (Table 79-1). As the infectious etiologies are discussed elsewhere, the focus of this chapter is on the noninfectious causes of chronic and recur-

TABLE 79-1. Noninfectious Causes of Chronic or Recurrent Meningitis

Mollaret's meningitis
Behçet's disease
Vogt-Koyanagi-Harada syndrome
Granulomatous diseases
   Sarcoidosis
   Wegener's granulomatosis
   Lymphomatoid granulomatosis
   Primary angiitis of the central nervous system
Other autoimmune vasculitides
   Systemic lupus erythematosus
   Sjögren syndrome
   Systemic necrotizing vasculitides
Drug-induced meningitis
Meningeal carcinomatosis
Spinal arachnoiditis
Migraine

rent meningitis, including the vasculitides (which are also discussed in detail in other chapters).

MOLLARET'S MENINGITIS

Mollaret's meningitis is a form of recurrent meningitis marked by episodic attacks of fever and myalgia, associated with the signs and symptoms of meningeal irritation. No other organ systems are involved. The attacks are self-limited, resolving without sequelae in 2 to 7 days. Other than the signs of meningeal irritation, the neurologic examination during attacks is usually normal; however, seizures, facial nerve palsies, anisocoria, and positive Babinski signs have been reported. The disease duration averages from 3 to 5 years, with the longest reported duration being 28 years. The meningeal attacks are of variable intensity and frequency. There is no sex predilection. Although rare in children, patients as young as 1 year old have been reported.

In Mollaret's meningitis, the CSF cell count ranges from 200 cells/mm^3 to thousands of cells, which are predominantly lymphocytes with a few polymorphonuclear cells and distinguishing endothelial cells intermixed. This endothelial cell is the histologic hallmark of Mollaret's meningitis; however, they are not pathognomonic. They are mononuclear cells with irregular and poorly differentiated nuclear and cytoplasmic membranes. They are only present during the first few days of the attack and then degenerate into a lytic or ghostlike cell before they clear completely. The CSF protein is mildly elevated, and the glucose level is normal to slightly low. Oligoclonal bands may be present. The CSF returns to normal within 1 week of the attacks, and between attacks the CSF is normal. The laboratory findings outside of the CSF are nonspecific, such as an elevated erythrocyte sedimentation rate or peripheral eosinophilia.

The etiology of Mollaret's meningitis is unknown but is felt to be autoimmune or allergic in nature. No microorganisms have been identified. Recently, herpes simplex type 2 DNA was detected by a polymerase chain reaction assay in the CSF during the acute illness, suggesting that this virus may play a major role in the pathogenesis.

Owing to the self-limited nature of this disease and lack of sequelae, treatment is symptomatic. The unpredictability of the disease makes treatment efficacy in Mollaret's meningitis difficult to assess.

BEHÇET'S DISEASE

Behçet's disease is a multisystem disorder that causes aseptic chronic or recurrent meningitis, sometimes as a presenting feature, and is also characterized by the classic triad of recurrent oral ulcerations, genital ulcerations, and inflammation of the eye. The disease, though global, is much more common in Japan, the Middle East, and the Mediterranean countries, where its prevalence can reach 10 per 100,000 population. One study in the United States showed a prevalence of 0.3 per 100,000 population. Men are affected two to three times more often than women. The average age of onset is approximately 28 years. The cause is unknown but most likely is autoimmune in nature.

As no combination of historical or laboratory findings are specific for Behçet's disease, the diagnosis remains clinical. According to the clinical diagnostic criteria established in 1990 by the International Study Group for Behçet's disease, the diagnosis depends on the presence of oral ulcerations plus two of the following: genital ulcerations, typical defined eye lesions, typical defined skin lesions, or a positive pathergy test. These oral lesions are aphthous or herpetiform ulcerations, which typically heal within several days without scarring, and recur at least three times in one 12-month period. They may be very painful. The recurrent genital lesions consist of pustules or painful ulcerations that may scar. Ocular manifestations, which may lead to blindness within 5 years, include retinal vasculitis; hypopyon and iritis, resulting from an anterior uveitis; and, in the late stage, optic atrophy and secondary glaucoma. The recurrent skin lesions include erythema nodosum, nonpruritic pseudofolliculitis, and subcutaneous thrombophlebitis. A positive pathergy test is 90 percent specific but only approximately 60 percent sensitive for Behçet's disease. This test for cutaneous hypersensitivity is positive when a sterile pustule with redness forms by 24 to 48 hours at the site of a sterile needle prick to the skin.

Behçet's disease also affects many other systems. Neurologic involvement is common, occurring in up to 30 percent of patients, usually within 5 years of disease presentation; in 5 percent, it may be the initial manifestation. The intermittency of the neurologic features is one of the most characteristic findings. Owing to the frequency and severity of neurologic involvement, the term ''neuro-Behçet's'' was coined in the literature. The mortality rate associated with neuro-Behçet's disease has been reported as high as 50 percent, with most deaths occurring within 1 year of neurologic symptom onset. However, with improved treatment modalities, mortality rates as low as 13 percent have been recently reported. Any portion of the neuraxis may be involved, and neurologic complications can vary from one relapse to the next. Three common patterns of central neurologic involvement are noted: a brainstem syndrome affecting many cranial nerves, a meningoencephalitic syndrome, and an organic confusional state. Meningoencephalitis can occur in up to 12 percent as the presenting neurologic picture and can vary from an uncomplicated aseptic meningitis to a fulminant and fatal meningoencephalomyelitis. Typically, fever, headache, meningismus, and CSF pleocytosis are present. Cerebral infarctions caused by meningeal vessel involvement may occur. The organic confusional state may lead to severe dementia, personality changes, or delirium. CSF pleocytosis may accompany the psychiatric symptoms; however, clinical findings of meningeal irritation are usually absent.

In acute meningitis, cell counts may exceed 500 cells/mm^3, but, with chronic manifestations, 60 cells or less are usually noted. Although these cells are usually lymphocytes, polymorphonuclear cells may be seen. The total protein level is normal or slightly elevated. The CSF glucose level in the active stages is typically normal. CSF IgG and IgA levels are increased with IgA oligoclonal bands but not IgG. The presence of these bands may be used to monitor disease activity. Serum laboratory findings in Behçet's disease are nonspecific, but suggestive of an inflammatory reaction. Cranial computed tomography (CT) and magnetic resonance imaging (MRI) may show signs of infarction or edema and are useful to distinguish neuro-Behçet's from multiple sclerosis, which may also present with a relapsing and remitting course, and from tumors and abscesses.

Treatment for Behçet's disease has been difficult to evaluate owing to the relapsing nature of the disease. Both local and systemic treatment is advocated. Topical steroids for oral, genital, and ocular lesions are recommended. Oral ulcers may also respond to topical tetracycline. Corticosteroids remain the mainstay of systemic treatment and are used alone or in conjunction with other immunosuppressant agents, such as azathioprine or chlorambucil. High-dose prednisone (1 mg/kg/day) may be required to control the ocular and neurologic manifestations. Other drugs tried in Behçet's disease include cyclophosphamide, cyclosporine, colchicine, thalidomide, levamisole, and dapsone. Plasmapheresis in acute situations has been helpful in some patients.

VOGT-KOYANAGI-HARADA SYNDROME

Another uveomeningoencephalic syndrome that may be difficult to differentiate from Behçet's disease is Vogt-Koyanagi-Harada syndrome (VKH). Like Behçet's disease, this syndrome is more common in Japanese patients and rare in whites. Its onset is typically later than that in Behçet's disease, peaking in incidence in the fourth to fifth decade. Unlike Behçet's disease, in which the blood vessels are affected, the etiology of VKH appears to be an autoimmune reaction to melanocytes. Melanocytes are located in the skin, uvea and retinal choroid, membrane of the inner ear, and leptomeninges, particularly at the base of the cerebrum, thus accounting for the particular limited pattern of involvement seen in this syndrome.

In VKH, the ocular findings are usually more pronounced than the otologic or neurologic manifestations, although involvement of the latter are a rather constant feature. In the early active stage, the ophthalmologic involvement consists of bilateral uveitis and choroidal inflammation, which may result in retinal detachment. In the recovery stage, the retina has a characteristic sunset glow appearance owing to depigmentation. Later ocular findings consist of cataracts, glaucoma, and globe atrophy. In the early active phase, the meningeal involvement usually follows the onset of the uveitis; however, meningeal involvement may precede ocular involvement. The meningeal involvement may lead to encephalopathy, seizures, myelopathy, or other focal signs. In some cases, the meningitis is subclinical. CSF lymphocytic pleocytosis ranges from less than 20 to 500 cells/mm^3. Elevated CSF protein level, averaging 49 mg/dl in one series, occurs in approximately 50 percent of patients. Opening CSF pressure is usually normal. CSF immunoglobulins have only been studied in a few patients, with occasional elevations of CSF IgG noted. Other manifestations of VKH include dysacousia with hearing loss and tinnitus, alopecia, poliosis (whitening of the eyebrows and lashes), and vitiligo. Unlike Behçet's disease, the cutaneous involvement is not ulcerative but rather characterized by depigmentation.

The treatment of VKH consists of systemic and local corticosteroid administration. Few studies using other immunosuppressant agents have been done, and their efficacy remains to be proved.

SARCOIDOSIS

The prevalence of sarcoidosis in the United States is 10 to 40 per 100,000. It is more frequent in women than in men and appears to be 10 to 20 times more common in blacks than in whites. The peak age of onset is 25 to 30 years of age, and it is rare below age 15 years. The etiology of sarcoidosis is unknown.

Sarcoidosis is responsible for multiple neurologic presentations, including an aseptic chronic or recurrent meningitis. Symptomatic neurosarcoidosis occurs in 4 to 14 percent of patients, usually within the first 2 years of disease onset, and may be the presenting feature. Spontaneous remissions occur in approximately two-thirds of patients with neurologic involvement, whereas one-third show a progressive course. The shorter the history and the younger the patient, the more likely is the resolution of symptoms. The most common central nervous system (CNS) involvement in sarcoidosis is the granulomatous infiltration of the meninges, particularly at the base of the skull. This causes cranial nerve entrapments and subsequent palsies, most commonly of the facial nerve. Facial nerve palsies also occur in approximately 50 percent of those who develop other CNS manifestations. Ocular involvement occurs in 30 percent of patients with neurosarcoidosis, ranging from iriditis and uveitis to papilledema as a result of meningeal involvement of the casing of the optic nerve and subsequent swelling. Meningeal involvement can occur in all regions of the CNS and may lead to obstructive hydrocephalus owing to scarring. Involvement over the surface of the brain may act as a seizure focus or, if generalized, may present with clinical meningitis. Rarely, space-occupying parenchymal lesions caused by granulomas may occur. Focal involvement of the arachnoid or dura of the spinal cord is unusual but can occur, presenting as transverse myelitis. Involvement of the hypothalamic-pituitary axis is not uncommon, and diabetes insipidus is the most frequent result.

The peripheral nervous system is involved in up to 50 percent of patients, in a pattern varying from symmetric polyneuropathy to mononeuritis multiplex. In these patients, CSF pleocytosis tends to be slight, and the CSF protein level is higher, as opposed to that in patients with CNS disease, but the glucose level is normal. Myopathy clinically occurs in up to 50 percent of patients with sarcoid; however, granulomas are often found on muscle biopsy even in asymptomatic patients.

The CSF findings in neurosarcoidosis show an elevated cell count, usually less than 100 mononuclear cells/mm^3, and an increased protein level, up to 200 mg/dl. Approximately one-half of the patients have elevated CSF IgG levels, derived mostly from serum. Rarely, oligoclonal bands are present. A low CSF glucose level may be present, especially when obvious meningeal signs are found. Patients with isolated hypothalamic or pituitary involvement may have normal CSF. CSF angiotensin-converting enzyme (ACE) levels are increased in approximately 50 percent of patients with neurosarcoidosis and only 8 percent of patients with systemic sarcoid. However, this is not specific, as the ACE level may also be increased with tumors or bacterial meningitis.

The diagnosis of sarcoidosis is based on the histologic findings of noncaseating granulomas containing large epithelial cells. There is no necrosis within the granulomas. Variable numbers of giant cells are present, either of the Langerhans or foreign body type.

Clinically, sarcoidosis is suspected by hilar adenopathy on chest radiograph. Additional suspicion is aroused by demonstrating impairment of the delayed-type skin hypersensitivity response to appropriate antigenic stimulation. Other immunologic alterations include elevation of serum immunoglobulins, particularly IgG, and a positive response to the Kveim-Siltzbach antigen, which is derived from a sarcoidosis-involved lymph node. In approximately 75 percent of patients with sarcoidosis, a nodule showing the histologic changes resembling sarcoidosis occurs when this antigen is injected intradermally. Elevation of ACE levels in the blood and CSF may help to establish the diagnosis or monitor disease activities. However, elevations of the serum ACE level occur in only 60 percent of patients and in 10 percent of controls.

Approximately 90 percent of symptoms improve with steroid therapy, though treatment must often continues for months. Oral steroids are usually adequate, such as prednisone 60 to 80 mg/day, with a slow switch to alternate-day therapy and then a gradual taper, monitoring for recurrent disease. Other immunosuppressive agents are of possible, but unproven, benefit.

WEGENER'S GRANULOMATOSIS

Wegener's granulomatosis is characterized by granulomatous lesions of the upper and lower respiratory tract, focal segmental glomerulonephropathy, and necrotizing vasculitis. The overall incidence of Wegener's granulomatosis is unknown, but it occurs 1.5 times more frequently in men than in women, and its peak incidence is in the fourth or fifth decade. Its etiology is also unknown.

Neurologic involvement occurs in up to 30 percent of patients with Wegener's granulomatosis and can include aseptic chronic meningitis similar to that seen in sarcoidosis, with granulomatosis in the basilar meninges. However, vascular involvement of the meninges can also occur. CSF may reveal lymphocytosis and elevated protein levels, particularly with meningeal involvement. No laboratory findings are specific for Wegener's granulomatosis. The diagnosis of Wegener's granulomatosis can be recognized on a clinical basis by the presence of upper and lower respiratory tract lesions, although pathologic diagnosis (biopsy) is mandatory. Recognition of Wegener's disease is important because it is universally fatal if left untreated, with an average survival of 5 months. However, a remission rate of over 90 percent has been reported with immunosuppressive treatment using cyclophosphamide.

LYMPHOMATOID GRANULOMATOSIS

Another systemic granulomatosis very similar to Wegener's granulomatosis is lymphomatoid granulomatosis. Again, the lungs are primarily involved, but unlike Wegener's granulomatosis the upper respiratory tract is usually spared. Neurologic manifestations occur in approximately 30 percent of cases. The most common CNS finding is necrotizing inflammatory masses within the brain parenchyma; however, the meninges are frequently involved, resulting in multiple cranial nerve palsies, encephalopathy, or radiculopathy with a picture of aseptic chronic meningitis. The etiology of lymphomatoid granulomatosis is unknown. It appears to be a mixture of granulomatosis and a lymphoproliferative disorder. It progresses to lymphoma in approximately 13 percent of patients.

No consistent laboratory abnormalities are typical. However, in contrast to Wegener's granulomatosis, leukopenia is very common. The CSF is abnormal in up to 50 percent of patients, with findings similar to those of sarcoidosis and Wegener's granulomatosis, except that the mononuclear cells seen are chiefly reticular cells with some plasma cells and lymphocytes. These cells simulate those found in meningeal lymphoma and other diffuse meningeal neoplasms. Diagnosis is based on the clinical presentation and tissue histology. Treatment is with prednisone and cyclophosphamide.

ISOLATED CENTRAL NERVOUS SYSTEM ANGIITIS

The fourth of the noninfectious granulomatous diseases that affects the meninges and can present as an aseptic chronic meningitis is isolated or primary angiitis of the CNS (PACNS). PACNS occurs twice as often in males as in females. It is a rare granulomatous vasculitis of unknown etiology, which is restricted for the most part to the CNS. The average age of onset is 48 years of age, although it has also been reported in the pediatric population. The mortality rate may exceed 85 percent.

PACNS may involve the entire neuraxis, but it predominantly affects the intracranial structures. It is usually asymmetric in distribution and, at times, may be remarkably focal. It most commonly involves the small vessels of the leptomeninges; however, larger vessels are involved in up to one-third of the cases. Clinically, PACNS is subacute in onset. It presents with headache and mental status changes, which progress to confusion and disorientation followed by lethargy and focal signs. Focal or generalized seizures occur in approximately one-fourth of patients. Cerebral edema is frequently massive. Among untreated persons, 90 percent eventually develop focal CNS signs.

The electroencephalogram is abnormal in approximately 80 percent of patients, most frequently showing generalized or focal slowing. The erythrocyte sedimentation rate is elevated in approximately 70 percent, usually in the low range and rarely exceeding 100 mm/h. Tests for autoantibodies such as antinuclear antibody are consistently negative.

CSF abnormalities are seen in 80 percent of patients. An increased opening pressure is frequent. The protein concentration is elevated in 80 percent of patients with a mean of 160 mg/dl, and the CSF IgG level is elevated in some patients. CSF lymphocytic pleocytosis is noted in approximately two-thirds of patients, with up to 250 cells/mm^3. Some erythrocytes (less than 1,000/mm^3) may also be seen in one-third of patients. CT and MRI studies show patchy areas of ischemia and edema. Angiography is normal in many patients; however, the remaining patients show arterial beading, aneurysms, or arterial branch occlusions. Leptomeningeal biopsy is the most useful method to establish the diagnosis. Histologic findings include angiitis, segmental intimal proliferation, vascular narrowing, and intensive inflammatory infiltrates with granulomas consisting of lymphocytes, plasma cells, multinuclear cells, and fibrinoid necrosis. However, owing to the focal nature of the disease, a negative biopsy does not exclude the diagnosis.

The mean duration from onset of symptoms to death is 6 months in untreated patients. Corticosteroids with another immunosuppressant, particularly cyclophosphamide, is the treatment of choice.

OTHER AUTOIMMUNE VASCULITIDES

Systemic Lupus Erythematosus

Neurologic involvement can be documented in 25 to 75 percent of patients with systemic lupus erythematosus (SLE) at some point in their disease. Psychiatric symptoms or seizures are the most common complications and sometimes are accompanied by CSF lymphocytic pleocytosis. However, clinical aseptic meningitis is rare in SLE, especially as a presenting manifestation. Aseptic meningitis has also been reported in SLE with elevated serum antiphospholipid antibodies.

Sjögren's Syndrome

Sjögren's syndrome is characterized by keratoconjunctivitis sicca, xerostomia, and a connective tissue disorder (usually rheumatoid arthritis). It is associated with anti-SSa and anti-SSb antibodies, which are autoantibodies to extractable components of nuclear cytoplasm. Peripheral nerve involvement is far more common than CNS involvement. However, CNS abnormalities occur in 20 percent of patients in some series and may mimic multiple sclerosis, with abnormal CSF findings and multiple lesions on MRI. A recurrent aseptic meningoencephalitis has also been noted. When present, CNS involvement is associated with cutaneous signs of vasculitis in over 70 percent of patients, which in turn is highly correlated with anti-SSa antibodies. The CSF shows an elevated IgG index in nearly 100 percent of Sjögren's syndrome patients with CNS disease.

Systemic Necrotizing Vasculitides

Polyarteritis nodosa, Churg-Strauss syndrome, temporal arteritis, Takayasu's arteritis, and drug abuse–associated vasculitis can also involve the meningeal blood vessels. Approximately 20 percent of patients with these diseases may have clinical or laboratory evidence of aseptic meningitis at some time during their illness. Aseptic meningitis has similarly been reported in other systemic vasculitides such as mixed connective tissue disease and Kawasaki disease.

DRUG-INDUCED ASEPTIC MENINGITIS

Aseptic meningitis can also occur as a reaction to a wide variety of drugs taken systemically. Whether this results from a direct toxic effect from diffusion of the drug across the blood–brain barrier or from a hypersensitivity reaction of the cerebral blood vessels is unknown. Medications known to cause drug-related aseptic meningitis include high-dose intravenous immunoglobulins, nonsteroidal anti-inflammatory drugs, co-trimoxazole, azathioprine, trimethoprim sulfate, and carbamazepine. Aseptic meningitis caused by nonsteroidal anti-inflammatory drugs occurs primarily in patients with connective tissue disorders, especially those with SLE and mixed connective tissue disease. Clinically, patients develop the classic signs of meningitis, usually including fever. In most cases, this reaction occurs within hours to 1 day of exposure and is reproducible upon re-exposure to the offending agent. CSF studies in general show lymphocyte-predominant pleocytosis unless the fluid was collected early in the course, at which time polymorphonuclear cells may predominate. Eosinophils may also be present. The CSF protein level is mildly elevated, and the glucose concentration is normal in most patients. Generally, the symptoms resolve without sequelae, and only supportive therapy is required. On the first exposure, of course, a full evaluation for other causes of aseptic meningitis is usually warranted.

MENINGEAL CARCINOMATOSIS

Meningeal carcinomatosis commonly presents with headache, cranial nerve signs, back pain, focal weakness, or seizures. Unlike most other chronic meningitides, nerve roots, including the cauda equina, are often involved with carcinomatous meningitis. This type of meningitis must be distinguished from the remote effects of cancer, toxicity of treatment, or infections. Malignant meningeal involvement can occur as a primary diffuse infiltration, either from CNS lymphoma or meningeal gliomatosis, or as an extension from a primary brain tumor such as a glioblastoma, astrocytoma, or medulloblastoma. However, a metastasis may also cause meningeal carcinomatosis, most commonly with breast cancer, lung cancer, melanoma, leukemia, and lymphoma.

Increased CSF pressure is generally present except in the early stages of the disease. The CSF protein level may be normal but is usually elevated. Cell counts are typically elevated but may be normal in up to one-third of patients. Large-volume samples or multiple CSF samples may need to be examined cytologically before the malignant cells can be identified. However, the presence of malignant cells is not specific for direct meningeal involvement, as they are often found in the CSF when brain tumors, particularly involving the ventricular wall or cortex, are present. Hypoglycorrhachia generally reflects diffuse meningeal involvement rather than such localized diseases. In some cases, cisternal puncture may have a higher yield when the basilar meninges are involved. Elevated CSF immunoglobulins and abnormal CSF IgG index and oligoclonal bands are often present. Tumor markers, such as vasopressin, carcinoembryonic antigen, adrenocorticotropin, lactic dehydrogenase, and β-glucuronidase, may also be helpful. MRI or myelography may show thickened, nodular nerve roots or epidural tumors. Meningeal contrast enhancement on MRI or CT is sensitive but not specific for diffuse carcinomatosis. Treatment is dependent on the tumor type.

SPINAL ARACHNOIDITIS

Spinal arachnoiditis can be acute, subacute, or chronic. Chronic spinal arachnoiditis can cause chronic lymphocytic pleocytosis and should be considered a variant of chronic meningitis. It usually follows intrathecal injection of a foreign substance, such as contrast material, antibiotics, or anesthetic agents. However, prolapse of a vertebral disc, spinal injury or surgery, or infections have also been implicated. The presence of blood in the CSF increases the likelihood of developing arachnoiditis. The CSF pleocytosis is generally lymphocytic, but, in acute cases following recent foreign substance administration, polynuclear cells may be predominant, and a mild eosinophilia may develop. The CSF protein level is increased to a variable degree. In patients with chronic adhesive arachnoiditis, loculated CSF may occur with an extremely high protein concentration. The diagnosis of chronic arachnoiditis is confirmed by MRI or myelography. Treatment is surgical but is not always effective, as the arachnoiditis may recur.

MIGRAINES

Migraine headaches may be another cause of recurrent CSF lymphocytic pleocytosis. In general, CSF pleocytosis is uncommon in severe but uncomplicated migraines but can occur with elevated cell counts in the range of 15 to 100 cells/mm^3. However, patients with complicated or hemiplegic migraines have a higher frequency of CSF abnormalities, with cell counts around 300 cells/mm^3 and minor elevations in protein level.

OTHERS

Recurrent aseptic meningitis can also occur as a result of intermittent leakage of cystic contents from a craniopharyngioma, dermoid cyst, epidermoid cyst, teratoma, or malignant glioma. Cerebral MRI is helpful in establishing the etiology of the meningitis in such cases. Patients with familial Mediterranean fever have also been reported to have recurrent aseptic meningitis. One in 2,000 subjects who received mumps vaccination have developed aseptic meningitis in Japan and Germany.

CONCLUSION

The causes of culture-negative chronic or recurrent meningitis are diverse, and the diagnosis is often difficult to make, particularly early in the disease process. CSF pleocytosis, protein levels, glucose levels, and immunoglobulin studies are mostly nonspecific. Recognition of systemic manifestations of the baseline diseases that cause aseptic meningitis is, therefore, often crucial. Various laboratory tests, such as viral titers and other serologic tests, arteriography, CT, and MRI may provide important clues for a correct diagnosis. Pathologic diagnosis is sometimes required, particularly for the granulomatous diseases. Prognosis is variable, ranging from a self-limited benign course to a fatal outcome, depending on the cause. Treatment also depends on the underlying disease. Thus, chronic or recurrent aseptic meningitis often becomes a challenging problem for physicians and requires thorough clinical investigations.

SUGGESTED READINGS

Fishman RA: CSF findings in diseases of the nervous system. p. 253. In Fishman RA (ed): Cerebrospinal Fluid in Diseases of the Nervous System. 2nd Ed. WB Saunders, Philadelphia, 1992

Frederics JAM, Bruyn GW: Mollaret's meningitis. p. 627. In McKendall RR (ed): Handbook of Clinical Neurology. 56th Ed. Elsevier Science Publishing, New York, 1989

International Study Group for Behçet's Disease: Criteria for diagnosis of Behçet's disease. Lancet 335:1078, 1990

Iomata H, Kato M: Vogt-Koyanagi-Harada disease. p. 611. In McKendall RR (ed): Handbook of Clinical Neurology. 56th Ed. Elsevier Science Publishing, New York, 1989

Shannon KM, Goetz CG: Connective tissue diseases and the central nervous system. p. 389. In Aminoff MJ (ed): Neurology in General Medicine. 2nd Ed. Churchill Livingstone, New York, 1995

Silberberg DH: Sarcoidosis of the nervous system. p. 701. In Aminoff MJ (ed): Neurology in General Medicine. 2nd Ed. Churchill Livingstone, New York, 1995

Stratigos AJ, Laskaris G, Stratigos JD: Behçet's disease. Semin Neurol 12: 346, 1992

Tucker T, Ellner JJ: Chronic meningitis. p. 188. In Tyler KL, Martin JB (eds): Infectious Diseases of the Central Nervous System. FA Davis, Philadelphia, 1993

80. PRION DISEASES

EUGENE C. LAI

The prion diseases are sometimes also referred to as the transmissible spongiform encephalopathies or transmissible cerebral amyloidoses. They encompass several diseases affecting humans and animals; the human prion diseases include Creutzfeldt-Jakob disease, Gerstmann-Sträussler-Scheinker syn-

TABLE 80-1. The Human Prion Diseases

Disease	Etiology
Creutzfeldt-Jakob disease	
Sporadic	Unknown
Familial	Prion mutation
Iatrogenic	Transmission
Gerstmann-Sträussler-Scheinker syndrome	Prion mutation
Kuru	Transmission
Fatal familial insomnia	Prion mutation

drome, kuru, and fatal familial insomnia (Table 80-1). The unique feature common to these disorders is the sharing of a similar pathogenesis that involves the aberrant metabolism of the prion protein. The term "prion" was introduced in 1982 by Stanley Prusiner to mean "small, proteinaceous, infectious particles which resist inactivation by procedures that modify nucleic acids." Recent advances in the molecular biology of prions revealed that the prion protein is coded for by a gene located at the short arm of human chromosome 20. It codes for a normal host protein, but the function of the prion protein has not yet been identified. In human prion diseases, an abnormal form of this protein, which becomes proteinase resistant, accumulates in the brain. These diseases may be sporadic, dominantly inherited, or acquired by transmission. The prion protein, which of course contains no nucleic acids (DNA or RNA), can produce disease after injection into animals, thus fulfilling its definition as an infectious agent composed purely of protein.

CREUTZFELDT-JAKOB DISEASE

Creutzfeldt-Jakob disease (CJD) is a rare central nervous system disorder characterized by a relentlessly progressive course and an invariably fatal outcome. It constitutes about 75 percent of all the human prion diseases. Sporadic, familial, and iatrogenic forms of CJD have been described.

Clinical Features

CJD is usually a disease of late middle age, but its range can extend from 16 to 82 years. Both sexes are affected equally. The clinical manifestations encompass virtually the entire nervous system and may be confusing in the early stages of the disease (Table 80-2). Approximately one-third of patients present with mental deterioration that includes memory loss, behavioral abnormalities, and confusion; another third of patients have only physical complaints, most often cerebellar ataxia or visual disturbance; and the final third of patients present with

TABLE 80-2. Clinical Characteristics of Creutzfeldt-Jakob Disease (Percentage of Patients With Symptoms and Signs)

Symptoms/Signs	At Onset	During Course
Mental deterioration	69	100
Memory loss	48	100
Higher cortical functions	16	73
Behavioral abnormalities	29	57
Involuntary movements	4	91
Myoclonus	1	78
Cerebellar ataxia	33	71
Pyramidal weakness/hyperreflexia	2	62
Extrapyramidal rigidity	0.5	56
Periodic electroencephalogram	0	60
Visual/oculomotor disturbance	19	42

a mixture of both mental and physical symptoms. More than one-quarter of the patients report prodromal symptoms, consisting of fatigue, disturbance of sleep patterns or appetite, anxiety, or weight loss that may last for several weeks. As a rule, the disease progresses rapidly, and symptoms advance within weeks. Memory decline usually progresses to profound and global intellectual deficits, often with prominent grasp, glabellar, palmomental, and snout reflexes. Movement disorders, such as cerebellar ataxia, tremor, dysarthria, hypokinesia, rigidity, or choreoathetoid movements, may become pronounced. Myoclonus, often provoked by sensory stimuli, usually appears in midcourse and is especially characteristic of the disease. Pyramidal tract involvement is also common, as manifested by hyperreflexia, extensor plantar reflexes (Babinski signs), and clonus. Visual complaints include hallucinations, diplopia, dimming or blurring of vision, and visual distortions that may evolve into cortical blindness. The patient continues to deteriorate to mutism, complete helplessness, and a vegetative existence. The disease typically ends in death from respiratory or systemic infections, usually within 1 year of onset. Only 5 to 10 percent of patients have clinical courses of more than 2 years.

Epidemiology and Etiology

The disease occurs in adults throughout the world, with an annual incidence of 0.5 to 2.0 cases per 1 million population. Sporadic CJD constitutes most cases. Its exact etiology is unknown but has been hypothesized to involve a somatic mutation of the prion gene that causes a spontaneous conformational conversion of the normal host prion protein to an abnormal form. A small proportion of the cases, varying from 5 to 15 percent, according to various reports, are familial and may arise from a germline mutation in the prion protein gene. Familial CJD has been found to be prevalent among Libyan Jews. The disease is also transmissible, as demonstrated in cases of iatrogenic CJD. Human to human transmission has occurred inadvertently during corneal and cadaveric dura mater transplantation and during the use of contaminated brain electrodes. A few cases have also resulted from treatment with growth hormone prepared from pooled human cadaveric pituitary glands. No transmission of the disease by casual contact or among family members has been reported.

Diagnosis

The cerebrospinal fluid, although it may contain a transmissible agent, is usually unremarkable and of little diagnostic value. Although typically normal, a computed tomographic scan of the head may show nonspecific cortical atrophy. Magnetic resonance imaging of the brain is also typically normal, but increased signal intensity in the basal ganglia, without contrast enhancement, has been reported in later stages of the disease. The electroencephalogram is often helpful diagnostically. Although normal early in the course of the illness, in later stages, it may show generalized slow wave activity or background disorganization that progresses to a diagnostically characteristic pattern of periodic (1 to 2 cycles/s) sharp waves against a slow background. The diagnosis can only be confirmed by finding the typical spongiform vacuolar changes in brain tissue from a brain biopsy. No other specific test is available at this time.

The differential diagnosis should include progressive neurodegenerative diseases such as Alzheimer's disease, severe parkinsonism, and cerebellar degeneration. Acquired immunodeficiency syndrome, cerebrovascular disease with multi-infarct dementia, and drug toxicities should also be ruled out.

Pathology

The pathologic abnormalities in CJD are confined to the central nervous system. There is degeneration and disappearance of neurons and their processes together with widespread hypertrophy and proliferation of astrocytes. These changes result in microscopic vacuolation and spongy appearance of the gray matter, particularly the cerebral cortex, hence the term spongiform encephalopathy. In 5 to 20 percent of cases, prion immunopositive amyloid plaques have been observed. The white matter is usually preserved, and inflammatory reactions are absent.

Management

There is no effective treatment available, and the disease is uniformly fatal. In view of the transmissibility of the disease iatrogenically, certain precautions should be taken in the medical care and handling of materials from these patients. It should be noted that, because of the low and restricted infectivity of the responsible agent, affected patients present minimal risks to caretakers, and the handling of blood and tissue specimens is not dangerous if appropriate precautions are taken. Isolation of the patient is not necessary. Casual skin contacts are allowed, and hand washing with ordinary soap afterward is recommended. Gloves should be worn when handling blood, body fluids, and tissues, and accidental skin exposure to these samples should be washed with a 1:10 dilution of sodium hypochlorite (household bleach). Contaminated surgical and pathologic instruments can be cleaned by steam autoclaving at 132°C and 15-lb/in^2 pressure for 1 hour or by immersing for 1 hour in 5 percent sodium hypochlorite. Laboratory specimens should be disposed of as biohazard waste after decontamination.

GERSTMANN-STRAÜSSLER-SCHEINKER SYNDROME

Gerstmann-Straüssler-Scheinker syndrome (GSS) is a rare neurodegenerative disease that has an apparent autosomal dominant pattern of inheritance. There are approximately 30 known families with GSS in various parts of the world, including the Americas, Europe, and Japan. The clinical features are dominated by cerebellar ataxia, pyramidal signs, and dementia. The average age of onset is 40 years, and the average duration is approximately 5 years, with a range from 1 to 11 years. Its neuropathology is characterized by extensive multicentric prion-containing amyloid plaques and spongiform changes in the gray matter of the cortex. Mutations in the protein-coding region of the prion protein gene that result in amino acid substitutions have been found in several kindreds.

KURU

Kuru is now a disease of historic interest only. It is restricted to the Fore tribe of Papua, New Guinea and is transmitted by ritual cannibalistic practices during the care of the dead. Patients present with progressive emotional lability, mental slowing, and movement disorders, such as ataxia, tremor, and rigidity that progress to mutism and a vegetative state. Death occurs within 1 year of symptom onset. Kuru has virtually disappeared as a result of the cessation of the practice of cannibalism.

FATAL FAMILIAL INSOMNIA

Fatal familial insomnia is a progressive autosomal dominant disease with subacute onset that is characterized by untreatable insomnia, dysautonomia, motor disturbance, and severe selective atrophy of thalamic nuclei. Several Italian families have been studied, and fatal familial insomnia is also linked to a mutation in the prion protein gene.

SELECTED READINGS

Brown P, Gibbs CJ, Rodgers-Johnson P et al: Human spongiform encephalopathy: the National Institute of Health series of 300 cases of experimentally transmitted disease. Ann Neurol 35:513–29, 1994

Davanipour Z, Alter M, Sobel E: Creutzfeldt-Jakob disease. Neurol Clin 4: 415–26, 1986

Lantos PL: From slow virus to prion: a review of transmissible spongiform encephalopathies. Histopathology 20:1–11, 1992

Prusiner SB: Molecular biology of prion diseases. Science 252:1515–22, 1991

Prusiner SB, Hsiao KK: Human prion diseases. Ann Neurol 35:385–95, 1994

Webb RM, Leech RW, Brumback RA: Spongiform encephalopathies: the physician's responsibility. South Med J 83:141–5, 1990

81. RICKETTSIAL INFECTIONS OF THE NERVOUS SYSTEM

J. DOUGLAS LEE

Rickettsiae are obligate intracellular, small, gram-negative pleomorphic bacilli that normally cause infection in rodents and other mammals; humans are incidental hosts. The rickettsiae include the organisms of typhus, spotted fevers (Rocky Mountain spotted fever [RMSF]), Q fever, and ehrlichiosis. Until recently *Rochalimaea* was also included in this group. Typhus and RMSF, which cause central nervous system (CNS) involvement in virtually all infected humans, and Q fever, which does so on occasion, are the most important concerns in patients with neurologic disease.

Although these diseases seem to be rare, they actually are not, and they remain a diagnostic consideration in both rural and urban settings. Each year, 1 thousand cases of RMSF, and somewhat fewer cases of typhus and Q fever, are reported in the United States. There is undoubtedly much under-reporting because of a lack of consideration of the diagnosis.

PATHOPHYSIOLOGY

The organisms of typhus and the spotted fevers selectively infect vascular endothelial cells, producing microvasculitis with inflammation, vascular permeability, local hemorrhage, thrombosis, luminal obstruction, and microinfarction. Since systemic vessels are involved diffusely, a characteristic rash appears in most patients. The rash and the various CNS syndromes dominate the clinical picture—the word *typhus* is derived from a Greek word meaning hazy or smoky, referring to the delirium characteristic of the disease. In the CNS, perivascular glial nodules are almost always present and are considered pathognomonic of rickettsial infection. These are accumulations of enlarged endothelial cells, lymphocytes, and macrophages that contain the organisms, which appear 1 to 2 weeks after the illness.

In contrast, the organism of Q fever, *Coxiella burnetii,* has no such predilection for endothelium, and vasculitis is not seen; so the frequency of CNS involvement (meningitis) is less, and the clinical picture is usually characterized by fever with atypical pneumonia and abnormal liver enzyme levels, but no rash.

CLINICAL PRESENTATION

The presentation is related to the type of pathology involved. Patients with RMSF or typhus have an abrupt onset of fever, chills, headache, myalgia, and arthralgia. Restlessness, irritability, confusion, and lethargy are usual, often with photophobia and stiff neck. This picture of an acute severe meningitis may develop within hours and may precede the rash. Other neurologic signs are generally nonfocal but may include increased reflexes and Babinski signs, spasticity, and movement disorders, especially athetosis. Cranial nerve involvement can include facial weakness, gaze palsies, nystagmus, and dysphagia. Eye findings are frequent, including papilledema, retinal fasciculitis, and uveitis. In a small percentage of patients, transverse myelitis may develop, including paraplegia or quadriplegia and a neurogenic bladder. Seizures are common. Within 1 week, most patients have a petechial rash, which on occasion becomes confluent. When the rash is accompanied by disseminated intravascular coagulation (DIC), it rarely may cause skin or extremity gangrene. Prior to antibiotic therapy, cases of full-blown encephalitis and delirium had an 80 percent mortality rate.

Patients with Q fever most often have a febrile pneumonia, but with few pulmonary symptoms. Headache and constitutional and gastrointestinal symptoms are common, but rash is not a feature. A small number of patients develop meningitis, with headache, nuchal rigidity, and confusion. Some also develop a chronic disease, such as hepatitis, endocarditis, or osteomyelitis. In endemic areas, seroprevalence in the population is high, and undiagnosed Q fever is frequent.

LABORATORY ABNORMALITIES

The leukocyte count is usually normal or low, with a left shift. Thrombocytopenia is common, as is mild prolongation of the prothrombin time. DIC is not commonly documented.

In typhus and spotted fevers, as multisystem vasculitides, abnormalities of the liver and muscle enzymes are common with the degree of abnormality related to the level of overall illness. Hypoalbuminemia, hypocalcemia, and hyponatremia are also frequent, perhaps related to vascular leakage and third spacing. The cerebrospinal fluid in RMSF often shows a modest mononuclear pleocytosis with normal glucose and elevated protein levels; in typhus and Q fever, the cerebrospinal fluid is usually normal. Imaging studies have rarely been reported and are usually normal. The electroencephalogram in most cases shows diffuse slowing

In Q fever, the liver enzyme abnormalities are more prominent, as are chest radiographic findings; muscle enzyme and fluid electrolyte abnormalities are less.

DIAGNOSIS

The diagnosis of rickettsial infections is clinical, with confirmation by serology during convalescence in most settings. *Proteus* agglutinins (Weil-Felix reaction) are commonly present but are nonspecific, insensitive, and delayed (up to 10 to 14 days after the onset of symptoms) and so should not be relied upon. Specific rickettsial antibodies may be detected after they develop later in the illness, and it is useful to freeze serum during the acute phase of the illness to allow testing of paired sera later. A few laboratories offer direct immunofluorescent staining to demonstrate the organism in tissue such as skin biopsies.

The most important disease to differentiate in the febrile patient with rash is meningococcemia. Counterimmunoelectrophoresis and latex agglutination, in addition to routine cultures, may help make this differentiation.

TREATMENT

A tetracycline is the treatment for all rickettsial infections in adults. Doxycycline 100 mg bid or tetracycline 500 mg qid is adequate. In children younger than 8 years old and those allergic to tetracycline, chloramphenicol 50 mg/kg/d in four equally divided doses is also effective (maximum dose 4 g/d). Drugs should be administered for 3 days after the patient becomes afebrile, usually about 7 to 10 days total. The fatality rate in typhus and RMSF remains close to 5 percent, with patients in the oldest age groups faring the worst.

SPECIFIC INFECTIONS

The identification and diagnosis of specific rickettsial infections is based on the geographic area of exposure, potential vector exposure, and the distribution and spread of the rash (Table 81-1). Diseases with tick vectors cluster in seasons and around activities allowing tick attachment.

TABLE 81-1. Rickettsial Diseases of Humans: Differential Features

Disease	Organism	Geography	Vector/Route	Reservoir	Rash[a]	Severity[b] (treated mortality)
RMSF[c]	R. rickettsii	Western hemisphere Eastern/SE US	Dog tick Wood tick	Tick	Extremities to trunk[d]	Severe (4–8%)
Epidemic typhus	R. prowazekii	Worldwide Eastern US[f]	Louse feces	Human Flying squirrel	Trunk	Severe (4%)[e]
Murine typhus	R. typhi	Worldwide Southern US	Flea	Rodents	Trunk to extremities	Moderate (1–4%)
Q fever	C. burnetii	Worldwide	Inhalation[g]	Numerous mammals	None	Moderate (uncommon)

[a] Rash may be absent in any of these but is usually present.
[b] Mortality rate is dependent on pre-existing disease and severity. It is likely that subclinical disease is common, and significant neurologic disease is a poor prognostic indicator.
[c] Similar spotted fevers exist with different rickettsiae, vectors, and vertebrate hosts on various continents.
[d] Ninety percent of patients.
[e] Brill-Zinsser disease or recrudescent typhus is seen in individuals from endemic areas years after immigration. Disease is mild.
[f] Rare disease in US.
[g] Hardy organisms inhaled from residua of infected placental tissue of wild or farm animals or domestic pets.

SUGGESTED READINGS

Kirk JL, Fine DP, Sexton DJ, Muchmore HG: Rocky mountain spotted fever: a clinical review. Medicine (Baltimore) 69:35–45, 1990

Marrie TJ: Rikettsial infections of the central nervous system. Semin Neurol 12:213, 1992

Saah AJ, Marrie TJ, Dumler JS, Walker DH: Rickettsial diseases. pp. 1719–41. In Mandell G (ed): Principles and Practice of Infectious Diseases. 4th Ed. Churchill Livingstone, 1992

82. MYCOPLASMA INFECTIONS

STEVEN J. SPINDEL

The normal human oropharynx and genital tract are colonized by a class of bacteria that lack a cell wall, called Mollicutes, which includes the mycoplasmas and ureaplasmas. These are the smallest known free-living organisms. A few of these agents can cause diseases in humans and have central nervous system (CNS) manifestations, including *Mycoplasma pneumoniae*, *Mycoplasma hominis,* and *Ureaplasma urealyticum.*

M. pneumoniae is a bacterial organism that is responsible for pharyngitis, bronchitis, and pneumonia in children and young adults. Nervous system disease has been well recognized in association with this organism, and neurologic manifestations are the most frequently occurring extrapulmonary symptoms in patients with *M. pneumoniae,* especially in children.

EPIDEMIOLOGY

M. pneumoniae-associated CNS disease was originally observed during epidemic outbreaks of "primary atypical pneumonia" in the 1940s, when the organism's identity was not yet known. Transmission occurs via contaminated respiratory droplets, and the incubation period ranges from 16 to 32 days. Epidemic outbreaks of respiratory infection have been observed to occur in 4- to 7-year cycles in crowded conditions such as schools, colleges, and military institutions. CNS manifestations occur in 7 to 10 percent of patients hospitalized with infection due to *M. pneumoniae.* Neurologic involvement is mainly reported in the pediatric populations, probably because of the increased frequency of the organism in children and young adults. Similarly, the trend for nervous system disease is to manifest in younger individuals, although it is an unusual pathogen of encephalitis in infants younger than 1 year old. Much like pulmonary disease, *M. pneumoniae* infections of the CNS show no gender preference and occur more often in the late summer and fall.

CLINICAL FEATURES

Usually, *M. pneumoniae* causes an acute tracheobronchial pneumonia with fever, sore throat, and a severe cough, which may be difficult to distinguish, by clinical or radiographic criteria, from many other causes of pneumonia. The pulmonary disease generally runs its course in 2 to 4 weeks.

M. pneumoniae can cause a primary infection of the CNS and neurologic manifestations as a complication of pulmonary infection. The organism has been isolated from the cerebrospinal fluid (CSF), providing evidence that invasion of the CNS does occur and that *M. pneumoniae* can directly cause neurologic disease. Some investigators believe that other mechanisms are also at work because of the inability to detect the presence of *M. pneumoniae* in the CSF or brain tissue in several reported cases with CNS disease. An autoimmune process has been postulated whereby antibodies are produced against brain tissue in response to the infecting organism. Other theories include the production of a neurotoxin or a vasculitis affecting the CNS. Other *Mycoplasma* species have been shown in experimental animal models to produce CNS injury by these mechanisms, although they have not been demonstrated with *M. pneumoniae.* Postmortem examination of the brain occasionally reveals edema, hemorrhage, perivascular inflammatory infiltrates, microthrombi, and demyelination.

Up to 20 percent of patients with neurologic symptoms have no associated pulmonary disease, a situation especially likely to occur in children. In those patients who have antecedent respiratory symptoms, the average time to the onset of neurologic symptoms is 10 days (range 3 to 30 days). Symptoms then develop abruptly, often peaking in less than 24 hours (Table 82-1). Neurologic complications include the following:

Encephalitis
Meningitis
Hydrocephalus
Psychosis
Myelitis
Polyradiculitis

Encephalitis and meningoencephalitis are the most common manifestation of CNS disease in *M. pneumoniae* infection. Encephalitis can be diffuse or focal and frequently affects the cerebellum (producing ataxia) and the pons (producing cranial nerve damage). Most patients have fever and meningeal symptoms, including headache, nausea, vomiting, and neck stiffness. Other clinical manifestations such as seizures, altered mental status, lethargy, ataxia, and focal neurologic defects (such as hemiparesis) are more commonly seen with encephalitis. Spinal cord involvement usually presents as transverse myelitis. Cranial nerve palsies also occur, and the facial nerve is most frequently affected. *M. pneumoniae* has also been associated with approximately 5 percent of patients with Guillain-Barré syndrome. A significant number of patients also suffer damage in other organ systems (e.g., heart, liver, and bone marrow).

Mortality and morbidity rates approaches 10 and 23 percent, respectively, in some series. The time interval between respiratory symptoms and neurologic complications does not seem to

TABLE 82-1. Signs and Symptoms of *Mycoplasma*-Associated Encephalitis

Sign and Symptom	% of Patients
Meningeal signs/symptoms	78
Temp ≥39°C	53
Convulsions	46
Unconsciousness	35
Somnolence	42
Ataxia	20
Ocular findings	15
Respiratory symptoms	38
Carditis	6

(Adapted from Koshkiniemi M: CNS manifestations associated with *Mycoplasma pneumoniae* infections: summary of cases at the University of Helsinki and review. Clin Infect Dis, suppl. 1, 17:S52, 1993, with permission.)

affect the prognosis. Residual neurologic deficits occur more often after cases of encephalitis or polyradiculitis than after meningitis—in most published case series, meningitis results in very few or no neurologic complications or deaths. The neurologic sequelae of encephalitis include mental retardation, seizures, choreoathetosis, decreased visual acuity, and movement disorders.

DIAGNOSIS

The CSF appears normal in up to 60 percent of cases. When pleocytosis is present, mononuclear cells predominate (55 to 75 percent). CSF glucose values are almost always normal, and the protein level is normal to high. The opening pressure may be normal or slightly elevated. Electroencephalographic abnormalities are noted in three-quarters of patients but usually reveal only diffuse, nonspecific slowing of limited diagnostic value. Brain imaging studies (such as computed tomography or magnetic resonance imaging) are either normal or show mild diffuse edema.

The primary diagnosis of *M. pneumoniae*-associated CNS disease is frequently made on clinical grounds and serologies. Serum complement fixation titers are the best available diagnostic test. A fourfold rise from acute to convalescent (obtained 7 to 21 days later) is diagnostic for *M. pneumoniae*. A single high titer of 1:32 or more also suggests the diagnosis. Titers begin to rise 1 week after the onset of infection and peak at 3 to 4 weeks. This test has good specificity (which rises with an increase in the titer), but the sensitivity is only approximately 50 percent. Complement fixation titers of the CSF are nonspecific because of cross-reactivity with antigens normally present in the CSF.

Cold agglutinins for *M. pneumoniae* are positive in 30 to 50 percent of patients with pulmonary disease. A high titer of cold agglutinins, that is, more than 1:128, can be very suggestive for *M. pneumoniae*. Bedside cold agglutinins are positive at titers of more than 1:64 and, when present, this finding supports the diagnosis. However, a negative test does not exclude the presence of *M. pneumoniae,* and a low titer is nonspecific since other conditions can cause a weakly positive test (viruses, other causes of atypical pneumonias, collagen vascular disease, and myeloma). The peripheral leukocyte count may be normal or mildly elevated.

Cultures for *M. pneumoniae* are slow growing, and the organism requires a special media containing yeast and supplemental nutrients. These cultures are not routinely performed, and the physician with a clinical suspicion for *M. pneumoniae* should notify the microbiology laboratory so that these specific cultures can be done. There are also species-specific RNA probes available for the direct demonstration of *M. pneumoniae* in sputum, pharyngeal swabs, and throat washings. Similar probes for *M. pneumoniae* in the CSF or brain tissue have not been well studied clinically. Other rapid techniques for diagnosing *M. pneumoniae* in clinical samples include enzyme immunoassays and indirect immunofluorescence, but these are not widely available. The use of the polymerase chain reaction has detected *M. pneumoniae* in the CSF, but its diagnostic utility remains uncertain.

The diagnosis of *Mycoplasma* can also be supported by the exclusion of other pathogens that can cause a similar clinical picture and CSF findings. The differential diagnosis includes viruses such as measles, mumps, varicella zoster, herpes simplex, adenovirus, other respiratory viruses, and enteroviruses.

TREATMENT

It is unclear whether the use of conventional antibiotic therapy for *M. pneumoniae* provides any benefit for CNS disease. Neurologic complications have been reported in patients receiving adequate antimicrobial therapy. Erythromycin and tetracycline for 2 to 3 weeks are the drugs of choice for infections due to *M. pneumoniae*. There are not enough data to support a longer duration of therapy for extrapulmonary symptoms. Other effective antibiotics include the new macrolides and the fluoroquinolones. Although these new agents do not penetrate into the CSF very well, the correlation between achieving adequate antimicrobial CSF levels and clinical outcome is uncertain. Note that tetracyclines and fluoroquinolones cannot be used in children, adolescents, or pregnant women. Additional therapies directed at CNS disease have included corticosteroids, anti-inflammatory medications, antidiuretics, and plasma exchange. There have been no prospective randomized trials of these modalities.

OTHER MYCOPLASMAS AND UREAPLASMAS

M. hominis and *U. urealyticum* have been identified as causes of meningitis in neonates. In one series, *M. hominis* and *U. urealyticum* caused 2.8 and 1.5 percent of neonatal meningitis, respectively. These infections may occur more commonly in newborn infants born to women in lower socioeconomic groups and those with little or no prenatal care. The neonatal meningitis caused by these organisms is as likely to occur in term infants as in premature infants. Infants become exposed to these organisms in the birth canal during delivery, and up to 30 percent subsequently become colonized. There are rare case reports of adults with ventriculoperitoneal shunt and ventriculostomy infections due to *M. hominis*. There are no reports of *U. urealyticum* causing CNS disease in adults.

SUGGESTED READINGS

Cassell GH, Cole BC: Mycoplasmas as agents of human disease. N Engl J Med 304:80, 1981

Clyde WA Jr: Clinical overview of typical *Mycoplasma pneumoniae* infections. Clin Infect Dis, Suppl. 1, 17:S32, 1993

Couch RB: *Mycoplasma pneumoniae* (primary atypical pneumonia). p. 1446. In Mandell GL, Douglas RG, Jr., Bennett JE (eds): Principles and Practices of Infectious Diseases. 3rd Ed. Churchill Livingstone, New York, 1990

Koshkiniemi M: CNS manifestations associated with *Mycoplasma pneumoniae* infections: summary of cases at the University of Helsinki and review. Clin Infect Dis, Suppl. 1, 17:S52, 1993

Maida E, Kristoferitsch W: CSF findings in *Mycoplasma pneumoniae* infections with neurological complications. Acta Neurol Scand 65:524, 1982

Ponka A: CNS manifestations associated with serologically verified *Mycoplasma pneumoniae* infection. Scand J Infect Dis 12:175, 1980

SPINAL CORD AND PERIPHERAL NEUROMUSCULAR DISEASE

PART **IV**

SECTION 1. DISEASES OF THE SPINAL CORD

83. CLINICAL APPROACH TO DISEASE OF THE SPINAL CORD

MARK H. LIBENSON

The spinal cord is the simplest portion of the central nervous system in terms of its functional anatomy, yet spinal cord disorders challenge the clinician with a full range of clinical presentations from a wide variety of causes. Disease processes encountered in the spinal cord include some with a slow onset of symptoms, such as metabolic or neurodegenerative disease of the spinal cord, and some that present as catastrophic neurologic emergencies requiring rapid diagnosis and treatment, such as spinal cord compression or trauma. The well understood arrangement of tracts and cell columns in the spinal cord allows for precise neuroanatomic localization of signs and symptoms, yet this same orderly anatomic organization is notorious for the production of falsely localizing signs that can lead the unwitting clinician astray.

GROSS ANATOMY OF THE SPINAL CORD

The spinal cord (medulla spinalis) represents the caudal continuation of the lower brain stem (medulla oblongata), beginning at the foramen magnum and tapering over its 45-cm adult length to end in the filum terminale, a narrow connective tissue band that anchors the spinal cord to the coccyx. Over most of its course, the diameter of the spinal cord is 1 cm or less, except for expansions at the levels of the cervical and lumbar plexuses reflecting the increased number of entering and exiting neurons relating to the limbs. In cross section, the spinal cord is generally somewhat oval in shape, wider in its transverse diameter, especially in its uppermost portions and at the cervical and lumbar enlargements. Below the level of T12, the substance of the cord tapers rapidly, forming the conically shaped *conus medullaris* (Fig. 83-1).

Viewed with the naked eye, this critical communication link between the body and the brain is strikingly frail. The unprotected spinal cord is a fragile structure and would undoubtedly be a yet more frequent site of injury were it not surrounded by an elaborate system of osseous, ligamentous, and fluid defenses that provide for the great flexibility of the spinal column while protecting the spinal cord itself from outside injury. Thus, the spinal cord is encircled by a series of bony vertebral rings, stabilized by a complex ligamentous system, sheathed in a tough connective tissue covering (the dura), and surrounded by a fluid cushion (the cerebrospinal fluid). Unlike the situation within the cranium where the dura is closely adherent to the cerebral hemispheres and plays an additional role as the inner periosteal lining of the cranial bones, the dural covering of the

spinal cord is situated away from the spinal cord, forming a permanent rather than "virtual" subdural space (Fig. 83-2).

Examined in cross section, a central, distinctive butterfly-shaped gray matter core is seen surrounded by white matter tracts. The central gray contains neuronal cell bodies; the white

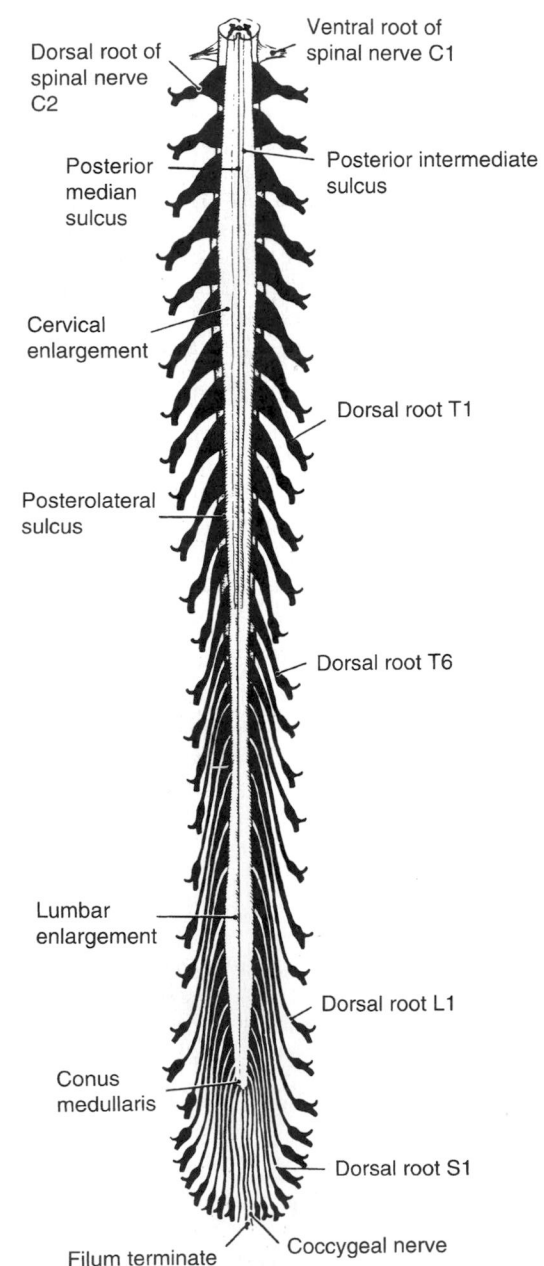

FIG. 83-1. Posterior view of the spinal cord showing attached dorsal root filaments and spinal ganglia. (From Carpenter MB: Core Text of Neuroanatomy. 3rd Ed. Williams & Wilkins, Baltimore, 1985, with permission.)

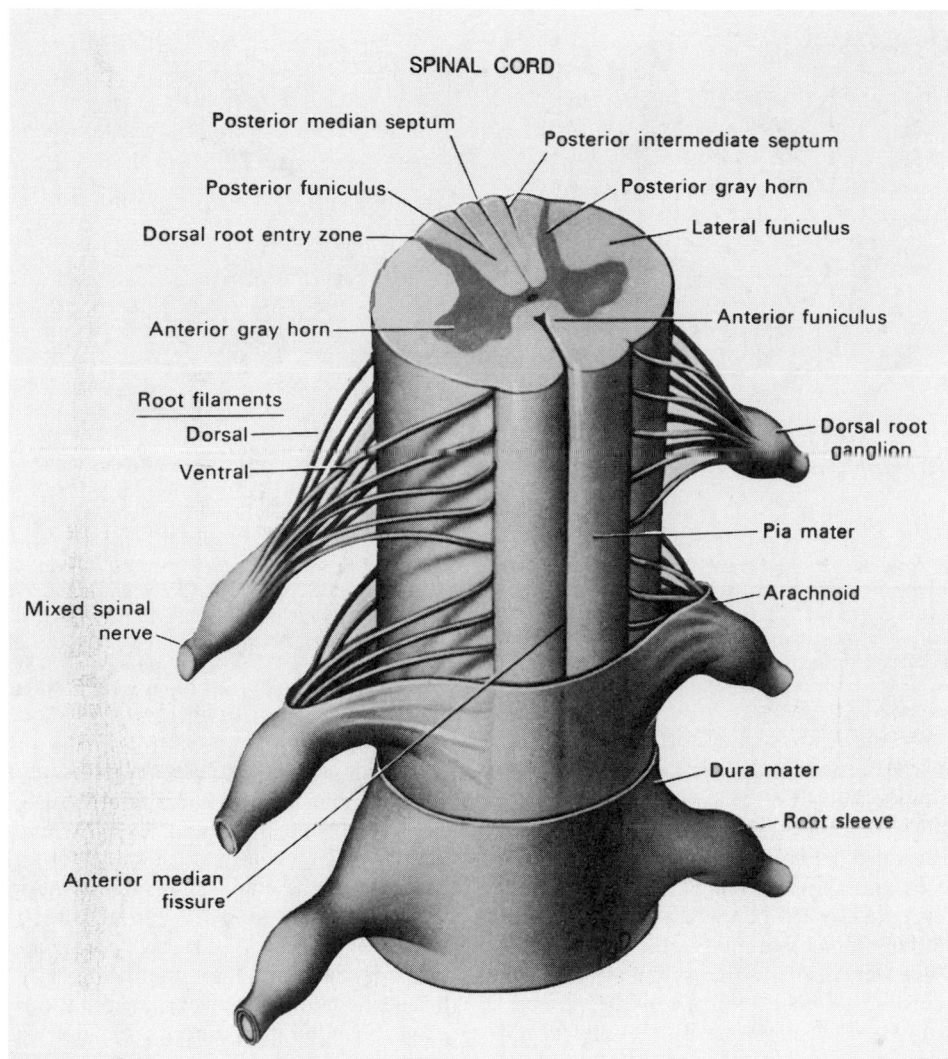

SPINAL CORD

FIG. 83-2. Anterior view of the spinal cord and its coverings. The pia mater is seen closely adherent to the spinal cord compared to the overlying arachnoidal and dural layers. Dorsal and ventral spinal rootlets are seen coalescing to form the spinal nerves. The dorsal root ganglia are seen just distal to this junction. (From Carpenter MB: Core Text of Neuroanatomy, 3rd Ed. Williams & Wilkins, Baltimore, 1985, with permission.)

matter consists of the ascending and descending myelinated tracts of the spinal cord. A small, ependyma-lined central canal runs the whole of the cord's length, and nearly all neurons that cross from one side of the spinal cord to the other do so in the commissure that lies anterior to this canal.

Reflecting the organization seen in the central nervous system as a whole, there is a general tendency in the spinal cord for motor structures to be located anteriorly and sensory structures posteriorly. Thus, the posterior gray matter of the spinal cord receives the dorsal (sensory) root, and the anterior gray of the spinal cord contains the anterior horn cells (motor neuron cell bodies), which give rise to the anterior (motor) root. The dorsal and anterior roots join together outside the cord to form each segment's spinal nerve, which pierces the dura and exits through its corresponding intervertebral foramen. The location of the white matter tracts represents an important exception to the anterior-posterior organizational rule, that is, the descending motor (corticospinal) tracts are located posterolaterally, and the sensory white matter tracts are located both anteriorly and posteriorly (dorsal and ventral spinothalamic tracts and dorsal columns) (Fig. 83-3).

Each spinal nerve is named for its adjacent vertebral body. This leads to two problems in nomenclature. Because there is an additional pair of spinal nerve roots compared to the number of vertebral bodies, the first seven spinal nerves are named for the first seven cervical vertebrae, each exiting through the intervertebral foramen *above* its correspondingly named vertebral body. The spinal nerve exiting below the level of C7, however, is referred to as the C8 spinal nerve (the "extra" spinal root), though no eighth cervical vertebra exists. Because of this "additional" nerve root, all subsequent roots exit *below* the vertebral body for which they are named, beginning with T1 (Fig. 83-4). The 8 cervical roots, 12 thoracic roots, 5 lumbar roots, 5 sacral roots, and 1 coccygeal root total 31 spinal nerve root pairs. All of these contain both motor and sensory roots with the exception of C1, which lacks a sensory component (explaining the absence of a "C1 dermatome").

The second problem in spinal root nomenclature arises from the relative positions of the spinal nerves with respect to their vertebral bodies. During the third embryonic month, the spinal segments are closely aligned to their corresponding vertebral segments, but, after this point in fetal development, the bony

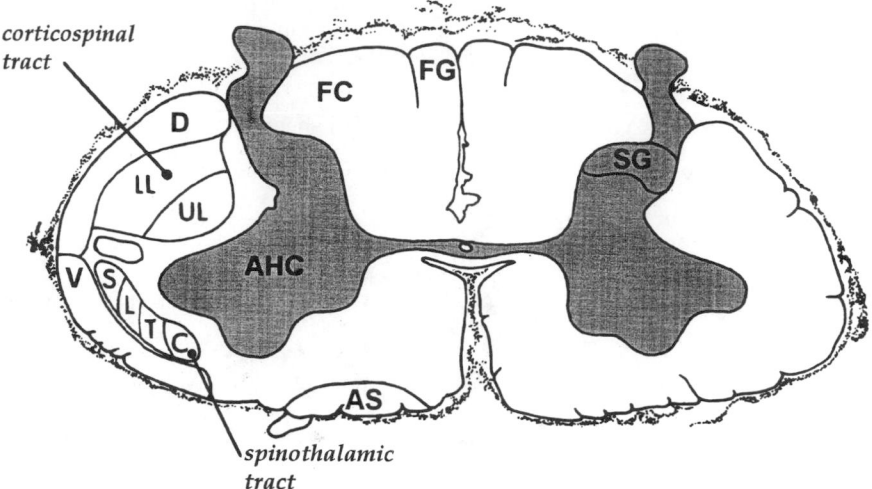

FIG. 83-3.   Cross section of the cervical spinal cord showing white and gray matter areas in cross section, including the lamination of the corticospinal and lateral spinothalamic tracts. *D,* dorsal spinocerebellar tract; *V,* ventral spinocerebellar tract; *LL,* portion of corticospinal tract serving lower limbs; *UL,* portion of corticospinal tract serving upper limbs; *S* (sacral), *L* (lumbar), *T* (thoracic), and *C* (cervical) mark portions of spinothalamic tract that carry sensory information from these areas; *AHC,* anterior horn cells; *FC,* fasciculus cuneatus; *FG,* fasciculus gracilis; *SG,* substantia gelatinosa; *AS,* anterior spinothalamic tract. (Adapted from Watson C: Basic Human Neuroanatomy, An Introductory Atlas. 2nd Ed. Little, Brown, Boston, 1977, with permission.)

spinal column's downward growth outpaces that of the spinal cord. This gives the impression that the lower portion of the spinal cord has "risen" in the spinal canal relative to the vertebral column. Indeed, because the adult spinal cord ends as the conus medullaris at approximately the L1 level, the lumbar and sacral roots must plunge downward below the termination of the spinal cord to find their respective intervertebral foramina, forming the distinctive *cauda equina* (horse's tail). As a consequence, a pathologic process at the level of the L4 vertebral body would be potentially in close proximity to both the L4 nerve root and the lower spinal roots that have arisen from the conus medullaris at the approximate level of L1 but have destinations caudal to the L4 vertebral body.

The vascular supply to the spinal cord consists of a single, larger anterior spinal artery and two smaller posterior spinal arteries. The anterior spinal artery is formed from a contributing branch from each vertebral artery, both of which join together at the level of the foramen magnum to form the anterior spinal artery, which accepts branches from segmental vessels of varying sizes as it descends the anterior surface of the spinal cord. This artery serves the anterior two-thirds of the cord. One or two smaller posterior spinal arteries also arise from the vertebral arteries and course down the dorsal aspect of the spinal cord, serving a wedge-shaped area constituting the posterior third of the cord.

FUNCTIONAL NEUROANATOMY OF THE SPINAL CORD

While a large number of ascending and descending tracts have been identified and mapped in the spinal cord, the three most important of these in terms of neuroanatomic localization of cord lesions are the corticospinal tracts, spinothalamic tracts, and the dorsal columns.

The *corticospinal tract* is formed from neurons the cell bodies of which are located in the motor areas of cerebral cortex, including the giant cortical motor neurons referred to as Betz

cells. The axons of these "upper motor neurons" reach the anterior horn cells of the spinal cord by passing through the internal capsule, the peduncles of the midbrain, and the belly of the pons. They continue caudally, forming a distinctive paired structure on the anterior surface of the medulla, the pyramids, from which the term "pyramidal tract" is derived. Without synapsing, nearly all of these pyramidal axons cross at the level of the medulla and the uppermost cervical spinal cord to form the decussation of the corticospinal tracts. Once crossed, the axons abandon their anterior location and move posteriorly to the posterolateral funiculi of the spinal cord. Most of these neurons are destined to synapse on the anterior horn cells of the anterior gray of the spinal cord, the "lower motor neurons." Furthermore, these neurons are laminated in a clinically important arrangement, with fibers destined for the lower limbs traveling more superficially in the cord and fibers destined for upper limbs traveling more deeply in the cord.

Damage to these corticospinal tract neurons (upper motor neurons) in the spinal cord results in ipsilateral clinical findings such as spastic weakness, increased deep tendon reflexes, and a Babinski sign (Table 83-1). When there is damage to the anterior horn cells (lower motor neurons), ipsilateral clinical findings occur at the level of the affected segments, including flaccid weakness, muscle wasting, decreased deep tendon reflexes, and fasciculations (in addition to a distinctive group of electrophysiologic findings in peripheral nerve and muscle seen during nerve conduction testing and electromyography, such as decreased compound muscle action potential amplitude, polyphasic motor units, fibrillation potentials, and decreased F-waves and H-reflexes, described more fully in Ch. 30). Thus, unilateral spinal cord damage causes ipsilateral motor findings on neurologic examination, possibly of the mixed upper motor neuron and lower motor neuron type.

There are two major ascending systems that transmit conscious sensory information: the spinothalamic tracts and the dorsal columns. The first neurons of both of these afferent systems begin as sensory structures situated in target organs (e.g.,

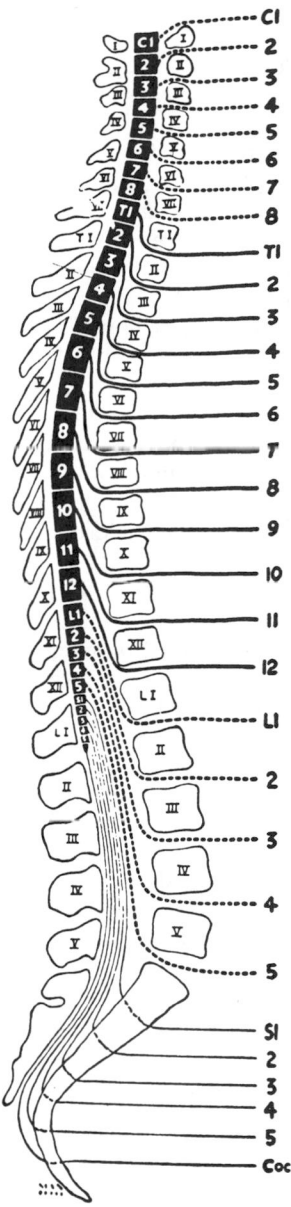

FIG. 83-4. Spinal cord root levels in relation to the vertebral body. Note the close association of vertebral and nerve root levels in the cervical cord compared to the lumbar cord. (From Haymaker W, Woodhall B: Peripheral Nerve Injuries. 2nd Ed. WB Saunders, Philadelphia, 1953, with permission.)

sensory receptors in skin and stretch receptors in muscle) with their cell bodies located in the dorsal root ganglia of the spinal nerves. These ganglia are seen as distinctive prominences on the dorsal nerve roots just proximal to the point where the anterior and dorsal branches join in the intervertebral foramen to form the peripheral spinal nerve.

The *spinothalamic tracts* transmit pain and temperature sensation, usually tested at the bedside in the form of pinprick and cold sensation. As the axons of these neurons enter the spinal cord, most rise one or two levels (in the dorsolateral tract of Lissauer) before entering the dorsal gray of the spinal cord (substantia gelatinosa) where they synapse with the second neuron of the spinothalamic system. This second neuron crosses immediately in the anterior commissure of the spinal cord and ascends in the anterolateral funiculus as the lateral spinothalamic tract. (A small number of spinothalamic fibers may remain uncrossed and ascend as the clinically less important anterior spinothalamic tract.) As a result, when the anterolaterally located spinothalamic tract is damaged in the spinal cord, the patient experiences sensory symptoms in the contralateral half of the body. This is contrary to the case of the motor system described above. Again, there is a clinically important lamination of this tract where, *like the corticospinal tract,* sensory neurons arising from the lower body travel more superficially in the tract and neurons arising from higher levels travel more deeply in the tract.

The *dorsal columns* transmit vibration and proprioceptive information, tested at the bedside by placing a vibrating tuning fork on bone and by testing the patient's ability to detect changes in joint position on passive motion. These neurons enter the spinal cord via the dorsal root alongside pain and temperature neurons, but, instead of making an immediate synapse as do the latter neurons, these axons enter the ipsilateral dorsal column immediately and do not synapse until they reach the gracile or cuneate nuclei of the medulla. Because this long, single neuron does not cross the midline until it passes through the foramen magnum, a lesion involving one side of the dorsal columns of the spinal cord causes ipsilateral loss of vibration and joint position sense. Because the sensory modality of light touch is transmitted through both the spinothalamic tracts and the dorsal columns, this type of sensation is not completely lost unless both the spinothalamic and dorsal column systems are affected.

SPINAL CORD LOCALIZATION

Determining the location of a lesion in the spinal cord begins with the question, ''Is the lesion in the spinal cord?'' In general, neurologic localization begins with the attempt to explain all of a patient's findings by a single lesion before invoking multiple lesions to explain a particular pattern of findings. While the concept may seem self-evident, it is worth repeating here, that is, spinal cord lesions do not disturb cortical or brainstem functions. Therefore, findings such as aphasias, disturbances of vision, eye movement, swallowing, or consciousness are not consistent with a simple spinal cord localization; the presence of such findings leads the search for the lesion above the level of the foramen magnum. Apparent exceptions to this rule include the presence of a Horner syndrome (the first-order neuron of the sympathetic innervation of the pupil, eye, and upper face

TABLE 83-1. Effects of Damage to the Major Functional Anatomic Units of the Spinal Cord

	Corticospinal Tracts	Anterior Horn Cells	Spinothalamic Tracts	Dorsal Columns
Modality	Motor	Motor	Pain and temperature	Joint position sense and vibration
Symptoms	Spastic paralysis, hyperreflexia	Flaccid paralysis, decreased reflexes	Loss of pain and temperature, sensation, numbness, anesthesia	Loss of proprioception, vibration sense, paresthesias, Romberg sign
Distribution of symptoms in relation to spinal cord lesion	Ipsilateral, below level of lesion	Radicular distribution according to levels involved	Contralateral, below level of lesion	Ipsilateral, below level of lesion

TABLE 83-2. Selected Spinal Cord Syndromes by Anatomic Location

Extradural	Vascular (ischemic/infarct)
Osteoarthritis	Arteriovenous malformation
Disc herniation	Intramedullary abscess
Epidural abscess	Paraneoplastic myelitis
Bony/meningeal metastases	Tumors (ependymoma, astrocytoma,
Epidural hematoma	oligodendroglioma, lipoma,
Cervical spondylosis	epidermoid, dermoid, teratoma,
Rheumatoid arthritis	hemangioma, hemangioblastoma,
Ankylosing spondylitis	metastatic carcinoma)
Other degenerative spine	Electrical injuries
disease	Spinal arachnoiditis
Paget's disease	Baló's concentric sclerosis
Craniocervical junction	*Select tracts/cell columns*
abnormalities:	Amyotrophic lateral sclerosis
Mucopolysaccharidosis	Primary lateral sclerosis
Klippel-Feil	HIV-associated vacuolar myelopathy
Achondroplasia	Adrenomyeloneuropathy/
Platybasia/basilar	adrenoleukocystrophy
invagination	Spinocerebellar degenerations
Pott's disease	Vitamin B$_{12}$ deficiency (subacute
Atlantoaxial dislocation	combined degeneration)
Foramen magnum tumor	Familial spastic paraparesis
Intradural	Werdnig-Hoffmann disease
Neurofibroma (schwannoma)	Kugelberg-Welander disease
Meningioma	Tabes dorsalis
Leptomeningeal carcinoma	Poliomyelitis infection
Sarcomas	HTLV-I–associated tropical spastic
Vascular tumors	paraparesis
Central cord syndrome	Lathyrism
Syringomyelia	*Malformative*
Hematomyelia (trauma)	Spinal dysraphism
Intramedullary tumors	Spinal bifida
Demyelinating disease	Meningocele
Infarcts	Myelocele
Diffuse/focal/multifocal	Myelomeningocele
Spinal cord trauma	Caudal regression syndrome
Hematomyelia	Diastematomyelia
Multiple sclerosis	Diplomyelia
Radiation myelitis	Hydromyelia
Transverse myelitis	Arnold-Chiari malformation type II
Viral myelitis	Tethered cord
Autoimmune (postinfectious)	
myelitis	

Abbreviations: HIV, human immunodeficiency virus; HTLV-I, human T-cell leukemia virus type I.

descends from the hypothalamus ipsilaterally in the spinal cord as low as T1). A second such apparent exception is pain and temperature abnormalities in the face (some trigeminal neurons subserving pain and temperature enter the pons and descend into the upper cervical cord as low as the C2 to C4 levels before synapsing in the nucleus of the spinal tract of V and ascending to the contralateral thalamus). Table 83-2 lists a selection of spinal cord syndromes by anatomic site.

Spinal cord localization is suggested when a patient presents with one of the hallmark spinal cord syndromes. While patients in clinical practice rarely present with textbook descriptions of these distinctive syndromes, recognition of partial expressions or fragments of these classic syndromes is often the first step in correct diagnosis.

Complete Spinal Cord Transection Syndrome

Transection of the spinal cord results in interruption of the long motor and sensory tracts with concomitant complete loss of voluntary motor and conscious sensory function below the level of the transection. Damage to sensory and motor roots at the level of the transection results in complete abolition of reflexes at the level of the lesion. Minutes after a complete cord transection, there follows a period of spinal cord hypoexcitability referred to as "spinal shock," which may last days to weeks. During this period, there is complete absence of reflex and

autonomic activity below the level of the injury with flaccid paralysis. In some cases, reflexes above the level of the transection are depressed, too. When the stage of spinal shock passes, hyperreflexia with spastic paralysis below the level of the injury supervenes.

Transections at high cervical levels result in tetraplegia. Transection at the level of C2 results in sensory loss over the whole body and the occipital area (indeed, all body regions except the trigeminal nerve's sensory distribution). Lesions at the level of C4 and below may allow for enough preserved phrenic nerve function (C3, C4, and C5) to allow eventually for adequate diaphragmatic function after the period of acute injury. Lesions from C6 to T1 involve diminishing subgroups of the muscles innervated by the brachial plexus and allow for increasing function of the arms and hands. Horner syndrome (ptosis, miosis, anhidrosis, and absence of facial flushing) is seen in cervical cord transection owing to disruption of descending sympathetics. Full diaphragmatic innervation compensates for loss of intercostal muscle and other auxiliary respiratory muscle innervation.

Spinal cord transection below the level of T1 allows for complete use of the upper extremities, including the hands. With lesions above T6, the abdominal reflexes are absent. With lesions at T10, the upper abdominal reflexes are preserved; with those at T12, all abdominal reflexes are present. With transection levels from L1 to S2, there are decreasing amounts of involvement of the lower extremities. With spinal cord levels below S2, innervation to the lower extremity muscles is preserved, but bowel and bladder function is affected, as described below.

During the initial stage of spinal shock after cord transection at any level, reflex emptying of the bladder is lost, resulting in urinary retention and bladder distention. In lesions that occur above the sacral level, leaving the spinal bladder center in the conus medullaris and the roots of the pudendal nerve (S2, S3, and S4) intact, automatic, reflex emptying of the bladder returns days to weeks after the injury. In sacral lesions that interrupt the bladder center, the bladder becomes autonomous with feeble, inefficient, and incoordinated contractions of the detrusor muscle. Combinations of these spastic and atonic bladder syndromes may occur in partial cord lesions at the sacral level.

Similarly, bowel function ceases immediately after complete cord transection at any level, with loss of rectal tone and the anal "wink" reflex. Spontaneous bowel peristalsis returns within a few days as a rule, as do the anal and bulbocavernosus reflexes when the cord lesion lies above the sacral level. Later, in the hyperreflexic stage, anal tone may actually become significantly increased. In lesions of the lumbosacral cord, however, the anus remains patulous. Complete spinal cord transection may be caused by trauma; severe compression from tumor, hematoma, or abscess; or transverse myelitis (viral or demyelinative), among other causes.

Syndrome of Spinal Cord Hemisection: The Brown-Séquard Syndrome

Hemisection of the spinal cord results in the distinctive syndrome of ipsilateral motor paralysis and contralateral pain and temperature loss below the level of the lesion, known as the Brown-Séquard syndrome. Although often not as prominent clinically, ipsilateral vibration and proprioceptive loss also occurs (on the same side as the motor symptoms). In the complete syndrome, the ipsilateral anterior horn cells and dorsal roots are also affected at the level of the transection. Thus, a complete hemisection of the cord on the right results in paralysis with increased reflexes (after the acute phase) and loss of joint position and vibration sense on the right side below the level of the lesion and loss of pain and temperature sense on the left side. If the lesion happens to occur at the level of the lumbar or cervical plexuses, lower motor neuron involvement at that level may be more easily observed with loss of segmental reflexes and, later, wasting and other signs of denervation in the muscles of that root level's distribution. Likewise with a right-sided spinal cord hemisection, an isolated area of complete sensory loss to both dorsal column and spinothalamic tract modalities is seen on the right in the dermatome(s) at or just below the level of the hemisection. This occurs as a result of interruption of all sensory neurons entering the cord on the right side at that level. Spinal cord hemisection may be caused by partial expressions of the causes of complete cord transections.

Syndrome of Extrinsic Spinal Cord Compression (Cord-Root Syndrome)

Lesions that compress the spinal cord from a location outside the dura produce symptoms in the outermost long pathways first. Owing to the specific lamination of the corticospinal and spinothalamic tracts, as described above (lower extremity fibers most superficial and upper extremity fibers deepest), cervical compressive lesions may cause motor and sensory symptoms to appear first in the lower extremities; symptoms then appear to "ascend" as compression increases. This anatomy is notorious for producing falsely localizing signs, for example, a distinct level of sensory loss may then be discernible at the level of the umbilicus (T10) in the case of a compressive tumor at the foramen magnum! The unwary clinician obtaining a magnetic resonance imaging scan of the thoracic cord might be falsely reassured by a normal result that misses the lesion completely. Therefore, sensory levels produced by extrinsic, compressive cord lesions only mark the lowest possible level of the lesion; the actual pathology may lie anywhere between the level of sensory loss and the foramen magnum.

In addition to affecting the long tracts of the spinal cord, extrinsic compressive lesions often involve motor and sensory roots at the level of the lesion. Identification of a root level can be a very helpful sign; the rostral limit of long tract (motor and sensory) loss only marks the lowest possible location of the lesion in the spinal cord. When, in addition, a focus of back pain is present or distinct lower motor neuron signs are found at a specific level, the level of the lesion may be pinpointed.

Lateral compressive lesions, though not causing a spinal cord hemisection *per se,* can very much resemble the Brown-Séquard syndrome. In cases of lateral compression rather than hemisection, the ipsilateral half of the spinal cord is usually more symptomatic than the contralateral half. Except in the case of early compressive lesions, some bilaterality to the signs and symptoms is common.

Central (Intramedullary) Spinal Cord Syndrome

The clinical syndrome caused by smaller intramedullary lesions is characterized by the destruction of the anterior commissure of the spinal cord, which contains crossing spinothalamic tract neurons. This results in a capelike distribution of anesthesia at the level of the lesion in the case of cervical lesions. Further symptoms caused by the lesion depend especially on the addi-

tional cord regions the lesion involves in the transverse plane. Lesions that include the anterior gray matter of the spinal cord may destroy the anterior horn cells, causing weakness and wasting of muscles at the involved levels. Further enlargement of the affected area may result in involvement of the spinothalamic tracts. Because fibers traveling to sacral areas travel most superficially in the spinal cord (see above), expanding intramedullary lesions cause increasing areas of analgesia, but with a tendency to *sacral sparing,* as these fibers are most distant from the center of the cord. Thus, an expanding cervical central cord lesion may begin by causing capelike anesthesia involving the arms but with progressively descending sensory involvement to the point that only the saddle area is spared. Larger lesions may similarly affect the descending corticospinal tracts. The most common causes of such lesions are syringomyelia, hematomyelia, and intrinsic cord tumors.

Syndromes of the Cauda Equina and Conus Medullaris

Because the cauda equina is composed of the lumbosacral roots as they descend into the thecal sac below the termination of the spinal cord, pathologic processes in this area may cause a patchy distribution of symptoms, depending on which nerve roots are involved. Pain is often prominent. Lesions of the conus medullaris may involve a similar array of nerve roots, but, because this region of the cord contains important reflex centers, disorders of bowel, bladder, and sexual function are more prominent.

Other Spinal Cord Syndromes

Anterior horn cell syndromes occur, sometimes with associated upper motor neuron involvement. The most important disorder among adults associated with this pattern is amyotrophic lateral sclerosis, in which there is a progression of both upper and lower motor neuron signs. Spinal muscular atrophy (Werdnig-Hoffmann disease) is a pure anterior horn cell degeneration usually presenting in infancy, though more slowly progressive forms are recognized. Infection with the poliomyelitis virus, now rare, shows a predilection for the anterior horn cell and produces asymmetric motor involvement and a cerebrospinal fluid pleocytosis after a febrile illness. Cervical and lumbar degenerative spine disease may result in stenosis of the spinal canal at those levels. This syndrome of *spinal cord stenosis* may mimic amyotrophic lateral sclerosis by causing both upper motor neuron signs from spinal cord compression and lower motor neuron signs at multiple levels owing to loss in height of the intervertebral foramina at multiple levels.

Occlusion of the anterior spinal artery produces a distinctive *anterior spinal artery syndrome* with loss of spinothalamic and corticospinal tract function. Dorsal column functions are preserved. Thus, the patient is paralyzed to a varying degree below the level of the lesion with complete loss of pain and temperature sensation, but with preservation of vibration and joint position sense.

Certain patterns of spinal cord involvement, though not anatomically confluent, are characteristic of specific disease processes. *Tabes dorsalis* occurs as a late complication of syphilitic infection. There is marked degeneration of the posterior columns, which produces an ataxia based on sensory loss. Loss of the posterior roots in the lumbosacral area is responsible for abnormal bowel, bladder, and sexual function caused by loss of sensory inputs and probably also explains the lancinating pains characteristic of this disorder. *Subacute combined degeneration* is the term used for the myelopathy associated with vitamin B_{12} deficiency (or rather failure to absorb vitamin B_{12} from the gut owing to lack of intrinsic factor in patients with pernicious anemia). Corticospinal, spinothalamic, and dorsal column tracts of the cord are all affected, with the posterior column findings being most prominent.

DIAGNOSTIC TESTING IN SPINAL CORD DISEASE

Careful history taking and a methodical neurologic examination frequently strongly suggest a specific diagnosis; electrophysiologic and radiologic testing often confirm the diagnostic impression. Spine radiographs give an idea of the caliber of the spinal canal, the height of the intervertebral foramina, or the presence of bony spurs. Plain radiographs of the spine may also show evidence of spine instability, fracture, or dislocation in cases of trauma. Flexion and extension views of the cervical spine may demonstrate the atlantoaxial subluxation that is common in individuals with Down syndrome. Plain radiographs may also show degenerative disease of the spine suggestive of disc or spondylitic disease. The appearance of lytic vertebral lesions may lead to a diagnosis of metastatic disease. Certain spinal cord malformations may be suspected when certain findings, such as spina bifida occulta, butterfly vertebrae or hemivertebrae, or a bony spur traversing the cord (diastematomyelia) are present.

Lumbar puncture allows for analysis of the cerebrospinal fluid and measurement of its pressure. Spinal fluid culture and serology may help pinpoint the etiology of infectious causes of spinal cord disease, such as spinal abscess. The isolated finding of very high protein levels in the spinal fluid is suggestive of spinal block, usually from tumor. More modest increases in spinal fluid protein are observed in cases of myelopathy that are associated with polyradiculopathy. Cytologic studies of spinal fluid may help make a specific diagnosis of malignancy. Cell counts in spinal fluid may point toward infection or other inflammatory processes. Measurement of spinal fluid IgG, myelin basic protein, and oligoclonal bands may help establish the diagnosis of multiple sclerosis.

After lumbar puncture, myelography may be performed by injecting contrast material through a spinal needle. The contrast medium outlines the subarachnoid space and allows visualiza-

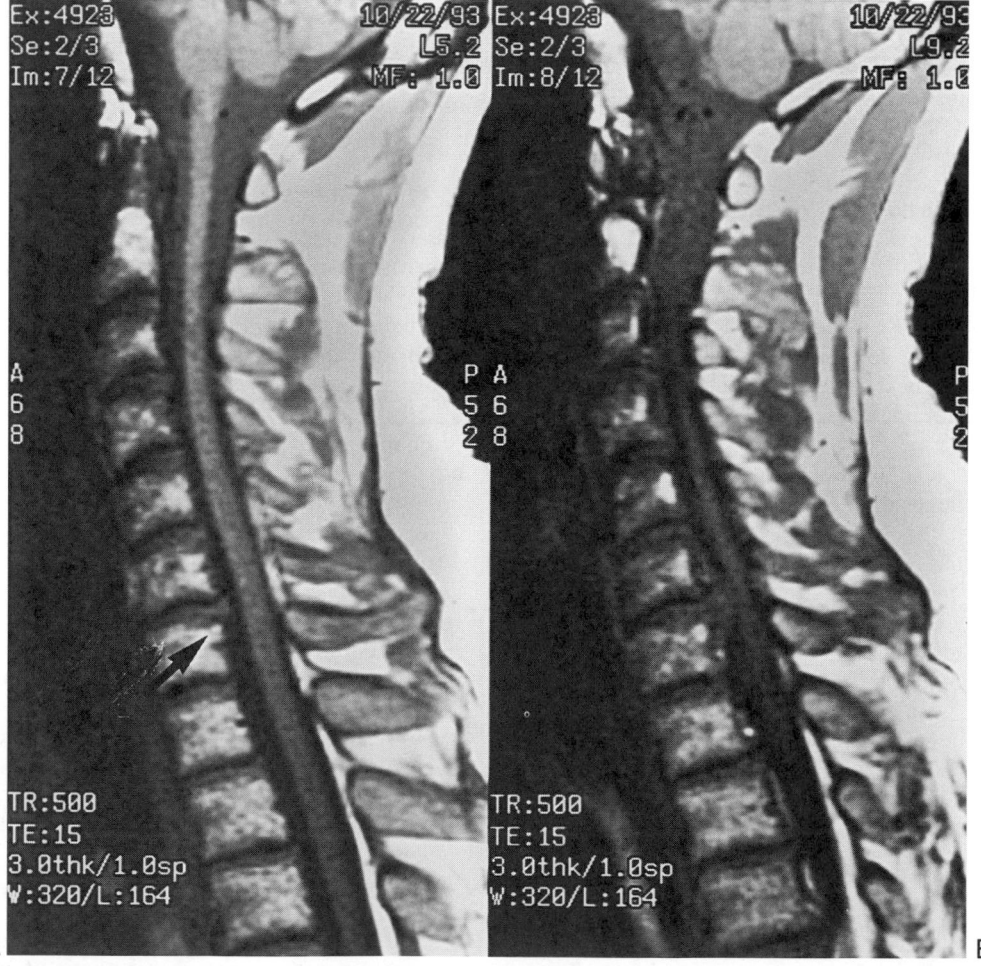

FIG. 83-5. (A & B) T1-weighted MRI scans of the cervical spine showing a herniation of the C6–C7 intervertebral disc. In Fig. A (midsagittal plane), the spinal cord appears gray and is surrounded by cerebrospinal fluid, which appears black. The vertebral bodies appear as a column of rectangles anterior to the cord and show a bright signal because of increased fat content in the marrow. The C6–C7 disc can be see protruding posteriorly (arrow). Fig. B shows the same scanning sequence but the plane of the scan is now just to the left of the midline. A larger portion of the disc can be seen herniating posteriorly and appearing to impinge on the spinal cord. (*figure continues.*)

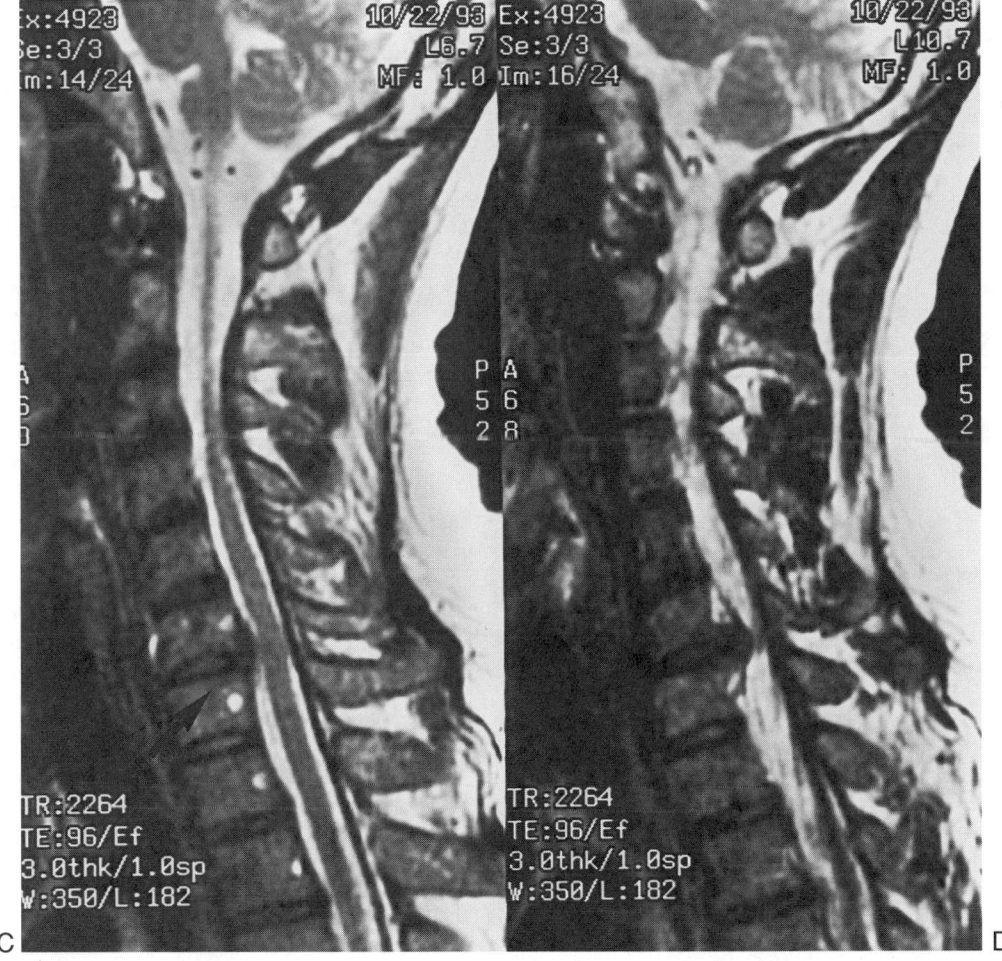

FIG. 83-5 (*Continued*). **(C & D)**, T2-weighted scans of cervical spine of the same patient. The cerebrospinal fluid now appears white in this sequence, surrounding the darker spinal cord. Fig. C is a Scan in midsagittal plane showing the same disc obliterating the subarachnoid space anterior to the spinal cord. There is no abnormal (bright) signal in the spinal cord to suggest damage to the spinal cord itself. Fig. D is a T2-weighted with scan plane again just left of the midline. The substance of this left-sided cervical disc herniation is better seen in this scan, extending posteriorly and to the left, impinging on the area traversed by the left C6 nerve root.

tion of the spinal cord, nerve roots, or intradural lesions, which appear as shadows or defects in the column of injected contrast. Extradural compressive lesions appear as an indentation on the thecal sac. Computed tomographic scan of the spinal cord, a so-called computed tomographic myelogram, may be performed after such an injection.

Use of both plain and computed tomographic myelography has, for the most part, been supplanted by magnetic resonance imaging of the spinal cord, which has revolutionized the diagnosis of spinal cord disease. Magnetic resonance imaging shows better detail, distinguishes better between normal and abnormal soft tissues, and has significantly improved the imaging of both extrinsic and intrinsic spinal cord disease (Fig. 83-5).

SUGGESTED READINGS

Adams RD, Victor M: Diseases of the spinal cord. pp. 1078–116. In Principles of Neurology. 5th Ed. McGraw-Hill, New York, 1993

Carpenter MB: Core Text of Neuroanatomy. 3rd Ed. Williams & Wilkins, Baltimore, 1985

Gray H: Gray's Anatomy. 23rd Ed. Revised and Edited by Warren H. Lewis. Lea & Febiger, Philadelphia, 1936

Hughes JT: Disorders of the spine and spinal cord. In Adams JH, Duchen LW (eds): Greenfield's Neuropathology. 5th Ed. Oxford University Press, New York, 1992

Ludwig G: Clinical symptomatology of spinal cord lesions. pp. 178–216. In Vinken PJ, Bruyn GW (eds): Handbook of Clinical Neurology. Vol. 2. John Wiley & Sons, New York, 1969

Williams PL, Warwick R: Functional Neuroanatomy of Man. WB Saunders, Philadelphia, 1975

84. SYRINGOMYELIA AND RELATED CONDITIONS

PATRICK A. ROTH
ALAN R. COHEN

Syringomyelia is a term used to describe a fluid-filled cavity in the spinal cord. It may be associated with several distinct conditions or may occur as an isolated entity. Syringomyelia has fascinated clinicians for years as the symptoms are often

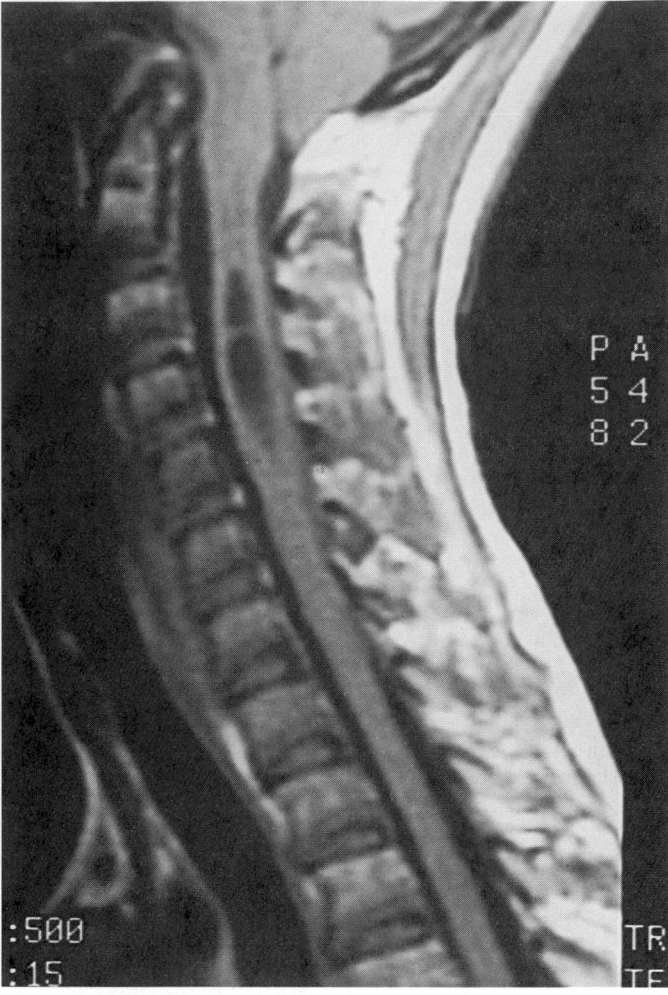

FIG. 84-1. Syrinx of the cervical cord with a septation.

a striking recapitulation of those predicted from a centrifugal distortion of the normal cross-sectional anatomy of the spinal cord. The diverse etiologies of this entity have generated a great deal of interest in its pathogenesis. The advent of magnetic resonance imaging (MRI) has revolutionized our understanding of this disease by improving diagnostic capabilities, providing precise anatomic information both preoperatively and postoperatively, and improving our understanding of the pathogenesis (Fig. 84-1).

The natural history of syringomyelia has never been adequately characterized. It appears to be variable, and it is thus difficult to predict the rate or extent of progression in any individual case. Most studies that have looked at the natural history of syringomyelia are retrospective and involve either many different treatments for a population of patients or several sequential treatments for an individual patient so that a predicted tempo or extent of progression cannot be reliably extracted to provide a sense of risk in any given case. These complex retrospective studies also limit our ability to evaluate critically and compare the various treatment modalities used.

Since a substantial portion of patients that are symptomatic will develop progressive problems, most surgeons initiate some form of treatment in cases of symptomatic syringomyelia.

HISTORY

The earliest report of syringomyelia is that of Étienne in 1564. He compared the cavitation of the spinal cord to the ventricles of the brain. The term syringomyelia was derived by Ollivier d'Angers in 1824 from the Greek words syrinx "to become hollow" and myelia "marrow." Virchow, in 1863, suggested the alternative term, hydromyelia, as he believed that the central canal was the source of the abnormal fluid within the canal. In 1875, Simon proposed that the term syringomyelia be used to describe a fluid collection within the substance of the cord separate from the central canal and that the term hydromyelia be used to describe a dilation of the central canal.

Several authors continue to distinguish syringomyelia from hydromyelia by using the two terms separately; others use the terms syringohydromyelia or hydrosyringomyelia to group the two entities into one category and thus avoid the distinction. We use the traditional term syringomyelia to include both of these theoretic anatomic variants, as the distinction is often difficult to display pathologically and there is no clinical relevance in separating the two entities on the basis of pathogenesis, natural history, or appropriate treatment modalities (Fig. 84-2).

PATHOGENESIS

The development of theories of the pathogenesis of syringomyelia is fascinating. Gardner proposed a "hydrodynamic" theory for the pathogenesis of a syrinx. According to his theory, the formation of a syrinx was the result of a communication between the fourth ventricle and the central canal of the spinal cord coupled with a relative obstruction in the outlets of the fourth ventricle, resulting in a "water-hammer" effect with cerebrospinal fluid (CSF) being propelled into the central canal with each systolic pulsation of the brain. Williams, alternatively, suggested that a syrinx was formed as a result of "craniospinal pressure dissociation." He postulated that a normal Valsalva maneuver results in flow of CSF from the intraspinal compartment into the intracranial compartment followed by a return flow back into the intraspinal compartment after the Valsalva. With an obstruction at the foramen magnum, there would be a relative impedance to this bidirectional flow, and alternative conduits would be utilized, such as flow between the central canal of the spinal cord and the fourth ventricle. Both the theories of Gardner and Williams are based on the existence of a communication between the fourth ventricle and the central canal of the spinal canal.

Recent evidence based on both autopsy and MRI studies suggests, however, that most syrinxes do not communicate with the fourth ventricle. This has lent some support to different theories of pathogenesis. Ball and Dayan in 1972 suggested that the syrinx was the result of flow across the spinal cord from the spinal subarachnoid space through Virchow-Robin spaces. Similarly, Aboulker in 1979 postulated that the syrinx was the result of flow across the spinal cord from the spinal subarachnoid space through the dorsal nerve root entry zone of the spinal cord. Milhorat et al. in 1993 suggested that the syrinx might result from a block of the normal cephalad-directed flow of CSF in the central canal, originating within the spinal cord parenchymal extracellular space. They pointed out that the central canal of the thoracic and lumbar segments of the spinal cord is normally obliterated in adults and that this might explain the predominance of cervical or cervicothoracic syrinxes in

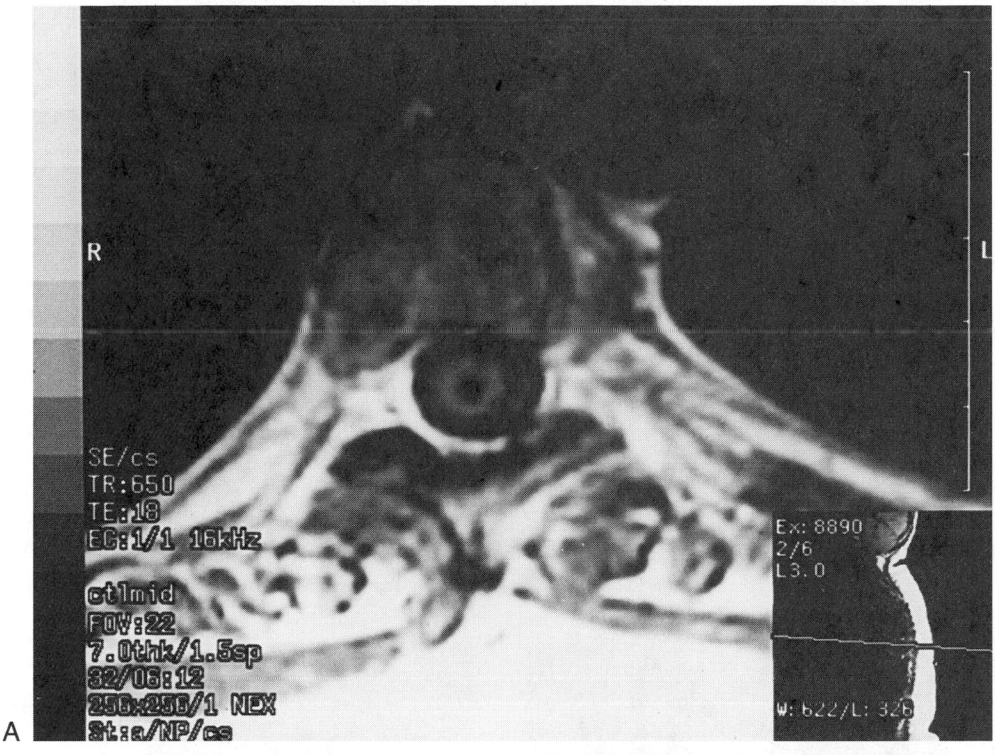

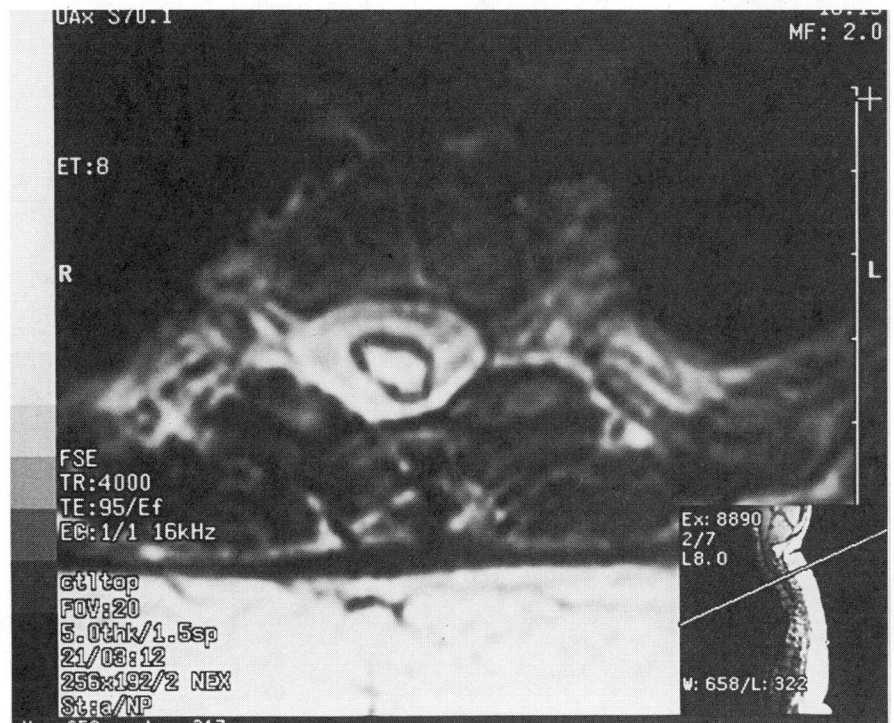

FIG. 84-2. **(A)** T1-weighted axial MRI of the spinal cord showing a syrinx that is symmetric and central in location. **(B)** T2-weighted axial MRI of the spinal cord showing a more eccentric and asymmetric syrinx.

adults and the holocord syrinxes more commonly seen in children.

EPIDEMIOLOGY

Many of the modern classification schemes have divided syringomyelia into a communicating and noncommunicating form. The ''communication'' refers to that of the syrinx with the basal cisterns and ventricular system. The term *communicating* may also imply that the syrinx is an extension of a collection of CSF that is not being adequately absorbed. In other words, communicating syringomyelias may be subsumed under the category of hydrocephalus. In other nomenclatures, the term *hydromyelia* is used synonymously with communicating syringomyelia.

Noncommunicating syringomyelias are much more common than communicating syringomyelias and typically include all of the common conditions associated with syringomyelia such as the Chiari I and Chiari II hindbrain malformations (which account for about one-half of all syrinxes identified by MRI), intramedullary tumors, trauma, arachnoiditis, and compression of the spinal cord or brainstem by either extradural or intradural masses (Fig. 84-3). When no cause for the syrinx is discovered, the term *idiopathic syringomyelia* is often applied. MRI has

helped identify many concurrent conditions in cases of syringomyelia and has thus resulted in a marked reduction in the perceived prevalence of idiopathic syrinxes. Syringomyelia is so commonly associated with these other related conditions that it is impractical to consider it as an isolated entity when describing its clinical presentations.

CLINICAL PRESENTATION

Syringomyelia Associated With a Hindbrain Malformation

The symptoms and signs associated with a syrinx are logically remembered if one bears in mind the cross-sectional anatomy of the spinal cord. Often juxtaposed on the symptoms and signs caused by the syrinx are the symptoms and signs caused by the associated hindbrain malformation.

The most common presenting symptoms of a syrinx with the Chiari I hindbrain malformation (Fig. 84-4) are difficulty using the hands and disturbances of gait. These symptoms generally have their onset in adolescence or early adulthood. Patients typically complain of weakness or loss of agility in their hands. Occasionally, patients describe their hand symptoms as numbness. The abnormalities of gait are often perceived initially as

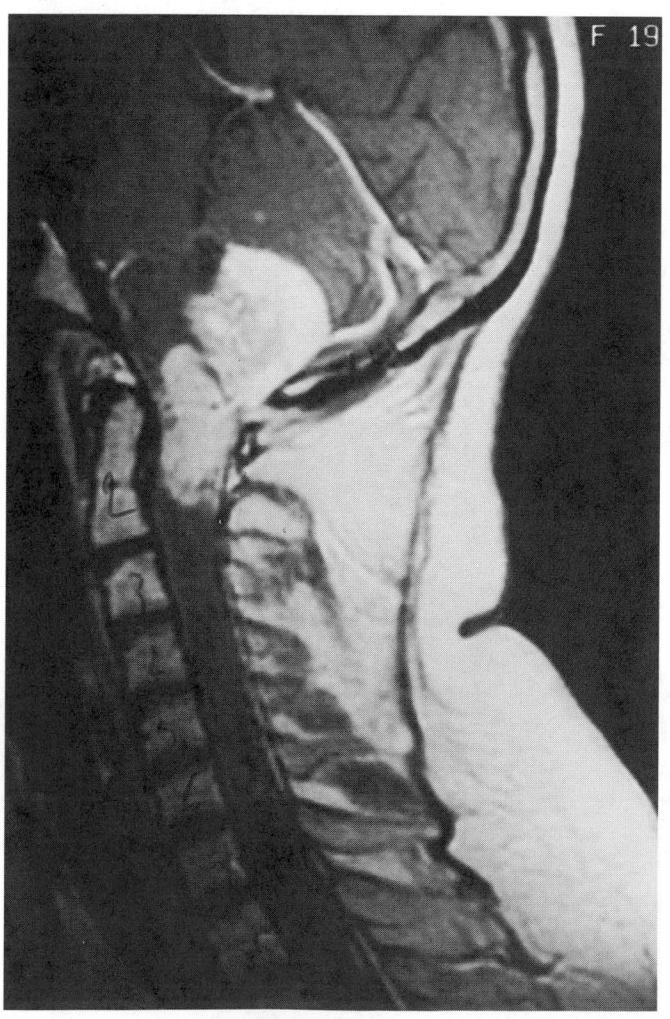

FIG. 84-3. Contrast-enhanced sagittal MRI of the cervicomedullary junction showing a hemangioblastoma with an associated cervical syrinx.

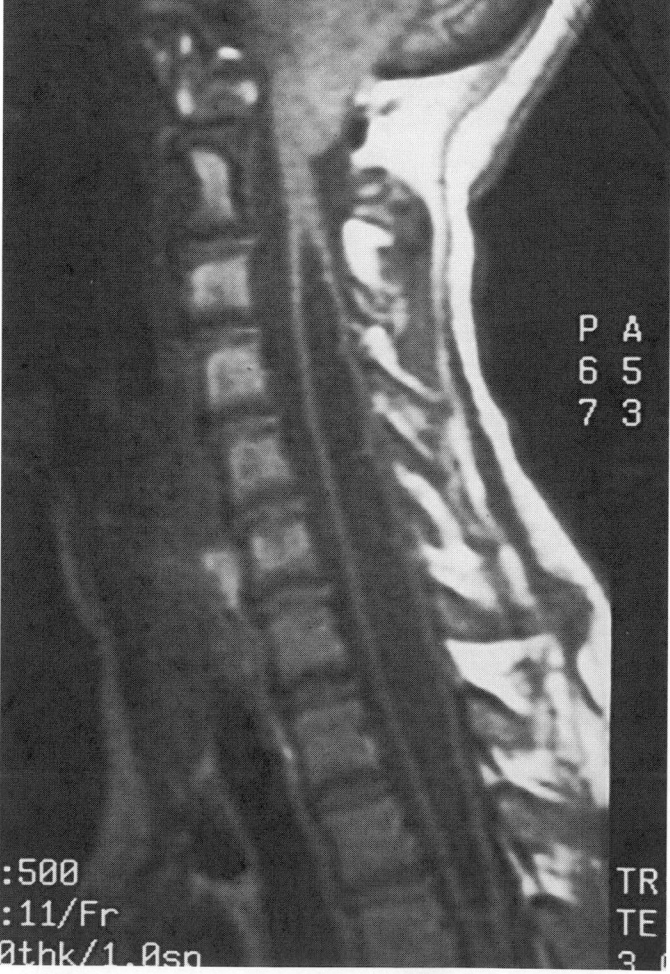

FIG. 84-4. Sagittal T1-weighted MRI of the cervical spinal cord showing tonsilar herniation characteristic of the Chiari I malformation. There is also an associated syrinx that does not communicate with the fourth ventricle.

weakness, stiffness, or fatigue. These symptoms are often asymmetric early.

Pain is the next most common presenting symptom. It is most often suboccipital in location. Typically, patients describe intensification of the pain with coughing or sneezing. This is also the case with the Chiari I malformation without syrinx, however. Occasionally, the pain has a radicular component in addition. Infrequently, the pain radiates into the arms or scapulae with a nonradicular, poorly localized, boring character, refered to as "funicular" pain. Bowel and bladder dysfunction are not prominent complaints early in the disease.

In some patients, atrophy is apparent, particularly in the hands; others develop noticeable scoliotic spine deformities, causing them to seek medical attention. Some patients seek medical attention for repeated unrecognized burns of their hands.

On examination, many of these patients demonstrate atrophy of the upper extremities. This typically involves the hands most prominently. Over time, contractures can occur in the hand causing a *main en griffe* (French for griffin-claw hand) appearance. This term has an interesting derivation; a griffin is a mythological monster that possesses the body and hind legs of a lion and the head, wings, and claws of an eagle. Scoliosis, when present, is typically centered on the cervicothoracic junction and can precede other neurologic symptoms by years.

The classic neurologic sign encountered is a suspended, cape-like, dissociated sensory loss involving the thorax and upper extremities. The presence of this sign on examination strongly localizes the lesion to within the parenchyma of the spinal cord. This finding is the result of disruption of the crossing spinothalamic tracts in the central portion of the cord. Sensation above and below the level of the syrinx can be normal if only the crossing fibers are affected. This forms the basis for the deficit being suspended. In addition, if the process involves only the spinothalamic tract, pain and temperature alone, and not fine touch or proprioception, are affected. This forms the basis for the deficit being dissociated.

As the syrinx enlarges, it next affects the anterior horn cells, first the more central anterior horn cells that supply the axial musculature and then the more peripheral anterior horn cells that affect the appendicular musculature. This is the presumed basis of the scoliosis (axial muscle weakness) and segmental atrophy and weakness of the distal arm, respectively. Further progression of the syrinx involves the intermediolateral cell column of the cord (when the syrinx extends into the thorax). This manifests as a Horner syndrome. Finally, the corticospinal tract and posterior columns are affected, resulting in spasticity and difficulty with fine touch and joint position sense.

Interestingly, the motor and sensory disturbances associated with a syrinx nearly always begin asymmetrically, although they end up affecting both sides. More chronic findings on examination include painless ulcerations of the fingers, edematous hands, and Charcot joints.

The presentation of syringomyelia with the Chiari II malformation is often more subtle. These patients come to medical attention at birth. There is essentially always an associated myelomeningocele, which causes a variable amount of extremity and bowel/bladder dysfunction, depending on the level of the myelodysplasia. Hydrocephalus is also a very common finding so that most of these patients require a ventricular shunt early in life.

Most syrinxes found with the Chiari II malformation are asymptomatic. Sometimes, the syrinx extends the entire length of the spinal cord, and yet signs attributable to the syrinx are difficult to elicit. The syrinx may appear along with other signs of shunt malfunction. The syrinx has even been reported to appear prior to ventricular dilation in cases of shunt malfunction.

Patients with the Chiari II malformation may present with a variety of symptoms and signs attributable to brainstem dysfunction during the neonatal period. These babies feed poorly, with choking, vomiting, and aspiration. They can become stridorous or apneic. Radiographic investigation may reveal hydrocephalus, a syrinx, a tight posterior fossa, or a combination of the above. It can be difficult to sort out which of the findings is contributing to the problem or whether the presentation is the result of an intrinsically disordered brainstem. The most common cause of a symptomatic Chiari II malformation is a shunt malfunction. This possibility should be entertained even if the initial imaging of the brain does not reveal enlarged ventricles as the ventricles will occasionally not change early in the course because of decreased compliance or displacement of CSF into a syrinx or into a bulging myelomeningocele repair site.

In rare cases, the syrinx extends cephalad into the brainstem and is thus referred to as syringobulbia. This typically occurs in the tegmentum, eccentrically to one side or the other. Patients may experience changes in their voice and dysphagia. On examination, atrophy and ipsilateral deviation of the tongue and ipsilateral pain and temperature sensation loss of the face may be found. In addition, nystagmus or Horner syndrome may be present. Often, the symptoms and signs can be difficult to separate from the associated Chiari malformation and direct brainstem compression.

Syrinx Associated With Spinal Cord Tumor

Intramedullary cord tumors account for 2 to 4 percent of all central nervous system tumors. Syrinxes have been found with all of the commonly occurring intramedullary spinal cord tumors and are thought to occur in 25 to 50 percent of these tumors. Syrinxes are more likely to occur in conjunction with cervical spinal cord tumors than with thoracic or lumbar spinal cord tumors. Astrocytomas, ependymomas, and hemangioblastomas account for more than 90 percent of these tumors. The CSF protein level is often increased in the syrinxes associated with spinal cord tumors. The syrinx can extend cephalad or caudad to the tumor or both.

Since the symptoms attributable to both the intramedullary tumor and syrinx are caused by disruption of the spinal cord, the clinical relevance of the syrinx, as distinct from that of the tumor, is often hard to assess. Often, the sensory level corresponds to the location of the tumor and not the syrinx even if the syrinx extends multiple segments above or below the tumor.

The most common presenting symptom in adults is pain. It is a complaint in up to 90 percent of all adults with intramedullary tumors. The pain is described as a poorly localized ache in the midline corresponding to level of the tumor. Often, the pain radiates into an extremity in a nonradicular pattern and is characterized as a poorly localized deep ache. Syrinxes that occur in conjunction with spinal cord tumors may also affect the motor and sensory modalities. Motor problems often begin asymmetrically and are usually most profound in the hands when the tumors are located in the cervical spine. Difficulties with gait can also develop later. Examination often reveals proximal weakness and, occasionally, atrophy. Distally, there

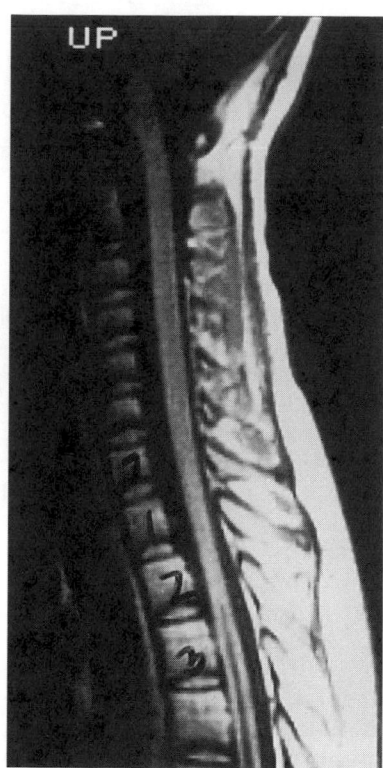

FIG. 84-5. Sagittal T1-weighted MRI of the cervicothoracic spinal cord showing a syrinx and an atrophic spinal cord. Previously, this patient had sustained a gunshot wound of the cervical spinal cord.

may be diminished fast finger motion and agility. Sensory disturbances also tend to start asymmetrically and distally. These disturbances may spread proximally and then cross to the other side. The classic finding of a suspended, dissociated sensory loss is uncommon but, when present, is highly suggestive of an intramedullary process.

Surgical removal of the tumor often also serves to eliminate the associated syrinx. The presence of a syrinx confers a better prognosis for complete surgical resection of the spinal cord tumor.

Post-traumatic Syringomyelia

Post-traumatic syringomyelia is a syndrome characterized by progressive deficits corresponding to a portion of the spinal cord remote from a previous injury. It usually manifests several years following the spinal cord injury. The incidence of post-traumatic syringomyelia is thought to be between 0.3 and 3.2 percent (Fig. 84-5).

The most common presenting symptom is pain. The pain can occur in the torso or extremity and may be related to movement of the head when cervical in location or to straining. Later findings include paresthesias, weakness, and hyperhydrosis. These symptoms typically are related to superiorly located segments of the spinal cord. Interestingly, the symptoms can skip segments of the cord. The paresthesias and motor findings usually start, and remain, asymmetric. Occasionally, the pain is replaced with hypalgesia.

DIFFERENTIAL DIAGNOSIS

The differential diagnosis of syrinx includes a large spectrum of pathologic processes. One must consider the inflammatory

myelopathies that affect the spinal cord. These may be infectious or idiopathic. Normally, the clinical course is more fulminant, evolving over a period of days. Likewise, the demyelinating diseases usually evolve over a time course too short to be mistaken for the more chronically evolving syrinxes.

Spinal arteriovenous malformations can present with a more chronic myelopathy. These malformations are most commonly dural malformations and are the result of a fistula or fistulae supplied by a radicular artery or arteries. The pathophysiology is thought to be a myelopathy from venous hypertension as the result of the fistula. On imaging studies, large serpiginous arterialized veins are seen in the subarachnoid space. The eponym *Foix-Alajouanine* has been used to describe a vascular disorder characterized by a necrotizing myelitis believed to be secondary to venous thrombosis involving a spinal cord vascular malformation. Occasionally, sudden deterioration is superimposed on a more chronic condition. Clinically, these malformations have a very variable presentation. The myelopathy is less likely to be a "central cord"-like syndrome, and paraparesis or quadriparesis is more likely to be an early finding.

Tethered spinal cord syndrome can present with a slowly progressive myelopathy much like the syrinx. Often, symptomatic tethered cords present with an orthopaedic deformity. This more frequently involves the thoracolumbar or lumbar spine and/or lower extremities, as opposed to the deformities typical of the syrinx, which primarily affect the cervical or cervicothoracic spine and/or upper extremities. The orthopaedic abnormalities associated with the tethered cord can be varus, valgus, or cavus changes of the foot; recurrent dislocations of the hip; or rotational abnormalities of an extremity or extremities. An isolated presentation of scoliosis is not uncommon. Patients can occasionally present with progressive isolated gait abnormalities such as spastic or wide-based gaits. Sometimes patients develop a peculiar change in posture, consisting of flexion of the knees and increased lumbar lordosis. In addition to orthopaedic deformities, patients with tethered cords may present with spinal cord and or, less commonly, root dysfunction. Again, this typically affects the lower extremities and can involve pain, weakness, sensory changes, or bowel/bladder dysfunction.

The tethered cord is often associated with a host of lesions, including myelomeningocele, myelocystocele, lipomyelomeningocele, spinal lipoma, meningocele, split cord malformation (diastematomyelia), and a thickened filum terminale. The presence of any of these conditions along with a low-lying conus medullaris should alert the clinician to the possibility of the tethered cord syndrome. Of interest is the myelomeningocele that is often associated with a syrinx and is nearly always associated with a low-lying conus in children. When these children present with progressive myelopathy and/or orthopaedic abnormalities, it is sometimes difficult to decide whether the predisposing condition is the syrinx, the tethered cord, or both.

Finally, *lesions extrinsic to the spinal cord* can mimic intramedullary processes. This is epitomized by the central cord injury, which typically results from a hyperextension injury, usually at C4–C5 or C5–C6, and leaves the patient with weakness predominantly affecting the hands bilaterally and relative sparing of the legs. Sensory disturbances are variable but, when present, can occur as a suspended, dissociated sensory loss, as in syrinxes. The central cord syndrome can also occur in a much more chronic form, presumably from repeated minor trauma to the cord from an extrinsic lesion, usually arthritic spurs. On MRI, there is often a bright spot on T2-weighted images. Experimental compression of the upper cervical spine in monkeys can produce pathologic changes in the central parts of the spinal cord in the area of C8 and T1. This is thought to be the result of venous stasis and has been proposed as the etiology of the central cord syndrome form extrinsic compression.

Finally, extrinsic lesions that occur at the foramen magnum can present similarly to the extrinsic lesions of the mid cervical spine. Patients with anterior cervicomedullary compression can present with a disproportionate amount of hand weakness. Sensory changes are often minimal unless the compression is dorsal at the cervicomedullary junction. This selective hand involvement is thought to occur because the decussation of the corticospinal tract destined for the hand occurs slightly more superior and ventral to the decussation of fibers destined for the lower extremities and can thus be selectively disturbed. This entity has been described as a "cruciate palsy," referring to the compression at the crossing of fibers.

DIAGNOSTIC EVALUATION

In cases of suspected syringomyelia, the study of choice is an MRI scan. MRI is the most sensitive study and the most informative. In cases of known Chiari malformation (type I or II) and suspected syrinx, a cervical MRI either confirms or rules out the diagnosis in virtually all cases. If the presence of a syrinx is confirmed, it is also necessary to look at ventricular size.

If a syrinx is found on MRI and there is no associated hindbrain malformation, history of trauma, or extramedullary spinal canal mass, it is important to administer contrast medium to search for a spinal cord tumor. If localization suggests that the syrinx is more caudal than the cervical spine, the MRI should extend down to the level of the conus to look for the many causes of tethered cord or to look for a vascular malformation.

For patients who cannot undergo MRI, the myelogram followed by a computed tomographic (CT) scan is sensitive and informative. The initial CT displays the syrinx as a dilated spinal cord and may also show stigmata of the Chiari malformations or an extramedullary mass in the spinal canal. A delayed CT of 6 to 12 hours may show contrast within the syrinx itself.

TREATMENT

Many techniques to treat syringomyelia have been developed by neurosurgeons over the past several years. These include posterior fossa bony decompression for the associated Chiari malformation with or without duraplasty, subpial tonsilar resection, lysis of adhesions, myelotomy, and plugging of the obex. In addition, simple percutaneous aspiration of the syrinx, terminal ventriculostomy (sectioning of the "terminal ventricle" or proximal filum terminale), syrinx-to-subarachnoid shunts, syrinx-to-peritoneum shunts, and subarachnoid-to-peritoneum shunts have been utilized.

The treatment to a large extent depends on the radiographic features of the syrinx. If there is hydrocephalus and the syrinx appears to communicate with the fourth ventricle or basal cisterns, the procedure of choice is a shunt. In cases of spinal cord tumors, the treatment is removal of the tumor.

In the other cases of syrinx, the most effective treatment is more controversial. When a syrinx is associated with a Chiari I malformation, most neurosurgeons perform some type of posterior fossa decompression. In addition to the bone removal, there is a wide variation in technique, as mentioned above. No studies substantiate the superiority of any one method over

another. We choose not to plug the obex because of its potential danger and because of recent evidence suggesting a lack of communication of the syrinx and the fourth ventricle in most cases. In cases in which there is a concomitant ventral compression of the brainstem (e.g., basilar invagination), it as been suggested that the anterior disease be corrected first to avoid settling of the cerebellum through the enlarged foramen magnum and subsequent exacerbation of the ventral compression.

Most neurosugeons reserve shunting of the syrinx to the subarachnoid space or other body cavities for cases of syrinx without hindbrain abnormalities or cases with progression of symptoms and radiographic persistence of syrinx despite posterior fossa decompression. Some neurosurgeons use shunting of the syrinx as a first line of treatment. Regardless of which method is used, around 20 percent of patients continue to deteriorate despite treatment. In addition, there is a subset of patients that do not progress, even without treatment. The inability to separate these two groups prospectively or retrospectively makes an analysis of the different treatments difficult. There is some suggestion that age greater than 40 years at presentation and a long duration of preoperative symptoms each confer a poor prognosis for successful treatment.

CONCLUSION

Syringomyelia is an important part of the differential diagnosis for subacute spinal cord dysfunction. It is a subject with a rich history and an evolving theory of pathogenesis. A lack of insight into the natural history of the disease has hampered our ability to evaluate different treatment modalities. The advent of MRI is likely to revolutionize our understanding of syringomyelia and clarify both its natural history and the treatments that are most appropriate.

SUGGESTED READINGS

Abouker J: La syringomyelie et les liquides intra-rachidiens. Neurochirurgie, suppl. 25:1–144, 1979
Ball MY, Dayan AD: Pathogenesis of syringomyelia. Lancet 2:799–801, 1972
Gardner WJ: Hydrodynamic mechanism of syringomyelia. J Neurol Neurosurg Psychiatry 28:247–59, 1965
Milhorat TH, Johnson WD, Miller JI et al: Surgical treatment of syringomyelia based on magnetic resonance imaging criteria. Neurosurgery 31:231–45, 1992
Milhorat TH, Miller JI, Johnson WD et al: Anatomical basis of syringomyelia occurring with hindbrain lesions. Neurosurgery 32:748–54, 1993

85. SPONDYLOSIS AND DISC DISEASE

DAVID S. GECKLE
MARY LOUISE HLAVIN

A careful clinical history and physical examination are critical for the diagnosis, localization, and treatment of degenerative spinal diseases, be it spondylosis or disc herniation. The combination of clinical symptoms and signs guides decision making regarding the need for diagnostic testing and appropriate therapy. Only a small fraction of patients with degenerative disease of the spine have a surgically significant disc herniation or spondylosis. History and physical examination remain the cornerstones to identifying these individuals and optimizing diagnosis and treatment for individuals with nonsurgical pathology.

Neurologic diagnosis begins with a comprehensive history and a review of past medical problems. Chronic diseases (diabetes mellitus, arthritis, and collagen vascular diseases), prior spinal trauma or surgery, metabolic disturbances (acromegaly, hypoparathyroidism, and renal osteodystrophy), malignancy, intravenous drug abuse, and vascular disease are just a few of the factors that can predispose a patient to spinal disease. The presence or absence of such factors can aid in the differentiation of a benign disc or spondylotic disease from neuropathies, plexopathies, infection, metastasis, or other etiologies.

LUMBAR DISEASE

Lumbar spinal disease consists primarily of two entities: disc herniation and spinal stenosis. Herniations occur approximately equally among men and women; stenosis appears more common among females than males. Approximately 95 percent of lumbar disc herniations occur at the L4-L5 and L5-S1 levels where most of the flexion, extension, and lateral bending occur. Manual labor or prolonged periods of riding in motor vehicles predispose people to lumbar disc disease. Spinal stenosis, or narrowing of the lumbar spinal canal and foramina sufficient to result in compression of the neural structures, is caused by congenital or degenerative hypertrophy of vertebral facets and the ligamentum flavum. It may be focal or throughout the entire lumbar spine.

Clinical Features

Low back pain is the most common manifestation of the herniated lumbar disc. Typically, the pain is a dull ache of gradual onset, which is worsened by exertion and relieved by rest. With acute herniations, it can frequently be a severe spasmodic pain of sudden onset exacerbated by any movement. Over time, the back pain usually progresses to sciatica, a progressive boring pain that radiates to the buttocks and/or down the posterolateral leg but may extend to the ankle or foot with lower disc herniations. This pain may be chronic or relapsing in nature and is frequently associated with sensory disturbances, typically paresthesias. The distribution of pain and sensory disturbances is useful in localizing the site of the lesion. Typical findings associated with lumbar root syndromes are summarized in Table 85-1. With far lateral disc herniations, the symptoms tend to be particularly severe.

Lumbar stenosis generally presents with a slowly progressive course spanning several years. The patient typically complains of leg pain, frequently bilateral, which may be sharp and lanci-

nating, dull and cramping, or burning in nature. It is usually triggered by walking, but standing or sitting for prolonged periods may exacerbate the condition. Generally, the pain is rapidly and dramatically relieved by lying down or sitting. Complaints of numbness, paresthesias, and leg heaviness or weakness during ambulation are common and may outweigh the pain component, though pain typically precedes their onset. Patients often report that they must walk in short stages, with frequent breaks to rest.

Although the symptoms of lumbar stenosis are caused by neural compromise, they are clinically similar to those of vascular insufficiency. Therefore, the term *neurogenic claudication* is frequently used. It is imperative to evaluate for the presence of true vascular claudication in these patients. One should always examine for the presence of diminished femoral or pedal pulses or trophic changes of vascular insufficiency. Since the two conditions may occur simultaneously, one must consider the diagnosis of lumbar stenosis when pain persists following successful vascular reconstruction.

Bladder dysfunction, though rarely the sole manifestation of a herniated disc, is typically, but not always, associated with conus or cauda equina compression. When associated with severe acute motor weakness, a massive central disc herniation is suggested. Sacral involvement leads to a cauda equina syndrome in 10 percent of patients with lumbar stenosis. It is important always to document a history of urinary retention or incontinence, impotence, and saddle sensory loss.

Patients with a herniated lumbar disc tend to have slow, deliberate, limited movements. Often, they hold their lower back. Inspection of the spine in patients with disc herniation usually reveals a flattening of the normal lordotic curve and paravertebral muscle spasm.

Approximately 50 percent of patients demonstrate a scoliosis to minimize traction on the affected nerve root, as seen in Figure 85-1. The seated patient tends to slide the hips forward to avoid the normal axial loading of the lower spine. The hip and knee of the symptomatic leg are frequently held in slight flexion to relieve tension on the affected root. Gait is often antalgic, with minimal weight bearing on the affected leg. With far lateral disc herniations, patients are often unable to walk and hold their leg in extreme flexion, with pain on minimal movement. Patients with lumbar stenosis tend to assume a stooped posture since forward bending often relieves the pain. Lumbar extension, which may significantly narrow the neural foramina, frequently leads to acute bilateral sciatica in patients with lumbar stenosis.

Percussion over the involved vertebrae frequently causes pain. Palpation along the sciatic nerve and into the sciatic notch, while generally causing pain, can rule out the presence of a peripheral nerve sheath tumor. With long-standing spinal disease, decreased muscle tone or bulk in the lower extremities may be seen. Circumferential measurements of thigh and calf can be used to verify this.

TABLE 85-1. Common Lumbar Root Syndromes

Root	Pain Location	Sensory Disturbance	Weakness	Reflex Change
L3	Anterior thigh, groin	Anterior thigh	Iliopsoas, (quadriceps)	(Patellar)
L4	Anterior thigh	Medial calf, medial foot	Quadriceps	Patellar
L5	Posterolateral thigh and calf, extending into great toe and dorsum foot	Dorsum foot, great toe, lateral calf	Tibialis anterior, extensor hallucis longus	None
S1	Posterolateral thigh and calf, extending into lateral toes and heel	Lateral foot, posterior calf	Gastrocnemius, toe flexors	Achilles

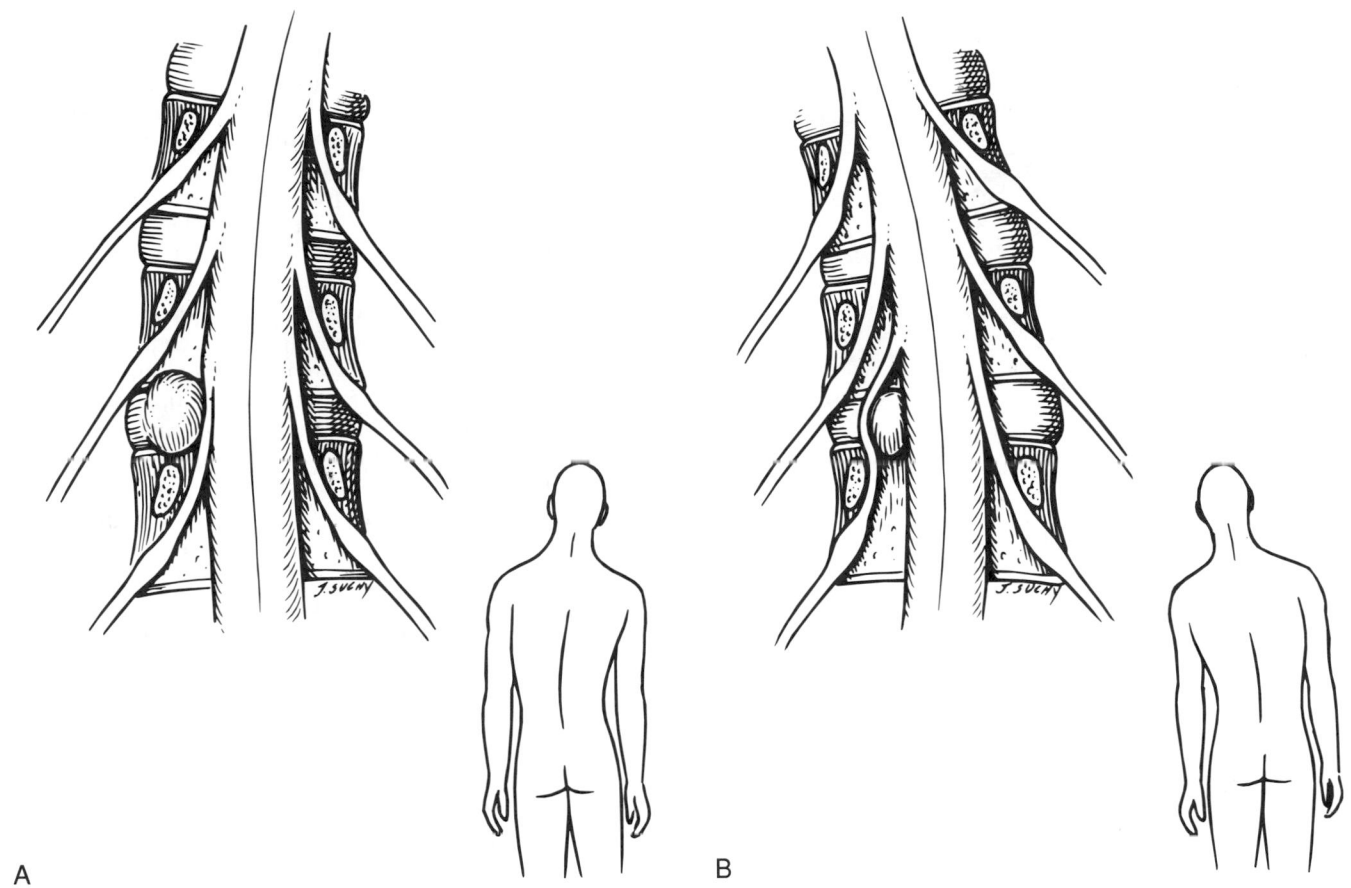

FIG. 85-1. Scoliosis minimizes traction on the affected lumbar nerve root. **(A)** In laterally placed herniations, the patient leans away from the affected side. **(B)** In medially located herniations, the patient leans towards the symptomatic side. (From Hlavin ML, Hardy RW, Jr: Lumbar disc disease. Neurosurg Q 1:29, 1991, with permission.)

Straight leg–raising maneuvers usually do not exacerbate symptoms of lumbar stenosis but are useful in the diagnosis of disc disease. Lasègue's sign, or the classic straight leg–raising test, is positive in up to 95 percent of true disc herniation cases (Fig. 85-2). The bowstring sign, a straight leg raising until pain is elicited with subsequent flexion of the knee resulting in relief of pain, may be added for confirmation. A positive crossed straight leg–raising test, or pain on raising the asymptomatic leg, is seen in approximately 30 percent of cases. This test produces pain as the involved root is dragged over a large or medially placed herniation (Fig. 85-3). Upper lumbar disc herniations produce pain with leg extension rather than flexion, providing the basis for the extensor sign or femoral nerve traction test. Tension on the upper nerve roots caused by this maneuver generally causes pain to the knee with L3 root impingement and below the knee with L4 root impingement. Patrick's sign, or the figure-four maneuver, may be useful in excluding hip disease, which can also result in pain referred to the low back (Fig. 85-4).

Sensory examination is the most subjective part of the physical examination. While generalizations regarding the patterns of sensory loss can be made, marked variations exist because of normal anatomic variation of dermatomal pattern, involvement of more than a single nerve root, or migration of a disc fragment. A far-lateral disc herniation typically causes compression of the root one level higher than usually expected (Fig. 85-5). Table 85-1 reports the sensory changes most typically associated with lumbar root compression. Rectal sensory examination is critical because many patients are unaware of this deficit.

Motor weakness, though the least frequently seen sign of disc herniation, provides another important adjuvant to lesion localization (Table 85-1). Testing, however, may be limited given that exertion causes pain. Testing muscle groups that do not stretch irritated nerve roots can help to overcome this problem (Table 85-2). Given the inherent strength of the lower extremities, weakness on routine static testing may be difficult to perceive. Subtle weakness can be unmasked using active motor testing, that is, having the patient heel-and-toe walk, squat, or climb up onto a stool. Since symptoms associated with lumbar stenosis may vary with exertion, it is important to perform motor testing both at rest and after activity.

Deep tendon reflex changes are the most objective sign of disc disease. For good results, it is essential for the patient to be as relaxed as possible. Reinforcement maneuvers, such as isometric pulling of clasped hands, may be of use. Having the patient kneel on a chair is a useful trick in eliciting an ankle jerk. It is also important to recall that the deep tendon reflexes diminish with advancing age. While diminution of the deep tendon reflexes is classically associated with disc herniation at a single level (Table 85-1), this pattern is not entirely reliable. For instance, a diminished patellar reflex is most frequently seen with a ruptured L3-L4 disc, but it can also be seen with a lesion at L2-L3. A decreased ankle jerk is most common with L5-S1 herniations; however, this finding may also be caused by compression of the S1 root by a large L4-L5 disc.

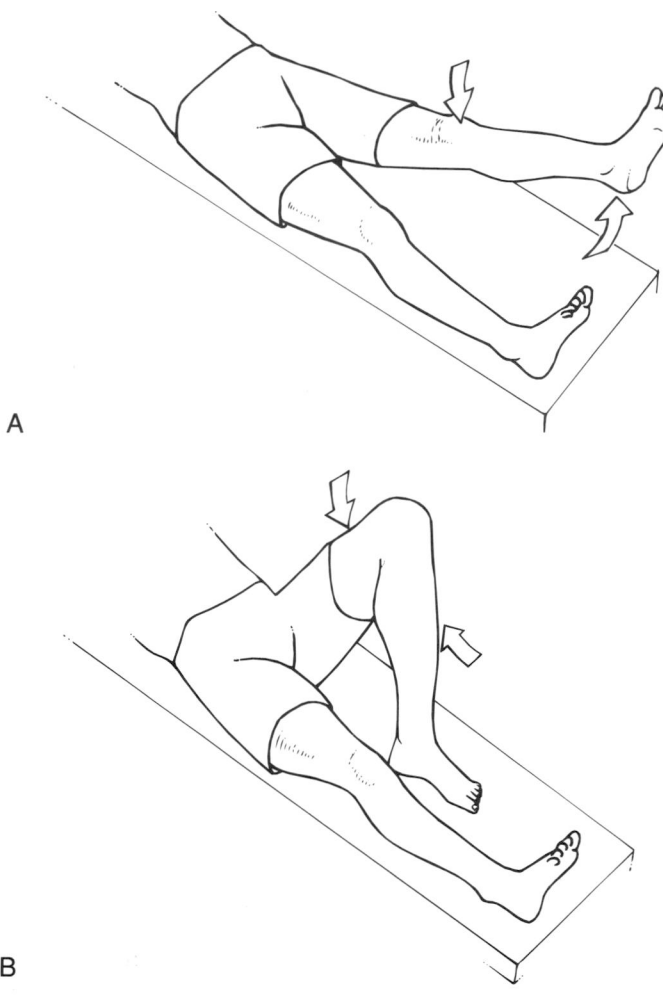

FIG. 85-2. The classic straight leg–raising test consists of two parts. **(A)** A straight leg raising followed by **(B)** a second lift with knee flexed. The first should cause radiating pain (not merely tightness in the posterior thigh!), the latter should not. (From Hlavin ML, Hardy RW, Jr: Lumbar disc disease. Neurosurg Q 1:29, 1991, with permission.)

The neurologic examination is often normal in patients with spinal stenosis, although occasionally diminution of reflexes or distal sensory loss, suggesting multiple root compression, can be seen with advanced disease.

Diagnosis

The value of plain spine radiographs in the diagnosis of lumbar disc disease remains controversial. Clearly, the plain spine film is the most effective method of evaluating alignment, an important consideration in preoperative planning for spondylotic disease. A narrowed disc space can be indicative of disc degeneration or protrusion; osteophyte formation suggests a more chronic process. Decrease of the anteroposterior and transverse diameters of the spinal canal, which is seen with severe developmental stenosis, can frequently be documented. In addition, plain films are invaluable in distinguishing disc disease from other conditions, which may present with similar symptoms, such as spondylolisthesis, spinal metastasis, fracture, infection, osteoarthritis, and vertebral hemangioma. Finally, radiographs can alert the surgeon to an occult spina bifida or spondylolysis preoperatively.

Myelography provides an indirect means of evaluating disc

herniation, while simultaneously excluding other intradural pathology, such as tumors, arachnoiditis, and vascular malformations. It is important to visualize the thoracolumbar junction (T10 to L1) to avoid missing a conus lesion or the occasional thoracic disc presenting with sciatica. In stenotic patients with a complete myelographic block, flexion views may convert the block to partial, allowing visualization of the distal levels. When combined with postcontrast computed tomographic (CT) imaging, myelography provides the most accurate demonstration of bony anatomy.

CT imaging is useful in evaluating the spine and surrounding structures. With the addition of intrathecal contrast, it can demarcate the thecal sac, cauda equina, and exiting nerve roots. CT is particularly helpful in far-lateral herniations and delineating bony anatomy. It is able to detect abnormalities of canal shape, lateral recess size, and neural foramina size, which are essential in evaluating patients with spinal stenosis.

Magnetic resonance imaging (MRI) allows for simultaneous noninvasive imaging of the spine, intervertebral discs, thecal sac, conus, cauda equina, exiting nerve roots, and surrounding structures in multiple planes. It has emerged as the primary imaging technique in the diagnosis of spine disease. The addi-

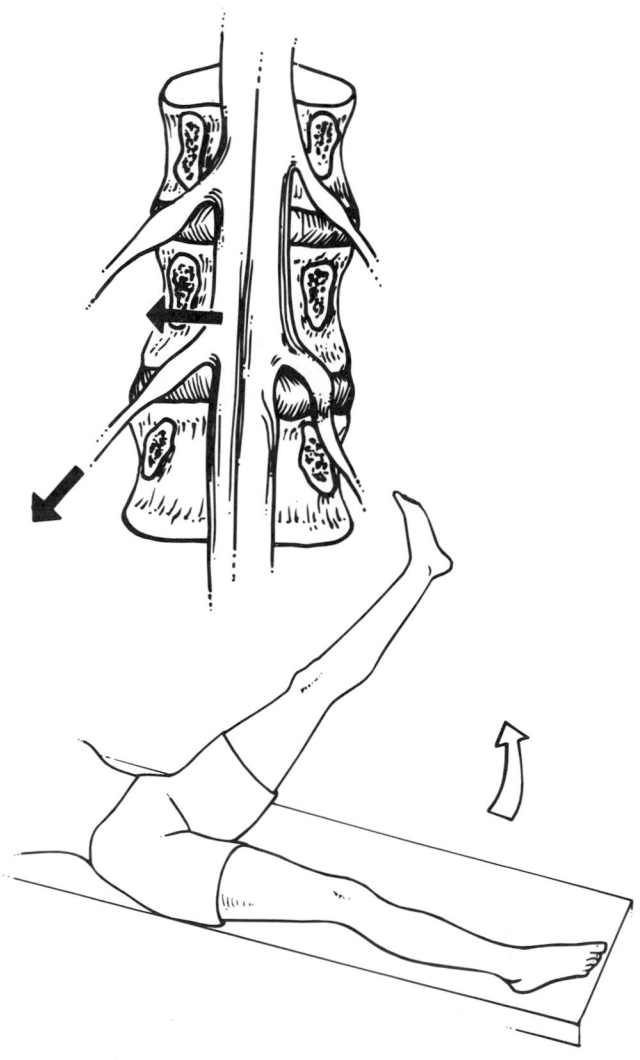

FIG. 85-3. The crossed straight leg raising produces pain with a large medial disc but not one located laterally. (From Hlavin ML, Hardy RW, Jr: Lumbar disc disease. Neurosurg Q 1:29, 1991, with permission.)

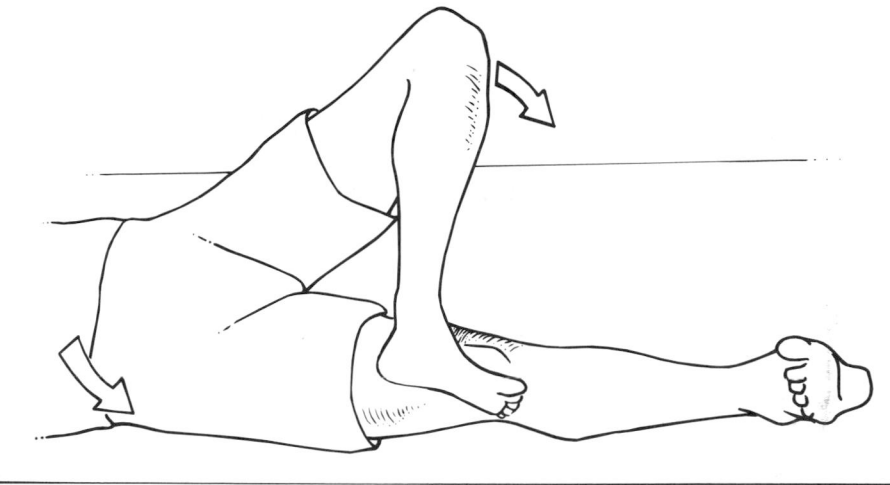

FIG. 85-4. Patrick's sign is elicited by externally rotating the hip with both the hip and knee flexed. This should not cause pain in the patient with disc herniation but rather suggests hip pathology. (From Hlavin ML, Hardy RW, Jr: Lumbar disc disease. Neurosurg Q 1:29, 1991, with permission.)

tion of intravenous gadolinium has been shown to be accurate in distinguishing postoperative scarring from recurrent disc herniation.

Although rarely indicated in straightforward cases of radiculopathy or stenosis, electromyography (EMG) may provide a useful adjunct in complex cases. For maximal benefit, EMG should be performed 3 to 5 weeks after symptom onset to allow for development of fibrillation potentials. Radiculopathy findings may disappear over time; so it is equally important not to

wait too long. One must always correlate the EMG findings with the clinical setting. Do not allow positive EMG results to dictate surgical intervention when appropriate clinical symptoms and radiologic findings are not present.

Treatment

Since more than 50 percent of patients with lumbar disc herniations respond to medical management, it is important to give nonsurgical therapy a trial in almost all patients. Clear indications for urgent surgical intervention include advanced neurologic deficit, cauda equina compression, sphincter dysfunction, neurologic deterioration with conservative management, and recurrent incapacitating episodes of pain. Persistent unacceptable disability from pain with nonoperative therapy represents the most common indication for surgery. One must carefully weigh the psychosocial factors (litigation, secondary gain, depression, and so forth) involved in the patient's disability prior to surgical intervention.

Nonoperative therapy for disc herniation consists of bed rest with the use of selected analgesics, anti-inflammatory agents, and muscle relaxants to reduce symptoms caused by irritation and edema of the affected root. When symptoms have resolved, instruction in posture, back exercises, and moderation of daily activities (''low back school'') are important. Unless neurologic deterioration occurs, most physicians advocate at least 2 to 3 weeks of nonsurgical therapy. Occasionally, a brief course of oral steroids (such as a methylprednisolone dose pack) is useful in relieving symptoms of acute herniation.

Although bed rest with lumbar flexion may provide temporary relief of painful radiculopathy, severe lumbar stenosis rarely responds to long-term nonsurgical management. In mild

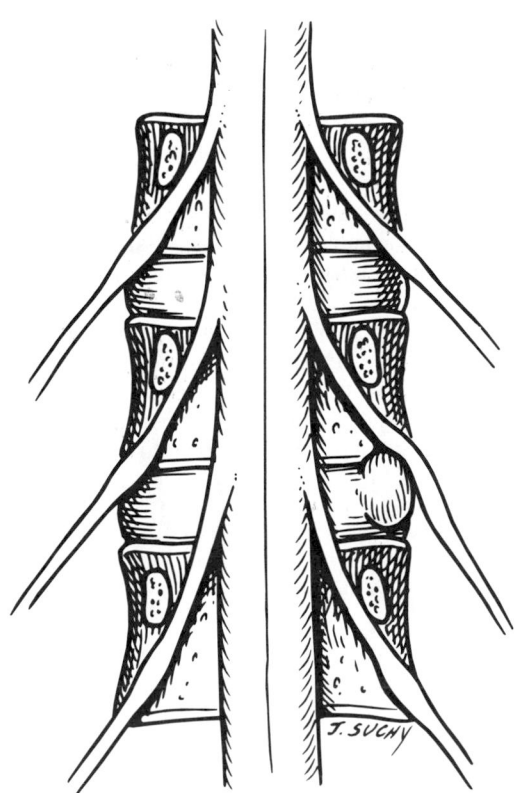

FIG. 85-5. Far-lateral disc herniations often compress the root above the disc space rather than that usually expected. (From Hlavin ML, Hardy RW, Jr: Lumbar disc disease. Neurosurg Q 1:29, 1991, with permission.)

TABLE 85-2. Muscle Groups Allowing Testing Without Root Stretching

Roots	Muscle Group
L2, L3, L4	Thigh adductors
L4, L5	Thigh abduction
L4, L5	Foot inversion
L5, **S1**	Foot eversion

cases, flexion exercises and a lumbar corset or brace may result in relief by facilitating postural correction. Analgesics, anti-inflammatory agents, and muscle relaxants are useful in treating the radicular symptoms while awaiting surgical decompression.

Definitive treatment for lumbar stenosis involves wide laminectomy with foraminotomies over the level of spinal compression. Discectomy is rarely indicated with adequate posterior decompression and may contribute to postoperative spinal instability. Inadequate decompression is a frequent cause of continued symptoms. Chronic cases of lumbar stenosis with advanced muscle atrophy or sphincter dysfunction are least likely to have full recovery. In patients with persistent postoperative mechanical low-back pain, spinal instability must be considered. In most cases, persistent nonradicular pain can be managed medically. In some, supplemental posterolateral spinal fusion may be needed.

The decision to operate is based on the combination of clinical findings, the physician's assessment, and the patient's input, given all the options. The goal should be the most cost-effective and expeditious management to return each individual safely to full, productive activity.

CERVICAL DISEASE

Benign cervical spine disease generally falls into one of two categories: radiculopathy or cervical myelopathic syndrome. The pathogeneses of these, however, differ somewhat and are essentially a result of two types of cervical disc anomalies: disc rupture (which results primarily but not exclusively in radiculopathy) and cervical arthrosis and spondylosis (which may result in radiculopathy, myelopathic syndrome, or both). The distinction between these two is essential as one is generally a self-limited condition while the other is progressive, and operative approaches to the two can vary significantly. While there is no sex predilection to cervical disc disease, predominantly male patients are affected by spondylotic myelopathy. Cervical disc disease is less common than lumbar disease, accounting for only about one in seven spinal herniations. Like lumbar disc disease, most cervical herniations occur at one of two levels that bear the brunt of spinal motion and stress, either C5-C6 or C6-C7. Multiple simultaneous levels of involvement are rare in acute cervical disc herniation but are common with spondylitic disease. Approximately 5 percent of cervical disc herniations are recurrent. Spondylosis in the cervical spine is typically generated by bony marginal spurring stimulated by bulging discs and is usually located posteriorly or intraforaminally. In contrast, in the lumbar region, this lipping is almost exclusively anterolateral in location and rarely results in foraminal encroachment. Hypertrophy of the ligamentum flavum rarely causes symptoms in the cervical spine, although hypertrophy and ossification of the posterior longitudinal ligament (OPLL) is a well-defined problem. Patients with cervical spondylosis

are twice as likely to have lumbar stenosis than the general population. Although generally not causative in and of itself, shallowness of the cervical canal predisposes patients to spondylotic myelopathy. Work-related stress, spasmodic torticollis, and congenital segmental defects such as Klippel-Feil undoubtedly play a role in the generation of cervical disease. The role of antecedent trauma is less clear.

Clinical Features

Pain, paresthesias, motor and sensory deficits are the hallmarks of cervical radiculopathy, although occasionally there may be a significant discrepancy between sensory and motor symptoms, resulting in either profound painless arm weakness with atrophy or severe incapacitating pain without other neurologic findings. The pain is typically proximal in distribution; the paresthesias are distal. Compression of the lower cervical roots produces very similar pain at the neck base, interscapular region, and shoulder and cannot be used to distinguish radiculopathies. However, cervical paraspinous or superior shoulder pain without radiation to the arm or scapular region should suggest C3-C4 disc herniation. A C6 radiculopathy sometimes causes chest pain, mimicking angina. Paresthesias are generally more accurate in localizing pathology, as summarized in Table 85-3. In addition to the more classic "pins-and-needles" paresthesia sensations, patients may complain of their hand or arm feeling "odd," sometimes described as cool and other times just as "not their own." Occasionally, a large centrally herniated disc results in acute quadriparesis with bowel or bladder dysfunction.

While the symptoms of bony spondylotic nerve root compression are similar to those of disc herniation, the course is often much more indolent. Although spastic paraparesis is the single most common presentation of cervical spondylotic myelopathy, it is distinctly unusual for symptoms to appear full blown or rapidly. Occasionally, however, symptoms can rapidly evolve after hyperextension. Early stages are typified by complaints of weakness and easy fatigability of the legs. The patient may note a painless pseudoglovelike sensory loss, which prompts a futile investigation for carpal tunnel or peripheral neuropathy. Electric-like sensations with neck motion (Lhermitte's phenomenon) are common, especially with neck extension. Neck or occipital pain and loss of temperature or pain sensation may be late symptoms.

Patients with cervical radiculopathy typically hold their head rigid secondary to spasm. Extension of the head, like extension of the back in lumbar disease, often causes pain by compressing the exiting root against the facets. The Spurling maneuver, axial spine loading in conjunction with contralateral head rotation and extension, can be used to elicit pain much in the same manner as Lasègue's sign. Flexion and extension may yield Lhermitte's phenomenon in patients with myelopathy.

TABLE 85-3. Common Cervical Root Syndromes

Root	Pain Location	Sensory Disturbance	Weakness	Reflex Change
C3, C4	Paraspinous muscles, superior shoulder	Neck	Diaphragm, nuchal muscles, strap muscles	None
C5	Neck, shoulder, anterior arm	Shoulder	Deltoid, supraspinatus, infraspinatus	(Biceps)
C6	Neck, shoulder, anterior upper arm, extending to antecubital fossa	Thumb, index finger, radial forearm	Biceps, brachioradialis, (extensor carpi radialis, pronator teres)	Biceps, brachioradialis
C7	Neck, shoulder, dorsum of forearm	Middle finger	Triceps, latissimus dorsi, pectoralis major, supinator, pronator teres	Triceps
C8	Neck, shoulder, ulnodorsal forearm	Ring, little fingers, hypothenar eminence	Intrinsic hand muscles, finger extensors	None
T1	Neck, shoulder, ulnar arm	Ulnar forearm	Intrinsic hand muscles (Horner syndrome)	None

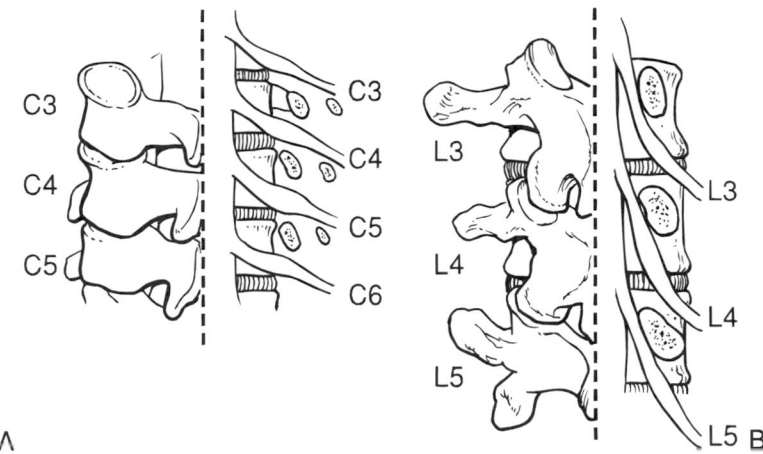

FIG. 85-6. Comparison of (**A**) cervical and (**B**) lumbar root anatomy. The left half of each drawing depicts the bony anatomy; the right side demonstrates the intradural and foraminal course of the nerve and how they are numbered. Note the closer application of the lumbar roots to the pedicle, which is found more laterally in the cervical region.

As in the lumbar spine, motor and reflex changes are most specific for localizing pathology. These are summarized in Table 85-3. In the cervical region, in contrast to the lumbar region, roots are numbered by the vertebrae to which they are cephalad (e.g., the C6 root exits at the C5-C6 disc space level, just above the C6 pedicle and slightly superior to the disc space). Cervical roots exit laterally and ventrally and are held snugly against the disc while coursing toward the inferior pedicle while lumbar roots wrap more closely under the inferior pedicle. This is demonstrated in Figure 85-6. Subtle signs of C7 compression include weakness of the latissimus dorsi and pectoralis major. Latissimus function is evaluated by having the patient cough deeply while palpating these accessory muscles of respiration from behind. Unequal contractions are indicative of weakness. Pectoralis function is best tested using a "pseudo" Froment's sign or book test. Patients supports a book between their palms with elbows extended, and the examiner then attempts to withdraw the book. Failure to maintain the humerus in adduction and involuntary elbow flexion indicates compensation for pectoralis weakness.

Motor, sensory, and reflex changes are rare in early phases of spondylotic myelopathy. Severe arthrosis, however, results in obvious sensory losses, paraparesis, hyperreflexia, spasticity with scissoring of gait, and even upper extremity weakness. Long-term pathology may also be accompanied by anterior horn cell damage or exiting root injury (radiculopathy), resulting in a mixed picture of lower motor neuron findings (hyporeflexia, atrophy, and fasciculations) in the upper extremities combined with upper motor neuron findings in the lower extremities.

Diagnosis

Plain spine films can be important in the evaluation of cervical spine disease. Lateral views may demonstrate depth of canal, pedicle size, facets, and subluxation. As a general rule, the depth of the canal should equal the width of the body at its midportion and should be no more than 15 to 25 percent smaller than the body (Fig. 85-7). Absolute measurements of 14 mm or less are indicative of a narrow canal. Spurs and retrolisthesis may produce further impingement on canal size. It is important to remember, however, that evidence of degenerative spine dis-

ease (disc space narrowing, osteophyte formation, and so forth) occurs in 25 to 50 percent of the population by age 50 and in 75 to 85 percent by age 65. These findings are most often incidental and asymptomatic in nature. Oblique views may be used to assess neural foramina. Dynamic flexion and extension films are important to assess for anterolisthesis and retrolisthesis.

MRI is rapidly supplanting CT myelography for assessment of cervical spine disease. However, definition and evaluation of bony anatomy, including osteophyte encroachment on foramina and OPLL, can be inadequate with this imaging modality. CT scanning with intrathecal contrast may be required for planning operative intervention, particularly with multilevel disease. It is important to remember that involvement at multiple levels can produce additive effects.

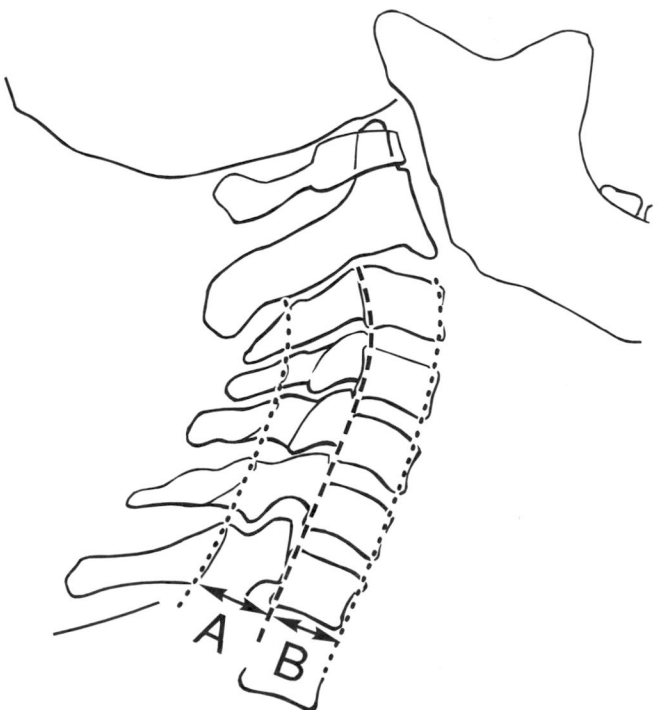

FIG. 85-7. Distance *A* represents canal width and should be no more than 15 to 25 percent smaller than *B,* the vertebral body width.

Treatment

As with lumbar radiculopathy, conservative therapy plays an important role in the management of cervical radiculopathy. Cervical disc herniations are usually self-limited, and patients respond to nonoperative management, consisting of rest, local heat, modulation/limitation of neck activity (through use of a cervical collar), traction, and pharmaceuticals, including anti-inflammatory agents, muscle relaxants, pain relievers, and occasionally steroids. It is imperative to ensure that there is no evidence of cord compromise before initiating traction to prevent cord injury. Head halter traction devices may be used, with initial weights starting at 5 lb and gradually increased as needed to no more than 5 lb per cervical level.

In cases of severe pain or significant radicular weakness or sensory loss, urgent surgery is indicated. Acute cord compression from disc herniation, as manifested by rapidly progressive paresis, sensory level, or bowel/bladder involvement, also warrants emergency decompression. It is important to remember that long-standing compression with prolonged conservative treatment may lead to pain abatement with persistent weakness or numbness. Failure of return of strength or sensation is an indication for surgical intervention.

Cervical myelopathy is, in most cases, a progressive disease with little room for conservative management. Early diagnosis and surgery are key in preventing irreversible spinal cord injury. Cervical collars and nonsteroidal anti-inflammatory drugs may temporarily alleviate pain but do not address the underlying disease.

Multiple surgical approaches exist for the treatment for both cervical disc and spondylotic disease. These include anterior cervical discectomy with or without fusion, posterior laminectomy and foraminotomy, multiple anterior discectomies with fusion, anterior corpectomy with fusion, and multiple level laminectomies. The ideal approach can be highly variable and individualized, both from patient to patient and surgeon to surgeon, discussion of the scope of which is beyond this text.

SELECTED READINGS

Ehni B, Ehni G, Patterson RH Jr: Extradural spinal cord and nerve root compression from benign lesions of the cervical area. p. 2878. In Youmans JR (ed): Neurological Surgery. 3rd Ed. WB Saunders, Philadelphia, 1990

Garfin SR, Rydevik BL, Lipson SJ et al: Spinal stenosis. p. 791. In Rothman RH, Simeone FA (eds): The Spine. 3rd Ed. WB Saunders, Philadelphia, 1992

Hlavin ML, Hardy RW Jr: Lumbar disc disease. Neurosurg Q 1:29, 1991

Walton J, Gilliatt RW, Hutchunson M et al: Aids to the Examination of the Peripheral Nervous System. New ed. Bailliere Tindall, London, 1986

86. VASCULAR DISEASE OF THE SPINAL CORD

JOSEPH H. FRIEDMAN

Vascular disorders of the spinal cord are rare, and most occur in the inpatient setting. Diagnosis may be difficult, and vascular etiologies for cord syndromes are often not considered. Spinal cord syndromes may be misdiagnosed as "laboratory-nega-

TABLE 86-1. Vascular Spinal Cord Syndromes

Acute
  Transient ischemic attack
  Infarct
  Subarachnoid hemorrhage
  Intramedullary hemorrhage
Rapidly progressive
  Epidural hematoma
  Subdural hematoma
Slowly progressive
  Arteriovenous malformation (dural or intradural)

tive" multiple sclerosis or postencephalitic demyelination. Statistics on the incidence and prevalence of vascular cord syndromes are not very reliable as a result. Probably the most commonly recognized vascular disorder of the spinal cord is stroke associated with aortic surgery. Stroke however also occurs in other settings and, as in the brain, is either ischemic or hemorrhagic. Spinal cord vascular syndromes are more difficult to evaluate radiologically owing to the small diameter and length of the cord, greater bone encasement, and the frequent problem with localization in which identical corticospinal signs can be caused by lesions anywhere in the thoracic cord. Table 86-1 lists vascular spinal cord syndromes.

The spinal cord is supplied by the single midline anterior spinal artery, which runs the length of the cord, and the two posterior spinal arteries (Fig. 86-1). The posterior spinal arteries, unlike the anterior spinal artery, form a plexus, and often the artery becomes so small that it appears to be discontinuous. The vascular supply to the anterior and posterior spinal arteries varies with the level (Fig. 86-2). The cervical anterior and posterior spinal arteries are supplied by the vertebral arteries. At lower levels, there are variable numbers of segmental arteries that arise from the aorta and enter the cord via the nerve root sheaths. One vessel, larger than the others, supplies the lower thoracic and lumbar cord is called the artery of Adamkiewicz. This artery arises from the aorta and generally enters the spinal canal on the left side.

The anterior spinal artery provides blood to about two-thirds of the cord, including the anterior horns, the lateral spinothalamic tracts, and the corticospinal tracts, but not the posterior columns. The posterior spinal arteries supply the posterolateral portion of the cord, including the posterior columns on each side. The venous system draining the cord is composed of multiple small networks rather than particular large vessels with well-defined territories.

The dura is supplied by dural branches of the intercostal or lumbar arteries that supply the cord. The pia is supplied by intramedullary spinal cord arteries. The subarachnoid space contains some vessels but fewer than the dura mater.

STROKE AND TRANSIENT ISCHEMIC ATTACK

Clinical Features

Ischemia of the spinal cord usually occurs in the distribution of the anterior spinal artery. Since the anterior portion is supplied by a single midline artery, in contrast to the paired posterolateral vessels and their plexus-type network that supply the dorsal portion, there is no collateral circulation in cases of hypoperfusion. Anterior cord ischemia typically causes the abrupt onset of radicular or diffuse back pain, flaccid weakness, sphincter dysfunction, and a sensory level for pain and temperature with preservation of the posterior column sensations of touch and position sense (Table 86-2). Obviously, the limbs

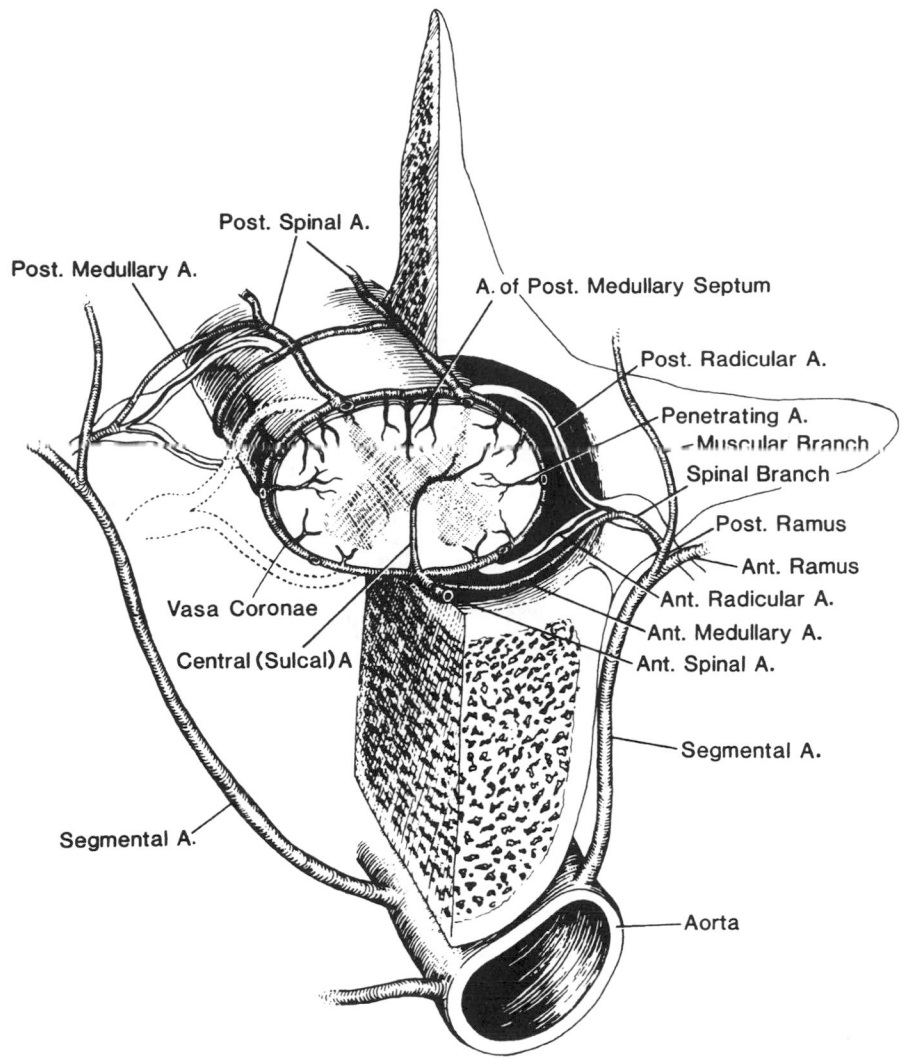

FIG. 86-1.   Arterial supply to the spinal cord. (From Sliwa JA, MacLean IC: Ischemic Myelopathy: a review of spinal vasculature and related clinical syndromes. Arch Phys Med Rehabil 73:365–72, 1992, with permission.)

involved and the sensory level depends on the level at which the ischemia occurs. While the region of the cord most at risk because of poor collateral circulation is T5-T7, any region of the cord can become ischemic. Sulcal artery occlusion can produce a Brown-Séquard syndrome or other partial cord syndromes, whereas sustained hypotension or aortic dissection is more likely to produce a symmetric anterior cord syndrome.

Posterior arterial and venous infarctions are very rare. Venous thrombosis can produce either bland or hemorrhagic infarction of the cord. Hemorrhagic infarcts tend to be sudden in onset, of rapid progression, and associated with back pain. Nonhemorrhagic infarcts are more insidious and indolent, developing over hours to days, without back pain. Embolic occlusion of veins is sudden in onset and often painful. Venous infarctions have a wider range of presentations than arterial occlusions owing to less well-defined vascular territories. Motor or sensory dysfunction or even central cord syndromes, such as dissociated sensory loss, can be seen, and the length of cord involved can be long.

Posterior artery occlusions produce motor involvement in all cases, but of a variable degree. The sensory loss also is variable

and may be limited to posterior column sensation. Bowel and bladder dysfunction are common.

Etiology

Aortic disease is the most likely etiology for cord ischemia but cardiac emboli, coagulopathies, vasculitides, and so forth are also potential causes. Syphilitic aortitis was the most common cause for cord stroke in the prepenicillin era, but atherosclerosis is thought to be the most common current cause. A rare cause of arterial emboli includes fibrocartilage. Atherosclerosis can cause spinal cord transient ischemic attacks (TIAs), infarcts, and slowly progressive syndromes. Aortic dissection may cause spinal cord ischemia and is typically associated with severe pain, probably from the vascular dissection itself independent of cord effects. Although cord infarcts may occur in a typical setting of atherosclerosis and peripheral vascular disease, it may occur in rare circumstances such as focal atherosclerosis following radiation treatment of a malignancy, aortic thrombosis, or a coagulopathy from an anticardiolipin antibody. A rare cause for cord stroke is sustained hypotension in a person who is

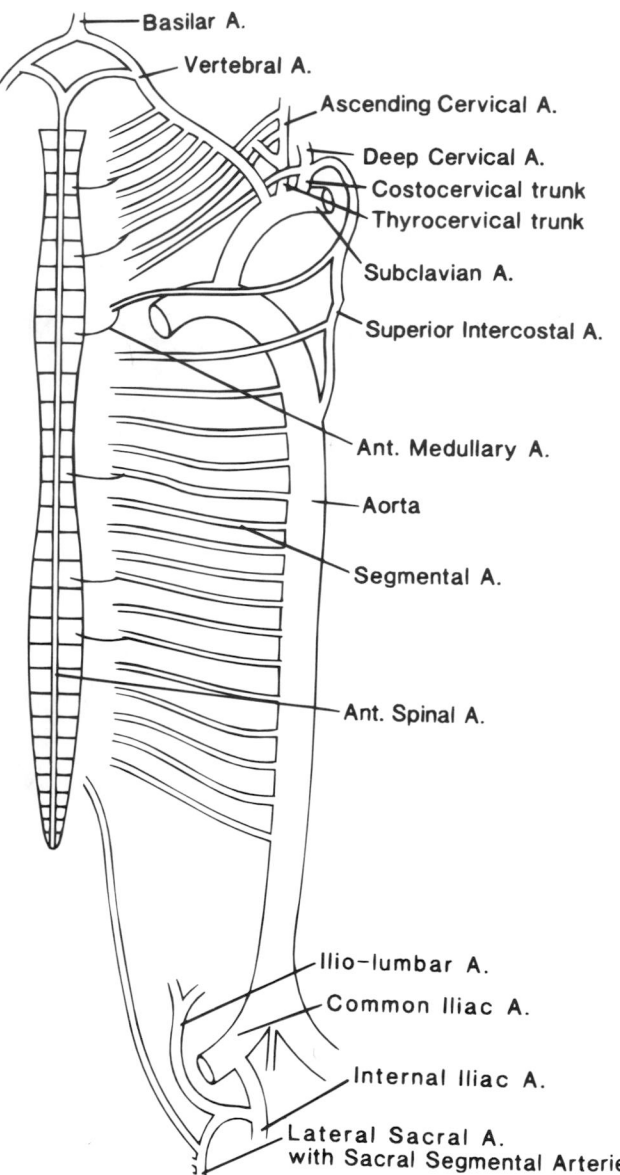

FIG. 86-2. Origin of the segmental arteries. (From Sliwa JA, MacLean IC: Ischemic myelopathy: a review of spinal vasculature and related clinical syndromes. Arch Phys Med Rehabil 73:365–72, 1992, with permission.)

maintained in an upright position, as may occur with a drug overdose in someone seated upright. Venous thrombosis may be idiopathic or associated with any thrombotic condition.

Spinal cord TIAs may result from arterial narrowing, emboli, or transiently increased venous pressure. Steal phenomena may also cause a TIA and occurs typically with an arteriovenous malformation (AVM) but has been observed with aortic coarctation.

The differential diagnosis for transient cord dysfunction must

TABLE 86-2. Features of Spinal Cord Stroke

Acute back and radicular pain
Flaccid leg weakness (occasionally arm and leg)
Loss of pain and temperature below lesion
Preservation of touch and position senses
Urinary retention

TABLE 86-3. Differential Diagnosis

Spinal cord transient ischemic attack
  Demyelinating disease
  Tumor
  Spinal stenosis/claudication
Spinal cord stroke
  Tumor
  Epidural hematoma
  Subdural hematoma
  Syringomyelia
  Abscess, infection
  Demyelination
  Transverse myelitis
  Disc herniation
  Arteriovenous malformation

include tumors, especially epidural metastases (Table 86-3). It is hypothesized that tumors cause transient neurologic dysfunction by a steal phenomenon, by arterial compression, or by increased venous pressure. Demyelinating diseases may also cause transient neurologic dysfunction and are frequently associated with pain, similar to that present with ischemia. If the episode is thought to be a TIA, then the proper evaluation depends on the clinical circumstances.

Evaluation

The evaluation of a spinal cord stroke or TIA should certainly include a two-dimensional echocardiogram and probably also a transesophageal echocardiogram (Table 86-4). Whether an aortic angiogram or a spinal angiogram should be performed needs to be determined by the clinical circumstances. Evaluations for syphilis, a coagulopathy, or a vasculitis need to be considered. Magnetic resonance imaging (MRI) of the spinal cord, including a contrast examination, should be considered mandatory to exclude a tumor masquerading as ischemia. There are two main problems in diagnosing spinal TIA and stroke. First, because they are so uncommon, they are not considered on the differential diagnosis. The second problem is in confirming the diagnosis once suspected. As with cerebral TIAs, the diagnosis is made on history, risk factors, and exclusion of alternative diagnoses. Unlike cerebral strokes, cord infarcts can rarely be visualized on computed tomography (CT) and only uncommonly with MRI. Spinal angiography is available only at centers with specialized neurosurgical services, is potentially harmful, may not reveal an occlusion if the embolus has dislodged or fragmented after causing infarction, and, finally, probably will not alter therapy, making it a questionable proposition. Thus, spinal cord infarct is often a diagnosis of exclusion. Spinal angiography probably has a morbidity rate of about 5 percent as a result of the dye load and the small, atherosclerotic vessels involved. It should be performed in cases of suspected spinal AVMs (see below) or other conditions in which a definitive diagnosis would alter management in a tangible fashion. Aortic dissection is a life-threatening diagnosis and, if considered possible, should be excluded with an MRI of the aorta if

TABLE 86-4. Evaluation of Ischemic Spinal Cord Syndromes (Transient Ischemic Attack and Stroke)

Magnetic resonance imaging of cord with and without gadolinium
Coagulation studies
Rapid plasma reagin test to exclude syphilis
Routine and transesophageal echocardiograms
Consider computed tomography of aorta and aortic and spinal cord angiogram
Vasculitis evaluation

the patient is stable or with a dynamic contrast CT scan of the aorta if the patient is unstable.

Treatment

Treatment for cord ischemia is presumably identical to that of cerebral ischemia, but no data exist. The risk of re-embolization should be reduced by using anticoagulants for cardiac emboli and aspirin when atherosclerosis is the presumed mechanism. Treatment of any other identified etiology such as a vasculitis, hypercoagulable state, and so forth should be implemented. There are no data to support or counter the use of heparin either in an acute infarct or shortly following a TIA. The author is concerned that the increased risk of hemorrhage into such a small structure as the spinal cord precludes its use except for treating a known thrombotic or cardiac embolic disorder.

When the stroke etiology is an aortic dissection, then this should be addressed as soon as possible. Obviously, these are the patients most at risk from surgery and from cautious waiting.

The prognosis for cord stroke is unclear. As with strokes in the cerebral circulation, the prognosis is highly variable and unpredictable in any particular individual. In one series of eight cases, the patients who survived were all able to walk out of the hospital. However, a different series reported significantly worse results, with most patients making little improvement and remaining unable to walk. Almost all patients in the second study suffered chronic limb pain for several months.

HEMORRHAGES AND VASCULAR MALFORMATIONS

Epidural Hematomas

Spontaneous hematomas into the epidural space occur more frequently than into the subdural space owing to their relative differences in vascularity. They both cause severe localized pain at the site of the hemorrhage, followed shortly by radicular pain. A few hours to a few days later, focal spinal cord deficits develop, which include paraparesis, quadriparesis, a sensory level, and bladder dysfunction. Syndromes such as the Brown-Séquard syndrome may also occur.

Most patients with spontaneous hematomas have a bleeding diathesis caused by excessive anticoagulation, liver failure, or use of antiarthritic drugs, which interfere with platelet function. The ictus may be triggered by sudden major changes in intra-abdominal or intrathoracic pressure but may also be precipitated by mundane activities such as straining to defecate or calisthenics.

Intradural Hematomas

Subdural hematomas may localize to any level of the cord but tend to be rostral and dorsal. In contrast, epidural hematomas are mostly anterior. The neurologic clinical features are similar for subdural and epidural hematomas, making a clinical distinction difficult prior to imaging. Progression of deficits is the rule until the bleeding abnormality is corrected and the clot evacuated.

The differential diagnosis is that of a rapidly progressive, painful cord syndrome. This includes sudden disc herniation, epidural cord compression from cancer, spinal cord ischemia, arterial dissection, epidural abscess, intraparenchymal tumor, and cyst. If the patient is evaluated when the pain is the only symptom, then an epi- or subdural hematoma should be considered only if a bleeding abnormality is known.

Since deficits progress over hours in the presence of a coagulopathy and outcome depends on the severity and duration of the deficits, this must be considered a neurosurgical emergency. An immediate MRI scan is the diagnostic test of choice while the coagulopathy is being reversed, followed by an emergency surgical decompression.

Dural Arteriovenous Malformation

Spinal AVMs are anatomically divided into intradural and nonintradural. Intradural AVMs can present with subarachnoid hemorrhage (SAH) or with progressive neurologic deficits.

Dural AVMs occur near the nerve root sheath and, unlike most other spinal cord vascular syndromes, tend to be slowly progressive and may not be painful. Dural AVMs are more common in elderly men than in women. The symptoms vary, depending on location. The legs are the most affected. Sensory levels, paraparesis, bladder dysfunction, and radicular pain are common. Diagnosis is difficult because of problems of imaging sensitivity. A careful dorsal myelogram is more sensitive than a spinal MRI scan, but even so an AVM may be missed. Spinal angiography is the most sensitive test.

The differential diagnosis of a progressive cord syndrome in older patients must include a demyelinating disease and tropical and familial spastic paraparesis. When the signs are primarily motor, then motor neuron disease or a peripheral neuropathy is considered. Depending on the rapidity of progression, a cord tumor must be excluded.

A ruptured spinal AVM causes severe spinal and radicular pain at the site of rupture followed by the usual signs of a SAH, meningismus and obtundation. If the history of pain is not obtained, a distinction from the usual cause of SAH, namely a ruptured berry aneurysm, cannot be made. Spinal AVMs make up only a small fraction of the total of SAH but should be considered when the cerebral angiogram is unrevealing, especially if a history is obtainable and points to a focal spinal onset. Since these malformations may rebleed, identification and treatment is important. There appears to be a predilection for SAH from spinal AVMs to affect women, particularly in pregnancy.

Both subdural and dural AVMs may induce slowly progressive cord syndromes and must be considered in cases of otherwise unexplained cord disease. Weakness and sensory changes in the legs are the most common presenting features, rather than pain, as is true of other vascular disorders of the spinal cord. Pain may be present, either early in the course or on a chronic basis but has no particular features to distinguish it from the more common low-back pain radicular syndromes. Bladder and sexual dysfunction may also occur.

Symptoms tend to occur in older patients, although the malformations are thought to be congenital. Since diagnosis may be difficult, it is possible that presentations at younger ages are thought to be due to laboratory-negative multiple sclerosis, an entity that becomes increasingly rare with age.

SUGGESTED READINGS

Caplan LR, McKee AC: Case records of the Massachusetts General Hospital: a 65 year old woman with an abrupt paralysis of the legs and impairment of bladder and bowel function. N Engl J Med 324:322–32, 1991

deToffol B, Cotty P, Gaymard B, Velut S: Progressive necrosis of the conus medullaris: magnetic resonance imaging and surgical findings. Neurosurgery 26:147–9, 1990

Kim RC, Smith HR, Henbest ML, Choi BH: Nonhemorrhagic venous infarction of the spinal cord. Ann Neurol 15:379–85, 1984

Koenig E, Thron A, Scharder V, Dichgans J: Spinal arteriovenous malformations and fistulae: clinical, neuroradiological and neurophysiological findings. J Neurol 236:260–6, 1989

Mattle H, Sieb JP, Rohner M, Mumenthaler M: Nontraumatic spinal epidural and subdural hematomas. Neurology 37:1351–6, 1987

Rosenblum B, Oldfield EH, Doppman JL, DiChira G: Spinal arteriovenous malformations: a comparison of dural arteriovenous fistulas and intradural AVM's in 81 patients. J Neurosurg 67:795–802, 1987

Sandson TA, Friedman JH: Spinal cord infarction: report of 8 cases and review of the literature. Medicine (Baltimore) 68:282–92, 1989

Satran R: Spinal cord infarction. Curr Concepts Cerebrovasc Dis Stroke 22: 13–7, 1987

Shephard RH: Spinal arteriovenous malformations and subarachnoid haemorrhage. Br J Neurosurg 6:5–12, 1992

Sliwa JA, MacLean IC: Ischemic myelopathy: a review of spinal vasculature and related clinical syndromes. Arch Phys Med Rehabil 73:365–72, 1992

SECTION 2. MOTOR NEURON DISEASES

87. AMYOTROPHIC LATERAL SCLEROSIS

JEREMY M. SHEFNER

Amyotrophic lateral sclerosis (ALS) is a progressive neurodegenerative disease of unknown etiology. While there has been an explosion of research in recent years relating to the possible etiology and treatment of ALS, the underlying cause has remained elusive. For approximately 10 percent of patients, an autosomal dominant pattern of inheritance has been determined, and, in about one-half of this group, the genetic mutation has been found. For the remaining 90 percent of patients, no genetic predisposition has been identified, and viral, immunologic, and neurotoxic hypotheses are all still under current consideration.

For years, ALS has represented a special challenge for neurologists, who were confronted with intellectually intact, often young patients for whom only symptomatic care was available. Despite detailed knowledge of the pathophysiology, epidemiology, and clinical course of the disease, therapeutic options were and are limited, and the most important role of the neurologist is often to provide information and emotional support. As of this writing, however, a number of promising new drugs are undergoing clinical trials, and it is hoped that the immediate future will bring an expansion of our ability to affect the natural course of this disease.

This chapter focuses on the diagnosis and care of patients with ALS. Hypotheses regarding the etiology of the disease and detailed discussion of potential therapeutic agents are deferred, although a brief summary of the most promising agents is presented.

DEFINITION

ALS is defined as a disease involving progressive upper and lower motor neuron deterioration at multiple levels of the neuraxis. At presentation, patients may have signs and symptoms related to just upper motor neuron or lower motor neuron disease, but the diagnosis can only be made with certainty if both types of abnormalities are present. The World Federation of Neurology has established criteria for the diagnosis of ALS; on purely clinical grounds, a diagnosis of ALS requires the presence of both upper and lower motor neuron signs in the bulbar musculature and concurrent upper and lower motor neuron involvement in two of the three spinal regions (cervical, thoracic, and lumbosacral). Lower motor neuron signs include weakness, muscle wasting, and fasciculations; upper motor neuron signs include increased deep tendon reflexes, spasticity, pseudobulbar features, extensor plantar responses, and other abnormal stretch reflexes.

When patients fulfill the criteria discussed above, the physician is left with little in the way of differential diagnosis, even in the absence of confirmatory diagnostic tests. Most commonly, however, patients present with fragments of the above syndrome, and the clinician must make appropriate use of neurophysiologic and radiologic tests to eliminate other possible diseases. Common initial presentations are discussed below; in time, most patients who present with partial syndromes will show spread of abnormalities; so the diagnosis becomes more obvious.

However, some patients present with some features of ALS but not others and demonstrate progression that does not seem consistent with the diagnosis of classic disease. A small subgroup of patients presents with a purely spastic disorder, involving increased tone in bulbar and spinal musculature, slow and clumsy movements, but little muscle wasting or weakness. This syndrome has been named *primary lateral sclerosis* and was described in the 1800s shortly after the original descriptions of ALS. Almost from its initial description, there was argument about whether primary lateral sclerosis represented a separate disease or an atypical presentation of ALS. It is generally believed that, in most cases, patients presenting initially with pure upper motor neuron signs will eventually develop classic ALS. However, a small subgroup of patients appear to have disease restricted to the descending cortical pathways. These patients have a more benign clinical course with expected survival greater than 15 years.

Another subgroup of patients presents with purely lower motor neuron signs; in these patients, reflexes are usually either absent or reduced. Often, the presenting complaint is limited to weakness in one limb; with time, weakness spreads to involve multiple extremities. Some of these patients will develop signs of upper motor neuron dysfunction and thus be classified as having classic ALS. Others will remain with only lower motor neuron signs, showing increasing weakness and atrophy in multiple areas of the neuraxis. Formerly, these patients were said to have *progressive muscular atrophy* and were distinguished from ALS patients on the basis of their lack of upper motor neuron signs and their slow progression. With increasing electrophysiologic sophistication, however, many of these patients are now known to have a motor neuropathy rather than an anterior horn cell disease; these patients are discussed in Chapter 106.

A final group of patients that should be mentioned are those that present with signs limited to the bulbar musculature. Usually, by the time they are initially seen, both upper and lower motor neuron signs are seen together; most often, speech is spastic, and fasciculations of the tongue are obvious. Historically, this presentation was called *progressive bulbar palsy* and was distinguished from classic ALS. It is now generally believed, however, that these patients will develop classic disease, and their clinical course is indistinguishable from that of other ALS patients.

EPIDEMIOLOGY

ALS is a rare disease. Its incidence of 1.5 in 100,000 population is fairly constant worldwide, except for some specific foci of higher incidence that probably represent toxic exposure. In the United States, this incidence implies that approximately 3,600 patients will be diagnosed with ALS every year. Given an average life span of 3 years after diagnosis, one would expect that there are approximately 11,000 patients living with ALS in the United States. Men are more likely to contract the disease than women, with recent studies suggesting a male-to-female ratio of about 1.5. In general, ALS is a disease of middle to late life. Although cases have been documented of onset in the teenage years, most studies show the average age of onset ranging from 55 to 60 years. The incidence appears to rise steadily until approximately age 65 and then declines slowly. The incidence does not vary according to race, environment, or occupation.

Approximately 10 percent of patients report a family history of ALS. A clear autosomal dominant pattern of inheritance has been documented in some families, and, in a subgroup of these families, a genetic defect on chromosome 21 involving a gene called *SOD1* has been identified. This gene encodes a protein (superoxide dismutase) that acts to reduce the concentration of toxic free radicals; how a defect in this gene acts to produce a disease specific for motor neurons has not been determined. Except for a slightly lower average age of onset, patients with familial ALS are indistinguishable from those with sporadic disease.

As mentioned above, there are some areas in the world where the incidence of ALS is much higher than in the United States. On Guam, a small peninsula in Japan, and parts of New Guinea, incidence rates are up to 100 times higher than elsewhere in the world. Many studies have attempted to determine why these areas have such high rates of ALS; the most likely cause seems to be a toxin in the food supply.

CLINICAL FEATURES

Although patients with classic ALS involving both the extremities and the bulbar musculature present with a very characteristic clinical picture, most patients with early disease have focal signs and symptoms. The most common initial symptom is that of arm weakness; about one-half of all ALS patients present in this fashion. A wrist drop is a characteristic early sign, often noted concurrently with intrinsic hand muscle wasting. For unclear reasons, flexor compartment forearm muscles are usually

affected later in the disease. Because of this asymmetry of forearm involvement, the hand often assumes a clawed posture. The disease usually spreads regionally, going from the distal to the proximal arm; biceps and deltoid muscles are usually affected before the triceps.

About one-quarter of patients present with lower extremity symptoms, most commonly a unilateral foot drop. As in the upper extremity, weakness tends to spread regionally, first to more proximal muscles in the same leg and then to the opposite leg, before ascending to involve the arms.

Most of the remaining patients present with symptoms of bulbar dysfunction or bulbar dysfunction in combination with other symptoms. Changes in the clarity of speech are often the first bulbar symptom, with difficulty swallowing also noted early. Patients notice that telephone communication is more difficult and often report that speech is more slurred late in the day. Swallowing liquids becomes difficult before solids; carbonated and alcoholic liquids are likely to be the least well tolerated, with thicker liquids tolerated better.

Most of the signs and symptoms mentioned above are related to lower motor neuron dysfunction; while upper motor neuron signs may be appreciated by the examining physician early in the course of ALS, they rarely are the cause of symptoms. Occasional patients present with initial complaints of limb stiffness and slowed movements, but such patients clearly are the exception. Even as the disease progresses and upper motor neuron signs become more flagrant, lower motor neuron loss continues to be the most important factor affecting disability.

Other less common presentations of ALS are isolated respiratory failure and diffuse fasciculations. Fasciculations are a relatively common symptom in the general population and can precipitate a visit to a neurologist. In the absence of clear signs of motor neuron loss, however, fasciculations are almost never a harbinger of ALS. Physical examination of patients with isolated fasciculations is usually sufficient to provide reassurance. Electromyography documents the presence of fasciculations but cannot distinguish between those that are benign and those that are associated with ALS. Muscle cramps are commonly reported by patients, but almost always in association with significant upper motor neuron disease; they are not usually seen in otherwise normal limbs.

There are a number of symptoms that should make the physician doubt the diagnosis of ALS. Although end-gaze nystagmus and mild abnormalities of rapid eye movements can be seen, diplopia or vertigo are extremely uncommon. Vague sensory symptoms are frequently reported by patients, but objective sensory loss is rare and should be a signal to consider alternative or concurrent disease processes. Often patients complain of a dysesthetic feeling; it is unclear whether this represents a true sensory symptom or muscle soreness from overuse. Bowel or bladder incontinence is also said not to occur in ALS. However, constipation is a frequent complaint, perhaps related to loss of abdominal muscle tone. In addition, urinary urge incontinence is frequently reported, more often by women than by men. Urinary dysfunction is seen most often in two patient groups. Female patients who recall having temporary urgency incontinence after childbirth are likely to have recurrence of such symptoms. In addition, women (and occasionally men) with a prominent upper motor neuron component to their disease may also report episodes of incontinence.

In the last 10 years, a number of carefully performed studies have yielded new information about how ALS progresses. Although patients report that periods of relative stability are interrupted by episodes of rapid deterioration, quantitative strength measurements have not confirmed these impressions. In several recent studies, patients were studied at regular intervals over a period of years using a battery of tests, including quantitative measurements of individual muscle strength and pulmonary function tests of vital capacity and inspiratory/expiratory force. It was found that, if measurements from local body areas were combined to produce separate scores for arms, legs, bulbar, and pulmonary performance, strength declined linearly in any given area. The rate of decline varied within the same patient for different body areas, so that, for example, pulmonary function could decrease more rapidly than lower extremity strength. However, if a certain body area declined in strength slowly initially, the decline tended to remain slow throughout the course of the disease.

The observation that ALS progresses in a predictable manner within local body regions for individual patients has a number of important implications. First, it allows physicians to give patients some way of evaluating how fast they are progressing and, to some extent, what the future will hold. Obviously, this information is more reassuring to slowly progressing patients, but most patients appreciate realistic appraisals of their disease course. In addition, the ability to predict with some accuracy the course of an individual patient is important in the design of therapeutic trials, offering the potential to decrease the size of control groups by reducing random variability of the population.

Another important recent observation is that the deficits in ALS tend to progress in a regional manner. Thus, patients presenting with distal leg weakness are likely to experience proximal spread of weakness or symptoms in the contralateral leg before cranial nerve or pulmonary symptoms are noted. Along with the observation discussed above that different body regions progress at different rates, the phenomenon of regional spread suggests that local conditions within the central nervous system affect the course of the disease.

LABORATORY EVALUATION AND DIFFERENTIAL DIAGNOSIS

Fully established classic ALS requires little in the way of laboratory support. However, in patients who present with focal complaints, a wide differential diagnosis must be considered. Compressive spinal and root pathology must be ruled out in patients without bulbar signs; concurrent cervical myelopathy with multiple root entrapments can produce a syndrome of combined upper and lower motor neuron dysfunction that is very difficult to distinguish from ALS. Clinically, the presence of sensory symptoms should help in leading to the correct diagnosis, but radiologic study is crucial. Currently, magnetic resonance imaging of the spine is the diagnostic modality of choice. Often, it is necessary to image the entire spine before concluding that a compressive syndrome is not present.

For patients who present with prominent upper motor neuron signs in the bulbar musculature and/or the extremities, such entities such as multiple strokes, mass lesions, and multiple sclerosis must be considered. Magnetic resonance imaging of the head in such patients is indicated and is usually a sufficient tool to rule out these diseases.

Historically, lumbar puncture has been performed frequently on patients with a probable diagnosis of ALS. Extremely high cerebrospinal fluid protein levels occasionally led to an unsuspected diagnosis of spinal cord compression, and the possibility

of infection was frequently discussed. With improved radiologic modalities, however, the utility of lumbar puncture in patients with classic signs has declined, and it is not necessary to perform this test routinely.

Blood tests do not play a major role in the diagnosis of classic ALS. However, some patients may present with only lower motor neuron signs, early age of onset, or other atypical features such as superimposed extrapyramidal or cerebellar signs. Such patients require specific laboratory tests based on their particular presentation. In patients who present primarily with lower motor neuron signs, the differential diagnosis includes motor neuropathy, plexopathy, toxic exposure, metabolic dysfunction, infection, and muscle disease. The syndrome of multifocal motor neuropathy with conduction block can mimic ALS with primarily lower motor neuron involvement; diagnosis is established through careful nerve conduction studies and clinical examination. In addition, antibodies to gangliosides are often present in peripheral blood; gangliosides are an essential component of nerve membranes. Thus, blood should routinely be sent for ganglioside antibodies in patients with a question of ALS and predominant lower motor neuron signs. Details of this syndrome are discussed elsewhere in this book.

A screen for heavy metal intoxication is frequently performed but rarely contributes to the diagnosis in patients with lower motor neuron signs. Both lead and mercury intoxication has been reported to be associated with ALS-like syndromes; however, the more usual presentation of toxicity is a predominantly motor neuropathy with some sensory abnormalities but absent upper motor neuron signs. Aluminum toxicity has been invoked as a possible cause of ALS in areas where the incidence of ALS is high, but evidence that it causes a significant neuropathy or ALS-like syndrome in the United States is essentially lacking. In general, unless there is a history of prior exposure, blood and urinary screens for heavy metals are not likely to be contributory.

One rare inherited metabolic disease can occasionally be mistaken for ALS. Hexosaminidase deficiency is usually a severe multisystem disease of childhood; however, occasionally it can present as late as age 40 years with a progressive disease that can closely mimic ALS. Hexosaminidase deficiency is inherited as an autosomal recessive trait, two genotypes of which have been associated with motor neuron syndromes. However, both types also involve other brain systems, frequently causing extrapyramidal or cerebellar signs and seizures. In general, screening for hexosaminidase deficiency is not warranted in patients with classic ALS presenting after age 40; however, in younger patients or in patients with atypical features, a blood test is available.

Infections rarely are a source of confusion in the diagnosis of motor neuron diseases. However, a few possibilities should be kept in mind. Lyme disease, caused by the infectious agent *Borrelia burgdorferi,* commonly causes a neuropathy or radiculopathy as a secondary effect. Usually, this neuropathy has both sensory and motor features, but occasionally motor dysfunction is noted in isolation. In patients with a predominantly lower motor neuron syndrome who live in endemic areas, Lyme titers should be obtained; however, as the incidence of incidental positive titers is high in such patients, determination of antibody type should also be performed, and a lumbar puncture to determine whether there is central nervous system antibody production may be necessary. Human T-cell leukemia virus type I (HTLV-I) is a neurotropic virus associated with a progressive spastic disorder sometimes associated with a neuropathy, making it very difficult to distinguish from ALS. If patients are from areas in which HTLV-I is endemic and have any atypical features such as back pain, bladder dysfunction, or absent bulbar signs, blood and cerebrospinal fluid tests for antibodies to HTLV-I are available.

ELECTROPHYSIOLOGIC FEATURES

Electromyography

The electromyogram (EMG) has proved to be an important tool both in establishing the diagnosis of ALS and in providing insight into its pathophysiology. The abnormalities seen in ALS are similar to those seen in other forms of neurogenic disease. Evidence of ongoing denervation is derived from the presence of abnormal spontaneous activity such as fibrillation potentials. As a consequence of denervation, surviving motor axons reinnervate muscle fibers, producing characteristic abnormalities in motor unit morphology, as recorded by conventional concentric EMG electrodes and by newer techniques such as single-fiber and macro-EMG. While the abnormalities seen in ALS resemble those present in other diseases of the anterior horn cell and motor axon, the distribution of abnormal findings and the pace of disease progression are often useful in distinguishing ALS from other diseases.

Fibrillation potentials, and positive sharp waves, reflect activity of individual muscle fibers that have lost their synaptic contact with motor neurons. The frequency with which fibrillations are observed in ALS varies according to the amount of weakness or atrophy of the muscle being studied, the duration of the disease, and the location in the body. In addition, fibrillation potentials are more likely to be seen in certain muscle groups than others. In the limbs, fibrillations are present more often in distal than in proximal muscles, with facial and tongue muscles being less likely than limb muscles to show fibrillations. Interestingly, fibrillations are noted in thoracic paraspinal muscles in most patients. Diagnostically, this is a useful finding as spondylosis of the thoracic spine is uncommon compared to cervical and lumbar spondylosis and abnormalities noted in the thoracic region are thus less likely to reflect root compression.

One of the most characteristic abnormalities seen in patients with ALS is the presence of fasciculations. Clinically, they are seen in most patients; electrophysiologically, they are noted almost without exception, even in sites where involuntary movements are not appreciated. It should be noted, however, that clinical and electrophysiologic fasciculations may be entirely benign and that there is no way to distinguish between benign fasciculations and those that represent motor neuron disease.

The changes seen in motor unit morphology in patients with ALS are qualitatively similar to those that occur as a consequence of any form of neurogenic atrophy. As anterior horn cells are lost, viable motor axons establish synaptic contact with muscle fibers that have been denervated. The electrical correlate of this process is an increase in amplitude of the motor unit action potential. On average, motor unit amplitude is increased by about a factor of 4 over normal, with units in severely involved muscles having amplitudes of approximately 10 times normal and amplitudes from units in only slightly affected muscles increased somewhat less.

The increase in size of individual motor unit potentials reflects reinnervation by viable motor axons after the death of other anterior horn cells. Thus, the number of functioning motor units in a given muscle should decrease with disease progres-

sion. A number of methods for estimating the number of motor units have been developed for distal muscles and have more recently been extended to larger proximal muscles. In general, the number of motor units present in a given muscle is estimated by determining the maximum amplitude of the compound muscle action potential and then recording potentials from many single motor units. The total number of motor units is estimated by dividing the average amplitude of the single motor unit potentials into the amplitude of the compound motor action potential.

Motor unit counting provides a very useful way to measure disease progression objectively. By sequential performance of this test on individual patients over time, it has become clear that there is very substantial motor unit dropout before patients report loss of strength in a muscle and before the amplitude of the compound motor action potential has declined below normal. The most rapid dropout of motor units actually occurs very early in the disease, often before a muscle is symptomatically weak. In patients whose disease follows a chronic course, motor unit counts may remain stable for years after dropping to approximately 10 to 20 percent of normal.

Nerve Conduction Studies

While many ALS patients report vague sensory symptoms, clinical sensory examination is usually normal. It is not surprising, therefore, that routine sensory nerve conduction studies are normal or nearly normal in most patients. However, just as very careful computerized tests of sensation have shown mild alterations in multimodal sensory function in ALS patients, so precise recordings of slower conducting sensory fibers have shown frequent mild abnormalities in the compound sensory action potential. This is consistent with autopsy studies, which have found up to 30 percent reductions in the number of dorsal root ganglion cells.

In studies of motor function, conduction velocity in ALS patients has consistently been shown to be normal or near normal until muscle atrophy becomes extreme. However, even when motor conduction velocity is normal, distal motor latency is often prolonged. Distal latencies that are prolonged out of proportion to proximal conduction velocity is a finding frequently associated with dying-back neuropathies in which the terminal axon is more affected than the cell body or proximal axon. Although ALS primarily causes a motor neuronopathy, recent morphologic studies suggest a component of dying-back axonopathy.

Diagnostic Electrophysiologic Criteria

ALS is primarily a clinical diagnosis. However, EMG and nerve conduction studies can be extremely important in establishing the diagnosis when insufficient clinical evidence is available. A number of criteria for the electrophysiologic diagnosis have been suggested. As in many other diseases, the rigid application of criteria is often more a hindrance than a help; however, certain guidelines should be remembered. First, evidence for muscle denervation should be diffuse, that is, fibrillation potentials and large motor units should be present in multiple muscles of multiple extremities. Most published criteria require denervation to be present in three of four areas of the neuraxis, with the four areas being bulbar, cervical, thoracic, and lumbosacral. Second, there should be no evidence of motor conduction block. While a formal discussion of conduction block is beyond the scope of this chapter, conduction block implies that there is an area of axon through which action potentials are not conducted, even though viable axon exists both proximal and distal to that area. Third, motor and sensory conduction velocity and compound sensory action potential amplitudes should be normal or nearly so from both arm and leg. If these conditions are fulfilled, the diagnosis of lower motor neuron disease can be considered confirmed. To make a diagnosis of ALS, however, clinical evidence of upper motor neuron disease must also be present.

TREATMENT

Presently, treatment of patients with ALS is supportive. There are currently no treatments that have been shown conclusively to alter the course of disease progression, although a number of very encouraging therapeutic trials are now being conducted. The agents being studied are of two types. One treatment strategy is based on the as yet unproved hypothesis that ALS is related to local overaccumulation of the excitotoxic neurotransmitter glutamate. This hypothesis is based primarily on observations that glutamate transport is focally reduced in areas of the brain and spinal cord important for motor function. In addition, in vitro studies have shown that motor neurons are very susceptible to pharmacologic manipulations that reduce glutamate transport. A number of drugs that antagonize the effects of glutamate are now being evaluated in clinical trials.

A second group of agents currently being evaluated is the newly isolated and cloned human nerve growth factors, which have been shown in vitro and in animal models to be protective of motor neurons and to slow the progression of several inherited diseases involving motor nerve degeneration. One agent is ciliary neurotrophic factor, which is present in Schwann cells and may act, under normal circumstances, to protect neurons from external trauma. Other factors that have been shown to be specifically neuroprotective for motor neurons are brain-derived neurotrophic factor and insulin-derived factor. All three of these agents are currently undergoing human clinical trials. Although it is not likely that deficiencies in any of these substances are related etiologically to ALS, they may prove to be effective in slowing the course of the disease.

Until one of these agents or another as yet untested drug is found to be effective in treating patients with ALS, the job of the neurologist is to treat complications of disease without treating the underlying illness. A number of specific problems can often be, at least temporarily, ameliorated. Focal weakness can produce early gait problems, often caused by unilateral or bilateral foot drop. Ankle-foot orthoses can return many patients' gait to almost normal. In patients with more significant lower extremity weakness, the involvement of a physical therapist with experience in neurologic disorders is essential. While it may seem trivial, the right kind of cane, or an appropriately modified walker can make a major difference in the life of a patient whose livelihood depends on the ability to ambulate. Similarly, disability from relatively focal upper extremity weakness can often be treated with either supports, braces, or modified instruments of daily living such as spoons or toothbrushes. A close association with a sophisticated occupational therapist provides patients with assistance that neurologists by themselves cannot give.

Another problem that must be addressed on a repeated basis is that of nutrition. ALS patients often lose a large percentage of their body weight even before swallowing becomes difficult. Some of this is unavoidable because of loss of muscle bulk from motor neuron loss. However, loss of appetite from inactivity or depression often plays a role. Patients must be counseled that rapid weight loss will produce weakness above and beyond their disease. If prior eating habits are not sufficient to maintain weight, dietary supplements should be added early in the disease course. Often, frequent smaller meals are better tolerated than three meals per day.

As disease progresses, good nutrition is made more difficult by the inevitable development of bulbar weakness and dysphagia. In many patients with early bulbar involvement, this may occur while the patient is ambulatory and otherwise still able to lead a relatively active life. In such patients, early consideration of jejunostomy or gastrostomy placement can greatly improve the patient's quality of life. Such procedures should be performed before patients become significantly malnourished. Beyond providing an alternative pathway for caloric intake, the presence of a gastrostomy tube can be of great emotional benefit. By the time such procedures are performed, meals have usually become times of great stress for patients, as they desperately try to eat enough to sustain themselves. Caloric supplementation via an alternative route gives patients the ability to eat without such pressure and to use mealtimes for enjoying the company of family.

Vitamin supplementation has become an issue for ALS patients, especially since the discovery that many patients with familial ALS have a potential disorder involving the reduced ability to detoxify free radicals. Vitamin E and β-carotene act to scavenge free radicals and therefore have been proposed as potentially delaying the progression of ALS. While no data currently exist to support this hypothesis, moderate vitamin supplementation is not likely to be harmful for patients, and some benefit may accrue. Many neurologists therefore recommend supplementation with vitamins C and E and β-carotene. Doses vary from neurologist to neurologist; as no therapeutic end point is clear, it is impossible to make a definite dose recommendation.

Ongoing evaluation of a patient's ability to communicate is also a necessary part of the care of ALS patients. Many patients will develop dysarthria, leading to mutism at some point in their disease. Speech therapy has been of occasional benefit in such patients; in general, patients with primarily upper motor neuron bulbar symptoms will do better with speech therapy than those with lower motor neuron weakness. A trial of speech therapy is probably warranted in all patients with worsening dysarthria. When vocal language can no longer be used, a number of options can be explored, ranging from computerized voice production devices for patients who have remaining upper extremity facility to systems that employ eye movements. Early attention to this issue and detailed discussion with patients is crucial, as it is much easier to make an appropriate decision regarding the best assistive device before communication is lost.

Another inevitable and often fatal complication of ALS is respiratory insufficiency. Weakness of the muscles of respiration will ultimately occur in all patients but may present early when the patient is otherwise functional or late in the setting of severe bulbar weakness and quadriplegia. In the second instance, assisted ventilation is not often seen as a reasonable option either by patients, their families, or their physicians. However, patients who retain the ability to speak and ambulate may derive a significant prolongation of life that is of reasonable quality. A number of devices can assist ventilation without the requirement of intubation; these include continuous positive airway pressure that can be provided by face mask and rocking beds that use gravity to assist inspiration and expiration. Such devices can delay the necessity for artificial respiration via endotracheal tube or tracheostomy.

If patients elect mechanical ventilation, the capability now exists for this to be performed at home. Respirators can be fitted to the backs of wheelchairs or sometimes attached to wheeled walkers in patients who retain the ability to walk. Patients can therefore choose this option without being hospitalized or even homebound. In a recent study of 24 patients who elected home ventilation, 90 percent reported that they would make the same decision again; approximately 50 percent of the patients' caregivers said they would choose such an option for themselves should the need arise. Such care is very expensive; in the same study, the average cost of home ventilation for 1 year was about $150,000.

One problem that patients often report that is not well treated is spasticity. This is obviously more of a problem for patients with prominent upper motor neuron disease; while this is the case for the minority of ALS patients, for some, it can be a significant problem. Baclofen is the most commonly used antispasticity drug for other neurologic disorders; however, it in general produces disappointing results in ALS patients. The major reason for this appears to be that doses high enough to produce reductions in spastic tone also produce significant added weakness in this patient population. Benzodiazepines are occasionally useful but must be employed very carefully in this group of patients already at risk for respiratory decompensation. Dantrolene, the other drug commonly used to treat spasticity, is almost always associated with unacceptable weakness in ALS patients.

An extremely important and overlooked component of the treatment of ALS patients is attention to the patient's emotional well-being. ALS is a devastating disease, producing progressive disability and dependence in the absence of intellectual deterioration. Depression in ALS patients is nearly universal and is at least partially treatable. Patients and family members nearly always benefit from referral to local support groups and frequently from individual therapy. In addition, pharmacologic treatment is often useful. While, in the past, most commonly used antidepressant medications were associated with side effects such as fatigue and dry mouth that were particularly distressing to ALS patients, the recently developed serotonin-selective reuptake inhibitors do not have these side effects and are much faster acting than older antidepressants.

SUGGESTED READINGS

Bradley WG: Recent views on amyotrophic lateral sclerosis with emphasis on electrophysiological studies. Muscle Nerve 10:490–502, 1987

Koliatsos VE, Clatterbuck RE, Winslow JW et al: Evidence that brain-derived neurotrophic factor is a trophic factor for motor neurons in vivo. Neuron 10:359–67, 1993

Korsching S: The neurotrophic factor concept: a reexamination. J Neurosci 13: 2739–48, 1993

Moss AH, Casey P, Stocking CB et al: Home ventilation for amyotrophic lateral sclerosis patients: outcomes, costs, and patient, family, and physician attitudes. Neurology 43:438–43, 1993

Munsat T, Andres PL, Finison L et al: The natural history of motoneuron loss in amyotrophic lateral sclerosis. Neurology 38:409–13, 1988

Rosen DR, Siddique T, Patterson D et al: Mutations in Cu/Zn superoxide dismutase gene are associated with familial amyotrophic lateral sclerosis. Nature 362:59–62, 1993

Rothstein JD, LJ Martin, Kuncl RW: Decreased glutamate transport by the brain and spinal cord in amyotrophic lateral sclerosis. N Engl J Med 326: 1464–8, 1992

Tyler HR, Shefner JM: Amyotrophic lateral sclerosis. pp. 169–216. In Vinken P, Bruyn G, Klawans H (eds): Handbook of Clinical Neurology. Vol. 59. Elsevier Science Publishing, New York, 1991

88. SPINAL MUSCULAR ATROPHY

KATHRYN N. NORTH
LINDA A. SPECHT

DEFINITION

Spinal muscular dystrophy (SMA) is a lower motor neuron disorder characterized pathologically by degeneration of the anterior horn cells, particularly in the spinal cord and bulbar motor nuclei. The clinical hallmarks of the disorder are symmetric muscle weakness and atrophy of limb muscles with clinical, electrophysiologic, and pathologic evidence of denervation.

The best described and most common form of the disorder presents predominantly in infancy and childhood and is linked to chromosome 5q. It is inherited in an autosomal recessive fashion. In the western world, acute SMA constitutes the most common genetic cause of infantile death and is the second most common serious neuromuscular disorder after Duchenne's muscular dystrophy. *The gene for classic SMA has recently been characterized.* Other disorders, sometimes referred to as SMA in the literature but not linked to 5q, are clinically and molecularly heterogeneous. These rare, non-5q SMAs are mentioned briefly.

CLINICAL FEATURES

Degeneration of the anterior horn cells in the spinal cord and lower brainstem results in a lower motor neuron pattern of weakness and muscle wasting in the limbs and tongue. The pattern of weakness in the limbs is symmetric, more proximal than distal, and more severe in the lower limbs. A "piano-playing" tremor of the outstretched hands is prominent in many patients. The muscles of the trunk are involved with intercostal weakness, and bulbar involvement results in atrophy and fasciculation in the tongue. Deep tendon reflexes are decreased or absent, and plantar reflexes, if present, are downgoing. Typically, the diaphragm is spared until late in the disease (in severe forms), and there is no involvement of cardiac or smooth muscle. Clinical exclusion criteria for SMA include the presence of arthrogryposis, sensory disturbance, intellectual impairment, or sphincter disturbance. Extraocular muscle weakness, marked facial weakness, respiratory failure at birth, cardiac involvement, and loss of hearing or vision are not associated with SMA (Table 88-1).

CLASSIFICATION/SUBTYPES

Classic Spinal Muscular Atrophy

Childhood-onset SMA is usually classified into three groups on the basis of age of onset and clinical severity (Table 88-2). Types I, II, and III are usually inherited in an autosomal recessive manner with genetic localization to chromosome 5q13 (see

TABLE 88-1. Diagnostic Criteria of Spinal Muscular Atrophy

Inclusion criteria
Symmetrical muscle weakness, proximal greater than distal
Lower limbs affected more than upper limbs
Trunk muscles involved, with poor head and trunk control in severe cases
Intercostal weakness but sparing of the diaphragm
Evidence of denervation, either clinical (fasciculations or tremor) or laboratory (EMG or muscle biopsy)

Exclusion criteria

Clinical	*Laboratory*
Central nervous system dysfunction	High creatine kinase
Arthrogryposis	Aminoaciduria
Abnormalities of other organ systems	Organic aciduria
	Hexosaminidase A or B deficiency
Sensory loss	Monoclonal gammopathy
Severe facial or extraocular muscle weakness	Biopsy evidence of lipid or glycogen storage disease or mitochondrial abnormality
Hypertonia or hyperreflexia	Abnormally slow nerve conduction velocity

(Adapted from Munsat TL: Workshop report. International SMA Collaboration. Neuromuscul Disord 1:81, 1990, with permission.)

below). The acute infantile form (Werdnig-Hoffmann or type I) presents before 6 months of age. Many infants are normal to examination during the first few months of life, although some are noted to be hypotonic at birth or to have exhibited decreased fetal movements. Children with this form of the disorder never attain the ability to sit. Progression to generalized paralysis of the limbs and trunk is rapid, and bulbar involvement, with fasciculations and wasting of the tongue, is a useful diagnostic sign. Although the infant remains visually alert, feeding difficulties, respiratory failure with aspiration, and recurrent respiratory infections usually lead to death by 2 years of age.

An intermediate form of SMA (type II or "chronic" Werdnig-Hoffmann disease) has its onset between 6 and 18 months of age. These children may be assessed as normal during the first 6 months of life and attain the ability to sit. Subsequent motor development is arrested, and they are unable ever to stand unassisted. Bulbar dysfunction is less marked, and tongue fasciculation is less common than in type I, but the peripheral tremor may be more marked. Survival, as in type I, is linked to respiratory function, and death is usually secondary to overwhelming respiratory infection. Prolonged survival into the third or fourth decade, with or without the need for artificial ventilation, may occur in this group of patients.

The mildest form of childhood-onset SMA (Kugelberg-Welander or type III) usually presents between 18 months and 17 years of age with proximal symmetric muscle weakness, predominantly affecting the legs. These patients usually, but not always, retain the ability to walk, although joint contractures and scoliosis may become evident. Bulbar function is usually preserved, and these patients survive into adulthood. As in type II, tremor is common and may be the presenting feature. This form of SMA is the most difficult to differentiate from the muscular dystrophies, and diagnosis may rely on evidence of denervation on electromyography (EMG), and muscle biopsy.

TABLE 88-2. Classification of Spinal Muscular Atrophy

Type	Onset	Missed Milestones	Age at Death
I (acute)	Birth–6 months	Never sit	Usually <2 years
II (intermediate)	<18 months	Never stand	>2 years
III (mild)	>18 months	—	Adult
IV (adult)	Adulthood	—	Adult

(Adapted from Munsat TL: Workshop report. International SMA Collaboration. Neuromuscul Disord 1:81, 1990, with permission.)

Other Forms

Other forms of so-called SMA are much more heterogeneous, clinically and genetically. They do not conform to the diagnostic criteria in Table 88-1, and there is thus far no evidence for linkage to chromosome 5q. Familial and sporadic forms have been identified that present with muscle weakness and evidence of denervation. Often, these disorders have a relatively mild course with no loss of ability to walk. Childhood forms include diffuse denervation in association with ophthalmoplegia, central nervous system malformation, pyramidal tract signs, or sensory involvement. A segmental or focal form results in localized weakness, particularly of the shoulder and hand, which may be associated with tremor. It is usually sporadic and briefly progressive, resulting in a fixed, localized deficit; progressive cases have been reported. Segmental atrophy of the spinal cord may be seen on magnetic resonance imaging.

The best understood form of non-5q SMA is known as Kennedy syndrome. This X-linked recessive disorder typically has its onset in the third decade with slow progression and involvement of the facial and bulbar muscles in addition to wasting of the proximal and, in some cases, distal musculature. There is usually asymmetry of clinical signs, with consistent and abundant fasciculations predominantly in the perioral muscles and intention tremor in the limbs. Striking gynecomastia is the first clinical sign in association with decreased fertility. Sensory abnormalities have been reported in some patients. The gene has been characterized at Xq12 and is an androgen receptor gene with an expansion of a tandem trinucleotide repeat (CAG) in the first exon.

NATURAL HISTORY/CONTROVERSIES

Russman et al. (1992) studied 141 patients with SMA with diagnosis based on onset of weakness before 18 years, evidence of denervation on EMG or muscle biopsy, normal nerve conduction velocities, and no sensory deficits. All familial cases were recessive. Their results challenged the current classification system with regard to the prognostic implications of age of onset relative to function, rational rehabilitation, and life expectancy. Thirty-nine percent of their patients were type I (weakness noted prior to 6 months of age); 73 percent of patients had been able to sit independently, and 8 percent could walk independently at one time. One patient in this group was 31 years old. Some children acquired new milestones after diagnosis. Forty-four percent had type II disease (onset between 7 and 24 months) with age range at evaluation from 1 to 38 years; 43 percent of this group had been able to walk at some time.

Age of onset criteria have thus proved to be too arbitrary and too dependent on observer variability; ultimate prognosis correlates better with best milestone achieved. In our experience, it is difficult to prognosticate for an infant with SMA who is not yet sitting. While most such infants never achieve the ability to sit and succumb to their illness by age 2 years, others eventually learn to sit during the latter half of their first year and go on to exhibit a stable course over many years or decades.

The second important observation in Russman et al.'s study was that, although strength in SMA patients did not increase with age, their absolute strength did not decrease. However, cross-sectional data convincingly revealed loss of function with time, independent of age of onset. This observation is consistent with reports from families and clinical observation. It has been suggested that SMA may not be a degenerative disease resulting from the death of anterior horn cells. An alternative hypothesis is that a fetal defect of the anterior horn cell is responsible for SMA and that the defect is limited and develops later in patients with late-onset disease. Progressive loss of function may be related to factors such as increased body mass, rather than an ongoing neurodegenerative process.

GENETICS AND DIAGNOSTIC TESTING

SMA is inherited in an autosomal recessive pattern. There is no evidence of effects of birth order, parental age, social class, or seasonal influences. Carriers are normal clinically and on laboratory testing. Type I SMA has an incidence of 1 in 20,000 to 25,000 live births, with a carrier frequency of 1 in 60 to 80. The chronic forms affect 1 in 24,000. In some Moslem countries, because of the high rate of consanguinity, the disease incidence is at least 40-fold greater.

In 1990, the genetic abnormality in the recessive forms of SMA was localized to chromosome 5q11.2–13.3, and the locus was subsequently narrowed to the region 5q13. All three types of childhood SMA are linked to the same locus in a number of studies. Analysis of SMA 5q families supports the view that, with certain exceptions, there is little phenotypic intrafamilial variability; occasional sibling pairs may have divergent courses and different survival characteristics. Some families have been studied who did not display linkage to 5q markers, raising the possibility of genetic heterogeneity or disease misclassification.

If the index patient satisfies the inclusion criteria for SMA, over 90 percent of all SMA families currently appear to be linked to chromosome 5q markers. The proportion of acute SMA families (type I) linked to 5q13 is higher and may approach 100 percent. At present, prenatal diagnosis from chorionic villous biopsy or amniocentesis using linkage studies is useful for informative families. With polymorphic markers close to the SMA locus, over 99 percent of 5q-linked families are informative. Appropriate allowances must be made in genetic counseling for sporadic cases owing to noninherited causes and for linkage heterogeneity or misdiagnosis.

In January 1995, the SMA-determining gene (termed the survival motor neuron or *SMN* gene) was identified, and mutation analysis was carried out in 229 patients with 5q SMA (types I, II, and III) (Lefebvre et al., 1995). The gene was homozygously deleted in 226 patients, and in the remaining three patients one allele was deleted with a point mutation or short deletions in the other. The function of the gene protein is not yet known, but it is expressed in a wide variety of tissues, including the spinal cord. No phenotype-genotype correlation between the gene defect and the type of SMA was observed, although deletions of contiguous segments of DNA appeared to be more frequent in type I than in type III patients. The latter observation is important in the light of simultaneous identification of a gene involved in motor neuron apoptosis, which maps close to but outside the critical SMA region (neuronal apoptosis inhibitory gene or *NAIP*). Parts of this gene were deleted in approximately 67 percent of type I SMA chromosomes, suggesting that this gene may also contribute to the SMA phenotype. Although the exact nature of the genetic mechanisms resulting in the SMA phenotype remains to be clarified, the identification of the SMA gene will obviate the need for complex linkage analysis in clinical testing for this disorder and in prenatal diagnosis.

DIAGNOSIS

Serum biochemistry is usually normal, although mild elevations of creatine kinase (up to five times normal levels) and aldolase may be present in severe cases. It should be noted that creatine kinase levels may be transiently elevated in normal newborns, limiting the value of this test as a diagnostic finding in early infancy.

The diagnosis of SMA rests primarily on the electrophysiologic and muscle biopsy findings. EMG typically shows evidence of denervation with fibrillations and fasciculations. The

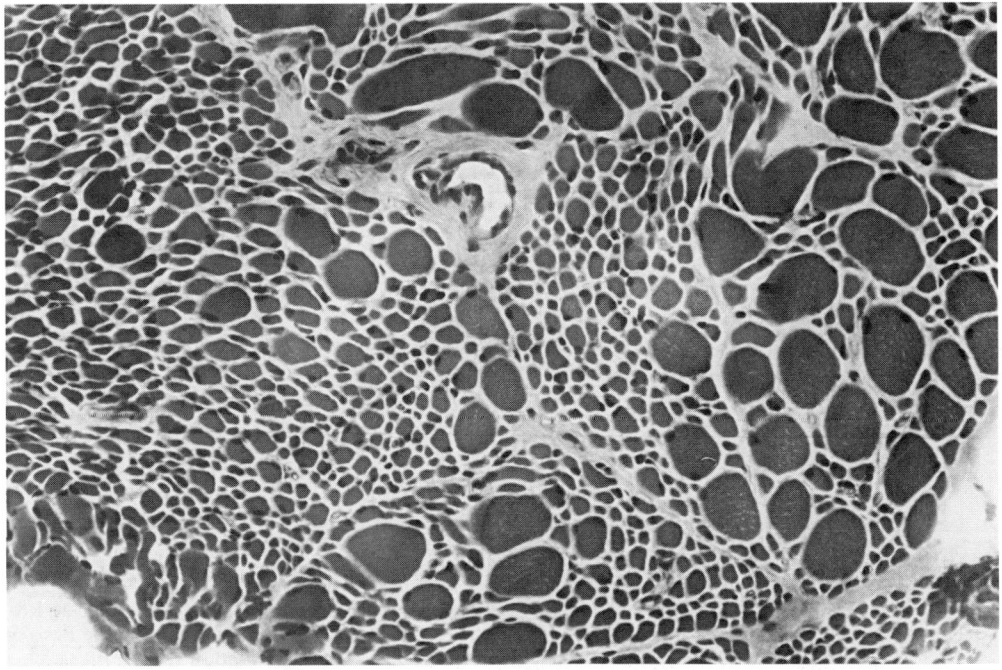

FIG. 88-1.   Muscle biopsy from a patient with spinal muscular atrophy type I demonstrating denervation atrophy with residual hypertrophic fibers. (Mn × 300.)

finding most specific for the disease is the presence of spontaneous rhythmic muscle activity at 5 to 15 Hz. This is observed in 75 percent of cases, irrespective of age or severity of disease, and can be activated by voluntary effort. Residual motor unit potentials are polyphasic and increased in amplitude and duration. The frequency of discharge shows little increase with increased muscular effort, and recruitment is impaired. Nerve conduction studies are usually normal, although conduction velocity in motor nerves may be decreased in the more severely affected children.

Muscle biopsy demonstrates denervation atrophy with large patches of small atrophic fibers and residual fibers that are normal or increased in size (Fig. 88-1). Fiber-type grouping is evident on adenosine triphosphatase stains and is due to compensatory reinnervation.

The presentation of acute infantile form of SMA must be differentiated from other causes of ''the floppy infant,'' which generally have different prognostic implications. In this setting, the presence of tongue fasciculations may be the major clinical diagnostic feature suggesting involvement of the anterior horn cells. Atonic cerebral palsy is usually associated with upper motor neuron signs such as hyperreflexia and cognitive impairment. Primary muscle disorders such as the congenital myopathies, congenital muscular dystrophy, congenital myasthenia gravis, and infantile mitochondrial myopathies may be differentiated by family history, biochemistry, EMG, or muscle biopsy. Disorders of the peripheral nerves include hypomyelinating neuropathies and polyneuritis; in such cases, nerve biopsy may also be required. Other disorders of infancy to be considered include botulism, poliomyelitis, spinal cord transection, and the hypotonia associated with Down syndrome, Marfan syndrome, and Prader-Willi syndrome.

There are undoubtedly other genetic syndromes in which involvement of the anterior horn cells may be a component and in which muscle biopsy may show a similar pathology to Werdnig-Hoffmann disease. Additional clinical features such as marked facial weakness, cognitive dysfunction, the presence of other exclusion criteria (Table 88-1), and nonlinkage to chromosome 5q should alert the clinician to consider alternative diagnoses.

Later-onset SMA, especially those forms without bulbar involvement, may present a more difficult diagnostic dilemma. Slowly progressive, symmetric proximal muscle weakness may be similar to the muscular dystrophies. EMG and muscle biopsy evidence of denervation provides the most important diagnostic clue as to the primary site of pathology. If the diagnosis remains unclear, then dystrophin assays on muscle biopsy may definitively exclude selected muscular dystrophies. Clinical evidence of denervation may be the primary presenting feature of amyotrophic lateral sclerosis; however, this disorder is differentiated from the late-onset forms of SMA by the eventual development of upper motor neuron signs.

TREATMENT

There is no specific therapy for SMA. In the infantile-onset forms of the disorder, management should focus on the symptomatic treatment of respiratory dysfunction and feeding difficulties. These patients are fragile and markedly hypotonic; orthopaedic treatment is limited to daily range-of-motion exercises for the joints. The early implementation of nasogastric feeds or insertion of a gastrostomy tube will minimize the risks of aspiration, ensure adequate nutrition, and facilitate the day-to-day care of the child. Chest physical therapy, in the later stages of the disease, may help to prevent pneumonia and aid in prolonging survival. Respiratory infections should be treated early with antibiotics. However, an individualized approach to severe respiratory infection or compromise should be developed with the child's family with regard to the use of artificial ventilation in the terminal stage of the illness.

The aim of treatment for the later onset or mild forms of SMA should be aimed at preserving mobility and minimizing respiratory complications. Specific and relatively early intervention can be helpful in maximizing the individual's potential. Physical therapy may be required on a regular basis to minimize joint contractures and maintain mobility. The major orthopaedic problems are scoliosis and hip dislocation; the age of onset and rate of progression appears to be directly related to the severity of muscle weakness.

Scoliosis almost always begins in the first decade of life in types II and III SMA, and the curves invariably progress over time. In patients who are unable to walk, spinal bracing may improve sitting stability. The decision regarding operative intervention (spinal arthrodesis) is easier to make if frequent pulmonary function studies have been done to establish a profile for the individual patient. In our clinic, surgery is recommended for patients over 10 years of age who have a flexible curve of 40 degrees or more and a forced vital capacity of more than 40 percent. Since worsening is invariable, the decision to intervene early should maximize the eventual result.

Proximal muscle weakness also predisposes these patients to progressive subluxation and dislocation of the hip. In nonambulant patients, it is important to prevent the hips from dislocating for reasons of comfort, good sitting balance, and maintenance of pelvic alignment; again, operative intervention may be required. Patients who have type III SMA and are still able to walk present a difficult management problem even though they have the mildest form of the condition. These patients are also prone to subluxation of the hip owing to proximal muscle weakness; however, surgical intervention with proximal femoral varus osteotomy results in additional weakening of the abductor muscles, and the physician should be cautious in recommending such a procedure in a patient who still walks. Although scoliosis is less marked, it does occur. Since these patients rely to a great extent on lumbar lordosis and a side-to-side waddle to walk, bracing or spinal arthrodesis may worsen their gait. It is therefore recommended that, in this small subset of patients, arthrodesis is postponed until the patient can no longer walk.

Specific therapies for SMA will only become a reality when there is better understanding of the underlying pathogenesis and the mechanism of anterior horn cell degeneration. The cloning of the SMA gene will be an important step in revealing the nature of the gene product so that we can begin to understand the biology of this disorder and eventually devise a rational approach to therapy.

SUGGESTED READINGS

Evans GA, Drennan JC, Russman BS: Functional classification and orthopaedic management of spinal muscular atrophy. J Bone Joint Surg [Br] 63B: 516–22, 1981

Gilliam TC, Brzustowicz LM: The molecular and genetic basis of the spinal muscular atrophies. pp. 883–7. In Rosenburg RN, Prusiner SB, DiMauro S et al (eds): The Molecular and Genetic Basis of Neurological Disease. Butterworth-Heinemann, Boston, 1993

Gilliam TC, Brzustowicz LM, Castilla LH et al: Genetic homogeneity between acute and chronic forms of spinal muscular atrophy. Nature 345:823–5, 1990

Iannacone ST, Browne RH, Samaha FJ et al: Prospective study of spinal muscular atrophy before age 6 years. Pediatr Neurol 9:187–93, 1993

Lefebvre S, Burgien L, Reboullet S et al: Identification and characterization of a spinal muscular atrophy-determining gene. Cell 80:155–65, 1995

Liu GT, Specht LA: Progressive juvenile segmental spinal muscular atrophy. Pediatr Neurol 9:54–6, 1993

MacKenzie AE, Jacob P, Surh L, Besner A: Genetic heterogeneity in spinal muscular atrophy: a linkage analysis based assessment. Neurology 44: 919–24, 1994

Munsat TL: Workshop report. International SMA Collaboration. Neuromuscul Disord 1:81, 1990

Roy N, Mahadevan MS, McLean M et al: The gene for neuronal apoptosis inhibitory protein is partially deleted in individuals with spinal muscular atrophy. Cell 80:167–78, 1995

Russman BS, Iannacone ST, Buncher CR et al: Spinal muscular atrophy: new thought on the pathogenesis and classification schema. J Child Neurol 7: 347–53, 1992

Shapiro F, Specht LA: The diagnosis and orthopaedic treatment of childhood spinal muscular atrophy, peripheral neuropathy, Friedreich ataxia and arthrogryphosis. J Bone Joint Surg 75A:1699–714, 1993

89. POSTPOLIO SYNDROME

DAVE HOLLANDER
THEODORE L. MUNSAT

The development of the Salk and Sabin polio vaccines represents one of the great triumphs of modern medicine. With the introduction of widespread vaccination programs, paralytic polio, the very name of which once conjured fear in both parents and physicians, has virtually disappeared in modern industrialized countries. Most physicians currently in practice have never seen a case of acute polio. There remain, however, thousands of survivors of the great polio epidemics of the past. For them, the memory of their acute illness is very real, and is evidenced by the residual amyotrophy and muscle weakness their limbs bear. The infirmities acquired by the victims of polio were initially believed to be static and nonprogressive. In the past few years, however, it has become evident that although the initial polio infection was monophasic in nature, the survivors of such infections may be prone to further progression of their symptoms, decades after their original illness. This progression is referred to as postpolio syndrome.

The onset of postpolio syndrome typically occurs about 30 years after the original bout of polio. It is conservatively estimated to develop in 25 percent of polio survivors, but the true figure may in fact be much higher. In the United States alone, there are estimated to be more than 500,000 polio survivors. Thus, the number of potential patients with postpolio syndrome is very significant. The core of postpolio syndrome consists of the triad of pain, fatigue, and progressive weakness. About one-third of patients with postpolio syndrome will display all these symptoms. Other less common features include the development of fasciculations and new muscle atrophy. The risk of developing these late sequelae is related to the severity of the initial illness (i.e., patients with severe polio are at greatest risk, and severely affected muscles are more likely to develop late weakness than clinically spared muscles). Nonetheless, even patients with mild polio may develop typical postpolio syndrome.

The pain of postpolio syndrome is usually musculoskeletal in origin, arising from the muscles and joints. The muscle pains are exertion-induced, presumably related to the limited exercise capacity of previously denervated muscles. The joint pains are mechanical in nature, the result of the years of unbalanced forces and stresses placed on joints, tendons, and ligaments that have had to compensate for muscle and limb weakness. Such pains are particularly common in the large weight-bearing joints. Frank degenerative arthritis may develop in such joints and act as a further cause of pain. In addition, pain may also develop as a consequence of nerve or root entrapment. Degenerative disc disease of the spine or scoliosis may result in radiculopathies. The long-term use of braces and crutches may cause compressive neuropathies, such as ulnar neuropathy and carpal tunnel syndrome. Fatigue in postpolio syndrome may be mild and limited to individual, previously affected muscle groups, or may be generalized. Such generalized fatigue may be severe and overwhelming, developing even after minimal exertion.

Muscle weakness may develop in any muscle group, including those that had previously seemed spared. This is a reflection of the fact that infection with the poliovirus usually involves motor neurons in a generalized, rather than focal, manner. Although certain regions of the neuraxis may be most severely affected, there is in fact more widespread, subclinical involvement. This new weakness is typically very slowly progressive, but even so, there may be very significant functional consequences associated with it. Patients who had previously been ambulatory may now be forced to use assistive devices, and the ability to perform other activities of daily life may become impaired. Respiratory symptoms may develop in patients who had previous involvement of respiratory muscles. Muscle atrophy may develop in a minority of patients.

The examination findings in patients with postpolio syndrome are largely similar to those seen in polio patients. Muscle atrophy, weakness, and areflexia are typically present, although in patients who had very mild polio, muscle bulk may appear intact. The weakness need not be limited to the amyotrophic limbs. Fasciculations may be present and there may be atrophy of muscles that were originally unaffected. Bulbar findings are rare. Upper motor neuron findings are also extremely uncommon but may occur, presumably as a consequence of the meningoencephalitis associated with the original polio infection. Before ascribing these findings to polio, however, other possible causes, such as cervical myelopathy or stroke, must be ruled out, especially if the upper motor neuron signs are prominent. Sensory changes are not a feature of postpolio syndrome but may occur secondarily, such as in cases of nerve entrapment.

The diagnosis of postpolio syndrome is based on clinical grounds; laboratory tests help confirm the diagnosis but are not in and of themselves diagnostic. The most useful tests in this regards are electromyography (EMG) and muscle biopsy. Nerve conduction studies will demonstrate reduced compound muscle action potentials in affected muscles, but are otherwise normal. The needle component of the EMG may demonstrate widespread active and chronic denervative changes, even in muscles seemingly unaffected, reflecting the more widespread subclinical involvement at the time of the original infection. The active changes consist of fibrillation potentials and positive sharp waves. Fasciculations may also be present. The chronic changes are due to denervation and subsequent reinnervation of muscle fibers. Motor unit potentials may be enlarged and prolonged, and there may be an increase in the number of polyphasic motor unit potentials. Recruitment is reduced. Single fiber EMG studies demonstrate increased fiber density and jitter, and blocking. Muscle biopsies may show a mixture of myopathic and neurogenic changes. The myopathic changes consist of variation in fiber size, central nuclei, fiber splitting, and increases in connective tissue. The neurogenic changes consist of fiber type grouping, group atrophy (suggestive of chronic denervation), and small angulated fibers (suggestive of acute denervation). The diagnostic usefulness of these tests is limited by the fact that similar EMG and biopsy findings may be seen in polio patients who do not suffer any of the late sequelae. Their main value lies in confirming the diagnosis of postpolio syndrome and helping to rule out other differential diagnostic considerations. This is particularly true in cases in which a clear antecedent history of polio is not available.

Diagnostic criteria for postpolio syndrome have been suggested. These consist of a history of acute polio and subsequent recovery, a prolonged period of functional stability (longer than 10 to 20 years), followed by the development of new neuromuscular symptoms. When these criteria are all present, the diagnosis of postpolio syndrome is straightforward. However, care must be taken to not overdiagnose postpolio syndrome. The development of musculoskeletal pain alone does not necessarily constitute postpolio syndrome PPS; such pains may develop in any patient with chronic disability from whatever cause. For this reason, there should also be evidence of new neuromuscular symptoms, such as weakness, fatigue, and so forth. In some cases, the initial symptoms, particularly if restricted to one limb, may resemble a radiculopathy or peripheral neuropathy. Imaging studies of the spine may be helpful in deciding whether a radiculopathy is present. EMG is less useful, as it is often difficult to diagnose radiculopathies by EMG in the face of the widespread denervative changes that may already be present as a consequence of the initial polio infection. Entrapment neuropathies, on the other hand, may often be diagnosed by EMG studies. Further diagnostic pitfalls arise in patients in whom there is no known history of polio. Diagnoses such as chronic inflammatory demyelinating polyneuropathy and myasthenia gravis may be entertained in some of these patients. In such cases, the EMG studies are extremely important in ruling out these diagnoses. The picture of new onset weakness, possibly associated with fasciculations and new atrophy, and without sensory involvement, may be mistakenly diagnosed as early amyotrophic lateral sclerosis. Although the diagnosis of amyotrophic lateral sclerosis requires the presence of both upper and lower motor neuron findings, many cases will initially present with just lower motor neuron findings, and may resemble postpolio syndrome. (In those rare instances of postpolio syndrome associated with upper motor neuron findings, the similarity to amyotrophic lateral sclerosis is of course even greater.) EMG and muscle biopsy will not be helpful in distinguishing between these two entities, as similar changes may be seen in both conditions. In such cases, it is the slow rate of progression and lack of development of significant bulbar and respiratory symptoms, as well as the failure to develop upper motor neuron signs, that will ultimately point to the diagnosis of postpolio syndrome. Occasionally, patients previously afflicted with polio will subsequently develop amyotrophic lateral sclerosis. In these cases, the reverse features (i.e., rapid progression, and development of bulbar and respiratory symptoms and upper motor neuron signs) lead to the correct diagnosis.

The management of postpolio syndrome is largely symptomatic. Pain can often be alleviated by the judicious use of orthotics and other assistive devices. Exercise is important in helping restore faulty postural alignment and may also help build up endurance, but fatiguing exercise may be detrimental in postpolio syndrome and should be avoided. Patients should be referred to a physical therapist for guidance in these matters. Anti-inflammatory medications may be used, as needed. Fatigue is best managed by frequent resting periods. Some patients may respond to anticholinergic therapy. There is little that can be done at this time to prevent the progression of weakness in postpolio syndrome, although clinical trials of neurotrophic agents are being planned and hold out some hope for the future. Patients should be reassured that progression is slow and rarely life-threatening. The exception of this is in patients who have previously had significant respiratory involvement. Such patients may have minimal respiratory reserve and may decompensate years after their initial illness. They may require ventilatory support, especially at night. Even for the majority of patients who do not develop respiratory symptoms, however, deficits and loss of function will occur, often necessitating adjustments in lifestyle. This loss of function can be especially disheartening and difficult to accept for polio patients who have had to overcome disabilities in the past, often by pushing themselves to the very limits of their ability. They may now become profoundly depressed. Their depression and sense of frustration may be exacerbated by the fact that their symptoms, which by their very nature may be mild and vague, especially early on, are often not taken seriously by others. Some patients may undertake unreasonably strenuous rehabilitation programs that may, if anything, aggravate their symptoms. Patient management in postpolio syndrome requires a thoughtful, supportive approach on the part of the treating physician.

SUGGESTED READINGS

Dalakas M, Illa I: Post-polio syndrome: concepts in clinical diagnosis, pathogenesis, and etiology. pp. 495–511. In Rowland LP (ed): Amyotrophic Lateral Sclerosis and Other Motor Neuron Diseases. Raven Press, New York, 1991

Jubelt B, Cashman NR: Neurologic manifestations of the post-polio syndrome. Crit Rev Neurobiol 3:199–220, 1987

Munsat TL: Post-Polio Syndrome. Butterworth-Heinemann, Boston, 1991

90. ATYPICAL MOTOR NEURON DISEASE

BARBARA E. SHAPIRO

There are several disorders that primarily affect the motor system but may be distinguished from amyotrophic lateral sclerosis (ALS) on clinical, laboratory, electrophysiologic, and/or pathologic grounds. These disorders are referred to in this chapter as atypical motor neuron diseases. ALS is a disorder characterized by selective destruction of upper motor neurons in the brain, and lower motor neurons (anterior horn cells, cranial nerve nuclei) in the brainstem and spinal cord. Patients typically present with focal weakness and more widespread lower motor neuron signs (atrophy, fasciculations). Spasticity and pathologic reflexes (upper motor neuron signs) may or may not be apparent on presentation, but will eventually develop. In contrast, the atypical motor neuron disorders comprise a group of diseases that often lack upper motor neuron signs completely. Moreover, the site of lower motor neuron pathology in a large subset of these disorders, believed to be immune-mediated, is thought to be at the level of the motor nerve itself, rather than the anterior horn cell. Furthermore, the motor nerve pathology may be demyelinating, axonal, or a combination of both. In addition, some atypical motor neuron disorders are known to affect the motor system in combination with cerebellar, extrapyramidal, cognitive, and/or mild sensory dysfunction. The motor system may also be affected in the setting of neoplasms, metabolic disorders, toxins, drugs, and as a result of electrical injuries, radiation, infections, and old polio and spinal cord lesions. Whereas these do not strictly speaking constitute atypical motor neuron diseases, they are briefly discussed below.

The atypical motor neuron disorders are important to identify for several reasons, including the possibility of uncovering a potentially treatable disorder, or one that is inherited, or one that may not carry the same grave prognosis that ALS currently carries. This chapter focuses on the important clinical clues that suggest an atypical motor neuron disorder, and then discusses some of the major disorders that should be considered in the differential diagnosis of uncommon presentations of motor neuron disease. Important laboratory, electrophysiologic, and pathologic findings are discussed.

CLINICAL CLUES

Most clinicians use pertinent clues on the neurologic examination and in the history to identify those patients with an atypical motor neuron disorder. Some clues, more valuable than others, are discussed first in the following sections and include:

Nonmyotomal pattern of weakness
Absence of muscle wasting in chronically weak limbs
Lack of concurrent upper and lower motor neuron signs in the same spinal segments
Nonregional spread of weakness
Presence of sensory symptoms and/or signs
Bladder or bowel dysfunction
Extraocular movement dysfunction
Cerebellar, extrapyramidal, cognitive, and/or psychiatric dysfunction
Onset of illness before age 35
Duration of illness longer than 5 years
Lack of bulbar involvement after 1 year
Positive family history
History of spontaneous remissions
History of malignancy, especially lymphoma

Nonmyotomal Pattern of Weakness.   Weakness in patients with ALS typically involves all muscles in a particular myotome, or spinal segment, as the site of lower motor neuron pathology is at the level of the anterior horn cell. Thus, both the biceps and deltoid tend to be weak at the same time, both being innervated by the same spinal segment, although by different motor nerves. In contradistinction, a disorder of the motor nerves themselves may produce a very different picture: the biceps may be weak, whereas the deltoid muscles are strong. Such a selective pattern of weakness, in the distribution of named nerves rather than myotomes, may serve as an extremely important clue pointing toward a disorder of motor nerves rather than anterior horn cells. This may easily be missed if muscle groups are not carefully and meticulously tested in isolation.

Absence of Muscle Wasting in Weak Limbs.   Preserved muscle bulk in the face of chronic weakness may suggest that the weakness is a consequence of demyelination, in the form of a conduction block, through segments of motor nerves. Muscle wasting may not be seen if the axon remains intact. This again places the pathology at the level of the motor nerve itself, rather than the anterior horn cell. Electrophysiologic testing is of paramount importance to confirm the presence of a conduction block. Whereas the definition of conduction block remains controversial, most would agree that a drop in the area of the compound muscle action potential by more than 50 percent between proximal and distal stimulation sites constitutes a true conduction block.

Lack of Concurrent Upper and Lower Motor Neuron Signs in the Same Spinal Segment.   Whereas lower motor signs often predominate early in the course of ALS, one usually finds preserved or brisk reflexes in the same distribution as those muscles that are weak and wasted. Failure to find concurrent upper and lower motor neuron signs in the same spinal segments should prompt a search for another disorder. In cervical spondylosis, for example, brisk reflexes are noted at segments below the weakness and hyporeflexia, resulting from nerve root as well as spinal cord compression. Thus, the arms may be weak and wasted, whereas the legs are spastic. Such a pattern should alert one to the possibility of a spinal lesion.

Nonregional Spread of Weakness.   Weakness in ALS tends to spread in a regional fashion. For example, if the right arm is initially weak, it is more common for the right leg or the left arm to become involved next, but not the left leg. Whereas this is not an absolute rule, any deviation from such a pattern of weakness should serve as a reasonable basis to investigate another cause of weakness.

Presence of Sensory Symptoms and Signs.   Whereas ALS does not involve sensory pathways, it is not uncommon for a patient to misinterpret a weak limb as numb, dead, or having altered sensation; however, a finding of true sensory loss on neurologic examination is a very important clue, and should prompt the clinician to search for another explanation of the patient's weakness.

Bladder or Bowel Dysfunction.   In practice, it is not uncommon for patients with ALS to report mild bladder incontinence or constipation. However, pronounced bladder or bowel dysfunction, especially early in the course of weakness, should prompt a search for another disorder.

Extraocular Muscle Weakness.   A finding of blurred or double vision or eye muscle weakness on examination should precipitate a search for another disorder.

Cerebellar, Extrapyramidal, Cognitive, and/or Psychiatric Dysfunction.   Progressive weakness accompanied by one or more of the following—incoordination, ataxia, tremor, dystonia, rigidity, depression, manic episodes, or dementia—should raise one's suspicion for a multiple system disorder. A detailed family history should be obtained, as many of these disorders are familial.

Unusual Time Course of Illness.   Onset of illness before age 35, duration of illness for more than 5 years, absence of bulbar involvement after 1 year, or history of spontaneous remissions are all unusual findings that should alert the clinician to the possibility of an atypical motor neuron disorder.

CLINICAL SYNDROMES

Atypical motor neuron diseases that can be differentiated from ALS and its variants are discussed in the following sections (Table 90-1).

Presumed Immune-Mediated Motor Neuropathies

These disorders affect the motor nerves themselves, and are characterized by progressive, asymmetric, predominantly lower motor neuron weakness. There is a presumed immunologic basis. Various names have been ascribed to these disorders, including multifocal motor neuropathy, multifocal motor conduction block neuropathy, and motor neuropathy with multifocal conduction blocks. In general, these patients are males with an age of onset less than 45 years, and present with chronic asymmetric weakness, often in distal upper extremity muscles, although proximal upper extremity weakness may predominate. Two key elements have been associated with these disorders, and help in differentiating them from ALS: (1) the finding of demyelination, generally in the form of conduction block, on electrophysiologic testing of motor nerves (Fig. 90-1) and (2) the presence of high serum titers of antibodies directed against nerve gangliosides. Gangliosides are glycolipids that contain lipid and carbohydrate moieties and are found in great quantity on the exterior surface of the plasma membranes of nerve fibers. The major antiglycolipid antibodies that have gained attention with respect to the motor neuropathies are those directed against GM-1 gangliosides that share the Gal(β1-3)GalNAc epitope. These may take the form of monoclonal or polyclonal IgM or IgG antibodies, but the majority are polyclonal IgM. There have

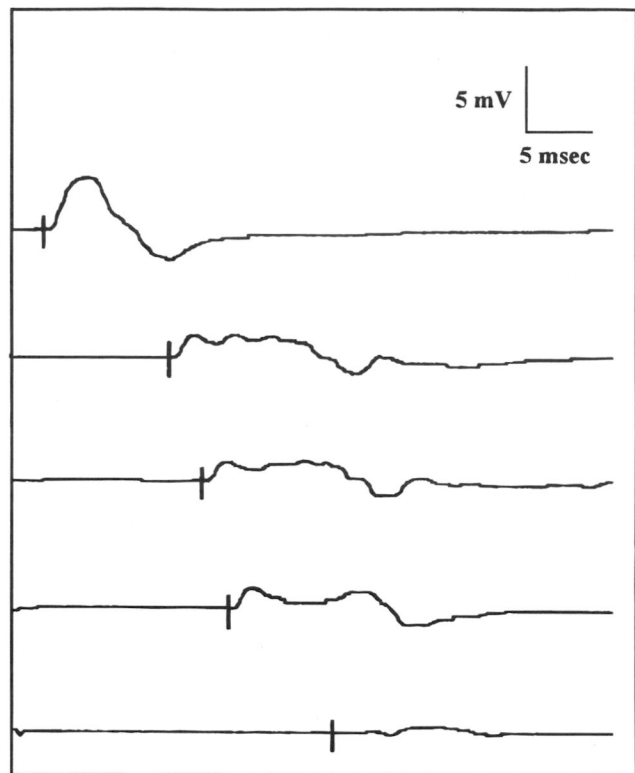

FIG. 90-1.   Conduction block and temporal dispersion in a patient with immune-mediated multifocal motor neuropathy. Motor nerve conduction of the ulnar nerve recording at the abductor digiti minimi muscle. Stimulation sites from top to bottom: wrist, below groove, above groove, axilla, and brachial plexus. Note drop in the area of the compound muscle action from wrist to brachial plexus.

been recent reports of selective antibody binding to a panel of white matter and nuclear protein antigens that may add specificity in differentiating immune-mediated lower motor neuron disorders from ALS.

Many patients with immune-mediated motor neuropathies have been successfully treated with immunomodulating therapies. Those patients most likely to respond to treatment present with chronic asymmetric distal upper extremity weakness, with minimal sensory signs and evidence of conduction block through segments of motor, but not sensory, nerves on nerve conduction studies. Elevated antiglycolipid antibodies are present in about one-half of cases. Such patients may have a remarkable response to intravenous human immunoglobulin treatment at a dose of 400 mg/kg/d for 5 consecutive days, which is generally a safe first-line mode of treatment. Patients with an absolute deficiency of IgA must receive globulins that contain no IgA. Pretreatment with 50 mg Benadryl (diphenhydramine hydrochloride) and two Tylenol an hour before the infusion begins is recommended, to prevent an allergic response. The treatment is generally repeated at the above dose for 1 to 3 days a month every month, depending on the treatment response. Quantitative motor testing is a useful way to follow the progression of the disease and treatment response. Some patients may require a full 5-day treatment course every month. Patients who do not respond, or do not receive a sustained effect, can be given a trial of cyclophosphamide, either as an oral daily dose of 2 mg/kg/d or monthly intravenous infusion of 1 to 3 g/M^2, following the white blood cell count and urinalysis weekly. The oral dose is halved if the white blood cell count falls below

TABLE 90-1.   Atypical Motor Neuron Disorders

Immune-mediated motor neuropathies

Non-immune-mediated lower motor neuron syndromes
  Benign focal amyotrophy
  Progressive muscular atrophy
  Progressive bulbar palsy
  Spinal muscular atrophy
  X-linked bulbospinal muscular atrophy
  Fazio-Londe disease

Multiple system disorders with motor signs
  Adult hexosaminidase A deficiency
  Spinocerebellar degenerations
    Machado-Joseph's disease
    Autosomal dominant cerebellar ataxias
  Other multiple system disorders
    Shy-Drager syndrome
    Guamanian Parkinson–amyotrophic lateral sclerosis
    Hallervorden-Spatz disease
    Creutzfeldt-Jakob disease
    Huntington's disease
    Pick's disease

Hyperparathyroidism

Paraneoplastic disorders with motor system dysfunction

Toxins/drugs

Electrical injury associated with motor neuron disease

Postradiation motor neuron disease

Infectious/postinfectious
  Chinese paralytic syndrome
  Retrovirus-associated disorders

Radiculopathy/myelopathy
Postpolio syndrome

4,000/mm³, and stopped if below 3,000/mm³, until it comes back to 4,000/mm³. If hematuria develops, the medication must be stopped immediately and should not be reintroduced. Treatment response may take 6 months to 1 year. The risks and benefits of cyclophosphamide must be carefully explained, including the need for weekly laboratory testing, and the increased risk of developing a malignancy after a lifetime dose of approximately 85 g. There has been less success with prednisone at 1 mg/kg/d.

There are rare reports of individuals with lower motor neuron syndromes and highly elevated anti-GM1 antibody titers, but no conduction block through motor nerves, who have shown improved strength with monthly intravenous cyclophosphamide treatment in combination with plasma exchange. These patients present with chronic asymmetric weakness in distal muscles greater than that in proximal muscles, usually in the upper extremities. Whereas there is no evidence of demyelination by nerve conduction studies, needle EMG examination reveals axonal loss in the form of active and chronic denervation and reinnervation. In some individuals who respond to treatment, there is a concomitant fall in antibody titers. Such patients are extremely important to recognize because of their potential response to treatment, yet there may be no way to distinguish them clinically or by EMG/nerve conduction studies from patients with either a progressive muscular atrophy variant of ALS or benign focal amyotrophy (discussed below).

Specific features that should alert the clinician to an immune-mediated motor neuropathy include weakness in the distribution of named nerves rather than myotomes; notable absence of muscle wasting in weak limbs; absence of upper motor signs, although there have been rare reported cases of patients with preserved or brisk reflexes in weak limbs; and minor sensory signs and symptoms. Thus, any patient presenting with a predominantly lower motor neuron syndrome should have careful, thorough electrophysiologic testing to look for features of demyelination: the presence of motor conduction block, marked conduction velocity slowing, prolonged distal motor latencies, and/or prolonged late responses. Screening should be done for the presence of elevated titers of antiglycolipid antibodies, as well as a monoclonal or polyclonal protein in serum and urine. It should be emphasized, however, that the pathogenic role of antiglycolipid antibodies in immune-mediated lower motor neuron syndromes remains unclear for several reasons. As noted above, many patients who respond to treatment have progressive weakness and motor conduction block on electrophysiologic testing but do not have elevated antiglycolipid antibody titers. Although response to treatment is often accompanied by a drop in antibody titers, this is not a consistent finding. In addition, elevated antiglycolipid antibody titers are nonspecific, and mild to moderately elevated titers can be seen in classical ALS, polyneuropathies, and other neurologic and autoimmune disorders. Furthermore, there is variation among laboratories as to what is considered an "elevated" titer. Response to treatment in patients presenting with distal weakness without motor conduction block or elevated antiglycolipid antibodies, or in patients with predominantly proximal weakness without conduction block, with or without elevated antibody titers, has not yet been established.

Non-Immune-Mediated Lower Motor Neuron Syndromes

Benign Focal Amyotrophy. A syndrome of slowly progressive weakness, benign focal amyotrophy occurs predominantly in males, most commonly affects distal hand muscles unilaterally, and generally presents in the second to fourth decades of life. It has been reported most commonly in Japanese and Asian Indian populations. Like ALS, the weakness tends to affect all muscles in the same spinal segment. However, weakness tends to stabilize after 1 or 2 years, and there is a conspicuous lack of upper motor neuron involvement. Electrophysiologic testing reveals chronic neurogenic changes on needle EMG in affected muscles, without evidence of conduction block. There is often mild involvement of the same spinal segments in the contralateral limb. Weakness will occasionally present in the lower extremities or proximal upper extremity muscles. The clues to this disorder are lack of upper motor neuron involvement, younger age of onset, predilection for distal hand muscles, and lack of progression over several years. However, it may be impossible to distinguish this disorder from classic ALS in its early presentation.

Progressive Muscular Atrophy. Patients with a progressive muscular atrophy variant of ALS present with an asymmetric pure lower motor neuron syndrome of weakness, wasting, and fasciculations that may progress for many years before death, with no upper motor neuron signs. Needle EMG examination reveals active and chronic denervation and reinnervation. Pathologic involvement of corticospinal tract involvement has been noted in some autopsied cases, confirming a diagnosis of ALS.

Fazio-Londe Disease. Fazio-Londe disease is a rare disorder that generally presents in the first decade of life with progressive bulbofacial weakness that may eventually spread to the extremities. Unlike typical motor neuron disease, ocular muscles are also affected. Inheritance in the majority of cases is autosomal recessive, although some cases appear to be sporadic. Death commonly occurs as a result of respiratory failure within 2 years of onset. At autopsy, loss of anterior horn cells and brainstem motor nuclei is found, but the corticospinal tracts are unaffected.

Multiple System Disorders With Prominent Motor Signs

Adult Hexosaminidase A Deficiency. The adult form of hexosaminidase A deficiency is a rare inherited disorder in which long-standing, progressive lower motor neuron findings, including weakness, wasting, and fasciculations, are invariably present in varying degrees. Whereas lower motor neuron signs usually predominate, upper motor neuron findings of weakness and spasticity, cerebellar findings of tremor and ataxia, and cognitive and psychiatric dysfunction (recurrent psychosis, depression) are common. Extrapyramidal findings are minimal. Onset of symptoms is most commonly in childhood, usually before the third decade, with survival often into adulthood. Because lower motor neuron findings predominate, such individuals have often been misdiagnosed with one of the spinal muscular atrophies, usually the Kugelberg-Welander type. The disorder, which is most prevalent (over 90 percent) in the Ashkenazi Jewish population, is inherited in an autosomal recessive fashion. Electrophysiologic testing usually yields normal nerve conduction studies. Needle EMG examination reveals large, prolonged polyphasic motor units with abnormal spontaneous activity in the form of fibrillation potentials, positive sharp waves, fasciculations, and, in some patients, complex repetitive discharges.

Hexosaminidase A is composed of an α and β subunit, located on chromosomes 15q and 5q, respectively, whereas hexosaminidase B is comprised of two β subunits. An activator protein, GM2 activator, located on 5q, enhances the activity of both enzymes. Hexosaminidase deficiency results in lysosomal accumulation of GM2 ganglioside, resulting in degeneration of nerve cells. Unlike the infantile form (Tay Sachs disease), where hexosaminidase A is absent and patients do not survive beyond infancy, these patients have a mutation in the α subunit of the hexosaminidase A enzyme, resulting in a severe deficiency, but not total absence, of hexosaminidase A activity. Rare cases of patients with a β subunit mutation (combined hexosaminidase A and hexosaminidase B deficiency) have been reported.

Clues that should alert the clinician to this disorder include the slow progression of a predominant lower motor neuron syndrome with onset before the third decade, a positive family history, spasticity, and signs outside the motor system including tremor, ataxia, dystonia, dementia, and/or psychosis. There is often a wide variation in phenotype and severity of disease within the same family. The pattern of weakness may be unusual, with a remarkable sparing of some muscle groups, whereas others, such as triceps, are involved early. In one retrospective study of a large population of patients with a diagnosis of ALS, 50 patients with at least one atypical feature (duration of illness >7.5 years, age of onset of illness <35 years, or positive family history of ALS) were screened for abnormal levels of hexosaminase A activity in peripheral blood leukocytes. No patient had hexosaminidase A deficiency, and less than 1 percent had white blood cell hexosaminidase A activity in the range of obligate heterozygotes.

Whereas the disorder is rare, patients with an atypical motor neuron presentation, especially those with cerebellar, extrapyramidal, cognitive, or psychiatric dysfunction that cannot be explained on another basis should be screened for hexosaminidase A and B deficiency. Although there is no known treatment, prenatal testing is available, and genetic counseling is important in families carrying the genetic defect.

Spinocerebellar Degenerations. Several multiple system disorders with ataxia as the salient feature have been described, often with accompanying lower motor neuron signs, and autosomal dominant inheritance. Many of these were at one time subsumed under the more general category of olivopontocerebellar atrophy.

MACHADO-JOSEPH'S DISEASE.   The primary features of Machado-Joseph's disease, incoordination and ataxia, are often accompanied by motor system dysfunction, including spasticity, muscle wasting, and fasciculations. When motor system signs predominate, an atypical motor neuron disorder may be suggested. However, other features of this disorder, including large-fiber sensory loss, external ophthalmoplegia, extrapyramidal signs, and spinal deformities, including pes cavus and scoliosis, should suggest this disease. Onset is generally in the third decade of life, although onset before age 10 and after age 50 have been reported. The inheritance is autosomal dominant with a wide phenotypic variability. Whereas it was originally described only in individuals of Portuguese-Azorean descent, it has now been noted in several other ethnic backgrounds and has been linked to chromosome 14q.

AUTOSOMAL DOMINANT CEREBELLAR ATAXIAS.   In autosomal dominant cerebellar ataxias, a group of heterogeneous multiple system disorders, ataxia is the predominant presenting symptom. Prominent motor system degeneration, including weakness, spasticity, wasting, and fasciculations, may develop. When motor system involvement is severe, the clinical picture may be confusing. However, other features, including large fiber sensory loss, optic atrophy, retinopathy, supranuclear ophthalmoplegia, extrapyramidal dysfunction, and cognitive impairment, should point the clinician toward a multiple system disorder. These patients generally present in their third to fourth decades, although onset may be as early as the second decade or as late as the seventh. The disorder has an autosomal dominant inheritance that has been linked to chromosomes 6p, 12q, and 14q. A fourth locus is known to exist. The 14q locus is located within the same gene locus as Machado-Joseph's disease, and may well represent a mutation of the Machado-Joseph gene.

Other Multiple System Disorders.   Several other multiple system disorders may have prominent upper and lower motor neuron signs as part of their symptom complex. These disorders, including the Shy-Drager syndrome, Guamanian Parkinson–ALS, and Hallervorden-Spatz, Creutzfeldt-Jakob, Huntington's, and Pick's disease, each have unique clinical presentations.

Hyperparathyroidism

Primary hyperparathyroidism has been historically associated with a classic neuromuscular syndrome characterized by proximal weakness and fatigue, with occasional atrophy, tongue fasciculations, and hyperreflexia that may suggest a motor systems disease. Muscle cramps are not uncommon. A variety of clinical and EMG findings have been reported in the past, including those associated with disorders of muscle, neuromuscular junction, and nerve. However, more recent prospective investigations of patients with primary hyperparathyroidism have failed to substantiate either the clinical or EMG findings previously reported. Discrepancies with earlier reports from the 1960s and 1970s that suggested a relationship between hyperparathyroidism and muscle and nerve disease may be due to more accurate and earlier testing for hyperparathyroidism currently available. In one recent case report, a patient with primary hyperparathyroidism secondary to hyperplasia presented with a 1-year history of weakness, dysarthria, dysphagia, and leg cramps. On examination, she was weak and wasted, with fasciculations, hyperreflexia, and spasticity. Some resolution of weakness and dysarthria occurred within a month of removal of the parathyroid tissue. When she died within a month from complications of bronchopneumonia, postmortem examination of the brain and spinal cord showed classic changes consistent with ALS. However, such case reports do not establish a causal relationship. Nevertheless, patients who present with true weakness and no other known cause should have calcium levels screened.

Paraneoplastic Disorders With Motor System Dysfunction

Paraneoplastic disorders are those that occur as a remote effect of cancer, but are due to neither direct tumor infiltration nor metastases. Reports of typical ALS as well as atypical motor neuron disorders have been described in association with several neoplasms, most commonly in association with malignant lymphoma. However, because the incidence of motor neuron disease is so high in the general population, its finding in the setting of cancer may be purely coincidental. Epidemiologic studies do not support an increased co-occurrence of typical ALS and cancer. Whereas a small number of individual case reports have reported improvement or stabilization of patients with clinically typical ALS after treatment of their neoplasm, these cases are extremely rare and differ pathologically from classical ALS. Associations have been found with lung and renal cancer, thymoma, lymphoma, and macroglobulinemia.

Malignant lymphoma has been associated with atypical as well as typical motor neuron disease presentations. In atypical cases, patients present with a predominant lower motor neuron syndrome of subacute progressive weakness, wasting, and fasciculations in the absence of pain. The weakness is often asymmetric, with predominant involvement of the lower extremities. Minor sensory signs and symptoms may be present. Rarely, demyelination in the form of motor conduction block is noted on nerve conduction studies. The weakness may precede the lymphoma, or vice versa. Cerebrospinal fluid (CSF) studies may reveal a slightly elevated protein and/or lymphocyte count and a monoclonal protein may be found in the serum. The spectrum of weakness ranges from stabilization and complete recovery to progressive weakness resulting in death. Outcome does not appear to be systematically related to treatment of the lymphoma. For practical purposes, all patients who present with a chronic pure lower motor neuron syndrome, and certainly those with a monoclonal protein, should be screened for a lymphoproliferative disorder. A skeletal survey and bone marrow biopsy are recommended. Patients with acquired demyelination on nerve conduction studies and elevated lymphocytes in the CSF should be evaluated for such. Some would suggest screening all patients with clinically typical ALS for lymphoma.

Toxins/Drugs

Investigations into the possible role of environmental and industrial toxins and drugs in motor neuron disorders have taken the form of epidemiologic studies and case reports. Most investigators have focused on the possible role of heavy metals, including lead, manganese, and aluminum. Chronic exposure to lead may result in a predominantly lower motor neuron syndrome of weakness, wasting, depressed reflexes, and occasional fasciculations. The upper extremities, specifically wrist and finger extensors and intrinsic hand muscles, are generally most affected. Rare cases of weakness with hyperreflexia have been reported. Constitutional symptoms, including weight loss, abdominal pain, constipation, anorexia, and fatigue, as well as minor personality and mood changes, are not uncommon. Needle EMG studies may show evidence of active and chronic denervation. Whereas some epidemiologic studies have shown an increased incidence of lead exposure in patients with typical ALS, these studies do not necessarily prove causality. However, a careful history of occupational exposure is mandated in any patient with ALS, as chronic lead exposure can result in a motor system disorder with upper and lower motor neuron signs and symptoms. In particular, atypical features with constitutional symptoms and central nervous system (CNS) changes as described above should raise one's suspicion. Although chronic exposure to lead vapor is rare, it can be seen in the setting of battery workers and car radiator repairers. The diagnosis of lead toxicity rests on finding elevated levels in the urine, blood levels being too insensitive to long-term exposure. Other laboratory values of help include a mild microcytic anemia with basophilic stippling. Diagnosis is confirmed by the use of chelating agents and measuring an increase in urine lead levels.

There have been rare reports of elevated aluminum levels in the CNS tissue of patients with Guamanian Parkinson–ALS, which is thought to be diet-related. Rarely, a predominantly lower motor neuron syndrome of distal weakness and wasting

has been noted with prolonged exposure to dapsone for various dermatologic disorders. The site of pathology is thought to be distal motor axon, with denervation noted on needle EMG. The effect is believed to be dose-related. Weakness generally reverses with withdrawal of the drug. Nitrofurantoin very rarely causes a predominantly motor neuropathy with axonal features.

Electrical Injury Associated With Motor Neuron Disease

There are rare reports of children and adults who develop a syndrome comprising upper and lower motor neuron signs following electrical injuries from either lightning, high-voltage power lines, or shorted household circuits. Weakness begins at the original site of trauma, days to months after the shock, usually in the upper extremity. Later, the contralateral upper extremity and then the bulbar musculature and lower extremities become involved. There is a tendency for symptoms to spread in a regional fashion, as in classic ALS. Eventually weakness, atrophy, and fasciculations develop, with spasticity and hyperreflexia. Sensory loss may be noted in the original area of shock, although sensory potentials are normal on electrophysiologic testing. In those rare cases that have come to autopsy, the pathology was classic for ALS. Whereas a few studies of patients with classic ALS have shown a higher than expected incidence of prior electrical and other types of injury compared to controls, causality has not been established. The relationship between electrical injuries and motor neuron syndromes is poorly understood, and at this point there is no known recommended treatment.

Postradiation Motor Neuron Disease

Very rarely, patients exposed to ionizing radiation for the treatment of a neoplasm have been known to develop a pure lower motor neuron syndrome. These patients typically present with progressive weakness, wasting, and fasciculations in the lower extremities 3 months to several years following radiation. There is a notable absence of pain, sensory symptoms, or bladder or bowel dysfunction. Reflexes are usually depressed or absent in weak limbs. The lower extremity muscles are preferentially involved, although radiation may involve the entire neuraxis, with typically 40 to 50 Gy. Needle EMG reveals fibrillation potentials and fasciculations with reduced recruitment of large, prolonged, polyphasic motor units in weak muscles. In some cases, muscle biopsy has shown chronic neurogenic changes, including fiber-type grouping and small angulated fibers. Spinal fluid protein may be elevated. The weakness generally ceases after several months, though rare patients will continue to progress over years. The site of pathology is thought to be at the anterior horn cell, although the mechanism of cell damage is poorly understood. Suggestions have included ischemic injury to vessels feeding the anterior horn cells, activation of a latent virus, and a direct toxic effect of the radiation on the anterior horn cells themselves.

Infectious/Postinfectious

A pure motor syndrome has been reported characterized by symmetric progression of weakness over days to weeks, usually in the setting of a preceding gastrointestinal illness. Reflexes in weak muscles may be lost, retained, or brisk. There are no accompanying sensory signs or complaints and CSF shows an elevated protein with normal cell count. Nerve conduction studies reveal low-amplitude compound muscle action potentials

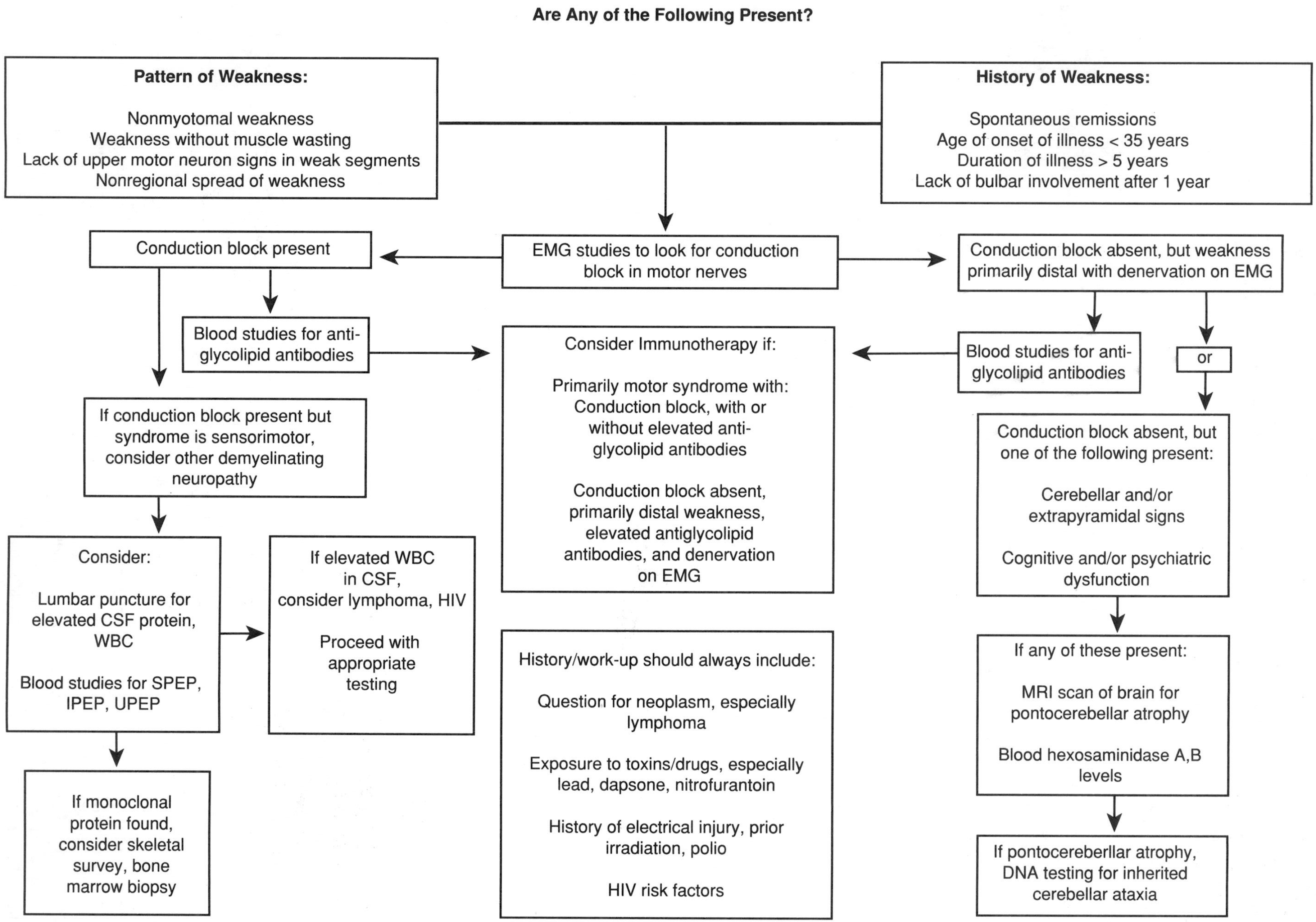

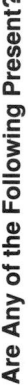

Are Any of the Following Present?

History of Weakness:

Spontaneous remissions
Age of onset of illness < 35 years
Duration of illness > 5 years
Lack of bulbar involvement after 1 year

Pattern of Weakness:

Nonmyotomal weakness
Weakness without muscle wasting
Lack of upper motor neuron signs in weak segments
Nonregional spread of weakness

EMG studies to look for conduction block in motor nerves

Conduction block absent, but weakness primarily distal with denervation on EMG

or

Blood studies for anti-glycolipid antibodies

Conduction block absent, but one of the following present:

Cerebellar and/or extrapyramidal signs

Cognitive and/or psychiatric dysfunction

If any of these present:

MRI scan of brain for pontocerebellar atrophy

Blood hexosaminidase A,B levels

If pontocereberllar atrophy, DNA testing for inherited cerebellar ataxia

Consider Immunotherapy if:

Primarily motor syndrome with: Conduction block, with or without elevated anti-glycolipid antibodies

Conduction block absent, primarily distal weakness, elevated antiglycolipid antibodies, and denervation on EMG

History/work-up should always include:

Question for neoplasm, especially lymphoma

Exposure to toxins/drugs, especially lead, dapsone, nitrofurantoin

History of electrical injury, prior irradiation, polio

HIV risk factors

Conduction block present

Blood studies for anti-glycolipid antibodies

If conduction block present but syndrome is sensorimotor, consider other demyelinating neuropathy

If elevated WBC in CSF, consider lymphoma, HIV

Proceed with appropriate testing

Consider:

Lumbar puncture for elevated CSF protein, WBC

Blood studies for SPEP, IPEP, UPEP

If monoclonal protein found, consider skeletal survey, bone marrow biopsy

FIG. 90-2. Algorithm for the diagnostic approach to patients with atypical motor neuron disease. SPEP, serum protein electrophoresis; IPEP, immunoprotein electrophoresis; UPEP, urine protein electrophoresis.

with normal distal motor latencies, F-wave latencies, conduction velocities, and sensory potentials. Needle EMG reveals fibrillation potentials with reduced recruitment of motor units. The site of pathology is thought to be distal motor axon or anterior horn cell. Several cases have been described in China (Chinese paralytic syndrome), although more recent reports have been described in the United States. Presentation of these patients differs from that of classic Guillain-Barré syndrome patients in that there is an absence of sensory complaints or signs, and reflexes may be preserved or even brisk, especially during the recovery stages of the illness. Recovery may take weeks to months.

Retrovirus-Associated Motor Neuron Disorders. Human immunodeficiency virus (HIV) infection has been associated with a variety of nerve and muscle disorders. Infrequent cases of HIV-infected young adults with a classic presentation of ALS both clinically and by electrophysiologic testing have been reported. Even rarer cases of a pure upper motor neuron syndrome have been reported. Any young adult presenting with an ALS-type syndrome and HIV risk factors should be screened, as early intervention of the HIV infection may be important. Human T cell leukemia virus type I has been associated with a progressive upper motor neuron syndrome consisting of spastic paraparesis and bladder and sensory dysfunction. The sensory findings and bladder dysfunction should alert the clinician to the presence of a disorder other than ALS.

Radiculopathy/Myelopathy

One must always consider spinal lesions in patients presenting with progressive motor dysfunction. Cervical spondylosis, for example, may result in compromise of the cervical roots and spinal cord. In this situation, lower motor signs of weakness, atrophy, and fasciculations are seen at the level(s) of the root compression, whereas upper motor neuron signs of hyperreflexia and spasticity are seen at levels below, from cord compression. This specific pattern of involvement—upper motor neuron signs at levels below lower motor neuron signs—should suggest the possibility of a spinal lesion. This condition should be suspected especially when there is a history of arthritis, neck pain, or neck spasm. A magnetic resonance imaging (MRI) scan of the cervical spine is useful in such a presentation. Other important clinical clues include sensory loss in the same root distribution as the weakness, and vibratory and joint position loss in the lower extremities, presumably from posterior column dysfunction. There may be bladder or bowel dysfunction from cord compromise, which is unusual in motor neuron disease. Needle EMG can be very helpful in documenting the extent of lower motor neuron involvement from cervical root compression, which should not be present at sites below the root compromise, unless there is a coexisting process such as ALS. However, the coexistence of lumbosacral radiculopathy may also confuse the picture, with findings of denervation in leg muscles on needle EMG. There are also rare reported cases of fasciculations in the lower extremities in cases of cervical spondylosis with myelopathy, although clearly, this should be considered an exception. Careful clinical and electrophysiologic examination are warranted to look for fasciculations and denervation/reinnervation in muscles outside the cervical and lumbosacral regions, such as bulbofacial and thoracic paraspinal muscles. These findings are extremely useful in clarifying a potentially confusing clinical situation. Some patients with

ALS and severe cervical spondylosis may derive temporary benefit from cervical decompression.

CONCLUSIONS

Over the next several years, a greater understanding of the atypical motor neuron disorders in particular the pathogenesis of the presumed immune-mediated disorders, will undoubtedly emerge. Further clarification of these disorders will guide the workup and treatment. For the present, any patient who presents with an atypical form of motor neuron disease, either by clinical history or examination, should have a careful and thorough workup to screen for the presence of a treatable or inherited disorder, or one that has a more favorable course than typical ALS (Fig. 90-2). The evaluation should include at the very least thorough electrophysiologic testing to look for evidence of conduction block through segments of motor nerves, blood testing for elevated antiglycolipid antibody titers, serum and urine immunoprotein electrophoresis, and a careful family history. Patients with motor conduction block on electrophysiologic testing, with or without elevated antibody titers, or elevated antibody titers in the proper clinical context, may well benefit from immunosuppressive therapy. The finding of a monoclonal protein in the blood or urine should lead to a skeletal survey and bone marrow biopsy. A positive family history with cerebellar, extrapyramidal, cognitive, or psychiatric dysfunction should alert one to the possibility of a multiple system disorder. In such situations, evaluation should include at the very least an MRI scan of the brain to look for pontocerebellar atrophy, DNA testing to screen for an inherited cerebellar ataxia, and blood testing for abnormal levels of hexosaminidase A and B. All patients should be questioned for any history of toxin exposure, especially lead, as well as a history of prior electrical injury, radiation, or polio, or constitutional symptoms that may suggest a neoplasm. Patients with spasticity and hyperreflexia at levels below lower motor neuron signs should have imaging of the appropriate spinal segments, preferably with an MRI scan, to look for evidence of combined root and cord compression that can be treated.

SUGGESTED READINGS

Harding AE, Deufel T: Advances in Neurology. Vol. 61. Inherited Ataxias. Raven Press, New York, 1993

Navon R, Argov Z, Frisch A: Hexosaminidase A deficiency in adults. Am J Med Genet 24:179–96, 1986

Pestronk A: Invited review: motor neuropathies, motor neuron disorders, and antiglycolipid antibodies. Muscle Nerve, 14:927–36, 1991

Pestronk A, Chaudhry V, Feldman E et al: Lower motor neuron syndromes defined by patterns of weakness, nerve conduction abnormalities, and high titers of antiglycolipid antibodies. Ann Neurol 27:316–26, 1990

Preston DC, Kelly JJ: Atypical motor neuron disease. In Brown WF, Bolton CF (eds): Clinical Electromyography. 2nd Ed. Butterworths-Heinemann, Stoneham, MA, 451–76, 1993

Rosenfield M, Posner J: Paraneoplastic motor neuron disease. pp. 445–59. In Rowland LP (ed): Advances in Neurology. Vol. 56. Amyotrophic Lateral Sclerosis and Other Motor Neuron Diseases. Raven Press, New York, 1991

Sadiq S, Latov N: Monoclonal gammopathy and motor neuron disease. Adv Neurol 413–20, 1991

Sadowsky CH, Sachs Jr E, Ochoa J: Postradiation motor neuron syndrome. Arch Neurol 33:786–87, 1976

Thomas PK: Separating Motor Neuron Diseases from Pure Motor Neuropathies. pp. 381–4. In Rowland LP (ed): Advances in Neurology. Vol. 56. Amyotrophic Lateral Sclerosis and Other Motor Neuron Diseases. Raven Press, New York, 1991

Younger DS, Rowland LP, Latov N et al: Lymphoma, motor neuron diseases, and amyotrophic lateral sclerosis. Ann Neurol 29:78–86, 1991

SECTION 3. DISEASES OF PERIPHERAL NERVE

91. APPROACH TO AND CLASSIFICATION OF PERIPHERAL NEUROPATHY

ERIC L. LOGIGIAN

Nerve injury has a relatively limited repertoire of clinical expression (Table 91-1) but hundreds of possible causes. Therefore, recognizing neuropathy is not usually difficult, whereas determining etiology frequently is. The best chance of making an etiologic diagnosis is through systematic classification of the neuropathy as shown in Table 91-2.

The questions appearing in Table 91-2 are answered with the help of several tools, the most important of which are the patient history, physical examination, and electrophysiologic studies, followed by various laboratory tests and examination of family members. The clinician can then decide if knowledge of nerve histology would likely be useful enough to justify the performance of a nerve biopsy. A simplified paradigm illustrating this approach to the evaluation of polyneuropathy is shown in Figure 91-1.

FIBER TYPES

Signs and symptoms of a peripheral neuropathy reflect the fiber types (sensory, motor, and autonomic) that are affected. Dysfunction of each fiber type results in "negative" and "positive" symptoms and signs (Table 91-1). As the patient's medical history unfolds, the nature of the symptoms tell us which fiber types are involved. Inquiry into what the patient can or cannot do is often useful. For example, motor fiber involvement of distal limb muscles may cause trouble with unscrewing jar lids from weakness of hand muscles or a tendency to trip when walking owing to footdrop. Involvement of proximal limb muscles may cause trouble in reaching above the head to comb or dry the hair, getting out of a chair, or walking upstairs. Sensory loss often results in infacility in the performance of fine motor tasks (out of proportion to distal muscle weakness) such as in buttoning, zipping, knitting. In the lower extremities, sensory loss may lead to balance trouble, making it difficult to walk in the dark or put on stockings while standing on one foot. Pain is a common sensory manifestation of peripheral neuropathy. One should determine its quality using the patient's own

TABLE 91-1. Signs and Symptoms of Peripheral Nerve Disease

Nerve(s) Involved	Negative	Positive
Motor	Weakness, wasting, clumsiness, areflexia, hypotonia, deformities (pes cavus, kyphoscoliosis)	Muscle twitches (fasciculations, myokymia), cramps
Sensory	Sensory loss, ataxia, clumsiness, areflexia, hypotonia	"Tingling," "pins and needles," "burning"
Autonomic	Postural hypotension, anhidrosis, impotence, bowel or bladder disturbance	Hyperhidrosis, gustatory sweating
Trophic		Foot ulceration, Charcot arthropathy

TABLE 91-2. Etiology of Neuropathy

Facet to Be Examined	Considerations
Anatomy	What fiber types (sensory, motor, autonomic) are involved? How is the neuropathy evolving in space?
Chronology	How is the neuropathy evolving in time?
Family history	Are there clues to an inherited neuropathy?
Associated conditions	Is there evidence of an underlying systemic disease, malnutrition, or exposure to neurotoxins (e.g,. medicines, solvents)?
Physiology	Is there predominant axon loss or demyelination?
Pathology	Are there distinctive pathologic features?
Severity	What is the functional severity?

words—where it is centered, whether it radiates, what exacerbates or improves it.

The physical examination affords the opportunity to quantitate the negative deficits in the three fiber systems; positive motor or autonomic phenomena may also be observable. With respect to motor fibers, disease of this fiber population is based on the presence of muscle atrophy and weakness. Particular attention should be paid to the tongue, spinati, deltoid and interossei muscles of the hand, the extensor digitorum brevis muscles of the feet, the calf, and tibialis anterior and quadricep muscles. Quantitating muscle strength is usually performed with the confrontation method, but in powerful leg muscles such as the hip abductors and ankle plantar flexors, more subtle weakness may be elicited by standing on one foot (to elicit pelvic tilt) and by attempting to walk on tiptoes, respectively. With confrontation muscle testing, the 0- to 5-point MRC scale is most useful for severe muscle weakness, but not for more subtle weakness in the 4− to 5− range. This is because the

FIG. 91-1. A scheme for the diagnostic evaluation of polyneuropathy. CIP, critical illness polyneuropathy; CIDP, chronic inflammatory demyelinating polyradiculoneuropathy; GBS, Guillain-Barré syndrome; HIV, human immunodeficiency virus; HMSN, hereditary motor and sensory neuropathy; HPPP, hereditary predisposition to pressure palsy; MFMN, multifocal motor neuropathy; MGUS, monoclonal gammopathy of undetermined significance. (Modified from Logigian EL: Peripheral neuropathy. pp. 325–31. In Feldman E (ed): Current Diagnosis in Neurology. CV Mosby, Boston, 1994, with permission.)

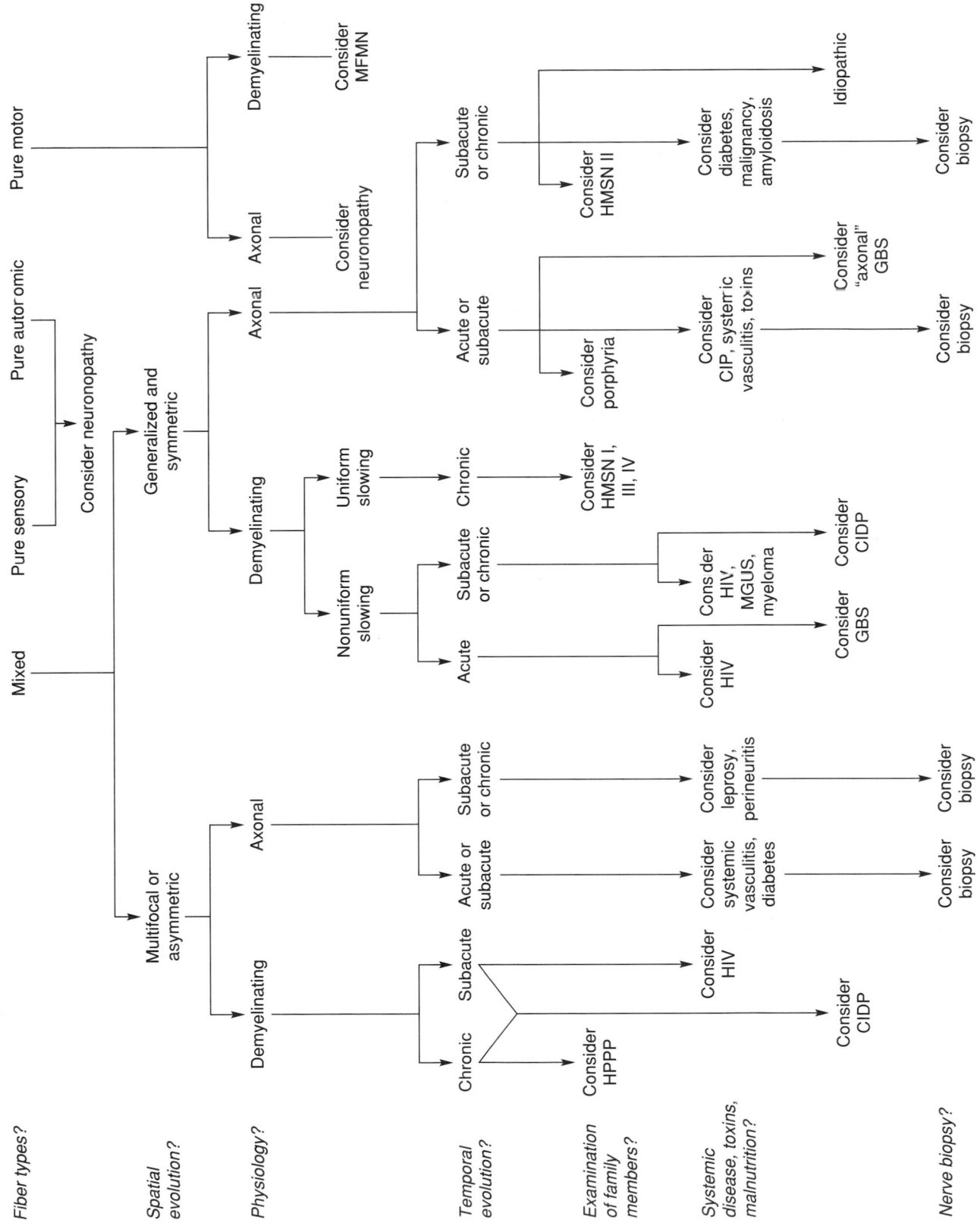

MRC scale is nonlinear and the range from 4 to 5 represents the upper 50 percent of the range of muscle force. For that reason, in patients with milder weakness, muscle strength is better estimated as a percentage of normal. In any case, limb muscles are tested along a proximal to distal axis from the shoulder/hip girdle muscles to those acting across the elbow/knee, to those acting at the wrist/ankle, and finally to the intrinsic hand and foot muscles. Most polyneuropathies selectively involve the longest nerve fibers and preferentially affect distal muscles, more in the legs than the arms. In the mildest cases, only the intrinsic foot muscles may be affected. In the severest, all muscles may be affected, including axial muscles innervated by short nerves such as the neck flexors and rectus abdominis.

With respect to sensory fibers, the two most useful bedside tests are sharp-dull discrimination (for small-fiber sensory function) and vibratory sense (for the large-fiber sensory system). The clinician establishes areas of reduced sensation in symptomatic areas (usually the toes and fingers) relative to more proximal asymptomatic areas. The more proximally the sensory disturbance extends, the more severe the neuropathy. In addition, since station, gait, and limb coordination are dependent on large-fiber sensory feedback, Romberg sign and ataxia of gait and limb can be manifestations of sensory neuropathy and should be specifically elicited.

The reflex examination, particularly the tendon jerks, is an easily performed and objective aspect of the physical examination. The presence of tendon areflexia in symptomatic limbs strongly supports the diagnosis of neuropathy affecting either the sensory afferents or motor efferents subserving the reflex arc. The presence of a plantar extensor response in a patient with symptoms consistent with polyneuropathy suggests that the correct diagnosis may be a central nervous system lesion, usually of the spinal cord. However, it should be remembered that there are certain diseases in which both the central and peripheral nervous systems are affected. The most important of these is vitamin B_{12} deficiency.

The autonomic nervous system is difficult to assess even in the laboratory. At the bedside, one is generally limited to checking for orthostasis, for anhydrotic skin in the extremities, and for abnormal pupillary responses.

Most polyneuropathies involve all three fiber types, particularly the sensory and motor populations. At onset, however, the only abnormalities may be positive sensory phenomena. Given time, significant motor and autonomic fiber involvement may occur. With more severe, longer-standing neuropathy, if only one fiber type appears to be involved, the clinician should consider one of the neuronopathies as a diagnosis. Sensory neuronopathy may be a paraneoplastic manifestation of small cell carcinoma with elevated anti-Hu antibody, an autoimmune manifestation of Sjögren's disease, or a toxic manifestation of pyridoxine abuse. For motor fibers, the diagnosis of motor neuron disease of some type should be considered. An alternative diagnosis in a patient with only lower motor neuron findings is multifocal motor neuropathy with conduction block, a disorder that should not be missed since, in contrast to the motor neuronopathies, it can be effectively treated.

SPATIAL EVOLUTION

The spatial distribution of the neuropathy is crucial in determining if the disease is localized to one body part (e.g., limb, trunk, cranial-innervated structure) as in a radiculopathy, mononeuropathy, or plexopathy, or if it is a more generalized process. If the disease is generalized, the next question is whether its pattern of evolution is asymmetric/multifocal or symmetric/diffuse. By asking which body part was affected first, second, and so on, it can be learned if the neuropathy evolved symmetrically or asymmetrically. For example, most acquired neuropathies present with a symmetric sensory disturbance in the feet, which then "ascends" to the knees, followed by the fingertips, forearms, anterior chest wall, and top of head. Neuropathy that begins only in one leg, for example, or in both hands, sparing the feet, is more unusual and suggests an asymmetric or multifocal process. The patient history is most important in making this distinction, since cumulative multifocal deficits may eventually become confluent and appear on physical examination later in the course to be symmetrically, diffusely distributed when in fact they accrued asymmetrically. Still, the physical examination may show that some nerves are affected out of proportion to others by the presence inter- and intralimb asymmetries in nerve function.

Asymmetric or multifocal polyneuropathy suggests the syndrome of mononeuropathy multiplex. This syndrome has a differential diagnosis that includes many treatable forms of neuropathy (e.g., vasculitic neuropathy, leprosy, chronic inflammatory demyelinating polyradiculoneuropathy [CIDP], multifocal conduction block). Its recognition is therefore of key importance in the evaluation of patients with polyneuropathy.

Finally, in generalized symmetric polyneuropathy, there are some exceptions to the usual pattern of selective distal involvement. For example, in Guillain-Barré syndrome, CIDP, or porphyric neuropathy, the girdle muscles may be as weak or weaker than the distal limb muscles.

TEMPORAL EVOLUTION

The temporal evolution of signs and symptoms is gathered in parallel with the spatial data. Only the history can provide precise temporal information about the disease, although the physical and electrophysiologic examinations may provide some clues to disease chronicity. The two key points to ascertain are (1) the time from onset to nadir or from onset to the current state if the nadir has not been reached and (2) the "slope" of the descent—smooth, stepwise, or relapsing-remitting.

Acute sensorimotor neuropathy with a time to nadir of less than 6 weeks is caused by only a few conditions, the most common being Guillain-Barré syndrome; others to consider are porphyric neuropathy, rapidly progressive vasculitic neuropathies, various acute toxic neuropathies (e.g., ingestion of large amounts of thallium or arsenic) and critical illness polyneuropathy. Severe, subacute progressive, or stepwise sensorimotor polyneuropathy with a time to nadir of 2 to 12 months has a broader differential diagnosis. The main treatable neuropathies to exclude are CIDP and vasculitic polyneuropathy. The former sometimes has a relapsing-remitting course.

FAMILY HISTORY

Patients with inherited polyneuropathy may remain asymptomatic for decades before seeking medical attention. Such patients typically have signs of neuropathy on examination but are unaware of their neuropathy (or those of family members) because of its slow progression. When such a patient does finally seek medical attention, clinicians may assume that the neuropathy is acquired unless they pay attention to three clues. The first is that long-standing neuropathy may produce characteristic deformities of the foot (pes cavus) and of the spine (kyphoscoliosis). The second is that in comparison to most acquired neuropathies, typical hereditary sensorimotor neuropathy has little in the way of positive sensory phenomena. The third is that examination of family members, even when asymptomatic, may reveal polyneuropathy. Recently, genetic tests have become available for the diagnosis of the most common demyelinative hereditary neuropathies (hereditary motor and sensory neuropathy, type IA; hereditary predisposition to pressure palsy). The nonresearch indications for these tests are still not clear, but they are occasionally useful in the evaluation of patients with an atypical presentation for these disorders or for genetic counseling.

SYSTEMIC DISEASE, MALNUTRITION, TOXINS

In the review of systems, the clinician must exclude diabetes, connective tissue disease, underlying malignancy, infection, malnutrition, megavitaminosis, and exposure to drugs, alcohol, or toxins at the workplace. On physical examination, signs of malnutrition (cheilosis, tongue depapillation) should be sought in addition to skin rash, adenopathy, thyromegaly, joint swelling, breast masses, and stool guaiac.

Various blood studies are sometimes helpful in documenting the presence of a systemic disease associated with neuropathy. In general, when the history and physical examination do not provide a clue to the presence of these diseases, the screening tests designed to detect their presence are usually negative. Certainly a fasting blood sugar should be obtained in any patient whose neuropathy is undiagnosed. However, given the vagaries of glucose tolerance testing, this test can be difficult to interpret. Electrolytes, in particular, creatinine and blood urea nitrogen should be obtained. A vitamin B_{12} level and complete blood count should be obtained, particularly in patients with a predominantly sensory neuropathy with or without corticospinal findings. Thyroid function tests are usually obtained, though they are rarely helpful. Similarly, detailed ''connective tissue screens'' in the absence of any symptoms or signs of connective tissue disease are rarely positive, and detailed testing to detect underlying neoplasia is usually fruitless. The exception is a patient with sensory neuronopathy and anti-Hu antibody in whom small cell carcinoma of the lung is likely. Otherwise, simple chest x-ray, breast examination, and stool guaiac testing is usually enough.

As many as 10 percent of patients with polyneuropathy have a monoclonal spike on serum electrophoresis. In many cases, the monoclonal protein appears to cause the neuropathy. It is therefore useful to obtain serum and urine protein and immunoelectrophoresis in a patient with otherwise idiopathic polyneuropathy. If a monoclonal paraprotein is found, then bone marrow biopsy and bone survey should be considered. The majority of such patients have no underlying hematologic disease and have what is now termed monoclonal gammopathy of undetermined significance (MGUS) neuropathy. Approximately 50 percent of these patients have an IgG or IgA monoclonal protein; the remainder have IgM. In about one-half of the IgM patients, the IgM cross-reacts to myelin-associated glycoprotein (MAG); the other epitopes are not yet known. Patients with IgM monoclonal protein are more likely to have demyelinative physiology than are those with IgG or IgA, although there is a large overlap. There are occasional patients with an anti-MAG polyneuropathy who lack a monoclonal protein. Therefore, in a patient with predominantly sensory demyelinative polyneu-

ropathy (characteristic of anti-MAG), it is reasonable to order this test even in the absence of an IgM or IgG spike.

Although leprosy is the most common cause of neuropathy worldwide, in Western culture, infectious causes of neuropathy are rare. The two to consider are human immunodeficiency virus (HIV) and *Borrelia burgdorferi* infections. Early on in infection with HIV, Guillain-Barré syndrome and CIDP can occur. Later, a painful sensory neuropathy may develop. In a patient with these kinds of neuropathies who is at risk for HIV, it is reasonable to obtain HIV titers. Lyme disease produces an acute painful radiculoneuropathy often in association with facial palsy and meningitis in addition to a more chronic milder sensory neuropathy. In patients with these syndromes who live in areas endemic for the organism, it is reasonable to obtain a serum Lyme titer. Otherwise, Lyme disease testing is more likely to yield false positives than true positives.

An underused test is examination of spinal fluid. In a patient with a chronic or subacute progressive polyneuropathy in whom other studies are not particularly helpful, the spinal fluid is useful in excluding cytoalbuminologic dissociation. This is seen most commonly in patients with diabetes or inflammatory demyelinating neuropathy. If cerebrospinal fluid protein is very high and the patient does not have diabetes, the diagnosis of CIDP should be considered even if electrodiagnostic and nerve biopsy studies are indeterminant.

PHYSIOLOGY

The electrophysiologic examination is very useful in several respects. It helps to confirm the presence of polyneuropathy and differentiate it from other related disorders. It provides objective data concerning the severity, side-to-side symmetry, and chronicity of the neuropathy. Most importantly, physiologic studies are critical in localizing entrapment mononeuropathies, or in determining whether or not polyneuropathy is primarily demyelinative or axonal. Further, it can often differentiate acquired from hereditary demyelinating neuropathy by the presence of nonuniform slowing of nerve conduction. Since acquired demyelinating neuropathy is caused by a short list of treatable diseases (CIDP, some forms of MGUS neuropathy, multifocal conduction block, and osteosclerotic myeloma), and hereditary neuropathy by a short list of genetic diseases (hereditary motor and sensory neuropathies I, III, IV; hereditary predisposition to pressure palsy), electrophysiologic studies to exclude predominant demyelination are central to the evaluation of polyneuropathy. Still, it should be remembered that there are some problems with these tests. Unless special studies are performed, results may be negative in (1) the rare pure autonomic or ''small fiber'' sensory neuropathy (since routine electrophysiologic studies detect medium and large-fiber abnormalities of the motor and sensory populations) and (2) mild sensory neuropathy with only paresthesia and no (or minimal) negative signs, since routine sensory studies document only negative phenomena.

NERVE BIOPSY

Nerve biopsy is virtually never performed to simply confirm nerve disease. The history, physical examination, and electrodiagnostic studies can almost always do that. Rather, nerve biopsy is reserved for diagnosis of a few relatively rare diseases with a characteristic histologic signature, such as vasculitic neuropathy, followed by leprosy, sarcoidosis, amyloidosis, and the leukodystrophies. It may also be employed in progressive polyneuropathies in which the diagnosis remains uncertain despite complete workup. In such cases, the clinician would be looking for histologic evidence of inflammatory neuropathy or possibly demyelination in a patient who does not meet demyelinative criteria electrophysiologically.

SEVERITY

Negative and positive symptoms of peripheral nerve disease result in functional problems that may range in severity from annoying paresthesia, mild gait ataxia, or minimal loss of hand dexterity without functional impairment to quadriplegia, deafferentation, or autonomic failure that leaves the patient bedbound and helpless. In determining disease severity, one should address both the "primary" symptoms and signs (Table 91-1) as well as the patient's unique functional problems produced by the neuropathy on activities of daily living or on occupational tasks. Thus, the same polyneuropathy that is of minor severity for a sedentary executive could be debilitating for an athlete or a musician. Naturally, the pace of the workup and the aggressiveness of treatment depends on the functional severity of the neuropathy.

PROBLEMS IN DIAGNOSIS OF NEUROPATHY

Pseudoneuropathy

Taken one by one, almost all physical findings that we commonly consider to be indicative of neuropathy in fact are not. For example, distal muscle wasting and weakness is seen in the rare cases of distal myopathy or spinal muscular atrophy. Stocking sensory loss can be seen in patients with dorsal column lesions, as in spinal multiple sclerosis. Ankle areflexia can be seen in patients with spinal cord disease. The bedside diagnosis of polyneuropathy is most secure when a number of these signs occur together in the absence of signs suggesting disease elsewhere. Even then, it can be difficult to differentiate root from nerve disease clinically, as in a patient with spinal stenosis of the lumbosacral spine (e.g., polyradiculopathy) versus a patient with progressive sensorimotor polyneuropathy. Both may have distal sensory loss, muscle weakness, and ankle areflexia. Clinically, the two may be differentiated by the presence of pseudoclaudication or radicular back pain in spinal stenosis and distal "burning" pain in neuropathy. The electrophysiologic clue is the presence of normal sensory potentials in spinal stenosis and low-amplitude potentials in polyneuropathy.

Occasionally, cervical transverse myelitis and spinal shock together (e.g., flaccid areflexic paralysis) are confused with an acute polyneuropathy such as Guillain-Barré syndrome. Clinically, the spinal cord patient is distinguished by the presence of a sensory and motor level, a brisk cerebrospinal fluid pleocytosis and the absence of demyelinative physiology.

Pseudoradiculopathy

Cervical radiculopathy due to disc disease is common; brachial "plexopathy" (better referred to as brachial neuritis) is not. It is no surprise, therefore, that the latter is not infrequently misdiagnosed as the former. This mistake has important implications, since the diagnosis of radiculopathy typically prompts a magnetic resonance imaging study of the spine. It is rare for such studies to be totally normal, and inappropriate disc surgery is the unfortunate outcome. Clinically, the disorders are separa-

ble by the nature and location of the accompanying pain (usually centered in the neck with radiation to the arm and exacerbated by head movement in radiculopathy and centered in the shoulder without radiation or worsening with head movement in brachial neuritis) and the presence of characteristic neurologic deficits in the distribution of one or more cervical roots in radiculopathy and in one or more characteristic nerves (long thoracic, suprascapular, axillary, anterior interosseous) in brachial neuritis. In the lower extremity, a similar scenario may occur in patients with diabetic amyotrophy, herpes zoster, or lumbosacral neuritis who may be misdiagnosed as lumbosacral radiculopathy due to disc disease. Again, one of the major distinguishing features is the presence of radiating back pain and mechanical exacerbation of pain in lumbosacral radiculopathy versus the other conditions in which the pain is typically more severe, and not centered in the back or worsened by back range of motion.

Pseudostroke

Acute mononeuropathies of the radial, proximal median, and peroneal nerves may initially be confused with plexus or root lesions and even stroke! Armed with an analytic approach and knowledge of anatomy, the clinician recognizes that all the deficits are in the territory of one nerve.

"Negative" Family History

Hereditary neuropathy is very slowly progressive and does not have much in the way of positive sensory phenomena. Therefore, it may not be noticed by the patient (or by affected family members) until late in life. Particularly with a "negative" family history and the absence of pes cavus deformity, examination of family members may be helpful in clinching the diagnosis of hereditary neuropathy in a patient with long-standing "idiopathic" neuropathy.

"Indeterminate" Physiology

There are occasional patients with possible CIDP whose nerve conduction studies do not meet criteria for demyelinative physiology. Since this neuropathy is often progressive, severe, and treatable, a nerve biopsy to carefully search for demyelinative histology with teased fiber analysis and a spinal tap to exclude a high cerebrospinal fluid protein should be considered.

Underlying Diabetes

The most common cause of neuropathy in Western culture is diabetes. The spectrum of diabetic neuropathy is broad. It can present as a mononeuropathy multiplex or as a symmetric polyneuropathy involving single or multiple fiber types. Therefore, when a patient has neuropathy and diabetes, it is often assumed that the two are related. Most of the time, this is the case. However, there are occasional patients with very mild diabetes but very severe progressive neuropathy who may have some variant of CIDP. It is important to keep this in mind, since these patients are often responsive to immunosuppressive drugs.

Atypical Amyotrophic Lateral Sclerosis

In a similar vein, there are occasional patients with a distal sensory disturbance in the feet who have in addition severe, progressive muscle wasting and weakness. Initially, such patients may be assumed to have a severe, predominantly motor polyneuropathy. Over time the correct diagnosis of atymotrophic lateral sclerosis with a coincidental minor sensory neuropathy becomes obvious.

SUGGESTED READINGS

Asbury AK, Gilliat RW: Peripheral Nerve Disorders. Butterworths, London, 1984

Barohn RJ, Kissel JT, Warmolts JR, Mendell JR: Chronic demyelinating polyradiculoneuropathy: clinical characteristics, course, and recommendations for diagnostic criteria. Arch Neurol 46:878–84, 1989

Brown WF, Bolton CF: Clinical Electromyography. Butterworths, Boston, 1987

Dyck PJ, Lais AC, Ohta M et al: Chronic inflammatory polyradiculoneuropathy. Mayo Clin Proc 50:621–37, 1975

Dyck PJ, Oviatt KF, Lambert EH: Intensive evaluation of referred unclassified neuropathies yields improved diagnosis. Ann Neurol 10:222–6, 1981

Dyck PJ, Thomas PK, Griffin JW et al: Peripheral Neuropathy. 3rd Ed. WB Saunders, Philadelphia, 1993

Kelly JJ, Kyle RA, O'Brien PC: Prevalence of monoclonal protein in peripheral neuropathy. Neurology 31:1480–3, 1981

Lewis RA, Sumner AJ: The electrodiagnostic distinctions between chronic familial and acquired demyelinative neuropathies. Neurology 32:592–6, 1982

Logigian EL: Peripheral neuropathy. pp. 325–31. In Feldmann E (ed): Current Diagnosis in Neurology. CV Mosby, Boston, 1994

Logigian EL, Kelly JJ, Adelman LS: Nerve conduction and biopsy correlation in over 100 consecutive patients with suspected polyneuropathy. Muscle Nerve 17:1010–20,

Ropper AH, Wijdicks EFM, Truax BT: Guillain-Barré Syndrome. FA Davis, Philadelphia, 1991

Schaumberg HR, Berger AR, Thomas PK: Disorders of Peripheral Nerves. FA Davis, Philadelphia, 1991

92. RADICULOPATHIES AND PLEXOPATHIES

MICHAEL T. HAYES

One of the common problems encountered in the emergency room or in an outpatient setting is that of weakness and/or numbness or pain in an extremity. The differentiation of sensory or motor dysfunction in a limb is daunting. As with most neurologic problems, careful clinical evaluation can result in an accurate anatomic localization of the lesion, which will usually narrow the differential diagnosis significantly. Lesions involving the central nervous system and the individual named nerves are discussed elsewhere in this text; radiculopathies and plexopathies are discussed here.

RADICULOPATHIES

Radiculopathies are the result of any process that affects the nerve at the level of the root. Disc disease, spondylosis, avulsion, metastasis, or any process that infiltrates the root may result in radicular symptoms.

The clinical diagnosis of a lesion involving a specific root is based on a determination of the motor, sensory, and reflex abnormalities. Sensory findings are of great importance in the diagnosis of a named nerve or plexus lesion, but are of less importance in a root lesion, as there are so much overlap and

TABLE 92-1. Signs and Symptoms of Radiculopathy

Root Lesion	Signs and Symptoms
C5	Interscapular pain, proximal arm weakness (biceps, deltoid, infra- and suprascapular muscles), loss of biceps reflex
C6	Pain radiating down the arm into thumb, proximal arm weakness, loss of biceps reflex
C7	Pain radiating into third finger, triceps weakness (often triceps is innervated almost solely by C7), loss of triceps reflex
C8	Pain radiating into fourth and fifth fingers, weakness of small muscles of the hand (median and ulnar innervated), if sensory loss will extend from the fourth and fifth fingers up the ulnar aspect of the forearm (above the wrist as opposed to ulnar nerve lesions, in which sensory abnormalities do not extend above the wrist)
T1	Pain radiating down the inner aspect of the arm, weakness of hand muscles, Horner syndrome
L4	Weakness of knee extension and hip adduction, pain radiating from knee to medial malleolus, loss of knee reflex. If the root is entrapped, radicular pain may sometimes be elicited by "reverse straight leg raising"
L5	Pain radiating down posterior aspect of leg into great toe, often significant weakness of ankle dorsiflexion (tibialis anterior is often predominantly innervated by L5), normal reflexes
S1	Pain radiating down posterior aspect of leg and into lateral aspect of foot, weakness of foot eversion, loss of ankle reflex

variability of dermatomes. Motor and reflex changes are better localizing signs in radiculopathy (Table 92-1).

Cervical

Injury to the roots in the cervical region may occur for a number of reasons. Radiculopathy from disk herniation in the cervical region is less common than in the lumbosacral region. The C6 and C7 roots are the most frequently affected. In cervical spondylosis (in which bony overgrowth of a vertebra occurs after degeneration of a disk, forming a bar posteriorly), the C5 and C6 roots are most commonly involved. It is important to keep in mind that cervical spondylosis may also cause a myelopathy as the bar compresses the spinal cord. Whereas the radicular symptoms may be the patient's major complaint, it is important to look for long tract signs such as spasticity and hyperreflexia below the level of the radiculopathy.

Root avulsion is an important and debilitating cause of radiculopathy. It is the tearing of a root secondary to neck and shoulder injuries. The deficit that results is permanent. Two classic syndromes of avulsion are Erb's palsy (Duchenne-Erb syndrome) and Klumpke's palsy.

Erb's palsy occurs with downward traction of the shoulder forcing an extreme angle between the head and shoulder and causing tearing of the C5 and C6 roots. This has been most frequently described with forceps deliveries where the head is forcibly pulled away from the undelivered shoulder. The clinical picture is a patient with minimal sensory changes but who is unable to abduct the shoulder or supinate the forearm and thus, though the hand remains strong, the use of the limb is severely limited.

Klumpke's palsy results from tearing of the C8 and T1 roots. The injury occurs with forceful upward traction on the arm. This type of injury may occur, for instance, with a fall in which the patient grabs for a ladder rung or some other support and wrenches the arm that is extended overhead. The patient suffers sensory loss in the fourth and fifth fingers and the ulnar aspect of the hand and forearm. All the intrinsic muscles of the hand are severely affected. The injury to the T1 root may be accompanied by a Horner syndrome (miosis, ptosis, and occasionally impaired facial sweating on the ipsilateral side to the injury) as sympathetic fibers that travel with the T1 root are also injured.

Diagnosis of root avulsion is made after careful elicitation of the patient history and a thorough examination along with myelography, electromyography (EMG), and sensory evoked potentials. Myelography can be helpful in demonstrating avulsed roots, but it is not infallible. After an injury, a psuedomeningomyelocele can form. This gives the radiologic impression of an avulsed root, but the root is actually intact. EMG, because it is a measure of actual nerve function, is crucial in the diagnosis of complex cases in which plexopathy and radiculopathy are possible diagnoses.

Infiltration of the meninges or invasion of the vertebrae by metastatic cancer may cause single or multiple radiculopathies.

Lumbosacral

Disc herniation is a more common problem in the lumbosacral region. The L4–L5 and L5–S1 discs are the most frequently involved (causing symptoms referable to the L5 and S1 roots, respectively). The L3–L4 disc or L4 root is far less commonly involved. Table 92-1 lists common signs and symptoms associated with each of the above. In addition to the sensory, motor, and reflex changes noted above, patients should be questioned about what precipitates pain. Coughing, straining, and standing often worsen radicular pain caused by root entrapment. In L5 and S1 root entrapments, radicular symptoms (not merely low back pain) are worsened by straight leg raising. This is tested by having the patient lie supine and the examiner raising the patient's leg by the heel until symptoms are produced. In L4 entrapments, radicular symptoms may be produced with reverse straight leg raising. The patient is prone and the examiner extends the hip to attempt to elicit symptoms.

Exact anatomic localization of lumbosacral roots lesions are more difficult than cervical root lesions because the lumbosacral roots have such a long subarachnoid course as they form the cauda equina. Also, lesions of the cauda equina can be confused with lesions of the conus of the spinal cord.

Cauda equina lesions usually involve more than one root. They may be caused by large, centrally herniated disks, severe spinal stenosis, or metastatic disease (commonly prostate cancer, leukemia, lymphoma, lung cancer, and some pinealomas). These lesions are usually exquisitely painful and involve sensation and reflexes above the sacral dermatomes early in the course. Sensory, motor, and reflex abnormalities are almost always asymmetric. This asymmetry is very important to demonstrate clinically, in making an early and accurate diagnosis.

Lesions of the conus, which are most commonly caused by ependymomas, dermoid cysts, lipomas, arteriovenous malformations, lymphomas, and less commonly by other metastatic disease, begin with a constant, dull backache. The earliest sensory abnormalities are in the lowest sacral dermatomes and involve the genital and perianal areas because the lesion starts at the base of the conus and ascends. The patellar reflexes are spared until very late and the neurologic abnormalities are very symmetric as opposed to cauda equina lesions.

Workup of suspected cauda equina or conus injuries include radiologic assessment and neurophysiologic studies. Magnetic resonance imaging (MRI) is the most effective test to visualize the lumbosacral region. If MRI is not possible (if the patient has a pacemaker, is claustrophobic, etc.), then myelography followed by computed tomography is also effective. Plain radiographs are not sufficient to assess these lesions, even if they demonstrate an abnormality (such as a lytic lesion), because they do not demonstrate anatomy of the process compressing or infiltrating the roots or conus. Nerve conduction tests and EMG are extremely useful in demonstrating the extent and severity of the lesion in a way not possible with techniques that demonstrate anatomy but not neural function.

Infectious entities like cytomegalovirus (predominantly in patients infected with human immunodeficiency virus) may cause an exquisitely painful and debilitating polyradiculopathy.

PLEXUS LESIONS

Lesions of the brachial and lumbosacral plexus may occur as a result of traumatic, inflammatory, neoplastic, or ischemic lesions. Sensory deficits may be much more pronounced and weakness in single or multiple named nerve distributions is noted. The main entities in the differential diagnosis are usually root lesions or injuries to individual or multiple named nerves.

Brachial

The brachial plexus is formed by the anterior rami of the C5–T1 roots, although the C4 and T2 rami may be involved in some individuals. The C5 and C6 roots form the upper trunk, the C7 root becomes the middle trunk, and the C7 and C8 roots become the lower trunk. All three trunks split into anterior and posterior divisions. The posterior divisions of all three form the posterior cord, which gives rise to the axillary and radial nerves. The anterior division of the lower trunk becomes the medial cord and gives off the ulnar nerve and the C8 innervated median nerve muscles. The anterior divisions of the upper and middle trunks become the lateral cord, from which originate the musculocutaneous nerve and the remainder of the median nerve. The trunks pass through the supraclavicular fossa under the cervical and scalene muscles. The cords form just above the clavicle and first rib and pass, with the subclavian artery, through the thoracic outlet. A good rule of thumb is that injuries occurring above the clavicle injure the trunks, below the clavicle injure the cords, and injuries occurring in the axilla injure the named nerves.

Traumatic injuries to the brachial plexus occur with bullet or stab wounds or with blunt injury to the shoulder as with firearm recoil or the football injury called "the stinger," in which one player drives his helmet into the shoulder of another player. The latter two injuries produce clinical pictures not unlike an Erb's palsy. Prolonged anesthesia with a patient's arm held in a suboptimal position may result in plexus lesions. Pressure under the arm as when patients use crutches may also result in injury. Brachial plexus injuries may be seen as a complication of sternotomy, angiography done by the brachial artery approach, and rarely, as a complication of an internal jugular catheterization. It is very important to differentiate plexus from root injury in traumatic injuries (which often involve both the neck and shoulder), as the former may be more amenable to surgical repair.

Brachial neuritis, also called Parsonage-Turner syndrome or neuralgic amyotrophy, is believed to be an inflammatory lesion of the brachial plexus. It tends to occur in the third decade of life and affects males more than females by a 2:1 ratio. Whereas it may be idiopathic, it has been described as a sequela of a viral infection or vaccination. It may also be seen postoperatively. Initially, there is a deep boring pain in the shoulder, rapidly followed by weakness, generally in the proximal arm. Frequently, the process is bilateral. This is an important point, as few processes affect the brachial plexus bilaterally. Sometimes the abnormalities in the unaffected arm are subclinical and are appreciated only on electrophysiologic studies. The branches of the plexus that are frequently affected are the axillary, radial, long thoracic, phrenic, suprascapular, and accessory nerves, although any part of the plexus may be affected. Occasionally, the lesion is very focal, as may be seen with isolated injury to the long thoracic without any history of trauma. Rarely, the paraspinal muscles may be affected. This is not so much because this is not a true plexus lesion, but rather because the lesion is inflammatory and may affect, on infrequent occasions, the posterior rami of the motor roots. A course of steroids has been advocated by some in the treatment of brachial neuritis; it is not unreasonable, as long as the patient has no contraindications to steroids, but there is no good evidence that they are effective. Treatment is mainly supportive, putting the limb in a sling initially and then recommending a course of physical therapy as the patient improves. Usually the patient recovers over the course of 6 months to a year, occasionally with some residual effects.

The brachial plexus may be affected by neoplasms. Pancoast syndrome or tumor occurs with local extension of a tumor growing in the apex of the lung to involve the first and second rib and the lower trunk (C8 and T1 and occasionally T2). The lesion is manifested by pain under the upper portion of the scapula and pain and numbness of the inner aspect of the arm and hand. There is weakness of C8 and T1 innervated muscles. Other lesions that frequently metastasize to the brachial plexus include lymphomas, melanomas, and breast cancers.

Patients are often treated with radiation for neoplasms of the chest, neck, or plexus, and there may be secondary radiation damage to the brachial plexus. Radiation damage to the plexus may occur days to years after the course of radiation. There are several clinical points that help distinguish radiation injuries from recurrent cancer. Painless lesions of the upper plexus are more likely to be radiation-induced, whereas painful lower plexus lesions are more likely to be neoplastic. Myokymic discharges (a nonspecific marker of neuron injury manifested by brief tetanic contractions of repetitively firing motor units) seen on EMG evaluation of the plexus are much more likely to be seen with radiation-induced lesions of the brachial plexus. MRI evaluation of the plexus may also help in the differentiation.

One somewhat controversial form of brachial plexopathy is thoracic outlet syndrome. Thoracic outlet syndrome encompasses cases that have a demonstrable neurologic deficit (true or neurogenic thoracic outlet syndrome) and those with less well defined syndromes with normal examination results or results suggesting vascular rather than brachial plexus compromise. The neurogenic form occurs when the lower trunk/medial cord is compromised. This may occur with the presence of an anomalous fibrous band attached to a rudimentary rib off of the C7 transverse process or a more well defined cervical rib. There are cases when an anatomic abnormality is not evident on imaging studies. The value of EMG is disputed in thoracic outlet syndrome. One school of thought suggests that normal study results are common with true thoracic outlet syndrome. The EMG, when abnormal, is clear with abnormalities in the ulnar sensory potential and denervation in the thenar and hypothenar muscle groups (C8 and T1 distribution muscles). Clinically, there should be sensory symptoms in the territory of the ulnar and medial cutaneous nerve of the forearm. Weakness should be demonstrable in the intrinsic muscles of the hand, and atrophy in those muscles may be seen. In fact, thoracic outlet syndrome is a rare entity compared with other nerve compression syndromes. Both intra- and extramedullary spinal

cord syndromes may mimic the syndrome. Long tract signs suggesting a myelopathy and Horner syndrome should be specifically looked for. If the syndrome is still suspected and no definite abnormalities on neurologic examination are found and there is no evidence of vascular insufficiency of the arm, a course of physical therapy emphasizing improvement in posture (keeping shoulders from drooping) should be prescribed. We believe that surgery should not be contemplated in patients without definite evidence of nerve compression (atrophy and an appropriately abnormal EMG) or vascular compromise in which arteriography demonstrates a surgically correctable abnormality in the shoulder. The failure rate, rate of recurrence, and risk of serious neurologic complications are relatively high.

Tomaculous neuropathy, in which patients suffer bouts of localized demyelination with pressure on a nerve, may present with a brachial plexus lesion. These patients also suffer multiple mononeuropathies of the same nature. Treatment is supportive.

Mononeuritis multiplex of any etiology may mimic a brachial plexopathy early on but will eventually involve single nerves in multiple limbs.

Lumbosacral

It is important to keep in mind that the lumbosacral plexus is actually two plexuses, the lumbar and the sacral. Injuries to the lumbar plexus can very often mimic symptoms of a femoral nerve lesion with weakness of hip flexion and knee extension. Clinically and electrophysiologically, it is important to test the hip adductors, which get their innervation through the lumbar plexus also, but by way of the obturator rather than the femoral nerve.

Lesions of the sacral plexus can be confused with lesions to its largest branch, the sciatic nerve. In addition to symptoms such as lower leg and hamstring weakness and sciatic distribution pain and paresthesias, there may be weakness of the gluteal muscles, the tensor fasciae latae, and the anal sphincter that can be demonstrated clinically or on EMG.

Injuries to the lumbosacral plexus may occur as a result of traumatic, metastatic, inflammatory, ischemic, or hemorrhagic etiologies.

Traumatic injuries to the lumbosacral plexus occur with crush injuries to the pelvis or with pelvic fractures. They may occur interoperatively with orthopaedic surgeries to the hip (generally sacral plexus) or when retractors are used in abdominal procedures (lumbar plexus).

Neoplasms that may invade the plexus include rectal, prostate, or cervical cancers or leukemias and lymphomas. Any mass, benign or malignant, in the pelvis may compress the plexus. Radiation injuries may also be a cause of lumbosacral plexopathies, as radiation to these tumors is fairly common. As opposed to neoplastic invasion, radiation injuries tend to be painless. Because the radiation field is usually in the midline when treating these cancers, the symptoms are often bilateral. Even when the symptoms are not bilateral, findings on EMG may be bilateral, helping to differentiate radiation injury from metastatic invasion, which tends, at least early in its course, to be unilateral. Myokymic discharges are seen on EMG in about 50 percent of radiation-induced lumbosacral plexopathies.

Ischemic injuries to the lumbosacral plexus are seen with diabetes and in cases of mononeuritis multiplex. These tend to be apoplectic in nature and exquisitely painful initially. In diabetes, injuries to the femoral nerve or lumbar plexus result in the syndrome of diabetic amyotrophy with intense burning pain in the thigh and weakness in the distribution of the femoral and/or the obturator nerves.

Inflammatory lumbosacral plexopathies are considerably less common than inflammatory brachial plexopathies, but they have been described, including a number of cases of painful lumbosacral plexopathies with high sedimentation rates that appeared to respond to steroids. A number of these cases were diabetic, however, and distinguishing them from ischemic plexopathies is difficult.

In patients on anticoagulants or with hemophilia, bleeding into the iliopsoas muscle may cause a compressive femoral nerve or lumbar plexus lesion.

APPROACH TO THE PATIENT

The approach to working up a case initially depends on whether the symptoms and examination are more consistent with a radiculopathy or plexopathy. If a radiculopathy is suspected, then MRI is most helpful in determining the cause of root injury. Gadolinium is useful in cases in which there is suspicion of meningeal inflammation or infiltration as a cause of radiculopathy. EMG is a complimentary study in that it helps characterize the severity of the root injury. Patients with clear radiculopathies, especially those demonstrated on EMG, who have no obvious lesion on radiologic studies may benefit from a lumbar puncture in assessing the patient for inflammatory, infectious, and neoplastic entities.

In cases of suspected plexus lesions, EMG is most effective in determining the location and extent of a lesion. MRI may be helpful but is negative in cases of inflammatory, ischemic, traction-induced, or even some metastatic lesions.

SUGGESTED READINGS

Adams R, Victor M: Principles of Neurology. 5th Ed. McGraw-Hill, New York, 1993

Dawson D, Hallett M, Millender L: Entrapment Neuropathies. 2nd Ed. Little, Brown, Boston, 1990

Kimura J: Electrodiagnosis in Diseases of Nerve and Muscle. 3rd Ed. FA Davis, Philadelphia, 1993

Oh S: Clinical Electromyography Nerve Conduction Studies. University Park Press, Baltimore, 1984

93. INFLAMMATORY DEMYELINATING POLYNEUROPATHIES

JAMES W. ALBERS

The inflammatory demyelinating polyneuropathies are acquired disorders of peripheral nerves and nerve roots. The precise etiologies are unknown, but immunologic mechanisms play a major role. These disorders are among the most common neuropathies evaluated in neuromuscular clinics, and up to 25 percent of idiopathic polyneuropathies are estimated to have an autoimmune basis. Acute and chronic forms of inflammatory demyelinating polyneuropathy exist, differing primarily in their onset and relapse rate. Most are considered idiopathic, but the frequent association with a systemic disorder such as plasma cell dyscrasia is important in directing the clinical evaluation and may eventually clarify the underlying pathophysiology. The acute and chronic inflammatory demyelinating neuropathies are discussed separately in this chapter, although they have many clinical, electrodiagnostic, and therapeutic similarities.

ACUTE INFLAMMATORY DEMYELINATING POLYNEUROPATHY

Clinical Features

Acute inflammatory demyelinating polyneuropathy (AIDP), also known as Guillain-Barré syndrome, acute inflammatory polyneuritis, or postinfectious polyneuritis, has an incident of slightly less than 2/100,000. AIDP presents with progressive weakness, usually symmetric, in the setting of areflexia, reduced distal sensation, frequent evidence of dysautonomia, and elevated cerebrospinal fluid (CSF) protein without pleocytosis. Most patients recall an antecedent illness, commonly a respiratory tract infection or gastroenteritis, within the 4 weeks preceding onset. Other illnesses and events associated with AIDP include hepatitis B, Epstein-Barr virus, cytomegalovirus, Lyme disease, toxoplasmosis, campylobacter enteritis, immunization, and surgery. Additional systemic illnesses, including human immunodeficiency virus (HIV) infection, Hodgkin's disease, non-Hodgkin's lymphoma, and systemic lupus erythematosus, are associated with neuropathy, but have neurologic presentations atypical for AIDP and are better classified among the chronic forms of demyelinating polyneuropathy.

Weakness in AIDP progresses rapidly and usually plateaus within 2 to 3 weeks of onset. Progression exceeding 4 weeks should suggest an alternative diagnosis. Weakness typically begins distally, but may begin proximally or in facial or bulbar muscles. An ascending paralysis as described in the older literature is uncommon. Prominent facial weakness occurs in about 50 percent of patients, but examination of orbicularis oculi muscles demonstrates weakness in virtually all hospitalized AIDP patients. Respiratory insufficiency requiring mechanical ventilation occurs in 20 to 30 percent of patients, usually within 2 weeks of onset. Occasional patients with marginal respiratory function require intubation later during their hospitalization if decompensation occurs in response to aspiration or infection. Whereas respiratory impairment is considered a major risk in AIDP, cardiac dysrhythmia and blood pressure abnormalities result from dysautonomia, as do impairment of bowel, bladder, and thermoregulation. The syndrome of inappropriate secretion of antidiuretic hormone occasionally occurs, attributed to abnormalities of autonomic afferents from vascular stretch receptors.

Fisher syndrome is thought to be a variant of AIDP consisting of ophthalmoplegia, ataxia, and areflexia. The temporal profile and CSF studies in Fisher syndrome are indistinguishable from AIDP, and some patients have electrodiagnostic evidence of a demyelinating polyneuropathy, whereas others have findings suggestive of a brainstem encephalitis.

Electrophysiologic Features

The electrophysiologic evaluation in AIDP provides evidence of an acquired demyelinating polyneuropathy. Because evaluations usually are performed early when the diagnosis is in question, the variety of findings reported reflect temporal changes associated with cumulative demyelination and axonal degenera-

TABLE 93-1. Representative Electrodiagnostic Protocol for Evaluating Suspected Demyelinating Polyneuropathy

Nerve conduction studies[a]
1. Test most involved site if mild or moderate, least involved site if severe.
2. Evaluate peroneal motor nerve (extensor digitorum brevis); stimulate ankle, below fibular head and knee. Measure F-wave latency.[b]
3. If abnormal, evaluate tibial motor nerve (abductor hallucis); stimulate ankle and knee. Measure F-wave latency.
4. If no responses, evaluate:
   a. Peroneal motor nerve (anterior tibialis); stimulate below fibular head and knee.
   b. Ulnar motor nerve (hypothenar); stimulate wrist and below elbow. Measure F-wave latency.
   c. Median motor nerve (thenar); stimulate wrist and elbow. Measure F-wave latency.
5. Evaluate sural nerve (ankle); stimulate calf.
6. Evaluate median sensory nerve (index finger); stimulate wrist and elbow. If response is absent or focal entrapment is suspected, record from wrist and stimulate midpalm; evaluate ulnar sensory nerve (fifth digit); stimulate wrist.
7. If distal CMAP amplitude substantially larger (>15%) than proximal CMAP amplitude, evaluate for abnormal temporal dispersion or partial conduction block.
   a. Measure CMAP duration (distal and proximal) to identify abnormal dispersion.
   b. Evaluate CMAP amplitude and duration over short segments (few mm) to identify partial conduction block.
   c. If capability exists, measure CMAP negative phase area (distal and proximal).
8. Evaluate additional nerve if findings are equivocal. Definite abnormalities should result in:
   a. Evaluation of contralateral extremity.
   b. Evaluation of specific suspected abnormality.

Needle examination
1. Examine anterior tibialis, medial gastrocnemius, abductor hallucis, vastus lateralis, biceps brachii, first dorsal interosseous (hand), and lumbar paraspinal muscles.
2. Any abnormality should be confirmed by examination of at least one contralateral muscle, looking for symmetry.

Abbreviation: CMAP, compound muscle action potential.

[a] Muscles in parentheses indicate recording site for conduction studies.

[b] All F-wave latency measurements are for distal stimulation sites. Record as absent if no response after 10 to 15 stimulations.

(Modified from Albers JW, Donofrio PD, McGonagle TK: Sequential electrodiagnostic abnormalities in acute inflammatory demyelinating polyradiculoneuropathy. Muscle Nerve 8:528–39, 1985, with permission.)

TABLE 93-2. Electrodiagnostic Criteria Suggestive of Chronic Acquired Demyelination

Evaluation should satisfy at least three of the following in motor nerves (exceptions explained in footnotes):
1. Conduction velocity less than 75% of the lower limit of normal (two or more nerves).[a]
2. Distal latency exceeding 130% of upper limit of normal (two or more nerves).[b]
3. Evidence of unequivocal temporal dispersion (increase in negative component duration exceeding 15% for proximal versus distal stimulation) or a proximal to distal amplitude ratio less than 0.7 (one or more nerves).[b,c]
4. F-wave latency exceeding 125% of upper limit of normal (one or more nerves).[a,b]

[a] Excluding isolated ulnar or peroneal nerve abnormalities at the elbow or knee, respectively.

[b] Excluding isolated median nerve abnormality at the wrist.

[c] Excluding the presence of anomalous innervation (e.g., median to ulnar nerve crossover).

(Modified from Albers JW, Donofrio PD, McGonagle TK: Sequential electrodiagnostic abnormalities in acute demyelinating polyradiculoneuropathy. Muscle Nerve 1985, 8:528–39, with permission.)

velocity slowing greater than can be explained by axonal loss is suggestive of demyelination, but abnormal dispersion of motor responses or unequivocal conduction block are the cardinal features of acquired demyelination (Fig. 93-1). The earliest abnormalities include absent F- and H-waves and decreased motor unit recruitment, all nonspecific findings. Only during subsequent examinations does evidence of segmental conduction block and conduction slowing become apparent. Some patients with normal conduction velocities have prolonged distal latencies, whereas other patients have normal distal latencies and reduced conduction velocities. These different presentations reflect the site of major abnormality, and most patients presenting with only prolonged distal latencies subsequently develop partial conduction block, abnormal temporal dispersion, and reduced conduction velocities.

The electrodiagnostic features of acquired demyelination are imprecise and depend upon identification of findings that cannot be explained by axonal degeneration alone (Table 93-2). During the first 2 weeks of illness, about 50 percent of AIDP patients fulfill strict criteria for demyelination, compared to almost 85 percent by the third week of illness. During these first few weeks, an unusual pattern of abnormal median but normal sural sensory responses occurs in almost 50 percent of AIDP patients. The extreme pattern of an absent median but present sural response in the appropriate clinical setting occurs almost exclusively in AIDP and is unusual in other types of neuropathy. A small percentage of patients never fulfill criteria

tion. The evaluation is similar to that of any polyneuropathy, the goal being to obtain sufficient information to document the presence of a peripheral disorder and to identify the predominant pathophysiology. This requires evaluation of sensory and motor nerves in the upper and lower extremities, including proximal stimulation of motor nerves and F-wave studies. A representative protocol is shown in Table 93-1.

The hallmark of all acquired demyelinating neuropathies is evidence suggestive of multifocal demyelination. Conduction

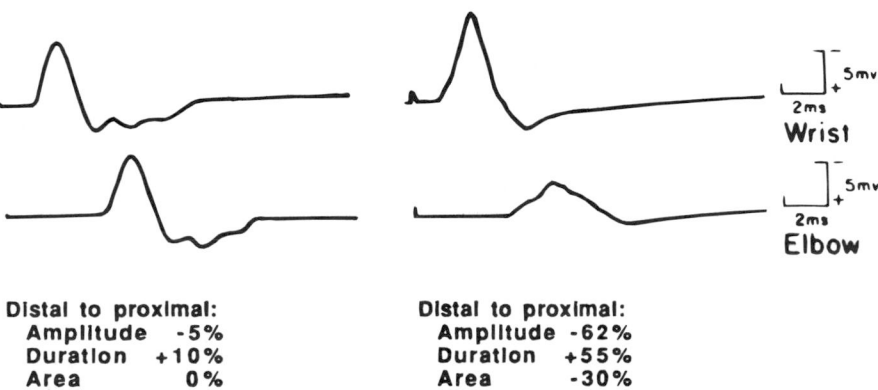

FIG. 93-1. Motor nerve conduction studies from a normal subject (left) and from a patient with an acquired inflammatory demyelinating polyneuropathy (right), demonstrating abnormal temporal dispersion and/or partial conduction block.

for demyelination, some because responses are unobtainable, obscuring any evidence of demyelination. In others, findings suggest only cumulative axonal degeneration, perhaps representing an axonal form of AIDP.

The needle electromyography (EMG) examination has a limited role in evaluating patients with AIDP. The occasional demonstration of myokymic discharges during the first few weeks of illness may be helpful in establishing the diagnosis, and ultimate demonstration of profuse fibrillation potentials may be helpful in defining the magnitude and extent of denervation in establishing prognosis.

Other Laboratory Features

Other than CSF and electrophysiologic evaluations, laboratory studies have limited use in AIDP. Abnormal white blood count and liver function tests occur frequently, but are nonspecific and thought to reflect an antecedent illness. Occasionally, elevated antibody titers to viral antigens help identify a specific antecedent event, but have no therapeutic implications. The most important role of laboratory studies is in identifying a systemic problem mimicking AIDP. For example, any patient with acute neuropathy and abnormal liver function studies, profound sensory loss, and unexplained leukopenia should be evaluated for arsenic intoxication (24-hour urine heavy metal screen and fingernail or hair arsenic analyses). Porphyric neuropathy also should be considered in patients with suspected AIDP, particularly if there is limited electrophysiologic evidence of demyelination, a history of recurrent episodes, or of the triad of abdominal pain, psychosis, and polyneuropathy. CSF pleocytosis, although not incompatible with AIDP, should suggest an alternative diagnosis such as human immunodeficiency virus-associated neuropathy. The association of AIDP with systemic lupus erythematosus exists, so serologic evaluation for collagen vascular disease or vasculitis is appropriate. Sural nerve biopsy may identify an underlying vasculitis or other systemic illness, but generally is not indicated.

Treatment

The advent of respiratory intensive care units dramatically reduced mortality in AIDP to its current rate of approximately 2 to 5 percent. All patients require observation for respiratory deterioration, and pulmonary therapy is important in limiting atelectasis. Frequent monitoring of forced vital capacity (FVC) is important, and the decision of whether to intubate depends upon both the extent and rate of respiratory deterioration. Intubation is indicated if the FVC falls below 15 ml/kg, but a rapid decline of FVC should result in elective intubation independent of the absolute measurement, as should aspiration with poor tracheal toilet, pulmonary infection with shunting, or early signs of respiratory fatigue. Arterial blood gases are poor indicators of impending respiratory failure, and increasing restlessness, tachycardia, tachypnea, and sleepiness, frequently precede blood gas changes. A low PO_2 and lower than normal PCO_2 may indicate early atelectasis with shunting. Hypercapnia generally precedes hypoxia, but is a relatively late finding of respiratory failure and a dangerous criterion for elective intubation.

Most deaths relate to medical complications of respiratory paralysis, but about 50 percent are sudden and presumably related to cardiac dysrhythmias or hypotension. Although dysautonomia is not directly related to the extent of weakness, catastrophic cardiac dysrhythmias or blood pressure lability are unusual in patients with mild functional impairment. Any suspicion of autonomic instability requires monitoring in an intensive care setting. Minor cardiac dysrhythmias occur in about 20 percent of hospitalized patients, but arrhythmias sufficiently severe to affect blood pressure or require medication occur in about 5 percent of patients. Most commonly, these are second- or third-degree atrioventricular blocks, for which a temporary pacemaker insertion is required. Autonomic instability resulting in hypotension or new hypertension occurs in 10 to 15 percent of AIDP patients. Hypotension is best managed by the rapid infusion of fluid, and sympathomimetics usually are not required. Most agree that hypertension should not be treated unless severe and persistent. Medications with a short half-life such as nitroprusside or propranolol are the drugs of choice.

Medical management includes prompt identification of infection. Almost 40 percent of hospitalized AIDP patients develop infections requiring antibiotic treatment, most commonly related to respiratory or urinary tracts. Urinary retention occurs frequently, related either to primary neurologic dysfunction or bed confinement. Urinary output should be monitored and retention treated with intermittent catheterization rather than an indwelling catheter to reduce the risk of infection. Hyponatremia is treated with fluid restriction. Nonambulatory patients require antiembolic protection, including support stockings and low-dose heparin (5,000 U subcutaneous twice daily). Early referral to physical therapy for passive or active exercise reduces the incidence of contractures and facilitates recovery.

Corticosteroids are of unproven efficacy and their use controversial in AIDP. Of the few controlled studies, most are inconclusive and at least one concluded that prednisone slowed recovery and increased the likelihood of relapse.

The demonstrated importance of humeral factors in AIDP suggested that therapeutic plasma exchange (TPE) might alter the course of illness. Several multicenter randomized studies, including the North American study of plasmapheresis and acute Guillain-Barré syndrome, confirmed the clinical, statistical, and economic efficacy of TPE in AIDP when initiated within the first few weeks after onset. In the North American study, TPE patients underwent exchange of a total of 200 to 250 ml plasma/kg body weight over 7 to 14 days, typically exchanging 40 ml/kg every other day. For respirator-dependent patients who received TPE, the median time of respiratory support was reduced by 11 days and the time to unassisted ambulation was shortened by more than 2 months compared to the control group, without a significant increase in the nature or frequency of complications.

Relapse occurred in only 4 (1.6 percent) of 245 patients in the North American study, 2 in each study arm. As TPE became the standard treatment, being initiated as soon after the diagnosis of AIDP was established, some centers observed an unexpectedly high relapse rate. Relapse usually occurred 1 to 6 weeks after completing TPE and responded to a second series of TPE, suggesting premature discontinuation of treatment. Whenever the initial series of five exchanges is completed before the fourth week of illness, we recommend continued interval exchanges (usually 1 or 2 per week) through the fourth or fifth week to reduce the likelihood of limited relapse (Table 93-3).

A randomized trial comparing intravenous immunoglobulin (IVIG) to TPE suggested that IVIG is at least as effective as plasma exchange in AIDP. Subsequent uncontrolled trials suggested that IVIG is associated with an increased incidence of relapse in patients with AIDP, and many feel that TPE remains the treatment of first choice in AIDP. Nevertheless, for some

TABLE 93-3. Suggested Therapeutic Plasma Exchange Schedule in AIDP[a]

Interval from onset of neurologic symptoms
  <3 weeks: five exchanges of 1 plasma volume each over 7 to 14 days[b]
  3–4 weeks: no exchange if stable or improving with mild impairment; otherwise, five exchanges of 1 plasma volume, as above
  >4 weeks: no exchange unless progressing

Interval from onset to completion of TPE
  <4 weeks: additional interval exchanges every 3 to 5 days through the end of week 5 to prevent limited relapse
  >4 weeks: no further exchanges

Abbreviations: AIDP, acquired inflammatory demyelinating polyneuropathy; TPE, therapeutic plasma exchange.

[a] For patients in whom the diagnosis of AIDP is secure and there is at least moderate motor impairment (may be ambulatory). The schedule is an approximation, and the actual timing depends upon availability of TPE, stability and condition of patient, coagulation factors, and other considerations.

[b] Some protocols begin with daily exchanges for 2 days, switching to an every-other-day or every-3-day schedule depending upon coagulation factors (e.g., if pre-exchange fibrinogen level <100 mg/100 ml, consider postponing exchange or using plasma products as part of replacement solution).

TABLE 93-4. Systemic Illness Occasionally Identified in Patients Presenting With CIDP

MGUS
Amyloidosis
Osteosclerotic myeloma (POEMS syndrome)
Multiple myeloma
Waldenström's macroglobulinemia
γ-Heavy-chain disease
Cryoglobulinemia
Lymphoma
Systemic lupus erythematosus
Castleman's disease
HIV infections
Vasculitis (confluent mononeuritis multiplex) ?
Occult malignancy ?

Abbreviations: CIDP, chronic inflammatory demyelinating polyneuropathy; HIV, human immunodeficiency virus; MGUS, monoclonal gammopathy of undetermined significance; POEMS, polyneuropathy, organomegaly, endocrinopathy, M protein, and skin changes.

patients such as those with poor venous access who require central lines for TPE, IVIG offers a particular advantage.

Prognosis

Most patients with AIDP ultimately recover, but neither TPE nor IVIG represents the ideal treatment, and prolonged hospitalizations and rehabilitation remain common, with 15 percent of patients having severe residual weakness. In general, clinical findings are poor predictors of outcomes in AIDP. Rapid evolution of weakness, advanced age, ventilator dependency, and a prolonged plateau prior to the onset of recovery suggest a poor prognosis. The best physiologic indicator of poor prognosis is an average motor evoked amplitude less than 20 percent of the lower limit of normal at plateau, although sequential recordings may be important in defining prognosis.

CHRONIC INFLAMMATORY DEMYELINATING POLYNEUROPATHY

Clinical Features

Chronic inflammatory demyelinating polyneuropathy (CIDP) resembles AIDP, but has a more prolonged course, usually with slow progression, often is relapsing, and generally is steroid-responsive. Diagnostic criteria for CIDP differ minimally from those used for AIDP, and the only reliable method for differentiating the two disorders early in their course is by an arbitrary judgment regarding the evolution of initial symptoms. CIDP patients usually have an interval between onset and peak impairment exceeding 4 weeks, averaging approximately 3 months. Whereas AIDP is a monophasic illness, CIDP includes monophasic, relapsing, and progressive forms. The term *chronic relapsing polyneuropathy* describes patients with clear relapses and remissions. Limited information exists about the natural course of patients with CIDP. Most patients receive some form of treatment, and relapses may occur in response to changes in medical therapy, masking the natural history. Ignoring whether relapses occur spontaneously or reflect changes in therapy, over 40 percent of patients have a relapsing course. Less than 15 percent of patients demonstrate progression despite treatment.

CIDP is characterized by diffuse weakness, abnormal reflexes, elevated CSF protein, and electrophysiologic evidence of multifocal demyelination with or without superimposed axonal degeneration. Sensory signs occur in over 85 percent of CIDP patients, probably more frequently than in AIDP. Identifiable antecedent events are relatively uncommon, occurring in less than 30 percent of patients. Symmetric motor or sensory symptoms are the initial manifestation in the majority of patients. Occasionally, gait ataxia is the presenting complaint. Facial weakness is common, particularly orbicularis oculi weakness, but is less prominent than in AIDP. Weakness usually begins in the distal lower extremities, and a proximal to distal gradient persists in most patients. About 50 percent of patients are nonambulatory during their most severe episode. Areflexia occurs in about 75 percent of CIDP patients, and most patients have absent Achilles reflexes. Symptomatic dysautonomia is uncommon. Impairment is typically less than that experienced by AIDP patients, but over 75 percent of CIDP patients develop at least moderate disability, preventing independent existence. Approximately 5 percent of CIDP patients require respiratory support at some time during their illness.

A major difference between AIDP and CIDP is the frequent association of an systemic illness in CIDP. The term *CIDP* is reserved for patients with idiopathic disease who do not have an associated illness. Nevertheless, at initial evaluation, it is impossible to distinguish idiopathic CIDP patients from those with an associated systemic illness, and patients with idiopathic CIDP may develop a systemic illness after a negative initial examination. The most common associated disease is a monoclonal gammopathy of undetermined significance (MGUS), but a variety of other associations exist, including those shown in Table 93-4.

Electrophysiologic Features

Electrophysiologic features in CIDP resemble those described late in the course of AIDP. For all practical purposes, patients with monophasic, relapsing, or progressive courses are electrodiagnostically indistinguishable. The electrodiagnostic criteria used as suggestive of acquired demyelination in CIDP differ little from those described for AIDP, being slightly more stringent to reflect changes related to chronic axonal stenosis or regeneration, both of which produce conduction slowing. Although strict criteria for demyelination are not always fulfilled, at least partial evidence of acquired demyelination is present in virtually all CIDP patients, and most clinicians consider this an important part of the diagnosis. Findings include slowing of motor conduction velocities, prolonged or absent F-waves, abnormal temporal dispersion, and partial conduction block. Sensory conduction study results are abnormal, and the combination of absent or abnormal median sensory responses with normal sural responses occurs in approximately 30 percent of patients, a somewhat lower rate than in AIDP. Needle EMG abnormalities occur in most patient with CIDP, consistent with superimposed axonal degeneration and regeneration.

Other Laboratory Features

Because a subset of patients with otherwise typical CIDP have an underlying systemic illness, and because some patients with idiopathic CIDP later develop a systemic illness, the laboratory evaluation of CIDP is important. Depending upon their presentation, the evaluation should include investigation for systemic lupus erythematosus and other collagen vascular diseases, vasculitis, diabetes, HIV infection, or malignancy. Suggested laboratory studies are listed in Table 93-5, but additional evaluations may be indicated in special situations. All patients with presumed idiopathic CIDP should be evaluated for a plasma cell dyscrasia, beginning with a serum protein electrophoresis. Patients with mild CIDP and a normal serum protein electrophoresis who respond to treatment do not require immunologic re-evaluation unless they relapse. If the evaluation remains normal after an initial relapse that responds to treatment, only relapses refractory to therapy require re-evaluation. For patients with progressive CIDP, re-evaluation should be performed 6 months after the initial diagnosis and then yearly. Re-evaluation should

TABLE 93-5. Recommended Laboratory Investigations in CIDP

All patients
  ANA
  Complete blood count
  ESR
  Glucose (random or fasting)
  Hepatitis antigen
  HIV antibody
  Liver function studies
  Serum protein electrophoresis
  Serum immunoelectrophoresis (or immunofixation)
  Urine immunoelectrophoresis

Additional evaluations (depending upon the severity of neuropathy, response to treatment, and clinical suspicion)
  Anti-MAG
  Anti-Gm$_1$
  Angiotensin-converting enzyme
  Cryoglobulins
  ENA
  Lyme antibodies
  Thyroid function studies
  Urine
    Porphyrins and δ-levulinic acid
    Heavy metals, including arsenic
  Imaging
    Chest and abdominal CT
    Radiologic skeletal survey
  Biopsy
    Sural nerve
    Bone marrow

Prior to beginning immunosuppressive treatment
  Chest x-ray
  PPD

Re-evaluation in progressive CIDP
  Repeat immunologic evaluation in 6 months and then yearly serum immunoelectrophoresis (or immunofixation)
  Radiologic skeletal survey
  Sural nerve biopsy

Abbreviations: ANA, antinuclear antibody; CIDP, chronic inflammatory demyelinating polyneuropathy; CT, computed tomography; ENA, extractable nuclear antigen; ESR, erythrocyte sedimentation rate; HIV, human immunodeficiency virus; MAG, myelin-associated glycoprotein; PPD, purified protein derivative.

include a serum immunoelectrophoresis (or immunofixation), urine immunoelectrophoresis, and radiologic skeletal survey. The skeletal survey is performed because of the occasional identification of a plasmacytoma in a patient without evidence of a monoclonal gammopathy.

Sural nerve biopsy is of proven usefulness in identifying acquired demyelination, but lack of specificity does not justify routine use. Biopsy is useful in identifying vasculitis, amyloid deposits, cytoplasmic inclusions, neurofilamentous swollen axons, or evidence of other specific pathology.

Because most patient with CIDP require immunosuppression, all patients should be evaluated for a response to purified protein derivative and undergo a chest x-ray prior to initiation of treatment with prednisone or other cytotoxic agents, if a recent evaluation has not been performed.

Treatment

The supportive treatment of patients with CIDP is identical to that described for AIDP, although respiratory distress requiring intubation is less common and symptomatic dysautonomia unusual. Unlike in AIDP, corticosteroids are of established efficacy in CIDP. The demonstrated efficacy of TPE, and the purported efficacy of a variety of immunosuppressants including azathioprine, cyclophosphamide, melphalan, total lymphoid irradiation, and, most recently, IVIG has resulted in numerous treatment protocols reflecting individual physicians' preferences for specific treatments depending upon disease duration, rate of progression, and severity. Unfortunately, there are no guidelines for selecting one protocol over another. Because treatment-related complications with prednisone and other forms of immunosuppression are not inconsequential, there is some optimism that IVIG will assume an increasing role in the future.

Most CIDP patients (70 of 77) evaluated at the University of Michigan over a 12-year period received treatment during their initial episode. Therapies reflected the collective experience of the neuromuscular faculty and available treatments during the interval of review (1979 to 1991). Initial treatments included oral prednisone (32 patients), TPE plus prednisone (24), TPE alone (11), TPE plus azathioprine (2), and IVIG (1). Prednisone was given at 60 mg/d in adults for 1 to 3 months, followed by a gradual taper. TPE schedules included five exchanges of 1 plasma volume each over 10 to 14 days. Azathioprine was given at 1 to 3 mg/kg/d when prednisone was contraindicated. Eleven patients received TPE alone, and response to TPE sometimes was taken as evidence supportive of the diagnosis. These and additional protocols are summarized in Table 93-6.

Patients receiving prednisone require interval weight, blood pressure, serum glucose, and potassium measurements, and should be placed on a high-protein, low-salt, low-fat diet. Laboratory tests initially should be performed every 2 to 4 weeks. Those who are purified protein derivative–positive require concurrent antituberculosis therapy. Patients treated with azathioprine should undergo liver function studies and complete blood counts repeated weekly for the first month, and then at longer intervals if the medication is continued.

Prognosis

Most patients with CIDP have a good clinical outcome. Occasional patients with mild impairment improve spontaneously. For the more severely impaired patient requiring treatment, re-

TABLE 93-6. Alternative Protocols for the Treatment of Chronic Inflammatory Demyelinating Polyneuropathy

Treatment	Advantages	Disadvantages
Therapeutic plasma exchange[a] 5 exchanges over 7–14 days Weekly exchanges for 10 weeks 2 exchanges/week for 3 weeks[b] QOD exchanges for 2 weeks[c]	Rapid response, usually in 7–14 days Few complications	Response short-lived (weeks to months) Central line if poor venous access Likely require concurrent immunosuppression Expense
Prednisone 60 mg/d until response or 3 months; reduce alternate day dose by ~15% of total 2-day dose ever 2 weeks until 20 mg QOD, then slow taper[d] 120 mg/d for 1 week, reduce by 20 mg/week for 5 weeks to 20 mg/day, then slow taper[e]	Established efficacy Response within weeks to months Fewer side effects once QOD schedule achieved Brief period of high-dose prednisone	Relative high incidence of complications (weight gain, fluid retention, hypertension, hyperglycemia, insomnia and mood changes, cataracts, skin changes, osteoporosis, aseptic necrosis of hip, infection) Daily schedule
Azathioprine Initiate at 1–2 mg/kg/d (50–100 mg); increase by 0.5 mg/kg increments as tolerated to 2.5 mg/kg; taper to maintenance dose of 1–2 mg/kg/d, monitoring for mild leukopenia	If tolerated and effective, maintenance schedule simple	Efficacy unproven, slow response (months) Drug fever, nausea and vomiting, bone marrow depression, hair loss, hepatitis, theoretic risk of neoplasia, infertility, birth defects (contraindicated in childbearing years), drug interaction (allopurinol)
Intravenous immunoglobulin 1 g/kg/d for 2 days (loading dose), followed by 1 gm/kg/d at 2 & 4 weeks, and then monthly (several), depending on response 0.3–0.4 g/kg/d for 3 or 4 days; treat relapse with intermittent intravenous immunoglobulin infusions[f]	Rapid response, usually in days Proven efficacy Few complications	Requires interval treatments Expense Possible transmission of hepatitis
Initiate therapeutic plasma exchange and prednisone concurrently	Avoid interval relapse after therapeutic plasma exchange	Steroid complications, as above
Initiate therapeutic plasma exchange and azathioprine	Avoid interval relapse after therapeutic plasma exchange	Azathioprine complications, as above

[a] All exchanges refer to one plasma volume each.

[b] Data from Dyck PJ, Daube J, O'Brien P, Pineda A: Plasma exchagne in chronic inflammatory demyelinating polyradiculoneuropathy. N Engl J Med 314:461–465, 1986.

[c] Data from Ropper AH, Weinberg D: Chronic immune demyelinating polyneuropathy (CIDP). Neurol Chron 1:1–8, 1992.

[d] Example switch to QOD (every-other-day) schedule: 60/60, 60/45, 60/30, 60/15; 60/0, 50/0, 45/0, 40/0, 30/0, 25/0, 20/0.

[e] Data from Dyck PJ, O'Brien PC, Oviatt KF et al: Prednisone improves chronic inflammatory demyelinating polyradiculopathy. N Engl J Med 314:461–5, 1986.

[f] Data from Faed JM, Day B, Pollock M, Taylor PK, Nukada H, Hammond-Tooke GD: High-dose intravenous human immunoglobulin in chronic inflammatory demyelinating polyneuropathy. Neurology 39:422–5, 1989.

sponse to initial treatment occurs in about 80 percent, typically within 1 to 3 weeks after initiation of TPE, and somewhat longer after starting prednisone. Treatment with a second or third modality in "poor responders" increases the response rate to almost 90 percent. At 5 years after onset, over 85 percent of patients have mild or no disability, with less than 10 percent of patients demonstrating a moderate to moderately severe impairment. Mortality related to CIDP or its treatment during the first 5 years after diagnosis is less than 5 percent. Unlike AIDP, relapse is common, with over 45 percent of patients relapsing after initial response to treatment, usually within the first year, and averaging four relapses within the first 5 years.

Most patients (approximately 75 percent) require chronic treatment for their CIDP. The most common treatment is prednisone, usually a low-dose alternate-day schedule of 5 to 20 mg every other day. A smaller percentage of patients are maintained on azathioprine (1 to 2 mg/kg/d). Rare patients with a relapsing course demonstrate TPE dependence. Current experience with IVIG is insufficient to justify its long-term use.

CONCLUSION

Patients with inflammatory demyelinating polyneuropathies comprise a substantial portion of patients with undiagnosed neuropathy presenting for evaluation. The acute and chronic forms of inflammatory demyelinating polyneuropathy have characteristic presentations, and the electrophysiologic features are easily recognized. The importance of these neuropathies is

disproportionate to their numbers, since the majority are treatable, some are associated with unrecognized but treatable systemic disorders, and they provide clues to the pathogenesis of other obscure neuropathies.

SUGGESTED READINGS

Albers JW, Kelly Jr. JJ: Acquired inflammatory demyelinating polyneuropathies; clinical and electrodiagnostic features. Muscle Nerve 12:435–51, 1989

Bleck TP: IVIg for GBS: potential problems in the alphabet soup. Neurology 43:857–8, 1993

Dyck PJ, Daube J, O'Brien P, Pineda A: Plasma exchange in chronic inflammatory demyelinating polyradiculoneuropathy. N Engl J Med 314:461–5, 1986

Dyck PJ, Lais AC, Ohta M et al: Chronic inflammatory polyradiculoneuropathy. Mayo Clin Proc 50:621–37, 1975

Dyck PJ, O'Brien PC, Oviatt KF et al: Prednisone improves chronic inflammatory demyelinating polyradiculoneuropathy more than no treatment. Ann Neurol 11:136–41, 1982

Guillain-Barré Syndrome Study Group: Plasmapheresis and acute Guillain-Barré syndrome. Neurology 35:1096–1104, 1985

Lisak RP, Brown MJ: Acquired demyelinating polyneuropathies. Sem Neurol 7:40–8, 1987

McKhann GM, Griffin JW, Cornblath DR et al: Plasmapheresis and Guillain-Barré syndrome: analysis of prognostic factors and the effect of plasmapheresis. Ann Neurol 23:347–53, 1988

Ropper AH, Weinberg D: Chronic immune demyelinating polyneuropathy (CIDP). Neurol Chron 1:1–8, 1992

Simmons Z, Albers JW, Bromberg MB, Feldman EL: Presentation and initial clinical course in patients with chronic inflammatory demyelinating polyradiculoneuropathy: comparison of patients without and with monoclonal gammopathy. Neurology 43:2202–9, 1993 van der Meche FGA, Schmitz PIM, The Dutch Guillain-Barré Study Group: A randomized trial comparing intravenous immune globulin and plasma exchange in Guillain-Barré syndrome. N Engl J Med 326:1123–9, 1992

94. DIABETIC NEUROPATHY

ASA WILBOURN
ROBERT W. SHIELDS, Jr.

Diabetes mellitus is probably the most common serious metabolic disorder that afflicts humans. In the United States alone, its estimated prevalence is almost 7 percent. It is generally considered under two main groups: (1) insulin-dependent diabetes mellitus (IDDM) and (2) non-insulin-dependent diabetes mellitus (NIDDM) (Table 94-1).

Diabetes mellitus has four major complications: neuropathy, nephropathy, retinopathy, and vascular disease. *Diabetic neuropathy* is a generic term for any diabetes mellitus-related disorder of the peripheral nervous system (PNS), the autonomic nervous system (ANS), and some of the cranial nerves:

1. Diabetic generalized sensorimotor polyneuropathy
2. Diabetic autonomic neuropathy
3. Diabetic polyradiculopathy
   a. Involving L2–L4 roots: diabetic amyotrophy
   b. Involving T4–T12 roots: diabetic thoracic radiculopathy
   c. Involving L5, S1 roots
   d. Involving C5–C7 roots
4. Diabetic limb mononeuropathies
5. Diabetic mononeuropathy multiplex
6. Diabetic cranial neuropathies

The more common types of diabetic neuropathy are reviewed in this chapter, beginning with the generalized disorders, then progressing to the regional and, ultimately, the focal ones.

Before diabetic neuropathy is discussed, however, the following two points need to be emphasized. First, diabetes mellitus is such a common disorder, particularly in the elderly, and its neurologic complications are so frequent, that it should always be included in the differential diagnosis whenever patients present with any of a multitude of neurologic complaints. Vigilance in this regard can prevent not only the performance of unnecessary, expensive diagnostic procedures, sometimes fruitlessly repeated at intervals, but also unneeded and potentially harmful treatments, including operations. Conversely, it is equally important to avoid reflexively attributing any neuromuscular abnormality that develops in a diabetic patient to diabetes mellitus, because neurologic disease not related to diabetes mellitus occurs in the same incidence in both the diabetic and nondiabetic populations.

DISTAL SENSORIMOTOR POLYNEUROPATHY–AUTONOMIC NEUROPATHY

Of the various subgroups of diabetic neuropathy, generalized sensorimotor polyneuropathy of diabetes mellitus (GSMP-DM) is by far the most common. Because autonomic fiber involvement is almost invariably associated with the sensorimotor features, it is reasonable to consider involvement of both fiber groups as a common entity. In general, the presence of GSMP-DM is related to the duration and severity of hyperglycemia. However, this form of diabetic neuropathy can occasionally be the presenting symptom of occult diabetes, and significant sensorimotor and autonomic abnormalities can be found in patients with only mild degrees of hyperglycemia. GSMP-DM increases in prevalence with advancing age and tends to correlate with diabetic retinopathy and nephropathy.

Many patients with GSMP-DM are essentially asymptomatic, or have only minimal symptoms. When present, these tend to be predominantly sensory in nature. Although some patients will report loss of feeling, most complain of distal lower extremity paresthesias and pain. The latter may be constant or episodic and may assume a wide variety of forms including burning, stabbing, or dull aching discomfort. Many patients complain of skin hypersensitivity, sometimes so severe that the mere touch of bedsheets produces extreme discomfort. Paresthesias (typically "pins and needles" or tingling sensations) may occur spontaneously, or with contact. These sensory complaints are often accentuated at night and frequently interfere with sleep. Sensory symptoms typically develop and evolve slowly. They

TABLE 94-1. Classification of Primary Diabetes Mellitus

Characteristics	Insulin-Dependent Diabetes Mellitus	Non-Insulin-Dependent Diabetes Mellitus
Synonyms	"Brittle" diabetes mellitus, juvenile-onset diabetes mellitus, type 1 diabetes mellitus	Stable diabetes mellitus, adult/mature-onset diabetes mellitus, type 2 diabetes mellitus
Genetic defect	High	High
Human leukocyte antigen and autoimmune associations	Yes	No
Concordance rate for identical twins	±50%	±100%
Possible cause	Immune-mediated β-cell destruction	Dysfunctional β-cell, with end-organ insulin resistance
Percentage of diabetes	5–10%	90–95%
Female/male ratio	1:1	1.4 to 1.8/1
Age of onset (years)	usually <40–45	usually >30–40
Body habitus	Lean or normal	Obese (>80%)
Mode of onset	Often abrupt	Usually insidious
Plasma insulin levels	Low/unmeasurable	Normal to high
Major cause of death	Diabetic coma; diabetic nephropathy	Cardioavscular disease
Types of diabetic neuropathy commonly associated	All except polyradiculopathy; in young, only distal symmetric polyneuropathy and autonomic neuropathy	All; often several coexisting

(From Wilbourn AJ: Diabetic neuropathies. p. 479. In Brown WF, Bolton CF (eds): Clinical Electromyography. 2nd Ed. Butterworth-Heinemann, Boston, 1993, with permission.)

may begin unilaterally or asymmetrically but ultimately they become bilateral and relatively symmetric. Characteristically, the sensory symptoms begin in the toes and feet and evolve in a distal-to-proximal gradient in the lower extremities. Thus, the symptoms of GSMP-DM manifest a length-dependent pattern, with the longest axons demonstrating involvement at their distal-most point. Consequently, patients with progressive lower extremity sensory symptoms generally do not experience similar symptoms in their fingertips or hands until the lower extremity symptoms are at or above the level of the knees. In severe progressive cases, sensory symptoms may appear over the anterior chest and abdomen. In most patients, the distressing painful component of GSMP-DM is self-limited and spontaneously improves after many months, whereas in some patients it progresses, or at least persists indefinitely. Although the typical mode of evolution of GSMP-DM is slow and insidious, a more fulminant acute painful polyneuropathy, often associated with profound weight loss, also occurs. In the majority of patients with GSMP-DM, motor fiber involvement is rather minimal and is typically confined to weakness and atrophy of the intrinsic foot muscles. Uncommonly, foot weakness may be prominent and with progressive extension proximally, bilateral footdrop may result.

ANS involvement is frequently subclinical in the early stages of the polyneuropathy, although it may be detected using sensitive methods to measure and quantitate autonomic function. In general, involvement of autonomic nerves also obeys a length-dependent pattern. In most patients, multiple organ systems are affected simultaneously. The sympathetic pupillodilator fibers may be involved relatively early, causing small pupil size and sometimes difficulties with dark adaptation. Cardiovascular involvement typically begins with reduced vagal function and an asymptomatic increase in resting heart rate. With more advanced sympathetic cardiovascular dysfunction, orthostatic hypotension may occur. Autonomic sudomotor fiber involvement often results in asymptomatic distal lower extremity anhidrosis. Some patients note compensatory hyperhidrosis involving the face and upper torso. In advanced cases, generalized anhidrosis may occur. Autonomic involvement of the gastrointestinal system frequently results in constipation and, paradoxically, episodic nocturnal diarrhea. Gastric atony often causes postprandial nausea and bloating, along with early satiety. Involvement of genitourinary autonomic fibers may produce a ''neurogenic bladder,'' resulting in reduced sensation of bladder fullness and incomplete emptying; the latter may lead to recurrent urinary tract infections. Sexual dysfunction is commonly encountered with diabetic ANS involvement. In males, decreased erectile function, sometimes associated with retrograde ejaculation, is common, whereas in women, reduced vaginal secretions and lubrication may occur. When ANS dysfunction is more advanced, the adrenal gland may be denervated, which may result in unawareness of hypoglycemia. This is caused by failure of the adrenal gland to release catecholamines in the setting of hypoglycemia and consequently the loss of sweating and tachycardia that typically alerts the patient to hypoglycemia.

The neurologic examination with GSMP-DM often reveals reduced superficial sensory perception to light touch, pinprick, and temperature sensation in a stocking distribution. Usually, joint position sense and vibratory sense are relatively preserved. On occasion, even in patients with rather severe sensory symptoms, tendon reflexes may be preserved and no atrophy or muscular weakness can be detected. This pattern of clinical involvement suggests that GSMP-DM may preferentially involve the smaller diameter peripheral nerve fibers that subserve the superficial sensory modalities. This is sometimes referred to as diabetic small-fiber neuropathy. Much less commonly, patients may present with imbalance of gait, due to sensory ataxia, in the absence of small-fiber symptomatology, suggesting preferential large-fiber involvement. Frequently, both large and small fibers appear to be equally involved, producing sensory deficits to all modalities, loss of deep tendon reflexes, and modest distal muscle weakness and atrophy. Typically, atrophy of the extensor digitorum brevis or minimal signs of toe extensor and flexor weakness may be the only signs of mild motor fiber involvement. Infrequently, rather severe motor fiber involvement occurs, producing bilateral footdrop and significant lower extremity weakness. In a few patients, acrodystrophic changes may occur, with accompanying foot ulcerations. Neuropathic arthropathy or Charcot joints are rare manifestations of GSMP-DM, and when present, are almost always confined to the bones of the foot.

Because GSMP-DM produces a rather nonspecific type of generalized sensorimotor dysfunction, its differential diagnosis includes a wide range of sensorimotor polyneuropathies. Consequently, the mere occurrence of a sensorimotor polyneuropathy in a diabetic patient does not automatically indicate that the polyneuropathy is caused by the diabetes. In this respect, the diagnosis of GSMP-DM is one of exclusion. Some of the polyneuropathies included in the differential diagnosis of GSMP-DM are easily differentiated from GSMP-DM by various clinical features and/or laboratory studies:

1. Uremia
2. Alcoholic/nutritional
3. Connective tissue disorders
4. Vasculitis
5. Vitamin B_{12} deficiency
6. Hypothyroidism
7. Toxic (e.g., metals, drugs, solvents)
8. Paraneoplastic
9. Paraproteinemia
10. Amyloidosis
11. Hereditary

Electrodiagnostic studies are extremely valuable in confirming the presence of GSMP-DM, and in characterizing its underlying pathophysiology of axon loss. With mild GSMP-DM, electrodiagnostic abnormalities are found only in the lower extremities. These typically consist of unelicitable H-responses, low-amplitude or unelicitable sensory (sural, superficial peroneal sensory) nerve conduction study (NCS) responses, mild slowing of conduction velocities on motor (peroneal, tibial) NCS, and fibrillation potentials in the intrinsic foot muscles, appearing either alone or in various combinations. With more advanced disease, the amplitudes of the motor NCS responses recorded from the intrinsic foot muscles decrease, and motor unit potential dropout is seen in those muscles on needle electrode examination. In about two-thirds of patients studied in the electrodiagnostic laboratory, the process is severe enough that abnormalities are found in the upper extremity, the initial ones usually being diminution of the sensory (median, ulnar, radial) NCS amplitudes. Whereas these electrodiagnostic features are characteristic of a primarily axon loss polyneuropathy, they are not diagnostic of GSMP-DM. Instead, they are rather nonspecific in nature, and are consistent with a wide variety of etiologies. Nonetheless, the presence of primarily axonal loss findings excludes the acquired or familial demyelinating polyneuropathies. In a small percentage of patients with GSMP-DM, essentially restricted to those who have predominantly small-fiber symptomatology, the electrodiagnosis is normal or only minimal abnormalities are seen. This is because the electrodiagnostic examination assesses only large myelinated nerve fibers.

Examination of the cerebral spinal fluid is rarely indicated in the evaluation of patients with suspected GSMP-DM. Typically, it is entirely normal, although a modest increase in CSF protein, rarely above 100 mg percent, can be seen. Nerve biopsy is also rarely performed, except to exclude a vasculitic neuropathy or amyloidosis. The biopsy findings in GSMP-DM are those of a nonspecific, primarily axon-loss, polyneuropathy. Depending upon the clinical circumstances, a variety of laboratory tests are often obtained to exclude treatable causes of polyneuropathy that may be occurring in the setting of diabetes mellitus. Usually, these include a complete blood count; chemical profiles of the blood; vitamin B_{12}, folic acid, and thyroid function studies; serum and urine for immunoelectrophoresis, sedimentation rate, and antinuclear factor.

A wide variety of autonomic tests can be performed on diabetic patients with GSMP-DM to assess for associated ANS involvement. Noninvasive cardiovascular tests, such as heart rate variability with deep breathing or Valsalva maneuver, are relatively sensitive methods for detecting early cardiovagal impairment. Various sudomotor function tests, including sympathetic skin response, thermoregulatory sweat testing, and quantitative sudomotor axon reflex test, may reveal abnormalities. Diabetic patients with symptomatic autonomic neuropathy require a specific evaluation of the particular organ system involved. Hemodynamic tilt tests are often valuable when orthostatic hypotension is present. Gastrointestinal atony is frequently evaluated with various radiographic techniques. Urinary bladder dysfunction can be assessed by quantitating the postvoiding residual urine, which typically is increased in diabetic cystopathy; cystoscopy and urodynamic studies are required to document and quantitate the degree of bladder dysfunction. Male sexual dysfunction, including erectile impotence, can be differentiated from psychogenic impotence with various tests, including penial tumescence studies during rapid eye movement sleep.

Traditionally, optimal glycemic control has been the foundation for the treatment of GSMP-DM and autonomic neuropathy. The results of the Diabetes Control and Complications Trial have confirmed the long-held clinical belief that aggressive treatment with relatively tight glycemic control can have a beneficial effect on the development and/or progression of GSMP-DM and autonomic neuropathy. A variety of other treatments have been proposed for GSMP-DM, including myo-inositol supplementation, aldose reductase inhibitors, gangliosides, and vitamin supplementation, all without significant clinical benefit.

The symptomatic management of GSMP-DM is primarily directed at the painful component, which is present in so many patients. Although hyperglycemia is known to have a direct effect on lowering pain tolerance, improvement in glycemic control rarely decreases pain appreciably. Minor analgesics are often prescribed, but seldom are of significant benefit. Narcotics may control GSMP-DM pain, but are inappropriate for management in most patients because of the chronic nature of the disorder. Anticonvulsants, especially phenytoin and carbamazepine, have been used successfully to treat painful GSMP-DM. These drugs are typically prescribed in conventional doses until "therapeutic" levels are obtained. Failure to respond once therapeutic levels are obtained should prompt discontinuation of these drugs.

Many tricyclic antidepressant medications also have been used to treat painful GSMP-DM. These appear to be as effective in patients who are not depressed as in those who are. The particular antidepressant employed is often determined by the need for sedation to assist in sleep and the presence of symptomatic autonomic neuropathy that might be exacerbated by the anticholinergic side effects of the drug. Amitriptyline (Elavil) is a particularly effective drug. It is rather sedating and can thereby provide the patient with the additional benefit of improved sleep. Unfortunately, anticholinergic side effects are rather common and can exacerbate underlying autonomic neuropathy, causing worsening of urinary bladder dysfunction and/or constipation. An alternative to amitriptyline is desipramine, a tricyclic antidepressant drug with a low anticholinergic side effect profile. This medication often can be tolerated at the higher doses that may be required to provide the maximum pain control. However, it is much less sedating than amitriptyline. In addition to their anticholinergic side effects, these drugs can potentiate orthostatic hypotension. Customarily, tricyclic antidepressant medications are started at relatively low doses (e.g., 25 mg qhs) because a small percentage of patients may have a very favorable response to such low doses. Usually, however, the dose must be increased slowly to more conventional levels of 100 to 150 mg qhs. Phenothiazines, alone, or in conjunction with antidepressants, have been reported to be effective in the treatment of painful GSMP-DM. However, it is difficult to justify the risk of tardive dyskinesia against the limited potential benefit of these drugs. The serotonin re-uptake inhibitor antidepressant medications, fluoxetine hydrochloride (Prozac) and paroxetine (Paxil), have also been used, in conventional antidepressant dosages. It is unclear whether these drugs are effective analgesics in these patients, or whether they are simply treating an underlying depressive reaction that is commonly present.

Mexiletine (Mexitil), an oral lidocaine derivative, has proven beneficial in the treatment of diabetic painful neuropathy. Beginning slowly with low doses of 150 mg/day for the initial 3 days, then progressing to 300 mg/d for the next 3 days and finally giving 10 mg/kg body weight daily in divided doses thereafter allows patients to tolerate the drug's frequent side effects of gastrointestinal disturbance, dizziness, and tremor. Mexiletine has a distinct advantage over the tricyclic antidepressants: it has no anticholinergic side effects that can potentiate underlying autonomic neuropathy. However, it can conceivably aggravate underlying cardiac arrhythmia, and thus should be used with caution in patients with such disturbances. The topical use of creams containing capsaicin (a component of certain hot pepper plant species), has reportedly provided pain relief in some patients. Capsaicin's mechanism of action has been attributed to depletion of substance P, a neurotransmitter for nociceptive afferent fibers and type C fibers. The depletion of substance P is likely to be secondary to its release from nerve terminals, a process that often initially produces sensations of local burning, warmth, and pain. This side effect, as well as the limitations of applying the cream over larger areas of the lower extremities that may be affected by painful symptoms, has tempered enthusiasm for this drug.

Clonazepam and Clonidine, an α_2-adrenergic agonist have also been proposed as effective treatment for painful diabetic neuropathy. Neither drug has been studied sufficiently to determine its precise role, if any. Treatments such as soaking feet in ice cold water and using transcutaneous electrical nerve stimulation (TENS) units usually are not effective or practical therapies.

Fortunately, for most patients with painful GSMP-DM, the intense, severe pain is self-limited and resolves spontaneously over a period of several months. This is an important point to emphasize to those who are undergoing treatment, especially if initial therapies are not effective.

DIABETIC POLYRADICULOPATHY

GSMP-DM constitutes approximately 75 percent of all diabetic neuropathies. The other 25 percent is composed of a variety of entities; the one often responsible for the most disabling symptoms is diabetic polyradiculopathy.

Diabetic polyradiculopathy, similar to *diabetic neuropathy,* is an umbrella term; it includes several diabetes-induced clinical disorders that affect predominantly the proximal PNS limb and trunk fibers, frequently in an asymmetric fashion. Included under this group designation are what were formerly considered independent syndromes (e.g., diabetic amyotrophy and diabetic thoracic radiculopathy), some neuropathic processes responsible at times for the lower extremity weaknesses associated with diabetes mellitus (e.g., diabetic footdrop), and some more diffuse disorders. Diabetic polyradiculopathy frequently appears in classifications of diabetic neuropathy under such terms as *asymmetric* or *symmetric proximal motor neuropathy.*

Although diabetic amyotrophy, the most common subgroup of diabetic polyradiculopathy, was well described by Garland and Taverner in 1953, it was not until 1981 that Bastron and Thomas proposed a unifying concept linking all the subgroups. They suggested that several of the non-GSMP-DM types of diabetic neuropathy have a common, underlying basis: injury, often sequential, of various lumbar, thoracic, and occasionally cervical roots due to diabetes mellitus. This hypothesis has not been universally accepted, primarily because there is considerable controversy regarding the exact site of nerve fiber damage (e.g., roots, plexus, peripheral nerves) in diabetic amyotrophy. Nonetheless, it has considerable appeal because it permits what appears to be a number of independent neuropathic syndromes linked only by underlying diabetes mellitus to be viewed in a coherent manner, with regard to clinical features and prognosis.

Diabetic polyradiculopathy affects the motor and sensory root fibers, causing axon degeneration, presumably from ischemia. Characteristically, it severely involves one root, or two or more contiguous roots. Although the process may remain focal, it frequently spreads to additional root(s), either contiguous ones ipsilaterally or, particularly, the corresponding contralateral root(s). This "territorial extension" occurs in nearly 70 percent of patients. The L2, L3, and L4 roots are the ones most likely to be affected, producing the clinical syndrome termed *diabetic amyotrophy.* The next most common subgroup is the syndrome of diabetic thoracic radiculopathy, in which one or more thoracic roots, usually the lower ones (e.g., T6–T12), are affected. GSMP-DM frequently coexists with diabetic polyradiculopathy. The simultaneous occurrence of these two independent diabetic PNS disorders can create confusion regarding the nature of the underlying pathophysiology.

Diabetic polyradiculopathy involving the L2–L4 roots (diabetic amyotrophy) has a variable mode of onset and evolution. Typically, it occurs in patients over the age of 60 who have relatively mild diabetes mellitus, often NIDDM. Most commonly, it begins unilaterally in the anterior aspect of the proximal lower extremity with severe pain, followed by significant weakness and atrophy of the anterior thigh muscles. The pain typically subsides after several weeks, although it may last much longer. Weakness, however, persists and is often accompanied by a relatively profound inexplicable weight loss, sometimes reaching 10 percent of body weight or greater. This constellation of symptoms often raises suspicion of an underlying malignancy.

Neurologic examination frequently discloses atrophy of the anterior thigh muscles and a reduced or absent patellar tendon reflex. Muscle testing usually reveals weakness of hip flexors, knee extensors, and thigh adductors. The presence of abnormalities in the distribution of both the femoral and obturator nerves suggests, on clinical grounds, that the responsible lesion involves the lumbar plexus or L2–L4 roots. Many patients also have clinical evidence of GSMP-DM of varying severity.

Diabetic amyotrophy may also present in a bilaterally symmetric, painless fashion, with clinical features identical to those described above. Intermediate syndromes of bilateral but asymmetric painless weakness as well as other variations may occur.

The differential diagnosis of diabetic polyradiculopathy affecting the L2–L4 roots includes a lumbar intraspinal lesion causing L2–L4 root compression, a lumbar plexopathy, and a femoral mononeuropathy.

Electrodiagnostic studies usually are very helpful in documenting motor axon loss in the L2–L4 myotomes, including the thigh adductors, thereby excluding femoral mononeuropathy. The high or midlumbar paraspinal muscles typically show prominent active denervation, making a lumbar plexopathy less likely. It is usually necessary to perform imaging studies on the lumbar spine, either a magnetic resonance imaging scan or computed tomography myelogram, to exclude a compressive lesion in the lumbar intraspinal canal. In certain patients, cerebrospinal fluid examination to exclude inflammatory lesions or infiltration of the subarachnoid space with malignant cells is also advisable. In patients with the painless symmetric syndrome, the electrodiagnostic studies are helpful in excluding myopathy, as are serum creatine kinase and aldolase assays.

Diabetic polyradiculopathy may also involve the lower lumbar and sacral (L5–S2) roots, although this usually occurs in conjunction with higher lumbar (L2–L4) root involvement. One of the prominent clinical features of diabetic L5 radiculopathy is footdrop. Bilateral footdrop from bilateral diabetic L5 radiculopathy is often mistakenly attributed to severe GSMP-DM. Diabetic, rather than compressive, L5 radiculopathy should be suspected whenever a patient with diabetes mellitus develops substantial L5 myotomal weakness and pain that is not relieved by bed rest and is more severe at night.

Diabetic thoracic radiculopathy results when diabetic polyradiculopathy affects thoracic roots, either in isolation or by territorial extension from ipsilateral L2–L4 involvement. Usually, one or more of the T6–T12 roots is involved unilaterally or, less often, bilaterally. The characteristic symptom is severe, persistent pain in the mid- or lower thoracic region, radiating to the upper or midabdomen. A dermatomal sensory loss is often demonstrable. The thoracic motor, as well as sensory, fibers are sometimes affected, but generally this is subclinical and discovered only upon needle electrode examination of the thoracic paraspinal and/or abdominal muscles. The symptoms of diabetic thoracic radiculopathy frequently are attributed to an intra-abdominal disorder. Many asymptomatic gallstones have been removed in an attempt to treat the pain caused by diabetic thoracic radiculopathy. Even when it is appreciated that the lesion is at the root level, other causes for thoracic radiculopathies must be excluded. Neuroimaging studies, and sometimes other tests as well, are indicated.

Rarely, diabetic polyradiculopathy may involve cervical roots. Typically, the midcervical roots, particularly C5–C7, are bilaterally affected. This usually occurs in combination with L2–L4 root involvement.

Diabetic polyradiculopathy has a favorable ultimate prognosis. Approximately three-quarters of patients will show satisfactory functional recovery after 1 year. Therapy consists primarily of pain management and an aggressive physical therapy program for gait training, to prevent falls and injuries and eventually to assist during the recovery phase.

PERIPHERAL MONONEUROPATHIES

Whether compression/entrapment mononeuropathies have a higher incidence in diabetic patients who do not have GSMP-DM than in nondiabetics is debated. Nonetheless, it is indisputable that some mononeuropathies occur with a markedly increased frequency in diabetics with GSMP-DM.

Median neuropathy at the wrist, or carpal tunnel syndrome and ulnar neuropathy at the elbow, both often bilateral, are particularly common in patients with GSMP-DM. An important point is that patients with GSMP-DM whose lower extremity symptoms are strictly distal to the knees are not likely to develop sensory complaints in their hands due to the polyneuropathy. Consequently, patients with known mild GSMP-DM who complain of hand pain and paresthesias usually have superimposed median and/or ulnar mononeuropathies. Neurologic examination of the upper extremities will often provide evidence of this, and electrodiagnostic studies are very useful in confirming the presence of these superimposed lesions. Carpal tunnel syndrome and ulnar neuropathy at the elbow should be managed aggressively in order to preserve nerve function in the hand. This requires carpal tunnel release or ulnar nerve transposition in patients with severe, progressive symptoms. There is good evidence that these lesions respond as well to surgical treatment as similar lesions do in patients who do not have underlying GSMP-DM.

A syndrome of neuroneuritis multiplex is occasionally observed in patients with diabetes mellitus. Typically, patients note acute pain associated with a sensorimotor deficit in the distribution of the affected nerve. This mode of onset is suggestive of an acute ischemic mechanism. Multiple nerves may be affected in a random, stuttering fashion. Differential diagnosis includes vasculitic neuropathy.

CRANIAL MONONEUROPATHIES

Isolated cranial neuropathies affecting the third, sixth, and occasionally the fourth cranial nerves occur with increased frequency in diabetic patients. The most common cranial nerve syndrome is diabetic oculomotor (third nerve) neuropathy. This typically affects patients over the age of 50 years and is quite rare in children. Usually, it develops abruptly; in approximately one-half of these patients, the oculomotor weakness is preceded by pain, frequently severe, located in the periorbital region. Occasionally, the pain precedes the weakness by several days. The clinical examination typically discloses oculomotor palsy with sparing of the pupillary fibers. This contrasts with compressive lesions of the oculomotor nerve, in which the pupillary fibers usually are the first to be affected. Pupillary sparing has been attributed to ischemia occurring centrally within the third nerve, resulting in the peripherally located parasympathetic pupilloconstrictor fibers being preserved. Nevertheless, the differential diagnosis of diabetic oculomotor palsy must include mass lesions causing third-nerve compression, including aneurysms of the posterior communicating artery. Evaluation of a patient with diabetic oculomotor neuropathy usually requires brain imaging, and sometimes lumbar puncture and angiography are indicated.

Much less often, an isolated palsy of the abducens nerve may result from diabetes mellitus. Isolated diabetic trochlear neuropathies are rare; more often they occur in conjunction with third- or sixth-nerve palsies. The differential diagnosis of these, as for oculomotor palsy, includes space-occupying lesions and inflammatory disorders. Idiopathic facial neuropathy (Bell's palsy) may occur with increased frequency in diabetic subjects, but the evidence for this is somewhat inconclusive.

Diabetic cranial neuropathies are occasionally recurrent; nonetheless, they are usually associated with a favorable prognosis and a good functional recovery.

SUGGESTED READINGS

Bastron JA, Thomas JE: Diabetic polyradiculopathy. Mayo Clin Proc 56:725, 1981

Brown MJ, Asbury AK: Diabetic neuropathy. Ann Neurol 15:2, 1984

Brown MJ, Greene DA: Diabetic neuropathy: Pathophysiology and management. p. 126. In Asbury AK, Gilliatt RW (eds): Peripheral Nerve Disorders. Butterworths, London, 1984

Dejgard A, Petersen P, Kastrup J: Mexiletine for treatment of chronic painful diabetic neuropathy. Lancet i:9, 1988

Diabetes Control and Complications Trial Research Group: The effect of intensive treatment of diabetes on the development and progression of long-term complications in insulin-independent diabetes mellitus. N Engl J Med 329:977, 1993

Garland H, Taverner D: Diabetic myelopathy. Br Med J 1:1405, 1953

Greene DA, Pfeifer MA: Diabetic neuropathy. p. 223. In Olefsky JM, Sherwin RS (eds): Diabetes Mellitus: Management and Complications. Churchill Livingstone, New York, 1985

Greene DA, Sima AAF, Albers JW et al: Diabetic neuropathy. p. 4. In Rifkin H, Porte D (eds): Diabetes Mellitus: Theory and Practice. Elsevier, New York, 1990

Halter JB, Porte D: The clinical syndrome of diabetes mellitus. p. 3. In Dyck PJ, Thomas PK, Asbury AK et al (eds): Diabetic Neuropathy. WB Saunders, Philadelphia, 1987

Max MB, Lynch SA, Muir J et al: Effects of desipramine, amitriptyline, and fluoxetine on pain in diabetic neuropathy. N Engl J Med 326:1250, 1992

Mulder DW, Lambert EH, Bastron JA et al: The neuropathies associated with diabetes mellitus. Neurology 11:275, 1961

Wilbourn AJ: Diabetic neuropathies. p. 477. In Brown WF, Bolton CF (eds): Clinical Electromyography. 2nd Ed. Butterworth-Heinemann, Boston, 1993

95. METABOLIC NEUROPATHY

DAVID H. WEINBERG

Peripheral nerves diseases are commonly encountered in both primary care and specialized neuromuscular medical practices. A seemingly endless list of diagnostic considerations confronts the thoughtful practitioner. The array of metabolic disorders

TABLE 95-1. Critical Features of Metabolic Diseases Associated with Neuropathies[a]

Disease States	Medical Associations	Additional Neurologic Signs	PN Type	Frequency	Miscellaneous
Nutritional/gastrointestinal disorders and neuropathy					
Vitamin B$_1$ deficiency (beriberi)	Alcoholism	Wernicke's encephalopathy	A	U	Usually chronic; rare acute or subacute PN
Vitamin B$_6$ deficiency	Drug-induced pernicious anemia or gastrointestinal disease (gastric or ileum)		A	R	Chapter 116
Vitamin B$_{12}$ deficiency		Myelopathy, encephalopathy	A	C	Megaloblastic anemia; myeloneuropathy distinctive
Folate deficiency	Malabsorption/diet		?	R	Sensory PN—unlikely
Vitamin B$_2$ deficiency	Malabsorption/diet	Possible "burning feet" syndrome	?	R	PN—unlikely
Niacin deficiency (pellagra)	Malabsorption/diet		R		PN—unlikely
Vitamin E deficiency	Malabsorption	Central nervous system prominent, myopathy and ophthalmoplegia	A	R	Red blood cells: acanthocytes PN small part of syndrome
Hypophosphatemia	Hyperalimentation	Subacute, severe PN	A?	R	Can simulate Guillain-Barré syndrome; <1 mg/dl
Chronic renal failure and neuropathy					
Uremia	End-stage CRF		A	C	Rare acute PN; CC < 5 ml/min
CTS	CRF	Mononeuropathy	M	C	CTS and UN usually
Shunt ischemia	Arteriovenous fistula	Mononeuropathy	A	R	Median and UN usually
Endocrine and neuropathy					
DM	Overt glucose intolerance		A	C	Chapter 111
Hypothyroidism	Myxedema	CTS or rare PN	M	U	
Hyperthyroidism	Overt Graves' disease	Rare "Basedow's paraplegia" or CTS or rare PN	A / PN	M / R	Common NMJ and muscle involvement
Acromegaly	Overt acromegaly DM			R	Mild PN; late onset
Hyperparathyroidism		MND-like syndrome: resolves with medication	?	R	Hypercalcemia
Psychiatry and neuropathy					
Porphyrias	Psychaitric Gastrointestinal: abdominal pain Variegate porphyria: cutaneous involvement	Subacute PN	A	R	Acute recurrent attacks; adolescent onset or frequent latent state; + FH
Metabolic neuromuscular disease in the intensive care unit					
Critical illness PN	Sepsis, encephalopathy, respiratory failure	Subacute PN	A	C	Motor signs dominate
NMJ blockade	NMJ blockers + steroids	Not PN	*	U	Pure motor
Myopathy	Renal ± hepatic insufficiency	Not PN	*	U	Pure motor

Abbreviations: A, axonal; M, mixed; U, uncommon; R, rare; C, common; CC, creatinine clearance; UN, ulnar neuropathy; CTS, carpal tunnel syndrome; PN, polyneuropathy; NMJ, neuromuscular junction; DM, diabetes mellitus; CRF, chronic renal failure.

[a] Disorders not covered in this chapter are referenced for the appropriate chapter.

that affect the peripheral nerves superficially appear the most formidable. This chapter presents a systematic approach for the consideration of these diseases.

First, it is essential to remember that the generalized polyneuropathies associated with metabolic diseases are almost exclusively of the axonal type with clear systemic manifestations of the underlying disease. Additionally, with the possible exception of an unusual case of vitamin B$_{12}$ deficiency or diabetes mellitus (Ch. 94), metabolic polyneuropathies are unlikely to be identified on a screening laboratory battery of tests for an axonal polyneuropathy in the absence of key systemic manifestations. Table 95-1 presents the conditions covered in this chapter with the critical associated medical symptoms or common laboratory abnormalities that should "raise the red flag" and direct the focus of the medical workup to identify these metabolic disorders.

Within the constraints of a such a broad chapter, whenever possible, the major topics are organized to reflect the symptoms or defining features of the associated metabolic disease to facilitate the pattern recognition necessary for diagnosis.

NUTRITIONAL AND GASTROINTESTINAL DISORDERS

The mechanism for the development of nutritional neuropathies in the United States and other industrialized countries occurs as a result of malabsorption, chronic alcoholism, dietary faddism, or drug toxicity (e.g., isoniazid). Usually dietary imbalance rather than starvation is active and conditions that increase the metabolic demands for the vitamin are often present (e.g., pregnancy, surgery, infection, growth).

Vitamin B$_1$ (Thiamine) Deficiency

In the United States, most thiamine deficiency cases occur in alcoholics. In chronic gastrointestinal diseases that can lead to reduced thiamine (such as vomiting and malabsorption), Wernicke's encephalopathy has occurred, but not commonly polyneuropathy. The predominant manifestation of thiamine deficiency in alcoholics is also Wernicke's encephalopathy. There is still much debate about the etiology of the peripheral neuropathy that is also seen. Some believe it is a direct toxic affect of alcohol, whereas others contend it is a manifestation of thiamine deficiency (beriberi). In third world regions where the diet is based on machine-milled rice, beriberi is still a common disease.

Clinical Features.   The onset of the polyneuropathy tends to be chronic (or subacute) with dominant sensory complaints: paresthesias, numbness, and dysesthesias. Pain and cramps in the calves are often present and the majority have edema of the face and ankles. The examination reveals graded distal limb sensory abnormalities typical of axonal "dying back" polyneuropathies. Most have a modest degree of distal weakness and depressed ankle jerks. Some patients have enlarged hearts and others modest elevations in the serum creatine kinase levels. Both the signs and symptoms are potentially reversible following replacement.

Treatment.   Intravenous thiamine is recommended initially at doses of 10 to 100 mg/day for 3 days, then 2.5 to 25 mg/day orally until the circumstances promoting the deficiency are reversed.

Vitamin B$_{12}$ (Cobalamin) Deficiency

There is great variability in the clinical presentation of this deficiency state. The most common manifestations are hematologic (megaloblastic anemia), gastrointestinal (gastric or terminal ileum disease) and neurologic. Spinal cord involvement represents the classic neurologic syndrome; however, a sensorimotor polyneuropathy is becoming more frequently appreciated. It is rarely isolated from spinal cord disease, making the clinical appearance distinctive (myeloneuropathy). The earliest symptoms could represent both central and peripheral neuropathic components: paresthesias, distal loss of proprioception, and to a lesser extent, impaired superficial sensation, depressed deep tendon reflexes and occasionally mild distal weakness. Signs of a myeloneuropathy subsequently develop with Babinski signs and, at times, brisk knee jerks. Impaired cognitive function can also occur with confusion, irritability, depression, memory impairment, or an altered state of arousal.

The diagnosis of cobalamin deficiency is often delayed, especially when the megaloblastic changes are absent or mild. Central nervous system signs and symptoms are often misinterpreted as multiple sclerosis or other central processes, and the peripheral nerve abnormalities are subtle. Folic acid supplementation can abolish the anemia and suppress the megaloblastic changes but not protect the central or peripheral nervous system from damage.

The great majority of B$_{12}$-deficient patients have pernicious anemia, the antibody-mediated destruction of intrinsic factor. Dietary inadequacies and local gastric or terminal ileum diseases preventing absorption are less likely etiologies.

Laboratory Features.   Most patients with B$_{12}$ deficiency have megaloblastic anemia, but those without it do have megaloblastic bone marrow changes. Serum B$_{12}$ levels represent the principal diagnostic test but it is neither completely sensitive nor specific. If clinical suspicion is high with a normal or equivocal B$_{12}$ value, further testing should be done. Methylmalonic acid is a critical cobalamin-requiring precursor involved in DNA synthesis that is increased in B$_{12}$ deficiency. Both serum and urine levels are elevated in most patients. More recently, holo-trans-cobalamin II, a necessary B$_{12}$ transport protein, has been found to be deficient in the serum of these patients. The role of this latter test is still being defined. If B$_{12}$ deficiency is diagnosed, a Schilling's test is necessary to evaluate intrinsic factor function by determining the absorptive capacity of B$_{12}$. Impaired B$_{12}$ absorption due to deficient intrinsic factor is characteristic of pernicious anemia. Intrinsic factor antibodies are fairly specific for pernicious anemia but not very sensitive, since upward of 40 percent of patients will have negative test results. Antiparietal cell antibodies are more sensitive but considerably less specific, limiting their usefulness.

Treatment.   The conventional protocol is 1,000 μg cyanocobalamin intramuscularly daily for the first week, followed by weekly injections for 1 month, then monthly injections lifelong. Oral cyanocobalamin is felt to be equally efficacious at 1 mg daily, but it has never gained general acceptance. Rapid improvement is noted almost immediately after treatment is begun, and a more gradual recovery will follow over the next 4 to 6 months. Adequate folate intake is also necessary.

Vitamin B$_6$ (Pyridoxine) Deficiency

In the adult, the pyridoxine deficiency polyneuropathy is seen exclusively in patients on specific medications (i.e., isoniazid, penicillamine, cycloserine, hydralazine). This is expanded further in Chapter 115 (toxic neuropathy).

Other Water-Soluble Vitamin Deficiency States

A limited number of reports have proposed a predominately sensory polyneuropathy associated with folate deficiency. Riboflavin (vitamin B$_2$) is alleged to be responsible for "burning feet" syndrome seen in some malnutrition/malabsorption states. Pellagra is caused by niacin deficiency, but it is unclear if there is an associated polyneuropathy syndrome. If so, it is certainly mild and not a major element of the disease.

Vitamin E Deficiency

There is increasing evidence that a profound vitamin E deficiency during childhood and adolescence may be responsible for a distinctive combination of central nervous system (CNS), peripheral nervous system, and muscle dysfunction. Again, the only recognized acquired human cause is malabsorption, and there can be a latency of many years before these rare neurologic problems slowly develop.

Clinical Features.   The earliest and most consistent neurologic findings are a loss of deep tendon reflexes, large-fiber sensory loss and sensory ataxia. The appreciation of pain and temperature are usually spared. Muscle weakness and atrophy occur, often in a proximal myopathic distribution. Many patients have a progressive external ophthalmoplegia. The peripheral neuropathy is usually overshadowed by CNS, ocular and systemic (gastrointestinal) involvement.

Laboratory Features.   A defining abnormality on the red blood cell smear is the presence of acanthocytes. Muscle and nerve biopsies are consistent with a large-fiber axonal polyneuropathy. Autopsies have also demonstrated a loss of spinal cord sensory fibers in the posterior columns and spinocerebellar tracts. Although a myopathy seems minimal in human disease, it is a prominent feature in all animal models.

Treatment.   Vitamin E replacement may prevent progression of the neuropathy. Oral doses of up to 5,000 to 10,000 mg/day are recommended, but parenteral intramuscular doses of 50 to 100 mg are preferred.

Hypophosphatemia

Hypophosphatemia, an unusual electrolyte abnormality, occurs almost exclusively in patients on hyperalimentation. The symptoms begin with tingling paresthesias on the tongue, fingers, and toes, but it can acutely progress to severe generalized areflexic weakness with impaired sensation and cranial mononeuropathies simulating Guillain-Barré syndrome. The serum phosphate level is always under 1 mg/dl.

RENAL INSUFFICIENCY

There are no clear peripheral nerve effects of acute renal failure; the neuromuscular problems are entirely from the muscle's response to altered electrolyte concentrations. In contrast, chronic renal failure (CRF) patients can suffer three potentially severe neuropathic consequences: (1) uremic polyneuropathy, (2) carpal tunnel syndrome and other compressive mononeuropathies, and (3) ischemic mononeuropathies.

Uremic Polyneuropathy

Clinical Features.   The symmetric, predominantly sensory symptoms of a slowly progressive polyneuropathy develop in end-stage disease when the creatinine clearance is less than 5 ml/min. The pattern of slowly ascending positive sensory phenomenon followed by distal numbness, and distal muscle atrophy and weakness is typical of the entire class of "dying back" axonal polyneuropathies. Other common but nonspecific symptoms include multifocal muscle cramping and the "restless legs" syndrome. The earliest signs of polyneuropathy include loss of vibration appreciation in the toes and depressed ankle reflexes. The early studies defining these features were done prior to hemodialysis, excluding an etiologic role for this procedure in the development of the polyneuropathy. Despite the fact that laboratory autonomic testing is often abnormal, the clinical correlate is usually not functionally significant.

A more rapidly progressive polyneuropathy with prominent motor features has been associated with CRF, with or without concomitant diabetes mellitus. Diabetes alone, critical illness polyneuropathy, or an inflammatory polyneuropathy would not explain all of the published cases. It would appear to be rare event relative to the common slowly progressive axonal polyneuropathy described above.

Laboratory Features.   Electromyelography (EMG) demonstrates an axonal polyneuropathy in most patients with CRF despite the fact that one-half have no symptoms. Some authorities recommend routine monitoring of the nerve conduction studies with an adjustment of dialysis to prevent the polyneuropathy, but most contend clinical observation and serum values of blood urea nitrogen and creatinine are adequate.

The sympathetic skin response and the R-R interval variation testing serve to evaluate sympathetic and parasympathetic autonomic function, respectively. Either or both of these tests can be abnormal in subpopulations of uremic patients. The sympathetic skin response correlates with the presence of a clinical dysautonomic syndrome of postural hypotension and impotence.

Course.   Adequate hemodialysis and peritoneal dialysis both halt the progression of uremic polyneuropathy, but improvement is rarely seen. Renal transplantation, however, results in a marked amelioration in the paresthesias within a few days or weeks. A more gradual resolution is seen in the fixed neurologic deficits over a period of weeks to months. As expected, the severity of the atrophy, weakness, and sensory loss predicts the pace and completeness of the recovery. The compressive mononeuropathies also improve. Renal rejection leads to a recurrence of the polyneuropathy; however, recovery is still expected if future transplantation is successful.

Carpal Tunnel Syndrome

Carpal tunnel syndrome and other mononeuropathies (such as an ulnar mononeuropathy) are commonly seen in these patients. At least in carpal tunnel syndrome, amyloid deposition (β_2-microglobulin) is often found in the wrist synovial and tendon tissues, leading to median nerve compression. Treatment is similar to that for the idiopathic mononeuropathy syndrome (see Ch. 100). The success of therapy depends upon the degree of axonal damage at the time it is rendered.

Ischemic Mononeuropathy Associated with Arteriovenous Fistulae

The most common vascular access for chronic hemodialysis is through a Brescia-Cimino arteriovenous fistula in the forearm (between the radial artery and the cephalic vein). The shunting of blood through the forearm results in variable degrees of ischemia distal to the fistula, which is exacerbated during hemodialysis. Thus, ischemic mononeuropathies can occasionally develop in either the median or ulnar nerves in the forearm, although it appears to be uncommon compared with the compressive lesions referred to above. The incidence and severity of this nerve damage appears higher for the less frequently used proximal arm fistulae. The development of symptoms or signs of a median, ulnar, or even a radial mononeuropathy in conjunction with the formation of one of these shunts justifies vascular ligation to prevent nerve damage.

ENDOCRINE NEUROPATHIES

With the exception of diabetes mellitus, which is covered in Chapter 94, peripheral nerve problems are uncommon in association with endocrinopathies.

Thyroid Disease

Hypothyroidism.   The majority of patients complain of distal paresthesias, but it is usually isolated to the hands and due to a compressive median nerve mononeuropathy (carpal tunnel syndrome). The symptoms often improve with thyroid replacement therapy, obviating the need for surgery. Infrequently, a mild axonal polyneuropathy or an EMG showing subclinical polyneuropathy is demonstrated. Rare case reports of a more severe large-fiber polyneuropathy have been published with predominantly demyelinating features on EMG and nerve biopsy.

Hyperthyroidism (Graves' Disease).   Hyperthyroidism is commonly associated with disorders of muscle and the neuromuscular junction but peripheral nerve dysfunction is usually quite modest. In clinically evident Graves' disease, the description of a flaccid paraplegia dates back to the nineteenth century (''Basedow's paraplegia''). It must be exceedingly rare, as is a distal axonal polyneuropathy, which may improve following treatment.

Acromegaly

Acromegaly is most commonly seen with a growth hormone–secreting tumor in the pituitary gland. The neurologic manifestations include both carpal tunnel syndrome, similar to that seen in hypothyroidism, and an axonal polyneuropathy. The early cases relating acromegaly and a polyneuropathy probably had concomitant diabetes mellitus (a common acromegaly complication). Symptoms usually occur late in the illness, are mild, and occur in the distribution of an typical axonal polyneuropathy.

Hyperparathyroidism

Weakness and fatigability are common presenting complaints of patients with hyperparathyroidism. At times, the weakness can be quite severe and dominates the sensory complaints. There are few systematic evaluations. The combination of generalized weakness, easy fatigability, atrophy, hyperreflexia, and limited, if any, sensory abnormalities suggests a motor neuron disease. It appears unlikely that the secondary hypercalcemia is responsible for the weakness.

Removal of the etiologic parathyroid adenoma is uniformly associated with rapid improvement in strength as well as the other associated signs.

PSYCHIATRY AND NEUROPATHY: THE PORPHYRIAS

The porphyrias are a group of seven hereditary disorders of heme biosynthesis, four of which can have an associated polyneuropathy (Table 95-2). Each form is associated with a specific enzymatic defect causing the accumulation of porphyrin precursors in its own unique patterns (Fig. 95-1). All of the ''neuroporphyrias'' (except plumboporphyria) have autosomal dominant inheritance but the penetrance is low. Thus, many ''asymptomatic'' relatives of an index patient will have the genetic defect and the potential to both develop and transmit the disorder. The key points in the identification of these conditions are the association with psychiatric (and often gastrointestinal) symptoms uniformly preceding the development of the polyneuropathy and the episodic nature of many symptoms.

Clinical Features. Acute intermittent porphyria, plumboporphyria, hereditary coproporphyria, and variegate porphyria all have similar neurologic manifestations, with hereditary coproporphyria and variegate porphyria also demonstrating photocutaneous lesions. Acute intermittent porphyria serves as the prototypic neuroporphyria by virtue of its frequency (yet all forms are rare).

The onset of symptoms is unusual before adolescence. There

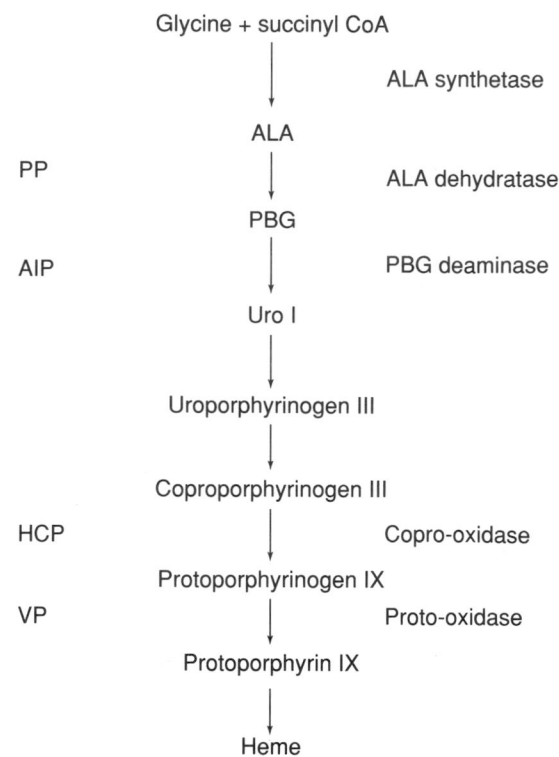

FIG. 95-1. Heme biosynthetic pathway with the neuroporphyrias listed on the left at the level of their respective enzymatic defects. PP, plumboporphyria; AIP, acute intermittent porphyria; HCP, hereditary coproporphyria; VP, variegate porphyria.

is great variability in the phenotypic expression, with clinically latent disease at times being associated with vague mood disorders. Early attacks usually consist of colicky abdominal pain with constipation, vomiting, and fevers. Attacks typically last days to weeks and recur intermittently. Psychiatric symptoms can accompany or precede the abdominal attacks, with many patients having long and complex psychiatric histories. The severity of the psychiatric episodes can vary considerably, but they often include psychotic behavior, visual hallucinations, and frank delirium.

Episodes are often associated with a defined group of established precipitating factors (Table 95-3) and symptoms can be

TABLE 95-3. Precipitating Factors Associated with Acute Porphyric Attacks

Drugs		Other Factors
Barbiturates	Methyldopa	Alcohol
Chlordiazepoxide	Phenytoin	Nutritional
Chlorpropamide	Rifampin	Hormonal
Ergotamines	Sulfonamides	Fever
Estrogens	Tricyclic antidepressants	Fasting
Griseofulvin		Sleep

TABLE 95-2. Nosology of the Porphyrias

Porphyria Types	Clinical Involvement	Diseases	Nomenclature (This Chapter)
Neuroporphyrias	Neuropsychiatric and gastrointestinal (autonomic)	AIP, PP	Neuroporphyrias
Neurocutaneous porphyrias	Mixed neuropsychiatric, gastrointestinal and cutaneous	HCP, VP	Neuroporphyrias
Cutaneous porphyrias	Cutaneous	PCT, EP, CEP	Not discussed

Abbreviations: ALA, δ-aminolevulinic acid; PBG, porphobilinogen; AIP, acute intermittent porphyria; PP, plumboporphyria; HCP, hereditary coproporphyria; VP, variegate porphyria; PCT, porphyria cutanea tarda; EP, erythropoietic porphyria; CEP, congenital erythroporphyria.

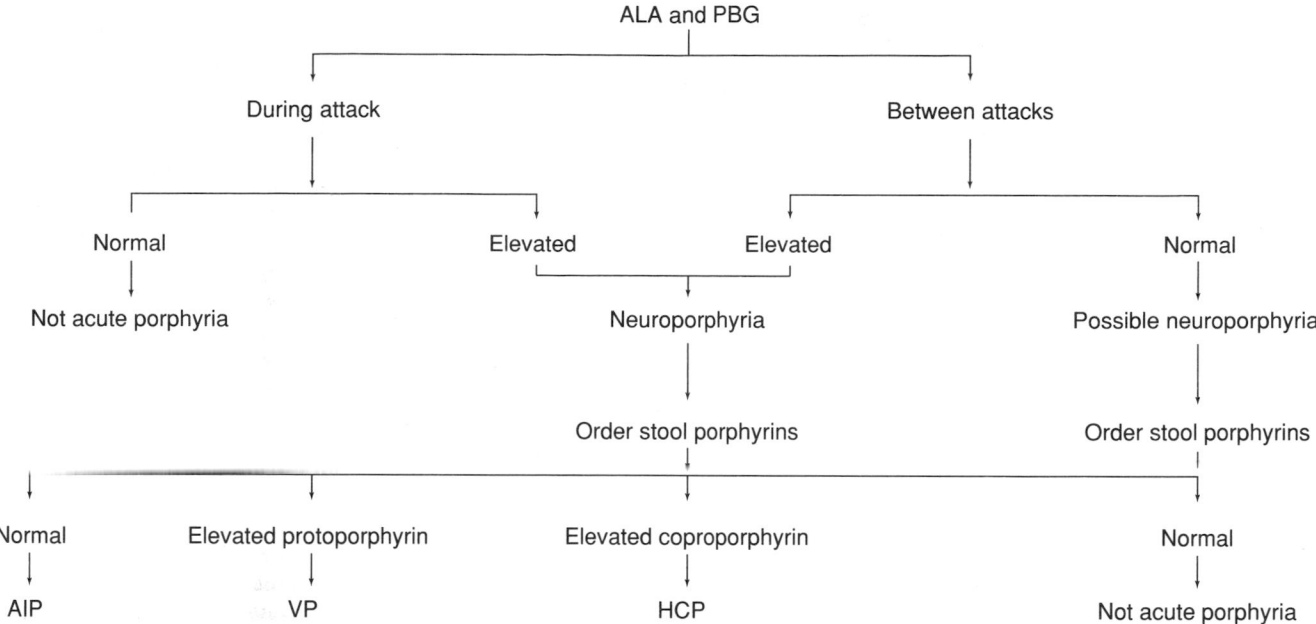

FIG. 95-2.   Laboratory flow diagram for suspected neuroporphyria starting with urinary ALA and PBG. ALA, δ-aminolevulinic acid; PBG, porphobilinogen; AIP, acute intermittent porphyria; HCP, hereditary coproporphyria; VP, variegate porphyria. (Modified from Tefferi A, Colgan JP, Solberg CA et al: Acute porphyrias: diagnosis and management. Mayo Clin Proc 69: 289–91, 1994, with permission.)

lessened by sleep or an intake of sugar. The porphyria-associated polyneuropathy rarely presents without prior bouts of abdominal pain and/or a psychiatric history. Unlike the majority of axonal polyneuropathies, the onset with porphyria is acute or subacute. Pain in the extremities or back can be significant, but weakness usually predominates. The weakness can begin either distally or proximally, with both asymmetric and symmetric distributions. Severe cases can progress to a flaccid quadriparesis with respiratory failure. Muscle tenderness and cramps are common, as are autonomic dysfunction and weakness in cranial musculature (ophthalmoplegia, ptosis, anisocoria, etc.).

Diagnostic clues to a porphyric polyneuropathy include an associated psychiatric and/or gastrointestinal illness, a positive family history, a relationship to specific precipitating factors (Table 95-3) and dark urine discoloration (porphobilinogen).

Laboratory Features.   Urine testing for heme biosynthetic intermediates is the best screening procedure for the neuroporphyrias. Figure 95-2 outlines the appropriate responses and interpretations, starting with the urine δ-aminolevulinic acid (ALA) and porphobilinogen (PBG) levels. If ALA and PBG are normal during an acute episode, those symptoms are not from one of the neuroporphyias. In acute intermittent porphyria, both ALA and PBG are usually increased, even between attacks. Enzyme measurements are reserved for confirmation of the diagnosis or to identify asymptomatic family members whose urine ALA and PBG are normal.

Neurophysiologic assessment of peripheral nerve function demonstrates predominantly axonopathy features, but changes of secondary demyelination may be present. This is distinct from Guillain-Barré syndrome, which the subacute motor course may simulate.

Course.   Typically, there is progression of the polyneuropathy over about 6 weeks. Attacks often involve all extremities,

cranial nerves, and respiratory muscles. Recovery begins within about 2 months of peak weakness, and although slow, it is usually complete.

Treatment.   Prevention is the most important intervention by avoiding provocative factors (Table 95-3). When an index patient is identified, it is crucial to search for carriers and asymptomatic patients so that education can prevent unnecessary exposures.

The development of a severe polyneuropathy requires an intensive care unit (ICU) setting. Hematin and glucose prevent ALA synthetase induction and are felt by some to alleviate symptoms over several days. One recommended protocol is initiated with intravenous glucose at 10 to 20 g/h. If there is no clinical change within 48 hours, hematin is added intravenously at 2 mg/kg/d. Potential systemic complications include hyponatremia, hypomagnesemia, azotemia, and autonomic instability.

METABOLIC NEUROMUSCULAR DISEASE IN THE INTENSIVE CARE UNIT (THE CRITICALLY ILL PATIENT)

Seriously ill ICU patients present a difficult problem for the consulting neurologist. Weakness has over the years been attributed to the metabolic demands of systemic illness, disuse, the concomitant development of Guillain-Barré syndrome, or the unmasking of unrecognized illnesses such as myasthenia gravis, motor neuron disease, and porphyria, among others. An enlarging and somewhat contradictory group of reports has recently been published describing weak patients in the ICU setting that do not fit these delineations. The following summary must be viewed as a work in progress with many of the subtleties yet to be defined.

When confronted with a weak patient in the ICU, the differential diagnosis is divided into four broad groups: (1) critical illness polyneuropathy, (2) neuromuscular junction blockade, (3) toxic myopathy, and (4) miscellaneous infrequent disorders that need to be considered.

Critical Illness Polyneuropathy

Critical illness polyneuropathy is a recently described disorder of surprising frequency in respirator-bound critically ill ICU patients. Many cases come to attention when unexplained ventilator dependency occurs in a patient during a complicated medical illness. Sepsis and multiple organ system failure appear to be necessary concomitants for the development of critical illness polyneuropathy, and usually a significant (septic) encephalopathy precedes the polyneuropathy. The encephalopathy complicates the diagnostic evaluation by limiting the sophistication of the neurologic examination during its evolution.

Clinical Features. Critical illness neuropathy represents an acute axonal polyneuropathy that is dominated clinically by motor signs with weakness, depressed, or absent reflexes and respiratory insufficiency. Sensory loss can be mild or absent clinically, although sensory nerves are usually involved pathologically and on neurophysiologic testing. About one-half of the cases can be demonstrated electrophysiologically before the clinical syndrome is evident.

Laboratory Features. EMG and spinal fluid evaluations are important to separate this condition from Guillain-Barré syndrome (in which demyelinating features on nerve conduction studies and an elevated spinal fluid protein are major differentiating points) and myopathy (in which the sensory potentials are normal). Low motor and sensory amplitudes are usually seen on nerve conduction studies, whereas the needle EMG examination characteristically contains fibrillation potentials and positive sharp waves in both the limb muscles and the diaphragms. These findings are consistent with an axonal degeneration disease mechanism. Neither demyelinating nor inflammatory features have been present on nerve biopsies.

Prognosis. The prognosis is fairly good if the patient survives the primary illness. Most patients gradually recover over weeks to months, often with a normal EMG at 6 to 12 months. No specific treatment has been demonstrated to hasten recovery.

Neuromuscular Junction Blockade

Following protracted exposure to certain nondepolarizing neuromuscular junction blocking agents (especially pancuronium and vecuronium), some patients have had prolonged and often severe weakness with depressed reflexes and normal sensation. Most of these patients have elevated levels of the drug, and in the case of vecuronium, elevated levels of the active metabolite (3-desacetylvecuronium). Renal insufficiency with or without hepatic insufficiency appears to be the critical associated feature responsible for the prolonged neuromuscular blockade.

The neuromuscular junction transmission defect is best demonstrated neurophysiologically with repetitive stimulation (decremental response), but many of the literature studies test mechanically with twitch tensions. The prognosis tends to be quite good, with recovery in hours to weeks. Treatment involves discontinuation of the offending agent, medical support, and treatment of associated illnesses such as renal failure.

Toxic Myopathy

Another group of patients has recently been identified who also develop acute, severe weakness following prolonged exposure to specific nondepolarizing neuromuscular junction blocking agents (again, usually pancuronium and vecuronium) but with normal neuromuscular junction function. The majority of these patients present with status asthmaticus and have also been given large doses of corticosteroids. Although similar patients have been described after high-dose steroids or neuromuscular junction blockers alone, the numbers are small compared with those following both. The combination of severe generalized weakness, respiratory failure, and depressed reflexes fits the phenotype of critical illness polyneuropathy and has been confused with this entity in the literature, but a myopathy has been convincingly demonstrated in some patients on both EMG and muscle biopsy. Thick myofilament (myosin) loss has been noted in several reports, but others have stressed a panfascicular muscle fiber necrosis. In these latter cases, the creatine kinase is markedly elevated, with the risk of rhabdomyolyis, but this has not been the case in all reports. The weakness tends to resolve over weeks to months. No specific treatment is known.

Miscellaneous Conditions

A series of other diagnoses are considered in the ICU setting, but retrospective and prospective studies suggest they must be quite uncommon. They include Guillain-Barré syndrome, myasthenia gravis, motor neuron disease, porphyria, nutritional neuropathies, spinal cord syndromes, and antibiotic toxicity, among others.

SUGGESTED READINGS

Aminoff MJ: Neurology and General Medicine. Churchill Livingstone, New York, 1989

Bolton CF: The polyneuropathy of critical illness. J Intensive Care Med 9: 132–8, 1994

Bolton CF, Young GB: Neurological Complications of Renal Disease. Butterworths, Boston, 1990

Joynt RJ: Baker and Baker's Clinical Neurology. JB Lippincott, Philadelphia, 1993

Schaumburg HH, Berger AR, Thomas PK: Disorders of Peripheral Nerves. FA Davis, Philadelphia, 1992

Swanson JW, Kelly JJ, McConahey WM: Neurological aspects of thyroid dysfunction. Mayo Clin Proc 56:504–12, 1981

Zochodne DW, Bolton CF, Wells GA et al: Critical illness polyneuropathy. Brain 110:819–42, 1987

96. INFECTIOUS AND GRANULOMATOUS NEUROPATHY

JONATHAN S. KATZ
WILSON W. BRYAN
RICHARD J. BAROHN

The infectious disorders that can produce a peripheral neuropathy include those that have been recognized for some time, such as leprosy and varicella-zoster, as well as more recently discovered conditions, such as Lyme disease and human immunodeficiency virus (HIV) infection. Whereas sarcoidosis does not have a proven infectious basis, it can produce an inflammatory neuropathy with granuloma formation, and therefore is included in this chapter.

LEPROSY

Leprosy is the most common cause of peripheral neuropathy in the world. Whereas leprosy has been a Third World health problem for centuries, cases in developed nations are becoming more common as immigration from endemic areas increases. The neurologic manifestations of this disease are also discussed in Chapter 54.

Mycobacterium leprae bacilli divide most actively between the temperatures of 27 and 30°C. Superficial tissues such as the anterior one-third of the eye, the testes, the upper respiratory tract, the skin, and the peripheral nerves, which are slightly below core body temperature, are preferentially infiltrated. The form of the disease that occurs in an individual patient depends on the host's T-cell-mediated immune response to *M. leprae*. Lepromatous (multibacillary) and tuberculoid (paucibacillary) leprosy are the two classic clinical presentations of the disease. Borderline leprosy is an intermediate form between lepromatous and tuberculoid leprosy.

Because of a strong host immune response, the disease manifestations in tuberculoid leprosy are relatively minimal when compared to lepromatous leprosy. A small number of sharply demarcated, hypopigmented, and slowly enlarging skin lesions are usually located on the extensor surfaces of the limbs, the face, or the buttocks. The lesions are anesthetic and dry, owing to involvement of small cutaneous nerves. Involvement (or invasion) of sensory or motor nerves that course below the skin lesions may produce a mononeuropathy. The sensory nerves most often affected are the digital, sural, radial, and posterior auricular nerves. The ulnar, median, peroneal, and facial nerves are the most susceptible sensorimotor nerves.

If the host immune response is deficient, there may be hematogenous spread of the bacillus, resulting in lepromatous leprosy. Because this form of the disease is known for its debilitating complications, early diagnosis is essential. The nodular, plaquelike skin changes and a sensory neuropathy occur symmetrically over the coolest surface areas, where the bacilli are abundant. The dorsal surfaces of the extremities and the pinnae of the ears are initially involved. If left untreated, the process spreads so that only the scalp, the crurae, and the axillae are spared. Invasion of superficial mixed nerves may produce palpable enlargements of the nerves and weakness. The ulnar nerve above the elbow is usually the first nerve affected, followed by the peroneal nerve. Eventually, a mononeuritis multiplex pattern becomes superimposed on the symmetric sensory neuropathy. Involvement of the superficial branches of the facial nerve creates a distinctive "buccinator smile" with characteristic series of wrinkles extending from the corner of the mouth, which results from sparing of the deep buccinator muscle. In addition, the patient is able to elevate only the lateral portion of the frontalis muscle. Repetitive trauma, skin ulcerations, and burns occur as the result of insensitivity to pain.

In cases where a peripheral neuropathy is accompanied by skin changes, the physician should consider the diagnosis of leprosy. Clues that help differentiate the neuropathy of leprosy from more common forms of peripheral neuropathy result from sparing of deeper and warmer tissues, where the bacilli are inactive. Muscle stretch reflexes are often preserved. Sensory loss spares the palms and soles, and autonomic modalities other than sweating are not involved. Nerve conduction studies may be normal if only small sensory nerves are involved; with more extensive disease, an axonal sensorimotor neuropathy can be documented.

Diagnosis is generally dependent on skin scrapings. Abundant bacilli in the subcutaneous tissues, which grow easily given the absence of a host immune response, are seen in the lepromatous form. In tuberculoid leprosy, in which the host reaction to the bacillus is intense, skin biopsy of the edge of a lesion shows granuloma formation and destruction of involved tissue, but the organisms are difficult to demonstrate. The lepromin skin test is positive in tuberculoid leprosy, but not in lepromatous leprosy.

For tuberculoid leprosy, the World Health Organization recommends dapsone and rifampin treatment for 6 months. In lepromatous and borderline forms, clofazimine is added and treatment is continued for at least 2 years or until skin smears show no evidence of bacteria. However, treatment may be required for many years, or even for life, in patients with extensive disease due to lepromatous leprosy.

Treatment is often accompanied by "leprosy reactions," also known as lepra type 1 and lepra type 2 reactions. The lepra type 1 reaction is caused by acceleration of the host immune response. Indolent skin and nerve lesions may suddenly become inflamed and tender and there may be a low-grade fever. In the more severe lepra type 2 reaction, the release of bacterial antigens causes immune complex deposition, producing erythema nodosum leprosum. Lepra type 2 complications include progression and formation of new nerve injuries, orchitis, arthritis, and iridocyclitis. Leprosy reactions may occur in untreated patients, often in the setting of a superimposed systemic illness. Treatment with prednisone may be necessary for severe type 2 reactions. Type 1 reactions should be treated with prednisone only if they threaten to cause nerve damage or disfiguring skin lesions. Treatment should be carried out for several months because reactions tend to recur when the prednisone is stopped.

Management of the insensitivity to pain involves the appropriate use of footwear and gloves. Splinting may be necessary to protect the wounds until healing is complete. Artificial devices to alert patients to pain have been ineffective.

LYME DISEASE

Lyme disease is caused by the spirochete *Borellia burgdorferi* that is transmitted by *Ixodes* ticks. Lyme disease is the most common vector-borne infection in the United States. However, although over 40,000 cases of Lyme disease have been reported to the Centers for Disease Control and Prevention over the last decade, the disease is restricted to the geographic regions where the vector is found. Endemic areas in the United States include the coastal Northeast, the upper Midwest, and the Pacific Coast. Whereas the disease has been reported year-round, the majority of cases occur in the spring and summer when ticks are most active.

There are early and late clinical stages of Lyme disease. The early stage can be further subdivided into localized and disseminated disease. Early localized Lyme disease includes the development of erythema chronicum migrans. This red macular rash usually expands from the center and develops a bull's-eye appearance. The rash is typically noted on the groin, axilla, or thigh and persists for 3 to 4 weeks. However, only 50 to 70 percent of patients infected by the organism after a tick bite develop erythema chronicum migrans. Flulike symptoms, including mild headache, chills, lymphadenopathy, or fever, may accompany the rash or occur alone.

Neurologic abnormalities eventually occur in 15 to 20 percent of patients with untreated early Lyme disease. Diffuse or focal meningeal inflammation characterizes the early disseminated form of the disease and occurs within days to weeks after the initial infection. Ten to 20 percent of cases involving the central nervous system are not preceded by erythema chronicum migrans. Meningitis occurs in 80 percent of patients with neurologic involvement. Meningeal symptoms may be mild or may fluctuate and consist of severe headache, nuchal rigidity, and malaise. Increased cerebrospinal fluid (CSF) protein and lymphocytosis are common. Cranial neuropathies, most often unilateral or bilateral Bell's palsy (although essentially any cranial nerve can be affected), occur in 50 percent of patients with neurologic abnormalities. Recovery is spontaneous and usually complete. Cardiac abnormalities (heart block, carditis, cardiomyopathy) can occur in up to 8 percent of patients in this stage of the disease. Chapter 59 gives a more detailed discussion of the general neurologic aspects of this disease.

Peripheral nerve involvement in the early disseminated stage usually takes the form of a radiculoneuritis. The initial manifestation is pain over a limb, the trunk, or the spine that begins subacutely and lasts for several days to months. The upper extremities are involved more often than the lower extremities. This eventually gives way to sensory and motor loss in the distribution of a nerve root, plexus, or peripheral nerve. The lesions may spread to involve multiple nerve distributions in a mononeuritis multiplex pattern. In addition, cases have been reported that appear similar to Guillain-Barré syndrome.

The chronic or late form of the disease occurs months to years after the onset of Lyme disease and is marked by the development of chronic arthritis. Diffusely aching muscles, psychiatric disturbances, and encephalomyelopathy may also occur at this stage. A peripheral neuropathy occurs in 30 to 50 percent of patients and is marked by painful paresthesias in a radicular distribution or a stocking-glove sensory loss. Electrophysiologic studies demonstrate an axonal sensorimotor neuropathy that may have a multifocal distribution.

The diagnosis of Lyme disease should be suspected in patients with a disorder of the peripheral nervous system following erythema chronicum migrans, or associated with aseptic meningitis. The diagnosis should also be considered in cases of mononeuritis multiplex and multiple cranial nerve palsies. If the only symptom is painful mononeuropathy, radiculopathy, or individual cranial nerve palsy, suspicion depends on whether the patient is from an endemic area. A history of a tick bite, outdoor work or activities, travel to an endemic area, or summer onset is also useful. However, Lyme disease is frequently overdiagnosed in patients with chronically aching muscles or subjective sensory problems, and this is largely due to the overinterpretation of abnormal serologic information (see below).

Because the spirochete is difficult to isolate from tissue, serologic testing has become the mainstay of diagnosis. Serum and spinal fluid testing for antibody to B. burgdorferi are commercially available. False-positive serum titers occur in 5 percent of healthy subjects; therefore, in nonendemic areas, the positive predictive value of the test extremely low. False positives have also been reported in syphilis, autoimmune diseases, and other neurologic disorders. Diagnosis depends on proving one of the following factors: previous physician-documented erythema chronicum migrans, specific CSF antibodies to B. burgdorferi,

a rise in convalescent serum antibody titer, or seroconversion from a negative titer. In patients with positive serum antibodies who do not meet the above criteria, Western blot analysis is useful as an adjunct to increase diagnostic specificity. False-negative results occur in the first 6 weeks of the infection before the patient has mounted a specific antibody response. Polymerase chain reaction may increase sensitivity in early infection prior to seroconversion, but this is available at only a few centers. In the chronic form of the disease, virtually 100 percent of patients should have serum antibodies to B. burgdorferi.

Most patients with neurologic involvement from Lyme disease require parenteral antibiotics. The exceptions to this are patients with early Lyme disease with isolated Bell's palsy or a mild neuropathy and normal CSF. For these patients, oral antibiotic therapy can consist of either 200 mg doxycycline twice a day or 500 to 1,000 mg amoxicillin three times a day for 30 days. For all other patients with neurologic manifestations, or if the CSF is abnormal, intravenous ceftriaxone, 2 g/d for 2 to 3 weeks, is considered the treatment of choice. Penicillin G, ampicillin, cefotaxime, doxycycline, and chloramphenicol are parenteral alternatives.

Patients with meningitis and radiculitis in the early stage of Lyme disease usually improve within days after beginning antibiotics. On the other hand, antibiotics probably do not affect the course of Bell's palsy due to Lyme disease, and patients with late neurologic involvement may respond very slowly over a period of months after therapy has been completed.

SARCOIDOSIS

Sarcoidosis is a generalized granulomatous process that typically affects the lungs, eyes, and parotid gland. Only in 5 percent of the cases is the central nervous system involved. In 50 percent of these patients, the neurologic manifestation is facial nerve paralysis. Involvement of other cranial nerves, including the optic, glossopharyngeal, vagus, and acoustic, may occur alone, or as part of a cranial mononeuritis multiplex (see Ch. 185).

Peripheral neuropathy occurs in only 8 percent of patients with neurosarcoidosis. The neuropathy may take one of several forms, including a sensorimotor axonal polyneuropathy, mononeuritis multiplex, cranial or unusual (e.g., phrenic nerve) mononeuropathy, lumbar plexopathy, or Guillain-Barré syndrome. A chronic, symmetric, sensorimotor axonal polyneuropathy was the most common presentation in a recently published small series of sarcoid neuropathy patients (see Zuniga et al., 1991). These patients complain of paresthesias and numbness in the toes and fingers, often associated with burning, dysesthetic pain. On examination, there is a stocking-glove loss to all sensory modalities, distal areflexia, and some patients may have distal weakness. Neurosarcoidosis may also present as mononeuritis multiplex with involvement of spinal roots or individual nerves. These patients often have cranial mononeuropathies as well. Patients may have unusual mononeuropathies, including patches of sensory loss on the trunk or phrenic nerve involvement, resulting in diaphragm paralysis and respiratory symptoms. Lumbar plexopathy and Guillain-Barré syndrome have been reported as individual case reports, but it is not clear whether the diagnosis is part of, or coincidental with, sarcoidosis.

Even patients without clinical evidence of neuropathy may show a reduction in sensory nerve action potential amplitudes in one or more nerve. The cerebrospinal fluid in patients with neuropathy may show a mononuclear pleocytosis, elevation of protein, or may be normal.

In 50 percent of patients with neurosarcoidosis, neurologic symptoms are the presenting complaint. The chest x-ray will usually demonstrate hilar adenopathy or diffuse pulmonary involvement, and pulmonary function tests will reveal decreased lung volumes and diffusion capacity. The serum angiotensin-converting enzyme is often elevated, but lacks specificity and sensitivity. Ocular examination may show granulomatous uveitis. Definitive diagnosis requires tissue biopsy, usually of an enlarged lymph node. Up to 40 percent of muscle biopsies demonstrate granulomas, even in patients lacking specific signs and symptoms. Sural nerve biopsies may shown infiltration of the epineurium by inflammatory cells and granulomas with evidence of axon loss.

Patients with mild distal sensory or sensorimotor neuropathies may not warrant immunosuppressive therapy. However, in patients with significant weakness, mononeuritis multiplex, or cranial nerve palsies, a trial of oral prednisone is recommended. The initial prednisone dose is typically in the range of 60 mg/d and then is slowly tapered. Although isolated mononeuropathies often improve, very little is known about prognosis of distal symmetric neuropathy in patients with sarcoidosis.

HERPES ZOSTER RADICULITIS

Herpes zoster radiculitis or cranial neuritis (shingles) results from a reactivation of varicella-zoster virus infection. After primary infection, the virus presumably becomes latent in sensory ganglia, and over 90 percent of adults are seropositive for antibodies against varicella-zoster virus. Other relevant aspects of varicella-zoster virus infection are covered in Chapter 67.

There are generally no identifiable factors that precipitate reactivation of the infection. The reactivation produces a vesicular rash in a dermatomal distribution. The thoracic dermatomes are involved in over one-half of cases, but the eruption can also occur in cranial nerve distributions (especially trigeminal nerve branches) and along cervical and lumbosacral dermatomes. The vesicular rash may be preceded by pain and paresthesias in the dermatome region by a week or more. Systemic signs such as fever, malaise, and headache can occur. In the majority of patients who are not immunocompromised, the vesicles dry up and resolve within 2 to 3 weeks and there are no sequelae. Herpes zoster occurs at all ages, but the incidence increases with age. By the ninth decade of life, the incidence reaches approximately 1 percent per year. In addition, immunosuppression secondary to cytotoxic drugs and malignancy increases the risk of developing shingles and disseminated zoster.

In immunocompetent patients, oral acyclovir (800 mg five times/d for 10 days) significantly reduces the time for cutaneous healing and resolution of acute pain, but has no effect on the development of post-herpetic neuralgia. Intravenous acyclovir is highly effective in preventing dissemination of the rash in immunocompromised patients. The role of corticosteroids is more controversial. Since acyclovir has become available, there are no clear-cut indications for corticosteroids in the treatment of shingles, and they should especially be avoided in immunocompromised patients.

Post-herpetic neuralgia is generally defined as the persistence of pain for longer than 4 to 12 weeks after the onset of the rash. Post-herpetic pain develops in 10 to 20 percent of patients, and is significantly more common in patients who are immunocompromised or over 60 years old. The pain is most often continuous and burning, but lancinating pains occur frequently. The pain may be so severe as to be disabling. Pain persists in only 22 percent of patients at 1 year and in only 2 percent at 5 years.

Amitriptyline is an effective therapy for post-herpetic neuralgia. Other antidepressants such as desipramine are also effective and may be better tolerated. Carbamazepine is not effective in treating the constant burning neuralgia seen in these patients, but may be useful for lancinating pains. If tricyclics are not effective, the short-term use of narcotics should be considered. Topical application of capsaicin cream applied three or four times a day for 2 to 4 weeks may be effective in some patients. Capsaicin should not be applied while the vesicular rash is still present.

Less common delayed complications of zoster infection include encephalitis, cranial arteritis, cranial nerve palsies, transverse myelitis, urinary retention, and focal weakness. Focal weakness in an extremity or in a cranial nerve distribution occurs in 5 to 10 percent of shingles cases and usually begins 2 to 4 weeks after the onset of the rash. The most common example of focal motor paresis is the onset of facial palsy following herpes zoster otiticus (Ramsey Hunt syndrome). Weakness in cervical and lumbar root distributions also occurs. Thoracic muscle involvement is common, but is seldom clinically apparent. These complications occur more frequently in patients with underlying malignancies. CSF in patients with focal motor weakness may show a pleocytosis with elevated protein, but this finding is also seen in 50 percent of patients who have uncomplicated shingles. Recovery from focal weakness is expected in 70 to 80 percent of patients and is usually complete.

HIV-RELATED NEUROPATHIES

Clinical evidence of a peripheral neuropathy occurs in 15 to 30 percent of HIV-infected patients who have acquired immunodeficiency syndrome (AIDS). Subclinical evidence of neuropathy, either by electrophysiologic studies or on nerve pathology, is present in 50 to 90 percent of severely immunosuppressed patients. HIV patients who develop neuropathy usually have CD4 counts of fewer than 200 cells/mm^3 and other manifestations of severe immunosuppression, although a few of the various neuropathies associated with HIV infection have a tendency to occur earlier in the course of the disease. Other neurologic aspects of HIV infection are covered in Chapters 76 and 77.

The types of peripheral neuropathies that can occur in HIV-infected individuals are as follows:

Distal symmetric polyneuropathy
Lumbosacral polyradiculopathy/cauda equina syndrome
Mononeuritis multiplex
Inflammatory demyelinating polyneuropathy
Facial nerve palsy (Bell's palsy)
Herpes zoster radiculitis
Autonomic neuropathy
Sensory ataxia/ganglioneuronitis

As a general rule, inflammatory demyelinating neuropathies occur early, mononeuritis multiplex occurs at intermediate stages, and distal symmetric polyneuropathy and the lumbosacral polyradiculopathy/cauda equina syndrome occur late in the course of infection. Although there is no cure for AIDS, various therapeutic interventions that may provide relief for the patient are available for each type of neuropathy.

Distal Symmetric Polyneuropathy

Of the HIV-related neuropathies, distal symmetric polyneuropathy is the most common. As previously noted, it occurs in the late stages of HIV infection. The cause of the neuropathy is unknown. Whereas the HIV virus has been cultured from the peripheral nerve of several patients with this neuropathy, other toxic, metabolic, or nutritional factors (e.g., vitamin B_{12} deficiency) may play a role.

Patients with distal symmetric polyneuropathy first note numbness and paresthesias in the toes, and this later progresses to the fingers. Lancinating or burning pain occurs in many patients. On examination, there is a stocking-glove sensory loss to all modalities, although touch and vibration are more affected than proprioception. Muscle stretch reflexes are often lost only at the ankles. Some patients are actually hyperreflexic in the arms and at the knees, and this most likely reflects a coexistent HIV myelopathy. Of course, the sensory abnormalities can be due to either process, and electrophysiologic studies are needed to confirm the presence of neuropathy in these cases. Eventually, patients with the distal symmetric polyneuropathy can develop weakness in the feet and hands.

The primary pathologic process is sensorimotor axonal degeneration. Electrophysiologic findings consist of low-amplitude motor and sensory potentials on nerve conduction study. Conduction velocities are normal or only mildly reduced. Needle electromyelography (EMG) often reveals fibrillation potentials in distal extremity muscles and neurogenic motor units.

An HIV patient may be taking medication that can also produce distal symmetric polyneuropathy. Such medications include vincristine (for Kaposi sarcoma), dapsone (for pneumocystis pneumonia), and isoniazid and ethambutol (for mycobacterial infections). However, the most common drug-induced neuropathy in these patients is caused by the nucleosides dideoxycytidine (ddC) and dideoxyinosine (ddI) that are used for the treatment of HIV-infected patients. Peripheral neuropathy occurs in up to 50 percent of patients who receive ddC or ddI, and this is their primary limitation. A patient with an HIV-related distal sensory polyneuropathy may have worsening symptoms and signs when one of these neurotoxic drugs is added. Determining whether the neuropathy is HIV- or drug-related can be difficult, and often a trial-and-error approach of discontinuing the drugs and looking for improvement is necessary. However, even this approach is problematic, as some patients who have a nucleoside neuropathy will continue to worsen for up to 6 weeks after discontinuing the drugs, the so-called coasting period. Patients with an underlying HIV-related neuropathy seem to be predisposed to developing nucleoside neuropathies.

A review of the patient's medications for any potentially neurotoxic drugs that might contribute to the neuropathy should be made, and if possible, such drugs should be stopped or the dose decreased. Symptomatic treatments include tricyclic antidepressants, carbamazepine, phenytoin, nonsteroidal anti-inflammatory agents (NSAIDs), capsaicin cream, and transcutaneous electrical nerve stimulation (TENS).

Lumbosacral Polyradiculopathy/Cauda Equina Syndrome

The HIV-related lumbosacral polyradiculopathy or cauda equina syndrome is most often due to cytomegalovirus (CMV) infection. Weakness and sensory loss in the legs begin asymmetrically and progress rapidly over days or several weeks. Patients become profoundly weak in the legs and often lose the ability to walk. A lumbar sensory level and a neurogenic bladder usually develop. Patients may complain of back pain that radiates into the legs.

CSF findings include a polymorphonuclear pleocytosis, elevated protein, and a reduced glucose. CSF cultures will grow CMV, but this may require 5 to 10 days. Gadolinium-enhanced lumbosacral magnetic resonance imaging scans have demonstrated striking root enhancement of the cauda equina roots.

Electrophysiologic studies are not necessarily required for accurate diagnosis and therapeutic intervention of these patients. If nerve conduction studies are done, the initial findings are a loss of peroneal and tibial motor and sural sensory amplitudes. As the weakness becomes profound, the responses often become unobtainable. After 2 weeks of weakness, the needle EMG will show profuse fibrillation potentials in proximal and distal lower extremity muscles and motor units will have a neurogenic recruitment pattern.

Intravenous ganciclovir therapy should be initiated immediately, even before CSF culture results are available. If the patient fails to improve with ganciclovir, or is already on ganciclovir for CMV infection elsewhere (retinitis, pneumonia, hepatitis), foscarnet can be used as a second-line agent. Intravenous ganciclovir or foscarnet is continued for the remainder of the patient's life. Early institution of anti-CMV therapy in this disorder can improve strength and ameliorate sensory symptoms and pain in some patients. However, the long-term prognosis is poor, and most do not survive 6 months.

The differential diagnosis for the lumbosacral polyradiculopathy syndrome in AIDS patients consists of neurosyphilis, mycobacterium infections, and leptomeningeal lymphomatosis. These disorders are diagnosed by specific CSF studies for each disease (e.g., Venereal Disease Research Laboratory test [VDRL], mycobacterial culture, cytology) and the absence of confirmatory evidence for CMV infection.

HIV-Related Mononeuritis Multiplex

Mononeuritis multiplex is an uncommon HIV-related neuropathy. Patients present with asymmetric patches of sensory loss on the face, trunk, or extremities. Alternatively, symptoms can begin as footdrop or hand weakness or a cranial motor neuropathy. Symptoms may resolve spontaneously or they may progress to a more severe generalized neuropathy.

Patients with mononeuritis multiplex often can be placed into one of two groups: (1) patients earlier in the course of HIV infection with relatively preserved CD4 counts without evidence of CMV infection in other organs, and (2) those late in the course of HIV infection with very low CD4 counts who usually have evidence of CMV infection in other organs. Patients in the first group seem to have benign courses with spontaneous stabilization or improvement of the neuropathy. In the latter group, either the neurologic deficits may progress or the neuropathy may stabilize as the patient is treated for the extraneural CMV infection. This implies that at least some mononeuritis multiplex patients have CMV as the etiology of the neuropathy. However, the CSF in these patients does not show the dramatic abnormalities seen in the HIV-related cauda equina syndrome.

Electrophysiologic studies confirm either isolated mononeuropathies or an asymmetric sensorimotor axonal neuropathy. In general, electrophysiologic findings have not helped to distinguish this heterogenous group of patients.

Reports regarding the pathology have varied. Some investigators, especially in France, have found dramatic vasculitis of endoneurial and epineural nerve vessels. In the large collection of mononeuritis multiplex patients seen at San Francisco General Hospital, this was not the finding. Some component of axonal degeneration is found in most patients. CMV inclusion bodies have been reported in endothelial cells of peripheral nerves by some authors. The presence of vasculitis in some patients raises the possibility that the mononeuritis multiplex in some HIV-infected patients has an immune-mediated mechanism. There are reports of improvement with prednisone therapy in the patients with vasculitis. One patient was reported to have cryoglobulinemia and responded to plasmapheresis therapy.

One approach to diagnosis and treatment is as follows. First, assess the stage of HIV infection and the CD4 count. If the patient is early in the course of the infection, with a CD4 count of more than 200 cells/mm^3, the approach is more conservative, as many of these patients may spontaneously improve. EMG and nerve conduction studies can determine the distribution and extent of the neuropathy. A serum VDRL and FTA-ABS and a test for the presence of cryoglobulins should be obtained. If the neuropathy is predominantly sensory and limited in distribution, as it often is in this stage, following the patient closely is reasonable. A more aggressive approach is justified in a patient with a CD4 count of fewer than 200 cells/mm^3, who usually has a history of AIDS-related complications. CSF studies are necessary to test for mycobacterial, cryptococci, syphilis, or CMV infection and for lymphomatous meningitis. The patient should be evaluated for evidence of CMV infection in other organs (eye, gut, lung); if infection is present, anti-CMV drugs should be started. If there is no evidence for neural or extraneural CMV infection, a sural or superficial peroneal nerve biopsy should be considered. This is probably the only clinical situation in which it is necessary to obtain a nerve biopsy in an HIV-infected patient. If CMV inclusions are observed, treat the patient with the appropriate antiviral agent(s); if vasculitis is present and there is no evidence for CMV, consider immunosuppressive treatment with prednisone. If cryoglobulinemia is present, consider plasmapheresis.

Inflammatory Demyelinating Polyneuropathy in HIV-Infected Patients

Both acute (Guillain-Barré syndrome) and chronic (chronic inflammatory demyelinating polyradiculopathy) forms of inflammatory demyelinating polyneuropathy have been reported in HIV-infected patients. The clinical and electrophysiologic presentations of these disorders are similar to the non-HIV-related demyelinating neuropathies. The only distinguishing feature in HIV-infected patients is the presence of CSF pleocytosis (white blood cell count usually > 25/mm^3). Nerve biopsies are not necessary, but have revealed demyelination, remyelination, and inflammatory cells.

Inflammatory demyelinating polyneuropathy may occur more often early in the course of HIV infection, but this is controversial. Cases have been reported to begin at the time of presumed HIV seroconversion. However, a number of cases of demyelinating neuropathy presenting in AIDS patients have been reported.

Treatment is similar to that given to non-HIV-infected pa-

tients. Guillain-Barré syndrome patients receive either intravenous immunoglobulin (IVIG) or plasmapheresis. As there is a general reluctance to give immunocompromised patients corticosteroids, initial treatment of chronic inflammatory demyelinating polyradiculopathy with IVIG or plasmapheresis is reasonable. If these are not effective, prednisone can be used. In general, HIV-infected patients with inflammatory demyelinating polyneuropathy improve with time and therapy. Whether their recovery is worse than non-HIV-infected patients with similar neuropathies is unknown.

Facial Nerve Palsy (Bell's Palsy)

Bell's palsy occurs at the time of seroconversion, in the setting of AIDS or AIDS-related complex, or in the setting of Guillain-Barré syndrome and chronic inflammatory demyelinating polyradiculopathy. In most cases, the etiology is unknown.

Herpes Zoster Radiculitis

Up to 10 percent of HIV-infected patients develop herpes zoster radiculitis (shingles). Immunocompromised HIV-infected patients who develop shingles may have sustained periods of new lesion formation and a failure of existing lesions to heal in the absence of antiviral therapy. All HIV-positive patients who develop herpes zoster limited to a dermatome are treated with oral acyclovir. However, in more widespread or disseminated outbreaks, intravenous acyclovir should be administered.

Autonomic Neuropathy

HIV-infected patients can develop symptoms of presyncope, syncope, diminished sweating, diarrhea, impotence, and bladder dysfunction presumably due to an autonomic neuropathy. Most of these patients have AIDS and they often have a coexistent distal symmetric polyneuropathy.

Sensory Ataxia Due to Ganglioneuronitis

Four cases of subacute sensory ataxia have been reported in HIV-infected patients. These patients had profound proprioceptive deficits and areflexia without weakness. Autopsy findings revealed inflammatory infiltrates in the sensory ganglia and proximal roots. One case occurred at the time of HIV seroconversion, one case was in an asymptomatic HIV-positive patient, and two cases were patients with AIDS. As so few of these cases have been reported, the exact place of this condition in the spectrum of HIV-related neuropathies is uncertain.

SUGGESTED READINGS

Barohn RJ, Gronseth GS, LeForce BR et al: Peripheral nervous system involvement in a large cohort of human immunodeficiency virus-infected individuals. Arch Neurol 50:167, 1993

Bazan III C, Jackson C, Jinkins JR, Barohn RJ: Gadolinium-enhanced MRI in a case of cytomegalovirus polyradiculopathy. Neurology 41:1522, 1991

Coyle PK: Neurologic complications of Lyme disease. Rheum Dis Clin N Amer 19:993, 1993

Delaney P: Neurologic manifestations in sarcoidosis: review of the literature, with a report of 23 cases. Ann Int Med 87:336, 1977

Gelber RH: Hansen's disease. West J Med 158:583, 1993

Greenberg MK, McVey AL, Hayes T: Segmental motor involvement in herpes zoster: an EMG study. Neurology 42:1122, 1992

Halperin JJ, Little BW, Coyle PK, Dattwyler RJ: Lyme disease: cause of a treatable peripheral neuropathy. Neurology 37:1700, 1987

Heck AW, Phillips II LH: Sarcoidosis and the nervous system. Neurol Clin 7:641, 1989

Logigian EL, Steere AC: Clinical and electrophysiologic findings in chronic neuropathy of Lyme disease. Neurology 42:303, 1992

Max MB: Treatment of post-herpetic neuralgia: antidepressants. Ann Neurol (suppl.)35:S50, 1994

Miller RG, Parry GJ, Pfaeffl W et al: The spectrum of peripheral neuropathy associated with ARC and AIDS. Muscle Nerve 11:857, 1988

Miller RG, Storey JR, Greco CM: Ganciclovir in the treatment of progressive AIDS-related polyradiculopathy. Neurology 40:569, 1990

Parry GJ: Peripheral neuropathies associated with human immunodeficiency virus infection. Ann Neurol (suppl.)23:S49, 1988

Sabin TD, Swift TR, Jacobson RR: Leprosy. p. 1354. In Dyck PJ, Thomas PK, Griffin JW et al (eds): Peripheral Neuropathy. 3rd Ed. WB Saunders, Philadelphia, 1993

So YT, Olney RK: Acute lumbosacral polyradiculopathy in acquired immunodeficiency syndrome: experience in 23 patients. Ann Neurol 35:53, 1994

Steere AC: Lyme disease. N Engl J Med 321:586, 1989

Thomas JE, Howard Jr. FM: Segmental zoster paresis—a disease profile. Neurology 22:459, 1972

Wood MJ: Current experience with antiviral therapy for acute herpes zoster. Ann Neurol (suppl.)35:S65, 1994

Zuniga G, Ropper AH, Frank J: Sarcoid peripheral neuropathy. Neurology 41:1558, 1991

TABLE 97-2. Hematologic Diagnosis of 28 Patients With Plasma Cell Dyscrasias and Polyneuropathy

Diagnosis	Number
Monoclonal gammopathy of undetermined significance	16
Primary systemic amyloidosis	7
Multiple myeloma (includes osteosclerotic myeloma)	3
Waldenström's macroglobulinemia	1
γ-heavy-chain disease	1

(From Kelly JJ Jr, Kyle RA, O'Brien PC et al: Prevalence of monoclonal protein in peripheral neuropathy. Neurology 31:1480, 1981, with permission.)

97. DYSPROTEINEMIC POLYNEUROPATHY

JOHN J. KELLY, JR.

One of the major advances in our understanding of polyneuropathies since the 1980s has been the realization that dysproteinemias or plasma cell dyscrasias and their accompanying monoclonal proteins (M-protein) or immunoglobulins are frequently associated with neuromuscular diseases. These syndromes may be distinctive and in several cases, appear to be due to the direct effects of the M-protein on peripheral nerve. For instance, M-proteins have been found to react with a variety of neuronal antigens found in myelin sheaths and axonal membranes. This review outlines our current knowledge in this rapidly advancing field and provides a clinical approach to these patients.

EPIDEMIOLOGY

Based on prevalence surveys, it is estimated that up to 5 percent of all polyneuropathy patients have a monoclonal gammopathy. The majority of these are likely to be polyneuropathies associated with monoclonal gammopathy of undetermined significance (MGUS) (Tables 97-1 and 97-2), with lower percentages of other syndromes. Based on these estimates, although inexact, these disorders are undoubtedly underdiagnosed.

HEMATOLOGIC EVALUATION

A plasma cell dyscrasia or monoclonal gammopathy (Table 97-1) is defined as a proliferation of a single clone of plasma cells, either neoplastic or non-neoplastic, usually associated with the production of a monoclonal serum protein that can be measured in the serum, urine, or both. Monoclonal proteins, or more properly immunoglobulins, consist of a single heavy chain (IgM, IgG, IgD, or IgA) and a single light chain (κ or λ). Polyclonal gammopathies comprise both light chains and generally more than one heavy chain. Occasionally, only the light chain or heavy chain may be secreted by the clone of plasma cells. Until recently, M-proteins were thought to have no biologic activity. It is now known that these proteins are secreted by expanded clones of immunoglobulin-secreting cells with activity directed at specific antigens. Many have idiotypically specific biologic activity, accounting for the remote effects of these monoclonal gammopathies.

The M-protein is most commonly detected by screening patients with serum cellulose acetate electrophoresis. In cases in which a spike is seen on serum cellulose acetate electrophoresis and in all cases in which a monoclonal gammopathy is suspected, such as idiopathic polyneuropathy or atypical motor neuron disease, immunoelectrophoresis or immunofixation should be performed, regardless of the results of serum cellulose acetate electrophoresis. These tests are more sensitive than serum cellulose acetate electrophoresis for the presence of a small M-protein and allow characterization of the single heavy and light chain, thus verifying the monoclonal nature of the immunoglobulin. Of the two, immunofixation is more sensitive and will detect M-proteins occasionally when immunoelectrophoresis is negative but is more expensive and technically more demanding. Urine should also be examined since monoclonal light chains (Bence-Jones proteinuria) may occasionally appear only in the urine, where their presence suggests either a malignant plasma cell dyscrasia or light-chain amyloidosis.

After identification and characterization of a M-protein in serum or urine, further studies should be done to classify the plasma cell dyscrasia (Table 97-1). If a diagnosis of MGUS is made, M-protein levels should be monitored on a yearly basis since a sudden increase could indicate malignant transformation

TABLE 97-1. Classification of Common Plasma Cell Dyscrasias

Disorder	Diagnostic Criteria
Monoclonal gammopathy of undetermined significance	Monoclonal protein in serum <3 g/dl and no malignancy or amyloid
Osteosclerotic myeloma	Solitary or multiple plasmacytomas with osteosclerotic features
Multiple myeloma	>10% abnormal plasma cells in bone marrow or plasmacytoma and monoclonal protein in serum or urine or osteolytic lesions
Waldenström's macroglobulinemia	IgM-monoclonal protein >3 g/dl; >10% lymphs or macroglobulinemia plasma cells in bone marrow
Primary systemic amyloidosis	Light-chain amyloid by histology
γ-Heavy-chain disease	Monoclonal heavy chain in serum or urine

(From Kelly JJ Jr, Kyle RA, O'Brien PC et al: Prevalence of monoclonal protein in peripheral neuropathy. Neurology 31:1480, 1981, with permission.)

of a formerly benign plasma cell dyscrasia, which can occur in up to 20 percent of cases.

POLYNEUROPATHY SYNDROMES

MGUS-Associated

MGUS-associated polyneuropathy syndromes comprise the largest number of polyneuropathies associated with plasma cell dyscrasias and is best approached by division into IgM-associated and non-IgM-associated types. The IgM group can be further separated into those with and without apparent antinerve activity. Table 97-3 presents the main neurologic features of these disorders.

IgM Monoclonal Gammopathy With Antinerve Activity. By far the most common member of the group with antinerve activity is the neuropathy with antibody activity against myelin-associated glycoprotein (MAG), a glycoprotein with neural adhesion properties located on the myelin sheath of peripheral (PNS) and central nervous system (CNS) myelin. This syndrome was first described by Latov and colleagues in 1980. Since then, multiple studies have shown that approximately 50 percent of all polyneuropathies associated with plasma cell dyscrasia are of IgM type and, of these, about 50 percent have anti-MAG activity. Other antinerve antibodies (Table 97-4) are much less common and are less clearly etiologically related to the polyneuropathy.

Neuropathy associated with anti-MAG activity (anti-MAG neuropathy, Latov syndrome) is the most firmly established and best characterized of the antinerve antibody neuropathy syndromes. Since 1987, since we began systematically testing all appropriate polyneuropathy patients, we have seen over 20 patients with this syndrome. The frequency has been increasing steadily, probably due to better recognition of the syndrome by referring physicians and the wider availability of the anti-MAG antibody test. Based on our experience and that of others, a fairly consistent clinical picture has emerged. These patients present with the slow and insidious onset, after months to years, of progressive ascending numbness, usually without pain or autonomic involvement, and sensory gait ataxia. Intention tremor may be prominent in some. Weakness is usually much less pronounced and indeed, early on, the clinical picture may resemble the sensory neuronopathy syndrome with predominant discriminatory sensory loss and preserved power. The findings tend to be quite symmetric and progress in a slow and steady proximal fashion, suggesting a length-dependent axonopathy. Most patients have thickening of the nerves in the upper arms, a finding generally absent in axonopathies.

Neurodiagnostic laboratory studies, especially electromyography (EMG) (Table 97-5), are helpful in suggesting the diagno-

TABLE 97-4. Antibody Activities of Monoclonal IgM in Peripheral Nerve Disorders

Antibody Activity	Clinical Syndrome	Type of Pathology
MAG	Sensory > motor polyneuropathy	SD
Acidic glycolipids	Polyneuropathy	?
Gangliosides GM$_1$ and GD$_{1b}$	Motor neuron disease	SD, possible AD
Chondroitin sulfate C	Sensory polyneuropathy	AD
Intermediate filaments	Polyneuropathy	SD
Neurofilament	Polyneuropathy	AD
Sulfatide	Sensory polyneuropathy	AD

Abbreviations: MAG, myelin-associated glycoprotein; SD, segmental demyelination; AD, axonal degeneration.

(Adapted from Steck AJ, Murray N, Dellagi K et al: Peripheral neuropathy associated with monoclonal IgM autoantibody. Ann Neurol 45:711, 1988, with permission.)

sis. Sensory nerve action potentials are absent or severely attenuated. Despite the fact that weakness is generally not pronounced in these patients, there is often marked slowing of motor conduction velocity and very prolonged distal latencies in the "demyelinating" range. Cerebrospinal fluid examination may disclose increased protein (>100 mg/dl) in advanced cases. Although these studies can suggest the diagnosis in the proper clinical setting, the keys to diagnosis are the nerve biopsy and serologic studies. Nerve biopsies show combined axonal degeneration and demyelinating features, and most patients display positive immunostaining of the nerve for the M-protein, which is deposited on the surface of the myelin sheath. Ultrastructural studies show splitting and widening of the outer lamellae of myelin, possibly due to the disadhesion activity of the anti-MAG antibodies, although the exact mechanism of antibody action is unknown. IgM has been demonstrated in the region of myelin lamellar widening, although macrophages thus far have not been demonstrated to play a role in the myelin damage. Immunmoblot and enzyme-linked immunosorbent assay (ELISA) studies disclose the anti-MAG antibodies in high titer in serum of these patients. These tests are now commercially available from a number of sources. The IgM appears to react with a carbohydrate epitope that is shared by MAG and other glycoproteins and glycolipids in the PNS and CNS. Recognition of these patients is important, since treatment that lowers anti-MAG levels with plasmapheresis or cytotoxic drugs promotes recovery.

The pathophysiology of this neuropathy is not completely understood. When anti-MAG antibody-containing sera were injected directly into peripheral nerves, intense complement dependent demyelination resulted. However, the morphologic picture was different from that observed in patients and more characteristic of the Guillain-Barré syndrome, with inflamma-

TABLE 97-3. Main Neurologic Features of Dysproteinemia Polyneuropathy Syndromes

Type of PN	Topography	Weakness	Sensory	Autonomic	Course	CSF	MNCV		Pathology
MGUS-IgM	Distal	+	+++	−	Prog	++	Very slow		SD
MGUS-IgG, MGUS-IgA	Distal	++	++	−	Prog	+	Slow		SD, AD
Amyloidosis	Distal	+/++	+++	+++	Prog	+	Mild slow		AD
OSM	Distal	+++	++	−	Prog	+++	Very slow		SD
WM	Distal	++	++	−	Prog	++	Very slow		SD, AD

Abbreviations: PN, polyneuropathy; CSF, cerebrospinal fluid protein concentration; MNCV, motor nerve conduction velocity; MGUS, monoclonal gammopathy of undetermined significance; OSM, osteosclerotic myeloma; WSM, Waldenström's macroglobulinemia; Prog, chronic progressive; SD, segmental demyelination; AD, axonal degeneration.

(From Kelly JJ Jr, Kyle RA, Latov N: Polyneuropathies Associated with Plasma Cell Dyscrasias. Martin-Nihjoff, Boston, 1987, with permission.)

TABLE 97-5. Major Electrodiagnostic Features of PN Associated with PCD

Type of PN	Demyelinating	Axonal	CTS	Pure Sensory	Other
MGUS-IgM	+ + +	+	−	+ +	+
MGUS-IgG, MGUS-IgA	+ +	+ +	−	+	+
OSM	+ + +	+	−	−	−
PSA	−	+ + +	+ +	+	+ + +[a]
MM	+	+ +	+	+	+ +[b]

Abbreviations: PN, polyneuropathy; PCD, plasma cell dyscrasia; CTS, carpal tunnel syndrome superimposed on polyneuropathy; MGUS, monoclonal gammopathy of undetermined significance; OSM, osteosclerotic myeloma; PSA, primary systemic amyloidosis; MM, multiple myeloma.

[a] Autonomic involvement.

[b] Root involvement and polyradiculopathies superimposed on PN.

(From Kelly JJ Jr: Peripheral neuropathies associated with monoclonal proteins: a clinical review. Muscle Nerve 8:138, 1985, with permission.)

tion and macrophage-induced demyelination. However, an animal model induced by systemic administration of anti-MAG enriched serum, which has the attributes of human anti-MAG neuropathy, has recently been described.

Treatment in these patients is difficult. They are often elderly and tolerate immunosuppressive drugs poorly. In addition, they are often poorly responsive to steroids and require more powerful drugs such as cyclophosphamide. Plasmapheresis is probably effective but requires prolonged treatment. It is unclear whether intravenous immunoglobulin will be effective, but if so, it will undoubtedly also require prolonged treatment. In our experience, a 6- to 9-month course of oral cyclophosphamide, designed to lower the M-protein level by at least one-half, allows recovery in the majority of patients, who attain clinical remission for months to several years. After therapy is stopped, the M-protein level gradually rises to pretreatment levels and the deficit begins to reaccumulate, but thus far, we have not had to retreat anyone. Whether pulse therapy with monthly intravenous doses of cyclophosphamide will be equally efficacious while sparing the patient from drug side effects is as yet unknown.

MAG-nonreactive IgM neuropathies are much less common and less well characterized than anti-MAG neuropathy. IgM antibodies in these patients may react with a variety of antigens (Table 97-4) but these reactions are, for the most part, less clearly related to disease activity. Some have axonal polyneuropathy by EMG. However, many have demyelinating features and are difficult to distinguish from anti-MAG polyneuropathy. In this group, immunofluorescent studies are generally negative and myelin lamellar splitting is not observed. These patients may, however, respond to treatment with steroids, plasmapheresis, or immunosuppressants and cytotoxics. In other cases, these patients resemble in clinical course, laboratory study results, and response to treatment those with chronic inflammatory demyelinating polyradiculopathy (CIDP).

IgG and IgA MGUS-Associated Polyneuropathies. The nature of IgG and IgA M-protein polyneuropathies is much less clearcut. Many of these patients have axonal polyneuropathies that are chronic and mild. Antinerve antibody activity of unclear significance is only occasionally demonstrated and, in general, these patients respond poorly to therapy. In comparative studies, these patients were found to have less evidence of sensory loss than those with IgM gammopathies and less evidence of demyelination on electrophysiologic studies. It is important to exclude amyloidosis, however, in these patients, especially when there is a recent onset, rapid progression, and pain or autonomic symptoms. Less commonly, these patients have a CIDP-like

picture with demyelination on EMG. In these, osteosclerotic myeloma and the Crow-Fukase syndrome should be excluded be excluded by appropriate tests.

PRIMARY SYSTEMIC AMYLOIDOSIS

Primary systemic amyloidosis is perhaps the best characterized of the polyneuropathies associated with M-proteins and accounts for up to one-quarter of cases in some series. This neuropathy characteristically occurs in older men and is very rare prior to the sixth decade of life. Most cases are unassociated with an underlying illness, but a few are associated with hematologic malignancies, such as myeloma and Waldenström's macroglobulinemia. Primary systemic amyloidosis generally presents as a multiple system disease due to the deposition of fragments of the variable portion of a monoclonal light chain, most often λ in tissue. Patients present with a medical disease with associated (sometimes incidental) polyneuropathy (60 percent) or severe polyneuropathy with minimal organ involvement (40 percent). A similar illness can occur in a variety of inherited amyloid polyneuropathies, owing to an abnormal circulating prealbumin (transthyretin) protein due to a single amino acid substitution. Polyneuropathy does not occur in amyloidosis secondary to chronic inflammatory disease or familial CNS amyloidosis.

Medical syndromes (Table 97-6) include the nephrotic syndrome due to amyloid infiltration of the kidneys, cardiac failure due to amyloid cardiomyopathy, chronic diarrhea with wasting due to amyloid infiltration of the gut wall, and autonomic neuropathy with prominent orthostatic hypotension. General laboratory studies reflect the medical syndromes with proteinuria occurring in a high percentage, elevated erythrocyte sedimentation rate in about one-half and a mild increase in benign-appearing plasma cells in bone marrow in many. Up to 90 percent have a M-protein in serum or a monoclonal light chain in urine when thoroughly screened with serum and urine immunofixation. Those patients lacking a M-protein, if not inherited, are

TABLE 97-6. Medical Syndromes in Amyloid Polyneuropathy

Syndrome	Frequency (%)
Orthostatic hypotension	42
Nephrotic syndrome	23
Cardiac failure	23
Malabsorption	16

(From Kelly JJ Jr, Kyle RA, O'Brien PC et al: The natural history of peripheral neuropathy in primary systemic amyloidosis. Ann Neurol 5:271, 1979, with permission.)

called nonsecretory, although immunocytologic studies of their tissue disclose that the amyloid derives from single (monoclonal) light chains. Presumably, the serum concentration is too low in these patients to allow detection. The light chains are deposited in tissue, where they are digested by macrophages with the production of amyloid fibrils, which are then insoluble.

The polyneuropathy has been well characterized. Sensory symptoms are typically most prominent and the earliest to appear. Almost all such patients present with numbness of the hands and legs, with complaints such as burning, aching, stabbing, and shooting pains being most common. In more than one-half of patients, cutaneous sensations (light touch, pain, temperature) are more frequently and severely affected than discriminative sensations (vibration and position sense). Occasional patients (about 20 percent) present with the typical symptoms of carpal tunnel syndrome before distal neuropathy symptoms appear, owing to amyloid infiltration of the flexor retinaculum of the wrist. Rare patients present with symptoms of autonomic dysfunction without symptoms of somatic sensory dysfunction. Symptoms and signs of weakness generally follow. These are usually less prominent than the sensory findings. Exceptions are rare patients with amyloid infiltrative myopathy with proximal muscle weakness and patients with malignant plasma cell dyscrasias, such as myeloma, who may present with compressive radiculopathies that can mimic mononeuropathies or plexopathies. The findings tend to be symmetric and predominant distally, with gradual proximal spread. Most patients soon complain of autonomic dysfunction with orthostatic lightheadedness and syncope, bowel and bladder disturbances, impotence, and sweating disturbances. Hypoactive pupils and orthostatic blood pressure drop with a fixed heart rate are the most easily detected autonomic signs at the bedside.

Electrophysiologic studies (Table 97-5) confirm the presence of a distal axonopathy that is maximal in the legs. Motor conduction velocities in the ''demyelinating'' range (<60 percent of the mean normal for that nerve) occur rarely, and then only in unreliable nerves, where the evoked compound muscle action potential is very low in amplitude. Sensory nerve action potentials are usually unobtainable. Often, there is evidence of disproportionate median nerve conduction slowing across the wrist due to carpal tunnel syndrome, which can suggest the diagnosis. Needle EMG shows the changes expected of a distal axonopathy, with abundant signs of distal denervation and reinnervation. Cerebrospinal fluid is usually acellular and there are generally mild elevations of protein levels, generally in the range of 50 to 70 mg/dl.

Diagnosis is dependent on the discovery of amyloid in tissue. Sural nerve biopsy is very useful in detection of amyloid in virtually all cases, although occasionally, it has to be sought through multiple sections. Amorphous deposits of amyloid on Congo red or cresyl violet stains typically appear in the perivascular regions of the epineurium or occasionally in the endoneurium. Amyloid is classically defined, however, by its appearance under polarized light when the Congo red–stained deposits emit an apple-green birefringence. Electron microscopy can also be used to identify the characteristic fibrils. In some hands, immunofluorescent staining for monoclonal light-chain fragments is useful, but it is technically difficult. Other useful tissues to biopsy (Table 97-7) include rectum, fat pad, and other affected organs.

Teased fiber studies show predominantly axonal degeneration. The reason for nerve fiber damage, however, is not always readily apparent in all cases. In some instances, marked axonal

TABLE 97-7. Results of Biopsy in Primary Amyloidosis With Neuropathy

Site	No. Patients	Positive (%)
Rectum	25	88
Kidney	4	75
Liver	2	100
Small intestine	2	100
Bone marrow	21	33
Sural nerve	10	100
Other (skin, gingiva)	2	100

(From Kelly JJ Jr, Kyle RA, O'Brien PC et al: The natural history of peripheral neuropathy in primary systemic amyloidosis. Ann Neurol 5:271, 1979, with permission.)

denervation can be evident with minimal amyloid infiltration. This has led to many theories of the pathogenesis of the neuropathy, including vascular and pressure changes by the amyloid deposits. However, direct toxic effects of the amyloid fibrils on nerve fibers and dorsal root ganglion cells seems more likely.

Treatment is problematic. The amyloid fibrils are insoluble once deposited in tissue. Thus, it is unlikely that improvement would appear, even with cessation of deposition of amyloid. Thus far, the neuropathy has resisted all attempts to halt its progression with combinations of anti-inflammatory medications such as steroids, alkylating agents such a melphalan and cyclophosphamide designed to slow production of the light chains, and even prolonged plasmapheresis designed to lower the light-chain concentration in serum. However, the nephropathy due to light-chain deposition has been shown to be at least partially reversible with a combination of melphalan and prednisone. Thus, these patients progress inexorably with increasing numbness and pain, autonomic failure, and weakness with added organ failure. Death usually occurs in 2 to 4 years from time of diagnosis and is generally due to major organ failure, cardiac most commonly. Patients with relatively pure neuropathies without significant organ failure survive (or suffer) the longest.

MULTIPLE MYELOMA NEUROPATHY

Multiple myeloma is a malignant plasma cell dyscrasia with high serum and urinary concentrations of M-proteins, infiltration of bone marrow by malignant plasma cells, and multiple bony lesions due to plasma cell infiltration. Most neurologic complications are due to secondary effects of the tumor (hypercalcemia, infections) or to malignant infiltration of nerve roots or secondary compression of spinal cord or nerve roots due to vertebral fractures. Polyneuropathies are uncommon. They occur in only a few percent of multiple myeloma patients and are diverse in nature, similar to the polyneuropathies associated with other malignancies. The exception is osteosclerotic myeloma, discussed separately below.

Neuropathies associated with typical lytic multiple myeloma include distal sensorimotor axonopathy, a CIDP-like picture, and a sensory neuropathy resembling the carcinomatous sensory neuropathy. In addition, these patients may also develop plasma cell dyscrasia polyneuropathy due to deposition of light-chain fragments in tissue. In one series, 20 percent of neuropathies associated with multiple myeloma were due to plasma cell dyscrasia. Superimposed root involvement may mistakenly suggest a picture of mononeuritis multiplex, which we have not seen in our patients with amyloidosis with the exception of carpal tunnel syndromes. The root and cord compressive syndromes should be managed by conventional means, but like nonmalignant primary systemic amyloidosis, the amyloid neuropathy does not respond to chemotherapy.

OSTEOSCLEROTIC MYELOMA POLYNEUROPATHY AND RELATED SYNDROMES

Osteosclerotic myeloma is a rare and relatively benign variant of multiple myeloma. Less than 3 percent of untreated myeloma patients have sclerotic bony lesions. In addition, whereas polyneuropathy is rare with typical multiple myeloma, it is quite common with osteosclerotic myeloma, occurring in 50 percent or more of reported cases. Also, patients with osteosclerotic myeloma are usually not systemically ill and usually present because of the neuropathy or other remote effects of the malignancy rather than as a direct effect of the malignancy as usually occurs in multiple myeloma. Anemia, hypercalcemia, and renal insufficiency are uncommon is osteosclerotic myeloma, bone marrows are rarely infiltrated with malignant plasma cells, and the serum M-protein concentrations are low. Finally, the course of osteosclerotic myeloma is indolent and these patients have prolonged survivals even without treatment. Thus, there is something singular about the syndrome of osteosclerotic myeloma and its paraneoplastic accompaniments. The syndrome can be difficult to diagnose even by experienced physicians.

The polyneuropathy accompanying osteosclerotic myeloma is distinctive and homogeneous. Deficits are mainly motor and slowly progressive without sudden changes in severity or tempo of progression. Patients present with the onset of weakness, mostly in distal limbs initially, with gradual proximal spread accompanied by reflex loss. Sensory loss is typically less striking and tends to disproportionately affect the larger sensory fibers, with greater loss of discriminative sensation than cutaneous sensation. Pain and autonomic dysfunction, with the exception of impotence (actually due to endocrine dysfunction), is very uncommon. Nerves are often palpably thickened. The deficit is usually very symmetric and the tempo of progression very slow, often over months to years. In keeping with the nature of the underlying disorder, general laboratory studies are usually relatively uninformative. The best clue to the diagnosis is the presence of a serum M-protein, which is present in about 75 to 80 percent of patients. However, the M-protein may be very small and obscured by the normal serum protein components in the electrophoresis, emphasizing the importance of immunoelectrophoresis or immunofixation in all patients with idiopathic polyneuropathy. The M-protein is characteristically IgG or IgA (never IgM), λ light chain (rarely κ), and rarely present in the urine, in contrast to multiple myeloma.

Neurodiagnostic studies are helpful but nonspecific. Nerve biopsy studies disclose a reduced concentration of myelinated fibers with changes of mixed demyelination and axonal degeneration. There may be mild foci of mononuclear cells in the epineurium surrounding blood vessels. These changes are nonspecific and characteristic of a number of neuropathies, including CIDP and diabetic polyneuropathy. The EMG (Table 97-5) reveals a mixed axonal and demyelinating picture that again is nonspecific but helpful in categorizing the neuropathy into the group with clear-cut demyelinating features and thus making it more likely to be diagnosable. Cerebrospinal fluid typically reveals a normal cell count but a very high protein concentration, generally higher than 100 mg/dl and sometimes as high as several hundred milligrams per deciliter. Since all these findings are nonspecific, the diagnosis often hinges on the discovery of the characteristic bony lesions and subsequent bone biopsy.

The osteosclerotic lesions may be solitary or multiple. They tend to affect the axial skeleton and very proximal long bones but spare the distal long bones and skull. They may be pure sclerotic or mixed sclerotic and lytic. Radioactive bone scans, although more sensitive than x-rays as a rule in detecting myeloma and other bony metastases, are not as sensitive as x-rays in detecting osteosclerotic myeloma lesions, probably due to the indolent nature of these plasmacytomas. Thus, all patients with unexplained polyneuropathies that fit the clinical profile as described above should be screened with a radiographic skeletal survey. On occasion, these lesions are misinterpreted by radiologists who are unfamiliar with their appearance and significance. Three of our patients were believed to have benign osteosclerotic lesions (fibrous dysplasia in a rib in two and a vertebral hemangioma in one) with negative radionuclide bone scans. We insisted on biopsy because of the clinical picture, and the presence of a serum M-protein and plasmacytomas were discovered, leading to effective treatment. Thus, if there is any question of the significance of a bony lesion in a patient with a suggestive clinical picture, the x-rays should be reviewed by the neurologist with the radiologist and the lesion should be biopsied if doubt remains. Open biopsy is generally preferable to needle biopsy, in our experience.

The diagnosis of this disorder is of more than academic interest, since these patients may be helped by tumoricidal treatment. Patients with solitary lesions do best. Radiotherapy in tumoricidal doses to the lesion results in elimination of the M-protein from the serum and gradual recovery of the neuropathy over the ensuing months in most patients. However, these patients should continue to be followed since they have a tendency to relapse with the development of new lesions months to years later. This is usually heralded by the return of the neuropathy and other symptoms and the reappearance of the serum M-protein. Patients with multiple lesions are more difficult to treat. Radiotherapy is generally not an option. In some cases, aggressive chemotherapy can help these patients, but in general, the outcome is not as favorable as for solitary lesions. Treatment usually requires large doses of steroids and alkylating agents. Treatments that are usually effective in autoimmune inflammatory neuropathies, such as steroids alone or azathioprine, are usually ineffective in these patients.

The cause of the polyneuropathy is not known, but most theories of pathogenesis have focused on some secretory product of the tumor, most likely the M-protein itself and specifically some component of the λ light chain. However, other secretory or autoimmune products are possible. Studies of antinerve antibody activity in the serum of these patients have been negative to date, including immunocytochemical studies of nerves. The pathogenesis of nerve damage in this disorder and whether it is an axonopathy or a primary demyelinating disorder remains unresolved at this time.

This disorder is also of considerable interest, since many of these patients develop a multiple system syndrome that goes by a variety of names, including POEMS syndrome (polyneuropathy, organomegaly, endocrinopathy, M-protein, skin changes) or Crow-Fukase syndrome. These patients have, in addition to polyneuropathy, other features (Table 97-8) suggesting the presence of an underlying endocrinopathy or even malignancy. The reason for the endocrinopathy is unclear. Limited data suggests a disturbance of the hypothalamic-pituitary axis rather than primary end-organ failure, possibly due to antibody activity against pituitary tissue. The organomegaly is usually nonspecific pathologically. Biopsy of affected lymph nodes

TABLE 97-8. Non-neurologic Abnormalities in 16 Patients with Osteosclerotic Myeloma and Polyneuropathy

Abnormality	Patient Number															
	1	2	3	4	5	6	7	8	9	10	11	12	13	14	15	16
Gynecomastia	+												+			
Hepatomegaly		+	+			+	+						+			
Splenomegaly				+		+										
Hyperpigment		+						+	+				+			+
Edema		+	+					+								
Lymphadenopathy		+		+												
Papilledema		+	+				+							+		
Digit clubbing		+									+		+			
White nails													+			+
Hypertrichosis			+					+					+			
Atrophic testes								+					+	+		
Impotence	+							+					+	+		
Polycythemia	+					+			+			+				+
Leucocytosis	+										+			+		
Thrombocythemia	+		+			+	+		+	+	+	+	+	+	+	+
Low plasma testosterone		+	+					+					+	+		
High estrogen		+						+						+		
Low thyroxine		+												+		
Hyperglycemia			+													

(From Kelly JJ Jr, Kyle RA, Miles JM et al: Osteosclerotic myeloma and peripheral neuropathy. Neurology 33:202, 1983, with permission.)

generally discloses hyperplastic changes, sometimes resembling the pathologic findings in the syndrome of angiofollicular lymph node hyperplasia (Castleman's disease), which is a benign localized or generalized hyperplastic lymph node syndrome of unknown etiology. Of interest, patients with generalized angiofollicular lymph node hyperplasia without bony lesions may also have the manifestations of Crow-Fukase syndrome associated with serum M-proteins or polyclonal gammopathies. Thus, it is likely that the main pathogenetic determinant of these syndromes is the presence of a serum product, most likely the IgG or IgA λ M-protein or polyclonal antibodies with similar specificity, directed against neural and other tissue.

The term *POEMS syndrome* for these patients is not entirely accurate and focuses attention on a small number of these patients to the exclusion of others. For example, of the patients with osteosclerotic myeloma polyneuropathy, most have features other than neuropathy that are fragments of a multiple systemic disorder, but only a few would qualify for the term *POEMS* (Table 97-8). Thus, we prefer the term *Crow-Fukase syndrome* when referring to patients with polyneuropathy and multisystemic disorder, as suggested by Nakanishi et al.

MISCELLANEOUS SYNDROMES

Waldenström's Macroglobulinemia

It is sometimes difficult to separate Waldenström's macroglobulinemia from IgM-MGUS, and the latter may evolve into Waldenström's macroglobulinemia over time. Thus, similar polyneuropathy syndromes occur. The most frequent polyneuropathy encountered is probably that associated with anti-MAG antibodies. This syndrome has the same features and clinical course as in IgM-MGUS. Other patients may have either a CIDP-like picture, a distal axonal neuropathy, typical amyloid polyneuropathy, or even the sensory neuronopathy syndrome usually seen with small cell cancer of the lung.

Cryoglobulinemia

This disorder is usually divided into three types. In type 1, the M-protein itself is a cryoglobulin in the setting of a plasma cell disorder. In type 2, the cryoglobulin is a mixture of an M-protein of IgM type with rheumatoid factor activity against polyclonal immunoglobulins, usually occurring in the setting of a lymphoproliferative disorder. Type 3 occurs in the setting of a collagen-vascular or other chronic inflammatory disease, and the cryoglobulin consists of polyclonal immunoglobulins. The polyneuropathy in all these syndromes is painful, symmetric or asymmetric, and sensorimotor and axonal in nature. Purpura occurs in distal limbs in a high percentage of patients and the neuropathy is generally considered to be due to a vasculopathy or vasculitis of skin and vasa nervorum.

Lymphoma, Leukemia, and Cancer

These disorders can be associated with M-protein and polyneuropathy. In lymphoma with IgM M-protein, the IgM may have anti-MAG activity with the usual clinical and pathologic features. Other syndromes without clear antinerve activity in the M-protein fraction may respond to ablation of the malignancy. Still other have an unclear relation to the malignancy and show little response to tumoricidal treatment or to lowering of the M-protein concentration in serum.

CONCLUSION

The field of plasma cell dyscrasias and neuromuscular diseases has been a fruitful area for active research since the mid-1980s. It is very important to recognize patients with these diseases since treatment may lead to remission. Also, careful study of these patients may lead to a better understanding of the pathogenesis of polyneuropathies and possibly motor neuron disease. This may in turn lead to effective treatment for conditions for which there are now no effective treatments. Therefore, despite their relative infrequency, increased recognition of these disorders will continue to be a high priority for both peripheral nerve specialists and for general neurologists.

SUGGESTED READINGS

Kelly JJ Jr: Peripheral neuropathies associated with monoclonal proteins: a clinical review. Muscle Nerve 8:138, 1985

Kelly JJ Jr., Adelman LS, Berkman E et al: Polyneuropathies associated with IgM monoclonal gammopathies. Arch Neurol 45:1355, 1988

Kelly JJ Jr, Kyle RA, Latov N: Polyneuropathies Associated with Plasma Cell Dyscrasias. Martinus-Nijhoff, Boston, 1987

Kelly JJ Jr, Kyle RA, Miles JM et al: Osteosclerotic myeloma and peripheral neuropathy. Neurology 33:202, 1983

Kelly JJ Jr, Kyle RA, Miles JM et al: The spectrum of peripheral neuropathy in myeloma. Neurology 31:24, 1981

Kelly JJ Jr, Kyle RA, O'Brien PC et al: Prevalence of monoclonal protein in peripheral neuropathy. Neurology 31:1480, 1981

Kelly JJ Jr, Kyle RA, O'Brien PC et al: The natural history of peripheral neuropathy in primary systemic amyloidosis. Ann Neurol 5:271, 1979

Kyle RA: Plasma cell dyscrasias. pp. 1–35. In Spitell JA Jr (ed): Clinical Medicine. Harper & Row, Philadelphia, 1981

Latov NR, Hays AP, Sherman WH: Peripheral neuropathy and anti-MAG antibodies. Crit Rev Neurobiol 3:301, 1988

Latov N, Sherman WH, Nemni R et al: Plasma cell dyscrasia and peripheral neuropathy with a monoclonal antibody to peripheral nerve myelin. N Engl J Med 303:618, 1980

Nakanishi T, Sobue I, Toyokura Y et al: The Crow-Fukase syndrome: a study of 102 cases in Japan. Neurology 34:712, 1984

Steck AJ, Murray N, Dellagi K et al: Peripheral neuropathy associated with monoclonal IgM autoantibody. Ann Neurol 45:711, 1988

Suarez GA, Kelly JJ Jr: Polyneuropathy associated with monoclonal gammopathy of undetermined significance: further evidence that IgM-MGUS neuropathies are different than IgG-MGUS. Neurology 43:1377, 1993

98. NEUROPATHIES OF CONNECTIVE TISSUE DISEASES

RICHARD K. OLNEY

Peripheral neuropathies of several types develop in the clinical context of known diffuse connective tissue diseases. Also, certain presentations of peripheral neuropathy raise the distinct concern that the neuropathy may be the initial manifestation of a previously unsuspected connective tissue disease. To facilitate the recognition of these latter neuropathies, the first section of this chapter reviews each type of neuropathy and comments on the known or possibly unsuspected connective tissue diseases that may be associated. To facilitate recognition of neuropathy in a patient with a known connective tissue disease, the second section reviews certain diffuse connective tissue diseases and comments on their associated neuropathies.

PERIPHERAL NEUROPATHIES ASSOCIATED WITH CONNECTIVE TISSUE DISEASES

The peripheral neuropathies that are associated most closely with diffuse connective tissue diseases are as follows:

1. Vasculitic neuropathy
2. Distal axonal polyneuropathy
3. Trigeminal sensory neuropathy
4. Sensory neuronopathy
5. Entrapment or compression neuropathy

Among these neuropathies, the diagnosis and initiation of treatment is most important to accomplish in a timely manner for vasculitic neuropathy, because it is the most rapidly evolving and potentially fatal, so its diagnosis is particularly emphasized.

Vasculitic Neuropathy

Vasculitic neuropathy is defined by the pathogenetic mechanism that produces injury to the nerve fibers: inflammatory occlusion of blood vessels produces ischemic infarction of one or more nerves. The probability of vasculitic neuropathy is usually suspected clinically when it presents as a mononeuropathy multiplex in a patient with a known connective tissue disease. However, the possibility of vasculitic neuropathy is also important to consider in many other patients. This neuropathy may be the initial manifestation of connective tissue disease, particularly polyarteritis nodosa. Furthermore, vasculitic neuropathy often presents as a generalized polyneuropathy with little or no asymmetry rather than as a mononeuropathy multiplex. Thus, the possibility of vasculitic neuropathy needs to be considered in many patients with neuropathy of undefined cause, especially in those patients in whom symptoms and signs have developed with asymmetry or without following a length-dependent distribution (this distribution is typical for distal axonal polyneuropathy and is discussed further under that heading) or in whom functionally significant deficits have developed rapidly (that is, over weeks or months). In other words, the possibility of vasculitic neuropathy needs to be considered in many patients with neuropathy of undefined cause, if there are clinical features that are atypical for the more common distal axonal polyneuropathy.

When vasculitis produces acute ischemia of a nerve, the patient usually experiences an immediate deep aching pain in a poorly localized but proximal distribution within the affected limb. Several hours to several days after this proximal deep aching pain, the patient develops a burning pain in the cutaneous distribution of the affected nerve. In patients with less acutely evolving vasculitic neuropathy, the proximal deep aching pain may be overshadowed by a more prominent distal burning pain that develops over days or several weeks. On neurologic examination, most patients have weakness and abnormal sensation for pain and temperature, whereas a minority of patients have impairment of vibration and position sense. This sensory loss and weakness typically develop over several hours to several days in the distribution of the affected nerve in the acutely evolving cases, or over days to weeks in a more confluent distal distribution in the more slowly evolving cases. In patients who present with the more obvious mononeuropathy multiplex, some nerves are more predisposed to involvement than others. The peroneal nerve is the most frequently affected by vasculitis, and the ulnar nerve is the most commonly involved in the upper limb. The nerve infarctions are typically located at "watershed" zones of relatively poor perfusion, which are at the midthigh level for the peroneal division of the sciatic nerve and at the mid–upper arm level for the ulnar nerve. If affected, the tibial and median nerves are also usually infarcted at these same levels.

After eliciting the patient history and conducting the physical examination, the first step in the diagnostic workup is electrodiagnostic evaluation. The electromyographic (EMG) and nerve conduction studies assess the severity and pathophysiologic basis for the clinical symptoms and signs. In vasculitic neuropathy, acute axon loss is the predominant pathophysiology identified. Thus, EMG studies reveal reduced recruitment of motor unit action potentials that parallels the clinical weakness, and fibrillation potentials are seen in affected muscles 1 to 4 weeks after onset of weakness. Nerve conduction studies document decreased amplitude of sensory nerve and compound muscle action potentials, with normal or mildly reduced conduction velocities. In patients with clinically obvious multifocal nerve involvement, a further purpose of these studies is to distinguish multifocal nerve infarction from multifocal entrapment. Whereas focally decreased conduction velocity or partial conduction block is seen at common entrapment sites with multifocal entrapment, signs of multifocal axonal degeneration distal to the midthigh or mid–upper arm levels are seen in vasculitic mononeuropathy multiplex. In patients without clinically obvious multifocal nerve involvement, a further purpose of these studies is to seek signs of multifocal or non-length-dependent axonal degeneration that are not obvious clinically. With sensory or motor nerve conduction studies, these signs include finding (1) a more than twofold difference in the amplitude between the right- and left-sided responses of the same nerve (i.e., bilateral asymmetry), (2) a low-amplitude response for one but not another nerve within a limb, or (3) a low-amplitude response for an upper limb nerve, if amplitude is normal for at least one lower limb nerve (i.e., non-length-dependence). With needle EMG studies, non-length-dependent axonal degeneration is identified by finding acute partial denervation (reduced recruitment of motor unit action potentials with or without fibrillation potentials) in some but not other proximal muscles that seem normal clinically.

The second step in the diagnostic evaluation is obtaining laboratory tests and possibly a nerve or muscle biopsy. The connective tissue diseases that are associated with vasculitic neuropathy are as follows:

1. Polyarteritis nodosa—usually not previously diagnosed
2. Rheumatoid arthritis—usually an established diagnosis
3. Others infrequently (either unsuspected or known):
    a. Systemic lupus erythematosus
    b. Systemic sclerosis
    c. Sjögren syndrome
    d. Churg-Strauss syndrome
    e. Wegener's granulomatosis

The two most common causes are polyarteritis nodosa and rheumatoid arthritis with vasculitis. The extent of laboratory testing, however, depends very much on the clinical context. The least extensive workup is indicated in a patient with a mononeuropathy multiplex, electrodiagnostic evidence suggestive of vasculitic neuropathy, a previously known diagnosis of rheumatoid arthritis, and the laboratory signs of a highly elevated erythrocyte sedimentation rate and rheumatoid titer. In such a patient, treatment may be initiated with reasonable confidence in the diagnosis of vasculitis, without performing a biopsy or other tests. The most extensive testing is indicated in a patient without a previously known connective tissue disease or in a case with a more confluent neuropathy in whom the possibility of vasculitis is less certain. In these patients, laboratory tests often include complete blood count with differential and platelet count, erythrocyte sedimentation rate, antineutrophil cytoplasmic antibody, antinuclear antibody, rheumatoid titer, complement levels, hepatitis B surface antigen, chemistry tests of renal and liver function, and urinanalysis. If the clinical suspicion of vasculitic neuropathy is sufficiently high, biopsy of nerve or muscle is

requested at the same time the preceding tests are ordered. This request is often made the same day as the clinical and electrodiagnostic evaluation, with the biopsy performed within 1 to 3 days as an emergency procedure. If the possibility of vasculitic neuropathy becomes reasonable only after some or all of the laboratory tests return—for example, in a more slowly evolving neuropathy that is partially or fully confluent—then biopsy of nerve or muscle is arranged when the possibility becomes reasonable as an urgent procedure.

Treatment of vasculitic neuropathy is usually initiated with glucocorticoids, either oral 1 mg/kg/day prednisone or intravenous 1 g/day methylprednisolone for 3 days followed by oral prednisone. If the vasculitis is restricted to peripheral nerve and muscle (which is as common as polyarteritis nodosa and rheumatoid vasculitis), treatment may be limited to prednisone for 4 to 12 months or 2 mg/kg/day azathioprine may be added and continued for 1 to 2 years. If the vasculitis is systemic and necrotizing, 2 mg/kg/day oral cyclophosphamide is often added and continued for 1 or more years. Recovery from the sensory and motor deficits is likely in survivors, with meaningful improvement in 28 percent at 3 months, 60 percent at 6 months, and 86 percent at 1 year.

Distal Axonal Polyneuropathy

This type of neuropathy develops in most types of diffuse connective tissue disease, which include the following:

1. Rheumatoid arthritis—a mild one in a majority with known rheumatoid arthritis if carefully sought
2. Systemic lupus erythematosus—in 6 to 21 percent with known systemic lupus erythematosus
3. Systemic sclerosis—in 10 to 15 percent with known systemic sclerosis
4. Sjögren syndrome—in 10 to 15 percent with known primary disease
5. Mixed connective tissue disease—in 10 percent with known mixed connective tissue disease
6. Giant cell arteritis—in 7 percent with known giant cell arteritis

The presenting complaints are usually sensory symptoms in the toes or feet. Paresthesias and symptoms of sensory loss are characteristic. The paresthesias are often described as tingling, but other adjectives referring to nonpainful extra sensations are not unusual. Symptoms of sensory loss include diminished awareness of pain (e.g., awareness of cut on foot only when blood seen), temperature (e.g., toes cannot sense when water in bathtub is hot), touch (e.g., noticed while clipping toenails), or position (e.g., difficulty getting toes in socks or stockings). Loss of position sense also may be noticed as imbalance. Partial sensory loss is occasionally described as feeling as if walking on sand or marbles. Pain in the toes or feet is a common symptom, too, but less characteristic if not associated with paresthesias or sensory loss. Sharp stabbing and lancinating pain, as well as more constant burning pain, is usually due to neuropathy. Dull aching or pressurelike pain are nonspecific.

With distal axonal polyneuropathy, sensory symptoms begin in the toes or feet symmetrically and gradually spread proximally over time in a length-dependent manner. At the time when distal lower limb symptoms have spread up to the midcalf level, similar symptoms usually begin in the fingertips symmetrically. Often, near this point in time, weakness at the ankles becomes an additional complaint. Symptoms that are due to ankle weakness include slapping of the feet with walking, tripping over steps or thick carpet, or having to step higher consciously to avoid tripping.

To distinguish distal axonal polyneuropathy from vasculitic neuropathy, the length-dependency and symmetry of symptoms and signs are important concepts. In distal axonal polyneuropathy, nerve fibers that are the same distance from the nerve cell bodies (or the same distance from the spinal cord) should be affected to a similar degree. Thus, both feet should be symptomatic near the same point in time (roughly within a month of each other) and fingers should not be affected until the lower legs are affected. If symptoms begin in one or both hands before involvement between the ankle and knee, this strongly suggests either vasculitic neuropathy or a superimposed compression neuropathy.

The neurologic signs of distal axonal polyneuropathy parallel those of the symptoms, but may be quantitatively different (either more or less severe than the complaints). The initial signs are usually a decreased threshold for perception of vibration in the toes and at the ankle, and depressed or absent ankle tendon reflexes. A decreased threshold for perception of pain (pinprick) and temperature (warm is usually more useful than cold, as feet themselves are often cool) is often observed as well. Wasting of intrinsic foot muscles and weakness of toe movements is occasionally seen early in the course of distal axonal polyneuropathy, but is usually delayed until the upper edge of the stocking decrease in sensation is up to the midcalf level. A decreased threshold for perception of pain, temperature, or vibration is seen in the fingers at about the same time the lower limb sensory level has spread up to the midcalf level.

The first step in the diagnostic workup is electrodiagnostic evaluation to assess the severity and pathophysiologic basis for the clinical symptoms and signs. In distal axonal polyneuropathy, signs of axon loss are seen most prominently in a distal and symmetrical distribution. Thus, EMG studies reveal reduced recruitment of motor unit action potentials in distal more than proximal muscles, and in intrinsic hand muscles no more severely than in muscles of anterior and posterior compartments of the lower leg. Reduced recruitment of motor unit action potentials is usually accompanied by signs of chronic partial denervation with reinnervation (an increased incidence of long-duration, large-amplitude, or polyphasic motor unit action potentials) and, in more rapidly progressive cases, signs of acute denervation (reduced recruitment associated with fibrillation potentials). Nerve conduction studies document symmetrically decreased amplitude of sensory nerve and compound muscle action potentials, with normal or mildly reduced conduction velocities. If axon loss is not in a symmetric and length-dependent distribution, then subsequent evaluation is refocused for a possible vasculitic neuropathy.

The second step in the diagnostic evaluation is obtaining laboratory tests. In a patient with a known connective tissue disease, these usually include complete blood count with differential and platelet count, erythrocyte sedimentation rate, antibody titers that correlate with activity for that particular connective tissue disease, chemistry tests of renal and liver function, vitamin B_{12} level, thyroid function tests, serum protein electrophoresis, and urinanalysis. The latter tests are obtained to evaluate the possibility of a cause for the polyneuropathy that is less directly related to the connective tissue disease. Distal axonal polyneuropathy is rarely the first sign of an unsuspected connective tissue disease.

The treatment of distal axonal polyneuropathy is often symptomatic or rehabilitative. Symptomatic treatments are usually for pain and commonly include tricyclic antidepressants (usually amitriptyline, nortriptyline, or desipramine) or membrane-stabilizing drugs (usually mexiletine or carbamazepine). Rehabilitative treatments often include orthotic shoe inserts for activity-related pain or plastic ankle-foot orthoses for ankle weakness. Potentially curative treatment is usually limited to those cases in which symptoms and signs turn out to be due to a confluent vasculitic neuropathy.

Trigeminal Sensory Neuropathy

Trigeminal sensory neuropathy is characterized by slowly progressive facial sensory symptoms, either unilaterally or bilaterally. The sensory symptoms often begin with a small unilateral patch of numbness that is around the mouth or on the cheek. This small patch typically expands gradually and unilaterally. The deficit is typically maximal over 6 to 24 months. Contralateral sensory symptoms do not develop in many patients, but may develop in some, often after a delay of several years. Facial numbness is often associated with paresthesias or pain.

The neurologic examination is abnormal for impaired perception of pain, temperature, or light touch in the symptomatic distribution. The corneal reflex is blunted or absent in many patients. The severity of sensory involvement can be objectively documented in a quantitative manner with blink reflex studies. An afferent delay (i.e., delayed ipsilateral R1 and bilateral R2) or an absent response is seen in about one-half of patients.

Trigeminal sensory neuropathy presents in two manners:

1. Trigeminal neuropathy as initial or early manifestation:
   a. Systemic sclerosis
   b. Mixed connective tissue disease
2. Trigeminal neuropathy also associated with:
   a. Sjögren syndrome
   b. Systemic lupus erythematosus
   c. Rheumatoid arthritis
   d. Dermatomyositis
   e. Undifferentiated connective tissue disease

It also has been reported in association with many other connective tissue diseases, including Sjögren syndrome, systemic lupus erythematosus, rheumatoid arthritis, dermatomyositis, and undifferentiated connective tissue disease.

Based on a limited amount of pathologic data that is available, trigeminal sensory neuropathy appears to result from degeneration of peripheral myelinated axons due to fibrosis or low-grade perivascular inflammation or vasculitis involving, or distal to, Gasser's ganglion. Even if caused by vasculitis, the development of systemic vasculitis is unusual. Furthermore, less than 10 percent of patients have even a subjective response to treatment with prednisone. Thus, trigeminal sensory neuropathy does not generally indicate the need to initiate prednisone or immunosuppressive therapy. However, trigeminal sensory neuropathy is important to recognize, because this often leads to the diagnosis and treatment of systemic sclerosis or mixed connective tissue disease.

Sensory Neuronopathy

Sensory neuronopathy is associated primarily with Sjögren syndrome. Most patients are middle-aged women who present with symptoms of sensory neuronopathy and are not known to have Sjögren syndrome. Although any limb may become symptomatic first, most patients present with symptoms in both legs and have gait ataxia. Other common chief complaints are clumsiness, incoordination, decreased awareness of limb position, or numbness. The onset is often insidious, but may be acute or subacute.

On neurologic examination, signs are usually most prominent in the lower limbs, but can be most severe in one arm. Sensory impairment is usually greater for vibration and proprioception than for pain and temperature. Deep tendon reflexes are usually depressed or absent in affected limbs. Strength is normal but may seem mildly reduced owing to the severity of incoordination. Romberg's sign is positive if lower limbs are affected. Pseudoathetosis may be prominent if the upper limbs are involved.

The first step in the diagnostic evaluation is electrodiagnostic testing. Sensory nerve action potentials are typically absent in affected limbs, but, if recordable, have normal conduction velocities unless the amplitude is severely reduced. EMG and motor nerve conduction studies have normal results or mild abnormalities in such a limited distribution as to be of doubtful clinical significance. These results then confirm that the neuropathy is a sensory neuronopathy and that the differential diagnostic possibilities are limited to Sjögren syndrome, a paraneoplastic syndrome, a short list of toxic exposures, or unknown cause.

If the patient has symptoms of dryness of eyes or mouth, the second step in the diagnostic evaluation includes those directed at documenting Sjögren syndrome. Reduced lacrimation by Schirmer's test, signs for keratoconjunctivitis sicca by the rose bengal test, evidence for Sjögren syndrome in minor salivary gland biopsy specimens, and elevated titers to antinuclear antibody or rheumatoid factor are usually present, whereas anti-Ro antibodies or arthritis are present in less than one-third. Other testing may be performed to look for a primary or recurrent tumor and include anti-Hw antibody.

The pathogenesis of sensory neuronopathy in Sjögren syndrome is a dorsal root ganglionitis; dorsal root ganglia biopsy specimens have revealed lymphocytic infiltration with degeneration and loss of the neurons in the few patients that have undergone this procedure. Because of this pathogenetic mechanism, immunosuppressive treatment with cyclophosphamide or other drugs is often used, but the benefit of such therapy is not established. About one-half of patients stabilize and functionally improve during immunosuppression, but objective signs of improvement (as with larger sensory nerve action potentials) are not usually seen.

Entrapment or Compression Neuropathies

An increased incidence of entrapment or compression neuropathies is generally accepted in association with some connective tissue diseases. The association of the carpal tunnel syndrome and rheumatoid arthritis has been most thoroughly studied. During the course of rheumatoid arthritis, one-quarter to one-third of patients are likely to develop symptoms for the carpal tunnel syndrome and have a positive Tinel sign. One-fifth to one-quarter of patients with Sjögren syndrome or systemic sclerosis may also develop the carpal tunnel syndrome. The predominant electrophysiologic abnormality in such cases is the prolongation of sensory and/or motor latency through the carpal tunnel. This electrodiagnostic feature is useful in

distinguishing entrapment or compression from ischemic neuropathy.

An increased incidence of ulnar neuropathy at the elbow and peroneal neuropathy at the fibular head has also been reported in rheumatoid arthritis. However, this seems to be based primarily on anecdotal reports rather than on prospective studies, and so may represent a simple chance association rather than a predisposition.

Other Neuropathies

Acute inflammatory demyelinating polyneuropathy, chronic inflammatory demyelinating polyneuropathy, and brachial neuritis have been described in patients with known systemic lupus erythematosus and, rarely, in patients later found to have systemic lupus erythematosus. These associations may represent the chance occurrence of two diseases or may possibly reflect an abnormal immunologic mechanism that predisposes to both diseases. Only speculative information presently addresses the nature of the association.

CONNECTIVE TISSUE DISEASES ASSOCIATED WITH PERIPHERAL NEUROPATHIES

The diffuse connective tissue diseases that are commonly associated with peripheral neuropathies are as follows:

1. Rheumatoid arthritis
2. Systemic lupus erythematosus
3. Systemic sclerosis
4. Sjögren syndrome
5. Mixed connective tissue disease
6. Systemic necrotizing vasculitides
   a. Polyarteritis nodosa
   b. Allergic granulomatosis (Churg-Strauss syndrome)
   c. Giant cell arteritis
   d. Wegener's granulomatosis

Rheumatoid Arthritis

Rheumatoid arthritis is the most common connective tissue disease. It affects 1 to 2 percent of adults worldwide and over 10 percent of the population that is above age 65 years. A definite diagnosis of rheumatoid arthritis requires the documentation of at least four of seven criteria in the 1987 revision. The neuropathies associated with rheumatoid arthritis are as follows:

1. Vasculitic neuropathy in less than 10 percent
2. Distal axonal polyneuropathy in majority
3. Trigeminal sensory neuropathy
4. Entrapment or compression neuropathies, especially carpal tunnel syndrome

Systemic necrotizing vasculitis complicates rheumatoid arthritis in 8 to 25 percent of cases by the time of death, usually after arthritis has been present for an average of 14 years. However, systemic necrotizing vasculitis is, on rare occasions, the major presenting feature of rheumatoid arthritis. Weight loss, rheumatoid nodules, and cutaneous lesions are usually seen with systemic necrotizing vasculitis. Clinically apparent vasculitic neuropathy develops in about one-half of patients with systemic necrotizing vasculitis. Although the majority of rheumatoid patients develop a mild sensory polyneuropathy, clinically significant vasculitic neuropathy develops in less than 10 percent. With rheumatoid vasculitis, the erythrocyte sedimentation rate is usually elevated and the rheumatoid factor typically has a high titer. The development of vasculitis in rheumatoid arthritis patient results in a poor prognosis. Even with steroid and immunosuppressive therapy, the 6-month survival rate is 80 percent and the 5-year one is 60 percent, similar to that for polyarteritis nodosa.

Although clinically significant vasculitic neuropathy develops in less than 10 percent, a majority of rheumatoid patients have evidence for a mild sensory distal axonal polyneuropathy when detailed clinical and electrodiagnostic examinations are performed. If nerve biopsies are performed on these patients, variable amounts of intimal thickening and less frequent perivascular mononuclear infiltration are often seen in endoneurial and epineurial vessels. Similar changes are frequent in peripheral nerves taken at autopsy from patients who had rheumatoid arthritis without clinically evident neuropathy. Thus, a low-grade vasculitis is one possible explanation for the mild sensory polyneuropathy, although there is no convincing evidence that immunosuppressive treatment is beneficial for it. Exposure to toxic medications and other undefined factors may also be important in the pathogenesis of the mild sensory distal axonal polyneuropathy.

Systemic Lupus Erythematosus

Systemic lupus erythematosus is a common connective tissue disease in young women. Its general prevalence in adults is about 1/2,000, but its prevalence is 1/250 in black women under 65 years and 1/1,000 in white women of comparable age. Women are five times more likely to be affected than men. Systemic lupus erythematosus is diagnosed by the cumulative occurrence of at least 4 of 11 multiple system or laboratory criteria. Although central nervous system involvement fulfills 1 of these 11 criteria, peripheral neuropathy does not. The neuropathies associated with systemic lupus erythematosus are as follows:

1. Vasculitic neuropathy—rarely
2. Distal axonal polyneuropathy in 6 to 25 percent
3. Trigeminal sensory neuropathy
4. Other neuropathies (rarely):
   a. Acute inflammatory demyelinating polyneuropathy
   b. Chronic inflammatory demyelinating polyneuropathy
   c. Brachial neuritis

About 6 to 21 percent of patients develop polyneuropathy, typically a distal axonal polyneuropathy with predominantly sensory symptoms and subacute or chronic evolution. Most are not caused by low-grade vasculitis; however, vasculitic neuropathy and demyelinating polyneuropathy are well described in occasional patients. When the neuropathy is produced by a systemic necrotizing vasculitis, improvement usually results from treatment with plasmapheresis, steroids, and immunosuppressive drugs. Steroids or other immunotherapies are not clearly beneficial in cases with distal axonal polyneuropathy.

Systemic Sclerosis

Systemic sclerosis usually presents initially with Raynaud's phenomenon. Some patients rapidly develop diffuse cutaneous signs with symmetric, widespread thickening of the skin and have early visceral involvement. Others have limited cutaneous signs with symmetric, distal limb and facial thickening and late visceral involvement. These latter patients usually have the CREST syndrome (calcinosis, Raynaud's phenomenon, esophageal dysmotility, sclerodactyly, and telangiectasias). The association of systemic sclerosis with trigeminal sensory neuropathy has been recognized for a long time. Although systemic sclerosis was once though not to be associated with neuropathies in the limbs, recent observations suggest that 10 to 15 percent of patients may have a distal axonal polyneuropathy.

Sjögren Syndrome

Sjögren syndrome may develop as a primary connective tissue disease or may be secondary to another one, usually rheumatoid arthritis, systemic lupus erythematosus, or systemic sclerosis. Women are nine times more likely to affected than are men. Sjögren syndrome is characterized by the dryness of the mouth (xerostomia) and the eyes (xerophthalmia). There are no universally agreed upon criteria for its diagnosis. One recent proposal that is as well accepted as any requires four of the following six criteria for a definite diagnosis and three of six for a probable diagnosis:

1. Specific symptoms of dry eyes
2. Specific symptoms of dry mouth
3. Evidence for keratoconjunctivitis with either a positive Schirmer's test or a positive result on the rose bengal dye test
4. Objective evidence for diminished salivary gland flow or salivary gland involvement
5. An abnormal minor salivary gland biopsy
6. The presence of autoantibodies (SS-A, SS-B, antinuclear antibody, or rheumatoid factor)

Peripheral neuropathy is present in 10 to 15 percent of cases of primary Sjögren syndrome, usually a distal symmetric one that begins with paresthesias in the feet. Although clinical symptoms and signs are limited to the sensory fibers initially, electrodiagnostic studies provide evidence for distal loss of sensory and motor axons in most patients. The erythrocyte sedimentation rate and the titer for rheumatoid factor are elevated in a majority of patients with neuropathy, and many have elevated titers for antinuclear antibody or Sjögren syndrome A (Ro) antibody. In patients with neuropathy, signs of cutaneous vasculitis are common, sensory loss may be asymmetric, and biopsy of sural nerves often suggests vasculitis. Thus, a low-grade vasculitis may be the usual pathogenetic explanation for the mild distal axonal polyneuropathy in Sjögren syndrome. However, systemic necrotizing vasculitis is rare, and convincing evidence of a beneficial effect of steroid or immunosuppression is lacking for most patients with Sjögren syndrome and neuropathy.

Mixed Connective Tissue Disease

Mixed connective tissue disease is an overlap syndrome of systemic lupus erythematosus, systemic sclerosis, and polymyositis, in which there is a high titer of extractable nuclear antigen and its ribonucleoprotein component. Although it was initially described in 1972, it is still not accepted as a specific diagnosis by many rheumatologists. Among those who accept its diagnosis, mild distal axonal polyneuropathy may be seen in about 10 percent of patients. Trigeminal sensory neuropathy is also associated with it.

Polyarteritis Nodosa

Polyarteritis nodosa is the most common type of systemic necrotizing vasculitis that produces vasculitic neuropathy, with involvement of small- and medium-size arteries. It is usually seen in middle-aged or older adults, with male predominance. Peripheral neuropathy develops in about one-half of patients. The neuropathy usually presents as a mononeuropathy multiplex or at least with asymmetry and is almost always due to vasculitis. The vasculitic neuropathy is the major presenting symptom in over one-third of cases and clinically apparent at presentation in most of the remainder. In the one-half who develop vasculitic neuropathy, it is usually present within the first year of polyarteritis.

In patients with polyarteritis nodosa, symptoms and signs of systemic disease are usually present. Weight loss and fever are each present in two-thirds to three-quarters of patients. Arthralgias and rash each occur in one-half. Less common clinical features include hypertension and renal, cardiac, or gastrointestinal involvement. An elevated erythrocyte sedimentation rate occurs in all but 5 to 10 percent. Anemia, leukocytosis, or abnormal urinalysis is found in most patients. Hepatitis B surface antigen is positive in a significant minority and may be causally related to polyarteritis nodosa in those cases.

The diagnosis requires the pathologic documentation of necrotizing vasculitis or the arteriographic demonstration of aneurysms at vessel bifurcations. Although arteriography of the renal, hepatic, or mesenteric vessels may support the diagnosis in many cases, similar abnormalities may be seen in Wegener's granulomatosis, left atrial myxoma, and infective endocarditis. The highest sensitivity and specificity from invasive testing in patients who present with neuropathy are achieved with biopsy of an electrophysiologically abnormal cutaneous nerve or with a muscle biopsy. In 1990, the American College of Rheumatology proposed criteria for the diagnosis and classification of vasculitis due to polyarteritis nodosa, whether presenting with or without neuropathy. In this study, an 82 percent sensitivity and a 87 percent specificity were achieved by satisfying 3 or more of the following 10 criteria:

1. Weight loss ($\geq$ 4 kg)
2. Livedo reticularis
3. Testicular pain or tenderness
4. Myalgias
5. Neuropathy
6. Hypertension (diastolic > 90 mmHg)
7. Elevated blood urea nitrogen or creatinine
8. Presence of hepatitis B surface antigen
9. Characteristic arteriographic abnormality
10. Pathologic evidence for necrotizing vasculitis

Untreated patients with polyarteritis nodosa have a 6-month survival of 35 percent and a 5-year survival of 13 percent. Steroid therapy improves survival to 68 percent at 6 months and 50 percent at 5 years. The early use of cyclophosphamide allows up to a 94 percent 6-month survival. Either cyclophosphamide or other cytotoxic therapy permits up to an 80 percent 5-year survival. Although there is a trend for cyclophosphamide to improve survival, this difference has not proven to be statistically significant, so some authors do not recommend the routine addition of cyclophosphamide. Although adversely affected by visceral involvement, the prognosis does not seem to be influenced by the occurrence of vasculitic neuropathy.

Allergic Granulomatosis (Churg-Strauss Syndrome)

The Churg-Strauss syndrome, or allergic granulomatosis, has been considered a variant of polyarteritis nodosa by some. It may be diagnosed with 85 percent sensitivity and 99.7 percent specificity by the presence of four or more of the following six criteria:

1. Asthma
2. Peripheral eosinophilia
3. Nonfixed pulmonary infiltrates
4. Paranasal sinus abnormality
5. Neuropathy
6. A biopsy with a blood vessel that contains extravascular eosinophils.

As with polyarteritis nodosa, vasculitic neuropathy is the only associated neuropathy. The prognosis and treatment of Churg-Strauss syndrome are essentially the same as polyarteritis nodosa.

Giant Cell Arteritis

Giant cell arteritis is perhaps the most common form of vasculitis, typically involving medium and large arteries that are branches of vessels originating from the aortic arch. Patients are usually over age 50 years, present with headache, and have an erythrocyte sedimentation rate elevated to 50 mm/h or more. It is diagnosed most specifically by a temporal artery biopsy that documents a necrotizing arteritis with giant cells. In contrast to the approximate 50 percent prevalence of neuropathy in polyarteritis nodosa or Churg-Strauss syndrome, neuropathy has been found in only 14 percent of patients with giant cell arteritis, with about one-half being diffuse peripheral neuropathies. Although the mechanism is uncertain, an immune-mediated cause for the neuropathy is implied by the majority of patients having improvement in neuropathic deficits with steroid therapy. Even though a small number of patients have developed an acute mononeuropathy or multiple mononeuropathies that suggest vasculitis, nerve ischemia seems related to thrombosis of nutrient or larger vessels, because the size of vessels involved with giant cell arteritis are larger than the epineurial arterioles that are affected in vasculitic neuropathy.

Wegener's Granulomatosis

Wegener's granulomatosis is diagnosed by identifying granulomatous vasculitis of small vessels in the upper and lower respiratory tracts and a segmental necrotizing glomerulonephritis. Peripheral neuropathy develops in 11 to 16 percent, with the majority being vasculitic mononeuropathy multiplex. In the minority of these patients with distal symmetric polyneuropathy, coincidental renal failure is common and offers an alternative explanation.

SUGGESTED READINGS

Arnett FC, Edworthy S, Block DA et al: The 1987 revised ARA criteria for rheumatoid arthritis (abstracted). Arthritis Rheum 30:S17, 1987

Chalk CH, Dyck PJ, Conn DL: Vasculitic neuropathy. p. 1424. In Dyck PJ, Thomas PK, Griffin JW et al (eds): Peripheral Neuropathy. 3rd Ed. WB Saunders, Philadelphia, 1993

Lightfoot RW, Michel BA, Bloch DA et al: The American College of Rheumatology 1990 criteria for the classification of polyarteritis nodosa. Arthritis Rheum 33:1088, 1990

Masi AT, Hunder GG, Lie JT et al: The American College of Rheumatology 1990 criteria for the classification of Churg-Strauss syndrome (allergic granulomatosis and angiitis). Arthritis Rheum 33:1094, 1990

Olney RK: Neuropathies in connective tissue disease. Muscle Nerve 15:531, 1992

Schumacher HR: Primer on the Rheumatic Diseases. 10th Ed. Arthritis Foundation, Atlanta, 1993

Tan EM, Cohen AS, Fries JF et al: The 1982 revised criteria for the classification of systemic lupus erythematosus. Arthritis Rheum 25:1271, 1982

Vitali C, Bombardieri S, Moutsopoulos HM et al: Preliminary criteria for the classification of Sjögren's syndrome. Arthritis Rheum 36:340, 1993

99. TOXIC PERIPHERAL NEUROPATHIES

ALAN R. BERGER

A variety of toxic substances can affect the human nervous system. Many cause combined dysfunction of the central nervous system (CNS) and peripheral nervous system (PNS) or affect the CNS alone. Peripheral neuropathy is the most common PNS reaction to neurotoxin exposure. Toxic neuropathies are occasionally pharmacological and iatrogenic; the recognition of these entities usually poses no diagnostic difficulty. The identification of a sporadic toxic peripheral neuropathy resulting from toxin exposure in the occupational setting may be more difficult, however, as the exposure history is frequently unclear, and clinical manifestations usually resemble those of naturally occurring neuropathies. Clinically relevant and reliable toxicologic tests are often unavailable or unhelpful, either because the necessary laboratory tests are not available, or the substance is undetectable because of the delay between exposure and examination. Consequently, when a naturally occurring medical cause is not readily apparent, there is an unfortunate tendency for many peripheral neuropathies to be misdiagnosed as toxic in nature. The result is that necessary treatment of a potentially remedial condition is delayed, or a baseless lawsuit initiated.

Our limited knowledge of the biochemical and pathophysiologic mechanisms of most neurotoxins has led to a simplistic classification system according to compound class (e.g., solvents, metals). Such a classification is clinically unhelpful and potentially misleading. A compound cannot be presumed to be neurotoxic because of a superficial resemblance to a related known toxin of similar class; all compounds within the same class are not neurotoxic (e.g., acrylamide monomer is capable of producing a devastating peripheral neuropathy, while the polymer is innocuous). Structure-toxicity relationships are clear for only a few classes of substances, such as organophosphates and hydrocarbons.

The following questions should be explored when an occupational or environmental toxin is suspected of causing a neuropathy in an individual or group.

1. *Is the pattern of clinical manifestations compatible with neurotoxic disease and, particularly, with the known neurotoxicity of the suspected compound?*

Neurotoxins rarely cause focal or asymmetric peripheral nerve disease. Since most neurotoxins cause diffuse neuronal and/or axonal dysfunction, their related symptoms and signs are usually widespread and symmetric and mimic naturally occurring metabolic, degenerative, nutritional, and demyelinating neuropathies. The majority of toxic peripheral neuropathies are of the distal axonopathy type; the remainder are mixed axonal/demyelinating. Only a very few toxic neuropathies are predominantly demyelinating in nature. Clinical manifestations should therefore obey a length-dependent relationship characteristic of symmetric distal axonal dysfunction. Symptoms and signs should begin in the feet and, with continued exposure, progress proximally. Strikingly asymmetric or multifocal deficits are unlikely to be due to neurotoxic insult.

2. *Is there a dose-response relationship between toxin exposure and the onset and severity of neuropathy?*

Neurotoxic symptoms usually coincide with or soon follow toxin exposure. Clinical symptoms due to toxic illness do not begin months to years after exposure, and, although some progression may continue for weeks to a few months after exposure (*coasting*), once exposure is terminated, clinical deficits should plateau and eventually improve. Prolonged, progressive deterioration after removal from exposure is usually incompatible with a toxic etiology. The extent and severity of neuropathic damage is usually commensurate with the degree of toxin exposure. It is therefore unlikely that a single, brief, low-level exposure will result in devastating peripheral neuropathy, unless there are multiple toxic insults or a preexisting neuropathy.

3. *Is the clinical pattern of neurologic dysfunction consistent among individuals similarly exposed to the suspected toxin?*

The type of clinical dysfunction that results from a single toxin may be remarkably variable, depending on the intensity and duration of exposure. A similar and consistent illness should, however, result in all individuals with identical exposure. As long as the dose and duration of exposure duration are similar, there is little variance of individual susceptibility or resultant clinical deficits. Idiosyncratic reactions to neurotoxins are unusual. A peripheral neuropathy is thus unlikely to be of toxic origin if it has occurred in only one member of a group similarly exposed. Likewise, neurotoxicity should he doubted when substantially different clinical manifestations occur within in a group of individuals whose chemical exposure is identical.

The suspicion of a toxic neuropathy is initially raised by particulars of the clinical history. In many cases, it alone may establish or strongly suggest the possibility of neurotoxicity. Since many toxic intoxications involve prolonged, low-level exposure, many patients are unable to discern a relationship between the insidious onset of their symptoms and toxin exposure. Inquiry should be directed to possible occupational, environmental, and iatrogenic exposures.

Attention to a patients' individual habits often proves diagnostically important. Does the patient wear protective devices and are the clothes changed before coming home? Are meals eaten in the workplace and are the hands washed prior to eating? Are coworkers similarly affected? Do symptoms improve when the patient is away from the potential toxin, such as on weekends or holidays? Do workplace conditions (ventilation, drainage) predispose workers to an unacceptably high risk of toxin exposure? Answers to these questions may, in some cases, be obtained only by a visit to the workplace. When domestic poisoning or substance abuse is suspected, home visits may be needed to check hobby workshops, medicine cabinets, and food and water sources. Inquiry should be made about recent pesticide applications and illnesses in pets and neighbors.

This chapter addresses those industrial and environmental compounds that have been shown to consistently cause peripheral neuropathy in humans. The scope of the chapter prevents coverage neuropathies due to pharmaceutical and therapeutic agents. In most instances, known or suspected pathogenetic mechanisms are not covered; further information may be obtained from one of the many excellent comprehensive neurotoxicology texts.

ACRYLAMIDE

Acrylamide compounds are used in flocculators and grouting agents. Only the monomer is neurotoxic; acrylamide polymer is innocuous, although it commonly is contaminated by monomer (up to 2 percent in flocculators). Acrylamide is absorbed readily by inhalation, ingestion, or dermal contact. Most occupational intoxications occur via the dermal route.

The rapidity and extent of acrylamide intoxication determines the nature of the clinical manifestations. Subacute, high-dose exposure causes a toxic encephalopathy, seizures, and severe truncal ataxia, followed by a peripheral neuropathy of variable severity. Prolonged, low-level exposure to acrylamide monomer causes a neuropathy of the central-peripheral axonopathy type (see below). Repeated dermal contact causes a contact dermatitis, which usually precedes the onset of neuropathy. Acrylamide neuropathy is characterized by excessive sweating of feet and hands and negative, rather than positive, sensory symptoms. Toe numbness is usually the initial symptom; pain and paresthesias are much less common. The large fiber modalities of vibration and proprioception are most severely affected. Hand clumsiness, out of proportion to sensory loss, gait ataxia, and an occasional intention tremor, may be evident. Widespread areflexia is an early finding. Even when there are only sensory symptoms, the clinical examination almost always demonstrates additional motor and cerebellar deficits (due to degeneration of cerebellar efferent and afferent fibers). Except for distal limb sweating, autonomic function is preserved and cranial nerves are normal.

Electrodiagnostic studies demonstrate an axonal sensorimotor neuropathy. Sensory potentials are either absent or diminished in amplitude, but motor and sensory conduction velocities are relatively preserved. Reduced sensory potential amplitudes may be an early indicator of subclinical neuropathy. Sural nerve biopsy shows diminished numbers of large diameter, thickly myelinated axons. Satisfactory clinical recovery is usual if toxin exposure is stopped before the neuropathy becomes severe, although vibration appreciation may remain impaired. If the neuropathy is severe, recovery may be incomplete with residual sensory loss, lower extremity spasticity, truncal ataxia, and memory loss.

Acrylamide neuropathy is an example of a toxic central-peripheral distal axonopathy. The initial pathologic dysfunction occurs at the distal ends of the longest peripheral nerve fibers, but as the neuropathy progresses, similar changes occur in proximal nerve segments, including distal segments of dorsal column, corticospinal, and spinocerebellar tracts. Residual sensory loss is probably due to incomplete regeneration of these CNS axons. Spasticity, due to degeneration of corticospinal tract, may emerge as PNS function improves.

ALLYL CHLORIDE

Allyl chloride is a halogenated hydrocarbon used in the manufacture of pesticides, epoxy resin, and monomers of polyacrylonitrile and glycerin. It is a volatile, colorless liquid at room temperature. Prolonged, high-level atmospheric exposure may produce a peripheral neuropathy of the distal axonopathy type. The initial symptom is numbness of the feet, but eventually a more extensive neuropathy ensues with pansensory loss in a stocking-glove distribution, distal weakness, and diminished Achilles reflexes. Recovery from mild neuropathy is usual once exposure is terminated. Experimental animals exposed to allyl chloride display multifocal accumulations of axonal neurofilaments with axonal degeneration of distal nerve segments in the PNS and dorsolateral columns of the spinal cord.

ARSENIC (INORGANIC)

Arsenic compounds are by-products of copper and lead ore smelting. Human intoxication is usually the result of acute, high-level poisoning due to suicidal or homicidal ingestion, chronic occupational exposure in smelting plants or mines, arsenic-laced illicit drugs, and arsenic-contaminated well water. Neurotoxicity is greatest with trivalent arsenic (arsenite); the pentavalent form (arsenate) is less toxic.

Arsenic polyneuropathy may have a subacute or chronic course. Environmental or occupational exposure usually involves prolonged, low-level intoxication. In contrast to more acute intoxication, in which neuropathy and bone marrow changes are the predominant abnormalities, the dominant clinical signs in chronic exposure involve the skin. These include hyperkeratosis and hyperpigmentation, Mee's lines (white transverse striae of nails), pitting edema of the distal extremities, and mucous membrane irritation. Weakness, malaise, anorexia, and vomiting may be early symptoms. Early on, an asymptomatic neuropathy may be demonstrated by careful clinical and electrodiagnostic examination. Eventually, with continued exposure, an overt clinical neuropathy develops with prominent numbness and burning of the hands and feet. Arsenic intoxication causes a sensory greater than motor neuropathy, and, although both large- and small-fiber sensory modalities are affected, proprioceptive function may be especially impaired. Weakness is usually mild and confined to the foot extensors and intrinsic hand muscles. Eventually a severe stocking-glove sensorimotor neuropathy develops. The degree of recovery is inversely related to the severity of the neuropathy at the time exposure is terminated. Mild cases recover satisfactorily, but those with severe deficits may have marked residua.

Subacute arsenic neuropathy begins within weeks of high-dose exposure. The ingestion of a large dose of arsenic causes abdominal pain, diarrhea, tachycardia, hypotension, vasomotor collapse, and occasionally death, all within a day. The patient may become somnolent and stuporous; an organic psychosis may develop, but usually clears rapidly. In a few patients, cognitive and behavioral impairments become permanent. If the patient survives, there frequently follows peripheral neuropathy, bone marrow depression, and skin changes. Neuropathy usually develops within 10 days to 3 weeks of acute or subacute exposure to arsenic. One report described neuropathic symptoms beginning as late as 8 weeks following exposure. Deterioration may continue for up to 5 weeks following cessation of exposure. The initial neuropathic symptoms are sensory. Numbness and painful paresthesias start in the feet but eventually affect the hands. Unlike acrylamide neuropathy, positive sensory symptoms such as aching, tingling, and burning, predominate. Weakness initially affects the feet, then the arms. The severity of the neuropathy depends on the dose ingested and the effect of early treatment. In some cases, respiratory muscles may be involved, and the disease course may mimic acute inflammatory demyelinating polyneuropathy (AIDP).

Electrodiagnostic examination performed early in the course of the neuropathy, may show what appears to be a demyelinating polyradiculoneuropathy. With time, however, there is evidence of widespread axonal degeneration with denervation in distal leg muscles, reduced sensory potential amplitudes, and relatively normal motor conduction studies. Subacute intoxication, in contrast to chronic exposure, tends to lack the prominent nail and skin changes. Recovery is gradual and, although sensory function may improve over a 2-year period, there is often substantial residual deficit.

Routine laboratory results are usually normal. With prolonged exposure there may be elevated arsenic levels in hair, fingernail clippings, and urine. In subacute intoxications these findings may be less impressive. Urine arsenic levels may remain elevated for weeks; levels greater than 25 μg per 24-hour specimen are abnormal unless there was recent seafood ingestion, a source of pentavalent arsenic. The rapid clearance of arsenic from the blood makes serum levels less reliable. The spinal fluid is acellular with normal protein. Sural nerve biopsy shows a reduction in the number of myelinated fibers. There is neither segmental demyelination nor inflammatory changes.

Treatment of both subacute and chronic arsenic neuropathy involves chelation therapy with either BAL (British antilewisite) or penicillamine. Once the neuropathy is fully developed, chelation therapy is of doubtful efficacy. Some have suggested that, for optimal results, chelation therapy should be continued for months following exposure.

CARBON DISULFIDE

Carbon disulfide (CS_2), a clear, colorless liquid that is a vapor at room temperature and readily absorbed by the lungs and, to a lesser extent, the skin. It is used in the production of viscose rayon fibers and cellophane films. Urinary levels of its metabolite, 2-triothiazolidine-4-carboxylic acid have proved to be a sensitive measure of CS_2; exposure. Occupational exposure to CS_2 is invariably via the respiratory route.

The predominant manifestation of acute and subacute, high-level exposure is CNS dysfunction. Prolonged, low-level exposure causes both PNS and CNS dysfunction. CNS abnormalities include anxiety, depression, and memory impairment, spasticity, hemiparesis, and extrapyramidal deficits. Chronic exposure to CS_2; in the 10 to 40 ppm range, causes asymptomatic slowing of motor nerve conduction in the legs. Higher concentrations (40 to 60 ppm) produce an overt, progressive, distal symmetric sensorimotor neuropathy. This neuropathy is characterized by impaired pain, touch and vibration appreciation, distal weakness, and areflexia in the legs. With continued exposure the arms are similarly affected. Once exposure is terminated, almost complete recovery from neuropathy, and most of the CNS abnormalities, can be expected. Occasionally, CNS recovery is incomplete, probably due to residual spinal cord damage.

Intoxication by CS_2 should be suspected when individuals in the proper clinical setting present with both a sensorimotor neuropathy and CNS dysfunction. Spinal fluid protein is normal. Electrodiagnostic studies in workers exposed to CS_2; are remarkable for showing mildly slowed motor conductions in the legs. In the early stages of neuropathy, the only physiologic abnormalities may be slight slowing of sensory conduction to the digits. Needle electromyography reveals acute and chronic denervation changes in distal leg muscles reflecting axonal degeneration and chronic motor unit reinnervation.

CYANIDE

Although chronic industrial cyanide poisoning is rare, repeated exposure to thiocyanate occurs in populations that consume cassava. Cassava is the tuber of the manioc shrub and ingestion results in elevated plasma thiocyanate levels. Chronic cassava consumption results in a distal symmetric sensorimotor neuropathy, characterized by ataxia, painful paresthesias, and severe proprioceptive deficits. The ataxia is probably due to peripheral neuropathy rather than cerebellar disease. Rapid, high-level ingestion results in a marked degree of spasticity, visual disturbances with eventual optic atrophy, and cochlear dysfunction.

ETHYLENE OXIDE

Ethylene oxide is used in the sterilization of heat-sensitive medical equipment in most hospitals and as an alkylating agent in industrial chemical synthesis. It is a gas at room temperature. Clinically significant occupational exposure most commonly has involved sterilization equipment operators who were exposed to high atmospheric levels and failed to use proper ventilatory equipment. A severe, but transient, encephalopathy results from acute, high-level intoxication. Headache, nausea, and eye irritation may precede mental status changes. Prolonged, low-level exposure results in both cognitive impairment and a reversible, distal, symmetric, sensorimotor axonopathy.

Initial neuropathic symptoms include numbness and weakness in the distal extremities and gait unsteadiness. Tendon reflexes, especially the Achilles, are diminished. Cranial nerve function is usually normal. Cognitive impairment may coexist with peripheral neuropathy. Electrodiagnostic studies demonstrate a diffuse axonopathy. The spinal fluid is usually acellular and the protein level normal. Axonal degeneration was the predominant pathology in one reported sural nerve biopsy. Complete recovery can be expected once exposure is terminated.

HEXACARBONS

The hexacarbons *n*-hexane and methyl *n*-butyl ketone (MnBK) will be considered together, as both are metabolized to 2,5-hexanedione, the responsible toxic agent. Methyl ethyl ketone, is not neurotoxic by itself, but is present in many solvent mixtures and may potentiate the neurotoxicity of *n*-hexane and MnBK. *n*-Hexane is used as a solvent and component of glues and lacquers. Intoxication is usually due to occupational exposure or deliberate inhalation abuse (glue sniffing).

Acute single exposure to high-dose hexacarbons results in narcosis and CNS depression. Massive repeated inhalation, usually due to recreational inhalation abuse, causes a predominantly motor neuropathy that may mimic AIDP because of its subacute progression and cranial nerve dysfunction. There may be prominent autonomic dysfunction with distal hyperhidrosis or anhidrosis, vasomotor instability, and impotence. Prolonged, lower-dose exposure to *n*-hexane or MnBK, usually in the occupational setting, causes a slowly progressive central-peripheral axonopathy. Sensory loss to touch, pin, vibration, and thermal sense is initially limited to the feet but, with continued exposure, progressively moves proximally. An early finding is diminution or loss of the Achilles reflex. Other tendon reflexes may be remarkably preserved despite marked sensory loss. Distal leg and arm muscles may be weak, and, with neuropathy progression, weakness and atrophy may become the prominent complaint. Cranial nerve and autonomic functions remain normal. In severe cases, the neuropathy is complicated by malaise, weight loss, abdominal pain, and leg cramps.

The electrodiagnostic studies of *n*-hexane neuropathy are unusual because of the profound slowing of distal motor conduction, a finding most unusual for toxic neuropathies but characteristic of severe hexane polyneuropathy. Slowed nerve conductions have also been reported in asymptomatic workers employed in factories with documented cases of solvent polyneuropathy. Visual, brainstem, and somatosensory evoked potentials may be abnormal. The spinal fluid protein is usually normal, although it may rarely be elevated due to spinal root involvement. The severity of the neuropathy dictates the completeness and rapidity of recovery. Patients with mild neuropathy usually make a complete and satisfactory recovery. The phenonemon of coasting, in which neuropathic deterioration continues despite cessation of exposure, is common with solvent neuropathies. Residual distal atrophy, weakness, and sensory loss is not uncommon with severe neuropathies. Signs of CNS dysfunction, such as spasticity and long-tract weakness, are due to degeneration in distal motor and sensory tracts, and may only become evident once the neuropathy improves.

LEAD

Overt clinical cases of lead neuropathy are now rare in North America and Europe, especially since the elimination of lead-containing paints. The potential for occupational exposure still exists, however, in smelting factories, the manufacture of batteries, demolition work, and automobile radiator repair. Environmental sources of lead include paint ingestion and consumption of moonshine whiskey. Some sporadic cases of lead poisoning relate to individuals burning lead-containing batteries for heat and lead exposure in indoor firing ranges.

Lead intoxication in children usually causes CNS, rather than PNS, dysfunction. In adults, peripheral neuropathy is a well-described complication of chronic lead intoxication. Prolonged exposure to lead is necessary before the neuropathy becomes symptomatic. In many cases, by the time neuropathy is evident there are a number of systemic features, including weight loss, anorexia, fatigue, constipation, and episodic abdominal pain. A microcytic, hypochromic anemia usually is present in cases of clinically overt neuropathy and renal insufficiency, and gout may occasionally occur.

Unlike most other toxic neuropathies, lead neuropathy is predominantly motor, with few, if any, sensory symptoms or signs. There is tremendous variability in the severity of the neuropathy. Although the older literature suggests that lead may produce a number of focal neurologic deficits, in adults, the most common neuropathic expression is a progressive, symmetric axonopathy that may prominently involve the arms. Weakness is accompanied by distal atrophy, reflex loss, and occasionally fasciculations. In children, weakness usually begins in the legs, often with marked atrophy. Needle EMG shows active and chronic denervation in weakened muscles. Conduction velocities are relatively spared, and, despite a paucity of sensory complaints, sensory potential amplitudes may be diminished.

Associated laboratory abnormalities include a mild anemia due to decreased hemoglobin synthesis, basophilic stippling of erythrocytes due to retained ribosomes, and elevated urine coproporphyrin. The spinal fluid is usually acellular, and the protein level is normal. Urine lead levels greater than 0.2 mg/l are usually regarded as abnormal. Serum lead levels are often clinically unhelpful due to the rapid clearance of lead from the circulation and uncertainty over normal lead levels. Since large amounts of lead are sequestered in soft tissues, the diagnosis can be confirmed by an increased urinary lead excretion after administration of a chelating agent. Calcium ethylenediaminetetraacetic acid (Ca-EDTA), BAL, and penicillamine all can be used for chelation, although Ca-EDTA is the usual recommended agent. Urine lead levels greater than 1 mg per 24-hour specimen, following chelation therapy, indicates excessive lead stores in soft tissues.

Eliminating further lead exposure is the initial step in treating lead intoxication. Since lead can be stored in bone, any condition that demineralizes bone will release lead into the blood. Chelation therapy binds soft tissue lead, promoting its excretion. In mild cases, penicillamine is used; alternatively, Ca-EDTA can be used. Both penicillamine and EDTA are administered in short courses. Recovery may begin within 2 weeks of beginning therapy and, except in advanced cases, is usually complete.

MERCURY

The atomic form of mercury and an individual's susceptibility and age determines, in part, the clinical symptoms of mercury intoxication. Exposure may be to metallic mercury, mercury vapor, inorganic mercury salts, complex organic mercurials, or short-chain alkyl mercurials. Mercury poisoning frequently occurs in the occupational setting, for example, in battery factories, mercury processing plants, and electronic applications factories. Since mercury metal is volatile with low vapor pressure at room temperatures, inadvertent spillage in enclosed poorly ventilated rooms may produce excessively high levels of mercury vapor. Despite the recent media concern, mercury-containing dental amalgam appears to pose little risk.

Although mercury intoxication mainly causes CNS dysfunction; the PNS, especially the dorsal root ganglia, may also be affected. Metallic mercury and mercury vapor have been reported to cause clinical polyneuropathy. It is unclear if organic mercury definitely produces neuropathy. Mercury metal vapor has been reported to cause a subacute, diffuse, predominantly motor neuropathy that may mimic AIDP. Evidence from electrodiagnostic studies and sural nerve biopsy suggest an axonal neuropathy with relative sparing of sensory axons. Recovery gradually ensues once exposure is terminated. Occupational exposure to elemental mercury may also cause a mild subclinical sensorimotor neuropathy.

Tremor and ataxia occasionally result from exposure to all types of mercury compounds. The tremor is usually of the intention type and has a large amplitude. Prominent and widespread CNS dysfunction is more a feature of intoxication with organic mercurials than inorganic or elemental mercury. CNS dysfunction includes hearing loss, dysarthria, ataxia, constricted visual fields, tremor, chorea, myoclonus, and cognitive impairment. Evidence of corticospinal tract dysfunction with hyperreflexia and Babinski signs may be present. Full recovery of CNS function is unusual.

A number of different systemic abnormalities may accompany neurologic symptoms. Elemental mercury produces red skin, blushing, dermatographia, and excessive perspiration. Skin changes and autonomic dysfunction are especially common in children with direct contact with mercurial compounds. Mild anemia, proteinuria, and glycosuria result from elemental and inorganic mercury intoxication. Complex organic mercurials cause nephrotoxicity; ingestion of inorganic mercury salts may cause acute gastrointestinal dysfunction. Rapid inhalation of high-level mercury vapor may cause acute pneumonitis.

METHYL BROMIDE

Methyl bromide is a gas used as a fumigant, fire extinguisher, refrigerant, and insecticide. Acute high-level exposure produces a reversible encephalopathy with visual and speech disturbances, delirium, and seizures. Prolonged, low-level exposure results in peripheral neuropathy, along with corticospinal and cerebellar dysfunction. The pattern of neuropathic deficits suggests that the underlying nature is axonal, but there are neither morphologic studies of human tissue nor experimental animal models to confirm this. Sensory and motor dysfunction develops only after months of exposure. Prominent complaints include unsteady gait and clumsy hands. Clinical examination demonstrates a stocking-glove distribution of pin and touch loss and flaccid weakness of distal leg muscles. Prominent calf tenderness may mistakenly suggest a diagnosis of myositis. Achilles hyporeflexia is common. Spinal fluid protein levels are normal. Electrodiagnostic studies show impaired sensory conduction studies and denervation in distal muscles. Improvement is gradual once exposure is terminated.

ORGANOPHOSPHATE ESTERS

Organophosphate esters are used as insecticides, petroleum additives, modifiers of plastics, lubricants, antioxidants, and flame retardants. Despite the multiple uses of organophosphate esters, occupational group exposure is rare; most cases of intoxication result from accidental exposure to pesticides, either during or after agricultural spraying. Fortunately, most organophosphate esters are quickly degraded in the environment.

Organophosphate esters may be absorbed via the skin or respiratory and gastrointestinal tracts; they phosphorylate and thereby inhibit acetylcholinesterase (AChE), which is located in nervous tissue and erythrocytes. The resultant accumulation of acetylcholine (ACh) causes excessive stimulation of muscarinic and nicotinic receptors.

Excessive ACh stimulation of muscarinic receptors is responsible for the acute cholinergic effects (type I syndrome), which are always apparent within a day of exposure, often within hours. The nature of the individual organophosphate and the degree of intoxication determines the intensity of the cholinergic state. Cholinergic symptoms include tachy- or bradycardia, diarrhea, vomiting, fasciculations, sweating, salivation, and micturition. Excessive exposure causes emotional irritability, nervousness, fatigue, diminished alertness, cognitive impairment, coma, and convulsions. On rare occasions, behavioral changes may be the only indication of organophosphate exposure. Atropine is usually effective in counteracting the muscarinic effects, but unless treatment is continued, cholinergic symptoms may recur, occasionally with fatal consequences. Patients should be adequately ventilated before atropine is given to minimize the risk of ventricular arrhythmias. The administration of pralidoxime may accelerate reactivation of inhibited AChE.

Excessive nicotinic receptor stimulation with depolarizing block underlies the type II or intermediate syndrome, which occurs within 12 to 96 hours of exposure. Its nomenclature reflects the fact that, when present, it follows the acute muscarinic effects, but precedes the later peripheral neuropathy. The initial feature is usually respiratory insufficiency, followed by weakness of neck flexors and proximal limb muscles. Distal strength is usually preserved. Weakness of palatal, facial, and extraocular muscles may be present, and dystonic posturing may occasionally be evident. Sensory function remains normal. Recovery begins 5 to 15 days after the onset of weakness and progresses from cranial nerves to respiratory muscles, proximal muscles and, finally, neck flexors. Atropine is ineffective, and there is no correlation between development of type II syndrome and the likelihood of later developing peripheral neuropathy.

Some organophosphate esters cause a central-peripheral axonopathy. It has been labeled the organophosphate-induced delayed polyneuropathy (OPIDP) because its onset may be delayed for 7 to 21 days following exposure. The neuropathy is a source of great morbidity; fortunately, most agricultural organophosphates do not produce neuropathy. Its development is independent of the degree of AChE inhibition. The most dramatic examples of neuropathy often result from compounds subtle or unappreciated cholinergic symptoms, especially when exposure is prolonged and low-level.

Cramping calf pain and painful paresthesias in the feet are usually the earliest symptoms of OPIDP. The neuropathy is predominantly motor. Weakness appears early and initially involves distal leg muscles before those of the hands. Despite the paucity of sensory complaints, objective evidence of sensory loss is almost always present. Gait ataxia, out of proportion to the degree of weakness, may be present. Tendon hyporeflexia is common. The ankle jerks are invariably absent; activity of the remaining reflexes depends on the degree of CNS dysfunction. Cranial nerve and autonomic functions are usually spared.

OPIDP tends to progress rapidly in contrast to the slower course of most other toxic axonopathies. Maximal clinical deficits usually develop within 2 weeks. A rare case of rapid-onset motor neuropathy after exposure to merphos has been reported, although it is not easy to separate such cases from naturally occurring AIDP. As with many other toxic neuropathies, evidence of CNS derangement becomes evident once the neuropathy improves. Patients with mild neuropathy have a good prognosis for satisfactory recovery. Severe deficits may not recover completely; there may be residual claw hand deformity, persistent atrophy, and footdrop, as well as spasticity and ataxia. Residual dysfunction is more often due to unresolved CNS abnormalities than unresolved neuropathy. Presently, there is no specific treatment to prevent the development of OPIDP.

Routine laboratory studies are usually normal. Diminished levels of erythrocyte AChE indicate recent organophosphate exposure. Early, severe weakness is often associated with AChE levels below 20 percent normal. The clinical significance of a single reading is uncertain due to the wide range of normal erythrocyte AChE levels; serial determinations that show progressive AChE depression are of greater clinical significance in documenting organophosphate intoxication. Low AChE levels, however, do not predict the development of OPIDP. Since erythrocyte AChE levels regenerate at the rate of 1 percent per day, levels may return to normal by the time the patient is medically examined. Pseudocholinesterase levels have little diagnostic value. The cerebrospinal fluid is usually acellular, and protein levels are either normal or slightly elevated.

Electrodiagnostic studies of OPIDP demonstrate an axonal neuropathy with acute and chronic denervation in distal and occasionally proximal limb muscles. Sensory potentials are usually unobtainable in the arms and legs. Despite having predominantly motor symptoms, diminished sensory potential amplitudes appear to be more sensitive than motor conduction changes in screening for organophosphate neuropathy. Motor conduction studies are either normal or minimally slowed.

POLYCHLORINATED BIPHENYLS

Polychlorinated biphenyls can be found in industrial insulation and transformer moldings. Ingestion of polychlorinated biphenyl contaminated food may cause a distal, symmetric sensory neuropathy with distal sensory loss and hyporeflexia. Accompanying skin changes include a brown acneform skin eruption and brown-pigmented nails. Electrodiagnostic studies show abnormal sensory conductions in the legs. Peripheral neuropathy is not definitively associated with the polychlorinated biphenyls used as fire retardants, although distal numbness has been reported.

THALLIUM

Although the use of thallous salts as rodenticides and insecticides is less common now than in the past, instances of poisoning continue to arise from homicidal or accidental ingestion, especially in children. Thallium intoxication produces a painful, sensory greater than motor, distal axonopathy with predominant involvement of large-diameter sensory fibers.

There are three distinct syndromes of thallium polyneuropathy, differing primarily by their temporal course. The most common scenario results from acute high-dose poisoning in which symptoms begin within 1 to 2 days of massive ingestion. The subacute variety begins within weeks of a less massive single-dose intoxication. Chronic thallium intoxication is the rarest and occurs after prolonged exposure to moderate levels. A symmetric distal axonopathy results from all three types of exposures, the only differences being the temporal course and associated systemic features.

Massive, acute exposure is followed within hours by severe gastrointestinal distress within hours. On rare occasion, vomiting, diarrhea, and abdominal pain are delayed by a day. Severe burning paresthesias in the feet, with intense joint pains, begins about 2 to 5 days following ingestion. Sensory symptoms occasionally involve the hands and trunk and both large- and small-fiber sensory modalities are involved. Although weakness is not a prominent complaint, it is usually evident on clinical examination. Tendon reflexes are usually preserved early in the disease course. Massive intoxication may result in lethargy, cardiac and respiratory failure, coma, and death. In survivors, recovery is gradual, usually incomplete, and frequently complicated by anoxia-induced CNS dysfunction. Alopecia, the classic sign of thallium poisoning, appears about 15 to 39 days after ingestion and therefore is of little diagnostic help early on. Renal insufficiency may complicate acute thallium poisoning.

Subacute thallium neuropathy develops 1 week or more after exposure, has a slower evolution, and may be marked by scalp alopecia. Other associated clinical features include hyperkeratosis, Mee's lines (white striae of nails), ataxia, chorea, and cranial nerve palsies. Subacute thallium intoxication produces a sensory greater than motor neuropathy. There is distal impairment of pin, light touch, and proprioception over the distal legs. Painful paresthesias of the feet may interfere with walking. Weakness is rarely severe, although there is usually some degree of distal weakness. Tendon reflexes may he either normal or slightly depressed. Autonomic dysfunction, primarily tachycardia or hypertension, may be present. The prognosis for the subacute neuropathy is excellent with most recovering within 6 months following termination of exposure. Hair regrowth is within 10 weeks after withdrawal. Spinal fluid protein is normal. Electrodiagnostic studies show a symmetric axonopathy with sensory potentials reduced more than motor, and nerve conduction velocities only mildly slowed.

Thallium exposure is established by demonstrating its deposition in urine or body tissues. Since alopecia is not present in every case, it cannot be fully relied upon as a marker of thallium intoxication. Treatment with potassium chloride or Prussian blue to bind thallium has been reported to promote survival.

TRICHLOROETHYLENE

Trichloroethylene (TCE) is an industrial solvent and degreasing compound used in the dry cleaning business and in the manufacture of rubber. Its euphoriant properties underlie its potential for recreational abuse. Rapid higher-dose intoxication usually occurs in an industrial setting and is characterized by trigeminal nerve dysfunction. Sensory deficits begin initially over the snout and then progresses outward. The rapidity and severity of the sensory impairment depends on the total dose. Severe numbness of the face, mouth, and oral pharynx may begin within 12 hours of exposure. Continued exposure causes motor deficits of mastication, facial expression, ptosis, dysarthria, vocal cord paralysis, and dysphagia. Central and paracentral scotomas have been reported. Although a somatic peripheral neuropathy has been reported to accompany the cranial nerve dysfunction, it has never been conclusively proven, and many doubt its existence. Recovery is usually complete within 2 years of stopping exposure. Occasional residua of facial numbness, pupillary disturbances, and disabling dysphagia may be present.

Chronic low-level TCE exposure has been reported to produce cognitive impairment and visual loss. A distal symmetric peripheral neuropathy has been suggested, but validation has been complicated by the fact that most chronic exposures are not to chemically pure TCE. The ability of TCE to cause a somatic polyneuropathy remains unproven.

VACOR

Vacor (N-3-pyridylmethyl-N'-p-nitrophenylurea [PNU]) is a rodenticide that is a structural analogue of nicotinamide. Its ingestion results in rapid-onset, severe, distal sensorimotor axonopathy with prominent autonomic dysfunction. Peripheral neuropathy is accompanied by acute diabetes mellitus, secondary to necrosis of pancreatic β cells. Ingestion of large amounts of vacor are followed by limb weakness, loss of postural reflexes, cranial nerve deficits, urinary retention, and diabetic ketoacidosis. Recovery is marked by a gradual return of strength over many months. Patients may remain diabetic with variable degrees of autonomic dysfunction.

SUGGESTED READINGS

Albers JW, Cariender D, Levine SP et al: Asymptomatic sensorimotor polyneuropathy in workers exposed to elemental mercury. Neurology 32: 1168–1174, 1982

Albers JW, Kallenback LR, Fine LI et al: Neurological abnormalities associated with remote occupational elemental mercury exposure. Ann Neurol 24: 651–659, 1988

Altenkirch H, Mager J, Stoltenburg G et al: Toxic polyneuropathies after sniffing a glue thinner. J Neurol 214:137–152, 1977

Andersen O: Clinical evidence and therapeutic indications in neurotoxicology, exemplified by thallotoxicosis. Acta Neurol Scand 70:185–192, 1984

Chang YC: Neurotoxic effects of n-hexane on the human central nervous system: evoked potentials abnormalities in n-hexane polyneuropathy. J Neurol Neurosurg Psychiatry 50:269–274, 1987

Chia L, Chiu F: Neurological studies on polychlorinated biphenyls (PCB)-poisoned patients. Am J Ind Med 5:117–121, 1984

Corsi G, Maestrelli P, Picotti G et al: Chronic peripheral neuropathy in workers with previous exposure to carbon disulfide. Br J Ind Med 40:209–211, 1983

Crystal HA, Schaumburg HH, Grober E et al: Cognitive impairment and sensory loss associated with chronic low level ethylene oxide exposure. Neurology 38:567–569, 1988

Donofrio PD, Wilbourn AJ, Albers JW et al: Acute arsenic intoxication presenting as Guillain-Barré-like syndrome. Muscle Nerve 10:114–120, 1987

Estrin WJ, Bowler RM, Lash A et al: Neurotoxicological evaluation of hospital sterilizer workers exposed to ethylene oxide. J Toxicol Clin Toxicol 28: 1–20, 1990

Feldman RG, Niles CA, Kelly-Hayes M et al: Peripheral neuropathy in arsenic smelter workers. Neurology 29:939–944, 1979

Fisher JR: Guillain-Barre syndrome following organophosphate poisoning. JAMA 238:1950–1951, 1977

Gross JA, Haas ML, Swift TF: Ethylene oxide neurotoxicity: report of four cases and review of literature. Neurology 29:978–983, 1979

He F, Zahng S: Effects of allyl chloride on occupationally exposed subjects. Scand J Work Environ Health 11:43–51, 1985

Lambert EH, Bunge RP: Peripheral Neuropathy. Vol. 2. WB Saunders, Philadelphia, 2133–2161, 1984

LeQuesne PM, McLeod JG: Peripheral neuropathy following a single exposure to arsenic. J Neurol Sci 32:437–451, 1977

Schaumburg HH, Spencer PS: Recognizing neurotoxic disease. Neurology 37: 276–278, 1987

Senanayake N, Karralliede L: Neurotoxic effects of organophosphorus insecticides: an intermediate syndrome. N Engl J Med 316:761–763, 1987

Windebank AJ, McCall JT, Dyek PJ: Metal neuropathy. Ann Neurol 10:38, 1981

100. INHERITED NEUROPATHY

GUILLERMO A. SUAREZ

The inherited neuropathies are a group of heterogeneous disorders. Some are related to known metabolic derangements (e.g., Fabry's disease), while others have no known cause (Table 100-1). A useful way to classify this latter group is based on the inheritance pattern, populations of neurons affected, natural history, and electrophysiologic and histopathologic findings. In the last few years, the tremendous advances in our understanding of the genetics of these disorders through gene mapping by linkage analysis and gene isolation by positional cloning and other techniques have provided new ways to classify these disorders.

An attempt to classify these conditions with a reference point is to consider which population (system) of neurons is predominantly affected. Selective degeneration of lower motor neurons, is classified as hereditary motor neuropathy or, simply, spinal muscular atrophy. Degeneration of motor and sensory neurons indicates hereditary motor and sensory neuropathies (HMSN). Degeneration of sensory and autonomic neurons is categorized as hereditary sensory and autonomic neuropathies (HSAN).

Inherited neuropathies are probably the most common undiagnosed neuropathies. Dyck and colleagues reported that 42 percent of a series of 205 patients with undiagnosed neuropathies were found to have an inherited neuropathy when an appropriate kinship history was obtained (recording skeletal abnormalities such as high arches), and relatives were appropriately examined. It must be emphasized that a critical part of the examination is obtaining an appropriate family history by specifically asking whether the relatives have foot deformities, high arches, gait problems, muscle atrophy, trophic ulcers, or neuropathic symptoms.

HEREDITARY MOTOR AND SENSORY NEUROPATHY

Originally, the term *peroneal muscular atrophy* or Charcot-Marie-Tooth disease was believed to be specific for one disorder. It is now known that this is not the case. Peroneal muscular atrophy occurs in several inherited neuromuscular disorders. Charcot and Marie emphasized the following features: pes cavus, progressive atrophy of distal leg muscles (legs resemble an inverted champagne bottle), tightness of Achilles tendons, hammertoes, and a steppage gait. Tooth emphasized that the disorder was inherited and concluded that it was due to disease of the peripheral nerves.

Landmark genetic, clinical, electrophysiologic, and pathologic studies of large kindreds by Dyck and Lambert allowed a separation in two main groups: (1) the hypertrophic or demyelinating form, later called hereditary motor and sensory neuropathy type I (HMSN I), characterized by diffusely low motor nerve conduction velocities associated with nerve biopsy findings of axonal atrophy, demyelination, and onion bulb formations, and (2) the neuronal form of Charcot-Marie-Tooth disease, subsequently named hereditary motor and sensory neuropathy type II (HMSN II), characterized by normal or near-normal motor conduction velocity without hypertrophic neuropathy on nerve biopsy.

The first group, hypertrophic type I, can be subdivided into (1) patients with a classical phenotype as described by Charcot, Marie, and Tooth, and (2) patients with recessively inherited or sporadic varieties, referred to as hereditary motor and sensory neuropathy type III (HMSN III) or Dejerine-Sottas disease. This is usually a more severe demyelinating neuropathy with onset at infancy or early childhood, and with very low conduction velocities; and HMSN IV or Refsum's disease with increased serum phytanic acid levels.

The mode of inheritance is generally autosomal dominant in both HMSN I and II. However, in a minority of cases, the disorder is sporadic or affects siblings but not their parents. These cases have been attributed to probable autosomal recessive inheritance or (1) a new mutation of a dominant gene, (2) autosomal inheritance with nonpenetrance or reduced penetrance in the parents, or (3) false paternity. X-linked inheritance has been established in four families by genetic studies.

HMSN I

Genetic Transmission. The mode of inheritance of HMSN I is autosomal dominant in the majority of families. The pattern of inheritance on genetic linkage analysis suggests that there are at least four varieties (Fig. 100-1):

1. HMSN IA: In most families with autosomal dominant inheritance, the HMSN I locus maps to a band (p11.2-p12) on the short arm of chromosome 17.

TABLE 100-1. Inherited Neuropathies

Disorder	Genetic Transmission	Clinical Features	Electrophysiologic Findings	Pathologic Findings
Hereditary motor and sensory neuropathies				
Type I				
IA: chromosome 17 (p11.2-p12); PMP22 gene	AD	Distal leg weakness and sensory loss	Slow NCV, reduced or absent SNAP	Hypertrophic neuropathy
IB: chromosome 1 (Duffy locus)	AD	Distal leg weakness and sensory loss		Hypertrophic neuropathy
X: X chromosome (q12-q21); connexin32 gene	X-linked	Distal leg weakness and sensory loss		Hypertrophic neuropathy
Type II Chromosome 1 (p site)	AD	Onset later in life	Near-normal NCV, absent SNAP	Reduction in large MF, axonal atrophy
Type III Dejerine-Sottas disease Point mutations on PMP22 and P0 genes	AR, AD, sporadic	Onset in infancy; delayed motor skills	Very slow NCV	Demyelination, axonal atrophy
Type IV Refsum's disease	AR	Retinitis pigmentosa, peripheral neuropathy, ataxia, skeletal malformations	Motor and sensory polyneuropathy	Demyelination and onion bulb formation
Hereditary sensory and autonomic neuropathies				
Type I	AD	"Painful feet," decreased pain and temperature sensation	Abnormal small nerve fiber function	Reduction of small MF and UF
Type II	AR	Onset in early childhood, plantar ulcers, mutilation of digits and toes	SNAP generally absent	Reduction of myelinated and UF
Type III Familial dysautonomia Linkage to chromosome 9	AR	Prominent autonomic manifestations, absence of fungiform papillae and defective lacrimation	Reduced SNAP, abnormal small nerve fiber function	Marked reduction of UF
Type IV	AR	Congenital insensitivity to pain, anhidrosis	Normal SNAP	Reduction of small MF
Inherited tendency to pressure palsies, deletion of 17p11.2-p12	AD	Recurrent mononeuropathies, mild distal polyneuropathy	Multiple mononeuropathies	Demyelination, thickening of myelin sheath (tomaculous)

Abbreviations: PMP, peripheral myelin protein; AD, autosomal dominant; AR, autosomal recessive; NCV, nerve conduction velocity; SNAP, sensory nerve action potential; MF, myelinated fibers; UF, ummyelinated fibers.

2. HMSN IB: In a minority of patients, the HMSN I locus is borne on the long arm of chromosome 1, linked to the Duffy blood group.
3. HMSN C: Families with autosomal dominant HMSN and not linked to either chromosome 1 or 17.
4. HMSN X: In some kindreds, linkage analysis localized the locus to the proximal long arm of the X chromosome. A recent study isolated a gap junction protein, connexin32, as the candidate gene that, if abnormal, can cause HMSN X.

Lupski and coworkers reported that a segment band of chromosome 17 (17p11.2-p12) was duplicated in affected members of families with HMSN IA. The human peripheral myelin protein 22 gene (PMP22) is found in the region of the duplication. PMP22 encodes for the synthesis of a peripheral nervous system myelin protein. Recent studies have found missense mutations of PMP22 in patients with HMSN IA without the duplication. Most patients with genetically defined HMSN IA have either a gene dose effect (duplication of 17p11.2-p12) or a mutation affecting the PMP22 gene on chromosome 17.

Interestingly, the human PMP22 gene is deleted in patients with inherited tendency to pressure palsies (ITPP) (discussed below). Recently, two allelic mutations of the PMP22 gene have been found to produce a demyelinating neuropathy in mice. These observations strongly suggest that alterations in PMP22 expression, alone or in combination with yet unknown environmental factors, are responsible for this group of neuropathies. These hypotheses are currently being investigated.

Clinical Features. Typically, only a small percentage of people with HMSN I seek medical attention for neuromuscular symptoms; many actually have no symptoms. Patients have difficulty pinpointing the onset of neurologic problems, and presenting symptoms are usually difficulty in running, stumbling, slapping of the feet in walking, and muscle atrophy; they might not be aware of their problems until a relative or friend mentions that "their gait is funny." Parents may report that children have weakness of ankles or running difficulty. Another common scenario is the incidental discovery of an indicator of neuropathy, such as an abnormal nerve conduction study (NCS): the electromyographer reports a more generalized nerve conduction abnormality, consistent with an inherited neuropathy, in patients who presented with low back pain, carpal tunnel syndrome, or other related disorders.

The symptoms in HMSN mainly relate to deficits, that is, weakness and atrophy of distal muscles. Sensory symptoms are those of a deficit-of-function "dead feeling." Positive symptoms, such as "prickling" or "asleep numbness" and painful paresthesias, are not typical and should alert the physician to a possible acquired neuropathy. Autonomic symptoms are usually not reported by patients. Muscle cramps in the lower extremities, especially after exercise, are common.

On clinical examination, the feet and legs are more affected than the hands. Inspection of the feet reveals pes cavus and hammertoes in approximately 70 percent of adult patients (Fig. 100-2). Kyphosis of the spine might be present in a small per-

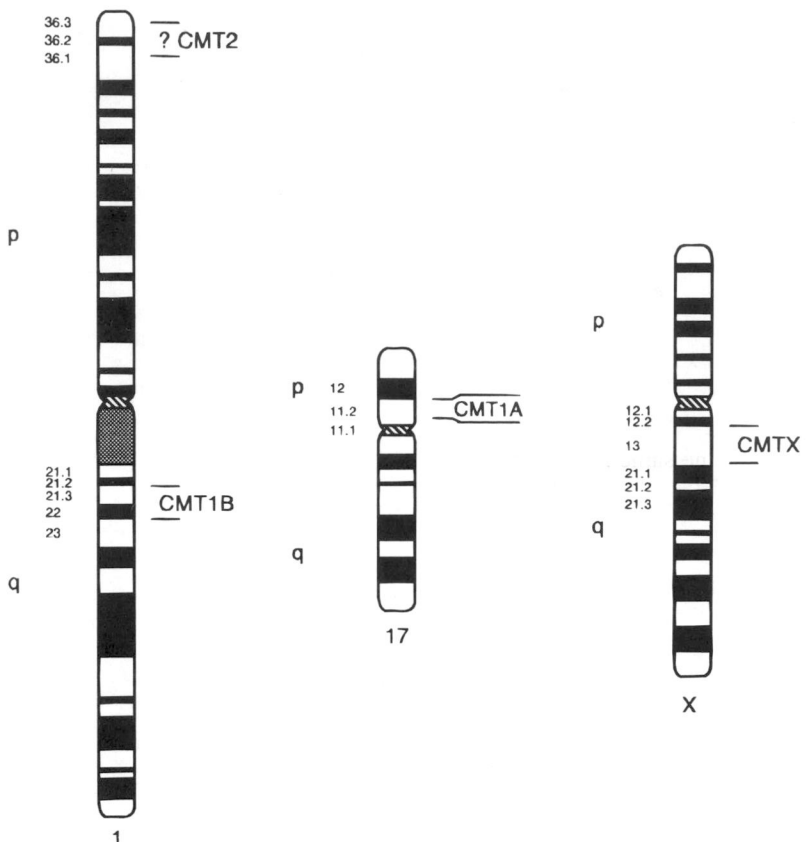

FIG. 100-1.   Idiogram of human chromosomes 1, 17, and X showing approximate localizations of HMSN IB (chromosome 1), HMSN IA (chromosome 17), HMSN IB and HMSN II (chromosome 1), and HMSN X (chromosome X) loci.

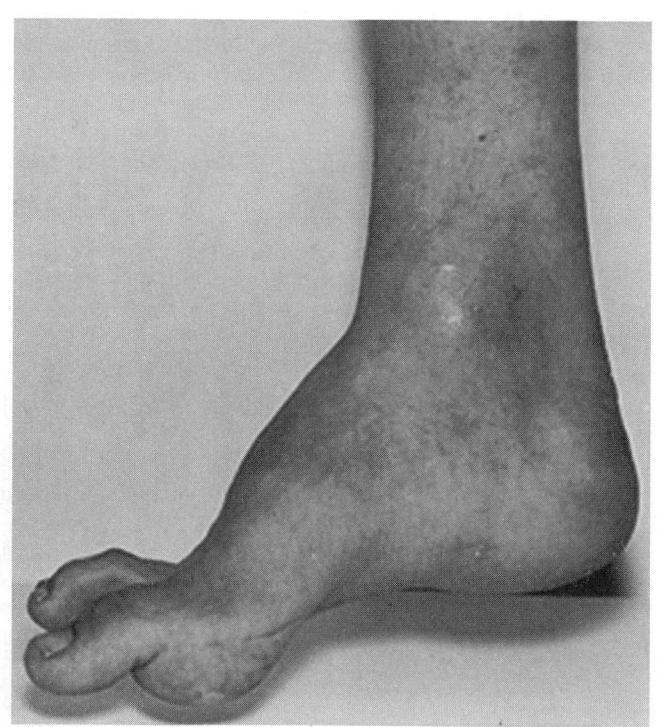

FIG. 100-2.   Typical pes cavus and hammertoes of a patient with HMSN IA.

centage of patients. Clinical enlargement of peripheral nerves or excessive firmness is present in 25 percent of patients. The nerves between the axilla and the elbow should be assessed and palpated for enlarged nerves. Entrapment points, such as the ulnar nerve at the elbow, should be avoided because the nerve is normally thickened at that point. Muscle weakness and wasting affects muscles of the feet, peroneal, and anterior tibial muscles, usually in a symmetric fashion. Later, in the upper limbs, a similar distal involvement occurs, first affecting intrinsic hand muscles. Deep tendon reflexes are usually diminished or absent in the lower and upper extremities, but there is significant variability in this sign. Classically, patients do not volunteer sensory symptoms, but sensory examination reveals distal impairment of sensation, usually affecting vibration and light touch in the feet and hands. Using quantitative sensory examination, an unequivocal abnormality of all sensory modalities is demonstrated. Occasionally, due to the sensory loss, high arches, atrophy of foot muscles, and calluses, ulcers develop over the metatarsal heads and over the tips of toes.

In some patients, there is a prominent upper limb tremor with the typical features of an essential tremor, associated with the classical phenotype of HMSN I. These cases have been labeled as Roussy-Lévy syndrome, but there is no evidence that this is a distinct clinical or genetic disorder. There is significant variability in respect to severity of neuropathic deficits among individuals, even from the same kinship. There are asymptomatic cases, with slow nerve conduction values, and sometimes minimal changes on sural nerve biopsy.

Laboratory Features. The nerve conduction and electromyographic features are useful to separate HMSN I from HMSN II. There is uniform slowing of motor conduction velocity in virtually all nerves tested in patients with HMSN I. There is good concordance of conduction velocity values within affected kindreds. Ulnar and median motor nerve conduction studies show the characteristic reduction in conduction velocity, but conduction studies in the lower extremities may not be very useful because of the more severe distal nerve fiber degeneration. A. E. Harding and P. K. Thomas proposed a criterion that a motor conduction velocity below 38 m/s be used as the cutoff value for HMSN I. This is a useful criterion provided that (1) the compound muscle action potential (CMAP) is at least 0.5 mV in the nerve where the conduction velocity is calculated, and (2) the mean values of conduction velocity for the same nerve of all affected individuals in the same kindred are used. If temporal dispersion of the CMAP or conduction block is found, an alternative diagnosis such as chronic inflammatory demyelinating polyneuropathy (CIDP) should be considered. Sensory nerves are also affected. Sensory nerve action potentials are uniformly reduced or unrecordable using standard electrophysiologic techniques. Routine laboratory studies, including cerebrospinal fluid (CSF), studies provide normal results.

Pathologic Features. Pathologic studies (especially of sural nerves) show the typical features of a hypertrophic neuropathy, including onion bulb formation, made up of circumferentially directed Schwann cell processes, marked reduction in large myelinated fibers, increase in transverse fascicular area, and increased frequency of paranodal and segmental demyelination and remyelination. Extensive morphometric studies by P.J. Dyck and colleagues have provided evidence for a primary axonal abnormality. There is clustering of demyelinating changes, increased frequency of demyelination and remyelination in distal segments, distal predominance of onion bulbs, and reduction in axon caliber relative to the number of myelin lamellae. These observations lend support to the hypothesis that axonal atrophy occurs first, and segmental demyelination may be secondary to it. This does not exclude a concomitant abnormality of Schwann cells.

HMSN IA and HMSN IB

The inheritance pattern, clinical features, electrophysiologic findings, course, and natural history of HMSN IA and HMSN IB overlap. Only molecular genetic techniques allow separation into these two groups. HMSN IA appears to be a less severe disorder than HMSN IB.

Treatment. There is no specific treatment for HMSN IA and IB. Clinical, genetic, and symptomatic counseling is important. Because of the high arches and foot deformities, proper foot care should be emphasized to avoid foot ulcers. Shoes should be comfortable, well-made, and protective. Visual inspection of the shoes and feet for injury should be carried out on a daily basis. Calluses must not be trimmed with a razor blade. If the patient develops a plantar ulcer, weightbearing should be avoided until the ulcer has healed. Foot braces may be tried, but they are not necessary for every patient. If gait is not improved by the brace, then it should not be worn. Foot surgery is usually reserved for those patients who begin to develop valgus deformity of the ankle or severe degrees of pes cavus. It should be fully discussed with the patient that surgery is not

going to cure the other manifestations of the disorder such as sensory loss and muscle weakness. Most affected individuals are able to work full time, and there is no evidence that the prognosis for life expectancy is any different than from the general population. Because of the distal weakness, training in an occupation that does not require fine motor skills may be recommended.

HMSN II: Neuronal Form

Genetic Transmission. Linkage analysis has recently localized the chromosomal locus responsible for HMSN II in four kindreds to the telomeric region of 1p on chromosome 1 (Fig. 100-1). In addition, evidence for genetic heterogeneity has also been documented.

Clinical Features. The clinical features of patients with HMSN II are similar to those with HMSN I. However, there are some differences. Patients with HMSN II are usually asymptomatic until later in life. Peripheral nerves are usually not clinically enlarged, and weakness of feet and leg muscles predominate; hands are less severely affected. Sensory loss is present in the distal extremities and foot deformities (pes cavus) tend to be less marked. On the basis of the clinical phenotype, it is very difficult or impossible to separate HMSN II from HMSN I.

Laboratory Features. Motor nerve conduction velocities are near normal or normal in patients with HMSN II. The mean conduction velocity of ulnar nerves in the kindred studies was about 38 m/s. Sensory nerve action potentials are uniformly reduced or absent.

Pathologic Findings. Sural nerve biopsies in patients with HMSN II have shown reduction of large myelinated fibers, particularly distally, without significant demyelination on teased fibers. Small onion bulbs may be seen.

HMSN II With Diaphragm and Vocal Cord Weakness

A large kindred with autosomal dominant HMSN II has been reported with a classical neuropathic phenotype, but, in addition, 50 percent of the affected individuals had vocal and diaphragm weakness. Death has been attributed to respiratory weakness, and intracurrent infections have been observed.

HMSN II: Autosomal Recessive

R. A. Ouvrier reported a more severe form of HMSN II with onset in infancy or early childhood and recessive inheritance. The treatment of HMSN II is similar to that of HMSN I.

HMSN III: Dejerine-Sottas Disease

HMSN III is a rare hypertrophic neuropathy of infancy, inherited in some cases as an autosomal recessive trait. Recent genetic studies have identified missense and point mutations in the PMP22 gene and in the P_0 gene (an important structural protein of peripheral nerve myelin). The clinical features are those of a severe neuropathy with onset in early childhood. Motor development is delayed. Motor skills such as jumping and running are impaired. There is progressive muscular weakness affecting legs and arms. General areflexia, with prominent

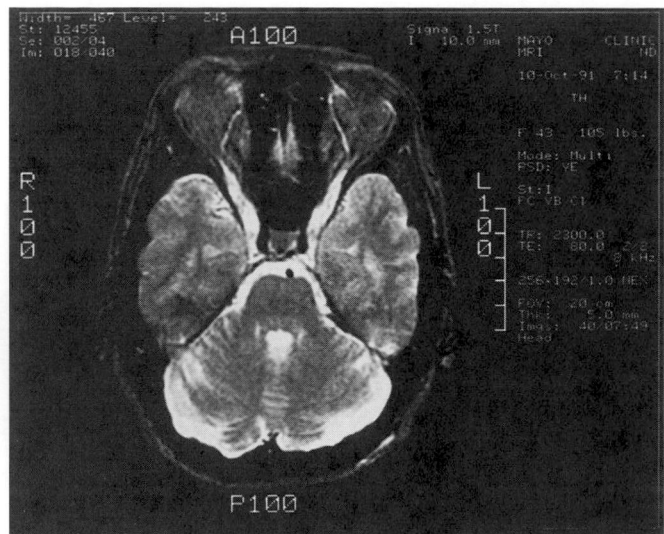

FIG. 100-3. Magnetic resonance imaging (MRI) of the brain showing an enlarged and hypertrophied fifth cranial nerve in a patient with Dejerine-Sottas syndrome.

enlarged peripheral or cranial nerves is typical (Fig. 100-3). There is definite sensory loss and some patients have marked sensory ataxia. The course is progressive with significant disability. Some patients are wheelchair-bound in early adulthood. Motor conduction velocity is markedly reduced, usually below 10 m/s. CSF protein levels are frequently elevated. Pathologic studies have shown enlargement of the transverse fascicular area, onion bulb formation (Fig. 100-4), segmental demyelination, reduction in the number of myelinated fibers, and axonal atrophy.

Other cases reported as congenital hypomyelinated neuropathy probably represent a variant of HMSN III. The differential diagnosis includes acquired and inherited demyelinating neuropathies occurring in children. In those patients labeled as having acquired neuropathy, the differential diagnosis must consider acute and chronic inflammatory demyelinating polyradiculoneuropathy; in those with inherited neuropathy, the

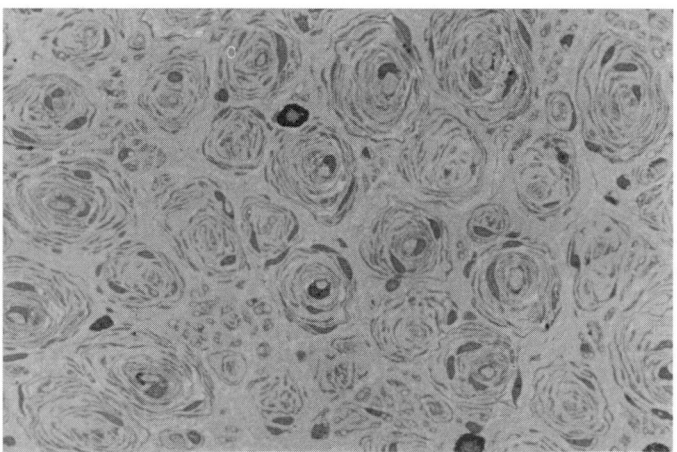

FIG. 100-4. Sural nerve biopsy of a patient with HMSN III (Dejerine-Sottas disease). Transverse section embedded in epon and stained with methylene blue. Note prominent onion bulb formations and reduction in the number of myelinated fibers. (Courtesy of C. Giannini, M.D., Department of Pathology, Mayo Clinic, Rochester, MN.)

differential diagnosis includes HMSN I and II, metachromatic leukodystrophy, Cockayne syndrome, inherited tendency to pressure palsies, and other rare neuropathies.

HMSN IV

HMSN IV (hypertrophic neuropathy associated with increased phytanic acid levels or Refsum's disease) also called Refsum's neuropathy—is discussed in Table 100-1.

HMSN With Associated Features

There are families with the clinical phenotype of peroneal muscular atrophy, and they present with additional distinct features such as spastic paraparesis (HMSN V), optic atrophy (HMSN VI), retinitis pigmentosa (HMSN VII), deafness, and cardiomyopathy. The inheritance pattern was, in most family studies, autosomal dominant.

HEREDITARY SENSORY AND AUTONOMIC NEUROPATHIES

The main feature of hereditary sensory and autonomic neuropathies (HSAN) is the prominent involvement of sensory and autonomic fibers. The primary pathologic foci of this disorder are mainly small-diameter pain and thermal sensory neurons (axons) and autonomic neurons. There is significant clinical and genetic heterogeneity. It would be desirable to classify these disorders by the altered cellular or genetic mechanism, but for most HSAN, this is not known. For practical purposes, a classification based on the inheritance pattern, clinical features, and the system of neurons predominantly affected is used (Table 100-1). The loss of pain sensation and sensory loss predisposes to the development of foot complications, including plantar ulcers, secondary infections such as cellulitis, and osteomyelitis, which may lead to osteolysis, eventually resulting in acral mutilations.

HSAN I

HSAN I is a genetically heterogeneous disorder, dominantly inherited in most cases. No genetic loci has yet been established by linkage studies. Neuropathic symptoms may begin in the second or fourth decade of life and slowly progress over time. Spontaneous neuropathic pain is typically burning, aching, or lancinating in quality, affects mainly the feet and legs, and is aggravated by heavy walking or weightbearing. Sometimes pain is related to local events such as calluses or plantar ulcers. Neurologic signs include sensory loss predominantly involving pain and temperature sensation, but all modalities may be affected. The decreased sensation typically affects feet and legs in a symmetric fashion. Deep tendon reflexes are absent at the ankles but present in the upper extremities. In some kindreds, a variable degree of motor involvement with peroneal muscular weakness may be seen. High arches of the feet with frequent corns and calluses of the soles of the feet may have gone unnoticed for years. Foot complications such as the typical plantar ulcer in the metatarsal head region or sole of the foot is a late manifestation of HSAN I. Plantar ulcers are not only caused by sensory loss, but other risk factors play a critical role. These include excessive use and abuse of feet, neglect of foot care, overweight, and neglect of foot injury. Men, particularly those involved in heavy physical activity, tend to develop ulcers more frequently than women. If foot ulcers are not recognized and treated promptly, a sequence of events occurs, leading to local infection, osteomyelitis, and loss of foot or leg.

Electrophysiologic studies reveal absence of sensory nerve action potentials (SNAPs). The neuropathologic features are those of a chronic neuropathic process affecting small myelinated and unmyelinated fibers with axonal atrophy, myelin remodeling, and axonal degeneration. The differential diagnosis includes other varieties of HSAN (discussed below). Three features are helpful to separate these conditions. (1) age of onset: HSAN I begins in the second or even later decades of life, but the other varieties (HSAN II to V) probably are congenital, with onset at birth; (2) progression of deficits: in HSAN I there is slow progression over the course of years, which is seldom the case in the other varieties; and (3) pattern of involvement: HSAN I tends to affect the lower extremities, while in the other varieties the lower and upper extremities and trunk are generally affected.

Spinocerebellar degeneration (i.e., Friedreich's ataxia) is separated from HSAN I by the following main features: (1) sensory loss that predominantly affects proprioception and vibratory sensation, (2) cerebellar ataxia, and (3) minimal autonomic and small-fiber dysfunction. Familial amyloidosis are separated clinically by the presence of sexual and sphincter dysfunction.

HSAN II

HSAN II is a rare recessively inherited condition with onset early in life. Unlike HSAN I, all sensory modalities are involved, affecting not only the lower extremities, but hands, face, and trunk are affected as well. Children with this disorder are at risk for ulcers of the feet, hand, lips, and tongue, and mutilation of fingers and toes may occur. Repeated paronychia, plantar ulcers, and stress foot fractures are usually present.

Neurologic examination reveals sensory loss that affects all modalities of sensation involving legs and hands. Reflexes are diminished or absent throughout. There is distal anhidrosis with sphincter dysfunction and impotence in men. Sensory nerve action potentials are absent. Pathologic studies of sural nerves have shown marked reduction to absence of myelinated fibers with a reduction in unmyelinated fibers as well. M. Donaghy reported the association of retinitis pigmentosa, spastic paraplegia, and neurotrophic keratitis with sensory neuropathy.

HSAN III: Familial Dysautonomia

Initially described by C.M. Riley (Riley-Day syndrome), HSAN III is a rare autosomal recessively inherited sensory neuropathy with autonomic manifestations, which affects mainly Ashkenazi Jews, with an estimated gene frequency in North American Jews of less than 1:100,000. The genetic locus has been established by linkage analysis and is located on chromosome 9q31-q33. This important discovery will undoubtedly lead to the identification of the specific abnormal gene(s) and eventually gene product(s) in familial dysautonomia.

The clinical manifestations are usually present at birth and consist of deficient lacrimation, poor sucking, episodic hyperthermia, frequent respiratory infections, vomiting, and failure to thrive. Emotional stimulation usually provokes autonomic crises with hypertension, profuse sweating, and excessive mottling of the skin. Constant clinical features helpful in the diagnosis are the absence of fungiform papillae on the tongue, defective lacrimation (alacrima), and corneal insensitivity. Hyporeflexia, decreased pain sensation, and kyphoscoliosis become apparent later in life.

Electrophysiologic studies reveal reduction in SNAPs with relatively preserved motor conduction velocities. Sural nerve biopsies demonstrate a marked reduction in the number of unmyelinated fibers. Postmortem examinations have shown marked reduction in the number of neurons in autonomic and spinal ganglia.

HSAN IV

A. G. Swanson originally described two affected siblings with insensitivity to pain, mild mental retardation, defective temperature control, and anhidrosis. Subsequent case reports have been documented. Pathologic findings include loss of unmyelinated fibers and lesser reduction of small myelinated fibers. This disorder is recessively inherited.

HSAN V

Low and colleagues reported a 6-year-old child with congenital loss of pain sensation with normal muscle strength, reflexes, and normal light touch and vibratory sensation. Sensory nerve action potentials were normal, but sural nerve biopsy revealed marked loss of small myelinated fibers. Additional cases have also been reported.

Treatment and Management

Emphasis on prevention of foot ulcers is the most important aspect of treatment for HSAN. Instructions along the lines described above for HMSN should be provided. Patients should be instructed not to abuse their feet. Children should avoid jumping from heights and certain sports like parachuting or kicking sports should be deemphasized. Careful foot care with daily inspection of feet and shoes is of utmost importance. Patients should wear shoes even inside the house. Feet care with daily soaks, followed by Vaseline lotion, is in order. Calluses should not be trimmed, rather should be rubbed off after soaking. If a plantar ulcer develops, weightbearing must cease until it is healed. Prompt debridement with antibiotic coverage is usually required. In most cases, acromutilations are seen in patients who abused their feet and neglected the injuries for a long time, until it was too late to salvage the foot or leg.

INHERITED TENDENCY TO PRESSURE PALSIES

Inherited tendency to pressure palsies (ITPP) is an autosomal-dominant neuropathy with susceptibility to pressure palsies. Genetic studies using linkage analysis have localized the abnormality to band 17p11.2-p12 on chromosome 17. In contrast with HMSN IA, this segment is deleted in ITPP. The human PMP22 gene, which is normally found in this region is deleted in ITPP and duplicated in HMSN IA. There are reports of a few families without linkage to chromosome 17, suggesting genetic heterogeneity.

Usually, the clinical manifestations start in the second or third decade of the patient's life. Onset of symptoms follows trivial trauma, compression, or sleeping on a limb. The resulting palsy, usually painless, persists for days or weeks instead of resolving in minutes or hours. Typically, a mononeuropathy with sensory loss and weakness develops in the appropriate anatomic distribution. The most commonly affected nerve trunks are the peroneal nerve at the fibular head, the radial nerve in the spiral groove of the humerus, and the ulnar nerve at the elbow. The history of minor compression or trauma is not always present. On examination, a mononeuropathy with

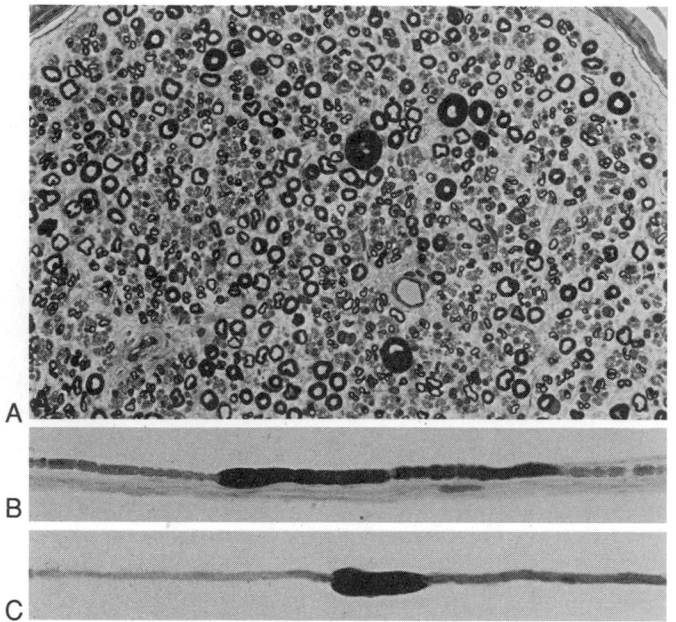

FIG. 100-5. Sural nerve biopsy of a patient with inherited tendency to pressure palsies (ITPP). **(A)** Transverse section embedded in epon and stained with methylene blue. Note several profiles showing focal thickenng of the myelin sheath "sausages or tomaculous." **(B, C)** Teased fiber preparation showing distinctive focal thickening of the myelin sheath "sausages." (Courtesy of C. Giannini, M.D., Department of Pathology, Mayo Clinic, Rochester, MN.)

the corresponding sensory loss and weakness in the distribution of the affected nerve is the rule. An important point, not always described in the literature, is that many patients have signs, albeit minor, of a distal, more generalized, neuropathy. There is mild distal symmetric sensory loss and depressed or absent ankle reflexes. In some patients, the telltale signs of an inherited neuropathy (high arches, hammertoes) are present.

Nerve conduction studies are helpful to detect conduction slowing or block at one or more entrapment sites. A more diffuse motor and sensory polyneuropathy affecting both clinically affected and unaffected nerves is a helpful clue to the diagnosis.

Pathologic studies, mainly of sural nerve biopsies, have shown segmental demyelination and remyelination with distinctive focal thickening of the myelin sheath, referred to as "sausages" or "tomaculous" (Fig. 100-5). Uncompacted axonal myelin and reduplicated segments of myelin have been demonstrated by electron-microscopy studies (Fig. 100-6). These observations suggest that a primary abnormality of myelin formation underlies this disorder, which may predispose myelinated fibers to be more susceptible to environmental factors, such as local trauma or compression. It should be emphasized that establishing heredity is critical in taking the clinical history in a patient who presents with pressure palsy. Family history is only revealed after detailed and often specific questioning.

The presence or recurrence of pressure palsies with associated mild signs of a generalized neuropathy are helpful clues to separate ITPP from individual cases of pressure palsy. To separate ITPP affecting the brachial plexus from sporadic brachial plexus neuropathy, the following features are helpful. In ITPP, the onset is usually painless, in contrast to the intensively severe pain found at onset in brachial plexus neuropathy. The relationship to trauma and the presence of a generalized neuropathy are helpful clues to the diagnosis of ITPP. The differential diagnosis of other multiple mononeuropathies associated with diabetes, leprosy, sarcoidosis, Lyme disease, or necrotizing vasculitis are considered in the differential of ITPP but usually do not present major diagnostic problems.

There is no specific treatment for this condition. The major point in management is education for the prevention of nerve injury by avoiding pressure damage. Individual pressure palsies are treated by appropriate splinting and physical therapy. Recovery may be prolonged, but the prognosis for return of function is good.

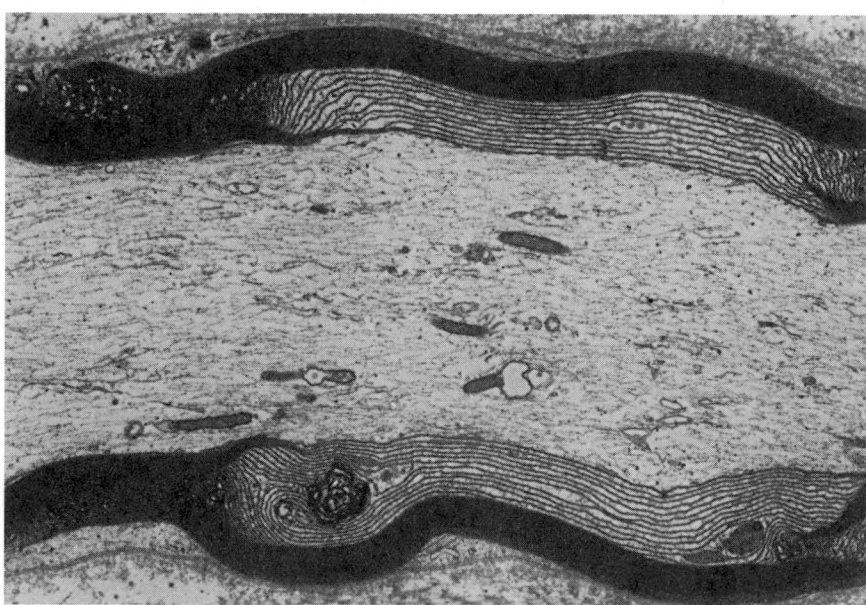

FIG. 100-6. Longitudinal section of large myelinated fiber from sural nerve of a patient with inherited tendency to pressure palsy showing uncompacted inner lamellae of myelin characteristic of the disorder (bar = 1 μm). (From Yoshikawa H, Dyck PJ: Uncompacted inner myelin lamellae in inherited tendency to pressure palsy. J Neuropathol Exp Neurol 50:649, 1991, with permission.)

FAMILIAL AMYLOID POLYNEUROPATHY

Inherited amyloidoses are autosomal-dominant disorders characterized by deposition of amyloid in peripheral nerves and other tissues. The clinical phenotypes of hereditary amyloidosis frequently have in common peripheral neuropathy with prominent autonomic manifestations, which differ in age of onset, genetic defect, clinical patterns of neuropathy, and other tissue involvement. The first familial amyloid polyneuropathy (FAP) to be described was the Portuguese variety reported by C. Andrade in 1952; it is the most common type, and the amyloid is derived from a point mutation on the transthyretin (TTR) molecule, formerly known as prealbumin. The first mutation reported was the methionine for valine substitution at position 30. Since then, more than 30 point mutations of the TTR gene have been identified.

FAP I (Andrade)

Originally described by Andrade in northern Portugal, familial amyloid polyneuropathy type I (FAP I) is dominantly inherited. It is the most common of FAP and has also been described in Brazil, Japan, Sweden, and elsewhere. Onset of symptoms is usually in the third or fourth decade but may occur later in life. Neuropathic symptoms are pain and paresthesias affecting the feet and legs first, which are often associated with marked sensory loss, mainly affecting pain and temperature sensation. Initially, a syndrome that mimics lumbosacral syringomyelia develops in the patient, and other sensory modalities are affected later. Autonomic symptoms are prominent and sometimes dominate the clinical picture, especially postural dizziness and hypotension, distal anhidrosis, impotence, urinary retention, and dysfunction of gastrointestinal motility with alternating episodes of diarrhea and constipation. Pupillary abnormalities with escalloped margins are also present.

The sensory abnormalities with loss of pain and temperature may predispose to the occurrence of foot ulcers or inadvertent burns. Neuropathic joint degeneration is a late complication. Sensory loss progresses to involve the upper extremities, usually affecting all sensory modalities in later stages. Muscle weakness and areflexia appears as the disease advances. Infiltration of other organs, such as kidneys, heart, and eyes, is typical in this disorder. The disease runs a progressive course, and patients usually die of renal failure or cardiac complications 10 to 20 years after onset. Electrophysiologic studies in the early stages of the disease show an axonal predominantly distal sensory polyneuropathy with reduced or absent SNAP and relative preservation of motor conduction velocity and CMAP.

Sural nerve biopsies revealed marked reduction in small myelinated and unmyelinated fibers with widespread amyloid deposits throughout. Immunohistochemical studies of the amyloid deposits with monoclonal antibodies are helpful in providing evidence for hereditary amyloidosis. Inherited amyloidosis specifically reacts with antiserum against TTR (Plate 100-1). Amyloid deposits are also found in sensory and autonomic ganglia. The mechanism of nerve damage is unknown. Asymptomatic carriers of the mutant TTR gene can be detected by radioimmunoassay of serum. Treatment is mainly supportive and symptomatic.

FAP II (Rukavina or Indiana)

Onset of FAP II symptoms is in the early midlife with carpal tunnel syndrome and "numbness" in the median innervated fingers. Amyloid deposits may be found in the flexor retinaculum overlying the median nerve at the wrist. Amyloid infiltration of the vitreous, resulting in vitreous opacities, is common. A more generalized sensory polyneuropathy may occur later, but the outlook is not as severe as a FAP I. Treatment of carpal tunnel syndrome by surgical decompression usually produces relief of symptoms.

Different point mutations at position 58 and 84 in the TTR

TABLE 100-2. Other Inherited Neuropathies Associated With Known Metabolic Defects

Disorder	Genetic Transmission	Clinical Features	Metabolic Abnormality	Pathologic Findings
Metachromatic leukodystrophy	AR	Infantile and adult forms; CNS involvement with mental retardation, blindness, deafness, hypertonic tetraplegia; PNS involvement with weakness, areflexia and slow NCV	Arylsulfatase A	MF loss, demyelination, and Schwann cell cytoplasm metachromatic granules
Globoid cell leukodystrophy (Krabbe disease)	AR	Onset at infancy; CNS white matter involvement with regression of motor skills, hypertonicity, seizures, and optic atrophy; PNS involvement with hyporeflexia and slow NCV	Galactosylceramidase	Segmental demyelination, inclusion material within Schwann cell cytoplasm
Adrenoleukodystrophy (ALD) and adrenomyeloneuropathy (AMN)	X-linked	Young males; spastic paraparesis, peripheral neuropathy, and signs of adrenal insufficiency	Abnormal β-oxidation of VLCFA	Loss of MF and UMF and Schwann cell inclusions
Fabry's disease	X-linked	Young males; painful small fiber neuropathy, anhidrosis, skin angiokeratomas, kidney, and vascular disease	α-Galactosidase	Small fiber neuropathy; glycolipid granules in vessels
Tangier disease	AR	Three types: (1) asymmetric polyneuropathy with normal NCV, (2) slowly progressing symmetric polyneuropathy, mainly in the lower extremities, (3) polyneuropathy with a syringomyelialike syndrome; orange tonsils	Abnormal catabolism of high density lipoproteins (HDL); very low plasma cholesterol	Clear vacuoles in Schwann cell cytoplasm; de- and remyelination and axonal degeneration
Abetalipoproteinemia	AR	Large fiber peripheral neuropathy, proprioceptive loss, ataxia, pes cavus, atypical retinitis pigmentosa, acanthocytosis	Absence of lipoproteins containing apolipoprotein B	Reduction of MF
Porphyric neuropathy (AIP, VP, and HCP)	AD	Porphyric attacks: painful crisis, progressive motor neuropathy, and/or encephalopathy	Abnormalities in regulation of heme synthesis	Wallerian degeneration

Abbreviations: AD, autosomal dominant; AR, autosomal recessive; CNS, central nervous system; PNS, peripheral nervous system; AIP, acute intermittent porphyria; VP, variegate porphyria; HCP, hereditary coproporphyria; NCV, nerve conduction velocity; VLCFA, very long-chain fatty acids; MF, myelinated fibers; UF, unmyelinated fibers.

gene have been demonstrated. Asymptomatic carriers could be identified using recombinant DNA techniques.

FAP III (Van Allen or Iowa Type)

The clinical manifestations of FAP III are similar to those of FAP I except for early renal involvement and high incidence of duodenal ulcers. Autonomic involvement is not as florid as in FAP I. Amyloid in FAP III is not derived from TTR. The amyloid fibrils consist of a variant of apolipoprotein A1.

FAP IV (Meretoja)

Originally described in Finland, FAP IV is characterized by ocular manifestations. Corneal opacities due to amyloid infiltration, referred to as lattice corneal dystrophy, is a cardinal clinical feature. A slowly progressive facial palsy with facial skin changes usually supervenes later. A mild generalized peripheral neuropathy without autonomic features may occur later.

OTHER INHERITED NEUROPATHIES ASSOCIATED WITH KNOWN METABOLIC DEFECTS

Other inherited neuropathies are summarized in Table 100-2.

SUGGESTED READINGS

Ben Othmane K, Middleton LT, Loprest LJ et al: Localization of a gene (CMT2A) for autosomal dominant Charcot-Marie-Tooth disease type 2 to chromosome 1p and evidence of genetic heterogeneity. Genomics 17: 370, 1993

Bergoffen J, Scherer SS, Wang S et al: Connexin mutations in X-linked Charcot-Marie-Tooth disease. Science 262:2039, 1993

Chance PF, Pleasure D: Charcot-Marie-Tooth syndrome. Arch Neurol 50:1180, 1993

Dyck PJ: Neuronal atrophy and degeneration predominantly affecting peripheral sensory and autonomic neurons. p. 1065. In Dyck PJ, Thomas PK, Griffin JW et al (eds): Peripheral Neuropathy. 3rd Ed. Philadelphia, WB Saunders, 1993

Dyck PJ, Chance P, Lebo R, Carney JA: Hereditary motor and sensory neuropathies. p. 1094. In Dyck PJ, Thomas PK, Griffin JW, et al (eds): Peripheral Neuropathy. 3rd Ed. WB Saunders, Philadelphia, 1993

Dyck PJ, Litchy WJ, Minnerath S et al: Hereditary motor and sensory neuropathy with diaphragm and vocal cord paresis. Ann Neurol 35:608, 1994

Fischbeck KH, ar Rushdi N, Pericak Vance M et al: X-linked neuropathy: gene localization with DNA probes. Ann Neurol 20:527, 1986

Hayasaka K, Himoro M, Sawaishi Y et al: De novo mutation of the myelin P$_0$ gene in Dejerine-Sottas disease (hereditary motor and sensory neuropathy type III). Nat Genet 5:266, 1993

Lupski JR, de Oca Luna RM, Slaugenhaupt S et al: DNA duplication associated with Charcot-Marie-Tooth disease type 1A. Cell 66:219, 1991

Roa BB, Dyck PJ, Marks HG et al: Dejerine-Sottas syndrome associated with point mutation in the peripheral myelin protein 22 (PMP22) gene. Nat Genet 5:269, 1993

101. COMMON ENTRAPMENT AND COMPRESSION NEUROPATHIES OF THE UPPER EXTREMITY

DAVID M. DAWSON

CARPAL TUNNEL SYNDROME

Carpal tunnel syndrome is the result of compression of the median nerve within the carpal canal, a closed space bounded on the volar surface by the thick transverse carpal ligament.

The normal cause of carpal tunnel syndrome is enlargement or hypertrophy of the nine flexor tendons that pass through this closed space. Both vascular effects on the median nerve, and the affects of chronic recurring compression appear to play a role in the pathogenesis of the nerve disorder. Briefly stated, it appears that the demyelinative lesion of the nerve, which accounts for the focal nerve conduction slowing, and probably in the end for the neurologic symptoms, is a result of compression of the myelin sheaths, distortion of the nodes of Ranvier, and interruption of normal saltatory conduction. Some intermittent symptoms, such as the nocturnal tingling, may be due to interference with blood supply to the nerves, since these symptoms are so easily reversible by change in wrist position.

Carpal tunnel syndrome is important in two ways that are unique to this disorder. It was the first clinical physiologic correlation to be well put together in the earliest days of clinical electromyographic (EMG) testing in the 1960s, and it is the one entrapment neuropathy for which a major occupational role has been defined. For this reason, it is in the forefront of legal and compensation systems calculations, based on an industrywide effort to reduce the high incidence of this disorder in workers. In a review of medical records in Rochester, Minnesota, incidence of 125 per 100,000 population was calculated in the late 1970s. In a recent survey in the Netherlands, 8 percent of the interviewees reported nighttime paresthesias of the hand, and of these about one-third were found to have carpal tunnel syndrome, an incidence of 220 persons per 100,000. The prevalence of carpal tunnel syndrome in those who work with their hands is many times these baseline figures. The highest reported incidence thus far is 15 percent, in a group of meat cutters. The incidence of carpal tunnel syndrome is increased among electronic parts assemblers, musicians, dental hygienists, and of course those who use their hands in nonoccupational ways such as those who knit, do carpentry, or filet fish.

In the nonoccupational group of patients with carpal tunnel syndrome, middle-aged women predominate, while of those who have an occupational basis for the condition, younger men are the peak population.

Clinical Features

The clinical features of carpal tunnel syndrome are known to most practitioners. The most frequently occurring and easily recognized clinical variant of the illness is slowly progressive nocturnal paresthesias, typically burning and unpleasant, located mostly in the hand. There may be some proximal radiation of the pain into the forearm and arm, rarely above the level of the shoulder. Many patients notice that some wrist positions exacerbate the symptoms, for example, when they drive with the wrist extended on the steering wheel or when they hold a newspaper. In the earliest stages of the illness the symptoms are intermittent, and there are no neurologic findings on examination. As the condition progresses, symptoms become more persistent, and there may be decreased tactile sensation over the fingertips, typically over the index and middle fingers. Two-point discrimination over the fingertips is a reliable method of testing, as is light pinprick sensation over the dorsum of the fingers. Testing over the palmar surface of the fingers is often difficult, and it should be noted that the palm itself is spared, owing to the anatomy of the median nerve (i.e., the palmar cutaneous nerve arises proximal to the carpal tunnel).

Other clinical variants of carpal tunnel syndrome are known. Some patients have pronounced autonomic disorder from the very beginning, for example, sweating and dry skin or features that resemble Raynaud's phenomenon. A few patients appear to have primary axonal damage from the beginning and present with dense sensory loss and atrophy of the thenar muscles; complain of weakness, which is most often due to clumsiness and lack of discriminative ability of the sensory nerve fibers, but a few have weakness of thumb abduction and opposition. Not all patients with carpal tunnel syndrome present with slowly progressive illness; some present with acute loss of function, probably due to vascular factors.

The prevalence of carpal tunnel syndrome during pregnancy is well known, typically beginning in the sixth or seventh month and returning to baseline following delivery in over 90 percent of individuals. A few women in whom this disorder develops during pregnancy do not recover sufficiently and have persistent problems.

Occupational Considerations

Efforts have been made to define the exact occupational exposures that increase the incidence of carpal tunnel syndrome. These efforts have not been highly successful because there has been disagreement about the necessary features for the diagnosis, some investigators using primarily neurophysiologic data, which have been unreliable in this setting for reasons that are discussed below.

Highly repetitive wrist movement, vibrating tools, awkward wrist positions, and forceful movements of the hand seem to correlate with a high incidence of carpal tunnel syndrome. Workers whose occupation requires forceful repetitive movement of the hand have an increased incidence of carpal tunnel syndrome—at least tenfold above that observed in workers who use the wrist without repetition and force. The matter remains under investigation. Some experts have not been able to find these correlations and believe that obesity, age, presence or absence of diabetes, and other nonergonomic factors are equally important. Nevertheless, major efforts are being made throughout the relevant industries to reduce the incidence of carpal tunnel syndrome and its major impact on the cost to productivity and of medical care for those workers affected.

Electrophysiologic Features

The electrophysiologic demonstration of carpal tunnel syndrome shows focal slowing of the median nerve at the wrist. This was first demonstrated by Simpson in 1956 and has been a mainstay of the investigation since that time. Distal motor studies across the wrist are easily performed but have a sensitivity of only about 50 percent. Prolongation of distal latency and conduction block between the palm and wrist are the two abnormalities commonly observed. When an inching technique is used across the palm, the exact area of neurophysiologic abnormality can be seen very clearly, and the sensitivity of the area is increased. The neurophysiologic disorder is localized within the palm, 2 to 4 cm distal to the wrist crease, which is at the distal edge of the volar carpal ligament. The most sensitive criterion for diagnosis of carpal tunnel syndrome is the demonstration of slowing of sensory or mixed nerve conduction at the wrist. Sometimes it is useful to test several digits in order to detect the abnormality. The use of an internal control, comparing a median conduction study to the analogous ulnar study, increases the electrophysiologic sensitivity to above 90 percent. A comparison of the median mixed palmar latency to the ulnar

mixed palmar latency across the wrist may prove useful. Likewise, a comparison of the median sensory latency of digit 4 to the ulnar sensory latency of digit 4 (digit 4 is usually dually innervated) is very sensitive in detecting subtle abnormalities of slowing.

Comparison of the symptomatic and asymptomatic hands in the diagnosis of carpal tunnel syndrome is often not helpful, since the asymptomatic hand is electrically affected in a high proportion of cases. Electromyography (EMG) is often used, primarily in the differential diagnosis. In patients with severe carpal tunnel syndrome and axonal loss, the abnormalities shown by EMG should be seen in the opponens muscle and the abductor pollicis brevis.

Approximately 95 percent of patients with clinically apparent carpal tunnel syndrome have definable neurophysiologic abnormalities. A few patients whose nerve conduction test appears to be normal respond to carpal tunnel release, which constitutes a false negative rate. Inevitably, there are also false positives, of which the most likely is the incidence of abnormality in the asymptomatic hand, but there are also confounding false positives produced by other diseases, such as peripheral neuropathy, amyotrophic lateral sclerosis, and cervical spine disease. A well-planned individualized investigation can usually manage these difficulties.

Differential Diagnosis

The most common differential diagnosis to be considered in a patient with apparent carpal tunnel syndrome is cervical radiculopathy—usually cervical root 6—which can often be recognized by the presence of neck pain, by pain that radiates to the arm in response to coughing or sneezing, and by a preponderance of pain proximally as opposed to distally (the opposite is true of carpal tunnel syndrome). When neurologic features are present, reflex loss, muscle atrophy, and sensory loss over the dorsum of the hand may be seen.

Thoracic outlet syndrome (discussed below), is most quickly recognized by showing that the symptoms occur with elevation and abduction of the arm, or by showing that the neurologic deficit spans the territories of C8 and T1 nerve roots, rather than the median nerve. Proximal median nerve dysfunction is most easily recognized by testing for the function of the flexor pollicis longus, which produces flexion of the distal joint of the thumb, or other flexor muscles, or the pronation of the wrist.

Transient ischemic attacks, affecting the contralateral cerebral hemisphere, usually do not produce anything the patient would describe as pain.

Treatment

Conservative management of carpal tunnel syndrome involves splinting the wrist in a slightly extended position, reduction of activity that might have caused the syndrome to develop, and steroid injection underneath the volar carpal ligament. The steroid injection technique can be performed by any practitioner, provided the median nerve is avoided and the steroid is injected several centimeters proximal to the wrist creases so that it can diffuse among the flexor tendons to reduce swelling and inflammation. The objective of conservative management is to reduce the tissue pressure within the carpal canal, which will rise with wrist extension or flexion or as a consequence of inflammation of the flexor tendons.

The patients who have progressive symptoms and have not

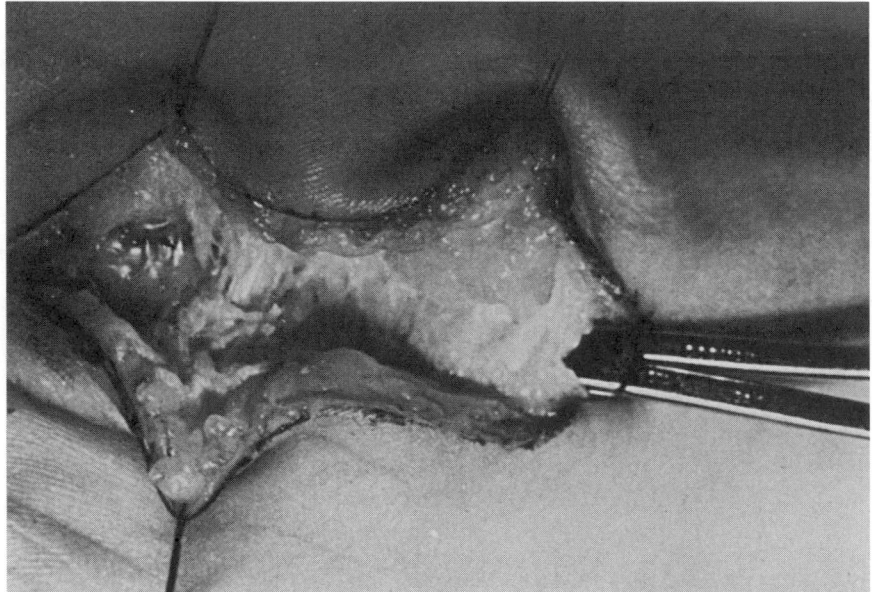

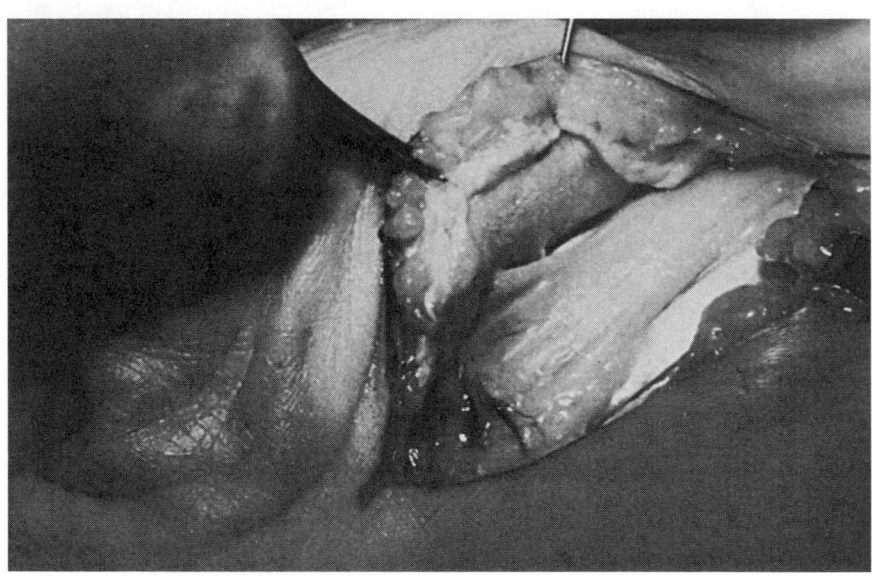

FIG. 101-1. Carpal tunnel syndrome. **(A)** A hemostat has been placed under the transverse carpal ligament. The patient's fingers are to the left, and the wrist is to the right. **(B)** The ligament has been incised exposing the median nerve directly beneath it. (From Dawson D, Hallet M, Millender L: Entrapment Neuropathies. p. 44. Little, Brown, Boston, 1983, with permission.)

responded to simple conservative measures (Fig. 101-1) should be referred to a surgeon for volar carpal tunnel release. Repeated steroid injections are to be avoided because they can lead to complications.

Patients who have late-stage carpal tunnel syndrome with advanced atrophy, sensory loss and few symptoms do not respond to surgery. The rare patients who have acute development of symptoms should be seen as an emergency and operated on promptly, since they can have irreversible loss of function. The responses to treatment are generally quite satisfactory. Patients who use their hands for heavy labor will not be able to return to work for 3 to 4 months after surgery. Those who have a sedentary lifestyle can go back to work with a bulky dressing on the wrist within a week. Many patients have some postoperative pain, produced either by local pressure on the wrist or use of

the wrist, and this may last for several months. The long-term effects of carpal tunnel syndrome surgery are good, but 10 percent of patients are worse after surgery.

ULNAR NEUROPATHY AT THE ELBOW

Ulnar neuropathy at the region of the elbow is second only to carpal tunnel syndrome in incidence of entrapment neuropathy of the upper extremity. The patient usually presents with tingling into the little finger, accompanied by some degree of weakness of the hand. With advancing disease, the motor symptoms predominate, and in the end a patient with ulnar neuropathy may lose considerable hand function, including digital control and grip. This is in contrast to carpal tunnel syndrome where the sensory symptoms and pain tend to predominate throughout.

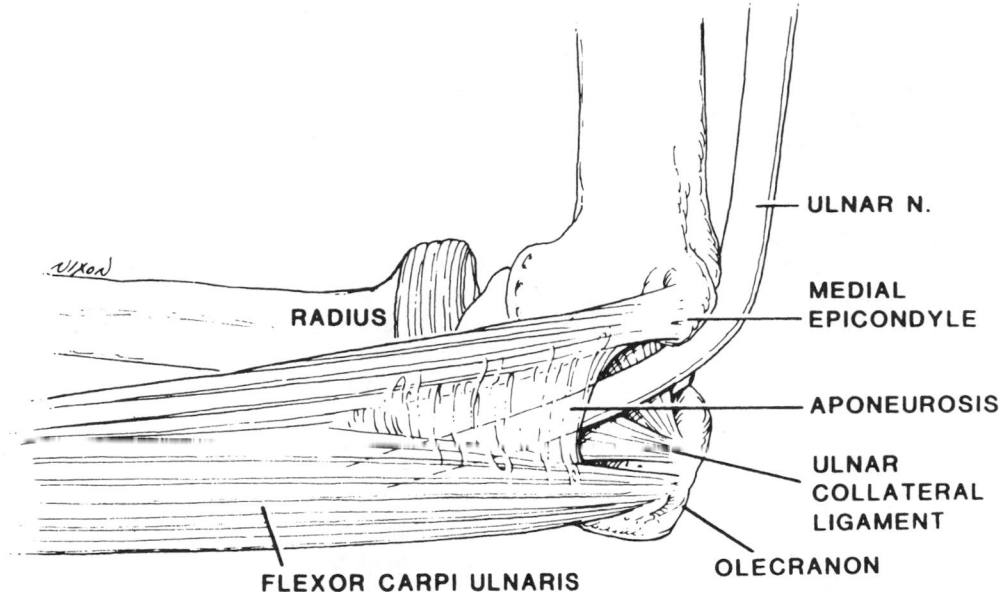

FIG. 101-2. View of the medial side of the right arm, showing the course of the ulnar nerve past the medial epicondyle and entering the cubital tunnel under the edge of the aponeurosis of the flexor carpi ulnaris. (From Kincaid JC: The electrodiagnosis of ulnar neuropathy at the elbow. Muscle Nerve 11:1005–15, 1988, with permission.)

The causes of ulnar neuropathy at the elbow are varied. An effort should be made when examining patients to ascertain the cause of the problem, but it must be recognized that even after careful neurophysiologic investigation and a surgical procedure, the exact cause of nerve compression can be difficult to corroborate. Probably the commonest cause of ulnar compression at the elbow, particularly in the milder cases and in those associated with repetitive elbow flexion, is the cubital tunnel syndrome (Fig. 101-2). In this abnormality the ulnar nerve is compressed by the edge of the aponeurosis of the flexor carpi ulnaris, located about 2 cm distal to the tip of the elbow when the elbow is flexed. Sometimes a Tinel sign can be elicited at that exact point or an inching technique with nerve conduction testing can show that as the point of compression.

In some patients, chronic trauma to the nerve, especially when the ulnar groove is shallow, can lead to symptoms. Recurrent subluxation of the nerve, which then rides up over the medial epicondyle, can be associated with ulnar nerve disorder, but it should be recognized that subluxation also occurs in patients who have no symptoms. In previous decades, prior fracture of the olecranon or other damage to the elbow joint would lead to slow progressive scarring of the nerve, and was called tardy ulnar palsy. This condition is rarely observed nowadays.

Clinical Features

Although sensory complaints are very frequent in patients with ulnar nerve disorder at the elbow, the sensory loss is usually slight and is located over the little finger and adjacent parts of the palm. Sometimes the split down the ring finger showing that the medial side is innervated by the ulnar nerve is a helpful diagnostic point.

The motor loss in ulnar nerve compression is important to verify correctly. Some patients, for example, musicians, who require careful digital control, may be more aware of the motor disability than the examination can show. Use of the long-finger flexors and extensors, innervated by radial and median muscles, can compensate for many movements of the digits but not all.

Finger abduction, especially abduction of the fifth and index fingers, are easily tested. Adduction is testable as well, especially adduction of the ring finger for which long-finger flexors and extensors cannot substitute. If there is marked weakness of lumbricals and interosseus muscles, power grip may be reduced; the patient may be aware of this and it can be measured and demonstrated.

An important muscle to test in the presence of an ulnar nerve lesion is the long flexor for the fifth finger. This is innervated in the forearm by the ulnar nerve and is the only reliably testable muscle in the forearm that is so innervated. The flexor digitorum profundus for digit 5 controls the terminal phalanx, producing flexion, which can be compared to other flexors in that hand or the comparable muscle on that side. Once that muscle has been shown to be abnormal, the site of the lesion is much better defined, since ulnar nerve compression at the wrist is thereby excluded.

Occupational Considerations

There is no clear-cut occupational exposure that leads to ulnar nerve disorder. Compression of the ulnar nerve can occur in the postoperative period. It is not a rare event to discover a patient with new weakness and sensory loss in the hand after a period of anesthesia. The mechanism for this is not well known, but sometimes pronounced prolonged flexion of the elbow or, contrariwise, extension on an armboard, or compression by an external sharp edge of the table can be confirmed.

Musicians seem particularly susceptible to ulnar nerve compression, and it has been observed particularly in violinists and flutists, both of whom practice many hours per day with one arm or both in a flexed position.

Differential Diagnosis

The differential diagnosis of ulnar nerve compression at the elbow differs from that of carpal tunnel syndrome. However, the two conditions may be easily confused or confounded, since at least one-half of the patients interviewed cannot reliably report which digits are affected by paresthesias. Thoracic outlet syndrome (discussed below), may occur in a form in which there is pronounced disorder of the C8 and T1 nerve roots. Usually this is associated with a fibrous band or other structural abnormality of the brachial plexus. Such patients may resemble those with ulnar neuropathy, but can be distinguished by the following facts: with C8-T1 root disorder, sensory loss is present over the medial side of the hand but extends upward over the territory of the medial antebrachial cutaneous nerve in the forearm. This does not occur with ulnar nerve palsies. Also, the muscle atrophy in neurogenic thoracic outlet syndrome includes all of the muscles in the hand and may in fact begin in the median territory producing "ulnar sensory loss" and "median weakness."

Other problems with the brachial plexus need to be considered on occasion and metastatic carcinoma or stretch injuries of the plexus can resemble ulnar neuropathy as well. This is sometimes seen, for instance, in the postcardiac surgery patient, in whom the disorder appears to be related to the position of the arm during surgery, producing intrinsic muscle weakness and ulnar sensory loss, usually due to brachial plexus stretch injury.

Treatment

Treatment of ulnar neuropathies at the elbow is less satisfactory than that of carpal tunnel syndrome. Early mild cases may respond to a simple restriction of elbow flexion, using a bivalve cast or orthosis, which can be manufactured by an occupational therapist and worn during periods of rest or at night. Steroid injection therapy plays no role. Inflammatory medication may occasionally be helpful.

With advancing motor or sensory loss or pain, a surgical approach is indicated. In some patients, especially those with mild early nerve compression, a simple release of the flexor carpi ulnaris aponeurosis, that is, a cubital tunnel release, may be sufficient. Beyond that point, surgeons can choose from several procedures. Some surgeons prefer an epicondylectomy, allowing the nerve to ride anteriorly into the bed of the removed epicondyle. Other surgeons prefer a transposition of the nerve in front of the epicondyle. The results of surgery are more commensurate with the degree of preoperative nerve disorder than they are with the choice of procedure. Generally speaking, the pain is relieved, and some return of function can be anticipated in most cases.

Electrophysiologic Features

The techniques for neurophysiologic investigation resemble those for carpal tunnel syndrome. Generally, the search is for an area of focal slowing near the elbow. It is quite common to be able to show that there is an abnormality of the ulnar nerve, either by a reduction of the ulnar sensory action potential from the fifth finger, or by general slowing and dispersion of the motor action potential. Sometimes these occur without a discernible focal slowing or conduction block at the elbow, unless there is careful attention to technique.

The neurophysiologic differential diagnosis is rather extensive. Neurogenic thoracic outlet syndrome must be excluded, primarily by showing that there is no focal slowing of the ulnar nerve, and that some median nerve innervated muscles are also

affected. Again, comparison with the opposite ulnar nerve may not be an effective technique, since the other side can be affected as well. The presence of generalized peripheral neuropathy can be ascertained by showing a reduction in another sensory action potential, such as the radial or the sural nerves.

THORACIC OUTLET SYNDROME

The diagnosis of thoracic outlet syndrome appears to carry a very high rate of error and does not have the neurologic or electrophysiologic support that exists for other entrapment neuropathies. There are a few patients who have the so-called "true" neurogenic thoracic outlet syndrome, commonly due to a fibrous band traversing the brachial plexus. These patients present with weakness, pain, and numbness in the hand according to a very specific neurologic pattern. These patients are very rare and even recognized experts in the field have seen no more than a handful of cases.

The second type of thoracic outlet syndrome is much more common, although the limits of the syndrome are very poorly defined. Patients present with numbness, tingling, and pain in the hand, without demonstrable neurologic deficit. The symptoms are often dependent on arm or shoulder position. In some centers in the United States the patients are operated on, typically with a removal of the first rib through a transaxillary approach. Many patients operated on in this way have persistent or increased symptoms postoperatively, and most neurologists do not usually recommend first rib removal in these circumstances. It may be that the syndrome is produced by shoulder or arm position and is related to muscular spasm. Often it will respond to physiotherapy over a period of several months, attesting to the reversible positional nature of the deficit.

Electrophysiologic investigation of patients with neurogenic thoracic outlet syndrome demonstrates reduced sensory action potentials in the little finger and medial forearm, as well as denervation changes in many of the intrinsic muscles of the hand (both ulnar and median) and sometimes in the muscles of the forearm that contain a C8 component. Earlier reports that slowing can be demonstrated across the thoracic outlet syndrome in the brachial plexus by nerve conduction testing are now believed to be erroneous. Likewise somatosensory testing, using an electrode over the spinal cord, does not appear to contribute to a diagnosis.

RADIAL NERVE ENTRAPMENT

The radial nerve can be affected by a compression or entrapment neuropathy in its proximal portions in the forearm. This produces a clinical picture consisting of partial weakness of extensors of the fingers. Since the nerve most commonly compressed is the branch of the radial known as the posterior interosseus nerve, the extensor carpi radialis is not affected, and the patient will retain the ability to dorsiflex the wrist, typically with some deviation of the wrist toward the radial side. The other muscles extending the thumb and the fingers may be sequentially or partially affected, often starting on the ulnar side of the hand. This may produce a most unusual appearance, which, once seen, can be subsequently recognized, but is often confusing at first.

Entrapment of the posterior interosseous nerve typically does not produce a sensory loss, since the superficial radial nerve leaves the parent nerve prior to the point of the constriction.

The radial tunnel syndrome is another version of radial entrapment at the elbow, in which there is pain at the site where this constriction occurs, typically 5 to 10 cm distal to the elbow joint itself. Tenderness there or radiating pain produced by compression during examination may suggest that the radial nerve is affected. This may occur with only minimal weakness of the hand.

The electrophysiologic investigation of radial tunnel syndrome or radial nerve compression depends on attempting to show slowing to distal radial innervated muscles or electromyographic changes restricted to radially innervated muscles. The manner is somewhat controversial and there appear to be patients who have the syndrome with barely detectable electrophysiologic abnormalities.

MEDIAN NERVE COMPRESSION IN THE FOREARM

A number of syndromes have been described in which the median nerve is affected near the elbow, typically within the mass of the pronator muscle. For this reason these syndromes are often collectively called pronator syndrome. A blow on the arm at that point, anomaly of the muscle or an arterial supply at that point, possibly hypertrophy of the pronator muscle, or compression by the arch of the flexor sublimis muscle have all been described. Since the entire median nerve is affected at that point, one would theoretically expect sensory loss throughout the median nerve territory in the palm and fingers, and weakness of finger flexion, wrist flexion, some thumb abduction, and so on. In fact, these findings are quite rare; the pronator syndrome is a rarely authenticated diagnosis, and even when found, the deficits in the median nerve seem to be very incomplete or partial.

A branch of the median nerve just distal to the pronator muscle is the anterior interosseus nerve. This is a nerve without a cutaneous sensory supply, supplying motor fibers to the flexors of the thumb and index finger. This rarely is involved in compressive lesions within the pronator muscle, and a subcategory of pronator syndrome consists only of anterior interosseus nerve palsy. However, a more prevalent version of anterior interosseus nerve deficit is not compressive at all. It is a subcategory of idiopathic brachial neuritis, also known as Parsonage-Turner syndrome. For some reason such patients very often have weakness of deltoid, biceps, serratus anterior, and the muscles innervated by the anterior interosseus nerve.

In summary, patients with a proximal median neuropathy in the region of the elbow should be viewed with skepticism. An anterior interosseus nerve palsy is usually due to idiopathic brachial neuritis rather than to compressive etiologies, and surgical exploration is not indicated. In those few patients in whom a pronator syndrome of some type exists, watchful waiting appears to be the best course in view of the vague nature of the syndrome in most instances and its unknown prognosis.

SUGGESTED READINGS

Dawson DM, Hallett M, Millender LH: Entrapment Neuropathies. 2nd Ed. Little, Brown, Boston, 1990
Dellon AL: Review of treatment results for ulnar nerve compression at the elbow. J Hand Surg [Am] 14:688–699, 1989
Dellon AL, Hament W, Gittelshon A: Nonoperative management of cubital tunnel syndrome: an 8-year prospective study. Neurology 43:1673–1677, 1993
Kaplan SJ, Glickel SZ, Eaton RG: Predictive factors in the nonsurgical treatment of carpal tunnel syndrome. J Hand Surg [B] 15:106–108, 1990
Katz JN, Larson MG, Sabra A et al: The carpal tunnel syndrome: diagnostic utility of the history and physical examination findings. Ann Intern Med 112:321–327, 1990
Miller RG: Ulnar neuropathy at the elbow. Muscle Nerve 14:97–101, 1991
Nathan PA, Myers LD, Keniston RC et al: Simple decompression of the ulnar nerve: an alternative to anterior transposition. J Hand Surg [Br] 17:251–254, 1992
Rosenbaum RB, Ochoa JL: Carpal Tunnel Syndrome and Other Disorders of the Median Nerve. Butterworth-Heinemann, Boston, 1993
Silverstein BA, Fine LJ, Armstrong TJ: Occupational factors and carpal tunnel syndrome. Am J Ind Med 11:343–358, 1987
Stock SR: Workplace ergonomic factors and the development of musculoskeletal disorders of the neck and upper limbs: a meta-analysis. Am J Ind Med 19:87–107, 1991
Szabo RM, Chidgey LK: Stress carpal tunnel pressures in patients with carpal tunnel syndrome and normal patients. J Hand Surg [Am] 14:624, 1989

102. COMMON ENTRAPMENT AND COMPRESSIVE NEUROPATHIES OF THE LOWER EXTREMITY

BASHAR KATIRJI

Although not as prevalent as their counterparts in the upper extremity, focal peripheral neuropathies of the lower extremity can be a diagnostic challenge, since they are commonly confused with lumbosacral radiculopathies or plexopathies. This is particularly true in elderly patients where lumbosacral radiculopathies, due to lumbar spine disease, are common, and incorrect diagnoses may lead to unnecessary spinal surgery.

PERONEAL NEUROPATHY AT THE FIBULAR HEAD

Anatomy

In the upper thigh, while sharing a common sheath with the tibial nerve (also called medial popliteal nerve), the common peroneal nerve (also called lateral popliteal nerve) innervates the short head of biceps femoris, the only hamstring muscle it innervates (Fig. 102-1). After separating from the tibial nerve in the upper popliteal fossa, the common peroneal nerve gives off the lateral cutaneous nerve of the calf, which innervates the skin over the upper third of the lateral aspect of the leg. It then winds around the fibular neck, lying in close contact with it, and passes through a tendinous tunnel between the edge of the peroneus longus muscle and the fibula, sometimes referred to as the fibular tunnel. Near that point, the common peroneal nerve divides into superficial and deep branches. The superficial peroneal nerve innervates the peroneus longus and brevis and the skin of the lower two-thirds of the lateral aspect of the leg and the dorsum of the foot. The deep peroneal is primarily motor; it innervates the ankle and toe extensors (tibialis anterior, extensor hallucis, extensor digitorum longus and brevis) and peroneus tertius in addition to the skin of the web space between the first and second toes.

Etiology

Peroneal neuropathy at the fibular head is the most common compressive neuropathy in the lower extremity, although its

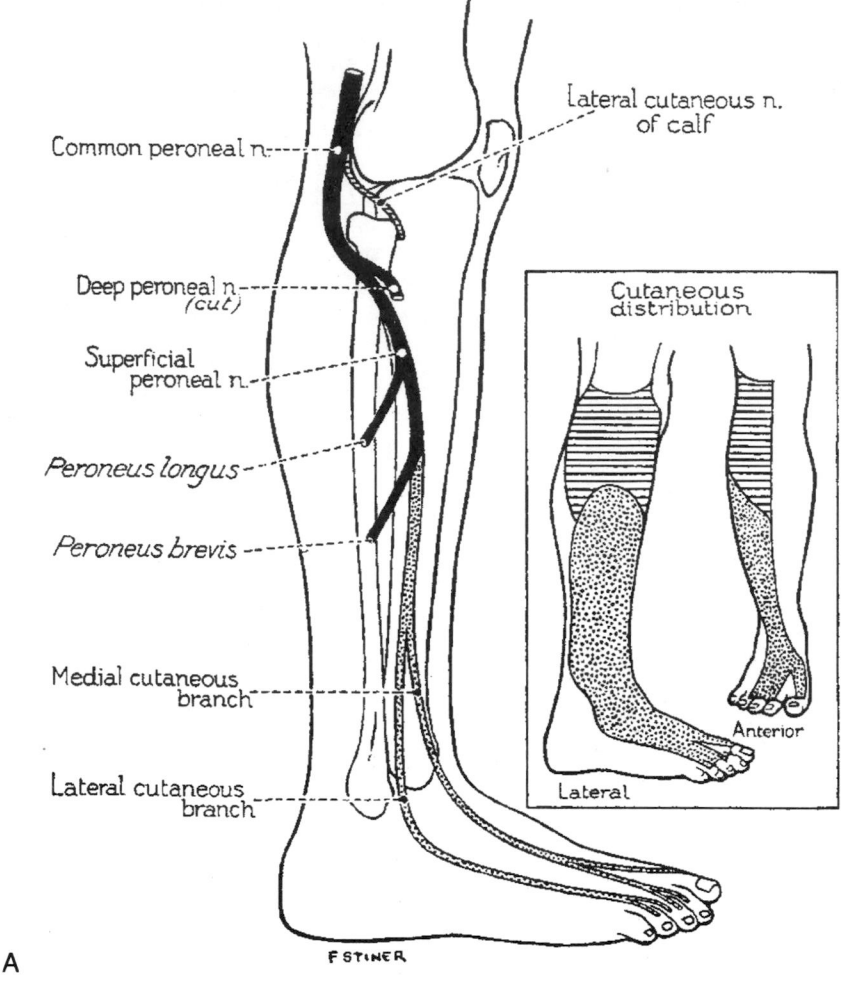

A

F STINER

FIG. 102-1.   Course and distribution of **(A)** the deep and **(B)** superficial peroneal nerves. (From Haymaker W, Woodland B: Peripheral Nerve Injuries. 2nd Ed. WB Saunders, Philadelphia, 1953, with permission.) (*Figure continues.*)

exact incidence and prevalence are unknown. In most cases, it results from prolonged compression of the peroneal nerve between an external object and the fibular head. The common predisposing factors for acute compression at the fibular head are as follows:

Recent surgery (such as anesthesia for coronary bypass)
Weight loss
Recent prolonged hospitalization (including bed rest, coma)
Habitual leg-crossing (combined with weight loss)
Diabetes
Peripheral polyneuropathy
Others (prolonged squatting, braces, plaster casts)

Following perioperative compression, the second most common cause of acute peroneal neuropathy at the fibular head is trauma, including fracture of the fibula, knee dislocation, knee surgery, and arthroscopy, lacerations, and blunt injuries. Stretch injuries of the peroneal nerve may occur following severe inversion sprains of the ankle. Extrinsic masses (osteomas, ganglia, lipomas, Baker cysts) or intrinsic nerve sheaths tumors are more rare. True peroneal entrapment at the fibular tunnel, usually caused by an anomalous firm fibrous arch overlying the nerve, is extremely rare.

Clinical Features

The onset of peroneal neuropathy is acute in perioperative compression and trauma, although in patients with weight loss or in those hospitalized for a grave illness, the onset is more subacute and, at times, difficult to determine. When peroneal palsy is progressive, a mass lesion, nerve tumor, or, rarely, true entrapment should be suspected. While the deep peroneal nerve is frequently more affected than the superficial nerve, selective deep peroneal nerve involvement is rare. The disorder is usually unilateral but can be bilateral. Peroneal neuropathies in the thigh (i.e., sciatic nerve lesions affecting the common peroneal nerve exclusively) are rare, accounting for less than 5 percent of all peroneal neuropathies. Defined as severe weakness of ankle dorsiflexion, footdrop is the most common presentation of peroneal neuropathy. Footdrop can be complete, that is, failure to dorsiflex the ankle and toes, or it can be partial; the foot may drag behind, get trapped, or cause the patient to fall. Because of weak eversion and unopposed inversion, patients often sprain their ankles. While numbness of the leg, usually involving the dorsum of the foot and lower lateral leg, is common, pain is rare. When present, it is deep and ill-defined, usually located around the knee. On examination, weakness is restricted to ankle and toe dorsiflexion and to ankle eversion. Ankle inver-

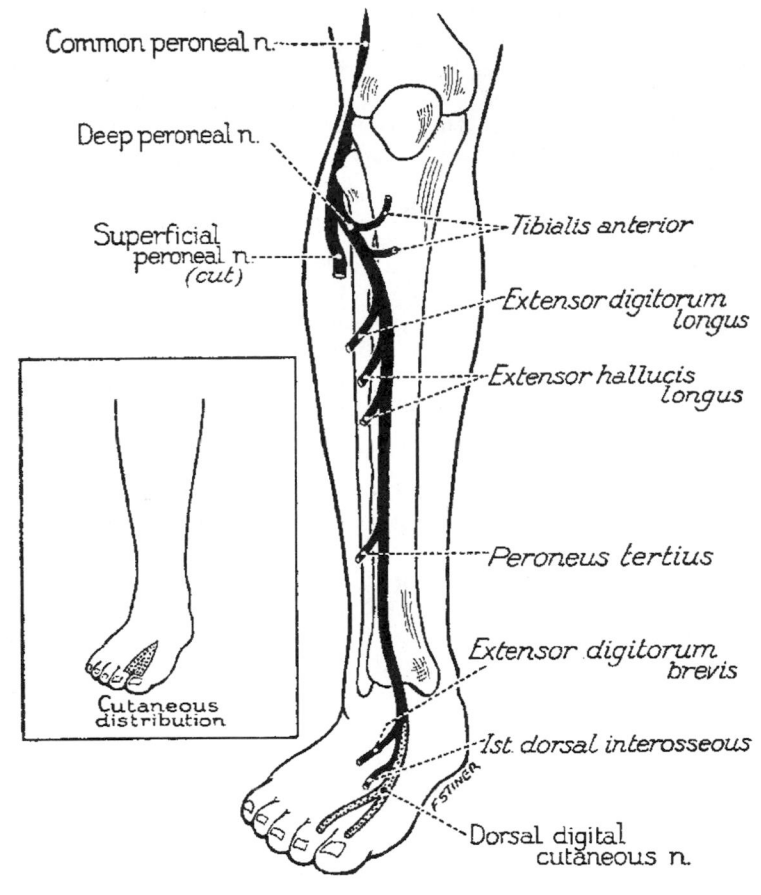

FIG. 102-1. (Continued).

TABLE 102-1. The Differential Diagnosis of Common Causes of Footdrop

	Peroneal Neuropathy at the Fibular Head	L5 Radiculopathy	Lumbar Plexopathy (Lumbosacral Trunk)	Sciatic Neuropathy (Mainly Peroneal)
Differential diagnosis				
Common causes	Compression (weight loss, perioperative), trauma	Disc herniation, spinal stenosis	Pelvic surgery, hematoma, prolonged labor	Hip surgery, injection injury, coma
Ankle inversion	Normal	Weak	Weak	Normal or mildly weak
Toe flexion	Normal	Weak	Weak	Normal or mildly weak
Plantar flexion	Normal	Normal	Normal	Normal or mildly weak
Ankle jerk	Normal	Normal (unless S1)	Normal (unless S1)	Normal or depressed
Sensory loss distribution	Peroneal only	Poorly demarcated, predominantly big toe	Well demarcated to L5 dermatome	Peroneal and lateral cutaneous of calf
Pain	Rare, deep	Common, radicular	Common, can be radicular	Can be severe
Electrodiagnosis				
Peroneal motor study to EDB and/or Tib ant	Low in amplitude or conduction block across fibular head	Usually normal but can be low in amplitude	Low in amplitude	Low in amplitude
Superficial peroneal sensory study	Low or absent[a]	Normal	Low or absent	Low or absent
Peroneal muscles[b]	Abnormal	Abnormal	Abnormal	Abnormal
Tibial L5 muscles[c]	Normal	Abnormal	Abnormal	Normal or abnormal
Other L5 muscles[d]	Normal	Normal or abnormal	Normal or abnormal	Normal
Biceps femoris (short head)	Normal	Usually normal	Usually normal	Abnormal
Paraspinal muscles fibrillations	Absent	May be absent	Absent	Absent

Abbreviations: EDB, extensor digitorum brevis; Tib Ant, tibialis anterior.
[a] Can be normal in purely demyelinating lesions or lesion of the deep peroneal nerve only.
[b] Below the knee: tibialis anterior, extensor digitorum longus, extensor digitorum brevis, extensor hallucis, and peronei.
[c] Tibialis posterior and flexor digitorum longus.
[d] Gluteus medius and tensor fascia lata.

sion, toe flexion, and plantar flexion are normal, but pseudoweakness, especially of ankle inversion, is common when the footdrop is complete. To avoid pseudoweakness, the ankle should be dorsiflexed passively to 90 degrees before testing these muscles. Hypoesthesia to touch and pain is limited to the lower two-thirds of the lateral leg and dorsum of the foot. The Tinel sign is sometimes elicited by percussion of the peroneal nerve at the fibular neck. Knee and ankle reflexes and the hamstrings, glutei, and quadriceps are normal. In deep peroneal neuropathy, the sensory manifestations are lacking (except occasionally in the first web space), and ankle eversion is normal.

Differential Diagnosis

Footdrop may result from an upper or lower motor neuron lesion. The lower motor neuron lesions include common and deep peroneal neuropathy, sciatic neuropathy (especially when affecting the common peroneal nerve predominantly or exclusively), lumbosacral plexopathy (particularly with lumbosacral trunk lesion), or L5 radiculopathy. Their clinical manifestations are shown in Table 102-1. Weakness of ankle inversion, toe or plantar flexion, or absent/depressed ankle jerk are not consistent with peroneal nerve lesion. Radicular pain and positive straight-

leg test (Lasègue test) are common in L5 radiculopathy and may be present in plexopathy or sciatic neuropathy. In a large study of common peroneal neuropathy, 43 percent of cases were clinically misdiagnosed by physicians, including neurologists. This was usually due to the difficulty in assessing ankle inversion and eversion in the presence of footdrop.

Electrodiagnosis

Nerve conduction studies and needle electromyography (EMG) are essential for both diagnostic and prognostic purposes. Even when the clinical situation is clear, the electrodiagnostic studies help confirm the site of the lesion (fibular head, thigh, deep branch), estimate the extent of injury (based on the conduction studies data) and its nature (demyelinating vs axonal vs mixed), and hence predict the expected course of recovery (weeks or months).

Nerve Conduction Studies.   The peroneal motor and sensory conduction studies should be obtained bilaterally for comparison. In addition to the usual practice of recording extensor digitorum brevis, it is essential to include the peroneal motor studies, recording the tibialis anterior, for two reasons. First, since

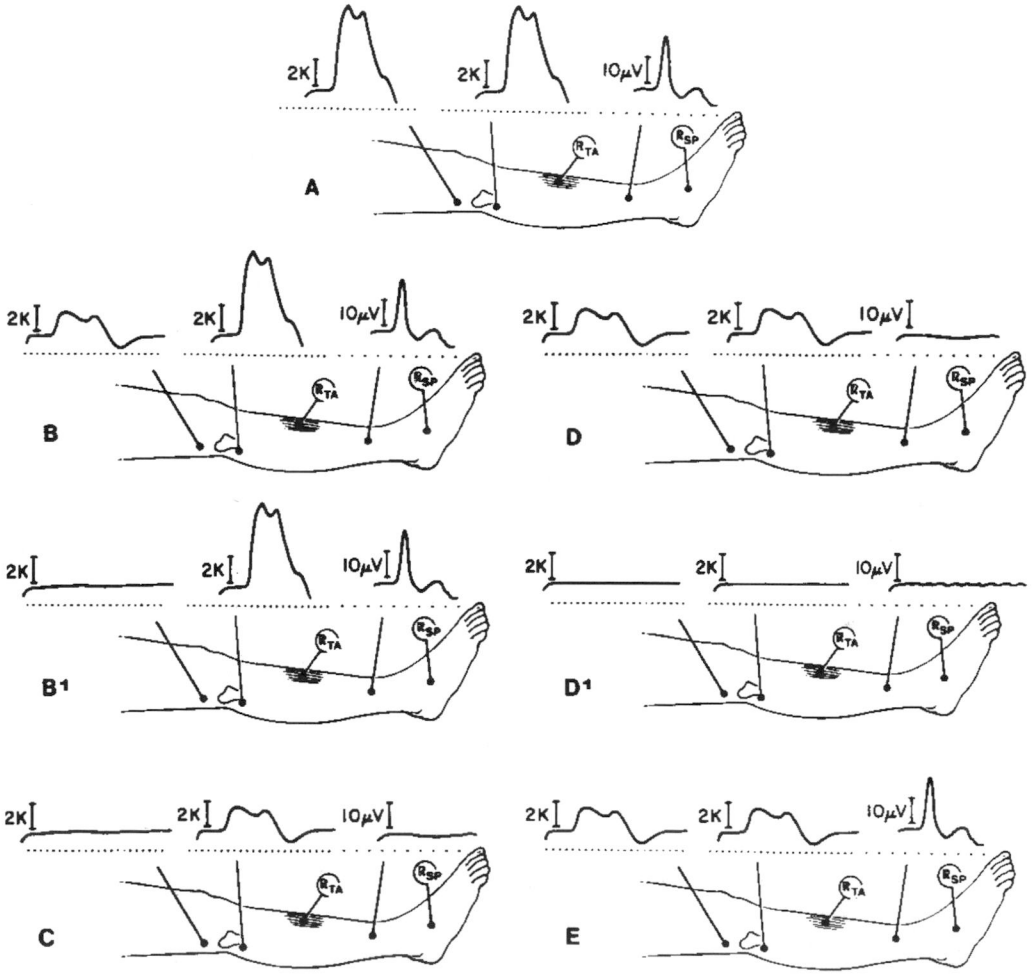

FIG. 102-2.   Diagrams of the nerve conduction studies in peroneal mononeuropathies. *A,* normal; *B* and *B*[1] "pure" conduction block, partial and complete; *D* and *D*[1] "pure" axonal loss, partial and complete; *C,* mixed; *E,* deep peroneal; *RTA,* peroneal motor response, recording tibialis anterior; *RSP,* recording site of the superficial peroneal sensory response. Proximal latencies are not drawn to scale. (From Katirji MB, Wilbourn AJ: Common peroneal mononeuropathy: a clinical and electrophysiologic study of 116 lesions. Neurology 38:1726, 1988, with permission.)

the tibialis anterior is the principal ankle dorsiflexor, establishing whether the disorder is demyelinating or axonal (and thus prognosis) should be performed using this most clinically relevant muscle. Second, the extensor digitorum brevis is not uncommonly atrophic (presumably due to tight shoes), resulting in an erroneous conclusion that the lesion is axonal and severe. The findings on nerve conduction studies, shown in Figure 102-2, can be divided into six patterns: conduction block (complete and partial), axonal loss (complete and partial), mixed lesions (conduction block and axonal), and selective deep peroneal lesions. Focal slowing is present in a minority of patients, usually associated with conduction block. Low-amplitude or absent motor responses (consistent with pure axonal loss) is observed in 50 percent of cases, pure conduction block in 20 percent, and mixed lesions in 30 percent. Thus, significant axonal loss is present in at least 80 percent of the lesions, including those in patients with perioperative compression. The superficial peroneal sensory amplitude is low to absent, except when the lesion is purely demyelinating or restricted to the deep peroneal branch; it is normal in radiculopathy but usually low or absent in lumbosacral plexopathy, sciatic neuropathy, or peripheral polyneuropathy. Therefore, to exclude these possibilities, the tibial motor and sural sensory studies and H reflex study should be performed.

Needle EMG. At least two deep and one superficial peroneal innervated muscles should be sampled. In all cases, fibrillation potentials are seen in the affected muscles when studied at least 3 weeks after the onset of footdrop. Sampling nonperoneal muscles such as the tibialis posterior, flexor digitorum longus, or gluteus medius is essential. As shown in Table 102-1, these are normal in peroneal lesions, but abnormal in L5 radiculopathy and lumbosacral plexopathy. In axonal peroneal neuropathies, unlocalizable by nerve conduction studies, sampling the short head of biceps femoris is mandatory to rule out a high peroneal lesion (sciatic neuropathy affecting the peroneal predominantly or exclusively). In these lesions, the short head of the biceps femoris is abnormal, and when the tibial component of the sciatic nerve is involved, the other hamstrings, gastrocnemius, and abductor hallucis are also affected, but the glutei are spared.

Prognosis

It is difficult to prognosticate based on clinical evaluation only. In general, as with other peripheral nerve injuries, partial lesions fare better than complete lesions, since local sprouting reinnervates muscle fibers effectively. The prognosis depends on the pathologic nature of the lesion, as shown in Table 102-2. In a large study of peroneal neuropathy, the vast majority of patients had prominent axonal loss: purely axonal lesions without demyelination was present in half of the patients and significant axonal loss in 80 percent. In contrast to common belief, this applies equally to the perioperative peroneal neuropathies, including the subgroup following anesthesia for coronary bypass surgery.

Management

In acute compressive lesions, patients should be observed to allow for improvement by remyelination or reinnervation. Conduction block lesions recover spontaneously in 2 to 3 months as long as further compression is prevented. Proper padding of beds, prevention of leg crossing, and arrest or reversal of intentional weight loss should be initiated promptly. A knee pad is helpful in ambulating patients. Ankle bracing is important when the footdrop is profound to prevent ankle contractures and sprains. Surgical intervention is appropriate in certain situations:

1. When the nerve is lacerated and visibly discontinuous. This repair could be primary (at the time of laceration suturing) or secondary (if local infection is feared).
2. When clinical or EMG evidence for reinnervation has not been established in the tibialis anterior despite 4 to 6 months from injury. Here, the nerve lesion is likely severe, at least of the third degree.
3. In slowly progressive peroneal neuropathies, a nerve tumor, ganglion, cyst, or, rarely, true entrapment, is suspected and the nerve explored after appropriate electrodiagnostic localization. Imaging studies, particularly magnetic resonance imaging, are particularly helpful in these special situations.

FEMORAL NEUROPATHY IN THE PELVIS OR AT THE INGUINAL LIGAMENT

Anatomy

The femoral nerve (also called the anterior crural nerve) is formed by the combination of the posterior divisions of the ventral rami of L2, L3, and L4 spinal roots (the anterior divisions of the same roots form the obturator nerve) (Fig. 102-3). It immediately gives branches to the psoas muscle before it enters its substance. Then, covered by a tight iliac fascia, the femoral nerve passes between the psoas and iliacus muscles where it innervates the latter. After passing underneath the rigid inguinal ligament, the femoral nerve branches widely into its terminal motor branches (to the quadriceps and sartorius) and sensory branches (to the anterior thigh), including the saphenous sensory nerve that innervates the medial half of the leg.

TABLE 102-2. Classification and Degrees of Peripheral Nerve Injury

Sunderland	First Degree	Second Degree	Third Degree	Fourth Degree	Fifth Degree
Seddon	Neurapraxia	Axonotmesis	Neurotmesis	Neurotmesis	Neurotmesis
Electrophysiology	Conduction block	Loss of axons	Loss of axons	Loss of axons	Loss of axons
Pathology	Segmental demyelination	Loss of axons with intact supporting structures	Loss of axons with disrupted endoneurium	Loss of axons with disrupted endoneurium and perineurium	Loss of axons with disruption of all supporting structures (discontinuous)
Prognosis	Excellent, recovery is usually complete in 2–3 months	Slow recovery, dependent on sprouting and reinnervation	Protracted and can fail due to misdirected axonal sprouts	Unlikely without surgical repair	Impossible without surgical repair

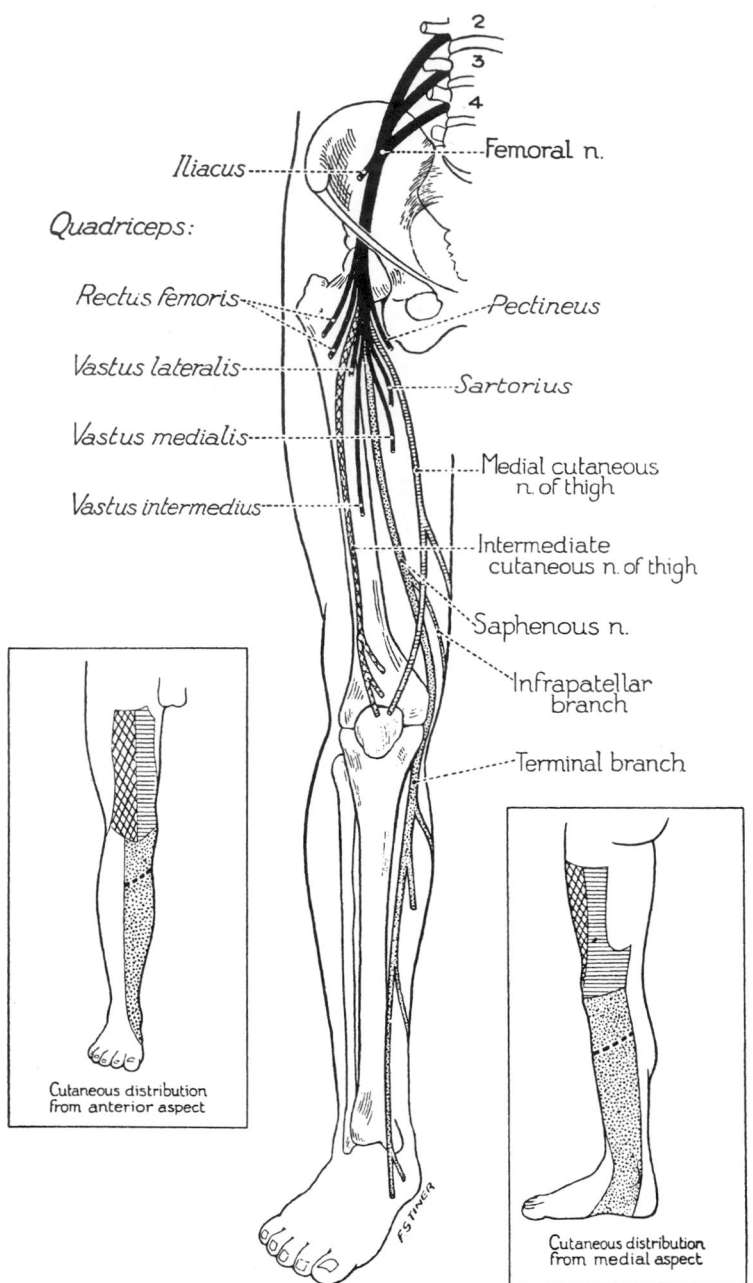

FIG. 102-3. Course and distribution of the femoral nerve. (From Haymaker W, Woodland B: Peripheral Nerve Injuries. 2nd Ed. WB Saunders, Philadelphia, 1953, with permission.)

Etiology

The femoral nerve can be compressed at the inguinal region or in the retroperitoneal pelvic space. The most common causes of femoral neuropathy are as follows:

1. Compression in pelvis by
   (a) Retractor blade during pelvic surgery: abdominal hysterectomy, radical prostatectomy, renal transplantation
   (b) Iliacus or psoas retroperitoneal hematoma: anticoagulation (systemic or subcutaneous abdominal heparin), hemophilia, coagulopathy, ruptured abdominal aneurysm, femoral artery catheterization
   (c) Pelvic mass: tumor, abscess, cyst, aortic or iliac aneurysm

2. Compression in the inguinal region by
   (a) Inguinal ligament during lithotomy position: vaginal delivery, laparoscopy, vaginal hysterectomy, urological procedures
   (b) Inguinal hematoma: femoral artery catherization such as for coronary angiography and total hip replacement
   (c) Inguinal lymphadenopathy
3. Stretch injury: hyperextension, dancing, yoga
4. Others: radiation, laceration, misplaced injection, ?diabetes

By far the most commonly reported causes are those related to pelvic surgery, such as following abdominal hysterectomy or radical prostatectomy. During these surgical procedures, the femoral nerve is compressed between the retractor's blade and the pelvic wall. Compression at the inguinal ligament during prolonged lithotomy positioning for various procedures, including vaginal delivery and laparoscopy, is not uncommon and is likely underestimated. Acute hemorrhage in the retroperitoneal space within the iliacus muscle, and, less commonly, the psoas muscle, result in a compartmental syndrome and secondary severe femoral nerve damage. Although diabetes has been reported to cause selective femoral neuropathy, most cases are actually due to more extensive disease affecting the lumbar plexus and roots (diabetic radiculoplexopathy or amyotrophy).

Clinical Features

Most femoral neuropathies present acutely with lower extremity weakness. Patients report buckling of the knee and frequent falls, particularly when they attempt to partially flex the knee. When the hip flexors are weak, patients cannot climb steps, since they are unable to clear the foot of the weak leg from the tread of stairs. Sensory symptoms over the anterior thigh and medial leg are common. Groin or thigh pain is mild (except with retroperitoneal hematomas). The neurologic examination reveals weakness of the quadriceps muscle (knee extension) with absent or depressed knee jerk. Thigh adduction is, however, normal. The iliopsoas muscle (hip flexion) is usually weak when the lesion is pelvic. It should be noted that the quadriceps assist in flexing the hip; Thus, mild hip flexion weakness can be falsely attributed to the iliopsoas weakness. Hypesthesia over the anterior thigh and medial calf is common.

The presentation of patients with acute iliacus or psoas hematoma is unique. Usually, they experience acute severe pain in the groin, thigh, and sometimes lower abdomen. They frequently keep the hip flexed to minimize pain, since hip extension (such as on reversed straight leg test) is extremely painful. In most cases, the neurologic deficit is restricted to the femoral nerve, but extensive hematomas may result in damage to the lumbar, and even the entire lumbosacral, plexus.

Differential Diagnosis

Femoral neuropathy should be differentiated from L2, L3, and L4 radiculopathy and from lumbar plexopathy (Table 102-3). Weakness of the thigh adductors, innervated by the obturator nerve, excludes a selective femoral lesion. Positive reversed straight-leg test is common in lumbar radiculopathy, but may occur with plexopathy and femoral nerve lesion due to retroperitoneal hematoma. In plexopathy or L4 radiculopathy, weakness of ankle dorsiflexion (tibialis anterior) is common. In patients with femoral neuropathy and severe pain, particularly in the setting of anticoagulation or coagulopathy, a retroperitoneal hematoma should be suspected and pelvic computed tomography scan obtained urgently.

Electrodiagnosis

The role of electrodiagnosis is primarily confirmative in typical cases, but is very helpful when true clinical weakness is not clear because of pain associated with recent surgery or delivery. In addition, the nerve conduction studies play an important role in predicting prognosis.

Nerve Conduction Studies. The femoral motor and saphenous sensory studies should be performed bilaterally for comparison. The saphenous sensory studies are technically difficult in the elderly patient, or if there is leg edema. Since the femoral motor response, recording rectus femoris, can only be evoked at one site (the groin), the pathophysiologic process and prognosis is dependent on the size (amplitude and/or area) of the response. In addition, since most femoral lesions are acute, care should be taken in accounting for the time for wallerian degeneration. The drop in sensory amplitudes lag behind motor amplitudes: the former reach their nadir in 8 to 11 days, and the latter in 4 to 5 days. Thus, beyond the period required for wallerian degeneration (i.e., after 10 to 11 days), the femoral motor amplitude is low and the saphenous sensory response is absent in axonal lesions, while they remain normal in demyelinating lesions.

Needle EMG. The quadriceps and iliacus muscles should be sampled in all patients with suspected femoral neuropathy. Fibrillation potentials and impaired recruitment is seen in affected muscles. The motor unit potentials are normal unless sprouting has occurred; in that case, they become large (increased in duration, high in amplitude and polyphasic). If the iliacus is abnormal, the lesion is pelvic, that is, not at the inguinal ligament. The thigh adductors and tibialis anterior are normal in femoral lesions (Table 102-3).

Prognosis

In general, femoral neuropathy carries a relatively good prognosis, even when the lesion is due to axonal loss. Sprouting and reinnervation are optimal, since the target muscle (quadriceps) is both proximal and relatively near the site of injury. The only exception is severe femoral neuropathy due to retroperitoneal compartmental hematoma, which, in most cases, does not recover well with time. Demyelinating lesions, such as those following lithotomy positioning, recover completely in 3 to 4 months. The femoral motor amplitude, recording rectus femoris, is essential in prognosticating these lesions.

Management

In order to prevent compression at the inguinal ligament, prolonged lithotomy positioning with extreme hip flexion and external rotation should be avoided. Most cases of femoral neuropathy are treated conservatively. The management of retroperitoneal hematoma (observation versus evacuation) is controversial. Obviously, stopping anticoagulation and/or correcting coagulopathy is mandatory. Physical therapy is recom-

TABLE 102-3. Differential Diagnosis of Femoral Neuropathy

	Femoral Neuropathy	Lumbar Plexopathy	Lumbar Radiculopathy
Thigh adductors	Normal	Abnormal	Abnormal
Tibialis anterior (ankle dorsiflexion)	Normal	Abnormal	Abnormal[a]
Saphenous sensory nerve action potential	Usually low or absent[b]	Low or absent	Normal
Paraspinal fibrillations	Absent	Absent	May be absent

[a] Abnormal in L4 radiculopathy only.
[b] Normal in purely demyelinating lesions.

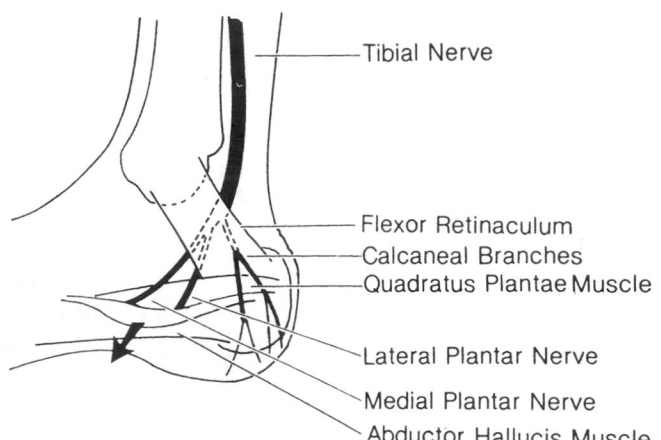

FIG. 102-4. The tibial nerve at the ankle with its three terminal branches. (From Dyck PJ, Thomas PK: Peripheral Neuropathy. 3rd Ed. WB Saunders, Philadelphia, 1993, with permission.)

mended in all patients. A knee brace is indicated in patients with severe weakness of the quadriceps to prevent falls.

TARSAL TUNNEL SYNDROME

Anatomy

After innervating the gastrocnemius, soleus, tibialis posterior, flexor digitorum profundus, and flexor hallucis longus in the calf, the tibial nerve passes through the tarsal tunnel at the medial aspect of the ankle and innervates the skin and muscles of the sole of the foot (Fig. 102-4). The roof of the tarsal tunnel is composed of a thin fascia, the flexor retinaculum, which connects the medial malleolus to the calcaneus. There, the tibial nerve is accompanied by the tibial artery and the tendons of the flexor digitorum longus and flexor hallucis longus. At, or

slightly distal to the tunnel, the nerve divides into its three terminal branches: (1) the calcaneal branch, a purely sensory nerve, that innervates the skin of the sole of the heel; (2) the medial plantar nerve, which innervates the abductor hallucis, flexor digitorum brevis, and flexor hallucis brevis, in addition to the skin of the medial sole, and, at least, the medial three toes; and (3) the lateral plantar nerve, which innervates the abductor digiti quinti pedis, flexor digiti quinti pedis, adductor hallucis, and the interossei, in addition to the skin of the lateral sole and two lateral toes.

Etiology

Tarsal tunnel syndrome is an uncommon disorder, caused by compression of the tibial nerve or any of its three terminal branches under the flexor retinaculum. Many reported cases lack objective neurologic signs or electrophysiologic confirmation. Most well-documented cases are unilateral, caused by remote trauma to the ankle (sprain or fracture/dislocation), tenosynovitis with or without rheumatoid arthritis, thrombophlebitis, or mass lesion within the tunnel (ganglion, lipoma, schwannoma).

Clinical Features

The most common symptom of tarsal tunnel syndrome is burning pain of the foot and ankle, which worsens after prolonged standing or walking. Paresthesias in the sole are less common, and weakness or imbalance are extremely rare. The neurologic examination should document sensory impairment in the sole in the distribution of one or all of the terminal branches. The Tinel sign, induced by percussion of the tibial nerve at the flexor retinaculum, is present in most patients. Muscle atrophy in one sole may be detected. Weakness is rare, since the long toe flexors are intact. The ankle jerk and sensation of the dorsum of the foot are normal.

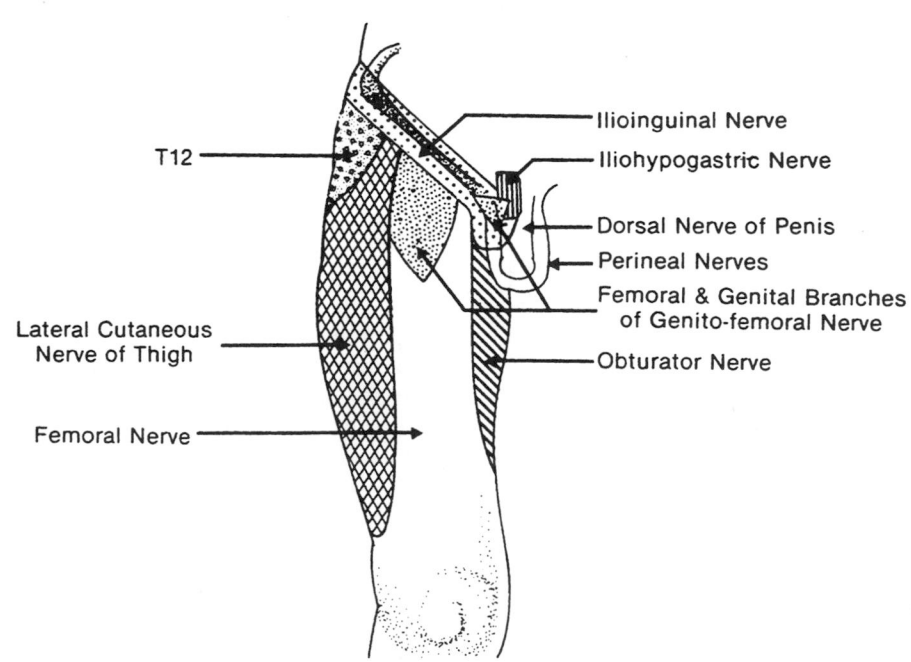

FIG. 102-5. Innervation of the skin of inguinal area and the upper thigh. (From Stewart JD: Focal Peripheral Neuropathies. 2nd Ed. Raven Press, New York, 1993, with permission.)

Electrodiagnosis

Similarly, the electrodiagnostic evaluation of the plantar nerves can be difficult for two reasons: (1) Sensory nerve action potentials, using surface stimulations and recordings, are technically difficult to elicit, especially in elderly patients with foot calluses or ankle edema. They are frequently be absent in asymptomatic individuals. (2) Needle examination of the muscles of the sole is painful, and may show denervation changes in controls, especially of the older age group.

Nerve Conduction Studies. Both the motor and sensory studies should be attempted bilaterally for comparison. In addition to the routine tibial motor studies, recording abductor hallucis, the tibial motor study recording the abductor digiti quinti pedis should also be performed. The former evaluates the medial plantar nerve, and the latter evaluates the lateral plantar nerve. The amplitudes are low and latencies slow in less than half of the patients. The plantar sensory studies can be performed by stimulating the toes or the sole, while recording orthodromically at the ankle slightly proximal to the flexor retinaculum. Asymmetric slowing or asymmetrically absent responses are diagnostic. Near-nerve needle recordings and stimulations have been advocated, but are invasive, painful, and may result in foot infection.

Needle EMG. Sampling of the abductor hallucis and abductor digiti minimi pedis may show chronic neurogenic changes with or without fibrillations.

Differential Diagnosis

The diagnosis of tarsal tunnel syndrome is difficult, since foot pain can be seen in a variety of orthopaedic, rheumatologic, and neurologic conditions, including stress fracture, bursitis, arthritis, plantar fascitis, lumbosacral radiculopathy, peripheral polyneuropathy, and reflex sympathetic dystrophy. This is particularly difficult in patients with a prior history of trauma where differentiating tarsal tunnel syndrome from reflex sympathetic dystrophy can be challenging. Careful evalua-

TABLE 102-4. Other Entrapment and Compressive Neuropathies in the Lower Extremity[a]

Nerve	Etiology	Clinical Manifestations	Differential Diagnosis	Management
Uncommon syndromes				
Lateral femoral cutaneous (Meralgia paresthetica)	Entrapment at the inguinal ligament (pregnancy, obesity, diabetes, belt, beeper), pelvic mass or hematoma or surgery	Paresthesia and pain (deep and superficial) in lateral thigh; exam: well-demarcated sensory impairment of the lateral femoral cutaneous nerve	L3 or L2 radiculopathy; femoral neuropathy	Conservative, since most resolve in months; local steroids are sometimes helpful; decompression at the inguinal ligament is rarely required
Ilioinguinal (inguinal neuralgia)	Inguinal hernia repair, appendectomy, retroperitoneal mass or incision	Burning pain in the lower abdomen, groin radiating to the scrotum and upper thigh, worse with walking; exam: sensory disturbance along inguinal ligament	Genitofemoral neuropathy (diagnostic nerve block might be required), L1 or L2 radiculopathy, hip joint disease	Analgesia and nerve blocks in postoperative cases; rarely, surgical exploration
Genitofemoral	Appendectomy, inguinal hernia repair	Painful paresthesia in upper thigh, scrotum, and medial groin; exam: sensory disturbance in scrotum and upper thigh, absence of cremasteric reflex	Ilioinguinal neuropathy (diagnostic nerve block might be required), L1 or L2 radiculopathy, hip joint disease	Conservative
Iliohypogastric	Retroperitoneal mass or incision (nephrectomy)	Asymmetrical abdominal wall bulging and trivial sensory loss in suprapubic area	Ilioinguinal or genitofemoral neuropathy, L1 or L2 radiculopathy	Conservative
Saphenous	Surgery for varicose veins or removal of saphenous vein for arterial graft, knee surgery, entrapment at Hunter's canal	Numbness with medial thigh with variable pain; exam: sensory loss in medial thigh	L4 radiculopathy, mild femoral neuropathy	Conservative; exploration of Hunter's canal is rarely indicated
Obturator	Hip surgery, pelvic fracture, obturator hernia, malignant neoplasm	Leg weakness, pain and paresthesia in thigh and inner leg; exam: weakness of thigh adductors	L2 and L3 radiculopathy, lumbar plexopathy, femoral neuropathy	Dependent on primary cause; surgical exploration is rarely required
Disputed syndromes				
Piriformis syndrome	Compression of the sciatic nerve by the overlying piriformis muscle	Pain in the buttock and leg with ill-defined paresthesia; normal neurologic and EMG examinations	Lumbosacral radiculopathy, particularly L5 and S1, hip joint disease, bursitis	Conservative with physical therapy; surgical exploration is rarely indicated
Anterior tarsal tunnel syndrome	Compression of the terminal segment of the deep peroneal nerve by the superficial fascia of the ankle (tight shoes, fractures, sprains)	Trivial; usually foot paresthesia and deep ankle pain; exam: atrophy of extensor digitorum brevis and hypesthesia in 1st web	Asymptomatic atrophy of the extensor digitorum brevis, common or deep peroneal neuropathy at fibular head, L5 radiculopathy, arthritis	Conservative with foot orthosis or local steroids

[a] See also Figure 102-5.

tion of the ankle and foot, including radiographs, bone scan, tomogram, and EMG, is often necessary for correct diagnosis. Electrodiagnostically, the tarsal tunnel syndrome should be differentiated from peripheral polyneuropathy and S1-S2 radiculopathies. The sural sensory and/or H reflex studies are abnormal in polyneuropathy and the findings are usually symmetrical. In S1 radiculopathy, other muscles innervated by the S1 root (such as the gastrocnemius) are usually affected, and the H reflex study is abnormal.

Prognosis

Most patients improve without any sequelae. Unfortunately, some patients, especially those associated with ankle trauma, may develop chronic pain and features of reflex sympathetic dystrophy.

Management

Conservative treatment should be initiated in all patients first. Sources of pressure, such as ill-fitting shoes, should be identified and eliminated. Other conservative measures include minimizing ankle edema by elevation and special stockings, medial arch support or bracing the foot with a light orthosis, anti-inflammatory agents, or local injection with long-acting corticosteroids. Only a small proportion of patients will require surgical decompression with variable results. Good results can be achieved by selecting patients with documented entrapment

who failed conservative treatment or those with identifiable mass.

Less common compressive and entrapment neuropathies in the lower extremity are summarized in Table 102-4 and shown in Figure 102-5.

SUGGESTED READINGS

Al Hakim M, Katirji MB: Femoral mononeuropathy induced by the lithotomy position: a report of 5 cases and a review of the literature. Muscle Nerve 16:891–895, 1993

Dawson DM, Hallett M, Millender LH: Tarsal tunnel syndromes. p. 291. In: Entrapment Neuropathies. 2nd Ed. Little, Brown, Boston, 1990

Devi S, Lovelace RE, Duarte N: Proximal peroneal nerve conduction velocity: recording from anterior tibial and peroneus brevis muscle. Ann Neurol 2: 116–119, 1977

Katirji MB, Lanska DJ: Femoral mononeuropathy after radical prostatectomy. Urology 36:539–540, 1990

Katirji MB, Wilbourn AJ: Common peroneal mononeuropathy: a clinical and electrophysiologic study of 116 lesions. Neurology 38:1723–1728, 1988

Katirji MB, Wilbourn AJ: High sciatic lesions mimicking peroneal neuropathy at the fibular head. Neurol Sci 121:172–175, 1994

Kvist-Poulsen H, Borel J: Iatrogenic femoral neuropathy subsequent to abdominal hysterectomy: incidence and prevention. Obstet Gynecol 60:516–520, 1982

Pickett JB: Localizing peroneal nerve lesions to the knee by motor conduction studies. Arch Neurol 41:192–195, 1984

Sourkes M, Stewart JD: Common peroneal neuropathy: a study of selective motor and sensory involvement. Neurology 41:1029–1033, 1991

Stewart JD: Focal Peripheral Neuropathies. 2nd Ed. Raven Press, New York, 1993

Young MR, Norris JW: Femoral neuropathy during anticoagulant therapy. Neurology 26:1173–1175, 1976

SECTION 4. DISEASES OF NEUROMUSCULAR TRANSMISSION

103. MYASTHENIA GRAVIS

DAVID C. PRESTON

The neuromuscular junction (NMJ) forms essentially an electrochemical link transmitting the nerve action potential to muscle. A variety of disorders are known to impair the NMJ either at the presynaptic or postsynaptic membrane. Among these disorders, myasthenia gravis (MG) is the most common with an incidence of 2 to 10 cases/100,000 cases per year. Over the last thirty years, the autoimmune pathophysiology of MG has been well elucidated with the recognition of antibodies directed against the nicotinic acetylcholine receptor. As this disorder is quite treatable and potentially curable, prompt recognition, especially early in the clinical course, is important. Mortality and morbidity, once not unusual in patients with MG, have been

dramatically reduced in the modern era with early diagnosis and the use of immunosuppression, plasma exchange, and thymectomy.

CLINICAL FEATURES

Patients with MG present with muscle weakness and fatigue. As the disorder is limited to the NMJ, there is no abnormality of mental state, sensory function, or autonomic function. Myasthenic weakness characteristically affects the extraocular muscles, bulbar muscles, proximal limb muscles, or a combination of these. Eye findings are the most common with ptosis and extraocular muscle weakness occurring in more than 50 percent of patients at the time of presentation and developing in more than 90 percent at some time during their illness. Frequently, extraocular weakness may begin asymmetrically with one eye involved and the other spared. A very small amount of extraocular weakness will be subjectively noticed by the patient as visual blurring or frank double vision. Myasthenic weakness has been known to mimic third, fourth, and sixth cranial nerve palsies as well as, rarely, an intranuclear ophthalmoplegia. Unlike third nerve palsies, however, MG never affects pupillary function. Fixed extraocular weakness tends to occur later. After extraocular weakness, bulbar muscle weakness is most common, with difficulty in chewing, swallowing, and speaking. Some patients experience severe fatigability and weakness of mastication, and are unable to keep the jaw closed after chewing. Myasthenic speech is nasal (from weakness of the soft palate) and slurred (from weakness of the tongue, lips, and face) but without any difficulty with fluency. When limb weakness develops in patients with MG mainly the proximal musculature is affected, and it is symmetric. Patients usually complain of difficulty arising from chairs or going up and down stairs, reaching with their arms, or holding their head up. Rare patients will present with a "limb-girdle" form of myasthenia gravis alone, and weakness of eye movement or bulbar muscle never develops.

The hallmark of MG is *pathologic fatigability,* that is, progressive muscle weakness with use. Patients typically improve after rest or upon arising in the morning, with worsening as the day passes. Generalized fatigue is a common complaint in many neurologic and nonneurologic disorders. In MG and other disorders of the NMJ, fatigue is limited to muscular fatigue alone and often progresses to frank muscle weakness. Patients with MG do not generally experience a sense of mental fatigue, tiredness, or sleepiness.

The clinical examination in a patient suspected of having MG is directed at muscular strength and demonstrating pathologic fatiguability. When trying to assess subtle weakness, it is frequently more useful to observe the patient performing functional tasks, such as arising from a chair or from the floor, and walking, rather than relying on manual muscle strength testing. Pathologic fatigability may be demonstrated by having the patient look up for several minutes (looking for ptosis or extraocular weakness) and count aloud to 100 (looking for nasal or slurred speech), or by repetitively testing the proximal limb or neck muscles. The remainder of the neurologic examination is normal. Reflexes are generally preserved or are reduced in proportion to the amount of muscle weakness.

MG may develop at any age, although it is more common in younger and middle-aged adults; women slightly outnumber men among younger patients, but more men are afflicted among middle-aged and older patients. In patients with MG, there is a well-recognized association of abnormalities of the thymus gland. Thymic hyperplasia is found in as many as 60 to 70 percent of all cases, and thymoma is found in 11 percent. Although the role of the thymus is not completely understood in MG, it is likely important in initiating and maintaining the autoimmune response (see below). Another interesting group of patients with MG is the 15 percent who have the ocular form of the disease whose symptoms remain restricted to the extraocular and eyelid muscles. When patients first present with fluctuating extraocular weakness, it is not possible to predict from either clinical or laboratory testing whether the disease will subsequently generalize or remain in the relatively benign restricted ocular form. If a patient has had restricted ocular myasthenia for 1 to 2 years, there is a high likelihood that the myasthenia will never generalize and will remain restricted to the extraocular muscles. This has some implications for treatment (see below), as patients with ocular MG do not develop crises or other severe complications of generalized MG.

Autoimmune MG may be seen in two other groups. Transient neonatal MG is recognized in 21 percent of neonates born to mothers with MG. Maternal immunoglobulin G (IgG) antibodies directed against the acetylcholine receptor are passed through the placenta, resulting in the same clinical syndrome. The illness is usually mild and self-limited, disappearing over the first few months of life as the maternal antibodies are degraded. Finally, MG may be seen as a complication of patients treated with penicillamine. The clinical syndrome is similar except that many patients will slowly improve once the penicillamine has been withdrawn.

DIAGNOSIS

The diagnosis of MG is usually straightforward and based primarily on the recognition of the clinical pattern of the disease followed by the appropriate laboratory, electrophysiologic, and radiologic evaluations. The laboratory evaluation of a patient suspected of having MG is as follows:

Tensilon test (preferably double blinded with cardiac monitoring)
Acetylcholine receptor antibodies
Antinuclear antibody
Thyroid function tests
Routine nerve conduction studies and EMG followed by repetitive nerve stimulation of both distal and proximal nerves
Single-fiber EMG if repetitive nerve stimulation is negative or equivocal
Chest imaging (computed tomography scanning or magnetic resonance imaging)

Tensilon Test

The Tensilon is a simple and quick test that can be used to evaluate the possibility of neuromuscular junction disease. Tensilon (edrophonium hydrochloride), a short-acting acetylcholinesterase inhibitor, is given intravenously, which may quickly reverse myasthenic weakness. It is most useful when there is an obvious objective clinical parameter to follow (e.g., degree of ptosis or extraocular muscle weakness). The clinician cannot rely on subjective improvement by the patient. When performing a Tensilon test, a double-blinded study is preferable. Two 1-ml syringes are drawn up: one with 10 mg of Tensilon and the other with saline. The syringes are coded with the physician performing the test unaware of which one contains the Tensilon. One syringe is selected. A test dose of 2 mg is given and flushed with normal saline. If no response is seen within 1 minute, the additional 8 mg is given, followed by a saline flush. A response is looked for over the next 3 minutes. The procedure is then repeated with the second syringe. Side effects of Tensilon are those of cholinergic excess (salivation, bradycardia, tearing, etc.). Atropine should be readily available if needed to counteract these side effects. Although Tensilon is generally considered a safe test, care must be exercised in all patients, especially older patients with cardiac disease, as, infrequently, bradycardia may lead to syncope, and, in exceptional cases asystole has been documented.

Acetylcholine Receptor Antibodies

Acetylcholine receptor antibodies are detected in greater than 75 to 85 percent of patients with generalized MG. Antibodies are much less frequent in patients with restricted ocular MG, occurring in only 50 percent of cases. Acetylcholine receptor antibodies are highly specific for MG with few false-positive results. In general, myasthenic patients with circulating antibodies have a high incidence of thymic abnormalities. Autoantibodies against other tissues including thyroid and gastric tissues are also frequently present. Autoimmune thyroid disease is particularly common and will eventually develop in 5 to 12 percent of patients.

Repetitive Nerve Stimulation

Repetitive nerve stimulation (RNS) is an effective way to fatigue the NMJ and cause depletion of acetylcholine. These studies are abnormal in more than 60 to 70 percent of myasthenic patients. A decremental response on RNS is the electrical correlate of clinical muscle fatigue and weakness in myasthenic patients. In normal subjects, slow RNS (2 to 3 Hz) results in little or no decrement, but in cases of MG, a decrement of the compound muscle action potential of 10 percent or more is characteristically seen. Both distal and proximal nerves can be tested. Although distal nerves (e.g., the ulnar nerve) are technically easier to perform, the diagnostic yield increases with stimulation of proximal nerves (i.e., spinal accessory, musculocutaneous, or facial nerves), which is not unexpected as the proximal muscles are often much more involved clinically than the distal ones. Every patient undergoing RNS also needs to have routine nerve conduction studies and EMG performed. Although RNS is a sensitive test for MG, there are a variety of other disorders that can also cause a decremental response that will be missed unless a complete study is performed (e.g., any severe denervating disease such as amyotrophic lateral sclerosis, the myotonic disorders, severe myopathies, and the Lambert-Eaton myasthenic syndrome).

Single-Fiber EMG

Normally, when a motor axon is depolarized, the action potential travels distally and excites all the muscle fibers within that motor unit at more or less the same time. The variation in the time interval between the firing of adjacent muscle fibers from the same motor unit (jitter) can be measured with single-fiber EMG (SF-EMG). Jitter is typically prolonged in disorders of the NMJ even without overt clinical weakness. In addition, SF-EMG may demonstrate "blocking" of muscle fibers (i.e., the endplate potential of one muscle fiber of a motor unit falls below threshold, and subsequently its muscle fiber action potential is not generated). The clinical correlate of blocking is muscle weakness. In patients who have difficulty cooperating with the examination, stimulated SF-EMG can be done. Often the extensor digitorum communis muscle is selected for study. If possible, it is always useful to study a clinically involved muscle. Indeed, a normal single-fiber examination in a clinically weak muscle effectively rules out the diagnosis of MG. SF-EMG is the most sensitive test to demonstrate impaired neuromuscular junction transmission (abnormal in 95 to 99 percent of patients with generalized MG). However, it must be emphasized that SF-EMG, although quite sensitive, is not specific, and it is typically abnormal in neuropathic and myopathic disease. Although it might be tempting to consider having any patient with fatigue undergo SF-EMG, the test is best reserved for those patients in whom the diagnosis of MG is strongly suspected, and other tests have been negative or equivocal. SF-EMG is

often a technically demanding examination for the patient as well as the electromyographer.

Chest Imaging

Every patient with MG should undergo routine chest imaging with either computed tomography scans (CT) or magnetic resonance imaging (MRI) to look for evidence of thymic hyperplasia or thymoma. The presence of a thymoma is a clear indication for subsequent thymectomy. Early diagnosis of thymoma is important before invasion of the tumor beyond its capsule has occurred with likely metastasis.

ETIOLOGY

The pathophysiology of MG is now well understood. MG is an autoimmune disease caused by sensitized T-helper cells and an IgG-directed attack on the nicotinic acetylcholine receptor of the NMJ. Thus, it is a disorder caused predominantly by antiacetylcholine receptor antibodies. A variety of experimental steps supports this hypothesis:

1. Antibodies are present in the serum of most patients with MG.
2. Antibodies can be passively transferred to animals producing experimental myasthenia.
3. Removal of antibodies allows recovery.
4. Immunization of animals with an acetylcholine receptor produces antibodies and can provoke an autoimmune disease (experimental autoimmune MG), which closely resembles the naturally occurring disease.

The mechanism of antibody damage to the receptor and motor endplate probably involves several steps. First, there is a complement-directed attack with destruction of the acetylcholine receptor and the junctional folds. Second, binding of the antibody to the receptor can cause stearic hindrance of acetylcholine binding at a neighboring site. Third, antibody binding can also result in increased removal of acetylcholine receptor from the membrane (modulation). Finally, the antibody can bind rarely to the acetylcholine receptor binding site itself and directly block acetylcholine binding. As mentioned above, there is a high incidence of thymic abnormalities in patients with MG. The role of the thymus in initiating and maintaining the autoimmune response in MG is unclear. However, it is notable that mammalian thymus expresses an acetylcholine receptor similar to that of embryonic muscle, and it is possible that this intrathymic acetylcholine receptor is the primary antigen-provoking antibody formation in the pathogenesis of MG.

The abnormal and reduced numbers of acetylcholine receptors lead to impaired NMJ transmission. When a nerve action potential invades and depolarizes the presynaptic junction, voltage-dependent calcium channels are activated allowing an influx of calcium. The influx of calcium then results in release of acetylcholine from the presynaptic terminal. Acetylcholine is packed and released in discrete amounts known as quanta. Acetylcholine quanta then diffuse across the synaptic cleft and bind to acetylcholine receptors in the postsynaptic membrane, resulting in an endplate potential. Normally, the endplate potential is well above threshold and causes the generation of a muscle action potential. With slow repetitive stimulation (2 to 3 Hz), the number of quanta is greatly depleted during the first several seconds, and, subsequently, fewer are released. The corresponding endplate potential falls in amplitude, but normally remains above threshold to ensure generation of a muscle action potential with each stimulation (i.e., the normal safety factor of NMJ transmission). In postsynaptic disorders such as MG, the number of quanta released by each stimulus is normal, but the effect of each quantum on its receptor is reduced. The net result is a lower endplate potential and a reduced safety factor of transmission at the NMJ. Thus, with slow repetitive stimulation in postsynaptic disorders, the endplate potential in some fibers may fall below threshold, with a resulting lack of a muscle fiber action potential. Clinically this manifests as signs and symptoms of weakness and fatigability, with a corresponding decrement during slow RNS.

TREATMENT

The treatment of patients with MG has improved substantially. Many options are available. Treatment consists of symptomatic agents (acetylcholinesterase inhibitors), immunosuppressives (steroids, azathioprine, cyclosporine), plasma exchange, intravenous immunoglobulin, and thymectomy.

Acetylcholinesterase Inhibitors

Symptomatic treatment consists primarily of giving acetylcholinesterase inhibitors, such as pyridostigmine (Mestinon). These agents slow the degradation of acetylcholine in the synaptic cleft and effectively increase the amount of neurotransmitter available at the postsynaptic junction. Mestinon has a short half-life and must be dosed every 4 to 6 hours. The optimal dose will vary widely between patients. Patients are typically begun on half a tablet (30 mg) of Mestinon every 6 hours and slowly titrated to a higher dose or more frequent dosing interval. There is no correct dosage. Some patients improve substantially on 3 to 4 tablets a day; others require far more. The major side effects are those of cholinergic excess, especially abdominal cramping and diarrhea, excessive perspiration, and salivation. Of course, excessive amounts can also cause weakness (cholinergic crisis). Most patients with MG will respond well, at least initially, to these meditations. Restricted ocular MG tends to be more refractory than generalized disease. For patients who have difficulty upon awakening in the morning, a slow release form (Mestinon Timespan) is available as a 180-mg dose to be taken at bedtime.

Immunosuppressives

Although acetylcholinesterase inhibitors are effective in most patients, the response is generally not completely satisfactory and most patients have a better long-term response by attacking the primary pathophysiology of the disease, the immune mechanism. This consists of immunomodulating treatments, such as steroids, other immunosuppressives, intravenous immunoglobulin, plasma exchange, and thymectomy.

Steroids are the mainstay of therapy in MG. Improvement, including remission, can usually be obtained with oral steroids. The typical dose of prednisone is 1 mg/kg/day taken as a single dose in the morning. Patients are often started on a low dose (10 to 20 mg qd) while under close supervision, or in the hospital because steroids, especially in high doses, may cause transient worsening of myasthenia during the first 2 to 3 weeks. The dose is slowly titrated up by 5 mg/day every 3 to 7 days until clinical benefit is obtained or a dose of 1 mg/kg is obtained. Improvement often begins in 1 or 2 months with maximal im-

provement occurring at 6 to 12 months. After remission, patients can be switched to alternate-day steroids with the same total dose, and then slowly tapered. The chance of a successful taper is improved when the steroid dose on the "on day" is tapered no faster than 5 mg/day/month. When the dose reaches 40 to 50 mg every other day, tapering is best slowed to 2.5 mg/day/month. Often patients will relapse several months after a successful taper and subsequent discontinuance. Many patients require the chronic administration of a low dose of steroids every other day to sustain a remission. The goal is to determine the lowest dose of every-other-day therapy that will prevent a relapse. Unfortunately, when patients relapse, they often require a higher dose of steroids dosed daily in order to go back into remission, which must then be followed by another long, slow, tapering process.

Many patients, especially the elderly, cannot tolerate the side effects of steroids (hypertension, weight gain, glucose intolerance, osteoporosis, cataracts, ulcers, etc.) and may require other types of immunosuppression. Azathioprine (AZA, Imuran) has gained wide acceptance in the treatment of myasthenia, and in many patients is now the drug of choice. The concomitant use of AZA therapy commonly allows steroids to be tapered or discontinued. Clinical improvement is commonly delayed for 2 to 3 months, but may not reach maximal benefit until the first year or two. Patients are typically started on 50 mg qd as a single morning dose and slowly increased to 2 to 3 mg/kg/day over the following several weeks. However, adverse reactions may occur with AZA. The most common is hematologic (anemia, leukopenia, thrombocytopenia) which require close monitoring of blood counts during therapy (every 1 to 2 weeks initially). A typical hematologic endpoint is to let the white blood cell (WBC) count drop to 3,500 to 4,000/mm^3 or the absolute lymphocyte count to drop to 5 to 10 percent. In addition, gastrointestinal disturbance elevation of liver enzymes (2 to 3 times normal), and susceptibility to serious infections may occur. Most of these complications can be dealt with by reducing the dose (hematologic and liver enzyme abnormalities) or dividing the dose with meals (gastrointestinal disturbance). Rarely, patients develop an acute, toxic hypersensitivity reaction to AZA with fever, abdominal pain, and rash, which requires prompt and permanent discontinuance of the drug. Also of concern is the slight increased risk of malignancy, especially lymphoma, which has been reported in nonmyasthenic patients treated with AZA.

Cyclosporin A (CSA), a drug that inhibits interleukin-2 and subsequently blocks cytotoxic lymphocytes and the proliferation of T-helper cells, is effective in preventing rejection in organ transplantation. This drug has also been found effective in several small studies of patients with MG. A typical induction dose is 5 mg/kg given as a divided dose in the morning and evening. After remission, the dose may be gradually reduced to a maintenance dose of 2 to 3 mg/kg. As with the other immunosuppressives, the goal is to determine the lowest dose that prevents a clinical relapse. Trough CSA levels need to be closely followed to maintain a level in the 100 to 200 ng/ml range. Blood pressure and renal function must be carefully followed. In regard to side effects, CSA is superior to other immunosuppressives in not suppressing the bone marrow. The major risks involve nephrotoxicity and hypertension. In addition, there are many potential drug interactions, most importantly, the high likelihood of nephrotoxicity with the concurrent use of nonsteroidal anti-inflammatory drugs (NSAIDs).

Prednisone, AZA, and CSA are first-line therapies in the

treatment of MG. The choice among the three is primarily based on the experience of the treating physician, with special emphasis on the side-effect profile for the individual patient. Each of these agents has potential serious side effects. Obviously, they should never be used in any patient unless adequate compliance and follow-up are possible. The major errors in using these agents are in prescribing a dose that is too low, for a duration that is too short, or nonaggressive treatment of side effects.

Plasma Exchange

Removal of antibody allows clinical recovery in patients with MG. Often 3 to 5 large-volume plasma exchanges are required to sufficiently reduce the antibody level. Plasma exchange is most appropriately performed when a patient has suddenly deteriorated and is in crisis, or before major surgery such as thymectomy. It is in this situation, when rapid reversal of clinical weakness is required, that plasma exchange is most useful in minimizing further worsening or serious complications, such as intubation or pneumonia. However, as routine treatment for MG, plasma exchange is invasive and only temporary, and is best reserved for those unusual patients who do not respond to other immunomodulating therapy.

Intravenous Immunoglobulin

Recently, intravenous immunoglobulin has been used successfully in a variety of autoimmune diseases. At present, the experience in patients with MG is small, although some patients have responded well. Intravenous immunoglobulin has the advantage of far fewer potential side effects than prednisone and the other immunosuppressives. Like plasma exchange, it may be most useful when a patient with MG has suddenly deteriorated and rapid reversal of the weakness is important. Typically, patients in this situation receive a dose of 400 mg/kg/day for 5 days.

Thymectomy

Using the above approach, most patients are successfully treated. The disease can be controlled in most patients, and it is now rare for patients to die of their illness. The disease tends to be lifelong, and patients usually require prolonged therapy. Spontaneous remissions can occur, but relapses often occur again in the future.

Although there has never been a prospective trial, thymectomy may lead to a complete remission or substantial improvement in 70 to 75 percent of patients. Clinical improvement commonly is delayed 6 to 12 months after the operation and may continue for 5 years or more. Patients with milder disease and relatively recent onset of symptoms (less than 3 years), without thymoma, tend to respond best with thymectomy. Young patients with early myasthenia tend to do particularly well (95 percent improvement or complete remission in one series). The surgical technique (transcervical vs transsternal) has been debated by many clinicians. Most agree that, for thymectomy to be effective, the entire thymus gland must be removed, which usually necessitates a transsternal incision. In the modern era, the morbidity and mortality associated with thymectomy has been dramatically reduced, making routine use of this therapy much more attractive. Unless the myasthenia is in complete pharmacologic remission prior to surgery, patients should routinely undergo several days of plasma exchange before thymectomy to reduce the likely worsening as a consequence of the stress of surgery, and to promote early postoperative extubation.

In addition, patients who relapse years after thymectomy, or who never obtained a complete remission from their initial thymectomy, may benefit from repeat thymectomy, even if imaging studies do not demonstrate residual thymus tissue. As 20 percent of normal individuals have some ectopic thymus tissue in the anterior mediastinum, some surgeons have advocated the use of extended thymectomy, removing all thymic, fat, and lymphatic tissue from the anterior mediastinum. In one study, five of six patients with chronic refractory myasthenia improved with repeat thymectomy using this technique.

The other indication for thymectomy, of course, is the presence of a thymoma. The myasthenia of patients with thymoma tends to be more severe, compared to other myasthenic patients, and often require the combination of surgery and aggressive medical therapy.

Restricted Ocular Myasthenia

Patients with restricted ocular myasthenia represent a therapeutic challenge, responding as well to immunosuppressive therapy and thymectomy as patients with generalized MG. However, there remains a controversy regarding how aggressively to treat these patients. Patients with ocular myasthenia may be treated very differently among major centers. Some investigators argue that ocular myasthenia is not a serious illness, and the risks of immunosuppression and/or surgery cannot be justified. In these centers, patients with restricted ocular myasthenia are treated with acetylcholinesterase inhibitors and local ophthalmologic therapy, such as eyelid crutches or eye patches. On the other hand, many clinicians would argue that when a patient first presents with myasthenia involving only the extraocular muscles, it is not possible to know if the disease will progress to generalized myasthenia (indeed, most will) and that nearly all treatments are most effective if begun early in the illness. Many patients with restricted ocular myasthenia consider themselves nearly disabled from diplopia alone. These issues need to be discussed with each patient before embarking on a path of aggressive or nonaggressive therapy.

Myasthenic Crisis

Rarely, the initial presentation of MG may be a myasthenic crisis. Crisis, of course, may also occur in patients with known myasthenia. Recognition and treatment of myasthenic crisis is one of the most important neuromuscular emergencies. In the 1960s, the mortality rate of myasthenic crisis was 50 percent. Now with modern intensive care units, early diagnosis, and effective theraphy, mortality from crisis is a rare event.

Patients with moderate to severe MG may develop increasing bulbar and respiratory weakness. Often, this is the result of a concurrent infection, or the addition of a new medicine. Several drugs are well known to exacerbate MG:

Aminoglycosides
Clindamycin
Colistin
Erythromycin
Lithium
Phenytoin

Polymyxin B
Procainamide
Propranolol and other β-blockers
Quinine
Quinidine
Tetracycline
Verapamil and other Ca^{2+} channel blockers

In response to worsening weakness, patients take more and more anticholinesterase medicines. Excessive anticholinesterase treatment can itself lead to increased weakness (cholinergic crisis). If not recognized early, the patient may succumb to primary respiratory collapse or aspirate from increasing bulbar weakness.

Patients in crisis, whether cholinergic or myasthenic, must be managed aggressively. Any myasthenic patient who reports sudden worsening of symptoms must be evaluated immediately. Although the literature stresses the difference between myasthenic crisis and cholinergic crisis, it is frequently impossible to tell them apart. Miosis, fasciculations, diarrhea, sweating, abdominal cramping, excessive salivation, and bradycardia all suggest cholinergic overdosage. Many clinicians will use a Tensilon test to try to distinguish between the two. However, it is frequently difficult to assess improvement in a patient who is in severe distress.

The treatment of myasthenic crisis is straightforward:

1. Admit to intensive care unit.
2. Stop all anticholinesterases.
3. Rule out and treat concurrent infection.
4. Identify and correct any electrolyte abnormality.
5. Follow respiratory status closely and intubate if vital capacity is falling and reaches 15 ml/kg, or higher, if patient is at risk of aspiration.
6. Administer plasma exchange (5 to 6 times every 2 weeks).

The major risk to life is respiratory failure. Patients should be watched carefully and intubated early to avoid later pulmonary complications. Anticholinesterases should be stopped. They can be restarted in a few days, and likely can be used at lower dosages. Plasma exchange in myasthenic crisis is very useful in lowering antibody titers and rapidly reversing weakness. If a patient had not previously been on steroids or other immunosuppressants, and no electrolyte imbalance or infection is discovered to explain the decompensation, then these will likely need to be used to prevent further crisis. It is then reasonable to begin prednisone in the hospital while the patient is intubated and receiving plasma exchange.

SUGGESTED READINGS

Brooke MH: A clinician's view of neuromuscular diseases. Williams & Wilkins, Baltimore, 1986

Drachman DB: Present and future treatment of myasthenia gravis. N Engl J Med 316:743–745, 1987

Drachman DB: Myasthenia gravis. N Engl J Med 390:1791–1810, 1994

Engel AG: Myasthenia gravis and myasthenic syndromes. Ann Neurol 16: 519–534, 1984

Hankins JR, Mayer RF, Satterfield JR et al: Thymectomy for myasthenia gravis: 14-year experience. Ann Surg 201:618–625, 1985

Lanska DJ: Indications for thymectomy in myasthenia gravis. Neurology 40: 1828–1829, 1990

Miano MA, Bosley TM, Heiman-Patterson TD et al: Factors influencing outcome of prednisone dose reduction in myasthenia gravis. Neurology 41: 919–921, 1991

Miller RG, Filler KA, Kiprov D, Roan R: Repeat thymectomy in chronic refractory myasthenia gravis. Neurology 41:923–924, 1991

Papatestas AE, Genkins G, Kornfeld P et al: Effects of thymectomy in myasthenia gravis. Ann Surg 206:79–88, 1987

Tindall RSA, Rollins JA, Phillips JT et al: Preliminary results of a double-blind, randomized, placebo-controlled trial of cyclosporine in myasthenia gravis. N Engl J Med 316:719–724, 1987

104. LAMBERT-EATON MYASTHENIC SYNDROME

H. ROYDEN JONES, JR.

CLASSIFICATION

The Lambert-Eaton myasthenic syndrome (LEMS) is the most prominent example of a presynaptic defect of neuromuscular transmission to occur in adults. LEMS was first defined as a paraneoplastic syndrome, usually associated with smokers who have small cell lung cancer (SCLC), but it may rarely occur with other malignancies. If no neoplasm is identified within 4 years, a paraneoplastic cause is less likely, especially with a nonsmoker. LEMS has an autoimmune basis that is not necessarily associated with a malignancy. The primary autoimmune, nonparaneoplastic form of LEMS now occurs with about equal frequency. An association with other autoimmune processes including vitiligo, thyroid disorders, rheumatoid arthritis, and pernicious anemia is noted in 34 percent of LEMS patients. LEMS occurs infrequently, perhaps at 10 percent the frequency of myasthenia gravis. It most commonly presents after age 40, although the primary autoimmune form of LEMS may occur in younger adults or, very rarely, in children. The youngest reported case had initial symptoms at age 1 but was not diagnosed until age 7. Recent studies demonstrate no particular sexual predominance. Most patients with LEMS are symptomatic less than a year; however, diagnostic recognition has been delayed 8 to 25 years after initial symptoms.

The neurophysiologic and immunologic characteristics of LEMS typify a presynaptic lesion of the neuromuscular junction. This is a mirror image of the more common postsynaptic defect, myasthenia gravis. Repetitive motor nerve stimulation (RMNS) at 2 to 3 Hz may produce a decremental response in both LEMS and myasthenia gravis. The facilitation of the typical low-amplitude compound muscle action potential, to brief voluntary exercise is characteristic of LEMS and provides the basis for electromyographic (EMG) diagnosis. Physiologic and immunologic investigations have identified that the primary site of immunopathology involves the voltage-gated calcium channels (VGCC). An immunoglobulin G (IgG) antibody adheres to the peripheral cholinergic nerve terminals blocking the calcium influx that normally occurs with nerve depolarization. This results in an inadequate release of acetylcholine quanta from motor and autonomic cholinergic nerve terminals. The VGCC present in the membrane of SCLC provides the presumed antigenic stimulus for antibody production in the paraneoplastic form of LEMS. The precise antigenic stimulus in the nonparaneoplastic varieties of LEMS remains to be identified.

CLINICAL DIAGNOSIS

The diagnosis of LEMS can often be suspected on clinical grounds. The patient's presentation is similar with either the primary autoimmune or secondary paraneoplastic form of LEMS. Ideally the electromyographic (EMG) and antibody results serve as confirmation of the initial diagnosis. Patients with LEMS characteristically present with weakness, vague numbness in the thighs, and various signs of autonomic dysfunction including dry mouth and impotence. However, LEMS is well known to have protean clinical manifestations, which may mimic myasthenia gravis, polymyositis, multiple sclerosis, occult malignancies, or functional disorders, including hysteria. LEMS may be associated with other paraneoplastic disorders, including cerebellar ataxia or primary sensory neuropathy; 23 of 50 LEMS patients seen at Queen Square (U.K.) and 14 of 17 seen by me at the Lahey Clinic were referred with another diagnosis.

The muscle weakness of LEMS mimics most myopathies with a typical proximal preponderance characterized by difficulties arising, walking, or climbing stairs. Although the proximal arm and neck muscles are often weak on examination, this is rarely noted by patients. Fatigue is a prominent symptom; it may be the initial manifestation of LEMS. At times initial neurologic examination may suggest that such individuals do not have true weakness, because of presumed inconsistency. The facilitative component of their weakness is mistaken for "give way" weakness typical of nonorganic processes leading to an initial consideration of psychological mechanisms (as noted in 3 of 17 LEMS patients seen here). Bulbar symptoms are less prominent than with myasthenia gravis: however, their presence should not exclude LEMS from diagnostic consideration, especially noting that 14 of our 17 patients had some form of bulbar difficulty; ptosis was noted in 54 percent and facial weakness in 16 percent of another LEMS study. With sustained upgaze, a paradoxical lid elevation may occur secondary to facilitation in LEMS. This contrasts with myasthenia gravis where this maneuver evokes increased ptosis. Occasionally muscle stiffness or tightness are prominent LEMS symptoms.

A pseudoataxia may occur secondary to paraspinal and very proximal leg girdle muscle weakness. Some patients with LEMS have a true gait ataxia secondary to a concomitant paraneoplastic cerebellar degeneration. In two patients, this led to an initial diagnosis of multiple sclerosis. Rarely, a primary sensory neuropathy presenting with stocking numbness may be the initial symptom of LEMS. An ataxia or neuropathy, in a patient with concomitant proximal limb weakness, should suggest a possible diagnosis of LEMS.

Autonomic symptoms, such as dryness of the mouth or in men a lack of penile erection, may provide important clues leading to a clinical diagnosis of LEMS; patients often need to be directly questioned to gain this information. Other patients may report a feeling of vague numbness, especially prominent in the thighs. The combination of vague weakness, dry mouth, and paresthesias at times has mimicked hyperventilation.

When patients with suspected LEMS do not have detectable weakness on neurologic examination, subtle weakness may be enhanced by watching the person arise from a chair or climb stairs. Deep tendon reflexes are typically absent or depressed; however, 4 of our 17 patients had normally active DTRs. In 78 percent of patients who have either areflexia or sluggish deep tendon reflexes, the characteristic postexercise facilitation, also found with muscle weakness, was demonstrated. Sluggish pupillary light responses, a sign of autonomic dysfunction, were noted in 12 percent of patients with LEMS.

DIFFERENTIAL DIAGNOSIS

Early in its course the diagnosis of LEMS can be elusive. Of our 17 patients, 14 had an "atypical" clinical presentation or an imprecise EMG performance, which led to erroneous impressions at the previous initial neurologic evaluations. Preceding diagnoses had included MG in 5 patients, myopathy in 5, depression in 2, functional or hysteria in 1, cerebellar degeneration or multiple sclerosis in 2, peripheral neuropathy in 1, and occult malignancy in 1.

The major clinical difference between MG and LEMS relates to the preponderance of bulbar symptoms at the onset with MG. Cranial nerve symptoms occur with LEMS, are usually mild, sometimes transient, and not the presenting symptom. Additionally, MG lacks the autonomic symptoms found with LEMS. Uncommonly, LEMS and MG may occur in the same patient confirmed by the presence of VGCC and acetylcholine receptor antibodies. Other rare presynaptic NMTDs (e.g., botulism and magnesium intoxication) present acutely. Only rarely do LEMS patients have sudden clinical onset.

Although proximal and neck weakness are common to both LEMS and inflammatory myositis, deep tendon reflexes are preserved with inflammatory myositis, and these patients lack the autonomic and vague sensory symptoms found in LEMS. In the young adult, metabolic myopathies, such as McArdle's disease, should be considered, noting the presence of muscle tightness, stiffness, and pain in 36 percent of patients with LEMS. These patients do not have myoglobinuria. Both inflammatory myositis and metabolic myopathies have elevated levels of serum creatine kinase, which is uncommon with LEMS, and, if present, is very modest.

Chronic inflammatory demyelinating polyneuropathy (CIDP), with its insidious onset of proximal weakness and areflexia, also enters the LEMS differential diagnosis. No clinical evidence of facilitation of muscle strength or deep tendon reflexes is found with CIDP. Rarely, a patient with LEMS presents with distal paresthesias and has a concomitant paraneoplastic primary sensory neuropathy. An ataxic gait may at first suggest multiple sclerosis or another coexistent paraneoplastic process of cerebellar degeneration.

The diagnosis of LEMS also needs to be considered in any person considered to be depressed, hysterical, or possibly malingering, who presents with vague weakness, paresthesias, or (male) sexual dysfunction. At times, about other characteristic symptoms or observing for subtle signs of proximal weakness or facilitation of strength or reflexes, may provide the initial clues to the correct diagnosis. This will alert the electromyographer to carefully test for LEMS.

DIAGNOSTIC TESTS

Tensilon Testing

Because the clinical presentation of some patients with LEMS may have many similarities to MG, some patients may require Tensilon (edrophonium hydrochloride) testing. The Tensilon test was positive "subjectively or objectively" in 14 of 21 patients with LEMS in one study. It cannot be utilized as a means to differentiate MG from LEMS.

Electromyography

Although LEMS can be clinically suspected, EMG provides the diagnostic standard for this illness. Because neuromuscular transmission defects can be demonstrated by RMNS in many motor unit disorders, it is necessary to perform standard motor and sensory nerve conduction studies with needle electromyography to exclude other lesions between the anterior horn cell and the muscle. Typically motor nerve stimulation demonstrates very diminished CMAPs in LEMS, often no more than 10 percent of normal. One must be aware with early LEMS the compound muscle action potentials may be normal as noted in 2 of 50 patients. Sensory nerve action potentials (SNAPs) are normal except when there is a concomitant primary sensory neuropathy when SNAPs are absent or of very low amplitude.

The key to the neurophysiologic diagnosis of LEMS is the facilitation defined by RMNS. Initially, at rest, RMNS demonstrates a significant NMTD, averaging a 27 percent decrement, with 2 to 3 Hz stimulation. In contrast to MG, wherein documentation of a decrement may require testing of multiple nerves, particularly proximal or bulbar, the NMTD in LEMS patients is usually present in all motor nerves tested. The crucial differentiation between a pre- and postsynaptic NMTD is the finding that high-frequency (20 to 50 Hz) RMNS or brief voluntary exercise will prompt a marked facilitation in patients with LEMS but not those with MG. High-frequency RMNS is painful and prone to movement artifact. Therefore testing for postexercise facilitation is preferred. In order to make an EMG diagnosis of LEMS, a postexercise facilitation greater than 100 percent, that is, twice the baseline, is necessary. Usually patients with LEMS will have a 400 to 1,000 percent compound muscle action potential facilitation (Fig. 104-1) except early in the illness when it is still near normal. It is very important for the electromyographer to have the suspected LEMS patient exercise for only 10 and absolutely no more than 15 seconds to achieve maximal postexercise facilitation and prevent its being masked. A previous improperly performed EMG may have contributed to failure to detect postexercise facilitation in three patients who were exercised too long (i.e., 30 to 60 seconds) at another EMG laboratory. The shorter period of exercise proved to be critical for our diagnosis of LEMS. Clinical examination and RMNS in 29 patients with SCLC and no symptoms of LEMS, did not detect subclinical cases.

Conventional needle EMG in LEMS patients demonstrates an increased number of low-amplitude, short duration motor unit potentials as seen with other myopathies. Their amplitude may enlarge with sustained contraction.

Antibody Tests

The development of VGCC antibody tests provides a means to confirm the clinical impression in both the paraneoplastic and the primary autoimmune forms of LEMS. These antibodies are present in 20 to 40 percent of SCLC patients who do not have LEMS. Thus, a positive VGCC antibody test per se does not diagnose LEMS. One needs the typical clinical and EMG findings for this diagnosis.

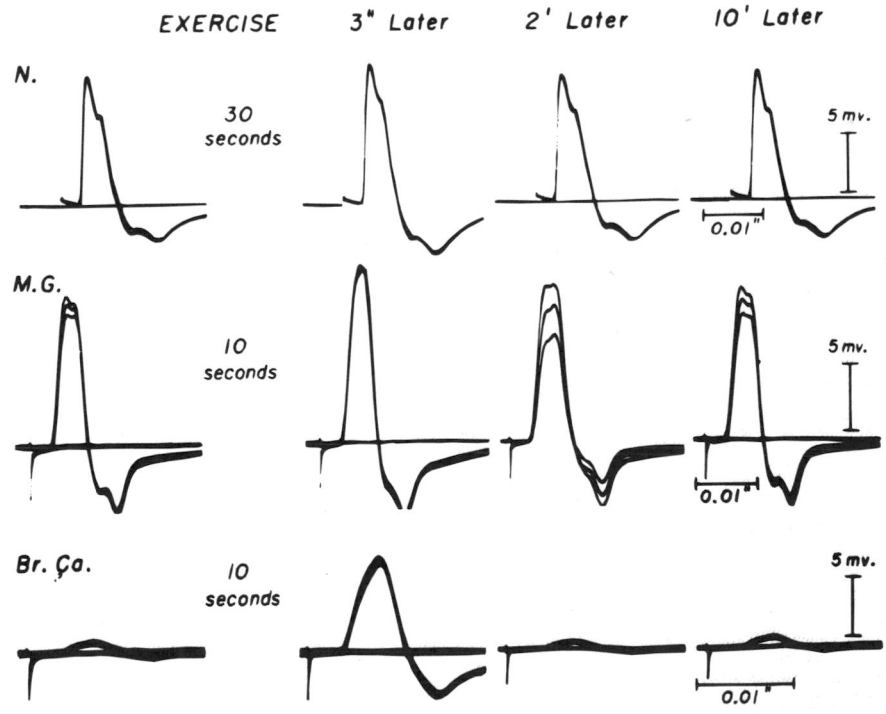

FIG. 104-1. Effects of exercise on the compound muscle action potential (CMAP) of the hypothenar muscles evoked by maximal stimulation of the ulnar nerve at the wrist. The response of the rested muscle as recorded on the left is compared with responses at 3 seconds, 2 minutes, and 10 minutes after the end of a maximal voluntary contraction of this muscle for 10 to 15 seconds. Each record consists of superimposed CMAPs evoked at a rate of 3 Hz *N*, normal patient; *MG*, patient with generalized myasthenia gravis, *Br. Ca*, LEMS patient with small cell lung cancer. The important finding in LEMS is the low-amplitude CMAP and the marked facilitation after brief voluntary exercise with an associated neuromuscular transmission defect. (From Rooke ED, Eaton LM, Lambert EH, Hodgson CH: Myasthenia and malignant intrathoracic tumor. Med Clin North Am 44:972, 1960 with permission.)

Chest Radiographs, Computed Tomography, and Magnetic Resonance Imaging

Only 3 of our 17 patients had abnormal chest radiographs prior to diagnosis of LEMS: two with SCLC and the other with a lymphoma. The LEMS-type EMG findings led to a chest radiograph, which demonstrated a perihilar mass in two others; biopsy diagnosed SCLC. By contrast, in 12 other patients, the chest radiograph was normal (11 patients) or not diagnostic (1 patient); computed tomography (CT) scan later diagnosed SCLC in 4 of 7 in this group. When LEMS is diagnosed and the initial chest radiograph is normal, chest CT or magnetic resonance imaging (MRI) needs to be performed. In some, this study will lead to the diagnosis of SCLC. However, when the CT scan is negative, pulmonary cytologic studies, including sputum analysis and bronchial washings, are also occasionally of value for the diagnosis of occult lung tumors in some LEMS cases. Repeat chest CT scan and MRI, in LEMS patients without documented SCLC, particularly middle-aged smokers, needs to be performed intermittently—possibly every 3 to 6 months—for at least 4 years after the initial LEMS diagnosis.

THERAPY

Two therapeutic modalities are utilized for LEMS, one directed to symptomatic improvement of neuromuscular transmission and the other for modifying the autoimmune process. Historically, guanidine, a drug that enhances ACh release from motor nerve terminals, was used effectively; however, its inherent renal and hematologic toxicity halted its use except in rare instances when all other therapies have failed. Another drug, 3,4-diaminopyridine (3,4-DAP), which also promotes acetylcholine release, by prolonging the VGCC time, is available for LEMS treatment in Europe, but only on a research basis in the United States. This medication has provided significant clinical and neurophysiologic improvement in patients with LEMS; it is equally effective in the patient with SCLC as with the idiopathic autoimmune form. Dosage is variable, starting at 5 mg tid to a maximum of 25 mg qid. Caution is advised using 3,4-DAP because its side effects include central nervous system irritability, usually manifested by seizures, which may occur with low doses, although more likely above 80 mg/day.

The anticholinesterase medication pyridostigmine (Mestinon), also improves neuromuscular transmission. However, it is not as effective in presynaptic disorders, such as LEMS, as with MG. It has been suggested that when 3,4-DAP is widely available—at times combined with Mestinon—it will be the first line of LEMS therapy, providing there is no history of seizures. Mestinon and 3,4-DAP provide only symptomatic therapy and do not address the autoimmune mechanisms responsible for both paraneoplastic and primary autoimmune LEMS.

Of the various forms of immunomodulation, prednisone is the drug of choice. In general, a dose of 40 to 100 mg/day is given until improvement begins, which may require a few months before switching to an alternate-day dosage decreasing by 10 to 20 mg every 10 to 15 days until a schedule of 40/10 to 80/20 mg is achieved. Then the high dose is gradually decreased to a maintenance level of 10/0 to 30/15 mg/day. Other clinicians suggest starting with the alternate-day schedule of prednisone at a dose of 1.0 to 1.5 mg/kg every other day. Azathioprine, starting with 50 mg daily and gradually increasing to 2.0 to 2.5 mg/kg daily, has also been suggested if prednisone alone is not effective.

Other forms of immunotherapy for LEMS have included plasmapheresis, which produces a temporary and often less effective result than with myasthenia gravis. Intravenous immunoglobulin IV Ig therapy for LEMS, with or without SCLC, has been limited to date. With an intravenous IV Ig dosage of 400 g/kg/day for 5 days, or 1 g/kg on two consecutive days, the four patients treated had return of strength beginning 2 to 3 days after infusion; the improvement lasted 3 or more weeks, and relapses were controlled by repeat courses.

Some researchers caution that immunomodulation therapy of LEMS may enhance the potential for previously unrecognized SCLC to become clinically manifest sooner than if host defenses were not compromised. This is an interesting thought, and if 3,4-DAP becomes available for general use and is proven to provide good symptomatic control, this hypothesis can be more widely tested.

Chemotherapy was the primary treatment modality in five SCLC patients found to have a tumor after their LEMS diagnosis. One patient also had a pneumonectomy. He did very well with the chemotherapy with resolution of the LEMS and no sign of the lung tumor for 6 years. However, he then was found to have SCLC in the opposite lung and died a few months later. One patient's illness has been stable for 1 year. Another patient treated primarily with chemotherapy died in a few months, and the other two SCLC patients with LEMS and similarly treated were lost to follow-up. Another person initially treated with prednisone had chemotherapy added when chest CT finally became positive 1 year after LEMS diagnosis, He died 6 months later.

Contraindicated Medications in LEMS

It is important to note that certain common medications have the propensity to exacerbate LEMS symptoms. Cardiac drugs, including β-adrenergic and calcium channel blocking agents and the antiarrhythmic agents procainamide, and quinidine also require cautious use in LEMS. The aminoglycoside antibiotics, quinine, and magnesium citrate cathartics may also potentiate the LEMS neuromuscular transmission defect by increasing weakness. Anesthesiologists need to be aware of a LEMS diagnosis, as it is important they select medications that will not prolong postoperative respiratory depression. On rare occasions, this may be the initial manifestation of LEMS.

PROGNOSIS/FOLLOW-UP

In a study conducted by J. H. O'Neill and colleagues, within 32 months of tumor diagnosis 18 of 23 patients with LEMS and SCLC died with a median survival of 8.5 months. There were five survivors; three had remission of LEMS with no detectable tumor from 2.9 to 4.2 years. In contrast, the prognosis in patients with LEMS but without SCLC was excellent in 21 patients, with a median follow-up of 6.9 years. Among our 17 patients with LEMS, 9 were found to have SCLC; 4 died at 2 and 3 months, 1.5 years, and 6 years after the initial diagnosis of LEMS. Two are now receiving 3,4-DAP and are stable. The remaining four with SCLC were lost to follow-up. Eight of our 17 patients have not developed SCLC. One died in 3 months, and autopsy failed to demonstrate a malignancy despite positive VGCC and anti-Hu antibodies. Another patient with LEMS, lymphoma, and cerebellar ataxia initially improved, but later worsened. The other cerebellar ataxia patient was improved 2 years after LEMS diagnosis. One patient initially believed to have myasthenia gravis has done very well on 3,4-DAP. She later developed both breast and ovarian carcinoma. Another patient with LEMS but not SCLC, initially diagnosed here 15 years ago, is doing very well now off prednisone. Three of our non-SCLC patients with LEMS have been lost to follow-up.

CONCLUSION

The early clinical signs of LEMS may mimic a number of neurologic syndromes, including MG, polymyositis, and multiple sclerosis. Evidence of muscle weakness may not always be present early on; one has to take care to not attribute reports of recent onset fatigue or muscle tightness to psychological mechanisms such as depression or hysteria. Bulbar symptoms suggesting MG or brainstem stroke may also be present. At times LEMS patients may have a positive Tensilon test, but the acetylcholine receptor antibodies are usually negative. Some patients with LEMS may have symptoms mimicking other paraneoplastic syndromes, including cerebellar ataxia and primary sensory neuropathy. A complete EMG, including search for an NMTD and postexercise facilitation within 10 to 15 seconds of maximal voluntary exercise, is essential for the appropriate differential diagnosis. A SCLC is found in 50 percent of patients with LEMS; these have a generally poor prognosis in contrast to those with the more benign idiopathic primary autoimmune form.

SUGGESTED READINGS

Bird SJ: Clinical and electrophysiologic improvement in Lambert-Eaton syndrome with intravenous immunoglobulin therapy. Neurology 42: 1422–1423, 1992

Blumenfeld AM, Recht LD, Chad DA et al: Coexistence of Lambert-Eaton myasthenic syndrome and subacute cerebellar degeneration: differential effects of treatment. Neurology 41:1682–1685, 1991

Breen LA, Gutmann L, Brick JF, Riggs JR: Paradoxical lid elevation with sustained upgaze: a sign of Lambert-Eaton syndrome. Muscle Nerve 14: 863–866, 1991

Brown JC, Johns RJ: Diagnostic difficulty encountered in the myasthenic syndrome sometimes associated with carcinoma. J Neurol Neurosurg Psychol 37:1214–1224, 1974

Gutmann L, Phillips LH, Gutmann L: Trends in the association of Lambert-Eaton myasthenic syndrome with carcinoma. Neurology 42:848–850, 1992

Howard JF, Sanders DB, Massey JM: The electrodiagnosis of myasthenia gravis and the Lambert-Eaton syndrome. Neurol Clin North Am 12:305–330, 1994

Jones HR: Lambert-Eaton myasthenic syndrome: enigmas in early clinical and electromyographic diagnosis: review of 12 cases. The New York Academy of Sciences, Myasthenia Gravis and Related Disorders: Experimental and Clinical Aspects. PIII-45; Washington, DC, April 12–15, 1992

Lambert EH, Eaton LM, Rooke ED: Defect of Neuromuscular conduction associated with malignant neoplasms. Am J Physiol 187:612–613, 1956

Lundh H, Nilsson O, Rosen I: Current therapy of the Lambert-Eaton myasthenic syndrome. Prog Brain Res 84:163–170, 1990

Lundh H, Nilsson O, Rosen I, Johansson S: Practical aspects of 3,4-diaminopyridine treatment of Lambert Eaton myasthenic syndrome. Acta Neurol Scand 88:136–140, 1993

McEvoy K: Diagnosis and treatment of Lambert Eaton myasthenic syndrome. Neurol Clin North Am 12:387–399, 1994

Newsome-Davis J, Leys K, Vincent A et al: Immunological evidence for the co-existence of the Lambert-Eaton myasthenic syndrome and myasthenia gravis in two patients. J Neurol Neurosurg Psych 1991,:452–453.

O'Neil JH, Murray NMF, Newsom-Davis J: The Lambert Eaton myasthenic syndrome: a review of 50 cases. Brain 111:577–596, 1988

Rooke ED, Eaton LM, Lambert EH, Hodgson CH: Myasthenia and malignant intrathoracic tumor. Med Clin North Am 44:977–988, 1960

Sanders DB, Howard JF: High dose intravenous immunoglobulin treatment in Lambert-Eaton myasthenic syndrome. The New York Academy of Sciences. Myasthenia Gravis and Related Disorders: Experimental and Clinical Aspects; PIII-44, Washington, D.C., April 12–15, 1992

Streib E: Adverse effects of magnesium salt cathartics in a patient with the myasthenic syndrome (Lambert-Eaton syndrome). Ann Neurol 2: 175–176, 1977

Ueno S, Hara Y: Lambert-Eaton myasthenic syndrome without calcium channel antibody: adverse effect of calcium antagonist diltiazem. J Neurol Neurosurg Psychiatry 55:409–410, 1992

105. TOXIC AND METABOLIC DISORDERS OF THE NEUROMUSCULAR JUNCTION

JACKSON PICKETT

There are many toxic and metabolic disorders of neuromuscular transmission. This chapter focuses on some of the more common disorders seen in the United States.

BOTULISM

There are four types of botulism (Table 105-1); all are rare. The four forms of botulism have similar signs and symptoms but vary in the source of the toxin. The toxin acts by binding to autonomic and motor nerve terminals. After being taken up by nerve terminals, the toxin reduces the number of quanta of acetylcholine released by a nerve stimulus. Recovery from the toxin involves sprouting of nerve terminals which form new synapses. This process can take months.

Infant Botulism

Clinical Features. The most common form of botulism is infant botulism. Most of the cases occur in the United States, but are also seen in Canada, South America, Australia, and Europe. Over 90 percent of the affected infants are less than 6 months of age; the remaining 10 percent are under 1 year of age. The sexes are equally involved. The spectrum of infant botulism (Table 105-2) varies from the sudden infant death

TABLE 105-1. The Number of Cases of Botulism Reported in the United States Each Year

Type	No. of Cases/Year
Infant botulism	50
Foodborne botulism	15–25
Undetermined source	7
Wound botulism	1

TABLE 105-2. Spectrum of Infant Botulism

Asymptomatic carriers of organism in stool
Mild cases
    Constipation
    Feeding difficulties
    Mild weakness
    Failure to thrive
Moderate-to-severe cases
    Hospitalized patients
    Sudden infant death syndrome

TABLE 105-3. Possible Factors in the Development of Infant Botulism

Source of spores
  Geographic location: 50% of the U.S. cases found in California, Pennsylvania, and Utah
  Nature of soil
  Parents who work in soil
  Rural living for infant less than 2 months of age
  Honey or corn syrup consumption
Susceptibility of host
  Age: 1 week to 1 year
  Breastfeeding
  Switch from mild to solid foods
  Less than one bowel movement per day for 2 months

syndrome to an otherwise healthy infant that has a change in stool character. Most of the reported cases have been severe enough to require hospital admission. Epidemiologic studies have identified many factors in the development of infant botulism (Table 105-3). It is assumed that infants consume spores that germinate in the gut, forming organisms that produce toxin. In most of the cases the source of the spores is not found.

The signs and symptoms of infant botulism severe enough to require hospitalization are shown in Table 105-4. Initial symptoms include constipation, poor feeding, weak cry, and a loss of head control. These symptoms last from 5 hours to 1 week before admission. When fully developed, the disorder causes weakness of cranial and limb muscles and abnormalities of the autonomic, mainly parasympathetic, nervous system. Symptoms and signs have usually peaked in 1 to 2 weeks. Recovery starts after 3 to 5 weeks and often takes 1 to 4 months.

The sequence of muscular involvement in infant botulism is as follows:

Autonomic nervous system
Cranial muscles
Proximal limb muscles
Distal limb muscles
Diaphragm

Local production of toxin in the gut may explain why constipation is often the first symptom. Cranial muscle weakness leads to difficulties with feeding and breathing. Breathing difficulties are first caused by weakness of bulbar muscles leading to airway obstruction and later by weakness of respiratory muscles. Proximal limb and neck muscles are often weaker than distal muscles; the diaphragm is involved late in the course of the disease. A symmetrical descending paralysis is typical.

Diagnosis. The combination of an infant who develops constipation, then feeding and respiratory difficulties and later

TABLE 105-4. Signs and Symptoms of Infant Botulism

Site	Sign/Symptom
Autonomic nervous system	Constipation
	Sluggish pupils
	Flushed appearance
	Decreased tearing or salivation
	Bradycardia or tachycardia
	Hypotension or hypertension
	Urinary retention
Cranial nerves	Poor feeding
	Reduced gag or suck reflex
	Facial weakness or ptosis
	Assisted ventilation
	Poor cry
Somatic nerves	Weakness
	Reduced stretch reflexes
	Decreased activity

TABLE 105-5. Differential Diagnosis of Infant Botulism

Infections
  Sepsis
  Meningitis
  Encephalitis
Metabolic
  Abnormalities of cations and glucose
  Disorders of amino acid metabolism
  Hypothyroidism
  Metabolic encephalopathy
  Reye syndrome
  Subacute necrotizing encephalomyelitis (Leigh disease)
Toxins
  Alcohols
  Anticholinergics
  Heavy metals
  Narcotics
  Organophosphates
Neuromuscular
  Congenital myasthenia gravis
  Congenital myopathy
  Diphtheritic neuropathy
  Guillain-Barré syndrome
  Infantile spinal muscular atrophy (Werdnig-Hoffman disease)
  Muscular dystrophy
  Poliomyelitis
  Tick paralysis

weakness of the neck and limbs should suggest the diagnosis of infant botulism. Disorders to consider in the differential are shown in Table 105-5. This differential can be reduced by screening for treatable infectious, metabolic, and toxic disorders; performing an electromyogram and nerve conduction studies; searching for a tick; and sending blood and stool to be analyzed for botulinal toxin and organism. The usual results of the electromyogram and nerve conduction studies are shown in Table 105-6. The conduction studies reveal a small compound muscle action potential that reflects an abnormality of motor unit, or motor neuron and the muscle fibers it innervates. An increment in compound muscle action potential amplitude with rapid repetitive stimulation localizes the disorder to the neuromuscular junction and would favor disorders such as botulism where the number of quanta released by a nerve stimulus is markedly reduced. An increment lasting many minutes may be diagnostic of botulism. Small and short motor unit potentials are as common as an increment but only localize the disorder to the distal nerve terminals, neuromuscular junctions, or muscle fibers. Electrodiagnostic studies usually localize the disorder to the distal part of the motor unit or to the neuromuscular junction.

The diagnosis of infant botulism depends on the demonstration of the organism or toxin in the stool and the absence of toxin in any food. Toxin can be found in the serum in up to 12 percent of cases. In the United States the type A toxin is most common in the west and type B in the east. The organism is usually *Clostridium botulinum,* but *C. butyricum* (type E toxin)

TABLE 105-6. Electrodiagnostic Studies Infant Botulism

EDx Study	Result
Conduction studies	
Motor conduction velocities and latencies	Normal
Compound muscle action potential amplitude	Reduced
Sensory conduction studies	Normal
Rapid repetitive stimulation (>10 Hz)	
Increment	92%
Decrement	47%
Electromyography	
Positive sharp wave and fibrillation potentials	54%
Small and short motor unit potentials	92%

(Data from Cornblath DR, Sladky JT, Sumner AJ: Clinical electrophysiology of infantile botulism. Muscle Nerve 6:448, 1983.)

TABLE 105-7. Treatment of Infant Botulism

Support respiratory
   Monitor for apnea
   Prevent airway obstruction
   May need respirator for months
Maintain nutrition
   May need tube feeding if unable to cough, gag, suck, or swallow
   Feed upright
Urinary retention
   Credé's maneuver
   Treat urinary infections
Of uncertain value
   Antibiotics
   Drugs to increase strength
   Human-derived antitoxin
   Laxatives and enemas

and *C. barati* (type F toxin) have been reported. To identify the toxin, mice are injected with serum or a stool extract, with and without antitoxin, and observed for death due to paralysis. Both toxin and organism can be excreted in the stool for months, even as the infant recovers. Infants can improve before the toxin in the stool peaks.

Management. The treatment of infant botulism in the hospital often involves intubation and mechanical ventilation, tube feedings and Credé's maneuver to empty the bladder (Table 105-7). The hospital course varies from a few days to 6 months; about 5 percent of infants relapse. It is important to anticipate respiratory problems. A respiratory arrest occurs in about 30 percent of infants. All infants with difficulty coughing, gagging, or swallowing should be observed for apnea. Antitoxin has not been used because no toxin was detected in the serum in about 90 percent of cases, and serious allergic reactions occurred when the horse serum was given. The use of a human-derived antitoxin may soon clarify whether antitoxin is effective. If antibiotics are needed, drugs that inhibit neuromuscular transmission, such as aminoglycosides, should be avoided.

With a mean hospital stay of 1 month and 80 percent of hospitalized infants on a respirator, complications of treatment are expected (Table 105-8). Most involve the respiratory system or are due to infections. Despite these problems in management and the presence of severe paralysis, only 2 to 3 percent of infants die, and the rest recover completely.

Foodborne Botulism

Clinical Features. Foodborne botulism differs from infant botulism in that a source of toxin is present and more than one-half the cases occur in outbreaks. Type A toxin is the most

TABLE 105-8. Complications Seen in the Treatment of Infant Botulism

All patients
  Apnea
  Autonomic instability
  Pneumonia
  Sepsis
  Urinary tract infection
Intubated patients
  Plugged endotracheal tube
  Postextubation stridor
  Recurrent atelectasis
  Subglottic stenosis
  Syndrome of inappropriate secretion of antidiuretic hormone
  Tracheal granuloma
  Tacheitis
  Tracheomalacia
  Unintended extubation

TABLE 105-9. Types of Distribution of Foodborne Botulism

Toxin Type	Fraction of Cases	Geographic Sites
A	70%	West of Mississippi
B	20%	East of Mississippi
C	10%	Alaska and Great Lakes

common (Table 105-9) and U.S. western states report more cases of botulism. The usual source of types A and B toxin is home-canned food; marine life is the typical source of type E toxin. Most patients with botulism are older than 10 years, and the median age is 30 to 40 years. The toxin does not cross the placenta, so the fetus of a mother with botulism is not at risk. The sexes are equally involved. The incubation period can vary from 2 hours to 8 days, but usually is 12 to 36 hours.

Typical initial signs and symptoms are blurred vision, diplopia, ptosis, dysarthria, dysphagia, and generalized weakness (Table 105-10). As with infant botulism, paralysis in foodborne botulism descends and is usually symmetric, although 20 percent of the cases can be asymmetric. Proximal muscles are weaker than distal and arms are more involved than legs. Autonomic involvement includes blurred vision, orthostatic hypotension, urinary retention, constipation, dry mouth, and dilated, fixed pupils. In addition to weakness and autonomic dysfunction there may be evidence of acute gastroenteritis with nausea, vomiting, abdominal pain, and diarrhea. The deficits peak in 4 to 5 days and most improvement occurs in months, although 2 years later some patients still report dyspnea, fatigue, dry mouth, constipation, or impotence.

Diagnosis. A symmetric descending paralysis with a mixture of autonomic, especially parasympathetic, dysfunction should suggest the diagnosis of botulism. The diagnosis would be supported by other cases with common food source for the toxin. The diagnosis of botulism is confirmed by detecting the toxin in serum or toxin or organism in the stool and its foodborne etiology is demonstrated by finding the source of the toxin.

Since the mouse assay is slow, electromyography may give more rapid support for the diagnosis. The changes in foodborne botulism are similar to those in infant botulism (Table 105-11). Milder cases may show more of an increment and findings may vary with the limb studied.

The differential diagnosis of foodborne botulism is as follows:

TABLE 105-10. Signs and Symptoms in Foodborne Botulism

Symptoms
  Abdominal cramps or pain
  Blurred vision
  Constipation
  Diarrhea
  Diplopia
  Dizziness
  Dysphagia
  Dysphonia
  Nausea or vomiting
  Photophobia
  Sore throat
  Urinary retention or incontinence
  Weakness
Signs
  Abnormal eye movement
  Ataxia
  Dilated and fixed pupils
  Dry mouth
  Nystagmus
  Postural hypotension
  Weakness

TABLE 105-11. Electrodiagnostic Studies in Foodborne Botulism

EDX Study	Result
Conduction studies	
Motor conduction velocities and latencies	Normal
Compound muscle action potential amplitude	Reduced in 85%
Sensory conduction studies	Normal
Repetitive stimulation	
Increment with rapid stimulation	62%
Decrement with slow stimulation	8%
Electromyography	
Small and short motor unit potentials	
Increased jitter and blocking with single-fiber electromyography	

(Data from Cherington M: Electrophysiologic methods as an aid in diagnosis of botulism: a review. Muscle Nerve 5:S28, 1982.)

Guillain-Barré syndrome
Tick paralysis
Shellfish poisoning
Myasthenia gravis
Lambert-Eaton syndrome

Guillain-Barré syndrome is an ascending, mainly motor, polyneuropathy. It can be distinguished from botulism by the presence of sensory abnormalities, ascending weakness, and a high cerebrospinal fluid protein. A search for a tick is reasonable. Shellfish poisoning develops over minutes, and usually sensory symptoms and signs are present. Myasthenia gravis and Lambert-Eaton syndrome usually develop more slowly than botulism.

Management. The key to successful management of a patient with severe botulism is the support of respiration. Respiratory failure may develop insidiously. Patients with a vital capacity of less than 30 percent of predicted value will usually need to be intubated. Antitoxin is often given, but its efficacy is uncertain and allergic reactions to horse serum can occur in 10 to 20 percent of patients. A human-derived antiserum should produce fewer allergic reactions. If gastrointestinal function permits, toxin can be removed with ipecac, gastric lavage, or enemas. Guanidine and 4-aminopyridine can improve strength in some patients but do not reverse respiratory paralysis. With current management only about 5 percent of patients will die, although infectious complications are common.

Wound Botulism

Clinical Features. Wound botulism favors young men involved in outdoor activities during the spring to fall seasons. Usually the wound is obvious with a compound fracture or crash injury. Wound botulism has been associated with intranasal cocaine administration, causing sinusitis, and a parenteral drug abuse, resulting in skin lesions. The symptoms and signs of wound botulism are similar to foodborne botulism. Patients with wound botulism lacks the nausea, vomiting, and diarrhea seen with foodborne botulism, but may have fever and sensory abnormalities due to the wound or its infection. About two-thirds of patients with wound botulism will require a respirator, and 10 to 15 percent will die.

Diagnosis. The combination of a wound and a descending paralysis should suggest the diagnosis of wound botulism. Circulating toxin in the serum is only found in about 40 percent of patients, and the organism is grown from the wound in 50 to 60 percent of cases. About three-fourths of the cases where the toxin type is identified are due to type A and the rest are due to type B. The most sensitive test for wound botulism is repetitive stimulation. An increment with repetitive stimulation is usually present and localizes the disorder to the neuromuscular junction.

The differential diagnosis of wound botulism is as follows:

Tetanus
Rabies
Myonecrosis
Acute cranial polyneuritis

Tetanus differs from wound botulism by the presence of trismus and spasms of facial and somatic muscles. Rabies has a much longer incubation period, 30 to 70 days after an animal bite, extreme excitability, hydrophobia, and a cerebrospinal fluid pleocytosis. Myonecrosis spares the cranial nerves. Acute cranial polyneuritis has less autonomic involvement, can have abnormal conduction studies or an elevated cerebrospinal fluid protein level, and lacks and increment with repetitive stimulation.

Management. Management focuses on supportive measures and local wound care. About two-thirds of wounds appear to be clean, although cultures often reveal the organism. Antibiotics and antitoxin are often used, but their efficacy is unknown.

Botulism From an Unknown Source

Clinical Features. Some cases of botulism occur in patients over the age of 1 year where no wound or food is the source of the toxin. In some of these cases the food source was missed or the wound was not apparent. But other cases have the same mechanism as infant botulism where the organism produces toxin in the gut. Production of the toxin in the gut, or autointoxication, is favored by gastrointestinal disease or surgery, gastric achlorhydria, or antibiotic treatment. Autointoxication should be suspected when (1) the patient has consumed food that contains *C. botulinum,* but not its toxin, and (2) a long incubation period is present.

DRUGS

Drugs can impair neuromuscular transmission by (1) unmasking or worsening an existing neuromuscular junction disorder, (2) causing a neuromuscular junction disorder in a previously normal patient, or (3) inducing the immune system to cause a syndrome resembling myasthenia gravis. Drugs that can induce an immune-mediated syndrome resembling myasthenia gravis are as follows:

Chloroquine
D-Penicillamine
Pyrithioxin
Thiopronin
Trimethadione

The resemblance to myasthenia gravis with some of these drugs is close and includes a decrement with slow repetitive stimulation, increased jitter with single-fiber electromyography and antibodies to the acetylcholine receptor. Most drugs aggravate,

TABLE 105-12. Drugs That Can Impair Neuromuscular Transmission by Their Direct Effect

Antibiotics	Calcium channel blockers
Aminoglycosides	Verapamil
Amikacin	Lidocaine
Dihydrostreptomycin	Procainamide
Gentamicin	Quinidine
Kanamycin	Trimethaphan
Neomycin	Hormones
Netilmicin	Adrenocorticotropic hormone
Streptomycin	Corticosteroids
Tobramycin	Estrogen
Fluoroquinolones	Progesterone
Ciprofloxacin	Thyroid hormone
Monobasic amino acids	Neuromuscular blocking drugs
Clindamycin	Ophthalmic drugs
Lincomycin	Betaxolol
Penicillin	Echothiophate
Ampicillin	Timolol
Polypeptides	Psychotropic drugs
Colistimethate	Lithium
Colistin	Monamine oxidase inhibitors
Polymyxin B and E	Phenelyzine
Sulfonamides	Phenothiazines
Tetracyclines	Chlorpromazine
Oxytetracycline	Promazine
Rolitetracycline	Rheumatologic drugs
Anticonvulsants	Chloroquine
Barbiturates	Miscellaneous drugs
Mephenytoin	Aprotinin
Phenytoin	Azathioprine
Trimethadione	Diuretics
Cardiovascular drugs	D,L-cranitine
β-Blockers	Emetine
Nadolol	Methoxyflurane
Oxprenolol	Sodium lactate infusion
Pindolol	Trihexyphenidyl
Practolol	X-ray contrast agents
Propranolol	
Bretylium	

produce, or unmask a neuromuscular junction disorder by their direct effect (Table 105-12).

The diagnosis of drug-induced neuromuscular junction disorders requires an accurate history of drugs taken by the patient. Renal or liver failure often accentuates the effects of drugs. The diagnosis can be confirmed by withdrawing the drug and observing the return of the patient to their previous state. Recovery from neuromuscular junction blocking agents can be prolonged and take several months.

HYPERMAGNESEMIA

Hypermagnesemia usually occurs in patients with renal failure who are given antacids or laxatives containing magnesium or treated for eclampsia with magnesium. The signs and symptoms of hypermagnesemia are as follows:

Amnesia
Ataxia
Cardiac arrest
Cutaneous flushing
Dry mouth
Hypotension
Loss of stretch reflexes
Nausea and vomiting
Nystagmus
Pupillary dilation
Respiratory arrest
Slurred speech
Urinary retention
Weakness

These findings should suggest the diagnosis and magnesium levels will confirm this impression. Electrodiagnostic studies reveal a small compound muscle action potential amplitude after a single stimulus, which increases in amplitude after exercises or repetitive stimulation. These abnormalities reflect a reduction in the release of acetylcholine at neuromuscular junctions.

The treatment of hypermagnesemia involves reducing magnesium intake, intravenous calcium or hemodialysis, depending on the severity of the findings. Support of respiration may be needed.

ORGANOPHOSPHATE INTOXICATION

Exposure to organophosphate compounds is usually accidental but can be part of a suicide attempt. They cause acute symptoms and signs (see Table 105-13) by irreversibly inhibiting acetylcholinesterase. This leads to an accumulation of acetylcholine

TABLE 105-13. Acute Signs and Symptoms Seen With Organophosphate Compounds

Muscarinic
  Abdominal pain
  Aching of eyes
  Airway obstruction
  Anorexia
  Blurred vision
  Bradycardia
  Bronchial contraction and secretion
  Conjunctival hyperemia
  Coughing
  Cyanosis
  Diarrhea
  Hypotension
  Involuntary defecation and micturition
  Lacrimation
  Laryngeal spasms
  Nasal hyperemia
  Nausea and vomiting
  Pulmonary edema
  Pupillary constriction
  Runny nose
  Salivation
  Sweating
  Urinary frequency
Nicotinic (including autonomic ganglia)
  Areflexia
  Fasciculations
  Fatiguability
  Hypertension
  Muscle cramps
  Ophthalmoparesis
  Pallor
  Respiratory failure
  Tachycardia
  Proximal > distal weakness
Central nervous system
  Anxiety
  Apathy
  Ataxia
  Cheyne-Stokes respiration
  Confusion
  Coma
  Decreased concentration and memory
  Depression
  Emotional lability
  Excessive dreaming
  Failure of central respiratory drive
  Insomnia
  Nightmares
  Restlessness
  Seizures
  Slurred speech
  Tension
  Tremor
  Withdrawal

at peripheral muscarinic and nicotinic synapses and at central nervous system synapses. Early findings consist of miosis, fasciculations of the eyelids, face, and calves, and excess secretion. Acute symptoms start in 5 minutes to 1 day and usually peak in one-half hour to 6 hours and last 1 to 5 days. Diagnosis is aided by a history of exposure, signs such as miosis and fasciculation, improvement with atropine and pralidoximine, and a reduction of cholinesterase activity in the serum or red blood cells.

Laboratory tests may aid in the diagnosis. Serum and red blood cell cholinesterase activity is inhibited early and for prolonged periods after exposure. For this reason cholinesterase levels do not correlate with clinical severity. After a single stimulus to a motor nerve the initial compound muscle action potential is followed by repetitive potentials. These repetitive potentials reflect an accumulation of acetylcholine at neuromuscular junctions, which depolarizes motor nerve terminals. Depolarized motor nerve terminals backfire and activate other muscle fibers via an axon reflex. Repetitive potentials are not diagnostic of organophosphate intoxication and can be seen in congenital myasthenic syndromes due to a deficiency of acetylcholinesterase and prolonged open time of sodium channels as well as with other drugs that inhibit acetylcholinesterase reversibly. Repetitive potentials are the earliest and most frequent change seen with electrodiagnostic studies. Repetitive stimulation may reveal a decrement. The decrement is due to a combination of collision of the orthodromic action potentials with the backfiring action potentials from earlier stimuli and desensitization of acetylcholine receptors due to a buildup of acetylcholine. A decrement with repetitive stimulation predicts the need for respiratory support.

The treatment of acute organophosphate intoxication involves supporting respiratory function, giving atropine to reverse the inhibition of acetylcholinesterase, and terminating exposure.

SNAKE BITES

A wide variety of snakes can inflict a bite that is potentially neurotoxic; some of these are listed below:

Australian elapids
Cobras
Coral snakes
Kraits
Mambas
North American rattlesnakes
Old world vipers
Sea snakes
South American rattlesnakes

Snake venom is a complex mixture, and it is unusual for neurotoxic features to dominate. In the United States bites by the Eastern coral snake and the Mojave rattlesnake can result in cranial and somatic muscular paralysis. Most snake bites involve young men bitten in summer. Usually the diagnosis is obvious although 15 percent of patients may lack fang marks and neurotoxic symptoms can be delayed for up to a day. Treatment includes antivenom, support of respiration, and treatment of other complications due to the venom.

SPIDER BITES

The black widow spider generates most of the neurotoxic spider bites. A typical case involves the female spider biting a young

TABLE 105-14. Signs and Symptoms of Black Widow Spider Bite

Common
  Pain
  Muscle cramping and rigidity
  Abdominal rigidity
  Sweating
  Anorexia, nausea, and vomiting
  Hyperesthesia of skin
  Headache
  Restlessness
Occasional
  Arrhythmias
  Bradycardia or tachycardia
  Bronchorrhea
  Cyanosis
  Delirium
  Fear of death
  Hypertension
  Increase or decrease in temperature
  Opisthotonos
  Piloerection
  Priapism and ejaculation
  Psychosis
  Salivation
  Seizures
  Shock
  Trismus
  Urinary retention

man on an extremity in the late summer or early fall. The bite may be painless or feel like a pinprick. Later a cramping pain develops and muscle contractions ensue often causing a rigid abdomen, trismus, and paroxysms of pain. The symptoms and signs seen after a black widow spider bite are shown in Table 105-14. Usually symptoms peak in a few hours, although in occasional cases may peak in the second day. Most symptoms resolve in one to two days. Patients can feel weak or lethargic for up to 1 month.

The diagnosis is based on knowing the patient was bitten by a spider and identifying the type of spider. This is usually easy to do although occasional patients may be bitten during sleep and 20 percent of patients do not show evidence of a bite.

The usual treatment consists of intravenous calcium gluconate, which often relieves the pain transiently. Patients are also given muscle relaxants such as methocarbamol or diazepam and narcotics for pain. An antivenom is available and effective but is derived from horse serum. Serious allergic reactions to the horse serum occur in about 3 percent of patients. For this reason the antitoxin is most likely to be given to the young, the old, pregnant women, and patients with cardiovascular disease.

SCORPION STINGS

Most scorpion stings are painful but otherwise spare the nervous system. In the United States the main neurotoxic scorpion is *Centruroides,* which mainly resides in the Southwest, and its sting leaves no visible mark. Signs and symptoms of a *Centruroides* sting are as follows:

Local pain and paresthesia
Pain and paresthesia remote to sting bite
Jerking or shaking of limbs or trunk
Blurred vision
Wandering eye movements
Hypersalivation
Trouble swallowing
Tongue fasciculations

Compromise of upper airway
Slurred speech

Patients with a severe sting should be hospitalized, sedated, given supportive care, and considered for antivenom therapy.

BEE AND WASP STINGS

The main danger of bee and wasp stings is an allergic reaction to their venom. In rare cases, myasthenia gravis has developed after a wasp sting.

TICK PARALYSIS

Tick paralysis is an uncommon disorder seen within the United States in the Pacific northwest, and Rocky Mountain and southern states. The tick season starts in March and ends in August with a peak in May and June. The most common ticks in the United States are *Dermacentor andersoni* and *D. variabilis.* Tick paralysis is usually due to a gravid female tick that has fed for 4 to 7 days. About 80 percent of cases are children, and two-thirds of the children are girls, which reflects their long hair where the tick hides. About 20 percent of cases are in adults, and 80 percent of these are men.

The disease starts with a day-long prodrome of irritability, lassitude, or generalized weakness. Over the next day or two a symmetric flaccid paralysis develops in the legs and ascends to the arms and then the neck, pharyngeal, and respiratory muscles. Weakness can be proximal more than distal. Areflexia and paresthesia are common, but objective sensory loss is unusual. Early on and in mild cases ataxia may be more prominent than weakness. From 10 to 12 percent of cases, almost entirely children, die.

Most laboratory tests are normal. Nerve conduction studies reveal involvement of motor and sensory nerves with mild slowing of conduction velocity, a reduced amplitude of the evoked response, and prolonged distal latencies.

The diagnosis of tick paralysis is suggested when a young girl develops an ascending areflexic paralysis in the spring or summer. These abnormalities resemble the Guillain Barré syndrome. The correct diagnosis hinges on finding and removing a tick, found on the head or neck in 60 to 70 percent of the cases. The tick should be removed by steady traction. Once the tick is completely removed, improvement is usually rapid.

SUGGESTED READINGS

Allen C: Arachnid envenomations. Emerg Med Clin North Am 10:269, 1992

Arnon SS: Infant botulism. Annu Rev Med 31:541, 1980

Cherington M: Electrophysiologic methods as an aid in diagnosis of botulism: a review. Muscle Nerve 5:S28, 1982

Cornblath DR, Sladky JT, Sumner AJ: Clinical electrophysiology of infantile botulism. Muscle Nerve 6:448, 1983

Gold BS, Barish RA: Venomous snake bites: current concepts in diagnosis, treatment and management. Emerg Med Clin North Am 10:269, 1992

Pascussi RM: Disorders of neuromuscular transmission. Semin Neurol 10:1, 1990

Rivner MH, Swift TR: Electrical testing in disorders of neuromuscular transmission. In Brown WF, Bolton CF (eds): Clinical Electromyography. 2nd Ed. Butterworth-Heinemann, Boston, 1993

Spach DH, Liles WC, Campbell GL et al: Tick-borne diseases in the United States. N Engl J Med 329:936, 1993

Spika JS, Shaffer N, Hargrett-Beam N et al: Risk factors for infant botulism in the United States. Am J Dis Child 143:828, 1989

Swift TR: Disorders of neuromuscular transmission other than myasthenia gravis. Muscle Nerve 4:334, 1981

SECTION 5. DISEASES OF MUSCLE

106. MUSCULAR DYSTROPHIES

BASIL T. DARRAS

Muscular dystrophies are genetically determined primary diseases of muscle, characterized pathologically by muscle fiber degeneration. As expected, the main symptom and sign of muscular dystrophies is weakness. Pathologic, clinical, and genetic criteria have been used as the basis for their classification. Table 106-1 lists the principal forms of muscular dystrophy and their mode of inheritance.

DUCHENNE AND BECKER MUSCULAR DYSTROPHIES (DYSTROPHINOPATHIES)

Duchenne muscular dystrophy (DMD) and Becker muscular dystrophy (BMD) are progressive myopathies, inherited as X-linked recessive traits. DMD is the most severe form of muscular dystrophy, with an incidence of about 1 in 3,500 live male births, and a prevalence rate in the total population of about 3 per 100,000. BMD has a similar presentation but a relatively milder clinical course. The incidence of BMD is about 1 in 30,000 male births. In addition, there is an intermediate group of patients with either mild DMD or severe BMD, who are also known as "outliers." It is now well known that all three types of muscular dystrophy are allelic, resulting from mutations of a single gene, called dystrophin gene.

Clinical Features

Duchenne Muscular Dystrophy. In children with DMD, although there is histologic and laboratory evidence of myopathy from birth, the onset of weakness usually occurs between 2 and 3 years of age; in some cases, it may be delayed. The child usually has difficulty with running, jumping, going up steps, and other similar activities; an unusual waddling gait, lumbar lordosis, and calf enlargement are also observed. Muscular weakness selectively affects proximal limb muscles before the distal, and the lower extremities before the upper. Early on, the

TABLE 106-1. Muscular Dystrophies

Form of Dystrophy	Inheritance
Duchenne Becker Emery-Dreifuss	X-linked recessive
Early-onset "Duchenne-like" Limb-girdle (Erb) Congenital	Autosomal recessive
Facioscapulohumeral Distal Oculopharyngeal Myotonic	Autosomal dominant

patient may complain of leg pains. Jumping and running are almost impossible in most cases, and, in arising from the floor, affected boys use hand support to push themselves to an upright position (Gower's sign). Cardiac muscle is also affected. Children with DMD often have varying degrees of mental retardation, although an occasional child may have average or above-average intelligence.

Physical examination shows pseudohypertrophy of the calf muscles (Fig. 106-1) and, in some instances, quadriceps muscles, lumbar lordosis, waddling gait, shortening of the Achilles

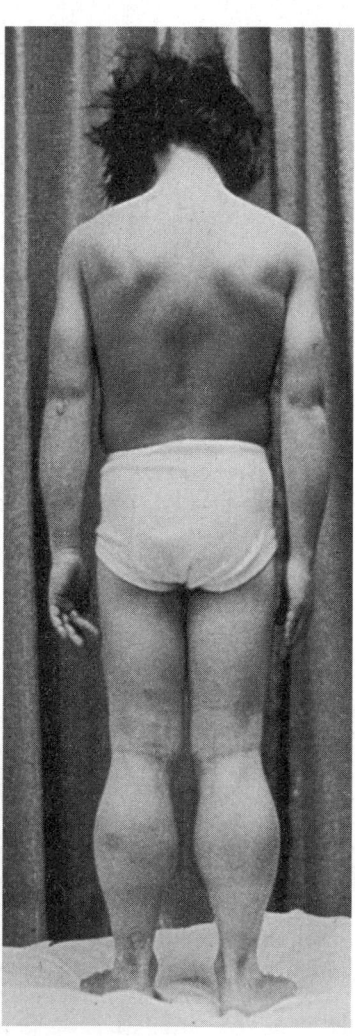

FIG. 106-1. Pseudohypertrophy of the calf muscles in a patient with Duchenne muscular dystrophy. (Courtesy of Theodore Munsat, M.D., New England Medical Center, Boston, MA.)

tendons (Figure 106-2), and hyporeflexia or areflexia. Between 3 and 6 years of age there may be some evidence of improvement, which is gradually followed by relentless deterioration, leading to wheelchair confinement by the age of approximately 12 years. Wheelchair-bound children tend to develop scoliosis and deterioration of pulmonary function. Most die in their late teens or twenties from respiratory insufficiency or arrhythmia secondary to cardiomyopathy. In some cases, the immediate cause of death is not apparent.

Becker Muscular Dystrophy. In BMD the age of onset of symptoms is usually later, and the degree of clinical involvement is milder; cardiac disease and mental retardation are not as common or as severe as in the Duchenne variety. Also contractures are not as likely to develop in BMD. In addition, in Becker and intermediate types of muscular dystrophy there is relative preservation of neck flexor muscle strength. Patients with BMD typically remain ambulatory beyond the age of 16 years and into adult life; they usually survive beyond the age of 30 years. The intermediate group of patients with mild DMD or severe BMD (outliers) usually become wheelchair-bound between the ages of 12 and 16 years. Creatine kinase values are usually highly increased in Becker dystrophy and, therefore, cannot be used as a way of differentiating between the two types of dystrophy. Further, the distinction between Becker dystrophy and limb-girdle dystrophy is often hard to make in cases with a negative family history for BMD. However, the calf muscle pseudohypertrophy is usually not as striking in limb-girdle dystrophy as it is in the Duchenne/Becker dystrophies.

Genetics

Dystrophin Gene. The DMD/BMD gene, now known as the dystrophin gene, was isolated recently; it is the largest gene yet identified in humans, spanning approximately 2.3 megabases at Xp21. The protein product dystrophin has a total molecular weight of 427 kD and is recognized on Western blots of human skeletal muscle proteins using polyclonal antidystrophin antibodies. With the use of immunocytochemistry, dystrophin has been localized to the cytoplasmic face of the plasma membrane of muscle fibers. It has also been shown that dystrophin is part of a large, tightly associated glycoprotein complex containing five other proteins. It is believed that in normal cells the dystrophin stabilizes the glycoprotein complex and protects it from degradation; in the absence of dystrophin, the complex is digested by proteases. The loss of associated membrane proteins as a result of dystrophin deficiency may initiate the degenerative changes seen in muscular dystrophy.

Dystrophin Gene Mutations. Of the DMD/BMD mutations identified so far, most are deletions, detected with the dystrophin cDNA in approximately 55 percent of DMD patients and 70 percent of BMD patients. Partial gene duplications have also been reported in a small percentage of patients (about 5 percent). In the remaining 30 to 35 percent of patients without detectable deletions or duplications, the nature of the molecular lesions leading to the DMD or BMD phenotype remains unknown. Some of the lesions could represent point mutations or splicing errors. Furthermore, some patients with "Duchenne-like" or "Becker-like" phenotypes, but without a clear-cut X-linked pattern of inheritance, may have defects in other genes, possibly those encoding the dystrophin-associated glycoproteins.

Published studies have failed to reveal any apparent correlation between the size of dystrophin gene deletions and the sever-

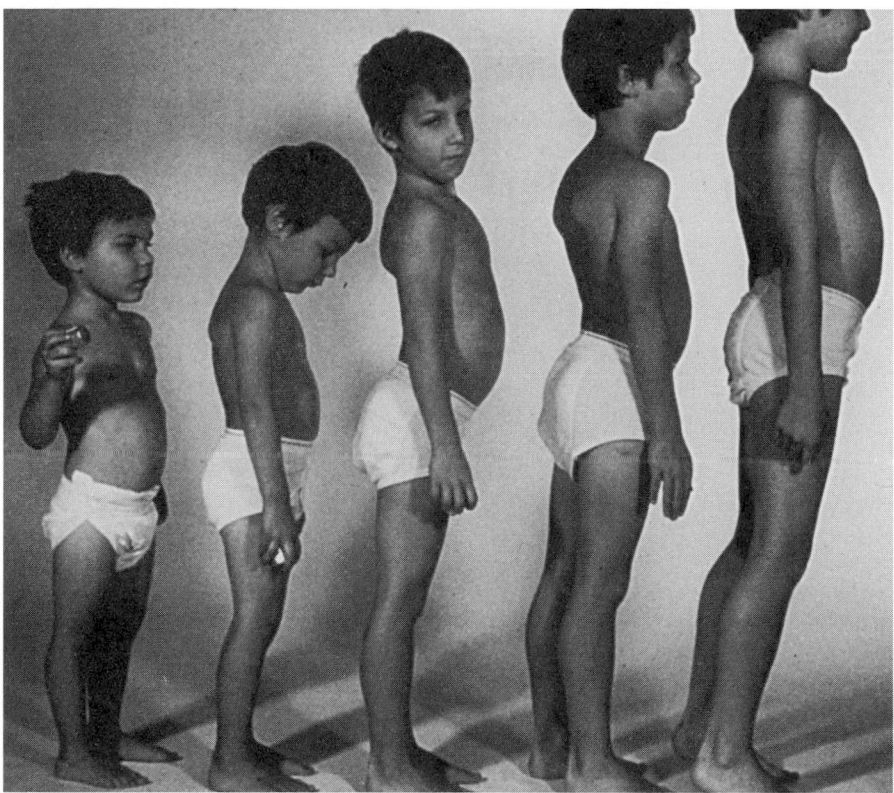

FIG. 106-2. A family of five brothers, all with Duchenne muscular dystrophy. Note the calf pseudohypertrophy, scapular winging, and the associated lumbar lordosis, which, combined with the forward pelvic tilt and heel cord tightening, lead to toe walking or even standing, as seen in the oldest boy. (Courtesy of Danilo A. Duenas, M.D., Miami Children's Hospital, Miami, FL.)

ity and progression of the DMD/BMD phenotype. The molecular basis of DMD versus BMD seems to be related to the disruption or preservation of the amino acid reading frame by the deletion mutations. The latter either disrupt or preserve the reading frame in most cases of DMD or BMD, respectively.

Dystrophin. Dystrophin can easily be detected on immunoblots of 100 μg of total muscle protein by using antidystrophin antibodies. The quantity and quality of dystrophin can be evaluated either visually or by using densitometry. If the 427-kD dystrophin protein is normal in size and amount, the diagnosis of DMD or BMD can almost be excluded. More than 99 percent of DMD patients display complete or almost-complete absence of dystrophin in skeletal muscle biopsy specimens. Most patients with BMD (about 85 percent) have dystrophin of abnormal molecular weight, either smaller (80 percent) or larger (5 percent), in gene deletion of gene duplication cases, respectively, which quite often is reduced in quantity. About 15 percent of the BMD patients, however, have normal-sized protein of reduced quantity. The test is very specific, because patients with neuromuscular diseases other than DMD/BMD have normal dystrophin. Dystrophin immunoblotting can be used in predicting quite accurately the severity of the evolving muscular dystrophy phenotype. It seems that what determines the severity of the disease is the quantity of the dystrophin molecule, rather than its size. DMD patients have less than 3 percent of the normal quantity of dystrophin. Patients with dystrophin levels between 3 and 10 percent of normal, regardless of protein size, seem to develop an intermediate phe-

notype (mild DMD or severe BMD). Patients with mild to moderate Becker phenotype usually have levels above 20 percent.

Diagnosis

Until a few years ago, the diagnosis of DMD/BMD was based on myopathic symptoms and signs, highly increased serum creatine kinase values, myopathic changes on electromyography and muscle biopsy, and sometimes a positive family history. Before the age of 5 years, the serum creatine kinase levels are usually 10 to 20 times the upper limit of normal, or even higher. The serum creatine kinase level is elevated even during the first year of life, when the patient is totally asymptomatic. The concentration of creatine kinase, however, tends to decline with age, at a rate of about 25 percent per year. The electromyogram (EMG) shows myopathic changes, usually small polyphasic potentials, and the muscle biopsy demonstrates degeneration, regeneration, isolated "opaque" hypertrophic fibers and significant replacement of muscle by fat and connective tissue. The cloning of the gene defective in DMD/BMD and the characterization of its protein product, dystrophin, have provided molecular diagnostic tools for accurate diagnosis of this disorder.

Sporadic Cases. In sporadic cases (i.e., family history negative for DMD/BMD), a muscle biopsy should be pursued first, especially when the clinical expression is not yet apparent (Fig. 106-3). Western blot analysis of dystrophin (step A of Fig. 106-3) derived from a muscle biopsy specimen can confirm the clinical diagnosis of DMD/BMD and be used to predict quite

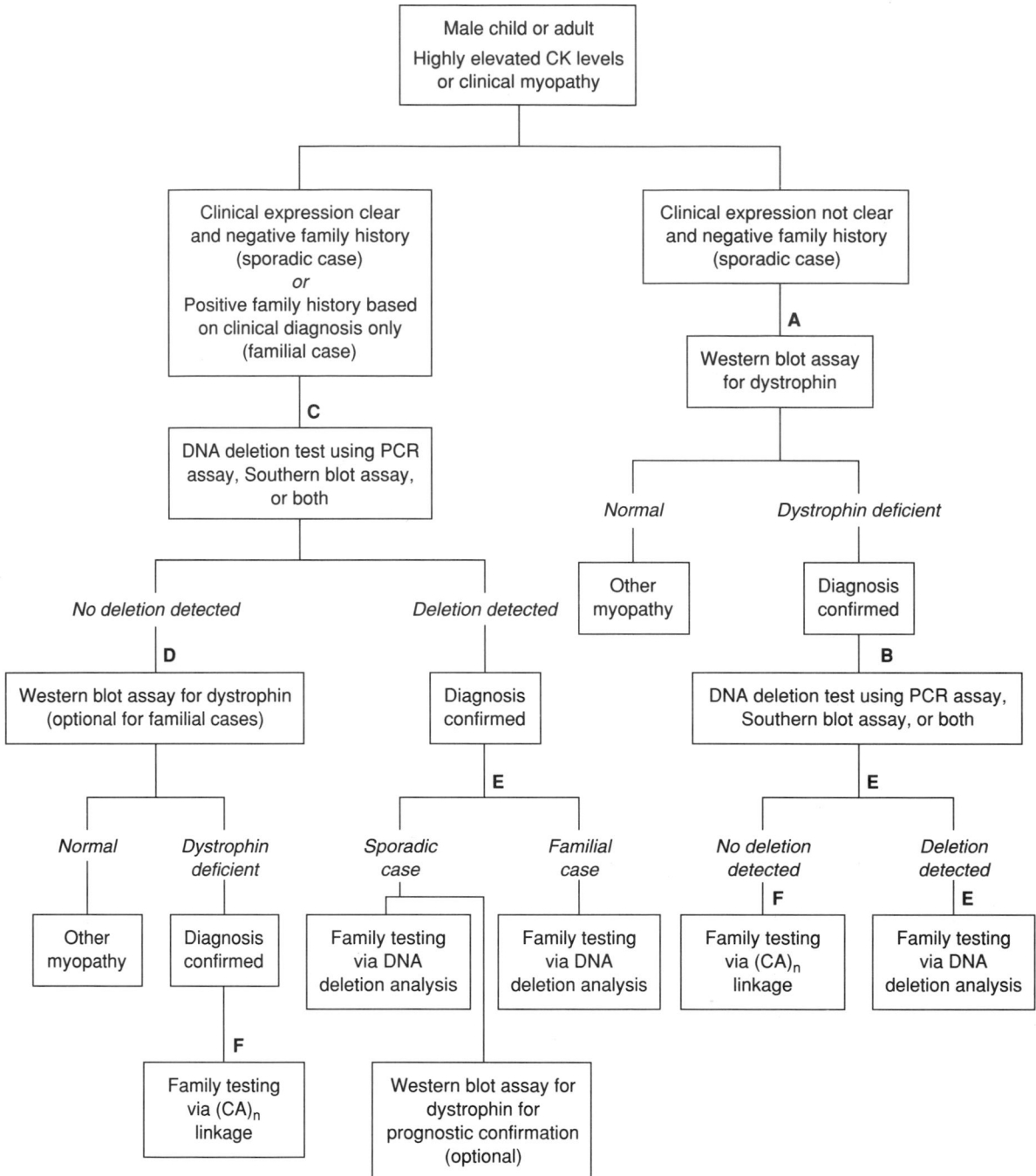

FIG. 106-3. Algorithm for the laboratory diagnosis of sporadic and familial cases of Duchenne muscular dystrophy and Becker muscular dystrophy, and for family testing (carrier detection and prenatal/presymptomatic diagnosis). (Modified from Darras BT: Duchenne/Becker muscular dystrophy. Scientific American Medicine. Vol. 3 (Neurology). Scientific American, 1993, with permission.)

accurately the severity of the disease, based on the amount of detectable dystrophin. When this test is normal, autosomal-recessive, Duchenne-like muscular dystrophy and/or other neuromuscular diseases (e.g., acid maltase deficiency) should be considered.

If the dystrophin assay result is abnormal, the next step (step B of Fig. 106-3) should be DNA-based analysis by multiplex polymerase chain reaction (PCR) or Southern blot to identify the molecular basis of the disorder. When the clinical phenotype is apparent at presentation of a sporadic case, the blood-based PCR test can be performed independently, and will confirm the

diagnosis of DMD/BMD if a deletion/duplication is detected (step C of Fig. 106-3). However, failure to detect a deletion will not exclude the diagnosis of DMD or BMD, in which case a Western blot assay should be performed to exclude or confirm the diagnosis (step D of Fig. 106-3). Upon documentation of a mutation in the dystrophin gene, it can be used as a marker for testing other at-risk family members. Carrier detection of at-risk females and prenatal diagnosis, by means of amniocentesis and/or chorionic villus biopsy, becomes possible following the detection of a DNA deletion or duplication (step E of Fig. 106-3). In the event that no deletion or duplication is found in the proband, linkage analysis (step F of Fig. 106-3) can be attempted for detection of at-risk female relatives and for prenatal diagnosis. Linkage analysis, which 30 to 35 percent of the families must consider, requires the cooperation of several family members.

Familial Cases. In cases of typical DMD or BMD with a family history of X-linked myopathy (i.e., familial cases), molecular diagnosis may not be necessary if the clinical diagnosis has been confirmed in another affected family member by analysis of the dystrophin protein or DNA, or both. In such familial cases, the clinical course in the older affected relative rather adequately, although not always, predicts the severity of the evolving muscular dystrophy for other family members. It should be remembered, however, that extragenic factors may

modify the clinical progression of DMD/BMD, even among members of the same family with the same mutation. If the diagnosis has not previously been confirmed by analysis of dystrophin or DNA in the proband, the PCR-based DNA deletion test (step C of Fig. 106-3) should be attempted first, since it is less invasive than protein testing. If such analysis fails to detect a dystrophin gene abnormality, a muscle biopsy for dystrophin assay (step D of Fig. 106-3) should be considered, particularly in clinically atypical cases, families without a clear-cut X-linked pattern of inheritance, and families with affected male and female siblings, suggesting an autosomal-recessive form of muscular dystrophy.

In a small number of cases, when using a single antibody, the Western blot dystrophin test result does not correlate with the clinical picture. Approximately 5 percent of patients with

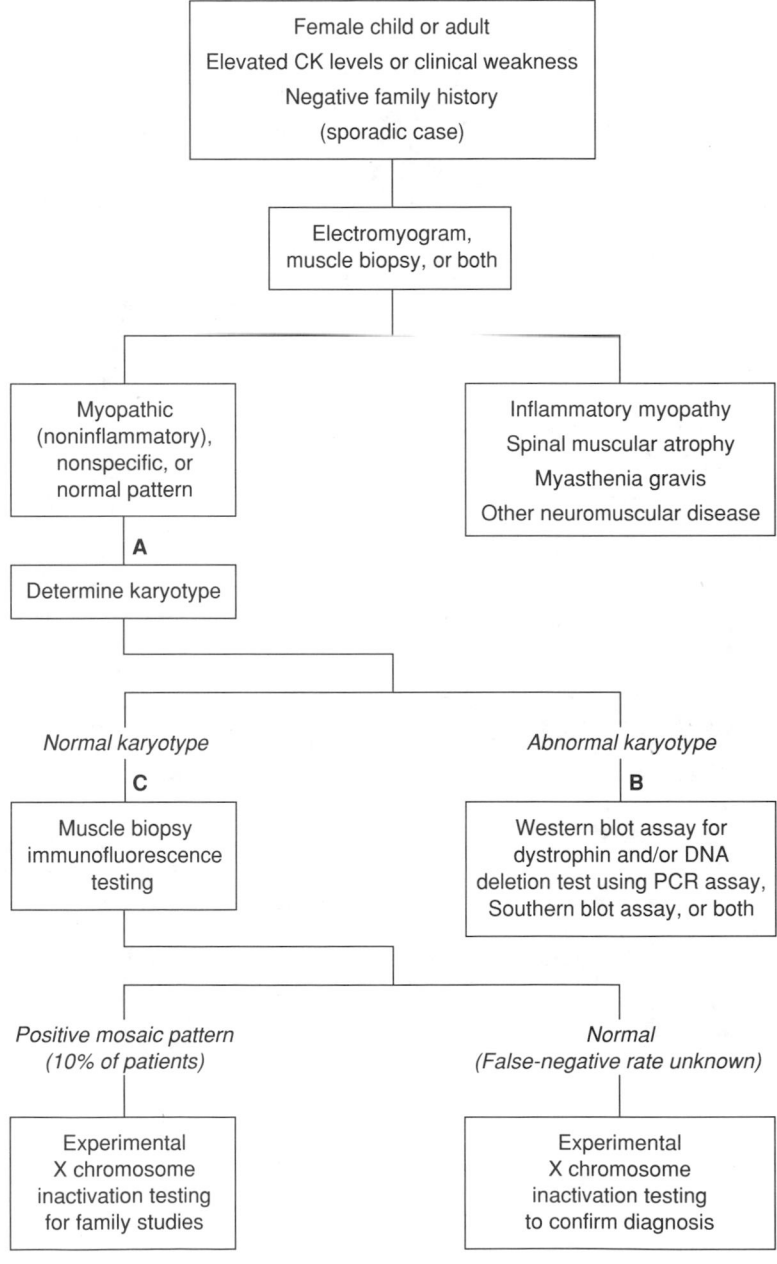

FIG. 106-4. Algorithm for diagnostic testing in females with elevated creatine kinase levels or clinical weakness and a negative family history for an inherited neuromuscular disease. (Modified from Darras BT: Duchenne/Becker muscular dystrophy. Scientific American Medicine. Vol. 3 (Neurology). Scientific American, 1993, with permission.)

classic BMD have been found to have no detectable dystrophin when assayed with the 60-kD antibody. In some of these cases, DNA analysis revealed large deletions, encompassing the epitopes to which the antibody used in the Western blot was raised. False-negative Western blot results can be avoided by incorporating the 6-10 and carboxy terminus antibodies in the Western blot analysis.

Females with Dystrophinopathy. Female patients can have an early-onset, progressive muscular dystrophy and, therefore, be symptomatic, if they have: (1) 45X, 46XY, or Turner mosaic karyotypes; (2) apparently balanced X/autosome translocations with breakpoints in Xp21, within the dystrophin gene, and preferential inactivation of the normal X, and (3) a normal karyotype but nonrandom X-chromosome inactivation leading to diminished expression of the normal dystrophin allele. Therefore,

chromosomal analysis (step A of Fig. 106-4) is indicated in all symptomatic females, especially the ones with highly elevated serum creatine kinase levels, following the exclusion of other neuromuscular diseases (e.g., polymyositis, spinal muscular atrophy) by electromyography and/or muscle biopsy. Further study with a dystrophin assay and/or a DNA deletion test (step B of Fig. 106-4) may be diagnostic in a symptomatic female, especially in cases with 45X, 46XY, or Turner mosaic karyotypes.

Dystrophin Immunostaining. In muscle biopsies derived from DMD patients, there is no detectable staining with antidystrophin antibodies, but in BMD patients, either normal or partial staining of the sarcolemma is observed. In patients with other neuromuscular diseases, there is homogeneous staining of the plasma membrane (Fig. 106-5). The test (step C of Figure 106-

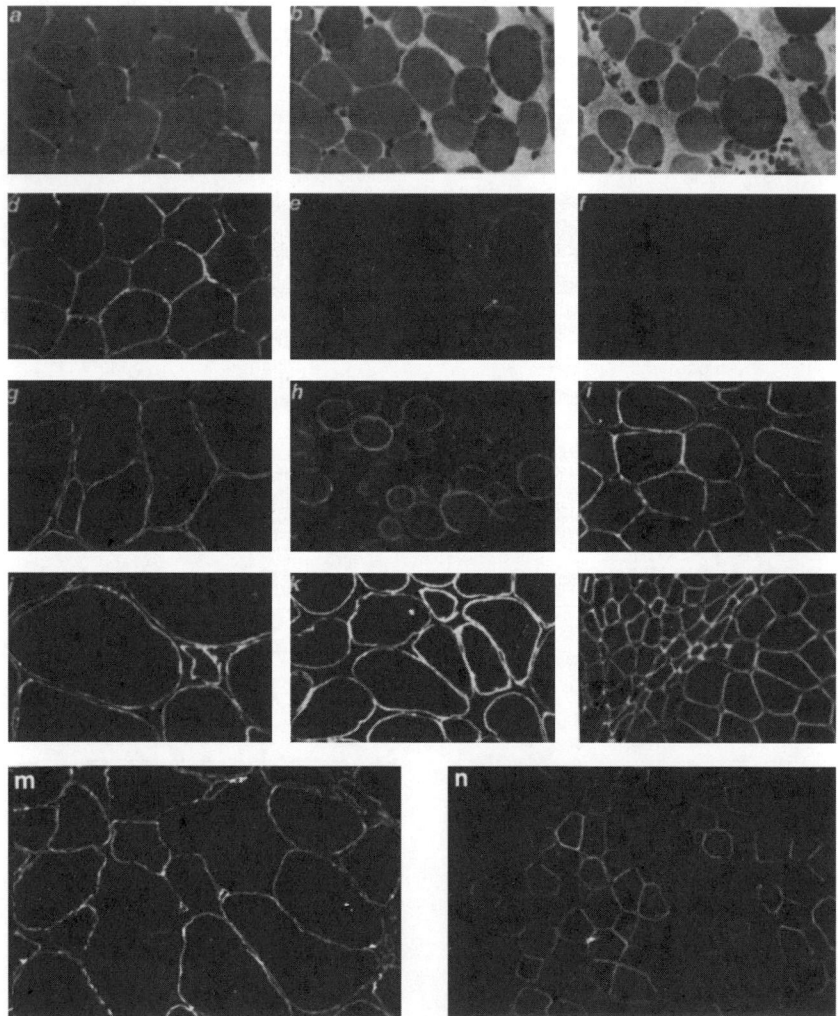

FIG. 106-5.   **(A–N)** Immunostaining of frozen sections of skeletal muscle biopsies. Figs. D–N show antidystrophin antibodies using indirect immunofluorescence. Figs. A, B, and C display hematoxylin & eosin-stained sections corresponding to Figs. D, E, and F, respectively. There is complete absence of immunofluorescence at the sarcolemma in a muscle section from a patient with Duchenne muscular dystrophy (DMD)(Figs. C & F), compared with the homogeneous staining of the plasma membrane in normal muscle (Figs. A & D) and in muscle biopsies from patients with Emery-Dreifuss muscular dystrophy (Fig. G). Fukuyama type of congenital muscular dystrophy (Fig. H), limb-girdle muscular dystrophy (Fig. I), fascioscapulohumeral muscular dystrophy (Fig. J), myotonic dystrophy (Fig. K), and Kugelberg-Welander type of spinal muscular atrophy (Fig. L). In a frozen section of muscle from a BMD patient (Fig. B), partial staining of the sarcolemma is observed (Fig. E). Note the mosaic pattern of immunostaining in muscle biopsies from a symptomatic (Fig. M) and an asymptomatic (Fig. N) DMD carrier. (Modified from Arahata K et al: Nature 333:861, 1988; Arahata K et al: N Engl J Med 320:138, 1989; Darras BT: J Pediatr, 117:1, 1990; Fig. M, courtesy of E. Bonilla, M.D., Columbia University, New York, NY.)

4) appears useful in identifying sporadic cases of symptomatic females with high levels of serum creatine kinase or clinical weakness, or asymptomatic female DMD carriers in families without a male proband or in families with no detectable deletion/duplication and uninformative linkage analysis results. Symptomatic and asymptomatic DMD carriers with elevated serum creatine kinase values may exhibit a characteristic mosaic pattern of dystrophin immunostaining (Figure 106-5). A negative (normal) result, however, does not exclude carrier status, due to the possibility of nonrandom X-chromosome inactivation, and also the possible selective loss of dystrophin-negative fibers. The dystrophin immunostaining and X-chromosome inactivation tests are not commercially available at this point, but they can be performed in selected clinical or research laboratories.

Treatment

Therapeutic interventions in DMD/BMD are aimed at maintaining function, preventing contractures, and providing psychological support. Passive stretching exercises to prevent contractures of the iliotibial band, the Achilles tendons, and flexors of the hip are the mainstays of physical therapy. Lightweight plastic ankle-foot orthoses (AFOs) should be applied if the foot remains in plantar flexion during sleep. Standing and/or walking can be maintained by using long-leg braces. Surgery can be performed to release contractures of the hip flexors, iliotibial bands, and Achilles tendons. Standing and ambulation seem to prevent scoliosis. After the age of 12 years, pulmonary function studies, electrocardiography, and chest radiographs should be performed yearly to monitor the pulmonary and cardiac functions. Overnight mouth intermittent positive pressure can be used to treat symptomatic nocturnal hypoventilation, and respiratory assistance may be used during periods of respiratory infection. Recent studies provide evidence that prednisone improves the strength and function of patients with DMD. This improvement begins within 10 days, requires a single dose of 0.75 mg/kg/day of prednisone for maximal improvement and reaches a plateau after 3 months. Observed side effects include weight gain, hypertension, behavioral changes, growth retardation, and cataracts. Prednisone may be recommended for selected ambulatory patients over the age of 5 years and continued if the side effects are not severe. Immunosuppression with azathioprine does not have a beneficial effect. Cyclosporin has been reported to improve clinical function in children with DMD who received the medication for 8 weeks. However, because of the rare reports of cyclosporin-induced myopathy in patients receiving the medication for other reasons, the use of cyclosporin in DMD remains controversial.

Myoblast transfer has been attempted recently in humans, but the results, so far, have not been encouraging. This and other experimental gene therapies are currently under evaluation.

EMERY-DREIFUSS DISEASE (HUMEROPERONEAL MUSCULAR DYSTROPHY)

Emery-Dreifuss disease is an X-linked type of muscular dystrophy with onset of symptoms usually in the first or second decade. The muscle weakness and wasting has a humeroperoneal distribution, often starting in the arms, with weakness of both the biceps and triceps and relative preservation of the deltoid muscles. Later on, distal leg weakness with atrophy of the peroneal muscles is noted. In some cases mild facial weakness may be observed as well. The myopathy tends to be slowly progressive. Contractures at the elbows are noted early, often associated with toe-walking as the first manifestations of the disease. Contractures of the posterior aspect of the neck and the Achilles tendons also occur. Cardiac involvement is common and consists of a cardiomyopathy, with atrioventricular (AV) block and often atrial paralysis. The electrocardiogram (EKG) may show varying degrees of AV block, small T waves, and atrial arrhythmias. The cardiomyopathy may lead to sudden death in approximately 50 percent of the affected individuals, usually early in adult life.

Laboratory studies show modest elevation of creatine kinase, which is rarely above a few hundred units per liter. While the electromyogram (EMG) usually displays myopathic features, it may also reveal evidence of denervation. The muscle biopsy usually shows mild myopathic changes with internal nuclei, variation in fiber size, focal connective tissue proliferation, and occasional necrotic fibers.

The differential diagnosis includes the rigid spine syndrome, which, in addition to the elbow and ankle contractures, is usually associated with limited flexion of the spine and relatively mild and slowly progressive myopathy. Cardiomyopathy, however, has not been observed.

Because the cardiac involvement in Emery-Dreifuss muscular dystrophy is potentially fatal, the cardiac status of the patient should be investigated even if he or she is asymptomatic. Installation of a cardiac pacemaker may be lifesaving in patients with evidence of AV block. Holter monitoring should be considered in patients with normal electrocardiograms.

MYOTONIC DYSTROPHY

Clinical Features

Myotonic dystrophy is the most common form of muscular dystrophy among Caucasians, with a prevalence estimated as 3 to 5 per 100,000 population and an incidence of 1 in 8,000. Myotonic dystrophy is a multisystem disorder, transmitted by autosomal-dominant inheritance, with variable penetrance. In the classical form, myotonic dystrophy has its onset in adolescence or adulthood, but a neonatal form also occurs. The main clinical features are myotonia (delayed muscle relaxation after contraction), weakness and wasting affecting facial muscles and distal limb muscles, frontal balding (in males), cataracts, cardiomyopathy with conduction defects, multiple endocrinopathies, and low intelligence or dementia. The face is long, with wasting of the masseter and temporal muscles; there is also variable ptosis and facial diplegia (Fig. 106-6). The neck is thin, because of wasting of the sternocleidomastoids. There may be associated dysarthria, swallowing difficulties, and mild external ophthalmoplegia. Myotonia can be an early symptom, demonstrated by percussion of muscles, usually of the thenar eminence, and by the difficulty with releasing the grasp. Later in the course of the disease, the progressive muscle weakness and wasting become the predominant features, leading to severe distal weakness in the hands and feet. Endocrinopathies include hyperinsulinism, rarely diabetes, adrenal atrophy, infertility in women, testicular atrophy, and growth-hormone secretion disturbances. Smooth and cardiac muscle involvement are usually expressed by disturbed gastrointestinal mobility and cardiac conduction defects.

The congenital form of the disease occurs in children born to mothers with myotonic dystrophy and presents with profound hypotonia at birth, associated with facial diplegia, feeding and respiratory difficulties, and skeletal deformities, such as club-

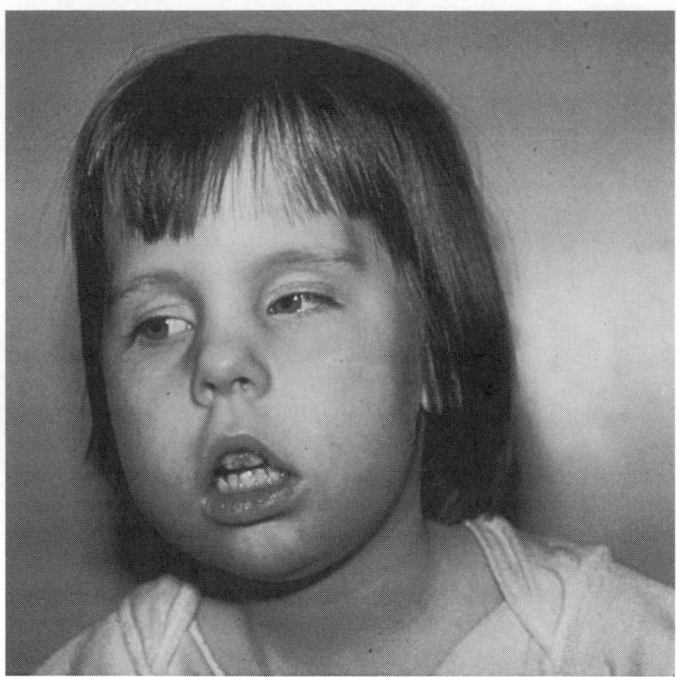

FIG. 106-6. Congenital myotonic dystrophy. The facial diplegia, ptosis, temporal, and masseter muscle wasting and the characteristic appearance of the mouth (like an inverted V) are to be noted. (Courtesy of N. Paul Rosman, M.D., New England Medical Center, Boston, MA.)

feet. Later, during childhood, delayed developmental progression is noted.

Until recently, the diagnosis of myotonic dystrophy was based on clinical features, family history, EMG, and muscle biopsy findings. EMG demonstrates myopathic potentials and myotonia. Muscle histology may reveal internal nuclei, type I fiber atrophy, and ring fibers. The diagnosis, however, could not be confirmed easily in many cases, especially mildly affected ones. The recent identification of the myotonic dystrophy mutation has provided molecular diagnostic tests for almost 100 percent accurate diagnosis of this disorder in both symptomatic and asymptomatic individuals.

Genetic Diagnosis

The myotonic dystrophy locus was mapped by linkage analysis to chromosome 19q13.3; this genetic localization finally led to the recent identification of the genetic defect, which is thought to be an amplified trinucleotide CTG repeat, located in the 3′ untranslated region of a gene, which putatively encodes a serine-threonine protein kinase (myotonin-protein kinase [DMK]). Although this CTG repeat is quite polymorphic, it is stable in normal individuals. In contrast, the CTG repeat in myotonic dystrophy chromosomes is unstable and can become significantly large. In normal individuals, the 2 alleles contain between 5 and 50 copies of the CTG repeat. However, normal individuals with 38 to 49 copies of the repeat are classified in a borderline category, because of the small possibility of

expansion of the CTG repeat in their offspring or family members. Mildly affected individuals or asymptomatic premutation ''carriers'' have 50 to 99 CTG repeats, while severely affected subjects have between 100 and 2,000 or more copies (full mutation) (Table 106-2). To date, a large number of affected individuals have been assessed by both Southern blot and PCR, and an increase in CTG copy number has been documented in over 99 percent of the subjects.

Amplification of the CTG repeat has been proposed to be the molecular mechanism for genetic anticipation, which is the increasing severity of the disease phenotype in successive generations; in myotonic dystrophy families, the CTG copy number increases during successive generations. A positive correlation has been observed between increased number of CTG repeats and earlier age of disease onset. Conversely, in a few families, reduction in size of the trinucleotide repeat mutation has been observed during transmission, with a decrease in disease severity. It is not possible, however, to predict the age of onset of the disease in a particular patient on the basis of the CTG copy number. For a given number of repeats (above 100), a wide range in disease severity may be observed. Nonetheless, infants with severe congenital myotonic dystrophy as well as their mothers, are shown to have, on average, a greater amplification of the CTG repeat. The greater the CTG repeat expansion in the mother, the higher the probability of a myotonic dystrophy offspring being affected with the congenital form of the illness. Unfortunately, these new developments do not explain the exclusive maternal inheritance in cases of congenital myotonic dystrophy. Genomic imprinting or the presence of a maternal intrauterine factor have been proposed as two possible mechanisms.

The amplification is detectable by Southern blotting in most cases utilizing DNA extracted from peripheral blood leukocytes. However, this type of analysis may fail to detect expansions where the CTG copy number is less than 100 to 150; in some of these cases, which are usually mildly affected, analysis by PCR is important. Conversely, some very large expansions may fail to amplify by PCR. Therefore, both techniques need to be employed in the molecular diagnosis of myotonic dystrophy.

Treatment

The treatment of myotonic dystrophy is currently symptomatic. As patients develop distal weakness, braces for footdrop are usually helpful. The myotonia frequently responds to medications that stabilize membranes, such as phenytoin, carbamazepine, quinidine, procainamide, and acetazolamide. Theoretically, it is better to start with phenytoin, carbamazepine, or acetazolamide, because procainamide and quinine prolong the conduction intervals, which are already abnormally prolonged in many patients with myotonic dystrophy. As these patients, however, are primarily troubled by the weakness and less by the myotonia, they may benefit more from mechanical devices like ankle supports than from membrane stabilizers.

LIMB-GIRDLE MUSCULAR DYSTROPHY

Limb-girdle dystrophy (LGD) was first described by W. H. Erb in 1884; the term embraces a number of conditions with

TABLE 106-2. CTG Repeat Expansion in Myotonic Dystrophy

Category	Normal	Borderline Normal	Premutation "Carriers"	Full Mutation
Number of repeats	5–37	38–49	50–99	Above 100
Clinical phenotype	Normal	Normal	Mildly symptomatic or no symptoms	Symptomatic

heterogeneous etiologies; it is still used as a generic term to describe those patients with muscular dystrophy of girdle distribution. Most cases are inherited in an autosomal recessive fashion and, as is to be expected, are sporadic. However, families with an autosomal dominant pattern of inheritance have been described as well.

The age of onset of LGD varies from early childhood to adulthood. In some cases, weakness may be noted early, leading to significant disability during childhood; in other cases the weakness may not be apparent until early in adult life. With the exception of a few cases with rapid progression, the course is usually slowly progressive. The weakness may be affecting the shoulder girdle (scapulohumeral type) or the pelvic girdle (pelvifemoral type) or both. Most childhood-onset cases have a pelvifemoral distribution of weakness. In many adult patients, the disease involves both shoulder and pelvic girdles with gradually increasing proximal limb weakness leading to restriction of mobility and eventually to wheelchair confinement. Neck flexor and extensor muscles may be involved concomitantly. Facial weakness is usually mild and, in some cases, totally absent. Even in mild cases, there is preferential weakness and atrophy of the biceps muscle (Fig. 106-7A). Distal muscle strength is usually preserved, even at the late stage of the disease. Low back pain may be a prominent symptom in patients with LGD. Intellect is usually normal and cardiac or other systemic involvement is not seen.

The Kugelberg-Welander variety of spinal muscular atrophy may mimic limb-girdle dystrophy of the pelvifemoral type. The differentiation might require a muscle biopsy and EMG to show evidence of denervation. Differentiation from BMD may be difficult in the absence of a positive family history, suggesting X-linked inheritance in BMD. Similarly, in females, the distinction from manifesting heterozygotes for BMD and DMD may be problematic as well. The prominent calf pseudohypertrophy and the usually greater elevation of creatine kinase levels in patients with BMD and in manifesting heterozygous females maybe helpful. Recently, blood DNA deletion analysis and also dystrophin analysis of muscle biopsies has been shown to differentiate conclusively between these conditions. Chronic polymyositis and myopathies related to thyrotoxicosis, Cushing's disease, or other metabolic etiologies may often present like LGD. The sparing of the pelvic girdle in early stages of facioscapuloperoneal dystrophy and the prominence of facial weakness in the latter help in the differential diagnosis from LGD. Nonetheless, the differentiation between facioscapulohumeral dystrophy and the scapulohumeral type of limb-girdle dystrophy may be hard to make on both clinical and pathologic grounds; the preferential atrophy of the biceps in LGD may be useful.

Creatine kinase levels are usually modestly elevated, not to the levels seen in patients with DMD and BMD. Electromyography shows myopathic changes with small polyphasic potentials; a muscle biopsy reveals dystrophic changes with degeneration and regeneration of muscle fibers, fiber-splitting, internal nu-

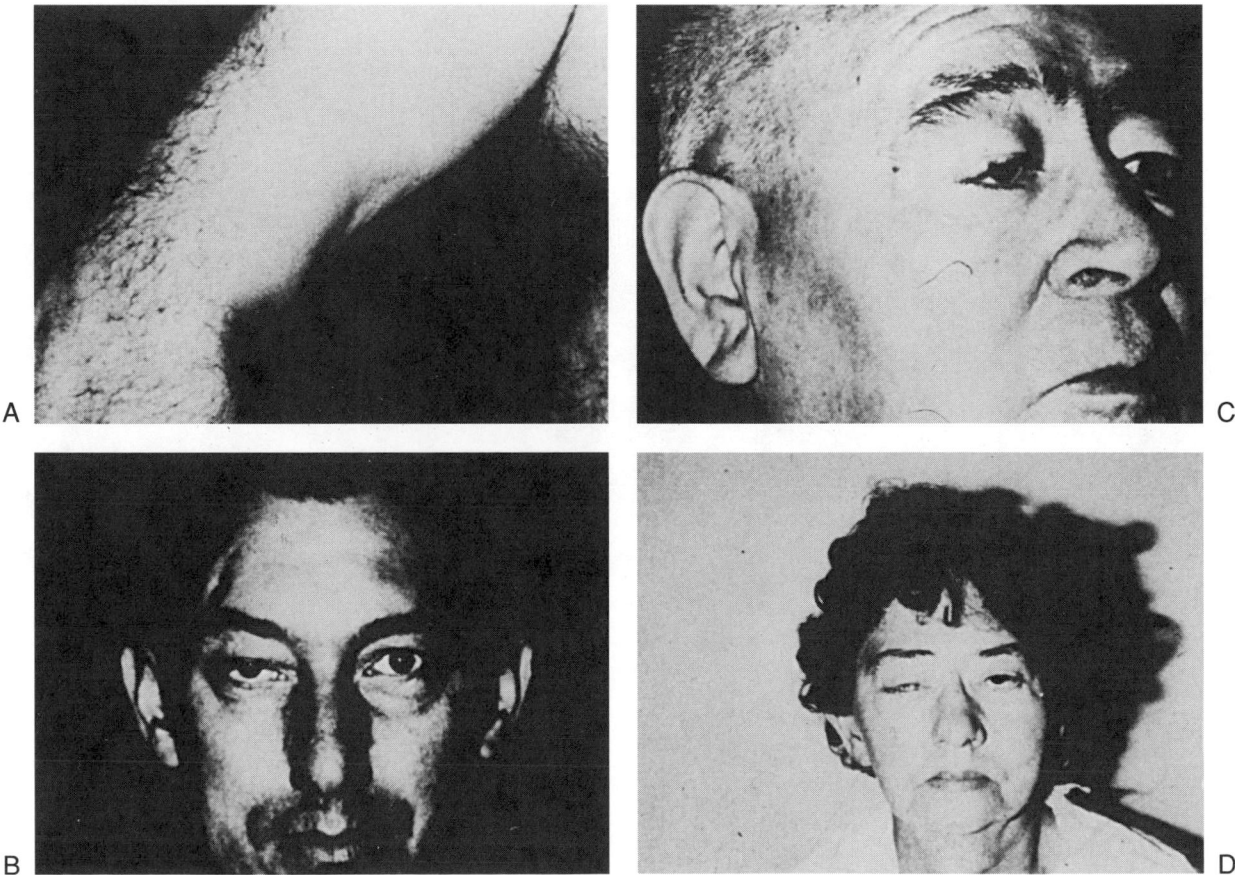

FIG. 106-7. **(A)** Selective atrophy of the biceps muscle, frequently seen in limb-girdle dystrophy. **(B–D)** Ptosis and extraocular muscle weakness in patients with oculopharyngeal dystrophy. The ptosis is bilateral but often asymmetric. (Adapted from M. Brook: A Clinician's View of Neuromuscular Disease. Williams & Wilkins, Baltimore, 1986, with permission.)

clei, fibrosis, and moth-eaten and whorled fibers. Therapy is supportive.

FACIOSCAPULOHUMERAL MUSCULAR DYSTROPHY

Facioscapulohumeral (FSH) muscular dystrophy was first described by Duchenne (1872) and, subsequently, by Landouzy and Dejerine (1884). The classical form is inherited in an autosomal dominant fashion. Although FSH muscular dystrophy is usually slowly progressive, it can be extremely variable in its severity and even the age of onset. The infantile variety has a very early onset (usually within the first few years of life) and is rapidly progressive with wheelchair confinement by the age of 9 to 10 years in most cases; this form is often sporadic. There is profound facial weakness, inability to close the eyes in sleep, and inability to smile and to show any evidence of facial expression. The weakness rapidly involves the shoulder and hip girdles with lumbar lordosis, pronounced forward pelvic tilt, and hyperextension of the knees and the head upon walking. Marked weakness of the wrist extensors may result in a wrist drop.

In the classical form of FSH muscular dystrophy the onset is usually in the second or third decade, and the progression is slow with almost normal life span. The facial muscles are involved initially with inability to close the eyes tightly, smile, or whistle; a pouting appearance of the lips, smooth face, and mild dimpling in the areas lateral to the angles of the mouth are characteristic (Fig. 106-8A,B). The facial weakness, however, can be mild early on and may remain mild for many years. The muscles of the shoulders and upper arms are also involved with marked atrophy of the biceps and triceps, but relative preservation of the deltoid muscles (Fig. 106-8C). There is significant scapular winging and characteristic appearance of the

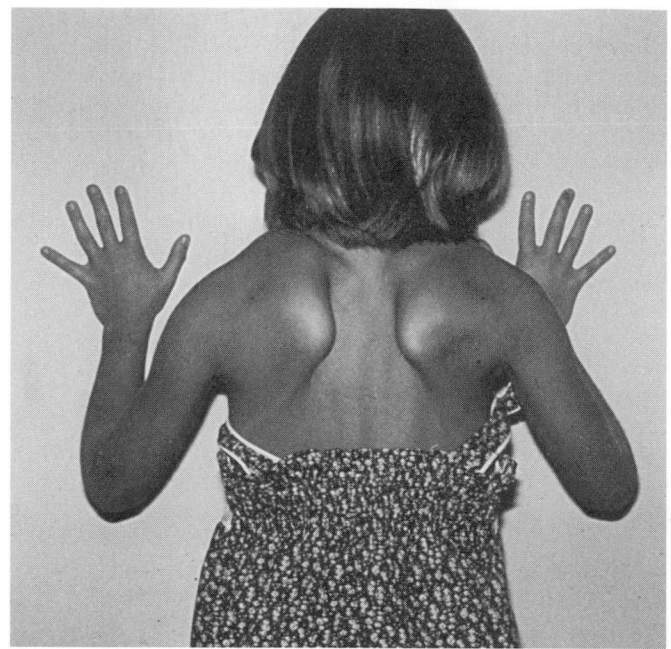

FIG. 106-9. Facioscapulohumeral muscular dystrophy. Profound scapular winging with rising of the scapulae upward and laterally. (Courtesy of N. Paul Rosman, M.D., New England Medical Center, Boston, MA.)

shoulders with bulging of the trapezii muscles (Fig. 106-8A), riding of the scapulae upward and over the lateral parts of the thorax (Fig. 106-9) and forward jutting of the medial ends of the clavicles, when the arms are abducted. Distal muscles of the upper extremities are usually spared, but a footdrop may

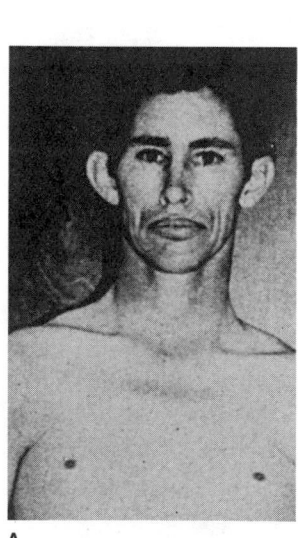
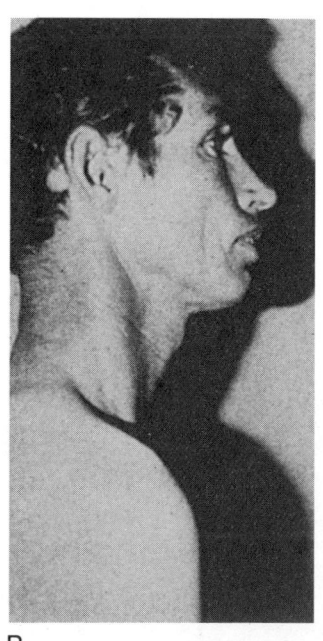
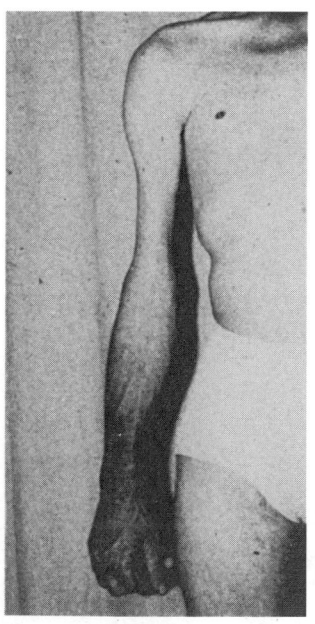
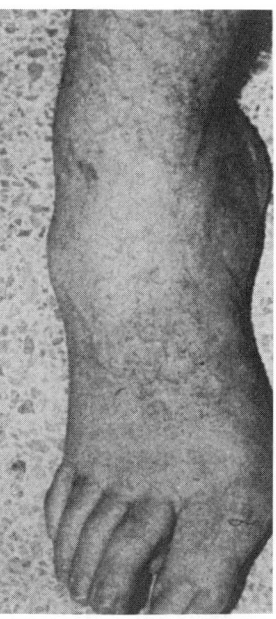

A   B   C   D

FIG. 106-8. Facioscapulohumeral muscular dystrophy. **(A)** The horizontal and widened appearance of the mouth with vertical dimpling on either side of the mouth are to be noted. The rest of the face is relatively unlined. **(B)** Pouting appearance of the lips, when viewed from the side **(C)** Atrophy of the arm due to wasting of the biceps and triceps. The deltoid and muscles of the forearm are relatively preserved ("Popeye" arm). **(D)** Hypertrophy of the extensor digitorum brevis (EDB) muscle, in spite of marked footdrop, seen as bulging on the lateral aspect of the foot. (Adapted from M. Brook: A Clinician's View of Neuromuscular Disease. Williams & Wilkins, Baltimore, 1986, with permission.)

occur (scapuloperoneal variety). In a number of cases, the disease progresses rapidly in middle age leading to significant disability. Exudative telangiectasia of the retina (Coats syndrome) with an associated sensorineural hearing loss has been described to occur in some cases of FSH muscular dystrophy.

The involvement of the facial muscles is usually more severe than in early myotonic dystrophy. The sternocleidomastoids are not so selectively involved as in myotonic dystrophy; also, there is absence of myotonia in FSH dystrophy. The scapuloperoneal variety is similar to the X-linked Emery-Dreifuss syndrome, but significant elbow contractures and cardiomyopathy are lacking. In addition, the mode of inheritance is different (autosomal dominant versus X-linked recessive). Differentiation from hereditary motor neuropathies may be hard to make in patients with weakness limited to the peroneal and anterior tibial muscle groups. In these cases, however, inspection of the extensor digitorum brevis (EDB) muscle is helpful because it is usually hypertrophic in FSH muscular dystrophy (Fig. 106-8D); atrophy of the EDB muscle is common in peripheral motor neuropathies. In limb-girdle dystrophy there is selective weakness of the biceps and involvement of the deltoid; the latter muscle is relatively spared in FSH muscular dystrophy.

The EMG displays myopathic features; the muscle biopsy shows variability in fiber size with a lot of rather large hypertrophic fibers, a few angulated atrophic fibers and quite often a significant inflammatory response. Histologic differentiation from polymyositis is based on the fact that hypertrophy of the muscle fibers is not seen in the latter. Creatine kinase levels are only mildly elevated and are rarely elevated in patients presymptomatically.

Treatment of FSH muscular dystrophy is primarily supportive. There is need to examine the eyes for evidence of Coats syndrome, which is usually treatable with photocoagulation of the abnormal vessels. Because the deltoid muscles are usually preserved, patients with significant weakness may show some improvement by surgical fixation of the scapulae. Because loss of scapular fixation may recur after surgery, it would be advisable to recommend surgery on one side and, if successful, to consider fixation of the other side later. Wrist and ankle supports may be useful also. In spite of the pronounced inflammatory response in muscle biopsies, therapy with corticosteroids is not advocated.

OCULOPHARYNGEAL MUSCULAR DYSTROPHY

Oculopharyngeal muscular dystrophy (OPD) is common in French-Canadian families in Quebec, and also in Spanish-American families in the southwestern United States. The inheritance of this dystrophy is autosomal dominant. The onset of OPD is in adult life, usually not until middle age; the initial features are ptosis, which is frequently asymmetric, and progressive extraocular weakness (Fig. 106-7B–D). Later on, difficulty with swallowing, which is variable in severity, as well as weakness of the neck, jaw, and facial muscles are noted. Generalized involvement may be seen also.

OPD is distinguished from FSH muscular dystrophy by the fact that the extraocular weakness in OPD is far more severe; it is also distinguished by the distribution of weakness. OPD can also be confused with myotonic dystrophy, but myotonia is absent in OPD; ocular muscle involvement is rarely severe in early myotonic dystrophy. The differentiation from a mitochondrial myopathy might pose a problem. However, the associated features of retinitis pigmentosa, ataxia, elevated cerebrospinal fluid protein, cardiac conduction defects, and developmental delay often seen in mitochondrial myopathies help in the differentiation. Muscle biopsy shows variation of fiber size and "rimmed" vacuoles. Creatine kinase levels may be elevated. In a small number of patients cricopharyngeal myotomy has been attempted with improvement of the dysphagia.

DISTAL MUSCULAR DYSTROPHY

Distal muscular dystrophy common in Sweden and less frequently in other parts of the world; it is inherited as an autosomal dominant trait. The onset of the symptoms is usually between 40 and 60 years of age; onset early in life has also been observed, however, often leading to generalized weakness with a more rapid progression. Initially, weakness of the hands is noted followed by slow involvement of the anterior tibial group of muscles. Proximal weakness is seen in less than 2 percent of the cases. EMG and the muscle biopsy reveal myopathic changes. Serum creatine kinase level may be normal or mildly elevated. Cardiomyopathy is rare.

CONGENITAL MUSCULAR DYSTROPHY

The term congenital muscular dystrophy has been applied to infants who are hypotonic and weak at birth and in whom muscle biopsies show changes consistent with muscular dystrophy. Arthrogryposis is commonly seen in the newborn period. The Fukuyama type of congenital muscular dystrophy, is more common in Japan, and it is characterized by hypotonia, generalized weakness, severe developmental delay, seizures, and microcephaly. A combination of congenital muscular dystrophy and demyelination of the cerebral hemispheres (leukodystrophy) has been described in white children. When congenital muscular dystrophy is associated with ocular dysplasia, hydrocephalus, and cerebral malformations the term cerebro-ocular dysplasia is applied. Ocular abnormalities include cataracts, optic nerve hypoplasia, corneal clouding, and retinal dysplasia or detachment. Therefore, congenital muscular dystrophy is not a single entity, but embraces a number of conditions in which evidence of muscular dystrophy is evident at birth. Serum creatine kinase levels may be normal or elevated and muscle biopsy is characteristically abnormal with extensive fibrosis, degeneration and regeneration of muscle fibers, and proliferation of fatty and connective tissue. In some cases, the clinical course is static, but in most patients it progresses very slowly. In a few cases, however, actual improvement has been seen. No definitive treatment is available for this disorder.

SUGGESTED READINGS

Dystrophinopathies

Arahata K, Ishiura S, Ishiguro T et al: Immunostaining of skeletal and cardiac muscle surface membrane with antibody against Duchenne muscular dystrophy peptide. Nature 333:861–863, 1988

Darras BT: Molecular genetics of Duchenne and Becker muscular dystrophy. J Pediatr 117:1–15, 1990

Darras BT, Koenig M, Kunkel LM, Francke U: Direct method for prenatal diagnosis and carrier detection in Duchenne/Becker muscular dystrophy using the entire dystrophin cDNA. Am J Med Genet 29:713–726, 1988

Dubowitz V: Muscle Biopsy: A Practical Approach. pp. 289–339. Baillière Tindall, London, 1985

Hoffman EP: Genotype/phenotype correlations in Duchenne/Becker dystrophy.

In Partridge TA (ed). Molecular and Cell Biology of Muscular Dystrophy, Chapman and Hall, London, 1990

Hoffman EP, Brown RH Jr, Kunkel LM: Dystrophin: the protein product of the Duchenne muscular dystrophy locus. Cell 51:919–928, 1987

Hoffman EP, Fischbeck KH, Brown RH et al: Characterization of dystrophin in muscle-biopsy specimens from patients with Duchenne's or Becker's muscular dystrophy. N Engl J Med 318:1363–1368, 1988

Hoffman EP, Kunkel LM, Angeline C et al: Improved diagnosis of Becker muscular dystrophy by dystrophin testing. Neurology 39:1011–1017, 1989

Monaco AP, Bertelson CJ, Gallati-Liechti S et al: An explanation for the phenotypic differences between patients bearing partial deletions of the DMD locus. Genomics 2:90–95, 1988

Griggs RC, Moxley RT, Mendell JR et al: Duchenne dystrophy: randomized, controlled trial of prednisone (18 months) and azathioprine (12 months). Neurology 43:520–527, 1993

Mendell JR, Moxley RT, Griggs RC et al: Randomized, double-blind six-month trial of prednisone in Duchenne's muscular dystrophy. N Engl J Med 320:1592–1597, 1989

Sharma KR, Mynhier MA, Miller RG: Cyclosporine increases muscular force generation in Duchenne muscular dystrophy. Neurology 43:527–532, 1993

Emery-Dreifuss Disease

Hopkins LC, Jackson JA, Elsas LJ: Emery-Dreifuss humeralperonal muscular dystrophy; an X-linked myopathy with unusual contractures and bradycardia. Ann Neurol 10:230–237, 1981

Rowland LP, Fetell M, Olarte M et al: Emery-Dreifuss muscular dystrophy. Ann Neurol 5:111–117, 1979

Myotonic Dystrophy

Aslanidis C, Jansen G, Amemiya C et al: Cloning of the essential myotonic dystrophy region and mapping of the putative defect. Nature 355:548, 1992

Brook JD, McCurrach ME, Harley AJ et al: Molecular basis of myotonic dystrophy: expansion of a trinucleotide (CTG) repeat located at the 3′ end of a transcript encoding a protein kinase family member. Cell 68:799, 1992

Brunner HG, Nillesen W, van Oost BA et al: Presymptomatic diagnosis of myotonic dystrophy. J Med Genet 29:780–784, 1992

Dubowitz V: Muscle Biopsy: A Practical Approach. pp. 380–395. Baillière Tindall, London, 1985

Griggs RC, Davis RJ, Anderson DC, Dove JT: Cardiac conduction in myotonic dystrophy. Am J Med 59:37–42, 1975

Harley HG, Rundle SA, Reardon W et al: Unstable DNA sequence in myotonic dystrophy. Lancet 339:1125–1128, 1992

Harper PS: Myotonic Dystrophy. 2nd Ed. WB Saunders, London, 1989

Suthers GK, Huson SM, Davies KE: Instability versus predictability: the molecular diagnosis of myotonic dystrophy. J Med Genet 29:761–765, 1992

Limb-Girdle Muscular Dystrophy

Brooke MH: Limb-girdle dystrophy. pp. 178–181. In: A Clinician's View of Neuromuscular Diseases, Williams & Wilkins, Baltimore, 1986

Dubowitz V: Muscle Biopsy: A Practical Approach. pp. 289–339. Baillière Tindall, London, 1985

Fascioscapulohumeral Muscular Dystrophy

Carroll JE, Brooke MH: Infantile fascioscapulohumeral dystrophy. In Serratrice G, Roux H (eds): Peroneal Dystrophies and Related Disorders. Masson, New York, 1979

Dubowitz V, Brooke MH: Muscle Biopsy: A Modern Approach. WB Saunders, Philadelphia, 1973

Ketenjiam AU: Scapulocostal stabilization for scapular winging in fascioscapulohumeral dystrophy. J Bone Joint Surg [Am] 60A:476–480, 1978

Munsat TL, Piper D, Cancilla P, Mednick J: Inflammatory myopathy with fascioscapulohumeral distribution. Neurology 22:335–347, 1972

Taylor DA, Carroll JE, Smith ME et al: Fascioscapulohumeral dystrophy associated with hearing loss and Coats syndrome. Ann Neurol 12:395–398, 1982

Oculopharyngeal Muscular Dystrophy

Victor M, Hayes R, Adams RD: Oculopharyngeal muscular dystrophy: a familial disease of late life characterized by dysphagia and progressive ptosis of the eyelids. N Engl J Med 267:1267–1272, 1962

107. INFLAMMATORY MYOPATHY

ISABELITA R. BELLA
DAVID A. CHAD

The term inflammatory myopathy refers to a spectrum of disorders that have in common the presence of lymphocytic infiltration of muscle tissue. Included in the clinical spectrum are infectious myopathies, sarcoid myopathy, and some dystrophic and toxic myopathies that have an inflammatory component. In this chapter, we focus our attention on a group of uncommon, immunologically mediated inflammatory myopathies that include three distinct conditions: polymyositis, dermatomyositis, and inclusion body myositis. Despite their rarity, they demand our attention for several reasons. First, for many patients the myopathy (polymyositis or dermatomyositis) is eminently treatable, but a positive response to immunotherapy depends on early diagnosis and prompt initiation of therapy. (Inclusion body myositis appears relatively resistant to treatment, but accurate diagnosis is crucial so that long-term therapy with potent immunosuppressive drugs is avoided.) Second, because an inflammatory myopathy (notably polymyositis or dermatomyositis) may be the first manifestation of a systemic disorder such as malignancy or collagen-vascular disease, accurate diagnosis of the myopathy allows the physician to recognize these complicating disorders when they are at an early and relatively manageable stage of their course. Third, because many different myopathic (and some nonmyopathic) disorders resemble the inflammatory myopathies, early and accurate recognition that weakness is caused by polymyositis, dermatomyositis, or inclusion body myositis allows the physician to avoid costly tests and procedures. Last, when clinicians have confidently established the diagnosis of one of these three conditions, they can enroll patients in clinical trials of new, more selective immunosuppressant agents that may provide our patients with a better quality of life.

CLINICAL FEATURES

The inflammatory myopathies are uncommon, with only 5 to 10 new cases per million per year in the United States. Peak incidence of polymyositis and dermatositis occurs in patients between the ages of 45 and 64, and there is a female predominance. Dermatomyositis, however, has a bimodal age distribution with a smaller peak in the juvenile age group (5 to 14 years). Inclusion body myositis occurs more often in men (male:female ratio of 2:1) with a predilection for the older patient (usual age of onset: over 50).

The clinical features of polymyositis and dermatomyositis are as follows:

Onset is subacute (weeks to months).

Distribution involves proximal muscles including limb girdles and neck flexors; dysphagia in 30 to 50 percent.

Rash (in dermatomyositis; may be subtle).

Other organs involved include lung and heart.

Associated conditions include malignancy (especially dermatomyositis) and collagen-vascular disorders. Dermatomyositis is associated with scleroderma and mixed connective tissue disease.

Diagnostic process is straightforward for dermatomyositis, broad differential for polymyositis. The polymyositis differential includes toxic, metabolic, endocrine, and dystrophic myopathies.

Response to treatment is gratifying.

Polymyositis and dermatomyositis are characterized by the subacute development of proximal muscle weakness with progression of symptoms over weeks to months. Muscle pain and tenderness may occur early in the course of these illnesses and are more often seen in dermatomyositis. Sensation is normal and tendon reflexes are preserved unless the muscle is severely weak and atrophic. Neck flexor, pharyngeal, and esophageal muscles are also frequently involved. Dysphagia is present in 30 to 50 percent of patients.

The clinical features of inclusion body myositis are as follows:

Onset is chronic (months to years).

Distribution involves proximal muscles including limb girdles and neck flexors; dysphagia in 30 percent; predilection for the quadriceps; affects distal muscles early in the course; tends to be asymmetrical.

Associated conditions on occasion include collagen-vascular disorders.

Diagnostic process is difficult; long interval between onset and diagnosis; may resemble amyotrophic lateral sclerosis.

Response to treatment is poor.

In contrast to polymyositis and dermatomyositis, inclusion body myositis progresses over many years and, in addition to proximal muscles, affects distal muscles early in its course. The quadriceps muscle can be selectively involved, leading to severe weakness and atrophy to the point that the patellar reflex may be lost (see Dalakas, 1991). Asymmetries in the distribution of weakness are also common. The average duration of symptoms from onset to diagnosis is 3 to 5 years. Inclusion body myositis is frequently misdiagnosed, most often as polymyositis resistant to treatment, but neurogenic features may prompt the diagnosis of amyotrophic lateral sclerosis. In all the inflammatory myopathies, facial and extraocular muscles are rarely affected; indeed, involvement of cranial muscles should raise the possibility of another diagnosis.

Skin Manifestations of Dermatomyositis

Dermatomyositis is distinguished by its characteristic rash, which usually accompanies, but may precede, the onset of weakness. The typical cutaneous manifestations of dermatomyositis are the heliotrope rash and Gottron sign. The heliotrope rash is a lilac discoloration of the periorbital skin, especially the upper eyelids, and is usually associated with periorbital edema. The Gottron sign (also known as Gottron's papules or plaques) refers to erythematous, violaceous raised papules and plaques occurring over bony prominences, especially the knuckles and proximal and distal interphalangeal joints (see Sto-

necipher, 1993), but can also be seen on the elbows, knees, and ankles. Another cutaneous manifestation is a flat, erythematous, sometimes photosensitive rash seen in the malar, perioral, forehead, anterior neck, and chest areas. Periungual telangiectasias, cuticular overgrowth, and nailfold infarcts may also be seen and the fingers may be cracked and rough with "dirty" horizontal lines. Another distinguishing feature is the presence of subcutaneous calcification located on the hands or arms; it is more often seen in juveniles (up to 40 percent). Breaks in the skin created by extruded calcification may lead to secondary infection.

Pulmonary and Cardiac Involvement

There are several causes of lung involvement in polymyositis and dermatomyositis. Weakness of pharyngeal muscles and an ineffective cough due to respiratory muscle weakness may cause aspiration pneumonia. In advanced cases, marked respiratory muscle weakness may lead rarely to respiratory insufficiency. In 10 percent of patients with polymyositis and dermatomyositis interstitial lung disease occurs; dyspnea and a nonproductive cough are the most common symptoms. Interstitial lung disease is present in 50 percent of patients with the anti-Jo-1 antibody (see below).

Cardiac abnormalities in polymyositis and dermatomyositis are common, occurring in more than 50 percent of patients. The most frequent abnormalities are nonspecific ST-T wave changes. Other abnormalities include heart block, bundle branch block, congestive heart failure, arrhythmias (tachyarrhythmias and sick sinus syndrome), myocarditis, and myocardial fibrosis. Fibrosis of the conduction system may be responsible for the electrocardiographic conduction defects. The muscle-brain fraction of creatine kinase is not useful in predicting the presence or absence of cardiac involvement. Pathologically, the myocardium resembles skeletal muscle (see below) with the presence of interstitial inflammatory cell infiltrates, necrosis, variation in myocyte size, degeneration of myocytes, and fibrosis. In one autopsy series (see Haupt et al., 1982) an active myocarditis was found in 25 percent of patients, all of whom had clinical evidence of congestive heart failure and ongoing skeletal muscle involvement. In two-thirds of patients with cardiac involvement, an antibody reacts to tissue ribonucleoproteins, suggesting a pathogenic role for humeral immunity in cardiac damage. Cardiac involvement is probably an important cause of death (approaching 20 percent) in poly- and dermatomyositis, sometimes occurring suddenly even as skeletal muscle function seems to be improving.

Association With Malignancy

It is likely that there is an increased frequency of malignancy in patients with inflammatory myopathy, but the risk has been difficult to define precisely. A recent population-based study (see Sigurgeirsson et al., 1992) found that there is a definite increased risk of cancer in patients with dermatomyositis; patients with polymyositis had a higher risk of cancer than the general population, but it is questionable whether the risk is real. A recent review of the literature suggests that approximately 25 percent of patients with dermatomyositis already have a malignancy or will be afflicted later, while the incidence of malignancy in polymyositis probably occurs at a lower rate and may not be different from the general population (see Callen, 1993). Although malignancy appears to be more common in older patients, young adults can have cancer-associated myositis. Many types of malignancies have been reported to occur with polymyositis and dermatomyositis, including carcinoma of the breast, stomach, lung, pancreas, skin, colon, and prostate. There is a suggestion that gynecologic malignancies, particularly ovarian cancer, may be encountered more frequently than other tumors. Overall, however, it appears that the types of malignancies correspond to the type typically found for a particular age group. Muscle weakness may occur 1 month to 6 years before discovery of the tumor or 4 months to 5 years after the discovery of malignancy. Several case reports suggest that the symptoms of myositis parallel the course of malignancy, with improvement following treatment of the tumor and recurrence of symptoms with development of metastasis.

In patients with polymyositis or dermatomyositis who have no extramuscular symptoms we recommend, and most investigators agree, that a directed search for a malignancy is indicated for the reasons given above. We perform a complete history and physical examination (with rectal, pelvic, and breast examinations), and our laboratory testing includes stool for occult blood, urinalysis, complete blood count and differential, electrolytes, chest radiograph, mammography, prostate specific antigen (in older men), and follow-up of any abnormalities found.

Inclusion body myositis does not appear to have an association with malignancy; only 8 cases of malignancy have been reported in over 100 patients described in the literature.

Association With Connective Tissue Disease

Polymyositis and dermatomyositis can occur as isolated entities, but up to 24 percent are associated with a connective tissue disorder, usually systemic lupus erythematosus, rheumatoid arthritis, Sjögren syndrome, systemic sclerosis, and mixed connective tissue disease, and may also be associated with systemic autoimmune disorders such as ulcerative colitis, primary biliary cirrhosis, and chronic graft versus host disease. Ranitidine and lupron therapy has also been reported as a causative factor. Inclusion body myositis may also be associated with collagen-vascular disorders such as Sjögren syndrome and systemic lupus erythematosus.

Association with Autoantibodies

Several autoantibodies to nuclear and cytoplasmic antigens involved in protein synthesis—found in 35 to 40 percent of patients with polymyositis and dermatomyositis—are referred to as *myositis-specific autoantibodies* (MSAs) because they occur most commonly or exclusively in these disorders (see Targoff, 1992). These MSAs can arise many months before the development of myositis symptoms, and they correlate with disease activity, disappearing as the myositis enters remission. Approximately a dozen MSAs have been described; the most common is an antisynthetase, anti-Jo-1, an autoantibody directed at histidyl-tRNA synthetase (the enzyme responsible for catalyzing the formation of histidyl-tRNA from histidyl and its cognate tRNA). Anti-Jo-1 is seen in 15 to 20 percent of all myositis patients, but most frequently in polymyositis. Patients with anti-Jo-1 often have a constellation of clinical features that has been termed the *antisynthetase syndrome*. These features include myositis, interstitial lung disease (found in 50 to 75 percent of patients with anti-Jo-1), arthritis, and Raynaud's phenomenon (see Targoff, 1992). They tend to have myositis in the spring, have a 5-year survival rate of 70 percent, with most dying of pulmonary complications.

Antibodies to nuclear antigens are frequently found in myositis patients, the most common pattern being nucleoplasmic. Anti-Mi-2 is exclusive to myositis patients, and occurs in 15 to 20 percent of patients with dermatomyositis. Anti-PM-Scl is seen frequently in myositis-scleroderma overlap.

Most assays for MSA are still research techniques and not commercially available except for the anti-Jo-1 antibody. MSAs may be helpful in predicting the clinical course and prognosis of patients.

LABORATORY FEATURES

The key laboratory features of the inflammatory myopathies are summarized in Table 107-1. Creatine kinase levels are elevated up to 50 times above normal in patients with polymyositis and dermatomyositis, while in those with inclusion body myositis, these levels are not usually elevated more than 10-fold; however, 4 to 5 percent of patients with active myositis can have normal levels. The erythrocyte sedimentation rate is elevated in approximately 50 percent of patients with polymyositis and dermatomyositis. Antinuclear antibodies are present in 15 to 47 percent of patients, usually those with associated connective tissue disorders.

Needle electromyography (EMG) studies in polymyositis and dermatomyositis reveal myopathic-appearing motor unit potentials (brief, small amplitude, polyphasic), which are recruited early, along with increased insertional activity, fibrillation potential activity, positive sharp waves, complex repetitive discharges, and usually normal nerve conduction studies (except in severe or long-standing disease when there are low motor amplitudes). While needle EMG abnormalities (fibrillation potentials) may be restricted to the paraspinal muscles, a completely normal needle EMG study is unusual and should prompt reconsideration of the diagnosis. Needle EMG studies in inclusion body myositis are more heterogeneous, often disclosing both myopathic and neurogenic features.

DIFFERENTIAL DIAGNOSIS

Many different conditions may simulate the inflammatory myopathies. Table 107-2 lists the more common disorders and their key differentiating features.

PATHOLOGY

Muscle biopsy examination is an important diagnostic tool in evaluating a patient suspected of having an inflammatory myopathy. Not only does it help exclude other potential causes for

TABLE 107-1. The Laboratory Diagnosis of Inflammatory Myopathy

Laboratory Feature	Finding(s)
Serum creatine kinase	Elevated[a]
Electromyography	Fibrillation potential activity Early recruitment Brief, low-amplitude, polyphasic motor units[b]
Muscle biopsy	Inflammation Necrosis and regeneration Perifascicular atrophy[c] Rimmed vacuoles[d]

[a] Mild elevation in inclusion body myositis, moderate to severe in polymyositis and dermatomyositis.
[b] In inclusion body myositis and chronic polymyositis and dermatomyositis also see high-amplitude, long-duration motor units.
[c] Seen in dermatomyositis.
[d] A characteristic of inclusion body myositis.

TABLE 107-2. Conditions That May Simulate the Inflammatory Myopathies

Disorder	Key Differentiating Feature(s)
Corticosteroid myopathy	EMG: no fibrillation potentials Normal creatine kinase
Hypothyroid myopathy	Psychomotor slowing, myoedema High thyroid-stimulating hormone
Toxic myopathy[a]	Positive history Vacuolar myopathy/scant inflammation
Acid maltase deficiency	EMG: myotonia Vacuolar myopathy Biochemical confirmation on muscle
Periodic paralysis	Positive history of episodic weakness Abnormal potassium concentration
Myotonic dystrophy[b]	Clinical and electrical myotonia Extramuscular manifestations
HIV myopathy	HIV serum positivity HIV positivity in muscle macrophages
Amyotrophic lateral sclerosis	Muscle atrophy with fasciculations Hyperreflexia Neurogenic atrophy
Multifocal motor neuropathy	EMG: conduction block Normal (or slightly elevated) creatine kinase
Diabetic polyradiculopathy	EMG: polyneuropathy Abnormal serum glucose and hemoglobin A_{1c}
Myasthenia gravis	Ptosis and opthalmoparesis Weakness if fatigable Positive Tensilon test
Lambert-Eaton syndrome	Autonomic component EMG: postexercise facilitation

Abbreviations: EMG, electromyography; HIV, human immunodeficiency virus.
[a] Especially cholesterol-lowering agents, such as chloroquine and colchicine.
[b] Distal weakness reminiscent of inclusion body myositis.

the patients' symptoms, it is important to differentiate between the various types, as prognosis, treatment, and association with malignancy differ for each type.

Pathologically, all the inflammatory myopathies are characterized by mononuclear inflammatory cell infiltrates, myofiber necrosis, and regeneration. (Because inflammatory infiltrates in muscle may be randomly scattered, a single biopsy may miss the inflammatory cells despite multiple sections. Therefore, rarely, patients with inflammatory myopathies are found to have normal muscle biopsies.) Differences in histologic appearance exist between the various forms, which help differentiate one from another.

In polymyositis, inflammatory infiltrates made up of lymphocytes, monocytes, and possibly plasma cells are found within fascicles in the endomysial connective tissue. Also commonly seen in polymyositis and inclusion body myositis is the invasion of nonnecrotic myofibers by mononuclear inflammatory cells.

Dermatomyositis is characterized histologically by the presence of atrophic fibers localized to the periphery of their fascicles, a feature designated as perifascicular atrophy and found in approximately 90 percent of juvenile patients and 50 percent of adult patients (Fig. 107-1). Occasionally the entire fascicle may be composed of atrophic myofibers, a pattern probably due to microvascular ischemia. Unlike polymyositis, the inflammatory cells are found in a perivascular distribution and in the perimysial connective tissue rather than the endomysium. Microvascular changes are prominent in this disorder. There is a marked decrease in the number of capillaries per unit area within areas of perifascicular atrophy. Capillary necrosis, thrombosis, and endothelial hyperplasia may be seen. A highly characteristic electron microscopic finding is the presence of undulating tubular arrays in the endothelial cells of intramuscular capillaries. More recently, complement C5b-C9 membrano-

lytic attack complex (MAC) deposition has been found in capillaries (Fig. 107-2).

In inclusion body myositis (Fig. 107-3), the inflammatory infiltrate is located in the endomysium, similar to polymyositis, but differentiated from it by the presence of rimmed vacuoles (basophilic material lines the vacuoles and by electron microscopy is shown to consist of membranous whorls) and small groups of angulated fibers. Although these small fibers are reminiscent of neurogenic atrophy, the atrophy affects both fiber types, and fiber type grouping suggestive of reinnervation is rare. Additionally, there is a marked variation in fiber size (hypertrophic as well as atrophic fibers) and an increase in endomysial fibrosis highlighting the chronic nature of this myopathy. Pathognomonic of inclusion body myositis is the presence of 15- to 18-nm nuclear and cytoplasmic filamentous inclusions that appear tubular and are found near the periphery of vacuoles and membranous whorls. Recently, rimmed vacuoles were found to be immunoreactive to ubiquitin and B-amyloid protein.

PATHOGENESIS

Although the exact mechanism for fiber damage is not completely known, there is increasing evidence for an immune pathogenesis. In dermatomyositis, the intramuscular microvasculature is believed to be the primary target of humeral processes mediated by complement C5b-C9 MAC. Complement deposition leads to necrosis and thrombosis of capillaries, small arteries, and venules found predominantly in the periphery of the fascicle, resulting in ischemia, myofiber destruction, and perifascicular atrophy. Consistent with the notion that dermatomyositis is mediated largely by humeral immunity is that the inflammatory infiltrate is composed mainly of B cells and helper T cells.

In polymyositis and inclusion body myositis a cell-mediated immune mechanism is highly suspected because the majority of inflammatory cells are made up of T cells and macrophages. These cytotoxic T cells are thought to recognize antigenic targets associated with major histocompatibility complex 1 (MHC-1) antigen in muscle fibers, as they surround and destroy healthy, nonnecrotic fibers. A viral pathogenesis has also been implicated in inclusion body myositis as the filamentous inclusions resemble myxovirus nucleocapsids. A chronic virus infection was supported by the isolation of a strain of adenovirus type II in two successive muscle-biopsy specimens from a patient with the disease; no additional reports of successful viral isolation have since appeared, however. In another study, immunoreactivity for mumps-virus antigens in the nuclear and cytoplasmic inclusions suggested that a persistent mumps virus infection could be the cause of the disease, but negative mumps-virus in situ hybridization studies have cast doubt on this theory.

TREATMENT AND PROGNOSIS

The natural history of polymyositis and dermatomyositis without therapy has never been formally studied. It is possible that in some patients these diseases would improve or resolve spontaneously. It has been our practice, however, to institute immunotherapy (corticosteroids) in patients who are impaired in their daily activities. On occasion, we encounter mildly affected elderly patients in whom we do not institute corticosteroids. Rather, we follow these patients closely and manage to avoid side effects of corticosteroids.

A number of unfavorable prognostic factors have been identi-

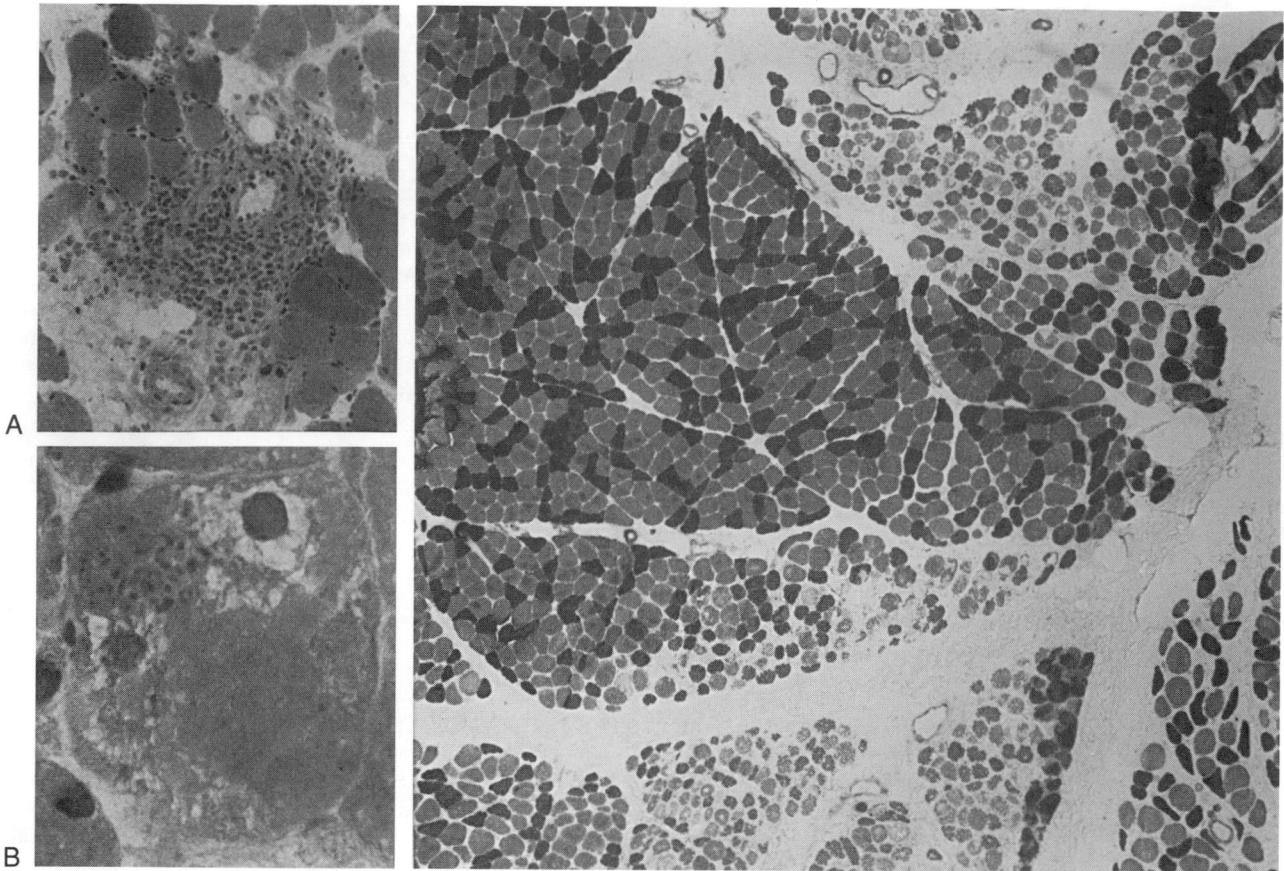

FIG. 107-1. Dermatomyositis. Perifascicular atrophy is typical of dermatomyositis and at times involves the entire fascicle (Frozen section; ATPase; pH 9.6; × 10). (Inset A) Perivascular inflammation (Frozen section: hematoxylin-eosin; × 25). (Inset B) Degenerating muscle fiber showing vacuoles and cytoid bodies. (Frozen section; hematoxylin-eosin; × 150.)

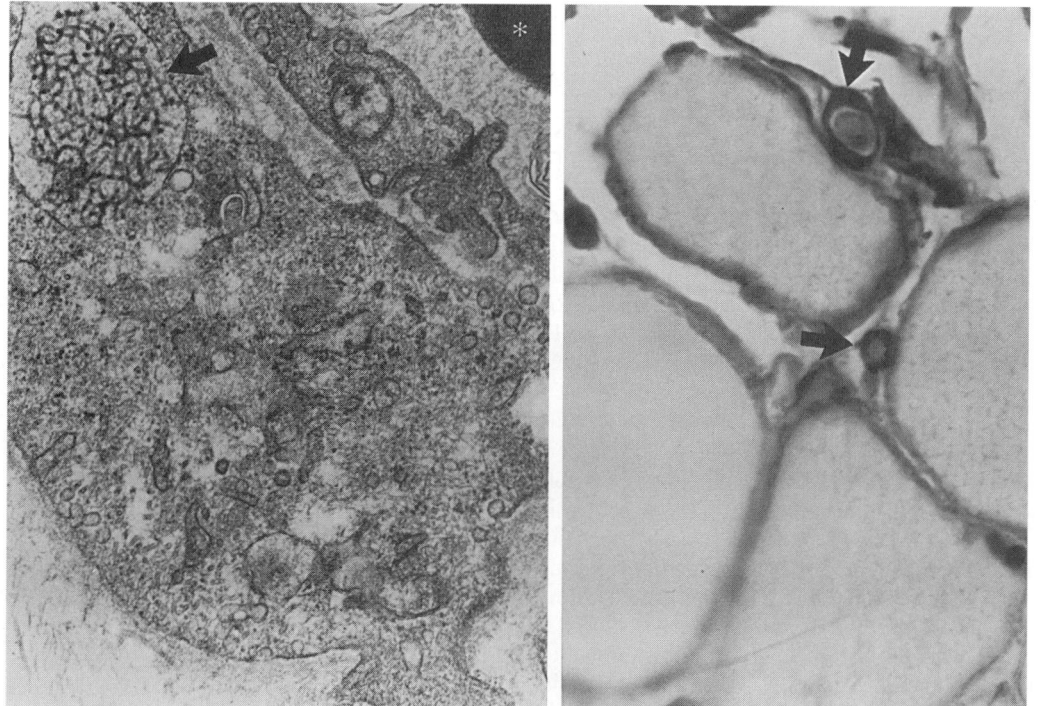

FIG. 107-2. Dermatomyositis. **(A)** Electron micrograph showing undulating tubular arrays in a capillary endothelial cell; *-Red blood cell (× 8,000). **(B)** Membranolytic attack complex (MAC) deposition in capillaries. (Frozen section; MAC antibody; × 150.)

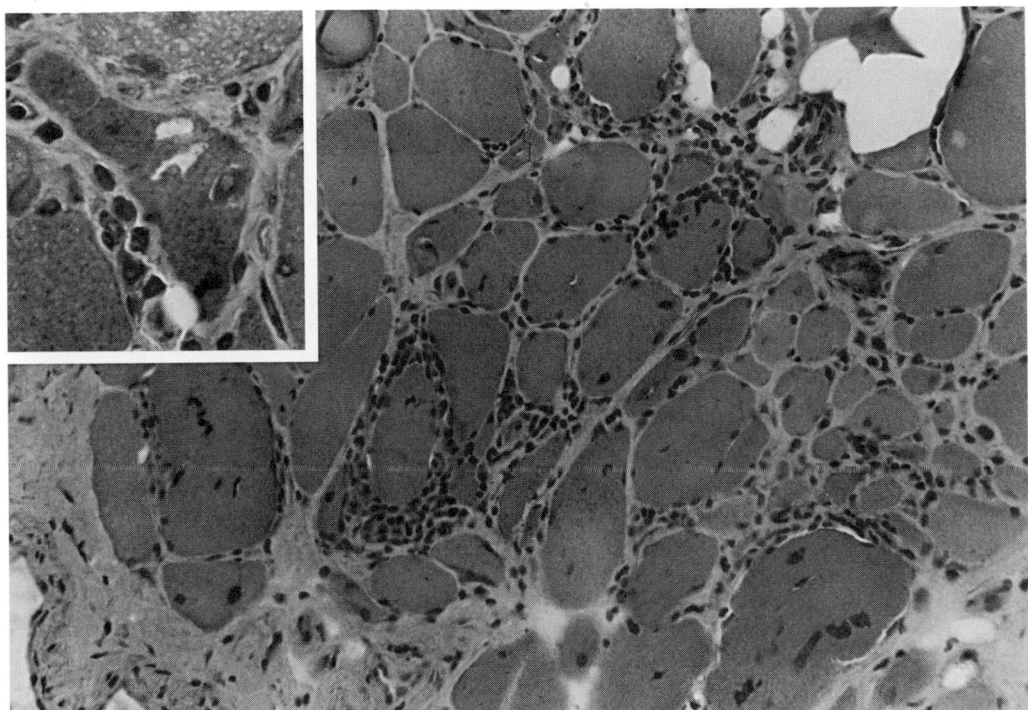

FIG. 107-3. Inclusion body myositis. Endomysial inflammatory infiltrate (lymphocytes, macrophages) surrounds nonnecrotic fiber. Chronic myopathic changes are also seen: variation in fiber size, split fiber, internalized nuclei, small groups of atrophic fibers. (Frozen section; hematoxylin-eosin; × 50.) (Inset) Rimmed vacuole in a small angulated fiber. (Frozen section; Gomori trichrome; × 150.)

fied. These include the presence of an underlying malignancy or an established collagen-vascular disorder, advanced age, and delay in the institution of adequate doses of corticosteroids soon after onset of clinically significant weakness interfering with daily activities. Other features such as the severity of the weakness at onset of the disease, degree of elevation of the creatine kinase level, and extent of abnormality of the muscle biopsy do not necessarily correlate with outcome.

Because of the presumed autoimmune pathogenesis of these disorders, the mainstay of pharmacologic therapy is immunosuppression. Treatment with corticosteroids has been based on empirical evidence and not on adequately controlled trials. Nonetheless, we join most investigators in the view that corticosteroid therapy is beneficial in polymyositis and dermatomyositis; inclusion body myositis differs in that it responds poorly to any type of therapy and probably accounts for polymyositis cases previously believed to be treatment-resistant. Two-thirds of the corticosteroid-treated patients with polymyositis and dermatomyositis improve to the point of no functional disability after 3 years of therapy (see Devere and Bradley, 1975). Many patients will require a low dose of corticosteroids to remain asymptomatic, although a few may be able to completely discontinue all medications.

We recommend treating patients with polymyositis or dermatomyositis whose weakness interferes with activities of daily living. In Table 107-3 we summarize our management strategies. High-dose prednisone is maintained for 6 to 8 weeks, followed by a gradual taper if improvement is sustained for several weeks. Improvement usually occurs 2 to 8 weeks after initiation of therapy. Patients who respond well have a substantial return of function in the first 4 to 6 months of treatment. Some patients will not improve even after 3 months of corticosteroid therapy. At that point, addition of cytotoxic immunosup-

pressive agents such as azathioprine, cytoxan, and methotrexate is probably indicated, but, while successful in some, in many patients improvement may be only partial and slow in coming. Plasmapheresis and total body low-dose irradiation have also been used in these disorders. In refractory cases of dermatomyositis, intravenous immunoglobulin produces short-lived improvement.

Although inclusion body myositis has been recognized for some time as a disorder refractory to immunosuppressant treatment, some investigators have reported improvement with corticosteroids. It has been our practice to carefully weigh the risks and benefits of corticosteroids and recommend a 3-month

TABLE 107-3. Management of Inflammatory Myopathies

Specific Therapy	Guidelines for Use
Corticosteroids (prednisone) 60 mg PO qd for 6–8 weeks If sustained improvement for several weeks, taper slowly to qod schedule (taper by 10 mg/month) Once on qod schedule, taper by 5 mg/month At 30 mg/day, taper by 2.5 mg/month schedule	Supplement vitamin D and calcium Low-salt diet, antacids Follow weight, glucose, lytes Exercise program
Azathioprine[a] If no response to prednisone after 6–8 weeks Begin with 50 mg PO qd[b] Increase by 50 mg/week to total daily dose of 2–3 mg/kg	Monitor complete blood count, white blood cells, platelets, and transaminases weekly until reach maintenance dose Goal is absolute lymphocyte count of 1,000 and mean corpuscular volume greater than 100 Follow laboratory studies every 2 months

[a] We prefer azathioprine; others choose methotrexate or cyclophosphamide.
[b] This is a test dose; 10% develop a severe flulike reaction and the drug must be stopped.

treatment trial with prednisone if the patient is otherwise healthy and is at a relatively early stage of the disease. In our experience, a positive response to therapy is unusual.

In patients on long-term corticosteroid therapy, corticosteroid-related myopathy is a consideration when an increase in weakness occurs without a major change in the creatine kinase levels, especially if the urinary creatine level is elevated. If a trial of reduced corticosteroid therapy leads to improvement in strength, the diagnosis of corticosteroid-related myopathy is confirmed. An EMG study may also help to distinguish corticosteroid-related myopathy from an exacerbation of inflammatory myopathy: in the latter we expect abundant fibrillation potential activity in weak muscles, while in the former these potentials are generally absent.

CONCLUSION

The inflammatory myopathies include three rather distinct entities: polymyositis, dermatomyositis, and inclusion body myositis. Diagnosis of dermatomyositis is usually fairly straightforward because there are very few other conditions that present with weakness and a rash. In addition, the muscle histopathology of perifascicular atrophy and capillary damage is characteristic. The diagnosis of polymyositis is more challenging because the differential diagnosis of proximal muscle weakness is extensive. When weakness, however, is joined by elevation in the level of serum creatine kinase, myopathic EMG with fibrillation potentials, and inflammatory cells surrounding nonnecrotic muscle fibers in a biopsy specimen, the diagnosis becomes more secure. When the clinician suspects polymyositis or dermatomyositis, a careful assessment of cardiac and pulmonary function should be undertaken because of the propensity of these diseases to affect the heart and lung. In addition searches for associated collagen-vascular disorders and malignancy (especially in dermatomyositis), are warranted. The diagnostic process is most difficult in inclusion body myositis because it evolves so slowly with features that may suggest a chronic neurogenic disorder. The serum creatine kinase level may be only minimally elevated, and the EMG may show a complex pattern of mixed myopathic and neuropathic changes. The muscle histopathology of rimmed vacuoles and filamentous inclusions is, however, fairly specific and establishes the diagnosis.

The inflammatory myopathies are felt to be immune-mediated disorders with humeral immunity playing an important role against the microvasculature in dermatomyositis, while lymphocytes are directed against the myofibers in polymyositis and inclusion body myositis. Although still predominantly used as a research tool, the recently discovered myositis-specific autoantibodies will help identify patients with associated pulmonary and connective tissue disorders and possibly help predict their clinical course.

The treatment of polymyositis and dermatomyositis with prednisone is usually gratifying, especially if it has been instituted relatively early in the courses of these diseases. Unfortunately, inclusion body myositis is often refractory to any of the traditional immunotherapies, but it is critically important to recognize this condition, thereby avoiding prolonged use of potentially toxic therapies.

SUGGESTED READINGS

Bohan A, Peter JB, Bowman RL et al: A computer-assisted analysis of 153 patients with polymyositis and dermatomyositis. Medicine (Baltimore) 56: 255, 1977

Callen JP: Dermatomyositis and malignancy. Clin Dermatol 11:61, 1993
Carpenter S, Karpati G: The major inflammatory myopathies of unknown cause. Pathol Annu 16:205, 1981
Dalakas MC: Polymyositis, dermatomyositis, and inclusion-body myositis. N Engl J Med 325:1487, 1991
Devere R, Bradley WG: Polymyositis: its presentation, morbidity and mortality. Brain 98:637, 1975
Haupt HM, Hutchins GM: The heart and cardiac conduction system in polymyositis-dermatomyositis: a clinicopathologic study of 16 autopsied patients. Am J Cardiol 50:998, 1982
Mastaglia FL, Ojeda VJ: Inflammatory myopathies. Ann Neurol 17:215,317, 1985
Rowland LP, Clark C, Olarte M: Therapy for dermatomyositis and polymyositis. p. XVII:451. In Griggs RC, Moxley RT (eds): Advances in Neurology. Vol. 17. Raven Press, New York, 1977
Sigurgeirsson B, Lindelof B, Edhag O et al: Risk of cancer in patients with dermatomyositis or polymyositis. N Engl J Med 326:363, 1992
Stonecipher MR, Callen JP, Jorizzo JL: The red face: dermatomyositis. Clin Dermatol 11:261, 1993
Targoff IN: Autoantibodies in polymyositis. Rheum Dis Clin North Am 18: 455, 1992

108. ENDOCRINE, NUTRITIONAL, AND DRUG-INDUCED MYOPATHIES

JOSHUA J. SUNSHINE
HENRY J. KAMINSKI
ROBERT L. RUFF

This chapter describes the skeletal muscle disorders associated with hyper- and hypofunction of the adrenal, thyroid, parathyroid, and pituitary glands. Iatrogenic steroid myopathy and its differentiation from inflammatory myopathy are discussed. Muscle weakness associated with osteomalacia, alcohol abuse, and as side effects from medication are also discussed. The muscle disorders associated with endocrine disorders are summarized in Table 108-1 and the toxic myopathies, in Table 108-2.

ADRENAL DYSFUNCTION AND IATROGENIC STEROID MYOPATHY

Glucocorticoid and Adrenocorticotropic Hormone

Between 50 and 80 percent of patients with Cushing's disease and up to 21 percent of patients treated with glucocorticoids for more than 6 months develop weakness and myalgias insidiously. Proximal leg weakness and myalgias are most common, while cranial nerve–innervated muscles and sphincters are usually spared. Serum levels of muscle-associated enzymes (lactate dehydrogenase [LDH], serum glutamic oxoloacetic transaminase [SGOT], creatine kinase, and aldolase) are usually normal. Patients with Cushing's disease and iatrogenic steroid myopathy share similar clinical and biochemical profiles. Patients with glucocorticoid-induced myopathy usually manifest one of the following signs of glucocorticoid excess: moon facies, buffalo hump, fragile skin, or osteoporosis.

Large-dose glucocorticoid treatment for asthma may result

TABLE 108-1. Summary of Endocrine Myopathies

Metabolic Disorder	Pattern of Weakness	Serum Level of Muscle Enzymes	Electromyographic	Other
Glucocorticoid excess	Proximal	Normal	Motor unit potentials are of low amplitude and short duration	Buffalo hump, fragile skin, osteoporoses
Inflammatory	Generalized but greater proximally	Elevated		
Adrenal insufficiency	Generalized and cramping	Normal	Normal	Exercise or excessive K$^+$ intake may result in flaccid quadriparesis
Hyperthyroidism	Proximal weakness out of proportion to atrophy; bulbar involvement	Usually normal; may be elevated in thyroid storm	80% have short-duration motor unit potentials	May be associated with myasthenia gravis
Thyrotoxic periodic paralysis	Flaccid generalized weakness	Normal	Impaired muscle fiber excitability	Usually associated with hypokalemia
Endocrine ophthalmopathy	Restricted to extraocular muscles	Usually normal or mildly elevated		May be unilateral or bilateral; patient may be hyper-, eu-, or hypothyroid
Hypothyroidism	Proximal weakness	Elevated	Usually normal, but low-amplitude polyphasic motor unit potentials, increased insertional activity, and positive waves may be seen	Myoedema
Growth hormone excess	Proximal weakness with minimal atrophy	Slightly elevated	50% of patients have myopathic changes; hypertrophic neuropathy and nerve entrapment of median nerve may also be present	Nerve entrapments are common
Hypopituitarism	Severe weakness and fatigability	Usually normal		
Hyperparathyroidism	Proximal and atrophic bulbar and sphincter muscles are spared	Normal	Decreased motor unit potential sizes; increased frequency of polyphasic potentials with activity	Primary hyperparathyroidism has increased [Ca^{2+}] and alkaline phosphatase, reduced [PO$_4^{2-}$] and brisk reflexes
Osteomalacia	Proximal weakness, wasting, myalgia	Usually normal	Short duration, low-amplitude polyphasic motor unit potentials	
Hypoparathyroidism	Tetanic mild weakness	Mildy elevated		Decreased [Ca^{2+}] and [Mg^{2+}] and distal numbness

in an acute myopathy that develops within a few days of administration. Several factors appear to contribute to the rapid onset of weakness and wasting in this population: (1) immobility may accelerate the onset of myopathy, (2) curarelike agents may potentiate the action of glucocorticoids, and (3) concurrent sepsis may accelerate muscle proteolysis.

Electromyographic (EMG) findings are variable. Typically, insertional activity is normal and the motor unit potentials are of low amplitude and short duration.

Glucocorticoids alter muscle carbohydrate and protein metabolism and may interfere with intracellular calcium homeostasis. Although the exact interaction of steroid-induced metabolic and physiologic changes in the production of steroid myopathy is not precisely known, it appears that the net result of glucocorticoids is to induce muscle protein catabolism.

Steroid myopathy is treated by decreasing the steroid dosage to the lowest possible level, adapting an alternate-day dosing schedule and converting to a nonfluorinated steroid. Exercise may be useful in preventing and treating muscle weakness and wasting in patients receiving glucocorticoids. Recovery may take many weeks.

Elevated levels of adrenocorticotropic hormone (ACTH) may be myopathic. Some patients treated for Cushing's disease with bilateral adrenalectomy develop hyperpigmentation and either clinical, EMG, or biopsy evidence of myopathy in spite of adequate glucocorticoid replacement. Their myopathy differs pathologically and clinically from steroid myopathy. Proximal weakness and wasting may develop up to 1 year after adrenalectomy. The exact mechanism of ACTH-induced myopathy is not known at this time.

Glucocorticoid Versus Inflammatory Myopathy. Steroid myopathy may be difficult to distinguish from inflammatory myopathy; however, some clinical clues may help. Weakness that occurs within 4 weeks of the onset of steroid treatment is likely from a flare in the inflammatory process and is best treated by continuing or increasing the dose of glucocorticoid. Elevated muscle enzymes suggest a flare-up of inflammatory myopathy. However, normal enzyme levels do not rule out a flare-up of an inflammatory myopathy. Weakness without any other stigmata of steroid use is likely from inflammation. Muscle biopsy will distinguish inflammatory myopathy from steroid myopathy only if active inflammation is found.

Adrenal Insufficiency

Adrenal insufficiency may cause severe generalized weakness, muscle cramping, and fatigue in approximately 25 to 50 percent of patients. Addison's disease may also produce respiratory muscle weakness and precipitate myasthenia gravis. The weakness and fatigue usually correct rapidly with glucocorticoid replacement. The serum levels of muscle-associated enzymes are usually normal, as is the EMG. Muscle biopsy is unremarkable except for diminished glycogen content.

TABLE 108-2. Summary of Toxic Myopathies

Toxic Etiologies	Pattern of Weakness	Serum Level of Muscle Enzymes	Other Considerations
Prescribed medications and vitamins			
Clofibrate, bezafibrate, etofibrate, biclofibrate, lovastatin, and gemfibrozil (hypocholesterolemic drugs)	Weakness, cramps, tenderness, painful proximal myopathy	Elevated	Myotonia may develop with clofibrate and related agents; lovastatin and clofibrate myopathies most likely to occur with renal failure or hypothyroidism
Labetalol	Generalized	Elevated	Other β-adrenergic agents can exacerbate myasthenia gravis (blockers) or myotonia (β₂-agonists or blockers)
ε-Amino caproic acid	Axial and proximal muscles	Elevated	Therapy duration more than 4 weeks; disseminated proximal muscle fiber necrosis on biopsy
Chloroquine	Progressive proximal muscle wasting	Elevated	Myopathy after patients take at least 500 mg/d for at least 1 year
Emetine	Proximal and axial	Elevated	Reversible and related to dose and duration of therapy
Colchicine	Proximal	Elevated	Associated with sensory neuropathy
Vincristine	Proximal	Usually not elevated	Neuropathy is a more common side effect of this agent
D-Penicillamine	Proximal myopathy	Elevated	Resembles polymyositis; may involve myocardium
Procainamide	Proximal	Elevated	Interstitial myositis as part of drug-induced lupus syndrome
Azidothymidine (AZT)	Proximal	Mild elevation	Mitochondrial myopathy with ragged red fibers
Cyclosporine	Generalized	Usually mild elevation	Myopathy may be severe when used with lovastatin or colchicine
Hypervitaminosis E	Proximal and painless	Elevated	Usually occurs when the patient overuses an over-the-counter preparation
Vitamin E deficiency	Generalized, including extraocular	Mild elevation	Usually associated with lipid malabsorption
Etretinate	Proximal	Usually mild elevation or normal	Myalgias present; may need to distinguish from psoriatic arthritis
Isotretinoin	Proximal	Usually mild elevation or normal	Arthralgias may also be present
Nonprescription drugs			
Cocaine	May be focal or generalized	Elevated	Myoglobinuria may develop from myoischemia
Heroin	May be focal or generalized	Elevated	Muscle necrosis usually develops as a consequence of pressure necrosis
Phencyclidine (PCP)	Generalized	Elevated	Muscle injury may be a consequence of overactivity
Ethanol			
Acute necrotizing myopathy	Generalized or focal; pain is prominent	Elevated	Myoglobinuria may result in renal failure in severe cases
Acute hypokalemia myopathy	Generalized flaccid weakness	May be normal or slightly elevated	May be painful when associated with hypomagnesemia
Other			
Chronic myopathy	Proximal	Elevated	May represent a combination of ethanol-induced damage and poor nutrition

Patients with primary adrenal insufficiency may develop flaccid quadriparesis associated with hyperkalemia. The disorder is triggered by intake of potassium or by exercise and resolves with lowering the serum potassium by glucose administration or glucocorticoid replacement.

Contributing factors to muscle weakness and fatigability in adrenal insufficiency are circulatory insufficiency (exercise-induced hypotension), fluid and electrolyte imbalance (hyponatremia, hyperkalemia, and hypovolemia), impaired carbohydrate metabolism, and starvation. The treatment for Addisonian myopathy is glucocorticoid and mineralocorticoid replacement.

THYROID DISEASE

Hyperthyroidism

Hyperthyroidism can cause weakness that usually begins several months after the onset of thyrotoxicosis. Proximal weakness is common and is often out of proportion to muscle atrophy. Arms may be affected more than legs, which results in scapular winging and shoulder girdle wasting. Distal weakness can occur but usually develops later and is less severe than proximal weakness. Severe atrophy can occur in some patients.

Thyrotoxic patients commonly complain of fatigue, exercise intolerance, myalgias, and breathlessness. Respiratory insufficiency requiring ventilatory support may occur. Bulbar muscles and the esophagus may be involved. Sphincters are usually spared. Serum levels of creatine kinase, SGOT, LDH, and myoglobin are usually normal or low. However, in thyroid storm, serum creatine kinase may be extremely high in association with rhabdomyolysis. Weakness and atrophy are proportional to the duration of illness and not the severity of the thyrotoxicosis. Thyrotoxicosis causes biochemical and electrophysiologic derangements in muscle that result in reduced efficiency of contraction, which is consistent with the clinical observation that weakness is usually more severe than atrophy. Weakness generally resolves when thyroid hormone levels are normalized.

The sudden onset of generalized weakness with bulbar palsy in thyrotoxic patients may be acute myasthenia gravis and a Tensilon test and antiacetylcholine receptor antibody titers are warranted.

There is a significantly greater incidence of thyroid disorders in patients with myasthenia gravis than expected by chance: 5.7 percent of myasthenic patients are hyperthyroid, 5.3 percent are hypothyroid, and 2.1 percent have nontoxic goiter. In addition, 8 to 17 percent of euthyroid myasthenic patients have circulating antithyroid antibodies. The incidence of thyroid disease in the general population is only approximately 1.5 percent. Conversely, approximately 0.35 percent of patients with hyperthyroidism have myasthenia gravis, which is 30 times higher than the prevalence of myasthenia gravis in the general population. Thyrotoxicosis usually precedes or develops simultaneously with myasthenia gravis. Rarely, signs of thyrotoxicosis will appear after myasthenia gravis is diagnosed. Both hyperthyroidism and hypothyroidism worsen the course of myasthenia gravis.

Thyrotoxic myopathy is treated by returning the patient to the euthyroid state. β-Adrenergic blocking agents may improve muscle strength, especially of respiratory muscles. Glucocorticoids block the peripheral conversion of thyroxine to triiodothyronine and may be useful in the acute treatment of thyrotoxicosis.

Thyrotoxic Periodic Paralysis

Thyrotoxic periodic paralysis, a complication of thyrotoxicosis, is clinically manifested as weakness lasting minutes to days that is either generalized (proximal > distal) or involves groups of muscles that were recently exercised or cooled. Bulbar and respiratory muscles are involved later or are spared. Occasionally, respiratory function may be compromised during severe attacks. Sphincters are usually spared. Serum potassium is usually decreased during the attack. However, normokalemia has been reported. Serum phosphate may also be reduced.

Most cases of thyrotoxic periodic paralysis are sporadic, whereas the majority of cases of familial hypokalemic periodic paralysis are familial. The age of onset is over 20 in over 90 percent of cases of thyrotoxic periodic paralysis compared with 60 percent of patients with familial hypokalemic periodic paralysis having their first attack before 16 years of age. The male/female ratio is approximately 6:1 in thyrotoxic periodic paralysis compared with 3:1 in familial hypokalemic periodic paralysis. Most of the reported cases of thyrotoxic periodic paralysis have occurred in Oriental patients and Native Americans, whereas familial hyperkalemic periodic paralysis is uncommon in Orientals.

The mainstay of treatment of thyrotoxic periodic paralysis is to return the patient to a euthyroid state. Propranolol alone successfully prevented paralytic attacks in some cases. Mild exercise may abort an impending attack. The treatment for acute paralytic attacks is potassium replacement, respiratory support, and airway protection.

Endocrine Ophthalmopathy

Graves' disease is manifested by a triad of goiter, restrictive ophthalmopathy, and infiltrative dermopathy. The ophthalmopathy is secondary to inflammation, edema, and fibrosis of the extraocular muscles and orbital fat. Enlargement of the orbital contents frequently results in exophthalmos and diplopia. Exophthalmos, usually painful, is commonly bilateral. However, Graves' ophthalmopathy is the most common cause of unilateral exophthalmos. Vision may be impaired by exposure-induced corneal ulceration and keratitis or optic nerve compromise by retro-orbital mechanical congestion and vascular compromise. The ocular changes of Graves' disease may precede thyroid dysfunction by months or years, occur concurrently with hyperthyroidism, or become apparent when the pa-

tient becomes hypothyroid in the course of treatment. Multiple muscle involvement with fusiform expansion and smoothly tapering margins into tendon insertions and uniform contrast enhancement are typical features on computed tomography (CT). Magnetic resonance imaging (MRI) reveals muscle enlargement in the majority of patients with Graves' disease. Some patients with high-grade ophthalmopathy manifest areas of increased signal on T2-weighted images consistent with orbital edema.

Mild ocular changes usually respond to topical adrenergic blocking agents. Guanethidine eye drops (5 percent) can be used for prolonged periods without systemic side effects. Exposure keratitis can be prevented by protecting the eye during the day with glasses and ophthalmic ointment and taping the eyelids at night. Surgery may be required for lid retraction that does not respond to adrenergic blocking agents. Edema of the lids and conjunctiva will often respond to local injections of glucocorticoids.

Indications for orbital decompression surgery are (1) compressive optic neuropathy not responsive to glucocorticoids, (2) exposure keratopathy, and (3) cosmesis. Extraocular muscle operations are sometimes required to correct diplopia or severe limitation of movement and are successful in relieving diplopia in 90 percent of patients.

Hypothyroidism

The primary manifestations of myopathy in hypothyroidism are insidious onset of proximal weakness, fatigue, decreased reflexes, slowed movements, myalgia, myoedema (painless, electrically silent local contraction produced by tapping or pinching the muscle), and less commonly, cramps and/or muscle enlargement. Respiratory muscle weakness occurs in a few cases. Muscle disease can occur without myxedema. Myoedema occurs in about one-third of hypothyroid patients but is also seen in a variety of disorders associated with malnutrition and wasting.

Serum creatine kinase activity is elevated in most hypothyroid patients whether or not other evidence of muscle disease is present. In symptomatic patients creatine kinase activity may be more than 10-fold higher than normal. Creatine kinase levels correct rapidly with thyroid replacement.

Distal paresthesias and entrapment neuropathy are common in hypothyroidism. However, neuropathy is not responsible for the weakness. EMG usually reveals myopathic changes.

Impaired energy metabolism may limit force generation in hypothyroidism. Repair and replacement of myofibrillar proteins may be restricted by reduced protein turnover. Slow contraction and relaxation appear to reflect diminished myosin adenosine triphosphatase activity and impaired calcium uptake by the SR. Diminished cardiac output and reduced β-adrenergic sensitivity may contribute to exercise intolerance. As in hyperthyroidism, multiple biochemical and physiologic derangements reduce muscle efficiency in hypothyroidism.

The only effective treatment is to restore the patient to a euthyroid state. Weakness improves slowly and can persist up to 1 year after a euthyroid state is achieved.

Pituitary Dysfunction

Growth Hormone Excess. Acromegalic patients may develop an insidious onset of proximal weakness with minimal muscle wasting. Serum levels of creatine kinase or aldolase may be slightly elevated. Approximately 50 percent of acromegalic patients have myopathic changes on EMG. Diffuse hypertrophic neuropathy and/or nerve entrapment, usually of the median nerve, develops in about half of the acromegalic patients. Thus, it is possible to find myopathic changes in the deltoid and neuropathic changes in the opponens pollicis. The neuropathy and myopathy develop independently and follow separate courses.

In spite of increased fiber diameter, acromegalics have decreased force-generating capacity. Decreased sarcolemmal excitability and reduced myofibrillar adenosine triphosphatase activity may contribute to the weakness. Impaired carbohydrate metabolism and possibly restricted muscle blood flow may also partially explain the fatigability. The exact etiology of growth hormone excess myopathy is not clear.

The myopathy usually resolves after growth hormone levels return to normal. Surgical removal is the currently preferred treatment for growth hormone–secreting pituitary tumors. Focused α-radiation is an alternative treatment, particularly for large tumors. Bromocriptine may be useful as an adjunct to surgical therapy or radiotherapy.

Pituitary Insufficiency.   Pituitary failure in adults (Simmonds disease) causes severe weakness and fatigability with disproportionate preservation of muscle mass. Thyroid and adrenal cortex hormone loss are primarily responsible for the myopathy, with less of a contribution from growth hormone loss. The causes of adult panhypopituitarism include thrombosis of the pituitary circulation, pituitary or hypothalamic tumors, head injury, granulomatous destruction, and meningitis.

In adults, the major deficits stem from loss of thyroid and adrenal corticohormones, and treatment is therefore appropriate replacement. Children, however, require growth hormone for normal muscle development.

PRIMARY AND SECONDARY HYPERPARATHYROIDISM AND METABOLIC BONE DISEASE

Primary Hyperparathyroidism

Primary hyperparathyroidism commonly results in symmetric proximal weakness and atrophy. Patients often complain of weakness and fatigability, and severely affected patients may have a waddling gait or be unable to walk. The bulbar muscles and sphincters are usually spared. Tendon reflexes may be brisk. Significant laboratory findings include elevated urinary creatine excretion and normal levels of creatine kinase and aldolase. Serum alkaline phosphatase and calcium concentrations are increased, and the serum phosphate is low. The severity of the weakness does not correlate with serum calcium or phosphate concentrations. In addition to myopathy, a peripheral neuropathy occurs in some patients with hyperparathyroidism. Parathyroidectomy appears to alleviate symptoms and improve strength.

Secondary Hyperparathyroidism

A resistance to the metabolic actions of parathyroid hormone results in secondary hyperparathyroidism. This may lead to a myopathy that is indistinguishable from primary hyperparathyroidism. Chronic renal insufficiency is also a common cause for secondary hyperparathyroidism and myopathy. Parathyroid hormone excess, uremic toxins, vitamin D deficiency, aluminum toxicity, and carnitine deficiency have all been implicated in the pathogenesis of this myopathy.

Osteomalacia secondary to malnutrition, malabsorption of vitamin D, or abnormal vitamin D metabolism may present as proximal muscle weakness, atrophy, and myalgias. The clinical presentation is also similar to that of primary hyperparathyroidism.

Despite their diverse etiologies, the muscle disorders associated with primary or secondary hyperparathyroidism and osteomalacia appear to result from either elevations in parathyroid hormone (primary and secondary hyperparathyroidism) and/or impaired action of vitamin D (secondary hyperparathyroidism and osteomalacia). Treatment of these disorders is directed at removing the primary cause. Consequently, patients with primary hyperparathyroidism improve with removal of the adenoma, and the myopathy of osteomalacia improves with vitamin D replacement. Patients with chronic renal failure may benefit from partial removal of hyperfunctioning parathyroid glands and treatment with $1,25(OH)_2D_3$ or $1\text{-}OH\text{-}D_3$, which can be converted in the lung to $1,25(OH)_2D_3$. Renal transplantation may improve weakness.

Hypoparathyroidism and Pseudohypoparathyroidism

Hypoparathyroidism is most commonly caused by surgical excision of the parathyroid glands or damage to their vascular supply. Idiopathic hypoparathyroidism can exist as an isolated entity, in association with thymic agenesis (DiGeorge syndrome), or as part of a familial condition associated with deficiency of adrenal, thyroid, and gonadal function. Pseudohypoparathyroidism is a defective cellular response to parathyroid hormone associated with either a normal or elevated level of parathyroid hormone. It is characterized by signs of hypoparathyroidism in association with distinctive skeletal anomalies and frequently intellectual impairment. In both pseudo- and true hypoparathyroidism, patients are hypocalcemic and hypomagnesemic, and the most frequently associated muscle disorder is tetany. Hypomagnesemia or hypocalcemia results in hyperexcitability of nerve fibers. This is manifested as perioral and distal paresthesias, carpopedal spasm, and diffuse muscle cramping. In severe cases, laryngeal muscle spasm can occur.

The treatment of choice is intravenous infusion of calcium 15 to 20 mg/kg body weight over 4 to 6 hours. In severe cases accompanied by seizures, 1 to 2 ampules of calcium gluconate can be administered by slow intravenous push with simultaneous monitoring of heart rate and blood pressure. If hypomagnesemia is present, 1 g magnesium sulfate can be given by slow intravenous push. The magnesium dose must be reduced in the presence of renal insufficiency.

Chronic treatment of hypocalcemia requires dietary supplementation of 2 to 5 g/day of elemental calcium, and vitamin D. Magnesium supplementation is required for hypomagnesemia. Myopathy rarely complicates hypoparathyroidism. Weakness and CPK elevation may be relatively mild, and muscle biopsy may be normal or show atrophic fibers. In addition to correcting hypocalcemia, hypomagnesemia, and hyperphosphatemia, calcium supplementation and vitamin D treatment help correct the myopathy. A similar syndrome has been described in patients with pseudohypoparathyroidism who had elevated serum creatine kinase and LDH activity without weakness. The serum levels of muscle-associated enzymes normalized with calcium and vitamin D treatment. The relation between these syndromes and hypoparathyroidism or pseudohypoparathyroidism is unclear. Some patients with mitochondrial myopathy have associated hypoparathyroidism.

TOXIC MYOPATHIES

Prescription Medications

Myalgias or muscle cramping has been reported with a large number of medications, including captopril, cimetidine, clofibrate, clofibride, colchicine, cytotoxic agents (particularly in a setting of cachexia), danazol, diuretics (particularly in association with hypokalemia), D-penicillamine, enalapril, ethylchorvynol, gold, isoetharine, labetalol, lithium, L-tryptophan, mercaptopropionylglycine, metolazone, nifedipine (and other similar calcium channel blockers), pindolol, procainamide (with or without a drug-induced lupus syndrome), rifampicin, salbutamol, suxamethonium, azidothymidine (AZT), and zimeldine. Myopathic conditions associated with specific medication are discussed below.

Hypocholesterolemic Drugs. Lovastatin, a 3-hydroxy-3-methylglutaryl-coenzyme A reductase inhibitor, will rarely cause a myopathy when used alone. However, when used with either gemfibrozil or cyclosporine, myopathy will more likely develop. Patients with severe hepatobiliary dysfunction or renal insufficiency may be at a higher risk of developing a myopathy when using lovastatin alone.

Clofibrate and related agents, bezafibrate, etofibrate, biclofibrate, lovostatin, and gemfibrozil, may induce a myopathy characterized by the acute onset of cramps, weakness, and tenderness with an elevation of serum transaminases and creatine kinase. Myotonia may develop in some patients in response to hypocholesterolemic agents, especially clofibrate. Accumulation of the active metabolite of clofibrate, chlorophenoxyisobutyric acid, may occur in renal failure, nephrotic syndrome, and hypothyroidism and may be the etiology of the myopathy. Some patients may also have an associated peripheral neuropathy. Decreasing the dose or halting the drug will be followed by gradual recovery.

Medications That Act on the Autonomic Nervous System. Labetalol, a selective α_1- and nonselective β-adrenergic receptor blocker, may produce a severe generalized myopathy with markedly elevated creatine kinase that improves with discontinuation of the medication. β-Adrenergic blockers may interfere with neuromuscular transmission and exacerbate myasthenia gravis. Some β_2-selective blockers or agonists can exacerbate myotonia.

ϵ-Aminocaproic acid inhibits fibrinolysis and has been used in different bleeding disorders. A myopathy affecting axial musculature whose symptoms begin 4 or more weeks after initiation of treatment is an uncommon complication. The etiology may be altered muscle membrane function or ischemia to the muscles.

Chloroquine is an antimalarial agent that may cause a myopathy after treatment with at least 500 mg/day for at least 1 year. Progressive painless proximal muscle wasting and weakness is characteristic. An associated neuropathy and cardiomyopathy may occur. The myopathy is slowly reversible following discontinuation of the medication.

Emetine has been used as an amebicide, as an emetic in acute poisoning, and in alcoholic aversion therapy. Proximal limb and trunk muscles are primarily affected, but a generalized myopathy may also ensue. The degree of muscle damage depends on the dose of emetine and the duration of exposure. Emetine myopathy is reversible.

Colchicine may induce a proximal myopathy, especially in patients with renal insufficiency. Distal sensory involvement secondary to axonal neuropathy is common. Plasma colchicine and creatine kinase are usually elevated. Discontinuation of colchicine improves strength and the sensory neuropathy.

Although vincristine commonly causes an axonal peripheral neuropathy, some patients develop a proximal myopathy. These side effects are dose-related and usually disappear 6 weeks after finishing treatment. Some patients, however, continue to have symptoms for a prolonged period of time.

D-Penicillamine may cause an inflammatory myopathy indistinguishable from polymyositis. Immunoregulatory mechanisms may be altered by this medication. Myocardial involvement may be fatal. Halting use of the drug results in recovery.

Procainamide may cause interstitial myositis as part of a lupuslike vasculitic reaction.

AZT causes a progressive, painful mitochondrial myopathy. Creatine kinase is normal or only moderately elevated. A clear distinction between AZT myopathy and human immunodeficiency virus myositis is sometimes difficult to make. Human immunodeficiency virus myositis can resemble polymyositis with inflammatory infiltrates. AZT myopathy may be due to impaired mitochondrial function. Ragged red fibers can be found in AZT myopathy, but inflammatory infiltrates are usually not present.

Cyclosporine by itself may result in a mild myopathy; however, cyclosporine in combination with lovastatin or colchicine may produce a more severe myopathy with rhabdomyolysis.

Vitamins and Related Agents. Hypervitaminoses E may result in proximal muscle weakness and elevated serum creatine kinase. Etretinate is a vitamin A derivative that is used in treating psoriasis. Skeletal muscle damage is an uncommon side effect and is manifested as proximal muscle weakness and tenderness. Isotretinoin is used for treatment of severe acne. Mild and transient arthralgias and myalgias can occasionally be seen.

Miscellaneous Agents. Organophosphate exposure usually results in a neuropathy; however, a myopathy may also result secondary to increased neurotransmitter in the neuromuscular junction.

Hypokalemic myopathy may be a consequence of numerous etiologies. Weakness, hypotonia, and depressed deep tendon reflexes from hypokalemia may result from treatment with laxative overdose, thiazide diuretics, mineralocorticoids, and toluene abuse. Weakness in the proximal muscles can develop quickly and can progress to flaccid paralysis of the limbs. Serum creatine kinase is usually elevated. Potassium replacement usually results in complete recovery.

Illicit Drugs

Cocaine results in myoglobinuria. This is either a direct toxic effect from cocaine or secondary to cocaine-induced ischemia. Excessive amounts of sympathomimetic drugs may produce acute rhabdomyolysis, myoglobinuria, and renal failure.

Heroin ingestion commonly results in alteration in consciousness and subsequent pressure-induced damage to skeletal muscle.

Phencyclidine (PCP) ingestion may cause myoglobinuria and acute renal failure. Excessive isometric motor activity may be the cause of PCP myopathy, as PCP does not have a direct toxic effect on muscle.

Ethanol-Associated Myopathies

Ethanol is myotoxic and acute, hypokalemic, and possibly chronic forms of alcoholic myopathy exist. Acute necrotizing myopathy commonly occurs on the background of chronic alcohol abuse. Excessive ingestion of alcohol results in noninflammatory muscle necrosis characterized as an acute onset of severe muscle pain, cramps, weakness, swelling, and tenderness. This myopathy may be generalized or focal. When occurring in the calves, this myopathy can resemble venous thrombophlebitis. Recovery depends on the extent of muscle destruction and may take several months. Severe cases may result in acute renal failure.

Acute hypokalemic myopathy is a complication of chronic alcoholism. The acute onset of painless weakness in the proximal limb muscles and/or limb girdle muscles without muscle cramps, tenderness or swelling is characteristic. Serum creatine kinase and aldolase are elevated and serum potassium is low. The loss of potassium may occur through vomiting and diarrhea. Hypokalemia can also develop from alcohol-induced hypomagnesemia. When the patient is hypokalemic and hypomagnesemic, the myopathy is often painful. Strength improves with potassium and magnesium replacement.

The existence of a chronic alcoholic myopathy is controversial. Some feel that chronic alcohol use results in the insidious onset of painless proximal muscle weakness and wasting. Others feel this is secondary to a peripheral neuropathy. Patients with a history of acute alcoholic myopathy will experience an elevated serum creatine kinase and myoglobin more so than those who have not had alcoholic myopathy after the same amount of alcohol is consumed. Chronic drinkers who occasionally binge will experience elevated serum creatine kinase and myoglobin without clinical evidence for an acute myopathy. This is an asymptomatic form of chronic alcoholic myopathy that may progress to permanent proximal muscle weakness.

Nutritional Myopathies

The impact of vitamin D deficiency/osteomalacia on skeletal muscle is discussed above. Vitamin E deficiency may result in generalized muscle weakness, including ocular muscles.

Acute Myonecrosis Including Bites and Stings

Severe myonecrosis can occur as a consequence of general anesthesia, status epilepsy, or prolonged unconsciousness, and in the latter case, it is probably due to pressure necrosis. In addition, a large number of agents, including the venoms of several snakes and spiders, have been implicated in causing acute myonecrosis with myoglobinuria. This condition is associated with extreme elevation in serum levels of muscle-associated enzymes and myoglobinuria. Extreme muscle swelling may produce compartment syndromes, leading to nerve entrapments and limb ischemia. Numerous snake venoms are myotoxic at the bite site. However, others have more widespread effects, causing muscle necrosis and myoglobinuria. Snake venoms that are associated with diffuse rhabdomyolysis are the tiger snake, Tiapan, Mulga, and seasnake. The venom of the Arkansas and Honduran tarantulas causes irreversible injury to the muscle fiber plasma membranes, leading to diffuse myonecrosis.

ACKNOWLEDGMENTS

This work was supported by the Office of Research and Development, Medical Research Service of the Department of Veterans Affairs (Drs. Kaminski and Ruff). Dr. Kaminski was also supported by National Institutes of Health Grant EY-00332 and an Osserman fellowship from the Myasthenia Gravis Foundation. Dr. Ruff was also supported by the Muscular Dystrophy Association.

SUGGESTED READINGS

Delbridge L, Marshman D, Reeve T et al: Neuromuscular symptoms in elderly patients with hyperparathyroidism: improvement with parathyroid surgery. Med J Aust 149:74, 1988

Floyd M, Ayyar D, Barwick D et al: Myopathy in chronic renal failure. Q J Med 63:509, 1974

Hosten N, Sander B, Cordes M et al: Graves ophthalmopathy: MR imaging of the orbits. Radiology 172:759, 1989

Jamal G, Kerr D, McLellan A et al: Generalized peripheral nerve dysfunction in acromegaly: a study by conventional and novel neurophysiological techniques. J Neurol Neurosurg Psychiatry 50:886, 1987

Kaminski HJ, Ruff RL: Endocrine myopathies (hyper- and hypofunction of adrenal, thyroid, pituitary glands and iatrogenic glucorticoid myopathy). p. 1726. In Engel AG, Franzini-Armstrong C (eds): Myology. 2nd Ed. McGraw-Hill, New York, 1994

Kissl JT, Mendell JR: The endocrine myopathies. p. 527. In Rowland LP, DiMauro S (eds): Myopathies. Vol. 62. Handbook of Clinical Neurology. Elsevier, New York, 1992

Martinez F, Bermudez-Gomez M, Celli B: Hypothyrodism. A reversible cause of diaphragmatic dysfunction. Chest 96:1059, 1989

Mastaglia FL: Toxic Myopathies. p. 595. In Rowland LP, DiMauro S (eds): Myopathies. Vol. 62. Handbook of Clinical Neurology. Elsevier, New York, 1992

McElvaney G, Wilcox P, Fairbarn M et al: Respiratory muscle weakness and dyspnea in thyrotoxic patients. Am Rev Respir Dis 141:1221, 1990

Miller D, Delcastillo J, Tsang T: Severe hypokalemia in thyrotoxic periodic paralysis. Am J Emerg Med 7:584, 1989

Mouritis M, Koorneef L, Van Mourik-Noordenbos A et al: Extraocular muscle surgery for Graves' opthalmopathy: does prior treatment influence surgical outcome. Br J Opthalmol 1990:481, 1990

Nora N, Berns A: Hypokalemic, hypophosphatemic thyrotoxic periodic paralysis. Am J Kidney Dis 13:247, 1989

Ruff RL: Acute viral myositis, virus-induced complex myositis and myoglobinuria. p. 193. In McKendall RR (ed): Viral Disease. Vol. 56. Handbook of Clinical Neurology. Elsevier, Amsterdam, 1989

Ruff RL, Gordon AM: Disorders of muscle: The periodic paralyses. p. 59. In Andreoli TE, Fanestil DD, Hoffman JF, Schultz SG (eds): Physiology of Membrane Disorders. Plenum, New York, 1986

Shee C: Risk factors for hydrocortisone myopathy in acute severe asthma. Respir Med 84:229, 1990

Turken S, Cafferty M, Silverberg S et al: Neuromuscular involvement in mild, asymptomatic primary hyperparathyroidism. Am J Med 87:553, 1989

109. METABOLIC MYOPATHIES

ZIAD RIFAI
ROBERT C. GRIGGS

The metabolic myopathies consist of a group of disorders associated with genetically determined biochemical defects and characterized clinically by weakness or exercise intolerance. In some of these disorders, other organ systems may be involved. Age of onset and severity of symptoms are variable. A single metabolic defect may be associated with a wide clinical spectrum, and different biochemical defects may have similar clinical manifestations. Nonetheless, for diagnostic purposes, it is useful to divide the metabolic myopathies into two groups: disorders presenting with exercise-induced myalgias, cramps, and fatigue, with or without myoglobinuria, and disorders associated with fixed or progressive muscle weakness.

The chromosomal localization and gene product have been identified in a large number of metabolic myopathies, improving accuracy of diagnosis and making genetic counseling and prenatal diagnosis feasible.

METABOLIC MYOPATHIES ASSOCIATED WITH EXERCISE INTOLERANCE

Metabolic myopathies associated with exercise intolerance are characterized by recurrent bouts of exercise-induced muscle pain, cramps, and stiffness. Severe episodes of muscle pain may be associated with weakness, muscle swelling, and tenderness. These findings reflect acute muscle fiber necrosis (rhabdomyolysis), as evidenced by the release into serum of large amounts of myoglobin and creatine kinase. Myoglobinuria occurs in extreme situations and may result in acute tubular necrosis and renal failure. The urine becomes amber in color owing to the presence of myoglobin.

The metabolic causes of recurrent episodes of myoglobinuria include defects of carbohydrate metabolism, defects of fatty acid metabolism, defects of the respiratory chain, and myoadenylate deaminase deficiency (Table 109-1). However, in about 50 percent of cases, a biochemical defect is not detected. Some of these patients are found to have an X-linked myopathy with abnormal dystrophin.

Disorders of Carbohydrate Metabolism

Deficiencies of several enzymes involved in glycogen metabolism have been associated with exercise intolerance and myoglobinuria (Table 109-1). Because glycogen is the major source of energy in the acutely exercising muscle, symptoms usually appear during intense physical activity.

Myophosphorylase Deficiency (McArdle's Disease). McArdle's disease is inherited as an autosomal recessive trait. The disease is restricted to skeletal muscle. Males are more frequently affected than females. Complaints of fatigue, exercise intolerance, and myalgias often start in childhood, but severe exercise-induced painful contractures, often called cramps by patients, usually do not occur until adolescence or early adulthood. Myoglobinuria occurs in about 50 percent of cases. The

TABLE 109-1. Differential Diagnosis of Recurrent Episodes of Exercise-Induced Muscle Pain and Myoglobinuria

Disorders of carbohydrate metabolism
  Myophosphorylase deficiency (McArdle's disease, type V glycogenosis)
  Phosphofructokinase deficiency (Tarui's disease, type VII glycogenosis)
  Phosphoglycerate kinase deficiency (type IX glycogenosis)
  Phosphoglycerate mutase deficiency (type X glycogenosis)
  Lactate dehydrogenase deficiency
  Phosphorylase b kinase deficiency

Disorders of fatty acid metabolism
  Carnitine palmitoyl transferase deficiency
  Long-chain acyl-coenzyme A dehydrogenase (LCAD) deficiency
  Short-chain 3-hydroxyacyl-coenzyme A dehydrogenase (SCHAD) deficiency

Defects of the respiratory chain
  Defects of complex I, complex III, and complex IV
  Coenzyme Q_{10} deficiency

Myoadenylate deaminase deficiency
X-linked myopathy with abnormal dystrophin
Idiopathic

onset of pain is typically associated with strenuous activity and is limited to the muscles that are being exercised. Rest may rapidly relieve the aching unless exercise is intense and prolonged, when pain may persist for several days. Slowing down at the first sign of fatigue may enable the patient to sustain exercise at a slower pace for a longer period, the so-called second-wind phenomenon.

Examination in between episodes is usually normal, but during a bout of rhabdomyolysis, muscle swelling, tenderness, and weakness may be present. After repeated attacks of myoglobinuria, fixed proximal weakness, may develop later in life.

LABORATORY TESTS. Resting serum creatine kinase is increased in the majority of patients and rises manyfold after exercise. Myoglobin may be detected in the urine during severe episodes of muscle pain. The forearm exercise test (described below) shows minimal or no rise in venous blood lactate, indicating a block in the glycolytic pathway. Muscle biopsy demonstrates the absence of myophosphorylase by a histochemical reaction. Periodic acid-Schiff-positive, glycogen-filled subsarcolemmal blebs are usually present. Necrotic and regenerating fibers can be seen following an episode of rhabdomyolysis. Biochemical analysis of a muscle specimen confirms the deficiency of myophosphorylase and usually demonstrates increased glycogen content.

EXHAUSTIVE FOREARM EXERCISE TEST. This test is used to narrow the differential diagnosis in a patient presenting with exercise intolerance. A catheter is introduced retrogradely into an antecubital vein and connected to a three-way stopcock. Blood samples are drawn through the side port and the patency of the catheter is maintained with a slow infusion of normal saline. The forearm muscles are exercised by squeezing a hand dynamometer to 50 percent of maximum grip strength until exhaustion (usually about 10 minutes). Ischemia, produced by inflating a sphygmomanometer cuff above arterial pressure, is often used, but is unnecessary and can cause severe muscle necrosis. Blood samples obtained at baseline, immediately after exercise, and 1, 3, 5, and 10 minutes after exercise are analyzed for lactate and ammonia determinations. In a normal person, venous lactate increases three to five times with exercise and ammonia doubles. Minimal or no rise in venous lactate indicates a block in the glycolytic pathway. Failure of ammonia to rise is associated with myoadenylate deaminase deficiency. Failure of either lactate or ammonia to increase may also indicate suboptimal exercise.

MANAGEMENT. There is no specific treatment. High-carbohydrate meals and unduly strenuous exertion should be avoided. Patients should stop exercise when their muscles start aching. The management of episodes of rhabdomyolysis includes bed rest and vigorous hydration. If myoglobinuria is present, sodium bicarbonate and fluids should be administered intravenously to alkalinize the urine and prevent acute tubular necrosis. Furosemide (40 to 80 mg intravenously) is also indicated in severe myoglobinuria.

Phosphofructokinase Deficiency (Tarui's Disease). The clinical presentation of phosphofructokinase deficiency is similar to that of myophosphorylase deficiency. Inheritance is autosomal recessive. Exercise-induced fatigue and cramps usually start in childhood. Severe episodes can be accompanied by nausea, vomiting, and myoglobinuria. Some patients have an associated mild hemolytic anemia due to reduction of the enzyme level in erythrocytes. The examination is normal during symptom-free intervals.

Abnormal laboratory tests include an elevated creatine kinase and an increased reticulocyte count. Bilirubin and uric acid levels may be increased owing to hemolysis. Venous lactate does not rise following forearm exercise. Muscle biopsy may show subsarcolemmal and intermyofibrillar accumulation of periodic acid-Schiff-positive material consisting mostly of normal glycogen. In some patients, an abnormal polysaccharide also accumulates in skeletal muscle. A specific histochemical reaction demonstrates the absence of phosphofructokinase. A biochemical assay confirms the enzyme deficiency. Management is similar to that of McArdle's disease.

Other Defects of Glycolysis Associated With Exercise Intolerance.　Deficiences of phosphoglycerate kinase, phosphoglycerate mutase, lactate dehydrogenase, and phosphorylase b kinase have been described in patients presenting with exercise-induced cramps, fatigue, and myoglobinuria. Inheritance of phosphoglycerate kinase is X-linked recessive. The other disorders are autosomal recessive. In each of these disorders, the specific enzyme deficiency is established by biochemical analysis of a muscle biopsy specimen.

Disorders of Fatty Acid Metabolism

Carnitine Palmitoyl Transferase Deficiency.　Carnitine palmitoyl transferase deficiency is inherited as an autosomal recessive trait localized to chromosome 1. This deficiency is the most common hereditary cause of myoglobinuria. Males are more frequently affected than females. Carnitine palmitoyl transferase is an enzyme involved in shuttling fatty acids across the inner mitochondrial membrane. Deficiency of the enzyme results in defective use of free fatty acids, which are the main source of energy during prolonged exercise. Muscle pain and cramps usually start after low-intensity sustained exercise and are often associated with myoglobinuria. Fasting exacerbates the symptoms and may even precipitate an attack. The muscles can become swollen, tender, and weak during an episode of myoglobinuria. Severe attacks may be associated with respiratory failure. Examination is normal in between episodes.

Serum creatine kinase is usually normal but may increase dramatically after exercise. The forearm exercise test demonstrates a normal rise of venous lactate and ammonia. Histologically, the muscle may be either normal or show a slight increase in the number and size of lipid droplets. The enzyme deficiency is demonstrated by a biochemical assay performed on a muscle biopsy specimen. A high-carbohydrate diet may benefit some patients. Myoglobinuria is managed as in McArdle's disease.

Defects of β-Oxidation.　A syndrome of recurrent myoglobinuria and hypoglycemic encephalopathy, usually beginning in childhood or adolescence, has been associated with deficiency of two other enzymes involved in fatty acid metabolism: long-chain acyl-coenzyme A dehydrogenase (LCAD) and short-chain 3-hydroxyacyl-coenzyme A dehydrogenase (SCHAD). Muscle weakness and cardiomyopathy can be present. Biochemical analysis of a muscle biopsy specimen confirms the diagnosis. Dietary treatment and administration of L-carnitine (50 to 100 mg/kg/d in divided doses) or riboflavin (100 mg/d) may be beneficial.

Defects of the Respiratory Chain.　Defects of complex I (reduced nicotinamide adenine dinucleotide-ubiquinone oxidoreductase), complex III (ubiquinone-cytochrome c oxidoreduc-

tase), and complex IV (cytochrome c oxidase) have each been associated with myopathy characterized by exercise intolerance and premature fatigue. Fixed weakness affecting the proximal limb muscles and, in some cases, the respiratory muscles may develop later in the course of the disease. Symptoms may first appear in childhood or adulthood. Myoglobinuria occurs in some patients. Lactic acidosis is usually present at rest and is exaggerated by exercise. Muscle biopsy shows ragged red fibers. The specific enzymatic defect is established by biochemical analysis of a muscle specimen, but in some instances, molecular genetic studies are also necessary.

Myoadenylate Deaminase Deficiency.　Myoadenylate deaminase deficiency occurs in about 1 percent of the general population and has been identified in patients with exercise-induced pain and cramps. Some of these patients also have recurrent myoglobinuria. It is not always clear whether the enzyme deficiency is the cause of the symptoms or the association is coincidental. Examination is normal. Venous ammonia does not rise following forearm exercise, but lactate does. The enzyme deficiency is demonstrated by a specific histochemical stain, and the diagnosis is confirmed by a biochemical assay showing less than 5 percent residual enzyme activity. There is no specific treatment.

METABOLIC MYOPATHIES ASSOCIATED WITH FIXED OR PROGRESSIVE WEAKNESS

Patients who present with fixed or progressive weakness, with or without other organ system involvement, may have one of several identifiable metabolic defects. Clinical severity and age at onset are variable, reflecting the severity and distribution of the biochemical abnormality. This group of disorders includes mitochondrial diseases and defects of carbohydrate and lipid metabolism (Table 109-2). Mitochondrial myopathies and encephalomyopathies are discussed in Chapter 194. The following review focuses on disorders of carbohydrate and lipid metabolism.

Disorders of Carbohydrate Metabolism

Acid Maltase Deficiency (Type II Glycogenosis).　Acid maltase is a lysosomal enzyme involved in glycogenolysis. Deficiency of this enzyme is inherited as an autosomal recessive trait and is probably genetically heterogeneous. The gene for acid maltase is localized to chromosome 17. Phenotypically, a severe infantile form (Pompe's disease) and milder childhood and adult forms have been recognized.

The severe infantile form presents in the first few months of life with hypotonia, generalized weakness, macroglossia, hepatomegaly, and cardiomegaly. Death occurs in infancy due to cardiorespiratory failure.

TABLE 109-2.　Metabolic Defects Causing Muscle Weakness

Disorders of carbohydrate metabolism
　Acid maltase deficiency (type II glycogenosis)
　Debrancher enzyme deficiency (type III glycogenosis)
　Brancher enzyme deficiency (type IV glycogenosis)
　Phosphorylase b kinase deficiency
　Phosphofructokinase kinase deficiency (rare)
　Myophosphorylase deficiency (rare)

Disorders of lipid metabolism
　Muscle carnitine deficiency
　Systemic carnitine deficiency

Mitochondrial myopathies (see Ch. 194)

Patients with the milder childhood form have delayed motor milestones, proximal weakness, and respiratory insufficiency. The muscles have a firm, rubbery consistency. Calf enlargement can be present and may lead to an erroneous diagnosis of Duchenne dystrophy. Enlargement of the liver and heart are infrequent findings. Death usually occurs before the end of the second decade of life from respiratory failure.

The adult-onset form presents in the third or fourth decade of life with slowly progressive proximal weakness affecting predominantly the pelvic girdle and mimicking limb girdle dystrophy or polymyositis. About one-third of patients have severe selective involvement of the respiratory muscles and may present with respiratory insufficiency. In these patients, restless sleep and early morning headaches may indicate impending respiratory failure.

The diagnosis of acid maltase deficiency should be considered in infants and children with weakness and organomegaly. The diagnosis should also be considered in adults presenting with limb girdle weakness, especially if respiratory muscle weakness is disproportionately severe.

In all three forms of the disease, creatine kinase is elevated and the electromyogram shows frequent spontaneous activity, including myotonia and pseudomyotonic discharges, which are particularly prominent in the paraspinal muscles of adult patients. Myopathic, short-duration, small motor unit potentials are recorded from proximal muscles. In the infantile and childhood forms, the electrocardiogram may show high-voltage QRS complexes and a short P-R interval. Muscle biopsy reveals a vacuolar myopathy. The vacuolar changes are most marked in the infantile form. The vacuoles are periodic acid-Schiff and acid phosphatase-positive. The diagnosis of acid maltase deficiency is confirmed by biochemical analysis of a muscle biopsy specimen.

There is no effective treatment. Forced vital capacity should be monitored periodically in children and adults. When respiratory decompensation is suspected, oximetry and capnography monitoring will help determine the need for ventilatory assistance, especially during sleep. Nasal positive pressure ventilation may be used in some patients, but others will require ventilation through a tracheostomy. Adult patients with respiratory failure may live for many years if appropriately supported.

Debrancher Enzyme Deficiency (Type III Glycogenesis). The gene for debrancher enzyme has been localized to chromosome 1. The enzyme deficiency is inherited as an autosomal-recessive trait. The disease may present in infancy, with hepatomegaly and fasting hypoglycemia associated in some cases with hypotonia, weakness, and cardiomegaly. As the child grows older, the hepatic manifestations improve but the weakness may progress. In adults, progressive weakness is the major symptom and may affect both proximal and distal muscles. Patients may complain of fatiguability, but myoglobinuria does not usually occur. Peripheral neuropathy may contribute to distal weakness and wasting. In some cases, the disorder resembles a motor neuron disease. The presence of associated cardiomyopathy and hepatomegaly is diagnostically useful.

Creatine kinase is elevated. The electrocardiogram shows biventricular hypertrophy. The electromyographic findings of frequent spontaneous activity and myopathic potentials are similar to those seen in acid maltase deficiency. Nerve conduction velocity may be slowed. Venous lactate production following forearm exercise is reduced. The muscle biopsy shows period

acid-Schiff-positive vacuoles. Biochemical analysis reveals increased glycogen content and confirms the enzyme deficiency.

There is no proven effective treatment for the myopathy. Fasting hypoglycemia in infants can be prevented by frequent low-carbohydrate, high-protein meals.

Brancher Enzyme Deficiency. Inheritance of brancher enzyme deficiency is autosomal recessive. In infants, the disease presents with hepatosplenomegaly, hepatic failure, and growth retardation, sometimes associated with weakness and cardiomegaly. Affected children do not survive beyond the first few years of life. In adults, the enzyme deficiency may cause a limb girdle myopathy.

Brancher enzyme deficiency has been reported in some cases of adult polyglucosan body disease characterized by upper motor neuron dysfunction, neurogenic bladder, and peripheral neuropathy. Dementia is present in about 50 percent of patients.

Other Disorders of Muscle Carbohydrate Metabolism Causing Weakness. Deficiency of myophosphorylase, phosphorylase b kinase, and phosphofructokinase usually presents with exercise intolerance and myoglobinuria in adults. However, deficiency of each of these enzymes has also, on rare occasions, been associated with late-onset myopathy characterized by progressive limb weakness. In addition, deficiency of either myophosphorylase or phosphofructokinase has been identified as a cause of rapidly progressive fatal weakness in infants.

Disorders of Lipid Metabolism (Carnitine Deficiency Syndromes)

Carnitine plays an essential role in the metabolism of fatty acids by muscle fibers. Primary carnitine deficiency is inherited as an autosomal-recessive trait and is associated with a lipid storage myopathy. The clinical manifestations are variable, but two forms can be recognized.

In systemic carnitine deficiency, carnitine content is reduced in plasma, heart, skeletal muscle, and liver. The disease presents in early childhood with episodes of hypoglycemic encephalopathy, metabolic acidosis, and evidence of liver damage. The episodes may resemble Reye syndrome and can be precipitated by fasting. A progressive lipid storage myopathy involving cardiac and skeletal muscles is usually present. Untreated, the disease is fatal.

In muscle carnitine deficiency, the major manifestation is slowly progressive axial and proximal limb weakness starting in childhood or occasionally in adulthood. Cardiac involvement may occur. Some patients also complain of exercise-induced myalgias. Plasma carnitine is normal.

Creatine kinase is normal or slightly elevated. The electromyogram is myopathic. The electrocardiogram may reveal biventricular hypertrophy or conduction abnormalities. Muscle biopsy shows abundant large lipid droplets that are best demonstrated by the oil-red-O stain for neutral lipids. The diagnosis is made by biochemical determination of muscle and plasma carnitine levels. Secondary causes of carnitine deficiency such as renal failure, cirrhosis, valproate therapy, organic acidurias, and defects of the respiratory chain should be excluded.

The standard treatment in both forms consists of replacement with 50 to 100 mg/kg/d of oral L-carnitine in divided doses. Systemic carnitine deficiency usually improves, but muscle carnitine deficiency may not. If carnitine treatment is ineffective, riboflavin (100 mg/d) or prednisone (0.5 to 1.5 mg/kg/d) can be considered. Severe episodes of hypoglycemic encephalopathy are treated with parenteral infusion of glucose and L-carnitine.

SUGGESTED READINGS

Di Donato S: Disorders of lipid metabolism affecting skeletal muscle: carnitine deficiency syndromes, defects in the catabolic pathway, and Chanarin disease. p. 1587. In Engel AG, Franzini-Armstrong C (eds): Myology. 2nd Ed. Vol. 2. McGraw-Hill, New York, 1994

DiMauro S, Tsujino S: Nonlysosomal glycogenoses. p. 1554. In Engel AG, Franzini-Armstrong C (eds): Myology. 2nd Ed. Vol. 2. McGraw-Hill, New York, 1994

Dubowitz V: Metabolic and endocrine myopathies. p. 465. In Dubowitz V (ed): Muscle Biopsy: A Practical Approach. 2nd Ed. Baillière Tindall, London, 1985

Engel AG, Hirschhorn R: Acid maltase deficiency. p. 1533. In Engel AG, Franzini-Armstrong C (eds): Myology. 2nd Ed. Vol. 2. McGraw-Hill, New York, 1994

Griggs RC, Mendell JR, Miller R: Metabolic myopathies. In: Evaluation and Treatment of Myopathies. FA Davis, Philadelphia, 1994

Griggs RC, Mendell JR, Miller R: Mitochondrial myopathies. In: Evaluation and Treatment of Myopathies. FA Davis, Philadelphia, 1994

Morgan-Hughes JA: Mitochondrial diseases. p. 1610. In Engel AG, Franzini-Armstrong C (eds): Myology. 2nd Ed. Vol. 2. McGraw-Hill, New York, 1994

Zierz S: Carnitine palmitoyl transferase deficiency. p. 1577. In Engel AG, Franzini-Armstrong C (eds): Myology. 2nd Ed. Vol. 2. McGraw-Hill, New York, 1994

110. CONGENITAL MYOPATHIES

JAMES A. RUSSELL

The congenital myopathies are incompletely understood disorders, currently recognized and defined by a combination of clinical and histologic criteria. These disorders usually have a neonatal or infantile onset and a slowly progressive or nonprogressive course. Proximal or generalized weakness with hypotonia are the usual presenting signs, with frequent involvement of facial, ventilatory, extraocular, and cardiac muscle. A wide variety of dysmorphic skeletal abnormalities that provide clues to the diagnosis may occur. A normal or mildly elevated serum creatine kinase concentration and a normal or mildly "myopathic" electromyogram (EMG) are the most likely results of commonly performed tests. Muscle biopsy in most instances reveals the distinctive histopathologic features that have historically defined these disorders. Muscle inflammation, necrosis, and regeneration are notable for their absence.

The application of molecular genetic techniques will undoubtedly lead to more accurate classification and understanding of these conditions as the responsible genes and gene products are identified. The following observations provide insight into the limitations of contemporary classifications and serve to emphasize the heterogeneity of these disorders.

1. Phenotypic features may prompt clinical suspicion of a congenital myopathy but are usually inadequate to predict a specific congenital myopathic type. Patients who have similar muscle histopathology (i.e., features on muscle biopsy)

may have different patterns of clinical involvement and different clinical courses.

2. Although the "typical" case is recognized in infancy and follows a relatively benign course, a wide spectrum of clinical presentations occur, including infantile mortality and cases initially recognized in adulthood.

3. The characteristic histologic features of the congenital myopathies are not specific. The initial hope and impression that an individual "disease" would be histologically distinct has not been realized. Identical histologic features may be seen in disorders arising from separate gene loci (e.g., the X-linked and autosomal dominant forms of myotubular myopathy). Muscle biopsies may manifest more than one of the features supposedly characteristic of a singular entity (e.g., rods and cores in the same biopsy). The same histologic features observed in heritable congenital myopathies may be seen in experimental or acquired pathologic conditions (e.g., nemaline rods in zidovudine therapy). Clinically affected relatives may have different pathology from the proband. In certain circumstances, muscle biopsy findings would appear to change over time in the same patient (although sampling error remains a plausible explanation for this phenomenon).

This chapter focuses on the more common of the currently recognized congenital myopathies. Clinical presentation and distinguishing clinical features, laboratory evaluation, and practical management are emphasized. Congenital muscular dystrophy and the mitochondrial myopathies are considered in Chapters 106 and 109, respectively.

CLASSIFICATION

Until such time that the molecular genetics and molecular biology of the congenital myopathies provide precise diagnostic parameters, nosologic definition remains an uncertain exercise. The classification in Table 110-1 separates these disorders into two groups, those with and those without the characteristic architectural changes of individual myofibers that currently define these conditions. In the former group, these architectural

TABLE 110-1. Classification of Congenital Myopathies

Congenital Myopathies With Architectural Changes of Individual Myofibers	Congenital Myopathies Without Architectural Changes of Individual Myofibers
Central core disease	Congenital fiber type disproportion
Multicore/minicore disease	Type I fiber predominance
Myofibrillar lysis myopathy	Uniform type I fiber myopathy
Selective myosin degeneration myopathy	Microfiber myopathy
Cap disease	Type II muscle fiber hypoplasia
Trilaminar fiber myopathy	Type I myofiber hypotrophy
Nemaline rod myopathy	
Mitochondria-jagged Z-line myopathy	
Z-band plaque myopathy	
Cytoplasmic body myopathy	
Spheroid body myopathy	
Mallory body myopathy	
Sarcoplasmic body myopathy	
Granulofilamentous body myopathy	
Centronuclear/myotubular myopathy	
Fingerprint body myopathy	
Zebra body myopathy	
Reducing body myopathy	
Tubulomembranous inclusion myopathy	
Cylindric spirals myopathy	
Sarcotubular myopathy	
Tubular aggregate myopathy	
Honeycomb myopathy	
Rimmed vacuole myopathy	
Granulovacuolar lobular myopathy	

TABLE 110-2. Congenital Myopathies for Which Gene Loci Are Known

Disorders	Location of Chromosome	Mode of Inheritance	Protein Product
Central core disease (malignant hyperthermia)	19q13.1	Autosomal dominant, reduced penetrance, variable expression	Probably ryanodine Receptor-1 gene
Nemaline myopathy	1p13-q25	Autosomal dominant reduced penetrance, variable expression	Unknown
Myotubular myopathy[a] (X-linked)	Xq28	X-linked recessive	Unknown

[a] Autosomal dominant, and perhaps recessive, forms of myotubular myopathy also exist for which the defective chromosome has not been identified.

(From Stirpe N: Neuromuscular disease gene search—status report. MDA Clinic Director's Report, April 1994, with permission.)

changes occur in addition to abnormalities in the proportion, size, and distribution of fibers of specific histochemical myofiber types. In the latter group, abnormalities in the proportion, size, and distribution of fibers of a specific histochemical myofiber type are the only finding. The congenital myopathies occurring with the greatest frequency are listed in Table 110-1. A number of these disorders have been identified by single case reports. Whether they represent distinct entities will require future verification.

GENETICS

The inheritances of the congenital myopathies are thought to include autosomal dominant, autosomal recessive, and possibly recessive and sporadic patterns of transmission. Identification of the inheritance pattern in an individual family may be complicated, as these disorders may not be phenotypically homogeneous within families. Infantile and ''adult-onset'' cases have been described within the same family in some of these disorders. In addition, a clinically unaffected parent of a child with a seemingly sporadic case may have an abnormal biopsy, implying carrier status or dominant inheritance with incomplete penetrance. Disorders in which the gene locus has been identified can be found in Table 110-2.

PATHOGENESIS

Many speculative mechanisms have been suggested relating to the pathogenesis of the congenital myopathies. All remain unproven. It has been postulated that the congenital myopathies occur secondary to maturational arrest of muscle. This consideration applies to centronuclear myopathy in particular. This disorder was originally labeled as myotubular myopathy owing to the resemblance of the affected muscle fibers to fetal myotubes. The myotubular stage of muscle ontogenesis occurs between 8 and 15 weeks of gestation, prior to any histochemical differentiation of muscle fibers. In contrast, centronuclear myopathy is associated with histochemical differentiation of myofiber types. Therefore, maturational arrest during the myotubular stage of muscle fiber development appears to be an unlikely mechanism. In the X-linked form of centronuclear myopathy, there appears to be persistence and overexpression of the fetal cytoskeletal proteins vimentin and desmin, proteins that normally disappear by term. It is hypothesized that the persistence of these proteins prevents the normal migration of myofiber nuclei and maintains them in a central position. Vimentin and desmin are found in normal concentrations in the autosomal-dominant form of the disorder, once again emphasizing the heterogeneity of these disorders.

Another proposed pathophysiologic mechanism for the congenital myopathies suggests that they develop secondary to central nervous system (CNS) disorders and are not true myopathies. The muscle histopathology would therefore represent the secondary effects of abnormal CNS system influences occurring at a critical time in muscle ontogenesis. A potential relationship between central core disease and cerebellar hypoplasia has provided one clue to this possibility, with the bulbospinal tracts providing the speculative link between cerebellum and muscle. It has also been pointed out that experimentally produced cores do not develop in the presence of muscle denervation, supporting the importance of the CNS in influencing the developing muscle.

CLINICAL FEATURES

All Congenital Myopathies

Although there are certain clinical features that occur more frequently in individual congenital myopathies, there is sufficient overlap to preclude a definite diagnosis of a specific congenital myopathy type on clinical grounds alone. Affected individuals are usually recognized in the neonatal period or in infancy but late onset or late recognition of many of these disorders may occur. In infancy, the child is usually hypotonic and ''floppy.'' Diminished or absent deep tendon reflexes are the norm and help to separate the congenital myopathies and other neuromuscular disorders from central causes of hypotonia. As the child develops, weakness in limb and axial muscles is manifested by an associated delay in motor milestones and with failure to match the performance of peers or older siblings at a similar age. Weakness is usually generalized or proximally predominant. Facial, masticatory, and pharyngeal weakness, footdrop, and scapular winging may occur. Neck weakness is common. Ptosis and ophthalmoparesis, commonly associated with centronuclear myopathy, may be a feature of other congenital myopathies as well. In most individuals, these disorders follow nonprogressive or slowly progressive courses. Cardiomyopathy, ventilatory muscle weakness, or restrictive lung disease secondary to kyphoscoliosis are factors that may lead to premature mortality either in infancy or later in life.

A wide variety of skeletal dysmorphisms are associated with the congenital myopathies. A list of recognized skeletal deformities associated with the congenital myopathies includes dolichocephaly, temporomandibular ankylosis, high-arched palate, micrognathia, kyphoscoliosis, congenital dislocation of hips, pes cavus/planus, rigid spine, equinovarus/valgus, pseudohypertrophy of calves, joint contractures, torticollis, pectus excavatum, increased lumber lordosis, ectomorphic habitus short stature, and hip dysplasia.

Individual Congenital Myopathies

There are few if any clinical features that allow, for certain, specific distinction between individual congenital myopathies and other neuromuscular disorders. Certain clinical features ap-

TABLE 110-3. Clinical Features That May Help to Identify Individual Congenital Myopathies

Feature	Disorders in Which Reported
Demographics	
"Delayed recognition"	Central core, centronuclear, cytoplasmic body, nemaline rod, reducing body
Infantile mortality	Centronuclear[a,b] (cm), central core, multi-/minicore, CFTD, cytoplasmic body, nemaline
Central Nervous System and Neuromuscular	
Calf hypertrophy	Cytoplasmic body, CFTD
Cramps/myalgias/rigidity	Central core, cytoplasmic body, tubular aggregate, honeycomb, cylindric spirals, spheroid body, trilaminar
Dysphagia	Centronuclear,[a,b] spheroid, cytoplasmic body, granulofilamentous, nemaline
Facial weakness	Central core, multi-/minicore, cap, trilaminar fiber, nameline, cytoplasmic body, Mallory body, tubulomembranous, tubular aggregate, Z-line disorganization, CFTD, uniform type I, centronuclear, reducing body, sarcotubular
Footdrop or scapular winging	Nemaline, centronuclear, sarcotubular, myofibrillar lysis
Mental retardation	CFTD, nucleodegenerative, fingerprint
Ptosis and ophthalmoparesis	Centronuclear,[a] nemaline, multi-/minicore, CFTD, reducing body
Seizures	Centronuclear,[b] fingerprint
Skeletal	
Rigid spine syndrome	CFTD
Skeletal abnormalities	Central core,[a] centronuclear,[a] multi-/minicore,[a] CFTD,[a] cytoplasmic body,[a] cap, myosin degeneration myopathy, tubulomembranous, uniform type 1
Temporomandibular ankylosis	Nemaline rod[a]
Systemic	
Cardiac involvement	Centronuclear[a,b] (cm), multi-/minicore (cm, cd, sd) nemaline (cm), reducing body, Mallory body, granulofilamentous, cytoplasmic body
Malignant hyperthermia	Central core,[a] multi-/minicore
Polyhydramnios	Centronuclear[b]
Ventilatory difficulties	Centronuclear,[b] central core, multi-/minicore, CFTD, cytoplasmic body, reducing body, nemaline

Abbreviations: cm, cardiomyopathy; cd, conduction defects; sd, septal defects; CFTD, congenital fibertype disproportion.
[a] Frequent feature.
[b] X-linked recessive form.

(Modified from Goebel HH, Lenard, HG: Congenital myopathies. p. 331. In Vinken PJ, Bruyn GW, Klawans HL (eds): Handbook of Clinical Neurology. Vol. 18. Elsevier, Amsterdam, 1992, with permission.)

pear to manifest more frequently in some congenital myopathies than others. These features are outlined in Table 110-3.

DIFFERENTIAL DIAGNOSIS

Differential diagnostic considerations vary, depending upon the age of onset and the clinical features of the individual patient. This discussion is limited to the most typical presentation, that of the floppy infant. Most floppy infants have CNS pathology as the apparent cause of their hypotonia. Distinguishing between a child with CNS pathology and a child with a congenital myopathy is not easy. It is often stated that children with hypotonia secondary to CNS disease are not weak. In my estimation, this is a clinical distinction that is difficult to recognize. Cognitive abnormalities, normal EMG examination results and creatine phosphokinase determinations, and joint contractures can be features common to both. Hyporeflexia or areflexia, although favoring a neuromuscular etiology, are not pathognomonic. Muscle biopsy is often required for diagnostic distinction.

The neuromuscular causes for the floppy infant syndrome include other myopathies, anterior horn cell diseases, rare congenital neuropathies, and neuromuscular transmission disorders. Other myopathies that may present clinically as congenital hypotonia include congenital muscular dystrophy, myotonic muscular dystrophy, glycogen and lipid storage disorders, and the mitochondrial disorders. Clinical features may be helpful but are rarely distinctive. Contractures are common, for example, in congenital muscular dystrophy. Examination of the mother provides the usual means of diagnosis in neonatal myotonic dystrophy. An abnormal EMG and elevated creatine kinase are more likely to occur in the "noncongenital" myopathies presenting in infancy with the exception of centronuclear/myotubular myopathy, in which an abnormal EMG is common. Definitive diagnosis often requires muscle biopsy.

Infantile spinal muscular atrophy (Werdnig-Hoffman disease) is the most common neuromuscular cause of hypotonia in most institutions. EMG and nerve conduction studies almost always identify this disorder as neurogenic in a laboratory with adequate pediatric experience. The same holds true for congenital hypomyelinating neuropathy and Dejerine-Sottas disease, in which abnormal sensory potentials on nerve conduction studies accompany widespread evidence of denervation on EMG. The congenital myasthenic syndromes are uncommon. Edrophonium testing, repetitive stimulation techniques, or the observation of stimulus-linked repetitive compound muscle action potential on motor conduction studies aid in the diagnosis of these disorders. Polio, Guillain-Barré syndrome, infantile botulism, and the inflammatory myopathies are rare causes of the floppy infant syndrome that are unlikely to be confused with the congenital myopathies because of their more typical acute or subacute clinical course.

DIAGNOSIS

At the present time, a blend of clinical and histopathologic findings is required for diagnosis of the congenital myopathies. Predictably, diagnostic confirmation and definition of the clinical boundaries of the congenital myopathies will be made by DNA testing in the foreseeable future.

Creatine Kinase

Creatine kinase is typically normal or mildly elevated in all of the congenital myopathies. A creatine kinase value in excess of two times normal should suggest an alternative diagnosis. With the exception of occasionally low-amplitude compound muscle action potentials, nerve conduction study results are normal. Early recruitment of motor unit potentials and motor units of short duration and low amplitude (the so-called myopathic pattern) has been described as a common finding in the congenital myopathies. In the experience of the EMG laboratory at Children's Hospital of Boston, many biopsy-proven congenital myopathies are associated with normal EMG study results when evaluating the floppy infant. Distinction between pathologically small motor unit potentials and normal small motor unit potentials of infancy is understandable. This problem may predispose to both false-positive and false-negative study results. Fibrillation potentials are common in centronuclear myopathy and have been reported in nemaline myopathy, congenital fiber type disproportion, cytoplasmic body myopathy, and reducing body myopathy. Myotonia and complex repetitive discharges have been reported in centronuclear myopathy and cytoplasmic body myopathy.

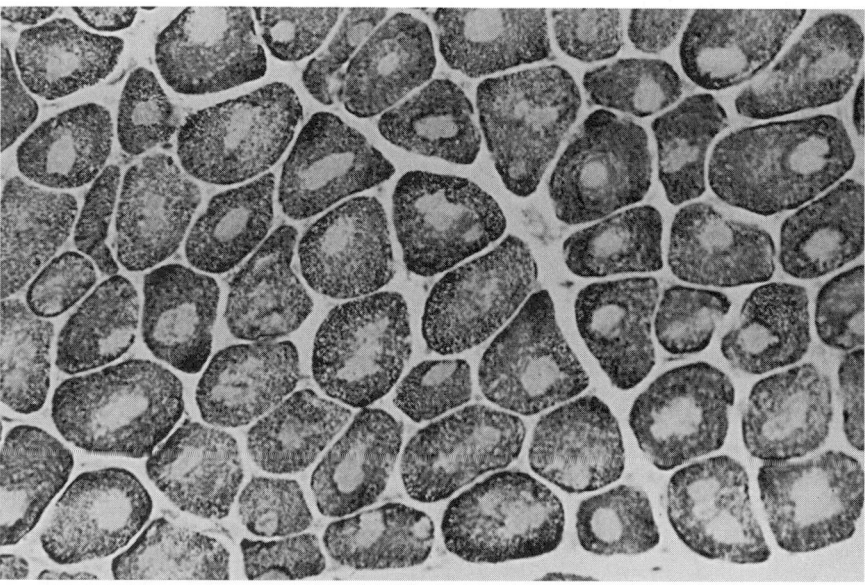

FIG. 110-1. Central core disease. A muscle biopsy from a 7-year-old boy with lifelong developmental delay associated with heel cord shortening. A cross section stained with reduced nicotinamide adenine dinucleotide demonstrates that the majority of myofibers lack oxidative activity in a corelike configuration, usually in a central location. (Courtesy of Thomas Smith, M.D., University of Massachusetts Medical Center, Worcester, MA.)

Muscle Biopsy

Muscle histopathology remains the cornerstone of diagnosis (Figs. 110-1 through 110-5). Unfortunately, there is no single pattern of abnormality that will define a specific congenital myopathy. Congenital fiber type disproportion (i.e., type 1 fiber predominance and type 1 fiber atrophy) is common to virtually all of the congenital myopathies but may not be apparent in a given individual or in a particular biopsied location. Many of the histologic characteristics that have historically defined a particular congenital myopathy type may occur together at a single biopsy site (e.g., the concurrence of central cores and nemaline rods). Histologic abnormalities are not uniformly dis-tributed and sampling error as well as changes in the histologic finding may occur over time. It is the predominant histopatho-logic finding when coupled with the appropriate clinical presen-tation that forms our current basis of diagnosis.

The biopsy specimen is usually obtained from the quadriceps on the side not invaded by the EMG needle. An alternative site might be chosen if the quadriceps seemed clinically spared or if the muscle seemed so severely afflicted that an "end-stage" biopsy might be expected. If the distal musculature seemed preferentially involved, the gastrocnemius would be the muscle of choice. If an upper extremity muscle were required, the bi-ceps would be chosen. In myopathies in which EMG examina-

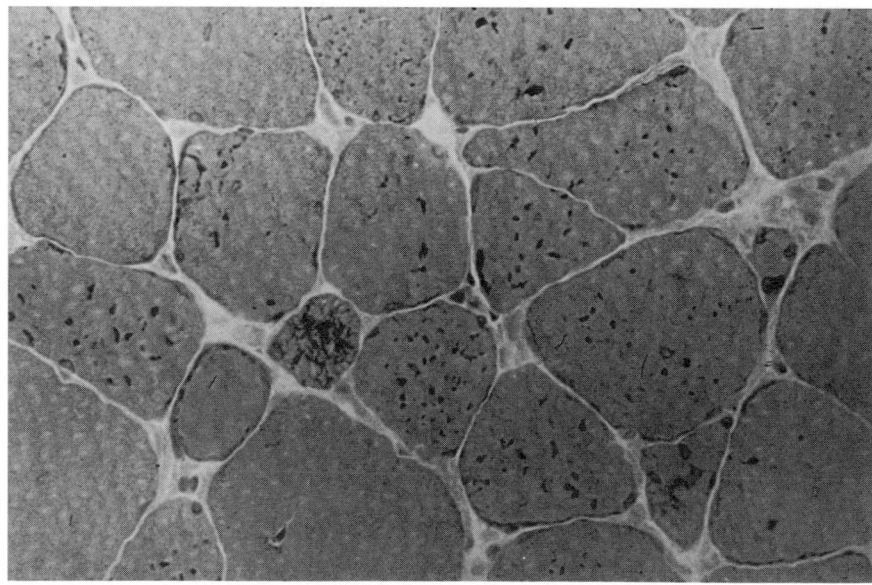

FIG. 110-2. Nemaline rod disease. A muscle biopsy from a 63-year-old man with a few years of recognized proximal weakness associated with long-standing inability to fully open his mouth and heel cord tightness. A modified Gomori trichrome-stained cross section demonstrates darkly stained rodlike structures scattered throughout the majority of myofibers.

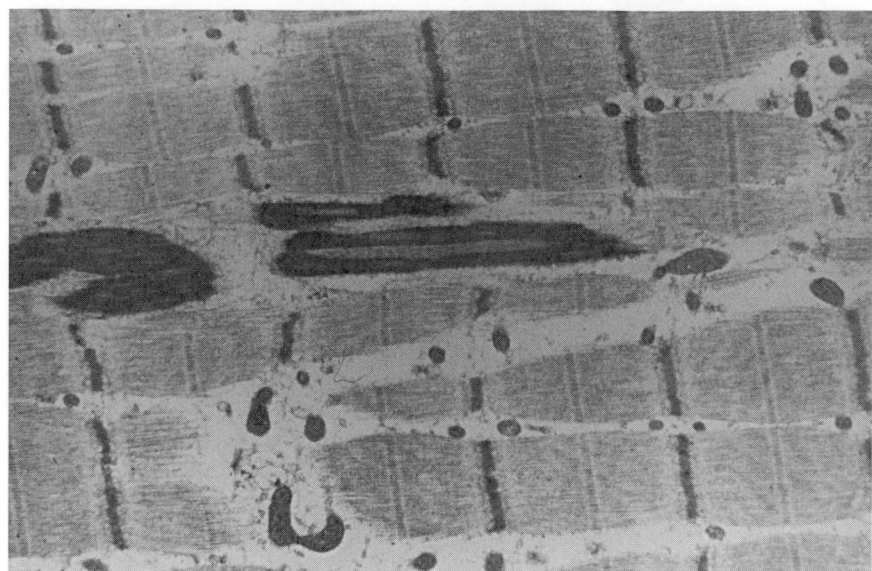

FIG. 110-3. Nemaline rod disease. A longitudinally oriented electron micrograph from a muscle biopsy of a child with nemaline myopathy demonstrating the longitudinal orientation of the rods and their relationship to the Z-discs.

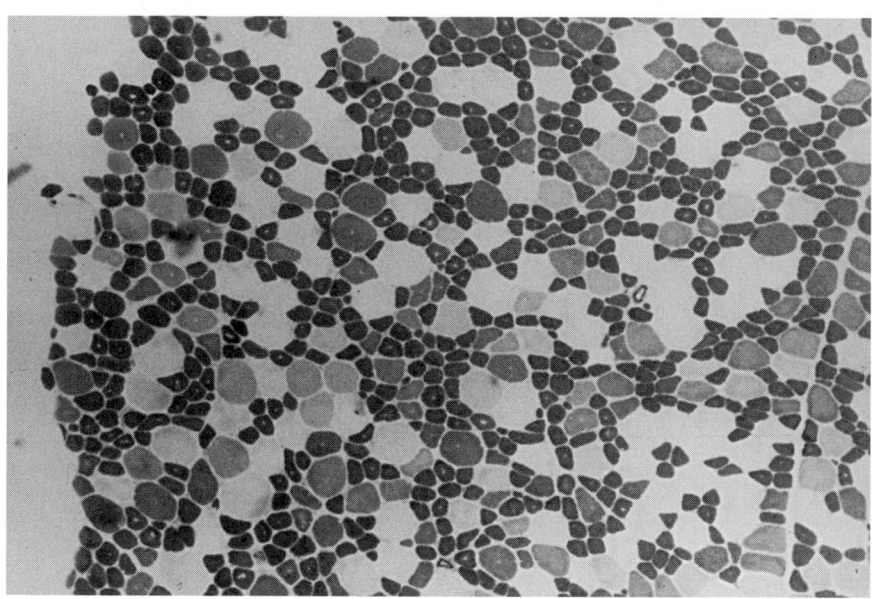

FIG. 110-4. Centronuclear myopathy with fiber type disproportion. A muscle biopsy from a 12-year-old girl with ptosis, distal weakness greater than proximal weakness, and tight heel cords. An adenosine triphosphatase—stained cross section (ph 4.3) demonstrates type 1 fiber atrophy and predominance as well as numerous fibers with absent central staining representing the locations of unstained nuclei. (Courtesy of Douglas Anthony, M.D., and Natasha Lec, M.D., Boston Children's Hospital, Boston.)

TABLE 110-4. Histopathology of the Common Congenital Myopathies[a]

Myopathy	Congenital Fiber	Other Abnormalities	Stains That Accentuate Disproportion
CFTD	Yes	No	ATPase
Central core	Yes	Central cores: circumscribed areas extending the length of the myofiber with a disrupted myofibrillar network and absent mitochondria; may occupy 20–100% of fibers in a given biopsy	NADH, SDH, PAS, phosphorylase, ATPase (areas of absent staining)
Nemaline rod	Yes	Nemaline rods: thin rodlike structures that appear to arise from the Z-disc based on their contiguity, a similar lattice structure, and their make-up (α-actinin)	Modified trichrome (red "bacillary" structures)
Centronuclear	Yes	Central nuclei: a single large central nucleus with surrounding halo seen in 50% or more of fibers	H&E, trichrome (central nuclei visualized), ATPase (central hole unstained)

Abbreviations: ATPase, adenosine triphosphatase; NADH, reduced nicotinamide adenine dinucleotide; SDH, succinate dehydrogenase; PAS, periodic acid-Schiff, CFTD, congenital fiber type disproportion; H&E, hematoxylin and eosin.
[a] See also Figs. 110-1 through 110-5.

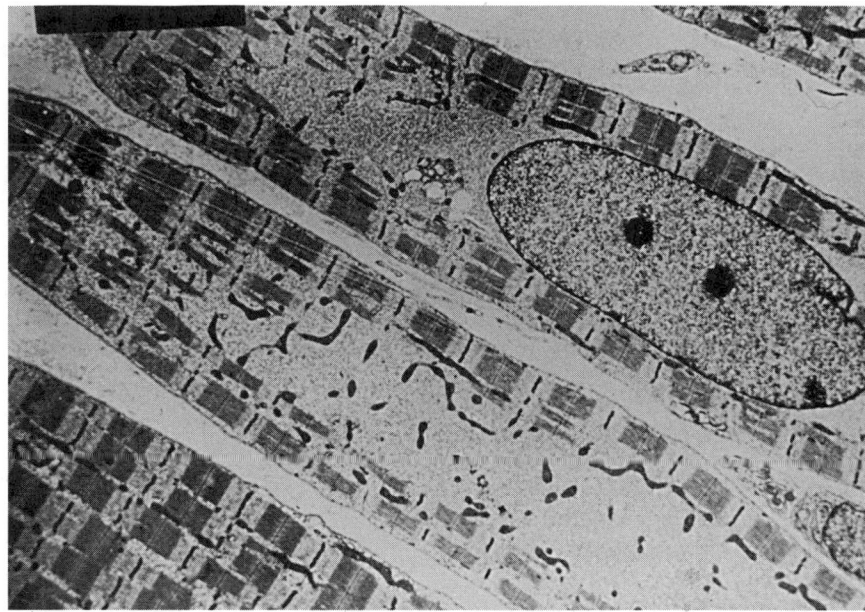

FIG. 110-5. Centronuclear myopathy. A longitudinally oriented electron micrograph from the muscle biopsy of a 2-day-old infant with hypotonia, facial weakness, micrognathia, and contractures of the elbows and knees. A centrally placed nucleus surrounded by an area of myofibrillar disruption is demonstrated. The peripherally located myofibrillar architecture is relatively preserved.

tions are more helpful, I use EMG data to aid in biopsy site selection. I prefer an open biopsy technique, although other laboratories experienced in needle biopsy techniques have been equally successful. As with all muscle biopsies, severely affected muscles are to be avoided as biopsy sites.

A description of the histologic abnormalities in the more common forms of congenital myopathies and the stains that accentuate them are listed in Table 110-4. It should be emphasized that with the exception of centrally located nuclei, frozen sections and histochemical stains are required for diagnosis. Paraffin sections by themselves are inadequate for diagnosis in the majority of these disorders.

There has been recent interest in the use of magnetic resonance imaging in the diagnosis of muscle disease. Its primary use has been to supplant the role of electromyography in the documentation of myopathy and in the choice of biopsy site. Although its usefulness in individual cases of certain types of myopathy has been well illustrated, it is not clear that its specificity and sensitivity are adequate to be routinely used in the diagnosis of the myopathies as a whole or in the congenital myopathies specifically.

MANAGEMENT

There are no specific treatments for the congenital myopathies. The management goals are for the most part similar to those for other chronic neuromuscular conditions:

1. Maintenance of optimal, independent neuromuscular function for as long as possible, with particular attention to ambulation
2. Reduction in the risk of falls and injury
3. Maintenance of patient comfort
4. Prevention or correction of joint contractures, particularly spine deformities and kyphoscoliotic cardiopulmonary disease
5. Maintenance of appropriate nutrition (adequate calories in

those with feeding difficulties; caloric restrictions in those with a propensity to obesity)
6. Provision of genetic counseling where needed
7. Prevention or prompt treatment of aspiration and other forms of pneumonia (when appropriate)
8. Recognition and treatment of associated congestive heart failure, symptomatic cardiac conduction defects, and pulmonary hypertension
9. Avoidance of malignant hyperthermia
10. Identification of patient and parental goals and provision of adequate counseling in situations in which the severity of the illness may be anticipated to significantly shorten the patient's life expectancy
11. Reassurance of patient and parents that in the majority of cases, neither significant progression or mortality is anticipated

The development of a uniform management protocol for patients with congenital myopathy is impeded by the clinical heterogeneity and variable natural history of these disorders as well as by the absence of controlled data pertaining to the management of these disorders. A brief review of the therapeutic options is provided below. It is beyond the scope of this chapter to provide detailed management guidelines concerning the numerous orthopaedic problems that may complicate these disorders (see Shapiro and Specht, 1993). Surgical intervention requires an orthopaedist skilled in corrective neuromuscular procedures. The goals of the surgery and the likelihood of success should be understood by all involved parties. Prolonged immobilization after any surgery is to be avoided.

There is little controlled data pertaining to the management of the congenital myopathies. Recommendations presented here are in large part extrapolated from the more systematically studied Duchenne's muscular dystrophy.

Contractures may be present at birth (i.e., arthrogryposis multiplex congenita) or may be acquired, concomitant to the development of weakness of muscle groups affecting the joint(s) in question. The goals of treatment are to restore or maintain function in a joint still capable of independent movement, to maintain comfort, or on occasion to allow improved hygienic care. Restoration of passive mobility to a joint whose surrounding muscles are incapable of effective movement serves little purpose.

Contractures that may occur in the upper extremities include adduction of the shoulder, flexion and pronation of the elbow, flexion and ulnar deviation of the wrists, and flexion of the metacarpophalangeal and proximal interphalangeal joints. The foundation of prevention and treatment is daily passive range-of-motion exercises. If passive range of motion becomes limited, nocturnal orthoses particularly for the wrist and fingers should be considered. Tendon releases and transfers are uncommonly performed.

Prevention of lower extremity and spinal contractures is best accomplished by keeping the patient ambulatory. Canes, crutches, and walkers may be useful if adequate upper extremity strength permits their use. Long leg braces (i.e., knee-ankle-foot orthoses with knee locks) are not readily embraced by patients in part owing to their weight and in part to the severity of falls that may occur with their use. When used, they are almost always in conjunction with a walker. Common contractures include flexion and abduction of the hip, flexion of the hip, and equinovarus posturing of the ankle. Daily passive range-of-motion exercises and orthoses are usually the first line of treatment. A variety of tendon-lengthening, -release, and -transfer procedures have been used for all of the aforementioned contractures. Shapiro prefers an individualized approach, avoiding for the most part both prophylactic and palliative surgical intervention. Lengthening of the hamstring and Achilles tendons and posterior tibial tendon transfers are the most frequently performed procedures and should be undertaken primarily in patients with incentive to continue walking. Although surgical procedures have been performed after a child has lost ambulatory capability, it is unlikely that they will lead to restored walking if the child has been in a wheelchair for 6 months or more. Most—if not all—surgical procedures, following this 6-month window should be undertaken for comfort considerations only.

The management of kyphoscoliosis involves wheelchair adaptions, spinal orthoses, and surgical intervention. Unfortunately, none of these procedures has slowed the progression of restrictive lung disease in patients with Duchenne's muscular dystrophy. Wheelchair seating systems using narrow frames, firm seats and backs, dual seat belts, and lateral chest wall supports are chosen primarily for comfort. Spinal arthrodesis enhanced by metallic instrumentation has been used to stabilize spinal curves in patients with congenital myopathy. In Duchenne's dystrophy, in which the natural history is better understood and progression is inevitable, intervention may take place when the curve is as small as 10 percent. In the congenital myopathies, in which significant kyphoscoliosis is rare, it is prudent to document progression prior to surgical intervention, ideally acting before the curve exceeds 40 percent.

Scapular fixation techniques are of little use in those congenital myopathy patients with significant scapular winging. Unlike facioscapulohumeral dystrophy, concomitant weakness of the deltoids and other shoulder girdle muscles precludes any functional benefit in the majority of congenital myopathy patients. Congenital dislocation of the hip may be treated successfully with closed reduction and spica casting in infancy but may require femoral osteotomy in those over than 18 months of age.

Patients with any degree of cardiopulmonary compromise should be immunized against influenza and pneumococcus. Baseline forced vital capacity and negative inspiratory force measurements (age permitting) and electrocardiograms should be obtained. An echocardiogram is obtained if there is any clinical suspicion of cardiac involvement or if the type of congenital myopathy, involved puts the patient at increased risk of cardiomyopathy.

ACKNOWLEDGMENTS

I would like to thank Dr. Thomas Smith of the University of Massachusetts Medical Center, Department of Pathology, for his permission to use the pathologic material in Fig. 110-1; Drs. Douglas Anthony and Natasha Lec of Boston's Children's Hospital, Department of Pathology, for their permission to use Fig. 110-4; and Drs. Anthony, Fred Shapiro of Boston Children's Hospital, Department of Orthopedics, and Roy Jones of the Lahey Clinic for their helpful review of the manuscript.

SUGGESTED READINGS

Banker BQ: The congenital myopathies. p. 1527. In Engel AG, Banker BQ (eds): Myology. 1st Ed. Vol 2. McGraw-Hill, New York, 1986
Bodensteiner JB: Invited review: congenital myopathies. Muscle Nerve 17: 131, 1994
Goebel HH, Lenard HG: Congenital myopathies. p. 331. In Vinken PJ, Bruyn GW, Klawans HL (eds): Handbook of Clinical Neurology. Vol. 18. Elsevier, Amsterdam, 1992
Jones Jr HR: EMG evaluation of the floppy infant: differential diagnosis and technical Aspects. Muscle Nerve 13:338, 1990
Sarnat HB: New insights into the pathogenesis of congenital myopathies. J Child Neurol 9:193, 1994
Shapiro F, Specht, L: The diagnosis and orthopaedic treatment of inherited muscular diseases of childhood. J Bone Joint Surg 75-A:439, 1993
Stirpe N: Neuromuscular disease gene search—status report. MDA Clinic Director's Report, April 1994

111. MYOTONIA AND PERIODIC PARALYSIS

ROBERT H. BROWN, JR.

In recent years, several lines of investigation have delineated the molecular basis for an expanding family of disorders of ion channels or receptors, including six inherited muscle diseases: hypokalemic periodic paralysis, hyperkalemic periodic paralysis, paramyotonia congenita, myotonia congenita, potassium-aggravated myotonia, and myotonic dystrophy. To a remarkable degree, it is now possible to integrate the clinical features of these diseases with an understanding of the mutant channel proteins at the molecular level. This chapter provides an overview of these diseases, with an emphasis on their clinical management and laboratory diagnostic testing.

CLINICAL DISORDERS

Myotonia

Myotonia is a disorder of skeletal muscle characterized by excessive electrical irritability of the muscle membrane. Clini-

TABLE 111-1. Classification of Periodic Paralyses and Myotonias

Disease	Gene	Chromosome
Nondystrophic		
Hyperkalemic periodic paralysis	Na channel	t17
Paramyotonia congenita	Na channel	17
Potassium aggravated myotonia	Na channel	17
Hypokalemic	Ca channel	1
Myotonia congenita		
Autosomal dominant (Thomsen's)	Cl channel	7
Autosomal recessive (Becker's generalized)	Cl channel	7
Schwartz-Jampel		?
Dystrophic		
Myotonic dystrophy	Myotonin (protein kinase)	19

cally, it causes muscle stiffness that typically worsens in the cold. On electromyography (EMG), myotonic muscle demonstrates abnormally long bursts of muscle fiber action potentials following discrete stimuli such as percussion. It is useful to distinguish between dystrophic and nondystrophic myotonic disorders (Table 111-1). The major disorder in the former category is myotonic dystrophy, whereas nondystrophic myotonias are hyperkalemic periodic paralysis, paramyotonia congenita, myotonia congenita, and potassium-aggravated myotonia (Table 111-2). Hypokalemic periodic paralysis is not generally associated with myotonia.

Hypo- and Hyperkalemic Periodic Paralysis

As the name implies, the central clinical problem in the periodic paralyses is episodic weakness. This may be profound, causing virtually total limb paralysis. Fortunately, it usually spares diaphragmatic and cardiac function as well as mentation. During hypokalemic periodic paralysis, serum potassium levels are low, whereas the converse is true during hyperkalemic periodic paralysis. Other clinical features distinguish these disorders. Hypokalemic paralysis is rarely associated with myotonia, whereas this is common in the hyperkalemic form. Hypokalemic paralysis typically begins in adolescence and affects

males more severely than females. It is provoked by ingesting carbohydrates. Hyperkalemic paralysis usually begins in early childhood and shows no influence of gender on severity. It is also triggered by fasting and may be aborted with ingestion of sweets. On the other hand, several clinical attributes are common to both entities. In either disorder, attacks may be frequent, may last up to several hours, and may be triggered by rest after exertion. During paralysis, skeletal muscle is depolarized and electrically silent in both diseases. Particularly in hyperkalemic paralysis, exercise may ameliorate symptoms of an impending attack of weakness; conversely, long periods of inactivity may provoke attacks. Some patients with hyperkalemic or hypokalemic periodic paralysis may develop slowly progressive, irreversible proximal muscle weakness.

Paramyotonia Congenita

Patients with paramyotonia congenita also develop episodes of paralysis, usually in response to sustained exposure to cold. The EMG of such patients is normal at rest, shows increased electrical irritability and myotonia with mild cooling, and becomes electrically silent during paralysis. In general, serum potassium levels are normal in these patients during attacks, although challenge with infusions of potassium may cause a reduction in the amplitudes of compound muscle action potentials similar to that seen in hyperkalemic periodic paralysis. In paramyotonia congenita, repeated muscle contractions may worsen the myotonia; this *para*doxic myotonic (hence *paramyotonia*) response is opposite that usually seen with myotonia. The distal limbs and facial muscles tend to be particularly affected by cold exposure in these patients. Thus, there may be difficulty opening the eyes or rapidly releasing grip.

Myotonia Congenita

Patients with myotonia congenita do not develop episodes of paralysis but are continuously stiff. In effect, myotonia congenita muscle is often in a state of isometric contraction. As a result, the muscles of these patients acquire a robust, hypertro-

TABLE 111-2. Features of the Periodic Paralyses and Nondystrophic Myotonias

	Periodic Paralyses		Paramyotonia Congenita	Potassium-Aggravated Myotonia	Generalized Myotonia	Myotonia Congenita	Myotonic Dystrophy
	Hypokalemic	*Hyperkalemic*					
Clinical							
Recurrent weakness	Yes	Yes	Rarely	No	No	No	No
Onset	Puberty	Infancy	Infancy	Infancy	Childhood	Childhood	Childhood
Attack duration	Hours to days	Minutes to days	Minutes to days				
Interictal interval	Hours to days	Minutes to days	Minutes to days				
Myotonia	No	Yes	Yes	Yes	Yes	Yes	Yes
Systemic features	No	No	No	No	No	No	Yes
Triggers	Cold, rest after exercise, carbohydrates	Cold, rest after exercise, fasting	Cold, rest after exercise, fasting	Cold	Cold	Cold	Cold
Ameliorators	Potassium, exercise	Carbohydrates, exercise	Warming, exercise	Warming	Warming	Warming	
Therapy							
Prevent paralysis	Acetazolamide	Acetazolamide	Acetazolamide				
Reduce myotonia	Mexiletine	Mexiletine	Mexiletine	Mexiletine	Mexiletine	Mexiletine	
Genetic							
Inheritance pattern	Autosomal dominant	Autosomal dominant	Autosomal dominant	Autosomal dominant	Autosomal recessive	Autosomal dominant	Autosomal dominant
Gene	Ca channel	Na channel	Na channel	Na channel	Cl channel	Cl channel	Myotonin kinase

phied appearance. Despite this, normal function is significantly impaired by the excessive stiffness. One form of this disease begins in early childhood and is dominantly inherited; this was first described by Thomsen, who was himself affected. Another form, designated as generalized myotonia, was described by Becker. This begins in later childhood and is inherited as an autosomal-recessive trait.

Potassium-Aggravated Myotonia

At least two features distinguish potassium-aggravated myotonia from myotonia congenita. In potassium-aggravated myotonia, but not myotonia congenita, myotonia is exacerbated by measures that increase serum potassium; in addition, myotonia in potassium-aggravated myotonia is relatively less cold sensitive. Two forms of potassium-aggravated myotonia have been distinguished on the basis of the degree of variability of the myotonia. In myotonia fluctuans, myotonia but not weakness is provoked by rest after exercise and by potassium ingestion. Patients with this disorder may go very long periods (months) without any symptomatic myotonia. By contrast, patients with myotonia permanens experience severe, unremitting myotonia, at times sufficient to impair breathing.

Myotonic Dystrophy

By contrast with the nondystrophic myotonic disorders, the pathology in myotonic dystrophy is not confined solely to skeletal muscle. Rather, myotonic dystrophy is a multiple system disorder that may involve skeletal muscle, the brain, the cardiac conducting system, and the endocrine system (insulin-resistant diabetes and testicular atrophy are common). These patients have a characteristic facial appearance with thinning of the temporalis and masseter muscles, frontal balding, ptosis, and a tendency toward slackness of muscle tone around the mouth. Most strikingly, over time, myotonic dystrophy patients can develop extreme distal limb weakness and wasting. As the name implies, these patients usually have some degree of myotonia, although it is less severe than in the nondystrophic myotonias. Myotonic dystrophy patients may not volunteer complaints of muscle stiffness, but on questioning may describe such manifestations of stiffness as difficulty releasing the hand from a doorknob on a cold day. Newborn infants with this disease may be strikingly hypotonic and floppy. Often the diagnosis of mild myotonic dystrophy in a mother is established only after she gives birth to a floppy newborn.

MUSCLE BIOPSY

Microscopic analysis of skeletal muscle in the periodic paralyses, paramyotonia congenita, and myotonia congenita, is normal early in the illness. In individuals with a long history of protracted paralytic episodes, there may be vacuoles within the muscles. After several decades, severely affected individuals develop irreversible proximal muscle weakness. These relatively subtle features contrast with the more myopathic findings in myotonic dystrophy muscle, which may show fiber size variation, fibrosis, central nuclei, ring fibers, and chains of nuclei. Electron microscopic evaluation sometimes shows duplication of t-tubules as an early manifestation of the vacuolar change.

PATHOPHYSIOLOGIC STUDIES

In normal nerve and muscle at rest, the intracellular compartment is hyperpolarized by about 90 mV with respect to the extracellular milieu. The resting conductances for potassium and chloride are large compared to that for sodium, and thus the resting potential (V_m), is determined largely by the Nernst potentials for potassium and chloride. An action potential occurs when the membrane is depolarized beyond the threshold for all-or-nothing excitation. In this circumstance, the conductance for sodium increases rapidly such that V_m approaches E_{Na}. Repolarization occurs for two reasons. The abrupt "activation" or rise in g_{Na} is self-terminating, because the depolarized sodium (Na) channel rapidly closes or inactivates. Slightly thereafter, an outward, repolarizing potassium (K) current is activated. Thus, g_{Na} falls and g_K rises. Both factors will drive V_m back toward E_K and E_{Cl}. In muscle, an additional factor affects the rate at which V_m relaxes back to the normal resting potential. Much of the outflow of K ions across the membrane is into the muscle cell transverse tubules (t-tubules), whose interiors are topographically outside the muscle cell. Because the t-tubules are extremely narrow, a small, outwardly flowing K current can lead to significant increases in the effective extracellular K inside the t-tubule. As indicated by the Nernst potential, this will increase in E_K across the t-tubule membrane and slow restoration of V_m, closer to the threshold for all-or-nothing firing. Fortunately, even with repetitive firing of the muscle cell, g_{Cl} is sufficiently large that it can "clamp" V_m, counteracting the change in E_K. As noted below, this clamping of V_m by the chloride channel is critical for normal, stable excitability of the muscle fiber.

Numerous investigations indicate that in the nondystrophic myotonias, the phenomena of myotonia and paralysis are closely related, reflecting different degrees of the same abnormality: conductance changes that slightly depolarize V_m, rendering V_m closer to the firing threshold. In theory, this could arise either by an increase in g_{Na} or a decrease in either g_K or g_{Cl}. With mild depolarization of V_m (failure of full restoration of V_m after excitation), the muscle cell initially becomes more readily excitable (more myotonic). As the degree of pathologic depolarization increases, the muscle ultimately becomes inexcitable and thus unable to contract to generate force. This phase corresponds to the paralytic phase of periodic paralysis.

Hyperkalemic Periodic Paralysis

In 1963, experimental data from periodic paralysis patients led Creutzfeld and colleagues to speculate that hyperkalemic periodic paralysis arises from excessive membrane depolarization because of a defect in Na conductance. This possibility has subsequently been examined by several investigators, prominently including Lehmann-Horn, Rudel, Ricker, and others. In muscle from hyperkalemic periodic paralysis patients, they documented that increasing extracellular K increases total inward current and simultaneously depolarizes the membrane potential in excess of the depolarization predicted by the Nernst equation. Both the increment in background current and the depolarization induced by elevated bath K were reversed by the addition of a sodium channel-blocking agent, tetrodotoxin. Cannon et al. extended these observations in patch clamp studies of muscle grown in culture from biopsies of a hyperkalemic paralysis patient. In this system, a fraction of the sodium channels showed imperfect inactivation; the fraction increased with increasing extracellular potassium concentrations. These and many other studies implicate a defect in Na conductance in the pathogenesis of hyperkalemic paralysis.

Myotonia Congenita

It is observed experimentally that reduction of g_{Cl} in normal skeletal muscle produces a tendency toward easily triggered, sustained, repetitive membrane firing. In the 1960s, reports documented that membrane chloride conductance is reduced in muscle of patients with Thomsen's disease. Two animal models lend credence to the role of an abnormal chloride conductance in myotonia. Bryant documented that congenital goat myotonia arises because of a reduction in skeletal muscle chloride permeability. In an elegant analysis, Adrian and Bryant demonstrated that sustained, repetitive myotonic firing of this goat muscle requires both a reduced chloride conductance and the accumulation of K^+ ions in an intact t-tubule system. In 1991, Steinmeyer and colleagues cloned a mammalian, voltage-dependent chloride channel "ClC-1" and demonstrated that this is disrupted in a myotonic mutant mouse (*adr/adr* mouse).

Hypokalemic Periodic Paralysis

The ionic pathophysiology of hypokalemic periodic paralysis has not been as precisely delineated as that of hyperkalemic periodic paralysis or myotonia congenita. Lehmann-Horn and associates established in the 1980s that affected muscle becomes depolarized and demonstrates an augmented net inward current on exposure to medium with low potassium. However, a single type of ion channel is not clearly incriminated by these or other physiologic investigations.

GENETIC AND MUTATION ANALYSIS

Hyperkalemic Periodic Paralysis, Paramyotonia Congenita, and Potassium-Aggravated Myotonia

The dominantly inherited disorders of hyperkalemic periodic paralysis, paramyotonia congenita, and potassium-aggravated myotonia arise from mutations in the α subunit of the skeletal muscle sodium channel; indeed, at least 15 different mutations have now been identified in the gene for this subunit in affected individuals. These mutations produce relatively minor amino acid changes that typically affect residues that are highly conserved across multiple species. Some fall into well-defined functional domains of the channel.

Myotonia Congenita

Both genetic linkage and mutation analyses have now established the fact that mutations in the ClC-1 gene on chromosome 7q underly two types of myotonia congenita: Becker's autosomal-recessive generalized myotonia and dominantly inherited myotonia congenita (Thomsen's disease).

Hypokalemic Periodic Paralysis

More recently, genetic linkage was established between hypokalemic periodic paralysis, a dominantly inherited disease, and a locus in human chromosome 1 encoding the α subunit of a voltage-sensitive, muscle calcium channel, the so-called dihydropyridine receptor. Two different mutations have been identified in most families with these diseases.

Myotonic Dystrophy

Myotonic dystrophy is also dominantly inherited. In 1992, Brook and associates described a new protein kinase named "myotonin" encoded by the myotonic dystrophy gene. The defect in patients with myotonic dystrophy is an expansion of a CTG repeat in the 3', noncoding region of this gene. This defect is genetically unstable, tending to expand even between single generations from a slightly enlarged "premutation" to much larger forms; in general, there is a strong correlation between the length of the (CTG) repeat and the severity of the myotonic dystrophy. Detailed analyses of the function of myotonin and levels of its activity in myotonic dystrophy patients have not yet been reported. The functional significance of these mutations is not well defined; one possibility is that myotonin produces myotonia by modulating the phosphorylation state of skeletal muscle ion channels, and that the degree of phosphorylation may be abnormal in patients with myotonic dystrophy. Alternately, it may be that the expanded CTG alters expression of the gene in some manner.

DIFFERENTIAL DIAGNOSIS AND EVALUATION

An algorithm for the evaluation of these patients is outlined in Figure 111-1. Perhaps the most useful initial question is whether the problem is recurrent weakness, myotonia, or both. Recurrent weakness with low and high potassium levels rapidly defines distinct entities: hypo- and hyperkalemic paralysis. Recurrent weakness with normal potassium can be seen either as a variant of hyperkalemic paralysis, in which case the serum potassium may rise within the normal range during attacks, or as paramyotonia congenita, in which case cold provokes the attacks of weakness. Myotonia without periodic weakness, if aggravated by potassium, usually reflects a defect in the sodium channel, in potassium-aggravated myotonia. Myotonia without periodic weakness, which is neither potassium sensitive nor part of a multiple system disease, typically arises from defects in the muscle chloride channel, in myotonia congenita. The presence of multiple system defects argues strongly in favor of the diagnosis of myotonic dystrophy. There are few other disorders in this differential evaluation. In Schwartz-Jampel syndrome, children with a distinctive facial appearance, including low-set ears, are myotonic but do not have recurrent paralysis. Patients with recurrent weakness with disturbed serum potassium levels but no clear family history of periodic paralysis merit a thorough evaluation for alternate causes of hypo- or hyperkalemia. Particularly striking is the conjoining of hypokalemic periodic paralysis with thyrotoxicosis, an entity more prevalent in Japan than in the United States.

If there is diagnostic ambiguity, provocative testing may be helpful. Thus, one may provoke hypokalemic weakness by administering oral glucose (5 g/kg, to a total of 100 g); if the diagnosis is strongly suspected and the oral glucose challenge is ambiguous, one may infuse intravenous glucose (3 g/kg over 1 hour), possibly with added insulin. During this procedure, the serum potassium should be monitored three or four times per hour, with close ECG monitoring as well. Provocative testing for hyperkalemic paralysis can be performed using oral potassium loading (1 mEq/kg), with frequent potassium monitoring and ECG surveillance for at least 3 hours after loading. Cooling of a limb while monitoring the EMG may assist in establishing the diagnosis of paramyotonia congenita. In these patients, cooling to 30°C induces fibrillations; additional cooling may produce electrical silence concurrently with clinical paralysis of the cooled muscles. It may be useful to monitor the amplitude of the compound muscle action potential during this process;

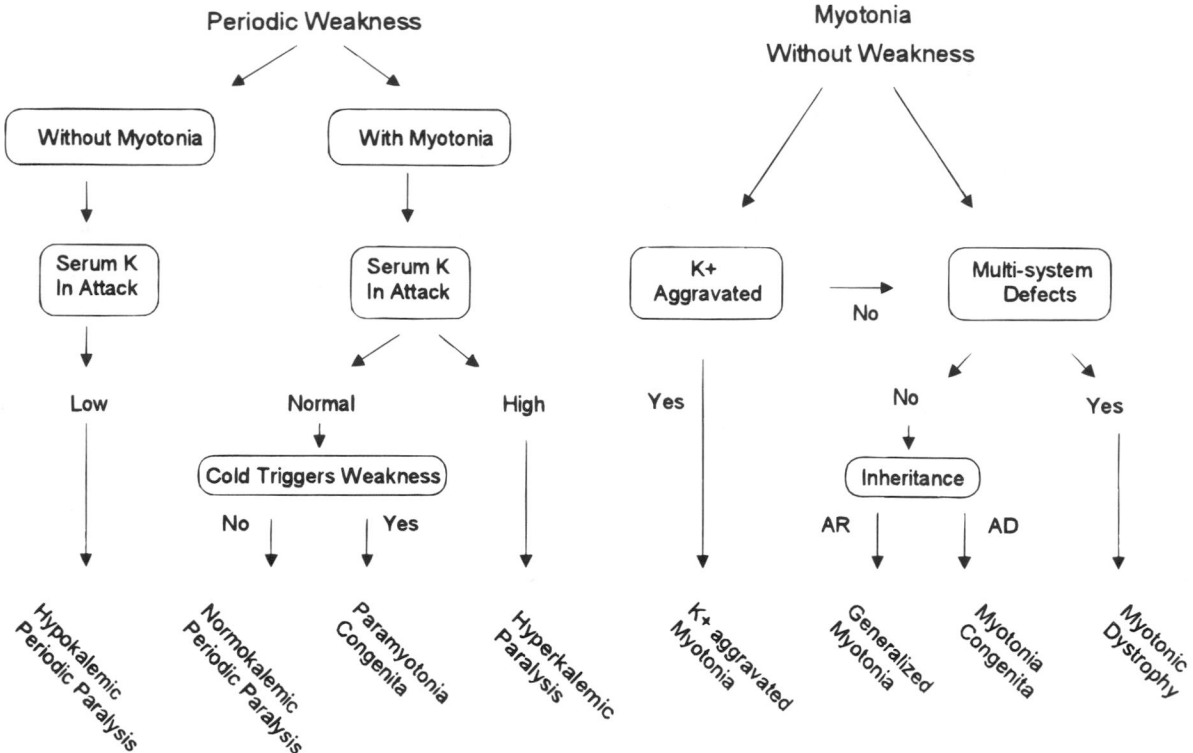

FIG. 111-1. Evaluation of the patient with periodic paralysis and myotonia.

the amplitude may drop dramatically with cooling in paramyotonia congenita patients.

The mainstay of laboratory investigations of these patients is screening of blood DNA for mutations in genes now established to be defective in each disorder (Tables 111-1 and 111-2). These studies require only a small blood sample and can be rapidly performed. The selectivity of the specific mutations for each disorder is close to 100 percent; the rate of false negatives is probably less than 10 percent. For these reasons, an accurate DNA diagnosis is cost-effective, obviating muscle biopsy in most cases.

TREATMENT

Myotonia associated with these disorders may be somewhat difficult to treat. In our experience, the most consistently helpful drug is mexilitine, a sodium channel-blocking lidocaine derivative. Benefit may also be seen with other "membrane-active" compounds such as phenytoin. Attacks of weakness may be reduced in frequency with the carbonic anhydrase inhibitor, acetazolamide; a related, more potent inhibitor, dichlorphenamide, is currently under evaluation. In hypokalemic paralysis, there appears to be little benefit from chronic (daily) potassium administration. On the other hand, some patients with hyperkalemic paralysis report benefit from chronic use of a potassium-wasting diuretic. Acute attacks of weakness in periodic paralysis usually respond to management of the serum potassium abnormality. In hypokalemic paralysis, it almost always suffices to administer potassium orally. If intravenous fluids are administered to patients with hypokalemic paralysis, high-sodium solutions may exacerbate weakness. For this reason, some authors suggest the use of mannitol solutions for intravenous infusion.

SUGGESTED READINGS

Brook JD, McCurrach ME, Harley HG et al: Molecular basis of myotonic dystrophy: expansion of a trinucleotide (CTG) repeat at the 3′ end of a transcript encoding a protein kinase family member. Cell 69:385–95, 1992

Bryant SH: Myotonia in the goat. Ann NY Acad Sci 317:314–25, 1979

Cannon SC, Brown Jr. RH, Corey DP: A sodium channel defect in hyperkalemic periodic paralysis: potassium induced failure of inactivation. Neuron 6:619–26, 1991

Catterall W: Structure and function of voltage-sensitive ion channels. Science 242:50–61, 1988

Creutzfeld OD, Abbott BC, Fowler WM et al: Muscle membrane potentials in episodica adynamia. Electroencephalogr Clin Neurophysiol 15:508–15, 1963

Engel AG: Evolution and content of vacuoles in primary hypokalemic periodic paralysis. Mayo Clin Proc 45:774–851, 1970

Fontaine B, Khurana T, Hoffman E et al: Hyperkalemic periodic paralysis and the adult muscle sodium channel alpha-subunit gene. Science 250:1000–2, 1990

Hoffman EP, Lehmann-Horn F, Rudel R: Overexcited or inactive: ion channels in muscle disease: Cell 80:681–6, 1995

Jurkat-Rott K, Lehmann-Horn F, Elbaz A et al: A calcium channel mutation causing hypokalemic periodic paralysis. Hum Molec Genetics 3:1415–19, 1994

Lehmann-Horn F, Grzeschik KH, Jentsch TJ: Tight linkage of recessive and dominant forms of human myotonia to skeletal muscle chloride channel gene. Science 257:797–800, 1992

Lipicky RJ, Bryant SH, Salmon JH: Cable parameters, sodium, potassium and chloride and water content and potassium efflux in isolated external intercostal muscle of normal volunteers and patients with myotonia congenita. J Clin Invest 50:2091–103, 1971

Ptacek L, Tawil R, Griggs RC et al: Dihydropyridine receptor mutations cause hypokalemic periodic paralysis. Cell 77:863–8, 1994

Roses AD: Myotonic dystrophy. pp. 633–46. In: The Molecular and Genetic Basis of Neurologic Disease. Rosenberg RN, Prusiner SB, DiMauro S et al (eds): Butterworth-Heinemann, Boston, 1993

Rudel R, Ricker K, Lehmann-Horn F: Genotype-phenotype correlations in human skeletal muscle sodium channel diseases. Arch Neurol 50:1241–8, 1993

1993

Rudel R, Lehmann-Horn F: Membrane changes in cells from myotonia patients. Physiol Rev 65:310–56, 1985

Steinmeyer K, Ortland C, Jentsch TJ: Primary structure and functional expression of a developmentally regulated skeletal muscle chloride channel. Na-

112. ABNORMAL MUSCLE ACTIVITY

LUDWIG GUTMANN

MYOKYMIA

Myokymia is a clinical phenomenon characterized by undulating, vermicular, rippling, and wavelike movements spreading across the muscle surface. The facial muscles are more commonly involved than those of the extremities, but whether they are depends on the nature of the underlying problem. It occurs as a manifestation in a number of disorders, the most common of which are Guillain-Barré syndrome, multiple sclerosis, radiation plexopathy, brain stem tumors, and timber rattlesnake (Crotalus horridus horridus) envenomation.

The disorders that most commonly produce myokymia and myokymic discharges affect the axon membrane microenvironment through such mechanisms as demyelination, radiation changes, direct toxic effects, ischemia, hypoxia, hypocalcemia, and edema. Axon compression is an uncommon cause of myokymia. One may see occasional isolated myokymic discharges involving a single motor unit in compressive neuropathies (e.g., carpal tunnel syndrome) and radiculopathies, but these are not sufficiently widespread to be noted clinically.

The clinically observable myokymia is associated with characteristic electromyographic (EMG) activity referred to as myokymic discharges. The myokymic discharges are typically short bursts of motor unit potentials. The motor unit potentials within the burst most often fire at a rate of 5 to 62 Hz and appear as doublets, triplets, or multiplets (Fig. 112-1). The number of times the motor unit fires within a multiplet may range from 4 to well over 100 per burst. Each myokymic burst usually fires recurrently at 2 to 10 Hz in a rhythmic or semirhythmic fashion. Occasionally, bursts may fire much less frequently, such as once every 20 to 30 seconds. Myokymic bursts with more spikes generally fire at a slower frequency. The actual rate of firing of myokymic bursts varies from one neighboring unit to the next, resulting in a complex firing arrangement within the muscle. The discharges may originate in the intramedullary portion of the motor axon, as in multiple sclerosis and pontine gliomas. They may arise peripherally in the motor axons, as in Guillain-Barré syndrome and radiation plexopathy.

Disorders in which myokymia has been reported include the following (asterisk indicates those in which it is regularly seen):

Guillain-Barré*
Multiple sclerosis*
Radiation plexopathy*
Intramedullary/extramedullary pontine tumors/masses*
Timber rattlesnake envenomation*
Chronic inflammatory demyelinating polyneuropathy
Neoplastic/inflammatory meningoradiculitis
Anoxic/ischemic rhombencephalopathy
Syringobulbia
Basilar invagination
Gold therapy
Cardiopulmonary rest
Subarachnoid hemorrhage

Facial myokymia, at times subtle, with its associated myokymic discharges, occurs in 15 percent of patients with Guillain-Barré syndrome. Myokymia in the extremities also occurs, but is much less frequent. In the Guillain-Barré syndrome, the facial myokymia is frequently bilaterally and often associated with mild facial weakness. It appears within the first 3 weeks of the illness and is present up to 1 month before clearing. The limb myokymia in this disorder is also transient. Its occurrence in the extremities in chronic inflammatory demyelinating polyneuropathy is occasionally seen.

In multiple sclerosis, myokymia also involves facial muscles much more frequently than those of the extremities. In the face, it is usually unilateral, transient, and present for only a few weeks. Recurrent episodes occasionally occur and may be either on the same or opposite sides. It may be associated with mild facial weakness, and at times, the myokymia is sufficiently prominent to result in a persistent contraction of the involved side of the face.

Facial myokymia in the presence of a posterior fossa tumor or mass is most often seen with a pontine glioma. It has been reported with other masses, including cerebellar astrocytomas, metastatic tumors, and acoustic neuromas. The myokymia is unilateral and may persist for many months to years. A persistent contraction of the involved side of the face has been reported in a number of cases.

Brachial and lumbosacral plexopathy due to radiation are often associated with myokymia. Myokymia is usually present in only one or a few muscles of the involved extremity, but occurs in 60 to 70 percent of cases. The myokymia may be present decades after the radiation occurred. It is often associ-

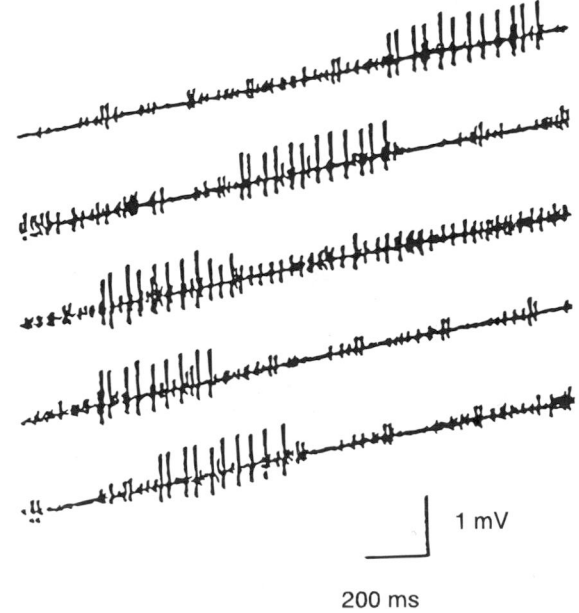

1 mV

200 ms

FIG. 112-1. Myokymic discharge appearing as a recurrent multiple once in each sweep. Other smaller myokymic discharges occur in the background.

ated with other neurogenic changes. Myokymia is unlikely to be due to tumor infiltration or traumatic plexopathy. Its presence, therefore, suggests radiation as a cause.

Timber rattlesnake envenomation is invariably associated with bilateral facial myokymia and myokymia of the extremities. The facial myokymia occurs as a result of a hematogenous spread of the toxin and disappears within several hours of the patient receiving antivenin therapy. The myokymia in the bitten extremity persists several days before clearing.

NEUROMYOTONIA

Neuromyotonia involves a continuous, albeit somewhat irregular, movement of the muscles associated with neuromyotonic discharges. Neuromyotonic discharges are prolonged bursts of motor unit potentials, often firing at a frequency of 40 to 200 Hz for up to a few seconds, usually beginning and ending abruptly (Fig. 112-2). The potential amplitude may wane but can easily be distinguished from myotonia. Unlike myokymia, the bursts do not recur repetitively in a rhythmic fashion and may be initiated by needle movement, voluntary effort, or nerve percussion. At times, neuromyotonia may be interspersed with myokymic discharges.

In 1961, Isaacs described the syndrome, now named after him, characterized by continuous muscle fiber activity with stiffness, cramps, and increased sweating. Neuromyotonia is the underlying electrophysiologic abnormality for the syndrome. The neuromyotonia arises from ectopic generators in the peripheral nerve. The discharges continue during complete proximal nerve blocks and are abolished by curare blockade. Neuromyotonia is often associated with underlying fibrillation potentials and fasciculations and, in addition to the above characteristics, continues during sleep and general anesthesia. Carbamazepine and phenytoin may have a beneficial effect in alleviating the symptoms.

In a recent review, Newsom-Davis and Mills reported five cases that had associated autoimmune manifestations, including oligoclonal bands in cerebrospinal fluid and improvement following plasma exchange. Additional cases in the literature have been associated with thymoma, myasthenia gravis, elevated acetylcholine receptor antibody titers, and penicillamine ther-

apy. At West Virginia University (my institution), there have been two cases of neuromyotonia with chronic inflammatory polyneuropathy and one case with amyloidosis associated with a monoclonal IgG κ spike. It has been suggested that neuromyotonia may result from antibody-mediated autoimmune mechanisms, possibly directed at peripheral nerve K^+ or Na^+ channels.

COMPLEX REPETITIVE DISCHARGES

Complex repetitive discharges are a rather dramatic but nonspecific EMG abnormality seen in a variety of myopathic and neurogenic processes. These include muscular dystrophies, polymyositis, motor neuron disease, radiculopathies, chronic polyneuropathies, and myxedema. Their presence implies chronicity of the disorder, but otherwise provides little diagnostic or other useful information. The appearance of CRDs on the EMG screen is invariably sudden and dramatic. Their complex and somewhat bizarre appearance resulted in the previously used term of *bizarre high-frequency discharges*.

Complex repetitive discharges represent the relatively synchronous firing of a group of muscle fibers. The complexes recur at rates of 5 to 100 Hz. The complex wave form of each individual discharge remains uniform, the shape may change suddenly within a train of discharges, and the train of discharges begins and ends abruptly (Fig. 112-3). The appearance and sound of complex repetitive discharges are distinctly different from myokymia, neuromyotonia, myotonia, and cramps: the sound is that of a machine gun firing.

Altered muscle membrane properties are in large part the pathophysiologic basis for complex repetitive discharges. It has been proposed that each individual complex within a complex repetitive discharge is composed of a series of individual muscle action potentials linked together by ephaptic transmission between involved muscle fibers. In some cases, nerve blocks and curare failed to abolish the complex repetitive discharges, whereas in other cases, they persist despite curare. Their precipitation by a nerve action potential has been described by Besser and Gutmann.

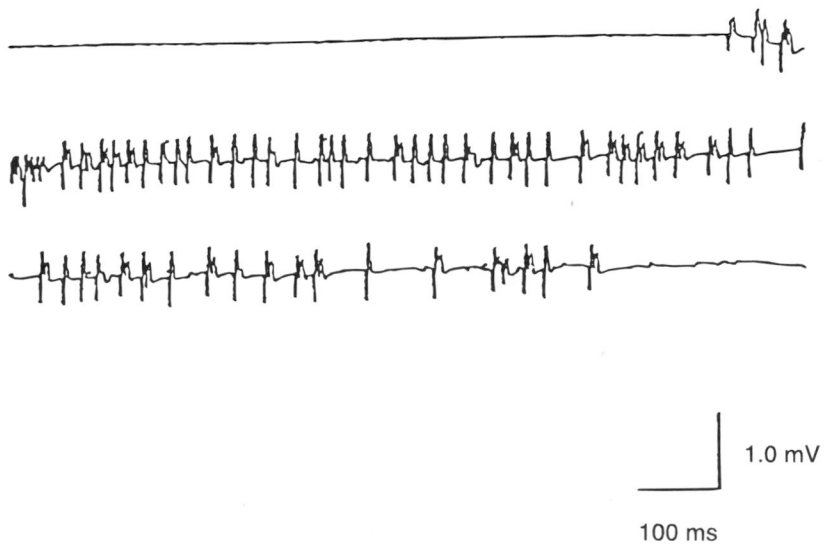

1.0 mV

100 ms

FIG. 112-2. Single neuromyotonic discharge.

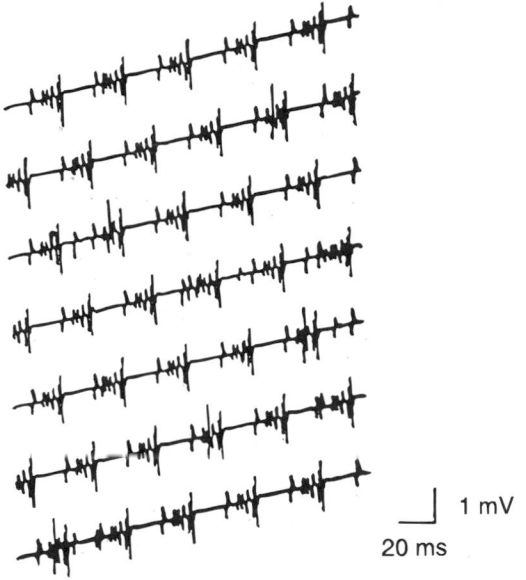

FIG. 112-3. Complex repetitive discharge.

CRAMPS

Cramps represent involuntary—usually painful—contractions of a group of muscle fibers that last seconds to minutes. They may occur in otherwise normal individuals in any muscle, but most commonly occur in the calves often at night. They may be precipitated by contraction of the involved muscle and alleviated by stretching the muscle. Pathologic states that predisposed to cramps include hyponatremia (as in athletes undertaking strenuous activities in hot weather), and a variety of neurogenic disorders including the motor neuron diseases, radiculopathies, and polyneuropathies. A cramp-fasciculation syndrome has been described in association with myalgias, stiffness, and exercise intolerance. This may be present for years either on a sporadic or hereditary basis and unassociated with any other neurogenic changes.

Cramps involve the spontaneous and synchronous firing of multiple motor units. The rate of motor unit discharges are irregular and occur at high frequencies, usually ranging from 40 to 60 Hz. The physiologic origin of cramps has not been clearly defined. It has been postulated that there may be both central and peripheral mechanisms. They have been precipitated by repetitive nerve stimulation distal to nerve blocks in some patients predisposed to cramps but not in others.

Quinine and carbamazepine have been reported to help alleviate cramps. The effect of diazepam and baclofen, γ-aminobutyric acid$_A$ and γ-aminobutyric acid$_B$ agonists, respectively, in patients with motor neuron disease, has lead to the suggestion that some cramps may result from impaired function of suppressive interneurons mediated by γ-aminobutyric acid as the neurotransmitter.

HEMIFACIAL SPASM

Hemifacial spasm is characterized by clonic contractions of unilateral facial muscles, usually beginning about the eye and then spreading to other muscles of the involved side of the face. This is based on the synchronous intermittent firing of multiple

motor units, with the generator being located proximally in the facial nerve. Despite the often dramatic appearance of the hemifacial spasm, it is unlikely to be associated with any serious underlying disorder in the posterior fossa. It is thought that most cases are due to an aberrant blood vessel compressing the facial nerve shortly after it exits the pons. The intermittent clonic activity involving the orbicularis oculi may interfere with vision and the cosmetic aspect of the problem may be distressing. Neuroimaging of the posterior fossa is unlikely to be helpful.

Carbamazepine and phenytoin are occasionally helpful in decreasing or abolishing the hemifacial spasm. Botulinum toxin injections are useful in decreasing the clonic contractions, especially in the orbicularis oculi. Posterior fossa exploration to remove the aberrant blood vessel, compressing the nerve, or altering its location is the most definitive therapy, but such surgery has a number of potential postoperative complications.

MYOTONIA

Myotonia is the delayed relaxation of a muscle after voluntary contraction or percussion. The delayed relaxation is accompanied by myotonic discharges. The latter are repetitive discharges at 20 to 80 Hz of single muscle fibers having the appearance of a positive wave or fibrillation potential. The waxing and waning quality of the discharges provides the "dive bomber" sound. The discharges originate in the muscle membrane, since neither nerve block or neuromuscular junction block with curare alter the myotonia.

In most of the myotonic syndromes, the myotonia improves as the muscle warms up with repeated use. In paramyotonia, it worsens with repeated muscle contractions. The myotonic disorders include myotonic dystrophy, the sodium channel disorders (hyperkalemic periodic paralysis, paramyotonia congenita, and potassium-sensitive myotonia congenita), and myotonia congenita.

SUGGESTED READINGS

Besser R, Gutmann L: Muscle action potential precipitated complex repetitive discharge. Muscle Nerve 11:1190–1, 1988

Denny-Brown D, Foley JM: Myokymia and the benign fasciculation of muscular cramps. Trans Assoc Am Physicians 61:88–96, 1948

Gutmann L: AAEM minimonograph #37: facial and limb myokymia. Muscle Nerve 14:43–9, 1991

Isaacs H: Continuous muscle fibre activity in an Indian male with additional evidence of terminal motor fibre abnormality. J Neurol Neurosurg Psychiatry 30: 126–33, 1967

Newsom-Davis J, Mills KR: Immunological associations of acquired neuromyotonia (Isaacs' syndrome). Brain 116:453–469, 1993

Nix WA, Butler NJ, Roontga S et al: Persistent unilateral tibialis anterior muscle hypertrophy with complex repetitive discharges and myalgia: report of two unique cases and response to botulinum toxin. Neurology 42:602–6, 1992

Obi T, Mizoguchi K, Matsuoka H et al: Muscle cramp as the result of impaired GABA function—an electrophysiological and pharmacological observation. Muscle Nerve 6:1228–31, 1993

Ptacek LJ, Johnson KJ, Griggs RC: Genetic and physiology of the myotonic muscle disorders. N Engl J Med 328:482–9, 1993

Rasminsky M: Ephaptic transmission between single nerve fibers in the spinal nerve roots of dystrophic mice. J. Physiol (Lond) 305:151–69, 1980

Tahmoush AJ, Alonso RJ, Tahmoush GP, Heiman-Patterson TD: Cramp-fasciculation syndrome: a treatable hyperexcitable peripheral nerve disorder. Neurology 14:1021–4, 1991

Trontelj J, Stalberg E: Bizarre repetitive discharges recorded with single fiber EMG. J Neurol Neurosurg Psychiatry 46:310–16, 1983

MOVEMENT DISORDERS

PART **V**

113. PARKINSON'S DISEASE: RECOGNITION, DIAGNOSIS, AND MANAGEMENT

LEWIS R. SUDARSKY

Parkinson's disease is among the most common of the movement disorders. Its prevalence is roughly 120 in 100,000 in the United States and in other parts of the industrialized world where it has been surveyed. Onset of Parkinson's disease is uncommon before age 40. Thereafter, the incidence increases sharply with age, ultimately affecting 1.5 percent of the population over 65, and 2.5 percent over 85. The illness was first described as a "shaking palsy" by James Parkinson in the early nineteenth century. There has been an explosion of knowledge since the early 1960s, with improvements in therapeutics that have fundamentally altered the natural history of the disease.

Neuropathologic examination in Parkinson's disease reveals a loss of pigmented neurons from the pars compacta of the substantia nigra. These cells contain neuromelanin and make neurotransmitter dopamine. Microscopic examination reveals pigmented neurons in various stages of decay; some contain a characteristic eosinophilic inclusion (Lewy body). The dopaminergic projections from the substantia nigra influence motor processing in the basal ganglia: dopaminergic neurons facilitate execution of movement and help suppress unwanted movement. Loss of 50 to 60 percent of these cells from the substantia nigra results in critical deficiency of dopamine in the striatum. Excess inhibitory output of the basal ganglia complex produces the bradykinesia and rigidity of Parkinson's disease.

The etiology of Parkinson's disease is not presently known. There are few epidemiologic clues to help define the cause. In studies of young-onset patients, rural residence, drinking well water, and exposure to pesticide chemicals have been associated with increased risk. Some cases of familial Parkinson's disease have been described with autosomal dominant inheritance, but surveys of twins suggest that Parkinson's is not primarily a genetic disorder. The current literature favors a complex multifactor hypothesis, with metabolic predisposition, exposure to exogenous toxins, and endogenous oxidant stress all playing a role.

RECOGNITION OF PARKINSON'S DISEASE

Parkinson's disease is appreciated on clinical grounds; no laboratory tests are used routinely to establish the diagnosis. The cardinal clinical features are bradykinesia, rigidity, and tremor. Shuffling gait and flexed posture are also characteristic, and are sometimes listed together as a fourth principal sign. Bradykinesia—slowness of movement—is the most disabling aspect of Parkinson's disease. Patients describe it as stiffness, weakness, or a pervasive slowness that affects every aspect of movement. Dressing, eating, and other activities of daily living take extra time. There is also paucity of movement (akinesia) and difficulty initiating movement. Patients experience some loss of dexterity for buttoning, handwriting, and fine finger movement. Many describe difficulty getting up from a chair or getting out of the car, movements that require truncal mobility and complex postural adjustments. This same difficulty is likely to be reflected in the patient's tennis serve, golf swing, or bowling score. It is difficult for patients with Parkinson's disease to perform two complex motor acts at the same time, so many such activities acquire a slow, deliberate character. Arrests of ongoing movement sometimes occur (freezing).

Rigidity is uniform through the range of movement, and can be palpated in the neck as well as about the wrist. Rigidity is often associated with cogwheeling, a ratchety quality appreciated during passive movement. The tremor of Parkinson's disease is a resting tremor, greatest in repose and less active during movement. It is a presenting feature of the illness for up to 70 percent of patients. Resting tremor is prominent when the patient is seated, but will often subside when full relaxation is achieved, as in sleep. The tremor has a frequency of 3 to 5 cycles/s. It is typically a pronation-supination tremor of the forearm, with wrist and finger flexion (pill-rolling). Tremor may also involve the lower limbs or jaw, though it does not typically produce a whole head or vocal tremor. Some patients with Parkinson's disease have an action tremor as well as a resting tremor, whereas others have no discernable tremor. (Isolated occurrence of an action tremor should not be confused with Parkinson's disease).

There is a lot of variability in the presentation, and two of the three cardinal manifestations are usually required for a definite diagnosis. The most typical case begins asymmetrically in the limbs with a resting tremor. A flexed posture and marche á petit pas both evoke the impression of Parkinson's disease, but are nonspecific. Flexion bias in postural and limb muscles can be seen with other basal ganglia disorders. A shuffling gait is nonspecific, reflecting injury to frontal/subcortical systems.

Beyond these core features, Parkinson's disease is a diagnosis of impressions. Associated features contribute to the clinical picture. There is a paucity of facial expression—sometimes a blank stare, occasionally a look of consternation. Reduced blinking gives way to blepharospasm as the eyes are approached. There is inability to inhibit blinking with tap on the glabellar prominence. A curious transformation of handwriting is regularly described, with involution into a tiny scrawl (micrographia). In stance, the patient is bent forward at the neck and back, resulting in a simian posture. The arms do not swing naturally in gait, and there is a tendency to turn en bloc, "as if the joints were soldered" (Charcot's description).

Dysarthria in Parkinson's disease is distinctive: speech is hypophonic and rapid, without normal prosody (emotional expression). There is sometimes stammering or palilalia (perseverative repetition of syllables). Patients are frequently unaware of their speech unintelligibility and need to make a specific effort to slow down. Drooling is a bothersome feature for some patients, with reduced swallowing and accumulation of saliva. Seborrhea is also characteristic of Parkinson's disease, with increased oil production from the sebaceous glands of the skin. Sensory symptoms are not typical, but are described. Many patients experience migratory discomfort associated with muscle stiffness. Loss of olfactory acuity is consistently present, and may be an early indicator. Slight edema is occasionally observed in an affected limb, a finding that has been attributed to venous stasis from akinesia. Dementia occurs in 10 to 20 percent of patients with Parkinson's disease, but is not typically a presenting feature. (Mental change in Parkinson's disease is discussed in a separate chapter.)

Positron emission tomographic studies using ^{18}F-fluorodopa demonstrate reduced uptake in the striatal complex in Parkinson's disease, particularly marked in the putamen. Quantitative analysis may reveal deficiencies in a very early, or even preclinical dopamine deficiency state. In practice, magnetic resonance imaging is sometimes obtained in atypical cases to rule out systems degeneration or ischemic change in the basal ganglia as a cause of symptomatic parkinsonism.

DIFFERENTIAL DIAGNOSIS

Unfortunately, the features that permit recognition and diagnosis of Parkinson's disease are not entirely specific. Fifteen to 25 percent of patients followed in a Parkinson's clinic will turn out to have a related disorder rather than idiopathic Parkinson's disease. In the London Brain Bank project, patients were examined during life by senior neurologists applying rigorous diagnostic standards. Despite extra effort and attention to the problem of diagnosis, more than 20 percent of cases did not meet pathologic criteria for Parkinson's disease at postmortem examination.

Table 113-1 lists the various causes of parkinsonian syndromes. Some patients presenting with a symmetric akinetic/rigid disorder have a related neurodegenerative disorder with involvement of the striatum. Progressive supranuclear palsy, multiple system atrophy, and corticobasal ganglionic degeneration can all present with parkinsonism. With time, other manifestations (abnormal eye movements, cerebellar, or corticospinal tract signs) emerge that help characterize the disorder. These less restricted degenerative disorders are known collectively as atypical parkinsonism or parkinsonism-plus syndrome.

A parkinsonian syndrome may also be the result of encephalitis, trauma, or toxic/metabolic injury to the nervous system. Postencephalitic parkinsonism of the kind illustrated in the film *Awakenings* is now rare. Drug-induced parkinsonism is important to recognize, as it is relatively common and fully reversible. The syndrome results from the motor effect of medications that depress dopaminergic function, most typically neuroleptic, antipsychotic drugs. These drugs are highly tissue bound, and symptoms often persist weeks after the offending medication has been discontinued.

Some patients with vascular disease develop Parkinson syndrome after lacunar infarction of the basal ganglia. The phenomenon of "atherosclerotic parkinsonism" has been controversial, as basal ganglia lacunae are often asymptomatic, but widespread, ischemic injury to the striatal complex will ultimately produce bradykinesia and rigidity. The extrapyramidal syndrome is not pure: mental change, corticospinal and corticobulbar tract findings are often associated. Most such patients have hypertension, and findings of small-vessel disease can be appreciated on imaging studies.

TABLE 113-1. Parkinsonism-Plus Syndromes

Progressive supranuclear palsy

Multiple system atrophy
 Shy-Drager syndrome
 Striatonigral degeneration
 Olivopontocerebellar atrophy

Parkinson's-amyotrophic lateral sclerosis-dementia of Guam

Generalized Lewy body disease

Corticobasal ganglionic degeneration

Alzheimer's/Parkinson's overlap syndrome

Huntington's disease: rigid variant

Hallervorden-Spatz disease

Gerstmann-Strausler syndrome

Causes of Secondary Parkinsonism
 Toxic
  MPTP (methyl-4-phenyl-tetrahydropyridine)
  Manganese
  Carbon monoxide

 Drug-induced
  Neuroleptic drugs
  Metaclopramide, prochlorperazine
  Reserpine

 Vascular disease ("arteriosclerotic parkinsonism")
  Basal ganglia lacunae
  Binswanger's disease

 Hydrocephalus

 Trauma

 Tumor

 Chronic hepatocerebral degeneration

 Wilson's disease

Infectious
  Postencephalitic parkinsonism
  Cruetzfeldt-Jakob disease
  Acquired immunodefiency disease

In the London Brain Bank study, asymmetry at onset and presence of a typical resting tremor were findings more likely to be associated with a diagnosis of Parkinson's disease at autopsy. There is always a degree of uncertainty when confronted with a symmetric akinetic/rigid disorder. In those cases characterized by axial rigidity, postural instability, and a shuffling gait, the diagnostic uncertainty is particularly high. These features have been observed to cluster with older age at onset and the presence of dementia in clinical studies. Some such patients have evidence of hydrocephalus or periventricular white-matter disease on magnetic resonance imaging. Postural instability is typically a late feature of Parkinson's disease, whereas it occurs early with progressive supranuclear palsy and related disorders.

A dramatic initial response to levodopa/carbidopa may be helpful in separating Parkinson's disease from the related disorders in Table 113-1. Many of these parkinsonian syndromes respond partially to levodopa, but a dramatic initial response and the emergence over time of levodopa dose dependence suggest the diagnosis of idiopathic Parkinson's disease.

MEASUREMENT OF PARKINSONISM

It is sometimes helpful to quantify the impairment produced by Parkinson's disease. Duration of the illness and total duration of levodopa therapy are helpful parameters of disease status, but direct measurement of Parkinson's-related disability is useful as a basis for comparison and clinical follow-up. As many patients are depressed, the subjective complaints do not always parallel the evolution of the illness over time. It is essential to have an objective measure for clinical trials (drug trials and surgical intervention studies). The degree of parkinsonism is not always

TABLE 113-2. Fourteen Motor Elements of the Unified Parkinson's Disease Rating Scale[a]

Speech[b]
Facial expression
Tremor at rest[b]
Action tremor
Rigidity[b]
Finger taps[b]
Hand movement
Pronation-supination of the hands
Leg agility
Getting out of a chair[b]
Posture
Gait[b]
Postural stability[b]
Body bradykinesia[b]

[a] These 14 standard elements are scored on the motor section of the UPDRS.
[b] Some items are redundant; the scale can be collapsed to these 8 items without loss of validity, according to Van Hilten et al. (1994).

well reflected in the standard neurologic examination and case recording. Because measurement is an important issue in a disease defined by its clinical syndrome, some of the approaches to quantitative assessment, ranging from rating scales to physiologic performance measures, are reviewed here.

In their landmark paper on the natural history of Parkinson's disease in the prelevodopa era, Hoehn and Yahr recognized five stages of the illness. In stage 1, the disease manifestations are principally unilateral. Stage 2 applies to the patient with bilateral symptoms and signs, but good preservation of balance. In stage 3, the disease remains mild to moderate and the patient is fully independent, but manifestations of postural instability are observed. The stage 4 patient is more severely disabled, but still able to walk about unassisted. In stage 5, the patient is not independently able to stand and walk. The Hoehn and Yahr global staging system is widely accepted and easy to apply. It characterizes the major landmarks of disease progression, but does not distinguish small degrees of change. Loss (or gain) of one stage implies a large change in clinical status.

Subsequent efforts to measure the impairment of Parkinson's disease, such as the Webster scale and its successor, the unified Parkinson's disease rating scale, separately score major disease manifestations. The unified scale was constructed by a committee of experts as a standard for clinical research. It includes sections on mental status, activities of daily living, motor performance, and side effects of therapy. In the motor section of the scale, 14 items are scored from 0 to 4 for severity (Table 113-2). Resting tremor, for example, is scored based on its amplitude and consistent presence. In this sort of rating scale, a patient's score may vary considerably over the course of the day with the medication cycle. There is a growing literature on the validity and reliability of the unified scale, and a videotape has been produced to standardize its application. The motor section of the scale is currently the most widely used clinical assessment instrument.

After 5 to 8 years of levodopa therapy, a majority of patients have developed fluctuations in response. For these patients, separate scores can be recorded in the ''on'' and ''off'' state. (For research purposes, ''off'' scores are generally recorded after an overnight washout.) It is useful to record the total daily ''off'' time, usually obtained from the patient's history. Some patients are able to keep a daily log of on, off, and on/dyskinesia for each waking hour, which is a great help in adjusting their medication. The percent of waking hours in the ''on'' and ''off'' state is a useful index of treatment efficacy.

The other major dimension of Parkinson's-related disability is the gradual loss of independence in activities of daily living. Schwab and England constructed an activities of daily living scale to measure disability in this context. The scale ranges from 100 percent (fully independent in activities of daily living) to 0 percent (bedridden, needing to be fed). It largely measures the time required to complete daily chores, and the ability to do them without assistance. Scoring of activities of daily living is based on the patient's subjective reporting. The Schwab and England scale focuses on advanced disability, whereas patients with Parkinson's disease now maintain independence much longer. The Unified Parkinson's disease rating scale looks at particular tasks problematic in moderate to advanced Parkinson's disease, such as cutting food and handling utensils, dressing, and washing. It also scores walking, falling, and freezing, again based on the patient's report.

All the rating scales described above suffer an important limitation, which is that the variability among different observers introduces a degree of imprecision to the measurement. The scales are also insensitive to mild degrees of impairment, and cannot define the point at which Parkinson's disease is first expressed. For research purposes, these semiquantitative clinical assessments are sometimes supplemented with direct measures of motor performance. Bradykinesia (slowness of movement) and akinesia (paucity of movement) are the major cause of disability in Parkinson's disease. Timed tests of movement are most commonly used to quantify bradykinesia. Pronation-supination of the wrist, alternately tapping the palm and dorsum of the hand against the knee, can be timed for 10 or 20 cycles. Likewise, two targets can be placed 12 in. apart, instructing the patient to alternate finger taps between the two targets. This test can be administered at the keyboard, or using a pencil and paper: total taps in 10 seconds, or time to complete 10 cycles.

In the neurophysiology lab, initiation and execution of a movement can be recorded with great precision. Reaction time is the interval between presentation of a ''go'' signal and the first agonist electromyographic burst. Movement time is the interval between initial muscle activity and completion of the movement. Both reaction time and movement time are prolonged in Parkinson's disease. Tremor amplitude and frequency can be documented in the laboratory by surface electromyography or accelerometric recording.

The disturbance in postural control and locomotion in Parkinson's disease can likewise be measured quantitatively. Most informative is a timed ''get up and go'' test. The patient is seated in a flat, hard chair without arms. He or she is instructed to stand up, walk a fixed distance, turn around, return, and sit down. The entire complex performance can be timed. Start hesitation, freezing, turn hesitation, and difficulty getting out of a chair are all reflected in the measurement. Platform tests of balance are relatively insensitive to postural instability in Parkinson's disease until the problem is at an advanced stage.

SUGGESTED READINGS

Hoehn M, Yahr M: Parkinsonism: onset, progression and mortality. Neurology 17:427–42, 1967.

Hughes AJ, Daniel SE, Kilford L, Lees AJ: Accuracy of clinical diagnosis of idiopathic Parkinson's disease: a clinico-pathological study of 100 cases. Neurol Neurosurg Psychiatry 33:181–4, 1992

Marsden CD: Parkinson's disease. Lancet 1:948–52, 1990

Pallis CA: Parkinsonism: natural history and clinical features. BMJ 3:683–90, 1971

Stern MB, Koller WC: Parkinsonian, Syndromes. Marcel Dekker, New York, 1994

Van Hilten JJ, van der Zwan AD, Zwinderman AH, Roos RAC: Rating impairment and disability in Parkinson's disease: evaluation of the UPDRS. Mov Disord 9:84–88, 1994
Watts RL, Mandir AS: Quantitative methods of evaluating Parkinson's disease. In Olanow CW, Lieberman AN (eds): The Scientific Basis for the Treatment of Parkinson's Disease. Parthenon, Park Ridge, NJ, 1992

$$Dopamine + O_2 + H_2O \xrightarrow{\text{MAOB}} 3,4\ Dihydroxyphenylacetaldehyde + H_2O_2$$

$$H_2O_2 + Fe^{2+} \longrightarrow Fe^{3+} + OH + OH^-$$

FIG. 114-1. Oxidation of dopamine.

114. SELEGILINE AND ANTIOXIDANTS: INITIAL THERAPY OF PARKINSON'S DISEASE

MARIE SAINT-HILAIRE
ROBERT G. FELDMAN

In the past few years, the treatment of Parkinson's disease in its early stage has been modified by the emphasis on prescribed neuroprotective therapy rather than on purely symptomatic treatment. This notion is based on the results of studies supporting the concept of oxidative stress in the pathogenesis of Parkinson's disease and the role of free radicals in the degenerative process. Free radicals are molecules with unpaired electrons that can react with polyunsaturated fatty acids in cellular membranes, producing lipid peroxidation and membrane damage, and that are able to interfere with the mitochondrial respiratory chain, leading to cell death. The interest in the role of free radicals in neurodegenerative disorders has led to the use of certain medications that could have a neuroprotective effect by reducing their formation, in particular selegiline. In order to understand new therapies of this type, it is important to review the concept of oxidative stress and its relation to Parkinson's disease.

ROLE OF OXIDATIVE STRESS

The concept of oxidative stress as a factor in nigral cell degeneration derives mainly from the observations that the oxidation of dopamine produces free radicals, and that 1-methyl-4-phenyl-1,2,3,6-tetrahydropyridine (MPTP) is neurotoxic for the nigral cells by oxidation into 1-methyl-4-phenyl-pyridinium ion (MPP$^+$).

Dopamine Oxidation

Dopaminergic neurons are susceptible to oxidative stress because the auto-oxidation of dopamine to form neuromelanin produces quinones and semiquinones, which are oxygen free radicals, and potentially neurotoxic. The observation that dopaminergic neurons containing the highest amount of neuromelanin are the earliest to be involved in Parkinson's disease suggests that dopamine turnover may play a role in nigral cell death. Dopamine is also oxidized by monamine oxidase-B (MAO-B). This reaction produces hydrogen peroxide (Fig. 114-

1), which, in the presence of free iron, can be transformed into highly reactive hydroxyl radicals and induce lipid peroxidation. The basal ganglia contain high concentrations of iron, and in Parkinson's disease, there is a marked increase in the iron level in the substantia nigra. This increased iron load would contribute to the formation of free radicals, especially in the presence of increased MAO-B, as seen with aging as well as Parkinson's disease. Protective mechanisms consisting of enzymes and vitamins are present, but there is still some controversy about the extent to which they may be impaired in Parkinson's disease. Catalase and glutathione peroxidase detoxify hydrogen peroxide, and their levels decrease or do not change in Parkinson's disease.

In addition to the role of endogenous dopamine, it has been suggested that the exogenous source of dopamine, given as levodopa for therapy of Parkinson's disease, could accelerate the death of nigral neurons through the same oxidative mechanisms. So far, there is no pathologic or clinical evidence to support that theory. Chronic levodopa therapy has not been shown to increase nigral death in animals or patients. Clinical studies suggest that introducing levodopa early in Parkinson's disease does not accelerate the progression of the disease and may even improve survival.

It has also been frequently mentioned that the onset of motor fluctuations is related to early use of levodopa in high doses. This is still a matter of controversy, because patients with more severe disease and rapid progression have early onset of motor fluctuations. These patients are likely to need higher doses of levodopa and to be treated more aggressively especially because they tend to be younger and more active. The earlier intervention in these patients might be related to the more severe disease rather than the opposite. However, several studies have indicated that low doses of levodopa combined with a dopamine agonist, such as bromocriptine, early in the course of disease, have less adverse reactions and decrease long-term complications of fluctuations and dyskinesias. This is the approach commonly used by neurologists.

Exogenous Neurotoxins

Another hypothetic cause of oxidative stress in Parkinson's disease is exposure to an environmental toxin. Interest in this hypothesis is based on the discovery that MPTP causes a syndrome similar to Parkinson's disease through oxidation into MPP$^+$ by MAO-B. Some epidemiologic studies have suggested that farming, pesticide, and insecticide use are associated with an increased risk of Parkinson's disease, although it is more likely that the development of Parkinson's disease depends on a combination of genetic predisposition, aging, and environmental factors. Both idiopathic Parkinson's disease and toxicity from MPP$^+$ are associated with a specific inhibition of complex I of the mitochondrial respiratory chain. The reason for this decrease is not clear. Inheritance of a mitochondrial defect is unlikely, because there is no evidence that Parkinson's disease

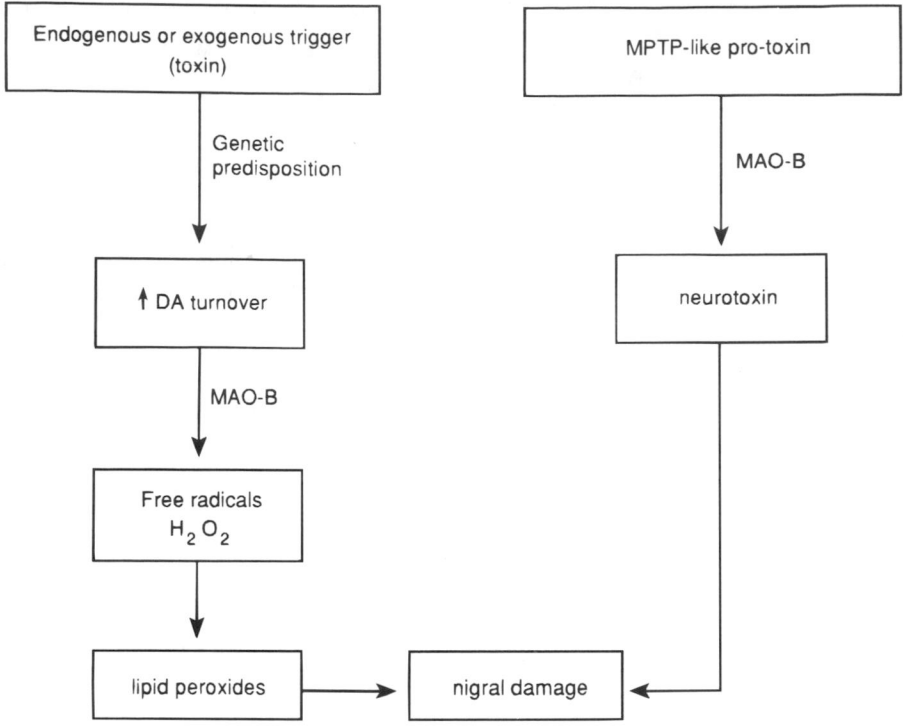

FIG. 114-2. Possible pathogenesis of Parkinson's disease.

is maternally inherited. Although there are reports of specific complex I subunits deficiency in the striatum of Parkinson's disease patients, or deletion of mitochondrial DNA, other researchers have been unable to reproduce these results. This suggests that perhaps the abnormality of complex I in Parkinson's disease is caused by the action of a toxin.

In summary, Parkinson's disease may be caused by an increase in cell death triggered by an endogenous or exogenous neurotoxin. The damage may occur through an increase in dopamine turnover facilitated by increased iron and MAO-B (Fig. 114-2). These observations provided the basis for studying selegiline in the progression of Parkinson's disease in the hope that it could (1) moderate the oxidative damage by preventing the oxidation of dopamine by MAO-B and (2) prevent the toxicity by MPTP-like exotoxins.

USE OF SELEGILINE

Selegiline (Deprenyl/Eldepryl) is an irreversible MAO inhibitor that is specific for MAO-B and does not potentiate the pressor effects of tyramine at doses below 20 mg/d. Studies on blood platelets have shown that a single oral dose of selegiline will inhibit 90 percent of the platelet MAO-B 2 hours after its administration. Postmortem studies in parkinsonian patients who received short-term selegiline showed that 88 percent of MAO-B was inhibited, but that MAO-A was unaffected. There is evidence that selegiline has value in Parkinson's disease because of its neuroprotecive, neurotrophic, and symptomatic effect.

Neuroprotective Effect

The potential neuroprotective effect of selegiline was first suggested by Birkmayer, who reported that patients receiving sele-

giline and levodopa lived longer than patients not receiving selegiline. Prospective studies were subsequently done in patients newly diagnosed with Parkinson's disease who were not yet receiving treatment. The most publicized study, known as deprenyl and tocopherol antioxidative therapy of parkinsonism (DATATOP), involved 800 patients randomly assigned to treatment with selegiline or placebo. The end point was defined as when patients were considered clinically to need to start levopopa therapy. Detailed statistical analysis of the data showed that selegiline slowed the rate of symptom development and delayed the need for levodopa by 50 percent. This study and others also showed that selegiline had a symptomatic effect, which might explain the delay in the need for levodopa. Long-term follow-up of the patients, however, showed that even patients who did not have any symptomatic benefit still had a delayed need for levodopa, suggesting a neuroprotective effect. Another prospective study on 100 patients, designed to minimize confounding symptomatic effect, supported this observation. Patients were randomized to receive selegiline or placebo, and Sinemet or bromocriptine. After 14 months of treatment, the patients were re-evaluated, 8 weeks after washout of selegiline or placebo, and 1 week after washout of Sinemet or bromocriptine. Deterioration of the parkinsonian score between baseline and the final visit was significantly greater in the placebo-treated group than the selegiline-treated group.

Postmortem analyses of nigral neurons showed that in patients treated with selegiline and levodopa, the number of neurons in the medial substantia nigra was greater than in those treated with levodopa alone. These pathologic observations also suggest that selegiline has neuron-saving effects.

Neurotrophic Action

There is evidence that selegiline can have some neuroprotective and neurotrophic effects independent from inhibition of MAO-

B. Experiments using DSP-4, a noradrenergic neurotoxin, demonstrated that selegiline has an action which is not related to MAO-B inhibition. Given 1 hour before DSP-4, selegiline blocked its norepinephrine-depleting effect. This protection declined sharply when N-(2-chloroethyl)-N-ethyl-2-bromobenzylamine (DSP-4) was given 24 hours or 4 days after selegiline, although MAO-B activity was still inhibited by 90 percent at 24 hours and by 70 percent after 4 days. The different time courses observed for the neuroprotective and MAO-B inhibitory effects suggested that the two phenomena were not linked. It is possible that selegiline acts by blocking the uptake of a toxic metabolite into the neurons.

The potential neurotrophic action of selegiline was experimentally demonstrated in mice, by administering selegiline for 3 weeks, starting 3 days after injection of MPTP. The 3-day delay allowed MPTP to be metabolized into MPP$^+$ by MAO-B, but selegiline reduced the loss of tyrosine hydroxylase in the substantia nigra, suggesting a protective effect not related to inhibition of MAO-B. Chronic selegiline treatment also increased the number of facial motoneurons surviving axotomy from 24 to 52 percent, possibly by compensation for the loss of target-derived trophic support.

Symptomatic Effect

In addition to the DATATOP study, other studies have shown that selegiline can have a symptomatic effect. The French Selegiline Multicenter Trial was especially designed to verify the efficacy of 10 mg/d of selegiline as monotherapy in de novo parkinsonian patients over a period of 3 months. This study demonstrated improvement of motor disability and mood in the patients on selegiline. There was no change on the Hoehn and Yahr scale, the Schwab and England disability scale, or the activities of daily living score. Selegiline was very well tolerated, as it was in the DATATOP study.

ROLE OF ANTIOXIDANT VITAMINS

Vitamins C and E have antioxidant and free radical scavenging properties that may help prevent the putative toxic effects of levodopa or other toxins in dopaminergic neurons.

Vitamin C penetrates into the brain, where it acts as a neuromodulator, antioxidant, and enzyme cofactor in catecholamine synthesis. It scavenges oxygen-containing radicals and participates in the enzymatic reduction of lipid peroxides. Vitamin C can reduce Fe^{3+} by converting it to Fe^{2+} and was shown to prevent levodopa toxicity and quinone formation in a human neuroblastoma line. Selegiline had only a partial protective effect and did not decrease quinone formation. These results indicated that levodopa toxicity in that cell line was mediated by two main mechanisms: generation of free radicals and formation of quinones. Because vitamin C and selegiline reduce levodopa toxicity by unrelated mechanisms, their combination could provide additional protection.

Vitamin C might also have a "trophiclike" effect. High concentrations of ascorbic acid can produce an increase in neurite growth and tyrosine hydroxylase activity, and enhance dopamine uptake and catecholamines levels in mesencephalic cultures.

Vitamin E blocks lipid peroxidation by donating a hydrogen ion to peroxy radicals. It appears that the midbrain has a unique ability to concentrate vitamin E during damage. However, levels of vitamin E are normal in the substantia nigra of parkinsonian patients, suggesting that the brains of these patients are not more susceptible to oxidative stress because of a lack of vitamin E.

Uncontrolled clinical studies have supported the protective effect of vitamins E and C. A retrospective study found that patients with Parkinson's disease who were self-supplementing with large daily doses of vitamin E for an average of about 7 years had significantly less severe disease than matched controls. In a pilot study, patients with early Parkinson's disease who received high daily intakes of vitamins C (3,000 mg/day) and E (3,200 U/d) went 2.5 years longer than unsupplemented patients before requiring levodopa to treat symptoms. However, DATATOP, a prospective double-blinded trial, did not find any beneficial effect of 2,000 U/d of vitamin E alone or in combination with selegiline in slowing down the progression of Parkinson's disease. The researchers concluded that despite this lack of benefit, studies of other antioxidants in Parkinson's disease are still warranted.

Therapeutic Recommendations

In the treatment of a newly diagnosed Parkinson's disease patient, selegiline is introduced to provide initial benefit, presumably by optimizing the effect of the patient's endogenous dopamine and for its potential neuroprotective action. The symptomatic benefit can be noticed in some patients at doses as low as 2.5 mg twice a day. Seldom is more than 10 mg/d required. The cardinal features of Parkinson's disease—rigidity, tremor, and bradykinesia—often produce mild to moderate impairment that lasts for several weeks to months, before clinical impairment demands more potent and specific therapy. In our practice, it is commonly recommended that the patient receive one-half a tablet (2.5 mg) of selegiline upon awakening, and another one-half tablet 4 to 6 hours later. If symptoms are unchanging, the dosage is increased to 1 tablet (5 mg) upon awakening and 1 again 4 to 6 hours later (for example, at 8:00 A.M. and 2:00 P.M.). Selegiline is usually not given in the late afternoon or evening, because the amphetamine metabolites can cause insomnia. Other potential side effects include skin rash and peptic ulcer disease because selegiline increases the gastric secretion of histamine. Selegiline is specific for MAO-B at the dose of 10 mg/d, and no specific diet is required. Interaction has been described with meperidine, causing hypertension and delirium.

Despite the differences in opinions about early or late introduction of levodopa, neurologists agree that it should be started when the patient's symptoms interfere significantly with activities of daily living, bimanual skills, and occupation, and that the lowest effective dose should be used. We start with one-half a tablet of Sinemet 25/100 at the first dosing (upon awakening) and again 4 hours after that. We always recommend that levodopa be given 30 minutes to 1 hour before food. If gastrointestinal symptoms are a problem, taking the Sinemet with crackers and orange juice may help. If the peripheral dopaminergic side effects are severe, additional carbidopa (Lodosyn) is added before each dose of Sinemet. Observations of reduction of rigidity, tremor, and bradykinesia in relation to a given dose are responded to by adjusting the amount of medication throughout the day. If the patient is already on selegiline, lower doses of levodopa will be necessary. Careful titration of the medications is important to prevent signs of excessive levodopa effect.

CONCLUSION

Oxidative stress is a plausible major factor in nigral cell degeneration in Parkinson's disease, based on the findings of increased iron content in the substantia nigra, decreased glutathione levels, and impairment of complex I of the mitochondria. It may be related to oxidation of dopamine with or without the influence of an MPTP-like toxin. Selegiline appears to have mild neuroprotective and symptomatic effects, and because it is also well tolerated, is now recommended in the early treatment in Parkinson's disease. There is also evidence that vitamins E and C have antioxidant and neuroprotective effects, but so far there has been no controlled study demonstrating that high doses can clinically slow down the progression of the disease. The use of levodopa is necessary when Parkinson's disease symptoms interfere significantly with activities of daily living, work, or hobbies. The symptomatic effects of selegiline act adjunctively with levodopa and dopamine agonists to reverse the symptoms of dopaminergic deficiency in Parkinson's disease. Careful titration is necessary to avoid the adverse effects of excessive levodopa. In addition, the potential interactions of selegiline with certain narcotic agents must be avoided.

SUGGESTED READINGS

Allain H, Pollak P, Neukirch HC and members of the French Selegiline Multicenter Trial: Symptomatic effect of selegiline in de novo parkinsonian patients. Mov Disord (Suppl)8:S36, 1993

Diamond SG, Markham CH, Hoehn MM et al: Multicenter study of Parkinson mortality with early versus late dopa treatment. Ann Neurol 22:8, 1987

Factor SA, Sanchez-Ramos J, Weiner WJ: Vitamin E therapy in Parkinson's disease. p. 457. In Steifler MB, Korczyn AD, Melamed E, Youdim MBH (eds): Parkinson's Disease: Anatomy, Pathology and Therapy. In: Advances in Neurology. Vol. 53. Raven Press, New York, 1990

Fahn S: A pilot trial of high-dose alpha-tocopherol and ascorbate in early Parkinson's disease. Ann Neurol 32(suppl):128, 1992

Grimes JD, Hassan MN: Evidence to support the simultaneous initiation of dopamine agonist and levodopa therapy in the management of patients with Parkinson's disease. Arch Neurol 45:206, 1988

Langston JW, Irwin I, Langston EB, Forno LS: 1-methyl-4-phenyl-pyridinium ion (MPP$^+$): identification of a metabolite of MPTP, a toxin selective to the substantia nigra. Neurosci Lett 48:87, 1984

Olanow CW, Koller W, Hauser R et al: A prospective, longitudinal controlled study of Deprenyl in Parkinson's disease (abstract). Neurology (suppl. 2)44:258, 1994

The Parkinson Study Group: Effects of Tocopherol and Deprenyl on the progression of disability in early Parkinson's disease. New Engl J Med 328:176, 1993

The Parkinson Study Group: Effect of deprenyl on the progression of disability in early Parkinson's disease. N Engl J Med 321:1364, 1989

Riederer P, Youdim MBH, Rausch WD et al: On the mode of action of L-Deprenyl in the human central nervous system. J Neurol Transm 43:217, 1978

Tanner CM, Langston JW: Do environmental toxins cause Parkinson's disease? Neurology (Suppl. 3)40:17, 1990

115. MANAGEMENT OF LEVODOPA RESPONSE FLUCTUATIONS

PETER LeWITT

Parkinson's disease is unique among neurodegenerative disorders for the near-complete relief of signs and disabilities that can be achieved with dopaminergic therapy. Restoration of dopaminergic neurotransmission by administration of the precursor of dopamine, levodopa, is efficacious even when there is extensive dropout of nigrostriatal projections. Most patients achieve immediate and satisfactory symptomatic control of parkinsonism with levodopa alone. While certain clinical features (such as resting tremor or imbalance) sometimes are unresponsive to levodopa therapy, the drug's overall effectiveness continues to be the standard by which other antiparkinsonian therapy can be judged.

At the advent of the levodopa era, few suspected the range of problems that would become common after long-term management of Parkinson's disease with this drug. Many clinicians in the 1970s regarded levodopa as almost the equivalent of a cure. At that time, only a few voices recognized its shortcomings. Oleh Hornykiewicz, one of the developers of levodopa, observed that, while levodopa was the "most natural substance" for treating the 'striatal dopamine deficiency syndrome'," it was "far from perfect as a drug." It was not long before the limitations of sustained levodopa therapy became evident, sometimes within 2 years after its initial use in a patient. For reasons that are still unknown, continued use of levodopa often fails to provide the same degree of benefit that most patients with Parkinson's disease experience in the first 2 years of treatment.

Several factors limit the usefulness of levodopa. Acute effects such as nausea and hypotension usually lessen over time but can be lasting problems. These dose-related problems are generally governed by the rate at which the drug is introduced and by a maximally tolerated upper limit of dose. In contrast, the problems of chronic therapy are idiosyncratic in that they are delayed in onset, occur in a wide range of doses, and do not develop for every subject. Some of the problems of long-term levodopa therapy are dose related. Among the undesired outcomes are the development of involuntary movements, resembling dystonia, chorea, motor restlessness, or a combination of these. With more sustained use of levodopa, the number of affected patients has tended to increase, at least in the view of some investigators. Others have not seen any relationship between the use of levodopa and the incidence of these problems. Another common pattern of change in levodopa response over time is that patients begin to experience varying effects from each dose of the drug on an hour-by-hour basis. After several years of therapy, it is common for patients to report an overall decline in the maximal effects derived from the drug. Psychic effects such as hallucination, delusional thoughts, and psychotic ideation become increasingly frequent, especially in an older patient population.

Pharmacologic research has explored many options for dealing with the limitations of levodopa therapy. Parkinsonism can be managed in several ways to extend the action of this drug or to augment its effects. A variety of options have been explored in the past decade, although understanding of the responsible mechanisms is only fragmentary. In this chapter, several issues of practical importance for managing complicated parkinsonism are discussed. Doctors treating patients with complications in the management of parkinsonism can benefit from reviewing the topics that are listed in Table 115-1 and discussed in detail in the following paragraphs.

MAXIMAL UTILIZATION OF ALTERNATIVES TO LEVODOPA

While levodopa may be the "gold standard" of antiparkinsonian therapy, other drugs can be efficacious for relieving mild

TABLE 115-1. Problem-Oriented Checklist for Monitoring
Levodopa Therapy

Has there been maximal utilization of alternatives to levodopa?
Are the timing and amounts of levodopa therapy optimal for achieving maximal benefit?
Are patients likely to benefit from strategies to extend effects from each dose of levodopa?
Are there new patterns of drug response warranting a change in the treatment regimen?
Have adverse effects evolved that call for a change in the regimen?
Do the responses to medications suggest an alternative diagnosis?
Has the medication regimen been assessed for cost-effectiveness?
Have supportive services for patients and their families been utilized to their maximum?

disabilities such as tremor, decreased arm swing, or other manifestations of mild bradykinesia. For many years, it has been controversial whether long-term levodopa therapy might have ill effects with respect to progression of disease or causation of motor fluctuations and dyskinesias. While there is no conclusive evidence to withhold levodopa from a patient with significant disability, many clinicians have adopted a conservative attitude regarding the start of such treatment for the minimally symptomatic patient. Since anticholinergics and amantadine may permit a delay in the use of levodopa or a smaller dose when this latter drug is used, these adjunctive drugs may be helpful even if they increase the number of medications taken and add to the possibility of side effects.

For some patients, the symptom most indicative of advance in the disease or its disability can be resting tremor. The cosmetic effects of tremor and its possible impact on livelihood or comfort cannot be underestimated, even though it typically does not interfere with movement of the limbs. In some instance, anticholinergic drugs and amantadine can be distinctively more effective for this symptoms than levodopa or they can substitute partially for levodopa.

Tremor can be unresponsive to conventional antiparkinsonian medications. In such situations, especially if tremor is unilateral (or unilateral relief would greatly help the patient's particular disabilities), Vim thalamotomy may be beneficial. These operations are now being carried out at a number of centers in the United States with a high degree of competence and a low risk for adverse outcomes. A new pharmacologic means for treating tremor is clozapine, an "atypical" neuroleptic with anticholinergic properties that also has an apparently unique (and uncharacterized) mode of action in reducing parkinsonian tremor. Botulinum toxin–selective denervation of affected forearm muscle has also been effective for some patients. A third pharmacologic approach is the use of β-blocking drugs or primidone. These drugs are especially useful for postural or action tremors occurring in patients with parkinsonism, just as they can help essential tremor.

TIMING AND AMOUNTS OF LEVODOPA THERAPY OPTIMAL FOR ACHIEVING MAXIMAL BENEFIT

Levodopa therapy often requires periodic adjustment in order to determine if the amounts and scheduling of doses are giving the best possible results. The features of parkinsonism can change over time, as can the patterns of drug response. For many patients, the most obvious change is a regular onset and decline in the antiparkinsonian effects from each dose of levodopa. This variability can be shown to follow closely the timing of the rise and fall of plasma levodopa concentrations. Analysis of the relationships between the drug's pharmacokinetics and clinical actions has suggested that the central nervous system

response to the drug is subject to a fixed delay and can be modeled as a system unable to store the drug after its delivery from the bloodstream. Neuroimaging of the brain with respect to levodopa uptake has also been informative. Patients with parkinsonism and typical wearing-off fluctuation patterns have been studied by administration of [18]Fluoro-dopa in tracer amounts for positron emission tomography studies. After intravenous injection of this labeled levodopa analogue, the rise in striatal activity of the parent tracer (or its metabolites) in the subjects with Parkinson's disease was diminished and was much briefer than that in controls. Similar results came from experiments modeling levodopa metabolism in a lesioned nigrostriatal system. These studies have provided an in vivo view of the transient nature of dopaminergic stimulation derived from each dose of levodopa. In these findings are evidence that patients may require more constancy in levodopa delivery to the brain for optimal control of parkinsonism.

A typical patient with Parkinson's disease responds to a regimen of levodopa between 300 and 800 mg/day, taken in divided doses three to six times daily at intervals of at least 3 hours between doses. However, there can be several reasons for patients to differ from these norms. Some individuals manifest marked improvement from as little as 200 mg/day. For this reason (as well as for the opportunity of developing tolerance to levodopa at its introduction), a levodopa regimen can be started with 150 to 200 mg/day for a few weeks to determine the extent of improvement that can be achieved. Sometimes, 200 mg/day (or less) of levodopa intake is the maximally tolerated dose because of adverse effects such as confusion or nausea. Small doses of carbidopa levodopa may contain less than optimal amounts of the peripheral decarboxylase inhibitor, and so carbidopa supplementation may be necessary (see below).

For patients with a great deal of sensitivity to each dose of levodopa, it may be necessary to divide carbidopa levodopa pills into small fragments in order to minimize the amount absorbed at any one time. Preparation of carbidopa levodopa in a suspension form is another way that patients can ingest precisely measured fractions of a carbidopa levodopa tablet's levodopa content. The precise mixture of this formula, either for use orally or through a per-gastric feeding tube, is as follows:

500 mg of levodopa (either as carbidopa/levodopa 10/100 or 25/100)
500 mg of ascorbic acid
250 ml of water

After grinding the tablets to powder, the ingredients can be mixed in a motorized blender for a short period. The resulting suspension has a concentration of 2 mg/ml. Despite the acidification of the ascorbic acid, the pH achieved does not permit the levodopa to enter into solution, and carbidopa is even less soluble in these conditions. However, the suspension is adequate for purposes of volume measurements in determining the levodopa dose. The ascorbic acid content provides some protection against oxidation of levodopa (which can be evident from a blackening of the solution with a flocculent precipitate). It is also possible for patients to prepare the suspension from levodopa tablets. In this situation, carbidopa can be taken separately in tablet form.

The timing of levodopa intake can be a critical determinant of optimal drug effect. Like their physicians, patients should become familiar with the pharmacokinetic profile of conventional levodopa, as illustrated in Figure 115-1. This curve can be contrasted with the more delayed rise and fall of levodopa with Sinemet CR, a sustained-release preparation that has been

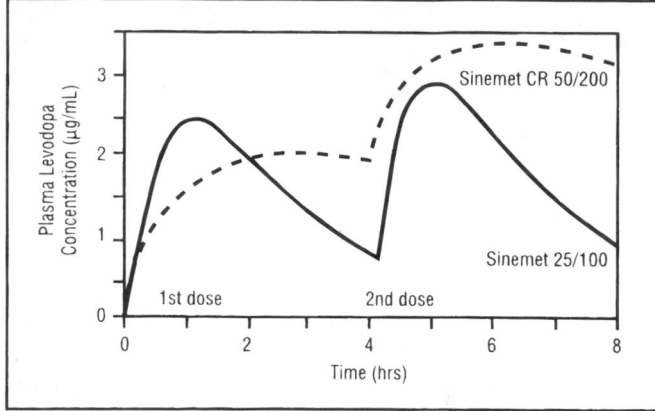

FIG. 115-1. Pharmacokinetics of plasma levodopa concentration after two doses of Sinemet 25/100 and Sinemet 50/200 CR, each given at 4-hour intervals.

available for several years. These curves of levodopa plasma concentration represent the net effects of drug absorption, distribution, and clearance under ideal conditions. Although measurements of plasma levodopa levels are not practical for management decisions in the usual clinical setting, such measurements have been an integral part of studies investigating the patterns of irregular levodopa response that can evolve with time. The pharmacokinetics of levodopa are subject to marked variability from dose to dose. Factors such as gastrointestinal (GI) transit time and meals can influence the response pattern by altering the absorption profile. However, the loss of the brain's "buffering" capacity for limiting motor consequences from the rise and fall of peripheral levodopa concentrations may become a critical determinant of antiparkinsonian effect after several years of treatment.

For patients with little storage capacity for the effects of levodopa, dosing with conventional carbidopa levodopa preparations at 2 to 2.5-hour intervals can improve the constancy of the effect. A decrease in the spacing to 1-hour intervals usually does not add further benefit. Such a strategy may result in an excessive intake, or, if sufficiently small levodopa amounts are ingested, inadequate levodopa levels to trigger an antiparkinsonian effect. Usually, the failure of significant improvement from 2-hour dosing with levodopa indicates another pattern of motor fluctuations that may need management by means other than extension of the drug's effect.

Most patients have found that taking the drug without food gives them the best chance for absorbing each dose levodopa. Hence, doses 0.5 hour before meals or 1 hour afterward can be advised, if patients do not develop nausea or other GI distress (which can often be alleviated with as little as a few crackers or a slice of bread). Absorption of levodopa can also be subject to interference by the protein intake in the diet. The entrance of levodopa into the bloodstream is controlled in part by mechanisms governing active uptake of L-neutral amino acids. There can be interference with this facilitated amino acid uptake, resulting from competition by the bulk of meals or their protein content. Some studies have claimed that protein-derived amino acids that compete with levodopa uptake are a common reason for fluctuation in the control of parkinsonism, which can be remedied by restriction of dietary protein intake. Most clinical experience, however, indicates that competition for levodopa uptake by protein in meals is of clinical significance for only

a small number of patients. It is often possible to test for this possibility by encouraging patients to compare outcomes from eating a high-protein content lunch for several days in a row, followed by several days of a low-protein lunch. Products that offer "controlled" protein intake do not offer an advantage over measured intake of protein for the rare patient sensitive to the competitive effects of dietary protein against the benefits of levodopa.

The absorption of levodopa is subject to complex influences. Since levodopa absorption occurs in the duodenum and jejunum, gastric retention of ingested levodopa can be a limiting factor of absorption and subsequent delivery to the central nervous systems. Irregular uptake of levodopa, because of vagaries in the stomach's release of the drug, can add 1 hour or more to the usual delay of 15 to 30 minutes between pill ingestion and the onset of clinical effect. Delayed uptake has been described to occur after the midday meal (the syndrome of the "siesta stomach") or in other patterns of seemingly random failure in achieving regular benefits from this drug. A sustained acid pH in the stomach interferes with uptake of ingested levodopa, and so measures such as antacid treatment have been proposed (but not proved) to increase levodopa's bioavailability. The drug's passage past the pylorus may be irregular on occasion. If decarboxylation of levodopa occurs in the stomach, the dopamine produced tends to inhibit release of stomach contents to the small intestine. In some instances, this problem may be helped by metoclopramide or, better, the peripherally acting dopamine inhibitor domperidone. Another drug that promotes gastric emptying, cisapride, may also be useful.

Some studies have shown that carbohydrate intake facilitates levodopa absorption. Based on this, a nutritional supplement with a fixed ratio of carbohydrate to protein has been marketed, though its likelihood of benefiting the average patient with motor fluctuations has not been established.

STRATEGIES TO EXTEND EFFECTS FROM EACH DOSE OF LEVODOPA

Sustained-Release Levodopa Preparations

Patients with a variation in their response to levodopa should be assessed critically as to how much discomfort and disability are present when the drug's effect is at its best. If the degree of improvement at such times is satisfactory, then another way to optimize the effects of the drug is by pharmacologic methods for prolonging the effect from each dose. The most obvious approach is to utilize a sustained-release preparation of levodopa. These preparations were developed in response to clinical experience that indicated that more constancy of levodopa's effect was desirable, especially for patients with abrupt "wearing-off" responses. Several controlled-release oral preparations of levodopa have been tested, and two are marketed. Madopar CR (formerly Madopar HBS) is a capsule transformed into a gelatinous diffusion body that floats on the fluid contents of the stomach. This preparation, which contains 100 mg of levodopa and 25 mg of benserazide, is not available in the United States. However, another preparation designed for delayed release of its contents has been marketed as Sinemet CR (formerly, Sinemet CR-4). Sinemet CR is a mixture of 50 mg of carbidopa and 200 mg of levodopa embedded in a polymeric matrix. Another Sinemet CR form contains 25 mg of carbidopa and 100 mg of levodopa. With each of these controlled-release preparations, there is a delayed onset of peak levodopa concentrations, as compared to conventional preparations. Both Sinemet CR and Madopar CR have been effective for decreasing end-of-dose and other types of motor fluctuations in some patients. Some comparisons have been conducted between the two, which suggest their pharmacokinetics profiles are similar. However, many clinicians comparing the utility of Sinemet CR to Madopar CR have found Sinemet CR to achieve a much more reliable extension of levodopa's effect.

Less levodopa is absorbed from both the Sinemet and the Madopar CR preparations, as compared to conventional forms of levodopa. In one study that compared the same group of patients who were receiving sustained-release and conventional Sinemet, bioavailability decreased by a mean of 28 percent. Another investigation found only an 11 percent decrease. However, the latter study found that the mean levodopa intake had to be augmented from 1,340 to 1,782 mg/day to achieve the same degree of optimal control with the use of the sustained-release product. The basis for the increased levodopa intake may be due in part to the larger quantity of levodopa in each Sinemet CR tablet (which contain carbidopa levodopa 50 mg/200 mg), for which the smallest unit of dosing is one-half tablet. Patients converting from a conventional formulation to the sustained-release product can achieve an increase in duration as well as improved consistency of effect. Sometimes, the switch to the sustained-release product leads to more simplicity in the medication schedule or better likelihood of compliance in a setting such as a nursing home.

With patients experiencing levodopa response fluctuations, most studies have shown that Sinemet CR produced clinical improvement, as characterized by more "on" time and fewer "off" periods. Used in combination with the conventional rapid-release preparations of Sinemet, the clinical effect can be tailored to produce both rapid actions and several hours of sustained effect. Since Sinemet CR is associated with a delayed onset of antiparkinsonian action, as compared to conventional levodopa preparations, the first dose of the day may require both forms to be given together for optimal effects. Many patients receiving Sinemet CR have also used booster doses of the conventional form for producing small increments of increased levodopa effect. Breaking of the Sinemet CR tablet in half does not abolish its sustained-release properties but somewhat hastens its absorption. A patient in need of more rapid effects from Sinemet CR might chew a fraction of the tablet and swallow the rest in an intact form.

The abruptness of wearing-off responses can be lessened with the sustained-release preparations. Comparisons to Sinemet 25/100 showed that, with wearing-off fluctuations, the total disability profile was improved with Sinemet CR, that is, a typical patient's total daily "on" time was increased, though the occurrence of dyskinesia was also enhanced. The overall disability profile also differentiated the two preparations. During "on" time, patients reported no difference in their functioning, though their motor disabilities when medication levels were below optimal effect ("off" states) were significantly less on the Sinemet CR regimen. The more gradual rise in plasma levodopa concentration may also be associated with a less abrupt onset of peak-effect dyskinesia or dystonia (which typically occurs 30 to 60 minutes after a dose of levodopa). The greater period of drug effect with Sinemet CR can be useful for patients with frequent awakening during the night because of dystonic cramping, tremor, or difficulty in attaining a comfortable sleeping position. Though sustained-release levodopa's more gradual rise and fall in drug concentration might seem to be beneficial for all patterns of motor fluctuation, some patients are not

helped. This has been recognized with the "diphasic" (dyskinesia-improvement-dyskinesia pattern) of levodopa's response. Trials of Sinemet CR have actually seemed to exacerbate the duration of dyskinesias experienced by such patients. Patients with increased occurrence of dyskinesias or other levodopa-related side effects as the day progresses may need to have the amount of the controlled-release preparation reduced in the afternoon doses because of its possible cumulative effects.

Monoamine Oxidase-B Inhibition

Another approach for lessening wearing-off responses involves inhibition of monoamine oxidase (MAO). This enzyme is the initiating step in the major pathway of dopamine catabolism. MAO has been differentiated into two forms on the basis of substrate specificity. In the therapeutics of Parkinson's disease, drugs with a broad-spectrum inhibition of MAO would pose a problem because MAO-A inhibition permits hypertensive reactions from tyramine to occur. However, inhibition of MAO-B can potentiate the effects of dopamine without the risks of adverse reactions from dietary amine. A selective and irreversible inhibitor of MAO-B, selegiline (deprenyl, Eldepryl), has been used to augment levodopa's effects. Because of its high selectivity for MAO-B, selegiline can be used safely at doses of 10 mg/day in chronic therapy for Parkinson's disease. Evidence for the augmentation of dopamine's effect has come from research in the rodent brain and in measurements of striatal dopamine concentrations in patients with parkinsonism who were treated with selegiline shortly before their death. In these postmortem studies, selegiline treatment achieved an inhibition of more than 90 percent of striatal MAO-B with 10 mg/day. This dose of selegiline has been widely adopted in using the drug for adjunctive therapy, though it is likely that chronic treatment with a lower dose would also achieve full inhibition of MAO-B. Brain MAO-B is synthesized at a relatively slow rate, and, for this reason, it would seem that lasting inhibition of MAO-B requires no more selegiline than an amount titrated against newly generated enzyme. Studies that have investigated regimens of up to 40 mg/day yielded no additional antiparkinsonian actions over those achieved with 10 mg/d. Another important factor in the clinical pharmacology of selegiline is that, on discontinuation of the drug, its effects as an MAO-B inhibitor linger for several weeks.

Selegiline has no effect on the absorption or peripheral metabolism of levodopa. Several additional properties besides MAO-B inhibition are unlikely to contribute to its pharmacologic profile in augmenting dopamine's action. The metabolites of selegiline may be a cause for some of the adverse effects some patients can experience from this drug. A conventional daily dose of selegiline is converted to small quantities of L-amphetamine and L-methamphetamine. It is unlikely that these have any direct effect on parkinsonism.

Administered with levodopa, selegiline augments both the magnitude as well as the duration of levodopa's effects. This can occur even with sustained-release levodopa preparations. Extensive clinical experience with selegiline supports the use of selegiline as a means for potentiation of levodopa's clinical effects. In some instances, selegiline therapy can lessen the problem of wearing-off decline in levodopa's action. Not all patients experiencing wearing-off will respond, however. Other types of motor fluctuations such as start hesitancy or sudden "off" states do not improve with selegiline, nor is selegiline useful in the management of patients with involuntary movements. A common problem with the addition of selegiline to a levodopa regimen is an exacerbation of dyskinesias, as well as hallucinations and other levodopa-induced adverse events. By retardation of the breakdown of dopamine, selegiline can produce increased peak-effect problems during the first hour following each dose of levodopa.

Adjunctive therapy with selegiline can be beneficial for patients who are undermedicated with levodopa. Sometimes the same types of improvement with selegiline could also be achieved by an increased dose or closer spacing of levodopa intake (or by a switch to a sustained-release form of levodopa). For patients already receiving levodopa at a maximally tolerated dose, addition of selegiline calls for a reduction in levodopa intake by 20 percent or more to avoid peak-dose side effects. Based on its action as an irreversible inhibitor of MAO-B, it would seem that the actions of selegiline should be lasting, although some studies have shown that, even when there is benefit, this can decline after several months.

As an MAO-B inhibitor, selegiline should be regarded as having an all-or-none effect. In trials investigating selegiline monotherapy, side effects were uncommon, and most adverse experiences with selegiline result from a potentiation of levodopa's effects. Among its reported side effects are jitteriness, insomnia, nausea, and, less commonly, dysphoric reactions. These adverse effects may be related to the L-amphetamine metabolites, since a reduction in the selegiline dose may lessen them. No dietary restrictions are needed with the use of selegiline at a daily dose of 5 to 10 mg/day. When daily intake exceeds 30 mg/day, however, the drug loses its selectivity for MAO-B and can produce tyramine-induced hypertensive reactions. A few serious adverse drug interactions have been described with selegiline. With meperidine (Demerol, also known as pethidine in other countries), a reaction resembling opiate overdosage has been described. Other opiate compounds might conceivably produce similar adverse reactions with selegiline. An adverse reaction between the selective serotonin reuptake blocker fluoxetine (Prozac) and selegiline has been described that resembles that described with meperidine.

Enteral Infusion of Levodopa

While the pharmacokinetic profiles of sustained-release levodopa preparations can improve the constancy of levodopa's effect, irregularities in gastric emptying can still govern the absorption of the drug. Domperidone does not always increase gastric emptying for the purpose of enhancing levodopa's uptake. Even if the stomach regularly delivers the drug to the upper GI tract, some irregularity in its uptake is inevitable owing to the influences of meals, GI circulation, and other factors. For some patients, the therapeutic window for levodopa can be so narrow that the only means for adequate control is through an invariant plasma blood concentration. Intravenous infusions of levodopa, adjusted to an optimal drug delivery rate for symptomatic relief, have shown that antiparkinsonian control can be improved by constant plasma levodopa concentrations. Similarly, methods for direct enteral infusion of levodopa suspensions have been shown to improve on the dose-by-dose variability associated with the drug taken in tablet form. A permanent route of enteral access can be installed with a minimum of discomfort, sometimes on an outpatient surgical basis. This method of per-gastric jejunal infusion makes use of a small-bore feeding tube inserted through the abdominal wall and connected to a portable pump. This procedure has few complications, in contrast with the problems associated with the

insertion of tubes by jejunostomy. The carbidopa/levodopa suspension can be prepared daily by the patient.

For patients unable to improve their clinical state by adjusting their oral intake of levodopa or adjunctive medications, jejunal infusion can offer great benefits. The use this physical means for bypassing the pylorus also provides an opportunity for a rate-controlled delivery of the drug to its primary absorptive site in the duodenum and jejunum. The use of levodopa in pill form constrains patient to the available dose sizes (or their fractions). In contrast, the infusion permits precise adjustment to either the optimal rate of delivery or the bolus dose needed for desired effects. The portable pumps currently available permit the levodopa delivery needed to achieve either stable or readily altered plasma concentrations of levodopa. The infusion rate can be adjusted in extremely small increments of drug delivery as titration proceeds in search of optimal effect. The clinical effect from each change of infusion rate becomes evident within 5 minutes. Constant infusion avoids the occurrence of peak concentrations and the consequent surge of dopaminergic effect that are associated with use of conventional levodopa preparations. The infusion technique also permits a patient to reduce or discontinue drug delivery at the start of dose-related adverse effects (such as dyskinesia). While the constant infusions can, in some instances, result in increased daily needs for levodopa, the net effect can be a marked improvement in the control of motor fluctuations. Other applications include improved control of dyskinesia, myoclonus, and pain syndromes associated with medication effect wearing off.

Additional Pharmacologic Strategies

Other approaches to extend the duration of levodopa's effect have been sought in inhibitors of catechol O-methyltransferase (COMT). Though COMT is not the part of the major route for dopamine catabolism, dual inhibition of both MAO and COMT have been proposed as a means for enhancing the effects of levodopa. A study exploring this possibility has shown that such a combination does not result in toxic dopaminergic effects. Another result of COMT inhibition is to decrease levodopa clearance by eliminating its conversion peripheral to an O-methylated derivative. Much of an administered dose of levodopa is converted to this inactive metabolite, which achieves greater plasma concentrations than the parent drug. The decreased availability of levodopa for the brain might be a source of variability in levodopa's effect.

Recently, several new and highly potent COMT inhibitors have entered into clinical investigation. One of them, entacapone (OR-611), has predominantly peripheral effects. In pharmacokinetic studies, entacapone extends the duration of levodopa's presence in the bloodstream without increasing its peak concentrations, an effect which has been recognized in clinical trials. Studies have been done with a COMT inhibitor highly similar in peripheral actions to entacapone but also possessing central actions. This compound, tolcapone (Ro 40-7592), may help to answer whether the additional inhibition of central COMT adds to any improvements in clinical outcome.

Like decarboxylase inhibition, blockade of COMT results in more delivery of levodopa to the brain with a longer duration. The extension and increased consistency of clinical effect resulting from COMT inhibition might result in better control of variability in the peripheral pharmacokinetics of levodopa. The ongoing clinical trials with entacapone and tolcapone will allow comparisons of clinical outcomes to be made to learn of any further advantage from central COMT inhibition.

Another means for extending the duration of levodopa's effect is by adjunctive use of amantadine. Although this application has not undergone a formal clinical trial, many clinicians have found this to be a prominent effect, even in patients who have lost benefit from this drug as a monotherapy. Its mechanism of action in this application has not been characterized.

PATTERNS OF DRUG RESPONSE WARRANTING CHANGE IN TREATMENT REGIMEN

With chronic therapy of parkinsonism, changes in clinical control of symptoms over time may herald new targets for treatment. Involuntary movements, dystonic postures, painful spasms, and sudden "freezing" may develop as inevitable consequences despite regular doses of levodopa. Attempts to alter levodopa intake may be unsuccessful at modulating these problems, and the use of dopaminergic agonists may now need to be considered [Table 115-2].

Therapy with either pergolide or bromocriptine may help to improve symptomatic control by partially substituting for levodopa, but only rarely are these ergot dopaminergic agonists useful as monotherapies. Together with an agonist, levodopa intake can be decreased to as little as 200 mg/day, though any further reduction usually lessens the overall degree of response. Both drugs have similar efficacy, and a switch from one to the other generally produces similar effects. However, some patients have better symptomatic control with either pergolide or bromocriptine, which differ in per-milligram potency by a factor of 10:1 to 15:1. These drugs need to be introduced gradually to ensure a minimum of adverse effects. To avoid the occurrence of nausea and hypotension, tolerance often takes weeks to develop.

Although not all patients improve from (or tolerate) dopaminergic ergots, these drugs can offer improvements for many problems of complicated parkinsonism. Doses in excess of 0.75 mg/day for pergolide and 25 mg/day for bromocriptine, if tolerated, should be assessed before concluding that this strategy is not likely to be beneficial. The titration of dose should be undertaken without a reduction of levodopa intake so that the independent actions of the agonist can be assessed directly.

For both bromocriptine and pergolide, there is a very wide range of optimal dose. In some patients, maximal effect is limited by a dose that produces adverse effects, which are the same

TABLE 115-2. Situations That May Require Use of Dopaminergic Agonists

When there is declining benefit over time from a levodopa regimen in excess of 750 mg/day.

With the occurrence of start hestitation or unpredictable episodes of "freezing" in place.

As partial substitution for levodopa when intolerable dyskinesias have occurred with levodopa therapy.

With early morning dystonia (the occurrence of dystonic foot cramping, usually unilateral.

With other end-of-dose dystonic reactions, as well as for relief of dystonic features that may have preceded the onset of parkinsonism or its treatment.

To provide a substitute for levodopa as an alternative for treating the diphasic (dyskinesia-improvement-dyskinesia) pattern of levodopa response.

For extension of levodopa's effect, even when other strategies may have failed.

Rarely, when there are certain parkinsonian features minimally responsive to levodopa treatment (such as tremor or imbalance) or when little overall effect from levodopa has occurred.

Rarely, in situations in which levodopa therapy is not well tolerated (because of nausea, hallucinations, sleep disturbance, or dyskinesias and despite the increased potency of the dopaminergic agonists).

that can occur with levodopa, that is, nausea and vomiting, postural lightheadedness, vivid dreams, confusion, delusions, or hallucinations. The best way to avoid adverse effects or to minimize their severity is to introduce the drug at a slow, gradual rate of increasing dosage. The best results come from adding no more than 2.5 mg of bromocriptine or 0.25 mg of pergolide per week. In such a manner, it may be weeks to several months before a patient reaches a daily intake that produces optimal effects (7.5 to 50 mg/day for bromocriptine and 0.75 to 5.0 mg/day for pergolide). This build-up schedule is more gradual than advocated in the product literature for either of these drugs. After consideration of the equivalence between bromocriptine and pergolide, the latter drug is available in tablets that permit a more gradual increment of dose. Apart from this advantage, the two drugs are similar in actions, although some patients derive more benefit from one or the other.

The dopaminergic agonists present another solution for managing the wearing off in levodopa effect. Because of their longer plasma half-lives, bromocriptine and pergolide regimens lessen the tendency for abrupt loss of clinical effect in levodopa-treated patients. Another situation in which dopaminergic agonists can improve antiparkinsonian control is when peak-effect dyskinesias are present. Patients whose disabling involuntary movements develop at the height of levodopa's antiparkinsonian actions sometimes can be helped by a decrease in the levodopa dose and the addition of bromocriptine or pergolide. The combination regimen (especially if levodopa can be reduced to one-half or less of its previous intake) often has less propensity for initiating dyskinesias, despite the same overall degree of antiparkinsonian control.

Other problems related to advanced Parkinson's disease can also be responsive to dopaminergic agonists. The tendency for falling as a result of retropulsion is usually not helped, but gait hesitancy, causing imbalance, can be improved by adding a dopaminergic agonist to a levodopa regimen. Dopaminergic agonists can be useful for early morning dystonia, a problem in which the feet are subject to painful spasms related to the gradual loss of dopaminergic effect over the course of the night. The extended duration of effect from dopaminergic agonists can, like sustained-release levodopa, avert this problem when these medications are taken at bedtime. Apart from this indication, antiparkinsonian medications are not generally advisable for use during sleeping hours, because they can cause vivid dreams and sometimes enhance nocturnal myoclonus.

In the past decade, there has been little formal investigation of drug "holidays," the notion that abrupt discontinuation of levodopa and other antiparkinsonian medications might lessen levodopa-induced adverse effects. While there has been limited support for the concept in terms of outcomes for several weeks after a drug holiday, the abrupt stopping of antiparkinsonian medications can be uncomfortable and dangerous (potentially precipitating a neuroleptic malignant syndrome–like response as well as the risk for aspiration pneumonia or deep vein thrombosis from marked rigidity). It is possible that the claimed benefits might also be achieved by partial reductions of drug, especially if the levodopa intake previously was excessive.

ADVERSE EFFECTS THAT CALL FOR A CHANGE IN REGIMEN

The occurrence of the following problems may be indications for changes in medications.

Peak-Effect Dyskinesias or Dystonia

The total intake of levodopa or the amount in each dose may need to be decreased if troublesome dyskinesias or dystonia occur. If these problems are more prominent in the afternoon and evening, there may be cumulative effects of levodopa from earlier in the day. Sometimes an increase in the intensity of peak-effect involuntary movements is a consequence of the previous addition of selegiline or a dopaminergic ergot. If so, these adjunctive medications (or their concomitant levodopa dose) can be decreased. Dyskinesias can be blocked with neuroleptic medications. With the use of small doses (e.g., 2.5 to 5 mg of molindone [Moban], a selective D^2 receptor blocker), it might be possible to lessen involuntary movements without much interference with levodopa's antiparkinsonian actions. Another approach to lessen levodopa-induced dyskinesias has been the use of clozapine. A recent study found that this "atypical" neuroleptic substantially reduced the amount of time patients spent in a dyskinetic state. While other neuroleptics would antagonize the control of bradykinesia, clozapine does not.

Vivid Dreams, Hallucinations, Psychotic Thinking

All forms of dopaminergic therapy and amantadine can cause these problems, sometimes in a dose-related pattern. A reduction in the amounts of these drugs taken at the end of day can improve quality of sleep by lessening the extent of disruptive dreams. Occasional hallucinations or illusions that are not "believed" (i.e., they are not associated with delusional thinking) may be tolerable for some subjects. While they can be forerunners to the eventual development of more psychotic overtones, benign hallucinations may be regarded by some patients as an acceptable tradeoff for the benefits of the medications. (The management of psychosis is reviewed in Ch. 116.)

Forgetfulness

Sometimes an accompaniment of too much dopaminergic therapy, decreased memory function can also develop in patients receiving anticholinergic medication. Even if this problem is not recognized initially, forgetfulness always calls for reducing and stopping anticholinergic agents, and this should be carried out from time to time to assess both benefits and possible contributions to impaired cognitive abilities.

Pleural Inflammatory Reactions

An extremely rare, idiosyncratic reaction occurring during therapy with pergolide, bromocriptine, and other dopaminergic ergots is pleural thickening with effusion. While this usually develops asymptomatically, the extent of this reversible reaction can be severe in pulmonary impairment. Annual chest radiographs are advisable for screening purposes, and pergolide or bromocriptine needs to be stopped if this reaction is found.

Erythromelalgia-Like Reactions

Another extremely rare idiosyncratic reaction is a painful, warm swelling, which typically occurs in the feet or shin regions. Resembling cellulitis, this inflammatory reaction can be severe. It seems to result from sustained use of dopaminergic ergot drugs, which need to be discontinued rapidly.

Postural Hypotension

Often asymptomatic, postural hypotension is seen in patients with Parkinson's disease who are receiving dopaminergic therapy. The extent of postural blood pressure drop can be alarming even if the patient is experiencing no lightheadedness. It may be that, with chronic orthostatic change in blood pressure, the recordings made in the arm cease to represent core blood pressure to the brain. Symptomatic hypotension may be a cause for reduction in the regimen of antiparkinsonian drugs. However, a trial of alternative medications can be undertaken to counter the blood pressure drop. These include salt loading, fludrocortisone, and indomethacin. Low-dose regimens of clonidine or propranolol have been described to elevate blood pressure. Slight elevation of the head of the bed has benefits for lessening the diuresis of salt retained during the day. In addition, the more chronic stimulation of the renin-angiotensin system may help to counter any tendency for orthostatic hypotension.

RESPONSES TO MEDICATIONS SUGGESTIVE OF AN ALTERNATIVE DIAGNOSIS

When a levodopa regimen of 750 mg/day (with carbidopa) has been unable to improve parkinsonism, the problem might be an incorrect diagnosis. There are several other neurodegenerative disorders (including progressive supranuclear palsy, Shy-Drager syndrome, and olivopontocerebellar degeneration) that have prominent parkinsonism but minimal or no effect from a trial of levodopa. Since these disorders may be difficult to distinguish from typical Parkinson's disease (especially in their early stages), the failure of response to levodopa may be the first clue for an alternative diagnosis. Rarely, cases of acquired parkinsonism (such as brainstem or striatal lesions, certain toxic exposures, or increased intracranial pressure) show a response to levodopa.

It is also important to recognize that, even in typical Parkinson's disease, features such as resting tremor, micrographia, and imbalance may fail to respond to levodopa or other medications.

COST-EFFECTIVENESS?

The medications for Parkinson's disease are expensive burdens for patients and health care systems. The effectiveness of drugs at relieving discomfort and disability should be questioned from time to time as to whether the costs represent a good value. As mentioned above, there are several alternative ways for relieving certain problems in Parkinson's disease therapeutics. For example, while controlled-release levodopa preparations can offer convenience and more sustained antiparkinsonian effects, their increased cost may lead patients to chose conventional levodopa, which is taken on a more frequent basis. Dopaminergic ergots can help against the wearing off of levodopa's effect (as can selegiline) but sustained-release levodopa preparations may be more cost-effective for solving this particular problem.

Some patients may wish to undergo a trial of reducing medication intake in order to determine the benefits versus the cost of therapy. In this way, patients can derive a sense of how much change in disability is achieved from each increment in medication. The question of whether chronic regimens of medications are continuing to help is particularly appropriate for reassessment of amantadine. This drug can lose effectiveness over time. Though some patients have continued benefit from 300 mg/day, others achieve the same results with 100 or 200 mg/day. A trial of reducing the dose of amantadine (over the course of 2 weeks) can be used to reassess its current value.

The same questions can be asked of other adjunctive medications. Like amantadine, dopaminergic agonists and sustained-release levodopa preparations may be helpful against the wearing off of effect. Sometimes, combination-regimen medications have evolved that duplicate each other at targeting the wearing-off problem. Trials of reducing medication intake might help to discover the minimum of medications needed for adequate symptomatic control. Since patients sometimes are unaware if starting a new medication has actually led to any benefit, a trial reduction might help to clarify this issue.

Generic equivalents for Sinemet (carbidopa/levodopa) and Parlodel (bromocriptine) have recently become available in addition to amantadine (Symmetrel) and levodopa. These preparations offer substantial savings to patients and are not known to differ in clinical actions from the brand-name products.

SUPPORTIVE SERVICES FOR PATIENTS AND FAMILIES

A wide range of information sources and services await patients and their families. Six national and several statewide Parkinson's disease support organizations provide newsletters, fact sheets, advisory services, and support group meetings. A number of well-written and accurate books describe the experience of living with parkinsonism. Some communities have geriatric services that can be utilized to great advantage by patients with parkinsonian and their families.

Rehabilitation approaches to parkinsonism include gait training, equipping the home for impaired ambulation and balance, and increasing endurance in the face of disabling bradykinesia and other aspects of impaired motor control. Learning "tricks" for overcoming freezing and implementation with walkers or canes for enhancing independent ambulation are all reasonable goals for rehabilitation services. Some patients feel that particular exercise programs have had a major impact on their well-being. Although the best form of exercise varies on the basis of age, level of physical conditioning, and gait/balance disturbance, most patients can benefit from a variety of exercise programs that have been developed (such as one available from the United Parkinson Foundation and a videotape entitled "Get Up and Go!"). Patients often need reassurance that the temporary exacerbation of tremor and slowness after exercise is not "bad" for their parkinsonism.

The recognition of depression in Parkinson's disease can be difficult since the motor aspects of the disorder can both hide and create the image of the disorder. Encouragement of outlets for communication in the setting of support groups, family discussions, or with mental health professionals is important. Many patients with Parkinson's disease, like others with physical disability in the "golden" years of retirement, are extremely frustrated and frightened by the impact of the disorder on their lives. To the extent that unrealistic perceptions of Parkinson's disease govern their thoughts, reassurance of the current status of this disorder is often important. Practitioners should acquaint themselves with studies in which the "natural" history of Parkinson's disease has been explored since benign outcomes of this disease are well known and the rate of disability in others can be realistically described. Many patients with Parkinson's disease are alarmed about the possible impact of the disorder on their mind. Though many patients to develop dementia or other types of impairment, many patients have retained full mental capabilities even after 10 or more years with the disorder. Patients may need frank assessments of their condition from time to time, not just optimistic reassurance from their physician.

Finally, patients can draw a great deal of optimism from the active realm of research into the causes and treatments of Parkinson's disease. For some individuals, involvement in clinical trials has provided major assistance in their coping with this disorder.

SUGGESTED READINGS

Calne DB (ed): Drugs for the Treatment of Parkinson's Disease. In: Handbook of Experimental Pharmacology. Vol. 88. Springer-Verlag, Berlin, 1989

Cedarbaum JM: The promise and limitations of controlled release oral levodopa administration. Clin Neuropharmacol 12:147, 1989

Cedarbaum JM, Gancher ST (eds): Parkinson's disease. Neurol Clin 10:1992

Jankovic J, Tolosa E (eds): Parkinson's Disease and Movement Disorders. 2nd Ed. Williams & Wilkins, Baltimore, 1993

Koller WC (ed): Handbook of Parkinson's Disease. (2nd ed.) Marcel Dekker, New York, 1992

Kurth MC, Tetrud JW, Irwin I et al: Oral levodopa/carbidopa solution versus tablets in Parkinson's patients with severe fluctuations: a pilot study. Neurology 43:1036, 1993

LeWitt PA: Treatment strategies for extension of levodopa effect. Neurol Clin 10:511, 1992

LeWitt PA, Ward CD, Larsen TA et al: Comparison of pergolide and bromocriptine therapy in parkinsonism. Neurology 33:1009, 1983

Nutt JG: On-off phenomena: relation to levodopa pharmacokinetics. Ann Neurol 22:535, 1987

Quinn N, Parkes JD, Marsden CD: Control of on/off phenomenon by continuous intravenous infusion of levodopa. Neurology 34:1131, 1984

116. MENTAL CHANGES IN PARKINSON'S DISEASE

JOSEPH H. FRIEDMAN

Two types of mental changes occur in Parkinson's disease that can be very broadly categorized as behavioral changes without cognitive impairment and dementia. Dementia is increased in Parkinson's disease compared to age-matched controls. It usually occurs after several years of the illness and correlates with disease severity; ultimately it affects about 30 percent of patients. The mental changes that are common in these patients are as follows:

1. Depression occurs in about 50 percent of parkinsonian patients and is medication responsive.
2. Fatigue occurs as a major problem in 30 percent of parkinsonian patients, correlating better with depression than disease severity.
3. Sleep disorders are very common, manifested mainly by difficulty staying asleep and falling back to sleep once awake, leading to daytime somnolence and sleep fragmentation. Vivid dreams and yelling in sleep are very common.
4. Visual hallucinosis occurs in 20 percent of drug-treated patients.
5. Psychosis occurs in 5 to 10 percent of drug-treated patients.
6. Dementia occurs in 30 percent of parkinsonian patients, brought on by the usual causes of dementia as well as by Parkinson's disease itself.

DEMENTIA

Parkinsonian patients are subject to the same dementing illnesses as other individuals. Dementia of the Alzheimer's type, vascular dementia, and other conditions presumably develop at the same rate as in an age-matched population without Parkinson's disease. In addition, Parkinsonian patients develop a dementia that is thought to be part of their primary Parkinson's disease pathology. Mild dementia can be difficult to recognize in Parkinson's disease owing to the confounding effects of motor dysfunction and medication. The DSM IV criteria defining dementia are difficult to apply strictly to Parkinson's disease.

There is no specific "Parkinson's dementia." Pathologically, there is a large overlap between Parkinson's disease with dementia, Alzheimer's disease, and diffuse Lewy body disease. Similarly, there is a large overlap between the clinical aspects of all of the dementias. Although one can statistically discriminate discrete populations having a "subcortical" dementia, characterized by deficits in memory, ordering, verbal fluency, problem solving, and visual perception tasks, from those with a "cortical" or Alzheimer's type dementia, with memory problems and aphasia, agnosia, or apraxia, individual cases are often more difficult to categorize.

It is possible that the subcortical type of dementia in Parkinson's disease is more slowly progressive than dementia of Alzheimer's type, but this is unknown. Tacrine, a cholinesterase inhibitor, enhances memory in patients with dementia of Alzheimer's type, but has not been tested in the dementias of Parkinson's disease. It may worsen the parkinsonism seen in advanced dementia of Alzheimer's type, as might be expected from its cholinergic properties. Theoretically at least, tacrine and other cholinergic drugs may worsen the cholinergic dopaminergic imbalance in Parkinson's disease, leading to worsening motoric dysfunction, and should therefore be used cautiously—if at all—in Parkinson's disease.

DEPRESSION

The incidence of depression is also increased in Parkinson's disease. Whether this is intrinsic to the disease or reactive is debated. Most studies have demonstrated an increase in depression in Parkinson's disease compared to age-matched controls, but one often-cited study found no difference in prevalence between parkinsonian patients and a cohort matched for disability with rheumatoid arthritis. There is some data to suggest that the quality of depression Parkinson's disease is somewhat different than that in idiopathic depression, with fewer suicide attempts and less feelings of guilt and failure but with more irritability and pessimism about the future.

Regardless of the epidemiology or theoretic aspects of depression, each patient must be approached in an individualized manner. Recognizing depression may be difficult. Since interpreting the affect of most parkinsonian patients' facial expression is problematic, it takes experience or long-term knowledge of one particular patient to use facial expression as a guide. Occasional patients complain that they are thought to be depressed or angry when they are not because of the masked facial expression. Loss of motivation, feelings of sadness in particular, loss of appetite, loss of libido, and anhedonia are the symptoms most important to evaluate. Fatigue, sleep disturbances, declining social interactions, and weight loss, which are guides to depression in non-parkinsonian patients, are so common in nondepressed Parkinson's disease that although

they are increased in depressed parkinsonian patients, they are not good guides to the diagnosis of depression. Depression also must be distinguished from apathy, which is often present with dementia and is probably untreatable. Apathy may be seen in Parkinson's disease itself without dementia, but is not common. A person with advanced Parkinson's disease may be unable to do much for enjoyment and may be resigned rather than apathetic or depressed. Complicating the diagnosis of depression is the possibility that the patient will deny feeling depressed even when depression is present. Information from family members can be very helpful in making the diagnosis.

Treating depression in Parkinson's disease is made difficult by the frailty of the patients and the frequent problem of drug intolerance, especially in patients already taking several psychoactive medications. There have been at least five double-blinded placebo-controlled trials of different antidepressants in Parkinson's disease, all finding the drugs to be effective in ameliorating depression and some noting concomitant improvement in parkinsonism. There are no studies comparing one antidepressant to another. What appears to be the case is that antidepressants are as effective in treating depression in Parkinson's disease as in the non-parkinsonian population. Therefore, the choice of drug should depend on the individual patient and the physician's degree of comfort with the various medications.

Coexisting problems that may help guide an antidepressant drug choice are drooling, prostatism, urinary urgency, insomnia, daytime somnolence, confusion, dementia, cardiac rhythm abnormalities, orthostatic hypotension, and so forth. Tricyclics are useful for a patient who may benefit from an anticholinergic agent, especially if insomnia is present. So, a patient who drools and has tremor or a spastic bladder may experience improvement in affect from the antidepressant actions of a tricyclic such as amitriptyline, imipramine, and so on, and physical improvement from the anticholinergic side effects. A patient with insomnia and anxiety may respond better to trazodone. The new class of serotonin re-uptake blockers is thought to be "activating" and may help patients with excessive somnolence and "inertia" during the day. They also have few side effects and are well tolerated in general. They should be given in the morning, unlike the other antidepressants, which are usually given at night, to avoid inducing or exacerbating insomnia. The serotonin re-uptake inhibitors can cause restlessness or akathisia, and on rare occasion may induce or worsen parkinsonism. Although these possibilities should not reduce the use of those drugs, these potential adverse effects should be recognized should they occur.

Selegiline has important theoretic drug interactions. Because meperidine (Demerol) can interact fatally with the antidepressant monamine oxidase inhibitors via an unexplained mechanism, it is recommended that meperidine and selegiline not be given together. In addition, concern has been raised about the use of selegiline and the serotonin re-uptake-inhibiting antidepressants because the nonspecific monamine oxidase-inhibitors, phenelzine and tranylcpromine, have caused a "serotonin syndrome" in patients taking the serotonin re-uptake inhibitors. Since serotonin is metabolized via monoamine oxidase-A, selegiline presumably should not cause this syndrome. Only a few cases have been reported in which the drugs have been used safely together, and there are no reports of interaction. However, caution is advised, as the data are scant.

Electroconvulsive therapy is another option for treating depression in Parkinson's disease and is probably underused. Electroconvulsive therapy is generally recommended for patients who are either refractory to antidepressant medications or who fail to tolerate them. Electroconvulsive therapy has a beneficial effect on the motor aspect of Parkinson's disease independent of effect on mood. The motoric benefit usually lasts days to weeks, but can last longer. About 75 percent of electroconvulsive therapy-treated parkinsonian patients improve motorically and a higher percentage improve psychiatrically. Following electroconvulsive therapy for depression, oral antidepressants are still required, but lower doses are needed to maintain a patient in remission than to achieve remission.

ANXIETY, OBSESSIVE-COMPULSIVE TRAITS, FATIGUE

Anxiety and obsessive compulsive personality traits may be increased in Parkinson's disease. Fatigue is another common problem that does not correlate with disease severity.

DRUG-RELATED MENTAL EFFECTS

The mental side effects of the antiparkinsonian drugs are legion and, aside from depression, most mental abnormalities occurring in Parkinson's disease are in fact drug induced. Sleepiness, mania, hypersexuality, confusion, personality changes, visual hallucinosis, vivid dreams, psychosis, and even depression itself have been reported as drug effects. These problems occur in a large percentage of patients. Older patients, especially demented ones, are more likely than others to experience mental side effects. The anticholinergic drugs, such as trihexyphenidyl (Artane), benztropine (Cogentin), and so forth are so likely to cause mental side effects, particularly memory loss, confusion, and hallucinations, that they should be used extremely cautiously in the elderly and almost never in the demented.

Sleep Disorders

Levodopa and the dopamine agonists frequently cause various sleep abnormalities. The most common are vivid dreams and sleep talking. Patients report dreams so realistic that only their content reveals to the patient that the phenomena experienced were dreams and not reality. In the case of the confused patient, the dream is mistaken for reality. In patients who are slightly demented, the vivid dream is sometimes interpreted as real when the content is believable—for example that a car accident had occurred during the night on the street below the house. More confusing to the patient is waking up in the middle of a dream, thinking it is real, and waking the spouse. It is important to distinguish dream phenomena from confusion, as the former can usually be treated simply with an explanation and reassurance, whereas the latter requires a reduction in Parkinson's disease medications. Parkinson's disease patients frequently yell, laugh, curse, or scream in their sleep. This is almost always a problem for the spouse or the rest of the household and not for the patient, since it causes awakening only uncommonly. Equally problematic is the almost as frequent jerking, hitting, and kicking that occurs during sleep, again without awakening the patient. A less common phenomenon is "REM (rapid eye movement) sleep disorder," induced by levodopa, in which patients will sometimes not be hypotonic during dream—or rapid eye movement—sleep, and will act out their dream, leading to falls and family complaints about nocturnal confusion. It is important, therefore, to take a complete history about altered behavior, because episodic behavioral alterations may turn out to be relatively benign drug effects on sleep rather than the beginning of a dementing or psychotic process. Nightmares are infrequent and are more common in people with a premorbid history of them. Unfortunately, the levodopa may exacerbate these by making them more vivid and better remembered in addition to causing the sufferer to cry and yell during sleep.

Visual Hallucinosis

Visual hallucinosis occurs in about 20 percent of drug-treated patients followed long term. This phenomenon refers to the experience of seeing real-appearing images in the presence of a clear sensorium. At first, the images are perceived as real, but after the first few attempts to touch them cause them to disappear, the patient learns to distinguish the hallucination from reality and usually is not much bothered by it. Hallucinations tend to be people, frequently children or small adults. These are strangers in most cases, but may be relatives, friends, or deceased acquaintances and are absolutely silent even when ostensibly conversing, closing doors, or performing other tasks that should make noise. The visions are free of emotional content, very much unlike the situation in primary psychoses, such as schizophrenia, in which the hallucinations (almost always voices) say demeaning or nasty things or behave in ways to excite or engage the person. In levodopa-induced hallucinosis, the visions appear at any time of day and tend not to upset the patient. Light does not abort their appearance, nor does darkness increase them. They frequently occur when the individual is alone or engaged in a routine social activity such as watching television with a spouse, and appear only rarely when involved in absorbing activities such as entertaining guests, playing with grandchildren, or visiting a doctor's office. They most commonly watch the patient, showing no emotion themselves. Visual hallucinations must be distinguished from visual delusions, which are misperceptions, with something seen as other than what it is. These usually occur in shadowy or dark areas and tend to take on a menacing aura. Visual delusions are not seen clearly, whereas visual hallucinations are seen as clearly or even more so than real objects. Occasionally, objects rather than people are hallucinated, but friendly animals such as dogs, horses, and cats may be perceived as well. The hallucinations may persist for seconds, minutes, or hours but tend to last minutes and to recur. They usually disappear when "touched" and will usually ignore attempts to engage them in conversation (they do not usually move their lips, attempt sign language, or write on paper pads). The same person or group will usually visit the patient repeatedly.

When the patient is demented or psychotic, the hallucinations are perceived as real, and may cause serious behavioral disturbances, especially if they are threatening. Auditory, tactile, or olfactory hallucinations are exceedingly rare, but may occur in psychosis.

Treatment usually requires a reduction in drug dose, but for some patients, the loss of motor function that ensues is more difficult to tolerate than the hallucinosis and some patients will choose to continue to suffer from them.

Psychosis

Psychosis, a "major" mental disturbance in which reality is significantly misperceived, causing a marked decline in psychosocial functioning, occurs in 5 to 10 percent of long-term treated patients. It is more common in the elderly and the demented but occurs in previously mentally intact parkinsonian patients with no prior psychiatric history. On formal neurologic examination, they score perfectly on the minimental status examination unless there is an attention deficit.

The psychosis induced by levodopa and the dopaminergic drugs tends to be relatively stereotypic. Visual hallucinations occur along with paranoid delusions. Most common is the delusion that the spouse is having a sexual affair. In the case of single patients, a common delusion is that their savings are being looted by the children or the caretaker is plotting to place them in a nursing home. Unfortunately, the appearance of psychosis in fact makes management at home more difficult and is the single most important predictor of nursing home placement in parkinsonian patients. Some patients believe they are about to die, are dead already, that loved ones have just died, and so forth.

Phenomena that are rare in primary psychoses, such as Capgras syndrome, the syndrome of reduplication in which the caretaker or some other significant person or even objects have been replaced by replicas that look and behave like the original, may occur. Unlike schizophrenia, dopaminergic psychosis has only "positive" phenomena. There is no loosening of associations, anhedonia, poverty of thought, loss of ego boundaries, or blunting of affect. A delirious or encephalopathic state may also occur, in which attention span is diminished and disorientation occurs.

Usually psychosis develops insidiously, although it may appear suddenly after a new medication is begun or an old one increased. Psychosis onset, however, in a patient on a stable medication schedule is common and the early features are frequently overlooked if not asked about at routine evaluations. It is common, for example, for psychosis to be present for months before being brought to the physician's attention.

Until recently, management of psychosis was almost impossible. One could reduce medication, attempt a drug holiday, or start a neuroleptic antipsychotic when a dose reduction was not sufficient. Since the commercial release of clozapine, the situation has changed dramatically. Management of psychosis is now a fairly straightforward problem in most cases. It is important to keep in mind that the neurologically impaired frequently suffer exacerbations and mental adverse effects when affected by an intercurrent non-neurologic process. Therefore, it is important to exclude medical problems such as infection, renal failure, thyroid dysfunction, or a new, non-neurologic medication as the underlying problem. However, this is usually not the case, and structural lesions are not worth looking for without a clear indication, such as a new focal sign or head trauma. Electroencephalography is virtually useless in this situation.

Once the physician feels comfortable that the problem is a drug-induced psychosis, then whichever drugs can be eliminated should be. Anticholinergic drugs have the highest mental adverse effect profile of the anti-Parkinson's disease medications and should be stopped at the onset of psychosis. Other anti-Parkinson's disease medications should then be tapered and discontinued, if possible, without jeopardizing motor function. The general approach is to reduce and then discontinue a single drug rather than reducing several drugs, with the aim of reducing polypharmacy as much as possible. There appears to be better tolerance for a single drug at a high dose than for multiple drugs at low to midlevel doses, although no data exists to support this widely held tenet. If a recent medication change precipitated the psychosis, then it should be reversed; otherwise, the order of drug discontinuation should be as follows: anticholinergics, selegiline, amantadine, dopamine agonist, and then levodopa. Once a lower limit of motor function has been reached, clozapine should be started if psychosis has not been ameliorated. Clozapine is an "atypical" neuroleptic that causes no parkinsonian side effects. Numerous studies now attest to its efficacy and tolerability when used properly. Although some specialists advocate hospitalizing psychotic parkinsonian patients, I try to avoid this if possible, as I believe the hospital environment worsens the problem. However, if the patient cannot be managed at home owing to patient or caretaker problems, then hospitalization is certainly justified. Clozapine should be initiated at 6.25 mg/ day, given at bedtime. This is only one-quarter of the smallest available tablet. The usual effective daily dose is in the 6.25 to 50-mg range, with some patients requiring 100 mg. This is in contrast to the doses used in schizophrenia, which are 300 to 900 mg daily.

In general, the dose is increased depending on response and adverse effects. Unlike schizophrenics, psychotic parkinsonian patients may respond within 1 or 2 days. It seems that once the dose is sufficient to keep the patient sleeping through the night, the psychosis remits. Therefore, it is suggested that the dose be increased daily until the patient sleeps through the night. If this does not improve the psychosis, the dose needs to be increased. Most patients do best if the dose is given at bedtime, alone, to reduce the sedative side effects. The major adverse effects are sedation, hypersalivation, weight gain, and orthostatic hypotension. Granulocytopenia, which occurs in under 2 percent, is not dose related, so weekly blood counts are mandated by the U.S. Food and Drug Administration regardless of dose. Outside the United States, the blood tests are reduced to monthly after the first few months. Confusion, possibly due to central anticholinergic effects, may occur in the demented psychotic patient, but occurs rarely—if at all—in the nondemented. If clozapine is not tolerated, then older methods, such as further drug reductions, must be instituted.

An alternative treatment for dopaminergic psychosis is electroconvulsive therapy, but very few reports about it have been published. Since electroconvulsive therapy does improve parkinsonism in the majority of patients and improves some primary psychoses, including mania, depression, and schizophrenia, it should be considered in clozapine-refractory or -intolerant patients. Unfortunately, the main population in this group will be demented psychotic patients, who are also the most likely to experience an electroconvulsive therapy delirium.

How long patients need to remain on clozapine is unknown. Most patients, once on clozapine, can have their anti-Parkinson's disease medications increased without problem. If psychosis recurs when anti-Parkinson's disease drugs are increased, then the clozapine dose is increased.

A new antipsychotic drug, risperidone, has a very low extrapyramidal syndrome profile, but unlike clozapine, may cause acute dystonic reactions and parkinsonism. Its role in the treatment of psychosis in Parkinson's disease remains to be elucidated.

SUGGESTED READINGS

Cummings JL: Depression and Parkinson's disease: a review. Am J Psychiatry 149:443–54, 1992
Faber R, Trimble MR: Electroconvulsive therapy in Parkinson's disease and other movement disorders. Mov Dis 6:293–303, 1991
Factor SA, Brown D, Molho ES, Podskalny GD: Clozapine: A 2 year open

trial in Parkinson's disease patients with psychosis. Neurology 44:544–6, 1994

Friedman JH: The management of the levodopa psychoses. Clin Neuropharmacol 14:283–95, 1991

Friedman JH, Friedman H: Fatigue in Parkinson's disease. Neurology 43: 2016–18, 1993

Hughes AJ, Daniel SE, Blankson S, Lees AJ: The clinicopathologic study of 100 cases of Parkinson's disease. Arch Neurol 50:140–8, 1993

Reid WG: The evolution of dementia in idiopathic Parkinson's disease: neuropsychologic and clinical evidence in support of subtypes. Int Psychogeriatr (Suppl. 2):147–60, 1992

Starkstein SE, Mayberg HS, Prezioi TJ, Robinson RG: A prospective longitudinal study of depression, cognitive decline, and physical impairments in patients with Parkinson's disease. J Neurol Neurosurg Psychiatry 55: 377–82, 1992

Stein MB, Heuser IJ, Juncos JL, Uhde TW: Anxiety disorders in patients with Parkinson's disease. Am J Psychiatry 147:217–20, 1990

117. MULTIPLE SYSTEM ATROPHY: STRIATONIGRAL DEGENERATION AND SHY-DRAGER SYNDROME

PAULA RAVIN

The term *multiple system atrophy* generally refers to a broad class of parkinsonian syndromes with features not normally seen in idiopathic Parkinson's disease. It has been noted in numerous neuropathologic studies that multiple system atrophy is found in 8 to 10 percent of patients diagnosed with idiopathic Parkinson's disease in life and, in some, is clinically indistinguishable. However, the postmortem examination of such patients reveals variable degrees of neurodegenerative changes in cerebellar, striatal, nigral, and subcortical structures such as the thalamus, nucleus accumbens, septal nuclei, hypothalamus, locus ceruleus, and a variety of parasympathetic nuclei (dorsal vagal nucleus, Edinger-Westphal nucleus, Onufs nucleus of the sacral cord, and so on). Hence, the term *multiple system,* though atrophy is not the only anatomic change. A number of reports give evidence for focal gliosis, neuronal loss, glial cytoplasmic inclusions, depletion of specific neurotransmitters (γ-aminobutyric acid, dopamine, norepinephrine, glutamate), and functional changes in metabolism of glucose or dopamine binding characteristics on positron emission tomographic scan.

Oppenheimer and Graham coined the term multiple system atrophy in a paper in 1969 broadly categorizing patients into three subclasses: Shy-Drager syndrome, striatonigral degeneration, and olivopontocerebellar atrophies, the latter of which is further subdivided into familial or sporadic forms. The syndrome of Steele-Richardson-Olszewski or progressive supranuclear palsy is not included since it represents a distinctive clinical picture of supranuclear downgaze palsy, axial dystonia, cognitive impairment, and mild parkinsonism and has discrete pathologic changes associated with the diagnosis.

CLINICAL DIAGNOSIS

Correct identification of multiple system atrophy in life presents a challenge to even the experts in movement disorders. The relevance of distinguishing these disorders early on pertains to prognosis, predicted responses to medication, possibility of a genetic association that can be identified (and may soon be tested with marker gene) and to referring patients to research centers with special interest in multiple system atrophy.

The typical signs and symptoms of Parkinson's disease are not always found in multiple system atrophy early on or may be insignificant clinically compared to other features. Classical resting tremor, for example, is found in 30 percent of idiopathic Parkinson's disease initially but only 5 percent or so of multiple system atrophy cases, with sustension or intention tremor seen in another 40 percent idiopathic Parkinson's disease initially and 10 percent of multiple system atrophy cases. Rigidity with akinesia/bradykinesia is common to both disorders, but postural instability is often seen early on in multiple system atrophy, whereas it is usually found in more advanced or late-onset idiopathic Parkinson's disease and does not evolve as rapidly. Recent papers attempting to distinguish idiopathic Parkinson's disease and multiple system atrophy retrospectively on clinical grounds have suggested certain other distinguishing features or red flags to look for in making an initial differential diagnosis and refining it over the first 2 to 3 years of observation.

To start with, the mean age of onset of multiple system atrophy (all subtypes) is 53, with progression of disability to death in an average of 7 to 10 years, as opposed to idiopathic Parkinson's disease with a mean age of onset at 60 and progression over, 10 to 20 years. The male/female ratio of multiple system atrophy appears to be 1.8:1.0 in familial olivopontocerebellar atrophy, 2.0:1.0 in Shy-Drager syndrome, and unclear in striatonigral degeneration, in which cumulative data would suggest a slight male predominance as in idiopathic Parkinson's disease (1.2:1.0).

Another red flag for multiple system atrophy is the presence of cerebellar signs such as truncal or limb ataxia, a positive Romberg's test, dysarthria and scanning speech, or lateral nystagmus with square-wave jerks. These symptoms are prominent early on in the majority of olivopontocerebellar atrophies, less so in striatonigral degeneration, and rare in Shy-Drager syndrome. However, the presence of cerebellar signs often excludes a diagnosis of Parkinson's disease and may lead to neuroimaging studies for diagnostic purposes. Computed tomography scans are unreliable for viewing posterior fossa structures, but may show widened hemispheric cerebellar sulci, enlarged prepontine and lateral cerebellar cisterns and vermian atrophy, as well as generalized cortical atrophy in advanced cases. Magnetic resonance imaging has proven to be very useful in demonstrating focal increased signal intensity in the pallidum and/or putamen and cerebellar atrophy of the hemispheres and peduncles. Positron emission tomography data can corroborate the presence of selective pathologic changes in these areas as evidenced by hypometabolism predominantly in the cerebellum for olivopontocerebellar atrophy and in the pallidum-putamen complex for striatonigral degeneration.

Autonomic dysfunction is a cardinal feature of multiple system atrophy in all forms early in the course but is found in only 10 percent of idiopathic Parkinson's disease late in the disease, often as an adverse effect of dopaminergic medication. Shy-

Drager syndrome is the most extreme example with incapacitating orthostatic hypotension, causing the patient to become wheelchair-bound within 5 to 7 years of diagnosis. More subtle signs such as impotence in males and sudden flushes or spontaneous blood pressure fluctuations, heat intolerance, and loss of sweating in the axilla, groin, and palms can precede the clinical diagnosis of multiple system atrophy by as much as 10 years.

Response to levodopa is often considered pathognomonic of idiopathic Parkinson's disease but may also be seen transiently in many cases of multiple system atrophy. Usually the benefit is less than would be expected for moderate doses of levodopa (300 to 500 mg/qd), and motor fluctuations correlating to the timing of medication can appear within 1 year of treatment initiation—an unusual response in idiopathic Parkinson's disease. Shy-Drager syndrome patients may experience improvement in rigidity and bradykinesia with levodopa but often cannot tolerate dose increases after several years, owing to exacerbation of orthostatic hypotension. Striatonigral degeneration patients, on the contrary, may respond quite dramatically to moderate or high doses of levodopa (>750 mg/d) but show progressive loss of responsivity over the first 5 to 7 years of treatment rather than fairly stable responses in the same time frame for Parkinson's disease patients. Abnormal involuntary movements often appear in multiple system atrophy patients after a few years of levodopa therapy and may be dose-limiting. Olivopontocerebellar atrophy shows variable degrees of parkinsonian symptoms with proportionate degrees of response to levodopa therapy for many years, though not to dopamine agonists, in several studies. The discriminating factor in these cases may be the preservation of striatal morphology and loss of nigral cells on neuropathologic examination, as seen in the familial form more often than the sporadic form of olivopontocerebellar atrophy.

Additional features that are noted to distinguish between multiple system atrophy and idiopathic Parkinson's disease include a symmetric presentation (45 versus 25 percent), infrequent development of cognitive dysfunction (<10 percent) in multiple system atrophy patients as opposed to more than 25 percent in Parkinson's disease, presence of pyramidal tract signs in olivopontocerebellar atrophy or striatonigral degeneration and absence in idiopathic Parkinson's disease, and prominent symptoms of a neurogenic bladder, including urinary retention, urgency, incontinence or bladder dyssynergia, in all forms of multiple system atrophy. Table 117-1 summarizes the variety of signs and symptoms that may be useful in making an *early* clinical diagnosis of multiple system atrophy most accurately.

Cognitive dysfunction is a variable feature of multiple system atrophy patients, though the test substrates for this have not been well defined or corroborated extensively. For the most part similar deficits to those in Parkinson's disease, described as a "subcortical dementia," may be seen in striatonigral degeneration or Shy-Drager syndrome but with qualitative differences on discrete tasks associated with frontal lobe dysfunction. Frontal lobe function tests are often subdivided into those associated with orbitofrontal, dorsolateral frontal, or frontostriatal pathways. No correlation has been made yet between degree of pathologic involvement of the striatum and severity of subcortical dementia or with the course of the motor disorder in either striatonigral degeneration or Shy-Drager syndrome.

In olivopontocerebellar atrophy, by way of contrast, several specific patterns of cognitive dysfunction have been noted to parallel the severity of disease, especially in familial autosomal-dominant forms, such as type V by the Konigsmark and Weiner classification. Changes in mood and affect with irritability, lability, and depression were commonly noted in this type, and hallucinations, psychosis, and memory loss were also reported in several family pedigrees. Tasks sensitive to dorsolateral frontal versus orbitofrontal dysfunction point to loss of cerebello-frontal connections as the disease progresses in these forms of olivopontocerebellar atrophy. The end result is behavioral and cognitive dysfunction similar to that seen in Alzheimer's disease.

NEUROPATHOLOGIC FEATURES

As noted before, the definitive diagnosis of multiple system atrophy is most accurately determined by the postmortem pathology. Histologically, the putamen shows marked loss of nerve cells with associated gliosis in the posterior and lateral portions. The anteromedial putamen and head of the caudate may evidence lesser changes in some cases, similar to the pa-

TABLE 117-1. Signs and Symptoms of Multiple System Atrophies

| | PD | MSA | | | PSP |
		SND	SD	OPCA	
Age of onset	60 ± 7	53 ± 7	52 ± 6	28 ± 4 (FOPCA) 49 ± 6 (SOPCA)	70 ± 6
Duration of disease (years)	10–20	7–10	5–10	10–25 (FOPCA) 6–15 (SOPCA)	6–10
Rigidity	+	+	+ +	±	+
Bradykinesia	+	+	+ +	±	+ +
Orthostasis	−	−	+ + +	±	−
Neurogenic bladder	−	−	+ +	±	−
Response to levodopa	+ +	+	+	±	−
Dyskinesia, dystonia	+ (young onset)	+ +	−	±	+
Tremor	+ +	+	+	+	−
Rapid progression	−	+	+ +	±	+ +
Cognitive dysfunction	+ ("subcortical")	+ ("subcortical")	±	+ + + (FOPCA) + (SOPCA)	+ + +

Abbreviations: FOPCA, familial olivopontocerebellar atrophy; SOPCA, sporadic olivopontocerebellar atrophy; PD, Parkinson's disease; SND, striatonigral degeneration; SD, Shy-Drager syndrome; OPCA, olivopontocerebellar atrophy; PSP, progressive supranuclear palsy; −, absent; +, mild; + +, moderate; + + +, marked.

thology of Huntington's disease. Melanin pigment or siderin granules are left behind from the degenerated putamen neurons and may also accumulate in the globus pallidus and substantia nigra-pars reticulata (not the pars compacta). Varying degrees of neuron loss are found in pontine nuclei, the inferior olives, Purkinje cells of the cerebellar hemispheres, and the intermediolateral columns of the thoracic and lumbar spinal segments or Onufs nucleus in the sacral cord.

Lewy bodies have long been considered the sine qua non for the diagnosis of idiopathic Parkinson's disease. They are identified as intracytoplasmic eosinophilic inclusions of 5 to 25 μm in diameter with a dense core and smudgy halo antigenically similar to neurofilament. In multiple system atrophy, they may be found at a slightly higher frequency than in normal aging controls but not to the extent seen in idiopathic Parkinson's disease. The distribution of Lewy bodies in both multiple system atrophy and idiopathic Parkinson's disease is generally the same, whereas the degree of gliosis, nigral cell degeneration, and pigmented deposits (melanin, lipofucsin, or siderin) is much greater in all the brainstem nuclei involved in multiple system atrophy.

The familial olivopontocerebellar atrophies tend to have an even more widespread neuron loss and reactive changes (gliosis and demyelination, axonal thinning, or gross atrophy) involving all the same areas affected by sporadic olivopontocerebellar atrophy. In addition, there is often a neuron wipe-out in the dentate nuclei, locus ceruleus, corticospinal tracts, Clarke's columns and spinocerebellar tracts, posterior column, and anterior gray horns. These extensive lesions explain the diversity and severity of clinical signs found in most cases of familial olivopontocerebellar atrophy, whereas spontaneous olivopontocerebellar atrophies are fairly stereotypic in appearance. The observation of extremely dense deposits of lipofucsin in all areas of neuron loss seen in a patient with familial olivopontocerebellar atrophy and glutamate dehydrogenase deficiency has been a confounding factor in trying to characterize the neuropathologic features of olivopontocerebellar atrophies uniformly. It seems that there are a variety of look-alikes in this subdivision of multiple system atrophies that may differ in their primary metabolic defect(s) but lead ultimately to a characteristic pattern of cellular loss.

THERAPEUTIC STRATEGIES

The therapy for multiple system atrophy depends on which systems degeneration presents the most troublesome symptoms, since parkinsonian features are usually not the predominant ones. Also, as noted earlier, response to dopaminergic drugs is poorly sustained and may include worsening of orthostatic hypotension. Dyskinesias often occur with levodopa therapy after an average of 2.5 years of replacement with low to moderate doses and can be seen simultaneously with axial rigidity, resting tremor, bradykinesia, and bulbar dysfunction (dysphagia and dysarthria). A slight response to levodopa may in fact be evident only in up to 40 percent of multiple system atrophy patients when clinical deterioration occurs after withdrawal of dopaminergics (e.g., for a "drug holiday") and failure of an enhanced response to levodopa after reintroduction a few weeks later.

Vague feelings of unsteadiness and overt falls early in the course of disease are common to all forms of multiple system atrophy and may be aggravated by treatment with neuroleptic-type drugs given for presumed "vestibulopathy"—bringing

out the parkinsonian aspects of these disorders instead. If postural changes in systolic pressure of greater than 20 mm Hg are found without dopaminergic therapy, further assessment of the autonomic nervous system can help define appropriate choices of drug therapy. Testing of the baroreceptor arc includes measurement of Valsalva ratio, the cold pressor test, and observing changes in blood pressure and electrocardiogram rhythm with hypoventilation and slow, steady breathing. These are simple physiologic tests of the integration of both the afferent and efferent limbs of the arc as well as vagal tone. More sophisticated testing of catecholamine responses and pharmacologic rechallenge tests are best performed in a dedicated laboratory setting where the exact conditions of the tests and their responses can be measured and interpreted accurately.

Mild orthostatic hypotension can be remedied with a combination of support hose or Jobst stockings (if tolerated) and volume expansion by adding salt to the diet. Often low-dose fludrocortisone (0.1 mg/d to 0.2 mg tid) is helpful if not contraindicated by a history of congestive heart failure Indomethacin at 25 to 50 mg tid or ibuprofen at 400 to 800 mg tid can indirectly result in higher mean arterial pressures, whereas a newly released α-agonist, midodrine, increases sympathetic tone sufficiently to overcome the postural drop in blood pressure but may lead to problematic supine hypertension.

Patients should be advised to avoid standing abruptly after prolonged sitting, and to try to stay well hydrated and avoid overexposure to hot and humid environments. They should prevent vasovagal responses due to consuming large meals, excessive alcohol, and straining at bowel movements. Sleeping in an elevated position (HOB up 30 degrees) in "reverse Trendelenburg" can ameliorate early morning hypotension by increasing the renin secretion overnight. The use of cardiac pacing or implantable devices for noradrenergic replacement therapy (an "autonomic pacing system") are still under investigation and show promise for the more refractory condition of primary autonomic failure without central nervous system involvement.

When dopaminergic therapy is no longer tolerated for extrapyramidal symptoms, anticholinergics may be beneficial in controlling tremor, rigidity, and bradykinesia at doses comparable to those used in idiopathic Parkinson's disease. A coincidental benefit is mild urinary retention as a side effect of these drugs in the face of urgency and incontinence seen in mild to moderate multiple system atrophy. However, acute or severe urinary retention may ensue if the multiple system atrophy patient also has detrusor dyssynergia.

The neurogenic bladder problems of multiple system atrophy can vary from incomplete voiding leading to recurrent infections from urinary stasis to involuntary urethral sphincter relaxation with incontinence of small or large volumes. This is, on rare occasions, accompanied by the same phenomenon in the anal sphincter, causing "double incontinence" in advanced multiple system atrophy. Treatment includes standard precautions such as urinary acidification and episodic to chronic antibiotic treatment plus using a postvoiding Credé maneuver and toileting schedules. Judicial limitations of fluid intake at night, and protective garments or condom catheters can improve urinary hygiene as well. Chronic constipation may parallel the course of the bladder disturbance and is addressed with bulk agents, stool softeners, increased daytime fluid intake and laxatives or enemas when all else fails. Cisapride, a novel drug for gastric atony, can also improve bowel motility without worsening parkinsonism at doses of 10 mg bid to 20 mg qid.

The gait disorder of multiple system atrophy is typically multifactorial and should in any case be evaluated by experienced physical and occupational therapists. Loss of postural reflexes presents the most dangerous component and is not remediable with medication. Teaching safety awareness and when to use assistive devices for ambulation is key to maintaining patient independence. Other factors such as extrapyramidal tone, postural hypotension, and limb ataxia may be diminished by the addition of amantadine (50 to 100 mg tid) to anticholinergic therapy at least for the first 1 or 2 years after diagnosis, but often not beyond that.

Finally, speech and swallowing disturbances in multiple system atrophy are quite refractory to pharmacologic therapy but need to be evaluated to reduce the risk of aspiration and fatal choking. Vocal pacing, respiratory exercises, and language boards can help patients communicate effectively when speech quality is grossly impaired. Standard aspiration precautions combined with cisapride or an H_2-blocker may also delay serious problems with pneumonia or reactive airway disease.

CONCLUSIONS

Multiple system atrophy is an apt term for a class of diseases that have in comon parkinsonism and the following atypical features:

1. Extrapyramidal signs like those of idiopathic Parkinson's disease but less responsive to dopaminergic therapy initially or within 2.5 years of using moderate doses of levodopa
2. Additional symptoms and signs of pathology in the cerebellum, pyramidal tract, autonomic nervous system, and numerous brainstem nuclei
3. Frequent development of spontaneous or dopa-induced dystonia and dyskinesia, also within a few years of presentation
4. Earlier mean age of onset and more rapid progression to disability than idiopathic Parkinson's disease
5. Characteristic pathologic changes on postmortem examination, with neuron loss and gliosis but without prominent Lewy bodies

Current research in multiple system atrophy relates to early diagnostic discrimination between idiopathic Parkinson's disease and the striatonigral degeneration variant by positron emission tomography and single photon emission computed tomography scanning with selective markers, identifying a common metabolic derangement that may cause the "systems" breakdown, and gathering enough epidemiologic data to identify a possible genetic precursor or environmental exposure contributing to these diseases. Whereas multiple system atrophy is far less common than idiopathic Parkinsin's disease, its "atypical" features often lead to families and physicians pursuing further studies both pre- and postmortem. The opportunity for better understanding of all parkinsonian disorders, therefore, lies in identifying multiple system atrophy patients and offering them specialized care and, ultimately, by encouraging their participation in research studies.

SUGGESTED READINGS

Bannister R, Oppenheimer D: Parkinsonian system degenerations and autonomic failure. In Marsden CD, Fahn S (eds): Movement Disorders. Butterworth, London, 1981

Hughes AJ, Colosimo C, Kleedorfer B et al: The dopaminergic response in multiple system atrophy. J Neurol Neurosurg Psychiatry 55:1009–13, 1992

Hughes A, Daniel S, Kilford L, Lees A: The accuracy of the clinical diagnosis of Parkinson's disease: clinicopathological study of 100 cases. J Neurol Neurosurg Psychiatry 55:181–4, 1992

Penny JB: Multiple system atrophy and non-familial divopontocerebellar atrophy are the same disease. Ann Neurol. 37:553–4, 1995

Polinsky RJ: Multiple system atrophy: clinical aspects, pathophysiology and treatment. In Jankovic J (ed): Neurologic Clinics. Vol. 2. WB Saunders, Philadelphia, pp. 487–98 1984a

Quinn N: Multiple system atrophy—the nature of the beast. J Neurol Neurosurg Psychiatry (special Suppl.) 78–89, 1989

118. PROGRESSIVE SUPRANUCLEAR PALSY

DOUGLAS G. COLE

Steele, Richardson, and Olzewski described progressive supranuclear palsy in 1964, and the disorder has since become a well-established clinicopathologic entity. Its dominant clinical feature is parkinsonism. Although relatively rare, it may be the most common clinicopathologically defined atypical parkinsonian disorder.

CLINICAL FEATURES

Patients generally present in their fifties and sixties, less often in their forties, seventies, or eighties. The presentation may include imbalance, loss of manual dexterity, visual disturbances, dysarthria, dysphagia, altered intellectual function, personality changes, or insomnia. All features are not invariably present in every patient, but most evolve eventually during the course of the illness.

Postural instability and visual disturbances are particularly characteristic and often early symptoms of progressive supranuclear palsy. Some patients begin to fall suddenly and without apparent explanation ("paroxysmal disequilibrium"). Most develop a tendency to fall backward, but they may fall in any direction. Some describe difficulty walking on an incline or on uneven surfaces, maintaining balance when lifting a heavy object, or arising from a chair or getting out of a car.

Visual difficulties primarily reflect impaired voluntary control of eye movements. Patients may describe difficulty navigating when walking down stairs or problems reading a book or trying to find food on a plate. They often complain of blurred vision and occasionally of diplopia. They may describe difficulty opening or closing the eyes. Some say that they simply cannot see.

Establishing the presence of early imbalance or visuomotor impairment in the history of a patient with parkinsonism strongly favors the diagnosis of progressive supranuclear palsy; sustained absence of either of these symptoms makes its diagnosis unlikely.

Speech and swallowing commonly deteriorate. Choking develops insidiously but eventually becomes a major source of morbidity. Most patients develop cognitive impairment (i.e., a modest loss of cognitive function compared with their baseline). Fewer are believed to develop dementia (i.e., a more profound and widespread decline of memory and other cognitive functions that alone is sufficient to compromise social and vocational abilities). Depression and personality changes are frequent. As in many parkinsonian disorders, sleep disturbances are common.

Examination of patients with progressive supranuclear palsy reveals symmetric, axially predominant parkinsonism, abnormal eye movements, gait instability, and pseudobulbar palsy. Axially predominant parkinsonism is characterized by rigidity and hypokinesia that is most prominent in the muscles of the neck and trunk. On casual observation, the examiner may note that the patient moves his or her head abnormally slowly, or en bloc with the trunk. Passive motion of the neck, especially to flexion and extension, reveals rigidity. The magnitude of this rigidity may vary, but neck tone is rarely normal, even in the early stages of progressive supranuclear palsy. When severe, it can be associated with retrocollis and dystonic extension of the entire trunk.

Patients with progressive supranuclear palsy lose facial expressiveness. Some patients develop rigidity of the limbs, but others have normal limb tone despite severe axial rigidity. Loss of manual dexterity is common. Fine movements of the fingers and hands become slow and uncoordinated. This loss of precise motor control may occasionally be exacerbated by apraxia, but prominent apraxia is uncommon.

Abnormal eye movements are a critical feature of progressive supranuclear palsy. The most typical abnormality is impaired voluntary gaze. The examiner may suspect a defect in eye movements when calling the patient's name in the waiting room: instead of turning the eyes briskly towards the sound of his or her name, the patient slowly turns the head, or even the whole body. On more formal examination, one can observe that when the patient holds his or her head still and tries either to follow a moving object with the eyes or to move the eyes in a particular direction without a visual target, the eye movements are incomplete, absent, slow, or fractionated. When the patient fixes the eyes on a stationary object while allowing the examiner to move his or her head, however, the eyes display a full range of motion (intact oculocephalic reflex or "doll's head response"). The ability to converge the eyes is lost. Typically, gaze remains conjugate.

Usually, the voluntary eye movement most prominently affected in progressive supranuclear palsy is downgaze. Although impaired voluntary downgaze strongly suggests the diagnosis of progressive supranuclear palsy in the correct context, it is not pathognomic for the disease. For example, impaired downgaze and parkinsonism can be seen in central nervous system Whipple's disease, which, though exceedingly rare, is eminently treatable. Furthermore, some patients with progressive supranuclear palsy display more involvement of horizontal or upgaze than downgaze. In this regard, one should note that decreased range of voluntary upgaze is common in elderly people. This eye movement finding alone is rarely sufficient for suspecting that a patient has progressive supranuclear palsy.

The severity of eye movement abnormalities in progressive supranuclear palsy is variable. When dramatic, supranuclear gaze palsy is easy to appreciate. When subtle, it may be detectable only through close observation. For example, some patients may have only slowing of the fast phase of opticokinetic nystagmus. The presence of square wave jerks and inability to suppress the vestibulo-ocular reflex can bolster suspicion of progressive supranuclear palsy.

Other patterns of eye movement abnormalities occasionally develop in patients with this disease. Several patients have been described with an internuclear ophthalmoplegia. Other patients lose all eye movements, including reflex eye movements. Rare

patients retain normal eye movements throughout the course of the disease.

Exceptional cases notwithstanding, the importance of a careful visuomotor examination in any patient with parkinsonism cannot be overemphasized. The combination of prominent impairment of voluntary eye movements and parkinsonism suggests progressive supranuclear palsy until proven otherwise.

In this disease, visual function can also be compromised by abnormal opening and closing of the eyes. Many patients with the disease have retracted upper eyelids, which gives them a characteristic staring expression. Decreased blink frequency, common in many parkinsonian disorders, makes patients susceptible to corneal injury. Alternatively, some patients with progressive supranuclear palsy find that they are unable to open their eyes voluntarily. This so-called apraxia of eyelid opening, when severe, can produce functional blindness. Visual acuity, however, is not primarily affected in progressive supranuclear palsy.

Patients with the disease typically have difficulty arising from a chair, and when they try to sit down, they often begin to topple backward uncontrollably. When standing, they may hold the trunk erect. They stand and walk with a normal base, bilateral symmetric diminution of arm swing, and en bloc turning. Their steps may be shuffling or festinating. The ability to walk in tandem or hop or stand on either foot is lost. Some patients display retropulsion when pulled from behind. Others fall spontaneously. Eventually, patients become entirely unable to walk.

Dysarthria and dysphagia in progressive supranuclear palsy reflect pseudobulbar palsy. Speech is slurred and quiet. Some patients develop difficulty initiating speech or irregular, halting speech or festinating speech. They may eventually become anarthric. Drooling is prominent. The gag reflex may be hyperactive or hypoactive. Aspiration is frequent. Primitive reflexes and frontal release signs, such as the glabellar response, root response, snout reflex, grasping, and palmomental responses are common. Utilization behavior, echolalia, pallilalia, or perseveration can be dramatic. Emotional incontinence can evolve.

Evidence of intellectual deterioration with the disease includes generalized cognitive slowing, inattentiveness, and memory loss. In some patients, the magnitude of intellectual decline equals that of the loss of voluntary motor control, and true dementia ensues. In others, however, intellectual involvement remains mild for years, despite disabling loss of motor function. Because motor dysfunction can progressively compromise a patient ability to communicate, establishing the intellectual status of a patient with progressive supranuclear palsy often requires careful and patient questioning. One should not assume, however, that a patient with the disease is demented on the basis of physical debility.

Rest tremor is rare in progressive supranuclear palsy. Absence of such a tremor by history or on examination is an important clue to the diagnosis. Strength, primary sensation, and cerebellar function are preserved. Occasional patients develop mild hyperreflexia or an extensor plantar response, but pyramidal tract dysfunction is not a prominent feature of the illness.

DIFFERENTIAL DIAGNOSIS

The major diagnostic considerations in a patient who may have progressive supranuclear palsy are other parkinsonian neurodegenerative disorders, most importantly Parkinson's disease. It has been estimated that about 5 percent of patients diagnosed with Parkinson's disease actually have progressive supranuclear palsy. Several clues are especially helpful in differentiating the two disorders. In contrast to progressive supranuclear palsy, imbalance and impaired vision are rare in the initial stages of Parkinson's disease. The eye movement defects so typical of the former are not seen in the latter. Whereas axial parkinsonism is the rule in progressive supranuclear palsy, appendicular predominance typifies Parkinson's disease. The symmetric distribution of parkinsonism in progressive supranuclear palsy contrasts with the asymmetric parkinsonism usually found in Parkinson's disease. Retrocollis, erect posture, and dystonic extension of the trunk are uncommon in patients with Parkinson's disease; mild anteroflexion of the neck and hunched posture are more typical. Rest tremor is almost always present at some point during the course of illness in patients with Parkinson's disease. Finally, patients with Parkinson's disease usually experience sustained and dramatic benefits from levodopa. This is not the case for patients with progressive supranuclear palsy (see below).

Other atypical parkinsonian disorders that respond poorly to levodopa may resemble progressive supranuclear palsy. Corticobasal-ganglionic degeneration produces asymmetric parkinsonism associated with severe apraxia and parietal sensory deficits. Multiple systems atrophies, such as striatonigral degeneration, Shy-Drager syndrome, and the olivopontocerebellar atrophies, produce varied patterns of deficits reflecting involvement of the corticospinal system, the cerebellar system, the autonomic nervous system, and the peripheral nerves. Some of these disorders are hereditary.

Normal pressure hydrocephalus is a poorly understood syndrome in which patients can develop gait ataxia followed by urinary incontinence and dementia. This syndrome should rarely, if ever, be confused with progressive supranuclear palsy. It is important to keep in mind in any patient who presents with impaired gait, however, because occasional patients with early stages of normal pressure hydrocephalus will improve following drainage of cerebrospinal fluid. Clues to the diagnosis of normal pressure hydrocephalus include the temporal evolution of symptoms (which is critical), the presence of hydrocephalus on imaging, normal cerebrospinal fluid pressure, and the absence of any atypical features.

Multiple cerebral infarctions can produce pseudobulbar palsy, but we have not seen infarctions alone mimic the entire syndrome of progressive supranuclear palsy. A history of stepwise decline is a clue to the presence of vascular disease. Spongiform encephalopathies sometimes enter into the differential diagnosis, but tend to produce evidence of cortical dysfunction, such as myoclonus, and tend to progress rapidly. The clinical pictures of Alzheimer's disease and Pick's disease may overlap with that of progressive supranuclear palsy. Usually, the relative prominence of dementia compared with motor involvement indicates the correct diagnosis, but sometimes, the scenario can confound even the most experienced observer. Wilson's disease and central nervous system Whipple's disease are both rare but important to consider because they are treatable. Uncommon hereditary disorders, such as adult onset Niemann-Pick disease and Joseph's disease, can, on rare occasions, mimic progressive supranuclear palsy.

DIAGNOSIS

The diagnosis of progressive supranuclear palsy rests on recognition of the characteristic syndrome. In a typical case, a single imaging study of the brain, ideally a magnetic resonance scan, is appropriate to screen for coexistent disorders, such as cerebral infarctions. This study may reveal prominent atrophy of the midbrain, with enlargement of the third ventricle, but these are not reliable findings. Patients who may have disorders with a biochemical signature, such as Wilson's disease, should be evaluated accordingly.

In some patients, a firm diagnosis cannot be made at the time of presentation. Rarely, characteristic abnormalities on positron emission tomography (PET) or single photon emission computed tomography (SPECT) can support a suspected diagnosis of progressive supranuclear palsy (see below). Generally, however, the most important step is to follow patients over time. Usually, the diagnosis of progressive supranuclear palsy will become readily apparent.

BIOLOGIC BASIS

The brains of patients with progressive supranuclear palsy show pronounced subcortical and midbrain atrophy with varying degrees of cortical atrophy. The substantia nigra is depigmented. Light microscopic examination reveals neuronal loss, gliosis, and globose neurofibrillary tangles. Neuronal loss and gliosis are severe in the substantia nigra, the subthalamic nucleus, the globus pallidus (especially the internal portion), and the superior colliculus. In some cases, neuronal loss is so severe in these areas that little remains but a skein of glia. Neuronal loss is slightly less prominent in the pretectum, locus ceruleus, periaqueductal gray matter, and substantia innominata. The brains of many patients show additional involvement of the motor nuclei in the brainstem (in particular, the ocular motor nuclei), the striatum, the thalamus, the dentate nucleus of the cerebellum, and the basal forebrain. The globose neurofibrillary tangles are composed of straight filaments, distiguishing them structurally from the flame-shaped neurofibrillary tangles of Alzheimer's disease, which are composed of paired helical filaments. The distribution of globose neurofibrillary tangles largely parallels that of neuronal loss, but no efforts have been made to establish a quantitative correlation between the two findings. Subtle pathologic changes may be found in the cortex, especially in the frontal regions.

The dopamine system is markedly abnormal. PET and postmortem studies have shown that dopamine in the striatum is profoundly depleted. Dopamine is relatively preserved in the cortex, however, indicating sparing of the mesocortical dopamine projections. PET and postmortem autoradiographic studies indicate that pharmacologically defined D2 dopamine receptors are decreased in the striatum, but striatal D1 dopamine receptors are preserved. This situation contrasts with that found in Parkinson's disease, in which striatal dopamine loss is associated with normal or increased numbers of striatal D2 receptors.

Levels of choline acetyl transferase, a marker of cholinergic activity, have been found to be moderately diminished in subcortical structures by some observers, but not by others. Levels of serotonin and norepinephrine have been found to be normal, but these neurotransmitters have been studied in only a few patients.

PET and SPECT have demonstrated decreased metabolic activity of the cortex, especially the frontal cortex, as well as the basal ganglia, thalamus, and pons. The observed abnormalities of the frontal cortex on these studies contrasts with its relative sparing by light microscopic analysis.

Degeneration of the striatonigral axis likely contributes to parkinsonism in progressive supranuclear palsy, but may not fully explain motor impairment: in the striatum, changes in ^{18}F-6-fluorodopa uptake measured with PET, an index of the integrity of nigrostriatal dopaminergic nerve terminals, do not correlate with the Hoehn and Yahr scale score, an index of parkinsonian disability. Loss of voluntary eye movements indicates compromise of the supranuclear brain structures, such as the superior colliculi and the frontal lobes, that regulate eye movements. Preservation of the reflex eye movements indicates sparing of the neuromuscular apparatus directly responsible for eye movements (i.e., the ocular motor nuclei and their associated nerves and muscle). Internuclear ophthalmoplegia suggests involvement of the medial longitudinal fasciculus. Loss of reflex eye movements indicates that pathology has extended to the ocular motor nuclei themselves. Pseudobulbar palsy arises from bilateral degeneration of extrapyramidal structures.

TREATMENT

Efforts to treat progressive supranuclear palsy have sought to exploit the strategy of neurotransmitter replacement that has been successful in Parkinson's disease. Some patients derive modest benefit from levodopa, but this benefit is rarely as dramatic as for patients with Parkinson's disease, and it wanes rapidly. Nevertheless, when used judiciously, there is little risk to a trial of levodopa. The patient's unsatisfactory response to levodopa over time often provides an important clue to the diagnosis of progressive supranuclear palsy.

Three factors are likely to account for the failure of dopamine replacement in progressive supranuclear palsy: (1) loss of striatal D2 dopamine receptors may compromise dopamine's benefits; (2) the output of the basal ganglia is funneled through the internal globus pallidus—because the internal globus pallidus degenerates in progressive supranuclear palsy, any benefits of restoring striatal activity would likely be limited because striatal signals could not be transmitted to the rest of the brain; (3) widespread degeneration of subcortical structures besides the basal ganglia decreases the likelihood that simply normalizing basal ganglia function would restore normal brain function.

Other approaches to treatment have included the use of direct dopamine receptor agonists, cholinergic agents, serotonin agonists or antagonists, and tricyclic antidepressants. These trials have been disappointing. The α^2-adrenergic antagonist idazoxan was shown in a double-blinded, placebo-controlled crossover study to ameliorate imbalance and manual dexterity in a small number of patients, but the magnitude of improvement was small. The use of idazoxan is also hampered by side effects and limited availability.

Treatment is otherwise palliative. Insomnia responds well to low doses of trazodone. Focal areas of dystonia or painful rigidity can be treated with injections of botulinum toxin. Precautions to prevent falls and aspiration are important.

COURSE

The syndrome of progressive supranuclear palsy worsens inexorably. Typical life expectancy from time of onset is about 5 years, although the range varies from 1 year to over 2 decades. Patients are at risk for bone fractures and brain trauma from falls, sepsis, wound infections, and aspiration pneumonia. They eventually become unable to walk, speak, or swallow, and often develop a fixed posture of dystonia in extension. Death is due to intercurrent illness or inanition.

It is important to provide patients and families with accurate information regarding the course and complications of progressive supranuclear palsy in order to help them make realistic plans for treating the secondary complications of the disorder when they occur.

UNRESOLVED ISSUES

Careful observation since the 1960s has firmly established progressive supranuclear palsy as a clinicopathologic entity. Nevertheless, many issues regarding the disease are unresolved. For example, the nature and true extent of dementia in patients with the disease must still be determined. The status of the cholinergic, noradrenergic, serotonergic, and amino acid neurotransmitter systems must be clarified. Understanding of the potential involvement of neurotransmitter systems must incorporate new information provided by molecular biologic identification of multiple, previously unrecognized receptor subtypes. The significance, if any, of globose neurofibrillary tangles must be established.

Beyond these phenomenologic issues are several more perplexing enigmas. Current understanding of the pathophysiology of basal ganglia disorders suggests that loss of dopamine produces parkinsonism by allowing overactivity of the inhibitory input from the internal globus pallidus to the thalamus. Experimental and human studies suggest that destruction of the subthalamic nucleus or internal globus pallidus can restore normal thalamic activity, and therefore ameliorate parkinsonism. Parkinsonism in progressive supranuclear palsy, a disorder in which there is concurrent degeneration of the substantia nigra, the subthalamic nucleus, and the internal globus pallidus, is not consistent with this scheme. This apparent paradox remains to be reconciled. It suggests, however, that pallidotomy, which may be useful to treat intractable Parkinson's disease, will not help patients with progressive supranuclear palsy.

Furthermore, the pathophysiology of dementia in progressive supranuclear palsy, when it occurs, is obscure. Some suggest that degeneration of subcortical structures alone can cause dementia by deafferenting the cortex. Others believe that dementia occurs only when the brain is subject to a second, independent process, such as Alzheimer's-type degeneration or infarction. A third possibility is that the subtle cortical pathology in progressive supranuclear palsy observed by some bespeaks functionally significant pathology sufficient to impair cognition.

Most importantly, the cause of neuronal degeneration in the disease is unknown.

In short, the recognition and characterization of progressive supranuclear palsy have raised more questions than they have answered. Efforts to treat, and ultimately reverse, the effects of the disease will require answers to these questions. No experimental model of the disease exists. For the time being, at least, new insights into the disease will come from clinically based investigation. Patients should be informed about available research studies and encouraged to participate in them when appropriate.

SUGGESTED READINGS

Agid Y, Javoy-Agid F, Ruberg M et al: Progressive supranuclear palsy: anatomoclinical and biochemical considerations pp. 191–206. Advances in Neurology. Yahr MD, Bergmann KJ (eds): Vol. 45. Raven Press, New York, 1986

Hughes AJ, Daniel SE, Kilford L, Lees AJ: Accuracy of clinical diagnosis of idiopathic Parkinson's disease: a clinico-pathological study of 100 cases. J Neurol Neurosurg Psychiatry 55:181–4, 1992

Steele JC: Progressive supranuclear palsy. Brain 95:693–705, 1972

Steele JC, Richardson JC, Olszewski J: Progressive supranuclear palsy. Arch Neurol 10:333–58, 1964

Troost BT, Daroff RB: The ocular motor defects in progressive supranuclear palsy. Ann Neurol 2:397–403, 1977

119. SECONDARY PARKINSONISM

JEFFREY D. MACKLIS

In addition to idiopathic Parkinson's disease, a wide variety of relatively common and more rare disorders can present with similar symptoms of parkinsonism, mimicking the clinical presentation of Parkinson's disease to varying degrees. Depending on the age of the patient, relevant concurrent illness, clinical circumstances, time course, and specifics of the neurologic examination, investigation of these possibilities may require only clinical awareness or in-depth laboratory and neuroimaging evaluation. This chapter briefly reviews some of the more relevant etiologies of secondary parkinsonism, roughly in the order of decreasing probability in most practice settings.

The complex of parkinsonian symptoms, including cogwheel rigidity, bradykinesia, rest tremor, and postural instability, can result in part from dysfunction at a variety of levels within the nigrostriatal system, most commonly resulting in functional dopamine deficiency. Because of this, disruption of this system by drugs or infarction in the striatum, imbalance of dopaminergic versus cholinergic striatal innervation, or toxic or viral injury to nigral neurons themselves can cause symptoms that alone can often be difficult to differentiate from the idiopathic nigral neuron degeneration of Parkinson's disease. In general, neurodiagnostic studies are most helpful in ruling out various secondary parkinsonian syndromes and other distinct diseases. In the current climate of health-care cost containment, it is not warranted and will not be possible to investigate all possibilities in all patients; this chapter may provide a framework in which to choose how extensive a diagnostic evaluation to pursue and in which direction to pursue it.

DRUG-INDUCED PARKINSONISM

Almost as common as idiopathic Parkinson's disease itself is parkinsonism resulting from prescribed medication, most commonly the antipsychotic and antiemetic phenothiazines (chlorpromazine and related compounds), butyrophenones (haloperidol and related compounds), metoclopramide, and extremely rarely and typically only at very high doses, potentially both antihypertensives reserpine and methyldopa. Although case reports of parkinsonism from piperazine derivative calcium channel-blockers and the antiarrhythmic amiodarone exist, the significance is uncertain, and these agents are rare in most clinical settings. The former neuroleptic compounds exert their action via dopaminergic blockade within the striatum, and the latter two antihypertensives via dopamine depletion. Drug-induced parkinsonism can occur at all ages and is usually readily treated by dosage adjustment or withdrawal.

Diagnosis is by careful elicitation of medication history and by diagnostic/therapeutic dosage reduction. It may not be possible to eliminate all parkinsonian features while maintaining successful antipsychotic treatment, but diagnosis can sometimes help with choices among alternative antipsychotic or sedative medications. The atypical antipsychotic clozapine has a much lower incidence of parkinsonian side effects but requires complex monitoring for the risk of neutropenia.

Although the occurrence of parkinsonian side effects in a population is not clearly dose dependent, on an individual basis the effects of all of these compounds are dose dependent and fully reversible. Resolution of symptoms takes days to weeks following discontinuation and should leave no residual symptoms or signs (although rarely months to years must pass until full resolution). Of course, idiopathic Parkinson's disease may exist as an underlying illness and may be worsened by pharmacotherapy with these agents, in which case small doses may cause pronounced symptoms.

VASCULAR PARKINSONISM

Vascular infarction or compromise within the striatum or subcortical white matter can mimic some aspects of idiopathic Parkinson's disease. Most often, this takes the form of small-vessel disease, resulting in multiple lacunar infarctions. Since the average age of onset for Parkinson's disease (approximately 60) falls within the range common for stroke, the clinical circumstances, presentation, and constellation of clinical signs are central to correct diagnosis. In addition, it is not uncommon for small-vessel disease and multiple appropriately placed lacunae to coexist with idiopathic Parkinson's disease. Although the diagnosis of the primary etiology of parkinsonism in these mixed cases can be imperfect, highly dependent on the relative progression of pyramidal and extrapyramidal signs over time and aided by observing the response to dopaminergic medication, more commonly, the clinical onset and signs are more easily differentiated between idiopathic Parkinson's disease and parkinsonism resulting from multiple infarctions.

This diagnosis was initially used to suggest a presumed etiology for Parkinson's disease in the late nineteenth century, continued through periods of favor and disfavor over the next century, and now is used more generically to describe secondary parkinsonism resulting from vascular disease. Although controversial in the past, this broader use provides a framework in which to view an important and relatively common part of the differential diagnosis of secondary parkinsonism. Attention to diagnosis of vascular disease and management of underlying risk factors can be important in avoiding complications of occult hypertension and cardiovascular disease, in addition to avoiding largely ineffective dopaminergic therapy with potentially important cardiovascular side effects.

Vascular parkinsonism most commonly occurs in patients with multiple risk factors for small-vessel disease, especially hypertension and prior history of stroke. Because lacunar infarctions in the striatum and subcortical white matter (or less frequently the brainstem or cerebellum) can occur either in relative clinical silence in a diffuse bilateral distribution or with a clearly ictal onset, the presentation is typically either subacute and symmetric (unlike the typically asymmetric presentation for idiopathic Parkinson's disease) or acute and unilateral. Stepwise progression can occur, but such a clear history is uncommon given the often subtle initial symptoms of these small infarctions. Rest parkinsonian tremor, festination, and seborrhea are uncommon, whereas associated pyramidal signs and superimposed gegenhalten rigidity are frequently present. Dementia, pseudobulbar palsy, and cerebellar signs can also be present, depending on the distribution of vascular infarction. Diagnosis can be aided by neuroimaging, especially by magnetic resonance imaging to look for an appropriate distribution of lacunar infarctions or small-vessel disease. The most common imaging findings are multiple infarcts in the caudate, putamen, or globus pallidus. Response to levodopa is frequently not as successful as in Parkinson's disease, since the lack of dopamine processing by nigral neurons is not typically the limiting pathology. Frequently, as with other subtle stroke symptoms and signs, gradual resolution can occur in the absence of specific therapy, or vascular parkinsonism can progress along with findings of more diffuse cerebrovascular disease.

Sinemet or direct dopaminergic agonists can be somewhat effective at alleviating symptoms in some cases. However, reducing the risk factors for stroke, especially hypertension, and initiating antiplatelet therapy are the most effective interventions to slow progression. Cognitive changes resulting from diffuse Binswanger's encephalopathy can exacerbate cognitive changes from dopaminergic medication and complicate treatment.

STRUCTURAL PARKINSONISM

Although usually easy to differentiate from idiopathic Parkinson's disease, a variety of structural lesions can cause a subset of parkinsonian features, including gait abnormalities and bradykinesia. Usually, other historical or clinical features will be present to aid in differential diagnosis. Basal ganglionic or midbrain mass lesions, normal-pressure or obstructive hydrocephalus, and chronic subdural hematoma can all lead to such variable presentations. Gait abnormalities are usually the presenting symptom, and atypical tremor or rigidity are common. Parkinsonian rest tremor is rarely present, pyramidal signs are the rule, and symptoms suggestive of individual diagnoses are frequently present and helpful. For example, headache or seizure with a mass or subdural hematoma, cognitive dysfunction and incontinence with normal-pressure hydrocephalus, and subacute progression all raise suspicion for one of these disorders.

Neuroimaging can frequently rule out or confirm one of these clinically suspected disorders. The pathology is thought to involve either direct striatal compression and compromise, periventricular white-matter compromise, or direct midbrain injury with nigral dysfunction, depending on the location of the mass lesion or the type and extent of the hydrocephalus. This is one of the few situations in which imaging is indicated in parkinsonian syndromes; in combination with vascular parkinsonism, these disorders present with atypical signs for parkinsonism and often lateralized pyramidal tract findings, pointing the way for neuroimaging.

Response to dopaminergic therapy is variable, with some thought that good response indicates midbrain compromise from the mass or hydrocephalus and poor response reflects primary striatal compromise. In cases of normal pressure hydrocephalus, mass, or subdural hematoma, appropriate further neurodiagnostics and possible surgical intervention are warranted. In many cases, dopaminergic therapy can be used symptomatically prior to or following primary therapy.

TOXIC PARKINSONISM

Although 1-methyl-4-phenyl-1,2,3,6-tetrahydropyridine (MPTP) has emerged as the most recently important and scientifically illuminating toxic cause of secondary parkinsonism, a variety of industrial and agricultural toxins, frequently occupation-related, can cause parkinsonism. Many of these toxins are mitochondrial poisons that interfere with electron transport. Others cause diffuse neurotoxicity with a marked effect on the basal ganglia. Careful elicitation of occupational and chemical exposure history is crucial to diagnosis, since laboratory confirmation is only possible in relatively few situations. Although modern industrial standards and safeguards have drastically reduced the toxin levels in modern U.S. work settings, older workers, immigrants from developing countries, and patients with subtle syndromes may still require diagnosis of these toxin exposures.

The best-known industrial toxin that can cause parkinsonism is manganese, which can be found in mine ore or, potentially, in vapors from unventilated welding. Such industrially related parkinsonism was much more common in the nineteenth and earlier twentieth century ("manganese madness"), and now is quite uncommon in this country. Manganese absorption occurs via the respiratory and gastrointestinal tracts and reaches high brain levels. Initial dementia and behavioral changes are the cardinal features, including agitation, psychosis, and aggression, following a time course from months to many years, depending on the exposure level. These classically make the transition to a more subdued affect and parkinsonian features over time. In addition to quite typical but symmetric parkinsonian findings, except rare rest tremor, patients can present with dystonia. Diagnosis is by careful elicitation of the patient history, with confirmation by serum and/or cerebrospinal fluid levels available but infrequently required. Elimination of the manganese exposure can reduce or stabilize symptoms and signs over a period of months.

A more modern toxin that produces a pathologic and clinical syndrome nearly identical to idiopathic Parkinson's disease is the synthetic narcotic contaminant MPTP, which caused a localized epidemic of toxic parkinsonism among intravenous drug abusers using the synthetic heroin analog 1-methyl-4-phenyl-4-propionoxypiperidine (MPPP) near San Jose, California, in the early 1980s. Monoamine oxidase-B (MAO-B) converts MPTP to 1-methyl-4-phenyl-pyridinium ion (MPP$^+$) a mitochondrial electron transport poison, responsible for the specific degeneration of dopaminergic substantia nigra neurons in this disorder. This neurotoxicology was one of the early indications for application of selegiline as an MAO-B inhibitor in Parkinson's disease. Although a few industrial exposure cases have been suggested, this should be extremely limited in most practice situations. The clinical presentation, apart from the typically much younger age at onset of these patients, can mimic Parkinson's disease remarkably, although rest tremor can be absent or less striking than other clinical signs. Diagnosis is by patient history, although circumstantial support via toxic screen may be helpful. In experimental settings, positron emission tomography has demonstrated striatal dopamine reduction strikingly similar to that in Parkinson's disease. Response to standard dopaminergic therapy has been quite beneficial, although the severity of many cases and the frequency of "freezing" as a limiting symptom have made treatment of many patients less satisfactory. In limited experimental trials of fetal nigral neuron transplantation, good therapeutic response has been obtained, thought to be especially long-lasting in MPTP cases since this is a static insult without ongoing degenerative disease.

A number of organic solvents, most notably, carbon disulfide, used in rayon and cellophane production, and less frequently, methanol, have been associated with secondary parkinsonism. Exposure to carbon disulfide and other industrial solvents is largely via the respiratory tract, although cutaneous absorption is also possible. Methanol exposure is usually via illicit ingestion. The clinical presentation, progression, and complex of symptoms and signs are very similar to those for manganese intoxication noted above. Although largely a problem of the nineteenth and earlier twentieth centuries in the United States lax industrial safeguards in less developed countries make these organic toxins relevant with some patient populations. Neuropathologically, necrosis in both the substantia nigra and globus pallidus could account for the parkinsonian findings appearing in combination with diffuse encephalopathy and peripheral neuropathy with carbon disulfide, and methanol results in degeneration in the putamen.

Carbon monoxide intoxication can also result in parkinsonian features, along with the diffuse encephalopathic, ataxic, and often dystonic findings that result from injury to the globus pallidus, hippocampus, cerebellar Purkinje cells, and deep cortical regions. Rarely would such a presentation be confused for idiopathic Parkinson's disease. Similarly, a variety of organic toxins including cytosine arabinoside (ara-C), pyridines, amines, nitrides, sulphatides, and excitatory amino acid analogs have been reported to cause parkinsonian features in rare cases. Some agricultural pesticides and herbicides, including paraquat, diquat, and other mitochondrial poisons, have been associated with toxic parkinsonism. Response of most of these toxic syndromes to standard dopaminergic therapy is variable, but typically unsatisfactory.

POST-TRAUMATIC PARKINSONISM

Both significant, isolated head trauma and more chronically acquired pugilistic parkinsonism from career-long boxing can result in partially parkinsonian syndromes. The pathology in the acute cases is thought to involve a combination of rotation shearing axonal injury and the hemorrhagic petechial microvascular disease associated with such rotation forces. Because the midbrain can be the site of maximal rotation in these cases, even injuries resulting in only subtle changes elsewhere can result in clinical parkinsonism. Alternatively, the parkinsonian symptoms and signs can be a small part of a complex of multifocal central nervous system injury that becomes clearly delineated only after partial recovery from the acute post-traumatic hospital course. In boxers with a history of repetitive head blows associated with less dramatic rotation injuries, the same pathology is thought to underlie the clinical syndrome. Although mild concussive injuries are common in all boxers, professionals without head protection and with more numerous episodes of loss of consciousness are thought to accumulate the most clinically marked parkinsonian pathology.

In the former isolated injury cases, a history of serious head trauma with concussion or coma is the rule, and parkinsonism is typically accompanied by cognitive changes, pyramidal and/or cerebellar signs, and frequently localizing midbrain signs on examination. Unlike many other secondary parkinsonian syndromes, rest tremor is common. Pugilistic parkinsonism is centrally related to occupation as a boxer or prior history of repeated low-level head injury. Dementia and parkinsonism, including rest tremor, are the central features, although ataxia and superimposed pyramidal signs from the same pathology or from unrelated prior subdural hematoma are not uncommon.

Neuroimaging most typically shows diffuse cerebral atrophy, and can reveal diffuse, bilateral basal ganglia calcifications from microhemorrhage, subtle midbrain white-matter changes on magnetic resonance imaging, or no additional definitive pathology. Imaging is also indicated to rule out chronic subdural hematoma as an atypical cause of secondary parkinsonism. Other neurodiagnostic studies, including electroencephalography and neuropsychological testing, are indicated depending on the clinical setting, but other studies are rarely helpful.

Response to standard dopaminergic therapy can be beneficial, although most commonly patients are not much improved because of the broader underlying pathology. Because of the spectrum of neurologic symptoms in addition to parkinsonism, treatment is symptomatic on an individualized basis. Often, not much can be done therapeutically beyond providing appropriate social supports and community services.

ENCEPHALITIC PARKISONISM

Although quite prevalent following the epidemic of Economo's encephalitis (or encephalitis lethargia) from approximately 1915 to approximately 1935, few survivors remain, and no more recent equivalent encephalitic epidemic has been associated with such parkinsonian features. Other viral encephalitides and syphilitic encephalitis have been associated with secondary parkinsonism in a much more limited number of cases. The parkinsonian symptoms and signs could develop over a wide period following the acute illness, from almost immediately to more than 10 years later. The parkinsonian findings usually lacked typical rest tremor. Dystonia, tics, and diffuse cognitive changes were common as well, along with other neurologic findings that were variable among patient populations studied. Pathologically, dopaminergic nigral neurons were strikingly reduced in number, without Lewy body formation, along with more diffuse neuronal injury and gliosis responsible for other elements of the syndrome. Although patients initially responded well to levodopa therapy when it was introduced in the 1960s, they were found to be extremely sensitive to toxic side effects with relatively small doses, and especially prone to both dyskinetic and cognitive complications.

METABOLIC DISEASES WITH PARKINSONIAN FEATURES

A few well-recognized metabolic disorders can include parkinsonian features among their broader and more defining clinical symptoms and signs. Although it is beyond the scope of this chapter to describe each of these disease states in individual detail, it is useful to keep these disorders in mind in the broadest differentiation of atypical parkinsonism in correctly aged and appropriate patients. Because the parkinsonism associated with these disorders is not isolated even at the onset, confusion with idiopathic Parkinson's disease is unlikely in most cases. Specific elements of the family or personal histories can direct appropriate use of diagnostic testing in individual circumstances.

Wilson's disease, a copper metabolism disorder with autosomal recessive inheritance and reduced ceruloplasmin levels resulting in hepatic and central nervous system copper deposition, can present with prominent basal ganglionic and/or cerebellar symptoms and signs. Parkinsonism is rarely found in isolation, as dystonia, dysarthria, and nonrest tremor are common initial symptoms. Onset is typically in the teens and twenties, but patients in early school age through their fifties have been described. Because this range begins quite a bit earlier than most idiopathic Parkinson's disease, especially young patients with parkinsonian findings should have this diagnosis considered. Diagnosis is by family history, slit-lamp examination for Kayser-Fleischer rings, and assay of abnormal copper metabolism with decreased serum ceruloplasmin in 95 percent of cases and increased urinary copper excretion. Hepatic biopsy for increased copper deposition is definitive in combination with other findings. Treatment is centrally via limitation of copper intake and absorption, and via chelation therapy. Dopaminergic symptomatic therapy could potentially confound observation of the clinical response to therapy and is rarely useful.

Other rare disorders can present with parkinsonian features among more diffuse neurologic findings. Acquired hepatocerebral degeneration can display a clinical picture similar to that of Wilson's disease, with mixed extrapyramidal findings, infrequent rest tremor, and prominent cognitive changes. Pathology typically includes prominent degeneration within the globus pallidus, caudate, and putamen. Both hypoparathyroidism and pseudohypoparathyroidism can result in bilateral basal ganglia calcification and symmetric parkinsonian features, including rest tremor, rigidity, and gait disturbance, along with dystonia and chorea. Parkinsonism is not found in isolation, with paresthesias, tetanic contractures, and seizures being the most common accompanying features. Hallervorden-Spatz disease, an autosomal recessive illness with iron deposition and degeneration of the globus pallidus, substantia nigra, and red nucleus, typically presents in childhood or adolescence and progresses over 1 or 2 decades. Parkinsonian features are mixed with prominent pyramidal and cognitive changes. Symptomatic dopaminergic therapy has been attempted with variable, limited results. Both pancreatic encephalopathy and central pontine myelino-

lysis can result in basal ganglionic lesions and have been described with parkinsonian features during the course of the illness. Attention to such rare associations may allow early diagnosis in some of these atypical parkinsonian disorders.

CONCLUSION

Although idiopathic Parkinson's disease is often straightforward to diagnose in its classic age range of onset, clinical features, progression, and response to dopaminergic therapy, a broader differential diagnosis should be considered when atypical features are present or when parkinsonism occurs in younger patients. A range of secondary parkinsonian syndromes exist, some of which are fully or partially reversible with appropriate diagnosis and management. Because of the protean nature of many parkinsonian syndromes, the history is often more helpful in specific diagnosis than the neurologic examination; specialized neurodiagnostic studies can be used to support or confirm a suspected diagnosis, but a broad laboratory screen is rarely indicated. Although most of the secondary parkinsonian syndromes are relatively rare, they represent an important class of pathologies within the nigrostriatal system that have illuminated the underlying basis of Parkinson's disease and its potential therapies.

SUGGESTED READINGS

Adams JH, Duchen LW: Greenfield's Neuropathology. 5th Ed. Oxford University Press, New York, 1992
Adams RD, Victor M: Principles of Neurology. 5th Ed. McGraw-Hill, New York, 1993
Rowland LD: Merritt's Textbook of Neurology. 8th Ed. Lea & Febiger, Philadelphia, 1989
Stern MB, Koller WC: Parkinsonian Syndromes. Marcel Dekker, New York, 1993

SECTION 2. NON-PARKINSONIAN MOVEMENT DISORDERS

120. PROGRESSIVE ATAXIA

DAVID M. DAWSON

The progressive ataxias of adult life are a complex and heterogeneous group of illnesses. In many instances, a cell-specific hereditary degeneration is present. Particular tracts and nuclei gradually disappear, typically by "dying back" without evidence of tissue reaction to the process. After many decades of effort by clinicians and neuropathologists, a number of classifications have been proposed all of which suffer from one or another problem. Finally, these cases are beginning to be understood on a genetic basis.

Nongenetic, idiopathic, or sporadic ataxia of adult life is a challenging clinical problem. Imaging studies will rapidly diag-

nose those cases due to tumor or infarction, and most of those due to multiple sclerosis. A few patients will present with ataxia, usually subacute and disabling, as a paraneoplastic illness. Rare diseases, such as progressive multifocal leukoencephalopathy, or Creutzfeldt-Jakob disease, may begin with ataxia, or brainstem signs. Many types of pathologic change in the nervous system need to be considered when a patient with progressive ataxia appears to have a nongenetic basis for the illness. Therefore, the first task in diagnosis of a case of progressive ataxia is to decide, if possible, if it is genetic or not.

The earliest detectable sign in patients with adult-onset cerebellar syndromes is gait disorder. Normal persons, even into advanced age, can walk tandem without undue efforts at balancing; therefore, heel-and-toe gait is the most sensitive test for early ataxia. It is, however, not specific, and patients with myelopathy, frontal gait disorder, vertigo, and even visual loss, will present diagnostic difficulty. The patient without dizziness who staggers is the most likely to have cerebellar disease.

Many other symptoms occur in the progressive ataxias, and their character can sometimes help establish a diagnosis. Nystagmus occurs with cerebellar disorder, but oscillopsia indicates pontine or mesencephalic disease, and is especially characteristic of tumors and multiple sclerosis. Diplopia usually means internuclear ophthalmoplegia or ocular palsy, whereas marked dysphagia, dysarthria, impaired cough, and altered respiratory reflexes occur with pontine disease and are especially seen in hereditary olivopontocerebellary atrophy and in paraneoplastic brainstem encephalitis. Extrapyramidal syndromes are seen in both sporadic and genetic forms of progressive ataxia. They can include rigidity, chorea, or dystonia of limbs, face, or trunk. Often, these features will not be present early in the course of an illness, and what appears originally to be a pure cerebellar syndrome will gradually acquire parkinsonian features as the illness progresses.

It is rare for the clinical features of a progressive ataxia to be diagnostically unequivocal. Data must be sought from radiologic, neurophysiologic, genetic, and biochemical sources, and one should not rely too much on clinical appearances.

INHERITED ATAXIC DISORDERS

An explosion of genetic data since 1990 promises to bring order in the disorganized world of inherited ataxias (Table 120-1). Five versions of autosomal-dominant cerebellar ataxia are now known, with firm chromosomal localizations and reasonably good clinical correlation. Two of the five are known to be trinucleotide repeating sequences, a genetic defect also at the basis of Huntington's disease and myotonic muscular dystrophy. Variability of severity, anticipation, and linkage of early onset cases to the gender of the parent are three genetic features shared by "trinucleotide repeat diseases."

The pathogenesis of the cell death in each instance still remains unknown.

Friedreich's Ataxia

Friedreich's ataxia is the most common hereditary ataxia, and is usually easy to recognize. Friedreich himself described a primarily spinal degeneration, affecting posterior and lateral columns, including spinocerebellar tracts; only in advanced cases are the Purkinje cells reduced.

Some patients have scoliosis. Many demonstrate cardiac conduction defects, or septal hypertrophy as a result of cardiomyopathy.

The cardinal features of the disease are onset before age 25,

TABLE 120-1. Chromosome Linkages as of July 1, 1994 Relevant to Hereditary Ataxia

Disease	Chromosome	Inheritance
Friedrich's typical ataxia	9q13	Recessive
Friedrich's late-onset ataxia	9 ?	Recessive
Freidrich's vitamin E deficiency	8 q	?
SCA-1 (olivopontocerebellar atrophy)	6p24	Dominant
SCA-2 (Wadia's ataxia)	12q	Dominant
Machado-Joseph disease (probably SCA-3)	14q24	Dominant
SCA-4 (with sensory loss)	16q	Dominant
Charcot-Marie-Tooth disease		
Type 1A	17p11	Dominant
Type 1B	1p22	Dominant
Type 2b	1p35	Dominant
Type x	x413	X-linked

autosomal recessive inheritance, absent tendon reflexes, and progressive ataxia.

Most patients develop dysarthria within 5 years of onset. Nerve conduction studies show evidence of axonal neuropathy. This latter point can be helpful in distinguishing hereditary motor sensory neuropathy, which in childhood cases may bear clinical resemblance to Friedreich's ataxia but produces motor and sensory slowing to less than 60 percent of normal values (at least type I Charcot-Marie-Tooth disease). Typical Friedrich's has a localization on chromosome 9q.

Variants of Friedreich's Ataxia

Among many variants of the clinical picture, onset of typical Friedreich's ataxia past age 25 is recognized. Such patients may live, usually wheelchair-bound, into the sixth or seventh decade, the degree of cardiomyopathy being the limiting factor in life span.

Optic atrophy, deafness, hypogonadism, mental retardation, retinopathy, and other clinical features have all been recorded in early onset ataxic syndromes. Further data from genetics laboratories are needed before these variant illnesses can be sorted out.

Autosomal-Dominant Cerebellar Ataxia (SCA-1)

SCA-1 corresponds to hereditary olivopontocerebellar atrophy, Schut-Haymaker syndrome, Menzel-type spinocerebellar degeneration, Marie's ataxia, and so on. The chromosomal localization is on the short arm of chromosome 6, near the human leukocyte antigen gene, and consists of a trinucleotide CAG repeat sequence.

The clinical features are quite heterogenous, and in common with other dominant ataxias, one sees considerable variation in the findings, depending on age of onset, pace of the illness, and duration. What began as a mild gait ataxia may decades later show up as a parkinsonian/dementia syndrome with autonomic failure, distinguishable at a late stage as a hereditary ataxia only by the undue amount of nystagnus. Most patients show early signs of spasticity, with increased tendon reflexes at an early stage.

Magnetic resonance imaging scans of patients with autosomal-dominant cerebellar ataxia show atrophy of the basis pontis, wide dilation of the fourth ventricle, and shrinkage of the medulla and cervical cord. The cerebellum shows mild variable changes, especially in the vermis.

Nerve conduction studies may show a symmetric, usually asymptomatic, axonal neuropathy.

"Cuban Ataxia" Wadia's Ataxia (SCA-2)

"Cuban ataxia," also called Wadia's ataxia, has been reported from India, Cuba, Canada, Scotland, and elsewhere. It has one distinctive clinical feature: saccadic velocity is markedly reduced, producing the syndrome of "ocular motor apraxia," in which head turning precedes lateral eye movement. Nystagmus is not observed. Pathologic descriptions do not differ from other olivopontocerebellar degenerations. The clinical features of most patients are about the same as those with autosomal-dominant cerebellar ataxia. The genetic localization is on the short arm of chromosome 12.

Machado-Joseph's Disease (SCA-3, Probable)

Originally described in families of Portuguese-Azorean background, Machado-Joseph's disease is now recognized to be world-wide in occurrence and is one of the most common of hereditary ataxias. It has been recorded in Japan, northern Australia, Brazil, several European countries, and among American blacks, all possible sites along Portuguese trade routes of several centuries ago.

The illness begins with gait ataxia, and produces progressive ataxia without dementia. In large families, one often sees early onset dystonia in some individuals, and up to one-third of patients may show lid retraction with prominent eyes, a characteristic sign. Some patients have diplopia at a distance due to abducens palsy.

When eye signs or dystonia are present in a family, recognition as Machado-Joseph's disease is possible, but in at least one-half of individual patients, the neurologic signs closely resemble those of other dominant ataxias.

The chromosome localization is on the long arm of chromosome 14 in both Japanese and Portuguese-American families. The nature of the gene defect is unknown at this time but by parallelism with Huntington's disease and autosomal-dominant cerebellar ataxia, a repeating trinucleotide sequence is expected to be found. The term SCA-3 has been used by French workers for a specific family, probably—but not yet proven to be—Machado-Joseph's disease.

SCA-4

Described in 1994 from Utah, SCA-4, associated with a trinucleotide repeat on chromosome 16q, features a prominent widespread sensory loss.

Dentatopallidoluysian Atrophy

A rare condition that is practically unknown in the United States, dentatopallidoluysian atrophy has been observed in Japan and Europe. Patients have ataxia with chorea, myoclonus, epilepsy, and dementia. In this instance, geneticists used a new approach and searched through genes known to have repeating trinucleotide sequences. They established a correlation on chromosome 12 for this disease.

Other Hereditary Ataxias

Many other less well defined familial conditions exist. Late-onset pure cerebellar degeneration (Holmes ataxia) is probably a recognizable syndrome, as is hereditary ataxia with retinal degeneration. Further information, beyond that known from clinical or neuropathologic data, is required. Most instances are observed in small family units or as sporadic cases.

NONGENETIC PROGRESSIVE ATAXIAS

Development of progressive ataxia in adult life may generate diagnostic and management problems for the clinician. In spite of modern diagnostic methods, uncertainties may persist. The following categories are those most often encountered.

Multiple System Atrophy

Idiopathic olivopontocerebellar atrophy, strionigral degeneration, Shy-Drager syndrome, and other entities are now grouped together under the title of multiple system atrophy since their neuropathologic changes overlap extensively. These are sporadic diseases of middle age, with no known cause, progressing over 10 or 15 years. Rigidity, subcortical dementia, and postural hypotension coexist with ataxia, dysarthria, and nystagmus. There are no distinctive laboratory or radiologic abnormalities.

Some patients with olivopontocerebellar atrophy have reduced glutamate dehydrogenase levels in blood or tissues, but a majority do not.

Multiple Sclerosis

Among the less common variants of demyelinating disease is one that produces progressive ataxia. The clinician should search for evidence of asymmetric loss of visual acuity, for internuclear ophthalmoplegia, or for asymmetric acquired pendular nystagmus, which are clues pointing toward multiple sclerosis. Magnetic resonance imaging scans may fail to show characteristic lesions in as many as 5 percent of multiple sclerosis patients, depending on technique. Evoked potential testing or cerebrespinal fluid examination may be helpful. Establishing a diagnosis of multiple sclerosis obviously has therapeutic implications.

Paraneoplastic Cerebellar Degenerations

Often searched for, paraneoplastic cerebellar degenerations remain very rare. Two main varieties occur.

Subacute Cerebellar Degeneration Associated With Anti-Purkinje Cell Antibodies. Most patients have an ovarian cancer, some have breast cancer or Hodgkin's disease, a few have no cancer. A few also have weakness due to associated Lambert-Eaton syndrome. The Purkinje cell antibody (Yo antibody) is specific. In clinical terms, patients develop a disabling pancerebellar syndrome over months, with little or no recovery even if the tumor is extirpated.

Neuron Cell Antibodies React With Neurons. Neuron cell antibodies (Hu antibodies) react with many neurons, including dorsal root ganglia, cells of the brainstem, and cerebellar cells. A bewildering variety of neurologic signs may result, with ataxia, dyparthria, and a subacute sensory neuropathy being common. Most patients have small cell lung cancers, but not all. Hu antibodies are more common than Yo antibodies.

Measurement of the serum antibodies should be undertaken whenever unexplained adult ataxic syndromes occur, since many cases are recorded in which the relevant neoplasm was discovered in this way.

Alcoholic Cerebellar Degeneration

Heavy exposure to alcohol, especially when combined with nutritional deprivation, has been associated with a degeneration of the anterior vermis of the cerebellum. The classic clinical syndrome is that of an ataxia of gait, with abnormalities of foot tapping or heel-knee-shin coordination testing, but without nystagmus or dysarthria. Most authorities would now classify this as a subcategory of Wernicke-Korsakoff syndrome, with identical causation and prognosis.

The clinical issue in the modern era is whether to accept alcohol as the cause when a patient has developed ataxia. It is probably best to restrict this diagnosis to those patients with the classic syndrome, atrophy of the anterior vermis on magnetic resonance imaging, and be alert to the possibility of diagnostic error.

SUGGESTED EVALUATION SCHEME

The following scheme is meant to outline the evaluation of a patient with progressive ataxia of unknown cause. An explanation of each step is added.

Clinical Features of Interest

Dementia. Significant cognitive disorder is seen with many progressive ataxic syndromes. Dementia is absent in Machado-Joseph's disease and cerebellar cortical degeneration.

Symmetry. Most degenerative diseases are nearly symmetric.

Improvement. Improvement at any stage, unless related to motivation changes in the patient, or to treatment, points toward vascular disease or demyelination.

Ocular Movements. Ocular dysmetria, nystagmus, large or small refixation movements, and slowing of saccadic velocity are all characteristic of cerebellar disease. Diplopia is not, and INO, monocular nystagmus, or pendular nystagmus may point to some as yet undiagnosed inflammatory or infiltrative process.

Extrapyramidal Signs. Dystonia, rigidity, tremor or other extrapyramidal signs may point toward a diagnosis.

Presence or Absence of Tendon Reflexes. Presence or absence of tendon reflexes is important. In Freidrich's ataxia, the reflexes are absent. They are also absent in demyelinating polyneuropathy, and one should be certain that an ataxic syndrome is central in origin, not due to a peripheral neuropathy that is causing a sensory ataxia. Testing for Romberg's sign and for position sense loss will help here; both are present with sensory ataxia.

Most of the adult-onset dominant ataxias produce hyperreflexia.

Telangiectasia or Sclerae. Search for telangiectasia on lips or sclerae, a clue to ataxia/telangiectasia.

Imaging Studies

Computed Tomography. Computed tomography scans show the posterior fossa poorly.

Magnetic Resonance Imaging. Magnetic resonance imaging is vital for showing tumors, infarctions, Chiari malformation, arachnoid cysts, multiple sclerosis, and a long list of other space-taking conditions. Owing to unusual presentations sometimes seen with these conditions that can be slowly progressive, a magnetic resonance image is mandatory.

Midsagittal images are best for noting the position of the cerebellar tonsils, and the size of the pons, fourth ventricle, and midline cerebellar cortex.

Evoked Potential Tests. Evoked potential testing is useful chiefly for the added information one may obtain from visual evoked responses. Some ataxic syndromes, such as Friedrich's, produces moderate symmetric delay of the P100 wave; marked slowing, or asymmetry, suggest another diagnosis.

Cerebrospinal Fluid Examination. Cerebral spinal fluid examination is rarely helpful; chronic granulomas or meningitis are occasionally a consideration.

Laboratory Evaluation. Laboratory tests should be done as follows:

1. Hu and Yo antibodies, especially in patients with subacute ataxia.
2. Ceruloplasmin below the age of 35. Usually Wilson's disease presents with upper extremity tremor, not with ataxia. It is clinically treatable.
3. Electrocardiography and/or echocardiography, to detect cardiomyopathy, seen in Friedrich's and some other ataxias.
4. Serum protein electrophoresis to detect IgA deficiency of ataxia-telangiectasia, usually a childhood illness, but worth considering.
5. Hexosaminadase level. Low hexosaminodase levels are a rare cause.
6. Vitamin E level. Vitamin E deficiency as a cause of spinocerebellar degeneration is seen in a number of different syndromes. Some of these are inherited, such as abetalipoproteinemia; others are acquired defects in lipid absorption, storage, or transport. Vitamin E levels are a consequence, then, of disordered metabolism.
7. Pyruvate and lactate levels. No good way has yet been devised for screening for mitochondrial disease such as MELAS (mitochondrial encephalopathy, lactic acidosis, and strokelike episodes) and myoclonus epilepsy, ragged red fibers (MERRF); it may be that direct DNA analysis will be best. In the meantime, pyruvate levels may help. One also needs to consider a group of childhood intermittent ataxias that are metabolic in origin and may be picked up in this way.
8. Toxic screen. Such screens will exclude factitious disease, inadvertant intoxication with barbituates, and so forth.
9. Low-density lipoprotiens. Testing for these will exclude acanthocytoxins as a cause of ataxia.
10. Phytanic acid. The presence of this indicates Refsum's disease.
11. In children, amino acid screen, blood ammonia, organic acids.

TREATMENT

In general, treatment of ataxic disorders is disappointing. Efforts to replace putative neurotransmitters by the use of γ-aminobutyric acid agonists or cholinergic agents have not been successful, nor has the use of tryptophan derivations. Those patients with rigidity or Parkinsonian features may respond to levodopa. Baclofen may be helpful if spasticity is present, but overall functional performance rarely improves.

The advice of a rehabilitation specialist or physiotherapist may contribute to gait training; patients do better with a wheeled or weighted walker.

The genetic advances in the field of inherited ataxias contain great promise for the future availability of specific replacement therapy, or for agents designed to prevent advance of disability.

SUGGESTED READINGS

Coutinho P, Andrade C: Autosomal dominant system degeneration in Portuguese families of the Azores Islands: a new genetic disorder involving cerebellar, pyramidal, extrapyramidal, and spinal cord motor functions. Neurology 28:703–9, 1978

Furneaux HM, Rosenblum MK, Dalmau J et al: Selective expression of Purkinje cell antigens in tumor tissue from patients with paraneoplastic cerebellar degeneration. N Engl J Med 322:1844–51, 1990

Hammack JE, Kimmel DW, O'Neill BP et al: Paraneoplastic cerebellar degeneration: a clinical comparison of patients with and without Purkinje cell cytoplasmic antibodies. Mayo Clin Proc 54:1423–41, 1990

Harding AE, Matthews S, Jones S et al: Spinocerebellar degeneration associated with a selective defect of vitamin E absorption. N Engl J Med 313:32–5, 1985

Posner JB: Cerebellar disorders. pp. 75–82. In Hildebrand J (ed): Neurological Adverse Reactions to Antineoplastic Chemotherapy. Springer-Verlag, Berlin, 1990

Posner JB, Dalmau J, Furneaux HM et al: Paraneoplastic ''anti-Hu'' syndrome: a clinical study of 47 patients. Neurology 40:165, 1990

Posner JB, Furneaux HM: Paraneoplastic syndromes. pp. 187–219. In Waksman BH (ed): Immunologic Mechanisms in Neurologic and Psychiatric Disease. New York, Raven Press, 1990

Orr HT et al: Expansion of an unstable trinucleotide CAG repeat spinocerebellar ataxia type 1. Nat Genetics 4:221–6, 1993

Takijanie Y, Nishizawa M, Tanaku H et al: The gene for Machado Joseph disease maps to human chromosome 14q. Nat Genet 4:299–304, 1993

Zoghbi HY: The spinocerebellar degenerations. Curr Neurol 13:87–110, 1993

121. TREMORS

FRISSO POTTS

Tremor is an involuntary, rhythmic oscillation of a body part produced by synchronized contraction of antagonist muscles. These oscillations tend to have a consistent frequency, and can be made to appear and disappear by postural adjustments of the body part. These characteristics, which will be discussed later in this chapter, allow us to differentiate tremors from other kinds of movement disorders.

DIAGNOSIS

The easiest way to classify tremors clinically is as follows:

Tremor at rest
  Parkinson's disease
Tremor during voluntary activity (action tremors):
  Physiologic tremor
  Enhanced physiologic tremor
  Essential or familial tremor
  Neuropathic tremor
  Writing tremor
  Orthostatic tremor
  Cerebellar tremor

Tremors at rest are most obvious when the affected body part is in repose and are abolished or much diminished during voluntary movement. The opposite is true of action tremors.

The clinical examination of the tremulous patient usually starts with visual inspection while the individual sits on a straight-backed, armless chair. The forearms resting supinated at the thighs and the hands allowed to rest between the slightly abducted knees. This position will bring out most tremors at rest. In some cases, it may be necessary to ask the patient to perform complex silent calculations, or cause other types of mild mental stress (e.g., asking the patient who the fifth vice-president of the United States was) in order to distract the patient and bring out the tremor. This is especially true if the patient has become adept at ''hiding'' the tremor. As a general rule, the less attention the patient pays to a resting tremor, the more likely it is to occur.

Asking the patient to hold the arms outstretched with fingers spread will activate most action tremors. In some cases, it may be necessary to ask the individual to perform a maneuver requiring precision, such as holding a pencil point close to, but not touching, a small target. Other provocative maneuvers are discussed further under specific tremors, below.

Clinical observation may be further refined by electrophysiologic studies,—such as electromyography (EMG),—that record the frequency and amplitude of the tremor, as well as the pattern of underlying muscle activity. These tremor tests are painless, easily performed, and increase diagnostic accuracy, especially in cases of mixed tremor types or in tremors that fail to respond to treatment. Figure 121-1 demonstrates the patterns seen in some commonly encountered tremors.

TREMOR AT REST

Rest tremor is seen exclusively in Parkinson's disease and in drug- or toxin-induced parkinsonism. Most frequently, the tremor involves the muscles of the forearm, giving the characteristic ''pill-rolling'' appearance. The tremor may also be seen in other parts of the body, although it is unusual for this to happen without some involvement of the upper extremities. Voluntary movement abolishes or markedly decreases the amplitude of the tremor. Thus, it rarely contaminates the patient's writing or interferes severely with activities of daily living. There are patients, however, in whom the severity of the tremor makes it more than a cosmetic nuisance. As many as 20 percent of patients with resting tremor of Parkinson's disease may have a superimposed action tremor (see Essential Tremor, below).

A tremor recording in Parkinson's disease demonstrates alternating EMG bursts in antagonist muscles at a frequency of 3 to 7 Hz (Fig. 121-1). The tremor appears to be generated by rhythmic activity of the lower motor neuron caused by descending rhythmic discharges from the hemispheres and uninfluenced by segmental stretch reflexes, since dorsal rhizotomy does not affect the tremor. The recording has the appearance of voluntary flexion-extension, pronation-supination movements of the hand; with little effort, a normal subject may generate a tremor recording indistinguishable from an affected individual.

The supranuclear origin of the tremor is also supported by the presence of rhythmic neuronal bursts in the contralateral sensorimotor cortex and ventrolateral thalamus in monkeys with 1-methyl-4-phenyl-1,2,3,6-tetrahydropyridine (MPTP)-induced parkinsonism. Similar activity has been recorded from the thalamus of patients with Parkinson's disease. These bursts are not affected by deafferentation, and can be eliminated by lesions of the appropriate thalamic nuclei with consequent resolution of the tremor.

The tremor usually improves with dopaminergic treatment for Parkinson's disease. Occasionally, the decrease in rigidity brought about by these drugs will uncover or enhance the resting tremor. For these cases, and for those who fail to respond to dopaminergic treatment, concomitant therapy with anticholinergic agents should be tried. A daily dose of 1 to 6 mg/day of benztropine mesylate or 2 to 12 mg trihexyphenidyl hydrochloride, may be useful. The medication should be given in three or four divided doses, and the least amount required for beneficial effect used.

When pharmacotherapy fails, severe cases of tremor at rest may be approached surgically. Stereotactic thalamotomy of the ventral intermediate nucleus as well as chronic electrical stimulation of this site without thalamotomy have shown encouraging results. Lately, stereotactic pallidotomy and cerebellar stimulation have gained increased acceptance. See the Suggested Readings for further discussion of surgical procedures.

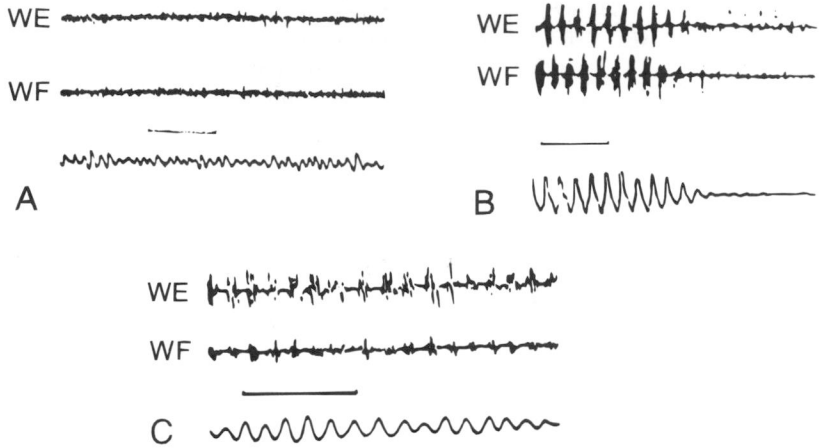

FIG. 121-1. Tremor recordings in **(A)** physiologic tremor, **(B)** Parkinson's disease, and **(C)** essential tremor. Surface electromyographic tracings are from wrist extensors (WE) and from wrist flexors (WF). The accelerometric tracing from the index finger is at the bottom of each tracing. Note diminution of tremor as subject goes from rest to reaching for an object in Fig. B. Time base is 1 second.

ACTION TREMORS

Not every investigator agrees with the use of the term *action tremor*. There are those who prefer the term *postural tremor*, whereas others prefer to divide these tremors into *kinetic* (those occurring during movement) and *static* (those occurring while the limb is held in a relatively fixed position). Further categorization introduces the term *task-specific tremor*, referring to tremors that occur only during a specific movement or task. I have chosen not to burden the reader with multiple subdivisions and I discuss each action tremor under this fairly broad term.

Tremors, in general, are very sensitive to changes in metabolic or emotional states. Anxiety tends to increase the amplitude of tremors, especially of action tremors; and it may be the precipitating cause in some cases. Many medications are known to produce or enhance action tremor. Some of these agents are as follows:

Corticosteroids
Methylxanthines
Lithium
Heavy metals
Thyroid hormone
Glutamates
Catecholamines
Neuroleptics
Tricyclics
Nicotine
Bromides
Valproic acid

Physiologic Tremor

Physiologic tremor is the most ubiquitous of the tremors discussed above. All individuals have it to a greater or lesser extent. It can be easily demonstrated by having a subject hold out an arm with fingers outstretched. The tremor is usually so slight that it cannot be seen on the fingers; but if a piece of paper is laid across the hand, the oscillations are amplified and become obvious. The genesis of this tremor is probably the combination of such disparate elements as individual motor unit recruitment rates and the intrinsic elastic properties of joints and other bony and connective tissue components. Mechanical perturbations caused by circulatory pulse waves may also contribute to the tremor.

No treatment is required.

Enhanced Physiologic Tremor

Enhanced physiologic tremor is easily seen in the outstretched fingers; it is of considerably larger amplitude than physiologic tremor and it can be quite disabling. Although it does not affect gross movements such as tracking an object, it affects writing and other tasks requiring precision. This tremor not only may be seen but also heard, since it may affect the speech apparatus. Tremor recording shows a regular rhythm at about 10 Hz and the surface EMG activity shows alternating bursts in antagonist muscles. The tremor is associated with muscle fatigue and may be induced in normal subjects by the administration of epinephrine or its congeners. Expectedly, it is the tremor of fear and anxiety—notably, of stage fright. This tremor may also be occur as a result of metabolic derangements. It is the tremor of hyperthyroidism, Cushing's disease, and of withdrawal from alcohol and from minor sedatives. Thus, it is important to look for underlying conditions causing a hyperadrenergic state. This is especially true if the tremor is continuous rather than intermittent; as would be the case in anxiety. See the above list of some commonly available drugs that may produce or enhance this tremor.

The catecholamines' effect is mediated by peripheral β-adrenergic receptors. That the locus of action of these drugs is outside of the central nervous system has been demonstrated by intra-arterial infusion experiments. Conversely, blockade of these drugs with propranolol diminishes or abolishes the tremor. It appears that these receptors are instrumental in producing synchronous α motor neuron discharges by enhancing the stretch reflex arc. What is not known is the exact location of the receptors and how they go about modulating neural activity.

Removal of underlying causes (environmental or metabolic) is the best management. When this is not possible, single doses of 20 to 40 mg propranolol will provide relief several hours. This is especially useful in the prophylactic treatment of performing artists. If there is concern over the potential bronchoconstrictive or hypoglycemic effect of propranolol's β$_2$-blockade, pure β$_1$-blockers (Metoprolol) may be used. These are not as effective and may require higher doses.

Essential Tremor

Also known as familial, rubral, or static tremor, essential tremor is most frequently seen affecting the upper extremities while a patient carries out tasks that require precision. It may involve other body parts, however, and gives the voice a quavering sound when it affects pharyngeal and laryngeal muscles. It is most common in older age groups and is responsible for most cases of so-called senile tremor. Although 60 percent of patients with essential tremor have a family history, sporadic cases abound. Transmission appears to be autosomal dominant, but the gene locus has not been found.

An important diagnostic point is that this tremor rarely, if ever, affects a body part without affecting the upper extremities first. The literature is replete with cases of "isolated essential tremor" involving neck muscles, a single digit, or a foot. In the vast majority of these cases, closer examination would find a focal dystonia presenting as tremor.

In general, patients with essential tremor have no other neurologic symptoms or signs. However, this tremor frequently coexists with acquired dystonias, such as writer's cramp and torticollis. As many as 20 percent of patients with Parkinson's disease have a superimposed essential tremor This does not necessarily mean that patients who develop essential tremor are at a higher risk than the general population for developing Parkinson's disease.

The frequency of the tremor ranges between 5 and 10 Hz, being faster in younger age groups and decreasing with age, even in the same individual. Surface EMG recordings demonstrate synchronous bursts in antagonist muscles (Fig. 121-1). In cases of dystonia presenting as tremor (the nodding head of torticollis is a classic example), or in cases of dystonia and tremor coexisting, the EMG pattern would nicely tease out the complex interaction between the participating muscles.

This tremor is most likely suprasegmental in origin, since manipulation of segmental reflex arcs has little effect on its amplitude or rhythm. Positron emission tomography studies using radioactive water or carbon-15–labeled carbon dioxide suggest that abnormal activation of the cerebellum and red nucleus may be playing a role in its genesis. At present, its pathophysiology is unknown.

A remarkable feature of this tremor is its response to alcoholic beverages. Within minutes of ingesting .5 to 1 ounce of ethanol, patients experience a decrease in tremor amplitude that may last for several hours. As the effect dissipates, a transient worsening may occur. Well-controlled studies have confirmed this effect and have shown that its action is within the central nervous system, since intra-arterial injection of ethanol has no effect on the tremor.

β-Blockers also have a beneficial effect on the tremor, but unlike ethanol, a single intravenous or oral dose has no effect; their efficacy may not become apparent unless administered for several days. As a general rule, nonselective β-blockers are more effective than selective β_1- or β_2-blockers. Lipophilic β-blockers are more effective than nonlipophilic ones because of their greater penetration of the blood–brain barrier. Some patients may respond to as little as 30 mg/day propranolol in divided doses; others may require ten times that much. The same warnings about β-blockers discussed above for enhanced physiologic tremor apply here.

Because of β-blockers' side effects, Primidone is fast becoming the drug of choice. Again, the dose needs to be individually adjusted. As little as 5 mg/day will be useful for some, whereas others will require nearly toxic doses. With either drug, optimal response requires starting at a very low dose with weekly increments to tolerance. Some patients respond to β-blockers and some to Primidone. Combination therapy is rarely useful. Those who do not respond to these drugs may benefit from Methazolamide in doses of 100 to 300 mg/day, or Nicardipine in doses of 30 to 60 mg/day.

When pharmacotherapy fails, a patient may find relief from surgical ablation of the ventralis lateralis, or ventral intermediate thalamic nucleus. Chronic stereotactic stimulation of the ventral intermediate nucleus or chronic cerebellar stimulation may also be useful in those who fail drug therapy.

Neuropathic Tremor

Neuropathic tremor is seen in a variety of acquired neuropathies. It is important to differentiate it from the essential tremor associated with hereditary sensorimotor neuropathy type I. The acquired neuropathies most likely to produce a tremor are chronic relapsing demyelinating polyneuropathy and IgM-associated paraproteinemic neuropathy. Causality is suggested by the fact that in a single patient, changes in the amplitude of the tremor vary directly with changes in the severity of the neuropathy. The tremor is generally irregular at a rate of 6 to 8 Hz. The EMG from antagonist muscles demonstrates bursts of varying amplitude and duration without a consistent pattern.

The presence of the tremor is not related to the degree of weakness or sensory loss. Slowing in motor conduction velocity is frequently seen in neuropathic tremor, but the degree of slowing is not related to severity. The pathophysiology of these tremors is unclear, and there probably are multiple mechanisms involved in their genesis. One of these may be desynchronization of afferent volleys from muscle spindles and Golgi tendon organs. The demyelinative features of the neuropathy probably play an important role, since in primarily axonal neuropathies (e.g., alcohol, diabetes), tremor is absent or barely noticeable, whereas the tremor may appear during recovery from Guillain-Barré syndrome.

Some patients may respond to propranolol or Mysoline, but therapy is best directed at the neuropathy.

Writing Tremor

Any action tremor may contaminate penmanship, but some individuals demonstrate a tremor predominantly during writing. The tremor is most often unilateral and shows no familial tendency. It may occur as an isolated symptom, or accompany other tremors or focal dystonias. It has been dubbed primary writing tremor; but it seems that it is the pronated, slightly extended position of the wrist rather than the act of writing itself that produces the tremor. This tremor may also be triggered by eliciting stretch reflexes from muscles responsible for forearm pronation. Tremor recordings vary from individual to individual. In some patients, bursts of EMG activity at a rate of 4 to 6 Hz can be recorded from antagonist muscles. The pattern may be synchronous or alternating, and the bursts in a single recording may vary in amplitude and duration. In some cases, a single muscle will show tonic activity, and its antagonist, a pattern of bursts.

All this suggests that this tremor has more in common with acquired dystonias, or the so-called occupational cramps, than with the above-mentioned tremors. As is generally true of dystonias, its pathophysiology is unknown.

Systemic therapy for this tremor relies mainly on the use of anticholinergic drugs in doses describe under tremor at rest. Atropine and Scopolamine in the usual cardiac doses have been tried, but have not produced encouraging results. β-Blockers, alcohol, levodopa, or neuroleptics are not useful. Biofeedback and other forms of therapeutic self-hypnosis have been used with varying success. These treatments are quickly giving way to intramuscular botulinum toxin injection. Upon identifying the muscles most active in the tremor, minute amounts of the toxin are injected in order to produce selective weakness or paralysis of the offending muscles. The number of injections necessary will depend as much on the severity of the tremor as on the skill of the administering physician.

Orthostatic Tremor

Although the true incidence of orthostatic tremor is not known, it is much less common than other types of action tremor. It is seen primarily in older age groups and occurs during the act of standing. The tremor appears after a latent period of several seconds or minutes upon assuming the standing posture, and is abolished by walking. It involves mainly the lower extremity and trunk muscles, although some weightbearing tasks in the upper extremities may produce tremor in susceptible individuals. The vast majority of patients suffering from this tremor have no other neurologic complaint, but there are reports of an association with essential tremor and painful cramp syndromes. One case associated with aqueductal stenosis and another with chronic relapsing demyelinating polyneuropathy have been reported.

The upright posture itself is not responsible for the tremor; rather, it appears that the isometric muscle activity required for weightbearing is the trigger. Surface EMG recording shows synchronous bursts in antagonist muscles occurring at rates as high as 30 Hz in some patients and as low as 7 Hz in others. Some authors have proposed that the tremor is due to impaired feedback from muscle spindles. However, its physiologic and pharmacologic underpinnings remain unknown.

Primidone in the doses cited above or Clonazepam in daily doses of 4 to 6 mg may improve some patients.

Cerebellar Tremor

Also known as cerebellar outflow tremor, cerebellar tremor is seen in late cortical atrophy of the cerebellum and in lesions of the cerebellar outflow tract, such as occur in multiple sclerosis. It is different from the appendicular dysmetria and ataxia associated with hemispheric cerebellar lesions. The tremor is manifested as regular oscillations of the trunk or limbs while maintaining a posture. The axial and proximal limb muscles demonstrate an alternating pattern of EMG bursts at about 3 Hz. The tremor also affects goal-directed movement, since as a limb approaches a target, the more distal muscles start to show the alternating bursts and the tremor increases in amplitude. The subjects show less tremor if they maintain their eyes open and observe the limb during the task, a phenomenon called visual stabilization. The mechanism for the tremor is unknown; it appears to be unrelated to abnormalities of stretch reflex or proprioceptive input.

Pharmacotherapy has yielded disappointing results. There has been some success using high doses (600 to 1,200 mg/day) of isoniazid hydrochloride. However, at these levels, liver toxicity is common. Carbamazepine has also been helpful for some patients. As in many other devastating tremors, stereotactic ablation of the ventral intermediate thalamic nucleus may be useful.

SUGGESTED READINGS

Bain PJ, Findley LJ, Thompson PD et al: A study of hereditary essential tremor. Brain 117:805, 1994

Busenbark K, Pahwa R, Hubble J et al: Double-blind controlled study of methazolamide in the treatment of essential tremor. Neurology 43:1045, 1993

Caparros-Lefebvre D, Blond S, Vermesch P et al: Chronic thalamic stimulation improves tremor and levodopa induced dyskinesias in Parkinson's disease. J Neurol Neurosurg Psychiatry 56:268, 1993

Cardoso FEC, Jankovic J: Hereditary motor-sensory neuropathy and movement disorders. Muscle Nerve 16:904, 1993

Deiber MP, Pollak P, Passingham R et al: Thalamic stimulation and supression of parkinsonian tremor. Evidence of cerebellar deactivation using positron emission tomography. Brain 4:267, 1993

Elble RJ, Moody C, Higgins C: Primary writing tremor: a form of focal dystonia? Mov Disord 5:118, 1990

Fitzgerald PM, Jankovic J: Orthostatic tremor: an association with essential tremor. Mov Disord 6:60, 1991

Garcia Ruiz PJ, Garcia de Yebenes Prous J, Jimenez Jimenez J: effects of nicardipine on essential tremor: brief report. Clin Neuropharmacol 16:456, 1993

Goldman MS, Ahlskog JE, Kelly PJ: the symptomatic and functional outcome of stereotactic thalamotomy for medically intractable essential tremor. J Neurosurg 76:924; 1992

Jenkis IH, Bain PG, Colebatch JG et al: A positron emission tomography study of essential tremor: evidence for overactivity of cerebellar connections. Ann Neurol 34:82, 1993

Koller WC, Vetere-Overfield B: Acute and chronic effects of propanolol and primidone in essential tremor. Neurology 39:1587, 1989

Nguyen JP, Degos JD: Thalamic stimulation and proximal tremor. A specific target in the nucleus ventrointermedius thalami. Arch Neurol 50:498, 1993

Speelman JD, VanManen J: Stereotactic thalamotomy for the relief of intention tremor of multiple sclerosis. J Neurol Neurosurg Psychiatry 47:596, 1984

Walker FO, McCormick GM, Hunt VP: Isometric features of orthostatic tremor. Muscle Nerve 13:918, 1990

Wills AJ, Jenkins LH, Thompson PD, Findley LJ, Brooks DJ: Red nuclear and cerebellar but no olivary activation associated with essential tremor: a positron emission tomography study. Ann Neurol 36:636, 1994

122. HUNTINGTON'S DISEASE

WALTER J. KOROSHETZ

Huntington's disease is an autosomal dominant neurodegenerative disease that leads to marked atrophy of basal ganglia structures, the caudate, and putamen, as well as less marked atrophy of other brain nuclei. It is thought to be the most common inherited adult neurodegenerative disease, affecting 1 in 15,000 in the United States. The average age of onset is approximately 38 years old; much younger-onset cases and onset in elderly patients also occurs less commonly. The hallmark of the illness is an involuntary movement disorder, chorea. Some patients have little or no chorea and instead appear slow and rigid (i.e., with parkinsonian characteristics). The illness leads to death, with an average duration of symptoms of about 20 years. The gene that causes the disease has been identified. The Huntington mutation is an expanded trinucleotide $(CAG)_n$ repeat that causes an excessively long polyglutamine stretch located in a novel protein called *huntingtin*. How the mutation leads to the onset of a disorder of motor, emotional, and cognitive control in persons who have matured normally until middle age is still a mystery. The gene discovery has made genetic diagnosis commonplace, both in neurologically normal individuals (presymptomatic testing) as well as neurologically or psychiatrically impaired individuals (diagnostic testing). It is hoped that research will soon uncover the cause of the slow neuronal loss, which is stimulated by the mutation and underlies the tragic illness.

CLINICAL MANIFESTATIONS

Huntington's disease is characterized by progressive impairment of an individual's cognitive, emotional, and motor control caused by neuronal death in the central nervous system, primarily in the caudate and putamen of the basal ganglia. Primary sensory pathways do not appear to be affected. Cerebellar function is affected only in an atypical Huntington's disease variant with signs usually beginning in childhood. The psychological effects of the disease are magnified by the fact that it is autosomal dominantly inherited and affected individuals have usually witnessed the entire course of the disease in their parent by the time they begin to show signs. Older siblings may also be severely disabled or have already died.

Because it is an autosomal dominant disorder, the thorough taking of a family history is essential to make the clinical diagnosis. Care is needed to avoid errors of incorrectly attributing any neurologic/psychiatric symptom to Huntington's disease in the presence of a family history. A negative family history that is taken as absolute, without investigation, can also lead to errors in not diagnosing Huntington's disease in an affected individual.

The disease progresses slowly and often in a pattern consisting of three phases. Early on, affected individuals have difficulty maintaining their premorbid level of function at work, school, or home. Emotional disorders may be prominent, there is disability owing to poor motor control, and chorea is usually present. In this stage, individuals can maintain their own activities of daily living. Toward the end of stage 1 the person loses the ability to remain employed or drive an automobile and becomes reliant on family or society for some level of support. In stage 2, dysarthria affects communication, and dysphagia may occur. Disordered motor control may lead to falls; chorea may be prominent; mentation is dulled. Such individuals require supervision to avoid self-injury; to prevent poor financial decisions; and even to maintain adequate nutrition, housing, and cleanliness. In stage 3, dystonia and rigidity may set in, choreoathetosis may be continuous, and the person becomes eventually bedridden and unable to speak or swallow. The course of the disease progresses fairly linearly down the Boston Independence and Physical Disability Scales (Table 122-1). The Total Functional Capacity Score, which is presented in Table 122-2, is more sensitive to progression of the disease in stages 1 and 2.

Presenting Signs and Symptoms

Persons with Huntington's disease present with a variety of clinical syndromes. Most commonly, an individual at risk for

TABLE 122-2. Total Functional Capacity Scale (Shoulson inventory)

Occupation
  0 = unable
  1 = marginal work only
  2 = reduced capacity for usual job
  3 = normal
Finances
  0 = unable
  1 = major assistance
  2 = slight assistance
  3 = normal
Domestic chores
  0 = unable
  1 = impaired
  2 = normal
Activities of daily living
  0 = total care
  1 = gross tasks only
  2 = minimal impairment
  3 = normal
Care level
  0 = full time skilled nursing
  1 = home or chronic care
  2 = home

this disease begins to fall behind in performance at work or home in the fourth or fifth decade of life. Slowness in executing tasks, inflexibility, forgetfulness, poor judgment, or increased irritability may impair their usual level of ability. They may present with a history of recent change in the degree of difficulty of their job or recent job loss. Family members often report that a change in personality has occurred in the 3 to 5 years preceding clinical symptoms. Increased numbers of motor vehicle accidents may occur. Increased irritability is common; occasionally florid psychiatric disorders predominate for years before the motor signs of Huntington's disease appear.

Symptoms of a motor disorder in early-stage Huntington's disease are not specific but are very suspicious if definite slow worsening occurs in an individual with a known affected parent. The spouse may report that the affected individual began to have sudden jerking movements during sleep over the past few years. These must be distinguished from the sleep-onset myoclonus that occurs in normal individuals but is often incorrectly assumed to be a sign of Huntington's disease in at-risk individuals. Clumsiness of fine finger movements is detected by some individuals (i.e. typists, musicians, and carpenters). A deterioration in baseline handwriting skills is common. Unexplained falls, dropping of objects, and a change in the usual pattern of walking or speaking are other common symptoms that may herald the onset of clinical Huntington's disease.

Because the mutation is inherited and individuals are clearly normal during childhood and throughout early adulthood and

TABLE 122-1. Boston Independence and Physical Disability Scales

Boston Independence Scale	*Boston Physical Disability Scale*
100: No special care needed	100: Normal no disease evident
090: No physical care needed if difficult tasks are involved	090: Onset-minimal signs, slight facial or extremity movement disorder
080: Predisease level of employment changes or ends; cannot perform household chores to predisease level; may need help with finances	080: Normal daily activity with effort, gait disturbance, stumbling, slurred speech
070: Self-care maintained for bathing, limited household duties (cooking and use of knives), driving terminates; unable to manage finances	070: Limited activity, occasional falls, overt chorea, less speech with dysarthria, occasional dysphagia
060: Needs minor assistance for dressing, toileting, bathing; food must be cut for patient	060: Can be left alone for short period of time, several falls, can walk up to 1 block outside of home
050: 24-hour supervision appropriate; assistance required for bathing, eating, toileting	050: Needs assistance in walking, limited ambulation at home, difficulty communicating and swallowing
040: Chronic care facility needed; limited self-feeding, liquefied diet	040: Limited ability to walk assisted; single-word utterances
030: Patient provides minimal assistance in own feeding, bathing, toileting	030: Confined to wheelchair, unintelligible speech, frequent choking
020: No speech, must be fed	020: Completely bedridden, anarthria
010: Tube fed, total bed care	010: Fixed posture requiring total care, gastrostomy, catheterization

slowly develop the clinical syndrome in early to middle adulthood, there can be no true "onset" of illness. Huntington's disease is inexorably progressive, though individuals accumulate disability at various rates. Diagnosis is usually made when chorea without other cause becomes evident. However, studies of at-risk individuals and newly diagnosed patients reveal that, even before chorea occurs, certain "soft signs" may appear. The speed of saccadic eye movements is slowed, and there may be an abnormal delay before the production of a saccadic eye movement to a command. Repetitive fine finger movements, repetitive tongue movements, or repetitive lingual pronunciations may be slow and clumsy. Individuals may have difficulty learning a sequence of motor acts (Luria three-step test). Restless movements may occur that resemble normal repositioning movements but at increased frequency. Stereotyped "habit" movements may be more apparent, or small-amplitude flicks of the fingers may be seen while the individual holds hands outstretched or walks.

Neuropsychological evaluation may reveal deficits in memory or in the ability to respond to changing instructions (changing sets). Clinical depression is common in the years just preceding or encompassing the time of clinical diagnosis. The suicide rate in this time period is markedly increased.

Chorea

The combination of fluid or jerky, writhing, torsional movements in all extremities resembles a form of primitive dance, and the word chorea is from the Greek, meaning to dance. In the early stages of the illness, the movements are often quick flicks of the fingers or muscles about the mouth or ankles. One common variant in which the fingers are quickly extended resembles the motion of "flicking the ashes off a cigarette." The movements in the face may resemble "winking" or quick, wry "smiling" movements. As indicated above, there is often an increased frequency and constancy of movements that are seen commonly in normal individuals and associated with "restlessness." A small proportion of affected individuals never demonstrate chorea. In most individuals, chorea is unsightly but not truly disabling. It can affect function in that patients may spill liquids, hit extremities against sharp or hot objects, or drop objects owing to a choreic movement. However, in some, chorea becomes so pronounced (large-amplitude continuous writhing movements) that it interferes with all normal motor activity. Chorea is inhibited by neuroleptic agents and enhanced by dopamine agonists. Treatment with neuroleptic drugs is problematic because it may worsen the voluntary movement disorder in a dose-dependent fashion (see below).

As the disease progresses, the involuntary movements change in form. In some individuals, the movements increase in amplitude and frequency so that the person is in constant motion while awake. The person may walk grotesque contortions of both axial and appendicular musculature. As the illness progresses, some individuals demonstrate a slowing of writhing movements to "choreoathetosis." In the late stages of the illness, the predominant disorder is dystonia, a fixed, abnormal, usually twisted posture. Progression to rigidity and dystonia can be iatrogenically produced by treating chorea overaggressively with neuroleptic drugs.

Disordered Motor Control

Major disability comes from the disordered voluntary motor disorder in Huntington's disease. This aspect of the disease progresses until there is almost no ability to make goal-directed purposeful movements to the extent that swallowing, speaking, and even sitting are no longer possible. Huntington's disease contains much of the bradykinesia found in Parkinson's disease without the same rigidity or tremor but instead with overlying chorea. This is not surprising because both diseases cause a dysfunctional striatum. In the motor control sphere, the old teaching that Parkinson's and Huntington's diseases cause opposite nervous system effects is incorrect. In the early stages, the motor disorder is characterized by slowness and incoordination. There is usually trouble in making rhythmic movements or fast, repetitive, fine movements with the tongue or fingers. When patients are asked to tap the index finger to the thumb or tap the tongue to the top lip repetitively, the movements are made more slowly than normal, and there are occasional deviations from the desired pattern. Patients have a peculiar inability to time fast tapping movements with the hand regularly. A test that demands changing the motor program is very difficult. To test these patients, they are asked to tap out a sequence of three motor acts (tap thigh alternately with a fist, then the side of the hand, and then the palm of the hand; then repeat the sequence). A similar disability is seen when the patient is asked to tap the front and back surface of their dominant hand on the palm of their nondominant hand alternately (disdiadochokinesia).

A change in the pattern of speech occurs, and some family members consider this to be the first sign of the disease. An alteration in pronunciation and in the normal phrasing and timing of speech is likely to be what is noticed early. On examination, repetitive lingual sounds are pronounced poorly (i.e., la, la, la, la, la) whereas repetitive buccal sounds are performed better (i.e., me, me, me, me, me). Swallowing movements are unfortunately also affected by the motor control disorder in Huntington's disease. Patients often begin with trouble swallowing dry foods such as crackers, cookies, or dry cereals. They are unable to strip such food pieces from the pharynx and may inhale them instead. Next, thin liquids such as water and soda are trouble; this can sometimes be remedied by the use of a straw to deliver the fluid straight to the back of the mouth, as the tongue coordination necessary to do so may not be present. Thicker liquids are easier to propel out of the mouth and are usually the easiest to swallow, even in the later stages of the illness.

Gait and posture are severely affected by the disease as it progresses. Gait may become wide based, and the steps are irregular in both timing and placement of the feet. Because of the combination of gait disorder and slurred speech, patients are not uncommonly misdiagnosed as inebriated by law enforcement officials. Postural instability occurs over time, and affected individuals will not be able to balance on one foot or walk tandem in a straight line. In the early or middle stage of the disease, they may exhibit retropulsion when given a light shove backward. Falling becomes a serious issue in the middle and later stages of the illness. A number of patients with Huntington's disease suffer subdural hematomas or orthopaedic injuries owing to falls. As the disease progresses into the later stages, all lose the ability to walk and even to maintain balance for the standing or upright sitting position.

There is an apraxia, which affects functional movement in patients with Huntington's disease. Occasionally a patient is misperceived as lazy or depressed because they are seen as not performing even the most simple tasks about the house. On examination, they may be unable to mimic the most basic hand postures, and it is clear that they do not have the ability to learn or produce the movement necessary for their activities of daily living. Because of slowness, incoordination, apraxia, and chorea, patients with Huntington's disease in the middle stage of the disease lose the ability to write, use keys, button clothing, tie shoelaces, wash dishes, feed themselves without spilling food, and so forth. In the later stages, affected individuals are totally dependent on others for feeding, clothing, and bathing because of the total lack of voluntary control of movement.

Death caused by Huntington's disease is usually triggered by aspiration pneumonia owing to pharyngeal dysfunction. Speech patterns change early in the illness, with slurring and poor modulation of volume and tone. As the illness progresses, dysarthria becomes more severe, and, in the later stages, speech becomes unintelligible. Individuals with end-stage Huntington's disease can do little more than moan or produce incoordinated vowel sounds. Swallowing dysfunction also occurs throughout the course of the illness. Choking spells usually do not occur until the later stages, though some patients have had occasional coughing or choking with swallowing in the early stages. As the disease progresses, the texture of food must be altered to allow effective swallowing. Thickening liquids and softening and moistening solid foods (puréed) is usually necessary as the disease progresses. Pharyngeal dysfunction eventually becomes so severe that nutritional needs cannot be met orally in the late stage of the illness. Aspiration of oral contents occurs as a final event, leading to pneumonia.

Reflexes are usually hyperactive, there may be clonus at the ankle. Tone is increased in the late stages of the illness coincident with dystonia, and tone is increased in the bradykinetic/rigid juvenile cases. In early-stage Huntington's disease, the tone in an extremity can be normal until the examiner attempts to produce passive movement or the patient produces active movement in another extremity. In these cases, the tone becomes activated by these stimuli. Despite severe dementia, frontal lobe signs are usually not seen (grasp, suck, and rooting reflex). Vertical eye movements can be limited in end-stage disease. With middle- to late-stage disease, horizontal eye movements are linked to unsuppressible head turn or blinks. No deficits in pupillary reflexes, hearing, visual acuity, visual fields, or primary sensation are apparent in Huntington's disease. Muscular wasting is seen, but the cause is not clear. Cerebellar signs such as dysmetria and nystagmus are not usually seen.

Autonomic abnormalities are not usually noted in this disease. Patients in its end stage become incontinent, usually associated with considerable dementia. Some patients with Huntington's disease have experienced unusual episodic sweating. In the late stages, we have seen occasional patients with recurrent high fevers, elevated creatine phosphokinase levels, and diaphoresis. A source of infection should be looked for in such cases but may not always be uncovered.

Psychiatric Disorders

Depression is extremely common in persons with Huntington's disease, and it may become apparent before the neurologic signs enable the clinical diagnosis. The suicide risk is increased in at-risk and affected individuals. Depressed mood usually responds to antidepressants, but the response is often a partial one. Depression may occur in the context of a mixed psychiatric disorder, or there may be cycling of mania and depression. An

unusual feature of some patients with Huntington's disease is an overwhelming "apathetic" disorder, usually with a less pronounced dysthymic disorder. Patients frequently are poor at generating spontaneous, constructive activity. It is not uncommon for patients with Huntington's disease to become extremely sedentary and spend most of the day in the house, either in bed or watching television. With structure and guidance, a much more productive level of activity can be sustained longer into the illness.

A disorder of emotional control is seen commonly in patients with Huntington's disease. This is often manifested by an increased level of irritability, with or without an underlying anxiety disorder. Angry outbursts in the home can be extremely disruptive and are one of the main causes for institutionalization of persons with Huntington's disease. These outbursts often occur suddenly and without warning. They are usually short-lived (minutes), but their repercussions for other family members may be longer lasting, especially if they are associated with physical violence. The individual with Huntington's disease may be contrite when confronted with the history but unable to alter the pattern of behavior. The trigger for emotional outbursts is not uncommonly a demand for assistance that is not met immediately or a request by the individual with Huntington's disease that is not considered reasonable by a caregiver or family member. Occasionally, emotional dyscontrol is a manifestation of delusional thought or severe depression. We have seen some individuals in whom episodes of emotional dyscontrol coincide with intense feelings of hunger occurring prior to a scheduled meal. Cigarette smoking also appears to be exceedingly common in persons with Huntington's disease, and the urge to smoke is often magnified to the extreme. Episodes of anger often occur in the context of some obstruction to smoking. In some very severe cases, hitting out or an angry outburst appears almost reflexive and triggered by most interactions. One must inquire into the safety of children or elderly individuals living in the home with a patient who suffers from emotional dyscontrol.

A true psychotic disorder with hallucinations occurs rarely as part of Huntington's disease. Paranoia, delusional thought, bizarre behavior, and anxiety disorders occur more commonly in combination with disordered emotional control. Obsessive compulsive behavior is not uncommon in patients with Huntington's disease. Fear of being alone or removed from the family, fear of bathing, fear of leaving the house, fear of heights, and fear of choking are not uncommon and may complicate the care of the patient.

Cognitive Disorders

In Huntington's disease, there is early memory impairment. This is progressive over time and is accompanied by impaired attention, distractability, and inflexibility. Previous mental tasks may take considerably longer and may be accompanied by more frequent errors. Reasoning ability, simple arithmetic processes, temporal ordering, and abstract thought all become severely impaired. Patients do most poorly on tests that require a change in strategy. They have trouble with tasks that require visual spatial integration of input, which may contribute to their driving disability. They have difficulty in generating and executing plans necessary to accomplish even relatively simple goals at work or in the home.

The dementia of Huntington's disease is a "subcortical dementia." Unlike Alzheimer's disease, the memory disorder does not progress to amnesia. It appears that new memories can be made and old memories recalled, but this occurs less often as the disease progresses. There is eventually a poverty of thought; only a small proportion of events can be recalled. Perseveration and impersistence are prominent as the disease progresses. Patients with Huntington's disease have severe impairment of motor skill learning. We have found a special inability for such patients to learn sequence information. In end-stage disease, either very limited and primitive communication or no apparent communication with the patient is possible.

Sleep Disorders

Patients may complain of inability to sleep or daytime drowsiness. Sleep studies often demonstrate abnormal sleep architecture, with frequent awakenings associated with motor jerks. Some patients improve with the use of clonazepam at bedtime. Amitriptyline at bedtime may also be helpful.

Nutritional/Metabolic Disorder

Many physicians caring for patients with Huntington's disease suspect that there is a hypermetabolic disorder. Weight loss is common and can be extreme and rapid. Institutionalized patients who are sedentary except for their chorea and dystonia can require huge caloric intake (3,000 to 4,000 cal/day) to maintain their body weight. It is our impression that patients do worse clinically as their weight decreases and sometimes improve as they gain weight. In our study of factors associated with slow progression of illness, with the exception of late-onset age, increased weight at the time of diagnosis was the most statistically significantly associated variable. No particular food group is known to be of special benefit. High-calorie nutritional supplements are often necessary to maintain body weight.

Clinical Variants

In most cases, symptoms and signs of Huntington's disease occur as outlined above, with soft signs and chorea first becoming manifest around age 40. The disease progresses over 20 years. The Boston Independence and Physical Disability Scales (Table 122-1) provide a means to chart the progression of the disease in an almost linear fashion from onset to end-stage disease. However, some individuals exhibit significant deviations from the more common clinical course.

Juvenile cases of Huntington's disease occur uncommonly, and they are usually inherited from an affected father or from a mother who was also affected as a juvenile. The genetic cause of this paternal sex effect is discussed below. Juvenile disease often presents as an akinetic/rigid syndrome without chorea. The saccadic eye movement velocity is usually very slow. Myoclonic tremor is common. Seizures may occur. Persons with juvenile Huntington's disease often present with failing grades and a deterioration in their coordination. Their disease tends to progress more rapidly, and our data suggest that the rate of progression is closely associated with onset age.

Persons without signs of Huntington's disease until their seventh or eighth decade usually have a very slow progression of disability. They often present with chorea without dementia and are frequently misdiagnosed as suffering from senile chorea. Unfortunately, the transmission of the *HD* gene is associated with "anticipation," the children of individuals with old age–onset Huntington's disease can develop signs of the illness much earlier than their parents.

In some patients, severe, disabling psychiatric disorders may cause disability years to decades before physical signs of the disease become evident.

RADIOLOGIC FEATURES

There is progressive atrophy of the caudate and putamen in persons with Huntington's disease. The caudate nucleus normally protrudes into the ventricle so that atrophy is easily observed as an increase in the width of the lateral ventricle. There is loss of the usual convexity of the lateral wall of the ventricle owing to caudate atrophy, leading to the so-called boxcar ventricular shape on computed tomography. Generalized brain atrophy is commonly seen along with caudate atrophy in the later stages of the illness. In individuals with elderly onset, the caudate atrophy is often considered proportional to the cortical atrophy, and the diagnosis is not apparent by imaging alone. In juvenile Huntington's disease, there may be an increased T2-weighted signal in the caudate on magnetic resonance imaging.

PATHOLOGIC FEATURES AND CLUES TO PATHOGENESIS

The brain weight in end-stage Huntington's disease is considerably reduced, but the cerebellar weight is often normal. The caudate in end-stage disease is severely atrophic and may consist only of a tissue paper–thin layer of glial cells with occasional neurons intermixed. The progression of the clinical signs of the disease appears to correlate with the pathologic grading of the degree of caudate atrophy. Interestingly, from a neurobiologic viewpoint, the neuronal death that occurs in Huntington's disease is cell-type specific. In the atrophic caudate, neurons that stain for nicotinamide adenine dinucleotide phosphate diaphorase and somatostatin are preferentially spared, and the spiny neurons are preferentially affected. There is also a gradient of cell death that occurs. The wave of cell death as the disease progresses seems to march from dorsal to ventral and medial to lateral in the caudate nucleus. There is a fine structure to the caudate and putamen neural architecture, which also exhibits region-specific changes as the disease progresses.

The pathologic features of Huntington's disease have been mimicked to some degree by animal model studies using toxins. Intrastriatal injection of chemicals that activate the N-methyl-D-aspartate type of glutamate receptor in the brain cause degeneration of spiny neurons in animals and selective sparing of the diaphorase-staining aspiny neurons. More interestingly, chemicals that block mitochondrial function also lead to the pattern of neuronal death seen in the brain of a patient with Huntington's disease. In addition, selective striatal damage is seen when these chemicals are administered systemically. There is also a described clinical syndrome in humans who have accidentally ingested one such mitochondrial inhibitor, 3-nitropropionic acid, which is characterized by striatal damage and dystonia. These observations have led to speculation that a mismatch between the energy demand caused by glutamate neurotransmission and the energy supply, as determined by mitochondrial function, leads to neuronal death, preferentially in the striatum and especially in spiny neurons. In further support of this theory, it has been found that the brain lactic acid levels are increased by excessive glutamate neurotransmission and by mitochondrial failure. Most importantly, brain lactate levels have been found to be elevated in patients with Huntington's disease.

MOLECULAR GENETICS

The gene mutation that causes Huntington's disease was identified in 1993. With the use of polymorphic DNA markers and linkage analysis in multiple large pedigrees, the gene was localized to the short arm of chromosome 4 in 1983. It was the first case of location of a disease gene based on DNA analysis of affected families, so-called reverse genetics.

The *HD* mutation is an expansion of a trinucleotide repeat $(CAG)_n$, which codes for a polyglutamine stretch of amino acids in a novel protein. In unaffected individuals, the *HD* gene can contain up to 33 (CAG) repeats, the average number of repeats in this gene in the normal population is approximately 22. In persons with Huntington's disease, there are greater than 38 (CAG) repeats in the *HD* gene that was inherited from an affected parent. Individuals with Huntington's disease usually also have a normal *HD* gene allele with less than 33 (CAG) repeats.

The discovery of the gene mutation led to the explanation of a number of puzzling issues in the genetics of Huntington's disease. Persons with juvenile Huntington's disease were found to have inherited exceedingly long $(CAG)_n$ repeats. Whereas most individuals with Huntington's disease have an allele with 40 to 55 (CAG) repeats, persons with the juvenile form have greater than 60 and as many as 80 (CAG) repeats in their *HD* gene. As discussed above, persons with juvenile Huntington's disease usually inherited the disease from an affected father. It was found that the length of the expanded $(CAG)_n$ repeat could further expand in father-to-child transmissions. Indeed the $(CAG)_n$ length was fairly constant in all tissues except in the sperm, where it was found to be unstable. Sperm from affected men contained a wide variety of $(CAG)_n$ repeat numbers. It is thought that fertilization by a sperm with a very high $(CAG)_n$ repeat length in the *HD* gene gives rise to an offspring with juvenile Huntington's disease. With the exception of the juvenile cases [$(CAG)_n$ greater than 60], the actual $(CAG)_n$ repeat length in persons with Huntington's disease has little or no predictive value.

Are there new *HD* mutations? We and others have followed individuals and families in whom a person with a clinical syndrome identical to Huntington's disease was found in the absence of a family history of affected parents. We wondered whether these cases represented new mutations or manifestations of another disease. After the discovery of the *HD* mutation, we found that the suspected individuals did have the *HD* gene. More interestingly, family members who were elderly and not affected by Huntington's disease had $(CAG)_n$ repeats in the intermediate range (33 to 38), greater than those found in the general population but less than those found in persons with the disease. The appearance of "de novo" cases was explained by expansion of an *HD* allele in the intermediate $(CAG)_n$ zone into the *HD* gene range (more than 38) during transmission from father to child.

NEUROBIOLOGY OF THE HUNTINGTON'S DISEASE PROTEIN

It is expected that a great deal will be learned about the pathogenesis of Huntington's disease from studies of the *HD* mutation. The development of transgenic mouse strains containing the *HD* mutation, it is hoped, will provide a faithful model of the disease to develop strategies aimed at preventing the progression of neuronal death. Homozygous knockout of the *HD* gene is reported to be fatal in a transgenic mouse model. Heterozygous knockout of the *HD* gene in a transgenic mouse model caused neuronal loss in the subthalamic nucleus and a disorder on certain learning tasks. The *HD* gene messenger RNA and protein are not confined to nervous tissue but have been found in all tissues. *HD* gene message and protein are also found in all brain regions, in brain tissue from persons affected with the illness, as well as in brain tissue from normal individuals. There does not seem to be a differential localization of the messenger RNA or the protein to the striatum.

GENETIC TESTING

Presymptomatic testing for Huntington's disease became available with the use of linkage analysis in appropriate families in 1983. The discovery of the gene mutation has simplified the genetic diagnosis, and it is now available in a variety of clinical laboratories. Because of the absence of a treatment that could prevent or slow down progression of the illness, there is no health benefit to early diagnosis. Many individuals wish to know their gene status to plan their careers, families, and finances. However, because of the tragic nature of the illness and the occurrence in loved ones, many individuals live in constant fear of inheriting the illness. The emotional stress of living at risk can motivate individuals to seek presymptomatic testing. A favorable outcome can be a great relief, but there is generally a 50 percent chance that the result will be unfavorable. The stress of living with the knowledge that one has the *HD* gene can be considerably more severe than that of living with a 50 percent risk. During the process of genetic counseling, many persons (30 to 50 percent) realize that the stress of living at risk is preferable to the stress of learning about an unfavorable gene status and drop out of testing. For this reason, it is recommended that presymptomatic testing be performed with careful counseling and with some delay between the request for testing and the actual DNA analysis. This allows the individual at risk to weigh carefully the potential personal effects of knowing that they will surely inherit the disease that had previously disabled their parent, siblings, or other relatives. Because of the high prevalence of depression in the years preceding diagnosis, it is also considered wise to screen persons coming for genetic testing for depressive disorder and especially suicidality since the stress of an unfavorable test result in the context of a uncontrolled depressive disorder may be tragic.

TREATMENT

There is no treatment that is known to slow down the progression of the neuronal degeneration in Huntington's disease. Medical treatment is tailored to specific issues that arise and affect the patient's functional level.

Depression

Depressive symptoms are common in patients with Huntington's disease. They may be very much tied to despair arising from situational issues such as declining function in the workplace, inadequate supports in the home, financial difficulties, and social isolation. Psychological counseling and guidance in managing the disability that comes with this disease can cause remarkable change. Maintenance of structured activities for the affected individual, either at home, through local Huntington's disease societies, in long-term care institutions, or in day care programs is also frequently very helpful in assisting the affected person to maintain a sense of self-worth.

Antidepressant medications can be of great help in those with a serious mood disorder. Tricyclic antidepressants (amitriptyline, imipramine, and nortriptyline) or serotonergic agents (fluoxetine or sertraline) have been used most commonly. Initially, relatively low doses are prescribed and changes in dose made at 3-week intervals until depression responds or toxicity develops. Amitriptyline before bedtime is also useful in some patients for their sleep disorder. Unlike patients with Alzheimer's or Parkinson's disease, patients with Huntington's disease do not have increased sensitivity to the anticholinergic side effects of the tricyclics. Fluoxetine can suppress appetite; so weight should be carefully monitored. The tricyclics may also be useful because of a tendency to stimulate appetite.

Occasional patients respond poorly to all attempts to treat their severe depression. In many cases, a partial improvement occurs, but some chronic dysthymic disorder persists for decades. In occasional patients with severe incapacitating depression, monoamine oxidase inhibitors or electroshock therapy has been successful.

Depressed patients with Huntington's disease may also suffer from emotional dyscontrol disorders. Suicide is not rare, and patients should be questioned about suicidal intent. In patients with a history of suicidal thought or with impulsive behavior, care should be taken to limit the amount of antidepressant and other medications prescribed at one time. When appropriate, a family member or caretaker should administer the medications.

Chorea

Chorea does decrease in frequency, speed, and amplitude with dopamine blocking agents but often at the price of increased incoordination, dystonia, and bradykinesia. In many cases, chorea is overmedicated with neuroleptic drugs to the patient's disadvantage. It is therefore important to determine whether treatment is actually leading to a functional improvement, as opposed to a cosmetic improvement, in chorea at the cost of decreasing motor function. In general, doses of haloperidol greater than 5 mg/day are met with worsening motor function, though exceptions to this rule occur commonly. In some patients, benzodiazepines such as clonazepam are helpful.

Emotional Dyscontrol

Management of the emotional outbursts is perhaps the most difficult and important task for the caregiver. Sudden verbal or physical abuse of self or others is the most common reason for institutionalization of patients with Huntington's disease.

Patients should first be evaluated for those events in their environments that trigger the outbursts. Common-sense but creative changes such as adjustments in the time of feeding if outbursts are triggered by hunger; a relaxation strategy when anxiety occurs; setting schedules and safe havens for smoking; and so forth can be very helpful. In some, there is an underlying depression or mania, and treatment with antidepressants, carbamazepine, valproate, or lithium is helpful. In some, there is a chronic sleep disorder, and irritability is related to sleep deprivation and improves with more restful sleep. Clonazepam, carbamazepine, and valproate may be helpful in limiting the level of increased irritability that underlies the emotional dyscontrol. Some patients are inappropriately fixated on specific concerns or demands. These are often the most difficult to manage; a trial of antidepressants that are useful in treating obsessive compulsive disorder (fluoxetine or clomipramine) can be of some help.

In some instances, a delusional thought disorder underlies the outbursts, and this may not always be apparent owing to the patient's communicative disability. Neuroleptic agents such as haloperidol, thioridazine (more sedating), and clozapine (less dystonia and bradykinesia) are in some instances effective, but their psychiatric benefits are balanced by their tendency to cause increased bradykinesia and rigidity. The motor control side effects of the neuroleptic medications tend to increase as the disease progresses.

In difficult-to-control patients, often a combination of medications is used. In addition to antidepressants and neuroleptics, valproate or carbamazepine should be tried in an attempt to level mood; high-dose propranolol and lithium can be effective in some severe dyscontrol disorders.

Motor Control Disorder

No medical treatment is known to have a major effect on this very disabling aspect of the disease. Emphasis should be placed on maintenance of safe ambulation and swallowing as long as possible. Physical therapy and conditioning exercises can improve a patient's safety and function. Some patients are thrown off balance by their chorea, and a very small dose of haloperidol may decrease the rate of falling. However, haloperidol worsens the postural stability; so it also increases the rate of falling in some. In some rare patients with a parkinsonian variant of Huntington's disease, a small dose of a dopamine agonist is helpful. Alterations in diet are necessary to prevent aspiration, with a soft thick moist substance being the most easily swallowed.

CONCLUSION

There is hope that scientific and clinical research will offer promising therapies based on new knowledge about the pathogenesis and effects of the gene mutation in Huntington's disease. At present, the families and patients afflicted by Huntington's disease often live a life that is very different from that of the "average American." There is a great need for understanding and knowledgeable physicians, social workers, genetic counselors, physical therapists, and so forth to help affected individuals maintain their self-worth and dignity throughout the process of neurodegeneration.

SUGGESTED READINGS

Bittenbender JB, Quadvasel FA: Rigid and akinetic forms of Huntington's chorea. Arch Neurol 7:275, 1962

Duayao M, Ambrose C, Myers R et al: Trinucleotide repeat length instability and age of onset in Huntington's disease. Nat Genet 4:387–92, 1993

Gusella JF, Wexler NS, Conneally PM et al: A polymorphic DNA marker genetically linked to HD. Nature 306:234, 1983

Hersch S, Jones R, Koroshetz W, Quaid K: The neurogenetics genie: testing for the Huntington's disease mutation. Neurology 44:1369–73, 1994

Haydon MR: Huntington's Chorea. Springer-Verlag, New York, 1981

Huntington G: On chorea. Med Surg Reporter 26:317–21, 1872

Huntington's Disease Collaborative Research Group: A novel gene containing a trinucleotid repeat that is expanded and unstable on Huntington's disease chromosomes. Cell 72:971–83, 1993

Myers RH, MacDonald M, Koroshetz W et al: De novo expansion of a (CAG)$_n$ repeat in sporadic Huntington's disease. Nat Genet 5:168–73, 1993

Myers RH, Vonsattel JP, Stevens TJ et al: Clinical and neuropathologic assessment of severity in HD. Neurology 38:341–7, 1988

Nasir J, Floresco S, O'Kusky JR et al: Targeted disruption of the Huntington's disease gene results in embryonic lethality and behavioural and morphological changes in heterozygotes. Cell 81:811, 1995

Ranen NG, Peyser CE, Folstein SE: A Physician's Guide to the Management of Huntington's Disease. Huntington's Disease Society of America, New York,

Young AB, Shoulson I, Penney JB et al: Huntington's disease in Venezuela: neurological features and functional decline. Neurology 36:244–9, 1986

123. TARDIVE DYSKINESIA AND OTHER DRUG-RELATED MOVEMENT DISORDERS

EDISON MIYAWAKI
DANIEL TARSY

Tardive dyskinesia is a clinically diverse syndrome in which choreatic, athetoid, dystonic, orofacial, lingual, or other abnormal involuntary movements manifest relatively late in the course of neuroleptic treatment. The advent of "atypical" neuroleptics with spectra of activity that differ from more traditional dopamine receptor antagonists has made the term *neuroleptic* so all-embracing as to be vague, but for the purposes of this discussion, "neuroleptics" (agents that produce an effect on the nervous system) will refer to "traditional" dopamine receptor antagonists used in various clinical contexts, including psychosis, affective disorder, antiemesis, pain syndromes, and others.

Nominal definitions of tardive dyskinesia cite as criteria for diagnosis a minimum of 3 months' exposure to a neuroleptic, persistence of involuntary movements 1 month after stopping the offending drug, and exclusion of other identifiable causes for the movement disorder. The first published reports of what would eventually be termed tardive dyskinesia appeared some years after the introduction of chlorpromazine for treatment of psychotic disorders, and used descriptive designations, including "buccolinguo-masticatory syndrome," "persistent dyskinesia," and "terminal extrapyramidal insufficiency syndrome." Controversy over a cause-and-effect relationship between neuroleptics and late-appearing movement disorders arose in light of observations, dating to Kraeplin's monographs (1896) on schizophrenia, that strange and excessive stereotypic behaviors ("parakinesia," "bizarrery," "grotesquery") manifested in catatonic and other psychiatric disturbances. Over time, however, it has become clear that tardive dyskinesia represents a problem apart from sporadic dyskinesias in psychotic or elderly patients, and a recent American Psychiatric Association Task Force Report (1992) underlines the importance of heightened awareness and early detection as prevention against what can be permanent disability.

PHENOMENOLOGY AND NATURAL HISTORY

The clinical manifestations of tardive dyskinesia are various. The most commonly described syndrome involves orofacial and lingual movements. Onset is insidious, and early features are subtle restless movements of the tongue, patterned (thus, tic-like) facial movements, and increased blink frequency. Later manifestations include chewing or lip "smacking," tongue movements in and out of the mouth, and writhing of the tongue at rest. Not all facial movements in the context of neuroleptic treatment are tardive dyskinesia, as in the case of the perioral tremor ("rabbit syndrome") that is thought to be a variant of drug-induced parkinsonism, and may be ameliorated with anticholinergic agents and neuroleptic discontinuation. Older patients may be particularly vulnerable to the development of orofacial dyskinesia per se, and although edentulism in the aged can be confused with tardive dyskinesia, some investigators have thought that loss of proprioceptive input from the mouth in edentulism may contribute to the development of tardive orofacial or other dyskinesias. Accompanying motor movements of the extremities and trunk may be of large amplitude and high velocity so as to suggest shrugs, tics, or even ballism, but more distal limb movements are as characteristic, such as "piano-playing" or "air-guitar" fingers, foot tapping, and extension of the great toe. Movements may achieve bizarre proportions, as in the case of "copulatory" pelvic thrusting movements. "Choreoathetosis" is applied to many of these manifestations, since the velocity of movements is similar to chorea and writhing can be athetoid and dancelike. In traditional neurologic nomenclature, however, chorea and athetosis are of random or flowing nature, somewhat different from the stereotypy and repetitiveness that seems characteristic in tardive dyskinesia. Terms like *tardive stereotypy* and *rhythmic chorea* have been applied as a consequence, but *tardive dyskinesia* has become the commonly accepted usage. As with other movement disorders, the involuntary movements of tardive dyskinesia usually worsen with emotional stress and sleeplessness, diminish with sedation, and disappear with sleep.

Younger patients may be particularly vulnerable to tardive dystonia, a phenomenologically distinct tardive dyskinesia variant that may coexist with stereotypic or choreoathetoid movements. Mean age of onset according to the literature, is approximately 40, although tardive dystonia may manifest at any age. Unlike in idiopathic dystonia, tardive dystonia does not appear to exhibit a clear bimodal distribution (with peaks in early childhood and in adulthood). Sustained abnormal postures of limbs, neck, head, or trunk that may be exacerbated with activating movements are typical; the face and jaw in isolation may be affected. Examples include torticollis, retrocollis, oromandibular dystonia, and truncal dystonia (in some cases with striking lateral flexion and backward twisting of the trunk at the waist that may occur in acute or tardive fashion, termed *Pisa syndrome*). Tardive dystonic manifestations are often the most debilitating aspects in tardive dyskinesia, and have been associated with often striking morbidity (e.g., gait disturbance, dystonia-induced rib fractures, eating-induced dystonia, others). Older patients may be predisposed to focal or segmental dystonias, particularly of cranial structures.

Additional tardive syndromes have been described. Akathisia, a subjective (inner) or objective (overtly motor) restlessness that is partially relieved by volitional activity, is a well-described acute effect of neuroleptics, but has also been described as a tardive syndrome. Recurrent oculogyric crises over the course of months have been observed after discontinuation of long-term antipsychotic treatment. Sporadic reports of tardive respiratory dyskinesia underscore the concept that any voluntary muscle may be affected in tardive dyskinesia. Periodic tachypnea, irregular respirations, grunting, and problems with speech and eating (often, but not exclusively in association with orofacial dyskinesia) have been described. It has been said that rhythmic tremor is not a tardive dyskinesia manifestation, though rare cases have been reported of 3- to 5-Hz resting and postural tremor—in the context of neuroleptic treatment—that worsened with withdrawal of the drug and responded to dopamine-depleting agents.

Although research definitions of tardive dyskinesia suggest a minimum of 3 months of neuroleptic exposure, dyskinesias may manifest after a shorter time course, and seemingly persistent movements may, on rare occasions, appear after a very brief exposure. Research definitions disagree on the definition of ''persistent'' dyskinesia, and there has been an increasing trend over time to identify tardive dyskinesia as a syndrome that will attenuate in most cases if neuroleptics are promptly discontinued or if dosage is reduced. Long-term studies in tardive dyskinesia suggest that the lessening or resolution of dyskinesia is correlated with length of follow-up; studies with follow-up for longer than 5 years show the greatest number of patients with clinical improvement.

Natural history studies suggest that tardive dyskinesia is not a progressive disorder. Once it is diagnosed, there are compelling data to suggest that reduction in drug dosage is associated with improvement over time, but in clinical practice, neuroleptic discontinuation is not always an option, and naturalistic studies may reflect changes in neuroleptic dosage deemed necessary to treat psychiatric exacerbations. Tardive dyskinesia can remit completely, especially when neuroleptics are discontinued promptly upon diagnosis.

DIFFERENTIAL DIAGNOSIS

Tardive dyskinesia must first be distinguished from other neuroleptic-induced extrapyramidal syndromes and from other drug-induced dyskinesias. In patients still receiving neuroleptics, more than one drug-related movement disorder may manifest. Acute or subacute parkinsonism (with or, more typically, without tremor), dystonia, or akathisia may coexist with tardive manifestations in one-quarter to one-third of patients. Dyskinesias similar to those seen in tardive dyskinesias have been reported following routine use of or toxic exposure to a number of commonly used drugs, though the associated movement disorder typically will resolve with discontinuation of the agent. A list of medications associated with hyperkinetic dyskinesias is provided in Table 123-1.

In general, tardive dyskinesia distinguishes itself by its persistence on discontinuation of the neuroleptic. The sporadic dyskinesias described in schizophrenia seem to differ from tardive dyskinesia, but they may also persist. They are less rhythmic, more variable and complex, and are rarely choreoathetoid or dystonic. Mouthing movements in the elderly, associated with dementia and edentulism, may also mimic persistent tardive dyskinesia. Neuroleptic withdrawal may itself ''unmask'' dyskinesias that can take days, weeks, or months to resolve. So-called withdrawal dyskinesia may share pathophysiologic mechanisms with tardive dyskinesia, and dyskinesias that are still manifest on neuroleptic discontinuation may be placed along a continuum from transient to permanent.

TABLE 123-1. Drugs Associated with Hyperkinetic Dyskinesia (Other Than Traditional Neuroleptics)

Drugs not commonly recognized as dopamine antagonists
  Prochlorperazine
  Metoclopramide
  Amoxapine (7-OH metabolite)
  Tetrabenazine
  α-Methyl-p-tyrosine

Drugs associated with dyskinesia in idiopathic Parkinson's disease
  Levodopa/carbidopa
  Parlodel
  Pergolide

Drugs associated with dyskinesia without major activity at dopamine receptors
  Anticholinergics
  Antihistamines
  Flunarizine (and other calcium channel blockers)

Drugs associated with chorea, sterotypy, or dyskinesia during acute use and/or withdrawal
  Amphetamine
  Other stimulants
  Alcohol
  Oral contraceptives
  Anabolic steroids
  Chloroquine-based antimalarials
  Phenytoin
  Carbamazepine
  Ethosuximide
  Methsuximide
  Buspirone
  Benzodiazepines
  Cimetidine
  Methyldopa
  Diazoxide
  Digoxin
  Methadone
  Fentanyl (on withdrawal)
  Baclofen
  Flecainide
  Mianserin
  Clebopride

Other drugs and other movements
  Ceftazidine (asterixis)
  Morphine/meperidine (myoclonus)
  Monoamine oxidase inhibitors (tremor, myoclonus)

Drugs and therapies that may aggravate existing tardive dyskinesia
  Tricyclic antidepressants
  Lithium
  Benzodiazepines
  Cannabis
  Possibly electroconvulsive therapy

Since tardive dyskinesia shares clinical features of other movement disorders, it is not surprising that differential diagnostic considerations embrace a number of putatively basal ganglionic diseases. Meige syndrome is an idiopathic focal dystonia characterized by blepharospasm and oromandibular dystonia that typically begins in middle age and may be clinically indistinguishable from orofacial tardive dyskinesia. Idiopathic torsion dystonia, young-onset parkinsonism, and dopa-responsive dystonia—all diseases with predilection for the young—may also mimic tardive dystonia. Facial tics and grimacing characterize Tourette syndrome, although childhood onset, absence of neuroleptic exposure, and the characteristically fluctuating course in Tourette help to differentiate it from tardive dyskinesia. Idiopathic disorders are typically progressive and are not associated with antecedent neuroleptic exposure, in contradistinction to the static or slowly resolving course seen in tardive dyskinesia. Other differential diagnostic considerations include systemic disorders with choreoathetosis: hyperthyroidism, hypoparathyroidism, hyperglycemia, Sydenham's or lupus chorea, antiphospholipid antibody syndrome, Henoch-Schönlein purpura, chorea gravidarum, neuroacanthocytosis, and rare cases of brain tumor or other space-occupying lesions manifesting as a dyskinesia. Stereotyped mannerisms manifest in mental retardation, autism, pervasive developmental disorder, viral encephalitis, and storage and metabolic diseases (e.g., ceroid lipofuscinosis, phenylketonuria). Unusually bizarre stereotypy characterizes Rett syndrome, an idiopathic disorder of girls characterized by autism and hand- and self-clasping.

Other basal ganglia disorders have neuropsychiatric manifestations that may be the herald of disease as well as movements that may be confused with tardive dyskinesia. Clinical history and associated objective features aid in proper diagnosis. Huntington's disease, familiar as an autosomal dominant disorder linked to chromosome 4, is a progressive movement disorder and dementia with prominent choreic manifestations early in the course. Unlike in Huntington's disease, pure chorea is an unusual manifestation in tardive dyskinesia. Wilson's disease is an autosomally recessive disorder associated with a high rate of consanguinity and with onset of symptoms in childhood, adolescence, or early adulthood. Various clinical presentations, which take two major forms, have been identified. Rigidity characterizes the "dystonic" variety, whereas tremor, dysarthria and speech abnormalities, reduced dexterity, and unsteady gait characterize a "pseudosclerotic" variety. Both forms are progressive, and manifest systemic evidence of abnormal copper deposition (in Descemet's membrane at the limbus of the cornea, liver, or lenticular nucleus). Hemochromatosis and alcoholic cirrhosis with portosystemic shunting have been associated with a non-Wilsonian form of hepatolenticular degeneration. Hallervorden-Spatz disease is an autosomal recessive disorder with childhood onset. Progressive spasticity, dystonia, choreoathetosis, and dementia accompany pathologic deposition of iron in the globus pallidus and brainstem. In general, the presence of neurologic signs other than dyskinesia or dystonia (pyramidal signs, gait ataxia, prominent dementia, among other things) suggests a diagnosis other than tardive dyskinesia.

Tardive dyskinesia remains a clinical diagnosis, and there is no confirmatory diagnostic test. Analysis of gross brain specimens at autopsy have found no consistent anatomic findings in tardive dyskinesia. Controversial literature suggests that increased ventricular size, described in schizophrenia in general, may be a marker for tardive dyskinesia. Magnetic resonance data offer mixed suggestions that prolonged T1 and shortened T2 relaxation times (the latter, particularly in left caudate) may occur in the basal ganglia. Shortening of T2 relaxation may relate to iron deposition or other mineralization in basal ganglia, as has been described in other movement disorders. Positron emission tomography studies with attention to both glucose metabolism and postsynaptic D2 receptor binding have been inconclusive. Striatal metabolic rates appear normal, though increases have been observed in globus pallidus, precentral motor cortex, and thalamus and bilateral cerebellar cortices. No differences were found between controls and affective disordered patients with tardive dyskinesia in a study using ^{76}Bromine-labeled spiperone, a marker for striatal (postsynaptic) D2 receptors. Diagnostic tests may not as yet be confirmatory for tardive dyskinesia, but there is a burgeoning interest in radiographic and functional correlates to tardive dyskinesia by way of elucidating mechanisms of dyskinetic disorders in general.

RISK FACTORS, PREVALENCE, AND INCIDENCE

Age (greater than 40 years), female gender, diagnosis of an affective disorder, and a history of prior neuroleptic-associated movement disorder have been identified as risk factors for the development of tardive dyskinesia. Even for the schizophrenic index patient, a history of affective illness in a first-degree relative confers greater risk for tardive dyskinesia. With advancing age in normal, nonpsychiatric cohorts, prevalence of spontaneous dyskinesia rises. Neuroleptic-associated dyskinesia prevalence rates seem to peak into the sixth decade of life and to plateau by the age of 70. Investigators are quick to caution that not all that moves in the elderly is tardive dyskinesia, though in the aggregate, patients greater than 60 years of age may be particularly at risk for tardive dyskinesia even when rates of spontaneous dyskinesia are taken into account.

Other patient-related risk factors are more controversial or are as yet unconfirmed in prospective studies or metanalyses. Tobacco use, history of cannabis or alcohol use, "non-right-handedness," a history of obstetric complications, edentulism, negative schizophrenic symptomatology (flat affect, social isolation), a history of response to electroconvulsive therapy, and indices of cognitive impairment that hint at "organic" brain dysfunction have been identified in the still-growing literature, but have yet to be corroborated. An interesting set of observations suggests that changes in body iron status may predispose to a number of neuroleptic-associated movement disorders. Phenothiazines chelate iron, and may predispose to tardive dyskinesia by two mechanisms: iron deposition in the brain has been associated with dopamine receptor supersensitivity; neuroleptic and metal ion ligands may predispose to free radical–mediated cell damage. Diabetes mellitus has been cited as a risk factor for tardive dyskinesia. Use of metoclopramide for gastroparesis, a common dysautonomic manifestation in diabetes, may be responsible, but animal studies suggest that hyperglycemia may worsen neuroleptic-induced dyskinesia. Metoclopramide may result in concomitant parkinsonism and tardive dyskinesia relatively early in the course of treatment.

Somewhat surprisingly, length of neuroleptic treatment and lifetime dosage have not been consistently demonstrated as risk factors in tardive dyskinesia. Advancing age confounds the effect of cumulative lifetime neuroleptic exposure. Drug "holidays" and other interruptions of neuroleptic treatment increase risk of psychiatric relapse and may increase the risk of tardive dyskinesia. Early reports noted a possible relationship between neuroleptic-associated parkinsonism and later tardive dyskinesia, but other reports have claimed that patients with early so-called hyperkinetic features (tremor or akathisia) were more likely to develop tardive dyskinesia than patients who exhibit early "hypokinetic" parkinsonism. Acute dystonic reactions have also been identified as a potential risk factor.

Patients who experience early parkinsonian or acute dystonic side effects are more likely to receive anticholinergic medications in concert with a neuroleptic, and it has been speculated that anticholinergic exposure may increase tardive dyskinesia risk. On the whole, however, the literature on anticholinergic drugs and tardive dyskinesia risk is mixed. Most studies have concluded that concomitant anticholinergic therapy does not represent a treatment-related risk factor for tardive dyskinesia. Nevertheless, anticholinergics do appear to worsen existing dyskinetic, and sometimes to alleviate dystonic, tardive manifestations. The varying anticholinergic properties of different neuroleptics do not appear to confer lesser or greater risk for tardive dyskinesia.

Psychopharmacologic practice has seen a trend in recent years to treat with lower "maintenance" neuroleptic dosage, and although advisable in general to treat with the lowest dose possible with the idea of reducing *risk,* it is by no means clear whether such a trend would necessarily result in lower *incidence* of tardive dyskinesia, given that neuroleptics can mask tardive manifestations. Prior to the appearance of atypical agents in practice, the specific type of neuroleptic had not been identified as a treatment-related risk factor in tardive dyskinesia. Risk is not convincingly increased with depot preparations of high-potency agents. An anecdotal experience with some theoretic justification has held that the low-potency agent thioridazine was associated with lower long-term risk for TD. Among "typical" neuroleptics, thioridazine exhibits a slightly different profile of affinities for dopamine receptor subtypes that had been thought to confer it a relatively greater effect on mesolimbic than neocortical and striatal dopamine pathways. "Atypical" agents, including clozapine and the substituted benzamide derivatives (remoxipride, sulpiride, and tiapride), have been thought to have greater mesolimbic specificity and thus the theoretic advantage of lesser risk for motor sequelae. One report of long-term experience with clozapine (1 year's treatment) demonstrated a lower risk of tardive dyskinesia in the clozapine-treated group when compared to a cohort treated with "typical" neuroleptics, but could not exclude the possibility that clozapine caused tardive dyskinesia in two patients. Experience with the substituted benzamide derivatives and with an even newer generation of partial dopamine agonists in the treatment of psychotic disorders is in its infancy, though single-blind and guardedly favorable studies of sulpiride and remoxipride as treatment for tardive dyskinesia have emerged.

Methodologic and conceptual problems would seem to make estimates of prevalence and incidence in tardive dyskinesia problematic or unreliable. Among various studies, diagnostic criteria and tardive dyskinesia rating scales differ, and there is significant variability in psychiatric patient populations (acute and chronic inpatient, private and public hospital, and so forth). Tardive dyskinesia is a disorder that paradoxically is both caused and ameliorated by neuroleptic treatment, so a commonly recognized problem in epidemiologic studies is the notion that ongoing treatment may obscure true prevalence. Provisos notwithstanding, a large recent metanalysis reported a mean prevalence rate of 24 percent. There has been a trend for increasing prevalence since the 1970s (13.5 to 28.6 percent). Long-term prospective studies suggest that length of neuroleptic treatment correlates in nearly linear fashion over the first 6 years with rising incidence of tardive dyskinesia 5 percent each year for the first 4 years, rising to 25 percent by the end of the sixth year).

MECHANISMS

Neuroleptic-induced postsynaptic dopamine receptor supersensitivity has been implicated in the pathogenesis of tardive dyskinesia. But criticisms of the dopamine supersensitivity hypothesis in tardive dyskinesia have arisen in light of several lines of empiric evidence. Acute dopamine receptor blockade results in receptor upregulation with reliable consistency in vivo and in vitro, but the long-term receptor state is less clear. Changes in neuroleptic binding site density are not clearly different between chronically psychotic patients with and without movement disorder, and upregulation of dopamine receptors has not been demonstrated in patients with tardive dyskinesia in receptor labeling studies. Neuroleptic exposure would be expected to give rise to changes in receptor density or in postsynaptic transduction mechanisms in all patients, but only 20 percent

will manifest tardive dyskinesia. The Cebus monkey is the nearest animal model that replicates the clinical manifestations of tardive dyskinesia in humans, particularly with respect to the potential for nearly persistent dyskinesias on neuroleptic withdrawal. Reductions in glutamic acid decarboxylase and γ-aminobutyric acid (GABA) in the globus pallidus and subthalamic nucleus were the salient findings in animals with persistent dyskinesia. Changes in GABA-ergic neurotransmission may represent epiphenomena of neuroleptic exposure, but such observations nevertheless support the notion that transmitters other than dopamine may be implicated in the pathophysiology of tardive dyskinesia.

Basal ganglia connections have been elucidated in primate models, and provide a framework for understanding mechanisms in hypokinetic and hyperkinetic movement disorders that embraces the role of multiple neurotransmitters. Glutaminergic cortical efferents innervate two striatal GABA-ergic pathways; peptides are cotransmitters in both pathways. An "indirect" basal ganglia–thalamocortical circuit, perhaps of central importance in the pathophysiology of tardive dyskinesia, receives somatotopically organized, excitatory afferents from cortex, but is also inhibited by dopaminergic projections (associated with D2 receptors) arising from the substantia nigra pars compacta. In what constitutes two serial inhibitions, a striatal GABA–enkephalin–neurotensin pathway inhibits activity of lateral globus pallidus, and pallidal GABA-ergic neurons in turn inhibit excitatory glutaminergic outflow from the subthalamic nucleus directed at GABA/substance P/dynorphin–containing neurons in the medial globus pallidus. Projections from medial globus pallidus inhibit thalamic outflow. The net effect of the indirect pathway is inhibition of thalamic outflow, and the functional corollary may be suppression of unwanted movements. Although disturbances in indirect pathway activity may disinhibit thalamic outflow and result in dyskinesia, changes at the level of the striatal dopamine receptor need not be the sole determining factor of the "downstream" pallidofugal effects that result in dyskinesia.

TREATMENT

Therapeutic strategies in tardive dyskinesia attempt to exploit newer understanding of pathophysiologic mechanisms, though the multiplicity of treatment options in tardive dyskinesia speaks to the fact that no one treatment has been wholly satisfactory. Reviews of treatment studies are replete in the literature, but many trials have been limited in duration and in sample size. A practical approach, however, may be enlisted in accord with some widely accepted guidelines:

1. Since prevention is fundamental, the indications for neuroleptic treatment should be clear, and ongoing assessment of need and benefit for neuroleptic treatment should be conducted.
2. Chronic treatment should enlist the minimum effective dose.
3. The ideal of treatment in tardive dyskinesia is neuroleptic discontinuation, but if other treatment is necessary, an attempt should be made at dosage reduction, since improvement or remission may occur at lower dosage.
4. Clozapine may be a promising neuroleptic alternative.
5. In general, relatively benign agents should be added initially if there is a need for suppression of dyskinesia.

Treatment of tardive dyskinesia beyond dose reduction or neuroleptic discontinuation is usually directed at specific tardive manifestations (e.g., choreoathetoid, dystonic, and akathisic tardive dyskinesia).

Choreoathetoid Tardive Dyskinesia Options

Neuroleptic-induced neuronal damage, perhaps mediated by free radical formation, has been a recent focus in tardive dyskinesia no less than in other movement disorders. The antioxidant vitamin tocopherol may be of benefit, and at doses employed (400 to 1,200 IU/day) is not associated with significant side effects. Agents that putatively share an ability to augment GABA neurotransmission represent a second category of treatment. Clonazepam and diazepam are the most commonly used benzodiazepines, though sedation is often a limiting side effect, and tolerance with respect to anti dyskinetic effect often manifests within months. Baclofen (up to relatively high doses of 80 mg/day has been used with effect, though drug-induced parkinsonism has been described as a sequela, and sedation is common. Sodium valproate and γ-vinyl GABA have been of inconsistent use. The use of electroconvulsive therapy in tardive dyskinesia is controversial, since early reports suggested that it may increase risk for the syndrome.

Dopamine-depleting agents, reserpine and tetrabenazine in particular, currently appear to be popular choices, although orthostatic hypotension and depression are major side effects that temper enthusiasm for their use. High doses may be required and therapeutic effect may not manifest for weeks to months into treatment. Since tetrabenazine has modest dopamine receptor antagonist activity, its use is theoretically disadvantageous in the treatment of tardive dyskinesia.

Dystonic Tardive Dyskinesia Options

Reserpine, tetrabenazine, baclofen, clonazepam, and electroconvulsive therapy have been tried with limited success. Muscarinic antagonists (trihexyphenidyl, benztropine, others) are a mainstay in treatment of dystonic tardive dyskinesia manifestations, though controversy arises as to whether these agents may potentially exacerbate accompanying choreoathetosis. Intramuscular botulinum toxin, a widely accepted treatment in focal and segmental dystonias, may represent an effective treatment modality, though the complexity of tardive dystonias may necessitate injection at multiple sites.

Akathisic Tardive Dyskinesia Options

Tardive and acute akathisia mimic each other, and acute treatments have been tried in treatment of the tardive condition. In acute akathisia, anticholinergics may have lackluster effect, except in those cases in which there is coexisting parkinsonism. In tardive akathisia, anticholinergics are not useful. β-Blockers may be an option, but in general reserpine and tetrabenazine seem most effective in open clinical trials.

DRUG-INDUCED PARKINSONISM

Any or all of the cardinal signs of Parkinson's disease—resting tremor, bradykinesia, rigidity, and postural instability—may be produced by neuroleptics. As a consequence, the diagnosis of a parkinsonian syndrome is made problematic in the face of known recent neuroleptic exposure. Unlike in tardive dyskinesia, differences in neuroleptic type relate to greater or lesser likelihood of acute extrapyramidal reactions. In general, agents with higher potency (e.g., haloperidol, fluphenazine, thiothix-

ene) are associated with greater risk, and those with lower potency (e.g., thorazine, thioridazine) with lesser risk. Other medications have been associated with drug-induced parkinsonism, including reserpine, metoclopramide, and amoxapine; less commonly, chronic use of cocaine and withdrawal from alcohol, diltiazem, and other calcium channel-blockers used principally in Europe for management of vertigo (cinnarazine and flunarazine) have been implicated in drug-induced parkinsonism. Among the serotonin re-uptake inhibitors, fluoxetine may worsen motor disability in idiopathic Parkinson's disease. Fluoxetine has also been associated with worsening parkinsonism and other extrapyramidal syndromes alone and in the setting of concomitant neuroleptic treatment—in the latter instance, probably as a result of an idiosyncratic drug–drug interaction. Increased serotonergic neurotransmission may also exert inhibitory effect on midbrain dopaminergic neurons projecting to the forebrain and striatum. Sertraline, unlike other serotonergic agents, exhibits mild dopamine reuptake inhibition in vitro.

Ninety percent of cases develop within the first 3 months of treatment, but many patients will manifest parkinsonism within the first 3 weeks. Elderly women on high-potency agents are particularly at risk. In a nonpsychiatric geriatric population, parkinsonism was identified in nearly 10 percent of cases, one-half of which were thought to be drug induced. In a cohort of young psychiatric patients, a large proportion (nearly 60 percent) had some form of extrapyramidal reaction; nearly one-half of the 60 percent (29 percent) exhibited drug-induced parkinsonism. Bradykinesia or akinesia may be the only manifestation of drug-induced parkinsonism; rigidity and reduced arm swing are early and frequent findings. Mutism and dysphagia may be prominent. Tremor is less common in drug-induced parkinsonism than in idiopathic Parkinson's disease, and when present in the limbs may be either of postural, action, or resting type. But series have cited tremor in up to 35 percent of cases, and recent tremor recordings with Fourier analysis of frequency spectra suggest that low-frequency tremor, often of lateralized nature, may be more common in early drug-induced parkinsonism than is clinically appreciated. Perioral tremor (rabbit syndrome) should be considered a focal manifestation of drug-induced parkinsonism.

Several lines of evidence point to a relationship between drug-induced parkinsonism and vulnerability to parkinsonism independent of drug exposure. Drug-induced parkinsonism has reported in the setting of neuroleptic withdrawal, and although it tends to improve within weeks of drug discontinuation, persisting parkinsonism has been described for as long as 18 months in small numbers of patients. In an elderly population, 25 percent of patients with drug-induced parkinsonism developed signs of idiopathic Parkinson's disease within 41 months of drug discontinuation. Such observations have prompted speculations that drug-induced parkinsonism may manifest in patients "vulnerable" to the development of basal ganglia disease. Individual sensitivity to neuroleptics has been invoked to explain the absence of a clear dose–response relationship in drug-induced parkinsonism. As in idiopathic parkinsonism, the drug-induced syndrome is more common with advancing age. Two clinicopathologic cases have appeared in the literature in which drug-induced parkinsonism resolved with neuroleptic discontinuation, but nigral degeneration, Lewy bodies, and neurochemical evidence for loss of striatal dopamine was documented at autopsy.

Drug-induced parkinsonism should be managed with reduction in neuroleptic dosage or change to a lower potency agent when feasible from a psychiatric viewpoint. When such conservative interventions fail to have a positive effect, use of additional agents may be necessary; anticholinergics are a mainstay of treatment. Trihexyphenidyl and benzotropine are commonly used agents. Amantadine has been used in drug-induced parkinsonism with limited success. For some years, clinicians understood there to be a reciprocal relationship between dopamine and acetylcholine in basal ganglia, as supported by the observations that anticholinergics were effective treatments in drug-induced parkinsonism (though less dramatic in their use in that syndrome when compared to their use in acute dystonic reactions) and that physostigmine, a parasympathomimetic, exacerbated phenothiazine-induced parkinsonism. Yet concomitant use of high-potency neuroleptics and anticholinergics commonly results in drug-induced parkinsonism to a greater degree than is observed with isolated use of low-potency agents such as thioridazine. The implication of such empiric evidence is that dopamine receptor activity and perhaps regional differences in basal ganglia are responsible for a predisposition to the development of drug-induced parkinsonism. More recent investigations have observed that dopamine receptor blockade is qualitatively different from catecholaminergic depletion states, such as occurs with reserpine therapy. Levodopa reverses drug-induced parkinsonism in animals and humans exposed to reserpine, but doses of levodopa to as high as 1 g have not been effective in treatment of neuroleptic-induced parkinsonism.

ACUTE DYSTONIA

Acute dystonic reactions are the earliest motor manifestations of neuroleptic treatment. Nearly all cases will manifest within 5 days of initiating treatment. Clinical phenomenology is no less various than in tardive dyskinesia. Oculogyric crises, blepharospasm, trismus, oromandibular dystonia, grimacing or lip distortions, tongue protrusions in or out of the mouth (in the former case, giving rise to the so-called bon-bon sign), myoclonic contractions of face, neck, and extremities, and glossopharyngeal contractions (which may present with stridor and respiratory embarrassment) may all manifest in combination or isolation. Spasmodic torticollis or retrocollis is common, and, in children, even more dramatic truncal presentations (opisthotonos, tortipelvis) may occur. Recent reports of recurrent oculogyric crises describe accompanying obsessional thoughts and hallucinations that recall the psychiatric concomitants of oculogyria in encephalitis lethargica. Some acute dyskinesias may be indistinguishable from the dyskinesias seen in tardive dyskinesia.

Overall incidence of acute dystonic reactions is approximately 10 percent, though males of African-American or Asian-American descent may be particularly vulnerable. Prevalence rates have been quoted as high as 39 percent. High-potency agents are prone to result in acute dystonia, though dose relationship with other neuroleptics is unclear, since very low and very high doses seem to associated with less dystonia. Patients treated with serial depot injections may present with recurrent episodes, often within 72 hours of administration. Neuroleptic use in any medical or psychiatric context may result in acute dystonic reactions, although there are no well-documented cases of acute dyskinesia after reserpine treatment.

The observation that anticholinergic administration typically aborts acute dystonic reactions has fueled the notion that acute dopaminergic blockade is mechanistically responsible for acute dystonic reactions. By that formulation, use of anticholinergics

restores the dopamine–acetylcholine imbalance produced by acute dopamine antagonism. Synthesis and release of dopamine increase acutely in response to dopamine receptor blockade, and this compensatory increase, which manifests over the course of days, may be more directly responsible for acute motor manifestations, which tend to occur over the same time period. Increased dopamine turnover in the setting of repeated neuroleptic administrations tends to attenuate with time, and, in turn, patients who experience acute dystonic reactions often develop ''tolerance'' in the face of continued neuroleptic administrations. Enhanced dopamine turnover in the setting of partial dopamine receptor blockade and a relatively upregulated dopamine receptor population may therefore be responsible for acute reactions.

In patients at risk, prophylactic use of anticholinergics may be indicated, since acute adverse reactions in psychotic patients can present formidable problems in compliance. Acute dystonic reactions are treated with parenteral anticholinergics as a first line, and with parenteral benzodiazepines as an alternative measure. The latter option is less desirable, owing to the risk of respiratory depression.

AKATHISIA

Akathisia (from the Greek, ''not sitting'') refers to a disorder in which patients exhibit excessive movements (forced marching, changes in leg position, rocking in place, even moaning) associated with an inwardly felt discomfort (a pulling or drawing sensation in the legs, tension, or anxiety) relieved by the motor acts. Movements may be voluntarily suppressed for a time, but unease will mount, and patients eventually relapse into a restlessness that may mimic worsening psychosis. Haskovec first described akathisia in hysteria in 1901, though later authors observed similar clinical presentations in Parkinson's disease, encephalitis lethargica, and postencephalitic parkinsonism. Soon after the introduction of neuroleptics, numerous reports surfaced, and Deniker emphasized the association between akathisia and drug-induced parkinsonism by his designation of a ''hyperkinetic-hypertonic syndrome.'' Additional experience that neuroleptic-induced acute akathisia responded to anticholinergic medications prompted the notion, now widely held, that acute akathisia represents an extrapyramidal reaction, though others have proposed that akathisia represents an affective reaction to the ''chemical strait-jacketing'' that results from the use of neuroleptics. Case reports have recently appeared linking akathisia with the serotonin re-uptake inhibitor fluoxetine. Though a rare side effect, the degree of subjective dismay, described as a feeling that one were ready to ''jump out of one's skin,'' has been thought to contribute to suicide attempts in several cases. High doses of fluoxetine and rapid dose escalation may increase risk. Mechanism is unknown, though serotonin-mediated down regulation of dopamine has been proposed.

The subjective experience of akathisia may help to distinguish acute akathisia from the tardive form, whose motor manifestations may be the same as in the acute state or may resemble the stereotypies and other adventitious movements of tardive dyskinesia. Akathisia shares some features with restless legs syndrome, but in the latter, symptoms are typically restricted to the legs, tend to manifest only in recumbency, and are relieved with walking. Associated periodic movements of sleep, myoclonus, and dystonic postures in the evening also serve to distinguish restless legs from acute akathisia. So-called pseudoakathisia refers to motoric features without associated subjective distress. It has been said that inner tension drives movement in acute akathisia, whereas movements cause ''secondary'' dismay in tardive states, though the distinction is often difficult to draw in clinical practice.

Acute akathisia should be suspected in any patient who exhibits both subjective and objective restlessness in the setting of first neuroleptic exposure, change to a higher potency agent, or increase in dosage of a standing neuroleptic. Akathisia may manifest more commonly in middle-aged women. Worsening ''psychotic'' agitation in the setting of escalating dosage should be a clue to neuroleptic-induced akathisia. ''Cyclic'' akathisia has been described in patients who receive regular depot injections. Since akathisia has been thought to be a dose- and potency-related phenomenon, conservative use of low-potency agents has been advocated as a first step in management.

Pharmacologic treatments have met with inconsistent results, and therapeutic options have been limited by an incomplete understanding of pathophysiology in akathisia. Traditionally, anticholinergics have been a mainstay, though their efficacy in akathisia is far less compelling that in neuroleptic-induced acute dystonia and drug-induced parkinsonism. When akathisia is accompanied by parkinsonism, anticholinergics may be a reasonable first-line agent. More recent literature suggests that lipophilic β-adrenergic agents may be most effective. Benzodiazepines provide some relief for subjective distress. Trials of amantadine, clonidine, and opiates have been limited or disappointing.

NEUROLEPTIC MALIGNANT SYNDROME

Neuroleptic malignant syndrome is an uncommon complication of neuroleptic therapy, thought to occur in less than 1 percent of patients. Hyperthermia (greater than 37°C) and muscle rigidity are cardinal features that manifest soon after neuroleptic exposure or after an increase in neuroleptic dosage. Associated phenomena include changes in mental status (principally an acute confusional state), evidence of autonomic instability (tachycardia, blood pressure fluctuation, tachypnea), elevations in creatine phosphokinase, leukocytosis, and metabolic acidosis. Acute withdrawal of levodopa or dopamine agonist in the setting of Parkinson's disease may also induce an neuroleptic malignant syndrome–like condition. Infection, dehydration, use of high-potency agents, and withdrawal of anticholinergic agents may predispose to the development of neuroleptic malignant syndrome. Mortality typically results from pulmonary embolism associated with deep venous thrombosis, renal failure, cardiovascular collapse, or pneumonia, and has been quoted at 10 to 25 percent of cases. The syndrome can manifest at any age, independent of gender and psychiatric diagnosis, though young men may be more commonly afflicted. Neuroleptic malignant syndrome may manifest after brief or even single exposure to neuroleptics. Though generally not associated with extrapyramidal reactions, the dibenzodiazepine clozapine has also been linked with neuroleptic malignant syndrome in several case reports.

Differential diagnosis includes meningitis, encephalitis, intercurrent systemic infection, heat stroke, anticholinergic toxicity, and malignant hyperthermia. Neuroleptic malignant syndrome resembles lethal catatonia, a rare condition described before the advent of neuroleptics, characterized by mutism, akinesia, fixed abnormal postures, and rigidity often in patients with a recent history of psychotic agitation. Profoundly catatonic patients may exhibit fever and dysautonomia. In light of data indicating that reintroduction of neuroleptic in patients with past neuroleptic malignant syndrome will precipitate another bout in only 25 percent of cases (but in up to 50 percent of cases in which the same neuroleptic or one of similar potency is used), it has been proposed that concomitant factors must predispose to neuroleptic malignant syndrome. Intercurrent illness, psychotic agitation, and dehydration have been suggested as possible predisposing causes. Other authors have suggested that lithium may act synergistically with neuroleptics to induce neuroleptic malignant syndrome by inhibition of dopamine-sensitive adenylate cyclase, inhibition of striatal dopamine, or prolonged blockade at dopamine receptors. A recently described ''serotonin syndrome'' associated with the concomitant use of serotonin re-uptake inhibitors and monoamine oxidase inhibitors presents with changes in mental status, including confusion and restlessness, diaphoresis, shivering, tremor, myoclonus, and hyperreflexia, and may mimic neuroleptic malignant syndrome. It has been suggested that neuroleptic malignant syndrome may be one entity in a spectrum of disorders in which muscular hypermetabolism and hyperthermia constitute a final common pathway. Comparison with malignant hyperthermia is often invoked in understanding pathophysiologic mechanisms in neuroleptic malignant syndrome. The connection between the two entities has been supported by similarities in muscle biopsy specimens in neuroleptic malignant syndrome and malignant hyperthermia. However, unlike malignant hyperthermia, anesthetic agents do not predispose to neuroleptic malignant syndrome, and patients with malignant hyperthermia are not at greater risk for neuroleptic malignant syndrome after neuroleptic exposure. Malignant hyperthermia is a hereditary disorder in which succinylcholine and inhalant anesthetics produce muscle contraction by triggering calcium influx of calcium into muscle cytoplasm. Though mechanistically distinct, malignant hyperthermia and neuroleptic malignant syndrome share similar clinical phenomenology, suggesting that different triggers may exist for the development of hypermetabolic ''stress'' in skeletal muscle.

Theories regarding mechanism in neuroleptic malignant syndrome invoke dopaminergic blockade, perhaps at the level of hypothalamus. An interesting recent observation of reduced serum iron levels in a prospective study of 32 episodes of neuroleptic malignant syndrome over 9 years has led to the notion that reduced serum iron may result in changes in central dopamine receptor sensitivity, thereby increasing vulnerability to neuroleptic malignant syndrome.

Treatment is largely supportive. Neuroleptic, anticholinergic, and lithium salts are discontinued, and special attention is paid to fluid status, control of blood pressure and fever, and treatment of concurrent infection. Subcutaneous heparin is used to prevent deep venous thrombosis. Bromocriptine, dantrolene, and levodopa may each have a role in refractory cases, but their efficacy is unclear, and their routine use is not universally accepted practice.

SUGGESTED READINGS

American Psychiatric Association Task Force on Tardive Dyskinesia: Tardive dyskinesia: a task force report of the American Psychiatric Association. APA Press, Washington, DC, 1992

Ayd FJ: A survey of drug-induced extrapyramidal reactions. JAMA 175:1054, 1961

Casey DE: Neuroleptic-induced acute extrapyramidal syndromes and tardive dyskinesia. Psychiatr Clin North Am 16:589, 1993

Jeste DV, Caligiuri MP: Tardive dyskinesia. Schizophr Bull 19:303, 1993

Kane JM, Smith JM: Tardive dyskinesia: prevalence and risk factors, 1959–1979. Arch Gen Psychiatry 39:473, 1982

Kane JM, Woerner M, Lieberman J: Tardive dyskinesia: prevalence, incidence, and risk factors. J Clin Psychopharmacol 8:525, 1988

Kang UJ, Burke RE, Fahn S: Natural history and treatment of tardive dystonia. Mov Disord 3:193, 1986

Khot V, Wyatt RJ: Not all that moves is tardive dyskinesia. Am J Psychiatry 148:661, 1991

Lang AE, Weiner WJ: Drug-Induced Movement Disorders. Futura, Mt. Kisco, NY 1992

Lazarus A, Mann SC, Caroff SN: The neuroleptic malignant syndrome and related conditions. APA Press, Washington, D.C., 1989

Marsden CD, Tarsy D, Baldessarini RJ: Spontaneous and drug-induced movement disorders in psychotic patients. p. 219. In Benson DF, Blumer D (eds): Psychiatric Aspects of Neurologic Disease. Grune & Stratton, New York, 1975

Rupniak NMJ, Jenner P, Marsden CD: Acute dystonia induced by neuroleptic drugs. Psychopharmacology 88:403, 1986

Tarsy D: Akathisia. p. 88. In Joseph AB, Young RR (eds): Movement Disorders in Neurology and Neuropsychiatry. Blackwell Scientific Publications Boston, 1992

Tarsy D, Baldessarini RJ: Tardive dyskinesia. Ann Rev Med 35:605, 1984

Yassa R, Jeste DV: Gender differences in tardive dyskinesia: a critical review of the literature. Schizophr Bull 18:701, 1992

124. PRIMARY AND SECONDARY GENERALIZED DYSTONIAS

JOSEPH JANKOVIC

Dystonia is a neurologic syndrome dominated by involuntary, sustained (tonic), or spasmodic (rapid or clonic), patterned, and repetitive muscle contractions, frequently causing twisting and other abnormal movements or postures. The most frequent forms of dystonia include blepharospasm, an involuntary closure of eyelids caused by forceful contractions of the orbicularis oculi; oromandibular dystonia, manifested by jaw closure (trismus, bruxism) or jaw opening; cervical dystonia, manifested by torticollis, retrocollis, anterocollis, and other twisting movements of the neck; and writer's cramp. Because of its variable presentation and fluctuating intensity, dystonia is often wrongly attributed to psychological causes. Traditional desriptions of dystonia emphasize that the muscle contractions are sustained; hence, rapid movements are often not recognized as dystonic. These rapid movements resemble myoclonus, which is a jerk-like movement produced by brief muscular contractions (positive myoclonus) or inhibitions (negative myoclonus). Some patients have both dystonia and myoclonus (dystonia-myoclonus syndrome). The latter disorder often improves with alcohol intake. One of the most characteristic features of dystonia, which helps differentiate it from the other hyperkinetic movement disorders, is that dystonic movements, whether slow or rapid, are repetitive and patterned (involving the same group of muscles). This is in contrast to chorea, which consists of brief movements that flow randomly from one body part to another. Tics are abrupt movements (or sounds) that are usually more intermittent and coordinated than dystonia or myoclonus, more easily suppressable, and are often preceded by premonitory symptoms such as an urge or a "tension" that is temporarily relieved by the execution of the tic. Some tics are more sustained and are referred to as dystonic tics.

Although dystonic movements are usually continual, the timing and intensity of the movements can be influenced by various factors, including emotion, fatigue, relaxation, motor activity, sensory tricks, and sleep. Rarely, dystonia can fluctuate so much that it might be absent in the morning and become pronounced and disabling in the afternoons and evenings. This diurnal dystonia usually occurs in children and young adults, may be associated with parkinsonian features in the patients and their relatives, and usually improves dramatically with levodopa. Not all patients with dopa-responsive dystonia have diurnal variations, and many patients with dopa-responsive dystonia are initially misdagnosed as having cerebral palsy. Another type of noncontinual dystonia are the paroxysmal dystonias. These are characterized by an abrupt onset or an exacerbation of dystonic movements lasting seconds to hours. They may be induced by a sudden movement (kinesigenic dystonia) or may occur spontaneously (nonkinesigenic dystonia). Paroxysmal dystonia may be sporadic or inherited, but head trauma, certain metabolic disorders, and other causes can produced paroxysmal dystonia. An example of secondary paroxysmal dystonia is the "oculogyric crisis" characterized by a sudden, intermittent, conjugate eye deviations, sometimes seen in patients with postencephalitic parkinsonism, Tourette syndrome, and drug-induced dystonia.

The severity of dystonia varies from a barely noticeable and often unrecognized symptom to disabling muscle contractions rendering the patient unable to ambulate or fully participate in activities of daily living. In several of the patients at my institution, the dystonic muscle contractions were so severe they produced muscle breakdown and myoglobinuria. Primary idiopathic dystonia often starts as a task-specific dystonia (e.g., writer's cramp). With increasing severity, however, the dystonic movements may occur in other, less specific activities and at rest and may eventually overflow to adjacent or other muscles. If left untreated, dystonia may evolve into fixed postures and contractures. Secondary dystonia usually is present at rest, even at onset.

Dystonia is often associated with either dystonic or essential-type tremor. Dystonic tremor is actually a rhythmic dystonia, most evident when the patient voluntarily attempts to move in the direction opposite to the force of dystonia. Thus, a patient with torticollis to the right, when attempting to maintain primary head position, may develop lateral irregular tremor that disappears when the patient "allows" the head to turn to the right (in the direction of the torticollis). In contrast, patients with coexistent essential-type tremor continue to have the oscillatory movement regardless of the direction of the force of the dystonia. Although the two types of tremor usually can be identified clinically, the differentiation may be aided by the use of electromyography. It is not yet clear whether the postural tremor associated with dystonia, such as the hand flexion-extension tremor seen in 25 percent of patients with cervical dystonia, is a form of essential tremor or whether it is an expression of some dystonia-related physiologic abnormality. A pathogenetic relationship between dystonia and essential tremor is suggested by the frequent ocurrence of essential-type postural tremor in family members of patients with dystonia. In some patients, head and trunk tremor (2- to 5-Hz frequency) may precede the onset of dystonia and may be the initial manifestation or forme fruste of dystonia (dystonic tremor). Certain task-specific tremors (e.g., primary writing tremor) may actually represent forms of focal dystonia. Some patients with primary writing tremor voluntarily contract their forearm muscles in an attempt to control the hand tremor. This compensatory muscle contraction is sometimes wrongly attributed to dystonia. Although the frequent coexistence of essential tremor and dystonia suggests that there is a pathogenetic link between the two disorders, linkage analyses have excluded the dystonia gene (DYT1) on chromosome 9 in hereditary essential tremor. This suggests that the genes for these two disorders are on separate loci or that the relationship between the two types of tremor is physiologic rather than genetic. Besides essential tremor and myoclonus, dystonia is occasionally also associated with other movement disorders, including parkinsonism.

The epidemiology of dystonia has not been studied by appropriate methods, but it has been estimated that there is at least 100,000 individuals with dystonia in the United States. If dystonic writer's cramp were included, the true prevalence would be much greater because the vast majority of patients with dystonic writer's cramp do not seek medical attention.

CLASSIFICATION

There are many ways to classify dystonia, but it is convenient to categorize dystonia according to its age at onset, etiology, and anatomic distribution.

Age at Onset

Age at onset is one of the most predictable determinants of future course and prognosis. Dystonia may start at any age and may be categorized as either infantile (less than 2 years), childhood (2 to 12 years), juvenile (13 to 20 years), or adult onset (older than 20 years). Childhood-onset dystonia, particularly common among Ashkenazi Jews, is often characterized by caudal-rostral progression, with legs being more involved early in the course. Whereas childhood-onset dystonia usually becomes generalized, adult-onset dystonia usually remains focal or segmental. A typical presentation of childhood-onset dystonia is inversion of one foot while running; the best examples of adult-onset dystonia are blepharospasm and torticollis.

Etiology

Dystonia is either a symptom of an underlying disorder (secondary dystonia) or a specific disease entity, in which case it is referred to as primary or idiopathic torsion dystonia. Primary torsion dystonia can be either sporadic or inherited, and it is not associated with any cognitive, pyramidal, cerebellar, or sensory abnormalities. The most important advance in our knowledge about genetic dystonia has been the identification of a gene marker for idiopathic Jewish and non-Jewish autosomal-dominant dystonia in the q34 region on chromosome 9. In about one-third of those carrying the gene, it is expressed clinically (30 to 40% penetrance). Using markers that are closely linked to the dystonia gene, several studies have demonstrated that many cases thought to be sporadic are acutally inherited. This is particularly true among dystonic patients of Ashkenazi Jewish origin. The gene for the dopa-responsive dystonia has been localized to the 14q chromosome.

Not all dystonias are of genetic origin; some are sporadic and others are secondary to some specific causes (Table 124-

1). Of the secondary dystonias, Wilson's disease is particularly important to recognize because early treatment of this autosomal recessive disease can result in a complete or near complete abolishment of neurologic and liver problems. Virtually any metabolic or structural lesion of the brain, particularly if it involves the putamen, other basal ganglia, and rostral brainstem structures, can produce dystonia.

About 40 percent of all patients with dystonia have been previously misdiagnosed as having a psychogenic illness. In actuality, however, less than 5 percent of all dystonias seen in a movement disorders clinic are of psychogenic origin, and the frequency is even lower in general neurologic practice. The differentiation between psychogenic and neurologic dystonia represents one of the most formidable challenges facing the clinical neurologist. Because primary dystonia is not associated with any laboratory abnormalities, the diagnosis of psychogenic dystonia must be based on positive criteria; it is not sufficient to merely exclude other causes. Certain clues usually provide evidence of a psychogenic etiology. These include false weakness, false sensory symptoms, multiple somatizations, self-inflicted injuries, bizarre movements or pseudoseizures, obvious psychiatric illness, and other features that are incongruous with typical dystonia. Relief of dystonia with psychotherapy, powerful suggestion, placebo, or physiotherapy virtually excludes a neurologic etiology because complete and permanent remissions are rare in "organic" forms of dystonia. Improvement under hypnosis or with amobarbital is not particularly helpful since both can ameliorate even neurologic dystonia. On the other hand, acute exacerbation and relief of the dystonia by a powerful suggestion coupled with intravenous or oral placebo provides important support for the diagnosis of psychogenic dystonia.

Besides Wilson's disease, another important cause of secondary dystonia is drug-induced dystonia. The dopamine receptor-blocking drugs (neuroleptics, such as the major tranquilizers, and gastrointestinal drugs, such as metoclopramide) can cause not only an acute transient dystonic reaction, but a persistent dystonic disorder (tardive dystonia). Besides central etiologies, which presumably account for the vast majority of dystonias, peripherally induced dystonia caused by an injury to a nerve or a nerve root, often associated with reflex sympathetic dystrophy, is being increasingly recognized as an important cause of focal and segmental dystonia.

Distribution

Dystonia is classified according to its anatomic distribution as focal, segmental, multifocal, generalized, and unilateral (hemidystonia).

Cranial Dystonia. Craniocervical structures are most frequently affected in adult-onset dystonia. Blepharospasm, an involuntary bilateral eye closure produced by spasmodic contractions of the entire (pretarsal, preseptal, and periorbital) orbicularis oculi muscles, is often accompanied by dystonic movements of the eyebrows and of the paranasal, facial, masticatory, labial, lingual, oral, pharyngeal, laryngeal, and cervical muscles. Blepharospasm is often exacerbated by exposure to bright light, wind, and air pollution, as well as by activity and stress. In most patients with blepharospasm, the onset is often heralded by increased frequency of blinking associated with a "sandlike" feeling of irritation in the eyes. Blepharospasm usually starts with clonic contractions of the eyelids, gradually

TABLE 124-1. Etiologic Classification of Dystonia

Primary dystonia
  Sporadic (idiopathic torsion dystonia)
  Inherited (hereditary torsion dystonia)
    Classic idiopathic torsion dystonia (pure dystonia, autosomal dominant, DYT1 [dystonia] gene)
    Non-classic idiopathic torsion dystonia (autosomal dominant)
    Atypical dystonia (autosomal dominant)
    Myoclonic dystonia (alcohol-responsive, autosomal dominant)

Secondary dystonia
  Associated with neurodegenerative disorders
    Sporadic
      Parkinson's disease
      Progressive supranuclear palsy
      Multiple system atrophy
      Multiple sclerosis
      Central pontine myelinolysis
    Inherited
      Dopa-responsive dystonia (gene on chromosome 14)
      Rapid-onset dystonia-parkinsonism
      Early-onset dystonia with parkinsonism
      Paroxysmal dystonia (kinesigenic, nonkinesigenic)
      X-linked recessive (dystonia-parkinsonism, in Philipinos)
      Wilson's disease
      Huntington's disease
      Juvenile parkinsonism-dystonia
      Progressive pallidal degeneration
      Hallervorden-Spatz disease
      Joseph's disease
      Ataxia telangiectasia
      Neuroacanthocytosis
      Rett syndrome
      Intraneuronal inclusion disease
      Infantile bilateral striatal necrosis
      Familial basal ganglia calcifications
      Spinocerebellar degeneration
      Olivopontocerebellar atrophy
      Hereditary spastic paraplegia with dystonia
  Associated with metabolic disorders
    Amino acid disorders
      Glutaric acidemia
      Methylmalonic acidemia
      Homocystinuria
      Hartnup's disease
      Tyrosinosis
    Lipid disorders
      Metachromatic leukodystrophy
      Ceroid lipofuscinosis
      Dystonic lipidosis ("sea blue" histiocytosis)
      Gangliosidoses
        GMI variant
        GM2 variants
      Hexosaminidase A and B deficiency
    Miscellaneous metabolic disorders
      Mitochondrial encephalopathies
        Leigh's disease
        Leber's disease
        Lesch-Nyhan syndrome
        Triosephosphate isomerase deficiency
        Vitamin E deficiency

Due to a known specific cause
  Perinatal cerebral injury and kernicterus
    Athetoid cerebral palsy
    Delayed-onset dystonia
  Infection
    Viral encephalitis
    Encephalitis lethargica
    Reye syndrome
    Subacute sclerosing panencephalitis
    Creutzfeldt-Jakob disease
    Acquired immunodeficiency syndrome
  Other
    Tuberculosis
    Syphilis
    Acute infectious torticollis
  Paraneoplastic brainstem encephalitis
  Cerebral vascular or ischemic injury
  Brain tumor
  Arteriovenous malformation
  Head trauma and brain surgery
  Peripheral trauma
  Toxins
    MN
    CO
    CS2
    Methanol
    Disulfiram
    Wasp sting
  Drugs
    Levodopa
    Bromocriptine
    Antipsychotics
    Metoclopramide
    Fenfluramine
    Flecainide
    Ergot
    Anticonvulsants
    Certain calcium channel-blockers
    Ergots

Psychogenic

Pseudodystonia
  Atlantoaxial subluxation
  Syringomyelia
  Arnold-Chiari malformation
  Trochlear nerve palsy
  Vestibular torticollis
  Posterior fossa mass
  Soft tissue neck mass
  Congenital postural torticollis
  Cojngenital Klippel-Feil syndrome
  Sandiffer's syndrome
  Stiff-person syndrome

(Modified from Jankovic J and Fahn S: Dystonic disorders. pp. 337–74. In Jankovic J, Tolosa E (eds): Parkinson's Disease and Movement Disorders. 2nd Ed. Williams & Wilkins, Baltimore, 1993, with permission.)

progressing to more sustained and forceful eye closure. Eventually, patients have difficulty reading, watching television, driving, and performing other daily activities that depend on normal vision. If left untreated, up to 15 percent become functionally blind. Various maneuvers such as wearing dark glasses, pulling on an upper eyelid, pinching the neck, talking, humming, or singing, can transiently relieve the involuntary eye closure in some patients. Afflicted women outnumber men 3 to 1 and in the vast majority, symptoms commences by 50 years of age.

Oromandibular dystonia consists of involuntary spasms of jaw, mouth, and tongue muscles producing jaw closure and trismus (jaw clenching) and bruxism (tooth grinding), often causing secondary dental wear and temporomandibular joint syndrome. In addition, involuntary tongue movements, jaw opening, or jaw deviation may cause difficulties with chewing, speaking, and swallowing. Oromandibular dystonia should be differentiated from hemifacial or hemimasticatory spasm, tardive dyskinesia, tetany, tetanus, and mechnanical disorder of the temporomandibular joint. Focal cranial and oromandibular dystonias are also discussed in Chapter 126.

Cervical Dystonia. Cervical dystonia is the most common form of focal dystonia encountered in a movement disorder clinic. Although torticollis, lateral rotation of the head, is the most frequent abnormal posture, the majority of patients have a combination of torticollis, laterocollis, retrocollis, and anterocollis. In addition to cervical involvement, at least one-third all patients with cervical dystonia have scoliosis, suggesting additional involvement of the thoracic muscles. Local pain accompanies cervical dystonia in more than one-third of all patients. The pain can be caused by intense muscular spasms or by associated cervical spondylotic radiculomyelopathy.

Cervical dystonia is often exacerbated during periods of stress or fatigue and is usually relieved by relaxation and various sensory maneuvers. Up to 20 percent of patients achieve spontaneous remission, but the dystonia usually recurs after a period of several months. In the vast majority of patients, cervical dystonia is a lifelong disorder, and in about 20 percent of patients, it progresses to a segmental or a generalized dystonia. Similar to other forms of dystonia, the abnormal muscle contractions that produce head deviation can be temporarily controlled by a variety of sensory tricks, such as touching the chin, face, or back of the head. Whereas this observation suggests that cervical dystonia can be influenced by altering the proprioceptive input, the exact mechanism of the "counterpressure," "sensory trick," or "geste antagoniste" phenomenon is not known. Focal cervical dystonia is discussed in more detail in Chapter 125.

Laryngeal Dystonia (Spasmodic Dysphonia). The career of a teacher, a trial attorney, or a professional singer can be prematurely ended with the development of spasmodic dysphonia. Despite growing evidence in support of neurologic origin, the symptoms are still too often attributed to psychogenic causes. Dystonia of the larynx may cause excessive and uncontrolled closing of the vocal folds (adductor spasmodic dysphonia), producing effortful and strained voice interrupted by frequent breaks in phonation. The abductor form of spasmodic dysphonia is much less common and it consists of prolonged vocal fold openings, producing breathy and whispering voice and phonatory pauses extending into vowels. The adductor spasmodic dysphonia is caused by hyperadductions of the thyroarytenoid vocalis complex, and the abductor form of spasmodic dysphonia is due to contractions of the posterior cricoarytenoid muscle. Whereas nearly all cases of adductor spasmodic dysphonia are thought to represent a form of focal dystonia (see also Ch. 125), many cases of abductor dysphonia are thought to be of psychogenic origin. Many patients with spasmodic dysphonia also have voice tremor, and in some cases, isolated voice tremor precedes the onset of spasmodic dysphonia by several years.

Limb Dystonia. Idiopathic limb dystonia usually starts as an action dystonia. In contrast, secondary dystonia, caused either by central (brain) or peripheral (nerve or root) injury or lesion, is often present at rest, even at the onset. The task-specific focal dystonias seen in many occupational cramps (e.g., graphospasm or writer's cramp) is the most common example of idiopathic arm dystonia. The task- or position-specific dystonias often occur with writing, typing, and feeding, during certain sports-related activities, and while playing musical instruments.

Similar to other forms of dystonia, hand and arm dystonias are often associated with either dystonic or essential type tremor. For example, some patients with writer's cramp may display involuntary supination of the hand away from the desk and when the patient volitionally pronates the hand in the act of writing, a twisting, jerking movement may appear. Such dystonic tremor occurs only during a specific action and the tremor may not be evident when arms are outstretched in front of the body or when placed in any other position. However, about one-third of patients with focal, task-specific dystonia experience a coexistent postural, essential-like tremor manifested by a flexion-extension oscillation of the hand during posture holding. When dystonia affects the foot in an adult, the possibility of

Parkinson's disease or a parkinsonian syndrome as the cause of the foot dystonia should be considered. Besides the striatal foot, some Parkinson's patients have a striatal hand deformity, often confused with rheumatoid arthritis. In children, the foot can twist into an equinovarus posture when the patient is running or walking, or the leg might kick during walking. The foot and leg dystonia may evolve into a fixed dystonic posture, commonly causing plantar flexion, extension at the knee, and flexion-adduction at the hip.

Trunk Dystonia. Trunk dystonia can result in scoliosis, lordosis, kyphosis, tortipelvis, and opisthotonic posturing. At onset, abnormal movements of the trunk may be seen during walking or running, but in the advanced stages of the disease, the trunk deformities become fixed and present even when the patient is sitting or lying. Many patients with trunk dystonia have a bizarre gait resembling the gaits of various animals; hence the terms *dromedary-, monkey-,* and *ducklike gait.* Various sensory tricks, such as placing the hands in the pockets, behind the neck or back, or on the hip, might enable the patient to walk relatively normally. Also, running, walking backward, or dancing might improve the truncal dystonia and dystonic gait.

Hemidystonia. In contrast to other types of dystonias, which are usually idiopathic, about 85 percent of patients with hemidystonia have computed tomography or magnetic resonance imaging evidence of contralateral basal ganglia lesion, a history of hemiparesis, or both. Besides ischemic or hemorrhagic strokes, other causes of hemidystonia include perinatal or other head trauma, thalamotomy, encephalitis, neurodegenerative disorders, arteriovenous malformation, and porencephalic cyst. Whereas a relatively long delay of several year between injury and onset is rather typical for dystonia related to perinatal injury, the latency between the acute lesion and subsequent onset of dystonia is often less than 6 months in adult patients.

ANATOMY, BIOCHEMISTRY, AND PATHOPHYSIOLOGY

Although in most patients with dystonia no specific abnormality can be identified by neuroimaging or autopsy studies, there is convincing evidence supporting central origin (basal ganglia, brainstem, or both) for this movement disorder. Some brains of patients with atypical dystonia have been found to have a mosaic pattern of striatal gliosis. Studies of patients with secondary dystonia have identified lesions involving the basal ganglia, particularly putamen, and the rostral brainstem. The involvement of basal ganglia in dystonia is also supported by the finding of reduced glucose metabolism, as demonstrated by position emission tomography scans, in the basal ganglia, the frontal projection field of the mediodorsal thalamic nucleus, and in the frontal cortex of patients with idiopathic torsion dystonia. No consistent abnormalities have been demonstrated in the few brains of patients with dystonia examined at autopsy. Neurophysiologic studies in patients with dystonia showed prolonged firing of electromyelographic activity with co-contraction of antagonist muscles, repetitive and slow spasms of 1 to 2 seconds each and separated by equal periods of relative electromyelographic silence (previously termed "myorhythmia"), postural 6- to 10-Hz frequency tremor, reduced reciprocal inhibition, and abnormal H reflex and blink reflex recovery cycle. These findings have been interpreted as being indicative of enhanced excitatory drive to the rostral brainstem or reduced spinal and brainstem inhibition.

TREATMENT

Despite paucity of knowledge about the cause and pathogenesis of most dystonic disorders, the symptomatic treatment of dystonia has markedly improved, largely as a result of the introduction of botulinum toxin. This therapeutic intervention is discussed in Chapter 125. Before contemplating symptomatic therapy, potentially curable causes of dystonia, such as certain drug-induced dystonias or Wilson's disease, should be considered. Physical therapy, including well-fitted braces, may be helpful to some dystonic patients, but are usually unsatisfactory when used alone.

Although there is little scientific rationale for the drugs used in the treatment of dystonia, about one-third of patients have been found to benefit from some pharmacologic therapy (Table 124-2). The selection of a particular choice of therapy is largely guided by personal clinical experience and by empiric trials. The first treatment of choice is usually determined by its low potential for adverse effects and by the anatomic distribution of dystonia (Table 124-3). Although only less than 10 percent of all children with dystonia have dopa-responsive dystonia, all patients with childhood-onset dystonia should be first treated with levodopa/carbidopa (Sinemet). Anticholinergic medications such as trihexyphenidyl have been found to be most effective for generalized dystonia. This therapy is generally well tolerated when the dose is increased slowly. It is generally recommended to start with a 2-mg preparation, one-half tablet at bedtime and advancing up to 12 mg/day over the next 4 weeks, eventually switiching to sustained-release preparations such as Artane Sequels (5 mg). Some patients require up to 60 to 100

mg/d, but may experience dose-related drowsiness, confusion, memory difficulty, and hallucinations. Pyridostigmine, a peripherally acting anticholinestarase, and eye drops of pilocarpine (a muscarinic agonist) often ameliorate at least some of the peripheral side effects such as dry mouth, urinary retention, and blurred vision.

Many patients require a combination of several medications and treatments. Benzodiazepines (clonazepam or lorazepam) may provide additional benefit for patients whose response to anticholinergic drugs is unsatisfactory. Baclofen may be helpful for oromandibular dystonia, but is only minimally effective for generalized dystonia. In selected cases of severe axial and generalized dystonia, however, continuous intrathecal infusions of baclofen may be useful. Dopamine receptor-blocking drugs or neuroleptics (e.g., fluphenazine) have been used in the treatment of dystonia, often in conjunction with anticholinergics. The use of dopamine receptor-blocking drugs in the treatment of dystonia, however, should be discouraged because of the potential for development of tardive dyskinesia. This risk may be possibly minimized by coadministrating reserpine or tetrabenazine. Tetrabenazine, a presynaptic dopamine-depleting drug, has been useful in some patients with dystonia, but its availability in the United States is limited. Attacks of kinesigenic paroxysmal dystonia may be controlled with anticonvulsants (e.g., carbamezapine, phenytoin), but the nonkinesigenic forms of paroxysmal dystonia are less responsive to pharmacologic therapy, although clonazepam and acetazolamide may be beneficial.

Surgical approaches, such as local denervation, muscle excision, and thalamotomy may be recommended to those patients who continue to have disabling dystonia despite other less invasive therapies.

TABLE 124-2. Pharmacologic Therapy for Dystonia[a]

Generic Name	Trade Name	Daily Dosage (mg)	Mechanism of Action
Trihexyphenidyl	Artane	6–40	Anticholinergic
Benztropine	Cogentin	4–15	Anticholinergic
Orphenadrine	Norflex	200–800	Anticholinergic
Clonazepam	Klonopin	1–12	Serotonergic; relaxant
Lorazepam	Ativan	1–16	Relaxant
Diazepam	Valium	10–100	Relaxant
Cyclobenzaprine	Flexeril	20–60	Relaxant
Chlodiazedoxide	Librium	10–100	Relaxant
Baclofen	Lioresal	40–120	Antispastic; γ-aminobutyric acid agonist; substance P antagonist
Primidone	Mysoline	50–800	Antiepileptic; antitremor
Valproate	Depakote	500–1,500	Antiepileptic; γ-aminobutyric acid-T inhibitor
Carbamazepine	Tegretol	1,600–1,600	Antiepileptic
Levodopa/carbidopa	Sinemet (CR)	75/300–200/2,000	Dopamine precursor
Bromocriptine	Parlodel	10–60	Dopamine agonist
Lisuride		1–10	Dopamine agonist
Pergolide	Permax	0.5–5	Dopamine agonist
Pimozide	Orap	2–10	Dopamine blocker
Lithium	Lithobid	600–1,800	Antidopaminergic
Tetrabenazine	Nitoman	50–300	Monoamine depleter and blocker
Combination Tetrabenazine		75	
Pimozide		6–25	
Trihexyphenidyl		6–30	
Botulinum toxin	Botox	5–400	Blocks acetilcholine release at neuromuscular junction units

[a] Surgical therapies include myectomy, peripheral denervation, or thalamotomy.

TABLE 124-3. A Guide for Symptomatic Treatment of Dystonia

Focal dystonias
  Blepharospasm
    Clonzepam, lorazepam
    Trihexyphenidyl
    Botulinum toxin injections
    Orbicularis oculi myectomy
  Oromandibular dystonia
    Baclofen
    Trihexyphenidyl
    Botulinum toxin injections
  Spasmodic dysphonia
    Botulinum toxin injections
    Voice and supportive therapy
  Cervical
    Trihexyphenidyl
    Diazepam, lorazepam, clonazepam
    Botulinum toxin injections
    Tetrabenazine
    Cycobenzaprine
    Carbamazepine
    Baclofen
    Peripheral surgical denervation
  Task-specific dystonias (e.g., writer's cramp)
    Benztropine, trihexyphenidyl
    Botulinum toxin injections
    Occupational therapy

Segmental and generalized dystonias
  Levodopa (in children to young adults)
  Trihexyphenidyl, benztropine
  Diazepam, lorazepam, clonazepam
  Baclofen (oral, intrathecal)
  Carbamazepine
  Tetrabenazine (with lithium)
  Triple therapy: tetrabenazine, fluphenazine, trihexyphenidyl
  Thalamotomy

SUGGESTED READINGS

Brewer GJ, Yuzbasiyan-Gurka V: Wilson's disease. Medicine 71:139–64, 1992

Ceballos-Baumann AO, Passingham RE, Warner T et al: Overactive prefrontal and underactive motor cortical areas in idiopathic dystonia. Ann Neurol 37:363–72, 1995

Deuschl G, Heinen F, Kleedorfer B et al: Clinical and polymyographic investigation of spasmodic torticollis. J Neurol 239:9–15, 1992

Fahn S, Williams D: Psychogenic dystonia Adv Neurol 50: 431–55, 1988

Grandas F, Elston J, Quinn N, Marsden CD: Blepharospasm: review of 264 patients. J Neurol Neurosurg Psychiatry 51:767–72, 1988

Jankovic J: Tardive syndromes and other drug-induced movement disorders. Clin Neuropharmacol 18:197–214, 1995

Jankovic J, Leder S, Warner D, Schwartz K: Cervical dystonia: clinical findings and associated movement disorders. Neurology 41:1088–91, 1991

Jankovic J, Fahn S: Dystonic disorders. pp. 337–74. In Jankovic J, Tolosa E (eds): Parkinson's Disease and Movement Disorders. 2nd Ed. Williams & Wilkins, Baltimore, 1993

Jankovic J, Hallett M: Therapy with Botulinum Toxin. pp. 1–608. Marcel Dekker, New York, 1994

Rivest J, Quinn N, Marsden CD: Dystonia in Parkinson's disease, multiple system atrophy, and progressive supranuclear palsy. Neurology 40:157–8, 1990

Tanaka H, Endo K, Tsuji S et al: The gene for hereditary progressive dystonia with marked diurnal fluctuation maps to chromosome 14q. Ann Neurol 37:405–8, 1995

125. FOCAL DYSTONIA: TREATMENT WITH BOTULINUM TOXIN

DANIEL TARSY

By contrast with generalized dystonia, which usually begins in childhood (see Ch. 124), adult-onset idiopathic dystonia usually remains localized to one body part without progression or spread to neighboring body regions. Whereas childhood-onset dystonia usually begins in the lower extremities, most adult dystonias begin in muscles of the face, neck, or upper extremities, where they remain focal. Occasionally, dystonia may spread to adjacent body parts to become segmental. Focal dystonias are listed in Table 125-1 together with their more common names. Adult-onset focal dystonias are considered to be focal manifestations of idiopathic torsion dystonia. The involuntary movements and abnormal postures of focal dystonia also occur in generalized dystonia, and focal dystonias in adults sometimes spread to adjacent body regions to produce segmental dystonia. Examples of segmental dystonia include the association of blepharospasm with oromandibular dystonia (Meige syndrome) and spasmodic torticollis with dystonic writer's cramp.

Adult-onset focal dystonia is far more common than childhood generalized dystonia. The reported prevalence of idiopathic adult-onset dystonia is 295/1,000,000, compared with 34/1,000,000 for generalized dystonia, but is undoubtedly underestimated in current studies. Recent prevalence estimates have indicated at least 250,000 cases of idiopathic dystonia in the United States. Since in many cases focal dystonia is incorrectly attributed to psychological causes, underdiagnosis is common and long delays in diagnosis and appropriate treatment result.

Dystonia is a syndrome of sustained muscle contractions that cause repetitive torsional movements and abnormal postures. Dystonic movements may either be slow and sustained (tonic) or rapid (clonic), are typically repetitive, and are patterned, by contrast with choreic movements, which are more random and unpredictable, and myoclonus, which is rapid, rhythmic, and unassociated with alterations in posture. In some cases, rapid dystonic movements are difficult to distinguish from myoclonic jerks; thus, the term *myoclonic dystonia* has been introduced. Some of these result from voluntary attempts to resist an abnormal posture, such as the patient with torticollis whose head pulls slowly to the right and jerks intermittently to the left. Essential tremor may coexist with focal dystonia to produce an associated tremor of the head and upper extremities. Dystonic movements in primary dystonia are characteristically made worse during voluntary movements. *Action dystonia* refers to involuntary movements that occur only during voluntary use of a group of muscles and are absent at rest. Some are task specific, such as writer's and other occupational cramp disorders; vocal cord, jaw, or tongue spasms activated by speech; pharyngeal contractions during swallowing; and foot dystonia while walking. As the dystonia progresses, it appears more spontaneously and may be precipitated by movements in other body parts. In severe cases, the dystonia may progress to a

TABLE 125-1. Focal Dystonias

Dystonia	Common Name(s)
Cranial dystonia	Blepharospasm
	Oromandibular dystonia
	Jaw opening
	Jaw closing
	Spasmodic dysphonia
	Adductor dysphonia
	Abductor dysphonia
	Pharyngeal dystonia
	Lingual dystonia
Cervical dystonia	Spasmodic torticollis
Arm dystonia	Writer's cramp
	Occupational cramps
Leg dystonia	Inversion foot dystonia

permanent fixed posture with or without contractures. Dystonia usually increases with fatigue or stress and improves or is abolished with relaxation and sleep. Some patients acquire sensory tricks or compensatory postures that partially suppress the dystonic movements and postures but complicate the appearance of the movement disorder.

Botulinum toxin has radically changed the management of adult-onset focal dystonia; its use in cranial and cervical dystonia is the subject of this chapter. The use of botulinum toxin in focal limb dystonia is discussed in Chapter 126. In many cases, botulinum toxin has become the treatment of first choice. Botulinum toxin works by inhibiting calcium-dependent release of acetylcholine at the neuromuscular junction and has been especially effective in the treatment of oculomotor disorders, blepharospasm, spasmodic dysphonia, and spasmodic torticollis. Botulinum toxin is the treatment of choice in blepharospasm and produces benefit in 70 to 80 percent of patients. Oromandibular dystonia of the jaw-closing and jaw-opening types both benefit from botulinum toxin, but injection requires special attention to anatomic details, and in the case of pterygoid and digastric injections for jaws-opening dystonia, carries the risk of causing dysphagia. Botulinum toxin is currently used in spasmodic torticollis after preliminary trials with medication have been undertaken, but is increasingly being used as a treatment of first choice in this situation as well. Botulinum toxin is also the treatment of choice for spasmodic dysphonia, a condition in which medications and speech therapy are ineffective.

CRANIAL DYSTONIA

Cranial dystonia refers to a combination of dystonic movements of the eyelids, face, and jaw that is also known as Meige syndrome. Onset is usually between ages 40 and 60 and more commonly occurs in women than men. Blepharospasm is the most common manifestation of cranial dystonia and produces involuntary forced closure of the eyelids and increased eyeblink frequency. Differential diagnosis includes secondary forms of blepharospasm due to neuroleptic drugs, Parkinson's disease, progressive supranuclear palsy, Wilson's disease, and lesions of the brainstem. Local irritative disorders of the eyes and eyelids would be expected to cause transient rather than chronic blepharospasm.

Blepharospasm is bilateral although sometimes asymmetric in distribution. Unilateral blepharospasm is usually due to hemifacial spasm, which is not a dystonia but an irritative disorder of the facial nerve that causes myoclonic facial muscle contractions limited to one side of the face. The contractions of the orbicularis oculi in blepharospasm may either be brief, causing repetitive blinking, or persistent, causing prolonged, forced closure of the eyes. Some patients manifest apraxia of eyelid opening, resulting in difficulty opening the eyes in the absence of orbicularis oculi spasm. Driving, bright lights, watching television, and reading are frequent aggravating factors. During examination, patients often display more prominent blepharospasm while relating their history than while quietly listening or being examined. Sensory tricks used to suppress blepharospasm are limited but may include jaw or neck movements, coughing, chewing gum, or placing a finger or hand near or on the upper lids. Eyebrow lifting and ticlike movements of the lower face and mouth may occur, representing attempts to control the blepharospasm; these movements do not necessarily warrant a diagnosis of Meige syndrome.

Pharmacologic treatment is usually unsatisfactory but has included anticholinergic drugs, benzodiazepines, baclofen, and tetrabenazine. Surgical interventions such as myectomy and selective facial nerve section have been used with limited lasting success and often produce cosmetically unacceptable facial muscle weakness. Botulinum toxin is currently the treatment of choice in patients unresponsive to medication and results in significant improvement in a majority of patients both in terms of eyeblink frequency and intensity of blepharospasm. Botulinum toxin is injected in doses of 2.5 units subcutaneously into medial and lateral upper eyelid, lateral lower eyelid, and intramuscularly into lateral canthus. The medial lower eyelid can also be injected but this is usually unnecessary and carries with it the risk of impaired lacrimal drainage and vertical diplopia due to diffusion into the inferior oblique muscle. Diffusion into the middle portion of the upper eyelid must be avoided to prevent levator palpebrae weakness. Therapeutic effect is usually evident within several days and lasts approximately 3 months. Unwanted effects include ptosis, ecchymosis, diplopia, ectropion, blurred vision, and dry eyes. Excessive weakness may prevent normal eye closure during sleep and should be managed with appropriate ophthalmic lubrication.

Oromandibular dystonia is the second most common manifestation of cranial dystonia. It may occur alone but is often associated with other cranial dystonias such as blepharospasm, lingual or pharyngeal dystonia, or spasmodic dysphonia.

Differential diagnosis includes tardive dystonia, edentulous jaw movements, and bruxism. Jaw muscles may be involved asymmetrically or even unilaterally and produce involuntary jaw opening, jaw closing, or jaw deviation. Associated movements of the lower face are common and may include contractions of the platysma, pursing movements of the lips, tongue protrusion, and spasmodic contractions of the mouth and pharynx. Blepharospasm, oromandibular dystonia, and spasmodic movements of the face and neck typically occur synchronously in repetitive and sometimes rhythmic fashion. In early stages, they may be triggered by speaking or chewing; later, they are precipitated by other facial movements; eventually, they become continuous. Oromandibular dystonia produces major disability, including pain, speech impairment, difficulty eating, and trauma to oral and dental structures. Pharmacologic therapy is usually ineffective, but similar to blepharospasm, has included anticholinergic drugs, benzodiazepines, baclofen, and tetrabenazine given alone or in combination.

Botulinum toxin has been used with some success in oromandibular dystonia, but administration requires more detailed anatomic knowledge and is more prone to complication owing to spread of toxin than treatment of blepharospasm. Combined management with an otolaryngologist and speech pathologist is strongly recommended. Jaw-closing oromandibular dystonia is technically easier to treat and less frequently associated with dysphagia. Injections are made into masseter and temporalis muscles and, if necessary, medial pterygoids. Jaw-opening dystonia requires injection into lateral pterygoids and anterior digastrics. Pterygoid injections must be done under electromyographic guidance and can usually be injected extraorally by someone experienced in the anatomy of this region. Other muscles can usually be located by palpation but are also best injected under electromyographic guidance. Doses of botulinum toxin vary considerably, and when the patient is initially treated, should begin with small doses titrated according to response over several treatment sessions. Typical doses for masseter are 25 to 75 units; temporalis, 15 to 75 units; pterygoids, 5 to 50 units; and anterior digastrics, 2.5 to 30 units. Two to three injections are administered per muscle in relatively small volumes per injection to reduce potential for regional spread. Dysphagia is the most common adverse effect and is more common following injection of jaw-opening than jaw-closing muscles. Nasal dysarthria, weakness of chewing, and local pain are other occasional adverse effects.

SPASMODIC DYSPHONIA

Spasmodic dysphonia, also referred to as laryngeal dystonia, is an action dystonia in which there is involuntary adduction or abduction of the vocal cords activated by speech, resulting in abnormal voice production. Adductor dysphonia accounts for approximately 90 percent of cases of laryngeal dystonia and consists of involuntary approximation of the vocal cords due to contraction or tensing of the thyroarytenoid and vocalis muscles during speech. This results in a characteristic voice disorder in which patients speak in an effortful, strained, and staccato pattern with frequent short breaks in vocalization. In abductor dysphonia, involuntary separation of the vocal cords due to contraction of the posterior cricoarytenoid muscles produces a characteristic breathy or whispered voice pattern with loss of volume. Some patients with adductor dysphonia compensate for adduction by whispering, whereas in a few patients, adductor and abductor dysphonia coexist, with one predominating over the other in most cases. Spasmodic dysphonia is often misdiagnosed as psychogenic in origin, but there is no evidence to support this view and patients with spasmodic dysphonia can usually be distinguished from patients with truly psychogenic voice disorders by appropriate otolaryngologic examination and voice-evaluation techniques.

Differential diagnosis includes voice tremor as a manifestation of essential tremor, extrapyramidal disorders affecting voice production, structural abnormalities of the vocal cords, and chronic inflammatory vocal cord conditions. Pharmacologic treatment is entirely unhelpful in this disorder and, by contrast with other focal dystonias, is not worth undertaking prior to the use of botulinum toxin. Vocal therapy techniques may be worthwhile in some cases, especially when there seems to be a nondystonic contribution to the voice disorder. Recurrent laryngeal nerve section can produce relief of symptoms, but adverse effects are common, and follow-up studies have shown a high relapse rate. Surgical techniques designed to relax or tighten the vocal cords are currently under investigation but are too new to assess. Prior to use of botulinum toxin, patients should undergo neurologic, otolaryngologic, and voice evaluation. Fiberoptic laryngoscopy to exclude anatomic abnormalities and to confirm hyperadduction or hyperabduction is desirable. Voice recording and videostrobolaryngoscopy are sometimes indicated to exclude other voice disorders that may be difficult to differentiate from spasmodic dysphonia.

Early treatment of spasmodic dysphonia with botulinum toxin used injections of 15 to 30 units into a single vocal cord. However, currently bilateral injections are usually given in a dose range of 1.5 to 7.5 units per cord. Following administration of appropriate local anesthesia, the cricothyroid membrane is penetrated with a 27-gauge electromyographic injection needle, with the patient in a supine position. The needle is directed 30 degrees laterally and superiorly into the vocal cord. The vocal cord is identified electromyographically by increased spontaneous activity or activation with phonation and botulinum toxin is injected into one or two injection sites on each side. In some centers, botulinum toxin has been injected by an indirect laryn-goscopic approach, which has the advantage of not requiring electromyographic guidance. An initial dose of 2.5 to 5.0 units bilaterally is recommended, with the understanding that there is a wide variability in response. Some patients will experience insufficient therapeutic effect and require an additional injection, whereas others may experience excessive effect manifested by a period of breathy or aphonic speech lasting for as long as several weeks. When benefit occurs, it usually appears within several days. The most common adverse effect is breathy speech or aphonia, which will dictate future dose adjustments. Dysphagia is relatively uncommon and is usually limited to subjective difficulty drinking liquids without aspiration. Once the appropriate dose is determined for individual patients, it should be expected that nearly all patients will experience significant improvement in speech. Duration of benefit is highly variable and ranges between 6 weeks and 6 months, with an average duration of 3 to 4 months.

Abductor dysphonia is treated by posterior cricoarytenoid injection. Injection technique is more difficult than with thyroarytenoid injection and requires positioning of the electromyographically guided needle posterior to the lamina of the thyroid cartilage. Only one posterior cricoarytenoid muscle is injected at a time because of the risk of compromising the airway by bilateral abductor paralysis. Overall success with this method is less than for adductor dysphonia and sometimes requires careful bilateral injections, cricothyroid injection, or thyroplastic procedures.

CERVICAL DYSTONIA

Cervical dystonia, also known as spasmodic torticollis, is the most common focal dystonia that comes to medical attention. Symptomatic forms may result from a variety of orthopaedic, neurologic, and infectious disturbances of the craniocervical junction, but most of these occur in children or young adults, are related to obvious underlying causes, and do not produce the characteristic features of idiopathic cervical dystonia as it presents in adults. Similar to other focal dystonias, cervical dystonia was once believed to be psychogenic in origin, but psychological studies and general clinical experience do not support this view. Onset is usually between ages 30 and 50 and women are affected slightly more often than men. Symptoms usually begin with mild neck stiffness or subtle postural deviations of the head. A small number of patients report neck pain at onset, although with the exception of post-traumatic cases, onset is usually unrelated to immediate antecedent trauma. As the disorder progresses, pain and discomfort become prominent in 75 percent of patients and is usually localized to the posterior paracervical region and shoulder. Pain is much more prominent than in other focal dystonias and is likely of musculoskeletal or radicular origin. Pain is typically located in the posterior cervical region ipsilateral to the direction of head rotation or head tilt and almost never occurs in the affected sternomastoid muscle. Symptoms of cervical spondylosis and radiculopathy may complicate the clinical picture after several years of persistent cervical dystonia.

Several abnormal head postures occur, consisting of various combinations of rotation (torticollis), lateral tilt (laterocollis), hyperextension of the head (retrocollis), and forward flexion (antecollis). Torticollis and laterocollis are the most common postures, whereas pure retrocollis and antecollis are relatively uncommon in idiopathic cervical dystonia. Retrocollis is particularly common as a manifestation of tardive dystonia due to neuroleptic drugs. Most patients display a combination of these postures, with the most common head position consisting of rotation of the head to one side with upward deviation of the chin and lateral tilt of the head to the opposite side. Symptoms often increase with fatigue and tend to be worse late in the day. Patients use a variety of sensory tricks, which are usually more effective early than later in the course. These begin with a light touch on the chin, but in more severe cases, require a hand on the back or side of the neck or head for relief. Head support while lying down usually reduces torticollis, but some patients experience an exacerbation of symptoms when in a reclining position. Some patients gain relief with use of a high-backed chair or recliner and will drive with the assistance of a head rest. Fixed deformities, such as sternomastoid hypertrophy and elevation or anterior displacement of one shoulder, may appear with time. Most patients exhibit tonic deviation of the head, but in some cases clonic jerks are prominent. In many cases, these are due to the patient's effort to suppress the abnormal posture. Head tremor is common and is due either to dystonic tremor or an associated essential tremor. The clinical course is usually one of slow progression over the first several months to years followed by a static course afterward. Spontaneous but usually temporary remissions have been reported in 5 to 10 percent of patients and will usually occur within 5 years of onset.

Most patients with cervical dystonia do not benefit from oral medications. Ordinary muscle relaxants are typically ineffective and have usually been tried prior to neurologic referral. The drugs of choice for treatment of cervical dystonia are anticholinergic drugs such as trihexyphenidyl, with which there has been the greatest experience. As many as 15 to 20 percent of patients respond to low or moderate doses of 4 to 10 mg. Although the percentage of responders is low, the response may be good enough to obviate the need for botulinum toxin treatment. Unfortunately, adverse effects are common even at low doses and include nausea, dry mouth, drowsiness, visual disturbance, forgetfulness, urinary retention, and glaucoma. Some patients manifest mild choreiform dyskinesias that clear after discontinuation of treatment. Sensitivity to side effects in adults usually precludes high-dose anticholinergic treatment. Benzodiazepines such as diazepam, lorazepam, or clonazepam are often helpful for symptomatic pain management but carry the risk of dependency and susceptibility to withdrawal symptoms after chronic use. Baclofen and carbamazepine are of little or no benefit, whereas dopamine receptor antagonists such as haloperidol are contraindicated for chronic use because of risk of tardive dyskinesia.

Nonpharmacologic therapies used to treat cervical dystonia have included hypnosis, biofeedback, relaxation techniques, psychotherapy, acupuncture, and braces, but in the majority of cases these are unhelpful. Physical therapy plays a limited role in the management of cervical dystonia but is useful as an adjunct to maximize range of motion and for pain management in patients who have partially benefited from other treatments.

Currently, patients with cervical dystonia are diagnosed earlier and are seeking treatment sooner than patients treated in the early years of botulinum toxin therapy. It is important to understand the ways in which cervical dystonia is disturbing, since all symptoms or signs are not equally benefited. Involuntary movements and pain are the two major manifestations. Involuntary movements are disturbing because of the jerking head movements, the cosmetic effect produced by postural deformities, difficulties in carrying out routine activities of daily living such as working, driving, reading, and watching television, subjective gait disturbance, fatigue related to constant efforts to suppress the involuntary movements, and head tremor. Chronic pain, social withdrawal, and reactive depression are common consequences. It is worthwhile to review these areas of disability in detail both before and after treatment so that expectations before treatment and gains after treatment can be more readily identified.

It is important to understand the anatomy of neck muscles and the way in which abnormal postures relate to contractions of specific cervical muscles (Table 125-2). The need for electromyography to assist botulinum toxin injection of cervical muscles is controversial and depends largely on the skills of the treating physician. Observed abnormal head postures can usually be correlated with a predictable pattern of muscle involvement. Careful observation and analysis of the patient's posture, involuntary movements, and voluntary movements, together with palpation of often hypertrophied muscles, usually allows for appropriate selection of muscles for injection.

Rotational torticollis is produced by the combined effect of sternomastoid contraction rotating the head contralaterally and contraction of ipsilateral posterior cervical muscles—splenius capitis, longissimus capitis, and oblique capitis inferior—rotating the head ipsilaterally. Although some authors include trapezius as a head rotator, it primarily tilts the head ipsilaterally, is extremely thin in the paracervical region, and in most cases does not require injection. Splenius capitis is a considerably thicker muscle and, in patients with cervical dystonia, is often hypertrophied and easily palpable in the posterior cervical triangle behind and below the mastoid, where it emerges from under the trapezius. In most cases, injection of ipsilateral splenius and contralateral sternomastoid is sufficient and electromyography is unnecessary. Since the semispinalis is a posterior cervical muscle that rotates the head contralaterally, it may be worth injecting this muscle with electromyographic guidance on the side contralateral to head rotation in cases resistant to routine patterns of injection. The oblique capitis inferior is a small and much deeper muscle that cannot be identified without electromyography and may also require injection in some cases.

Laterocollis is produced by contraction of the ipsilateral sternomastoid (clavicular more than sternal head), levator scapulae, scalenus muscles, splenius, and trapezius. In this case, electromyography is useful in estimating the degree to which each muscle contributes to head tilt. In most cases, weakening of ipsilateral sternomastoid, levator scapulae, and splenius is suffi-

TABLE 125-2. Action of Commonly Injected Cervical Muscles

Muscle	Action
Sternomastoid	Contralateral rotation Ipsilateral tilt Anterior flexion
Trapezius	Shoulder elevation Ipsilateral tilt Neck extension
Splenius capitis	Ipsilateral rotation Ipsilateral tilt Neck extension
Levator scapulae	Shoulder elevation Ipsilateral tilt
Scalenus group	Ipsilateral tilt Head flexion
Deep postvertebrals (semispinalis, longissimus capitis)	Ipsilateral tilt Head extension

cient. Injections into the scalenus group are usually avoided since they are deep, more likely to be associated with dysphagia, and in close anatomic relationship to the brachial plexus and lung.

Retrocollis is probably the easiest form of cervical dystonia to treat and requires injections into splenius capitis, trapezius, and sometimes deeper posterior cervical muscles such as semispinalis. Side effects are rare and limited to occasional excessive neck extensor weakness. Antecollis is often resistant to treatment with botulinum toxin. Although sternomastoid muscles, scalenes, and platysma contribute to anterior head flexion and are easily injected, the more important prevertebral head flexors longus colli and longus capitis are more powerful muscles that require intraoral injection, which is associated with a high risk of severe dysphagia and occasional bacterial sepsis. If electromyography indicates a significant contribution by sternomastoid and scalenes, bilateral injection of these muscles may be considered but will be associated with a higher incidence of dysphagia.

Typical initial injections into the sternomastoid are 50 to 70 units; splenius capitis, 80 to 100 units; trapezius, 60 to 80 units; levator scapulae, 30 to 50 units; scalenus muscles, 20 to 40 units; and deeper posterior cervical muscles, 80 to 100 units. Women, patients with smaller neck muscles, or patients with previous surgical denervation and patients given bilateral injections should receive lower doses to reduce the incidence of dysphagia and excessive neck muscle weakness.

Botulinum toxin has been demonstrated to be safe and effective in a number of open and controlled trials. Although subjective improvement sometimes seems to exceed objective measures of benefit, published studies have uniformly shown significant improvement for both abnormal head posture and pain in 60 to 80 percent of patients. Initial response to treatment should be documented carefully in order to justify follow-up treatments. The degree of torticollis observed in the examining room may not adequately represent the amount of improvement. Although in many cases improvement in head posture is apparent, family members are sometimes better observers than the patient, who is often less aware of head position. Improvement in pain, increased range of motion, reduced dystonic tremor, reduction in the need to voluntarily suppress abnormal postures, and resultant improvements in mood are useful indicators of treatment response. The cause of primary resistance is uncertain, but 20 to 25 percent of patients fail to respond to treatment. Patients treated relatively early may respond more favorably than patients with chronic cervical dystonia, possibly owing to muscle contractures and fixed postures. A change in the pattern of muscle activity whereby uninjected, deeper posterior cervical muscles develop increased spasm may account for other treatment failures.

The use of botulinum toxin in cervical dystonia is remarkably safe. Immediate side effects are limited to occasional small subcutaneous hematomas and rare occurrence pneumothorax. When possible, patients should discontinue aspirin for several days prior to injections. Patients anticoagulated with Coumadin (warfarin) with prothrombin times in therapeutic range can be safely injected. Occasional, brief pain may occur if the needle encounters the greater occipital nerve in the suboccipital region or the brachial plexus during scalene injection. Later-appearing adverse effects include dysphagia, neck weakness, and new patterns of cervical pain. Dysphagia is relatively uncommon if doses in sternomastoid muscles are kept below 60 units. Higher injections closer to the mastoid and into the posterior aspect

of this muscle also minimize this side effect. When it occurs, dysphagia appears 5 to 6 days after injection and lasts for 2 to 4 weeks. Dysphagia is primarily for solid foods and relatively easily managed with soft solids or thick liquids and modification of swallowing techniques such as turning the head toward the weak side. Aspiration is possible but is relatively rare in botulinum-induced dysphagia. A modified barium swallow with fluoroscopy may demonstrate unilateral pharyngeal weakness but is not necessary for routine management in most cases. Excessive weakness in neck muscles is uncommon, but patients may experience difficulty elevating their head from a bent position or turning in bed, owing to excessive posterior cervical muscle weakness. Occasionally, patients experience increased pain at the injection sites or a new distribution of cervical or shoulder pain within the first several weeks of injection. This usually occurs in patients with pretreatment cervical pain and may be due to new patterns of muscle use and ligamentous stretch. Generalized fatigue, myalgia, and weakness are uncommon and in controlled studies have not exceeded similar effects following placebo. Although single-fiber electromyographic studies may show evidence for neuromuscular blockade in muscles distant from the injection site and minor abnormalities of autonomic cardiovascular reflexes have been demonstrated, clinical manifestations of these laboratory observations have not been apparent.

BOTULINUM TOXIN

Clostridium botulinum produces seven antigenically distinctive toxins that are all potent paralytic agents. These are designated as A, B, C, D, E, F, and G. These toxins are polypeptides with a molecular mass of 150,000 Dal. When the single-chain toxin is cleaved, it yields a dichain molecule in which a heavy chain of about 100,000 Dal is linked by a disulfide bond to a light chain of approximately 50,000 Dal. In this form, botulinum toxin is capable of producing neuromuscular junction blockade. Botulinum toxin produces weakness by blocking acetylcholine release. The steps involved in this process include binding to the preterminal membrane, internalization of the toxin, and blockade of neurotransmitter release. The heavy chain of the toxin is responsible for binding to the presynaptic nerve terminal, whereas the light chain is responsible for blockade of acetylcholine release. Botulinum toxin A has been shown to exert its effect by cleaving the synaptic protein SNAP-25, which is a constituent of the synaptic vesicle membrane. As a result of this cleavage, the presynaptic vesicle loses its ability to fuse with the nerve terminal membrane in order to initiate exocytosis.

In animal studies, botulinum toxin has been shown to reach the central nervous system, where it binds to brain synaptosomes. However, the toxin's clinical effect in botulism or local muscle paralysis following injection is not believed to be due to central nervous system mechanisms. After injection into a muscle, the toxin diffuses up to 4.5 cm from the injection site. Since the radius of spread appears to be determined by the dose and volume injected, injections of smaller doses and volumes may reduce spread to adjacent muscles, thereby reducing incidence of unwanted weakness in adjacent muscles. Clinical studies comparing efficacy of multiple and single injections have produced inconsistent results, and it is currently recommended that 2 to 4 injections be given into each treated muscle.

Long-term effects of intramuscular botulinum toxin have been studied widely in animals, but only occasionally in humans. In experimental animals, botulinum toxin causes denervation atrophy, whereas in human studies of orbicularis oculi muscles, atrophy and fibrosis persist up to 4 months after exposure to botulinum toxin. Botulinum toxin produces sprouting of motor axon terminals in both animal and human studies. Some of these sprouts end blindly, whereas others appear to terminate on muscle motor endplates. Although it is uncertain whether axonal sprouting is responsible for recovery of muscular strength after botulinum toxin injection, most histologic studies show incomplete sprouting unlikely to represent functionally effective reinnervation. The dose of botulinum toxin capable of producing significant systemic toxicity in humans is not known. In monkeys, the median lethal dose for botulinum toxin A is estimated at 40 U/kg. This would amount to approximately 3,000 units in a 75-kg man. The lethal oral dose is also not known with certainty but has been estimated to be in the vicinity of 10^4 to 10^6 times the parenteral dose.

In recent years, the appearance of secondary resistance has emerged as an increasing problem in botulinum toxin clinics. It is presumed that many if not all of these cases are due to the appearance of blocking antibodies to botulinum toxin A. Interestingly, experience with botulism food poisoning has failed to show antibodies to botulinum toxin in surviving patients. Unfortunately, there is no simple and readily available assay for botulinum antibodies. A difficult in vivo mouse neutralization assay is available and enzyme-linked immunosorbent assay (ELISA) has also been used for detection of botulinum antibodies but has not been correlated with the presence of secondary resistance. In several studies, the frequency of detectable botulinum antibodies has been in the range of 3 to 5 percent, with evidence that increased dose and reduced interval between injections are related to the presence of antibodies. Currently, there is increased interest in the development of alternative botulinum toxin serotypes such as type F and type B, which are beginning to undergo clinical evaluation.

Botulinum toxin should be administered by a physician well acquainted with the diagnosis and treatment of disorders characterized by excessive and inappropriate muscle spasm. It is important to carefully review the anatomy relevant for the body part being injected. Although not necessary in every case, electromyography is often helpful in the use of botulinum toxin for cranial and cervical dystonias. Since its introduction into clinical practice, significant adverse effects have been extremely rare. Despite its extreme potency, it is a remarkably safe drug increasingly used to treat spasmodic muscles in a wide variety of body locations. Although there is no information regarding potential adverse effects in pregnancy, it is recommended that botulinum toxin not be used in pregnant or lactating women. Primary muscle disorders such as myasthenia gravis, Lambert-Eaton syndrome, motor neuron disease, and primary myopathies are relative contraindications to the use of botulinum toxin. However, since the amount of toxin that reaches the systemic circulation following local intramuscular injection is minute, this may not necessarily constitute an absolute contraindication in a dystonia for which no other treatment is available. Experience in children has been limited and safety has not been studied in detail. Preliminary studies have not demonstrated a different side effect profile but, because of the absence of information on long-term exposure, children should probably not be treated chronically except for unusual, extenuating clinical circumstances.

SUGGESTED READINGS

Blasia J, Chapman ER, Link E et al: Botulinum neurotoxin A selectively cleaves the synaptic protein SNAP-25. Nature 365:160, 1993

Blitzer A: Botulinum toxin injection for the treatment of oromandibular dystonia. Ann Otol Rhinol Laryngol 98:93, 1989

Blitzer A, Brin MF: Laryngeal dystonia: a series with botulinum toxin therapy. Ann Otol Rhinol Laryngol 100:85, 1991

Blitzer A, Brin MF, Stuart C et al: Abductor laryngeal dystonia: a series treated with botulinum toxin. Laryngoscope 102:163, 1992

Comella CL, Buchman AS, Tanner CM et al: Botulinum toxin injection for spasmodic torticollis: increased magnitude of benefit with electromyographic assistance. Neurology 42:878, 1992

Conference Report: Clinical use of botulinum toxin. NIH Consensus Development Conference Statement. Arch Neurol 48:1294, 1991

Dutton JJ, Buckley EG: Botulinum toxin in the management of blepharospasm. Arch Neurol 43:380, 1986

Girlanda P, Vita G, Nicolosi C et al: Botulinum toxin therapy: distant effects on neuromuscular transmission and autonomic nervous system. J Neurol Neurosurg Psychiatry 55:844, 1992

Greene P, Kang U, Fahn S et al: Double-blind, placebo-controlled trial of botulinum toxin injections for the treatment of spasmodic torticollis. Neurology 40:1213, 1990

Jankovic J, Brin MF: Therapeutic uses of botulinum toxin. N Engl J Med 324:1186, 1991

Jankovic J, Schwartz KS: Longitudinal experience with botulinum toxin injections for treatment of blepharospasm and cervical dystonia. Neurology 43:834, 1993

Ludlow CL: The treatment of speech and voice disorders with botulinum toxin. JAMA 264:2671, 1990

Marsden CD: The focal dystonias. Clin Neuropharmacol (suppl. 2):S49, 1986

Marsden CD: The problem of adult-onset idiopathic torsion dystonia and other isolated dyskinesias in adult life. Adv Neurol 14:259, 1976

Report of the Therapeutics and Technology Assessment Subcommittee of the American Academy of Neurology: Assessment: the clinical usefulness of botulinum toxin-A in treating neurologic disorders. Neurology 40:1332, 1990

Schantz EJ, Johnson EA: Properties and use of botulinum toxin and other microbial neurotoxins in medicines. Microbiol Rev 56:80, 1992

Weiner WF, Lang AE: Movement Disorders: A Comprehensive Survey. Futura, New York, 1989

Zuber M, Sebald M, Bathien N et al: Botulinum antibodies in dystonic patients treated with type A botulinum toxin: frequency and significance. Neurology 43:1715, 1993

126. OCCUPATIONAL CRAMP

MARJORIE H. ROSS
MICHAEL E. CHARNESS

DEFINITION

Focal dystonia, the involuntary sustained contraction of muscles of a single part of the body, can affect the neck, the facial muscles, and the limbs. Involvement of the upper extremity is more common than involvement of the lower extremity and is often task specific. When the dystonia is elicited by the highly skilled movements of certain occupations, the disorder is termed occupational cramp. Occupational cramp has been associated with a wide variety of such tasks, including writing, typing, and playing a musical instrument. Occupational cramp can be subdivided into simple cramp, initiated by a single task; dystonic cramp, initiated by several tasks; and progressive cramp, denoting a transition from simple cramp to dystonic cramp. The first accounts of occupational cramp date back 400 years. The sometimes bizarre nature of this disorder has led to confusion about its etiology, and occupational cramp was often labeled a psychiatric condition. However, the clinical and electrophysiologic evidence gathered in recent years points to a disturbance of central nervous system motor processing.

EPIDEMIOLOGY

The prevalence of focal dystonia has been estimated from a Mayo Clinic database to be 295 patients per million. This may be an underestimate, since occupational cramp is probably underdiagnosed. In most series, 8 to 14 percent of musicians who present to performing arts clinics have occupational cramp. Musician's cramp is twice as common in men as in women. There is an increased frequency of focal dystonia among family members of patients with inherited torsion dystonia. Some degenerative neurologic diseases, such as Parkinson's disease or Wilson's disease, may, on rare occasions, present as focal dystonia, but exact incidence and prevalence data are unknown.

CLINICAL FEATURES

Occupational cramp usually presents insidiously, first manifesting as a loss of speed or dexterity. Musicians commonly complain of the uncharacteristic effort required to perform previously automatic technical feats. Writers note slowness, a deterioration in penmanship, and fatigue. Later, a variety of involuntary stereotyped movements are sometimes reported. In writer's cramp, this typically consists of overgripping the pen as a result of exaggerated flexion of the index finger and thumb, so that the pen rides up or rolls out of the writing position. Conversely, sometimes the thumb or index finger will actually lift off the pen. Writing on a horizontal surface may be severely compromised, but forming the same letters on a vertical surface, such as a blackboard, may remain unaffected. In musician's cramp, flexion of the ring and little fingers and extension of the middle or index finger are two of the many patterns observed (Fig. 126-1). The movements are not painful, although many

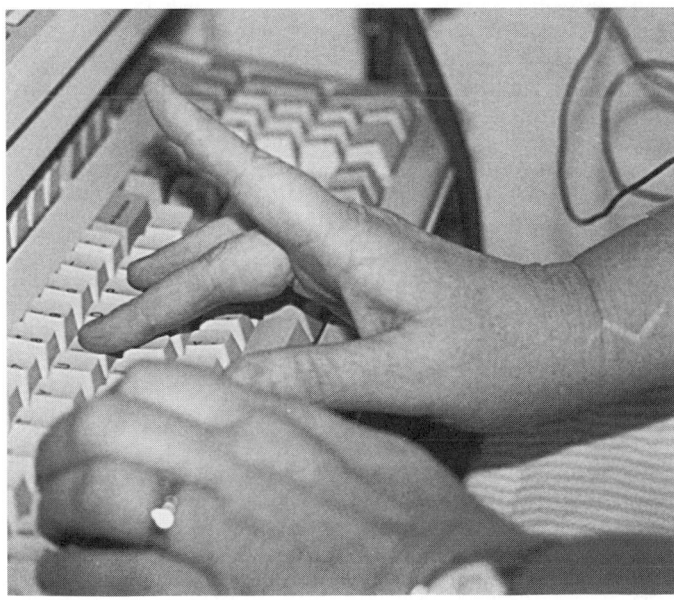

FIG. 126-1.   Dystonic index finger extension.

patients develop uncomfortable tightness in their hand, forearm, and arm while attempting to overcome the dystonic movements. The dystonia may generalize to other tasks and may even occur at rest. It may also spread to other muscles in the same extremity or to the neck. Like patients with torticollis, patients with writer's cramp attempt to compensate for their disorder by changing hand position or the size of the writing instrument. Some patients even attempt to change handedness for the task, which in a minority of cases may lead to dystonia in the previously unaffected side.

There may be a history of previous injury to the extremity or of specific nerve entrapment, such as carpal tunnel syndrome or cubital tunnel syndrome. Entrapment may cause concomitant symptoms of numbness, tingling, pain, or weakness.

Neurologic examination is usually normal, except in cases associated with nerve injury. Subtle abnormalities such as tremor are sometimes seen. Since the disorder may be entirely task specific, it is imperative to watch the patient perform the affected task. It is helpful to videotape the patient to document progression or improvement with therapy. In mild cases, the abnormal movements may be difficult to discern; it may be apparent only that the hand is stiff, awkward, and slow.

Spontaneous remission is rare and recurrence after remission is common.

PATHOPHYSIOLOGY

Focal dystonia results from involuntary co-contraction of antagonist muscles, as demonstrated by polygraphic electromyography. Electrophysiologic studies also reveal reduced activation of selective muscles and overflow contraction in adjacent muscles. The generator for the alternation of antagonist muscles is believed to reside in the central nervous system, implying dysfunction at this level in focal dystonia. Nondystonic patients with ulnar neuropathy can also exhibit co-contraction of antagonist muscles, which suggests that peripheral nervous system injury may precipitate abnormal central nervous system processing in some patients.

Focal dystonia has also been evaluated by electrophysiologic testing of the monosynaptic reflex arc. In normal subjects, an H reflex, the electrical correlate of the monosynaptic reflex, can be obtained by stimulating the median nerve and recording from the flexor carpi radialis. A prior or simultaneous stimulation of the radial nerve, which innervates the wrist extensors, will inhibit the median H reflex. Reciprocal inhibition of the H reflex is reduced in the affected, resting limb in patients with focal dystonia.

DIAGNOSIS

Diagnosis is based largely upon medical history and physical examination. Polygraphic electromyography is an investigational technique and is not required to make the diagnosis.

If the dystonia progresses to involve other limbs or additional neurologic symptoms and signs develop, additional workup is warranted to explore the possibility of a degenerative neurologic disease. The long differential diagnosis of symptomatic dystonia includes Parkinson's disease, Wilson's disease, and spinocerebellar degeneration. Most adult patients with focal dystonia beginning in adult life will not have an identifiable cause and structural imaging studies of the brain are not routinely obtained.

If there is a history of injury to the extremity or symptoms and signs of nerve entrapment, the patient should have nerve conduction studies and electromyography.

TREATMENT

Occupational cramp can be a devastating disorder. Musician's cramp has ruined the careers of many performing artists, including the great pianist Leon Fleisher. Writer's or typist's cramp can render a patient unemployable and dependent on disability insurance. Rest and avoiding the activity that precipitates the cramp, the mainstays of treatment in overuse injury, are uniformly unhelpful. Anticholinergic and dopaminergic medications, which can improve segmental and generalized dystonia, are relatively ineffective in occupational cramp and are poorly tolerated, owing to side effects.

Hypnotherapy, biofeedback, and motor retraining have been reported to be of some benefit in occupational cramp. Our experience is that these modalities alone are ineffective in most patients. Attempts at strengthening antagonist muscles may be somewhat helpful. Writing devices that change hand position have produced significant improvement in selected patients with writer's cramp. We have also observed improvement in musician's cramp when instruments are modified to alter hand position.

The most recent therapeutic advance in the treatment of focal dystonia has been the selective weakening of dystonic muscles by the injection of botulinum toxin A. Botulinum toxin is injected through a hollow electromyographic needle, which is first used to electrically identify the target muscles. Botulinum toxin disrupts neuromuscular transmission by preventing the presynaptic release of acetylcholine. The goal of botulinum toxin injection is the production of sufficient weakness to prevent dystonic contraction without disabling the task by causing excessive weakness. The effect is always reversible and the duration of beneficial effect is 1 to 6 months. There is always a tradeoff between weakness and reduced dystonia; however, functional improvement may be quite dramatic, especially when one particular muscle is involved, such as extensor indicis proprius in writer's cramp. However, selective weakening of dystonic muscles does nothing to address the failure of other muscles to contract at appropriate times. This problem and the susceptibility of highly skilled tasks to mild weakness makes it unrealistic to expect a return to premorbid levels of musical performance.

Side effects are generally limited to weakness in adjacent muscles related to local diffusion of the toxin; there is no systemic weakness. Repeated injections over years may cause the formation of antibodies to botulinum toxin and resistance to therapeutic effect.

Surgical correction of an associated nerve entrapment may sometimes be associated with improvement in occupational cramp. We recommend peripheral nerve surgery only when the peripheral nerve symptoms and signs independently warrant this treatment.

SUGGESTED READINGS

Cohen LG, Hallett M: Hand cramps: clinical features and electromyographic patterns in a focal dystonia. Neurology 38:1005–12, 1988
Cohen LG, Hallett M, Geller BD, Hochberg F: Treatment of focal dystonias of the hand with botulinum toxin injections. J Neurol Neurosurg Psychiatry 52:355–63, 1989
Lederman RJ: Focal dystonia in instrumentalists: clinical features. Medical Problems of Performing Artists 6:132–36, 1991
Marsden CD, Sheehy MP: Writer's cramp. Trends Neurosci 13:148–153, 1990
Ross MH, Charness ME, Lee D, Logigian EL: Does ulnar neuropathy predispose to focal dystonia? Muscle Nerve 18:606–611, 1995

127. TICS AND TOURETTE'S DISORDER

FREDERICK J. MARSHALL
ROGER KURLAN

In 1885, Gilles de la Tourette embarked on the task of cataloging and organizing the disorders of movement at the suggestion of his mentor, Charcot. Having earlier translated Beard's article on the peculiar "Jumping Frenchmen of Maine," the 28-year-old Tourette struck out to find evidence of their progenitors on the wards of the Salpetriere in Paris. Instead, he came on a small group of patients who suffered from multiple motor and vocal tics. Of the nine patients described in his original article, five suffered from scatologic outbursts, a symptom that provoked them to self-imposed social isolation and prompted generations of physicians, including Charcot himself, to presume a functional etiology for the disorder.

The syndrome of Gilles de la Tourette, now properly referred to as Tourette's disorder, has captured the imagination of clinicians ever since. It was not until the 1960s, however, that Tourette's disorder emerged from its status as a rare curiosity. With the introduction of haloperidol treatment and the demonstration that chronic motor and vocal tics could be suppressed medically, the disorder became the concern of neurologists as well as psychiatrists. More than any other advance, the success of phenothiazine treatment placed Tourette's disorder firmly in the center of an emerging understanding of the links between brain and behavior.

DEFINITION, PHENOMENOLOGY, AND NATURAL HISTORY

Despite compelling evidence of its hereditary nature, and of the genetic linkage with a spectrum of other neurobehavioral disorders such as obsessive-compulsive disorder and attention deficit hyperactivity disorder, there remains no disease-specific biologic marker for Tourette's disorder. As such, the diagnosis of Tourette's disorder rests upon recognition of its characteristic signs and symptoms. DSM-IV (*Diagnostic and Statistical Manual of Mental Disorders,* fourth edition) criteria include (1) presence of both multiple motor tics and one or more vocal tics at some time during the illness (not necessarily concurrently); (2) duration longer than 1 year, during which time there is no tic-free interval longer than 3 months; (3) onset prior to age 18; (4) marked distress or significant impairment in social, occupational, or other important areas of functioning; and (5) absence of possible confounding agents or conditions (e.g., stimulants, Huntington's disease, postviral encephalitis).

The remaining primary tic disorders include chronic multiple tic disorder, and transient tic disorder. The former differs from

Tourette's disorder in that *either* motor *or* vocal tics (but not both) must be present for more than 1 year. Transient tic disorder differs from both chronic tic disorder and Tourette's disorder in that symptoms must be of less than 1 year's duration. It is now widely suspected that these disorders exist on a continuum of severity; the underlying genetic defect in Tourette's disorder expresses itself in milder form as both chronic and transient tic disorders.

There are also a number of secondary causes of tics. Tics may occur in hereditary neurologic disorders such as Huntington's disease, the neurocutaneous syndromes, dystonia musculorum deformans, and neuroacanthocytosis. Perinatal encephalopathy, stroke, head trauma, carbon monoxide poisoning, and central nervous system infections (e.g., encephalitis lethargica, Sydenham's chorea) have all been reported as causes of tics. Drugs that have been implicated include amphetamines, anticonvulsants (carbamazepine, phenobarbital, and Dilantin), cocaine, methylphenidate, and levodopa. The antipsychotics themselves may cause tardive tics.

Among the hyperkinetic movement disorders, tics may be differentiated on several grounds. In addition to being abrupt in onset and duration, they are characterized by a tendency to spontaneously fluctuate, to be multifocal and migratory, and to be at least temporarily suppressible. Often, the patient may describe premonitory symptoms of a sensory nature, such as a "tickle" or "urge", which are then relieved by the movement itself. Tics tend to increase during times of stress. To the extent that they are suppressed for any length of time, however, tics generally re-emerge in force once the patient relaxes The physical and emotional burden of suppressing tics is frequently overwhelming, and patients describe a feeling of exhaustion attendant on efforts to keep their tics from emerging. Most patients say their tics tend to become less severe during intense concentration on or distraction by some other activity.

Tics may be subdivided into simple and complex types, as well as motor and vocal forms. Simple motor tics are defined as abrupt contractions of a single muscle group, such as eye blinking, head jerking, or wrist flicking. By contrast, complex motor tics involve the coordinated contractions of a series of muscle groups. The resultant movements may take on an almost purposeful appearance, as exemplified by touching or stroking behaviors, dancelike movements, or copropraxia (obscene gestures).

Vocal tics may be thought of as a particular variety of motor tic involving contractions of the laryngeal, pharyngeal, respiratory, or oronasal musculature. Simple vocal tics are inarticulate noises that do not convey meaning. Examples include snorting, grunting, barking, and clicking. Complex vocal tics are generally words or fragments of words. Despite the emphasis placed upon coprolalia (obscene speech) as a symptom of Tourette's disorder, less than 20 percent of patients ever actually suffer from this symptom. Although it is perhaps the most socially stigmatizing manifestation of Tourette's disorder most patients may be reassured that the symptom tends to be transitory.

Many patients with Tourette's disorder demonstrate a tendency to repeat their own words (palilalia) or the last words that they hear (echolalia). Similarly, they may mimic or copy the gestures and movements of others (echopraxia). These behaviors may be manifestations of the underlying tic disorder, or may blend into the realm of obsessive-compulsive disorder. One important means of differentiating complex tics from compulsions is to question the patient about the meaning, if any, he or she ascribes to the behavior. Whereas tics are not associated with any preformed ritualistic set of notions about their significance, compulsions invariably are. For example, compulsive acts are often performed according to specific rules, such as repeating acts a certain number of times or in a particular order. Complex motor tics, on the other hand, do not have such ritualistic qualities.

Tourette's disorder and the related primary tic disorders generally have their onset in the childhood years. As many as 20 percent of school-aged children develop some sort of transitory tic. These are often either altogether ignored by the family and other care providers, or are attributed to the passing mannerisms of a "childish" nature. Estimates of the lifetime risk of full-blown Tourette's disorder vary widely, but a likely assessment would be 30 to 50 cases per 100,000 people. There is a 3:1 ratio of males to females with the syndrome. It occurs in all races and socioeconomic classes. The clinical picture is relatively uniform across cultural groups, save for a decreased incidence of coprolalia among Japanese. The most likely location for the initial tic to present is the face and eyes, with decreasing incidence of tics occurring in a rostral-caudal fashion throughout the remainder of the body. Approximately 12 to 37 percent of subjects with Tourette's disorder present with simple vocal tics (e.g., throat clearing) as the initial symptom, with a far fewer number presenting with complex vocal tics.

There have been a number of studies to establish the long-term prognosis of the disorder. When tics alone are considered, the general consensus is that approximately one-third of patients will enjoy complete remission by late adolescence or early adulthood. Another one-third will have a significant decrease in both the amount and severity of their tics. The final one-third of patients will remain symptomatic throughout early adulthood and middle age. Little is known about Tourette's disorder in the geriatric age range. The most famous of Tourette's original patients, the Marquise de Dampièrre, is said to have lived out her life in seclusion, dying at the age of 86. Collective experience would indicate, however, that tics as well as obsessive-compulsive disorder tend to diminish with advanced age.

RELATED DISORDERS

The genetic association between Tourette's disorder and obsessive-compulsive disorder is now widely accepted. Approximately 50 percent of Tourette's disorder patients suffer from symptoms of obsessive-compulsive disorder. Typical compulsions relate to ritualistic cleaning and grooming behaviors (e.g., hand washing, showering, teeth brushing), ordering and arranging objects, checking and rechecking objects in the environment (e.g., locks, switches, electrical outlets, stoves), counting, hoarding, and repeating certain actions (e.g., walking though a doorway, touching a piece of furniture). Common obsessions include fear of contamination, fear of thinking evil or sinful thoughts contrary to one's religion, fear of losing potentially vital objects or loved ones, recurring thoughts of doing harm to self or others, and recurring sexual thoughts and images that are ego-dystonic.

Evidence for the hypothesis that obsessive-compulsive disorder is an alternative expression of the genetic trait for Tourette's disorder comes from family studies demonstrating an increased incidence of obsessive-compulsive disorder among first-degree relatives of Tourette's disorder probands. Segregation analyses of Tourette's disorder families implicate an autosomal-dominant inheritance pattern with variable expression of Tourette's, obsessive-compulsive, and chronic tic disorders. There appears to be a gender-specific penetrance of these traits, with males showing almost complete penetrance when considering Tourette's and chronic tic disorders alone. Females, on the other hand, show a 56 percent penetrance for Tourette's and chronic tic disorders alone, increasing to 70 percent when obsessive-compulsive disorder is added.

Between 20 and 60 percent of children with Tourette's disorder have symptoms compatible with a diagnosis of attention deficit hyperactivity disorder, including decreased attention span, poor impulse control, difficulty concentrating, and restlessness. Indeed, the symptoms of attention deficit hyperactivity disorder often predate the onset of tics, prompting treatment with stimulant medications that themselves may trigger or worsen the underlying tic disorder.

The association between attention deficit hyperactivity and Tourette's disorders, however, is generally less well documented than that between obsessive-compulsive and Tourette's disorders. Some family studies demonstrate that attention deficit hyperactivity disorder segregates separately from Tourette's disorder; in any event, an etiologic relationship is difficult to establish with certainty.

In addition to attention deficit hyperactivity and obsessive-compulsive disorders, patients with Tourette's disorder frequently suffer from other comorbid behavioral difficulties, including depression, anxiety, and conduct disorder. Personality characteristics such as irritability, argumentativeness, and impulsivity all may occur, either as a part of the disorder itself, or as a reaction to it.

TREATMENT

Tourette's disorder is multifaceted, requiring an individualized assessment and treatment plan for each patient. In general, one or another aspect of the disorder emerges as most troublesome. Thus, one patient may find that the tics are disabling, whereas another may be incapacitated by obsessive fears. Once identified, the patient's primary problem may be specifically targeted.

It is important to bear in mind that most Tourette's disorder patients have only mild to moderate symptoms. Such patients are typically well adapted to their social, educational, and family environments, and may ideally avoid medication altogether. If interventions are to be made, they are often most useful in the context of a restructured environment. This is particularly true in the case of school, where patients may benefit from such simple measures as supportive counseling, self-paced learning, one-on-one tutorials, and small group teaching. We regard the home as a place of refuge, where it is not necessary for the patient to expend energy in the taxing effort to suppress tics. Family and individual supportive counseling may be of benefit here as well.

Treatment with medications should be reserved for patients with disabling disease, as defined with regard to maladaptations in home, work, or school environments. A large variety of agents are currently available for the treatment of tics, obsessive-compulsive symptoms, attention deficit, hyperactivity, and other related behavioral disorders (Table 127-1). Agents must be selected on the basis of target symptoms and potential side effects. Dosages should be titrated slowly, seeking the least amount of drug that is both effective and tolerable.

Haloperidol was introduced as a highly effective tic-suppressing agent in the late 1960s. Prior to its introduction, clini-

TABLE 127-1. Pharmacologic Treatments of Tourette's Disorder

Problem	Agent
Tics	Clonidine
	Neuroleptics
	Tetrabenazine, reserpine
	Other drugs
	Botulinum toxin injections (for dystonic tics)
Obsessive-compulsive symptoms	Selective serotonin re-uptake inhibitors
Attention deficit hyperactivity disorder	Clonidine
	Stimulants

cians had tended to view Tourette's disorder as a psychological disorder. The remarkable response rate (75 to 80 percent) forced a new understanding of the syndrome in terms of a derangement in brain dopaminergic systems. With the more recent clarification of the link between obsessive-compulsive and Tourette's disorders, this formulation has expanded to include serotonergic models as well. The major action of the neuroleptics in tic suppression is thought to rest upon their blockade of dopamine D2 receptors. The antipsychotic agent, clozapine, with its predominant action at the D4 receptor, has not been effective in Tourette's disorder patients previously responsive to haloperidol.

Although haloperidol is the most commonly prescribed medication for Tourette's disorder, it is important for clinicians to avoid the reflexive use of this agent. We favor starting at a very low dosage, 0.25 mg nightly, and working up slowly by 0.25 to 0.5 mg every 4 to 7 days until symptoms are relieved or side effects appear. Most patients respond at dosages of 5 mg/d or less. We prefer not to exceed 15 mg/d. In an effort to avoid the worst effects of sedation, we aim for a single bedtime dosing schedule.

Motor side effects of haloperidol include acute dystonic reactions, drug-induced parkinsonism, akasthisia, and tardive dyskinesia. In addition, patients may develop disabling drowsiness, depression, increased appetite with attendant weight gain, and school and social phobias.

Pimozide is the only neuroleptic currently marketed specifically for the treatment of Tourette's disorder. It has been shown to be equally as effective as haloperidol for suppressing tics. The motor side effect profile is similar to that of the other neuroleptics, including haloperidol, fluphenazine, and trifluoperazine. Like the latter agents, however, it is possibly less sedating than haloperidol. Any of these neuroleptics can be used satisfactorily to suppress tics. The most serious potential side effect of pimozide is prolongation of the Q-T interval. There are rare reports of sudden death at dosages in excess of 60 mg/d (which is much higher than the dosages typically employed to treat tics). An electrocardiogram should be obtained prior to starting this medication, and it should be monitored during the period of dosage adjustment. Patients may begin treatment at 1.0 mg (one-half a tablet) nightly. Medication should be slowly titrated to achieve the minimum effective dosage. Maximum recommended dosage is 0.2 mg/kg/day, generally not in excess of 10 mg/day.

A number of non-neuroleptic tic-suppressing agents have gained adherents among clinicians treating patients with Tourette's disorder. In general, these agents are less reliably effective than the neuroleptics, but their side effect profiles are favorable.

The centrally acting antiadrenergic agent, clonidine, has been used extensively for the suppression of tics. Although our experience has been favorable, recent double-blinded studies have failed to establish uniform efficacy. The comorbid occurrence of behavioral difficulties often prompts consideration of clonidine therapy, as this agent is frequently used for treatment of attention deficit hyperactivity disorder. Side effects include drowsiness, orthostatic symptoms, anticholinergic effects, and irritability. Acute withdrawal may lead to rebound hypertension as well as agitation and tachycardia. Effects of treatment may take up to 3 months to manifest. Clonidine is started in dosages of 0.05 mg (one-half a tablet)/day, and gradually increased until thrice-daily dosing is achieved. We prefer the brand-name drug, Catapress, as generic formulations have had variable bioavailability. Dosages generally do not exceed 0.5 mg/day total. A transdermal delivery system, Catapress-TTS (Boehringer Ingelheim, Ridgefield, CT), allows dosing once a week, and is useful in children who may find it difficult to swallow pills. The patches come in sizes of 3.5, 7.0, and 10.5 cm^2 (corresponding to 0.1, 0.2, and 0.3 mg/d).

Clonazepam has not been studied in any large, double-blinded, clinical trials, but has received a number of favorable reports with regard to control of motor tics. The diffuse projections of the γ-aminobutyric acid-ergic system make it difficult to precisely characterize clonazepam's locus of action. Efficacy in tic suppression is not thought to be secondary to sedative effects, as other benzodiazipines show no significant benefit in Tourette's disorder. The recommended starting dosage is 0.25 to 0.5 mg/d, with gradual increases over 3 to 6 months to a maintenance dose of 2 to 6 mg/d. More rapid titration commonly yields difficulties with sedation. Side effects include drowsiness and poor concentration; ataxia, dizziness, and headache may occur.

Other agents that have been reported to have a role in the management of tics include reserpine, tetrabenazine, and the calcium channel-blockers. Case reports of carbemazipine, lithium, corticosteroids, estrogens, and clomiphene have been conflicting. Trials of the opiate antagonist naloxone have not confirmed earlier reports of success with this agent. Local intramuscular injections of botulinum toxin can be used to treat patients with painful dystonic (consisting of muscle tightening or twisting) tics.

Treatment of obsessions and compulsions associated with Tourette's disorder has rested primarily upon the use of serotonin re-uptake inhibitors. The first of these that was widely used for the treatment of obsessive-compulsive disorder was clomipramine. There have been several head-to-head trials demonstrating the superior efficacy of clomipramine when compared with other tricyclic antidepressants that do not selectively inhibit serotonin re-uptake. Major improvement or complete suppression of obsessive-compulsive disorder symptoms can be expected in up to 50 percent of patients. Patient compliance with drug initiation may represent a challenge if the obsessional framework extends to fear of medication. The most common side effects are those of the other tricyclic antidepressants, including anticholinergic effects such as xerostomia, constipation, and orthostasis. Seizures may occur slightly more commonly than with other tricyclics. Prolongation of the P-R and Q-T intervals on the electrocardiogram may occur. Treatment with clomipramine generally commences with 25 mg nightly, and is titrated gradually to the lowest effective dosage. A maximum of 250 mg/day in adults or 3.0 mg/kg/d in children should not be exceeded, owing to concerns about cardiotoxicity and lowered seizure threshold. Administration with food may allay the nausea commonly associated with serotonin re-uptake inhibition.

Another serotonin re-uptake inhibitor, fluoxetine, has also proven to be beneficial in the suppression of obsessive-compulsive disorder symptoms in roughly one-half of patients treated.

This has been demonstrated in primary obsessive-compulsive disorder, as well as obsessive-compulsive disorder associated with Tourette's disorder. Major side effects appear to be dose dependant and include anxiety, insomnia, motor restlessness, and social disinhibition. Suicidality has been reported in a small number of adults and children taking fluoxetine, but a causal relationship remains unclear. The best prevention entails close monitoring of adverse effects within the context of a supportive clinical alliance between physician and patient. Liquid formulation enables dosage to start low (2.5 to 5.0 mg/d in children). The drug is titrated slowly to a range of 20 to 80 mg/d in divided doses.

A variety of other serotonin re-uptake inhibitors are currently being evaluated in the treatment of obsessive-compulsive disorder. These include sertraline, fluvoxamine, and paroxetine. The short-acting 5-HT 1a receptor agonist, buspirone, enhances serotonin transmission while inhibiting dopaminergic transmission. Unfortunately, results of studies using this agent in isolation to treat symptoms of obsessive-compulsive disorder have been equivocal. There is perhaps a brighter role for buspirone when used in conjunction with the serotonin re-uptake inhibitors to augment their effects.

Treatment of attention deficit hyperactivity disorder has been dominated by the use of stimulants. The most common medication prescribed is methylphenidate, which has been shown superior to dextroamphetamine and pemoline in comparative studies. Side effects include agitation, insomnia, headaches, anorexia, weight loss, and lowered seizure threshold. Although psychological dependence can occur with long-term use of high-dose methylphenidate, it has not been reported in children treated for attention deficit hyperactivity disorder. This agent is contraindicated in patients with glaucoma. The typical dosage range for methylphenidate is 0.1 to 0.3 mg/kg bid. Pemoline enables once-a-day dosing, but its longer half-life narrows the therapeutic window.

Tic exacerbation is possible when using stimulants to treat attention deficit hyperactivity disorder associated with Tourette's disorder. It should be remembered, however, that a mild worsening of tics may be well worth it to a patient who is debilitated in the classroom by symptoms of attention deficit hyperactivity disorder. The addition of a low dosage of a neuroleptic may be required to suppress tics that are significantly worsened by stimulant therapy for attention deficit hyperactivity disorder.

An attractive alternative to the stimulant medications mentioned above is clonidine, itself effective against both tics (see above) and attention deficit hyperactivity disorder. We frequently use this drug as a first-line agent for youngsters with Tourette's disorder whose school performance is impaired by hyperactivity and attention problems.

The tricyclic agent desipramine has been shown to be effective in controlling the symptoms of attention deficit hyperactivity disorder associated with Tourette's disorder. Usual dosage ranges from 25 to 75 mg/d. Rare reports of sudden death in children treated with this tricyclic, however, raise concern about its potential cardiotoxicity. Close monitoring of the electrocardiogram both before and during treatment with desipramine is mandated.

As noted above, Tourette's disorder patients frequently suffer from poor interpersonal relationships on the basis of behavior disturbances. These may range from simple character traits such as defensiveness and argumentativeness, to full-blown personality disorders. The underlying link between these problems and Tourette's disorder is difficult to establish with certainty.

Whether they are specific to Tourette's disorder or merely a result of the emotional, social, and personal difficulties associated with living with the disease is not well understood. In any case, these behavior disturbances have proven extremely difficult to treat with medications. Rather, a coordinated approach, involving supportive counseling, family therapy, and school and community interventions, appears most useful. As always, it remains important to maintain a low threshold of suspicion for depression, which can often be extremely difficult to assess in children.

SUMMARY

Tourette's disorder represents one end of the spectrum of primary tic disorders. Recognition of the clinical heterogeneity of the syndrome has represented a major advance in recent years, and has enabled a more rational approach to therapy based upon targeting of dominant symptoms. With knowledge that Tourette's disorder is inherited has come hope that the underlying genetic defect will soon be unraveled. Genetic counseling has become an integral part of management in these patients, as has a multidisciplinary approach to supportive treatment.

SUGGESTED READINGS

Bruun RD, Budman CL: The natural history of Tourette's syndrome. Adv Neurol 58:1, 1992

Devinsky O, Geller BD: Gilles de la Tourette's syndrome. p. 471. In Joseph AB, Young RR (eds): Movement Disorders in Neurology and Neuropsychiatry. Blackwell Scientific, Oxford, 1992

Golden GS: Treatment of attention deficit hyperactivity disorder. p. 423. In Kurlan R (ed): Handbook of Tourette's Syndrome and Related Tic and Behavioral Disorders. Marcel Dekker, New York, 1993

Jankovic J: Diagnosis and classification of tics and Tourette syndrome. Adv Neurol 58:7, 1992

King RA, Vitulano LA, Riddle MA: The treatment of obsessive-compulsive disorder in Tourette's syndrome. p. 401. In Kurlan R (ed): Handbook of Tourette's Syndrome and Related Tic and Behavioral disorders. Marcel Dekker, New York, 1993

Kurlan R: Tic disorders: an overview. p. 465. In Joseph AB, Young RR (eds): Movement Disorders in Neurology and Neuropsychiatry. Blackwell Scientific, Oxford, 1992

Kurlan R: Tourette's syndrome: current concepts. Neurology 39:1625, 1989

LeWitt PA: Pharmacotherapy beyond the catacholaminergic systems. p. 389. In Kurlan R (ed): Handbook of Tourette's Syndrome and related tic and behavioral disorders. Marcel Dekker, New York, 1993

Pauls DL: The inheritance pattern. p. 307. In Kurlan R (ed): Handbook of Tourette's Syndrome and Related Tic and Behavioral disorders. Marcel Dekker, New York, 1993

Shapiro AK, Shapiro E: Neuroleptic drugs. p. 347. In Kurlan R (ed): Handbook of Tourette's Syndrome and Related Tic and Behavioral Disorders. Marcel Dekker, New York, 1993

Tourette Syndrome Classification Study Group: Definitions and classification of tic disorders. Arch Neurol 50:1013, 1993

128. MYOCLONUS

DENNIS E. WILKINS

The traditional and deceptively concise term *myoclonus* actually encompasses a wide variety of clinical expressions, pathophysiologies, etiologies, and classifications. It is an uncommon neurologic phenomenon, less frequently encountered in the office than in the hospital. For these reasons, a simplified, pragmatic approach is used here in discussing myoclonus as it presents in adults in an outpatient setting. Basic concepts and a classification scheme are highlighted by details of some of the more common or more notorious clinical disorders. The complete and definitive treatise on myoclonus, written by Marsden, Hallett, and Fahn, is recommended for further information.

DEFINITION

The convoluted history of *myoclonus* precludes a succinct definition. Terminology has been based sometimes on clinical manifestations (e.g., "minipolymyoclonus"), sometimes on pathophysiology (e.g., "reticular reflex myoclonus"), and sometimes on etiology (e.g., the myoclonus of Creutzfeldt-Jakob disease). There is general agreement that *myoclonus* applies to shocklike twitches or jerks of muscles generated by the central nervous system, but attempts at more specific descriptions become bogged down in contradictions and inconsistencies. For example, myoclonus can be normal or abnormal; associated with an otherwise normal or abnormal neurologic status; familial or not familial; subtle, involving a motor unit, or prominent, involving the the entire body; represented by an individual jerk or a series or jerks; acute and transient, or chronic and persistent; rhythmic or arrhythmic; intimately related to epilepsy or not; spontaneous or reflex-sensitive or movement-induced or state-dependent; without need for treatment or treatment-responsive or treatment-refractory. Any definition of myoclonus must also be concerned not only by what it is, but by what it is not. Many neurologic phenomena can twitch and jerk in potentially confounding, similar ways: fasciculations, blepharospasm, hemifacial spasm, tics, chorea, ballismus, tremor, asterixis, normal startle reflex, abonormal startle syndromes, psychogenic movements. Ultimately, myoclonus can be functionally defined as a quick, involuntary muscle movement arising in the central nervous system and not conforming to the nonmyoclonic disorders listed immediately above.

Specifics of the clinical history and context supplemented by examination will most often delineate a clinical syndrome that, once recognized, allows for accurate diagnosis. Situations may exist, however, when the most expert clinicians hesitate or err even after careful analysis of involuntary movements as to distribution, speed and abruptness, rhythmicity, and sensitivity to posture, movement, sensory stimuli, or physiologic state. In such a case, if the question of myoclonus is important for patient management, one possible approach would employ specialized electrophysiologic techniques. Technical details are beyond the scope of this chapter, but they can range from a straightforward surface recording of muscle activity to sophisticated, computerized, jerk-locked averaging of electroencephalographic data. At best, a clinical neurophysiologist experienced in movement disorders and the use of related diagnostic technology can differentiate myoclonus from nonmyoclonus, localize the anatomic origin within the central nervous system, and characterize the degree of reflex sensitivity.

CLASSIFICATION

We will classify myoclonus into four groups: (1) normal myoclonus, (2) abnormal myoclonus in an otherwise normal patient, (3) abnormal myoclonus in an epileptic but otherwise normal patient, and (4) abnormal myoclonus with or without epilepsy in a patient with other neurologic abnormalities.

Normal Myoclonus

As an individual falls asleep, a sudden jerk of all or part of the body may accompany a vivid sensory experience, especially a sense of falling. This is the presumptively universal hypnic jerk, rivaled in frequency only by a similarly ubiquitous myoclonic expression, the hiccough.

Abnormal Myoclonus in an Otherwise Normal Patient

The most common example of abnormal myoclonus in otherwise normal patients is periodic movements in sleep, a potentially disruptive disorder discussed in Chapter 129.

Quite rare, but more traditionally definitive of this category, is ballistic movement overflow myoclonus. In this familial disorder with onset in the first decade of life, rapid voluntary movements are imperfectly generated, leading to variable degrees of disability. For a given movement, relevant muscles are excessively activated, and extraneous muscles are inappropriately incorporated into the movement. The result is a too-vigorous, incoordinated, jerky motion. Those afflicted are otherwise normal neurologically and exhibit an unremarkable electroencephalogram. Attempted therapies fail to be consistently effective in this lifelong problem.

Abnormal Myoclonus in an Epileptic but Otherwise Normal Patient

It is estimated that 7 percent of all patients with epilepsy—a significantly higher percentage if only adults are considered—have a specific electroclinical syndrome termed juvenile myoclonic epilepsy (of Janz). The importance of this disorder lies in its relatively high prevalence, its classical myoclonic symptoms, and its frequent misdiagnosis in the face of highly effective therapy. The hallmark is the onset of myoclonus near puberty, between 12 to 18 years of age, with a peak at age 14. The myoclonus tends to emphasize the upper extremities and is characteristically most active shortly after awakening. The motor phenomena may present subtly with a twitchy, clumsy "jitteriness" of the hands or dramatically with a flinging of a bar of soap from the shower or a cup of coffee across the breakfast table. A generalized tonic-clonic convulsion may arise from a brief series of myoclonic jerks or occur unheralded; in either event, 80 percent of individuals will be so afflicted at some point. A smaller fraction, 25 percent, may experience true absence seizures in childhood. Juvenile myoclonic epilepsy is a primary generalized epilepsy, idiopathic in origin, and unassociated with other neurologic abnormalities. As with many epilepsies, sleep deprivation and overuse of alcohol can be aggravating factors. One clinical point to emphasize is that these patients may not recognize their morning motor manifestations (i.e., myoclonus) as being related to other seizure events. Unless the clinician specifically seeks this historical diagnostic key, the syndromic diagnosis may be missed, and a suboptimal therapy initiated. Such a situation is not rarely encountered in young adults in the office. Valproic acid is totally effective in up to 86 percent of patients but must be maintained indefinitely, since a relapse rate approaching 91 percent has been reported with attempted anticonvulsant withdrawal. The most characteristic but not necessarily the most common electroencephalographic component of this electroclinical syndrome consists of a bilaterally symmetric polyspike-and-wave discharge, the slow wave occurring at 4 to 6 cycles/s. Interictal recordings, however, may be normal, especially in successfully treated patients.

Abnormal Myoclonus with Other Abnormalities and With or Without Epilepsy

Initially, when a neurologically normal child or adolescent exhibits myoclonus and generalized motor seizures, juvenile myoclonic epilepsy (discussed immediately above) must be considered. Over a number of years, however, a progressive myoclonic epilepsy syndrome may instead develop, characterized by increasingly refractory epileptic manifestations in association with an evolving dementia, ataxia, or other neurologic abnormalities. Such a scenario is fortunately quite rare. But in spite of this rarity, the drama of progressive neurologic devastation coupled with a daunting array of at least 15 specific recognized causes for this syndrome has historically commanded much attention. Some of the more noteworthy etiologies include the degeneration of Unverricht-Lundborg syndrome, the storage diseases of ceroid lipofuscinosis and Lafora body disease (polyglucosan inclusions), and the mitochondrial disorder termed MERRF—myoclonic epilepsy and ragged red fibers. Although the syndromic diagnosis derives from the clinical course, the overall context, combined with a variety of neurologic details, usually act as clues pinpointing a more specific diagnostic entity. These incurable processes are typically inherited in an autosomal-recessive pattern. At first, valproate and clonazepam may effectively treat myoclonus and seizures, whereas phenytoin may occasionally aggravate circumstances.

The progressive myoclonic epilepsy syndrome may, indeed, culminate in a form of myoclonic dementia, but emphasis upon the young age of its victims and upon the prominent epileptic features are important identifying characteristics. The more frequent occurrence of myoclonic dementia in the middle-aged and in the elderly presents the probability of a much more restricted differential diagnosis (i.e., Creutzfeldt-Jakob disease versus Alzheimer's disease). These two disorders may exhibit substantial overlap of clinical and laboratory findings. Creutzfeldt-Jakob disease, also known as subacute spongiform encephalopathy, does not present with myoclonus, but 88 percent of patients will eventually twitch and jerk sometime in the course of their disease. Similarly, the majority will also develop a periodic electroencephalogram at some point. In fact, the persistent absence of both myoclonus and a periodic electroencephalogram should force serious reconsideration of the diagnosis of subacute spongiform encephalopathy. The high prevalence of Alzheimer's disease, combined with observations suggesting that one-quarter of closely followed patients may display myoclonus by 8 years after onset, indicates that Alzheimer's disease may be the more common cause of myoclonic dementia. Given that senile dementia of the Alzheimer type may also, on rare occasions, generate a periodic electrocephalogram and have an atypically fast course, and given that subacute spongiform encephalopathy may have an atypically slow course, an accurate etiologic diagnosis for myoclonic dementia—short of the pathologist's bench—may be prohibited.

Most clinicians will have more than a passing acquaintance with the medical state known as a toxic-metabolic encephalopathy. Patients with this condition may present in the office in the earlier stages of confusion, delirium, or stupor. A spectrum of agitated muscular activity can be associated: fasciculatory twitching, trembling tremors, asterixis, myoclonus, and the ultimate generalized motor convulsion. Distinguishing among the various phenomena may be obvious or difficult; recognizing them as the hyperactive expression of a stressed neuromuscular system is crucial. Some of the more frequent etiologies would include withdrawal from alcohol or benzodiazepines, hyponatremia, uremia, and lithium intoxication.

A particular metabolic derangement requires special note. Nonketotic hyperglycemia can generate a prolonged series of myoclonic jerks limited to one part of the body, a scenario often referred to as "epilepsia partialis continua." Approximately 60 percent of these patients will have an underlying structural lesion, often old and static, anatomically correlating with the distribution of the repetitive myoclonus. Uncommon but not rare, this disorder can actually be the presenting symptom for the new diagnosis of diabetes. Patients may be alert or minimally encephalopathic. The myoclonus is typically resistant to therapy with anticonvulsants but will eventually respond to the correction of the hyperglycemia. Singh and Strobos (1980) reported an average blood glucose of 690 mg percent (range, 321 to 1,509) in their patients; hyponatremia and hyperosmolality were less prominent but probably contributing metabolic imbalances.

This book focuses upon office practice, and it undeniably would require the most exceptional circumstances to encounter a comatose patient in that setting. Yet, a rare disorder that permeates the literature on myoclonus should be briefly mentioned for completeness. Anoxic encephalopathy, of course, is one of the more common causes of "metabolic" myoclonus within the hospital. Among those who recover with moderate residual damage—as evidenced by cognitive deficits, emotional lability, dysarthria, ataxia, and so on—a chronic, more circumscribed form of myoclonus can be seen, evoked reliably by precise, voluntary movements and less reliably by sensory stimuli. Here, arrhythmic jerks of variable intensity can disrupt important daily functions such as speech, eating, and dressing. Even walking can be disabled by sudden lapses of leg tone, perhaps representing a "negative" myoclonic phenomenon. Clonazepam may aid the myoclonus, though obviously the damaged central nervous system substrate remains limiting.

Focal injury to certain structures within the brainstem or spinal cord gives rise to a special form of myoclonus termed "segmental" myoclonus. Although a spectrum of clinical manifestations have been reported, the most representative example would simulate a tremor with persistent rhythmicity at 1 to 3 cycles/s, unaltered by voluntary actions, different physiologic states, or sensory stimuli. The prototypical entity here is palatal myoclonus, arising when axons from the dentate nucleus of the cerebellum are interrupted in their passage to the inferior olivary nucleus of the brainstem. Lesions resulting in such a disconnection would most often result from ischemic infarction, followed in frequency by demyelinating inflammation or shearing trauma. Palatal myoclonus expresses itself through the muscles of the soft palate, pharynx, and larynx, with more prominent cases overflowing into physiologically related cervical muscles and the diaphragm. Clonazepam has been reported as helpful in some instances. This entire picture of palatal myoclonus can be mimicked at the spinal level when one or more contiguous cord segments become injured by any of a number of insults, such as physical or electrical trauma, infection, or demyelination.

CONCLUSION

To thoroughly explore myoclonus would demand a journey into remote recesses of the neurologic world, burdened by the irregularities of generations of accumulating knowledge and requiring occasional use of sophisticated modern neurophysiologic techniques. In the present context, such a journey is neither practical nor worthwhile. Instead, this chapter attempts to offer real help to the clinician faced with an adult patient in the office with whom the question of myoclonus arises. A working definition of myoclonus is complemented by a pragmatic classification, and basic information regarding carefully selected disorders is provided.

SUGGESTED READINGS

Berkovic SF, So NK, Andermann F: Progressive myoclonic epilepsies: clinical and neurophysiological diagnosis. J Clin Neurophysiol 8:261, 1991
Brown P, Cathala F, Castaigne P, Gadjusek DC: Creutzfeldt-Jakob disease: clinical analysis of a consecutive series of 230 neuropathologically verified cases. Ann Neurol 20:597, 1986
Dreifuss FE: Juvenile myoclonic epilepsy: characteristics of a primary generalized epilepsy. Epilepsia (suppl.) 4:S1, 1989
Hallett M, Chadwick D, Marsden CD: Ballistic movement overflow myoclonus: a form of essential myoclonus. Brain 100:299, 1977
Jankovic J, Pardo R: Segmental myoclonus: clinical and pharmacologic study. Arch Neurol 43:1025, 1986
Lance JW, Adams RD: The syndrome of intention or action myoclonus as a sequel to hypoxic encephalopathy. Brain 86:111, 1963
Marsden CD, Hallett M, Fahn S: The nosology and pathophysiology of myoclonus. p. 196. In Marsden CD, Fahn S (eds): Movement Disorders. Butterworth Scientific, London, 1982
Mayeux R, Stern Y, Spanton S: Heterogeneity in dementia of the Alzheimer type: evidence of subgroups. Neurology 35:453, 1985
Singh BM, Strobos RJ: Epilepsia partialis continua associated with nonketotic hyperglycemia: clinical and biochemical profile of 21 patients. Ann Neurol 8:155, 1980

129. MOVEMENT DISORDERS IN SLEEP AND RESTLESS LEGS SYNDROME

BRUCE EHRENBERG

BACKGROUND

Thomas Willis in 1685 was the first to describe patients troubled by restless leg movements, and he noted that they often had insomnia. Ekbom published a series of articles about restless legs syndrome (RLS) in 1940s, and for a time his name became synonymous with the disorder (Ekbom syndrome). Symonds described abnormal twitches during sleep—"nocturnal myoclonus"—which he distinguished from "common nocturnal jerks." The latter are now called sleep-onset myoclonus, hypnic jerks, or sleep starts and are considered normal, as are the twitches of various skeletal muscles without synchrony, periodicity or symmetry, usually seen during rapid eye movement (REM) sleep. Symonds's patients with nocturnal myoclonus all had insomnia, and at least one case had periodic arousals at 1-minute intervals, consistent with the modern definition of periodic limb movements disorder of sleep (PLMS; this terminology has replaced nocturnal myoclonus). The current definition also allows for the fact that at least as many patients may present with hypersomnia as with insomnia.

Lugaresi et al. were first to polygraphically record periodic leg movements in sleep from patients with PLMS. They recorded similar nocturnal phenomena from patients with RLS, thus indicating that these two disorders may be physiologically linked. His group also studied the sleep manifestations of various other forms of pathologic myoclonus and found that (1) spinal myoclonus and facial spasms often persist during sleep; (2) cortically mediated epileptic myoclonus (rhythmic jerks of epilepsia partialis continua, repeated partial motor seizures of Jacksonian epilepsy, and spasms of subacute sclerosing leucoencephalitis) gradually decreases with onset of sleep; and (3) movements of extrapyramidal origin (choreoathetosis, hemiballismus) or subcortical and brainstem origin (palatal myoclonus, opsoclonus) reliably disappear in sleep. Nevertheless, these disorders must be carefully differentiated from PLMS, as should the myoclonic manifestations of Alzheimer's and Creutzfeldt-Jakob disease. Also, the fasciculations of amyotrophic lateral sclerosis and other diseases of the anterior horn cell or lower motor neuron are mediated at the spinal cord level and do not disappear in sleep. The REM behavior disorder is a nocturnal syndrome with movements ranging from fragmentary myoclonus to rather extreme gross body movements during REM sleep, often involving widespread motion of limbs in an "acting out" fashion, as though the patient were physically involved in a dream; this may be seen in an "idiopathic" form, or with degenerative disorders such as olivopontocerebellar degeneration, and may be related to a loss of the generalized motor inhibition normally found in human REM sleep.

The tremor of Parkinson's disease diminishes during sleep. Because of the age group involved, PLMS is common in Parkinsonian patients, though this was originally thought to be from levodopa treatment. However, considering the short half-life of levodopa (as used in the early studies), it is likely that most of the observed movements occurred after the dopaminergic effects had worn off. Indeed, levodopa is now a first-line treatment for the leg movements of RLS and PLMS. Similarly, dopaminergic blockers such as chlorpromazine or haloperidol are known to cause akathisia, which, as Walters and Hening have noted, is strikingly similar to RLS, and these patients often have PLMS-like activity during sleep as well.

Sleep bruxism (nocturnal teeth-grinding) and fragmentary myoclonus of non-REM (NREM) sleep are two other movement disorders found in sleep that share some common features with RLS and PLMS, and may be "distant cousins" physiologically. Table 129-1 summarizes the relations of movement disorders with sleep.

DEFINITIONS AND METHODOLOGIES
Clinical Features

Periodic Limb Movements Disorder of Sleep. PLMS is defined by the characteristic repetitive episodes of stereotyped limb movements. Although the arms can be involved, the vast majority of patients have only leg movements, usually consisting of big toe extension sometimes combined with partial flexions of the ankle, knee, and hip (it has been noted that there may also be fanning of the smaller toes, thus mimicking the Babinski and "triple flexion" responses; however, this is not a common presentation). Unlike most other movement disorders, which are abolished during sleep, PLMS activity appears with the onset of sleep. The movements are usually associated with disturbances of sleep ranging from full awakenings to minimal electroencephalographic (EEG) arousals, and the percentage of movements associated with any such sleep disruption can vary from 0 to 100 percent, but usually is about 35 percent. Patients are unaware of all but the most prominent movements and arousals, and the movement activity can vary greatly from night

TABLE 129-1. Movement Disorders and Sleep

Type of Movement	NREM	REM	Awake
Tremor (essential or Parkinson's)	−	−	+
Choreoathetosis (including Huntington's)	−	±	+
Hemiballismus	−	−	+
Spinal myoclonus	+ +	±	+
Palatal myoclonus and epileptic myoclonus	±	±	+
Opsoclonus	−	−	+
Epilepsia partialis continua	±	−	+
Other sleep-related epilepsy	+	Rare	±
Spasms of SSPE	±	?	+
Torsion dystonias	±	−	+
Paroxysmal nocturnal dystonia	+	−	−
REM behavior disorder	−	+	−
PLMS	+	Rare	+
RLS	+	Rare	+
Sleepwalking (somnambulism)	+	−	−
Sleep bruxism (teeth-grinding)	+	±	−
Fragmentary non-REM myoclonus	+	+ (normal)	−
Benign neonatal sleep myoclonus	+	Rare	−
Sleep starts	+	−	−
Rhythmic movement disorder (head-banging)	+	Rare	−

Abbreviations: PLMS, periodic limb movements of sleep; REM, rapid eye movement (sleep); RLS, restless legs syndrome; NREM, non-rapid eye movement (sleep).

to night, making it difficult to diagnose PLMS by patient history alone. Bed partner reports of leg kicking can be helpful, and if periodic movements are carefully timed, the diagnosis may be made. The movements generally have a duration of 0.5 to 5 seconds (most patients average 2 seconds) and a repetition interval of 5 to 90 seconds (most patients repeat at 20- to 40-second intervals). The limbs are immobile between episodes.

The amplitude of the movements can be crudely measured on the PSG by comparing the electromyogram (EMG) in the anterior tibialis muscles during voluntary contractions while awake, to the EMG bursts in the same muscles during sleep. However, since volitional muscle activation varies, there is no reliable way to calibrate the EMG output for all patients; some patients may have repeated arousals in association with very small EMG bursts that are difficult to distinguish from background noise. Perhaps these recording problems account for those cases where the apparent movements are too few in number to explain a particular patient's daytime sleepiness. Indeed, the polysomnogram (PSGs, all-night sleep EEG) of some hypersomniacs without leg movements show numerous arousal and subarousal EEG patterns with the same periodicities seen when leg movements are present, thus implying that the movements are only an epiphenomenon of a fundamental central nervous system (CNS) disturbance during sleep; some clinicians believe that these nonmovement arousals (sometimes called α intrusions) are equal in impact to the disturbance of sleep seen in full-blown PLMS.

Contrariwise, there are patients with PLMS who have very large numbers of leg movements, but few or no EEG arousals. These patients may have less prominent daytime fatigue, but some may develop degenerative arthritis. Some patients have very violent kicks, and may injure their bed partners or themselves. (Two PLMS patients in our clinic developed knee injuries while asleep, eventually requiring surgery.)

The distribution of leg movements over the various sleep

stages can vary; some patients have the largest amounts of leg movement activity in stages 3 to 4, but most have the maximum activity in stage 2. One study showed the relationship between RLS and PLMS in nine members of one family; the leg movements were recorded in wakefulness as well as sleep and showed a periodicity similar to that seen in PLMS, with the intermovement intervals gradually increasing as the patients became drowsy and entered stage 2 sleep; the authors concluded that RLS and PLMS "represent two clinical manifestations of the same CNS dysfunction."

When scoring PSG recordings, the sleep stages are delineated first, so that leg movements can be assessed according to the sleep stage in which they occur (including brief periods of wakefulness). Leg movements associated with the end of an apnea or hypopnea are thought to be hypoxia-induced, and are counted separately, since they may be abolished by treatments for sleep apnea. It is useful to note the number of times a leg movement is followed by a full awakening usually defined as the appearance or an occipital α (8 to 12 Hz) rhythm for at least 60 seconds; an incomplete awakening, α for 15 to 60 seconds; or an arousal, which can be defined as the appearance of occipital α activity for 3 to 15 seconds. (Occasionally, there are large amounts of generalized 7 to 11-Hz activity during NREM sleep—the so-called "α δ" pattern—in patients with the fibrositis-fibromyalgia syndrome, although these patients can have α δ without PLMS.) Further, it may be difficult to differentiate some "normal" features of NREM sleep from subtle arousal patterns: (1) prolonged spindle-β (12 to 18 Hz) activity, (2) bursts of δ (1 to 3 Hz) activity, (3) K complexes. Subtle arousals can be surmised when a physiologic event such as a leg movement is closely associated with a vertex V wave or K complex, EEG phenomena that are known to occur normally when externally applied stimuli disturb sleep.

Carskadon et al. found that PLMS is common in the "normal" elderly, and even though their subjects complained of neither nocturnal insomnia nor daytime sleepiness, there was a substantial amount of daytime sleepiness on objective testing (Multiple Sleep Latency Test); Coleman remarked that this "indicates that the concept of having a sleep-wake complaint is very subjective." Indeed, patients with PLMS may present with either insomnia (sleep maintenance type*) or hypersomnia. This looks like a paradox, but working diagnoses are usually based on presenting complaints, even though objective (PSG/ Multiple Sleep Latency Test) findings may not fully explain the patient's symptoms. Indeed, the line distinguishing insomniacs from hypersomniacs is blurred on close examination: both groups have poor-quality sleep of which they are aware to various degrees, and the primary difference is the ability of the insomnia patients to maintain alertness—appropriately in the daytime, but *too* well at night—whereas the hypersomnia patients have similarly poor quality sleep at night and much more difficulty staying awake in the day.

Restless Legs Syndrome. Restless legs syndrome is "characterized by disagreeable leg sensations, usually prior to sleep onset, that cause an almost irresistable urge to move the legs." The main symptom is often difficult for the patient to describe, and sometimes the words used—*itching, tingling*—suggest the

dysesthesias of peripheral neuropathy; whereas at other times, the patient will describe severe pains in the legs, suggesting sciatica, diabetic nerve infarct, or radiculopathy due to root encroachment. All of these must be ruled out before a diagnosis of RLS can be comfortably considered, although it is likely that some patients (e.g., those with diabetic or uremic neuropathies) can have both RLS and a neuropathy at the same time. The sensations are usually deep-seated, bilateral, and restricted to the lower legs, but can involve the thighs, and rarely may be unilateral or involve the arms.

The disorder can begin at any age and may wax and wane over the years. In familial cases, there may be earlier age onset in each successive generation. The inheritance pattern may be autosomal dominant but the variable penetrance can make cases from small families appear to be sporadic until a detailed family history is obtained (including data on nocturnal movements). There is a tendency for exacerbation in times of stress, and many women with RLS may have their initial bout during the latter half of their first pregnancy.

The restlessness or discomfort begins toward evening, and increases further with sitting or lying down, making television- or movie-watching difficult. The symptoms are nearly always relieved by walking or pacing, or by exercise of any kind, including stretching, cycling, swimming, and running. However, when the patient sits back down, the symptoms tend to return quickly unless the exercise has been extensive. Montplaisir et al. have developed simple laboratory methods to diagnose RLS using only surface EMG electrodes applied to the anterior tibialis muscles during a 30-minute evening recording. This test was called the suggested immobilization test because patients were asked to sit on a stretcher or bed with eyes open and try to remain motionless. This method yielded positive results (periodic EMG bursts on the recordings) in about 67 percent of patients if recorded on two consecutive nights. To increase the sensitivity of testing, the forced immobiliaztion test was developed. This test is similar to the suggested immobilization test except that patients sit on the stretcher with their legs tied down in the extended position.

Nearly all patients with RLS also have PLMS in sleep, as demonstrated by polysomnography. However, RLS patients can also be shown to have periodic leg movements while awake if they are closely observed after being asked to avoid voluntary leg movements. The periodicity is often briefer in the awake state (typically 15 seconds apart) than during sleep (usually 20- to 40-second intervals, as previously described for PLMS). Montplaisir et al. showed that the intermovement interval in familial RLS/PLMS with insomnia lengthens from 24 seconds in stage 1 sleep, to 35 seconds upon entering stage 2 of sleep. Patients with severe RLS/PLMS may not be able to sleep at all, but those who are able to sleep usually can enter stage 2 within 30 to 60 minutes, and although there may be abundant periodic leg movements, their sleep is usually no worse than the average patient with PLMS alone, and there is a tendency for the RLS patient to have fewer leg movements toward morning. Some of the severely afflicted patients are phase-delayed; that is, they stay awake for several hours, and then fall asleep when the leg movements have diminished, as though their sleep mechanism was suspended until the circadian phase was right for the movements to drop out. These patients may then sleep later into the morning in order to "catch up" on the number of hours they need, whereas still others are unable to obtain more than 4 to 5 hours total sleep per night.

As with PLMS, RLS patients may complain of either insom-

---

*It should be noted that sleep maintenance insomnia is usually associated with a physiologic sleep disorder, whereas sleep onset insomnia is most often associated with a psychological or psychiatric condition.

nia or excessive daytime sleepiness. The RLS patients with excessive daytime sleepiness are often older, but young adults with it may require more therapeutic effort, since employability may be an issue. Excessive daytime sleepiness was studied by Coleman et al. in a small group of older PLMS patients; the number of arousals per hour of sleep correlated with the subsequent day's degree of sleepiness as measured on the Multiple Sleep Latency Test. Another study showed differences in the sleep disruption patterns of insomniac and hypersomniac PLMS patients: the sleepy patients had longer histories of poor sleep (average 22.4 versus 14.3 years), but more total arousals that were short in duration and concentrated in clusters. The reasons for these findings are not clear, but Rosenthal et al. suggest two hypotheses: (1) the insomniacs are more sensitive to awakening stimuli during sleep (such as the leg movements may represent), whereas the hypersomnolent patients tend to sleep through the stimuli; or (2) the two groups represent two points on a continuum, with the hypersomnolent patients being at a more advanced stage.

Coleman et al. looked at the final diagnosis among sleep disorders patients whose PSGs showed PLMS; in one early study of 441 sleep-clinic patients, they found more than 40 periodic movements in 19 percent of insomniacs, 15 percent of sleep apnea patients, 10 percent of narcoleptics, 12 percent of patients with "other hypersomnias," and 9 percent of patients with other disorders, including parasomnias and sleep–wake schedule disorders. This seems to indicate that PLMS is either a nonspecific finding among patients with a variety of sleep complaints, or that PLMS may be a contributing factor in many different sleep disorders. The latter concept is supported by the fact that many patients with daytime hypersomnolence have only PLMS as a sleep-disturbing factor on their PSGs. In addition, there are several studies that show an increased incidence of PLMS in narcolepsy, but other studies dispute the importance of the finding, or show no increase; it is likely that PLMS is hereditary and its determinants may turn out to be loosely linked to the human leukocyte antigen-DR2 locus that has been found prevalent among narcoleptics. However, no matter how sleepy, PLMS patients do not have the REM-onset tendency diagnostic of narcolepsy.

Conditions found with RLS (but not usually with PLMS alone) include iron- and folate-deficiency anemias, neuropathies with diabetes, amyloid or uremia, and normal pregnancy. PLMS was found prevalent among childhood leukemics in remission; the patients had all received cranial irradiation and intrathecal methotrexate, which may have altered central dopamine and serotonin function. Cold feet may trigger attacks of RLS, according to Ekbom, whereas a fever sometimes abolishes the movements. Although these same factors have not all been reported in association with PLMS, there is a report of improvement in PLMS in a patient using thermal biofeedback, and one PLMS-insomnia patient whom I observed had her best sleep during treatment with α-interferon (an agent that induces fevers and sleep).

Fibromyalgia/fibrositis syndrome has been related to PLMS and "α-δ" sleep. The latter involves the appearance of large amounts of α activity during deep NREM sleep (stages 3 and 4, often called "δ sleep"), and can be found in patients with other disorders, including hypersomnolence, eating disorders, and schizoid or affective disorders. Some fibrositis patients may respond to chlorpromazine or amitriptyline, but antipsychotics can cause akathisia (which Walters and Hening have argued is

a form of RLS) and PLMS, whereas tricyclics may worsen both daytime sleepiness and PLMS.

A study of three patients with atypical depression found that each had PLMS. Other disorders in which PLMS or RLS may play a part include attention deficit hyperactivity disorder (pediatric and adult forms), migraine, toxemia of pregnancy, epilepsy, premenstrual syndrome, and pseudodementia. Treatment of the sleep problem in each of these disorders may be helpful, but larger, controlled studies are needed to confirm these findings.

EPIDEMIOLOGY

PLMS and RLS together may affect up to 5 percent of the population, but the incidence of PLMS increases with age and is most prevalent in the elderly (see Coleman et al., 1983). A survey of healthy seniors over age 60 found PLMS in 57 percent, although one-half had fewer than five movements per hour. In other studies, PLMS/RLS incidences of 37 to 53 percent have been found among sleep disorder patients over 60 years of age, and 18 percent in one study had PLMS or RLS as their primary diagnosis, whereas longitudinal follow-up showed an increasing prevalence of nocturnal movements with aging. On the other end of the age spectrum, children as young as 1 year have been diagnosed with PLMS and RLS.

Among patients of all ages, 3 to 26 percent of insomniacs and 1 to 12 percent of hypersomnolent patients can be diagnosed with PLMS/RLS. Given the high prevalence among the elderly, the rate of sleep complaints seems low compared to younger age groups. Perhaps many seniors accept the prevailing geriatric stereotype of slowed function or lowered expectations of sleep quality.

ETIOLOGY

As mentioned above, PLMS is almost invariably present in cases of familial RLS. Montplaisir et al. noted an elevation of dopamine metabolites in the CNS and suggest that dopamine receptors may be reduced in sensitivity in these disorders.

Askenasy et al. thought that PLMS/RLS in Parkinson's disease patients results from basal ganglia dysfunction, but this conclusion was based on improvement from levodopa. Wechsler et al. showed that PLMS patients have hyperexcitable blink reflexes, somatosensory evoked responses, long-latency motor responses, and H reflexes, indicating possible pontine dysfunction. However, PLMS may still be either the cause—through sleep deprivation—or the result of such hyperexcitability.

Referring to Smith's work on the Babinski-like appearance of the lower extremities during the movements of PLMS, Walters and Henig have questioned whether there is pyramidal tract dysfunction in PLMS, causing a release of central inhibitory activity.

The antigravity muscles of the legs (gastrocnemii, quadriceps, glutei) can overpower the opposing muscles, causing contractures in immobilized patients when a stroke or spinal cord lesion blocks upper motor neuron outflow. There may be an innate drive for the opposing muscles to be exercised, and this need may be genetically greater in the PLMS/RLS patients, such that internal mechanisms supervene whenever daytime activity levels have been insufficient. Exercise in normals has been shown to improve stage 3 to 4 sleep (possibly protective against PLMS); exercise may reduce the central drive for PLMS and is known to reduce the symptoms of RLS. In two women athletes accustomed to 5 hours of strenuous exercise daily, the sudden cessation of all exercise led to marked PLMS and sleep disruption, plus daytime hypersomnolence within a week's time. By extension, it is possible that in the elderly the deterioration in stages 3 to 4 sleep and the great prevalence of PLMS are both caused by age-related reductions in exercise levels. This does not account for the occasional case of severe PLMS found in young adults or children, but such early-onset cases may be due to genetic factors, as can be clearly seen in familial RLS.

Coleman et al. noted that patients with PLMS may have altered circadian rhythms, and postulated that this might be an underlying causative factor in PLMS. RLS symptoms also show a marked circadian pattern, with most patients having maximum restlessness during the evening and first part of the night. It has been suggested that these disorders may be caused by dysfunction of the circadian rhythm pacemaker in the suprachiasmatic nucleus. The suprachiasmatic nucleus is well supplied with α-aminobutyric acid (GABA) receptors, perhaps explaining the response to benzodiazepines, and also valproate, which is thought to enhance activity at these receptors. Another intriguing aspect of the circadian hypothesis is the known association of the daily temperature curve with the sleep–wake cycle; since many PLMS patients note ''cold feet,'' this suggests altered thermoregulation in the hypothalamus, perhaps in turn caused by suprachiasmatic nucleus dysfunction.

Some argue that instead of causing poor sleep, PLMS may be a normal phenomenon. Bixler et al. found a 6 percent incidence of PLMS (with a PSG showing at least 3 clusters of 30 or more consecutive leg movements) in a normal population (mean age, 40 years). However, their subjects had arousals with only 10 percent of the leg movements. This may explain why there were no sleep complaints; patients with insomnia or hypersomnolence usually have arousals in association with more than 30 percent of the leg movements.

TREATMENT

Only since the early 1980s have effective pharmacologic treatments for PLMS/RLS emerged. Drugs that affect the GABA-receptor have been popular, including the benzodiazepines, baclofen and valproate. However, the benzodiazepines are most commonly used as sleep-inducing medications in the general practice treatment of insomnia, and more recently, clonazepam use has become widespread among psychiatrists treating various affective disorders, including depression. Indeed, since PLMS/RLS causes 15 percent of insomnia, there may well be many undiagnosed PLMS/RLS patients who are fortuitously receiving an appropriate treatment. However, hypersomnolent PLMS patients may have great difficulty with the sedative effects of benzodiazepines, even in very small doses. The other major problem with benzodiazepines is the gradual development of tolerance to the beneficial effects. This can be a vexing problem when attempts are subsequently made to withdraw the medication, since the underlying sleep disorder will be severely exacerbated. Other withdrawal effects include tremors, headaches, nausea, and even seizures (all partly brought out by the sleep disruption as well as the ''denervation hypersensitivity'' of the GABA receptor). This could account for patients who are so addicted that they cannot tolerate being weaned. Indeed, PLMS/RLS patients (and other patients with chronic severe sleep disturbances) may gravitate toward benzodiazepines when obtainable (or to alcohol as an alternative) and then develop addiction after initially obtaining relief.

Since there is no clear mechanism of action for benzodiazepines other than sedative/hypnotic effects, and no evidence that the leg movements are significantly reduced, the search has continued for more effective, less problematic therapies. Baclofen was found effective in one study, but interestingly, it also did not decrease the leg movements, but seemed to improve sleep by decreasing the number of arousals associated with the leg movements. One problem with this drug is its short half-life. Another class of agents that affects GABA receptors but has not been formally studied in PLMS is the barbiturates, including phenobarbital, among the most widely prescribed sleep agents for decades. Ekbom found phenobarbital helpful in only milder cases, mainly as a sedative, and again, the problems of tolerance and abuse are well recognized with this class of drugs.

Valproate is a medication whose mechanism of action is not understood, but studies have suggested that its anticonvulsant property involves enhancement of GABA-receptor activity. This medication is not known to produce addiction, and tolerance to its antiepileptic effects has not been seen. Valproate has been used as a sleep-inducing agent in Europe. At my institution, valproate in low to moderate doses at bedtime improves nocturnal sleep and daytime alertness in 40 percent of PLMS patients. PLMS patients with hypersomnolence may be extremely sensitive to the usually mild sedative effects of valproate, so we give small doses only at bedtime, aiming for a low serum level in the morning; patients who return with high levels may complain of excessive morning fatigue, headaches, and moodiness, probably related to a ''hangover.'' However, in some patients, after a few weeks it may be appropriate to increase the dose to maintain the beneficial effect.

The most effective medications for RLS, and also quite useful for PLMS, are the dopaminergic agents levodopa, bromocriptine, pergolide, and α-hydroxybutyrate (which has a prodopaminergic effect during withdrawal). The slow-release form of levodopa/carbidopa has been most beneficial for RLS patients and also in intractable cases of PLMS. Studies by Coleman et al. originally speculated that levodopa might be an exacerbating factor for PLMS, but work by Montplaisir et al. has demonstrated that the effects of the short-acting form only last 2 hours, after which there is rebound, causing exacerbation of the PLMS. Thus, regular levodopa/carbidopa may work for patients whose symptoms occur only at bedtime, but is suboptimal for RLS or PLMS patients whose worst sleep occurs in the latter half of the night, when bouts of leg movement activity increase in intensity in the lighter stages of NREM sleep. For these patients, one slow-release 50/200-mg tablet at bedtime constitutes a major improvement in therapy, since this form lasts 4 to 6 hours, allowing most patients to experience a better night's sleep. This long-acting form is also a boon to RLS patients with diurnal leg symptoms that begin early in the day. Indeed, many patients experience their first morning RLS symptoms only after initiating an evening dose of levodopa, as a rebound phenomenon. Rebound is more severe with higher daily doses of levodopa, and can be counteracted by using the long-acting form in evenly divided 24-hour dosing schedules, plus adding medications with alternative mechanisms of action to the regimen, so as to reduce the total daily levodopa intake.

Another long-acting dopaminergic agent is pergolide, in doses of 0.05 to 0.1 mg, usually given at bedtime. Bupropion is touted as a dopamingergic-serotonergic antidepressant, and in daily doses of 75 to 150 mg may be helpful when levodopa/

carbidopa is not tolerated. In any case, for depressed RLS patients, it is a good alternative to tricyclic and SSRI antidepressants, since members of both these classes may exacerbate RLS/PLMS. (Of the other antidepressants, only trazodone and monoamine oxidase inhibitors are tolerable to these patients.)

Pemoline, methylphenidate, and D-amphetamine have long been used as daytime stimulants in patients with hypersomnolence, and each may act as a dopaminergic agonist. Although some patients who take stimulants report improved nocturnal sleep quality, it is not known how many of these patients might have PLMS/RLS; in any case, most patients develop insomnia if the stimulant doses are high enough.

Narcolepsy patients have a 10 to 75 percent incidence of PLMS (increasing with advancing age). Valproate, levodopa, or α-hydroxybutyrate produce better quality nocturnal sleep, leading to a decrease in daytime sleepiness, allowing reductions in stimulant dosage.

Opiates (including propoxyphene) can be very helpful in PLMS/RLS; codeine was used in one study, and despite the potential for tolerance and abuse, the authors state that their patients tend to follow the prescribed regimens. Compared to valproate, levodopa, or benzodiazepines, the opiates have a longer and better record of safety in pregnancy, and may be especially useful when PLMS or RLS become severe early in the first trimester.

Adrenergic blockers have limited use in patients with sleep disorders. An occasional patient with PLMS may respond to an α-adrenergic blocker such as phenoxybenzamine. Studies have shown a moderate—but not necessarily long-lasting—response to the β-blocker propranolol in RLS, akathisia, and narcolepsy. Clonidine, an α_2-adrenergic agonist, has been used in RLS.

Serotonergic agents such as I-tryptophan and 5-hydroxytryptophan have been used with rare success in RLS, but have not been found useful in PLMS. Other therapies useful in treating RLS that have not worked for PLMS patients include iron and folate (both helpful in RLS even in the absence of a deficiency), vitamin E, vasodilators, and aldehydes, but none of these is currently in widespread general use, although clearly any RLS patient with anemia should be evaluated and treated appropriately.

Aside from valproate, another anticonvulsant that has been tried in PLMS/RLS is phenytoin. Carbamazepine has been used in RLS, but in my institution has mostly caused exacerbations, probably owing to its tricyclic structure.

Patients with PLMS/RLS sometimes are awakened by leg cramps, but most patients with recurrent nocturnal cramps do not have PLMS. Nevertheless, quinine, long used for nocturnal cramps, may benefit PLMS patients.

Other drugs that can bring out or exacerbate RLS or PLMS include lithium, caffeine, terbutaline, and nifedipine (all calcium channel-blockers are suspect; they can cause parkinsonism and akathisia, probably by reducing dopaminergic neurotransmission). As mentioned earlier, antipsychotic-neuroleptic drugs commonly cause akathisia, which is similar to RLS and can be associated with a sleep disturbance that may be the same as PLMS.

In treating PLMS, it must always be kept in mind that subtle forms of sleep apnea may cause the clinical appearance of periodic leg movements on PSG without obvious changes in respiration or oxyhemoglobin saturation. Therefore, in cases where the PLMS seems intractable to all medications, a trial of nasal (continuous positive airway pressure) or a dental device (a

"snore guard") may be warranted if snoring has been a concomitant.

SUGGESTED READINGS

The ASDA Atlas Task Force: Recording and scoring leg movements. Sleep 16:749–59, 1993

Coleman RM, Bliwise DL, Sajben N et al: Epidemiology of periodic movements of sleep. pp. 217–29. In Guilleminault C, Lugaresi E (eds): Sleep/Wake Disorders: Natural History, Epidemiology, and Long-Term Evolution. Raven Press, New York, 1983

Diagnostic Classification Steering Committee, Thorpy MJ, Chairman: International Classification of Sleep Disorders: Diagnostic and Coding Manual. pp. 69–71, 291–3. American Sleep Disorders Association, Rochester, MN, 1990

Ehrenberg BL: Sleep Pathologies associated with nocturnal movements pp. 634–48. In: Joseph AB, Young RR (eds): Movement Disorders in Neurology and Neuropsychiatry. Blackwell Scientific, Boston, 1992

Ekbom KA: Restless legs syndrome. Neurology 10:868–73, 1960

Montplaisir J, Godbout R, Pelletier G, Warnes H: Restless legs syndrome and periodic limb movements during sleep. pp. 589–97. In Kryger MH, Roth T, Dement WC (eds): Principles and Practice of Sleep Medicine. WB Saunders, Philadelphia, 1994

Walters A, Hening W: Clinical presentation and neuropharmacology of restless legs syndrome: a review. Clin Neuropharmacol 10:225–37, 1987

130. STIFF-MAN SYNDROME

KATHLEEN McEVOY

Stiff-man syndrome is a rare disorder of motor function characterized by involuntary stiffness of axial muscles and superimposed painful muscle spasms. The etiology is unknown, but there are clinical and laboratory associations with autoimmune diseases, and it is becoming increasingly apparent that stiff-man syndrome may form a spectrum of diseases with some types of encephalomyelitis. In addition, some cases of the syndrome may be paraneoplastic. Whether these atypical cases of stiff-man syndrome are varying manifestations of the same pathologic entity or phenotypically similar but pathophysiologically distinct from typical stiff-man syndrome remains to be defined.

Stiff-man syndrome is also known as Woltman-Moersch syndrome, acknowledging the neurologists who first recognized and described this condition in the 1950s. They published a report of 14 patients with progressive and fluctuating rigidity and spasms seen over a 35-year period at the Mayo Clinic. In the years following this report, numerous other patients were recognized throughout the world. By 1990, about 100 patients had been reported in the literature.

EPIDEMIOLOGY AND THE AT-RISK POPULATION

Stiff-man syndrome is clearly rare, but its true prevalence cannot be known, owing to poor ascertainment. Diagnosis can be made only if it is suspected, and physician recognition of this rare and unusual disorder is very low, especially in the primary-care setting. Misdiagnosis as a psychiatric disorder is common. Since stiff-man syndrome can be a devastating and sometimes life-threatening condition when untreated, its recognition is critical.

The index of suspicion for diagnosis of stiff-man syndrome

should be elevated in certain patient populations, particularly those with a personal or family history of organ-specific auto-immune diseases or organ-specific autoantibodies. Women may be more likely to develop the syndrome. The age of onset of symptoms is usually in the fifth decade of life but ranges from the third through at least the seventh decade, with cases in children rarely reported. No antibody-positive cases have been reported in children.

SYNDROME RECOGNITION

Clinical Manifestations

Typical stiff-man syndrome is well characterized by the diagnostic criteria laid out by Lorish et al. in 1989: (1) a prodrome of stiffness and rigidity in axial muscles; (2) slow progression of stiffness to include proximal limb muscles, making volitional movement and ambulation difficult; (3) a fixed deformity of the spine; (4) superimposed episodic spasms precipitated by sudden movement, jarring, noise, and emotional upsets; (5) normal findings on motor and sensory examinations; (6) normal intellect; and (7) typical electromyographic findings of continuous muscle activity abolished by intravenous diazepam, or a positive therapeutic response to oral diazepam. Although these criteria remain valid for the diagnosis of typical stiff-man syndrome, reflex asymmetry and enhancement are common, and extensor plantar responses may be seen in otherwise typical patients. Symmetry of stiffness is the rule, to which there are exceptions.

The spinal deformity is a most helpful feature in recognizing stiff-man syndrome and in distinguishing it from common back pain. Symptoms usually develop over a period of months, beginning in the low back muscles, producing pain and stiffness, and also deformity of the spine, with exaggerated lumbar lordosis. Paraspinal muscle spasm is pronounced and lumbar range of motion is severely limited. Lordosis is usually maintained even with forward bending, which is done almost completely at the hips. Abdominal muscles are often rigid. Many patients describe abdominal protuberance, which is really due to the spinal deformity. After months or years, paraspinal hypertrophy develops and may be striking. Whereas the muscular activity is generally noted to abate during sleep, the spinal deformity may become fixed and persistent.

In some patients, the muscular hyperactivity and spinal deformity are more rostral, producing cervical tightness and hunching of the shoulders. In most patients, disease is predominant at one level so that either the lumbar or cervical level is symptomatic. Stiffness and rigidity may extend to the anterior neck muscles, but trismus is not seen in typical stiff-man syndrome, and would suggest the possibility of tetanus as the cause of muscle stiffness.

Stiffness and simultaneous contraction of agonists and antagonists may spread to the proximal extremities. In lumbar patients, this produces a characteristic stiffness of gait not unlike that of Frankenstein's monster. Ambulation is slow and difficult, and may be punctuated by "freezing" episodes. Falls are common. Postural reflexes are overridden by stiffness, so the patient falls "like a tin soldier," and the risk of fracture is high. Fear of falling exacerbates the gait disorder, since emotional stimuli potentiate the abnormal muscle stiffness. Most patients experience increased stiffness in social situations or in public places. Stressful situations and exposure to cold temperatures also aggravate stiffness and spasms.

Not surprisingly, any activity requiring truncal flexibility is performed slowly and awkwardly, if at all. This includes arising from chairs, getting out of bed, tying shoes, and arising from a fall. Mobility and ability to perform activities of daily living may be severely limited. This and the aggravation of symptoms in public places or social situations render many patients essentially house-bound.

Painful muscle spasms are a universal feature of stiff-man syndrome, and they are generally more amenable to treatment than the underlying stiffness and rigidity. Their absence in an untreated patient renders the diagnosis suspect. The spasms occur primarily in axial muscles, but may spread to involve the limbs as well. They may arise spontaneously, but are usually induced by movement, startle, or emotional stimuli. Common examples include an unexpected tap on the shoulder, the sound of a doorbell or telephone, or excessive activity producing back pain. These spasms may be herculean in strength, sufficient to break bones and to bend the pins used for repair.

Autoimmune Associations

The autoimmune pathogenesis of stiff-man syndrome is strongly supported by (1) the presence of antibodies to glutomic acid decarboxylase (anti-GAD) or anti-islet cell antibodies (anti-ICA) in most patients, (2) the common presence of other organ-specific autoimmune diseases or autoantibodies in stiff-man syndrome patients and first-degree relatives, and (3) the response to immunosuppressive therapy. The target of autoimmune attack within the central nervous system is not known with certainty, nor is it known whether the antibodies detected are pathogenic or merely markers of disease. Passive transfer of the syndrome to animals via patient serum has not yet been demonstrated, and there is no animal model of the disease.

Anti-GAD antibodies have been detected in significant numbers of patients reported to have stiff-man syndrome in several series. Anti-ICA are nearly identical to anti-GAD, with differences only in the N-terminal epitopes and are adequate as a screening test for the diagnosis. This antibody is present in low titer in many patients early in the course of development of type I diabetes mellitus. Anti-ICA are present in high titer in the majority of patients diagnosed with typical stiff-man syndrome in recent years at the Mayo Clinic, independent of the presence of diabetes. Titers have not fallen with time, and are present in patients with long-standing stiff-man syndrome. This antibody is very rare in persons with neither diabetes nor stiff-man syndrome, but may occasionally be detected in intermediate titers in patients with multiple autoimmune endocrinopathies. Recent reports describe a new antibody in patients with breast cancer and stiff-man syndrome.

Most patients with autoimmune stiff-man syndrome harbor other autoantibodies, most commonly antithyroid antibodies. Many have other autoimmune diseases, as do their first-degree relatives. Type I diabetes is present in a approximately 30 percent of patients. Most patients have antimicrosomal thyroid antibodies, and some have had clinical autoimmune thyroid disease, either Hashimoto's or Graves'. Other autoimmune endocrinopathies and organ-specific autoimmune diseases from the "thyrogastric cluster" of autoimmunity may be seen, including pernicious anemia, vitiligo, premature ovarian failure, premature gray hair, autoimmune adrenal failure, and myasthenia gravis.

The presence of anti-GAD or anti-ICA, other autoantibodies, or other autoimmune diseases in the patient or family, help to support the diagnosis of stiff-man syndrome in a patient with the appropriate clinical presentation, but are not necessary for the diagnosis. An association with epilepsy has been postulated, but is not supported by the literature.

Stiff-man syndrome is frequently misdiagnosed as a psychiatric disorder. Until recent years, there was considerable doubt in the medical community as to the existence of the syndrome. In fact, many patients with it do have coexisting psychiatric conditions, generally anxiety or affective disorders, and some overuse alcohol and other medications, in part to control their disease.

The combination of the unusual nature of the symptoms, the limited findings on neurologic examination despite significant disabilities in function and gait, the lack of findings on routine laboratory testing, the exacerbation by emotional stimuli, the frequency of accompanying anxiety or affective disorder, and probably also the relative frequency of the disease in women all contribute to the common error of attributing symptoms solely to psychiatric disease. Even the efficacy of treatment with benzodiazepines may be taken to support this error in diagnosis.

Other Laboratory Testing

The diagnosis of stiff-man syndrome is made on clinical grounds based on the patient history and examination results. The clinical index of suspicion is raised in patients with known tendencies to autoimmune disorders. The presence of anti-GAD or anti-ICA strongly supports the diagnosis in patients with appropriate signs and symptoms. Other laboratory testing may provide specific support for the diagnosis of stiff-man syndrome but largely serves to rule out other diseases.

Electrophysiologic testing in stiff-man syndrome includes routine electromyography (nerve conduction studies and needle electrode examination), as well as specialized surface electrode studies documenting the pattern of muscle activity in axial and limb muscles and the response to stimuli. Nerve conduction study results are generally normal, including long-loop reflexes. Routine electromyographic testing shows continuous activation of normal-appearing motor unit potentials in affected muscles despite attempts to relax. Surface electrode demonstration of widespread continuous muscle activity in axial muscles is important as a tool for to documenting that inability to relax is not simply due to discomfort from the recording needle. Additional studies may be done to document simultaneous activation of agonists and antagonists in limbs, and exaggerated response to startle stimuli in many patients.

Brain and spinal imaging is typically normal, as is spinal fluid examination. Occasional patients show inflammatory cerebrospinal fluid (CSF) changes, including mild pleocytosis, elevated IgG index, or oligoclonal bands. These changes may be more likely in atypical patients, such as those with cerebellar signs, and may represent an inflammatory phase in the development of stiff-man syndrome, or in some cases, true encephalomyelitis. In such patients, as in those with inflammatory changes on magnetic resonance imaging, it is particularly important to exclude demyelinating disease.

ATYPICAL SYNDROME FORMS

Atypical forms of stiff-man syndrome may be seen. Some patients have findings that are otherwise typical of the syndrome except for the presence of mild brainstem or cerebellar signs such as ophthalmoparesis, nystagmus, or dysmetria. Jerking

stiff-man syndrome, or stiff-man syndrome with prominent myoclonic jerks, has been described. The presence of significant sensory disturbance or significant primary sphincter dysfunction suggests an alternate diagnosis, such as demyelinating disease, other causes of myelopathy, or central nervous system disease.

Symptoms of stiff-man syndrome usually develop over a period of months. More rapid onset—a period of 6 to 8 weeks or less—suggests encephalomyelitis as the underlying cause. In these cases, other neurologic manifestations are commonly present, especially brainstem or cerebellar signs. Anti-GAD antibodies have been detected in patients with pathologically proven encephalomyelitis with rigidity.

Encephalomyelitis With Rigidity

The pathogenic mechanisms of typical stiff-man syndrome are not known with certainty. Some forms of encephalomyelitis may produce progressive stiffness and rigidity. Since the original description of the syndrome, several cases have been reported with clinical features highly suggestive of stiff-man syndrome but with additional focal neurologic signs atypical for the diagnosis, including cerebellar signs, oculomotor disturbances, facial or bulbar weakness, extensor plantar responses, vertigo, or epilepsy. Autopsies have shown inflammatory infiltrates in the gray matter of the spinal cord and brainstem, with perivascular lymphocytic infiltration and microglial proliferation. These cases were called progressive encephalomyelitis with rigidity. Anti-ICA and anti-GAD antibodies have been detected in several nondiabetic patients with confirmed encephalomyelitis with rigidity. In a patient with symptoms of stiff-man syndrome, the possibility of underlying encephalomyelitis is suggested by any of the following: onset of symptoms over less than 6 to 8 weeks, the presence of fever or clouding of consciousness, inflammatory CSF changes, or focal neurologic signs.

Paraneoplastic Stiff-Man Syndrome

Most stiff-man syndrome is not paraneoplastic. Thorough evaluations and long follow-up reveal no evidence of cancer in the vast majority of patients. In a few cases, the syndrome has been associated with carcinoma; however, most well-documented cases have features suggestive of underlying encephalomyelitis, as outlined above. Antibodies against a separate antigen and a distinct clinical picture, with predominantly proximal lower extremity rather than axial involvement, have been described in patients with stiff-man syndrome associated with breast cancer.

DIAGNOSIS

The overlap between the clinical entities of typical stiff-man syndrome, progressive encephalomyelitis with rigidity, and paraneoplastic stiff-man syndrome suggests that stiff-man syndrome, as originally described by Moersch and Woltman, may be part of a spectrum of disease, with the syndrome perhaps resulting from a more confined form of spinal encephalomyelitis. Occasional focal neurologic signs and CSF changes might then be expected even with typical stiff-man sydrome, and additional focal signs, a more fulminant onset, and more inflammatory CSF would be the rule in more extensive cases of encephalomyelitis. Paraneoplastic inflammation might produce still a different distribution of involvement. Alternatively, stiff-man syndrome and progressive encephalomyelitis with rigidity may be different diseases with similar signs and symptoms.

The diagnosis of typical stiff-man syndrome remains primarily clinical, using the diagnostic criteria as previously outlined, with support from serologic and electrophysiologic tests. Further testing, including magnetic resonance image scanning and spinal fluid examination, may be necessary to exclude other neurologic disease. The time course of the ''slow'' progression should be longer than 8 weeks. A clinical classification of stiff-man syndromes might be extended beyond typical stiff-man syndrome to include (1) cases of atypical stiff-man syndrome that have focal neurologic signs and (2) cases that are atypical in that they have focal neurologic signs and also either rapid onset and progression of symptoms or myoclonus.

A differential diagnosis should include multiple sclerosis, other causes of myelopathy, extrapyramidal syndrome including Parkinson's disease, bilateral frontal lobe dysfunction (e.g., due to hydrocephalus, vascular disease, trauma, or malignancy), degenerative disorders producing spasticity, tetanus, other causes of primary muscle stiffness or continuous muscle fiber activity such as Isaacs syndrome, and other orthopaedic or rheumatologic causes of reduced spinal range of motion.

MANAGEMENT

For nearly a decade after stiff-man syndrome was first described, there was no known effective treatment for this disorder. In 1963, Howard discovered the efficacy of diazepam, and benzodiazepines have remained a mainstay of treatment. As in other autoimmune disorders, although pharmacologic manipulations may be directed at the physiologic defect (e.g., benzodiazepines for stiff-man syndrome, anticholinesterase drugs for myasthenia gravis), immunosuppressive therapy may be necessary for optimal management. In recent years, immunosuppression has proven effective in some cases; however, despite a combined approach to treatment with both directly neuroactive drugs and immunosuppressive agents, symptomatic control is sometimes marginal. Patient education and supportive care are essential.

Pharmacologic Manipulation of Spinal Mechanisms of Stiffness

Diazepam was the first drug shown to be effective in stiff-man syndrome, and it has been the most widely used. Its efficacy is unquestionable. The exact mechanism by which it relieves stiffness and spasms in stiff-man syndrome is not known, but it is believed to act at the spinal level via the γ-aminobutyric acid receptor system to reduce abnormal motor activity. Whereas modest antianxiety doses of diazepam are of some benefit and have often been administered even prior to diagnosis, stiff-man syndrome patients frequently require and tolerate very large doses. Many patients take 40 to 60 mg/day, a few take more than 100 mg/day, and doses over 300 mg/day have been reported. A reasonable starting dose is 5 mg tid, but this may need to be escalated rapidly. Equivalent doses of other benzodiazepines are also effective. Sedation may occur transiently but is usually not a dose-limiting side effect. Mood and personality changes are common and frequently limit the dose. Abuse and dependence on these and other agents may develop in stiff-man syndrome, despite claims to the contrary. Care should be taken to ensure that the drugs are being used to treat symptoms of stiff-man syndrome rather than anxiety per se.

Baclofen is also efficacious in stiff-man syndrome. As with benzodiazepines, very large doses may be needed, sometimes over 100 mg/d. An initial dose of 5 mg bid or tid may be increased every few days as tolerated. Since strength is normal in stiff-man syndrome, there is no unmasking of underlying muscle weakness as may be seen in multiple sclerosis or other forms of spasticity. Dosage is therefore limited by other side effects, mainly sedation. Intrathecal administration allows high spinal levels with much lower brain levels, and is thus an attractive consideration in this syndrome. Initial experience with intrathecal baclofen is promising. Although the pump implantation and drug titration entail risk, expense, and effort, the benefits may be significant.

Sodium valproate in anticonvulsant doses and vigabatrin may also provide at least modest benefit. Alcoholic beverages relieve symptoms but medicinal use is not recommended, especially as affective disorders and substance abuse are common in stiff-man syndrome.

Pharmacologic manipulation of spinal mechanisms of stiffness frequently provides less than satisfactory control of stiff-man syndrome, at least with oral administration. Spasms may be eliminated, but relieved stiffness and improved mobility are often possible only with high doses and significant medication side effects. Intrathecal baclofen may circumvent this, but is expensive, invasive, somewhat cumbersome, and not generally available. Immunosuppression is therefore often indicated.

Immunosuppression and Related Therapies

Corticosteroids and azathioprine are dearly effective in reducing disease activity in stiff-man syndrome. Isolated reports of response to corticosteroids antedate the discovery of antibodies in stiff-man syndrome, and even the suspicion that the syndrome was autoimmune. The possibility of a direct effect on mechanisms of stiffness has been raised. The comparable efficacy of other immunoactive treatments suggests that any direct effect of steroids on syndrome-related stiffness must be small.

Prednisone may be administered in a regimen similar to that used in myasthenia gravis. Initial doses of 60 mg/d generally take effect within a few weeks. A switch or rapid taper to alternate-day therapy and then a slow taper of the dose is usually well tolerated. Experience thus far is too limited to predict the likely lowest tolerated dose, especially as many patients are concurrently treated with azathioprine. Unlike myasthenia gravis, in which immunosuppression often obviates the need for anticholinesterase medications, stiff-man syndrome seldom responds so well to immunosuppression that diazepam can be withdrawn.

Some side effects of corticosteroid treatment are of particular concern in stiff-man syndrome. Diabetes mellitus is present in about 30 percent of these patients; this complicates corticosteroid treatment but is not an absolute contraindication. Steroid-induced osteoporosis may increase the risk of fractures due to falls. If intrathecal baclofen is to be used, the increased infection risk with any immunosuppression is of concern.

Azathioprine appears to be an effective steroid sparing agent in stiff-man syndrome, and may allow steroids to be tapered completely. Again following the pattern of treatment of myasthenia, an initial dose of 50 mg once per day may be increased over 1 month to 2 to 2.5 mg/kg/d in three divided doses. Liver enzymes and a complete blood count must be checked weekly for the first month and monthly thereafter. A normal level of thiopurine methyltransferase activity in patients' red blood cells ensures that they are not among the 1 in 300 who are severely deficient in this enzyme, which participates in azathioprine metabolism. A normal level of thiopurine methyltransferase does not, however, rule out the possibility of severe leukopenia or hepatic dysfunction.

Hepatic intolerance usually occurs early, within the first week. The white blood cell count may drop at any time. High doses of steroids may falsely elevate the white blood cell count early in the course of azathioprine treatment. As steroids are tapered, the leukopenia then becomes apparent. About 5 percent of persons are intolerant of azathioprine, owing to a febrile serum sickness type of response. Others note gastrointestinal upset, which may respond to dividing the daily doses into six rather than three. The long-term risk of promoting the development of neoplasms with azathioprine appears to be very small, and is almost certainly less than the overall risks of prolonged steroid treatment.

Plasma exchange is effective in some cases, and has rescued some severely affected individuals from crisis situations. Other patients do not improve with plasma exchange, but may still respond well to steroids and azathioprine. Experience with intravenous IgG in stiff-man syndrome is limited but promising.

Nonpharmacologic treatments may significantly augment the effects of pharmacotherapy in stiff-man syndrome. Physiatric intervention may provide symptomatic relief of muscle discomfort and stiffness, as may aids and instruction in mobility and gait safety. Stretching exercises benefit some patients. Behavioral medicine and biofeedback may also be helpful in managing the psychological factors that can aggravate symptoms. Good patient education allows patients and their families to understand the organic nature of the syndrome and the role of stress and psychological factors. As in other rare disorders, patients very much appreciate the chance to speak with others suffering from the same disorder.

In addition to managing stiff-man syndrome itself and watching for side effects and complications of treatment, treating physicians must be vigilant for development of associated conditions, such as diabetes and multiple endocrine failure.

SUMMARY

The diagnosis of stiff-man syndrome has been primarily clinical, supported by electrophysiologic findings. Clinical criteria for diagnosis have thus necessarily been strict and exclusive in order to ensure accurate diagnosis of the specific syndrome. A number of neurologic and musculoskeletal disorders can resemble the syndrome in some aspects. Differentiation from demyelinating disease is essential.

Diazepam and other drugs that act on the γ-aminobutyric acid receptor system are effective in stiff-man syndrome. Anti-GAD and anti-ICA have been found in many patients with stiff-man syndrome, lending support to the autoimmune hypothesis. Immunosuppression with corticosteroids or azathioprine ameliorates symptoms in most patients. Plasma exchange is sometimes helpful.

With the advent of improved neuroimaging to exclude demyelinating or structural disease, and with serologic testing to lend positive support to the diagnosis of stiff-man syndrome in questionable cases, we are now able to reapproach the issue of defining the diagnosis of stiff-man syndrome, and may consider a wider spectrum of clinical manifestations and etiologies, including primary autoimmune stiff-man syndrome, stiff-man syndrome associated with encephalomyelitis, paraneoplastic stiff-man, syndrome, and atypical clinical manifestations.

SUGGESTED READINGS

Auger RG: AAEM mini-monograph: diseases associated with excess motor unit activity. Muscle Nerv (in press)
Lorish TR, Thorsteinsson G, Howard FM: Stiff-man syndrome updated. Mayo Clin Proc 64:629, 1989
McEvoy KM: Stiff-man syndrome. Semin Neurol 11:3, 1991

BEHAVIORAL
NEUROLOGY
AND EPILEPSY

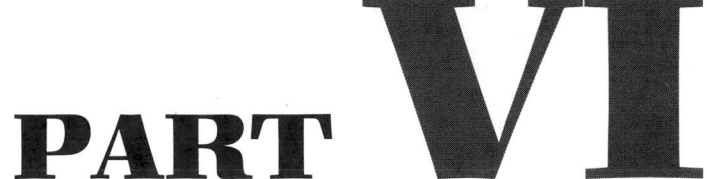

SECTION 1. BEHAVIORAL NEUROLOGY

131. EXAMINING MENTAL STATE

SANDRA WEINTRAUB

Cognitive and behavioral abnormalities commonly result from structural brain damage or from temporary physiologic disruption of the brain's normal function. The mental state examination detects abnormalities and characterizes them in a way that is of relevance for predicting the nature and locus of disease. Brief mental state screening tests have been developed to assist the clinician, but these tests have limited usefulness because of their ceiling effects and also because many of them do not include tests for some important functions such as language and reasoning. This chapter describes how to examine a patient in order to identify a clinical profile. The primary domains of attention, mood, memory, language, visual perceptual functions, executive functions, and comportment form the basis of the examination. Each of these neurocognitive systems is well-defined in terms of its component elementary mental operations and also with respect to its underlying anatomic affiliations. Specific tests are discussed, but the emphasis here is on interpretation.

THEORETIC FRAMEWORK

Mesulam proposed that mental functions can be divided into two general groups. The state-dependent functions rely on neuronal networks that project diffusely throughout the cortex and serve to set and rapidly modify the information processing state. Examples of the domains of mental processes that are mediated in this way include arousal, attention, and mood. The channel-dependent functions, by contrast, rely on discrete neuroanatomic pathways. Domains of mental functioning mediated in this way include language, complex visuoperceptual and spatial processes, and explicit memory. Deficits in the state-dependent functions, such as impaired attention, are not of strict localizing value, but the clinician must note them, since they can cause general disruption of performance on the examination. Conversely, deficits in the channel-dependent functions (e.g., aphasia) are typically of localizing value, especially when they occur in a patient who is alert, attentive, and cooperative.

Based on this classification, Fig. 131-1 presents a conceptual framework within which performance on the examination of mental state can be interpreted. At the basis of all conscious mental activity is wakefulness or arousal. Diminished arousal will color all mental acts. Normal wakefulness does not guarantee, however, that a patient can allocate attentional resources effectively. Altered attention will also affect performance on all types of mental tasks. Mood disturbance and diminished motivation are also mechanisms whereby mental operations are affected in a pervasive manner. Thus, deficits in arousal, attention, mood, and motivation—all state-dependent functions—may not be of localizing value, but their presence alerts

the clinician to the possibility that other deficits may be traceable to these more elementary problems. This distinction is critical to differentiating between true diffuse primary impairments and the *impression* of diffuse impairment.

Two major domains of channel-dependent functions that weigh heavily in the examination of mental state are language and complex visual-perceptual and spatial abilities. These functions are of interest not only because of their intrinsic localizing value but also because many tests of mental state require that patients be able to comprehend language, speak, and draw normally. Language functions include auditory and reading comprehension, repetition, naming, writing, and spontaneous speech. In most individuals, these are all dependent on a well-characterized network in the left cerebral hemisphere. Complex perceptual processes in the visual modality, such as object/form recognition and spatial perception, rely on ventrofugal pathways from visual cortex to the inferior temporal regions and dorsofugal pathways to the posterior parietal regions, respectively. The spatial distribution of attention is subserved by a large-scale network involving frontal, parietal, and cingulate components and their subcortical connections in the right cerebral hemisphere.

Explicit (or conscious, volitional) memory, another domain with distinctive mental operations, requires the integrity of limbic circuitry. Comportment (a shorthand term for the complex processes that underlie our ability to adapt our behavior to the social context) and related "executive functions" (reasoning, judgment, decision making) are subserved by the frontal lobes and their extensive connections throughout the brain (frontal networks).

The goal of the mental state examination is to identify the primary domain of impairment. A major obstacle to this goal is the fact that most of the tests we use at bedside or in the office are multifactorial—they were not designed on the basis of current knowledge about the functional organization of the brain and do not address single mental operations or even isolated domains. To illustrate the problem of interpretation, take the task of mental calculations, a staple in the mental state examination of most neurologists. Although we are asking the patient to perform calculation, successful completion of this task *also* requires preserved language comprehension, sustained attention, a normal level of motivation and cooperation, and normal speech output. If one were to perform functional imaging of the brain while a person were carrying out this task, it is likely that the entire brain would "light up." Therefore, if the patient suceeds at this task, the examiner can be satisfied that all these functions (and their underlying anatomic networks), including calculation skill, are probably intact. However, if the patient fails this task, then there are a number of possible explanations, each of which has different implications for the underlying pathophysiology. Table 131-1 lists the primary domains, important component functions, and the repercussions of primary deficits on other areas of the examination.

TESTS

Numerous tests are available to assess relevant functions, and in many cases, clincians prefer tests with which they have had

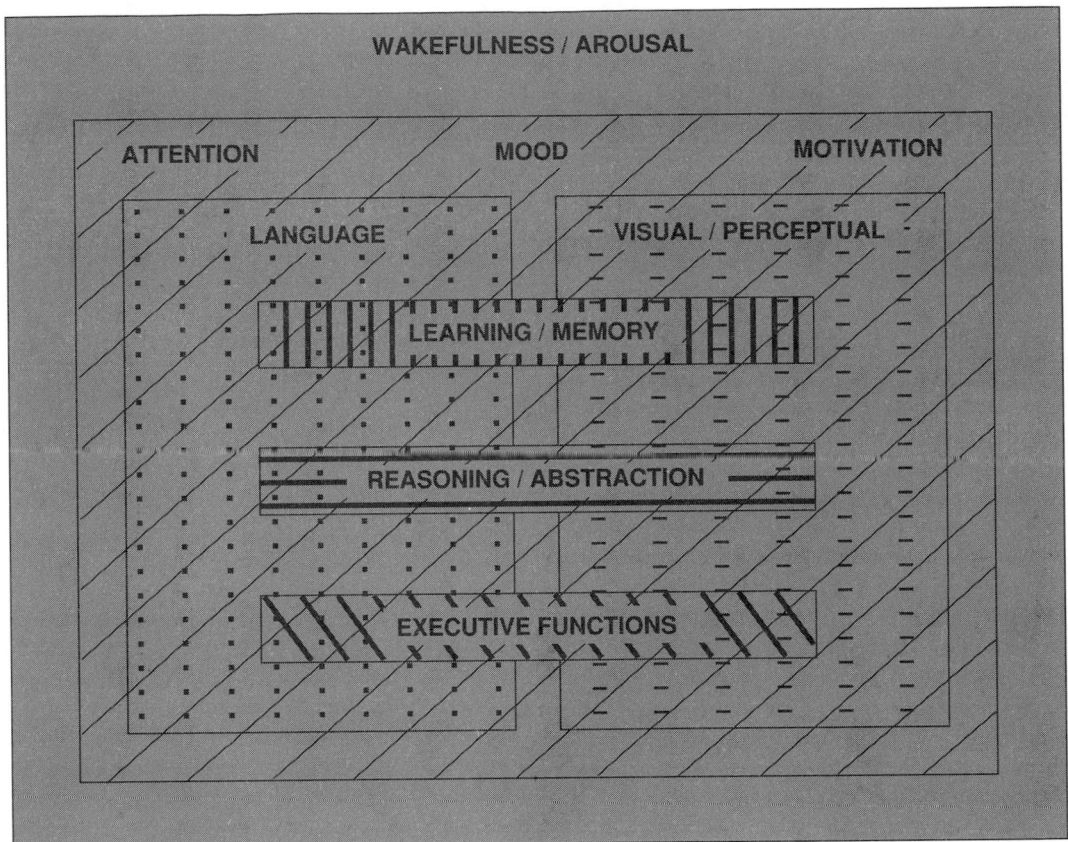

FIG. 131-1. Each rectangle represents a primary mental domain. Attention, mood, and motivation are individual processes but are grouped together because they are all state-setting functions. The transparency between domains indicates that tests of one domain typically enlist additional mental processes from other domains for performance. For example, reciting a list of words from memory after a 3-minute delay (Learning/Memory test) also requires normal language, attention, mood, motivation, and arousal. If any of these processes are abnormal, then failure at this task cannot be definitively attributed to a true amnesia.

experience. Test selection should be guided by two general principles: first, the test should be as selective as possible with respect to the primary neurocognitive domain addressed and with respect to the number of mental processes actually enlisted; second, the test shoud be appropriate to the patient's level of education, cultural background, and level of life accomplishment. This chapter highlights some simple tests that are convenient to administer at bedside. More complete descriptions and references to some of the tests can be found in Weintraub and Mesulam (1985).

Table 131-2 suggests some tests and presents general guidelines for interpreting performance in high school–educated individuals over the age of 65. Some of these tests require more time than the examiner may have available, and it is recommended that the examiner either sample these behaviors with more abbreviated versions or use equivalent tests addressing these functions and then use clinical judgment to rate the *relative* level of performance (normal, mildly, moderately or severely impaired) among the primary domains.

Wakefulness

Use the level of wakefulness as a guideline to interpret performance on other tasks. If arousal is sufficiently impaired, it may even be advisable to terminate the examination until such time as arousal is normal. Diminished arousal implies interruption of neuronal projection systems, at either their origin or their termination points at multifocal sites or throughout the cortex, by chemical or structural lesions.

Mood/Motivation

As is also the case with impaired arousal and attention, a disturbance of mood can color the patient's performance in all areas of the examination, yielding an impression of widespread cognitive deficiencies. Mood disturbances are often biochemically based, but can also be seen in individuals with psychological disorders, and in these latter patients, it is usually the psychosocial history that helps the clinician decide upon the direction of the diagnosis.

In some patients with focal cerebral lesions, there may be a dissociation between the experience of mood and the ability to convey it in the form of speech prosody and facial and body gestures. Some patients with right cerebral strokes may appear to be depressed on this basis. The converse may be true—that is, patients who are depressed may be unable to convey affect through their tone of voice or facial expressions. Some patients with bilateral cerebral disease may display "pseudobulbar affect" or emotional incontinence, an exaggerated display of emotion that lacks the accompanying feeling state.

Attention

One of the most important pieces of information derived from the mental state examination is whether there is a primary defect

TABLE 131-1. Effects of Primary Deficits in Neurocognitive Domains on Other Portions of the Examination

Cognitive Domain (Network) Components	Repercussion of Deficits on Other Parts of the Examination
Arousal (state-dependent)	Pervasive: affects performance on all tasks
Mood/motivation (state-dependent)	Pervasive: poor cooperation invalidates test results. Tendency to respond "Don't know" when capable of responding correctly.
Attention (state-dependent)	Pervasive: attention is required for all conscious mental operations. Interpret other deficits cautiously.
Vigilance	Pervasive: affects performance on all tasks
Span	Limits the amount of information the patient can absorb—reduced number of story elements or words that can be learned. If sentences are too long, patient may appear to have language comprehension or repetition deficits.
Perseverance	Patient gives up easily: diminished spontaneous recall on memory tests; appearance of hemispatial "neglect" on drawing and cancellation tests due to failure to persist.
Response inhibition	Tendency to respond impulsively to all types of instructions
Language: linguistic components (channel-dependent)	In general, deficits affect all tasks that involve language processes
Spontaneous speech	Interferes with all tasks that rely on speech output, including memory recall, digit span, similarities, orientation, etc.
Auditory comprehension	Interferes with performance of all tasks that require comprehension of oral instructions
Repetition	Difficulty repeating word lists, number series, stories
Naming	Difficulty performing similarities or recalling specific words after a delay interval
Reading comprehension	Difficulty performing tasks where instructions are printed
Writing	Difficulty performing tasks where writing is a component (calculations, memory recall)
Complex visual/spatial perceptual processes (channel-dependent)	In general, deficits interfere with any task that requires visual perception, such as constructions, nonverbal memory tasks, etc.
Object/form perception	Difficulty on drawing tasks, naming tasks
Spatial perception	Difficulty on tasks requiring looking at or reproducing figures
Spatial distribution of attention (channel-dependent)	Difficulty processing information stimuli in the unattended field
Learning and explicit memory	In general, deficits may interfere with memory for task instructions
Executive functions/comportment (frontal networks)	Deficits are most apparent in activities of daily living rather than on formal testing. However, deficits can interfere with testing in a pervasive manner owing to inability to formulate or organize a plan of action.

of attention. Once it is established that attention is impaired, other deficits may not be valid for interpretation. There are several distinct components of attention, each of which entails different cognitive operations and some of which may be selectively affected by frontal lobe lesions. Vigilance, closely linked to arousal, refers to the ability to sustain attention over time. The Continuous Performance Paradigm is the simplest test of this function, which is often impaired in patients with toxic or metabolic encephalopathy, brainstem or midbrain injuries, and multifocal cortical lesions. Present a string of random letters—one per second—orally and ask the patient to respond each time the letter *A* occurs. Short versions of this task are sensitive only in severely impaired patients. In patients with more subtle vigilance impairment, a longer version of the test may be more helpful (e.g., 300 letters over 5 minutes).

The digit span is a measure of the immediate attention span. Normal individuals can repeat 5 to 7 digits in sequence. A reduced digit span will mean that the patient will not be able to process normal amounts of information. For example, if the examiner tests memory in a patient with a digit span of 4 and tells the patient a short story with 10 elements of information, it is almost certain that the patient will not initially register the entire story after a single presentation. Five minutes later, when the patient remembers 3 or 4 elements, the examiner cannot conclude beyond a reasonable doubt that this represents an accelerated rate of forgetting, a conclusion necessary to diagnose the amnestic syndrome and an underlying limbic lesion. As in the case of diminished vigilance, the examiner needs to be cautious when interpreting task failure in patients with a reduced span.

Perseverance, or the ability to sustain relevant behavioral output, is another component of attention and can be measured with the use of series generation tasks. Serial seven's are difficult even for individuals with a college education, so other types of tasks (Table 131-2) may be more appropriate. The F-A-S test measures the ability to generate lists of words beginning with these letters, each for a 60-second interval. Patients with diminished perseverance may be impaired on memory recall tests and other types of tasks due to the more primary inability to sustain behavioral output. Abulia is one manifestation of a defect in perseverance; perseveration is another.

Patients with impaired attention are often easily distracted. Some patients may, in addition, be unable to inhibit an overt response to the distracting stimulus. Response inhibition is a component of attention that can be selectively affected by lesions in the frontal lobe or along its numerous connections to cortical and subcortical regions (frontal networks). One measure of this function is the Stroop interference procedure (Fig. 131-2). The patient is first asked to name the colors in a series of colored dots. Next, the patient is asked to read printed color words. In the interference condition, the patient is presented with 50 color names, each of which is printed in an opposing color (i.e., *black* is written in gray letters, *gray* in white, and so on), and the task is to name the color of the letters as quickly as possible. Patients with deficits in response inhibition will perform the interference condition far more slowly than normal individuals and will also tend to read the word rather than name the color of the letters (i.e., make errors of commission).

A simpler bedside test is the motor "Go—No Go" procedure, based on clinical techniques originally described by the Russian neuropsychologist, A. R. Luria. The patient is asked to place her hand flat on a table surface and to raise and immediately lower the index finger in response to a single loud tap of a pencil. The patient is next instructed to refrain from respond-

TABLE 131-2. Guidelines for Testing Primary Domains and Suggested Interpretation of Performance for Patients Over Age 65

Domain Components	Tests[a]	65–69 Years[a]	70–74 Years[a]	75+ Years[a]
Arousal (state-dependent)	Rate level of arousal: normal, drowsy, stuporous, comatose; use to interpret performance on other parts of examination	Normal	Normal	Normal
Mood/motivation (state-dependent)	Assess from interview and observation; use to interpret performance on other parts of examination	Appropriate to situation; stable	Appropriate to situation; stable	Appropriate to situation; stable
Attention (state-dependent)				
Vigilance	Auditory Continuous Performance: 300 letters presented orally in random sequence, 30 targets ("A")	29/30	28/30	27/30
Span	Digit Span: Present strings of random digits of increasing length, two trials at each length; span is longest sequence that can be repeated without error	6–7 forward	6–7 forward	5–6 forward
Perseverance	Series Generation Tasks: Easy: Count backward from 20 to 1 Intermediate: Months in reverse Hard: F-A-S-word list generation	10 seconds 9–15 seconds Total: 36–56 seconds	15 seconds 25 seconds Total: 32–52 seconds	15 seconds 30 seconds Total: 30–50 seconds
Response inhibition	Stroop Interference Test: Read 50 color dots Name 50 color words Name 50 colors in interference condition Motor Go—No Go: 50 trials, 20 "Go", 30 "No Go," randomly administered	25–35 seconds 15–24 seconds 52–80 seconds 4 commission errors	24–37 seconds 16–24 seconds 47–80 seconds 4 commission errors	27–33 seconds 20–27 seconds 50–94 seconds 4 commission errors
Language (linguistic; channel-dependent: left cerebral hemisphere)				
Spontaneous speech	Examine speech for disturbances in rate, intonation, melody, articulation, word-finding, word formation, grammaticality	Normal	Normal	Normal
Auditory comprehension	Ask patient to respond "yes" or "no" to these questions: "Do dogs fly?" "Do you put on your shoes before your socks?"	No errors	No errors	No errors
Repetition	Ask patient to repeat: Easy: The red book is on the table. Intermediate: Near the table in the dining room. Hard: No if's and's, or but's.	No errors	No errors	No errors
Naming	Boston Naming Test: Administer 30 even- or odd-numbered items	26–30/30	25–29/30	26–29/30
Reading comprehension	Ask patient to read sentence silently and to point to correct item to complete its meaning: "The first meal of the day is called . . . morning lunch breakfast eggs	Correct	Correct	Correct
Writing	Ask patient to write his/her name and address and a sentence about the weather	Correct	Correct	Correct
Prosody (right cerebral hemisphere)	Ask patient to repeat the following sentences, placing stress as indicated: "*Steve* drove the car home." "Susan baked a cake??!!"	Accurate repetition	Accurate repetition	Accurate repetition
Complex visual/spatial perceptual judgments (channel-dependent)				
Object/form perception	Facial Recognition: short form	Age-corrected total score: 41–54	Age-corrected total score: 41–54	Age-corrected total score: 41–54
Spatial perception	Judgment of Line Orientation: Administer 15 odd- or even-numbered items	11/15 minimum	11/15 minimum	9/15 minimum
Spatial distribution of attention (channel-dependent)	Random Letter Cancellation Test: Allow patient 2 minutes to find all the "A's" (30 per side of the page)	29/30 left; 29/30 right	28/30 left; 28/30 right	27/30 left; 27/30 right
Learning and explicit memory	Three Words Three Shapes Test: Immediate incidental recall Trials to criterion 5 minutes 15 minutes 30 minutes Multiple choice	Copy is accurate. Incidental recall minimum of 4 items. Criterion (5/6 items) usually reached at this point but may require 1 additional study-recall trial. After 5, 15, and 30 minutes, recall is a minimum of 5 and there may be minor variations from the original stimuli (e.g., one design is lacking one element). On multiple choice, recall is 6/6 correct.		
	Drilled Word Span Procedure	Most individuals will have a word span of 5–7 (digit span minus 1). The list can be learned within 3 trials; older subjects may require 4–5. At 60 seconds with no distraction, recall is complete. At 60 seconds with no distraction, recall is complete. At 60 seconds with distraction, 3 minutes, and 10 minutes, older patients may lose 1 word. Multiple choice recognition is complete.		
Executive functions/comportment (frontal networks)	Conceptual Flexibility: Ask patient to split objects in Figure 131-3 into two groups and then to form two different groups with the same objects	Patients should be able to form two groups on the basis of shape and then two groups on the basis of color		

[a] Guidelines for interpretation are based on a limited control sample of subjects with at least a high-school education and average estimated intelligence. Adjustments should be considered for individuals with less education and/or less-than-average intelligence.

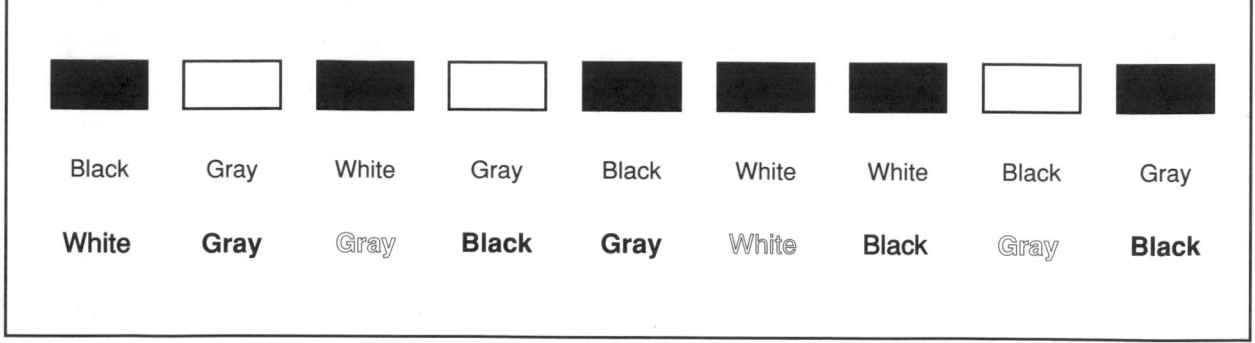

FIG. 131-2. A modification of the Stroop procedure. First ask the patient to name the colors (white, black, gray). Next, ask the patient to read the words in the second line. Finally, ask the patient to name the color of the letters in the words on the bottom line. The classic stimuli are usually the colors red, green, and blue. However, this variation lends itself to being easily reproduced and brought to bedside.

ing if the examiner taps twice. The examiner then delivers a series of one or two taps in random order. Patients with an impairment of response inhibition will be unable to keep from raising the index finger when two taps are delivered. A more subtle impairment exists when a patient does not make the more overt finger response but the examiner notices muscle flickers in the forearm. Impaired response inhibition can manifest itself as a more general tendency to "jump the gun," leading patients to make careless errors.

Language

The classification of aphasia syndromes is based on the profile of deficits among a number of basic language modalities. The patient's spontaneous speech should be scrutinized for problems with articulation, melody, pitch, fluency, rate, grammaticality, and word-finding. Auditory comprehension should be tested with simple questions that can be answered with either yes or no. Lengthy questions may exceed a patient's immediate attention span and commands that require a physical action may penalize patients with normal comprehension who have apraxia. Repetition should be tested by having the patient repeat a grammatically complex but short sentence, such as "No if's, and's, or but's." Reading comprehension can be tested by asking the patient to silently read a short sentence and select from multiple choice a word that correctly completes it (Table 131-2). Writing is a complex activity that can be disrupted in the absence of structural lesions in the language network of the left cerebral hemisphere. For example, patients in acute confusional states may have a disturbance of writing despite an intact language system, presumably due to the more primary disruption of arousal and attention encountered in those states (Chedru and Geschwind, 1972). Naming of objects is a very sensitive test of the integrity of the language system, since this ability is affected by lesions almost anywhere in the language network. Administering alternate odd- or even-numbered items from the Boston Naming Test provides an objective measure of naming. If the examiner uses objects easily available at bedside, the patient should be asked to name the less common parts of the object (i.e., lapel of a jacket or hem of a skirt).

Genuine aphasic symptoms are of great localizing value. In addition, their presence alters the interpretation of performance on tests, such as similarities or list learning, that requires the integrity of the language system.

The melodic features of speech production, or prosody, can be affected by selective lesions in the right cerebral hemisphere. Such alterations may make a patient incapable of conveying affect in his tone of voice, or using emphatic prosody in conversation (e.g., uttering "*Margo* plays the piano" versus "Margo plays the *piano*"). Asking the patient to repeat sentences that vary in their emphasis or affective tone can serve as a test of this function.

Complex Visual Perceptual and Spatial Processes

Tests of constructions are often used to assess complex visual perceptual and spatial processes. However, constructions can also be disrupted by other factors. For example, impulsive patients with frontal lobe disease may have difficulty drawing a clock or assembling puzzles despite integrity of their basic perceptual processes or drawing skill. In this instance, it would not be accurate to conclude that impaired constructions imply parietal lobe damage. However, if an alert, attentive, and cooperative patient cannot decide if two photographs of faces are the same or different or if one geometric figure is in the same plane as another, then localization of these deficits to the occipitotemporal and parieto-occipital areas, respectively, is more certain.

The short version of Facial Recognition and an alternate item (15 items) administration of Judgment of Line Orientation provide concise measures of these functions (Benton et al, 1989). If time is limited, the first 6 items of the former and the practice items of the latter can be used for quick screening.

A disturbance of the spatial distribution of visual attention can be measured in the visual modality with target cancellation tasks. Note the point of origin of the patient's search. Patients with right cerebral lesions may begin on the right side of the page and search in an erratic fashion. Hemispatial neglect may be apparent, but the examiner should also make sure that failure to explore one side of the page is not due to a more general disturbance of perseverance.

Learning and Memory

The examiner should test orientation and make sure to ask the patient about the examiner's rather than the patient's identity, since even severely amnestic patients remember their own names. The essence of memory testing is to document either a defect of storage or an accelerated rate of forgetting in the absence of attentional, language, and other primary deficits.

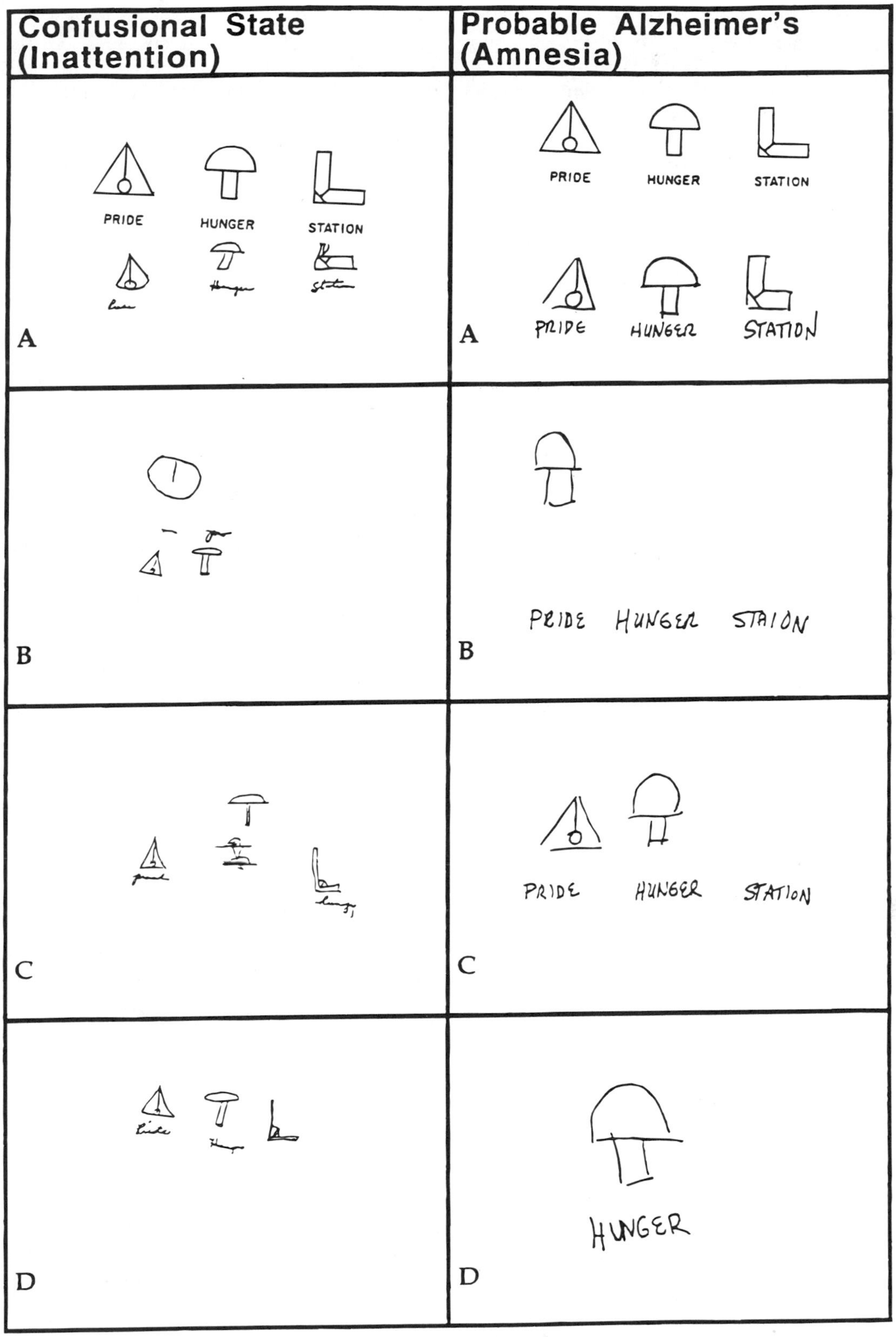

FIG. 131-3. Three Words Three Shapes Test. Left column: sample taken from a 75-year-old woman in an acute confusional state due to medication effects. Right column: sample taken from a 64-year-old man with a progressive decline in memory subsequently confirmed as Alzheimer's disease on postmortem. A, copy; B, incidental recall; C, recall after three additional study-recall trials for the confused patient and only one such trial for the amnestic patient; D, spontaneous recall after a 30-minute delay. The confused patient took longer to learn the stimuli but then retained them well. The amnestic patient required only one additional trial to learn the stimuli but then lost the information over time.

The Three Words Three Shapes Test (Fig. 131-3) was designed to control for attentional problems, language deficits, and constructional impairments and to enable the examiner to assess if memory is impaired at the stage of learning, retention, or retrieval. Having the patient first copy the 6 stimuli focuses attention on them. It also allows the examiner to note whether there are any primary constructional or language deficits that could alter interpretation of this memory task. The patient is not forewarned that this is a memory test and incidental recall is tested next. If 5 of the 6 stimuli are reproduced (criterion), delayed recall is tested 5, 15, and 30 minutes later. If the patient recalls fewer than 5, the examiner presents the original again for the patient to inspect for a 30-second interval, after which the patient is asked to immediately draw them again (study-recall trial). Drilling proceeds in this manner until 5 stimuli are reproduced or 5 study-recall trials are exhausted. This procedure is necessary to ensure that the information for which memory will be tested has first been acquired. Then delayed recall is tested as above. Following the last delay trial, multiple-choice recognition is tested. Spontaneous recall after each of the delays can provide a measure of the rate of forgetting and can be compared with recognition.

Another strategy to test learning is the Drilled Word Span procedure. Select a list of words equal in length to the digit span minus one (i.e., the word span). Drill these words until the patient can repeat them succesfully three times in a row. If the patient still has difficulty with this list length, drop to the next level at which the patient can repeat the list without error. Test recall after 60 seconds without distraction, after another 60 seconds with distraction, and then again after 3 minutes. Multiple-choice recognition can also be tested.

Patients with a true amnesia will show a loss of information after distraction and after a delay interval. Patients with inattention may have difficulty initially learning information but should then not show any loss of what they have learned over time (Fig. 131-3). Occasionally, however, severely inattentive or abulic patients may be unable to spontaneously retrieve information despite remembering it, and this is often confirmed by their accurate performance on multiple choice.

Comportment and Executive Functions

The complex domain of comportment and executive functions is characterized by mental operations that serve to orchestrate behavior and make it adaptable to the social setting and mo-ment-to-moment demands. The component functions are notoriously difficult to objectively measure with tests. However, derangements of these functions are among the most common mental state symptoms encountered in clinical practice. Observations of the patient's level of insight into his or her illness, decision making, and reasoning about everyday issues and health-care decisions can provide clues about the integrity of this domain. Examiners should also question caregivers about these issues in the patient's daily life. Asking a patient what to do in the event of a fire in a movie theater is helpful to assess judgment only if the patient provides the wrong answer. However, if the answer is correct, this does not guarantee that the patient would act in that manner in the real situation, in which there are many contingencies and alternative options.

Proverb interpretation is commonly tested but the explanations are usually highly overlearned, so that a correct response does not necessarily imply intact reasoning. Reasoning tests that emphasize categorization and mental flexibility, such as object-sorting tasks (Fig. 131-4), are often difficult for patients with a primary deficit in this domain.

The frontal lobes and their extensive connections with other cortical and subcortical regions (frontal networks) provide the neuronal substrate for these complex behaviors. The fact that the frontal lobes are so heavily interconnected with many brain regions explains why so many illnesses that affect the brain in a multifocal fashion (e.g., toxic and metabolic encephalopathies, multiple bilateral strokes, hydrocephalus) result in ''frontal'' symptoms. Comportment and executive function deficits can affect test performance in two general ways: a patient may perform normally on all other parts of the examination; alternatively, patients may do poorly on all tasks due to distractibility and poor planning.

CLINICAL PROFILE

When the examination is completed, the clinician should be able to identify the domain in which the primary clinical deficit exists. In many patients, it will be possible to pinpoint one salient domain of impairment. In others, there may be one domain of impairment and additional symptoms that are secondary to the primary deficit. In yet others, there may be multiple domains of impairment. The clinician should decide if there is one primary deficit or more and what the relative contribution of each domain is to the overall clinical picture: normal, mildly

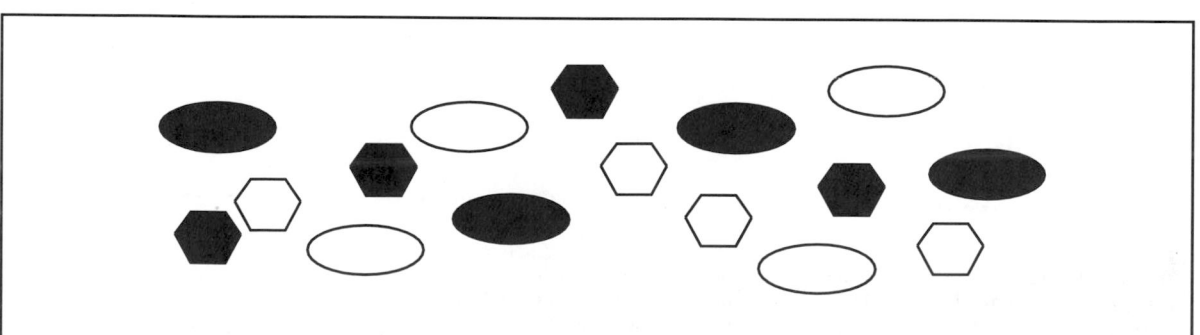

FIG. 131-4. Object-sorting task. Ask the patient to divide the objects into two groups based on some similarity. Once this has been done, ask the patient to think of a way to divide the objects into two different groups. One strategy is to group all the ovals and all the hexagons. Another strategy is to group all the white objects and all the black objects.

TABLE 131-3. Profiles of Common Neurobehavioral Syndromes on Mental State Testing

Syndrome	Primary Neurocognitive Domains						Underlying Anatomy
	Attention	Mood	Language	Complex Visual Perception	Explicit Memory	Comportment/ Executive Functions	
Aphasia syndrome			+ +				Left cerebral hemisphere
Hemispatial neglect	#	#		+ +			Right cerebral hemisphere
Balint syndrome				+ +			Bilateral parieto-occipital
Acute confusional state	+ +		*	*	*		Frontal networks
Dyslexia			+ +				Left cerebral hemisphere
Probable Alzheimer's disease	#	#	#	#	+ +		Limbic system
Progressive aphasia			+ +		*		Left cerebral hemisphere
Depression	#	+ +	*	*	*	*	Projection systems
Schizophrenia	+ +	#				+ +	Frontal networks

Abbreviations: + +, salient domain of impairment on examination; #, impairment may be present; *, performance of tests of this domain may suffer secondary to primary impairment.

impaired, moderately impaired, or severely impaired. The profile thus derived can be used to generate a list for the differential diagnosis.

Table 131-3 illustrates some common neurobehavioral syndromes and their associated clinical profiles on mental state testing. Attentional deficits are prominent in patients with toxic/metabolic encephalopathies and mutifocal structural brain disease. Disturbances of mood also follow this pattern; this may explain why many depressed patients also have prominent attention deficits. Language deficits are prominent in patients with focal lesions of the left cerebral hemisphere, in patients with the behaviorally focal dementia syndrome of primary progressive aphasia, and in patients with developmental dyslexia. Visual Perceptual and spatial deficits are primary in patients with lesions in the parieto-occipital and temporo-occipital regions bilaterally. Primary amnesia is always associated with bilateral damage to the limbic system. Alterations in reasoning, judgment, insight, and comportment often accompany frontal lobe lesions, focal dementias affecting the frontal lobes, or frontal networks disease (i.e., multifocal lesions).

This approach is useful not only in patients with focal lesions but also in individuals with developmental syndromes, degenerative diseases, and psychiatric syndromes with well-known pathophysiology, such as some forms of mood disorders and schizophrenia. Since a single mental state symptom can be associated with a number of possible underlying causes, this approach makes no assumptions about pathophysiology but rather emphasizes the definition of a clinical profile with implications for the underlying neuroanatomic mechanism. The medical history, age of the patient, neurologic examination, and ancillary laboratory data contribute to narrowing the various possibilities outlined in the differential diagnosis.

SUGGESTED READINGS

Benton A, Hamsher KdeS, Varney N, Spreen O: Contributions to Neuropsychological Assessment. Oxford University Press, New York, 1989

Chedru F, Geschwind N: Writing disturbances associated with acute confusional states. Cortex 3: 1972

Kaplan E, Goodglass H, Weintraub S: The Boston Naming Test. Lea & Febiger, Philadelphia, 1983

Mesulam M-M: Large-scale neurocognitive networks for language, memory and attention. Ann Neurol: 28:597–613, 1991

Mesulam M-M: Attention, confusional states and neglect, p. 125. In: Principles of Behavioral Neurology. FA Davis, Philadelphia, 1985

Weintraub S, Mesulam M-M: Mental state examination of young and elderly adults in behavioral neurology. p. 73. In: Principles of Behavioral Neurology. FA Davis, Philadelphia, 1985

132. DIFFERENTIAL DIAGNOSIS OF DEMENTIA

BRUCE H. PRICE

Dementia implies the insidious onset of progressive mental decline that gradually interferes with activities of daily living appropriate for age and background. It is an acquired condition that persists in an otherwise alert patient. Cognitive deficits may occur in comportment, attentional matrix, recent memory, language, or visuospatial functions. The term does not suggest an etiology. It may be reversible or irreversible, dramatically progressive or indolent, and characterized by multiple or isolated cognitive deficits. Table 132-1 summarizes basic points concerning dementia.

TABLE 132-1. Dementia

Dementia is a generic term that does not suggest etiology.

Dementia implies the insidious onset of progressive mental decline that gradually interferes with activities of daily living appropriate for age and background.

Situational stress cannot explain the changes. Dementia occurs in the context of clear consciousness.

Dementia is a clinical syndrome that may be reversible or irreversible, dramatically progressive or indolent, and characterized by multiple cognitive deficits or isolated disturbances of affect, motivation, and personality.

Deficits may occur in one or more of the following:
Comportment
Attentional matrix
Recent memory
Language
Visuospatial functions

Because there are few specific, sensitive laboratory tests, the diagnosis of dementia relies heavily upon clinical criteria. Brain tissue is usually necessary for definitive diagnosis.

The patient's history, elementary neurologic examination, and neuropsychological profile usually suggest the underlying disease process.

INITIAL CONSIDERATIONS

When a patient is referred for assessment of cognitive decline, the first necessity is to differentiate dementia syndromes from normal aging, psychiatric disease, focal neurologic syndromes, and acute confusional states.

Although aging is associated with increased susceptibility to dementia, confusion, and depression, major mental decline is not the natural course of old age. Normal cognitive aging, even into the ninth decade, is compatible with independent living. Cognitive functions that should remain preserved over the lifespan include temporal orientation, immediate attention, vocabulary, and certain visuospatial skills. Mild age-related decrements involve sustained attention, difficulties with visual greater than verbal memory recall, confrontation naming, mental flexibility, and response speed. These losses may be counterbalanced by improvements in vocabulary, judgment, insight, and wisdom.

The incorrect diagnosis of degenerative dementia instead of depression occurs in 8 to 15 percent of patients referred for assessment of mental decline. Depressed patients may exhibit poor attention and memory, apathy, social withdrawal, even mutism and incontinence. Particularly in patients 60 years or older, sadness may not be openly expressed and somatic concerns and excessive fatigue may displace neurovegetative features. The differentiation from other dementias can be challenging. The problem is compounded by the coexistence of depression in 20 to 30 percent of patients with degenerative dementias.

Helpful clues include a history of prior depression in the patient or family, onset over days to several weeks, marked agitation with pacing and persecutory delusions, precipitation by a serious life event, and persistent complaints of memory difficulty. Cognitive testing reveals variability of performance and impaired attention with insufficient mental effort during memory encoding. Once successfully embedded, memories tend to remain available. Inquiries are often met with the response, ''I don't know.'' Language and praxis are spared. Normal encephalographic (EEG) and neuroimaging results are characteristic findings.

The dementia of depression is potentially reversible with antidepressants or even electroconvulsive therapy. Highly anticholinergic antidepressants may worsen cognitive deficits. If the possibility of concomitant depression exists, aggressive therapy should be attempted. Mania, schizophrenia, conversion reactions, and malingering are usually more readily apparent.

Focal lesions of the frontal, temporal, or parietal lobes may produce restricted cognitive deficits that mimic dementia. Aphasia, dyscalculia, amnesia, and inattention may occur in the wake of stroke, tumor, or infection. Usually only one major area of cognition is disordered, sparing other intellectual activities. A sudden or stepwise course, accompanying neurologic deficits, and focal EEG and neuroimaging abnormalities help in making the differential diagnosis.

The most important feature distinguishing acute confusional states from dementia is the patient's inability to maintain a coherent stream of thought. The patient is awake but attention is impaired. This situation is usually accompanied by distractibility, perseveration, thought intrusions, even florid hallucinations. Secondary cognitive deficits involve language, memory, and visuospatial skills. Confusion often fluctuates throughout the day and night. Affect may range from apathy to agitation. A multitude of medications, failure of almost any organ system, and systemic inflammatory or neoplastic diseases are important diagnostic considerations. The elderly are more prone to toxic/metabolic encephalopathies; recovery may gradually occur over weeks. It is particularly gratifying when the simple withdrawal of a medication returns the patient to a normal baseline.

Onset within hours to days, disruption of sleep–wake cycle, florid hallucinations, asterixis, primitive reflexes, postural tremor, and myoclonus are suggestive of acute confusional states. If the EEG does not show characteristic diffuse background slowing, then the diagnosis of a toxic-metabolic encephalopathy is unlikely. Many elderly patients may present in an acute confusional state, the underlying dementia exacerbated by an intercurrent infection. As the treated infection resolves, dementia surfaces and is confirmed by the family's history.

GENERAL CONSIDERATIONS

Table 132-2 presents a formidable list of the causes of dementia in adults. It is necessarily incomplete. Every dementia preferentially involves certain cell and/or neurotransmitter systems. Not all mental faculties are affected simultaneously. The cognitive profile is dictated more by neuroanatomic lesion site than specific histopathology. Although often anatomically incorrect, the differentiation between cortical and subcortical dementia profiles is clinically useful. Deficits caused by subcortical disease include slowed and inefficient cognitive processing and alterations in personality, mood, or behavior. Parkinson's, Huntington's, and Wilson's diseases; progressive supranuclear palsy; normal pressure hydrocephalus; demyelinating diseases; leukodystrophies; and acquired immunodeficiency syndrome dementia are representative of this subtype. Salient deficits in patients with cortical dementias include language and praxis skills. Alzheimer's and Pick's diseases are prototypes of this subtype. Other disorders such as Creutzfeldt-Jakob and diffuse Lewy body diseases or neurosyphilis may equally involve both cortical and subcortical structures. Amnesia, cognitive disorganization, and impaired visuospatial skills can be caused by either cortical or subcortical lesions.

In general, most patients with dementia do not refer themselves. Relatives or associates usually note the onset first. Referrals often occur in crisis settings either on Monday mornings after a family reunion or Friday afternoons when a family is seeking weekend respite.

The detection of dementia in its early stages can be difficult. In the elderly, routine activities may be less taxing; therefore, disruption of daily living activities may not be as apparent. Normal aging is associated with intrinsic mental decline of a mild degree, enabling the uninformed family's acceptance of ''senility'' as the normal aging pattern. Pre-existing asymptomatic lesions in limbic and association cortex can become symptomatic with normal aging. Highly functioning individuals may be able to mask the symptoms of dementia for a protracted time. Most mental status examination have a ceiling effect. Results within the normal range may still reflect considerable decline compared to the individual's superior baseline talents.

PATIENT HISTORY

A detailed patient history can narrow the differential diagnosis (Table 132-3). Since cognitive impairment must be measured against that person's baseline, their highest degree of formal education, life achievements, and normal personality traits should be established first. The family is often, but not always,

TABLE 132-2. Causes of Dementia in Adults

Degenerative disorders
  Alzheimer's disease
  Pick's disease
  Nonspecific neuron loss
  Parkinson's disease
  Diffuse Lewy body disease
  Huntington's disease
  Progressive supranuclear palsy
  Spinocerebellar degenerations
  Idiopathic basal ganglia calcification
  Striatonigral degeneration
  Wilson's disease
  Hallervorden-Spatz disease
  Thalamic dementia
  Motor neuron disease

Vascular dementias
  Multiple large vessel occlusions
  Lacunar state (multiple subcortical infarcts)
  Binswanger's disease
  Mixed cortical/subcortical infarctions
  Mitochondrial encephalomyopathies

Myelinoclastic disorders
  Demyelinating
    Multiple sclerosis
    Marchiafava-Bignami disease
  Dysmyelinating
    Metachromatic leukodystrophy
    Adrenoleukodystrophy
    Cerebrotendinous xanthomatosis
    Ceroid lipofuscinosis (Kufs disease)
    Polyglucosan body disease
    Tay-Sachs disease
Traumatic conditions
  Subdural hematoma
  Dementia pugilistica

Neoplastic dementias
  Meningioma (particularly subfrontal)
  Glioma
  Metastatic lesions
  Meningeal carcinomatosis
  Paraneoplastic

Hydrocephalic dementias
  Communicating
    Normal pressure hydrocephalus
  Noncommunicating
    Aqueductal stenosis
    Intraventricular neoplasm
    Intraventricular cyst
    Basilar meningitis

Inflammatory conditions
  Systemic lupus erythematosus
  Temporal arteritis
  Sarcoidosis
  Sjögren-Larsson syndrome
  Granulomatous arteritis

Infection-related dementias
  Syphilis
  Lyme disease
  Chronic meningitis (tuberculosis, fungal)
  Brain abscess
  Progressive multifocal leukoencephalopathy
  Whipple's disease
  Human immunodeficiency virus encephalopathy/opportunistic infections
  Creuzfeldt-Jakob disease
  Gerstmann-Straussler disease
  Subacute sclerosing panencephalitis

Metabolic disorders
  Cardiopulmonary failure—hypoxia, hypercapnia
  Uremia
  Hepatic encephalopathy
  Endocrine disorders
    Thyroid
    Adrenal
    Parathyroid
  Anemia and other hematologic conditions
  Deficiency states (vitamin B_{12}, folate, niacin)
  Porphyria
  Hypoglycemia

Toxic exposures
  Alcohol-related syndromes
  Polydrug abuse
  Heavy metals
  Industrial solvents

Psychiatric disorders
  Depression
  Mania
  Schizophrenia
  Conversion reaction
  Malingering

TABLE 132-3. Patient History Survey

1. Highest degree of formal education, life achievements; baseline personality traits?

2. Impact of decline on activities of daily living?
   Work performance
   Financial accountability
   Walking, driving skills
   Grocery shopping
   Household chores
   Repetition of conversations
   Misplacement of personal belongings

3. When did cognitive difficulties begin? What was the initial feature? Were the changes abrupt or insidious in onset? Did they resolve, persist without change, or worsen over time? In what sequence were deficits noted?

4. Changes in self-care, personality, behavior? Altered language, including word-finding difficulties, paraphasias, diminished fluency, comprehension, or writing? Ataxia, incontinence, seizures?

5. Underlying illnesses, current medications?

6. History of poor nutrition, head trauma, cardiac disease, strokes, artherosclerotic risk factors, subarachnoid hemorrhage, meningitis?

7. Exposure to alcohol, illicit drugs, industrial toxins, human immunodeficiency virus, Lyme disease, syphilis?

8. Past or present depression in the patient or patient's family?

9. Family history of dementia such as Alzheimer's, Pick's, Huntington's, Parkinson's diseases; spinocerebellar degenerations; Tay-Sachs disease? Confirmed by laboratory tests or brain autopsy?

a more reliable historian than the patient. However, family members may disagree as to time of onset, initial deficits, and sequence of events. Some tend to use calendar landmarks to date onset, but subtle decline preceding these events can often be elicited. After further reflection, usually during the follow-up examination, a more accurate history may be forthcoming.

Pattern recognition in the differential diagnosis of dementia is essential. A patient with insidious onset of progressive amnesia over months to years suggests the possibility of Alzheimer's disease. Language involvement in Alzheimer's disease is common and is characterized by anomia, paraphasias, and diminished comprehension over time. Nonfluent aphasias such as Broca's are hardly ever seen. Language impairments are unusual in normal pressure hydrocephalus. Subacute onset with rapid deterioration accompanied by myoclonus and pyramidal and extrapyramidal signs is more typical of Creutzfeldt-Jakob disease. A previously fastidious person who over months to years suffers a decline in personal hygiene, comportment, and planning with relative sparing of recent memory and language is more likely to have Pick's disease or nonspecific neuron loss.

In the era we live in, abuse of drugs such as toluene or cocaine, and the possibility of transmissible diseases such as human immunodeficiency virus, Lyme disease, or syphilis must be explored. Past history of head trauma, subarachnoid hemorrhage, or meningitis is associated with the emergence of hydrocephalus. Patients with recurrent cardiac-induced syncope can develop hippocampal gliosis with subsequent amnesia.

Past history of depression in the patient or their family suggests the need for further inquiries regarding the possibility of a current mood disorder. Given their genetic implications, a family history of Alzheimer's, Huntington's, Parkinson's, *or Tay-Sachs diseases* or spinocerebellar degenerations should influence the investigation. Autopsy or biochemical confirmation is helpful.

ASSOCIATED NEUROLOGIC DEFICITS

The recognition of dementia and associated focal elementary neurologic deficits can guide the differential diagnosis and subsequent investigations (Table 132-4). Impaired visual and/or auditory acuity can be misinterpreted by patients and their families as cognitive decline. On occasion, it is rewarding to witness the dramatic effects of improved sight and hearing. Normal elementary neurologic examination results in the context of dementia favors Alzheimer's, Pick's, or nonspecific neuron loss diseases. Pseudobulbar affect suggests multiple deep lacunae or motor neuron disease, such as amyotrophic lateral sclerosis. Gait abnormalities suggest Parkinson's disease, frontal network lacunae and normal pressure hydrocephalus. Visual field cuts, hemiparesis, or hemineglect are most consistent with cortical infarcts, but adult polyglucosan body disease can present this way as well. Supranuclear gaze paresis suggests progressive supranuclear palsy, among other possibilities. Fasciculations, distal atrophy, and bulbar signs in the context of a frontal network dementia point to motor neuron disease. Dementia occurs in 20 percent of such patients. Accompanying sensory abnormalities, myoclonic jerks, or tremors yield helpful clues in the differential diagnosis. Choreiform movements are not seen in every patient with Huntington's disease, particularly in those with onset after age 60. Cerebellar signs in the face of dementia constitute a different set of considerations. Dysarthria, tremors, or ataxia suggest the possibilities of ceroid lipofuscinosis (Kufs), Tay-Sachs, and Gerstmann-Straussler diseases.

LABORATORY INVESTIGATIONS

Every patient with a suspected dementia syndrome requires comprehensive evaluation. The first goal is to discover remediable causes. The second goal is to establish the correct diagnosis in order to counsel the patient and family regarding possible intervention and prognosis. The next goal is education and support of the patient and family with the help of other disciplines, including management of the patient's ongoing primary health care. Finally, persuasion of the family regarding the value of definitive diagnosis by autopsy and possible genetic counseling should be considered.

In up to 20 percent of patients referred for evaluation of intellectual deterioration, there may be treatable causes. Depression, intracranial masses, subdural hematomas, hydrocephalus, thyroid disease, and nutritional deficiencies constitute the majority of these cases. Further deterioration may be prevented in other diseases. For instance, multi-infarct dementia can be stabilized with treatment of underlying stroke risk factors and prevention of further ischemic events. Despite careful clinical assessment, laboratory investigations are required to establish the underlying cause. Unexpected findings are not uncommon. Table 132-5 lists those investigations necessary to discover remediable causes and identify etiology of the underlying dementia.

Some investigations require special comment. Bedside mental status testing can be a valuable screen to establish the proba-

TABLE 132-4. Dementias Associated With Elementary Neurologic Abnormalities

Abnormality	Associations
Pseudobulbar affect	Bilateral strokes Demyelinating diseases Motor neuron disease
Gait and station	Parkinson's disease Vascular dementias Normal pressure hydrocephalus Neurosyphilis Progressive supranuclear palsy Tay-Sachs disease
Adventitial movements	Huntington's disease Parkinson's disease Cruetzfeldt-Jakob disease Wilson's disease Striatonigral degeneration
Visual fields	Mass lesions Cortical strokes Brain abscess Adult polyglucosan body disease
Extraocular movements	Progressive supranuclear palsy Wernicke-Korsakoff encephalopathy Strokes Multiple sclerosis
Dysarthria	Progressive supranuclear palsy Multiple sclerosis Motor neuron disease Parkinson's disease Paraneoplasia
Pyramidal/motor system	Stroke Motor neuron disease/amyotrophic lateral sclerosis Parkinson's disease with dementia Tay-Sachs disease Hallervorden-Spatz disease
Extrapyramidal	Parkinson's disease Progressive supranuclear palsy Huntington's disease Wilson's disease Striatonigral degeneration
Sensory	Metachromatic leukodystrophy Vitamin B_{12}, folate deficiencies Thyroid disease Neoplasia Paraneoplasia
Cerebellar	Creutzfeldt-Jakob disease Paraneoplasia Spinocerebellar degenerations Tay-Sachs disease Gerstmann-Straussler disease Hallervorden-Spatz disease

TABLE 132-5. Laboratory Investigation of Dementia

Essential	Optional
Neuropsychological examination	Electroencephalograph
Head computed tomography or magnetic resonance imaging	Cerebrospinal fluid analysis VDRL, rapid plasma reagin
Chest x-ray	Human immunodeficiency virus
Electrocardiogram	ANA
Complete blood count	Urinalysis
Electrolytes	Small bowel biopsy
Calcium	Nerve biopsy
Blood urea nitrogen	Brain biopsy
Liver, thyroid function tests	Genetic studies
Vitamin B_{12}, folate levels	

bility of dementia. Formal neuropsychological tests administered by trained personnel are more precise and quantitative, given their highly standardized, age-related norms. Specific tests of attentional matrix, frontal network functions, and memory, language, and visuospatial abilities provide useful profiles. These results also help exclude the possibilities of normal aging, acute confusional states, and psychiatric diseases.

Among the degenerative dementias, three patient groups can be identified by neuropsychological profile: (1) those with amnesia as the primary deficit; (2) those in whom aphasic, agnosic, or apraxic difficulties are most outstanding; and (3) those whose salient deficit involves motivation and comportment. The great majority of patients in the first group will be found, on postmortem examination, to have had Alzheimer's disease. The second group will show a mixture of pathology, with a preponderance of Alzheimer's and Pick's disease changes. Pathology in the third group is more heterogenous but includes Pick's disease and nonspecific neuron loss with primary involvement of prefrontal cortex.

Magnetic resonance imaging or computed tomography brain scan is an essential laboratory aid. They are relatively easy, safe tests that may detect most intra- and extracranial mass lesions, ischemic infarcts, gliosis, hydrocephalus, demyelination, and leukodystrophies. However, problems with interpretation are common: (1) sulcal widening and ventricular dilation are found in many elderly cognitively intact individuals; (2) some dementia patients may have normal scan results such as in Alzheimer's disease; (3) Some nondemented patients may have multiple lesions without cognitive impact; (4) the degree of atrophy is not a reliable predictor of dementia severity; and (5) T2 pulse sequence abnormalities on magnetic resonance imaging bear an unclear relationship to type and severity of dementia. As with all other tests, they must be interpreted within the clinical framework.

When the patient's history, neuropsychological and neurologic profiles, and laboratory test results are entirely consistent with a particular dementia syndrome, then further special investigations are not necessary. Cerebrospinal fluid analysis remains an important part of the investigation of atypical dementias when looking for evidence of infection, demyelination, paraneoplasia, or vasculitic disease. The usefulness of routine EEG is questionable. In many degenerative dementias such as Alzheimer's and Pick's diseases, the EEG results may be normal until moderate to advanced stages. Minor changes, such as reduced amplitude and minimal Θ slowing, are nonspecific. EEG abnormalities do not consistently correlate with the degree of impairment. However, the EEG becomes generally slowed soon after onset of diffuse Lewy body disease. Preserved EEG background rules out toxic-metabolic encephalopathies.

The question of brain biopsy is sometimes pertinent. The procedure is usually driven by the possibility of treatable causes. Histologic diagnosis is not necessarily reliable, false-positive and -negative results may occur, seizures can subsequently develop, and anesthesia may worsen the patient's mental state. However, at times it can be useful in diagnosing Whipple's disease, carcinomatous meningitis, or vasculitic diseases. Small bowel biopsy may obviate the need for brain biopsy in the diagnosis of Whipple's disease. Sural nerve biopsy may be required to diagnose Kufs disease.

Dementia in later childhood and early adult life is rare. It poses a different set of diagnostic possibilities and investigations. Psychiatric problems are far more common in this age group. However, inherited metabolic disorders can manifest themselves by behavioral and emotional changes that may precede by months or years the incipient onset of cognitive and neurologic decline. Remediable causes in this age group include tumors, hydrocephalus, and Wilson's, Lesch-Nyhan, and thyroid diseases. Leukodystrophies, subacute sclerosing panencephalitis and other chronic encephalitides, Huntington's disease, and spinocerebellar degenerations also occur in this age group.

PRINCIPLES OF MANAGEMENT

Once the diagnosis of irreversible dementia has been established, the physician should continue to involve the patient and his or her family. It is my practice to inform the patient and their families about the diagnosis, reducing the need for family secrets while encouraging a team approach. Social workers can be invaluable in anticipating and addressing the psychosocial and financial needs of the family.

The functional characterization of dementia stages is helpful. Patients with mild dementias are capable of most activities of daily living. Those with moderate involvement may require some daily assistance. Patients with advanced disease need nearly total assistance. Serial neurologic and neuropsychological follow-ups 4 to 6 months after initial evaluation often clarify the nature and course of the disease. Sudden deterioration after gradual decline suggests ''beclouded dementia,'' a dementia worsened by superimposed toxic-metabolic or systemic insults. Mild to moderately demented patients who develop congestive heart failure or urinary tract infections usually respond to proper treatment over the course of several weeks with improved mental functions.

Simplifying the patient's surroundings can improve his or her behavior. Familiar circumstances are most comfortable; novelty can be disconcerting. Crowds or family gatherings with multiple, loud stimuli can temporarily worsen the patient's mentation. Medications and their intake should be simplified, avoiding psychoactive drugs if possible. This is where the role of a primary doctor assumes great importance. Polypharmacy and/or highly anticholinergic drugs can be prescribed by multiple unsuspecting physicians, with dire consequences. The possibility of coexistent depression must be kept in mind. Low-dose benzodiazepines or neuroleptics may be required in agitated patients. Autopsy verification establishes the definitive diagnosis and often allows the family to achieve closure and move on.

We are entering a remarkable new era in the assessment and treatment of dementia. Dementias thought to be hopeless in the recent past are no longer approached with such therapeutic nihilism. Neurotransmitter trials in Alzheimer's disease, early genetic detection and family counseling in Huntington's disease, and genetically engineered enzyme replacement therapies for type 1 Gaucher's disease offer promise. Emerging neurobiologic developments now mandate early diagnosis, allowing early intervention. The assessment of dementia is no longer a sterile intellectual exercise. It represents a diligent effort that will increasingly offer hope to many patients.

SUGGESTED READINGS

Cummings JL, Benson DF: Dementia: A Clinical Approach. 2nd Ed. Butterwort, Stoneham, MA, 1992

Heilman KM, Valenstein E: Clinical Neuropsychology. 3rd Ed. Oxford University Press, New York, 1993

Katzman R, Rowe JW: Principles of Geriatric Neurology. Contemporary Neurology Series. Vol. 38. FA Davis, Philadelphia, 1991

Mesulam MM: Principles of Behavioral Neurology. FA Davis, Philadelphia, 1985

Terry RD, Katzman R, Bick KL: Alzheimer Disease. Raven Press, New York, 1994

133. ALZHEIMER'S DISEASE AND RELATED DISORDERS

KIRK R. DAFFNER

Alzheimer's disease has been characterized as "the coming plague of the twenty-first century." The prevalence of the disease has risen steadily as the average age of the population has increased. It has been estimated that up to 10 percent of Americans 65 and older suffer from the disease, whereas for the population 85 and older, estimates of the prevalence have been as high as 47 percent. As many as 4 million Americans may suffer from Alzheimer's disease, and the cost of caring for them is over $80 billion per year. Based on current rates, it is estimated that in 50 years, there will be as many as 14 million cases of Alzheimer's disease in the United States alone.

Given these numbers, it is not surprising that the evaluation of dementia is a significant component of most practices in neurology. In the early 1980s, one study suggested that neurologists were seeing one case of dementia for every two cases of stroke. In general, the tendency in medicine has been to diagnose Alzheimer's disease in any elderly individual with a significant deterioration in cognitive status. Although Alzheimer's disease is the major cause of dementia in America, it accounts for only 55 to 70 percent of cases. Unfortunately, autopsy series have revealed that the accuracy of the clinical diagnosis of Alzheimer's disease can be as low as 55 percent. Given the prevalence of this disease, such a low "hit rate" suggests a diagnostic accuracy close to chance. Neurologists in research settings who have closely followed the established diagnostic criteria, reviewed below, have achieved much higher accuracy. Such precision in diagnosis will become increasingly important as new treatments are made available, especially if intervention at an early stage yields the best prognosis. Even before such time, diagnostic accuracy is crucial for ensuring that a patient's dementia is not due to a reversible etiology, as is estimated to be the case in 10 to 15 percent of patients, and for educating family members and caregivers about the illness and allowing them to make appropriate plans based on prognosis.

The diagnosis of Alzheimer's disease, Pick's disease, diffuse Lewy body disease, and so on is ultimately a histopathologic one, made at autopsy or, on rare occasions, upon brain biopsy. Few if any patients enter our offices carrying slides of the histology of their diseased brains. Yet, we often speak of living patients as, for example, having "Alzheimer's disease." Our diagnostic nomenclature and the thinking behind it often muddies the crucial distinction between clinical diagnosis and final pathology. As neurologists, we practice within the realm of clinical syndromes. The different clinical patterns or profiles observed can be used by us to provide reasonably accurate estimates of the likelihood of the underlying neuropathology. Figure 133-1 illustrates the relationship between the clinical and neuropathologic planes. Rather than starting with a named pathologic entity and noting all of the clinical features that have been associated with it, this chapter begins with the salient clinical patterns seen in degenerative dementia that are most useful in predicting underlying pathology. The chapter emphasizes the degenerative dementias that do not have prominent motor findings and thus does not include such entities as Huntington's disease or Parkinson's disease. The major clinical profiles reviewed are (1) progressive amnestic dementia, (2) progressive comportmental dementia, and (3) progressive focal neuropsychological deficits (such as primary progressive aphasia).

PROGRESSIVE AMNESTIC DEMENTIA

In patients with progressive amnestic dementia, a decline in memory functions is the salient or core feature. The clinical pattern is most often insidiously progressive, with memory impairments being the initial source of disruption of activities of daily living. Family members may note that the patient is increasingly forgetful of appointments or events, repeats the same stories or questions, and tends to misplace items. Early in the course of the disease, mental state testing tends to reveal relatively preserved autobiographic information, variable recall of recent events, and subtle disorientation. Even in the mildest cases, acquisition of bits of information that exceeds digit span is impaired. There is difficulty retrieving newly learned information even after short delays. Such patients tend to perform better with recognition tasks. Over time, patients exhibit increasing problems with encoding as well as recognition of even simple material.

To make the diagnosis of progressive amnestic dementia, the problems with the storage, retention, or retrieval components of memory must be primary. They cannot be explained by impairments in attention, motivation, language, or visuospatial functioning. For example, one must ensure that the patient is not in a confusional state, with markedly disrupted attentional abilities, that would make it impossible to accurately encode new information. Nor can the medical history or serial examinations suggest a static insult to limbic structures (e.g., a hypoxic-ischemic event, herpes encephalitis, or Korsakoff syndrome) without evidence of a progressive decline.

Although memory dysfunction is prominent in patients with this pattern of dementia, they also exhibit impairments of language, attention, visuospatial functioning, reasoning, and judgment. Language disturbances are extremely common. Patients tend to have naming difficulties and empty, fluent speech consistent with features of anomic, transcorticosensory, or Wernicke's aphasia. The ability to generate lists of words is frequently impaired. The addition of such a task to mental state tests has been shown to enhance the sensitivity of diagnosis. Whereas the performance of simple tasks of vigilance and automatic attentional processing is relatively well preserved, many patients exhibit disruption of more complex aspects of attention that require controlled information processing, response selectivity and inhibition, and appropriate exploration of extrapersonal space. This kind of impaired attention may be the first nonmnestic function to be disturbed. Many patients show abnormalities in visuospatial functioning, both the visuoconstructive (e.g., drawing cubes or intersecting pentagons) and visuop-

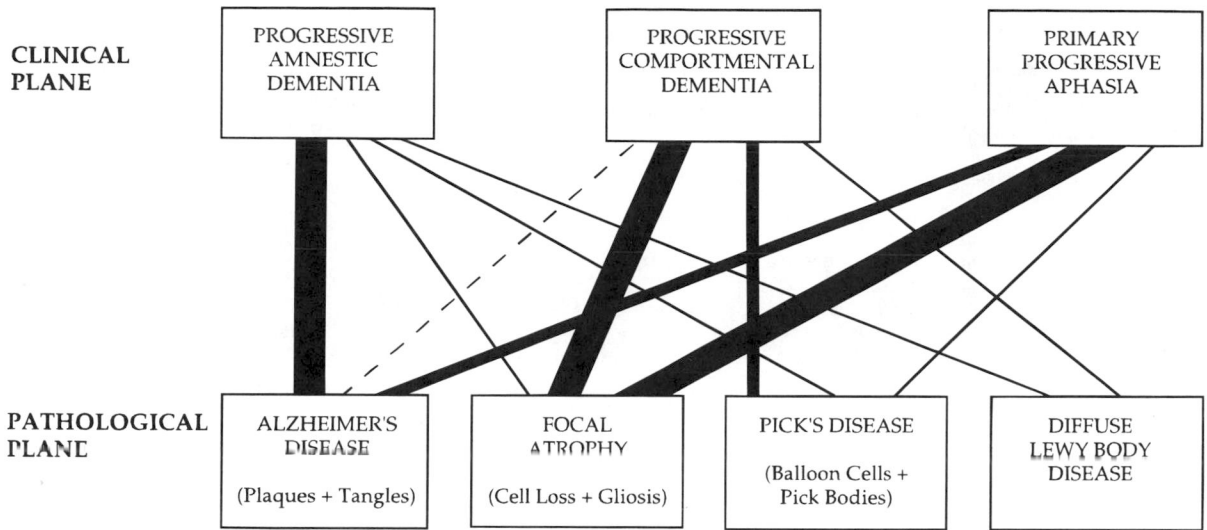

FIG. 133-1. Relationship between clinical and pathologic planes in degenerative dementia. The clinical plane designates the prominent feature of different dementia profiles as reviewed in the text. The pathologic plane represents different salient histologic findings. The thickness of the lines indicates the relative probability that a particular clinical profile will be associated with a particular underlying pathologic process. (Adapted from Weintraub S, Rubin NP, Mesulam MM: Primary progressive aphasia: longitudinal course, neuropsychological profile, and language features. Arch Neurol 47: 1329–35, 1990, with permission.)

erceptual (e.g., matching the angles made by pairs of lines) aspects. Insight is frequently undermined, especially as the illness progresses, and may reflect increasing disruption of frontal networks by the pathology of the disease.

The dementia profile of progressive amnestic problems in combination with other cognitive deficits is the most common one seen in the elderly. On a pathologic plane, this clinical syndrome is most often associated with the plaques and tangles that define Alzheimer's disease. The National Institute of Neurological and Communicative Disorders and Stroke–Alzheimer's Disease and Related Disorders Association (NINCDS–ADRDA) Work Group codified the clinical criteria associated with a high likelihood of Alzheimer's pathology. Criteria for "probable Alzheimer's disease" includes (1) the presence of dementia, (2) progressive worsening of memory and other cognitive functions, (3) deficits in two or more areas of cognition, (4) no disturbance of consciousness, (5) age of onset between 40 and 90, and (6) the absence of systemic or central nervous system disorders that could account for the dementia. (See Table 133-1 for details of the NINCDS–ADRDA criteria.)

Use of these clinical criteria has yielded diagnostic accuracy in autopsy series of better than 80 percent. In our dementia clinic, which adhered to strict NINCDS–ADRDA criteria for probable Alzheimer's disease and closely attended to the neuropsychological profiles in dementia described in this chapter, the diagnosis of probable Alzheimer's disease was accurate approximately 95 percent of the time. Other neuropathologic causes of this pattern of progressive amnestic dementia cited in the literature that are much less frequent than Alzheimer's disease include diffuse Lewy body disease, Pick's disease, and focal, nonspecific neuronal degeneration.

The cognitive profile seen most typically in Alzheimer's disease is consistent with the distribution of pathology in this disease and well-established brain–behavioral relationships. In the early stages of the illness, pathologic changes, especially the accumulation of neurofibrillary tangles, tend to involve limbic

regions and over time spread to neocortical areas. The temporolimbic system has been shown to play a central role in memory processing. Thus, pathology in this region helps to explain the salient memory disturbance observed in most cases of Alzheimer's disease (see Ch. 137).

Alzheimer's disease pathology is characterized by neurofibrillary tangles (composed of paired helical filaments that contain an abnormally phosphoralated τ protein), senile plaques (composed of dystrophic neurites and a central core of extracellular deposits of amyloid), significant loss of neurons, and diminished synaptic density. The limbic system is particularly ravaged, but the process is multifocal, involving widespread regions of the central nervous system, with the relative sparing of primary motor and sensory cortex. The cholinergic system, arising from the basal forebrain, is significantly disrupted; many other neurotransmitter systems are damaged, as well. Given the wide range of pathology affecting multiple ascending neurotransmitter systems and multifocal areas of cortex involved in different aspects of cognition, it is not surprising that a simple pharmacologic intervention for Alzheimer's disease has not proven successful.

As of yet, there is no single securely established theory to account for the array of neuropathologic findings in Alzheimer's diseases. This is an area of very active research in neuroscience. The debate continues over whether β-amyloid is derived from neuron or vascular sources. In either case, β-amyloid is likely to be the result of altered processing of the amyloid precursor protein, although the reduced capacity to clear minor products of amyloid precursor protein degradation remains a possibility. β-Amyloid appears to be toxic to mature neurons in vitro, perhaps by interfering with the normal inhibition of protease activity. Senile plaque formation seems to involve stages of development from noncompacted, diffuse deposits of amyloid not associated with neuronal degeneration to dense core-type plaques that are almost always associated with dystrophic neurites. The exact relationship between β-amyloid and neurofibrillary tangles remains to be established, although brain

TABLE 133-1. NINCDS–ADRDA Criteria for Clinical Diagnosis of Alzheimer's Disease

I. The criteria for the clinical diagnosis of *probable* Alzheimer's disease include:
  1. Dementia established by clinical examination and documented by the Mini-Mental State Test, Blessed Dementia Scale, or some similar examination, and confirmed by neuropsychological tests
  2. Deficits in two or more areas of cognition
  3. Progressive worsening of memory and other cognitive functions
  4. No disturbance of consciousness
  5. Onset between ages 40 and 90, most often after age 65
  6. Absence of systemic disorders or other brain diseases that in and of themselves could account for the progressive deficits in memory and cognition

II. The diagnosis of *probable* Alzheimer's disease is supported by:
  1. Progressive deterioration of specific cognitive functions such as language (aphasia), motor skills (apraxia), and perception (agnosia)
  2. Impaired activities of daily living and altered patterns of behavior
  3. Family history of similar disorders, particularly if confirmed neuropathologically
  4. Laboratory results of:
    a. Normal lumbar puncture as evaluated by standard techniques
    b. Normal pattern or nonspecific changes in EEG, such as increased slow-wave activity
    c. Evidence of cerebral atrophy on CT with progression documented by serial observation

III. Other clinical features consistent with the diagnosis of *probable* Alzheimer's disease, after exclusion of causes of dementia other than Alzheimer's disease, include:
  1. Plateaus in the course of progression of the illness
  2. Associated symptoms of depression, insomnia, incontinence, delusions, illusions, hallucinations; catastrophic verbal, emotional, or physical outbursts; sexual disorders; and weight loss
  3. Other neurologic abnormalities in some patients, especially those with more advanced disease and including motor signs such as increased muscle tone, myoclonus, or gait disorder
  4. Seizures in advanced disease
  5. CT normal for age

IV. Features that make the diagnosis of *probable* Alzheimer's disease uncertain or unlikely include:
  1. Sudden, apoplectic onset
  2. Focal neurologic findings such as hemiparesis, sensory loss, visual field deficits, and incoordination early in the course of the illness
  3. Seizures or gait disturbances at the onset or very early in the course of the illness

V. Clinical diagnosis of *possible* Alzheimer's disease:
  1. May be made on the basis of the dementia syndrome; in the absence of other neurologic, psychiatric, or systemic disorders sufficient to cause dementia; and in the presence of variations in the onset, presentation, or clinical course
  2. May be made in the presence of a second systemic or brain disorder sufficient to produce dementia, which is not considered to be the cause of the dementia
  3. Should be used in research studies when a single, gradually progressive, severe cognitive deficit is identified in the absence of other identifiable cause

VI. Criteria for diagnosis of *definite* Alzheimer's disease are:
  1. The clinical criteria for probable Alzheimer's disease
  2. Histopathologic evidence obtained from a biopsy or autopsy

VII. Classifications of Alzheimer's disease for research purposes should specify features that may differentiate subtypes of the disorder, such as:
  1. Familial occurrence
  2. Onset before age 65
  3. Presence of trisomy-21
  4. Coexistence of other relevant conditions such as Parkinson's disease

Abbreviations: NINCDS–ADRA, National Institute of Neurological and Communicative Disorders and Stroke–Alzheimer's Disease and Related Disorders Association; CT, computed tomography; EEG, electroencephalogram.

(From McKhann G, Drachman D, Folstein M et al: Clinical diagnosis of Alzheimer's disease: report of the NINCDS-ADRDA work group under the auspices of Department of Health and Human Services task force on Alzheimer's disease. Neurology 34: 939–44, 1984, with permission.)

regions with a high density of plaques tend to receive projections from tangle-laden neurons.

The relationship between observed pathology and the clinical profile of dementia also requires further investigation. Some studies have reported a correlation between dementia severity and number of senile plaques. Others have correlated dementia severity with the number and distribution of neurofibrillary tangles and not plaques. Recently, investigators have emphasized that cognitive decline in Alzheimer's disease reflects reduced synaptic density in the prefrontal cortex due to loss of neurons projecting from distant regions in the parietal and temporal cortices. Another challenge is sorting out the connection between "normal aging" and Alzheimer's disease. Although there have been reports of individuals over 80 without evidence of neocortical plaques and tangles, this is a rare finding. Many would argue that there is no qualitative distinction between the histologic features associated with Alzheimer's disease and aging.

Researchers have not yet determined what triggers the pathophysiologic process. Age is the most important risk factor for developing Alzheimer's disease. Genetic factors play a role, with individuals who have first-degree relatives with Alzheimer's disease being at greater risk (three- to fourfold) for developing the disease. The autosomal-dominant form of familial Alzheimer's disease accounts for a small percentage of cases and presents with early onset. Up to 70 percent of these cases may be due to a recently identified gene on chromosome 14. Apolipoprotein E (Apo E), which is coded for on chromosome 19, has 3 allelic variants (E2, E3, E4). The E4 allele has been shown to be a major susceptibility factor in late-onset familial and sporadic cases of Alzheimer's disease, lowering the mean age of onset. As a group, patients with E4/4 present with Alzheimer's disease on average 15 years before those without an E4 allele. E4/4 may serve as a "pathologic chaperone" for β-amyloid, which promotes the formation of amyloid filaments. Other factors that may increase the risk of developing Alzheimer's disease include a history of head trauma, lack of education, increased maternal age at the time of the patient's birth, and a family history of Down syndrome. A causal link between Alzheimer's disease pathology and an infectious or toxic agent (e.g., aluminum) has not been established.

Workup for a patient suspected of having Alzheimer's disease should follow the guidelines reviewed in Chapter 132. A good history from a reliable informant about the patient's baseline and changes in cognitive and behavioral status is invaluable. A detailed mental state examination, as reviewed in Chapter 131 is essential for establishing a patient's current level of cognitive functioning and for illuminating a profile of salient deficits. As noted early, formal mental status evaluation and neuropsychological assessment are among the most useful tools for establishing the diagnosis of probable Alzheimer's disease. The most challenging cases are the ones that present either very early or very late in the course of the illness. Very early on, activities of daily living may not yet be clearly disrupted and it can be difficult to distinguish this pattern from age-associated memory impairments. It is essential to follow dementia patients longitudinally to establish a clearly progressive course. In cases of very late and severe dementia, it may be impossible to adequately test a patient, and no salient pattern of deficits may emerge. In fact, the end stages of a wide range of dementing illnesses tend to have a very similar appearance.

Clinical neuroimaging with computed tomography (CT) or magnetic resonance imaging (MRI) is appropriate to rule out lesions such as tumors or strokes that could account for or contribute to the dementia profile. Scattered foci of increased T2 signal or even more definitive areas of infarction should not automatically yield a diagnosis of "vascular dementia," especially in patients whose clinical profile points to a progressive amnestic dementia. Assessing the potential role of presumed infarctions in the cognitive decline of patients requires clinical judgment and awareness of how the anatomic distribution of such lesions might plausibly disrupt cerebral networks subserving specific neuropsychological functions. Furthermore, patients presumed to have vascular dementia often have coexistent Alzheimer's pathology. Recently, research protocols have employed MRI morphometric analysis of the hippocampal region and demonstrated significant focal atrophy in patients with probable Alzheimer's disease. In the future, such technology may aid in diagnosis. Functional neuroimaging with, for example, single photon emission computed tomography (SPECT) has suggested the most typical pattern in Alzheimer's disease is bilateral temporo-parietal hypoperfusion, which, if present in a patient, can be interpreted as consistent with the diagnosis of probable Alzheimer's disease. Currently, there is no noninvasive, diagnostic test for Alzheimer's disease that has acceptable sensitivity and specificity. However, since such a test would be enormously useful, it is being actively pursued.

Whereas the cognitive abnormalities in Alzheimer's disease tend to be emphasized, changes in affect, personality, and behavior are also major sources of suffering for patients and their caregivers. Fifteen to 20 percent of patients with Alzheimer's disease develop symptoms of major depression, most often early in the course of their illness. Such depression may further erode daily functioning and cognitive performance and can be responsive to treatment with antidepressant medication. Alzheimer's disease patients with depression have been shown at autopsy to have increased pathology in brainstem locus ceruleus, dorsal raphe nucleus, and substantia nigra and to exhibit evidence of reduced catecholamine levels.

Delusions or fixed false beliefs are common in Alzheimer's disease, occurring in up to 40 percent of cases, probably more often in midcourse. They often involve the patients' conviction that someone is stealing from them, that they are not in their own home, or that their spouse is not faithful. Hallucinations have been reported in approximately 25 percent of Alzheimer's disease patients. Psychotic symptoms in Alzheimer's have been associated with a more rapidly deteriorating course. Diminished engagement or withdrawal from social and physical surroundings is common. Anxiety, irritability, wandering, and aggressive behaviors are frequently observed and may become more likely as the severity of the dementia increases. Incontinence becomes increasingly prevalent as the dementia progresses, with the majority suffering from this problem in the late stages of the illness.

Management of patients with probable Alzheimer's disease is challenging. The rewards come in supporting a patient and his or her family through the different stages of the illness that can last many years. It is essential to establish a therapeutic relationship with the caregiver and, if possible, the patient. Education of families and caregivers about the illness can enhance their empathy for the patient, increase their tolerance for a range of maladaptive behaviors, establish more realistic expectations, and allow them to prepare for the future. It is important to ensure that the home environment is safe (e.g., limited access to dangerous appliances or utensils) and to establish daily routines for the patient. Typically, disruption of routines leads to confusion and a deterioration in functional status. When unwanted behaviors emerge, it is worthwhile reviewing the context in which they arose to see if simple manipulations of the patient's schedule or environment can be beneficial. Medications need to be employed judiciously, clearly identifying target symptoms, using the lowest doses possible, and watching closely for side effects. Treatment of depression with medications that have low anticholinergic side effects is usually preferable. Low doses of neuroleptic medications (e.g., haloperidol), short-acting benzodiazepines (e.g., oxazepam), or sedating antidepressants (e.g., trazodone) may be necessary to treat anxiety, agitation, or behavioral outbursts. It is important to rule out intercurrent illnesses or problems if a patient demonstrates more rapid decline in status and exhibits what has been called a "beclouded dementia." Communication with the patient's internist and other physicians is crucial. We have also found that social work input is extremely helpful to caregivers for increasing services at home, finding appropriate day programs, providing supportive counseling, and reviewing long-term plans for the patient.

New medications are being developed to treat patients with probable Alzheimer's disease. Recently, tacrine (Cognex), an acetylcholinesterase inhibitor, received U.S. Food and Drug Administration approval. Some have argued that Cognex does "too little, too late, and is too toxic". The most recent data suggest that in the small percentage of patients who can tolerate very high doses (160 mg/d), there is a measurable improvement in cognitive test scores and global assessment by clinical observers. Better tolerated products are being developed. Regardless, it seems unlikely that enchancing single neurotransmitters such as acetylcholine is likely to have a major, lasting impact on the course of the illness. Promising new strategies for treatment include efforts to augment the survival and functioning of degenerating neurons (e.g., with nerve growth factor), and to slow the degenerative process by blocking the potential neurotoxicity of β-amyloid or manipulating the processing of the amyloid precursor protein. Numerous drugs are in or about to enter clinical trials, and thus we are approaching a very exciting period in this field.

PROGRESSIVE COMPORTMENTAL DEMENTIA

Patients with progressive comportmental dementia exhibit salient changes in personality and behavior, accompanied by compromised attention, motivation, judgment, insight, and other executive functions. The abulia, apathy, or withdrawal exhibited by these patients may be mistaken for depression, whereas their inappropriate, embarrassing, and impulsive behaviors may be misinterpreted as symptoms of mania. Often, the diagnosis of a dementing illness may not be entertained for years.

The impairment of executive functioning is the major source of disruption of activities of daily living. The relative preservation of memory functions helps to distinguish this pattern of dementia from that of probable Alzheimer's disease. Interpretation of mental state testing can often be very challenging. Some patients will perform normally on routine cognitive tests and especially brief mental state screening examination that emphasize orientation, memory, language, and visuospatial skills. In such cases, the clinician must rely heavily on the caregivers' observations of personality changes, inappropriate behaviors, or poor judgment. Other patients may do poorly on all formal cognitive tests including those of memory, not because of primary disruptions in memory functions but owing to markedly impaired attention, engagement, or motivation. Providing encouragement or patiently waiting for responses may allow the demonstration of preserved recall of current or personal events that helps to confirm relatively intact memory functions. Attempts to overcome diminished motivation or attention by drilling information may also be necessary. Most often, patients exhibit deficits in tasks requiring complex attention that are mediated by frontal networks. Deficits can be seen in tasks such as word list generation, the motor Go–No Go Test, the Trail Making Test, the Stroop paradigm, the Wisconsin Card Sort,

TABLE 133-2. Features of the Different Degenerative Dementia Syndromes

	Progressive Amnestic Dementia[a]	Progressive Comportmental Dementia	Primary Progressive Aphasia
History and neuropsychological profile	Salient, progressive memory deficits (that are primary) along with impairments in language, attention, and visuospatial functions	Salient changes in personality and behavior accompanied by impairments in executive functioning, complex attention, insight, and judgment; memory relatively well preserved	Progressive impairments in language functions; memory relatively well preserved
Language characteristics	Fluent, wtih features of anatomic, transcorticosensory or Wernicke's aphasia	Diminished spontaneous verbal output and initiative; concrete formulations; inappropriate statements	One-half of patients exhibit progressive nonfluent aphasia
Age of onset	Senile > presenile[b]	Presenile[b] > senile	Presenile[b] > senile
Gender	Female > male	??[c]	Male > female
Single-photon-emission computed tomography	Bilateral temporoparietal hypoperfusion	Anterior hypoperfusion	Left frontal and perisylvian hypoperfusion
Most common underlying pathology	Alzheimer's disease (plaques and tangles)	Focal atrophy (cell loss and gliosis)	Focal atrophy (cell loss and gliosis)
Other associated pathologies	Picks' disease, focal atrophy, diffuse Lewy body disease	Pick's disease, diffuse Lewy body disease, (Alzheimer's disease)	Alzheimer's disease, Pick's disease
Prominent distribution of pathology	Limbic regions and association areas	Frontal lobes and anterotemporal lobes	Left frontal and perisylvian regions

[a] Clinical diagnosis of probable Alzheimer's disease (see text).
[b] Presenile = under the age of 65.
[c] There is controversy in the literature regarding the male to female ratio associated with this syndrome.

and the Visual-Verbal Test. These tests are reviewed in Chapter 131.

This pattern of decline has received several names in the literature, including dementia of the frontal lobe type, frontal lobe degeneration of non-Alzheimer type, or progressive comportmental dementia. It is a relatively common syndrome, accounting for between 10 and 20 percent of cases of degenerative dementia. Age of onset tends to be younger than with probable Alzheimer's disease (mean age, mid-fifties) (Table 133-2.) There appears to be a higher proportion of male patients than female observed with Alzheimer's disease. SPECT scans tend to show hypoperfusion in anterior regions, as opposed to the temporoparietal pattern more typically seen in probable Alzheimer's. CT or MRI may show disproportionate frontal atrophy. Such abnormalities involving frontal lobes are consistent with the profile of neuropsychological and behavioral deficits observed in these patients.

On the pathologic plane, autopsy studies suggest that this clinical pattern is most commonly associated with marked atrophy of the frontal lobes and anterotemporal regions, which is associated histologically with the nonspecific degenerative changes of neuron loss and gliosis. A much smaller percentage (approximately 20 percent) of cases has had histologic features pathognomonic for Pick's disease, including ballooned cells and argentophilic intracytoplasmic inclusions (i.e., Pick bodies). There is controversy in the literature regarding whether the presence of Pick bodies is necessary to make the diagnosis of Pick's disease. Without requiring such criteria, the distinction between the two major pathologic entities associated with progressive comportmental dementia may become blurred. Of note, this pattern of dementia is rarely associated with the plaque and tangle pathology seen in Alzheimer's disease.

Diffuse Lewy body disease (in which there is widespread distribution of Lewy bodies in brainstem, basal forebrain, and cortex) can present with prominent behavioral changes and has recently been reported as a fairly common form of degenerative dementia. This syndrome has been associated with fluctuating cognitive impairment, transient episodes of marked confusion, and a high incidence of visual and/or auditory hallucinations and delusions. It is most often accompanied by extrapyramidal signs or heightened sensitivity to neuroleptic medication. Progressive subcortical gliosis is a rare cause of this pattern of

dementia and manifests itself with major changes in personality and behavior and a range of psychiatric symptoms. Creutzfeldt-Jakob disease has been associated with this profile of dementia, reportedly with pathology predominating in the frontal lobes. Although this chapter focuses on degenerative diseases, it is important to point out that the dementias that exhibit prominent impairments in attention and executive functioning probably have the widest differential diagnosis and constitute many of the potentially reversible conditions. These conditions include space-occupying lesions, hydrocephalus, toxic-metabolic insults (e.g., vitamin B_{12} deficiency, hypothyroidism, side effects from medications, alcohol abuse), multiple infarctions that disrupt frontal networks, infections (e.g., human immunodeficiency virus, syphilis), and depression. Most of these conditions have other associated neurologic or medical features. Also of note, the degenerative dementias that have prominent motor symptoms (e.g., Huntington's disease, Parkinson's disease, progressive supranuclear palsy) often exhibit salient alterations in behavior, personality, executive functioning, and psychiatric status.

PROGRESSIVE FOCAL NEUROPSYCHOLOGICAL DEFICITS

There is a set of degenerative diseases that present with salient progressive neuropsychological deterioration that is relatively circumscribed, at least in the first years of the illness. Such ''dementia'' patterns are orders of magnitude less common than progressive amnestic dementia (i.e., probable Alzheimer's disease), and to qualify for the diagnosis of one of these disorders, patients cannot have prominent impairments in memory. Clinical symptomatology can be interpreted as reflecting the relatively focal distribution of pathologic damage within the nervous system. This category of dementia includes progressive visuospatial dysfunction, progressive apraxia, and the entity on which the final section of this chapter focuses, primary progressive aphasia.

Initially described by Mesulam in the early 1980s, the syndrome of primary progressive aphasia has an insidious onset and progressive deterioration of language functions over many years. About one-half of the reported cases present with nonfluent aphasia, a pattern not seen in patients with a diagnosis of probable Alzheimer's disease. Language disturbance is the major source of disruption of activities of daily living. Acalculia, apraxia, and construction problems often coexist, but memory functions are relatively preserved, particularly if evaluated by nonverbal tasks or assessment of activities of daily living. Nonverbal cognitive abilities (e.g., visuospatial skills, reasoning) often can be shown to be intact, especially in patients suffering from a nonfluent aphasia syndrome, in which comprehension of task demands is adequate. Social skills, interpersonal conduct, self-comportment, judgment, and insight are well preserved. Patients often develop their own compensatory strategies for dealing with their communication deficits. In the later stages of the illness, patients may begin to demonstrate deterioration in other areas of cognition or behavior.

The average age of onset is in the early sixties and there is a higher proportion of men than seen in patients with probable Alzheimer's disease (Table 133-2.) Evidence suggests a relatively selective degeneration of the left perisylvian region that is consistent with the clinical syndrome of progressive language dysfunction. Neuroimaging with CT or MRI tends to show greater atrophy of this region than that in the right hemisphere. Functional neuroimaging, with PET or SPECT, has pointed to diminished activity in the left frontal and perisylvian regions with relative sparing of the right hemisphere.

On the neuropathologic plane, autopsies of 13 cases of patients with primary progressive aphasia have revealed that most do not have the plaque and tangle pathology of Alzheimer's disease, which was seen in only 31 percent of cases. The majority (54 percent) exhibited focal atrophy with neuronal loss, gliosis, and spongiform changes, and 15 percent had neuropathologic changes consistent with Pick's disease. The most severe pathology in this illness is often seen in the left perisylvian and frontal regions.

Although primary progressive aphasia may be the most extensively studied of the degenerative diseases presenting with progressive focal neuropsychological deficits, an analogous entity involves progressive visuospatial dysfunction. Such patients can present with disorders of the so-called dorsal visual pathway (Balint syndrome [simultagnosia, ocular apraxia, optic ataxia], spatial disorientation, dressing problems), or the ventral visual pathway (object agnosia, prosopagnosia, alexia without agraphia). Although often there are ''neighborhood signs'' (e.g., Gerstmann syndrome), memory is relatively well preserved, distinguishing these syndromes from progressive amnestic dementia. The few autopsied cases have suggested a range of pathologic entities, including Alzheimer's disease, nonspecific neuron loss and gliosis, Creutzfeldt-Jakob disease, and adult-onset glycogen storage disease. As would be predicted from the clinical profile, the pathology tends to predominate posteriorly, in the occipitotemporal or occipitoparietal regions.

CONCLUSION

In summary, the degenerative dementias are a major public health problem. Although Alzheimer's disease is clearly the most common disorder, many cases of dementia are not due to this entity. Neurologists need to distinguish between the clinical and the pathologic planes. A medical history from observant informants, a thorough elementary neurologic examination (looking for sensorimotor and extrapyramidal findings), and a detailed mental state examination (to capture the salient pattern of cognitive and behavioral impairments) are extremely helpful. Such an approach allows us to make an appropriate clinical diagnosis, from which we can derive estimates of the relative likelihood of an underlying neuropathologic disease. Good neurologic care is essential for allowing patients with degenerative dementia to maintain as much independence and dignity as possible within their communities or specialized facilities. The future is likely to bring increasing success with pharmacologic interventions aimed at slowing or reversing the degenerative process in these devastating diseases.

ACKNOWLEDGMENTS

I would like to thank Dr. Leonard Scinto for his helpful comments on this manuscript and Ms. Pat Lyall for her expert technical assistance. I have appreciated the ongoing support of Drs. Mesulam, Weintraub, and Price, who have been superb colleagues.

SUGGESTED READINGS

Cummings JL, Benson DF: Dementia: A Clinical Approach. 2nd Ed. Butterworth-Heinemann, Boston, 1992

McKhann G, Drachman D, Folstein M et al: Clinical diagnosis of Alzheimer's disease: report of the NINCDS-ADRDA work group under the auspices of Department of Health and Human Services task force on Alzheimer's disease. Neurology 34:939–44, 1984

Terry RD, Katzman R, Bick KL: Alzheimer Disease. Raven Press, New York, 1994

Weintraub S, Mesulam MM: Four neuropsychological profiles in dementia. pp. 253–82. In Boller F, Grafman J (eds): Handbook of Neuropsychology. Vol. 8. Elsevier, Amsterdam, 1993

Whitehouse PJ: Dementia. FA Davis, Philadephia, 1993

134. CONFUSIONAL STATES AND METABOLIC ENCEPHALOPATHY

MICHAEL RONTHAL

Confusion may be defined as a disorder of higher cognitive function characterized by loss of the normal coherent stream of thought or action. In attempting to elicit the history it soon becomes apparent that the patient is distractible and inattentive. These two disorders are consistently present in all confused patients. Conversely, distractibility and inattention do not always imply confusion, but are often encountered in the course of daily living. What leads to a diagnosis of confusion is the inability of the patient to interact with the examiner in an orderly, goal-directed, and coherent fashion, making it impossible to ''stay on track.'' When attention is ''low,'' distractibility is ''high.''

Inattention in these patients is a global dysfunction and does not imply a loss of directed attention to hemibody or hemispace. One cause of global inattention is dysfunction of the subcortical arousal mechanisms in the brainstem—failure in this system may result in drowsiness, progressing to coma. This syndrome, however, is not the subject of this chapter; rather, dysfunction in the supratentorial compartment is explored.

PSYCHOLOGY OF ATTENTIONAL SYSTEMS

Basic attentional mechanisms function at a subconscious level to allow for normal cognitive and motor function. The system has survival value and is present in humans and animals during consciousness. The following characteristics can be defined.

Selectivity. We are subject at all times to multiple external and internal environmental stimuli. If effective learning or action is to take place, only a limited number of these can be handled at any particular moment. Thus the predatory animal following the trail of his prey must pay selective attention to that trail at the expense of many other surrounding stimuli. The nursing mother selects stimuli originating from her newborn infant at the expense of other environmental cues.

Coherence. Coherence implies the ability to maintain selective attention over time.

Distractibility. Although selectivity and coherence allow for effective thought and action, at the same time other coincident and simultaneous stimuli need to be monitored. The animal must be capable of screening the environment and have a set of rules to determine the criteria that lead to a shift of focus. Thus, at a cocktail party, one is capable of a one-on-one conversation—the background bustle is filtered out. Yet if one's name is spoken softly, one's attention shifts automatically to the sound. The rules for distraction are complex and depend on the immediate state of the animal and upon previous learning.

Universality. The monitoring system must register as many environmental stimuli as possible.

Sensitivity. The rules that determine shift of focus depend sensitively on the state of the organism.

PATHOPHYSIOLOGY OF CONFUSION

A confused patient is distracted by trivial stimuli yet fails to react to stimuli of importance. He or she may suddenly shift attention at an inappropriate moment, yet may maintain attention after it has become inappropriate. We are not dealing with a simple rise or fall in the arousal level, but rather a more profound disruption of the normal hierarchy of rules. Action and thought lose their normal coherence, the patient responds in an inappropriate manner, and the line of thinking becomes dramatically jumbled.

PHYSICAL SIGNS

As in any syndrome of disordered function, the diagnosis is made on the basis of examination and the eliciting of physical signs: here the signs are to be found in the mental status examination. Not all patients will exhibit all the signs decribed, but at various times one or more of the following signs will be found.

All confused patients are *inattentive.* Usually a few simple tests of the attentional system will suffice to establish abnormalities. Tests of attention are discussed in Chapter 131. Repeating months or days of the week backward, counting forward in threes, and repeating seven numbers forward or five backward are good screening tests.

Loss of Coherence

Loss of coherence is established upon attempting to elicit a consecutive history. The dialogue becomes bizarre—the topic shifts abruptly or the patient may persist with a topic long since thought abandoned. Fragments of the program of action are preserved, but, although individual movements are executed correctly, the overall program is lost. This represents one kind of "ideational apraxia," as originally described by Hugo Liepmann.

Disorders of Memory

Although patients are usually amnestic for the episode of confusion when they recover, memory is sometimes distorted rather than lost during the confusional state. A *paramnesia* is an error of memory in which the answers to the questions are incorrect, but the elements of the correct answer are present. Geographic paramnesia is the most frequent. Here the patient, when asked for orientation, may state that he is in another city or town, yet may correctly identify the building or hospital. When confronted with his previous answer he may state that he is, for example, in the "branch office" in the other town.

Propagation of Error

Once the error has been made, the patient will persist in the delusion and will bring other environmental elements into apparent coherence. For example, the stand to which the apparatus for intravenous infusion is attached may be interepreted as being a lamp in his living room.

Inattention to Environmental Stimuli

In true amnestic syndromes, the patient is hyperattentive to environmental cues and relies upon them in order to function. The confused patient, in the example quoted above, will deny that he is in a hospital or doctor's office, even though the evidence is all around him.

Occupational Jargon

The patient may use language reminiscent of his work place. Occasionally he speaks in "military" or "legalistic" style. When asked to name, say, a pair of spectacles, he may describe them as "an optical instrument for the purpose of increasing visual acuity"

Isolated or Predominant Disturbance of Writing

Spoken language is usually relatively well preserved, although an occasional anomia or neologism may be seen. Conversely, writing is often disrupted, sometimes severely. Writing may degenerate to a scrawl; it frequently does not stay on the line, but moves upward, and there are often perseverations of loops. The deficit cannot be ascribed to an aphasia, but rather represents a breakdown in writing secondary to the basic attentional deficit.

Unconcern With or Denial of Illness

Confused patients may be fully aware of their illness, but show unconcern or denial, a feature shared with patients who have right hemisphere lesions but are not confused.

Unconscious Humor or Playful Behavior

Confused patients are often unconsciously funny. The apparent wit is the chance result of an incoherent stream of thought that results in the apposition of incongruous or inappropriate phrases and ideas. One patient who believed that he was at home, when confronted with the undeniable evidence of another patient in the next bed thought for an instant and stated ''I'm going to charge them rent''!

Gait Disorder

This is probably the most frequently missed sign: having established the diagnosis of ''confusion'' we rarely get the patient up to walk. The gait disorder may be nonspecific in type, but occasionally asterixis may involve the lower limb muscles, resulting in sudden loss of tone with a sudden lurch downward.

Hyperactivity

The patient may be hyperactive to the point of requiring four-point restraints. He may be described as ''wild'' or ''psychotic'' and may be admitted to a psychiatric ward in ''delirium.'' Delirium tremens is one such hyperactive form of confusional state or encephalopathy characterized by the appearance of formed hallucinations, sometimes of animals, which may elicit fear.

CAUSES OF CONFUSION

Intoxication

The most common cause of a diffuse encephalopathy or confusional state is some sort of ''brain intoxication.'' The toxin may be exogenous, that is, alcohol, street drugs, or pharmaceutical preparations, or it may be endogenous, that is, organ failure or some other dysmetabolic state. Thus failure of virtually any of the body systems is a possible cause of confusion and must be assiduously sought. Sepsis—acute, subacute, or chronic—in any anatomic organ is a likely culprit. In these patients, treatment of the underlying systemic illness or withdrawal of the exogenous toxin is the treatment of the disordered cognitive state. It should be appreciated that recovery of brain function may be delayed for some days after correction of the causative abnormality.

Patients with borderline or very mild dementia are particularly vulnerable to metabolic or toxic encephalopathy. In the presence of severe inattention and confusion it may not be possible to establish a true baseline, and it is only after recovery that the fixed or progressive deficits can be established. Some authors have referred to this vulnerable brain syndrome with confusion as ''beclouded dementia.'' At the bedside, the clue to an intoxication is the presence of asterixis, or, more rarely, multiple myoclonus.

Cerebrospinal Fluid Pleocytosis

The presence of cells in the spinal fluid is a potent cause of confusion. The cells may be red cells, white cells, bacteria or some other infecting agent, or even malignant cells. A spinal tap is mandatory in the workup of these patients, even when a metabolic abnormality is suspected.

Seizure

Patients may be confused either as part of a partial seizure, or in the postictal state. On occasion anticonvulsant drugs themselves may be the culprit, but ordinarily confusion secondary to a seizure disorder will respond to anticonvulsants. Because the seizure may not be immediately clinically apparent at the bedside, an EEG is part of the essential workup of these patients.

Head Injury

Confusion may be the presenting syndrome in the immediate post-head-injury state. It may be transient, as after a minor concussion, or it can be prolonged as part of the recovery phase of more serious injuries. Because there may be no clear history of head injury, a careful examination of the skull and scalp are essential in the evaluation of these patients.

Structural Brain Lesions

An acute or fairly rapidly progressive structural brain lesion may be the cause. In general these lesions, whether they be stroke, focal inflammatory, or some surgical pathology, are usually to be found in the right hemisphere. The elementary examination may or may not demonstrate left body signs, and an imaging procedure is sometimes the only way to demonstrate the focal pathology.

As we noted above, all confusional patients are inattentive and it has been suggested with fairly good evidence that the right hemisphere is dominant for the function of attention. The predominance of right hemisphere lesions in this subgroup of patients may therefore reflect a disturbance of the basic underlying attentional matrix. It has been argued that confusion cannot be diagnosed in patients with left hemisphere lesions because they are aphasic. With sophisticated neuropsychological testing it can usually be shown, even in the presence of aphasia, that the patient is attentive, and does not lack coherence.

Patients with lesions of the under surface of either the right or left occipital lobe may present with a hyperactive confusional state, sometimes to the degree that they may require physical restraint. In such cases it is impossible to examine the visual fields, and imaging is the only way to demonstrate the lesion. Agitation may also occur after infarction in the right middle cerebral artery territory.

WORKUP

Confusional state or *diffuse encephalopathy* is simply a label used to describe a clinical syndrome. That syndrome, as can be seen from the above discussion, has many and varied causes. The true test of the astute clinician is to find and treat the cause. The cause may be as mundane as a urinary tract infection or as obscure as an inborn error of metabolism which becomes apparent at a time of stress. The workup may therefore be long, arduous and expensive! Table 134-1 lists some common causes of confusional states and the appropriate tests. All patients will require a blood screen for organ failure, a workup for sepsis, an imaging process, an EEG, and a spinal tap for the reasons given above. A urine and blood toxic screen will be added in suspicious circumstances. Some confused patients may require

TABLE 134-1. Common Causes of Confusional States and the Appropriate Tests

Cause	Site	Test
Infection	Urinary tract	Urinalysis/culture
	Lung/bronchi	Sputum analysis, radiograph
	Meninges	Spinal tap
	Brain	Spinal tap
	Other organ	As appropriate
Meningeal irritation		Spinal tap
Toxin	Exogenous	Blood/urine toxic screen
	Endogenous	
	Renal	BUN/creatinine
	Respiratory	Blood gases
	Cardiac	Exam, radiograph, ultrasound
	Liver	Liver function tests
	Endocrine	As appropriate
	Porphyria	Urine screen
	Withdrawal	
	Alcohol	
	Barbiturate	
Electrolyte disorder		Electrolyte screen
		Calcium
		Magnesium
		pH
		Glucose
Vitamin deficiency	B_1	Red cell transketolase
	B_6	
	B_{12}	Blood level
Other system dysfunction		As appropriate
Seizure		EEG
Migraine		
Stroke		Imaging study
Miscellaneous	Occult neoplasm	Imaging study
	Blood diseases	Complete blood count
	Space-taking lesion	Imaging study
	Postoperative state	

a more extensive workup, searching for the cause which may remain occult and a challenge to diagnostic skill

CHRONIC CONFUSION

On occasion, especially after an acute right hemisphere stroke the patient becomes confused and does not recover. The basic defect of attention persists and the patient lapses into a "chronic confusional state." It might be argued that these patients are essentially demented. The essential difference between *dementia* and *chronic confusional state* is that the dementia is progressive and the chronic confusional state is static.

SUGGESTED READINGS

Amit R: Acute confusional state in childhood. Childs Nerv Syst 4:255–8, 1988
Chedru F, Geschwind N: Writing disturbances in acute confusional states: Neuropsychologia 10:343–53, 1972
Devinsky O, Bear D, Volpe BT: Confusional states following posterior cerebral artery infarction: Arch Neurol 45:160–3, 1988
Geschwind N: Disorders of attention: a frontier in neuropsychology. Philos Trans R Soc Lond [Biol] 298:173–85, 1982
Gnanamuthu C: Confusional states and seizures: when are they related? Postgrad Med 84:149–52, 154, 156–8, 1988
Lipowski ZJ: Delirium (acute confusional states). JAMA 258:1789–92, 1987
Mesulam MM, Waxman SG, Geschwind N, Sabin TD: Acute confusional states with right middle cerebral artery infarctions: J. Neurol Neurosurg Psychiatry 39:84–9, 1976
Mulalley WJ, Ronthal M, Huff K, Geschwind N: Chronic confusional state. NJ Med 86:541–4, 1989
Pousada L, Leipzig RM: Rapid bedside assessment of postoperative confusion in older patients: Geriatrics 45:59–64, 66, 1990
Schmidley JW, Messing RO: Agitated confusional states in patients with right hemisphere infarctions: Stroke 15:883–5, 1984

135. SPEECH AND LANGUAGE DISORDERS

HOWARD S. KIRSHNER

Speech and language disorders have long attracted interest because human communication is the function that sets us apart most clearly from the animals. These disorders provide a window on the mind-body connection and link neurology to cognitive psychology, linguistics, and philosophy. Speech and language disorders, however, also have practical usefulness. They are among the most common of serious neurologic maladies. About 20 percent of strokes produce language disturbance, and a greater number affect speech articulation. Language deficits are common in patients with traumatic brain injuries, brain tumors, dementias, neurodegenerative diseases, and infections of the nervous system such as acquired immunodeficiency syndrome (AIDS). Disorders of communication frustrate patients and families and challenge the abilities of physicians.

In recent years, knowledge about language and the brain has expanded greatly. New developments include brain imaging modalities such as computed-tomography (CT) and positron emission tomography (PET) scanning and magnetic resonance imaging (MRI); electrical stimulation mapping of the language cortex for epilepsy surgery; and sophisticated linguistic models of the cognitive operations involved in language function.

MOTOR SPEECH DISORDERS

Motor speech disorders are abnormalities of the motor production of speech, or articulation, in the absence of abnormal language. Patients with motor speech disorders can comprehend both spoken and written language, and their speech output, if comprehensible at all, can be transcribed into normal language. These disorders include. (1) dysarthrias, disorders of speech articulation; (2) dysphonias, abnormalities of voice; (3) apraxia of speech; and (4) stuttering.

Dysarthrias

Dysarthrias involve abnormal articulation of sounds or phonemes, especially distortions of consonant sounds, errors in the place of articulation, voicing, or opening of the velum. For example, production of a "p" sound and a "b" sound differ only in the initial voicing of the "p"; a dysarthric patient might consistently substitute "b" for "p." Dysarthrias can be caused by mechanical difficulty in the larynx or vocal cords or by neurologic diseases. Neurogenic dysarthrias are classified into six categories: (1) flaccid (2) spastic, (3) ataxic, (4) hypokinetic, (5) hyperkinetic, and (6) mixed.

Flaccid dysarthria is associated with lower motor neuron disorders affecting the bulbar muscles, neuromuscular junction, cranial nerves, or brainstem anterior horn cells. Examples include polymyositis, myasthenia gravis, and bulbar poliomyelitis. Flaccid dysarthria is characterized by breathy, nasal speech, with consonant errors. *Spastic* dysarthria is seen in patients with bilateral lesions of the motor cortex or corticobulbar tracts, such as bilateral strokes. The speech has a harsh, "strain-strangle" quality, with slow rate, low pitch, and imprecise consonants. *Ataxic* dysarthria or "scanning speech," associated with cerebellar disorders, involves irregular or slow rhythm of speech, with pauses and abrupt explosions of sound and abnormal or excessively equal stress on specific syllables. *Hypokinetic* dysarthria, seen in Parkinson's disease, is associated with decreased and monotonous loudness and pitch, increased rate with occasional pauses, and some consonant errors. *Hyperkinetic* dysarthria, seen in Huntington's disease, is characterized by excessive variation in rate, loudness and timing, with distorted vowels. In dystonia, hyperkinetic dysarthria can also include harsh, strain-strangle speech with imprecise consonants. The final category, *mixed* dysarthria, involves combinations of the other types. Common examples include multiple sclerosis, which often combines spastic and ataxic characteristics, and amyotrophic lateral sclerosis, which links spastic and flaccid elements. With practice, a clinician can use speech patterns to confirm suspected neuroanatomic diagnoses.

Dysphonias

Dysphonias, or disorders of voicing, are part of dysarthria. Hoarseness can result from laryngitis or a paralyzed vocal cord. Neurogenic dysphonias include the breathy voice of myasthenia gravis and the whispered voice of Parkinson's disease.

Apraxia of Speech

Apraxia of speech is an inability to program sequences of phonemes, especially consonants. Consonants are substituted rather than distorted, as in dysarthria. The misarticulations increase with polysyllabic words that require multiple consonant shifts. Difficulty with initial consonants makes the speech hesitant and groping. Errors are inconsistent from one attempt to the next, in contrast to the more regular distortion of phonemes seen in dysarthria; for example, a patient attempting to repeat the word "artillery" five times might produce five different utterances.

Apraxia of speech is rare in isolated form, but it frequently contributes to the aphasic deficit of Broca's aphasia. Speech apraxia as part of an aphasia is defined by the inconsistent articulatory errors in the presence of preserved comprehension, and by the ability of the patient to write better than speak.

Stuttering

Stuttering is a frequently hereditary disorder characterized by initial pauses and dysfluency of speech production, without other articulatory or language disorders. Stuttering is usually a childhood, developmental disorder, but a close imitation can occur in acquired brain lesions, usually involving the left hemisphere.

APHASIAS

Language disorders, or aphasias, are defined as abnormalities of symbolic communication, or language, acquired as a result of brain disease. This definition distinguishes aphasias from motor speech disorders, from congenital or developmental language disorders (often called "dysphasias"), and from psychi-

TABLE 135-1. Bedside Language Examination

Speech expression
  Spontaneous speech
  Automatic sequences
Naming
Auditory comprehension
Repetition
Reading
  Aloud
  Comprehension
Writing
  Spontaneous
  Dictation
  Copying

atric thought disorders. Psychotic patients express bizarre, illogical language content in well-articulated, syntactically correct sentences; the abnormality lies in thought, not in its expression in language.

Aphasia is diagnosed by a six-part bedside language evaluation (Table 135-1), used in conjunction with a neurologic history and examination. The first test item, spontaneous speech, can be ascertained during the clinical interview. Automatic sequences, such as the days of the week, are helpful in provoking speech output. The most important variable is fluency, the free-flowing quality of the utterances. The presence of articulatory errors or dysarthria should be noted, along with circumlocutions, word-finding pauses, and paraphasic errors. These errors can be of the literal or phonemic type, involving substitution of an incorrect sound ("ben" for "pen"); or of the verbal or semantic type, involving substitution of an incorrect word ("spoon" for "fork"). "Jargon speech" is so replete with paraphasic errors that the meaning cannot be interpreted. Naming is evaluated with objects, body parts, colors, and parts of objects. Auditory comprehension is tested by asking the patient to follow spoken commands of one, two, and three steps. Care must be taken to exclude hearing loss, motor paralysis, or apraxia as the cause of a failure to follow commands; if doubt exists, comprehension can be tested by yes/no questions or by commands that require only a pointing response. Repetition is tested with polysyllabic words and phrases such as "Methodist Episcopal," which are sensitive to dysarthria, and with sentences, especially grammatically complex, unfamiliar phrases such as "no ifs, ands, or buts," which are sensitive to aphasia. If apraxia of speech is suspected, the patient is asked to repeat "artillery" five times. Reading is tested by asking the patient to follow printed commands or to read paragraphs for meaning. Writing, the final element, is tested by spontaneous generation of sentences, writing to dictation, or copying.

Muteness, or absence of speech, can be difficult to interpret. A mute patient may be aphasic, but may suffer instead from severe dysarthria, a frontal lobe syndrome such as abulia or akinetic mutism, a basal ganglia disorder such as parkinsonism, a psychiatric disorder such as catatonia, or a mechanical disorder of the larynx. In general, a mute aphasic cannot write or comprehend language normally.

The physician uses the bedside language examination, together with the neurologic examination, to localize diseases in the nervous system. The history provides clues as to the etiology of the disorder. For example, the sudden onset of fluent aphasia heralds an embolic stroke, whereas a slowly developing anomia may indicate an early dementia or a left hemisphere brain tumor. More detailed examination of language function can be obtained by consultation with a speech/language pathologist or neuropsychologist. Standard language testing batteries such as the Boston Diagnostic Aphasia Examination or the Western Aphasia Battery are helpful in quantitating a language deficit, in supporting a syndrome classification, and in following progress during rehabilitation. Finally, neurodiagnostic and brain imaging studies confirm the medical diagnosis. CT scanning and MRI detect brain lesions such as strokes or brain tumors. PET and single photon emission computed tomography (SPECT) show the metabolic activity or blood flow of brain regions; activation of these regions can be be studied during language tasks.

Handedness and Cerebral Dominance

Approximately 99 percent of right-handed patients and most left-handed patients have relative left-hemisphere dominance for language. Both autopsy studies and measurements based on CT scans and MRI have shown anatomic brain asymmetries, especially a larger superior temporal plane in the left cerebral hemisphere. Left-hemisphere language dominance appears to be genetically programmed, since temporal lobe asymmetries are found even in newborns and in illiterate people. Further knowledge of language dominance is emerging from testing of epilepsy patients in preparation for surgical resection; the areas important for language are determined by the Wada test, in which sodium pentobarbital is injected into the internal carotid artery, or by intraoperative stimulation mapping of the language cortex.

Occasionally, aphasia develops in right-handed patients with right-hemisphere lesions (''crossed aphasia''). Aphasia in left-handers may be seen with lesions of either hemisphere, but most commonly the left. Recent studies have shown less difference in initial language profiles or ultimate recovery between right- and left-handers than previously thought. Atypical syndromes are occasionally seen in left-handers, such as preserved comprehension in a patient with a large left-hemisphere lesion, suggesting right-hemisphere comprehension ability.

Classification and Diagnosis

Aphasias have been classified into eight traditional syndromes: Broca's, Wernicke's, global, conduction, anomic, and three transcortical aphasias. In addition, two single-modality deficits, aphemia and pure word deafness, and syndromes of alexia and agraphia deserve attention. Finally, a category of subcortical aphasia has been added from brain imaging studies.

Broca's Aphasia. Broca's aphasia is characterized by nonfluent speech, varying from mutism to hesitant, struggling efforts to speak (Table 135-2). The patient utters the meaningful items of a sentence, omitting pronouns, prepositions, and arti-

cles, a phenomenon referred to as ''telegraphic speech'' or ''agrammatism.'' Patients hesitate on names, but can often indicate some knowledge of the word (''tip-of-the-tongue'' phenomenon). Repetition is effortful and slow. Auditory comprehension is adequate for simple conversations and commands but breaks down on complex grammatical constructions, which are also difficult for the patient in expressive speech. Reading is often more affected than auditory comprehension. Writing is impaired, even with the nonparalyzed left hand. Patients with Broca's aphasia are aware of their deficits, often becoming frustrated and depressed. The lesions of Broca's aphasia involve the left frontal lobe, classically the posterior portion of the inferior frontal gyrus, anterior to the motor face area. Small lesions of Broca's area permit nearly compete recovery, whereas larger left frontoparietal lesions produce an early global aphasia, which evolves gradually into Broca's aphasia. Associated damage in the subcortical and periventricular white matter may be necessary to produce lasting loss of expressive speech.

Aphemia is a transitory syndrome of muteness or nonfluent speech, with preserved writing and comprehension. Some authorities equate aphemia with isolated apraxia of speech. Lesions involve the face area of the motor strip, sometimes with extension into the inferior frontal gyrus and underlying white matter.

Wernicke's Aphasia. In contrast to the nonfluent speech of Broca's aphasia, patients with Wernicke's aphasia speak fluently, but with empty phrases, circumlocutions, and paraphasic errors of both literal and verbal type (Table 135-2). Naming may provoke bizarre, paraphasic substitutions. Auditory comprehension is severely impaired. Reading is affected much like auditory comprehension, but some patients show sparing of one or the other modality. Writing is well formed but contains spelling and word choice errors; in mild cases, writing may serve as a sensitive clue. Patients with Wernicke's aphasia are usually not depressed, but they may be unaware of their deficits and may become angry when not understood. Motor and sensory findings are usually absent in patients with Wernicke's aphasia, though some have right hemianopia. The lesion typically involves the classical Wernicke's area in the posterior left superior temporal gyrus. Destruction of most of Wernicke's area appears necessary for lasting loss of comprehension, but there is often associated damage in the supramarginal and angular gyri.

Pure word deafness is a rare syndrome of inability to understand or repeat spoken language, in the absence of expressive language difficulty or deafness for nonverbal sounds. Classically, pure word deafness results from bilateral temporal lesions that disconnect Wernicke's area from both auditory cortical

TABLE 135-2. Language Features of the Eight Classical Aphasias

Syndrome	Speech	Naming	Comprehension	Repetition	Reading	Writing
Broca	Nonfluent	Anomic	Mild	Hesitant	Mild	Poor
Wernicke	Fluent	Paraphasic	Poor	Paraphasic	Impaired	Poor spelling
Global	Nonfluent	Anomic	Poor	Poor	Poor	Poor
Conduction	Fluent	±Impaired	Normal	Poor	±Impaired	±Impaired
Anomic	Fluent	Anomic	Normal	Normal	Normal	Normal
TCMA	Nonfluent	±Impaired	Normal	Normal	±Impaired	±Impaired
TCSA	Fluent	Paraphasic	Poor	Normal	Poor	Poor spelling
MTCA	Nonfluent	Poor	Poor	Normal	Poor	Poor

Abbreviations: TCMA, transcortical motor aphasia; TCSA, transcortical sensory aphasia; MTCA, mixed transcortical aphasia.

areas. The syndrome also occurs with unilateral left temporal lesions.

Global Aphasia.   Global aphasia may be thought of as the sum of Broca's and Wernicke's aphasia, a loss of all six major language functions (Table 135-2). Spontaneous speech is non-fluent or mute, and the patient cannot name, repeat, understand, read, or write. Most patients have extensive left-hemisphere damage and profound neurologic deficits of right hemiplegia, right hemisensory loss, and right hemianopsia. When less severe deficits involve all language functions, the syndrome is called "mixed aphasia."

Conduction Aphasia.   Conduction aphasia is an unusual syndrome in which repetition is affected out of proportion to other language modalities (Table 135-2). Speech is fluent but may be interrupted by pauses to correct literal paraphasic errors. Auditory comprehension is intact. Conduction aphasia was traditionally explained as a disconnection between Wernicke's and Broca's areas. Others have explained the repetition difficulty as a deficit of auditory verbal short-term memory. Lesions involve either the left temporal lobe, without destruction of Wernicke's area, or the inferior parietal lobule.

Anomic Aphasia.   Anomic aphasia is a selective deficit of naming. Speech is fluent, except for word-finding pauses and circumlocutions, and the other language modalities are intact. This syndrome is less localizing than other types of aphasia. Anomic aphasia is seen with focal lesions of the left temporal or inferior parietal region but is also common in encephalopathies, aging, and dementia.

Transcortical Aphasias.   The transcortical aphasias have in common the preservation of repetition. The word "transcortical" refers to disruption of centers that project onto the perisylvian language cortex, rather than of the language cortex itself. Transcortical motor aphasia (TCMA) resembles Broca's aphasia, in that there is marked dysfluency or difficulty initiating speech, but the patient with TCMA repeats normally. The lesions of TCMA spare Broca's area but involve the adjacent left frontal cortex or subcortical white matter. Transcortical sensory aphasia (TCSA) resembles Wernicke's aphasia except for the sparing of repetition. The lesions involve the posterior left temporo-occipital region. This syndrome also occurs in Alzheimer's disease. Mixed transcortical aphasia (MTCA), also called the "syndrome of the isolation of the speech area," resembles global aphasia except that repetition is not only spared but may be excessive or palilalic. Some patients mimic and learn new song lyrics or complete poems if given the first lines. Reported cases have had large, watershed infarctions sparing the perisylvian language area, or advanced dementing illnesses.

Subcortical Aphasias.   Unlike the other aphasia syndromes, subcortical aphasias are diagnosed by the location of the brain lesion rather than by language features. In recent years, aphasia syndromes have increasingly been associated with subcortical lesion sites. First, lesions of the left thalamus produce fluent aphasia, usually with better comprehension and repetition as compared to Wernicke's aphasia. Patients may fluctuate between periods of drowsiness, with severe aphasia, and periods of alertness, with improved language function. Second, lesions of the left putamen, anterior limb of internal capsule, and caudate nucleus produce syndromes of dysarthria and nonfluent

TABLE 135-3. Language Features of the Classical Alexias

Feature	Alexia With Agraphia	Pure Alexia Without Agraphia
Speech	Fluent, often paraphasic	Normal
Naming	± Impaired	Color anomia
Repetition	Normal	Normal
Comprehension	Intact, or mildly impaired	Intact
Reading	Severely impaired	Impaired, ± sparing of letters
Writing	Severely impaired	Normal
Associated signs	Right hemianopsia	Right hemianopsia
Localization	Left angular gyrus	Left occipital lobe, splenium

speech, with less abnormality of phrase length and repetition as compared to Broca's aphasia. Lesions extending into the deep temporal white matter or "temporal isthmus" may impair comprehension, producing subcortical equivalents of Wernicke's and global aphasia.

Alexias.   Alexia with agraphia is an acquired illiteracy, with intact spoken language modalities except for anomia and mild fluent, paraphasic speech (Table 135-3). The syndrome is associated with focal lesions of the left angular gyrus. Associated deficits include the "Gerstmann syndrome" of agraphia, inability to calculate, right-left confusion, and "finger agnosia", an inability to name or point to specific fingers on the patient's or examiner's hand.

Pure alexia without agraphia (Table 135-3) is an isolated inability to read. The lesions involve the left posterior cerebral artery territory, including the left medial occipital and medial temporal lobes and the splenium of the corpus callosum. Some patients have difficulty naming colors. Most have at least a partial right hemianopia. Another frequent association is with short-term memory loss, explained by damage to the hippocampus and adjacent medial temporal structures. Pure alexia has been explained as a disconnection between the intact right occipital visual cortex and the left hemisphere centers for decoding of visual language symbols.

Alexia is also seen as part of the language deficit of aphasia. The alexia of Broca's aphasia is called the "third alexia." Neurolinguists have described four separate patterns of alexia: "deep," "phonological," "surface," and "letter-by-letter" alexia. Letter-by-letter alexia is identical to the syndrome of pure alexia without agraphia. Both deep and phonological alexia involve the visual recognition of whole, familiar words, without ability to decode graphemes into phonemes; surface dyslexia involves the opposite ability to convert graphemes laboriously into phonemes, without any recognition of words or phrases at a glance. Similarly, agraphias can be divided into pure agraphias, which are rare, and agraphia associated with aphasia.

Language in Dementias.   Aphasia is usually the result of focal, destructive lesions of the brain, but language disturbances also occur in acute encephalopathies and dementias. In dementia of the Alzheimer type, language deteriorates along a generally predictable gradient: naming of people and objects is deficient early in the course, along with simplification of discourse and language content; reading, writing, and auditory comprehension deteriorate during the middle stages; in the terminal phase, articulation and expressive speech begin to fail. A less common pattern, called "primary progressive aphasia," often begins with loss of fluency in patients who may not develop a generalized dementia for several years. This syndrome is seen in patients with Pick's disease, a few other atypical dementing diseases, and occasionally Alzheimer's disease.

Language and the Right Hemisphere

The right hemisphere, although dominant for language in only a small minority, plays an important role in communication. The elements of communication most affected by right hemisphere disease are "prosody," or cadence and intonation of speech, and "pragmatics," or practical, extralinguistic messages that normal speakers convey. Patients with right-hemisphere disease sound flat in their intonation, and they may fail to comprehend emotional nuances, irony, sarcasm, and humor in the speech of others. They understand what is said, but not how it is said. The communication deficit of right-hemisphere lesions, although it does not meet the definition of aphasia, is socially disabling to patients, hindering readjustment to family and work environments.

Recovery and Therapy

Patients with aphasia from acute brain injury or stroke improve spontaneously for several months. The aphasia type often changes during recovery; global aphasia evolves into Broca's aphasia, and Wernicke's aphasia may recover toward the profile of conduction or anomic aphasia. Early recovery of language function may involve resolution of edema or reactivation of partially damaged tissue in the language cortex, but later recovery likely requires the reorganization of new cortical areas for language function, either in adjacent left-hemisphere or analogous right-hemisphere regions. In general, such recovery is much more complete in children than in adults.

Speech therapy, carried out by trained speech/language pathologists, aims to facilitate language recovery by a variety of methods. In traditional therapy, repeated practice is carried out to improve performance in the major communication modalities of speech, auditory comprehension, reading, and writing. The therapist focuses on specific language operations that are deficient, working first in an artificial language task, and then applying these functions to communication in the real world. A number of new speech therapy techniques have been developed. Melodic intonation therapy entrains musical intonation into speech, theoretically involving the right hemisphere in speech production. Visual action therapy employs simple gestures to convey meaning. Computer techniques originally developed for primate communication have enabled even severely aphasic patients to combine pictures of nouns and verbs, creating simple sentences that can be printed or transmitted to a voice synthesizer. Other "augmentative speech devices" permit simple, stereotyped language expression. Finally, pharmacologic agents are beginning to be used in language rehabilitation. Bromocriptine, a dopamine agonist used in Parkinson's disease, increases speech production in some patients with transcortical motor aphasia. Although the medical profession often considers speech therapy as an unproved treatment, large, randomized trials have clearly established that speech therapy is effective in promoting better communication in aphasic patients.

SUGGESTED READINGS

Alexander MP, Benson DF: The aphasias and related disturbances. pp. 1–58. In: Joynt RJ (ed): Clinical Neurology. Vol. 1. JB Lippincott, Philadelphia, 1993

Alexander MP, Naeser MA, Palumbo CL: Correlation of subcortical CT lesion sites and aphasia profiles. Brain 110:961–91, 1987
Kirshner HS: Handbook of Neurological Speech and Language Disorders. pp. 1–532. Marcel-Dekker, New York, 1995
Kirshner HS: Behavioral Neurology: A Practical Approach. Churchill Livingstone, 1986:1–230.
Kirshner HS, Casey PF, Henson J, Heinrich JJ: Behavioral features and lesion localization in Wernicke's aphasia. Aphasiology 3:169–76, 1989
Ojemann GA: Cortical organization of language. J Neuroscience 11:2281–87, 1991
Posner MI, Petersen SE, Fox PT, Raichle ME: Localization of cognitive operations in the human brain. Science 240:1627–31, 1988
Sarno MT: Acquired Aphasia. 2nd ed. Academic Press, San Diego, CA, 1991
Weintraub S, Rubin NP, Mesulam M: Primary progressive aphasia: longitudinal course, neuropsychological profiles, and language features. Arch Neurol 47:1329–35, 1990
Wertz RT, Weiss DG, Aten LJ et al: Comparison of clinic, home and deferred language treatment for aphasia: a VA cooperative study. Arch Neurol 43:653–8, 1986

136. HIGHER-ORDER VISUAL IMPAIRMENT

MICHAEL P. ALEXANDER

Higher-order visual impairments are those that cannot be accounted for by deficits in visual acuity, visual fields, or gaze mechanisms. Most higher-order visual impairments are due to lesions in visual association cortex (Brodmann's areas 18 and 19) or to the outflow from those regions to multimodal association cortex in temporal lobe (particularly area 37) and hippocampus or in parietal lobes (particularly areas 7, 39, and 40). The clinical approach to these impairments is facilitated by the fact that the higher-order deficits are readily divided along three separate dimensions. First, deficits in processing visual stimuli for language content or associations are due to lesions of the left hemisphere. Deficits in processing visual material for spatial content, for some perceptual properties, and for some aspects of emotional content are usually due to right-hemisphere lesions. Second, deficits in visual processing for discrimination and identification are due to lesions in inferior (temporo-occipital cortex) visual association cortex. Deficits in visual processing for attentional, spatial, and kinesthetic properties of the stimulus are due to lesions in superior (parieto-occipital) visual association cortex (Table 136-1). Third, deficits in the spatial manipu-

TABLE 136-1. Classification of Higher-Order Visual Impairments According to Whether the Lesion Is in the Superior or Inferior Visual Association Cortex

Inferior (temporo-occipital cortex) visual system disorders	
Pure alexia	Left occipitotemporal
Object agnosia	Bilateral inferior occipitotemporal Large left inferomedial occipitotemporal
Prosopagnosia	Bilateral inferior occipitotemporal Large right inferomedial occipitotemporal
Superior (parieto-occipital cortex) visual system disorders	
Neglect	Contralateral parieto-occipital (left neglect more severe)
Visually guided movements	Contralateral parieto-occipital
Balint syndrome	Bilateral parieto-occipital
Primary dressing disorder ("dressing apraxia")	Right superior parieto-occipital
Ideational apraxia	Left parietal
Visuoconstructive disorders	Either left or right parietal

lation of visual stimuli are usually associated with parietal lesions, but the error patterns of right and left brain lesions may differ substantially. These three dichotomous patterns operate simultaneously.

This chapter reviews the common higher-order deficits, attempting to place them in relation to the three dimensions just outlined. For each disorder, clinical assessment methods, treatment strategies (if any), and natural history are discussed.

SYNDROMES OF IMPAIRED IDENTIFICATION OF COMPLEX VISUAL STIMULI

Disorders of deficient identification are produced by lesions in the inferior visual association cortex.

Pure Alexia

Pure alexia is characterized by an inability to read despite preservation of adequate acuity, fields, and attention and despite no other impairment in spoken language or in writing (thus, ''pure'' alexia and alexia without agraphia). Pure alexia is caused by lesions in the language-dominant (usually left) hemisphere's occipitotemporal lobes (Table 136-2). It is not specific to any etiology, described after infarcts, hemorrhages, tumors abscesses, and even focal degenerative disorders. Most cases in clinical practice will be due to left posterior cerebral artery territory infarctions. Few cases are totally ''pure.'' Right hemianopia is common—damage to geniculocalcarine pathways or to calcarine cortex. Anomic aphasia is also common, although usually mild—damage to inferior temporal gyrus. A particularly severe color-naming deficit may be observed. The general naming deficit may be much more severe with visual presentation of objects than with either tactile presentation or spontaneous speech, so-called optic aphasia or visual anomia. Large lesions may produce object agnosia (see below). Lesions that involve the hippocampus, parahippocampal gyrus, or the deep medial temporal white matter will cause significant memory problems. The alexia is independent of any of these associated deficits. Patients are quite aware of their reading impairment but may be less aware of the associated deficits.

Alexia testing is straightforward. Present stimuli in an uncrowded field to eliminate attentional, perceptual, and scanning problems. Begin with single letters and move to single words and then short, connected text. Ask the patient to read targets aloud. If unsuccessful, present an array of four to six written stimuli (letters or words) and ask the patient to point to them as you name them. All patients with suspected pure alexia must be tested for other language deficits, especially writing, and for visual recognition, or at least naming to visual presentation, of other stimuli—colors, common objects, etc., The same approach can be followed: (1) naming colors or objects to visual presentation and then pointing to a specified color or object in

TABLE 136-2. Pure Alexia

Examination
  Oral reading
    Single letters
    Words
    Connected text
    Words
  Forced choice comprehension
Commonly associated signs
  Right visual field defect
  Color anomia
  Verbal memory deficits

an array of four to six; (2) if impaired at the latter, naming objects that are palpated or described.

The most common lesion anatomy of pure alexia is a large medial occipitotemporal lesion producing right hemianopia and damaging the posterior callosal projections preventing processed visual information from passing from the right inferior association cortex to the left, at least via the most efficient pathways, thus impairing extraction of language information. White matter lesions subjacent to that area can also cause alexia by disrupting the input of left and right visual association cortex into a critical cortical node for visual-language processing. Lesions in the left inferior occipitotemporal junction (areas 37 and 19) can also produce alexia, identifying that area as the critical site for visual-language associations.

Patients with severe pure alexia cannot read or recognize single letters, although they may still recognize iconic written stimuli, such as advertising signs, traffic signs, menu items, or their own names. When forced to choose among written words, they can show considerable capacity to recognize words, but they are not aware of that capacity. Improvement follows a typical course. Letter recognition improves, and as it does, patients begin to read letter-by-letter, assembling words by slowly reading off the letters. This becomes faster, and they seem to recognize short words in their entirety. With more improvement, the letter-by-letter strategy will not be evident to an observer except on very long and unfamiliar words. At this point, the patient is no longer truly alexic, but reading is such an effort that it is rarely pursued. Furthermore, any impairment in verbal memory from medial temporal damage will make it virtually impossible for the patient to recall what he so effortfully reads.

Treatments are unproven. Most treatments have been attempted on only single patients and are of unknown general efficacy. If the patient cannot read single letters, there may be no reasonable treatment. Letter-by-letter reading will improve with simple practice. Patients should probably use visually uncrowded text with well-marked margins. The content of the therapy material should be familiar to the patient so that he does not have to struggle additionally for meaning beyond the individual words. Rapid, forced choice word selection tasks may help the patient improve word recognition without resorting to the laborious letter-by-letter strategy. Recall that therapy should be tempered if the patient also has verbal memory deficits.

Object Agnosia

Object agnosia is characterized by an inability to recognize common objects despite adequate acuity, and so on. There are two prototypical forms of visual agnosia. In apperceptive agnosia, patients are able to recognize colors and movement. The patients complain of impaired vision, not impaired recognition. Their corrected acuity is reduced, and visual fields are very hard to establish but are usually full to perimetry techniques. The usual etiology of apperceptive agnosia is anoxia or carbon monoxide poisoning, and the lesion anatomy has, therefore, been laminar necrosis of the striate cortex. The agnosia is not specifically a deficit in recognition of well-perceived stimuli. It is a form of elemental perceptual impairment that precludes recognition.

Patients with associative visual agnosia much more accurately meet the defining criteria. The patients complain of impaired recognition, not impaired vision. The usual etiology is

TABLE 136-3. Associative Visual Agnosia

Examination
  Objects
    Naming
    Identification by description
    Categorization
    Matching to name
Commonly associated signs
  Bilateral lesion
    Superior attitudinal visual field defect
    Prosopagnosia
    Achromatopsia
    Amnesia
  Left lesion
    Right visual field defect
    Alexia
    Anomic aphasia
    Semantic memory deficits
    Verbal memory deficits

infarction, but traumatic contusions, tumors, and focal degenerative disorders have been described. The usual lesion anatomy is bilateral lesions in inferior temporo-occipital association cortex, but large left temporo-occipital lesions may also produce associative agnosia (Table 136-3).

Depending upon the lesion configuration, associated signs are somewhat variable. Patients with bilateral lesions usually have superior altitudinal visual field deficits. Disturbed color vision (achromatopsia) and impaired facial recognition (prosopagnosia) are common (see below). If lesions extend into the medial temporal structures, including hippocampus, there may be significant memory impairments. Alexia and anomic aphasia may be present, depending on the extent of the left-sided lesion.

Patients with large unilateral left lesions present a clinical problem of distinguishing agnosia from several boundary syndromes (Fig. 136-1). Very large left occipitotemporal lesions

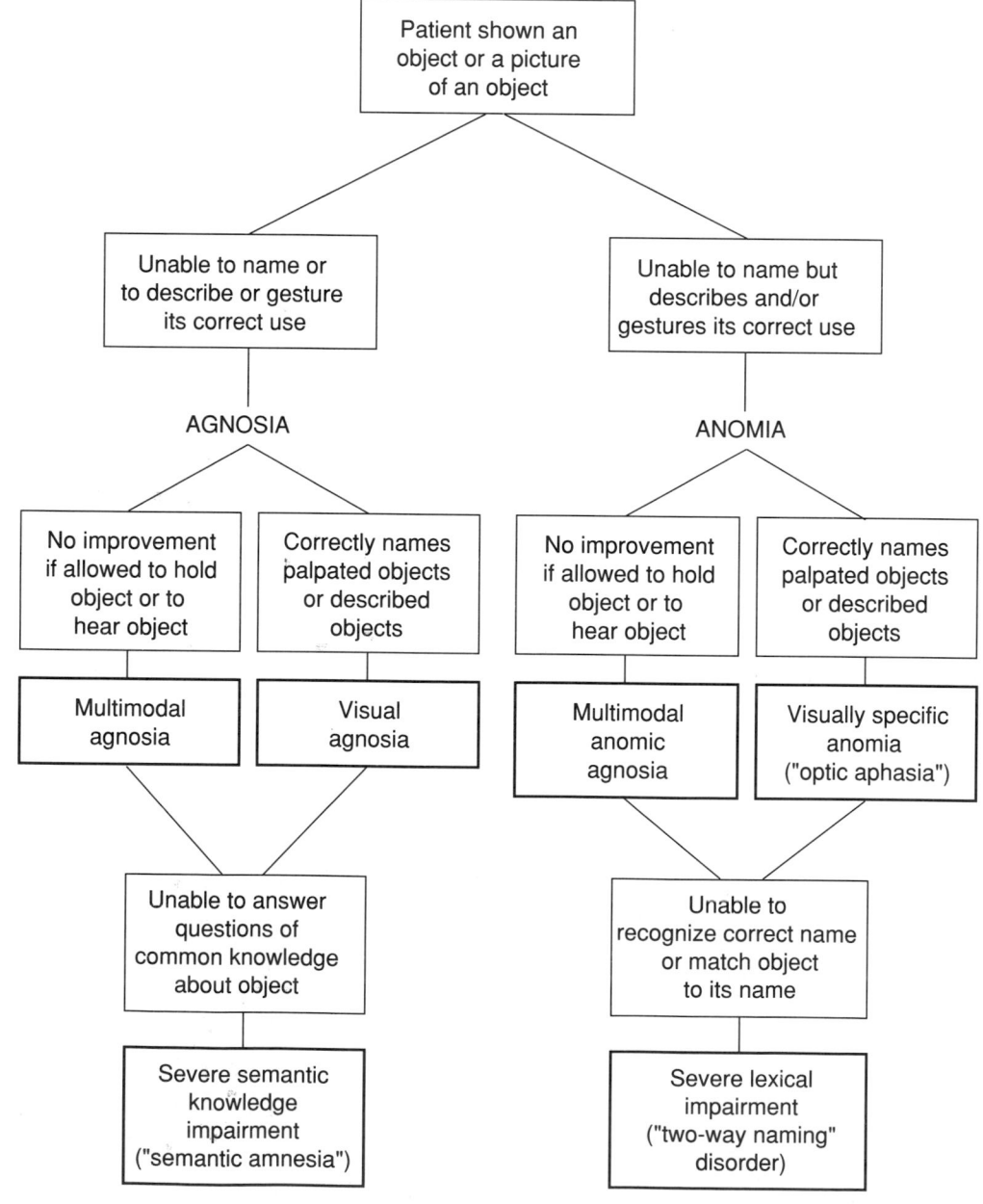

FIG. 136-1.   Flowchart showing the method by which agnosia may be distinguished from boundary syndromes that may resemble it.

produce alexia and anomic aphasia, and, as described above, may produce optic aphasia, in which patients recognize objects, are able to describe their use, usually recognize their names and can name them from a description, but are unable to *name* them from vision alone. Patients with object agnosia should be unable to identify an object presented visually and thus be unable to describe its use or match it to its name. It is uncertain if there is an unambiguous boundary between these syndromes. Many allegedly agnosic patients have actually been able to select a named object from an array, suggesting that the problem is not only visual recognition but also name retrieval.

Another boundary condition for associative agnosia is semantic amnesia or multimodal agnosia. Associative visual agnosia should be marked by preserved recognition and knowledge of objects in any format except visual. Thus, they could define a described object, describe a named object, provide information about the object's use, construction and common location, and name an object placed in their hands. Many patients with large left lesions, usually large posterior cerebral artery infarctions, are, however, unable to recognize an object through any sensory route (thus, multimodal agnosia) or to provide any associated commonly known information about the object (semantic amnesia). While relatively rare, this loss of semantic knowledge has been described after herpes encephalitis or posterior cerebral artery territory infarctions. Loss of semantic memory is a hallmark of Alzheimer's disease and Pick's disease. There is no suggestion that knowledge of objects (or faces, letters, etc.) are housed in particular cells. It is believed that the occipitotemporoparietal association cortices house the mechanisms critical to activate knowledge.

Agnosia testing is designed to define the level of recognition impairment and its modality-specificity (Table 136-3). The patient is shown simple objects or pictures of objects (visually more challenging) and asked to name them. If he cannot, he may be simply anomic, so he is asked to describe the object's function. If he can, he is anomic, but he should be asked to name it from description and palpation. This resolves whether he has a general anomia or visual anomia or both. If he cannot provide any associated information about an object, but can name it with tactile input, he should be asked to point to the named object in an array. If he can, he presumably has simply a very severe lexical-semantic deficit. If he cannot, he should be asked to sort objects or pictures into natural categories. If he cannot, he has definite agnosia, but categorization through other modalities should be probed—"Is a hammer a carpentry tool?", "Is a camel a type of fish?" If impaired, he has multimodal agnosia and general semantic knowledge loss.

Cases of visual agnosia and all of its boundary conditions have produced enormous information about how the brain organizes knowledge, in part by the sensory modality through which it is experienced and in part by the abstract (and verbal) categories. There are critical cortical regions for modality-specific and modality independent associational networks.

Treatments of visual agnosia, multimodal agnosia, and semantic memory loss have not been reported. Many patients improve. Patients with bilateral inferior occipitotemporal lesions may be left with recognition deficits in areas that are particularly demanding perceptually: distinguishing faces (see below), recognizing photographs, line drawings or video clips. Patients with large left unilateral lesions may have remaining more clear-cut visual-language deficits (alexia and optic apha-

sia) and general language deficits (anomic aphasia), and less perceptual recognition impairment.

Prosopagnosia

Prosopagnosia is defined by an inability to recognize familiar faces despite preservation of adequate acuity. Prosopagnosia is usually caused by bilateral lesions in inferior temporo-occipital cortex, and patients will have superior altitudinal visual field deficits (Table 136-4). Achromatopsia is also commonly seen. Depending upon lesion extent in medial temporal regions there may be considerable memory impairment. Some patients have only large right temporo-occipital lesions. They usually have left hemianopia and impaired topographical memory. With either lesion configuration impairments in other perceptually demanding visual discriminations have been reported, most notably a farmer unable to distinguish between the cows in his dairy herd. Note that by the discussion above, prosopagnosia can be considered a modality-specific loss of knowledge. It has been demonstrated in normal subjects that the right hemisphere is faster and more reliable at recognizing familiar faces than the left. That lasting prosopagnosia after unilateral right lesions occurs less frequently than after bilateral injuries also suggests that the right association cortex is the critical processing node but that in most patients the left association cortex can extract enough perceptual information for recognition, even if slowly.

Testing for prosopagnosia requires some planning. Because it is a visual modality-specific deficit, the examiner must be careful to provide only visual information. Magazine pictures or family pictures are useful. If real people (i.e., family members) are used for testing, they must be cautioned not to speak or to wear distinctive clothing items. This is not a test of perception that happens to use faces. It is a test of recognition of familiar, known faces. Patients with bilateral lesions may be anomic, but descriptions of the target's occupation, relationship, and so on suffice to eliminate prosopagnosia. Semantic memory deficits can be differentiated from prosopagnosia by performance on strictly verbal tasks. A patient with prosopagnosia will have abundant knowledge of named people.

No treatment has ever been proposed. Patients with large bilateral lesions usually improve through a stage of profound object agnosia. Perhaps because it is perceptually more demanding, facial recognition usually recovers less well than object agnosia, but the relative recoveries depend on lesion site, size, and laterality. Some patients have recovered from proso-

TABLE 136-4. Prosopagnosia

Examination
  Famous and familiar faces
    Naming
    Identification by description
    Categorization
    Matching to name
Commonly associated signs
  Bilateral lesion
    Superior attitudinal visual field defects
    Achromatopsia
    Amnesia
  Right lesion
    Left visual field defect
    Topographic amnesia

pagnosia but remained unable to recognize emotional expressions.

SYNDROMES OF IMPAIRED VISUAL ATTENTION

The disorders that result from impaired visual attention are produced by lesions in the superior visual association cortex and its outflow to parietal and frontal lobes, and by lesions in parietal heteromodal association cortex. Directed attention, to be sure, is a very complex operation that utilizes a network that includes structures far from visual cortex.

Neglect

Failure to attend to stimuli in extrapersonal space constitutes neglect. Neglect can be seen in either right or left hemispace after lesions in the contralateral hemisphere. Left hemispatial neglect is much more severe than right hemispatial neglect after comparable lesions, one of many pieces of evidence that the right hemisphere is dominant for attentional functions. Neglect may be seen after any structural lesions of any etiology. Within the hemisphere, neglect can been seen with dorsolateral frontal, dorsolateral striatal, anterior cingulate, posterior thalamic, or parietal lesions. The manifestations and mechanisms of neglect differ for these different lesion sites. Large lesions, damaging more than one of those regions, produce the most severe neglect. In clinical practice large infarctions in middle cerebral artery territory produce the most dramatic neglect. Large posterior cerebral artery territory infarctions involving posterior thalamus and extensive parieto-occipital cortex also produce very dramatic neglect. The associated signs may be quite varied, depending on lesion size and site. Neglect is however, independent of visual field deficits. Any combination of field deficits and neglect can be seen, depending on lesion site.

Testing for neglect is readily accomplished at the bedside with paper and pencil. Although not the cause of, or necessary for, neglect, primary sensory deficits, including sensory extinction, should be defined. Among the many proposed tests of neglect, line bisection and line or object cancellation are most easily performed and sensitive. For line bisection the patient is given a sheet of paper, presented in his midline, with numerous horizontal lines of various lengths distributed to the right and the left of the paper's midline. He is asked to bisect each line; neglect is measured as systematic deviation from the midline. For cancellation tasks, the patients is given a sheet of paper with randomly arrayed lines or objects, and he is told to mark out each line or designated target object. Failure to cancel lines in parts of space defines neglect. Neglect may be apparent in other tests. When reading aloud, the patient may fail to read one end of each line of text. When quickly shown compound words (e.g., doghouse), he may neglect one side of the word. If asked to copy complex figures, he may start the copy far to one side and fail to copy or disproportionately miscopy one side. For all tests of neglect, patients with right-sided lesions will show much more left neglect than patients with comparable left-sided lesions will show right neglect.

Patients with parietal lesions seem to show neglect because they fail to pay attention to contralateral hemispace. Thus, when a competing stimulus is available in right space, attention will turn to the right. Patients with dorsolateral frontal and dorsolateral striatal lesions appear to show neglect because they fail to form an intention to move attention to the contralateral hemispace. As long as stimuli are available to draw attention, the patient may move into the impaired hemispace. Only if the task requires the patient to generate his own strategy to move attention, for instance, on copying tasks, will he fail. For parietal or frontal lesions, left hemispatial neglect is always much more noteworthy than right neglect after comparable lesions. A variety of experimental tests have demonstrated that the right brain carries out complex processing of the left visual field stimuli that are neglected, demonstrating the distinction between attention and perceptual processes.

Treatment of left hemispatial neglect has been attempted in a variety of ways. The primary motivation for these treatments has been the frequent observation that left hemineglect is a significant factor in a bad functional outcome after rehabilitation for stroke. Treatments have included both direct and compensatory. In direct treatments, microcomputer presentation has been used to direct attention to the impaired side before presentation of stimuli. Patients can also be given practice in directing gaze in the horizontal plane to specific points in the impaired hemifield. Compensatory treatments are all techniques of providing a perceptual anchor in the neglected hemispace, such as, a brightly colored marker down the left margin of books or on the bathroom mirror, with the patients instructed to always look to the marker. Both techniques seem to improve patients' function in test circumstances and perhaps in self-care activities.

Right hemispatial neglect recovers quite quickly. Left hemispatial neglect, in addition to being more severe is much slower to recover. Several studies in patients with stroke indicate that most recovery occurs within 4 to 6 weeks of onset. Patients with persistently severe neglect 4 weeks after onset may have incomplete long-term recovery and often do very poorly in rehabilitation. In Massachusetts, only visual fields and acuity are considered relevant to driving, but patients with any degree of hemispatial neglect, regardless of their visual fields, should not drive. Significant neglect also probably precludes cooking at open stove tops and using power tools.

Visually Guided Movement

As noted above, the superior visual associate cortex is involved in mechanisms of hemispatial attention—detection of the *presence* of a stimulus, its distance, and direction of movement—not in mechanisms of visual recognition. This is commonly expressed as the view that dorsal visual systems (occipitoparietal) are concerned with the "where" of an object, and the ventral visual systems (occipitotemporal) are concerned with "what" of an object.

One implication of that dichotomy is that the parieto-occipital regions are concerned with the generation of movements toward a detected object. This could involve eye movements to obtain fixation (the better to facilitate discrimination in the ventral systems) or limb movements to capture the object. For eye movements, active fixation must be inhibited, presumably by frontal to occipital projections, allowing new fixations to be made. For limb movements, there must be a cerebral representation of location that allows for size (large objects at a distance have the same retinal space as small objects that are near) and movement and that can represent space in both visual and kinesthetic forms so that rapid movement to a visually detected point can occur. The superior parietal lobe contains cells that serve this purpose, and projections to frontal cortex guide these movements. White matter pathways in the parietal lobe between the frontal gaze center (area 8) and the occipital gaze center (area

19) allow the fixation changes. All these mechanisms only work in contralateral space, depending on parietal callosal connections to drive movement of limbs to a target in the field contralateral to the arm used (i.e., the left arm into right space). Damage to these parietal systems, produces a deficit in directing gaze toward an object in space contralateral to the lesion and a deficit in directing the hand toward the object. These two deficits disappear as soon as the object is in central fixation because now both hemispheres have spatial information and guide the limbs.

The eye movement deficit is well known to clinicians, especially for patients with right brain lesions, as gaze preference, poor fixation or tracking into the impaired field, and impaired optokinetic nystagmus. The limb movement deficit, often called impaired visually guided reaching or optic ataxia, is not as well known because all bedside reaching tasks are done to a fixated target. If the patient is forced to reach to a target in the peripheral field, they will be unable to direct movement to the target. This is easily tested at bedside. First, proprioceptive deficits and visual field loss must be detected. If they are absent, visually guided reaching can be tested by having the patient maintain central fixation on the examiner's nose and then asking him to reach to a fingertip held a few degrees into the impaired side of space. Most patients, and in fact most neurologists, are amazed at how easily this is normally accomplished on the intact side.

Any structural lesion in the posterior parietal lobe may produce these deficits, but because the superior parietal lobule (area 7) is particularly critical for visually guided reaching, the usual middle cerebral artery territory infarction may not cause a problem, even if it does not cause hemiparesis or proprioceptive loss. Most reported cases have been tumors.

There is no known treatment for these deficits, but their prognosis is generally favorable because of the instantaneous correction produced by central fixation. The same techniques described as direct treatment of neglect may be useful in accelerating recovery.

Balint Syndrome

The Balint syndrome represents the effects of bilateral parietal lesions in which central visual fixation cannot compensate because neither hemisphere can generate normal visual attention or visual control of movement. Thus, it is as though patients have bilateral neglect, attending only to what is fixation, neglecting nonfixated targets on either side. Furthermore, they may be trapped in fixation, unable to direct volitionally gaze to any other target. Finally, they have severe bilateral optic ataxia, even to targets in fixation because neither hemisphere can represent location or spatially guided movement. These three elements—visual inattention, so-called "psychic paralysis" of gaze, and optic ataxia—are Balint syndrome. Some patients have partial inferior altitudinal visual field defects.

The disorder requires bilateral parietal lesions. Not surprisingly, most reported cases have been through-and-through gunshot wounds. Some patients have had butterfly gliomas. Bilateral posterior parietal strokes also can produce Balint syndrome.

No treatment has been suggested. The prognosis is quite poor, and patients may actually function better if blindfolded because they will rely on proprioception exclusively.

RELATED DISORDERS OF SPATIAL-MOTOR CAPACITY

There are several cognitive disorders related to these deficits that are not usually considered in this context that should be briefly mentioned.

Limb Praxis

Apraxia is almost universally covered in papers on aphasia for several reasons. First, both are common after left brain lesions, and they commonly co-occur. Second, both have a communicative intent, at least as praxis is usually tested. Third, both apraxia and aphasia are viewed as related to handedness. In the context of this chapter it is only important to note that praxis involves learning to use the arm and hand for a large number of tasks. The constraints of the tasks are spatial and kinesthetic, not communicative. To throw a ball requires activating a series of movements designed to bring the hand and fingers to a particular point where the ball can serve as a substitute for the hand to travel to a point specified in visual space. Stirring a cup of coffee is highly restricted by the spatial limits of the cup and the implications of that space for the restrictions of movement. Thus, limb praxis, as usually tested, simply probes the preservation of the movement patterns unconstrained by space. Deficits in these movement patterns that are facilitated by spatial cues (such as a real object) are usually referred to as ideomotor apraxia. Lesions can be in the praxis-dominant parietal lobe, usually the left, at least in right-handers, or they can be anywhere in the projections from the parietal lobe to the motor systems for the movement, whether the ipsilateral or contralateral hand. In fact, large corona radiata lesions often produce the most persistent ideomotor apraxia.

There are other patients who are able to demonstrate correct movement patterns but cannot place them correctly in space. Thus, they cannot actually throw a ball, stir a cup, and so on. This has been called "tool use apraxia" but is now considered the most transparent manifestation of ideational apraxia. It is also associated with lesions in the praxis-dominant hemisphere, usually large and including superior parietal lobe and deep white matter. Many patients clearly have both ideational apraxia and ideomotor apraxia so severe that they do not improve with the actual object.

The clinical assessment is straightforward. Once the patient's comprehension is established, he is requested to pretend to carry out a number of learned movements. If he fails, he is given actual objects to use. Nurses and therapists will usually be aware of isolated ideational apraxia before the neurologists.

No treatment is known. The prognosis is usually good especially for very familiar movements of everyday care.

Dressing Apraxia

Most patients who are unable to dress themselves fail for neurologically mundane reasons, severe weakness, visual neglect, or confusion. A very small number have trouble dressing because they cannot represent the spatial, kinesthetic problems of visually guiding their limbs into the clothes. This is primary dressing disorder (dressing apraxia is a confusing term). Lesions producing this deficit are found in the right superior parietal region. Any etiology can cause this. No treatment has been suggested, but selecting clothes that are not visually confusing and laying them out in a mannikinlike manner are both helpful. The prognosis is usually favorable.

Needless to say, patients with Balint syndrome have both ideational apraxia and dressing apraxia.

Drawing Impairments

The topic of drawing impairments is too complex to address completely. It should, nevertheless, be clear that parieto-occipital lesions would produce deficits that would make drawing or copying quite difficult. Lesions of either hemisphere produce disturbances in these visuoconstructive tasks. The tasks require at a minimum integration of movement with perception, complete attention to the entire visual target, and the ability to direct attention to subcomponents of the target. Probably because of coincident neglect and subsequent inability to register the configuration of the entire target, right posterior lesions produce much worse drawings and constructions than left posterior lesions. Patients with left parieto-occipital lesions usually conserve the overall design of the target, whether drawing from memory or copying. Patients with right lesions may lose the overall design, attempting to place individual subparts without respect to the total configuration. Patients with right-sided lesions may also start from the middle of the object and work to the right, never or incompletely returning to the left side.

These differences in visuoconstructive deficits can be brought out by having the patient draw familiar but complex figures (house, flower, etc.) from memory and also complex geometric figures to copy. This part of the examination, combined with neglect tests, takes no more than a few minutes and may be a much clearer window into the patients' deficits than any other testing.

CONCLUSION

The clinical classification of higher-level visual disorders follows from the distinctions between impairments in discrimination or recognition and impairments in attention or visuospatially controlled movement and between language-based and nonlanguage-based tasks. These disorders have been extraordinarily informative vehicles for construction of theories of how the brain carries out complex mental operations. Although something of this fascinating scientific question has been addressed here, the primary focus has been clinical. In clinical practice these disorders are not uncommon, and this chapter has summarized the etiologies and clinical settings in which they will be encountered and the most direct strategies of bedside diagnosis. To the extent that they are treatable, current treatment has been reviewed.

SUGGESTED READINGS

Benson DF, Greenberg JP: Visual form agnosia. Arch Neurol 20:82–89, 1969
Coslett HB, Saffran E: Simultanagnosia. Brain 114:1523–45, 1991
D'Esposito M, McGlinchey-Berroth R, Alexander MP et al: Dissociable cognitive and neural mechanisms of unilateral visual neglect. Neurology 43: 2638–44, 1993
Damasio A, Damasio H: The anatomical basis of pure alexia. Neurol 33: 1573–83, 1983
Damasio AR, Benton AL: Impairment of hand movements under visual guidance. Neurol 29:170–4, 1979
Damasio AR, Damasio H, Van Hoesen GW: Prosopagnosia: anatomic basis and behavioral mechanisms. Neurology 32:331–41, 1982
DeRenzi E: Disorder of Space Exploration and Cognition. pp. 237–254. Wiley, Chicester, UK, 1982
DeRenzi E: Prosopagnosia in two patients with CT scan evidence of damage restricted to the right hemisphere. Neuropsychologia 24:385–9, 1986

Feinberg T, Heilman KM, Rothi LG: Multimodal agnosia after unilateral left lesion. Neurology 36:864–7, 1986
Mesulam MM: A cortical network for directed attention and unilateral neglect. Ann Neurol 10:309–25, 1981
Tyler HR: Abnormalities of perception with defective eye movements. Cortex 4:154–77, 1968

137. DISORDERS OF MEMORY

RONALD C. PETERSEN

SCOPE OF THE PROBLEM

Memory complaints are encountered commonly in clinical practice, especially as the patient population ages. Memory is an essential cognitive function, and even a relatively mild impairment can disrupt one's professional and social life. Occasionally memory disorders constitute the sole complaint of the patient and can be very disabling. Among cognitive complaints, memory dysfunction is the most frequent problem brought to the clinician's attention; yet, it can be perplexing for the clinician as to how to pursue an evaluation. The task for the clinician becomes one of determining the following: (1) Does a memory problem exist? (2) What is the anatomic localization of the problem? (3) What is the mechanism of the disorder? (4) What treatments are available for a memory disorder?

DOES A MEMORY DISORDER EXIST?

It can be difficult to determine whether a memory disorder exists. Patients and families will often attribute any type of cognitive or emotional disorder to a memory problem. It is as if memory function is the final common pathway for a variety of cognitive complaints. The clinician must be certain that the patient is not referring to difficulties with attention, concentration, naming, or language. For example, it is typical for an older patient to complain of word-finding difficulties and attribute this to a poor memory.

A major problem exists in the literature on memory with respect to terminology. Memory functions are quite complex, and, consequently, a variety of terminology has developed over the years to describe various aspects of learning and recall performance. While several sets of terminology relating to multiple theoretical models have evolved, there are certain commonalties among the various theoretical approaches. These features can perhaps be best appreciated by considering a classic amnestic syndrome such as that resulting from bilateral amygdalohippocampectomies or the alcoholic Wernicke-Korsakoff syndrome. In these examples, the primary cognitive dysfunction is one of impaired learning or acquisition of new information. The neurologic process thought to be disrupted in this disorder is *consolidation* or the actual formation of a more permanent memory trace. Failure of the consolidation process is also known as *anterograde amnesia,* referring to the inability to lay down new memories after the onset of the memory disorder.

In dramatic cases of the amnestic syndrome, the clinician may spend considerable time interviewing and examining the patient with a seemingly normal interpersonal interaction. The clinician may then leave the room to return 5 minutes later and have the patient be unaware of the previous interview or of having met the clinician. This dramatic amnesia results from a failure of consolidation.

In the typical amnestic syndrome, information acquired prior to the onset of the memory disorder is variably recalled. Older memories may be better preserved than the more recently experienced events. This gradient may reflect an ongoing consolidation failure in recent days and months, which may degrade the more recently acquired information. When a patient does not recall information learned previous to the onset of the memory disorder, this is termed *retrograde amnesia.*

While these abnormalities in memory function are quite prominent, patients with the amnestic syndrome have relatively preserved general intellect, attention, and language. These preserved functions allow the patient to carry on a reasonably normal conversation in the immediate time frame, but when patients are required to recall information encountered in the recent past, they have great difficulty. In this sense, the amnestic syndrome represents a rather pure disruption of memory function.

Information-Processing Model

Why does the amnestic syndrome occur? This question can be addressed by analyzing an information-processing model. Most information is received in the brain through sensory processing systems and is stored for a brief period of time in these systems. These processing networks are initially modality-specific and then converge to bring together information regarding a perceptual event from a variety of different sensory modalities. The sensory information is held in a temporary register, which is dependent on attention and serves the function of holding the information for subsequent processing. As shown in Fig. 137-1, the temporary processing registry is of limited capacity, and the information persists in this store for only a short period of time (seconds). While information is in this temporary register, some of it is selected for further processing depending on the experience of the individual and the requirements of the learning situation. For example, if one were to process information regarding a soft-drink can, certain visual features of its cylindrical nature, the shading of the can, and its overall size would

be held in a visual information register briefly. If the can were held in the hand, there would be somatosensory information that would also be retained, and if one manipulated the can to hear the sound of bending aluminum, auditory information would also be held in a register for a brief period of time. All of this information would ultimately coalesce, but in its initial processing phase would be held in the modality-specific stores. This relatively limited processing temporary store can be assessed clinically by asking patients to recite a digit span such as a telephone number. Typically, most individuals will be able to process up to approximately 7 independent items of information and hold them for a matter of up to a minute without rehearsal. However, if the material is not rehearsed or further encoded, the information decays relatively rapidly.

The actual learning process requires this information to be encoded in terms of previous experiences and transferred to a more permanent memory register. This transfer process, which has been referred to previously as consolidation, is the primary site of dysfunction in most organic amnesias. In the amnestic syndrome, the patients are able to recite a normal digit span but are unable to transfer information from this temporary store to a more permanent memory register. The transfer of information from the temporary store to the more permanent register can be assessed by providing the patient with a list of items, such as words, which exceeds the immediate memory span of approximately 7 units or by requiring the patient to recall the information after a delay interval filled with intervening activities that prevent rehearsal. For example, to use the latter technique the clinician could present five or six words to the patient and ask him or her to remember them over a series of three or four learning trials. The clinician could then engage in other activities for perhaps 15 minutes and ask the patient to try to recall the five or six words after a 15-minute delay. This technique can be useful to the clinician for assessing this critical aspect of information processing involved in consolidation. Figure 137-1 presents a schematic of this information-processing model and provides some terminology that corresponds to various aspects of the scheme as well as tasks that can be used to assess the various aspects of processing.

Most investigators accept these features of memory function as reasonably universal but employ a variety of terms to discuss

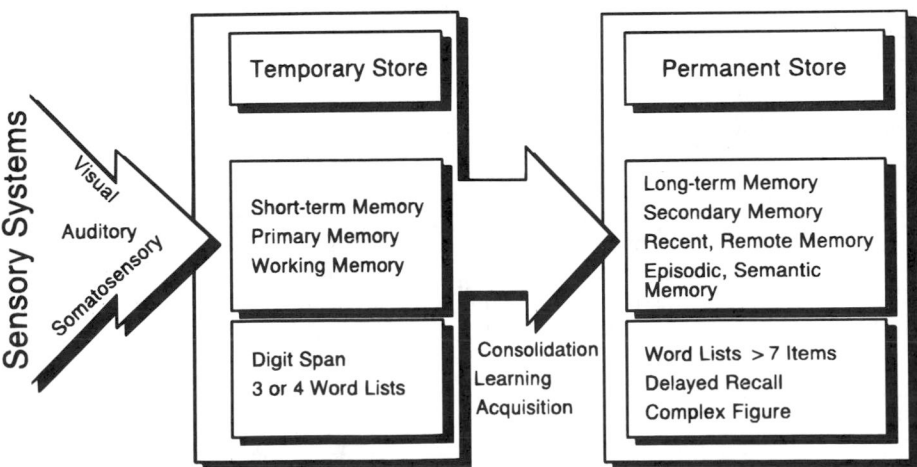

FIG. 137-1. Information processing scheme depicting a temporary store and a more permanent store. For each store, alternative terminology in various theoretical models and office testing procedures are indicated.

these concepts in various theoretical models. This theorizing results in myriad confusing terminology. Some of the more commonly used terms in various theoretical discussions of memory are defined below.

Glossary

Short-Term Memory. Short-term memory refers to the limited-capacity temporary storage buffer shown in Figure 137-1. It has a finite capacity and information remains in the store for a relatively brief period of time (seconds to a minute) without rehearsal. This type of store would hold a telephone number for a short time. It reflects an attentional rather than a memory process. This term is often used loosely in clinical practice and, without a specific definition, may best be avoided.

Long-Term Memory. The long-term aspect of memory function refers to the more permanent large-capacity memory store also outlined in Figure 137-1. Long-term memory usually refers to our knowledge base of previously learned information. Occasionally, this store is divided into two components: recent memory and remote memory. These terms are defined imprecisely along a temporal dimension with recent memory typically referring to memories in hours to days in duration and remote memory referring to distant past memories of many years. However, these terms are not specific.

Primary Memory. Primary memory is similar in the temporal domain to the concept of short-term memory. Primary memory refers more to the processing nature of this type of memory than to the actual storage function. It tends to deemphasize a precise temporal gradient and describes the type of processing performed on material held in the temporary store.

Secondary Memory. In a similar fashion, the term secondary memory refers to memory processes that support retention across long retention intervals. It is somewhat similar to the long-term memory notion, but once again, emphasizes the processes involved in the storage and retrieval of previously learned information rather than the temporal dimension.

Working Memory. The concept of working memory refers to material held in primary memory on which further elaboration is done. The term refers to the selection of material in the temporary store for further processing and encoding into the more permanent memory store. Working memory refers to encoding processes and the use of strategies for facilitating the consolidation process. This is a dynamic aspect of memory and can be impaired in attentional disorders.

Episodic Memory. Episodic memory refers to memory for events that are related to a specific spatial or temporal context. There is no temporal dimension to this type of material but rather this concept incorporates the specific situation in which an event was remembered. For example, when an individual tries to learn a list of words in a particular setting, this material would be referred to as existing in episodic memory. This type of memory is severely affected in pathologic processes involving the medial temporal lobes and diencephalic structures and is impaired in most organic amnesias.

Semantic Memory. The term semantic memory is typically used in contrast to episodic memory to refer to information that

is stored in the more permanent knowledge base without any reference to the specific learning context. For example, information that we have learned about a concept such as gravity would be incorporated into our semantic memory store in spite of the fact that we do not remember the specific context in which we acquired this information. This type of information forms our knowledge of the world and is relatively resistant to disruption in many memory disorders.

Declarative Memory. Declarative memory refers to memory that is directly accessible to consciousness and is also significantly affected in most organic amnesias. Declarative memory refers to recently experienced information about which we are aware and often includes remembering the circumstances in which this information was learned. Damage to medial temporal and diencephalic structures can disrupt this type of memory.

Procedural Memory. In contrast to declarative memory, procedural memory refers to skills and procedural operations. Certain overlearned motor skills and mechanical sequences are part of procedural memory. This type of memory is often spared in many organic amnesias and presumably involves structures in the basal ganglia rather than the medial temporal lobe or diencephalic structures.

Summary. As one can see, there are many terms that refer to multiple aspects of memory function. These terms are not mutually exclusive and at times refer to very similar concepts. The individual differences among the terms are derived from the theoretical background from which they are derived and pertain to one theoretical model or another. Each of these terms can be useful in specific instances, but the overall concept of temporary and more permanent memory stores may be ultimately more useful.

Conclusion

Based on the information presented in this conceptual frame, the clinician can then decide whether the patient's problem involves memory primarily or other cognitive functions. If the patient appears to be describing a failure of consolidation with preservation of attention, language, and other cognitive processes, then it is likely that the clinician is dealing with an organic memory disorder and an evaluation is appropriate.

WHAT IS THE LOCALIZATION OF THE PROBLEM?

To a certain extent, the information processing scheme outlined in Figure 137-1 has anatomic analog. For example, as is shown in Figure 137-2, the primary sensory receiving areas and the unimodal (modality-specific) association areas corresponding to each sensory modality provide the substrate for the input processing of sensory information. Superimposed upon this sensory-processing scheme is the role of attentional functions that are largely subserved by frontal and subcortical structures. The role of attention in the sensory processing is to preserve the incoming information in the temporary holding store. In addition, certain association areas in the right hemisphere (temporoparietal and frontal association areas) may also contribute to the selective preservation of information in these temporary memory registers.

Following initial processing in the primary sensory and unimodal association areas, the information is elaborated upon and

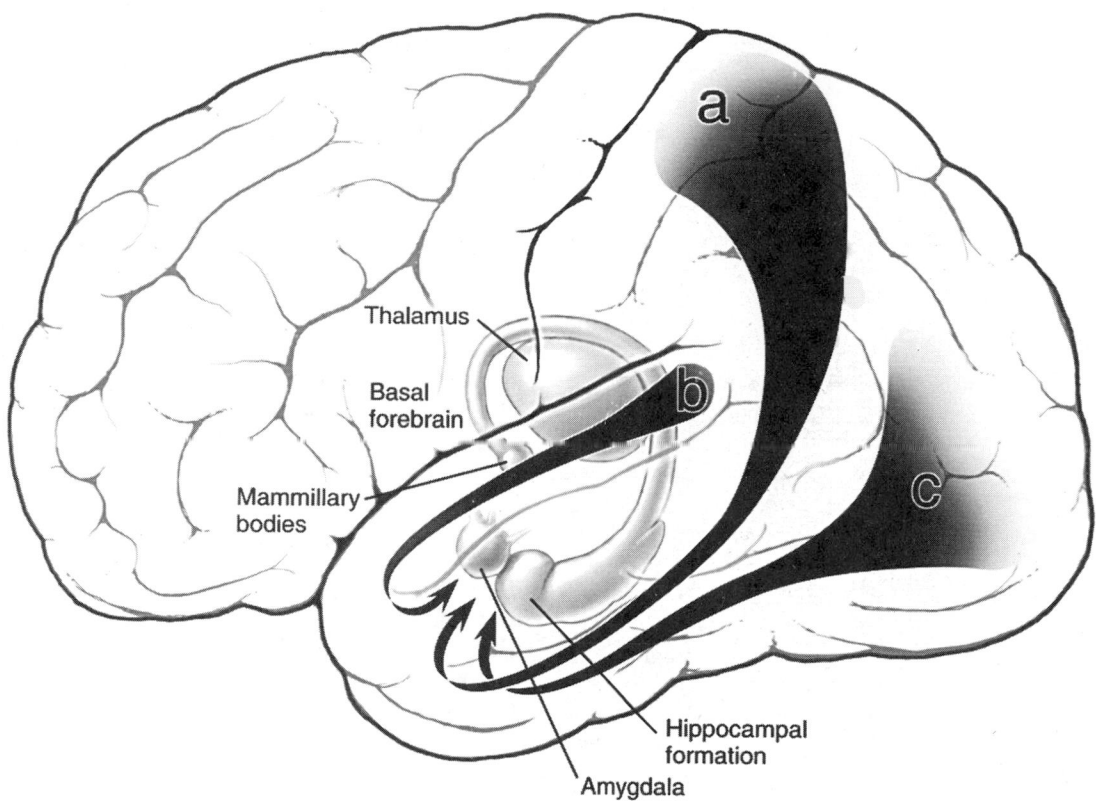

FIG. 137-2. Anatomic localization of the flow of information from sensory association areas to temporolimbic structures for memory acquisition. *a,* Somatosensory association area; *b,* auditory association area; *c,* visual association area.

transferred through multimodal association areas residing largely in temporoparietal and frontal regions. These areas serve to combine the individual modality-specific aspects of the stimulus to be remembered and further enrich the elaboration of the information. Using the example of a soft-drink can cited earlier, all of the properties of the individual modalities such as the visual, somatosensory, and auditory aspects of the can itself would coalesce into the multimodal sensory areas to provide a richer perception of the individual sensory experiences. The soft-drink can would not only have visual features of a cylinder of a certain size but would also have somatosensory features of a smooth object and auditory features of an aluminum can. The information is then transferred from the multimodal association areas to the limbic system largely through the entorhinal cortex and parahippocampal regions (Fig. 137-2). It is then processed through the perforant pathway from the entorhinal cortex to the hippocampal formation and limbic system, which constitutes the anatomic basis for major aspects of the consolidation process. It is important to realize that the information is not stored in the hippocampal formation and limbic system but rather is processed in these regions and ultimately transferred back to cortical association areas where the neural networks that embody the remembered information are located. The actual neural representation of the information to be remembered is diffusely distributed in neocortical regions, and these areas correspond to the more permanent aspects of storage in the information processing model. This interaction between the association areas and the limbic system is a dynamic process and is ongoing constantly with the remodeling of information in the more permanent stores taking place on a regular basis. Conse-

quently, memory should be viewed as a dynamic process with constant reorganization of information rather than as a passive system of storage of facts and information.

Returning to our soft-drink can example, it is at the point of the limbic system involvement that the soft-drink can now takes on meaning as a soft-drink can based on our previous knowledge. In addition, if we have had previous personal experiences with certain types of soft-drink cans, these aspects of the sensory event are also brought to bear on remembering this particular perceptual event.

In this model, while many areas of cortex and subcortical regions are involved in the acquisition process, the temporolimbic system is the critical focus of much of the consolidation activity. The clinician needs to focus on the temporolimbic system as a site of impairment in most organic amnesias with significant acquisition or consolidation defects. Most commonly encountered amnestic syndromes will involve dysfunction of these structures.

In summary, when encoding or acquisition processes are primarily involved, the most likely structures implicated are the medial temporal lobe, including the entorhinal cortex, perforant pathway, hippocampal formation, thalamus, hypothalamus, surrounding third ventricular structures, basal forebrain, and the multiple interconnecting pathways. Most disease processes that affect memory significantly will involve these structures anatomically or pharmacologically. For severe memory disorders, the involvement needs to be bilateral. However, unilateral lesions can give material-specific deficits such as verbal or nonverbal processing difficulties.

The anatomic localization of retrieval processes is less clear but likely involves some aspect of limbic system processing as well as other regions of the cerebral cortex, such as the prefrontal region, which may be involved in attention and retrieval strategy generation, and the temporoparietal neocortex, including higher-order association areas where the neural networks that actually embody the material to be remembered reside. These structures subserve the anatomic localization of the more remote memories or knowledge base and consequently are relatively preserved except in the setting of diffuse or advanced disease processes.

WHAT IS THE MECHANISM OF THE DISORDER?

As with all neurologic disorders, the temporal course of the development of the symptoms is of paramount importance. This factor coupled with other features of the history, such as trauma, alcohol use, concomitant cancer, vascular disease, or psychiatric illnesses, may all give the clinician an insight into possible mechanisms (Table 137-1).

Acute Memory Loss

From a temporal perspective, if the memory disturbance has come on acutely, the clinician should consider a vascular etiology. Since many of the central limbic structures that subserve memory are in the distribution of the vertebrobasilar arterial system, these structures should be investigated. For example, ischemia to the medial temporal lobes or the thalamus can present with the acute onset of a memory impairment.

Other conditions that can produce an acute memory loss include transient global amnesia, about which the precise mechanism is not known, but presumably some type of temporary dysfunction of these limbic structures is involved. In certain other medical contexts, hypoxia, hypoglycemia, migraine, intracerebral hemorrhages—particularly resulting from anterior communicating artery aneurysm rupture, drug ingestion, or toxic exposure could produce an acute memory loss. In addition, psychogenic causes of amnesia need to be considered in the appropriate context.

Initially, an imaging study may be helpful to evaluate a possible infarct, hemorrhage, mass, or infection. A head computed tomography (CT) scan with and without contrast is helpful initially; however, a negative scan does not eliminate all considerations. Many of the structures involved in memory function may not be visualized well by CT, since they reside in close proximity to the calvarium of the middle cranial fossa, which can produce artifacts on CT. Magnetic resonance imaging (MRI) may be preferred because of its increased sensitivity to detect small lesions in critical structures. Recently, magnetic resonance scans, using certain acquisition procedures, have been particularly useful at detecting lesions, including atrophy in the medial temporal lobe region. If an infarct is detected in the thalamus, medial temporal lobe, or limbic system structures, then an investigation regarding the etiology of this event as discussed in Chapter 42 would need to be considered.

If the patient complains of multiple acute episodes of loss of memory, a complex partial seizure disorder of temporal lobe origin should be considered and pursued. As mentioned, if there is a history of trauma or psychiatric disease, then these etiologies need to be evaluated as well. Occasionally, transient ischemic attacks of the vertebrobasilar artery circulatory system can present with memory impairment, although usually other neurologic symptoms also occur.

Transient global amnesia is a rather unique condition involving a relatively pure amnestic problem of short duration; typically, individuals suffering from this disorder will be unable to lay down any new memories for a period of several hours and will have a retrograde amnesia of variable extent. The individual otherwise looks well and is neurologically intact. However, because of their inability to consolidate any new information, they will ask the same question repeatedly, since they are unable to retain the answer that was given to them previously. The precise etiology of this condition is not known, but it is likely that it involves medial temporal lobe and limbic system structures on a transient basis. Other causes of temporary dysfunction of the temporolimbic system must be considered also such as ischemia or a seizure disorder, but if there are no other features of these alternative conditions, transient global amnesia may be the best explanation.

Finally, nonorganic or psychogenic conditions can present with an acute memory loss. Often these amnesias have certain features that distinguish them from organic memory problems. Typically, a retrograde amnesia is a prominent feature of the symptom complex, often in the setting of relatively preserved learning and acquisition, that is, no anterograde amnesia. These individuals may claim to have forgotten their names, family information, and occasionally emotion-laden experiences. While prominent isolated retrograde amnesia cases have been reported, they are quite uncommon. In evaluating suspected nonorganic amnesias, there are often clues from the performance of the patient. The patient may give inconsistent responses on tests with "failure" on easier memory tasks, such as recognition tests, with relatively normal free recall performance. Patients may "forget" information that is distinctly resistant to loss such as personal identity. However, the clinician should also seek supporting psychiatric evidence for nonorganic amnesias before concluding that the memory deficit has no organic basis.

TABLE 137-1. Onset of Memory Disorder

	Time	Etiology

Acute	Seconds to minutes	Vascular[a]
		  Ischemic
		  Hemorrhagic
		Transient global amnesia[a]
		Seizure disorder[a]
		Migraine[a]
		Hypoxia
		Psychiatric

Subacute	Days to weeks	Infectious Inflammatory Metabolic Toxic Neoplastic Psychiatrics
Chronic	Months to years	Degenerative Neoplastic Deficiency state Psychiatric

[a] Can be episodic.

Subacute Memory Loss

A subacute (days to weeks) evolution of a memory disorder would raise the consideration of infections, inflammations, or toxic or metabolic etiologies. Other features of the history and examination should alert the clinician to consideration of infectious possibilities and consideration of a cerebrospinal fluid analysis. Herpes simplex encephalitis should be considered, especially in the setting of altered cognition with seizures, since this is a treatable condition. Some inflammatory conditions may present with a memory disorder, including multiple sclerosis, central nervous system sarcoidosis, or Sjögren syndrome. Finally, in the appropriate clinical context, meningeal carcinomatosis or limbic encephalitis can present with a memory impairment, although usually with additional cognitive and neurologic findings. As always, a psychiatric explanation should be considered.

Chronic Memory Loss

Finally, if the memory disorder has evolved over months to years, a degenerative disorder such as Alzheimer's disease becomes much more likely in the appropriate age group. Other considerations include a neoplasm, particularly of the limbic system, deficiency state, or psychiatric conditions including depression. In a degenerative disease such as Alzheimer's disease, acquisition processes and retrieval processes are affected early and may be the only manifestation of disease in the initial stages. Later, however, other cognitive functions become impaired, and memory is no longer an isolated defect.

Occasionally, distinctions are drawn between predominantly cortical dementias such as Alzheimer's disease and predominantly subcortical dementias such as those seen in Parkinson's disease, vascular disease, progressive supranuclear palsy, or multiple sclerosis. In subcortical dementias, the patient also often needs additional effort to learn the material, but once it has been learned, it is recalled reasonably well, especially with cues. In cortical dementias, learning is impaired despite adequate effort, and recall with cues is also significantly impaired. The subcortical dementias may also have impaired attention, which contributes to the learning difficulties. The cortical-subcortical distinction needs to be made with some caution because there is often significant overlap. Investigations of chronic memory disorders include imaging studies, MRI or CT scan, and laboratory studies more typical of those associated with a dementia evaluation, as discussed in Chapter 132.

EVALUATION OF MEMORY DISORDERS

History

The history from a patient with a memory disorder can be very important. Typically, the history should focus on the recall of recent events rather than recall of remote memories that may be preserved. In the course of taking a history, the patient can be asked about recent events in the news, including events of the past few days or significant news items of recent months, such as natural disasters, major crimes, or prominent political events. This line of questioning presumes that the patient has been exposed to these events and a family member can be asked to corroborate these issues. Typically, most people are aware of major weather events such as hurricanes, earthquakes, or floods that are commonly in the news. If a person is a sports fan, recent events can be tested by asking about the performance of the patient's favorite teams. These questions are meant to assess the acquisition of significant information most people would demonstrate if they have been exposed to the events. Often patients with memory problems will be vague about the answers to these questions and provide little detail.

The clinician needs to be certain that the patient is attentive and does not have a significant language problem, aphasia, when assessing memory. Many people, as they age, are aware of word-finding problems usually for names of people. They will often attribute this to a failing memory and this needs to be assessed, since some naming deficits are a part of normal aging and represent a retrieval failure for previously learned information rather than an acquisition or learning problem.

Occasionally, in taking a history from a patient, certain details of the history itself may be lost. The clinician can get an impression of the severity of the problem by asking the patient to recount events of the past day or two in terms of travel, activities with family members, or how they got to the clinician's office. While not necessarily quantitative, these questions can be quite informative as to the possibility of a significant memory problem.

Mental Status Evaluation

An accurate mental status examination is an essential component of evaluating someone with a memory disorder. As indicated, it is important to determine if memory is in fact impaired or other cognitive deficits contribute to the problem. A complete discussion of mental status testing is found in Chapter 131.

The clinician can use one of the standard mental status examinations available such as the Mini-Mental State Examination or the Short Test of Mental Status but must be aware of the limitations of these instruments. These tests usually use three or four word lists with a relatively short recall interval and may underestimate early memory deficits. Alternatively, if the patient has difficulty with delayed recall with three or four words, there is likely a significant memory problem. The Short Test of Mental Status also assesses an element of learning by taking into account the number of trials the subject requires to learn the four words accurately.

In general, office testing of memory should include sets of verbal and nonverbal materials which are presented over several learning trials. This will give an index of learning or acquisition. A several-minute delay, usually 15 to 30 minutes, should be interposed to assess delayed recall. Recent evidence indicates that, in addition to acquisition deficits, delayed recall performance may be a sensitive index of early impairment. Based on the findings of the clinician in the office, specific recommendations can be made to the neuropsychologist for further, more extensive, memory testing.

The mental status examination should also include evaluation of attention and language functions (see Chs. 131 and 135) to be certain that the patient is not significantly inattentive, leading to poor learning or acquisition or that the patient does not have a significant aphasia with profound anomia. If the patient performs reasonably well in the general assessment of cognitive function but performs poorly with respect to acquisition or delayed recall then the clinician needs to pursue an investigation of the etiology of the problem. Inconsistencies or a depressed affect may alert the clinician to psychiatric contributions to the cognitive impairment such as those found in depression. It may be helpful to augment the mental status examination with an inventory of psychiatric symptoms.

Neuropsychological Testing

Neuropsychological testing can be viewed as an extension of the mental status examination. The same principles involved in evaluating mental status in the office can be used in interpreting the results of neuropsychological testing. In general, the clinician will be primarily interested in the results of the memory tests. The testing should involve acquisition of verbal material that exceeds the primary memory capacity and requires the

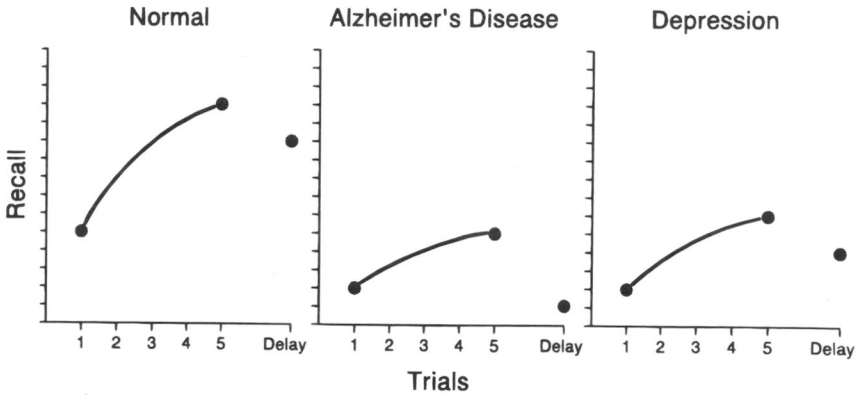

FIG. 137-3. Hypothetical learning curves in normal aging, Alzheimer's disease, and depression. The significant differences pertain to the slopes of the learning curves and the relation of performance on delayed recall to the final learning trial.

transfer of information from the temporary memory store to the more permanent memory store. This usually will involve multiple learning trials of a list of 10 to 15 words. A delay of approximately 15 to 30 minutes should be interposed between the final acquisition trial and a later recall test. The clinician should assess the patient's ability to generate a learning curve, that is, improve recall on each successive learning trial. Ultimately, the patient should recall more than 5 or 6 items over the several learning trials. That is, one should see evidence that the patient has transferred some information from the temporary memory store to the permanent memory store. As shown in Figure 137-3, learning curves can take on characteristic features of underlying disorders. Ideally, performance on these instruments should be assessed relative to age and education appropriate norms. After the delay interval, free recall for the material should be assessed and recall performance of at least 50 percent of the initially acquired material should be achieved. This, however, will vary with the age and education of the patient as well. Some neuropsychological learning instruments also involve the use of semantic cueing and facilitated recall. These measures are meant to assess the patient's ability to use provided acquisition strategies and subsequent recall through the use of these semantic cues. These can be very sensitive tools to detect very early memory impairments involving damage to medial temporal lobe structures.

An analogous set of materials that is largely nonverbally mediated, such as a complex geometric figure, should be used as well. There are various instruments for assessing the learning and recall of visuospatial materials. The same principles as applied to verbal learning should be used in the assessment of nonverbal recall.

As with the mental status examination, neuropsychological testing should also assess other aspects of cognitive function including attention, language, visuospatial skills, higher reasoning processes, praxis, and constructions. This will help the clinician determine if memory is the sole cognitive function impaired or is impaired out of proportion to other mental abilities. It will also help the clinician determine if other cognitive functions such as attention and language are having an impact on memory performance, thereby requiring qualification of the memory test results.

The combination of the clinician's history, mental status examination, general neurologic examination, and neuropsychological testing should provide adequate information for a deter-

mination of a memory deficit. Occasionally if performance is equivocal, some of the tests may need to be repeated at an appropriate interval, using alternate test forms to determine the stability of the findings.

Evaluations of Memory Disorders

Neuroimaging.   Table 137-2 outlines the studies that may need to be done in the evaluation of memory disorders. If memory function is the primary cognitive disorder affected, limbic system structures need to be imaged. A CT scan with and without contrast is helpful, but MRI is more sensitive. Since the relevant structures are often difficult to visualize on CT images, magnetic resonance scans evaluating temporal lobe structures, the thalamus, basal forebrain, and interconnecting pathways can be particularly useful. Occasionally, contrast agents are helpful in bringing out subtle lesions or in characterizing possible infarctions. In some instances, functional imaging scans such as positron emission tomography (PET) or single photon emission computed tomography (SPECT) are helpful in delineating certain memory disorders. In the early course of some diseases, structural changes may not be evident, and a functional abnormalities may be the only imaging index of impairment. To a certain extent, these scans are limited by the resolution of the particular instrument, but with improved spatial resolution, these techniques are becoming increasingly sensitive at evaluating medial temporal lobe structures. Due to their limited availability and expense, they should be reserved for selected cases.

Electroencephalogram.   Since complex partial seizure disorders of temporal lobe origin can present with episodic memory disturbances and occasional persistent memory deficits, an awake and asleep electroencephalogram may be necessary to assess a possible epileptogenic etiology of the memory disorder. Careful attention to seizure foci in medial temporal and inferior frontal regions should be made with this examination. The medial temporal lobe structures, including the amygdala and hippocampus, are among the most epileptogenic structures in the brain, and since they subserve memory, occasionally a subtle complex partial seizure disorder can be the etiology of a memory deficit. Ideally, this study should be done with sleep deprivation.

Laboratory Evaluation.   As indicated above, a number of laboratory studies that assess various processes that are not neces-

TABLE 137-2. Evaluation of Memory Disorders

Imaging studies
   CT
   MRI
   PET, SPECT
Electroencephalogram
Cerebrospinal fluid analysis
   Microbiology
      Gram stain
      Bacterial cultures
      Fungal cultures
      AFB cultures
      Viral cultures
      PCR—herpes simplex encephalitis; *Borrelia burgdorferi*
   Chemistry
      Protein
      Glucose
      VDRL
      FTA-Abs
      IgG index
      Oligoclonal bands
   Cell count
   Cytology
Blood studies
   Chemistry group including glucose
   Hematology group
   Sedimentation rate
   Vitamin B_{12}, folic acid
   Thyroid function studies
   Syphilis serology
   Toxicology screen
   Alcohol level
   Optional
      ANA
      ENA
      Heavy metal screen
      HIV
      Lyme serology
      Copper
      Ceruloplasmin
      Anticardiolipin antibody
      Lupus anticoagulant
      Anti-Purkinje cell antibody
      Antineuronal nuclear antibody
      Arterial blood gas

Abbreviations: CT, computed tomography; MRI, magnetic resonance imaging; PET, positron emission tomography; SPECT, single-photon-emission computed tomography; AFB, acid-fast bacillus; PCR, polymerase chain reaction; VDRL, Venereal Disease Research Laboratory; FTA-Abs, fluorescent treponemal antibody-absorption; ENA, extractable nuclear antigens; ANA, antinuclear antibodies; HIV, human immunodeficiency virus; IgG, immunoglobulin G.

sarily specific for a memory dysfunction but can affect cognitive performance should be considered. Among these would be a chemistry group, hematology group, sedimentation rate, B_{12}, folic acid, thyroid function studies, syphilis serology, antinuclear antibody, extractable nuclear antigen, 24-hour urine for heavy metals, HIV, Lyme serology, toxicology screen, alcohol level, copper, ceruloplasmin, anticardiolipin antibodies, lupus anticoagulant, anti-Purkinje cell antibody, antineuronal nuclear antibody, and an arterial blood gas can be considered in the appropriate clinical context. In addition, a cerebrospinal fluid analysis for possible bacterial, fungal, mycobacterial, or viral infections, cell count, total protein, glucose, syphilis serology, IgG index, IgG synthesis rate, oligoclonal bands, and polymerase chain reaction for herpes simplex virus or *Borrelia burgdorferi* along with a cytologic examination for neoplastic cells can be considered. All these tests need to be evaluated in the appropriate clinical context, and, as indicated above, vascular studies may be necessary as well as other evaluations for systemic diseases.

Psychiatric Consultation. In the appropriate clinical context, a psychiatric consultation may be useful. Since many psychiatric conditions that may account for or contribute to a memory disorder are treatable, this aspect of the evaluation should be considered. The psychiatrist should be particularly attentive to disorders of mood and anxiety.

TREATMENT

If a treatable cause of a memory impairment is disclosed during the evaluation of the imaging or laboratory tests, the offending process should be treated. For example, if a seizure disorder is found, appropriate antiepileptic drugs can be used. Similarly, if a neoplasm, infarct, inflammatory process or an infection such as herpes simplex encephalitis is identified, strategies aimed at treating the underlying disorder should be considered.

Often, however, a specific etiology is not found or a single insult has occurred, and the patient is left with a significant memory problem. The two major approaches to treating memory disorders involve pharmacologic agents and/or behavioral measures. The overall state of treatment of these disorders is not particularly advanced, and consequently, most of the measures are meant to be palliative.

Pharmacologic Treatments

Most of the drugs designed to aid memory are modulators of one or more neurotransmitter systems. Since the cholinergic system is intimately involved in attention and memory functions by virtue of its projections in the limbic system, most of the early work on memory disorders has involved drugs designed to enhance cholinergic function. The Food and Drug Administration approved a drug recently for the treatment of Alzheimer's disease, and this agent is an acetylcholinesterase inhibitor (tacrine or Cognex). Numerous other drugs have been developed in an attempt to augment cholinergic function such as cholinergic precursors (lecithin or phosphatidylcholine), acetylcholinesterase inhibitors (tacrine, velnacrine, E2020), or direct cholinergic agonists (arecoline). The most effective strategy thus far has involved the use of acetylcholinesterase inhibitors.

A variety of other drugs operating on other mechanisms have been used, for example, adrenergic agents, serotonergic compounds, peptides, nootropics, calcium channel antagonists, and antioxidants. Most of these have been studied in the context of Alzheimer's disease. Occasionally agents designed to augment catecholaminergic functioning have been helpful in treating attention and memory disorders. Compounds such as methylphenidate, pemoline, or bromocriptine have been marginally successful in some conditions in which attention is the primary cognitive function impaired.

Occasionally memory is affected in depression, and consequently treatment of the primary underlying psychiatric disorder can secondarily augment memory function. Some of the newer antidepressants such as fluoxetine, sertraline, or paroxetine can be helpful. These tend to be activating agents as well and may augment attention, which secondarily improves memory. These drugs need to be considered in the appropriate medical context with respect to contraindications and side effects. In addition, psychotherapy may be helpful in the appropriate context. The pharmacologic treatment of memory disorders is in its infancy and a great deal remains to be learned about successful drug treatments.

Behavioral Treatments

Most of the behavioral treatments for memory and other cognitive disorders occur in the setting of the treatment of traumatic brain injury. From a practical standpoint, individuals with memory disorders can be taught to use external aids such as schedule books, diaries, watch alarms, or to keep a notepad and thereby circumvent many of the problems arising from memory disorders. Alternatively, internal strategies such as mental imagery, semantic elaboration, and mentally retracing one's steps can also be useful. Often these techniques require a reasonable amount of training and effort to become skillful at them. Detractors of this position claim that cognitively impaired individuals may be incapable of mastering these complex mnemonic strategies. However, in certain instances, these techniques can be helpful.

Recently, several computer-assisted techniques have been developed to assist patients at learning new cognitive skills. Some patients can achieve success at acquiring domain-specific knowledge for learning job-related skills. For example, some amnestic patients can be taught the vocabulary and techniques necessary to operate a computer. In certain training settings, cognitive rehabilitation can be quite successful at enhancing memory and other cognitive functions.

SUMMARY

Memory disorders are found commonly in clinical practice and their identification, evaluation, and treatment can be very rewarding for both the patient and the clinician. Principles of memory function can be applied to the assessment and evaluation of patients with a memory disorder. Certain anatomic structures are known to be involved in various types of memory disorders, and the evaluation of these structures can be revealing. If a particular problem is disclosed through the evaluation process, remedial steps can be made. Alternatively, treatment strategies involving certain drugs and behavioral techniques can be helpful to patients with memory disorders.

ACKNOWLEDGMENTS

I would like to thank Drs. Neill Graff-Radford and M-Marsel Mesulam for their suggestions on this chapter. I would also like to thank Ms. Ellen Ptacek for her superb secretarial assistance in preparation of this manuscript.

SUGGESTED READING

Buschke H: Cued Recall in Amnesia. J Clin Neuropsychol 6:443–450, 1984

Folstein MF, Folstein SE, McHugh PR: "Mini-Mental State": a practical method for grading the cognitive state of patients for the clinician. J Psychiatr Res 12:189–198, 1975

Ivnik RJ, Malec JF, Smith GE et al: Mayo's Older Americans Normative Studies: WAIS-R, WMS-R, and AVLT Norms for Ages 56 Through 97. Clin Neuropsychologist 6:1–104, 1992

Kokmen E, Smith GE, Petersen RC et al: The Short Test of Mental Status: correlations with standardized psychometric testing. Arch Neurol 48: 725–728, 1991

Lezak MD: Neuropsychological Assessment. 3rd Ed. Oxford, New York, 1995.

Petersen RC: Memory Assessment at the Bedside. In Yanagihara T, Petersen RC (eds): Memory Disorders: Research and Clinical Practice. New York, Marcel Dekker, 1991

Petersen RC, Smith GE, Ivnik RJ et al: Memory function in very early Alzheimer's disease. Neurology 44:867–872, 1994

Petersen RC, Smith GE, Kokmen E et al: Memory function in normal aging. Neurology 42:396–101, 1992

Squire LR, Butters N: Neuropsychology of Memory. 2nd Ed. Guilford, New York, 1992

Weintraub S, Mesulam M-M: Mental status assessment of young and elderly adults in behavioral neurology. In M-M Mesulam (ed): Principles of Behavioral Neurology. FA Davis, Philadelphia, 1985.

Yanagihara T, Petersen RC: Memory Disorders: Research and Clinical Practice. Marcel Dekker, New York, 1991

138. LEARNING DISABILITIES

DAVID K. URION

Learning disorders and disorders of tonic and selective attention represent some of the most common clinical issues in pediatric behavioral neurology. Many clinicians find working in this area somewhat frustrating, since it is marked by few trustworthy clinical landmarks, little helpful basic research, dogmatic statements from any of a number of authorities, and much sociopolitical controversy. Various disciplines within medicine have laid territorial claim to the areas and continue to promulgate models adapted from their own experience. Hence, developmental and behavioral pediatricians have offered "input/output" models, which most neurologists allege ignore the last 20 years of cognitive neuroscience. Child psychiatrists have offered up a symptoms/signs checklist approach, in the various incarnations of the *Diagnostic and Statistical Manual of Mental Disorders* (DSM-IV), which are straightforward although without a fundamental model that can be investigated and proved or disproved. Child neurologists have introduced models based upon research in adults, which may or may not prove valid in developing brains, or which are based upon neurolinguistic precepts. Developmental neuropsychologists have offered a triaxial model of developing human cognition that posits a relationship between cognitive functions and brain structures.

Faced with these myriad ideas, what is the clinician to do? This chapter uses a model of developing human cognitive function that is heavily based upon the triaxial model and influenced by insights from the field of adult behavioral neurology. It is the model that is fundamentally used in the daily function of the Learning Disabilities/Behavioral Neurology Program at Children's Hospital, Boston, and as such has been refined in daily clinical practice over the past 20 years. It has all the potential pitfalls noted above, but it also makes certain assertions that in time will be proved or disproved and therefore may lead to further insights into brain–behavior relationships in children.

This area of clinical practice is potentially quite large. It has been estimated that between 5 and 7.5 percent of the childhood population of North America has a diagnosable disorder of selective attention, and roughly 5 percent may suffer from some form of a learning disorder. Many families will therefore seek consultation regarding these issues in their children; if rational support and evaluation is not available from the orthodox medical community, people will seek comfort and succor elsewhere. As advocates for children's well-being, the medical community has a responsibility to deal with such problems as they arise in an appropriate and reasoned matter, just as it would when children are referred for evaluation of a much less common disorder such as one of the childhood epilepsies. It is therefore incumbent upon the clinician to develop some sort of approach to these disorders. One such approach is proposed in this chapter.

DEFINITIONS

Disorders of selective attention are frequently encountered in clinical practice, and have a long history in Anglo-Saxon medicine. The first recognized English-language description of attention disorders comes from Sir George Frederic Still's 1902 Coulstonian lectures, "On Some Abnormal Psychical Conditions in Children." Still's description of such children has not been improved upon over the years. He believed that these children, given to "passionate" swings of emotional behavior, "wanton mischievousness," and an inability to respond to punishment in an appropriate fashion, had some "defect in moral control" that was based upon brain dysfunction. Alfred Tredgold recognized a strong hereditary component to this disorder, and suggested that it was the morbid inheritance of some minimal brain damage that led to this condition. He believed that slums were the consequence of the repeated intermarriage of such individuals, and favored voluntary sterilization as treatment.

Whereas my opinion is less eugenic, the current categorization in the DSM-IV recapitulates many of these same observations (Table 138-1). This definition, while far from perfect, is useful in clinical practice, if for no other reason than it is now so widely accepted and available. It is not particularly useful in clinical practice as a diagnostic tool, however, since the notion of a characteristic being present more prominently than would be expected for a child of similar developmental age and stage is difficult for most clinicians in practice.

We have therefore favored tools that embed such knowledge of child development in the instrument itself. That is, rating scales that take the child's age into account in their scoring are more useful in clinical practice. Many such scales are available. I have favored the use of Conners' Rating Scales (in parent and child versions) (Fig. 138-1), because of its demonstrated validity, ease of administration and scoring, as well as its broad age range (3 through 17 years) (Conners, 1973). It should be noted that such rating scales do not make a clinical diagnosis, but help the clinician define a child with a high likelihood of such a diagnosis, or conversely lead one to look elsewhere for the origin of the child's troubles.

Whereas the Conners' Scales help define certain target behaviors in a patient history closely associated with attention, anxiety, and conduct disorders, the clinician may find it useful to expand the history gathering to elicit other psychiatric symptoms. Instruments such as Achenbach's Child Behavior Checklist (Achenbach, 1978) (Fig. 138-2) are useful in this regard, and again have the advantage of easy administration and scoring. They do not replace patient evaluation and interview, but may help the clinician direct the interview, or lead to further evaluation in a more appropriate setting.

Adult models of selective and tonic attention have yet to establish validity in research on developing brain. However, current research in children strongly suggest that subtypes of attention disorders exist in childhood, and may parallel those in the adult. At present, in clinical practice one recognizes the syndromic nature of the "diagnosis" of an attention deficit disorder, and may be influenced in treatment choice by some provisional subtype definition. It is difficult to support a more elaborated approach in clinical practice at present.

Learning disorders represent an even more complex situation, and have been likened by some exasperated researchers to pornography—hard to define, but known when seen. In this regard, a reasonable working definition of a childhood learning disorder would be a dysfunction in one or several, but not many, cognitive domains that is not due to primary sensory deficits or lack of language fluency. The crux of this definition lies in

TABLE 138-1. Diagnostic Criteria for Attention-Deficit/ Hyperactivity Disorder

A. Either (1) or (2):
  (1) Six (or more) of the following symptoms of inattention have persisted for at least 6 months to a degree that is maladaptive and inconsistent with developmental level:

    Inattention
    (a) Often fails to give close attention to details or makes careless mistakes in schoolwork, work, or other activities
    (b) Often has difficulty sustaining attention in tasks or play activities
    (c) Often does not seem to listen when spoken to directly
    (d) Often does not follow through on instructions and fails to finish schoolwork, chores, or duties in the workplace (not due to oppositional behavior or failure to understand instructions)
    (e) Often has difficulty organizing tasks and activities
    (f) Often avoids, dislikes, or is reluctant to engage in tasks that require sustained mental effort (such as schoolwork or homework)
    (g) Often loses things necessary for tasks or activities (e.g., toys, school assignments, pencils, books, or tools)
    (h) Is often easily distracted by extraneous stimuli
    (i) Is often forgetful in daily activities

  (2) Six (or more) of the following symptoms of hyperactivity-impulsivity have have persisted for at least 6 months to a degree that is maladaptive and inconsistent with developmental level:

    Hyperactivity
    (a) Often fidgets with hands or feet or squirms in seat
    (b) Often leaves seat in classroom or in other situations in which remaining seated is expected
    (c) Often runs about or climbs excessively in situations in which it is inappropriate (in adolescents or adults, may be limited to subjective feelings of restlessness)
    (d) Often has difficulty playing or engaging in leisure activities quietly
    (e) Is often "on the go" or often acts as if "driven by a motor"
    (f) Often talks excessively
    Impulsivity
    (g) Often blurts out answers before questions have been completed
    (h) Often has difficulty awaiting turn
    (i) Often interrupts or intrudes on others (e.g., butts into conversations or games)

B. Some hyperactive-impulsive or inattention symptoms that caused impairment were present before age 7 years

C. Some impairment from the symptoms is present in two or more settings (e.g., at school [or work] and at home)

D. There must be clear evidence of clinically significant impairment in social, academic, or occupational functioning

E. The symptoms do not occur exclusively during the course of a pervasive developmental disorder, schizophrenia, or other psychotic disorder and are not better accounted for by another mental disorder (e.g., mood disorder, anxiety disorder, dissociative disorder, or a personality disorder)

Code based on type
  314.01 Attention-deficit/hyperactivity disorder, combined type, if both criteria A1 and A2 are met for the past 6 months
  314.00 Attention-deficit/hyperactivity disorder, predominantly inattentive type, if criterion A1 is met but criterion A2 is not met for the past 6 months
  314.01 Attention-deficit/hyperactivity disorder, predominantly hyperactive-impulsive type, if criterion A2 is met but criterion A1 is not met for the past 6 months

Coding note: For individuals (especially adolescents and adults) who currently have symptoms that no longer meet full criteria, "in partial remission" should be specified.

(From American Psychiatric Association Staff: Diagnostic and Statistical Manual of Mental Disorders: DSM-IV. 4th Ed. American Psychiatric Association, New York, 1995, with permission.)

delineating what a "cognitive domain" might be, and how one measures dysfunction.

Extreme cases help define some working limitations. Society, and especially the child's environment in school, determine certain important elements. I have utterly no musical abilities whatsoever, and possess what is commonly referred to as a "tin ear"; since twentieth-century American society does not demand that I do anything musical, I am not considered disabled. In Tonga, however, where all responsible and educated citizens are expected to master the nose flute and compose original material for it, I would be considered profoundly disabled.

The stance of the practicing physician, then, must be to help families identify a pathway through this morass, and follow it. The physician has a role as advocate for the child, reminding the family and school that any individual's needs must be met

Teacher's Questionnaire

Name of Child   Grade

Date of Evaluation

Please answer all questions. Beside *each* item, indicate the degree
of the problem by a check mark (√)

	Not at all	Just a little	Pretty much	Very much
1. Restless in the "squirmy" sense.				
2. Makes inappropriate noises when he shouldn't.				
3. Demands must be met immediately.				
4. Acts "smart" (impudent or sassy).				
5. Temper outbursts and unpredictable behavior.				
6. Overly sensitive to criticism.				
7. Distractibility or attention span a problem.				
8. Disturbs other children.				
9. Daydreams.				
10. Pouts and sulks.				
11. Mood changes quickly and drastically.				
12. Quarrelsome.				
13. Submissive attitude toward authority.				
14. Restless, always "up and on the go."				
15. Excitable, impulsive.				
16. Excessive demands for teacher's attention.				
17. Appears to be unaccepted by group.				
18. Appears to be easily led by other children.				
19. No sense of fair play.				
20. Appears to lack leadership.				
21. Fails to finish things that he starts.				
22. Childish and immature.				
23. Denies mistakes or blames others.				
24. Does not get along well with other children.				
25. Uncooperative with classmates.				
26. Easily frustrated in efforts.				
27. Uncooperative with teacher.				
28. Difficulty in learning.				

FIG. 138-1. Example of Conners' Teacher's Rating Scale Questionnaire.

as circumstances best allow and that the focus should be on that child's unique gifts and needs. The role of the physician is also to protect child and family from the gurus, charlatans, and experts who populate this arena, and prey, unconsciously or premeditatedly, upon parents' deepest fears and vulnerabilities.

The practicing physician, then, requires some rational, systematic approach to this area, just as in any area of difficult clinical practice where experience and judgment are difficult and the scientific basis is the thinnest. What follows is one such approach, used in our unit, which the practicing physician may find useful.

PATIENT HISTORY

In addition to the standard medical history taken in clinical pediatric neurologic practice, certain other items in the child's background prove useful. A detailed developmental history is obviously important, as are detailed observations of the child's function in two rather different settings: home and school. Our unit has relied heavily upon structured, historical questionnaires to obtain certain pieces of this history. This allows the encounter to be a bit more efficient, and also allows direct access to teacher observations, without demanding that the teacher be present or communicated with on a constant basis.

ASSESSMENT

In addition to the standard neurologic examination, the physician needs to have certain measures of cognitive function available in order to make an appropriate diagnosis in a patient. Standardized intelligence testing is beyond the ken of most physicians. Language screening, however, is crucial to this area, as is some determination of a child's ability to manipulate complex visuospatial material.

TEACHER'S REPORT FORM FOR AGES 5–18

Please Print

For office use only
ID #

Your answers will be used to compare the pupil with other pupils whose teachers have completed similar forms. The information from this form will also be used for comparison with other information about this pupil. Please answer as well as you can, even if you lack full information. Scores on individual items will be combined to identify general patterns of behavior. Feel free to print additional comments beside each item and in the spaces provided on page 2.

PUPIL'S FULL NAME	FIRST	MIDDLE	LAST	PARENTS' USUAL TYPE OF WORK, even if not working now (*Please be as specific as you can—for example, auto mechanic, high school teacher, homemaker, laborer, lathe operator, shoe salesman, army sergeant.*)

PUPIL'S SEX ☐ Boy ☐ Girl

PUPIL'S AGE

ETHNIC GROUP OR RACE

FATHER'S TYPE OF WORK: _____

MOTHER'S TYPE OF WORK _____

TODAY'S DATE
Mo. _____ Date _____ Yr. _____

PUPIL'S BIRTHDATE (if known)
Mo. _____ Date _____ Yr. _____

THIS FORM FILLED OUT BY:

☐ Teacher (full name) _____

☐ Counselor (full name) _____

GRADE IN SCHOOL

NAME AND ADDRESS OF SCHOOL

☐ Other (specify position & give full name): _____

I.   For how many months have you known this pupil? _____ months

II. How well do you know him/her?   1. ☐ Not Well   2. ☐ Moderately Well   3. ☐ Very Well

III. How much time does he/she spend in your class or service per week?

IV. What kind of class or service is it? (Please be specific, e.g., regular 5th grade, 7th grade math, learning disabled, counseling, etc.)

V.   Has he/she ever been referred for special class placement, services, or tutoring?
     ☐ Don't Know   0. ☐ No   1. ☐ Yes—what kind and when?

VI. Has he/she repeated any grades?
     ☐ Don't Know   0. ☐ No   1. ☐ Yes—grades and reasons

VII. Current school performance—list academic subjects and check box that indicates pupil's performance for each subject:

Academic subject	1. Far below grade	2. Somewhat below grade	3. At grade level	4. Somewhat above grade	5. Far above grade
1. _____	☐	☐	☐	☐	☐
2. _____	☐	☐	☐	☐	☐
3. _____	☐	☐	☐	☐	☐
4. _____	☐	☐	☐	☐	☐
5. _____	☐	☐	☐	☐	☐
6. _____	☐	☐	☐	☐	☐

A

FIG. 138-2. Examples of the Achenbach Child Behavior Checklist. **(A)** Teacher's checklist. **(B)** Parent's checklist. (© Thomas M. Achenbach Center for Children, Youth, and Families, University of Vermont, Burlington, VT. Reprinted with permission.)

Please Print

Below is a list of items that describe pupils. For each item that describes the pupil *now or within the past 2 months,* please circle the *2* if the item is *very true or often true* of the pupil. Circle the *1* if the item is *somewhat or sometimes true* of the pupil. If the item is *not true* of the pupil, circle the *0*. Please answer all items as well as you can, even if some do not seem to apply to this pupil.

0 = Not True (as far as you know)   1 = Somewhat or Sometimes True   2 = Very True or Often True

0 1 2   1. Acts too young for his/her age
0 1 2   2. Hums or makes other odd noises in class

0 1 2   3. Argues a lot
0 1 2   4. Fails to finish things he/she starts

0 1 2   5. Behaves like opposite sex
0 1 2   6. Defiant, talks back to staff

0 1 2   7. Bragging, boasting
0 1 2   8. Can't concentrate, can't pay attention for long

0 1 2   9. Can't get his/her mind off certain thoughts; obsessions (describe): _____

0 1 2   10. Can't sit still, restless, or hyperactive

0 1 2   11. Clings to adults or too dependent

0 1 2   12. Complains of loneliness

0 1 2   13. Confused or seems to be in a fog
0 1 2   14. Cries a lot

0 1 2   15. Fidgets
0 1 2   16. Cruelty, bullying, or meanness to others

0 1 2   17. Daydreams or gets lost in his/her thoughts
0 1 2   18. Deliberately harms self or attempts suicide

0 1 2   19. Demands a lot of attention
0 1 2   20. Destroys his/her own things

0 1 2   21. Destroys property belonging to others
0 1 2   22. Difficulty following directions

0 1 2   23. Disobedient at school
0 1 2   24. Disturbs other pupils

0 1 2   25. Doesn't get along with other pupils
0 1 2   26. Doesn't seem to feel guilty after misbehaving

0 1 2   27. Easily jealous
0 1 2   28. Eats or drinks things that are not food—*don't* include sweets (describe):_____

0 1 2   29. Fears certain animals, situations, or places other than school (describe): _____

0 1 2   30. Fears going to school

0 1 2   31. Fears he/she might think or do something bad
0 1 2   32. Feels he/she has to be perfect

0 1 2   33. Feels or complains that no one loves him/her
0 1 2   34. Feels others are out to get him/her

0 1 2   35. Feels worthless or inferior
0 1 2   36. Gets hurt a lot, accident-prone

0 1 2   37. Gets in many fights
0 1 2   38. Gets teased a lot

0 1 2   39. Hangs around with others who get in trouble
0 1 2   40. Hears sounds or voices that aren't there (describe):

0 1 2   41. Impulsive or acts without thinking
0 1 2   42. Would rather be alone than with others

0 1 2   43. Lying or cheating
0 1 2   44. Bites fingernails

0 1 2   45. Nervous, high-strung, or tense
0 1 2   46. Nervous movements or twitching (describe):

0 1 2   47. Overconforms to rules
0 1 2   48. Not liked by other pupils

0 1 2   49. Has difficulty learning
0 1 2   50. Too fearful or anxious

0 1 2   51. Feels dizzy
0 1 2   52. Feels too guilty

0 1 2   53. Talks out of turn
0 1 2   54. Overtired

0 1 2   55. Overweight
56. Physical problems *without known medical cause:*
0 1 2   a. Aches or pains (*not* stomach or headaches)
0 1 2   b. Headaches
0 1 2   c. Nausea, feel sick
0 1 2   d. Problems with eyes (*not* if corrected by glasses) (describe):

0 1 2   e. Rashes or other skin problems
0 1 2   f. Stomachaches or cramps
0 1 2   g. Vomiting, throwing up
0 1 2   h. Other (describe):_____

FIG. 138-2. (A) *(Continued).*

CHILD BEHAVIOR CHECKLIST FOR AGES 4–18

Please Print

For office use only
ID #

CHILD'S FULL NAME   FIRST   MIDDLE   LAST

PARENTS' USUAL TYPE OF WORK, even if not working now. *(Please be specific—for example, auto mechanic, high school teacher, homemaker, laborer, lathe operator, shoe salesman. army sergeant.)*

SEX   ☐ Boy   ☐ Girl

AGE

ETHNIC GROUP OR RACE

FATHER'S
TYPE OF WORK: _____

TODAY'S DATE   Mo. _____ Date _____ Yr. _____

CHILD'S BIRTHDATE   Mo. _____ Date _____ Yr. _____

MOTHER'S
TYPE OF WORK: _____

GRADE IN SCHOOL _____

NOT ATTENDING SCHOOL ☐

Please fill out this form to reflect *your* view of the child's behavior even if other people might not agree. Feel free to print additional comments beside each item and in the spaces provided on page 2.

THIS FORM FILLED OUT BY:

☐ Mother $\left(\begin{smallmatrix}\text{full}\\\text{name}\end{smallmatrix}\right)$ _____

☐ Father $\left(\begin{smallmatrix}\text{full}\\\text{name}\end{smallmatrix}\right)$ _____

☐ Other—full name & relationship to child: _____

I. Please list the sports your child most likes to take part in. For example: swimming, baseball, skating, skate boarding, bike riding, fishing, etc.

☐ None

	Compared to others of the same age, about how much time does he/she spend in each?				Compared to others of the same age, how well does he/she do each one?			
	Don't Know	Less Than Average	Average	More Than Average	Don't Know	Below Average	Average	Above Average
a. _____	☐	☐	☐	☐	☐	☐	☐	☐
b. _____	☐	☐	☐	☐	☐	☐	☐	☐
c. _____	☐	☐	☐	☐	☐	☐	☐	☐

II. Please list your child's favorite hobbies, activities, and games, other than sports. For example: stamps dolls, books, piano, crafts, cars, singing, etc. (Do *not* include listening to radio or TV.)

☐ None

	Compared to others of the same age, about how much time does he/she spend in each?				Compared to others of the same age, how well does he/she do each one?			
	Don't Know	Less Than Average	Average	More Than Average	Don't Know	Below Average	Average	Above Average
a. _____	☐	☐	☐	☐	☐	☐	☐	☐
b. _____	☐	☐	☐	☐	☐	☐	☐	☐
c. _____	☐	☐	☐	☐	☐	☐	☐	☐

III. Please list any organizations, clubs, teams, or groups your child belongs to.

☐ None

	Compared to others of the same age, how active is he/she in each?			
	Don't Know	Less Active	Average	More Active
a. _____	☐	☐	☐	☐
b. _____	☐	☐	☐	☐
c. _____	☐	☐	☐	☐

IV. Please list any jobs or chores your child has. For example: paper route, babysitting, making bed, working in store, etc. (Include *both* paid and unpaid jobs and chores.)

☐ None

	Compared to others of the same age, how well does he/she carry them out?			
	Don't Know	Below Average	Average	Above Average
a. _____	☐	☐	☐	☐
b. _____	☐	☐	☐	☐
c. _____	☐	☐	☐	☐

B

FIG. 138-2. (B) *(Continued).*

Below is a list of items that describe children and youth. For each item that describes your child *now or within the past 6 months*, please circle the *2* if the item is *very true or often true* of your child. Circle the *1* if the item is *somewhat or sometimes true* of your child. If the item is *not true* of your child, circle the *0*. Please answer all items as well as you can, even if some do not seem to apply to your child.

Please Print

0 = Not True (as far as you know)   1 = Somewhat or Sometimes True   2 = Very True or Often True

0 1 2	1.	Acts too young for his/her age		0 1 2	31.	Fears he/she might think or do something bad
0 1 2	2.	Allergy (describe): _____				
		_____		0 1 2	32.	Feels he/she has to be perfect
				0 1 2	33.	Feels or complains that no one loves him/her
0 1 2	3.	Argues a lot				
0 1 2	4.	Asthma		0 1 2	34.	Feels others are out to get him/her
				0 1 2	35.	Feels worthless or inferior
0 1 2	5.	Behaves like opposite sex				
0 1 2	6.	Bowel movements outside toilet		0 1 2	36.	Gets hurt a lot, accident-prone
				0 1 2	37.	Gets in many fights
0 1 2	7.	Bragging, boasting				
0 1 2	8.	Can't concentrate, can't pay attention for long		0 1 2	38.	Gets teased a lot
				0 1 2	39.	Hangs around with others who get in trouble
0 1 2	9.	Can't get his/her mind off certain thoughts; obsessions (describe): _____		0 1 2	40.	Hears sounds or voices that aren't there (describe): _____
		_____				
0 1 2	10.	Can't sit still, restless, or hyperactive				_____
				0 1 2	41.	Impulsive or acts without thinking
0 1 2	11.	Clings to adults or too dependent				
0 1 2	12.	Complains of loneliness		0 1 2	42.	Would rather be alone than with others
				0 1 2	43.	Lying or cheating
0 1 2	13.	Confused or seems to be in a fog				
0 1 2	14.	Cries a lot		0 1 2	44.	Bites fingernails
				0 1 2	45.	Nervous, highstrung, or tense
0 1 2	15.	Cruel to animals				
0 1 2	16.	Cruelty, bullying, or meanness to others		0 1 2	46.	Nervous movements or twitching (describe):
						_____
0 1 2	17.	Day-dreams or gets lost in his/her thoughts				_____
0 1 2	18.	Deliberately harms self or attempts suicide		0 1 2	47.	Nightmares
0 1 2	19.	Demands a lot of attention		0 1 2	48.	Not liked by other kids
0 1 2	20.	Destroys his/her own things		0 1 2	49.	Constipated, doesn't move bowels
0 1 2	21.	Destroys things belonging to his/her family or others		0 1 2	50.	Too fearful or anxious
0 1 2	22.	Disobedient at home		0 1 2	51.	Feels dizzy
0 1 2	23.	Disobedient at school		0 1 2	52.	Feels too guilty
0 1 2	24.	Doesn't eat well		0 1 2	53.	Overeating
0 1 2	25.	Doesn't get along with other kids		0 1 2	54.	Overtired
0 1 2	26.	Doesn't seem to feel guilty after misbehaving		0 1 2	55.	Overweight
0 1 2	27.	Easily jealous			56.	Physical problems *without known medical cause:*
0 1 2	28.	Eats or drinks things that are not food — *don't* include sweets (describe): _____		0 1 2		a. Aches or pains (*not* stomach or headaches)
				0 1 2		b. Headaches
		_____		0 1 2		c. Nausea, feels sick
				0 1 2		d. Problems with eyes (*not* if corrected by glasses) (describe): _____
0 1 2	29.	Fears certain animals, situations, or places, other than school (describe): _____		0 1 2		e. Rashes or other skin problems
				0 1 2		f. Stomachaches or cramps
		_____		0 1 2		g. Vomiting, throwing up
0 1 2	30.	Fears going to school		0 1 2		h. Other (describe): _____

FIG. 138-2. (B)   *(Continued).*

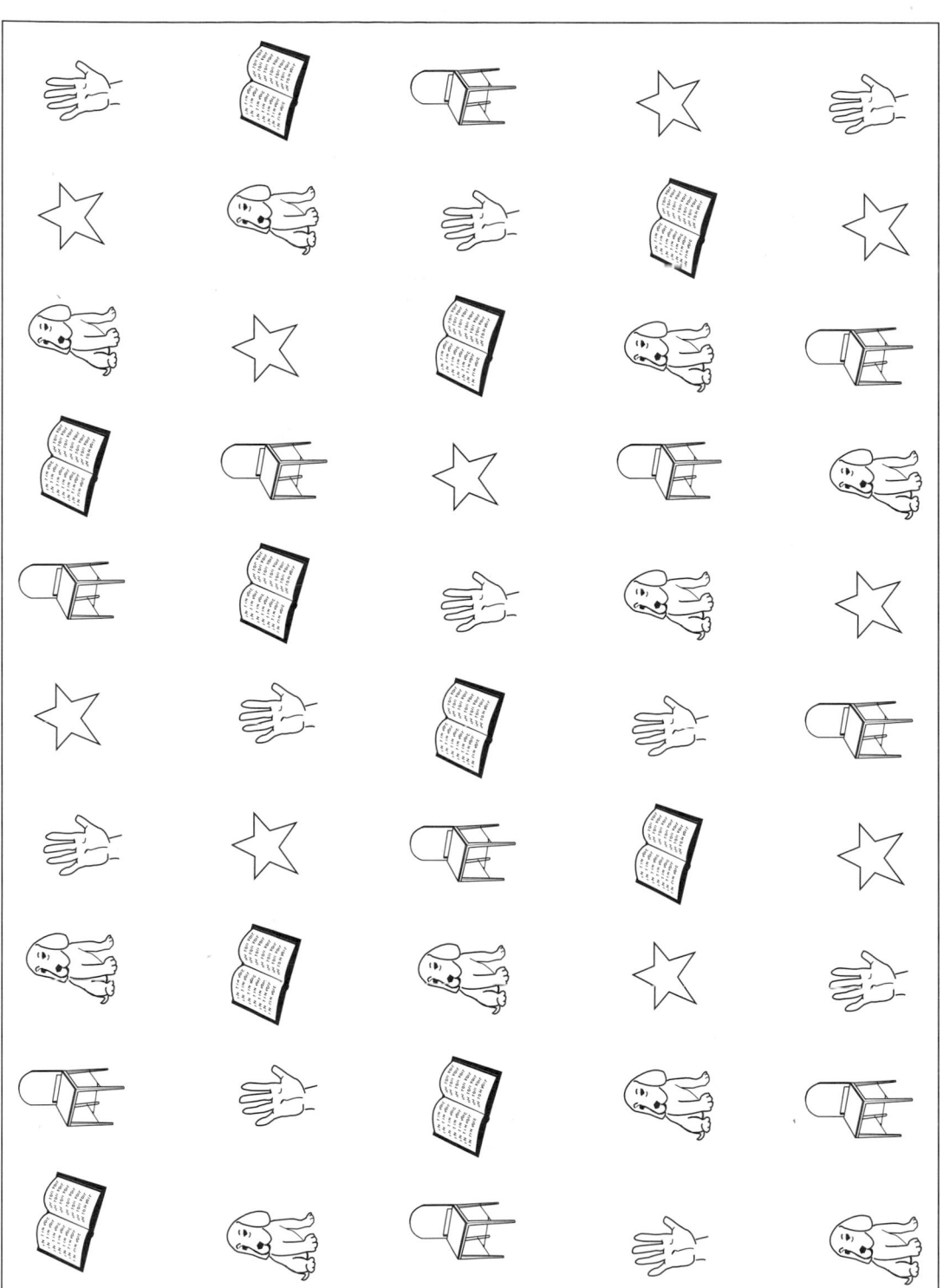

FIG. 138-3. An example of the Rapid Automatized Naming Battery.

Language Screening

Language screening in the office is best done through a combination of informal assessment (when all else fails, talk to the patient) and standardized measures. In office practice, assessment should include vocabulary, word retrieval, word fluency, and automaticity of recall measures.

Vocabulary can be assessed in most school-age children by the Peabody Picture Vocabulary Test, which asks the child to identify a vocabulary item from a set of four related pictures (Dunn, 1970). The test is standardized, and relatively uninfluenced by cultural or ethnic origins.

Word retrieval is best assessed using the Boston Naming Test (Goodglass and Kaplan, 1983; Kaplan et al., 1983), which is standardized for children over the age of 5, and also free of cultural bias. The task here is to identify a presented picture, offered in a series of line drawings arranged in their order of use, in colloquial North American English. The score generated is the last item answered correctly before six consecutive errors, minus the scattered early errors. In addition to the quantitative aspect of the test, the presence of paraphasic errors can also be noted qualitatively. Semantic paraphasias (*hippopotamus* for *rhinoceros*) are common in childhood language disorders; literal paraphasias (*pellet* for *palette*) less so and thus of more interest to the clinician.

Word fluency, the ability to sort vocabulary by phonologic category, is an important foundation skill for literacy, and thus should be assessed. The NCCEA Word Fluency Task is standardized for children over the age of six, and thus has great advantage in clinical practice. The patient is asked to list as many words as he or she can remember in one minute that start with a given letter; proper nouns are excluded. The letters used for the English-language version of this test are *F, A,* and *S.* The score generated is the number of legitimate responses for each letter, summed together, minus the disallowed responses. The test is normed beginning at age 6.

Some investigators have demonstrated that the automaticity of retrieval is the best predictor of later reading ability in young children; hence, measuring this in a first-grader who is having trouble learning to read is an important screening evaluation for the physician. The child who can perform this task adequately is at lower risk than the child who struggles. ''Watchful waiting'' may be appropriate for the child who performs such tasks well; it is an unacceptable stance for a child who does this task poorly. The Rapid Automatized Naming Battery and Rapid Alternating Stimulus Battery are standardized for children 5 years of age and older (Fig. 138-3). The task here is to name the stimuli in order as rapidly as possible. The score generated is the time required to complete the task. Errors are also noted as a qualitative observation. The test is normed beginning at age 5.

These language screening measures will help the physician determine which children require further language or reading assessment, and those whose issues may be more developmental in nature. Many young children struggle with early reading. The child who struggles with reading but performs well on all these tasks should receive some follow-up screening to ensure that reading levels are improving steadily. The child who has poor word retrieval skills, who has reduced automaticity, or who has a poor knowledge of phonology is a child at risk and should be referred for further evaluation.

Visuospatial Screening

Visuospatial skills are also central to the child's experience of school. We have preferred the Rey-Osterreith Complex Figure

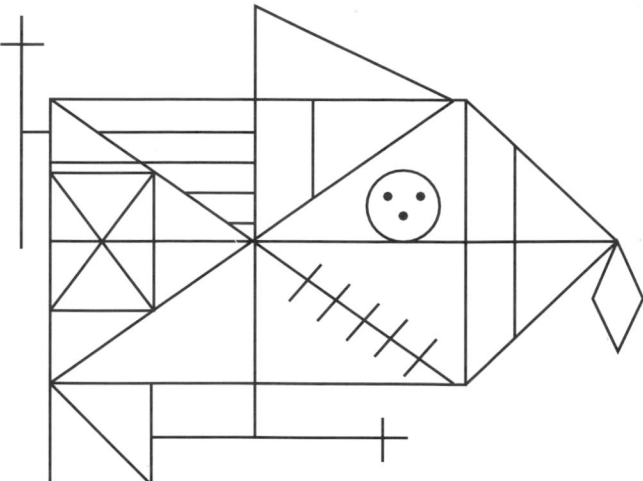

FIG. 138-4. The Rey-Osterreith Complex Figure.

(Fig. 138-4) as the most useful tool for assessment in this area. It has been standardized, and thus allows for some rational measurement of this capacity; like the Boston Naming Test, it is a rich task, with much qualitative information available as well. A child who is said to be struggling with the integration of complex material in school and who performs poorly on this task is probably not suffering from an attention deficit disorder, but rather from some form of a learning disorder that is unlikely to respond to medication. This situation may require more involved academic testing to determine how the patient might better approach complex material.

The examination, then, consists of a series of screening maneuvers to evaluate language and visuospatial function, two commonly encountered areas of dysfunction in childhood. If the child has strong historical evidence of attention problems and no difficulties on most of these tasks, then a diagnosis of an attention deficit disorder may be made in isolation. It is likely that such a child will have a favorable response to medication (see Treatment, below), and further academic testing may be held until response to medication is determined. If the child has no evidence of attention problems by patient history, and significant difficulties on these screening maneuvers, or evidence of attention problems with concomitant problems on screening, then further evaluation should be undertaken before any medical management is proposed.

TREATMENT

Treatment represents the most vexatious area of clinical practice. Beyond straightforward decisions such as treating a seizure disorder discovered in the course of evaluation, the real decision rests with trials of medication for attention problems.

Choice of medication is crucial. For all the controversy in the lay press, stimulants (methylphenidate, dextroamphetamine, pemoline) are still the mainstays of such therapy.

Methylphenidate (Ritalin)

Methylphenidate is available in short-duration and sustained-release preparations. Whereas each child's metabolism of these compounds varies, the average half-life of the regular formulation compound is 4 to 6 hours, and of sustained release is 6 to 8. Dosing should begin at 0.5 mg/kg/day, and proceed stepwise as indicated by clinical response. Doses above 1.5 mg/kg/day are of dubious clinical benefit. Common side effects include insomnia, appetite suppression, headache, nausea, and motor tics. These are treatment-related, and cease after medication is withdrawn. Tourette syndrome may be exacerbated, or even potentiated, by the administration of stimulants; thus, a careful elicitation of a family history is important, and other medications should be chosen if a strong family history of tics or obsessive-compulsive disorders is discovered.

Dextroamphetamine (Dexedrine)

Dextroamphetamine is an alternative to methylphenidate. The functional half-life of this medication is somewhat shorter than methylphenidate's in many children, and thus may require more frequent dosing. It exists in regular and extended-release forms (the latter known as spansules). Potency is roughly twice that of methylphenidate, and so dosing ranges for children are between 0.25 and 0.75 mg/kg/day.

Side effects are similar to those of methylphenidate; cross-reactivity to side effects is not complete, and hence offering dextroamphetamine to a child who has experienced anorexia on methylphenidate is rational.

Pemoline (Cylert)

Pemoline is the third stimulant available in the United States for the treatment of attention disorders. It has a long half-life, and thus allows for once-daily dosing. Given its pharmacokinetics, onset of action is slower than with the other two stimulants, and thus may be limiting for some children who still have difficulties in the early stages of treatment. Dosing regimens are usually between 1 and 3 mg/kg/day.

Side effects are similar to those of methylphenidate and dextroamphetamine; the *Physician's Desk Reference* advocates periodic examination of the transaminases, because of early, rare reports of hepatotoxicity. This has not been an issue in children in my 10-year experience with this medication, and may be more of an issue for adults.

Tricyclic Agents

Tricyclic agents, particularly of the desmethylated imipramine derivative group (such as desipramine or nortriptyline), have a demonstrable efficacy in the treatment of attention disorders. They are good choices when coincident depression is diagnosed, and may be more helpful in older children and adolescents with attention disorders. Given their long half-lives, they allow for once- or twice-daily dosing. The usual dosing range for attentional problems is 1 to 3 mg/kg/day; blood levels are

poorly correlated with clinical efficacy in this usage, and thus are often not measured.

The potential cardiotoxicity of these medications has led to great concern. Several deaths, apparently from arrhythmias, have been alleged. It is therefore prudent to obtain pretreatment electrocardiograms to assess whether any abnormalities of the Q-T interval exist, as well as to take a careful family history for any potential inherited signs of sudden cardiac death.

Clonidine

Clonidine has demonstrated efficacy in the treatment of attention disorders. It is also beneficial in the treatment of motor and vocal tics, and may therefore be a good choice in the individual with Tourette syndrome and attention disorder, a common comorbid pattern. The dosing regimen is 0.005 to 0.01 mg/kg/day, and the medication is available in pill and transdermal patch forms. The latter is useful when sedation, the most commonly encountered side effect of clonidine, is an issue.

Other Medications

A plethora of other agents are in use for the treatment of attention disorders. Research has yet to establish a strong foundation regarding the efficacy of many of these other medications in the current clinical literature. In children with impulsivity that is not attributable to mental retardation, the use of clonidine or busiprone has yielded beneficial results. The dosage range for the latter agent is 0.25 to 10 mg/kg/day.

SUGGESTED READINGS

Achenbach TM: The child behavior profile: I. Boys aged 6–11. J Consult Clin Psychol 46:478–88, 1978
Conners CK: Rating scales for use in drug studies with children, Psychopharmacol Bull 9:24–84, 1973
Dunn LM: Expanded Manual for the Peabody Picture Vocabulary Test. American Guidance Services, Minneapolis, 1970
Goodglass H, Kaplan E: The Assessment of Aphasia and Related Disorders. 2nd Ed. Lea & Febiger, Philadelphia, 1983
Kaplan E, Goodglass H, Weintraub S, Segal O: Boston Naming Test. Lea & Febiger, Philadelphia, 1983
Levine MD: Attentional variation and dysfunction. pp. 468–76. In Levine MD, Carey WB, Crocker AC (eds): Developmental-Behavioral Pediatrics. 2nd Ed. WB Saunders, Philadelphia, 1992
Levine MD: Neurodevelopmental variation and dysfunction among school-aged children. pp. 477–90. In Levine MD, Carey WB, Crocker AC (eds): Developmental-Behavioral Pediatrics. 2nd Ed. WB Saunders, Philadelphia, 1992
Osterreith P: Le test de copie d'une figure complexe. Arch Psychol 30:206, 1994
Rey A: L'examen psychologique dan les cas d'encéphalopathie traumatique. Arch Psychol 28:112, 1941
Weintraub S, Mesulam M-M: Mental state assessment of young and elderly adults in behavioral neurology. pp. 84–99. In Mesulam M-M (ed): Principles of Behavioral Neurology. FA Davis, Philadelphia, 1985

SECTION 2. EPILEPSY

139. EPILEPSY IN CHILDREN

GREGORY L. HOLMES

Epilepsy is one of the most frequently encountered neurologic problems presenting in childhood. Children with seizures differ from adults in a number of ways, including the type of epileptic syndrome, prognosis, and therapy. In this chapter some of the unique features of seizures in children are discussed.

The history and neurologic examination remain the cornerstone of the diagnosis in epilepsy. It is important to determine by history whether the patient had a seizure and, if so, what type. The clinician evaluating the child with a history of a paroxysmal disorder must differentiate a seizure disorder from other episodic disorders such as breath-holding attacks, syncope, night terrors, or movement disorders such as tics or choreoathetosis. A careful history or observation of the event usually is sufficient to distinguish seizures from nonepileptic events. For example, breath-holding attacks are invariably preceded by an upsetting event that causes the child to cry. Night terrors occur during slow-wave sleep, as opposed to nocturnal seizures, which typically occur during transitions from wakefulness to sleep or vice versa. If there is uncertainty about the diagnosis, it is usually better to withhold treatment and wait for another attack before embarking on an extensive workup and initiation of antiepileptic drugs.

The electroencephalogram (EEG) can be useful in supporting the clinical suspicion of epilepsy. Epileptiform activity is defined as any paroxysmal discharges containing spikes or sharp waves, either localized or generalized. Spikes refer to transient electrical events lasting less than 70 msec. They typically have a biphasic or polyphasic form, exceed the amplitude of the background activity in the region and are usually followed by a surface-negative slow wave. Sharp waves have a duration of 70 to 200 msec, and, like spikes, are clearly delineated from background activity. Generalized epileptiform discharges consist of spike-and-wave, sharp-and-slow waves, and multiple spikes.

Epileptiform activity on the EEG is rarely diagnostic of epilepsy. For example, in large studies of normal children up to 9 percent will have epileptiform activity on EEG. Conversely, a normal EEG does not rule out the possibility of epilepsy, since patients with well-documented seizures may have normal EEGs. This is particularly important when dealing with partial seizures. It is not uncommon for children with either simple or complex partial seizures to have a normal EEG, sometimes even during the ictal event. The "yield" of the EEG is increased by recording during sleep, hyperventilation, and photic stimulation. If the record is normal sleep deprivation may be useful.

Once the diagnosis of a seizure disorder is established, the clinician should determine the seizure type. The classification of the seizures is given in Chapter 140. The next step is to try to determine whether the child has an epileptic syndrome. A syndrome is defined as a cluster of signs and symptoms customarily occurring together. Identification of an epileptic syndrome

may allow the physician to determine genetic risk, that is, certain epileptic syndromes are associated with specific genotypes. In addition, syndrome identification helps determine the type of evaluation that is necessary, the appropriate therapy, and prognosis.

Epilepsy is defined as two or more unprovoked seizures. Seizures that are precipitated by such factors as fever, head trauma, hypoglycemia, or an intracranial infection are considered to be provoked seizures. The child who has multiple seizures induced by fever would not be considered to have epilepsy.

In this chapter the common clinical and EEG features of childhood seizures and the epilepsies will be discussed (Table 139-1). When the epileptic conditions occur predominantly or exclusively in children, recommendations regarding drug therapy are provided.

PARTIAL SEIZURES IN CHILDREN

Partial seizures in children can vary from those that are quite benign to more malignant conditions. Partial seizures frequently generalize, and most generalized tonic-clonic seizures are partial seizures that secondarily generalize. Often the generalization occurs so quickly that the focal onset is not seen.

Simple Partial Seizures

The signs or symptoms of the simple partial seizure depend on the focus of the seizure. Seizures involving the motor cortex occur most commonly consist of rhythmic to semirhythmic clonic activity of the face, arm, or leg. There is usually no difficulty in diagnosing this type of seizure. Seizures with somatosensory, autonomic, and psychic symptoms (hallucinations, illusions, deja vu) may be more difficult to diagnose. Psychic symptoms usually occur as a component of a complex partial seizure.

Complex Partial Seizures

Complex partial seizures (CPS), formerly called temporal lobe or psychomotor seizures, are one of the most common seizure types encountered in both children and adults. CPS, while commonly beginning in the temporal region, may start elsewhere. The clinical manifestations vary as a function of the seizure onset. CPS may be preceded by a simple partial seizure, which may serve as a warning to the patient (i.e., aura) of a more severe seizures. It is important to recognize that the aura may enable the clinician to determine the cortical area in which the seizure is beginning. Common auras in children include fear, a rising sensation in the abdomen, dizziness, or a feeling that cannot be described.

By definition, all patients with CPS have impaired consciousness; thus the patient does not respond to commands, or responds in an abnormally slow manner. While CPS may be characterized by simple staring and impaired responsiveness, behavior is usually more complex during the seizure. Automatisms (involuntary motor activity) are common during the pe-

TABLE 139-1. Epileptic Syndromes: Typical EEG Features and Treatment

Syndrome	EEG Features	Treatment
Febrile convulsions	Variable	Oral diazepam at time of fever
West syndrome (infantile spasms)	Hypsarrhythmia; modified hypsarrhythmia	ACTH or prednisone
Partial seizures	Focal spikes or sharp waves	Carbamazepine, phenytoin, valproic acid
Childhood absence	Generalized spike-and-wave activity	Ethosuximide
Juvenile absence	Generalized spike-and-wave activity	Valproic acid
Lennox-Gastaut syndrome	Slow (<2.5 Hz) spike waves; slow background, multifocal spikes	Valproic acid, phenytoin, clonazepam, phenobarbital
Benign partial epilepsy with centrotemporal spikes of childhood (benign rolandic epilepsy)	Blunt, high voltage centrotemporal spikes; activated by sleep; rare generalized spike waves	Carbamazepine, phenytoin, valproic acid
Juvenile myoclonic epilepsy	Rapid (3.5–6 Hz) generalized spike wave; frequent photoparoxysmal response	Valproic acid

riod of impaired consciousness in CPS. Automatic behavior is quite variable and may consist of activities such as facial grimacing, gestures, chewing, lip smacking, snapping fingers, and repeating phrases; the patient does not recall this activity following the seizure. Although variable, CPS usually last from 30 seconds to several minutes. This should be contrasted to absence seizures, described below, which usually last less than 15 seconds. Most patients have some degree of postictal impairment, such as tiredness or confusion.

CPS may arise in a variety of locations. Temporal lobe onset, especially in mesial structures (hippocampus and amygdala) often begins with an aura, followed by staring and automatic behavior such as chewing, swallowing, and aimless movements of the hands. CPS beginning in the frontal lobe are more likely to have prominent motor components such as tonic posturing or clonic activity. In addition, these seizures are frequently nocturnal and short in duration.

CPS can be caused by a variety of factors including tumors, trauma, congenital abnormalities, vascular malformations, and infection. A history of a prolonged febrile seizure early in life is often obtained.

Although some children with CPS may "outgrow" their seizure, some patients have seizures that are poorly controlled and continue into adulthood. When medically intractable, surgery should be considered.

Benign Rolandic Epilepsy

Benign rolandic epilepsy (BRE) is an epileptic syndrome that is characterized by nocturnal generalized seizures and diurnal partial seizures arising from the lower rolandic area. The disorder is associated with a striking EEG pattern consisting of midtemporal-central spikes. BRE is a familial disorder with an apparent autosomal dominant pattern with variable penetrance. Siblings of children with BRE may have a similar EEG pattern but never develop seizures.

The patient may present with either nocturnal generalized tonic-clonic seizures or daytime simple partial seizures. The syndrome is termed *rolandic* epilepsy because of the characteristic clinical and electroencephalographic feature of partial seizures involving the region around the lower portion of the central gyrus of Rolando. The characteristic features of benign rolandic epilepsy include an aura of tingling or numbness in the oral-buccal cavity; speech arrest because of motor involvement of the mouth; preservation of consciousness; excessive drooling; and tonic or tonic-clonic activity of the face. In nocturnal seizures the initial event is typically clonic movements of the mouth with salivation and gurgling sounds from the throat.

Secondary generalization of the nocturnal seizure is common. The initial focal component of the seizure may be quite brief, and it is surmised that this portion of the seizure may not be seen by the parents.

The disorder is characterized by a very distinctive, dramatic EEG pattern. The characteristic interictal EEG correlate is distinct high amplitude, usually diphasic spike with a prominent following slow wave in the (rolandic) region.

Despite the dramatic EEG, the disorder was an excellent prognosis with almost all children having a remission of the disorder by age 16 years. Interestingly, despite the dramatic EEG features, the EEG is not predictive of when the child will go into remission.

Evaluation of Children With Partial Seizures

All patients with partial seizures, whether simple or complex, should have an EEG, which should include periods of sleep and wakefulness, hyperventilation, and photic stimulation. The EEG, while not diagnostic of epilepsy, can provide supporting evidence for the diagnosis. Focal spikes and sharp waves, termed epileptiform activity, suggest an epileptic region. Patients with BRE should have spikes in the midtemporal or central region. While patients with active BRE should always have an abnormal EEG, the lack of epileptiform activity does not eliminate the possibility of other types of partial seizures. For example, patients with complex partial seizures beginning in the mesial aspects of the temporal lobe (hippocampus or amygdala) frequently have normal EEGs.

Patients with BRE and normal neurologic examinations need no further diagnostic tests. Other patients with simple or complex partial seizures should have neuroimaging to rule out a structural lesion such as a tumor. While computed tomography (CT) scanning will usually eliminate the possibility of a malignant lesion, magnetic resonance imaging (MRI) is more sensitive for scar tissue and congenital brain anomalies.

Treatment of Children with Partial Seizures

In the recent past it was not unusual for children or adults to be placed on both phenytoin and phenobarbital for their first generalized tonic-clonic seizure or partial seizure. There are now an increasing number of physicians deciding not to treat the first seizure with antiepileptic drugs (AEDs) at all. In a prospective study, 238 children with a first unprovoked seizure were closely followed for a mean of 30 months by Shinnar and his colleagues in the Bronx. The vast majority of the children were not treated with AEDs. Subsequent seizures occurred in only 36 percent. The cumulative risk for recurrence was 60 percent at 36 months in children with a history of a static neurologic insult (termed *remote symptomatic* by the authors) versus 36 percent in children with an idiopathic seizure. The EEG was the most important predictor of recurrence in children with idiopathic seizures. Children with an idiopathic seizure and a normal EEG had a cumulative recurrence risk of 26 percent at 36 months. Age at the time of the first seizure and duration of the seizure did not affect recurrence risk. This study of largely untreated children demonstrated that the recurrence risk following a first unprovoked seizure is low.

There are many factors that must be considered when deciding whether to start AED therapy and each child must be evaluated as an individual. However, in view of the not insignificant risk encountered with AEDs, in most children it appears reasonable to wait for a second seizure before subjecting the child to years of drug therapy. In the case of BRE, where the prognosis is uniformly good, some clinicians do not recommend treatment until the child has had three or even more seizures.

In children there are a variety of drugs that are effective in the treatment of partial seizures, including the established drugs carbamazepine, valproate, and phenytoin. While not extensively studied in children, felbamate and gabapentin appear to be effective in the treatment of partial seizures.

GENERALIZED SEIZURES IN CHILDREN

Generalized seizures are those that begin suddenly, and without warning, and involve bilateral cortical structures from onset. Seizure severity varies from dramatic generalized tonic-clonic seizures to more subtle absence seizures.

Generalized Tonic-Clonic Seizures

As noted above, most generalized tonic-clonic seizures are partial seizures that generalize. Children that have primary generalized tonic-clonic seizures usually have other types of generalized seizures such as absence or myoclonic, or both. Typically these patients have normal development and neurologic examinations and have a positive family history for epilepsy. EEGs typically demonstrate generalized bursts of spike-and-wave.

Absence Seizures

Formerly termed *petit mal,* typical absence seizures are usually characterized by an abrupt cessation of activity, and a change of facial expression with a "blank" gaze. The seizures are short, rarely lasting over 30 seconds, and are never associated with an aura or postictal impairment. Typical absence seizures almost always begin during childhood, with the usual age of onset between 3 and 6 years. While they occasionally continue into adulthood, they are most prevalent during the first 10 years of life. In the majority of patients with typical absence seizures the neurologic examination is normal.

Hyperventilation is a very useful technique when typical absence seizures are suspected. Three minutes of hyperventilation in an untreated child is quite likely to induce an absence seizure. Photic stimulation, usually administered during the EEG, may also precipitate an absence seizure. The EEG signature of a typical absence seizure is the sudden onset of 3 Hz generalized symmetrical spike- or polyspike-and-slow wave complexes. A normal EEG during the awake and sleep states as well as during hyperventilation and photic stimulation in an untreated child makes the diagnosis of absence epilepsy very unlikely.

There are three syndromes in which absence seizures are one of the seizure types; childhood absence (pyknolepsy) epilepsy, juvenile absence epilepsy, and juvenile myoclonic epilepsy (JME). *Pyknolepsy* describes typical absence seizures (i.e., both simple and complex) in children between the ages of 3 and 5 years and puberty, who are otherwise normal. There is a strong genetic predisposition, and girls are more frequently affected. The absences are very frequent, occurring at least several times daily, and tend to cluster. The absences may remit during adolescence, but generalized tonic-clonic seizures may develop. *Juvenile absence epilepsy* begins around puberty, and differs from pyknolepsy in that the seizures are more sporadic and generalized tonic-clonic seizures somewhat more common.

Juvenile myoclonic epilepsy (JME) is a familial disorder that typically begins in the second decade of life and is characterized by mild myoclonic seizures, generalized tonic-clonic or clonic-tonic-clonic seizures, and occasionally absence seizures. The myoclonic seizures are usually mild to moderate in intensity and involve the neck, shoulders, and arms. The movements involve an entire extremity or body part rather than an isolated muscle contraction. They can occur either singularly or repetitively and may cause the patient to drop objects. They are generally bilateral, although sometimes asymmetric with changing left-right accentuation. Rarely, the jerks may involve the legs and cause the patient to fall to the ground. The interictal EEG in this disorder is reported to be distinctive and easily distinguished from other forms of generalized epilepsies. The characteristic interictal feature of the EEG is the fast (3.5 to 6 Hz) spike-and-wave and multiple spike-and-wave complexes. This pattern contrasts with the 3-Hz spike-and-wave complexes seen in classic absence and the slow (1.5 to 2.5 Hz) spike-and-wave complexes seen with atypical absence seizures.

Atypical absence seizures are characterized as having a less abrupt onset or cessation, more pronounced changes in tone, and longer duration than typical absence. They usually begin before 5 years of age and are associated with other generalized seizure types and mental retardation. The ictal EEG is more heterogeneous, showing 1.5 to 2.5 Hz slow spike-and-wave or polyspike-and-wave discharges that may be irregular or asymmetric. The interictal EEG is usually abnormal, with slowing and multifocal epileptiform features.

Patients with a history suggestive of childhood, juvenile, or JME with typical EEG findings do not require any additional workup. Children with atypical absence seizures often have the Lennox-Gastaut syndrome (see below), a disorder that requires more extensive evaluations, including MRI and metabolic testing.

Treatment of Primarily Generalized Seizures

Because of the very high recurrence risk, it is recommended that any child presenting with absence seizures begin treatment immediately. In children presenting with a single primary generalized tonic-clonic seizure it is reasonable to wait until the second seizure to begin therapy. Valproate and ethosuximide are most commonly used for the treatment of absence seizures. In patients that also have generalized tonic-clonic seizures valproate is the drug of choice.

Infantile Spasms

Infantile spasms or West syndrome is a unique, and frequently malignant, epileptic syndrome confined to infants. The usual characteristic features of this syndrome are tonic or myoclonic seizures, hypsarrhythmic EEGs, and mental retardation. Infantile spasms are an age-specific disorder beginning only in children during the first 2 years of life. The spasms can be classified into three major groups: flexor, extensor, and mixed flexor-extensor types. Flexor spasms consist of flexion of the neck, trunk, arms, and legs. Spasms of the muscles of the upper limbs result either in adduction of the arms in a self-hugging motion or in adduction of the arms to either side of the head with the arms flexed at the elbow. Extensor spasms consist of a predominance of extensor muscle contractions, producing abrupt extension of the neck and trunk with extensor abduction or adduction of the arms, legs, or both. Mixed flexor-extensor spasms include flexion of the neck, trunk, and arms and extension of the legs or flexion of the legs and extension of the arms with varying degrees of flexion of the neck and trunk. Infantile spasms frequently occur in clusters, and the intensity and frequency of the spasms in each cluster may increase to a peak before progressively decreasing.

On the basis of past history, physical examination, and laboratory studies, cases of infantile spasms have been conventionally classified into those in which there is no apparent preceding neurologic disorder or identified etiologic factor (idiopathic) and those in which a prior, presumptively responsible, pathologic event or disorder is demonstrated (symptomatic cases). The majority of infants who have development infantile spasms have developmental delay, neurologic deficits, or both, before the onset of the spasms, unfortunately, even in children with normal development before the onset, the disorder is associated with slowing or regression of development.

Infantile spasms are usually associated with markedly abnormal EEGs, the most common of which is hypsarrhythmia. This pattern consists of high-amplitude slow waves mixed with spikes and sharp waves. The EEG background activity is completely disorganized and chaotic. A large number of etiologic factors have been associated with infantile spasms. These include hypoxic-ischemic injuries, tuberous sclerosis, congenital brain anomalies, infection, and head injury. Virtually any agent that can harm the brain has been associated with infantile spasms. Why some children with these conditions develop spasms is unclear.

The workup of a child with infantile spasms should include an MRI to look for a congenital anomaly, evidence of tuberous sclerosis or a congenital infection, metabolic evaluation, and a spinal tap. While recommendations for treatment of infantile spasms are controversial, the most common therapy is adrenocorticotropic hormone ACTH. Standard antiepileptic drugs such as carbamazepine, phenytoin, or phenobarbital are usually not effective. While some children rapidly respond to ACTH and develop normally, a significant number of infants either continue to have spasms or develop other seizure types. Some infants progress into the Lennox-Gastaut syndrome (LGS).

Because of the poor prognosis in most infants with infantile spasms, there recently has been interest in the early surgical treatment of these children. In some infants, regional cortical abnormalities have been resected with resolution of the spasms. Positron emission tomography (PET) has been used in some centers to help identify these regional abnormalities. Unfortunately, only a few children with infantile spasms have an identifiable focal lesions.

Lennox-Gastaut Syndrome

LGS is characterized by a mixed seizure disorder in which tonic seizures are a major component, and a slow spike-and-wave EEG pattern. The syndrome always begins in childhood and the vast majority of children have mental retardation. Patients with the LGS typically have very frequent seizures. A mixture of seizure types is the rule in LGS. The most frequently occurring are tonic, tonic-clonic, myoclonic, atypical absences, and "head drops," which represent a form of atonic, tonic, or myoclonic seizures. Tonic seizures are a major component of this syndrome. They are typically activated by sleep and may occur repetitively throughout the night.

The sine qua non of the EEG findings in the LGS is the slow spike-and-wave discharge superimposed on an abnormal, slow background. The slow spike-and-wave or sharp-and-slow-wave complexes consist of generalized discharges occurring at a frequency of 1.5 to 2.5 Hz. Although sleep increases the frequency of the discharges, hyperventilation and photic stimulation rarely activate these discharges.

As with infantile spasms, LGS is associated with a variety of etiologic agents that cause brain injury. The evaluation of the child should include an EEG, MRI, and metabolic screening. Treating children with LGS is very difficult since the seizures are often quite intractable to AEDs. When possible the physician should strive to avoid treating the child with multiple AEDs, since this typically leads to drug toxicity without satisfactory treatment of the seizures. Valproate and felbamate appear to be the most efficacious drugs in the treatment of this disorder. In patients with medically intractable seizures corpus callosotomy may be useful.

Febrile Seizures

A febrile seizure is a seizure occurring in infancy or childhood that occurs between 3 months and 5 years of age, in association with a fever, but without evidence of intracranial infection or defined cause. Febrile seizures must be differentiated from epilepsy, which is characterized by recurrent, afebrile seizures. Patients with epilepsy, however, are often more susceptible to seizures during fever. Unfortunately, when a child has a seizure with fever, there is no definitive way to determine whether the seizure is secondary to the fever or is the first manifestation of epilepsy.

The first febrile seizure in the majority of children occurs before 3 years, with the average age of onset between 18 and 22 months. Most studies have demonstrated a higher incidence in boys. Febrile seizures may be of any type, although they are usually generalized tonic-clonic in type. Febrile seizures are associated with a very low mortality rate. When deaths do occur they are usually secondary to the agent causing the fever or antecedent neurologic disorder. Prospective studies have shown a very low incidence of acquired motor or intellectual abnormalities following a febrile seizure.

While relatively few children who experience febrile seizures develop epilepsy, many children experience recurrences of febrile seizures. Approximately a third of the children will have at least one recurrence. Three-fourths of recurrences take place within 1 year of the first febrile seizure and 90 percent within 2 years. Recurrence risk is not uniform for all children with febrile seizures. The most important factor appears to be age of onset of the first febrile seizure. The younger the child at the first attack, the more likely are further febrile seizures. While children who have one or more febrile seizures are at increased risk for the development of epilepsy the risk is quite small. The risk for developing epilepsy appears to be increased by several factors. If the febrile seizure duration is greater than 15 minutes, occurs more than once in 24 hours, or has focal features, the risk increase significantly.

When evaluating a child with febrile seizures the physician must first determine whether there is an underlying illness that requires immediate, specific treatment. The most urgent diagnostic decision is whether to do a lumbar puncture. One of the earliest signs of meningitis may be a seizure, which like a febrile seizure, is usually short and generalized tonic-clonic in type. While meningitis usually results in meningismus, in patients under the age of 2 years clinical signs of meningitis may be minimal or absent.

In the absence of specific clinical indications, there is little evidence in the literature indicating that other tests are helpful in determining the etiology of seizures associated with fever. Although frequently ordered by physicians, skull films, serum glucose, calcium, blood urea nitrogen (BUN), and electrolytes are not routinely recommended. Brief, single, self-limited febrile seizures from which the child fully recovers are seldom due to conditions such as hypoglycemia or toxins. Unless the physical examination points to a possible structural lesion, A CT or MRI scan is *not* warranted in the evaluation of febrile seizures. Somewhat surprisingly, the EEG has not been found to be useful in the evaluation of a child with febrile seizures. While there remains some controversy, in general, most authorities feel that the EEG is a poor predictor of either febrile or afebrile seizure recurrence.

Since febrile seizures are benign events, there are few compelling reasons to place the child on chronic AEDs, since all the AEDs have side effects. While most studies demonstrate that phenobarbital is effective in reducing recurrence risk, the behavioral disturbances seen in some children taking the drug limits its usefulness. Valproic acid, while effective, carries a small risk for hepatic dysfunction. Carbamazepine and phenytoin are not effective in reducing seizure frequency.

An effective way to reduce recurrence risk is to administer diazepam, 0.3 mg/kg every 8 hours when the child has a fever or appears to be developing an illness. This form of intermittent therapy has proven to be effective in reducing, but not eliminating febrile seizure recurrences.

Withdrawing Antiepileptic Drugs in Children

In general, once a child goes 2 years without a seizure the physician should consider withdrawal of AEDs. While certain factors such as age at onset greater than 12 years, a positive family history, slowing on the EEG prior to AED withdrawal, and mental retardation increase the risk of recurrence, even in these children the physician and parents may wish to consider withdrawal of AEDs. A withdrawal period of 6 to 8 weeks is recommended.

SUGGESTED READINGS

Annegers JF, Hauser WA, Shirts SB et al: Factors prognostic of unprovoked seizures after febrile convulsions. N Engl J Med 316:493–8, 1987
Berg AT, Shinnar S, Hauser WA et al: Predictors of recurrent febrile seizures: a metaanalytic review. J Pediatr 116:329–37, 1990
Cavazzuti GB: Epidemiology of different types of epilepsy in school age children of Modena, Italy. Epilepsia 21:57–62, 1980
Chugani HT, Shewmon DA, Sankar R et al: Infantile spasms: II. Lenticular nuclei and brain stem activation on positron emission tomography. Ann Neurol 31:212–19, 1992
Chugani HT, Shields WD, Shewmon DA et al: Infantile spasms: I. PET identifies focal cortical dysgenesis in cryptogenic cases for surgical treatment. Ann Neurol 27:406–13, 1990
Eeg-Olofsson O, Petersen I, Sellden U: The development of the electroencephalogram in normal children from the age of 1 through 15 years: paroxysmal activity. Neuropediatrie 2:375–404, 1971
Farwell JR, Lee YJ, Hirtz DG et al: Phenobarbital for febrile seizures-effects on intelligence and on seizure recurrence. N Engl J Med 322:364–9, 1990
Hirtz DG, Nelson KB: The natural history of febrile seizures. Annu Rev Med 34:453–71, 1983
Snead OC III, Benton JW, Myers GL: ACTH and prednisone in childhood seizure disorders. Neurology 33:966–970, 1983

140. DIAGNOSIS AND CLASSIFICATION OF EPILEPSY

EDWARD B. BROMFIELD

Epilepsy, a tendency toward recurrent unprovoked seizures, is among the most common of neurologic conditions, affecting 0.5 to 1.0 percent of the population at any given time. Furthermore, up to 10 percent of individuals at some time in their lives experience at least one seizure, either provoked or unprovoked. These high prevalence rates are related to the fact that epilepsy is not a specific disease, but rather a symptom of brain dysfunction, a "final common pathway" of many different cerebral insults. Because of the variety of causative conditions and clinical manifestations, classification systems are necessary for appropriate diagnosis and treatment.

SEIZURES AND SEIZURE CLASSIFICATION

Physiologically, an epileptic seizure is an uncontrolled, abnormally synchronous discharge of a collection of neurons. This excessive discharge causes a transient abnormality in brain function, the specific nature of which is determined by the brain region(s) involved. Motor cortex, for example, typically produces stiffening or rhythmic jerking of the corresponding limb; somatosensory cortex, tingling or "electricity"; primary visual cortex, flashing lights or spots; auditory cortex, ringing or buzzing; and olfactory or gustatory regions, hallucinations of smell or taste. Cortical association areas may give rise to more complex phenomena such as formed hallucinations in the appropriate modalities, and limbic cortex may produce emotional experiences or memory phenomena (e.g., vivid recall of a specific event or déja vu experience). Because the pathophysiologic process is one of too much rather than too little neuronal activity, epileptic brain dysfunction often takes the form of what Hughlings Jackson called "positive symptoms," as illustrated above. "Negative symptoms," such as paralysis or sensory loss, are much less common in epileptic seizures than in processes that lead to decreased neuronal activity, such as brain ischemia.

If enough of the brain is involved in the abnormally synchronous discharge, consciousness is lost, and the patient cannot report any further phenomena. Seizures that spread from one to the other hemisphere often impair consciousness. Automatic-appearing movements, such as chewing, swallowing, or picking with one's hands are commonly seen after consciousness is lost. If most or all of the cerebrum is involved, a stereotypic event known as a generalized tonic-clonic seizure (synonyms: grand mal or major motor seizure; generalized convulsion) occurs. This consists of widespread stiffening (tonic phase—increase in muscle tone) followed by rhythmic jerking (clonic phase). The entire event seldom takes longer than 1 to 2 minutes. Return to normal mental state occurs gradually, however, over minutes to hours, during the phase of "postictal" recovery.

Implicit in the above discussion is the paradigm of a seizure starting locally and then spreading throughout the brain, with successive impairments reflecting the involvement of additional brain regions. This sequence applies to partial seizures, which may occur without or with loss of consciousness (simple or complex partial seizure), and may or may not culminate in a generalized tonic-clonic seizure (partial seizure secondarily generalized). For classification purposes, consciousness is defined operationally as the ability to respond appropriately to the environment, or to remember events during any time period in which response is impaired because of a motor or language disturbance.

Seizures may also be primarily generalized, that is, involve the entire cerebrum apparently simultaneously without evidence of focal onset. Such seizures can take the form of a tonic-clonic convulsion or be less severe. A primarily generalized seizure that consists only of brief staring is called an absence seizure (formerly "petit mal"). A myoclonic seizure consists of a single rapid movement or series of such movements. When generalized, these are bilateral, although not always symmetrical. Clonic seizures are manifested by rhythmic, repetitive jerking movements. Generalized tonic seizures consist of sudden stiffening, usually in an abnormal but symmetrical posture. Tonic-clonic seizures typically have tonic and clonic phases, as described above. Atonic seizures result in sudden loss of muscle tone and falling, or in milder form, head nods or jaw drops. (Sudden falls may also occur with myoclonic, tonic, or clonic seizures if legs are involved.) Below is a simplified version of the International Classification of Epileptic Seizures, last revised in 1981.

I. *Partial* seizures (seizures beginning locally)
   A. Simple partial seizures (consciousness not impaired)
      Motor
      Somatosensory or special sensory
      Autonomic (e.g., rising epigastric sensation, flushing)
      Psychic-cognitive (e.g., déja vu, fear, aphasia)
   B. Complex partial seizures (consciousness impaired)
      Beginning as simple partial seizures (see above)
      With impairment of consciousness at onset
   C. Partial seizures secondarily generalized (can start as simple, complex, or simple evolving to complex partial)
II. *Generalized* seizures (bilaterally symmetrical and without local onset)
   A. Absence
      Typical (petit mal)
      Atypical
   B. Myoclonic
   C. Clonic
   D. Tonic
   E. Tonic-clonic (grand mal)
   F. Atonic
III. *Unclassified* epileptic seizures (inadequate or incomplete data)

The advent of long-term video-electroencephalographic (EEG) recording was one of the key factors behind revision of the classification. Currently, this technique is generally reserved for especially difficult cases, so that diagnosis typically depends primarily on history and interictal EEG findings. Other than those with motor manifestations, simple partial seizures can be diagnosed only on the basis of the patient's history. For complex partial seizures, the patient's history should be supplemented by that of other observers. Descriptions of automatisms, defined as complex behaviors of which the patient has no awareness or memory, and other evidence of altered consciousness are extremely important. The term "aura," coined initially by Galen for the "breeze" that some individuals felt just before their seizures, currently refers to whatever the patient recalls experiencing before consciousness is lost, that is, the simple partial seizure that precedes a complex partial or secondarily generalized event. Interictal physical examination and neuroimaging studies can indicate focal or global abnormalities that may predispose to seizures, but are only indirectly relevant to diagnosis and classification.

Several conditions may present with events resembling either partial or generalized seizures. These include cerebral ischemia, syncope, migraine, movement disorders, sleep disorders, metabolic disturbances, and psychiatric conditions, which are discussed elsewhere in this volume. There are several characteristic features related to onset, progression of symptoms, stereotypy, duration, and postictal changes that help to distinguish seizure types from each other and from nonepileptic events.

Almost all seizures begin abruptly; indeed, it is their very unpredictability that is responsible for much of the associated functional impairment. While some patients may have a prodromal feeling that may last hours or more, the seizure itself is usually sudden. Although certain psychosocial or lifestyle factors, most commonly sleep deprivation and, less often, stress, may increase the likelihood of seizures occurring on a given day, most seizures have no clear precipitant. Furthermore, the sequence of events that follows seizure onset is quite stereotyped for a given patient. Certain sequences tend to be stable even across patients; a symptom that can be associated with simple partial seizures, such as abdominal upset or déja vu, is not of diagnostic help if it follows rather than precedes alteration in consciousness. In generalized tonic-clonic seizures, the clonic movements almost always slow progressively before they stop. Duration of seizures is also surprisingly consistent across patients for a given seizure type (Table 140-1). Simple partial seizures last seconds to a few minutes, and complex partial seizures usually slightly longer. The duration of either primarily or secondarily generalized tonic-clonic seizures is rarely longer than 2 minutes. Bilateral tonic posturing or clonic movements are usually (though not always) associated with loss of consciousness. Another characteristic of motor activity arising from an epileptic mechanism is that it cannot generally be stopped by stimulation or gentle restraint. Finally, postictal confusion and/or somnolence is characteristic of most seizures manifested by loss of consciousness. (Exceptions are typical absence seizures and certain complex partial seizures, especially those of frontal lobe origin.)

While ictal EEG recording with synchronized video is the "gold standard" for seizure classification, routine interictal studies can also be extremely helpful. As discussed in Chapter 19, the majority of patients prone to either partial or generalized seizures eventually show a confirmatory interictal epileptiform abnormality, particularly if sleep is obtained. Often, a focal interictal EEG abnormality is the only indicator that a general-

TABLE 140-1. Selected Clinical and EEG Features of Different Seizure Types

Seizure Type	Clinical Features	Typical Duration	Postictal Period	Interictal EEG
Simple partial	Motor, somatosensory, special sensory, autonomic, or psychic symptoms	10–180 s	Mild and brief if any	Spikes or sharp waves over appropriate area, with or without associated slowing
Complex partial	Altered consciousness, often beginning with stare and followed by automatisms; may be immediately preceded by simple partial	15–300 s	Highly variable (none to many minutes)	Same as above
Partial secondarily generalized	Simple and/or complex partial seizure followed by tonic posturing evolving to repetitive, bilateral muscle contractions	30–120 s (exclusive of partial seizure at onset)	Minutes to hours	Same as above
Absence (typical)	Arrest of activity, staring with loss of awareness; may have subtle tonic, clonic, myoclonic, or atonic features; automatisms occur rarely	5–20	None	Generalized 2.5–4/s spike-wave or multiple-spike-and-slow-wave complexes
Absence (atypical)	Altered awareness, perhaps incomplete; variably abrupt onset and cessation	5–180 s	Variable	Slow (<2.5 Hz) spike wave and/or multiple spike-and-slow-wave complexes, abnormal background
Myoclonic	Sudden isolated or multiple jerks, usually involving upper > lower body, restricted or extensive	<1 s if isolated	None	Multiple spike-and-slow-wave complexes
Clonic	Rhythmically repetitive myoclonic jerks, usually with altered consciousness	Variable	Variable	Generalized spike-wave and/or multiple-spike-and-slow-wave complexes
Tonic	Bilateral tonic posturing, usually involving trunk and face; loss of consciousness	5–20 s; may cluster	Seconds to minutes	Generalized spike-wave or multiple spike-and-slow-wave complexes; bursts of multiple spikes
Tonic-clonic	Tonic posturing followed by clonic jerking bilaterally	30–120 s	Minutes to hours	Generalized discharges as above
Atonic	Altered awareness and loss of muscle tone accompanied by sudden falling, or, when milder, head nod or jaw drop	Seconds; rarely >1 min	Variable	Slow spike-wave, multiple spike-and-slow-wave complexes, abnormal background

ized tonic-clonic seizure was actually a partial seizure, which secondarily generalized. Clinical features that can contribute to this diagnosis include symptoms compatible with a simple partial seizure immediately preceding loss of consciousness, a witnessed complex partial seizure before generalization, or a postictal (Todd's) paralysis. As described in succeeding chapters, this distinction has implications for treatment.

CLASSIFICATION OF EPILEPSY SYNDROMES

While alternatives have been proposed (see Lüders and colleagues, 1993), the International Classification of Epileptic Seizures has achieved wide acceptance and application. The task of classifying epileptic syndromes, while equally important clinically, has been more difficult. The schema proposed in 1989 by the Commission on Classification and Terminology of the International League Against Epilepsy is likely to remain the standard for the foreseeable future, and will be summarized here.

As in any other medical discipline, a syndrome refers to a collection of signs and symptoms that go together; in the case of "the epilepsies," syndrome definitions may include seizure type(s), age of onset, presumed etiology, physical characteristics, neurological status, family history, and EEG and neuroimaging findings. Certain syndromes are sufficiently well characterized to provide reliable information about prognosis and response to treatment. Epileptic syndromes may be broadly grouped along two dimensions, regarding presumed etiology (idiopathic vs symptomatic) and seizure type (partial vs generalized). *Idiopathic*, as used here, refers to the absence of an underlying brain insult and in general implies a genetic cause. A genetic etiology may be present without a positive family history, as family members may have the trait (sometimes apparent on EEG) without the clinical syndrome, and in other individuals

the syndrome may result from a spontaneous mutation. *Symptomatic* refers to the presence of a specific brain insult thought to be the cause of the tendency toward recurrent seizures. The equivalent terms "primary" and "secondary" have been dropped because of the potential confusion with the concept of primarily and secondarily generalized seizures. *Cryptogenic* refers to cases in which a specific insult is presumed but not identified. An abbreviated and slightly modified form of the international classification follows in outline form.

I. Partial epilepsies and syndromes (also called focal, local, or "localization-related")
   A. Idiopathic (with age-related onset)
      Benign epilepsy with centrotemporal spikes
      Childhood epilepsy with occipital paroxysms
      Primary reading epilepsy
   B. Symptomatic
      Chronic progressive epilepsia partialis continua of childhood
      Syndromes with seizures precipitated by sensory stimuli or activities ("reflex" epilepsies)
      Temporal lobe epilepsies (mesial and lateral)
      Frontal lobe epilepsies (multiple subareas)
      Parietal lobe epilepsies
      Occipital lobe epilepsies
II. Generalized epilepsies and syndromes
   A. Idiopathic (with age-related onset, in order of age)
      Benign neonatal familial convulsions
      Childhood absence epilepsy
      Juvenile absence epilepsy
      Juvenile myoclonic epilepsy
      Epilepsy with grand mal seizures on awakening
      Other idiopathic generalized epilepsies
      Reflex epilepsies with generalized seizures

B. Cryptogenic or symptomatic
   Infantile spasms
   Lennox-Gastaut syndrome
   Epilepsy with myoclonic-astatic seizures
   Epilepsy with myoclonic absences
C. Symptomatic—many inborn errors of metabolism and congenital malformations
III. Epilepsies and syndromes undetermined whether focal or generalized
   A. With both generalized and focal seizures
   B. With unclassifiable seizures
IV. Special syndromes
   A. Situation-related seizures
      Febrile convulsions
      Isolated seizures or isolated status epilepticus
      Seizures precipitated by acute systemic metabolic or toxic disturbance

These and other syndromes are described in Chapter 139 and in several of the Suggested Readings. Some of the more important syndromes are displayed in tabular form (Table 140-2), which may better highlight the relationships among them. Briefly mentioned in the table is the unusual but conceptually important group of syndromes known as reflex epilepsies, which may be either idiopathic or symptomatic and either partial or generalized. These are not simple reflex responses as the term may imply, but refer to reproducible elicitation of seizures by stereotyped sensory stimuli or activities. In selected individuals, seizures may be precipitated by such elementary stimuli as flashing lights or such complex activities as reading or eating.

Of particular interest to the adult neurologist are the several (presumed) symptomatic partial epilepsies, particularly temporal and frontal. *Temporal lobe epilepsies* typically include simple partial seizures characterized by autonomic, psychic, and/or certain special sensory phenomena. Examples are a rising epigastric sensation, sudden fear, déja vu, unpleasant olfactory or gustatory hallucinations, or visual distortions of size or distance. (None of these, however, is pathognomonic for temporal lobe origin.) Complex partial seizures arising from the temporal lobe often begin with a motionless stare followed by oroalimentary automatisms and later by a postictal state gradually resolving over minutes. Secondary generalization occurs but usually with only a minority of seizures. Other clinical features often include a history of febrile seizures, onset in childhood or adolescence, and temporal discharges on EEG. Associated personality traits have been demonstrated in some studies, but their diagnostic usefulness is controversial (see Ch. 143). Lesions are not typically visualized on neuroimaging, although careful magnetic resonance imaging (MRI) analysis often shows signs of hippocampal sclerosis, and positron emission tomography studies demonstrate unilateral temporal lobe hypometabolism. Response to medical treatment is often unsat-

isfactory, but surgery may be an excellent option in appropriately selected candidates (see Ch. 142). Temporal lobe epilepsies are the most common epilepsy syndromes seen in adults.

Frontal lobe epilepsies have been increasingly recognized in recent years due to improvements in neuroimaging and intracranial EEG studies. While the clinical distinction from temporal lobe syndromes may not always be clear, complex partial seizures associated with frontal lobe pathology are typically shorter in duration, more often lack postictal confusion, and are more prone to secondarily generalize. Isolated simple partial seizures occur less often, and motor manifestations are more common and dramatic, sometimes leading to diagnostic confusion with psychogenic episodes. Seizures often occur several times a day, especially during sleep, and may evolve into status epilepticus. EEG may be normal or nonspecifically abnormal, even ictally (when artifact often obscures the tracing). For patients uncontrolled by medication, the likelihood of surgical success is less than in the case of temporal lobe epilepsies, unless a resectable structural lesion is present. The frontal lobes are very large and include a variety of functionally distinct areas, including primary and supplementary motor, cingulate, frontopolar, orbitofrontal, dorsolateral, and opercular regions. Delineating characteristics of seizures arising from each of these areas is an active area of study.

Occipital and *parietal lobe epilepsies* are less common than frontal and especially temporal lobe syndromes. The expected contralateral visual or somatosensory phenomena do not always occur, and rapid spread to other areas may mimic seizures of temporal or frontal origin. Forced contraversion of head and/or eyes, at times with retained consciousness, is common in occipital lobe epilepsies, as is a history of migraine. Because of proximity to the posterior frontal lobe, parietal lobe seizures often include motor phenomena, and language disturbances are typical if the seizure arises in the dominant hemisphere. Structural lesions are frequently but not always seen.

The most important idiopathic generalized syndrome seen in adults is that of *juvenile myoclonic epilepsy*. While onset is typically in adolescence, the syndrome remits in less than 20 percent of cases. The cardinal symptom, that of bilateral but not always symmetric rapid jerks, is often not remarked upon by the patient without specific questioning. Rare patients actually have unilateral myoclonus, though usually involving either side at different times, which may further obscure the diagnosis. In many cases, myoclonic seizures have been occurring for years before the patient comes to medical attention, most often at the time of his or her first generalized tonic-clonic seizure. The patient may regard the morning myoclonus as merely "shakiness" or "nerves." In other patients, however, myoclonus involving the lower extremities can result in sudden falls or injuries. In addition to myoclonic and generalized tonic-clonic seizures, a substantial minority of patients also have absence seizures, clinically similar to but less frequent than those associated with childhood absence epilepsy. Another important feature is extreme sensitivity to sleep deprivation and alcohol; lifestyle adjustments in these areas are important adjuncts to drug therapy. Examination and imaging studies are normal, but EEG usually demonstrates generalized spike-wave or multiple-spike-and-slow wave complexes, often faster than 3 Hz. Photosensitivity, manifested by an abnormal EEG response or even a clinical seizure during strobe light stimulation, is also common. Response to medical treatment is usually excellent, although, as noted, relapse is common if medications are withdrawn following a seizure-free period.

TABLE 140-2. Selected Epilepsy Syndromes

Seizure Type	Etiology	
	Idiopathic (primary)	Symptomatic (secondary)
Partial	Benign rolandic Childhood occipital	Temporal lobe[a] Frontal lobe[a] Parietal lobe[a] Occipital lobe[a]
Generalized	Childhood absence Juvenile myoclonic[a] Other idiopathic generalized	Lennox-Gastaut syndrome

[a] Discussed in text.

USE OF SEIZURE AND SYNDROME CLASSIFICATION IN TREATMENT DECISIONS

Of nearly two dozen drugs marketed for epilepsy in the United States, less than 10 are commonly used. On the basis of animal testing, clinical experience, and a few large, controlled clinical studies, a rough consensus has been reached regarding drugs of choice for specific seizure types and syndromes. In general, drugs that are effective in treating partial seizures, such as phenytoin and carbamazepine, are also effective for generalized tonic-clonic seizures, but not for other generalized seizures. Valproate can be used for virtually all seizure types and is especially helpful in the idiopathic generalized syndromes with more than one seizure type, such as juvenile myoclonic epilepsy; although effective for partial seizures, it is regarded by some as a second choice in partial epilepsies. Barbiturates are still in use, mainly for partial and generalized tonic-clonic seizures; the phenobarbital precursor primidone is also an important alternative to valproate for juvenile myoclonic epilepsy. Ethosuximide is the most selective antiepileptic drug, ineffective for partial or generalized tonic-clonic seizures but highly efficacious in treating absence seizures. Benzodiazepines can be useful in treating myoclonic and some other seizure types. More detail regarding drug treatment is provided in Chapter 141. As discussed in Chapter 142, consideration for surgery is highly dependent on accurate syndrome classification, particularly as regards localization of the seizure focus. Finally, for those rare syndromes in which seizures occur only or mainly in response to a specific activity or stimulus, therapy can sometimes be based on behavioral techniques. In general, then, accurate diagnosis and classification provide the foundation for effective treatment.

SUGGESTED READINGS

Commission on Classification and Terminology of the International League Against Epilepsy: Proposal for revised classification of epilepsies and epileptic syndromes. Epilepsia 30:389; 1989

Commission on Classification and Terminology of the International League Against Epilepsy: Proposal for revised clinical and electrographic classification of epileptic seizures. Epilepsia 22:489, 1981

Dam M, Gram L: Comprehensive Epileptology. Raven Press, New York, 1991

Engel J Jr: Seizures and Epilepsy. FA Davis, Philadelphia, 1989

Lüders HO, Burgess R, Noachtar S: Expanding the international classification of seizures to provide more localizing information. Neurology 43:1650, 1993

Wyllie E: The Treatment of Epilepsy: Principles and Practice. Lea & Febiger, Philadelphia, 1993

141. MEDICAL TREATMENT OF SEIZURES

STEVEN C. SCHACHTER

The management of patients with epilepsy has always been a challenge for clinicians. Over time, the concept of optimum therapy has evolved from complete control of seizures in spite of side effects and without regard for psychosocial problems to treatment that enables the patient to lead a lifestyle consistent with his or her capabilities. Consequently, those patients who were unable to function according to their abilities because of medication side effects or psychosocial difficulties, now can anticipate a full and useful life with the help of new medications and epilepsy surgery.

Designing and implementing a management plan to maximize the quality of life for the patient with epilepsy requires an accurate, objective measurement of the patient's seizure type(s), frequency, and severity; medication side effects; and psychosocial problems. This is an ongoing, often lengthy process that can test the strength of the doctor-patient relationship, but it is streamlined by a working knowledge of available antiepileptic drugs (AEDs), AED pharmacokinetics, drug-drug interactions, and drug side effects.

INITIAL TREATMENT

The first step is to establish the seizure type(s) within the framework of the seizure classification of the International League Against Epilepsy, as discussed in Chapter 140. Most patients experience more than one type of seizure, for example, complex partial and secondary generalized, and identification of seizure type(s) helps to select AED therapy. Direct questions are often necessary to probe for identification of seizure triggers, such as sleep deprivation, alcohol intake, and stress, since measures to limit exposure to these triggers may successfully augment AED therapy.

Complete seizure control with minimal side effects can be achieved in approximately 70 to 80 percent of patients with single drug therapy; with combinations of anticonvulsants in only an additional 10 to 15 percent of patients can significant seizure control be expected without significant side effects. Even before therapy has begun, the physician should enlist the additional cooperation of the patient's significant others in tracking seizure frequency and severity. By encouraging the patient to keep track of seizures, seizure triggers, and medications on a calendar the clinician can ascertain whether seizures correlate with triggers such as stress or menses, and also monitor compliance with the AED regimen. If the patient experiences any side effects, he or she can record the time of day they occur, Similarly, the clinician should monitor AED serum levels if an AED is started or stopped, if an AED dose is changed, or if the patient experiences side effects or increased seizures.

Table 141-1 shows the recommended initial treatment for the different types of seizures. If one AED is unsuccessful be-

TABLE 141-1. Recommended Treatment for Different Seizure Types

Seizure Type	Initial Therapy	Second-Line or Adjunctive Therapy
Primary generalized tonic-clonic seizures	Carbamazepine Phenytoin Valproate	Primidone Phenobarbital
Partial seizures with or without secondary generalization	Carbamazepine Phenytoin	Valproate Phenobarbital Gabapentin Primidone Lamotrigine
Secondary generalized seizures	Carbamazepine Phenytoin Valproate	Primidone Phenobarbital Gabapentin Lamotrigine
Absence seizures	Ethosuximide Valproate	
Myoclonic seizures	Valproate	Clonazepam
Mixed seizures (myoclonic and tonic-clonic)	Valproate	Phenytoin Primidone

TABLE 141-2. Common and Rare Side Effects of Antiepileptic Drugs

Drug	Trade Name	Systemic Side Effects	Neurotoxic Side Effects	Rare Idiosyncratic Reactions
Phenytoin	Dilantin	Gingival hypertrophy, body hair increase, rash, lymphadenopathy	Confusion, slurred speech, double vision, ataxia, neuropathy (with long-term use)	Agranulocytosis, Stevens-Johnson syndrome, aplastic anemia, hepatic failure, dermatitis/rash, serum sickness
Carbamazepine	Tegretol	Nausea, vomiting, diarrhea, hyponatremia, rash, pruritus, fluid retention	Drowsiness, dizziness, blurred or double vision, lethargy, headache	Agranulocytosis, Stevens-Johnson syndrome, aplastic anemia, hepatic failure, dermatitis/rash, serum sickness, pancreatitis
Valproate	Depakote	Weight gain, nausea, vomiting, hair loss, easy bruising	Tremor	Agranulocytosis, Stevens-Johnson syndrome, aplastic anemia, hepatic failure, dermatitis/rash, serum sickness, pancreatitis
Felbamate	Felbatol	Nausea, vomiting, anorexia, weight loss	Insomnia, dizziness, headache, ataxia	Aplastic anemia, hepatic failure
Gabapentin	Neurontin	None known	Somnolence, dizziness, ataxia	Unknown
Primidone, phenobarbital	Mysoline (primidone)	Nausea, rash	Alteration of sleep cycles, sedation, lethargy, behavioral changes, hyperactivity, ataxia, tolerance, dependence	Agranulocytosis, Stevens-Johnson syndrome, hepatic failure, dermatitis/rash, serum sickness
Ethosuximide	Zarontin	Nausea, vomiting	Sleep disturbance, drowsiness, hyperactivity	Agranulocytosis, Stevens-Johnson syndrome, aplastic anemia, dermatitis/rash, serum sickness
Lamotrigine	Lamictal	Rash, nausea	Dizziness, somnolence	Stevens-Johnson syndrome, hypersensitivity syndrome

cause of ineffectiveness or side effects, then a second AED may be tried. In general, it is preferable to maintain a patient on a single AED. When the initial medication is determined to be ineffective, the second drug should be titrated to therapeutic level or dosage before the first AED is tapered. As previously stated, combinations of AEDs may be necessary in some patients. Virtually all combinations of medications have been tried, although certain combination should be avoided, for example, phenobarbital, primidone, and diazepam, since all three drugs are central nervous system (CNS) depressants.

Side effects are a major cause of medication intolerance and noncompliance. Table 141-2 shows the common and rare side effects of the most prescribed AEDs. Information on the contraindications for each medication is available to the clinician from the manufacturer, and should be consulted before prescribing. The AEDs differ in how easily and rapidly a loading dose can be administered as shown in Table 141-3. This consideration is particularly important for patients with frequent seizures. Table 141-3 also presents the likely mechanism of action for each AED. Table 141-4 gives pharmacokinetic information, including frequency of dosing, number of days needed to achieve steady state, and frequency of initial monitoring (serum levels, liver function tests, renal function tests, and complete blood counts). The information presented in Table 141-4 applies to adults; therefore, physicians who treat children with epilepsy should consult prescribing information for correct dosing regimens.

NONCOMPLIANCE WITH ANTIEPILEPTIC DRUG THERAPY

When a patient's seizures are uncontrolled, the clinician must consider whether the patient is noncompliant, which is the most

TABLE 141-3. Loading and Initial Dosing, Mechanism of Action Antiepileptic Drugs

Drug	Trade Name	Intravenous Loading Dose	Oral Loading and Maintenance Dose	Mechanism of Action
Phenytoin	Dilantin	15 mg/kg (not more than 50 mg/min)	15 mg/kg in three divided doses over 9–12 hours; 5 mg/kg/day maintenance	Blocks sodium-dependent action potentials; reduces neuronal calcium uptake
Carbamazepine	Tegretol	N/A	Start at 2–3 mg/kg/day; increase dose every 3–5 days to 10 mg/kg/day; dose may need to be further increased to 15–20 mg/kg/day after 2–3 months because of hepatic autoinduction	Blocks sodium-dependent action potentials; reduces neuronal calcium uptake
Valproate	Depakote	N/A	15 mg/kg/day in three divided doses; increase by 5–10 mg/kg/day every week as needed and tolerated	Reduces high-frqeuency neuronal firing; (?) blocks sodium-dependent action potentials; enhances GABA effects on CNS
Gabapentin	Neurontin	N/A	300 mg first day, 300 mg bid second day, 300 mg tid third day; increase as needed to 1,800 mg/day in three divided doses	Unknown
Ethosuximide	Zarontin	N/A	20–40 mg/kg/day in 1–3 divided doses	Modifies low-threshold or transient neuronal calcium currents
Barbiturates	Mysoline (primidone)	90–120 mg every 10–15 minutes as needed to maximum of 1,000 mg	1–5 mg/kg/day	Prolongs GABA-mediated chloride-channel openings; decreases CNS excitability
Lamotrigine	Lamictal	N/A	For patients taking and enzyme-inducing AED: 25 mg bid titrated upward by 50-mg increments every 1–2 weeks as needed. For patients taking VPA: 25 mg every other day with increases of 25 to 50 mg every 2 weeks as needed to a maximum of 300 to 500 mg/day. The maximum dosage used in US open-label drug trials is 700 mg/day.	Inhibition of voltage-dependent sodium channels, resulting in decreased release of the excitatory neurotransmitters glutamate and aspartate

TABLE 141-4. Pharmacokinetic Information for Antiepileptic Drugs

Drug	Percent Bound to Plasma Protein	Elimination Half-Life (h)	Time to Steady State (days)	Frequency of Dosing	Frequency of Initial Monitoring	Therapeutic Level (μg/ml)
Phenytoin	90	15–30	5–15	qd or bid	2–3 weeks	10–20
Carbamazepine	70–80	11–17 (chronic therapy)	3–10	bid, tid, or qid	3, 6, 9 weeks	4–12
Valproate	60–95 (decreases with serum levels over 100 μg/ml)	6–18	2–4	bid or tid	1–2 weeks	50–150
Felbamate	25	20–23	5–10	bid or tid	(CBC, LFTs)	32–137
Gabapentin	0	5–7; increases with decreased creatinine clearance (see prescribing information)	1–2	tid	None	2–3
Ethosuximide	0	40–50	6–12	qd, bid, or tid	2–3 weeks	40–100
Phenobarbital	40–60	30–50	16–21	qd or bid	3–4 weeks	10–40
Lamotrigine	50–55	10–15 with enzyme-inducing AED; 40–60 with VPA	5–15	bid	none	not established

Abbreviation: AEDs, antiepileptic drugs.

common reason for incomplete seizure control. Up to half of patients treated for epilepsy may not take their medications as directed, and over half of patients seen in emergency rooms because of recurrent seizures are noncompliant. Clinicians should suspect noncompliance if a patient does not accept the diagnosis, has limited financial means, has difficulty tolerating side effects, or forgets when or how to take medication because of frequent seizures or associated memory impairment. As is true of patients with other chronic illnesses, compliance on the part of patients with seizures decreases with increasingly long intervals between clinic visits and increasingly complicated medication regimens. Serum levels may help to monitor compliance, but the clinician should be aware that these levels may vary if medications are stored in or near a humid environment, if the patient takes generic medications from different manufacturers, or if there is a significant change in the patient's weight. Further, serum levels may fluctuate during the day, particularly those for valproate, and may vary for women during the menstrual cycle.

SIDE EFFECTS

For most patients, monotherapy enhances compliance, provides a greater therapeutic window, and is more cost effective than combination therapy—that is, there are usually fewer side effects, idiosyncratic reactions, and teratogenic effects, and no risk of AED-AED interactions. Within the first 6 months of AED therapy, systemic toxicity and neurotoxicity are as likely to contribute to meditation failure as lack of efficacy. As shown in Table 141-2, the neurotoxic effects of commonly used AEDs includes diplopia, nystagmus, dysarthria, ataxia, incoordination, tremor, sedation, mood alteration, dizziness, headache, and cognitive impairment. The extent to which patients complain about side effects—for example, cognitive side effects—depends on the level of functioning of the patient and the patient's perception of the physician's willingness to listen. Detailed neuropsychological testing may help determine whether a patient's complaint of memory loss or trouble concentrating is medication-related and also whether a patient is functioning up to full potential.

Adding an AED to an existing AED, that is, changing a patient from monotherapy to polytherapy, may result in increased AED side effects. For example, adding carbamazepine to phenytoin offers little benefit over either drug alone and may increase mean total phenytoin serum levels by 35 percent and decrease phenytoin clearance by 37 percent. The effects of adding one AED to another are outlined in Table 141-5. Combinations of anticonvulsants and other types of medications may also cause side effects. For instance, giving propoxyphene or erythromycin to a patient who is taking carbamazepine often elevates carbamazepine levels. The common AED–non-AED interactions are shown in Table 141-6.

For patients who have peak-level side effects from a particular AED, the usual strategy is to modify the medication regimen or treatment schedule to minimize side effects while maximizing seizure control and compliance, such as spreading out the dosage—more frequent, smaller doses over the day. The physician should attempt to correlate drug serum levels with the patient's side effects before abandoning that medication. Specifically, levels should be obtained when a patient is experienc-

TABLE 141-5. The Common Antiepileptic Drug–Drug Interactions

	Carbamazepine	Phenytoin	Valproate	Amotrigine	Neurontin	Phenobarbital
AEDs that increase AED levels	Valproate Felbamate (increases carbamazepine epoxide)	Valproate Diazepam (these may increase free and/or total phenytoin levels) Ethosuximide Felbamate	Felbamate	Valproate	None	Valproate
AEDs that decrease AED levels	Phenobarbital Phenytoin Primidone Felbamate	Carbamazepine	Carbamazepine	Phenytoin Carbamazepine	None	Carbamazepine

Abbreviations: AEDs, antiepileptic drugs.

TABLE 141-6. The Common Antiepileptic Drug–Nonantiepileptic Drug Interactions

	Carbamazepine	Phenytoin	Valproate	Phenobarbital
Drugs that increase AED levels and/or enhance effects	Erythromycin Cimetidine Propoxyphene Isoniazid Calcium channel blockers Fluoxetine Valproate (may increase free level)	Chloramphenicol Dicumarol Disulfiram Tolbutamide Isoniazid Phenylbutazone Aspirin Chlordiazepoxide Phenothiazines Estrogens Halothane Methylphenidate Sulfonamides Trazadone Cimetidine	Aspirin Dicumarol	Antihistamines Tranquilizers Corticosteroids MAO inhibitors Amitriptyline Imipramine
Drugs that decrease AED levels	Warfarin Doxycycline Theophylline Haloperidol Oral contraceptives	Isoniazid Chronic alcohol use	None	None

Abbreviations: AED, antiepileptic drug; MAO, monoamine oxidase.

ing side effects and then compared with levels when the patient is free from symptoms. This comparison may help to prove a cause-and-effect relationship. Serum levels that are associated with neurotoxicity vary from one patient to another and may occur within the so-called "therapeutic range." Free-serum phenytoin and valproate levels have clinical significance in managing patients with low albumin levels or patients who are taking multiple drugs that are tightly protein-bound and should be multiplied by 10 to approximate the "effective" total serum level. Woman with catamenial exacerbation of seizures should have their serum AED levels checked in the premenstrual period and compared with midcycle levels, since anticonvulsant levels tend to drop during the menses.

When AEDs are withdrawn, special caution is warranted. Abrupt discontinuation of an AED may increase the risk of seizures and status epilepticus. Withdrawal from CNS depressants, such as phenobarbital, and the benzodiazepines should be accomplished over weeks to months.

A full discussion of the teratogenicity of AEDs is beyond the scope of this chapter. In general, women who take an AED have double the risk of bearing a malformed infant. The risk is even higher for women who take multiple AEDs or who have a personal or family history of malformations. Features of the fetal anticonvulsant syndrome include limb abnormalities, craniofacial abnormalities, and growth and development abnormalities. Women planning a pregnancy should begin to take folic acid, 0.4 mg/day, before conception and throughout pregnancy. Women with a previous pregnancy complicated by a fetal malformation, such as a neural tube defect, should take 4 mg/day of folic acid and should probably avoid valproate and carbarmazepine. Congenital malformations have been reported in association with all of the "older" AEDs; clinical experience with felbamate, gabapentin and lamotrigine has not bean sufficient yet to determine risk. As in every clinical situation, the physician must weigh the risk/benefit ratio for treating epilepsy in a pregnant woman.

PSYCHOSOCIAL ISSUES

The comprehensive management of patients with epilepsy includes dealing with the psychosocial aspects of this disorder. Even patients with infrequent seizures may be significantly affected by their disorder, particularly with regard to employment, driving, and insurance. These effects may be better appreciated and addressed if the physician attempts to uncover the

psychological and social problems that adversely affect the patient's quality of life. This process begins with the clinician's taking a complete psychosocial history, including previous psychiatric illness or treatment, education, employment, driving, insurance, interpersonal relationships, and attitude toward having epilepsy. A number of questionnaires have bean developed for this purpose that supplement the psychosocial history and provide a quantifiable means of assessing and following patients as pharmacotherapeutic and psychosocial interventions are implemented. Uncovering a source of psychosocial stress may lead to an effective strategy toward reducing the impact of that stress on the patient, which in turn may help reduce seizure frequency.

ADJUNCTIVE THERAPIES

Women with catamenial seizure exacerbation often have associated neuroendocrine disorders, such as polycystic ovarian syndrome, premature menopause, and inadequate luteal phase. Hormonal therapy may improve seizure control in these women. Specifically, drugs, such as oral or intramuscular medroxyprogesterone and oral progesterone, should be tried after being evaluated in a neuroendocrine facility. Similarly, patients with stress-induced seizures may benefit from stress reduction, biofeedback, and relaxation instruction from professionals with experience in teaching these techniques to patients with epilepsy.

CONCLUSIONS

The successful management of epilepsy is based on accurate seizure diagnosis and early recognition if a patient's epilepsy is refractory because of seizure frequency or severity, medication side effects, psychosocial factors, or, as is most common, combinations of these factors. The clinician should closely monitor the patient as anticonvulsants are adjusted and should make available appropriate resources such as support groups, individual or family counseling, educational guidance, and stress reduction techniques. In selected cases, hormonal treatments, investigational anticonvulsants, or epilepsy surgery may be appropriate. As new drugs with known mechanisms of action are introduced, the range of options for patients will further increase and a rational approach to polypharmacy may emerge. Until then, cautious use of medications alone and in combination will minimize side effects and enable patients to achieve their potential within the limits of current therapy. As Lennox and Markham wrote over 40 years ago, physicians who treat patients with epilepsy must "match modern drug and surgical therapy with practical sociopsychological therapy."

SUGGESTED READINGS

Lennox WG, Markham CH: The sociopsychological treatment of refractory epilepsy. JAMA 152:1690–4, 1953

Lindhout D, Omtzigt GC: Teratogenic effects of antiepileptic drugs: implications for the management of epilepsy in women of childbearing age. Epilepsia 35:S19–S28, 1994

Pellock JM: Standard approach to antiepileptic drug treatment in the United States. Epilepsia 35:S11–S18, 1994

Schachter SC: Advances in the assessment of refractory epilepsy. Epilepsia 34:S24–S30, 1993

142. STATUS EPILEPTICUS

FRANK W. DRISLANE

Fortunately, most epileptic seizures stop within minutes. If a patient has continuous seizures or does not recover between recurrent seizures there is "a condition characterized by an epileptic seizure that is so frequently repeated or so prolonged as to create a fixed and lasting condition," and this is called status epilepticus (SE). Operationally, the term is reasonable after 30 minutes. Status epilepticus has been recognized for centuries, but until the last few decades the term has been applied primarily to generalized convulsive seizures. Just as there are many types of epileptic seizures, there are many forms of SE. The simplest classification is that of convulsive or nonconvulsive status, but a description of syndromes based on partial (focal) or generalized onset of seizures provides more insight into pathophysiology and clinical management (Table 142-1).

GENERALIZED CONVULSIVE STATUS EPILEPTICUS

Generalized convulsive status epilepticus (GCSE) is the most dramatic, best-studied, and most dangerous form of SE. It is potentially life-threatening, but treatable in most cases, so it is important for the clinician to have an appreciation for the etiology, electro- and pathophysiology, progression, and consequences of GCSE. A plan for medical management and pharmacotherapy is crucial.

Convulsive SE is readily recognizable. GCSE may start with focal or complex partial seizures but often begins with a generalized convulsion. Convulsions recur, and most last but a few minutes, with intervals of persistent unresponsiveness. Each convulsion may begin with a tonic phase with tensing of extensor muscles and forced expiration, followed after several seconds by a clonic phase with gradually slowing clonic movements. Both phases are usually bilateral and symmetric, although there may be a focal onset with head or eye deviation even when there is not a unilateral motor onset in the limbs. Consciousness is impaired, at least from the time of tonic seizures.

Less often, movement is continuous; in this case clonic movements eventually diminish, often with replacement by repetitive jerking movements of the eyes, eyelids, or facial muscles alone, sometimes with intermittent limb jerking. This constitutes "subtle" SE and implies continuing epileptic brain activity with a progressive "decoupling" of electrical and motor systems.

Most estimates of the incidence of convulsive SE suggest about 60,000 cases each year in the United States, but population-based surveys indicate that it may occur several times as often. Less is known about the incidence of other forms of SE.

Convulsive SE is not a disease itself, but rather a life-threatening manifestation of some underlying cause. Table 142-2 lists several causes of SE and is an amalgamation of several studies. Causes vary tremendously because of the different populations examined, for example, the incidence of alcohol and drug-related SE is generally greater in studies from urban hospitals. Causes or precipitants of convulsive SE also differ depending on whether one studies patients with known epilepsy or those presenting with acute, new illness. Table 142-2 focuses on adult cases. Congenital abnormalities and infection increase in importance in children, and SE occurs more often in children.

Often, there is an interaction between an acute systemic illness and prior neurologic disease, including prior epilepsy and other earlier neurologic insults. Prior epilepsy is often assumed but is actually the case in a minority of patients. Approximately one-third of cases occur in patients with prior epilepsy, and 1 percent of patients with a diagnosis of epilepsy will have an episode of SE in a given year. Anticonvulsant withdrawal is often assumed in patients with prior epilepsy, although this may be less frequent than presumed. Physician-changed medication regimens may be responsible for withdrawal seizures as often

TABLE 142-1. Types of Status Epilepticus

Type	Description
Generalized	
Generalized tonic-clonic	"Grand mal" may be secondarily generalized from a focus
Absence	"Petit mal," "spike-wave stupor"
Myoclonic	
Tonic	Pediatric; often with Lennox-Gastaut syndrome
Clonic	Infants
Partial (focal) onset	
Simple partial	Motor; epilepsia partialis continua
	Sensory: rare, or rarely diagnosed; can be visual
	Autonomic: rare, or rarely diagnosed
	Psychic: fear, emotional content
	Aphasic
Complex partial	Includes impairment of consciousness
Special types	
Neonatal/pediatric	Includes electrographic status epilepticus of sleep, infantile spasms
"Subtle" status	

TABLE 142-2. Causes of Status Epilepticus

Factor	% Patients[a]
Anticonvulsant withdrawal	25
Alcohol withdrawal	25
Cerebrovascular: including stroke, anoxia, hemorrhage	22
Metabolic: acute encephalopathy, e.g., hypoglycemia, systemic infection	22
Trauma	15
Drug toxicity	15
CNS infection	12
Tumor	8
Congenital lesion	8
Prior epilepsy	33
Idiopathic, no cause found	30

[a] Percentages add to >100% due to multiple causes, e.g., a patient with a congenital lesion and chronic epilepsy with anticonvulsant withdrawal or infection.

as patient noncompliance. Infections may have a direct role in epileptogenicity, but several antibiotics can also precipitate seizures and alter anticonvulsant metabolism. New anticonvulsants may also alter the metabolism of others and lead to subtherapeutic levels of prior medications.

The epidemiology of convulsive SE provides several important clinical lessons. First, there is usually an identifiable cause of SE, and this should be sought. Trauma, new or prior vascular disease, metabolic derangements, drug toxicity (whether prescribed or ''recreational''), and infection not only help to explain the SE but often determine the subsequent course and must be found to be treated appropriately. Alcohol abuse and benzodiazepine withdrawal are other common contributors. Second, there is often more than one cause or precipitant, and medication withdrawal, infection, or sleep deprivation may add to an earlier illness and precipitate convulsive SE. In some series up to 50 percent of patients have either an infection or a recent medication change. Conversely, even with an acute illness convulsive SE occurs more often in people with prior neurologic deficits. Third, despite the many known causes of SE, patients may present in status as the first sign of neurologic disease. This is especially true in children where up to 10 percent of initial seizures may be SE, particularly with febrile seizures.

Convulsive SE can lead to numerous complications (Table 142-3). Autonomic changes can be severe and include hypertension, tachycardia, arrhythmias, diaphoresis, hyperthermia, and vomiting; many of these are due to increased circulating catecholamines. Hyperthermia may be a result of the excessive convulsive muscle contractions as well as a hypothalamic effect. The electrocardiogram (ECG) may show conduction abnormalities or ischemic patterns. Autonomic dysfunction and cardiac arrhythmias may explain much of the mortality of SE and some other unexplained sudden death in epilepsy patients.

Blood flow and cerebral metabolism are elevated in early SE but decline eventually, and the excessive metabolic rate of discharging neurons may outstrip the oxygen and glucose supply. As seizures continue, autoregulation may break down and contribute to cerebral edema, particularly in children. Many physiologic changes of early SE appear to reverse after about 30 minutes, with subsequent hypotension, hypoxemia, hypoglycemia, and increasing acidosis and hyperkalemia. Hypotension and bradycardia may be worsened by anticonvulsant and other medications. Cardiac arrhythmias may be precipitated by lactic acidosis and catecholamines. Hypotension or volume depletion may complicate medical and metabolic disorders or lead to venous stasis and even cerebral venous thrombosis.

SE prompts cortisol and prolactin release, although prolactin may become exhausted and return to normal levels in prolonged SE. Leukocytosis and spinal fluid pleocytosis may occur, but this should not be attributed to the SE itself until infection or other inflammation has been excluded. Aspiration pneumonia is common if airway protection is not assured. Respiratory failure is probably more often due to medications than to SE itself.

Patients with SE may have subsequent intellectual impairment, but studies are generally retrospective and include only prolonged status and subjects with prior and substantial neurologic and intellectual impairment and those on several anticonvulsant drugs. SE may worsen chronic epilepsy.

Abundant experimental animal evidence shows that convulsive SE leads to neuronal damage due directly to the neuronal epileptic activity, but systemic complications, especially hypotension, respiratory failure, and hypoxia, worsen the prognosis and contribute to cerebral damage. This is more difficult to substantiate in humans. Experimental work using convulsant agents and electrical stimulation suggests that SE can lead to hippocampal damage and a subsequent recurrent seizure disorder. The cellular activity of SE releases excitatory amino acids, which are, in turn, neurotoxic in excessive amounts. Electrical stimulation produces similar effects after 30 minutes or so—the same time at which human homeostasis appears to deteriorate during convulsive SE. Thus, both clinical and experimental data implicate 30 minutes as a critical time before which convulsive status should be interrupted.

Patients may also exhibit an orderly sequence of electroencephalographic (EEG) changes in SE, including discrete seizures, then merging seizures and eventual interruptions by flat periods, and finally, periodic discharges. Clinical convulsions abate as the EEG progresses. Patients in later EEG stages have seizures particularly refractory to the usual anticonvulsants medication and have a worsened prognosis. This suggests that these signs of SE warrant aggressive treatment as the sign of continuing and damaging SE even without motor phenomena. The EEG can show whether comatose patients are in a postictal state or are still having seizures.

Despite the many complications, the underlying disease is the most important factor in determining the prognosis of GCSE. No morbidity or mortality numbers are worth reporting without a precise description of the population studied. Nevertheless, the mortality rate has declined in recent decades, and the mortality rate of the SE itself should be below 1 to 2 percent with reasonable treatment; that of the condition causing GCSE may be substantially higher. Anoxia, stroke, drug toxicity, central nervous system infection, and severe metabolic derangements predict a worse outcome. Tumors and head injury vary in prognostic gravity, depending on the series. SE caused by alcohol abuse or drug withdrawal has a better outcome. A long duration of SE, especially with systemic complications of hypothermia and hypotension, and delayed effective treatment also worsen outcome. Patients unresponsive to initial treatment with one or two anticonvulsant drugs (patients with ''refractory'' SE) have a worse prognosis.

It has become increasingly clear that SE is almost two different conditions in patients with prior epilepsy and in those with a new diagnosis. Patients with prior epilepsy, and those with a precipitation by anticonvulsant or other medication withdrawal,

TABLE 142-3. Complications of Status Epilepticus

Systemic
Cardiac:	Hypertension, tachycardia (reversing after 30 min), arrhythmias, cardiac arrest
Pulmonary:	Apnea, respiratory failure, hypoxia, neurogenic pulmonary edema, aspiration pneumonia
Autonomic:	Fever, sweating, hypersecretion (including tracheobronchial), vomiting
Metabolic:	Hyperkalemia, hyperglycemia, then, hypoglycemia, volume depletion and venous stasis and possible thrombosis
Endocrine:	Increased prolactin and cortisol
Other:	Leukocytosis, CSF pleocytosis, vertebral and other fractures, physical injury, rhabdomyolysis, renal failure, disseminated intravascular coagulation

Brain
Neuronal damage similar to that of hypoxia, hyperthermia: cortical layers 3 and 5, cerebellum, and hippocampus
Cerebral edema, raised intracranial pressure
Cortical vein thrombosis

Neurologic sequelae
Increased seizure frequency, recurrent status epilepticus
Decreased cognitive function (?)
Drug effects; increased exposure to anticonvulsants

respond far better to treatment; this may be due to earlier detection and diagnosis, partial treatment from earlier anticonvulsant administration, or the absence of acute insults that worsen the prognosis in the other patients. Children also fare far better than adults; older patients are often prey to underlying illnesses with higher morbidity and mortality rates.

Clinical lessons also emerge from the pathophysiology and prognostic studies of convulsive SE. First, the longer the SE, the more refractory it becomes and the more neuronal damage occurs. Second, although systemic factors, including hypotension, hypoxia, and acidosis, may add to the neurologic complications, some damage appears to accrue from the synchronized discharging neural activity itself. Persistent EEG discharges are generally an indication for treatment, so an EEG is necessary when convulsions have ended but the patient has not yet awakened. Third, clinical and experimental data suggest that 30 minutes of convulsive SE is a critical duration in neurologic function and probably in prognosis. This duration is far less certain in other, particularly nonconvulsive, forms of SE.

OTHER TYPES OF STATUS EPILEPTICUS

Convulsive SE is rarely a diagnostic problem, but other forms of SE may present less dramatically on general wards or even in the outpatient setting, and diagnosis becomes more important. Management is often similar but less urgent. Other forms of SE can be divided into generalized seizures and those with a partial or focal onset.

Generalized Forms of Status Epilepticus

Absence (Petit Mal). Terminology in this area is confusing, with descriptions of ''spike-wave stupor'' and ''epileptic twilight states.'' Absence status implies generalized epileptiform EEG discharges (Fig. 142-1).

Because of the difficulty of detection it is hard to know how often absence status occurs. It may be a quarter as frequent as convulsive SE. It typically occurs in patients with prior genetic primary generalized epilepsy, but patients may be otherwise healthy, seizure-free, and off medication for years. It may well present to the office physician as confusion and limited responsiveness in an older person with a remote history of epilepsy and no recent treatment, sometimes with infection or other systemic illness. Older patients have more de novo absence SE. Metabolic and pharmacologic precipitants exist, and benzodiazepine withdrawal is particularly common. Persistent epileptic unresponsiveness with generalized EEG discharges also explains some persistent coma following generalized convulsions.

Onset may be sudden or gradual. Patients may be awake, walking and talking, though they are often confused. Motor activity may be preserved but clumsy. There is occasionally some blinking or sporadic myoclonus. Absence SE can persist for days or weeks without recognition. The earlier history of epilepsy should be suggestive. It is entirely possible that most cases are missed, although the diagnosis is readily confirmed by EEG. Some show generalized 3-Hz epileptiform discharges, and some may be secondarily generalized from a focus.

Benzodiazepine treatment is often successful rapidly, especially in younger patients with primary generalized epilepsies. Valproic acid may be more efficacious in preventing recurrences. Most patients return to normal, although recurrence of absence SE is relatively common. Response to anticonvulsant therapy can be delayed in older patients and those with a less certain cause. The typical absence status of patients with prior epilepsy is not known to be life-threatening although occasional episodes end with a generalized convulsion.

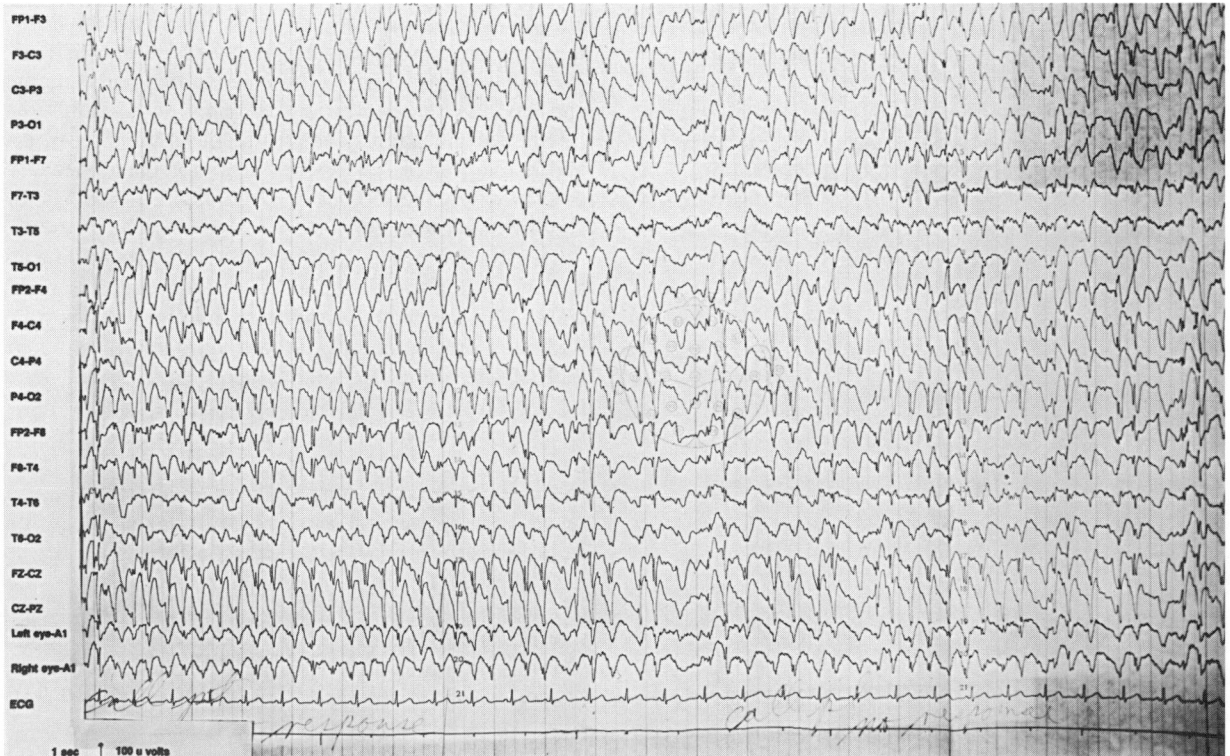

FIG. 142-1. EEG of a 33-year-old woman with a history of epilepsy who was ambulatory and speaking but confused at the time of an office visit. The EEG showed approximately 3-Hz generalized spike-and-slow-wave discharges with a frontal and central emphasis, consistent with absence SE.

Myoclonic Status Epilepticus.   Myoclonic status epilepticus (MSE) also comes in several forms. The most severe is that following anoxia, essentially always a fatal condition. Persistent myoclonus due to a severe encephalopathy without MSE is potentially reversible. The EEG helps to determine whether myoclonus is the sporadic sign of an encephalopathy or part of MSE; the former has a better prognosis. At least following anoxia, MSE is best considered the sign of a severely damaged brain rather than a treatable epileptic condition. MSE may have motor manifestations limited to ''subtle'' status, also an ominous sign after anoxia.

MSE as a manifestation of generalized epilepsies such as in juvenile myoclonic epilepsy, on the other hand, may include prolonged epileptic myoclonus without loss of consciousness. The EEG shows generalized polyspike and slow-wave discharges with a normal background between episodes. Episodes may go on for hours (with preserved consciousness), but the prognosis is excellent given the prior normal neurologic function. Similarly, patients can return to baseline in the MSE of progressive myoclonus epilepsies, although this may be part of a progressive, debilitating, neurologic disease. In all of these conditions the EEG can help to distinguish MSE from encephalopathies with less rhythmic abnormalities.

Tonic Status Epilepticus.   Tonic SE is rare and is seen primarily in children, particularly with Lennox-Gastaut syndrome. Treatment of the potentially injurious seizures is often frustrating, as is the associated mental retardation. Rarely, benzodiazepines have been cited as triggering tonic status. Tonic (and atonic) SE is distinctly uncommon in adults and certainly in those with normal neurologic function interictally. Similarly, generalized clonic SE is a pediatric condition. Clonus is often of low amplitude; both sides of the body are usually involved but may move asynchronously.

Status Epilepticus With a Partial (Focal) Origin

Epilepsia Partialis Continua.   The most readily recognized focal SE is continuous regular muscle jerking or epilepsia partialis continua (EPC). EPC signifies involvement of motor cortex. Focal SE implies focal pathology, and tumors, acute vascular disease (such as vasculitis or new strokes) and infectious diseases, particularly encephalitis, are among the most common causes. Old epileptogenic lesions can be activated by a new metabolic, infectious, or other stress, such as hyponatremia or renal failure. Nonketotic hyperglycemia is particularly common. Trauma and mitochondrial disorders are other possible causes, and occasional children with rolandic epilepsy have continuous motor symptoms with a presumed genetic origin. Some episodes are seen in progressive lesions such as a Rasmussen's encephalitis, presumed due to a slow viral agent and generally limited to children and adolescents. Most episodes of focal SE do not generalize. Whether EPC leads to significant neuronal damage is controversial.

Other Forms of Partial Status Epilepticus Without Motor Activity.   Other forms of partial status without motor activity are rarely diagnosed. It is unclear whether the neural substrates involved are less vulnerable to epileptic processes or whether this is a failure in diagnosis. Perhaps the best reported cases are those of aphasic status. Patients may appear extremely similar to those with Wernicke's aphasias of embolic vascular origin. Continuous EEG discharges are almost always in the left

hemisphere, particularly in posterior temporal (or frontal) areas. Speech arrest, however, occurs in many different types of seizures, particularly of frontal lobe origin.

Persistent visual hallucinations and eye movements may be seen with occipital SE. Prolonged sensory symptoms, including autonomic, can also occur in partial SE, but ictal discharges may be difficult or impossible to record. A high index of suspicion, ready use of the EEG, and a response to anticonvulsants are the keys to diagnosis and treatment.

Complex Partial Status Epilepticus.   Complex partial status epilepticus (CPSE) implies an impairment of consciousness from seizures with a focal origin, sometimes called fugue states or ''psychomotor status.'' Confusion is the most common symptom. A sudden alteration in behavior, particularly in a patient with prior epilepsy, should raise this possibility; although the diagnosis is frequently invoked to explain bizarre behavior, it is actually relatively rare. Some patients may also have complex partial seizures with a prolonged postictal phase. CPSE may be continuous or include discrete seizures so frequent that recovery does not occur between them. CPSE can go on for weeks. The usual site of origin is assumed to be mesial temporal structures with limbic connections, but implanted electrode recording has shown that frontal lobe onset is common. The EEG may show the seizure clearly (though less likely in frontal areas without implanted electrodes) or may have just persistent focal slowing. Seizures may spread rapidly, and nonconvulsive SE with generalized discharges (absence SE) may actually arise from a focus.

CPSE can be very difficult to distinguish from absence SE; these patients may exhibit more bizarre behavior during confusional states, leading to confusion with psychiatric disease or metabolic encephalopathies with delirium. CPSE should be stopped, but not as urgently as GCSE. Most CPSE responds relatively rapidly to anticonvulsants but may recur even with adequate anticonvulsant therapy.

Nonconvulsive Status Epilepticus.   Nonconvulsive status epilepticus (NCSE) includes many of the syndromes described above. Most patients have absence SE; far fewer have CPSE. SE with simple partial sensory or autonomic symptoms and all SE without convulsions are included.

Electrographic Status Epilepticus.   There are also patients with electrographic status epilepticus (ESE) where the significance of the continuous epileptic discharges on EEG is unknown or controversial. Children with continuous ESE during sleep (ESES) may have no clear clinical concomitant, but most have mental retardation and epilepsy, generally attributed to a static encephalopathy. Many have markedly impaired language function. In waking, the children tend to be healthier than those with a Lennox-Gastaut syndrome. Medications may improve the EEG without affecting overall clinical condition or behavior. At times, ESES is associated with neuropsychological regression after previously normal development.

ESE may also be seen in adult patients, in some cases representing absence SE or following convulsive status. In other cases it may be an unexpected finding in patients with severe medical illness with encephalopathies and with uncertain clinical significance. Some patients have subtle motor phenomena, but in others coma is the only manifestation. Diagnosis rests on the EEG. Anticonvulsant treatment is occasionally helpful but may be unrewarding primarily due to the severe underlying illness.

TREATMENT

As in all areas of medicine, effective treatment is facilitated tremendously by the correct diagnosis. Convulsive SE is rarely a diagnostic difficulty, but nonconvulsive status epilepticus (NCSE), including after generalized seizures, may be difficult to recognize and may even be missed altogether. Conversely, not all that shakes and responds poorly is status epilepticus (Table 142-4). Movement disorders, including chorea, myoclonus, tremors, and tics, have been treated as SE with potentially greater harm from the treatment than from the disease.

Pseudostatus is particularly troublesome. Further complicating diagnosis, these nonepileptic episodes often occur in patients with epileptic seizures, as well. Out-of-phase limb movements and more complicated vocalizations correlate with nonepileptic spells. Iatrogenic morbidity is common in these patients, and spells may persist until treatment causes respiratory arrest. Recurrence is common. Psychiatric management is appropriate but not always successful.

Clinical Evaluation

The history often provides some reason for SE (Table 142-2). A history of trauma, drug overdose, alcohol use, medical illness, stroke, or epilepsy may be available through family members, companions, medical bracelets, and personal possessions. Physical examination focuses on the underlying cause of SE and localization of the neurologic abnormality. Vital signs are crucial, given the cardiovascular complications; respiratory failure is an occasional complication of SE but more often results from medications. The general examination can show signs of infection (e.g., fever, nuchal rigidity, or skin lesions) or systemic illness such as kidney or liver disease. Signs of head injury or coagulopathy are also important. The neurologic examination also assesses whether seizures are actually continuing in subtle ways.

Laboratory Studies

Appropriate laboratory studies include a search for metabolic abnormalities, particularly of sodium, calcium, magnesium, and glucose; kidney, liver, and coagulation assays are also important. Toxicology screen, anticonvulsant drug levels, and arterial oxygen tension are often helpful, but treatment must begin before these levels are known. The blood gas and prolactin level can be useful in the consideration of pseudoseizures. Women

of childbearing age should have a pregnancy test, in part for counseling with regard to the effects of SE and medications. When pregnant, women should be assessed for eclampsia. Urgent computed tomography scans are prompted by concerns for head injury, an asymmetric neurologic examination or by seizures with a focal origin. Any source of infection must be found. Lumbar puncture is mandatory with any suggestion of central nervous system infection, or when SE is of unknown cause or difficult to control.

GCSE is diagnosed without an EEG, and treatment begins without it. An EEG is necessary for diagnosis of NCSE, although treatment may begin based on clinical suspicion. It is mandatory when a patient does not respond to initial treatment, as it may be impossible to ascertain clinically whether the patient is postictal or still seizing.

Medical Management

Treatment begins as in other emergencies—with attention to airway, breathing, and circulation (ABC). Patients with GCSE or coma from other forms of SE usually need intubation, at least for airway protection. Physical safety and prevention of further injury must be assured. A soft oral airway is reasonable, but forced insertion or use of hard objects is not. Thiamine and a bolus of 50 percent glucose should be infused after establishment of a reliable normal saline intravenous line. Cardiac monitoring should continue for patients with GCSE or other coma, with attention to arrhythmias and ischemia. Medical management attempts to normalize blood pressure, volume status, temperature, ventilation, and oxygenation. For alcoholic or malnourished patients, 2g of magnesium is appropriate; hypomagnesemia may worsen seizures, although magnesium is not an anticonvulsant. Drug overdoses may prompt gastric emptying or even hemodialysis.

Anticonvulsant Therapy

The choice of anticonvulsant drugs in SE is still controversial. Relatively few studies have compared different medications, and it is important to stress that most series describe GCSE alone. Generalized nonconvulsive status following convulsive seizures should probably be considered as much of an emergency as GCSE, but other forms of SE are of less certain morbidity and urgency in treatment. Almost all published protocols and guidelines refer to GCSE; differences regarding other forms of SE will be pointed out. Medication use is generally similar but with less urgency. Nevertheless, other forms of SE can lead to convulsive seizures, and a casual approach is inappropriate.

Rather than trying to decide on "the best" anticonvulsant drug it may be more useful to consider medications in two classes. One is that of very rapidly acting anticonvulsants, largely limited to benzodiazepines, which are often necessary for the interruption of SE, especially when the physiologic and pathologic consequences of GCSE are imminent. Benzodiazepines are invaluable in interrupting continuous seizures but may not be necessary when seizures are discrete, if with incomplete recovery. The other medications (led by phenytoin and phenobarbital, but including most other anticonvulsants) work less rapidly but provide continued protection against the reemergence of SE and are almost always necessary after the first few minutes. The goal must be to stop continuous convulsions or other symptoms and to interrupt continuing EEG discharges.

TABLE 142-4. Differential Diagnosis of Apparent Status Epilepticus

With prominent motor abnormalities
Movement disorders: myoclonus, tremors, chorea, tics, dystonic reactions
Structural disease: decerebrate, decorticate posturing
Psychiatric: pseudoseizure/conversion, acute psychosis

Usually "nonconvulsive"
Epilepsy-related: postictal state, periodic lateralized epileptiform discharges, with acute structural lesions
Acute encephalopathies: toxic: drug and alcohol related; metabolic, e.g., hypoglycemia, delirium related to drugs, alcohol, or infection
Psychiatric: catatonia, acute psychosis
Sleep disorders: narcolepsy, cataplexy, parasomnias
Syncope: cardiac, vagal, hypovolemia, medication toxicity
Vascular: strokes, transient ischemic attacks
Head injury: stupor, coma, amnesia
Transient global amnesia

TABLE 142-5. Anticonvulsant Properties in the Treatment of Status Epilepticus

Medication	Doses	Kinetics	Complications	Comment
Phenytoin	15–20 mg/kg <50 mg/min Maint. level ≈20 μg/ml	Effect: 10–30 min Peak effect: 1 h Elim. $t_{1/2}$: 24–48 h	Cardiac arrhythmias Hypotension	Bolus lasts 6–24 h Best in following level of consciousness Worst for cardiac disease
Phenobarbital	10–20 mg/kg <100 mg/min Maint. level ≈40 μg/ml	Effect: 5–20 min Peak: 1 h Elim. $t_{1/2}$: 120 h	Respiratory depression, hypotension (possible synergy with benzodiazepines)	Slower than benzodiazepines Depression of consciousness can be prolonged after loading
Diazepam	10 mg (.2 mg/kg) Repeat q15 min; up to ?40 mg <5 mg/min	Effect: 1–2 min Peak: 20–30 min Metabolite $t_{1/2}$: 36 h	Sedation, respiratory depression, hypotension Recurrent seizures as it wears off	Very rapid interruption of convulsions Needs to be followed by maintenance anticonvulsants
Lorazepam	4–8 mg (.1–.2 mg/kg) <2 mg/min	Effect: 2–5 min Peak: 15–30 min Elim. $t_{1/2}$: 12–15 h	Same as diazepam; less sudden	More prolonged protection; up to 12 h, against seizure recurrence No active toxic metabolites
Pentobarbital	Load 3–5 mg/kg Maintenance 1–4 mg/kg/h	Effect: minutes Elim. $t_{1/2}$: 20–40 h	Respiratory depression More severe hypotension Hypothermia	Uniformly effective High mortality due to underlying disease Duration of treatment unknown (?24 h)

Phenytoin. Phenytoin is probably the most frequently used anticonvulsant for SE but is often given in inadequate doses. Its major disadvantage is the long time required for a loading infusion (Table 142-5) although it may be beneficial before reaching "therapeutic levels." The advantage of minimal sedation from medication alone is generally overstated but may be pertinent with head trauma, hemorrhage, or raised intracranial pressure where it is important to monitor alertness. Patients with GCSE are unconscious, and the most immediate concern is stopping the seizures. In the absence of acute structural lesions, phenytoin may be successful alone in as many as 80 percent of patients with GCSE. It can then become a long-term maintenance medication without changing or adding drugs. Patients may need adjunctive benzodiazepines to interrupt convulsions if they occur during the phenytoin infusion. Many authorities recommend phenytoin as the primary treatment of GCSE, sometimes after initial interruption of convulsions with a benzodiazepine.

A usual loading dose is 15 mg/kg, but 20 mg/kg is reasonable before concluding that phenytoin is insufficient. It should be given by intravenous bolus or in saline solution at a maximum rate of 50 mg/min; it may precipitate in glucose solutions. Intramuscular phenytoin is poorly absorbed and should not be used.

Conduction defects are the primary cardiac toxicity, but hypotension is not rare. Cardiac monitoring is appropriate during phenytoin infusion. Elderly patients or those with cardiac disease may not tolerate phenytoin as well as phenobarbital. Acute toxicity is more closely related to the infusion rate than to total dose; patients with possible complications may tolerate greater doses in slower infusions. A new prodrug, without the propylene glycol carrier, may obviate some toxicity.

Phenobarbital. Phenobarbital is often used if phenytoin is insufficient. It is frequently avoided for fear of sedation, but its advantages include a relative lack of cardiac toxicity until very high doses are reached. Aside from phenytoin it is the major anticonvulsant available intravenously for longer term management. Its loading is faster than that of phenytoin, but its lipid solubility is lower and brain penetration slower. Up to 20 mg/kg is reasonable. Nevertheless, phenobarbital may act quickly, even before therapeutic levels have been established. In addition, while some SE may be refractory to phenytoin, high enough doses of phenobarbital will control almost all seizures. Very high doses require artificial ventilation and may cause hypotension, but they may also be tolerated better than expected. Sedation is expected with high doses of phenobarbi-

tal, but levels below 40 μg/ml should not produce prolonged coma.

Phenobarbital has been compared favorably to a combination of diazepam and phenytoin in one prospective trial; clinical response was actually faster with phenobarbital. Barbiturates and benzodiazepines may have a particularly severe effect on respiratory depression and hypotension when used together.

Diazepam. Diazepam can be very efficacious in the rapid interruption of convulsive SE but should not be used alone. Usual practice administers 10 mg intravenously over a few minutes, repeating if necessary. Rectal administration has been effective, particularly in children. Intramuscular diazepam is absorbed slowly. Diazepam is very lipid-soluble, enters the brain rapidly, and may have an anticonvulsant effect within a minute. Nevertheless, it redistributes to many tissues, and its central nervous system effect declines in 20 to 30 minutes; recurrent seizures or SE are common when longer acting anticonvulsants do not follow early diazepam administration. Repeated doses may lose effectiveness but produce metabolites with prolonged elimination half-lives and potential toxicity, including prolonged coma. Continuous infusion of diazepam (generally 4 to 8 mg/h) is often discussed for the management of SE but is rarely practiced, probably because the best doses have not been established clearly, and rapid acute tolerance may develop. Continuous infusion should only be used in intensive care units. Iatrogenic apnea can occur suddenly; it is often ascribed to seizures or to "tongue swallowing."

Benzodiazepines are particularly effective in typical absence SE, and subsequent longer term anticonvulsants may be unnecessary. For patients with continuous generalized discharges and coma, however, they are not as efficacious. Diazepam is a very common first treatment for SE, but conservative management would restrict it to patients with continuing convulsions or those having another convulsion during infusion of a maintenance medication. Different reviews have found diazepam effective in up to 83 percent of SE, or as low as 38 percent.

Lorazepam. Lorazepam has several advantages over diazepam. It may be rapid enough to interrupt seizures quickly and still have a more prolonged anticonvulsant effect; some feel that it satisfies the requirements for both the acute interruption of SE and prolonged protection against recurrence. Doses are approximately half that of diazepam. Its lipid solubility is half that of diazepam, and its brain penetration is slower, but it is still rapid. Its effect declines less rapidly than the effect of diazepam, but it has no active, troublesome metabolites.

Many epileptologists prefer lorazepam because of its favorable pharmacokinetics, but direct comparative studies are few. A double-blind, randomized trial found lorazepam marginally more effective in controlling SE than diazepam, with an onset of action not significantly different. Adverse effects of lorazepam are similar to those of diazepam, though perhaps less sudden. Lorazepam may provide 12 hours of anticonvulsant effect, but acute tolerance may occur and reduce its maintenance value.

Midazolam. Midazolam has proved successful in some particularly refractory cases of SE after failure of other benzodiazepines and phenytoin. In such cases it may avoid the adverse effects of barbiturate-induced coma. Its action is extremely rapid due to high lipid solubility, but its effect is short-lived, and recurrences of seizures may be expected. It may be utilized in 0.2 mg/kg (5 to 20 mg) intravenous boluses. It may be the best intramuscular treatment of SE when this is the only available route.

Clonazepam. Clonazepam appears similar to other benzodiazepines and is popular in Europe but is not available in intravenous form for the treatment of SE in the United States.

Paraldehyde. Paraldehyde has fallen out of favor in clinical trials but remains a popular alternative, especially in patients with allergies to other anticonvulsants and in whom intravenous access is limited: 5 to 10 ml may be given rectally mixed with mineral oil. Intramuscular use yields a faster effect but may produce sterile abscesses. The physical preparation is important because of its rapid decomposition and reaction with plastic and rubber tubing. Its onset of action is slower than for medications described earlier. Its effective half-life is 6 hours. It may be more effective in the treatment of SE prompted by alcohol withdrawal, but this has not been studied well. Oral administration in the setting of possible aspiration can lead to serious pulmonary toxicity. Its smell accounts for some of its unpopularity.

Valproic Acid. Valproic acid is generally available in rectal form only in the treatment of SE. Rectal doses of 17 mg/kg were recommended. Peak concentrations may lag by hours, and the effect may be even more delayed. Many patients never achieve therapeutic levels. It may be a useful adjunct in the long-term treatment of refractory or intermittent SE and is helpful in preventing the recurrence of absence SE. Currently, there is little role for valproic acid in the acute management of SE.

Carbamazepine. Enteral carbamazepine may be useful in long courses of refractory seizures, but it is not available intravenously or helpful acutely in SE. Felbamate, gabapentin, and lamotrigine are not currently available intravenously and have not been well studied for SE.

Pentobarbital. When GCSE has continued for 30 to 45 minutes or when other forms of SE must be stopped (though no one knows exactly when that is) pentobarbital (or thiopental) can provide a definitive treatment. Short-acting barbiturates are rapid but require intensive care unit treatment. Loading doses of 3 to 5 mg/kg followed by infusion of 1 to 4 mg/kg/h are typical; some studies suggest that many patients need at least

3.5 mg/kg/h. Effectiveness is assayed by effect on the EEG, with an attempt to either eliminate seizures or aim for a "burst suppression" or flat recording; most reviewers aim for a burst suppression pattern. The half-life of pentobarbital is approximately 20 hours but may be extended at higher levels. Accordingly, prolonged coma after pentobarbital treatment should not be attributed to a destroyed or "burnt out" brain before the medication has had time to dissipate. Levels are more useful to indicate residual toxicity than they are in assessing therapeutic effect.

All SE should be suppressible with adequate pentobarbital doses, but hypotension is very common. Usually, volume replacement and low doses of vasopressors are sufficient. Myocardial function and temperature regulation can be impaired. Most reports of pentobarbital use show a very high mortality, usually attributed to severe underlying diseases, causing SE refractory enough to require pentobarbital. An advantage of pentobarbital, besides its invariable effectiveness when used in large enough doses, is a reduction of cerebral metabolism and blood flow. The infusion is also easy to adjust. The optimal duration of barbiturate-induced coma has not been established; recommendations range from 4 to 72 hours. Patients should probably have therapeutic levels of two other anticonvulsants before pentobarbital withdrawal. Currently, pentobarbital should be considered the definitive treatment of GCSE after 30 to 45 minutes of convulsions or when earlier medications have failed or are unavailable.

Inhaled Anesthetics. Inhaled anesthetics are less well studied and far less convenient but may have a role in patients allergic to pentobarbital. Most increase cerebral blood flow, a theoretical disadvantage. Isoflurane is possibly the most effective anesthetic with the least cardiovascular effect in the setting of SE. Halothane is used relatively frequently, but isoflurane may produce a burst suppression EEG tracing with less severe cardiovascular effects. Both may require vasopressors. Nitrous oxide does not appear effective. Enflurane can precipitate convulsions.

Lidocaine. Lidocaine can also cause convulsions and must remain a last resort. It can produce a rapid effect without significant respiratory depression.

Propofol. Intravenous propofol, a nonbarbiturate anesthetic, is extremely lipid-soluble and very rapid. It can cause severe respiratory depression and nonepileptic involuntary movements and can also precipitate seizures.

Neuromuscular Blocking Agents. Neuromuscular blocking agents eliminate motor activity, but it must be understood that they are not anticonvulsants. They may provide false reassurance when SE continues on an electrical, cellular, and metabolic basis. They can help when excessive motor activity impairs oxygenation, acid-base balance, or temperature regulation, but adequate doses of anticonvulsants, particularly pentobarbital, will obviate these problems.

Steroids and Osmotic Agents. Steroids and osmotic agents may be used to treat cerebral edema that results from prolonged SE, particularly in children, but efficacy has not been established. Rarely, a persistent seizure focus causing refractory partial SE may be resected surgically.

Summary. Most medication trials have studied patients with GCSE. Other forms of SE may benefit from the same medications with somewhat less urgency. Intravenous benzodiazepines usually interrupt absence SE, and subsequent treatment may be unnecessary. For partial or nonconvulsive SE, enteral valproate and carbamazepine are more valuable, although the response may take days. Rarely will pentobarbital or anesthetics be necessary there; medications with a greater toxicity, including those with a potential for worsening seizures, are even less appropriate. In children, phenobarbital is often preferred to phenytoin for reasons of absorption, efficacy, and longer term side effects.

Electroencephalography

EEG use in SE depends on the seizure type and vigor of treatment. It is generally unnecessary with generalized convulsions or other motor phenomena, but is mandatory when motor activity has ceased and the patient has not returned to normal; the clinician needs to know if seizures are actually continuing. The EEG is necessary in assessing medication effect with high doses of anticonvulsants, particularly pentobarbital. Certainly, with neuromuscular blocking agents the EEG is required to tell whether SE has been treated at all.

Protocol

Protocols for the treatment of SE emphasize the ABCs of cardiorespiratory support in acutely ill patients followed by one of several orders of standard anticonvulsants, often emphasizing diazepam, lorazepam, phenytoin, and phenobarbital. Rather than choose one protocol for all patients it might be best to keep in mind the principles listed below:

1. Be sure of the diagnosis. Distinguish from myoclonus, other movement disorders, decerebrate posturing, and pseudoseizures. Blood gases and EEG may be helpful.
2. Determine the cause of SE through history, examination, and appropriate laboratory tests.
3. Attention to airway, respiration, blood pressure, and cardiac rhythm. Most patients with GCSE require intubation. Patients with other forms of SE generally do not. Establish an intravenous line with saline, thiamine, and glucose. Antibiotics are given when infection is considered. Blood should be drawn for metabolic studies, anticonvulsant levels, and toxic screens.
4. A long-acting medication is necessary. Phenytoin is the most frequently used maintenance medication and should be given in saline at 50 mg/min, with attention to the cardiogram, to a dose of 15 to 20 mg/kg rather than the commonly used 1,000 mg. Phenobarbital is more often used for children and for elderly patients or those with cardiac rhythm disturbances, at 10 to 20 mg/kg, up to 100 mg/min, with attention to blood pressure.
5. Rapidly acting anticonvulsants (i.e., benzodiazepines) should be given if GCSE has lasted 30 minutes, if convulsions are continuous, if convulsions occur during the infusion of phenytoin or phenobarbital, or if phenytoin or phenobarbital are not successful. Lorazepam, 4 to 8 mg in adults, can be given at a rate of 2 mg/min and repeated if necessary.
6. Definitive treatment with pentobarbital should be used after 30 to 45 minutes or if the above agents are unsuccessful. This should be done in the intensive care unit after intubation. Induction is with 3 to 5 mg/kg and an attempt to eliminate epileptiform activity on the EEG; many clinicians proceed to burst suppression EEG tracings. Maintenance is with 1 to 4 mg/kg/h as needed to control seizures and attain the desired EEG recording.
7. When used, pentobarbital might be discontinued after 24 to 48 hours, assuming clinical and electrographic seizures have ceased and that two longer acting anticonvulsants are at high therapeutic levels.
8. Continued reassessment of clinical and EEG activity, as well as attention to the diagnosis and medical complications, is necessary until the patient returns to normal.
9. Maintenance medications must be chosen and established at therapeutic levels. Attention is given to complications such as hypothermia, acidosis, hypotension, rhabdomyolysis, renal failure, infection, and cerebral edema.

Continual reassessment of the patient's clinical condition and EEG are necessary, as is questioning about the diagnosis, underlying disease, and medication effectiveness. When SE does not respond to treatment as expected attention should refocus along several lines. First, be sure the diagnosis of SE was correct. Second, the underlying cause is crucial, and SE can continue especially when trauma, hemorrhage, or infections such as encephalitis remain untreated. Third, medications are often given in inadequate doses, such as the 1,000-mg standard phenytoin infusion. Fourth, medication absorption may be insufficient if there are problems with intravenous access or if given by another route. Finally, SE may be treated successfully and then recur, most often due to inadequate attention to maintenance levels of longer acting anticonvulsants or to lack of treatment of the underlying disease.

SUGGESTED READINGS

Barry E, Hauser WA: Status epilepticus: the interaction of epilepsy and acute brain disease. Neurology 43:1473–8, 1993
Hauser WA: Status epilepticus: epidemiologic considerations. Neurology 40(suppl. 2):9–13, 1990
Lothman EW: The biochemical basis and pathophysiology of status epilepticus. Neurology 40(suppl. 2):13–23, 1990
Meldrum BS, Horton RW: Physiology of status epilepticus in primates. Arch Neurol 28:1–9, 1973
Schomer DL: Focal status epilepticus and epilepsia partialis continua in adults and children. Epilepsia 34(suppl. 1):S29–S36, 1993
Tomson T, Lindbom U, Nilsson BY: Nonconvulsive status epilepticus in adults: thirty-two consecutive patients from a general hospital population. Epilepsia 33:829–35, 1992
Van Ness PC: Pentobarbital and EEG burst suppression in treatment of status epilepticus refractory to benzodiazepines and phenytoin. Epilepsia 31:61–7, 1990
Walton NY: Systemic effects of generalized convulsive status epilepticus. Epilepsia 34 (Suppl. 1):S54–S58, 1993

143. SURGICAL TREATMENT OF EPILEPSY

DONALD L. SCHOMER

Surgical approaches to epilepsy are useful mainly in forms of medically intractable partial epilepsy. Partial seizures are those that have a focal neocortical onset. They remain partial, either simple or complex, or secondarily generalized. The surgical approach aims to remove the area of brain that generates the onset of the ictal event, called the "epileptic zone," or, in cases of identifiable "lesions," to remove the lesion and the surrounding area that is necessary to initiate convulsive behavior. Surgery, in the partial epilepsies, attempts to either make the disorder controllable medically or to produce a "cure." Callosotomy, however, aims to reduce the occurrence of a certain specific type of seizure, the drop attack, and is used in patients with mixed seizures. At a recent international meeting of the major epilepsy surgical centers in Palm Desert, California, the need for surgical approaches was delineated. It is estimated that the incidence of epilepsy in the United States is between 0.5 and 1.0 percent, which translates as between 1.25 and 2.5 million people with all forms of epilepsy. Somewhere between 40 and 60 percent of the total population of people with epilepsy have partial or focal onset seizures. This represents 500,000 to 1.5 million people. Approximately 50 percent of this latter group will achieve good control with medication, leaving between 250,000 and 750,000 people with poorly controlled forms of partial epilepsy. Of this group, it is estimated that 30 percent would benefit by a surgical procedure. This translates to approximately 75,000 people in the United States with potentially surgically amenable or treatable forms of partial epilepsy. Approximately 5,000 new cases are added to this number every year. While these figures probably represent a slight overestimate of the number of cases where surgery may help, given the fact that only between 1,500 and 2,500 cases are surgically treated on a yearly basis in this country, there is a tremendous underutilization of this approach.

Difficulties in dealing with a surgical approach are multiple. There needs to be better primary care physician recognition that surgical approaches are reasonable. Patients need to be evaluated by groups experienced in the diagnosis and management of the surgical patients. While there are probably an adequate number of facilities available in the United States to make this form of treatment a viable and more frequently used alternative, the expense to implement such an approach could be enormous. There needs to be a recognition of the importance for funding surgical treatment, since the payoff in a successful outcome is a productive individual. These issues have significant psychosocial and fiscal ramifications.

IDENTIFYING THE POPULATION AT RISK

In 1975 two pioneers in the surgical treatment of epilepsy, McNaughton and Rasmussen wrote that "Without doubt, the proper evaluation and selection of patients for surgical management of the symptom, epilepsy, is the most important single factor in determining the success or failure of this form of treatment in reducing the seizure tendency." In the United States, most patients presenting with epileptic seizures are seen and treated by pediatricians, internists, and general medical physicians. Most patients with new onset seizures have a routine EEG evaluation and some form of imaging study, that is, computed tomography (CT), or magnetic resonance imaging (MRI). If patients continue to have seizure events for more than 3 months following adequate trials with at least one or several antiseizure drugs, they should be referred to a neurologist. Most practicing neurologists are quite capable of reevaluating such a patient. They first confirm that the continuing events are epileptic in nature and then identify additional reasonable medical alternatives. Most neurologists are comfortable in prescribing additional antiseizure medications in a controlled fashion and dealing with some of the known provocations. However, if, after several additional medical trials, the patient is still having seizures, he or she should be considered for formal evaluation at one of the nation's epilepsy centers.

Epilepsy centers are multidisciplinary diagnostic and treatment units. Patients are usually first screened by an epileptologist, that is, a neurologist specializing in epilepsy. Most epilepsy centers try to coordinate their efforts with those of the referring MD/neurologist. If a surgical approach is to be considered, it must be weighed in the context of the relative refractoriness to medication, identification of the focal onset of the events, an understanding of the natural history of the specific seizure syndrome if identifiable, and the impact that the workup, surgery, and postoperative care will have on the individual and his family.

Refractoriness is itself a difficult concept to define. Patients should, as a minimum, have clinical breakthrough seizures while on "adequate" medications. The events must be disturbing enough that the patient's lifestyle is adversely affected by their occurrence. Consider a patient who has only an occasional nocturnal generalized seizure that may occur at intervals of 4 to 8 weeks. The consequence of those seizures is profound fatigue the following day. That fatigue may constitute relative refractoriness if it subsequently adversely affects the patients' economic independence or social or psychiatric well-being. Some patients may have complex partial seizures reduced by medication to simple partial events. In some cases, the simple partial seizures may be manifested by minor unpleasant smells or a feeling of nausea, but in other cases they may be associated with profound feelings of doom that makes the person distraught and anxious for many hours. In the one case, the patient may be appropriately willing to live with these experiences, but in the other case the subject may find them so disturbing that surgery becomes a real alternative. Many patients are adversely affected by their antiseizure medicines and would consider a surgical approach if it meant fewer medicines, lower doses of medicines, or possible withdrawal altogether from drugs.

The epileptologist makes every attempt to identify a "seizure syndrome." This is helpful when considering counseling patients for surgery because there is now an understanding of the expected natural history of the disorder. It is important, for instance, to identify the "benign" syndromes like rolandic or occipital epilepsy where, even if the disorder is somewhat resistant to treatment, it has an excellent long-term prognosis. This can be compared to mesial temporal sclerosis where, if the patient is refractory to medicines, the natural history would support a more aggressive approach surgically. In the cases of symptomatic partial epilepsy, where the seizures are secondary to a structural lesion, the lesion and the epilepsy need to be dealt with together. With the advent of improved imaging and EEG recording techniques, many patients can now be defined as having one of these syndromes early on in their treatment.

Medication compliance is another major issue. In order for a patient to be deemed medically refractory there must be clear, well-documented trials with several medicines that have failed to produce control.

INVESTIGATION OF SURGICAL PATIENTS

Figure 143-1 illustrates the protocol for evaluating potential surgical patients.

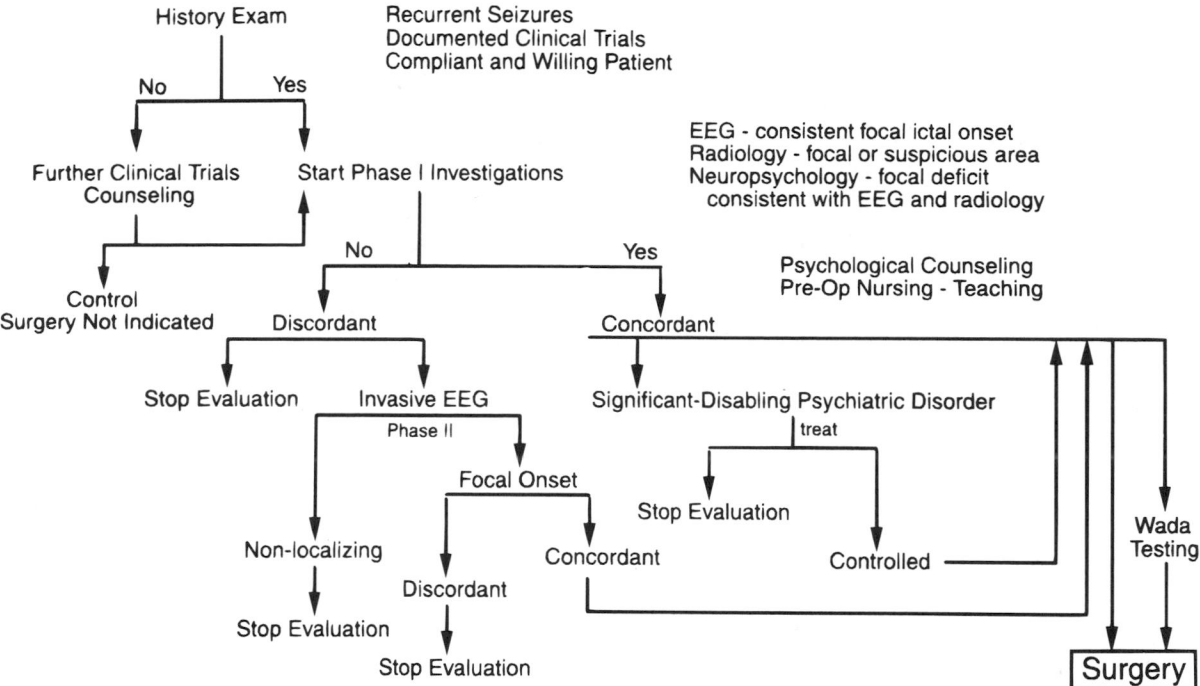

FIG. 143-1. The evaluation and decision-making process that would ultimately lead to a focal cortical resection for either temporal or frontal lobe. Phase I EEG investigations are noninvasive, while Phase II investigations require the use of at least one type of invasive electrode as defined.

History

It is important to review with the patient and relevant family members the history of the onset and course of the patient's seizure disorder. It is worth noting the first event and the circumstances surrounding that event, such as head injuries, fevers, loss of sleep, unusual stress, exposures to medicines, drugs, or toxins. The subsequent evolution of the seizure disorder is equally important in assessing the natural history as well as outlining the historical response to medications and side effects. It is always worth checking original data obtained early in the course of the disorder, including neurologically relevant findings, physical abnormalities, abnormal imaging studies, or electroencephalograms (EEGs). If available, the early imaging studies and EEG should be reviewed and compared to more recently acquired studies to better define the natural history of the disorder in the individual. Historically, it is important to note any abnormalities or changes in the psychosocial or educational development that may give clues to either medication side effects or progressive neurologic disease. Detailed developmental histories are invariably obtained on patients by the epileptologists. These questions not only outline the prospective patient's birth history and development but also outline the family's response to the disorder. This serves two purposes. First, in attempting to define any seizure syndrome, it is important to note trends that exist in biologically related individuals and their families. These observations are not only relevant to identifying and detailing others with specific syndromic forms of epilepsy but also in defining other conditions that have familial tendencies and may be either part of the epileptic syndrome or misdiagnosed as seizures. Potential confounding disorders include manic depressive disease, seasonal affective disorder, or schizophrenic disorders just to mention a few. Second, this type of detailed history lays the groundwork for all future personal and family counseling that will be necessary before surgery can be attempted. The patient's response to his seizures as well as the family's reaction to him and his seizures are necessary to understand if the patient is going to express anger, frustrations, and fears as well as hopes for a surgical procedure. For instance, if a patient's surgical procedure is successful and he has no more seizures postoperatively, but remains in a socially and psychologically over protected environment, he may not be, in the end, significantly better, from the psychosocial or educational perspective, for having undergone surgery. As a corollary to this observation is the fact that many successful surgical patients end marriages that were based on their illness or on their role as a "sick person."

Physical Examination

The physical examination includes a general examination looking for major medical problems such as cardiac murmurs or arrhythmias as well as significant neurocutaneous stigmata that would indicate an underlying hereditary familial disorder where epilepsy may be playing a part. The neurologic examination should be detailed. Subtle differences in cortical sensory function need to be tested, subtle motor coordination asymmetries noted, and subtle reflex asymmetries documented. These become more important when trying to find corresponding imaging abnormalities or EEG findings.

Investigative Testing

Telemetered EEG is one of the mainstays in the evaluation of an individual for surgery. Baseline EEG studies are important in noting the presence of interictal epileptic activity. If present, it is important to note whether the discharges are consistently focal, multifocal, or generalized in appearance. Slowing on the EEG, either focal or generalized, is also an important observation. The former pattern suggests a structural abnormality that may correlate with seizure onset. The latter may reflect either a more widespread diffuse disease process or a secondary effect from medication. When considering someone for focal cortical resection, however, the most important EEG data is that which is recorded during "an event." The EEG onset of a seizure usually occurs before the patient is aware of the "event." If the EEG changes occur after the patient is aware of the onset of the seizure, the EEG may not be showing the area of onset but rather an area into which the epileptic physiologic event has spread. In order to enhance the spatial capabilities of the EEG, sphenoidal electrodes are frequently used when exploring for focal onset in the inferior temporal regions or posterior inferior frontal areas. It is also best to record spontaneous seizures that occur without alterations in medication dosing or associated with behavioral manipulations. If seizure frequency is such that it would be statistically unlikely to capture an event while doing EEG recording, drugs can be withdrawn in a controlled environment. Advances in technology allow for computer-assisted detections of seizures and interictal epileptic abnormalities. This allows the investigator to find abnormalities that might otherwise go either unnoticed or unseen. It is necessary to capture several typical seizures on EEG before making a decision regarding the completeness of this part of the evaluations. It is also reasonable to record the behavior of the patient on video. If there is a clear focal onset seen on the EEG that correlates with the onset of the clinical activity and the events are typical for the patient, this part of the evaluation can be considered complete. If no such clear correlation is seen, the patient may then become a candidate for more invasive EEG (discussed below).

Parallel to the EEG evaluation, patients usually undergo imaging procedures. The most helpful studies now are done with magnetic resonance techniques. Subjects should have T1- and T2-weighted images with coronal, anteroposterior, and sagittal views. Obvious lesions and malformations are looked for depending on the seizure semiology. Evidence for sclerosis is looked for in mesial temporal regions and in frontal areas when appropriate clinically. Thin cuts are also useful when looking for subtle cortical migration abnormalities where congenital asymmetries are noted. Gadolinium enhancement is also useful when trying to define vascular or neoplastic abnormalities. A more recent adjunct to MRI are the magnetic resonance volumetric studies, which are particularly useful in hippocampal regions when evaluating patients with hippocampal sclerosis. If an atrophic hippocampus can be demonstrated with this technique and it is on the same side as EEG onset, this is extremely helpful in prognosticating a successful long-term response to surgical removal of that area as well as predicting the lack of cognitive consequences from the removal.

Dynamic imaging is gaining popularity in some centers and includes single photon-emitted computed tomography (SPECT), positron-emitted tomography (PET), and functional MRI (fMRI). In all three techniques, it is important to know the state of the patients while they are being studied. The results, if obtained during the seizure, show the effects of increased neuronal activity focally that may be manifest by increased blood flow as noted through SPECT or PET techniques, increased metabolic activity as demonstrated on specific forms of PET scans, or changes in the oxy- to deoxyhemoglobin ratios seen on fMRI. The opposite findings are also noted if done during interictal periods, with a few minor exceptions.

Detailed neuropsychological testing is done preoperatively to assess general level of cognitive capability as well as to assess for focal areas of relatively inadequate performance. In patients undergoing evaluation for focal cortical resections, an additional localizing finding is a deficit in cognitive performance that is in the same region as the EEG and imaging procedures.

The neuropsychologist can also provide necessary counseling, which is relevant to the surgical and postoperative care but also addresses the anxieties and fears that surround the procedure. Identifying major psychiatric disorders is important, since the presence of major psychosis or suicidal depression are both contraindications to going forward with surgery. If identified and successfully treated, many patients can continue their workups. The neuropsychologist also addresses issues related to the family or work that must be resolved before an operation.

The neuropsychologist is the individual who is responsible for assessing hemispheric specialization for memory and language. This is confirmed, when necessary, by doing a Wada procedure which involves injecting relatively small doses of sodium amytal into the carotid artery (intracarotid amytal procedure) while assessing cognitive function during the time of transient medication-induced deficit.

Invasive EEG

There are occasions where the scalp recording of seizures does not afford sufficient information so that a surgical decision can be made. Under those conditions, invasive EEG may be helpful. A variety of electrodes is tailored to the specific surgical questions asked. Foramen ovale electrodes are perhaps the least invasive of invasive electrodes. They are placed through the foramen ovale and are directed along the mesial aspects of each temporal lobe. These electrodes can remain in place for many weeks and are often coupled with surface/scalp electrodes or other more invasive electrodes. Recording with the foramen ovale electrodes is useful in localizing seizures that, by seizure semiology, are suspected of originating in mesial temporal structures. While this electrode is relatively noninvasive, the major complication, tic douloureux, is relatively high. Epidural pegs are likewise relatively noninvasive with respect to brain penetration. Multiple electrodes can be placed through small twist drill holes, and their recording contacts are in the epidural space. Both hemispheres can be investigated through this multiple electrode placement procedure. Since the electrodes are on the inside of the skull, recordings show higher amplitude and much less artifact than scalp recordings do. These electrodes are often useful in investigating patients where frontal or central seizure foci are suspected. Electrode strips or grids can be placed either by burr holes or through a craniotomy. From the patient's perspective, this is relatively invasive; however, very little neocortical damage occurs with these procedures. These electrodes are useful in investigating patients where neocortical onset of seizures is suspected and where the hemisphere of onset can be identified. An additional advantage of the grid electrodes is that they allow for the investigator to stimulate the brain and identify eloquent cortex before planning the surgical procedure. Depth electrodes are perhaps the most invasive of the recording procedures. These electrodes are placed so that they penetrate the brain substance and are targeted for deep limbic sites; they are most helpful in investigating patients where, with surface and sphenoidal electrodes, seizure onset cannot be clearly determined, but the events are believed to be of limbic origin. Since each of the electrodes has multiple contacts, the physiologic evolution of the seizure can be reasonably detailed. Today most epilepsy centers use depth electrodes primarily in the investigation of patients with a suspected deep mesial frontal seizure onset, although there are still some temporal cases where they are appropriate.

SURGICAL STRATEGIES

Focal Excision of Epileptic Tissue, Temporal Lobe

The focal excision of epileptic tissue of the temporal lobe is the most frequently performed procedure for epilepsy, and accounts for 60 to 70 percent of the focal removals. The decision to operate is outlined in Figure 143-1. If patients with temporal lobe onset seizures make it to the surgical procedure, the most frequently performed operation is a corticoamygdalohippocampectomy, which is carried out with relatively significant variation, depending on the specific epilepsy center. Some centers perform a standardized en bloc removal, where 5 to 6 cm of the nondominant temporal lobe and up to 5 cm of the dominant hemisphere temporal lobe is removed. The measurement is made from the tip of the temporal fossa along its lateral extent. Variable amounts of mesial tissue are removed. Some centers remove only mesial structures, leaving the lateral temporal neocortex relatively intact. Most centers, however, tailor their procedure to the specifics of the patient's physiology. Removal may be more or less on lateral or mesial aspects, depending on seizure physiology. The more lateral removals are done primarily in patients with temporal neocortical seizure onset, while

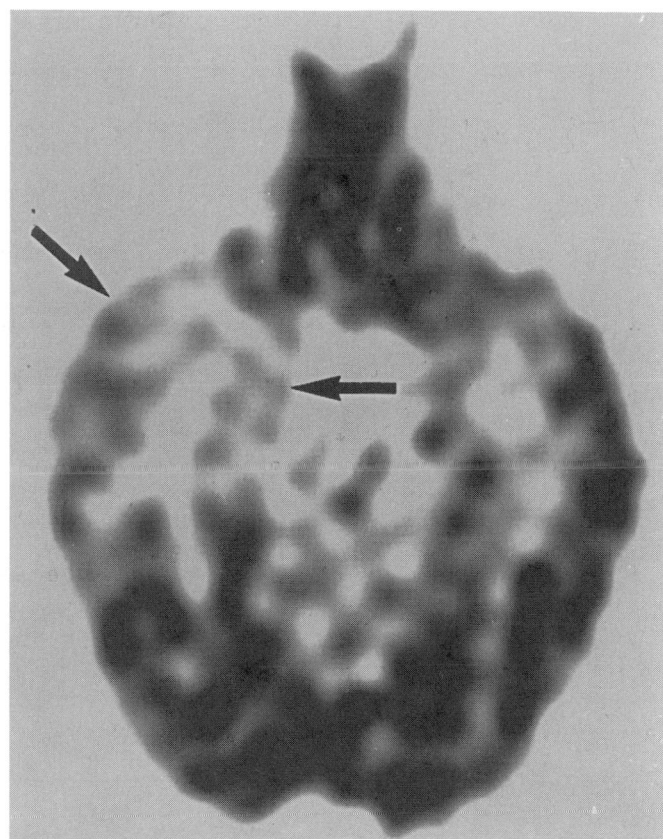

FIG. 143-3. FDG PET study showing an area of significant decreased metabolic activity in the region of the right temporal lobe that is more prominent along the mesial structures (*arrows*).

more significant mesial removals are done in patients where mesial sclerosis is found. Results of this type of surgery are quite good—overall success rate between 80 and 90 percent. Half of the responders are seizure-free or have rare auras, while the other half have significant improvement in seizure frequency, having only perhaps a few auras or rare seizures. Of the patients undergoing this procedure, 10 to 20 percent do not benefit significantly by it. If patients respond, there is frequently noted improvement in testable cognition. This probably has multiple etiologies. The absence of seizures probably allows for the individual to better formulate new memories. The reduction in medication coincident with seizure control also allows for better attention to cognitive processes.

Frontal Removals

Focal cortical excision is next most frequently applied to seizures of frontal lobe origin. The epileptic zones that are approachable are primarily in the area of the prerolandic dorsolateral cortex and anterior mesial frontal cortex. Since seizures that originate in these areas often have rapid secondary generalization, investigations are often complicated by depth electrode investigations. The outcome for focal frontal removals does not seem to be statistically as good as for temporal removals. Overall success is more in the range of 60 to 70 percent compared to 80 to 90 percent for temporal cases. The responders, like patients with temporal lobe seizures, also have noted improvements in cognition for the same reasons.

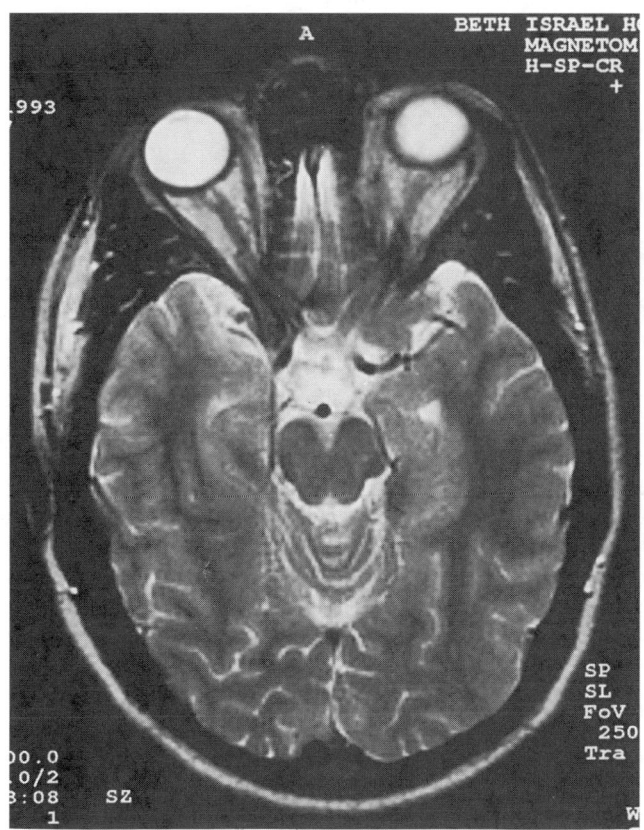

FIG. 143-2. MRI showing thin cuts through the temporal lobes that were considered to be normal.

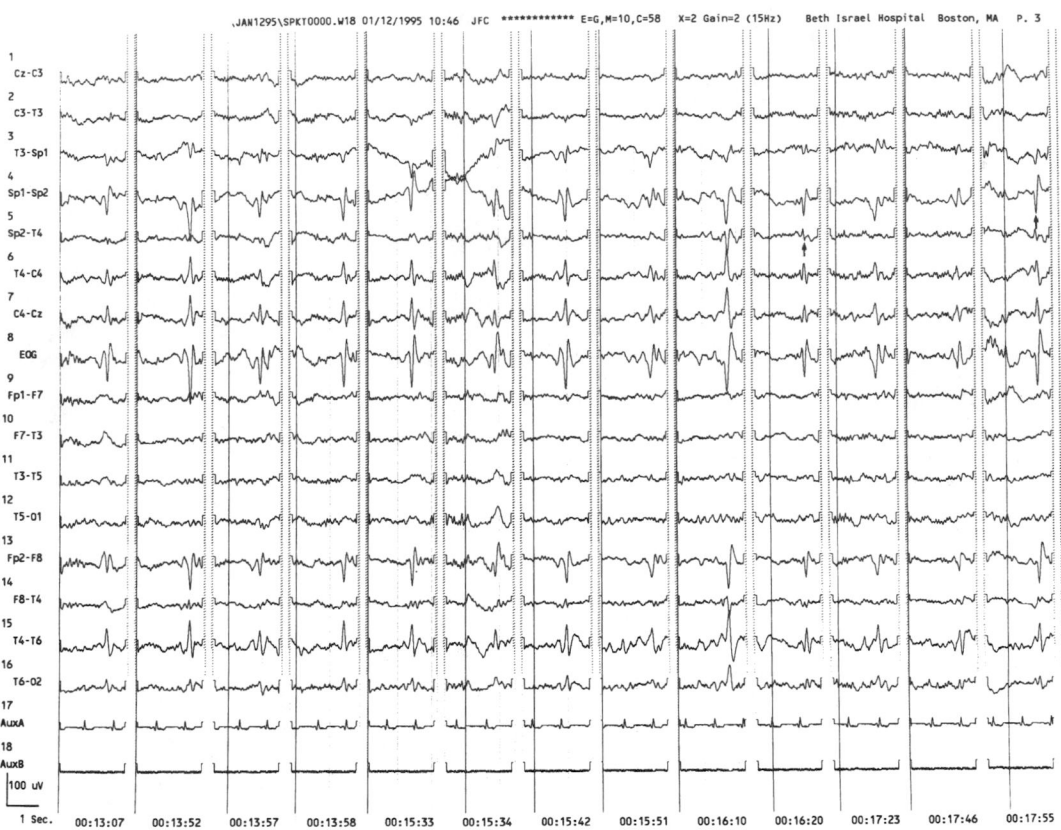

FIG. 143-4. Automated interictal spike detection algorithms detected multiple sleep-enhanced epileptic spike and wave discharges seen from the right inferior temporal leads Sp2 and more broadly from the right inferior temporal surface where there is a zone of isopotentiality between Sp2 and T4. Phase-reversing discharges are noted by arrows.

Multiple Lobectomies and Hemispherectomy

These procedures are considered reasonable alternatives in the setting of a patient with regional or hemisphere-wide onset seizure activity and concomitant severe neurologic impairment. Many of these patients have early damage to a hemisphere or to multiple lobes within one hemisphere and have associated hemiparesis, loss of visual field, and sensory deficit. Multiple disorders are commonly encountered when dealing with this surgical subpopulation; the most common is perhaps the chronic progressive encephalitis described by Rasmussen. Other etiologies include the Sturge-Weber syndrome and hemimegalencephaly. Children presenting with the hypsarhythmia EEG pattern and intractable seizures, who also have lateralized or localized PET abnormalities, are now being considered candidates for this procedure if medications fail. The procedure includes either multiple lobectomies or an entire hemispherectomy. The latter may be either complete or modified. In the modified approach, both the frontal and occipital poles are left in place with their pial blood supply untouched. They are, however, deafferented by undercutting the neocortex through its underlying white matter. In so doing, the cortex, while left intact, is nonfunctional. It is believed that this approach reduces the long-term sequelae of hemosiderosis that was described by early investigators performing this procedure. The outcome from this procedure in many cases is dramatic. Overall, about 75 percent of patients undergoing this procedure become seizure-free or develop medical tractability. There is often a significant improvement in behavior and occasionally an improvement in cognition and in the hemiparesis. In children

with infantile spasms and the hypsarhythmic EEG pattern, there may often be dramatic improvement in cognition and neurologic development.

Subpial Transections

Patients with clear focal seizure onset from essential cortical areas such as the primary motor or sensory cortex or language areas such as Broca or Wernicke may be candidates for this procedure. In these cases, "subpial sectioning of the cortex is carried out at 5-mm intervals with a blunted knife that passes around the gyrus transverse to the axis of the gyrus. This procedure sections the gray matter connections that run horizontally and, in turn, connect functional columns to each other." It is believed that this inhibits the functional columns from being pathologically synchronized and leading to a clinical event. Overall, the functional state of the column remains intact. The procedure is not commonly employed, but, where it is, the majority of patients have significant reduction in seizure frequency and have very little or no worsening of their functional capacity.

Lesionectomy

In patients with identifiable lesions, the area of epileptogenesis is usually near or surrounding the lesion. This fact, however, needs to be proven during the presurgical evaluation. If the lesion is in the anterior or middle temporal lobe, this is usually the case. The surgical approach therefore would be to tailor the temporal lobectomy to include the lesion and epileptogenic

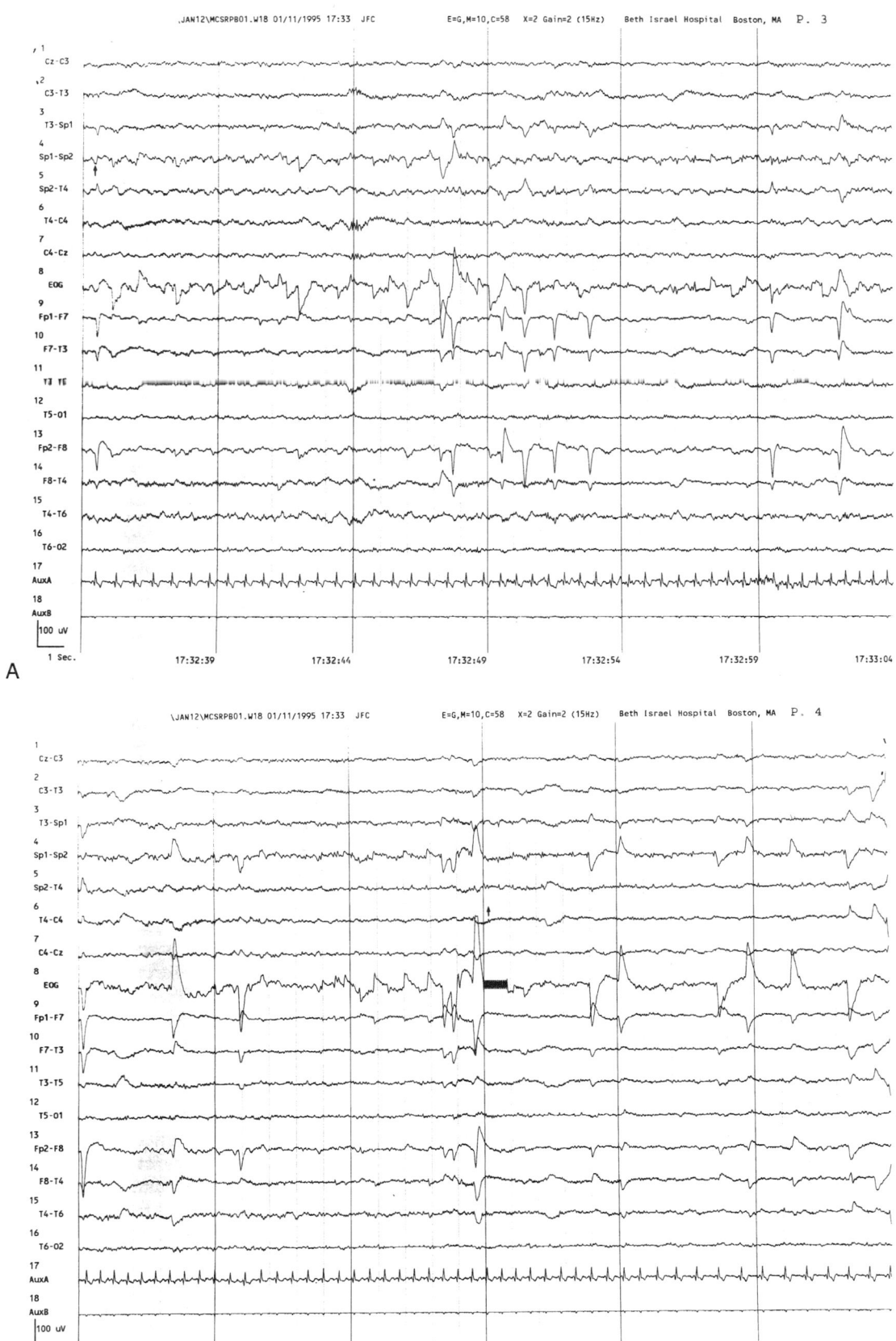

FIG. 143-5. **(A–C)** The patient had multiple ''events'' where he had a warning of an ascending sense of nausea followed by loss of consciousness, during which time he repeated ''déja vu.'' The arrow depicts the physiologic onset of the ictus. There is rhythmic delta activity starting at 17:32:35, followed by an attenuation of activity at 17:33:19, followed by rhythmic 2 to 6-Hz spikes at 17:33:39.

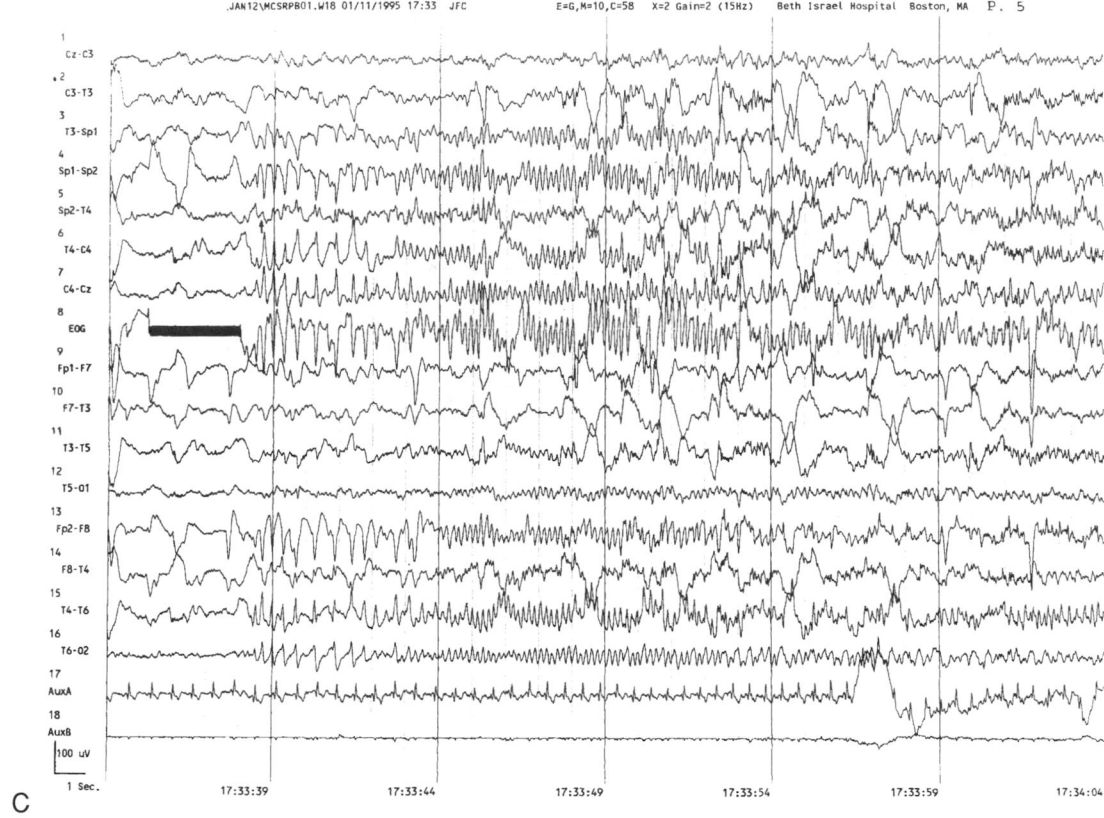

FIG. 143-5.   *(Continued)*

zone. However, if the lesion is nontemporal, the surgical approach must again be tailored to two separate issues: first, whether the epileptic zone can be removed surgically, and second, whether the lesion can be removed. Outcome measures for lesionectomy relate to both the control of epilepsy and treatment for the lesion. The surgical outcomes with respect to epilepsy are very similar to responses for focal cortical removals, that is, temporal lobe removals tend to fare better than frontal removals. The excision of the lesion and the response to that procedure relates directly to the nature of the pathology of the lesion itself.

Callosotomy

Callostomy is the only epilepsy surgical procedure that is never considered to be curative—best, it is palliative. It is considered where the patient's seizure type is predominantly "drop attacks." This type of seizure is seen primarily in patients who have widespread brain pathology and multiple seizure types. Drop attacks remain quite resistant to medications, although with some of the newer drugs there are some successes. Drop attacks are frequently associated with repeat head and body injury. Callosotomy is now frequently done as a two-step approach. Patients who qualify for it will have an anterior two-thirds callosotomy section done initially. In most cases, this is sufficient, and no further procedure is necessary. It is also beneficial from the perspective of cognitive impairment, since leaving the posterior third of the callosum intact seems to reduce the unusual complications noted in the early description of this technique. A posterior one-third section can be done in a separate setting if the anterior two-thirds section has failed. If this

procedure is successful in controlling the drop attacks, patients often times show some improvement in their cognitive capability. More important, however, is that it seems to positively affect the long-term outcome of this patient population and reduce some of the problematic difficulties encountered in caring for them.

CONCLUSION

The surgical approach to patients with medically intractable forms of epilepsy is a relatively underutilized technique. The proper choice of patients for this form of treatment is perhaps the single most important facet in determining the outcome. While this approach may be expensive, the results, if successful, far outweigh the initial investment. The evaluation is best done in one of the major epilepsy centers. The following case study provides an example of such an evaluation.

CASE STUDY

The patient was a 26-year-old, left-handed man. His first seizure occurred on February 20, 1991 after several days of heavy drinking. There was no warning. He lost consciousness, fell, and developed tonic followed by tonic-clonic movements. A second seizure occurred in the hospital on the same day. The patient was hospitalized with a normal MRI and EEG by history. Treatment with carbamazepine controlled the generalized seizures, but the patient continued to have small events heralded by an ascending sense of nausea, a staly taste, and an unpleasant smell, followed by a loss of consiousness during which he repeated the phrase "déja vu."

Treatment with valproate, phenytoin, Gabapentin, chlorazepate, felbamate, and lamotrigine was tried, all without success. The events occur with a frequency of 1 to 10 a week and significantly affect the patient's work and personal relationships.

The patient had been adopted as a newborn. Several episodes of short-duration febrile convulsions had occurred between the ages of 6 and 18 months. Childhood physical and cognitive development were normal. The patient has had difficulty with memory retrieval since the onset of the seizures, which is felt to be secondary to medication.

The physical examination showed slight discoloration of the iris of the left eye. The neurologic examination showed decreased olfaction in the right nostril and a decrease in cold sensation and two-point discrimination on the left side of the face and the left arm and hand. Reflexes were normal and symmetric. In terms of neuropsychological testing, the patient underwent the Wechsler Adult Intelligence Scale test, the digit span and visual span tests, the F-A-S test, the Stroop Interference test, the alternating writing sequences test, the motor go-no-go test, Trail Marking, the Dichotic Digit Listening test, the Wechsler Memory Scale, the Rey Auditory Verbal Learning test, the Rey Complex Figure test, the Warrinton Recognition Memory test, the Boston Naming test, the Revised Wide Range Achievement test, the Facial Recognition test, the visual cancellation test, tests of judgment, the Short Category test, the finger tapping task, the Grooved Pegboard task, complex gait testing, and the Beck Depression Inventory. These tests suggested a marked impairment in visual, nonverbal memory for both encoding and retrieval tasks.

Wada testing (ICA) revealed left hemisphere dominance for language despite the patient's left handedness. There was a mild deficit in nonverbal retrieval with the right hemisphere injection. Figures 143-2 through 143-5 show the radiologic and EEG findings.

SUGGESTED READINGS

Blume HW, Schomer DL: Surgical approaches to epilepsy. Annu Rev Med 301–13, 1988

Engel J: Surgical Treatment of the Epilepsies. 2nd Ed. Raven Press, New York, 1993

Luders HO: Epilepsy Surgery. Raven Press, New York, 1992

Theodore WH: Surgical Treatment of Epilepsy. Elsevier, Amsterdam, 1992

144. EPILEPSY AND BEHAVIOR

SHAHRAM KHOSHBIN

To the practicing neurologist, the issue of epilepsy and behavior presents two distinct complex and difficult management problems: (1) diagnosis and management of cognitive and behavior changes in patients with different types of epilepsy, and (2) diagnosis and management of patients presenting with behavioral symptoms or symptom complexes akin to those seen in epileptic patients but without classical ictal or electroencephalographic (EEG) manifestations of seizures. The latter has been referred to as *temporolimbic dysfunction,* as the manifestations

of these symptoms and symptom complexes are similar to those described in the literature as being associated with complex partial epilepsy and/or focal lesions in the temporal lobe, frontal lobe, the limbic system, and their connections. Although these problems have been recognized since antiquity, and have been the subject of numerous anecdotal reports and small and large prospective and retrospective studies, for a number of reasons, including the multifactorial etiologies of behavioral symptoms, varied theories of pathophysiology, and methodological difficulties in carrying out behavioral research, they have remained controversial. Specifically, correlation between these symptom complexes and epilepsy, particularly temporal lobe epilepsy, has not been clearly established. However, patients suffer from significant morbidity because of these symptom complexes. In this chapter we discuss neuropsychiatric behavioral disorders presumed to be related to epilepsy with an emphasis on management rather than pathophysiology.

In the management of patients with epilepsy, it is helpful to keep a general view of the disorder in the form of what we shall refer to as the *patient care diamond* (Fig. 144-1), with major aspects of patients' problems constituting the different points of the diamond with reciprocal relations between each point. In this section, we particularly emphasize those symptoms related to reciprocal relationships between seizures and psychiatric symptomatology, and those behavioral symptoms related to the use of antiepileptic drugs and surgical treatment of epilepsy.

The overview considers the following:

1. Behavioral changes and seizures can be separate but related manifestations of the same underlying pathology.
2. Abnormal behavior can develop as a result of partial inhibition or enhancement of activity in neighboring or distant regions of the brain (postictal and interictal symptoms).
3. Seizures as a behavior can be positively or negatively reinforced, resulting in other behaviors mimicking seizures (pseudoseizures) and/or abnormal psychological adaptation (personality disorders).
4. The unpredictable and disruptive nature of seizures produces psychological stress.
5. Behavioral abnormalities can be a result of a chronic illness with its social limitations and cultural stigmatization.
6. Cognitive and behavioral abnormalities can be secondary to the effects of treatment with anticonvulsant drugs.

Many pathophysiologic mechanisms have been suggested to explain these reciprocal relationships. Mechanisms underlying the epileptic focus and ictal behavioral manifestations related to these focal lesions (such as paroxysmal depolarizing shift) are now well understood. There is also good evidence for propagation of these focal dysrhythmias to adjacent and distant areas via excitatory and inhibitory circuits, causing additional behavioral manifestations. However, mechanisms underlying symptoms not temporally related to the ictal discharge have been less clearly understood. Suggestions have been made of processes such as "hyperconnectivity" or "misconnectivity." Some aspects of the animal model of kindling have provided interesting possible mechanisms for these spatially and temporally distant manifestations.

CLASSIFICATION OF BEHAVIORAL CHANGES

Many recent studies have utilized psychiatric classifications of disease to address these behavioral manifestations. Although the symptoms seen in patients with epilepsy or temporolimbic

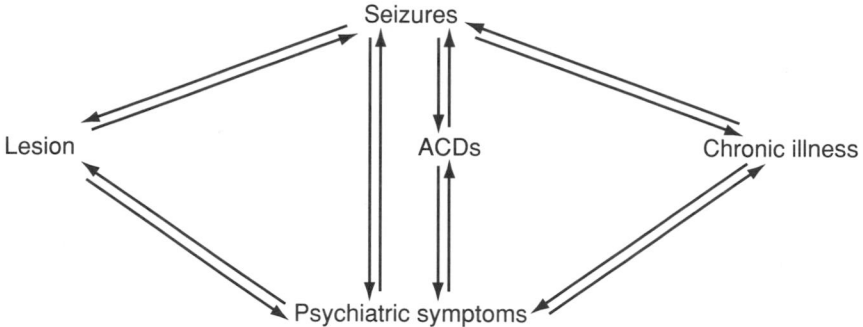

FIG. 144-1. The behavior and epilepsy patient care diamond.

dysfunction do not exactly correspond to the criteria set for these diagnoses in the different versions of the Diagnostic and Statistical Manual, this classification offers a practical model for the practicing clinician. The major categories are as follows:

1. Cognitive disorders (disorders of attention, memory, and learning)
2. Psychoses (ictal, interictal, and forced normalization)
3. Affective disorders (depression, mania and bipolar symptoms)
4. Anxiety disorders (panic attacks and phobias)
5. Personality disorders (hypergraphia, hyperreligiosity, viscosity, altered sexuality, and aggressivity)
6. Pseudoseizures (somatoform disorders and conversion)
7. Hypothalamic disorders (neuroendocrine disorders and eating disorders [anorexia])

Symptoms in each one of these categories can be seen in different stages in relationship to the seizure, and can be grossly classified as shown in Table 144-1.

COGNITIVE DISORDERS

Both in the pediatric as well as the adult population, major issues of management related to cognitive difficulties are raised. Complaints are primarily of attention and concentration, and memory problems. As with other symptoms, in the evaluation of cognitive disorders multiple factors must be considered: biologic factors (cognitive function as a result of the site of the original lesion and/or as a result of clinical and subclinical seizures); psychiatric factors (as a result of affective disorders,

primarily depression); iatrogenic factors (side effects of antiepileptic medication); and social factors (secondary to lack of educational opportunities and school environment acceptability of the seizure patient).

For the younger patient in school, issues surrounding learning can be evaluated by direct contact with the school or the school psychologist, although many studies have shown reduced global intelligence in patients with epilepsy. This is certainly not true for all forms of epilepsy. Earlier age of onset of seizures and frequency of generalized seizures have been correlated with reduced intelligence quotient (IQ). Neuropsychological testing, specifically Wexler Intelligence Scale for Children and Wechsler Adult Intelligence Scale for the older patient are the two most commonly used tests in the evaluation of these patients.

Memory disorders are the most common cognitive complaint of patients. Laterality has been considered, although most patients with memory complaints show bilateral-temporal foci; as expected, problems with verbal memory is more prominent in patients with left temporal lesions. In patients who complain of memory problems, the EEG is helpful to rule out the possibility of frequent subclinical discharges. Sedation and cognitive difficulties secondary to anticonvulsant drugs should also be considered. Attempts to use monotherapy and to use lower dosages of antiepileptic medication helps to improve memory function.

Language dysfunction, mostly in the form of word-finding difficulty, is another common cognitive disorder. Word-finding difficulty is more prevalent among patients with left temporal lesions. However, patients with right temporal lesions seem to have language difficulties, mainly as a result of aprosody.

Clearly, achievement in school and college may be affected by the speed of responding to timed tests (slowed reaction time). Patients either due to frequent subclinical seizures or antiepileptic drug side effects have slowness of response and show abnormality on routine vigilance tests. To improve the patient's academic performance, the physician could request that additional time be provided to the patient when taking timed tests. Clearly, patient advocacy by the physician proves to be the most effective intervention technique in this case. In younger children with school difficulty, neuropsychological testing by an experienced educational neuropsychologist may be needed for the possibility of specific learning disabilities.

PSYCHOSIS

The oldest, and one of the most controversial, correlations of abnormal behavior in epilepsy is with psychosis. Many investigators have questioned the correlation between seizures and psychotic symptoms. A number of studies, however, have

TABLE 144-1. Stages of Seizure Symptoms

Relationship to Seizure	Stage	Symptomatology
Temporal	Prodromal	Long duration, noted 2–3 days before seizure
	Ictal	Brief duration Alterations of consciousness Motor automatisms Sensory disturbances Autonomic symptomatology
	Postictal	From immediately after to 1–3 days after seizure Confusion
Nontemporal	Interictal	Intermittent, episodic, or persistent, associated with the epileptic focus
	Forced normalization	After cessation of seizures and normalization of EEG Remission when EEG shows recurrence of abnormalities

shown an unequivocal increase in the prevalence of psychosis among epileptic patients. To distinguish the behavioral abnormality of interictal psychosis from functional psychosis, the term *schizophrenialike psychoses of epilepsy* has been used. Certain findings have been considered to be more common among patients with epilepsy who show psychosis. These are left-handedness or ambidexterity, left-sided or bilateral temporal foci, left-hemisphere tumors or other structural lesions, especially in women. As in other behavioral disorders, psychosis can be seen during the prodromal, ictal, and postictal periods in temporal relation to the seizure, or interictally. Interictal psychosis is suspected in the epileptic who develops persistent hallucinations and paranoid delusions, with an onset in middle age. Certain factors are more prevalent in ictal and postictal psychosis, where hallucinations are mostly olfactory and gustatory. In the interictal psychosis, visual and auditory hallucinations are more prevalent, particularly visual hallucinations. These hallucinatory experiences are usually stereotypic as opposed to functional psychosis. In both ictal and interictal psychoses, affect is preserved as opposed to the flat affect seen with functional psychosis. The sensorium is usually cloudy in ictal psychosis and clear in interictal psychosis. The presence of autonomic signs and symptoms and motor automatisms are indicative of ictal psychosis. The EEG in patients with postictal or ictal psychoses is usually positive, showing epileptogenic discharges. However, with interictal psychosis, negative EEGs and/or borderline findings are more common. Psychosis associated with normalization of the EEG and reduction or remission in clinical seizures has been referred to as "forced normalization" described by Landolt. This is not a very frequent phenomenon; however, it is reminiscent of the old observation of antagonism between psychosis and epilepsy when an improvement in psychosis was noted when seizures are more frequent, and when seizure control resulted in worsening of psychosis. This was the observation that led to Von Meduna's use of electroconvulsive therapy in psychosis. Psychosis can be seen with all forms of epilepsy. However, most studies have shown a higher prevalence among patients with complex partial seizures, specifically patients with left-sided temporal lesions. Also, history of early cerebral lesions, birth trauma, perinatal encephalopathy, or infections in childhood are more prevalent among patients with epilepsy and psychosis. Certain chromosomal anomalies, such as Klinefelter syndrome, have been associated with both seizures and psychosis. Prolonged fugue states with wandering and multiple personalities in patients with complex partial seizures have been the subject of a number of anecdotal reports.

Management

Treatment of psychosis, whether interictal or ictal and postictal, still requires the use of neuroleptic medication. However, since most neuroleptic drugs are known to induce seizures, there has been a reluctance to treat psychosis vigorously. Haloperidol (Haldol), in doses not to exceed 6 mg/day, and molindone (Moban), not to exceed 225 mg/day, have been helpful. Some reports have suggested that B_{12} and folate deficiency is seen more frequently among patients with psychosis, and the correction of this should be included in the therapy. Carbamazepine (Tegretol) has been the anticonvulsant drug of choice in these patients. The addition of benzodiazepines such as clonazepam (Klonopin) has been helpful in some patients with interictal psychosis. However, it has been reported that benzodiazepine

withdrawal could itself trigger a psychotic episode in patients with epilepsy. In surgical series, conflicting results have been seen with regard to psychosis. Some series show an improvement in the ictal and postictal psychotic periods. There have also been indications for what is known as postoperative psychosis, which seems to occur in patients who have a family history of psychiatric disease.

ANXIETY DISORDERS

Ictal fear is one of the most common symptoms of complex partial seizures. When present, it has been associated with increasing prevalence of interictal behavioral disorders and psychopathology. Prodromal anxiety is also quite common. Prolonged periods of heightened anxiety is seen in the postictal period. Interictally, patients report anxiety as frequently as depressive episodes. Panic attacks also occur with greater frequency among patients with epilepsy, and are clinically difficult to distinguish from complex partial seizures. Many studies have tried to distinguish between the two disorders. Hyperventilation, which may occur with both disorders, may result in symptoms in patients with panic that one usually associates with seizures, such as loss of consciousness, dizziness, and depersonalization. Panic attacks, as opposed to seizures, are associated with family history of neuroses and history of childhood phobias, are usually slow in buildup, and last longer than seizures. Panic attacks can also be precipitated by provocation tests, and motor automatisms seen with seizures are usually not seen with panic.

Phobias have also been reported in patients with epilepsy. Most patients with frequent seizures may exhibit agoraphobia. Phobias for sharp objects and driving may be a result of concern regarding self-injury during a seizure.

Management

Benzodiazepines, particularly clonazepam (Klonopin), but also clorazepate (Tranxene), lorazepam (Ativan), and alprazolam (Xanax) have been used; carbamazepine (Tegretol) and propranolol (Inderal) have also been used with some success. Buspirone (Buspar), in our experience, has been a very effective antianxiety medication when benzodiazepines could not be used.

AFFECTIVE DISORDERS

As in the other behavioral manifestations, depression in epilepsy is multifactorial. Ictal depression is usually sudden in onset and resolves spontaneously. However, both prodromal and postictal depression have been reported to last over 2 or 3 days. Interictal depression is seen in association with the other interictal disorders, and the prevalence seems to be higher among patients with complex partial seizures, with a suggestion of a predominance of left temporal focus on EEG.

The issue of suicide and epilepsy has received much attention in the literature. Studies claim that the rate is 5 to 25 times higher than in the general population. These patients usually overdose on anticonvulsant drugs. A number of factors should warn against increased risk of suicide, especially (1) family history of depression, (2) presence of interictal psychosis, (3) past history of repeated suicide attempts, and (4) left-sided lesions.

Mania is not uncommon among patients with epilepsy.

Mostly patients exhibit hypomanic episodes, sometimes referred to in the literature as "epileptic excitement." These episodes are usually seen postictally. An association with right temporal lobe foci has been made in these cases. Bipolar illness is also more frequent among patients with temporal lobe epilepsy, creating yet another difficult point of differential diagnosis. Here, the EEG can be very useful in distinguishing atypical bipolar disease from temporal lobe epilepsy.

Management

Tricyclic antidepressants have been known to reduce seizure threshold and therefore should be used with caution, although in our experience, in regular therapeutic doses an increase in seizures is not usually seen. Amitriptyline, imipramine, and doxepine have been the most frequently used. Fluoxetine (Prozac) and MAO inhibitors have also been known to produce seizures, and therefore do not necessarily offer a better alternative. Lithium, especially at toxic levels, has been strongly associated with seizures as well as epileptiform discharges on the EEG. Carbamazepine, valproate, and phenytoin are believed to be superior to barbiturates in the treatment of patients with depressive symptomatology. In general, monotherapy is preferred in these patients.

PERSONALITY DISORDERS

The issue of interictal personality disorders has been the subject of much controversy. The diagnosis is difficult clinically, and standard neuropsychological tests for personality disorders, such as the Minnesota Multiphasic Personality Inventory, fail to measure some of the traits known to be associated with epilepsy.

Some of these personality characteristics may actually constitute a positive aspect in the life of a patient, like deepened philosophical interests and hypergraphia, while others may be the causes of morbidity and social maladjustment, like altered sexuality, aggressivity, and viscosity. It is also clear that these symptoms and symptom complexes are not present in all patients with epilepsy, and although primarily associated with complex partial seizures, they are only seen in a small percentage of patients with temporal lobe epilepsy. References to these symptoms have been present in the literature for many years. They became the focus of recent attention since the report of Waxman and Geschwind on hypergraphia in patients with temporal lobe epilepsy. Subsequently, these authors described a symptom complex of varied and interesting personality characteristics, including religiosity, deep concern with religious and philosophical issues, feelings of deepened emotionality, hyposexuality, tendency to adhere to certain thoughts and actions (viscosity), and aggressivity. Certain aspects of this cluster appear to be opposite to symptoms observed in animals with bilateral temporal lobectomies manifesting placidity and hypersexuality, known as the Klüver-Bucy syndrome. Bear and Fedio devised a new personality inventory to quantify the presence of these symptoms in patients with temporal lobe epilepsy. This personality inventory has been used in many different studies with mixed results as to the prevalence of these symptoms, individually or in clusters, in patients with different forms of epilepsy. The original syndrome described by Geschwind, constituting hypergraphia, hyperreligiosity, altered sexuality, aggressivity, and viscosity, has been recognized in the behavioral neurology literature as "Geschwind syndrome" since our original reference to the presence of this syndrome in the case of Dutch painter Vincent Van Gogh.

Hypergraphia

As opposed to disorders of spoken language, disorders of writing are relatively less explored in the neurologic literature. The correlation between agraphia and aphasias was made much later than the original descriptions of aphasias. However, disorders of writing in psychiatric disease has been long recognized, specifically, compulsive writing in schizophrenia. Studies comparing hypergraphia in patients with schizophrenia and temporal lobe epilepsy have shown a greater prevalence of this symptom among patients with epilepsy. Waxman and Geschwind's article brought attention to this interesting symptom in patients with temporal lobe epilepsy. They described extensive writing with attention to great detail and multiple repetitions, and also indicated an association with religiosity and deep philosophical interests. Patients usually make copious notes and keep detailed diaries. They also show great interest in writing fiction and poetry, again usually with great attention to detail and tendency to repetition. Hypergraphia has been reported to be of sudden onset in some hospitalized patients after surgery for epilepsy, and the patients describe a compulsion and urge for writing. These patients describe more frequently ictal symptoms of ecstasy, elation, and déja vu. EEG studies in patients with hypergraphia shows the presence of bitemporal abnormalities; however, there is a predominance of right-sided foci.

Religiosity

Commonly associated with hypergraphia, an unusual and deep interest in religion has been described in patients with complex partial seizures. Ictal religious auras and more prolonged feelings of ecstasy associated with religious aspects have been reported in the prodromal phase and during ictus. Interictal symptoms have been described—during times of increased seizure frequency and also in periods of forced normalization—as sudden religious conversions, and periods of heightened interest in religion in patients previously not so inclined. Other associated personality traits are hypermoralism, deep philosophical interests, and feelings of personal destiny. Anticonvulsant treatment has not been known to affect these symptoms, but changes in hypergraphia and religiosity have been seen after temporal lobectomy.

Viscosity

Patients with temporal lobe epilepsy have been reported to have a tendency to engage in long conversations and verbal exchanges, showing an inability to terminate and perceive messages and cues for termination of such exchanges from others. In certain cases, the speech may be without informational content, and circumstantiality has been described. Viscosity has been noted to be more prevalent among patients with left temporal foci.

ALTERED SEXUALITY

Hyposexuality is common among patients with epilepsy. It is of interest, however, that unless the physician inquires, patients usually exhibit a lack of concern and do not complain. Both female and male patients report not only lack of sexual activity, but also reduction in masturbation and sexual fantasy. Prevalence of infertility is higher among epileptic patients, and in males with frequent seizures, impotence has been reported, with improvement in both drive and potency after anticonvulsant therapy and after lobectomy. Females report failure to reach orgasm; however, this may be associated with the use of some anticonvulsants, particularly barbiturates and benzodiazepines. Hypersexuality has also been reported, particularly in temporal lobe epilepsy. Reports of exhibitionism, masochism, transvestism, and fetishism have all been anecdotal.

Abnormalities of sex hormones, including gonadotropins, testosterone, estrogen, and progesterone have been reported in all forms of seizures, particularly temporal lobe epilepsy. Association between these abnormalities and hyposexuality, and also an increased prevalence of homosexuality among patients with complex partial seizures, has been postulated.

Ictal sexual excitement (orgasmic seizures) is rare and is mostly seen in women. However, masturbatory behavior is seen ictally as well as postictally in both sexes.

Management

Ictal and postictal sexual symptoms, as well as interictal complaints of decreased libido, seem to improve with anticonvulsant therapy. In patients with hyposexuality, barbiturates and benzodiazepines should be avoided. Marriage counseling, psychotherapy, and group therapy should be offered to the patients.

AGGRESSIVITY

The issue of aggression and epilepsy has received a great deal of attention, both in the early literature and in the most recent studies. In the prodromal stage, most patients and their families report increased irritability and, at times, explosive behavior, but this is quite different from the more common reports of rage and explosive behavior seen during the ictus or in the immediate postictal period usually associated with restraining the patient during motor automatisms. The latter are usually nondirected and brief, and the patient may be amnestic for these events. However, interictally, an increase in irritability, aggressivity, and an intermittent rage reaction similar to the so-called "episodic dyscontrol syndrome" is noted, patients have periods of heightened anxiety and irritability during which minor provocations may result in directed explosive behavior disproportionate to the situation. These episodes are also seen in periods of forced normalization.

The issue of ictal aggression in epilepsy has been the subject of a detailed review by the Committee on Violence and Epilepsy, which found ictal aggression to be extremely rare. Self-mutilatory behavior and suicidal attempts by violent means have been seen during ictus and postictally, particularly in temporal lobe epilepsy, but these are seen less frequently in epileptics than among patients with psychosis. EEG studies in prison populations have shown a higher incidence of abnormalities. Most of these studies were done at a time when certain nonspecific EEG patterns were still considered as abnormal because of the lack of large normal population studies. The validity of these original studies is now in question. However, among patients with temporal lobe epilepsy exhibiting aggressivity, a higher prevalence of left temporal discharges and evoked potential abnormalities lateralizing to the left hemisphere have been reported.

Management

Carbamazepine and clonazepam (Klonopin) have been used in the treatment of interictal aggressivity. We have used propranolol successfully in these patients in addition to an anticonvulsant regimen. When aggressivity has been associated with periods of mania, lithium has also been prescribed. However, lithium levels require careful monitoring in patients with epilepsy, and this treatment is generally discouraged. Tricyclic antidepressants have also been used in some of these patients. In children, barbiturates ought to be avoided, and there is some indication that the new anticonvulsant drug Gabapentin (neurontin) may result in increased irritability and aggressivity, similar to behavior associated with barbiturates. As with all other behavioral syndromes, the clinician should consider that aggressive behavior has multifactorial etiology and the patient's background, family history, and social milieu should be considered. Individual counseling, psychotherapy, and group therapy should be offered to these patients.

PSEUDOSEIZURES

The presence of psychogenic seizures in patients with epilepsy, especially those with onset in childhood, has been reported in both generalized as well as partial and complex partial seizures. This presents not only a diagnostic difficulty but produces problems with management specifically leading to polytherapy in patients who report continuation of seizures despite adequate control of epileptic fits. Many recent reports have tried to outline clinical means of distinguishing pseudoseizures from epileptic fits. These have been aided by the use of closed-circuit TV monitoring now available in most EEG laboratories. Behavioral seizures should be suspected when patients with frequent daily seizure episodes show persistently normal EEG findings, and when the patient reports frequent seizures but this does not correspond to the family's report of frequency of seizures. In generalized seizures, atypical movements, such as alternating movements of the limbs, flailing of the arms, and side-to-side movements of the head, are indicative of pseudoseizures. When generalized seizures are not followed by confusion and autonomic signs, pseudoseizures should be considered. However, the distinction of psychogenic seizures in patients with complex partial epilepsy is by far more difficult than in generalized seizures. These patients may require inpatient evaluation with closed-circuit TV monitoring and with telemetry. We have found that with the increased availability of portable video cameras, one could request family members to make video recordings of the events taking place at home. A review of these tapes has made it increasingly easy to distinguish psychogenic seizures.

Psychopathology seen with patients with pseudoseizures ranges from conversion disorders to factitious (Munchausen syndrome) to malingering. An early history of physical and sexual abuse and history of frequent seizures in childhood has been associated with all of the above. Careful EEG monitoring and measurements of prolactin levels after seizures have been helpful (prolactin levels may be only minimally elevated after partial complex seizures). Individual psychotherapeutic intervention is needed in these patients, and monotherapy is preferred in anticonvulsant therapy.

EVALUATION OF BEHAVIORAL DISORDERS IN EPILEPSY

Electroencephalography

EEG remains the mainstay of evaluation of patients with epilepsy, although interictal EEG, if positive, can only be supportive of the diagnosis. Presence of epileptiform abnormalities can be quite helpful. A normal EEG does not rule out correlation between behavior and seizures, as most mesial temporal foci cannot be seen on a regular surface EEG. However, caution must also be used in overinterpreting some of the atypical findings seen in EEG, which in large normal studies have been found to be present in patients with no complaints of seizures or behavioral disorders. In this regard, findings of 14 and 6 positive spikes and psychomotor variants and benign epileptiform transience of sleep, which previously were considered as signs of abnormality, have now come into question. After sleep deprivation, special EEG electrode placements such as nasopharyngeal electrodes, sphenoidal electrodes, and maxillary electrodes clearly increase the yield of findings in patients with mesial temporal lesions. However, EEG and closed-circuit TV monitoring have been particularly helpful in the evaluation of the behavioral aspects of epilepsy. Monitoring units are now available in most centers and the evaluation of patients with high morbidity due to their behavioral symptoms in these centers is quite cost effective. Computerized processing of EEG data and evoked potentials to form probability maps provide a sensitive method for evaluation of functional disorders. In addition, they allow comparison to maps of large normal populations. However, because of excessive statistical manipulation of the raw data, artifacts abound. However, in combination with standard EEG and other functional studies such as positron-emission tomography (PET), single-photon-emission computed tomography (SPECT), and functional magnetic resonance imaging (MRI), these techniques increase the sensitivity in diagnosis of seizure-related behavior.

Neuroimaging

Neuroimaging studies have been most helpful in the diagnosis of epilepsy, and also have elucidated the changes underlying behavioral aspects. MRI is clearly a preferred technique to computed tomography (CT) scan in the evaluation of patients with epilepsy and behavioral disorders. The lack of bone artifact, and the availability of coronal and sagittal sections allow for better evaluation of the temporal lobes. MRI can show us the presence of mass lesions, especially small, low-grade tumors, and small vascular malformations. Also, areas of cortical dysplasia can be evaluated with greater accuracy than with other techniques. In the evaluation of behavioral changes, ventricular size, and most recently through utilization of thinner slices and special angles of the coronal section, volumetric measurements of the hippocampal region have been quite useful. Bilateral nonspecific increase in T2-weighted signal intensity in the hippocampal region and the white matter adjacent to these areas have also been reported in patients with temporal lobe disorders. Functional MRI, which is still in its infancy, may soon become the most sensitive test in the evaluation of behavioral disorders. Rapid succession acquired MRI slices show signal changes caused by variations in the oxygenation state of venous vasculature during functional activation. PET and SPECT have demonstrated interictal changes of hypometabolism in patients with complex partial seizures. Hypermetabolism is seen during the seizure and at times in association with a surrounding area of hypometabolism in complex partial seizures. Both PET and SPECT show areas of hypoperfusion, not only surrounding the area of the ictus but also at distant areas, giving further evidence to the distant effects of the epileptic focus.

BEHAVIORAL DISORDERS AND QUALITY OF LIFE IN EPILEPSY

Recently, different scales for assessing quality of life in patients with epilepsy have been devised, similar to those for other chronic neurologic illnesses. These scales address the issues affecting the whole patient, especially the psychosocial aspects, which are of great importance in the evaluation of behavioral symptoms. As more data from these studies become available, prognostic evaluation as well as therapeutic mediation in all aspects of behavioral disorders related to epilepsy will become more accurate and will allow a reevaluation of the controversial aspects of behavior and epilepsy.

SUGGESTED READINGS

Bear DM, Fedio P: Quantitative analysis of interictal behaviour in temporal lobe epilepsy. Arch Neurol 34:454–86, 1977

Blumer D: Hypersexual episodes in temporal lobe epilepsy. Am J Psychiatry 126:1099–106, 1970

Delgado-Escueta AV, Mattson RH, King L et al: Special report: the nature of aggression during epileptic seizures. N Engl J Med 305:711–6, 1981

Devinsky O: Clinical uses of the quality of life in epilepsy inventory. Epilepsia 34 (suppl. 4):S39–S44, 1993

Flor-Henry P: Psychosis and temporal lobe epilepsy: a controlled investigation. Epilepsia 10:363–95, 1969

Geschwind N: Pathogenesis of behaviour changes in temporal lobe epilepsy. In Ward A, Penry J, Purpura D (eds): Epilepsy. Raven Press, New York, 1983

Henry TR, Mazziotta JC, Engel J: Interictal metabolic anatomy of mesial temporal lobe epilepsy. Arch Neurol 50:582–9, 1993

Herzog AC, Russell V, Vaitukaitis JL: Neuroendocrine dysfunction in temporal lobe epilepsy. Arch Neurol 39:133–5, 1982

Khoshbin S: Van Gogh's malady and other cases of Geschwind's syndrome. Neurology 36(suppl. 1):213–4, 1986

Khoshbin S: Seizure disorders. pp. 730–43. In Branch WT (ed): Office Practice of Internal Medicine. WB Saunders, Philadelphia, 1994

Khoshbin S, Kim DH: Cortical auditory evoked potential mapping in females with panic disorder. Neurology 39(suppl. 1):226, 1989

Khoshbin S, Levin AL: Cortical evoked potential mapping in the episodic dyscontrol syndrome. Neurology 36(suppl 1)348–9, 1986

Khoshbin S, Levin L, Milrod L et al: Cortical evoked potential mapping in complex partial seizures. Neurology 34(suppl):219, 1984

Landolt H: Serial encephalographic investigations during psychotic episodes in epileptic patients and during schizophrenic attacks. pp. 91–133. In de Hass L (ed): Lectures on Epilepsy. Elsevier, Amsterdam, 1958

Slater E, Beard AW: The schizophrenia-like psychoses of epilepsy. Br J Psychiatry 109:95–150, 1963

Spiers PA, Schomer DL, Blume HW, Mesulam M-M: Temporolimbic epilepsy and behavior. In Mesulam M-M (ed): Principles of Behavioral Neurology. Contemporary Neurology Series. pp. 289–326. F.A. Davis, Philadelphia, 1985

Stevens JR: Neuropathology of schizophrenia. Arch Gen Psychiatry 39:1131–9, 1982

Taylor DC: Sexual behavior and temporal lobe epilepsy. Arch Neurol 21:510–16, 1969

Waxman SG, Geschwind N: Hypergraphia in temporal lobe epilepsy. Neurology 24:629–36, 1974

SECTION 3. DISORDERS OF SLEEP

145. DISORDERS OF SLEEP

JEAN K. MATHESON

Sleep is an active, clinically important behavior during which the entire physiology of the organism changes. This physiology has a temporal organization under cerebral influence. Sleep pathology may represent a primary disorder of mechanisms regulating sleep or failure within a specific organ system manifesting in a unique way during sleep. Sleep complaints should not be ignored or treated empirically with pharmacologic agents. More often than not, disordered sleep is a symptom of underlying disease.

PHYSIOLOGY

Rapid eye movement (REM) and non-REM (NREM) are the two sleep states. REM sleep was discovered by Aserinsky and Kleitman in the early 1950s. By waking subjects during REM, they also established that vivid dreaming occurs during this state. Soon thereafter Dement recognized that episodes of REM sleep alternate with NREM sleep in cycles lasting approximately 90 minutes throughout the night.

Recordings derived from electroencephalograms (EEG), electro-oculograms to determine eye movements, and electromyograms (EMG) of chin tone are necessary to distinguish sleep states. Polysomnography is the technique used to record multiple physiologic variables during sleep. In clinical practice several other physiologic measures are typically recorded, including respiratory effort from the chest and abdomen, oral and nasal airflow, cardiac rhythm, and EMG activity in the anterior tibialis muscles of the legs.

NREM sleep is divided into four stages, I, II, III, and IV. The waking EEG with the eyes closed reveals the characteristic *α-rhythm,* which is a posteriorly predominant 8- to 12-Hz rhythm that attenuates with eye opening. Stage I sleep is characterized by the gradual disappearance of the alpha rhythm, which is replaced by slower, 2-to 7-Hz activity and some fast 12-to 14-Hz low-voltage activity. Stage II is distinguished by the presence of spindles (bursts of 12- to 14-Hz activity, lasting at least 0.5 seconds, with a spindle appearance) and K complexes (high-voltage biphasic negative/positive waves best seen at the vertex, usually associated with spindles). Stages III and IV are defined by the presence of high-voltage slow-wave activity of 2 Hz or less. An epoch of 30 seconds is measured: if 20 to 50 percent of the record shows high-voltage slow-wave activity, it is termed stage III; more than 50 percent high-voltage slow-wave activity is termed stage IV. Stages III and IV are often described together as *slow-wave sleep* or *delta sleep.* Delta sleep can be characterized as deep sleep, because during this stage subjects are difficult to arouse. Detailed dreaming does not occur, but subjects awakened during this sleep stage have reported ''thinking.'' The normal subject descends in an orderly progression through the four NREM sleep stages. Delta sleep appears 30 to 45 minutes after sleep onset. The first REM period follows this delta sleep, about 70 to 90 minutes after sleep onset.

The polysomnogram during REM shows dramatic changes. A sudden loss of EMG values is seen in the chin muscles, which reflects generalized skeletal muscle atonia. Except for the eye muscles and respiratory muscles, the subject is paralyzed. Rapid eye movements occur in phasic bursts. The EEG shows mixed frequencies similar to those of stage I and waking. Characteristic sawtooth waves sometimes occur during eye movements. Respirations and heart rate are irregular.

The first REM period is short, approximately 10 minutes. The end of the first REM period completes the first sleep cycle. Thereafter NREM continues to alternate with REM; the healthy young adult goes through four to six cycles (Fig. 145-1). Sleep architecture is the organization of sleep stages and cycles. The normal young adult spends approximately 5 percent of the night in stage I, 50 percent in stage II, 12 percent in stage III, 13 percent in stage IV, and 20 percent in REM. Delta sleep is concentrated in the first third of the night, whereas REM episodes become progressively longer later in the night. Delta sleep decreases as a function of age, but REM percentage is relatively

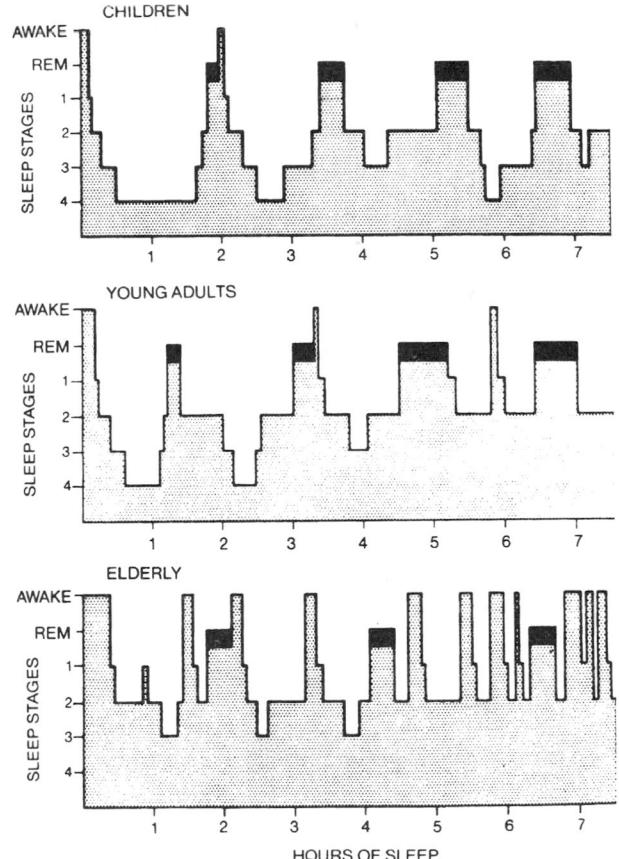

FIG. 145-1. Sleep architecture. REM sleep alternates with NREM in cycles approximating 90 minutes in all age groups. Delta sleep is prominent in childhood and decreases in the elderly as awakenings and wake time increase. (From Kales A, Kales JD: Sleep disorders: recent findings in the diagnosis and treatment of disturbed sleep. N Engl J Med 290:487, 1974, with permission.)

decreases as a function of age, but REM percentage is relatively stable after early childhood. Of the newborn's daily 17 to 18 hours of sleep, 50 percent is REM. Children and early adolescents sleep 10 to 11 hours. Most adults prefer to sleep 7 to 8 hours a day, but sleep needs vary. Short sleepers are classified as those individuals who feel adequately rested with less than 6 hours of sleep; long sleepers require more than 9 hours.

Sleep efficiency is defined as the time spent asleep divided by the time spent in bed. Sleep efficiency decreases in old age, as both the number of arousals and the time spent in bed increase. This does not necessarily represent "normal" aging. Arousals usually have a cause (see Sleep Disorders). If there are frequent external or internal disrupters of sleep, the sleep patterns change. After arousal, the patient develops stage I sleep, followed by stage II sleep, repetitively, and the percentages of delta sleep and REM sleep decrease. Drugs can also inhibit REM and delta sleep. Monoamine oxidase inhibitors and tricyclic antidepressants, for example, decrease the percentage of REM sleep dramatically. Alcohol and caffeine increase arousal. If patients are deprived of either REM or delta sleep, "rebound" is usually seen on recovery nights. REM rebound can be intrusive and frightening, with an abundance of vivid dreams. Chronic partial sleep deprivation results in inattentiveness in monotonous tasks, deterioration of mood, irritability, and even mild paranoia.

REM sleep and NREM sleep differ physiologically. REM sleep is characterized by both phasic and tonic changes. The drop in baseline EMG correlates with a tonic change. Rapid eye movements correlate with phasic changes. Tonic physiologic changes also include impaired thermoregulation, hypotension, bradycardia, increased cerebral blood flow and intracranial pressure, increased respiratory rate, and penile erection. Intercostal and upper-airway muscles become atonic, but the diaphragm maintains activity. Phasic changes include vasoconstriction, increased blood pressure, tachycardia, and further increases in cerebral blood flow and respiratory rate. During NREM, the physiologic state is more stable, but blood pressure, heart rate, cardiac output, and respiratory rate decrease. Growth hormone is secreted during stages III and IV, in the first third of the night. Many other rhythms occur, but these need not be directly tied to sleep, as discussed later.

REM sleep can be abolished by lesions restricted to the pons, but the generator of REM/NREM cycling has not been established. The neurotransmitters serotonin, norepinephrine, and acetylcholine all appear to play some role in the regulation of sleep. "Hypnogenic" peptides have been isolated, including delta sleep-inducing peptide, substance S, a muramyl peptide, and interleukin-1.

Chronobiology is the science of the temporal organization of physiologic processes. Circadian rhythms are bodily rhythms that occur approximately every 24 hours. Sleep is the most obvious example of a circadian rhythm. Many other circadian rhythms exist, including body temperature, growth hormone secretion, and cortisol secretion. In an environment free of external time cues, human beings have a "free-running" period of approximately 25 hours; the subject tends to go to bed 1 hour later each day. This means that if a regular schedule is maintained, circadian clocks are "reset" backward approximately 1 hour each day by environmental cues. It follows that it is easier to delay, rather than to advance bedtime, because circadian rhythms move in the direction of daily delay. In the free-running environment, rhythms that usually occur together may desynchronize. The sleep/activity cycle can become longer than the body temperature rhythm, which remains at about 25 hours. Two separate pacemakers emerge, termed X (body-temperature drive) and Y (rest/activity drive). REM sleep and cortisol secretion follow the X pacemaker, whereas slow-wave sleep and growth hormone follow the Y pacemaker. The Y pacemaker is thought to reside in the suprachiasmatic nucleus of the hypothalamus. The location of the X pacemaker is unknown.

SLEEP DISORDER CLASSIFICATION

In 1972 the Association of Sleep Disorders Centers established a diagnostic classification system of sleep and arousal disorders. The nosology served to unify clinical definitions across medical and research disciplines. The disorders were classified by presenting complaint rather than by etiology into four major categories: disorders of initiating and maintaining sleep, or insomnias; disorders of excessive somnolence; disorders of the sleep-wake schedule; and dysfunctions associated with sleep, sleep stages, or partial arousal (parasomnias.) This organization is helpful in approaching differential diagnosis. However, for statistical and research purposes the classification is inadequate because one disorder may present with more than one symptom. Thus, the classification was revised in 1990, as the International Classification of Sleep Disorders (ICSD) (Table 145-1) and is now based on broadly defined pathophysiologic mechanisms rather than presenting symptoms. The major divisions of the ICSD classification are the (1) dyssomnias, (2) parasomnias, (3) sleep disorders associated with medical and psychiatric disorders, and (4) proposed sleep disorders.

DYSSOMNIAS

The dyssomnias are primary sleep disorders that produce either *difficulty initiating and maintaining sleep* or *excessive daytime sleepiness.* Within the classification of the dyssomnias, the sleep abnormalities must be fundamental to the existence of the disorder. Psychiatric and medical disorders that influence sleep, as only one component of the clinical presentation, are not included in the ICSD definition of dyssomnia. The dyssomnias are further divided into three groups: the intrinsic, the extrinsic, and the circadian rhythm sleep disorders. Intrinsic sleep disorders are thought to originate within the body, (e.g., narcolepsy or obstructive sleep apnea). Extrinsic sleep disorders originate outside of the body (e.g., poor sleep hygiene or environmental disruption). Circadian rhythm sleep disorders represent disorders in timing of the sleep-wake cycle within the 24-hour day.

Difficulty Initiating and Maintaining Sleep (Insomnia)

Inability to sleep may take the form of prolonged initial latency to sleep, recurrent nocturnal awakenings, or early morning awakening without the ability to return to sleep. Insomnia is an extremely common complaint that causes high levels of frustration and significant misery. For reasons that are inexplicable, insomnia is frequently trivialized by the clinician and treated pharmacologically without attention to the underlying etiology of the complaint. Inability to initiate or maintain sleep is a symptom that must be explored with the same approach the clinician uses to assess other medical complaints. As in most disorders, a careful history is the most significant diagnostic tool. Exploring the patient's daily schedule in an orderly fashion is often markedly revealing. A sleep log helps document patterns that suggest specific disease. The schedule of daily activi-

TABLE 145-1. International Classification of Sleep Disorders

1. Dyssomnias
   A. Intrinsic sleep disorders
      1. Psychophysiologic insomnia
      2. Sleep state misperception
      3. Idiopathic insomnia
      4. Narcolepsy
      5. Recurrent hypersomnia
      6. Idiopathic hypersomnia
      7. Posttraumatic hypersomnia
      8. Obstructive sleep apnea syndrome
      9. Central sleep apnea syndrome
      10. Central alveolar hypoventilation syndrome
      11. Periodic limb movement disorder
      12. Restless legs syndrome
      13. Intrinsic sleep disorder not otherwise specified
   B. Extrinsic sleep disorders
      1. Inadequate sleep hygiene
      2. Environmental sleep disorder
      3. Altitude insomnia
      4. Adjustment sleep disorder
      5. Insufficient sleep syndrome
      6. Limit-setting sleep disorder
      7. Sleep-onset association disorder
      8. Food allergy insomnia
      9. Nocturnal eating (drinking) syndrome
      10. Hypnotic-dependent sleep disorder
      11. Stimulant-dependent sleep disorder
      12. Alcohol-dependent sleep disorder
      13. Toxin-induced sleep disorder
      14. Extrinsic sleep disorder not other specified
   C. Circadian rhythm sleep disorders
      1. Time zone change (jet lag) syndrome
      2. Shift work sleep disorder
      3. Irregular sleep-wake pattern
      4. Delayed sleep phase syndrome
      5. Advanced sleep phase syndrome
      6. Non-24-hour sleep-wake disorder
      7. Circadian rhythm sleep disorder not otherwise specified
2. Parasomnias
   A. Arousal disorders
      1. Confusional arousals
      2. Sleepwalking
      3. Sleep terrors
   B. Sleep-wake transition disorders
      1. Rhythmic movement disorder
      2. Sleep starts
      3. Sleep talking
      4. Nocturnal leg cramps
   C. Parasomnias usually associated with REM sleep
      1. Nightmares
      2. Sleep paralysis
      3. Impaired sleep-related penile erections
      4. Sleep-related painful erections
      5. REM sleep-related sinus arrest
      6. REM sleep behavior disorder
   D. Other parasomnias
      1. Sleep bruxism
      2. Sleep enuresis
      3. Sleep-related abnormal swallowing syndrome
      4. Nocturnal paroxysmal dystonia
      5. Sudden unexplained nocturnal death syndrome
      6. Primary snoring
      7. Infant sleep apnea
      8. Congenital central hypoventilation syndrome
      9. Sudden infant death syndrome
      10. Benign neonatal sleep myoclonus
      11. Other parasomnia not otherwise specified
3. Sleep disorders associated with medical/psychiatric disorders
   A. Associated with mental disorders
      1. Psychoses
      2. Mood disorders
      3. Anxiety disorders
      4. Panic disorders
      5. Alcoholism
   B. Associated with neurologic disorders
      1. Cerebral degenerative disorders
      2. Dementia
      3. Parkinsonism
      4. Fatal familial insomnia
      5. Sleep-related epilepsy
      6. Electrical status epilepticus of sleep
      7. Sleep-related headaches
   C. Associated with other medical disorders
      1. Sleeping sickness
      2. Nocturnal cardiac ischemia
      3. Chronic obstructive pulmonary disease
      4. Sleep-related asthma
      5. Sleep-related gastroesophageal reflux
      6. Peptic ulcer disease
      7. Fibrositis syndrome
4. Proposed sleep disorders
      1. Short sleeper
      2. Long sleeper
      3. Subwakefulness syndrome
      4. Fragmentary myoclonus
      5. Sleep hyperhidrosis
      6. Menstrual-associated sleep disorder
      7. Pregnancy-associated sleep disorder
      8. Terrifying hypnagogic hallucinations
      9. Sleep-related neurogenic tachypnea
      10. Sleep-related laryngospasm
      11. Sleep choking syndrome

(From Thorpy MJ (chairman): ICSD—International Classification of Sleep Disorders: Diagnostic and Coding Manual. Diagnostic Classification Steering Committee, American Sleep Disorders Association, Rochester, MN, 1990, with permission.)

ties gives insight into the patient's personality and discloses habits that contribute to poor sleep hygiene. All medical history is relevant, and illnesses that may cause nocturnal arousal are particularly important. A family history of sleep disorder and history of childhood sleep behavior is useful. A review of drug use is critical, including prescription medications, home remedies, caffeine, alcohol, and illicit drugs.

Excessive Daytime Sleepiness

Excessive daytime sleepiness is defined as the tendency to fall asleep inappropriately when sedentary. Patients with excessive daytime sleepiness may or may not demonstrate hypersomnolence (i.e., excessive sleep during a 24-hour period). Patients with chronic disorders of excessive daytime sleepiness often accept sleepiness as normal. The clinician should look for a history of excessive daytime sleepiness in any situation presenting as chronically reduced performance, including dementia or depression or in situations suggesting episodic inattention, such as automobile accidents. Instead of sleepiness, many patients cite blackouts, forgetfulness, poor concentration, automatic be-

havior, or amnestic spells. Children may have poor school performance or behavioral problems. These situations require the taking of a sleep history that includes questioning whether or not sleeping occurs during sedentary activities, social activities, driving, and eating. Sleepiness needs to be distinguished from fatigue and disorders of consciousness secondary to encephalopathy. On careful study most patients with excessive daytime sleepiness will prove to have either sleep-disordered breathing or narcolepsy.

Intrinsic Sleep Disorders

"*Psychophysiologic insomnia* is a disorder of somatized tension and learned sleep-preventing associations that results in a complaint of insomnia and associated decreased functioning during wakefulness." (This definition and those that follow are taken from the *ICSD Diagnostic and Coding Manual*.) Such patients usually do not have evidence of underlying psychiatric disease, but they may be highly focused on their insomnia. Overconcern with the process of going to sleep is alerting, induces increased tension, and becomes a sleep-preventing association. The precipitant for this disorder may be a period of acute insomnia associated with an external stress (adjustment sleep disorder; see below.) A characteristic pattern emerges: inability to obtain satisfactory sleep for a few nights induces fear that another sleepless night will follow. Patients report that they feel alert as soon as they try to initiate sleep. They toss and turn, watch the clock, and become frustrated and angry that they are unable to sleep. Often, sleep is better in a new environment free of the usual external sleep-onset associations.

Psychophysiologic insomnia can be treated with relaxation techniques in combination with methods that decondition the patient's negative associations with sleep onset. A technique known as *stimulus-control therapy,* proposed by Bootzin, is highly effective. The patient is instructed to (1) go to bed only if sleepy; (2) use the bed only for sleeping and sexual relations, not as a place to read, write, or watch television; (3) get up and leave the bedroom if sleep is not obtained within 10 to 15 minutes and engage in a nonstimulating activity until sleepiness is perceived; (4) repeat this step as many times as necessary throughout the night; (5) maintain a fixed schedule of awakening each morning; and (6) not nap during the day.

"*Sleep state misperception* is a disorder in which a complaint of insomnia or excessive sleepiness occurs without objective evidence of sleep disturbance." Underestimation of the actual amount slept is common in insomniacs. Some patients complain of absolute lack of sleep. Polysomnographic recording reveals a normal sleep latency, a normal number of arousals and awakenings, and normal sleep duration, but the patient perceives poor or absent sleep. This disorder needs to be distinguished from the phenomenon of paradoxical improvement in sleep during overnight recording in the sleep laboratory, which occurs in patients with psychophysiologic insomnia. In the latter disorder (discussed above) sleep may improve in a novel environment, including the sleep laboratory, and this improvement is appreciated by the patient.

Sometimes patients report sleepiness that cannot be verified on objective testing with the multiple sleep latency test (MSLT; see below); this may be a sleep state misperception. Sleepiness, however, is more difficult to measure than the presence or absence of sleep. Many patients who report near absence of sleep are mistakenly treated with hypnotic medications for years, without improvement. The existence of this disorder underscores the usefulness of polysomnographic evaluation of patients with chronic sleep complaints.

"*Idiopathic insomnia* is a lifelong inability to obtain adequate sleep that is presumably due to an abnormality of the neurological control of the sleep-wake system." This disorder may also be termed childhood-onset insomnia. Unlike "short sleepers" who feel rested despite short sleep durations, patients with this disorder complain of chronically poor performance because of poor sleep. Polysomnographic evaluation reveals increased sleep latency, decreased efficiency, and increased arousals, but the etiology of the disrupted sleep is not apparent. Because of the chronicity of the disorder, patients often develop secondary sleep disorders such as psychophysiologic insomnia and hypnotic dependence. There is no effective treatment except directing attention to conditions that may aggravate the underlying insomnia.

"*Narcolepsy* is a disorder of unknown etiology which is characterized by excessive sleepiness that typically is associated with cataplexy and other REM sleep phenomena such as sleep paralysis and hypnogogic hallucinations." Narcolepsy was first defined as a distinct disorder in 1880 by Gelineau,

who described the syndrome as a "rare, little known neurosis characterized by imperative need to sleep." It is now known that the disorder is not rare. The prevalence is estimated at between 2 and 16 in 10,000 persons. The onset of symptoms occurs typically in the second or third decades, and both sexes are equally affected. A family history is noted in approximately one-third of cases.

The discovery of REM sleep was followed by the finding that patients with narcolepsy have abnormal REM physiology. It is now accepted that the major manifestations of narcolepsy represent a disorder of control mechanisms that regulate REM sleep. Episodes of REM occur at the wrong time, intruding on wakefulness, and the physiologic components of this sleep state dissociate and appear independently. These major symptoms are referred to as the narcolepsy tetrad: (1) excessive daytime sleepiness, (2) cataplexy, (3) hypnogogic hallucinations, and (4) sleep paralysis. Few patients report all of these symptoms, especially in the early stages of the disorder, but almost all patients have evidence of excessive daytime sleepiness.

The cardinal symptom of narcolepsy is excessive daytime sleepiness, and approximately 10 percent of patients complain of this symptom alone. The tendency to sleep inappropriately may have a gradual or an abrupt onset. History taking typically reveals that patients remember brief lapses of attention in sedentary situations years before presentation to a physician. With time, sleepiness is evident in clearly inappropriate situations, such as driving, attending business conversations, eating, or engaging in sexual intercourse. Patients are frequently able to recognize impending drowsiness and take measures to alert themselves. Irresistible sleep attacks are characteristic, however, and tend to occur when the urge to sleep has been delayed. Two features are unique to the naps of narcoleptics: (1) dreaming during naps is common and (2) brief naps of 5 to 10 minutes duration are remarkably refreshing.

Cataplexy is a sudden, usually brief, loss of muscle tone induced by emotion. The presence of cataplexy is considered diagnostic of narcolepsy, but only 60 to 80 percent of patients experience this symptom, and it may occur years after the onset of sleepiness. Rarely, cataplexy is the presenting symptom of the disorder. Idiopathic cataplexy may exist but is poorly described. Laughter and anger are the most common precipitants, but the emotional trigger may be specific to the patient. The weakness that develops usually involves the muscles of the face or the supporting muscles of the legs; it may be so mild as to give only the sense that the face will not move properly or so profound as to cause a sudden fall. The appearance of facial tremulousness can be confused with seizure activity. Occasionally, patients have difficulty speaking. Consciousness is maintained during a cataplectic episode, but prolonged episodes may be immediately followed by REM sleep. Cataplexy is the result of sudden skeletal muscle atonia sparing extraocular eye movements and diaphragm. Deep tendon reflexes during the episode are absent. This atonia is similar to that which occurs during normal REM sleep. Cataplexy thus seems to represent a dissociation of normal REM phenomena, occurring inappropriately during waking.

In hallucinations occurring at the onset of sleep, referred to as hypnogogic hallucinations, the sensory events associated with normal dreaming occur during perceived wakefulness. These hallucinations are a manifestation of the sudden onset of inappropriate and dissociated REM sleep. Hallucinations may involve any sensory system and are frequently visual, auditory, or vestibular.

Sleep paralysis is an inability to move skeletal muscles voluntarily during sleep-wake transitions. Normal subjects may experience the sensation on awakening from REM, but narcoleptics typically complain of sleep paralysis at sleep onset. The episodes can be associated with extreme fear, especially when they are associated by threatening hypnogogic hallucinations. Sleep paralysis is thought to be another manifestation of REM-related atonia.

Two other symptoms are typical of narcolepsy: automatic behavior and disrupted nighttime sleep. Patients with automatic behavior complain that they perform complex, often routine activities "automatically," with partial amnesia and evidence of inattention during the behavior. "Microsleeps" or poor attentiveness caused by sleepiness may be the cause of this behavior. Just as patients have difficulty maintaining alertness because of intrusion of sleepiness during the day, narcoleptics complain of inability to maintain sleep at night. The narcoleptic's sleep tends to be punctuated by frequent awakenings and vivid dreams. Periodic movements in sleep syndrome and sleep apnea are more common in narcoleptics and contribute to poor-quality sleep. Cataplexy, hypnogogic hallucinations, and sleep paralysis are episodic symptoms that may resolve. Complaints of automatic behavior, poor memory, and disturbed sleep often worsen with age. The degree of sleepiness remains relatively constant over the years.

The underlying pathogenesis of narcolepsy is not understood. Polysomnographic studies demonstrate two major features: (1) excessive daytime sleepiness, as measured by multiple daytime naps; and (2) the tendency to develop REM sleep within minutes of sleep onset in daytime and nocturnal recordings. Normal patients do not show sleep-onset REM unless they are sleep deprived, on an irregular sleep-wake cycle, or withdrawing from REM-suppressing medication. Recordings during periods of cataplexy and sleep paralysis show the sudden onset of muscle atonia characteristic of REM sleep.

More than 90 percent of patients with narcolepsy carry the HLA-DR2/DQw1 antigens, specifically the DRw15 subtype of DR2 and the DQw6 subtype of DQw1. A specific allele of DQw6, DQB1-0602, is the best marker across ethnic groups, but need not be present. Patients negative for the DQB1-0602 allele are more likely to represent familial than sporadic cases. DR2-DQw1-positive monozygotic twins may be discordant for narcolepsy, suggesting an environmental influence independent of the genetic contribution.

Occasionally narcolepsy or cataplexy, or both, occur in association with other neurologic disorders, in which case the condition is called symptomatic narcolepsy. Both narcolepsy and cataplexy have been described in patients with tumors in the region of the third ventricle and upper brainstem. Cataplexy has also been described in Niemann-Pick disease. Occasionally narcolepsy is said to follow head trauma and encephalitis. Patients with symptomatic narcolepsy have also been reported to have a high prevalence of the DR2 antigen.

The diagnosis of narcolepsy is secure if excessive daytime sleepiness is associated with unequivocal cataplexy. The diagnosis can be confirmed in these patients—especially in those without a clear history of cataplexy—with polysomnographic studies. The current standard of diagnosis is the MSLT, which measures the tendency to sleep and the type of sleep the patient obtains in brief naps scheduled throughout the day. The mean latency to sleep is usually less than 5 minutes. The diagnosis of narcolepsy requires that two of five naps demonstrate REM sleep. A polysomnogram on the night preceding the MSLT is preferred, to exclude sleep deprivation as a cause of short daytime latencies and sleep-onset REM and to identify other sleep disorders.

Excessive daytime sleepiness is treated with central nervous system (CNS) adrenergic stimulant medication. Nonamphetamine stimulant medications, such as pemoline and methylphenidate, have fewer side effects than do amphetamines and are effective in most patients. The goal of treatment is to use the lowest effective doses of stimulant medication that will maintain adequate alertness to perform day-to-day activities. Stimulants used late in the day may increase nocturnal sleep deprivation and, paradoxically, increase excessive daytime sleepiness.

Cataplexy is best treated with tricyclic antidepressant drugs, particularly those with prominent anticholinergic properties. The effectiveness of these drugs appears to derive from the synergistic effect of uptake inhibition of norepinephrine and serotonin combined with their anticholinergic properties. Clomipramine is the most effective anticataplectic drug currently available. Protriptyline is also highly effective, widely used, and better tolerated. Fluoxetine may be used in patients who are intolerant of tricyclic drugs, but it is less effective.

Nonpharmacologic techniques include the use of *strategic napping*. Brief naps during the day, during periods of maximum fatigue, or before periods of required alertness result in decreased sleepiness and decreased total daily dose of stimulant medication. Attention is directed to maintenance of nocturnal sleep by avoidance of stimulant drugs, caffeine, and alcohol in the evening. Because patients with narcolepsy have a higher incidence of sleep-disordered breathing than normal individuals, the clinician should remain vigilant to the possibility that sleep-disordered breathing is contributing to excessive daytime sleepiness and should treat that disorder appropriately.

Recurrent hypersomnia is a disorder characterized by recurrent episodes of hypersomnia that typically occur weeks or months apart." Kleine-Levin syndrome is the prototype of these disorders. This is usually thought of as a disorder of young men, but young women are also affected, with a male/female sex ratio of 3:1. In a large series, median age of onset was 16.0 for men and 19.5 for women. Daily sleep durations of 18 to 20 hours are associated with behavioral abnormalities including hyperphagia and lack of sexual inhibition. During periods of wakefulness, the patient appears apathetic and irritable. Delusions and hallucinations occasionally occur. EEGs may show background slowing and bursts of high-voltage slow waves. Spontaneous remission is typical. A thorough neurologic evaluation is appropriate to exclude structural abnormalities of brain.

"Idiopathic hypersomnia is a disorder of presumed central nervous system cause that is associated with a normal or prolonged major sleep episode and excessive sleepiness consisting of prolonged (1–2 hours) sleep episodes of non-REM sleep." This disorder has also been termed non-REM narcolepsy and CNS hypersomnolence. Patients demonstrate excessive sleepiness on the MSLT, but there is no evidence of sleep-onset REM. The all-night polysomnogram should not show nocturnal disruption induced by sleep-disordered breathing, leg movements, or other causes. Psychiatric and medical conditions that might contribute to sleepiness are absent. Thus, the diagnosis is one of exclusion. However, a group of these patients, when restudied, have been shown to demonstrate subtle evidence of sleep-disordered breathing (see below) that has been termed *upper airway resistance syndrome*. Brain tumors, especially those in the region of the third ventricle may induce sleepiness as a

primary symptom. Magnetic resonance imaging or computed tomography of the brain is an appropriate screening technique in patients whose hypersomnia is unexplained.

"*Posttraumatic hypersomnia* is excessive sleepiness that occurs as a result of a traumatic event involving the central nervous system." Subtle derangements of neurologic function often follow head trauma, and there may be disruption of usual sleep patterns. It is critical, however, to exclude life-threatening conditions such as subdural hematoma and atlantoaxial dislocation. The latter condition has been associated with sleep attacks that may be secondary to brainstem ischemia or involvement of medullary respiratory centers.

"*Obstructive sleep apnea syndrome* is characterized by repetitive episodes of upper airway obstruction that occur during sleep, usually associated with a reduction in blood oxygen saturation.

"*Central sleep apnea syndrome* is characterized by a cessation or decrease of ventilatory effort during sleep usually with associated oxygen desaturation."

"*Central alveolar hypventilation syndrome* is characterized by ventilatory impairment, resulting in arterial oxygen desaturation that is worsened by sleep, which occurs in patients with normal properties of the lung."

Obstructive sleep apnea inexplicably was not identified as a clinical entity until 1965 when Gastaut described repetitive obstructive apneas in obese, somnolent patients with cardiovascular abnormalities. Since that time sleep-disordered breathing has emerged as an important clinical problem with varied clinical presentations that affects multiple organ systems. The absence of attention to this disorder during the medical training of a large percentage of currently practicing physicians has contributed to continued delay in the appreciation of its importance. The cardinal features of the sleep-disordered breathing syndromes are sleep-related respiratory irregularity, oxygen desaturation, sleep disruption, and excessive daytime sleepiness. Considerable confusion exists in the evolving terminology. Initial clinical descriptions focused on the presence of either obstructive or central apneas. An apnea is defined as absence of airflow for a period of 10 seconds. The apnea is termed obstructive if evidence elists of continued respiratory effort. Central apnea is characterized by absence of respiratory effort throughout the 10-second episode. Although the underlying pathophysiology may be different, the outcome is similar, and the repetitive presence of either type of apnea can cause arousals and oxygen desaturation. The presence of 5 apneas/h of sleep was initially defined as necessary to establish the presence of both syndromes. It has became clear, however, that either incomplete obstructions or central hypoventilatory episodes without apnea, both termed hypopneas, are also important in causing similar physiologic changes and symptoms. Thus, the term sleep-disordered breathing is used as a more accurate description of a phenomenom often characterized by a combination of respiratory patterns. Specific characterization of the predominant abnormalities during sleep, however, remains important in understanding the individual pathophysiology and in designing treatment. Ironically, the term *obstructive sleep apnea syndrome* now refers to a disorder characterized by recurrent airway obstructions during sleep, resulting in functional impairment, even if true apnea is not present.

Sleep-disordered breathing is a ubiquitous problem. An epidemiologic study of employed men and women aged 30 to 60 years generated estimated prevalences of 9 percent for women and 24 percent for men using the definition of a minimum combined apnea/hypopnea index of 5/h of sleep. The prevalence of sleep apnea syndrome defined as an apnea/hypopnea index of at least 5 associated with daytime sleepiness is 2 percent for women and 4 percent for men in the same group, (as noted by Young et al. in 1993). The prevalence in older age groups is thought to be significantly higher. Prevalence rates for children are unknown, but the disorder is not uncommon in this age group.

Most sleep-disordered breathing comes about through repetitive upper airway obstruction caused by collapse at the level of the pharynx, usually at the soft palate or posterior to the base of the tongue. The mechanism of collapse is thought to be complex. Sleep relaxes upper airway dilator muscles and impairs reflexes that are critical to maintaining airway patency against the negative pressures induced by the chest wall muscles. Anatomic narrowing because of tonsils, low soft palate, macroglossia, vascular congestion, fat, or structural abnormalities such as micrognathia, predisposes to collapse. Dilator muscle activity is inhibited by alcohol and sedating drugs such as benzodiazepines. Conditions that induce pharyngeal motor or sensory impairment such as myasthenia, muscular dystophy, stroke, or other brainstem pathology can be predisposing factors.

Patients with predominantly obstructive events usually come to medical attention because of excessive daytime sleepiness, often only after an episode of sleep while driving or at work. Apneas are frequently noted by the bedpartner in association with loud chronic snoring. Obesity is a strong risk factor, but it need not be present, especially in patients with structural abnormalities of the upper airway. Morning headache, inattentiveness, and pseudodepression are common neurologic symptoms. Some evidence shows that stroke risk is increased in this group. Hypoxia contributes to nocturnal seizures, and sleep deprivation may induce poor seizure control in the epileptic. Systemic and pulmonary hypertension, nocturnal arrhythmias, and right heart failure are accepted cardiovascular consequences. Polycythemia may indicate severe nocturnal hypoxia with daytime hypoxia. Impotence and enuresis are seen, more often in severe patients.

Central sleep apnea episodes often represent Cheyne-Stokes (or periodic) breathing. In this familiar respiratory pattern recurrent episodes of hyperventilation are followed by apneic periods in a waxing and waning pattern. This type of central apnea is characterized by a normal or low PCO_2. Control of breathing during sleep is dependent on the chemical responses to PCO_2 and PO_2. The set-point for response to PCO_2 increases variably at sleep transition. If the PCO_2 is lower than this new set-point, an apnea follows. Hypoxia or transient wakefulness induced by the apnea, or both, can increase the PCO_2 responsiveness, inducing hyperventilation and a PCO_2 that again falls below threshold values for sleep. Delays in circulation time in congestive heart failure induce similar instability in this feedback system. Periods of central apnea predispose to obstruction as well, in part because absence of airflow contributes to airway collapse and probably because central input to the upper airway muscles is desynchronized in relation to chest wall and diaphragmatic activation. Combined episodes of central and obstructive apnea are called mixed apneas.

Central sleep apnea other than periodic breathing is uncommon. Nocturnal hypercarbia is characteristic and indicates alveolar hypoventilation. Bilateral medullary lesions from tumor or infarct, syringobulbia, and surgical cordotomy represent lesions in the pathways involved in automatic breathing that are known to induce this type of central apnea. Autonomic dysfunction including Shy-Drager syndrome, familial dysautonomia, and diabetic neuropathy induces chemoreceptor dysfunction and failure of respiratory control. Central sleep apnea may also be seen in neuromuscular disease inducing severe respiratory muscle dysfunction such as phrenic nerve paralysis, myopathies, myasthenia gravis, and motor neuron disease.

The patients with central sleep apnea syndrome usually present with difficulty initiating and maintaining sleep and nocturnal restlessness. In the case of hypercapnic central sleep apnea signs of respiratory failure including cor pulmonale are often present. Central sleep apnea with a Cheyne-Stokes pattern is a common cause of disrupted sleep in the elderly and in patients with congestive heart failure or metabolic disorders such as renal failure. A wide variety of neurologic disorders predispose to this breathing pattern including stroke and degenerative diseases.

Diagnosis of sleep-disordered breathing requires all-night polysomnography. Severity of disease is measured by degree of sleep disruption, oxygen desaturation, cardiovascular abnormalities associated with apneas, and respiratory events per hour of sleep (apnea/hypopnea index).

Nasal constant positive airway pressure (CPAP) is the mainstay of treatment for obstructive sleep apnea and for some patients with predominantly central apneas. CPAP should be titrated during a night of polysomnography. Airway pressure acts as a pneumatic splint to maintain upper airway patency during sleep. Tolerance is generally good, and the response to treatment is often dramatic. Its effectiveness in central sleep apnea is not understood, but many of these patients have some degree of obstruction that may exacerbate the tendency to breathe periodically. Bilevel positive airway pressure (BiPAP) is a newer, similar technique that allows for independent manipulation of inspiratory and expiratory pressures as well as timed nasal pressure ventilation. BiPAP is sometimes better tolerated in purely obstructive apnea and is used especially in patients with neuromuscular weakness and central sleep apnea. Intermittent positive pressure volume ventilation delivered by nasal mask is necessary in more severe cases of neuromuscular weakness and hypoventilation. Periodic breathing may respond to low-flow oxygen, especially if hypoxia or congestive heart failure is present. Severe oxygen desaturation in obstructive sleep apnea patients can be treated with oxygen, especially if there is intolerance to CPAP. Obstructive sleep-disordered breathing improves with removal of alcohol and sedating drugs that decrease upper airway tone. Protriptyline, a stimulating tricyclic can be used to increase daytime alertness and upper airway tone. In the obese patient weight loss is always advised but success is generally not long-lived. When obvious upper airway anatomic abnormalities are present, surgical correction is considered depending on the patient's age, tolerance of CPAP, and complexity of surgery. Children often benefit from tonsillectomy. Uvulopalaopharnygoplasty produces success rates significantly lower than CPAP.

"*Periodic limb movement disorder* is characterized by periodic episodes of repetitive and highly stereotyped limb movements that occur during sleep."

"*Restless legs syndrome* is a disorder characterized by disagreeable leg sensations, usually prior to sleep onset, that cause an almost irresistible urge to move the legs." Restless legs is an extremely annoying, aching, crawling sensation affecting predominantly the legs when sedentary, especially when trying to initiate sleep. The subject feels the overwhelming urge to continually move the legs to abort the sensation. All patients with restless legs syndrome have another disorder, periodic limb movement disorder (also termed periodic leg movements or nocturnal myoclonus). Periodic limb movement disorder may also exist without the complaint of restless legs. These patients show recurrent, periodic leg jerks involving flexor muscles of the legs, analogous to the withdrawal reflex. Upper extremity movements may also occur. Leg twitches occur approximately every 20 to 40 seconds episodically throughout the night. Hundreds of leg jerks may occur, unknown to the patient but often witnessed by the bed partner. The repetitive movements result in arousal. Patients with these disorders may present with either difficulty initiating and maintaining sleep or excessive daytime sleepiness. Restless legs syndrome is sometimes familial. Periodic limb movements can be exacerbated and possibly induced by drugs, especially tricyclic antidepressants. Both disorders may be intermittent and related to an underlying metabolic abnormality, such as uremia, iron deficiency, and chronic alcohol use. Symptoms may be worse during pregnancy. Periodic limb movements may also accompany other primary sleep disorders, including sleep apnea and narcolepsy. Often, no etiology is discovered. Carbidopa-levodopa and dopamine agonists both reduce leg movements and ameliorate the sensation of restless legs. A small dose of the controlled-release formulation of carbidopa-levodopa before bedtime is often effective, but a pattern of withdrawal restlessness during the day develops. Clonazepam and codeine may also be used with moderate success.

Extrinsic Sleep Disorders

"*Inadequate sleep hygiene* is a sleep disorder due to the performance of daily activities that are inconsistent with the maintenance of good quality sleep and full daytime alertness." Many daily behaviors are inconsistent with obtaining good-quality sleep. Frequent daytime napping, inattention to maintenance of regular sleeping hours, caffeine, nicotine, and alcohol are the most common offenders. Poor sleep secondary to this or another disorder may perpetuate the maladaptive habits. For example, insomniacs frequently insist on maintaining caffeine intake or daytime naps to counteract the effects of sleep deprivation.

The presence of at least one of the following behaviors is necessary for the diagnosis of inadequate sleep hygiene by ICSD standards: (1) daytime napping at least two times each week; (2) variable wake-up times or bedtimes; (3) frequent periods (two to three times par week) of extended amounts of time spent in bed; (4) routine use of products containing alcohol, tobacco, or caffeine in the period preceding bedtime; (5) scheduling exercise too close to bedtime; (6) engaging in exciting or emotionally upsetting activities too close to bedtime; (7) frequent use of the bed for nonrelated activities (e.g., television watching, studying); (8) sleeping on an uncomfortable bed (poor mattress, inadequate blankets, and so forth); (9) allowing the bedroom to be too bright, too stuffy, too cluttered, too hot, too cold or in some way nonconductive to sleep; (10) performing activities demanding high levels of concentration shortly before bed; and (11) allowing such mental activities as thinking, planning, reminiscing, and so forth to occur in bed.

"*Environmental sleep disorder* is a sleep disturbance due to a disturbing environmental factor that causes a complaint of either insomnia or excessive sleepiness." External physical factors are temporally associated with the development and resolution of the sleep complaint. The elderly appear to be at more risk for this disorder. Attention to the quality of the sleep environment may avoid needless trials of hypnotic medication. Perhaps nowhere is this more apparent than in the hospitalized setting.

''*Altitude insomnia* is an acute insomnia, usually accompanied by headaches, loss of appetite and fatigue, that occurs following ascent to high altitudes.'' This insomnia is associated with a periodic (Cheyne-Stokes) respiratory pattern caused by low inspired oxygen pressure. Arousals are associated with the hyperventilatory phase of the periodic breathing (see discussion on sleep-disordered breathing above).

''*Adjustment sleep disorder* represents sleep disturbance temporally related to acute stress, conflict, or environmental change causing emotional arousal.'' Inability to initiate sleep in the face of an acute stressor is a nearly universal experience. Occasionally the opposite is true: patients note excessive sleepiness in response to a stressful situation. Symptoms are generally short lived and resolve with removal of the stressor.

''*Insufficient sleep syndrome* is a disorder that occurs in an individual who persistently fails to obtain sufficient nocturnal sleep required to support normally alert wakefulness.'' A large percentage of the population suffers from self-imposed sleep deprivation. Sleep logs help document the disorder for the patient who is often unwilling to recognize the problem. A history reveals that symptoms resolve during vacations and weekends when sleep duration increases. Symptoms resolve if the patient chooses to prolong nocturnal sleep.

''*Limit setting disorder* is a predominantly childhood disorder that is characterized by the inadequate enforcement of bedtimes by a caretaker, with resultant stalling or refusal to go to bed at an appropriate time.'' The disorder is characterized by persistent struggle between the caretaker and child, with sleep disruption for both. Irregular sleep-wake cycles may develop. The disorder resolves with the institution of firm limits. The underlying psychosocial factors that may foster the lack of limit setting are multiple and deserve exploration.

''*Nocturnal eating (drinking) syndrome* is characterized by recurrent awakenings with the inability to return to sleep without eating or drinking.'' This disorder occurs predominantly in early childhood and is associated with breast or bottle feeding. Consuming large amounts of fluid during the night contributes to repeated awakenings because of excessive urination. An adult variant of this disorder is unusual but striking in its presentation. Patients wake fully and engage in uncontrolled binge eating without evidence of similar behavior during daytime hours.

''*Hypnotic-dependent sleep disorder* is characterized by insomnia or excessive sleepiness that is associated with tolerance to or withdrawal from hypnotic medications.'' Hypnotic medications are to be avoided whenever possible. The benzodiazepines and benzodiazepine receptor agonist drugs are the safest sleep-inducing medications but should be reserved for short-term use in patients with transient, usually situationally induced insomnia. Hypnotics are discouraged for several reasons. The underlying etiology of the insomnia may be masked or exacerbated, as in sleep-disordered breathing. Tolerance to the benzodiazepines develops with regular use, and the medication becomes ineffective, resulting in escalation of dose. Half-lives of the benzodiazepines and their active metabolites vary widely. Drugs with long half-lives result in accumulation and impaired performance during waking, especially in the elderly. Withdrawal effects are more evident with shorter-acting drugs. Rebound insomnia follows withdrawal, leading the patient to overestimate the underlying sleep disorder.

''*Stimulant-dependent sleep disorder* is characterized by a reduction of sleepiness or suppression of sleep by central stimulants and resultant alterations in wakefulness following drug abstinence.'' Stimulants are an obvious cause of difficulty initiating and maintaining sleep, but they can easily be overlooked if not pursued in the history. Caffeine is the most common stimulant, in the form of coffee, tea, soft drinks, or chocolate. Decongestants and bronchodilators are often forgotten offenders. Nonamphetamine stimulants prescribed for attention deficit disorder and narcolepsy (such as pemoline and methylphenidate) may produce insomnia as a major side effect, usually because of dosing too late in the day. Prolonged periods of sleeplessness followed by excessive sleep are seen in amphetamine and cocaine abuse.

''*Alcohol-dependent sleep disorder* is characterized by the assisted initiation of sleep onset by the sustained ingestion of ethanol that is used for its hypnotic effect.'' Alcohol usually results in fragmentation of sleep and frequent arousal, contrary to the popular belief that it helps induce sleep. Alcohol also exacerbates sleep-disordered breathing. Many patients become alcohol dependent in attempting to treat insomnia of other etiologies with nocturnal alcohol. Instead, alcohol exacerbates the problem.

Circadian Rhythm Sleep Disorders

The activities of modern society allow for marked variations in the patterns of day-to-day activity. Air travel and shift working are common. Nighttime activities are no longer limited by darkness. Continuous activity with the potential for disrupting sleep-wake cycles is particularly evident in the hospitalized setting. When the timing of sleep is disrupted, the patient is said to have a circadian rhythm sleep disorder.

''*Time zone change (jet lag) syndrome* consists of varying degrees of difficulties in initiating or maintaining sleep, excessive sleepiness, decrements in subjective daytime alertness and performance, and somatic symptoms (largely related to gastrointestinal function) following rapid travel across multiple time zones.''

''*Shift work sleep disorder* consists of symptoms of insomnia or excessive sleepiness that occur as transient phenomena in relation to work schedules.'' An abrupt change in the sleep schedule induced by travel across time zones or a change in work shift results in transient disorders of the sleep-wake cycle. Circadian rhythms are out of phase with the imposed sleep schedule. Subjects note difficulty in both initiating and maintaining sleep, as well as sleepiness during waking hours. Schedules that result in an ''advance'' of the sleep cycle, as in eastward flight, are more poorly tolerated. A natural endogenous rhythm of 25 hours makes it easier to delay, rather than advance, bedtime. Symptoms resolve after circadian rhythms entrain to the new schedule, which may take more than a week. If the sleep-wake cycle changes constantly, because of either travel or shift work, no entrainment occurs and the circadian rhythm disorder becomes persistent.

''*Irregular sleep-wake pattern* consists of temporally disorganized and variable episodes of sleep and waking behavior.'' The sleep pattern of the patient with an irregular sleep-wake cycle is erratic. Unlike patients with non-24-hour sleep-wake syndrome (see below), sleep logs reveal no underlying periodicity. This disorder usually occurs in patients with developmental abnormalities of the brain. Prolonged illness with enforced bed rest and absence of attention to daily routines, may be precipitating factors. Patients complain of chronic fatigue. Neither sleep nor wakefulness is well maintained. This disorder is treated by external reinforcement of a normal sleep-wake cycle, but it usually recurs.

''*Delayed sleep phase syndrome*'' is a disorder in which the major sleep episode is delayed in relation to the desired clock time that results in symptoms of sleep-onset insomnia or difficulty in waking at the desired time.'' Patients habitually adopt a late bedtime and wake late in the day. The amount of sleep and its quality are normal. The patient is symptomatic when attempts to advance the bedtime to an earlier hour fail. These patients appear to be less able to advance their circadian rhythms to reset the body's natural tendency to delay endogenous rhythms, or to compensate for occasional schedule changes. Bright-light therapy is the most effective treatment. Patients are exposed to bright light in the range of 2,500 to 10,00 lux during morning hours, which serves to advance endogenous rhythms and allow for earlier sleep onset.

''*Advanced sleep phase syndrome* is a disorder in which the major sleep episode is advanced in relation to the desired clocktime, that results in symptoms of compelling evening sleepiness, an early sleep onset, and an awakening that is earlier than desired.'' This disorder is commonly seen in the elderly. Advanced sleep phase may explain the physiologic changes seen in endogenous depression, including early REM latency and early morning awakenings. Patients with advanced sleep phase syndrome alone generally do not complain of the disorder. When symptoms are bothersome, patients can be treated with progressive delay of bedtime, or bright-light therapy in the evening.

''*Non-24-hour sleep-wake syndrome* consists of a chronic steady pattern comprised of 1–2 hour daily delays in sleep onset and wake times in an individual living in society.'' Patients with this disorder present with what appears to be an erratic sleep-wake cycle. Sleep logs demonstrate, however, that there is a non-24-hour periodicity in the sleep-wake cycle. This disorder mimics the prolongation of the sleep cycle that can be seen in experimental environments in which subjects are isolated from time cues and are said to be ''free-running.'' Patients who do not attend to environmental cues, including the blind, may develop this syndrome.

PARASOMNIAS

The term *parasomnia* refers to undesirable physical events that occur during sleep or are exacerbated by sleep. These phenomena are often sleep-stage-specific. Subdivisions of the parasomnias are (1) the arousal disorders, (2) the sleep-wake transition disorders, (3) the parasomnias usually associated with REM sleep, and (4) the other parasomnias.

Arousal Disorders

The term *Disorders of arousal* refers to behaviors characterized by confusion and automatic behavior following sudden arousal from delta sleep. Broughton established the uniqueness of these disorders in a classic paper in 1968. He noted that arousal from delta sleep in both normals and to an exaggerated extent in patients with this disorder was associated with the following factors: (1) body movements, (2) autonomic activation, (3) mental confusion and disorientation, (4) automatic behavior, (5) relative nonreactivity to external stimuli, (6) poor response to efforts to provoke behavioral wakefulness, (7) amnesia for many intercurrent events, and (8) fragmentary recall of dream-

like mentation. The tendency to arouse spontaneously from delta sleep tends to be a familial trait with first presentation in childhood and resolution by adolescence. However, episodes may occur for the first time or recur with greater severity in adolescence or adulthood. Stress, sleep deprivation, and any factors that may contribute to sleep disruption are clear exacerbants. Sleep apnea and alcohol are frequent causes of adult recurrence. Occasionally seizure activity may induce the arousal. There is a long-standing debate as to the contribution of emotional factors. Anxiety, depression, and obsessive-compulsive personality may be over-represented in this patient population, but at least half of the patients show no diagnosable psychiatric disorder.

''*Confusional arousals* consist of confusion during and following arousals from sleep, most typically from deep sleep in the first part of the night.'' These episodes are most commonly seen in forced arousals from delta sleep, particularly in individuals with a family or personal history of sleepwalking or sleeptalking, and in children under the age of 5. Amnesia for the events during the arousal is typical. This is predominantly a problem for individuals such as physicians who are called at night and must react appropriately.

''*Sleepwalking* consists of a series of complex behaviors that are initiated during slow wave sleep and result in walking during sleep.'' Sleepwalkers characteristically arouse during the first third of the night from delta sleep, leave the bed in a confused state, and perform complex, automatic acts. Some episodes of sleepwalking are initiated by sleep terror (see below), in which case the behaviors exhibited may be violent, as the subject tries to combat a perceived threat. More routine behaviors, such as eating and urinating, may be performed in a remarkably stereotyped fashion idiosyncratic to the subject. The patient may awaken during the behavior embarrassed and bewildered. Most often the patient returns to bed and has no memory of the episode. Patients are at risk of injuring themselves and their bedpartners. The typical inability to awaken the patient fully and stop the behaviors is particularly frightening and dangerous to the bedpartner. Attack specifically directed at the bedpartner is frequent and can raise difficult legal issues. It is thought that murders have been committed. Care must be taken to secure the sleep environment to prevent falling from heights. Occasionally dangerous objects, such as knives and guns, need to be made inaccessible.

''*Sleep terrors* are characterized by a sudden arousal from slow wave sleep with a piercing scream or cry, accompanied by automatic and behavioral manifestations of intense fear.'' Typically, the individual arouses within the first 2 hours of sleep, sits bolt upright, and screams. Marked tachycardia, mydriasis, and sweating may be evident. The subject is agitated, confused, and difficult to console or arouse fully. Dream recall is not detailed, but a single terrifying image, such as a demon, insect, or intruder, may be reported. Generally sleep is resumed in a few minutes with amnesia for the entire event.

Occasional parasomnic episodes with typical family and personal histories need not require further evaluation. The distinction between these disorders and a REM-related nightmare (see below) can usually be made on the basis of history. In the latter the patient can recount detailed dream activity, whereas in the disorders of arousal only fragmentary images or fears are recalled. Motoric activity associated with detailed dream recall indicates REM behavior disorder (see below) rather than sleepwalking. Atypical features may suggest nocturnal seizure (see below.)

Polysomnographic study and sleep-deprived full-montage EEGs are recommended in patients with violent behavior, frequent disruptive episodes, atypical clinical features, or excessive daytime sleepiness. Polysomnograms may confirm sudden arousal from delta sleep, even in the absence of an episode; some sleep laboratories induce arousal with a buzzer to precipitate the clinical syndrome. More importantly, the polysomnogram may identify another cause of arousal, such as sleep apnea, that precipitates the behavior in the predisposed patient. Seizure activity, although not frequent, may induce arousal, or seizure itself may mimic the clinical syndrome (see below).

The first line of treatment is removal of the possible underlying precipitants of arousal or delta sleep rebound, or both. Improved sleep hygiene helps, with avoidance of sleep deprivation, irregular sleep/wake cycles, caffeine, and alcohol. Stress reduction by relaxation techniques appears to be useful. Hypnosis has been tried with success. Coincident sleep apnea should be treated, even if not severe. The mainstay of treatment for recurrent injurious or disruptive episodes is clonazepam, qhs. Many patients use the medication intermittently in settings that are either dangerous, embarrassing, or known to precipitate their episodes. Clonazepam and other benzodiazepines appear to increase the arousal threshold.

Sleep-Wake Transition Disorders

"*Rhythmic movement disorder* comprises a group of stereotyped, repetitive movements involving large muscles, usually of the head and neck, which typically occur immediately prior to sleep onset and are sustained into light sleep." This disorder is predominantly recognized as headbanging or rocking in children, with onset at about 6 months and resolution, in most cases, by the age of 4. Persistence into adulthood is sometimes seen. "*Sleep starts* are sudden, brief contractions of the legs, sometimes also involving the arms and head, which occur at sleep onset." Also called hypnic jerks, these episodes are often associated with the sensation of falling and are considered normal unless they occur so frequently as to interfere with sleep onset. When episodes are disruptive, sleep-onset epilepsy should be considered. Periodic limb movement disorder may induce arousal at sleep onset, but the movements are less generalized, and polysomnographic study reveals persistent movements during sleep.

Parasomnias Usually Associated With REM Sleep

"*Nightmares* are frightening dreams that usually awaken the sleeper from REM sleep." Because nightmares occur during REM sleep, the subject arouses easily and has detailed dream recall. Episodes typically occur in the last half of the night when REM is more predominant. The episodes may be recurrent in the same night, reflecting the periodicity of REM. Sleep-onset nightmares reflect abnormal REM sleep as in narcolepsy or drug withdrawal states. Nightmares are thought to occur normally in childhood. In adults recurrent nightmares may represent underlying psychiatric disorders, especially anxiety and depression. Medications should always be considered, especially antidepressants that cause REM suppression followed by REM rebound on withdrawal, centrally acting antihypertensives, and antiparkinsonian drugs. Physiologic disruptions occurring during REM sleep such as sleep-disordered breathing or arrhythmia may also induce nightmare.

"*Sleep paralysis* consists of a period of inability to perform voluntary movements either at sleep onset (hypnagogic or predormital form) or upon awakening either during the night or in the morning (hypnopompic or postdormital form)." Sleep paralysis represents a partial arousal or entry into REM sleep such that the atonia of REM sleep is present, but the cerebral cortex is awake. This is a common symptom of narcolepsy (see above) especially at sleep onset. Normal subjects may have occasional episodes of sleep paralysis on awakening. A familial disorder has been described with sleep-onset sleep paralysis without other features of narcolepsy. Sleep paralysis is particularly common in patients taking REM modifying drugs, especially monoamine oxidase inhibitors.

"*REM sleep-related sinus arrest* is a cardiac rhythm disorder that is characterized by sinus arrest during REM sleep in otherwise healthy individuals." Asystole may be prolonged, lasting as long as 9 seconds. This arrhythmia shows response to atropinergic drugs. Most patients have been treated with artificial pacemakers, because the natural history of the disorder and the risk of sudden death are unknown.

"*REM sleep behavior disorder* is characterized by the intermittent loss of REM sleep EMG atonia and by the appearance of elaborate motor activity associated with dream mentation." Lack of the usual atonia of REM sleep allows the patient to enact dreams. Patients typically run, punch, kick, or leap from bed. Vocalization consistent with the dream activity is usual. The patient may be able to correlate detailed dreaming with the witnessed motoric behavior. Sometimes the patient is able to incorporate ongoing conversation and activity into the dream, giving rise to the misperception that he is confused or hallucinating. This disorder occurs most frequently in older men, but all ages are represented. About one-third of patients have underlying neurologic disease, of varied type including but not limited to dementia, Parkinson's disease, olivopontocerebellar atrophy, brainstem tumor, and stroke. When looked for carefully, this disorder may be the presentation of early neurologic disease, especially Parkinson's disease. Medications, especially antidepressants, including fluoxetine, tricyclics, and monoamine oxidase inhibitors, and as well as drug withdrawal, can induce the syndrome. The violent content of dreams frequently suggests the misdiagnosis of post-traumatic stress disorder, especially in patients already treated with multiple antidepressants. Clinical descriptions consistent with this disorder were noted in patients with alcohol withdrawal years before the condition was described.

The diagnosis can be confirmed unequivocally if a full polysomnographic study is available. During episodes of REM sleep excessive tone and movements are noted, usually correlated with some manifestation of the clinical behavior. For unclear reasons clonazepam (0.5 to 2.0 mg qhs) is remarkably effective in treating REM sleep behavior disorder and results in resolution or significant attenuation of the clinical symptoms in most cases.

Other Parasomnias

"*Sleep bruxism* is a stereotyped movement disorder characterized by grinding or clenching of teeth during sleep." This is a common disorder that is sometimes correlated with stress. It results in disrupted nocturnal sleep, temporomandibular joint dysfunction, damage to teeth, and morning headache. Bruxism is inhibited by the use of a nocturnal tooth guard.

"*Sleep enuresis* is characterized by recurrent involuntary micturition that occurs during sleep." Bedwetting after the age

5 years is considered abnormal. There may be a delay in toilet training without the development of continence during sleep, termed primary enuresis. Secondary enuresis refers to the development of bedwetting after toilet training is complete. Symptomatic enuresis is secondary to underlying medical disease (e.g., urogenital disorder, nocturnal seizure, or sleep apnea). Some cases of enuresis follow arousal from delta sleep, but enuresis may occur in any sleep stage. If no underlying medical cause is identified, the disorder is treated with bladder training, behavioral techniques, and (if these fail) imipramine.

"*Nocturnal paroxysmal dystonia* is characterized by repeated dystonia or dyskinetic (ballistic, choreoathetoid) episodes that are stereotyped and occur during NREM sleep." Both short- and long-lasting episodes have been described and appear to have different mechanisms. Short episodes often respond to carbamazepine. Brief episodes of stereotyped dystonic, choreoathetoid, and/or ballistic movements may be associated with mumbling or crying. Episodes arise from all stages of NREM sleep. EEGs during the episodes are reportedly without evidence of seizure activity. A history of known generalized seizures is present in many of the patients. Recent cases suggest frontal lobe epileptic foci. Long-duration episodes have been observed in one patient who later developed Huntington's disease.

"*Sudden unexplained nocturnal death syndrome (SUND)* is characterized by sudden death during sleep in healthy young adults, particularly of Southeast Asian descent."

MEDICAL/PSYCHIATRIC SLEEP DISORDERS

Conditions Associated with Mental Disorders

Disordered sleep is typical of most psychiatric disorders. Unipolar depression characteristically presents with a disorder of initiating and maintaining sleep, most commonly early morning awakening. The patient may fall asleep easily but wake a few hours later, alert and unable to return to sleep. This can be the earliest symptom apparent to the patient. Sleep studies in some of these patients demonstrate an earlier-than-normal REM latency and increased phasic REM activity early in the night. By contrast, the sleep in bipolar depressive disease is characterized by prolonged periods of inability to sleep during the manic phase and excessive sleep during the depressive phase. Most actively psychotic patients have difficulty maintaining sleep, but some may be hypersomnolent at the onset of their psychosis. Patients with panic disorder may wake suddenly at night with panic; polysomnographic evaluation is sometimes useful to distinguish these episodes from sleep terror. The treatment of sleep disorders of psychiatric cause is directed to treatment of the underlying illness. Improvement in sleep is often a sensitive measure of the effectiveness of treatment.

Conditions Associated With Neurologic Disorders

Cerebral Degenerative Disorders, Dementia, Parkinsonism. Sleep disruption is a prominent, but not well studied, symptom in all of the degenerative diseases of brain. Patients with degenerative disease of brain are at particular risk of sleep-disordered breathing because of Cheyne-Stokes respirations, abnormal chest wall and upper airway muscle tone, brainstem dysfunction, and sedating medications. The resulting hypoxemia can contribute to episodes of nocturnal confusion. In the disorders involving motor systems, sleep fragmentation also occurs secondary to rigidity, tremor, myoclonus, and periodic limb movements. Brainstem involvement induces REM sleep abnormalities, including the REM sleep behavior. Circadian rhythm disorders are frequent and probably represent derangement of neurologic control mechanisms, coupled with the secondary effects of disrupted sleep and medication.

Sleep-Related Epilepsy. Seizures are facilitated by sleep, particularly stage II sleep. Hypoxia secondary to sleep apnea also precipitates seizures. Grand mal seizures are suggested by falls from bed, incontinence, bitten tongue, and morning confusion. In a patient with known seizure disorder, paroxysmal nocturnal behaviors of any sort are best considered seizure activity until proved otherwise. Atypical seizures with symptoms only during sleep may represent difficult diagnostic problems. Some types of seizure disorders, especially complex partial seizures with temporolimbic symptoms, closely mimic sleep terrors and sleep-walking. *Episodic nocturnal wandering* is a syndrome that may be indistinguishable from the disorders of arousal, but it usually has atypical features. The wandering tends to be less goal directed and organized than typical sleepwalking. Speech tends to be unintelligible. Automatisms may be noted. Rather than clustering in the first third of the night when delta sleep is abundant, episodes often recur frequently in the same night or appear late. There is a high prevalence of interictal EEG abnormalities in these patients, and episodes respond to anticonvulsants. A variety of paroxysmal nocturnal autonomic symptoms have been ascribed to the partial epilepsies, including breathing abnormalities, arrhythmias, and flushing. Standard polysomnography employs a limited EEG montage that is inadequate for the evaluation of seizure disorders. A full EEG montage with polysomnographic monitoring or EEG telemetry needs to be employed when the diagnosis is in doubt.

Sleep-Related Headaches. Cluster headache is a severe unilateral orbital headache associated with ipsilateral rhinorrhea and tearing. The headache is frequently nocturnal and appears to be exacerbated specifically by REM sleep. Chronic paroxysmal hemicrania, a similar headache disorder that is more frequent in women and responsive to indomethacin, is also REM related. Increased blood flow and hypoxemia during REM may be etiologic factors. Most patients note that migraine is improved by sleep, but occasionally the reverse is true. Sleep-related headache may be the presentation of raised intracranial pressure, exacerbated by the supine posture and episodic elevation in intracranial pressure during REM sleep. Morning headache is typical of sleep apnea syndrome and bruxism.

Conditions Associated With Other Medical Disorders

Just as medical illness disrupts the quality of life during the day, it also affects the maintenance of sleep. A careful consideration of possible systemic disease is important in every patient with a sleep disorder. Almost every disease, at some point in its course, may disrupt sleep. Most painful disorders cause nocturnal arousal, especially arthritis and peptic ulcer disease. Insomnia may be the presenting complaint of congestive heart failure with nocturia, paroxysmal nocturnal dyspnea, or arousal secondary to Cheyne-Stokes respirations. Pulmonary dysfunction is exacerbated during sleep and predisposes patients to sleep-disordered breathing. Sleep disruption is particularly prominent in hyperthyroidism and uremia.

PROPOSED SLEEP DISORDERS

"Menstrual-associated sleep disorder is a disorder of unknown cause, characterized by a complaint of either insomnia or excessive sleepiness, that is temporally related to the menses or menopause."* Premenstrual excessive sleepiness is a sometimes dramatic disorder that appears within the first 2 years after the onset of menstruation. Periodic episodes of hypersomnolence tend to occur 6 to 10 days before the onset of menses. The disorder is treated successfully with birth control pills. Menopausal insomnia is characterized by recurrent awakenings, often associated with hot flashes or night sweats. Premenstrual insomnia is common, characterized by difficulty in initiating and maintaining sleep; it is often associated with other symptoms attributed to the premenstrual syndrome.

"Sleep-related laryngospasm refers to episodes of abrupt awakenings from sleep with an intense sensation of inability to breathe, and stridor."* The disorder is frightening but usually benign. Otolaryngologic examination reveals no abnormality. The disorder tends to recur several times and then resolve. It is more common in smokers and patients with esophageal reflux. Sleep apnea and upper airway pathology need to be considered. Rarely, nocturnal seizure is the etiology.

SUGGESTED READINGS

Anch A, Browman, CP, Mittler MM, Walsh JK: Sleep: A Scientific Perspective. Prentice-Hall, Englewood Cliffs, NJ, 1988

Bootzin RR, Engle-Friedman, M, Hazelwood L: Insomnia. Pp. 81–115. In Lewinsohn PM, Teri L (eds): Clinical Geropsychology, New Directions in Assessment and Treatment. Pergamon Press, New York, 1983

Broughton RJ: Sleep disorders: disorders of arousal? Science 159:1070, 1968

Guilleminault C, Pool P, Motta J, Gillis AM: Sinus arrest during REM sleep in young adults. N Engl J Med 311:1006, 1984

Guilleminault C, Stoohs R, Quera-Salva M-A: Sleep-related obstructive and nonobstructive apneas and neurologic disorders. Neurology, suppl. 6. 42: 53, 1992

Kryger MH, Roth T, Dement W: Principles and Practice of Sleep Medicine. 2nd Ed. WB Saunders, Philadelphia, 1994

Lewy AJ, Sack RL, Miller S, Hoban T: Antidepressant and circadian phase-shifting effects of light. Science 235:352, 1987

Mahowald MW, Ettinger MG: Things that go bump in the night: the parasomnias revisited. J Clin Neurophysiol 7:119, 1990

Matheson JK: Sleep and its disorders. p. 1003. In: Internal Medicine. 4th Ed. CV Mosby, St. Louis, 1994

Matsuki K, Grumet FC, Lin A: DQ (rather than DR) gene marks susceptibility to narcolepsy. Lancet, 339:1052, 1992

Moore-Ede MC, Czeisler CA, Richardson GS: Medical progress: circadian timekeeping in health and disease. N Engl J Med, 309:469 and 530, 1983

Phillipson EA, Bradley TA: Clinics in Chest Medicine. Breathing Disorders in Sleep. WB Saunders, Philadelphia, 1992

Schenck CH, Bundlie SR, Patterson AL, Mahowald MW: Rapid eye movement behavior disorder. JAMA 257:1786, 1987

Thorpy MJ (chairman): ICSD—International Classification of Sleep Disorders: Diagnostic and Coding Manual. Diagnostic Classification Steering Committee, American Sleep Disorders Association, Rochester, MN, 1990

Thorpy MJ: Handbook of Sleep Disorders. Marcel Dekker, New York, 1990

Young T et al: The occurrence of sleep-disordered breathing among middle-aged adults. N Engl J Med 328:1230, 1993

SECTION 4. PSYCHIATRIC ISSUES IN NEUROLOGIC PRACTICE

146. PSYCHIATRIC ISSUES IN NEUROLOGIC PRACTICE

BARRY S. FOGEL

ANXIETY AND PANIC

Symptoms of anxiety are nearly universal among patients seen in neurologic practice, but the manifestations of anxiety differ widely among individuals. Anxiety, or behavioral symptoms related to anxiety, frequently represent complete or incomplete forms of anxiety disorders. These conditions, the most prevalent of mental disorders in the general population, are readily treated once diagnosed. This section of the chapter addresses the following themes: (1) identification of anxiety in neurologic patients, (2) assessment of the anxious patient, (3) general management, and (4) pharmacologic treatment.

Recognition and Characterization of Anxiety

The cognitive experience of anxiety is one of worry, fear, or apprehension, often accompanied by irritability or difficulty concentrating. The somatic experience of anxiety may include restlessness or a keyed-up feeling, fatigability, muscle tension, palpitations, sweating, trembling, dyspnea, choking sensations, chest discomfort, nausea, dizziness, paresthesias, and hot or cold feelings. Symptoms frequently are linked to hyperventilation or to overactivity of the sympathetic nervous system. The behavioral manifestations of anxiety may include seeking reassurance or comfort, avoiding a fearful stimulus, inhibition of action, physical hyperactivity, explosive behavior or speech in response to personal or environmental irritation, or repetitive speech or action. In a given patient, one or another dimension of anxiety—cognitive, affective, or behavioral—may predominate.

The predominance of a particular dimension of anxiety may be due to either disorder-specific or patient-specific factors. Typically, behavioral manifestations are the most prominent features of phobias and obsessive-compulsive disorder, whereas somatic manifestations predominate in panic disorder. Patients with dementia or severe mental retardation may display somatic or behavioral manifestations of anxiety but be unable to generate or express the cognitions associated with worry or apprehension. In particular, "agitation" in cognitively impaired persons in institutional settings can be a behavioral manifestation of anxiety. Patients with characterologic unawareness of their own feelings may similarly complain of or display somatic symptoms of anxiety while denying worry or stress. Such patients may reveal their anxiety behaviorally by showing unusual rigidity in their approach to dealing with their medical problems.

Anxiety may be well founded in the patient's objective situation or be completely endogenous. Often, there is a combination of causal factors. Emotional reactions to illness will tend to follow the patient's historical pattern of stress response, a pattern influenced by their level of trait anxiety or "neuroticism." Moreover, the cognitive and behavioral details of anxiety disorders can incorporate concerns related to neurologic disease, as when a patient with agoraphobia and epilepsy insists that she cannot go out alone because she might have a seizure.

Anxiety-related phenomena obviously require further assessment when they appear to be a major source of the patient's distress or disability, or when they interfere with the efforts of the patient, the physician, or caregivers to deal with the patient's neurologic disorder. When a patient has symptoms in excess of objective neurologic findings, amplification of neurologic symptoms by anxiety should be considered when the patient has some definite symptoms of anxiety, and the neurologic symptoms are amplified concurrently with an aggravation of those symptoms. Thus, aggravation of headache by anxiety would be supported by its worsening at time of muscle tension and worry. However, because anxiety disorders are highly prevalent in the general population, the mere presence of anxiety symptoms or an anxiety disorder should not be taken uncritically as an explanation for neurologic symptoms in excess of findings.

Diagnosis

The goals of initial assessment of the anxious patient are to determine (1) whether the patient has an immediate, remediable cause for the anxiety such as pain or misinformation; (2) whether there is a medical condition (e.g., hyperthyroidism) or an exogenous substance (e.g., caffeine) causing or aggravating the anxiety symptoms; (3) whether the patient has an anxiety disorder; (4) whether the patient has some other primary psychiatric disorder that can cause anxiety; and (5) whether there is relevant past history to guide management or treatment.

The inquiry about discomfort or worry is straightforward in the cognitively intact patient; in those with impaired cognition or communication, pain and discomfort may need to be inferred from the patient's facial expression and movements. In the office setting, the relative or other caregiver who accompanies the cognitively impaired or aphasic person to the office may be able to assist.

Exogenous Factor.   The most common exogenous causes of anxiety in office practice are caffeine and alcohol. As few as two cups of coffee or the equivalent daily is sufficient to produce clinically significant symptoms of anxiety in predisposed individuals, and patients do not necessarily make the connection between their caffeine habit and their anxiety symptoms. Alcohol, consumed in moderate to heavy quantities in the evening, can be associated with anxiety symptoms and elevated blood pressure the following day. Other frequent causes are sympathomimetic decongestant drugs, theophylline preparations taken for lung disease, and rebound anxiety from short-acting hypnotics taken at night only. A wide range of prescription drugs cause anxiety, nervousness, or insomnia in a small pro-

portion of patients who presumably have a pharmacodynamic vulnerability to those agents. For most of these, the time course of the prescription and the symptoms will permit the diagnosis. For long-term medications and over-the-counter drugs, a trial of discontinuation of the suspected drug may be needed.

Endocrinologic and Neurologic Assessment.   Although numerous systemic diseases can produce symptoms of anxiety, only the endocrine disorders commonly *present* with anxiety: hyperthyroidism, hypercortisolism, and hyperparathyroidism all can do so. For this reason, a screen of thyroid function, electrolytes, and calcium is part of the medical assessment for persistent symptoms of anxiety. Assessment of anxious patients for more unusual endocrine conditions, such as pheochromocytoma and insulinoma, is not routine.

The neurologic disease that most often presents with dramatic anxiety symptoms is partial epilepsy: fear is the most common ictal emotion, and there is considerable overlap between the phenomenology of panic attacks and the phenomenology of partial seizures with ictal fear. Evaluation for epilepsy is indicated for recurrent episodic anxiety with lateralized symptoms, alteration of consciousness or memory, or severe postattack fatigue or headache. Patients with apparently typical panic attacks should be evaluated for epilepsy only if they have a history of definite seizures, have a major risk factor such as a known cortical lesion, or have failed to respond to standard drug therapy for panic disorder. There are well-documented cases of antiepileptic drugs suppressing seizures with ictal fear, leaving "panic attacks" as a residual; the "panic attacks," which represent aborted seizures, may cease with more aggressive antiepileptic drug therapy.

Although it usually does not present with anxiety, Parkinson's disease is associated with an increased prevalence of anxiety symptoms and anxiety disorders. Other movement disorders associated with an increased prevalence of anxiety disorders are essential tremor and Tourette's disorder. In the early stages, the abnormal movements of these conditions sometimes are misattributed to anxiety. If an anxiety disorder is to be diagnosed later in the course, the neurologist should take care to indicate to the patient that this is a second diagnosis, and not a psychiatric explanation of the patient's neurologic disorder. Tourette's disorder is specifically associated with obsessive-compulsive disorder.

Nonparoxysmal anxiety symptoms are frequently encountered in patients in the early stages of degenerative neurologic diseases, where the patient experiences symptoms of dysfunction of the central nervous system but examination and test results are still negative or equivocal. These symptoms, if not due to direct effects of the degenerative disease on subcortical or limbic structures, may be a reaction to an altered sense of self or to functional impairment, or may reflect conscious worry about the diagnosis.

Symptoms

After excluding immediate concerns and exogenous causes for anxiety, the assessment proceeds to an inventory of symptoms of anxiety in the cognitive, somatic, and behavioral domains, determining how long the patient has been symptomatic and whether the symptoms are associated with distress, impaired function, or self-imposed limitations. An anxiety disorder is present when symptoms are persistent or recurrent, and of sufficient severity or multiplicity to have functional consequences.

Important distinctions among anxiety disorders are made according to whether the patient has panic attacks, avoidant behavior, obsessive thoughts, or compulsive rituals, and whether the anxiety symptoms are linked to a specific traumatic event. The corresponding anxiety disorders are panic disorder, phobias (agoraphobia, social phobia, and various specific phobias), obsessive-compulsive disorder, and post-traumatic stress disorder with anxious mood. Multiple anxiety symptoms lasting 6 months or more without these distinguishing features suggest a diagnosis of generalized anxiety disorder.

Clinically significant anxiety that occurs in close relation to a major life stressor may represent an adjustment disorder (i.e., a reaction to acute stress that temporarily exceeds the individual's ability to cope). A history of significant anxiety symptoms preceding the stressor suggests that a patient with stress-related anxiety actually suffers from a relapse or aggravation of a pre-existing anxiety disorder, rather than an adjustment disorder.

The anxiety disorders are distinguished from other psychiatric disorders in which anxiety may be a symptom, but for which other symptoms are more prominent, and define the syndrome. In neurologic office practice, the most important disorder to be distinguished is depression, which frequently is accompanied by symptoms of anxiety. The most distinctive feature of depression is loss of pleasure or interest in usual activities. Other symptoms not usually due to anxiety without depression are significant changes in weight, early morning awakening, and guilt feelings.

Anxiety due to early dementia is distinguished from a primary anxiety disorder by cognitive impairment disproportionate to the patient's level of anxiety. Anxiety secondary to thought disorder is discussed below in section on thought disorders; the distinguishing feature is disorganization of thinking beyond the mild distractability and inattentiveness that frequently accompany anxiety.

General Management

If the patient's anxiety appears related to physical discomfort or a remediable concern, such as a need for more medical information, these concerns are addressed concretely. When possible, exogenous substances that aggravate anxiety are eliminated. In the case of caffeine, a slow taper usually is better tolerated than abrupt withdrawal, which can cause headaches and influenza-like aches and pains. When alcohol is thought to contribute, the patient is asked to abstain for a specific time period to assess the contribution of alcohol to the symptoms; this may avert defensiveness about whether drinking is excessive.

If a patient has anxiety directly related to a recent stressor, and not associated with long-term problems with anxiety, the patient is likely to benefit from psychosocial interventions to help him or her deal with the stressor. These interventions include formal psychotherapy, support groups, pastoral counseling, or counseling by the physician or a member of the clinical care team. The choice of intervention is based both on the patient's preferred style of coping and the resources available locally. Psychotherapy from a mental health professional usually is preferable when it appears that the patient has personal concerns going beyond the evident stressor; support groups or counseling by the clinician often are satisfactory when the main issues are related to coping with a neurologic disease. Pharmacologic therapy for symptoms of anxiety should be considered if there is significant insomnia, irritability, or disruption of daily activity by anxiety. Benzodiazepines are the usual drug of choice in this situation.

Panic Disorder. Patients suffering from panic disorder usually respond best to a combination of psychological and pharmacologic therapy. Initially, the patient should be educated as to the benign significance of panic attacks, their origin in overactivity of the sympathetic nervous system, and their controllability with medication if desired. If the attacks are frequent and uncomfortable, treatment can be initiated with a benzodiazepine; clonazepam is particularly effective, with alprazolam being an alternative for those who find clonazepam too sedating. For longer-term therapy, a tricyclic antidepressant or serotonin re-uptake inhibitor is gradually substituted for all or part of the benzodiazepines. After pharmacologic therapy is offered, the patient is taught a method of relaxation for coping with the panic attacks: deep breathing, progressive muscular relaxation, self-hypnosis or visualization, or biofeedback are all effective methods. Further teaching or reading to reinforce thinking about the benign nature of the episodic anxiety symptoms is offered.

Patients who cannot achieve adequate suppression of panic attacks despite educational approaches and a trial of a benzodiazepine and an antidepressant in usual therapeutic dosage should be placed on a trial of a drug effective for partial epilepsy. Patients who do not want pharmacologic therapy, or whose panic attacks have an apparent relationship to specific interpersonal conflicts, should be referred to a psychotherapist.

Phobias. Patients with specific phobias must be repeatedly exposed to the feared stimulus to extinguish the fear. The usual treatment is to teach the patient a method of relaxation, and then expose the patient to progressively stronger stimuli while the patient practices the relaxation technique. Exposure is supplemented with education: people with fears of flying, for example, are taught about the principles of aviation and the basis of flight safety. When there is only an occasional need to confront the feared stimulus, a benzodiazepine and/or β-blocker can be given in anticipation of exposure to help control symptoms.

Patients with agoraphobia or social phobia usually require antidepressant drugs in addition to the techniques for specific phobias. For these two conditions, monoamine oxidase inhibitors are effective in some patients who do not respond to tricyclic antidepressants or serotonin re-uptake inhibitors. Socially maladroit individuals may require formal social skills training to address the realistic basis for their avoidance of social interaction.

Obsessive-Compulsive Disorder. Patients with obsessive-compulsive disorder respond specifically to drug therapy with serotonin re-uptake inhibitors. Compulsive rituals will also respond to behavior therapy in which patients practice inhibiting their compulsive behavior, using relaxation procedures to cope with the anxiety that emerges when the ritual is omitted.

Post-traumatic Stress Disorder. Patients with post-traumatic stress disorder virtually always requires formal psychotherapy that addresses the traumatic event and its emotional significance for the patient. Although there is no drug therapy known to be generally effective for this disorder, the use of antianxiety drugs to treat anxiety symptoms is well established. Recurrent panic attacks in post-traumatic stress disorder ordinarily would be treated with a benzodiazepine acutely and with an antidepressant over the longer term. Anecdotes suggest that antiepileptic drugs for partial seizures may be helpful in stabilizing mood and minimizing severe anxiety in patients with post-traumatic stress disorder.

Pharmacologic Treatment

Benzodiazepines. Benzodiazepines are the mainstay of short-term pharmacologic therapy for anxiety. They offer the benefit of virtually immediate action. The only significant medical contraindication is severe pulmonary disease with hypoventilation. However, two frequently occurring situations in neurologic practice require precautions. First, patients with gait disturbance can become significantly more unsteady on benzodiazepines. Their gait should be reassessed after starting a benzodiazepine, and again after steady state is reached with continued dosing. Second, patients with cognitive impairment, and especially patients with frontal system dysfunction, can show signficant disinhibition on the benzodiazepines. Behavior should be reassessed after the initial dose, and again at steady state.

For the treatment of anxiety in the context of an adjustment reaction, any benzodiazepine will do, but current fashion favors intermediate-acting agents without active metabolites—lorazepam or oxazepam. However, longer-acting agents such as diazepam may be more convenient and economical, provided that dosage is kept low and one is alert to accumulation of the drug—steady state may not be reached for over a week. For the treatment of panic attacks, clonazepam or alprazolam are preferred because they appear to suppress panic attacks better than other benzodiazepines, at dosages that have equal effect on anticipatory anxiety.

Optimum dosages of benzodiazepines for treatment of anxiety in neurologic patients vary widely for several reasons. First, there is considerable variation in benzodiazepine metabolism in the general population, and even more variation among persons with chronic diseases. Second, patients who have received antiepileptic drugs or antispasticity agents may be pharmacodynamically tolerant to some of the effects of benzodiazepines. Third, regional brain disease can influence drug response, as when frontal system disease increases the risk of disinhibition. Typical dose ranges for benzodiazepines are alprazolam 0.25 to 1.0 mg tid to qid; clonazepam 0.25 to 1.0 mg qhs to bid; lorazepam 0.25 to 1.0 mg tid; oxazepam 10 to 30 mg tid; and diazepam 2 to 10 mg qhs to tid.

To determine the optimum dose of a benzodiazepine for a given symptom in a given patient, start with a small initial dose. If the first dose is ineffective, a slightly higher dose is given the next time, until the patient receives noticeable benefit. The minimum beneficial dosage is given repeatedly until the pharmacologic steady state is reached; the situation is then reassessed. Doses are adjusted repeatedly until the desired effect is obtained. In this way, the mimimum dose to control symptoms is determined by approaching it from below. Patients who are responsible and cognitively intact may titrate benzodiazepine dosage for themselves within parameters specified by the physician.

Antidepressants. Virtually all of the chronic anxiety disorders can be treated with antidepressants rather than benzodiazepines, although the onset of therapeutic action is slower. Patients who are intolerant of the sedation or ataxia produced by benzodiazepines may prefer antidepressants, particularly the serotonin re-uptake inhibitors. However, when these drugs are used for anxiety disorders, they should be started at dosages well below the usual recommended dosages for depression, because they can transiently aggravate anxiety symptoms if they are started at standard antidepressant dosages. Typical starting doses would be paroxetine 5 to 10 mg/day or sertraline 12.5 to 25 mg/day. In patients with a history of extreme sensitivity to medication, fluoxetine liquid can be used, as it permits titration from an extremely low starting dose (e.g., 2 mg/day). Once it is established that a dose is tolerated, increases can be made every 2 to 3 days until symptoms are relieved or the full antidepressant range is explored.

Buspirone. Buspirone, a serotonin-1A partial agonist, is effective for generalized anxiety, but not for phobia or panic. It is less effective than benzodiazepines for the autonomic symptoms of anxiety, and, like the antidepressants, may require several weeks of continued dosage to attain maximal effectiveness. The chief advantage of buspirone is that for some patients, it is both effective and essentially free of side effects. When side effects do occur, they commonly are dizziness, tinnitus, or gastrointestinal upset, and not sedation or ataxia. The drug is safe in patients with chronic lung disease and hypoventilation, and it can be safely given to people with a history of alcohol abuse.

Effective use of buspirone is based on appreciating its widely variable pharmacokinetics, which are partially due to a large first-pass effect. Because of this, some patients will obtain therapeutic or adverse effects on as little as 10 mg/day, and others will need 60 mg/day or more to obtain any noticeable effect. Patients must therefore be instructed to start with 5 mg twice a day, and raise the dose in 5-mg increments every 1 or 2 days until they obtain a therapeutic benefit, experience limiting side effects, or reach a dose of 20 mg three times/day. The therapeutic dose should then be maintained for at least 4 weeks to attain maximum benefit. The relatively long titration period and latency for effect makes benzodiazepine therapy necessary in the interim for most patients with clinically signficant anxiety.

Patients who have been treated with benzodiazepines in the past rarely report satisfactory relief of anxiety from buspirone alone. However, concurrent administration of buspirone can make possible satisfactory relief at a lower dosage of benzodiazepines than would otherwise be needed. This strategy is particularly useful when concurrent neurologic disease makes the patient vulnerable to ataxia and falls at the dosage of benzodiazepines needed to control anxiety with single-drug therapy.

Neuroleptics. Anxious or agitated patients who voice paranoid, highly suspicious, or angrily accusatory ideas may benefit from neuroleptic treatment even if they do not suffer from a full-blown psychosis. Patients with early dementia, epileptic hyperemotionality, or unstable personalities may fit this description, particularly when under stress. Drugs of choice in this situation are neuroleptics with some intrinsic sedating or anxiolytic effect, given at dosages well below those used to treat schizophrenia. Options include thioridazine 25 mg one to three times daily; perphenazine, 2 to 4 mg one to three times daily; or risperidone 0.5 to 1 mg once or twice a day. High-potency nonsedating agents such as haloperidol may be less satisfactory in this situation because of their relative lack of anxiolytic effect, and the risk of akathisia.

Duration of Treatment. When benzodiazepines are given for relief of situational anxiety, they should be tapered gradually when the crisis is over and the patient is coping well. In fact, most patients given benzodiazepines for true situational anxiety will taper themselves, and a reluctance to do so suggests that there may be an underlying anxiety disorder. Duration of therapy for patients with anxiety disorders follows from the natural history of anxiety disorders—some patients have a relapsing-remitting course and others have a chronic course. When benzodiazepines or antidepressants are given for an anxiety disorder, the patient should be continued on the drug until free of symptoms, or adequately relieved, for at least 3 months. At that point, a gradual taper of the drug can be attempted. If symptoms recur, the patient is put back on the minimum dosage necessary to control symptoms for another 3 months, and a taper is tried again. Long-term maintenance should be considered if symptoms recur on each of three attempts to taper medication.

MOOD DISORDERS

Mood disorders, especially depression, are the most frequent psychiatric complication of chronic neurologic disease. The prevalence of clinically significant depression in clinical neurologic populations has been estimated at 30 to 50 percent among stroke patients, 10 to 20 percent among patients with Alzheimer's disease, 27 to 54 percent among patients with multiple sclerosis, 40 percent among patients with Parkinson's disease, and more than 33 percent among survivors of severe traumatic brain injury. Depressive phenomena can aggravate the primary symptoms of neurologic disorders, or make them less bearable to the patient. Furthermore, patients may seek neurologic consultation or treatment for neurologic symptoms of depression, such as cognitive impairment or somatic pain, particularly of the head, back, or neck. Because of the ubiquity of depression, its recognition and initial treatment have become part of the usual outpatient neurologic practice. This section of the chapter reviews (1) the symptoms of depression and mania, (2) assessment of patients with suspected mood disorder, (3) general management, and (4) pharmacologic treatment.

Symptoms

Depression.   The cardinal symptoms of depression are depressed mood and loss of interest or pleasure in life activities. However, the term *depressed* is not always accepted as an accurate description of the mood by patients with depression; some will prefer to describe their mood as irritable, sad, discouraged, or negative. Other patients will complain of or acknowledge a loss of interest or pleasure, while denying any negative mood. Patients' descriptions of their moods are influenced by cultural and personality factors, as well as by the effects of brain diseases. In particular, patients with right hemisphere damage frequently deny depressed mood even when their caregivers see them as visibly depressed, and the patients acknowledge a loss of interest and pleasure.

In depression of clinical significance, the cardinal symptoms are accompanied by persistent distress, or by mood-related impairment in social, occupational, physical, or cognitive functioning. In addition, patients have some combination of associated symptoms, including the following:

Weight loss/weight gain
Insomnia/hypersomnia
Psychomotor agitation or retardation
Fatigue or loss of energy
Feelings of worthlessness or guilt

Trouble concentrating or making decisions
Recurrent thoughts of death or suicide or self-injurious behavior

The concurrence of five or more symptoms of depression for most of the time over a 2-week period is the syndrome of major depression. Clinically significant depression need not meet diagnostic criteria for major depression. Patients with chronic neurologic disease can have a small number of depressive symptoms whose intensity makes them clinically important. Moreover, the persistence of depressive symptoms over time can contribute substantially to disability and distress even when the individual symptoms are not severe.

Mania.   The cardinal symptom of mania is a mood that is elevated, expansive, or irritable. A manic episode consists of such a mood persisting for 1 week or more, producing impairment in social or occupational function or disrupting relationships, and accompanied by a combination of associated symptoms—at least three if the mood is elevated or expansive, and at least four if the mood is irritable. These include the following:

Grandiosity or inflated self-esteem
Decreased need for sleep
Talkativeness
Erratic thought or speech patterns—jumping from topic to topic
Distractability
Agitation or increased goal-directed behavior
Excessive involvement in pleasureable but potentially dangerous activities (impulsive travel, sexual escapades, high-risk investments)

The diagnosis of hypomanic episode requires a duration of 4 days, a similar number of associated symptoms, and a lesser degree of functional impairment. Psychotic features such as delusions and hallucinations are frequently encountered in manic episodes. By definition, they are not compatible with a diagnosis of hypomanic episode.

As with depression, patients with neurologic diseases can have clinically significant hypomanic phenomena that fall short of diagnostic criteria for a hypomanic episode. For example, elevated, expansive, or irritable moods, accompanied by an accelerated rate of speech and action, can occur as a consequence of right hemisphere damage from stroke, tumor, or demyelinating disease, as a complication or dementing illnesses, or as a consequence of levodopa therapy for Parkinson's disease. Also, partial or full syndromes of hypomania can be induced by antidepressant or stimulant therapy.

Bipolar Disorders.   Mood disorders comprise a range of conditions, partially of genetic origin, in which patients have episodes of major depression, mania, or hypomania, combinations of depressed and hypomanic symptoms, or chronic symptoms of depression or hypomania falling short of a full syndrome for a major depressive episode or hypomanic episode. The more common of these disorders include major depressive disorder, bipolar (manic-depressive) disorder, and dysthymic disorder, or chronic depression that lasts 2 years or more. In the past several years, there has been increasing awareness of milder forms of bipolar disorder, in which recurrent episodes of depression alternate with hypomanic symptoms of lesser intensity. These conditions, referred to as bipolar spectrum conditions, include bipolar II disorder (recurrent major depressive episodes with hypomanic episodes) and cyclothymic disorder (multiple episodes of subsyndromal depressive and hypomanic periods, occurring over a span of 2 years or more.)

Depressive Symptoms in Neurologic Patients. Neurologic patients with impaired insight into their physical or cognitive deficits, such as those with frontal system or right hemisphere disease, also have impaired self-awareness of affective states. When assessing such patients for depressive symptoms, the observations of the family usually are needed to supplement the history. Also, systematic inquiry about the associated symptoms of depression may yield many positive symptoms even though depressed mood is denied or minimized.

Patients with aphasia and related communication problems may have difficulty articulating their mood. Such patients can be given a simple visual analogue scale of mood with a happy face at one end and a sad face at the other, and can be asked to describe their usual mood over the past week, or at the time of the interview. Patients' responses on the visual analogue scale show remarkable validity when tested against depression rating scales completed by caregivers.

When depressive symptoms are elicited, both the physician and the patient may be tempted to attribute some symptoms to the patient's neurologic or systemic illness, and others to depression. Such efforts tend to be unreliable, because symptoms like sleep disturbance or weight changes are multiply determined, and the presence of a specific medical problem does not exclude depression as an aggravating factor. The interpretation of symptoms as depressive versus medical, if attempted at all, is best done retrospectively in light of which symptoms respond to treatment for depression.

Pain as a Depressive Symptom. Pain itself is not regarded as an associated symptom of depression. However, depressed mood and its accompaniments are strongly associated with chronic pain, both in clinical samples and in the general population. In chronic pain samples, patients usually report that the pain preceded the depression, or that the onset was simultaneous.

The relationship between pain and depression in clinical practice appears to be circular. Increased pain leads to increased depression, which leads either to increased pain or decreased tolerance of whatever pain is present. There is little evidence that depression causes pain in the absence of a painful condition such as osteoarthritis, radicular disease, migraine, or tension headache. However, the latter conditions are so highly prevalent that the presentation of depression as back, neck, or head pain is an everyday occurrence. Diagnostically, however, the patient is most accurately seen as having two diagnoses, a somatic disease causing the pain and a mood disorder aggravating the pain.

Depression and Grief. The symptoms of normal bereavement overlap extensively with the symptoms of clinical depression. Whereas delusional guilt, suicide attempts, and incapacitating psychomotor retardation are not part of normal bereavement, virtually every other depressive symptom can occur, including death wishes and hallucinations of the lost person. Grief over lost function, as can occur in a patient recovering from a stroke or a spinal cord injury, produces very similar symptomatology. Grief becomes a clinical problem when its symptoms lead to a major loss of function, interfere with the patient's self-care or compliance with medical treatment, or are unbearable to the patient. In addition, psychosis and suicidal behavior define grief as a clinical problem. Grief that becomes problematic in this way, so-called complicated bereavement, effectively can be regarded as a mood disorder,

and is assessed and treated accordingly. When it is unclear whether a patient's bereavement will be complicated, closer medical follow-up is indicated until the situation declares itself.

Diagnosis

Assessment begins with a categorization of the patient's syndrome based on his or her history of mood changes. If the chronology of the symptoms is unclear from the medical history, the patient or caregiver can be asked to draw a graph showing fluctuation of mood above and below normal over the time since the onset of mood changes, and also indicating major life events. The history will distinguish between patients with depressive symptoms only, and those who also have had manic or hypomanic symptoms. The latter require different pharmacologic treatment and have a different prognosis. The history will also reveal whether the depression has been chronic, episodic but persistent, or relatively recent and apparently reactive to a life stress or illness-related problem. Detailed chronology of the relationship between the course of the patient's neurologic illness, drug treatments, and mood symptoms should help establish whether the mood symptoms are directly linked to disease activity or to a specific medication.

The historical review also includes a detailed alcohol and drug history, if this was not obtained earlier. If the patient is actively drinking alcohol or abusing drugs, or has just recently abstained after prolonged use, a mood disorder should not be diagnosed based on current symptoms. A confident diagnosis of a primary mood disorder requires the persistence of the mood syndrome after 1 or more months of total abstinence.

Patients are assessed for evidence of psychosis. Manic patients usually will volunteer their grandiose or persecutory delusional material or readily answer questions about their unusual perceptual experiences. Depressed patients may not volunteer symptoms of psychosis and will require direct questioning regarding concerns about guilt or persecution, or ''voices,'' particularly of a critical or punitive character. Patients should be assessed for current suicidal ideas or plans.

The patient's general medical problem list and medication list are reviewed for entities that can cause or aggravate mood disorder. If the patient has a new onset of major depression with weight loss and is middle-aged or older, appropriate screening is done for cancer.

Often the patient will be on medications sometimes associated with mood disturbance but without a clearly established connection to major depression, such as β-blockers or digoxin. These medications rarely are a sole cause of clinically significant depression, but they can augment depressive symptoms so that they become more distressing or disabling. Whereas the diagnosis of a drug-induced depression should not be made unless the drug is the primary or sole cause of the mood disturbance, there often is practical benefit in discontinuing the suspect drug and, if necessary, substituting a therapeutically equivalent agent with lesser effect on the central nervous system.

Patients' level of insight into their mood disturbance is assessed, as are general cognitive capacities, including memory and abstract reasoning. If the patient has suicidal ideas or plans or preoccupations with death, the reasons for not acting on these are elicited.

Management

Patients with psychotic features or active suicidal ideas are referred for specialized treatment by a psychiatrist. When feasible, a decision about immediate treatment of psychosis with neuroleptics, and a decision about hospitalization for the patient's protection, are made collaboratively with the psychiatrist who will assume responsibility for treatment. Patients with mood disorders of lesser severity may appropriately be treated by the neurologist. Treatment by the neurologist may be preferable when depression or hypomania complicates or is coincident with a chronic neurologic disease already being treated, or when a primary depression has presented with a headache or back or neck pain and the patient is more comfortable being treated in a purely "medical" context.

New Diagnoses of Depression. Patients diagnosed with a depression for the first time require education regarding the diagnosis and its meaning. They are told that they suffer from a disturbance of brain and endocrine physiology that has both mental and physical symptoms and that can be helped with medical treatment. If the patient has presented with a specific complaint such as back pain, an explanation is offered of how the physiologic changes of depression can aggravate the pain or make its pain less bearable. If the depression is related temporally to a specific external stress, bereavement, or aggravation of physical illness, the concept of depression as a form of stress response is emphasized (e.g., when stress exceeds the capacity to cope, or makes an excessively prolonged demand on coping resources, the syndrome of depression may develop). If the depression is accompanied by specific and treatable problems such as radicular pain, treatment for both the depression and the somatic problem are offered at the same time.

Virtually all patients with clinically significant depression are offered education and antidepressant drug therapy. Also, patients are referred for psychosocial therapy according to their situation. If the patient is coping with a new diagnosis of a major chronic neurologic disease, a referral for individual counseling is offered, as is information about support groups for patients and families. If the patient is dealing with grief, appropriate secular or religious support is offered. If the patient has an evident emotional or interpersonal conflict related to the depression, the patient is referred to a psychotherapist for at least brief psychotherapy. If the patient is chronically depressed, longer-term individual or group psychotherapy can work additively or even synergistically with drug therapy.

Recurrent Depression. Patients with recurrent depression will do best with maintenance antidepressant drug therapy and psychotherapy to address those maladaptive cognitions or interpersonal behaviors that lead to depressed moods or create unhappy situations. If patients have had apparently adequate maintenance dosages of antidepressant drugs and have relapsed despite compliance with the regimen, they should be treated with an antidepressant drug of a different therapeutic class. Patients who have not received psychotherapy or were referred in the past but did not establish rapport with the therapist should be offered a referral to a psychotherapist.

Hypomanic Symptoms. Patients with hypomanic symptoms may decline treatment because they may find their elevated mood and increased energy adaptive or enjoyable. However, when there is a history of crashes into depression, or of bad judgment while hypomanic leading to harm, the risks of the patient's hypomania are pointed out. It is explained that mood-stabilizing treatment does not prevent normal good moods, but only the excessive and risky expansiveness of hypomania. If

the patient has hypomania as a consequence of a specific lesion such as a right temporal stroke or tumor, mood-stabilizing medication can be described as routine treatment for the consequences of the lesion, and the potential benefits of mood stabilization for cognitive performance can be pointed out.

Pharmacologic Therapy

Pharmacologic therapy for primary mood disorders has been well established by a large number of controlled clinical trials. By contrast, very few studies have been done of antidepressants in specific populations with neurologic disease and mood disorders. The studies that have been reported in neurologic populations have used tricyclic antidepressants, drugs that are now less preferred for the treatment of depression in primary care because of their greater systemic toxicity than the selective serotonin re-uptake inhibitors. The recommendations given here are an extrapolation from studies done in populations without gross brain disease.

Major Depression. Major depression with prominent weight loss and sleep disturbance is treated with tricyclic antidepressants unless the patient has electrocardiographically confirmed heart block or has known or expected intolerance of anticholinergic effects. The secondary amine tricyclics, nortriptyline and desipramine, are preferred to the tertiary amines amitriptyline and imipramine because they have fewer anticholinergic and hypotensive effects, and because their blood levels are more easily monitored. Starting dosage in a frail, elderly, or chronically ill patient is 10 mg of nortriptyline at bedtime or 10 mg of desipramine bid to tid; the dosage is increased gradually as tolerated. The dosage is raised until symptoms are relieved; until limiting side effects of sedation, tachycardia, hypotension, or confusion develop; or until typical therapeutic doses are reached (50 to 75 mg of nortriptyline qhs or 50 mg bid to tid of desipramine). A blood level of the drug is obtained if the patient has neither benefit nor side effects when that level is reached; the therapeutic range is 50 to 150 ng/ml for nortriptyline and over 120 ng/ml for desipramine. Patients who are younger and without systemic illness will require higher dosage, as will those who smoke or those who have been on enzyme-inducing antiepileptic drugs, such as carbamazepine or phenytoin.

If the patient cannot take tricyclics or cannot tolerate them and has depression with insomnia and weight loss, alternative therapies are venlafaxine and nefazodone. Venlafaxine's most common side effects are sedation, sweating, and hypertension; although it occasionally causes orthostatic hypotension, it does not have quinidine-like effects that aggravate heart block. The starting dosage is 25 mg bid to tid; the dosage is raised gradually to a maximum of 100 mg. tid. Nefazodone can cause sedation or gastrointestinal upset, but is relatively free from major systemic side effects. It does, however, inhibit metabolism of many drugs, notably carbamazepine. If the drug is given to a patient on carbamazepine, the blood level of carbamazepine should be followed, and the dosage reduced as necessary. Nefazodone is started at 50 mg bid; it is gradually raised as high as 600 mg/day in two to four doses, as tolerated.

Patients in whom weight loss and sleep disturbance are less prominent than depressed or irritable mood are treated initially with selective serotonin re-uptake inhibitors: fluoxetine, sertraline, paroxetine, and fluvoxamine are all equally effective. They may be especially effective for chronic depression and for the chronic irritable states that can accompany limbic epilepsy or Parkinson's disease. Whereas the selective serotonin re-uptake inhibitors have few serious systemic side effects, they can produce neurologic side effects including tremors, sedation, myoclonic jerks, and apathy, and patients with pre-existing brain disease may be more senstive to these side effects. Starting doses are kept low to assess tolerance before advancing to more typical antidepressant dosage. All drugs can be given once a day. Starting doses are fluoxetine 5 to 10 mg; sertraline, 12.5 to 25 mg; paroxetine, 5 to 10 mg; fluvoxamine, 12.5 to 25 mg. The Dose is increased gradually to a maximum of four times the manufacturer's recommended minimum dose (i.e., fluoxetine, 80 mg; sertraline, 200 mg; paroxetine, 80 mg; fluvoxamine, 200 mg). Meaningful blood levels are not available for clinical use. However, most patients will either respond or develop limiting side effects before reaching the maximum doses listed. The selective serotonin re-uptake inhibitors have inhibiting effects on the cytochrome P450 system, and can cause increased antiepileptic drug levels. Levels of carbamazepine and phenytoin should be rechecked after initiating concurrent therapy with a selective serotonin re-uptake inhibitor.

If a patient's depression responds to a serotonin re-uptake inhibitor but a tremor develops, the tremor can be suppressed with either a benzodiazepine or a β-blocker in dosages similar to those that would be used for essential tremor. Myoclonic jerks, if disruptive, can be suppressed with a small dose of clonazepam (e.g., 0.5 to 1.0 mg/day), usually given at bedtime. Apathy complicating otherwise effective treatment with a re-uptake inhibitor can be managed with 5 to 10 mg of methylphenidate or dextroamphetamine once or twice a day.

Patients with depression characterized by prominent apathy need especially careful diagnostic assessment for such entities as metabolic encephalopathies (e.g., hepatic, hypothyroid), sleep disorders (especially obstructive sleep apnea), and early Parkinson's disease. If these entities have been excluded, one drug of choice is bupropion, a particularly stimulating antidepressant. Bupropion is started at 75 mg bid. If it is tolerated without excessive nervousness or agitation, it is raised to 75 mg tid, and eventually, in small steps, to a maximum of 150 mg tid. The most troublesome side effect of bupropion is seizures; the risk is approximately 0.4 percent at 450 mg/day for patients without specific risk factors for seizures. The risk rises substantially if more than 150 mg is taken at one time; patients should be cautioned not to make up missed doses. If the drug is to be tried in patients with risk factors for seizures, such as those with apathetic depression following traumatic brain injury, concurrent antiepileptic drugs should be given.

Other relatively stimulating antidepressants include desipramine and fluoxetine, the latter being the most stimulating of the selective serotonin re-uptake inhibitors. Monoamine oxidase inhibitors are effective and highly stimulating broad-spectrum antidepressants with substantial antianxiety and antiphobic effects; guidelines for their safe use are detailed in textbooks of psychopharmacology.

When treating neurologic patients for major depression, about 1 in 10 will develop hypomania, and a substantial proportion of those with pre-existing cognitive impairment will develop confusion. If hypomania develops on an antidepressant, the drug should be withdrawn. A mood-stabilizing drug is started, and the antidepressant is reintroduced afterward if still needed for depressive symptoms.

If confusion develops when treating major depression in a patient with cognitive impairment, the drug should be stopped.

Confusion developing on a tricyclic does not rule out future successful treatment with a selective serotonin re-uptake inhibitor. However, the rate of upward dosage titration should be particularly slow in patients with a history of antidepressant-induced confusion.

Patients treated for major depression with one of the above agents may have a partial response to treatment, with enough benefit to warrant continuation of the drug, but with enough residual symptoms to pursue further treatment. Augmentation of antidepressant treatment can be tried in this situation. Addition of lithium, 300 mg qd to tid, is one of the best established maneuvers in this situation. T_3 (triiodothyronine), 25 to 50 micrograms per day, is another option.

Hypomania and Bipolar Conditions.   Patients with hypomania, or with a history of hypomania and depression, require mood-stabilizing medication. The first mood-stabilizing medication of proven benefit was lithium, which remains the treatment of choice for bipolar disorder with prolonged manic and depressive episodes. It was subsequently discovered that carbamazepine and valproate were effective for bipolar disorder, and might be superior to lithium for patients with mixed manic and depressive symptoms, or with rapid alternation between hypomania and depression. The efficacy of antiepileptic drugs for mood disorders is not predicted by any electroencephalographic finding. The blood levels at which the drugs are effective for mood disorders is roughly the same as their therapeutic levels for the treatment of epilepsy, except that valproate levels of up to 150 μg/ml may be effective and tolerated in the treatment of acute mania.

The mood-stabilizing antiepileptic drugs carbamazepine and valproate also may be effective for fluctuating or unstable moods in patients with gross brain disease, including those recovering from traumatic brain injury or encephalitis, those with static encephalopathies, and those with dementing illnesses. However, the support for their use for this purpose is entirely anecdotal. Their use often is justified by the independent clinical need for an antiepileptic drug.

Guidelines for the clinical use of carbamazepine and valproate are found in Chapter 25. Lithium is given on twice daily to thrice daily schedule, aiming for a blood level of about 1.0. Higher levels, though in the published therapeutic range for treatment of bipolar disorder, tend to be poorly tolerated by neurologic patients. The starting dose in a patient without kidney disease is 300 mg tid. Lithium clearance is linked to creatinine clearance and dosage must be reduced in patients with renal insufficiency. Both diuretics and nonsteroidal anti-inflammatory drugs raise lithium levels by increasing its resorption in the proximal tubule; lithium dose must be reduced accordingly.

The prelithium workup consists of tests of kidney and thyroid function and an electrocardiogram. Renal insufficiency, thyroid disease, and sinus node dysfunction are all relative contraindications to lithium. Ongoing treatment is monitored with thyroid and kidney function tests every 3 to 6 months to screen for the development of hypothyroidism (a reversible side effect in about 10 percent of patients) and renal insufficiency (a problem of dubious relationship to lithium but affecting its safe use).

Patients on lithium, or their responsible caregivers, must be aware that lithium levels rise rapidly with dehydration and that the therapeutic index of lithium is very low; therefore, the drug must be discontinued if the patient develops vomiting or diarrhea, or if there is any question of dehydration due to decreased oral intake, unusual heat, or intercurrent systemic disease. Confusion or a flapping tremor are signs of lithium encephalopathy; the drug should be discontinued in a confused or coarsely tremulous patient, and a lithium level should be checked.

Patients receiving mood-stabilizing medications may develop major depression on their lithium or antiepileptic drugs, even though they are protected from hypomania. Antidepressants can be added to the regimens of such patients.

Duration of Therapy. Major depression tends to recur; continuation of treatment beyond the relief of symptoms minimizes the risk of recurrence. Treatment for a first episode of major depression should be continued for 6 to 9 months; an effort to taper and discontinue the antidepressant can be made at that time. If the patient has a recurrence of symptoms, the medication is resumed at a therapeutic level for another 3 months, and withdrawal is attempted again, with a similar approach. If a patient has failed three attempts to taper antidepressants, long-term maintenance therapy should be offered. There is no evidence that dosages for long-term maintenance are different than those for initial treatment of the depression.

Bipolar disorder is regarded as a chronic illness requiring long-term drug therapy for optimal outcome. However, some cases clearly ''burn out'' after several years of cycling. The natural history of hypomanic phenomena following gross brain disease is not known. The decision to discontinue mood-stabilizing medication in a case of primary bipolar disorder should be made in consultation with a psychiatrist. When mood stabilizers are used to control hypomania or mood fluctuations related to a gross brain lesion, they are continued until the physician finds it timely to see if the patient can do without them. Practically, the mood stabilizers used are antiepileptic drugs whose continued use may be justified as prevention for focal seizures. In this situation, the drugs are continued as long as one would continue the antiepileptic drug therapy for its conventional indication.

PERSONALITY DISORDERS AND REACTION TO DISEASE

Neurologic diseases pose unique challenges to patients' coping and self-image. In some cases, there are visible stigmata of disease, as in Tourette's disorder or muscular dystrophy. In others, the disease is invisible but disabling, as in poorly controlled epilepsy. Coping with these disorders challenges patients with normal personalities. When patients with maladaptive or rigid personality traits face the stress of neurologic disease, they frequently develop overt mental or behavioral symptoms. This section of the chapter deals with (1) stress and coping, (2) personality types and disorders in neurologic practice, and (3) practical management strategies.

Stress and Coping

Illness creates stress for patients through symptoms, disruption of life routines, changes in appearance or function, effects on interpersonal relations, and occupational or economic consequences. Illnesses require patients to change their behavior in ways contrary to their habits and inclinations.

When confronted with the stress of illness, patients employ coping mechanisms, a combination of conscious and unconscious strategies for either dealing with the stress or excluding it from conscious awareness. Highly adaptive coping mechanisms involve handling the situation in a way that maximizes the patient's satisfaction of legitimate needs and averts preventable conflicts and problems. These mechanisms include anticipation of problems (e.g., participation in patient education or studying the disease), affiliation with others (e.g., support group participation, sharing problems with family and friends), self-assertion (e.g., advance directives), self-observation, humor regarding the situation, and altruism (e.g., assisting others with the same illness or participating in clinical trials). At the opposite end of the spectrum are coping mechanisms that may exclude some painful thoughts from consciousness, but do so at the expense of problem solving, and may endanger one's health or network of supportive relationships. Such mechanisms include denial, projection (i.e., blaming), acting out (e.g., behaving in a violent, self-destructive, or provocative manner), apathetic withdrawal, help-rejecting complaining, and passive aggression (e.g., noncompliance with treatment accompanied by excuses).

Overt problems with depression and anxiety develop when the stress of illness exceeds the patient's ability to cope. Patients with more adaptive coping mechanisms are able to tolerate more stress for a longer period of time, but if stress is sufficiently severe and/or prolonged, most patients will develop emotional symptoms.

When patients display less adaptive coping styles, they either may be using their usual coping mechanisms or may have reverted to less adaptive behavior because they are overwhelmed by the severity of the stress or because cognitive impairment or a mood disorder has temporarily impaired their adaptive function. A common pattern is seen in patients with relapsing-remitting illnesses, such as multiple sclerosis or systemic lupus, wherein the patient shows more adaptive coping when in remission than during acute exacerbations.

Whereas coping styles, like personality, are generally stable over time, specific coping mechanisms can be learned or strengthened with practice. The habit of becoming educated about one's illness and anticipating problems can be learned, and can be promoted by an active teaching approach by the neurologist and care team. Affiliation, self-observation, and self-assertion can be strengthened by experiences in support groups, or by counseling of the patient together with family caregivers. Negative coping through such mechanisms as denial and blaming sometimes can be attenuated by psychotherapy if the patient can be engaged in a psychotherapeutic relationship sufficiently trusting to permit confrontation of these usually maladaptive behaviors.

Because regression to less adaptive coping can be triggered by stress, more effective coping can be promoted by regulating the amount of stress that patient must face in a given period of time. Practical methods for regulating stress include adequate pain control, pacing of diagnostic and therapeutic procedures to avoid overloading the patient, and more frequent contacts with the neurologist or other members of the professional care team when the patient is more severely ill. Formal relaxation exercises or structured physical exercise also have stress-reducing effects.

Personality Types and Disorders

Personality traits are characteristic, stable patterns of behavior and interpersonal interaction. Personality types are constellations of traits that occur together frequently enough to be recognizable by clinicians. Personality disorders are stable, lifelong constellations of personality traits that are sufficiently rigid and maladaptive that they cause the patient significant distress or impairment, and are recognized as deviating from the usual expectations of the patient's culture. The *Diagnostic and Statis-*

TABLE 146-1. Classification of Personality Disorders

Cluster A
   Paranoid personality disorder: a pattern of distrust and suspiciousness; interpreting others' motives as malevolent
   Schizoid personality disorder: a pattern of detachment from social relationships and a restricted range of emotional expression
   Schizotypal personality disorder: a pattern of acute discomfort in close relationships, cognitive or perceptual distortions, and eccentricities of behavior
Cluster B
   Antisocial personality disorder: a pattern of disregard for, and violation of, the rights of others
   Borderline personality disorder: a pattern of instability in interpersonal relationships, self-image, and affects, and marked impulsivity
   Histrionic personality disorder: a pattern of excessive emotionality and attention-seeking
   Narcissistic personality disorder: a pattern of grandiosity, need for admiration, and lack of empathy
Cluster C
   Avoidant personality disorder: a pattern of social inhibition, feelings of inadequacy, and hypersensitivity to negative evaluation
   Dependent personality disorder: a pattern of submissive and clinging behavior related to an excessive need to be taken care of
   Obsessive-compulsive personality disorder: a pattern of preoccupation with orderliness, perfectionism, and control

(From American Psychiatric Association: Diagnostic and Statistical Manual of Mental Disorders 4th Ed. American Psychiatric Association, Washington, D.C., with permission.)

tical Manual of Mental Disorders, fourth edition (DSM-IV), of the American Psychiatric Association recognizes 10 such personality disorders (Table 146-1).

These personality disorders are grouped into three clusters. Paranoid, schizoid, and schizotypal personalities (cluster A) share the feature of oddness or eccentricity. Antisocial, borderline, histrionic, and narcissistic personalities (cluster B) share the feature of being dramatic, emotional, or erratic. Avoidant, dependent, and obsessive-compulsive personalities (cluster C) include the feature of a high level of anxiety, particularly if patients with these personalities are prevented from carrying out their usual style of adaptation. Clinical classification of personality disorders into categories is limited by overlap between categories and general problems of reliability. However, assignment of a patient with problematic personality traits into one cluster or another tends to be more reliable, and may have some utility in planning clinical management strategy.

In addition to these personality disorders, neurologists frequently recognize characteristic personality types associated with regional brain dysfunction. Specifically, patients with frontal lobe lesions may show a personality characterized by impulsiveness, poor judgment and planning, and shallowness of affect. Patients with irritative temporal lobe lesions may show hyperemotionality and a "sticky" interpersonal style.

Personality disorders are determined partly by neurobiology and partly by early life experience. Definite genetic factors have been established for schizotypal personality and antisocial personality. Borderline personality has been repeatedly linked to traumatic early life experience—particularly physical and/or sexual abuse. Genetic studies suggest that schizotypal personality and schizophrenia occur in the same kindreds, as do obsessive-compulsive personality and obsessive-compulsive disorder. Similarly, avoidant personality is associated with social phobia.

Cluster B personality disorders are associated with substantially increased incidence of major depression and the various substance abuse disorders. They are also associated with an increased rate of suicide attempts and self-injurious behavior.

Personality Types and Disorders in Neurologic Practice. In the setting of practice, the formal diagnosis of personality disor-

der is far less relevant than recognition of patients with rigid or maladaptive personality traits, and understanding of their main behavioral themes. However, if a personality disorder diagnosis has been made after careful evaluation by a reliable psychiatrist or psychologist, it can be a useful guide to what to expect from the patient. When a patient presents a pattern of problematic interpersonal behavior, the possibility of a personality disorder should be considered. A provisional diagnosis of the personality disorder is suggested by the nature of the patient's interpersonal problem. However, since personality disorders are by definition long-standing patterns of behavior, further information about the patient's characteristic interpersonal style must be obtained to confirm the impression. The relevant data come from the educational, occupational, military, marital, and social history. These data can be collected de novo by the neurologist, but often are available from a primary care physician, a social agency, or a mental health professional.

Patients with cluster A diagnoses tend to be mistrustful, and become uncomfortable if the neurologist shows excessive familiarity or concern, or presumes a collaborative relationship. The forced intimacies of hospitals, rehabilitation centers, and nursing homes similarly cause these patients emotional distress. Under stress, they may become overtly paranoid or even delusional. Their life history typically shows a paucity of intimate relationships and avoidance of social activities; their pattern of interests may include some odd preoccupations.

Patients with cluster B diagnoses bring themselves to the attention of the neurologist by making demands or by challenging rules. Although they initially may be charming or engaging, they eventually become a burden to the practioner, directly or implicitly demanding special treatment. Angry outbursts or acting out can be evoked by disappointment of their expectations. The life histories of antisocial, borderline, and histrionic individuals are characterized by drama and instability, typically with many broken or unsatisfactory relationships. Narcissistic personalities may either brag about accomplishments or present detailed excuses for their lack of fulfillment of their talent.

Patients with cluster C diagnoses come to the attention of the neurologist through some form of noncompliance with treatment or requirement for special attention. Noncompliance results from anxiety or avoidance, rather than anger, and special requests arise not from a sense of entitlement but from needs to assuage their anxiety. Thus, a patient with an avoidant personality fails to attend educational groups despite a need for information; one with a dependent personality makes many calls to the office to reconfirm instructions; one with an obsessive-compulsive personality needs to review the diagnosis and therapeutic recommendations in exhaustive detail. Their life histories suggest that their characteristic style of avoidance, dependence, or compulsiveness began in their school years and continued as a feature of their marriage relations and work experience.

Patients with frontal lobe personality syndromes are brought to the attention of the neurologist by family members who are concerned about the patient's self-destructive or self-neglecting behavior. Typically, the behavior had its onset following the acquisition of a frontal lesion or came on insidiously in the case of a frontal lobe dementia. The patient might or might not acknowledge the behavior in question, but if the behavior is acknowledged, its significance will be minimized.

Patients with the personality syndrome of an irritative temporal lesion will make the neurologist aware of their emotional intensity. At times, it will be difficult to get the patient to leave the office. The behavior will have developed gradually over the course of years, in parallel with the course of the patient's limbic epilepsy.

Management

All maladaptive personality traits and coping mechanisms are aggravated by anxiety and by pain and discomfort. When a patient first is perceived as being "difficult," realistic sources of anxiety and worry should be identified and addressed to the extent feasible. Patients with personality disorders are less able to tolerate frustration and disappointment. Therefore, their appointments should be scheduled on days and at times when the neurologist is likely to be punctual. Sufficient time should be allowed for the appointment to minimize any sense of hurry.

Paranoid, Schizoid, and Schizotypal Personalities. Patients with paranoid, schizoid, or schizotypal personalities should be treated in a cool, polite, and professional manner that avoids any excessive warmth or familiarity. Because these patients often are uncomfortable in conversations, they should be given written information about their diagnosis and treatment and should be encouraged to ask questions in writing if concerns arise after the appointment.

When patients with these personalities become overtly paranoid under stress, they should be offered neuroleptic drugs. A low dose of a midpotency agent, such as 4 mg of perphenazine or 10 mg of molindone qd to tid, usually is tolerated and helpful. The drug should be given for the duration of the acute stress, then gradually tapered. Patients should be offered the drugs as an aid to coping with the specific stresses that triggered their paranoid symptoms (e.g., acute illness, surgery, grief). The drug can be described as an aid to organization of thought, or can be related to the patients' own descriptions of their emotional distress (e.g., "to help with nervousness").

Antisocial, Borderline, Histrionic, and Narcissistic Personalities. Patients with dramatic and often manipulative personalities can lead physicians into deviations from their own usual practice style almost before they know what is happening. As soon as the patient's personality type is recognized, three principles should be applied. First, all communications should be exceedingly clear and unambiguous. If a family member, a friend, a social agency, or another clinician is involved in the patient's treatment, they should be communicated with directly and should get the same message as the patient regarding diagnosis and treatment. Second, usual rules of one's practice regarding prescriptions and refills, telephone calls, billing, appointment length, and other details should be observed without deviation. Third, if patients impose upon the physician, or behave unacceptably in the office, limits should be set firmly and without anger.

When patients with these personalities become overwhelmed by stress, they may develop a brief psychosis or an intense anxiety state. Management of the former situation is described below in the section on thought disorders. Intense anxiety in a patient with one of the dramatic personality disorders is best treated with a low dose of a relatively sedating neuroleptic, such as thioridazine 10 to 25 mg tid or perphenazine 2 to 4 mg tid. Even though patients may request benzodiazepine antianxiety drugs, these agents are a risky choice because of the possibility of disinhibited behavior. The prescription of the neuroleptic in these circumstances is explained as a treatment for overwhelming anxiety; the specific drug choice is explained as motivated by safety considerations.

On occasion, the demands of patients with antisocial, borderline, or narcissistic personalities simply cannot be met, as when a patient wants the physician's cooperation with a disability claim the physician does not support, or when a patient wants refillable prescriptions for abusable drugs. When the patient will not accept the physician's limits and responds with an angry attack on the physician, the patient should be told that such behavior is not acceptable in the physician's practice. A referral to another physician is offered, and the encounter is documented in the record. The patient may threaten litigation, but this should not influence the limit-setting approach.

Avoidant, Dependent, and Obsessive-Compulsive Personalities. The avoidant personality presents problems in neurologic practice primarily by noncompliance with rehabilitation or with other treatment recommendations such as exercise or diet that require effort and at which the patient can fail. Patients' fear of failure or humiliation leads them to avoid any situation in which they may be judged. The symptoms of the avoidant personality overlap with those of social phobia and are aggravated by depression. Mobilizing the avoidant patient's cooperation begins by identifying and offering drug treatment for any clinically significant depression; selective serotonin re-uptake inhibitors are the usual drugs of choice. The patient's fear of failure is identified explicitly, and with the help of an appropriate therapist (e.g., occupational therapy, physical therapy) the task is broken into subtasks so small that it is difficult for the patient to fail.

Patients with dependent personalities may fail to solve illness- or treatment-related problems despite adequate intelligence, because their characteristic style is to be helpless until an authority figure tells them what to do. Pragmatic approaches to medical treatment with such personalities identify a support person upon whom the dependent patient can lean; the support person is then educated about the illness and its treatment. The dependent person who has become socially isolated may attempt to develop an emotional dependency upon the physician. In the short term, this can be managed by scheduling more frequent appointments but discouraging nonemergent telephone calls between appointments. In the longer term, a psychotherapist or social worker can be engaged to assist the patient in finding social supports unrelated to medical treatment.

Obsessive-compulsive personalities may have difficulty making treatment decisions because of obsessional indecisiveness, or may take up the physician's time with excessively detailed questions. Such patients' needs for information should be met realistically with handouts and suggested reading about the conditions from which they suffer. If they are truly paralyzed by indecision and uncomfortable about it, referral for psychotherapy or a trial of an selective serotonin re-uptake inhibitor are both reasonable options. Both interventions are framed as efforts to help the patient deal with the unpleasant moods of anxiety or depression or to help them come to a decision, rather than as a direct confrontation of their obsessional personality style.

Frontal Lobe Personalities. Managing the frontal lobe personality syndromes requires working with the patient and the family together. The family must learn to set limits and provide cues without anger or condescension, understanding that the patient's behavior is strongly determined by the environment.

If the patient has some capacity for insight, education is offered regarding the deficit and the need for external cuing to function at one's best. The patient's feelings of humiliation about being monitored by others are acknowledged empathically.

Temporal Lobe Personalities. In dealing with temporal lobe personalities, the neurologist should not overreact to the patient's intensity, particularly when feelings of anger or of despair are expressed. The transient nature of some of the patient's more painful feelings can be pointed out. If ''stickiness'' is a problem, the patient can be taught to recognize it as a feature of the illness rather than a moral defect, so that the neurologist can more easily point it out when it is interfering with a comfortable physician–patient relationship.

Somatization and Amplification of Illness

As suggested in the above sections, Anxiety and Panic and Mood Disorders, patients with depression or anxiety disorders may amplify the physical symptoms of systemic or neurologic disease. This amplification of symptoms can be alleviated, at least in part, by effective treatment of the mood disorder or anxiety disorder.

Patients with personality disorders may amplify somatic symptoms on a different basis, with a different management strategy implied. Patients with personalities in the odd cluster may incorporate medical diagnoses or somatic diagnoses into idiosyncratic beliefs about themselves or their bodies. If these beliefs lead to significant distress or disability, an effort should be made to treat them. Verbal challenge of these beliefs is not effective. If the beliefs are delusional or nearly so, a trial of neuroleptic therapy can be considered, as discussed below in the section on Thought Disorders. If the beliefs are strongly held but open to objective test, a trial of a selective serotonin reuptake inhibitor should be considered; these have been shown effective in body dysmorphic disorder, a condition in which the patient has a strong conviction of a bodily defect disproportionate to any objective finding.

Patients with personality disorders in the dramatic cluster may amplify symptoms or exaggerate diagnoses because their illnesses and symptoms function as claims on the attention of others. To extinguish amplification of symptoms in the physician–patient relationship, the attention given to the patient should depend as little as possible on the intensity of complaints or the drama with which they are expressed. Patients with this type of symptom amplification often belong to families in which illness complaints serve an important communicative function. Family therapy can enable some such families to communicate more straightforwardly, with the benefit of reduced somatic complaints.

Patients with avoidant personalities may amplify symptoms because their symptoms function as an excuse for an actual or feared poor performance. Since the patient has a strong need for this excuse, it is usually futile to expect complete symptom resolution. The efficacy of treatment should be monitored by objective signs, and by patients' comments on how bearable they find the symptoms.

Patients with dependent personalities, like those with dramatic personalities, may amplify symptoms because they function as a claim on the attention and care of others. Management is similar.

Patients with obsessive-compulsive personalities may amplify symptoms by expressing them in obsessional detail. This may pose difficulties for the neurologist in monitoring treatment response. Global self-ratings of symptoms, such as the visual analogue pain scale, are superior methods for getting useful feedback from such patients.

THOUGHT DISORDERS

Disordered thinking, as inferred from disordered speech and behavior, is the characteristic abnormality of schizophrenia and related psychotic disorders. It is also a feature of delirious states, an expression of several of the drug-induced encephalopathies, a potential complication of dementia, and a feature of the more severe forms of mood disturbance, both manic and depressive. Thought disorder usually is accompanied by impaired self-monitoring, and consequently by impairment in everyday function. Symptoms of thought disorder frequently can be alleviated with neuroleptic (antipsychotic) medication. For this reason, the recognition of thought disorder has particular importance for determining the pharmacologic treatment of patients with disturbances of mood or behavior. This section of the chapter with reviews (1) symptoms of thought disorder, (2) assessment of the patient with thought disorder, (3) management of the neurologic outpatient with thought disorder, (4) pharmacologic treatment, and (5) strategies for managing psychosis in dementia and psychosis in Parkinson's disease.

Symptoms

Thought disorder may present with abnormal content of thinking, abnormal process of thinking, or a combination. Evidence for these abnormalities of thinking, as inferred from the patient's speech and behavior, includes the following:

Hallucinations in any sensory modality
Delusions
Disorganized speech not accounted for by aphasia
Disorganized or bizarre behavior
Markedly abnormal motor behavior not accounted for by a movement disorder (odd posturing, stereotyped movements, prominent mannerisms, prolonged immobility, purposeless hyperactivity)

Thus, the presence of hallucinations can be inferred from either the patient's report of hallucinations or observed behavior suggesting response to a hallucinated voice.

Abnormal thinking can manifest in milder forms with symptoms that suggest but do not confirm the presence of a thought disorder. These symptoms include the following:

Vagueness and obscurity of speech
Idiosyncratic associations
Affect incongruous with the situation or subject of the conversation
Suspiciousness
Unusual beliefs held with great intensity

Paranoid thinking often accompanies thought disorder, but can occur in the presence of otherwise normal thought processes.

Assessment

The presence of thought disorder implies dysfunction of cortical association areas; when the patient acts on disordered thinking, there is an additional inference of impaired executive control functions. The differential diagnosis of thought disorder includes conditions that directly or indirectly influence the function of cortical association areas and executive control functions. These include the following:

Diffuse cortical dysfunction (delirium and dementia)
Focal temporal lobe dysfunction (Wernicke's aphasia, temporal lobe seizures)
Abnormal modulation of cortical function (mania, depression, amphetamines, cocaine, phencyclidine, hypercortisolism, hyperthyroidism)
Schizophrenia (frontotemporal dysfunction of obscure etiology)
Overactivation of association areas by extraordinary stress (brief psychotic disorder)

Assessment begins with establishing the full set of mental and behavioral symptoms from which the patient suffers, including mood symptoms and cognitive symptoms, such as disorientation and memory loss. The mental status examination frequently shows some cognitive impairment in the patient with current symptoms of thought disorder, so the examiner's aim is to determine whether the disturbance of speech and behavior is disproportionate to whatever cognitive impairment is found. Thought disorder disproportionate to cognitive impairment is evidence for a psychotic disorder rather than delirium or dementia.

The medical and drug history provides evidence for or against psychosis due to metabolic disturbance or an exogenous agent. However, laboratory testing and drug screening often are necessary to completely exclude the diagnosis of a drug-induced psychosis or metabolic encephalopathy, since the symptoms of exogenous and endogenous psychotic disorders do overlap.

The diagnosis of psychosis due to a focal cortical lesion requires both demonstration of the lesion and compatibility of the mental syndrome with the known effects of the lesion. The psychosis associated with Wernicke's aphasia is a paranoid state with irritability. The psychosis typically associated with long-standing and poorly-controlled temporal lobe seizures is characterized by paranoid thinking and hallucinations, with relative preservation of the capacity for interpersonal relationships and emotional expression.

The diagnosis of psychosis due to extraordinary stress (brief psychotic disorder) usually is easy because the stressor is known and the patient does not have a past history of chronic thought disorder. Characteristically, patients with a brief stress-induced psychosis show confusion and perplexity or evident emotional turmoil and affective lability. If a patient presents (usually brought by concerned relatives) with an acute change in mental status and evidence for thought disorder, a history of recent trauma or major stress should be sought.

A thought disorder not explained by neurologic or systemic disease, exogenous agents, or severe stress is either a primary psychotic disorder such as schizophrenia, or a mood disorder with psychotic features. To diagnose a mood disorder with psychotic features, definite evidence for depression or mania should be present in the history or on the examination. When the content of abnormal thought is congruent with the mood (e.g., delusions of guilt in depression; hallucinated commands from God in mania), the thought disturbance is regarded as a complication of the mood disorder, reflecting greater severity. Mood-congruent delusions are likely to resolve completely with successful treatment of the mood disorder.

When the content of abnormal thought is incongruent or bizarre, the patient may be suffering from a psychosis with combined features of schizophrenia and a mood disorder—so-called schizoaffective disorder. The delusions and other psychotic features of this disorder can persist despite normalization of mood.

Persistent symptoms of thought disorder associated with impairment in social or occupational function and lasting more than 6 months suggest the diagnosis of schizophrenia. Schizophrenia is a chronic disorder of brain function with heterogenous manifestations. Some patients present primarily with so-called negative symptoms of impaired range and intensity of emotional expression, impaired initiation of goal-directed behavior, and impaired productivity of thought and speech. Others show dramatic positive symptoms of hallucinations, delusions, paranoid ideas, and bizarre behavior. Patients can have chronic negative symptoms with intermittent episodes of positive symptoms or may have mainly one type of symptom throughout the course of their disorder.

The median age of onset of schizophrenia is in the early 20s for men and in the late 20s for women, but there is considerable variability, and the illness begins after age 40 in some patients. Such late-onset cases are more likely to present to neurologists, because of the appropriate suspicion that new-onset thought disorder later in life may be a sign of gross brain disease. Full evaluation for gross brain disease is appropriate for patients with symptoms typical of schizophrenia and less than 6 months' duration of illness. Patients who present with a long-standing psychotic disorder typical of schizophrenia would not require a full neurodiagnostic evaluation for gross brain disease unless there were additional features on the history or neurologic examination that suggested another diagnosis.

A psychotic disorder distinct from schizophrenia can develop in middle age or later life that is characterized by nonbizarre delusions and relatively little additional evidence of thought disorder or dementia. Patients with this condition, called delusional disorder, have a fixed false belief. Typical beliefs include delusions that one's partner is unfaithful, the delusional conviction that one suffers from a particular somatic disease, delusions of persecution, and delusions of romantic involvement with a person, usually of high status, with whom there is no actual connection. Delusional disorder is not associated with the general impairment in social functioning that is typical of schizophrenia. Patients with delusional disorder have an excess of white matter abnormalities on magnetic resonance imaging and may show mild impairment of executive cognitive functioning on neuropsychological testing, but they do not suffer from dementia.

Management

Once a patient is identified as having a thought disorder, management strategy depends on the context in which the neurologist is seeing the patient. If the patient is receiving psychiatric care or will be referred to a psychiatrist, the main aims of the neurologist are to exclude gross brain disease, systemic disease, or exogenous agents as causes of the thought disorder and to identify concurrent neurologic conditions in need of treatment. If the patient has been treated with neuroleptic drugs (see below), the neurologic assessment should include assessment for drug-induced movement disorder. The full neurologic evaluation of the patient with a psychotic disorder who is under psychiatric care includes magnetic resonance imaging of the brain and electroencephalography. The former offers the most definitive exclusion of frontotemporal anatomic lesions, and the latter screens the patient for paroxysmal brain electrical activity that may be relevant to subsequent treatment for the psychosis. Although the issue is controversial, many psychiatrists will consider the use of antiepileptic drugs as treatment adjuncts when a patient with psychosis has a paroxysmal electroencephalogram and the psychosis has been poorly responsive to standard treatment with neuroleptics.

When a thought disorder arises in a patient who will be continuing in treatment with the neurologist for dementia, epilepsy, Parkinson's disease, or another brain disease, the neurologist must first decide whether to involve a psychiatrist, and if so, how to divide responsibility between the neurologist and the psychiatrist. If care is to be divided, a specific decision should be made regarding who will prescribe which drugs, and who will be responsible for monitoring for side effects. Patients with mood disorders with psychotic features usually should be referred to a psychiatrist, as their severe mood disorders require aggressive biologic treatment, possibly including electroconvulsive therapy.

Patients with delusional disorder tend to resist direct confrontation regarding their delusions and may also resist referral to a psychiatrist. They may be more accepting of neuroleptic medication prescribed by the neurologist.

When initiating neuroleptic medication within the context of neurologic care, the initial prescription is accepted better by the patient if the goal of treatment is expressed in terms relevant to the patient's subjective concerns. Thus, for example, patients with schizophrenia may initially accept medication ''to help [them] organize [their] own thoughts better'' or ''to reduce the voices that are bothering [them].'' Ultimately, continuation of therapy must be based on fully informed consent by the patient, including discussion of the diagnosis.

The comprehensive management of schizophrenia goes well beyond the capabilities of the neurologic practitioner. The social and occupational impairments associated with the disorder and its usual early onset indicate a complex mix of family education, vocational rehabilitation, social skills training, and reality-oriented counseling. In addition, many patients require supportive environments separate from family members to attain their highest possible level of independence and well-being.

Comprehensive management of psychotic complications of chronic neurologic disease begins with education of the patient and family and provision or arrangement of assistance in addressing practical problems in coping with the illness that increase the patient's level of stress. Comprehensive psychiatric assessment can help identify priorities for psychological or environmental intervention, so it is valuable even when the diagnosis is not in doubt and the neurologist is committed to provide principal care for the patient. Specific advice on management strategy should be requested at the time of the referral.

Pharmacologic Therapy

Neuroleptics. Neuroleptic (antipsychotic) medications are the primary drug therapy of thought disorder. The neuroleptic drugs comprise several distinct pharmacologic classes, but all share the property of blocking dopamine receptors in both the striatum and the frontal and limbic cortex. Their benefits for the treatment of psychotic symptoms (thought disorder) have been attributed primarily to their effect on limbic and perhaps frontal cortical dopamine receptors. The effect of the drugs on striatal dopamine receptors is responsible for their many adverse effects on the motor system.

Typical neuroleptic agents are distinguished from one another by their potency in blocking dopamine receptors and by the extent of their actions on other neurotransmitter receptors such as the muscarinic cholinergic receptors. The less potent agents tend to be more anticholinergic, and to also have antihistaminic and α-adrenergic blocking properties. Newer, or atypical, neuroleptic agents, of which clozapine and risperidone are the first available in the United States, have significantly different pharmacodynamics. In addition to blocking dopamine receptors, they block S2 serotonin receptors. Clozapine is distinguished in addition by relatively less binding to striatal D2 dopamine receptors and greater binding to limbic cortical D3 receptors. All of the typical neuroleptic agents can cause drug-induced parkinsonism, with the incidence highest with the more potent, less anticholinergic agents. Risperidone also can do so, but with lower incidence than would be expected from its potency in blocking D2 receptors. Clozapine rarely causes drug-induced parkinsonism, and may even alleviate parkinsonian symptoms because of its anticholinergic effects.

Neuroleptic drugs have both immediate and delayed effects on thought disorder. Almost immediately, patients may show a reduction in such symptoms as agitation, emotional lability, and overtly paranoid behavior. Disorganized speech may become more coherent within hours to days. Resolution of delusions and hallucinations can occur in hours to days when they are acute symptoms of recent onset, as can be encountered in delirium or stress-related psychosis. Long-standing delusions, as occur in schizophrenia or delusional disorder, may take several weeks to improve, and may not resolve completely. Resolution of delusions associated with mood disorder tends to occur synchronously with the restoration of normal mood. The negative symptoms of schizophrenia, which do not improve much with typical neuroleptic therapy, can improve with the atypical neuroleptics. Response of negative symptoms occurs over weeks to months of therapy.

Neuroleptics are given as primary or sole therapy for schizophrenia, delusional disorder, and brief psychosis, for psychotic symptoms of delirium or dementia, and for psychotic states induced by drugs, metabolic disturbance, or gross brain disease. Neuroleptics are given together with mood-stabilizing drugs for mania or mixed manic-depressive states with psychotic features. They are combined with antidepressants to treat major depression with delusions. The psychosis of temporal lobe epilepsy is treated with neuroleptics in combination with antiepileptic drugs.

Choice and Dosage. Neuroleptic dosage differs according to the purpose of neuroleptic therapy. For acute behavioral emergencies in younger and relatively healthy adults, neuroleptics are given every hour until the patient is behaviorally stable; transfer to the care of a psychiatrist is generally arranged simultaneously. Typical doses are 5 mg/hr haloperidol 5 mg/hr or thiothixene either orally or parenterally. The neuroleptic is combined with a benzodiazepine (e.g., 1 to 2 mg of lorazepam each dose) for more rapid behavioral control. For acute behavioral emergencies in older or more frail individuals, the dose increments are haloperidol 0.5 to 1.0 mg per dose with lorazepam 0.5 to 1.0 mg. Haloperidol is usually given without lorazepam for emergencies in patients with dementia, because of the concern that lorazepam will induce a confusional state.

For ongoing treatment of schizophrenia or a related psychosis (e.g., the schizophrenia-like psychosis of temporal lobe epilepsy), typical daily doses of neuroleptics are 5 to 10 mg. of haloperidol or fluphenazine, 10 to 20 mg of thiothixene, or 25 to 50 mg of molindone. An equivalent dose of risperidone would be 3 mg bid.

For treatment of a chronic, lower-grade thought disorder, such as delusional disorder or paranoid symptomatology in early dementia, a lower dosage of neuroleptic may suffice. At these lower doses, lower-potency agents, despite their anticholinergic, sedating, and hypotensive effects, may be well tolerated and even liked by patients because of their anxiolytic and sleep-promoting actions. Typical doses are haloperidol or fluphenazine, 1 to 2 mg/day; molindone, 5 to 10 mg/day; perphenazine 4 to 12 mg/day; thioridazine 10 to 25 mg tid or 50 to 75 mg qhs; or risperidone, 0.5 mg qhs to 1.0 mg bid.

The atypical neuroleptic drug clozapine currently has a unique place in the treatment of psychosis. It is the single most effective agent for thought disorder and the one most likely to relieve negative symptoms of schizophrenia, and it also has the fewest extrapyramidal side effects and the lowest risk of tardive dyskinesia and neuroleptic malignant syndrome. However, it carries a 1 percent risk of agranulocytosis and a 3 to 5 percent risk of seizures. For this reason, it is not prescribed routinely to patients with psychotic disorders. Clozapine is indicated, however, for schizophrenia poorly responsive to conventional therapy, for schizophrenia with drug-induced movement disorders of unacceptable severity, and for the treatment of psychosis in Parkinson's disease. When used for schizophrenia, a typical dose of clozapine is 300 to 500 mg/day, approached over a slow dose titration.

When clozapine is administered, the patient must have a weekly white blood cell count; the drug is discontinued if the white blood cell count falls below 3,000/mm^3. Because of the seizure risk, patients with known epilepsy or risk factors for seizures (e.g., history of traumatic brain injury) should be treated with an anitepileptic drug concurrently. Phenytoin or valproate is preferred; carbamazepine is avoided because of concern about additive bone marrow suppression.

Neurotoxicity.   During the first several days after starting typical neuroleptic therapy, patients are at high risk of developing extrapyramidal motor symptoms. Younger patients, particularly young men, may develop acute dystonia. This usually involves the neck, with torticollis or opisthotonus. All patients are at risk of drug-induced parkinsonism. Some patients develop typical rest tremors, but rigidity and akinesia without noticeable tremor also can develop and are more likely to go undetected if muscle tone and voluntary movement are not systematically checked. Acute dyskinesia, involving either the orofacial region or the extremities, also occurs, although less commonly than drug-induced parkinsonism. Akathisia occurs frequently and when subtle can be mistaken for anxiety, agitation, or the purposeless hyperactivity of psychosis. Typically, the patient with akathisia will report physical discomfort if he or she attempts to remain still.

With the exception of akathisia, the acute extrapyramidal disorders will respond to antiparkinson medication. Dopamine agonists, either amantadine, 100 mg bid to tid, or bromocriptine 2.5 mg daily to tid, are more effective for rigidity and akinesia than anticholinergic antiparkinson drugs. Parenteral anticholinergic agents (e.g., benztropine 2 mg; trihexyphenidyl 5 mg; or diphenhydramine 50 mg) are immediately and decisively effective for acute dystonia. Akathisia usually responds to propranolol at a typical dose of 20 mg to 40 mg tid. Some patients with movement disorders due to neuroleptics can be withdrawn from antiparkinson drugs after several weeks of neuroleptic

therapy, without recurrence of the motor symptoms and signs. If withdrawal of antiparkinson drugs is attempted, the patient should be re-examined for recurrent signs, since not all patients with psychotic disorders will complain of their movement disorders, even when the signs are evident and the disorder is functionally relevant.

Use of neuroleptics for more than a few months is associated with the risk of movement disorders that will persist after the neuroleptics are withdrawn. These late complications of neuroleptic therapy, the tardive movement disorders, include tardive dyskinesia, tardive dystonia, and tardive akathisia. The dyskinesias include choreoathetosis, buccolingual movements, blepharospasm, respiratory dyskinesia, and dysphagia due to dyskinesia of the larnyx and pharnyx. Tardive dystonia usually involves flexion-extension movements of the trunk; torsion dystonia is less common. Tardive akathisia resembles acute akathisia. Both advanced age and female sex are risk factors for the tardive movement disorders, as is pre-existing gross brain disease and an indication for neuroleptics other than schizophrenia. Tardive movement disorders tend to remit over months to years, with an average of 50 percent improvement at 9 months. However, a substantial number of patients have permanent symptoms. There is no established treatment. Symptoms can be suppressed by dopamine blockers or by reserpine, but the former may aggravate the underlying condition, and the latter has many side effects, notably apathy and depression. Drugs reported in case histories to give partial relief to individual patients have included benzodiazepines, calcium channel-blockers, and buspirone.

The most life-threatening neurologic side effect of neuroleptic therapy is the neuroleptic malignant syndrome. This disorder, which tends to occur during the initiation of neuroleptic therapy, in relation to dose increases, or at times of intercurrent acute illness, is characterized by severe tremulous rigidity, autonomic instability, hyperthermia, and delirium. The patient appears to have an acute encephalopathy, and the most conspicuous laboratory finding is an elevated creatine kinase. Untreated, the disorder can lead to widespread rhabdomyolysis, myoglobinuria, and death. Treatment begins with discontinuation of the neuroleptic, hydration, and control of temperature and blood pressure. Specific therapies of reported benefit are dantrolene, used intravenously as for malignant hyperthermia, and bromocriptine, titrated to the point of relieving muscular rigidity. A starting dose of bromocriptine in this setting is 5 mg q8h.

Special Therapeutic Situations

Psychosis in Dementia.   When treating psychosis in dementia, the aims are to improve the patient's everyday function and to reduce the burden on caregivers. Therefore, neuroleptic therapy should aim to contain paranoid behavior, hallucinations, and agitation but to avoid adding disabling parkinsonian symptoms to the patient's pre-existing cognitive impairments. Office-based outpatient monitoring of neuroleptic therapy for psychosis in dementia should include an overview of the patient's functional dependencies and the caregiver's burdens at each visit.

The initial dose of a neuroleptic should be very low, to avoid overshooting the optimum dose. Typical doses are haloperidol, 0.25 to 0.5 mg/day; risperidone 0.25 to 0.5 mg/day; or thioridazine, 10 to 25 mg/day. In some patients, even these doses will unmask subclinical extrapyramidal signs. If there is no adverse or therapeutic effect at the initial dose, the dose can be increased in increments of similar size every 2 to 3 days until there is improvement in the target symptoms or until extrapyramidal symptoms develop. Drug therapy should be maintained for at least 4 weeks at the minimum dose that produces an early therapeutic action or at the highest dose that can be given without problematic motor side effects. Then, the overall balance of positive and negative effects of neuroleptic therapy should be assessed, to permit an informed decision about whether to continue it or to adjust the dosage.

If there is a good response of delusions or hallucinations to a neuroleptic, but there remains a persistent problem with insomnia or agitation, the latter problem should be treated with a non-neuroleptic therapy. Options include a low-dose sedating antidepressant at bedtime for insomnia, and a selective serotonin re-uptake inhibitor or β-blocker for agitation.

Psychosis in Parkinson's Disease.   The occurrence of delusions, hallucinations, paranoid ideas, and other psychotic symptoms in Parkinson's disease often limits effective levodopa therapy in the late stages of the disease. Reducing levodopa dosage or substituting direct agonists for part of the levodopa occasionally helps, but usually has no benefit for mental status except at the cost of worse motor disability. In this situation, treatment of the drug-induced psychosis with clozapine may permit relief of psychosis with maintained or even improved motor function.

Clozapine treatment for Parkinson's disease with psychosis is most likely to be beneficial when the patient is not demented, or has only mild cognitive impairment. Treatment should begin at a very low dose of clozapine (e.g., 6.25 mg/day). If the drug is tolerated, dosage can be increased at weekly intervals until there are limiting side effects (usually sedation or anticholinergic effects) or the patient has relief of psychotic symptoms. Doses rarely need to exceed 100 mg/day, and some improvement in motor disability is common.

Risperidone, though it is substantially less likely than typical neuroleptics to cause drug-induced parkinsonism in patients with schizophrenia, unfortunately does aggravate the motor symptoms of Parkinson's disease. It is not a viable substitute for clozapine in the situation of advanced Parkinson's disease with drug-induced psychosis.

Psychotic Symptoms in Limbic Epilepsy.   When a patient with limbic epilepsy develops a schizophreniform psychosis, drug therapy is similar to that for schizophrenia. In choosing a neuroleptic, there is reason to avoid the low-potency neuroleptics chlorpromazine and thioridazine: these agents may cause seizures. Evidence on which to base a preference for one higher-potency agent over another is limited, but molindone and fluphenazine appeared benign regarding precipitation of seizure activity in one in vitro study. More important than the choice of neuroleptic is optimal management of the seizures themselves. Barbiturates and primidone should be avoided, and vigorous efforts should be made with rational drug combinations or even surgery to control the seizures, since persistent seizure activity appears related to the development of psychosis. When patients are on multiple-drug regimens that include a neuroleptic, antiepileptic drug levels should be rechecked after changes in the psychotropic regimen, because of the possibility of drug interactions.

Another group of patients with limbic epilepsy do not have a chronic psychosis, but have emotional hyperintensity and idiosyncratic thinking that intermittently reaches the point of paranoia or near-delusional conviction. Such patients may suffer distress from their thoughts, or alienate employers or social supports with anger and accusations. Low-dose neuroleptic medication may mitigate the symptoms of thought disorder in these patients. Typical doses are haloperidol or fluphenazine 0.5 to 2 mg/day; molindone 5 to 15 mg/day; or risperidone, 0.5 to 1.0 mg/day.

SUGGESTED READINGS

Anxiety and Panic

Anxiety disorders. pp. 1287–1360. In Bloom FE, Kupfer DJ (eds): Psychopharmacology—The Fourth Generation of Progress. Raven Press, New York; 1995

Goldberg RJ, Posner DA: Anxiety in the medically ill. pp. 87–104. In Stoudemire A, Fogel BS (eds): Psychiatric Care of the Medical Patient. Oxford University Press, New York, 1993

Noyes R, Holt CS: Anxiety disorders. pp. 139–160. In Winokur G, Clayton PJ (eds): The Medical Basis of Psychiatry. 2nd ed. WB Saunders, Philadelphia, 1994

Wise MG, Taylor SE: Anxiety and mood disorders in medidally ill patients. J Clin Psychiatry 51:27–32; 1990

Mood Disorders

Akiskal HS: Mood disorders. pp. 365–80. In Winokur G, Clayton PJ (eds): The Medical Basis of Psychiatry. WB Saunders, Philadelphia, 1994

Cohen-Cole SA, Brown FW, McDaniel JS: Assessment of depression and grief reactions in the medically ill. pp. 53–70. In Stoudemire A, Fogel BS (ed): Psychiatric Care of the Medical Patient. Oxford University Press, New York, 1993

Mood disorders. In Bloom FE, Kupfer DJ (eds.): Psychophamacology—The Fourth Generation of Progress. Raven Press, New York, 1995

Starkstein SE, Robinson RG: Depression in Neurologic Disease. Johns Hopkins University Press, Baltimore, 1993

Stoudemire A, Fogel BS, Gulley LR, Moran MG: Psychopharmacology in the medical patient. pp. 155–206. In Stoudemire A, Fogel BS (eds): Psychiatric Care of the Medical Patient. Oxford University Press, New York, 1993

Personality Disorders and Reaction to Disease

American Psychiatric Association: Diagnostic and Statistical Manual of Mental Disorders. 4th Ed. pp. 629–74. American Psychiatric Association. Washington, D.C. 1994

Green SA: Principles of medical psychotherapy. pp. 3–18. In Stoudemire A, Fogel BS: Psychiatric Care of the Medical Patient. Oxford University Press, New York, 1993

Fogel BS: Personality disorders in the medical setting. pp. 289–306. In Stoudemire A, Fogel BS: Psychiatric Care of the Medical Patient. Oxford University Press, New York, 1993

Ratey JJ: Neuropsychiatry of Personality Disorders. Blackwell Science, Cambridge, MA 1995

Thought Disorders

American Psychiatric Association: Diagnostic and Statistical Manual of Mental Disorders. 4th Ed. pp. 273–316. American Psychiatric Association, Washington, D.C. 1994

Andreasen NC: Thought disorder. pp. 393–402. In Winokur G, Clayton PJ (eds): The Medical Basis of Psychiatry. WB Saunders, Philadelphia, 1994

Rich SS, Friedman JH: Treatment of psychosis in Parkinson's disease. pp. 151–82. In Stoudemire A, Fogel BS (eds): Medical-Psychiatric Practice. Vol. 3. American Psychiatric Press, Washington, D.C. 1995

Schizophrenia. pp. 1171–1286. In Bloom FE, Kupfer DJ (eds): Psychopharmacology—The Fourth Generation of Progress. Raven Press, New York, 1995

NEURO-ONCOLOGY

PART **VII**

SECTION 1. BRAIN TUMORS: GENERAL ASPECTS

147. CLASSIFICATION, EPIDEMIOLOGY, AND ETIOLOGY OF BRAIN TUMORS

DAVID SCHIFF

Brain tumors are clinically highly heterogeneous; they can be rapidly fatal or incidental and trivial. They include tumors of (1) the brain parenchyma itself, (2) the coverings (meninges) of the brain, (3) the nearby cranial nerves and skull base, (4) the ventricular system, and (5) the anatomically related pituitary and pineal glands. Certain space-occupying anomalies and malformations that are without neoplastic potential, such as lipomas and colloid cysts of the third ventricle, are usually also included among brain tumors. More than 100 different types of brain tumor are known, although gliomas (meaning all tumors that arise from astrocytic, oligodendroglial, or ependymal cells), metastases, and meningiomas constitute the majority. The terms benign, malignant, and cancerous lose their usual meanings within the skull, because relatively small, slowly growing, mitotically inactive tumors with little or no metastatic potential may be lethal if they are located in a region of the brain where they cannot be completely resected.

CLASSIFICATION

Precise classification is critical to guide treatment, to determine prognosis, to facilitate communication among physicians, and to ensure the validity of clinical treatment trials. Although some tumors are relatively easy to classify, others are a challenge in this regard. Several attempts have been made to provide a workable classification scheme, and much of the current nomenclature is derived from early classification systems. The most widely used classification of brain tumors is the World Health Organization (WHO) scheme. Like earlier systems, this scheme was based on the concept of grouping tumors according to their normal ontogenic counterparts. In 1993 this system was revised, taking advantage of the insights gained from immunohistochemistry, electron microscopy, and molecular biology regarding the origins of some of these tumors (Table 147-1).

The WHO classification recognizes histologic grades of malignancy of some tumor types. The four astrocytoma grades are as follows: grade 1, histologically distinct pilocytic astrocytomas, which are often surgically curable; grade 2 (''low-grade''), characteristically diffuse infiltrating lesions with nuclear atypia but little or no mitotic activity; grade 3 (''anaplastic''), lesions that typically have mitoses in addition to nuclear atypia; and grade 4, corresponding to glioblastomas with the additional histologic features of necrosis and/or endothelial proliferation. Because mortality rates generally correlate directly

with tumor grade, this system has biologic as well as histologic significance. Furthermore, it may be less subjective, with better interobserver reliability than earlier grading systems. (Anaplastic astrocytomas and glioblastomas are sometimes colloquially termed ''high-grade'' or ''malignant.'') Some pathologists continue to use older grading systems; thus, it is important to know not only the grade of an astrocytoma but the system on which the grading was based.

Similar grading criteria can be applied to oligodendrogliomas, mixed oligoastrocytomas, and ependymomas. Anaplastic oligodendrogliomas are characterized by nuclear pleomorphism and increased mitotic rate. Generally, these tumors behave more aggressively than do typical oligodendrogliomas. For some tumors, such as ependymomas, the relationship between their histologic features and biologic behavior is less clear.

As with gliomas, varying grades of malignancy are recognized within meningiomas. In addition to the histologically benign meningioma (which comprises most meningiomas), occasional tumors are termed ''atypical'' and others ''malignant'' or ''anaplastic.'' Atypical meningiomas may have hypercellularity, nuclear pleomorphism, increased mitotic activity, and foci of necrosis. Malignant meningiomas generally have these features to an even greater extent, although invasion of brain parenchyma or metastasis by a meningioma, even in the absence of these features, warrants the designation ''malignant.'' Both atypical and malignant meningiomas are more likely to recur after resection than are typical ones.

Finally, it is important to recognize that the WHO system is based solely on the histologic features of tumors and not on their location. Location is very important because some types of tumors have regional predilections (Table 147-2) and because resectability often depends as much (or more) on the location of the tumor as on its histology. For example, pilocytic astrocytomas frequently occur in the cerebellar hemispheres, hypothalamus, or optic pathways. Whereas pilocytic astrocytomas in the cerebellum typically are curable surgically, histologically identical tumors in the hypothalamus are incurable. Similarly, a large meningioma of the hemispheric convexity can be totally resected, with complete cure, but a much smaller meningioma of the skull base can have devastating consequences for a patient. Thus, from the clinical viewpoint, both histologic type and location are crucial determinants of management and prognosis.

EPIDEMIOLOGY

Primary Brain Tumors

Although primary brain tumors are second only to stroke as a cause of neurologic death in adults, the true incidence of these tumors is unclear. For example, autopsy-derived series include some tumors that were asymptomatic during life, generating relatively high rates, whereas series requiring histologic confirmation during life may exclude tumors that are rapidly fatal or difficult to biopsy. Changes in nomenclature and improvements

TABLE 147-1. World Health Organization Histologic Typing of Central Nervous System Tumors

Number	Type of Tumor	Number	Type of Tumor
1	**Tumors of neuroepithelial tissue**	3	**Tumors of the meninges**
1.1	*Astrocytic tumors*	3.1	*Tumors of meningiothelial cells*
1.1.1	Astrocytoma	3.1.1	Meningioma
1.1.1.1	Variants: Fibrillary	3.1.1.1	Variants: Meningothelial
1.1.1.2	Protoplasmic	3.1.1.2	Fibrous (fibroblastic)
1.1.1.3	Gemistocytic	3.1.1.3	Transitional (mixed)
1.1.2	Anaplastic (malignant) astrocytoma	3.1.1.4	Psammomatous
1.1.3	Glioblastoma	3.1.1.5	Angiomatous
1.1.3.1	Variants: Giant cell glioblastoma	3.1.1.6	Microcystic
1.1.3.2	Gliosarcoma	3.1.1.7	Secretory
1.1.4	Pilocytic astrocytoma	3.1.1.8	Clear cell
1.1.5	Pleomorphic xanthoastrocytoma	3.1.1.9	Chordoid
1.1.6	Subependymal giant cell astrocytoma (tuberous sclerosis)	3.1.1.10	Lymphoplasmacyte-rich
		3.1.1.11	Metaplastic
1.2	*Oligodendroglial tumors*	3.1.2	Atypical meningioma
1.2.1	Oligodendroglioma	3.1.3	Papillary meningioma
1.2.2	Anaplastic (malignant) oligodendroglioma	3.1.4	Anaplastic (malignant) meningioma
1.3	*Ependymal tumors*		*Mesenchymal, nonmeningiothelial tumors*
1.3.1	Ependymoma		
1.3.1.1	Variants: Cellular	3.2	*Benign neoplasms*
1.3.1.2	Papillary	3.2.1	Osteocartilaginous tumors
1.3.1.3	Clear cell	3.2.2	Lipoma
1.3.2	Anaplastic (malignant) ependymoma	3.2.3	Fibrous histiocytoma
1.3.3	Myxopapillary ependymoma	3.2.4	Others
1.3.4	Subependymoma		
			Malignant neoplasms
1.4	*Mixed gliomas*	3.2.5	Hemangiopericytoma
1.4.1	Oligo-astrocytoma	3.2.6	Chondrosarcoma
1.4.2	Anaplastic (malignant) oligo-astrocytoma	3.2.6.1	Variant: Mesenchymal chondrosarcoma
1.4.3	Others	3.2.7	Malignant fibrous histiocytoma
		3.2.8	Rhabdomyosarcoma
1.5	*Choroid plexus tumors*	3.2.9	Meningeal sarcomatosis
1.5.1	Choroid plexus papilloma	3.2.10	Others
1.5.2	Choroid plexus carcinoma		
		3.3	*Primary melanocytic lesions*
1.6	*Neuroepithelial tumors of uncertain origin*	3.3.1	Diffuse melanosis
1.6.1	Astroblastoma	3.3.2	Melanocytoma
1.6.2	Polar spongioblastoma	3.3.3	Malignant melanoma
1.6.3	Gliomatosis cerebri	3.3.3.1	Variant: Meningeal melanomatosis
1.7	*Neuronal and mixed neuronal-glial tumors*	3.4	*Tumors of uncertain histogenesis*
1.7.1	Gangliocytoma	3.4.1	Hemangioblastoma (capillary hemangioblastoma)
1.7.2	Dysplastic gangliocytoma of cerebellum (Lhermitte-Duclos)		
1.7.3	Desmoplastic infantile ganglioglioma	4	**Lymphomas and hemopoietic neoplasms**
1.7.4	Dysembryoplastic neuroepithelial tumor	4.1	Malignant lymphomas
1.7.5	Ganglioglioma	4.2	Plasmacytoma
1.7.6	Anaplastic (malignant) ganglioglioma	4.3	Granulocytic sarcoma
1.7.7	Central neurocytoma	4.4	Others
1.7.8	Paraganglioma of the filum terminale		
1.7.9	Olfactory neuroblastoma (aesthesioneuroblastoma)	5	**Germ cell tumors**
1.7.9.1	Variant: Olfactory neuroepithelioma	5.1	Germinoma
		5.2	Embryonal carcinoma
1.8	*Pineal parenchymal tumors*	5.3	Yolk sac tumor (endodermal sinus tumor)
1.8.1	Pineocytoma	5.4	Choriocarcinoma
1.8.2	Pineoblastoma	5.5	Teratoma
1.8.3	Mixed/transitional pineal tumors	5.5.1	Immature
		5.5.2	Mature
1.9	*Embryonal tumors*	5.5.3	With malignant transformation
1.9.1	Medulloepithelioma	5.6	Mixed germ cell tumors
1.9.2	Neuroblastoma		
1.9.2.1	Variant: Ganglioneuroblastoma	6	**Cysts and tumor-like lesions**
1.9.3	Ependymoblastoma	6.1	Rathke cleft cyst
1.9.4	Primitive neuroectodermal tumors (PNETs)	6.2	Epidermoid cyst
1.9.4.1	Medulloblastoma	6.3	Dermoid cyst
1.9.4.1.1	Variants: Desmoplastic medulloblastoma	6.4	Colloid cyst of the third ventricle
1.9.4.1.2	Medullomyoblastoma	6.5	Enterogenous cyst
1.9.4.1.3	Melanotic medulloblastoma	6.6	Neuroglial cyst
		6.7	Granular cell tumor (choristoma, pituicytoma)
2	**Tumors of cranial and spinal nerves**	6.8	Hypothalamic neuronal hamartoma
2.1	*Schwannoma (neurilemmoma, neurinoma)*	6.9	Nasal glial heterotopia
2.1.1	Variants: Cellular	6.10	Plasma cell granuloma
2.1.2	Plexiform		
2.1.3	Melanotic	7	**Tumors of the sellar region**
		7.1	Pituitary adenoma
2.2	*Neurofibroma*	7.2	Pituitary carcinoma
2.2.1	Circumscribed (solitary)	7.3	Craniopharyngioma
2.2.2	Plexiform	7.3.1	Variants: Adamantinomatous
		7.3.2	Papillary
2.3	*Malignant peripheral nerve sheath tumor (MPNST) (neurogenic sarcoma, anaplastic neurofibroma, "malignant schwannoma")*	8	**Local extensions from regional tumors**
2.3.1	Variants: Epithelioid	8.1	Paraganglioma (chemodectoma)
2.3.2	MPNST with divergent mesenchymal and/or epithelial differentiation	8.2	Chordoma
		8.3	Condroma
2.3.3	Melanotic		Chondrosarcoma
		8.4	Carcinoma
		9	**Metastatic tumors**
		10	**Unclassified tumors**

(From Kleihues P, Burger PC, Scheithauser BW: Histological Typing of Tumours of the Central Nervous System, World Health Organization, International Histological Classification of Tumours. Springer-Verlag, Berlin, 1993, with permission.)

TABLE 147-2. Most Common Brain Tumors by Location

Location	Tumor
Cerebral hemispheres	Astrocytoma, grades 1–4
	Metastasis
	Oligodendroglioma
	Meningioma
	Primary central nervous system lymphoma
	Ependymoma
	Sarcoma
	Ganglioglioma[a]
	Desmoplastic infantile ganglioglioma[a]
	Primitive neuroectodermal tumor[a]
Corpus callosum	Astrocytoma, especially high-grade
	Oligodendroglioma
	Lipoma
Lateral ventricle	Ependymoma
	Central neurocytoma
	Meningioma
	Subependymoma
	Choroid plexus papilloma[a]
	Choroid plexus carcinoma[a]
	Subependymal giant cell astrocytoma[a]
Third ventricle	Astrocytoma, especially pilocytic[a]
	Colloid cyst
	Ependymoma
	Subependymoma
Suprasellar cistern	Pituitary macroadenoma
	Craniopharyngioma[a]
	Germ cell neoplasm[a]
	Meningioma
	Optic glioma[a]
Optic chiasm and nerve	Astrocytoma, especially pilocytic[a]
	Meningioma
Pituitary region	Adenoma
	Craniopharyngioma[a]
	Meningioma
	Germ cell neoplasm[a]
	Dermoid cyst
	Metastasis
Pineal region	Germ cell neoplasm[a]
	Teratoma[a]
	Pineoblastoma[a]
	Pineocytoma[a]
	Astrocytoma
	Epidermoid cyst
Brainstem	Astrocytoma[a]
	Metastasis
Cerebellum	Metastasis
	Hemangioblastoma
	Astrocytoma, especially pilocytic[a]
	Medulloblastoma[a]
	Primary central nervous system lymphoma
Cerebellopontine angle	Acoustic schwannoma
	Meningioma
	Epidermoid cyst
	Schwannoma of other cranial nerves
	Chemodectoma
	Choroid plexus papilloma
	Ependymoma
	Metastasis
Fourth ventricle	Ependymoma[a]
	Choroid plexus papilloma[a]
	Subependymoma
Foramen magnum	Meningioma
	Schwannoma
	Neurofibroma

[a] Particularly in children.

(Modified from Okazaki H, Scheithauer BW: Atlas of Neuropathology. Gower Medical Publishing, New York, 1988, with permission of the Mayo Foundation.)

in noninvasive neuroimaging make trends over time difficult to interpret. In view of these factors, it is not surprising that the age-adjusted incidence of primary brain tumors in various studies ranges from 7.9 to 14.1 in 100,000 a year. To give these numbers perspective, the American Cancer Society estimated that 17,500 primary brain tumors (9,600 men and 7,900 women)

would be diagnosed in the United States in 1994, with 12,600 deaths. Most studies suggest that primary brain tumors are slightly more frequent in men than in women (male/female ratio, 1.2 to 1.4:1). Racial variation among brain tumors is generally small, although some studies have found that blacks have a decreased incidence of primary brain tumors in comparison with whites, whereas Japanese have an increased incidence of germ cell neoplasms and craniopharyngiomas. Data compiled from several tumor registries suggest that the peak incidence of primary brain tumors occurs around the age of 50 years; however, autopsy data from Rochester, Minnesota, suggest that the incidence grows continuously with increasing age.

Because of the wide range of tumor types and outcomes of the many different primary brain tumors, such "lumped" figures are not very meaningful. Data from cancer registries suggest that of all primary brain tumors, gliomas comprise 50 percent and meningiomas 28 percent. The findings from one series are shown in Table 147-3. Autopsy-derived series, by contrast, show an excess of meningiomas over gliomas; however, many of these meningiomas were clinically silent during life.

Gliomas show a male prevalence (male/female ratio, 1.5:1). The peak age of different gliomas varies; one study found that the median age for ependymomas was the mid-20s; for low-grade astrocytomas, age 38 years; and for high-grade astrocytomas, age 50 years. The median age of patients with oligodendrogliomas is the mid-40s. Unlike gliomas, meningiomas show a female predominance (male/female ratio, 0.6:1). The median age for symptomatic meningiomas is 52 years. However, as noted above, most meningiomas are diagnosed only at autopsy. (Between 1 and 2 percent of all autopsies disclose a meningioma.)

Tumor registry data based on clinically apparent lesions revealed that 19 percent of primary brain tumors were pituitary adenomas; these occurred more commonly in women than in men. Because as many as 27 percent of unselected autopsied patients have pituitary microadenomas, the importance of selection criteria is clear.

In children, primary tumors of the central nervous system are the most common solid malignancy, with about 1,500 cases

TABLE 147-3. Histologically Confirmed Primary Intracranial Neoplasms in Adults[a]: Frequency Distribution (Connecticut, 1935–1964)

Type	No.	%
Glioblastoma	1,105	52.1
Meningioma	389	18.4
Astrocytoma	214	10.1
Pituitary adenoma	122	5.7
Acoustic neuroma	46	2.2
Hemangioma	41	1.9
Craniopharyngioma	30	1.4
Medulloblastoma	27	1.3
Ependymoma	27	1.3
Oligodendroglioma	22	1.0
Sarcoma	19	0.9
Pinealoma	6	0.3
Chordoma	5	0.2
Others	66	3.1
Total	2,119	99.9

[a] Age 15 years and older.

(Modified from Schoenberg BS, Schoenberg DG, Christine BW, Gomez MR: The epidemiology of primary intracranial neoplasms of childhood: a population study. Mayo Clin Proc 51:51, 1976, with permission of the Mayo Foundation.)

TABLE 147-4. Malignant Brain Tumors in Children Younger Than 15 Years

Type	No.	%
Low-grade supratentorial astrocytoma	220	25
Medulloblastoma	204	23
Cerebellar astrocytoma	109	12
High-grade supratentorial astrocytoma	95	11
Brainstem glioma	80	9
Ependymoma	73	8
Unclassified	66	7
Oligodendroglioma	16	2
Mixed glioma	10	1
Cerebellar glioblastoma	8	1
Choroid plexus papilloma	3	0.3
Meningioma	2	0.2
Ganglioneuroma	1	0.1
Total	887	99.6

(Data from Duffner PK, Cohen ME, Myers MH, Heise HW: Survival of children with brain tumors: SEER program, 1973–1980. Neurology 36:597, 1986.)

diagnosed annually in the United States. After leukemia, they are the leading cause of cancer death in children. Rates of brain tumors in children are 2 to 2.5 in 100,000 a year. Some studies suggest that these tumors are slightly more common in boys (male/female ratio, 1.2:1). In contrast to adults, in whom most of the tumors are located supratentorially, most brain tumors in children occur infratentorially. Low-grade supratentorial astrocytomas and medulloblastomas each account for 20 to 25 percent of childhood tumors, with cerebellar astrocytomas, high-grade supratentorial astrocytomas, brainstem gliomas, and ependymomas each accounting for about 10 percent (Table 147-4). In contrast to adults, meningiomas are unusual in children. They are more likely to be found intraventricularly, to be associated with neurofibromatosis, or to be the biologically aggressive papillary type. The incidence of different types of tumors is strongly age dependent. In children younger than 2 years, medulloblastomas, ependymomas, and low-grade supratentorial astrocytomas of the visual pathways constitute a large fraction, whereas brainstem gliomas and cerebellar astrocytomas are rare.

Some evidence suggests that the incidence of primary brain tumors is increasing. Many neuro-oncologists have noted in recent years an increase in the number of immunocompetent patients with primary central nervous system lymphoma (PCNSL). Analysis of a cancer epidemiology database suggested an almost threefold increase in PCNSL between 1973 and 1984. This increase occurred in subgroups at very low risk for human immunodeficiency virus (HIV), suggesting that these were true sporadic cases and not related to immunodeficiency. With this same database, other investigators found that during the same time, the combined rates for *all* primary malignant brain tumors increased 5 percent a year for people 75 to 84 years old. The incidence of primary brain tumors in people younger than 75 years was fairly stable during this period. Similar trends have been noted in other industrialized countries. Whether such findings reflect better neuroimaging methods, a more aggressive approach to illness in the elderly, or other artifact, or whether they represent a genuine increase in primary brain tumors in the elderly is not known.

Metastatic Brain Tumors

Early studies suggested that the incidence of intracranial metastases was equal to that of primary brain tumors. However, au-

topsy studies have shown that these early studies, which were generally based on information from hospital records and death certificates, significantly underestimated the frequency of intracranial metastases. Several autopsy surveys of patients dying of systemic cancer showed that 20 to 25 percent of such patients harbor intracranial metastases. By applying these estimates to the 526,000 U.S. citizens dying of cancer annually, it is estimated that there are approximately 100,000 to 130,000 new cases of intracranial metastasis annually in the United States (greatly outnumbering symptomatic primary brain tumors). Intracranial metastases include intraparenchymal, leptomeningeal, and dural-based metastases. Fifteen percent of autopsied cancer patients had parenchymal metastases, 8 percent had leptomeningeal metastases, and 9 percent had dural-based metastases. Lung cancer is by far the most common cause of parenchymal metastases, accounting for almost one-half of all cases. Breast cancer is the second leading cause; melanoma, colon cancer, and renal cell carcinoma are also significant contributors. The acute leukemias are the most common cause of leptomeningeal metastases, although lymphoma commonly metastasizes to the subarachnoid space, as do breast cancer, melanoma, and lung cancer occasionally. Breast cancer, lymphoma, prostate cancer, and neuroblastoma are the most frequent causes of dural-based metastases. Viewed differently, the various autopsy series suggest that intracranial metastases are likely to develop in 34 percent of patients with lung cancer, 31 percent of those with breast cancer, and 73 percent of those with melanoma. Two-thirds of the "brain metastases of unknown primary" arise from primary lung tumors.

ETIOLOGY OF PRIMARY BRAIN TUMORS

In most cases, the cause of a primary brain tumor is unknown, but a few risk factors have been identified, including some heritable conditions, exposure to certain physical agents, and immunologic defects. As with malignancies elsewhere in the body, brain tumors generally consist of genetically altered clones of cells. In the widely accepted multihit hypothesis, an initially normal cell undergoes a genetic change that confers a survival or proliferative advantage; subsequently, cells derived from this clone undergo further genetic changes, conferring progressively greater growth as well as mitotic and (ultimately) malignant potential. In general, two such genetic mechanisms have been identified. One is an *alteration* of a normal cellular gene (the *proto-oncogene*) important in the control of cell growth, differentiation, and division. When such a gene is altered, it may become an *oncogene,* which produces a quantitatively or qualitatively altered protein resulting in uncontrolled cell proliferation. The second mechanism involves the *loss* of normal cellular genes important in suppressing cell proliferation. The absence of the products of such *tumor suppressor* genes, or *antioncogenes,* is an important factor in the development of some tumors. The relationship of these genetic mechanisms to human brain tumorigenesis is an active area of research.

The role of inherited genetic factors in the pathogenesis of primary brain tumors is exemplified by certain of the phakomatoses, although the mechanisms by which these factors produce tumors are only beginning to be understood. In neurofibromatosis 1 (von Recklinghausen's neurofibromatosis), an autosomal dominant disorder associated with defective production of the protein neurofibromin coded for by a gene on chromosome 17, approximately 15 percent of the patients have low-grade optic pathway gliomas; cerebellar astrocytomas, pilocytic astrocytomas of the third ventricle, and high-grade astrocytomas also occur. Neurofibromatosis 2, a much less common autosomal dominant disorder, manifests typically as bilateral eighth nerve schwannomas; other central nervous system tumors, including ependymomas, multiple meningiomas, and schwannomas of the trigeminal or other cranial nerves, may develop in these patients.

In tuberous sclerosis, an autosomal dominant trait with a high incidence of sporadic cases, the predominant cerebral lesion is hamartomatous, but occasionally subependymal giant cell astrocytomas develop. Glioblastomas, ependymomas, and ganglioneuromas have also been reported. In von Hippel-Lindau disease, an autosomal dominant disorder, retinal angiomatous tumors are associated with hemangioblastomas of the central nervous system. The hemangioblastomas may be solitary or multiple; although they typically are cerebellar, they are also commonly found in the spinal cord and medulla. As a familial syndrome, hemangioblastomas may also occur without retinal lesions. The nevoid basal cell carcinoma (Gorlin) syndrome is an autosomal dominant disorder characterized by multiple basal cell carcinomas at an early age in addition to variable congenital bony abnormalities. Medulloblastomas develop in 2 to 3 percent of the patients, and meningiomas and craniopharyngiomas have also been reported.

Several other rare syndromes highlight genetic influences on brain tumors. Bilateral retinoblastomas are inherited in an autosomal dominant fashion and are sometimes followed by pineoblastoma, the so-called trilateral retinoblastoma. Patients with this syndrome have one mutated and one normal germline *RB*1 gene. In retinoblastomas from these patients, somatic mutation has inactivated the previously normal allele. This is a typical example of a tumor suppressor gene. Tumor suppressor genes also play an important role in the Li-Fraumeni syndrome, which involves an autosomal dominant aggregation of osteosarcoma and soft tissue sarcomas, breast cancer, and, to a lesser extent, brain tumors (primarily gliomas). Some of the families with this syndrome have been shown to have a germline mutation within the p53 gene on chromosome 17, a well-known tumor suppressor gene that is frequently altered in sporadic human tumors. Turcot syndrome refers to an inherited adenomatous polyposis coli associated with astrocytomas and medulloblastomas. Paragangliomas (also known as *glomus tumors* or *chemodectomas*) are occasionally inherited in an autosomal dominant fashion; in such cases, the tumors tend to be bilateral. Curiously, these tumors are inherited almost exclusively through the paternal line, with offspring of affected females being unaffected, possibly reflecting the phenomenon of genomic imprinting. Finally, rare pedigrees have been reported in which several members have had gliomas, although the significance of these findings is uncertain.

The role of environmental exposures in the pathogenesis of human brain tumors is much less well understood than it is for tumors of other organ systems. The best established environmental carcinogen in humans is ionizing radiation, which predisposes to the development of meningiomas and gliomas. A large retrospective cohort study revealed a fourfold to ninefold increase in the relative risk of meningiomas developing in patients receiving scalp irradiation (estimated brain dose was as low as 70 to 175 cGy) for tinea capitis. In these cases, the scalp almost always showed trophic changes, and tumors always developed within radiation portals, with a mean latency of 37 years. Meningiomas in such patients are more likely to be multiple or malignant than in the general population. An increased

risk of developing meningiomas has also been reported in women with early exposure to radiation through full-mouth dental radiography. In patients receiving higher doses of cranial radiation (e.g., in the range of 5,000 cGy for pituitary adenomas), the latency period for another tumor to develop is shorter, and osteogenic sarcomas and fibrosarcomas have been reported in addition to meningiomas. Radiation also predisposes to the development of glial tumors. The relative risk of a glial tumor developing after low-dose scalp radiotherapy for tinea capitis is 2.6. Further evidence comes from follow-up evaluations of children who received prophylactic brain irradiation (usually about 2,000 cGy) for acute lymphoblastic leukemia. These children have a 22-fold excess of brain tumors, primarily astrocytomas.

Whereas tobacco, alcohol, and dietary factors have been shown to play a role in producing systemic malignancy, they have not been shown to be factors in the development of central nervous system neoplasms, although studies have demonstrated that dietary *N*-nitroso compounds cause brain tumors in animals. Case-control studies have suggested associations between other environmental exposures and the development of brain tumors; however, these studies were beset by recall bias and other methodologic problems. Among the substances linked to an increased incidence of brain tumors are petrochemicals, vinyl chloride, herbicides and pesticides, formaldehyde, and hair dyes and sprays. An increased death rate from brain tumors, primarily gliomas, has been noted among electrical industry workers, with the highest risk among workers thought to have the greatest exposure to electromagnetic fields. Some studies suggest an association between head trauma and the later development of meningioma. Case-control studies of childhood brain tumors have also suggested an increased risk in children who live near high-tension lines. More recently, anecdotal reports of brain tumors in people who use cellular telephones have captured the public's attention, but currently no solid epidemiologic evidence supports this association.

Immune defects, whether congenital, iatrogenic, or virally mediated, are important risk factors for PCNSL. Iatrogenic immunosuppression is a very powerful risk factor for this tumor; for example, in renal transplant recipients, the disease develops at a rate of 2.2 cases in 1,000 a year, at a relative risk of 300 compared with that of the general population. Congenital immunodeficiency syndromes such as severe combined immunodeficiency and Wiskott-Aldrich syndrome are also strongly associated with PCNSL. More recently, autopsy series have revealed that 2 to 5 percent of patients dying of the acquired immunodeficiency syndrome harbor PCNSL. Epstein-Barr virus genome can be found in the malignant lymphocytes of most HIV-associated cases of PCNSL and is found only occasionally within the tumors of immunocompetent patients with PCNSL. Although Epstein-Barr is known to immortalize a small percentage of the lymphocytes it infects, its precise role in the cause of PCNSL is uncertain. Viruses have not otherwise been demonstrated to play a role in the pathogenesis of other human primary brain neoplasms.

SUGGESTED READINGS

Devinsky O: Radiation-induced tumors of the central and peripheral nervous system. p. 79. In Rottenberg DA (ed): Neurological Complications of Cancer Treatment. Butterworth-Heinemann, Boston, 1991

Duffner PK, Cohen ME, Myers MH, Heise HW: Survival of children with brain tumors: SEER program, 1973–1980. Neurology 36:597, 1986

Eby NL, Grufferman S, Flannelly CM et al: Increasing incidence of primary brain lymphoma in the US. Cancer 62:2461, 1988

Greig NH, Ries LG, Yancik R, Rapoport SI: Increasing annual incidence of primary malignant brain tumors in the elderly. J Natl Cancer Inst 82:1621, 1990

Kleihues P, Burger PC, Scheithauer BW: The new WHO classification of brain tumours. Brain Pathol 3:255, 1993

Lopes MBS, VandenBerg SR, Scheithauer BW: The World Health Organization classification of nervous system tumors in experimental neuro-oncology. p. 1. In Levine AJ, Schmidek HH (eds): Molecular Genetics of Nervous System Tumors. Wiley-Liss, New York, 1993

Okazaki H, Scheithauer BW: Atlas of Neuropathology. Gower Medical Publishing, New York, 1988

Posner JB, Chernik NL: Intracranial metastases from systemic cancer. Adv Neurol 19:579, 1978

Ron E, Modan B, Boice JD Jr et al: Tumors of the brain and nervous system after radiotherapy in childhood. N Engl J Med 319:1033, 1988

Rosenfeld SS, Massey EW: Epidemiology of primary brain tumor. p. 121. In Anderson DW (ed): Neuroepidemiology: A Tribute to Bruce Schoenberg. CRC Press, Boca Raton, 1991

Russell DS, Rubinstein LJ: Pathology of Tumours of the Nervous System, 5th Ed. Williams & Wilkins, Baltimore, 1989

Wrensch M, Bondy ML, Wiencke J, Yost M: Environmental risk factors for primary malignant brain tumors: a review. J Neurooncol 17:47, 1993

148. CLINICAL PRESENTATION AND DIAGNOSIS OF BRAIN TUMORS

PATRICK Y. WEN

The presentation and diagnosis of brain tumors has changed considerably with increasing sophistication of diagnostic tools. As a result of the widespread availability of sensitive imaging techniques such as magnetic resonance imaging (MRI), tumors are being detected at an earlier stage and patients have increasingly subtle clinical symptoms and signs at diagnosis. This chapter discusses the clinical presentation and diagnosis of brain tumors in general. Chapter 149 discusses the general principles of management of brain tumors, and subsequent chapters discuss specific tumors in detail.

CLINICAL PRESENTATION

Patients with brain tumors typically present with headaches, seizures, nonspecific cognitive or personality changes, or focal neurologic signs.

Headaches

Headaches are the presenting symptom in approximately 35 percent of patients with brain tumors, and they develop during the course of the disease in 70 percent. Most of these headaches are intermittent and nonspecific. They are usually dull and non-throbbing and are often indistinguishable from tension headaches. The headaches are frequently on the same side as the tumor, although they can also be generalized. Supratentorial tumors usually produce headaches with a frontal location since most supratentorial pain-sensitive structures are supplied by the trigeminal nerve. The posterior fossa is innervated by cranial nerves IX and X as well as upper cervical nerves, and tumors in this area usually result in pain in the occipital region and

TABLE 148-1. Features of a Headache Indicating Possible Need for Cerebral Imaging

Most useful
Wakes patient up at night
Worse on waking and improves over the course of the day
Worse with postural change, coughing or exercise
Less useful
Recent onset
Different from the patient's usual headaches
Increased severity
Nausea or vomiting
Patients with headaches associated with papilledema or focal neurologic signs should always be imaged

neck. Occasionally posterior fossa tumors can produce headaches located at the vertex or in the retroorbital region.

Certain headache features are suggestive of an underlying tumor (Table 148-1). These include headaches that wake the patient at night or that are worse on waking and improve over the course of the day, headaches that are exacerbated by postural change, coughing, or exercise, headaches of recent onset that are different from or more severe than the patient's usual headaches, and the presence of nausea or vomiting, papilledema, or focal neurologic signs. Patients with these features usually require further evaluation with computed tomography (CT) or MRI. However, in this era of cost containment, it is important to be selective in obtaining cerebral imaging studies for patients presenting with headaches. Most patients with chronic headaches and a normal neurologic exam do not need imaging.

Papilledema

Papilledema is important evidence of increased intracranial pressure transmitted through the optic nerve sheath. The incidence of papilledema in older series of patients with brain tumors has been reported to be 50 to 70 percent. Because of advances in neuroimaging, many patients are diagnosed at an earlier stage, and the incidence of papilledema in patients with brain tumor today is probably much lower. In a recent review of 100 consecutive patients with malignant gliomas who underwent surgery at Brigham and Women's Hospital in Boston, only 8 percent had papilledema at the time of diagnosis. Papilledema tends to be more common in children and in tumors that are slowly growing or located in the posterior fossa. It is usually not a useful indicator of increased intracranial pressure in the elderly. Papilledema may interfere with optic nerve function and result in transient visual obscurations, especially with maneuvers that briefly increase intracranial pressure such as coughing and sudden postural change. Meningiomas involving the optic nerve may produce optic atrophy in the ipsilateral eye and (by increasing intracranial pressure) result in papilledema in the contralateral eye, giving rise to the Foster Kennedy syndrome.

Seizures

Seizures are the presenting symptom in approximately one-third of patients with brain tumors and are present at some stage of the illness in 40 to 60 percent of patients. Approximately half the patients have focal seizures and the other half have secondarily generalized seizures. In patients with gliomas, seizures occur in 59 percent of frontal tumors, 42 percent of parietal tumors, 35 percent of temporal tumors, and 33 percent of occipital tumors. Tumors in subcortical areas, such as the thalamus and posterior fossa, are much less epileptogenic. Slowly growing tumors and tumors located near the Rolandic fissure are particularly likely to cause seizures. Approximately 10 to 20 percent of adult patients with new-onset seizures have brain tumors, and these patients should always have CT or MRI as part of their evaluation, especially if they also have focal findings on examination or on electroencephalography (EEG). Patients with malignant gliomas who present with seizure tend to have a better prognosis since their tumors are usually diagnosed at an earlier stage.

Altered Mental Status

Mental status changes are the initial symptom in 15 to 20 percent of patients with gliomas and are frequently present in patients by the time of diagnosis (McKeran and Thomas 1980). These changes may range from subtle problems with concentration, memory, affect, personality, initiative, and abstract reasoning to severe cognitive problems and confusion. Changes in mentation are especially common in frontal lobe tumors but will also occur in patients with increased intracranial pressure from the mass effect of the tumor or hydrocephalus, or as a result of gliomatosis cerebri. With increasing intracranial pressure there is also depression of the level of consciousness, resulting in drowsiness and eventually leading to stupor and coma if treatment is not administered.

Focal Neurologic Symptoms and Signs

Whereas headaches, seizures, and altered mental status may be seen with tumors in many locations, certain clinical features have specific localizing value.

Cortical Tumors. Frontal lobe tumors are often clinically silent initially. As the tumor enlarges personality changes may occur such as disinhibition, irritability, impaired judgment, and lack of initiative (abulia). In addition hemiparesis, seizures, aphasia, urinary frequency and urgency, and gait difficulties may be present. Gaze preference and primitive reflexes, such as forced grasping and snout, may be present. Meningiomas of the olfactory groove may produce anosmia.

Temporal lobe tumors frequently cause seizures. These include simple partial seizures characterized by olfactory and gustatory hallucinations, déjà vu, and feelings of fear and pleasure, as well as complex partial seizures characterized by impairment of consciousness, repetitive psychomotor movements, and automatic behavior. Temporal lobe tumors may also cause memory disturbances, visual field defects (superior quadrantinopsia), and (when the dominant temporal lobe is involved) aphasia.

Tumors of the parietal lobe can produce contralateral sensory loss, involving particularly joint position sense, two-point discrimination, stereognosis, and graphesthesia, although other modalities may also be involved. Lesions in the dominant parietal lobe are associated with aphasia, whereas lesions in the nondominant parietal lobe may result in neglect of the contralateral side and the loss of ability to acknowledge deficits (anosognosia). Hemiparesis, homonymous visual defects (or neglect), agnosias, apraxias, sensory seizures, and disturbance of visual spatial ability, may also be present.

Occipital lobe astrocytomas may cause homonymous hemianopsia and, less commonly, visual seizures characterized by lights, colors, and formed geometric patterns. Tumors at the parieto-occipital junction may produce visual agnosias such as aprosopagnosia (inability to recognize faces) or Balint syndrome.

Diencephalic and Brainstem Tumors. Thalamic tumors may produce contralateral sensory loss, hemiparesis, cognitive impairment, and occasionally visual defects and aphasia. Obstruc-

tive hydrocephalus occurs commonly and is associated with headache, nausea, vomiting, gait unsteadiness, and urinary incontinence.

Brainstem tumors produce cranial neuropathies, weakness, numbness, ataxia, and occasionally vertigo, nausea, vomiting, and hiccups. As the tumor increases in size the aqueduct or fourth ventricle may be compressed, producing hydrocephalus.

Pineal Region and Third Ventricular Tumors. Pineal tumors present either with symptoms of hydrocephalus resulting from compression of the third ventricle and aqueduct or with symptoms produced by compression of the tectum of the midbrain. Midbrain compression may result in disturbance of extraocular function including Parinaud syndrome, characterized by impairment of upgaze and pupillary light reflex and convergence retraction nystagmus. Occasionally children may present with precocious puberty.

Tumors around the third ventricle may produce hydrocephalus. Valsalva maneuvers and positional changes may increase cerebrospinal fluid (CSF) obstruction and lead to severe headaches and occasionally leg weakness and syncope. Tumors in this region may also produce symptoms resulting from hypothalamic dysfunction, autonomic dysfunction, and impaired memory.

Cerebellar Tumors. Headaches and ataxia are the two most common symptoms in patients with cerebellar tumors. The headaches may be due to the tumor or hydrocephalus. They are often occipital and associated with nausea, vomiting, and occasionally neck stiffness. Some patients may experience vertigo. Midline cerebellar lesions may produce truncal ataxia, whereas lesions in the cerebellar hemispheres may cause appendicular ataxia, although frequently the findings are relatively subtle. Examination may also show nystagmus, hypotonia, and frequently cranial nerve and corticospinal tract signs from brainstem compression. Head tilt away from the lesion may occur with incipient tonsillar herniation.

False Localizing Signs

When tumors produce increased intracranial pressure, shifting of intracranial structures occurs, resulting in clinical features that suggest involvement of sites distant from the tumor—false localizing signs. Examples include abducens (sixth) nerve palsy resulting from compression of the nerve as it passes forward over the petrous ligament and compression of the cerebral peduncle by the free edge of the tentorium cerebelli contralateral to a herniating uncus, producing hemiparesis on the same side as the lesion.

DIFFERENTIAL DIAGNOSIS

Many conditions producing increased intracranial pressure or progressive neurologic deficits may mimic brain tumors clinically (Table 148-2). These include subdural hematomas, brain abcesses, hydrocephalus, benign intracranial hypertension, progressive multifocal leukoencephalopathy, multiple sclerosis, vascular malformations, cerebral infarctions, and Alzheimer's disease. Many of these conditions have characteristic radiologic appearances that enable them to be differentiated from brain tumors. However, some of these conditions cannot be distinguished from brain tumors on the basis of their radiologic appearances alone, and a definite diagnosis requires biopsy. These include some brain abcesses, inflammatory lesions, demyelinat-

TABLE 148-2. Differential Diagnosis of Brain Tumors

Conditions producing increased intracranial pressure and/or progressive neurologic
  deficits, or both
  Subdural hematomas
  Hydrocephalus
  Cysts
  Benign intracranial hypertension
  Brain abscesses
  Progressive multifocal leukoencephalopathy
  Multiple sclerosis
  Central nervous system vasculitis
  Vascular malformations
  Cerebral infarctions
  Degenerative diseases (e.g., Alzheimer's disease)
  Hamartomas
  Congenital anomalies (e.g., Chiari malformation)

ing lesions, hamartomas, and congenital anomalies. Even when the imaging characteristics of a lesion are highly suggestive of a tumor, a biopsy is usually indicated to obtain tissue for precise histologic diagnosis and grading of the tumor, since these factors will have a significant influence on treatment.

RADIOLOGIC DIAGNOSIS

The introduction of CT scanning and more recently MRI has revolutionized the diagnosis and management of brain tumors.

Skull Radiographs

Plain skull films are rarely necessary today with the widespread availability of CT and MRI. Occasionally they may be useful in demonstrating calcification, bony erosion, or hyperostosis.

Plain films may demonstrate calcifications related to tumors. The presence of calcifications usually indicates a relatively slowly growing tumor. Astrocytomas are the most common calcifying tumors. Although calcifications occur only in approximately 20 percent of astrocytomas, their overall frequency more than compensates. Other tumors that frequently calcify are craniopharyngiomas (70 to 80 percent), oligodendrogliomas (50 to 60 percent), ependymomas (50 percent), gangliogliomas (35 percent), and meningiomas (10 percent).

Persistent elevation of intracranial pressure can cause erosion of normally calcified structures. In children erosion of the inner table of the skull may lead to a "hammered metal" appearance. Pituitary tumors may produce erosion of the clinoid processes and sella turcica. Slowly growing tumors, such as meningiomas, may produce hyperostosis of the adjacent skull.

Tomography was previously used to demonstrate the double floor of the sella in pituitary tumors and enlargement of the internal auditory canal in acoustic tumors but is now rarely used; CT with bone windows will demonstrate these changes.

Computed Tomography

CT remains the most widely used form of neuroimaging for the diagnosis of brain tumors due to its wider availability and lower cost, although MRI is used with increasing frequency. CT scans will detect over 90 percent of brain tumors. Small tumors (less than 0.5 cm), tumors adjacent to bone (such as pituitary adenomas, clival tumors, and acoustic neuromas), brainstem tumors, and low-grade astrocytomas may be missed and are better detected by the more sensitive MRI. CT tends to be better tolerated than MRI because of its shorter scanning time, and it is also more sensitive for detecting calcification and bony involvement. Although CT is less sensitive than MRI, the CT appearance of certain tumors may be more specific. For example, small round cell tumors such as medulloblastomas

are isodense or hyperdense compared with brain parenchyma before contrast administration, whereas astrocytomas are almost always hypodense. Thus medulloblastomas can frequently be differentiated from cerebellar astrocytomas by CT. MRI appearances of tumors tend to be less specific, making similar differentiation with MRI more difficult.

The use of contrast enhancement is indispensable in the evaluation of brain tumors and may help to distinguish an isodense lesion from the surrounding parenchyma or disclose a hypodense lesion hidden within an area of edema. The introduction of nonionic contrast media has resulted in a four- to fivefold reduction in serious contrast reactions. Other recent advances in CT scanning include shorter scan times and increased sensitivity of detectors, resulting in decreased radiation dosage. Despite these advances, MRI is being used with increasing frequency because of its greater resolution and sensitivity.

Magnetic Resonance Imaging

MRI is a complex, rapidly evolving modality that has assumed an increasingly important role in the diagnosis of brain tumors. MRI has the advantage of being more sensitive than CT, allowing the detection of small tumors that may be missed by CT. It provides much greater anatomic detail in multiple planes and is especially useful for visualizing skull base, brainstem, and posterior fossa tumors. MRI is also superior to CT in detecting hemorrhage and solid and cystic components within tumors and in demonstrating the relationship of the tumors to intracranial vessels.

As with CT scans, the administration of a contrast agent, gadolinium diethylenetriaminepentaacetic acid, to T1-weighted MRI scans greatly increases the sensitivity of the test.

MRI is evolving rapidly. Newer imaging sequences are continually being developed, reducing scan times and improving the information obtained from the images. Newer techniques such as MR spectroscopy, which allows direct investigation of tumor metabolism, and echoplanar MRI, which can scan images in less than 100 ms and provide information on tumor perfusion and diffusion, are currently being evaluated for possible use in grading tumor and separating recurrent tumor from radiation change. Echoplanar MRI may also help to differentiate tumor from edema. MR angiography provides a means of displaying blood vessels in the brain in a noninvasive manner. It is increasingly replacing conventional angiography, although angiography has better resolution and is still necessary in certain situations. MRI is also being integrated with advanced image processing techniques to produce three-dimensional definition of brain tumors to aid in surgical planning.

Angiography

The importance of angiography has diminished significantly with the availability of CT and MRI. It is no longer used for the routine diagnosis of brain tumors. Its role is limited to (1) the preoperative evaluation of the vascular anatomy in certain patients (e.g., sphenoid wing meningioma encircling the carotid artery); (2) the assessment of the patency of venous sinuses in extracerebral tumors (e.g., falx meningioma); (3) the embolization of large tumors such as meningiomas, and (4) the search for arteriovenous malformations and aneurysms in patients who present with hemorrhage. However, even for many of these indications, MR angiography is increasingly taking the place of conventional angiography.

Positron-Emission Tomography

Positron-emission tomography (PET) is a versatile imaging modality that provides dynamic information regarding the metabolism and physiology of the brain and brain tumors. Its use is unfortunately limited by its high cost, restricted availability, and limited scanner resolution. PET is not used for the routine diagnosis of brain tumors, but it can provide important information complementing that obtained by CT and MR scanning. PET with (^{18}F) fluorodeoxyglucose to measure glucose metabolism can be used to tumor grade noninvasively determine in patients with malignant gliomas. PET can also be used to differentiate radiation necrosis from recurrent tumor and to study the metabolic effects of chemotherapy, radiotherapy, and steroids on tumor metabolism.

Single-Photon-Emission Computed Tomography

Single-photon-emissions computed tomography (SPECT) involves the intravenous administration of radiopharmaceuticals that are taken up by the brain and tumor cells. These radiopharmaceuticals emit photons that are detected by a rotating gamma camera. Standard tomography reconstruction algorithms are then used to generate cross-sectional images of the brain. Although SPECT is not used in the initial diagnosis of brain tumors, it is increasingly being used to complement information obtained by CT or MRI scanning. ^{201}Tl chloride, a potassium analogue that is taken up by viable tumor cells, has been used to differentiate low-grade from high-grade gliomas and to identify residual astrocytoma after radiotherapy. More recently it has been used in combination with ^{99m}Tc hexamethylpropylene amine oxime, a blood flow tracer that crosses normal blood–brain barrier, to differentiate radiation necrosis from recurrent glioma.

LABORATORY DIAGNOSIS

A number of laboratory tests may contribute to diagnosis and management.

Perimetry

Visual fields can be evaluated quantitatively by a combination of Goldmann kinetic perimetry and static perimetry using Humphries visual fields. Measurement of visual fields is especially important in the evaluation of tumors in the vicinity of the optic chiasm such as pituitary adenomas. Perimetry may be useful in confirming deficits found on examination, detecting subtle changes not found on confrontation, and monitoring the effects of treatment.

Electroencephalography

Seizures are the presenting symptom in approximately one-third of patients with brain tumors. The presence of focal slow waves and spikes or frank epileptiform activity on EEG may be the first indication of a focal lesion and the need for cerebral imaging. Large tumors producing mass effect and tumors involving the diencephalon may produce asynchronous generalized slowing. However, the EEG is often normal in patients with brain tumors and thus has limited value as a screening test.

Audiometry

Audiometry is a useful test for the diagnosis of cerebellopontine angle tumors. Ninety-eight percent of patients with acoustic neuromas have sensorineural hearing loss on pure tone audiometry. The most common pattern is high-frequency hearing loss together with reduced speech discrimination. Vestibular testing, including electronystagmography, may be positive in patients with cerebellopontine angle tumors but is rarely needed.

Evoked Potentials

Evoked potentials have a role in the diagnosis of acoustic neuromas. The brainstem auditory evoked potentials are abnormal in 92 to 96 percent of patients with acoustic neuromas and are a cost-effective screening test for patients with a low probability of these tumors. The most useful indications of compression of the auditory nerve are prolongation of the wave I to III and wave I to V interwave latencies. When wave I cannot be visualized, the ear-to-ear difference and the absolute latency of wave V may be useful. Compression of the anterior visual pathway by tumors can reduce the amplitude of visual evoked potentials. However these tumors are usually diagnosed by MRI, and visual evoked potentials are rarely necessary. Evoked potentials also have an important role in monitoring neurologic function during surgical resection of tumors.

Cerebrospinal Fluid Analysis

Examination of the CSF can be useful in the diagnosis of certain brain tumors and in evaluating the extent of leptomeningeal spread. However, it is important to recognize that lumbar puncture holds definite risks for patients with increased intracranial pressure and should be avoided in these patients.

Examination of the CSF is very useful in patients with primary central nervous system lymphoma. It helps to eliminate infections, which are often major considerations in the diagnosis, and may help make the diagnosis if tumor cells are identified. A positive cytology may also be helpful in the diagnosis of pineal region tumors, which are often difficult to biopsy. Examination of the CSF is important in postoperative staging of patients with medulloblastomas and primitive neuroectodermal tumors since the presence of leptomeningeal disease influences prognosis and treatment. Cytologic examination of the CSF may also be useful in the diagnosis of neoplastic meningitis in patients with metastatic brain tumors and occasionally in patients who have gliomas with leptomeningeal spread. CSF cytology is rarely useful in the initial diagnosis of gliomas.

Germ cell tumors arising in the pineal region may produce biologic markers such as α-fetoprotein, the β-subunit of human chorionic gonadotrophin, and placental alkaline phosphatase. The presence of these markers helps in the diagnosis and subsequent follow-up of these germ cell tumors (Table 148-3).

Endocrine Evaluation

Tumors in the region of the pituitary gland and hypothalamus may be associated with a variety of endocrine abnormalities. Evaluation of the hypothalmic-pituitary axis involves measurement of hormonal levels in the blood and urine, dynamic testing, and occasionally hormonal sampling of venous sinuses to help localize the tumor (see Ch. 156 on pituitary tumors).

TABLE 148-3. Tumor Markers in Patients With Pineal Tumors

Tumor Type	AFP	HCG	PLAP
Germinoma	−	±	+
Teratoma	−	−	±
Malignant teratoma	±	±	±
Undifferentiated germ cell tumor	±	±	±
Choriocarcinoma	−	+	±
Endodermal sinus tumor	+	−	±
Embryonal cell tumor	+	+	±
Pineocytoma	−	−	−
Pinealblastoma	−	−	−

Abbreviations: AFP, α-fetoprotein; HCG, human chorionic gonadotropin; PLAP, placental alkaline phosphatase.

SUMMARY

The diagnosis of brain tumors depends on careful clinical evaluation of the patient and judicious use of imaging and laboratory tests. Recent advances in imaging techniques have revolutionized the diagnosis of brain tumors and have allowed patients to be diagnosed at earlier stages of their illness. The challenge for the future lies not only in developing improved methods of diagnosis, but also in ensuring cost-effective evaluation.

SUGGESTED READINGS

Barkovich AJ: Neuroimaging of pediatric brain tumors. Neurosurg Clin 3: 739–69, 1992

Black PMcL, Wen P: Clinical, imaging, and laboratory diagnosis of brain tumors. p. 191. In Laws E, Kaye A (eds): Encyclopedia of Brain Tumors. Churchill Livingstone, London, 1995

Brody AS. New perspectives in CT and MRI imaging. Neurol Clin 9:273–86, 1991

Carvalho PA, Schwartz, RB, Alexander E et al: Detection of recurrent gliomas with quantitative thallium-201/technetium-99m HMPAO single-photon emission computerized tomography. J Neurosurg 77:565–70, 1992

Forsyth P, Posner J: Headaches in patients with brain tumors: a study of 111 patients. Neurology 43:1678–83, 1993

Hicks RJ, Hesselink JR, Wismaer GL et al: Brain: neoplasia. p. 483. In Edelman R, Hesselink JR (eds): Clinical Magnetic Resonance Imaging. WB Saunders, Philadelphia, 1990

Jaekle KA: Clinical presentation and therapy of nervous system tumors. p. 1008. In Bradley WG, Daroff RB, Fenichel GM, Marsden CD (eds): Neurology in Clinical Practice. Butterworth-Heinemann, Boston, 1991

Kilbanski A, Zervas NT: Diagnosis and management of hormone-secreting pituitary adenomas. N Engl J Med 324:822–31, 1991

Kingsley DPE: Neuroradiological imaging of brain tumors. p. 141. In Thomas DGT (ed): Neuro-oncology. Primary Malignant Brain Tumors. Johns Hopkins University Press, Baltimore, 1990

McKeran RO, Thomas DGT: The clinical study of gliomas. p. 194. In Thomas DGT, Graham DL (eds): Brain Tumors: Scientific Basis, Clinical Investigation and Current Therapy. Baltimore, 1980

Rozental JM: Positron emission tomography (PET) and single photon emission computed tomography (SPECT) of brain tumors. Neurol Clin 9:287–305, 1991

Segall HD, Destian S, Nelson HD et al: CT and MR imaging in malignant gliomas. p. 63. In Apuzzo MLJ (ed): Malignant Cerebral Glioma. American Association of Neurologic Surgeons, Park Ridge, IL, 1990

Thomas DGT, McKeran RO: Clinical manifestations of brain tumors. p. 94. In: Thomas DGT (ed): Neuro-oncology. Primary Malignant Brain Tumors. Johns Hopkins University Press, Baltimore, 1990

Weingarten S, Kleinman M, Elperin L, Larson EB: The effectiveness of cerebral imaging in the diagnosis of chronic headache. Arch Intern Med 152: 2457–62, 1992

Wen PY, Schiff D: Clinical evaluation of patients with astrocytomas. p. 26. In Black PMcL, Schoene W, Lampson LA (eds): Astrocytomas. Blackwell Scientific Publications, Oxford, 1993

149. GENERAL PRINCIPLES OF MANAGEMENT OF PATIENTS WITH BRAIN TUMORS

PATRICK Y. WEN

The management of brain tumor patients requires a multidisciplinary approach, involving the close collaboration of physicians from various specialties including neurology, neurosurgery, radiotherapy, medical oncology, internal medicine, and psychiatry. The management issues can be divided into the definitive treatment of the tumor itself and supportive care. Although neurologists and internists are usually not directly involved in the definitive treatment of brain tumors, they have a crucial role in providing supportive care for these patients.

TREATMENT

Observation

Occasionally, when the patient is asymptomatic and there is strong evidence on radiologic studies that the tumor is "benign" (e.g., a small convexity meningioma), it may be reasonable to observe the patient closely with serial computed tomography (CT) or magnetic resonance imaging (MRI) scans and consider intervention only if the tumor is enlarging or producing symptoms.

For most brain tumors, some form of treatment is usually necessary. As with other neoplasms, the optimal management of brain tumors may involve a combination of treatments including surgery, irradiation, and chemotherapy. By the time a brain tumor produces neurologic symptoms it is usually 20 to 50 g in size (2 to 5 $\times$ 10^{10} cells). Because of the confined intracranial volume, the tumor is usually lethal when it reaches 100 g (10^{11} cells). With some benign tumors, most or all of the tumor can be removed surgically, allowing the patient to be cured. However, for most malignant brain tumors, complete surgical resection is not possible. Even "gross total resection" removes only about 90 percent of the tumor, reducing the tumor burden to 2 to 5 g (2 to 5 $\times$ 10^9 cells). Radiation therapy may kill up to 2 logs of cells (leaving 2 to 5 $\times$ 10^7 cells), and chemotherapy may kill an additional log of cells (leaving 2 to 5 $\times$ 10^6 cells). Unfortunately current combined modality treatment cannot reduce the tumor burden of most malignant brain tumors sufficiently (to 5 $\times$ 10^5 cells) to allow the body's immune mechanisms to eradicate the remaining tumor. As a result, treatment for these tumors is rarely curative.

Surgery

The initial step in the treatment of most brain tumors is surgical resection of as much tumor as is neurologically safe. For some "benign" tumors such as meningiomas, acoustic neuromas, pituitary adenomas, and pilocytic astrocytomas, surgery alone may be curative. Recent advances in surgical techniques including the use of the operating microscope, the cavitron aspirator, intraoperative ultrasound, laser systems, CT- and MRI-guided stereotaxy, and intraoperative neurophysiologic monitoring have greatly improved the safety of surgery. For tumors that cannot be resected, surgery still has a very important role. In addition to allowing a precise histologic diagnosis to be made, it debulks the tumor, relieving any symptoms resulting from mass effect, and possibly increases the effectiveness of adjuvant therapies by reducing the number of cells that must be treated, altering cell kinetics, and removing radioresistant hypoxic cells and areas of tumor inaccessible to chemotherapy. Stereotactic biopsies should be reserved for deep or critically located tumors that cannot be safely resected.

Radiotherapy

Radiotherapy has an important role in the treatment of all malignant brain tumors, as well as some recurrent benign brain tumors. Ionizing radiation acts as a nonspecific cytotoxic agent by causing DNA damage, either directly, or more commonly, indirectly via generation of free radicals. Cell death usually results from the inability of damaged cells to reproduce and is usually seen during the first or subsequent attempts at division. The amount of radiation that can be delivered to the brain is limited by the tolerance of normal tissue. Current radiation doses and fractionation schedules for brain tumors have been developed to take advantage of the greater ability of normal cells to repair DNA damage, compared with tumor cells, and enables the maximum tolerated dose to be administered. Typically for malignant gliomas this is 6,000 cGy in 180- to 200-cGy fractions. Unfortunately most brain tumors are relatively radioresistant and the maximum tolerated doses are usually insufficient to eradicate the tumors completely.

In an attempt to improve on the results of conventional external beam irradiation, several novel strategies have been developed to sensitize tumors selectively to the effects of radiation using radiosensitizers and altered fractionation schedules. Studies are ongoing, but the results have been relatively disappointing. More promising approaches toward improving the effectiveness of radiotherapy are strategies directed at escalating the tumor dose while biologically or physically limiting the dose to normal brain. These include the use of stereotactic brachytherapy, stereotactic radiosurgery, and fractionated stereotactic radiotherapy.

Stereotactic Brachytherapy.   Stereotactic techniques can be used to place catheters containing radioactive isotopes accurately within brain tumors, enabling tumoricidal doses of radiation to be delivered to defined volumes without substantial risk of serious radiation injury to surrounding normal tissues. Typically brachytherapy delivers an additional 5,000 to 6,000 cGy of radiation, increasing the total dose of radiation delivered to the tumor bed above 11,000 cGy. This technique has been used primarily for the treatment of malignant gliomas. In selected glioblastoma patients, brachytherapy increases median survival from 9 to 12 months to 18 to 24 months. Many of these patients develop symptomatic radiation necrosis at the site of implantation and require surgical resection of the necrotic tissue.

Stereotactic Radiosurgery.   Small (less than 4 cm) radiographically well-defined tumors can be treated with a single high-dose fraction of ionizing radiation in stereotactically directed narrow beams. Radiosurgery may be performed using γ-rays from ^{60}Co sources in γ-knives, x-rays from linear accelerators, or charged particle beams from cyclotrons (Fig. 149-1). Like brachytherapy, it significantly increases the radiation dose delivered to the tumor bed while sparing normal brain (Fig. 149-2). Radiosurgery has the advantage over brachytherapy of being noninvasive, which allows patients with tumors in surgically inaccessible or eloquent areas of the brain or serious coexisting medical illnesses to be treated as outpatients. Promising results have been achieved with radiosurgery for the treatment of brain metastases, small malignant gliomas, and a variety of benign brain tumors, including skull base meningiomas, acoustic neuromas, and pituitary tumors not involving the optic chiasm.

Stereotactic Radiotherapy.   A novel technique involving the precise delivery of fractionated radiation to the tumor volume, stereotactic radiotherapy spaces surrounding brain. It combines the accuracy of stereotactic radiosurgery with the reduced toxicity of fractionated external beam irradiation and is likely to be a very useful therapy for a variety of brain tumors, including pituitary adenomas and acoustic neuromas.

Chemotherapy

Chemotherapeutic agents exert their effects primarily by interfering with cell multiplication. The mechanisms of action of the drugs most commonly used for the treatment of brain tumors are summarized in Figure 149-3. Because cell multiplication is a feature of many normal cells as well as tumor cells, most chemotherapeutic agents have toxic effects on normal cells, especially those with a high rate of turnover such as bone marrow. The goal of chemotherapy is to select drugs that inhibit the growth of tumor cells with minimal toxicity to the patient. In addition to the normal problems of drug resistance and toxicity, certain problems are unique to chemotherapy for brain tumors. The most important of these is the presence of the blood–brain

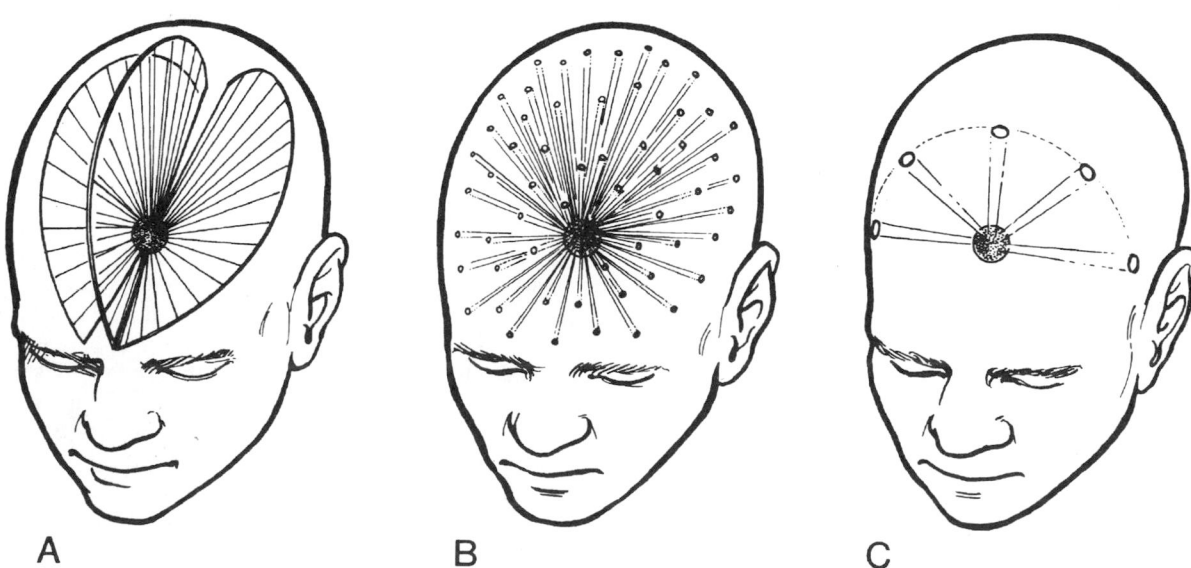

A   B   C

FIG. 149-1.   Points of beam entry into the patient's head with various radiosurgical techniques. **(A)** γ-Unit. **(B)** Linear accelerator with multiple non-coplanar converging arcs. **(C)** Proton beam.

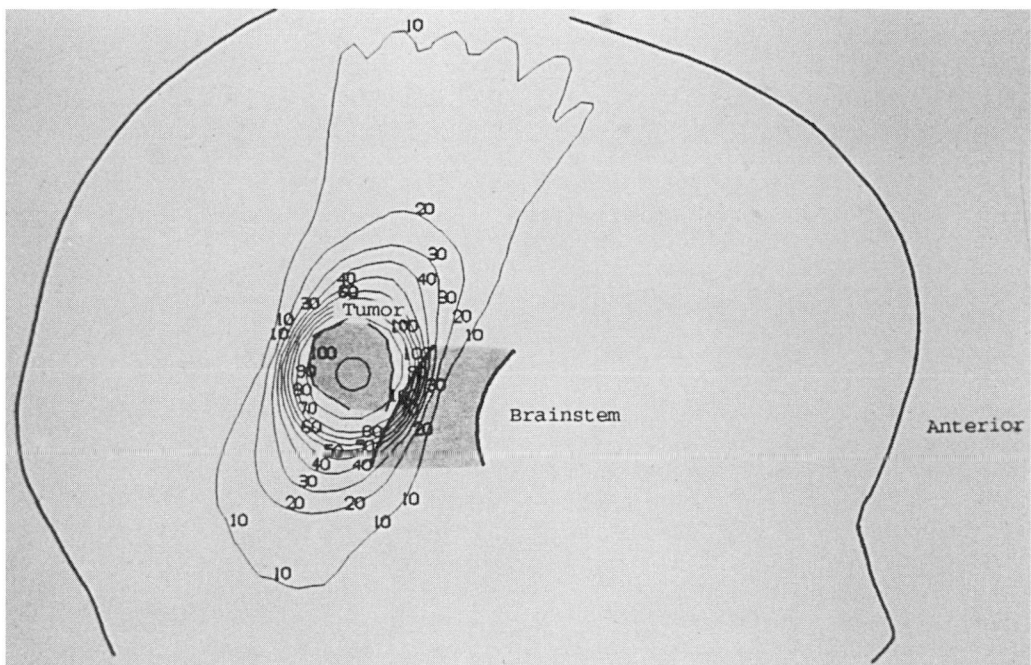

FIG. 149-2.   Diagram showing the isodose curves around a pineal tumor treated with radiosurgery. Note the rapid fall-off in radiation dose to surrounding structures, including the brainstem.

barrier, which limits the passage of water-soluble drugs into the brain. Strategies have been developed to disrupt the blood–brain barrier, using agents such as mannitol and leuco-trienes, to increase the passage of water-soluble drugs into the tumor. Unfortunately these approaches have had only a minimal effect in improving effectiveness of the chemotherapy. Other strategies to increase the effectiveness included the use of intra-carotid injections, administration of the chemotherapy before radiation (neoadjuvant therapy), high-dose chemotherapy with autologous bone marrow transplantation, a combination of chemotherapy with biologic response modifiers, and interstitial chemotherapy, in which a biodegradable polymer, impregnated with a chemotherapeutic agent, is implanted into the tumor bed, resulting in prolonged exposure of the tumor to the drug while minimizing systemic toxicity. Studies evaluating these approaches are currently in progress.

Novel Therapies

Recently, a number of promising new approaches for the treatment of brain tumors have been developed and are in the process of being evaluated in clinical trials. These include immunotherapy, hormonal therapy, differentiating agents, antiangiogenic agents, and gene therapy for malignant gliomas, as well as hormonal therapy for meningiomas.

Participation in Clinical Studies.   Progress in the treatment of patients with brain tumors has been slow, partly because of the rarity of certain tumors, and partly because of the widespread nihilism associated with the treatment of brain tumors: very few patients are enrolled in clinical trials. It is important that physicians caring for patients with brain tumors consider enrolling them in clinical trials so that promising new therapies can be evaluated more rapidly.

SUPPORTIVE THERAPY

In addition to providing definitive treatment, an important role of physicians is to provide effective supportive care. Despite the importance of these management issues, few formal studies exist to guide optimal management.

Anticonvulsants

The treatment of patients with gliomas who present with seizures is straightforward and involves the use of standard anticonvulsants. Electroencephalography may be useful if the diagnosis of seizures is in doubt, but it is not routinely needed for patients who give a clear history of seizures or do not have symptoms suggestive of seizures.

In addition to the usual complications of anticonvulsants, glioma patients experience an increased incidence of particular side effects. Approximately 15 to 20 percent of glioma patients treated with dilantin and undergoing cranial irradiation develop a morbilliform rash, and a small percentage will develop Stevens-Johnson syndrome. The mechanism is unknown but may result from depletion of suppressor T cells by the radiotherapy, allowing a hypersensitivity reaction to phenytoin to develop. Stevens-Johnson syndrome has also been described in glioma patients receiving carbamazepine, whereas patients receiving phenobarbital have an increased incidence of shoulder-hand syndrome.

As well as producing adverse effects, anticonvulsants also have clinically significant interactions with other drugs commonly used in brain tumor patients. Phenytoin induces the hepatic metabolism of dexamethasone and significantly reduces the half-life and bioavailability of this corticosteroid. Conversely, dexamethasone may also reduce phenytoin levels. A number of chemotherapeutic agents commonly used in brain tumor patients such as carmustine (BCNU) interact with phenytoin, causing the levels to fall and potentially leading to

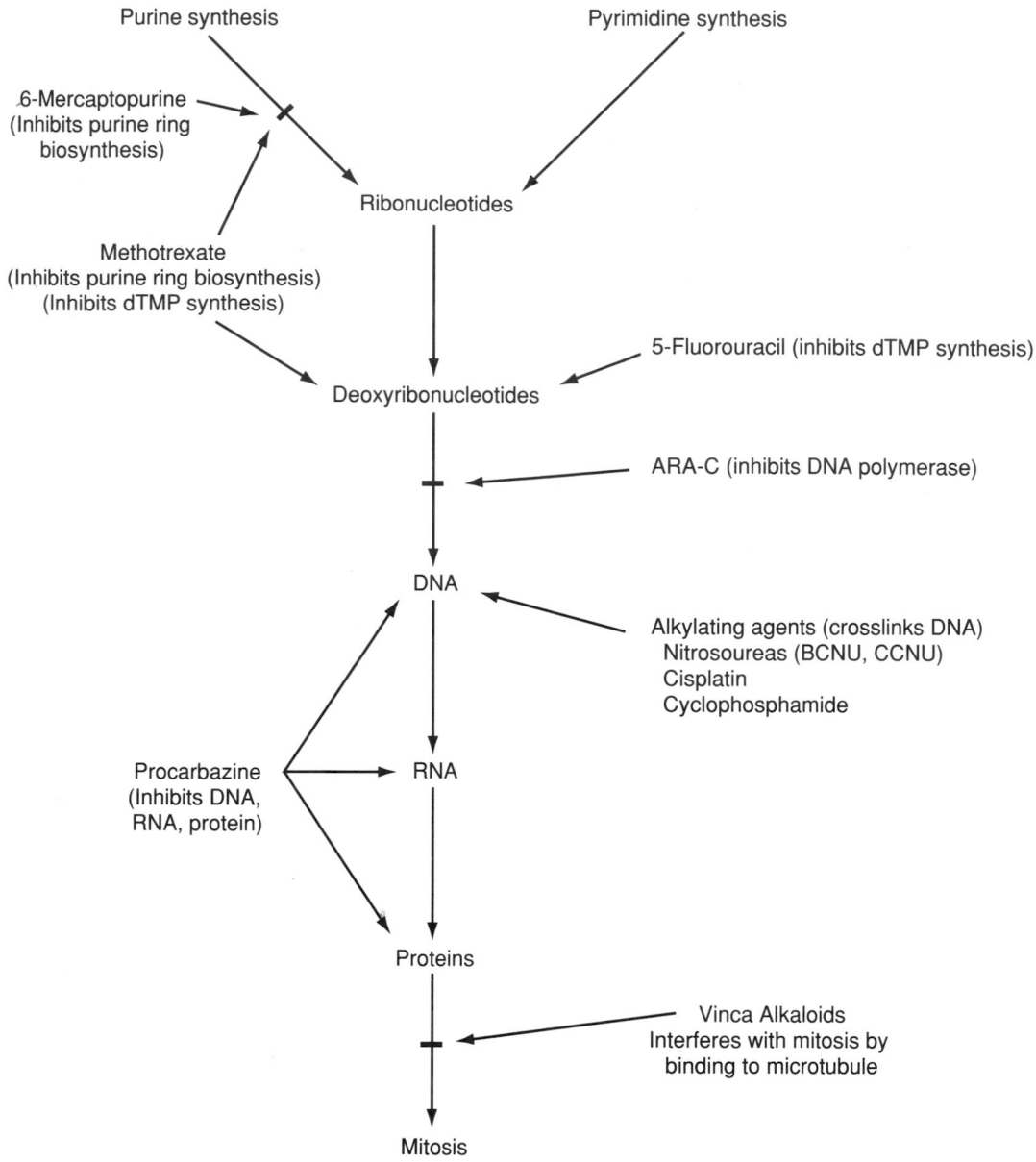

FIG. 149-3. Mechanisms of action of chemotherapeutic agents commonly used in brain tumors.

breakthrough seizures, while phenobarbital may interfere with certain chemotherapeutic agents.

The role of prophylactic anticonvulsant therapy in brain tumor patients who have not had a seizure is controversial. Because the risk of seizures in patients with infratentorial tumors is small, anticonvulsant therapy is usually not indicated. The role of anticonconvulsant therapy in patients with supratentorial tumors who have not had a seizure is unknown. Most of these patients are placed on prophylactic anticonvulsant therapy because they are perceived to be at high risk from seizures and because many of them will be undergoing surgery.

Two small retrospective studies have evaluated the usefulness of anticonvulsant therapy in glioma patients without a history of seizures and have produced conflicting results. Boarini et al. (1985) studied 68 patients, of whom 33 received prophylactic anticonvulsants. Seizures occurred in 39 percent of untreated patients and 21 percent of patients receiving anticonvulsants. Moreover, patients receiving anticonvulsants had fewer generalized seizures. By contrast, Mahaley and Dudka (1981) studied 59 patients and found that the incidence of seizures was higher (39 percent) in patients who received anticonvulsants than in patients who did not (28 percent).

The role of prophylactic anticonvulsant therapy for patients with brain metastases who have not had a seizure is also unknown. In 1988 Cohen et al. retrospectively reviewed 160 patients with brain metastases who had not had a seizure and found that those patients receiving prophylactic anticonvulsant therapy with dilantin had the same frequency of late seizures (10 percent) as patients receiving no treatment. More recently, Glantz et al. (1994) conducted a small prospective, placebo-controlled, randomized study evaluating the efficacy of valproic acid in protecting patients with newly diagnosed brain metastases from seizures. No significant difference in seizure frequency was found at 7 months (20 percent) between patients receiving valproic acid or placebo, suggesting that prophylactic anticonvulsants may not be effective in these patients.

Many brain tumor patients are treated with anticonvulsants partly because they have had a craniotomy. The issue of whether prophylactic anticonvulsant therapy reduces the frequency of seizures after craniotomy is unclear. Early studies such as that of North et al. (in 1983) found that prophylactic anticonvulsants reduced the frequency of postoperative seizures. However, analysis of their data showed that most of the increased seizure frequency in the patients receiving placebo occurred in the first postoperative week. More recently (1992) Foy et al. completed a prospective trial involving 276 consecutive supratentorial craniotomy patients who were randomized postoperatively to receive either carbamazepine or phenytoin, or no treatment. No difference in the incidence of seizures (37 percent) or death was found between the two groups, suggesting that prophylactic anticonvulsant therapy may not be routinely needed after craniotomy.

Because of the increased incidence of allergic reactions in patients with brain tumors receiving anticonvulsant therapy, and the lack of clear evidence that anticonvulsant therapy reduces the incidence of seizures, routine anticonvulsant therapy in brain tumor patients who have not experienced a seizure is probably unecessary. Possible exceptions are patients with brain metastases in areas of high epileptogenicity (e.g., motor cortex) and patients with tumors invading the cortex, such as melanoma. These patients probably have a higher incidence of seizures and may benefit from prophylactic anticonvulsant therapy. Patients who do a significant amount of driving may also benefit from prophylactic anticonvulsants. Several prospective randomized studies are currently in progress evaluating the role of prophylactic anticonvulsants in patients with newly diagnosed brain tumors. These studies will provide much needed guidance on the optimal use of anticonvulsants in these patients.

Treatment of Peritumoral Edema

The vasogenic edema surrounding many brain tumors contributes significantly to the morbidity associated with the tumors. This edema results from disruption of the blood–brain barrier, allowing protein-rich fluid to accumulate in the extracellular space. This breakdown of the blood–brain barrier is caused by the absence of tight endothelial cell junctions in tumor blood vessels and the production of factors such as vascular permeability factor, glutamate, and leukotrienes, which increase the permeability of tumor vessels.

Most brain tumor patients with peritumoral edema can be adequately managed with corticosteroids. Occasionally when significant intracranial pressure (ICP) and mass effect exist, other measures may be required.

Acute Treatment of Increased Intracranial Pressure. Corticosteroids may take several days to reduce ICP from peritumoral edema. Some brain tumor patients present acutely with significantly increased ICP and may require other measures to lower the pressure until corticosteroids have had a chance to take effect or until the patient undergoes a craniotomy and debulking procedure. These measures include:

1. Elevation of the head of the bed (more than 30 degrees). This displaces cerebrospinal fluid from the intracranial cavity and enhances cerebral venous outflow.
2. Fluid restriction (1 to 1.5 L/day).
3. Osmotic agents. Agents such as mannitol, which are relatively impermeable to the blood–brain barrier, are com-

monly used for the short-term treatment of increased ICP. These agents decrease ICP by reducing total brain water, creating an osmotic gradient toward the intravascular space. Mannitol may also decrease ICP by increasing erythrocyte deformability and hemodilution with decreased blood viscosity. Mannitol is usually given at an initial dose of 0.75 to 1.0 g/kg followed by 0.25 to 0.5 g/kg every 3 to 5 hours, aiming for a target osmolality of 300 to 310 mOsm/L. The effect of mannitol on ICP is usually achieved within 10 to 30 minutes after administration, with maximal ICP reduction within 20 to 60 minutes. Complications of therapy with osmotic agents include hypokalemia, hypochloremic alkalosis, dehydration, hypotension, nonketotic hyperosmolar state, and rebound intracranial hypertension after prolonged use.
4. Diuretics. These are effective for the short-term treatment of increased ICP, especially when used in combination with osmotic therapy. They produce a mild osmotic diuresis (resulting in an osmotic gradient toward the intravascular space), reduce cerebrospinal fluid formation, and remove sodium and water from the brain. Loop diuretics, such as furosemide (20 to 40 mg) are most commonly used. Administration of furosemide 15 minutes after administration of mannitol appears to be the most effective in lowering ICP. The main side effects of loop diuretics are electrolyte disturbance and systemic dehydration.
5. Hyperventilation is an effective short-term measure used to reduce ICP. It produces hypocarbia and lowers ICP by reducing cerebral blood volume. The reduction in ICP is rapid, although the maximal effect may follow the change in PCO_2 by 15 to 30 minutes. Usually the PCO_2 is gradually lowered to 25 to 35 mmHg to achieve the desired ICP. The ICP gradually returns to baseline despite hyperventilation, making this an effective treatment for increased ICP only in the short term.

Corticosteroids. Corticosteroids are usually indicated in any brain tumor patient who is symptomatic from peritumoral edema. They produce their antiedema effect by reducing the permeability of tumor capillaries, limiting the leakage of sodium, protein, and water into the peritumoral extracellular space. Corticosteroids may also increase the clearance of peritumoral edema by facilitating the transport of fluid into the ventricular system, from which it is cleared by cerebrospinal fluid bulk flow.

Most patients are usually started on dexamethasone (or an equivalent steroid) at a dose of 16 mg/d. Although this is often given in four divided doses, its biologic half-life is sufficiently long to allow the medication to be administered twice daily. Most patients improve within 48 to 72 hours. In general, headaches tend to respond better than focal deficits. If 16 mg of dexamethasone is insufficient, the dose may be increased up to 100 mg/d. Despite the usefulness of corticosteroids, they are associated with a large number of well-known side effects (Table 149-1).

Three complications of corticosteroid therapy are of particular concern to brain tumor patients. These include gastrointestinal complications, steroid myopathy, and opportunistic infections such as *Pneumocystis carinii* pneumonitis (PCP).

GASTROINTESTINAL COMPLICATIONS. Most brain tumor patients receiving corticosteroids are treated with H_2 blockers or antacids to prevent peptic ulceration and upper gastrointestinal hemorrhage. However, the relationship between corticosteroids

TABLE 149-1. Complications of Corticosteroid Therapy

Type	Complication
Neurologic	Common
	Behavioral changes, insomnia, myopathy, hallucinations, hiccups, tremor, reduced taste and smell, cerebral atrophy
	Uncommon
	Psychosis, dementia, seizures, dependence, paraparesis (epidural lipomatosis)
Dermatologic	Thin, fragile skin, purpura, echymosis; striae, hirsuitism; acne, inhibition of wound healing, Kaposi's sarcoma
Rheumatologic	Osteoporosis, avascular necrosis, growth retardation, tendinous rupture
Gastrointestinal	Increased appetite, abdominal bloating, gastrointestinal bleeding and perforation, pancreatitis, liver hypertrophy
Opthalmologic	Visual blurring, cataract, glaucoma, exopthalmos, uveitis
Cardiovascular	Hypertension, atheroscleosis, arrhythmia (with IV push).
Endocrine/metabolic	Hyperglycemia, hypokalemia, hypophosphatemia, hypernatremia, hyperlipidemia, redistribution of body fat (centripetal obesity, buffalo hump, and so forth), amenorrhea
Urogenital	Polyuria, genital burning (with IV push)
Miscellaneous	Opportunistic infections (including candidiasis, *Pneumocystis carinii* pneumonitis), hypersensitivity reactions, neutrophilia, lymphopenia, night sweats
Steroid withdrawal	Pseudorheumatism (very common), headache, lethargy, low-grade fever, adrenal insufficiency, pseudotumor cerebri

(Adapted from Delattre JY, Posner JB: Neurologic complications of chemotherapy and radiation therapy. p. 421. In Aminoff MJ (ed): Neurology and General Medicine. 2nd Ed. Churchill Livingstone, New York, 1994, with permission.)

and peptic ulceration and gastrointestinal bleeding remains controversial. The widespread impression that corticosteroids are potentially ulcerogenic originated from observations that stress produced acute ulcers, as well as anecdotal studies suggesting that corticosteroids increase and alter the composition of gastric acid secretion. Theoretically an association between corticosteroid therapy and peptic ulceration could be established by a prospective randomized clinical trial. However, such a trial is unlikely ever to occur because of the low incidence of peptic ulceration and the difficulty in recruiting sufficient patients. Several meta-analyses of placebo-controlled trials evaluating the use of corticosteroids in a variety of diseases have been conducted to determine if an association exists between corticosteroid therapy and peptic ulceration and gastrointestinal bleeding. The results have been conflicting, with some studies showing no statistically significant association between corticosteroid use and upper gastrointestinal tract bleeding, and others showing a small association.

At present, the available data do not definitively support an association between corticosteroids and peptic ulceration and gastrointestinal bleeding. Even if an association exists, the overall incidence of peptic ulceration and gastrointestinal bleeding is very low. Few data are available on the risk of peptic ulceration and gastrointestinal bleeding, or the effectiveness of prophylactic therapy with H_2-blockers in brain tumor patients, who often take high doses of steroids. Whereas these medications are relatively benign, some H_2-blockers (e.g., cimetidine) can produce central nervous system side effects such as confusion, and most H_2-blockers are expensive. In the absence of data from clinical studies guiding the use of H_2-blockers in brain tumor patients, the use of these medications should probably be restricted to the perioperative period and to patients receiving very high doses of corticosteroids. For most other patients, prophylactic therapy with H_2 blockers is probably unnecessary unless they are at high risk for developing peptic ulceration (previous history of peptic ulcers, anticoagulation or nonsteroidal anti-inflammatory drug administration, and old age).

A less well-recognized complication of steroid therapy is perforation of the gastrointestinal tract. This is frequently difficult to diagnose because clinical features of peritonitis may be masked by the steroids. Such perforation can often be averted by prevention of constipation. A high index of suspicion is also important since early diagnosis improves the outcome of this serious complication.

STEROID MYOPATHY. Myopathy is a common complication of steroid therapy and contributes significantly to the morbidity of patients with brain tumors. The reported incidences of steroid myopathy in brain tumor patients varies from 2 to 21 percent, with the largest series reporting clinically symptomatic steroid myopathy in 10.6 percent of patients. It can frequently be prevented by using the lowest possible dose of steroids needed to prevent symptoms resulting from peritumoral edema.

Steroid myopathy usually occurs with prolonged steroid therapy; most patients develop weakness between the 9th and 12th weeks of treatment. Variation of individual susceptibility is marked. Some patients become weak after using a low dose of steroids for a few weeks, whereas others never develop problems despite receiving large doses of steroids for months or years. Steroid myopathy has been especially associated with the use of 9-α-fluorinated corticosteroids such as dexamethasone, but the evidence supporting this relationship is relatively weak. Steroid myopathy usually has a subacute onset over several weeks. It is characterized by weakness and wasting in pelvifemoral muscles, especially the quadriceps, and may eventually spread to the pectoral girdle, neck, and trunk. Eventually all limb muscles may become weak, but a proximal emphasis persists. Muscle pain is not a feature and tendon reflexes are preserved.

Serum creatine phosphokinase, aldolase, and other muscle enzyme levels are almost invariably normal. Electromyography is commonly unrevealing. Occasionally mild myopathic changes may be seen without abnormal irritability or spontaneous discharges. Muscle biopsy results are nonspecific but may show atrophy, involving especially type IIb muscle fibers.

The precise pathophysiology of steroid myopathy is unknown. It is likely that steroids exert their effects through inhibition of protein synthesis and increased protein catabolism. Interestingly, the risk of developing steroid myopathy is significantly lower in patients taking phenytoin, for reasons that are unclear; possibly phenytoin induces hepatic metabolism of dexamethasone, reducing the effective exposure of muscle cells to the glucocorticoids.

Treatment of steroid myopathy is difficult. Ideally the steroid should be discontinued but if this is not feasible, the lowest possible dose should be used. Recovery after stopping steroid therapy can be expected in 2 to 3 months but may be much slower if treatment is continued at a reduced dose. Anecdotal reports suggest that weakness occurring during treatment with fluorinated corticosteroids improves when the drugs are replaced by an eqivalent dose of nonfluorinated steroid. Animal studies suggest that muscle activity may reduce steroid-induced wasting, raising the possibility that a program of physical therapy may potentially help to reduce the severity of myopathy in patients receiving long-term steroid therapy.

PNEUMOCYSTIS CARINI PNEUMONITIS. *Pneumocystis carinii* is a unicellular eukaryote capable of causing life-threatening pneumonitis in immunocompromised patients. It is most common in patients with the Acquired immunodeficiency syndrome but is also being seen with increasing frequency in other immunosuppressed patients such as organ transplant recipients and patients with hematologic malignancies.

PCP is rare in patients with solid tumors but may occur in these patients in the setting of steroid therapy. Increasing evidence shows that patients with brain tumors receiving corticosteroids may be at increased risk of PCP, especially during the steroid taper. The mechanisms by which steroids predispose to the development of PCP are poorly understood, but they involve suppression of cellular immunity, leading to reactivation of latent infection by *P. carinii.*

Physicians caring for brain tumor patients receiving steroids should maintain a high index of suspicion for PCP. Although the clinical features of PCP are usually those of an acute diffuse pneumonia, the presentation can be subtle and nonspecific, and the diagnosis should be considered in any patient developing respiratory symptoms. The diagnosis is usually made by visualization of the organism in sputum, fluid obtained by bronchoalveolar lavage, or transbronchial biopsy. Toluidine blue O, Gram-Weigert, and Grocott-Gomori methenamine silver nitrate stains are useful for detecting the cyst wall, whereas Giemsa stains detect the internal forms (sporozoites or trophozoites).

Trimethoprim sulfamethoxazole (TMP/sulfa) is the treatment of choice for PCP if the patient can tolerate it. The standard doses are trimethoprim (15 to 20 mg/kg) and sulfamethoxazole (75 to 100 mg/kg) IV or PO for 21 days. Intravenous pentamidine (3 to 4 mg/kg IV daily for 21 days) is as effective as TMP/sulfa but is less often used since it requires intravenous administration and is associated with greater toxicity. Patients with established PCP may paradoxically benefit from treatment with corticosteroids. The steroids reduce the inflammatory response of the alveolitis and result in clinical improvement and possibly reduced mortality.

Because of the risk of PCP, it may be prudent to consider prophylactic therapy against PCP for brain tumor patients re-ceiving prolonged courses of corticosteroids. Trimethoprim/sulfa is highly effective in the prophylaxis of PCP. The optimal dosage has not been established, but it is effective when administered either as a single dose daily (e.g., Bactrim DS (160 mg of trimethoprim plus 800 mg of sulfamethoxazole) or 3 days a week. Adverse reactions are infrequent in patients with brain tumors. For patients with allergic reactions to TMP/sulfa, aerosolized pentamidine is an effective alternative.

Venous Thromboembolic Disease

Venous thromboembolic disease is common in patients with brain tumors. In one recent study of patients with high-grade gliomas, all of whom were ambulatory and outside the perioperative period, 19 percent developed either deep vein thrombosis or pulmonary emboli. This risk is increased to 37 to 60 percent in the postoperative period and in hemiplegia. The incidence of venous thromboembolic disease is also increased in patients with other types of brain tumors such as meningiomas (72 percent), brain metastases (20 percent), and primary CNS lymphoma (18 percent).

The pathogenesis of venous thromboembolism in brain tumor patients is not completely understood. Contributing factors include venous stasis in hemiparetic limbs, as well as release of procoagulant substances (e.g., vascular endothelial growth factor) and fibrinolytic inhibitors from tumor tissue and surrounding cerebral tissue, leading to subclinical chronic disseminated intravascular coagulation.

The optimal therapy for venous thromboembolic disease in patients with brain tumors is unknown. These patients are often perceived to be at increased risk of intracranial hemorrhage with anticoagulation because of the vascularity of the tumors and anecdotal case reports of hemorrhage. Certain metastatic tumors, such as melanoma and choriocarcinoma, may have a

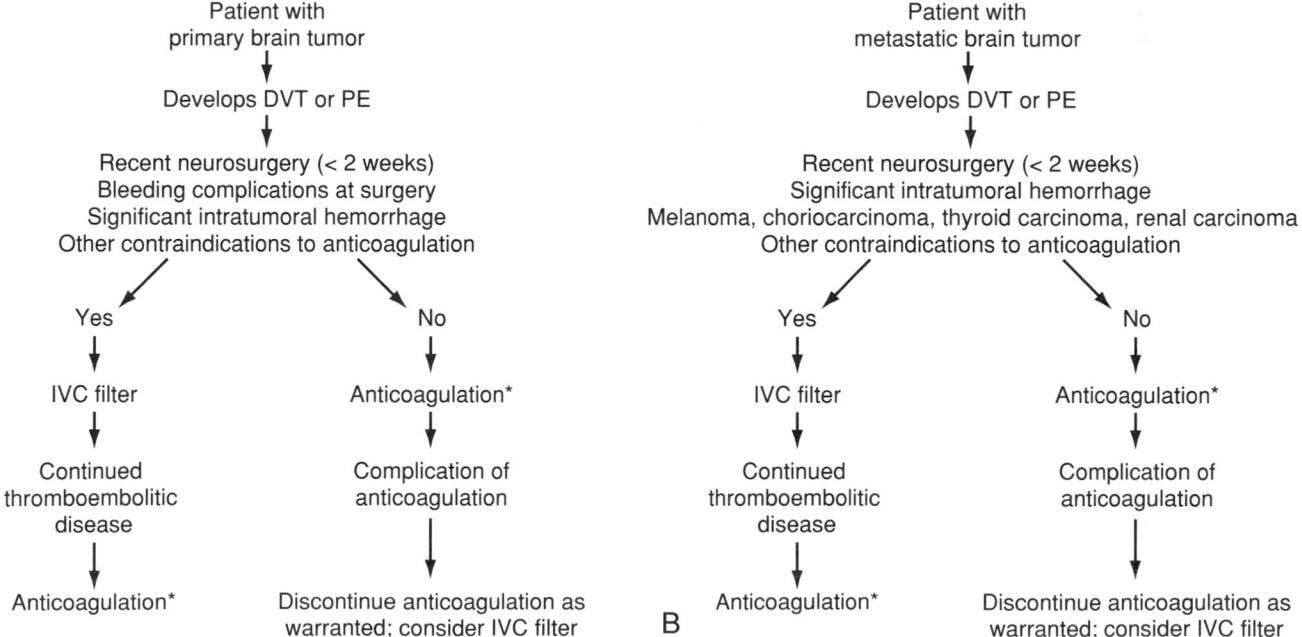

FIG. 149-4. Algorithm for treating patients with brain tumor and venous thromboembolism. **(A)** Treatment of patients with primary brain tumor. **(B)** Treatment of patients with metastatic brain tumor. Anticoagulation in both cases is performed initially with warfarin. If thrombosis or thromboembolism persists, treatment with subcutaneous heparin, 10,000 units two to three times a day, should be considered. The activated partial thromboplastin time should be twice the control level. DVT, deep venous thrombosis; IVC, inferior vena cava.

particularly high propensity for hemorrhage. As a result, most brain tumor patients with deep venous thrombosis and pulmonary emboli are managed with inferior vena cava filtration devices rather than anticoagulation.

However, several retrospective studies have suggested that the risk of intracranial hemorrhage in brain tumor patients receiving anticoagulation outside the immediate postoperative period may not be significantly increased (0 to 7 percent). Moreover, a recent study by Levin et al. (1993) suggests that brain tumor patients with venous thromboembolic disease treated with inferior vena cava filters experience a high percentage of complications (67 percent) such as recurrent deep venous thromboses and postphlebitic syndrome, which severely reduce the quality of life of the affected patients.

Because of the high complication rate in patients treated with inferior vena cava filters, as well as evidence suggesting that the risk of the anticoagulation in these patients is not increased, consideration should be given to treating venous thromboembolic disease in brain tumor patients with anticoagulation rather than such filters (Fig. 149-4).

Rehabilitation

Many brain tumor patients have significant neurologic deficits and benefit from physical, occupational, and speech therapy. The details of rehabilitation are discussed in greater detail in Chapter 228.

Emotional and Psychological Support

The diagnosis of a brain tumor inevitably has a profound and often devastating effect on patients and their families. An important aspect of care includes supplying information about the tumor and the therapeutic options in a compassionate manner, as well as giving emotional and psychological support. Patients and their families will frequently benefit from the help provided by patient support groups, psychiatrists, and societies such as the American Brain Tumor Association (3725 North Talman Avenue, Chicago, IL 60618; Tel: 312-286-5571; Patient Line: 1-800-886-2282), the Brain Tumor Society (60 Leo M. Birmingham Parkway, Brighton, MA 02135; Tel: 617-783-0340), and the National Brain Tumor Foundation (323 Geary Street, Suite 510, San Francisco, CA 994102; Tel: 1-800-934-CURE [2873]).

Terminal Care

Despite some important advances in recent years, most patients with malignant brain tumors eventually die from their disease.

When further therapy is no longer possible or not warranted because of the poor quality of the patient's life, all efforts should be directed toward keeping the patient comfortable and avoiding unnecessary prolongation of suffering.

SUGGESTED READINGS

Boarini D, Beck DW, Van Guilder JC: Post-operative prophylactic anticonvulsant therapy in cerebral gliomas. Neurosurgery 16:290–2, 1985

Cohen N, Strauss G, Lew R et al: Should prophylactic anticonvulsants be administered to patients with newly-diagnosed cerebral metastases? A retrospective analysis. J Clin Oncol 6:1621–4, 1988

Conn HO, Blitzer BL: Non-association of adrenocorticosteroid therapy and peptic ulcer. N Engl J Med 294:473–9, 1976

Conn HO, Poynard T: Adrenocorticosteroid administration and peptic ulcer: a critical analysis. J Chron Dis 38:457–68, 1985

Delattre J, Safai B, Posner JB: Erythema multiforme and Stevens-Johnson syndrome in patients receiving cranial irradiation and phenytoin. Neurology 38:194–8, 1988

Delattre JY, Posner JB: Neurologic complications of chemotherapy and radiation therapy. p. 421. In Aminoff MJ (ed): Neurology and General Medicine. 2nd Ed. Churchill Livingstone, New York, 1994

Dropcho EJ, Soong SJ: Steroid-induced weakness in patients with primary brain tumors. Neurology 41:1235–9, 1991

Eidelberg D: Neurological effects of steroid treatment. p. 173. In Rottenberg DA (ed): Neurological Complications of Cancer Treatment. Butterworth-Heinemann, Boston, 1991

Eidelberg D: Steroid myopathy. p. 185. In Rottenberg DA (ed): Neurological Complications of Cancer Treatment. Butterworth-Heinemann, Boston, 1991

Fadul CE, Lemann W, Thaler HT, Posner JB: Perforation of the gastrointestinal tract in patients receiving steroids for neurologic disease. Neurology 38: 348–52, 1988

Foy PM, Chadwick DW, Rajgopalan N et al: Do prophylactic anticonvulsant drugs alter the pattern of seizures after craniotomy. J Neurol Neurosurg Psychiatry 55:753–7, 1992

Glantz M, Friedberg M, Cole B et al: Double blind, randomized, placebo-controlled trial of anticonvulsant prophylaxis in adults with newly diagnosed brain metastases. Proc Annu Meet Am Soc Clin Oncol 13:A492, 1994

Hensen JW, Jalaj JK, Walker RW et al: *Pneumocystis carinii* pneumonia in patients with primary brain tumors. Arch Neurol 48:406–9, 1991

Labar DR: Prophylactic antiepileptic medications after craniotomy. Neurol Alert 11:27–8, 1992

Levin JM, Schiff, Loeffler JS et al: Complications of therapy for venous thromboembolic disease in patients with brain tumors. Neurology 43:1111–4, 1993

Mahaley M, Dudka L: The role of anticonvulsant mediciations in the management of patients with anaplastic gliomas. Surg Neurol 16:399–401, 1981

Messer J, Reitman D, Sacks HS et al: Association of adrenocorticosteroid therapy and peptic-ulcer disease. N Engl J Med 309:21–4, 1983

North JB, Penhall RK, Hanieh A et al: Phenytoin and postoperative epilepsy. J Neurosurg 58:672–7, 1983

Schiff D, DeAngelis LM: Therapy of venous thromboembolism in patients with brain metastases. Cancer 73:493–8, 1994

Spiro HM: Is the steroid ulcer a myth? N Engl J Med 309:45–7, 1983

Wen PY, Black PB: Clinical presentation, evaluation and preoperative preparation of the patient. In Berger MS, Wilson CB (ed): Textbook of Gliomas WB Saunders, Philadelphia (in press)

SECTION 2. BRAIN TUMORS: SPECIFIC TUMOR TYPES

150. LOW-GRADE GLIOMAS

RAUL F. VALENZUELA
FRED H. HOCHBERG

Low-grade gliomas account for approximately 10 to 20 percent of primary brain tumors in adults and a higher percentage in children. They are a heterogenous group of slowly growing tumors with a relatively good prognosis that usually appear as nonenhancing lesions on computed tomography (CT) or magnetic resonance imaging (MRI) (Table 150-1). Most low-grade gliomas are astrocytomas, with smaller numbers of oligodendrogliomas, oligoastrocytomas, and gangliogliomas (Table 150-1).

These tumors have differing radiologic and microscopic appearances and vary in their natural histories and response to treatment. For example, surgery may be curative for cerebellar pilocytic astrocytomas but is of little benefit for astrocytomas within the pons or medulla, whereas patients with oligodendrogliomas or mixed low-grade astrocytomas tend to respond to chemotherapy. Regardless of the precise histology, low-grade gliomas can produce significant morbidity in patients who are often in the prime of their lives.

DIAGNOSIS

Clinical Features

Patients with low-grade gliomas typically present with seizures, headaches, disorders of memory or personality, or focal neurologic signs. Seizures are the most common presenting symptom and occur in 60 to 90 percent of patients with low-grade gliomas. Conversely, the incidence of an underlying tumor in patients presenting with seizures is approximately 7 percent in adolescents and 20 percent in older adults. Frequently, patients will have experienced seizures for many years before the low-grade glioma is diagnosed. Occasionally patients will present with a more acute course as a result of hemorrhage or cystic degeneration within a long-standing mass.

Imaging

Low-grade gliomas appear as diffuse nonenhancing, hypodense masses on CT scans and as nonenhancing, low-signal-intensity masses on T1-weighted MRI images and high-signal-intensity masses on T2-weighted image (Table 150-1, Fig. 150-1). Frequently, the areas of abnormality distort normal anatomy. The cortical gyri are compressed, deformed, or thickened, and effacement of the ipsilateral ventricles may be noted. These appearances may be difficult to distinguish from an area of infarction, encephalomalacia, demyelination, inflammation, or infection. Some low-grade gliomas have characteristic appearances. Pilocytic astrocytomas of the cerebellum are characterized by cysts containing enhancing mural nodules. Calcification or hemorrhage are frequently seen within oligodendrogliomas and oligoastrocytomas. Enhancement usually suggests a more malignant pathology in most gliomas but is a frequent finding in patients with pilocytic astrocytoma and ganglioglioma. Increasingly, patients are being diagnosed with incidental low-grade gliomas on CT or MRI scans performed for the evaluation of head trauma or symptoms unrelated to the underlying tumor.

TABLE 150-1. Features of Low-Grade Gliomas

Tumor	Age Group (years)	Location	Appearance	Survival (years)	Therapy
Astrocytoma	35–40	Frontal, temporal	Nonenhancing mass	5–8	Biopsy Resection if possible Radiotherapy for incompletely resected tumor
Subependymal giant cell astrocytoma	10–20	Ventricular	"Candle dripping"	Extended	Observation Occasional surgery
Pleomorphic xanthoastrocytoma	10–30	Frontal, temporal	Enhancing superficial mass	Extended	Surgery
Oligodendroglioma	30–50	Subcortical	Calcified, nonenhancing mass AO usually enhances	6–10 3 (AO)	Surgery Radiotherapy for inoperable or incompletely resected tumor Chemotherapy for AO
Oligoastrocytoma	40–50	Subcortical	Nonenhancing mass May be calcified	6	Surgery Radiotherapy Chemotherapy (PCV)
Ganglioglioma	10–30	Temporal, frontal	Variably enhancing hypodense mass	Extended (>80% at 10 yr)	Surgery
Pilocytic astrocytoma	10–20	Cerebellum, optic nerve, hypothalamus	Cyst with enhancing nodule	Extended (> 20 yr)	Surgery if possible Radiotherapy for inoperable tumors

Abbreviations: AO, anaplastic oligodendroglioma; PCV, procarbazine, lomustine, and vincristine.

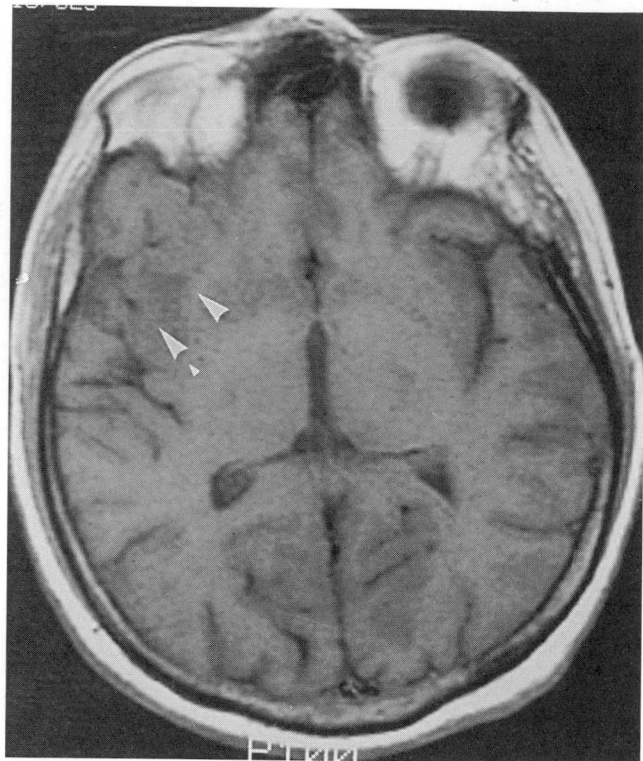

FIG. 150-1. Patient presented at age 31 with complex partial seizures. A CT scan showed a hypodense, non-contrast-enhancing lesion (*arrowheads*) and a needle biopsy demonstrated a well-differentiated oligoastrocytoma. Subsequent serial MRI studies continued to show a stable, non-contrast-enhancing lesion in the right temporal-frontal area as depicted here. He remained seizure-free under standard antiepileptic treatment.

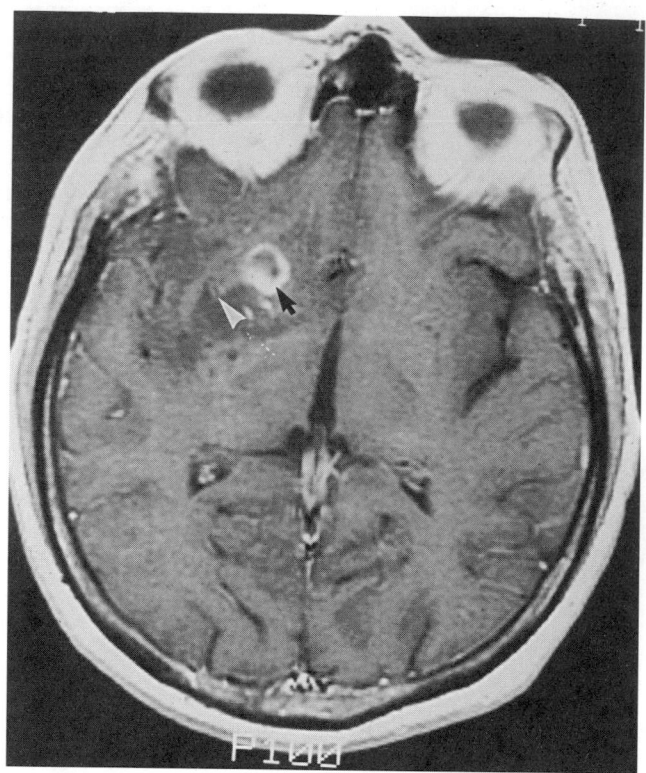

FIG. 150-2. The same patient as in Fig. 150-1 ten years after his original diagnosis. He presented with increasingly frequent partial complex seizures. MRI showed a new area of enhancement (*arrow*) within the original lesion (*arrowhead*). A needle biopsy showed progression to glioblastoma multiforme. The tumor still had a oligodendrocytic component.

Newer imaging modalities may be used to evaluate patients with low-grade gliomas, especially in helping to determine tumor grade. Positron emission tomography (PET) utilizing [18]fluorodeoxyglucose (FDG) measures glucose uptake within tumor. Low-grade gliomas usually have decreased glucose metabolism. Areas of increased glucose metabolism correlate with foci of aggressive change within benign masses and can be used to help neurosurgeons select targets for stereotactic biopsy. Single-photon-emission computed tomography (SPECT) utilizing [20]Tl has been proposed as a less expensive alternative to PET. Thallium uptake ratios (uptake of thallium in the tumor relative to a contralateral region) below 1.4 suggest a low-grade glioma. Measurement of cerebral blood volume (CBV maps) within tumors using ultrafast echoplanar MRI has also been used to grade gliomas. Sequential scans every second are performed following venous injection of gadolinium-diethylenetriamine pentaacetic acid or gadodiamide to provide measurements of tissue concentrations during its first pass through brain vasculature. These concentrations are proportional to the local vascular supply. High-grade foci of tumor within low-grade gliomas have elevated capillary CBV. CBV mapping correlates with both glucose uptake on PET scans and tumor histology as seen on biopsy.

PATHOLOGY

Low-grade astrocytomas are thought to arise from either type I astrocytes or O2A precursor cells, which can differentiate into type 2 astrocytes and oligodendrocytes. Oligodendrogliomas arise from oligodendrocytes or O2A cells.

Low-grade gliomas are well-differentiated glial neoplasms showing mild-to-moderate increase in cellularity and slight cellular atypia. They usually do not have features such as endothelial proliferation, a high degree of cellularity, mitoses, or necrosis, which are found in high-grade gliomas. Low-grade astrocytomas are usually classified as grade I or II in the World Health Organization or St. Anne-Mayo systems and grade I in the Modified Ringertz system. The classification of oligodendrogliomas and oligoastrocytomas is less well defined, but they are usually classified as grade I or II in the St. Anne-Mayo systems and grade A in the Smith system.

The Problem of Malignant Dedifferentiation

Although low-grade gliomas are often considered histologically ''benign'' tumors, they produce significant morbidity and usually result in a shortened life expectancy. Between 50 and 80 percent of patients with low-grade gliomas will eventually develop a malignant glioma (Fig. 150-2). This transformation usually occurs between 3 and 7 years after diagnosis and results from sequential genetic alterations. The early low-grade tumor stages usually involve mutations that inactivate the p53 tumor suppressor gene on the short arm of chromosome 17. Later on, loss of chromosome 10 results in the transformation to glioblastoma multiforme. Oligodendroglioma and oligoastrocytoma have a similar tendency to undergo malignant differentiation, but the genetic abnormalities involve chromosome 19. Once transformation to a higher grade occurs, the prognosis is generally very poor.

THERAPY

The optimal management of patients with presumed low-grade gliomas is controversial. Although patients with large, symptomatic, enlarging tumors clearly require surgery, the most appropriate treatment for patients who present with seizures or headaches and are found on imaging studies to have a nonenhancing, hypodense lesion is often unclear. The therapeutic options for these lesions, which are presumed to be low-grade gliomas, range from observation alone to surgery plus postoperative radiation.

Proponents of a conservative approach suggest observing the patient and considering surgery and radiotherapy only if the tumors are symptomatic or if evidence of tumor growth exists. Reasons cited for this approach include the indolent nature of these tumors, the lack of data from prospective studies supporting the superiority of aggressive early treatment, and concerns about the long-term neurotoxicity of radiation therapy. A study by Recht et al. provides some support for this conservative approach. In a retrospective review of patients with suspected low-grade gliomas, they found no difference in survival or quality of life between those who were treated immediately compared with those who received treatment only when clinical or radiologic evidence of tumor progression emerged. The projected median survival in both groups was 84 months. Most authors, however, favor early intervention. The reasons for this approach include uncertainty about a diagnosis based only on radiologic findings (approximately 4 to 10 percent of glioblastomas and 30 to 50 percent of anaplastic astrocytomas do not enhance; a cold PET scan or CBV map supports the diagnosis of low-grade glioma but is not definitive), the generally poor prognosis of patients with astrocytomas, and the tendency for these tumors to dedifferentiate to a more anaplastic state.

Surgery

The role of surgery varies with the location and histology of the low-grade glioma. The goals of surgery are to (1) establish a histologic diagnosis, (2) alleviate symptoms by debulking the tumor, (3) improve prognosis and potentially cure the patient, and (4) remove the epileptogenic focus if the patient is experiencing seizures. The specific kind of surgery depends on the objectives.

Stereotactic Biopsy. A stereotactic biopsy is usually performed to obtain tissue for histologic diagnosis from deep-seated tumors or tumors in eloquent areas or to obtain a histologic diagnosis prior to proceeding with a definitive resection of more accessible tumors. The risks of stereotactic biopsy are small, but sampling errors can occur, since gliomas typically have highly heterogeneous histologies, and areas of high-grade tumor may be missed by the stereotactic biopsy. The use of functional imaging (PET, CBV mapping) may be useful in helping the surgeon to biopsy areas of the tumor that are most likely to show a higher grade histology. However, the larger amounts of tissue available when tumor resection is carried out generally provide a more accurate diagnosis of histologic grade.

Craniotomy. Surgical resection allows the tumor to be debulked (relieving symptoms produced by mass effect), prolongs

survival, improves seizure control, and possibly reduces the risk of the tumor transforming to a higher grade. Surgery may be curative for pilocytic astrocytomas, but although it prolongs survival, it is rarely curative for patients with infiltrative tumors such as fibrillary or protoplasmic astrocytomas, oligdendrogliomas, or oligoastrocytomas. In one study, Laws et al. reported the results of 461 cases of low-grade glioma seen at the Mayo Clinic between 1915 and 1975 that were treated with maximal feasible removal. Surgical mortality (any death within 30 days of surgery) was 2 percent, and one in five patients experienced worsening of their preoperative deficit. The extent of surgery strongly correlated with survival. The 5- and 10-year survival rates for patients who had total tumor removal was double that of patients who had subtotal resection or biopsy. The longest survivors were patients below the age of 20 years, with complete resection, without premorbid disorders of consciousness or personality, and with minimal or no postoperative deficit. Although this was a retrospective study with a high rate of pilocytic tumors, it established the importance of surgical resection. In general, maximal surgical resection should be attempted when it can be done with acceptable morbidity.

Radiotherapy

The goals of radiotherapy are to prevent tumor recurrence and malignant dedifferentiation and to improve symptoms. The potential benefits of radiotherapy must be weighed against the side effects, which include radiation necrosis and neuropsychological and neuroendocrine dysfunction. These late sequelae are related to the dose of radiation, the volume of tissue treated, and the duration of survival. Most patients with low-grade gliomas are treated with conventional fractionated external beam radiotherapy, which takes advantage of the differential radiobiologic sensitivities of neoplastic and normal brain tissue. More focal forms of radiotherapy such as interstitial brachytherapy and stereotactic radiosurgery are seldom used to treat low-grade gliomas. However, stereotactic fractionated radiotherapy, which combines the accuracy of radiosurgery with the reduced toxicity of fractionated external beam radiotherapy, is likely to play an increasing role in the treatment of these tumors.

Chemotherapy

Increasing evidence shows that oligodendrogliomas and oligoastrocytomas are sensitive to chemotherapy (Fig. 150-3). The best results have been seen with the procarbazine, lomustine (CCNU), and vincristine regimen (PCV), but other agents such as melphalan have also shown activity. Although responses have been reported with both low-grade and high-grade tumors, chemotherapy should generally be reserved for patients with anaplastic oligodendrogliomas and anaplastic oligoastrocytomas because of the long-term risk of myelodysplasia and leukemia (about 5 percent at 5 years) with the use of nitrosureas. The response rate for patients with recurrent anaplastic oligodendrogliomas is approximately 70 to 80 percent, with a median duration of response of 12 to 15 months. The results are generally worse for patients with anaplastic oligoastrocytomas. Because of the encouraging results with chemotherapy in patients with recurrent anaplastic oligodendrogliomas, there is an increasing trend to treat newly diagnosed patients with either neoadjuvant or adjuvant chemotherapy. A multicenter study is currently under way that will evaluate the benefit of administer-

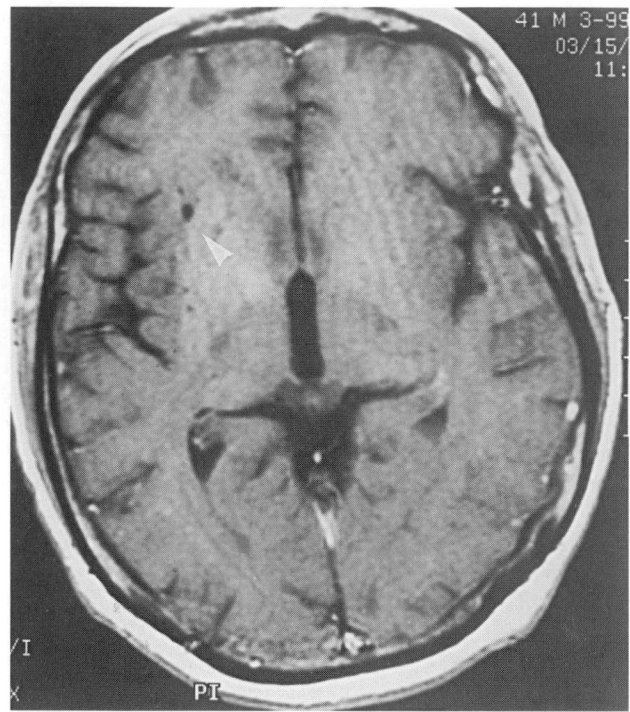

FIG. 150-3. The same patient as in Figs. 150-1 and 150-2 after treatment with chemotherapy, which produced a complete response with disappearance of the contrast-enhancing area. The patient has a normal neurologic examination and his seizures are controlled with standard antiepileptic monotherapy.

ing PCV chemotherapy before radiotherapy, compared with radiotherapy alone.

Chemotherapy may play a role in the treatment of selected patients (e.g., when the tumor behaves aggressively despite the apparent ''benign'' pathology, when the tumor is felt to be inoperable, and in an attempt to delay radiotherapy in very young children). Response rates of 50 to 60 percent have been seen in young children (less than 5 years old) with low-grade gliomas treated with the combination of carboplatin and vincristine.

SPECIFIC HISTOLOGIC SUBTYPES

Although the great majority of low-grade gliomas are fibrillary astrocytomas, several other histologic types of astrocytoma are seen that possess unique biologic behaviors and require specific forms of management.

Fibrillary and Protoplasmic Astrocytoma

Low-grade fibrillary or protoplasmic astrocytic tumors represent 10 to 15 percent of all brain tumors and 40 percent of all gliomas. They occur most commonly in younger patients and have a peak incidence between the ages of 30 and 40 years. The tumor usually involves the frontal (about 45 percent) and temporal (30 percent) lobes. Protoplasmic astrocytomas are much less common than the fibrillary type and tend to be located in the temporal lobes, usually at the cortical margin. Both forms of low-grade glioma diffusely infiltrate beyond CT or MRI margins. Biopsy of the edge of the tumor shows cells that may be confused with reactive astrocytes. Staining techniques utiliz-

ing glial fibrillary acidic protein are commonly used to exclude other tumor types.

Optimal management is controversial. Patients with small, asymptomatic tumors that are not increasing in size can often be followed with serial radiologic studies. Ideally some form of functional imaging (PET, CBV mapping) is performed to monitor tumor grade. Those patients with large, symptomatic, progressive tumors should be treated with complete surgical resection, if possible. Patients with ''complete'' resections can be closely observed and treated with radiotherapy only if evidence of tumor progression exists. Patients with large, symptomatic or progressive tumors that are inoperable or can only be partially resected, should undergo radiotherapy. The role of radiotherapy remains controversial, but several retrospective studies have shown that postoperative radiotherapy increases 5-year survival to 46 to 64 percent, compared with 19 to 34 percent for surgery alone. The radiotherapy usually consists of 50 to 55 Gy in 180 to 200 cGy fractions to the tumor volume and a 1 to 2-cm margin. Older patients (more than 40 years) appear to benefit more than younger patients. The increased accuracy of newer techniques such as stereotactic radiotherapy is likely to reduce the risk of long-term neurotoxicity. Several prospective, multicenter, randomized studies are in progress to evaluate the role of radiotherapy.

With standard treatment, the survival rate at 5 years is 50 to 60 percent and at 10 years 30 to 40 percent. Recent series, reflecting CT or MRI evaluations, show median survivals approaching 7.5 years, an improvement that probably represents diagnosis at an earlier stage in the natural history of these tumors rather than improved therapeutic efficacy. The most important prognostic factor is age; patients over 40 have a shorter survival than younger patients. Other favorable prognostic factors include good performance status, complete resection, and lower proliferative potential (as determined by bromodeoxyuridine labeling). Less well-established favorable prognostic factors include tumor location (e.g., frontal pole, temporal tip), long duration of symptoms, presentation with seizures, lack of neurologic deficits, and a cystic component to the tumor.

The role of chemotherapy for low-grade fibrillary astrocytomas is unproved. In one randomized study, by Eyre and colleagues, the addition of adjuvant lomustine (CCNU) to radiotherapy did not improve survival.

Pilocytic Astrocytoma

Pilocytic astrocytomas are predominantly juvenile tumors with a peak incidence in the second and third decade. They represent as much as one-fourth of all cerebellar tumors but only about 3 percent of cerebral hemisphere astrocytomas. The most common locations are the cerebellum, optic nerve and hypothalamus, but they can also be found in the cerebral hemispheres, especially in the temporoparietal region or lateral ventricles. (Hypothalamic and optic pilocytic astrocytomas are dealt with in Ch. 151). Genetic analysis of tumor tissue frequently shows loss of segments of the long arm of chromosome 17. In contrast to fibrillary astrocytomas, p53 gene abnormalities are almost never present. The typical appearance is that of a well-circumscribed cystic mass with a mural nodule. The tumors are composed of elongated, bipolar astrocytic cells with oval nuclei and fibrils lying in parallel rows. Microcysts are usually present and commonly degenerate into larger cysts. Pilocytic astrocytomas are well-circumscribed tumors that usually displace rather than infiltrate surrounding brain and can often be cured by resection.

For these tumors, an attempt at complete surgical resection is recommended, if possible. Incompletely resected tumors can usually be safely observed. When the tumor progresses, further resection should be performed, if possible, and if not, the tumor can be treated with focal external beam radiotherapy, stereotactic radiosurgery, or stereotactic radiotherapy. Chemotherapy using agents such as nitrosoureas, carboplatin and vincristine, or etoposide has some benefit in children but no proven role for adults.

The overall prognosis is generally very good for pilocytic astrocytomas. For patients whose tumor can be fully resected, survival rates are 80 percent at 10 years and 70 to 80 percent at 20 years, while for patients undergoing partial resection, survival rates are 70 to 80 percent at 10 years and 50 to 60 percent at 20 years. The survival rate is lower for patients undergoing biopsy alone (40 to 50 percent at 20 years). Neither Kernohan nor St. Anne-Mayo grading correlates with outcome.

Two rare astrocytomas, subependymal giant cell astrocytoma and pleomorphic xanthoastrocytoma, have distinguishing pathologic characteristics, but both behave like low-grade astrocytomas.

Subependymal Giant Cell Astrocytoma

Subependymal giant cell astrocytomas occur in patients with tuberous sclerosis and generally arise before adulthood in the subependymal layer of the lateral ventricle. These tumors are composed of giant astrocytes. They tend to grow very slowly and can often be managed by close observation.

Pleomorphic Xanthoastrocytoma

Pleomorphic xanthoastrocytomas are usually superficial tumors with giant multinucleated astrocytes and intracellular lipid. The presence of mitotic activity has no prognostic value, but if necrosis is present, the diagnosis should be questioned. Despite their pathology, many of these tumors have a relatively benign course, although some tumors will eventually behave more aggressively.

Oligodendroglioma

Oligodendrogliomas represent 5 percent of all intracranial gliomas. The tumors occur in two populations, young patients between 6 and 13 years and older patients between 25 and 50 years.

Oligodendrogliomas contain cells that resemble fried eggs (small, round cells with perinuclear halos) interspersed with zones of calicification and microcysts and a rich capillary network. The fried egg appearance is an artifact resulting from fixation of the tissue in formalin. Often tumors contain both oligodendroglial and astrocytic cells, which are probably derived from the same precursor cells. Patients with these "mixed" gliomas containing as few as 5 percent oligodendroglia may fare better than those with pure astrocytic tumors. The oligodendroglial component appears to convey both a sensitivity to chemotherapy and a survival advantage.

Most oligodendrogliomas are hypodense, calcified, nonenhancing, frontal lobe tumors that present with seizures or headaches. They may invade the cortex and leptomeninges or metastasize within the central nervous system (incidence, about 5 percent) and rarely to extracranial organs such as bone, lymph nodes, and lung.

The treatment of low-grade oligodendrogliomas is similar to that of low-grade astrocytomas. Small, asymptomatic tumors can be either observed and treated (only if radiologic or clinical evidence of progression exists), or they can be resected if a surgical cure is possible. Large, symptomatic, or enlarging tumors should be resected, if possible. Patients with complete resections can be observed and treated with radiotherapy when the tumor recurs. As with low-grade astrocytomas, the role of radiotherapy for incompletely resected tumors is unproved. While some retrospective studies show no benefit, others suggest that the addition of radiotherapy to surgery increases survival from 25 percent at 5 years for surgery alone to 60 percent at 5 years for patients treated with both surgery and radiotherapy. A small number of studies suggest that low-grade oligodendrogliomas may respond to chemotherapeutic regimens such as PCV.

With standard treatment, the prognosis is slightly better than that of low-grade astrocytomas (5-year survival rate of 60 to 80 percent and 10-year survival rate of 30 to 50 percent).

Anaplastic Oligodendroglioma

Anaplastic oligodendrogliomas account for approximately 3 percent of high-grade gliomas. Although they are clinically aggressive tumors, they have a better prognosis than other high-grade gliomas, with a 5-year survival rate of approximately 45 percent. As discussed above, these tumors are highly chemosensitive and respond to a variety of alkylating agents, especially the PCV regimen. In a recently completed study by Cairncross and colleagues using high-dose PCV (CCNU 130 mg/m^2 on day 1, vincristine 1.4 mg/m^2 on days 8 and 29, and procarbazine 75 mg/m^2 on days 8 to 21) for patients with both newly diagnosed and recurrent anaplastic oligodendrogliomas, a 75 percent response rate was observed. Oligodendrogliomas may be chemosensitive partly because they have very low levels of O^6 alkyl guanine-DNA alkyltransferase, a DNA repair enzyme implicated in nitrosurea resistance.

Standard therapy for newly diagnosed anaplastic oligodendrogliomas involves maximal surgical resection, followed by limited field radiotherapy to a total dose of 55 to 60 Gy. The role of adjuvant chemotherapy is unknown and is being evaluated in a multicenter study. Patients with recurrent tumors should be treated with PCV or another alkylating agent-based regimen.

Oligoastrocytoma

Oligoastrocytomas contain a mixture of oligodendroglial and astrocytic cells, the latter accounting for at least 25 percent of the tumor. These tumors are more common in men and have a peak incidence in the fifth decade. They represent up to one-fifth of supratentorial gliomas and are most frequently located in the subcortical white matter. Like pure oligodendrogliomas, oligoastrocytomas are chemosensitive tumors and respond to regimens such as PCV. In general, the prognosis tends to fall between that of fibrillary astrocytomas and oligodendrogliomas. Well-differentiated tumors (Kernohan grade 1 or 2) have a median survival of about 6 years and anaplastic tumors (Kernohan grade 3 or 4) have a median survival of about 3 years. Improved survival is associated with lower histologic grade, extent of surgical resection, postoperative irradiation (doses above 50 Gy), and younger age. The impact of chemotherapy on survival remains to be assessed.

Ganglioglioma

Gangliomas are rare tumors that account for 1 percent of primary brain tumors. They usually occur before the fourth decade and are located in the cerebral hemispheres, especially the temporal lobes. Histologically, gangliogliomas contain neoplastic neurons, which stain with synaptophysin, as well as a glial component. The prognosis for these tumors is very good. They tend to be well-differentiated, slowly growing tumors that can be surgically cured. The 5-year recurrence rate is 25 percent for hemispheric gangliogliomas and 50 percent for those in the spinal cord or brainstem. Fortunately, after a second resection, about 70 percent of patients remain free of further recurrences at 5 years. Overall survival is above 80 percent at 10 years, although dedifferentiation to high-grade ganglioglioma can occur. The prognosis tends to be worse with tumors located in the spinal cord or brainstem. Higher histologic grade and male gender are associated with a greater incidence of recurrence, but other prognostic factors are not well established due in part to the rarity of this tumor. Radiotherapy may benefit recurrent tumors that cannot be resected. A more detailed discussion of the signs, symptoms, and treatment of gangliogliomas is provided in Chapter 164.

SUGGESTED READINGS

Cairncross G, Macdonald D, Ramsay D: Aggressive oligodendroglioma: a chemosensitive tumor. Neurosurgery 31:78, 1992

Cairncross G, Macdonald D, Ludwin S et al: Chemotherapy for anaplastic oligodendroglioma. J Clin Oncol 12:2013–21, 1994

Eyre HJ, Crowley JJ, Townsend JJ et al: A randomized trial of radiotherapy versus radiotherapy plus CCNU for incompletely resected low-grade gliomas: a Southwest Oncology Group study. J Neurosurg 78:909–14, 1993

Forsyth P, Shaw E, Scheithauer B et al: Supratentorial pilocytic astrocytomas. A clinicopathologic, prognostic, and flow cytometric study of 51 patients. Cancer 72:1335, 1993

Glass J, Hochberg F, Gruber M et al: The treatment of oligodendroglioma and mixed oligodendroglioma-astrocytomas with PCV chemotherapy. J Neurosurg 76:741, 1992

Lang F, Epstein F, Ransohoff J et al: Central nervous system gangliogliomas. Part 2: Clinical outcome. J Neurosurg 79:867, 1993

Laws E, Taylor W, Clifton M et al: Neurosurgical management of low-grade supratentorial astrocytomas. J Neurosurg 61:665, 1984

Macdonald DR: Low-grade gliomas, mixed gliomas, and oligodendrogliomas. Semin Oncol 21:236–236, 1994

Miller D, Lang F, Epstein F: Central nervous system gangliogliomas. Part 1: Pathology. J Neurosurg 79:859, 1993

Packer R, Lange B, Ater J et al: Carboplatin and vincristine for recurrent and newly diagnosed low-grade gliomas of childhood. J Clin Oncol 11:850, 1993

Peterson K, Caincross JG: Oligodendroglioma. Neurol Clin 1995 (in press)

Recht LD: Low grade gliomas. Neurol Clin 1995 (in press)

Recht L, Lew R, Smith T: Suspected low-grade glioma: is deferring treatment safe? Ann Neurol 31:431, 1992

Rogers L, Morris H, Lupica K: Effect of cranial irradiation on seizure frequency in adults with low-grade astrocytoma and medically intractable epilepsy. Neurology 43:1599, 1993

Russell D, Rubinstein L: Pathology of Tumors of the Nervous System. 5th Ed. Wilkins & Wilkins, Baltimore, 1989

Shaw E, Daumas-Duport C, Scheithauer B et al: Radiation therapy in the management of low-grade supratentorial astrocytomas. J Neurosurg 70:853, 1989

Shaw E, Scheithauer B, O'Fallon J et al: Oligodendrogliomas: the Mayo Clinic experience. J Neurosurg 76:428, 1992

Shaw E, Scheithauer B, O'Fallon J et al: Mixed oligoastrocytomas: a survival and prognostic factor analysis. Neurosurgery 34:577, 1994

Smith M, Ludwig C, Godfrey A et al: Grading of oligodendrogliomas. Cancer 52:2107, 1983

Vecht C: Effect of age on the treatment decisions in low-grade glioma. J Neurol Neurosurg Psychiatry 56:1259, 1993

Vertosick F, Selker R, Arena V: Survival of patients with well-differentiated astrocytomas diagnosed in the era of computed tomography. Neurosurgery 28:496, 1991

151. OPTIC PATHWAY AND HYPOTHALAMIC GLIOMAS

NANCY J. TARBELL
PATRICK D. BARNES

Optic gliomas are rare and account for approximately 1 to 5 percent of intracranial gliomas. Their overall incidence is approximately 1 in 105,000 patients. They most frequently occur in children (75 percent in the first decade and 90 percent within the first two decades). The location is of significant therapeutic and prognostic importance. Tumors involving the optic nerve alone are associated with a better prognosis than intracranial gliomas involving the optic chiasm and tracts. Tumors involving the optic chiasm frequently cannot be separated from those arising in the hypothalamus, and for purposes of management, these tumors are generally considered together.

The occurrence of neurofibromatosis-1 in patients with optic glioma ranges from 10 to 50 percent. Conversely, the frequency of optic gliomas in patients with neurofibromatosis-1 has been estimated at 1 to 5 percent. However, a 15 percent incidence of enlargement of the optic nerve or chiasm on computed tomography (CT) or magnetic resonance imaging (MRI) has been reported in asymptomatic patients with neurofibromatosis type 1. These findings may represent an early optic glioma, gliosis, hamartoma, or (rarely), a neurofibroma. These uncertainties emphasize the need for clinical symptoms or biopsy, or both, prior to initiation of treatment in patients with imaging evidence of optic pathway abnormalities.

Because of the rarity of this tumor, the diagnostic and therapeutic approaches have been controversial. Anecdotal cases of spontaneous regression have been reported, supporting the view that these tumors may have an indolent course. However, a more aggressive natural history with tumor progression and death has been documented in most long-term reports. Untreated intracranial optic system tumors will progress locally or cause death in 75 percent of patients.

Most optic gliomas are slow-growing and histologically low-grade astrocytomas. The occurrence of high-grade astrocytomas or tumors with other histologies is unusual. Rarely, supratentorial low-grade astrocytomas of the chiasmatic/hypothalamic area have been reported to undergo malignant transformation.

Hypothalamic tumors have been reported to have a less favorable prognosis than tumors confined to the chiasm. However, with CT and MRI it is now clear that most chiasmic tumors involve the hypothalamus as well. Chiasmal gliomas are further chacterized according to their involvement of surrounding structures, including the optic nerves, optic tracts, and hypothalmus (Fig. 151-1).

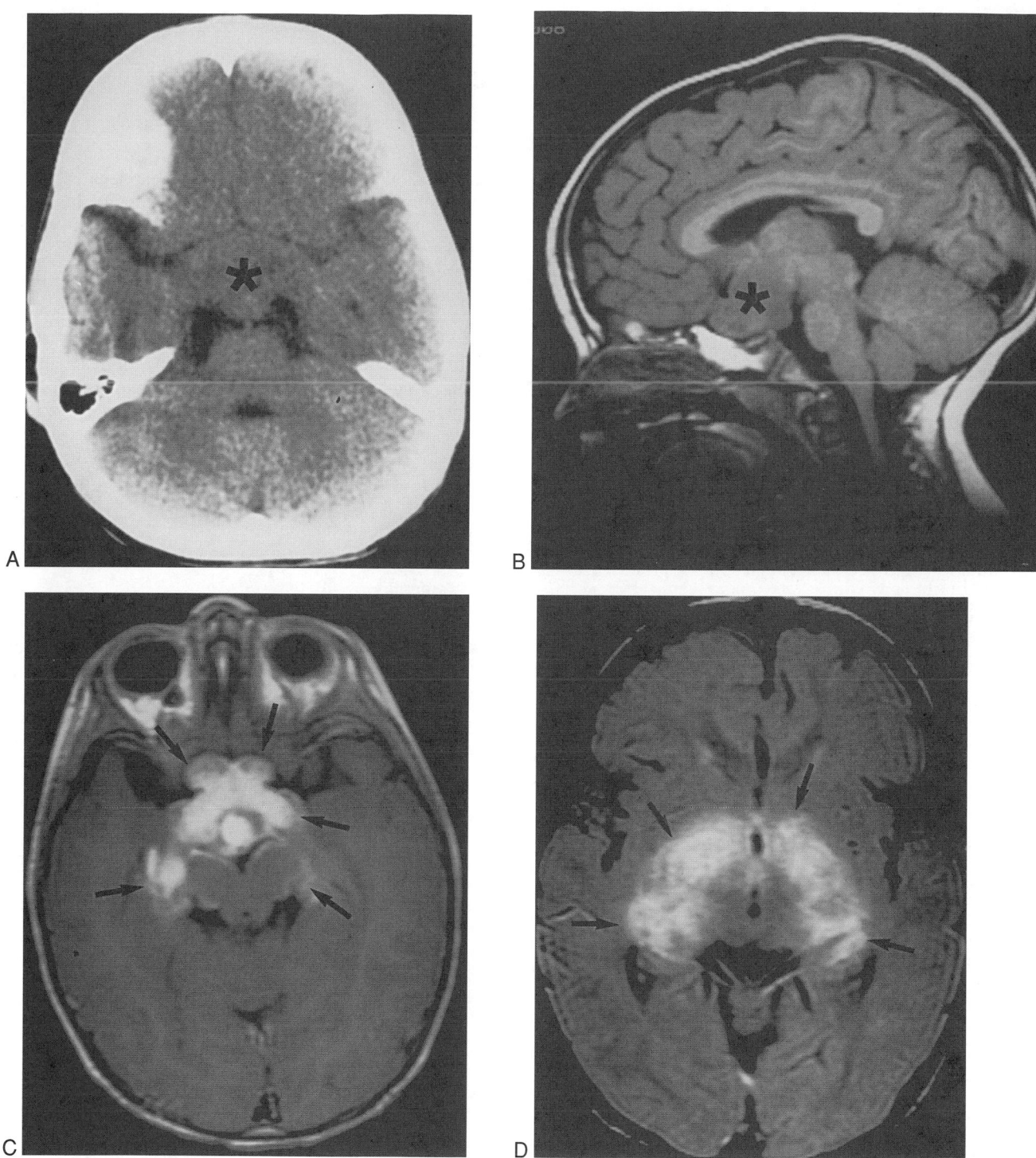

FIG. 151-1. A 2-year-old girl with optic hypothalamic astrocytoma. **(A)** CT shows a nonspecific suprasellar mass (*asterisk*). **(B)** Sagittal T1-weighted MRI demonstrates the optic/hypothalmic tumor (*asterisk*), which markedly enhances with gadolinium (*arrows*) on the axial T1-weighted MRI **(C)**. **(D)** Axial proton density and T2-weighted MRI show the optic tract involvement (*arrows*). In patients with neurofibromatosis-1, such involvement is difficult to distinguish from the dysplastic foci of neurofibromatosis.

CLINICAL PRESENTATION, STAGING AND WORKUP

Optic chiasm lesions present with unilateral or bilateral loss of vision and often with visual field cuts or hypothalamic dysfunction, or both. Funduscopic examination usually reveals a pale optic disc. Cranial nerve deficits and hydrocephalus may be present. Endocrine dysfunction, in particular precocious pu-

berty, is not uncommon. Typical presenting signs and symptoms are listed in Table 151-1. Visual abnormalities are almost always present.

The diencephalic syndrome (emesis, emaciation, and euphoria) may be associated with more posterior tumors centered at the hypothalamus. The clinical presentations of hypothalamic tumors are more varied and include gelastic epilepsy, visual

TABLE 151-1. Signs and Symptoms

	Approximate %
Visual abnormality	95
Visual acuity	50
Field cuts	25
Both	20
Endocrine	35
Precocious puberty	30
Diabetes insipidus	8
Neurologic	50
Ataxia	15
Headache	15
Seizure	15
Macrocephaly	10
Personality change	5
Papilledema	5
Cranial nerve palsy	5

TABLE 151-2. Survival and Visual Response After Radiation

Author	No. of Patients	Control (No./Patients)	10-Yr Survey (%)	Vision Improved (%)
Horwich, 1988	29	26/29	93	43
Pierce, 1990	24	21/24	100	30

deficits, increased intracranial pressure due to extension into the third ventricle and foramina of Monro, behavioral changes, and endocrine dysfunction. The history and general physical examination should involve a search for evidence of neurofibromatosis-1, and the workup should include baseline neuroendocrine studies and formal visual field testing.

RADIOLOGIC EVALUATION

MRI including contrast enhancement is now preferred to CT for initial and follow-up imaging evaluation (Fig. 151-1). Thin sections through the optic nerves and chiasm allow excellent definition of the extent of disease. Optic gliomas may cause concentric enlargement of one or both optic nerves, an enlarged chiasm, or abnormalities of the optic tracts. Most tumors exhibit contrast enhancement. Neurofibroma occurs rarely in children with neurofibromatosis, appearing as a large eccentric optic nerve mass. The differential diagnosis of a suprasellar mass in a child includes craniopharyngioma, germ cell tumors, ectopic pinealoma and (in older patients) a pituitary adenoma or meningioma. Serum and cerebrospinal fluid tests α-fetoprotein, and human chorionic gonadotrophin should be performed if germ cell tumors are considered. In patients with neurofibromatosis-1, dysplastic intensities are often present and may not be readily distinguished from extension of the optic tumor (Fig. 151-1).

THERAPY

Controversy over optimal therapy still exists. Alvord (1988) reviewed 623 cases in the literature and confirmed that most optic system tumors are low-grade astrocytomas with a variable but nonetheless continuous growth rate.

Surgery

Surgery for initial management of intracranial chiasmal/hypothalamic lesions is usually limited to biopsy, since resection is not possible without morbidity such as visual impairment and hypothalamic dysfunction. Placement of a ventricular catheter may be needed to relieve hydrocephalus. In special circumstances partial resection may be warranted, such as for exophytic and recurrent tumors. Although a biopsy is indicated in most patients, it may not be necessary in patients with neurofibromatosis-1, progressive symptoms, and characteristic imaging findings.

Radiotherapy

Most modern reports utilizing megavoltage radiotherapy document an advantage for patients with progressive chiasmal glio-

mas. Radiotherapy is generally the treatment of choice for symptomatic chiasmatic/hypothalamic gliomas in all but very young children. Many recent series report excellent survival after radiotherapy, generally 90 percent at 10 years (Pierce and colleagues, 1990; Horwich and Bloom, 1985). However, it is not uncommon for deaths to occur from disease progression many years after treatment. This emphasizes the need for long-term follow-up.

Visual outcome is an important measure of treatment success for chiasmal/hypothalamic gliomas. Following radiotherapy, an improvement in vision is seen in approximately one-third of patients, with most patients experiencing visual stabilization (Table 151-2). This success in maintaining or improving vision is only possible if treatment is initiated before severe visual damage has occurred. Therefore, documented visual deterioration is a major indication to initiate therapy promptly.

Chemotherapy

Chemotherapy has been increasingly used, particularly in the young child. Packer (1988) has updated the results of treatment with vincristine and actinomycin for recurrent tumors or newly diagnosed optic gliomas in children younger than 6 years of age. This regimen appears to stabilize disease and allows radiotherapy to be delayed in most of patients. Hopefully, the use of chemotherapy for very young patients (under 3 years of age) will allow a delay in radiotherapy and a reduction in the frequency and severity of radiation sequelae.

COMPLICATIONS

Retrospective studies of long-term radiotherapy complications have been confounded by the fact that many of these children have associated learning disabilities related to neurofibromatosis-1. Pierce et al (1990) reported some evidence of increased learning disabilities or decreased memory after treatment, in contrast to a smaller number of children who had definite evidence of learning disabilities prior to radiotherapy. Most but not all of these patients had neurofibromatosis-1. The occurrence of neurologic abnormalities associated with chiasmal/hypothalamic glioma after treatment is difficult to define. Visual abnormalities and psychological trauma undoubtedly contribute to learning difficulties, but they are difficult to quantify. Neuropsychological testing is recommended pre- and posttreatment to define the cognitive impairment better and to indicate the need for and timing of intervention.

Imaging findings of calcifications, white matter abnormalities, and atrophy have been reported in patients following radiotherapy. The clinical significance of these findings remains uncertain in most cases.

Neuroendocrine abnormalities may be the consequence of tumor involvement or treatment effects. Therefore, careful endocrine evaluation and monitoring is important, not only at presentation, but for many years after treatment. This is especially critical for children since hormonal replacement is crucial to normal development.

Another reported complication of radiotherapy is Moyamoya syndrome. This syndrome is named for the characteristic angiographic appearance (''puff of smoke'') of arterial collaterals at the base of the brain associated with progressive narrowing of one or both internal carotid arteries; it manifests as repetitive ischemic episodes. Potential late complications after radiotherapy also include hemorrhage and the rare risk of second malignancies. Patients with neurofibromatosis-1 already have an increased risk of malignant tumors, and this risk may be increased after radiotherapy.

CONCLUSIONS

Gliomas of the optic pathway and hypothalamus present with visual deterioration, endocrine disorders, and/or neurologic abnormalities. These are the most common tumors in children with neurofibromatosis-1. With rare exceptions the course is progressive, albeit variable. Radiotherapy appears to impact significantly on disease-free progression and overall survival. Most patients experience improvement or stabilization in vision, demonstrating a clear benefit to radiotherapy for progressive disease. The endocrine and neuropsychological consequences of the tumor and treatment are significant and warrant careful follow-up. Chemotherapy for the very young (less than age 3 and perhaps less than age 5) appears warranted to delay radiotherapy.

SUGGESTED READINGS

Alvord EC, Lofton S: Gliomas of the optic nerve or chiasm. J Neurosurg 68: 85–98, 1988

Barnes P, Kupsky W, Strand R: Cranial and intracranial tumors. p. 204. In Wolpert S, Barnes R (eds): MRI in Pediatric Neuro-radiology. Mosby Year St. Louis, Book, 1992

Eliason MJ: Neuropsychological patterns: neurofibromatosis compared to developmental learning disorders. Neurofibromatosis 1:17–25, 1988

Haugh RM, Markesbery WR: Hypothalamic astrocytoma: syndrome of hyperphagia, obesity, and disturbances of behavior in endocrine and asctronomic function. Arch Neurol 40:500–63, 1983

Horwich A, Bloom HJG: Optic gliomas: radiation therapy and prognosis. Int J Radiat Oncol Biol Phys 11:1067–79, 1985

Lewis RA, Gerson LP, Axelson RA et al: von ??? neurofibromatosis: II. Incidence of optic gliomata. Ophthalmology 91:929–35, 1984

Packer RJ, Sutton LN, Bilaniak LT et al: Treatment of chiasmatic/hypothlamic gliomas of childhood with chemotherapy: an update. Ann neurol 23: 79–85, 1988

Pierce SM, Barnes PD, Loeffler JS et al: Definitive radiation therapy in the management of symptomatic patients with optic glioma: survival and long-term effects. Cancer 65:45–52, 1990

Wisoff J, Abbott R, Epstein F: Surgical management of exophytic chiasmatic-hypothalamic tumors of childhood. J Neurosurg 73:661–67, 1990

152. BRAINSTEM GLIOMAS

DENNIS C. SHRIEVE

Brainstem gliomas are a heterogeneous group of tumors in terms of clinical presentation, histologic grade, and prognosis. The generic term *brainstem glioma* refers to neoplasms arising in the rhombencephalon (medulla or pons) or the mesencephalon (midbrain). Tumors of the diencephalon (thalamus or hypothalamus) are included by some authors. Historically these tu-

TABLE 152-1. Classification of Brainstem Gliomas

Intrinsic
  Location
    Midbrain/diencephalic
    Pontine/medullary
    Cervicomedullary
  MRI Appearance
    Focal
    Diffuse
    Cystic
Exophytic
  Tectal
  Fourth ventricular
  Anterolateral
  Posterolateral

mors were considered under a single heading because of similarities in presenting symptoms, poor definition on pre-computed tomography (CT) imaging tests, difficulty in obtaining tissue diagnosis, and overall poor prognosis. More recently, advances in neuroimaging and neurosurgical techniques as well as results from cooperative group studies have identified pretreatment characteristics that define distinct prognostic groups.

EPIDEMIOLOGY

Primary gliomas of the brainstem account for 10 to 15 percent of brain tumors in children, resulting in 250 to 300 cases each year in the United States. The incidence in adults is less well documented but probably accounts for less than 5 percent of primary adult gliomas. As such, brainstem gliomas are considered primarily a pediatric brain tumor. Median age at diagnosis in most studies is 5 to 7 years, with no clear male or female predominance. As is the case with other gliomas, the etiology is unknown, but there may be an association with known congenital syndromes, most commonly neurofibromatosis.

PATHOLOGY

Intrinsic brainstem gliomas are uniformly astrocytic in origin. All grades of astrocytoma may be found at biopsy: pilocytic astrocytoma, ordinary astrocytoma, anaplastic astrocytoma, and glioblastoma multiforme. Prognosis is, as expected, related to tumor grade. Unlike other astrocytomas, however, tumor grade is highly predictable based on appearance on magnetic resonance imaging (MRI) scan. Because of the often acute presentation and the limited role of surgery in many cases, biopsy is often not indicated.

CLASSIFICATION

Classification of brainstem gliomas may be made on the basis of tumor location and appearance on MRI scan (Table 152-1). Intrinsic brainstem gliomas are considered unresectable and may involve the midbrain, pons or medulla alone, or may span the entire brainstem. Tumors of the midbrain, with or without thalamic involvement, carry a relatively better prognosis compared with tumors of the pons or medulla. Exophytic tumors of the dorsal aspect of the medulla or tectal plate or tumors that fill the fourth ventricle are amenable to surgical resection and are nearly uniformly of low-grade histology. Exophytic tumors with more anterolateral extension into the cerebellar pontine angle or posterolateral extension into the cerebellum are commonly more invasive, high-grade tumors.

Tumors may be classified as either diffuse or focal based on

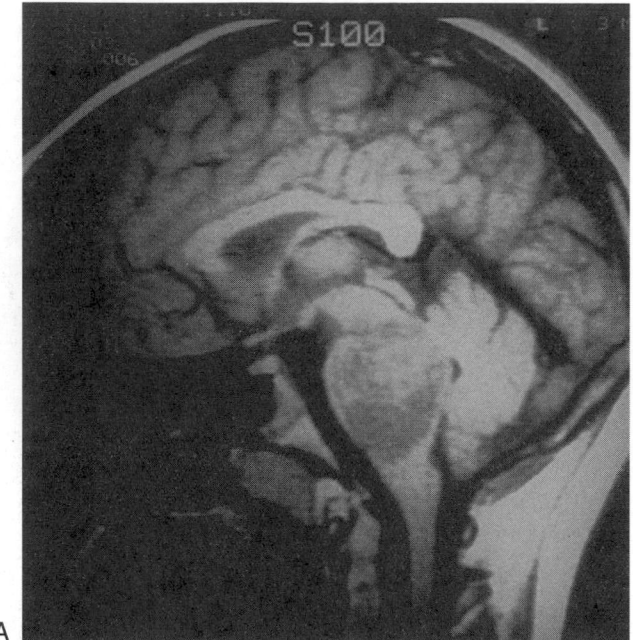
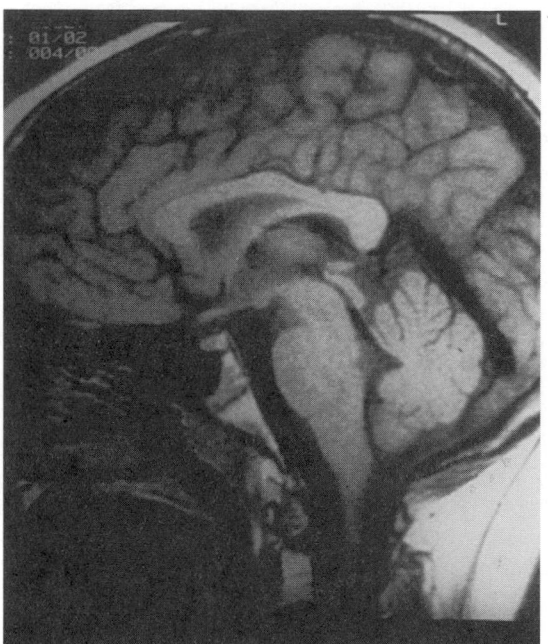

FIG. 152-1. **(A)** Diffuse pontine glioma in a 10-year-old boy. The patient received hyperfractionated radiotherapy (1 Gy twice daily to 7,200 cGy). **(B)** Postradiotherapy MRI showing response to treatment. Despite nearly complete radiographic response the patient died of local failure 15 months following radiotherapy.

MRI appearance. Focal tumors are confined to one anatomic subsite of the brainstem and are usually defined as nonexpansile and less than 2.5 cm in greatest dimension. Diffuse tumors expand the subsite or entire brainstem (Fig. 152-1). Intrinsic tumors of the cervicomedullary junction represent a distinct subclass of brainstem lesions that are amenable to surgical resection and are usually of low-grade histology (Fig. 152-2).

CLINICAL PRESENTATION

Most patients present with neurologic symptoms, including cranial nerve deficits, long tract signs, or ataxia. The classic presentation of a patient with an intrinsic brainstem tumor is multiple cranial nerve deficits and contralateral hemiparesis. Although patients may present with isolated cranial nerve findings, multi-

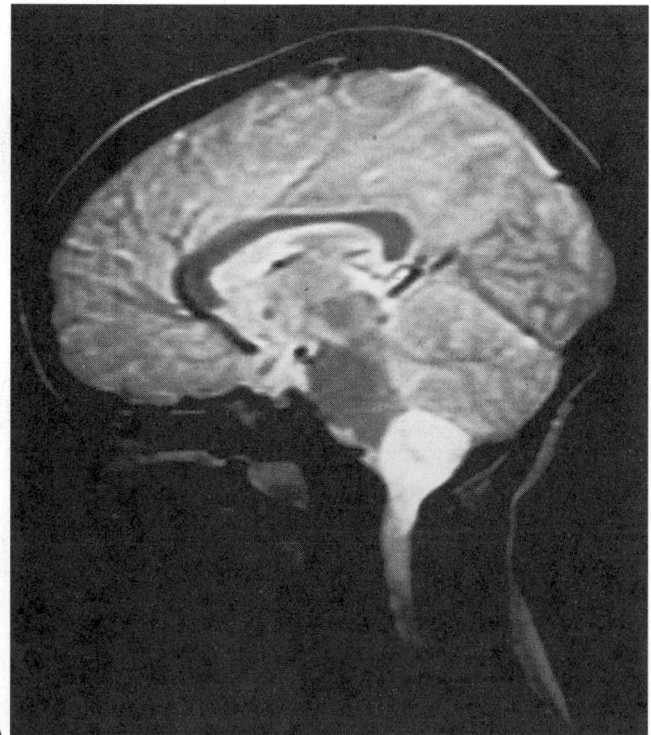
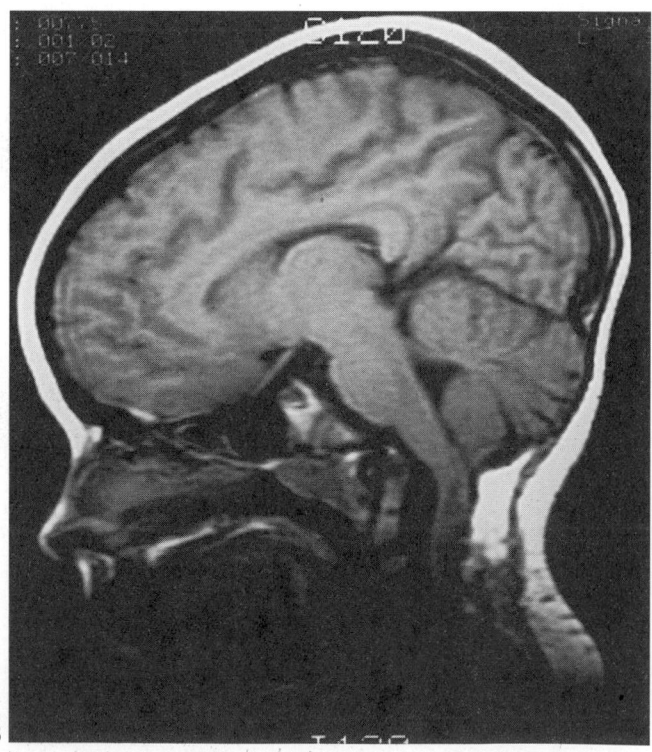

FIG. 152-2. **(A)** Cervicomedullary tumor in 4-year-old girl (March 1988). The tumor was resected and pathology studies showed pilocytic astrocytoma. **(B)** Follow-up scan 5 years after surgery showing no evidence of recurrence (August 1993).

ple or bilateral cranial neuropathies are present in 70 percent. The most commonly involved cranial nerves are VI and VII followed by III and V. Patients with dorsally exophytic tumors or tumors of the tectum may present with symptoms referable to hydrocephalus due to obstruction of the fourth ventricle or aqueduct.

The duration of symptoms at presentation is of prognostic value. Patients with a shorter history of symptoms have a poorer prognosis than those with a more protracted course. Most modern studies have found that a history of symptoms of 2 months or less is associated with a poorer outcome than a longer history.

DIAGNOSIS

Clearly any patient with cranial neuropathy, ataxia, or extremity weakness must be evaluated with whole-brain imaging. MRI with gadolinium is the examination of choice when brainstem glioma is suspected. The definition of the brainstem on axial, coronal, and sagittal sections is far superior to that obtained with CT. Sagittal MR images are especially helpful in radiotherapy treatment planning.

DIFFERENTIAL DIAGNOSIS

The distinct appearance of a diffuse pontine glioma on MRI scan is usually considered sufficient to make the diagnosis without histologic confirmation. Most institutions have a policy not to biopsy such lesions since the procedure is not without risk, the histology is nearly always malignant astrocytoma, and most patients present acutely and benefit from prompt treatment. Such patients treated without biopsy make up an extremely poor prognostic group, thus validating this approach.

Focal intrinsic brainstem lesions are usually associated with a more protracted history of symptoms, occur more commonly in older patients, and may be approached in a more conservative manner. Biopsy is usually recommended since the probability of the diagnosis of low-grade astrocytoma is great and the possibility of the presence of a non-neoplastic process exists. Differential diagnosis of a focal nonexpansive lesion of the brainstem includes vascular malformation, cysticercosis, encephalitis, tuberculoma, arachnoid cyst of the clivus, multiple sclerosis, post infectious encephalomyelitis, or other nonspecific inflammatory reactions (gliosis) (Fig. 152-3).

Exophytic lesions are usually approached surgically for diagnosis as well as resection. These are most often low-grade astrocytomas of the brainstem, but the differential diagnosis includes ependymoma and medulloblastoma. These tumors have in common a primary surgical approach. Adjuvant therapies are quite different depending on the histologic diagnosis and age of the patient.

TREATMENT

The role of surgery in the initial management of patients with brainstem glioma is limited. For diffuse pontine gliomas surgery has no role and biopsy is not usually recommended. Surgery may be indicated for cervicomedullary, focal, cystic, or exophytic tumors. Biopsy (open or CT-guided stereotactic) is indicated when the diagnosis of brainstem glioma is in doubt.

For most patients radiotherapy is the primary treatment modality. For diffuse lesions radiation fields encompass the entire brainstem with adequate margin around the tumor. For focal lesions, fields may be less extensive, covering the tumor with a 2-cm margin. "Standard" fractionated radiotherapy (1.7 to 2.0 Gy/day) was employed for many years with poor results. The addition of radiation sensitizers or chemotherapy, or both, has not improved survival in poor-prognosis patients. More re-

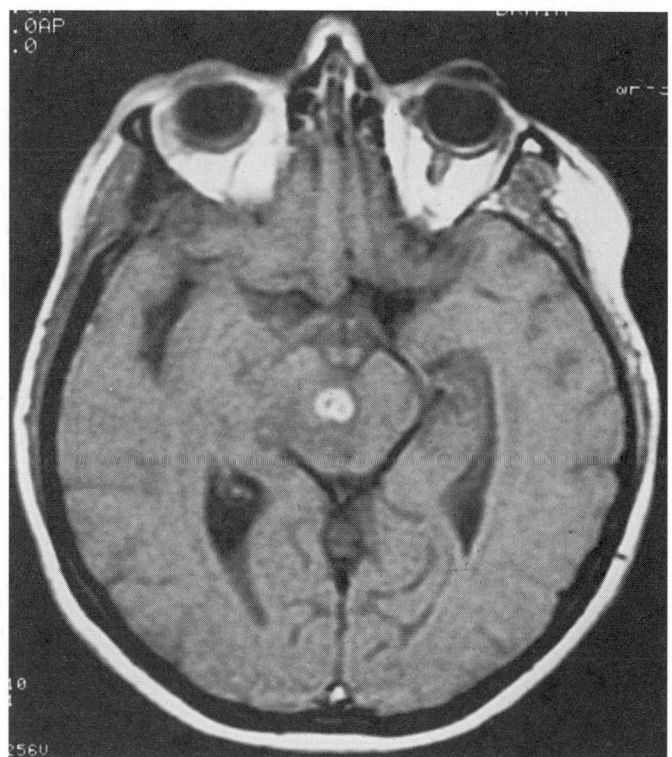

FIG. 152-3. Focal lesion of the pons in a 43-year-old woman found on workup for headaches. The lesion was biopsied and found to be inflammatory with no evidence of tumor. The patient was treated with a short course of steroids and the lesion has regressed slightly over a 6-month follow-up period.

cently hyperfractionated radiotherapy has been used by several groups in an attempt to increase the total tumor dose. Although these trials have resulted in escalation of the total dose up to 78 Gy, no clear benefit has accrued using this approach.

PROGNOSIS

As previously stated, brainstem gliomas are a heterogeneous group of tumors in terms of presenting symptoms, appearance on imaging studies, histology, appropriate workup, therapy, and prognosis. In children, pretreatment characteristics define two distinct prognostic groups (Table 152-2). The most common subtype is the diffuse pontine glioma, associated with a short (less than 2-month) history of symptoms, typically in a younger (less than 7-year-old) patient. This constellation of presenting characteristics is pathognomonic and biopsy is not warranted. Current treatment would be radiotherapy, conventional or hyperfractionated. Median survival for this group of patients is approximately 1 year, with only rare survivors at 2 years.

Focal brainstem lesions proved to be low grade on biopsy carry a much better prognosis. Intrinsic focal brainstem gliomas have up to 80 percent survival at 5 years following hyperfrac-

TABLE 152-2. Prognostic Factors in Children With Brainstem Gliomas

	Prognosis	
Characteristic	Poor	Better
Duration of symptoms	≤2 mo	>2 mo
Location	Pons/medulla	Midbrain
Appearance on MRI	Diffuse	Focal
Age	≤6 yr	>6 yr

tionated radiotherapy. Other special subtypes such as cervicomedullary tumors and dorsally exophytic lesions of the brainstem or tectum are amenable to surgery, and adjuvant radiotherapy may be withheld until the time of tumor regrowth.

Brainstem gliomas in adults are less well characterized by prognostic factors. Overall survival has been reported to be better compared with the pediatric group, probably because a higher proportion of poor-risk pediatric patients are entered on treatment protocols. Survival in adults appears to be correlated to histology and is comparable to survival of patients with similar astrocytic tumors of the cerebral hemispheres.

SUGGESTED READINGS

Albright AL, Guthkelch N, Packer RJ et al: Prognostic factors in pediatric brain-stem gliomas. J Neurosurg 65:751, 1986

Barkovich AJ, Krischer J, Kun LE: Brain stem gliomas: a classification system based on magnetic resonance imaging. Pediatr Neurosurg 16:73, 1990

Berger MS, Edwards MSB, LaMasters D et al: Pediatric brain stem tumors: radiographic, pathological, and clinical correlations. Neurosurgery 12:298, 1983

Edwards MSB, Prados M: Current management of brain stem gliomas. Pediatr Neurosci 13:309, 1987

Edwards MSB, Wara WM, Ciricillo SF, Barkovich AJ: Focal brain-stem astrocytomas causing symptoms of involvement of the facial nerve nucleus: long-term survival in six pediatric cases. J Neurosurg 80:20, 1994

Epstein F: A staging system for brain stem gliomas. Cancer 56:1804, 1985

Epstein F, Wisoff JH: Intrinsic brainstem tumors in childhood: surgical indications. J Neurooncol 6:309, 1988

Freeman CR, Suissa S: Brain stem tumors in children: results of a survey of 62 patients treated with radiotherapy. Int J Radiat Oncol Biol Phys 12:1823, 1986

Freeman CR, Krischer J, Sanford RA et al: Hyperfractionated radiotherapy in brain stem tumors: results of a pediatric oncology group study. Int J Radiat Oncol Biol Phys 15:311, 1988

Freeman CR, Krischer J, Sanford RA et al: Hyperfractionated radiation therapy in brain stem tumors. Cancer 68:474, 1991

Freeman CR, Krischer J, Sanford RA et al: Final results of a study of escalating doses of hyperfractionated radiotherapy in brain stem tumors in children: a Pediatric Oncology Group study. Int J Radiat Oncol Biol Phys 27:197–206, 1993

Halperin EC, Wehn SM, Scott JW et al: Selection of management strategy for pediatric brainstem tumors. Med Pediatr Oncol 17:116, 1989

Kretschmar CS, Tarbell NJ, Barnes PD et al: Pre-irradiation chemotherapy and hyperfractionated radiation therapy 66 Gy for children with brain stem tumors. Cancer 72:1404, 1994

Levin VA, Edwards MS, Wara WM et al: 5-Fluorouracil and 1-(2-chloroethyl)-3-cyclohexyl-1-nitrosourea (CCNU) followed by hydroxyurea, misonidazole, and irradiation for brain stem gliomas: a pilot study of the Brain Tumor Research Center and the Children's Cancer Group. Neurosurgery 14:679, 1984

Packer RJ, Allen JL, Goldwein JL et al: Hyperfractionated radiotherapy for children with brainstem gliomas: a pilot study using 7,200 cGy. Ann Neurol 27:167, 1990

Sanford RA, Freeman CR, Burger P, Cohen ME: Prognostic criteria for experimental protocols in pediatric gliomas. Surg Neurol 30:276, 1988

Shrieve D, Wara WM, Edwards MSB et al: Hyperfractionated radiation therapy for brainstem gliomas in children and adults. Int J Radiat Oncol Biol Phys 24:599, 1992

153. MALIGNANT GLIOMAS

PATRICK Y. WEN
HOWARD A. FINE
PETER McL. BLACK
JAY S. LOEFFLER

In 1994, an estimated 17,500 patients were diagnosed with primary brain tumors in the United States. Malignant gliomas are the most common type of primary brain tumor and account for nearly half the total. They are also responsible for most of the 2.5 percent of cancer deaths caused by primary brain tumors. Approximately 50 to 70 percent of malignant gliomas are glioblastomas and 20 to 40 percent are anaplastic astrocytomas, with smaller numbers of anaplastic oligodendrogliomas, mixed oligoastrocytomas, and ependymomas. This chapter focuses on anaplastic astrocytomas and glioblastomas. Anaplastic oligodendrogliomas and mixed oligoastrocytomas are discussed in Chapter 150, low-grade gliomas and ependymomas in Chapter 161.

EPIDEMIOLOGY

Malignant gliomas occur slightly more commonly in men than in women (1.5:1), and in whites compared with African Americans, Latinos, and Asians. Malignant gliomas tend to affect an older population than low-grade gliomas. Whereas low-grade astrocytomas are most common in patients between 20 and 40 years of age, anaplastic astrocytomas usually occur in patients between 30 and 50 years of age, and glioblastomas in patients 50 years or older. The incidence of malignant gliomas may be increasing in the elderly. Some studies have shown a 200 to 500 percent increase in the incidence of these tumors in patients 75 years and older between 1973 and 1985. Whether this finding is the result of improved detection or whether the number of cases has really increased is unclear.

Several genetic disorders are associated with an increased incidence of malignant gliomas. These include neurofibromatosis-1 and -2, tuberous sclerosis, Turcots syndrome (inherited adenomatous polyposis coli associated with astrocytomas and medulloblastomas), and the Li-Fraumeni syndrome, in which families have a dominantly inherited germline mutation within the p53 tumor suppressor gene on chromosome 17, resulting in an increased incidence of malignant gliomas as well as breast cancer, sarcomas, and leukemias. In addition to patients with these syndromes, increasing evidence shows that patients with malignant gliomas have an increased familial incidence of these tumors in general.

The role of environmental factors in the pathogenesis of malignant gliomas is largely unknown. The strongest association has been with ionizing radiation. Children treated with low-dose radiotherapy for tinea capitis have a 2.6-fold increase in gliomas, and children treated with prophylactic brain irradiation for acute lymphoblastic leukemia have a 22-fold excess of gliomas. An association exists between vinylchloride and gliomas but the significance of this is unknown. Anecdotal reports have recently suggested that exposure to electromagnetic radiation and cellular telephones may be associated with an increased incidence of gliomas. A large epidemiologic study looking into these associations is currently under way.

MOLECULAR BIOLOGY

Significant progress has recently occurred in understanding the molecular biology of malignant gliomas. As with other neoplasms, combinations of genetic alterations in proto-oncogenes and tumor suppressor genes are thought to be involved. A proto-oncogene is a normal cellular gene that through overexpression, mutation, or rearragement results in a protein that promotes the growth of the cell. Conversely, a tumor suppressor gene is a normal cellular gene that acts to check cell growth but becomes inactivated during the process of tumorigenesis. Malignant gliomas are a heterogenous group of tumors in which a number of pathways involving a variety of genetic alterations in proto-oncogenes and tumor suppressor genes are involved.

The genetic alterations that have been reported for astrocytomas include mutations in the p53 and retinoblastoma tumor suppressor genes, as well as putative tumor suppressor genes on chromosomes 17p, 10, and 19q. Proto-oncogenes frequently implicated in astrocytomas include the epidermal growth factor receptor (EGFR), *MDM2,* and platelet-derived growth factor receptor genes. Genes less often involved include N-*myc,* C-*myc, Gli,* N-*ras,* and K-*ras.*

It is believed that at least three different pathways lead to the formation of glioblastomas. The first pathway involves mutation in the p53 tumor suppressor gene at the astrocytoma stage, loss of tumor suppressor genes on chromosomes 9p, 13q, or 19q in the transition to anaplastic astrocytoma, and amplification of EGFR or *MDM2* genes or loss of tumor suppressor genes on chromosome 10 in the transformation to glioblastoma. A second de novo pathway does not involve mutations of p53, but instead loss of a tumor suppressor gene on chromosome 10 or amplification of the EGFR proto-oncogene, or both. A third pathway consists of genetic alterations that have not yet been identified.

The growth factors produced by genetic alterations in malignant gliomas have important effects not only on cell proliferation but also on other aspects of glioma biology. Basic fibroblast growth factor and vascular endothelial growth factor have an important role as angiogenic factors, stimulating the formation of new blood vessels critical for tumor growth. In addition, vascular endothelial growth factor alters the permeability of tumor blood vessels, leading to peritumoral edema, and acts as a procoagulant, contributing to the increased incidence of thromboembolic disease in patients with malignant gliomas.

CLINICAL FEATURES

Malignant gliomas and the associated peritumoral edema produce symptoms by a combination of compression and infiltration of surrounding brain, vascular compression, and increased intracranial pressure.

The presenting symptoms for malignant gliomas are similar to those for other brain tumors (see Ch. 148). They include headaches (30 to 50 percent), seizures (30 to 60 percent), focal neurologic deficits (40 to 60 percent), and mental status changes (20 to 40 percent). The headaches are often nonspecific and indistinguishable from tension headaches, although as the tumor enlarges, features of increased intracranial pressure may appear. Seizures occur in 59 percent of frontal gliomas, 42 percent of parietal gliomas, 35 percent of temporal gliomas, and 33 percent of occipital gliomas. The presentation of patients with malignant gliomas is becoming increasingly subtle as the widespread availability of cerebral imaging allows patients to be diagnosed at an earlier stage. The duration of symptoms tends to be fairly short (weeks or a few months), although patients whose tumors have developed from pre-existing low-grade gliomas may have a long history of seizures.

IMAGING

Computed Tomography and Magnetic Resonance Imaging

Malignant astrocytomas have variable appearances radiographically. In general they tend to be less circumscribed than low-grade astrocytomas and surrounded with more edema. On com-

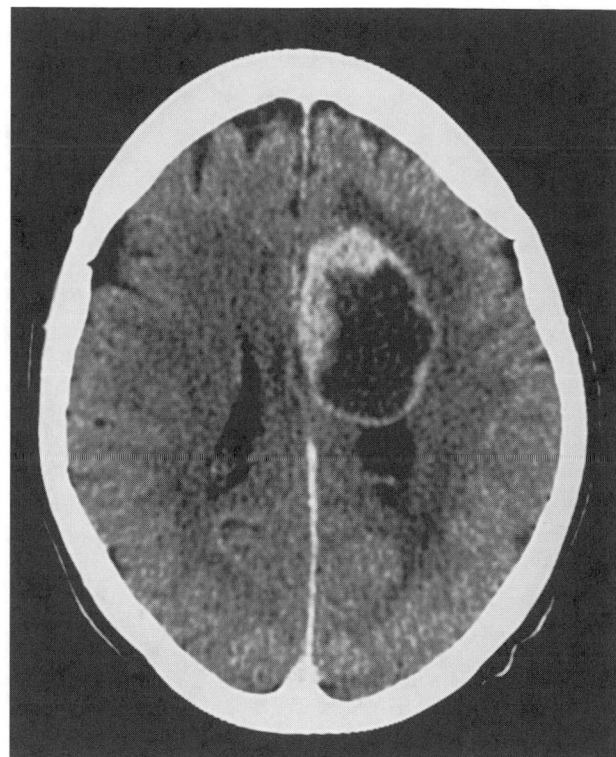

FIG. 153-1. CT scan of a 50-year-old woman with a left frontal glioblastoma, showing a ring-enhancing lesion with a central area of necrosis and surrounding edema. From Black P, Wen PY: Clinical, imaging and laboratory diagnosis of brain tumors. In Kaye A, Laws E, (eds): Brain Tumors. Churchill Livingstone, Edinburgh, 1995, with permission.)

puted tomography (CT) scans they appear as hypodense or isodense lesions that enhance variably with contrast (Figs. 153-1 and 153-2). Glioblastomas frequently have a central hypodense area of necrosis surrounded by a thick enhancing rim of tumor. Often extensive surrounding edema is seen. On magnetic resonance imaging (MRI) these tumors characteristically have low signal intensity on T1-weighted images and high signal intensity on T2-weighted images. Tumor cells extend at least as far as the margins of increased T2 signal. The appearance of contrast-enhanced T1-weighted MRIs is similar to that of contrast-enhanced CT scans. These tumors tend to infiltrate along white matter tracts and frequently involve and cross the corpus callosum. Hemorrhage may be present, but calcification is uncommon unless the malignant glioma arose from a pre-existing lower grade lesion.

Contrast enhancement results from extravasation of dye into the extracellular space through a disrupted blood–brain barrier. Thus it is a manifestation of a disturbed blood brain barrier rather than a true measure of tumor extent. Corticosteroids, by re-establishing the blood–brain barrier, can reduce tumor enhancement and lead to the erroneous conclusion that tumor size has been reduced. Although enhancing tumors tend to have a higher histologic grade than nonenhancing tumors, exceptions are frequent, and caution should be used when relating contrast enhancement to malignancy. Approximately 4 to 10 percent of glioblastomas do not enhance, whereas a higher percentage of low-grade gliomas show enhancement. Functional imaging techniques such as positron-emission tomography (PET) scanning using ^{18}F-fluorodeoxyglucose (FDG) and cerebral blood

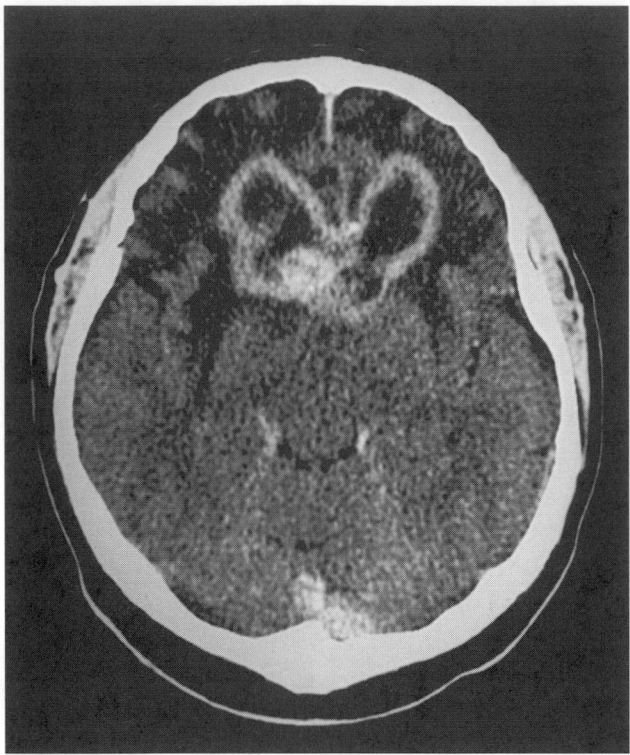

FIG. 153-2.   CT scan of a 30-year-old man with a "butterfly glioblastoma" involving the corpus callosum and both frontal lobes.

volume maps using echoplanar MRI may provide more accurate noninvasive methods of evaluating tumor grade.

Postoperative CT or MRI scans obtained to determine the amount of residual tumor (serving as a baseline for gauging response to further treatment) should be performed within 5 days of surgery. Postsurgical enhancement typically develops around the fifth postoperative day, peaks after approximately 2 weeks, and may persist for months.

In recent years the introduction of new treatment modalities such as stereotactic brachytherapy and radiosurgery, which deliver high focal doses of radiation to the tumor, have resulted in an increased incidence of radiation necrosis. This appears as contrast-enhancing lesions with surrounding edema on CT or MRI, developing 4 to 16 months after treatment. The radiologic appearance of radiation necrosis is indistinguishable from tumor recurrence on CT or MRI, posing a difficult management problem. Frequently, a definitive diagnosis can only be made by stereotactic biopsy. Functional imaging with FDG-PET and ^{20}T ^{99m}Tc hexame-hytpropyleneamine-oxime (HMPAO), single-photon-emission computed tomography (SPECT) scans are noninvasive methods that can be useful in differentiating radiation changes from tumor recurrence in some patients.

Positron Emission Tomography

PET provides dynamic information regarding the metabolism and physiology of brain tumors. It is not used for the routine diagnosis of brain tumors but can provide important information complementing CT and MRI. Most PET studies in brain tumors have used FDG to measure glucose metabolism, which is increased in tumor cells. FDG-PET has been used to determine tumor grade in patients with malignant gliomas noninvasively to localize areas of probable tumor for stereotactic bi-

opsy, to differentiate residual tumor after surgery from postoperative changes, to study the metabolic effects of chemotherapy, radiotherapy, and steroids on tumor metabolism, to identify tumor recurrence, and to diffentiate radiation necrosis from tumor recurrence.

Single-Photon-Emission Computed Tomography

SPECT is more widely available than PET and is used with increasing frequency to complement information obtained by CT or MRI scanning in patients with brain tumors. ^{201}Tl chloride, a potassium analogue that is taken up by viable tumor cells, has been used to differentiate low-grade from high-grade gliomas and to identify residual astrocytoma after radiotherapy. More recently it has been used in combination with ^{99m}Tc HMPAO, a blood flow tracer that crosses normal blood–brain barrier, to differentiate radiation necrosis from recurrent glioma.

DIFFERENTIAL DIAGNOSIS

As indicated in Chapter 148, many conditions that produce increased intracranial pressure or progressive neurologic deficits may mimic malignant gliomas clinically. These include other brain tumors (especially metastases, primary central nervous system lymphoma, and enhancing low-grade gliomas), and non-neoplastic conditions such as subdural hematomas, brain abscesses, hydrocephalus, benign intracranial hypertension, progressive multifocal leukoencephalopathy, multiple sclerosis, vascular malformations, cerebral infarctions, and Alzheimer's disease. Many of these conditions have characteristic radiologic appearances that differentiate them from malignant gliomas. However, some of these conditions, especially other types of tumor, can be difficult to distinguish from malignant gliomas on the basis of their radiologic appearances alone, and a definitive diagnosis requires histologic examination.

PATHOLOGY/HISTOLOGIC GRADING

Malignant gliomas are extremely heterogenous tumors characterized by increased cellularity, pleomorphism, mitoses, endothelial proliferation, and necrosis (Fig. 153-3). Because of their astrocytic origin, tumor cells are often glial fibrillary acidic protein positive.

The ideal tumor grading system combines the ability to predict behavior and prognosis with reproducibility and a minimum of interobserver variation. Several grading systems have been proposed for astrocytomas, most using three or four grades of malignancy. Unfortunately, the multiplicity of schemes contributes to a sense of confusion concerning the grading of astrocytomas and makes comparison of results between different studies difficult.

Earlier grading schemes such as the World Health Organization and Kernohan systems correlated poorly with patient survival. These systems have been replaced by four grading systems that have prognostic implications: (1) the modified Ringertz system, (2) the St. Anne-Mayo/Daumas-Duport system, (3) the University of California, San Francisco (UCSF) system, and (4) World Health Organization Classification (WHO) (Table 153-1).

The modified Ringertz system separates astrocytomas into three histologic grades: astrocytoma, anaplastic astrocytoma, and glioblastoma multiforme. Patients with anaplastic astrocy-

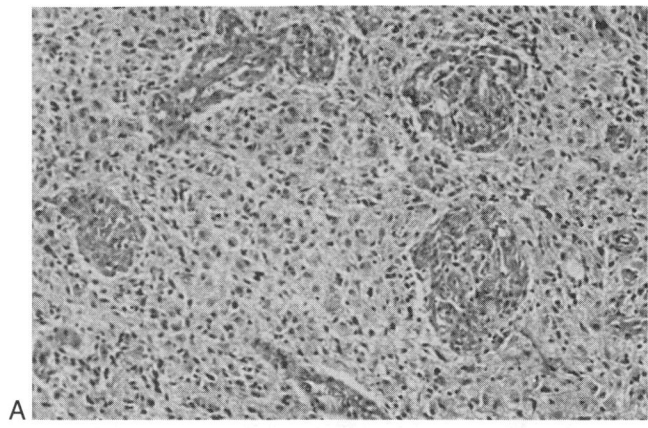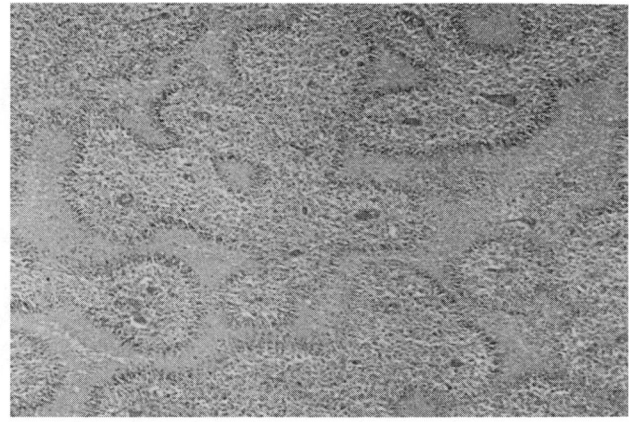

A   B

FIG. 153-3. **(A)** Histology of glioblastoma showing extensive areas of necrosis lined by pseudopalisading. **(B)** Areas of endothelial proliferation. (From Okazaki H, Scheithauer BW: Atlas of Neuropathology. CV Mosby, St. Louis, 1988, with permission.)

tomas have a significantly increased 1-year survival (60 to 73 percent) compared with glioblastoma (35 to 44 percent). Low-grade astrocytomas consist of a uniform population of glial fibrillary acidic protein-positive cells with a mild-to-moderate increase in cellularity and relatively little nuclear or cytoplasmic pleomorphism. Anaplastic astrocytomas are characterized by marked increase in cellularity, moderate pleomorphism, mitotic figures, and vascular endothelial proliferation (Fig. 153-4). Glioblastomas have areas of necrosis often surrounded by pseudopalisading in addition to the features present in anaplastic astrocytomas.

The St. Anne-Mayo (Daumas-Duport) scheme is based on the presence or absence of four histologic criteria: (1) nuclear atypia, (2) mitoses, (3) endothelial proliferation, and (4) necrosis. Grade I tumors have none of the criteria, grade II have one, grade III have two, and grade IV have three or four criteria present. Median survival for patients with grades II, II, and IV tumors were 4 years, 1.6 years, and 0.7 years, respectively. Very few patients have grade I tumors. An advantage of this grading scheme is that it is relatively easy to use and interobserver variation is small. The concordance among pathologists who use the St. Anne-Mayo system is reported to be as high as 94 percent.

The UCSF classification divides astrocytomas into a four-tiered system based on degree of cellularity, cytoplasmic and nuclear pleomorphism, vascular proliferation, and number of mitoses. The four grades of astrocytoma are mildly anaplastic, moderately anaplastic, highly anaplastic astrocytomas, and glioblastoma multiforme. Median survival for patients with moderately anaplastic astrocytoma is 220 weeks, for highly anaplastic astrocytoma 116 weeks, and for glioblastomas 66 weeks.

Recently, the WHO published a revised histologic classification of central nervous system tumors. In this classification, pilocytic astrocytomas corresponds to grade 1, astrocytomas to

grade II, anaplastic astrocytomas to grade III, and glioblastomas to grade IV (Table 1).

Malignant gliomas are extremely heterogeneous and the histology of tissues obtained by stereotactic biopsy are not always representative of the entire tumor. The larger amounts of tissue obtained by surgical resection usually allow a more accurate histologic diagnosis to be made. Even when sampling errors are taken into account, the grading of astrocytomas based on histologic appearance remains inexact. Although patients with higher grades tend to have a poorer prognosis, the outcome for individual patients within a single grade can be quite variable. Because of these limitations, there is increasing interest in improving tumor grading using techniques to determine the proliferative index of the tumors. These techniques include antibodies against bromodeoxyuridine (BUdR), Ki-67, and proliferating cell nuclear antigen.

The greatest experience has been with BUdR, a thymidine analogue, which is administered intravenously at surgery. The proportion of cells labelled with BUdR on histologic sections of tumor provides an indication of the cells in DNA synthesis. This BUdR labeling index correlates with patient survival. Mean labeling indices for glioblastoma, anaplastic astrocytoma, and astrocytomas are 9.3, 4, and 1 percent, respectively. Regardless of the pathologic diagnosis patients with a labeling index of greater than 5 percent had a much poorer prognosis than patients with indices below 5 percent. Similar results have been obtained with antibodies to Ki-67, which labels an antigen in all phases of the cell cycle except G_0, and with proliferating cell nuclear antigen.

UNCOMMON TYPES

Several less common histologic variants of malignant gliomas are seen. Gliosarcoma consists of a sarcomatous component

TABLE 153-1. Astrocytoma Grading Systems

Kernohan	Modified Ringertz	UCSF	St. Anne-Mayo	WHO	
Astrocytoma grade 1 Astrocytoma grade 2	Astrocytoma (grade 1)	Mildly anaplastic astrocytoma Moderately anaplastic astrocytoma	Astrocytoma grade 1 Astrocytoma grade 2	Pilocytic Astrocytoma Astrocytoma	grade I grade II
	Anaplastic astrocytoma (grade 2)	Highly anaplastic astrocytoma Gemistocytic astrocytoma	Astrocytoma grade 3	Anaplastic Astrocytoma	grade III
Astrocytoma grade 3 Astrocytoma grade 4	Glioblastoma multiforme (grade 3)	Glioblastoma multiforme	Astrocytoma grade 4	Glioblastoma	grade IV

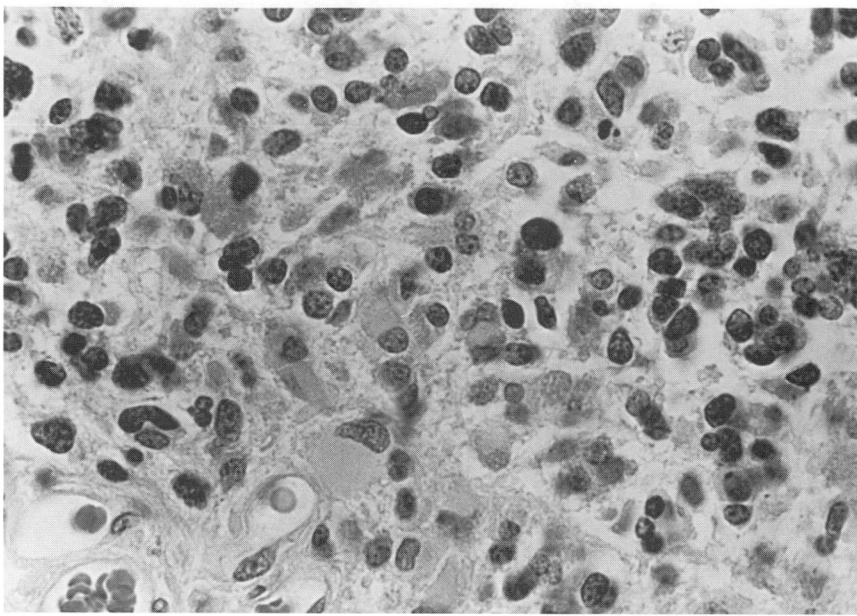

FIG. 153-4. Anaplastic astrocytoma showing hypercellularity and nuclear pleomorphism.

admixed with glioma. This is a variant of glioblastoma and has the same prognosis. Gemistocytic astrocytoma consists of cells with abundant eosinophilic cytoplasm, often occurring as foci within more usual fibrillary tumor, and has a prognosis similar to anaplastic astrocytoma. Gliomatosis cerebri is an uncommon form of malignant glioma characterized by diffuse infiltration of the brain by malignant astrocytes without the formation of a discrete mass. These tumors tend to have the same prognosis as glioblastoma. Pleomorphic xanthoastrocytoma is a rare tumor with a characteristic histologic appearance that arises in the temporal or parietal region of children and young adults and has a more indolent course than malignant glioma.

PROGNOSTIC FACTORS

Malignant gliomas are a prognostically heterogenous group of tumors. In addition to tumor histology, age at diagnosis and Karnofsky performance status are the most important prognostic factors. Young age, a histologic diagnosis of anaplastic astrocytoma, and a high Karnofsky score are favorable prognostic factors.

Age

Data from the Brain Tumor Cooperative Group studies show that younger patients live significantly longer than older patients, even when adjusted for other important prognostic factors. Patients under age 40 with glioblastomas have a 50 percent 18-month survival rate compared with 20 percent for those between 40 and 60 and 10 percent for those over 60. Age may be an even more important prognostic factor than histology. In one recent study, patients under 60 with anaplastic astrocytoma lived longer than those with glioblastoma, but patients over 60 had similar median survivals times regardless of the histology.

Histology

As previously discussed, patients with anaplastic astrocytomas have a significantly better prognosis than patients with glioblas-

tomas. Median survival for anaplastic astrocytoma is approximately 36 months compared with 10 months for glioblastomas.

Performance Status

The prognosis of patients with malignant gliomas decreases as the Karnofsky performance status decreases. Malignant glioma patients with a score of greater than 70 have a 34 percent 18-month survival compared with 13 percent for those with a score of less than 60.

Other favorable prognostic factors that have been observed with less consistency include a long duration of symptoms prior to diagnosis, presence of seizures, absence of mental status and personality changes at diagnosis, location of tumor (e.g., frontal and temporal pole), small preoperative tumor size, gross total resection, small postoperative and postradiation tumor size, and blood group O.

TREATMENT

As with other neoplasms, the optimal management of malignant gliomas involves cytoreduction through multimodality therapy including surgery, irradiation, and chemotherapy. Interpretation of the results of clinical trials involving patients with malignant gliomas has frequently been complicated by inadequate patient numbers, absence of appropriate controls, and failure to take into account prognostic factors such as patient age and tumor grade, which significantly influence patient survival.

Surgery

The optimal treatment of patients with malignant gliomas involves surgical resection of as much tumor as is neurologically safe. Stereotactic biopsies should be reserved for deep or critically located tumors that cannot be safely resected. The safety of surgery has been greatly improved in recent years by the use of the operating microscope, the cavitron ultrasonic aspirator, intraoperative ultrasound, laser systems, CT- and MRI-guided stereotaxy, and intraoperative neurophysiologic monitoring.

Operative mortality ranges from 0 to 3 percent and morbidity from 8 to 14 percent. In addition to debulking the tumor and relieving any symptoms resulting from mass effect, surgery allows a precise histologic diagnosis to be made and possibly increases the effectiveness of adjuvant therapies by reducing the number of cells that must be treated, altering cell kinetics, and removing radioresistant hypoxic cells and areas of tumor inaccessible to chemotherapy. The role of surgery in prolonging survival remains controversial. Although some studies suggest that patients undergoing resection live longer than those who only have biopsies, (suggesting that the extent of resection is important), other studies indicate that survival correlates more closely with the amount of residual tumor seen on postoperative CT scans than the actual amount of tumor resected.

Surgery plays an important role in the treatment of patients with recurrent tumor. In selected patients with a discrete tumor mass, reoperation can increase survival by as much as 9 months. Surgery has also assumed an increasingly important role in the patients who have been treated with stereotactic brachytherapy or radiosurgery. These patients frequently develop radiation necrosis, which is radiologically indistinguishable from tumor recurrence; surgical biopsy is often required for definitive diagnosis. In approximately 40 to 65 percent of patients treated with brachytherapy and 10 to 30 percent of patients treated with radiosurgery, the areas of radiation necrosis become symptomatic and require surgical resection.

Radiotherapy

Radiotherapy remains the most effective adjunctive therapy to surgery for the treatment of patients with malignant gliomas. The value of radiotherapy was demonstrated by Brain Tumor Study Group (BTSG) study 69-01 (reported by Walker and collegues), which showed that 50 to 60 Gy of whole-brain radiotherapy increased median survival in patients with malignant gliomas from 14 weeks after surgery alone to 36 weeks. Subsequent studies confirmed the benefit of radiotherapy and suggested that survival was related to to an increase in the dose of radiation up to 60 Gy. Administration of doses of radiation above 60 Gy at standard fractionation were associated with a significantly increased risk of radiation injury to normal brain tissue. Based on these studies the recommendation for conventional external beam radiotherapy is 60 Gy in single daily fractions of 1.7 to 2 Gy, five times a week. This is usually administered to a limited field that includes the enhancing volume on CT scans together with a 2- to 3-cm margin or a 1-cm margin beyond T2-weighted MRI changes. No survival advantage seems to exist for irradiating the whole brain compared with treating more limited fields, and whole-brain irradiation may be associated with a higher incidence of delayed neurotoxicity.

In an attempt to improve on the results of conventional external beam irradiation, several novel strategies have been developed to sensitize tumors selectively to the effects of radiation and escalate the tumor dose while biologically or physically limiting the dose to normal brain.

Radiosensitizers and Altered Fractionation Schedules

Hypoxic cell sensitizers, pyrimidine analogs, and perfluorochemical emulsions have been used to increase the sensitivity of glioma cells to ionizing radiation. Although studies are ongoing, the results so far have been disappointing.

Another approach uses hyperfractionation. This utilizes the greater capacity of normal brain tissue to repair sublethal damage, compared with glioma cells, and involves the administration of several small fractions of radiation a day to a higher total dose. To date no study has demonstrated a survival advantage using hyperfractionated schedules. Similarly disappointing results have been obtained with accelerated fractionation, which involves the administration of conventional fraction sizes over a shorter period, reducing the opportunity for tumor cells to repopulate during treatment.

Stereotactic Brachytherapy

Most patients with malignant gliomas treated with 60 Gy of standard external beam radiation have persistent disease, and 80 to 100 percent recur within 2 cm of the primary site. Brachytherapy uses stereotactic techniques to place catheters containing radioactive isotopes (e.g.,^{125}I) accurately within brain tumors, allowing tumoricidal doses of radiation to be delivered to defined volumes, while reducing the risk of serious radiation injury to surrounding normal tissues. Typically brachytherapy delivers an additional 50 to 60 Gy of radiation, increasing the total dose of radiation delivered to the tumor bed to more than 110 Gy.

Brachytherapy is limited to unifocal, well-defined, supratentorial tumors less than 4 cm in diameter that do not involve corpus callosum, brainstem, or ependymal surfaces. Because of these restrictions, only 20 to 30 percent of patients with malignant gliomas are suitable candidates.

Stereotactic brachytherapy produces a modest increase in survival in patients with glioblastomas when used as adjunctive therapy after surgery and standard external beam radiotherapy. Median survival in these patients is increased from 11 to 14 months to 18 to 27 months, with a significantly increased percentage of long-term survivors. By contrast, patients with anaplastic astrocytomas do not appear to benefit from brachytherapy.

Focal radiation necrosis occurs in most patients undergoing brachytherapy, and 40 to 65 percent of patients require resection of the necrotic mass 6 months to 2 years after the procedure. Despite the high reoperation rate, the quality of life of most patients undergoing brachytherapy appears to be satisfactory.

In an attempt to improve on the results of brachytherapy, several studies are under way evaluating the combination of brachytherapy with hyperthermia, hypoxic cell sensitizers, and pyrimidine analogs.

Stereotactic Radiosurgery

Stereotactic radiosurgery is a technique used to treat small (less than 4 cm) radiographically well-defined tumors with a large single fraction of ionizing radiation using stereotactically directed narrow beams. Like brachytherapy, it significantly increases the radiation dose delivered to the tumor bed while sparing normal brain. Radiosurgery has the advantage over brachytherapy of being noninvasive, which allows patients with tumors in surgically inaccessible or eloquent areas of the brain or serious coexisting medical illnesses to be treated as outpatients. Preliminary results, as reported by Loeffler and colleagues, appear promising; selected patients treated with external irradiation followed 3 weeks later by stereotactic radiosurgery delivering 1.2 Gy in a single fraction to the enhancing mass and a 2- to 4-mm margin had a median survival (for glioblastoma patients) of 26 months, with only 19 percent of patients requiring reoperation for radiation necrosis.

Stereotactic Radiotherapy

Stereotactic radiotherapy is a novel technique that involves the precise delivery of fractionated radiation to the tumor volume while sparing surrounding brain. It combines the accuracy of stereotactic radiosurgery with the reduced toxicity of fractionated external beam irradiation and is likely to be a highly useful adjunctive therapy for malignant gliomas as well as a variety of other brain tumors.

Although techniques such as brachytherapy and radiosurgery may improve local tumor control, they do not treat tumor cells infiltrating into the surrounding brain. Increasingly, patients are relapsing at distant sites, and a growing need exists for more effective medical therapy to complement the advances in surgery and radiation therapy.

Chemotherapy

Adjuvant Chemotherapy. Even though more than 20 randomized trials have been performed, the role of adjuvant chemotherapy for patients with malignant gliomas remains controversial. Chemotherapy probably has a modest but significant effect in increasing survival when administered following surgery and radiotherapy. In BTSG trial 69-01 (reported by Walker et al.) the median survival was not significantly prolonged, but at 18 months, 19 percent of patients receiving carmustine (BCNU), radiation, and surgery were alive compared with 4 percent of those receiving surgery and radiation alone. In BTSG trial 75-01 (reported by Green et al.) the addition of BCNU to surgery and radiotherapy significantly increased median survival from 40 weeks to 50 weeks and also increased the percentage of patients surviving 18 months to 24 percent. More recently, a meta-analysis of the major adjuvant chemotherapy trials showed a 10.1 percent increase in survival at 1 year and an 8.6 percent increase at 2 years for patients treated with both chemotherapy and radiation compared with radiation alone.

Currently, standard therapy for patients with newly diagnosed malignant gliomas involves maximum feasible surgical resection followed by limited field external beam radiation with or without adjuvant chemotherapy with BCNU (200 mg/m^2). For patients with anaplastic astrocytoma, procarbazine, lomustine, and vincristine (PCV) (lomustine 110 mg/m^2 on day 1; vincristine 1.4 mg/m^2 on days 8 and 28; procarbazine 60 mg/m^2 on days 8 to 21) appear to be superior to BCNU. Other chemotherapeutic agents have not proved to be any more effective than BCNU or PCV. Patients under 50 years of age and with good performance status benefit most from adjuvant chemotherapy.

The results of standard therapy remain poor. The median survival of patients with glioblastomas is approximately 9 to 12 months, whereas the median survival of patients with anaplastic astrocytomas is 24 to 39 months.

Chemotherapy for Recurrent Gliomas. Chemotherapy may play a palliative role in patients with recurrent malignant gliomas. Response rates of 20 to 50 percent have been reported with a variety of agents, although this is usually not associated with prolonged survival. One approach is to begin with nitrosourea-based chemotherapy (BCNU or PCV) if the patient has not been treated with these drugs before. In patients who recur after treatment with nitrosoureas, potentially useful agents include procarbazine, cyclophosphamide and vincristine, and carboplatin. When appropriate, patients with recurrent gliomas should be encouraged to participate in ongoing clinical trials so that more effective drug regimens can be developed.

New Approaches to Chemotherapy. The poor results with conventional chemotherapy have led to a search for new drugs with greater antiglioma activity as well as strategies to use currently available agents more effectively.

Several promising agents have recently become available and are entering clinical trials. These include temozolamide and topotecan (a topoisomerase I inhibitor), which have excellent central nervous system penetration, and paclitaxel (Taxol), a microtubule binding agent that acts both as a cytotoxic agent and a radiosensitizer.

Intra-arterial chemotherapy has been used in an attempt to deliver higher concentrations of drug to the tumor while avoiding systemic toxicities. This approach has produced slightly higher tumor response rates (27 to 60 percent), but patient survival is usually not significantly prolonged. In addition, intra-arterial administration of agents such as BCNU have been associated with significant ophthalmic and neural toxicity.

Attempts have also been made to increase the permeability of water-soluble drugs across the blood–brain barrier by transient disruption of the barrier with agents such as intra-arterial mannitol. Several studies combining blood–brain barrier disruption and intra-arterial drug administration have produced slightly increased response rates. However, the usefulness of this approach remains questionable, and agents such as mannitol expose normal brain to higher doses of chemotherapy, increasing the potential for neurotoxicity. The recent development of drugs that are more selective in disrupting the blood–brain barrier, such as leukotrienes, may increase the effectiveness of this approach.

Increasing interest has also arisen in overcoming the resistance of gliomas to alkylating agents by delivering higher doses accompanied by hematopoietic growth factors and autologous bone marrow transplantation (ABMT). Although several studies with ABMT have shown higher response rates in patients with recurrent gliomas, this has not generally translated into prolonged survival. Moreover, significant extramedullary toxicities, such as hepatotoxitiy and neurotoxicity, have been observed in some of these studies. Slightly more encouraging results have been observed when ABMT has been used in the adjuvant setting. Many of these studies used only single agents, and it is possible that the use of ABMT with combinations of chemotherapeutic agents that have nonoverlapping toxicities will be more effective.

Interstitial chemotherapy is a more promising approach that involves the implantation into the tumor bed of biodegradable polymers impregnated with a chemotherapeutic agent. This produces prolonged exposure of the tumor to the drug while minimizing systemic toxicity. A recently completed phase III study in patients with recurrent gliomas in involving reoperation and implantation of polymer wafers impregnated with BCNU into the tumor bed produced a median survival of 46 weeks. In addition to delivering chemotherapy, polymer wafers may also be useful for delivering steroids, antiangiogenic agents, and other novel therapies.

Another promising approach is the use of preradiation (neoadjuvant) chemotherapy. Radiation damages the tumor microvasculature, limiting the delivery of drug to the tumor, by producing tissue hypoxia and cellular growth arrest, it also reduces the effectiveness of chemotherapy. Treatment of patients with chemotherapy prior to radiotherapy potentially overcomes these problems. Recent studies using preradiation BCNU and cisplatin have shown encouraging results.

Despite these newer strategies, the therapeutic efficacy of radiotherapy and chemotherapy remains limited, partly because the final common pathway of cytotoxicity for both chemotherapy and radiotherapy is DNA damage, a relatively nonselective process that occurs in normal as well as neoplastic cells. This results in a low therapeutic ratio that prevents the use of the high doses of chemotherapy and radiotherapy necessary to kill tumor cells completely. As a result, increasing interest has arisen in finding new therapeutic methods for treating gliomas.

NEW THERAPIES

Immunotherapy

The results of immunotherapy in the past have been dissapointing, but the recent availability of more potent cytokines and advances in molecular biology have led to renewed interest in this form of treatment.

Clinical studies with cytokines such as interferon-α and -β as well as tumor necrosis factor have shown modest antitumor activity. Response rates of 0 to 20 percent have been reported for interferon-α and up to 50 percent for interferon-β, although the duration of responses has generally been short. A new generation of more potent cytokines, such as BG9015 (a nonmutated interferon-β), have been developed and are in clinical studies. Other cytokines such as interleukin-4 have shown promising antitumor activity in preclinical studies. Combinations of cytokines with chemotherapy appear to have synergistic effects and may be more effective than either modality alone.

Over the past few years, interest has arisen in adoptive immunotherapy using interleukin-2 and lymphokine-activated killer cells. Most studies in patients with gliomas have used direct injections of lymphokine-activated killer cells and interleukin-2 either into the parenchyma around the tumor at craniotomy or into tumor beds using indwelling catheters. The results of lymphokine-activated killer cell therapy have generally been disappointing, partly because these cells cannot migrate and kill infiltrating tumor cells.

Passive immunotherapy with monoclonal antibodies has been limited by significant technical problems including the lack of truly tumor-specific antigens, poor access of antibodies across the blood–brain barrier, and the development of neutralizing antibodies. Despite these problems, preliminary studies with radiolabeled antibodies against the epidermal growth factor receptor have shown encouraging antitumor activity. Current research is directed toward developing more specific, chimeric, and human antibodies. Whether these strategies will increase the effectiveness of monoclonal antibodies remains to be seen.

Antiangiogenesis

Gliomas produce specific angiogenic peptides (e.g., basic fibroblast growth factor and vascular endothelial growth factor) to stimulate the formation of new blood vessels, which are critical for tumor growth. There is increasing interest in angiogenesis inhibition as a new therapeutic strategy for gliomas. Several potent inhibitors of angiogenesis have been identified (e.g., platelet factor-4, TNP-470, and angiostatin) and will be evaluated in phase I studies in the near future.

Differentiation Agents

Another interesting approach involves the use of agents such as phenylacetate and retinoic acid, which are thought to produce antitumor activity by inducing differentiation of glioma cells. These agents are generally well tolerated and are being evaluated in clinical studies.

Growth Factor and Second Messenger Inhibition

Numerous therapeutic strategies have been developed based on our increased understanding of the influence of growth factors and second messengers on glioma growth. Among the more promising strategies are those involving inhibition of protein kinase C (PKC), epidermal growth factor, and platelet-derived growth factor autocrine systems.

PKC is a ubiquitous cell membrane-associated second messenger involved in the transduction of mitogenic signals from the cell surface to the nucleus. Recent studies suggest that inhibition of PKC activity suppresses growth of glioma cell lines. Tamoxifen is a potent inhibitor of PKC that produces a 40 percent response rate in patients with recurrent gliomas when used at very high doses (160 to 200 mg/d). More potent inhibitors of PKC have been developed and will be entering clinical trials in the near future.

Platelet-derived growth factor is probably involved in autocrine and paracrine loops in the growth of many gliomas. New therapeutic strategies are being investigated to break such loops, including use of the drug suramin, which inhibits the factor, and the development of dominant negative mutations of platelet-derived growth factor that inhibit the wild-type molecule.

Gene Therapy

The rapid advances in molecular biology have resulted in a number of novel therapies for malignant gliomas. One strategy uses genetically engineered thymidine kinase-negative mutants of herpes simplex virus-1. These viruses replicate and kill dividing cells such as glioblastoma but do not replicate in nondividing brain cells. Preliminary studies have shown that they have significant antitumor activity against gliomas in nude mice. Another strategy involves a gene encoding an enzyme that makes tumor cells more susceptible to chemotherapy. In this approach, the herpes simplex thymidine kinase gene is inserted into a replication-defective murine retrovirus. Murine fibroblast cell lines can be engineered to produce these recombinant retroviruses constitutively. When the murine fibroblasts are injected into gliomas, proliferating tumor cells become infected by the retroviral vector. These tumor cells produce thymidine kinase and become susceptible to attack by the antiherpes drug gancyclovir. Nondividing brain cells are not infected by the retroviral vectors and remain unaffected by gancyclovir. Animal studies using this strategy have shown promising results and clinical studies are in progress. Clinical studies using replication-defective adenovirus vectors to insert the thymidine kinase gene into glioma cells are also about to begin.

Many other strategies for gene therapy exist and are under active investigation. These include increasing the immunogenicity of tumors by transfection of antisense RNA, increasing local cytokine production, enhancing major histocompatibility complex antigen expression, and introducing tumor suppressor genes or genes inducing apoptosis into tumor cells. Hopefully, these novel approaches will lead to the long-awaited breakthroughs in glioma therapy.

SUPPORTIVE THERAPY

Despite some promising advances in the treatment of malignant gliomas, the prognosis for most of these patients remains poor. In addition to providing optimal treatment for the tumor, an important part of management is to provide compassionate and effective supportive care. Many of these patients require glucocorticoids to control cerebral edema and anticonvulsants to treat seizures (see Ch. 141). The use of prophylactic anticonvulsant therapy for glioma patients who have not had seizures remains controversial. Although most patients with gliomas are treated with prophylactic anticonvulsants, little evidence exists to support this practice (see Ch. 141 for details). Because of the increased incidence of allergic reactions in patients with brain tumors receiving anticonvulsant therapy (especially phenytoin), their routine use in those patients who have not experienced a seizure is probably unnecessary.

Many brain tumor patients have significant neurologic deficits and benefit from physical, occupational, and speech therapy. They may also require the emotional and psychological support provided by patient support groups, social workers, psychiatrists, and the various brain tumor societies (see Ch. 149).

TERMINAL CARE

Despite some important advances in recent years, almost all patients with malignant gliomas eventually die from their disease. When further treatment is no longer possible or not warranted because of the poor quality of the patient's life, all efforts should be directed toward keeping the patient comfortable and avoiding unnecessary prolongation of suffering.

SUMMARY

Despite intensive research, progress in the treatment of patients with malignant gliomas has remained slow. However, recent advances in our understanding of the biology of gliomas and in gene transfer techniques have resulted in exciting new therapeutic approaches that may lead to better treatments for patients with malignant gliomas in the near future.

SUGGESTED READINGS

Berger MS: Malignant astrocytomas: Surgical aspects. Semin Oncol 21: 172–85, 1994

Berger MS, Wilson CB: Textbook of Gliomas. WB Saunders, Philadelphia, (in press).

Black PMcL, Schoene W, Lampson LA (eds): Astrocytoma: Diagnosis, Treatment and Biology. Blackwell Scientific Publications, Boston, 1993

Bruner JM: Neuropathology of malignant gliomas. Semin Oncol 21:126–38, 1994

Fine HA: The basis for current treatment recommendations for malignant gliomas. Neurooncol 20:111–20, 1994

Green SB, Byar DP, Walker MD et al: Comparison of carmustine, procarbazine and high-dose methylprednisolone as additions to surgery and radiotherapy for the treatment of malignant glioma. Cancer Treat Rep 67:121–32, 1983

Hoshino T, Ahn D, Prados MD et al: Prognostic significance of the proliferative potential of intracranial gliomas measured by bromodeoxyuridine labelling. Int J Cancer 53:550–5, 1993

Kaye A, Laws E (eds): Encyclopedia of Brain Tumors. Churchill Livingstone, Edinburgh, 1995

Leibel SA, Scott CB, Loeffler JS: Contemporary approaches to the treatment of malignant gliomas with radiation therapy. Semin Oncol 21:198–219, 1994

Loeffler JS, Shrieve D, Wen PY et al: Radiosurgery for intracranial malignancies. Radiol Clin (in press).

Lesser GJ, Grossman S: The chemotherapy of high-grade astrocytomas. Semin Oncol 21:220–35, 1994

Levin VA, Gutin PH, Leibel S: Neoplasms of the central nervous system. P. 1674. In DeVita VT Jr, Hellman S, Rosenberg SA (eds): Cancer: Principles and Practice of Oncology. Vol. 2. (4th Ed. JB Lippincott, Philadelphia, 1993

MacDermott MW, Wilson CB: Management of primary brain tumors. P. 215. In Hatchinski V (ed): Challenges in Neurology. FA Davis Philadelphia, 1992

Nazzaro JM, Neuwelt EA: The role of surgery in the management of supratentorial intermediate and high grade astrocytomas in adults. J Neurosurg 73: 331–44, 1990

Packer RJ: Prognostic factors in patients with brain tumors. P. 275. In Salcman M (ed): Neurobiology of Brain Tumors. Williams & Wilkins, Baltimore, 1991

Prados MD: Treatment strategies for patients with recurrent brain tumors. Semin Radiat Oncol 1:62–8, 1991

Radhakrishman K, Bohnen NI, Kurland LT: Epidemiology of brain tumors. Brain Tumors. p. 1. In Morantz RA, Walsh JW (eds): Marcel Dekker, New York, 1994

Ram Z, Culver KH, Walbridge S et al: In situ retroviral-mediated gene transfer for the treatment of brain tumors in rats. Cancer Res 53:83–8, 1993

Scharfen CO, Sneed PK, Wara WM et al: High activity iodine-125 interstitial implant for gliomas. Int J Radiat Oncol Biol Phys 24:583–91, 1992

Shapiro WR: Chemotherapy of malignant gliomas: studies of the BTCG. Rev Neurol 148:428–34, 1992

Sneed PK, Larson DA, Gutin PH: Brachytherapy and hyperthermia for malignant astrocytomas. Semin Oncol 21:186–97, 1994

Walker MD, Alexander E Jr, Hunt WE et al: Evaluation of BCNU and/or radiotherapy in the treatment of anaplastic gliomas: a cooperative trial. J Neurosurg 49:333–43, 1978

Wong AJ, Zoltick PW, Moscatello DK: The molecular biology and molecular genetics of astrocytic neoplasms. Semin Oncol 21:139–48, 1994

154. PRIMARY CENTRAL NERVOUS SYSTEM LYMPHOMA

LISA M. DeANGELIS

Primary central nervous system lymphoma (PCNSL) used to be an extremely rare brain tumor. Known by a variety of names, including microglioma, reticulum cell sarcoma, perivascular sarcoma, and lymphosarcoma, PCNSL represented only about 1 percent of all intracranial tumors. However, since 1974, there has been a clear and dramatic increased incidence of this tumor among immunocompetent individuals. No obvious explanation has been found for this epidemiologic change. PCNSL is known to have a marked predilection for patients suffering from a variety of immunocompromised states including congenital (Wiskott-Aldrich syndrome) and acquired immunodeficiencies (renal transplant recipients). Patients with the acquired immunodeficiency syndrome (AIDS) have the highest incidence of PCNSL, which occurs in about 2 to 6 percent of human immunodeficiency virus type 1 (HIV-1)-infected patients and accounts for most patients with this neoplasm in some regions.

CLINICAL FEATURES

PCNSL occurs in all age groups, but the peak incidence is in the sixth and seventh decades of life. Immunocompromised patients are considerably younger, and the median age of onset among AIDS patients is about 40. There is a slight male predominance among immunocompetent patients, and 90 percent of AIDS-related PCNSL occurs in men.

PCNSL usually presents as a brain tumor. Patients develop headache, symptoms of increased intracranial pressure, and lateralizing signs appropriate to the area(s) of involvement. Because the most commonly affected region of the brain is the frontal lobe, and about 40 percent of patients have multifocal disease at diagnosis, most patients have cognitive or personality abnormalities, which may be the only clinical manifestation in some patients. PCNSL is usually a rapidly growing tumor, and symptoms are present for only a few weeks in most patients.

PCNSL is primarily a brain tumor, but it can involve all compartments of the central nervous system including the spinal fluid, spinal cord, and eye. It usually involves the deep periventricular regions of brain, and at least one lesion in almost every patient is adjacent to the ventricular system, which allows easy access of tumor into the cerebrospinal fluid (CSF). At autopsy virtually all patients have focal microscopic disease within the subarachnoid space overlying areas of brain involvement or in an adjacent ependymal area. It is the rare patient who has clinical symptoms or signs suggestive of leptomeningeal tumor and therefore, the physician can not rely on the clinical picture to indicate the presence or absence of subarachnoid spread of tumor. Widespread diffuse leptomeningeal seeding producing symptoms and signs can also be seen but this occurs in a small minority of patients.

In patients with PCNSL, leptomeningeal infiltration usually accompanies parenchymal brain lymphoma, but rarely patients develop primary leptomeningeal lymphoma in the absence of a brain mass. Patients present with cranial neuropathies, lumbosacral radiculopathies, increased intracranial pressure, or a combination of these symptoms. The diagnosis is established by demonstrating malignant lymphocytes in the CSF and by excluding the presence of widespread systemic lymphoma, which can occasionally present in the leptomeninges.

Primary spinal cord lymphoma is less common than primary leptomeningeal lymphoma. It can occur in isolation or can accompany brain lymphoma. Patients develop a painless progressive myelopathy, usually at the thoracic level. CSF may be normal, and enhanced magnetic resonance imaging (MRI) of the spine is the best means of establishing the diagnosis.

Unlike primary involvement of the leptomeninges or spinal cord, ocular involvement is quite common and may be the first indication of disease. Typically ocular lymphoma involves the vitreous or retina. Patients present with floaters, visual blurring, or segmental visual loss from a retinal detachment. Patients who first develop ocular lymphoma have a 50 to 80 percent chance of developing cerebral lymphoma. Frequently the latency between the onset of ocular and central nervous system disease is many years, and in some patients their long-standing visual symptoms are not accurately attributed to ocular lymphoma until their brain tumor is correctly diagnosed. Conversely, patients with PCNSL have a 12 to 18 percent incidence of ocular involvement at diagnosis and about half of these patients have no visual symptoms. Ocular lymphoma is best appreciated on ophthalmologic examination, particularly using the slit-lamp. It most often appears as a chronic vitritis but does not have a consistent and durable response to corticosteroids, which are usually effective for idiopathic vitritis. An initial response to steroids that wanes is often the first indication that the vitritis is caused by ocular lymphoma. Diagnosis can be confirmed with a vitreous biopsy, but some patients who have received corticosteroids may have a false-negative biopsy (see below). The incidence of ocular involvement among AIDS patients with PCNSL is unknown since most patients have not been studied routinely. Ocular lymphoma has been reported in AIDS patients occurring in isolation or in conjunction with cerebral tumor. Visual symptoms in AIDS patients may be particularly difficult to interpret because of the high incidence of cytomegalovirus (CMV) retinitis in this population, making careful ophthalmologic examination especially important.

PATHOLOGY

PCNSL is a diffuse non-Hodgkin's lymphoma typically of the intermediate or high-grade variety. The vast majority are of the large cell or large cell, immunoblastic subtypes, and 98 percent are B-cell neoplasms. They are identical histologically to com-

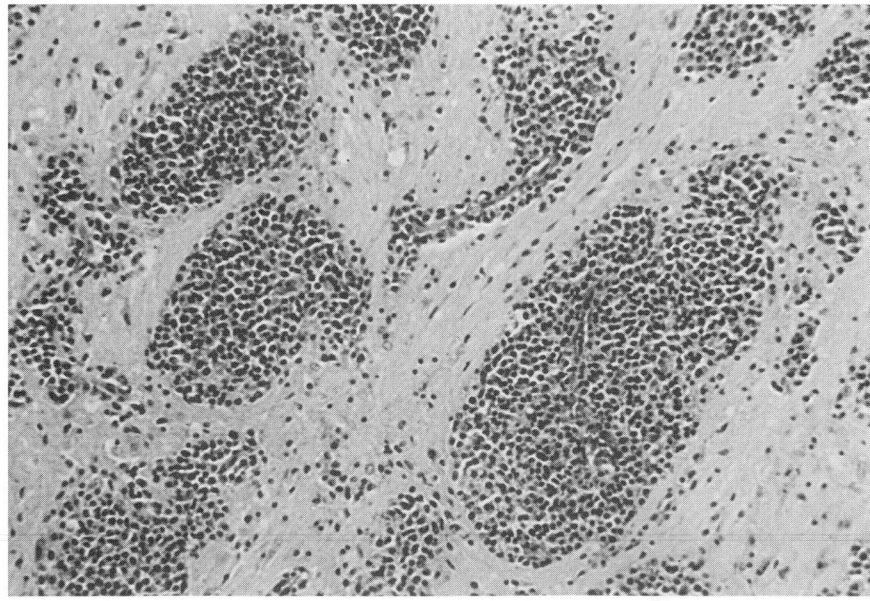

FIG. 154-1. Microscopic section showing the prominent perivascular growth pattern of PCNSL.

parable lymphomas found systemically. Pathologically they have a characteristic perivascular growth pattern (Fig. 154-1). Tumor cells tend to grow in the perivascular spaces, although they do not destroy or obliterate the vascular lumen. Tumor cells do infiltrate the brain parenchyma between vessels, and in the epicenter of the neoplasm they tend to grow in sheets of cells. Brain infiltration tends to be widespread and at autopsy is always more extensive than suspected on the basis of computed tomography (CT) or MRI. The multifocal nature of this tumor is particularly evident at autopsy, as seen in at least half of immunocompetent patients. However, almost 100 percent of AIDS patients have multifocal tumor at autopsy. Some patients have no detectable large focal mass and only widespread microscopic infiltration of the cerebrum. Tumor necrosis, hemorrhage, or calcification are not prominent pathologic features of PCNSL in immunocompetent patients, but necrosis is seen commonly in AIDS-related PCNSL.

Tumors in some patients are accompanied by a prominent reactive lymphocytosis. These reactive cells infiltrate PCNSL lesions and may cause diagnostic confusion. The reactive cells are T cells, and the neoplastic lymphocytes are almost always B cells, so lymphocyte typing can differentiate between the two cell populations. This is not necessary for routine processing or diagnosis of most PCNSLs. However, when patients have been treated with corticosteroids prior to biopsy and tumor lysis has occurred (see below), these reactive lymphocytes are left behind and the specimen is often misdiagnosed as an inflammatory process.

LABORATORY EVALUATION

Because patients with PCNSL present with central neurologic symptoms, the first test most patients undergo is a cranial scan. MRI is clearly superior to CT, but the radiographic appearance of PCNSL is similar on both. Prior to contrast administration PCNSL is usually iso- or hyperdense on CT and isointense on T1-weighted MRI. After contrast administration, the lesions enhance prominently and diffusely (Fig. 154-2). The borders of the lesions are usually indistinct and the amount of surrounding edema variable. Unlike malignant gliomas or brain metastases, no central necrosis is seen, and the typical periventricular location is also atypical for these more common causes of intracranial tumors.

At diagnosis authors have reported a variable incidence of positive CSF cytologic examinations ranging from 0 to 25 percent. When patients are examined routinely and more than one sample is available, we found that one-third of patients have malignant lymphocytes in their CSF and an additional one-third have suspicious cells.

The CSF usually shows other nonspecific abnormalities such as an elevated protein concentration in 85 percent of patients and a lymphocytic pleocytosis in 50 percent. An increased cell count may be due to the presence of malignant cells in the CSF or to a reactive lymphocytosis, which may accompany tumor cells or be present in isolation. Glucose concentration is almost always normal unless florid leptomeningeal tumor is present, in which case the concentration is low.

DIFFERENTIAL DIAGNOSIS

Immunocompetent Patients

Most patients with PCNSL present with a space-occupying intracranial lesion identified on CT or MRI, and the diagnosis is

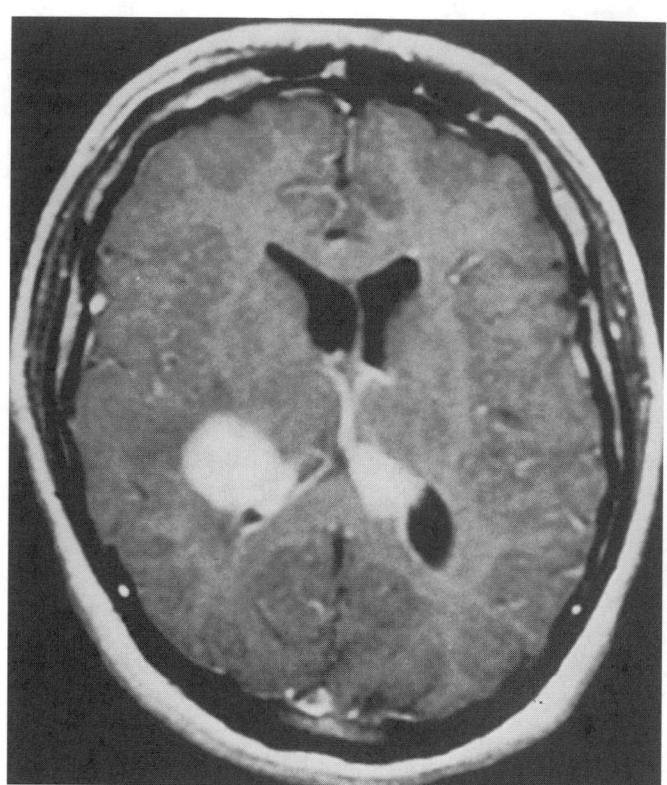

FIG. 154-2. Gadolinium-enhanced MR image demonstrating multifocal, periventricular, diffusely enhancing PCNSL in an immunocompetent patient.

clear on a biopsy specimen. However, in some situations the diagnosis is extremely difficult or is made so by early intervention with corticosteroids.

Patients who present with multiple intracranial lesions are frequently mistakenly diagnosed with brain metastases. Furthermore, approximately 13 percent of patients with PCNSL have a prior history of systemic cancer, which can further substantiate this clinical impression. If brain metastases are diagnosed on the basis of CT or MRI, patients frequently receive empiric therapy with palliative whole-brain radiotherapy. When tumor recurs or no systemic cancer becomes evident with further clinical follow-up, the diagnosis of PCNSL may become evident on a CSF examination or a subsequent brain biopsy. However, short-course radiotherapy (typically delivered to brain metastases) has cost the patient the opportunity of receiving more definitive and potentially curative treatment with chemotherapy and a less toxic fractionation schedule of radiotherapy.

More commonly, early administration of corticosteroids interferes with the opportunity to establish the diagnosis pathologically. Most patients who have space-occupying lesions identified by CT or MRI receive corticosteroids immediately to reduce perilesional edema and thus improve neurologic function. Unlike all other brain tumors, PCNSL may shrink and even disappear after corticosteroid administration. This shrinkage is due to a direct cytotoxic effect by the steroids on the malignant lymphocytes, resulting in resolution of the lesion. Resolution or significant shrinkage can occur in some patients within a few days of steroid delivery, although the prevalence of this response increases with prolonged administration. This effect, which is most dramatic in brain lesions, can also be seen in ocular and leptomeningeal lymphoma. Although tumor resolution with corticosteroid is characteristic of PCNSL, not all patients respond to steroids in this fashion. Therefore, the absence of tumor regression after steroid administration does not militate against the diagnosis of PCNSL.

More importantly, other neurologic processes that appear as diffuse contrast-enhancing lesions on CT or MRI can also appear to resolve with corticosteroids. Acute multiple sclerosis can produce periventricular enhancing lesions that disappear after steroids; central nervous system sarcoid can have a similar appearance. Multiple sclerosis can be particularly difficult to distinguish from PCNSL because both can be accompanied by a CSF pleocytosis and even oligoclonal bands.

Immunosuppressed Patients

The differential diagnosis of PCNSL in immunosuppressed patients is different from that in immunocompetent patients. From a practical point of view this section concentrates on the AIDS patient although it would apply to any immunocompromised individual with a space-occupying lesion.

In the AIDS patient PCNSL does not have the characteristic radiographic features seen in the immunocompetent patient. On CT or MRI PCNSL is usually a ring-enhancing lesion in AIDS patients, and a diffusely enhancing mass is rarely seen (Fig. 154-3). This ring-enhancing pattern correlates with the high incidence of tumor necrosis seen pathologically. Because the characteristic radiographic appearance of PCNSL is lacking in the AIDS patient, the lesion is indistinguishable from other CNS processes, specifically infection. Central nervous system toxoplasmosis is the most common cause of an intracerebral mass in AIDS, and PCNSL is the second. When an intracranial mass is identified on CT or MRI in an AIDS patient, empiric antitoxoplasmosis therapy is begun. Usually the patient is followed clinically and a scan is repeated in 2 to 3 weeks to assess response. If improvement is seen, antitoxoplasmosis treatment is continued, but if no improvement is evident brain biopsy is performed to ascertain the correct diagnosis. However, early biopsy should be considered in two groups of patients, those with a negative toxoplasmosis serology and those who deteriorate clinically during the 2-week observation period. These patients are likely to have PCNSL and early diagnosis before the patient has sustained significant clinical deterioration can improve their outcome when treated for lymphoma.

Brain biopsy is often avoided or delayed in AIDS patients even when clinically indicated. Because PCNSL is steroid sensitive, a short course of corticosteroids is often suggested as a ''diagnostic test'' in lieu of obtaining tissue. However, AIDS-related PCNSL does not usually regress after corticosteroids, and therefore steroids can not provide any useful diagnostic information.

The incidence of associated leptomeningeal seeding of PCNSL in AIDS patients is as high as that seen in the immunocompetent population. The CSF can offer an early and simple means of diagnosis. All AIDS patients with a space-occupying lesion should have a lumbar puncture with a CSF cytologic examination. Rarely must a lumbar puncture be avoided because of concern regarding cerebral herniation. In addition, if PCNSL is suspected even before tissue confirmation has been obtained, an ophthalmologic examination may also support the clinical impression if lymphocytes are seen in the vitreous.

Immunocompetent patients with PCNSL do not need a complete systemic evaluation to search for systemic lymphoma. However, AIDS patients with systemic lymphoma have a very high incidence of extranodal involvement, including central nervous system disease. A complete evaluation, including body CT scans and bone marrow biopsy, should be performed in all AIDS patients with apparent PCNSL to ensure that no systemic lymphoma is present, which would markedly change the therapeutic regimen.

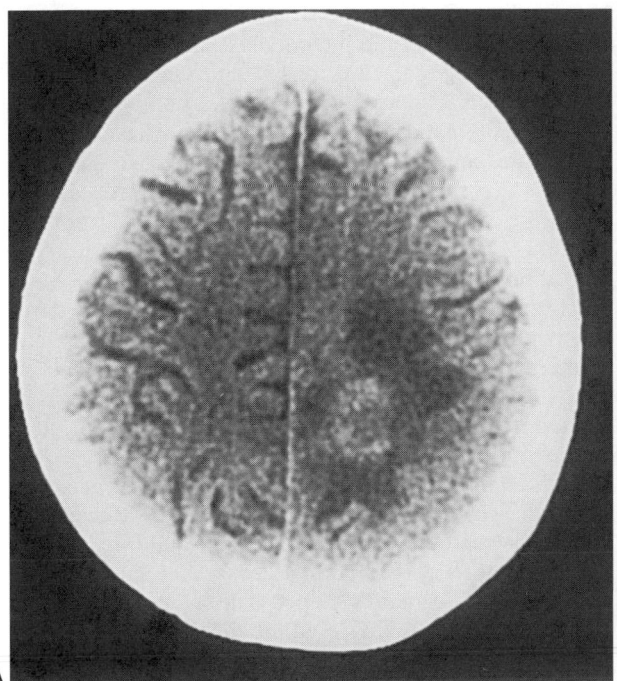 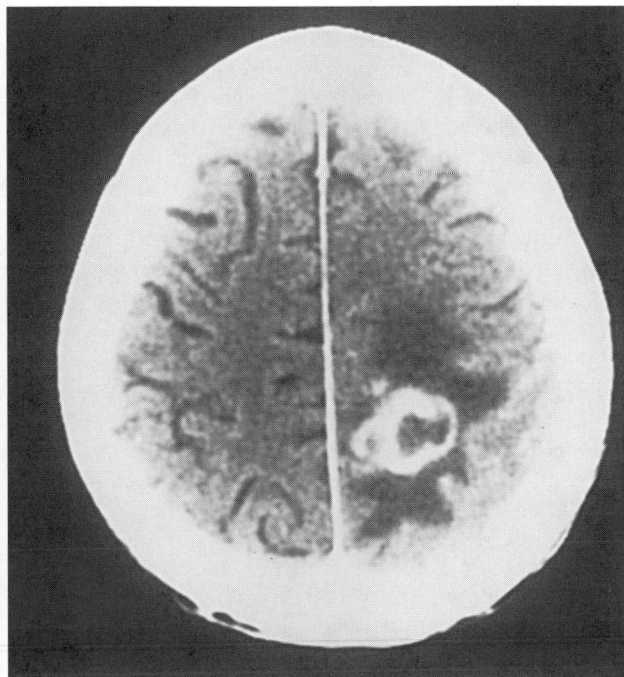

A   B

FIG. 154-3. Gadolinium-enhanced MRI demonstrating a ring-enhancing PCNSL in an AIDS patient. Note the relatively superficial location of the lesion.

TREATMENT

Immunocompetent Patients

PCNSL is a highly aggressive neoplasm, and the median survival of immunocompetent patients with supportive care alone is only 3 months. Surgical resection does not contribute to survival, and the median is increased to only 4 to 5 months with surgery alone. For decades, cranial radiotherapy (4,000 to 5,000 cGy) has been the cornerstone of treatment for PCNSL, increasing median survival to 12 to 18 months. Although highly effective at producing a complete remission in more than 90 percent of patients, tumor recurs within 1 year in most patients after radiotherapy, and 5-year survival is only 3 to 4 percent. These survival statistics are comparable to those for a glioblastoma multiforme. Unlike malignant gliomas, PCNSL frequently recurs in regions of the brain remote from the original area of involvement. Relapse usually occurs in the brain, but it may be accompanied by leptomeningeal or ocular relapse. Furthermore, tumor can recur in either of these locations in the absence of brain relapse. Therefore, patients need a complete neurologic restaging at the time of any documented relapse.

Chemotherapy was initially explored as a potential therapeutic option for patients with recurrent disease. Single agents, such as high-dose methotrexate and high-dose cytarabine, were able to induce short-duration remissions in several patients. These agents were then combined with radiotherapy and introduced as part of an initial therapeutic regimen. At Memorial Sloan-Kettering Cancer Center we used a regimen of preradiation high-dose methotrexate (1 g/m^2) combined with intra-Ommaya methotrexate to treat any leptomenigeal tumor present regardless of the CSF cytologic result. This was followed by radiotherapy and high-dose cytarabine. In the 31 treated patients the median disease-free survival was 41 months, significantly longer than the 10 months seen in patients treated with radiotherapy alone. In addition to this regimen, other chemotherapy schedules have also proved beneficial. The addition of procarbazine, lomustine, and vincristine to radiotherapy improves median survival to 30 months. Neuwelt et al. have a unique approach using blood–brain barrier disruption with intra-arterial mannitol followed by intra-arterial methotrexate as well as systemic cyclophosphamide, procarbazine, and dexamethasone. Their goal is to avoid radiotherapy, although 9 of their 16 evaluable patients required radiation as part of their initial treatment. Median survival was 44.5 months, clearly superior to radiation alone.

Standard chemotherapy regimens for systemic lymphoma have not proved advantageous in the treatment of PCNSL. Cyclophosphamide- and doxorubicin-based regimens, when combined with radiotherapy, give a median survival comparable to radiation alone. Patients develop rapid brain (and occasionally extensive leptomeningeal) relapse while on these chemotherapy programs. Despite the expected cytotoxic superiority of the agents in the systemic lymphoma regimens, these combinations do not perform as well because the drugs cannot penetrate the intact blood–brain barrier. Areas of bulky disease that are easily visualized on CT or MRI have an abnormal blood–brain barrier, and even water-soluble drugs can penetrate into these regions. However, this highly infiltrative disease always has microscopic tumor hiding behind an intact blood–brain barrier, and it is precisely these areas that often grow (while large contrast-enhancing masses are regressing) in response to systemic lymphoma regimens. Thus far, all the more successful chemotherapeutic programs for PCNSL employ agents with an intrinsic capability of penetrating an intact blood–brain barrier (e.g., procarbazine, lomustine) or are delivered in doses that facilitate drug delivery behind the barrier (e.g., high-dose methotrexate or cytarabine).

Ocular lymphoma requires specific treatment. Ocular irradiation to a total dose of 3,600 to 4,000 cGy is the most effective therapy, producing clinical improvement and regression of cells in most patients. When ocular involvement is present at diagnosis the ocular radiotherapy must be coordinated with any planned cranial irradiation to avoid overlapping ports. When ocular lymphoma is present in isolation, we irradiate the eyes only, although some have advocated concurrent cranial irradiation to reduce the risk of subsequent central nervous system relapse. However, no evidence shows that early brain irradiation reduces cranial recurrence, and the neurologic toxicity of cranial radiotherapy is considerable. Chemotherapy has limited efficacy against ocular lymphoma because most drugs penetrate poorly into the vitreous; however, high-dose cytarabine has proved effective.

Recurrent PCNSL often responds to additional treatment. Radiotherapy is effective if not delivered as part of the initial regimen. Additional chemotherapy, particularly using agents not previously administered, can also induce sustained remissions.

Immunosuppressed Patients

Treatment of PCNSL in AIDS patients is more difficult and less successful than comparable treatment in immunocompetent patients. Whole-brain radiotherapy alone gives a median survival of only 2 to 5 months in HIV-1-infected patients. Although most patients with AIDS-related PCNSL respond to radiotherapy with regression of tumor on CT or MRI, death occurs within months, usually from opportunistic infections. Most patients die from systemic infection, but at autopsy virtually all AIDS patients with PCNSL have coexistent central nervous system infections. The most common include HIV-1 encephalitis, CMV encephalitis, toxoplasmosis, cryptococcal meningitis, or multiple infections. These neurologic infections may not be recognized or possible to diagnose prior to death, but they often account for a patient's poor clinical condition. Many AIDS patients with PCNSL who have a good radiographic response to treatment fail to improve clinically, often because these other central nervous system processes are present. This makes an assessment of the efficacy of antitumor therapy very difficult.

Although some patients die from infectious processes, many die from uncontrolled or recurrent PCNSL. The use of chemotherapy in AIDS patients is complicated by their underlying immunosuppression and reduced ability to tolerate cytotoxic drugs. No large group of AIDS patients with PCNSL has been treated with combined modality therapy. However, individuals have been reported who appear to benefit from a vigorous approach and who have prolonged survival of 2 years or more. Often these are patients who have PCNSL as their AIDS-defining illness, and they have not suffered multiple systemic complications of HIV-1 infection. Because combined modality therapy appears to benefit a subpopulation, any AIDS patient with PCNSL should be considered for chemotherapy and radiotherapy at diagnosis or enrolled in a clinical trial studying this issue. Unfortunately many patients will not be eligible for such treatment, especially those in poor neurologic condition. These patients are best treated with palliative whole-brain radiotherapy, perhaps delivered in a short-course rapid fractionation schedule. Ocular lymphoma in the AIDS patient should be treated with ocular irradiation, and patients with malignant lymphocytes in the CSF should receive intrathecal chemotherapy.

SUGGESTED READINGS

Baumgartner JE, Rachlin JR, Beckstead JH et al: Primary central nervous system lymphomas: natural history and response to radiation therapy in 55 patients with acquired immunodeficiency syndrome. J Neurosurg 73:206, 1990

Chamberlain MC: Long survival in patients with acquired immune deficiency syndrome—related primary central nervous system lymphoma. Cancer 73:1728, 1994

DeAngelis LM: Primary central nervous system lymphoma imitates multiple sclerosis. J Neurooncol 9:177, 1990

DeAngelis LM: Primary central nervous system lymphoma. PPO Updates 6: 1, 1992

DeAngelis LM, Yahalom J, Heinemann MH: Primary CNS lymphoma: combined treatment with chemotherapy and radiotherapy. Neurology 40:80, 1990

DeAngelis LM, Yahalom J, Thaler HT et al: Combined modality therapy for primary CNS lymphoma. J Clin Oncol 10:635, 1992

Fine H, Mayer RJ: Primary central nervous system lymphoma. Ann Intern Med 119:1093, 1993

Formenti SC, Gill PS, Lean E et al: Primary central nervous system lymphoma in AIDS. Cancer 63:1101, 1989

Hochberg FH, Miller DC: Primary central nervous system lymphoma. J Neurosurg 68:835, 1988

Ling SM, Roach III M, Larson DA et al: Radiotherapy of primary central nervous system lymphoma in patients with and without human immunodeficiency virus. Cancer 73:2570, 1994

Murray K, Kun L, Cox J: Primary malignant lymphoma of the central nervous system. J Neurosurg 65:600, 1986

Nelson DF, Martz KL, Bonner H et al: Non-Hodgkin's lymphoma of the brain: can high dose, large volume radiation therapy improve survival? Report on a prospective trial by the radiation therapy oncology group (RTOG): RTOG 8315. Int J Radiat Oncol Biol Phys 23:9, 1992

Neuwelt EA, Goldman D, Dahlborg SA et al: Primary CNS lymphoma treated with osmotic blood-brain barrier disruption: prolonged survival and preservation of cognitive function. J Clin Oncol 9:1580, 1991

van den Bent MJ, Vanneste JAL, Ansink BJJ: Prolonged remission of primary central nervous system lymphoma after discontinuation of steroid therapy. J Neurooncol 13:257, 1992

155. MENINGIOMAS

PETER McL. BLACK

Meningiomas are the most common benign brain tumor and the second most common primary brain tumor overall after gliomas. They account for approximately 15 to 20 percent of intracranial tumors. The overall incidence of meningiomas is approximately 2.7 per 100,000 population, but it is likely that this is an underestimate of the true incidence because many meningiomas are asymptomatic. They occur twice as often in women as men and tend to occur in later life. The incidence rates peak in the sixth decade for men and the seventh decade for women. Rarely, meningiomas may occur in children. Meningiomas occur more commonly in patients who have neurofibromatosis or who have been exposed to previous cranial irradiation. The incidence of meningiomas is also slightly increased in patients with carcinoma of the breast. It has been suggested that head trauma may play a part but the evidence is not convincing. Approximately 5 to 15 percent of patients have multiple meningiomas, particularly in association with neurofibromatosis.

ETIOLOGY AND BIOLOGY

Meningiomas arise from the arachnoid cap cells, which form the outer lining of arachnoid granulations of the brain (Fig. 155-1) and compress cortex or cranial nerves as they grow. The cause of meningiomas is unknown, but 40 to 80 percent of these tumors have a loss of genetic material from the long arm of chromosome 22, at a locus separate from the gene for neurofibromatosis-2. Some evidence shows that a second tumor suppressor locus relevant to meningioma formation may be located on chromosome 22q. Malignant meningiomas are associated with deletion of loci on chromosomes 1p, 9q, and 17p. Other deletions may also contribute to the growth of meningiomas.

Meningiomas have receptors for sex hormones and other ligands, including progesterone, estrogen, androgen, dopamine, and the β-receptor for platelet-derived growth factor. Analysis of the contributions of these receptors to meningioma growth is intriguing and may have important implications for pathophysiology and future therapies. The presence of hormonal receptors may explain the tendency for some meningiomas to increase in size and become symptomatic during pregnancy.

In the 1970s interest arose in the estrogen receptor, since it appeared that some of these tumors had estrogen receptor activity on competitive inhibition tests. With more sensitive and specific immunohistochemical and molecular biologic techniques, it became clear that estrogen receptors are expressed in only a small percentage of these tumors. Progesterone receptors, however, are expressed in 70 to 80 percent of meningiomas.

Androgen and dopamine receptors are also expressed in a significant percentage of meningiomas, although in less robust quantities than the progesterone receptor. Dopamine receptors appear to be expressed equally in men and women; androgen receptors, like progesterone, are expressed more frequently in women.

The platelet-derived growth factor system, which seems important in many brain tumors, is found in abundance in meningioma tissue. The β-form of the receptor is expressed along with the B subunit of platelet-derived growth factor itself, creating the potential for an autocrine loop within meningioma tissue. The precise role these hormonal and growth factor receptors have on the growth of meningiomas is currently unclear.

CLASSIFICATION AND PATHOLOGY

The characteristic histologic features of meningiomas are whorls that form around a central hyaline material, eventually calcify, and form psammoma bodies or interlacing bundles of elongated fibroblasts with narrow nuclei. No pathologic marker is unequivocal for meningiomas. Epithelial membrane antigen and vimentin are positive in most of these tumors, and glial fibrillary acidic protein and anti-Leu7 are almost always negative.

The classification of meningiomas is quite confusing. The traditional World Health Organization classification divided them into meningiotheliomatous (syncytial), fibrous, transitional, psammomatous, and angiomatous types, but this distinction has little prognostic importance (Table 155-1 and Plate 155-1). Fatty degeneration, hemorrhage, calcification, and cyst formation may occur.

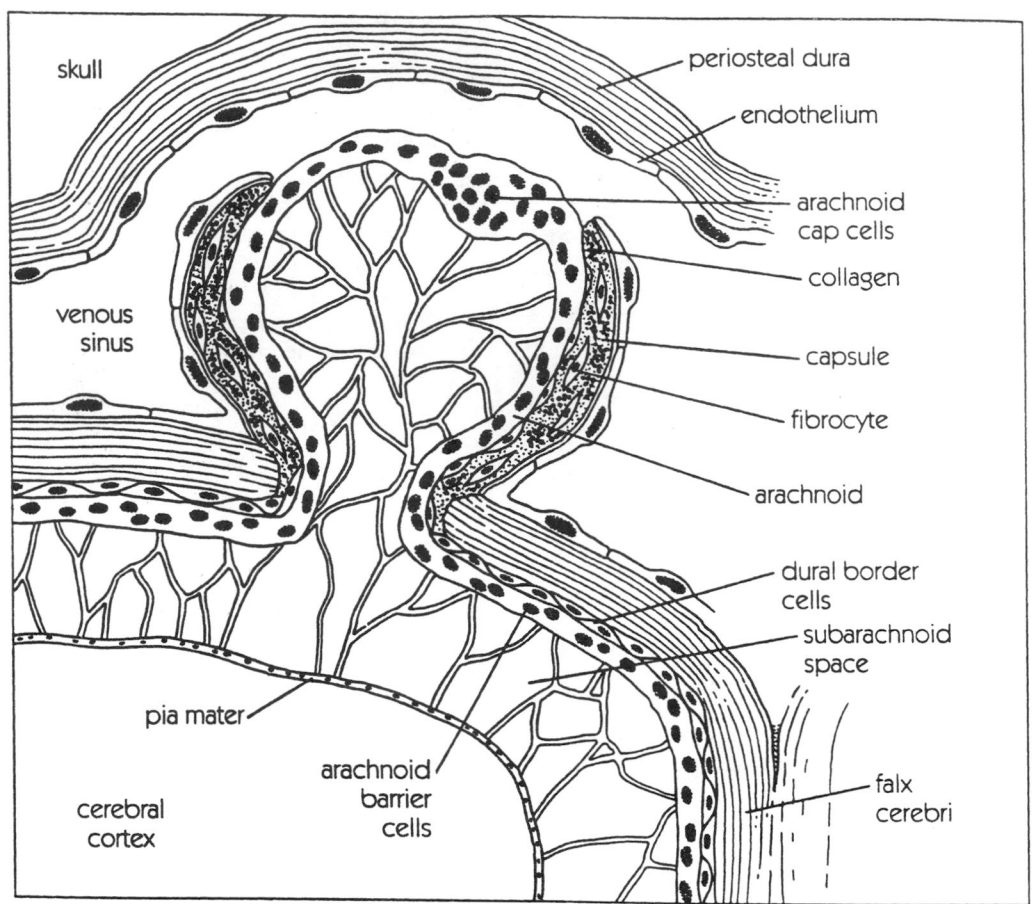

FIG. 155-1. Location of the arachnoid cap cells in the arachnoid villi. Meningiomas are thought to originate from these arachnoid cap cells. (From Al-Mefty O, Origitano TC: Meningiomas. p. 28. In Rengachary SS, Wilkins RH (eds): Principles of Neurosurgery. Wolfe Publishing, London, 1994, with permission.)

Papillary and angioblastic meningiomas are more aggressive variants. The angioblastic meningioma has in the past been thought to be similar to the hemangiopericytoma, but in fact is quite different from it because the hemangiopericytoma is more a sarcoma than a meningioma and arises from the pericytes around capillaries.

Malignant meningiomas are characterized by abundant mitosis, nuclear pleomorphism, necrosis, high nuclear-to-cytoplasmic ratio, loss of normal architecture, and invasion of surrounding brain. Aggressive meningiomas contain one or more anaplastic features but do not meet the criteria for malignancy.

In 1985 and 1986 Jaaskelainen and colleagues proposed a grading system that is predictive of outcome. This system uses points for loss of architecture, increased cellularity, nuclear pleomorphism, mitotic figures, focal necrosis, and presence of brain infiltration to establish whether a tumor is *benign* (0 to 2 points), *atypical* (3 to 6 points), *anaplastic* (7 to 11 points), or *sarcomatous* (12 to 18 points). For grade 1 tumors, the recurrence rate at 5 years is 3 percent, for grade II it is 38 percent, and for grade III it is 78 percent.

Several other methods have been used to help predict the behavior of meningiomas. The most useful is the bromodeoxyuridine (BUdR) labeling index. Bromodeoxyuridine is a thymidine analogue that is incorporated into cells undergoing DNA synthesis. The proportion of tumor cells on histologic sections labeled with BUdR (the BUdR labeling index) provides an indication of the proliferative potential of the tumor. Meningiomas with a labeling index of 1 percent have a higher recurrence rate than normal and for those with an index of 5 percent or higher the recurrence rate is 100 percent.

CLINICAL PRESENTATION

As with other brain tumors, meningiomas may present with seizures, headaches, and focal neurologic deficits. Patients frequently have subtle symptoms for a long period before the meningioma is diagnosed. Increasing numbers of patients are reported with asymptomatic meningiomas discovered by

TABLE 155.1. World Health Organization Classification of Meningiomas

Class	Subtype	Predominant Feature
Classic	Meningotheliomatous	Synctial cells with lobules
	Fibroblastic	Spindle cells with collagen
	Transitional	Mixture of above types
	Psammomatous	Exuberant psammoma bodies
	Angiomatous	Abundant sclerosing blood vessels
Angioblastic	Hemangioblastoma	Capillary endothelial cells with lipid stromal cells
	Hemangiopericytoma	Poorly differentiated pericytic cells with reticulin
Aggressive	Papillary	Papillary pattern with few anaplastic features
Malignant	Anaplastic	Invasion of brain parenchyma metastases

TABLE 155-2. Common Locations of Meningiomas

Location	%
Falx/parasagittal	25
Convexity	20
Sphenoid wing	20
Olfactory groove	10
Suprasellar	10
Posterior fossa (petrosal)	10
Intraventricular	2
Miscellaneous (optic nerve, clivus, and so forth)	3

neuroimaging studies performed for unrelated reasons. The precise clinical features vary depending on location. Ninety percent of meningiomas are intracranial, and of these 90 percent are supratentorial. Table 155-2 outlines the common sites of meningiomas.

Convexity meningiomas are usually located anterior to the central sulcus and may remain asymptomatic until they reach a large size. They typically present with seizures, focal neurologic deficits, or headaches. Falx and parasagittal meningiomas produce similar symptoms, but they often involve the sagittal sinus, making complete resection much more difficult. Large parasagittal meningiomas may result in bilateral leg weakness. Olfactory groove meningiomas also frequently grow to a large size before they become symptomatic since anosmia and mental status changes are often unrecognized. When the tumor becomes very large, visual loss may result from compression of the optic nerves and chiasm.

The presenting symptoms of sphenoid ridge meningiomas vary depending on their exact location. Medial sphenoid ridge meningiomas may involve the cavernous sinus, giving rise to occulomotor palsies and facial numbness (Fig. 155-2). The ca-

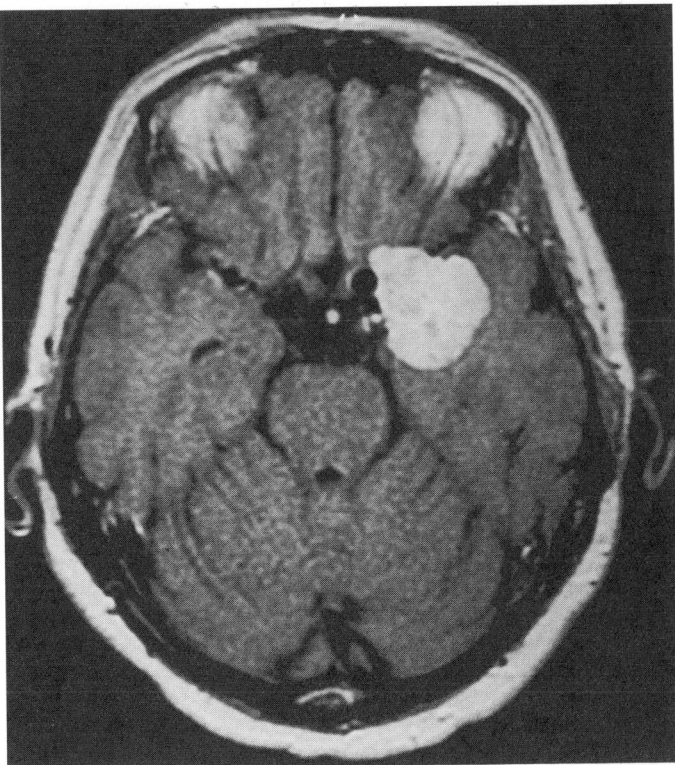

FIG. 155-2. Axial MRI with gadolinium showing an enhancing meningioma arising in the left sphenoid wing and involving the cavernous sinus and carotid artery. This tumor could not be completely resected and was treated with stereotactic radiotherapy. Follow-up 2 years later showed slight reduction in tumor size.

rotid artery may also be encased by the tumor, preventing complete surgical resection. As the tumor enlarges, the optic nerves may be affected. A large meningioma may produce atrophy of the ipsilateral optic nerve as well as papilledema in the contralateral optic nerve by increasing intracranial pressure, giving rise to the Foster Kennedy syndrome.

Posterior fossa meningiomas may produce a wide range of symptoms depending on the structures involved. Meningiomas arising from the petrous bone may compress cranial nerves, especially the eighth nerve, resulting in deafness. Petroclival meningiomas may cause trigeminal neuralgia and hemifacial spasms. Tentorial and foramen magnum meningiomas may produce headaches and symptoms of brainstem compression.

Intraventricular meningiomas usually present with headaches resulting from increased intracranial pressure. Intraorbital meningiomas may present with progressive painless visual loss and proptosis.

Spinal meningiomas account for less than 10 percent of meningiomas. They tend to occur in women (female/male ratio, 5:1), usually between the ages of 40 and 70. They are intradural, extramedullary tumors occurring predominantly in the thoracic spine. Initially they present with back and radicular pain, but as the tumor enlarges and compresses the spinal cord, pyramidal weakness and sensory loss may occur.

IMAGING

In 50 to 60 percent of patients with meningiomas, plain radiographs may show changes such as calcification and hyperostosis or thinning of the adjacent skull. However, with the availability of computed tomography (CT) and magnetic resonance imaging (MRI), skull radiographs are now rarely needed.

On non-contrast CT, meningiomas appear as well-defined, hyperdense masses often with coarse calcification (Fig. 155-3). They have a broad dural base and may expand the adjacent cerebrospinal fluid spaces. The underlying cortex may appear to be buckled from external compression by the tumor. Hyperostotic changes or blistering in the adjacent calvarium may occur. Meningiomas enhance brightly and homogeneously with iodinated contrast. The amount of peritumoral edema is variable and tends to be correlated with angioblastic histology, the presence of hormone receptors, and a high proliferation index.

On high-field-strength MRI, meningiomas are slightly hypointense on T1-weighted images and iso- to slightly hyperintense on T2-weighted images. At lower field strengths, they tend to be isointense on T1- and T2-weighted images, and therefore small meningiomas may be missed on noncontrast studies. Thus, small meningiomas are the only brain tumor better visualized on CT than MRI. Meningiomas often demonstrate a "speckled" pattern of signal intensity thought to be due to tumor vascularity, calcification, and/or cystic foci. Punctate or curvilinear signal voids may be present at the interface of the brain and the meningioma, representing pial vessels at the margin of the tumor. After the administration of gadolinium, intense enhancement is usually noted, and a tapered projection of enhancement or "dural tail" may be seen at the margin of the tumor (Fig. 155-4).

Indistinct margins, marked edema, mushroom-like projections from tumor, invasion deeply into brain, and heterogenous enhancement all suggest aggressive behavior. However, malignant meningiomas cannot be distinguished with certainty by radiologic studies. This is important to bear in mind when considering whether a patient should be observed.

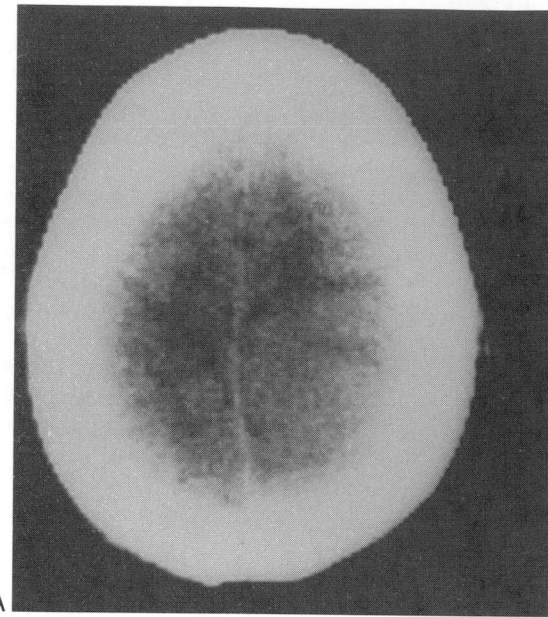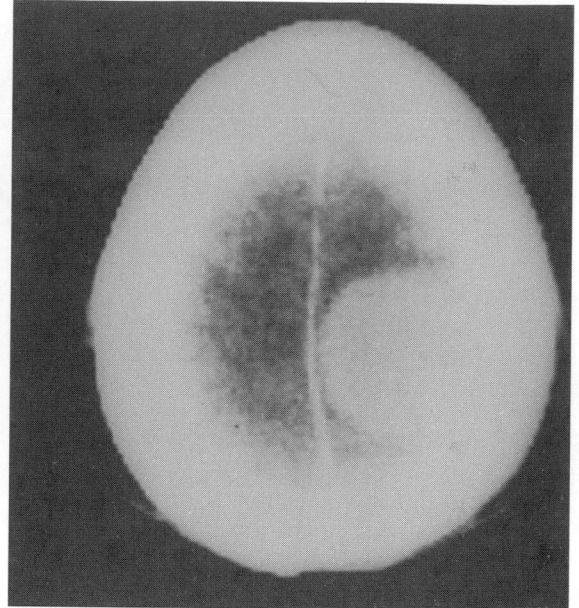

FIG. 155-3. **(A)** Unenhanced axial CT scan showing a large slightly hyperdense convexity meningioma. **(B)** Enhanced CT scan showing the tumor enhancing brightly. This tumor was resected completely.

Three-dimensional reconstruction from MRI can demonstrate the tumor's relationship to other structures including cerebral blood vessels, brainstem, and cranial nerves. MR angiography has largely replaced conventional angiography for imaging adjacent blood vessels, although angiography may be necessary when embolization of the tumor is being considered. For convexity meningiomas, MR venography is particularly helpful in evaluating the dural sinuses, which may be invaded by tumor.

Preliminary results suggest that positron emission tomography studies may be useful in determining whether a meningioma will be recur. Tumors with low glucose utilization have a lower risk of recurrence than tumors with a high glucose utilization.

TREATMENT

Surgery

The primary treatment for meningiomas is surgery. However, some tumors maybe asymptomatic, and those that present with seizures only can safely be observed. An approach this surgeon finds useful is to follow tumors less than 2 cm that are asymptomatic and not associated with edema. In these cases, observation means annual CT scans with contrast.

Surgery requires significant surgical judgment and skill. Total resection is usually possible with tumors of dura, falx, lateral sphenoid wing, frontal base, and cerebellar convexity. Complete resection may not be feasible in tumors involving the sagittal and cavernous sinuses, cerebellopontine angle, clivus (Fig. 155-5), tentorial notch or optic nerve sheath. However, better understanding of neuroanatomy and improved neurosurgical techniques are allowing many of these lesions to be surgically excised today. The complication rate should be less than 10 percent for new neurologic deficits in most meningiomas and the mortality rate less than 4 percent. These rates may be higher in elderly patients and those with skull-based tumors. As discussed below, there is an increasing trend to treat patients whose tumor cannot be completely excised with postoperative external beam radiotherapy or radiosurgery after aggressive but subtotal resection.

Meningiomas are not always curable even if they are completely excised. The recurrence rate depends on completeness of removal, site of tumor, and biologic aggressiveness. For complete removal the recurrence varies from 8 to 20 percent over 10 years; for patients with obvious residual tumor it is 29 to 55 percent over a 10-year period.

FIG. 155-4. Axial MRI with gadolinium showing an enhancing meningioma arising from the left frontal convexity and projecting into the sylvian fissure.

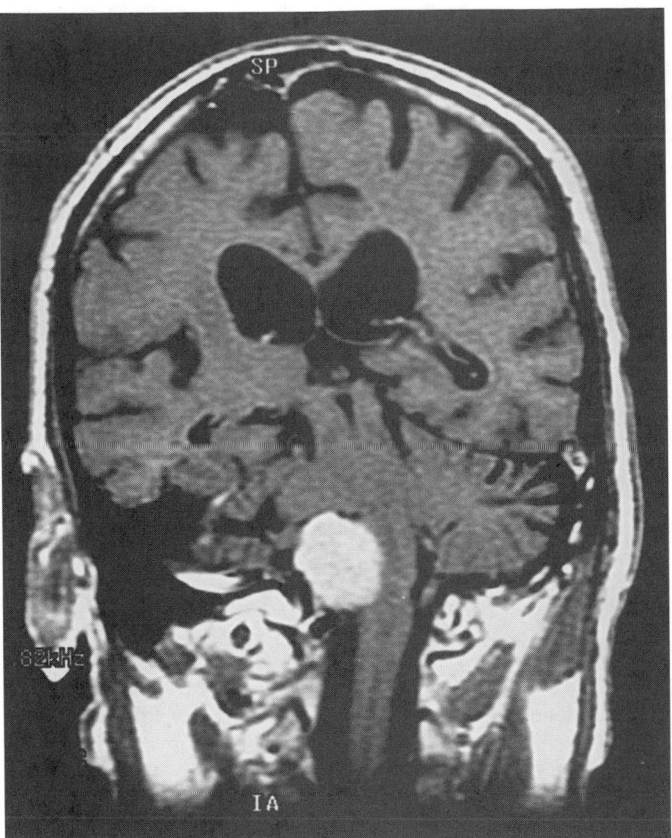

FIG. 155-5. Coronal MRI with gadolinium showing a clivus meningioma compressing the brainstem.

Patients with meningiomas have an increased mortality. The cumulative relative survival rates (ratio of observed rate to expected rate) at 1, 5, 10, and 15 years were 83, 79, 74, and 71 percent, respectively.

Radiotherapy

Until recently the use of external beam radiotherapy for meningiomas has been controversial because of concerns about long-term neurotoxicity, as well as conflicting evidence regarding efficacy. Early studies of external beam radiotherapy showed no therapeutic benefit, but several recent studies have shown tumor control rates of 50 to 90 percent at 10 years. Goldsmith et al. recently reported on 140 patients treated at the University of California, San Francisco between 1967 and 1990. The 5- and 10-year progression-free survival rates were 89 and 77 percent respectively. For patients treated after 1980, the 5-year progression-free survival rate increased to 98 percent. Only 3.6 percent of patients experienced complications, which included blindness, necrosis, and death. No second brain tumors were seen. The studies of Goldsmith and others suggest that external beam radiation may have a role in the treatment of selected patients with inoperable, partially resected, and recurrent meningiomas.

One of the traditional limitations of external beam radiation has been radiation to surrounding brain. This limitation is now considerably less because techniques of focused radiation have been developed using the linear accelerator or multiple cobalt sources (the γ-knife) that avoid exposure to brain outside the target area. Radiation may be given in one large fraction (stereotactic radiosurgery) or in multiple small fractions (stereotactic

radiotherapy). Early results with stereotactic radiosurgery have been promising although the follow-up in most studies is limited. In the largest reported series, Kondziolka et al. treated 94 patients who had benign meningiomas with stereotactic radiosurgery and reported 4-year tumor control rates of 92 percent, with tumor shrinkage in 33 percent of patients. Stereotactic radiotherapy offers the potential for treating meningiomas while avoiding injury to adjacent radiosensitive structures such as the optic chiasm. Preliminary results are encouraging, but follow-up is too short for firm conclusions to be drawn.

Medical Therapy

As indicated above, increasing evidence shows that the growth of meningiomas is influenced by hormones and growth factors, raising the possibility of medical therapy for meningiomas. Approximately 30 percent of meningiomas have estrogen receptors, and 70 to 80 percent have progesterone receptors. Treatment with antiestrogens such as tamoxifen and medroxyprogesterone acetate has been ineffective, but antiprogesterone agents have shown promise. In pilot studies with the antiprogesterone mifepristone (RU 486), response rates of 36 to 60 percent have been obtained. Based on these encouraging results, a multicenter study is currently in progress evaluating the efficacy of mifepristone. Meningiomas express a number of other receptors including those for dopamine D1, platelet-derived growth factor, and androgens. Antagonists of these receptors inhibit meningioma growth in vitro and may play a role in the treatment of meningiomas.

Chemotherapy for malignant meningiomas using standard regimens for soft tissue sarcomas has been uniformly disappointing; have been occasional responses have been reported to interferon-α.

Supportive Therapy

Corticosteroids are useful for treating peritumoral edema, but they do not change the growth pattern of the tumor and have significant long-term side effects. These include diabetes mellitus, osteoporosis, proximal muscle wasting, and obesity. They should not be used for longer than 1 month at a time unless they are absolutely necessary.

Anticonvulsants are generally not necessary for most skull-based meningiomas. The use of anticonvulsants for patients with convexity meningiomas who have not had a seizure remains controversial. Frequently, these patients are placed empirically on anticonvulsants for 6 to 12 months after the tumor has been resected. However, a study by Foy et al. suggested that postoperative anticonvulsant therapy may not be necessary.

Because patients with meningiomas have a significantly increased risk of venous thromboembolic disease, preventive measures such as pneumatic compression devices are important during the peri-and postoperative periods.

MALIGNANT MENINGIOMAS

Malignant meningiomas account for only 12 percent of meningiomas, but they pose a significant management problem. They have a very high recurrence rate after surgery and generally respond poorly to treatment with radiotherapy, chemotherapy, or hormonal therapy. Unlike other malignant brain tumors, systemic metastases may occur in up to 24 percent of patients with malignant meningiomas, usually to lung and bone.

SUMMARY

The diagnosis and management of meningiomas remain a major challenge to the clinical neurologist and neurosurgeon. With the advent of better imaging techniques, tumors are identified earlier and may be found in asymptomatic patients or patients with only a seizure as the presenting problem. Surgical techniques using the operating microscope, evoked potential monitoring, and improved understanding of anatomy have allowed tumors to be resected with better results. Radiotherapy appears to have substantial effect in limiting tumor growth, and the use of sex steroids may also have a significant adjunctive role. The overall care of patients with problematic meningiomas still requires considerable judgment and skill.

SUGGESTED READINGS

Al-Mefty O (ed): Meningiomas. Raven, New York, 1991
Al-Mefty O, Origitano TC: Meningiomas. Principles of Neurosurgery. p. 28,1. In Rengachary SS, Wilkins RH (eds): Wolfe Publishing, London, 1994
Black P.McL: Meningiomas. Neurosurgery 32:643–57, 1993
Carroll R, Glowacka D, Dashner K, Black PM: Progesterone receptor in meningiomas. Cancer Res 53:1312–6, 1993
Cushing H, Eisenhardt L: Meningiomas: Their Classification, Regional Behavior, Life History and Surgical End Results. Charles C Thomas, Springfield, IL, 1938
DeMonte F: Current management of meningiomas. Oncology 9:83–6, 1995
Foy PM, Chadwick DW, Rajgopalan N et al: Do prophylactic anticonvulsant drugs alter the pattern of seizures after craniotomy. J Neurol Neurosurg Psychiatry 55:753–7, 1992
Glaholm J, Bloom HJG, Crow JH: The role of radiotherapy in the management of intracranial meningiomas: the Royal Marsden Hospital experience with 186 patients. Int J Radiat Oncol Biol Phys 18:755–61, 1990
Goldsmith BJ, Wara WM, Wilson CB et al: Postoperative irradiation for subtotally resected meningiomas. J Neurosurg 80:195–201, 1994
Grunberg SM, Weiss MH, Spitz IM et al: Treatment of unresectable meningiomas with the antiprogesterone agent mifepristone. J Neurosurg 74:861–6, 1991
Jaaskelainen J: Seemingly complete removal of histologically benign intracranial meningioma: late recurrence rate and facts predicting recurrence in 657 patients. Surg Neurol 26:461–9, 1986
Jaaskelainen J, Haltia M, Laasonen E et al: The growth rate of intracranial meningiomas and its relationship to histology. An analysis of 43 patients. Surg Neurol 24:165–72, 1985
Kallio M, Sankila R, Hakulinen T et al: Factors affecting operative and excess long-term mortality in 935 patients with intracranial meningioma. Neurosurgery 31:2–12, 1992
Konziolka D, Lunsford LD: Radiosurgery of meningiomas. Neurosurg Clin North Am 3:219–30, 1992
Lunsford LD: Contemporary management of meningiomas: radiation therapy as an adjuvant and radiosurgery as an alternative to surgical removal? J Neurosurg 80:187–90, 1994
Mahmood A, Caccamo DV, Tomacek et al: Atypical and malignant meningiomas: a clinicopathological review. Neurosurgery 33:955–63, 1993
Mirimanoff RO, Dosoretz DE, Linggood RM et al: Meningioma: analysis of recurrence and progression following neurosurgical resection. J Neurosurg 62:18–24, 1985
Schmidek H (ed): Meningiomas and Their Surgical Management. WB Saunders, Philadelphia, 1991
Wilson CB: Meningiomas: genetics, malignancy, and the role of radiation in induction and treatment. J Neurosurg 81:666–75, 1994

156. PITUITARY TUMORS

GARY S. RICHARDSON

Tumors in the pituitary sella represent the most common clinical manifestation of the intersection between neurology and endocrinology. Whereas the most common pituitary tumor, the pituitary adenoma, typically has both endocrine and neurologic manifestations, many pituitary tumors (particularly those without autonomous endocrine function) present with isolated neurologic symptoms. As with other tumors, advances in imaging techniques permit recognition of pituitary tumors at an earlier point in their pathologic evolution, often in advance of clinically apparent neurologic or endocrine manifestations. Indeed, the sensitivity of magnetic resonance imaging (MRI) may now have made the incidental pituitary mass the most common clinical presentation of a pituitary adenoma for the neurologist. This trend makes it more important for the neurologist to be familiar with the pathology and presentation of pituitary tumors.

The differential diagnosis of a pituitary mass includes a number of pathologic processes and tumor histologies, many of which are reviewed elsewhere in this volume. This chapter is intended to provide an overview of pituitary pathology, with an emphasis on the pituitary adenoma, including a discussion of clinical presentation, diagnostic methods, and specific treatment approaches.

PITUITARY ANATOMY AND PHYSIOLOGY

Normal Anatomy

The normal pituitary gland lies in the sella turcica (Fig. 156-1). The gland consists of two parts, the anterior lobe (adenohypophysis) and the posterior lobe (neurohypophysis). Embryologically, the anterior lobe is derived from Rathke's pouch, an epithelial extension from the ventral neural ridges. In development, three components are recognized: the pars distalis, which develops into the anterior lobe; the pars intermedius, vestigial in adults, but which may be the source of some unusual pituitary tumors; and the pars tuberalis, which extends up to envelop the pituitary stalk and the median eminence. Perhaps the most important clinical manifestation of this embryologic origin is the occurrence of cysts arising from remnants of Rathke's pouch. The posterior pituitary gland arises from a ventral extension of the floor of the third ventricle, which forms the median eminence, the pituitary stalk, and the posterior lobe.

The normal human pituitary gland measures approximately $10 \times 13 \times 6$ mm and weighs between 0.5 and 0.9 g. It is significantly larger in girls at menarche and in women during pregnancy and lactation. It is bounded by the bony confines of the sella turcica except superiorly, where the diaphragma sella, an extension of the dura mater, separates the sella from the suprasellar cistern and the cranial cavity. Important anatomic relationships include the sphenoid sinus anteriorly and inferiorly, the cavernous sinuses laterally, and the optic chiasm superiorly.

The posterior pituitary gland arises from the ventral hypothalamus and consists of bundled axons from neurons in the magnocellular regions of the supraoptic and paraventricular hypothalamic nuclei. The normal posterior gland appears as a signal-intense area in the posterior aspect of the sella on T1-weighted MRI (Fig. 156-1). The high signal intensity is thought to represent accumulated secretory product within the axons and is decreased in clinical settings in which posterior pituitary hormone is depleted (e.g., diabetes insipidus).

Blood flow to the anterior pituitary is greater than for any other organ in the body (approximately 0.8 ml/g/min). The principal source of this blood flow is a portal system arising from the superior hypophyseal artery, including capillary beds in both the median eminence and the pituitary gland itself. The clinical significance of this unusual high-flow and low-pressure

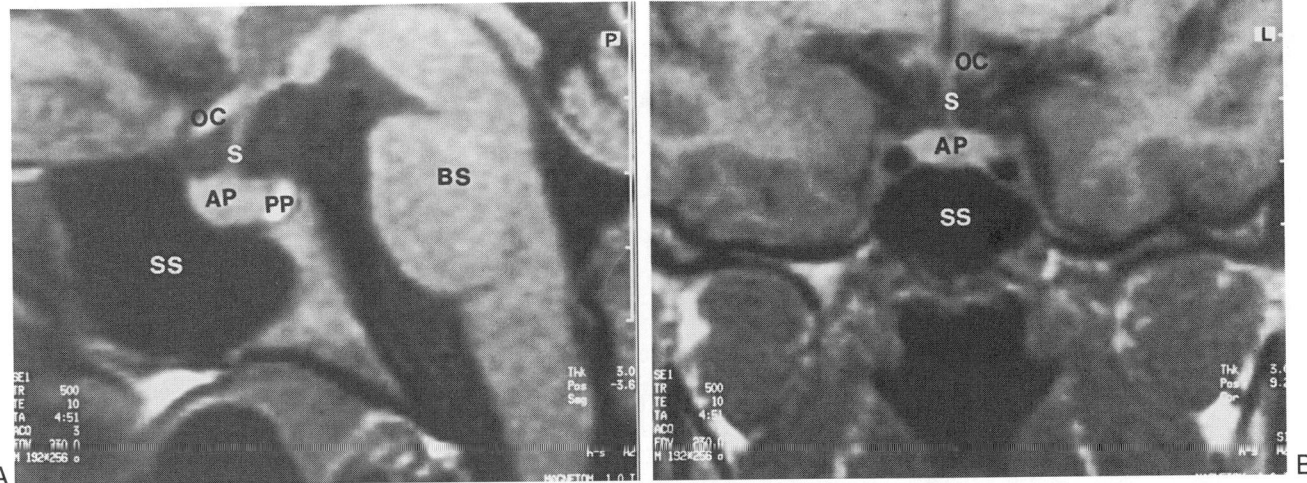

FIG. 156-1. **(A)** Magnified, T1-weighted, sagittal and **(B)** coronal MRI images of the pituitary gland in a 21-year-old woman referred for evaluation of mild hyperprolactinemia. While the concave enlargement of the gland is considered to be one sign of a microadenoma, the size and shape of the gland are within normal limits for young women. AP, anterior pituitary gland; PP, posterior pituitary gland; S, pituitary stalk; SS, sphenoid sinus; OC, optic chiasm (at the origin of the optic tracts in the coronal view).

vascular supply is that it predisposes the pituitary to infarction when the sella contents expand and compromise blood flow. This occurs in the setting of a pituitary tumor (pituitary apoplexy) or as a consequence of puerperal enlargement of the pituitary coupled with hypotension (Sheehan syndrome).

Normal Physiology

The anterior pituitary glands consist of five recognized secretory cell types, based on immunohistochemical characterization of their principal secretory products (Table 156-1). Whereas other peptides are found within the normal pituitary, most of these are felt to act as paracrine (local) factors within the gland. Some circumstantial evidence suggests that other pituitary hormones exist, but these have not been convincingly identified.

The secretory activity of the anterior pituitary gland is regulated by peptide factors synthesized in the hypothalamus and transported via the hypophyseal portal vasculature. Secretion of most pituitary hormones appears to be regulated primarily by specific stimulatory factors, with inhibitory factors playing a less important role. An exception to this is prolactin, for which inhibitory regulation by dopamine released by cells of the arcuate nucleus of the hypothalamus provides the principal regulatory influence. The significance of this distinction is that any

pathologic process that interferes with transport of dopamine to the pituitary can produce clinically significant hyperprolactinemia. This is most commonly seen in the setting of a intrasellar mass that deforms the pituitary stalk. The resulting hyperprolactinemia (stalk syndrome) is usually distinguishable in magnitude from the prolactin elevations produced by prolactinoma (i.e., less than 150 ng/ml) but may still be sufficient to produce clinically significant hypogonadism.

DIAGNOSIS OF PITUITARY TUMORS

Prevalence

When all histologies are taken together, the prevalence of pituitary tumors is very high. The increased use of sensitive imaging techniques including high-resolution computed tomographic (CT) scanning and MRI, particularly with gadolinium enhancement, has made the clinical recognition of pituitary masses much more common and has made the approach to the pituitary "incidentaloma" an important clinical problem. In one series of patients receiving CT scans for other reasons, 20 percent had pituitary lesions greater than 3 mm in diameter. Other estimates for the incidental finding of a pituitary mass on CT or MRI range from 3.7 to 6.5 percent.

Autopsy series are generally consistent with these estimates, demonstrating a prevalence for pituitary microadenomas (less than 10 mm diameter) of between 10 and 20 percent. There was no demonstrable influence of either age or gender. In all the available autopsy series, incidental macroadenomas (adenomas larger than 1 cm in diameter) are very uncommon, suggesting that the smaller tumors found in the younger patients do not typically progress in size, or that larger tumors are consistently recognized clinically. When histology is evaluated, most incidental pituitary tumors found at autopsy are microadenomas, with lesser numbers of cysts, metastases, and infarcts.

Differential Diagnosis

A number of pathologic processes can present as a mass within the pituitary sella (Table 156-2). As suggested by the autopsy

TABLE 156-1. Principal Secretory Products of Normal Pituitary

Cell Type	Secretory Products
Somatotroph	Growth hormone (GH)
	Human placental lactogen
Lactotrph	Prolactin
	Vasoactive intestinal polypeptide (VIP)
Corticotroph	Adrenocorticotropic hormone (corticotropin)
	β-Lipotropin hormone (β-LPH)
	α-Melanocyte-stimulating hormone (α-MSH)
Thyrotroph	Thyroid-stimulating hormone (TSH)
Gonadotroph	Luteinizing hormone (LH)
	Follicle stimulating hormone (FSH)
	Dynorphin
	Atrial natriuretic peptide

TABLE 156-2. Tumors of the Pituitary Sella

Tumors
  Pituitary adenoma
  Metastasis
    Breast
    Leukemia
    Lymphoma
    Lung
  Meningioma
  Craniopharyngioma
  Hamartoma
  Glioma
  Germinoma and teratoma
  Dermoid and epidermoid tumors
  Chordoma
  Neuroma
Cysts
  Rathke's cleft cyst
  Arachnoid cyst
Inflammation and infection
  Sarcoidosis
  Infection
    Bacterial abscess
    Tuberculosis
    Mycotic or viral infection
  Eosinophilic granuloma
  Lymphocytic and autoimmune hypophysitis
Vascular
  Aneurysm
  Carotid/cavernous fistula

series described above, by far the most common type is the pituitary adenoma, which may account for 10 to 20 percent of all intracranial tumors. The autopsy series suggest that, collectively, metastases form the second most common group of pituitary tumors. While involvement of the pituitary is common in metastatic disease, presumably reflecting the high blood flow though the gland, most of these tumors are incidental findings. It is unusual for a pituitary presentation to be the first manifestation of metastatic disease. When clinical differentiation is important, the more aggressive malignant tumor is commonly associated with earlier, more complete hypopituitarism, including hypoprolactinemia and diabetes insipidus, without the enlargement of the pituitary sella that typically accompanies slower growing adenomas.

The next most common single histology presenting clinically as a pituitary mass is the craniopharyngioma. The prevalence of these tumors is age dependent. In children, craniopharyngiomas are more common than pituitary adenomas, whereas the frequency decreases sharply in adulthood. Preoperative differentiation of craniopharyngioma from pituitary adenoma can be difficult. Craniopharyngiomas are more likely to be cystic, and half will have calcifications, which are more readily identified by CT than MRI. The typical origination of the craniopharyngioma from cell rests in the pituitary stalk results in a higher frequency of visual field compromise and diabetes insipidus than is seen with pituitary adenomas, and these clinical features can be helpful in the differential diagnosis.

Rathke's cleft cysts are also common findings at autopsy, but they constitute a small percentage of clinically detected pituitary masses. At the time of clinical presentation, the cysts can be quite large, and typically present with headache, hypopituitarism, and visual field disturbances. While the cystic nature of the tumor is often clear on T1-weighted MRI, the variable content of the mucoid cyst fluid makes the T1-weighted signal characteristics an unreliable diagnostic tool.

A variety of other tumor histologies can present in the parasellar region, including glioma, germinoma, and neuroma. Meningiomas are common tumors of the parasellar region, ac-

counting for approximately 10 percent of all tumors in the area of the chiasm, but they rarely invade far enough into the pituitary sella to be confused radiologically with a pituitary adenoma.

Inflammatory and vascular lesions can present as a sellar or parasellar mass. Systemic inflammatory and granulomatous disorders (e.g., sarcoidosis or histiocytosis) may include pituitary presentations. The pituitary stalk is commonly involved, and these disorders need to be considered in the differential diagnosis of an enlargement confined to the stalk on MRI. Diabetes insipidus is the most common endocrine manifestation (e.g., Hand-Schüller-Christian disease), and diagnosis is generally possible in the setting of the other systemic manifestations. Occasionally, inflammatory processes are confined to the pituitary. In lymphocytic hypophysitis, a disorder seen exclusively in women (most commonly in the postpartum setting), an autoimmune reaction to the anterior pituitary gland can result in hypopituitarism and a mass on MRI indistinguishable from a pituitary adenoma. In these cases, trans-sphenoidal biopsy may be necessary to establish the diagnosis.

Among vascular lesions, the most important are carotid artery aneurysms. These may extend into the pituitary and appear as an intrasellar tumor on CT scans. Differentiation of this rare presentation is important because of the potential for disaster during attempted trans-sphenoidal resection. MRI is generally sufficient to correctly identify a vascular lesion, although in complicated aneurysms or those with extensive thrombus, an angiogram is occasionally required.

Imaging

MRI is now the modality of choice for evaluation of the pituitary gland and adjacent structures. The greater resolution of MRI and improved delineation of soft tissue anatomy are required for sensitive recognition of intrapituitary tumors, particularly those less than 1.0 cm in diameter. In addition, the greater ease with which multiplanar imaging can be accomplished, and the absence of ionizing radiation, are important advantages of MRI over CT for routine imaging. Typically, MRI scans examining the pituitary are performed using T1-weighted sagittal profiles and thin T1-weighted coronal images with and without gadolinium enhancement. Under normal conditions, this approach allows delineation of the pituitary gland, the pituitary stalk, the optic chiasm, and other important adjacent neural structures (Fig. 156-1).

In specific situations, other imaging approaches may be appropriate. The greater resolution of bone allowed by CT scanning makes this approach useful in addressing the question of bony erosion by tumor. Angiography may be necessary to address definitively the possibility of aneurysm presenting as an intrasellar mass. Similarly, modified MRI or CT scanning protocols may be useful in distinguishing the specific tumor types within the sellar region. For example, CT scanning provides improved recognition of calcifications characteristic of craniopharyngioma.

Special Studies

Recently the diagnosis of small endocrine tumors has been enhanced by the development of radiologic methods designed to localize endocrinologically active tissue. In petrosal sinus sampling, catheters are positioned bilaterally in the petrosal sinuses to permit simultaneous sampling of blood from both sides of pituitary gland venous drainage. Theoretically, a gradient in hormone concentration between petrosal samples and simultaneous samples from the periphery (e.g., the inferior vena cava) serves to confirm the pituitary origin of hormone overproduction. Similarly, an interpetrosal gradient allows lateralization of the source to one side of the gland. This approach is particularly useful in the evaluation of patients with suspected Cushing's disease (see below), in which ectopic sources of hormone excess (e.g., pulmonary carcinoid) can be difficult to distinguish from small pituitary microadenomas that are commonly at the lower limit of reliable MRI detection. The amplitude of the petrosalperipheral and interpetrosal gradients can be increased by stimulation of corticotropin secretion with ovine corticotropin-releasing factor, which typically produces an exaggerated response from corticotrope adenomas.

Initial work with this method suggested that adequate localizing and lateralizing gradients predicted surgical cure by transsphenoidal resection (or hemihypophysectomy when tumor could not be found during surgery). However, subsequent data have raised serious questions regarding the reliability of lateralization, given the variability of venous anatomy, the localization of many tumors to the midline, and the paradoxical reversal of the interpetrosal lateralization gradient after ovine corticotropin-releasing factor stimulation. Whereas some authors recommend routine use of petrosal sampling in patients with suspected Cushing's disease without unambiguous MRI findings, others argue that the procedure is too difficult to interpret to be of clinical use.

Other recent developments include the use of single-photon-emission computed tomographic scanning in conjunction with radiotracers developed from peptides such as somatostatin to localize extrapituitary remnants of pituitary tumors.

CLINICAL PRESENTATION

The Pituitary Mass

The clinical presentation of patients with pituitary tumors can be broadly organized into symptoms of mass effect and symptoms of hormonal excess. With the exception of mild hyperprolactinemia occurring in nonfunctioning tumors (see above), the symptoms of hormone excess occur in patients with functional tumors, and the resultant syndrome depends on the hormone produced. Symptoms arising as a consequence of mass effects of the tumor itself are relatively independent of the pathologic process underlying the tumor, except that they are more likely to predominate in nonfunctional tumors, in which the absence of endocrine symptoms makes early detection less likely. Here, the specific anatomic relationships of the pituitary sella and the direction of tumor expansion dictate the nature of the clinical presentation (Fig. 156-2). In addition, the rapidity of tumor growth appears to play an important role. Cranial nerve compromise by a tumor extending laterally into the cavernous sinus is unusual in the setting of slowly expanding lesions such as pituitary adenomas but is more common with rapidly growing tumors such as metastatic carcinoma, or after sudden expansion of adenomas in the setting of infarction or hemorrhage (pituitary apoplexy, see below).

Neurologic Manifestations

The most common symptom due to mass effect of an intrasellar tumor is headache. Expansion of the pituitary contents with distention of the diaphragma sellae is the presumed mechanism for headache, which can occur even with smaller (i.e., less than 1 cm) intrasellar tumors. The prevalence of both headache and incidental small pituitary tumors (see above) makes the specificity of this association difficult to prove, but a causal relationship is supported by the common finding that larger tumors that have breached the diaphragma sella may paradoxically produce no headache symptoms.

Extension of pituitary tumors superiorly results in contact with the optic chiasm and visual field defects. Given the inverted organization of the visual efferents within the chiasm, compression of the chiasm from below results in typical presentation with bilateral superior temporal quadrantanopsia. As compression proceeds, the field defect progresses to bitemporal hemianopsia. The gradual growth of most pituitary tumors results in a subtle progression of the vision loss, and defects are commonly quite advanced at the time of clinical recognition.

Lateral extension of pituitary tumors into the cavernous sinus can result in compromise of cranial nerves along their course through the sinus (Fig. 156-2). The most commonly involved nerve is the oculomotor nerve (third), resulting in ophthalmoplegia, ptosis, and mydriasis. Less commonly, the abducens (sixth) or trochlear (fourth) nerves are involved, producing unilateral oculomotor weakness and diplopia. The first and second branches of the trigeminal nerve also pass through the cavernous sinus near the sella, and involvement of these nerves can present as facial pain or anesthesia. Finally, sympathetic branches traveling with V_1 may be may also be compromised, resulting in a central Horner syndrome.

Other structures within the cavernous sinus, most notably the carotid artery, are occasionally involved by lateral extension of a pituitary tumor. Significant compromise of the carotid artery at this point presents catastrophically, with hemispheric dysfunction and hemiplegia. In the absence of acute hemorrhage or infarction, this usually indicates a more aggressive histology such as metastatic carcinoma. Anterior extension of the tumor into the sphenoid sinus can result in cerebrospinal fluid rhinorrhea and meningitis.

Endocrine Manifestations

Endocrine manifestations of secretory pituitary adenomas are discussed below. The principal endocrine manifestation of a pituitary mass is hypopituitarism, the mechanism of which is often unclear. Whereas some pituitary deficits presumably arise as a direct consequence of tumor growth and infarction of the normal gland, this mechanism cannot account for the nature of the deficits that are commonly seen. Hormonal deficiency often occurs, although a large portion of the normal gland remains intact. Furthermore, growth hormone deficiency is the most common defect in this setting despite the preponderance of growth hormone-positive cells in the normal pituitary. Finally, significant hormone deficits are often reversed with surgical removal of the tumor. Taken together, these observations suggest that the mechanism responsible for most of the associated hormone deficiency involves interference with communication between the hypothalamus and the anterior pituitary gland, either at the level of the pituitary stalk or though disruption of local paracrine factors whose role in normal hormonal secretion remains incompletely defined.

Hypopituitarism due to a pituitary mass can involve any of the pituitary hormonal axes in any combination, but some systems appear to be more vulnerable. Gonadotropin (luteinizing hormone and follicle-stimulating hormone FSH) and growth

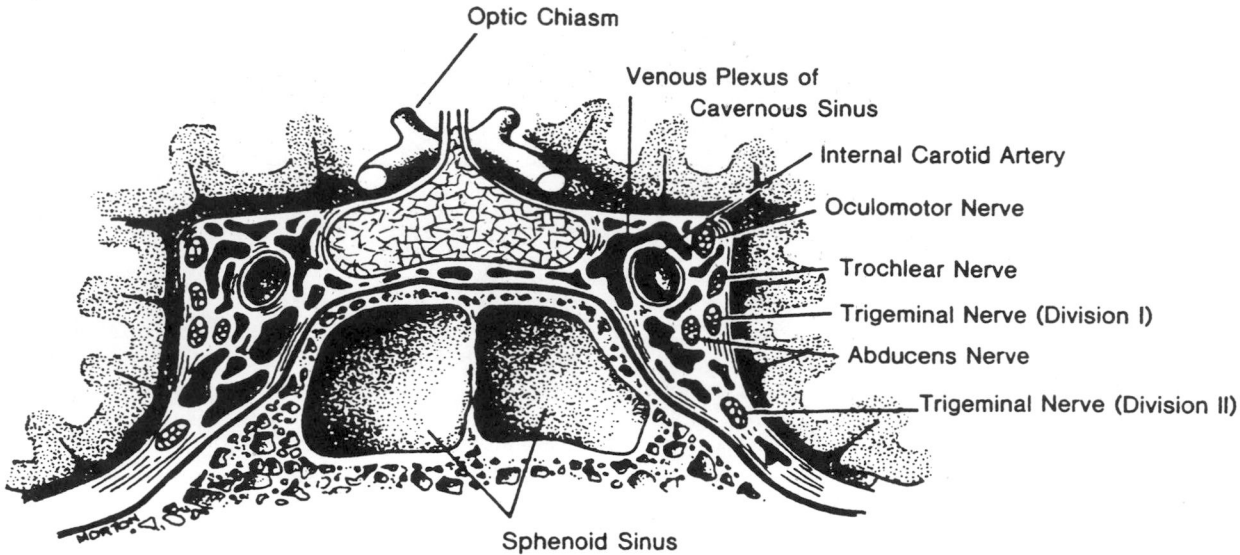

FIG. 156-2.   Anatomic relationships of the pituitary to adjacent structures. (From Reid R, Quigley M, Yen S: Pituitary apoplexy: a review. Arch Neurol 42:712–9, 1985, with permission.)

hormone function are affected most frequently, followed by the thyroid axis (thyroid-stimulating hormone), and then the adrenal axis (corticotropin). Hypoprolactinemia is a relatively rare manifestation of a pituitary mass. As noted above, whereas the other anterior pituitary hormones are controlled primarily through stimulation by hypothalamic factors, prolactin is principally under inhibitory control by dopamine. Thus, the effect of a pituitary mass on this axis is generally to increase prolactin secretion, producing clinical effects of hyperprolactinemia and occasionally mimicking a functional prolactinoma. When hypoprolactinemia is seen, it may indicate destruction of lactotropes by a more aggressive tumor histology (e.g., metastasis or previous hemorrhage).

Central diabetes insipidus is also an unusual manifestation of hypopituitarism due to a pituitary tumor, because the cell bodies responsible for secretion of vasopressin are located above the sella in the hypothalamus and are thus unaffected by intrasellar tumors. Diabetes insipidus is more common in parasellar tumors such as craniopharyngiomas or meningiomas arising at the level of the pituitary stalk or above.

Pituitary Apoplexy

Infarction and hemorrhage of the pituitary gland (pituitary apoplexy) is a neurologic emergency. The high metabolic demand of the normal gland, coupled with its tenuous blood supply through a portal (double-capillary) vascular system, predisposes the gland to infarction in situations where blood supply is compromised. Typically, pituitary apoplexy occurs in one of two clinical settings. In the first, pituitary tumors increase both metabolic demand and pressure within the sella, thereby reducing flow through the low-pressure blood supply. When tumor growth produces a critical reduction in blood flow, apoplexy with sudden onset of headache and neurologic symptoms may occur. The previous growth of the tumor and erosion of the bony sella determine the direction and extent of hemorrhage expansion, and the nature of the neurologic symptoms (see above).

Pregnant women can develop pituitary apoplexy at the time

of delivery (Sheehan syndrome). In this setting, the pituitary is probably normal (although women with pre-existing pituitary tumors may be at increased risk), but the physiologic hypertrophy of the gland associated with pregnancy produces predisposing conditions analogous to those seen with pituitary tumors. At delivery, transient hypotension probably precipitates the crisis, resulting in infarction and neurologic symptoms. With a normal gland and no erosion of the sella, the neurologic manifestations, other than headache, may be subtle or absent, and Sheehan syndrome may be unrecognized until hypopituitarism becomes evident after delivery with failure of lactation or postpartum amenorrhea.

Syndromes of Pituitary Hormone Excess

The most common pituitary tumors, pituitary adenomas are generally divided into those that secrete excess hormone and those that are nonsecreting. The alternate designation of ''nonfunctioning'' adenoma is less accurate, since many tumors that do not secrete significant amounts of hormone are nonetheless ''functioning'' in that they have been shown to produce peptide hormone or appropriate mRNA when examined using more sensitive methods. Approximately 25 to 30 percent of patients shown to have pituitary adenomas have no clinically detectable hormone overproduction. These tumors present as a pituitary mass, largely indistinguishable in their clinical manifestations from tumors of other, nonendocrine histology. The remaining 70 to 75 percent of adenomas are ''functional,'' producing specific hormones or hormone fragments in excess, and their clinical presentation typically reflects the specific action of those hormones (Table 156-3).

Hyperprolactinemia

The most common functional pituitary tumors secrete prolactin (''prolactinomas''). Clinically significant hyperprolactinemia occurs most commonly as a consequence of prolactin-secreting pituitary adenomas, but a variety of other causes need to be considered in the patient with an elevated prolactin level, including the following:

TABLE 156-3. Laboratory Evaluation of Suspected Secretory Pituitary Adenoma

Tumor Type	Clinical Syndrome	Laboratory Tests	Diagnostic Results
Somatotroph	Acromegaly	Somatomedin C (insulin-like growth factor)	More than upper limit of normal (e.g., 475 ng/ml; varies with assay)
		Oral glucose suppression of growth hormone	GH >5 μg/L at baseline, 1 h, and 2 h after 100-g oral glucose load
Lactotroph	Hyperprolactinemia Hypogonadism	Serum prolactin	>250 ng/ml is diagnostic
			100–250 ng/ml is ambiguous; need to consider renal status, medications (e.g., phenothiazines), pituitary stalk compression, and so forth
Corticotrph	Cushing's disease	Plasma cortisol and corticotropin	Elevated cortisol with loss of normal diurnal variation (i.e., AM level = PM level) and detectable or elevated corticotropin
		Plasma cortisol at 8 AM following 1 mg dexamethasone at 11 PM the night before ("overnight dexamethasone suppression test")	>5 μg/dl demonstrates inadequate suppression; multiple false positives to single-dose, single-determination test (e.g., depression) restrict this test to use as screening tool
		24-h urine for free cortisol and metabolites (17-hydroxycorticosteroids) at baseline and after low-dose dexamethasone (0.5 mg PO q6h × 8 doses) and high-dose dexamethasone (2 mg PO q6h × 8 doses)	Baseline 24-h urinary free cortisol more than upper limit of normal (e.g., 100 μg/24 h)
			Low-dose dexamethasone: plasma cortisol >5 μg/dl; urinary free cortisol and 17-hydroxycorticosteroids >50% of baseline value
			High-dose dexamethasone: plasma cortisol <5 μg/dl; urinary free cortisol and 17-hydroxycorticosteroids <50% of baseline value.
			Failure to suppress with high-dose dexamethasone suggests nonpituitary Cushing's syndrome (e.g., adrenal tumor)
Thyrotroph	Secondary hyperthyroidism	Thyroid-stimulating hormone (TSH), with thyroid function test (T_4, THBR)	Elevated thyroid function tests with elevated or normal TSH (≥1 miU/L)
Gonadotroph	Hypergonadotropic hypergonadism	Luteinizing hormone	Elevated gonadotropins with normal or elevated testosterone (male) or estradiol (female)

Functional pituitary tumor
Pituitary stalk compression
Hypothalamic disease
Primary hypothyroidism
Neurogenic factors
Pregnancy
Medications (e.g., phenothiazines)
Cirrhosis
Chronic renal failure
Severe stress
Idiopathic factors

As a general rule, a prolactin concentration above 150–200 ng/mL usually indicates the presence of a prolactin-secreting adenoma, since secondary causes of hyperprolactinemia rarely produce levels this high. Hyperprolactinemia of any cause generally presents with hypogonadism, either oligomenorrhea in a woman, or oligospermia and impotence in a man. Galactorrhea (nonpuerperal lactation) can occur in both men and women, but is much more common in women with hyperprolactinemia because of the dependence of milk production on co-stimulation of the breast glandular tissue by estrogen. It is important to note that galactorrhea is present at the time of diagnosis in less than half of patients with hyperprolactinemia due to a prolactinoma. This is because the sustained hypogonadism (and hypoestrogenemia) produced by the tumor also inhibits milk production.

Acromegaly and Gigantism

Growth hormone excess presents clinically as either gigantism or acromegaly, depending on whether the onset of growth hormone overproduction occurs before the closure of the long-bone epiphyses. By far the most common cause of either acromegaly and gigantism is a pituitary somatotrope adenoma secreting the hormone, but pancreatic islet cell tumors and hypothalamic gangliocytomas producing excessive growth hormone-releasing hormone and secondary pituitary somatotrope hyperplasia have been described. Regardless of mechanism, growth hormone excess leads to overproduction of growth factors such as somatomedin C (insulinlike growth factor 1). Through direct action and via these growth factors, growth hormone excess results in the clinical syndromes in which excessive growth of cartilage and soft tissue produce the typical changes in hands, feet, and facies associated with acromegaly or the elongation of long bones in gigantism. Insulin resistance is also commonly seen.

Diagnosis of pituitary growth hormone overproduction is most commonly made by demonstrating abnormal failure of the hormone to decrease in response to hyperglycemia (oral glucose load) in the setting of a pituitary abnormality on MRI or CT. Improvements in assays for circulating insulinlike growth factor 1 have permitted increasing reliance on this measure as a screening device, and as a means of following therapy. Plasma measurement of growth hormone-releasing hormone should be performed in patients with abnormal growth hormone measures but no clear pituitary tumor on MRI.

Recently, important advances have been made in understanding the pathogenesis of somatotrope adenomas. X-chromosome inactivation studies have established that most of these tumors are monoclonal, arising from a somatic mutation of a single cell. This makes the hypothesized role of abnormal hyperstimulation by hypothalamic growth factors less important, although a contributory role cannot be excluded. A subset of somatotrope adenomas has been shown to have altered forms of the G_s regulatory protein that controls adenylyl cyclase activity, resulting in autonomous growth hormone secretion and cell growth.

Cushing's Disease

Corticotropin excess is most commonly a consequence of a pituitary adenoma secreting the hormone and in this setting constitutes Cushing's disease, named for Harvey Cushing, the neurosurgeon who first described the relationship between the clinical syndrome and a pituitary tumor and who pioneered the trans-sphenoidal surgical approach. The broader term Cushing's syndrome is used to describe patients with cortisol excess from any cause (including iatrogenic steroid administration and functional adrenal tumors).

The clinical presentation of the patient with Cushing's disease is similar to that of other causes of cortisol excess, with characteristic obesity, muscle wasting, striae, insulin resistance, and hypertension. Hypokalemia is occasionally seen, but this is a mineralcorticoid effect that is usually more prominent in patients with functional adrenal tumors producing aldosterone. As with growth hormone excess and acromegaly, other causes of corticotropin excess must be excluded, including tumors of lung, pancreas, and thyroid that produce corticotropin-releasing hormone (CRH), leading to secondary corticotrope hyperplasia. Because the pituitary tumors responsible for Cushing's disease are often quite small, and may be at the lower limit of MRI detection, other localization techniques such as petrosal sinus sampling (see above) may be required to exclude extrapituitary causes.

Extraordinary elevations of corticotropin can be seen in patients with oat cell carcinoma of the lung. The levels of corticotropin in these patients are often sufficient to produce hyperpigmentation and hyperaldosteronism, features rarely seen in the patient with Cushing's disease. Obesity is usually not prominent in these patients, reflecting the opposing impact of other factors produced by the oat cell tumor.

Diagnosis of Cushing's disease is made by demonstrating the failure of cortisol production to decrease in response to exogenous steroid (dexamethasone). The impairment of feedback inhibition in Cushing's disease is a partial one, such that suppression will occur at higher dexamethasone doses. This allows differentiation of adrenal tumors, which are more resistant to suppression.

Secondary Hyperthyroidism

The clinical manifestations of thyroid-stimulating hormone hypersecretion are primarily those of hyperthyroidism and are generally indistinguishable from hyperthyroidism of any cause. With modern radioimmunoassays for this hormone, the causal role of the pituitary thyrotrope can usually be recognized by the inappropriate concentrations of the hormone for measured T_4 and T_3. In contrast to primary hyperthyroidism (e.g., Graves disease) in which levels of the hormone are suppressed by the excess thyroid hormones, in secondary hyperthyroidism arising as a consequence of a thyroid-stimulating hormone-secreting pituitary adenoma, levels of this hormone are elevated or inappropriately normal for the concentrations of T_4 and T_3.

Pituitary Hypergonadism

Follicle-stimulating hormone or luteinizing hormone hypersecretion (or both) due to a functional pituitary tumor occurs more frequently than was originally reported. With improved gonadotropin assays and MRI scans, this functional tumor is now felt to comprise up to 17 percent of functional macroadenomas in men. The tumor is more common in men than in women and typically occurs in middle age. Clinical manifestations of the hypersecretion itself are very subtle. Rarely, testosterone levels are significantly elevated in men with associated complaints of hypersexuality. More typically, sex steroid levels are normal, and, in the absence of clinical symptoms, the tumors present with manifestations of the pituitary mass. Preoperative diagnosis is made based on the presence of normal or elevated gonadal steroids combined with elevated gonadotropins.

Many tumors previously thought to be nonsecretory have been shown to secrete one of the subunits of the gonadotropin hormones. New radioimmunoassays specific for the β-subunit, which is unique to each of the three pituitary glycoprotein hormones (thyroid-stimulating hormone, luteinizing hormone, or follicle-stimulating hormone) or the α-subunit, which is common to all of them, can be secreted in excess by a functional pituitary tumor. The α-subunit is found free in normal plasma, but a function specific to the subunit has not been defined. These secretory tumors are also not associated with a recognizable clinical syndrome, and they typically present with large parasellar masses and symptoms related to the mass effects.

TREATMENT

Surgery is the initial treatment of choice for most tumors of the sella and parasellar regions. This is particularly true in the setting of optic chiasm compromise when rapid tumor decompression is necessary to limit or reverse a visual field defect. The exact location of the tumor, its likely histology, and its relationship to anatomic structures in the region together determine which surgical approach is required. Tumors within the pituitary sella, and those with limited extrasellar extension, can usually be approached via the trans-sphenoidal route with substantially reduced operative morbidity. In experienced hands, this approach has a high success rate and is the initial treatment of choice for most pituitary adenomas. Extension beyond the sella laterally, or superior extension with invasion or entrapment of the optic chiasm, typically necessitates a superior surgical approach through a transfrontal craniotomy.

Radiotherapy represents an alternative when surgery is not an appropriate initial step. In addition, postoperative radiation is used for certain tumor histologies for which remission and recurrence rates after operative resection can be reduced with combined therapy. Whereas postoperative radiation is still used to treat residual tumor after resection of pituitary adenoma, it is no longer routinely given to patients after resection of nonsecretory adenomas, or to those in whom endocrine measures are normal. The improved resolution available with MRI and newer endocrine measures permits an expectant approach in which radiation, and the attendant risk of hypopituitarism, can be reserved for patients with clear evidence of tumor growth, or endocrine evidence of recurrent hypersecretion.

The applicability of medical therapy for pituitary tumors depends entirely on the tumor histology. Besides chemotherapy, available medical therapy consists of endocrine manipulation of sensitive tumors. Somatostatin, an inhibitory peptide involved in the normal regulation of pituitary hormones, has been adapted for clinical use as octreotide. Administered subcutaneously, this medication has been shown to control growth hormone secretion in patients with acromegaly and to reduce the size and limit the growth of somatotropic tumors. Its principal application is in the control of unresectable residual tumor after surgery, or as primary therapy in patients who are not surgical candidates. In addition, it is now being used preoperatively to reduce the size of large tumors and improve the results of transsphenoidal resection. Octreotide has also been used in the management of other secretory tumors (e.g. those related to thyroid-stimulating hormone), but the response in this setting is more variable, reflecting the inconsistent expression of somatostatin receptors in other functional adenomas.

The most widely used medical therapy in this setting utilizes the oral dopamine (D_2) receptor agonists in the managment of prolactinoma. The most widely used of these drugs, bromocriptine, is generally effective as a means of limiting prolactin secretion and reducing tumor mass in prolactinomas. The impact on active tumors can be dramatic, and institution of bromociptine therapy is a viable alternative to surgery in the patient with a macroprolactinoma and vision loss. Reduction of tumor size and improvement of the visual fields can occur within hours of starting treatment, but the potential for a poor tumor response dictates that simultaneous preparation for surgical resection be made should bromocriptine not have the desired result.

In patients with small prolactinomas (less than 10 mm in diameter), the potential for cure with sustained use of bromocriptine remains controversial. This is because the natural history of these tumors remains incompletely defined. In macroprolactinomas, bromocriptine has been reported to produce sustained remissions in 5 to 15 percent of patients after treatment of 5 years. Use of bromocriptine is typically limited by the side effects, most notably nausea and orthostatic hypotension, and by the significant percentage of resistant or incompletely responsive tumors. Bromocriptine has also been shown to be effective in the management of some somatotropic tumors, but the response is much more variable than with prolactinomas, and dopamine receptor agonists are rarely sufficient as the primary treatment in these tumors.

SUMMARY

Tumors of the pituitary are common and represent an important intersection between neurology and endocrinology. Differential diagnosis of pituitary tumors includes a number of tumor histologies and pathologic processes involving the pituitary sella and the parasellar region. Identification and diagnosis of pituitary tumors has been enhanced by the development of new imaging technology, most notably MRI, which is now the imaging method of choice for tumors in this region.

Clinical manifestations of pituitary tumors are divided into manifestations of the tumor's mass effect and effects of overproduction of specific hormones. Mass effects include neurologic symptoms related to impingement upon adjacent structures, including headache and visual field compromise. Enlargement of a pituitary mass can also produce endocrine deficits. Excessive secretion of pituitary hormones by specific functional adenomas results in recognizable clinical syndromes including acromegaly, Cushing's disease, and hyperprolactinemia.

Treatment of pituitary tumors is dependent on size and histology, but surgery, typically through the trans-sphenoidal approach, is generally the initial treatment of choice. Medical therapy is also effective in specific settings, most notably in the treatment of prolactinoma, for which dopamine receptor agonists are now the treatment of choice.

SUGGESTED READINGS

Black PM, Hsu DW, Klibanski A et al: Hormone production in clinically nonfunctioning pituitary adenomas. J Neurosurg 66:244–50, 1987

Chambers E, Turski P, LaMasters D, Newton T: Regions of low density in the contrast-enhanced pituitary gland: normal and pathologic processes. Radiology 144:109–13, 1982

Chandler WF: Sellar and parasellar lesions. Clin Neurosurg 37:514–27, 1991

Chong BW, Newton TH: Hypothalamic and pituitary pathology. Radio Clin North Am 31:1147–53, 1993

El-Azouzi M, Black PM, Candia G et al: Trans-sphenoidal surgery for visual loss in patients with pituitary adenomas. Neurol Res 12:23–5, 1990

Grua JR, Nelson DH: ACTH-producing pituitary tumors. Endocrinol Metab Clin North Am 20:319–62, 1991

Klibanski A, Zervas NT: Diagnosis and management of hormone-secreting pituitary adenomas. N Engl J Med 324:822–31, 1991

Martin JB, Reichlin S: Clinical Neuroendocrinology. FA Davis, Philadelphia, 1987

Molitch ME, Russell EJ: The pituitary "incidentaloma." Ann Intern Med 112:925–31, 1990

Oldfield EH, Chrousos GP, Schulte HM et al: Preoperative lateralization of ACTH-secreting pituitary microadenomas by bilateral and simultaneous inferior petrosal venous sinus sampling. N Engl J Med 312:100–3, 1985

Peyster R, Adler L, Viscarello R et al: CT of the normal pituitary gland. Neuroradiology 28:161–5, 1986

Reid R, Quigley M, Yen S: Pituitary apoplexy: a review. Arch Neurol 42:712–19, 1985

Schwartzberg DG: Imaging of pituitary gland tumors. Semin Ultrasound CT MRI 13:207–23, 1992

Ur E, Mather SJ, Bomanji J, et al: Pituitary imaging using a labeled somatostatin analogue in acromegaly. Clin Endocrinol 36:147–50, 1992

Wolpert S, Molitch M, Goldman J, Wood J: Size, shape, and appearance of the normal female pituitary gland. AJR 143:377–81, 1984

157. CRANIOPHARYNGIOMA

R. MICHAEL SCOTT

Craniopharyngiomas are suprasellar tumors that commonly manifest in childhood. More than 50 percent of these tumors are diagnosed in patients under the age of 18 years, and the diagnosis in older patients is a relatively rare event. Craniopharyngiomas are the most common brain tumors of nonglial origin in children, representing approximately 3 to 6 percent of most patient series. A slight male preponderance is frequently seen, but many series report an equal male female incidence.

The biology of these tumors is fascinating. It is generally agreed that the tumor represents an embryonal rest of Rathke's pouch (the evagination of the oral pharyngeal mucosa through the skull base that is destined to form the anterior pituitary), and it is hypothesized that failure of complete involution of this hypophyseal pharyngeal duct tract leads to development of the craniopharyngioma. The tumor is therefore presumed to be congenital and to have been present and growing since birth. Nevertheless, an adult patient in my series was demonstrated by magnetic resonance imaging (MRI) to have no suprasellar pathology 6 years before the discovery of a tumor that became symptomatic during pregnancy. This suggests that additional stimuli may be important in provoking the growth of vestigial remnants of the hypophyseal pharyngeal duct to form a mass lesion.

The radiologic and gross appearances of these tumors are often quite dramatic. They frequently contain cysts that can assume giant size, insinuating themselves among the structures at the base of the brain or extending throughout the subarachnoid cisterns into the posterior fossa, sylvian fissures, or inferior frontal lobes. Their solid portions frequently contain calcification, a virtual *sine qua non* in radiologic diagnosis. These tumors commonly excite reactive change in adjacent brain and the tumor may become tightly adherent to structures around it, such as the arteries in the circle of Willis, the optic apparatus, and the undersurface of the hypothalamus. The cysts often contain a brownish yellow fluid that has been compared with machinery oil and that may glitter and shimmer because of cholesterol crystals resulting from breakdown of epithelial desquamation; this material may provoke the irritative response of tissues adjacent to the tumor.

The microscopic appearance of these tumors is also quite characteristic. They contain a mixture of squamous epithelium, loosely arranged cells, and cystic areas lined by epithelium. The squamous areas can become keratinized, form whorls, and show areas of calcification or ossification. Their striking histologic picture is very rarely confused with other intracranial neoplasms.

The clinical presentation of these patients can roughly be divided into three categories. One of the most common modes presents with symptoms related to endocrine dysfunction. Given that most tumors are adherent to and displace the pituitary stalk, it is not surprising that this would be the case. The endocrinologic symptoms can vary from growth retardation to more overt expressions of endocrine dysfunction, such as delayed or precocious puberty and diabetes insipidus. Symptoms related to hypothyroidism may be elicited, and menstrual irregularities, impotence, and other symptoms of pituitary dysfunction may be reported in older patients. A second mode of presentation involves visual disturbances. Because of the proximity of craniopharyngiomas to the optic apparatus and the tumor's relatively slow growth, severe visual deficits ranging from bitemporal hemianopsias to unilateral or bilateral blindness may develop without being noted by the patient. The third major category of tumor presentation involves symptoms related to increased intracranial pressure. In craniopharyngioma, intracranial hypertension is almost always due to obstructive hydrocephalus, which results when the tumor grows upward into the third ventricle, interfering with passage of cerebrospinal through the third ventricle to the aqueduct. These patients will develop acute or chronic hydrocephalus with papilledema and

all of the usual symptoms of increased intracranial pressure, including headache, vomiting, and altered mental status.

DIAGNOSIS AND PREOPERATIVE EVALUATION

In most patients with craniopharyngioma, the diagnosis is made primarily from the neuroradiologic studies. Before the common usage of computed tomography (CT) and MRI, plain radiographs of the skull were obtained to demonstrate the presence of calcification in the sellar or suprasellar region. The calcium frequently clumps into discrete areas but may consist only of calcification around the rim of cystic portions of the tumor. Currently, the CT scan is the most effective test for demonstrating the presence of calcification in these tumors (Fig. 157-1) and remains a helpful adjunct to diagnosis and surgical planning. Calcification is less well seen on MRI where it appears only as signal voids. MRI imaging has nevertheless become the essential study in the preoperative evaluation of these patients. No other study demonstrates so exquisitely the exact anatomic confines of the tumor and the displacement or invasion of the optic apparatus, hypothalamic structures, arteries of the circle of Willis, pituitary stalk, and so forth (Fig. 157-2). The surgeon will be greatly helped in patient evaluation by studies in sagittal, axial, and coronal planes, and gadolinium enhancement is imperative to determine if cysts are associated with bulk neoplastic tissue.

These patients need a thorough endocrinologic evaluation, although if they are ill with increased intracranial pressure or profound visual deficits, often not much time is available to obtain it. A careful history regarding the presence of symptoms suggesting diabetes insipidus should be obtained, and serum electrolytes and urine-specific gravities should be checked. Morning and evening serum cortisone levels, baseline thyroid

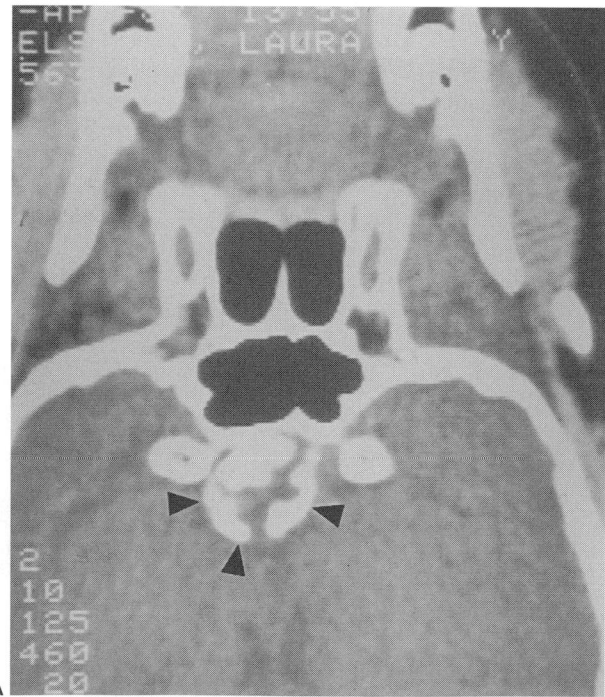
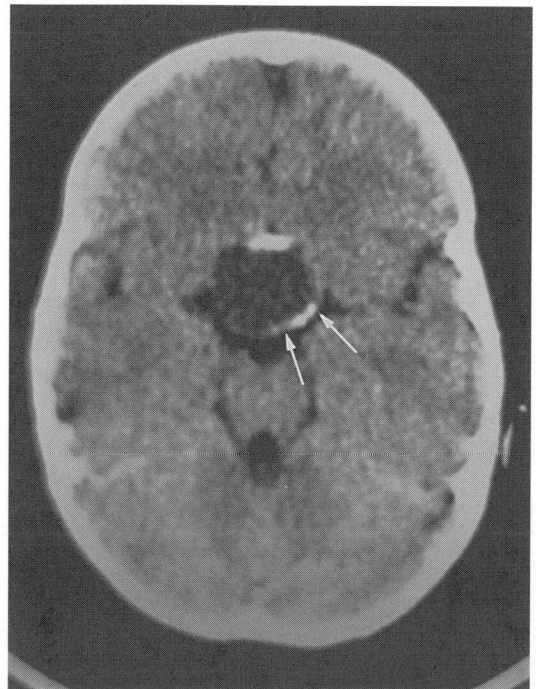

FIG. 157-1. **(A)** Noncontrast coronal CT scan, demonstrating circular intrasellar and suprasellar clumps of calcification (*arrowheads*) in a craniopharyngioma in an 8-year-old girl. **(B)** Nonenhance axial CT scan demonstrating a thin rim of calcification (*arrows*) bordering a large cystic craniopharyngioma in a 4-year-old girl. The calcifications could not be recognized as such on the MRI of this patient.

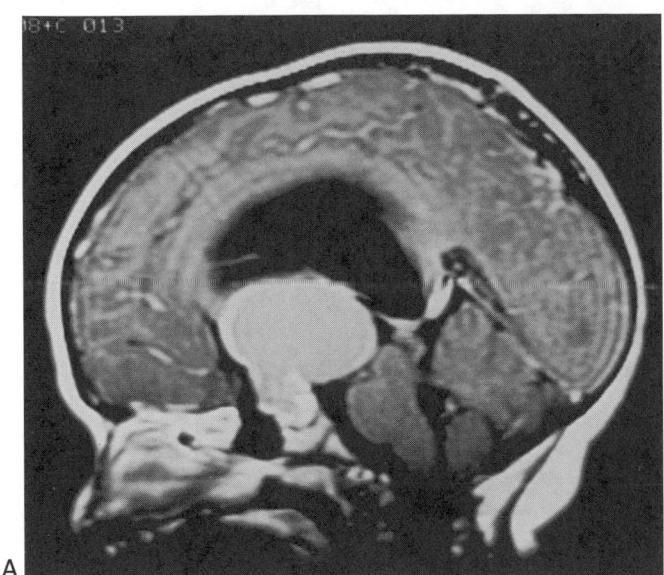
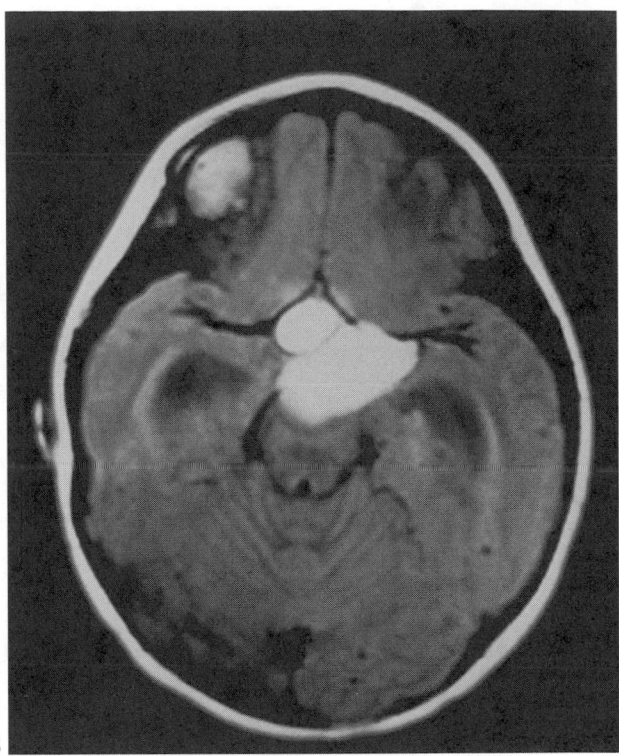

FIG. 157-2. **(A)** T1-weighted, gadolinium-enhanced sagittal MRI demonstrating an intrasellar and suprasellar mass filling the third ventricle, displacing the brain stem posteriorly, and causing massive obstructive hydrocephalus. **(B)** Proton-density, nonenhanced axial MRI in the same patient. The cyst is bright on MRI because of its high lipid content. The encroachment of the tumor cyst on the vessels in the circle of Willis, especially the left anterior and middle cerebral artery, can be clearly visualized, along with invagination of the tumor into the ventral midbrain.

function studies, growth hormone levels, and (in adolescent and postadolescent patients) luteinizing and follicle-stimulating hormone levels should be obtained. The endocrine evaluation is important as a baseline to aid in anesthetic management, to anticipate postoperative problems, and to assess treatment morbidity. All patients should receive an ophthalmologic evaluation to determine funduscopic appearance, the presence of peripheral visual field disturbance, and acuity changes. Concern has increased over the past decade for the neuropsychological deficits that result from this tumor's compression of the hypothalamus and distortion of limbic system structures, which result in changes in personality, disturbances in eating patterns, loss of memory, and so forth. For these reasons, I believe it is important to obtain neuropsychological testing of the patient before therapy of any type, if at all possible. Unfortunately, because of the urgency of the patient's symptomatology, it is often impossible to obtain these tests until well into the postoperative period, but, as noted above, they are an important part of the evaluation of the treatment morbidity of this tumor, and they aid in long-term postoperative management.

DIFFERENTIAL DIAGNOSIS

The differential diagnosis of tumors that occur in the suprasellar region (causing visual, endocrinologic, and intracranial pressure symptoms) can be problematic. Hypothalamic optic system gliomas infiltrate these structures and compress and elevate the floor of the third ventricle. Epidermoid and dermoid tumors are often midline tumors that can involve suprasellar structures and result in signs and symptoms similar to those of a craniopharyn-

gioma. Hypothalamic hamartomas can cause precocious puberty and present as masses on radiologic evaluation. Giant suprasellar carotid aneurysms can cause mass effect in the suprasellar region and present with rim calcification on radiologic studies. Pituitary tumors can expand the sella and grow upward into the third ventricle, causing endocrinologic deficits and visual disturbances. Rathke's cleft cysts, another lesion resulting from a residual of Rathke's pouch, can cause localized suprasellar mass effect along with endocrinologic deficits. Germ cell tumors such as germinoma can present with diabetes insipidus and masses in the suprasellar region. Infectious or inflammatory disorders such as lymphocytic hypophysitis or infundibulitis, sarcoidosis, or histiocytosis X can also mimic certain signs and symptoms of the craniopharyngioma. In virtually every case, however, the differential can be considerably reduced by careful interpretation of the radiographic studies. The classic findings on CT and MRI described above are rarely found in lesions other than craniopharyngioma.

TREATMENT

For decades, the preferred method of treatment for craniopharyngioma has been total extirpation of the tumor. The surgery can be extraordinarily challenging, since these tumors are frequently adherent to all of the structures with which they come in contact, including the optic apparatus, vessels in the circle of Willis, the pituitary gland and stalk, and the hypothalamus (Fig. 157-3). Injury to any of these structures can result in devastating complications such as stroke, blindness, or permanent endocrine dysfunction. These tumors excite an intense inflam-

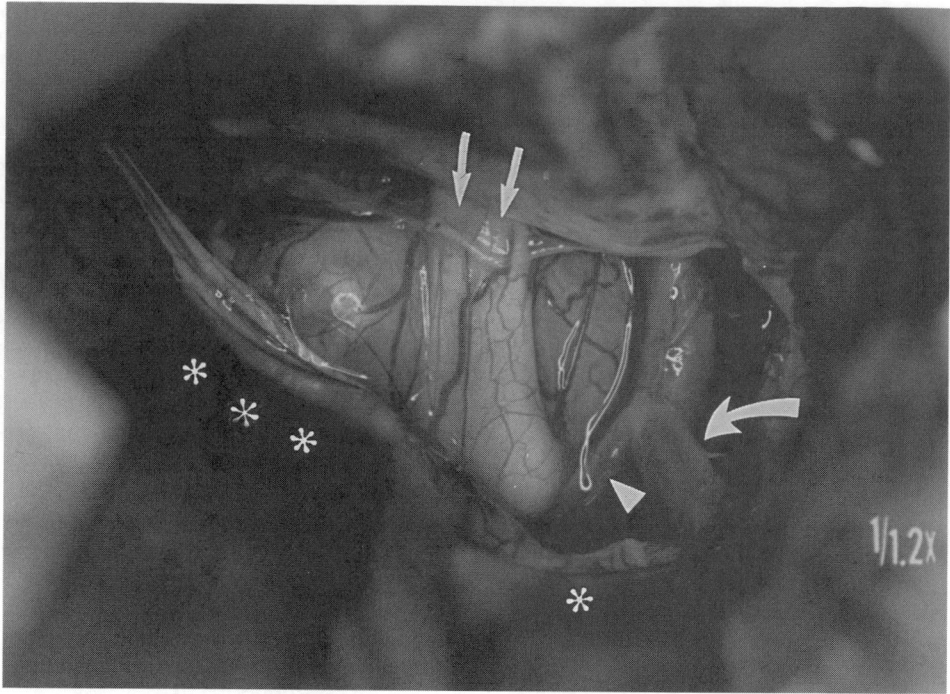

FIG. 157-3. A right subfrontal exposure of an intrasellar and suprasellar craniopharyngioma, as viewed from the surgeon's perspective. The frontal lobe is elevated by two retractors (*asterisks*). The mass is lifting and flattening the right optic nerve (*arrows*) and displacing the right carotid artery laterally. The right anterior cerebral artery (*arrowhead*) and the right middle cerebral artery (*curved arrow*) are also visualized.

matory response around themselves, possible because of their cholesterol-laden cyst contents, and the plane of cleavage between tumor and normal brain, optic nerve, or vessels may be difficult to develop. In most series in which total removal has been accomplished, the patients are virtually always hypopituitary. Nearly all patients require medication for diabetes insipidus, and most require treatment for hypothyroidism as well as steroid, growth, and sex hormone deficiency. If surgical removal has led to hypothalamic injury, the patients will frequently have significant problems controlling appetite and may become obese and apathetic. Learning disabilities are also common sequelae following surgical excision. These tumors often grow to considerable size, and damage to memory and learning centers and to the hypothalamic/pituitary axis may be a significant problem prior to any form of treatment. Surgery is often carried out on an urgent basis because of compression of the optic apparatus and visual compromise. However, surgery may fail to reverse preoperative deficits and may occasionally increase them, since many of these deficits are caused not only by compression of the optic system but also by vascular compromise of those structures—which tends to worsen when dissection along the optic system affects its vascular supply. In the hands of proficient surgeons, total removal, as determined by postoperative CT or MRI scanning, can be anticipated in approximately 50 to 90 percent of primary procedures, but only 65 percent of these patients can be expected to be free of recurrent tumor at 10-year follow-up.

Because of the complications that seem to follow attempts at total removal of craniopharyngioma, some surgeons have resorted to treatment regimens that involve combined surgery and radiotherapy. Radiotherapy for craniopharyngioma is an effective treatment for these lesions, with 10-year survival figures approaching 90 percent for patients so treated, either with

biopsy alone or with more aggressive surgery. However, radiotherapy has its own set of complications, including endocrinologic dysfunction similar to that seen after surgical excision (although usually to a lesser degree), radiation-induced vasculopathy (with the development of moyamoya syndrome leading to strokes or transient ischemic attacks), learning disabilities, and finally, the induction of second neoplasms such as glioblastoma or meningioma. Patients under the age of 3 or 4 seem particularly susceptible to the development of vasculopathy and learning difficulties. In the very young patient whose tumor cannot be totally removed, it is not unreasonable to consider observation alone following surgery, with radiation delayed until the child has reached age 4 or 5, or the tumor begins to regrow. In most series, tumor regrowth will have occurred by 40 months or so after the operation.

Recent advances in radiotherapy such as stereotactic radiotherapy promise to limit exposure of the normal brain to radiation and reduce the deleterious side effects of treatment, but these techniques are just beginning to be employed, and long-term results are as yet unknown. In certain patients in whom residual disease is located in a relatively circumscribed area, stereotactic radiosurgery can be utilized to deliver a single dose of high-energy ionizing radiation to the lesion to destroy it. This form of treatment can injure the optic nerves and tracts and cause other cranial nerve dysfunction, however, and cannot be employed where tumor abuts these structures unless permanent visual deficits are already present. When large nonremovable cysts are present, creating mass effect that recurs promptly despite needle or catheter drainage, radioisotopes such as ^{32}P can be instilled into the cyst to damage or destroy cyst wall epithelium and diminish or stop the production of cyst fluid. These treatment regimens are difficult to utilize because of issues of dosimetry and uniformity of dose delivery, particularly in patients in whom prior irradiation has been carried out or when multiple cysts are present. This treatment modality requires precise cannulation of the cyst and a delivery system that limits distribution of the isotope to the tumor cyst alone. Intracavitary bleomycin may also help in reducing cyst size and facilitating surgical removal of particularly difficult tumor cysts. Bleomycin is a chemotherapeutic agent that has the property of causing craniopharyngioma cysts to shrink, toughen, and thicken. These changes may permit surgical excision of a cyst that otherwise might fragment when its walls were grasped.

SUMMARY

The craniopharyngioma is a suprasellar neoplasm probably of congenital origin. It has a characteristic pathologic and radiographic appearance and a common mode of clinical presentation related to signs of endocrine or visual dysfunction, or else increased intracranial pressure from obstruction of cerebrospinal fluid flow through the third ventricle. The tumor can be treated by surgery and radiotherapy, alone or in combination. Each approach has its advocates, but both have the potential for significant long-term morbidity. Ongoing studies in neuropsychologic outcome and treatment side effects can be expected to shed additional light on this debate over the next several years.

SUGGESTED READINGS

Backlund EO, Axelsson B, Bergstrand CG et al: Treatment of craniopharyngiomas—the stereotactic approach in a ten to twenty-three years' perspective. I. Surgical, radiological and ophthalmological aspects. Acta Neurochir (Wien) 99:11–9, 1989

Epstein FJ, Handler MH (eds): Craniopharyngioma: the answer. Pediatr Neurosurg, suppl. 1.21:1–132, 1994

Fischer EG, Welch K, Shillito J et al: Craniopharyngiomas in children: long-term effects of conservative procedures combined with radiation therapy. J Neurosurg 73:534–40, 1990

Hetelekidis S, Barnes PD, Tao ML et al: Twenty-year experience in childhood craniopharyngioma. Int J Radiat Oncol Biol Phys 27:189–93, 1993

Hoffman HJ, DeSilva M, Humphreys RP: Aggressive surgical management of craniopharyngiomas in children. J Neurosurg 76:47–52, 1992

Pollack IF, Lunsford LD, Slamovits TL et al: Stereotaxic intracavitary irradiation for cystic craniopharyngiomas. J Neurosurg 68:227–33, 1988

Pusey E, Kortman KE, Flannigan BD et al: MR of craniopharyngiomas: tumor delineation and characterization. AJNR 8:439–44, 1987

Rutka JT, Hoffman HJ, Drake JM, Humphreys RP: Suprasellar and sellar tumors in childhood and adolescence. Neurosurg Clin North Am 3:803–20, 1992

Sorva R, Heiskanen D, Perheentupa J: Craniopharyngioma surgery in children: endocrine and visual outcome. Childs Nerv Syst 4:97–9, 1988

158. ACOUSTIC NEUROMA

DAVID M. VERNICK

Named after their most common presenting feature, acoustic neuromas are a benign tumor of the eighth cranial nerve. They are actually a Schwann cell tumor originating at the Schwann cell–glial cell junction of the vestibular portion of the nerve. Attempts to improve the accuracy of the name have resulted in their being called acoustic neurinomas, acoustic schwannomas, and vestibular schwannomas in some papers. They account for 8 percent of all intracranial tumors in adults and 80 percent of

all cerebellopontine angle tumors. Their overall incidence of occurrence clinically is about one tumor per 100,000 population per year. Histologic presence at autopsy examination shows an incidence of 0.8 to 2.7 percent in temporal bone studies. Most of the difference is due to small tumors that must lie relatively dormant for years.

Acoustic neuromas occur with equal frequency on the superior and inferior branches of the vestibular nerve. They are unilateral, except in cases of the genetic disorder neurofibromatosis type 2 (NF2) in which they are bilateral. There is no side predilection, nor is their a sex bias. Common age of presentation is 30 to 40 years, but all ages have been reported.

HISTORY

By the late 1800s, the diagnosis of cerebellopontine angle tumors was made by the presence of hearing loss, facial numbness, and headache. No diagnostic tests were available to confirm the findings. Audiometric, vestibular, and radiologic testing developed during the early 1900s allowed for earlier and more accurate diagnosis. Unilateral sensorineural hearing loss with decreased discrimination and unilateral decreased caloric response became the main diagnostic findings in patients with acoustic neuromas. Radiology could show widening of the internal auditory canal. Surgery was the best treatment at the time, with radiotherapy being in its infancy, but mortality and morbidity rates ran high.

Today the auditory and radiographic techniques have improved dramatically to allow for diagnosis of smaller tumors. Treatment options have been refined to reduce the morbidity and mortality rates of therapy markedly. Preservation of facial nerve function and, in small tumors, hearing are now expected results. Despite all of the advances, however, the average size of tumors detected has decreased minimally. The average time of onset of symptoms until the diagnosis of the tumor is 4 years. Although benign by histology, acoustic neuromas still present a diagnostic and therapeutic challenge to the physician.

PRESENTATION

The most common presenting feature of acoustic neuromas is unilateral hearing loss (Table 158-1). This is usually a progressive sensorineural loss, but in 10 percent of cases there is a sudden shift in the hearing. (Only 1 to 3 percent of all patients with sudden hearing loss have acoustic neuromas, however.) The loss is usually a high frequency loss but can be almost any configuration and may recover. In addition to the hearing loss, speech discrimination, the ability to understand words, is usually markedly reduced even when the hearing loss is mild. Only 1 to 3 percent of all patients with diagnosed tumors have normal hearing. This number probably will increase with the increased

TABLE 158-1. Presenting Symptoms of Acoustic Neuromas

Early	Hearing loss that is unilateral and may be sudden
	Tinnitus—unilateral
	Disequilibrium
Late	Hypesthesia or paresthesia of face
	Facial spasm or weakness
	Dysarthria
	Dysphagia
	Aspiration
	Hoarseness
	Headache
	Ataxia

sensitivity of magnetic resonance imaging (MRI) scanning in picking up small tumors.

Unilateral tinnitus can be an early presenting feature of acoustic neuromas. It is subjective (only heard by the patient) and can be almost any type of sound. Usually it is constant, not pulsatile. Workup may show an asymmetric hearing loss that accompanies the noise, but audiometry can be normal.

Disequilibrium is frequently present in patients with acoustic neuromas but is not a common presenting feature. Because the tumors are slow growing, the body has a chance to compensate for the gradual loss of one peripheral vestibular system. Patients usually have imbalance on questioning, but it is mild to moderate in nature. Acute vertigo is uncommon but can occur from a sudden change in the size of the tumor such as from hemorrhage into the tumor. Large tumors may press on the cerebellum or brainstem and give the patient ataxia late in the course.

Other presenting signs are uncommon unless the tumor is large. These result from pressure on adjacent cranial nerves. Hypesthesia or paresthesia of the face can occur with trigeminal nerve involvement. The earliest sign of this is decrease in the corneal reflex. Facial nerve palsy can occur, but more often facial nerve involvement presents with facial twitching. The functions of lower cranial nerves (nerves IX, X, and XI), such as speech and swallowing, can be impaired as well, leading to dysarthria, dysphagia, aspiration, and hoarseness. Long tract signs have been seen late in very large tumors. The brainstem can be compressed, or the cerebellar tonsils can herniate through the foramen magnum. Hydrocephalus and death can occur in untreated cases.

Asymptomatic cases account for less than 1 percent of present tumors found. Increased use of MRI scanning may increase this number substantially.

PHYSICAL EXAMINATION

After a thorough history has been taken, physical examination, not MRI scanning, should next be carried out. Otologic examination will show a normal-appearing ear. Gross auditory testing should confirm the presence of an asymmetric hearing loss. Tuning fork testing will confirm this. The Rinne test will show air conduction greater than bone conduction bilaterally. Weber testing will lateralize to the side of the better hearing ear.

Neurologic testing may show some cranial nerve deficits such as an absent corneal reflex or hypesthesia of the face. Facial twitching may be present. Other cranial nerve deficits are uncommon unless the tumor is large. Balance is usually grossly intact in the office.

LABORATORY TESTING

Audiometry has been and still is the best initial screening test for the diagnosis of acoustic neuromas. (Only 5 percent of acoustic neuromas will have a normal auditory evaluation.) Pure tone and speech audiometry should be performed. Test results will show an asymmetric sensorineural hearing loss, usually more prominent in the higher frequencies (Fig. 158-1). Typically the speech discrimination score is markedly reduced in the affected ear, being much lower than expected given the degree of hearing loss present.

Many other auditory tests have been used historically to try

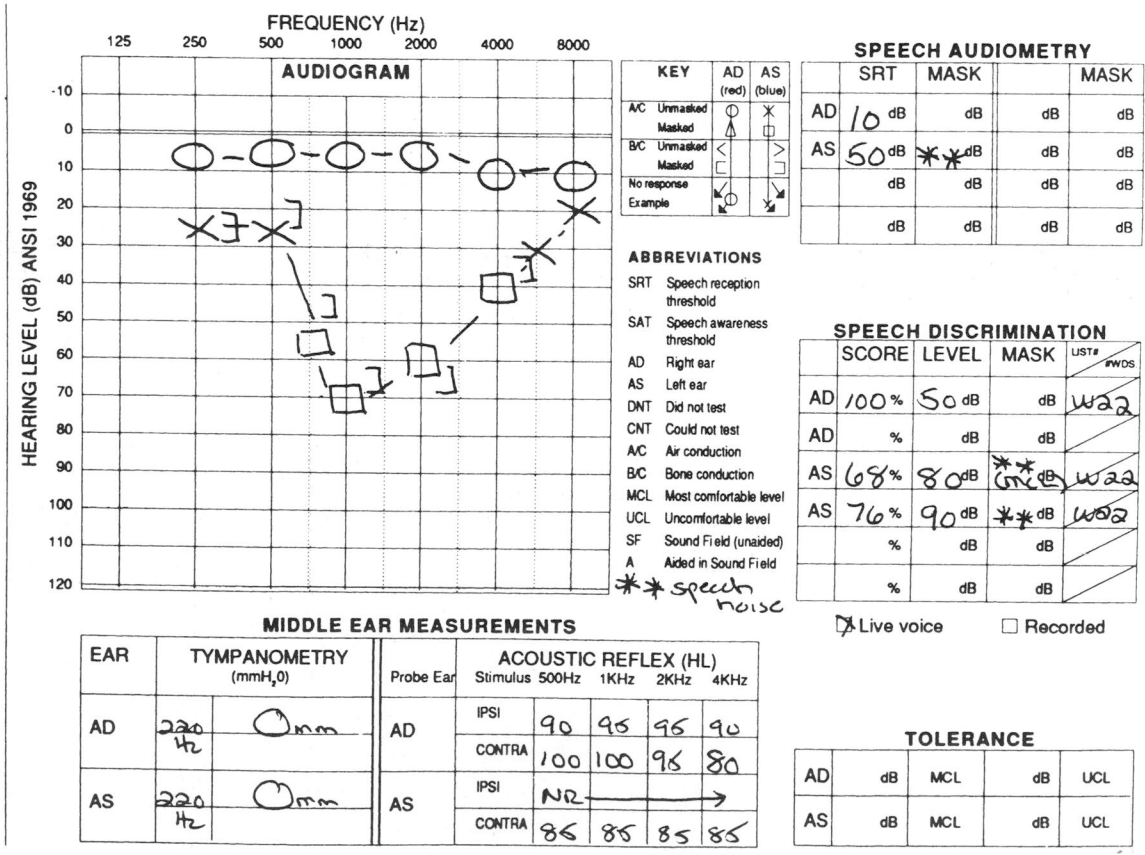

FIG. 158-1. Audiogram of patient with a left acoustic neuroma.

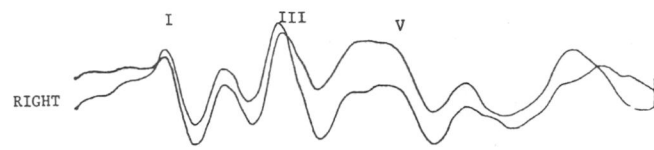

STIMULUS/ MASKING (dBnHL)	I	III	V	I-III	I-V
RIGHT	1.52	3.56	5.44	2.04	3.92
LEFT	1.60	3.80	5.72	2.20	4.12

LATENCIES (MSEC)

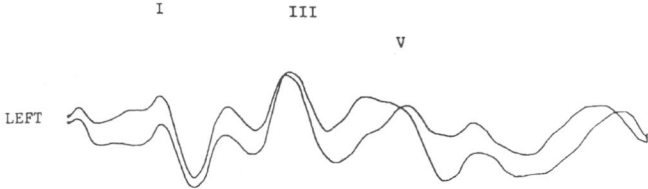

FIG. 158-2. Brainstem-evoked response audiometry of patient with a left acoustic neuroma.

to diagnose acoustic neuromas. These include acoustic reflex testing, impedance audiometry, and Bekesy audiometry. They all had limited accuracy and diagnostic value. Their utility has diminished with the advent of brainstem-evoked response audiometry.

Brainstem-evoked response audiometry should be done in anyone with an unexplained asymmetry in audiometric testing either in pure tone or in discrimination. This test will show abnormalities in 90 to 95 percent of patients with tumors. Although not all postive tests reflect the presence of a tumor, the test is a great screening device as it is quick, painless, inexpensive, and accurate. Test results will show a delay in nerve conduction time on the affected side, reflecting the probable presence of a tumor (Fig. 158-2).

Vestibular testing has lost its usefulness as a screening test for diagnosis of acoustic neuromas because of the accuracy of evoked response audiometry. When testing is performed, a decreased or absent caloric response on the affected side may be seen. This information is useful in predicting how dizzy a patient may be postoperatively if surgery is performed.

Radiologic testing has advanced through the years from plain films, polytomograms, posterior fossa myelography, and computed tomography (CT) with contrast agents to MRI. Improved accuracy and patient safety have accompanied the advances. When brainstem testing is abnormal or cannot be done because of the severity of the hearing loss or when suspicion is high, MRI scanning with gadolinium contrast should be performed. It will allow for the diagnosis of tumors larger than 1 to 2 mm in diameter (Fig. 158-3). If a patient cannot tolerate the MRI scan, CT scanning with contrast is almost as accurate.

Acoustic neuromas show up on CT and MRI scans as enhancing lesions. CT scans can show widening of the internal auditory canal. A soft-tissue mass can be seen in the widened canal, extending into the posterior fossa. This mass enhances with iodinated contrast material.

MRI scans show a soft tissue mass on T1-weighted images, which is brighter than cerebrospinal fluid. With gadolinium contrast, the tumors show up as bright masses. Rare false-posi-

tive scans have been reported in small lesions located laterally in the internal auditory canal. These are probably inflammatory lesions that resolve with time.

A cost-effctive approach to the workup of patients suspected of having an acoustic neuroma was proposed by Welling and Glasscock (Table 158-2 and Fig. 158-4). This approach uses MRI scanning for high-probability situations and brainstem-evoked audiometry testing for screening lower probability situations.

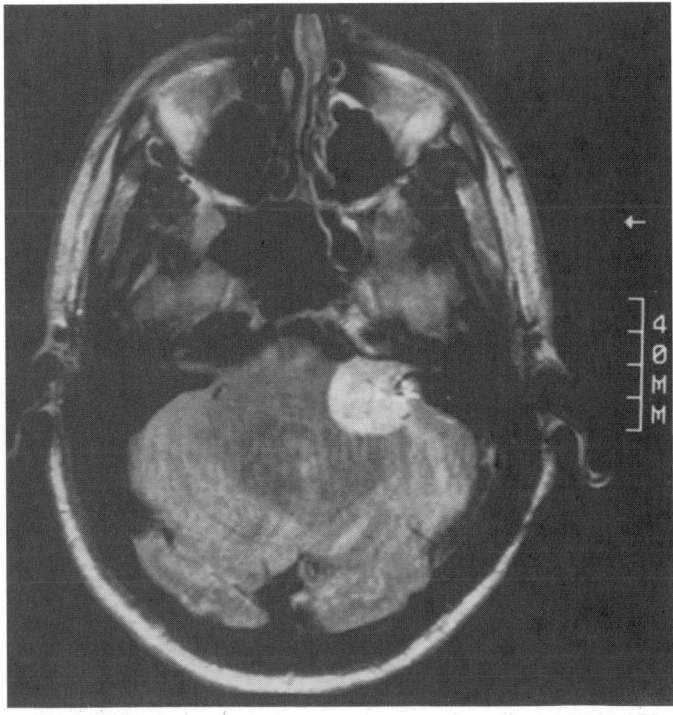

FIG. 158-3. Gadolinium-enhanced magnetic resonance image of acoustic neuroma.

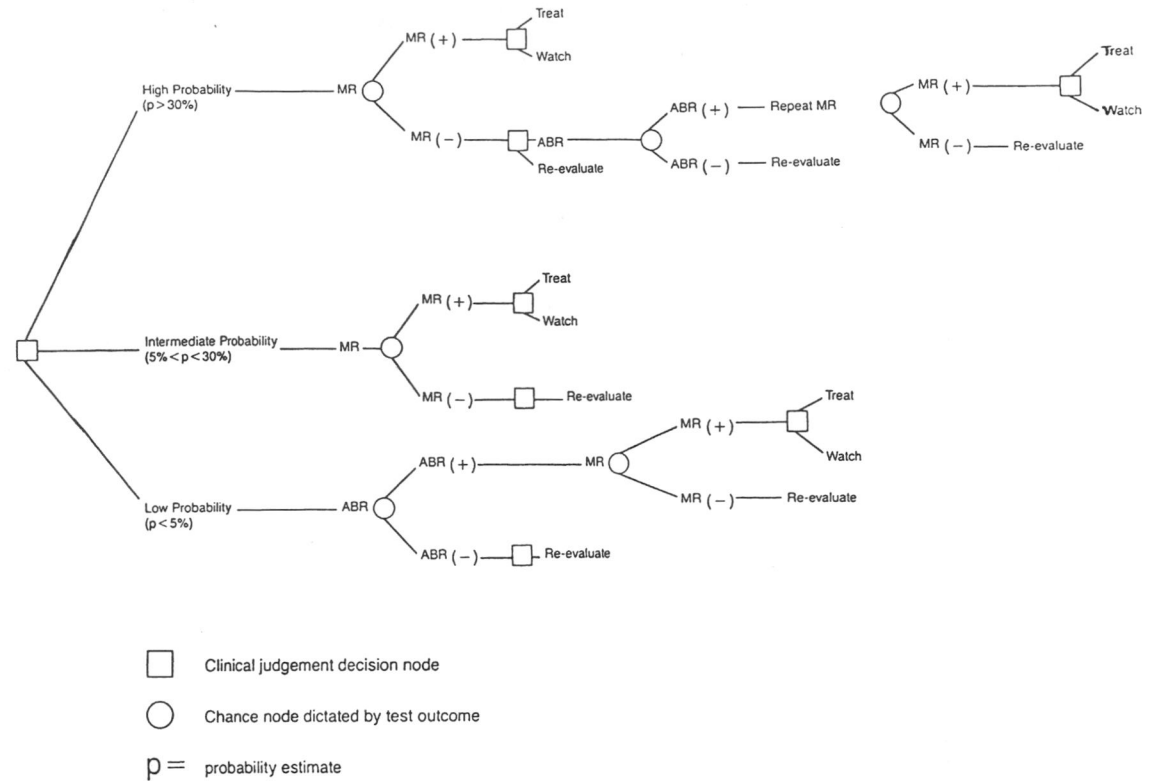

FIG. 158-4. Cost-effective workup of patient with possible acoustic neuroma. (From Welling BD, Glassock ME III et al: Otolaryngology—Head and Neck Surgery. Mosby-Year Book, St. Louis, 1990, with permission.)

DIFFERENTIAL DIAGNOSES

Although most of the tumors of the cerebellopontine angle are acoustic neuromas, other tumors do occur. Tumors presenting in the cerebellopontine angle include the following:

Acoustic neuroma
Meningioma
Glioma
Cholesteatoma
Hemangioma
Aneurysm
Arachnoid cyst
Lipoma
Metastatic tumor

Meningiomas are present 5 to 10 percent of the time. Cholesteatomas, gliomas, hemangiomas, aneurysms, arachnoid cysts,

TABLE 158-2. Probability That an Acoustic Neuroma Is Present in Relation to Symptoms

Symptoms	Probability	Category
"Classic" unilateral asymmetric sensorineural hearing loss, tinnitus, decreased discrimination	$P > 30\%$	High
Sudden sensorineural hearing loss	$5\% < P < 30\%$	Intermediate
Otherwise unexplained persistent unilateral tinnitus		
Isolated vertigo	$P < 5\%$	Low
Historically explained unilateral hearing loss, tinnitus		
Symmetric hearing loss		

(From Welling BD, Glassock ME III et al: Otolaryngology—Head and Neck Surgery. Mosby-Year Book, St. Louis, 1990, with permission.)

lipomas, and metastatic tumors are far less common but can present with symptoms similar to those of an acoustic neuroma. Imaging studies can help in the preoperative differential diagnosis.

TUMOR GROWTH

Acoustic neuromas are slow-growing, with an average growth rate of 2 mm/yr. Rates as high as 10 mm/yr have been seen in a few cases. Up to 40 percent of cases show no growth or even shrinkage on serial scans. There is no correlation between growth rate and tumor size at presentation. Growth rate tends to be constant over time, but sudden changes in tumor size can occur if there is hemorrhage into the tumor.

NEUROFIBROMATOSIS

Two major types of neurofibromatosis—NF1 and NF2—are recognized today. A thorough discussion of these disorders is presented in Chapter 159. The hallmark of NF2 is bilateral acoustic neuromas. In NF2, most patients present with the same symptoms as with other acoustic neuromas, i.e., with progressive hearing loss, tinnitus, or disequilibrium. Treatment options are basically the same as with unilateral acoustic neuromas but must be tempered because of the bilateral nature of the losses and the potential deafness that can result. Hearing preservation with surgery is possible but not as common as with the unilateral cases.

CHILDREN

Less than 20 cases of acoustic neuromas in children younger than 15 years of age have been reported. The ages range from

1 to 14, with a mean age of 9 years. Presenting symptoms many times included loss of other cranial nerve function in addition to hearing loss. This is likely due to the larger size of the tumors at the time of diagnosis. This larger size probably reflects lack of consideration of the diagnosis rather than any true biologic difference in the tumor's behavior. Treatment options are the same as for adults.

TREATMENT

Once the diagnosis of an acoustic neuroma has been made, treatment options need to be discussed. Three major paths of therapy are present—observation, surgery, and radiation therapy. Chemotherapy has not yet made an impact on treatment.

Since acoustic neuromas are slow-growing tumors and since up to 40 percent of them either do not grow or shrink in size, immediate active interventional therapy is not necessary in most cases. In patients who are older than 65 or who have other significant medical problems, follow-up MRI scans in 6- to 12-month intervals will allow for determination of the growth rate of the tumor and prognostic planning prior to intervention. One contraindication to this wait-and-see approach is in those patients with large tumors in whom brainstem compression or hydrocephalus may occur. A second contraindication is in those patients with good hearing. Delay in therapy may compromise the chances of hearing preservation.

Radiation therapy is a treatment option for patients. The mode of radiotherapy optimal for acoustic neuroma therapy is still under investigation. Current options include external γ therapy (γ knife), proton beam therapy, and stereotactic radiosurgery with cobalt-60, either in a single or a fractionated regimen. Cessation of tumor growth or tumor shrinkage can occur in up to 80 percent of cases in some series. Long-term complications do occur with therapy and include hearing loss and facial nerve injury as well as some major incranial problems. Surgery in patients who do not respond to radiation may be more difficult.

Surgery remains the main modality of therapy today for treatment of acoustic neuromas. The 1991 National Institutes of Health Consensus Development Conference reviewed all options of therapy and reached this conclusion. The approach can be via the translabyrinthine, suboccipital, or middle fossa routes, depending on the size of the tumor and whether hearing preservation is being attempted. In many institutions, this is done by a team consisting of a neurosurgeon and an otologist. Postoperative mortality and morbidity rates have been markedly reduced as microsurgical techniques have evolved and intraoperative monitoring has advanced. Facial nerve monitoring during the surgery has markedly reduced the incidence of postoperative facial nerve injuries. Hearing preservation can now be achieved in 40 to 50 percent of cases when the tumor is less than 1.5 cm, the preoperative hearing is better than 50 dB, and the discrimination is better than 50 percent. Hospital stays have also decreased secondary to better techniques.

Other complications such as a cerebrospinal fluid leak occur in 5 to 10 percent of individuals from the suboccipital approach and less than 5 percent from the translabyrinthine approach. Most of these close spontaneously with or without a lumbar drain after several days. Postoperative vertigo is more of an issue with smaller than with larger tumors. Since tumor removal requires sacrifice of the vestibular nerves, any function that remains is acutely lost. Small tumors have not destroyed most of the vestibular function and thus leave the patient vertiginous

for several days afterward. Mild imbalance usually resolved in 3 to 6 months. Injuries of other cranial nerves (V, VI, IX, X, and XI) can occur during tumor dissection. Brainstem-stroke and even death can occur from injury to the vertebrobasilar circulation. Fortunately the incidence of these complications has drastically decreased as surgical techniques have improved.

SUMMARY

Although benign in nature, acoustic neuromas have challenged physicians throughout history. Advancements in the diagnostic and therapeutic fields of audiology, medicine, radiology, radiation therapy, and surgery have greatly improved our ability to detect and treat these tumors. Morbidity and mortality rates have been substantially reduced. Room is still present, however, for even greater success in the years to come.

SUGGESTED READINGS

Chen TC, Maceri DR, Giannotta SL et al: Unilateral acoustic neuromas in childhood without evidence of neurofibromatosis: case report and review of the literature. Am J Otol 13:318–22, 1992

Curtin HD, Hirsch WL, Jr: Imaging of acoustic neuromas. Otolaryngol Clin North Am 25:553–607, 1992

Khanosary A, Rand RQ, Wilson GH: Stereotactic radiosurgery of acoustic neuromas. pp. 559–69. In Samii M (ed): Surgery in and around the Brain Stem and Third Ventricle. Springer, Berlin, 1986

Leksell D: Stereotactic radiosurgery. Neurol Res 9:59–68, 1987

Mirko T, Thomsen J: Management of acoustic neuromas. Acta Otolaryngol (Stockh) 111:616–32

Nedzelski JM, Schessel DA, Pfleiderer A et al: Conservative management of acoustic neuromas. Otolaryngol Clin North Am 25:691–705, 1992

NIH Consensus Development Conference, Acoustic Neuroma, Dec 11–13, 1991, No. 4, Vol. 9, pp. 1–24.

Roland PS, Glasscock ME, Bojrab DI et al: Normal hearing in patients with acoustic neuromas. South Med J 80:166–9, 1987

Roos KL: The neurofibromatoses. Ear Nose Throat J 71:512–9, 1992

Selesnick SH, Jackler RK: Clinical manifestations and audiologic diagnosis of acoustic neuromas, Otolaryngol Clin North Am 25:521–51, 1992

Welling DB, Glasscock ME, Woods CI et al: Acoustic neuroma: a cost-effective approach. Otolaryngol Head Neck Surg 103:364–70, 1990

159. THE NEUROFIBROMATOSES

BRUCE R. KORF

The neurofibromatoses are a set of at least two distinct disorders that have in common a predisposition to formation of tumors of the nervous system, both central and peripheral. These genetically determined disorders have been the subject of intense research in recent years, culminating in the discovery of the genes responsible for neurofibromatosis types 1 (NF1) and 2 (NF2). Although neither disorder can be cured, both are important to recognize clinically because of the potential for treatment of complications and the need to provide genetic counseling.

CLASSIFICATION OF THE NEUROFIBROMATOSES

There are two well-recognized forms of neurofibromatosis, referred to as NF1 and NF2. These are contrasted in Table 159-

TABLE 159-1. Comparison of Neurofibromatosis Types 1 and 2

	Neurofibromatosis Type 1	Neurofibromatosis Type 2
Frequency	1:4,000	1:40,000
Mode of inheritance	Autosomal dominant	Autosomal dominant
Features	Café-au-lait spots, neurofibromas, optic gliomas, learning disabilities, malignant schwannomas, etc.	Bilateral vestibular schwannomas, schwannomas, meningiomas, ependymomas, etc.
Chromosome locus	Chromosome 17	Chromosome 22
Gene product	Neurofibromin	Merlin (schwannomin)
Function	GTPase activating protein	Cytoskeletal protein

Abbreviation: GTPase, guanosine triphosphatase.

1. NF1 is the most common form, about 10-fold more frequent than NF2. The two disorders were not distinguished in earlier literature, but recent genetic studies have confirmed that they are entirely distinct entities. Correct diagnosis is important for clinical care. Individuals with NF1, for example, are not at increased risk for vestibular schwannomas, whereas this tumor is usually present in those with NF2. Conversely, complications such as learning disabilities and optic glioma are found in those with NF1, but not NF2.

There are rare individuals whose disease does not fit well into the classification scheme of NF1 or NF2. It is possible that there are variant forms of either disorder. Alternatively, there may be other types of neurofibromatosis besides NF1 and NF2, perhaps caused by mutations at other genes yet to be discovered. The disorders in these patients may be better understood as the genetic basis of the neurofibromatoses becomes more thoroughly explored.

NEUROFIBROMATOSIS TYPE 1

NF1 is the most common form of neurofibromatosis, occurring in about 1:4,000 individuals. NF1 affects individuals of all racial and ethnic groups worldwide. It is often referred to as von Recklinghausen neurofibromatosis, after the German pathologist who first noted that the characteristic tumors are derived from peripheral nerves. Although NF1 is sometimes referred to as "Elephant Man's disease," it has recently been determined that Joseph Merrick, who was known as the Elephant Man, actually had a different disorder called Proteus syndrome, which is associated with bony and cutaneous overgrowths, epidermal nevi, and café-au-lait spots. Individuals with NF1 should understand that the physical deformities of the Elephant Man do not occur in neurofibromatosis.

Diagnosis

The diagnosis of NF1 is based on clinical criteria; there is currently no laboratory test available. Diagnostic criteria are as follows:

1. Six or more café-au-lait spots larger than 5 mm prepubertal or 15 mm postpubertal
2. Freckles in skinfolds such as axillae or groins
3. Two or more neurofibromas or one plexiform neurofibroma
4. Two or more iris Lisch nodules
5. Optic glioma

6. Characteristic skeletal deformity such as tibial dysplasia or sphenoid dysplasia
7. First-degree relative with NF1 by above criteria

A person who satisfies any two of these criteria is generally agreed to have NF1. Many of the features, however, are age dependent, making diagnosis in young children a challenge.

Café-au-lait macules (Fig. 159-1) most commonly bring the disorder to attention. These are flat, brown spots that generally begin to appear in the early weeks of life and may continue to get darker and increase in number for the first several years. The diagnostic criteria for NF1 require six or more café-au-lait spots larger than 5 mm before puberty or 15 mm after puberty. Virtually all persons with NF1 fulfill this criterion, but there is no correlation between the number of café-au-lait spots and the severity of NF1 or between the location of spots and the location of complications of the disorder. Individuals in the general population may have one or two, or even up to six café-au-lait spots, and not have NF1. There is a rare hereditary trait of multiple café-au-lait spots without other signs of NF1 that is not linked to the NF1 gene.

Another cutaneous diagnostic sign is the occurrence of freckling in intertriginous areas, such as axillae and groins. This usually begins at around 3 to 5 years of age and, when it occurs, is highly specific to NF1. It is often the next sign of NF1 to

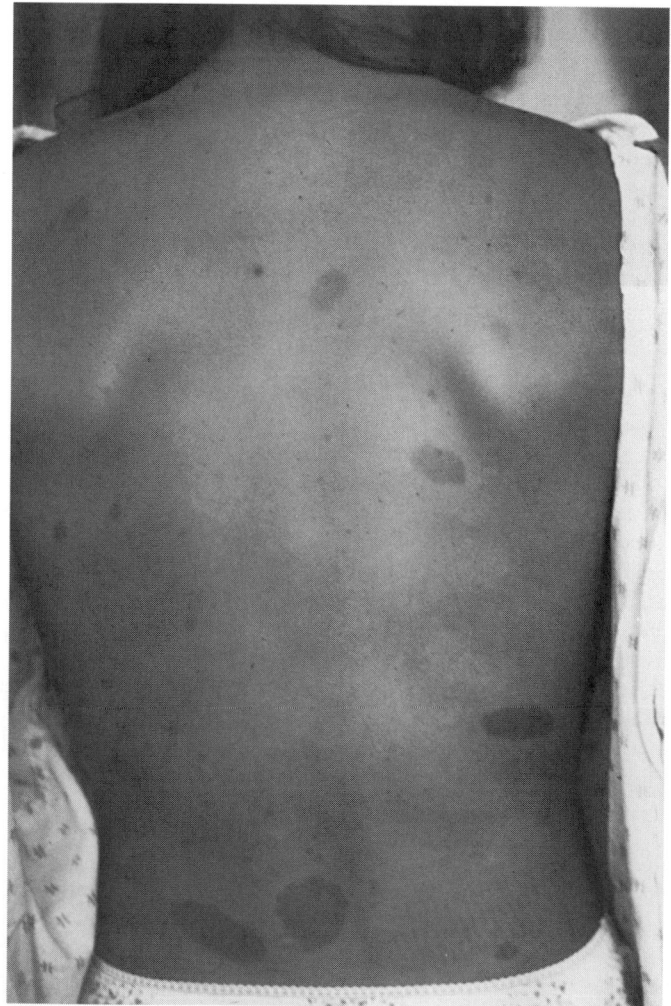

FIG. 159-1. Multiple café-au-lait spots in child with neurofibromatosis type 1.

be found in young children who first present with multiple café-au-lait spots. Freckling tends to increase with age and may occur throughout the body, lending an appearance of diffuse hyperpigmentation.

The neurofibroma is the lesion that gives the disorder its name. Neurofibromas most commonly appear on the skin as small papules, usually having a purplish hue. They may occur at any age but are most commonly seen in late childhood or puberty. Many women note an increase in the size and number of neurofibromas during pregnancy. Neurofibromas can occur any place in the body where there is a nerve. Usually they cause no symptoms other than cosmetic, although rarely symptoms of nerve compression may occur (see below).

Three diagnostic criteria involve the eye. Lisch nodules are tan melanocytic hamartomas of the iris. It is necessary to use the slit lamp to identify Lisch nodules and distinguish them from iris macules, which are not associated with neurofibromatosis. Lisch nodules are specific to NF1 and occur on at least 95 percent of individuals with NF1 past 6 years of age. As such, they are useful diagnostic markers but do not interfere with vision. Lisch nodules are not a feature of NF2.

Optic glioma, identified as thickening of the optic nerve, occurs in about 15 percent of children with NF1. Only rarely do optic pathway tumors become progressive and symptomatic. Anyone found to have an optic glioma should be examined for other signs of NF1, although at least 50 percent of optic gliomas occur in those without neurofibromatosis.

Orbital plexiform neurofibroma is a rare complication of NF1, involving neurofibroma growth in the orbit and upper eyelid. There is usually an associated dysplasia of the sphenoid bone. Orbital plexiform neurofibroma is clinically apparent in the early years of life. It is a congenital lesion that grows during the preschool years. It is clinically recognized as overgrowth of the upper eyelid, downward and outward or inward displacement of the eye, and transmission of venous pulsations to the globe. There may be glaucoma of the affected eye, but neurologic complications are rare.

Aside from sphenoid dysplasia, one other bone lesion is characteristic of NF1 and represents a diagnostic criterion. This is dysplasia of a long bone, most commonly the tibia. It is a congenital lesion, recognized by anterolateral bowing of the lower leg. There is substantial risk of fracture of the tibia, leading to pseudoarthrosis.

The final diagnostic criterion is based on family history. Since NF1 is inherited as a dominant trait, the existence of an affected first-degree relative satisfies one diagnostic criterion for NF1. About 50 percent of cases of NF1 are sporadic, however, owing to a new mutation.

A diagnostic evaluation for NF1 consists of physical examination, with careful attention to skin lesions, and an ophthalmologic examination with the slit lamp to look for Lisch nodules. A family history should be obtained, and, if possible, both parents should be examined for signs of neurofibromatosis.

Natural History and Management

Important complications of NF1 are listed in Table 159-2. The overall frequency of severe complications has been overstated in much of the medical literature, since severe complications are more likely to bring a person to medical attention or be published. Studies that have attempted to avoid this bias, including one population-based study, have shown that approximately two-thirds of individuals with NF1 have relatively mild in-

TABLE 159-2. Major Types of Complications of Neurofibromatosis Type 1

Cutaneous	Cosmetic impairment, itching
Neurologic	Nerve compression, spinal cord compression, headache, seizure, learning disability, developmental delay, brain tumor, aqueductal stenosis
Ophthalmologic	Orbital dysplasia, glaucoma, optic glioma
Orthopaedic	Long bone dysplasia, pseudoarthrosis, mandibular dysplasia or cysts, scoliosis, sphenoid wing dysplasia
Vascular	Hypertension caused by renal artery stenosis or pheochromocytoma
Growth	Macrocephaly, short stature
Gastrointestinal	Constipation, intestinal obstruction (caused by neurofibroma)

volvement, often never requiring medical attention. Life expectancy is only slightly reduced, mostly owing to malignancy.

Much of the medical burden associated with NF1 is due to the neurofibroma. There are three major types of neurofibromas. Cutaneous neurofibromas involve nerve endings in the skin. These usually first appear in late childhood or adolescence and can continue to appear throughout life. They are painless, although some people complain of itching. The number an individual will get is unpredictable. Cutaneous neurofibromas sometimes pose a cosmetic problem or may cause discomfort by rubbing against clothing. They can be removed with plastic surgery and probably do not grow back, although new ones can appear at any time.

Nodular neurofibromas represent neurofibromas that are attached to major nerves. Often they can be palpated as firm masses below the surface of the skin. These tumors may grow to large size but usually are asymptomatic unless they occur near a bone and cause nerve compression. It is difficult to remove nodular neurofibromas surgically because nerve fibers run through the entire mass, which is different from schwannomas in which the nerve is displaced by the tumor. Nodular neurofibromas involving nerve roots (Fig. 159-2) can grow across the neural foramen as dumbbell tumors and may cause nerve root compression or compression of the spinal cord. Unexplained pain in a patient with NF1 should prompt investigation for a nerve root tumor causing referred pain. Tumors of spinal nerve roots are treated surgically.

Plexiform neurofibromas are congenital lesions that involve diffuse enlargement of a major nerve and its branches. In infancy, only a subtle soft tissue asymmetry may be noticed, but often these neurofibromas grow rapidly during early childhood. It is rare for a plexiform neurofibroma to appear first in adulthood. Sometimes there is hyperpigmentation of the overlying skin, and early in life this may be the only clue that a plexiform neurofibroma is present deeper inside the body. Plexiform neurofibromas can lead to limb overgrowth (Fig. 159-3), facial deformity, or obstruction of internal organs. The only available treatment is surgical, but it is virtually impossible to remove a plexiform neurofibroma completely, so regrowth is common. Neither chemotherapy nor radiation therapy is effective in treating plexiform neurofibromas, unless malignant transformation has occurred.

Malignant tumors are relatively rare in persons with NF1, occurring in about 5 percent or fewer. Malignant schwannoma (neurofibrosarcoma) usually occurs in a pre-existing plexiform neurofibroma and presents with sudden growth of a portion of the lesion and/or unexplained pain. It is important to realize that growth and pain are common in plexiform tumors and usually do not indicate malignancy. Treatment involves surgery and/or radiation for local control and chemotherapy.

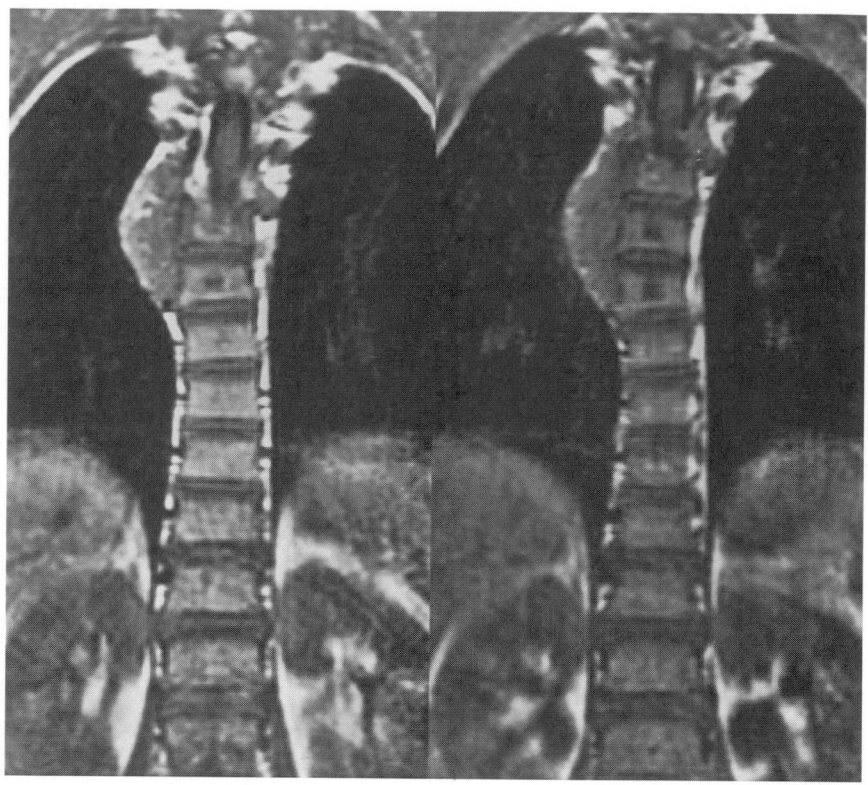

FIG. 159-2. MRI study of paravertebral neurofibroma involving several nerve roots in thoracic spine.

Brain tumors associated with NF1 include gliomas and optic gliomas. Optic gliomas are common in children with NF1, but only a small number, perhaps 1 percent, progress. Progression usually occurs in children aged 4 to 6 years. Gliomas of the orbital portion of the optic nerve lead to loss of vision, pain, proptosis, impaired ocular movement, and optic disc swelling. Chiasmatic gliomas (Fig. 159-4) cause visual field deficits, optic atrophy, and hypothalamic disturbance, particularly precocious puberty. Because of the indolent nature of the lesions, treatment should only be instituted after clear demonstration of progression. Biopsy is usually unnecessary, and surgery is indicated only for unilateral orbital tumors that have already caused complete blindness. The standard treatment is radiation therapy, although recently, encouraging results have been obtained in young children under 6 years of age treated with chemotherapy.

Gliomas can also occur anywhere in the brain at any age. They should be distinguished from areas of enhanced T2-weighted signal seen by magnetic resonance imaging (MRI) in children with NF1 (Fig. 159-5). These signals are commonly seen in the basal ganglia, internal capsule, brainstem, and cerebellum and are not malignant or premalignant lesions. They tend to disappear with age and may represent areas of abnormal myelination or, possibly, gliosis. There is evidence that these ''UBOs'' may occur more commonly in children with NF1 who have learning disabilities.

Learning disabilities are common in individuals with NF1, occurring in at least one-half. There does not appear to be a cognitive profile that is specific to the disorder, and management is the same as for learning disabilities seen in the general population. Only a small proportion have mental retardation. Some children with NF1 have attention deficit disorder, with or without hyperactivity, and respond to treatment similarly to those with similar problems in the general population. Other developmental problems, including hypotonia and motor developmental delay, may occur in association with NF1. Mental retardation occurs relatively rarely, affecting 5 percent or fewer.

Headaches occur commonly in individuals with NF1, particularly in young children. These are often accompanied by abdominal discomfort and probably represent migraine headaches. Treatment with migraine prophylaxis, such as with β-blocking medications, is often effective. Seizures, in contrast, are not common in NF1. It is rare for these to indicate the presence of a structural lesion, even in the case of partial seizures.

It is common to find macrocephaly in those with NF1. Often this is absolute macrocephaly, but sometimes head size is normal, though large in relation to body size. Macrocephaly in NF1 is usually benign, not associated with cognitive or neurologic problems. Rarely, hydrocephalus may occur due to aqueductal stenosis. This presents with typical signs of increased intracranial pressure. Many with NF1 have short stature relative to other nonaffected members of their families. No specific neuroendocrine dysfunction is found in most of these individuals.

Routine clinical management for individuals with NF1 should include a regular schedule for medical evaluation. This is usually offered once a year or more often if there are active problems. Medical tests, including imaging studies, are best reserved for specific clinical indications. There is no evidence that baseline imaging in the absence of signs or symptoms of neurologic disease is useful in clinical management.

Genetic Counseling

NF1 is transmitted as an autosomal dominant trait. An affected individual therefore has a 50 percent chance of passing the

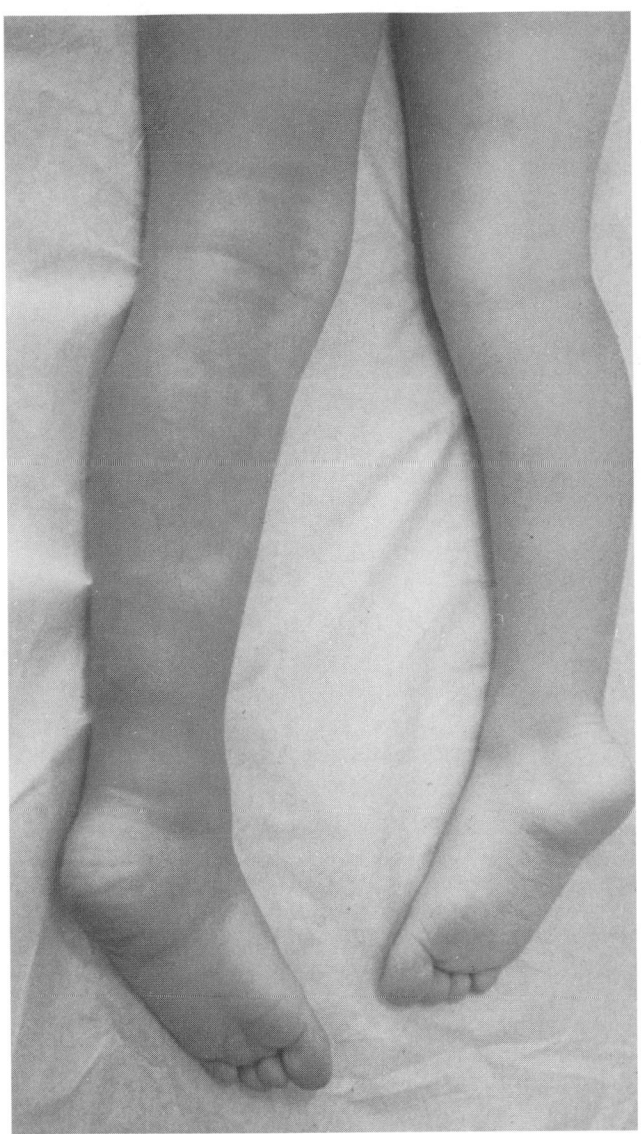

FIG. 159-3. Overgrowth of lower limb caused by plexiform neurofibroma. There is pigmentation along the course of the sciatic nerve.

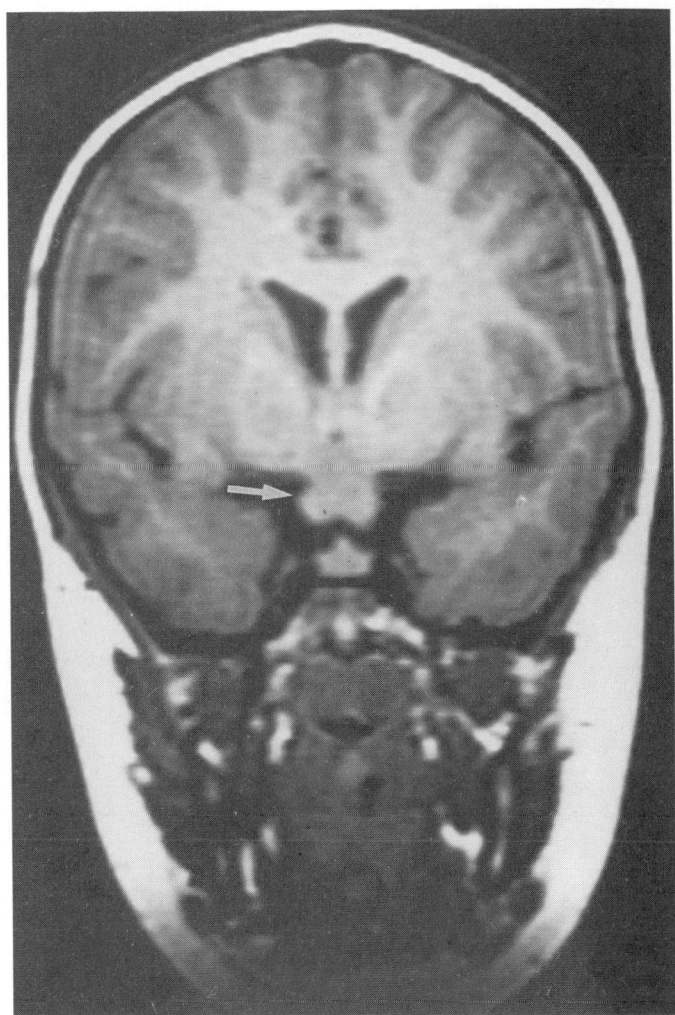

FIG. 159-4. Coronal MRI showing optic glioma of chiasm (*arrow*).

disorder on to any child. The expression of the disorder tends to vary from person to person in a family; so severity in the next generation cannot be predicted. About 50 percent of cases occur in the absence of a family history owing to a new mutation. The mutation rate of the NF1 gene is about 1:10,000, the highest rate known for any gene. No specific cause has been identified to explain these mutations.

The NF1 gene is located on chromosome 17 and encodes a protein known as neurofibromin. This appears to function as a regulator of the ras protein, which is involved in the control of cell division and differentiation. The mutations responsible for NF1 appear to be diverse, making mutation analysis difficult and, so far, unsuitable as a diagnostic test. Polymorphic genetic markers can be used to track the NF1 gene through a family if two or more generations are affected, enabling prenatal or presymptomatic diagnosis in such cases. Unfortunately, no means of genetic testing is available to diagnose NF1 in sporadic cases or to provide prenatal testing for sporadically affected individuals.

NEUROFIBROMATOSIS TYPE 2

NF2 is about 10-fold less frequent than NF1, occurring in about 1:40,000 individuals. It can be more difficult to diagnose at an early age but is more commonly associated with severe, often life-threatening, problems.

Diagnosis

Diagnostic criteria for NF2 are listed in Table 159-3. The defining lesion of NF2 is the presence of bilateral vestibular schwannomas. Rarely these may present in childhood, but more commonly they become symptomatic after the second decade. The tumors tend to arise from the vestibular branch of the eighth nerve and often present with vertigo or balance problems. Tinnitus and hearing loss occur with growth of the tumors. They are best detected and followed with MRI (Fig. 159-6), although audiograms and auditory brainstem-evoked responses can also reveal their presence. NF2 should be considered in any individual with a vestibular schwannoma, particularly in those whose tumors present before the third decade. It should be remembered, though, that sporadic unilateral vestibular schwannomas are much more common than NF2. Schwannomas of other cranial nerves, spinal nerve roots, and other peripheral nerves can also occur in individuals with NF2.

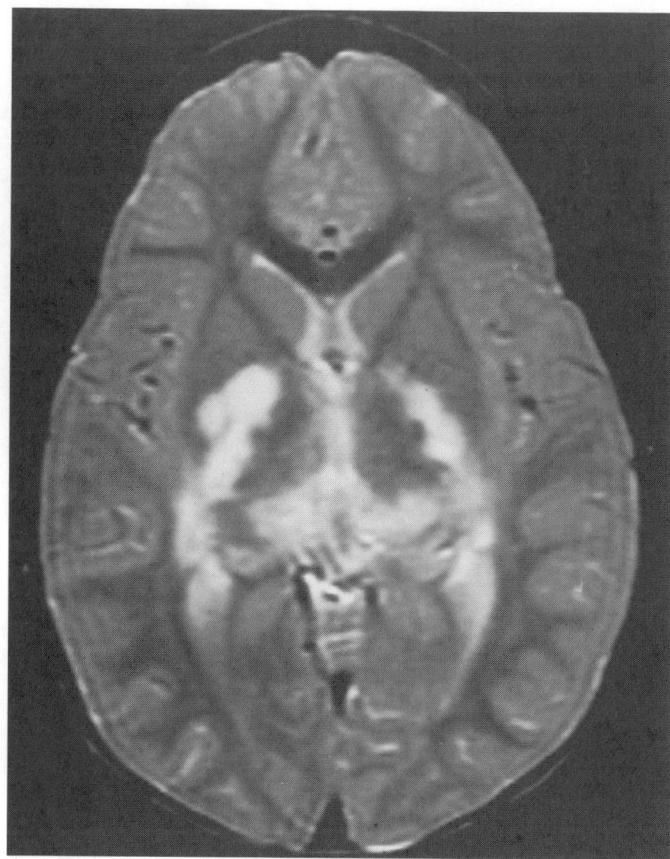

FIG. 159-5. Brain MRI showing multiple areas of T2-weighted signal intensity in basal ganaglia. The patient had no neurologic symptoms.

According to the National Institutes of Health diagnostic criteria, in the absence of bilateral vestibular schwannomas, NF2 can also be diagnosed in an individual with a first-degree relative with NF2 and some NF2-related features. These include unilateral vestibular schwannoma, meningioma, glioma (usually of the spinal cord), ependymoma, or cataract. The latter can be a helpful sign of NF2 in young children and consists of cortical wedge opacities or presenile posterior subcapsular cataracts.

Cutaneous manifestations are less common in NF2 than in NF1. Some individuals have café-au-lait spots and rarely may have as many as six. Skinfold freckles are not found in NF2. Skin tumors may occur in NF2, but typically are schwannomas rather than neurofibromas.

Like NF1, about one-half of cases of NF2 are sporadic. This presents a problem in diagnosis, since many young people with NF2 have neither bilateral vestibular schwannomas nor a family

TABLE 159-3. Diagnostic Criteria of Neurofibromatosis Type 2 Slightly Modified from Those Suggested by National Institutes of Health Consensus Development Conference on Neurofibromatosis, 1987

Bilateral vestibular schwannomas
  OR
First degree relative with NF2 and
  Unilateral vestibular schwannoma, or any two of following features:
    Schwannoma
    Neurofibroma
    Meningioma
    Glioma
    Cortical wedge opacity or juvenile posterior subcapsular cataract

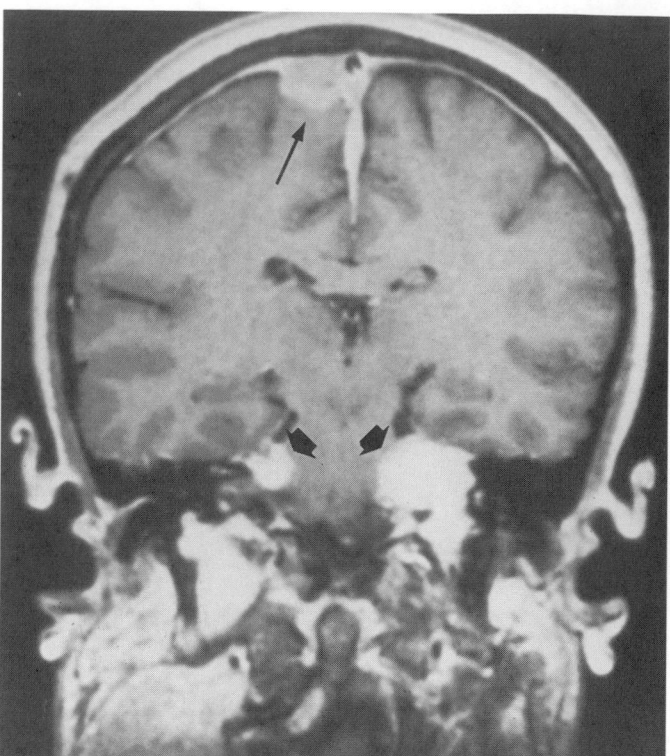

FIG. 159-6. Gadolinium-enhanced MRI from patient with neurofibromatosis type 2 showing bilateral vestibular schwannomas (*large arrows*) and meningioma (*small arrow*).

history of the disorder. Strict adherence to the diagnostic criteria would prevent one from diagnosing NF2 in a sporadically affected person with unilateral vestibular schwannoma, meningioma, and cataract, for example. NF2 should be strongly considered in an individual having two or more features listed in Table 159-3.

Natural History and Management

Unlike NF1, NF2 tends to "breed true" in families in terms of disease severity. Some families have relatively mild manifestations and later age of onset, whereas others have a more fulminant course. In NF2, death caused by complications of the condition is much more common than in NF1. In one recent study, the mean age of death was 36.25 years, with a range of 16 to 67 years.

Routine clinical care should focus on early detection of complications. Slit-lamp examination can detect cataracts in young children at risk of inheriting the disorder. These rarely cause major visual problems but can help in establishing the diagnosis. Audiologic testing should be offered to at-risk individuals and repeated every few years. Evidence of hearing loss or symptoms of vestibular schwannoma should be followed up with MRI, which can also be offered during adolescence and early adult life even in the absence of signs or symptoms, since early detection of vestibular schwannoma can help in following the lesion and providing genetic counseling.

The standard treatment of vestibular schwannoma is surgery. Small tumors are usually observed without treatment until definite growth or progressive symptoms occur; early surgery may not prevent later symptoms, since vestibular schwannomas tend to be multifocal and therefore can regrow after surgery. Major complications related to these tumors include hearing loss and facial nerve damage. Some centers have advocated stereotactic radiosurgery, but it is not clear that the outcome of treatment with this method is different from that of conventional surgery.

Spinal schwannomas can lead to nerve root compression or spinal cord compression. It is important to look for these tumors in a person with NF2 about to undergo surgery for vestibular schwannoma, since intraoperative cervical hyperextension is potentially dangerous in a person with a cervical schwannoma. Treatment of these tumors, and of meningiomas, is surgical. Malignant tumors are rare in NF2, and nontumor manifestations are likewise uncommon.

Genetic Counseling

NF2 is transmitted as a dominant trait, like NF1. Because most of the manifestations of NF2 are later in onset; however, it is often difficult to establish the diagnosis in at-risk children. These children are best followed clinically as though affected, unless genetic testing can be used to determine that they are not at risk. Currently, genetic linkage analysis can be offered in families with at least two generations of affected individuals. The NF2 gene has been cloned and encodes a cytoskeletal protein referred to as merlin or schwannomin. Mutation analysis is underway on a research basis, and eventually it may be a means of diagnostic testing. Laboratory studies have demonstrated that both copies of the NF2 gene are inactive in tumor cells of schwannomas and meningiomas, supporting the notion that the NF2 gene functions as a so-called tumor suppressor gene.

SUMMARY AND FUTURE PROSPECTS

Although NF1 and NF2 have been known as clinical enitities for many years, our understanding of the basis for these disorders is recent, since the cloning of the genes. In spite of this progress, however, clinical management is currently limited to anticipatory guidance, early detection of symptoms, symptomatic treatment, and genetic counseling. There is hope, however, that increased understanding of the pathogenesis will lead to improved diagnostic tests and advances in therapy. Affected individuals can be directed to the National Neurofibromatosis Foundation, Suite 7-S, 141 Fifth Avenue, New York, NY 10010 (phone 1-800-323-7938) for additional information.

SUGGESTED READINGS

Aoki S, Barkovich AJ, Nishimura K et al: Neurofibromatosis types 1 and 2: cranial MR findings. Radiology 172:527, 1989

DiMario FJ, Jr., Ramsby G, Greenstein R et al: Neurofibromatosis type 1: magnetic resonance imaging findings. J Child Neurol 8:32, 1993

Evans DGR, Huson SM, Donnai D et al: A clinical study of type 2 neurofibromatosis. QJM 84:603, 1992

Evans DG, Ramsden R, Huson SM et al: Type 2 neurofibromatosis: the need for supraregional care? J Laryngol Otol 107:401, 1993

Gutmann DH, Collins FS: Neurofibromatosis type 1: beyond positional cloning. Arch Neurol 50:1185, 1993

Hofman KJ, Boehm CD: Familial neurofibromatosis type 1: clinical experience with DNA testing. J Pediatr 120:394, 1992

Hofman KJ, Harris EL, Bryan RN, Denckla MB: Neurofibromatosis type 1: the cognitive phenotype. J Pediatr 124:S1, 1994

Housepian EM, Chi TL: Neurofibromatosis and optic pathways gliomas. J Neurooncol 15:51, 1993

Hughes RAC, Huson SM (eds): The Neurofibromatoses. Chapman and Hall, New York, 1994

Huson SM, Harper PS, Compston DAS: Von Recklinghausen neurofibromatosis. A clinical and population study in south-east Wales. Brain 111:1355, 1988

Korf BR: Diagnostic outcome in children with multiple café au lait spots. Pediatrics 90:924, 1992

Korf BR, Carrazana E, Holmes GL: Patterns of seizures observed in association with neurofibromatosis 1. Epilepsia 34:616, 1993

Martuza RL, Eldridge R: Neurofibromatosis 2. Engl J Med 318:684, 1988

Mautner VF, Tatagiba M, Guthoff R et al: Neurofibromatosis 2 in the pediatric age group. Neurosurgery 33:92, 1993

Narod SA, Parry DM, Parboosingh J et al: Neurofibromatosis type 2 appears to be a genetically homogeneous disease. Am J Hum Genet 51:486, 1992

North K: Neurofibromatosis type 1: review of the first 200 patients in an Australian clinic. J Child Neurol 8:395, 1993

North K, Joy P, Yuille D et al: Specific learning disability in children with neurofibromatosis type 1: significance of MRI abnormalities. Neurology 44:878, 1994

Riccardi VM, Eichner JE: Neurofibromatosis: Phenotype, Natural History, and Pathogenesis. Johns Hopkins University Press, Baltimore, 1992

Rubenstein AE, Korf BR: Neurofibromatosis. Thieme, New York, 1990

Stumpf DA, Alksne JF, Annegers JF et al: Neurofibromatosis. Arch Neurol 45:575, 1988

Trofatter JA, MacCollin MM, Rutter JL et al: A novel moesin-, ezrin-, radixin-like gene is a candidate for the neurofibromatosis 2 tumor suppressor. Cell 72:791, 1993

Viskochil D, White R, Cawthon R: The neurofibromatosis type 1 gene. Annu Rev Neurosci 16:183, 1993

Ward K, O'Connell P, Carey JC et al: Diagnosis of neurofibromatosis 1 by using tightly linked, flanking DNA markers. Am J Hum Genet 46:943, 1990

160. SKULL BASE TUMORS

EBEN ALEXANDER III

Skull base tumors present some of the most difficult management problems of any type of brain tumor. In spite of remarkable developments in clinical neurophysiology (including cortical mapping and evoked response monitoring), neuroradiology, and operative neurosurgery, skull base tumors remain a significant challenge. Advances in three-dimensional image reconstruction to assist in surgical planning, as well as the use of stereotactic radiosurgery and stereotactic fractionated radiotherapy, have provided some therapeutic benefit. This chapter discusses some of the less common skull base tumors (meningiomas, the most common skull-based tumors, are addressed in Ch. 155).

CHORDOMA

The chordoma, accounting for roughly 1 percent of intracranial tumors, arises from the remnants of the embryonic notochord. In spite of its origin, it is rare in children and usually presents in the fourth to sixth decades. There is a 2:1 male preponderance. Most occur in the sacrococcygeal region, but the second most frequent site of origin is the clivus (approximately 25 percent). Clivus and sphenoid sinus chordomas usually present with neck pain, headache, and a sensation of nasal obstruction. Visual disturbances caused by involvement of cranial nerves II, III, IV, and VI are present in one-half of cases. The so-called basisphenoidal chordomas, occurring in the more rostral clivus, usually present with upper cranial neuropathies and endocrine abnormalities secondary to involvement of the diencephalon. In contrast, basioccipital chordomas, arising from the lower clivus at the spheno-occipital synchondrosis, cause mainly lower cranial nerve palsies and long tract signs.

The tumor is often gray or colorless, lobulated, soft, and gelatinous in appearance. There may be areas of calcification, mucin, and hemorrhage. It usually arises in the midline of the clivus but often extends to one side, growing forward into the nasopharynx and sella turcica, the adjacent cavernous and sphenoid sinuses, or posteriorly and inferiorly into the brainstem. Growth always involves destruction of any restraining bone.

Histologically, the neoplastic cells exist in lobulations of variable size within a fibrous connective tissue stroma. Tumor cells, often very pleomorphic with occasional mitotic figures, are arranged in solid sheets or along interconnected or isolated strands. Some cells have a homogeneous eosinophilic cytoplasm, which is distinct from intercellular material; others contain various degrees of vacuolation. An extremely vacuolated cell known as the physaliphorous (bubble-bearing) cell is very characteristic of the chordoma. Some areas may consist of mesenchymal differentiation, including bone and cartilage. Tumors with cartilaginous foci are less likely to metastasize. Metastases increases with survival and occurs in 10 to 16 percent of cases.

One biologic variant is the chondroid chordoma, which usually consists of fibrous connective tissue, sparse tumor cells intertwined with cartilagenous foci, immature myxoid elements, and calcification. This form usually occurs in the basioccipital region and carries a longer median survival (20 to 30 years).

A magnetic resonance imaging scan of the chordoma shows irregular and extensive bone destruction with a mixed pattern of long and short T1- and T2-weighted patterns. Because of the very slow growth, chordomas are usually large at the time of presentation.

Chordomas are very difficult to remove completely, and even partial resection may result in significant morbidity owing to the deep central location and extent of spread at diagnosis. In one study, average survival for chordomas after surgical resection and radiation therapy was 4.1 years, and in a subgroup containing foci of chondrosarcoma, 15.8 years (Heffelfinger et al., 1973). In a more recent review, combination surgery and radiotherapy often led to prolonged tumor control, especially for those lower in the nasopharynx (Perzin and Pushparaj, 1986). One other long-term study suggests that radical surgery followed by fractionated radiation therapy to a dose of 6,000 to 6,500 cGy yields the best results and that marginal failures are likely in the absence of appropriate treatment volume selection (Lybeert and Meerwaldt, 1986). At the Stereotactic Radiosurgery/Radiotherapy Center of the Brigham & Women's Hospital, we have obtained reliable local control using linear accelerator-based stereotactic radiosurgery as an adjunct to surgical resection, with minimal peripheral tumor radiation doses of 1,500 to 1,700 cGy.

CHONDROSARCOMA

Chondrosarcomas represent roughly 6 percent of all skull-based tumors, with approximately three-fourths of all the chondrosarcomas of the cranium occurring around the skull base. This is most likely due to the fact that the skull base is derived through endochondral calcification of the cartilaginous matrix. These tumors are probably derived from the primitive mesenchymal stem cell of the matrix. Most patients present in their third and fourth decades, and there is an equal distribution between the sexes. A normal neurologic examination is more common in

patients with chordoma, whereas visual loss, facial numbness, and multiple cranial neuropathies are more common in patients with chondrosarcoma. This reflects the tendency of chordomas to originate from the clivus and chondrosarcomas to originate from the temporal bone.

Roughly two-thirds of the skull-based chondrosarcomas occur in the middle cranial fossa, followed by the anterior and the posterior fossa. These lesions are similar to the chordomas in that they are fairly slow growing and locally recurrent with significant bony destruction. Lesions in the parasellar region (the most common site of origin) typically compress optic nerves and disturb hypothalamic-pituitary function. Occasionally, they erupt through the nasal and paranasal sinuses penetrating the skull base. The degree of histologic anaplasia correlates somewhat with survival, with 5-year survival rates of 90 percent for grade I as opposed to 40 percent for grade III tumors. The mesenchymal subtype is a more malignant form with a higher tendency for recurrence, metastasis, and increased vascularity.

Biochemical composition of chondrosarcomas correlates with the prognosis of these lesions. Tumors with a hyaline extracellular matrix have a less malignant course than tumors with myxoid and fibrous extracellular matrix. This chemical categorization implies that more malignant chondrosarcomas have a more immature cartilage, indicating reversion to an embryonal state.

Magnetic resonance imaging scans of chondrosarcomas show that they commonly extend into the nasopharynx and the upper spinal canal and demonstrate regions of multiple calcifications (''popcorn'' areas of calcification). On computed tomographic scan, the chondrosarcoma contains regions of multiple calcifications throughout the chondroid matrix as well as a very irregular pattern of bony destruction and some local thickening of bone with a calcified cartilaginous cap, often combined with irregular bone destruction.

As with chordomas, chondrosarcomas are very difficult to treat because of their relative inaccessibility to surgical resection and their overall resistance to radiation therapy. It is unusual for the skull-base chondrosarcomas to metastasize; their course is usually one of local progression.

Total gross resection of these lesions has become possible on occasion through the evolution of lateral skull-base techniques. Postoperative radiotherapy enhances survival after radical surgical excision. Patients with chordomas or low-grade chondrosarcomas at the base of the skull treated with fractionated high-dose postoperative radiation delivered with a proton beam (median tumor dose 69 cobalt Gy equivalents) have a 5-year local control rate of 82 percent and disease-free survival rate of 76 percent. Patients with large tumors (more than 75 cc) and cervical spine disease have a higher recurrence rate.

GLOMUS TUMORS

Glomus tumors (glomus jugulare or glomus tympanicum) are the most common tumor of the region of the middle ear. This is also the second most common tumor to occur in the temporal bone after the neurilemmoma. Glomus tumors, also known as chemodectomas, arise from chemoreceptor cells normally found in the adventitia of the jugular bulb just inferior to the floor of the middle ear, as well as in the bony canals that transmit the tympanic branches of the glossopharyngeal and vagus nerves. They also occur in the bone adjacent to the mucosa of the middle ear (glomus tympanicum). These lesions usually present in the sixth decade, although they occasionally occur in patients as young as the midteens. There is a strong (six-fold) predilection for occurrence in women, and there is a definite tendency toward clusters within families, suggesting a genetic predisposition. Glomus tumors often demonstrate fairly slow growth and tend to extend along planes of low resistance, especially along the carotid artery to the carotid canal into the middle fossa or up to the jugular foramen and hypoglossal canal and posterior fossa. Although in general they demonstrate benign behavior, they can be invasive locally. Because of their extreme vascularity, there is a high propensity toward hemorrhage.

They often present with cranial nerve dysfunction, with the facial nerve being most commonly involved. They can also produce a conductive hearing loss, as well as an obvious mass detected by photoscopy or otoscopic examination of the external auditory canal, or they can present with pulsatile tinnitus. With progressive extension into the base of the brain, they produce fifth, sixth, ninth, and tenth nerve symptoms, as well as long tract signs from brainstem compression, and often hydrocephalus.

In advanced stages, they demonstrate widespread destruction of the local bony structures, enlarging the jugular foramen and carotid canal, ensuring significant bone destruction. Angiography often reveals their extreme vascularity; these lesions are composed mainly of a very thin wall of vessels within cords of epithelioid cells.

Glomus tumors may run a protracted course over decades. One-half of these tumors may recur within 3 years of their initial surgical management, and, because of their prolonged course, a 5-year survival does not indicate cure. Dissemination throughout the cerebrospinal fluid pathways can occur after the tumor has extended intracranially, but metastases to other parts of the body occur in less then 1 percent of cases. The most common cause of death is from intracranial compression of neural structures owing to extensive intracranial tumor growth.

The differential diagnosis is often straightforward because of the location and hemorrhagic tendency of these lesions. Their histologic appearance is characteristic, with small nests of round to polygonal cells, often dispersed around prominent dilated vascular channels. There is some variation in size of chromatin content of these nuclei with rare mitoses. They usually demonstrate a very complex and extensive network of reticulin because of the intricate pattern of small blood vessels.

Surgical management of glomus tumors can be challenging because of the extensive involvement of critical arterial and venous structures, as well as cranial nerves around the base of the brain. Because of their extreme vascularity, utilization of a neodymium: yttrium aluminum garnet laser is often useful in expediting safer resection. A cure is possible after complete surgical excision, but there is approximately a 33 percent recurrence rate after gross total resection, which indicates invasiveness or the possibility of multicentric origin of this tumor.

Fractionated radiation therapy (5,000 cGy in 25 daily fractions) offers additional tumor control after surgical resection and induces fibrosis of tumor vessels with a marked decrease in blood flow. Although radiographic evidence of decreased vascularity is not always documented, the patients usually demonstrate improvement in symptoms without further tumor growth over many years.

Complication rates for fractionated radiation therapy and surgical removal are similar, and combination therapy with both modalities is advisable when tumor removal is felt to be incomplete.

Stereotactic radiosurgery with peripheral tumor doses in the range of 1,500 to 1,700 cGy is very useful as a surgical adjunct, whether used several months preoperatively to devascularize the tumor or postoperatively to improve local control. The lower cranial nerves often found adjacent to the tumor capsule generally tolerate radiosurgical doses of 1,500 cGy over small portions of their length (e.g., 2 to 3 cm).

ESTHESIONEUROBLASTOMA

Esthesioneuroblastoma, otherwise known as olfactory neuroblastoma, generally originates from olfactory epithelium in the superior aspect of the nasal cavity near the cribriform plate. This tumor is rare and has a very poorly understood embryogenesis. Cells of origin are derived from the neural crest with a histologic resemblance to childhood neuroblastoma.

Esthesioneuroblastomas usually present in adolescents and young adults, although there is a later peak in the sixth and seventh decades. There is a 2:1 male preponderance, and there has been no demonstrable familial predispostion. Presenting symptoms are due to both the intrinsic high vascularity of the tumor and the location high in the nasal cavity, with epistaxis and nasal destruction being common presenting symptoms. As the tumor grows, it invades the cribriform plate and extends into the anterior cranial fossa with early complete anosmia.

The appearance on computed tomographic scan is one of homogeneous enhancement. Although the lesion does extend intracranially, it remains extra-axial without ever invading into the cerebral parenchyma. Angiography reveals mild vascularity, slightly more than is seen with other nasal tumors that may invade the floor of the anterior fossa.

As with many of the other tumors discussed in this chapter, the natural history is one of a fairly slow but insidious course. Local recurrence with intracranial invasion is common. Five-year survival rates are around 50 percent, but this decreases somewhat when the anterior skull base has been invaded. Tumor recurrence up to two decades after the original presentation may occur. Persistent local recurrences are very common. Esthesioneuroblastoma metastatic to local lymph nodes, as well as to the lungs and to bone, occurs in 20 to 40 percent of cases. The 5-year survival rate of 75 percent of patients without metastases is lowered to approximately 40 percent in those who have distant metastases. There is no obvious correlation between histologic grade of the primary and the propensity to metastasize.

Esthesioneuroblastoma is more sensitive to radiotherapy than most other skull-based tumors discussed here. Fractionated radiation doses of 5,000 to 6,000 cGy achieve tumor regression and tumor control with potential curability. Chemotherapeutic agents, such as cyclophosphamide, vincristine, and doxorubicin, have been useful. Responses to chemotherapy may be observed even in those patients who have failed prior radiation therapy. Even minimal responses often produce significant palliation of the pain involved with this tumor, as well as symptoms of nasal obstruction and epistaxis.

NASOPHARYNGEAL CARCINOMA

Nasopharyngeal carcinoma is uncommon in the Western World, although the frequency is 100 times as great in the Chinese population in southern Asia. Most of these tumors demonstrate squamous differentiation, with less frequent histologic variants consisting of lymphoepithelioma and nonkeratinizing carcinoma.

This carcinoma is frequently associated with a positive titer for the Epstein-Barr virus. Native Chinese living in other countries still have a greater risk of developing this carcinoma. The prevalence of nasopharyngeal carcinoma among Chinese born in the United States is slightly higher than the incidence in this country at large. Various environmental agents have been evaluated for their potential role in inducing nasopharyngeal carcinoma, including methylnitrosamines in salted fish and domestic inhaled carcinogens. The age distribution curves indicate that this environmental exposure must occur early in life.

Recent investigations have shown a correlation of certain histocompatibility antigen subtypes with the incidence of nasopharyngeal carcinoma and revealed occasional familial clustering of the disease. Overall, males are affected three times as often as females.

Patients usually present in the fifth decade, usually with local symptoms from tumors in the nasal fossa and palate. The tumor often spreads through the multiple regional lymphatic channels and often involves the skull base in one-fourth of cases. In those patients, cranial nerve palsies, mainly around the pons, are seen. In the average period of 7 months between onset of symptoms and diagnosis, approximately one-half of the patients have already developed regional metastases to the cervical lymph nodes.

The 5-year survival rate for this disease ranges from 20 to 40 percent and is worse with the more common histology of squamous cell carcinoma as opposed to patients with nonkeratinizing carcinoma or the lymphoepithelioma variant.

The lymphoepithelioma variant contains a predominantly lymphocytic component, which may very well represent an immunologic response to the tumor. These patients often present at an earlier age, and the tumor follows a more benign course.

The Epstein-Barr virus is a herpesvirus with proven oncogenic potential in other tissues that are part of the immune system. Increasing viral titers correlate with a decreased survival in patients with nasopharyngeal carcinoma. Those patients who have been in remission for several years tend to have lower viral titers.

Fractionated radiation therapy has been useful in treating these tumors. The treatment volume must include the sinuses at the base of the anterior fossa, including the ethmoid and the sphenoid sinus, as well as the cavernous sinus in the base of the skull out to the foramen ovale and spinosum and the carotid canal. The dose utilized ranges from 6,500 to 7,000 cGy over a 7- to 7.5-week period. Because the temporal lobes are usually included in the radiation fields, a minority of patients develop delayed radiation necrosis in these areas.

Chemotherapy with a combination of 5-fluorouracil and cisplatin has been shown to be effective in one-half of the cases. In other trials, single agents using either methotrexate, cyclophosphamide or bleomycin have produced responses in 40 percent of patients, although these are usually of brief duration. Human leukocyte interferon may also be of some value. The extensive spread along the skull base often makes this tumor a very difficult and challenging problem for surgery, as well as for stereotactic radiosurgery.

SUGGESTED READINGS

Applebaum EL, Mantravadi P, Haas R: Lymphoepithelioma of the nasopharynx. Laryngoscope 92:510–4, 1982

Austin JP, Urie MM, Cardenosa G, Munzenrider JE: Probable causes of recurrence in patients with chordoma and chondrosarcoma of the base of skull and cervical spine. Int J Radiat Oncol Biol Phys 25:439–44, 1993

Austin-Seymour M, Munzenrider J, Goitein M et al: Fractionated proton radia-

tion therapy of chordoma and low-grade chondrosarcoma of the base of the skull. J Neurosurg 70:13–7, 1989

Chetiyawardana AD: Chordoma: results of treatment. Clin Radiol 35:159–61, 1984

Decker DA, Drelichman A, Al-Sarraf M et al: Chemotherapy for nasopharyngeal carcinoma: a 10 year experience. Cancer 52:602–5, 1983

Elkton D, Hightower SI, Lim ML et al: Esthesioneuroblastoma. Cancer 44:1087–94, 1979

Gastpar J, Wilmese, E, Wolf H: Epidemiologic and immunologic aspects of nasopharyngeal carcinoma. J Med 12:257–84, 1981

Hassounah M, Al-Mefty O, Akhtar M et al: Primary cranial and intracranial chondrosarcoma. A survey. Acta Neurochir (Wien) 78:123–32, 1985

Heffelfinger MJ, Dahlin DC, MacCarty CS, Beabout JW: Chordomas and cartilagenous tumors at the skull base. Cancer 32:410–20, 1973

Kveton JF, Brackmann DE, Glasscock ME, 3d et al: Chondrosarcoma of the skull base. Otolaryngol Head Neck Surg 94:23–32, 1986

Lybeert ML, Meerwaldt JH: Chordoma. Report on treatment results in eighteen cases. Acta Radiol Oncol 25:41–3, 1986

Lybert MLM, Van Andel JG, Eykenboom WMH et al: Radiotherapy of paragangliomas. Clin Otolaryngol 9:105–9, 1984

Mankin HJ, Cantley KP, Lippiello L et al: The biology of human chondrosarcoma. I. Description of cases, grading and biochemical analyses. J Bone Joint Surg Am 62A:160–76, 1980

Mankin JH, Cantley KP, Schiller AL et al: The biology of human chondrosarcoma. II. Variation in chemical composition among types and subtypes of benign and malignant cartilage tumors. J Bone Joint Surg [AM] 62:176–88, 1980

Neel HB: Nasopharyngeal carcinoma: clinical presentation, diagnosis, treatment and prognosis. Otolaryngol Clin North Am 18:3, 1985

Newbill ET, Johns ME, Cantrell RW: Esthesioneuroblastoma: diagnosis and management. South Med J 78:275–82, 1985

Perzin KH, Pushpraraj: Nonepithelial tumors of the nasal cavity, paranasal sinuses, and nasopharynx. A clinicopathologic study. XIV: chordomas. Cancer 57:784–96, 1986

Sekhar LN, Schramm VL: Tumors of the Cranial Base: Diagnosis and Treatment. Futura, Mount Kisco, NY, 1987

Shah JP, Feghali J: Esthesioneuroblastoma. CA Cancer J Clin 33:154–9, 1983

Simko TG, Griffin TW, Gerdes AJ et al: The role of radiation therapy in the treatment of glomus jugulary tumors. Cancer 42:104–6, 1978

Spector GJ, Ciralsky RH, Ogura JH: Glomus tumors in the head and neck III. Analysis of clinical manifestations. Anal Otol 84:73–9, 1975

Spector GJ, Sobols S: Surgery for glomus tumors at the skull base. Otolaryngol Head Neck Surg 88:524–30, 1980

Suit HD, Goitein M, Munzenrder J et al: Definitive radiation therapy for chordoma and chondrosarcoma of the base of the skull and cervical spine. J Neurosurg 56:377–85, 1982

Volpe NJ, Liebsch NJ, Munzenrider JE, Lessell S: Neuro-ophthalmologic findings in chordoma and chondrosarcoma of the skull base. Am J Ophthalmol 115:97–104, 1993

Wade PM, Jr, Smith RE, Johns ME: Response of esthesioneuroblastoma to chemotherapy. Report of 5 cases in view of the literature. Cancer 53:1036–41, 1984

Waga S, Tochio H, Yamagiwa M, Nishioka H: Chondrosarcoma of the ethmoid sinus extending to the anterior fossa. Surg Neuro 16:324–8, 1981

161. EPENDYMOMAS

JOAO O. SIFFERT

Ependymomas are tumors of neuroepithelial tissue that arise from the ependymal or subependymal cells surrounding the ventricles and central canal of the spinal cord. Intracranial ependymomas represent approximately 10 percent of brain tumors in children and less than 5 percent of intracranial gliomas diagnosed in adults. The mean age at the time of diagnosis is 5 to 6 years, with approximately 60 percent of children younger than 5 years of age and 4 percent older than 15 years of age.

Spinal cord ependymomas affect primarily adults and account for approximately 50 percent of all ependymomas and 30 to 60 percent of all spinal cord tumors. Usually these tumors are of the myxopapillary histologic type. Spinal cord tumors are discussed in more detail in Chapter 166.

Ependymomas localize most commonly to the fourth ventricle, where they may extend through the foramina of Luschka and Magendie, as well as superiorly through the cerebral acqueduct and inferiorly toward the cervical spine. One-third of the intracranial ependymomas are localized above the cerebellar tentorium, involving the lateral and third ventricles, as well as the cerebral parenchyma. In the latter case, ependymomas are thought to originate from ependymal cell rests.

SIGNS AND SYMPTOMS

The localization of ependymomas in the central nervous system dictates the presenting clinical manifestations. Symptoms may precede tumor diagnosis by up to 12 months.

Posterior fossa tumors, which often lead to obstructive hydrocephalus, may cause headaches and vomiting, both signs of increased intracranial pressure. Papilledema is uniformly present in such cases. Tumor compression or invasion of the brainstem leads to cranial nerve palsies and long tract signs. Other signs such as gait ataxia, limb incoordination, and nystagmus constitute evidence of compromise of either cerebellum or brainstem. Tumors extending into the cervical spinal canal may produce torticollis and neck pain as the only clinical manifestations. Patients with cerebral hemisphere tumors may present with visual field deficits, weakness, hyper-reflexia, or seizures. Occasionally, patients with either large tumors or hydrocephalus caused by obstruction of the foramen of Monro may also present with signs of increased intracranial pressure. Very young children with long-standing hydrocephalus may present with enlargement of the head, developmental delay, and irritability as sole clinical manifestations.

NEUROIMAGING

The neuroimaging appearance of ependymomas reflects their often heterogeneous pathologic features. Posterior fossa ependymomas typically appear on computed tomographic scan as heterogeneous, often hyperintense, well circumscribed fourth ventricular masses, commonly associated with hydrocephalus. Supratentorial tumors are usually situated in periventricular regions but may extend into adjacent cerebral parenchyma. In both locations, contrast enhancement is heterogeneous. Cyst formation and calcifications are common. Magnetic resonance imaging (MRI) scans also demonstrate diverse signal intensities, with nonuniform gadolinium enhancement. In certain cases, the extension of ependymomas through the fourth ventricular foramina, in association with gadolinium enhancement, allows neuroimaging differentiation from medulloblastomas and cerebellar astrocytomas (Fig. 161-1).

PATHOLOGY

The macroscopic appearance of ependymomas demonstrates solid tumor areas that may contain areas with cysts, necrosis, edema, calcification, or hemorrhage. Microscopically, typical ependymomas consist predominantly of neoplastic ependymal cells that exhibit histologic patterns such as perivascular pseudorosettes and less frequently the pathognomonic ependymal rosettes (Fig. 161-2). Occasional mitoses, nuclear atypia and rare foci of necrosis may be seen and are not necessarily indicative of aggressive behavior.

Anaplastic ependymomas, in contrast, are characterized by the presence of significant cellular pleomorphism, necrosis, increased cellularity, frequent mitoses, multinucleation, and giant cells. Most often, anaplastic ependymomas are found in the cerebral hemispheres.

Subependymomas, another category of ependymal tumor, are formed by nests of ependymal cells in a dense glial fibrillary matrix. They are usually found in tissue surrounding the fourth

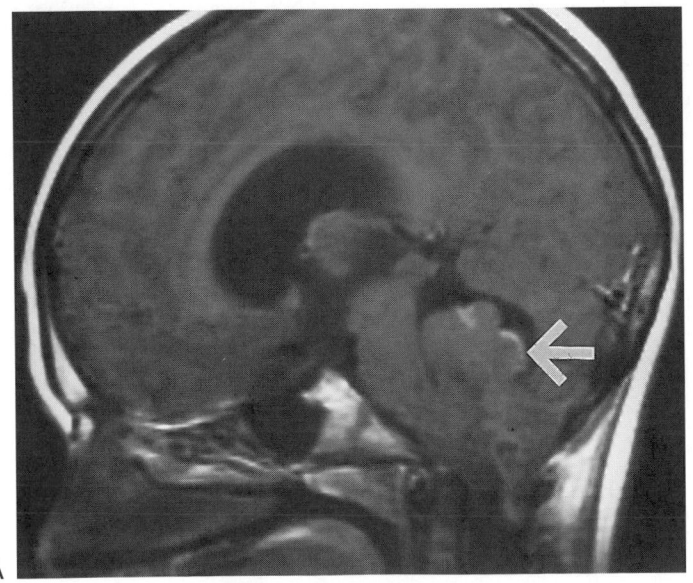
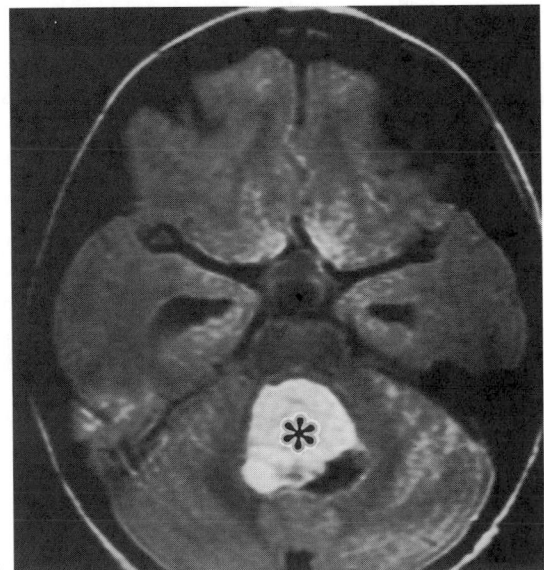

FIG. 161-1. Four-year-old girl with headaches and ataxia. **(A)** Sagittal T1-weighted MRI scan after gadolinium injection shows minor and irregular enhancement of the fourth ventricular ependymoma (*arrow*). Note extension of the tumor through the foramen magnum. **(B)** Axial proton-density MRI scan shows the tumor as a hyperintense mass (*asterisk*) surrounded by the hypointense CSF within the dilated fourth ventricle. (From Wolpert S, Barnes PD: MRI in Pediatric Neuroradiology. Mosby Year Book, St Louis, 1992, with permission.)

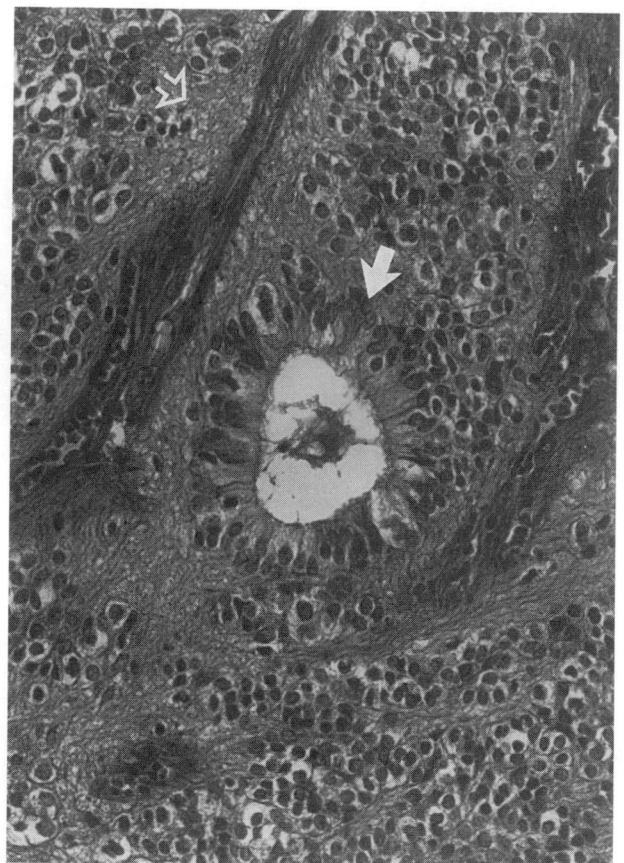
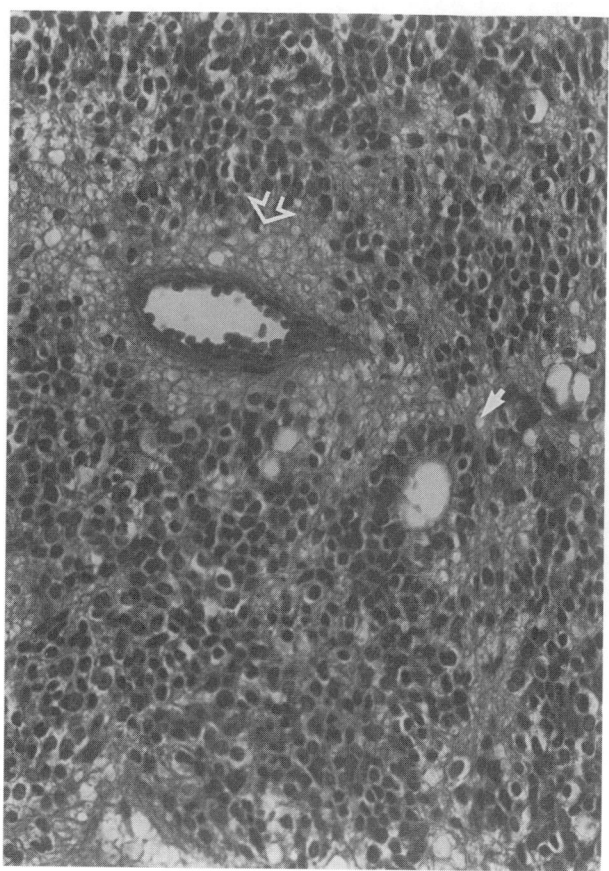

FIG. 161-2. (A & B) Histologic features of ependymoma. The figure shows essentially monomorphic meoplastic ependymal cells within a fibrillary background, perivascular pseudorosettes (*open arrows*), and ependymal rosettes (*solid arrows*).

ventricle, occasionally appearing in multiple foci. These tumors tend to have a benign, often asymptomatic, course.

THERAPY

Surgical resection and radiation therapy are mainstays of treatment for ependymomas. Gross total resection of intracranial ependymomas has been associated with higher survival rates and is the recommended initial treatment. External beam radiation therapy is used as adjuvant treatment following both gross total and partial surgical resections.

Patients with disseminated neuraxis disease at the time of diagnosis are treated with full craniospinal radiation. Therefore, initial investigation of patients with ependymoma should also include enhanced spinal MRI scan and cerebrospinal fluid (CSF) cytologic analysis. In contrast, the patients with low-grade nondisseminated tumors receive involved field radiation. The use of involved field radiation for patients with nondisseminated disease is based on the observations that up to 9 percent of patients may have CSF pathway dissemination and that tumor recurrence happens typically in the original site prior to distal sites. The volume of radiation utilized for treatment of patients with anaplastic nondisseminated tumors is controversial. Those who favor full craniospinal radiation argue that anaplastic tumors are more likely to have CSF pathway dissemination.

When delivered under conventional regimens, total doses of radiation to the original tumor bed greater than 4,500 cGy and generally between 5,000 and 5,500 cGy are thought to be associated with improved outcome. Current hyperfractionation regi-

mens allow even higher doses to be delivered with similar toxicity profile, but long-term survival data are not yet available.

The specific role of chemotherapy in the treatment of ependymomas has not been established. Tumor response to cisplatin alone, nitrosoureas, and cyclophosphamide in combination with vincristine, has been reported. Currently, chemotherapy is utilized in patients with recurrent ependymoma and in infants, in whom radiation is deferred until age 3 years.

PROGNOSIS

Adults have longer survival compared with children. The overall 5-year survival rate in children with ependymomas ranges from 28 to 58 percent, according to different series reported.

Factors associated with worse prognosis include young age at presentation (less than 2 to 3 years) and subtotal surgical resection, as measured by postoperative enhanced MRI scan. Among the supratentorial ependymomas, anaplastic features, particularly large numbers of mitoses and increased cellularity, seem to predict a worse prognosis in both children and adults.

Recurrence at the primary tumor site constitutes the main pattern of failure, irrespective of pathology, localization, therapy, and age of presentation. Extraneural metastases occur rarely. Thus, local disease control remains the most important therapeutic goal in attempts to improve survival of patients with ependymomas.

SUGGESTED READINGS

Cohen ME, Duffner PK: Brain Tumors in Children. Principles of Diagnosis and Treatment. 2nd Ed. Raven Press, New York, 1994

Dohrmann GJ, Farwell JR, Flannery JT: Ependymomas and ependymoblasto-mas in children. J Neurosurg 45:272–83, 1976

Healey EA, Barnes PD et al: The prognostic significance of postoperative residual tumor in ependymoma. Neurosurgery 28:666–72,

Kleihues P, Burger PC, Scheithauer BW et al: WHO International Histological Classification of Tumors. Histological Typing of Tumors of the Central Nervous System. 2nd Ed. Springer-Verlag, New York, 1994

Kricheff I, Becker M: Intracranial ependymomas: factors influencing prognosis. J Neurosurg 21:4–14, 1964

Lyons MK, Kelly PJ: Posterior fossa ependymomas: report of 30 cases and review of the literature. Neurosurgery 28:659–65, 1991

Moørk SJ, Loøken AC: Ependymoma. A follow up study of 101 cases. Cancer 40:907–15, 1977

Russell DS, Rubinstein LJ: Pathology of Tumors of the Nervous System. 5th Ed. Williams & Wilkins, Baltimore 1989

Shiffer D, Chiò A: Ependymoma: internal correlations among pathological signs. The anaplastic variant. Neurosurgery 29:206–10,

Sutton L, Goldwein G et al: Prognostic factors in childhood ependymomas. Pediatr Neurosurg 16:57–65, 1990–91

Tamura M, Ono N, Kurihara H et al: Adjunctive treatment for recurrent child-hood ependymoma of the IV ventricle: chemotherapy with CDDP and MCNU. Childs Nerv Syst vol. 6:186–9, 1990

Wolpert S, Barnes PD: MRI in Pediatric Neuroradiology. Mosby Year Book, St Louis, 1992

162. MEDULLOBLASTOMA

SCOTT L. POMEROY

Medulloblastoma, the most common malignant brain tumor of childhood, accounts for approximately 20 to 25 percent of all primary tumors of the central nervous system among children younger than 15 years old. The tumor arises within the cerebellum and has a slight male predominance. It occurs with maximum incidence in children 5 and 9 years old, with approximately 70 percent of patients diagnosed before the age of 20. A smaller peak incidence occurs between ages ranging from 20 to 24 years. The disease is rare after the fourth decade.

Since its early description by Bailey and Cushing, medulloblastoma has been believed to arise from an embryonal cell, possibly from the external granule cell layer of the developing cerebellum. Its etiology is not known. Greater than 90 percent of patients with the tumor have no known predisposing condition. Between 5 and 10 percent of patients have congenital anomalies or inherited genetic syndromes. The most common of these is the basal cell nevus (Gorlin) syndrome. Medulloblastoma may also arise in patients with ataxia-telangiectasia, xeroderma pigmentosum, Li-Fraumeni syndrome, or Turcot syndrome. For most patients, however, the tumor arises from either spontaneous mutations or extrinsic factors that alter the expression of growth-regulating genes. No environmental causes have been proved to date.

CLINICAL PRESENTATION

Medulloblastoma most commonly presents with signs of increased intracranial pressure, which include nocturnal or morning headache, nausea, vomiting, and alteration of mental status. The tumor usually arises in the cerebellar midline. It may occur in the cerebellar hemispheres of adults, but this is unusual for children. Owing to this localization, truncal ataxia, titubation of the head, and unsteady gait frequently accompany signs of elevated intracranial pressure.

Magnetic resonance imaging or computed tomography reveal a contrast-enhancing midline or, occasionally, paramedian tumor, which often distorts or obliterates the fourth ventricle. The enhancement may be heterogeneous owing to regions of necrosis, hemorrhage, or cystic changes. Tumor margins frequently are indistinct because of invasion of the cerebellum or its peduncles, or less often the brainstem. Because medulloblastoma has a strong tendency to metastasize throughout the central nervous system, contrast-enhanced imaging of the entire neuraxis, including the spine, should always be performed once the diagnosis is established. An example is shown in Figure 162-1. The tumor less commonly metastasizes outside the nervous system, most often to bone. Therefore, a radionucleotide bone scan and a bone marrow aspirate should also be performed at the time of diagnosis. Cytologic examination of the spinal fluid obtained by lumbar puncture completes the metastatic workup.

PATHOLOGY

At surgery, medulloblastoma is a soft, friable tumor, often with foci of necrosis. Microscopic examination reveals a highly cellular tumor with abundant dark staining round or oval nuclei. The cytoplasm of these cells is scanty and undifferentiated. Mitoses are abundant. Neuroblastic Homer Wright rosettes can be found in up to 40 percent of cases. Immunohistochemical analysis demonstrates neuronal markers, including synaptophysin and neurofilament proteins, in the majority of cases. Markers of glial lineage such as glial fibrillary acidic protein are found less commonly. A desmoplastic variant has been described, which may be associated with a better prognosis.

THERAPY

Surgical resection remains the first critical component in the management of medulloblastoma. Gross total surgical removal of tumors that have not infiltrated vital regions such as the brainstem and that are not metastatic at the time of the initial diagnosis can improve outcome. The goal of surgery should be to remove as much of the tumor as can be accomplished without inflicting incapacitating neurologic deficits such as persistent ataxia or cranial nerve deficits. A disorder of language production has been found to occur following surgery to the midline cerebellum. It is characterized by mutism in association with emotional lability. The most severely affected individuals also have varying degrees of inattention and difficulty initiating movements as well as language. These symptoms frequently resolve over the course of weeks to months, although some patients may not fully recover language skills.

External beam radiation therapy of the cranium and spine, with increased radiation dosage to the tumor site, is the second mode of therapy that has been found to be effective for medulloblastoma. Current practice standards recommend radiation dosages of 5,400 cGy to the posterior fossa and 3,600 cGy applied to the remainder of the cranium and the spine. This approach may be supplemented in some cases by boosts of radiation to residual nodules or metastatic lesions.

The role of chemotherapy in the treatment of medulloblastoma is less clear. Most large centers add chemotherapy to the therapeutic regimen either before or after radiation therapy. The

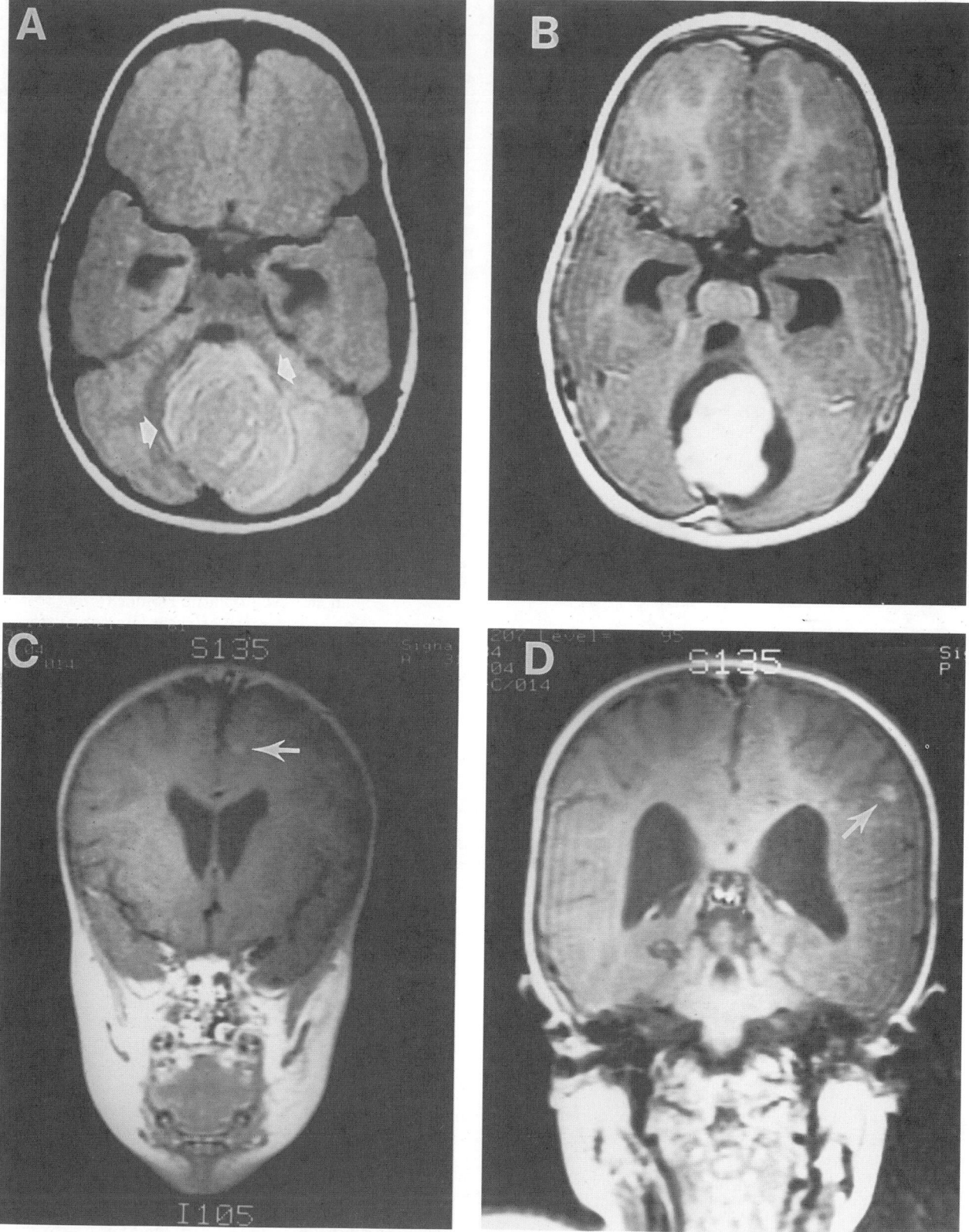

FIG. 162-1. Magnetic resonance imaging scans of a 2-year-old boy with the basal cell nevus syndrome and medulloblastoma. **(A)** A large midline mass (*arrows*) is evident in this transverse section through the posterior fossa taken without contrast enhancement. **(B)** Enhancement is evident after an intravenous injection of contrast dye. **(C & D)** Although no evidence for metastasis was found at the initial diagnosis, 5 months later, the patient had multiple enhancing nodules (*arrows*) in the cerebral hemispheres and in the spinal canal.

most commonly used agents include nitrosourea compounds, cyclophosphamide, cisplatin, and vincristine. For very young children, many centers recommend chemotherapy as a means to delay radiation of the craniospinal axis until the age of 2 to 3 years. This approach was developed based on a growing consensus that deleterious effects of radiation on neurocognitive function are most pronounced when the treatment is given during the first 3 years of life. It is too early to know whether the substitution of chemotherapy during these years will have less severe effects on cognitive function.

OUTCOME

The outlook for medulloblastoma has improved significantly in the past 20 to 30 years. Although this may be accounted for in part by improvements in neurosurgical technique, increased radiation doses probably have had the greatest role in extending survival rates. While 20 to 50 percent of patients survived 5 years after diagnosis in the 1960s, the 5-year survival rates of most major centers presently range from 50 to 75 percent. Survival rates 10 years after diagnosis, however, are still less than 50 percent, perhaps because increased radiation dosing is a relatively new advance. Unfortunately, the radiation dose is near the tolerated limit for normal brain and spinal cord. It is unlikely that additional increases in radiation dose will improve survival further. With improved local control in the central nervous system, the incidence of systemic relapse has apparently increased. Because of these complications, chemotherapy has assumed an increasing role in the therapy of medulloblastoma. Most current experimental treatment protocols continue the search for increasingly effective combinations of chemotherapeutic agents that may improve the survival of this malignancy without inducing further long-term neurologic sequelae.

SUGGESTED READINGS

Bailey P, Cushing H: Medulloblastoma cerebelli; a common type of midcerebellar glioma of childhood. Arch Neurol Psychiatry 14:192, 1925

Bergsma D: Birth Defects Compendium. Alan R Liss, New York, 1973, pp. 137–8

Berry MP, Jenkin RD, Colin MB et al: Radiation treatment for medulloblastoma: a 21-year review. J Neurosurg 55:43, 1981

Bloom HGJ, Wallace ENK, Henk JM: The treatment and prognosis of medulloblastoma in children: a study of 82 verified cases. AJR 105:43, 1969

Cohen ME, Duffner PK: Brain Tumors in Children. Raven, New York, 1994, pp. 193–6

Duffner PK, Horowitz ME, Krischer JP et al: Postoperative chemotherapy and delayed radiation in children less than three years of age with malignant brain tumors. N Engl J Med 328:1725, 1993

Evans AE, Jenkin RDT, Sposto R et al: The treatment of medulloblastoma. J Neurosurg 72:572, 1990

Evans G, Burnell L, Campbell R et al: Congenital anomalies and genetic syndromes in 173 cases of medulloblastoma. Med Pediatr Oncol 21:433, 1993

Friede RL: Developmental Neuropathology. Springer-Verlag, Berlin, 1989

Hughes EN, Shillito J, Sallan SE et al: Medulloblastoma at the Joint Center for Radiation Therapy between 1968 and 1984. The influence of radiation dose on the pattern of failure and survival. Cancer 61:1992, 1988

Kadin ME, Rubenstein LJ, Nelson JS: Neonatal cerebellar medulloblastoma originating from the fetal external granular layer. J Neuropathol Exp Neurol 29:583, 1970

Kleihues P, Burger PC, Scheithauer BW: Histological Typing of Tumours of the Central Nervous System. Springer-Verlag, Berlin, 1993

Kopelson G, Linggood RM, Kleinman GM: Medulloblastoma in adults: improved survival with supervoltage radiation therapy. Cancer 51:1334, 1982

Raimondi AJ, Tomita T: Medulloblastoma in childhood. Acta Neurochir 50:127, 1979

Rekate HL, Grubb RL, Aram DM et al: Muteness of cerebellar origin. Arch Neurol 42:607, 1985

Russell DS, Rubenstein LJ: Pathology of Tumors of the Nervous System. Williams & Wilkins, Baltimore, 1989

Tarbell NJ, Loeffler JS, Silver B et al: The change in patterns of relapse in medulloblastoma. Cancer 68:1600, 1991

Wisoff JH, Epstein FJ: Pseudobulbar palsy after posterior fossa operation in children. Neurosurgery 15:707, 1984

Wolpert SM, Barnes PD: MRI in Pediatric Neuroradiology. CV Mosby, St Louis, 1992

163. PINEAL TUMORS

DENNIS Y. WEN
WALTER A. HALL

Tumors arising in the region of the pineal gland are relatively rare. They account for up to 1 percent of brain tumors in adults and 8 percent of brain tumors in children. There is a higher incidence in Japan where pineal tumors account for 4 percent all intracranial tumors. In children, pineal tumors are several times more likely to occur in males than in females and usually present in the second decade of life.

PATHOLOGY

Over one-half of pineal region tumors are germ cell derived, and only 20 percent are derived from pineal cells (pineocytoma and pineoblastoma). The remainder of pineal region tumors include gliomas of the pineal gland and lesions arising from surrounding structures such as neuroectodermal, mesenchymal, and metastatic tumors; vascular malformations; as well as benign lesions such as lipomas, pineal, and arachnoid cysts (Table 163-1).

Intracranial germ cell tumors arise from developmental nests of primitive totipotential germ cells and are histologically indistinguishable from their counterparts in the gonads that occur in young adults. Germinomas account for almost two-thirds of pineal germ cell tumors, with teratomas being three times less common (Fig. 163-1). Malignant choriocarcinomas, endodermal sinus tumors, and embryonal carcinomas are three times rarer than teratomas. Germ cell tumors frequently have mixed histology, making definitive diagnosis and treatment difficult

TABLE 163-1. Tumors of the Pineal Region

Tumors of germ cell origin
Germinoma
Nongerminoma germ cell tumors (embryonic tissue)
Teratoma
Dermoid
Nongerminoma germ cell tumors (extraembryonic tissue)
Choriocarcinoma
Embryonal carcinoma
Endodermal sinus (yolk sac) tumor
Tumors of pineal parenchymal origin
Pineocytomas
Pineoblastomas
Tumors of support cells and adjacent structures
Astrocytomas
Ependymomas
Choroid plexus papillomas
Meningiomas
Non-neoplastic cystic and vascular lesions
Pineal cysts
Arachnoid cysts
Vascular lesions
Vein of Galen aneurysm
Cavernous malformation

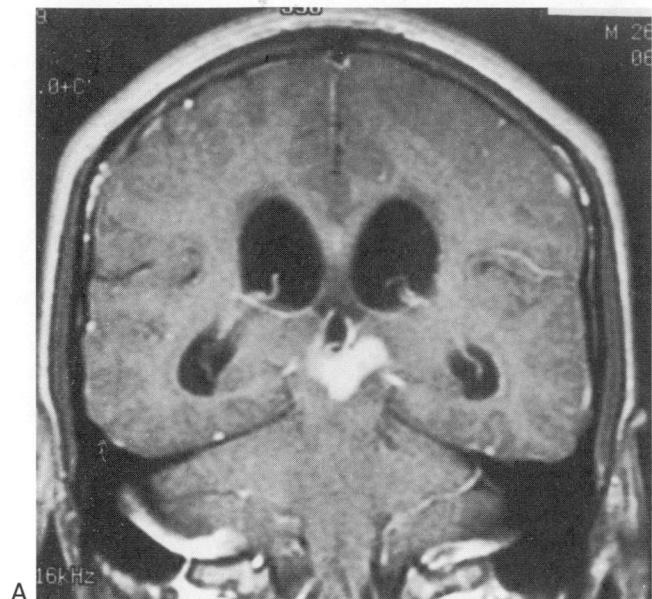
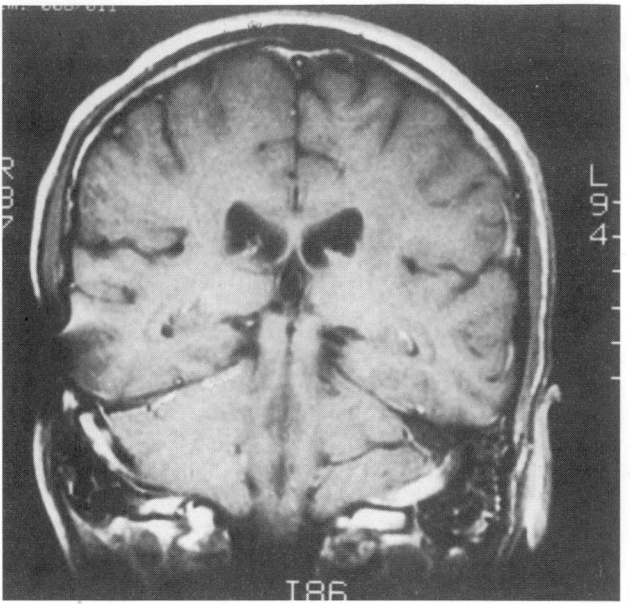

FIG. 163-1. **(A)** Coronal contrast-enhanced MRI of a 22-year-old man with an enhancing pineal region tumor with associated hydrocephalus. **(B)** Patient underwent ventricular shunting and radiation therapy with complete resolution of a stereotactic biopsy–proven germinoma. Note the normal ventricle size and disappearance of the enhancing mass after successful treatment.

(Fig. 163-2). Cerebrospinal fluid (CSF) spread may occur, but systemic metastases without prior surgical intervention are uncommon.

PRESENTING SYMPTOMS

Pineal region tumors may present with a variety of symptoms. However, the deep-seated location and close proximity to CSF outflow pathways adjacent to the midbrain and hypothalamus result in some characteristic syndrome complexes. Many patients present with a vague headache or mental and visual disturbances that make it difficult to diagnose pineal region lesions without an imaging study. A detailed neurologic examination may alert the astute clinician to the possibility of pineal pathology.

Intracranial Hypertension

Obstruction of the aqueduct of Sylvius or tumor extension into the posterior third ventricle results in noncommunicating hydrocephalus. Headaches, lethargy, mental status changes, nausea, and emesis may result. False localizing signs such as an abducens (sixth cranial nerve) nerve paresis with diplopia may develop, and papilledema may be present.

Local Effects

The close proximity of the tectum of the midbrain, lying inferior to the pineal gland, can cause Parinaud syndrome. Failure of upgaze is almost invariable, but other components of the syndrome, loss of convergence, pupillary abnormalities, and retractory nystagmus, occur less frequently. The oculomotor (third cranial nerve) nerve nucleus may be directly affected, and hyperacusis from disturbance of the inferior colliculus can occur with larger lesions. Further tumor expansion may cause vertigo and ataxia from disruption of corticocerebellar pathways and memory problems caused by mammillothalamic tract interruption.

Infiltration Surrounding Structures

The more malignant tumors may infiltrate the adjacent thalamus and cause hemibody sensory changes. Further lateral infiltration may affect the internal capsule and cause paresis, plegia, or

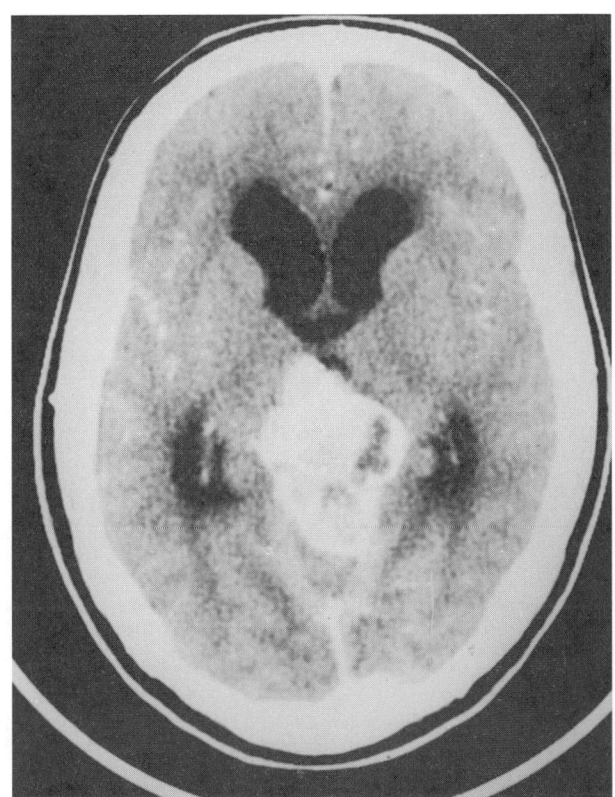

FIG. 163-2. Axial contrast-enhanced CT of a mixed germ cell tumor in the pineal region in a young female patient. There is marked ventriculomegaly from the obstructive hydrocephalus.

even visual field abnormalities. With hypothalamic infiltration, disturbances of water regulation and body temperature, weight gain, somnolence, or precocious puberty may result. Unilateral thalamic involvement can cause contralateral sensory or motor deficits, with bilateral infiltration causing bilateral motor and sensory symptoms.

DIAGNOSTIC STUDIES

Radiology

The advent of computed tomography (CT) and especially magnetic resonance imaging (MRI) has made the diagnosis of such tumors relatively straightforward. Skull films are usually unremarkable; however, the presence of intracranial hypertension or a large (more than 1 cm) calcified pineal mass is distinctly abnormal. Pineal calcification in a child younger than 10 years of age is highly suspicious for a tumor.

While CT demonstrates most lesions, the multiplanar imaging and superior tissue differentiation afforded by MRI makes this modality the diagnostic test of choice. MRI should be obtained with and without intravenous contrast administration. Different signal characteristics may help differentiate between teratomas, lipomas, dermoid tumors, and epidermoid tumors. Teratomas contain a mixture of fat, soft tissue, and calcification (present in teeth) compared with lipomas, which are hypodense on CT and hyperintense on MRI. On MRI, dermoid tumors possess fat and inhomogeneous areas from dermal structures compared with epidermoid tumors, which have wall calcification and intracystic material bearing CSF characteristics. Germ cell tumors tend to have marked homogeneous enhancement.

Infiltration into surrounding structures and tumor dissemination throughout CSF pathways is well demonstrated on MRI. In evaluating the spinal neuraxis for evidence of tumor spread, usually seen with pineoblastoma, spinal MRI is gradually supplanting myelography and postmyelography CT. If CSF tumor dissemination is suspected, spinal MRI with gadolinium should be considered and performed before surgical intervention.

Cerebral angiography may be necessary to diagnose a vascular lesion in the pineal region such as a vein of Galen aneurysm or vascular malformation. Occasionally, angiography is necessary to plan the optimal surgical approach to the pineal region lesion. Magnetic resonance angiography may eventually replace conventional angiography in this role.

Cerebrospinal Fluid Cytology

The close proximity of pineal tumors to the ventricular system may result in meningeal seeding with symptoms of nerve root or spinal cord compression. While less than 10 percent of all pineal region tumors seed the subarachnoid space, up to one-third of pineoblastomas and nongerminomatous germ cell tumors may do so. CSF dissemination portends a poor prognosis. CSF cytology may be useful in the initial evaluation of a patient, both for staging the disease and potentially to obtain a diagnosis. The diagnostic yield from lumbar CSF cytologic examination is greater than from CSF obtained from the ventricles, either by direct ventricular puncture or from accessing a shunt system. However, lumbar puncture is contraindicated in patients with obstructive hydrocephalus in whom there is a clear risk of herniation. If CSF is obtained, by whatever route, it should be carefully analyzed cytologically and for tumor markers. CSF should be obtained prior to any surgical procedure because the spillage of tumor cells at the time of surgery may occur and result in a false-positive cytologic examination result.

TABLE 163-2. Tumor Markers Associated With Pineal Tumors

Tumor Histology	AFP	β-HCG	PLAP
Germinoma	−	−	+
Undifferentiated germ cell tumor	±	±	±
Pineocytoma/pineoblastoma	−	−	−
Endodermal sinus (yolk sac) tumor	+	−	±
Embryonal cell tumor	+	+	±
Choriocarcinoma	−	+	±
Teratoma	−	−	±
Malignant teratoma	±	±	±

Abbreviation: PLAP, placental alkaline phosphatase.

(Modified from Baumgartner JE, Edwards MSB: Pineal tumors. Neurosurg Clin North Am 3:853–62, 1992, with permission.)

Tumor Markers

Pineal region tumors of the germ cell group may produce a variety of oncofetal antigens. α-Fetoprotein (AFP) is a glycoprotein normally produced in the yolk sac, fetal liver, or gastrointestinal tract. Tumors derived from yolk sac elements such as endodermal sinus tumors and embryonal carcinomas may express AFP on immunohistochemical staining and serum and CSF AFP levels may be elevated (Table 163-2). Undifferentiated germ cell tumors and malignant teratomas may also express AFP. Human chorionic gonadotrophin (β-HCG) is secreted by trophoblastic epithelium of the placenta. β-HCG is elevated in choriocarcinoma and embryonal carcinoma and may be present in other undifferentiated germ cell tumors or malignant teratomas. Pure germinomas rarely secrete any markers, although β-HCG can be present in up to 10 percent of germinomas. Placental alkaline phosphatase is a nondiagnostic marker associated with germinomas.

Overall, only 15 to 20 percent of pineal tumors secrete markers. It is unclear whether CSF or serum marker levels are more sensitive. The frequency of mixed histologic types of up to 40 percent with germ cell tumors makes the use tumor markers for diagnosis problematic. The presence of AFP alone, however, does support the diagnosis of a nongerminomatous tumor. A positive or negative β-HCG does not help direct therapy. The main value of these markers is to determine the effect of therapeutic intervention and to help detect early recurrence. There should be an elevated CSF-to-blood ratio in marker levels for pineal tumors, or other pathologic processes associated with elevated serum AFP and β-HCG levels should be suspected.

TREATMENT

Surgery

For many years, surgery for lesions of the pineal region was associated with considerable neurologic morbidity and mortality. Until the 1970s, many neurosurgeons advocated treatment of associated hydrocephalus with ventricular shunting and radiotherapy of the pineal lesion, often without diagnostic tissue. Advances in microneurosurgical techniques, neuroanesthesia, and more optimal neuroimaging in the last two decades have made such an approach unreasonable.

All pineal region tumors should be approached by controlling associated hydrocephalus and obtaining tissue for histologic diagnosis to guide subsequent therapy. The presence of tumor spread into surrounding local structures or into the CSF pathways should be determined by suitable imaging studies and CSF examination (Fig. 163-3).

Hydrocephalus may be treated with either temporary external ventricular drainage if definitive tumor resection with re-estab-

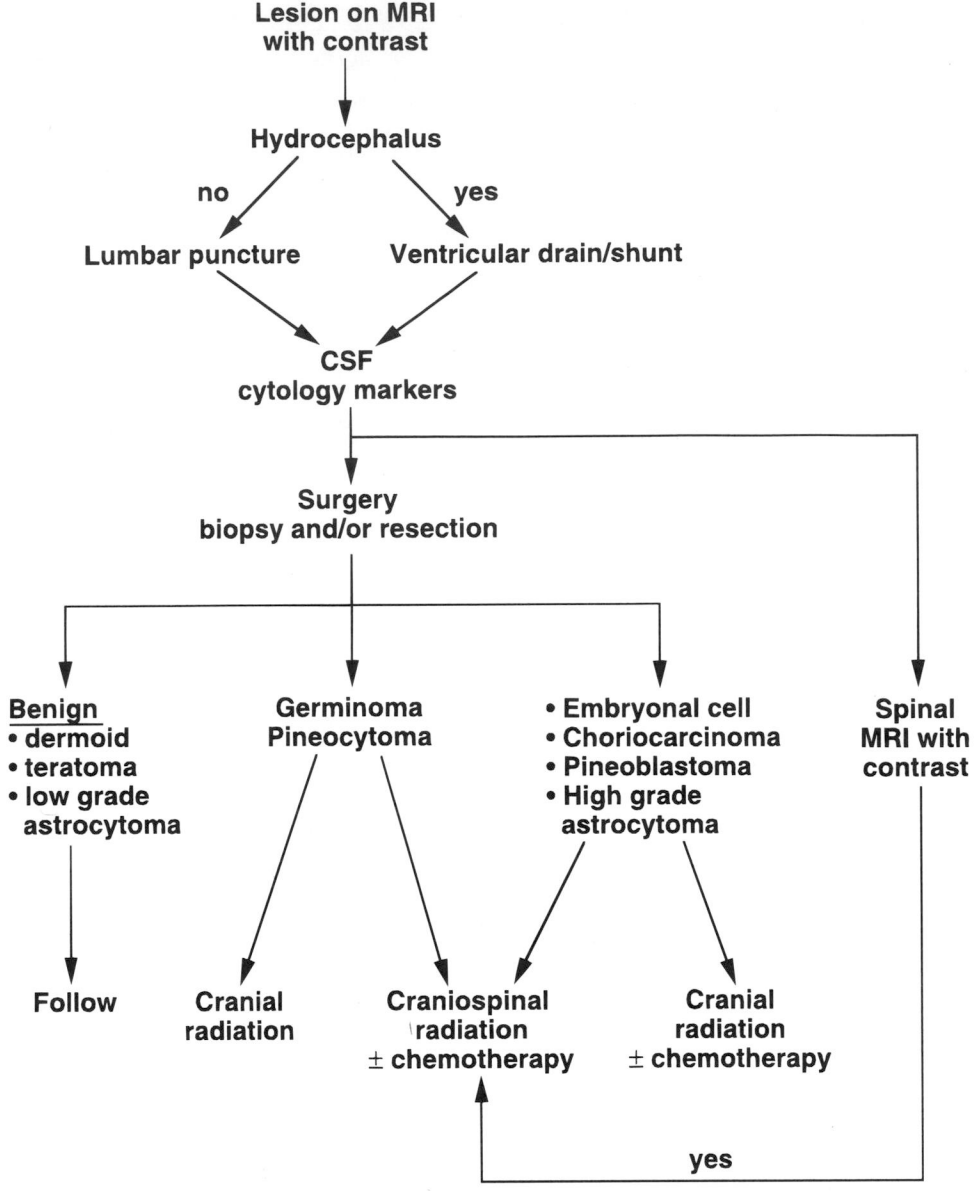

FIG. 163-3. Management plan for pineal region tumors.

lishment of CSF flow is planned or by permanent ventricular shunting if complete tumor removal is not possible. There is a potential for systemic tumor dissemination with CSF diversion.

Histopathologic diagnosis may be obtained by either percutaneous image-directed stereotactic needle biopsy or by a variety of open surgical approaches to the pineal region. The mixed histology of many pineal tumors (15 percent) and the small tissue samples obtained with stereotactic biopsy may result in misdiagnosis or even nondiagnosis, owing to sampling error. Nevertheless, stereotactic biopsy has been proved to be a relatively safe and effective procedure, and when there is documented CSF dissemination or CSF AFP levels are elevated it may be the procedure of choice.

Open biopsy allows simultaneously for more accurate tissue sampling and for more complete tumor resection, particularly if benign pathology is identified (dermoid, teratoma, cyst, or cavernous malformation). Debulking more malignant tumors that are less sensitive to adjuvant therapies when there is no disseminated disease may have a role but is controversial.

Radiation Therapy

Benign tumors should be treated with surgery alone. Radiation therapy has been used diagnostically when a germinoma was suspected, a dose of 20 Gy was given, and the response was measured. If a response was seen, the diagnosis of germinoma was confirmed, and further treatment to a total of 50 to 55 Gy was administered. This approach is no longer indicated now that tissue may be obtained with acceptable morbidity from stereotactic or open biopsy procedures. When patients have already received external beam radiation (50 to 60 Gy) to the primary site, new treatment modalities such as stereotactic radiosurgery, may allow a further boost to the primary site for control of recurrences. The role of radiosurgery for initial treatment of pineal tumors remains to be defined.

Germinomas, astrocytomas, pineocytomas, and pineoblastomas that have not disseminated should receive focal irradiation to the primary site alone. Germinomas in particular are very radiosensitive tumors. Craniospinal irradiation is reserved for those patients with documented CSF spread or for prophylaxis in patients with high-grade malignant tumors, particularly pineoblastomas and nongerminomatous germ cell tumors.

Chemotherapy

The pineal gland has no blood–brain barrier, and chemotherapeutic agents may be useful for a variety of pineal region tumors, especially germ cell tumors. Germinomas respond to chemotherapeutic regimens similar to those used for testicular tumors, such as cisplatin, vinblastine, and bleomycin. Recurrent or disseminated germinomas will respond to chemotherapy, unlike nongerminomatous germ cell tumors, which respond less well. There have been few reports of chemotherapy for pineal parenchymal tumors, but, if pineoblastomas are in fact similar to primitive neuroectodermal tumors, such as medulloblastomas, they may also be expected to respond.

PROGNOSIS

The prognosis for pineal tumors is related to histology. Tumors such as teratomas are benign and can be cured with surgery if resection is complete. Germinomas respond well to radiation therapy, and 10-year survival rates of 75 percent have been reported. By contrast, nongerminomatous germ cell tumors respond less well to treatment, and few patients survive 5 years.

SUMMARY

Pineal tumors are rare and may present with nonspecific symptoms and signs or classic neurologic syndromes. MRI with and without contrast is the imaging technique of choice, and preoperative staging should include CSF cytology and tumor marker analysis. Tissue diagnosis is essential to guide therapeutic intervention and may be accomplished safely by stereotactic or open biopsy procedures. Resection is indicated for benign lesions and may be useful in focal malignant disease. Subsequent radiation or chemotherapy is guided by the histopathology identified and the presence of dissseminated disease.

SUGGESTED READINGS

Allen JC: Controversies in the management of intracranial germ cell tumors. Neurol Clin 9:441–52, 1991
Allen JC, Ho KJ, Packer R: Neoadjuvant chemotherapy for newly diagnosed germ-cell tumors of the central nervous system. J Neurosurg 67:65, 1987
Baumgartner JE, Edwards MSB: Pineal tumors. Neurosurg Clin North Am 3:853, 1992
Casenti L, Colombo F, Pozza F et al: Combined radiosurgery and external radiotherapy for intracranial germinomas. Surg Neurol 34:79, 1990
Chao CK, Lee ST, Lin FJ et al: A multivariate analysis of prognostic factors in management of pineal tumor. Int J Radiat Oncol Biol Phys 27:1185, 1993
Dearnaley DP, O'Hern RP, Whittaker S et al: Pineal and CNS germ cell tumors: Royal Marsden Hospital experience 1962–1987. Int J Radiat Oncol Biol Phys 18:773, 1990
Edwards MSB, Davis RL, Laurent JP: Tumor markers and cytologic features of cerebrospinal fluid. Cancer 56:1773, 1985
Edwards MSB, Hudgins RJ, Wilson CB: Pineal region tumors in children. J Neurosurg 68:689, 1988
Hoffman HJ, Otsubo H, Hendrick EB et al: Intracranial germ cell tumors in children. J Neurosurg 74:545, 1991
Horowitz MB, Hall WA: Central nervous system germinomas. A review. Arch Neurol 48:652, 1991
Latchaw RE, Johnson DW, Kanal E: Primary intracranial tumors: tumors of congenital, pineal, and vascular origin and the phakomatoses. p. 561. In Latchaw RE (ed): MR and CT Imaging of the Head, Neck and Spine. Mosby Year Book, St. Louis, 1991
Linstadt D, Wara WM, Edwards MS et al: Radiotherapy of primary intracranial germinomas: the case against routine craniospinal irradiation. Int J Radiat Oncol Biol Phys 15:291, 1988
Russell DS, Rubenstein LJ: Pathology of Tumors of the Nervous System. 5th Ed. Williams & Wilkins, Baltimore, 1989
Sawaya R, Hawley DK, Tobler WD et al: Pineal and third ventricular tumors. p. 3171. In Youmans JR (ed): Neurological Surgery. 3rd Ed. WB Saunders, Philadelphia, 1990
Schiethauer BW: Neuropathology of pineal region tumors. Clin Neurosurg 32:351, 1985
Stein BM, Fetell MR: Therapeutic modalities for pineal region tumors. Clin Neurosurg 32:445, 1985

164. UNCOMMON BRAIN TUMORS AND INTRACRANIAL CYSTS

PATRICK Y. WEN
DAVID SCHIFF
LIANGGE HSU

In preceding chapters, the common brain tumors as well as some rarer brain tumors were discussed. This chapter describes some miscellaneous uncommon brain tumors and the more common intracranial cystic lesions that may mimic brain tumors clinically.

UNCOMMON BRAIN TUMORS

Ganglion Cell Tumors

Gangliogliomas or gangliocytomas are rare tumors containing large mature neurons. These tumors form a spectrum based on their glial cell content. The term *gangliocytoma* is reserved for lesions consisting of large neoplastic but well-differentiated neurons with minimal glial background; *gangliogliomas* also contain a neoplastic glial component.

Ganglion cell tumors occur most frequently in children and young adults. Eighty percent of these patients are under 30 years of age. They are found most commonly in the temporal lobes but may occur anywhere in the brain. The most common presentation is long-standing epilepsy. Headaches and focal neurologic deficits occur less frequently.

Computed tomographic (CT) and magnetic resonance imaging (MRI) appearances are often nonspecific. Typically they appear as poorly enhancing hypodense lesions (Fig. 164-1). Sometimes there is a contrast-enhancing mural nodule (which may be calcified) associated with a cyst. These tumors are often superficially located and may invade the subarachnoid space.

Ganglion cell tumors are usually well-demarcated and slow growing and are consistent with long survival if surgically accessible. Totally resected tumors do not recur. Even after subtotal resection, the prognosis is good. When gangliogliomas become anaplastic, which occurs in fewer than 10 percent of tumors, changes in the glial component are thought to be responsible. Radiotherapy is usually recommended for unresectable recurrent gangliogliomas and for subtotally resected gangliogliomas with an anaplastic component. It is generally deferred following subtotal resection of low-grade gangliogliomas.

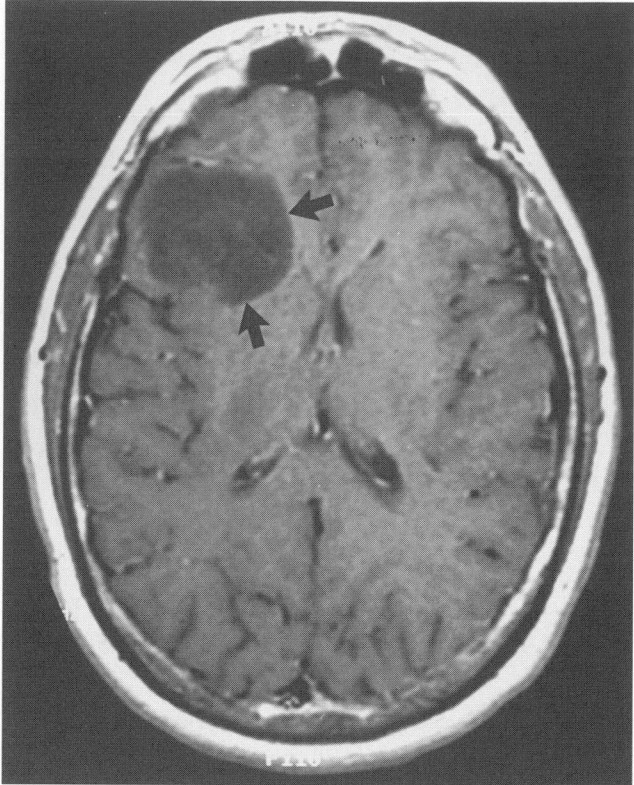

FIG. 164-1.   A 39-year-old man who presented with complex partial seizures. T1-weighted MRI scan shows a nonenhancing hypodense ganglioglioma in the right frontal lobe *(arrows)*.

Choroid Plexus Tumors

Choroid plexus tumors consist of choroid plexus papillomas (CPPs) and choroid plexus carcinomas (CPCs). CPPs histologically resemble normal choroid plexus and probably represent local hamartomatous overgrowths. CPCs are aggressive tumors with variable histologic features, including dense cellularity, mitoses, nuclear pleomorphism, focal necrosis, loss of papillary architecture, and invasion of neural tissue.

CPPs are very uncommon in children and are even rarer among adults. Most series show a male preponderance. In adults, about 80 percent are located in the fourth ventricle, with the remainder arising in the cerebellopontine angle. They are almost invariably associated with hydrocephalus as a result of cerebrospinal fluid (CSF) secretion by the tumor itself and obstruction of the ventricular system. Headache is the most common symptom. On CT scan, these tumors are often calcified and show contrast enhancement (Fig. 164-2); differentiation from ependymoma may be difficult. MRI scan may reveal flow voids, reflecting tumor vascularity.

The treatment for CPP is surgical resection. If completely excised, these tumors are unlikely to recur. Even subtotally resected CPPs have a benign course. Adjuvant radiotherapy is not indicated, but focal external beam radiotherapy may be useful for recurrent tumors that are inoperable. Leptomeningeal seeding may occur with histologically benign tumors.

Approximately 10 percent of all choroid plexus neoplasms are CPCs. Invasiveness usually precludes gross total surgical resection, and leptomeningeal dissemination frequently occurs. Radiotherapy and chemotherapy have not markedly improved prognosis, and most patients succumb within a few years. CPCs may be hard to distinguish from systemic metastasis (especially from lung cancer) to the choroid plexus, which occurs more commonly than CPC.

Central Neurocytoma

This tumor was not recognized until 1982, when Hassoun et al. reported on two patients in their thirties with slowly progressive calcified intraventricular tumors in whom electron microscopic findings of synapses and synaptic vesicles suggested a neuronal lineage. The patients' age and clinical course, intraventricular tumor location, the absence of Homer Wright rosettes, and mature appearance to the cells argued against these being neuroblastomas, an aggressive embryonic parenchymal pediatric tumor. In ensuing years, it became apparent that many tumors previously diagnosed as intraventricular oligodendrogliomas or, less commonly, ependymomas, were actually neurocytomas. About one-half of all intraventricular tumors in adults are central neurocytomas. Similar tumors are rarely found in spinal cord or in brain parenchyma (cerebral neurocytomas).

Most patients with central neurocytomas are in their third or fourth decades, although no age is entirely exempt. The clinical history is usually brief. Most patients have hydrocephalus and symptoms and signs of increased intracranial pressure at presentation. Thirty percent of patients have visual disturbances, and 25 percent have impaired cognitive function. Focal neurologic deficits are uncommon. A few patients have presented with intraventricular hemorrhage.

The typical CT appearance is a slightly hyperdense intraventricular mass, which enhances moderately with contrast (Fig. 164-3). The majority of central neurocytomas are multicystic and calcified, with a broad-based attachment to the superolateral ventricular wall. They are typically found in the lateral or

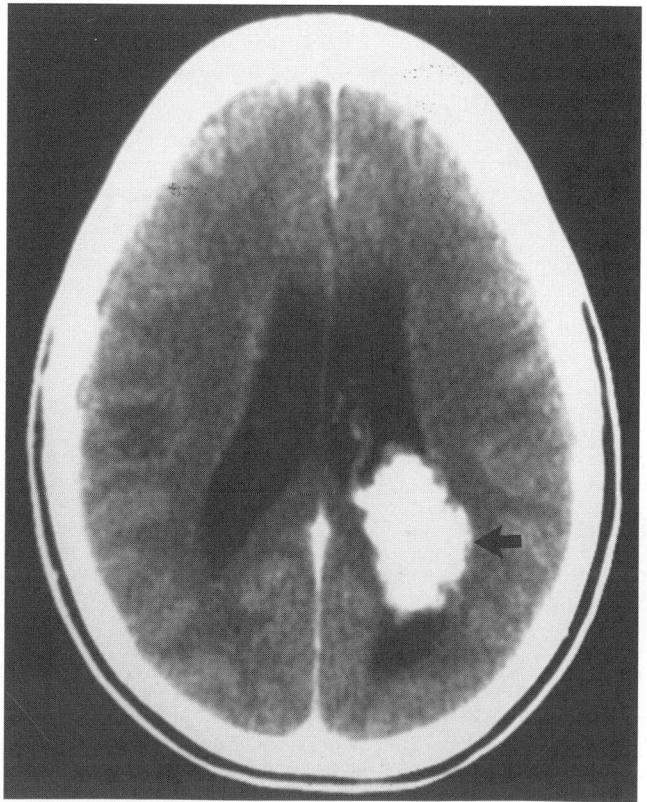

FIG. 164-2.   Axial CT scan with contrast showing a large enhancing choroid plexus papilloma in the right lateral ventricle *(arrow)*.

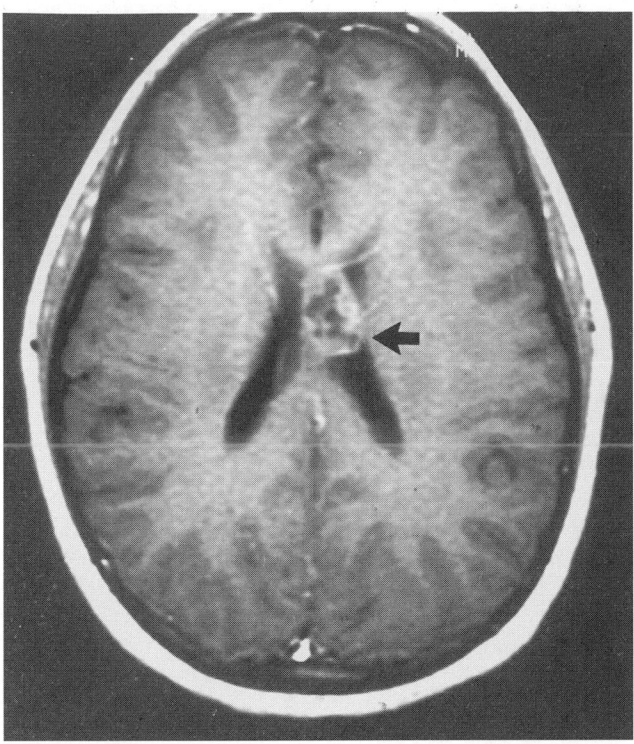

FIG. 164-3. Axial CT scan with contrast showing a slightly enhancing neurocytoma in the left lateral ventricle *(arrow)*. (From Schiff D, Wen P: Uncommon brain tumors. Neurol Clin, 1995 (in press), with permission.)

third ventricle, attached to the septum pellucidum or ventricular wall at the foramen of Monro. They spare the occipital and temporal horns. On MRI, the tumors are slightly hyperintense on both T1- and T2-weighted images and enhance with contrast.

The optimal treatment of these tumors is complete surgical resection. Frequently, however, only subtotal resection is possible. Even a subtotal resection is consistent with long-term survival, since these tumors usually regrow slowly. Reoperation should be considered for symptomatic recurrence. Focal external beam radiotherapy has a role in patients with recurrent or progressive disease. Leptomeningeal dissemination is extremely rare. The role of chemotherapy for central neurocytomas is unknown.

Dysembryoplastic Neuroepithelial Tumors

Like the central neurocytoma, dysembryoplastic neuroepithelial tumor (DNT) was only recently recognized. The specific pathologic features of DNTs include their supratentorial cortical location, the presence of neurons, foci of dysplastic cortical organization, multinodular architecture with components resembling astrocytoma, oligodendroglioma or oligoastrocytoma, and a columnar structure oriented perpendicular to the cortical surface. The histogenesis of these lesions is uncertain, but they may arise from the external granule layer of cortex.

Patients with DNTs usually present with long-standing, often refractory, seizure disorders, which frequently begin during childhood. These patients generally have normal intelligence and stable neurologic deficits. Rarely, mass effect and increased intracranial pressure are present. CT scans typically show a low-density lesion with little or no ring enhancement. When these tumors are superficial, the overlying calvarium may be deformed, a reflection of their slow growth. On MRI, DNTs appear as a T1-weighted hypointense, T2-weighted hyperin-

tense cortically based lesion, which focally expands the cortex. They are usually located either in the temporal or frontal lobes.

Irrespective of treatment, these tumors generally remain stable in size. Thus, the main indication for intervention is palliation of symptoms, particularly epilepsy that is resistant to medication. Surgically accessible lesions may be resected; lesions in eloquent cortex are best observed. There is no indication for radiotherapy.

Dysplastic Ganglioctyoma of the Cerebellum (Lhermitte-Duclos Disease)

This extremely rare and curious entity is characterized pathologically by loss of normal cerebellar cortical architecture and focal thickening of the folia. Light microscopy reveals abnormal hypertrophic ganglion cells, which superficially resemble Purkinje cells, and there is a reduction of the central cerebellar white matter.

This disease is typically diagnosed in adults (average age 34). The most common presentation is a slowly growing cerebellar mass with associated hydrocephalus. Some patients have macrocephaly and mental retardation. It has been found incidentally at autopsy, and rarely it has been associated with sudden death. On CT scan, the lesion is poorly defined and sometimes calcified. MRI shows a nonenhancing, isodense or hypodense lesion on T1-weighted images and alternating bands of signal on T2-weighted images. The only effective treatment is surgical resection, although a few cases have recurred after apparent gross total resection.

Several reports have recently noted an association between Lhermitte-Duclos disease and Cowden's disease, an autosomal dominant syndrome characterized by facial tricholemmomas, acral keratosis, oral papillomatosis, intestinal polyps, and an increased incidence of breast and thyroid cancer. Thus, Lhermitte-Duclos disease may be the central nervous system manifestation of Cowden's disease. Whether Lhermitte-Duclos disease is best considered a hamartoma or neoplasm is uncertain.

Hemangioblastomas

These tumors are most commonly located in the cerebellum, although they may be found in the spinal cord, medulla, and (rarely) the cerebrum. Histologically, they consist of endothelial and stromal cells and closely resemble renal cell carcinoma. About 10 percent of patients have polycythemia from tumor production of erythropoeitin.

Tumors may occur sporadically or as part of the autosomal dominant von Hippel-Lindau syndrome. Patients with von Hippel-Lindau syndrome often have multiple hemangioblastomas, which are frequently asymptomatic. In addition, they may have retinal angiomatosis, renal cell carcinoma, visceral cysts, and adrenal pheochromocytomas. Manifestations of this syndrome are likely to be related to changes in a tumor suppressor gene on chromosome 3. Approximately 23 percent of patients with hemangioblastoma have von Hippel-Lindau syndrome. With more thorough screening and development of gene probes, this incidence may turn out to be an underestimate.

Although hemangioblastomas can occur at any age, they are most commonly found in young and middle-aged adults, in whom they account for 7 percent of posterior fossa tumors. They have a tendency to form cysts with a mural nodule of tumor. The solid tumor nodule enhances homogenously, and flow voids from related blood vessels may be seen with MRI (Fig. 164-4). Hemangioblastomas are relatively well demar-

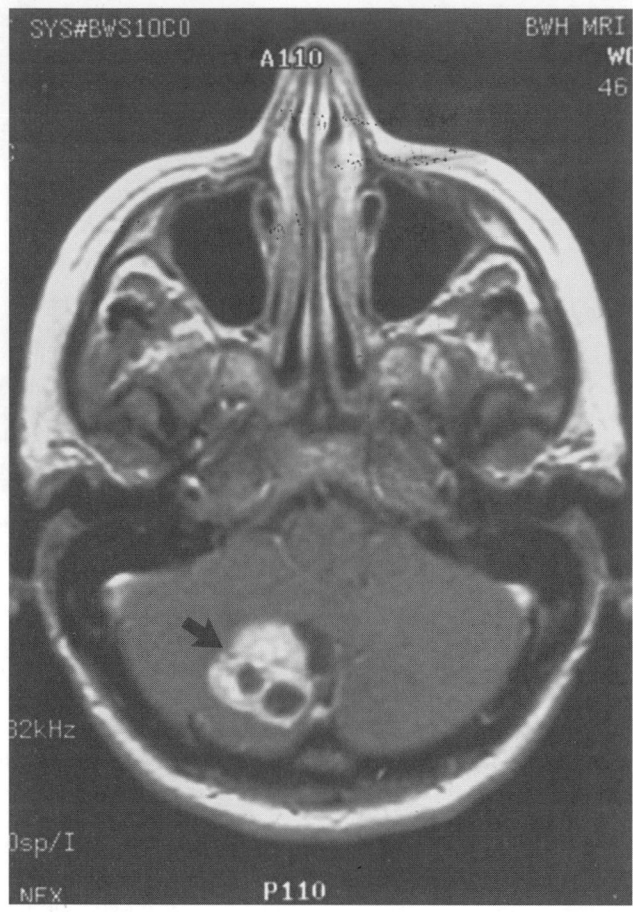

FIG. 164-4. Axial T1-weighted MRI with gadolinium showing cystic contrast-enhancing hemangioblastoma in the right cerebellar hemisphere *(arrow)*.

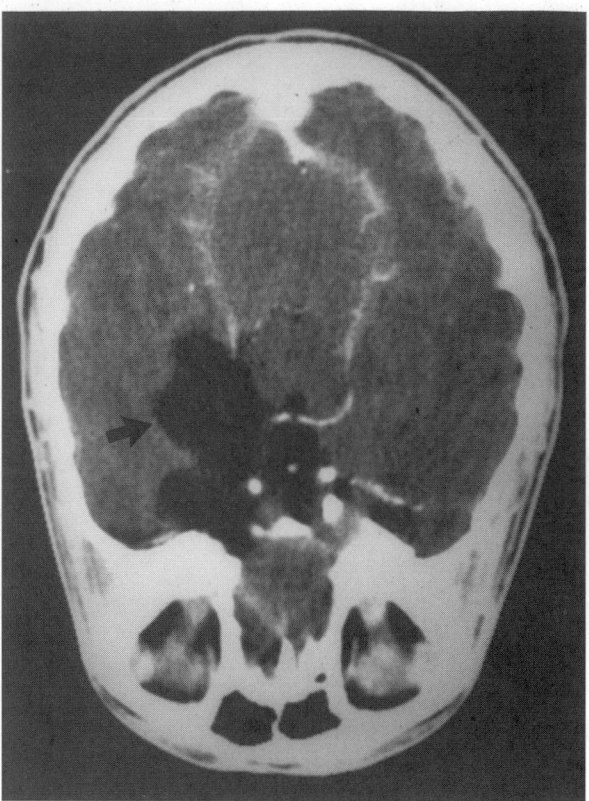

FIG. 164-5. Axial CT scan showing large hypodense epidermoid cyst in the left cerebellopontine angle *(arrow)*. (From Black P, Wen P: Clinical, imaging, and laboratory diagnosis of brain tumors. In Kaye A, Shaw E (eds): Encyclopedia of Brain Tumors. Churchill Livingstone, Edinburgh, 1995, with permission.)

cated, and invasion and remote metastasis are rare. Treatment consists of surgical resection of symptomatic lesions. Gross total resection is generally curative, although patients may develop multiple tumors. Radiotherapy, either fractionated external beam or radiosurgery, may be beneficial for unresectable or progressive residual tumors.

INTRACRANIAL CYSTS

Dermoid and Epidermoid Cysts

These epithelially lined developmental anomalies are thought to arise from inclusion of ectodermal elements during neural tube development. The distinction between dermoids and epidermoids is based on the presence of hair and sweat and sebaceous glands.

Dermoids occur most frequently in the posterior fossa, especially the midline vermis or fourth ventricle. The suprasellar cistern is another common site. Dermoids may produce symptoms from local mass effect, and rupture of their contents into the CSF can produce a fatal granulomatous meningitis. Cerebellar dermoids are sometimes associated with dermal sinuses of the occiput, which can predispose to bacterial meningitis. On CT scan, they appear as low-density midline lesions; on MRI scan, they are identical to lipomas with short T1- and T2-weighted values and minimal contrast enhancement. Treatment of symptomatic dermoids is surgical, although incompletely resected cysts may gradually recur.

Intracranial epidermoid cysts are more common than dermoids and occur most frequently in the cerebellopontine angle and petrous bone. The middle cranial fossa is also a common site. Patients may experience headaches or neurologic deficits from the mass effect of the cysts. Rarely, they develop recurrent aseptic meningitis from leakage of cyst contents. On CT scan, they appear as low-attenuation lobulated masses in characteristic locations (Fig. 164-5). The density is identical to CSF, making visualization of these lesions sometimes difficult. On MRI scan, they appear as extra-axial masses with prolonged T1- and T2-weighted values. As with dermoids, malignant transformation into carcinoma has rarely been reported. Treatment is surgical, although their tendency to insinuate along cranial nerves and tissue planes may make gross total resection of posterior fossa epidermoid cysts impossible. Postoperative aseptic meningitis from cyst leakage generally responds to steroids.

Colloid Cysts

These are spheric cysts located between the forniceal columns in the roof of the third ventricle. They account for approximately 1 percent of intracranial mass lesions. The incidence of colloid cysts may be increasing as more patients with small, asymptomatic cysts are found on routine neuroimaging for unrelated symptoms. The derivation of colloid cysts is uncertain, but they probably represent a developmental malformation and not a true neoplasm. Histologically they have an outer fibrous layer and an inner epithelium of ciliated or mucin-producing cells. Because of their location, even relatively small lesions may block the foramen of Monro, producing hydrocephalus.

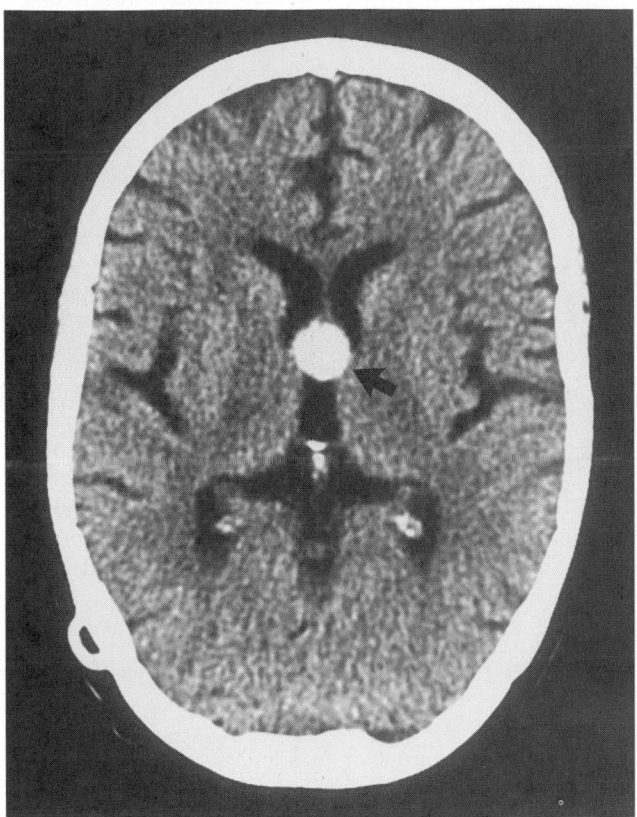

FIG. 164-6. Axial CT scan showing hyperdense midline colloid cyst in the region of the third ventricle *(arrow)*. The patient had a history of headaches and required ventriculoperitoneal shunting for hydrocephalus.

Men and women are affected with equal frequency. They can occur at any age but usually become symptomatic in the third to the sixth decades. Most symptomatic patients present with headaches, papilledema, and mental status and gait abnormalities related to hydrocephalus. The classic clinical description of intermittent headaches and drop attacks occurs in only one-third of patients.

Colloid cysts are iso- or hyperdense on precontrast CT and do not enhance (Fig. 164-6). On MRI scan, they may be hyperintense or have a hypointense center on T2-weighted MRI. With either modality, their location, shape, and lack of enhancement are virtually pathognomonic.

Patients with small asymptomatic colloid cysts without evidence of hydrocephalus may be followed by serial examinations and neuroimaging studies. Treatment of symptomatic lesions consists of surgical excision. This is curative but technically challenging, given the intimate relationship to the fornices. Ventricular peritoneal shunts may also be necessary in patients with hydrocephalus.

Arachnoid Cysts

These are intra-arachnoid collections of CSF, which account for 1 percent of intracranial mass lesions. Most of these cysts are congenital, and 75 percent of symptomatic arachnoid cysts occur in children.

Arachnoid cysts result from accumulation of CSF within a split or duplicated arachnoid memebrane. CSF may accumulate as a result of secretion by arachnoid cells lining the cyst or be trapped as a result of unidirectional flow into the cyst. As the cyst increases in volume, it may produce symptoms by com-

pressing adjacent brain or by obstructing CSF flow. The cysts usually contain clear CSF with normal cell count and protein. Occasionally, the protein content may be elevated if the cyst does not communicate freely with the CSF pathways. Xanthochromia may result from hemorrhage into the cyst. A markedly elevated protein level or pleocytosis should suggest the possibility of a cystic neoplasm rather than an arachnoid cyst.

Arachnoid cysts may arise from any part of the nervous system where arachnoid is found. The most common site is the sylvian fissure where one-half of all arachnoid cysts are located. Other sites include the cerebral convexity, interhemispheric fissure, suprasellar cistern, quadrigeminal cistern, cerebellopontine angle, midline of the posterior fossa, and the spine. The precise symptoms depend on the location of the cysts. Arachnoid cysts involving the sylvian fissure are more common in men and typically present with headaches, seizures, and less commonly with focal neurologic deficits. Subdural hematomas may occur following relatively minor head trauma. Suprasellar cysts usually cause obstructive hydrocephalus and occasionally visual and endocrine dysfunction. Quadrigeminal cysts and posterior fossa cysts may also cause hydrocephalus, as well as other brainstem symptoms. The incidence of patients with asymptomatic arachnoid cysts is increasing as more patients undergo neuroimaging procedures for unrelated symptoms.

The diagnosis of arachnoid cysts may be made either by CT or MRI. On CT scans, arachnoid cysts appear as nonenhancing, hypodense, extra-axial masses with smooth borders. Large cysts may compress adjacent brain and erode the overlying portion of the skull. Metrizamide CT cisternography and ventriculography may show delayed uptake of contrast in those cysts that communicate with the subarachnoid space. MRI is the radiographic

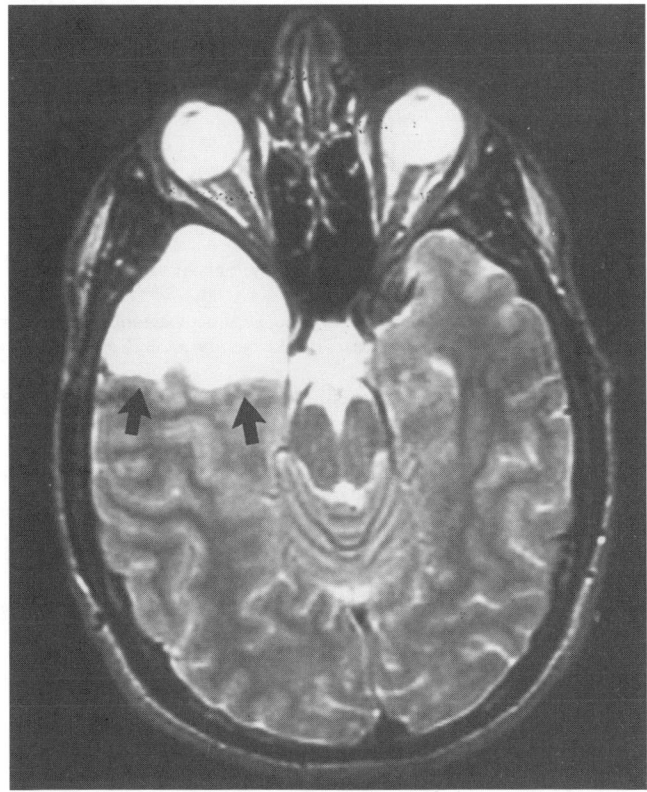

FIG. 164-7. Axial T2-weighted MRI scan showing large right middle cranial fossa arachnoid cyst, anterior to the temporal lobe *(arrow)*. The cyst fluid typically has the same signal intensity as CSF and appears as a high signal on T2-weighted images.

study of choice for arachnoid cysts. It allows better visualization of the relationship of the cysts to surrounding neural structures and the underlying pathology of the cyst. On MRI scan, the cyst fluid usually has the same signal characteristics as CSF (low density on T1-weighted and high density on T2-weighted images) (Fig. 164-7). The differential diagnosis of arachnoid cysts includes chronic subdural hygromas, infarcts, low-grade gliomas, gangliogliomas, epidermoids, and cerebellar hemangioblastomas.

The treatment depends on whether the cysts are producing symptoms. Asymptomatic cysts can be followed with serial examinations and imaging studies. Surgical intervention is indicated in patients with symptoms of increased intracranial pressure, seizures, focal neurologic deficits, or cognitive impairment. The surgical options include craniotomy for partial or complete cystectomy, fenestration into the subarachnoid space, or cyst-peritoneal shunting. Needle aspiration usually provides only temporary benefit and is not a good long-term treatment option.

SUGGESTED READINGS

Albrecht S, Haber RM, Goodman JC, Duvic M: Cowden syndrome and Lhermitte-Duclos disease. Cancer 70:869–76, 1992

Ashley DG, Zee C-S, Chandrasoma PT, Segall HD: Lhermitte-Duclos disease: CT and MR findings. J Comput Assist Tomogr 14:984–7, 1990

Burger PC, Scheithauer BW, Vogel FS: Surgical Pathology of the Nervous System and Its Coverings. Churchill Livingstone, New York, 1991

Camacho A, Kelly PI: Colloid cysts of the third ventricle. pp. 36.1–10. In Rengachary SS, Wilkins RH (eds): Principles of Neurosurgery. Wolfe, London, 1994.

Celli P, Scarpinati M, Nardacci B et al: Gangliogliomas of the cerebral hemispheres: report of 14 cases with long-term follow-up and review of the literature. Acta Neurochir (Wien) 125:52–7, 1993

Cirillo SF, Edwards MSB: Intracranial arachnoid cysts. pp. 51.1–11. In Rengachary SS, Wilkins RH (eds): Principles of Neurosurgery. Wolfe, London, 1994.

Daumas-Duport C: Dysembryoplastic neuroepithelial tumours. Brain Pathol 3: 283–95, 1993

Daumas-Duport C, Scheithauer BW, Chodkiewicz JP et al: Dysembryoplastic neuroepithelial tumor: a surgically curable tumor of young patients with intractable partial seizures. Neurosurgery 23:545–56, 1988

Dohrmann GJ, Collins JC: Choroid plexus carcinoma. J Neurosurg 43:225–32, 1975

Haddad SF, Moore SA, Menezes AH et al: Gangliogliomas: 13 years of experience. Neurosurgery 31:171–8, 1992

Hassoun J, Gambarelli D, Grisoli F et al: Central neurocytoma: an electron-microscopic study of two cases. Acta Neuropathol (Berl) 56:151–6, 1982

Hassoun J, Soylemezoglu F, Gambarelli D et al: Central neurocytoma: a synopsis of clinical and histological features. Brain Pathol 3:297–306, 1993

Krouwer HGJ, Davis RL, McDermott MW et al: Gangliogliomas: a clinicopathological study of 25 cases and review of the literature. J Neurooncol 17: 139–54, 1993

Lang FL, Epstein FJ, Ransohoff J et al: Central nervous system gangliogliomas. Part 2: clinical outcome. J Neurosurg 79:867–73, 1993

McGirr SJ, Ebersold MJ, Scheithauer B et al: Choroid plexus papillomas: long-term follow-up of a surgically treated series. J Neurosurg 69:843–9, 1988

Miller DC, Lang FF, Epstein FJ: Central nervous system gangliogliomas. Part 1: pathology. J Neurosurg 79:859–66, 1993

Nakagawa K, Aoki Y, Sakata K et al: Radiation therapy of well-differentiated neuroblastoma and central neurocytoma. Cancer 72:1350–5, 1993

Neuman HPH, Eggert HR, Weigel K et al: Hemangioblastomas of the central nervous system: a 10-year study with special reference to von Hippel-Lindau syndrome. J Neurosurg 70:24–30, 1989

Padberg GW, Schor JDL, Vielvoye GJ et al: Lhermitte-Duclos disease and Cowden disease: a single phakomatosis. Ann Neurol 29:517–23, 1991

Russell DS, Rubinstein LJ: Pathology of Tumors of the Nervous System. Williams & Wilkins, Baltimore, 1989

Wichmann W, Schubiger O, von Deimling A et al: Neuroradiology of central neurocytoma. Neuroradiology 33:143–8, 1991

165. BRAIN METASTASES

ROY A. PATCHELL

Brain metastases are neoplasms that originate in tissues outside the brain and spread secondarily to the brain. Metastases to the intracranial structures and cranium are the most common metastatic neurologic complications of systemic cancer. Although brain metastases usually indicate a poor prognosis for the patient, advances in treatment have made it possible to reverse most of the symptoms of brain metastases and give patients an extension of useful life. With proper therapy, less than one-half of all patients with brain metastases die as a result of their brain disease.

INCIDENCE

Modern neuroimaging techniques and autopsy studies on patients with cancer have demonstrated that metastases to the brain, as a group, are the most common intracranial tumors, considerably outnumbering primary brain tumors in the general population. Twenty to 40 percent of patients with cancer develop brain metastases, and there are as many as 170,000 new instances of brain metastases each year in the United States. The frequency may be higher in the future with improvement in the ability of magnetic resonance imaging (MRI) to detect small tumors. The real incidence of brain metastases may also be increasing because of longer survival times of patients with cancer in general.

The histologic type of the primary tumor strongly influences the frequency and pattern of intracranial spread (Table 165-1). In adults, the most common sources of brain metastases are the lung, breast, gastrointestinal tract, genitourinary tract, and skin (malignant melanoma). In patients younger than 21 years old, brain metastases arise most often from sarcomas (osteogenic sarcoma, rhabdomyosarcoma, and Ewing sarcoma) and germ cell tumors.

METHOD OF SPREAD AND DISTRIBUTION

Most tumor cells reach the brain by hematogenous spread, usually through the arterial circulation. Most commonly, the metas-

TABLE 165-1. Frequency of Metastatic Brain Tumors by Primary Site

Tumor Type	Percentage
Lung	64
Squamous cell	30
Adenocarcinoma	17
Small cell	15
Large cell	2
Breast	14
Unknown primary	8
Melanoma	4
Colorectal	3
Hypernephroma	2
Other	5

tasis originates in the lung from either a primary lung tumor or from a metastasis to the lung. In a few cases, tumor cells may reach the brain via the vertebral venous system (Batson's plexus).

Within the brain, metastases are most commonly found in the area directly beneath the gray-white junction. The predominance of metastases at this site is due to a change in the size of blood vessels at this point; the narrowed vessels act as a trap for emboli. Brain metastases also tend to be more common at the terminal "watershed areas" of arterial circulation (the zones on the border of or between the territories of the major cerebral vessels). The distribution of metastases among the large subdivisions of the central nervous system follows roughly the relative weight of and blood flow to each area. Therefore, approximately 80 percent of brain metastases are located in the cerebral hemispheres, 15 percent in the cerebellum, and 5 percent in the brainstem.

Recent experience with MRI shows that the frequency of multiple metastases is higher than was previously believed. Approximately two-thirds to three-fourths of patients with brain metastases have multiple lesions. The phrase *single brain metastasis* refers to an apparent single cerebral lesion; no implication is made regarding the extent of cancer elsewhere in the body. On the other hand, the phrase *solitary brain metastasis* is used properly to describe the relatively rare occurrence of a single brain metastasis that is the only known site of metastatic cancer in the body. Metastases from colon, breast, and renal cell carcinoma are often single, whereas malignant melanoma and lung cancer have a greater tendency to produce multiple cerebral lesions.

CLINICAL PRESENTATION

Metastases to the brain are usually symptomatic, and more than two-thirds of patients with brain metastases have some neurologic symptoms during the course of their illness. Over 80 percent of brain metastases are discovered *after* the diagnosis of systemic cancer has been made.

The clinical presentation of brain metastases is similar to that of other mass lesions in the brain (Table 165-2). Headache is a common presenting symptom, which may be followed after an interval of days or weeks by other focal symptoms or signs. Seizures, either focal or generalized, occur in approximately 10 percent of patients at presentation and are more common in patients with multiple metastases. Abnormalities of higher mental functions may take the form of a nonfocal encephalopathy (1 to 2 percent of patients with metastases) or may relate to localized dysfunction (e.g., aphasia). Focal weakness is second only to headache in frequency as a presenting symptom. Five to 10 percent of patients may present with acute neurologic symptoms caused by hemorrhage into the tumor or by cerebral

infarction from embolic or compressive occlusion of a blood vessel. Because the signs and symptoms related to cerebral lesions are varied, the presence of brain metastases should be suspected in all patients with known systemic cancer in whom new neurologic findings develop.

DIAGNOSIS

The best diagnostic test for brain metastases is contrast-enhanced MRI. Contrast-enhanced MRI is more sensitive than either enhanced computed tomographic (CT) scanning (including double-dose delayed contrast) or unenhanced MRI in detecting lesions in patients who may have intracranial metastases (Fig. 165-1). For both CT scans and MRI, multiplicity of lesions is a useful finding that usually distinguishes metastases from gliomas or other primary tumors. Because the treatment is different, single metastases must be carefully distinguished from primary brain tumors (benign or malignant), abscesses, and cerebral infarcts and hemorrhages. A biopsy may be needed to establish the diagnosis.

TREATMENT

Natural History

Brain metastases are associated with a poor prognosis, regardless of treatment. Untreated patients have a median survival of only about 1 month, and nearly all untreated patients die as a direct result of the brain tumor.

Newly Diagnosed Brain Metastases

A variety of treatments are available for patients with intracranial metastases. Corticosteroids, radiotherapy, and surgical therapy all have an established place in treatment. Chemotherapy is also useful for treating some patients with chemosensitive tumors. Several factors must be considered when determining the ideal treatment for each patient, including the extent of systemic disease, the patient's neurologic status at the time of diagnosis, and the number and sites of metastases. An approach to the patient with a suspected brain metastasis is given in Figure 165-2.

Corticosteroids. Most patients with brain metastases should be started on corticosteroid therapy at the time of diagnosis. For most tumors, steroids are not tumoricidal but act to reduce symptoms. The mechanism of action of corticosteroids is not completely understood, although a reduction in the edema surrounding the metastatic tumors is a frequent effect. More than 70 percent of patients improve symptomatically after starting steroid therapy. Symptoms reflecting generalized neurologic dysfunction or brain edema respond more consistently to treatment than do focal symptoms such as hemiparesis. The clinical effects of steroids are noticeable within 6 to 24 hours after the first dose and reach maximum effect in 3 to 7 days. The median survival of patients treated with steroids alone is approximately 2 months.

Radiotherapy. Whole-brain radiotherapy (WBRT) is the treatment of choice for most patients with brain metastases. WBRT increases the median survival to 3 to 6 months. Data from large retrospective studies have shown that more than one-half of patients treated with WBRT die ultimately of progressive systemic cancer and not as a direct result of brain metasta-

TABLE 165-2. Symptoms and Signs of Cerebral Metastases

Symptoms	Percentage of Patients	Signs	Percentage of Patients
Headache	50	Hemiparesis	62
Focal weakness	40	Impaired cognition	75
Behavioral and mental change	35	Unilateral sensory loss	25
Seizures	12	Papilledema	11
Ataxia	20	Ataxia	20
Aphasia	10	Aphasia	16

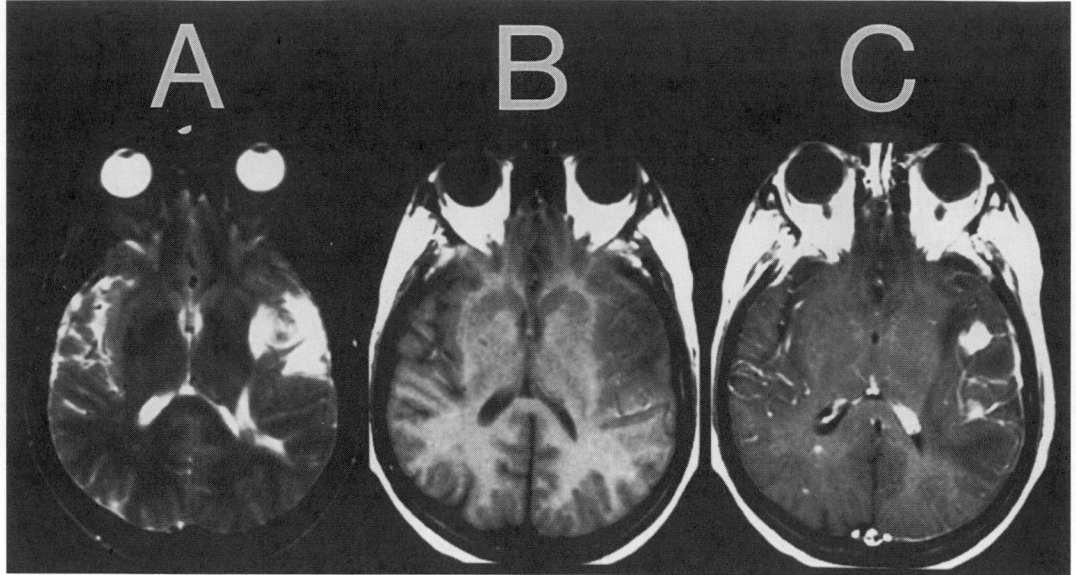

FIG. 165-1. Three MRI scans of the same anatomic level of a patient with brain metastases. **(A)** T2-weighted image showing edema in the right temporal lobe. **(B)** An unenhanced T1-weighted study showing a mass in the right temporal area and no other definite lesions. **(C)** A gadolinium contrast–enhanced scan showing the right temporal lobe mass and two additional lesions in the left occipital area.

ses. More favorable outcomes are associated with Karnofsky performance scores of 70 percent or above, absent or controlled primary tumor, patient age less than 60 years, and metastatic spread limited to the brain (true solitary metastasis).

Unfortunately, there is no consensus on the optimum radiation dose and schedule for the treatment of brain metastases. The best available data on the effect of dose and schedule for the treatment of brain metastases comes from several large-scale multi-institutional trials conducted by the Radiation Therapy Oncology Group. These studies have shown that there is no significant difference in the frequency and duration of response for conventional once-per-day radiation schedules with total radiation doses ranging from 2,000 cGy over 1 week to 5,000 cGy over 4 weeks. Regimens of 1,000 cGy in a single dose or 1,200 cGy in two doses were less satisfactory. Currently, typical radiation treatment schedules for brain metastases consist of short courses (7 to 15 days) of whole-brain irradiation using relatively high doses per single daily fraction (150 to 400 cGy/day) with total doses in the range of 3,000 to 5,000 cGy. Such schedules minimize the duration of treatment while still delivering adequate amounts of radiation to the tumor. Increased focal radiation to the tumor site in the brain has also not been demonstrated to be beneficial. A recent retrospective study has shown that giving a boost dose to the tumor site is no better than WBRT alone in preventing neurologic recurrences or increasing survival.

Radiotherapy has complications. In the short term, patients may have a transient worsening of symptoms while receiving therapy. Many physicians believe that maintaining patients on steroids during radiotherapy will minimize radiotherapeutic complications, although conclusive proof of this has not been produced. The long-term neurologic side effects of radiotherapy are usually not a significant issue in the treatment of patients with brain metastases because of the relatively short survival of these patients. However, some reports have suggested that over 10 percent of long-term survivors (more than 12 months) will develop symptoms such as dementia, ataxia, and urinary

incontinence. In these patients, imaging studies show cortical atrophy and hyperdense white matter changes. Although the pathogenesis of such alterations is unknown, it has been speculated that high-dose/large-fractionation schedules may be a factor. Therefore, in patients with anticipated long survivals, a more prolonged course of radiotherapy with smaller doses per fraction should probably be used. A reasonable schedule for patients with a good prognosis would be a total dose of 4,500 to 5,000 cGy given in fractions of no more than 200 cGy.

Surgery. Surgical therapy is usually not an option for most patients with brain metastases because of the presence of unresectable multiple lesions or extensive systemic cancer. In the subgroup of patients whose only metastasis is in the brain, however, death is more likely to be caused by the brain metastasis than by progressive systemic disease. Therefore, in patients with controlled systemic cancer in whom brain metastases develop, the treatment of the brain disease is the factor that will most influence the length of survival. In this group, the question of more aggressive therapy, particularly surgery, for the brain metastases is usually raised. Several advances over the past 20 years have decreased the risks associated with the surgical approach. Safer anesthesia, the widespread use of corticosteroids, the development of modern noninvasive cranial imaging technology, and the introduction of stereotactic surgery have been foremost among these changes.

Despite the possible advantages of surgical treatment, until recently, the role of surgery was unclear because of an absence of controlled trials. Many uncontrolled surgical series demonstrated longer survival rates for surgically treated patients than for nonrandomized or historical controls treated with WBRT alone.

Two published, prospective randomized trials have assessed the value of surgical removal of single brain metastases. In a prospective randomized trial performed at the University of Kentucky, 48 patients with known systemic cancer were treated with either biopsy of the suspected brain metastasis plus WBRT

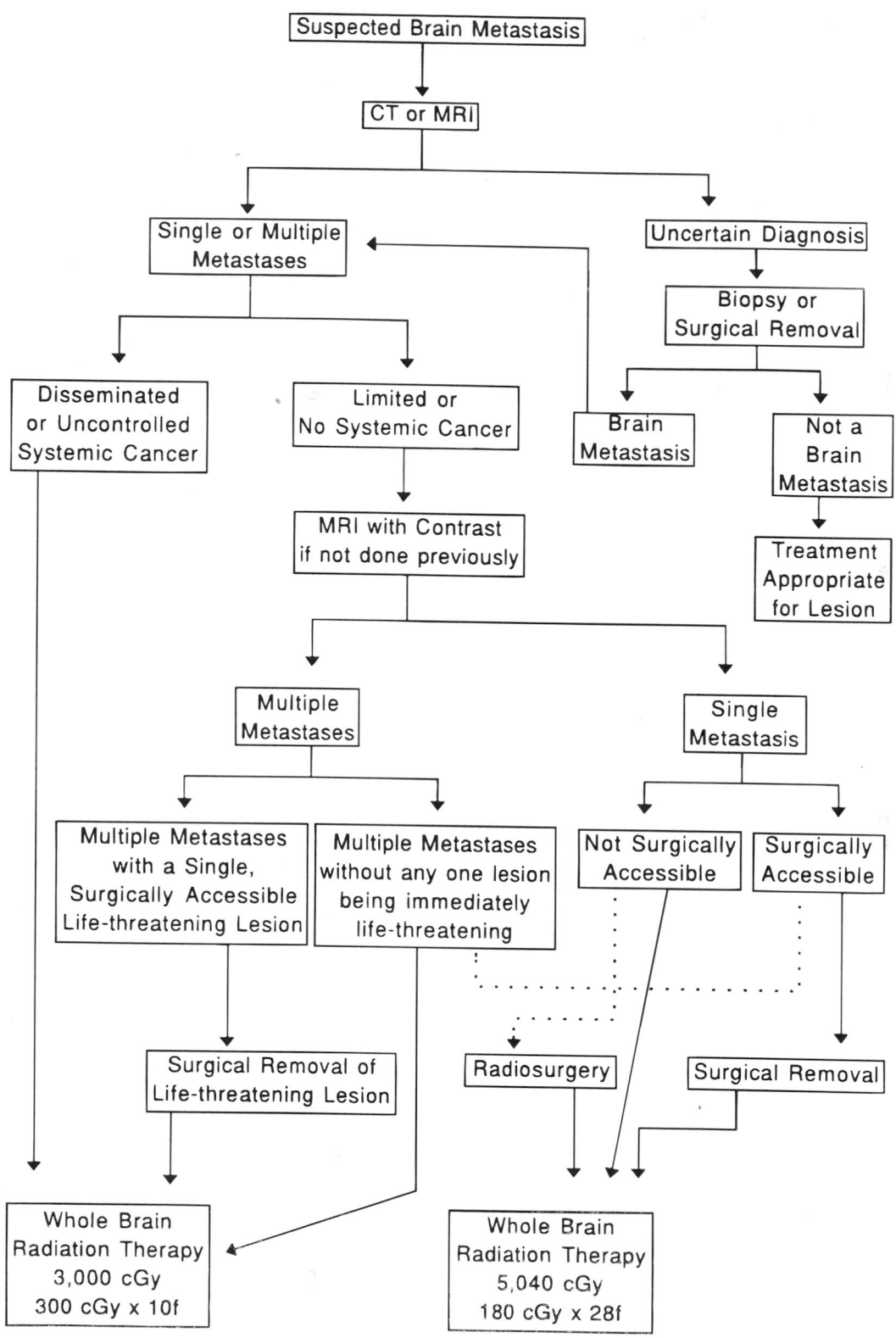

FIG. 165-2. An approach to the patient with suspected brain metastasis. Dashed lines indicate plausible but unproven therapies.

or complete surgical resection of the metastasis plus WBRT. The radiation doses were the same in both groups, consisting of a total dose of 3,600 cGy given as 12 daily fractions of 300 cGy each. A statistically significant increase in overall survival time was found in the surgical group (40 weeks versus 15 weeks), and a significantly smaller proportion of surgically treated patients died of neurologic causes. In addition, the time to recurrence of brain metastases and duration of functional independence were significantly longer in the group treated with surgical resection. The 1-month mortality rate was 4 percent in each group, indicating that the surgical procedure itself did not contribute to mortality rates. An important finding was that, despite screening with both contrast-enhanced MRI and CT scanning before patients were entered into the study, 6 of 54 (11 percent) patients with a known diagnosis of systemic malignancy were found *not* to have metastatic brain tumors when tissue was obtained at biopsy or at attempted resection. The nonmetastatic lesions consisted of three astrocytomas, two abscesses, and one sterile inflammatory lesion.

A second randomized study, conducted as a multi-institutional trial in the Netherlands, evaluated 63 patients randomized either to complete surgical resection plus WBRT or to WBRT alone. The WBRT schedules were the same for both treatment arms and consisted of 4,000 cGy given in a nonstandard fractionation scheme of 200 cGy twice per day for 2 weeks (10 treatment days). Survival was significantly longer in the surgical group (10 months versus 6 months), and a nonsignificant trend toward longer duration of functional independence was seen in the surgically treated patients. No data concerning recurrence of brain metastases were given. The 1-month mortality rates were 9 percent in the group treated with surgery and 0 percent in the group treated with WBRT alone.

Although diagnostic biopsies were not obtained in the group treated with WBRT alone, 1 patient (of 31) in that arm of the study was later found to have a malignant glioma when surgery was performed on the presumed metastatic brain lesion after it had progressed. The tumors of all 32 patients in the surgery group were verified as metastatic by tissue studies at operation. Two other patients were randomized into the study but excluded from the final analysis because they were found not to have metastatic tumors before the start of treatment. In all, of 65 patients, 3 (5 percent) did not have metastatic tumors.

The results from the two randomized trials clearly show that surgical resection is of benefit in selected patients. Surgical therapy plus postoperative WBRT is now the treatment of choice for patients with surgically accessible single brain metastases. However, WBRT alone remains the standard treatment for most patients with brain metastases. Single metastases occur in approximately one-third of patients. Unfortunately, nearly one-half of the patients in this group are not candidates for surgery because of inaccessibility of the tumor, extensive systemic disease, and other factors. Therefore, at most, only 15 to 20 percent of all patients with brain metastases will benefit from surgical resection. The rest should be treated with WBRT, although, stereotactic radiosurgery may be used to treat multiple metastases and may also have a place in the treatment of single brain metastases (see below).

The best results with surgery are achieved in those patients with a single surgically accessible lesion and either no remaining systemic disease (true solitary metastasis) or with controlled systemic cancer limited to the primary site only. One study suggested that survival rates are significantly increased for patients undergoing resection of brain metastases from nonsmall cell lung carcinoma if the primary lung disease is also completely resected. No correlation was demonstrated between survival rates and initial cancer stage per se. Also, surgical treatment may be indicated for those patients without known systemic cancer (to obtain a tissue diagnosis) and for patients for whom death is imminent because of impending cerebral herniation.

SURGERY FOR MULTIPLE LESIONS.   The efficacy of surgery in the management of multiple metastases remains to be demonstrated. Two published retrospective studies reached opposite conclusions regarding the safety and efficacy of surgical removal of more than one brain metastasis. A study from M. D. Anderson Cancer Center compared patients with multiple metastases who underwent resection of all their brain metastases with patients with multiple metastases who underwent resection of some but not all of their brain tumors. A further comparison was made with patients with single metastases who were treated with complete resection plus WBRT. The authors found that the group with completely resected multiple metastases did relatively well (median survival 14 months); their survival rates were similar to those of the group treated by resection of a single metastasis (median survival 14 months). The patients who did not undergo excision of all their brain tumors did less well (median survival 6 months). The 30-day mortality rate for the group with multiple metastases was only 4 percent. No comparison was made with patients treated with WBRT alone (the standard treatment for multiple metastases).

A second retrospective study, performed at the University of Colorado, reported a surgical series containing 18 patients with multiple metastases and 28 patients with single metastases. The group with multiple metastases had a median survival of 5 months; those with single metastases had a median survival of 12 months. For both groups combined, only 50 percent of patients had complete resections, and the percentage of complete resections in the multiple metastases group was not reported. The 30-day mortality rate in both groups was 0 percent.

The results of the studies cited above suggest that the postoperative morbidity and mortality rates for patients with multiple metastases treated with surgery are relatively low and are comparable to those reported for patients with single surgically resected metastases. However, it is not possible to draw a firm conclusion regarding the efficacy of surgery for multiple metastases from the studies published to date.

POSTOPERATIVE RADIOTHERAPY.   A controversy remains regarding whether postoperative radiotherapy should be given as WBRT (as opposed to focal radiation) or whether radiotherapy is necessary at all after complete resection of a single metastasis. There is no doubt that radiation therapy, when given as the only treatment for brain metastases, results in longer survival times. Postoperative WBRT is believed by some to be beneficial for treating residual tumor in the operative site or at other sites in the brain. However, brain metastases tend to be discrete masses that are theoretically capable of being totally removed. Although it is possible that other undetected microscopic metastases may exist elsewhere in the brain, this contention has never been proved either by autopsy analysis or by clinical studies (retrospective or prospective).

The usefulness of postoperative WBRT has not yet been tested in a randomized trial; however, several nonrandomized retrospective reports have compared surgery plus postoperative WBRT to surgery alone in the management of single brain metastases. The retrospective studies do not firmly establish the efficacy of postoperative WBRT in the treatment of single metastases, although they suggest that WBRT may decrease the recurrence rate. Little evidence exists to suggest that meaningful improvement in overall survival is achieved by the addition of WBRT. However, current practice is to use WBRT postoperatively.

Stereotactic Radiosurgery. The development of stereotactic radiosurgery, a new method of delivering intense focal irradiation by using a linear accelerator or multiple cobalt-60 sources (γ knife), has added a new method of treatment for brain metastases. Radiosurgery dosimetry is calculated to deliver a highly focused single dose of radiation to destroy tissue locally (Fig. 165-3). This is not the same as conventional radiotherapy, which uses much lower radiation doses calculated to be just below levels that are harmful to normal cells (but presumably lethal to tumor cells). Radiosurgery, therefore, is not a substitute for WBRT but may be a replacement for surgical therapy in selected patients.

Prospective clinical trials currently under way may help determine the role of radiosurgery both in the primary treatment of patients with single and multiple metastases and in the management of recurrent brain metastases. Several uncontrolled series of highly preselected patients have been published. These studies suggest that the local control rate for radiosurgery in the treatment of single metastases is about 80 percent and is similar to that achieved by conventional surgery. However, 5 to 15 percent of patients develop focal radiation necrosis and often require surgical removal of the necrotic debris. Unfortunately, the data presented so far are sketchy, with limited follow-up times and few quantitative data regarding survival or overall improvement in quality of life. To date, no controlled or randomized trials testing the efficacy of radiosurgery have been published. Therefore, no definitive conclusion can be drawn regarding its efficacy in the treatment of brain metastases.

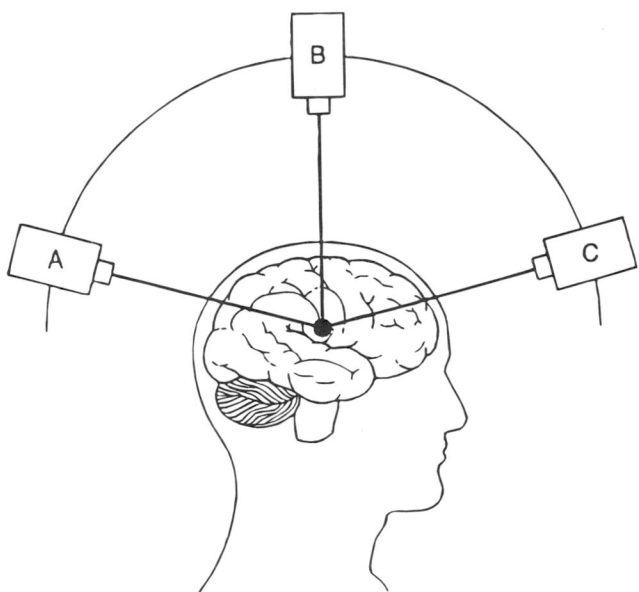

FIG. 165-3. Generalized overview of radiosurgical technique. Small-diameter, low-dose beams of γ radiation are given from many points outside the brain (*A, B, C*). The γ knife uses 201 cobalt-60 sources; the linear accelerator uses a single-beam generator that is repositioned to deliver each individual beam. The beams are focused on the intracranial lesion, and the total dose to the lesion is the sum of the individual beams.

Interstitial Brachytherapy. The use of interstitial brachytherapy, a technique involving the placement of radioactive implants within the area of tumor, has been advocated in selected patients. The implants allow the delivery of high-dose focal radiation to the tumor while minimizing the risk of significant radiation exposure to the surrounding normal brain tissue because of the rapid falloff of radiation intensity at the margins of the precalculated target area. Along with radiosurgery, brachytherapy may offer an additional treatment option for patients with unresectable metastases or for patients who have received previous maximal doses of WBRT. However, the role of brachytherapy in the primary management of brain metastases has yet to be determined.

Chemotherapy. The efficacy of chemotherapy in the management of brain metastases has not been demonstrated, although evidence has accumulated to suggest that chemotherapy may have a role in the treatment of selected patients. However, most systemically administered chemotherapeutic agents that have been proved to be effective against the primary cancer have been ineffective against cerebral metastases from the same cell population.

Chemotherapy has been used in the treatment of brain metastases from a variety of primary tumors; however, the results have generally been unimpressive, although some small, uncontrolled series of patients with certain highly chemosensitive tumors (breast, small cell lung cancer, and germ cell tumors) have been published. Chemotherapy is usually not the primary therapy for most patients, and it is seldom the only therapy. At present, chemotherapy should be used to treat only those metastatic brain tumors that are known to be chemosensitive. If progression occurs when the patient has received chemotherapy alone, more definitive treatment with surgery or radiation may be given.

Recurrent Brain Metastases

Another difficult and frequently encountered clinical problem is the treatment of recurrent brain metastases. The reappearance of brain metastases often occurs when patients also have extensive systemic disease. In general, the same types of treatment used for newly diagnosed brain metastases are also available for recurrences. However, the type and extent of previous therapy given may limit the therapeutic options available at this later time.

Commonly, patients with recurrences have already been treated with radiotherapy to the brain, which limits the amount of subsequent radiation that can be safely given. The amount of additional radiation that can be offered is usually in the range of 1,500 to 2,500 cGy, a dose usually too low to control tumor growth. Two uncontrolled studies found no meaningful increase in survival or control of neurologic symptoms in patients who underwent further radiotherapy after the recurrence of brain metastases. However, these studies consisted of relatively heterogeneous patient groups with extensive disease and a large proportion of radioresistant tumors. Reirradiation may be somewhat more beneficial in the subpopulation of patients who show an initial favorable response to radiotherapy and who remain in good general condition when the cerebral recurrence develops. Even in this favorable subgroup, however, only 42 percent of patients show symptomatic improvement, and the median survival after reirradiation is 5 months. Despite such relatively poor results, additional radiotherapy is frequently the only treatment option for patients with recurrent disease.

Conventional surgery for recurrent tumors is an option for patients who have a single recurrence and controlled systemic disease. The experience with reoperation is limited. A published report from Memorial Sloan-Kettering Cancer Center contained a series of 21 patients who were treated with craniotomy for their initial brain metastases and who underwent a second craniotomy for recurrence. After the second operation, two-thirds of the patients experienced neurologic improvement, and the median survival time after operation for the recurrence was 9 months. These patients were a select group with relatively little systemic disease and a single recurrent metastasis.

The outcome for patients who receive radiotherapy as the only treatment for the initial brain metastases and who are then treated with surgery at recurrence appears to be less favorable. A study from the Memorial Sloan-Kettering Cancer Center included patients who were treated with surgery after WBRT failed as the initial therapy. The median survival after operation for recurrence was 5 months. However, this group fared less well in overall survival time than comparable patients undergoing surgery plus WBRT as initial treatment for newly diagnosed brain metastases. Usually, additional radiotherapy is not given after surgery for a recurrence; however, brachytherapy with implantation of removable radioactive sources has been attempted in a few patients with incomplete resections. The value of brachytherapy for recurrent metastases is unclear.

Stereotactic radiosurgery has been used to treat patients with recurrent brain metastases. In these patients, radiosurgery has the theoretical advantage of being able to deliver large doses of additional radiation to small areas of the brain and may be used even if prior WBRT has been given. A large number of reports of stereotactic radiosurgery for recurrent brain metastases have now been published. The treated lesions are usually well controlled, with a decrease in size or stabilization after treatment in 80 to 90 percent of patients. This suggests that sterotactic radiosurgery may be a useful palliative treatment in the management of recurrent brain metastases.

CONCLUSION

Significant advances have occurred in the diagnosis and treatment of brain metastases, and the therapeutic nihilism of the past is not warranted for most patients with brain metastases. With currently available treatments, most patients do not die of their brain metastases and usually experience effective palliation of neurologic symptoms and meaningful extension of life.

SUGGESTED READINGS

Bindal RK, Sawaya R, Leavens ME et al: Surgical treatment of multiple brain metastases. J Neurosurg 79:210–6, 1993

Burt M, Wronski M, Arbit E et al: Resection of brain metastases from non-small-cell lung carcinoma. Results of therapy. Memorial Sloan-Kettering Cancer Center Thoracic Surgical Staff. J Thorac Cardiovasc Surg 103:399–411, 1992

DeAngelis LM, Mandell LR, Thaler HT et al: The role of postoperative radiotherapy after resection of single brain metastases. Neurosurgery 24:798–805, 1989

Delattre JY, Krol G, Thaler HT et al: Distribution of brain metastases. Arch Neurol 45:741–4, 1988

Dropcho EJ: Central nervous system injury by therapeutic irradiation. Neurol Clin 9:969–88, 1991

Gelber RD, Larson M, Borgelt BB et al: Equivalence of radiation schedules for the palliative treatment of brain metastases in patients with favorable prognosis. Cancer 48:1749–53, 1981

Graus F, Walker RW, Allen JC: Brain metastases in children. J Pediatr 103:558–61, 1983

Hazuka MB, Burleson W, Stroud DN et al: Multiple brain metastases are associated with poor survival in patients treated with surgery and radiotherapy. J Clin Oncol 11:369–73, 1993

Hoskin PJ, Crow J, Ford HT: The influence of extent and local management on the outcome of radiotherapy for brain metastases. Int J Radiat Oncol Biol Phys 19:111–5, 1990

Mehta WP, Werwie S, Levin AB et al: Surgery versus radiosurgery for metastases. Acta Neurochir (Wien) 122:157–8, 1993

Patchell RA, Tibbs PA, Walsh JW et al: A randomized trial of surgery in the treatment of single metastases to the brain. N Engl J Med 322:494–500, 1990

Seigers HP: Chemotherapy for brain metastases: recent developments and clinical considerations. Cancer Treat Rev 17:63–76, 1990

Smalley SR, Laws ER, Jr, O'Fallon JR et al: Resection for solitary brain metastasis. Role of adjuvant radiation and prognostic variables in 229 patients. J Neurosurg 77:531–40, 1992

Vecht CJ, Haaxma-Reiche H, Noordijk EM et al: Treatment of single brain metastasis: radiotherapy alone or combined with neurosurgery? Ann Neurol 3:583–90, 1993

SECTION 3. SPINAL CORD TUMORS

166. SPINAL CORD TUMORS

EUGENE ROSSITCH, Jr.

Tumors of the spinal cord can be divided into three groups based on their anatomic location: (1) extradural tumors; (2) intradural, extramedullary tumors; and (3) intradural, intramedullary tumors (Fig. 166-1 schematically depicts the relationship of the tumor to the spinal cord, subarachnoid space, and dura). The first category, extradural tumors, is discussed separately in Chapter 167. This chapter discusses intradural extramedullary and intradural intramedullary spinal cord tumors, as well as tumors arising from the cauda equina.

Intradural spinal cord tumors account for 2 to 4 percent of all central nervous system tumors and occur with an incidence of approximately 1.3 per 100,000. Extramedullary tumors (meningiomas and neurofibromas) account for approximately 80 percent of intradural tumors in adults and 50 percent of intradural tumors in children.

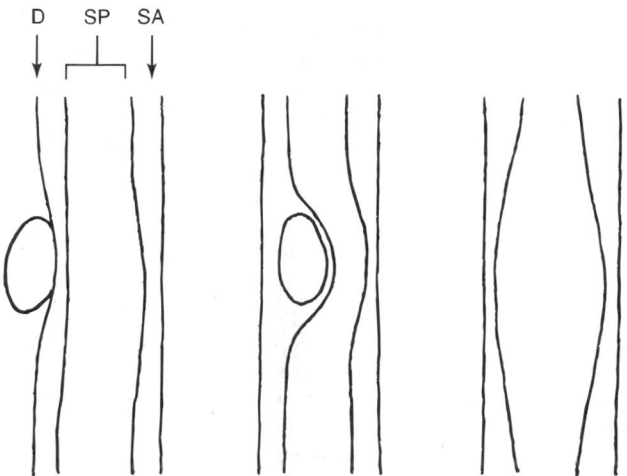

FIG. 166-1. Diagram showing **(A)** epidural tumor; **(B)** extramedullary, intradural tumor; and **(C)** intramedullary tumor. D, dura; SP, spinal cord; SA, subarachnoid space.

EXTRAMEDULLARY TUMORS

The two most common neoplasms in this category are neurofibromas and meningiomas. These occur with equal frequency.

MENINGIOMAS

Meningiomas occur throughout the spine but are most common in the thoracic region around T7. They occur more frequently in women than in men, with a ratio of 5:1. Most patients are middle aged, with the peak age of onset in the sixth decade. Meningiomas are usually located ventrolateral or lateral to the spinal cord. They presumably arise from arachnoid cluster cells and therefore are located at the exit zones of nerve roots or the entry zone of arteries into the spinal canal. In spite of this relationship, they can usually be separated from the roots at the time of surgery. These tumors usually occur singly, but they may be multiple in patients with neurofibromatosis.

Most patients present with slowly progressive symptoms, including radicular pain, weakness, numbness, and, in advanced cases, sphincter disturbance. Incomplete transection syndromes such as the Brown-Séquard syndrome are fairly common.

On magnetic resonance imaging (MRI), meningiomas are well-circumscribed tumors that are isointense with the spinal cord on T1-weighted and T2-weighted images and slightly increased in signal intensity on the long TR/short TE spin density images. They usually enhance uniformly following gadolinium administration (Fig. 166-2).

NEUROFIBROMAS

Neurofibromas arise from the dorsal nerve roots and occur at every level of the spine, although they are slightly more common in the thoracic region. They have an equal incidence in men and women. The tumors usually occur as single lesions but are frequently multiple when associated with neurofibromatosis. They are soft and avascular, and 25 percent extend through the vertebral foramina, giving rise to a dumbbell appearance. The root is involved in the matrix of the tumor and can rarely be completely spared during surgery.

Two-thirds of patients present with slowly progressive radicular pain. This pain is often worse at night and may be exacer-

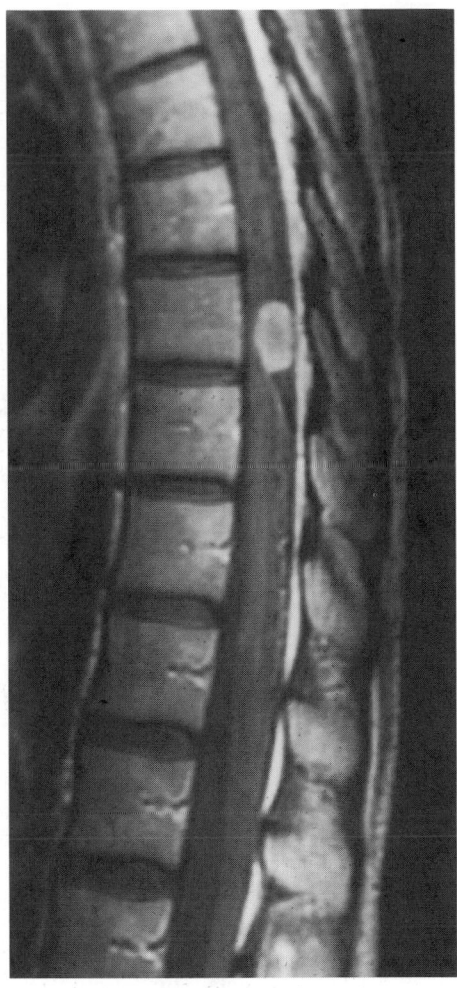

FIG. 166-2. Sagittal MRI scan of the thoracic spine with gadolinium (TR 600, TE 16). This image shows an extramedullary, intradural lesion. The patient was a young woman with a progressive myelopathy. At surgery, a meningioma was resected.

bated by postural changes, coughing, and straining. As the tumor enlarges, there may be paresthesia, weakness, depressed segmental reflexes, pyramidal signs, and autonomic dysfunction.

On MRI, these tumors appear as circumscribed, enhancing, intradural, extramedullary tumors. Unlike meningiomas, they frequently have increased signal on T2-weighted images.

INTRAMEDULLARY TUMORS

Intramedullary tumors account for 20 percent of intradural tumors in adults and 50 percent of intradural tumors in children. The most common intramedullary tumors are ependymomas, astrocytomas, malignant gliomas, and hemangioblastomas. The differential diagnosis of intramedullary tumors is summarized in Table 166-1.

EPENDYMOMAS

These are the most common intramedullary tumors in adults and the second most common intramedullary tumors after astrocytomas in children and adolescents. They occur twice as frequently in males as in females and have a peak incidence in the fourth decade. Ependymomas are fairly well circumscribed

TABLE 166-1. Differential Diagnosis of Intradural Spinal Cord Tumors

Common Tumors	Uncommon Tumors	Nontumorous Lesions
Extramedullary		
Meningiomas	Ependymoma	Arachnoid cyst
Neurofibromas	(filum terminale)	
	Dermoid	
	Epidermoid	
	Lipoma	
	Angioma	
	Metastases	
	Chordoma	
	Lymphoma	
	Myxoma	
	Sarcoma	
Intramedullary		
Ependymoma	Oligodendroglioma	Multiple sclerosis
Astrocytoma	Ganglioglioma	Cavernous angioma
Malignant glioma	Schwannoma	Infection
Hemangioblastoma	Metastatic tumors	Abscess
	Teratoma	Sarcoidosis
	Dermoid	
	Epidermoid	
	Lipoma	
	Neurenteric cyst	

and tend not to invade the surrounding brain. They can occur anywhere along the spinal cord but tend to have a slightly increased incidence in the cervical cord. Frequently, these tumors are associated with a cyst, which is usually located over the cranial pole. Histologically, they are made up of sheets of cells broken up by pseudorosettes.

The earliest symptom is usually a nonspecific dull aching pain in the region of the tumor. The pain gradually increases in severity, characteristically tends to be worse on lying, and improves when the patient is sitting or standing. In a minority of patients, the pain will wake the patient up from sleep. Some patients will develop a characteristic burning or lancinating pain. As the tumor enlarges, weakness, sensory loss, and paresthesias occur, but these may not develop until years after the onset of pain. Since these tumors are located near the center of the spinal cord, they tend to destroy crossing pain and temperature fibers, giving rise initially to segmental dissociated sensory loss that descends with time. This is often noticed early in the upper extremities when the patient may present with reduced pain and temperature sensation in the hands while retaining light touch and position sense. Unfortunately this classic picture occurs in less than one-quarter of patients with intramedullary spinal cord tumors. Because of the lamination of spinothalamic tracts, with fibers from the sacral region ascending in the periphery of the tracts and fibers from higher levels being added more centrally, ependymomas, which usually arise from the center of the spinal cord, frequently spare sensation from the perianal region ("sacral sparing"). In contrast, extramedullary tumors that compress the spinal cord from the outside tend to involve the sacral fibers first, producing sacral sensory loss. Rarely patients may present with acute pain and neurologic deficits following a hemorrhage within the tumor. Skeletal abnormalities such as scoliosis, and segmental contractures occur commonly in patients with ependymomas.

It can be difficult to differentiate an intramedullary tumor such as an ependymoma from syringomyelia since both can produce gradual progressive symptoms over many years and both have cysts on imaging studies. Syringomyelia, however, is often found with other abnormalities such as Chiari malformations, hydrocephalus, and congenital abnormalities of the cervical spine. MRI and computed tomographic myelography

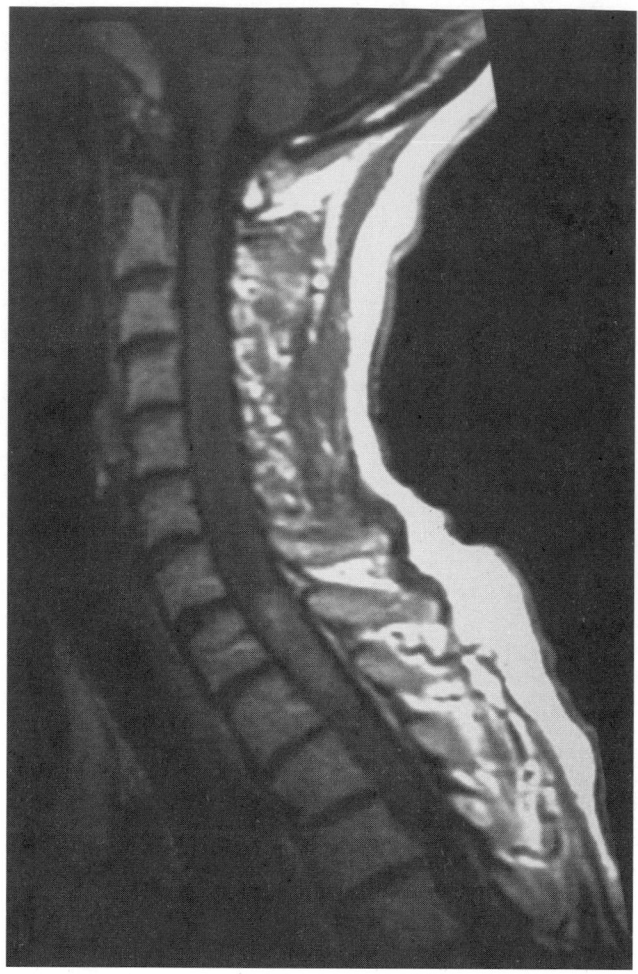

FIG. 166-3. Sagittal MRI scan of the lumbosacral spine with gadolinium showing a large, enhancing myxopapillary ependymoma in the cauda equina. The patient had neurofibromatosis type 2 and presented with right leg pain and weakness. The tumor was subtotally resected and then treated with external beam radiotherapy.

may be helpful in differentiating the two. On MRI scans, ependymomas appear as circumscribed enhancing lesions often associated with a nonenhancing cyst, whereas syringomyelias and hydromyelias will not enhance. On myelography, the tumor appears as a nonspecific widening of the spinal cord shadow. Unlike syringomyelia, the cystic cavity only fills occasionally with contrast in the postmyelogram computed tomographic scan.

ASTROCYTOMAS

Astrocytomas are more common in males than in females and have a peak incidence in the third to fifth decades. Ninety percent of spinal cord astrocytomas are low-grade tumors, which may either be diffusely infiltrating or pilocytic. Ten percent of intramedullary astrocytomas are high-grade astrocytomas.

Low-grade astrocytomas present with clinical features similar to those of ependymomas with back pain, slowly progressive weakness, sensory loss, and gait difficulties. High-grade astrocytomas present with more rapidly progressive symptoms, and leptomeningeal seeding may occur.

Infiltrating fibrillary astrocytomas present as diffuse nonenhancing masses on MRI. Occasionally there may be cysts associated with the tumor. Pilocytic astrocytomas appear as densely enhancing lesions on MRI. These are usually associated with a large peritumoral cyst.

Patients with low-grade astrocytomas have 80 percent 5-year and 50 percent 10-year survival rates. Patients with high-grade astrocytomas have a much worse prognosis and usually die within a few years.

OLIGODENDROGLIOMAS

Oligodendrogliomas account for only 1 percent of spinal cord tumors and have similar presenting features as astrocytomas.

HEMANGIOBLASTOMAS

Hemangioblastomas account for 3 percent of intramedullary spinal cord tumors and present either as slowly enlarging masses or, occasionally, as subarachnoid hemorrhage. Approximately 30 percent of patients have von Hippel-Lindaus syndrome.

MRI may show an enhancing mass or a nodule associated with a cyst. The protein content of the cysts is usually higher than cerebrospinal fluid on MRI. Myelography shows nonspecific enlargement of the spinal cord, which may extend beyond the borders of the tumor cysts. Large dorsal varices may be present.

METASTATIC TUMORS

The number of patients with intramedullary metastatic tumors is increasing as patients with cancer live longer (Fig. 166-3). They usually present with subacute, progressive, asymmetric weakness and sensory loss. Spinal cord metastases need to be differentiated from epidural spinal cord compression, radiation myelopathy, and paraneoplastic myelopathy. Although spinal cord metastases may respond to radiotherapy, the prognosis is generally poor.

TREATMENT

The optical treatment of most spinal cord tumors is surgical excision. Radiotherapy may have a role if excision is incomplete. Factors that determine whether a tumor can be completely resected include the histology of the tumor, the location and extent of the lesion, and the technical ability of the surgeon. Recent advances in surgery, including the operating microscope, lasers, intraoperative ultrasound, and intraoperative spinal cord monitoring, have greatly improved the safety and effectiveness of surgery. The operative mortality rate is now generally less than 5 percent. Most intramedullary tumors are approached through an incision made between the dorsal columns, although occasionally the tumor may be approached through the dorsal nerve root or even anteriorly.

Approximately 80 percent of ependymomas can be completely resected. Postoperatively, 5 to 10 percent have transient worsening of their deficits. The patients[7] postoperative neurologic status tends to be directly related to their preoperative neurologic condition. Even with a "complete resection," 5 to 10 percent of patients develop tumor recurrence after 5 years.

Astrocytomas are generally more difficult to remove completely, and their prognosis is usually worse. In general, children tend to do better than adults.

There is relatively little data concerning the effectiveness of radiotherapy. Radiotherapy is usually reserved for patients

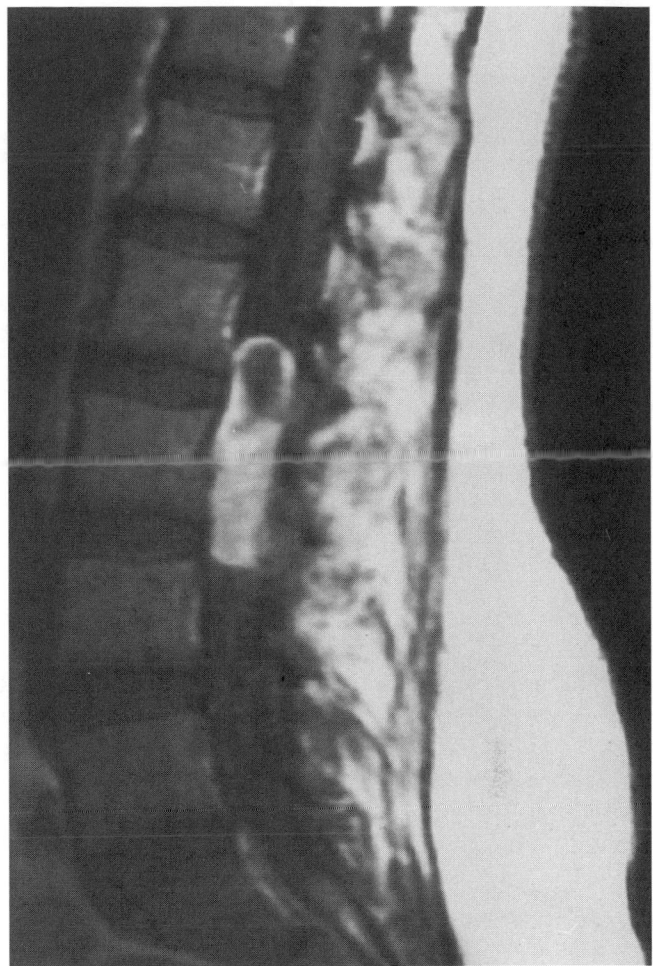

FIG. 166-4. Sagittal MRI scan of the cervical and upper lumbar spine with gadolinium (TR 500, TE 20) showing an enhancing intramedullary breast carcinoma metastasis at the level of T1. The adjacent cervical cord is expanded by edema.

whose tumors cannot be completely resected. The recommended dose is 4,500 to 5,000 cGy administered over 5 to 6 weeks. There is some evidence that radiotherapy may prolong the survival of patients with incompletely resected ependymomas and astrocytomas.

The role of chemotherapy for high-grade spinal cord gliomas is unproved.

TUMORS OF THE CAUDA EQUINA

The most common tumors in the cauda equina are ependymomas, neurofibromas, epidermoids, dermoids, meningiomas, lipomas, and metastatic tumors. Ependymomas of the cauda equina usually have a myxopapillary histology and account for nearly 60 percent of all spinal ependymomas (Fig. 166-4).

Pain is the most common presenting symptom of cauda equina tumors and may precede neurologic deficits by a long period of time. In one-half of the patients, the pain is worse at night or after lying down. Unlike musculoskeletal pain, this pain is usually not helped by changing positions and is usually only relieved when the patient sits or stands up. Less commonly, patients may present with painless, progressive leg weakness or numbness or sphincter disturbance.

Plain radiographs may show widening of the interpeduncular distance, erosion of the posterior vertebral body, or enlargement of a neural foramen. However, these tumors are easily diagnosed by MRI or myelography.

Approximately 50 percent of myxopapillary ependymomas can be successfully resected. Neurofibromas can also be removed, but injury to the nerve root is relatively common.

SUGGESTED READINGS

Abernathy C D: Intraspinal extramedullary tumors. pp. 38.1–8. In Rengachary SS, Wilkins RH (eds): Principles of Neurosurgery. Wolfe, London, 1994

Cooper PR: Outcome after operative treatment of intramedullary spinal cord tumors in adults: intermediate and long term results in 51 patients. Neurosurgery 25:855–9, 1991

Epstein FJ, Farmer JP, Freed D: Adult intramedullary astrocytomas of the spinal cord. J Neurosurg 77:355–9, 1992

Epstein FJ, Farmer JP, Freed D: Adult intramedullary spinal cord ependymomas: the results of surgery in 38 patients. J Neurosurg 79:204–9, 1993

Friedman A: Intramedullary tumors and tumors of the cauda equina. pp. 39.1–12. In Rengachary SS, Wilkins RH (eds): Principles of Neurosurgery. Wolfe Publishing, London, 1994

Levy W, Latchaw J, Hahn J et al: Spinal neurofibromas: a report of 66 cases and a comparison with meningiomas. Neurosurgery 18:331–4, 1986

McCormick P, Post K, Stein B: Intradural extramedullary tumors in adults. Neurosurg Clin North Am 1:591–608, 1990

McCormick P, Stein BM: Intramedullary tumors in adults. Neurosurg Clin North Am 1:609–30, 1990

McCormick PC, Torres R, Post KD et al: Intramedullary ependymoma of the spinal cord. J Neurosurg 72:523–32, 1990

Shaw EG, Evans RG, Scheithauer BW et al: Radiotherapeutic management of intraspinal ependymomas. Int J Radiat Oncol Biol Phys 12:323–7, 1986

Sonneland PRL, Scheithauer BW, Onofrio BM: Myxopapillary ependymoma: a clinicopathologic and immunocytochemical study of 77 cases. Cancer 56:883–93, 1985

Sundaresan N, Schmidek H, Schiller A, Rosenthal D: Tumors of the Spine. Diagnosis and Clinical Management. WB Saunders, Philadelphia, 1990

Sze G: Magnetic resonance imaging in the evaluation of spinal cord tumors. Cancer 67:1229–41, 1991

SECTION 4. NEUROLOGIC COMPLICATIONS OF SYSTEMIC CANCER

167. METASTATIC EPIDURAL SPINAL CORD COMPRESSION

HARRY S. GREENBERG

Metastatic epidural spinal cord compression is defined as compression of the spinal cord or cauda equina nerve roots from a metastatic lesion outside the spinal dura. It is an important cause of morbidity and mortality in patients with cancer.

CLINICAL MANIFESTATIONS

Back pain is the initial complaint in up to 96 percent of patients with epidural spinal cord compression. Pain may precede neurologic symptoms by days to 3 or more years. It is very unusual for patients with metastatic epidural spinal cord compression to present without pain, but cord compression from lung or renal metastases and lymphoma do so more frequently. The median duration of pain before development of neurologic signs has varied from 7 to 23 weeks. Duration of pain is probably related to tumor growth rate, being shortest for highly malignant tumors such as lung and kidney and longest for more typically less malignant tumors such as breast and prostate carcinoma. The majority of patients have local pain, secondary to stretching of the pain-sensitive cortical bone and periosteum. Local pain is usually constant and relentlessly progressive and exacerbated by coughing, sneezing, straining, or exercise. The worsening of pain on recumbency is the most distinctive feature of the pain of metastatic epidural spinal cord compression and differ-

entiates it from disc disease. Radicular pain is present in 90 percent of patients with lumbosacral, 79 percent with cervical, and 55 percent with thoracic metastatic epidural spinal cord compression. It is frequently bilateral in the thoracic area and unilateral or bilateral in the lumbosacral and cervical areas. Radicular pain is an important localizing sign.

Weakness is present in about 80 percent of patients with metastatic epidural spinal cord compression at presentation. Fifty percent of patients are ambulatory, 35 percent are paraparetic, and 15 percent are paraplegic at the time of diagnosis. Once weakness is present, progression is often rapid, and urgent investigation and treatment are crucial. Thirty percent of patients with weakness become paraplegic within 1 week. Rate of progression of weakness is dependent on the tumor growth rate. Weakness is usually bilateral and symmetric (87 percent). The degree of weakness and ability to ambulate at the time of diagnosis are important clinical predictors of outcome.

Bladder and bowel symptoms are also frequently present at the time of diagnosis (57 percent) and can take the form of frequency, urinary retention, or incontinence. Autonomic disturbance is a bad prognostic sign, as it implies bilateral cord or root damage and is usually associated with moderate to severe weakness. Objective sensory disturbance is found in 78 percent of patients at the time of diagnosis. The severity of sensory loss almost always mirrors the severity of motor weakness.

Care should be taken to examine lymph nodes, breasts, lungs, and kidneys and perform a rectal examination. Limited straight leg raising usually points to an epidural or intradural extramedullary lesion causing root compression; segmental pain and sacral sparing suggests intramedullary disease. Spinal cord, conus medullaris, cauda equina, or peripheral nerve lesions can produce a flaccid areflexic paralysis. Concurrent cerebral symptoms or signs favor performance of magnetic resonance imaging (MRI) when there is no risk of neurologic deterioration. If there are two spinal levels involved clinically or on a radiograph, then both sites must be clearly imaged.

ETIOLOGY

The epidural space is a true space that lies between spinal cord dura and the bony spinal canal. It contains fat, connective tissue and a rich paravertebral venous plexus, which drains the vertebrae and intervertebral spaces. The most common mechanism of metastatic epidural spinal cord compression is by hematogenous arterial spread to bone marrow, which results in vertebral body collapse and formation of an anterior epidural mass. A second mechanism is spread by direct invasion of tumor through the intervertebral foramina from a paravertebral source. This occurs in 75 percent of patients with epidural spinal cord compression caused by lymphoma and 15 percent of patients with metastatic epidural spinal cord compression from other solid tumors.

Another probable mechanism of metastatic epidural spinal cord compression is by retrograde venous spread from the primary site via Batson's paravertebral plexus. In humans, it is rare to find metastatic epidural spinal cord compression without bony involvement or direct spread through the bony foramina.

BIOLOGIC BASIS

Animal models have been used to demonstrate morphologic features of cord damage and subsequent recovery. Following 3 hours of cord compression in cats, selective demyelination without axonal disruption evolves over the subsequent 21 hours and continues for 1 week. Most demyelinated fibers show evidence of remyelination by 1 month. If compression is produced slowly over a 48-hour period and maintained for 7 days, it is still possible for the patient to recover from paralysis, suggesting that demyelination is a more important factor than cord ischemia. With more prolonged compression, there was cord ischemia and irreversible neurologic changes. If tumor cells are injected anterior to thoracic vertebra, they grow into the epidural space in rats. One of the earliest features of metastatic epidural spinal cord compression is breakdown of the blood–spinal cord barrier with vasogenic edema and an increase in prostaglandin E_2. Administration of steroids or nonsteroidal anti-inflammatory agents decreases the vasogenic edema and prostaglandin E_2, and produces objective improvement in weakness.

At autopsy, in humans with metastatic epidural spinal cord compression, there is vascular congestion, hemorrhage, and edema at the site of cord compression, suggesting that venous occlusion is an important factor in the pathogenesis of cord damage.

EPIDEMIOLOGY

The most common tumors causing epidural spinal cord compression are tumors of the breast, lung, prostate, lymphoma, sarcoma, and kidney, accounting for over 70 percent of cases. Spinal cord compression is the initial manifestation of malignancy in one-half of cases diagnosed in a general hospital but less than 8 percent diagnosed in cancer centers.

The median age at diagnosis of metastatic epidural spinal cord compression has varied from 53 to 63 years, with sex differences reflecting the primary neoplasm (e.g., breast and prostate).

The histology of the tumor may be more important in determining the prognosis than the type of treatment. Myeloma, lymphoma, and breast carcinoma have almost a 80 percent initial response rate, and 75 percent of patients with breast carcinoma who are still alive at 1 year remain ambulatory. Only 25 percent of patients with lung or renal carcinoma and melanoma respond to any treatment modality.

PREVENTION, RISK FACTORS, AND ASSOCIATED CONDITIONS

To improve clinical outcome, it is important to identify patients early in their illness or who are at high risk for metastatic epidural spinal cord compression before the appearance of neurologic symptoms or signs. Patients with malignancy should be advised to inform their physician if they develop new back pain, the initial complaint in up to 96 percent of patients who go on to develop metastatic epidural spinal cord compression. High-risk patients include those with known malignancy and recent-onset back pain and those who are not known to have malignancy but who have a new backache that is worse on recumbency or is radicular and that is situated in the thoracic region or associated with spinal tenderness. These patients will require anteroposterior and lateral plain radiographs of the involved areas (Fig. 167-1). Oblique radiographs are needed if there is radicular pain, as foraminal enlargement may be missed on standard views. If there is evidence of focal bony pathology, myelography will demonstrate an abnormality in approximately 60 percent of cases. If the spine radiographs are normal but the pain is characteristic, a spinal computer-assisted tomographic scan is recommended. Spinal computed tomographic (CT) scanning will accurately differentiate between bony metastases and benign bony disease. If CT demonstrates bony metastases or a paraspinal mass, then MRI or CT–myelography is indicated.

Radiation therapy is the treatment of choice for bony metastases without metastatic epidural spinal cord compression, as this provides very effective palliation for bone pain and will prevent progression of epidural metastases in most cases. In prostate cancer, irradiation of the lumbar spine coincidental to the irradiation of para-aortic nodes and the normally radiated pelvic area prevented or delayed the development of the lumbar spine metastases, which might significantly reduce cauda equina compression.

Rapid onset and quick progression are bad prognostic variables. Patients with a preoperative symptom duration greater than 2 months have better postoperative recovery of function than those with shorter histories. The duration of paraplegia before starting treatment is also important. It has been traditionally taught that, when paraplegia is present for greater than 24 hours before initiation of treatment, the chances of recovery are slight, although recent reports question this doctrine. In children with metastatic epidural spinal cord compression, prognosis for recovery from complete motor and sensory loss was significantly better than in adults, with 50 percent becoming ambulatory after surgical decompression and medical therapy.

DIFFERENTIAL DIAGNOSIS

Approximately 50 percent of adult patients presenting with an acute transverse myelopathy will be diagnosed as having meta-

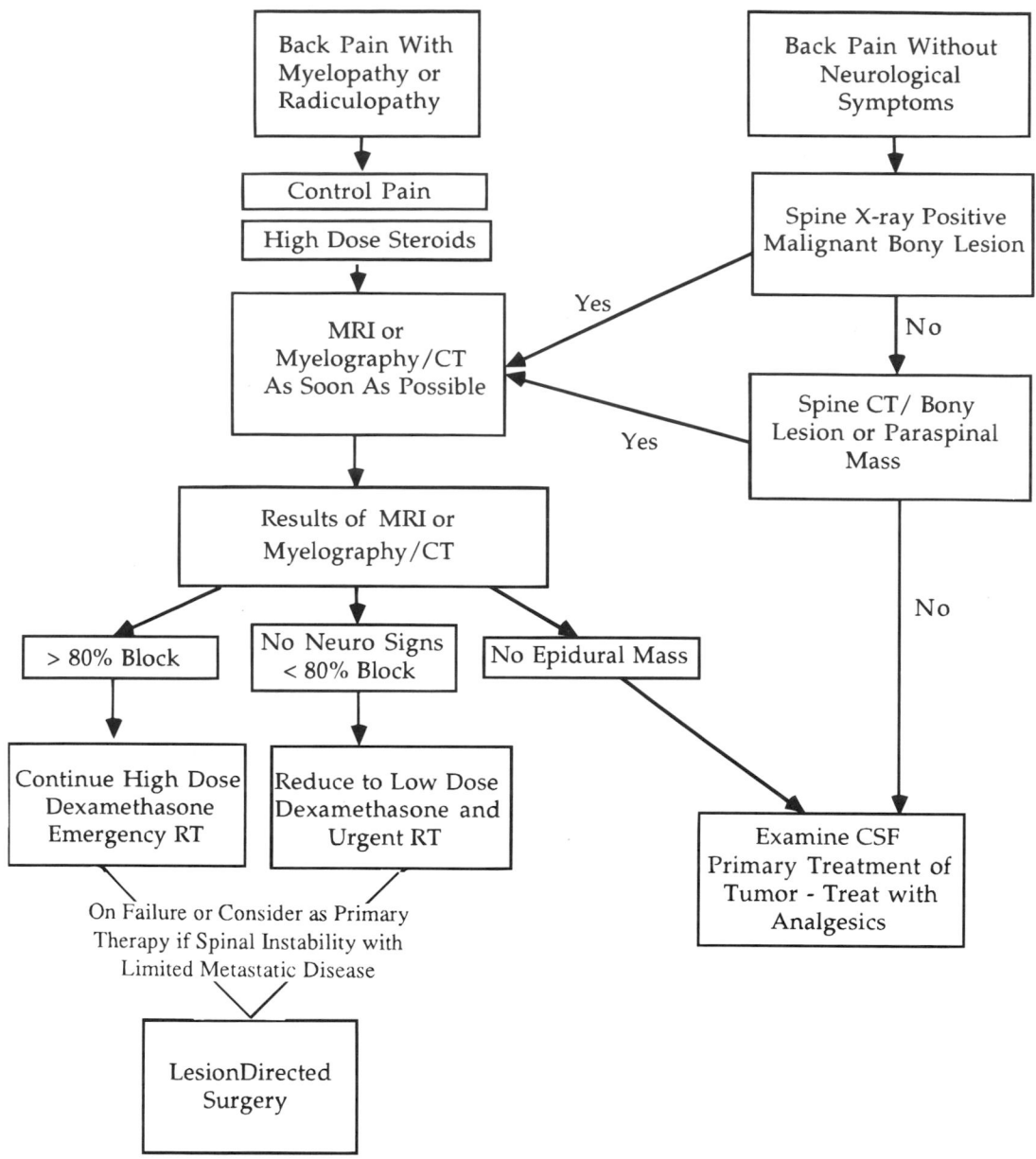

FIG. 167-1. Algorithm for the management of suspected metastatic epidural spinal cord compression with back pain with or without neurologic symptoms. RT, radiotherapy; CSF, cerebrospinal fluid.

static epidural spinal cord compression. In 47 percent of patients who develop metastatic epidural spinal cord compression, it is the initial presentation of their malignancy, and of these almost one-half will have lung carcinoma identified.

However, less than 50 percent of patients with malignancy, considered clinically to have metastatic epidural spinal cord compression, will have this diagnosis confirmed by myelography. Myelography in patients with cancer, back pain, and myelopathy is normal in 23 percent, and in those with back pain and radiculopathy it is normal in 37 percent.

A history of previous radiation therapy, trauma, vascular or disc disease, or infection is important. Patients taking anticoagulants have an increased risk of subdural hematoma following lumbar puncture. Chemotherapy increases the risk of infections and hemorrhage. Patients receiving chronic steroids may develop cord compression from epidural fat.

The differentiation between epidural abscess and metastasis is often difficult. Epidural abscess is more frequently posteriorly situated and will often cover multiple vertebral body segments. If there is vertebral collapse owing to an infective cause, the disc space is frequently destroyed; metastatic vertebral disease usually spares the disc space. Epidural abscess may be associated with increased systemic white blood cell count, fever, or cerebrospinal fluid pleocytosis, but, as the dura is an effective barrier, the cerebrospinal fluid may be normal. Blood cultures often yield the correct organism.

Arteriovenous malformations can produce myelopathy as a result of direct pressure or following hemorrhage. In the majority of cases, the arteriovenous malformation is at the thoracolumbar junction, either extradural or intradural; in approximately 10 percent, the arteriovenous malformation arises from the anterior spinal artery and is intramedullary in the cervical cord. They may be identified by their "snakelike" appearance on myelography or by demonstrating flow voids or characteristic signal changes of hemorrhage using MRI.

Carcinomatous meningitis occurs in approximately 5 percent of patients with cancer at autopsy. Intradural extramedullary or intramedullary metastases have frequencies of less than 4 percent that of epidural spinal cord compression. Noncompressive causes of neural involvement should also be considered. Vascular damage to the spinal cord may cause myelopathy as a result of direct pressure or compression of major feeding radicular arteries as they enter through the intervertebral foramina. Myelopathy secondary to radiation, intrathecal methotrexate chemotherapy, infectious diseases, coagulopathies, and paraneoplastic syndromes may occur in patients with cancer.

DIAGNOSTIC WORKUP

Plain radiographs are an essential, highly predictive, inexpensive, quick investigation that should be obtained if myelography or MRI is pending. Between 84 and 94 percent of patients with metastatic epidural spinal cord compression have an abnormal plain radiograph at the time of presentation.

Over 30 percent of patients will have radiographic evidence of multiple sites of vertebral involvement, and, if plain radiographs, CT, and surgical findings are combined, as many as 86 percent may have more than one vertebra involved. Multiple vertebral involvement is particularly common in breast and prostatic carcinoma. Metastatic epidural spinal cord compression most commonly occurs at the site of vertebral involvement on plain radiographs, especially when there is evidence of vertebral collapse. The primary compression of the spinal cord from metastatic deposits occurs in the thoracic region in approximately 70 percent of patients, in the lumbosacral spine in 20 percent, and in the cervical spine in 10 percent of patients. Multiple sites of metastatic epidural spinal cord compression occur in approximately 20 percent of all patients. This is particularly common in breast cancer and is uncommon in lung cancer.

In a review of 600 cases of spinal cord or nerve root compression, vertebral metastases occurred in 563 patients (Constans et al., 1983). The vertebral body was involved in 45 percent of these patients, the posterior arch in 41 percent, and the entire vertebra in the remaining 14 percent of patients. Epidural lesions without vertebral involvement occurred in 30 patients and intradural lesions in 7 patients. The location within the vertebra of metastatic involvement is important for the surgical treatment of epidural spinal cord compression but is not a good indicator of the primary site of neoplasm. Epidural metastases usually do not invade the dura. Posterior extradural tumor is easily accessible by laminectomy, but anterior extradural disease may require an anterior cervical, transthoracic, or transabdominal approach.

If there is back pain or a localizing sign and the spinal radiograph is abnormal, the probability of epidural disease is 0.9, but if the radiograph is normal, it is only 0.1. Spinal radiographs have a sensitivity of 91 percent for predicting epidural disease and a specificity of 86 percent. Bone scanning has a similar sensitivity but a specificity of only 53 percent. Particularly useful radiologic features for predicting epidural disease are greater than 50 percent vertebral collapse (85 percent) and pedicular erosion (31 percent).

Spinal CT is valuable in investigating patients with cancer and local back pain who have a normal examination and spinal radiographs. Two-thirds of these patients have spinal metastases on CT scan, but only 17 percent will have metastatic epidural spinal cord compression. In these cases rarely has there been a greater than 50 percent block. Patients without cortical disruption on CT, rarely develop metastatic epidural spinal cord compression at that site at a later date.

Different algorithms for the investigation of patients with cancer and back pain have resulted from recent clinical studies utilizing spinal radiographs, bone scanning, and spinal computer-assisted tomography. All advise MRI or myelography with CT if the spinal radiograph is abnormal.

MRI has replaced myelography as the procedure of choice, although there are no prospective trials comparing the two procedures. However, it is advisable to get the test that is readily available, as the patient may deteriorate while waiting for investigation.

MRI is noninvasive, effectively demonstrates metastatic epidural spinal cord compression, and gives a positive image of the spinal cord to diagnose intramedullary disease better. Intradural extramedullary metastases are equally well diagnosed by gadolinium-enhanced MRI or by myelography. Asymptomatic second areas of metastatic epidural spinal cord compression are identified with MRI and are important for radiation planning. Anatomic definition of vertebral and extraspinal disease on MRI is necessary when planning a surgical procedure. All patients with suspected metastatic epidural spinal cord compression should have their total spine imaged. It is helpful to per-

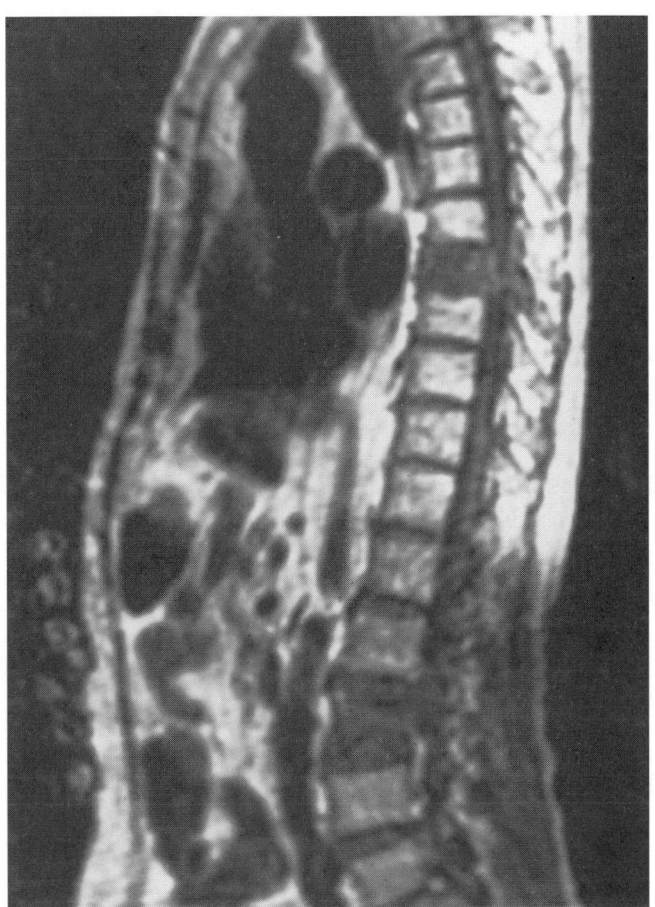

FIG. 167-2.   MRI scan (using the body coil) showing two areas of vertebral involvement, one with ESCC at T8 and another with asymptomatic L3 metastasis.

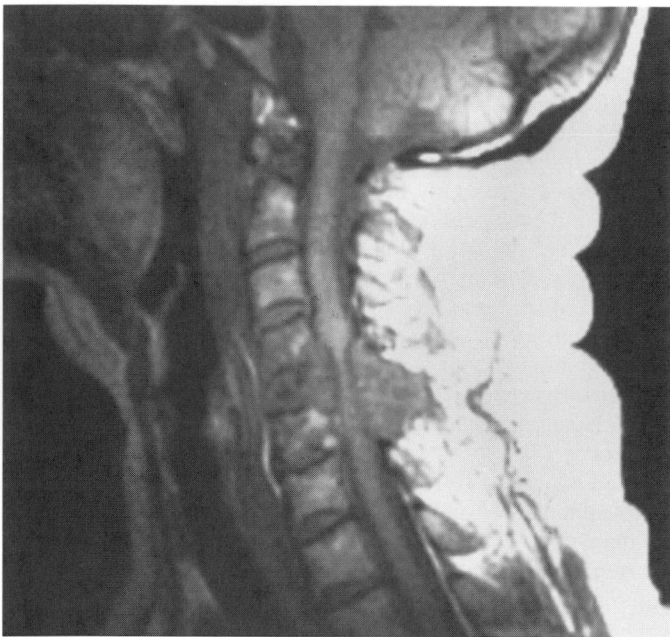

FIG. 167-3.   MRI scan (using local spinal cord) showing severe metastatic ESCC with collapse of C5 vertebral body and severe destruction of posterior elements and local invasion of C4 and C6 vertebral bodies.

TABLE 167-1.   Survival Times From Diagnosis of Epidural Spinal Cord Compression in Patients With Common Tumors Treated by Radiotherapy

Site	Mean	Standard Deviation	Median	Range
Lung	3.0	3.9	1.5	0–18
Breast	14.0	12.8	9.2	0.6–49.3
Kidney	8.5	13.4	3.7	0.5–70.8
Prostate	11.7	14.7	5.1	0.2–61.3
Lymph/myeloma	8.6	14.4	4.9	0.3–66.5
Other	6.3	8.2	3.5	0.1–28.9
All	8.1	11.8	3.1	0.4–70.8

(Fropm Sorensen PS, Borgesen SE, Rohde K et al: Metastatic epidural spinal cord compression: results of treatment and survival. Cancer 65:1502, 1990, with permission.)

form sagittal MRI ''scout scans'' using the body coil (Fig. 167-2), as they will often identify multiple vertebral deposits that can subsequently be studied in more detail using local spinal coils (Fig. 167-3). MRI has fewer risks than myelography in patients with intracranial mass lesions or bleeding tendencies. When there has been previous surgery or scoliosis, MRI sagittal images are difficult to interpret. Patients who are claustrophobic or who have a ferromagnetic implant cannot be scanned. Movement artifact may limit scan interpretation, and myelography would then be preferable.

Myelography is as sensitive as MRI to identify extradural lesions and has the added advantage of yielding cerebrospinal fluid, which may help to exclude or confirm alternative diagnoses (e.g., carcinomatous meningitis or abscess). The addition of spinal CT improves sensitivity for bony and paravertebral involvement. Clinical deterioration may occur directly following myelography; however, it is difficult to separate this from the natural history of the disease. If there is a complete block following lumbar injection, a second puncture for a cervical myelogram or MRI is necessary to visualize the upper limit of the block and to exclude second lesions.

If the cause of epidural spinal cord compression is uncertain, CT-guided biopsy of a paraspinal or epidural mass or percutaneous needle biopsy of a collapsed vertebral body may be helpful.

Simple investigations such as chest radiograph, prostate-specific antigen, mammography, abdominal ultrasound, or abdominal and chest CT scan may immediately demonstrate the primary malignancy in patients who present with metastatic epidural spinal cord compression.

PROGNOSIS AND COMPLICATIONS

The severity of weakness at presentation is the most significant prognostic variable for recovery of function. Eighty percent of patients who were ambulatory at presentation remain so after treatment. Between 30 and 45 percent of patients who are non-ambulatory with antigravity proximal leg function will regain ambulation, where as only 5 percent of patients who have no antigravity proximal function will walk again. The radiobiology of the tumor also plays an important role in response. In one study, 75 percent of patients with radiosensitive tumors who were nonambulatory but could raise their legs off the bed became ambulant after radiotherapy, but only 34 percent of comparable patients with radioresistant tumors became ambulant after radiotherapy (Gilbert et al., 1978). After treatment, the probability of ambulant patients surviving 1 year is 0.73, and the probability of nonambulant patients surviving 1 year is 0.09. Survival by tumor type is shown in Table 167-1. In selected series of paraplegic patients with anterior epidural spinal cord compression treated with anterior decompression and radiotherapy, between 50 and 90 percent of patients had an improvement in motor function.

MANAGEMENT

Emergency Measures

Patients with cancer, back pain, and an abnormal progressing neurologic examination, who demonstrate myelopathy or radiculopathy, should undergo emergency MRI or CT-myelography, whichever is the most readily available procedure (Fig. 167-1). Stable patients with uncertain neurologic findings can be scanned urgently over the next 24 hours. Control of pain prior to myelography or MRI may help to prevent movement artifact. High doses of steroids such as 100 mg of dexamethasone IV and 24 mg q 6 h will produce pain relief in 64 percent of patients within 24 hours and can also result in significant clinical improvement. High-dose intravenous dexamethasone can cause side effects, including vaginal burning, elevations in blood pressure, glucose intolerance, and electrolyte disturbance, and caution should be used in those suspected of having an infection or gastrointestinal symptoms. Doses should be tapered rapidly and immediately if there is less than 80 percent spinal block or gradually after 72 hours, following treatment with radiotherapy or surgery.

Patients with metastatic epidural spinal cord compression and abnormal neurologic examination with weakness should be monitored at frequent intervals with a neurologic examination. If patients develop a neurologic deficit during radiation therapy and it is unresponsive to steroid dose increase, directed surgical approach should be considered. If back pain is due to vertebral involvement with spinal instability and the patient has otherwise limited metastatic disease, spinal stabilization should be considered.

In experimental studies, dexamethasone can be identified in spinal cord within 5 minutes of intravenous injection and has a half-life of approximately 4 hours. A dexamethasone dose-response effect has been demonstrated in an animal model of metastatic epidural spinal cord compression, producing decreased spinal cord water content, reduced epidural swelling, and a transient clinical improvement. A prospective randomized double-blinded trial of a single high dexamethasone dose (100 mg IV) compared with a conventional initial dose (10 mg IV), both subsequently followed by 4 mg PO q6h did not demonstrate a significant difference in ambulation, bladder function, or control of pain at 24 hours (Vecht et al., 1989). Based on the half-life of dexamethasone, any effect of single high-dose dexamethasone would be expected to be of short duration, and a more prolonged course of high-dose steroids may be justified.

Patients with neoplastic spinal cord compression are at an increased risk of deep venous thrombosis and pulmonary embolus. Prophylactic subcutaneous heparin, antiembolic stockings, or compression pumps will help reduce morbidity and mortality rates. In the presence of urinary retention or constipation, intermittent or permanent catheterization should be considered, and laxatives/suppositories should be initiated early in the course of admission. Care should be taken when nursing patients with paraparesis or paraplegia to prevent pressure sores.

In 1978, a retrospective nonrandomized series of 235 patients with metastatic epidural spinal cord compression concluded that radiation therapy alone is as effective as decompressive laminectomy and radiation therapy (Gilbert et al., 1978). This study was instrumental in changing initial therapy for metastatic epidural spinal cord compression from surgery to radiation therapy. There has only been one randomized prospective comparison of laminectomy followed by radiation therapy versus radiation therapy alone (Young et al., 1980. This failed to reveal any different between the treatment arms; however, the sample size made it difficult to demonstrate a significant difference. Recently, a renewed interest in surgery has focused on a directed surgical approach based on the site and level of metastatic epidural spinal cord compression.

Radiotherapy

The response of epidural metastatic lesions to radiation is well documented. Lymphoma, seminoma, myeloma, Ewing sarcoma, and neuroblastoma are very radiosensitive; breast and prostate tumors are less so; and kidney, colon, and lung cancers and melanoma are frequently radioresistant.

Radiation therapy is still the generally accepted first line of treatment of metastatic epidural spinal cord compression in radiosensitive tumors. Its use in radioresistant tumors is more controversial. A large retrospective study reported that radioresistant tumors are as effectively treated with radiation therapy alone as with laminectomy and radiation therapy (Gilbert et al., 1978). The optimal dose and fractionation regimen for metastatic epidural spinal cord compression remains unknown. In fact, there may be no generally optimal plan. Each plan constructed represents a compromise between delivery of the highest dose achievable to improve tumor control, a desire to achieve palliation as expeditiously as possible, and the intrinsic radiosensitivity of the spinal cord; often a regimen of 30 Gy in 10 fractions is chosen as the best solution.

Traditionally, two vertebral bodies above and below the my-elographic block have been treated, taking into account other vertebral bodies with documented metastasis. Whether these volume recommendations will continue in the modern imaging era remains to be seen. The sensitivity of the spinal cord to radiation limits the prescribed amount of therapy, and the spinal cord dose should always be calculated as well as the dose to the involved vertebral body. The incidence of permanent radiation injury to the spinal cord directly correlates with the total dose and fraction size. Spinal cord tolerance has been considered to be between 45 and 50 Gy in 180-cGy fractions, between 35 and 37.5 Gy in 250-cGy fractions, and between 30 and 33 Gy in 300-cGy fractions. The size of the radiation field also plays an important role, and reductions in treatment volume allow a larger dose. Radiation therapy has recently been reported to produce a delayed recovery in ambulation (3 to 6 months) in patients paraplegic for up to 9 days. Recovery was more common in patients whose weakness had a gradual onset over weeks.

Surgery

The role of surgery is being re-evaluated. Surgery is a major undertaking in patients with metastatic disease who have limited life expectancy. Nevertheless, it has been advocated to obtain diagnostic material, to help the rapidly deteriorating patient, to decompress the spinal cord and nerve roots, to correct spinal instability, to relieve pain, and to promote early mobilization. Spinal instability is a potential cause of cord damage and is not affected by radiation therapy. Recently, spinal surgeons, extrapolating from traumatic spinal cord injury and using a similar framework, have divided the bony space into three columns: anterior column—anterior longitudinal ligament and anterior vertebral body; middle column—posterior longitudinal ligament, posterior vertebral body, and pedicles; and posterior column—facet joints, lamina, and interspinous ligaments. Spinal instability occurs most often if the cortical bone in more than one of three columns is involved, either by tumor or by previous surgery. Surgical relief of pain can be achieved in approximately 75 percent of patients.

Most old trials compared decompressive laminectomy with radiation therapy. Decompressive laminectomy for metastatic epidural spinal cord compression in the presence of vertebral body collapse is contraindicated. It has a 25 percent risk of major neurologic deterioration, 22 percent risk of spinal instability, and only 3 percent recovery of ambulation. The only indications for decompressive laminectomy are tissue diagnosis and removal of posteriorly situated epidural deposits, when vertebral body disease is absent. In a retrospective study of patients with rapidly progressing weakness developing over 48 hours or less, radiation therapy was shown to be superior to posterior decompressive laminectomy in the return of patients to ambulatory status. In this same series, radiosensitive lesions did better than radioresistant lesions regardless of treatment (surgery versus radiation), emphasizing that the type of tumor is prognostically more important than the type of therapy (Gilbert et al., 1978). Paraplegic patients traditionally have not improved with posterior decompressive laminectomy, but anterior vertebral body resection shows some promise in paraplegic patients. Problems with wound closure and infection, which may be increased with radiation therapy, produce significant morbidity. Longer term problems are spinal instability or nonfusion and worsening pain. Posterior stabilization may be required following decompressive laminectomy to prevent spinal instability.

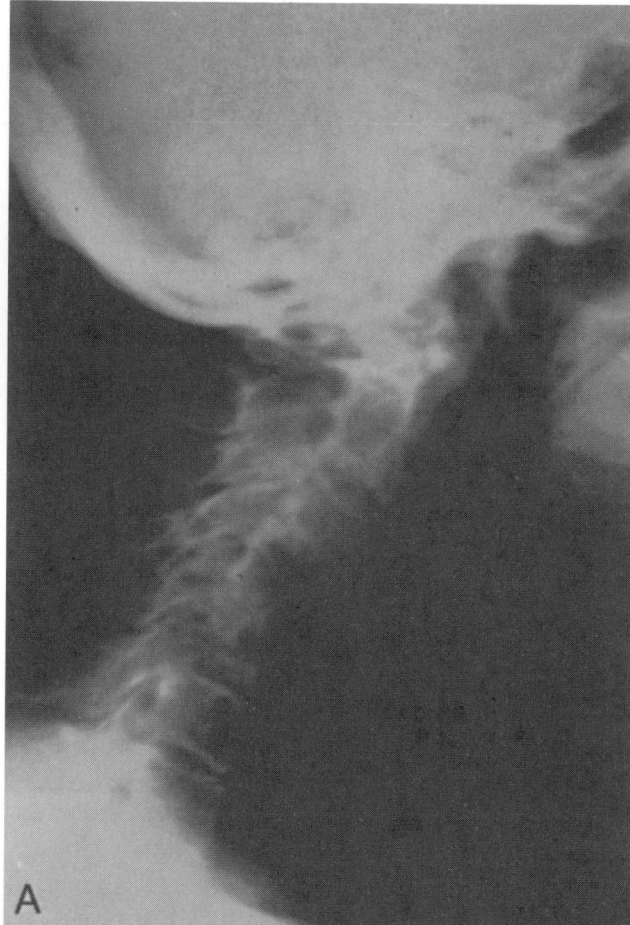
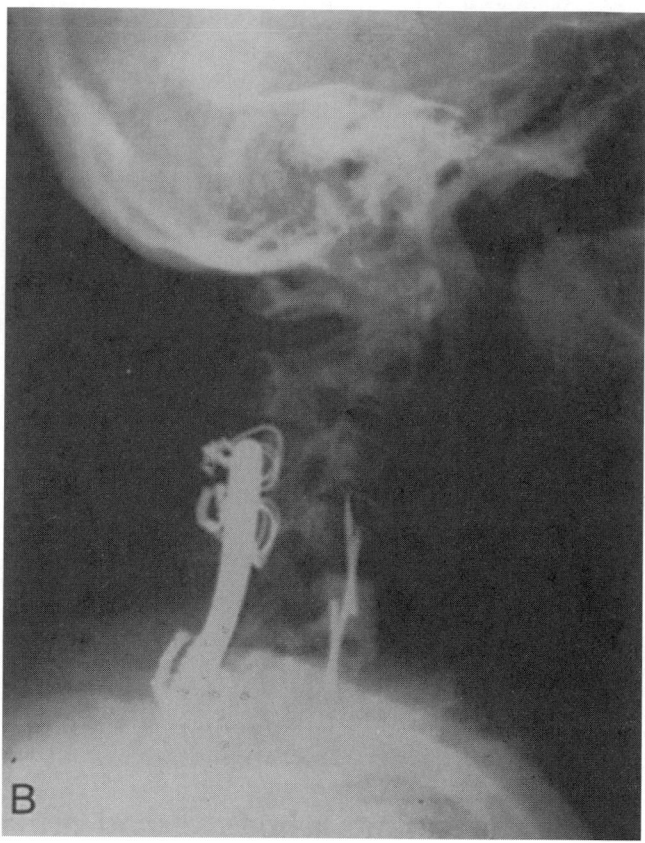

FIG. 167-4.   Plain radiographs (**A**) before and (**B**) after vertebral body resection with anterior and posterior stabilization.

In selected patients with spinal instability, anterior decompression should be considered before radiation therapy. Patients with vertebral compression with anteriorly placed epidural lesions will require a transthoracic, transabdominal, or retroperitoneal approach for vertebral body resection. Anterior stabilization is usually produced using Steinmann pins and methyl methacrylate or bone graft. Concomitant posterior stabilization may be necessary if the neural arch is also involved with tumor (Fig. 167-4).

Clinical outcome following anterior decompression in patients with a single anteriorly situated epidural metastasis is remarkably good. Fifty-two percent of these patients, who are in good general health and have either not responded to radiation or have a radioresistant tumor, will have an improvement in ambulation and a median survival of 16 months. The operative mortality rate is 7 percent, and the surgical morbidity rate is 11 percent. Transient neurologic worsening occurs in approximately 2 percent. Spinal instability develops in 5 percent of patients, and recompression at the initial site will eventually occur in 22 percent of patients.

In other surgical series of vertebral body resection, pain improved in 60 to 97 percent, and neurologic function improved in 55 to 97 percent. However, in one study, the postoperative mortality rate was almost 36 percent. Prior radiation therapy may also increase the morbidity and mortality rates of anterior decompression.

Single-stage synchronous anterior decompression by a posterolateral approach with posterior stabilization has been advocated in patients with vertebral collapse and destruction of the neural arch posteriorly. Initial results in selected patients are encouraging, with two-thirds of nonambulant patients in one series regaining the ability to walk. This combined procedure by a posterolateral approach may reduce respiratory or abdominal complications related to anterior transthoracic or transabdominal surgery.

The literature on metastatic epidural spinal cord compression is notable for the lack of good randomized studies dealing with clinical aspects and therapeutic options. There is, however, a randomized multi-institutional study in progress to investigate patients with metastatic epidural spinal cord compression who are ''surgical candidates'' to study the question whether lesion-directed surgery with stabilization and radiation is more effective than radiation alone.

Chemotherapy

Chemotherapy may have a place in treating patients who have metastatic epidural spinal cord compression, have previously had radiation, and are not surgical candidates or in those with widespread metastases. Complete resolution of paraparesis following intravenous chemotherapy has been reported in patients with breast cancer who have not responded to radiation.

SUGGESTED READINGS

Barron KD, Hirano A, Araki S, Terry RD: Experiences with metastatic neoplasms involving the spinal cord. Neurology 9:91–106, 1959

Black P: Spinal metastasis: current status and recommended guidelines for management. Neurosurgery 5:726–46, 1979

Byrne TN, Waxman SG: Spinal cord compression: diagnosis and principles of management. In Contemporary Neurology Series. FA Davis, Philadelphia, 1990

Constans JP, DeDivitis E, Donzelli R et al: Spinal metastases with neurological manifestations: review of 600 cases. J Neurosurg 59:111–8, 1983

Elsberg CA: Extradural spinal tumors—primary, secondary, metastatic. Surg Gynecol Obstet 46:1–20, 1928

Findlay GFG: The role of vertebral body collapse in the management of malignant spinal cord compression. J Neurol Neurosurg Psychiatry 50:151–4, 1987

Gilbert RW, Kim JH, Posner JB: Epidural spinal cord compression from metastatic tumor: diagnosis and treatment. Ann Neurol 3:40–51, 1978

Greenberg HS, Kim JH, Posner JB: Epidural spinal cord compression from metastatic tumors: results with a new treatment protocol. Ann Neurol 8: 361–6, 1980

Helweg-Larsen S, Rasmusson B, Soelberg Sorenson P: Recovery of gait after radiotherapy in paralytic patients with metastatic epidural spinal cord compression. Neurology 40:1234–6, 1990

Moore AJ, Uttley D: Anterior decompression and stabilization of the spine in malignant disease. Neurosurgery 24:713–7, 1989

O'Rourke T, George CB, Redmond J et al: Spinal computed tomography and computed tomographic metrizamide myelography in the early diagnosis of metastatic disease. J Clin Oncol 4:551–83, 1986

Portenoy RK, Galer BS, Salamon O et al: Identification of epidural neoplasms: radiography and bone scintigraphy in the symptomatic and asymptomatic spine. Cancer 64:2207–13, 1989

Redmond J, Friedl KE, Cornett P et al: Clinical usefulness of an algorithm for the early diagnosis of spinal metastatic disease. J Clin Oncol 6:154–7, 1988

Rodichok LD, Ruckdeschel JC, Harper GR et al: Early detection and treatment of spinal epidural metastases: the role of myelography. Ann Neurol 20: 696–702, 1986

Ropper AH, Poskanzer DC: The progress of acute and subacute transverse myelopathy based on early signs and symptoms. Ann Neurol 4:51–9, 1978

Ruff RL, Lanska DJ: Epidural metastases in prospectively evaluated veterans with cancer and back pain. Cancer 11:2234–41, 1989

Siegal T, Siegal TZ: Surgical decompression of anterior and posterior malignant epidural tumors compressing the spinal cord: a prospective study. Neurosurgery 17:424–32, 1985

Sorensen PS, Borgesen SE, Rohide K et al: Metastatic epidural spinal cord compression: results of treatment and survival. Cancer 65:1502–8, 1990

Stark RJ, Henson RA, Evans SJW: Spinal metastasis: a retrospective survey from a general hospital. Brain 105:189–213, 1982

Sundaresan N, Galicich JH, Lane JM et al: Treatment of neoplastic epidural cord compression by vertebral body resection and stabilization. J Neurosurg 63: 676–84, 1985

Vecht ChJ, Haaxma-Reiche H, van Putten WLJ et al: Initial bolus of conventional versus high dose dexamethasone in metastatic spinal cord compression. Neurology 39:1255–7, 1989

Young RF, Post EM, King GA: Treatment of spinal epidural metastases: randomized prospective comparison of laminectomy and radiotherapy. J Neurosurg 53:741–8, 1980

168. NEOPLASTIC MENINGITIS

STUART A. GROSSMAN

The disseminated and multifocal seeding of the leptomeninges by malignant cells is referred to as neoplastic meningitis. This disorder is also called carcinomatous meningitis, lymphomatous meningitis, or leukemic meningitis, depending on the histology of the underlying disease. Neoplastic meningitis occurs when tumor cells gain access to the cerebrospinal fluid (CSF) and are transported throughout the central nervous system (CNS) by the bulk flow of the CSF. This is a serious complication of cancer that results in substantial morbidity and mortality. A high index of suspicion and early diagnosis and treatment are key to the optimal management of this increasing common and devastating neuro-oncologic disorder.

ANATOMY AND PHYSIOLOGY

The neuraxis of an adult contains approximately 140 ml of CSF in the ventricles and the spinal and cortical subarachnoid space. Approximately five times that much CSF is produced daily by the choroid plexus in the lateral, third, and fourth ventricles. CSF flows through the CNS in a predictable fashion. It leaves the fourth ventricle through the foramina of Magendie and Luschka, traverses the spinal subarachnoid space, returns to the basilar cisterns, and passes over the cortical convexities into the superior sagittal sinus via the arachnoid granulations (Fig. 168-1). CSF flow along these pathways results from the continuous production of CSF and alterations in pressure within the subarachnoid space that result from arterial pulsations, changes in position, and Valsalva maneuvers.

INCIDENCE

Neoplastic meningitis was once thought to be rare and was uncommonly diagnosed before death. However, leptomeningeal metastases are now recognized with increasing frequency as a result of heightened awareness of the diagnosis, new neuroimaging techniques, and improved survival in some systemic malignancies. In large series, most patients with neoplastic meningitis have breast cancer (11 to 64 percent), lung cancer (14 to 29 percent), or melanoma (6 to 18 percent). It is currently estimated that leptomeningeal disease occurs in 5 percent of patients with breast cancer, 9 to 25 percent with small cell lung cancer, 23 percent with melanoma, 5 to 29 percent with non-Hodgkin's lymphomas, and 11 to 70 percent with leukemias. Autopsy studies demonstrate that 19 percent of patients with cancer and neurologic complications have meningeal involvement and that concomitant intraparenchymal or epidural metastases are common. Patients with lymphomas are at highest risk if they have bone marrow, testicular, or extranodal sites involved and if the tumors have a diffuse, lymphoblastic, or Burkitt's histology. Although neoplastic meningitis usually occurs in patients with advanced and progressive systemic cancer, it can present as the first manifestation of a malignancy.

PATHOGENESIS

Tumor cells most commonly gain access to the subarachnoid space by direct extension from pre-existing tumors or by hematogenous dissemination as listed below.

Direct extension from
  Pre-existing CNS tumors (epidural, subdural, or intraparenchymal)
  Pre-existing systemic tumors that advance along nerve roots to gain access to the subarachnoid space
Hematogenous
  Via arachnoid vessels or choroid plexus

Direct extension is best exemplified by the leptomeningeal involvement associated with some primary brain tumors. Ependymomas, pineoblastomas, and medulloblastomas, which are

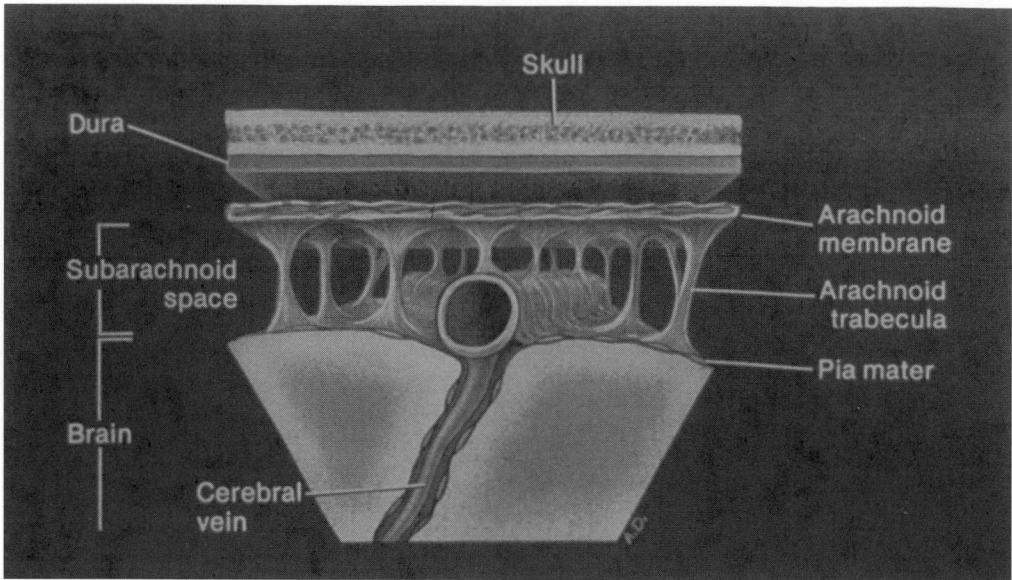

FIG. 168-1.   Anatomy of the leptomeninges. (Modified from Grossman SA, Moynihan TJ: Neoplastic meningitis. Neurol Clin North Am 9:843–56, 1991, with permission.)

contiguous with the CSF, frequently involve the CSF. However, symptomatic leptomeningeal disease is less common with intraparenchymal astrocytic brain tumors. Metastatic tumors can also reach the meninges by direct extension. Patients with solid tumors and neoplastic meningitis frequently have cerebral, cerebellar, or epidural metastases, which can provide direct access to the leptomeninges.

The leukemias provide a model for hematogenous dissemination to the leptomeninges. These malignant cells traverse the walls of the superficial arachnoid veins and surrounding adventitia en route to the CSF. They migrate through arachnoid vessels, seed the choroid plexus, and extend into the leptomeninges from hemorrhagic brain infarcts. This pattern of tumor dissemination into the leptomeninges has also been noted in solid tumors. Patients with small cell lung cancer and isolated leptomeningeal disease have been found to have tumor filling the Virchow-Robin spaces with perivascular extension, perineural and perivascular lymphatic involvement, invasion of endoneural and perineural sheaths of the intervertebral foramina, and choroid plexus involvement.

Solid tumors may also enter the subarachnoid space through the venous plexus of Batson, perivenous spread from bone marrow metastases, or direct extension along nerve sheaths. The latter has been noted in patients with squamous cell carcinoma of the head and neck.

Once malignant cells gain access to the CSF, they spread along the surface of the meninges of the brain and spinal cord. Exfoliated cells are carried by the flow of the CSF to distant regions of the CNS. Tumor deposits on leptomeningeal surfaces invade subpial parenchyma, penetrate spinal nerve roots, and produce masses in the subarachnoid space. The basilar cisterns, posterior fossa, and cauda equina are most commonly affected. Gravity may be responsible for the high risk for symptomatic involvement in these areas.

CLINICAL PRESENTATION AND DIAGNOSIS

Neoplastic meningitis may become clinically apparent in several ways (Table 168-1). Patients frequently present with signs

TABLE 168-1. Signs and Symptoms of Neoplastic Meningitis

Signs and Symptoms	Etiology
Increased intracranial pressure	CSF flow abnormalities
Focal neurologic abnormalities	Parenchymal invasion in Virchow-Robin space or along spinal cord Direct invasion of nerves in subarachnoid space Occlusion of penetrating pial blood vessels
Encephalopathy	Interference with normal CNS metabolism

Abbreviations: CSF, cerebrospinal fluid; CNS, central nervous system.

(Modified from Grossman SA, Moynihan TJ: Neoplastic meningitis. Neurol Clin North Am 9:843–56, 1991, with permission.)

and symptoms of increased intracranial pressure and hydrocephalus. These occur as a result of obstruction of normal CSF flow pathways. CSF flow abnormalities have been identified in up to 70 percent of patients with neoplastic meningitis using radionuclide CSF flow scans. Leptomeningeal tumor can also invade underlying brain and spinal parenchyma, nerve roots, and vessels that supply the CNS. These lesions can cause focal neurologic deficits or seizures. Some patients present with a diffuse encephalopathy, which may be secondary to tumor-induced changes in brain metabolism or regional cerebral blood flow.

A high index of suspicion is required to make an early diagnosis of leptomeningeal metastases. The diagnosis should be considered if signs and symptoms suggest multifocal involvement of the CNS. Multiple cranial nerve palsies that result in diplopia, dysphagia, dysarthria, and hearing loss are common presenting complaints. Headache, changes in mental status, back or radicular pain, incontinence, lower motor neuron weakness, and sensory abnormalities are also frequently reported. The vast majority of patients have a combination of cranial nerve, cerebral, and spinal signs and symptoms at the time of diagnosis.

LABORATORY STUDIES

Examination of the CSF is the most useful laboratory test for the diagnosis of neoplastic meningitis (Table 1681-2). Only

TABLE 168-2. Diagnostic Tests for Neoplastic Meningitis

Test	Parameter
Lumbar puncture	↑ Pressure (50%)
	↑ Protein (75%)
	↓ Glucose (40%)
	First cytology result positive (50%)
	One of ≥ three cytology results positive (85%)
Myelography/spinal MRI	Subarachnoid masses
Brain CT/MRI	Meningeal enhancement
	Enlarged ventricles

Abbreviations: CT, computed tomography; MRI, magnetic resonance imaging.

(Modified from Grossman SA, Moynihan TJ: Neoplastic meningitis. Neurol Clin North Am 9:843–56, 1991, with permission.)

3 percent of patients with leptomeningeal metastases have a completely normal lumbar puncture. A positive CSF cytology is found in approximately 50 percent of patients with this disorder on the initial lumbar puncture and in 85 percent of patients who undergo multiple diagnostic spinal taps. The CSF cytology is much more likely to be positive in the lumbar region than in the ventricle of the same patient with documented leptomeningeal involvement. A positive CSF cytology is virtually diagnostic of leptomeningeal metastases. However, differentiating reactive from malignant lymphocytes can be difficult and may lead to false-positive cytologies in patients with viral infections of the CNS. Elevations in opening pressure or CSF protein and a pleocytosis are common but nonspecific abnormalities. A low CSF glucose can occur with CNS infections or leptomeningeal metastases.

BIOCHEMICAL MARKERS

Numerous biochemical markers have been studied in the CSF of patients with neoplastic meningitis. Unfortunately, their utility is limited by poor sensitivity and specificity. Carcinoembryonic antigen (CEA), a high molecular weight glycoprotein produced by colon, breast, ovarian, bladder, and lung cancer cells, is not normally detectable in the CSF. A number of studies have demonstrated that an elevated CSF CEA level, in the absence of a markedly elevated serum level, is relatively specific for carcinomatous meningitis. This biomarker is not useful in patients with lymphomatous meningitis. CSF CEA levels tend to decline with successful therapy and can rise in patients before other findings of leptomeningeal relapse are evident.

Studies of CSF β-glucuronidase, lactate dehydrogenase, and β_2-microglobulin have been disappointing. Elevations of these markers are not specific for neoplastic meningitis, often fluctuate widely, and can be elevated as a consequence of antineoplastic therapy. As a result, they are rarely of use in the diagnosis or monitoring of this disorder.

RADIOLOGIC STUDIES

Radiologic studies are important in the diagnosis of neoplastic meningitis. Contrast-enhanced computed tomography or magnetic resonance imaging scans of the brain are routinely obtained in patients with cancer and worrisome neurologic signs or symptoms. These scans identify most intraparenchymal lesions and provide an estimate of the risk of herniation following lumbar puncture. Approximately one-half of patients with neoplastic meningitis have abnormal imaging studies. Some radiologic findings, such as multiple subarachnoid mass lesions, are virtually diagnostic of neoplastic meningitis. Others, such as those with hydrocephalus without an identifiable mass lesion,

are consistent with or suggestive of the diagnosis. Meningeal enhancement is of limited utility in the early diagnosis of leptomeningeal malignancy. Contrast enhancement of the basilar cisterns or cortical convexities is usually seen with advanced leptomeningeal involvement when the CSF cytology is likely to be positive. In addition, it is commonly associated with infections, inflammatory diseases, trauma, subdural hematomas, and recent neurosurgical procedures, making it a nonspecific finding.

TREATMENT

The goals of treatment in patients with neoplastic meningitis are (1) to improve or stabilize the neurologic status of the patient and (2) to prolong survival. Fixed neurologic deficits, such as paraplegia or cranial nerve palsies, usually do not improve with therapy, although a diffuse encephalopathy may resolve dramatically. Without therapy, the median survival of patients with this disorder is 4 to 6 weeks, and death usually results from progressive neurologic dysfunction. Occasionally patients with indolent tumors live significantly longer even without therapy. Appropriate therapy for neoplastic meningitis often provides effective local control. As a result, many patients succumb to systemic rather than neurologic complications of their neoplasm.

Treatment of neoplastic meningitis must encompass the entire nervous system, as tumor cells are disseminated widely by the flow of CSF (Table 168-3). Radiation should be administered to symptomatic regions of the neuraxis and to bulk disease identified on neuroimaging studies. Intrathecal chemotherapy is directed at subclinical leptomeningeal deposits and tumor cells floating in the CSF. Craniospinal irradiation is of limited benefit in solid tumors, which are not exceptionally radiosensitive. In addition, this is time consuming and myelosuppressive, especially in patients who have received prior antineoplastic therapy. High doses of systemically administered cytarabine, methotrexate, or thiotepa can yield therapeutic concentrations of these agents in the CSF for short periods of time. However, the systemic toxicities of these agents prohibit twice-weekly dosing, making this an inadequate approach for established leptomeningeal metastases.

Intrathecal chemotherapy is usually administered through an implanted subcutaneous reservoir and ventricular catheter (SRVC) (Fig. 168-2). These devices are associated with little morbidity or mortality when placed by an experienced neurosurgeon. Intraventricularly administered drugs reach the CSF reliably. They may also be more uniformly distributed and associated with a higher response rate and longer remissions than drugs administered in the lumbar CSF. Use of the SRVC is also less painful than repeated lumbar punctures. However, even when an SRVC is in place, periodic lumbar punctures are needed to determine the response to intraventricular chemotherapy. This is necessary because the ventricular CSF cytology is much less likely to be positive than a specimen taken from the lumbar region at the same time. In addition, the normal

TABLE 168-3. Standard Therapy for Neoplastic Meningitis

Radiation therapy to sites of symptomatic and bulk disease
Intrathecal chemotherapy
    Methotrexate (10 mg twice weekly)
    Thiotepa (10 mg twice weekly)
    Cytarabine (90 mg/week)
OPtimal treatment of systemic disease

(Modified from Grossman SA, Moynihan TJ: Neoplastic meningitis. Neurol Clin North Am 9:843–56, 1991, with permission.)

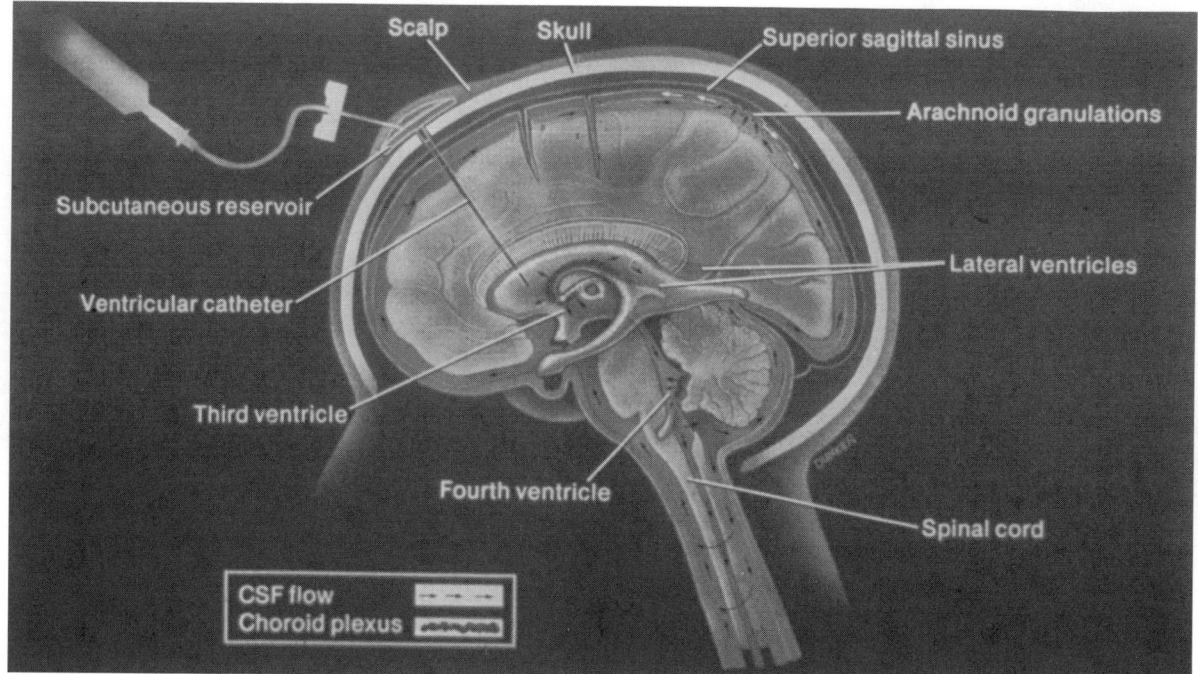

FIG. 168-2. CSF circulation in a patient with an Ommaya reservoir. (Modified from Grossman SA, Moynihan TJ: Neoplastic meningitis. Neurol Clin North Am 9:843–56, 1991, with permission.)

ventricular CSF glucose level is higher and the protein concentration is lower than lumbar samples.

CSF flow abnormalities are common in patients with neoplastic meningitis. Radionuclide ventriculography in patients with neoplastic meningitis has shown that up to 70 percent have ventricular outlet obstructions, abnormal flow in the spinal canal, or impaired flow over the cortical convexities. As a result, patients with neoplastic meningitis should undergo radionuclide ventriculography to determine if they have serious CSF flow disturbances. These can affect the distribution, efficacy, and toxicity of intrathecal chemotherapy and are potentially reversible with radiation therapy.

A limited number of antineoplastic agents are suitable for intrathecal administration. Fixed doses of these agents should be administered as the volume of CSF is not a function of surface area in adults. Although combination chemotherapy has led to substantial improvements in the treatment of systemic cancers, combination intrathecal regimens have yet to demonstrate superiority to any single intrathecal agent.

Methotrexate is the most widely used and thoroughly studied agent for intrathecal administration. Ten milligrams of preservative-free methotrexate mixed in artificial CSF or saline is usually given twice weekly for eight treatments or until the CSF clears. This is commonly followed by weekly and then monthly maintenance therapy if the patient remains free of progressive disease. These treatments will result in therapeutic concentrations (more than 10^{-6} M) that persist for 48 hours. Serum levels peak at 10^{-7} M and fall slowly. The low but prolonged systemic concentrations of this cycle-active agent may result in significant myelosuppression. With this treatment approach, approximately 50 percent of patients will stabilize or improve, but the median survival remains under 6 months even in patients with responsive malignancies.

Intrathecal cytarabine, a synthetic pyrimidine nucleoside, is commonly used in patients with leukemic and lymphomatous meningitis. This agent has limited activity in most solid tumors. The half-life of cytarabine is short in the serum but longer in the CSF because of the low levels of cytidine deaminase in the CSF. An intrathecal dose of 30 mg daily for 3 days results in therapeutic concentrations (more than 4×10^{-4} M) for more than 72 hours. The systemic toxicities of intrathecal cytarabine are minimal because of the drug is rapidly deaminated in the systemic circulation. Response rates in leukemic meningitis range from 50 to 70 percent.

Thiotepa, a potent alkylating agent with activity in many solid tumors, can be administered intrathecally. It is stored as a sodium salt and should be mixed with sterile water instead of artificial CSF to avoid injecting a hypertonic solution into the subarachnoid space. A recently reported randomized phase III trial comparing intrathecal thiotepa and methotrexate demonstrated identical survival with these agents. However, thiotepa appeared to be associated with fewer overall and neurologic toxicities than methotrexate.

TREATMENT-RELATED TOXICITIES

Significant toxicities can accompany therapy for neoplastic meningitis. These can result from placement of the SRVC and the administration of radiation and intrathecal chemotherapy. The primary toxicities seen with the SRVC include perioperative complications, migration of the ventricular catheter tip into adjacent brain tissue, or infections of the device. Many of the infections are secondary to *Staphylococcus epidermidis* and can be treated with local antibiotics rather than removal of the SRVC. Radiation for leptomeningeal disease can be fairly myelosuppressive. Myelosuppression is common if the treatment portals are large, the patient is receiving systemic antineoplastic therapies, or the marrow reserve is compromised by prior antineoplastic therapies or tumor in the bone marrow. Intrathecal methotrexate can result in acute arachnoiditis and seizures, which are associated with high CSF levels. Long-term administration of intrathecal methotrexate, especially following cranial irradiation, almost invariably results in radiologic and clinical manifestations of treatment-induced leukoencephalopathy. These white matter changes are initially seen in asymptomatic patients on routine neuroimaging studies. However, patients subsequently develop progressive neurologic signs and symptoms, which can be fatal. Although the pathogenesis of this toxicity has not been determined, recent data suggest that it may result from direct toxicity to neurons with secondary demyelination. Mucositis and myelosuppression, from intrathecal methotrexate, can be prevented with the systemic administration of folinic acid. The acute and chronic toxicities of intrathecal cytarabine and thiotepa are less well characterized.

NEW THERAPEUTIC APPROACHES

Several new intrathecal chemotherapeutic agents or delivery techniques are being evaluated to improve the efficacy or reduce the toxicity of therapy for neoplastic meningitis. Those in clinical trials now include 4-hydroxycyclophosphamide, an active metabolite of cyclophosphamide, liposomally encapsulated cytarabine, and antibodies conjugated to radioactive isotopes.

THERAPEUTIC DECISIONS

Many clinicians are hesitant to treat patients with neoplastic meningitis. Therapy can result in significant neurologic toxicities; fixed neurologic deficits rarely improve; most patients have extensive and progressive systemic disease; and survival, even with therapy, can be short. However, prompt evaluation of patients with cancer and neurologic signs and symptoms can result in a diagnosis of neoplastic meningitis before serious and permanent neurologic disabilities occur. A similar approach is recommended in the evaluation of epidural metastases in which a late diagnosis is often associated with permanent paraplegia. An early diagnosis of epidural metastases and prompt, appropriate therapy provides excellent local control, allowing most patients to die of progressive systemic disease with intact spinal cord function. Similarly, early diagnosis and treatment of leptomeningeal disease should provide excellent local control.

Once the diagnosis of leptomeningeal metastases is made, several factors should be considered in deciding how aggressive treatment should be (Table 168-4). Patients with an excellent performance status, an indolent systemic cancer that is potentially responsive to treatment, and minimal or no evidence of systemic disease should be considered for aggressive therapy. On the other hand, in patients with multiple, serious, fixed neurologic symptoms; a poor performance status; and extensive

disease from a poorly responsive tumor, deficits are unlikely to benefit from therapy.

Ideal treatment candidates should begin radiation to bulk and symptomatic sites of disease and placement of an SRVC should be considered. A CSF flow scan should be performed to obtain information on the distribution of intraventricularly administered drugs. Local radiation should be administered to sites of abnormal CSF flow. Intrathecal chemotherapy should be accompanied by optimal management of the patient's underlying systemic malignancy. Patients who are poor candidates for aggressive therapy may benefit from radiation therapy to symptomatic sites or supportive measures only. Local radiation therapy and a trial of intrathecal chemotherapy delivered by lumbar puncture may be appropriate in patients who are intermediate candidates. This approach allows time for the natural course of the disease to be manifest before committing to a more aggressive or conservative approach.

CONCLUSIONS

Neoplastic meningitis is a serious complication of systemic malignancies that appears to be increasing in frequency. Although it occurs with virtually any malignancy, it is recognized most often in patients with breast cancer, lymphomas, and small cell cancer of the lung. A high index of suspicion is required to make the diagnosis of leptomeningeal metastases. A careful history and physical examination usually reveals signs and symptoms that indicate involvement of more than one area of the CNS. The diagnosis of neoplastic meningitis is made by a positive CSF cytology, subarachnoid metastases identified on radiologic studies, or a compelling history and physical examination combined with an abnormal, but not diagnostic, examination of the CSF. Treatment should include radiation therapy to symptomatic areas of the CNS, intrathecal chemotherapy, and optimal therapy of the systemic cancer. Careful selection of patients for aggressive therapy is indicated. Despite the potential toxicities of therapy, many patients will receive substantial palliation, some will live for more than 1 year, and most will die of systemic tumor progression without symptomatic recurrence of their leptomeningeal metastases. New efforts are underway to decrease the toxicity and improve the efficacy of antineoplastic therapy for this devastating complication of cancer.

SUGGESTED READINGS

Bleyer WA, Drake JC, Chabner BA: Neurotoxicity and elevated cerebrospinal fluid methotrexate concentration in meningeal leukemia. N Engl J Med 289:770–3, 1973

Boyle R, Thomas M, Adams JH: Diffuse involvement of the leptomeninges by tumor—a clinical and pathological study of 63 cases. Postgrad Med J 56:149–58, 1980

Chamberlain MC, Sandy AD, Press GA: Leptomeningeal metastasis: a comparison of gadolinium-enhanced MR and contrast-enhanced CT of the brain. Neurology 40:435–8, 1990

Ettinger LJ, Chervinsky DS, Freeman AI, Creaven PJ: Pharmacokinetics of methotrexate following intravenous and intraventricular administration in acute lymphocytic leukemia and non-Hodgkin's lymphoma. Cancer 50: 1676–82, 1982

Gilbert MR, Harding BL, Grossman SA: Methotrexate neurotoxicity: in vitro studies using cerebellar explants. Cancer Res 49:2502–5, 1989

Glass JP, Melamed M, Chernik NL, Posner JB: Malignant cells in cerebrospinal fluid (CSF): the meaning of a positive CSF cytology. Neurology 29: 1369–75, 1979

Grossman SA, Finkelstein DM, Ruckdeschchel JC et al: Randomized prospective comparison of intraventricular methotrexate and thiotepa in patients

TABLE 168-4. Factors Influencing Treatment Decisions in Neoplastic Meningitis

	Good Treatment Candidate	Poor Treatment Candidate
Features of tumor	Indolent Treatment responsive	Aggressive Resistant
Extent of systemic tumor	Absent	Widespread
Degree of fixed neurologic deficits	None	Multiple, serious
Performance status of patient	Normal	Confined to bed

(Modified from Grossman SA, Moynihan TJ: Neoplastic meningitis. Neurol Clin North Am 9:843–56, 1991, with permission.)

with previously untreated neoplastic meningitis. J Clin Oncol 11:561–9, 1993

Grossman SA, Moynihan TJ: Neoplastic meningitis. Neurol Clin North Am 9: 843–56, 1991

Grossman SA, Trump DL, Chen DC et al: Cerebrospinal fluid flow abnormalities in patients with neoplastic meningitis. An evaluation using [111]indium-DTPA ventriculography. Am J Med 73:641–47, 1982

Gutin PH, Weiss HD, Wiernik PH, Walker MD: Intrathecal N, N′, N″-triethylenethiophosphoramide [thio- TEPA (NSC 6396)] in the treatment of malignant meningeal disease: phase I–II study. Cancer 38:1471–5, 1976

Krol G, Sze G, Malkin M, Walker R: MR of cranial and spinal meningeal carcinomatosis: comparison with CT and myelography. AJR Am J Roentgenol 151:583–8, 1988

Olson ME, Chernik NL, Posner JB: Infiltration of the leptomeninges by systemic cancer. A clinical and pathologic study. Arch Neurol 30:122–37, 1974

Schold SC, Wasserstrom WR, Fleisher M et al: Cerebrospinal fluid biochemical markers of central nervous system metastases. Ann Neurol 8:597–604, 1980

Shapiro WR, Young DF, Mehta BM: Methotrexate: distribution in cerebrospinal fluid after intravenous, ventricular and lumbar injections. N Engl J Med 293:161–6, 1975

Sze G, Soletsky S, Bronen R, Krol G: MR imaging of the cranial meninges with emphasis on contrast enhancement and meningeal carcinomatosis. AJNR Am J Neuroradiol 10:965–75, 1989

Twijnstra A, Ongerboer de Visser BW, van Zanten AP: Diagnosis of leptomeningeal metastasis. Clin Neurol Neurosurg 89:79–85, 1987

Wasserstrom WR, Glass JP, Posner JB: Diagnosis and treatment of leptomeningeal metastases from solid tumors: experience with 90 patients. Cancer 49:759–72, 1982

Yap HY, Yap BS, Tashima CK et al: Meningeal carcinomatosis in breast cancer. Cancer 42:283–6, 1978

Zimm S, Collins JM, Miser J et al: Cytosine arabinoside cerebrospinal fluid kinetics. Clin Pharmacol Ther 35:826–30, 1984

169. NEUROLOGIC COMPLICATIONS OF CHEMOTHERAPY

PATRICK Y. WEN

Neurologic complications are seen with increasingly frequency in patients with cancer as a result of aggressive antineoplastic therapy and prolonged patient survival. These complications may result from the direct toxic effects of the drug on the nervous system or indirectly from metabolic encephalopathies, infections, or cerebral vascular disorders induced by the drugs. It is important to recognize these complications since they may be confused with metastatic disease and because they may result in significant disability, requiring that the drug be discontinued before irreversible damage occurs.

In this review the neurologic complications of the more commonly used chemotherapeutic agents, hormones, and biologic response modifiers in patients with cancer are discussed. A list of these complications, along with the specific drugs that cause them, are also presented in Table 169-1.

CHEMOTHERAPY

Drugs That Commonly Cause Neurotoxicity

Cisplatin. Cisplatin is an alkylating agent frequently used in the treatment of ovarian, testicular, small cell lung, and head and neck cancers.

NEUROPATHY.   The main neurotoxicity of cisplatin is an axonal neuropathy affecting predominantly large myelinated sensory fibers. This usually occurs with doses greater than 400 mg/m^2 and is characterized by numbness, paresthesias, and occasionally pain in the extremities. Proprioception is impaired, and reflexes are lost, but pinprick, temperature sensation, and power are often spared. Nerve conduction studies show decreased amplitude of sensory action potentials and prolonged sensory latencies, compatible with a sensory axonopathy. Sural nerve biopsy shows both demyelination and axonal loss. It is unclear whether the primary site of damage is the sensory nerve, dorsal root ganglia, or both. After cessation of chemotherapy, the neuropathy may improve and even return to normal after many months. The main differential diagnosis is a paraneoplastic neuropathy. The latter tends to be progressive despite discontinuation of cisplatin and involves all sensory fibers.

There is no treatment for cisplatin neurotoxicity, but amifostine partially protects peripheral nerves from cisplatin, and a double-blind placebo-controlled study suggested that the adrenocorticotropic hormone (4–9) analogue, Org 2766, may prevent cisplatin neurotoxicity. Recently nerve growth factor has been shown to prevent cisplatin neuropathy in animals, and clinical trials using this agent are in progress.

Arterial infusions of cisplatin in the extremities or neck may produce focal neuropathies. Autonomic neuropathies have also been rarely observed.

CRANIAL NEUROPATHIES.   Cisplatin may cause ototoxicity, leading to high-frequency sensorineural hearing loss and tinnitus. The toxicity is due to peripheral receptor (hair loss) in the organ of Corti and is dose related. Audiometric hearing

TABLE 169-1. Neurologic Complications of Chemotherapy and Biologic Response Modifiers

Acute encephalopathy	Vasculopathies and "strokes"
Altretamine	Asparaginase
Asparaginase	Carmustine (IA)
5-Azacytidine	Cisplatin (IA)
Carmustine	Methotrexate
Cisplatin	
Cytarabine (HD)	Aseptic meningitis
5-Fluorouracil	Cytarabine
Glucocorticoids	Methotrexate
Ifosfamide	Levamisole
Interferons	
Interleukin-2	Headaches
Methotrexate	Glucocorticoids
Misonidazole	Retinoic acid
Procarbazine	Tamoxifen
Tamoxifen	
	Visual loss
Dementia	Carmustine (IA)
Carmofur	Cisplatin
Carmustine	Tamoxifen
Cytarabine	
α-Interferon	Cranial neuropathies
Fludarabine	Carmustine (IA) (ototoxicity)
Methotrexate	Cisplatin (ototoxicity, vestibulopathy)
	Vincristine (extraocular palsies)
Acute cerebellar syndrome	
Cytarabine (HD)	Myelopathies
5-Fluorouracil	Cytarabine (IT)
Procarbazine	Methotrexate (IT)
Vincristine	Thiotepa (IT)
Seizures	Neuropathies
Asparaginase	Altretamine
Busulfan (HD)	5-Azacytidine
Carmustine	Cisplatin
Cisplatin	Cytarabine
Dacarbazine	Misonidazole
Etoposide	Paclitaxel
Methotrexate	Procarbazine
Vincristine	Suramin
	Teniposide
	Vinca alkaloids

Abbreviations: HD, high dose; IT, intrathecal; IA, intra-arterial.

loss is present in 74 to 88 percent of patients receiving cisplatin, and symptomatic hearing loss occurs in 16 to 20 percent of patients. Cranial irradiation probably increases the likelihood of a significant hearing loss. The hearing loss tends to be worse in children, although they have a slightly greater ability to improve after the drug has been stopped. Cisplatin may also cause a vestibulopathy, resulting in ataxia and vertigo.

Rarely, cisplatin therapy may result in optic neuritis and retinopathy. These are more common after intracarotid administration of the drug.

SPINAL CORD INVOLVEMENT (LHERMITTE SIGN). This symptom, characterized by paresthesias in the back and extremities with neck flexion is seen in 20 to 40 percent of patients receiving cisplatin. Patients tend to develop this after weeks or months of treatment. Neurologic examination is usually normal, and the Lhermitte sign usually resolves spontaneously several months after the drug has been discontinued. It is thought to result from transient demyelination of the posterior columns. Very rarely, a true myelopathy has been reported.

UNCOMMON COMPLICATIONS. Rarely, cisplatin may produce an encephalopathy resulting in seizures and focal neurologic symptoms, including cortical blindness. The encephalopathy tends to be more common after intra-arterial administration of the drug. It has to be distinguished from a metabolic encephalopathy that may result from water intoxication caused by prehydration or from the renal impairment, hypomagnesemia, hypocalcemia, and syndrome of inappropriate antidiuretic hormone secretion (SIADH) that may follow treatment with cisplatin.

Cisplatin can also cause late vascular toxicity, resulting in strokes. Other rare complications include taste disturbance and a myasthenic syndrome.

Methotrexate. This is a dihydrofolate reductase inhibitor used in the treatment of a wide range of cancers, including leukemias, lymphomas, choriocarcinomas, breast cancer, central nervous system (CNS) lymphoma, and carcinomatous meningitis. The clinical expression of its neurotoxicity is determined by the dosage, route of administration, and use of other therapeutic modalities, such as irradiation, with overlapping neurotoxicities.

INTRATHECAL METHOTREXATE TOXICITY. Aseptic meningitis is the most common neurotoxicity associated with intrathecal methotrexate therapy. This complication occurs in approximately 10 percent of patients, although some series have reported incidences as high as 50 percent. It begins 2 to 4 hours after the drug is injected and may last for 12 to 72 hours. The clinical features are indistinguishable from other types of chemical meningitis and consist of headaches, nuchal rigidity, back pain, nausea, vomiting, fever, and lethargy. The cerebrospinal fluid (CSF) shows a pleocytosis and an elevated protein level. These symptoms resemble bacterial meningitis but occur too soon after injection of the drug to be due to an infection. The symptoms are usually self-limited and require no specific treatment. Aseptic meningitis can be prevented to some extent by injecting methotrexate with hydrocortisone. Some patients who developed aseptic meningitis have been retreated with methotrexate without subsequent problems.

Transverse myelopathy is a much less common complication of intrathecal methotrexate characterized by back or leg pain followed by paraplegia, sensory loss, and sphincter dysfunction. The symptoms usually occur between 30 minutes and 48 hours after treatment but may occur up to 2 weeks later. The majority

of cases show clinical improvement, but the extent of recovery is variable. This complication is more common in patients receiving concurrent radiotherapy or frequent treatments of intrathecal methotrexate.

Rarely, intrathecal methotrexate may produce an acute encephalopathy, subacute focal neurologic deficits, neurogenic pulmonary edema, and sudden death.

Accidental overdosage of methotrexate (more than 500 mg) usually results in myelopathy, encephalopathy, and death. The use of rapid CSF drainage, ventriculolumbar perfusion, high-dose leucovorin, and alkaline diuresis has allowed occasional patients to survive.

HIGH-DOSE METHOTREXATE NEUROTOXICITY. High-dose methotrexate may cause acute, subacute, or chronic neurotoxicity.

Acute high dose methotrexate neurotoxicity is characterized by somnolence, confusion, and seizures within 24 hours of treatment. Symptoms usually resolve spontaneously without sequelae.

Weekly treatments with high-dose methotrexate may produce a subacute "strokelike" syndrome characterized by transient focal neurologic deficits, confusion, and occasionally seizures. Typically the disorder develops 6 days after high-dose methotrexate, lasts 15 minutes to 72 hours, and resolves spontaneously without sequelae. Computed tomographic scans and CSF are usually normal, but the electroencephalogram shows diffuse slowing. Methotrexate may be subsequently administered without the encephalopathy recurring. The pathogenesis of this syndrome is unknown but may be related to reduced cerebral glucose metabolism.

Chronic leukoencephalopathy has also been reported in a number of patients following high-dose methotrexate.

LEUKOENCEPHALOPATHY. The major delayed complication of methotrexate therapy is a leukoencephalopathy. Although this syndrome may be produced by methotrexate alone, it is exacerbated by radiotherapy, especially if the latter is administered before or during methotrexate therapy. The clinical features are characterized by the gradual development of cognitive impairment, months or years after treatment with methotrexate. This may range from mild learning disabilities to severe progressive dementia, together with somnolence, seizures, ataxia, and hemiparesis. Computed tomographic and magnetic resonance imaging scans show cerebral atrophy and diffuse white matter lesions. Pathologic lesions range from loss of oligodendrocytes and gliosis to a necrotizing leukoencephalopathy. The clinical course is variable. Many patients stabilize or improve after discontinuation of the methotrexate, but the course is progressive in some patients and may lead to death. No effective treatment is available. The cause of the leukoencephalopathy is unknown. It is possible that cranial irradiation may either potentiate the toxic effects of methotrexate or disrupt the blood–brain barrier, allowing high concentrations of methotrexate to reach the brain.

Suramin. Suramin inhibits the binding of a number of growth factors to their receptors, including platelet-derived growth factor, basic fibroblast growth factor, and transforming growth factor-β. It also inhibits DNA polymerases and glycosaminoglycan catabolism. Suramin is used mainly for the treatment of refractory prostate cancer. It causes a severe peripheral neuropathy in 10 percent of patients. The neuropathy can resemble Guillain-Barré syndrome clinically. Some patients develop proximal weakness and paresthesias in the face and extremities, followed by more generalized weakness. The neuropathy usually improves after the drug is discontinued. Because the development of neuropathy correlates with blood levels of suramin, it can be prevented by monitoring blood levels of the drug (serious complications are uncommon at plasma levels less than 350 μg/ml).

Paclitaxel and Docetaxel. These are promising new agents used in the treatment of a variety of cancers, including ovary, breast, and nonsmall cell lung cancers. These are plant alkaloids that inhibit microtubule function, leading to mitotic arrest. Paclitaxel produces a dose-limiting peripheral neuropathy, which occurs in 60 percent of patients receiving 250 mg/m^2. The neuropathy is predominantly sensory and affects both large and small fibers. Symptoms usually begin after 1 to 3 weeks of treatment. Patients develop burning paresthesias of the hands and feet and loss of reflexes. Occasionally, perioral numbness, weakness, and autonomic neuropathies may occur. The neuropathy often does not progress, despite continued treatment, and there have been reports of patients even improving with continuing therapy. Some patients develop arthralgias and myalgias beginning 2 to 3 days after a course of paclitaxel and lasting 2 to 4 days. Docetaxel produces the same neuropathy as paclitaxel. Nerve growth factor prevents the neuropathy in mice and is being evaluated in clinical trials.

Vincristine. Vincristine is a vinca alkaloid used in the treatment of many cancers, including leukemia, lymphomas, sarcomas, and brain tumors. Its main toxicity is an axonal neuropathy resulting from disruption of the microtubules within axons and interference with axonal transport. The neuropathy involves both sensory and motor fibers, although small sensory fibers are especially affected. Virtually all patients have some degree of neuropathy, which is the dose-limiting toxicity. The earliest symptoms are usually paresthesias in the fingertips and feet. Muscle cramps are also common. These symptoms may occur after several weeks of treatment or even after the drug has been discontinued and progress for several months before improving. Children tend to recover more quickly than adults. Initially objective sensory findings tend to be relatively minor compared with the symptoms, but loss of ankle jerks is common. Occasionally there may be profound weakness, with bilateral foot drop and wrist drop, and loss of all sensory modalities. This occurs especially in older patients who are cachectic, patients who have received prior radiation to the peripheral nerves, or who have pre-existing neurologic diseases such as Charcot-Marie-Tooth syndrome. Vincristine may also cause focal neuropathies.

Neurophysiologic studies show a primarily axonal neuropathy. Although there are anecdotal reports that glutamine may help some patients with vincristine neuropathy, there is generally no effective treatment.

Autonomic neuropathy is common in patients receiving vincristine. Colicky abdominal pain and constipation occurs in almost 50 percent of patients, and rarely paralytic ileus may result. All patients receiving vincristine should receive prophylactic stool softeners and laxatives. Less commonly, patients may develop impotence, postural hypotension, and atonic bladders.

Cranial neuropathies may occasionally be caused by vincristine. The most common nerve to be involved is the oculomotor nerve, resulting in ptosis and ophthalmoplegia. Other nerves that may be involved include recurrent laryngeal nerve, optic nerve, facial nerve, and auditory nerve. Vincristine may also cause retinal damage and night blindness.

Rarely, vincristine may cause SIADH, resulting in hyponatremia, confusion, and seizures. CNS complications unrelated to SIADH may also occur. These include seizures, encephalopathy, transient cortical blindness, ataxia, athetosis, and parkinsonism.

The related vinca alkaloids vindesine and vinblastine have less neurotoxicity. This may be related to differences in lipid solubility, plasma clearance, and terminal half-life and different sensitivities of axoplasmic transport.

Drugs That Occasionally Cause Neurotoxicity

Carboplatin. Carboplatin is an alkylating agent used for a variety of cancers, including ovarian, cervical, testicular, lung, and head and neck. Unlike cisplatin, peripheral neuropathy and CNS toxicity occur only rarely at conventional doses. However, intra-arterial carboplatin may produce strokelike syndromes and retinal toxicity.

Cytarabine. This is a pyrimidine analogue used in the treatment of leukemias, lymphomas, and neoplastic meningitis. This agent has little neurotoxicity when used at conventional doses.

High doses (3 g/m^2 q 12 h) cause an acute cerebellar syndome in 10 to 25 percent of patients. Patients above the age of 40 with abnormal liver function and underlying neurologic dysfunction and receiving more than 30 g of the drug are especially likely to develop cerebellar involvement. Typically, the patient develops somnolence and occasionally encephalopathy 2 to 5 days after completing treatment. Immediately afterward the patient develops cerebellar signs. These may range from mild ataxia to inability to sit or walk unassisted. Rarely patients may experience seizures. The pathologic changes are localized to the cerebellum where there is widespread loss of Purkinje cells. In some patients the cerebellar syndrome resolves spontaneously, but it is permanent in others. No specific treatment is available, but avoidance of very high doses of the drug has led to a decline in the incidence of this syndrome.

High-dose cytarabine may occasionally cause peripheral neuropathies resembling the Guillain-Barré syndrome, brachial plexopathy, encephalopathy, lateral rectus palsy, and an extrapyramidal syndrome.

Intrathecal administration of cytarabine produces high levels of drug in the CSF for at least 24 hours and is used to treat neoplastic meningitis. It can cause a transverse myelopathy similar to that seem with intrathecal methotrexate. Rarely, it can also cause aseptic meningitis, encephalopathy, headaches, and seizures.

5-Fluorouracil. 5-Fluorouracil is a fluorinated pyrimidine, which disrupts DNA synthesis by inhibiting thymidylate synthetase. It is used in the treatment of many cancers, including colon and breast cancers and gliomas.

An acute cerebellar syndrome can occur in approximately 5 percent of patients. This usually begins weeks or months after treatment and is characterized by the acute onset of ataxia, dysmetria, dysarthria, and nystagmus. These symptoms usually resolve completely after the drug is stopped. The development of a cerebellar syndrome may be partly explained by the fact that 5-fluorouracil readily crosses the blood–brain barrier, with the highest concentrations being found in the cerebellum.

Rarely, 5-fluorouracil can cause an encephalopathy, optic

neuropathy, eye movement abnormalities, and a parkinsonian syndrome.

The combination of 5-fluorouracil and levamisole used for the treatment of colon cancer has been rarely associated with the development of an encephalopathy and ataxia resulting from multifocal demyelinating lesions in the periventricular white matter. The cause of these lesions is unknown, and they usually improve with steroids and discontinuation of the drugs. The importance of recognizing this syndrome is that the cerebral lesions may be mistaken for brain metastases.

The administration of 5-fluorouracil and other drugs may also increase the incidence of neurotoxicity. The coadministration of 5-fluorouracil and allopurinol, phosphonacetyl-L-aspartic acid (PALA), doxifluridine, carmofur, and tegafur have all been reported to cause encephalopathies and cerebellar syndromes.

Ifosfamide. This is an analogue of cyclophosphamide, with similar systemic toxicities. Unlike cyclophosphamide, it can also produce an encephalopathy in 20 percent of patients. The encephalopathy begins hours or days after administration of the drug and usually resolves completely after several days. This encephalopathy is thought to result from accumulation of choracetaldehyde, one of the breakdown products of ifosfamide. Patients at increased risk for the encephalopathy include those with renal dysfunction, low serum albumin, prior treatment with cisplatin, and previous encephalopathy with ifosfamide. There is no specific treatment for the encephalopathy. Ifosfamide may also rarely cause seizures, cerebellar ataxia, weakness, cranial nerve dysfunction, and an extrapyramidal syndrome.

Nitrosoureas. Nimustine nitrosoureas (carmustine BCNU, lomustine, PCNU, and ACNU) are lipid-soluble alkylating agents that rapidly cross the blood–brain barrier and are used for the treatment of brain tumors, melanoma, and lymphoma. These drugs generally have little neurotoxicity when used at conventional doses.

High-dose intravenous BCNU used in the setting of autologous bone marrow transplantation can cause an encephalomyelopathy and seizures, which develop over a period of weeks to months after the administration of the drug.

Intra-arterial BCNU produces ocular toxicity and neurotoxicity in 30 to 48 percent of patients. Patients often complain of headache and eye and facial pain, and retinopathy and blindness may occur. The neurotoxicity includes confusion, seizures, and progressive neurologic deficits. Imaging and pathologic studies show findings similar to radiation necrosis confined to the vascular territory perfused by the BCNU. Concurrent radiotherapy may increase the neurotoxicity of intracarotid BCNU. Injection of the drug above the origin of the ophthalmic artery reduces the incidence of ocular toxicity but increases the neurotoxicity.

Procarbazine This is a weak monoamine oxidase inhibitor that probably acts as an alkylating agent. It is used for the treatment of lung carcinoma, lymphoma, and brain tumors. At normal oral doses, it can cause a mild reversible encephalopathy and neuropathy and, rarely, psychosis and stupor. Procarbazine also potentiates the sedative effects of narcotics, phenothiazines, and barbiturates. Intravenous and intracarotid procarbazine produces a severe encephalopathy.

Asparaginase This is used mainly for the treatment of acute lymphocytic leukemia. Neurotoxicity with asparaginase is rare, but it affects coagulation and may cause hemorrhagic and thrombotic complications, including sagittal sinus thrombosis and cerebral infraction. These complications typically occur after several weeks of treatment. Patients usually present with seizures, headaches, or focal deficits. Asparaginase may also produce a reversible encephalopathy.

Drugs That Rarely Cause Neurotoxicity

Anthracycline Antibiotics (Doxorubicin, Daunorubicin, and Mitoxantrone). Apart from accidental intrathecal injection, which can cause a myelopathy and encephalopathy, these agents have little neurotoxicity.

Chlorambucil. This usually has little neurotoxicity but can cause an encephalopathy and seizures when taken in very high doses.

Etoposide. This is a topoisomerase II inhibitor used in the treatment of lung cancer, germ cell tumors, and refractory lymphoma. It generally has little neurotoxicity, even in high doses. Rarely, it can cause a peripheral neuropathy or mild disorientation and seizures.

Fludarabine. Fludarabine is an inhibitor of DNA polymerase and ribonucleotide reductase that is used to treat chronic lymphatic leukemia, macroglobulinemia, and indolent lymphomas. Neurotoxicity is uncommon, but it can cause headaches, somnolence, confusion, and paresthesias at low doses and seizures, visual loss, paralysis, and coma at high dose.

Hydroxyurea. This is an antimetabolite used for the treatment of resistant chronic myelogenous leukemia, and certain solid tumors, including melanoma; ovarian carcinoma; trophoblastic neoplasms; and cervical, head and neck, and prostate cancers. Rarely, it can cause headaches, drowsiness, confusion, and seizures.

Mechlorethamine (Nitrogen Mustard). This is an alkylating agent used for the treatment of Hodgkin's lymphoma and malignant pleural effusions. It may rarely cause sleepiness, headaches, and weakness. At the high doses used for bone marrow transplantation, it has been reported to cause confusion and seizures.

Plicamycin. This is used to treat refractory hypercalcemia and may cause headaches, lethargy, and irritability. These side effects tend to be dose dependent.

Thioguanine. This antimetabolite is used to treat leukemia nd brain tumors. It can rarely cause loss of vibratory sense and ataxia.

HORMONAL THERAPY

Aminoglutethimide

This inhibits the synthesis of steroid hormones and is used for the treatment of breast carcinoma, adrenocortical carcinoma, and ectopic Cushing syndrome. It frequently causes mild lethargy and rarely may cause vertigo and ataxia.

Corticosteroids

Corticosteroids are frequently used in patients with cancer for a variety of reasons. They reduce peritumoral edema in patients

TABLE 169-2. Neurologic Complications of Corticosteroids

Common	Uncommon
Myopathy	Psychosis
Visual blurring	Hallucinations
Tremor	Hiccups
Behavioral changes	Dementia
Insomnia	Seizures
Reduced taste and olfaction	Dependence
Cerebral atrophy	Epidural lipomatosis
	Neuropathy

with primary and secondary brain tumors and spinal cord edema in patients with epidural spinal cord compression. Corticosteroids have a direct cytolytic effect against neoplastic lymphocytes and is used in the treatment of leukemias and lymphomas. High-dose corticosteroids are frequently given with chemotherapy to reduce nausea and vomiting; low doses are used to improve the appetite and sense of well-being in some patients with cancer.

The side effects of prolonged steroid therapy are well known (see Table 149-1). The incidence of complications increases with higher doses and prolonged therapy, but there is also significant variation in individual susceptibility.

The systemic side effects include a cushingoid appearance, truncal obesity, hirsutism, acne, impaired wound healing, striae, easy bruising and capillary fragility, immunosuppression, hypertension, glucose intolerance, electrolyte disturbance, fluid retention, peripheral edema, increased appetite, gastrointestinal bleeding, osteoporosis, avascular necrosis, growth retardation, cataracts, glaucoma, and visual blurring.

The neurologic complications of corticosteroids are summarized in Table 169-2. The most common complication is steroid myopathy. This is characterized by weakness of the proximal muscles, affecting primarily the hip girdle. Patients typically complain of difficulty getting up from a chair or climbing stairs. In severe cases, the pectoral girdle and neck muscles may also be involved. Steroid myopathy tends to occur after prolonged use of high doses of steroids, but there is significant variation in patient susceptibility, and some patients will develop a myopathy after using low doses of steroids for a short period. Electromyography is usually normal, and creatine kinase levels are usually not elevated.

Corticosteroids often produce alterations in mood. An improved sense of well-being, anxiety, irritability, insomnia, difficulty concentrating, and depression are all relatively common. Occasionally, patients may develop steroid psychosis. This usually takes the form of acute delirium, but the psychosis may resemble mania, depression, or schizophrenia.

Other common neurologic complications of corticosteroids include tremors, visual blurring, reduced sense of taste and smell, and cerebral atrophy on neurimaging studies. Rare complications include hiccups, dementia, seizures, and cord compression as a result of epidural lipomatosis.

Steroid withdrawal can also produce a variety of symptoms, which can be fairly disabling. These include headaches, lethargy, nausea, vomiting, anorexia, myalgia and arthralgia (pseudorheumatism), fever, abdominal pain, postural hypotension, pseudotumor, and panniculitis.

Estramustine

This is used to treat prostate cancer and may occasionally cause headaches.

Leuprolide Acetate

This is a gonadotropin-releasing hormone analogue used for the treatment of prostate cancer and refractory breast cancer. Neurologic complications are uncommon, but this drug can cause headaches, dizziness, and paresthesias.

Mitotane

This drug, which suppresses adrenocorticosteroid production and is cytotoxic to adrenal cortical cells, is used for the treatment of adrenocortical carcinoma. It produces lethargy, sedation, and dizziness in 40 percent of patients.

Octreotide

This is a long-acting analogue of somatostatin used for the treatment of carcinoid tumors, vasoactive intestinal peptide–secreting tumors, and certain pituitary adenomas. It can cause headaches, dizziness, and rarely seizures.

Tamoxifen

This is an antiestrogen that is used for the treatment of breast cancer. It can produce retinopathy, encephalopathy, and ataxia, especially when used in high doses.

Other antiestrogens and antiandrogens, such as flutamide, are usually not associated with neurotoxicity.

BIOLOGIC RESPONSE MODIFIERS

In recent years, there has been increasing interest in the use of biologic response modifiers in the treatment of cancers. Frequently, they are used in combination with conventional chemotherapeutic agents.

α-Interferon

This is used therapeutically in a number of cancers, including hairy cell leukemia, Kaposi sarcoma, and myeloma. Systemic toxicities include flulike symptoms and myelosuppression. The flulike symptoms tend to be worse at the onset of therapy and usually improve with time. Neurotoxicity tends to be dose related and includes headaches, confusion, lethargy, hallucinations, and seizures. These are usually reversible, but occasionally a permanent dementia or a persistent vegetative state may result. Rarely, α-interferon has been associated with oculomotor palsy, sensorimotor neuropathy, brachial plexopathy, and polyradiculopathy.

Intrathecal administration of α-interferon has been evaluated for the treatment of meningeal and brain tumors, multiple sclerosis, amyotrophic lateral sclerosis, and progressive multifocal leukoencephalopathy. An acute reaction is usually seen within hours of the first injection and consists of headache, nausea, vomiting, fever, and dizziness. The symptoms usually resolve over the next 12 to 24 hours. A severe encephalopathy develops in a significant number of patients within several days of the onset of treatment. This is dose dependent and tends to be worse in patients who have received cranial irradiation.

β- and γ-Interferon

These have neurotoxicities similar to α-interferon, although intrathecal β-interferon appears to be better tolerated.

Interleukin-2

This has been used alone and in combination with lymphokine-activated killer cells and tumor-infiltrating lymphocytes in the treatment of a number of cancers, especially renal cell carcinoma and melanoma. Neuropsychiatric complications occur in 30 to 50 percent of patients. These include cognitive changes, delusions, hallucinations, and depression. In addition, there have been reports of transient focal neurologic deficits, acute leukoencephalopathy, and brachial neuritis. Interleukin-2 has been administered directly into the tumor bed in the treatment of gliomas and can cause significant cerebral edema.

Colony-Stimulating Factors (Granulocyte Colony-Stimulating Factor, Granulocyte–Macrophage Colony-Stimulating Factor)

These are used to increase the granulocyte count and reduce the incidence of infections in patients with nonmyeloid tumors receiving chemotherapy. Musculoskelatal symptoms such as cramps and bone pain occur commonly. Rarely, they may cause fatigue and headaches. Granulocyte–macrophage colony-stimulating factor has also been reported to cause confusion and neuropathies.

SUGGESTED READINGS

Barba D, Saris S, Holder C et al: Intratumoral LAK cell and interleukin-2 therapy of human gliomas. J Neurosurg 70:175–82, 1989

Delattre J-Y, Posner JB: Neurological complications of chemotherapy and radiation therapy. pp. 421–46. In Aminoff MJ (ed): Neurology and General Medicine. 2nd Ed. Churchill Livingstone, New York, 1994

Delattre JY, Vega F, Chen Q: Neurologic complications of immunotherapy. pp. 267–93. In Wiley RG (ed): Neurologic Complications of Cancer. Marcel Dekker, New York, 1995

Denicoff KD, Rubinow DR, Papa MZ et al: The neuropsychiatric effects of treatment with interleukin-2 and lymphokine-activated killer cells. Ann Intern Med 107:293–300, 1987

Feinberg WM, Swenson MR: Cerebrovascular complications of L-asparaginase therapy. Neurology 38:127–33, 1988

Forsyth PA, Cascino TL: Neurologic complications of chemotherapy. pp. 241–66. In Wiley RG (ed): Neurologic Complications of Cancer. Marcel Dekker, New York, 1995

van der Hoop G, Vecht CJ, van der burg MEL et al: Prevention of cisplatin neurotoxicity with an ACTH (4–9) analogue in patients with ovarian cancer. N Engl J Med 322:89–94, 1990

Herzig RH, Hines JD, Herzig GP et al: Cerebellar toxicity with high dose cytosine arabinoside. J Clin Oncol 5:927–32, 1987

La Rocca RV, Meer J, Gilliatt RW et al: Suramin-induced polyneuropathy. Neurology 40:954–60, 1990

Legha SS: Vincristine neurotoxicity. Pathophysiology and management. Med Toxicol 1:421–7, 1986

Lipton RB, Apfel SC, Dutcher JP et al: Taxol produces a predominantly sensory neuropathy. Neurology 39:368–73, 1989

Macdonald DR: Neurologic complications of chemotherapy. Neurol Clin 9:955–67, 1991

Meyers CA, Obbens EA, Scheibel RS et al: Neurotoxicity of intraventricularly administered alpha-interferon for leptomeningeal disease. Cancer 69:88–92, 1991

Meyers CA, Scheibel, Forman AD: Persistent neurotoxicity of systemically administered interferon-alpha. Neurology 41:672–77, 1991

Phillips PC: Methotrexate toxicity. pp. 115–34. In Rottenberg DA (ed). Neurological Complications of Cancer Treatment. Butterworth-Heinemann, Boston, 1991

Phillips PC, Reinhard CS: Antipyrimidine neurotoxicity: cytosine arabinoside and 5-fluorouracil. pp. 97–114. In Rottenberg DA (ed): Neurological Complications of Cancer Treatment. Butterworth-Heinemann; Boston, 1991

Rottenberg DA (ed): Neurological Complications of Cancer Treatment. Butterworth-Heineman, Boston, 1991

Young DF, Posner JB: Nervous system toxicity of the chemotherapeutic agents. pp. 91–129. In Vinken PJ, Bruyn GW (eds): Handbook of Neurology. Vol. 39. North Holland, Amsterdam, 1980

170. NEUROLOGIC COMPLICATIONS OF RADIOTHERAPY

EDWARD J. DROPCHO

The central nervous system (CNS) was once considered to be relatively resistant to high-energy radiation. With patients living longer after CNS radiotherapy and with the advent of sensitive neuroimaging techniques, it has become clear that the limits of tolerance of the CNS need to be revised downward. Table 170-1 summarizes the adverse effects of irradiation on the nervous system.

CEREBRAL INJURY

Acute Encephalopathy

Brain injury by therapeutic irradiation has traditionally been classified according to its time of onset into *acute, early delayed,* and *late* forms. The acute reaction to cranial irradiation usually occurs during the first several days of radiotherapy and consists of headache, nausea, fever, somnolence, and worsening of pre-existing focal symptoms. Fatal cerebral herniation has been reported but is rare. Acute radiotherapy encephalopathy tends to occur more frequently and to be more severe among patients with large intracranial mass(es) and in patients who receive large (greater than 300 cGy) daily dose fractions of whole-brain irradiation (WBRT). Increased cerebral edema is the most likely cause of symptoms, but this is rarely seen in neuroimaging studies. Acute toxicity generally responds well to increased doses of dexamethasone. Patients with large primary tumors or multiple metastases should be pretreated with dexamethasone for 24 to 72 hours prior to initiating cranial radiotherapy.

Early Delayed Encephalopathy

Early delayed encephalopathy typically consists of headache, somnolence, and/or deterioration in pre-existing deficits occur-

TABLE 170-1. Adverse Effects of Irradiation on the Nervous System

Cerebral injury
  Acute
  Early delayed
  Delayed
    Focal necrosis
    Diffuse injury
Neuroendocrine effects
Optic neuropathy
Cranial neuropathies
Spinal cord injury
  Transient myelopathy
  Delayed progressive myelopathy
  Motor neuron syndrome
Peripheral nerve injury
Cerebrovascular damage
Radiation-induced tumors

ring 1 to 4 months after the completion of WBRT. Corticosteroids usually produce symptomatic improvement, but the syndrome resolves after several weeks with or without corticosteroids. The very few neuropathologic descriptions of early delayed encephalopathy suggest damage to myelin, glial cells, or both. Early delayed encephalopathy is of particular clinical importance among patients with primary brain tumors, since the clinical and radiographic changes of early delayed neurotoxicity are indistinguishable from those of tumor recurrence or progression.

Another example of early delayed encephalopathy is the *somnolence syndrome,* which occurs in 40 to 60 percent of children with leukemia who receive 1,800 to 2,400 cGy of prophylactic WBRT. The syndrome occurs 3 to 8 weeks after completion of radiotherapy and consists of drowsiness, nausea, irritability, and less commonly fever or transient papilledema. The somnolence syndrome is probably more frequent and more severe in children younger than 3 years old. Symptoms resolve without sequelae within 3 to 6 weeks. Corticosteroids hasten recovery and may also prevent the syndrome if given during the course of WBRT. Occurrence of the somnolence syndrome does not presage the development of severe delayed neurotoxicity.

Focal Cerebral Necrosis

Delayed radiotherapy neurotoxicity can occur several months to 10 or more years after cranial radiotherapy. This may either take the form of *focal necrosis* or *diffuse cerebral injury.* Focal cerebral radiation necrosis occurs after focal radiotherapy or WBRT given for primary or metastatic brain tumors and after incidental irradiation of the brain during treatment of pituitary adenomas or other extraneural tumors of the head and neck. The incidence of cerebral necrosis after 5,000 cGy or more is generally quoted as 3 to 5 percent, but many reports do not provide the ''denominator'' of how many patients were treated, and many patients with brain tumors die before they are at risk for developing this complication. Recently, the incidence of focal cerebral necrosis has been increasing as more patients with brain tumors are being treated with brachytherapy and stereotactic radiosurgery, which deliver high doses of focal radiation to the tumor site.

When cerebral necrosis occurs in patients with primary brain tumors, it is most often located in close proximity to the tumor, even in patients who received a uniform dose of WBRT without a focal tumor ''boost.'' The frequent localization of cerebral necrosis within or close to the primary tumor site has led to speculation that peritumoral cerebral edema potentiates radiotherapy injury. Cerebral necrosis affecting both frontal lobes, temporal lobes, and/or brainstem is prone to occur following radiotherapy for pituitary tumors or for nasopharyngeal carcinoma.

Cerebral necrosis predominantly involves the white matter, with relative but not complete sparing of cerebral cortex and deep gray matter. In extreme cases, there are confluent foci of coagulative necrosis of all parenchymal elements. Demyelination and loss of oligodendrocytes are present in less severely affected areas, with variable axonal loss, axonal swellings, focal calcifications, fibrillary gliosis, and scattered perivascular infiltrates of mononuclear cells. Extensive vascular changes are a nearly constant feature of focal cerebral necrosis, including fibrinoid necrosis or hyaline thickening of vessel walls, thrombosis of small vessels, proliferation of adventitial fibroblasts, hyaline transudates surrounding affected vessels, and formation of telangiectasias.

The clinical presentation of focal cerebral necrosis is typically that of a subacute space-occupying lesion occurring with a peak onset 15 to 18 months following completion of cranial radiotherapy; the latent period may rarely be as short as 4 months or as long as 7 years. Computed tomography (CT) or magnetic resonance imaging (MRI) scans show a mass lesion with a combination of ''edema'' and patchy or ring enhancement. Neither the clinical features nor the routine neuroimaging studies distinguish cerebral necrosis from recurrent or progressive tumor. Definitive diagnosis of cerebral necrosis therefore requires pathologic confirmation, although, in patients with malignant gliomas, there is often an intermingling of active tumor with areas of cerebral necrosis, so that brain biopsies carry a risk of sampling error.

An alternative way of diagnosing cerebral necrosis is with metabolic imaging. Studies of positron emission tomography scanning in patients with malignant gliomas have shown that differences in uptake of ^{18}F-fluorodeoxyglucose can distinguish cerebral necrosis from recurrent tumor. Thallium-single photon emission CT scanning yields similar results. Positron emission tomography or single photon emission CT scans are not always unequivocal, however, especially in patients who have recurrent tumor intermingled with areas of necrosis.

Dexamethasone or other glucocorticoids produce at least partial clinical and radiographic improvement in most patients with cerebral necrosis. This improvement is usually temporary or patients become steroid dependent, but exceptional patients maintain their improvement even after the steroids are discontinued. There are anecdotal reports of definite clinical and radiographic improvement in patients anticoagulated with heparin or warfarin. Surgical debulking of necrotic brain tissue is probably worthwhile in patients who do not show adequate response to conservative measures and who have a focal accessible mass lesion. Unfortunately, some patients continue to deteriorate despite surgical debulking because of progressive necrosis adjacent or contralateral to the original site of cerebral necrosis.

Numerous and sometimes conflicting attempts have been made to determine the dose relationship of cerebral necrosis and to establish dose thresholds. There are several formulas based on total radiotherapeutic dose, daily dose, and treatment duration to calculate ''dose equivalents,'' such as the ret, neuret, and brain tolerance unit. This allows comparison of different dose-fraction treatment regimens. The dosimetric analyses of cerebral necrosis have led to several general conclusions. First, the radiotherapeutic dose per daily fraction is an important determinant of the risk of cerebral necrosis. Second, in most studies, the risk of cerebral necrosis as a function of the dose equivalent forms a sigmoid curve. Third, although the exact dose-risk curves differ among different studies, most agree that, above a critical exposure level, the curve is a steep one and that small increments in dose lead to a significantly higher risk of cerebral necrosis. Fourth, with ''safe'' radiotherapy regimens, the risk of cerebral necrosis is very low, but there is probably no absolute therapeutic dose ''threshold'' below which cerebral necrosis cannot occur.

Diffuse Cerebral Injury

The most frequent neurotoxic effect of cranial radiotherapy is not *focal* necrosis but *diffuse* cerebral injury. This may be classified according to the age of the patient and the setting in which cranial radiotherapy is administered, but, in all these groups (except patients with ''methotrexate leukoencephalopathy''), a common pathophysiology probably applies. For all of these patient groups, there is not a clear correlation between abnormalities in neuroimaging studies and the severity of clinical neurologic and neuropsychologic deficits.

Primary Brain Tumors in Adults.   There are several reports of serial neuroimaging studies in this population, but very little neuropsychologic data. This is at least partially due to the fact that only a small minority of adults with glioblastoma multiforme or other malignant primary brain tumors survive long enough for delayed diffuse cerebral injury to become an issue. Serial CT or MRI scans show diffuse cortical atrophy, ventricular dilation, and abnormal attenuation of hemispheric white matter in at least 50 percent of ''long-term'' (greater than 18 to 24 month) survivors with malignant gliomas following 4,000 to 6,000 cGy of WBRT. These changes may progressively worsen over time.

Some but not all patients with these radiographic abnormalities develop clinically important cognitive impairment. At least 30 to 50 percent of adults with malignant gliomas are unable to return to their premorbid employment and functional status because of moderate to severe diffuse cortical dysfunction. Neuropsychologic testing in these patients demonstrates particular difficulties with tasks requiring attention or problem solving. The more severely affected patients develop progressive dementia and prominent gait disturbance reminiscent of normal pressure hydrocephalus, but few patients benefit from ventriculoperitoneal shunting. Several autopsies of patients with malignant gliomas and symptomatic diffuse injury have shown marked cerebral atrophy with diffuse demyelination and ''spongiform'' changes in the hemispheric white matter, but with relative preservation of axons and blood vessels. Patients older than 50 years of age at diagnosis appear to be more likely to develop diffuse cerebral injury than younger patients. A potentiating effect of nitrosoureas or other chemotherapy on the neurotoxic effect of WBRT has been postulated but not proved. Recently there has been a trend toward treating malignant gliomas with focal radiotherapy ports rather than WBRT.

Brain Metastases.   Focal cerebral necrosis is a rare complication of WBRT given for brain metastases, since patients generally receive less than 4,000 cGy and few patients survive long enough to be at risk. On the other hand, at least one-half of patients who survive more than 1 year after WBRT for brain metastases develop abnormalities on serial CT scans, including diffuse cerebral atrophy, ventricular enlargement, and abnormal signal in the periventricular white matter. Most patients with abnormal neuroimaging studies do not have gross neurologic deficits or cognitive impairment, although there are very few detailed studies of serial neurologic and neuropsychologic examinations in this population. A proportion of long-term survivors with brain metastases, perhaps as many as 10 percent, develop a disabling syndrome of progressive dementia, psychomotor retardation, and gait disturbance appearing 6 to 18 months after WBRT. Autopsies in a few of these patients have shown diffuse injury to myelin sheaths with relative preservation of axons and blood vessels. The risk of ''radiotherapy dementia'' is probably increased among patients who receive daily doses of more than 200 cGy. Ventriculoperitoneal shunting produces a temporary and partial improvement in a

minority of patients, but to date there is no reliable way to predict which patients would benefit from a shunt.

Administration of prophylactic WBRT (2,000 to 3,000 cGy) to patients with small cell lung carcinoma decreases the overall incidence of brain metastases (from an average of 25 percent to about 5 to 8 percent), delays the median time of appearance of brain metastases, and reduces the incidence of brain metastases as a solitary site of relapse. Prophylactic WBRT continues to be controversial, however, because of its risk of neurotoxicity. CT and MRI scans show diffuse cerebral atrophy and abnormal hemispheric white matter in the majority of patients with small cell lung cancer who survive more than 1 year after prophylactic WBRT. These abnormalities often become progressively worse on serial imaging studies. Gross neurologic deficits are uncommon, but most patients have impairment of memory and cognitive functions on neuropsychologic testing, and a few patients develop progressive dementia with gait disturbance. Clinically overt diffuse cerebral injury is more likely to occur in patients who receive high daily dose fractions and/or concomitant systemic chemotherapy during prophylactic WBRT.

Primary Brain Tumors in Children.   The dilemma of treating primary brain tumors in children is that many tumors respond well to aggressive therapy, including cranial or craniosinal radiotherapy, but there is little doubt that the developing brain is more sensitive to radiotherapy than the adult brain. As with adult patients with brain tumors, there is a rather loose correlation between neuroimaging abnormalities and the findings of neuropsychologic evaluations. Serial CT or MRI scans show cerebral atrophy and periventricular white matter abnormalities in up to 50 percent of children following 2,500 to 4,000 cGy of WBRT. A distinctive pattern of intracerebral calcifications called ''mineralizing microangiopathy'' (see below) also occurs in up to 30 percent of patients. Several studies of disease-free survivors of childhood primary brain tumors have demonstrated significant declines in mean intelligence quotient (IQ) scores following WBRT (but not focal radiotherapy). The deficits described in prospective studies tend to be less severe than those in retrospective reports. Neurobehavioral problems and learning disabilities following WBRT are often present in children whose full-scale IQ still lies in the normal range. These abnormalities include short-term memory loss, attention deficit disorders, visual perceptual difficulties, and impaired fine motor coordination, which are reflected in poor school performance and the need for special education. There is general agreement that cognitive decline is more frequent and more severe among children irradiated when less than 3 to 5 years of age.

Childhood Leukemia.   Prophylactic WBRT (1,800 to 2,400 cGy) and intrathecal methotrexate in children with acute lymphoblastic leukemia are highly effective in reducing the incidence of leukemic meningitis, but CNS prophylaxis carries a significant risk of neurotoxicity. The most common finding on CT or MRI scans following CNS prophylaxis is diffuse cerebral ''atrophy,'' seen in 40 to 50 percent of patients in whom serial neuroimaging studies are done. In some of these patients, however, the neuroimaging abnormalities are reversible, and CT or MRI scan findings generally do not correlate well with the results of neuropsychologic testing. Most but not all neuropsychologic studies of survivors of childhood leukemia have demonstrated cognitive impairment developing 1 to 3 years after

CNS prophylaxis. In most studies, the IQ scores of children remained in the average range but were either less than the IQ of "controls" or showed a decline on serial testing. Performance IQ is more likely to be affected than verbal IQ. Significant neuropsychologic dysfunction and learning disabilities can be present in children with IQ scores in the average range. It is generally agreed that cognitive impairment is more frequent and more severe in children given CNS prophylaxis before 3 to 6 years of age. Cognitive impairment is more likely to occur after CNS prophylaxis with a combination of WBRT plus methotrexate than with methotrexate alone.

The second most common neuroimaging abnormality in long-term survivors of acute lymphocytic leukemia is the development in 4 to 30 percent of patients of calcifications in the basal ganglia, dentate nuclei, and cerebral gray–white matter junction within 5 years of WBRT. This is more common among younger children (less than 5 years old) and in children with overt leukemic meningitis. The pathologic correlate of these calcifications is *mineralizing microangiopathy,* consisting of calcification of the walls of small blood vessels, luminal occlusion, and a variable degree of microscopic necrosis. To date, all patients with mineralizing microangiopathy received WBRT, with or without intrathecal or intravenous methotrexate; it has not been reported in patients who received methotrexate but not WBRT. Many children with mineralizing microangiopathy do not have obvious concomitant neurologic deficits, but, as a group, these children probably have more severe cognitive impairment than patients with normal scans or with cerebral atrophy but no intracerebral calcifications.

The most devastating sequela of CNS prophylaxis is *delayed leukoencephalopathy,* which generally begins insidiously with personality changes, confusion, or somnolence 4 to 24 months after CNS prophylaxis. Some children show neurologic stabilization or improvement after cessation of methotrexate treatments, but many suffer a progressive course that, in the most severe cases, leads to profound dementia, spastic quadriparesis, seizures, and coma. Leukoencephalopathy is not restricted to children receiving CNS leukemia prophylaxis; it may also occur in adults who receive WBRT and intrathecal methotrexate for leptomeningeal metastases from breast carcinoma and other solid tumors. CT or MRI scans early in the course show decreased attenuation of deep hemispheric white matter with patchy areas of contrast enhancement, followed later by diffuse atrophy, ventricular dilation, and intracerebral calcifications.

The pathology of leukoencephalopathy features multiple foci of coagulative necrosis disseminated throughout the hemispheric white matter, with occasional lesions in the cerebellum and brainstem but generally sparing the cerebral cortex and basal ganglia. In severe cases, the lesions coalesce to produce massive destruction of the entire centrum semiovale. In addition to demyelination and severe loss of oligodendrocytes, striking axonal fragmentation and axonal swellings are present within and around the necrotic foci. Vascular changes such as fibrinoid necrosis and fibrin extravasation may be present but are not frequent or severe. These changes often coexist with mineralizing microangiopathy.

The exact pathogenesis of leukoencephalopathy remains unknown, but there is little doubt that the neurotoxic effects of cranial radiotherapy and methotrexate are synergistic. Leukoencephalopathy occasionally occurs after intrathecal or high-dose intravenous methotrexate *without* cranial radiotherapy, but WBRT clearly increases the likelihood of developing leukoencephalopathy manyfold. The risk of developing leukoencephalopathy is increased in several settings: (1) following high cumulative doses (intrathecal plus intravenous) of methotrexate; (2) when the methotrexate is given *during* or *after* the WBRT; (3) when WBRT and methotrexate are given for therapy of overt leukemic or carcinomatous meningitis rather than for prophylaxis; and (4) in patients with abnormalities of cerebrospinal fluid flow that result in delayed clearance of methotrexate from the CNS.

NEUROENDOCRINE EFFECTS

The hypothalamic-pituitary axis is clearly sensitive to cranial radiotherapy. In children, the most common neuroendocrine sequela to radiotherapy is growth failure; irreversible biochemical growth hormone deficiency is present in up to 90 percent of children within 12 months after irradiation of primary brain tumors, with clinical growth failure occurring in 50 to 90 percent. This occurs in children receiving WBRT as well as those irradiated for medulloblastoma or other posterior fossa tumors, in whom the radiotherapy ports encompass the posterior hypothalamus. Other factors contributing to short stature in some of these children include precocious puberty, poor nutrition, systemic chemotherapy, and failure of vertebral body growth following spinal axis radiotherapy. Children receiving prophylactic radiotherapy for CNS leukemia prophylaxis often have biochemical growth hormone deficiency but generally have normal growth rates. Most children are euthyroid after WBRT but show elevated thyroid-stimulating hormone levels or an exaggerated response to exogenous thyrotropin-releasing hormone. Clinical hypothyroidism is more likely to occur among children who receive craniospinal axis radiotherapy, as the thyroid gland is included in cervical spine radiotherapy ports.

In contrast with children, hypothyroidism is the most common neuroendocrine sequela of radiotherapy in adults. Free thyroxine levels are low in up to two-thirds of long-term survivors following WBRT for primary brain tumors; stimulation tests indicate defective hypothalamic thyrotropin-releasing hormone production as the primary abnormality. Mild to moderate hyperprolactinemia is found in 50 to 75 percent of adults irradiated for primary brain tumors. Hyperprolactinemia may be accompanied by impotence in men and decreased libido in both sexes. Oligomenorrhea in women probably reflects a combination of hyperprolactinemia and gonadotropin-releasing hormone deficiency. The pituitary-adrenal axis is relatively spared, both in children and adults. Diabetes insipidus is inexplicably rare.

OPTIC NEUROPATHY

Radiation injury to the optic nerve and chiasm most often occurs in patients treated for tumors of the orbit or paranasal sinuses, pituitary adenomas, or craniopharyngiomas. For many of these patients, it is impossible to spare the anterior visual system when irradiating tumors with curative intent. Optic neuropathy less commonly occurs following WBRT for primary or metastatic brain tumors. The median latency period from radiotherapy to the onset of symptoms is 12 months, without a clear relationship between the radiotherapeutic dose and latent interval. Radiotherapeutic regimens using a high daily dose fraction probably carry an increased risk of subsequent optic neuropathy. The pathology of radiation-induced optic neuropathy is a nonspecific mixture of axonal loss, demyelination, gliosis, and microvascular changes.

Patients with radiation-induced optic neuropathy generally present with painless monocular loss of acuity and/or visual field constriction. Funduscopic examination initially shows optic nerve head swelling with hyperemic discs, telangiectasias, hemorrhages, cotton-wool spots, and narrowed retinal arterioles. Fluorescein angiography shows retinal capillary nonperfusion. Less commonly, the fundus may appear relatively normal if the main injury is to the retrobulbar optic nerve. Visual field deficits include central scotoma, altitudinal loss, or quadrantic loss. Most patients progress over several weeks to severe, often bilateral vision loss and optic atrophy, although about one-third of involved eyes show partial improvement. Corticosteroids have no effect.

OTHER CRANIAL NEUROPATHIES

Other than the optic nerve, hypoglossal palsy is the most frequent radiotherapy-induced cranial neuropathy, occurring 2 to 10 years after treatment of primary head and neck tumors. The probable mechanism is entrapment of the nerve by fibrosis. Less common is unilateral palsy of the vagus nerve, spinal accessory nerve, or multiple lower cranial nerve palsies. Cranial nerves II to VII seem resistant to "ordinary" external photon beam radiotherapy but may be injured by proton beam irradiation of pituitary tumors. Hearing loss is a common complication of cranial radiotherapy but is generally due to a conductive loss or to cochlear damage rather than to damage to the auditory nerve itself.

SPINAL CORD INJURY

Transient Myelopathy

The most common form of radiotherapy-induced spinal cord injury is a transient syndrome occurring in 5 to 15 percent of patients who receive "incidental" radiotherapy to the cord during treatment of lymphoma or extraneural tumors of the head, neck, or thorax. The risk of transient myelopathy is higher in patients receiving more than 4,000 cGy to the spinal cord and in patients receiving high daily dose fractions. Transient myelopathy occurs after a latent period of 1 to 30 months after the completion of radiotherapy, with the peak onset at 3 to 6 months. The syndrome typically consists solely of paresthesias or "electric shock" sensations radiating down the spine (Lhermitte symptom) and frequently extending down the limbs as well. These symptoms are often precipitated by neck flexion or physical exertion. Patients rarely report other symptoms and almost never show any objective signs of spinal cord dysfunction. MRI scans and myelography are normal. The syndrome resolves gradually over 1 to 9 months, and affected patients are not at higher risk for developing severe delayed myelopathy. Transient myelopathy is generally believed to be caused by demyelination of the posterior columns, but there is no neuropathologic proof of this in humans.

Delayed Progressive Myelopathy

Delayed, severe myelopathy has been recognized for more than 40 years as a complication of radiotherapy given for a variety of neoplasms. The reported incidence figures for delayed radiation myelopathy range from 1 to 12 percent but are probably misleading because many patients do not survive long enough to be at risk for developing this complication. The peak time of onset of radiation myelopathy is 9 to 18 months after the completion of radiotherapy, but exceptional patients have latent intervals as short as 3 months or as long as 5 years after treatment.

The earliest symptoms of delayed radiation myelopathy are usually numbness or dysesthesias in the legs, followed by weakness and sphincter dysfunction, with the upper level of cord dysfunction ascending to lie within the irradiated area. A Brown-Séquard pattern is fairly common early in the course. In most patients, the neurologic deficit progresses over weeks to months in a steady or (less commonly) stepwise fashion, leading to paraplegia or quadriplegia in at least 50 percent of patients. Some patients stabilize or improve temporarily while receiving dexamethasone. The clinical features of radiation myelopathy do not reliably distinguish it from spinal metastases (extradural or intramedullary), paraneoplastic "necrotizing myelopathy," or other subacute myelopathies.

The cerebrospinal fluid in delayed radiation myelopathy is usually normal but may contain slightly elevated protein levels or a mild pleocytosis. Myelography is typically normal, but occasional patients have focal or diffuse fusiform spinal cord enlargement that is indistinguishable from an intrinsic cord tumor. MRI scans in the majority of reported patients show swelling of the affected cord and high T2-weighted signal intensity; most patients also have streaky areas of focal enhancement. The MRI abnormalities may extend beyond the radiotherapeutic ports and generally persist for several months, followed by spinal cord atrophy in long-term survivors.

The histopathology of delayed radiation myelopathy is somewhat variable, both between patients and in different areas of the spinal cord in the same patient. White matter is characteristically more severely affected than gray matter, with a predilection for the posterior columns and superficial lateral tracts. Coalescing foci of demyelination and axonal degeneration in these areas are accompanied by wallerian degeneration above and below the necrotic zones. There is a variable astroglial response. In cases in which gray matter is involved, the neurons may show central chromatolysis but are often remarkably preserved. In the most severe cases, there are foci of total coagulative necrosis. Vascular changes, including fibrinoid necrosis of the vessel walls, hyaline thickening and obliteration of lumens, telangiectasias, extravasation of hyaline material, and perivascular lymphocytic cuffing, are variable and may be mild compared with the degree of demyelination and parenchymal necrosis.

As with cerebral radiation necrosis, there have been numerous attempts to correlate retrospectively the risk of radiation myelopathy with a radiotherapeutic "dose equivalent" that allows comparison between different treatment regimens. Although the exact risk estimates from different series vary somewhat, several generalizations can be made. First, there is probably an inverse correlation between the equivalent dose of radiotherapy and the latent period of delayed radiation myelopathy. Second, after total spinal cord doses of 5,000 cGy or less, given in daily fractions of 200 cGy, the risk of radiation myelopathy is probably less than 5 percent. Third, this risk increases with a higher dose per daily fraction, higher total dose, shorter total treatment duration, and longer extent of spinal cord irradiated. Fourth, unexplained differences in individual sensitivity to radiotherapy result in the occurrence of delayed radiation myelopathy in a very small percentage of patients who receive a "safe" radiotherapeutic regimen. Anecdotal reports suggest increased sensitivity of the spinal cord in children, and a possible potentiating effect of concomitant chemotherapy on the risk of developing radiation myelopathy.

Motor Neuron Syndrome

A rare syndrome of selective damage to lower motor neurons may occur in patients following spinal radiotherapy for medulloblastoma or after paraspinal radiotherapy for lymphoma or germ cell tumors. Patients present with subacute, unilateral or bilateral leg weakness beginning 4 to 14 months after completion of radiotherapy. Examination shows muscle atrophy, fasciculations, normal or decreased tendon reflexes, flexor plantar responses, and no sensory or sphincter involvement. In most patients, the syndrome progresses slowly over several months and then stabilizes but does not improve. The cerebrospinal fluid is normal or shows slightly elevated protein levels, and electromyography confirms diffuse denervation. It is believed that lumbosacral anterior horn cells are the primary site of damage in these patients, but neuropathologic proof for this is lacking. It is possible that the syndrome represents selective damage to motor axons or roots.

Peripheral Nerve Injury

Effects of radiation on peripheral nerves, especially the brachial plexus, are discussed in Chapters 172, 176, and 177.

CEREBROVASCULAR DISEASE

The most common deleterious effect of radiotherapy on the cerebral circulation is development of occlusive disease of major extra- or intracranial vessels. Stenosis or occlusion of the extracranial carotid arteries has most commonly occurred after cervical or supraclavicular radiotherapy given for lymphomas, carcinomas of the breast or thyroid, or a variety of other head and neck tumors. Amaurosis fugax, transient ischemic attacks, or (less commonly) cerebral infarcts occur after an interval of 6 months to 57 years after radiotherapy, with a median latent period of approximately 19 years. Arteriograms show disease limited to the radiotherapy ports, including such "unusual sites" as the proximal common carotid artery and the internal carotid artery distal to the common carotid bifurcation. The reported morbidity of carotid endarterectomy or bypass grafting in these patients is low, despite the frequent presence of periarterial fibrosis. It is impossible from the anecdotal reports of this rare complication to make any confident statements about the relative merits of treatment with surgery, antiplatelet agents, or warfarin.

Radiotherapy-induced occlusive disease of intracranial vessels most often follows radiotherapy for optic glioma or pituitary or suprasellar tumors, mainly in children and young adults. The reported interval between radiotherapy and symptoms ranges from 2 to 20 years, with a median of 5 years. The single most frequent arteriographic finding is narrowing or occlusion of the supraclinoid internal carotid artery; approximately two-thirds of patients also have a "moyamoya" pattern.

Radiotherapy-induced arteriopathy appears to represent an acceleration of "ordinary" atherosclerosis. Most studies have postulated the endothelium as the primary site of injury, with a possible additional factor of injury to the vasa vasorum. Many of the reported patients have hypercholesterolemia or other hyperlipidemia, and diet-induced hyperlipidemia in animals is known to potentiate radiotherapeutic injury to major vessels.

RADIATION-INDUCED TUMORS

An increasing number of case reports and epidemiologic studies indicate that tumorigenesis can be a sequela not only of therapeutic doses of cranial radiotherapy given for brain tumors but also of much lower doses of brain irradiation. The most common radiotherapy-induced intracranial tumors are meningiomas, sarcomas, and gliomas. Meningioma following cranial radiotherapy for primary brain tumors occurs after a median latency of 15 years; meningioma following low-dose radiotherapy for fungal scalp infections occurs after a peak latency period of 35 to 40 years. This suggests an inverse relationship between the dose of cranial radiotherapy RT and the latent period for tumorigenesis.

Benign or malignant gliomas have been reported after cranial radiotherapy in a number of settings, including long-term survivors of medulloblastoma, pituitary adenomas, and suprasellar tumors and patients irradiated for extracranial diseases. The mean latent period to diagnosis of radiotherapy-induced gliomas is approximately 10 years, with no clear correlation between the latency and either the radiotherapy dose or the patients' age when irradiated. Three-fourths of post-radiotherapy gliomas are glioblastoma multiforme or anaplastic astrocytoma. There are no distinctive histologic features of the tumors, and no striking differences in clinical behavior compared with malignant gliomas in general. Approximately 40 percent of reported radiotherapy-induced gliomas occurred in long-term survivors of childhood leukemia who received prophylactic WBRT. Gliomas are the most common nonhematologic tumors occurring as second neoplasms in leukemia survivors, with an estimated incidence as high as 2.3 percent 5 years following CNS prophylaxis. There seems, however, to be an association between leukemia and glial tumors in addition to the tumorigenic effect of WBRT.

SUGGESTED READINGS

Asai A, Matsutani M, Kohno T et al: Subacute brain atrophy after radiation therapy for malignant brain tumor. Cancer 63:1962, 1989

Constine LS, Konski A, Ekholm S et al: Adverse effects of brain irradiation correlated with MR and CT imaging. Int J Radiat Oncol Biol Phys 15: 319, 1988

Constine LS, Woolf PD, Cann D et al: Hypothalamic-pituitary dysfunction after radiation for brain tumors. N Engl J Med 328:87, 1993

DeAngelis LM, Delattre JY, Posner JB: Radiation-induced dementia in patients cured of brain metastases. Neurology 39:789, 1989

Dropcho EJ: Central nervous system injury by therapeutic irradiation. Neurol Clin 9:969–88, 1991

Duffner PK, Cohen ME: The long-term effects of CNS therapy on children with brain tumors. Neurol Clin 9:479–95, 1991

Gallego J, Delgado G, Tunon T, Villanueva JA: Delayed postirradiation lower motor neuron syndrome. Ann Neurol 19:308, 1986

Gilbert HA, Kagan AR (eds): Radiation Damage to the Nervous System. Raven Press, New York, 1980

Goldwein JW: Radiation myelopathy: a review. Med Pediatr Oncol 15:89, 1987

Imperato JP, Paleologos NA, Vick NA: Effects of treatment on long-term survivors with malignant astrocytomas. Ann Neurol 28:818, 1990

Johnson BE, Becker B, Goff WB, Petronas N: Neurologic, neuropsychologic, and computed cranial tomography scan abnormalities in 2- to 10-year survivors of small cell lung cancer. J Clin Oncol 3:1659, 1985

Murros KE, Toole JF: The effect of radiation on carotid arteries: a review article. Arch Neurol 46:449, 1989

Packer RJ, Meadows AT, Rorke LB et al: Long-term sequelae of cancer treatment on the central nervous system in childhood. Med Pediatr Oncol 15: 241, 1987

Packer RJ, Sutton LN, Atkins TE et al: A prospective study of cognitive function in children receiving whole-brain radiotherapy and chemotherapy: 2-year results. J Neurosurg 70:707, 1989

Rottenberg DA (ed): Neurological Complications of Cancer Treatment. Butterworth-Heinemann, Boston, 1991

Rubinstein AB, Shalit MN, Cohen ML et al: Radiation-induced cerebral meningioma: a recognizable entity. J Neurosurg 61:966, 1984

Salvati M, Artico M, Caruso R et al: A report on radiation-induced gliomas. Cancer 67:392, 1991

Williams JM, Davis KS: Central nervous system prophylactic treatment for childhood leukemia: neuropsychological outcome studies. Cancer Treat Rev 13:113, 1986

171. PARANEOPLASTIC SYNDROMES

JOSEP DALMAU
FRANCESC GRAUS

When patients with cancer develop neurologic symptoms, metastasis is usually the cause. Other neurologic complications result from infections, vascular and metabolic disorders, and neurotoxicity from chemotherapy and radiotherapy. This chapter focuses on the remote effects of cancer on the nervous system, which refers to neurologic disorders of unknown cause that occur at higher frequency in patients with cancer than in the general population. The term *paraneoplastic syndromes* is used for this concept. The frequency of these syndromes is unknown and varies among studies depending on (1) how the paraneoplastic syndrome is defined, (2) the type of neurologic evaluation used for study (i.e., clinical examination alone, or associated with electrophysiologic studies), and (3) the care with which other possible causes of neurologic disability are excluded (i.e., advance neoplastic disease, loss of weight).

Clinically significant paraneoplastic syndromes occur in less than 1 percent of cancer patients (Table 171-1). Most of these

TABLE 171-1. Paraneoplastic Syndromes Affecting the Nervous System

Paraneoplastic syndromes of the central nervous system
 Paraneoplastic cerebellar degeneration
 Paraneoplastic encephalomyelitis[a]
  Limbic encephalitis
  Brainstem encephalitis
  Myelitis
 Paraneoplastic opsoclonus-myoclonus
 Paraneoplastic necrotizing myelopathy
 Motor neuron syndromes
  Amyotrophic lateral sclerosis
  Subacute motor neuronopathy
 Visual paraneoplastic syndromes
  Cancer-associated retinopathy
  Optic neuritis

Paraneoplastic syndromes of the peripheral nervous system
 Paraneoplastic sensory neuronopathy
 Acute polyradiculoneuropathy
 Brachial neuritis
 Multineuritis and vasculitis
 Subacute or chronic sensorimotor peripheral neuropathy
 Sensorimotor neuropathies associated with plasma cell dyscrasias
  Myeloma
  Waldenström's macroglobulinemia
 Autonomic neuropathy
 Neuromyotonia

Paraneoplastic syndromes of the neuromuscular junction and muscle
 Lambert-Eaton myasthenic syndrome
 Polymyositis/dermatomyositis
 Acute necrotizing myopathy
 Carcinoid myopathy
 Cachectic myopathy
 Carcinomatous neuromyopathy

[a] Can include cerebellar symptoms, autonomic dysfunction, and sensory neuronopathy.

disorders develop before the diagnosis of cancer; therefore, these patients are usually first seen by neurologists. Since syndromes can develop in patients without cancer, the ones that strongly suggest a paraneoplastic origin include the following:

Lambert-Eaton myasthenic syndrome
Subacute cerebellar syndrome
Subacute sensory neuropathy
Opsoclonus-myoclonus
Subacute autonomic dysfunction (postural hypotension, gastro-
 intestinal immotility)
Dermatomyositis (in older population)
Subacute encephalomyelitis
Subacute retinopathy
Subacute limbic encephalopathy
Subacute motor neuronopathy and atypical motor neuron dis-
 ease

The likelihood that a disorder is paraneoplastic will depend on (1) the type of syndrome; (2) the clinical exclusion of an underlying tumor; and (3) for some disorders, the presence of characteristic autoantibodies (Table 171-2). In many patients with paraneoplastic disorders, the neoplasm is small, remains localized along the course of the disease, and is difficult to demonstrate even with thorough, repetitive clinical studies.

For most paraneoplastic syndromes, the pathogenesis is unknown. However, in some disorders, the patient's serum and cerebrospinal fluid (CSF) contain antibodies directed against neuron proteins expressed by the associated tumor (Table 171-2). It is believed that the ectopic expression of these proteins leads to the development of an immunologic response against the tumor that cross-reacts with the nervous system, resulting in the paraneoplastic disorder. This autoimmune hypothesis has been proven for the Lambert-Eaton myasthenic syndrome and myasthenia gravis, but for other paraneoplastic syndromes, the role of the antibodies in the pathogenesis of the disease remains unclear. Clinically, the identification of these antibodies is important for two reasons: (1) their detection confirms the paraneoplastic origin of the neurologic dysfunction, and (2) their characterization directs the search for the tumor to one or a few organs. However, similar paraneoplastic syndromes may develop without the presence of antibodies; this situation almost always occurs when the associated tumor is different from the typical histologic type involved in the antibody-related disorder. For example, the anti-Hu antibody is almost always detected in the serum of patients with paraneoplastic sensory neuronopathy and small cell lung cancer, but the antibody is rarely present in paraneoplastic sensory neuropathy associated with other tumors. Conversely, some paraneoplastic disorders may be mediated by antibodies that are not detected by currently available techniques. Non-immune-mediated mechanisms such as competition for an essential substrate (i.e., carcinoid myopathy) or viral infection (i.e., subacute motor neuronopathy) have been proposed as the cause of other paraneoplastic disorders.

For most paraneoplastic syndromes, particularly those involving the central nervous system, treatment is usually unrewarding. In a few instances, prompt identification and treatment of the tumor and/or the paraneoplastic disorder may result in stabilization or improvement of the neurologic symptoms. A general diagnostic approach to a patient with neurologic dysfunction of possible paraneoplastic origin is shown in Table 171-3.

Paraneoplastic neurologic syndromes can involve any part of the central or peripheral nervous system, including neuro-

TABLE 171-2. Antibody-Associated Paraneoplastic Neurologic Disorders

Antibody	Antigen	Symptoms	Tumor[a]
Anti-Yo	34 and 62 kd (cytoplasm of Purkinje cells)	Cerebellar degeneration	Ovary, breast; fallopian tube
Anti-Ri	55 and 80 kd (nuclei of neurons)	Opsoclonus, ataxia	Breast
Anti-Hu	35–40 kd (nuclei of neurons)	Sensory neuronopathy; encephalomyelitis[b]	SCLC; neuroblastoma
Antiretinal	23, 65, 145, 205 kd (photoreceptors, ganglion cells)	Cancer-associated retinopathy	SCLC
Anti-voltage-gated calcium channel	Presynaptic calcium channels (MysB)	LEMS	SCLC
Hodgkin's disease	Purkinje cells	Cerebellar degeneration	Hodgkin's disease
Paraneoplastic stiff-man syndrome	128 kd (neuronal synapse)	Stiff-man syndrome	Breast

Abbreviations: LEMS, Lambert-Eaton myasthenic syndrome; SCLC, small cell lung cancer.
[a] Tumors most frequently associated.
[b] Encephalomyelitis may include some or all of the following symptoms: limbic encephalitis, cerebellar symptoms, brainstem encephalitis, myelitis, and/or autonomic dysfunction. Patients with isolated cerebellar degeneration or limbic encephalitis may be anti-Hu negative, even when the associated tumor is SCLC.

TABLE 171-3. Diagnostic Approach to a Patient with Neurologic Dysfunction of Possible Paraneoplastic Origin

Known Cancer	No Known Cancer
1. Rule out metastatic complications: (MRI of involved site, CSF cytology and appropriate tumor markers [CEA, etc.])	1. Workup for cancer detection: chest CT, pelvic examination, mammography, serum tumor markers (CEA, CA-125, CA-15-3, etc.)
2. Rule out nonmetastatic complications: (toxic effects of chemotherapy and radiotherapy, metabolic and nutritional deficits, coagulopathy, infection, post-traumatic nerve injury)	2. Study of CSF for cells, IgG ratio, oligoclonal bands, cytology
3. Study of CSF for cells, IgG ratio, oligoclonal bands	3. Presence of paraneoplastic antibodies in serum and CSF
4. Presence of paraneoplastic antibodies in serum and CSF	4. Follow up and search for cancer if steps 2 and 3 are positive

Abbreviations: CEA, carcinoembryonic antigen; CA-125, marker of ovarian cancer; CA 15-3, marker of breast cancer; CSF, cerebrospinal fluid; CT, computed tomography; MRI, magnetic resonance imaging.
(Modified from Posner JB: Paraneoplastic syndromes. In: Neurologic complications of cancer. FA Davis, Philadelphia (in press), with permission.)

muscular junction and muscle (Table 171-1). Some syndromes are mainly restricted to one area of the nervous system (paraneoplastic cerebellar degeneration), but the same type of symptoms may be observed as part of a more widespread syndrome (paraneoplastic encephalomyelitis) or in association with other paraneoplastic disorders (paraneoplastic cerebellar degeneration and Lambert-Eaton myasthenic syndrome). Even when symptoms appear restricted to one area of the nervous system (paraneoplastic cerebellar degeneration), minor signs of dysfunction of other regions are usually present (corticospinal tract involvement, mild cognitive dysfunction).

SYNDROMES OF THE CENTRAL NERVOUS SYSTEM

Paraneoplastic Cerebellar Degeneration

Patients with paraneoplastic cerebellar degeneration typically develop rapid progressive symptoms that evolve, over weeks or months, to a severe pancerebellar dysfunction. Symptoms include truncal and appendicular ataxia, dysarthria, and nystagmus. The main pathologic hallmark is extensive loss of Purkinje cells, accompanied by proliferation of Bergmann astrocytes in the molecular layer, loss of granule cells, and sometimes, in-

flammatory infiltrates in the deep cerebellar nuclei. Gynecologic tumors, breast cancer, lung cancer, and lymphomas are the most commonly associated neoplasms. Pure subacute cerebellar dysfunction in adult patients should be considered paraneoplastic until another cause is demonstrated. Paraneoplastic cerebellar degeneration may be subdivided into several disorders that appear to differ in prognosis and tumor association. Some subtypes are described in Table 171-4.

The most common and well characterized paraneoplastic cerebellar degeneration is defined by a subset of patients who harbor an antibody called anti-Yo, which reacts with 34- and 62-kd proteins expressed in the cytoplasm of Purkinje cells and tumor, usually gynecologic or breast cancer. If the presence of a tumor is not known, patients with anti-Yo-positive paraneoplastic cerebellar degeneration should have breast and pelvic examination, mammography, pelvic computed tomography (CT), and measurement of the ovarian tumor antigen CA-125. If no malignancy is revealed, repeat mammography, pelvic examination under anesthesia, and uterine dilation and curettage are recommended. When no cancer is evident, surgical exploration and removal of pelvic organs may be considered, particularly in postmenopausal women.

TABLE 171-4. Subtypes of Paraneoplastic Cerebellar Degeneration

Subclass	Sex	Tumor[a]	Onset[b]	Clinical Findings
Anti-Yo	F	Gynecologic, breast	Before	Subacute pancerebellar symptoms
Anti-Hu[c]	F > M	SCLC	Before	Sensory neuronopathy, encephalomyelitis
Anti-Ri	F	Breast	Before/after	Opsoclonus, truncal ataxia, myoclonus
PCD-HD	M > F	Hodgkin's disease	After	May remit; less severe than other subtypes
PCD-LEMS	M = F	SCLC	Before	Pancerebellar symptoms with proximal weakness; decreased reflexes in legs (LEMS may be overlooked)

Abbreviations: PCD, paraneoplastic cerebellar degeneration; SCLC, small cell lung cancer; HD, Hodgkin's disease; LEMS, Lamber-Eaton myasthenic syndrome.
[a] Indicates only the tumors most frequently associated.
[b] Onset of neurologic symptoms before or after tumor diagnosis.
[c] Anti-Hu associated encephalomyelitis may develop with predominant cerebellar symptoms that usually are associated with other symptoms, including sensory neuronopathy, limbic encephalitis, brainstem encephalitis, myelitis, and/or autonomic dysfunction. Patients with SCLC and PCD alone or associated with LEMS may be anti-Hu negative.

Paraneoplastic cerebellar degeneration has been reported in association with a large variety of neoplasms. However, when neoplasms other than breast and gynecologic tumors are involved, patients are anti-Yo negative. Patients with predominant truncal ataxia and oculomotor abnormalities may harbor an antibody called anti-Ri. In this subset of patients, the tumor is usually breast cancer or, much less frequently, gynecologic or small cell lung cancer. Opsoclonus is almost always present in the early stages of the disease and may evolve toward flutter, or resolve. In addition to paraneoplastic cerebellar degeneration, these patients may develop dementia, mixed peripheral neuropathy, and axial rigidity and myoclonus. If no tumor is identified, anti-Ri-positive patients should have close clinical follow-ups and repeated mammography every 6 months. Treatment with steroids and immunosuppressants (cyclophosphamide) may result in improvement of the neurologic disorder.

Paraneoplastic cerebellar degeneration may also be the presentation of anti-Hu-associated paraneoplastic encephalomyelitis. In this case, paraneoplastic cerebellar degeneration should be considered a fragment of paraneoplastic encephalomyelitis, since the cerebellar dysfunction rarely persists as the main neurologic symptom (see Paraneoplastic Encephalomyelitis, below). In those patients in which paraneoplastic cerebellar degeneration remains the only or major dysfunction, anti-Hu antibodies are usually negative, even when the associated tumor is small cell lung cancer.

In addition, there are two other anti-Yo negative subtypes of paraneoplastic cerebellar degeneration. One is characterized by the association with Hodgkin's disease. Paraneoplastic cerebellar degeneration-Hodgkin's disease predominates in men (6:1), and patients are usually younger (20 to 40 years) that other paraneoplastic cerebellar degeneration patients. By contrast with other subtypes of paraneoplastic cerebellar degeneration, cerebellar symptoms usually develop after the diagnosis of the lymphoma, sometimes heralding tumor recurrence, but occasionally during remission. Some of these patients develop antibodies that react with the cytoplasm of Purkinje cells; the antigen has not been characterized. Paraneoplastic cerebellar degeneration-Hodgkin's disease patients also differ from other paraneoplastic cerebellar degeneration patients in that cerebellar symptoms may remit spontaneously or respond to treatment with clonazepam.

Another anti-Yo-negative paraneoplastic cerebellar degeneration develops in association with Lambert-Eaton myasthenic syndrome, and is commonly associated with small cell lung cancer. Typically, patients develop neurologic symptoms either of Lambert-Eaton myasthenic syndrome or paraneoplastic cerebellar degeneration before the tumor is diagnosed. Unless Lambert-Eaton myasthenic syndrome develops first, its diagnosis may be overlooked.

For all subtypes of paraneoplastic cerebellar degeneration, either associated with antineuron antibodies or not, diagnostic tests including head CT and magnetic resonance imaging (MRI) are usually normal in the early stages of the disease, and evolve to cerebellar atrophy.

For most types of paraneoplastic cerebellar degeneration, particularly anti-Yo-associated degeneration, treatment of the tumor does not result in improvement of the neurologic symptoms. Autopsies of anti-Yo-positive patients demonstrate total or near total loss of Purkinje cells, which probably occurs early in the course of the disease, prior to diagnosis. Plasmapheresis, intravenous immunoglobulin (IgG) and immunosuppressants are usually ineffective. In a few patients with tumors other than breast and gynecologic cancers, resection of the tumor has resulted in neurologic improvement.

Patients with anti-Yo associated paraneoplastic cerebellar degeneration die as a result of the tumor or remain severely disabled. The course of the cancer in these patients appears to be more indolent than in patients without paraneoplastic disease.

Paraneoplastic Encephalomyelitis

Paraneoplastic encephalomyelitis describes patients with cancer who develop clinical signs of dysfunction of various parts of the nervous system and postmortem signs of inflammation within the brain, brainstem, spinal cord, dorsal root ganglia, and nerve roots. The distribution of pathologic findings along the neuraxis is variable, giving rise to several syndromes that can occur alone or in association. Neurologic symptoms of paraneoplastic encephalomyelitis include dementia (limbic encephalopathy), cerebellar degeneration, brainstem encephalopathy, myelopathy, and autonomic dysfunction. Many patients with paraneoplastic encephalomyelitis also have symptoms of sensory neuropathy. Paraneoplastic encephalomyelitis/paraneoplastic sensory neuropathy have been reported in association with almost all types of tumors, but in most patients (80 percent), the underlying tumor is carcinoma of the bronchus, particularly small cell lung cancer. The tumor usually remains small, its metastatic spread being limited to regional lymph nodes; in a number of patients, the tumor is not detected until autopsy. The subset of patients with paraneoplastic encephalomyelitis/paraneoplastic sensory neuropathy and small cell lung cancer have in their serum and CSF high titers of the antibody called anti-Hu. The anti-Hu antibody reacts with protein antigens of 35 to 40 kd expressed in neurons and small cell lung cancer cells. Anti-Hu-associated paraneoplastic encephalomyelitis has a mild predominance in women.

Anti-Hu-associated paraneoplastic encephalomyelitis/paraneoplasty sensory neuropathy develops before the diagnosis of the tumor in 80 percent of patients. Symptoms develop subacutely and progress until stabilization or death in a few weeks or months. Most patients (73 percent) have signs and symptoms of multifocal involvement of the nervous system; in these patients as well as in patients with unifocal involvement, the predominant disorder is paraneoplastic sensory neuropathy. Table 171-5 indicates the predominant and nonpredominant clinical findings in a series of 71 patients with anti-Hu-associated paraneoplastic encephalomyelitis/paraneoplastic sensory neuropathy. Paraneoplastic sensory neuropathy is described below, under Paraneoplastic Syndromes of the Peripheral Nerves.

Limbic encephalopathy predominates in 20 percent of paraneoplastic encephalomyelitis patients. Symptoms include confusion, depression, agitation, anxiety, memory deficits, dementia, and partial complex seizures. When limbic encephalopathy develops alone, the anti-Hu antibody may be absent even in patients with small cell lung cancer.

Motor neuron dysfunction predominates in 20 percent of paraneoplastic encephalomyelitis patients. Almost all patients have signs of involvement of other areas of the nervous system, which allows the differentiation from amyotrophic lateral sclerosis. In general, symptoms start with proximal loss of strength, affecting limbs in an asymmetric pattern. Neck flexor/extensor weakness may be the initial deficit. Distal involvement of extremities, fasciculations, and muscle atrophy are common. In those patients with predominant involvement of the anterior horn of the spinal cord or associated paraneoplastic sensory

TABLE 171-5. Clinical Findings in Anti-Hu-Associated Sensory Neuronopathy and/or Encephalomyelitis[a]

Symptoms	Percent
Unifocal	27
Sensory neuropathy	20
Limbic encephalopathy	6
Brainstem encephalopathy	1
Multifocal	73
Sensory neuropathy	54
Cerebellar degeneration	25
Limbic encephalopathy	22
Braintem encephalopathy	31
Motor neuronopathy[b]	45
Autonomic dysfunction	28
Visual loss	1
Lambert-Eaton myasthenic syndrome[c]	1
Myoclonus	1
Polymyositis	1
Diffuse encephalomyelitis	3

[a] Table shows the frequency of predominant and nonpredominant clinical findings in a series of 71 patients. Predominant symptoms are those that cause maximum disability to the patient; their frequency is indicated in text.
[b] Includes weakness, fasciculations, muscle atrophy.
[c] Incidence is probably underestimated, owing to the lack of routine electrophysiologic studies.

(Data from Dalmau J, Graus F, Rosenblum MK, Posner JB: Anti-Hu-associated paraneoplastic encephalomyelitis/sensory neuronopathy: a clinical study of 71 patients. Medicine 71:59, 1992.)

neuropathy, reflexes are decreased or abolished. Other patients have hyperreflexia, clonus, and extensor plantar responses.

Symptoms of cerebellar degeneration are predominant in about 15 percent of paraneoplastic encephalomyelitis patients. Gait ataxia is the usual presentation; however, most patients eventually develop a pancerebellar syndrome. A distinctive clinical feature of these patients, compared with those with other types of paraneoplastic cerebellar degeneration, is that almost all anti-Hu positive patients will develop signs of severe involvement of other areas of the nervous system.

Brainstem encephalopathy develops in one-third of paraneoplastic encephalomyelitis patients, but in only one-half is it predominant. The most frequent symptoms include oscillopsia, diplopia, dysarthria, dysphagia, gaze abnormalities—both internuclear or supranuclear (vertical and horizontal), subacute hearing loss, and facial numbness.

Approximately one-fourth of paraneoplastic encephalomyelitis patients develop autonomic nervous system dysfunction. In 10 percent, this is the first and predominant symptom(s), including postural hypotension, gastroparesis and intestinal immotility, sweating abnormalities, neurogenic bladder, and impotence. Abnormal (sluggish) pupillary responses is a common finding. Respiratory or autonomic failure due to severe neurologic dysfunction are frequent causes of death.

Routine CSF studies show increased protein concentration and/or pleocytosis in 80 percent of the patients; the ratio of CSF to serum IgG is elevated in most, and oligoclonal bands are frequently detected. If paraneoplastic sensory neuropathy is present, the electrophysiologic findings are suggestive of selective damage of the sensory pathways (see under Paraneoplastic Sensory Neuropathy, below) suggesting dorsal root ganglia involvement. Motor nerve velocities and F wave studies are normal. In some patients, signs of motor denervation secondary to myelitis and anterior horn involvement are also present. Only a minority of patients with paraneoplastic encephalomyelitis have MRI abnormalities, including atrophy of the cerebellum, and in some patients with limbic encephalopathy, increased signal on T2-weighted images involving the medial aspect of the temporal lobes. With time, these abnormalities may revert to normal, leaving only atrophic changes.

The most important diagnostic test is the detection of the anti-Hu antibody in serum and CSF. This assay must be done by immunohistochemistry and Western blot analysis of recombinant HuD protein or cerebral cortical neurons. The anti-Hu antibody is almost always present in patients with symptoms of paraneoplastic encephalomyelitis/paraneoplastic sensory neuropathy and small cell lung cancer. In patients with an unknown primary tumor, the detection of this antibody should prompt the search for a small cell lung cancer. Only a few patients with anti-Hu-associated paraneoplastic encephalomyelitis/paraneoplastic sensory neuropathy and tumors other than small cell lung cancer have been reported, including neuroblastoma, prostate cancer, and chondromyxosarcoma. If a careful workup, which must include CT or MRI of the chest and bronchoscopy, does not demonstrate the tumor, periodic (every 6 months) clinical follow-ups and CT of the chest are recommended. The anti-Hu antibody may be absent in patients with small cell lung cancer and pure or predominant symptoms of limbic encephalopathy and cerebellar degeneration.

Treatment with steroids, plasmapheresis, and immunosuppressants are usually ineffective. Intravenous immunoglobulin is usually unrewarding; the few patients reported who stabilized or improved with this treatment were receiving concomitant antitumor therapies. However, earlier detection and treatment of a small cell lung cancer with chemotherapy may result, if the paraneoplastic encephalomyelitis is not severe, in stabilization and improvement of the neurologic dysfunction. Anti-Hu-positive patients with mild to moderate nonprogressive sensory neuropathy should receive treatment only for the tumor. If a tumor is not detected, periodic clinical and radiologic follow-ups are recommended; immunosuppressants should be avoided. However, patients with rapidly progressive neurologic deterioration should be considered for aggressive immunosuppression. One patient improved with intravenous IgG, cyclosporin, and cyclophosphamide.

Limbic encephalopathy, either alone or associated with other symptoms of paraneoplastic encephalomyelitis, may resolve spontaneously; however, accompanying symptoms of paraneoplastic sensory neuropathy or paraneoplastic encephalomyelitis usually progress or stabilize but rarely improve.

Paraneoplastic Opsoclonus-Myoclonus

Opsoclonus is a rare disorder of ocular motility characterized by the presence of spontaneous, arrhythmic, large-amplitude conjugate saccades ocurring in all directions of gaze without a saccadic interval. Opsoclonus is frequently associated with myoclonus, and both can have a paraneoplastic origin. The tumors most frequently involved include neuroblastoma (in the pediatric population), lung cancer (particularly small cell lung cancer), and carcinoma of the breast.

Nearly 50 percent of children with paraneoplastic opsoclonus-myoclonus have neuroblastoma, and about 2 percent of children with this tumor develop paraneoplastic opsoclonus-myoclonus. Other symptoms include myoclonus of limbs and trunk, hypotonia, and irritability that cannot be differentiated from nonparaneoplastic opsoclonus-myoclonus. In one-half of patients, paraneoplastic opsoclonus-myoclonus precedes the diagnosis of neuroblastoma. Symptoms usually fluctuate and may have a prolonged course. Treatment of the neuroblastoma results in improvement of paraneoplastic opsoclonus-myoclonus in one-third of the patients. Paraneoplastic opsoclonus-myoclonus frequently responds to steroids, but may relapse with steroid withdrawal and with intercurrent infections. Spontaneous resolution has been observed. Patients with paraneoplastic opsoclonus-myoclonus have better tumor prognosis than patients without paraneoplastic symptoms.

In adults, paraneoplastic opsoclonus often develops in association with truncal ataxia, resulting in gait difficulty and frequent falls. Other symptoms include vertigo, dizziness, nausea, vomiting, myoclonus, dysarthria, dysphagia, and diplopia or blurry vision. Less frequently, patients develop confusion, decreased hearing, proximal muscle weakness, axial rigidity, and paroxysmal spams, including blepharospasm. Symptoms have sudden onset and reach their peak in 1 to 4 weeks. Spontaneous or therapeutic improvement of opsoclonus are usually followed by ocular flutter and dysmetria. In more than one half of the patients, paraneoplastic opsoclonus-myoclonus precedes the diagnosis of the tumor. The most common offender is small cell lung cancer.

In women, the detection of the anti-Ri antibody should prompt the search for a breast cancer, and less frequently, a gynecologic neoplasm. In rare instances of brainstem encephalopathy associated with opsoclonus, patients may harbor the anti-Hu antibody. In these patients, a search for small cell lung cancer is mandatory. No other antineuron antibodies indicative of a specific type of tumor have been identified in paraneoplastic opsoclonus-myoclonus patients.

In general, the CSF shows mild inflammatory changes and may have oligoclonal bands. MRI studies are usually normal, but may show hyperintense T2-weighted images in the dorsal midbrain. The electroencephalogram may be normal or demonstrate generalized slowing of the background activity, without epileptiform activity. There have been clinical responses to immunosuppressants, clonazepam, thiamine, and treatment of the tumor, but interpretation of these results is confounded by the possibility of spontaneous improvement.

Paraneoplastic Necrotizing Myelopathy

Paraneoplastic necrotizing myelopathy, a rare syndrome, has been reported in association with several carcinomas and lymphoma. There is no relationship between the neurologic disorder and the course of the neoplasm. The disorder develops acute or subacutely in the thoracic portion of the spinal cord, with progressive ascending or descending spinal cord deficits. Symptoms include sphincter dysfunction, segmental sensory deficits that may have an ascending progression, and flaccid or spastic paraplegia that evolve to tetraplegia or flaccid paraplegia. Back pain and/or radicular symptoms are rare. Symptoms progress over days or weeks and eventually result in respiratory failure and death. The CSF shows elevated protein and at times mild pleocytosis, but is usually acellular. A myelogram may be normal or demonstrate swelling of the cord. There are no MRI studies of patients with autopsy-proven paraneoplastic necrotizing myelopathy. There are no biologic markers of this disorder; therefore, a definitive diagnosis cannot be established without postmortem study.

In patients with solid tumors, the diagnosis of leptomeningeal, epidural and intramedullary metastasis, and postradiation myelopathy should always be entertained before the diagnosis of paraneoplastic necrotizing myelopathy. The differential diagnosis between these disorders is facilitated by considering (1) the presence of pain (present in leptomeningeal, epidural, and intramedullary metastasis, usually absent in paraneoplastic necrotizing myelopathy), (2) mode of onset (long and insidious for postradiation myelopathy; subacute for metastases and paraneoplastic necrotizing myelopathy), (3) history of radiotherapy (postradiation myelopathy occurs within the port of irradiation; regions of overlapping ports should be investigated), (4) initial myelopathic dysfunction (paraneoplastic necrotizing myelopathy usually starts in the thoracic spinal cord; leptomeningeal metastasis is multifocal; postradiation myelopathy often involves the cervical cord after irradiation of head and neck tumors), (5) extension of disease (metastasis to the brain is identified in two-thirds of patients with intramedullary metastasis), (6) presence of neoplastic cells in the CSF indicative of leptomeningeal metastasis, and (7) MRI of the involved site of the spinal cord, which usually demonstrates epidural and leptomeningeal metastasis and, less frequently, intramedullary metastasis. In patients with lymphoma and leukemia, a syndrome identical to paraneoplastic necrotizing myelopathy may be caused by viral infections, particularly of the herpes group, as well as by toxic effects of intrathecal chemotherapy or radiotherapy, and more rarely by septic infarcts.

There is no treatment for paraneoplastic necrotizing myelopathy. In patients with solid tumors, if the diagnosis of intramedullary metastasis cannot be ruled out, treatment with radiotherapy should be considered to stop progression of symptoms.

Motor Neuron Syndromes

Cancer and motor neuron syndromes can be separated into three groups: (1) typical amyotrophic lateral sclerosis, (2) subacute motor neuropathy, and (3) motor neuron dysfunction as a component of paraneoplastic encephalomyelitis (this latter group is discussed above).

Amyotrophic Lateral Sclerosis. Epidemiologic studies have demonstrated no significantly increased incidence of amyotrophic lateral sclerosis in patients with cancer. However, a few patients with cancer, usually of the lung or kidney, have had remission or improvement of amyotrophic lateral sclerosis after treatment of the malignancy. In addition, patients with Hodgkin's disease or other lymphoproliferative disorders can develop symptoms of involvement of upper and lower—or only lower—motor neurons. In some patients, electrophysiologic studies demonstrate multifocal conduction blocks. If no tumor is known, patients with amyotrophic lateral sclerosis, paraproteinemia, and increased CSF proteins with or without oligoclonal bands should be considered for bone marrow biopsy to rule out a lymphoproliferative disorder.

Subacute Motor Neuropathy. Subacute motor neuropathy is characterized by subacute, progressive, painless, often patchy and asymmetric muscle weakness that is more prominent in the lower extremities. Reflexes are decreased or abolished. There is usually sparing of bulbar muscles; fasciculations are rare. Sensory symptoms, if any, are mild and transitory. The neurologic symptoms usually have a benign course, independent of the activity of the neoplasm. Neurologic stabilization or spontaneous improvement is common. Tumors involved include Hodgkin's lymphoma and, less frequently, non-Hodgkin's lymphoma. CSF shows mildly increased proteins with a normal cell count. Electrophysiologic studies show denervation with normal or mild slowness of motor nerve velocities. The pathologic findings include neuron degeneration predominantly involving the anterior horn of the spinal cord. Inflammatory infiltrates are mild or absent. Patchy areas of segmental demyelination involving spinal roots and brachial and lumbar plexuses have been observed.

This disorder should be differentiated from a lower motor neuron syndrome secondary to radiotherapy. In these patients, the distribution of muscle weakness is more distal, and although symptoms stabilize, they do not improve. The tumor most commonly involved is seminoma. However, patients with Hodgkin's lymphoma treated with mantle radiation may develop slowly progressive (over several years) weakness and atrophy involving neck flexors and extensors and proximal muscles of the upper extremities. Characteristically, a strip of atrophy involving paraspinal muscles is also observed. Distal reflexes are usually preserved; sensation is normal. No pathologic studies have been reported. There is no treatment for this disorder.

Visual Paraneoplastic Symptoms

In patients with cancer, visual symptoms and blindness are usually related to metastatic infiltration of optic nerves by tumor, neurotoxicity from chemotherapy and radiotherapy, and anemia. On rare occasions, patients develop cancer-associated retinopathy and optic neuritis of paraneoplastic origin.

Cancer-Associated Retinopathy. Cancer-associated retinopathy is characterized by episodic visual obscurations, light-induced glare, photosensitivity, night blindness, and impaired color vision. Symptoms may begin unilaterally but become bilateral within days or weeks, and usually precede the diagnosis of the tumor. Small cell lung cancer is the most common underlying tumor; other tumors include melanoma and gynecologic neoplasms. Examination shows peripheral and ringlike scotomata, impaired visual acuity and color vision, and retinal arteriolar narrowing. Visual evoked responses are usually normal, but electroretinographic studies demonstrate reduced or flat photopic and scotopic responses. CSF is usually normal; in some patients elevated immunoglobulins and pleocytosis have been reported. Head CT and MRI are normal. Pathologic studies demonstrate loss of photoreceptors or ganglion cells, along with infiltrative macrophages with melanin granules and inflammatory infiltrates in the retinal arterioles. The serum of some patients may harbor antibodies that react with antigens contained in photoreceptors and ganglion cells; some of these antigens are also expressed by the tumor (Table 171-2). One of these antigens is a 23-kd calcium-binding protein, named recoverin, which is contained in photoreceptors.

Treatment with steroids may improve or stabilize the visual symptoms. Symptoms in antibody-positive patients that do not respond to steroids may be stabilized with plasmapheresis.

Paraneoplastic Optic Neuritis. Paraneoplastic optic neuritis is more rare than cancer-associated retinopathy. It may develop in isolation, but is usually associated with paraneoplastic encephalomyelitis. The onset is subacute, with painless, bilateral visual loss. The examination may show papilledema.

SYNDROMES OF THE PERIPHERAL NERVES

Paraneoplastic Sensory Neuropathy

The typical onset of paraneoplastic sensory neuropathy is pain and paresthesias asymmetrically involving one limb, which can be confused with a radiculopathy or multineuropathy. Usually, symptoms progress rapidly (over several weeks) to involve other extremities and sometimes the face and trunk. Other cranial nerves may be affected, resulting in loss of taste and sensorineural deafness. Eventually, there is severe loss of sensation, interfering with walking and movement of the extremities. More than 70 percent of patients with paraneoplastic sensory neuropathy develop symptoms of involvement of other areas of the nervous system, including muscle weakness, positional hypotension, seizures, or any other symptoms of paraneoplastic encephalomyelitis. There is involvement of all modalities of sensation, with predominant deficits of joint position and vibratory sensation. These deficits result in sensory ataxia involving legs (gait ataxia) and arms (pseudoathetotic movements). Deep tendon reflexes are asymmetrically decreased or abolished. When paraneoplastic sensory neuropathy is combined with other signs of paraneoplastic encephalomyelitis, the examination may demonstrate muscle weakness and atrophy, fasciculations (anterior horn involvement), cerebellar and brainstem dysfunction, and memory and cognitive deficits (limbic encephalopathy). Frequently, there are sluggish pupillary reactions and symptoms and signs of autonomic dysfunction (orthostatic hypotension, gastrointestinal immotility, bladder dysfunction, sweating abnormalities). Depending on the area of major involvement, the combination of paraneoplastic encephalomyelitis and paraneoplastic sensory neuropathy can be confused with a multiple mononeuropathy or subacute polyneuritis.

In more than 80 percent of patients with paraneoplastic sensory neuropathy, the associated tumor is small cell lung cancer. Sensory symptoms usually precede the diagnosis of the tumor. In patients with no known cancer, paraneoplastic sensory neuropathy should be clinically suspected when sensory symptoms develop asymmetrically or involve the trunk and cranial nerves. The CSF shows increased proteins with pleocytosis (in general, less than 100 cells/dl); oligoclonal bands and an increased IgG CSF to serum ratio are common. Electrophysiologic studies demonstrate decreased or abolished somatosensory evoked potentials and action potentials of sensory nerves. Motor conduction studies are normal; signs of motor denervation are absent unless there is a concomitant myelitis with anterior horn involvement.

The detection of the anti-Hu antibody in serum and/or CSF should direct the search for small cell lung cancer. If no tumor is detected, periodic (every 6 months) clinical follow-ups and CT of the chest are recommended (see Paraneoplastic Encephalomyelitis, above). Frequently in patients with paraneoplastic sensory neuropathy and the anti-Hu antibody, the tumor cannot be detected until late in the course of the disease or until autopsy.

If the anti-Hu antibody is negative and tests suggest sensory neuropathy (DRG involvement), the search for a neoplasm should have a wider spectrum, including other (non-small cell lunger cancer) lung tumors and breast cancer. In these patients, periodic follow-ups for at least the first 2 years after symptom development should include mammography and CT of the chest and abdomen.

In rare instances, paraneoplastic sensory neuropathy may have a chronic course (6 months to 3 years) and be mild to severe in intensity. In these patients the differential diagnosis must include Sjögren syndrome, which may develop with sensory neuronopathy and be negative for anti-Ro and anti-La antibodies. Some patients with Sjögren syndrome and sensory neuropathy harbor in their serum an antineuron antibody that immunohistochemically resembles the anti-Hu antibody. Western blot analysis of Hu recombinant antigens (HuD), which are positive for the presence of anti-Hu antibodies but negative in patients with Sjögren syndrome, helps to differentiate the disorders. Patients with sensory neuropathy of unknown cause who are anti-Hu-negative should be studied for Sjögren syndrome and undergo salivary gland biopsy.

Patients with carcinoma of the lung and lymphoma can develop an acute sensory neuropathy that may improve spontaneously. In these patients, the clinical and electrophysiologic findings suggest a sensory variant of the Guillain-Barré syndrome.

The treatment of paraneoplastic sensory neuropathy is discussed above, under Paraneoplastic Encephalomyelitis.

Acute Polyradiculoneuropathy

Acute paraneoplastic polyradiculoneuropathy resembling a typical Guillain-Barré syndrome is usually associated with Hodgkin's disease. The course of the neurologic syndrome is independent of the lymphoma, and symptoms can develop either during active disease or when the patient is in remission. These patients may respond to plasmapheresis.

In some patients with anti-Hu-associated paraneoplastic encephalomyelitis, a subacute involvement of the anterior horn of the spinal cord and DRG may mimic acute polyneuritis.

Brachial Neuritis

Patients with cancer may develop a clinical picture resembling the brachial neuritis observed in patients without cancer. The neoplasm most commonly involved is Hodgkin's lymphoma, and the causal mechanism is unknown. The differential diagnosis has to be made among the more common causes of brachial plexopathy, including tumor infiltration, radiation injury, ischemic neuropathy, and traumatic injury of the plexus.

Multineuritis and Vasculitis

There have been only a few reports of patients with paraneoplastic vasculitic neuropathy, usually associated with carcinoma of the lung, prostate, kidney, endometrium, or lymphoma. Patients with this disorder develop a progressive and often asymmetric and painful sensorimotor neuropathy (multiple mononeuropathy), which may antedate the diagnosis of the neoplasm. In addition to peripheral nerve vasculitis (epineural vasculitis), there is usually muscle vasculitis and sometimes symptoms of central nervous system involvement (paraneoplastic encephalomyelitis). Positive anti-Hu serology has been reported when small cell lung cancer is the associated tumor.

The course and response to treatment is variable. Spontaneous improvement and response to chemotherapy may occur. Steroids and cyclophosphamide have been effective in some patients.

Subacute and Chronic Sensorimotor Neuropathy

In patients with cancer, peripheral neuropathy is common, but a paraneoplastic origin is rare. Sensorimotor neuropathy can be caused by chemotherapeutic agents, diabetes, alcoholism, chronic illness, and metabolic and vitamin (B_{12}) deficits. In patients with no known cancer, the development of sensorimotor neuropathy is not often indicative of a paraneoplastic syndrome and has much less significance that the development of subacute sensory neuropathy or cerebellar degeneration. When

sensorimotor neuropathy is paraneoplastic, the most frequently associated tumor is lung cancer. Neurologic symptoms include symmetric distal paresthesias, numbness, and weakness. Deep tendon reflexes are abolished. Symptoms of neuropathy usually develop after the diagnosis of cancer, but sometimes precede the tumor by years. The course is usually slow and progressive; a subacute onset of symptoms raises the possibility of a paraneoplastic origin. Symptoms may have a remitting and relapsing course suggesting chronic inflammatory demyelinating polyneuropathy.

CSF studies are usually normal. Nerve conduction studies are consistent with axonal neuropathy, but a few patients may have decreased conduction velocities consistent with demyelination. Nerve biopsy commonly shows axonal degeneration and, less frequently, segmental demyelination or both. In some patients, particularly those with remitting relapsing symptoms, the symptoms may improve with steroids.

Patients with breast cancer can develop a slowly progressive sensorimotor neuropathy with predominant sensory symptoms. Initial symptoms include itching and muscle cramps, and may precede the tumor diagnosis. Proximal weakness and symptoms suggesting central nervous system involvement, such as hyperreflexia and extensor plantar responses, may be present. Patients usually remain functional. There is no known treatment.

Sensorimotor Neuropathies Associated With Plasma Cell Dyscrasias

Approximately 10 percent of patients with peripheral sensorimotor neuropathy of unknown origin have monoclonal gammopathy. Plasma cell dyscrasias associated with peripheral neuropathy include monoclonal gammopathy of uncertain significance (MGUS), multiple myeloma, Waldenström's macroglobulinemia, cryoglobulinemia, monoclonal gammopathy with solid tumors, monoclonal gammopathy with benign lymph node hyperplasia, γ heavy-chain disease, and POEMS syndrome (polyneuropathy, organomegaly, endocrinopathy, M-protein, skin changes).

Patients with myeloma can develop neuropathies in the three following clinical situations.

Osteolytic Multiple Myeloma Without Amyloidosis. In patients with osteolytic multiple myeloma without amyloidosis, the neuropathy resembles the sensorimotor type seen in patients with carcinoma. The incidence is probably less than 5 percent. Improvement of multiple myeloma with chemotherapy is not associated with improvement of neurologic symptoms.

Osteolytic Multiple Myeloma With Amyloidosis. The clinical picture for multiple myeloma with amyloidosis is similar to the neuropathy of amyloidosis, characterized by autonomic dysfunction and lancinating and burning dysesthesias. These sensory symptoms predominate over motor deficits. In addition, these patients can develop superimposed radicular pain and deficits secondary to involvement of the spine by multiple myeloma. Treatment of multiple myeloma does not modify the neurologic symptoms.

Osteosclerotic Myeloma. Approximately 50 percent of patients with osteosclerotic multiple myeloma have symmetric, distal sensorimotor neuropathy. Motor symptoms predominate, and become progressive and disabling unless the osteosclerotic lesion is treated. Electrophysiologic and pathologic studies are similar to those with chronic inflammatory demyelinating polyneuropathy. There are decreased motor nerve conduction velocities with evidence of conduction blocks. Increased proteins in the CSF may result in papilledema. Patients with osteosclerotic myeloma differ from those with osteolytic multiple myeloma in that they are younger, their bone marrow is rarely infiltrated with plasma cells, renal function is better preserved, and M components are low in serum and rarely present in urine. The disorder predominates among the Japanese. Seventy-five percent of these patients have detectable λ-light chain with IgG or IgA heavy chains. A radiologic survey always demonstrates a solitary or reduced number of osteosclerotic lesions, which tend to involve the axial skeleton (truncal and proximal long bones) and spare the skull. Radioisotope bone scans are usually less sensitive than radiographic skeletal studies.

Frequently, patients with osteosclerotic myeloma develop symptoms included in the POEMS syndrome: polyneuropathy, organomegaly (hepatosplenomegaly, lymphadenopathy), endocrinopathy (gynecomastia, impotence, testicular atrophy, low plasma testosterone, low serum thyroxine, high serum estrogen, hyperglycemia), M protein, and skin changes (hirsutism, thickening of the skin, hyperpigmentation, hyperhydrosis). Less frequently, some of these symptoms are also associated with plasma cell dyscrasias other than osteosclerotic myeloma.

Identification of this disorder is important because treatment of the osteosclerotic lesions with excision or radiotherapy can improve and reverse the neurologic and systemic symptoms.

Patients with Waldenström's macroglobulinemia may develop a demyelinating sensorimotor neuropathy with marked slowing of nerve conduction velocities. Sensory symptoms are prominent. The IgM paraprotein may react with myelin-associated glycoprotein (anti-MAG), but in some cases the IgM paraprotein may lack anti-MAG reactivity. A minority of patients have predominant axonal degeneration. Reduction of IgM levels can improve the neuropathy.

Autonomic Neuropathy

Paraneoplastic autonomic neuropathy may occur alone or associated with paraneoplastic encephalomyelitis/paraneoplastic sensory neuropathy; in this case, the autonomic dysfunction may be the first sign of paraneoplastic encephalomyelitis/paraneoplastic sensory neuropathy. Symptoms (see above) often precede the diagnosis of the tumor, which usually is small cell lung cancer. If small cell lung cancer is the underlying tumor, the anti-Hu serology is positive. In some patients, treatment of the tumor may stabilize or improve the autonomic symptoms.

Neuromyotonia

The most frequent causes of cramps in cancer patients include electrolyte imbalances, nerve compression and infiltration by the neoplasm, peripheral neuropathy, chemotherapy, and radiotherapy. Cramps may also occur in association with a much rarer disorder, namely paraneoplastic neuromyotonia. This disorder is characterized by progressive aching, stiffness, spasms, and rigidity, which prevent muscle relaxation. Myokymia, hyperhidrosis, and signs of sensorimotor neuropathy are common. The electromyogram is characterized by continuous high-frequency, bizarre, motor unit discharges that persists after stopping a voluntary effort. Small cell lung cancer and thymoma are the tumors more commonly involved. Treatment with phenytoin, carbamazepine, or diazepam, as well as plasmapheresis, can be effective.

Stiff-man syndrome, which is also associated with continuous muscle fiber activity but relatively normal motor unit potentials, may also have a paraneoplastic origin. The associated tumors are Hodgkin's lymphoma, lung cancer, thymoma, and breast cancer. Patients with stiff-man syndrome and breast cancer harbor in their serum and CSF an antibody against a 128-kd neuronal protein concentrated in synapses.

These disorders must be differentiated from myotonia, a manifestation that can be observed in polymyositis/dermatomyositis. Paraneoplastic mytonia is a rare disorder and may precede the diagnosis of the tumor (usually small cell lung cancer). It may improve spontaneously or after treatment of the tumor.

SYNDROMES OF THE NEUROMUSCULAR JUNCTION

Syndromes of the neuromuscular junction include myasthenia gravis associated with thymoma (discussed in Ch. 103) and the Lambert-Eaton myasthenic syndrome.

Lambert-Eaton Myasthenic Syndrome

Lambert-Eaton myasthenic syndrome is a disorder of neuromuscular transmission characterized by a defect in the presynaptic quantal relase of acetylcholine in response to a nerve stimulus. About 60 percent of patients with the syndrome have small cell lung cancer; neurologic symptoms usually develop before the tumor diagnosis. Patients complain of weakness and fatigability that appear to be greater than what the examiner finds. Symptoms improve at the beginning of muscle contraction, but prolonged exercise results in muscle discomfort, stiffness, and fatigability. Upper extremities are rarely affected at the onset of the disease; however, most patients eventually develop arm weakness. More than 50 percent of patients have cholinergic dysautonomia, including dry mouth, sexual impotence, and blurry vision. On examination, there is proximal muscle weakness, decreased or absent reflexes (particularly in the lower extremities), and mild and transitory—if any—cranial nerve involvement (diplopia, ptosis, difficulty swallowing). In addition to these clinical findings, the diagnosis of Lambert-Eaton myasthenic syndrome is based on electrophysiologic studies. Characteristically, nerve conduction studies show reduced amplitude of the compound muscle action potentials, which progressively increase in response to fast rates of repetitive stimulation (20 to 50 Hz) or after a short period of maximum voluntary contraction.

Lambert-Eaton myasthenic syndrome is the prototype antibody-mediated paraneoplastic disorder. Animals injected with serum or IgG from patients with the syndrome develop clinical and electrophysiologic signs of the disease. The antibodies of some patients immunoprecipitate a subtype of voltage-gated calcium channels of the presynaptic neuromuscular junction; this property is used as a serologic diagnostic test. The serum of some patients reacts with a cloned antigen (MysB) contained in the β-subunit of neuronal calcium channels.

Lambert-Eaton myasthenic syndrome usually responds to plasmapheresis and immunosuppressive therapy. The release of acetylcholine is facilitated by 3,4-diaminopyridine, resulting in symptomatic improvement. The concomitant treatment of the tumor may result in improvement or remission of the neurologic syndrome. Recurrence of the syndrome usually heralds recurrence of the tumor.

Lambert-Eaton myasthenic syndrome can develop in association with other paraneoplastic syndromes such as paraneoplastic cerebellar degeneration (usually with no detectable antibodies other than anti-voltage-gated calcium channel) and paraneoplastic encephalomyelitis (often with positive anti-Hu serology).

SYNDROMES OF THE MUSCLES

Polymyositis/Dermatomyositis

Polymyositis/dermatomyositis is an inflammatory disease of the muscle, probably autoimmune in nature. Its association with cancer is rare, and the existence of paraneoplastic polymyositis/dermatomyositis is controversial. However, most authors believe that in the older population, the incidence of dermatomyositis and cancer is much higher than in the noncancer population. Males and females are affected in equal numbers. Characteristic cutaneous changes and weakness usually precede the identification of cancer. Tumors commonly involved are lung, ovary, stomach, and breast. Patients typically present with proximal muscle weakness of subacute onset, elevated levels of serum creatine kinase, and electromyographic evidence of myopathy. Neck flexors, pharyngeal muscles, and respiratory muscles are commonly involved; their dysfunction may result in aspiration and hypoventilation and contribute to death. Reflexes and sensory examination are normal.

Clinical, eletromyographic, and pathologic findings are similar in patients with and without cancer. However, no laboratory test is specific. In some patients, the serum creatine kinase levels are normal. Characteristic skin changes may occur without muscle weakness; however, these patients may complain of fatigue and myalgias. Several autoantibodies have been identified in patients with polymyositis/dermatomyositis; the most specific, anti-Jo-1, is identified in a group of patients with associated interstitial lung disease. Low titer of antinuclear antibodies typical of other connective tissue diseases can also be detected. There are no specific markers indicative of the paraneoplastic origin of dermatomyositis.

Different immune mechanisms appear to be involved in polymyositis and dermatomyositis. Whereas polymyositis results from cell-mediated cytotoxic mechanisms, dermatomyositis appears to result from a humoral immunomediated vasculopathy.

The course of polymyositis/dermatomyositis is independent of the malignant disease. Treatment of the tumor may or may not improve the neurologic syndrome. Steroids and other immunosuppressants (azathioprine, cyclophosphamide, methotrexate) have been used successfully in paraneoplastic and nonparaneoplastic dermatomyositis. Intravenous immunoglobulin is proven to be effective in dermatomyositis refractory to other treatments. Patients with paraneoplastic disease usually die as a consequence of the tumor.

Myositis, similar to polymyositis, can be a symptom (rarely the only symptom) of graft-versus-host disease that some patients, usually with hematologic malignancies, develop after bone marrow transplant. Some of these patients also have skin abnormalities secondary to graft-versus-host disease that are easily differentiated from dermatomyositis. The myositis of these patients responds to prednisone, but treatment should be directed to the graft-versus-host disease.

In patients with solid tumors or hematologic malignancies, opportunistic infections such as toxoplasma can cause a focal or diffuse inflammatory myopathy that can mimic polymyositis.

Acute Necrotizing Myopathy

Acute necrotizing myopathy is a rare disorder that presents with painful proximal muscle weakness that rapidly progresses to involve respiratory, pharyngeal, and truncal muscles. Death usually occurs during the first 12 weeks. In most patients, the paraneoplastic disorder precedes the diagnosis of the tumor. Carcinoma of the lung, breast, colon, and bladder are most often associated. Serum creatine kinase is elevated and there is electromyographic evidence of myopathy. Pathologic studies demonstrate widespread muscle necrosis with mild or no inflammatory infiltrates. There is no effective treatment, but one patient improved after removal of the breast cancer.

Carcinoid Myopathy

Carcinoid myopathy typically develops years after the carcinoid syndrome. Symptoms include proximal muscle weakness, fatigability, and cramps. Pathologic studies demonstrate type 2 fiber atrophy with mild or no inflammatory infiltrates. Treatment with cyproheptadine is usually effective.

Cachectic Myopathy

Most patients with advanced cancer, as well as other debilitating diseases, develop general muscle wasting and weakness. Pathologic studies demonstrate a predominance of small fiber and grouped atrophy, with no inflammatory infiltrates. Treatment of the underlying disease may reverse the disorder.

Carcinomatous Neuromyopathy

Carcinomatous neuromyopathy is characterized by proximal muscle weakness, diminished reflexes, normal or mildly elevated serum creatine kinase, and mixed neuropathic-myopathic findings on electrophysiologic and pathologic studies. The cause of this paraneoplastic syndrome is unknown. The tumor most commonly associated is lung cancer. The observation of this disorder in well-nourished patients, along with the presence of clinical and laboratory findings of ''neuropathic'' involvement, indicates that the disorder is different from cachectic myopathy. Studies have demonstrated degeneration of intramuscular motor nerve fibers, which may explain the myopathic electromyographic findings.

SUGGESTED READINGS

Clouston PD, Saper CB, Arbizu T et al: Paraneoplastic cerebellar degeneration. III. Cerebellar degeneration, cancer, and the Lambert-Eaton myasthenic syndrome. Neurology 42:1944, 1992

Dalakas MC: Polymyositis, dermatomyositis and inclusion-body myositis. N Engl J Med 325:1487, 1991

Dalmau J, Graus F, Rosenblum MK, Posner JB: Anti-Hu-associated paraneoplastic encephalomyelitis/sensory neuronopathy: a clinical study of 71 patients. Medicine 71:59, 1992

Digre KB: Opsoclonus in adults. Report of three cases and review of the literature. Arch Neurol 43:1165, 1986

Hammack J, Kotanides H, Rosenblum MK, Posner JB: Paraneoplastic cerebellar degeneration. II. Clinical and immunologic findings in 21 patients with Hodgkin's disease. Neurology 42:1938, 1992

Jacobson DM, Thirkill CE, Tipping SJ: A clinical triad to diagnose paraneoplastic retinopathy. Ann Neurol 28:162, 1990

Kelly JJ: Peripheral neuropathies associated with monoclonal proteins. A clinical review. Muscle Nerve 8:138, 1985

Luque FA, Furneaux HM, Ferziger R et al: Anti-Ri: an antibody associated with paraneoplastic opsoclonus and breast cancer. Ann Neurol 29:241, 1991

Ojeda VJ: Necrotizing myelopathy associated with malignancy. A clinicopathologic study of two cases and literature review. Cancer 53:1115, 1984

O'Neill JH, Murray NM, Newsom-Davis J: The Lambert-Eaton myasthenic syndrome. A review of 50 cases. Brain 111:577, 1988

Peterson K, Rosenblum MK, Kotanides H, Posner JB: Paraneoplastic cerebellar degeneration. I. A clinical analysis of 55 anti-Yo antibody-positive patients. Neurology 42:1931, 1992

Posner JB: Paraneoplastic syndromes. In: Neurologic complications of cancer. FA Davis, Philadelphia, (in press)

Schold SC, Cho ES, Somosundaram M et al: Subacute motor neuronopathy: a remote effect of lymphoma. Ann Neurol 5:271, 1979

Younger DS, Rowland LP, Latov N et al: Lymphoma, motor neuron diseases, and amyotropic lateral sclerosis. Ann Neurol 29:78, 1991

172. NEUROLOGIC PAIN SYNDROMES IN CANCER PATIENTS

JULIE E. HAMMACK

Cancer pain is an enormous problem worldwide. It has been estimated that at least 70 percent of those patients with advanced cancer report moderate to severe pain during the course of their illness, necessitating the use of opioids. Applying these prevalence rates to U.S. cancer statistics from 1993, 368,000 of the 526,000 patients who died from cancer and 819,000 of those surviving cancer experienced moderate to severe cancer-related pain during that year. At least 25 percent of cancer patients experience neurologic complications related to their malignancies or antineoplastic therapy. Physicians involved in the care of these patients must be especially alert to pain, as it is the most common presenting symptom of malignant invasion of the nervous system. Indirect effects of malignancy including opportunistic infection, coagulopathy, and paraneoplatic disorders can be associated with pain. Moreover, these cancer-related pain syndromes must be differentiated from pain and neurologic disability resulting from antineoplastic therapies if appropriate treatment is to be administered. This chapter reviews some of the more common pain syndromes associated with malignancy and its treatment. Many of these syndromes involve the nervous system directly; others do so indirectly or not at all, but present with symptoms familiar to the consulting neurologist.

ESTABLISHING A "PAIN DIAGNOSIS"

There is limited clinical emphasis on cancer pain and its causes in most medical and neurology training programs. As a result, there is an unfortunate tendency to view cancer pain as a single diagnostic entity. In fact, the causes of cancer pain are myriad. Careful medical and neurologic evaluation of each pain complaint is essential to best treat the pain and to prevent the development of otherwise unsuspected complications. A comprehensive pain evaluation in one study revealed a previously undiagnosed etiology of pain in 64 percent of patients (Gonzales et al., 1991). New neurologic diagnoses were made in 36 percent, and an unsuspected infection was discovered in 4 percent of patients.

As with any medical history, the pain history emphasizes the onset, quality, severity, location, ameliorating and exacerbating

factors, and associated symptoms. The patient's response to previous analgesics and other treatments should be determined, as should the effect of pain on the patient's level of function and psychological state. The physical examination should include a complete neurologic examination in all patients. Diagnostic studies are directed by historical and physical findings.

CANCER PAIN MECHANISMS

Neurologic pain syndromes may be organized into three distinct mechanisms (Table 172-1). The most common is direct tumor

TABLE 172-1. Causes of "Neurologic" Cancer Pain Syndromes

Syndromes related to direct or indirect tumor involvement
  Bone metastases
    Vertebral syndromes
      C8–T1
      T12–L1
    Skull base syndromes
      Jugular foramen syndrome
      Clivus syndrome
      Orbital syndrome
      Parasellar and middle cranial fossa syndrome
      Occipital condyle syndrome
  Dural metastases
  Meningeal metastases
  Intraparenchymal metastases
  Retroperitoneal metastases
  Pseudotumor cerebri
    Dural sinus thrombosis
      Skull or dural metastases
      Coagulopathy
      Hyperviscosity syndromes
      Dehydration/sepsis
    Superior vena cava obstruction
  Cerebral hemorrhage
    Dural, meningeal, intraparenchymal metastases
    Coagulopathy
  Cervical, brachial, or lumbosacral plexopathy
  Peripheral neuropathy
    Tumor invasion
    Paraneoplastic
  Central pain syndromes from brain and spinal cord lesions
Syndromes related to antineoplastic therapy
  Postsurgery
    Postmastectomy pain syndrome
    Post-thoracotomy pain syndrome
    Postamputation pain syndrome
    Post–radical neck dissection pain syndrome
  Postradiotherapy
    Brachial and lumbosacral plexopathy
      Acute
      Chronic
    Radiation myelopathy
    Radiation-induced tumors
  Post-chemotherapy/other medications
    Peripheral neuropathy
      Vinca alkaloids
      Cisplatin
      VP-16
      Paclitaxel
      Suramin
      Misonidazole
      Hexamethylmelamine
    Corticosteroids
      Steroid pseudorheumatism
      Perineal burning
      Aseptic necrosis of the humeral and femoral heads
      Pseudotumor cerebri
    Phenobarbital pseudorheumatism
    Headache
      Retinoic acid
      Leuprolide
      Corticosteroids
  Other
    Infections
      Oral and lower gastrointestinal anaerobic bacteria
      Herpes varicella-zoster
      Acute and post-herpetic neuralgia
Pain syndromes unrelated to cancer or its treatment
  Diagnoses of exclusion after cancer or therapy-related causes have been excluded

invasion of nervous tissue (brain, spinal cord, or peripheral nerve) or adjacent structures, with resulting compression of nervous tissue (i.e., epidural spinal cord compression). Second, cancer treatments (surgery, radiation, chemotherapy) may injure the nervous system or adjacent structures and produce pain by activation of nociceptors or injury to nervous tissue with deafferentation. Finally, patients with cancer may have pain problems unrelated to cancer or its therapy (migraine headache, carpal tunnel syndrome). Patients in this third category are in a minority, and it is imperative that they be thoroughly evaluated to exclude a cancer-related pain syndrome.

Cancer pain may be further subdivided into nociceptive and neuropathic mechanisms. Nociceptive pain is produced by activation of peripheral nerve fibers sensitive to noxious stimuli. The nocioceptive stimuli travel through fibers innervating somatic structures (bone, muscle, dura, fascia, skin, blood vessels) or visceral structures (pleura, peritoneum, organ capsules, hollow visci) when these structures are stretched, obstructed, or otherwise injured. Nociceptive somatic pain is typically well localized, may be sharp or dull, and is made worse by maneuvers that stress the involved structure. Bone metastasis is the most common nocioceptive somatic pain syndrome. Visceral nocioceptive pain tends to be more diffuse and poorly localized. Depending on the viscera involved, it may be sharp, dull, or colicky. Visceral pain is typically accompanied by signs of visceral dysfunction (dyspnea, jaundice, nausea, abdominal distention, and so forth).

Neuropathic pain results from direct injury to the central or peripheral nervous system, with subsequent aberrant pain fiber transmission, deafferentation, and reorganization of central sensory processing. Neuropathic pain has unique features including lancination, anesthesia, paresthesiae, allodynia, itching, and hyperpathia. Depending on the site of involvement, neuropathic pain follows the referral pattern of a specific peripheral nerve, plexus, root, or sensory tract. Other signs of neurologic dysfunction, including weakness, reflex changes, and autonomic dysfunction, may be present. Many cancer pain syndromes involve more than one of the above mechanisms; for instance, epidural tumor produces nociceptive bone pain and neuropathic radicular pain.

PAIN SYNDROMES SECONDARY TO DIRECT TUMOR INVASION

It is estimated that direct tumor involvement of pain-sensitive structures is responsible for pain in at least two-thirds of cancer patients with pain. Invasion of somatic, visceral, and neural tissues produces pain characteristic to each structure. Visceral pain syndromes are not dealt with at length here, with the exception of pain from involvement of retroperitoneal structures (see below). The reader is directed to sources listed in the bibliography for a more complete discussion of visceral pain syndromes. The following sections describe some of the more common somatic-nociceptive and neuropathic pain syndromes.

Bone Metastases

Bony metastasis is the most common cause of cancer-related pain. Cortical bone is anesthetic, but the cancellous portion of bone and the investing periosteum are exquisitely pain-sensitive when injured or stretched. Bone pain is typically well localized, sharp, and constant. Bone metastases in some locations may produce pain radiating to distant sites (see Vertebral Syn-

dromes, below). Malignant bone pain is worse when the involved bone is stressed and is typically worse at night, often interfering with sleep. Local production of prostaglandins (e.g., PGE_2) may play a critical role in pain related to bony metastases. Although opioids are the mainstay of therapy for moderate to severe bone pain, corticosteroids and nonsteroidal anti-inflammatory medications (NSAIDs) may be useful secondary to their antiprostaglandin effects. Biphosphonates and calcitonin may also be useful adjuvants in the treatment of refractory pain related to bone metastases or primary bone tumors. Antineoplastic therapy, including radiotherapy, chemotherapy, and sometimes surgery, commonly reduces metastatic bone pain by cytoreduction and a resulting decrease in the pain stimulus.

There are a number of well-described pain syndromes secondary to bone metastases. The following are most common.

Vertebral Syndromes. The axial skeleton is especially vulnerable to metastatic involvement in patients with solid tumors. The proximity to the spinal cord and other important neural structures makes the early identification of vertebral metastases uniquely important to prevent the development of serious neurologic complications, such as epidural spinal cord compression. Malignant bone involvement typically produces pain located directly over the involved vertebra. This pain is worse with percussion or movements that stress the spine. Malignant spine pain is often worse at night secondary to the elongation of the spine (and stretching of injured periosteum) after several hours of maintaining a reclining posture. The vertebral body and pedicle are the most common sites of metastases. Plain x-ray of the spine may demonstrate sclerotic or lytic lesions, vertebral collapse, and loss of a pedicle (Fig. 172-1). Epidural extension of tumor may impinge upon adjacent nerve roots, producing neuropathic pain radiating into the arms (cervical spine), buttocks or legs (lumbosacral spine), or around the chest or abdomen "like a belt or band" (thoracic spine). Evidence of a myelopathy may or may not be present with epidural spinal cord compression. One should thus have a high index of suspicion for epidural cord compression in any cancer patient with

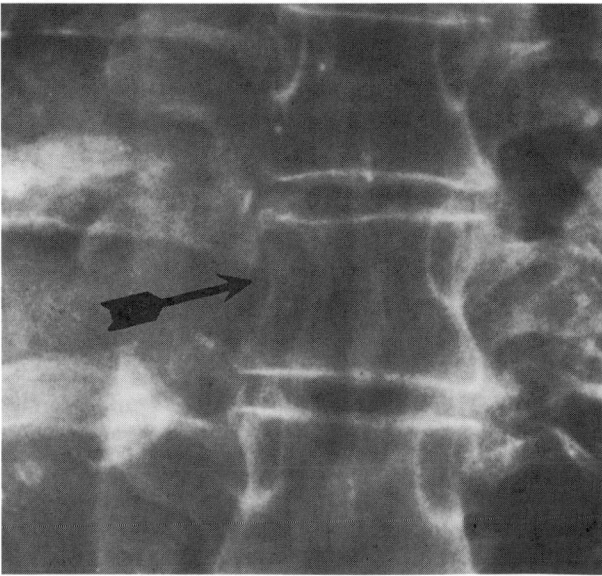

Fig. 172-1. Plain radiograph of the thoracic spine demonstrating loss of a pedicle secondary to a metastasis—the so-called winking owl sign *(arrow).*

persistent spine pain, especially if evidence of root or cord compromise is present; this constitutes a neurologic emergency requiring high-dose steroids, emergent imaging procedures, and emergent radiotherapy or neurosurgical intervention (see below, under Epidural Spinal Cord Compression).

Vertebral involvement at some levels produces pain that radiates to distant sites. Metastases to the T12 or L1 vertebrae may produce pain radiating to either iliac crest or to the ipsilateral sacroiliac joint. This may result in inappropriate imaging of the pelvis or sacrum and failure to diagnose the actual lesion, with resulting epidural progression. C8–T1 vertebral involvement may produce pain radiating into the interscapular region, which again may prompt imaging of the inappropriate spinal level.

Metastatic involvement of the C1–C2 vertebrae may simulate a skull base lesion and be associated with atlantoaxial subluxation or odontoid fracture. A severe occipital headache made worse by head movement is characteristic, often with associated torticollis. These patients are at high risk of developing a compressive cervical myelopathy with quadriparesis and sensory loss (usually beginning in the upper extremities), autonomic dysfunction, and respiratory arrest.

Expeditious diagnosis and treatment are essential. Magnetic resonance imaging (MRI) and/or myelography are the most sensitive diagnostic studies. C1–C2 spinal lesions are inherently unstable and neurosurgical and orthopaedic consultations are appropriate in addition to radiotherapy.

Skull Base Syndromes. Metastases to the base of the skull produce pain secondary to bony or soft tissue involvement and invasion or compression of neural structures. Cranial nerve dysfunction is frequently seen, depending on the site of involvement.

JUGULAR FORAMEN SYNDROME. The pain in jugular foramen syndrome is dull and constant and typically refers to the occiput or postauricular region. Occasionally, pain may refer to one or both shoulders. There may be associated sharp lancinating pain (glossopharyngeal neuralgia) in the throat or ear, and on rare occasions, syncope is present. The pain may be exacerbated by neck flexion or swallowing if glossopharyngeal neuralgia is present. Deficits of cranial nerves IX, X, and XI are common.

CLIVUS SYNDROME. Malignant invasion of the clivus produces a vertex headache that is worse with neck flexion. A number of cranial nerves (nerves VI through XII) pierce the dura in the vicinity of the clivus and thus may be compromised, depending on the location of the metastasis. Usually multiple cranial nerves are involved. Nasopharyngeal carcinoma, chordoma, meningioma, prostate cancer, and breast cancer are the most common malignancies associated with this syndrome.

ORBITAL SYNDROME. Orbital metastases produce pain that is localized behind the eye, supra- or periorbitally. It is dull and constant and may be worse on lying down or with eye movement. Visual loss; dysfunction of cranial nerves V1, V2, III, IV, and VI; and proptosis are common.

PARASELLAR AND MIDDLE CRANIAL FOSSA SYNDROME. Involvement of structures within the cavernous sinus produces symptoms that closely parallel those of the orbital syndrome. Proptosis and visual loss are less frequent, however. Ipsilateral neuropathic facial pain (usually periorbital or maxillary), diminished corneal reflex, and weakened muscles of mastication secondary to gasserian ganglion involvement is common.

OCCIPITAL CONDYLE SYNDROME. Occipital condyle syndrome is characterized by dull, constant occipital pain that is worsened by neck movements. Ipsilateral tongue weakness, fasiculations, and wasting are characteristic and secondary to involvement of the hypoglossal nerve within the hypoglossal canal. Tenderness to palpation of the occiput may be present, as may neck stiffness. On rare occasions, sternocleidomastoid weakness is present.

Appropriate imaging procedures for skull base lesions include plain x-ray and/or bone scan. Computed tomograpy (CT) with bone windows or MRI, including special skull base, orbital, or cavernous sinus views, is usually required to delineate the lesion.

Other Causes of Headache

Pain-sensitive structures in the head include periosteum, dura, soft tissues (skin, fascia, muscle, adipose tissue), extradural blood vessels, cornea, sclera, uvea, and cranial nerves (especially nerves V, VII, IX, and X). Malignant invasion or stretching of any of the above structures will produce head pain. Brain parenchyma itself is anesthetic.

Brain metastases (parenchmal, meningeal, and dural) are the most common neurologic complication of cancer, occuring in 15 to 20 percent of patients; headache is the most common presenting symptom. Parenchymal metastases produce head pain secondary to raised intracranial pressure and resulting dural traction. Supratentorial metastases typically produce frontal headache, whereas head pain from infratentorial metastases refers to the occiput, although variation in this referral pattern is common. The headache produced by brain metastases is worsened by maneuvers that increase intracranial pressure, such as cough, Valsalva maneuver, and lying flat. The pain is typically worse at night and may awaken the patient from sleep. Acute, severe headache may occur in the setting of hemorrhage into a cerebral metastasis. Vomiting and somnolence may occur in more advanced cases, indicating traction on brainstem structures secondary to a rostral-caudal herniation syndrome. Focal neurologic defects and seizures are variably present.

Meningeal tumor may produce headache by direct dural invasion, raised intracranial pressure (often from communicating hydrocephalus), or by invasion of pain-sensitive cranial nerves (nerves V, VII, IX, and X) or cervical roots. Neurologic signs and symptoms at multiple levels of the neuraxis is a cardinal feature of meningeal malignancy, and meningismus may be present. Gadolinium-enhanced MRI and myelography are helpful in diagnosis. Cerebrospinal fluid (CSF) examination is the definitive diagnostic test. Repeated lumbar punctures, however, may be required to isolate malignant cells.

Breast, prostate, lung, and hematologic malignancies may metastasize to the dura and can produce headache from direct stimulation of dural nociceptors or by mass effect and raised intracranial pressure. Dural metastases may hemorrhage, especially if a coagulopathy is present, producing acute or chronic subdural hematomas. Venous sinus occlusion may result from skull or dural metastases, producing pseudotumor cerebri and headache from raised intracranial pressure. Other causes of venous sinus occlusion include l-asparaginase administraion (which depletes plasma proteins involved in coagulation and fibrinolysis), polycythemias, paraproteinemias with hyperviscosity syndrome, and other hypercoagulable states. Contrast CT of the head demonstrates no enhancement within the clot-filled superior sagittal sinus, with enhancement of the walls of the sinus (delta sign). MRI of the head has supplanted digital sub-

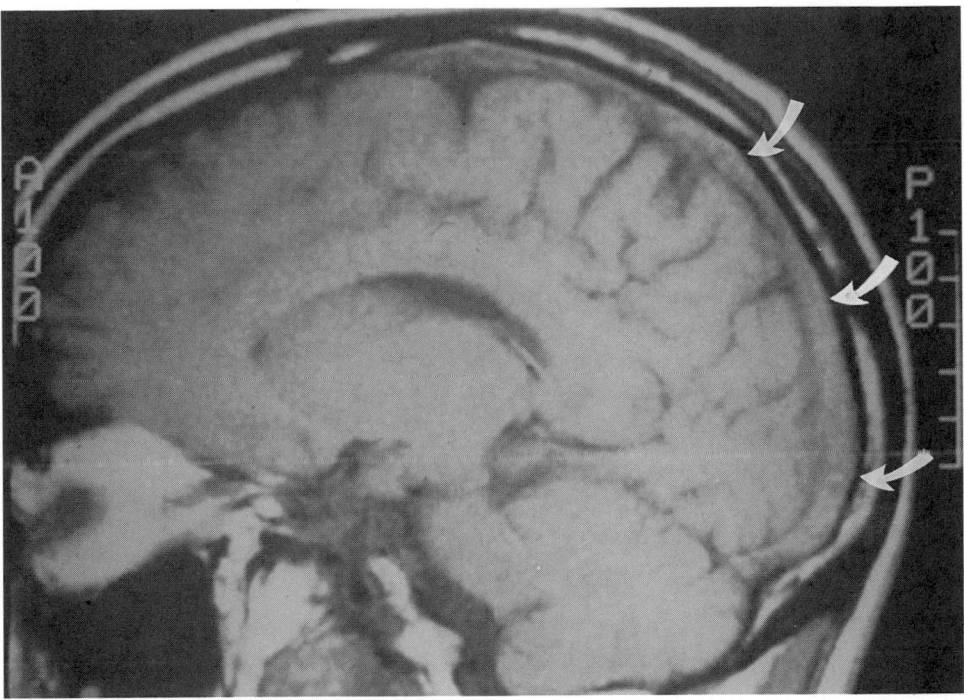

Fig. 172-2. Sagittal noncontrast MRI of the head demonstrating clot within the superior sagittal sinus *(arrows)*.

traction angiography as the standard diagnostic test for this disorder (Fig. 172-2).

Mediastinal tumors causing superior vena cava obstruction produce raised intracranial venous pressure and headache. Retinoic acid, used in the treatment of promyelocytic leukemia and other malignancies, may produce pseudotumor cerebri and headache without venous sinus occlusion. Leuprolide, a GnRH analogue used as an antiandrogen in the treatment of prostate cancer, on rare occasions produces migraine headaches.

Cranial neuropathies from extracranial malignant involvement are often painful. Squamous cell carcinoma of skin or oropharynx is notorious for perineural invasion with resulting pain and cranial nerve defects. Any primary or metastatic tumor, however, may injure somatic or neural structures of the head and neck. Pain syndromes from skull base malignant invasion are described above, under Bone Metastases. Trigeminal nerve invasion anywhere along its course produces pain referred to the face or ear. Injury to cranial nerves VII, IX, and X commonly produces pain felt in or around the external auditory meatus or helix. Otherwise asymptomatic head and neck tumors may present with lancinating pain referred to the ipsilateral ear, tongue, or throat from invasion of branches of cranial nerves IX and X. Hypotension and syncope may be associated with glossopharyngeal nerve involvement from stimulation of chemoreceptive and baroreceptive afferents originating in the carotid sinus and carotid body. *Evaluation of any patient with otherwise unexplained ear pain should include a careful examination of the oropharynx and larynx.*

Herpes zoster virus may remain latent in the trigeminal (cranial nerve V) and geniculate ganglia (cranial nerve VII) and reactivate in immunocompromised patients. Patients with hematopoietic malignancies, especially lymphoma, and those receiving potent immunosuppressant chemotherapy are especially vulnerable. Typically, the infection is heralded by an itching, burning discomfort in the cornea and forehead (V1) or ear and tongue (cranial nerve VII). Erythema of the conjuctiva,

forehead, or helix may precede the development of herpetic blisters. Ipsilateral facial nerve weakness may be present with geniculatate ganglion herpes zoster infection (Ramsay Hunt syndrome). Herpetic keratitis is a serious complication of trigeminal herpes zoster infection. These patients should be followed closely by an ophthalmologist during the acute phase of infection. A further discussion of acute herpes zoster infection and post-herpetic neuralgia may be found below under Pain Syndromes Related to Antineoplastic Therapy.

Visceral Pain Syndromes

Injury to organ capsules, pleura, peritoneum, or obstruction of hollow visci by malignancy typically produces pain and evidence of visceral dysfunction. There are myriad visceral pain syndromes that are not discussed here. The retroperitoneal pain syndrome, however, is occasionally encountered in cancer patients with back pain. The retroperitoneal space is richly innervated by the celiac plexus and spinal nerves, which may be encased by pancreatic, hepatobiliary, renal, and gastrointestinal tumors and lymphomas. The pain is usually localized to the epigastrium and radiates into the back in 25 to 30 percent of patients. Alternately, pain from retroperitoneal metastases may be felt exclusively in the upper lumbar spine and flank. Paraspinal retroperitoneal tumors may invade the epidural space via the intervertebral foramina or vertebrae. Neurologic defects may result from epidural extension or by invasion of the lumbosacral plexus, which is also located within the retroperitoneum. Evidence of visceral dysfunction is variably present depending on the location of tumor within the retroperitoneal space and abdominal cavity.

Pain from retroperitoneal tumors is worse with extension of the spine (as when lying supine) and is ameliorated by forward flexion. Consequently, many patients report that sleep is possible only while seated, flexed forward over a table or desk. This pain syndrome is most commonly seen in the setting of pancreatic cancer; jaundice and weight loss are thus usual accompaniments. Useful imaging procedures include CT and MRI of the abdomen and pelvis. Selected patients should also have imaging of the spine with MRI or myelography if tumor is noted to invade the vertebra or intervertebral foramen or if symptoms and signs suggest neurologic involvement of the cauda equina.

Neuropathic Pain Syndromes Secondary to Tumor Invasion

Tumor may infiltrate structures at all levels of the nervous system. Neuropathic pain is variably described as sharp, lancinating, and paroxysmal or dull, gnawing, and constant. *Burning, tingling, "pins and needles," "numbness," squeezing,* or *stretching* are frequent qualifiers used by patients. Allodynia (the perception of pain when a non-noxious stimulus is applied) is characteristic and causes the touch of garments or bedclothes to be excruciatingly uncomfortable. Itching is an underrecognized feature of neuropathic pain. Weakness, sensory loss, and autonomic dysfunction in the appropriate neural distribution may be present.

Brain and spinal cord parenchyma are anesthetic, although stretching (as with raised intracranial pressure secondary to cerebral metastases) or irritation of dural coverings (e.g., leptomeningeal metastases) may produce somatic nocioceptive pain (see Other Causes of Headache, above). Chronic pain from otherwise "anesthetic" central nervous system structures may result from disruption and presumed reorganization of central pain pathways. This type of deafferentation pain is rare in patients with brain or spinal cord tumors, as they often do not survive long enough for neural reorganization to occur. On rare occasions, a metastasis to the ventral posterior nucleus of the thalamus may produce a neuropathic pain syndrome (Dejerine-Roussy) affecting the contralateral hemibody.

Epidural Spinal Cord Compression. Epidural spinal cord compression is a neurologic emergency that presents initially with spine pain in over 90 percent of patients. Pain originating from vertebral body involvement may be referred to a site distant from its origin (see Vertebral Syndromes, above). Thoracic spine metastases are most common and often are associated with bilateral thoracic radicular pain described as a "tight band" around the chest or abdomen. This may prompt an inappropriate evaluation of the cardiac or gastrointestinal system. Cervical and lumbosacral epidural metastases usually manifest with unilateral radicular pain. Although pain is commonly the first symptom, most patients have some degree of motor, sensory, or autonomic dysfunction at the time of diagnosis. This is regrettable, as the neurologic outcome is inversely related to the degree of neurologic deficit at the time of diagnosis. Prompt diagnosis is imperative. Any patient in whom the diagnosis is suspected should receive 100 mg dexamethasone intravenously, and undergo plain films of the entire spine (Fig. 172-1) and an MRI or myelogram (Fig. 172-3) with postmyelography CT. Treatment consists of radiotherapy to the area of epidural involvement, with margins that usually encompass the two vertebrae above and below the level of epidural tumor. Surgery is reserved for those without a tumor diagnosis, for those with radiation-insensitive tumors, and for those with recurrent tumor within a previously irradiated field. A simple laminectomy is usually ineffectual, as most epidural tumors are located anterior to the spinal cord, which would not be decompressed by such

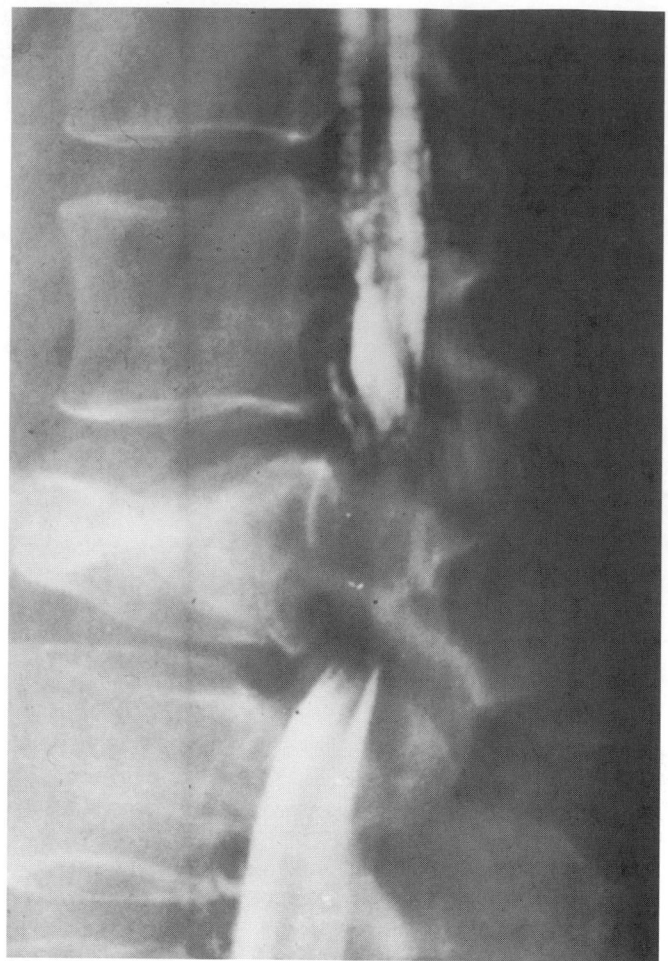

Fig. 172-3. Pantopaque myelogram demonstrating a block to flow of contrast within the lumbar spine secondary to epidural cord compression by tumor. Note the collapsed, sclerotic vertebral body.

an approach. The favored procedure is a combined anterolateral or posterior approach with vertebrectomy, bone graft, and rod stabilization.

Leptomeningeal Metastases. Solid tumors (especially breast, lung, and melanoma) and hematologic malignancies may metastasize to the meninges. Head and spine pain are the most common presenting symptoms. Pain may result from invasion of cranial or spinal nerves, raised intracranial pressure, or from direct invasion and irritation of the meninges. Neurologic findings are typically multifocal and localized to more than one level of the central nervous system. Multiple cranial neuropathies and a cauda equina syndrome are the most common clinical findings, presumably owing to the tendency of tumor cells to settle in the basal meninges of the posterior fossa and in the dural sac. Contrast CT and MRI of the head may demonstrate meningeal enhancement and communicating hydrocephalus. Gadolinium-enhanced MRI of the spine will usually demonstrate linear enhancement of the cord and roots. Myelography may be normal or show nodular filling defects along the course of the spinal roots. On rare occasions, a complete block to flow of contrast is present. Spinal fluid analysis provides the definitive diagnosis, although cytology may be negative despite repeated examinations. Usually, the CSF protein is elevated and a reactive pleocytosis is present. CSF glucose may be reduced.

CSF tumor markers, including carcinoembryonic antigen, β-glucuronidase, β_2-microglobulin, and lactate dehydrogenase may facilitate the diagnosis if cytology is negative.

Brachial Plexopathy. Brachial plexopathy from direct invasion by apical lung cancer (Pancoast syndrome) or by adjacent cervical lymph nodes involved by metastatic tumor (breast, lung, lymphoma, head and neck cancer) presents most commonly with aching ipsilateral scapular or shoulder pain followed by C8–T1 root distribution neuropathic pain. Lower trunk or medial cord distribution weakness and sensory loss (axilla, medial arm, and ulnar two fingers) is typical. Pain is present at diagnosis in over 95 percent of patients. Invasion of the upper plexus is less common and presents with aching pain in the shoulder radiating into the thumb and forefinger; weakness is in a C5–C6 root distribution. Symptoms may progress to a panplexopathy from either a lower or upper plexopathy. A supraclavicular mass may be palpable and a Tinel sign (paresthesiae felt in the arm and hand) thus elicited. An ipsilateral Horner syndrome or the presence of panplexus involvement indicates a high likelihood of extension of tumor into the cervical or upper thoracic epidural compartment with impending epidural cord compression.

CT or MRI both adequately visualize the brachial plexus (Fig. 172-4). MRI has the added advantage of visualizing the epidural compartment. Electromyography may be helpful, in selected cases, to delineate the extent of disease. In previously irradiated patients, this syndrome must be distinguished from radiation-induced injury (see Radiation Plexopathy, below).

Lumbosacral Plexopathy. Pain is present in 98 percent of patients at the time of diagnosis and is the most common presenting symptom of lumbosacral plexopathy. Tumor involves the plexus by direct extension in 75 percent, with remote metastases accounting for the remainder. Sarcomas, lymphomas, and tumors of the colon and genitourinary tract are most commonly implicated. Unilateral severe constant or lancinating pain in the buttock or leg is characteristic. There may be associated weakness, sensory loss, and reflex changes depending on the segments of the plexus involved. Lower plexus involvement (L4–S1) is most common. Differentiation from a lumbosacral radiculopathy may be impossible on clinical grounds. Bowel, bladder, and sexual dysfunction indicate either bilateral plexus involvement or extension of tumor into the spinal canal with an associated cauda equina syndrome. CT or MRI are adequate imaging modalities, neither one having a clear advantage over the other. Myelography or MRI of the spine should be considered in those patients with a paraspinal mass, electromyographic (EMG) evidence of radicular involvement, and in those with bowel, bladder, or sexual dysfunction.

Peripheral Neuropathy. Peripheral nerve involvement by tumor is less common than plexus involvement; intercostal neuropathies, however, are frequent with chest wall invasion by lung cancer. Similarly, retroperitoneal tumors may invade spinal nerves, producing radicular-like abdominal pain. Tumors of the limb (e.g., osteogenic sarcoma) may produce solitary or multiple mononeuropathies as a result of local extension.

Paraneoplastic neuropathies may be associated with both solid tumors and hematologic malignancies. A subacute sensory neuronopathy (anti-Hu syndrome) is seen in association with small cell lung carcinoma. The clinical presentation is dominated by profound sensory defects, although burning or lancinating neuropathic pain is a common associated feature. Dysautonomia—as manifested by bowel, bladder, and sexual dysfunction—xerostomia, and sweating abnormalities may be prominent. Nerve conduction studies reveal absent sensory nerve action potentials but no motor abnormalities. A characteristic serum antibody, anti-Hu, is diagnostic. Multiple myeloma, plasmacytoma, and Waldenström's macroglobulinemia may also be associated with an axonal or demyelinating painful sensorimotor polyneuropathy.

PAIN SYNDROMES RELATED TO ANTINEOPLASTIC THERAPY

Acute or chronic pain may result from surgery, radiotherapy, or chemotherapeutic agents used in the treatment of cancer. Although pain resulting from malignant invasion is more common, it is important that therapy-related pain be considered in the differential diagnosis of any cancer patient with pain. Pain resulting from cancer treatment will likely require different therapy than that required for malignant pain and may carry vastly different prognostic implications. Accurate diagnosis of treatment-related pain will prevent inappropriate antineoplastic therapy when metastases or tumor recurrence have been presumed responsible for the pain.

Postsurgical Pain Syndromes

Acute postsurgical pain results from injury to somatic, visceral, or neural structures. The features and treatment of this pain are no different in cancer patients than in the general population undergoing surgery. The following discussion, thus, is limited to chronic pain syndromes relating to surgery. There are four well-characterized postsurgical pain syndromes that result primarily from injury to a peripheral nerve or plexus.

Postmastectomy Pain Postmastectomy pain is a neuropathic pain syndrome occurring in 4 to 10 percent of women undergoing mastectomy, although it may occur following a simple lumpectomy or thoracotomy. In most cases, the pain results from post-traumatic neuroma formation on the intercostobrachial nerve, a cutaneous sensory branch of T1–T2. The discomfort is described variously as a burning, tingling, constricting, constant pain, sometimes with a paroxysmal component in the anterior chest wall, posterior arm, and axilla. The "phantom breast" phenomenon may be present. Sensory loss in the axilla and anterior chest is usual and there may be marked allodynia. A trigger point may be found along the mastectomy incision. Arm movement typically exacerbates the pain, predisposing to shoulder immobility and adhesive capsulitis (frozen shoulder). Postmastectomy pain usually develops within a few weeks of surgery, although on occasion may be delayed by as long as 6 months. As a rule, this pain syndrome is not associated with tumor recurrence.

Post-thoracotomy Pain. Post-thoracotomy pain is neuropathic pain, beginning soon after surgery, resulting from traction or section of one or more intercostal nerves with or without neuroma formation. Rib resection or traction on the rib and its neurovascular bundle are the usual mechanisms of injury. Pain is located along the incision, which may display exquisite point tenderness, and is often burning and constricting with or without a lancinating component. Allodynia may be present, making even the light touch of garments unbearably painful. Three

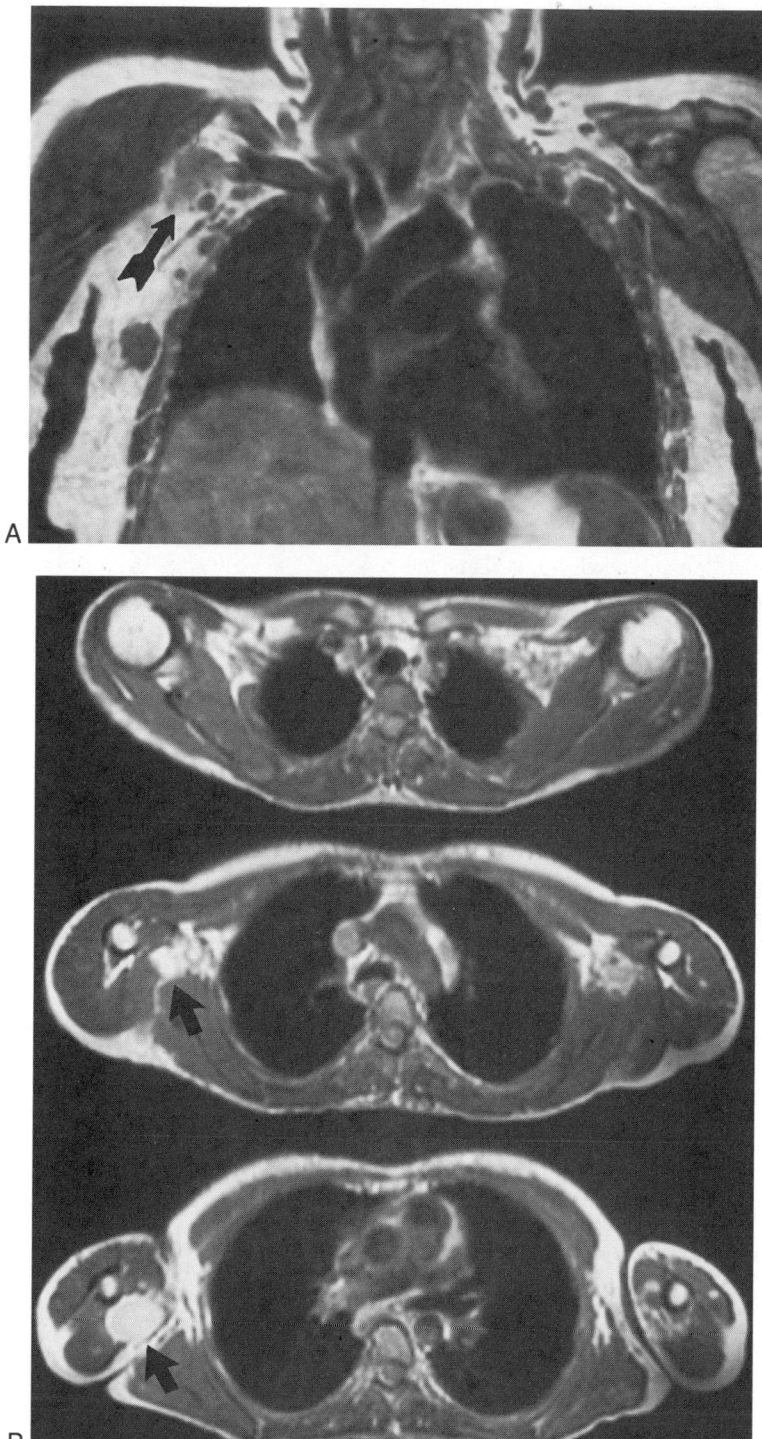

Fig. 172-4. **(A)** Coronal and **(B)** axial MRIs through the brachial plexus of two different patients with supraclavicular and axillary adenopathy from lymphoma. Both patients were symptomatic with medial cord plexopathies.

groups of patients with post-thoracotomy pain have been identified. The first and largest group were those patients in whom postsurgical thoracotomy pain resolved by 2 months after surgery. In those patients in whom incision pain recurred, all were found to have recurrent tumor. The second group contained patients whose post-thoracotomy pain steadily increased in intensity following surgery. In these patients as well, recurrent tumor or infection were the most likely causes. The third group consisted of patients whose pain was stable or decreasing over a protracted time period (8 months). Unless pain later increased in intensity, this pattern was not associated with recurrent malignancy in most patients. Clearly, a high index of suspicion must be maintained in patients undergoing thoractomy for malignancy whose incision pain increases in intensity or recurs after the initial postoperative period. A thorough search for infection or recurrent tumor should be made.

Postamputation Pain. The amputation of a limb, usually performed to treat sarcoma, may produce two distinct neuropathic pain syndromes. Stump pain is experienced in the distal stump along the incision and is usually secondary to traumatic neuroma formation. Trigger points are common along the incision. Pain is often burning, lancinating, or itching and may make the wearing of a prosthesis impossible. Treatments include administration of those medications commonly used in the treatment of neuropathic pain (tricylic antidepressants, anticonvulsants), trigger-point injection, and sometimes reoperation to resect or transpose the neuroma into muscle or soft tissues. Refitting of the prosthesis is often helpful. Phantom pain is a painful sensory experience in which pain localizes to the amputated limb. The ''limb'' may be felt to assume unusual positions and may feel swollen or misshapen. Pain is often severe, burning, tingling, or lancinating. Phantom pain is present in most patients in the immediate postoperative period and usually decreases with time. As the pain resolves, the phantom sensation typically shrinks or telescopes into the stump. The recurrence of phantom pain, in the absence of medication changes, should alert the clinician to the possibility of cancer recurrence or stump infection. The frequency of prolonged phantom pain varies considerably in the literature. Interestingly, severe phantom pain is more likely to occur if that limb is painful prior to the amputation. Preoperative epidural lumbar local anesthetic infusion significantly reduces the incidence of phantom pain. Once established, phantom pain may be refractory to even the most aggressive therapies; thus, every effort should be made to reduce the incidence by providing optimal preoperative analgesia to patients undergoing amputation.

Post–Radical Neck Dissection Pain. Post–radical neck dissection pain follows procedures for the removal of head and neck tumors and results from sectioning or traction of the cervical plexus and cervical nerves. The cervical plexus is formed by the anterior primary rami of C1–C4 and is located behind the sternocleidomastoid muscle. Branches of the cervical plexus supply sensation to the skin of the posterior and lateral head and the entire neck to the shoulders. Part of the external ear is also supplied by this plexus. Motor fibers supply the ansa hypoglossi, the spinal accessory nerve, and the nerve innervating the levator scapulae muscle. Pain resulting from cervical plexus injury is described as burning or constricting, with or without a lancinating component, and is generally localized to the sensory distribution outlined above. Pain may radiate to the helix of the ear or the external auditory canal. Myofascial

discomfort may result from removal of the sternocleidomastoid and strap muscles with an overuse syndrome of the contralateral neck musculature. Drooping of the shoulder following surgery may produce a traction injury of the suprascapular nerve with aching discomfort over the scapula and weakness of external rotation at the shoulder. Recurrent or escalating pain in a patient after radical neck dissection with or without episodes of syncope (secondary to carotid sinus involvement or glossopharyngeal neuropathy) suggests recurrent tumor or soft tissue infection. The latter may be surprisingly indolent, unassociated with fever, and respond dramatically to empiric antibiotic therapy directed against oral anaerobes. The diagnosis of soft tissue infection may be difficult in tissues already erythematous and indurated by radiation and surgery. Imaging studies (CT or MRI) assist in making the diagnosis, although they may not differentiate recurrent tumor from infection. Surgical exploration may be appropriate in some instances.

Postradiation Pain Syndromes

Acutely, radiotherapy may cause a self-limited pain syndrome related to cutaneous or mucosal injury. Oropharynx and esophageal mucositis is seen after radiation of head and neck tumors or cervical spine radiation. Radiation proctitis is a usual cause of rectal pain during or immediately after radiation for pelvic tumors. Viscous lidocaine oral swishes for oral mucositis and a low-fiber diet with use of rectal steroid for proctitis may be all that is required for relief, although opioids may be required if pain is more severe. An acute skin reaction during the course of radiation is common and is usually managed with moisturizing lotions and mild analgesics. Avoidance of ultraviolet exposure and use of sun block is said to lessen the risk of skin injury in the irradiated area. Necrosis of bone within the radiation field may occur as a delayed phenomenon and be an ongoing source of pain. Rarely, radiation-induced tumors may present many years later and manifest as a painful mass within the previous radiation port. Malignant sarcomas of the nerve sheath may be seen years after radiation to a plexus or peripheral nerve and present with neuropathic pain radiating along the course of the involved nerve or plexus. Radiation-induced meningiomas, sarcomas, and gliomas may be seen if the brain was included within the field of radiation.

Radiation may damage neural structures, including the brain, spinal cord, root, plexus, and peripheral nerve. With few exceptions, radiation injury to the central nervous system is painless, or pain is mild and overshadowed by the neurologic deficits. Radiation injury to the peripheral nervous system is often painful, however. The brachial and lumbosacral plexi are especially prone to radiation injury, presumably because of their proximity to common sites of malignant involvement (e.g., lung, lymph nodes, pelvic organs) and their consequent inclusion in irradiated fields. The brunt of radiation-induced injury falls on the cells with the highest rate of turnover—Schwann cells and vascular endothelial cells. The pathologic findings are characterized by demyelinization, hyalinized microvasculature, fibrosis, and sometimes frank necrosis of neural tissue.

Radiation Plexopathy. Radiation plexopathy presents from 6 months to 20 years after radiation. Unlike malignant invasion of the plexus, from which it must be differentiated, radiation plexus injury is painful in only 18 percent of patients. A mild aching discomfort in the shoulder or buttock is common (depending on the plexus involved). Radiation fibrosis of the

TABLE 172-2. Differences between Radiation and Malignant Brachial Plexopathy

	Malignant	Radiation-Induced
Pain	> 90%	18%
Location of pain	Shoulder, axilla, medial arm, ulnar two fingers	Shoulder, lateral arm, thumb and forefinger
Area of involvement	Lower trunk/medial cord	Upper trunk/lateral cord
Horner syndrome	Often present	Absent
Lymphedema	Usually absent	Often present
Electromyography	Decreased sensory and motor action potentials	Decreased sensory and motor action potentials
	Denervation on needle examination	Denervation on needle examination
	No myokymia	Myokymia present
Computed tomography/magnetic resonance imaging	Circumscibed mass	Normal or indistinct tissue planes
Clinical course	Progressive pain and weakness	Weakness may progress; pain may improve

plexus may, however, produce dysesthesias, sensory loss, and profound weakness, as in malignant plexopathy. The distribution of neurologic defects may be helpful in clinically differentiating radiation from malignant plexopathy (Table 172-2). Radiation-induced brachial plexopathy most commonly involves the upper trunk or lateral cord (C5–C6 segmental distribution), whereas malignant plexopathy usually involves the medial cord or lower trunk (C8–T1 distribution). The lower trunk and medial cord are relatively protected from the effects of radiation by the overlying clavicle but are more likely to be involved by tumors of the lung apex and malignant involvement of supraclavicular lymph nodes. Lymphedema of the upper extremity is more common in radiation plexopathy secondary to radiation fibrosis and obstruction of lymphatic channels. EMG will show myokymic discharges in C5–C6 innervated muscles in radiation plexopathy, although their presence does not exclude recurrent malignancy if the plexus has been previously radiated. A Horner syndrome is common in malignant plexopathy but rare in radiation-induced injury. CT or MRI is helpful in identifying recurrent tumor, which usually manifests as a circumscribed mass (Fig. 172-4). Imaging in radiation plexopathy is either normal or demonstrates nonspecific thickening of tissues with loss of distinct tissue planes. In selected cases, surgical exploration may be required to differentiate the two syndromes. Both radiation-induced and malignant plexopathy may coexist in the same patient making accurate diagnosis and appropriate management difficult. Table 172-2 summarizes the differences between radiation and malignant brachial plexopathy.

An acute reversible plexopathy may seen during or immediately after a course of radiotherapy encompassing the brachial plexus. This is characterized by aching shoulder pain and paresthesiae in the hand and forearm. Transient weakness may be present in C6–C7 innervated muscles. CT or MRI results are normal. Nerve conduction studies may show slowed conduction across the plexus. Needle examination may show reduced recruitment in C6–C7 innervated muscles but usually no motor unit changes. Presumably, this lesion results from acute radiation-induced demyelination. Symptoms typically resolve over weeks to months. This syndrome does not appear to predict the development of delayed radiation injury to the plexus.

Severe pain is similarly uncommon in radiation lumbosacral plexopathy, which usually presents with paresthesiae, sensory loss, and leg weakness with diminished deep tendon reflexes occuring 1 to 30 years following radiation treatment. Symptoms usually begin in L5–S1 segments and may be bilateral. Patients receiving intrapelvic (intracavitary) radiation—for cervical, uterine, or prostatic malignancies—in addition to external beam therapy may be especially at risk, secondary to the higher dose

of radiation administered and closer proximity to the plexus. Radionecrosis of the pelvic bone may accompany this syndrome. Imaging procedures and EMG show findings similar to those described in radiation brachial plexopathy.

Radiation Myelopathy. Radiation myelopathy typically presents as a Brown-Sequard syndrome with ipsilateral limb weakness and loss to vibration and joint position sense with crossed anesthesia to pinprick and temperature. Pain occurs in less than 30 percent of patients but may include focal spine pain, burning dysesthesiae, lancinating pain, and allodynia below the level of the lesion. Pain in a radicular pattern may also be noted. This entity must be differentiated from epidural, meningeal, or intramedullary spinal cord tumors with MRI of the spine or myelography.

Postchemotherapy Pain Syndromes

A variety of chemotherapy agents produce a painful peripheral neuropathy, often associated with distal sensory loss and weakness and/or autonomic dysfunction. Vincristine and other vinca alkaloids commonly produce a sensorimotor peripheral neuropathy that is usually asymptomatic but that may produce burning or tingling dysesthesiae of the distal extremities associated with allodynia. On occasion, vincristine may produce an acute painful mononeuropathy; acute severe jaw pain is a common example. Other isolated cranial nerve palsies have been reported. Vinca alkaloids may also cause an acute ileus secondary to autonomic neuropathy. Cisplatin, VP-16, procarbazine, misonidazole (a radiosensitizer), Suramin, and paclitaxil (Taxol) are other agents that may produce painful neuropathies. The symptoms resolve partially or completely with discontinuance of the responsible agent. Occasionally, neuropathic pain may persist and on rare occasions, the symptoms of peripheral neuropathy begin or progress after the chemotherapeutic agent has been stopped. Symptomatic relief of neuropathic pain from these toxic neuropathies may be obtained with adjuvant analgesics (including tricyclic antidepressants and anticonvulsants), opioids, or the use of transcutaneous electrical nerve stimulation (TENS).

Corticosteroids are commonly prescribed to cancer patients as components of chemotherapy regimens, as adjuvant analgesics, as antiemetics, and in the treatment of cerebral or spinal cord edema. Corticosteroids may have a number of psychological and neurologic effects, including psychosis, mania, depression, and hiccoughs. Several pain syndromes have been attributed to these medications as well. A burning sensation in the perineum is described by over 50 percent of patients given large intravenous bolus doses (100 mg) of dexamethasone administered in the treatment of epidural spinal cord compression. The etiology is unknown. The burning sensation lasts only minutes and treatment is neither available nor required. It is helpful to warn patients of this possible effect prior to administration of high-dose intravenous dexamethasone.

Steroid pseudorheumatism is characterized by diffuse myalgias and arthralgias during withdrawl of steroids. There are no abnormalities on EMG and no associated elevation of serum muscle enzymes. This adverse effect does not appear to be dependent on the dosage, length of therapy, or speed of withdrawl. Steroid pseudorheumatism is especially common in young muscular individuals. Although the exact pathogenesis is unknown, it has been postulated to be secondary to sensitization of joint and muscle nociceptors. Treatment consists of reinstituting steroids at a higher dose with slower withdrawl.

Aseptic necrosis of the femoral or humeral head may follow the intermittent or chronic daily use of glucocorticoids. Pain is localized to the joint or its referral zone (i.e., hip refers to the knee; shoulder refers to the elbow) and is exacerbated by weightbearing and movement of the involved joint. Symptoms usually precede radiographic changes by several weeks. A bone scan is useful in early diagnosis, as is MRI of the involved joint. If diagnosed early, treatment is conservative with appropriate opioid and nonopioid analgesics and discontinuation of the corticosteroids. Surgical intervention may be required in those patients with joint destruction or poorly controlled pain.

Phenobarbital, often used as an anticonvulsant in patients with primary or metastatic tumors to the central nervous system, may cause a pain syndrome characterized by shoulder discomfort and immobility. If diagnosed early, "phenobarbital pseudorheumatism" resolves with discontinuance of the drug. The pathogenesis is unknown but signs and symptoms are typical of an adhesive capsulitis. If severe, a superimposed sympathetically maintained pain syndrome (reflex sympathetic dystrophy) may develop, leading to a painful, useless limb. Many oncology patients seen by the neurologist are chronically maintained on both steroids and phenobarbital. The differential diagnosis of shoulder and arm pain in these patients should include bone metastases, cervical epidural tumor, brachial plexopathy, aseptic necrosis of the humeral head, and phenobarbital pseudorheumatism.

Herpes Zoster Virus Infection

Reactivation of latent herpes zoster virus is common in immunocompromised patients, including those receiving intensive chemotherapy with resulting impairment of humoral and cell-mediated immunity. Herpes zoster virus reactivation in cranial nerves is discussed above. Reactivation in cervical, thoracic, and lumbosacral dermatomes is more frequent than cranial involvement. Over 50 percent of reactivations occur in thoracic dermatomes. The blistering rash is usually preceded by itching, burning, and erythema in the affected dermatomes. Usually only a few contiguous roots are involved. Their selection is apparently random, although nerve root irritation, as by epidural tumor, may make herpes zoster virus reactivation more likely at that site. Occasionally, weakness in muscles supplied by the same nerve root may occur. Viral dissemination to lung, liver, and brain is a life-threatening complication more likely to occur in the immunocompromised patient. Pain related to herpes zoster virus infection is divided into acute (within 2 months of the skin eruption) and chronic (greater than 2 months). The acute

pain results from inflammation in neural and somatic structures. Chronic pain (post-herpetic neuralgia) occurs after the acute inflammation has resolved and is due to deafferentation resulting from destruction of fibers within the root and dorsal root ganglion. Post-herpetic neuralgia is characterized by a severe burning, itching, lancinating pain with allodynia and hyperpathia. The incidence of post-herpetic neuralgia is greatest in the elderly and it may be especially refractory to treatment in this age group (see below).

If the zosteriform eruption is present, the antiviral agent acyclovir should be administered. Acyclovir will speed healing, relieve acute pain, and lessen the risk of dissemination. Corticosteroids may also reduce acute pain, but should not be used in immunocompromised patients, as their use may increase the likelihood of viral dissemination. Neither antiviral agents nor corticosteroids has been shown to reduce the incidence of post-herpetic neuralgia in controlled trials. Opioids and nonsteroidal anti-inflammatory drugs should be used without hesitation in acute herpes zoster virus infection when pain is moderate to severe. Local anesthetic blockade of sympathetic fibers supplying the affected dermatomes may provide analgesia in both acute herpes zoster virus pain and in post-herpetic neuralgia. Other medications with reported analgesic activity in acute herpes zoster virus include levodopa and amantadine, by unknown mechanisms.

Tricyclic antidepressants are the first line therapy for postherpetic neuralgia. They have no effectiveness against the pain associated with acute herpes zoster virus. Amitriptyline, nortriptyline, doxepin, or imipramine are most commonly used for continuous dysesthetic pain. Anticonvulsants (including phenytoin, carbamazepine, valproic acid, and lioresal) are useful for paroxysmal lancinating pain. A trial of opioids may be indicated in selected, reliable patients when other medications have proved inadequate. These medications may be administered chronically with no significant toxicity and with minimal risk of psychologic dependence if closely supervised by a physician. Sympathetic blockade may provide partial analgesia in postherpetic neuralgia, although its precise role in treatment has not been established in controlled trials. TENS is occasionally helpful and should be tried in most patients. Topical application of capsacin, which depletes pain fiber endings of substance P, may occasionally be useful. Neurosurgical modalities for the treatment of selected patients include spinal cord stimulation, dorsal root entry zone lesioning, and deep brain stimulation. These procedures should be reserved for patients refractory to all other interventions who are experiencing severe, disabling pain.

CONCLUSION

The differential diagnosis of pain in the cancer patient is extremely varied. Just as early accurate diagnosis is essential to the management of any neurologic syndrome, so too is it in pain syndromes in cancer patients. There is a high frequency of occult neurologic disease in these patients. Pain may be the first symptom of a progressive disabling neurologic disorder in which early recognition will allow prompt and sometimes life- and function-preserving treatment. In addition to indicating appropriate primary therapy of the underlying malignancy, knowledge of cancer pain mechanisms will guide the clinician in selection of the best analgesic or neurosurgical/neuroanesthetic procedure. Moreover, cognizance of pain syndromes resulting from antineoplastic therapy may avoid the mistaken diagnosis of recurrent malignancy and subsequent inappropriate therapy.

SUGGESTED READINGS

Bach S, Noreng MF, Tjellden NU: Phantom limb pain in amputees during the first 12 months following limb amputation, after preoperative lumbar epidural blockade. Pain 33:297–301, 1988

Bruera E, McDonald N: Intractable pain in patients with advanced head and neck tumors: a possible role of local infection. Cancer Treat Rev 70:691–2, 1986

Clouston PD, DeAngelis L, Posner JB: The spectrum of neurological disease in patients with systemic cancer. Ann Neurol 31:268–73, 1992

Clouston PD, Sharpe DM, Corbett AJ et al: Perineural spread of cutaneous head and neck cancer. Arch Neurol 47:73–7, 1990

Elliot K, Foley KM: Neurologic pain syndromes in patients with cancer. Neurol Clin 7:333–60, 1989

Foley KM: Pain syndromes in patients with cancer. pp. 59–75. In Bonica JJ, Ventafridda V (eds): Advances in Pain Research and Therapy. Vol 2. Raven Press, New York, 1979

Forsyth PA, Posner JB: Headache in patients with brain tumors: a study of 111 patients. Neurology 43:1678–83, 1993

Gonzales GR, Elliot KJ, Portenoy RK, Foley KM: The impact of a comprehensive evaluation in the management of cancer pain. Pain 47:141–4, 1991

Granek I, Ashikari R, Foley KM: Postmastectomy pain syndrome: clinical and anatomic correlates. Proc Am Soc Clin Oncol 3:122, 1983

Kanner R, Martini N, Foley KM: Nature and incidence of postthoracotomy pain. Proc Am Soc Clin Oncol 1:152, 1982

Kori SH, Foley KM, Posner JB: Brachial plexus lesions in patients with cancer: 100 cases. Neurology 31:45–50, 1981

Portenoy RK: Cancer Pain: epidemiology and syndromes. Cancer 63:2298–2307, 1989

Portenoy RK, Duma C, Foley KM: Acute herpetic and postherpetic neuralgia: clinical review and current management. Ann Neurol 20:651–64, 1986

Portenoy RK, Lipton RB, Foley KM: Back pain in the cancer patient: an algorithm for evaluation and management. Neurol 37:134–8, 1987

Solomon L: Drug-induced arthropathy and necrosis of the femoral head. J Bone Joint Surg 55:246–61, 1973

173. NEUROLOGIC COMPLICATIONS OF BONE MARROW TRANSPLANTATION

KATHERYN SWOBODA
PATRICK Y. WEN

Bone marrow transplantation is now well established as a major treatment modality for a variety of disorders, including aplastic anemia, hematologic lymphoreticular malignancies, myelodysplastic syndromes, and severe combined immunodeficiency. More recently, it has shown promise in the treatment of certain metabolic disorders including Gaucher's disease and metachromatic leukodystrophy, as well as solid malignancies such as breast carcinoma. In patients with malignancies, bone marrow transplantation allows the administration of what would otherwise be lethal doses of chemotherapy. In others, it allows for replacement of pathologic marrow or serves to help correct an existing enzymatic deficiency. In many cases, it offers patients

the only chance for cure of the disease. In spite of the increasing efficacy of therapeutic regimens and improvements in the prophylaxis and treatment of infectious complications, the morbidity and mortality associated with bone marrow transplantation remains high. Most series have reported neurologic complications in more than one-half of all recipients, and severe neurologic compromise resulting in death occurs in approximately 5 to 8 percent. However, recent data suggests that such complications are decreasing, in part due to the increasing percentage of autologous transplants being performed.

In autologous marrow transplantation, the patient's own marrow is harvested and treated to remove abnormal cells, often via the use of specific monoclonal antibodies directed against tumor cells. In the case of allogeneic transplant, the replacement marrow is obtained from human leukocyte antigen–matched donors. The marrow is then reinfused following a preparatory regimen that includes both chemotherapy and myelotoxic doses of radiation (averaging 12 Gy). The chemotherapy regimen varies depending upon the underlying disease process and treatment center, but commonly used agents have included high-dose cyclophosphamide, etopside, carmustine, Lomustine, ifosfamide, busulfan, carboplatin, cytosine arabinoside, and daunorubicin. Recipients are then placed on a variety of immunosuppressive regimens in hopes of minimizing the chances of rejection or graft-versus-host disease (GVHD). Strict isolation procedures are required in the first 2 to 4 weeks after transplantation until engraftment takes place and marrow function is re-established. Potential sources of neurologic injury include cumulative exposure to toxic chemotherapy and radiation treatments, disorders of immunoregulation and immunodeficiency, and central nervous system (CNS) dysfunction secondary to failure of other organ systems (Table 173-1).

INFECTION

Infection following bone marrow transplantation is common, and accounts for 8 to 14 percent of complications. For the first month following transplantation, the recipient is severely immunocompromised and is susceptible to local and disseminated bacterial, viral, and fungal infections. Prior to engraftment, strict isolation procedures and prophylactic antibiotic regimens are crucial in ensuring good outcome. The use of granulocyte colony-stimulating factor and granulocyte-macrophage colony-stimulating factors, which increase the leukocyte count, have helped to lessen the risk of overwhelming sepsis. Aggressive treatment of fever in an empiric fashion with a stepwise succession of broad-spectrum antibacterial, antiviral, and antifungal agents has also dramatically improved survival and outcome in the immediate post-transplantation period. Unfortunately, cellular immunity is still persistently and perhaps indefinitely impaired, requiring continued vigilance for late parasitic, viral, and fungal infections. For the majority of patients, however, this risk seems to significantly decrease following the end of the first year.

CNS complications frequently occur as a result of overwhelming systemic infections in the first few weeks after transplantation. Disseminated infection can lead to disseminated intravascular or metabolic encephalopathy due to multisystem organ failure. Endocarditis from a variety of organisms may result in embolic events or mycotic aneurysms, with accompanying ischemic or hemorrhagic complications. Direct CNS involvement due to meningitis, encephalitis, or abcesses may also occur.

TABLE 173-1. Potential Sources of Neurologic Injury Following Bone Marrow Transplantation

Infection
  Primary
    Meningitis
    Encephalitis
    Cerebral abscesses
  Secondary
    Sepsis
    Disseminated intravascular coagulation
    Endocarditis

Treatment-related toxicities
  Primary
    Headache
    Seizures
    Ataxia
    Neuropathy
    Myelopathy
    Leukoencephalopathy
    Postirradiation somnolence syndrome
    Sensorineural hearing loss
  Secondary
    Metabolic encephalopathy
    Thrombocytopenia and hemorrhage
    Nutritional deficiencies
    Neuropsychiatric and cognitive difficulties
    Neuroendocrine disorders

Thrombotic complications
  Primary
    Large or small vessel cerebral arterial thrombosis
    Cerebral venous sinus thrombosis
  Secondary
    Nonbacterial thrombotic endocarditis
    Disseminated intravascular coagulation
    Acquired protein C deficiency
    Hepatic veno-occlusive disease

Immune-mediated disorders
  Acute graft-versus-host disease
    Headache
    Metabolic encephalopathy
  Chronic graft-versus-host disease
    Polymyositis
    Polyneuropathy
    Mononeuritis multiplex
    Myasthenia gravis
    Direct central nervous system involvement

The incidence of bacterial infections is greatest in the first months after transplantation, in keeping with the expected severe granulocytopenia. A wide variety of organisms has been implicated. Some of the more common have included *Staphylococcus, Streptococcus, Corynebacterium, Bacteroides, Clostridium, Listeria, Klebsiella, Enterobacteriae, Pseudomonas,* and *Haemophilus.* Meningitis has occurred with and without accompanying systemic infection, and may result form contiguous spread from a parameningeal focus such as a sinusitis or otitis. Organisms are often difficult to isolate, and broad-spectrum coverage to include *Listeria* and gram-negative organisms is necessary. In patients who are neutropenic, meningitis or meningoencephalitis may be present in the absence of a significant cerebrospinal fluid pleocytosis, and a low threshold for empiric CNS coverage in patients with either headache or subtle meningitic features is appropriate. Intracranial bacterial abscesses are surprisingly rare, although they are most likely to be found in the presence of disseminated disease.

Viral infections occur less commonly, and usually in the setting of disseminated systemic infection. However, focal reactivation of dermatomal herpes zoster virus is relatively common, and in one series, 29 percent of patients subsequently developed more generalized dissemination. Rare occurrences of post-her-

petic vasculopathy presenting as stroke have been described, usually following either ophthalmic zoster or disseminated disease.

The most common causes of a viral encephalitis are herpes simplex and cytomegalovirus. Occasionally, cases may be caused by adenovirus or Epstein-Barr virus. Symptoms are often atypical, characterized by subacute nonfocal encephalopathy or progressive obtundation in the absence of seizures. Cerebrospinal fluid (CSF) studies may be fairly unremarkable, or show only a mild pleocytosis or elevated protein. In the case of herpes encephalitis, the typical necrotizing lesions on imaging studies and characteristic frontotemporal electroencephalographic abnormalities may be absent. Polymerase chain reaction studies of CSF may improve the diagnostic yield in such patients, although empiric coverage with acyclovir is often warranted. Spread of viral agents occurs hematogenously from transfused blood products or systemic infection, reactivation of latent virus, or via nasopharyngeal or feco-oral transmission. Cytomegalovirus-negative and irradiated blood products are routinely used in bone marrow transplantation centers in hopes of avoiding the serious morbidity and mortality that can result from such infections.

Fungal infections reach the CNS via either hematogenous spread or direct extension from cranial sinuses. The most common organism involved is *Aspergillus fumigatus,* which has accounted for between 50 and 60 percent of all CNS infections in some series. CNS aspergillomas and sinonasal disease uniformly require surgical therapy for eradication. However, in spite of recent advances in combination therapy, invasive *Aspergillus* is usually lethal. Mucormycosis has a similarly poor prognosis, although selected patients with aggressive surgical debridement of sinonasal infection have had a good outcome. These organisms have a propensity for vascular invasion and tissue necrosis, frequently resulting in intraluminal thrombosis with resultant vascular occlusion, hemorrhage or embolic phenomena, and the formation of necrotizing abcesses. Nasal pain, epistaxis, and sinus congestion are common presenting complaints, with sinus x-rays or computed tomography (CT) scans often showing relatively nonspecific sinusitis. Prophylaxis with fluconazole has been disappointing, and infections are rarely eradicated with systemic antifungal therapy alone. Candidal meningitis, meningoencephalitis, and multiple brain abcesses have been reported, as have rare cases of disseminated *Torulopsis glabrata.* These infections have a better prognosis, and are more likely to respond to systemic antifungal therapy. In the future, earlier detection and new combinations of therapy and prophylactic regimens should lead to continued improvements in overall outcome in this group of patients.

Parasitic agents have been surprisingly uncommon, considering their frequency in other immunocompromised populations. Pulmonary infections with PCP are the most frequently encountered in the category. Cerebral toxoplasmosis may present either with focal abscesses or as a diffuse encephalopathy or meningoencephalitis. Stereotaxic biopsy of lesions may be diagnostic, although in the case of characteristic imaging studies, a trial of empiric therapy is often warranted. Subclinical infections are common in the general population, and in most cases are believed to be reactivation of a pre-existing infection. CSF and serologic antibody titers are variable and not always helpful, although toxoplasma infection is unlikely if the serology is negative.

TREATMENT-RELATED TOXICITIES

Toxicity resulting from the preparatory regimen is to be expected to some extent when the anticipated goal is cure. Acute or chronic effects may occur, and are often a result of the cumulative insults of chemotherapy, radiation, and the underlying disease process. Acute effects may include encephalopathy, thrombocytopemia, peripheral neuropathy, sensoneural hearing loss, ataxia, seizures, and nutritional disorders. Later on, leukoencephalopathy, neuroendocrine disorders, neuropsychiatric and cognitive difficulties, and ocular complications may occur.

Toxic or metabolic encephalopathy is common, and has accounted for up to 37 percent of neurologic complications in some series. This may be due to transient effects on renal, cardiac, pulmonary, or hepatic function, or as a result of direct CNS toxicity of the treatment regimen itself. Manifestations include confusion, personality changes, hallucinations, tremor, headache, somnolence, or seizures. High-dose cytosine arabinoside has been associated particularly with cerebellar dysfunction, and seems to have a selective toxic effect on Purkinje cells. Ifosfamide, which is used with increasing frequency in autologous transplants, particularly in patients with solid malignancies, may cause confusion and hallucinations or, more rarely, an akinetic mute state. Cyclosporin A, commonly used as an immunosuppressive agent after transplantation for the prevention of GVHD, has been associated with a wide variety of neurologic toxicities. These have included headache, seizures, tremor, neuropathy, myelopathy, encephalopathy, and focal neurologic deficits. More than 10 cases of cortical blindness have now been reported in patients on cyclosporin, at least 4 of them in bone marrow transplant recipients. Bone marrow transplantation (MRI) characteristically demonstrates signal abnormalities in the posterior white matter that are entirely reversible with reduction or discontinuation of cyclosporin dosage. The mechanisms of toxicity leading to this particular clinical presentation are poorly understood. Contributing factors that have been implicated to date include hypomagnesemia, concurrent treatment with high-dose steroids, hypertension, hypocholesterolemia, and microangiopathic hemolytic anemia.

Leukoencephalopathy is a relatively uncommon complication, occurring in less than 2 percent of patients undergoing bone marrow transplantation. Unfortunately, it often leads to severe progressive neurologic impairment and death. It seems to occur almost exclusively in those who receive both cranial irradiation and intrathecal chemotherapy. Particularly at risk are those who receive both pre- and post-transplantation intrathecal therapy with either cytosine arabinoside or methotrexate. Rare cases have also followed treatment with amphotericin B. Clinical effects include the progressive onset of lethargy, slurred speech, ataxia, confusion, dysphagia, and ultimately, quadriparesis with decerebrate posturing. Neuroimaging studies and pathology reveal diffuse confluent white matter degeneration and necrosis. In one review of 415 patients after bone marrow transplantation 7 patients developed leukoencephalopathy. Patients treated with more than four or five doses of intrathecal therapy after transplantation did not have lower rate of CNS relapse and the risk of leukoencephalopathy increased the number of doses of therapy administered. Methotrexate administered concurrently or following radiation are especially likely to result in serious neurologic sequelae. The time to onset of symptoms is extremely variable and may occur form 1 to 14 months after transplantation although symptoms are most often apparent in the first 6 months.

Postirradiation somnolence syndrome is a reversible phenomenon characterized by transient lethargy, headache, low-grade fever, gastrointestinal disturbances, and depression. It has been commonly observed in children treated for leukemia with prophylactic radiation. However, occasional adults have also been reported. It typically occurs several weeks after transplantation, and seems to respond to treatment with steroids and antidepressant therapy.

More subtle long-term neuropsychologic and cognitive deficits have not been well studied to date in adults. They are better documented than children, where poor school performance may bring them more quickly to attention. One recent study of adult patients undergoing bone marrow transplantation found a surprisingly large percentage of patients with significant impairments in a variety of areas. Memory seemed most significantly impaired, and more than 33 percent of patients scored in the impaired range in this domain. Measures of complex cognitive processing were also notably affected. Again, a history of cranial irradiation and intrathecal chemotherapy were predictors of poor test performance. This study illustrates the need for further research in this area, and suggests that cognitive impairment may be an important sequela of bone marrow transplantation.

Complications involving the spinal cord are infrequent, but may manifest in several ways. Rapidly ascending paralysis and more subtle chronologically progressive forms of myelopathy have been described. Myelopathies have been associated with cyclosporin and methotrexate and cytosine arabinoside. In other cases, the etiology is obscure. Pathologic findings have ranged from spongiotic degeneration preferentially involving the posterior columns to diffuse cord necrosis. Whether these cases represent a synergistic toxic effect due to the combination of chemotherapy, radiation, and borderline nutritional status, or to other poorly understood mechanisms is unclear. Rarely, patients may manifest Lhermitte sign, which has been classically associated with demyelinating disease. However, in this population, it seems to remit spontaneously and has a benign prognosis.

Mild peripheral neuropathies due to chemotherapy are common, but clinically disabling effects are rare. Patients with leukemia and prior chemotherapy seem more likely to be significantly affected. At least one case of an acute demyelinating polyneuropathy leading to reversible ventilory failure has been described in a patient with chronic myelogenous leukemia who had received high-dose cytosine arabinoside. The clinical course was consistent with Guillain-Barré syndrome. Patients with chronic inflammatory demyelinating neuropathy may develop severe exacerbations during the conditioning regimen for transplantation or immediately thereafter. Acute sensorineural hearing loss rarely occurs, but milder deficits are probably common. The use of aminoglycosides for treatment of post-bone marrow transplantation infection increases the risk of significant injury.

Mucositis and gastrointestinal distress are common in the first 2 to 3 weeks after transplantation and may lead to a compromised nutritional status. Total parenteral nutrition is often used during this period to offset potential complications. In one case, a 15-year-old boy with acute lymphoblastic leukemia developed onset of nystagmus, sixth nerve palsy, truncal ataxia, and progressive confusion and coma. He was subsequently diagnosed with Wernicke's encephalopathy and improved dramatically with thiamine but was left with residual symptoms, including memory deficit, nystagmus, and ataxia. Although such severe examples are rare, milder forms of nutritional deficiencies may be difficult to diagnose, and warrant consideration in the absence of other obvious factors.

Thrombocytopenia is an expected complication prior to engraftment of the new marrow in all bone marrow transplant recipients. Subarachnoid, subdural, and parenchymal hemorrhages sometimes occur and may lead to persistent neurologic compromise or death. Aggressive monitoring and replacement of platelets is mandatory, although hemorrhage is not necessarily associated with the degree of thrombocytopenia.

Late neuroendocrine abnormalities are also common after transplantation. The combination of total body irradiation and chemotherapy may induce a postmenopausal status in women and azoospermia in men. Thyroid dysfunction develops in up to 40 percent of patients. In children, growth retardation may occur; it sometimes responds to growth hormone replacement. These abnormalities are not clearly predictable, and periodic follow-up is indicated.

Ocular complications have become increasingly common as survival times after bone marrow transplantation continue to lengthen. Keratoconjuctivitis sicca seems to develop to some degree in the majority of patients following total body irradiation, although it is seen with increased frequency in GVHD. Without proper recognition and treatment, serious complications, including blindness, may result. Cataracts are common after transplantation, and the risk may exceed 80 percent after 4 years.

THROMBOTIC COMPLICATIONS

Cerebrovascular events are relatively common after bone marrow transplantation, accounting for between 6 and 28 percent of neurologic complications. A significant percentage of recipients develop a hypercoagulable state and as a group are prone to a variety of thrombotic complications. The most frequently encountered clinical manifestations include hepatic veno-occlusive disease, disseminated intravascular coagulation, nonbacterial thrombotic endocarditis, and thrombotic or embolic stroke. Superior vena cava and other large vessel thromboses, pupura fulminans, and small bowel infarction due to microvascular thrombosis have also been observed. The pathogenesis of this hypercoagulability state is not well understood. In the case of nonbacterial thrombotic endocarditis, it has been hypothesized that the preparatory chemotherapy and radiation regimens may damage cardiac endothelium and lead to degenerative changes in the connective tissue of the cardiac valves, thus creating a nidus for thrombosis. A similar mechanism has been proposed for veno-occlusive disease, with degeneration of venular endothelium as the originating event. In both of these examples, a significant portion of cases demonstrate concomitant low-grade disseminated intravascular coagulation. The direct infusion of marrow into the bloodstream may play a role in some cases, since it contains a large bolus of cells, platelets, and fibrin debris. Alternatively, the subsequent development of an immune-mediated process such as GVHD may predispose to ongoing cellular injury and release of thromboplastin into the circulation. Rarely, acquired protein C deficiency has also been implicated.

Regardless of the pathogenesis, strokes due to either embolic or thrombotic events remain an important cause of neurologic morbidity and mortality. Antemortem diagnosis of nonbacterial thrombotic endocarditis is rarely made since cardiac murmurs are unusual and endocardiography often misses small vegeta-

tions. Thus, detection of low-grade disseminated intravascular coagulation via the careful monitoring of platelet counts, prothrombin time, fibrinogen levels, and fibrin degradation products may help to prospectively identify patients at risk, and lead to improvements in our ability to prevent neurologic insult. It is only once patients at risk are identified that we can expect meaningful evaluation of therapeutic interventions such as antiplatelet agents and anticoagulation.

IMMUNE-MEDIATED DISORDERS

Immune-mediated disease in recipients of allogenic bone marrow transplantation is quite common, and represents one of the largest causes for diminished quality of life and morbidity among long-term survivors. Between 25 and 60 percent of patients develop some form of GVHD, a disorder believed to result primarily from the reaction of immunocompetent donor lymphocytes to non-human leukocyte antigen matched host antigens. Humoral mechanisms also likely play a role, as evidenced by the nearly universal deposition of immunoglobulin and complement along the dermal–epidermal junction in chronic GVHD. Given the frequency of systemic involvement, neurologic complications have been surprisingly infrequent. More often, neurologic dysfunction results as a consequence of widespread involvement with multiple system organ failure. However, GVHD-associated myositis, myasthenia gravis, and—rarely—central and peripheral nervous system involvement may occur.

Acute GVHD is typically manifested by rash, hepatic impairment, diarrhea, and abdominal pain. Primary CNS involvement in this syndrome has not been recognized to date, although common features in severe systemic involvement include an increased predisposition to infection, stroke, and metabolic encephalopathy. Chronic GVHD develops more frequently in older patients, and in those who have suffered from acute GVHD. In both disorders, diffuse lymphocytic infiltration is found in numerous tissues throughout the body. Chronic GVHD shares similar features with other autoimmune disorders including systemic lupus erythematosis, Sjögren syndrome, progressive systemic sclerosis, and lichen planus. In addition to skin changes, it is characterized by multiple organ involvement, including hepatic dysfunction, oral and esophageal mucositis and stricture, sicca syndrome, pulmonary insufficiency, limb contractures, and generalized wasting. A small number of patients have developed myositis as the sole or major presenting feature of their disease. Clinically, the syndrome is indistinguishable from idiopathic polymyositis. Muscle biopsies reveal a characteristic monocytic infiltration, with fiber necrosis and active phagocytosis. In at least four cases, the inflammatory infiltrates have been documented to be of donor origin. Infectious causes have not been apparent in these cases, but this bears careful consideration since rare cases of polymyositis have been linked to elevations in *Toxoplasma* IgM titers or with various viral agents including coxsackie, influenza, and hepatitis B. The patients with GVHD-associated myositis respond to treatment with prednisone or other immunosuppressive therapies.

Several cases of myasthenia gravis in bone marrow transplant recipients have now been described, and also seem to occur in association with chronic GVHD. These patients meet all criteria for the classic autoimmune mediated disorder, including proximal and bulbar fatigable muscle weakness, response to cholinesterase inhibitors, decremental response with repetitive nerve stimulation, and the presence of antibodies against the acetylcholine receptor. Discrete thymomas have not been observed, although thymic atrophy has been noted in some cases of GVHD. Some authors have hypothesized that autoantibodies might develop in response to subtle antigenic differences in the acetylcholine receptor between donors and recipient. However, others have noted that the presence of acetylcholine receptor antibodies may significantly precede the onset of clinical disease. In both GVHD myositis and myasthenia, the number of patients with the underlying diagnosis of aplastic anemia is greatly increased. Aplastic anemia is well known to have an association with a variety of other autoimmune disorders, as well as thymoma. This suggests that the pre-existing hematologic disorder somehow predisposes to the later development of these disorders. In one study, acetylcholine receptor antibodies were found in 21 of 51 bone marrow transplant recipients, especially those with aplastic anemia or acute nonlymphocytic leukemia, but not in other forms of leukemia or with the myelodysplastic syndromes. The disordered immunoregulation in these patients is complex and requires further study. Although it its clear that donor cells probably do play a role in the genesis of these syndromes, how these cells mediate their influence remains uncertain, and a certain predisposition to their development lies in the host as well.

Peripheral nerve involvement has only rarely been associated with GVHD. These have included several cases of generalized neuropathies, as well as guillain-barre syndrome, mononeuropathies, and mononeuritis multiplex. Nerve biopsies have also occasionally shown evidence of monocytic perineural infiltrates in the absence of clear-cut clinical symptoms. Although GVHD may rarely be implicated in such cases, a high degree of suspicion for an alternative cause of symptoms, particularly infection, should be maintained.

Direct CNS involvement secondary to GVHD has been reported in only a few cases. One patient had presumed GVHD-related encephalitis with mental status changes, dysphagia, progressive muscle atrophy, and cachexia. The disease was resistant to treatment with methylprednisone, cyclophosphamide, and high-dose immunoglobulin, and ultimately died of pneumonia more than 3 years after transplantation. Pathologic examination revealed diffuse perivascular lymphocytic infiltrates in meninges and brain parenchyma, similar to those seen in his other organs and in experimental GVHD. Two cases of subacute panenecephalitis, with symptoms beginning several months after transplantation in conjunction with GVHD have been described. An additional case involved an infant with complete heart block and respiratory insufficiency in the absence of pulmonary disease whose brain showed focal lymphohistiocytic infiltrates in the absence of obvious infection.

SECONDARY MALIGNANCY AND DISEASE RECURRENCE

Recurrence of the primary disease process or occurrence of secondary malignancy always remains a possibility. In the case of hematologic or lymphoreticular malignancies, the likelihood of CNS recurrence is directly linked to the underlying disease process. For instance, CNS relapse for acute lymphoblastic leukemia is between 16 and 20 percent in most series, whereas the risk for acute nonlymphocytic leukemia is less than 2 percent. Secondary malignancies are rare and the majority do not directly involve the CNS. However, at least two cases of glioblas-

toma multiforme have occurred as a second primary neoplasm. Rare cases of Epstein-Barr virus with lymphoma involving the CNS have also been reported.

SUMMARY

Neurologic complications are common following bone marrow transplantation and occur in more than one-half of all recipients. Approximately 5 to 6 percent of patients will die as a direct result of these complications. The differential diagnosis is often broad, and careful consideration must be given to a diverse range of factors, including the nature of the primary disease process, the specific preparatory regimen involved, prior exposure to potentially neurotoxic therapies, and current immunocompetence. Becoming familiar with the potential complications encountered and remaining vigilant to the fact that neurologic disease may present in an atypical or subtle manner can greatly facilitate early intervention and lead to improved outcome and quality of life.

SUGGESTED READINGS

Amato AA, Bahohn RJ, Sahenk Z: Polyneuropathy complicating bone marrow and solid organ transplantation. Neurology 43:1513, 1993

Anfrykowski MA, Schmitt FA, Gregg ME et al: Neuropsychologic impairment in adult bone marrow transplant candidates. Cancer 70:2288, 1992

Atkinson K, Biggs J, Darveniza P et al: Spinal cord and cerebellar-like syndromes associated with the use of cyclosporin in human recipients of allogenic marrow transplants. Transplant Proc 17:1673, 1985

Bleyer WA: Neurologic sequelae of methotrexate and ionizing radiation: a new classification. Cancer Treat Rep (suppl.)65:89, 1981

Bolger GB, Sullivan KM, Spence AM et al: Myasthenia gravis after allogenic bone marrow transplantation: relationship to chronic graft-versus-host disease. Neurology 36:1087, 1986

Davis DG, Patchell RA: Neurologic complications of bone marrow transplantation. Neurol Clin 6:377, 1988

Deeg HJ, Strob R, Thomas ED: Bone marrow transplantation: a review of delayed complications. Br J Haematol 57:185, 1984

Ghalie R, Fitzsimmons WE, Bennett D et al: Cortical blindness: a rare complication of cyclosporine therapy. Bone Marrow Transplant 6:147, 1990

Goldberg S, Tefferi A, Rummans T: Post-irradiation somnolence syndrome in an adult patient following allogeic transplant. Bone Marrow Transplant 9:499, 1992

Johnson NT, Crawford SW, Sargur M: Acute acquired demyelinating polyneuropathy with respiratory failure following high-dose systemic cytosine arabinoside and marrow transplantation. Bone Marrow Transplant 2:203, 1987

Majolino I, Caponetto A, Scime T et al: Wernicke-like encephalopathy after autologous bone marrow transplantation. Haematologica 75:282, 1990

Mohrmann R, Mah V, Vinters HV: Neuropathologic findings after bone marrow transplantation: an autopsy study. Hum Pathol 21:630, 1990

Nelson KR, McQuillen MP: Neurologic complications of graft-versus-host diseases. Neurol Clin 6:389, 1988

Openshaw H, Hinton DR, Slatkin NE et al: Exacerbation of inflammatory demyelinating polyneuropathy after bone marrow transplantation. Bone Marrow Transplant 7:411, 1991

Patchell RA, White CL, Clark AW et al: Neurologic complications of bone marrow transplantation. Neurology 35:300, 1985

Patchell RA, White CL, Clark AW et al: Nonbacterial thrombotic endocarditis in bone marrow transplant patients. Cancer 55:631, 1985

Reece DE, Frei-Lahr DA, Shepherd JD et al: Neurologic complications in allogenic bone marrow transplant patients receiving cyclosporin. Bone Marrow Transplant 8:393, 1991

Snider S, Bashir R, Bierman P: Neurologic complications after high dose chemotherapy and autologous bone marrow transplant for Hodgkins disease. Neurology 44:681, 1994

Thompson CB, Sanders JE, Flournoy N et al: The risks of central nervous system relapse and leukoencephalopathy in patients receiving marrow transplants for acute leukemia. Blood 67:195, 1986

Trigg ME, Meenzes AH, Giller R et al: Combined anti-fungal therapy and surgical resection as treatment of disseminated aspergillosis of the lung and brain following BMT. Bone Marrow Transplant 11:493, 1993
Wiznitzer M, Packer RJ, August CS et al: Neurologic complications of bone marrow transplantation in childhood. Ann Neurol 16:569, 1984

174. NEUROLOGIC COMPLICATIONS OF LYMPHOMA

LAWRENCE RECHT

The term *lymphoma* denotes a heterogeneous group of malignant neoplasms derived from lymphoreticular tissues. Approximately 30 percent of lymphomas are histologically characterized as Hodgkin's disease and distinguished by the presence of characteristic Reed-Sternberg cells; the remainder comprise a diverse group of neoplasms that are classified as non-Hodgkin's lymphoma. From the neurologist's viewpoint, this subdivision is clinically important because Hodgkin's disease only rarely infiltrates central nervous system (CNS) directly. By contrast, this phenomenon occurs frequently in certain types of non-Hodgkin's lymphoma.

Non-Hodgkin's lymphomas can be further subdivided according to the tumor's characteristic pathologic features. However, the terms used have often been confusing. In an attempt to allow correlation between the several histologic classifications of non-Hodgkin's lymphoma, the Working Formulation was developed; from a neurologic perspective, the higher the grade, the more likely the occurrence of direct CNS infiltration (Table 174-1).

The neurologic complications of systemic lymphomas can be grouped according to whether they result from either direct invasion of tumor or a remote effect of tumor or treatment.

TABLE 174-1. Characteristics of the Subtypes of Non-Hodgkin's Lymphoma According to the Working Formulation, Including Propensity to Invade the Central Nervous System

Subtype	Relative Frequency (%)	Growth Pattern	Incidence of Central Nervous System Invasion
Low grade			
Small lymphocytic	5	Diffuse	Rare
Follicular small cleaved cell	25	Follicular	Rare
Follicular mixed cell	10	Follicular	Rare
Intermediate grade			
Follicular large cell	5	Follicular	Rare
Diffuse small cleaved cell	10	Diffuse	Intermediate
Diffuse mixed cell	10	Diffuse	Intermediate
Diffuse large cell	20	Diffuse	Intermediate
High grade			
Immunoblastic	10	Diffuse	Intermediate
Lymphoblastic	5	Diffuse	High
Small noncleaved cell	5	Diffuse	High

DIRECT INVOLVEMENT OF THE CENTRAL NERVOUS SYSTEM BY LYMPHOMA

Lymphomas can invade the CNS at any time during the course of the disease; CNS involvement may be present at time of diagnosis, occur during the course of progressive disease, or most distressingly, be the first sign of a relapse after a complete remission. CNS invasion by lymphoma occurs frequently in non-Hodgkin's lymphoma and is one of the more commonly involved extranodal sites; approximately, 10 percent of these patients will develop this complication. In patients with acquired immunodeficiency syndrome, CNS invasion by lymphoma occurs in up to 25 percent, tends to be more aggressive, and is generally harder to treat than in otherwise normal individuals.

Lymphomas produce CNS symptoms directly by some combination of leptomeningeal infiltration, intraparenchymal mass lesions, epidural masses, or infiltration of blood vessels or peripheral nerves.

Systemic Lymphoma

Direct CNS infiltration is seen almost exclusively in non-Hodgkin's lymphoma; only occasional reports describe its occurrence in Hodgkin's disease. The likelihood of developing CNS involvement varies as a function of the particular non-Hodgkin's lymphoma histology. As a general rule, the more aggressive the grade of lymphoma, the higher the risk of developing leptomeningeal disease (Table 174-1); in the most aggressive lymphomas (i.e., lymphoblastic and small noncleaved cell types), this risk approaches 25 percent. Involvement of either bone marrow, testes, or leukemic transformation increases this risk further, as does receiving prior chemotherapy and younger patient age.

Most commonly, lymphomas gain access to the CNS via the meninges. Tumor implants are inhomogeneously distributed, being most pronounced at the base of the brain, and spinal cord and lymphoma cells often can be found infiltrating into Virchow-Robin's spaces. Less commonly, parenchymal invasion results in visible intraparenchymal masses. Certain lymphoma types, such as mycosis fungoides, although rarely invading CNS, seem to result in a disproportionately high incidence of mass lesions.

Meningeal Involvement

Meningeal involvement can occur at any time in the lymphomatous disease process; it may be present at time of diagnosis (when it may be clinically asymptomatic), can occur as a manifestation of relapse after a complete remission, or most commonly, can develop in the setting of progressive systemic disease. It may even be the sole manifestation of non-Hodgkin's lymphoma, although this is distinctly unusual. Moreover, there seems to be a correlation between the presence of intraocular non-Hodgkin's lymphoma and CNS lymphomatous mass lesions, which may represent either a multicentric or metastatic disease process.

Any neurologic symptom may be associated with meningeal lymphoma. Most commonly, patients present with symptoms of either general CNS dysfunction (i.e., headache, altered mental status), cranial nerve abnormalities (the abducens and facial being most often affected), or spinal cord dysfunction. Since more unusual syndromes can occur, the best approach is to maintain a high index of suspicion and to have a low threshold for performing confirmatory tests when a non-Hodgkin's lymphoma patient at risk develops neurologic symptomatology.

The diagnosis of meningeal lymphoma is made most definitively by identification of neoplastic cells in the cerebrospinal fluid (CSF). At least one CSF parameter is abnormal in virtually all patients with meningeal involvement. Cytologic examination should yield lymphoma cells in over 90 percent of these patients if three examinations are performed and adequate material is obtained. Because meningeal disease may be present at disease onset and associated with no symptoms, all patients with newly diagnosed non-Hodgkin's lymphoma of intermediate or aggressive histologic subtype should have a lumbar puncture performed as part of their staging procedure.

Sometimes, identification of neoplastic cells cannot be made despite a high index of suspicion. In these situations, other radiographic examinations may be helpful. The appearance of ventricularly based intraparenchymal masses or noncommunicating hydrocephalus on computed tomography or magnetic resonance imaging in a patient with non-Hodgkin's lymphoma suggests a meningeal process. Similarly, visualizing discrete gadolinium-enhancing nodules on nerve roots in the cauda equina or within the spinal cord itself strongly supports a diagnosis of meningeal disease. Even with these sensitive tests, a diagnosis may still be elusive despite a high degree of suspicion. Determination of β_2-microglobulin, analysis of lymphocyte markers, and in vitro gene amplification by polymerase chain reaction to demonstrate chromosome translocations on CSF material are all potentially useful in this situation.

The development of meningeal or parenchymal involvement by lymphoma is generally associated with a very poor prognosis. Median survivals after diagnosis are generally measurable in weeks, although this may reflect the failure to control CNS disease rather than CNS involvement per se. Nevertheless, an aggressive therapeutic approach using some combination of steroids, radiotherapy, and either local or systemic chemotherapy is warranted in order to minimize or prevent neurologic morbidity.

Although symptoms and signs may suggest a focal disorder, the finding of meningeal involvement connotes a diffuse process; therefore, the entire neuraxis needs to be treated to ensure that all tumor is eradicated. Unlike their effects on most other neoplasms, steroids are more than just palliative when used in lymphoma; sometimes, brisk oncolytic effects can be observed and even large bulky masses may quickly disappear.

Since this is a diffuse disease, radiotherapy ports can be extended to include the entire neuraxis; this can be associated with increased neurologic morbidity, however, and tends to produce myelosuppression which may limit tolerance to chemotherapy. For this reason, a preferred approach combines focal irradiation to areas of maximal involvement with chemotherapy. Focal symptoms such as cranial dysfunction are generally effectively ameliorated and lymphomatous parenchymal lesions also generally respond.

Although systemic chemotherapy using high-dose methotrexate or cytosine arabinoside has been used relatively effectively as a therapy for meningeal lymphoma, most workers recommend use of local chemotherapy via intrathecal or intraventricular routes either concomitantly or instead of radiotherapy. Either methotrexate or cytosine arabinoside can be used; lymphomas tend to respond to both agents more frequently than do other solid neoplasms. Although it has been difficult to demonstrate a clear superiority of intraventricular therapy, use of an Ommaya reservoir does combine the practical advantage of ease of administration with the theoretic one of better penetration into the entire neuraxis. Furthermore, in experienced hands, complication rates are low.

Using a combined modality approach, neurologic symptomatology can be controlled in approximately 80 percent of patients, although median survival length is still short, ranging from 1 to 8 months. Relatively favorable prognostic factors are young age, CNS involvement occurring as an isolated event, and receiving combined therapy. Furthermore, when meningeal lymphoma is present at the onset of disease, the outcome is not invariably fatal; up to 25 percent can attain long-term survival with intensive treatment.

Epidural Lymphoma

Approximately 5 percent of lymphoma patients develop epidural spinal cord compression secondary to their primary disease; this complication occurs with equal frequency in both Hodgkin's and non-Hodgkin's disease, although the latter is more commonly found when it occurs as a first disease manifestation.

When a presenting symptom, systemic lymphoma may be found during staging procedures, but in a large percentage, the spinal column may represent the sole site of involvement. Prognosis for these patients tends to be better than when disease occurs in the setting of established lymphoma; in approximately 20 percent, evidence of distant disease is never noted and patients may be cured.

Most epidural lesions are diagnosed when extranodal or extensive nodal disease already exists. Similar to other solid neoplasms, the thoracic cord is most frequently involved; by contrast, however, lymphomas frequently spread from paraspinous regions into the epidural space via intervertebral foramina. This results in a radiographically demonstrable complete block despite normal plain spine films, an important point for the clinician to remember in evaluating a lymphoma patient with spinal cord dysfunction.

Presenting signs and symptoms are similar to those produced by other cancers. Although technically symptoms are not an effect of direct CNS infiltration, the frequent coexistence of epidural and meningeal lymphoma makes the matter moot. Because it will alter the therapeutic approach, it is important to characterize exactly the pathologic process. Therefore, in a patient in whom epidural lymphoma is suspected, a CSF examination (when not contraindicated by complete spinal block) should be performed in addition to imaging of the entire spine.

The approach to treating lymphomatous epidural compression is similar to that delineated for other neoplasms. Because the administration of steroids can result in a brisk oncolytic response, however, it is possible to miss a lesion if undue delays occur before diagnostic testing after steroids are started.

When epidural lymphoma occurs as the presenting symptom, decompression is indicated, if only to make a diagnosis. Most lymphomatous lesions respond effectively to irradiation, however; surgery is then generally reserved if lesions progress or recur after irradiation. Overall, therapeutic results are generally favorable and the presence of epidural lymphoma probably does not impact much on the ultimate prognosis.

Neoplastic Angioendotheliomatosis (Intravascular Lymphoma)

Neoplastic angioendotheliomatosis, although a rare complication of non-Hodkin's lymphoma, frequently produces CNS symptoms. Originally believed to be a disorder of endothelial cells, recent immunohistochemical and molecular evidence indicate that the proliferative cells are actually of lymphocytic, primarily B cell origin. Therefore, the condition is more properly designated intravascular lymphomatosis or angiotropic large cell lymphoma.

Intravascular lymphoma is characterized by the presence of neoplastic cells within the lumina of small and intermediate-size blood vessels. The skin and CNS are preferentially involved. Its clinical features are related to vascular occlusion by neoplastic cells, which accumulate in small arterioles, capillaries, and venules and include progressive multifocal cerebrovascular events, paraparesis, a subacute encephalopathy, and peripheral or cranial neuropathies. Neurologic involvement is usually associated with a rapidly, albeit fluctuating, clinical course.

Because clinical and radiographic features are nonspecific, diagnosis is rarely made during life; when it is suspected, the only definitive method of diagnosis is by brain or meningeal biopsy. Anecdotal reports suggest that intravascular lymphomas may respond to steroids, plasmapharesis, or chemotherapy.

Neurolymphomatosis

Neurolymphomatosis refers to the condition when peripheral nerves are infiltrated by non-Hodgkin's lymphoma. It is a rare manifestation of non-Hodgkin's lymphoma that usually results in a rapidly progressive and fatal painful neuropathy that cannot be attributed to chemotherapy, Guillain-Barré syndrome, or a paraneoplastic syndrome.

When confined to the peripheral nerves, the diagnosis can be extremely difficult to make. At autopsy, however, predominant and exclusive infiltration of peripheral nerves is seen. The cause of the neuropathy is unknown. No treatment has been effective.

Should Central Nervous System Prophylaxis Be Administered to Lymphoma Patients?

Similar to the leukemias, early initial therapies for non-Hodgkin's lymphoma did not include CNS-directed treatment, and the subsequent development of CNS lymphoma was noted to be significant. Furthermore, it was noted that CNS involvement was more likely to occur in aggressive, extensive non-Hodgkin's lymphoma. When multivariate analyses were performed, the three most important factors predicting CNS invasion were histology (lymphoblastic and small noncleaved cell), younger age (< 40 years), and advanced stage; the estimated probability of developing meningeal metastases was as high as 60 percent when all three factors were present.

Despite the ability to define a high-risk patient, however, the case for CNS prophylaxis is not as clear-cut as it is in leukemia because isolated CNS relapse is an unusual occurrence in non-Hodgkin's lymphoma patients; data accrued from two large trials of the Eastern Cooperative Oncology Group indicated that only 1 percent of patients with diffuse histiocytic lymphoma (the most common form of non-Hodgkin's lymphoma) develop isolated CNS relapses. Therefore, since prophylaxis is associated with potential complications, the morbidities of treatment may outweigh any minimal benefits.

Few previous studies have specifically addressed the benefits of prophylaxis in non-Hodgkin's lymphoma, and differing conclusions have been drawn. Retrospective studies analyzing large non-Hodgkin's lymphoma patient cohorts suggest that the incidence of CNS involvement is similar whether or not patient receive prophylaxis in the form of radiotherapy or intrathecal chemotherapy. Furthermore, in a recent study comparing intensive chemotherapy with a standard CHOP (cyclophosphamide, hydroxyurea, vincristine [Oncovin], and prednisone) regimen in which CNS prophylaxis was excluded revealed similar survivals and outcomes, suggesting strongly that prophylaxis did not improve outcome.

PARANEOPLASTIC SYNDROMES ASSOCIATED WITH LYMPHOMA

Besides directly infiltrating the central and peripheral nervous systems, lymphomas may produce neurologic symptoms via a number of more indirect mechanisms. It is important for the clinician to be aware of these indirect complications both because they may be treatable and because mistaking them for tumor progression may result in the administration of incorrect treatments. Many of these complications are similar to those produced by other cancers and can be found detailed in other chapters of this book; here, however, the focus is on those syndromes that are grouped under the rubric *paraneoplastic* and exclusively or predominantly associated with lymphoma (see also Ch. 171).

A number of syndromes in cancer patients have been termed paraneoplastic because they are not due to either the cancer or any known treatment, infection, or vascular or metabolic aberration. In recent years, intensive research into these fascinating syndromes has indicated that many of them probably occur secondary to autoimmune mechanisms. Virtually any paraneoplastic syndrome can occur in a patient with lymphoma; certain ones seem especially frequent, however. A reported association exists between paraneoplastic cerebellar degeneration and Hodgkin's disease. Another peculiar syndrome that seems almost exclusively associated with lymphoma is subacute motor neuropathy. Seen in both Hodgkin's disease and non-Hodgkin's lymphoma patients, it is usually noted while the patient is in remission and its manifestations occur independent of the underlying neoplasm's activity. Painless and often patchy weakness of a lower motor neuron variety is encountered; it occurs subacutely and is progressive, and senory loss is mild. The electromyogram reveals denervation. Pathologically, degeneration of anterior horns and demyelination of anterior nerve roots is seen. The course is benign and generally stabilizes or improves spontaneously.

A syndrome that approximates more closely actual motoneuron disease, with both upper and lower motor neuron signs, has also been recently reported in patients with lymphoma; its occurrence is frequently associated with a coexistent paraproteinemia. This association is common enough to prompt some workers to suggest searching for such underlying conditions in all patients with otherwise typical amyotrophic lateral sclerosis.

Remote syndromes involving peripheral nerves seem particularly common in patients with either lymphoma or related diseases such as myeloma. An acute polyradiculopathy indistinguishable for classic Guillain-Barré syndrome has been associated with Hodgkin's disease; it may occur at any stage of the disease. Hodgkin's disease has also been associated with a painful brachial neuritis that seems to occur more frequently in the setting of proximate administration of radiotherapy.

Finally, a rare association between lymphoblastic lymphoma and myasthenia gravis has been reported, in which elevated anti-acetylcholine receptor antibody levels disappeared with successful treatment of the lymphoma.

SUGGESTED READINGS

Diaz-Arrastia R, Younger DS, Hair L et al: Neurolymphomatosis: a clinicopathologic syndrome re-emerges. Neurology 42:1136–41, 1992

Fisher RI, Gaynor ER, Dahlberg S et al: Comparison of a standard regimen (CHOP) with three intensive chemotherapy regimens for advanced non-Hodgkin's lymphoma. New Engl J Med 328:1002–6, 1993

Glass J, Hochberg FH, Miller DC: Intravascular lymphomatosis. A systemic disease with neurologic manifestations. Cancer 71:3156–64, 1993

Haddy TB, Adde MA, Magrath IT: CNS involvement in small noncleaved-cell lymphoma: is CNS disease per se a poor prognostic sign? J Clin Oncol 9:1973–82, 1991

Johnson GJ, Oken MM, Anderson JR et al: Central nervous system relapse in unfavourable-histology non-Hodgkin's lymphoma: is prophylaxis indicated? Lancet ii:685–7, 1984

Lokich J, Galbo C: Leptomeningeal lymphoma: perspectives on management. Cancer Treat Rev 8:103–10, 1981

Mackintosh FR, Colby TV, Podolsky WJ et al: Central nervous system involvement in non-Hodgkin's lymphoma: an analysis of 105 cases. Cancer 49:586–95, 1982

Malow BA, Dawson DM: Neuralgic amyotrophy in association with radiation therapy for Hodgkin's disease. Neurology 41:440–1, 1991

Perez-Soler R, Smith TL, Cabanillas F: Central nervous system prophylaxis with combined intravenous and intrathecal methotrexate in diffuse lymphoma of aggressive histologic type. Cancer 57:971–7, 1986

Perry JR, Deodhare SS, Bilbao JM, Murray D, Muller P: The significance of spinal cord compression as the initial manifestation of lymphoma. Neurosurgery 32:157–62, 1993

Recht L, Straus DJ, Cirrincione C et al: Central nervous system metastases from non-Hodgkin's lymphoma: treatment and prophylaxis. Am J Med 84:425–35, 1988

Schold SC, Cho ES, Somasundaram M, Posner JB: Subacute motor neuronopathy: a remote effect of lymphoma. Ann Neurol 5:271–87, 1979

Young RC, Howser DM, Anderson T et al: Central nervous system complications of non-Hodgkin's lymphoma. The potential role for prophylactic therapy. Am J Med 66:435–43, 1979

Younger DS, Rowland LP, Latov N et al: Lymphoma, motor neuron diseases, and amyotrophic lateral sclerosis. Ann Neurol 29:78–86, 1991

175. NEUROLOGIC COMPLICATIONS OF LEUKEMIA

KENDRA PETERSON

Leukemia is the most common cancer in children, and occurs in significant numbers of adults as well. Neurologic disorders in patients with leukemia are common (Table 175-1). They may result from direct leukemic infiltration of the nervous system, may be the indirect consequence of associated vascular events, or may result from complications of treatment. Familiarity with the specific neurologic disorders that occur in patients with leukemia can provide opportunities to prevent untoward complications; recognizing and distinguishing the various manifestations when they occur directs appropriate and specific therapy.

DIRECT NERVOUS SYSTEM INVOLVEMENT

Leukemia may directly invade any part of the central or peripheral nervous system. Meningeal leukemia is by far the most common manifestation of direct nervous system involvement.

TABLE 175-1. Neurologic Complications of Leukemia

Direct nervous system involvement by leukemia
  Meningeal leukemia
  Parenchymal leukemia
  Chloroma
  Peripheral nerve infiltration
Neurologic vascular complications of leukemia
  Hemorrhagic
    Blast crisis
    Thrombocytopenia
    Disseminated intravascular coagulation
    Hemorrhagic embolic infarcts
    Infection (*Aspergillus*)
  Ischemia/infarction
    Leukocytosis
    Disseminated intravascular coagulation
    Cortical vein thrombosis (L-asparaginase)
Treatment-related neurologic complications
  Acute/subacute
    Radiation-induced
      Somnolence syndrome
      Posterior column dysfunction
    Chemotherapy-induced
      Meningitis
      Myelopathy
      Encephalopathy
      Cerebellar dysfunction (cytosine arabinoside)
  Delayed/chronic
    Cognitive decline/dementia
    Radiation necrosis
    Necrotizing leukoencephalopathy
    Mineralizing microangiopathy
    Endocrine dysfunction
    Second malignancies

Meningeal Leukemia

The clinical problem of leukemic infiltration of the meninges has changed over the last several decades. Before the routine use of systemic chemotherapy, meningeal leukemia was only rarely reported. The development of effective combination chemotherapies achieved systemic remission in many patients and allowed longer survival, but subsequent meningeal relapse became common; the incidence of this complication increased 10- to 20-fold in the period from 1947 to 1970. About one-half to two-thirds of patients successfully treated for systemic leukemia in this period eventually developed central nervous system (CNS) relapse. The great majority of meningeal relapse occurred within the first year of systemic remission, though in rare patients was delayed for as long as 10 years. Recently, the routine use of CNS prophylactic therapy for many patients with leukemia has once again diminished the incidence of this complication, now to 5 to 10 percent of patients.

Meningeal involvement is typically a late manifestation of leukemia and is rarely detectable at presentation. Meningeal leukemia often occurs in isolation during systemic remission, but may herald the onset of bone marrow relapse. The current practice of routine surveillance of the cerebrospinal fluid (CSF) now allows subclinical diagnosis of meningeal leukemia in many patients prior to the development of neurologic symptoms.

Meningeal leukemia has been described as a complication of all forms of leukemia, although it occurs more commonly in some types than others. Meningeal involvement is more likely to complicate acute rather than chronic leukemia, lymphocytic rather than nonlymphocytic leukemia, and childhood rather than adult leukemia. Similar to the experience in childhood leukemia, the incidence in adult patients may be increasing as systemic therapies become more effective in maintaining prolonged systemic remission. The rare T-cell lymphocytic leukemias are more prone to CNS involvement and more resistant to treatment than the more common B-cell leukemias.

There has been some controversy as to the source of leukemic cells within the CNS. Prior hypotheses that leukemic cells arise directly from hematopoietic sources within the CNS (choroid plexus or meninges themselves), or by direct invasion from the bone marrow of the skull, have generally been displaced by the view that leukemic cells reach the CNS by hematogenous spread. Pathologically, there is a spectrum of involvement from invasion of the meningeal veins and superficial involvement of the arachnoid, to more extensive perivascular infiltration of the Virchow-Robin spaces and extension into the deep arachnoid, and finally to disruption of the pia-glial membrane and parenchymous infiltration of the brain, cranial nerves, and spinal nerve roots. Hematogenous metastasis to the meninges may occur early in the course of the disease but is ineffectively treated by systemic therapies, and therefore may be a reservoir for late relapse.

As noted, meningeal leukemia may be asymptomatic and diagnosed only by routine CSF evaluation. When meningeal leukemia is present, symptoms and signs referable to any level of the neuraxis may be present. Most typical are symptoms of increased intracranial pressure, with headache, nausea, and vomiting, and in younger children, separation of the cranial sutures. Papilledema is present in about one-half of patients. Optic nerve and chiasm infiltration may impair vision, and involvement of cranial nerves III and VI frequently causes ophthalmoplegia. Facial weakness due to involvement of cranial nerve VII is not infrequent. The lower cranial nerves are involved less commonly. Radicular symptoms resulting from spinal nerve root involvement are relatively uncommon in children but occur with increased frequency in adults. Rare parenchymal brain infiltration may precipitate seizures or focal deficits. Up to one-fourth of children with meningeal involvement by acute lymphoblastic leukemia develop a syndrome of hyperphagia, obesity, and somnolence as a result of hypothalamic infiltration.

Computed tomography or magnetic resonance image scans may be normal, though they frequently reveal mild to moderate increased ventricular size. Contrast-enhanced magnetic resonance imaging may detect diffuse meningeal enhancement, and, on rare occasions, focal nodular meningeal deposits.

The diagnosis of meningeal leukemia depends on the detection of malignant cells in the CSF. Cytocentrifugation is more sensitive than routine cytology in detecting leukemic cells. Leukemic cells are rarely present if the total CSF white blood cell count is less than $10/mm^3$. The presence of pleocytosis may be misleading, however, as it may be caused by infection or chemical meningitis following intrathecal chemotherapy or subarachnoid hemorrhage. Other abnormalities may include elevated pressure, mildly elevated protein, and sometimes hypoglycorrhachia. CSF markers such as β_2-microglobulin, β-glucuronidase, and polyamine levels are nonspecific but can support a clinical suspicion. Very rarely, patients are treated for meningeal leukemia without a definite pathologic diagnosis, but only when there is strong clinical and supporting laboratory evidence, and other meningeal processes have been excluded.

CNS prophylactic therapy is now routinely included in the initial treatment regimen of many patients with leukemia, particularly in childhood acute lymphoblastic leukemia and others considered at high risk of CNS relapse. The optimum CNS prophylactic regimen is still being defined; combination cranial radiotherapy and intrathecal methotrexate was used commonly in the past, though regimens that exclude cranial radiotherapy and use intrathecal methotrexate alone or combination intrathecal chemotherapies are more commonly used currently.

Treatment of meningeal leukemia typically includes multimodality therapy with neuraxis radiotherapy and combination intrathecal and systemic chemotherapy. Response to therapy depends on a number of variables, including the type of leukemia and the stage at which meningeal leukemia is diagnosed. As one might anticipate, patients with subclinical involvement generally respond to therapy more favorably than those with overt disease. Patients who develop meningeal relapse while in systemic remission fare better than those who relapse during initial therapy. Patients who have not received prior cranial radiotherapy respond at relapse better than those who relapse after radiotherapy. Overall, about 20 to 35 percent of patients treated for meningeal leukemia will achieve long-term remission.

Parenchymal Leukemia

Parenchymal infiltration of the nervous system occurs either diffusely or as isolated nodular deposits. There is debate as to whether parenchymal leukemic infiltration ever occurs without meningeal involvement. In the majority of cases parenchymal involvement is associated with, and probably results from, direct extension of meningeal disease. Pathologic examination has yielded occasional cases of parenchymal disease without evidence of meningeal disease; this may represent a different pathway of entrance into the CNS other than through meningeal veins, or may represent the resistance of parenchymal deposits in spite of successful treatment of meningeal disease.

Chloroma

Chloromas, which are green in color owing to the presence of myeloperoxidase, are rare complications of myelogenous leukemias. They are collections of myeloid cells that occur most commonly in skin, liver, and lymph nodes. They may also occur in bone and extend adjacent to bone to affect the nervous system by local compression of spinal cord, nerves, or other structures. On rarely occasions, they occur within brain parenchyma, typically as a single mass lesion, though they are occasionally multiple. Chloromas may present with focal neurologic dysfunction, though are asymptomatic and noted only at autopsy in as many as one-half of affected patients.

Peripheral Nerve Involvement

Leukemic peripheral nerve infiltration is a very rare event that usually occurs in patients with uncontrolled systemic disease. Patients may present with polyneuropathy or focal infiltration of individual nerves or nerve roots.

NEUROLOGIC VASCULAR COMPLICATIONS

Both hemorrhagic and ischemic vascular complications of leukemia occur frequently, either as a direct consequence of the disease or resulting from a number of commonly associated conditions. In some settings, hemorrhagic and ischemic complications occur simultaneously.

Hemorrhage

Intracranial hemorrhage is the most common neurologic vascular complication of leukemia; it is usually intracerebral and less often subdural or subarachnoid. It may occur in a single site or be multifocal. Intracranial hemorrhage may be massive and result in significant neurologic compromise, causing or contributing to death in 10 to 20 percent of leukemic patients. It may instead be small, subclinical, and diagnosed only on computed tomography or magnetic resonance imaging scans or at autopsy.

"Spontaneous" intracranial hemorrhage occurs most often in the setting of blast crisis, usually with a total white blood cell count of greater than 100,000/mm^3. This is associated more commonly with acute myelocytic than with acute lymphocytic leukemia, and probably results from direct vascular infiltration by leukemic cells. Intracranial hemorrhage also occurs in the setting of several associated problems: (1) thrombocytopenia, usually with a platelet count of less than 25,000/mm^3, associated with either leukemic bone marrow replacement or as a result of chemotherapy; (2) disseminated intravascular coagulation, most frequently seen in promyelocytic leukemia or associated with sepsis; (3) septic or nonseptic embolic hemorrhagic infarcts; and (4) specific infections such as *Aspergillus* commonly present with hemorrhagic lesions.

Spinal subdural and/or subarachnoid hemorrhage is a rare complication of leukemia, usually associated with diagnostic or therapeutic lumbar puncture in patients with platelet counts less than 50,000/mm^3. Platelet transfusion during and following lumbar puncture may be helpful in avoiding this complication. When it occurs, the condition is typically self-limited, though may occasionally require surgical intervention in order to prevent long-term neurologic compromise.

Ischemia/Infarction

Cerebral ischemia and infarction occurs in patients with leukemia as a result of either arterial or venous thrombosis, and may present with single, multifocal, or diffuse lesions. Typically, patients present with focal neurologic deficits referable to the involved brain region, though in some settings, patients may have more global cerebral dysfunction. Recognizing the particular clinical syndrome and associated etiology can direct appropriate therapy and prevent additional neurologic injury.

Ischemia may result directly from stasis and hypercoaguability in the setting of a significantly elevated white blood cell count. Patients with leukemia are also prone to develop small vessel thrombosis in the setting of disseminated intravascular coagulation, and typically present with fluctuating global encephalopathy or multifocal neurologic signs. Disseminated intravascular coagulation may be difficult to diagnose early in the course, as the patient may initially have normal measurable coagulation profiles; with strong clinical suspicion and serial coagulation studies, this diagnosis may be confirmed and then effectively treated with heparin anticoagulation. Cerebral infarction also results from septic embolic events (most often secondary to fungal infection such as *Aspergillus*) and, less commonly, nonseptic emboli. Embolic infarcts present clinically with focal neurologic deficits or seizures.

Cortical vein thrombosis resulting in venous infarcts (and sometimes hemorrhage) occurs as a result of leukemia-induced venous stasis, or following treatment with L-asparaginase chemotherapy, which results in the depletion of plasma proteins. Treatment of cortical vein thrombosis is controversial, but heparin anticoagulation is probably indicated if hemorrhage is not present. Replacement of plasma proteins with fresh frozen plasma has also been advocated in patients treated with L-asparaginase.

TREATMENT-RELATED NEUROLOGIC COMPLICATIONS

Neurologic complications of both radiotherapy and chemotherapy is discussed in detail in Chapters 169 and 170. Some of the vascular complications that result from chemotherapy-induced thrombocytopenia or L-asparaginase-induced thrombosis have already been discussed, and neurologic infections occurring in immunocompromised hosts are covered elsewhere. Highlighted here are some of the specific toxicities related to treatment of leukemia. These can be categorized as either acute/subacute or delayed/chronic complications affecting the brain or spinal cord, and result from radiotherapy, intrathecal or systemic chemotherapy, or combination therapy.

Acute/Subacute

Acutely, cranial irradiation is usually well tolerated without significant toxicity, except for mild fatigue, headache, and nausea occurring in some patients. Subacute radiation injury is more common, and typically presents with a "somnolence syndrome" sometimes with associated irritability, anorexia, and ataxia, developing a few weeks to months after finishing treatment. The pathophysiology is thought to be demyelinating, and is usually reversible within a few weeks. Corticosteroids may limit the severity and duration of this syndrome. A similar reversible subacute myelopathy may develop following spinal irradiation, often presenting with posterior column dysfunction and Lhermitte sign.

The most common neurotoxicity associated with intrathecal chemotherapy is chemical meningitis. Mild cases are often asymptomatic; symptomatic patients develop headache, fever, nausea, and meningismus usually within 12 hours of treatment. The CSF profile, with elevated protein and granulocytic pleocytosis, may be difficult to distinguish from bacterial meningitis. This is generally a self-limited condition without long-term sequelae.

Myelopathy is an uncommon acute complication of intrathecal chemotherapy with either methotrexate or cytosine arabinoside. Patients present with back pain, leg weakness, numbness, and incontinence, usually within a few hours of drug administration. Elevated CSF myelin basic protein in some patients treated with cytosine arabinoside has suggested that the initial event in the pathogenesis may be demyelination. Rare pathologic examinations have demonstrated noninflammatory necrosis of the spinal cord. The outcome of this condition is variable; some patients experience complete recovery, whereas others are left with significant neurologic dysfunction.

High-dose systemic chemotherapies may also have acute cerebral toxicity. Both high-dose methotrexate and cytosine arabinoside can cause a reversible syndrome of diffuse encephalopathy characterized by somnolence, confusion, or seizures, usually occurring within a few hours of treatment, though rarely it may be delayed for a few weeks. Subsequent doses of high-dose chemotherapy do not necessarily precipitate the same syndrome. It is more typical for high-dose cytosine arabinoside to cause a pancerebellar syndrome, presenting as ataxia, dysarthria, and nystagmus. Although it is unpredictable in which patients this uncommon syndrome will occur, the incidence is dose-dependent and perhaps occurs more commonly in older patients. The cerebellar dysfunction may be mild and transient, or have devastating permanent neurologic sequelae.

When cranial irradiation is combined with intrathecal methotrexate, very rare patients have been reported to develop, within hours of initial treatment, acute and severe encephalopathy with obtundation, seizures, and increased intracranial pressure. Although usually reversible, in severe cases, patients have progressed to coma or even death.

Delayed/Chronic

More common and troublesome than the acute and subacute neurologic complications of leukemia treatment are the delayed and chronic complications that can lead to a spectrum of disorders manifested by mild cognitive dysfunction at one extreme, to significant morbidity and long-term neurologic dysfunction or death at the other. Computed tomography and magnetic resonance imaging studies have demonstrated radiological abnormalities in as many as one-half of long-term survivors of leukemia, which may or may not represent clinically evident pathology. Radiologic findings include diffuse atrophy, white-matter T2-weighted hyperintensities that in many patients appear to improve over time, and gray-matter calcifications that may become more apparent over time. Radiologic abnormalities are significantly more prevalent in patients who have received cranial irradiation or combination radiotherapy and chemotherapy than in those who have received chemotherapy alone.

Cranial irradiation alone can cause cognitive decline or dementia, or result in areas of frank brain necrosis, typically delayed for months or years following therapy. The degree of late radiation effects is related to the age of the patient, and to the total dose and fractionation schedule. The mean overall intelligence quotient in irradiated children is 10 to 15 points lower than that of their siblings, or of children with leukemia who do not receive radiation.

When combined with intrathecal methotrexate cranial irradiation can precipitate potentially the most devastating neurologic complication encountered in this group of patients—necrotizing leukoencephalopathy. The incidence of necrotizing leukoencephalopathy appears to be much greater when methotrexate is administered concurrent with or following radiotherapy, and is much less when given prior to radiotherapy. It is rarely encountered in patients who have received a total radiation dose of less than 2,000 cGy. Usually within 6 months of completing treatment, patients present with lethargy, irritability, focal deficits, and seizures. The outcome is variable, with some patients stabilizing or improving, and others progressing to obtundation, coma, and death. Pathologically, the white-matter lesions demonstrate demyelination, axonal degeneration, and noninflammatory coagulative necrosis. Recognition of this complication in its severe form has prompted revision of treatment protocols for CNS prophylaxis, so that most patients are no longer treated with both cranial radiotherapy and intrathecal methotrexate prophylactically.

Patients treated with cranial irradiation may also develop a late complication confined to the gray matter, referred to pathologically as mineralizing microangiopathy. It is characterized by injury to the walls of the microvasculature with thrombosis and calcification. The role of chemotherapy in precipitating this condition is unknown. As in the other delayed radiation complications, younger children are more prone to this complication than older children or adults. The typical presentation is a focal neurologic deficit or seizures, usually milder than the syndrome associated with leukoencephalopathy.

Another common delayed treatment-related complication in long-term survivors of leukemia is hypothalamic-pituitary dysfunction. In children, growth retardation can occur as a result both of growth hormone deficiency and of the direct effects of radiation on the axial skeleton. Long-term survivors, especially those treated with radiotherapy, are also prone to develop CNS malignancies, including meningiomas and malignant gliomas.

SUGGESTED READINGS

Barcos M, Lane W, Gomez GA et al: An autopsy study of 1206 acute and chronic leukemias (1958 to 1982). Cancer 60:827–37, 1987
Bleyer WA: Biology and pathogenesis of CNS leukemia. Am J Pediatr Hematol/Oncol 11:57–63, 1989
Bleyer WA: Central nervous system leukemia. Pediatr Clin North Am 35:789–814, 1988
Brinch L, Evensen SA, Stavem P: Leukemia in the central nervous system. Acta Med Scand 224:173–8, 1988
Clark AW, Cohen SR, Nissenblatt MJ, Wilson SK: Paraplegia following intrathecal chemotherapy. Cancer 50.42–7, 1982
Collins RC, Al-Mondhiry H, Chernik NL, Posner JB: Neurologic manifestations of intravascular coagulation in patients with cancer. A clinicopathologic analysis of 12 cases. Neurology 25:795–806, 1975
Crosley CJ, Rorke BL, Evans A, Nigro M: Central nervous system lesions in childhood leukemia. Neurology 28:678–85, 1978
Feinberg WM, Swenson MR: Cerebrovascular complications of ι-asparaginase therapy. Neurology 38:127–33, 1988
Hansen PB, Kjeldsen L, Dahlhoff K, Olesen B: Cerebrospinal fluid beta-2-microglobulin in adult patients with acute leukemia or lymphoma: a useful marker in early diagnosis and monitoring of CNS-involvement. Acta Neurol Scand 85:224–7, 1992
Mulhern RK, Friedman AG, Stone PA: Neuropsychological status of children with acute lymphoblastic leukemia treated for central nervous system relaspe. Am J Pediatr Hematol/Oncol 11:106–13, 1989
Ochs JJ: Neurotoxicity due to central nervous system therapy for childhood leukemia. Am J Pediatr Hematol/Oncol 11:93–105, 1989
Price RA, Johnson WW: The central nervous system in childhood leukemia: I. The arachnoid. Cancer 31:520–33, 1973
Price RA, Jamieson PA: The central nervous system in childhood leukemia. II. Subacute leukoencephalopathy. Cancer 35:306–18, 1975
Walker RW: Neurologic complications of leukemia. Neurologic Clinics 9:989–99, 1991

176. NEUROLOGIC COMPLICATION OF LUNG CANCER

MICHAEL L. GRUBER

Primary cancer of the lung is the leading cause of cancer death for both men and women in the United States. The American Cancer Society projected 170,000 new lung cancer cases and 146,000 deaths for 1993, accounting for 18 percent of new cancers in men and 12 percent in women. The 5-year survival rate is reported to be 5 percent for stage 2 and 3 disease and 30 to 50 percent for stage 1.

Non-small cell lung cancers are the most common primary lung tumors and include adenocarcinomas and large cell anaplastic and epidermoid cell types (Table 176-1). Adenocarcinoma is the most common non-small cell lung cancer, and its incidence appears to be increasing. Small cell lung cancer accounts for approximately 25 percent of primary lung neoplasms and is generally nonresectable at the time of diagnosis. Non-

TABLE 176-1. Relative Incidence and Tendency to Metastasize of Primary Lung Cancers

Histologic Type	Incidence (% of All Primary Lung Cancers or % of All Non-Small Cell Primary Lung Cancers)	Percent With Metastasis at Diagnosis
Small cell	15–25	70
Non-small cell	75–85	
Adenocarcinoma	40	40
Epidermoid cell	30	17
Large cell	15	14

small cell lung cancer is more likely to be localized when discovered.

Table 176-2 summarizes the possible neurologic complications of lung cancer. The most common of these complications are the result of metastases to the brain, spinal cord, epidural space, and the leptomeninges. Metastases to more than one site in the central nervous system occurs in 20 percent of patients. Nonmetastatic neurologic complications include metabolic encephalopathy, infection, cerebrovascular events, symptoms due to organ failure and/or complications of therapy, and paraneoplastic disorders.

LOCAL INVASION

Local invasion in the thorax can result in compression of the recurrent laryngeal nerve, causing hoarseness, paralysis of the phrenic nerve, (producing elevation of the hemidiaphragm and dyspnea), and a Horner syndrome caused by sympathetic nerve involvement.

Pancoast syndrome is seen in 3 percent of lung cancer patients. Tumor in the superior sulcus erodes bone and compresses the lower portion of the brachial plexus. The eighth cervical nerve and the first two thoracic nerves are usually affected. This can result in posterior shoulder pain that radiates to the medial aspect of the arm and the fourth and fifth fingers. Numbness of the medial side of the arm, forearm, and hand and weakness and atrophy of the hand may develop. If the stellate ganglion is also involved, a Horner syndrome is noted. At times, in previously irradiated patients, symptoms of lower brachial plexus dysfunction are seen. The issue is whether the new symptoms are due to tumor recurrence or radiation plexopathy. In radiation-induced plexopathy, pain is not a prominent feature, Horner syndrome is uncommon, and the upper plexus appears

TABLE 176-2. Neurologic Complications of Lung Cancer

Local invasion
  Recurrent laryngeal nerve paralysis
  Phrenic nerve paralysis
  Sympathetic nerve paralysis
  Brachial plexus involvement—Pancoast syndrome
Complications of metastasis to:
  Brain
  Spinal cord
  Epidural space
  Leptomeninges
Nonmetastatic complications
  Metabolic/endocrine
  Cerebrovascular
  Central nervous system infections
  Side effects of treatment
  Paraneoplastic syndrome

to more involved. A magnetic resonance imaging (MRI) scan of the brachial plexus is the diagnostic procedure of choice.

BRAIN METASTASES

Primary lung cancer is the most common cause of brain metastasis, accounting for half of all cases. Small cell lung cancer is more likely to metastazise to the brain than non-small cell lung cancer. The apparent increase in the incidence of brain metastases is in large part due to the rising incidence of lung cancer. The brain is frequently the first site of recurrence and may be the only site of metastatic disease. Clinically manifested brain metastases occur in 25 to 30 percent of lung cancer patients. This is usually seen at the time of systemic relapse, but in 20 percent of patients, neurologic symptoms precede the discovery of the lung cancer. When the primary cancer is unknown and the patient presents with brain metastases, over one-half will eventually prove to have a primary lung tumor. Lung cancer spreads to the brain by hematogenous dissemination through the cerebral arterial circulation. The location of the deposits is related to the blood supply, with 80 percent of lesions ocurring in the cerebral hemispheres (usually at the gray and white matter junction), 17 percent in the cerebellum, and 3 percent in the brainstem.

The clinical presentation of brain metastasis is usually subacute, developing over days or weeks (Table 176-3). Headache is the most common symptom and focal weakness and change in mental status are the most frequent signs. In 2 to 5 percent of cases, an encephalopathy with depressed mood, agitation, decreased memory, and confusion is seen. Visual field loss, ataxia, and aphasia frequently occur. Seizures may herald the diagnosis in 15 percent of patients. Intratumoral hemorrhage and tumor embolus can result in the abrupt onset of neurologic symptoms that at times can resemble a stroke.

The number of metastatic brain tumors is best determined by a contrast-enhanced brain MRI scan. The lesions appear as solid or cystic masses that enhance with gadolinium and are surrounded by an area of peritumoral edema. In approximately 50 percent of cases, there is a single metastatic deposit in the brain. Surgical resection of a solitary brain metastasis followed by whole-brain radiotherapy is now the accepted treatment for patients with controlled primary disease. This approach has improved both survival and quality of life. When the diagnosis of lung cancer and a solitary brain metastasis is synchronous, surgical treatment of both tumors may result in a better outcome and, in some cases, a cure.

An alternative diagnosis needs to be considered in the setting of a known primary lung neoplasm and a solitary brain mass. Approximately 11 percent of cancer patients with a single brain lesion did not have a metastastatic tumor. One-half of these patients had potentially reversible infectious or inflammatory

TABLE 176-3. Symptoms and Signs of Brain Metastasis

Symptoms	% of Cases	Signs	% of Cases
Headache	53	Hemiparesis	66
Focal weakness	40	Impaired cognition	77
Mental/behavioral	31	Unilateral sensory loss	27
Seizures	15	Papilledema	26
Ataxia	20	Ataxia	24
Aphasia	10	Aphasia	19

(From Posner JB: Management of central nervous system metastases. Semin Oncol 4:81–91, 1977, with permission.)

conditions and the other one-half had astrocytomas. When aggressive therapy is considered, tissue should be obtained for a definitive pathologic diagnosis.

The management of brain metastses is evolving with improvement in the control of the primary disease, better imaging techniques, and more aggressive treatment. Surgical resection of multiple metastatic deposits (two or three) can be accomplished safely in a patient with controlled systemic disease and a high Karnofsky performance score. Resection of a large symptomatic tumor can be life-saving even when other lesions are present, and may provide the time that is necessary to treat the remaining tumors.

Stereotactic radiosurgery refers to a single high-dose radiation treatment to a small-volume target (<3 cm in diameter), using either a linear accelerator or the Leksell γ knife unit. This allows for a precise and very effective delivery of ablative radiation to the metastatic tumor, sparing normal brain tissue. The local control rate is more than 85 percent in most series. The majority of patients were able to discontinue or reduce their dependence on corticosteroid medication. Radiosurgery may offer reduced operative and neurologic morbidity for small lesions that are not located in eloquent areas. In a subset of patients (25 to 35 percent) whose performance status is good and who have controlled local disease and one to three brain lesions, surgery and/or stereotactic radiosurgery followed by whole-brain radiotherapy can extend survival and improve quality of life.

Palliative treatment is reserved for patients with poor Karnofsky performance scores, multiple lesions, or advanced systemic disease. Corticosteroids, anticonvulsants, and whole-brain radiotherapy (30 Gy/10 days) benefits 75 percent of those treated, resulting in a median survival of 3 to 4 months, with 10 to 15 percent of patients living 1 year. Whole-brain radiotherapy schedules are best determined by prognosis. Patients with a more favorable outlook (small cell lung cancer) should be treated with smaller fractions over a longer interval (40 Gy/4 weeks) to avoid radiation injury (dementia, endocrinopathy).

Small cell lung cancer patients who are complete responders (10 percent of patients) to initial therapy are often offered prophylactic cranial irradiation in the hope of decreasing the high incidence of brain metastases that is reported to occur in as many as 80 percent of patients living 2 or more years. However, there is no increase in survival in those treated.

Chemotherapy is investigative and is generally used when surgery and radiation fail. There are reports of patients with small cell lung cancer and brain metastases who have had excellent reponses to the chemotherapeutic agents commonly employed in the treatment of the the primary lung tumor.

SPINAL CORD METASTASES

Lung cancer, responsible for 50 percent of intramedullary spinal cord metastases, is seen clinically in 1 percent of patients. The disease is rapidly progressive and is almost always associated with sensory symptoms or signs (sensory level, spine or radicular pain) and weakness. A contast-enhanced MRI scan is the diagnostic procedure of choice. Radiotherapy may relieve symptoms and prolong life.

EPIDURAL SPINAL CORD COMPRESSION

Metastases to the epidural space surrounding the spinal cord and cauda equina is the second most common neurologic com-

plication of systemic cancer. There are approximately 18,000 new cases of epidural spinal cord compression annually in the United States. In most patients, the tumor metastasizes to the vertebral body or neural arch and extends anteriorly to compress the spinal cord or cauda equina. Lung cancer is the most common cause for epidural spinal cord compression in most series. It is more likely than other malignancies to present with spinal symptoms as the initial manifestation of the disease and generally is seen in the first 6 months. Compression occurs most frequently at the thoracic level (70 percent), then lumbar (20 percent), and least often in the cervical area (10 percent). In 20 percent of cases, there are multiple areas of involvement. Therefore, a MRI scan of the entire spine is the diagnostic study of choice. When MRI imaging is not an option, a complete myelogram should be done.

Back pain is the presenting symptom in more than 90 percent of cases and must be differentiated from the pain of degenerative arthritis. Radicular pain helps localize the level of involvement. Most patients have pain for weeks before neurologic symptoms develop. Once weakness occurs, there is a rapid progession to paraplegia with little likelihood (<5 percent) of reversibility. Therefore, prompt investigation is required in the cancer patient with back pain.

Emergency treatment consists of high-dose steroids (100 mg/day dexamethasone for 72 hours and then taper) and external beam radiotherapy. In patients whose primary disease is controlled, surgery, including vertebral body resection, tumor removal, and stabilization of the spine, should be considered. Laminectomy has little to offer, given the anterior location of the pathology. Radiotherapy is the initial treatment provided in neurologically intact patients (see Ch. 167).

CARCINOMATOUS MENINGITIS

Leptomeningeal or ''carcinomatous'' meningitis is less common than brain metastases or epidural spinal cord compression. There is widespread infiltration of the meninges, with a predilection for the cisterns, sylvian and hippocampal fissures, and the cauda equina. This results in symptoms and signs that reflect involvement of multiple sites in the nervous system. Altered mental status, headache, cranial nerve dysfunction, and radicular pain of cervical or lumbosacral origins are described alone or in combination. The diagnosis should be considered when multiple levels of the neuraxis are involved. Adenocarcinoma of lung and small cell lung cancer are the more common primary tumors that invade the meninges, ocurring in 2 to 3 percent of patients.

The presence of malignant cells in the cerebrospinal fluid (CSF) is diagnostic. The yield from the first CSF cytology is 50 percent but is over 90 percent after the third spinal tap. It is important to collect an adequate sample (6 to 10 ml) and deliver the CSF to the cytologist promptly. A contrast-enhanced brain scan may demonstrate enhancement of the meninges, parenchymal metastases (40 percent of cases), and hydrocephalus in one-half of patients. Biopsy of the leptomeninges should be considered when the CSF cytology is negative and a definitive diagnosis is required.

Treatment generally consists of irradiating the symptomatic area and administering chemotherapy via either an Ommaya reservoir or intrathecal injection. High-dose intravenous methotrexate followed by calcium leucovorin rescue is a consideration when CSF flow is compromised or nodular deposits are identified. The median survival of patients who have leptomeningeal metastases and lung cancer is 2 to 4 months, with 10 to 15 percent living 1 year (see Ch. 168).

NONMETASTATIC COMPLICATIONS

Of the nonmetastatic complications of lung cancer, metabolic encephalopathy is the most common and is usually due to multiple abnormalities rather than a single etiology. Abnormalities of fluid and electrolyte balance, hypercalcemia, and hepatic failure are the most frequent. The earliest symptom is change in mental status, which can be subtle at onset and then progress rapidly to stupor and coma. Asterixis, tremor, and myoclonus are often seen in this setting. Medications that sedate or alter mood should be stopped. Wernicke's encephalopathy is a consideration in some patients and thiamine should be provided empirically.

The syndrome of inappropriate secretion of antidiuretic hormone is reported in 11 percent of small cell lung cancer patients. This is related to the presence of neurosecretory granules and other structures that allow for the synthesis of hormones, biogenic amines, and a variety of growth factors. This may lead to confusion and seizures.

Cerebrovascular lesions are reported to occur in 15 percent of patients at autopsy. Marantic or nonbacterial thrombotic endocarditis is the most common cause of brain infarction in the cancer patient. It is seen most commonly with adenocarcinoma of the lung. On postmortem examination, sterile vegetations are present on the heart valves; these embolize and occlude small and medium-size cerebral arteries. Multiple infarctions are described, some being hemorrhagic. The presentation can mimic a cerebral infarction in one-third of patients, but more often will present with either a nonfocal encephalopathic picture or evidence of multiple-vessel involvement. Transesophageal echocardiography will identify the valvular vegetations. The use of heparin remains controversial.

Disseminated intravascular coagulation is seen in both small cell and non-small cell lung cancer. Occlusion of small vessels by fibrin emboli causes an encephalopathy with seizures and transient focal signs. Laboratory findings include thrombocytopenia, decresed fibrinogen, elevated fibrin split products, and the presence of D-dimer. The prothrombin and partial thromboplastin times are prolonged. Anticoagulation may benefit some patients. Disseminated intravascular coagulation is usually seen in the final stages of the illness.

Other cerebrovascular complications of lung cancer include hemorrhagic brain metastases, ruptured neoplastic aneurysm, superior sagittal sinus thrombosis, and subdural hematoma. Complications of cancer treatment include nervous system injury from radiotherapy, direct toxicity of chemotherapeutic agents, and infectious complications that are most often the result of treatment-induced myelosuppression.

PARANEOPLASTIC SYNDROMES

Paraneoplastic syndromes seen in lung cancer include limbic encephalitis, opsoclonus-myoclonus, retinopathy, brainstem encephalitis, subacute cerebellar degeneration, necrotizing myelopathy, subacute sensory neuronopathy, Lambert-Eaton syndrome, and dermatomyositis. Small cell lung cancer is more frequently associated with these syndromes. Many of these patients have the anti-Hu antibody. It is important to remember that paraneoplastic syndromes are very uncommon and may antedate the discovery of the tumor in one-half of cases. There-

fore, it is imperative to search for evidence of metastatic disease (see Ch. 171).

SUGGESTED READINGS

Adler Jr et al: Stereotactic radiosurgical treatment of brain metastases. J Neurosurg 76:444–9, 1992

Byrne TN: Spinal cord compression from epidural metastases. N Engl J Med 327:614–19, 1992

Coffey RJ et al: Radiosurgery for solitary metastases. Int J Radiat Oncol 20:1287–95, 1991

Graus F, Rogers LR, Posner JB: Cerebrovascular complications in patients with cancer Medicine (Baltimore). 64:16–35, 1985

Kelly P et al: Results of computed tomography based computer-assisted stereotactic resection of metastatic intracranial tumors. J Neurosurg 22:7–17, 1988

Kristjansen P: Should current management of SCLC include prophylactic cranial irradiation. Lung Cancer 10 (Suppl. 1):319–29, 1994

Loeffler JS et al: The treatment of recurrent brain metastases with stereotactic

Patchell RA et al: A randomized trial of surgery in the treatment of single metastases to the brain. N Engl J Med 322:494–500, 1990

Posner JB: Surgery for metastases to the brain. N Engl J Med 322:544–5, 1990

Posner J: Management of central nervous system metastases. Semin Oncol 4:81–91, 1977

Smalley SR et al: Resection for solitary brain metastasis. J Neurosurg 77:531–40, 1992

Sundaresan N et al: Treatment of neoplastic spinal cord compression. Neurosurgery 29:645, 1991

177. NEUROLOGIC COMPLICATIONS OF BREAST CANCER

LLOYD M. ALDERSON
JOHN W. HENSON

Breast cancer is diagnosed in over 150,000 women each year in the United States, making it the most common malignant neoplasm in women. One-third of patients with breast cancer will ultimately develop metastatic complications, often involving the nervous system. Focal infiltration or compression of neural structures by malignant cells is the most common mechanism, but nonmetastatic and treatment-related complications are also frequently seen. Most neurologic manifestations appear in patients with advanced systemic disease. However, since the median survival of patients with metastatic breast cancer is long (2 to 3 years), the early recognition and aggressive treatment of potentially disabling nervous system complications is crucial to preserving the quality of life. This chapter discusses the clinical presentation, diagnosis, and treatment of the neurologic manifestations of breast cancer. Although many of these issues are common to other cancers, this chapter emphasizes those aspects unique to cancer of the breast.

BRAIN METASTASES

Brain metastases are the most common neurologic complication of breast cancer, arising in 25 percent of all patients with metastatic disease. Among the cancers that frequently metastasize to brain, breast is second only to lung as a primary site. Patients with infiltrating ductal histology and patients who are younger (less than 55 years) are at the highest risk of brain metastases. It is rare for brain lesions to be the presenting sign of undiagnosed breast cancer.

Brain metastases arise from tumor cells that travel through the arterial circulation, and thus their distribution reflects the anatomy of the circulatory system of the brain. Lesions most commonly arise near the surface of the brain in the distal fields of the internal carotid arteries. Although the brainstem is an unusual site for metastases, recent magnetic resonance imaging (MRI)-based studies suggest that the incidence of cerebellar lesions is higher in patients with breast cancer than in patients with other carcinomas. As with other malignancies, brain metastases in patients with breast cancer are frequently multiple; only one-half of patients presenting with brain metastases will have a single lesion.

The symptoms of brain metastases from breast cancer usually develop over weeks. Cerebral hemisphere metastases can produce headache, hemiparesis, seizures, or language disturbance. Confusion, apathy, depression, and visual field defects often go unrecognized as symptoms of cerebral metastases located in less eloquent areas of the brain or of multiple small metastases. In the posterior fossa, metastases cause occipital headache, ataxia, nausea, vomiting, nystagmus, and diplopia.

When a brain metastasis is suspected, the diagnostic study of choice is a gadolinium-enhanced MRI, which is more sensitive for small lesions than enhanced computed tomography (CT). Lesions typically appear round with thick ring enhancement and edema infiltrating the surrounding white matter. Hemorrhage into a brain metastasis from breast cancer is uncommon.

In patients with breast cancer who have a single brain lesion and limited-stage systemic disease, etiologies other than metastases have to be considered. In 10% of patients with breast cancer and an enhancing brain lesion who undergo biopsy or resection, the diagnosis of metastasis will be incorrect. Meningioma is associated with breast cancer and should be considered when a brain lesion appears to be dural based. When meningiomas do develop in patients with breast cancer, metastasis into the meningioma is a well-described phenomenon. Venous and arterial infarctions are also associated with breast cancer (see below) and can present as an enhancing parenchymal brain lesion.

Patients with newly diagnosed brain metastases from breast cancer often benefit from the administration of glucocorticoids. Dexamethasone (4 mg every 6 hours) can give dramatic symptomatic improvement by reducing the edema that surrounds the lesion. The chronic administration of high doses of dexamethasone (more than 8 mg/day) significantly increases the risk of morbidity from side effects; therefore, the dose should be tapered in the weeks following diagnosis. However, some patients will experience neurologic deterioration even with small reductions in the dose of glucocorticoid and may remain steroid-dependent.

Anticonvulsants should be administered to patients who develop seizures. For those patients who do not present with seizures, anticonvulsants should be withheld until needed. Phenytoin is the anticonvulsant of choice because of its efficacy, ease of management and low cost. Physicians should be aware of an increased risk of Stevens-Johnson syndrome in patients who are receiving phenytoin during radiotherapy. Valproic acid, carbamezapine, and phenobarbitol are also effective anticonvulsants, but the latter may produce unacceptable sedation. It is important to monitor drug levels regularly, particularly during chemotherapy or changes in tamoxifen dose. Patients with hypoalbuminemia may experience symptoms of toxicity even when anticonvulsant levels are within the therapeutic range.

Radiation, surgery, and chemotherapy have all been used effectively in combination or alone in the treatment of brain metastases from breast cancer. Radiotherapy to the whole brain is recommended for the majority of patients with brain metastases. It provides symptomatic improvement in many patients and significantly prolongs patient survival. Radiation is administered either in 3-Gy fractions to a total of 30 Gy over 10 to 14 days, or in 2-Gy fractions to 40 Gy over 4 weeks.

Although the benefit of surgery in patients with radioresistant metastases has been convincingly demonstrated, its benefit in patients with breast cancer is less clear. However, in patients with one or two brain lesions and limited or indolent systemic disease, resection of brain lesions can result in long-term local control of disease, may result in significant improvement in neurologic defects, and can help to control seizures. Surgical resection may also be indicated in the patient with symptomatic progression of brain metastases following radiotherapy. Following surgical removal of the lesion, whole-brain radiotherapy should be administered.

A recent development in the therapy of brain metastases is stereotactic radiosurgery. In this technique, a radiation source is precisely focused to deliver a single dose of 9 to 25 Gy to a sharply defined region of the brain. The indications for radiosurgery are similar to those for surgery. Like surgical resection, radiosurgery provides local control in 85 to 95 percent of treated metastases while avoiding the risks associated with general anesthesia and craniotomy. With this procedure, there is a small risk the patient will require surgical evacuation of necrotic material 3 to 12 months after treatment, and the risk of severe radionecrosis limits this technique to lesions that are 3 cm or less in diameter.

Unlike most malignancies, breast cancer metastases in the brain often respond to chemotherapy. This is particularly important for the patient with a recurrent or progressive brain lesion who has already received maximum radiotherapy. Uncontrolled studies using a variety of protocols in highly selected patients have demonstrated complete or partial responses in over 50 percent. Those patients who respond can often be identified after the second course of chemotherapy.

SPINAL CORD COMPRESSION

Breast cancer is the most common primary tumor causing spinal cord compression. Tumor cells travel through the blood to the vertebral bodies, and spinal cord compression occurs when the tumor extends beyond the bone into the spinal canal, displacing the thecal sac. Metastatic deposits in the vertebral lamina or pedicle are less common but can also be the origin of epidural disease. Another important etiology of spinal cord compression is mechanical deformity of the spinal column associated with vertebral body collapse following replacement of bone by metastatic tumor.

Pain is the initial symptom in 95 percent of patients with cord compression and precedes the diagnosis by at least 1 week in the majority of patients. The pain is midline and localized to the spinal segment involved and there may be a radicular component. Localized back pain is usually dull and constant and is often more marked with bedrest. This is in contrast to back pain associated with most nonmalignant conditions, which improves with rest. Radicular pain can be sharp and exacerbated by movement. Motor symptoms usually follow pain by several weeks and the presence of weakness indicates an advanced degree of spinal cord compression. Weakness typically begins in the proximal lower extremities and is associated with hyperactive deep tendon reflexes and an extensor plantar response. These abnormal reflexes are important to help differentiate spinal cord compression from other causes of weakness such as steroid-induced myopathy, in which reflexes and plantar responses are normal. Sensory symptoms include numbness and paresthesias. A sensory level should be sought, as this finding helps to confirm the spinal cord as the site of neurologic injury. Bowel or bladder dysfunction is a late finding in patients with spinal cord compression, but it can be the presenting symptom when there is compression of the conus medullaris from a lesion arising in vertebral bodies T10–L1. With epidural compression of the conus medullaris or cauda equina, urinary retention is often accompanied by flaccid paralysis of both legs, low back pain radiating into the rectum, and perianal anesthesia. It is important to evaluate patients suspected of having spinal cord compression for the presence of bladder distention secondary to urinary retention. With sensory loss, patients may be unaware of urinary retention, and a history of frequent small voidings may be the only clue that bladder catheterization is needed.

Any patient with cancer who develops back pain should be considered to have spinal cord compression until it is proven otherwise. When cord compression is suspected, imaging of the spine must proceed with urgency. Plain films can be useful to identify involved vertebrae. A loss of vertical height in a vertebral body of greater than 50 percent or the loss of a pedicle strongly suggest epidural spinal cord compression. However, MRI or myelography is required to define the distribution and severity of disease. MRI is the study of choice, but myelography should be employed if a good-quality MRI cannot be obtained. MRI will define compression of the thecal sac and displacement of the cord as well as help define bony lesions, paraspinal disease, and intramedullary spinal cord tumors. Whether MRI or myelography is used, the entire spinal column must be examined in the initial study. Approximately 80 percent of patients with spinal cord compression will have vertebral metastases distant from the point of compression, and as many as 15 percent of patients with cord compression will have synchronous epidural metastases.

Corticosteroids are useful in the immediate management of spinal cord compression. An intravenous bolus of 96 mg dexamethasone, given at the time the diagnosis is suspected, followed by 96 mg/day in four divided doses over the following 3 days, is recommended. The drug can then be tapered over the following 2 weeks. Radiation is the principle therapy for most patients with breast cancer and spinal cord compression and should be initiated within 8 to 12 hours of making the diagnosis. In the majority of patients, radiation will maintain or improve neurologic function and provide control of pain. Radiation is administered as a 3- to 5-Gy fraction in each of the first 3 days, followed by 2 Gy daily to a total dose of 40 Gy. The treatment is given through a single posterior port that includes two vertebral bodies above and below the point of compression.

Although most patients with breast cancer and spinal cord compression will respond to radiotherapy, surgery is indicated in some situations. In patients with limited-stage systemic disease and symptomatic spinal cord compression from metastatic involvement of a single vertebral body, surgical resection of the lesion followed by radiotherapy can result in long-term local control. Those patients for whom radiation has failed or who require stabilization of the spinal column may also need surgery. Finally, surgery may be indicated when spinal cord compression results from vertebral body collapse with posterior herniation of disc fragments into the spinal canal. In patients with inoperable cord compression who cannot be treated with additional radiation, chemotherapy can be effective, particularly in those with responsive systemic disease.

The most important determinant of neurologic outcome is the functional status of the patient at diagnosis. In a study of 56 patients with breast cancer and spinal cord compression treated with radiation, 89 percent had improvement in pain control, 60 percent of those with motor dysfunction improved, and 4 of 6 (67 percent) with bladder dysfunction improved. Patients who cannot walk at the time of diagnosis of spinal cord compression have a much smaller chance of significant neurologic improvement, emphasizing the need for the physician to be consistently vigilant for cord compression in patients with known breast cancer. However, even in paraplegic patients, radiation should be administered to maintain spinal stability and to control pain.

LEPTOMENINGEAL METASTASES

Malignant cells invade the cerebrospinal fluid (CSF) in approximately 5 percent of all patients with metastatic breast cancer. The incidence of leptomeningeal metastases from breast cancer may be rising, owing to longer survivals afforded by more effective systemic therapies. Malignant cells gain access to the leptomeninges primarily from the blood vessels surrounding the CSF space, but can also spread directly from brain or epidural metastases. Malignant cells can then disseminate throughout the neuraxis, infiltrating brain, spinal cord, and nerve roots and block CSF resorption, resulting in communicating hydrocephalus. Symptoms and signs of leptomeningeal metastasis are the result of direct infiltration of malignant cells into nerve tissue or interference with the blood supply.

The diagnosis of leptomeningeal metastasis is suggested by the clinical presentation of multifocal dysfunction along the neuraxis. Headache occurs in one-third of patients with leptomeningeal metastasis and is usually bifrontal. Mental status changes include lethargy, confusion, and memory loss. Fifteen percent of patients with the condition develop focal or generalized seizures. Other symptoms include nausea and vomiting, lightheadedness, and diabetes insipidus.

The clinical presentation of leptomeningeal metastasis often reflects the involvement of both cranial and spinal nerves. Diplopia and oculomotor palsies are the most common cranial nerve findings, occurring in 20 percent of patients with the condition. Facial weakness, hearing loss, loss of vision, facial numbness, and tongue weakness are also common. Involvement of the tenth cranial nerve can result in hoarseness and dysphagia and can lead to aspiration pneumonia. The majority of patients with leptomeningeal metastases will also have signs referable to a spinal root. Weakness of a lower extremity is more common than of the upper extremity, and most of these patients will have reflex asymmetry. Patients rarely complain of sensory symptoms, but paresthesias, sensory loss, or radicular pain can occur. Bowel and bladder dysfunction occur in approximately 10 percent of patients with leptomeningeal metastases.

Diagnosis is made by the identification of malignant cells in the CSF. Malignant cells are found in only one-half of initial cytologic studies from patients with leptomeningeal metastases, but the chance of a positive cytology with three examinations is approximately 80 percent. The less specific indices of elevated total protein, elevated opening pressure, and decreased glucose concentration are suggestive of leptomeningeal metastasis in the appropriate clinical setting. It is rare for a patient with leptomeningeal metastases to have a completely normal CSF. Tumor markers in the CSF of cancer patients suffer from low specificity, but if a marker has been shown to be secreted by the primary tumor of a particular patient, elevated levels in the CSF can be diagnostic in the absence of positive cytology, particularly if the concentration in the CSF exceeds that in the blood. CA 15-3 is a marker of tumor progression in some patients with breast cancer and can be useful in the diagnosis of leptomeningeal metastasis.

Untreated, the course of leptomeningeal metastasis is one of progressive neurologic disability and death in a few weeks. Unlike patients with lung cancer or melanoma, however, over one-half of patients with leptomeningeal metastasis from breast cancer will respond to therapy, and some patients survive many months after diagnosis. Intrathecal methotrexate and radiation are the primary therapies. Glucocorticoids can help relieve acute symptoms.

Methotrexate is administered in 12-mg doses in preservative-free saline directly into the CSF through a surgically placed ventricular catheter (Ommaya reservoir) or by lumbar puncture. With this dose of methotrexate, therapeutic concentrations will remain in the CSF for 36 to 48 hours. To prevent mucositis and myelosuppression, leukovorin (10 mg) is given every 12 hours for four doses starting 24 hours after treatment. CSF cytology, cell count, and total protein are obtained with each treatment to follow the response to therapy. Methotrexate is given two times weekly for 3 weeks followed by three weekly treatments and then monthly for 4 months. Cytosine arabinoside and thiotepa can also be administered intrathecally as second-line agents.

Radiotherapy should be administered to symptomatic and radiographically detected areas of leptomeningeal metastases. A total dose of 30 Gy to the involved area given over 2 weeks is commonly employed. Craniospinal radiation is rarely employed because of its toxicity to the bone marrow.

The survival of patients with breast cancer and leptomeningeal metastases is dependent on their response to therapy. Among patients treated with intrathecal methotrexate, the overall median survival is approximately 12 weeks, but in the 50 percent of patients whose disease responds to therapy (with a clearing of malignant cells from the CSF or a significant reduction in CSF protein), the median survival is longer than 6 months.

CRANIAL AND PERIPHERAL NEUROPATHY

Cranial Neuropathy

Breast cancer can cause cranial neuropathies by neural compression from metastases to the base of the skull. Breast cancer is by far the most common primary tumor to do this, accounting for 17 of 43 cases in one large study. Cranial neuropathy can also occur as a result of cranial radiation, but in this situation the neuropathy is usually bilateral and symmetric.

A skull base metastasis should be considered when cranial neuropathies can be attributed to a lesion in a single location. Orbital metastases can compress the optic nerve or extraocular muscles and result in pain, proptosis, blurred vision, and diplopia. Involvement of the cavernous sinus or parasellar region results in unilateral frontal headache with ocular paresis without proptosis. With metastases to the temporal bone adjacent to the middle cranial fossa, patients have numbness, paresthesias, and pain in the distribution of the second and third division of the trigeminal nerve. Mental neuropathy can result from metastases to the mandibular bone, and breast cancer is the most common primary tumor among patients with this problem. Ipsilateral hearing loss and facial weakness suggest that the petrous portion of the temporal bone is involved. Bone metastases to the region adjacent to the jugular foramen can present with hoarseness, dysphagia, and pain in the posterolateral pharynx. Finally, metastasis to the occipital condyle results in unilateral occipital and neck pain with weakness of the tongue and sternocleidomastoid.

The diagnosis of metastases to the skull is made with plain films, CT with bone windows, and radionuclide bone scan. Leptomeningeal metastases should also be considered, particularly when more than one cranial nerve is involved. The treatment for all of these lesions is focal radiation.

Brachial Plexopathy

Sensory and motor symptoms referable to the ipsilateral brachial plexus occur in one-half of all patients with breast cancer. Many of these patients will have undergone surgery and radiotherapy to the region of the chest wall overlying the brachial plexus, making it difficult to determine whether the symptoms are caused by tumor invasion, radiation-induced brachial plexopathy, or nerve damage at the time of surgery (postmastectomy pain syndrome) (Table 177-1).

Compression of the plexus by tumor has clinical features that distinguish it from other etiologies of upper extremity sensory and motor disturbances. Pain is the initial and dominant symptom in 80 percent of patients with tumor invasion of the plexus, with the pain preceding motor dysfunction by weeks to months. The pain typically involves the posterior aspect of the arm and the fourth and fifth fingers of the hand, consistent with involvement of the lower trunk of the plexus (C8 or T1). A palpable axillary mass is sometimes present and tumor may be visualized with MRI or CT imaging of the brachial plexus. Compression of the upper trunk (C5, C6) by metastatic tumor to the cervical lymph nodes is less common than lower trunk involvement in patients with breast cancer. In this case, pain is localized to the lateral shoulder, radial forearm, and thumb. Horner syndrome may occur secondary to compression of the paraspinal sympathetic nerves by metastatic tumor in the cervical region.

Diagnosis may require surgical exploration and biopsy of the plexus when tumor invasion is suspected but a mass cannot be demonstrated radiographically. An aggressive diagnostic approach is warranted in the patient who can be treated with radiotherapy to the involved area. The treatment of invasive plexopathy is focal radiation, and pain control improves with treatment in the majority of patients. Narcotic analgesics are also useful in the control of debilitating pain.

Radiation-induced brachial plexopathy occurs in 10 percent of patients receiving radiotherapy to the chest wall. In this condition, the nerves are compressed by radiation-induced fibrosis of the soft tissue surrounding the plexus. These changes are often accompanied by lymphedema in the affected arm. Unlike compressive plexopathy, the typical presenting symptom is paresthesias referable to involvement of the upper trunk or whole plexus. Lower trunk involvement alone is rare. Patients with weakness as the predominant initial symptom of plexopathy are much more likely to have radiation-induced brachial plexo-

TABLE 177-1. Etiology of Upper Extremity Pain in Patients With Breast Cancer

	Metastatic Plexopathy	Radiation Plexopathy	Postmastectomy Pain Syndrome
Initial symptoms	Aching, severe pain followed by weakness	Paresthesia and weakness	Burning and constricting pain
Distribution	Posterior arm and fourth and fifth digits	Shoulder, radial forearm	Chest wall
Magnetic resonance imaging/computed tomography	Axillary mass	Loss of tissue planes	Normal
Treatment	Radiation, analgesics	Analgesics, dorsal root entry zone ablation	Topical anesthetic, analgesics

pathy than metastatic plexopathy. Symptoms begin soon after radiotherapy is complete and patients who have received radiation fractions of 2 Gy or more—to a total dose of 60 Gy or more—are more likely to develop radiation-induced brachial plexopathy than patients who have received a lower dose. The diagnosis is supported by a CT or MRI study showing loss of the normal tissue planes in the area adjacent to the plexus. In both radiation-induced brachial plexopathy and metastatic plexopathy, electromyography shows motor and sensory neuropathy of axonal type, but myokimic discharges are more common in radiation-induced brachial plexopathy. However, electromyography is rarely a useful diagnostic test for these conditions. There is no effective therapy for radiation-induced brachial plexopathy, and two-thirds of patients will lose some function of the involved arm with time. Surgical lysis of fibrotic tissue has not been helpful, but surgical ablation of the dorsal root entry zone in affected dermatomes can ease the disabling pain that can accompany radiation-induced brachial plexopathy.

Patients with postmastectomy pain syndrome can also present with pain in the upper extremity. The pain results from interruption of the intercostal brachial nerve at the time of surgery. A neuroma develops in the severed nerve ending and may serve as a sensitive trigger point for the pain. Symptoms usually begin within 6 months of surgery, and the pain is typically described as a burning and constricting sensation in the posterior aspect of the arm and axilla, radiating across the anterior chest wall. The pain is often exacerbated by movement and improves with immobilization. Pain may respond to therapies given for other neuropathic pain syndromes (tricyclic antidepressants, anticonvulsants, analgesics, and transcutaneous electrical nerve stimulation [TENS]), and topical anesthetic agents such as capsaicin may also be effective.

Two less common etiologies of neuropathy in the upper extremity are cervical disc herniation and radiation-induced nerve sheath tumors. Disc herniation commonly affects the C7 root in isolation. Nerve sheath tumors can occur as a result of radiation to the chest wall, often with a latency of several years. They can be detected with MRI, but surgical exploration is usually required to make the diagnosis.

Peripheral nerves supplying the lower extremities are much less commonly affected by breast cancer than those supplying the upper extremities. Bone metastases to the pelvis and sacrum can compress the sacral plexus or adjacent nerves, particularly the sciatic nerve. When bilateral signs or urinary incontinence is present, a careful evaluation for compression of the cauda equina is indicated.

CEREBROVASCULAR COMPLICATIONS

Cerebrovascular complications are associated with a variety of malignancies, including cancer of the breast. Although the most common etiology of hemorrhagic or ischemic infarction in patients with cancer is atherosclerosis, the cancer itself can sometimes cause neurologic dysfunction through direct or indirect affects on the blood, the heart, or on the vessels. When stroke occurs in a patient with breast cancer, it can be due to one of the paraneoplastic cerebrovascular syndromes. The three most common of these are intravascular coagulation, nonbacterial thrombotic endocarditis, and cerebral venous thrombosis. Early recognition and treatment of patients presenting with these syndromes can result in the prevention of further neurologic deterioration.

Intravascular coagulation results in fibrin deposits in the terminal branches of multiple cerebral arteries, resulting in small hemorrhagic or ischemic infarctions. Patients commonly present with fluctuating signs of diffuse cerebral dysfunction such as delirium, stupor, and generalized seizures, signs that are sometimes incorrectly ascribed to metabolic encephalopathy. Symptoms usually precede the laboratory abnormalities of decreased fibrinogen and platelets and elevated split-fibrin products. In patients who present with these symptoms and have laboratory evidence of disseminated intravascular coagulation, an evaluation for treatable etiologies such as occult infection should be made. The role of systemic anticoagulation remains controversial.

Nonbacterial thrombotic endocarditis occurs in patients with carcinoma of the breast and can precipitate stroke. In this syndrome, an aseptic vegetation, which can form a nidus for emboli to the brain and other organs, develops on the mitral or aortic valve. Patients present with an acute neurologic deficit or may have multiple transient deficits. Involvement of systemic organs is common, but the presenting signs are usually neurologic. Most patients will have elevated prothombin times and decreased platelets and one-third will have laboratory evidence of disseminated intravascular coagulation. Echocardiography and cerebral angiography can help make the diagnosis. Patients may improve with successful treatment of the primary tumor, and in patients with limited systemic disease, anticoagulation may prevent additional infarction.

Thrombosis in the dural venous sinuses is also associated with cancer of the breast. The presenting signs and symptoms include headache, seizures, hemiparesis, visual field defects, and mental status changes. Laboratory study results are often normal, but MRI or cerebral angiography demonstrate venous sinus occlusion. In patients with breast cancer, tumor involvement of dural or calvarial structures adjacent to the sinus can precipitate venous sinus thrombosis. It is important to identify this condition, as the dural metastasis is likely to respond to radiotherapy. Intravenous heparin therapy is also controversial in this syndrome, but the risk of hemorrhage in patients anticoagulated for this problem is low and is probably outweighed by the potential benefits.

Tumor embolus is a potential etiology of stroke in patients with breast cancer. The embolus originates in the lung, and stroke from this cause carries a particularly grave prognosis.

TABLE 177-2. Causes of Encephalopathy in Patients With Breast Cancer

Metabolic
  Hypoxemia
  Sepsis
  Hypoglycemia
  Uremia
  Electrolyte imbalance
  Hypercarbia (carbon dioxide narcosis)
  Hepatic failure
  Nutritional deficiency
  Thyroid disorder
Toxic
  Sedative or narcotic intoxication
  Glucocorticoids
  Alcohol or other drug overdose
  Chemotherapeutic agents
  Anticonvulsants
  Anticholinergics

METABOLIC ENCEPHALOPATHY

Diffuse encephalopathy with or without focal signs can be a prominent sign of many of the neurologic and systemic complications of breast cancer. In the majority of patients, diffuse encephalopathy is the result of multiple metabolic or nutritional abnormalities related to the underlying cancer. However, focal findings on neurologic examination should prompt a search for a structural brain lesion. Causes of metabolic and toxic encephalopathy in cancer patients are listed in Table 177-2.

PARANEOPLASTIC SYNDROMES

Paraneoplastic syndromes are disorders of unknown etiology that occur with increased frequency in patients with cancer. The identification of a neurologic paraneoplastic syndrome is important because the symptoms may precede the diagnosis of cancer by several months, allowing identification of the malignancy at an early stage. In breast cancer patients, the most common of these rare disorders is subacute cerebellar degeneration. The symptoms are ataxia, dysarthria, nystagmus, and vertigo. MRI of the brain fails to show a focal lesion but may demonstrate cerebellar atrophy. Pathologically, there is a strik-ing loss of Purkinje cells. In many of these patients a circulating antibody (anti-Yo) that binds to proteins shared by breast tumor cells and Purkinje cells can be identified. Another syndrome that occurs in patients with breast cancer is characterized by opsoclonus, ataxia, vertigo, and a vertical gaze palsy. Occasional patients with this latter syndrome harbor an antibody (anti-Ri) that reacts with tumor and neuron proteins. Other paraneoplastic syndromes that have been reported in patients with breast cancer include peripheral neuropathy, dermatomyositis, subacute myelopathy, and parkinsonism with degeneration of the substantia nigra. These syndromes are discussed in Chapter 171.

SUGGESTED READINGS

Anderson NE, Rosenblum MK, Posner JB: Paraneoplastic cerebellar degeneration: Clinical-immunological correlations. Ann Neurol 24:559–67, 1988

Boogerd W, Hart AA, van der Sande JJ, Engelsman E: Meningeal carcinomatosis in breast cancer. Cancer 67:1685, 1991

Boogerd W, Vos VW, Hart AA, Baris G: Brain metastases in breast cancer: natural history, prognostic factors and outcome. J Neurooncol 15:165, 1993

Byrne TN, Waxman SG: Spinal Cord Compression: Diagnosis and Principles of Management. FA Davis, Philadelphia, 1990

Coffey RJ, Flickinger JC, Bissonette DJ, Lundsford LD: Radiosurgery for solitary brain metastases using the cobalt-60 gamma unit. Int J Radiat Oncol Biol Phys 21:591, 1991

Graus F, Rogers LR, Posner JB: Cerebrovascular complications in patients with cancer. Medicine 64:16, 1985

Grossman SA, Finkelstein DM, Ruckdeschel JC et al: Randomized prospective comparison of intraventricular methotrexate and thiotepa in patients with previously untreated neoplastic meningitis. J Clin Oncol 11:561–69, 1993

Harris JR, Morrow M, Bonadonna G: Cancer of the breast. In Devita VT, Hellaman S, Rosenberg SA (eds): Cancer. Principles and Practice of Oncology. 4th Ed. JB Lippincott, Philadelphia, 1993

Henson JW, Posner JB: Neurological complications. p. 2268. In Holland JF (ed): Cancer Medicine. 3rd Ed. Lea & Febiger, Philadelphia, 1993

Hill ME, Richards MA, Gregory WM et al: Spinal cord compression in breast cancer: a review of 70 cases. Br J Med 68:969, 1993

Kori S, Foley KM, Posner JB: Brachial plexus lesions in patients with cancer: 100 cases. Neurology 31:45, 1981

Olsen NK, Pfeiffer P, Mondrop K, Rose C: Radiation-induced brachial plexopathy in breast cancer patients. Acta Oncol 27:885, 1993

Prados MD, Wilson CB: Neoplasms of the central nervous system. p. 1080. In Holland JF (ed): Cancer Medicine. 3rd Ed. Lea & Febiger, Philadelphia, 1993

NEUROLOGY IN GENERAL
MEDICINE

PART **VIII**

SECTION 1. CARDIOLOGY AND CARDIAC SURGERY

178. NEUROLOGIC COMPLICATIONS OF CARDIAC SURGERY

JON BRILLMAN

From the earliest days of cardiac surgery it has been apparent that neurologic complications represented the most serious sequelae of these procedures. Despite improvements in surgical technique and extracorporeal circulation, a variety of neurologic syndromes are still associated with the operations. Technologic advances have made it increasingly possible since the 1980s for older patients (older than 70 years) to undergo coronary artery bypass grafting (CABG) operations with low morbidity. The downside of this trend is that these patients have more advanced atherosclerosis and consequently suffer a higher incidence of cerebral sequelae.

Early reports of neurologic disorders associated with open-heart operations were attributed to hypotension and macroembolic events from diseased valves. It is now evident that the major central neurologic complications of stroke and/or encephalopathy are usually unpredictable, and that intraoperative hypotensive episodes or clear-cut embolic sources are not often found. Strokes, which occur with an incidence of 2 to 10 percent, are now known to result not only from cardiac emboli but from atheromatous emboli from an ectatic, rigid aorta during aortotomy or cross-clamping. The coexistence of carotid stenosis with coronary artery disease increases the risk of stroke to a minor degree, and how it should be handled preoperatively, as is discussed below, is still debated.

Severe encephalopathy, characterized by a delay in extubation and emergence from anesthesia, small reactive pupils, and restlessness or agitation, is a serious complication, occurring in 5 to 15 percent of cases and having a high mortality rate. Despite the fact that patients are on extracorporeal circulation with an artificial pump oxygenator for up to 2 hours, surgical factors may play a more important role in encephalopathy than does extracorporeal circulation.

Another issue, yet to be fully defined or explained, is that of minor cognitive changes after cardiopulmonary bypass procedures; such changes are found on neuropsychiatric testing in up to 25 percent of patients (Fig. 178-1). The extent to which these changes affect the lives of the increasingly elderly population undergoing heart operations is not yet known and is under intense study.

This chapter deals with the various neurologic complications in common cardiac operations and discusses what is known about their pathogenesis.

STROKE

In cardiopulmonary bypass procedures, stroke occurs with an incidence of 0.9 to 10 percent, depending on whether one examines prospective or retrospective studies. Territorial infarcts result from microemboli from diseased valves, left ventricular or atrial thrombi, and atheromatous emboli from a rigid aorta. Watershed strokes due to hypoperfusion have been reported, but are extremely rare. A review of the neuroimaging studies in 30 patients who suffered stroke following CABG surgery found that computed tomography (CT) scans along with results of 6 angiograms suggested that most of the infarcts resulted from microemboli from the heart. A retrospective analysis of 126 patients with a history of ischemic stroke who underwent open-heart surgery demonstrated a 13.4 percent incidence of new strokes or worsening of prior deficits, but a small percentage (3.2 percent) that were moderate or severe in degree. Accordingly, it is recommended that CABG surgery following a stroke be delayed for several months, if possible. An analysis of strokes occurring after CABG surgery in 54 patients found that the presence of a cervical bruit only slightly increased the risk of stroke (by 2.9 percent), and that a history of transient ischemic attack, prolonged pump times (more than 2 hours), atrial fibrillation, and congestive heart failure increased the risk of postoperative stroke.

Despite these studies, the cause of stroke following most cases of CABG surgery is often obscure and usually unanticipated. Pre-CABG endarterectomy remains a controversial procedure, and the clinician's judgment remains the most important factor in determining whether it should be carried out in the presence of a carotid bruit or Doppler-demonstrated carotid stenosis. Most recommend that endarterectomy be considered independently of cardiac considerations. That is, if a patient has a surgically accessible carotid stenosis that is more than 70 percent stenotic and is appropriate to the clinical symptoms, an endarterectomy should be performed earlier that the CABG procedure in accordance with the widely accepted data from NASCET (North American Symptomatic Carotid Endarterectomy Trial). Most studies have demonstrated that simultaneous endarterectomy and coronary revascularization procedures produce unacceptable rates of complications, which include stroke and vascular death.

Atheromatous emboli from the heart and ascending aorta are emerging as a significant risk for stroke and death in the increasingly aging population undergoing open heart surgery and CABG surgery. One group found a high correlation of cerebral atheromatous emboli and severe ascending aortic arteriosclerosis in autopsied individuals who underwent cardiac surgery. Others have found that intraoperative echocardiography may be able to identify patients at high risk for emboli from this source. Clearly, manipulation of a severely arteriosclerotic aorta with an aortotomy and aortic cross-clamping is a significant risk factor for stroke in this group of patients. In the future, surgeons may wish to use intraoperative echocardiography to identify portions of the aorta less calcified for the site of aortotomy or placement of cross-clamps. Accordingly, manipulation of the aortic arch, particularly during aortotomy, is a likely

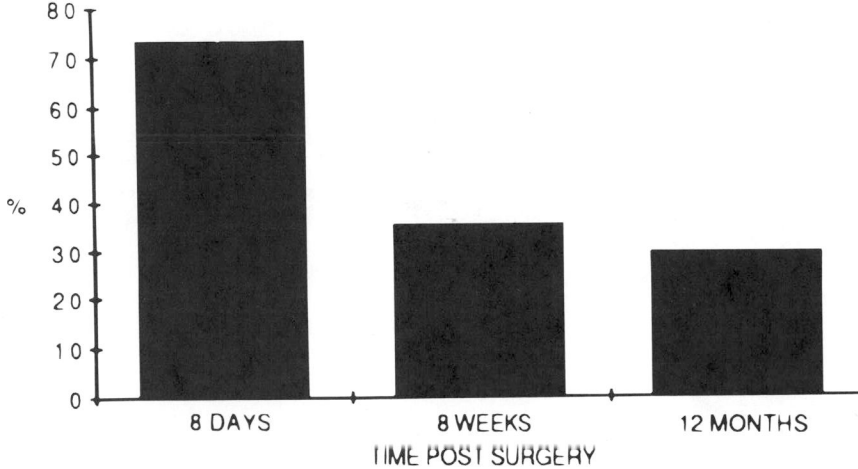

FIG. 178-1. A graph showing the persistence of neuropsychological deficits after coronary artery bypass graft surgery. (From Rodewald G: Introduction to the subject. p. 175. In Wyllner AE, Rodewald G (eds): Impact of Cardiac Surgery on the Quality of Life. Plenum Press, New York, 1990, with permission.)

source for embolic stroke in a significant number of patients undergoing cardiopulmonary bypass procedures.

Circulating prothrombotic factors are altered during cardiopulmonary bypass, as in the case of elevated levels of fibrinopeptide A and thromboxane B_2, but the extent to which this contributes to stroke is as yet unknown.

Open-heart procedures for valve replacement pose a special problem because of the possibility of air emboli. Intraoperative transcranial Doppler studies have demonstrated that these emboli are most likely to occur during the redistribution of blood from the heart-lung machine to the patient when the heart is reactivated and begins to eject actively. Air emboli do not cause large vessel occlusions, however, and the evidence suggests that they are more likely to be associated with encephalopathy owing to their extreme small size and widespread distribution during cardiopulmonary bypass procedures.

HYPOTENSION AND CEREBRAL BLOOD FLOW DURING CARDIOPULMONARY BYPASS PROCEDURES

Encephalopathy following cardiopulmonary bypass—both CABG encephalopathy and encephalopathy associated with open-heart procedures—mimics the result of bilateral diffuse frontal lobe ischemia. As the patient undergoing cardiopulmonary bypass procedures is on extracorporeal circulation for a period that may last 1 or 2 hours, one would suspect that impairment of perfusion of the brain would be an important mechanism of brain injury. Intraoperative hypotension during these procedures certainly may occur under extreme and unusual circumstances, but it is rare. Indeed, a perusal of the intraoperative records of patients who have suffered encephalopathy following heart surgery rarely reveals evidence of hypotension occurring during the procedures. Hypotension perioperatively may be related to left ventricular failure, arrhythmias or blood loss, but when the patient is on the pump, the circulatory status is relatively controlled by the perfusionist. Nevertheless, if hypotension occurs, it is attributable to decreased peripheral vascular resistance that may result from hemodilution with crystalloid prime, warming the hypothermic patient and anesthetic agents. Years of experience and animal experimentation have shown that 50 mmHg is a safe mean arterial pressure during cardiopul-

monary bypass procedures. Figure 178-2 shows that in over 300 patients studied, only 2 percent have pressures of less than 50 mmHg and the vast majority of pressures fall well within the safety margin that has been established over the years. In fact, under circumstances of hypothermia with the patient's body temperature cooled to 27 or 28°C, 30 mmHg has been shown to be a mean arterial pressure that is quite safe in terms of cerebral protection. Perfusion flow rates maintained by the perfusionist are usually at around 2.2 or 2.4 L/min/m² of body surface using a roller or centrifugal pump (nonpulsatile or pulsatile flow). Under hypothermic conditions, lower flows, even as low as flow rates of 1.2 to 1.4 L/min/m² have been shown to be safe, and in fact, have been believed to be protective by some investigators by reducing the likelihood of cellular edema of the brain. Investigations designed to determine if hypotension causes postoperative cerebral damage show conflicting results. Some have found that time-dependent hypotension (< 50 mmHg) tended to impair cerebral function and slow the electroencephalogram. Slogoff and colleagues, however, found no relationship between perfusion pressure, length of cardiopulmonary bypass, and neurologic dysfunction in a large number of patients.

Cerebral blood flow is reduced during moderate hypothermic cardiopulmonary bypass (Fig. 178-3). Following the induction of hypothermia to moderate levels (28°C), gases such as carbon dioxide go into solution. Because of this, two different strategies have evolved regarding PCO_2 management during hypothermic cardiopulmonary bypass. The first option of management, which is called α-stat management, maintains the PCO_2 and pH at 40 mmHg and 7.50, respectively, values that are temperature corrected. At body temperatures of 28.5°C, the pH-state approach increases PCO_2 by 50 percent and significantly increases cerebral blood flow. Evidence suggests, however, that neurologic outcome is not altered by this strategy and that cerebral autoregulation is best maintained by using the α-stat approach. Under this circumstance, the lower limit of autoregulation appears to be about 30 mmHg. Although the addition of carbon dioxide during the procedure will increase cerebral blood flow, most studies show that there is a corresponding fall in oxygen extraction in the brain and that the vasodilation that may occur may increase the risk of embolic load, which, as is

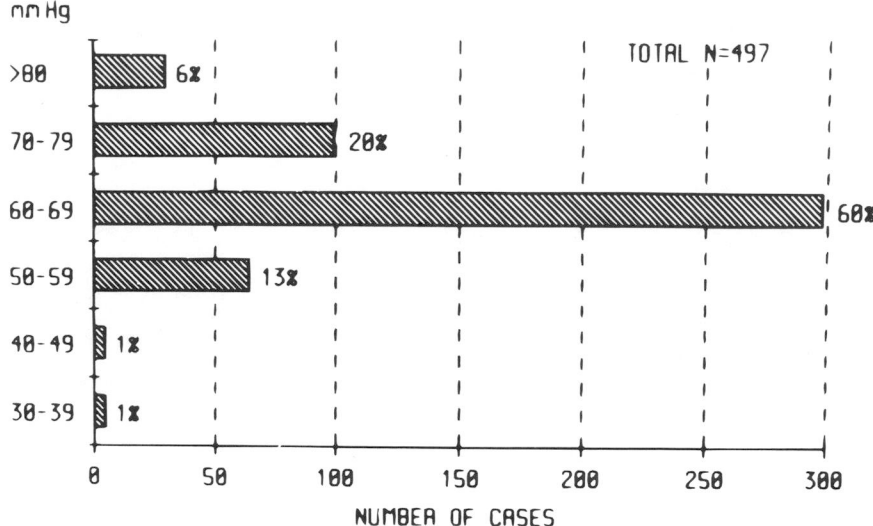

FIG. 178-2. Mean arterial blood pressures in a large group of patients during coronary artery cardiopulmonary bypass surgery. (From Rodewald G: Introduction to the subject. p. 175. In Wyllner AE, Rodewald G (eds): Impact of Cardiac Surgery on the Quality of Life. Plenum Press, New York, 1990, with permission.)

discussed below, may be a more important factor in neurologic sequelae. Cerebral blood flow, as determined by xenon washout and mean flow velocities as demonstrated by intraoperative transcranial Doppler technique, demonstrate a fall in cerebral blood flow and flow velocities following induction of anesthesia to a slight degree, followed by a rise after hemodilution. During hypothermic cardiopulmonary bypass, however, cerebral blood flow falls at an average of 1 percent per minute but then rises again during rewarming.

Therefore, despite reductions in cerebral flow at moderate

hypothermia during cardiopulmonary bypass, neurologic complications as a consequence of this appear to be rare, owing to intact autoregulation and increased oxygen extraction of the brain.

In summary, it would appear that hypotension is rarely seen during cardiopulmonary bypass in open-heart and CABG procedures. The decline in cerebral blood flow that occurs during hypothermia seems independent of neurologic outcome and the brain is not protected by the addition of carbon dioxide during the procedure.

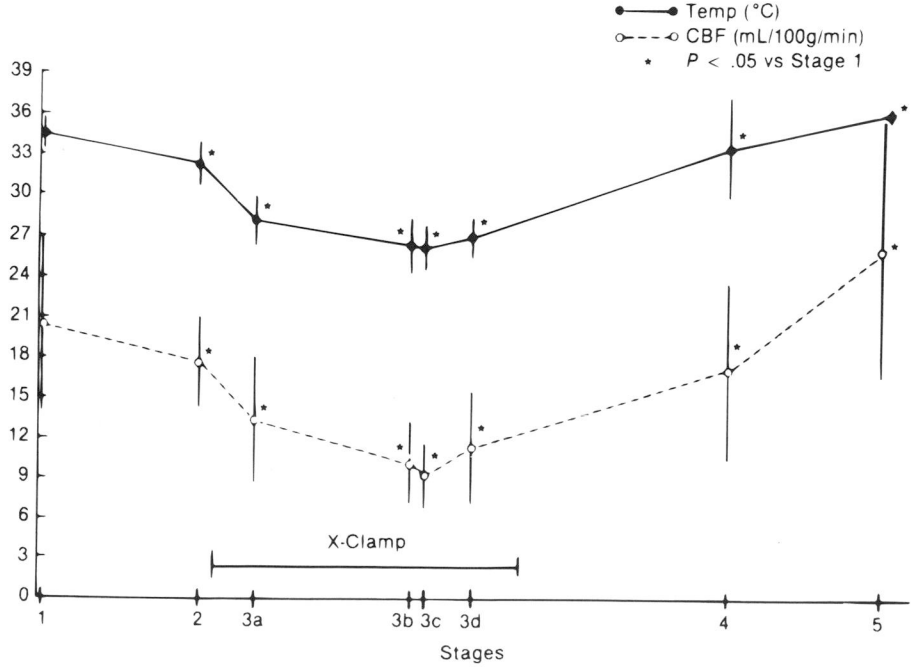

FIG. 178-3. The relationship between blood temperature and cerebral blood flow during cardiopulmonary bypass surgery. Note that hypothermia is associated with a reduction in cerebral blood flow. (From Rodewald G: Introduction to the subject. p. 175. In Wyllner AE, Rodewald G (eds): Impact of Cardiac Surgery on the Quality of Life. Plenum Press, New York, 1990, with permission.)

MICROEMBOLI

A unique neuropathologic observation by Moody *et al.* has provided significant information toward uncovering the pathogenesis of the cognitive decline following cardiopulmonary bypass procedures. These investigators demonstrated the presence of capillary and small arterial dilations in the penetrating vessels of the brain in patients after cardiac surgery and aortography. Using an alkaline phosphatase stain that reacts strongly with small arterioles and capillaries (5 to 50 μm), a map of the small intracerebral circulation was provided without the disruptive effects of intravascular injection. Millions of these vascular abnormalities, called small capillary arterial dilations appeared as sausagelike dilations, usually multiple, along the penetrating small vessels with intact capillary or arterial walls and empty lumens (Fig. 178-4). They were thought to represent the ghosts of microemboli that had either dissolved or passed on. The actual composition and source of these emboli remain unknown.

The real-time identification of cerebral microemboli may be accomplished by both retinal fluorescein angiography and transcranial Doppler examination. In 1971, emboli were observed in the retina during surgery on bypass. Using a fundus camera, investigators have demonstrated a 100 percent incidence of microvascular occlusions in the retina with fluorescein angiography, believed to be due to microemboli (less than 200 μm) during CABG surgery. As these microvascular occlusions were observed in patients who underwent cardiopulmonary bypass surgery using bubble oxygenators, it was conjectured that the bubble oxygenator was the source of the microemboli. Oxygenator type, therefore, plays a role in microembolic events.

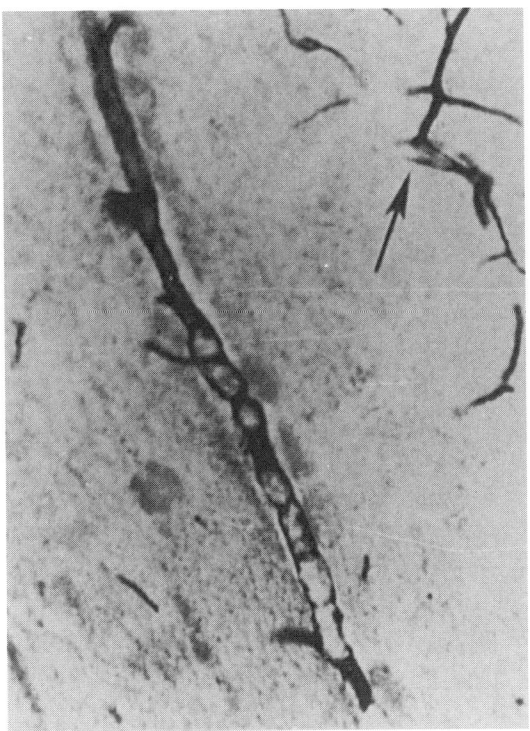

FIG. 178-4. A medium-size arteriole *(arrow)* in a patient who underwent cardiopulmonary bypass surgery, showing small capillary arterial dilations. The swollen areas are clear and have intact vascular walls. (From Moody DM, Bell MA, Challa VR et al: Brain microemboli during cardiac surgery or aortography. Ann Neurol 28:477–86, 1990, with permission.)

Accordingly, a brief discussion of the different types of oxygenators and bypass apparatus follows.

The basic cardiopulmonary apparatus is shown in Figure 178-5. Deoxygenated blood is drained by gravity from the right atrium into a large reservoir, where it is diluted to approximately 50 percent of its hematocrit value by crystalloid prime. A centrifugal or roller pump, which produces laminar nonpulsatile flow in most cases, directs the blood through the oxygenator. The blood is then returned to the patient through a 40-μm arterial line filter. Even now, arterial line filters are not always used. Oxygenated blood is circulated through the aortotomy to the various organs. Pumps are present that continually drain the left ventricle so that the surgeon may operate in a bloodless field for the decompressed heart.

Bubble oxygenators require that oxygen is bubbled directly into venous blood using a direct blood gas interface, and the gaseous exchange takes place at the surface of the bubbles. Membrane oxygenators, however, more closely simulate the capillary–alveolar membrane and are therefore more closely related to pulmonary capillaries. In this type of oxygenator, a semipermeable membrane is placed between the blood and gas and microbubbles are not formed. Certainly, most institutions that perform cardiopulmonary bypass procedures now recognize that membrane oxygenators are less likely to be a source of microbubbles, and therefore bubble oxygenators are currently in limited use.

Transcranial Doppler has proved to be an excellent tool in detecting microemboli, particularly during cardiopulmonary bypass surgery. Using a 2-mHz probe fixed over the temporal window, microemboli varying in size from 50 μm to several hundred micrometers in diameter may be consistently detected. These presumed microemboli have been found by numerous investigators and appear as high-amplitude flow disturbance signals that produce an audible blip and can clearly be distinguished from flow signal and artifact (Fig. 178-6). These signals are often called high-intensity transient signals. Clinically, emboli may be detected in patients who have biomechanical heart valves and are found three to five cardiac cycles after an intravenous injection of air for contrast-enhanced echocardiography. In patients with mechanical prosthetic heart valves, high-amplitude Doppler signals were identified in 54 percent of patients. Similar signals could not be found in patients who had received biologic prosthetic heart valves. Recent studies have shown that high-intensity transient signals are most common during precannulation; aortotomy; insertion and removal of the aortic cannula, vent, and cardioplegia needle; aortic cross-clamp (total and partial) and clamp removal; defibrillation; and displacement of the heart and other maneuvers. Hence, the widespread use of membrane oxygenators has removed the threat of many of these events coming from the heart-lung machine, but they still occur in great numbers as a result of surgical maneuvers. Studies have shown that high-intensity transient signals may be correlated with declining cognitive function postoperatively. We have found that neurologic complications with encephalopathic features are most commonly associated in patients who have had more than 60 microembolic events intraoperatively. Higher numbers of microemboli are also associated with neurocognitive decline from pre- to postoperative intervals in patients who appear to be asymptomatic. Microembolic events occur most commonly as a consequence of surgical maneuvers, particularly cardiac manipulation and aortotomy and cross-clamp application and removal. The emboli that result from these procedures are most likely to result in neurologic symptoms and

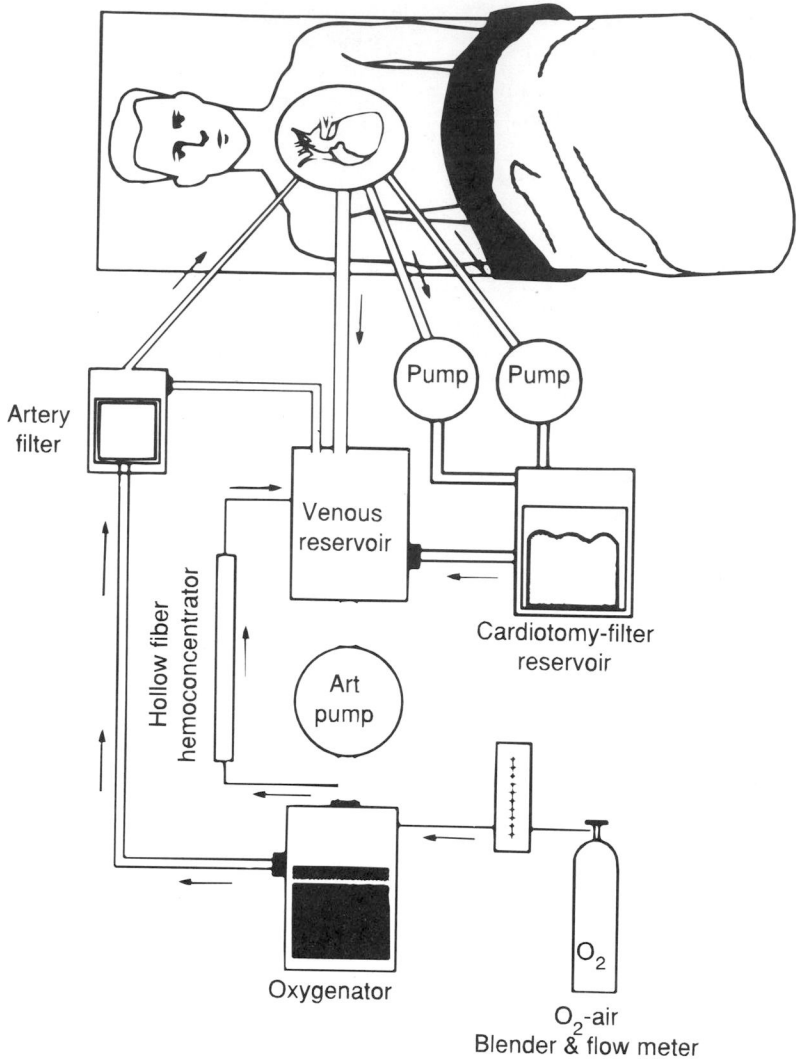

FIG. 178-5. Basic cardiopulmonary bypass apparatus. (From Casthely PA: The anatomy of cardiopulmonary bypass. pp. 23–35. In Casthely PA, Bregman D (eds): Cardiopulmonary Bypass: Physiology, Related Complications and Pharmacology. Futura, Mt. Kisco, NY, 1991, with permission.)

signs postoperatively. Emboli also occur from the perfusion apparatus, and although greater numbers of these are associated with neurocognitive decline, they do not appear to be as serious and produce less neurologic dysfunction than those from the surgical technique.

The use of membrane oxygenators, arterial line filtration, repeated de-airing of the heart, positioning of the patient, and reduced manipulation of the heart to inspect posterior anastomoses during CABG procedures may well be beneficial in reducing the number of these unwanted events.

As the microemboli are far too small to obstruct cerebral vessels, it is not completely understood how neurologic dysfunction may ensue. Evidence from experimental models in animals suggests that microemboli, which pass through even the smallest circulation, may reduce cerebral blood flow and impair neuron function, as is evidenced by reduced somatosensory evoked potentials.

Microemboli, therefore, occur in large numbers during cardiopulmonary bypass procedures and are readily detected by transcranial Doppler examination intraoperatively. As significant alterations in cerebral perfusion pressure are rare and poorly correlated with cognitive dysfunction or neurologic se-

quelae, it is likely that microemboli play a significant role in postoperative neurologic disorders.

OTHER POSSIBLE ETIOLOGIC FACTORS

The possibility that functional capillary closure in the brain may result from nonpulsatile flow during cardiopulmonary bypass procedures and that this may play a role in neurologic damage needs to be clarified further. One study found an increase in cerebral blood flow and cerebral metabolic rate for oxygen ($CMRO_2$) in 11 randomized patients who were switched from nonpulsatile to pulsatile flow using a pump-head interrupter. The reversal of the reduction of cerebral blood flow by the addition of pulsatile perfusion suggests that an increase in cerebral blood flow may result solely from changes in the arterial wave-form characteristics. Until now, the role of pulsatile perfusion in preserving brain function was not well understood, and some investigators have found that pulsatile perfusion does not correlate with improved neurologic outcome. Indeed, nonpulsatile or laminar flow is the preferred mechanism of ejecting blood during open-heart procedures.

Neuroradiologists have shown interest in patients undergoing cardiopulmonary bypass procedures. Reference has already

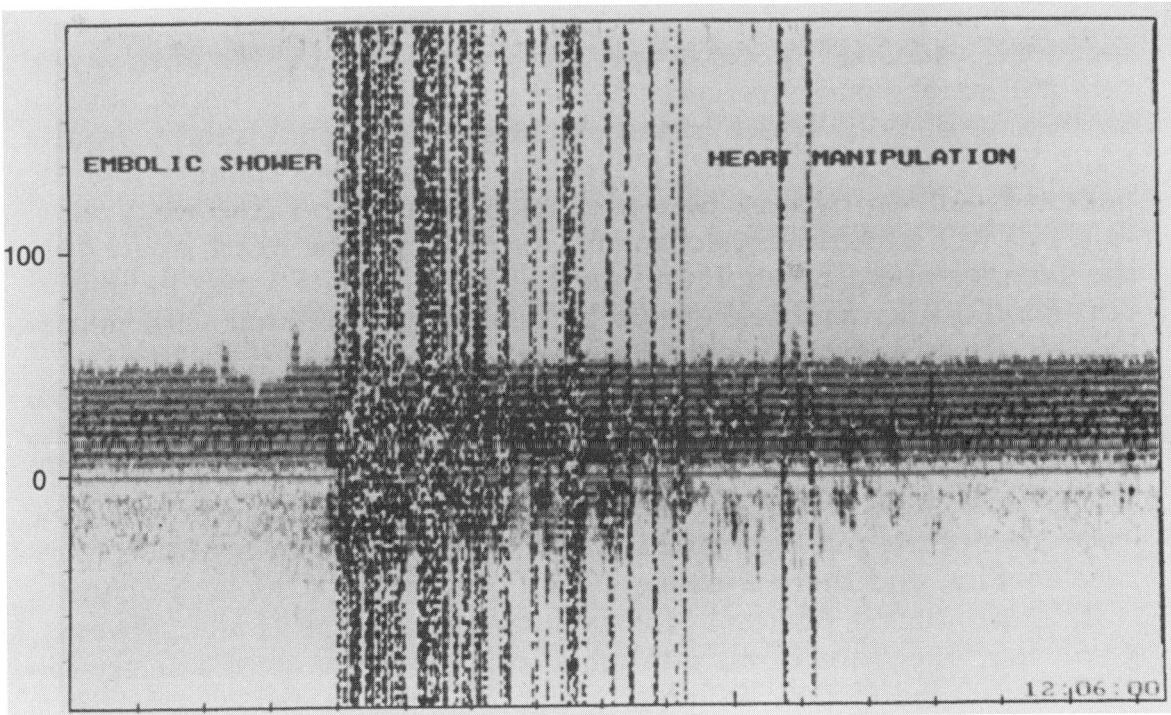

FIG. 178-6. Transcranial doppler monitoring shows a shower of microemboli coinciding with manipulation of the heart during graft inspection near the end of a coronary artery bypass graft procedure.

been made to the pattern of cerebral infarction on CT scanning, and examination of CT scans in stroke patients has confirmed that cerebral infarctions postoperatively are territorial in nature and are not due to diffuse perfusion deficits. Although diffuse cerebral edema has been demonstrated on magnetic resonance image scanning in the immediate period following CABG surgery, the significance of this is uncertain and its relation to neurologic or neurocognitive decline is unknown. Other investigators have found no new cerebral lesions on contrast-enhanced magnetic resonance imaging following cardiopulmonary bypass. It is likely that further investigations of brain functions such as measurement of high-energy phosphates using magnetic resonance spectroscopy and evaluation of cerebral blood flow and metabolism by position emission tomography scanning will shed further light on brain damage in this group of patients.

PERIPHERAL NERVOUS SYSTEM COMPLICATIONS OF CARDIOPULMONARY BYPASS PROCEDURES

The peripheral nervous system may be damaged in open-heart and CABG procedures. Fortunately, most of the neuropathies and plexopathies that result are transient and reversible.

The most common peripheral neurologic injury reported in cardiopulmonary bypass procedures is that of brachial plexus damage. In most cases, the lower trunk or medial cord fibers are involved as confirmed by clinical and electrodiagnostic evaluation. The mechanism of injury has been reported to be attributable either to traumatic cannulation of the internal jugular vein on the side of the injury or to excessive traction on the brachial plexus following sternotomy with fracture of the first cervical rib. Ulnar neuropathies, usually reversible after 4 to 6 weeks, are fairly common and result from compression of the nerve at the elbow, particularly during prolonged procedures. Peroneal neuropathies as well as saphenous neuropathies have

also been reported and are due to either direct compression of the peroneal nerve around the fibular head or stretching of the saphenous nerve. The extent to which hypothermia renders the peripheral nervous system susceptible to damage during these procedures is conjectural, but it is known that both axonal degeneration and myelin breakdown may occur during exposure to extreme cold.

An additional problem involving the peripheral nervous system with some more serious consequences is that of hemidiaphragmatic paralysis resulting from phrenic nerve injury, the result of exposure of the phrenic nerve to the topical ice-saline slush that is commonly used to maintain cardiac hypothermia during cardioplegic arrest. In one series, 54% of patients undergoing CABG surgery exhibited abnormal diaphragmatic motion. Postoperatively, phrenic nerve conduction studies demonstrated a high percentage of abnormalities ipsilaterally. Although some degree of diaphragmatic paresis may persist in up to one-quarter of the patients in this circumstance, it appears to have little morbidity, although prolonged hospital stays have been noted in individuals with phrenic nerve injuries. Care to insulate the nerve during these procedures may limit damage to the phrenic nerve.

SUGGESTED READINGS

Berger MP, Tegeler CH: Transcranial Doppler detection of emboli. pp. 232–41. In Babikian V, Weschler L (eds): Transcranial Doppler Ultrasonography. Clinical and Research Application. Mosby-Year Book, St. Louis, 1993

Blauth CI, Arnold JV, Schulenberg WE et al: Cerebral microembolism during cardiopulmonary bypass: retinal microvascular studies in vivo with fluorescein angiography. J Thorac Cardiovasc Surg 95:668, 1988

Brillman J: CNS complications of coronary artery bypass surgery. In Neurological Clinics. Neurocardiology 11:474–95, 1993

Clark RE, Brillman J, Davis DA: Microemboli during CABG: genesis and effect on outcome. J Thorac Cardiovasc Surg. 109:249–58, 1995

Coffey CE, Massey EW, Roberts KB et al: Natural history of cerebral complications of coronary artery bypass graft surgery. Neurology 33:1416, 1983

DeVita MA, Robinson LR, Rehder J et al: Incidence and natural history of phrenic neuropathy occurring during open heart surgery. Chest 103:850, 1993

Gilman S: Neurological complications of open heart surgery. Ann Neurol 28: 475, 1990

Hanson MR, Bever AC, Furian AJ et al: Mechanism and frequency of brachial plexus injury in open-heart surgery: a prospective analysis. Ann Thorac Surg 36:675, 1983

Harris DNF, Bailey SM, Smith PLC et al: Brain swelling in first hour after coronary artery bypass surgery. Lancet 342:586, 1993

Hise JH, Nipper ML, Schmitker JC: Stroke associated with coronary artery bypass surgery. Am J Neuroradiol 12:811, 1991

Lederman RJ, Brever AC, Hanson MR et al: Peripheral nervous systems complications of coronary artery bypass graft surgery. Ann Neurol 12:297, 1982

Moody DM, Bell MA, Challa VR et al: Brain microemboli during cardiac surgery or aortography. Ann Neurol 28:477, 1990

Reed GL, Singer DE, Picard EH, DeSanctis RW: Stroke following coronary-artery bypass surgery. N Engl J Med 319:1246, 1988

Rodewald G: Introduction to the subject. In Speidel H, Rodewald G (eds): Psychic and Neurologic Dysfunctions After Open Heart Surgery. Thieme, New York, 1980

Slogoff S, Girgis KZ, Keats AS: Etiologic factors in neuropsychiatric complications associated with cardiopulmonary bypass. Anesth Analg 61:903, 1982

Wareing TH, Davila-Roman VG, Brazilai B et al: Management of the severely atherosclerotic ascending aorta during cardiac operations: a strategy for detection and treatment. J Thorac Cardiovasc Surg 103:453–62, 1992

Willner, Rodewald G: Impact of cardiac surgery on the quality of life: neurological and psychological aspects. Plenum, New York, 1990

179. COMPLICATIONS OF CARDIAC CATHETERIZATION

CATHY A. SILA

Cardiac catheterization can be performed of the right heart or left heart. For adults, left-sided catheterizations are primarily performed for coronary arteriography, which remains the gold standard for the diagnosis of coronary artery disease and the basis of therapeutic interventional cardiology. The Sones technique of brachial artery catheterization and Judkins and Schoonmaker modifications of percutaneous femoral artery catheterization have their respective advantages and disadvantages. Common to both is that the majority of complications relate to the puncture site.

The Sones technique, described in 1958, employs an antecubital incision over the brachial artery, a procedure that requires skill and knowledge of the anatomy to avoid the proximal median nerve during dissection and necessitates an arteriotomy and arterial closure. The principle advantage of this technique lies in manipulating a single soft catheter. Percutaneous femoral arterial catheterization, originally described by Seldinger in 1953, was modified by Judkins in 1967. This technique is much easier to learn but requires accurate puncture of the common femoral artery below the inguinal ligament and requires several catheter changes over a guidewire. The Schoonmaker modification of 1968 combines the two techniques, producing a single-catheter percutaneous femoral approach.

Aggregate data from nearly 325,000 patients undergoing cardiac catheterization defines a major complication rate of 0.7 percent for death, myocardial infarction, ventricular fibrillation, cerebral embolization, infection, or arterial complications, including arterial stenosis or thrombosis, hematoma, pseudoaneurysm, or arteriovenous fistula formation. Neurologic complications can arise when the peripheral nervous system is injured by direct trauma during dissection or puncture, compression from hematoma, or ischemia from compromise of blood supply from a major limb artery. Central nervous system complications are primarily the result of embolism.

PERIPHERAL NERVOUS SYSTEM COMPLICATIONS

Although peripheral nerve complications are seen almost exclusively in the setting of vascular complications, their incidence is extraordinarily low, occurring in 0.01 percent in one series, and are mostly the subject of case reports. The risk of any complication depends upon the specific procedure and increases with a concomitant anticoagulation regimen and patient factors, including advanced age, congestive heart failure, or smaller vascular access, as seen with pre-existing peripheral vascular disease, smaller body surface area, or female gender. Most series have focused on severe complications requiring surgical repair or hemorrhage requiring blood transfusions. The incidence of complications by specific procedure is 0.5 to 1.0 percent for diagnostic coronary arteriography, 1.0 to 3.0 percent for percutaneous coronary angioplasty, 3.0 percent for coronary athererectomy, 7.5 percent for balloon valvuloplasty, and 11.0 percent for intracoronary stents. The complication rate increases with the complexity of the intervention, with the highest rates reported for intra-aortic balloon pump counterpulsation support. The contributions to the increased risk are multifactorial and related to manipulation of relatively stiff guidewires, larger sheath size, and need for prolonged sheath placement. Risk of pseudoaneurysm formation and hemorrhage has also been related to the complex antiplatelet and anticoagulant regimens used during stent placement. Inadvertant puncture of the superficial femoral artery, rather than the ideal cannulation of the common femoral artery, has also been related to increased risk of pseudoaneurysm or arteriovenous fistula formation, as the superficial femoral artery is smaller, lies closer to venous branches, and has less connective tissue support to aid in vascular compression after sheath removal.

Median Nerve Injuries

The median nerve in the antecubital region may be directly injured during the dissection required for the Sones technique, resulting in immediate pain, paresthesia in the median distribution in the hand, and weakness of median nerve–innervated hand muscles, including the median long flexors and intrinsic muscles of the thumb, radial wrist flexor, and pronator. Hemorrhage into the antecubital space or proximal forearm, if rapid, would produce the same symptoms, along with the local pain and obvious swelling. Slowly developing hematomas that cause a gradual increase in intracompartmental pressure can result in insidious median nerve compression with signs and symptoms that may be more difficult to diagnose. Owing to the anatomy of the forearm, hematoma formation is poorly tolerated by the median nerve and warrants early surgical exploration and decompression.

Pseudoaneurysm formation of the brachial artery can cause median nerve compression but is rare compared to its counterpart in the femoral artery.

The electromyographic (EMG) manifestation of median nerve injuries at the elbow is typically a main trunk involvement proximal to the origin of the anterior interosseous nerve, pronator teres, and flexor carpi radialis muscles. Median nerve motor and sensory conduction amplitudes were absent or reduced, with little change in conduction velocity. The needle electrode examination reveals fibrillation potentials and motor unit loss in various combinations, depending upon the severity or involvement of the particular fibers. Electrodiagnostic studies can be useful in localizing the lesion and determining its severity in all patients. Usually, an EMG at 3 weeks after the injury is sufficient, but in medicolegal cases in which there may be some pre-existing neuropathy that might confuse later interpretation, an early EMG study at the time of the injury is useful. Severe axon loss lesions known to be due to laceration with no evidence of recovery at 3 weeks should be considered for early exploration and grafting. Compressive lesions with some continuity present should be considered for grafting if there is no significant recovery after 6 months or so.

Ischemic monomelic neuropathy involving the upper extremity has been primarily described in the setting of brachial artery–cephalic vein arteriovenous fistulae created for the purpose of hemodialysis. Although conceivable, it has not been reported after heart catheterization.

Femoral Nerve Injuries

Laceration injuries to the femoral nerve are usually due to punctures at or slightly above the level of the inguinal ligament before the nerve undergoes extensive branching shortly after passing under the inguinal ligament on its way into the thigh. The symptoms and signs include pain and paresthesias over the anterior thigh and medial calf, weakness and atrophy of the quadriceps muscles, and reduction or loss of the patellar reflex. In milder lesions, burning paresthesias affecting the medial and intermediate femoral cutaneous nerves may occur.

Retroperitoneal hematoma formation due to inadequate hemostasis or concomitant antithrombotic regimens can cause compression of the femoral nerve or lumbar plexus, with respective involvement of the iliac or psoas muscles. Typically, these occur on the side of arterial puncture, but they have also been described contralaterally, where they are presumed to be due to the anticoagulant regimen alone. Hemorrhage is contained within fascial planes, and produces evolving nerve compressive symptoms commensurate with the rate of bleeding. Slowly evolving hemorrhages may produce insidious onset of symptoms, typically local pain in the groin, flank, or abdomen that typically radiates into the anterior thigh. Spontaneous hip flexion and external rotation may be seen along with pain upon hip movement. Numbness and paresthesias in the anterior thigh extends into the medial calf, along with weakness of the quadriceps muscles and diminution or loss of the patellar reflex. Hip flexor weakness is often hard to confirm because of pain. Cutaneous ecchymoses are frequent, but a palpable mass may be absent. Computed tomography (CT) of the pelvis is the most effective method of rapid diagnosis. A confirmed diagnosis of retroperitoneal hemorrhage necessitates discontinuation and reversal of anticoagulation and may warrant surgical exploration in some cases.

Pseudoaneurysms of the common femoral artery typically present with a painful, pulsatile groin mass in the absence of neurologic signs. Pseudoaneurysms of the profunda femoral artery may present solely as a compressive femoral neuropathy.

Duplex ultrasound scanning is particularly helpful in detecting the presence of blood flow into the perivascular hematoma and can also be used to guide obliteration by direct mechanical compression. Successful obliteration is less likely during anticoagulation, but does not necessarily require its discontinuation. Direct surgical repair may be necessary if neurologic symptoms are progressive or exacerbated by compressive techniques.

The lateral femoral cutaneous nerve can be injured by tight hemostatic pressure bandages if compression occurs where the lateral femoral cutaneous nerve passes through or underneath the upper lateral end of the inguinal ligament. Painful or burning paresthesias typical of meralgia paresthetica occur and can subside spontaneously. Local nerve blocks may be useful in the management of persistant pain.

Ischemic monomelic neuropathy of the lower extremity may occur, with acute occlusion of the superficial or common femoral artery. Patients typically complain of severe pain and numbness involving the foot, with decreased sensation and hyperpathia most prominent distally and shading proximally in a stocking pattern. Distal weakness predominantly involving intrinsic foot muscles is also present and may occur in the absence of cutaneous signs of limb ischemia. Many patients are initially misdiagnosed owing to a misconception that ischemia does not cause significant nerve injury in the absence of ongoing arterial insufficiency, especially in the absence of signs of muscle or skin necrosis. Also, symptoms are often much more prominent than the neurologic signs, which do not fit the pattern of a mononeuropathy. The EMG findings are characteristic, however, and suggest axon-loss lesions of motor and sensory nerves supplying the affected distal limb. Although the pattern is also consistent with a peripheral neuropathy, the axon loss is so disproportionate in the affected limb that a coexistant neuropathy should not pose a diagnostic dilemma.

CENTRAL NERVOUS SYSTEM COMPLICATIONS

The reported central nervous system complications of cardiac catheterization are uncommon, but are nearly 10 times more frequent than complications affecting the peripheral nervous system.

Diagnostic Coronary Angiography

Aggregate data encompassing 44,880 patients from four large series suggests an average risk of 0.16 percent for transient or permanent cerebral or retinal neurologic deficits. The risk for children appears to be higher—1.3 percent—with seizures occurring more frequently with cerebral ischemia than seen in adults. These data, collected primarily through retrospective review of neurologic consultation records, probably underestimate the true frequency of events, particularly the transient ones. Resolution of focal deficits within a few days occurs in more than one-half of the patients; however, visual defects are more likely to persist and some strokes have been fatal. The symptoms are often acute in onset and suggest a vascular mechanism. Indeed, embolism of air, catheter-related clot, or atheromatous material dislodged during manipulation of the relatively stiff guidewire are commonly accepted explanations. However, cerebral localization of these events have consistently shown a preponderance for involvement of the posterior circulation. Analysis of the 72 reported cases reveals that only 30 percent involve the anterior circulation commonly manifested as hemiparesis, hemisensory deficit, aphasia, gaze preference, or retinal visual defects. There is insufficient information to demonstrate any preponderance of the right or left carotid circulation. At least 53 percent of reported events clearly implicate the posterior circulation, manifested as brainstem syndromes, hemianopic visual field defects, confusional states with agitation or neglect, or prominent amnestic syndromes. Symptoms of uncertain vascular localization account for the remaining 17 percent, but when these case histories are carefully reviewed and forced into a posterioranterior classification scheme, the majority involve binocular visual complaints and mental status changes highly suggestive of posterior circulation involvement. There have been a number of explanations offered for the posterior circulation predominance, but none are very satisfactory. It was initially suggested that a retrograde brachial approach would more likely cause inadvertant right vertebral artery entry or embolization when traversing the subclavian curve, but subsequent series composed predominantly or exclusively of femoral artery catherizations have confirmed the same magnitude of posterior circulation predominance. Migraine or vasospasm have also been suggested as possible mechanisms, since transient visual disturbances are not uncommon during cerebral angiography and occur more frequently in migrane sufferers during coronary catheterization. The etiology of such evanescent symptoms remains in dispute, although it is unlikely that migraine or vasospasm could account for most of the infarcts. Embolization has been clearly documented as a mechanism, and animal studies of dogs undergoing aortography have demonstrated focal small capillary and arteriolar dilations or microaneurysms that are believed to be the residual of air or fat emboli. However, every other large clinical series of cardioembolic stroke has an anterior circulation predominance that reflects the relative supply of the cardiac output.

The neurologic approach has generally focused on cerebral localization of symptoms, diagnosis, and management of any persistant neurologic deficit. The use of anticoagulation should be considered to prevent re-embolization in the setting of atrial fibrillation or persistant thrombus within the cardiac chambers or perhaps within the aortic arch. Thrombolytic therapy has been used successfully to lyse cerebral emboli complicating coronary and cerebral angiographic procedures in a few case reports. However, this therapy carries with it a risk of cerebral hemorrhage, and until further information from multicenter trials is available, it should not be considered a standard of care.

Case Study 1. A 72-year-old farmer with multiple vascular risk factors underwent diagnostic coronary angiography prior to repair of an abdominal aortic aneurysm. During the arch injection, he suddenly developed a dense right hemiplegia with some mild hemisensory alterations in the hand and foot, sparing visual and other cranial nerve functions. An urgent brain CT scan and left carotid angiogram were normal. Three days later, his clinical examination results were consistent with a pure motor hemiparesis, and brain magnetic resonance imaging revealed a left paramedian pontine infarct. Although lacunar infarcts are conventionally attributed to intrinsic arteriolar disease, the clinical timing of symptoms suggested branch occlusion during basilar embolism (Fig. 179-1).

Therapeutic Coronary Catheterization

Focal neurologic complications following percutaneous transluminal coronary angioplasty, atherectomy, and stent placement have been recorded in 0.2 to 0.3 percent of patients and are

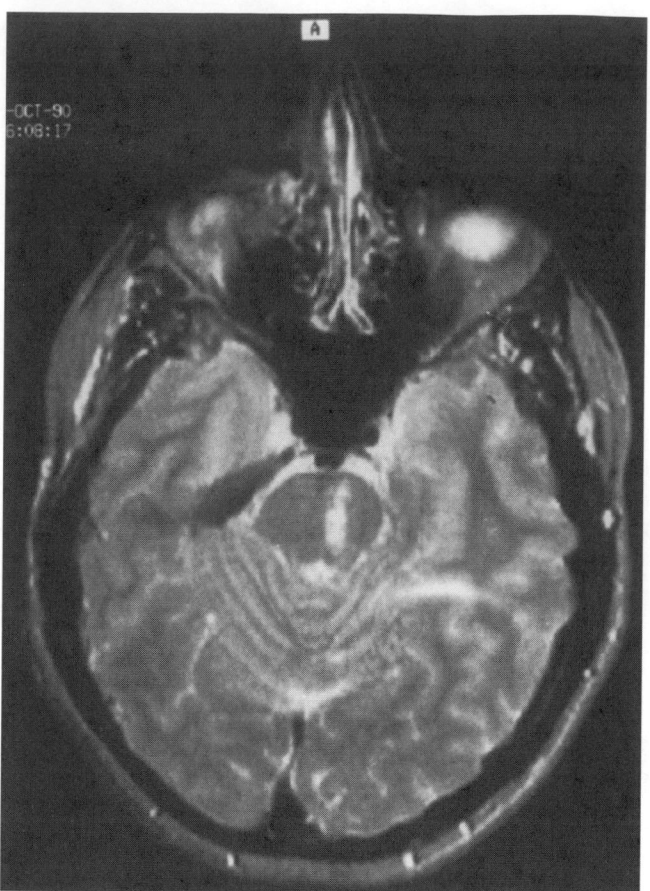

FIG. 179-1. Magnetic resonance imaging brain scan displaying a left paramedian pontine infarct in a 72-year-old man. This evidence, combined with the clinical timing of the patient's symptoms, suggests branch occlusion during basilar embolism.

clinically similar to those seen in diagnostic catheterization patients with presumed similar mechanisms. The observed reduction in complication rates of contemporary series when compared to earlier series is likely a reflection of numerous modifications in catheterization technique, catheter design, and use of antithrombotic drugs.

Percutaneous Transluminal Valvuloplasty

Percutaneous balloon valvuloplasty has emerged since the late 1980s as a nonsurgical treatment for mitral, aortic, and pulmonic valve stenosis in adults and children. The risk of cerebral embolism is 1.4 to 11 percent for aortic valvuloplasty and 0 to 4.2 percent for mitral valvuloplasty. Events during aortic valvuloplasty are often highly focal neurologic deficits suggesting branch embolization. Rare case reports of calcific material on fundoscopy or on brain CT scans implicate valvular debris. The risk of systemic embolization with mitral valvuloplasty appears linked with evidence for atrial thrombus that can be dislodged during the procedure. Transesophageal echocardiography should be performed prior to the procedure to search for evidence of thrombus. Three months of anticoagulation prior to treatment of potential thrombi has been recommended.

Case Study 2. A 52-year-old otherwise healthy schoolteacher with rheumatic mitral stenosis underwent transluminal balloon valvuloplasty. She had no history of atrial arrhythmias

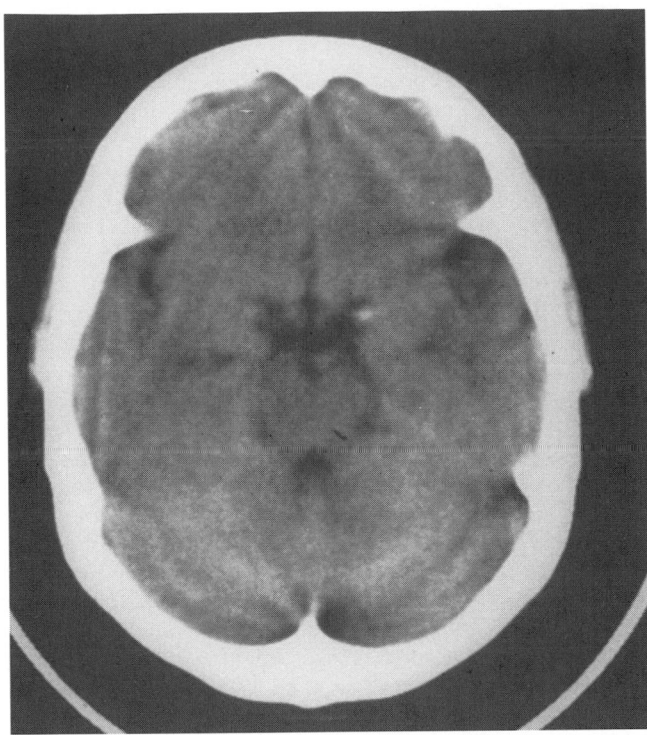

FIG. 179-2. Computed tomography brain scan demonstrating a hyperdensity in the left middle cerebral artery region of a 52-year-old woman. Although an embolus was suspected here, the patient's condition was rapidly improving and therefore no further diagnostic tests were recommended.

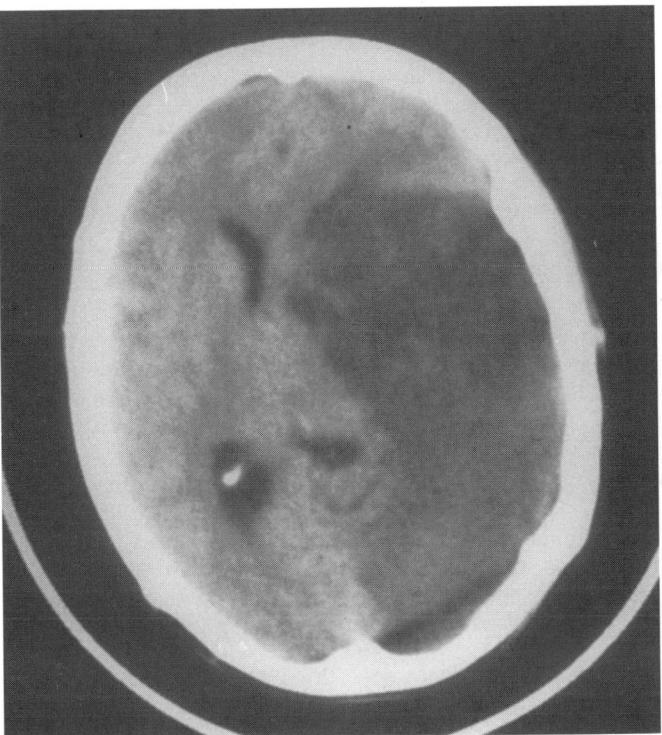

FIG. 179-3. Computed tomography brain scan demonstrating a fatal left, middle, and posterior cerebral artery infarct in the same patient as in Fig. 179-2.

and her preprocedure transthoracic and transesophageal echocardiograms were reported as negative for atrial thrombus. Five minutes after the procedure, she became acutely mute with a right hemiparesis. At 15 minutes, she was dysphasic with modest right-arm weakness. By 45 minutes, she had only occasional word-finding difficulties. Urgent brain CT demonstrated a hyperdensity in the region of the left middle cerebral artery suspicious for an embolus (Fig. 179-2), but since her clinical syndrome was rapidly and spontaneously improving, cerebral angiography was not recommended. Embolization of intraatrial thrombus was considered after rereview of the transesophageal echocardiogram was intrepreted by one observer to show spontaneous echo contrast, a marker for turbulence, and potential for clot formation. The risk of anticoagulation-related cardiac tamponade was felt to be unacceptable since the procedure involves right-heart catheterization and blind right-to-left atrial septal puncture that can be complicated by inadvent atrial wall puncture. That night, she became difficult to arouse, then hemiplegic and mute. Carotid ultrasound was normal, but transcranial Doppler failed to demonstrate left middle artery signal. A fatal left middle and posterior cerebral artery infarct evolved (Fig. 179-3). The proposed mechanism of infarction was middle cerebral embolism with early, partial recanalization but subsequent focal thrombosis perhaps triggered by reduced flow during sleep.

SUGGESTED READINGS

Alio J, Esplugas E, Arboix A, Rubio F: Cerebrovascular events in cardiac catheterization. Stroke 24:1264, 1993

Anstandig J, Wilbourn AJ: Iatrogenic median nerve lesions at the elbow: EMG features in twelve patients. Muscle Nerve 10:647, 1987

Davidson CJ, Skelton TN, Kisslo KB et al: The risk for systemic embolization associated with percutaneous balloon valvuloplasty in adults. Ann Intern Med 108:557–60, 1988

Dawson DM, Fischer EG: Neurologic complications of cardiac catheterization. Neurology 27:496–7, 1977

Galbreath C, Salgado ED, Furlan AJ, Hollman J: Central nervous system complications of percutaneous transluminal coronary angioplasty. Stroke 17:616–19, 1986

Ganglani RD, Turk AA, Mehra MR et al: Contralateral femoral neuropathy: an unusual complication of anticoagulation following PTCA. Cathet Cardiovasc Diagn 24:176–8, 1991

Habermann ET, Cabot WD: Median nerve compression secondary to false aneurysm of the brachial artery. Bull Hosp Joint Dis 35:158–61, 1974

Jacobs MJ, Gregoric ID, Reul GJ: Profunda femoral artery pseudoaneurysm after percutaneous transluminal procedures manifested by neuropathy. J Cardiovasc Surg 33:729–31, 1992

Keilson GR, Schwartz WJ, Recht LD: The preponderance of posterior circulatory events is independent of the route of cardiac catheterization. Stroke 23:1358–9, 1992

Kosmorsky G, Hanson MR, Tomsak RL: Neuro-ophthalmologic complications of cardiac catheterization. Neurology 38:483–5, 1988

Lockwood K, Capraro J, Hanson MR, Conomy JP: Neurologic complications of cardiac catheterization. Neurology 33(suppl. 2):143, 1983

Moody DM, Bell MA, Challa VR et al: Brain microemboli during cardiac surgery or aortography. Ann Neurol 28:477–86, 1990

Nishimura RA, Holmes DR, Reeder GS: Percutaneous balloon valvuloplasty. Mayo Clin Proc 65:198–220, 1990

Schaub F, Theiss W, Heinz M et al: New aspects in ultrasound-guided compression repair of postcatheterization femoral artery injuries. Circulation 90:1861–5, 1994

Sommer C, Ferbert A: Damage to the lateral femoral cutaneous nerve after transfemoral angiography. Nervenarzt 63:633–5, 1992

Vik-Mo H, Todnem K, Flling M, Rosland GA: Transient visual disturbance during cardiac catheterization with angiography. Cathet Cardiovasc Diagn 12:1–4, 1986

Warfel BS, Marini SG, Lachmann EA, Nagler W: Delayed femoral nerve palsy following femoral vessel catheterization. Arch Phys Med Rehabil 74:1211–15, 1993

Weissman BM, Aram DM, Levinsohn MW, Ben-Shachar G: Neurologic sequelae of cardiac catheterization. Cathet Cardiovasc Diagn 11:577–83, 1985

Wilbourn AJ, Furlan AJ, Hulley W, Ruschhaupt W: Ischemic monomelic neuropathy. Neurology 33:447–51, 1983

180. MYOCARDIAL DAMAGE AND CARDIAC ARRHYTHMIAS

WILLIAM T. TALMAN
PATRICIA H. DAVIS

Practitioners are often faced with the effects of the intimate relationship between cardiac and brain function. Although the critical reliance of the brain on normal circulation is obvious, the deleterious effects of neurologic disturbances on cardiac function are less well appreciated. This chapter briefly reviews both the neurologic complications of cardiac disturbances and cardiac complications of neurologic disease, focusing on cardiac arrhythmias as a cause and effect of neurologic conditions. Although this chapter deals exclusively with clinical issues, the reader is referred to recent reviews of the neuroanatomy and physiology of cardiac control by Talman and Benarroch (1992) and Talman and Kelkar (1993).

The heart is capable of generating a normal rhythm and maintaining normal cardiac output in the absence of innervation, but tight coupling of neural and cardiovascular activity plays a significant role in balancing cardiovascular responses to stimuli in health and disease. Despite the brain's important contribution to normal cardiac function, neural input to the heart may also have detrimental effects. Thus, neurologic disturbances may induce cardiac abnormalities in anatomically healthy hearts and complicate cardiac dysfunction in diseased hearts. The scope of these interactions may have far-reaching implications. Conversely, cardiac disease may lead to some of the same neurologic disorders that themselves could have induced the presenting cardiac abnormalities.

Interruption of all parasympathetic and sympathetic input to the heart leads to sinus tachycardia with a cardiac rate of approximately 90 beats/min. In addition, the heart no longer demonstrates spontaneous changes in its rate or changes in response to stimuli. Therefore, denervation, as may occur with autonomic neuropathies or in the transplanted heart, may lead to fixed tachycardia. Even if peripheral autonomic input to the heart is intact, imbalances between sympathetic and parasympathetic activity can disturb cardiac rhythm and output. In this way, primary neurologic disorders may promote potentially dangerous arrhythmias and electrocardiographic changes that may be difficult to distinguish from those due to myocardial ischemia and infarction.

ELECTROCARDIOGRAPHIC ABNORMALITIES

An important example of this phenomenon is the electrocardiographic evidence of myocardial ischemia or injury seen in association with numerous central nervous system lesions. Because it may be impossible to differentiate such changes from those of true atherosclerotic disease, the affected patient must be treated as if there were a primary cardiac event. Indeed, atherosclerotic coronary disease not only may coexist but may predispose the heart to coronary vasoconstriction as a result of a central process. On the other hand, in some patients, electrocardiographic (ECG) changes may occur in the absence of primary cardiac disease.

The most common ECG abnormalities associated with central lesions are prolongation of the Q-T interval, ST segment depression, flattening or inversion of the T wave, and U waves. Although less frequent, some other ECG changes may be even more disturbing. These include elevated, peaked, or notched T waves; ST segment elevation; increased P-wave amplitude; increased QRS voltage; and Q waves. Obviously, such changes might suggest severe metabolic disturbances or ischemic cardiac disease. Their evolution in a manner similar to ischemic changes and occasional elevation of cardiac enzymes in the absence of myocardial infarction further blurs the distinction. It should be clear that a physician would follow a potentially errant diagnostic and therapeutic approach if the only considered explanation for "ischemic" ECG changes and elevated cardiac enzymes accompanying an acute cerebrovascular event were acute myocardial infarction with cerebral embolization. Recognizing that the same changes might occur with a central lesion alone, the physician would be less likely to subject the patient to anticoagulation in the absence of other evidence of cardiogenic emboli. However, ECG changes suggesting ischemia, even in the absence of coronary disease, are associated with significantly increased mortality. Therefore, it is prudent to treat patients for their central disease in a monitored setting until a myocardial infarction has been excluded. The ECG and enzyme changes may, in fact, result from myocardial injury but not depend on coronary disease. The cardiac injury, like the ECG changes, may partially or totally reverse, leaving only U waves and Q-T prolongation.

No ECG pattern is pathognomonic for a particular central lesion, but some central conditions are more likely than others to produce ECG findings. ECG changes are most commonly seen in patients with subarachnoid hemorrhage, intracerebral hemorrhage, ischemic stroke, or head trauma. Less frequent causes include brain tumors, meningitis, multiple sclerosis, spinal cord lesions, hydrocephalus, and manipulation of the basal forebrain during neurosurgery.

Certain ECG changes, such as prolongation of the ST segment, may increase the patient's risk of developing cardiac arrhythmias. Both arrhythmias and changes suggesting ischemia are generally considered secondary to excess or imbalanced cardiac sympathetic nerve activity. Like other ECG changes, arrhythmias may be seen in a wide variety of disorders, including subarachnoid hemorrhage, head injury, cerebral ischemia, cerebral tumors, and seizures. Even neurosurgical manipulation of the brain may evoke arrhythmias. Although arrhythmias with central lesions may be transient and benign, some may portend a fatal outcome. The high incidence of sudden death in patients with subarachnoid hemorrhage is in large part due to fatal ventricular arrhythmias, but this grave complication is by no means restricted to that condition. It has been seen in patients with intracerebral hemorrhage, strokes, and other central lesions as well.

CARDIAC ARRHYTHMIA AS A COMPLICATION OF NERVOUS SYSTEM DISEASE

Of course, cardiac arrhythmias occur much more frequently as a result of primary cardiac disturbance than as a complication of central or peripheral nervous system disease. When the latter is the case, arrhythmias may affect the nervous system in one of two ways: (1) by altering global cerebral blood flow or (2) by causing embolization of a cardiac thrombus. Those arrhythmias that reduce cardiac output may lead to concomitant arterial hypotension. In the absence of cerebrovascular stenosis and with rapid return of cardiac output and blood pressure to normal, this condition is associated with syncope, a transient loss of consciousness without lasting neurologic sequelae. Because patients with such symptomatic arrhythmias have a significant risk of sudden death, they should undergo careful cardiologic evaluation and treatment if the tendency for an arrhythmia is found. The classic presentation in such a case is unprovoked sudden loss of consciousness with little to no warning and without respect to the patient's position at the time of the event. Palpitations and chest discomfort may certainly occur, but their absence does not preclude an arrhythmia.

The same arrhythmia in a patient with a critically stenotic cerebral vessel may lead to signs of focal cerebral ischemia with or without syncope or presyncope. It is very important to keep in mind that syncope is not a sign of cerebral ischemia alone. Therefore, if confronted with a patient who has had transient loss of consciousness, even if left with focal signs, the physician must aggressively seek the cardiac and hemodynamic cause of both events rather than considering the alteration of consciousness secondary to cerebral ischemia.

EMBOLIZATION FROM THE HEART

Another way in which arrhythmias may lead to cerebral ischemia is through embolization from the heart. Atrial fibrillation is the major arrhythmia associated with increased risk of cardioembolic stroke. Currently, nonvalvular atrial fibrillation is the most commonly encountered arrhythmia, and although atrial fibrillation associated with valvular heart disease or thyrotoxicosis also confers increased risk of stroke, management of patients with atrial fibrillation in these settings is not discussed further in this chapter. Nonvalvular atrial fibrillation is associated with a fivefold increase in risk of stroke. The prevalence of atrial fibrillation increases with age from 0.5 percent at 50 to 59 years of age to 8.8 percent at 80 to 89 years. The importance of nonvalvular atrial fibrillation as a risk factor also increases with age, so that between ages 80 and 89 years, it contributes to 24 percent of strokes and thus approaches hypertension (33 percent) as a risk factor. Although the overall risk of stroke in patients with nonvalvular atrial fibrillation is approximately 5 percent per year, not all patients with this arrhythmia are at increased risk of stroke. For example, patients under 60 years of age without associated cardiac disease, hypertension, or diabetes (lone atrial fibrillation) may have the same risk of stroke as age- and sex-matched controls. Whereas patients with none of the risk factors have an event rate of 1 percent per year, stroke risk increases significantly in patients with a history of hypertension, age over 65 years, diabetes, or a previous history of stroke or transient ischemic attack. Risk also increases if transthoracic echocardiography reveals left atrial enlargement or left ventricular dysfunction, but not all strokes in patients with nonvalvular atrial fibrillation are due to cardioembolism. About 12 percent of patients with atrial fibrillation have 50 percent or greater internal carotid stenosis on carotid duplex studies. In one population-based study, the prevalence of atrial fibrillation was 11 percent in those with primary intracerebral hemorrhage, as compared to 18 percent in those with ischemic stroke, suggesting that in at least some patients, the association is incidental. In addition, nonvalvular atrial fibrillation may occur as a result of the stroke.

Primary prevention of stroke with anticoagulants in patients with nonvalvular atrial fibrillation has been investigated in five clinical trials. A metanalysis of these trials has shown that the reduction in risk of stroke is 68 percent (95 percent confidence interval, 50 percent to 79 percent) in patients treated with warfarin. The risk reduction was 84 percent (95 percent confidence interval, 55 percent to 95 percent) in women and 60 percent (95 percent confidence interval 35 to 76 percent) in men. The international normalized ratios ranged from 1.5 to 4.0 in these studies; two were double-blind, placebo-controlled trials. The risk of major hemorrhage on warfarin was 1.3 percent per year, as compared to 1.0 percent per year in the placebo or control group. Results for aspirin therapy are less clear. An American study found that 325 mg/day of aspirin was more effective than placebo in preventing stroke, although the effect was not demonstrated in those over age 75. A Danish study did not show a significant effect of 75 mg of aspirin, but patients in this study had a higher mean age. When the results of these two studies were combined, reduction of risk of stroke was 36 percent (95 percent confidence interval 4 to 57 percent).

Recent recommendations include use of aspirin for those patients with none of the risk factors listed above, as the risk of ischemic stroke or systemic embolism is low. In patients under age 75 years with risk factors, warfarin would be the therapy of choice as long as there is no contraindication to anticoagulation (dementia, poor balance, recent bleeding, poorly controlled hypertension, and inability to correctly comply with the treatment regimen). In patients over age 75 years, the benefit of warfarin over aspirin in preventing ischemic stroke was negated by increased risk of intracranial hemorrhage.

It is also important to assess whether the patient with nonvalvular atrial fibrillation is a candidate for cardioversion to sinus rhythm. A recent analysis suggested that cardioversion followed by low-dose amiodarone to maintain normal sinus rhythm would be the preferred strategy for managing chronic nonvalvular atrial fibrillation because of a lower complication rate than with chronic warfarin therapy. Recommendations for cardioversion include warfarin therapy for 3 weeks for patients in nonvalvular atrial fibrillation for more than 2 days prior to cardioversion. The drug should be continued until sinus rhythm has been maintained for 4 weeks.

The therapy of choice in those with nonvalvular atrial fibrillation and a previous transient ischemic attack or stroke is warfarin. Warfarin (mean international normalized ratio, 2.9), with a 67 percent reduction of risk of recurrent stroke, is significantly more effective than aspirin (300 mg), which had a 14 percent risk reduction. The incidence of major bleeding was 2.8 percent per year on warfarin versus 0.9 percent per year on aspirin, but there were no intracranial hemorrhages. By treating 1,000 patients with nonvalvular atrial fibrillation and a previous stroke or transient ischemic attack for 1 year with warfarin, 90 vascular events could be prevented, as compared to 40 vascular events for those treated with aspirin. The optimum time for starting anticoagulation because of the risk of hemorrhagic conversion after a recent ischemic stroke in a patient with nonvalvular atrial fibrillation has not been addressed, but it is hoped that it will be determined when the results of ongoing trials of anticoagulation in acute ischemic stroke are available. Risk of early recurrent stroke (within the first month) appears to be low in patients with nonvalvular atrial fibrillation.

Future trials will address the level of anticoagulation necessary to prevent ischemic stroke. Lower international normalized ratios will be used, as well as low-dose warfarin combined with aspirin. At present, the American College of Physicians recommends a target international normalized ratio of 2.0 to 3.0 for patients with nonvalvular atrial fibrillation. In summary, warfarin is the therapy of choice for patients with nonvalvular fibrillation and other risk factors. For patients with no other risk factors, aspirin is the optimum therapy. However, decisions concerning anticoagulation have to be individualized. This is particularly true in elderly patients, who are at increased risk of intracranial hemorrhage.

SUGGESTED READINGS

Atrial Fibrillation Investigators: Risk factors for stroke and efficacy of antithrombotic therapy in atrial fibrillation: analysis of pooled data from five randomized controlled trials. Arch Intern Med 154:1449, 1994

Disch DL, Greenberg ML, Holzberber PT: Managing chronic atrial fibrillation: a Markov decision analysis comparing warfarin, quinidine, and low-dose amiodarone. Ann Intern Med 120:449, 1994

EAFT (European Atrial Fibrillation Trial) Study Group: Secondary prevention in non-rheumatic atrial fibrillation after transient ischaemic attack or minor stroke. Lancet 342:1255, 1993

Kanter MC, Tegeler CH, Pearce LA, Weinberger J et al: Carotid stenosis in patients with atrial fibrillation: prevalence, risk factors, and relationship to stroke. Arch Intern Med 154:1372, 1994

Kapoor WN, Karpf M, Wieand HS, Peterson JR et al: A prospective evaluation and follow-up of patients with syncope. N Engl J Med 309:197, 1983

Kopecky SL, Bersh BJ, McGoon MD: The natural history of lone atrial fibrillation. A population-based study over three decades. N Engl J Med 317:669, 1987

Laupacis A, Albers G, Dunn M, Feinberg W: Antithrombotic therapy in atrial fibrillation. Chest 102:426S, 1992

Ruff RL, Talman WT, Petito F: Transient ischemic attacks associated with hypotension in hypertensive patients with carotid artery stenosis. Stroke 12:353, 1981

Sandercock P, Bamford J, Dennis M, Byrne J et al: Atrial fibrillation and stroke: prevalence in different types of stroke and influence on early and long-term prognosis (Oxfordshire Community Stroke Project). BMJ 305:1460, 1992

The Stroke Prevention in Atrial Fibrillation Investigators: Warfarin versus aspirin for prevention of thromboembolism in atrial fibrillation: Stroke Prevention in Atrial Fibrillation II Study. Lancet 343:687, 1994

The Stroke Prevention in Atrial Fibrillation Investigators: Predictors of thromboembolism in atrial fibrillation: II. Echocardiographic features of patients at risk. Ann Int Med 116:6, 1992

Talman WT: Cardiovascular regulation and lesions of the central nervous system. Ann Neurol 18:1, 1985

Talman WT, Benarroch E: Neural control of cardiac function. In pp. 177–86 Dyck PJ, Thomas PK, Griffin JW, Low PA et al (eds): Peripheral Neuropathy. 3rd Ed. WB Saunders, Philadelphia, 1992

Talman WT, Kelkar P: Neural control of the heart. Neurol Clin 11:239, 1993

Vangerhoets F, Bogousslavsky J, Regli F, Van Melle G: Atrial fibrillation after acute stroke. Stroke 24:26, 1993

Wolf PA, Abbott RD, Kannel WB: Atrial fibrillation as an independent risk factor for stroke: the Framingham Study. Stroke 22:983, 1991

181. NEUROLOGIC COMPLICATIONS OF INFECTIVE ENDOCARDITIS

AMY PRUITT

Since William Osler's detailed description of infective endocarditis in 1885, reports of neurologic complications have appeared regularly. Most authors report a stable distribution of neurologic problems and concur that embolic stroke is the most common neurologic complication. There is also general agreement on the relatively constant frequency of total neurologic complications in about 30 percent of patients with infective endocarditis for about one-half of whom the neurologic problem is a presenting symptom of the disease. In most series, patients with neurologic complications have a mortality between 1.5 and three times that of patients without nervous system involvement. Table 181-1 details the percentage of neurologic complications and mortality in 879 patients from five recent series published since 1978, with patient accrual spanning three decades.

These stable incidence and mortality rates mask an evolving spectrum of conditions predisposing to infective endocarditis, causative organisms, and diagnostic and therapeutic techniques. The practicing neurologist should be familiar with the clinical settings in which infective endocarditis is likely to occur, the differential diagnosis of neurologic conditions resembling infective endocarditis, diagnostic procedures, and management of specific neurologic issues that arise frequently in consultation. This chapter outlines the demographic setting of endocarditis in the 1990s; the frequency, distribution, and timing of neurologic events in different types of native and prosthetic valve endocarditis; and current therapeutic recommendations based upon several recently published series as well as a series of 144 patients from my institution. Although the clinical distinction between acute and subacute infective endocarditis has been used for many decades, from the neurologist's perspective, the classification of infective endocarditis according to etiologic agent and underlying condition (native versus prosthetic valve infective) is a more practical formulation and is used in this discussion.

EPIDEMIOLOGY

Table 181-2 lists the conditions predisposing to infective endocarditis. In 20 to 27 percent of infective endocarditis cases, no underlying cardiac condition is apparent, whereas among identifiable predisposing conditions, mitral valve prolapse and degenerative changes greatly outweigh congenital heart disease and rheumatic heart disease. Along with the changing spectrum of underlying cardiac conditions, the age of the affected population is changing. In the recent series from the University of Pennsylvania, the mean ages of patients with and without neurologic complications were similar at 48 and 53, but the range was large (18 to 97) and there was a tendency for a "missing middle," with patient groups clustering among the old (over age 65) and young adults (under age 40). Other series report a higher mean age, probably reflecting local referral patterns.

Risk factors for infective endocarditis include those associated with underlying cardiac abnormalities, patient behavior, and medical and surgical therapies for other conditions. Intravenous drug abuse accounts for an increasing percentage of community-acquired infective carditis and stroke among young adults, whereas 10 to 20 percent of infective endocarditis cases may be hospital-acquired in patients over age 60. Iatrogenic risk factors include invasive instrumentation of the gastrointestinal and genitourinary tracts and indwelling devices such as arterioarterial fistulae, pacemakers, intra-aortic balloon pumps, and central intravenous catheters. Improved medical treatment of native valve infective endocarditis has led to an increasing population at risk for prosthetic valve endocarditis.

The above demographic changes, along with improved medical therapy of systemic malignancy, multiple organ failure, and sepsis, also alter the spectrum of organisms causing infective

TABLE 181-1. Neurologic Complications of Infective Endocarditis: Comparison of Recent Series

Author/Year	No. Patients	% Neurologic Complications	% Stroke[b]	Mortality With Neurologic Complications	Mortality Without Neurologic Complications
Pruitt et al. (1978)	216	39	17	58	20
Salgado et al. (1989)	175	36.5	17	20.6	14.6
Gransden et al. (1989)	178[a]	33	7		
Kanter and Hart (1991)	166[a]	35	20	35	19
Pruitt (1995)	144	29	18	32	13

[a] Series included only native valve endocarditis.
[b] Ischemic and hemorrhagic strokes are grouped together.

endocarditis. The distribution of causative organisms varies among institutions with disparate referral patterns, but several generalizations can be made. In native valve endocarditis, streptococci were responsible for up to 90 percent of infective endocarditis cases in the preantibiotic era. This frequency has declined to around 60 percent in recent studies. The most frequent streptococci are those of the viridans group. Group D streptococci, of which *Enterococcus faecalis* is the most common, account for up to 10 percent of the cases and are particularly resistant to bactericidal antibiotics. Another group D streptococcus, *S. bovis,* observed in association with digestive tract neoplasms, is increasing in frequency. Most recent series have shown an increasing incidence of *Staphylococcus aureus* infection, particularly among patients abusing intravenous drugs or subjected to recent surgery. *S. aureus* now accounts for up to 30 percent of infective endocarditis of cases in some institutions and valves with no apparent pre-existing lesions are involved in up to 30 percent of these cases. Patients with prosthetic valve endocarditis are prone to *Staphylococcus epidermidis* and *S. aureus* infections. Other patient populations, particularly the elderly with multiple system disease and immunocompromised hosts, display a wider range of causative organisms, including those of the *Haemophilus, Actinobacillus, Cardiobacterium, Eikenella,* and *Kinzella* (HACEK) bacterial group and fungal organisms. In heavily pretreated inpatient populations, the incidence of culture-negative endocarditis appears to be rising as well, and accounted for 5.5 percent of cases in my recent experience. From the neurologist's perspective, it is the increasing incidence of *S. aureus* and other virulent bacteria, such as enterococci, along with the less common fungi that alters the pace and severity of neurologic complications. Table 181-3 summarizes demographic characteristics, heart valve involvement, and microbiology in my recent series.

Pathophysiology

The major neurologic manifestations of endocarditis reflect focal, multifocal, or generalized brain malfunction and include stroke (ischemic or hemorrhagic), encephalopathy, and central nervous system (CNS) infection (meningitis, abscess). These complications arise by three major mechanisms: embolization to large and small arteries, infection of brain and meninges, and toxic or immune-mediated injury. Embolism of infected platelet/fibrin thrombi, the most commonly reported neurologic event in all series, can result in bland infarction, micro- or macroabscess formation, septic vasculitis, or mycotic aneurysm. These events represent a continuum of processes whose outcome depends on host defense factors, the involved cardiac valve, the timing and appropriateness of antibiotic therapy, and organism virulence. Continuous bacteremia can produce fever with delirium or metastatic infection of the brain (abscess) or meninges (meningitis). Encephalopathy, the presenting symp-

TABLE 181-2. Distribution of Cardiac Conditions Predisposing to Native Valve Endocarditis

Defect	Frequency (Range)
Mitral valve prolapse	20–29%
Congenital heart defects	13–20%
Degenerative changes	20–21%
Rheumatic heart disease	6–20%
Heart disease with no antecedent	20–27%

(Data from Terpenning MS, Buggy BP, Kaufmann CA: Infective endocarditis: clinical features in young and elderly patients. Am J Med 83:626, 1987; McKinsey DS, Ratts TE, Bisno AL: Underlying cardiac lesions in adults with infective endocarditis: the changing spectrum. Am J Med 86:681, 1987; and Aragon T, Sande MA: Infective endocarditis. p. 190. In Stein JH (ed): Internal Medicine. 4th Ed. Mosby-Year Book, St. Louis, 1994.)

TABLE 181-3. Comparison of Endocarditis Cases With and Without Neurologic Complications

	Patients with Complications (n = 42)[a] n	Patients with Complications (n = 42)[a] %	Patients Without Complications (n = 102)[b] n	Patients Without Complications (n = 102)[b] %
Sex				
Males	25	70	70	71
Females	12	30	28	29
Type of valve				
Native	37	88	93	91
Prosthetic	5	12	9	9
Valve affected				
Mitral	21	50	37	37
Aortic	11	26	20	20
Mitral and aortic	3	7	12	11.7
Tricuspid	2	4.7	9	8.8
Anticoagulation	2	4.7	10	10
Vegetations by echo	22/39	59[c]	35/84	40.6
Organism				
Staphylococcus aureus	18	43[c]	28	28
Streptococcus viridans	6	14	25	24
Enterococcus	4	9.6	18	17
Staphylococcus epidermidis	2	4.8	12	11.7
Culture-negative	1	2.4	7	6.8
Other	11	26[c]	12	11.7
Risk factor				
Intravenous drug use	18	50[c]	28	28
Rheumatic heart disease	4	11	6	6.1
Nosocomial	5	14	14	14
None identifiable	2	5.4	9	9
Outcome				
Improved without surgery	16	40	65	64
Improved, valve replaced	11	27.5	24	23.5
Death	13	32[c]	13	12.7
Due to neurologic complication	6	14	0	0

[a] Mean age, 48.
[b] Mean age, 53.
[c] P < 0.05.

(Data from Pruitt AA: Neurologic complications of infective endocarditis: a review of an evolving disease and its management issues for the 1990's. Neurologist 1: 20–34, 1995.)

TABLE 181-4. Neurologic Complications in 42 Episodes of Infective Endocarditis

	n	% of Total	% at Presentation
Stroke			
Cerebral embolism*	20	14	7
Single	9		
Multiple	11		
Hemorrhagic	3		
Hemorrhagic on warfarin	1		
Intracranial hemorrhage	6	4.1	2.8
Mycotic aneurysm	2		
Septic arteritis (?)	3		
Subdural hematoma and hemorrhagic infarction	1		
Central nervous system infection			
Brain abscess	3		
Meningitis	4		
Aseptic	2		
Purulent	2		
Miscellaneous			
Seizures	6	4.1	1.3
Paraspinal abscess	2	1.3	1.3
Visual obscurations	1		
Peroneal palsy	1		
Radial palsy	1		
Postoperative lower brachial plexopathy	1		
Delirium	2		
Herpes zoster	1		
Opiates	1		

[a] 13/20 emboli occurred within 48 hours of presentation at a time of uncontrolled infection (65%).
(Data from Pruitt AA: Neurologic complications of infective endocarditis: a review of an evolving disease and its management issues for the 1990's. Neurologist 1: 20–34, 1995.)

tom in 27 percent of elderly infective endocarditis patients in one series, poses a complex differential diagnosis, including microabscesses, meningitis, toxic reaction to drugs, and local cardiac complications such as congestive heart failure, perivalvular abscesses, and arrhythmias leading to a low-flow state. The continuous antigenic stimulation of infective endocarditis leads to formation of nonspecific humoral antibodies, such as rheumatoid factor and cryoglobulins, and of circulating immune complexes that may play a role in several less common neurologic sequelae, including late aneurysmal rupture and mononeuropathies.

Of most concern to the clinical neurologist are those CNS manifestations that precede diagnosis of infective endocarditis. In the series of Gransden et al. (1989), early neurologic events correlated with the causative organism of community-acquired native valve endocarditis. Of neurologic events associated with S. aureus infective endocarditis, 54 percent occurred at presentation of the disease, whereas only 19 percent of streptococcal patients experienced early neurologic problems. Salgado and others report that overall, 16 to 23 percent of neurologic complications occur at presentation and another 30 percent occur after initiation of antibiotic therapy but before bacteriologic cure. In my recent experience, 13 of 20 embolic strokes (65 percent) occurred with 48 hours of presentation at a time of uncontrolled infection. Of 144 patients with infective endocarditis, nearly one-fifth (19 percent) presented with a neurologic problem, only 3 of whom, however, had no other evidence of infective endocarditis. Table 181-4 summarizes the distribution and timing of neurologic complications of infective endocarditis.

Differential Diagnosis

Given the protean neurologic manifestations of infective endocarditis, the neurologist needs to consider the possibility of its presence in many patients. The readily recognizable situation of a febrile patient with focal neurologic deficit and heart murmur represents the minority of case presentations. With a declining frequency of underlying heart disease and a concomitant increase in virulent pathogens, a cardiac murmur may be detected at initial evaluation in only one-third of cases. The diagnosis of infective endocarditis should be considered in any febrile patient with a focal neurologic deficit or headache or with an intracranial hemorrhage unexplained by conventional atherosclerotic vascular risk factors. The host and environmental epidemiologic risk factors outlined above should be considered in weighing the possibility of infective endocarditis. Careful questioning of patients with underlying heart conditions should elicit omission of antimicrobial prophylaxis in patients undergoing surgical procedures for whom such treatment is recommended (congenital malformations, prostheses, previous bacterial endocarditis, rheumatic conditions, mitral valve prolapse, and hypertrrophic cardiomyopathy). Current recommendations for dental and surgical procedures at high risk for introducing bacteremia include teeth cleaning, tonsillectomy, intestinal or respiratory tract procedures, cholecystectomy, cystoscopy and other genitourinary manipulations, hysterectomy, prostate surgery, and vaginal childbirth with evidence of vaginal infection. However, the classic triad of neurologic involvement in infective endocarditis—fever, elevated erythrocyte sedimentation rate, and evidence of CNS embolism—can be seen with atrial myxoma, vasculitis due to polyarteritis nodosa or other collagen vascular disease, and nonbacterial thrombotic endocarditis. In many of these situations, prior diagnosis of vasculitis or neoplasia is absent. Therefore, blood cultures (at least two, separated by more than several hours) must be obtained in any suspicious clinical setting. In patients who have recently received antibiotics, additional cultures with, when appropriate, media supplemented with β-lactamase may be necessary. Longer incubation times are necessary for fungi and some fastidious bacteria.

Although the diagnosis of infective endocarditis rests primarily on clinical and microbiologic data, echocardiography plays an increasing role in early evaluation. Transesophageal echocardiography has proved superior to standard two-dimension echocardiography for detection of valvular abscesses and for evaluation of prosthetic valve endocarditis. Echocardiographic data are used as inclusionary criteria for endocarditis in recent series. A patient with a febrile illness and new vegetations on echocardiography should be classified and treated as having infective endocarditis. Several studies have shown an association between demonstrable valvular vegetations and risk of subsequent embolism as well as increased likelihood of valve replacement for congestive heart failure. Recent University of Pennsylvania data show that 74 percent of patients with cerebral emboli had demonstrable vavlular vegetations, whereas only 41 percent of those without neurologic involvement had positive echocardiographic findings. These figures agree with composite report by Lutas et al. (1986) of 11 studies in which the embolic rate was 36 percent for patients with demonstrable vegetations and 15 percent for those with normal echocardiograms. Vegetations larger than 10 mm are generally associated with a higher incidence of emboli than are smaller lesions (47 versus 19 percent). Although embolization may decrease the size of vegetations, re-embolization is also more common in lesions that initially were larger than 10 mm. The presence of vegetations larger than 10 mm and clinical evidence of embolism may lead to consideration of valve replacement, though at present, further prospective data are needed before management decisions can be based on presence and size of cardiac vegetations. Echocardiographic demonstration of vegetations in fungal and certain prosthetic valve infective endocarditis cases may be an indication for valve replacement.

SPECIFIC MANAGEMENT ISSUES

Table 181-5 summarizes the questions most frequently posed to neurologic consultants involved in the management of patients with diagnosed infective endocarditis. The following sections of this chapter address these issues, outline current recommendations for management of the most frequently encountered neurologic complications, and emphasize issues peculiar to prosthetic valve endocarditis.

Cerebral Emboli

Cerebral embolism is the most common neurologic complication of native valve endocarditis or prosthetic valve endocarditis. Aggregate data suggest that about 15 percent of all patients with native valve endocarditis present with brain ischemia and that this complication is extremely uncommon with tricuspid valve endocarditis. In recent series, there is a slight association of mitral valve infection, with a greater risk of cerebral emboli and a much stronger association of cerebral ischemia with causative organism. *S. aureus* infective endocarditis has been associated with roughly double the frequency of cerebral embolism compared to that of streptococcal infective endocarditis cases.

The incidence of emboli is roughly equal in reports pre- and postdating the advent of computed tomography (CT), but there is an increase in detected multiple emboli in the CT era (18 versus 50 percent). CT is the best diagnostic procedure for the acute investigation of sudden focal neurologic deficit in infective endocarditis and can differentiate bland from hemorrhagic infarctions. Magnetic resonance imaging (MRI) may be useful in follow-up of cerebral emboli and may be more sensitive in demonstrating evolution of microabscesses, cerebritis, and aneurysm formation (see discussion of mycotic aneurysms below). Current recommendations call for follow-up MRI if clinically feasible after 1 to 2 weeks of treatment.

Emboli tend to cluster at the time of presentation or during uncontrolled infection and may be associated with systemic emboli in nearly one-half of cases. Late embolism after infec-

TABLE 181-5. Questions Frequently Posed to Neurologic Consultants

Anticoagulation
  What are the risks and benefits of anticoagulation during an episode of endocarditis?
  Should anticoagulation be discontinued in patients with prosthetic valve endocarditis?
  When after an embolic stroke can anticoagulation be reinstituted safely in patients receiving antibiotic therapy for endocarditis?
  Is there a role for heparin or antiplatelet agents?
Cardiac surgery
  Is there a risk of increasing stroke deficit if the patient requires emergent valve replacement?
  Should cerebral emboli be an indication for valve replacement?
  Is there a subgroup of patients who will respond to valve repair surgery and avoid prosthetic valves?
Mycotic aneurysms
  To what extent should a search for aneurysms be undertaken in every patient with endocarditis?
  What is the proper management of mycotic aneurysms?
Antibiotics
  Does the choice of antibiotics or the duration of therapy change for various neurologic complications?

tion is controlled occurs largely in patients with prosthetic valves. A bout of cured native valve endocarditis does not change future stroke risk in patients with valvular heart disease. In a group of 140 patients followed for 22 months after bacteriologic cure, 15 developed stroke, 14 of whom had prosthetic valves. In other studies, stroke subsequent to cured infective endocarditis was readily explained by atherosclerotic risk factors, new infective endocarditis, prosthetic valves, or excessive anticoagulation.

The above data suggest that anticoagulation is not indicated for prevention of recurrent embolic stroke in cured native valve endocarditis. A more pressing question for the neurologic consultant is the role of anticoagulation *during* an episode of infective endocarditis. In the 1940s, it was argued that anticoagulation would improve antibiotic penetration into infected vegetations and prevent thrombi propagation. More recently, it has been argued that there is no role for anticoagulation in infective endocarditis because valvular vegetations are not propagating thrombi and can break off regardless of anticoagulation, with subsequent risk for cerebral hemorrhage.

Large series emphasizing the role of anticoagulation in producing intracranial hemorrhage in infective endocarditis have given rise to fears about using anticoagulants in the setting of infection. In one large series, one-half of the cerebral hemorrhages occurred in the 3 percent of patients anticoagulated at the time of embolism. Experimental evidence suggests that the "worsening" role of anticoagulants may be particularly pronounced when the cerebral emboli are septic. The data have led to confusing recommendations about instituting anticoagulants following cerebral emboli, withholding anticoagulants in prosthetic valve endocarditis, and reinstituting anticoagulants during the course of treatment of infective endocarditis in patients for whom chronic anticoagulation is otherwise indicated. I believe some of the confusion can be resolved by considering the issues of native valve endocarditis and prosthetic valve endocarditis separately.

In native valve endocarditis, the recurrence rate of emboli is low after infection is controlled. Since most emboli have occurred within the first 48 hours, particularly with virulent organisms, anticoagulation is of no benefit in preventing recurrent emboli. Should recurrent emboli develop, every effort to control infection should be instituted, including consideration of cardiac surgery for patients with large vegetations, and the neurologist should counsel withholding of anticoagulation until infection is more adequately controlled, or for at least 48 hours, to minimize risk of bleeding into infarcted cerebrum. Should emboli develop in an anticoagulated patient, the neurologist should advise cessation of anticoagulation for 48 hours for similar reasons. On the other hand, the development of native or prosthetic valve endocarditis without emboli does not dictate the cessation of otherwise indicated anticoagulation therapy. Though the platelet-fibrin thrombus is believed to play a role in formation and propagation of vegetations, the role of antiplatelet agents in preventing embolization has not been addressed in a prospective clinical study.

Cardiac Surgery

Patients with infective endocarditis come to cardiac surgery for a variety of reasons, and the presence of cerebral emboli may contribute to the decision about timing of valve replacement. The neurologist is frequently asked about the risk of bleeding into an ischemic stroke during bypass or the effect of nonpulsatile blood flow or hypotension on a recent infarction. What appears clear from various series is that valve replacement is not mandatory for patients with early embolism in the absence of other cardiac indications. If emergent cardiac surgery is required, several studies have suggested that in patients operated on within a few days of stroke the deficits may worsen. The complication rate in my series was 30 percent for patients who required valve replacement within 2 weeks. Another study suggested that emergent valve replacement conferred no special increased risk. Consensus suggests that if the physician has the luxury, he or she should wait until cerebral edema has subsided—thus, at least 5 days.

Prosthetic Valve Endocarditis

Patients with bioprosthetic or mechanical valves have a 1 to 4 percent incidence of infective endocarditis, conventionally divided into late (more than 60 days postoperatively) and early (less than 60 days following valve replacement). Though the incidence of prosthetic valve endocarditis cases in various series reflects hospital referral patterns, aggregate analysis of more than 200 patients in the literature suggests that inadequately anticoagulated patients with mechanical valves are at greatest risk of embolism. Thus, it would not be prudent to advise discontinuation of anticoagulation at the onset of prosthetic valve endocarditis in a high-risk mechanical valve. A recent study by suggests that heparin may be safer than Coumadin (warfarin) in this population. Of 16 patients treated with heparin, 15 were embolism free. There is general agreement that hemorrhage into embolism confers a high mortality; therefore, it is recommended that if an embolism occurs, anticoagulation should be discontinued for 48 hours, with repeat CT scanning performed prior to reinstitution of anticoagulation in high-risk valves.

Recommendations for Anticoagulants

Recommendations concerning anticoagulation for native and prosthetic valve endocarditis are as follows:

1. The development of native valve or prosthetic valve bacterial endocarditis does not dictate cessation of otherwise indicated warfarin therapy.
2. Anticoagulation is not indicated for the prevention of recurrent embolic stroke in native valve endocarditis.
3. If a cerebral embolic event occurs in an anticoagulated patient with infective endocarditis, withhold anticoagulation for 48 hours unless the patient has a high-risk prosthetic valve.
4. If fungal endocarditis is present, consider discontinuation of anticoagulation in all but the highest-risk prostheses.
5. Routine initiation of anticoagulation to prevent stroke in bioprosthetic valve endocarditis is not justified.

Areas of future study include the role of antiplatelet agents in preventing stroke, confirmation of the encouraging report of heparin's safety in prosthetic valve endocarditis, and refinement of echocardiographic data about vegetations and cardiac surgery. The role of valve repair surgery, used to avoid the long-term risk of prosthetic valves, needs to be clarified for patients with large vegetations and high embolic risk.

Intracranial Hemorrhage

Intracranial hemorrhage occurs in 3 to 6 percent of patients with infective endocarditis. Four mechanisms are responsible: ruptured mycotic aneurysm, septic arteritis, hemorrhagic transformation of initially bland embolic infarction, and, in rare instances, immune complex injury to vasculature resulting in aneurysmal formation months to years after the initial episode of infective endocarditis. Intracranial hemorrhage is associated with a high mortality and represents a spectrum of arterial injury from acute pyogenic necrosis to late rupture of an aseptic aneurysm. Hemorrhagic transformation of cerebral infarction is dealt with in this chapter under Cerebral Emboli, above. Septic arteritis, seen in three cases in my current series, occurs early in the course of virulent organism-related infective endocarditis and may have a higher rate of occurence when there is purulent meningeal inflammation.

Infectious intracranial aneurysms, more commonly known by the Oslerian term *mycotic aneurysms,* are recognized in 1 to 5 percent of infective endocarditis cases. The true incidence almost certainly exceeds the diagnosed numbers, as many aneurysms may heal after antibiotic therapy. Typical locations for mycotic aneurysms due to infective endocarditis are sites where septic emboli are likely to lodge and tend to be more peripheral than those associated with extravascular infectious sources. Fungal infective endocarditis, however, is associated with large proximal aneurysms. The original studies by Molinari et al. (1973) of mycotic aneurysm formation appear confirmed by subsequent neuropathologic investigation. His dog studies suggested that aneurysm formation depended on embolic site, host defenses, and efficacy and timing of antimicrobial therapy. Dogs developed mycotic aneurysms within 3 days if they were untreated, whereas antibiotics delayed the formation of aneurysms by 7 to 10 days or resulted in the formation of brain abscess. Invasion of the vessel wall occurred from the vasa vasorum of the adventitia, with weakening and subsequent rupture.

An eloquent debate has arisen in the literature about the aggressiveness indicated in the search for mycotic aneurysms. On the one hand, it has been argued that all patients with neurologic abnormalities not attributable to systemic toxicity, including cerebrospinal fluid pleocytosis, should undergo four-vessel cerebral angiography and that single accessible lesions in medically stable patients should be promptly excised. Opposing this view are others who emphasize the rarity of mycotic aneurysms, their symptomatic clustering in the early stages of infection, and the extremely low incidence of late rupture following bacteriologic cure of endocarditis. It is not surprising that there is a divergence of opinion, given the conflicting outcomes from large series. In the study by Ojemann et al. (1983) of 27 cases followed up with angiography during antibiotic treatment, 8 aneurysms disappeared, 5 decreased, 4 were unchanged, 6 increased, and in 4 cases, new aneurysms formed. Though there is ample documentation that aneurysms heal with antibiotic therapy alone, there is only one systematic study correlating CT and four-vessel angiography. Among the important findings in this study were the high frequency of multiple aneurysms and the high incidence of aneurysms (11/35 patients with neurologic signs). However, there were no mycotic aneurysms in patients with normal CT scan results. All 11 patients with aneurysms had abnormal CT scan results. A reasonable conclusion drawn by these authors was that CT is a practical screen for the possibility of aneurysm. These data need to be confirmed, however, and the role of MRI and magnetic resonance angiography remains unclear.

I prefer a compromise in approach to mycotic aneurysm. Recognizing that for many unfortunate patients with aneurysm, the rupture will occur at presentation or too early in the course for meaningful intervention, I recommend emergent CT for patients with neurologic symptoms. The presence of blood on CT should dictate four-vessel angiography; decisions about emergent surgery will depend on the patient's medical condition, the location and integrity of the aneurysm(s), and their multiplicity. Current techniques for excising mycotic aneurysms require ligation of the affected vessel, and the likelihood of severe neurologic deficit should be weighed in the management decision. Severe persistent headache or "sentinel" transient embolic symptoms with normal CT scan findings also dictate lumbar puncture. Since minimal aneurysm leakage can result in a focal meningeal reaction, cerebrospinal fluid pleocytosis would sway the decision in favor of four-vessel angiography.

Yet to be defined is the role of prophylactic angiography in high-risk patients who require acute valve replacement and short- or long-term anticoagulation. Some authors have advocated angiography in all such patients prior to surgery, as reports of aneurysm rupture perioperatively have raised concern, and the often young patients involved may receive lifelong anticoagulation with mechanical prostheses. It is possible that since one of the mechanisms of aneurysm formation is adventitial invasion, we should consider those patients with *S. aureus* meningeal reaction at particular risk and study them with angiography prophylactically. However, it is my opinion that available information on the low incidence of late hemorrhage even in this group does not justify routine angiography in this setting.

Current recommendations for the management of mycotic aneurysms are as follows:

1. Routine angiography for all patients with meningitis or evidence of cerebral emboli is not justified.
2. The indications for neurosurgical repair need to be individualized by organism; aneurysm location, number, and size; and the patient's medical condition.
3. Serial angiography is indicated for those mycotic aneurysms that are being treated medically.
4. Angiography is not recommended prior to anticoagulation of all patients requiring acute valve replacement.

Brain Abscess

A continuum exists between ischemic/hemorrhagic cerebrovascular disease in infective endocarditis and CNS infection, depending on host factors, organism, and antibiotic therapy. An increased incidence of radiographically demonstrable cerebritis and microabscess formation is apparent in the MRI era. However, the incidence of macroscopic brain abscess has remained low in all series. Allowing for more sensitive radiographic techniques, however, three abscesses were apparent in my recent series. All developed on antibiotic therapy and resolved without surgical intervention. CT- or MRI-guided needle aspiration proved useful in the management of two of these cases.

A recent clinicopathologic conference raises a cautionary tale about superinfection of cerebral embolic infarctions in the setting of central venous line–induced septicemia. A (presumably) initially bland infarction may have been seeded by *S. aureus* and resulted in the development of brain abscesses months after the patient completed a 17-day course of antibiotics. Patients with "uncomplicated" septicemia and recent cerebral infarction may deserve a full infective endocarditis course of antibiotics, and transesophageal echocardiography may disclose vegetations and dictate longer duration of therapy in patients with bacteremia.

SUMMARY

Despite earlier detection and better antibiotic therapy, the frequency of neurologic complications of bacterial endocarditis remains high, and patients with neurologic complications are distinguished from those without such sequelae by having more frequent angiographically demonstrable vegetations, a higher frequency of *S. aureus* as the pathogen, a rising rate of both nosocomial infections and intravenous drug abuse as the underlying risk factors for infective endocarditis, and twice the mortality rate. Mortality from infective endocarditis in the group with neurologic complications is due to the neurologic problem in about one-half and to cardiac compromise in the remaining one-half. The challenge in the diagnosis of patients with infective endocarditis involves an awareness of the evolving spectrum of host factors and organisms. The challenge in management of patients with endocarditis remains the establishment of criteria for identification of those few patients for whom early surgical or medical (anticoagulation) intervention can minimize neurologic morbidity.

Management Issues Requiring Further Study

Transesophageal Echocardiography. The role of transesophageal echocardiography in defining patients with clinical endocarditis who can have a shorter course of antibiotis, in selecting those who required full treatment for endocarditis, and in committing certain patients to valve replacement of repair needs to be developed further.

Anticoagulation. The role of heparin in preventing emboli in prosthetic valve endocarditis and the possible role of antiplatelet agents in reducing the risk of cerebral emboli are worthy of further study.

Magnetic Resonance Angiography. The sensitivity of magnetic resonance angiography in detecting unruptured mycotic aneurysms needs to be correlated with conventional angiography.

SUGGESTED READINGS

Barrow DL: Infectious intracranial aneurysms: comparisons of groups with and without endocarditis. Neurosurgery 27:472, 1990

Bertorini TE, Laster RE, Thompson BF: Magnetic resonance imaging of the brain in bacterial endocarditis. Arch Intern Med 149:815, 1989

Brust JCM, Dickinson PCT, Hughes JED et al: The diagnosis and treatment of cerebral mycotic aneurysms. Ann Neurol 27:238, 1990

Case Records of the Massachusetts General Hospital 31–1991. N Engl J Med 325:341, 1991

Davenport J, Hart RG: Prosthetic valve endocarditis 1976–1987. Antibiotics, anticoagulation and stroke. Stroke 21:993, 1990

Delahaye JP, Poncet PH, Malquarti V et al: Cerebrovascular accidents in infective endocarditis: role of anticoagulation. Eur Heart J 11:1074, 1990

Francioli PJ: Central nervous system complications of infective endocarditis. In Scheld WM, Whitley RJ, Durack DT (eds): Infections of the Central Nervous System. Raven Press, New York, 1991

Gransden WR, Eykyn SJ, Leach RM: Neurological presentations of native valve endocarditis. Q J Med 73:1135, 1989

Hart RG, Foster JW, Luther MF et al: Stroke in infective endocarditis. Stroke 21:695, 1990

Hart RG, Kagan-Hallet K, Joerns SE: Mechanisms of intracranial hemorrhage in infective endocarditis. Stroke 18:1048, 1987

Kanter MC: Cerebral mycotic aneurysms are rare in infective endocarditis. Ann Neurol 28:590, 1990

Kanter MC: Management of acute stroke in infective endocarditis. Neurology 40(suppl. 1):S417, 1990

Kanter MC, Hart RG: Neurologic complications of infective endocarditis. Neurology 41:1015, 1991

Keyser DL, Biller J, Coffman TT et al: Neurologic complications of late prosthetic valve endocarditis. Stroke 21:472, 1990

Leport C, Vilder JL, Bricaire F et al: Fifty cases of late prosthetic valve endocarditis: improvement in prognosis over a 15 year period. Br Heart J 58:66, 1987

Lutas EM, Roberts RB, Devreux RB et al: Relation between the presence of echocardiographic vegetations and the complication rate in infective endocarditis. Am Heart J 112:107, 1986

Maruyama M, Kuriyama Y, Sawada T et al: Brain damage after open heart surgery in patients with acute cardioembolic stroke. Stroke 20:1305, 1990

McKinsey DS, Ratts TE, Bisno AL: Underlying cardiac lesions in adults with infective endocarditis: the changing spectrum. Am J Med 82:681, 1987

Molinari GF, Smith L, Goldstein MN et al: Pathogenesis of cerebral mycotic aneurysms. Neurology 23:325, 1973

Ojemann J, Crowell RM: Infectious intracranial aneurysms. pp. 225–63. In Ojemann RG (ed): Surgical Management of Cerebrovascular Disease. Williams & Wilkins, Baltimore, 1983

Pruitt AA: Neurologic complications of infective endocarditis: a review of an evolving disease and its management issues in the 1990's. Neurologist 1: 20–34, 1995

Pruitt AA, Rubin RH, Karchmer AW et al: Neurologic complications of bacterial endocarditis. Medicine (Baltimore) 57:329, 1978

Salgado AV, Furlan AJ, Keys TF et al: Neurologic complications of endocarditis: a 12 year experience. Neurology 39:173, 1989

Stilhart B, Aboulker J, Khouadja F et al: Should the aneurysms of Osler's disease be investigated and operated upon prior to hemorrhage? Neurochirurgie 32:410, 1986

Terpenning MS, Buggy BP, Kaufmann CA: Infective endocarditis: clinical features in young and elderly patients. Am J Med 83:626, 1987

Ting W, Silverman N, Levitsky S: Valve replacement in patients with endocarditis and cerebral septic emboli. Ann Thoracic Surg 51:18, 1991

Zisbrod Z, Rose DM, Jacobwitz IJ et al: Results of open heart surgery in patients with recent cardiogenic embolic stroke and central nervous system dysfunction. Circulation 76(suppl. V):V-109, 1987

182. HYPERTENSIVE ENCEPHALOPATHY AND ECLAMPSIA

JAMES O. DONALDSON

Hypertensive encephalopathy is an acute or subacute cerebral disorder due to a sustained, substantial increase in blood pressure; it is largely reversible with treatment of hypertension. This condition occurs both in chronically hypertensive patients with an abrupt rise in an already increased blood pressure and in previously normotensive patients—most notably in young women with toxemia of pregnancy and among children and young adults with acute glomerulonephritis and other renal diseases. Other causes include use of sympathomimetic agents such as phenylpropanolamine ingested in conjunction with a weight control program, oral ingestion of phencyclidine, and high tyramine ingestion by depressed patients being treated with a monoamine oxidase inhibitor. Hypertensive encephalopathy has been reported both during rebound hypertension following withdrawal of clonidine hydrochloride and a few hours after an infusion of saralasin acetate during investigation of renin-dependent hypertension. Also, quadriplegics and paraplegics with complete spinal cord lesions above T5–T6 can develop a hypertensive crisis as part of autonomic hyper-reflexia due to a painful visceral stimuli including chronic constipation, bladder distention, and childbirth.

There is no one blood pressure above which hypertensive encephalopathy occurs because the critical blood pressure is relative to an individual patient's customary blood pressure. In customarily normotensive patients, a blood pressure of 140/90 mmHg *or lower* may suffice, whereas chronically hypertensive patients may require blood pressures in excess of 240/140 mmHg. The minimum duration of sustained relative hypertension required for the development of hypertensive encephalopathy in humans is undetermined. A few minutes of severe hypertension during sexual intercourse and during acute anxiety attacks are tolerated. However, mild pre-eclampsia can precipitously evolve into eclampsia with sustained rises in blood pressure lasting less than 1 hour.

PATHOLOGY

The microscopic hallmark of hypertensive encephalopathy is focal or segmental fibrinoid arteriolar necrosis with surrounding ring hemorrhages. These lesion tend to occur in the occipital lobes and in patches that often represent watersheds between the territories of major cerebral arteries. Arterial hyalinization will also be present in chronically hypertensive patients.

CLINICAL SYNDROME

The clinical manifestations are (1) headache, (2) alterations in mental functions and level of consciousness, (3) convulsions, (4) cortical disorders of vision, and, less frequently, (5) aphasia, vertigo, and tinnitus.

Headache

Headache is probably the earliest and most common symptom. At first nothing may distinguish it from an ordinary muscle-contraction headache. The location is nonspecific and more likely to be predominantly frontal, unlike the morning occipital headache often ascribed to poorly controlled chronic hypertension. Headache may be a more prominent symptom among previously normotensive patients than among those with chronic hypertension. Usually the severity of headache with unresponsiveness to simple analgesics and the development of nausea and encephalopathy suggest that the headache is more significant than originally was apparent.

Encephalopathy

The manifestations of altered cerebral dysfunction include confusion, agitation, lassitude, somnolence, and disorientation plus obtundation ranging from stupor to coma. Not part of this syndrome are asterixis and myoclonic jerks, which are more characteristic of uremia. It is of more than historical interest that, in 1914—soon after the clinical determination of blood urea and the introduction of the blood pressure cuff—Volhard used *pseudouremia* for the syndrome that Oppenheimer and Fishberg named *hypertensive encephalopathy* in 1928.

Seizures

The convulsions of hypertensive encephalopathy are characteristically generalized tonic-clonic seizures with the exception of simple focal seizures by some children with acute glomerulonephritis. As noted by Gowers and later by Oppenheimer and Fishberg, superimposed on generalized convulsions may be clinical features of multiple seizure foci irregularly punctuating either one prolonged convulsion or successive seizures. The author has observed aversive eye movements caused by a focus in one hemisphere with one eclamptic convulsion, as well as limb jerking caused by a focus in the other hemisphere during the next seizure.

Visual Disturbances

Visual disturbances of hypertensive encephalopathy among previously normotensive patients may differ from those in patients with chronic hypertension. In women with severe preeclampsia, photopsias herald the onset of eclamptic convulsions for 40 to 50 percent. Indeed, "eclampsia," which is derived from a Greek verb meaning "to shine forth," could have been named for this perception of a streak of light. Cortical blindness and Anton syndrome may occur in the absence of convulsions among young, previously normotensive patients with acute glomerulonephritis and severe toxemia of pregnancy. The typical finding on inspecting the optic fundi is severe arteriolar constriction and sometimes a serous retinal detachment. Blurred vision is a commonly recorded complaint among usually older, chronically hypertensive patients, but unlike the younger, previously normotensive group, the eye grounds are more likely to show hemorrhages and exudates, papilledema, and chronic arteriolar changes.

NEURODIAGNOSTIC TESTING

Although the diagnosis of hypertensive encephalopathy should be considered in anyone with severe hypertension, headache, and an altered mental status, the modern clinician must sort out hypertensive encephalopathy from other causes of brain dysfunction in hypertensive patients. Unlike our forebears, modern clinicians have the advantage of a variety of neurodiagnostic studies.

Cerebrospinal Fluid

Lumbar puncture can reveal that cerebrospinal fluid is under normal, or, more commonly, elevated pressure. The concentration of protein in cerebrospinal fluid is typically 50 to 150 mg/dl. A few red cells can be expected.

Electroencephalography

The electroencephalogram (EEG) reflects the status of the patient—from mild slowing of background activity in patients just having difficulty thinking to delta activity in stuporous patients, often prominently in the posterior regions in patients with cortical blindness. Trains of spike-wave and multispike-wave discharges occur during a convulsion. In the case of eclampsia, the EEG can be normal 24 hours beforehand and Jost has observed that EEG abnormalities decrease if blood pressure decreases.

Imaging

Both computed tomography (CT) and magnetic resonance imaging (MRI) can be normal, can demonstrate bleeding, or can indicate cerebral edema either focally or diffusely with slitlike ventricles. Edema is characteristically in the occipital lobes, in scattered loci in the white matter, deep gray matter, and brainstem—in essence mimicking the previously described neuropathology. Neuroradiologists often remark that zones of edema are in watersheds between the territories of major cerebral arteries. Of special interest is one otherwise rare pattern

consisting of arcuate hypodense bands through the external and internal capsules.

The timing of the appearance of this cerebral edema is important. Not infrequently radiologists interpret hypodense areas as cerebral infarctions without considering their timing. CT within hours of a standard ischemic stroke is usually normal. A hypodense wedge denoting cytotoxic cerebral edema with swelling of neurons and glia develops several days later. By contrast, CT soon after a hypertensive crisis may detect hypodense areas, which with adequate antihypertensive treatment may vanished within several days. This sequence is consistent with vasogenic cerebral edema from leakage of water and protein into brain through a leaky blood–brain barrier, as is the change in magnetic resonance after administration of gadolinium.

Single-photon-emission computed tomography utilizes radioactively labeled substances that are almost entirely bound up by the brain during their first transit through the cerebral circulation. In hypertensive encephalopathy this technique has demonstrated increased uptake, and thus presumably increased regional blood flow, in occipital regions where MRI demonstrated edema. The finding was also reversible.

PATHOGENESIS

The pathogenesis of hypertensive encephalopathy with its ring hemorrhages and fibrinoid necrosis can now be attributed to the failure of vasoconstriction at extremely high blood pressures to limit both perfusion through the capillary bed and the pressure exerted upon capillary endothelial cells. In pathophysiologic terms the upper limit of the autoregulation of cerebral blood flow is exceeded in hypertensive encephalopathy. The breakthrough occurs first in the occipital lobes and in the watersheds. At higher pressures the process operates throughout the brain and generalized vasogenic cerebral edema results. The upper limit of autoregulation of cerebral perfusion is directly dependent upon an individual's customary blood pressure. Thus those who usually have low blood pressures (e.g. children and pregnant young women) develop hypertensive encephalopathy at blood pressures that would be considered to be acceptable control for a patient with chronic hypertension.

TREATMENT

Hypertensive encephalopathy presents an emergency situation. The objectives are to decrease blood pressure to within the range of autoregulation, to control convulsions, and to manage cerebral edema. The cause of the hypertensive crisis can define the mode. For a quadriplegic with fecal impaction, enemas may be the ultimate cure although antihypertensive medication may be needed temporarily. In this case a drug such as labetalol, which blocks both α- and β-adrenergic receptors, is an excellent choice. Similarly, in the case of renin-dependent hypertension, angiotensin-converting enzyme inhibitors, such as captopril and enalaprilat, are effective.

Hypertension

The ideal antihypertensive drug for hypertensive encephalopathy would lower systemic blood pressure rapidly to within the range of autoregulation but in a controlled manner, to prevent overshooting that range. A ganglionic blocking agent such as trimethaphan is effective but too unpredictable for frequent use in an era with other available drugs. Furthermore, the agent should have minimal effect on cerebral vessels. For instance, although nitroglycerine decreases systemic resistance, it also dilates cerebral vessels and thereby could theoretically worsen hypertensive encephalopathy.

The targeted zone can be estimated from knowledge of a individual patient's customary blood pressure. If this is unknown, mean arterial blood pressure should be lowered by 20 to 25 percent. Determination of an acceptable range of blood pressures may require monitoring intracranial pressure for severely stuporous patients and those with extensive cerebral edema on CT or MRI.

Most often vasodilators are used to decrease peripheral resistance. Each has its advantages and disadvantages. Basically, doctors use the agent with which they are most familiar. Sodium nitroprusside is the drug of choice for many; however, it must be shielded from light and its administration requires constant nursing attention, which may not be practical. Bolus injections of diazoxide may be effective within 1 to 5 minutes and may last for 6 hours or more, but blood pressures lower than the target zone can occur and thereby cause end-organ ischemia. Hydralazine is the choice of many obstetricians. However, its onset of action even after intravenous administration is relatively slow, approximately 20 minutes. Nifedipine, a calcium channel blocker, has the advantage of oral administration if intravenous access is a problem. Sublingual and buccal nifedipine take effect within 5 to 10 minutes, oral doses after 15 to 20 minutes.

Seizures

The best prophylactic anticonvulsant in hypertensive encephalopathy is effective antihypertensive treatment. Obstetricians have traditionally preferred to use magnesium sulfate (10 mg IM or IV loading dose followed by 5 mg IM or IV every 4 hours). A recent study comparing magnesium sulfate with phenytoin showed that magnesium sulfate treatment was superior; however, patients were not controlled for blood pressure levels. Therefore, it is still fair to conclude that blood pressure management is the first line of attack in preventing eclamptic seizures. If convulsions occur, diazepam is a common choice for immediate control.

Cerebral Edema

The principles for treatment of the vasogenic cerebral edema of hypertensive encephalopathy rest on its pathophysiology. Usually the cerebral edema of hypertensive encephalopathy abates soon after blood pressure is controlled. However, in comatose patients with widespread cerebral edema, intracranial pressure monitoring and more aggressive treatment may be needed. A simple first measure is corticosteroid therapy, which limited research suggests to be effective for vasogenic cerebral edema of hypertensive encephalopathy just as it is for edema surrounding tumors metastatic to brain. Hyperventilation would also be predicted to help by both decreasing intracranial pressure and increasing the upper limit of autoregulation. It should be pointed out that mannitol can be predicted to be ineffective and potentially dangerous due to passage of the drug through a leaky capillary blood–brain barrier, thereby worsening cerebral edema.

SUGGESTED READINGS

Calhoun DA, Oparil S: Treatment of hypertensive crisis. N Engl J Med 323: 1177, 1990

Chester EM, Agamanolis DP, Banker BQ, Victor M: Hypertensive encephalopathy: a clinicopathologic study of 20 cases. Neurology 28:928, 1978

Dinsdale HB: Hypertensive encephalopathy. Neurol Clin 1:3, 1983

Donaldson JO: Eclamptic hypertensive encephalopathy. Semin Neurol 8:230, 1988

Hauser RA, Lacey M, Knight MR: Hypertensive encephalopathy, magnetic resonance imaging demonstration of reversible cortical and white matter lesions. Arch Neurol 45:1078, 1988

Jellenik EH, Painter M, Prineas J, Russell RR: Hypertensive encephalopathy with cortical disorders of vision. Q J Med 33:239, 1964

Lucas MJ, Leveno KJ, Cunningham FG: A comparison of magnesium sulfate with phenytoin for the prevention of eclampsia. N Engl J Med 333:201–5, 1995

Schwartz RB, Jones KM, Kalina P et al: Hypertensive encephalopathy: findings on CT, MR imaging, and SPECT imaging in 14 cases. AJR 9:379, 1992

183. AORTIC DISSECTION

CORMAC A. O'DONOVAN
JOHN P. CONOMY

Although aortic dissection is relatively uncommon, it is being recognized more often nowadays as a result of an increased awareness of its existence and the availability of new radiologic diagnostic methods. Clinical diagnosis remains a difficult problem and frequently occurs only when the physician has a high index of suspicion of the condition. The difficulty arises because many of the symptoms are usually associated with more common diseases. Sir William Osler said, "There is no disease more conducive to clinical humility than aneurysm of the aorta."

The term *aortic dissection* is used interchangeably with *dissecting aortic aneurysm*, but the presence of an aneurysm is not a prerequisite for the occurrence of dissection of the aorta. At the beginning of the century, aortic dissection was diagnosed mainly at autopsy, after the patient had presented in an obtunded state and had deteriorated rapidly to death. Although aortic dissection remains relatively uncommon and diagnosis can be difficult, early recognition is important because delays in instituting treatment have a significant impact on survival. At the other end of the spectrum, small aortic dissections are frequently discovered at autopsy, and only careful retrospective analysis of the medical record points to undiagnosed aortic dissection as the likely cause of symptoms that persisted for many years before the death of the patient. The marked improvement in outcome after treatment in recent years is related to early diagnosis in cases of atypical chest pain and other unexplained symptoms. Recognition of the differences between proximal and distal dissections in terms of symptoms, the temporal course of the disease progression, and outcomes from different treatment modalities is necessary for understanding this important condition.

The first case of dissecting aortic aneurysm described in the literature was that of George II of England, who died of it in 1761. The condition was not named until about 50 years later, when two more cases were described. Until the early 1930s, the diagnosis was rarely made before death. Catastrophic rupture of the aorta was the most commonly reported presentation. In those cases, profound shock from hemodynamic instability dominates the clinical picture, and death from shock rapidly supervenes. A small, contained rupture of a dissecting aortic aneurysm mimics the signs and symptoms of lesions more often associated with other structures in the vicinity of the aorta, and therefore aortic dissection is frequently undiagnosed as the cause. This difficulty in diagnosis is reflected in an 1843 statement by Peacock, who said ''nor are the symptoms which attend its formation and progress such as can be regarded as characteristic of its affection.''

INCIDENCE

The incidence of aortic dissection is difficult to establish from the reported series and is probably understimated because of the occurrence of sudden death with this condition. Population-based studies using data from angiography, surgical cases, and autopsy reports estimate 40 cases/1,000,000/year, which would mean an incidence rate of 10,000 cases annually in the United States. Historically, when aortic dissection was usually diagnosed postmortem, autopsy series showed an overall incidence of 4 percent. The enhanced awareness of the condition and the availability of newer radiologic methods for detection, not an increased incidence, is responsible for the extensive literature available today on the subject. Dissecting aortic aneurysm is said to be the second most common form of aneurysm affecting the aorta, after the dilated fusiform atherosclerotic form. However, it may prove to be the most common as our diagnostic ability improves. Antemortem diagnosis is made more readily when the ''tear'' is more severe and symptoms are more florid. Small dissections of the aorta in patients with less profound clinical symptoms are primarily detected today as a result of radiologic techniques. Aortic dissection is thought to occur most commonly in middle-aged hypertensive patients. Cases involving children are rare. The incidence of dissecting aneurysm at autopsy in patients younger than 20 years is low, approximately 1 in 2,500. Younger patients with dissection of the aorta show a higher incidence of the conditions that predispose the medial layer of blood vessels to weakness.

CAUSES

The association of different diseases with aortic dissection is difficult to assess for a number of reasons. Because the overall incidence is low, the possibility that aortic dissection is associated by chance with a given disease rather than being one of the cardinal features of it frequently exists. However, conditions featuring inherited defects in connective tissue formation, such as Ehlers-Danlos syndrome, are relatively common causes of aortic dissection. Marfan syndrome has the most well-known asssociation with aortic dissection, which is the most common cause of death in this syndrome. Other congenital conditions in which aortic dissection is sometimes seen include Turner syndrome, congenital bicuspid or tricuspid aortic valve, and Noonan syndrome. Systemic conditions giving rise to dedifferentiation of elastic tissue can cause overproduction of a mucoid substance, which subsequently accumulates in the medial layer of the aorta.

Aortic dissection commonly occurs in conditions in which the aorta has been previously dilated by any of several different pathologic processes. In many of these cases, the dissection is overshadowed by the distention of the aorta, especially when the dissection is relatively small and clinically silent. The classification of idiopathic cases under the category of *medial degeneration* occurs commonly and is most often seen in patients over 40 years of age. This term is applied when intimal tears are not evident and the only detectable lesion is the hematoma within the medial layer. Focal ischemic necrosis of muscle may be followed by degeneration of elastic tissue and collagen to produce clefts in the medial layer. In younger patients, abnormal accumulation of mucoid substance in the media caused by

excessive production may degrade the elastic tissue. Intimal tears, which are seen in almost 95 percent of cases, may occur as a result of weakening of the aortic wall through a defect in the media, rather than as a rupture of the intimal lining as the primary process. Elderly patients with aortic dissection have a history of hypertension, and they predominantly have distal lesions. However, the exact association between aortic dissection and hypertension is tenuous, given its low incidence in hypertensive patients in whom dilated, fusiform atherosclerotic aneurysms are the most frequently reported aortic lesion. Of women younger than 40 with aortic dissection, up to half are pregnant; despite the high frequency of this occurrence, the mechanism remains obscure. A number of vasculitides are associated with aortic dissection, including giant cell arteritis, relapsing polychondritis, systemic lupus erythematosus, Takayasu's arteritis, and rheumatic fever, but these associations are usually based on single case reports. If it affects the aorta, trauma to the chest wall usually causes transection but can occasionally cause aortic dissection. Aortic surgery involving either the aorta or the aortic valve can result in dissection postoperatively.

CLASSIFICATION SYSTEM

The systems used to classify aortic dissections are based on the location of the dissection. Determining the extent of the hematoma is of value for comparing results of various treatments so as to guide management of these patients. However, categorizing the different ''types'' solely on location of the dissection leaves out other important factors, such as location of the associated intimal tears and the extent of retrograde as well as anterograde progression of the dissecting process.

The most widely used classification system is probably that of DeBakey, who has extensive surgical experience with this disease (Fig. 183-1). This system is based on findings from the series of patients with aortic dissection on whom he operated. The system consists of three types; type 1 lesions occur in the ascending aorta to beyond the aortic arch (60 to 70 percent); type 2 lesions involve the ascending aorta only; and type 3 lesions arise beyond the subclavian artery (20 to 30 percent). The Stanford system, developed by Dailey and colleagues, classifies lesions on whether the ascending aorta is involved (type A) or not (type B). Further subdivision using this system is made according to the location of the associated intimal tear (site 1, ascending; site 2, arch; site 3, descending).

ANATOMIC CONSIDERATIONS

The human spinal cord is supplied with blood via a single anterior and two posterior spinal arteries (Fig. 183-2). The spinal arteries are terminal branches of the radiculomedullary arteries, which follow the anterior nerve roots through the intervertebral foramina. The radiculomedullary arteries are derived from the segmental arteries, which arise along the length of the aorta. The anterior spinal artery is formed at its rostral end by the union of two branches of the vertebral arteries. In the cervical region, the anterior spinal artery receives contributions from the costocervical and thyrocervical trunks, branches of the extracranial portion of the vertebral artery, the occipital branch of the external carotid artery, the deep cervical artery, and the ascending cervical artery, all of which have multiple anastomoses with each other (Fig. 183-3). As the anterior spinal artery descends caudally, it receives a variable number of feeders from the radiculomedullary branches of the segmental arteries. These

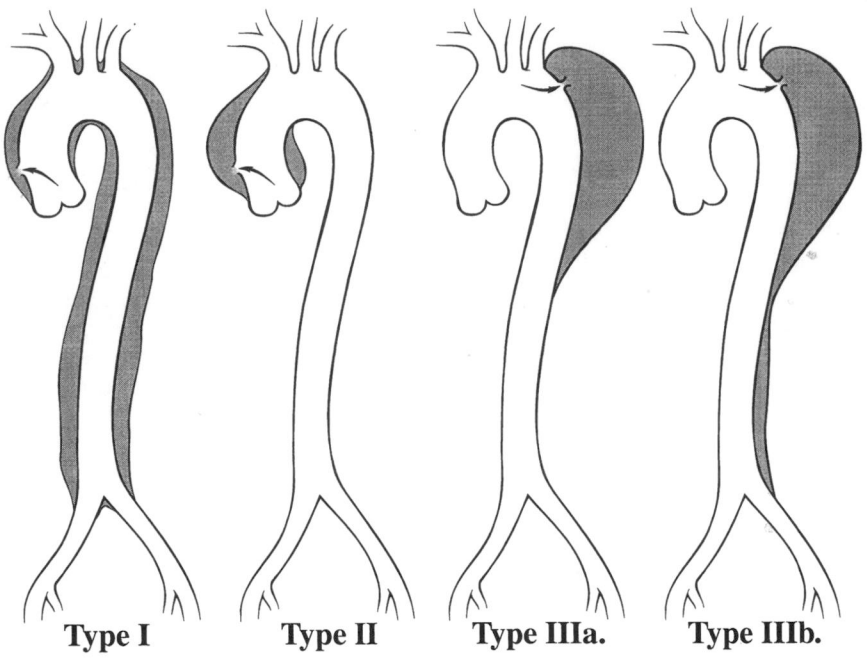

Type I **Type II** **Type IIIa.** **Type IIIb.**

FIG. 183-1. DeBakey's classification system of dissecting aortic aneurysms. (From DeBakey ME et al: J Thorac Cardiovasc Surg 49:130, 1965, with permission.)

segmental feeders are least developed in the upper to midthoracic region, where the anterior spinal artery may be discontinous, retelike, and narrow. In the midthoracic to upper lumbar region, the large artery of Adamkiewicz reinforces the blood supply of the anterior spinal artery and continues as the anterior median sulcal artery, which extends to the caudal region. There it joins

an anastomotic ring at the conus medullaris, which receives segmental branches from the lumbar and iliolumbar arteries and has a collateral circulation with the posterior spinal arteries in this region (Fig. 183-4). This circulation provides a relatively rich blood supply to the lumbosacral enlargement and the cauda equina. The posterior spinal artery, in contrast to the anterior

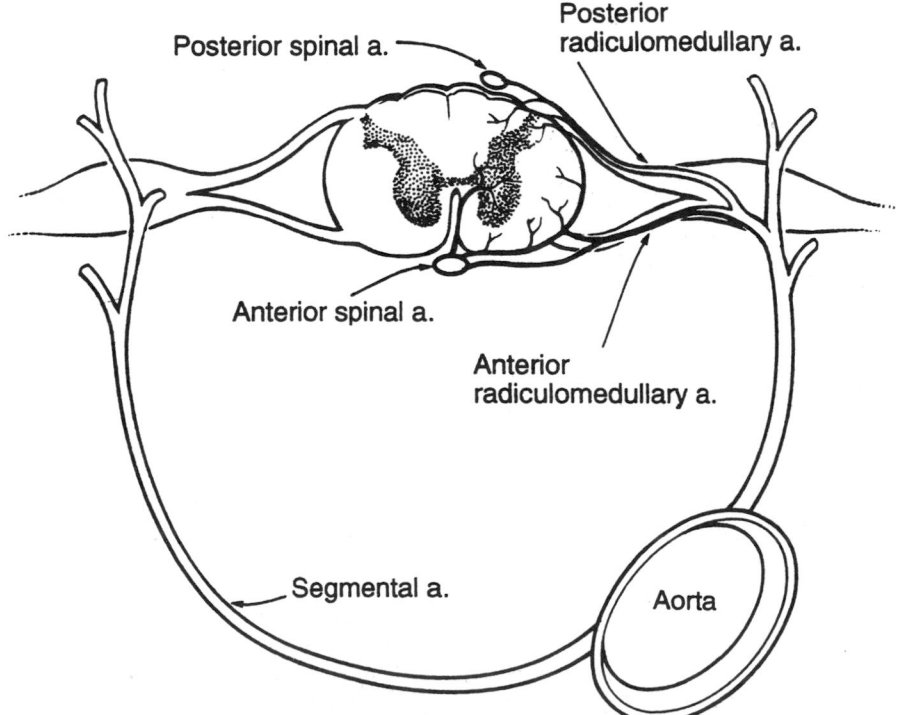

FIG. 183-2. Segmental arteries of the aorta giving rise to radiculomedullary and spinal arteries. (From O'Donovan CA, Conomy JP: Neurological complications of diseases of the aorta. p. 63. In Vinken PJ, Bruyn GW, Klawans HL (eds): Handbook of Clinical Neurology. Vol. 19. Elsevier-North Holland Publishing, Amsterdam, 1993, with permission.)

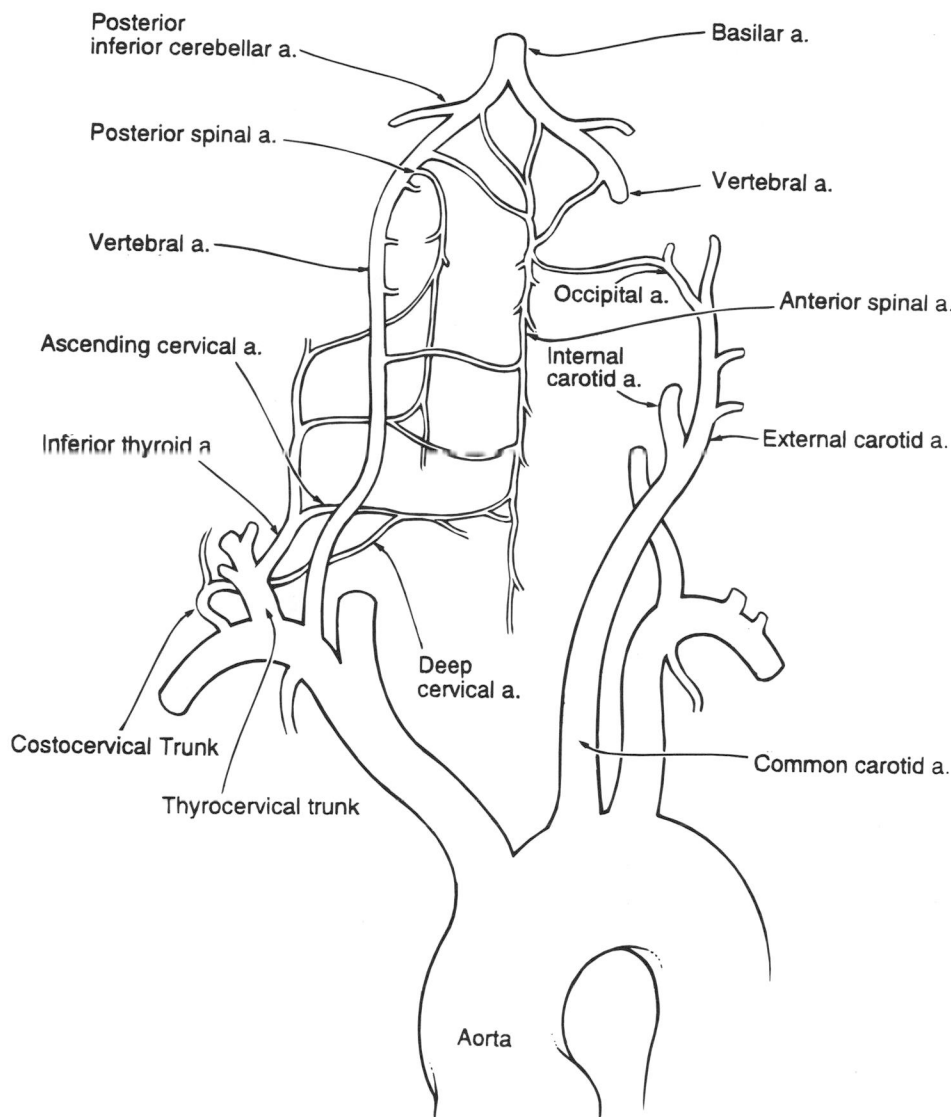

FIG. 183-3.   Rostral end of the anterior spinal artery formed by two branches of the vertebral arteries with multiple feeding vessels. (From O'Donovan CA, Conomy JP: Neurological complications of diseases of the aorta. p. 63. In Vinken PJ, Bruyn GW, Klawans HL (eds): Handbook of Clinical Neurology. Vol. 19. Elsevier-North Holland Publishing, Amsterdam, 1993, with permission.)

spinal artery, has an abundant supply of feeding radiculomedullary branches. This dual supply of the posterior third of the spinal cord segment is in stark contrast to the anterior aspect, where the sulcal branches of the single anterior spinal artery supply alternate halves of the spinal cord. Thus, the anterior spinal cord is more vulnerable to vascular insults, because the anterior spinal artery is an end artery with little anastomotic flow from the posterior artery. Clinical features of vascular lesions involving the anterior spinal cord are therefore relatively consistent.

PATHOPHYSIOLOGY

Whereas *aortic dissection* has been used synonymously with *dissecting aortic aneurysm* (as noted above), *dissecting aortic hematoma* is also appropriate to describe this condition. Pathologic examination of dissecting aortic hematomas after surgery or at autopsy may be unable to distinguish whether the abnormalities in the media and intima are primary or secondary. He-

matomas within the aortic wall are thought to arise from tears in the intima or disruption of the vasa vasorum within the media. Connective tissue disorders affect the integrity of the media of blood vessels and therefore predispose them to rupture of the vasa vasorum. However, they can also weaken vessel walls, which subsequently stretch, tearing the intimal lining. Atherosclerosis and systemic hypertension are thought to be the commonest causes of aortic dissection initiated by intimal tears.

The gap between the intima and media in aortic dissection causes symptoms through different mechanisms. The effects of the dissecting process depend not only on the extent of the dissection but also on the proximity to critical vessels supplying regions of the spinal cord that have poor collateral circulation. When aortic dissection causes symptoms of focal ischemia, blockage of the ostia of the aortic branches is the presumed mechanism. Ischemia of the spinal cord causes predominantly lower motor neuron signs because the gray matter requires more oxygen than the white matter does. Animal experiments have shown that the overall oxygen requirements of the spinal cord

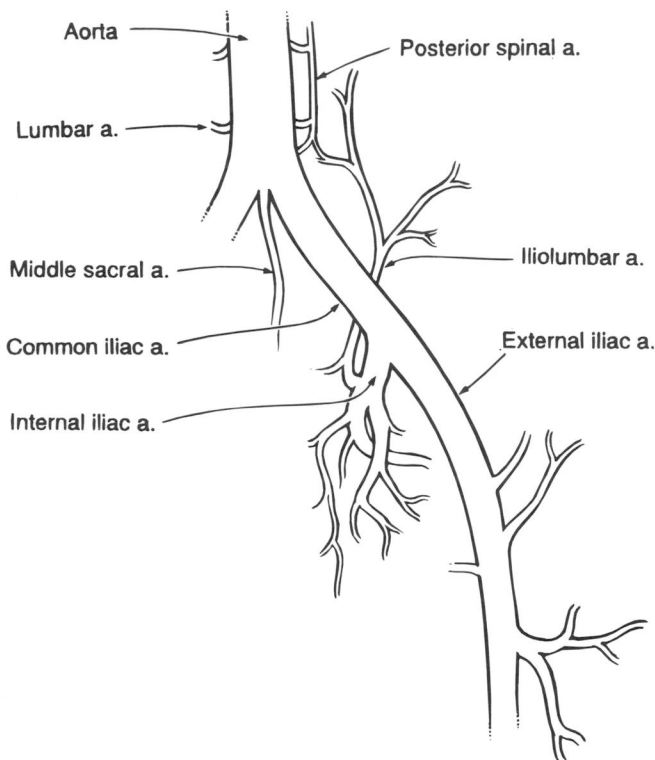

FIG. 183-4. Caudal end of the aorta demonstrating an anastomoses at the conus medullaris formed by the lumbar and iliolumbar arteries. (From O'Donovan CA, Conomy JP: Neurological complications of diseases of the aorta. p. 63. In Vinken PJ, Bruyn GW, Klawans HL (eds): Handbook of Clinical Neurology. Vol. 19. Elsevier-North Holland Publishing, Amsterdam, 1993, with permission.)

are about two-fifths that of cerebral tissue. Indeed, during aortic surgery, the spinal cord blood supply can be occluded for up to 30 minutes without causing postoperative neurologic deficits. This phenomenon may partly explain how extensive aortic dissections can cause either no symptoms or only transient ones.

Collateral circulation also determines whether ischemic symptoms result from occlusion of the ostia of the radicular branches. However, collateral circulation does not account for the relatively low incidence of clinical ischemic syndromes of the spinal cord compared with the cerebral circulation. The blood supply of the spinal cord was described in some classic works a few decades ago. Little is known about the frequency of anatomic variations between individuals because these studies have not been repeated recently owing to the tedious work involved in dissecting and identifying the various branches. The small size and number of vessels in the midthoracic region are frequently invoked to explain the high incidence of ischemia in this region of the spinal cord compared with others. When symptoms resolve rapidly without persistent neurologic deficits because the dissecting process is self-contained, the diagnosis can be extremely difficult. Nonvascular lesions close to the aortic dissection may be misdiagnosed as the cause of the symptoms. This misdiagnosis has sometimes resulted in inappropriate operations on these "incidental" lesions in an attempt to alleviate symptoms.

CLINICAL FEATURES

The difficulty in diagnosing aortic dissection clinically arises not from the unusual nature of the symptoms but from the close

resemblance to those occurring in more common conditions. Acute dissection is easily confused with myocardial infarction; chronic aortic dissection tends to be more associated with distal lesions, for which the differential diagnosis is much more extensive. Few large series of well-studied cases report on the clinical signs, because shock supervenes in many cases and obscures the details of the patient's history and physical examination. The most common symptom is pain, and most of the literature on the clinical features contains lengthy descriptions of the characteristics of the pain in an attempt to highlight the features peculiar to aortic dissection. Neurologic symptoms occur frequently and when present result in a much higher rate of antemortem diagnosis. Discussion of the clinical features of this condition may be easier to understand when seen in relation to different organ systems.

Cardiovascular Features

Pain. Chest pain is the most common symptom in aortic dissection, occurring in up to 90 percent of patients. Despite its frequent occurrence, the precise mechanism is unknown. Animal experiments suggest that the pain is caused by the diffusion of blood into surrounding tissues, and not by distention of the aortic wall. This mechanism explains the pain that occurrs when blood leaks from the dissection, but not that associated with small contained ruptures that do not extend to the external layers of the aortic wall.

The three most common characteristics of the pain in these descriptions are its severity, mode of onset, and radiation. The pain is usually described by patients as the most severe pain they have ever experienced, abrupt in onset, and of maximum intensity from the start, in contrast to that of myocardial infarction, which is frequently gradual in onset. The pain is described in many different terms, such as ripping, tearing, choking, sharp, constricting, stabbing, knifelike, or burning, as "something broken loose in the chest," and (rarely) as throbbing, pulsating, or colicky.

Location of the pain is also highly variable and has been described in the substernal area, precordium, and back of the chest, but it can occur in many other regions of the chest. The region of the chest to which the pain is referred does not appear to be consistently related to the area of dissection. Anterior thoracic pain is more frequently related to proximal dissection and posterior interscapular pain to distal dissections. Pain commonly radiates from anterior to posterior; however, it can also have a "wandering" or "migratory" character. The patient tends to shift positions without relief, and the pain may be aggravated by respiration.

Painless aortic dissection is unusual, occurring in only one-tenth of patients. Underecognition of pain may be due to altered mental status, particularly in those who subsequently experience cardiovascular collapse as a result of hypovolemic shock.

Murmur. A murmur in a patient with chest pain may provide a valuable clue for diagnosing aortic dissection. Diastolic murmurs in the region of the aortic valve are of greatest significance. Murmurs can be produced by either the dilation of the aortic ring or by alterations in the alignment of the aortic valve leaflets. Dilation of the aortic ring can occur from loss of tone secondary to hematoma formation in the medial layer or by disruption of the nerve endings in the outer adventitial layer. Alteration of alignment of the aortic valves can result from currents occurring in the region of intimal tears, and aortic insufficiency can result from blood flowing into the aneurysmal sac and returning to the lumen in diastole. Pulsations and thrills may also be detected in the thoracic and abdominal area and may provide other evidence of aortic dissection when chest pain is the only symptom.

Shock and Syncope. Shock may occur in up to 25 percent of patients with aortic dissection and varies in degree according to the rate and amount of blood loss. Half of these patients have severe shock, while the other half maintain a systolic blood pressure greater than 100 mmHg. Syncope at the onset of chest pain is thought to distinguish aortic dissection from myocardial infarction. Although the cause of syncope in aortic dissection may overlap with that of shock due to cerebral ischemia from blood loss, syncope can occur through other mechanisms, such as reflex neurogenic stimulation of the aortic depressor nerve by the pooling of blood in the false lumen after dissection occurs along the innominate or carotid arteries. Paradoxically, hypertension may occur as a result of ischemia of the kidney or the medullary region of the brainstem, destruction of the aortic depressor nerve, or aortic obstruction.

Congestive heart failure is not infrequent. Pericardial tamponade, which is the most common cause of death in aortic dissection, can be seen in some survivors. Pericardial friction rubs, venous distention (including the superior vena cava syndrome), and inequality of the pulses in the upper and lower extremities have also been reported.

Neurologic Features

The most comprehensive description of the neurologic aspects of aortic dissection was compiled by Weisman and Adams, who had examined 38 cases of aortic dissection in detail and confirmed the diagnosis postmortem. Neurologic symptoms and signs are present in 15 to 20 percent of patients with aortic dissection. The actual incidence is probably much higher because neurologic findings are frequently overlooked in the presence of other clinical features. In some cases, the only clinical manifestations described are neurologic. When symptoms and signs of aortic dissection include neurologic abnormalities, the antemortem diagnosis rate of aortic dissection increases considerably.

Cerebrum. Transient disturbances of cerebral function caused by aortic dissection can result in focal symptoms similar to a transient ischemic attack or to a more global cerebral hypoperfusion causing dizziness without prolonged loss of consciousness. These transient symptoms may resolve spontaneously due to a re-entrant tear. When symptoms progress to include coma, a focal neurologic deficit in the obtunded patient may reflect the effects of the initial phase of the dissecting process in a branch of the aorta. Dissection of the carotid arteries can result in unequal carotid pulses, increased amplitude of the carotid pulsations as a result of periarterial sympathectomy, or asynchrony of the pulses in the carotids as a result of velocity differences. Less commonly occurring cerebral manifestations include transient global amnesia, headaches caused by the superior vena cava syndrome, and hemorrhagic cerebral infarcts, which are thought to be caused by reperfusion after occlusion of vessels. Impingement of the aneurysmal sac on nerves in the neck may cause speech or voice changes from inferior or recurrent laryngeal nerve involvement. Horner syndrome secondary to sympathetic nerve dysfunction is occasionally caused by aortic dissection.

Spinal Cord. The occurrence of paraplegia after aortic surgery is well known, but it also occurs in aortic dissection. The same factors that cause paraparesis postoperatively also apply to aortic dissection. Infrarenal dissection of the aorta is less likely to cause paraparesis than a dissection located above the renal arteries, probably because of the location of the artery of Adamkiewicz. In fact, a number of intercostal arteries may dissect without clinical evidence of spinal cord damage. When paraplegia occurs as a result of aortic dissection, the role of ischemia of the peripheral nerves versus spinal cord is difficult to determine. As with all other vascular insults to the spinal cord, the findings in paraplegia are usually limited to those of anterior spinal artery occlusion. Aortic dissection may be difficult to distinguish from other causes of paraplegia associated with pain, such as spinal epidural abscess and spontaneous hematomyelia, in which widening of the aorta on a chest x-ray may be the only clue for differentiating between these conditions.

Peripheral Nerves. Ischemic necrosis of nerves in aortic dissection is said to be the most common neurologic complication of aortic dissection, occurring about three times as often as spinal cord or brain involvement. The clinical presentation is usually that of a cold, pulseless extremity with weakness, anesthesia, and loss of tendon reflexes. However, an aneurysmal dilation of the aorta, extending to involve a small nutrient branch artery and causing a mononeuropathy from compression or regional ischemia limited to one or two nerves, offers a greater diagnostic challenge. Proximal occlusion of vessels close to their origin at the aorta can result in ischemia of nerves distally with axonal loss in a condition known as *ischemic monomelic neuropathy*. Acute rupture of the aorta with hemorrhage and chronic contained rupture with hematoma formation are other mechanisms by which a compressive neuropathy may occur. Femoral, sciatic, and obturator nerves are the most commonly affected. Involvement of these nerves can occur in unusual combinations, which is sometimes explained by the occurrence in combination of a compartment syndrome from compression by extravasated blood, in addition to aneurysmal compression of a nerve at another site where the initial rupture occurred. Iliopsoas hematoma can cause the iliacus syndrome and compress the femoral nerve, whereas the psoas syndrome involves the obturator and lateral femoral cutaneous nerves, in addition to the femoral nerve. Pain radiating into the lower abdomen and inguinal regions may be caused by iliohypogastric nerve irritation, and when this pain is localized to the testes, the anterior scrotal branches of the inguinal nerve and the genital branch of the genitofemoral nerve are probably involved. Other unusual presentations of mononeuropathies can result from lateral popliteal nerve compression and from impingement on the lateral femoral cutaneous nerve of the thigh, causing buttock pain with numbness on the outer aspect of the thigh. Historically, radicular pain was a frequent occurrence in aortic dissection as a result of syphilitic aneurysms affecting the proximal aspect of aortic branches.

Miscellaneous Symptoms

Arrhythmias, fever, and cyanosis have all been reported in a minority of patients. Symptoms referable to the respiratory system are many and include cough, hemoptysis, altered breathing caused by tracheal tug, and pleural effusions. Gastrointestinal symptoms are also common, and almost half of these patients experience abdominal pain. Dysphagia caused by esophageal displacement can be the presenting symptom of aortic dissection in some cases. Gastrointestinal bleeding may occur with hematemesis as a result of rupture into the esophagus, and melena maybe caused by bowel infarction from mesenteric artery occlusion. Nausea and vomiting may result from stimulation of the mesenteric autonomic ganglia during acute rupture. Examination of the abdomen in these cases may reveal tenderness, rigidity, abdominal discoloration, or a mass. Chronic dissection may be associated with uremia and acidosis as a result of a contained dissection occluding the renal arteries. Clinical diagnosis of renal artery involvement by the dissecting process is difficult because the pain described in these situations is rarely typical of renal pain. Ocular complications include blindness from carotid artery dissection or hypertensive retinopathy.

DIAGNOSTIC TESTING

Abnormal laboratory test results are frequent in cases of aortic dissection; however, their clinical importance is overshadowed by the many different radiologic tests that have greater sensitivity and specificity. The laboratory test findings in aortic dissection are reported in more detail in earlier series of cases of aortic dissection at a time when chest x-ray was the only radiographic technique available. The abnormal laboratory test results reported were usually seen in a minority of patients and consisted of modest deviations from normal values. Results are nonspecific for aortic dissection and include findings such as leucocytosis, increased serum amylase and blood urea nitrogen concentrations, progressive elevation of the sedimentation rate over days, and hematuria. The development over several days of anemia and increased serum bilirubin as a result of progressive loss of blood into the aneurysmal sac and subsequent hemolysis may be useful as a diagnostic aid. Normal cardiac enzymes in a patient with sudden onset of severe chest pain should also alert the clinician to the diagnosis of aortic dissection.

The choice of radiologic test is determined both by the degree of suspicion of the diagnosis and the clinical condition of the patient. Although angiography may be the radiologic gold standard for diagnosing aortic dissection, the risk of complications, which is greatest with emergent angiography, still exists in elective procedures. Chest x-rays were used almost exclusively as a screening test for aortic dissection many decades ago, but newer radiographic techniques are more specific and delineate more accurately the extent of the dissection. Chest x-ray has a sensitivity of up to 90 percent. Although none of the chest x-ray findings are specific enough to allow a precise radiographic diagnosis of aortic dissection, they prove extremely useful in the acute setting in differentiating from conditions such as myocardial infarction, spinal cord lesions, or abdominal emergencies. The most pathogonomic finding is deformity of the supracardiac shadow, which is produced by extension of the dissection along the aortic arch branches (Fig. 183-5). Fluid is frequently seen in the left pleural cavity from rupture into this cavity. Other findings may include enlargement of the heart and displacement of the trachea and esophagus.

Computed tomography (CT) is frequently used because of its widespread availability and ability to visualize the site and extent of aortic dissection (Fig. 183-6). The intimal tear may be more readily identified with CT than with angiography because the scanning plane is perpendicular to the long axis of

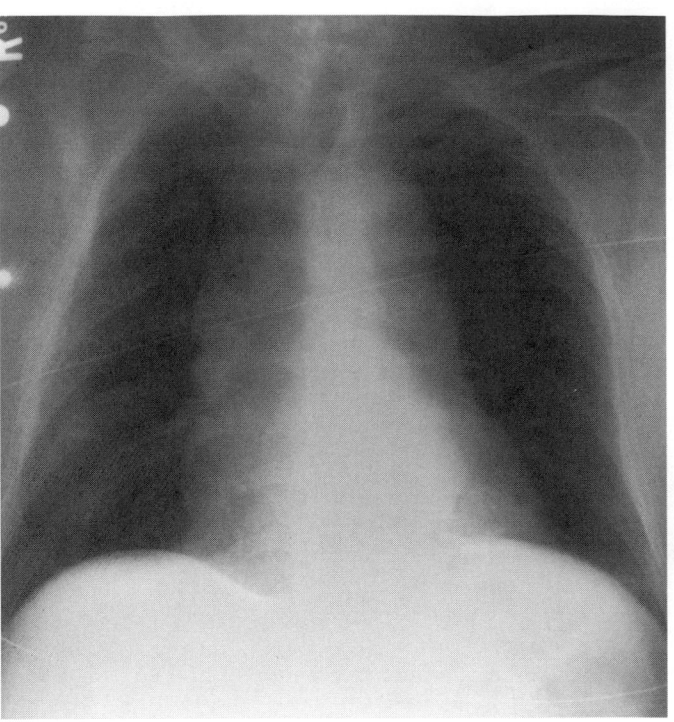

FIG. 183-5.   Chest radiograph showing tortuosity and prominence of the aorta and widening of the superior mediastinum in aortic dissection. (Courtesy of R. White, M.D., Cleveland Clinic Foundation, Cleveland, OH.)

the vessel and because calcifications can be seen in displaced intima. Aortic wall thickening is a feature of many processes, and aortic dissection can be differentiated from these conditions based on its appearance on CT. Fluid in the pleural, pericardial, and mediastinal spaces commonly accompanies aortic dissection and is readily recognizable by CT. One limitation of CT is its inability to determine which channels fill major vessels. Transesophageal echocardiography is in many ways the diagnostic procedure of choice, particularly in emergency situations, in which its sensitivity and specificity are almost 100 percent. Lesions of the arch of the aorta and (to a slightly lesser extent) the proximal ascending aorta are particularly well visualized. Distal lesions are not well seen, however, and other lesions such as thrombi may be interpreted incorrectly as aortic dissections.

Experience with magnetic resonance imaging (MRI) is less than with other procedures but is increasing rapidly. One of the main limitations of MRI in urgent situations is the increased length of time needed to carry out the scan compared with other radiologic tests. However, imaging can be carried out in many different planes without loss of spatial resolution. Furthermore, the different MRI signal characteristics of other vascular lesions, such as plaques, and the signals from various flow patterns and velocities are particularly useful in assessing aortic dissection for conditions such as a false lumen (Fig. 183-7).

Angiography remains the standard by which other diagnostic methods are assessed (Fig. 183-8). It continues to be widely used, especially where it is readily available and can be performed safely, even in acutely ill patients, by experienced radiologists. One of its advantages is in determining the relationship of the major aortic branch vessels to the dissection. Thrombosis of the false lumen is a possible source of false-negative angiographic studies, but other angiographic features can usually alert one to this misdiagnosis. In practice, trans-

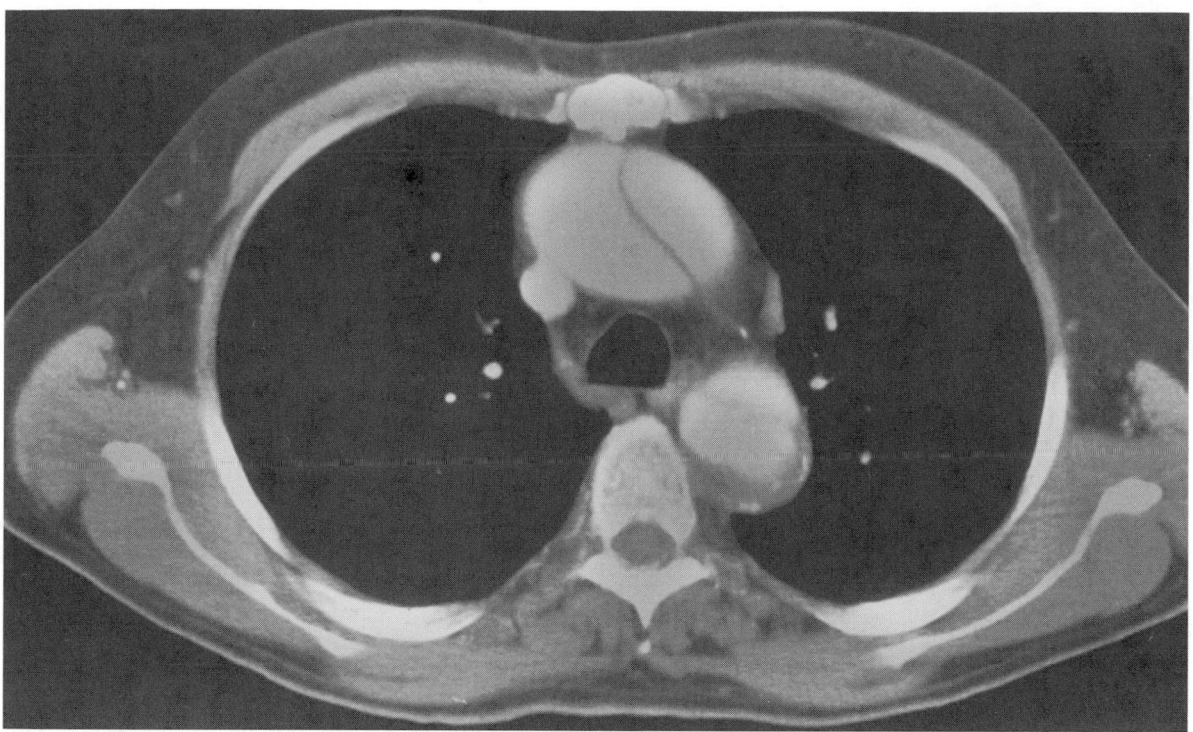

FIG. 183-6. CT scan of the chest showing thrombus in the false channel of the posterior aspect of the descending aorta. (Courtesy of R. White, M.D., Cleveland Clinic Foundation, Cleveland, OH.)

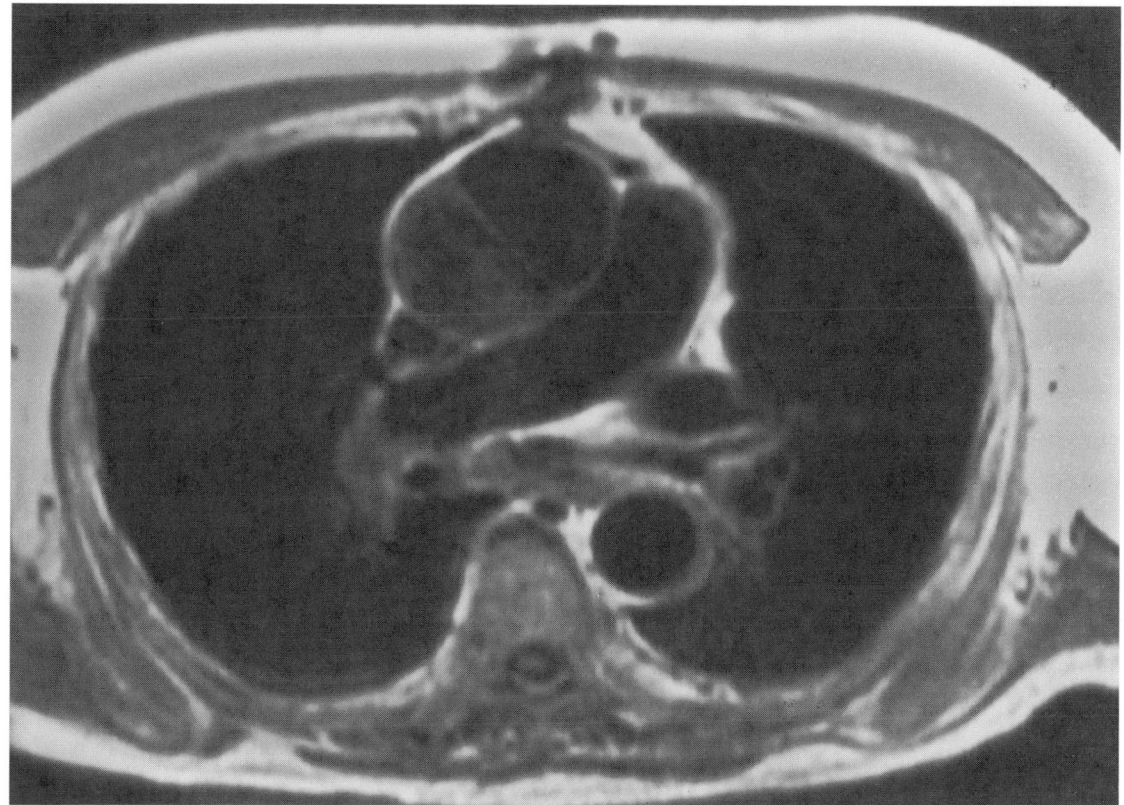

FIG. 183-7. MRI scan of DeBakey type 2 dissection in the ascending aorta showing signal changes consistent with slow flow in the false channel. (Courtesy of R. White, M.D., Cleveland Clinic Foundation, Cleveland, OH.)

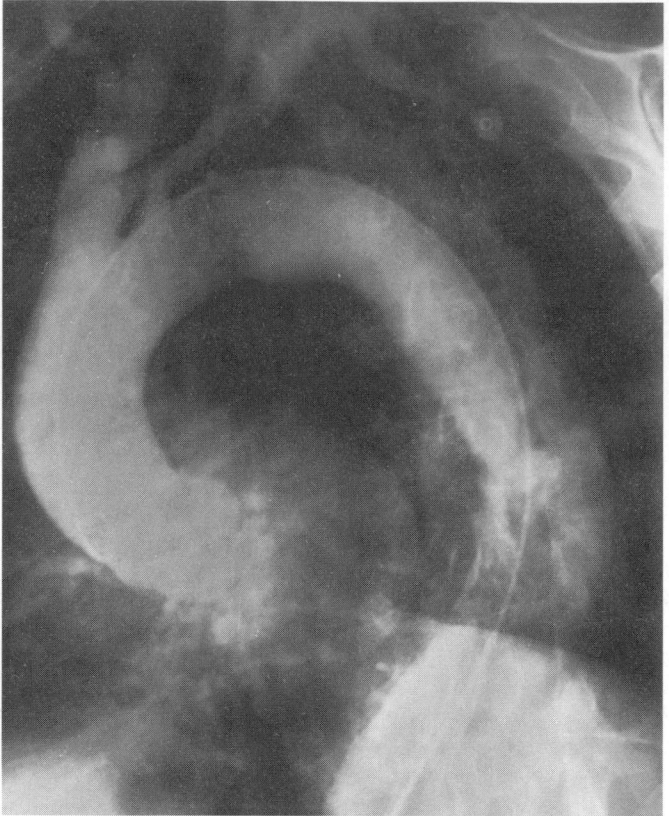

FIG. 183-8.   Angiogram of DeBakey type 3 dissection showing mild early enhancement of false channel, which extends to base of subclavian artery. (Courtesy of R. White, M.D., Cleveland Clinic Foundation, Cleveland, OH.)

esophageal echocardiography is probably the most frequently used emergency radiologic test. Echocardiography also allows aortic valve and cardiac function to be assessed (Plate 183-1). Surgeons tend to require angiography for preoperative planning, particularly if coronary artery disease coexists, but these strategies may change as experience with other procedures accumulates. CT is used when transesophageal echocardiography and angiography are unavailable. CT and MRI are best for distal dissections as they are useful in long-term follow-up of the progression of aortic dissection.

MANAGEMENT

Varying approaches to the management of aortic dissection are increasingly reported in the literature, paralleling the increased availability of diagnostic methods for early detection and increased experience with different surgical approaches. There is consensus on the general principles for treatment, based mostly on the location of the lesion. However, dissections warranting surgery in an otherwise healthy younger patient may be treated more conservatively by medical methods in an elderly patient. Proximal lesions are generally treated by surgery because the shearing forces of cardiac outflow speed the progression of the lesion and medical management is insufficient in these patients, who deteriorate rapidly without urgent surgical intervention. Medical treatment should begin even before a definitive diagnosis of aortic dissection is made.

Patients suffering aortic dissection are best treated in an intensive care unit with the cooperation of both medical and surgi-

cal services. The immediate goals of treatment are not only to lower the absolute blood pressure but also to reduce the rate of increase of the blood pressure. The drugs used must not only modulate these factors but also show high potency in this regard and have a short half-life for easy titration of dosages. Sodium nitroprusside, the most widely used hypotensive agent, is used in doses ranging from 25 to 300 μg/min. Diuretics increase the effectiveness of these hypotensive agents by decreasing fluid retention. However, agents with pure hypotensive effects increase heart rate and are probably best avoided. Therefore, simultaneous use of a β-adrenergic blocking drug is almost always necessary. Propranolol is the β-blocking agent most often used, but other agents, such as esmolol, which is cardioselective and ultra-short-acting, are also useful. β-Blocking agents may be used alone in normotensive patients. Trimethaphan camsylate, which reduces the rate of rise and absolute level of blood pressure, may be useful when β-blockers are contraindicated, but its side effects and tolerance building allow it to be used only for less than 48 hours. Calcium antagonists have also been used with some success when β-blockers are contraindicated. Reserpine was given intramuscularly many decades ago, but it has now been superseded by other agents.

A detailed discussion of surgical techniques and the rationale for choosing among them is beyond the scope of this text. The published indications for surgical treatment show a fair consensus. However, centers with a low surgical mortality rate advocate operative treatment for all types of aortic dissection and fail even to acknowledge the role of medical treatment early in acute proximal aortic dissection. Surgical therapy is warranted for all acute proximal dissections and also for arch dissections, which are complicated by rupture or localized aneurysm formation. Distal dissections are generally treated medically except when evidence exists of leaking, rupture, or rapid aortic enlargement. Acute distal dissections that may also require surgical therapy are those in which (1) medical therapy fails and blood pressure elevation persists, (2) there is retrograde extension into the ascending aorta, or (3) ischemia of an organ or limb develops. Less definitive indications include distal dissections in patients with conditions such as connective disorders that predispose them to aneurysm formation. Chronic dissections that result in aortic insufficiency or that show evidence of recurring invariably require surgical correction. Operating on chronic dissections may sometimes prove easier than during the acute stage because the tissues have more tensile strength after partial regeneration.

PROGNOSIS

The survival of patients with aortic dissection depends on many factors, including where the dissection is located, how rapidly treatment is instituted, how well hypertension is controlled, and whether re-entry tears develop. The increased survival rate in modern times is related not only to more aggressive management but also to earlier diagnosis. Rupture into the pleural, pericardial, and peritoneal cavities occurs in up to 80 percent of patients. The most common mechanism of death is pericardial tamponade. Long-term survival is usually associated with distal aneurysms, for which carefully monitored medical management has increased the favorable outcome rates considerably in recent years. Whereas 40 years ago antemortem diagnosis was rare and the survival rate low, aggressive treatment of this condition has improved survival rates to between 60 and 90 percent.

SELECTED READINGS

Anagnostopoulos CE: Acute Aortic Dissections. University Park Press, Baltimore, 1975

Cooke JP, Safford RE: Progress in the diagnosis and management of aortic dissection. Mayo Clin Proc 61:147, 1986

DeBakey ME, McCollum CH, Crawford ES et al: Dissection and dissecting aneurysms of the aorta: twenty year follow-up of five hundred twenty-seven patients treated surgically. Surgery 92:1118, 1982

Hirst AE Jr, Johns VJ Jr, Kime SW Jr: Dissecting aneurysm of the aorta: a review of 505 cases. Medicine 37:217, 1958

Moersch FP, Sayre GP: Neurologic manifestations associated with dissecting aneurysm of the aorta. JAMA 144:1141, 1950

O'Donovan CA, Conomy JP: Neurological complications of diseases of the aorta. p. 63. In Goetz CG, Tanner CM, Aminoff MJ (eds): Systemic Diseases, Part 1. In Vinken PJ, Bruyn GW, Klawans HL (eds): Handbook of Clinical Neurology. Vol. 19. Elsevier-North Holland Publishing, Amsterdam, 1993

O'Gara PT, DeSanctis RW. Aortic dissection. p. 931. In Loscalzo J, Creager MA, Dzau VJ (eds): Vascular Medicine: A Textbook of Vascular Biology and Diseases. Little, Brown, Boston, 1992

Slater EE, DeSanctis RW: The clinical recognition of dissecting aortic aneurysm. Am Jo Med 60:625, 1976

Weismann AD, Adams RD: The neurological complications of dissecting aortic aneurysm. Brain 67:69, 1944

Wolfe WG: Dissecting aneurysms of the aorta. p. 1548. In Sabiston DC Jr (ed): Textbook of Surgery. 14th Ed. WB Saunders, Philadelphia, 1991

SECTION 2. PULMONARY DISORDERS

184. NEUROSARCOIDOSIS

BARNEY J. STERN

Sarcoidosis affects the nervous system in 5 percent of patients with the disease. Patients typically present in their third or fourth decade, although they can be affected at any age. Neurologic symptoms are the presenting feature of sarcoidosis in one-half of individuals with neurosarcoidosis. Some three-quarters of patients destined to develop neurologic disease do so within 2 years of becoming afflicted with sarcoidosis. One-third to one-half of patients with neurosarcoidosis have more than one neurologic manifestation.

PATHOPHYSIOLOGY

The cause of sarcoidosis remains unknown. Inflammatory cells, particularly CD4 lymphocytes, are activated; these cells congregate at sites of disease activity and secrete various cytokines, including interleukin-2, interleukin-1, interferon-γ, and tumor necrosis factor. Monocytes/macrophages form granulomas, and ultimately irreversible fibrosis can develop. Small foci of ischemic necrosis can be found, presumably a result of vascular compromise from perivascular inflammation.

Meningeal inflammation is the most characteristic pathologic feature of central nervous system (CNS) sarcoidosis. Inflammation can extend to the cranial nerves, compromising these structures, and to the cerebrospinal fluid (CSF) pathways, leading to hydrocephalus. Brain or spinal cord disease can result from spread of inflammatory cells along the Virchow-Robin spaces, leading to the appearance of discrete granulomatous mass lesions or a diffuse encephalopathy/vasculopathy. Hypothalamic inflammation is the most common site for parenchymal disease. Finally, peripheral nerves and muscle can be involved in the inflammatory state.

CLINICAL MANIFESTATIONS AND DIAGNOSIS

The neurologic manifestations of sarcoidosis, together with their approximate frequencies, are outlined in Table 184-1.

Many of the diverse presentations of neurosarcoidosis can be best approached if they are thought of as fitting within one of these broad categories.

Patients with known systemic sarcoidosis who develop neurologic disease consistent with sarcoidosis should be evaluated for the reasonable exclusion of other disease entities, particularly infection and neoplasia. The patient can then be treated for neurosarcoidosis. If the patient does not respond as expected, the diagnosis should be questioned and a more extensive evaluation pursued to consider other diagnoses.

If a patient without known sarcoidosis develops a clinical

TABLE 184-1. Neurologic Manifestations of Sarcoidosis

Clinical Manifestation	Approximate Frequency (%)
Cranial neuropathy	50–75
Facial palsy	(25–50)
Meningeal disease	10–20
Aseptic meningitis	
Mass	
Hydrocephalus	10
Parenchymal disease	50
Brain	
Endocrinopathy	(10–15)
Mass lesion(s)	(5–10)
Encephalopathy/vasculopathy	(5–10)
Seizures	(5–10)
Vegetative dysfunction	
Spinal canal	
Extramedullary or intramedullary disease	
Cauda equina syndrome	
Neuropathy	15
Axonal neuropathy	
Mononeuropathy	
Mononeuropathy multiplex	
Sensorimotor	
Sensory	
Motor	
Demyelinating neuropathy	
Guillain-Barré syndrome	
Myopathy	15
Nodule	
Polymyositis	
Atrophy	

(Adapted from Stern BJ: Neurosarcoidosis. Neurol chronicle 2:1992 and Stern BJ, Schoufeld SH: Neurosarcoidosis. p. 289. In Arieff AI, Griggs RC (eds): Metabolic Brain Dysfunction in Systemic Disorders. Little, Brown, Boston, 1992, with permission.)

syndrome consistent with neurosarcoidosis, the diagnostic challenge can be considerable. Since corticosteroid therapy can mask signs of systemic disease, treatment should be postponed, if possible, while a search for systemic disease is initiated. An examination of the skin and lymph nodes may reveal abnormalities that can be biopsied. Sarcoidosis most frequently affects intrathoracic structures (87 percent of patients), followed by lymph node, skin, and ocular disease (15 to 28 percent of patients). Systemic disease can often be demonstrated if a comprehensive approach is followed, using the following tests:

Serum angiotensin-converting enzyme
Serum calcium
Chest x-ray
Pulmonary function tests including diffusing capacity
Ophthalmologic examination
Endoscopic nasal examination
Whole-body gallium scan
24-hour urinary calcium excretion
Anergy screen
Muscle magnetic resonance imaging (MRI)

If the patient has impaired smell or taste, nasal or olfactory nerve disease might be present. If dry eyes or mouth are noted, lacrimal, parotid, or salivary gland inflammation is possible.

Patients with possible CNS disease should be questioned about symptoms relating to neuroendocrinologic or hypothalamic dysfunction, since problems in these areas are the most common parenchymal disorders found in CNS sarcoidosis. Inquiry about alterations in menses, libido, and potency should be made as well as the presence of galactorrhea. Excessive thirst can be caused by resetting of the hypothalamic osmostat, diabetes insipidus, hypercalcemia, hypercalciuria, and corticosteroid-induced diabetes mellitus. Alterations in body temperature, sleep, and appetite can develop. Patients with CNS symptoms other than transient cranial nerve palsies or aseptic meningitis, should undergo neuroendocrinologic evaluation including tests for thyroid function (for consideration of hypothalamic hypothyroidism), prolactin, testosterone or estradiol, follicle-stimulating hormone, luteinizing hormone, and cortisol.

Although computed tomography (CT) scans can demonstrate abnormalities in CNS sarcoidosis, the preferred imaging technique is MRI with contrast enhancement. Rarely do brain T1-weighted images provide much information, although hydrocephalus and optic nerve and chiasm enlargement can be seen. With T2-weighted imaging, areas of increased signal intensity can be appreciated, especially in a periventricular distribution. Contrast administration can demonstrate leptomeningeal enhancement as well as parenchymal abnormalities. Spine MRI can visualize intramedullary disease, which appears as an enhancing fusiform enlargement, focal or diffuse enhancement, or atrophy. Enhancing nodules or thickened or matted nerve roots can be appreciated with images of the cauda equina.

CSF analysis can reveal an elevated pressure, increased total protein, hypoglycorrhachia, and a predominantly mononuclear pleocytosis. The IgG index can be elevated and oligoclonal bands may be detected. CSF angiotensin-converting enzyme can also be elevated in patients with CNS sarcoidosis, although abnormalities are also seen in the presence of infection and malignancy. A normal CSF angiotensin-converting enzyme assay does not exclude the diagnosis of neurosarcoidosis. The CSF CD4/CD8 ratio can be elevated.

Visual, auditory, or somatosensory evoked potentials can be abnormal in patients with optic nerve, eighth nerve, or spinal cord disease, respectively. Occasional patients with CNS sarcoidosis have evoked potential abnormalities without overt clinical disease in the area being studied. Furthermore, rare patients with sarcoidosis but no clinically evident CNS disease can have evoked potential abnormalities.

CNS tissue is rarely obtained for pathologic examination. Therefore, the clinician should always keep an open mind as to the diagnosis. Patients can be classified as having possible, probable, and definite CNS sarcoidosis based on the the certainty of the diagnosis of multisystem sarcoidosis, the characteristics of the CNS disease, and the patient's response to therapy. If the patient is not responding to therapy, consideration should be given to biopsy so as to exclude other diagnoses and confirm the clinical suspicion of sarcoidosis. Some other diagnostic considerations are listed below:

Multiple sclerosis
Sjögren syndrome
Systemic lupus erythematosus
Neurosyphilis
Neuroborreliosis
Human immunodeficiency virus infection
Behçet's disease
Vogt-Koyanagi-Harada disease
Toxoplasmosis
Brucellosis
Whipple's disease
Lymphoma
Germ cell tumors
Craniopharyngioma
Isolated angiitis of the CNS
Lymphocytic hypophysitis
Pachymeningitis
Low CSF pressure meningeal enhancement

Patients without known systemic sarcoidosis who develop a brain or spinal cord mass are usually biopsied. If pathologic examination suggests noncaseating granulomas, appropriate cultures should be obtained. Surgical excision should be avoided since surgery is rarely curative and patients can deteriorate from surgical excision of a granulomatous mass. As mentioned, corticosteroid therapy can mask systemic disease. If a patient with known sarcoidosis develops a CNS mass, an empiric trial of corticosteroid therapy is appropriate, especially if infection and malignancy can be reasonably excluded by CSF examination. If the patient does not respond to corticosteroid therapy, a biopsy should be pursued. In either of these scenarios, if a mass progressively enlarges in spite of corticosteroid therapy, surgical exploration should be strongly considered to evaluate the possibility of a malignancy.

Nerve conduction studies can characterize peripheral nerve disease as primarily axonal or demyelinating. Entrapment neuropathies can be demonstrated, especially at the carpal tunnel. Electromyography can help define the presence of a myopathy or further characterize the pattern of peripheral nerve compromise. Muscle or nerve biopsy is informative if the diagnosis of neuromuscular disease is in doubt.

If the patient is relatively functional, much of the diagnostic evaluation can be done on an outpatient basis. Patients need to be counseled as to the complexity of the evaluation and understand that a comprehensive and deliberate evaluation is time consuming; therefore answers may not be immediately forthcoming.

TREATMENT

No rigorous studies have defined the optimal treatment for neurosarcoidosis. Most authorities recommend corticosteroid therapy for patients without contraindications. Therapeutic decisions should be guided by the patient's clinical course, the expected natural history of the patient's clinical manifestations, and adverse treatment effects.

Some two-thirds of patients have a monophasic neurologic illness; the remainder have a chronically progressive or remitting-relapsing course. The former patients typically have an isolated cranial neuropathy, most often involving the facial nerve, or a bout of aseptic meningitis. Those with a chronic course usually have CNS parenchymal disease, hydrocephalus, multiple cranial neuropathies (especially involving cranial nerves II and VIII), peripheral neuropathy, and myopathy. It is not at all certain that treatment changes the natural history of the disease, though in the short term symptoms can often be alleviated with therapy. A goal of treatment is to diminish the irreversible fibrosis that can develop and minimize tissue ischemia that might result from perivascular inflammation. With time, the inflammatory process can "burn out," allowing immunosuppressive therapy to be withdrawn.

A peripheral facial nerve palsy usually responds to 2 weeks of prednisone therapy. The first week's prednisone dose is usually 0.5 to 1.0 mg/day (or 40 to 60 mg/day), followed by a taper over the second week. This approach can also be used as initial therapy for other cranial neuropathies and aseptic meningitis. However, even prolonged, aggressive therapy can fail to prevent irreversible optic and eighth nerve dysfunction.

Patients with a peripheral neuropathy or myopathy can respond to a short course of corticosteroid therapy. However, prolonged treatment is often necessary. Corticosteroids should be tapered slowly, as discussed below.

Asymptomatic ventricular enlargement probably does not require treatment. Mild, symptomatic hydrocephalus can respond to corticosteroid therapy, although prolonged treatment is often required. Life-threatening hydrocephalus or corticosteroid-resistant hydrocephalus require ventricular shunting. Unfortunately, patients can evolve from mild hydrocephalus to severe disease quite rapidly. Patients and caregivers must be educated as to when to seek emergent care. Shunt placement is not without risk in this patient population, which is why "prophylactic" shunting is not readily performed. Shunt obstruction from the inflamed CSF and ependyma is common and placement of a foreign object in the CNS of an immunosuppressed host predisposes to infection.

Corticosteroid therapy can improve the status of patients with a diffuse encephalopathy/vasculopathy or a CNS mass lesion. Only rarely does immunosuppressive treatment improve neuroendocrine dysfunction or vegetative symptoms. Seizures occur most commonly in patients with parenchymal disease or hydrocephalus. Control of seizures is usually not difficult if the underlying inflammatory process can be controlled.

Corticosteroid treatment for CNS parenchymal disease and other severe neurologic manifestations of sarcoidosis usually starts with prednisone 1.0 to 1.5 mg/kg/day. The higher doses are used in patients with particularly severe disease. These patients often require prolonged therapy and prednisone should be tapered very slowly. The patient might be observed on high corticosteroid doses for 2 to 4 weeks to ascertain the clinical response. The prednisone dose can then be tapered by 5-mg decrements every 2 weeks as the clinical course is monitored.

The disease tends to exacerbate at a prednisone dose approximating 10 mg daily. Patients often exhibit an individual dosage "floor" below which worsening can be expected. If a dose of prednisone of 10 mg daily can be achieved, the patient should be evaluated for evidence of subclinical worsening of disease. For patients with CNS disease, an enhanced MRI scan is useful. Intense enhancement suggests that disease is active and further decreases in corticosteroid dose may lead to a clinical exacerbation. On the other hand, persistent CSF abnormalities are usually not an indication for continuing high-dose corticosteroid therapy, since patients can remain quite functional in spite of an abnormal CSF. Efforts to "normalize" the CSF often require intense immunosuppression, with its attendant adverse effects. If the disease appears quiescent, the daily prednisone dose can be tapered by 1 mg every 2 to 4 weeks. If a patient has a clinical relapse, the dose of prednisone can be doubled (unless the dose is very modest, in which case prednisone 10 to 20 mg daily can be prescribed). The patient should be observed for approximately 4 weeks before another taper is begun. Patients may require multiple cycles of higher and lower corticosteroid doses. This effort is usually warranted since the disease can become quiescent and without attempts at withdrawing medication, patients may be needlessly exposed to the harmful side effects of corticosteroids.

A short course of methylprednisolone 20 mg/kg/day intravenously for 3 days, followed by high-dose prednisone for 2 to 4 weeks, is occasionally warranted. Patients with severe acute neurologic compromise can improve on this regimen. Furthermore, if it is unclear whether a patient might benefit from more intense immunosuppression, this protocol can be used to judge a response over a relatively short time. One or two target signs or symptoms can be used to judge the clinical response, for instance, the results of psychometric tests or a timed walk. One caveat should be noted: if the patient has a CNS mass lesion unresponsive to high-dose intravenous corticosteroids, surgical resection is probably appropriate in life-threatening situations.

Daily dosing of corticosteroids is usually superior to alternate-day therapy in patients with neurosarcoidosis. However, if a patient is doing very well on a modest dose of daily prednisone, an attempt can be made to wean the patient slowly onto alternate-day therapy.

Alternate Treatments

Alternate therapies are occasionally considered for neurosarcoidosis. Experience in this area is limited and firm recommendations are not available. Indications for the use of alternate treatments include the need to avoid corticosteroids as initial therapy, serious adverse chronic corticosteroid effects, and disease activity in spite of aggressive corticosteroid therapy.

Medications that have been used to treat sarcoidosis include cyclosporine, azathioprine, methotrexate, cyclophosphamide, and chlorambucil. None of these agents have been studied in a placebo-controlled manner, and none has been rigorously compared with others. Rarely is it possible to withdraw corticosteroid treatment completely; patients do best on a modest dose of corticosteroid combined with an alternate agent.

Cyclosporine or azathioprine are reasonable first-line agents that can be added to the patient's existing corticosteroid dose. After the alternate agent dose has been brought to the desired level, the corticosteroid dose can be slowly lowered as the clinical status is monitored. The patient needs to be closely monitored for adverse effects of the alternate agent. One way of

choosing among the various alternate agents is to note the organ
systems compromised by sarcoidosis and avoid drugs that have
notable adverse effects directed at the already compromised
organ. For instance, azathioprine, methotrexate, and chlorambucil are associated with liver toxicity, cyclosporine can cause
renal impairment, and methotrexate, cyclophosphamide, and
chlorambucil can cause pulmonary fibrosis. All these agents
except cyclosporine are implicated in causing malignancies.

If a patient with CNS disease fails or cannot tolerate two
alternate agents, consideration should be given to radiotherapy.
Patients may stabilize, at least in the short term. Ultimately,
immunosuppression often needs to be continued, at least in
modest doses.

General Supportive Care

Patients require close attention to their general medical condi-
tion. Potential adverse effects of treatment should be sought.
An exercise and dietary program are often highly beneficial.
Rehabilitation services should be utilized as appropriate.
Depression is not uncommon and treatment can be helpful.

Therapy of endocrinologic disturbances is important. In particular, hypothyroidism and hypogonadism should be treated.
Since patients are often on protracted, low-dose corticosteroid
regimens, a supplement of corticosteroid is appropriate during
periods of intercurrent illness.

Patients are at risk for osteoporosis. Screening should be
done on a regular basis. Treatment of osteoporosis is often a
challenge since sarcoidosis itself can cause hypercalcemia and
hypercalciuria. Since the management of osteoporosis is an
evolving science, it is best to work closely with an expert in
this area. Deflazacort, a corticosteroid preparation with a low
propensity for causing osteoporosis, is effective in treating sarcoidosis. Salmon calcitonin nasal spray is an effective osteoporosis prophylactic agent.

LONG-TERM COMPLICATIONS

Patients with refractory neurosarcoidosis not only are prone to
the primary effects of the inflammatory process but are also at
risk for the long-term complications of treatment. If a patient
is not doing well, the diagnosis of sarcoidosis should be ques-

TABLE 184-2. Selected Long-Term Complications of Neurosarcoidosis

Infection
  Cryptococcal meningitis
  Tuberculous meningitis
  Toxoplasmosis
  Progressive multifocal leukoencephalopathy
  Listeria monocytogenes
Spinal epidural lipomatosis
Corticosteroid myopathy
Lymphoma
Inclusion body myositis

(Adapted from Stern BJ: Neurosarcoidosis. Neurol Chronicle 2:1, 1992.)

tioned, and also a search for intercurrent complications should
ensue. Some potential complications are noted in Table 184-2.

SUGGESTED READINGS

Agbogu BN, Stern BJ, Sewell C, Yang G: Therapeutic considerations in patients with refractory neurosarcoidosis. Arch Neurol (in press)
Cheng TM, O'Neill BP, Scheithauer BW, Piepgras DG: Chronic meningitis: the role of meningeal or cortical biopsy. Neurosurgery 34:590, 1994
Edmonds LC, Stubbs SE, Ryu JH: Syphilis: a disease to exclude in diagnosing sarcoidosis. Mayo Clin Proc 67:37, 1992
Fidler HM, Rook GA, Johnson NM, McFadden J: *Mycobacterium tuberculosis* DNA in tissue affected by sarcoidosis. BMJ 306:546, 1993
Junger SS, Stern BJ, Levine SR et al: Intramedullary spinal sarcoidosis: clinical and magnetic resonance imaging characteristics. Neurology 43:333, 1993
Krumholz A, Stern BJ, Stern EG: Clinical implications of seizures in neurosar-coidosis. Arch Neurol 48:842, 1991
Peeples DM, Stern BJ, Jiji V, Sahni KS: Germ cell tumors masquerading as central nervous system sarcoidosis. Arch Neurol 48:554, 1991
Sherman JL, Stern BJ: Sarcoidosis of the CNS: comparison of unenhanced and enhanced MR images. AJNR 11:915, 1990
Soucek D, Prior C, Luef G et al: Successful treatment of spinal sarcoidosis by high-dose intravenous methylprednisolone. Clin Neuropharmacol 16:464, 1993
Stern BJ: Neurosarcoidosis. Neurol Chronicle 2:1, 1992
Stern BJ: Neurosarcoidosis. p. 535. In Evans RW, Baskin DS, Yatsu FM (eds): Prognosis of Neurological Disorders. Oxford University Press, New York, 1992
Stern BJ, Krumholz A, Johns C et al: Sarcoidosis and its neurological manifesta-tions. Arch Neurol 42:909, 1985
Stern BJ, Schonfeld SA: Neurosarcoidosis. p. 289. In Arieff AI, Griggs RC (eds): Metabolic Brain Dysfunction in Systemic Disorders. Little, Brown, Boston, 1992
Stern BJ, Schonfeld SA, Sewell C et al: The treatment of neurosarcoidosis with cyclosporine. Arch Neurol 49:1065, 1992

SECTION 3. NEPHROLOGY AND UROLOGY

185. NEUROLOGIC MANIFESTATIONS OF RENAL FAILURE AND DIALYSIS

CHARLES F. BOLTON
G. BRYAN YOUNG

In the United States, over 100,000 persons receive treatment for end-stage renal disease, 80 percent by various types of dialysis, a few with continued conservative treatment, and the rest by transplantation. Nervous system complications are common in all groups.

This review concentrates on the principal neurologic complications of renal failure and its treatment, as these would present in office neurologic practice, usually where the consultant is in proximity to a major hemodialysis center. Comments concerning the general principles of the clinical and laboratory approach are followed by a review of the main disorders of the central and peripheral nervous systems.

GENERAL PRINCIPLES

The Central Nervous System

Clinical Evaluation. Mental status changes are generally the earliest and most common central nervous system effects of renal failure or its treatment. The practitioner should ask the patient's companion about changes in behavior, speech, memory, and intellectual capabilities. The time course of such changes should be established. For example, progressive dialysis encephalopathy tends to fluctuate at first, then steadily progresses, and slowly resolves with effective treatment. Stroke, transient ischemic attacks, and seizures are of sudden onset and resolve quickly. A simple mental status examination, such as the Mini-Mental State Examination (Table 185-1), serves both to document specific deficits and to quantify the dysfunction for follow-up purposes.

Investigative Tests. Investigative tests depend on the history and physical examination. The indications and limitations of tests of function and structure should be clearly understood. Electrophysiologic tests of brain function include electroencephalography (EEG) and evoked responses. EEG is useful for assessing uremic encephalopathy, the adequacy of dialysis, and seizure disorders and in making the specific diagnosis of progressive dialysis encephalopathy. Quantitative tests, including frequency analysis and middle latency auditory evoked responses, are useful in assessing the adequacy of dialysis.

Tests of brain structure include computed tomography (CT) and magnetic resonance imaging (MRI) scans. These can detect specific structural lesions such as subdural hematomas, abscesses, or neoplasms. Because of the presence of bony artifact

TABLE 185-1. Mini-Mental State Examination

Maximum Score	Test
	Orientation
5	What is the (year) (season) (day) (month)?
5	Where are we (state/province) (country) (city) (building) (floor)?
	Registration
3	Name three objects (1 second to say each), then ask the patient to repeat all three. Give 1 point for each correct answer.
	Repeat until the patient learns all three. Count trials and record.
	Attention and Concentration
5	Serial 7 (counting backward by 7 from 100); stop after five answers. Alternatively, spell "world" backward.
	Recall
3	Ask for the three objects repeated above.
	Give 1 point for each correct answer.
	Language
9	Name a pencil and a watch (2 points).
	Repeat the following: "No ifs, ands, or buts" (1 point).
	Follow a three-stage command: "Take a paper in your right hand, fold it in half, and put it on the floor" (3 points).
	Read and obey: "Close your eyes" (1 point).
	Write (not copy) a sentence (1 point).
	Copy a design (1 point).

(From Folstein MF, Folstein SE, McHugh PR: Mini-Mental State: a practical guide for grading the cognitive state of patients for the clinician. J Psychiatr Res 12:189–98, 1975, with permission.)

in posterior fossa structures and the temporal lobes on CT, MRI is a more sensitive examination.

Peripheral Nervous System

Clinical Evaluation. Neuromuscular conditions associated with acute renal failure are uncommon and are usually confined to muscle weakness induced by disturbances of water and electrolyte metabolism. On the other hand, such conditions are common in chronic renal failure. The nature of these neuromuscular disorders will vary according to the stage of renal failure [during conservative treatment, during hemodialysis, or following successful renal transplantation (Table 185-2)]. These facts should be kept in mind, since it will help to focus questioning during

TABLE 185-2. The Main Disorders of the Peripheral Nervous System in the Management Stages of Uremia

Conservative Management	Dialysis	Renal Transplantation
Developing uremic polyneuropathy	Stabilizing uremic polyneuropathy	Recovery from uremic polyneuropathy
Diabetic mononeuropathy and polyneuropathy	Persisting diabetic neuropathy	Persisting diabetic neuropathy
Pressure palsies	Carpal tunnel syndrome and amyloidosis	
Cachetic myopathy	Ischemic neuropathy and shunts or fistulas	
	Primary myopathy and bone disease	

history taking and in the selection of the most appropriate tests on physical examination.

In taking a history, one should ask about muscle weakness or fatigue, cramps, the presence or absence of sweating in the hands and feet, disorders of bowel and bladder function, and problems in standing or walking. Impotence in the male can be clarified from the observation that it is likely psychogenic if early morning penile erections regularly occur, but is probably organic in their absence.

The patient's own words in describing symptoms should be noted and are important diagnostically. Thus, the sensory symptoms of neuropathy are characteristically not only numbness and tingling, but a tight or bandlike feeling about the ankles, a sensation on the soles of the feet as if the patient is wearing tight socks, and (rarely) pain or burning. The restless leg syndrome, which may or may not be associated with peripheral neuropathy, is often an indescribably unpleasant sensation that is relieved only by movement of the legs.

On physical examination, observe the location and type of surgical scars, particularly those related to the creation of arteriovenous fistulas in the upper limbs for access during chronic hemodialysis, since they may play a role in the development of upper limb mononeuropathies. The type and severity of muscle wasting is important diagnostically. Diffuse muscle wasting may be caused by disuse, secondary either to the cachexia associated with chronic renal failure or to diffuse pain from underlying bone or joint disease. In the bone disease induced by hyper-

parathyroidism or the toxic effects of aluminum, muscle pain and wasting are characteristically more severe in the proximal lower limbs but occasionally will involve the proximal upper limbs as well. Focal wasting may occur in the distribution of the nerves that are subject to compression or entrapment, particularly in carpal tunnel syndrome, in the proximal thenar, in wasting of the median nerve in the hand (Fig. 185-1), in the ulnar-innervated hand muscles in case of compressive neuropathy of the ulnar nerve at the elbow, and in anterior compartment wasting in compression of the common peroneal nerve at the fibular head. In my experience, fasciculations are not a manifestation of neuromuscular disease in renal failure.

Many patients in chronic renal failure are frail, and excessive force should be avoided when testing muscle strength. The deep tendon reflexes are usually preserved in primary myopathies and defects in neuromuscular transmission and are characteristically decreased in neuropathy. Reduced or absent ankle jerks are one of the early signs of uremic polyneuropathy. In eliciting deep tendon reflexes, it is important to use a hammer that is of sufficient length and heavy enough to move the tendon effectively with soft enough rubber not to cause undue discomfort.

In testing sensation, one should first ask the patient to outline carefully (with a finger) the areas of impaired sensation they have experienced. This is often more reliable than formal sensory testing in delineating areas of sensory loss. Light touch should be tested with a tissue, and pain with a sharp splinter from a tongue depressor. The splinter should be disposed of to

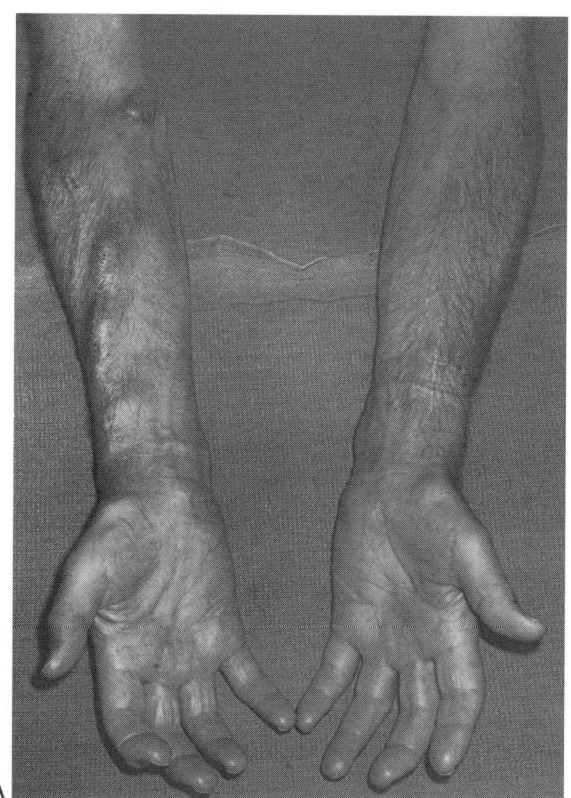
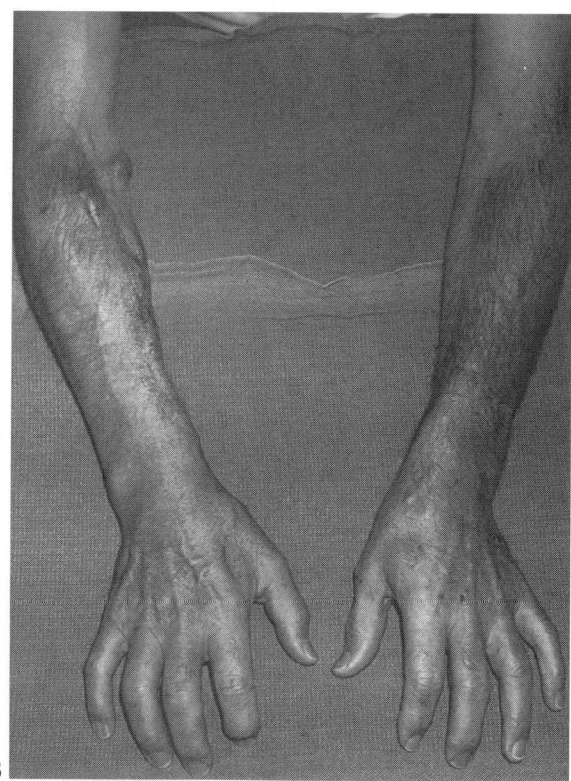

FIG. 185-1.   (A & B) The upper limbs of a patient who had β_2-microglobulin amyloidosis that caused bilateral carpal tunnel syndrome (note proximal thenar wasting) and a right ulnar neuropathy (note wasting of interosseus muscles). Tissue biopsy performed at the time of carpal tunnel surgery revealed infiltration of blood vessels by amyloid. The pain may have been caused by an arthropathy (note thickening and flexion contraction of interphalangeal joints) and periodic nerve ischemia. Repeated surgery for carpal tunnel syndrome provided only transient relief. (The Brescia-Cimino forearm fistula caused the dilated veins of the right forearm). (From Bolton CF, Young GB: Neurological Complications of Renal Disease. Butterworth, Boston, 1990, with permission.)

avoid transmitting an infectious agent. Vibratory sensation is tested with a 128 cycle/s tuning fork. Position sense first becomes abnormal at a distal digital joint in the hands or feet and is normally sensitive enough that the patient can detect even the smallest movement. Two-point discrimination can be measured with an instrument that has two well-defined, but not excessively sharp, points. Values greater than 3 mm in the fingertips of patients of all ages (and in the feet greater than 1 cm in the young and greater than 3 cm in the elderly) should be considered abnormal. I have found formal testing of temperature sensation of little practical value in this group of patients.

In testing stance and gait, look for a steppage gait due to predominant weakness of the feet and ankles. In proprioceptive loss involving the lower limbs, the gait will be ataxic and this phenomenon will be worse with the eyes closed. Early distal weakness in the lower limbs can be determined by asking the patient to walk on either the toes or heels; proximal weakness will be detected by having the patient attempt to rise from the squatting position.

Postural hypotension is common in patients on chronic hemodialysis due to fluctuations in fluid volume. However, postural hypotension is rarely caused by an autonomic neuropathy alone (see below). Autonomic insufficiency can be tested clinically by observing blood pressure and pulse in the recumbent position and then on standing. A significant postural hypotension is present if the systolic pressure drops 30 mm or more; the heart rate should normally increase by a factor of at least 1.04. Sweating can be crudely assessed by palpating the skin surfaces. Sweating in the axilla is mediated by apocrine glands that are stimulated by circulating catecholamines and hence are not affected by neuropathy.

Neurophysiologic Studies. After the history and physical examination, are complete, the nature of the underlying neuromuscular disorder is often still in doubt, and electrophysiologic studies are of great value. They will clearly identify the presence and severity of uremic polyneuropathy and are valuable in following the course of this neuropathy during the various stages of chronic renal failure (Table 185-2). They are also valuable in detecting the presence and severity of mononeuropathies, such as carpal tunnel syndrome and compressive neuropathy of the ulnar nerve at the elbow and of the common peroneal nerve at the fibular head. For example, in carpal tunnel syndrome, symptoms may be strongly suggestive of the disorder but the physical examination will be negative, with no evidence of muscle weakness or sensory loss. In my experience, Phalen's and Tinel's signs are unreliable. In cases of primary myopathy, if the cause is simply disuse atrophy, electrophysiologic studies will be entirely normal. Repetitive nerve stimulation studies will rule out neuromuscular transmission defects induced by antibiotic drugs.

Patients on chronic hemodialysis are understandably reluctant to undergo unnecessary painful procedures. However, standard motor and sensory nerve conduction studies cause little discomfort, particularly when performed by a sensitive and experienced electromyography (EMG) technician. On the other hand, needle EMG of muscle is clearly more uncomfortable and thus this type of testing should, in my opinion, be reserved for patients who have moderate or severe polyneuropathies and are likely to have evidence of denervation. Moreover, abnormal spontaneous activity, a sign of denervation, may be peculiarly absent in uremic neuropathy. (See below for this rather interesting aspect of uremic polyneuropathy.)

Nerve and Muscle Biopsy. Nerve and muscle biopsy may be necessary in only a few instances, when history, physical examination, and electrophysiologic studies are still inconclusive. This is most likely to occur in cases of primary myopathies, in which electrophysiologic studies may be normal in cases of metabolic disturbances of muscle or equivocal in other types of primary myopathies. In patients in end-stage renal failure, the usual indications for nerve biopsy are suspicion of underlying vasculitis or amyloidosis.

If nerve biopsy is decided on, it is usually best to take a longitudinal section of the entire cross section of a sural nerve. The biopsy should include adjacent muscle, subcutaneous tissue, and skin, particularly when a vasculitis is in question. Special stains will have to be performed in suspected amyloidosis. In cases of muscle biopsy, the muscle should be chosen from a muscle that is moderately weak and has not been needled by a previous electromyographic examination.

These biopsies should be performed only by an experienced and skilled surgeon. The neuropathologist should also be competent and will wish to be informed, in advance, about the nature of the suspected disorder, so that the tissue can be received in optimal condition and the appropriate testing and analysis carried out.

PRINCIPAL DISORDERS OF THE NERVOUS SYSTEM

Central Nervous System

Uremic Encephalopathy. The first symptoms of uremia include lethargy, slowness in thinking, general malaise, sleep disturbance, headache, and decreased libido. Personality changes include apathy, flatness of affect, depression, or irritability. Restlessness and impaired concentration, attention, and memory are common. Occasionally patients become frankly delirious. Symptoms are variably improved by hemo- or peritoneal dialysis, depending on their adequacy and frequency, but are completely reversed by successful renal transplantation.

Convulsive seizures are still occasionally encountered in chronic renal failure. If they are not caused by acute, severe metabolic derangement, the possibility of a complication such as a stroke, cerebral neoplasm or abscess, progressive dialysis encephalopathy, or drug-related cause should be considered.

Persistent focal signs are rare in uremic encephalopathy and should prompt the search for a structural lesion. Diffuse motor phenomena such as postural tremor, asterixis, and multifocal myoclonus are not uncommon in uremia. Tremor is found in mild renal failure, even when treated by dialysis; asterixis and multifocal myoclonus reflect a more severe or advanced metabolic disturbance.

Routine EEGs show mild, intermittent slowing in the θ frequency range (more than 4- but less than 8-Hz waves), more prominent in the anterior head (Fig. 185-2). Arousal from sleep is often abnormal, showing rhythmic δ-waves in adults. Spontaneous epileptiform activity is uncommon but may appear in a generalized fashion during photic stimulation. Triphasic waves or intermittent rhythmic δ patterns are usually features of more advanced uremia, sufficient to require hospitalization. Improvement in the EEG, quantitative EEG, and middle latency evoked responses parallels clinical improvement with adequate dialysis therapy or following renal transplantation.

The differential diagnosis of uremic encephalopathy includes drug intoxication [especially when renal excretion is a major determinant of the drug or its active metabolites (e.g., amantadine, opiates and β-blockers)]; degenerative conditions such as

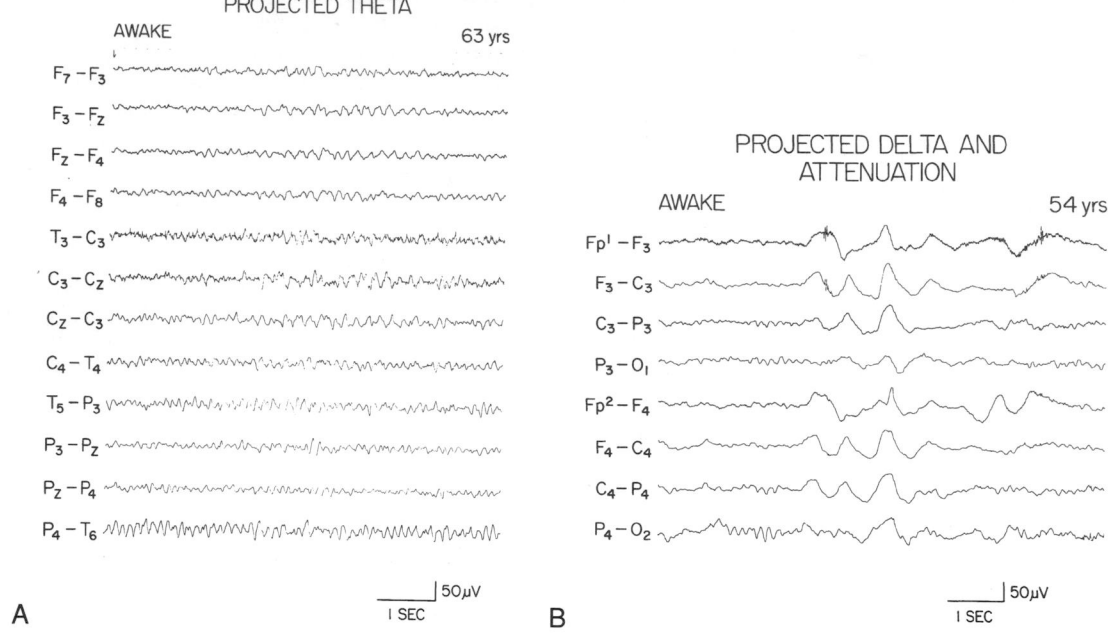

FIG. 185-2. EEGs from patients with mild uremic encephalopathy. (**A**) The 63-year-old man was less affected; his recording shows bursts of 4- to 5-Hz low-voltage waves in the anterior head. (**B**) The 54-year-old man's EEG contains a burst of less than 3 Hz medium voltage, frontally predominant rhythmic δ-waves, which is coincident with a reduction in normal, faster rhythms. Following this burst is a 2-second period of generalized flattening or attenuation. (From Bolton CF, Young GB: Neurological Complications of Renal Disease. Butterworth, Boston, 1990, with permission.)

Alzheimer's disease (usually associated with gradual decline in memory and then other intellectual functions in a steadily progressive manner—confusion and fluctuation in mental status are not early features, as they often are in metabolic encephalopathies such as uremia); complications of dialysis including subdural hematomas and progressive dialysis encephalopathy (see below); depressive illness; and conditions that may affect both the kidneys and the brain such as lead intoxication and certain collagen-vascular diseases.

Management includes adequate clearance of uremic neurotoxins (e.g., by increasing the frequency of dialysis treatments from twice to three times weekly).

Neurologic Complications of Dialysis.

PROGRESSIVE DIALYSIS ENCEPHALOPATHY. It has been shown that progressive dialysis encephalopathy, which is found in patients on chronic dialysis, relates to aluminum intoxication of the brain. The encephalopathy may be associated with symptomatic aluminum poisoning of other organ systems (e.g., vitamin D-resistant osteomalacia with a tendency toward fractures), proximal myopathy in the lower limbs, and a severe, refractory, noniron deficiency hypochromic microcytic anemia.

The main manifestations include (1) a prominent speech disturbance usually consisting of a nonfluent aphasia and dysarthria; (2) involuntary motor phenomena (myoclonus, tremor, asterixis, and seizures); (3) gait disturbance (ataxia or apraxia, or both, wide based or small stepped); and (4) general mental decline or dementia. The symptoms and signs fluctuate considerably early in the course of the illness and are more progressive later in the course. The tempo varies markedly among patients. The differential diagnosis includes chronic uremic encephalopathy, drug intoxication, subdural hematoma, degenerative conditions, and Creutzfeldt-Jakob disease.

The EEG can help to establish the diagnosis. Characteristically, generalized bursts of slow-frequency waves, triphasic waves, or irregular spike-and-wave patterns are seen. This occurs out of proportion to the uremia and, unlike uremic encephalopathy (see above), is not helped by increasing the frequency of dialysis treatments. Serum or bone aluminum concentrations and the desferoxamine infusion tests give estimates of the body burden of aluminum and offer indirect support of the diagnosis. Patients with PDE, progressive dialysis encephalopathy at least in the early stages, often respond to benzodiazepines, with prompt but temporary resolution of signs for several hours.

Treatment depends first on prevention. Epidemics related to high aluminum content in the tap water or dialysate have largely been eliminated, but it pays to remain vigilant. Aluminum-containing antacids, used to bind phosphate in the gut, are a source of aluminum exposure for some. Citrate increases aluminum absorption from the gastrointestinal tract. It is best to substitute calcium carbonate. Secondary treatment in the early phases includes eliminating aluminum exposure and the use of desferoxamine. Benzodiazepines have only a transient beneficial effect.

SUBDURAL HEMATOMA. Chronic subdural hematomas, probably related to the intrinsic coagulopathy of uremia and the iatrogenic anticoagulation, occur in 3 percent of patients on hemodialysis. A history of trauma may or may not be reported. Any adult age group is affected.

Patient often complain of headache and when they are brought to medical attention, the level of consciousness is often diminished. Focal signs such as lateralized motor weakness are often present but may be hard to detect if the patient is obtunded or poorly cooperative or if bilateral subdural collections are present. Gait disturbance is especially common (e.g., features of apraxia, ataxia, or hemiparesis may be found). Patients' signs and symptoms may fluctuate considerably.

Subdural hematomas are best confirmed by neuroimaging

using CT or MRI scans. The treatment is almost always surgical, with drainage or evacuation of the clot.

DIALYSIS DYSEQUILIBRIUM.   Full-blown dialysis dysequilibrium rarely presents in office practice, but some patients exhibit transient symptoms of a less severe nature. This condition occurs mainly in individuals with chronic renal failure who have just started on hemodialysis. It relates to osmotic shifts of water causing edema of the brain, especially of the cerebral cortex. It is associated with metabolic acidosis of the brain and cerebrospinal fluid.

Symptoms and signs include headache, anorexia, nausea, vomiting, dizziness, blurring of vision, and muscle cramps in milder cases; more severely affected patients may experience myoclonus, tremors, seizures, and coma. The EEG may show generalized, excessive rhythmic slowing. The incidence is higher in children, hypertensives, and those with pre-existing brain disease (e.g., trauma or recent stroke).

The syndrome should be recognized and differentiated from progressive dialysis encephalopathy, dementing illness, and threatened stroke. Dialysis dysequilibrium can be prevented by using hemofiltration (no osmotic gradients) rather than dialysis. Slower hemodialysis or substitution of hemodialysis for chronic ambulatory peritoneal dialysis will also prevent the syndrome. Alternatively, increase in osmolality of the dialysate by the addition of mannitol, glycerol, or glucose is effective. The substitution of bicarbonate for acetate in the dialysate has also been recommended.

HEMODIALYSIS HEADACHE.   Hemodialysis headache, which affects about 60 percent of patients on hemodialysis, begins within a few hours of dialysis, usually as a throbbing bifrontal or generalized headache, often with nausea or vomiting. Antimigraine treatment is often effective.

OTHER CONDITIONS.   Vitamin deficiencies are now uncommon, since supplements of water-soluble vitamins are provided to replace those lost from the body in dialysis. It is wise, however, to be on guard for the possibility of thiamine deficiency (which may cause a Wernicke's encephalopathy or a polyneuropathy, or both) and biotin deficiency (which may also produce a neuropathy with or without an encephalopathy characterized by myoclonic jerks, asterixis, and amnesia).

Neurologic Complications of Renal Transplantation.

COMPLICATIONS OF IMMUNOSUPPRESSIVE DRUGS.   Primary central nervous system lymphoma and opportunistic infections of the brain or meninges are now much less frequent than before the advent of Cyclosporin A. This drug is the main immunosuppressant used in transplants. It has better success and fewer severe adverse effects compared with earlier immunosuppressive agents, although a number of neurologic side effects are seen. These include postural tremors (22 percent of cases), seizures (up to 5 percent, often associated with hypomagnesemia), (less commonly) cerebellar intention tremors or ataxia, burning feet, myoclonus, hallucinations, encephalopathy, polyneuropathy, or spinal cord dysfunction (rare).

Stroke.   Cerebrovascular complications are increased in patients with chronic renal failure, whereas patients on dialysis are more prone to intracranial hemorrhage. Following transplantation, patients are more prone to ischemic stroke. The main risk factor is hypertension. Lipid abnormalities, diabetes mellitus, and secondary polycythemia may play a contributory role. Attending physicians should be aware of these complications, should reduce risk factors as much as possible, and should investigate promptly if patients have features of threatened stroke, such as transient ischemic attacks.

Peripheral Nervous System

Uremic Polyneuropathy.   In the early stages of chronic renal failure, during conservative management, uremic polyneuropathy is usually not clinically evident, although mild abnormalities may be detected with electrophysiologic studies, or very mild clinical signs may be evident. Only when end-stage renal failure has been reached, when the creatine clearance is less than 5 ml/min, does significant polyneuropathy occur. At that point 60 percent of patients will have some evidence of uremic polyneuropathy. The most common early symptoms are restless leg syndrome, cramps, numbness, tingling, and uncomfortable sensations, but these may be relatively nonspecific and may occasionally occur in the absence of clinical or electrophysiologic evidence of uremic neuropathy. They may be related to transient neural membrane dysfunction brought about by changes in water and electrolytes. The earliest clear-cut clinical signs are impaired vibratory perception in the toes and reduced ankle jerks. Rarely, the neuropathy is severe, with distal wasting and weakness, absent deep tendon reflexes, severe distal sensory loss to all modalities, and an inability to walk.

On occasion, uremic polyneuropathy seems to advance rapidly over a matter of weeks and may be predominantly of a motor variety. It is likely that this type of neuropathy is associated with underlying sepsis, possibly at the site of shunts or fistulas, or following intercurrent operation. The neuropathy is more properly called critical illness polyneuropathy. It will reverse satisfactorily once the sepsis is brought fully under control.

The autonomic nervous system is commonly involved in a mild form, detected only by testing of the cardiac R-R interval, in which the normal variation in this interval is lost or diminished. However, overt clinical evidence of autonomic nervous system dysfunction is uncommon. Any manifestations of autonomic neuropathy will stabilize during chronic hemodialysis and improve following successful renal transplantation.

In uremic polyneuropathy, electrophysiologic studies will show a primary axonal degeneration of motor and sensory fibers. Secondary segmental demyelination may be present, and thus conduction velocities may be moderately reduced and distal latencies prolonged. Compound muscle action potential amplitudes and sensory action potential amplitudes are the earliest to be involved, along with prolongation of H- or F-wave latencies. These electrophysiologic abnormalities may be present in up to 80 percent of patients on chronic hemodialysis, whether children or adults. Because of the discomfort, needle EMG need not be performed, except in polyneuropathies that are moderate or severe. We have recently observed that abnormal spontaneous activity, positive sharp waves, and fibrillation potentials may be strangely absent when clinical and histologic evidence of denervation of muscle is present. We have speculated that uremic toxins may in some way inhibit the production of this abnormal spontaneous activity.

Clinical and electrophysiologic assessment of the peripheral nervous system in patients on chronic hemodialysis is a valuable method of assessing how well controlled the uremic syndrome is by the particular dialysis techniques. Thus, if the polyneuropathy appears to be worsening (since it should normally stabilize during chronic hemodialysis), efforts should be made to optimize the hemodialysis. The nephrologist may do this in a variety of ways: increase the weekly frequency, change the type of dialyzer, and so forth. However, improvement in the neuropathy may not occur for a number of months or may not occur at all. Hence, if the uremic neuropathy continues to worsen, the patient should be strongly considered for successful renal transplantation. When this is done, one can expect prompt and progressive improvement in the uremic polyneuropathy, even in severe cases.

Peritoneal dialysis does not appear to be any more effective than chronic hemodialysis in controlling uremic polyneuropathy.

Uremic Mononeuropathy.   A variety of mononeuropathies may occur during chronic hemodialysis, since uremic toxins render nerves susceptible to damage from focal compression or ischemia.

CARPAL TUNNEL SYNDROME.   Carpal tunnel syndrome may occur in 31 percent of patients on chronic hemodialysis. It causes symptoms remarkably similar to those experienced by patients who are not in chronic renal failure. Thus, periodic numbness and tingling throughout the median nerve distribution and aching pain radiating proximally occur commonly and are characteristically worsened by acts such as reading a newspaper, repeatedly grasping objects, and so forth. These symptoms may seriously disturb the patient's sleep. However, a distinctive feature is that in patients in chronic hemodialysis with this syndrome, the symptoms are worse during each hemodialysis procedure. Moreover, the carpal tunnel syndrome is more likely to occur in the arm that contains the Cimino-Brescia fistula (Fig. 185-1). Physical signs of median nerve compression, such as wasting of the thenar eminence, are late signs, and hence electrophysiologic studies are usually necessary to establish the diagnosis. Abnormalities in sensory conduction are the first to appear.

In most cases, the carpal tunnel syndrome is of uncertain cause or is clearly secondary to the forearm Cimino-Brescia fistula. However, less commonly, patients will develop amyloidosis (Fig. 185-1) if they have been on chronic hemodialysis for longer than 10 years. This produces generalized arthropathy, in addition to carpal tunnel syndrome. This type of amyloidosis is seen only in chronic renal failure and is due to the accumulation of β-microglobulin, a substance normally present in the body in very small amounts but that accumulates in end-stage renal failure. At the time of carpal tunnel syndrome, appropriate stains for this type of amyloid must be performed to establish the diagnosis. Avoidance of cuprophan membranes for chronic hemodialysis may eliminate this serious complication.

Conservative management, such as splinting the wrists, is usually not effective in treating carpal tunnel syndrome, but sectioning of the flexor retinaculum is usually quite effective. If it appears that the Cimino-Brescia fistula is a significant contributing factor, it may ultimately be necessary to band or ligate the fistula.

MONONEUROPATHIES ASSOCIATED WITH ARTERIOVENOUS FISTULA OR SHUNTS.   The Cimino-Brescia fistula commonly used for access during chronic hemodialysis will occasionally produce periodic aching and burning in the hand; this is really a steal syndrome, causing periodic ischemia to the tissues. It can be successfully treated with either banding or ligation of the fistula. However, in other instances, true carpal tunnel syndrome develops due to vascular congestion and ischemia in the region of the carpal tunnel. The diabetic is particularly prone to this disorder. Again, surgical decompression of the carpal tunnel area may be beneficial.

In rare circumstances, an arteriovenous fistula or shunt placed more proximally in the upper arm may induce a sudden, severe, ischemic neuropathy affecting the median, ulnar, and radial nerves. This is an emergency situation that requires immediate surgical takedown of the fistula or shunt. Even then, severe and permanent neurologic dysfunction may result.

EIGHTH NERVE DYSFUNCTION.   Chronic renal failure, either through the toxicity of uremic toxins or the use of antibiotics or diuretics, may affect both cochlear and vestibular divisions. Improvement may occur, either through hemodialysis or by successful renal transplantation.

COMPARTMENT SYNDROMES.   Because of the tendency toward excessive bleeding in chronic renal failure, and particularly if anticoagulant drugs are being used, compartment syndrome may develop suddenly. A typical site is the psoas muscle. There may be sudden, severe pain and motor and sensory loss within the distribution of the femoral nerve. CT scan may demonstrate the acute hemorrhage and surgical decompression may be beneficial.

COMBINED DIABETIC AND UREMIC POLYNEUROPATHY.   In recent years, more diabetic patients have been accepted into dialysis and transplant programs, and thus the problem of combined diabetic and uremic polyneuropathy is being seen with increasing frequency. In both types of polyneuropathy, a symmetrical motor and sensory involvement is present, with reduced deep tendon reflexes, ataxia, and distal loss of sensation. However, diabetic polyneuropathy is more likely to induce compressive palsies, such as tardy ulnar palsy or carpal tunnel syndrome, and autonomic disturbances and multifocal denervation of muscle are more common. Also, in diabetic polyneuropathy, conduction velocities tend to be lower and attempts at collateral reinnervation are usually more successful than in uremia.

Each polyneuropathy also acts differently in response to organ transplantation. As already noted, uremic polyneuropathy improves promptly with successful kidney transplantation. On the other hand, pancreatic transplantation causes minimal improvement in diabetic polyneuropathy.

Disturbances of Muscle in Uremia.   Defects in neuromuscular transmission are quite uncommon and, when present, are caused by certain antibiotic drugs or high levels of magnesium. Such defects can readily be demonstrated in the EMG laboratory by repetitive nerve stimulation techniques. Severe disturbances of water or electrolytes may induce significant muscle weakness. Attacks of hyperkalemic periodic paralysis may occur in uremic patients and, in contrast to familial varieties, the serum potassium remains abnormal between attacks.

Tetany is a rare manifestation of chronic uremic and is caused by lowered serum levels of calcium or magnesium or is a result of respiratory alkalosis. Hypocalcemia occurs in renal failure as a result of the kidney's inability to synthesize I,25-dihydroxyvitamin D_3. It may also be due to poor mobilization of calcium salts from bone. The rarity of tetany in renal failure is likely due to the corrective action of the associated acidosis. Thus, it will only become manifest if patients are treated with large amounts of alkali. Tetany presents as numbness and tingling in the extremities, light-headedness, and carpopedal or laryngospasm. Percussion of a peripheral nerve may induce contraction of the muscle it supplies (Chvostek's sign). During electrophysiologic studies, needle EMG may reveal spontaneous repetitive

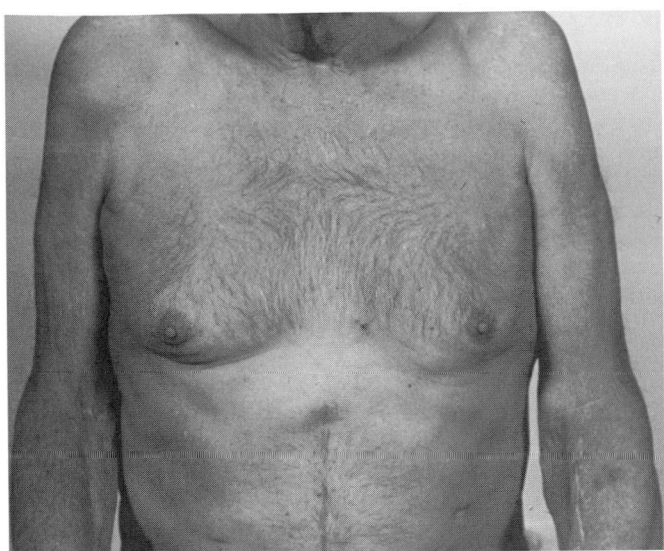

FIG. 185-3. Severe muscle wasting in a 67-year-old man who had received chronic hemodialysis for 7 years. It was associated with underlying pain secondary to progressive bone disease. He also had a progressive dementia, but aluminum intoxication was never proved. Although he had a mild uremic polyneuropathy, needle electromyography of shoulder girdle muscles revealed only an increased proportion of polyphasic units, consistent with a primary myopathy. (From Bolton CF, Young GB: Neurological Complications of Renal Disease. Butterworth, Boston, 1990, with permission.)

Bosch BA, Schlebush L: Neurophysiological deficits associated with uraemic encephalopathy. SAMJ 79:560–2, 1991

Folstein MF, Folstein SE, McHugh PR: Mini-Mental State: a practical guide for grading the cognitive state of patients for the clinician. J Psychiatr Res 12:189–98, 1975

Jablecki CK: Myopathies. p. 385. In Brown WF, Bolton CF (eds): Clinical Electromyopathy. Butterworth, Boston, 1987

Nielsen VK: Pathophysiological aspects of uraemic neuropathy. p. 197. In Canal N, Pozza G (eds): Peripheral Neuropathies. Elsevier/North-Holland, New York, 1978

O'Hare JA, Callaghan NM, Murnaghan DJ: Dialysis encephalopathy: clinical, electroencephalographic and interventional aspects. Medicine 62:129–41, 1983

Okada J, Yoshikawa K, Matsuo H et al: Reversible MRI and CT findings in uremic encephalopathy. Neuroradiology 33:524–6, 1961

Penn AS: Myoglobinuria. In Engel AG, Banker BQ (eds): Myology. 1st Ed. McGraw-Hill, New York, 1986

Shields RW, Root KE, Wilbourn AJ: Compartment syndromes and compression neuropathies in coma. Neurology 36:1370–4, 1986

Swift TR: Disorders of neuromuscular transmission other than myasthenia gravis. Muscle Nerve 4:334–53, 1984

Tegner R, Lindholm B: Vibratory perception threshold compared with nerve conduction velocity in the evaluation of uraemic neuropathy. Acta Neurol Scand 71:284–9, 1985

Tyler HR: Neurologic disorders in renal failure. Am J Med 44:734–48, 1968

Vallance P, Leone A, Calver A et al: Accumulation of an endogenous inhibitor of nitric acid synthetase in chronic renal failure. Lancet 339:572–5, 1992

Wyrtzes L, Markley HG, Fisher M, Alfred AJ: Brachial neuropathy after brachial artery-antecubital vein shunts for chronic hemodialysis. Neurology 37:1398–400, 1987

Zochodne DW, Bolton CF, Wells GA et al: Polyneuropathy associated with critical illness: a complication of sepsis and multiple organ failure. Brain 110:819–42, 1987

discharges appearing as double, triple, or multiple discharges with the typical appearance of motor unit potentials. Tetany can be successfully treated by correction of hypocalcemia and alkalosis.

In rare circumstances when high-dose steroids are used to treat certain forms of primary renal disease, a steroid myopathy may be induced. This is usually relatively mild and is characterized by normal levels of creatine phosphokinase and normal electrophysiologic studies, including needle EMG of muscle. Muscle biopsy may be normal or may reveal a type 2 fiber atrophy.

When bone is significantly affected by hyperparathyroidism or aluminum accumulation, it may induce painful and sometimes severe wasting of muscle, particularly in proximal muscles (Fig. 185-3). However, as in steroid myopathy, electrophysiologic and morphologic studies of muscle are often normal, or biopsy may reveal type 2 fiber atrophy, a nonspecific finding. These features are also present in patients who have muscle wasting caused by the cachexia of renal failure.

Myoglobinuria may be a cause of acute and severe renal failure requiring hemodialysis. The muscles may be weak, swollen, and painful; occasionally they are surprisingly normal on examination. The creatinine phosphokinase is invariably considerably elevated. With successful treatment, muscle strength usually promptly returns to normal.

SUGGESTED READINGS

Alfrey AC, LeGendre GR, Kaehny WD: The dialysis encephalopathy syndrome. Possible aluminum intoxication. N Engl J Med 294:184–8, 1976

Asbury AK, Victor M, Adams RD: Uremic polyneuropathy. Arch Neurol 8:413–28, 1963

Baker LRI, Brown AL, Byrne J et al: Head scan appearances and cognitive function in renal failure. Clin Nephrol 32:242–8, 1989

Bolton CF, Young GB: Neurological Complications of Renal Disease. Butterworth, Boston, 1990

186. NEUROLOGIC MANIFESTATIONS OF ELECTROLYTE DISORDERS

ROBERT LAURENO

Electrolyte disorders may manifest by neurologic problems ranging from coma to muscle cramps. In ambulatory medicine the neurologist typically encounters the less severe neurologic manifestations, and vigilance is necessary to diagnose such cases. When encountering patients with headache, depression weakness, and many other symptoms, the neurologist should consider electrolyte disorders in the differential diagnosis.

HYPONATREMIA

In normal volunteers, experimental hyponatremia causes cramps, weakness, decreased taste sensation, fatigue, and mental dullness. Hyponatremia may also cause tremor, dizziness, nausea, vomiting, headache, and altered mentation. Any one or combination of these problems may bring the patient to the doctor. Although delirium, coma, and convulsions are typically treated in the acute-care environment, less severe cerebral manifestations such as confusion and lethargy may be encountered in the ambulatory setting. The physician's level of suspicion for hyponatremia should be heightened when the patient is taking diuretics or carbamezipine.

Duration and rapidity of onset of hyponatremia are important determinants of the clinical manifestations. Over one-third of Daggett's patients with serum sodium below 120 mEq/L were without neurologic symptoms, perhaps because the hyponatremia evolved slowly. The implications of this data for outpatient practice is that a complaint of malaise, cramps, headache, and/or vomiting will occasionally have as its basis severe hyponatremia ([Na$^+$] less than 110 mEq/L). Sterns has shown that severe hyponatremia has a mortality rate of only 8 percent, primarily because of the underlying disease rather than the hyponatremia itself. The poor prognosis of severe hyponatremia reported in some other series may be in part due to myelinolysis, a disease caused by the correction of hyponatremia.

Myelinolysis Following Correction of Hyponatremia

When a physician discovers a severely hyponatremic patient in the office setting, the first inclination may be to admit the patient to a hospital for prompt correction of the extreme metabolic derangement. This impulse must be checked because correction of hyponatremia can cause central pontine and extrapontine myelinolysis. The outpatient clinician's awareness of this iatrogenic danger can ensure that appropriate precautions are taken when the patient is transferred to a hospital ward.

Myelinolysis is a dissolution of myelin disproportionate to any associated damage of neurons and axons. The lesions occur symmetrically in the center of the pons, the thalamocapsular regions, subcortical white matter, and elsewhere. This disease characteristically causes spastic tetraplegia and muteness in the acute phase. Cognitive, emotional, and movement disorders as well as other features may occur. Sometimes the lesions of myelinolysis can be seen on computed tomography scans, but they are more reliably seen on T2-weighted magnetic resonance imaging scans done 1 week or more after the onset of the symptoms.

Because the neurologic abnormalities usually appear 2 to 3 days after correction of hyponatremia, myelinolysis is basically an inpatient disease. The latency period may occasionally be a week or more. Under these circumstances a patient who has improved after correction of hyponatremia may be discharged from the hospital, only to develop muteness, paralysis, or other manifestations of myelinolysis as an outpatient.

Treatment of Hyponatremia

When admitting a hyponatremic patient to the hospital, the outpatient physician should remind the inpatient team to proceed with caution. Whenever possible the serum sodium should be elevated no more than 10 mEq/L over any 24-hour period to minimize the risk of myelinolysis. Such control of the rate of rise of serum sodium may not always be achievable due to the variables of a given case. Often simply eliminating diuretics, alcohol, or some other cause of hyponatremia will suffice to correct the serum sodium. Naturally coma, status epilepticus, or agitated confusion cannot be taken lightly. When these extreme neurologic manifestation suggest that life is in danger, hypertonic (3 percent) saline can be given in 100-ml boluses. However, corrective saline infusion should be moderated as soon as the patient is clinically improving, even though the serum sodium may still be at a severely low level. The serum sodium should be checked at least every 4 hours to monitor the rate of correction.

HYPERNATREMIA

In the outpatient clinic the encephalopathy of hypernatremia may be encountered as lethargy, mild confusion, or generalized weakness. More severe manifestations (rhabdomyolysis, seizures, or coma) are unlikely to be encountered outside the hospital. Although only 11 percent of patients remain fully alert when serum sodium exceeds 160 mEq/L, symptoms may be absent in chronic hypernatremia even when serum sodium exceeds 175 mEq/L. This adaptation to hypernatremia is caused by a compensatory increase in brain osmolality due to accumulation of potassium, amino acids such as taurine, and polyols. This beneficial increase in intracellular osmolality can be problematic when treatment is administered. If there is a rapid therapeutic decline of extracellular osmolality, the brain's increased osmoles cannot diminish as quickly. In other words, the extracellular fluid is relatively hypotonic to the brain, which, as a result, can swell. Aware of this danger of cerebral edema, the outpatient physician should remind the inpatient team to avoid rapid correction of hypernatremia. Certainly in children, and probably in adults as well, it is best to limit the decline in serum sodium to 0.5 mEq/L/h.

HYPOKALEMIA

Generalized weakness, the primary neurologic manifestation of hypokalemia, may be episodic or acute. However, the weakness is usually subacute or chronic. When serum potassium is greater than 2.5 mEq/L, prominent weakness is rarely seen. However, some patients with minimal depression of potassium (3.0 to 3.5 mEq/L) have malaise, fatigue, cramps, or restless legs. When potassium drops below 2.0 mEq/L, some weakness almost always exists. Although quadriparesis may occur with potassium less than 2.0 mEq/L, some patients are ambulatory with potassium at that level. The weakness is initially worse in proximal muscles. Tendon reflexes are often retained, but areflexia can occur when weakness is profound. Hypokalemic weakness is usually due to changes in muscle membrane polarization, but rhabdomyolysis may be a contributing or predominant cause of weakness in some cases.

Hypokalemia can cause tetany, usually but not always in the setting of alkalosis. Paradoxically, hypokalemia protects against tetany in the setting of hypocalcemia.

The physician's index of suspicion for hypokalemia must be high when the outpatient is taking diuretics or is in some other way at risk for hypokalemia.

HYPERKALEMIA

As opposed to the muscle disorder seen in hypokalemia, the generalized weakness of hyperkalemia appears to be a peripheral neuropathy. Depression of tendon reflexes, numbness, paresthesias, and retained mechanical irritability of muscle all point in this direction. Guillain-Barré syndrome has been incorrectly diagnosed in some cases. Usually no weakness occurs until the serum potassium exceeds 7 mEq/L. Weakness almost always occurs when potassium exceeds 9 mEq/L. Weakness may be gradually progressive or episodic; it may be mild or as severe as quadriplegia.

HYPOCALCEMIA

Tetany, the characteristic neurologic manifestation of hypocalcemia, is caused by peripheral nerve hyperirritability. Spontaneous discharge of motor and sensory axons cause a syndrome of sensory symptoms and muscle contractions that develop and abate in a characteristic sequence. Muscle contractions begin distally with carpopedal spasm. Eventually wrist flexion, elbow bending, arm adduction, and supination of the forearms are seen. Although tetany can culminate in opisthotonos, it is not always so severe. For years some patients have only occasional, brief attacks of stridor or carpopedal spasm.

In such patients, latent tetany may be detected by eliciting Chvostek sign, which is said to be present when percussion of the facial nerve anterior to the external auditory meatus results in contraction of ipsilateral facial muscles. Unless the orbicularis oculi contracts, Chvostek sign is not present. Whereas Chvostek sign is present in 8 percent of normal people, Trousseau sign is more specific for latent tetany. Trousseau sign, occurring in only 1 percent of normal individuals, is said to be present when a pneumatic cuff, inflated on the upper arm to 20 torr above systolic blood pressure, produces paresthesias and carpal spasm in that limb.

Central nervous system manifestations of hypocalcemia such as coma and convulsions will not be encountered in a physician's office, but confusion, dementia, and personality change will be. Headaches, presumably due to increased intracranial pressure, can also be the primary manifestation of hypocalcemia in the outpatient. Hypocalcemia sometimes causes cramps and uncommonly causes parkinsonism. Evidence shows that hypocalcemic patients are more vulnerable than normal individuals to phenothiazine-induced dystonia.

HYPERCALCEMIA

Hypercalcemia can cause a wide range of mental disorders. Confusion, drowsiness, depression, anxiety, paranoia, and mania have all been observed in the ambulatory patient. Generalized weakness, usually chronic but occasionally acute, can also occur. In these cases there may be brisk tendon reflexes, Babinski signs, and muscle atrophy. With or without these objective findings, hypercalcemia can cause cramps. Occasionally these features have suggested the misdiagnosis of amyotrophic lateral sclerosis. Rarely hypercalcemia causes parkinsonism.

HYPOMAGNESEMIA

Tetany has been reported inconsistently in hypomagnesemia. Although it has been suggested that hypomagnesemia induces tetany by decreasing the ionized calcium levels, the tetany is successfully treated with magnesium. As a rule, major manifestations such as delirium and convulsions will not be seen in office practice, but cramps, confusion, other mental disorders, Chvostek sign, tremor, and myoclonus will be encountered.

HYPERMAGNESEMIA

Typically weakness emerges when serum magnesium reaches the 7- to 9-mEq/L level; areflexia develops at 9 to 10 mEq/L. No sensory symptoms or mental features are present. Edrophonium injection transiently improves strength because magnesium causes its paralysing effect at the neuromuscular junction. The electrical manifestations resemble those of the Lambert-Eaton syndrome, namely, low-amplitude compound muscle action potentials, a progressive decline in amplitude at 2/s repetitive nerve stimulation, and an increase in amplitude after isometric exercise or with 50/s repetitive nerve stimulation. A slight increase in serum magnesium can aggravate pre-existing myasthenia gravis or Lambert-Eaton syndrome.

HYPOPHOSPHATEMIA

Hypophosphatemia is an inpatient problem that can cause apathy, confusion, and seizures. It may also cause two neuromuscular disorders, rhabdomyolysis or acute areflexic paralysis (which resembles Guillain-Barré syndrome), or both. Alcoholic patients often develop hypophosphatemia 2 to 4 days after hospitalization. When the outpatient clinician admits an alcoholic patient to the hospital, the inpatient team should be reminded to monitor for hypophosphatemia and treat it promptly to avoid these neurologic problems.

CONCEPTS

Electrolyte disorders manifest by effects at all levels of the nervous system. The central nervous system is affected by hyponatremia, hypernatremia, hypocalcemia, hypercalcemia, hypomagnesemia, and hypophosphatemia. Peripheral nerve is affected by hypocalcemia, hypomagnesemia, hyperkalemia, and hypophosphatemia. The neuromuscular junction is affected by hypermagnesemia. Hypokalemia and hypophosphatemia and sometimes sodium derangements affect muscle.

The major neurologic presentations of electrolyte disorders are generalized weakness, tetany, and encephalopathy. Generalized weakness occurs in hypokalemia, hyperkalemia, hypercalcemia, hypermagnesemia, and hypophosphatemia, and to a lesser extent in hyponatremia and hypernatremia. Ambulatory patients may complain of weakness when no conspicuous abnormality is seen on examination. Tetany occurs in hypocalcemia, hypomagnesemia, and hypokalemia. Because the tetany can be mild and episodic for years, patients may only mention these spasms in passing. Encephalopathy occurs in hyponatremia, hypernatremia, hypocalcemia, hypercalcemia, hypomagnesemia, and hypophosphatemia. In the outpatient setting lethargy, confusion, dementia, depression, anxiety, paranoia, and mania all necessitate that the physician measure electrolytes.

Other manifestations of electrolyte disorders include parkinsonism (hypocalcemia, hypercalcemia), cramps (hypokalemia, hyponatremia, hypocalcemia, hypercalcemia, and hypomagnesemia), and headache (hypocalcemia, hyponatremia).

When patients are taking particular medications, the neurologist should be attuned to the possibility of certain electrolyte disorders. For example, antacids can cause hypercalcemia, phosphate-containing cathartics can cause hypocalcemia, and diuretics can cause hypokalemia or hyponatremia. Carbamezipine-induced hyponatremia, which can manifest as breakthrough seizures in a previously well-controlled epileptic, is of particular importance to the neurologist.

Although most patients with metabolic encephalopathy have relatively symmetric neurologic manifestations, focal neurologic features are possible in any electrolyte-related encephalopathy. Such focal signs are usually seen in the acute care rather than the ambulatory setting.

Severe neurologic signs can emerge when an electrolyte disorder accentuates a mild, underlying, neurologic disease. For example, modest hypermagnesemia may greatly accentuate pre-existing Eaton-Lambert syndrome or myasthenia gravis.

For several reasons the severity of an electrolyte derangement does not correlate simply with the severity of the neurologic manifestation. First, some individuals are more sensitive than others to a given metabolic insult. Second, the electrolyte level measured is sometimes not the critical physiologic parameter. Whereas ionized calcium is the stronger correlate of neurologic dysfunction, total serum calcium is often routinely measured. Third, the duration and rapidity of onset of an electrolyte derangement are major factors determining severity of symptoms. An extreme electrolyte derangement may be virtually asymptomatic when the problem develops over weeks or months. On the other hand, a moderate electrolyte derangement may cause severe symptoms when the problem develops acutely. Finally, other variables may be interacting with the electrolyte in question. For example, when hypocalcemia and hypokalemia coexist, the latter disorder prevents the former from causing tetany.

Correction of electrolyte derangements can cause or precipitate neurologic disorders. Correction of hypokalemia may unmask tetany in a hypocalcemic individual. The rapid correction of sodium derangements can be even more perilous. Rapid correction of hypernatremia can cause brain swelling. Rapid correction of hyponatremia can cause central pontine and extrapon-tine myelinolysis. When admitting a vulnerable patient to the hospital, the neurologist should remind the inpatient team that caution in therapy lessens the incidence of these complications.

SUGGESTED READINGS

Comi G, Testa D, Cornelio F et al: Potassium depletion myopathy: a clinical and morphological study of six cases. Muscle Nerve 8:17, 1985
Fishman RA: Neurological aspects of magnesium metabolism. Arch Neurol 12:562, 1965
Henson, RA: The neurological aspects of hypercalcaemia: with special reference to primary hyperparathyroidism. J R Coll Physicians Lond 1:41, 1966
Karp BI, Laureno R: Pontine and extrapontine myelinolysis: a neurologic disorder following rapid correction of hyponatremia. Medicine (Baltimore) 72: 359, 1993
Krendel DA: Hypermagnesemia and neuromuscular transmission. Semin Neurol 10:42, 1990
Laureno R: Neurologic syndromes accompanying electrolyte disorders. p. 545. In Goetz CG, Tanner CM, Aminoff MJ (eds): Handbook of Clinical Neurology. Part I, Vol. 19(63): Systemic Diseases. 1993
Layzer RB: Neuromuscular Manifestations of Systemic Disease. FA Davis, Philadelphia, 1985
Sowden JM, Borsey DQ: Hyperkalaemic periodic paralysis: a rare presentation of Addison's disease. Postgrad Med J 65:238, 1989
Sterns RH: Severe symptomatic hyponatremia: treatment and outcome—a study of 64 cases. Ann Intern Med 107:656, 1987

SECTION 4. GASTROENTEROLOGY AND HEPATOLOGY

187. NEUROLOGIC EFFECTS OF MALABSORPTION AND VITAMIN DEFICIENCY

MARTIN A. SAMUELS

Intestinal malabsorption refers to an impairment of one or more of the steps involved in normal digestion and absorption of nutrients. The neurologic manifestations of malabsorption are mostly related to the vitamin deficiency that may result, regardless of the underlying disease causing the malabsorption. Vitamins are biologically active organic compounds that are essential for normal growth, development, and health and that cannot be synthesized by the body. The four fat-soluble vitamins are A, D, E, and K, and the nine water-soluble vitamins are B_1 (thiamine), B_2 (riboflavin), niacin, B_6 (pyridoxine), folic acid, B_{12} (cyanocobalamin), C (ascorbic acid), pantothenic acid, and biotin.

FAT-SOLUBLE VITAMIN DEFICIENCY

Fat-soluble vitamin deficiency is usually caused by disorders that lead to fat malabsorption and steatorrhea. The main neuro-logic complication of *vitamin A* deficiency is night blindness, usually associated with xerophthalmia (dryness of the conjunctivae). *Vitamin D* deficiency may result in diffuse bone pain or tetany related to the associated hypocalcemia. *Vitamin K* deficiency causes decreased prothrombin activity in the blood not associated with liver disease or the use of warfarin. Intracerebral, intraventricular, subarachnoid, subdural, and epidural hemorrhages may occur in patients with vitamin K deficiency. *Vitamin E* deficiency consists of ophthalmoplegia, retinal pigmentary degeneration, spinocerebellar ataxia, myopathy, and an axonal polyneuropathy.

WATER-SOLUBLE VITAMIN DEFICIENCY

The water-soluble vitamin deficiencies occur in a variety of circumstances.

Thiamine, Riboflavin, Niacin, and Pyridoxine Deficiency

Thiamine vitamin B_1 deficiency is usually caused by severe malnutrition, sometimes coupled with increased requirements (e.g., pregnancy, hyperthyroidism). In North America it is usually associated with alcoholism. Because it tends to be associated with generalized malnutrition, thiamine deficiency is often part of a multiple deficiency state, particularly including riboflavin and niacin. For this reason, some of the early, nonspecific effects of thiamine deficiency such as an axonal polyneuropathy cannot be strictly proved to be due to thiamine deficiency itself. However, acute Wernicke's encephalopathy has been clearly shown to be due to thiamine deficiency. It consists of an array of symptoms and signs usually including a mental abnormality (confusion, delirium, or amnesia), ataxia, and ocular abnormalities (e.g., nystagmus, cranial nerve palsies, ptosis). It is quite clear, however, from pathologic studies, that most patients suffering from thiamine deficiency do not show the entire classic triad (i.e., amnesia, ataxia, and ophthalmoplegia). For this reason, it is prudent to have a low threshold for treating patients with thiamine if the suspicion of malnutrition is raised. Failure to treat can lead to permanent deficits, the most disabling of which is chronic amnestic dementia (Korsakoff's psychosis). Red blood cell transketolase levels and careful magnetic resonance imaging focusing on the mammillary bodies may help in making the diagnosis, but any serious suspicion of malnutrition, particularly in alcoholic patients, should lead the clinician to replace thiamine, parenterally at first, followed by long-term oral supplementation.

Riboflavin (vitamin B₂) deficiency results from inadequate dietary intake of milk, liver, meat, eggs, and some green leafy vegetables. The major neurologic manifestation is photophobia, usually associated with excessive lacrimation and itching of the eyes.

Niacin deficiency (i.e., deficiency of either nicotinic acid or nicotinamide, or both) is usually related to malnutrition and alcoholism. The deficiency state, known as pellagra, causes the triad of dermatitis, diarrhea, and dementia. The dementia is characterized by memory loss and slowness of thought without the aphasic or apraxic phenomena commonly seen in Alzheimer's disease.

Pyridoxine (vitamin B₆) deficiency is caused by malnutrition or by the intake of a pyridoxine antagonist such as isoniazid. The major neurologic manifestation is a severe polyneuropathy.

Folic Acid and Vitamin B₁₂ Deficiency

Folic acid and *cobalamin (vitamin B₁₂)* deficiencies result in megaloblastic anemias. The term *megaloblastic anemia* refers to a characteristic pattern of morphologic abnormality in the blood and bone marrow that probably arises from impaired DNA synthesis. Clinically, this is usually the result of a deficiency of one of two factors, vitamin B₁₂ or folic acid, both of which are essential to the formation of the deoxyribosyl precursors of DNA. This deficiency results in abnormal development of erythroblasts in the marrow such that intramedullary hemolysis occurs, resulting in anemia. The peripheral blood contains macrocytic erythrocytes. The disordered DNA metabolism also affects the maturation of granulocytes and megakaryocytes, resulting in hypersegmented polymorphonuclear leukocytes in the peripheral blood. This disordered DNA metabolism is clearly not confined to the blood cells, since giant epithelial cells are found in many other organs including the mouth, stomach, and skin. The neurologic effects of the megaloblastic anemias are probably due to a primary metabolic derangement in neural tissue and are clearly not directly related to the anemia per se. Since the blood-forming organs are particularly sensitive to the effects of B₁₂ or folate deficiency, it is unusual to find the neurologic effects in patients in whom no disorders of the blood are found. Anemia is, however, only one and probably a relatively late sign of B₁₂ or folate deficiency, so it is possible to find a clear example of the neurologic effects of B₁₂ or folate deficiency without anemia. It is distinctly rare, however, to find

TABLE 187-1. Causes of Vitamin B₁₂ Deficiency

Defective diet (low in animal or bacterial products)
Defective absorption
  Deficiency of intrinsic factor
    Pernicious anemia
    Gastrectomy
  Intestinal disease
    Malabsorption (sprue, resection, bypass, or disease of terminal ileum)
    "Blind loop" syndrome
    Fish tapeworm infestation
Deranged metabolism or increased requirement (thyrotoxicosis, pregnancy, neoplasia)

no hematologic signs of B₁₂ or folate deficiency in a patient with proved neurologic effects of these vitamin deficiencies.

Vitamin B₁₂. Vitamin B₁₂ deficiency may be due to a number of causes which are summarized in Table 187-1. The most prevalent form, at least in North America, is pernicious anemia (or Addison's anemia, Biermer's anemia, primary anemia). It arises from failure of the gastric fundus to secrete adequate amounts of intrinsic factor to ensure intestinal absorption of cobalamin, a process that is usually immune mediated, but may be familial or result from gastric neoplasia. Histamine-fast achlorhydria is usually present in pernicious anemia, but this method of diagnosis will, of course, not be useful in other forms of vitamin B₁₂ deficiency. In disorders other than pernicious anemia, serum B₁₂ levels are required for diagnosis. Since vitamin B₁₂ is stored in various tissue in large amounts, the appearance of pernicious anemia after the cessation of B₁₂ absorption or intake is delayed by at least 3 years. Even though pernicious anemia is the most common cause of B₁₂ deficiency, it seems clear that vitamin B₁₂ deficiency from any of the causes listed in Table 187-1 may result in the identical clinical picture. The three neurologic manifestations of vitamin B₁₂ deficiency are subacute combined degeneration of the spinal cord, mental changes, and optic neuropathy.

PATHOGENESIS OF THE NEUROLOGIC COMPLICATIONS. The pathogenesis of the neurologic complications of vitamin B₁₂ deficiency is not entirely clear, but several facts are known. Cobalamin, a pyrol, is synthesized by microorganisms and ingested in meat, liver, fish, eggs, and milk. In a normal North American diet, 5 to 30 μg are ingested a day, of which 1 to 5 μg are absorbed. Two to 5 mg are stored in the body, of which about 1 mg is stored in the liver. It is thus very difficult to become vitamin B₁₂ deficient based on dietary deficiency. Only a pure lactovegetarian could perform such a feat and even then, the huge stores would forestall symptoms for 3 to 5 years.

Four forms of cobalamin exist in animals: hydroxocobalamin, its analogue cyanocobalamin, and its two coenzymes adenosylcobalamin and methylcobalamin. Cobalamin is bound to intrinsic factor, a 44,000-dalton mucoprotein secreted by the parietal cells of the stomach. This intrinsic factor/cobalamin complex is absorbed via specific receptors in the terminal ileum.

Cobalamin Enzyme Systems. Two major cobalamin-dependent enzyme systems exist, each using a different one of the two coenzymes methylcobalamin and adenosylcobalamin. The purpose of the methylcobalamin-dependent system is to generate tetrahydrofolate, which in turn is required for the conversion of uridylmonophosphate to thymidyl monophosphate, to be incorporated into DNA.

In the system, shown in Figure 187-1, methylcobalamin acts as a coenzyme for methyltransferase, otherwise known as methionine synthetase. Methylcobalamin acts as a methyl donor for the generation of methionine from homocysteine and then

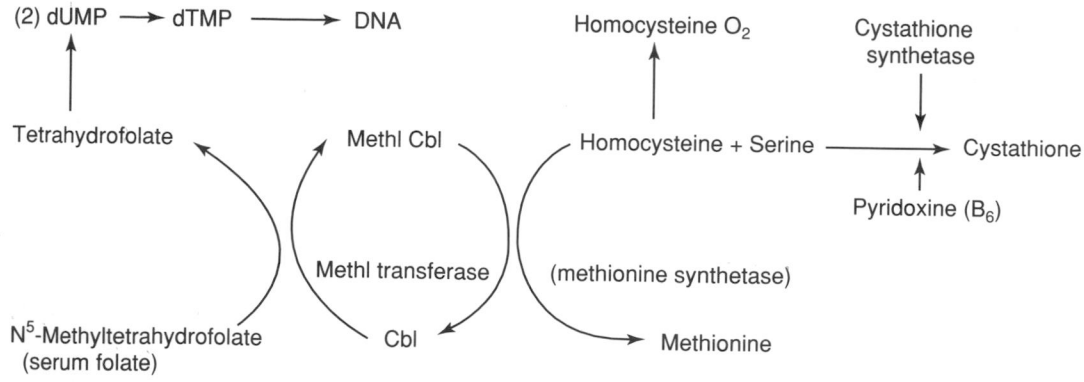

FIG. 187-1.   The methylcobalamin-dependent methyl transferase system.

acts as a methyl group acceptor for the conversion of N^5-methyltetrahydrofolate (serum folate) to tetrahydrofolate. Deficiency of methylcobalamin results in a low serum methionine and elevated homocysteine (i.e., greater than 16.2 μmol/L), which in turn is oxidized to homocystine. Thus, one form of homocystinuria is due to methylcobalamine deficiency. The other more common, inherited form of homocystinuria is due to deficiency in cystathione synthetase, the enzyme that combines serine with homocysteine to form cystathione.

In vitamin B_{12} deficiency, inadequate methyltransferase activity results in the so-called folate trap, meaning serum folate cannot be converted to tetrahydrofolate. This results in a high serum folate level and the incorporation of uridyl residues into DNA. This abnormal DNA is fragile, leading to all the manifestations of vitamin B_{12} deficiency seen in rapidly dividing cells, such as those in the bone marrow, skin, and intestinal tract. For these reasons, patients with vitamin B_{12} deficiency have hypersegmented polymorphonuclear leukocytes in the peripheral blood, macrocytosis, megaloblasts in the bone marrow, intramedullary hemolysis, and gastrointestinal symptoms. Since central nervous system neurons do not multiply, it has been traditionally considered unlikely that the methyltransferase system had anything to do with the neurologic manifestations of the disease. However, oligodendrocytes do multiply, so it is conceivable that failure of this system could lead to a disorder of myelin metabolism. One supporting bit of evidence for this hypothesis is the fact that nitrous oxide toxicity is known to produce all the manifestations of subacute combined degeneration of the nervous system and is known to be an inhibitor of methyltransferase activity.

The second vitamin B_{12}-dependent enzyme system utilizes the adenosylcobalamin coenzyme to help methylmalonyl coenzyme A (CoA) mutase catalyze the conversion of methylmalonyl CoA to succinyl CoA, as shown in Figure 187-2.

Deficiency of adenosylcobalamin will therefore result in ele-

vated methylmalonic acid (i.e., greater than 271 mnol/L) Evidence shows that methylmalonic acid is toxic to myelin because it will substitute for malonic acid, leading to long chain fatty acids with odd (rather than the normal even) number of carbon atoms. The abnormal myelin made of fatty acids with odd numbers of carbon atoms is fragile, leading to demyelination. Evidence from animal experiments supports this concept in that the addition of valine to the diet exacerbates latent vitamin B_{12} deficiency. As can be seen from Figure 187-2, valine is a precursor of the presumptive toxin, methylmalonic acid.

CLINICAL NEUROLOGIC SYNDROMES. The clinical neurologic syndromes of vitamin B_{12} deficiency are (1) subacute combined degeneration of the spinal cord, (2) mental abnormalities, and (3) optic neuropathy. They have in common an identical pathology consisting of a myelinopathy followed by axonal disease, which is probably secondary.

Subacute Combined Degeneration of the Spinal Cord. Subacute combined degeneration of the spinal cord (or subacute combined sclerosis, posterolateral sclerosis) is the term used to designate the spinal cord disease caused by pernicious anemia. Patients tend to complain of generalized weakness and paresthesias that begin distally and progress proximally. As these symptoms progress, stiffness and weakness in the limbs develops. Loss of vibration sense is the most profound sign, often joined later in the course of disease by joint position sense loss as well. The Romberg sign is positive and the gait is unsteady and awkward. Weakness and spasticity are usually worse in the legs than the arms and may progress to a spastic paraplegia if untreated. Babinski signs are present, but the deep tendon reflexes are variable. They may be grossly increased with clonus, absent, or show any intermediate degree of activity. Occasionally, a sensory level may be found on the trunk, implicating the spinothalamic tracts. This finding should always be viewed with the greatest skepticism and lead one to exclude other causes of spinal cord disease exhaustively. All the findings of

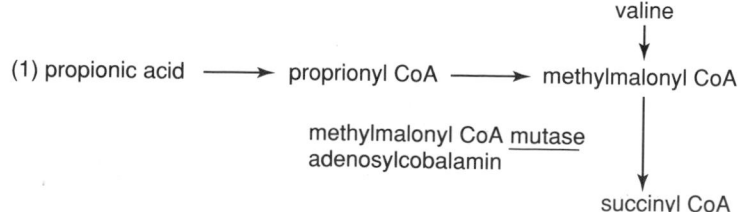

FIG. 187-2.   The adenosylcobalamin-dependent methylmalonyl coenzyme A (CoA) mutase system.

pure vitamin B_{12} deficiency may be attributable to myelopathy alone, and no convincing evidence shows that B_{12} deficiency itself causes a neuropathy. However, in practice, the frequent concomitant existence of folate and other vitamin deficiencies makes it difficult to be sure of this point. Many patients with vitamin B_{12} deficiency have distal symmetrical impairment of cutaneous sensation, absent deep tendon reflexes, and even slowed nerve conduction velocities, suggesting a neuropathic component. This is probably due to concomitant folate deficiency, but the outside chance that vitamin B_{12} deficiency itself may cause a peripheral neuropathy cannot be rigorously excluded.

Case Study. A 49-year-old right-handed junior high school teacher, who was in superb health and who had exceptional cognitive and intellectual skills, began feeling fatigued about 6 months before presentation. By her account, feelings of fatigue progressed and she felt a "tingling numbness" in her toes bilaterally. These symptoms worsened slowly for about 3 months, when she developed a flulike illness with myalgias, fevers to 103°, visual blurring, bilateral tinnitus, and lethargy. Following that illness, she presented to her primary physician, who began an evaluation for seemingly new symptoms of agitated depression and gait difficulty. *Haemophilus influenza* pneumonia was diagnosed and Augmentin begun in addition to Xanax and Pamelor. Despite these treatments she found her balance continually worsening, her thinking becoming less clear, and an increase of a "burning sensation" in her toes and fingers, with her right more than left leg feeling "heavy." She stopped driving and teaching. She had no localized weakness, asymmetric numbness, bowel or bladder dysfunction, episodic changes in consciousness, fever, stiff neck, or any acknowledged change in language. She noted that food had smelled and tasted different recently. Her brother noted that she had had some feelings of persecution and paranoia. She minimized her cognitive difficulties, although she acknowledged that her teaching skills had not been "up to snuff."

She had had no significant prior medical illnesses. A tetracycline allergy was present. She had had no operations or transfusions and neither smoked or drank. She is now off Xanax and Pamelor and has recently been taking only estrogen, based on a diagnosis of "menopausal changes." She denied a history of travel out of her home town or to regions endemic with encephalitis, and no contributory family history was present.

On examination, blood pressure was 100/58, heart rate 84, and respiratory rate 10; she was afebrile. She was a neatly dressed and extremely polite, quiet woman in no distress. She was somewhat flat in affect, and her behaviors and hand motions tended to mimic the examiner's words and actions. A mental status examination revealed normal attention to serial tasks, but difficulty attending to complex conversation or multistep concepts, in response to which she occasionally confabulated, missing details. Her language showed no abnormalities of fluency, repetition, naming, or comprehension. Praxis was normal. Visual spatial scanning was normal, without neglect. She was somewhat concrete in logic and abstractions. Digit span was 6–7 forward but only 2–3 in reverse. Following normal registration and immediate recall of a story with seven details, she could only recall two details, even with prompting, at 5 minutes. There were no clear signs of frontal release. Luria sequencing was poor.

Cranial nerve examination revealed normal smell, fundi, visual fields, and corrected acuity. Extraocular movements, pupillary function, facial sensation and movement, and hearing, palate, and tongue functions were all normal. Motor examination revealed gegenhalten tone, especially in the legs. Power was normal and symmetric. Reflexes were brisk although not clearly pathologic. However, bilateral Babinski signs were present. Coordination testing revealed bilateral discoordination (legs worse than arms), with rapid alternating movement difficulties but no clear dysmetria. Pain and temperature sensation was subjectively normal and symmetric without correlation to her paresthetic symptoms. Gait and stance were both abnormal, with a truncal ataxia, instability at rest, walking, and turning, and a positive Romberg sign. Evidence existed of severe loss of vibration and position sense in all four extremities (worse in the legs).

Laboratory evaluation revealed normal electrolytes, glucose, cholesterol, triglycerides, calcium, magnesium, and phosphate, as well as normal thyroid, renal, and liver function. Blood values were as follows: hematocrit 32.4 percent; hemoglobin, 11.1 g/dl (normal, 11.5 to 16.4); mean corpuscular volume, 113 μm^3 (normal, 80 to 90); mean corpuscular hemoglobin, 38.7 pg/cell (normal, 27 to 32); and mean corpuscular hemoglobin concentration, 34.2 percent (normal, 32 to 36). The blood smears (Plate 187-1) showed macrocytosis and multilobed polymorphonuclear leukocytes.

Other values were as follows: erythrocyte sedimentation rate, 70 mm/h; reticulocyte count, 4.3 percent (normal, 0.8 to 2.8); prothrombin time and activated partial thromboplastin times, normal; white blood count, 5,100 (84 percent polymorphonuclear leukocytes, 15 percent lymphocytes, 1 percent eosinophilic leukocytes); serum iron, 96 $\mu g/dl$ (normal, 45 to 173); total iron-binding capacity, 282 $\mu g/dl$ (normal, 195 to 395); ferritin, 73 $\mu g/L$ (normal, 10 to 300); spinal fluid, clear and under normal pressure; cerebrospinal fluid (CSF) glucose, 65 mg/dl (normal, 40 to 70) with simultaneous blood glucose of 91 mg/dl (normal, 70 to 112); CSF protein, 32 mg/dl (normal, 10 to 44), with no oligoclonal bands; serum folate greater than the assay range of 0 to 20 $\mu g/L$ (normal, 3 to 15); vitamin B_{12} serum level, 17 ng/L (normal, 240 to 1,200); vitamin B_6 (pyridoxine) level, 3.8 $\mu g/L$ (normal, 3.6 to 18).

Part I Schilling test using an orally ingested capsule containing^{57} Co (0.5 μCi) revealed urinary excretion of 0.58 percent of the total orally ingested activity (lower limit of normal, 10 percent). Antiparietal cell and anti-intrinsic factor antibodies were detected in the patient's serum. Upper endoscopy was grossly normal but biopsy revealed gastric fundus atrophy with no sign of malignancy. Magnetic resonance imaging of the head and spine were completely normal despite a special effort made to visualize the presumed spinal cord abnormality.

Neuropsychological testing estimated her premorbid IQ to be 120, based on her vocabulary, education, and achievement. She scored a full-scale IQ of 98 with a pathologically large gap between her verbal score (111) and her performance score (82). Her memory quotient was 83, greater than 2 standard deviations below expectations. Visual information storage was impaired, but less so than verbal storage. The Boston naming test was within the normal range (53/60), but she struggled and perseverated. Mood scales revealed anxiety but no depression. The neuropsychologist felt that the pseudodementia of depression was very unlikely and suggested the diagnosis of vitamin B_{12} deficiency based solely on the cognitive test results.

Clinical neurophysiologic studies showed normal motor nerve conduction velocities. The soleus H reflex was absent bilaterally. The right sural nerve potential amplitude was at the low end of the normal range with a normal conduction velocity. Electromyogram showed no spontaneous activity in the soleus, extensor hallucus longus, biceps femoris, or lumbar and sacral paraspinal muscles. Electroencephalogram showed generalized slowing in the θ range, most prominently in the left temporal region.

The patient was started on vitamin B_{12}, 1,000 μg/day. Within 1 day, her mental status and gait began to improve. By 3 days she was walking unaided and after 7 days she was transferred to a rehabilitation facility, where she stayed for 1 more week before returning home. One month from the time of her first B_{12} injection, she returned to work. She has been maintained on monthly B_{12} injections since. All hematologic indices have returned to normal and her mental state and gait are "supernormal" according to her and her brother, meaning that she is now functioning at a level higher than ever before.

Comment: This patient's history, laboratory findings, and clinical course are classic for subacute combined degeneration of the nervous system due to vitamin B_{12} deficiency caused by an autoimmune disease (i.e., pernicious anemia). Note that the serum B_{12} level was very low and the folate level high, due to the folate trap (see above). The illness is chronic but with a subacute phase and responds dramatically to appropriate therapy. The blood smear, neurologic examination, and neuropsychological profile are enough to suggest the diagnosis. This patient's return to a "supernormal" state probably indicates the very long-term nature of this insidious disorder, upon which was superimposed a dramatic subacute illness characterized by encephalopathy and gait disorder. Note the absence of polyneuropathy even in the face of this very severe vitamin B_{12} deficiency state.

In subtler situations, a serum homocysteine and methylmalonic acid level could be used to assay for intracellular vitamin B_{12} function. These were not required in this patient's case because of the obvious nature of her illness and the very low serum vitamin B_{12} level.

Pathologically the lesion in the nervous system is a degeneration of white matter in the spinal cord and occasionally the brain. The myelin sheaths and axons are both involved, the former more profoundly than the latter. These changes begin in the posterior columns of the lower cervical and upper thoracic segments and spread from there up and down and also laterally in the cord to involve the lateral columns. On microscopic study, early changes consist of swelling and destruction of the myelin sheath with subsequent axonal destruction. Later, a cribriform appearance develops. Eventually, white matter is lost and is replaced by gliosis. The focal lesions have a rough but not absolute symmetry, and they extend caudally and rostrally so that ultimately the entire area of the dorsal columns is involved. In the meantime, the lesions have begun in the lateral columns and extend into the other long tracts. The gray matter is spared. Similar changes can be seen in the cerebral hemispheres and optic nerves. The myelin of peripheral nerves may also be involved, but axons have not been shown to be unequivocally affected.

MENTAL CHANGES. Mental changes are frequent in patients with vitamin B_{12} deficiency. In most cases these changes reflect abnormalities in level of consciousness with inattention, confusion, somnolence, apathy, and delirium being the cardinal features. True dementia, defined as intellectual impairment in the absence of a disorder of level of consciousness, is certainly a relatively rare manifestation of pure vitamin B_{12} deficiency. Pure mental change as the only manifestation of vitamin B_{12}

deficiency is exquisitely uncommon. Case reports of true dementia and pure mental change as manifestations of vitamin B_{12} deficiency are contaminated with concomitant causes of dementia and disordered mental status.

OPTIC NEUROPATHY. Optic neuropathy (papillopathy and retrobulbar neuropathy) is the third and last major neurologic complication of vitamin B_{12} deficiency. It is characterized by bilateral involvement of the optic nerves resulting in loss of central visual acuity and depressed sensitivity greater for color than for white in the centrocecal area of the field of vision. This is the rarest of the three neurologic manifestations of vitamin B_{12} deficiency but may be the only or presenting manifestation of the syndrome. It may be subclinically present in many more cases than previously believed if very sensitive measurement of optic nerve function such as visual evoked responses is used. This syndrome is clinically similar to a number of other bilateral optic neuropathy syndromes including the so-called tobacco/alcohol amblyopia, diabetic optic neuritis, Leber's hereditary optic neuropathy, and tropical ataxic neuropathy. Some neurologists feel that the etiology of all of these syndromes, including vitamin B_{12} deficiency-induced optic neuropathy, is linked to an abnormality in metabolism due to a shortage of sulphur-donating amino acids. Recent evidence from an epidemic of optic neuropathy and myelopathy in Cuba has raised the question of whether a mitochondrial disorder, such as that known to cause Leber's hereditary optic neuropathy, may be present in patients whose metabolism is then stressed by vitamin B_{12} deficiency and perhaps cyanide toxicity (as might be acquired by eating large amounts of casava and/or smoking cigarettes or cigars, as is done in Cuba), leading to the expression of an optic neuropathy and myelopathy in people who otherwise would not have become ill were it not for the mitochondrial defect.

DIAGNOSIS. The diagnosis of vitamin B_{12} deficiency rests on various laboratory tests. The microbiologic assay with *Euglena gracilis* remains the gold standard against which other tests are measured, but the study is done in only a few laboratories and is not practical for routine use. The radioimmunoassay for vitamin B_{12} is now quite accurate. Formerly this test often yielded falsely high values compared with the microbiologic assay, but now all commercial kits use intrinsic factor itself, yielding an accurate result. In general, levels under 100 pg/ml are associated with neurologic disease. The Schilling test is now only used in patients who have received vitamin B_{12}. The best assays for intracellular cobalamin deficiency are the serum methylmalonic acid (normal, 73 to 271 nml/L), which tests adenosylcobalamin coenzyme activity, and the serum homocysteine (normal, 5.4 to 16.2 μmol/L), which tests methylcobalamin coenzyme activity. Elevated levels indicate vitamin B_{12} deficiency.

TREATMENT. Treatment consists of parenteral vitamin B_{12} injections. Shortly after vitamin B_{12} is begun, the folate trap will be released, causing a sudden drop in serum folate level. That must be replaced or a secondary folate deficiency will result. If one inadvertently treats a vitamin B_{12}-deficient patient with folate alone, this may partially correct the hematologic manifestations of the illness while masking the progression of the neurologic problems. Thus one should treat the patient with vitamin B_{12} initially and follow the serum folate. When it falls, folate may be safely replaced.

Folic Acid Deficiency. Folic acid (folate) deficiency accounts for nearly all the cases of megaloblastic anemia not due

TABLE 187-2. Causes of Folate Deficiency

Defective diet (low in vegetables and liver)
Defective absorption
   Intestinal malabsorption (sprue, steatorrhea, massive diverticulosis, short circuits of gastrointestinal tract)
   "Blind-loop" syndrome
Deranged metabolism
   Increased requirement (hemolytic anemia, pregnancy, neoplasia)
   Impaired utilization (liver disease, administration of folic acid antagonists or anticonvulsants)

to vitamin B_{12} deficiency. The causes of folate deficiency are summarized in Table 187-2:

Unlike vitamin B_{12}, the bodily stores of folic acid are quite limited. A folate deficiency syndrome may commence within several months of dietary deprivation, making it a much more common problem among the malnourished than is vitamin B_{12} deficiency. Folate, once absorbed through the entire small intestine, is reduced by specific liver enzymes to tetrahydrofolic acid, a compound that plays a major role in the metabolism of one carbon fragments by its synthesis and transfer of methyl groups. Via this mechanism folate is vital for the conversion of deoxyuridate to thymidylate, a precursor needed for DNA synthesis. Thus, tetrahydrofolate derivations are closely linked to vitamin B_{12}-dependent reactions, and the hematologic alterations in vitamin B_{12} and folate deficiency are indistinguishable. Deficiencies of the two vitamins have very similar effects and a deficiency of one may lead to faulty utilization of the other. For example, patients with vitamin B_{12} deficiency may have an initially elevated serum folate, which will plummet rapidly when vitamin B_{12} is administered, thus requiring concomitant treatment with folate lest a folate deficiency state, previously masked by the vitamin B_{12} deficiency, should become clinically significant. Many patients with vitamin B_{12} deficiency have concomitant folate deficiency, but the vast majority of those with the overwhelmingly more common folate deficiency state will have no vitamin B_{12} deficiency. Folic acid deficiency is almost never pure. Since it accompanies malnutrition it is nearly always associated with multiple vitamin deficiencies. The most common neurologic manifestation of this state is a polyneuropathy.

POLYNEUROPATHY. The symptomatology of nutritional polyneuropathy includes distal paresthesias, burning, and weakness. On examination, a distal loss of reflexes and sensation is found. The essential pathologic change is an axonal degeneration with "dying back" of the axons according to length. Some minor degrees of segmental demyelination may also occur, usually due to entrapment of metabolically weakened nerves. The common entrapment neuropathies (e.g., carpal tunnel syndrome, meralgia paresthetica, peroneal palsy, and ulnar palsy) are all more frequent in patients with an underlying metabolic axonopathy such as that due to vitamin deficiency. In circumstances in which the major vitamin deficiency is likely to be folic acid (i.e., when folate antagonists have been given), a mild polyneuropathy of the type described above occurs. No evidence shows that pure folate deficiency has any other neurologic manifestations.

Vitamin C and Biotin Deficiency

Ascorbic acid (vitamin C) deficiency is rarely seen in North America today. The resultant syndrome of scurvy may cause lassitude and irritability, but a specific neurologic syndrome is not known.

Biotin deficiency cannot result from inadequate intake alone since it is produced by the intestinal bacteria. Raw eggs contain avidin, which binds biotin, and large consumption can result in biotin deficiency. The neurologic syndrome is nonspecific and consists of lassitude, somnolence, depression, and hyperesthesia.

SUGGESTED READINGS

Beck WS: Neuropsychiatric consequences of cobalamin deficiency. Adv Intern Med 36:33–56, 1991
Harding AE, Muller DPR, Thomas PK et al: Spinocerebellar degeneration secondary to chronic intestinal malabsorption: a vitamin E deficiency syndrome. Ann Neurol 12:419–24, 1982
Healton EB, Savage DG, Brust JCM et al: Neurologic aspects of cobalamin deficienty. Medicine (Baltimore) 70:221–45, 1991

188. HEPATIC ENCEPHALOPATHY

EDWARD J. LEVINE
JEFFREY D. ROTHSTEIN

Hepatic encephalopathy is a common medical condition that faces the primary care physician and specialist alike. It is a neuropsychiatric syndrome characterized by abnormal mental status occurring in patients with hepatic insufficiency. It complicates both acute and chronic liver disease.

Subtypes of hepatic encephalopathy are classified by the rate of progression and nature of the underlying hepatic disease, as follows:

Portal-systemic encephalopathy
Fulminant hepatic failure
Hepatocerebral degeneration
Spastic paraparesis

Portal-systemic encephalopathy generally results from cirrhosis. It can run an acute, subacute, or chronic course. Fulminant hepatic failure is defined as the onset of hepatic encephalopathy within 8 weeks of the beginning of the illness in the absence of prior liver disease. Late-onset hepatic failure is similar to fulminant hepatic failure with the exception that encephalopathy occurs from 8 to 24 weeks following the onset of illness. Hepatocerebral degeneration and spastic paraparesis are irreversible conditions that may rarely occur in patients with chronic liver disease. Patients present with neurologic abnormalities similar to those seen in Wilson's disease or in those with spinal cord tumors, respectively. This chapter focuses primarily on portal-systemic encephalopathy, since it would be the most common condition encountered by the office practitioner. Fulminant hepatic failure will also be addressed briefly.

PORTAL-SYSTEMIC ENCEPHALOPATHY

Clinical Features

The syndrome is characterized by alterations in behavior ranging from diminished attention span to coma. Alterations in motor tone and posture, slowing of the electroencephalogram

TABLE 188-1. Signs and Symptosm of Hepatic Encephalopathy

Stage[a]	Mental Status/Behavior	Motor/Reflexes
1	Mild confusion Anxiety Irritability Agitation Diminished attention Impaired serial 7s Altered sleep patterns Depression	Fine postural tremor Slowed coordination
2	Drowsiness Lethargy Gross personality changes Disorientation (time) Poor recall Inappropriate behavior	Asterixis Dysarthria Primitive reflexes—suck, grasp Paratonia Ataxia
3	Delirium or profound confusion Paranoia Disorientation: time and place Incomprehensible speech Somnolent but arousable	Hyper-reflexia Seizures Babinski sign Hyperventilation Incontinence Hypothermia Myoclonus
4	Coma	Decerebrate posturing Brisk oculocephalic reflexes

[a] Signs and symtoms may vary within each stage.

(EEG) with characteristic triphasic slow waves, and characteristic elevations in fasting plasma ammonia and cerebrospinal fluid glutamine concentrations are also present.

The four general clinical stages of hepatic encephalopathy, based on severity, are shown in Table 188-1. Stage 1 encephalopathy consists of very mild changes and may be quite subtle. Findings range from mild confusion to reversal of sleep patterns and personality changes. In stage 2 hepatic encephalopathy the mental status worsens, and asterixis is seen. Asterixis is a transient loss of postural tone of the extensors of the wrist when the hands are outstretched. It is not specific for hepatic encephalopathy and may be seen with uremia, pulmonary disease, and malnutrition. Stage 3 encephalopathy signifies more profound and serious neurologic abnormalities. Focal or generalized seizures may develop. The patient may become somnolent or incontinent. Physical examination may reveal rapid deep respirations accompanied by hyperflexia with Babinski signs present. In stage 4 coma, diminished responsiveness to pain occurs. Also, irreversible decerebrate and decorticate posturing is seen.

Diagnosis

The diagnosis of hepatic encephalopathy is based on both clinical and laboratory details. It is easy to recognize encephalopathy in a patient with fulminant hepatic failure. When hepatic disease is not clinically obvious, the nonspecific nature of early hepatic encephalopathy may make the diagnosis more difficult. Abnormal laboratory tests of hepatic function may establish the presence of liver disease. An elevated plasma ammonia level may be useful in confirming the diagnosis, but a normal plasma ammonia concentration does not exclude this diagnosis. An elevation in cerebrospinal fluid glutamine concentration is the most specific and sensitive laboratory test for this disease and correlates well with the degree of hepatic encephalopathy. Unfortunately, glutamine assays are not performed in some clinical laboratories. The coagulopathy and thrombocytopenia that can accompany hepatic disease may make lumbar puncture unsafe. If a lumbar puncture is warranted in this situation, correction of the bleeding parameters with fresh frozen plasma or platelets may be necessary.

The EEG is abnormal in patients with hepatic encephalopathy, but the abnormalities are nonspecific. Triphasic slow waves, commonly attributed to hepatic encephalopathy, may occur in patients with head injury, subdural hematomas, uremia, cerebral anoxia, and electrolyte abnormalities. Psychometric testing, although not particularly helpful in diagnosing hepatic encephalopathy, provides a semiquantitative means of following response to therapy. Easy bedside evaluations include trail making (Reitan number connection) and tests using block designs or star constructions.

Differential Diagnosis. Since the neuropsychiatric manifestations of hepatic encephalopathy are nonspecific, it is important to exclude other causes of encephalopathy in patients with liver disease. Toxins, metabolic abnormalities, and structural lesions can cause similar clinical features. Focal neurologic signs are unusual in hepatic encephalopathy and should provoke a search for structural abnormalities, although patients with a stable, subclinical lesion (head trauma, chronic subdural hematoma, stroke) may develop focal neurologic signs or symptoms when hepatic encephalopathy develops. If concern exists for structural disease, a computed tomography scan of the head is indicated. Meningitis, subarachnoid hemorrhage, and intracerebral hemorrhage all need to be considered, since they are not rare conditions in patients with alcoholic cirrhosis.

Pathogenesis

Over the years multiple theories have attempted to explain the biochemical pathophysiology of hepatic encephalopathy. In general these theories are based on serum, cerebrospinal fluid, or brain tissue abnormalities measured in either patients or animal models. No single theory can account for all the behavioral, electrophysiologic, and biochemical changes found in patients or animal models. It is probably a multifactorial disorder, with several substances contributing to the altered mental status. The best test of a given theory should be that when the chemical abnormalities measured in patients are mimicked in animals, behavioral and electrophysiologic abnormalities are produced similar to those seen in hepatic encephalopathy. Too often, theories have been based on measurements in humans, without sufficient animal modeling to prove causation. Nevertheless, two major theories have the most experimental support: (1) the ammonia hypothesis and (2) the endogenous benzodiazepine hypothesis.

Ammonia Hypothesis. It has long been known that arterial blood concentrations are often elevated in patients with hepatic encephalopathy, although the actual value may not always correlate with the severity of the attack. In experimental animal models of hepatic encephalopathy, blood ammonia levels are often elevated. The mechanisms by which ammonia leads to disturbances of neural transmission have been extensively studied and it has been found that ammonia can inhibit both excitatory synaptic transmission and inhibitory postsynaptic potentials. In addition, it can alter the metabolism of brain glutamate and as a result could be responsible for the brain edema associated with fulminant hepatic failure (see below).

Endogenous Benzodiazepine Hypothesis. In the 1980s specific benzodiazepine receptor antagonists, such as flumazenil, were found to ameliorate hepatic encephalopathy in animal models, in anecdotal reports, and in uncontrolled clinical trials of human subjects. Because of the specificity of the benzodiazepine receptor antagonists, those observations suggested that the drug might be blocking the encephalopathic actions of a benzodiazepine-like substance. Subsequently, double-masked, placebo-controlled trials confirmed the anecdotal clinical observations, although only a small subset of patients improved with flumazenil treatment. The nature of the benzodiazepine-like substance present in hepatic encephalopathy is not entirely clear. At least two substances (together or separately) may be the causal agents. Small amounts of halogenated benzodiazepines, such as diazepam, have been found in excess in some patients, and even larger amounts of biologically active nonbenzodiazepine substances are present in the serum of hepatic encephalopathy patients. One such endogenous substance with benzodiazepine-like properties, endozepine-4, has been identified; it appears to be increased in plasma and cerebrospinal fluid from patients or animals with hepatic encephalopathy. The causal relationship of excess endozepine-4 to hepatic encephalopathy is not yet certain, but interestingly, very large increases of endozepine-4 (more than 1,000 times normal) have been found in a rare neurologic disorder of relapsing unconsciousness (idiopathic recurring stupor). This finding suggests that endozepine-4 could be responsible for, or contribute to, the encephalopathy in both diseases.

Treatment

Recognition of Precipitating Causes. Perhaps the most important aspect of treating hepatic encephalopathy is to treat the precipitating cause (Table 188-2). Agitated patients are often misdiagnosed and treated with sedatives, which obviously may worsen the situation. Use of sedatives (especially benzodiazepines) and narcotics should be avoided in stable cirrhotics to prevent encephalopathy. Excessive diuretic therapy may cause a hypokalemic alkalosis. Hypokalemia is a stimulus for the kidney to produce ammonia, and alkalosis favors the diffusion of ammonia in the central nervous system. Intravascular volume depletion from diuretic therapy reduces renal blood flow and increases the blood urea nitrogen concentration. Excess urea can then diffuse into the gut, leading to increased ammonia production by bacterial ureases. Bacterial infections can precipitate encephalopathy and are often unsuspected because patients with chronic liver diseases are frequently hypothermic. Cultures of blood, urine, ascites, if present, and cerebrospinal fluid should be obtained for all cases of unexplained encephalopathy.

Specific Therapies. The therapy for hepatic encephalopathy is based on the premise that substances in the gastrointestinal tract are acted on by intestinal bacteria and converted into "toxins" that are absorbed into the blood. These toxins bypass the liver via collateral circulation, enter the brain, and presumably induce encephalopathy. Based on these principles, therapy is directed at (1) decreasing the colonic substrate for these putative comagenic toxins, (2) reducing the bacteria capable of producing these toxins, (3) diminishing the influx of these compounds into the central nervous system, and (4) decreasing the effect these compounds have on neurotransmitter activity and metabolism.

Reduction of Gastrointestinal Protein and Toxins. Reduction of dietary protein is a simple method of reducing gastrointestinal protein and should be the first step in therapy. Protein intake can be withheld for the first 1 to 2 days, and is gradually increased in increments of 10 g/day. Dietary intake should not be less than 40 mg/day chronically, as negative nitrogen balance ensues with the subsequent risk of infection and with diminished hepatic regeneration. Optimally, the daily protein intake should be 1.5 g/kg/day in order to maintain positive nitrogen balance. Vegetable protein has been proved to produce less encephalopathy than animal protein diets. Patients with hepatic encephalopathy secondary to gastrointestinal hemorrhage, constipation, or large protein loads should be treated with tap water enemas and lactulose to evacuate nitrogenous substrates.

Lactulose is the mainstay of therapy to prevent or diminish encephalopathy. Its cathartic action increases ammonia elimination. Bacterial metabolism of lactulose acidifies the colonic contents and converts ammonia to its ionized and less absorbable form. Lactulose may be administered orally (30 ml per nasogastric tube hourly until a loose bowel movement occurs) or as a retention enema (300 ml in 700 ml water) in obtunded patients. For patients with recurrent hepatic encephalopathy, lactulose can be used chronically (15 to 45 ml orally two to four times a day), aiming for two to three soft bowel movements a day. In patients refractory to dietary protein restriction and lactulose therapy, the oral antibiotics neomycin and metronidazole have been used to promote colonic bacteriostasis.

Reduction of Gastrointestinal Bacteria. In patients who cannot be managed with dietary protein restriction and lactulose therapy, the elimination of gastrointestinal bacteria may prove useful. The premise of this therapy is that diminution of gastrointestinal flora diminishes the production of ammonia and other possible toxins. Neomycin can be taken orally in a dose of 1 to 2 g every 6 hours. Only small amounts of this drug can be absorbed, however, and since it is excreted primarily in urine, its use should be avoided in patients with renal insufficiency. Even in patients with normal renal function, prolonged therapy can produce ototoxicity and nephrotoxicity.

An alternative to neomycin is metronidazole. It is given 250 orally three times a day. Side effects include leukopenia, peripheral neuropathy, metallic taste, and disulfiram-like reaction.

Other Therapies. Because patients with hepatic encephalopathy have abnormal plasma and cerebrospinal fluid amino acid concentrations, it has been suggested that the increased plasma aromatic amino acids produced in these patients may interfere with normal neurotransmitter syntheses. Hence, trials with solutions enriched with branched-chain amino acids for transport into the central nervous system have been tried. The results of these studies are mixed and controversial. Because of the excessive cost of these solutions, the high osmolality and fluid

TABLE 188-2. Precipitants of Hepatic Encephalopathy

Drugs
    Sedatives
    Tranquilizers
    Narcotics
    Diuretics
Electrolyte imbalance
    Hyponatremia
    Hypokalemic alkalosis
    Hypovolemia
Excessive nitrogen load
    Gastrointestinal hemorrhage
    Excess dietary protein
    Azotemia
    Constipation
Infection

load, and the marginal benefit, this therapy is not routinely recommended.

An important, rare subset of patients with hepatic encephalopathy includes those suffering from inherited urea cycle defects (e.g., ornithine transcarbamylase deficiency). In these patients, primarily children, accumulation of ammonia is believed to be responsible for the encephalopathy, and attempts to lower serum ammonia have proved useful. Infusions of sodium phenylacetate may be employed to control potentially fatal hyperammonemia successfully. Alternative therapies include the use of arginine or citrulline, depending on the specific enzyme deficiency.

Flumazenil (Romazicon, RO 15-1788) is a benzodiazepine receptor antagonist widely used in Europe. It is reported to reverse hepatic encephalopathy in some patients, eliminate relapsing encephalopathy, and allow the resumption of normal protein intake in patients with chronic hepatic failure. This drug is available in the United States, but is used primarily for reversal of benzodiazepine overdose. At this time it is not approved for use in hepatic encephalopathy.

FULMINANT HEPATIC FAILURE

Unlike chronic disease, fulminant hepatic failure is associated with a high mortality rate (more than 50 percent). It is usually secondary to viral hepatitis or drug-induced liver disease, usually acetaminophen overdose. Patients have multiple metabolic abnormalities that can contribute to the encephalopathy. Of particular concern is hypoglycemia, which can be treated with infusions of 10 percent dextrose in water. Intensive care monitoring and particularly liver transplantation have been of benefit in decreasing overall mortality. In particular, attention needs to be paid to electrolyte disorders, acid-base balance, glucose, and coagulation defects, as well as pulmonary, cardiac, and renal status. Constant vigilance for infections must be maintained.

Cerebral Edema

Although this encephalopathy appears similar to that associated with chronic liver disease, the underlying mechanisms and the treatment may be quite different. Most importantly, fulminant hepatic failure is associated with lethal cerebral edema, which is the major extrahepatic lesion found at autopsy. Because papilledema may not be seen, no good clinical indices for cerebral edema exist. Sudden deterioration of consciousness and hyperactive reflexes, along with plantar reflexes and decerebrate/decorticate posturing may suggest increased intracranial pressure (ICP), but these can also be seen in patients with metabolic encephalopathy. Abnormal pupillary light responses and oculocephalic (''dolls'' eye maneuver) reflexes may be reversible; however, abnormal oculovestibular reflexes (cold caloric test) carry a poor prognosis. Computed tomography may reveal slit-like ventricles or other signs of an increased ICP. ICP transducers have been used by some to help monitor ICP, but their use may cause significant intracranial bleeding. Therapies aimed at controlling ICP, such as hyperventilation and furosemide therapy, can be employed. Mannitol has been used to reduce elevated pressure, but in patients with an ICP greater than 60 mmHg, it may be deleterious. Mannitol should be used only when ICP transducers are in place. The value of steroids has not been proved.

Treatment

Given the large number of metabolic problems, the approach to fulminant hepatic failure is not as effective as that used for chronic hepatic disease. Most patients are obtunded or comatose, and therefore little dietary protein is ingested. Lactulose can be used to remove nitrogen waste from the gut initially but can produce complicating electrolyte disturbances secondary to excessive diarrhea.

Orthotopic liver transplantation is the treatment of choice for stage 3 and 4 encephalopathy, assuming the patient is a candidate.

SUGGESTED READINGS

Basile AS, Jones, EA, Skolnick P: The pathogenesis and treatment of hepatic encephalopathy: evidence for the involvement of benzodiazepine receptor ligands. Pharm Rev 43:27, 1991

Butterworth RF: Pathophysiology of hepatic encephalopathy: the ammonia hypothesis revisited. p. 9. In Bengtsson F, Jeppsson B, Almdal T, Vilstrup H (eds): Progress in hepatic encephalopathy and metabolic nitrogen exchange. CRC Press, Boca Raton, FL, 1991

Cole M, Mullen KD: Hepatic coma and portal-systemic encephalopathy. p. 326. In Johnson RT, Griffin JW (eds): Current Therapy in Neurologic Disease. 4th Ed. BC Decker, St. Louis, 1993

Conn HO: Hepatic encephalopathy. p. 69. In Schiff L, Schiff ER (eds): Diseases of the Liver. Vol. 2. JB Lippincott, Philadelphia, 1993

Rothstein JD, Garland W, Puia G et al: Purification and characterization of naturally occurring benzodiazepine receptor ligands. J Neurochem 58: 2102, 1992

Rothstein JD, Guidotti A: Endozepines: non-benzodiazepine endogenous allosteric modulators of GABA$_A$ receptors. p. 115. In Izquierdo I, Medina J (eds): Naturally Occurring Benzodiazepines: Structure, Distribution and Function. Ellis Horword, London, England, 1993

Victor M, Rothstein JD: Neurologic manifestations of hepatic disease. p. 1442. In Asbury AK, McKhann GM, McDonald WI (eds): Diseases of the Nervous System. WB Saunders, Philadelphia, 1992

SECTION 5. HEMATOLOGY

189. NEUROLOGIC MANIFESTATIONS OF COAGULATION DISTURBANCES

KAREN FURIE
EDWARD FELDMANN

The neurologic manifestations of coagulation disorders primarily involve the central nervous system and take the form of cerebral ischemia and intracranial hemorrhage. The peripheral nervous system is rarely affected. A myriad of coagulation disorders may be responsible, some of which have unique features that aid in their recognition and diagnosis.

CLINICAL PRESENTATION

A neurologist in office practice usually encounters a patient with coagulation disorder after a thrombotic or hemorrhagic event. However, some coagulation disorders can be detected before they produce neurologic symptoms because of a strong family history or transient sentinel events such as migraine headaches, transient ischemic attacks (TIAs), or seizures.

The age of a patient with ischemic or hemorrhagic symptoms is a prime determinant of the aggressiveness with which coagulation disorders are sought. Hematologic abnormalities account for 2 to 5 percent of venous and arterial infarctions in adults under 45 years of age. Older patients with cerebral infarcts are more likely to have atherothrombotic disease or a cardiac source of embolism as the responsible mechanism. Similarly, older patients with intracranial hemorrhage are much more likely than younger patients to have bled secondary to hypertension, trauma, anticoagulation, or cerebral amyloid angiopathy, rather than an endogenous coagulopathy. However, older patients with a history of autoimmune disease, recurrent unexplained thrombotic events, or a family history of clotting abnormalities should also undergo a thorough evaluation for coagulation disorders (Table 189-1).

Features of the patient's history may suggest a particular diagnosis. For example, livedo reticularis, mitral valve prolapse, spontaneous abortions, deep vein thrombosis, and pulmonary emboli are associated with the antiphospholipid syndrome. A family history of venous or arterial thromboses early in life may point to a factor deficiency or inherited platelet disorder. Complaints of fatigue and weight loss may indicate an underlying malignancy. Unexplained fevers, arthralgias, myalgias, personality change, or seizures may be clues to systemic lupus erythematosus.

Thus, every patient with an atypical stroke presentation such as young age, absence of cardiovascular risk factors, positive family history of coagulation abnormalities, or past medical history of recurrent thrombotic or hemorrhagic events should undergo a hematologic evaluation to identify potentially re-

sponsible abnormalities. Whereas a neurologist should be comfortable ordering the studies listed in Table 189-1, patients with abnormal laboratory studies requiring complex management, or those in whom there is a high index of suspicion and no apparent hematologic explanation, should be seen by a hematologist. If neurosurgical intervention is required, hematologic consultation to establish proper hemostasis becomes crucial.

CEREBRAL INFARCTION

Factor Deficiencies

Figure 189-1 details the human coagulation cascade. Particular attention should be paid to the fibrinolytic roles of protein C, protein S, and antithrombin III (AT III). Congenital AT III, protein S, or protein C deficiencies are usually associated with venous infarction. Diagnosis is difficult because factor levels may be reduced as a consequence of a thrombotic event. In fact, low levels of protein C after an acute stroke may be predictive of a poor outcome. It is, therefore, essential to obtain a premorbid history of deficiency and screen family members before attributing the cause of stroke to a factor deficiency.

AT III binds to serine protease inhibitors of thrombin. Its activity is greatly increased by heparin. Heparin resistance is a clue to AT III deficiency. Congenital AT III deficiency is autosomal dominant with variable penetrance, occurring in one of every 2,000 to 5,000 individuals. Homozygous deficiency

TABLE 189-1. Hematologic Studies for Evaluation of Coagulation Abnormalities in Stroke Patients

Test	Comments
Prothrombin time (PT)	Prolongation indicates deficiency or inhibition (e.g., coumadin) of factors I, Ia, II, IIa, VII, X, or Xa, or dysfibrogenemia/afibrinogenemia
Partial thromboplastin time (PTT)	Prolongation may be the result of hemophilia A (factor VIII deficit), hemophilia B (factor IX deficit), dysfibrogenemia/afibrinogenemia, inhibition by antibodies (antiphospholipid antibody), or medication (heparin)
Platelet count	Diminished in congenital and acquired thrombocytopenias
Bleeding time	Prolonged in von Willebrand's disease, aspirin use
Plasma von Willebrand factor level	Reduced in von Willebrand's disease
Platelet aggregation test	Abnormal in heparin-induced thrombocytopenia, Glanzmann's thrombasthenia
Anticardiolipin antibody	Present in the antiphospholipid syndrome
Lupus anticoagulant	Present in the antiphospholipid syndrome
Protein C	Congenital or acquired deficiency
Protein S	Congenital or acquired deficiency
Antithrombin III	Congenital or acquired deficiency
Fibrinogen	Diminished in congenital deficiencies or disseminated intravascular coagulation
D-dimers	Increased in disseminated intravascular coagulation
Factor VIII	Reduced in hemophilia A
Factor IX	Reduced in hemophilia B

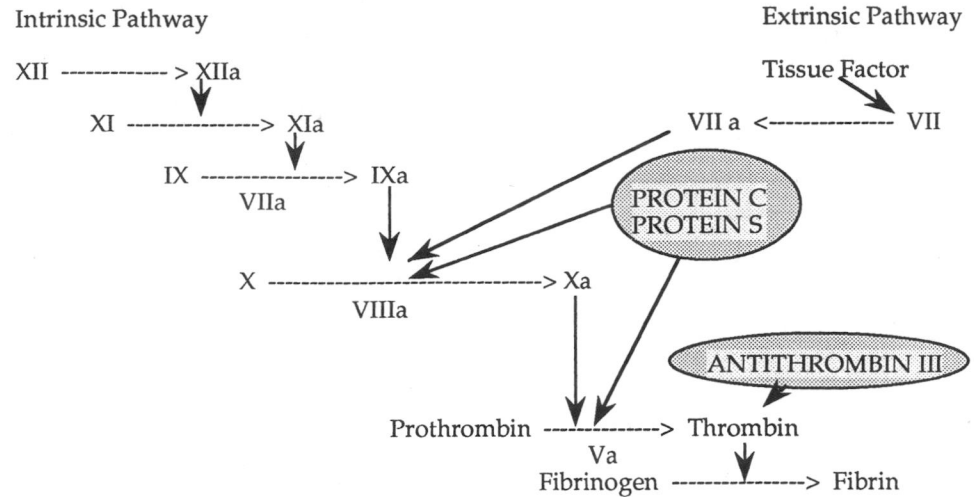

FIG. 189-1. The coagulation cascade.

is incompatible with life. However, heterozygotes have a 20 to 60 percent measurable decrease in enzyme levels. Patients may also be heterozygous or homozygous for a qualitative reduction in enzyme activity, which is only detectable by functional assays.

AT III deficiency may be acquired in patients with hepatic insufficiency, nephrotic syndrome, acute thrombotic consumption, heparin, oral contraceptives, or l-asparaginase treatment. Venous occlusive disease involving the sagittal sinus or cortical veins is the common mechanism of infarction. Arterial thromboses have rarely been reported with AT III deficiency. Patients with congenital deficiency benefit from long-term anticoagulation with warfarin. Patients with acquired deficiencies often have associated factor deficiencies or platelet abnormalities that preclude anticoagulation therapy.

Protein C is a vitamin K-dependent factor. It binds to thrombomodulin on endothelial cells and is converted to an active protease by thrombin. Once active, it inhibits factors V and VIII. Protein C deficiency is either a primary condition, an autosomal dominant trait, or a secondary condition caused by Coumadin use, disseminated intravascular coagulation, hepatic insufficiency, or acute thrombotic consumption.

Congenital protein C deficiency usually presents with venous infarction at a young age. Reports have been documented of adult venous infarction, but arterial infarcts are very rare. Homozygotes are subject to catastrophic neonatal venous infarctions. Approximately 1 in 200 individuals in the general population may be asymptomatic heterozygotes.

Protein S is a vitamin K-dependent protein that when unbound enhances the activity of protein C. In its bound form, protein S circulates in association with C4 binding protein, an acute-phase reactant. Levels are lower in women and blacks. Congenital protein S deficiency is transmitted in an autosomal dominant pattern or deficiency can be acquired through Coumadin therapy, nephrotic syndrome, or hepatic insufficiency. Deficiency is usually associated with venous infarctions, although cerebral arterial thrombotic events have been reported.

Although a congenital heparin cofactor II deficiency has been described, no causal relationship to cerebral ischemic events has been demonstrated.

Fibrinolytic Disorders

Hereditary plasminogen deficiency is a rare autosomal dominant disorder that can lead to arterial or venous infarcts. These patients are treated with heparin or Coumadin. Dysfibrinogenemia, a condition in which an abnormal, lysis-resistant fibrin clot forms, is not known to cause cerebral infarcts. Patients have been reported with factor 12 (Hageman factor) and prekallikrein deficiencies, but no clear evidence exists of an increased incidence of stroke in these patients.

Antiphospholipid Antibody

Antiphospholipid antibodies predispose to both venous and arterial thrombotic events. This family of antibodies includes the lupus anticoagulant, detectable in plasma, and anticardiolipin antibody, present in serum. Although normal, healthy individuals may harbor either antibody, they are also seen in association with thrombotic events and platelet disorders in patients with the primary antiphospholipid syndrome. They are present in up to half of patients with systemic lupus erythematosus and may be seen in other autoimmune disorders as well. In patients with lupus, the presence of antiphospholipid antibody increases the risk of stroke two- to fivefold. Phenothiazines, hydralazine, and phenytoin may caused drug-induced antiphospholipid antibodies, but these antibodies are usually not pathogenic.

Patients may present with transient ischemic attacks or stroke. Clues to the diagnosis include a history of deep vein thrombosis, migraine, mitral valve prolapse, recurrent miscarriages, thrombocytopenia, or livedo reticularis. Recurrent events may be more common in patients with other vascular risk factors such as hyperlipidemia and cigarette smoking.

The treatment of patients with antiphospholipid antibodies remains controversial. Retrospective data suggests a benefit from anticoagulation with warfarin to an international normalized ratio greater than 2.6. One uncontrolled prospective trial found a lower recurrent stroke rate in patients receiving combination aspirin and dipyridamole. Immunosuppressive therapy is of no clear benefit. Firm treatment recommendations cannot be made until prospective, randomized, controlled clinical trials have been completed. Many physicians treat patients with recurrent events or evidence of cardiac disease with long-term warfarin.

Platelet Abnormalities

Thrombocytosis is considered primary or "essential" when due to a myeloproliferative disorder. An elevated platelet count may also be a secondary phenomenon. Only essential thrombocytosis is associated with cerebral ischemic events. Abnormal platelet aggregability in essential thrombocytosis has been demonstrated by visualizing circulating platelet aggregates in symptomatic patients. Neurologic manifestations of essential thrombocytosis include transient ischemic attack, cerebral infarct, hemorrhage, headache, seizures, or vertigo. There have been three case reports of patients with essential thrombocytosis who had superior sagittal sinus thrombosis. A middle cerebral artery territory infarct that evolved slowly over months has also been described. Patients may be treated with either aspirin or dipyridamole.

Heparin-induced thrombocytopenia (HIT) is an idiosyncratic reaction that occurs in 1 to 2 percent of patients who receive heparin, usually in the postoperative setting. In type I, the platelet count declines 1 to 5 days after the initiation of heparin. It is believed to be due to a direct effect of heparin causing platelet clumping and is considered benign and reversible. Type II is an immune response usually seen after 5 days of therapy in patients given heparin for the first time, but in patients with prior heparin exposure it can occur within hours of the first dose. The proposed mechanism of type II is the binding of an IgG antibody to endothelial heparan, thus stimulating tissue factor production. This process is irreversible. Cerebral infarction is seen 5 to 10 days after the initiation of therapy. The infarcts may be caused by either venous or arterial occlusion. Heparin resistance can be an indicator of impending heparin-induced thrombocytopenia. The prognosis is poor, with 25 percent of patients dying or suffering severe disability. Treatment involves the discontinuation of heparin, which should lead to a rise in the platelet count within 5 days.

Secondary Hypercoagulable States

Hypercoagulable states may be a consequence of underlying medical conditions such as malignancies (Trousseau syndrome), pregnancy, nephrotic syndrome, Cushing syndrome, ulcerative colitis, and paroxysmal nocturnal hemoglobinuria. Their underlying pathophysiology is multifactorial and poorly understood. The mechanism of infarction in these patients is also multifactorial and may be caused by diffuse intravascular coagulation, nonbacterial thrombotic endocarditis with embolism, tumor embolus, or venous occlusion. Nonbacterial thrombotic endocarditis, associated with malignancies, is a marker of a prothrombotic state, with associated underlying valvular damage acting as the nidus for clot formation. Gastrointestinal adenocarcinomas are the tumors most commonly associated with thromboembolic complications. The hypercoagulable state of nephrotic syndrome is believed to be caused by an AT III deficiency acquired by urinary loss of protein, although other factor deficiencies and platelet hyperaggregability may also play a role. Normal pregnancy produces a physiologic state of low-grade disseminated intravascular coagulation that has the potential to decompensate and cause thrombotic events.

INTRACRANIAL HEMORRHAGE

Hemophilia

Hemophilia is an X-linked recessive disorder caused by deficiency of factor VIII (hemophilia A) or factor IX (hemophilia B). The risk of intracranial hemorrhage is 2.5 to 3 percent per year. Intracerebral hemorrhage in hemophilia has a mortality of 25 to 30 percent. Hemorrhage may be the result of trivial trauma or may occur spontaneously. Therapy consists of replacing factor VIII or IX. Factor VII, X, XI, or XIII deficiencies may also result in intracerebral hemorrhage, although these are very rare.

Disseminated Intravascular Coagulation

In disseminated intravascular coagulation, clotting factors become activated and consumed because of the inappropriate circulation of thrombin and plasmin as a secondary response to a number of medical conditions: pregnancy, sepsis, liver failure, malignancy, or trauma. It presents in severely ill patients with either thrombotic or hemorrhagic events anywhere in the body. Laboratory abnormalities include anemia, thrombocytopenia, decreased fibrinogen, and increased fibrin split products. Treatment should attempt to correct the underlying condition and provide replacement of consumed products.

Neonatal Hypoprothrombinemia

Intracranial hemorrhage is the presenting feature in up to 63 percent of patients with neonatal vitamin K deficiency. One-third of these are intracerebral hemorrhages. The mortality is 9 to 13 percent. Deficiency is particularly common in Eastern countries, more often in breast-fed infants. Patients usually present with symptoms of elevated intracranial pressure. The deficiency is believed to be caused by either inadequate maternal supply or impaired absorption of vitamin K following gastrointestinal infection or antibiotic use. Treatment is replacement of vitamin K.

Iatrogenic

Office-based neurologists will often encounter patients who have been treated with anticoagulants, fibrinolytics, and antiplatelet agents after documented myocardial infarction, atrial fibrillation, TIAs, or acute cerebral infarctions.

Anticoagulation with heparin or warfarin alone accounts for 10 to 20 percent of intracerebral hemorrhages. Heparin acts by accelerating the binding of AT III to serine proteases. Coumadin interferes with the carboxylation of vitamin K-dependent factors II, VII, IX, and X. The effects of either drug can be reversed, heparin with protamine sulfate and Coumadin with vitamin K and fresh frozen plasma. Thrombolytic agents activate plasmin to lyse the fibrin matrix of thrombus. Aspirin irreversibly acetylates cyclo-oxygenase, preventing production of thromboxane A_2, an inducer of platelet aggregation and vasoconstriction. Ticlopidine interferes with platelet glycoprotein receptors, inhibiting the binding of fibrinogen to activated platelets.

Heparin anticoagulation for acute myocardial infarction is associated with a minimal risk of intracerebral hemorrhage. Chronic warfarin therapy is not commonly used for myocardial infarction prophylaxis.

Trials of warfarin anticoagulation for the prevention of stroke in patients with myocardial infarction or atrial fibrillation have

TABLE 189-2. Intracerebral Hemorrhage in Clinical Trials of Warfarin Therapy for Stroke Prevention in Atrial Fibrillation and Myocardial Infarction

Study	Drug	Study Population	INR	No. of Patients	ICH (no.)	%/Yr
WARIS (Smith et al., 1990)	Warfarin	MI	2.1–4.8	607	5	0.27
	Placebo			607	0	0.00
AFASAK (Peterson et al., 1989)	Warfarin	AF	2.8–4.2	355	1	0.40
	Placebo			336	0	0.00
SPAF (Stroke Prevention in Atrial Fibrillation Investigators, 1994)	Warfarin	AF	2.0–3.5	393	1	0.40
	Placebo			723	0	0.00
BAATAF (Boston Area Anticoagulation Trial/Atrial Fibrillation Investigators, 1990)	Warfarin	AF	1.5–2.7	212	1	0.21
	Placebo			208	0	0.00
CAFA (Conolly et al., 1991)	Warfarin	AF	2.0–3.0	187	1	0.41
	Placebo			191	0	0.00

Abbreviations: INR, normalized ratio in all patients; ICH, intracerebral hemorrhage; MI, myocardial infarction; AF, atrial fibrillation.

(Adapted from del Zoppo GJ, Mori E: Hematologic causes of intracerebral hemorrhage. Neurosurg Clin North Am 3:637, 1992, with permission.)

shown that intracranial bleeding is relatively rare (less than 5 percent a year) in closely monitored patients (Table 189-2). An excessively prolonged prothrombin or partial thromboplastin time and hypertension (greater than 180/100 mmHg) increase the risk of hemorrhage. Prior ischemic infarctions do not increase the risk of hemorrhage in these patients. Hemorrhages tend to occur in the territories of the small vessels of the cerebellum, pons, and basal ganglia, vessels commonly diseased by hypertension. Those who bleed are slightly older (mean age of 73 versus 69). Hemorrhage due to anticoagulation may evolve gradually over hours to days, sometimes with associated headache, rather than presenting acutely.

Patients on anticoagulation for stroke prevention after carotid and vertebrobasilar transient ischemic attacks have an incidence of intracerebral hemorrhage of 1.14 in 100 patient years, compared with 0.31 in 100 patient years in the general population. It is not clear that anticoagulation in patients who present with cerebrovascular disease carries a greater risk of intracerebral hemorrhage than anticoagulation for other causes.

The risks of anticoagulation with heparin for acute strokes has been poorly studied. Uncontrolled studies document an increased risk of intracranial hemorrhage in anticoagulated patients. However, hemorrhagic conversion of infarcts in anticoagulated patients are often asymptomatic, and such hemorrhagic transformation commonly occurs in patients not treated with anticoagulants.

The administration of fibrinolytic agents such as streptokinase, urokinase, or tissue plasminogen activator after acute myocardial infarction has been associated with intracerebral hemorrhage, subarachnoid hemorrhage, and subdural hematoma, with an overall incidence of 0.3 to 0.4 percent. Risk factors for intracerebral hemorrhage in this setting are age over 70, diastolic blood pressure over 110 mmHg, female gender, prior neurologic history, and use of nonsteroidal anti-inflammatory drugs, propranolol, nitrates, or calcium antagonists. Most hemorrhages occur within 24 hours of therapy and, when intracerebral, are lobar in location. Patients with lobar hemorrhage require further investigation for an underlying lesion such as aneurysm or arteriovenous malformation. The mortality rate is high, approximately 50 percent for intracerebral and subarachnoid hemorrhage and approaching 75 percent for subdural hematoma.

The use of fibrinolytics for acute stroke is experimental. The rate of intracerebral hemorrhage in these studies ranges between 0 and 17 percent, but it must always be compared with the risk of spontaneous hemorrhagic conversion in untreated patients.

Antiplatelet agents such as aspirin, ticlopidine, and dipyridamole are often used for primary and secondary stroke prevention. Table 189-3 summarizes the rates of intracerebral hemorrhage in the large antiplatelet trials. The risk of intracerebral hemorrhage caused by antiplatelet agents may be minimally increased, but this should not preclude their use in the prophylaxis of myocardial infarction and stroke.

FIBRINOGEN DISORDERS

Afibrinogenemia is a rare autosomal recessive disorder that represents the extreme of a spectrum of fibrinogen disorders. More commonly, rather than having no fibrinogen, patients are heterozygous and hypofibrinogenemic, with greatly reduced levels of plasma fibrinogen detectable on sensitive assays. Homozygotes with afibrinogenemia usually manifest a bleeding tendency whereas heterozygotes may be asymptomatic.

In dysfibrogenemia, an autosomal dominant disorder, fibrinogen is quantitatively normal but dysfunctional. These entities may be distinguished by quantitative and functional serum determinations of fibrinogen. Dysfibrinogenemia may be asymptomatic or may result in a moderate bleeding tendency. Patients may present with intracerebral hemorrhage. In the setting of an acute hemorrhage, treatment consists of administering fresh frozen plasma, cryoprecipitate, or fibrinogen concentrates. In addition, dysfibrinogenemic patients may be at increased risk of thrombotic events due to a hypercoagulable state.

Platelet Dysfunction

Congenital thrombocytopenias are rarely the cause of intracerebral hemorrhage. Thrombocytopenia with absent radius syndrome is an autosomal recessive condition associated with renal, cardiac, and skeletal malformations. Infantile intracerebral hemorrhage is the usual cause of death. Wiskott-Aldrich is an X-linked recessive syndrome of thrombocytopenia, eczema, and chronic infections. It, too, carries a poor prognosis with a high incidence of infantile deaths due to intracerebral hemorrhage.

Acquired platelet disorders include thrombotic thrombocytopenic purpura (TTP), idiopathic thrombocytopenic purpura (ITP), and hemolytic uremic syndrome. TTP accounted for approximately 5 percent of a series of intracerebral hemorrhages associated with underlying hematologic abnormalities. TTP may be associated with a pentad of findings: microangiopathic hemolytic anemia, thrombocytopenic purpura, neurologic symptoms, renal disease, and fever. Only 30 percent of patients

TABLE 189-3. Intracerebral Hemorrhage in Antiplatelet Trials for Stroke Prevention

Study	Study Population	Antiplatelet Agent	Dose (mg)	No. of Patients	ICH (no.)	%/Yr
AICLA (Bousser et al., 1983)	TIA	ASA/DP	990/225	202	0	0.00
		ASA	990	198	1	0.17
		Placebo		204	2	0.34
UK-TIA (UK-TIA Study Group, 1988)	TIA	ASA	1,200	815	13	0.40
		ASA	300	806	0	0.00
		Placebo		814	3	0.09
TASS (Hass et al., 1989)	TIA	Ticlopidine	500	1,529	7	0.14
		ASA	1,300	1,540	7	0.14
CATS (Gent et al., 1989)	STR	Ticlopidine	500	525	2	0.27
		Placebo		528	0	0.00
ACCSG (American-Canadian Cooperative Study Group, 1985)	TIA	ASA/DP	1,300/300	448	2	0.30
		ASA	1,300	442	4	0.60
Swedish (Britton et al., 1987)	STR	ASA	1,500	253	3	0.59
		Placebo		252	2	0.40
ESPS (European Stroke Prevention Study Group, 1987)	TIA/STR	ASA/DP	975/225	1,250	3	0.12
		Placebo		1,250	0.12	
Dutch (The Dutch TIA Trial Study Group, 1991)	TIA/STR	ASA	30	1,555	13	0.32
		ASA	283	1,576	15	0.37
AFASAK (Peterson et al., 1989)	AF	ASA	75	336	0	0.00
		Placebo		723	0	0.00
SPAF (Stroke Prevention in Atrial Fibrillation Investigators, 1994)	AF	ASA	325	517	1	0.20
		Placebo		528	0	0.00
PHS (Steering Committee of the Physicians' Health Study Research Group, 1989)	ASX	ASA	163	11,037	23	0.04
		Placebo		11,034	12	0.02
Peto (Peto et al., 1988)	ASX	ASA	500	3,429	14	0.07
		No treatment		1,710	6	0.06

Abbreviations: ICH, intracerebral hemorrhage; TIA, transient ischemic attack; STR, stroke; ASX, asymptomatic; ASA, aspirin; DP, dipyridamole.

(Adapted from del Zoppo GJ, Mori E: Hematologic causes of intracerebral hemorrhage. Neurosurg Clin North Am 3:637, 1992, with permission.)

actually have all five features. TTP may occur secondary to pregnancy, immunologic disorders, malignancies, infections, or drugs. Schistiocytosis is prominent on the peripheral smear. The mainstay of therapy is plasma exchange, but immunosuppression with steroids and splenectomy are sometimes employed. Anticoagulation with heparin is contraindicated, as is platelet transfusion, the latter associated with sudden death and a protracted course in patients with TTP. Antiplatelet therapy with aspirin, dipyridamole, or sulfinpyrazone is recommended, with a reported improved outcome in 50 percent of patients. Mortality in treated patients is approximately 10 percent.

ITP is an immune-mediated consumptive platelet disorder, commonly caused by an underlying malignancy. Intracerebral hemorrhage occurs in less than 5 percent of patients with ITP. Patients who present with intracerebral hemorrhage caused by ITP are treated with platelet transfusion, which may be supplemented by immune therapy with methylprednisolone or immune γ-globulin. Emergency plasmapheresis or splenectomy have also been employed.

Hemolytic uremic syndrome is rarely a cause of intracerebral hemorrhage. Platelet dysfunction manifests through a prolonged bleeding time that cannot be corrected with peritoneal dialysis or hemodialysis. Cryoprecipitate and desamino-d-arginine vasopressin (DDAVP) may be effective in normalizing the bleeding time in 30 to 40 percent of patients.

In other disorders, platelets are quantitatively normal yet fail to provide hemostasis because of abnormalities of adhesion, producing intracranial hemorrhage. Examples include the Bernard-Soulier syndrome and Glantzmann's thrombasthenia, in which congenital absence of receptor glycoproteins results in an inability of platelets to bind to membrane receptors at injury sites. When patients present with a hemorrhage the treatment is platelet transfusion; however, a small proportion of patients

develops antibodies to the missing protein, which renders infused platelets dysfunctional.

Patients may have reduced levels of von Willebrand factor, an adhesion macromolecule released by platelets and endothelial cells, resulting in prolonged bleeding time and a tendency for spontaneous or post-traumatic hemorrhage. Patients with type I von Willebrand's disease have a moderate reduction in von Willebrand factor, whereas those with type II have normal levels of dysfunctional protein. Type III von Willebrand's disease is a severe autosomal recessive disorder with both quantitative and qualitative abnormalities. Treatment includes prophylactic therapy with cryoprecipitate before surgical procedures or following trauma, or as symptomatic therapy after a hemorrhagic event. DDAVP may be given to patients with a type I deficiency. However, it is ineffective in type II and type III disease and may actually exacerbate the condition.

Malignancy

Patients with cancer frequently have abnormal coagulation parameters and thrombocytopenia. Graus and collegues reported 88 intracerebral hemorrhages associated with coagulopathies in their autopsy series of 3,426 cancer patients. Most of these hemorrhages were supratentorial and located in the white matter. Most of these patients had leukemia, which is associated with depletion of coagulation factors and thrombocytopenia. Sixty percent of patients with promyelocytic leukemia die of intracerebral hemorrhage secondary to disseminated intravascular coagulation.

FEMORAL NEUROPATHY

Femoral neuropathy caused by iliopsoas hematoma has been reported in patients with hemophilia or those treated with anticoagulants. Computed tomography is the diagnostic imaging modality of choice. Treatment includes cessation of anticoagulation. Percutaneous decompression or surgical evacuation may be necessary as well. Most patients do not regain function.

SUGGESTED READINGS

Adams H, Butler M, Biller J et al: Nonhemorrhagic cerebral infarction in young adults. Arch Neurol 43:793, 1986

American-Canadian Cooperative Study Group: Persantine aspirin trial in cerebral ischemia. Part II. Endpoint results. Stroke 16:406, 1985

Anzola G, Magoni M, Ascari E et al: Early prognostic factors in ischemic stroke. Stroke 24:1496, 1993

Atrial Fibrillation Investigators: Risk factors for stroke and efficacy of antithrombotic therapy in atrial fibrillation. Arch Intern Med 154:1449, 1994

Benasi G, Ricci P, Calbucci F: Slowly progressive ischemic stroke as a first manifestation of essential thrombocythemia. Stroke 20:1271, 1989

Becker P, Miller V: Heparin-induced thrombocytopenia. Stroke 20:1449, 1989

Bhanchet P, Tuchinda S, Hathirat P: A bleeding syndrome in infants due to acquired prothrombin complex deficiency. Clin Pediatr 16:992, 1977

The Boston Area Anticoagulation Trial/Atrial Fibrillation Investigators: The effect of low-dose warfarin on the risk of stroke in patients with nonrheumatic atrial fibrillation. N Engl J Med 323:1505, 1990

Bousser MG, Eschwege E, Haguenaw M et al: "AICLA" controlled trial of aspirin and dipyridamole in the secondary prevention of atherothrombotic cerebral ischemia. Stroke 14:5, 1983

Britton M, Helmers C, Samuelsson K: High dose acetylsalicylic acid after cerebral infarction. A Swedish cooperative study. Stroke 18:325, 1987

Connolly SJ, Laupacis A, Gent M et al: Canadian atrial fibrillation anticoagulation (CAFA) study. J Am Coll Cardiol 18:349, 1991

del Zoppo GJ, Mori E: Hematologic causes of intracerebral hemorrhage. Neurosurg Clin North Am 3:637, 1992

The Dutch TIA Trial Study Group: A comparison of two doses of aspirin (30mg vs. 283mg a day) in patients after a transient ischemic attack or minor ischemic stroke. N Engl J Med 325:1261, 1991

Estol C: Anticoagulation. p. 83. In Feldmann E (ed): Intracerebral Hemorrhage. Futura, Armonk, 1994

Eyster M, Gill F, Blatt P: Central nervous system bleeding in hemophiliacs. Blood 51:1179, 1978

European Stroke Prevention Study Group: The European stroke prevention study (ESPS) principal endpoints. Lancet 2:1351, 1987

Gent M, Blakeley JA, Easton JD et al: The Canadian-American Ticlopidine Study (CATS) in thromboembolic stroke. Lancet 1:1215, 1989

Goodnough L, Saito H, Ratnoff O: Thrombosis or myocardial infarction in congenital clotting factor abnormalities and chronic thrombocytopenias: a report of 21 patients and a review of 50 previously reported cases. Medicine 62:248, 1983

Graus F, Rogers L, Posner J: Cerebrovascular complications in patients with cancer. Medicine 64:16, 1985

Greaves M: Coagulation abnormalities and cerebral infarction. J Neurol Neurosurg Psychiatry 56:433, 1993

Green D, Otoya J, Oriba H et al: Protein S deficiency in middle-aged women with stroke. Neurology 42:1029, 1992

Gustafsson C: Coagulation factors and risk of stroke. p. 31. In Kessler C, Rosengart A (eds): Hemostasis and Stroke. CRC Press, Boca Raton, FL, 1994

Hart R, Kanter, M: Hematologic disorders and ischemic stroke. Stroke 21:1111, 1990

Hass WK, Easton JD, Adams HP et al: A randomized trial comparing ticlopidine hydrochloride with aspirin for prevention of stroke in high risk patients. N Engl J Med 321:501, 1989

Hirsh J, Piovella S, Pini M: Congenital antithrombin III deficiency. Am J Med, suppl. 3B. 87:34, 1989

Kyritsis A, Williams E, Schutta H: Cerebral venous thrombosis due to heparin-induced thrombocytopenia. Stroke 21:1503, 1990

Laus M, Giunti A: Lumbosciatic pain and coagulopathies. Chir Organi Mov 76:229, 1991

Levine S, Brey R: Antiphospholipid antibodies and ischemic cerebrovascular disease. Semin Neurol 11:329, 1991

Levine S, Deegan M, Futrell N et al: Cerebrovascular and neurologic disease associated with antiphospholipid antibodies: 48 cases. Neurology 40:1181, 1990

Levine S, Brey R, Joseph C et al: Risk of recurrent thromboembolic events in patients with focal cerebral ischemia and antiphospholipid antibodies. Stroke, suppl. 1. 23:I-29, 1992

Maggioni A, Franzosi M, Santoro E: The risk of stroke in patients with acute myocardial infarction after thrombolytic and antithrombotic treatment. N Engl J Med 327:1, 1992

Martinez H, Rangel-Guerra R, Marfil L: Ischemic stroke due to deficiency of coagulation factors: report of 10 young adults. Stroke 24:19, 1993

Mayer S, Sacco R, Hurlet-Jensen A: Free protein S deficiency in acute ischemic stroke. A case control study. Stroke 24:224, 1993

McDonald T, Tatemichi T, Kranzler S et al: Thrombosis of the superior sagittal sinus associated with essential thrombocytosis followed by MRI during anticoagulant therapy. Neurology 39:1554, 1989

Merrick H, Zeiss J, Woldenberg L: Percutaneous decompression for femoral neuropathy secondary to heparin-induced retroperitoneal hematoma: case report and review of the literature. Am Surg 57:706, 1991

Miller V, Hart R: Heparin anticoagulation in acute brain ischemia. Stroke 19:403, 1988

Montgomery R, Natelson S: Afibrogenemia with intracerebral hematoma. Am J Dis Child 131:555, 1977

Natowicz M, Kelly R: Mendelian etiologies of stroke. Ann Neurol 22:175, 1987

Niakan E, Carbone J, Adams M et al: Anticoagulants, iliopsoas hematoma and femoral nerve compression. Am Fam Physician 44:2100, 1991

Olson J: Mechanisms of hemostasis. Stroke, suppl. 1. 24:I-109, 1993

Peterson P, Boysen G, Godtfredsen J et al: Placebo-controlled randomized trial of warfarin and aspirin in prevention of thromboembolic complications in chronic atrial fibrillation. The Copenhagen AFASAK study. Lancet 1:175, 1989

Peto R, Gray R, Collins R et al: A randomized trial of the effects of prophylactic daily aspirin among male British doctors. BMJ 296:313, 1988

Preston F, Martin J, Stewart R et al: Thrombocytosis, circulating platelet aggregates, and neurological dysfunction. BMJ 2:1561, 1979

Radberg J, Olsson J, Radberg C: Prognostic parameters in spontaneous hematomas with special reference to anticoagulation treatment. Stroke 22:571, 1991

Rosove M, Brewer P: Antiphospholipid thrombosis: clinical course after the first thrombotic event in 70 patients. Ann Intern Med 117:303, 1992

Rothrock J, Hart R: Antithrombotic therapy in cerebrovascular disease. Ann Intern Med 115:885, 1991

Sacco R, Owen J, Mohr J: Free protein S deficiency: a possible association with cerebrovascular occlusion. Stroke 20:1657, 1989

Samuels M, Thalinger K: Cerebrovascular manifestations of selected hematologic diseases. Semin Neurol 11:411, 1991

Seligsohn U, Berger A, Abend M: Homozygous protein C deficiency manifested by massive venous thrombosis in the newborn. N Engl J Med 310:559, 1984

Shih SL, Lin JCT, Liang DC et al: Computed tomography of spontaneous intracranial haemorrhage due to haemostatic disorders in children. Neuroradiology 35:619, 1993

Sloan M, Price T: Intracranial hemorrhage following thrombolytic therapy for acute myocardial infarction. Semin Neurol 11:385, 1991

Smith P, Arneses H, Holme I: The effect of warfarin on mortality and reinfarction after myocardial infarction. N Engl J Med 323:147, 1990

Steering Committee of the Physicians' Health Study Research Group: Final report on the aspirin component of the ongoing physicians' health study. N Engl J Med 321:129, 1989

Stern B, Kittner S, Sloan M: Stroke in the young (Part 1). Maryland Med J 40:453, 1991

Stern B, Kittner S, Sloan M: Stroke in the young (Part 2). Maryland Med J 40:565, 1991

Stroke Prevention in Atrial Fibrillation Investigators: Warfarin versus aspirin for prevention of thromboembolism in atrial fibrillation: stroke prevention in atrial fibrillation study II. Lancet 343:687, 1994

Thaler E, Lechner K: Antithrombin III deficiency and thromboembolism. Clin Haematol 10:369, 1981

Tran T, Marbet T, Duckert F: Association of hereditary heparin cofactor II deficiency with thrombosis. Lancet 2:413, 1985

UK-TIA Study Group: United Kingdom transient ischemic attack (UK-TIA) aspirin trial: interim results. BMJ 296:316, 1988

Warfel B, Marini S, Lachmann E et al: Delayed femoral nerve palsy following femoral vessel catheterization. Arch Phys Med Rehabil 74:1211, 1993

Wintzen A, Broekmans A, Bertina R: Cerebral haemorrhagic infarction in young patients with hereditary protein C deficiency: evidence for "spontaneous" cerebral venous thrombosis. BMJ 290:350, 1985

190. NEUROLOGIC COMPLICATIONS OF SICKLE CELL DISEASE

ROBERT J. ADAMS

Sickle cell diseases and thalassemias are relatively common medical conditions that predispose to a small but important list of neurologic problems. This chapter focuses on the neurologic complications most commonly encountered in these diseases, with emphasis on diagnosis and treatment. These hemoglobinopathies are genetic abnormalities involving the production of hemoglobin. Sickle cell disease (SSD) refers to any condition in which the production of an abnormal hemoglobin (Hb) causes in vivo distortion of the erythrocyte (sickling), which in turn causes hemolysis and intermittent vascular obstruction. Thalassemias are diseases in which one or both of the α- or β-chain are underproduced, leading to imbalanced globin chain synthesis, abnormal hemoglobin, and subsequent damage to the red blood cell or its precursor. Thalassemias are further characterized as to the degree of underproduction, with a 0 superscript indicating no production and one or two + symbols denoting partial production. In SSD the chains are abnormal; in thalassemia they are normal but the hemoglobin tetramer is abnormal.

The genes predisposing to these conditions are found primarily but not exclusively among certain ethnic populations. Individuals of African, Saudia Arabian, or Asian descent have a likelihood of carrying genes for SSD and α-thalassemia and persons with lineage from countries bordering the Mediterranean Sea and all parts of Asia have a predisposition to β-thalassemia. However, any of these conditions may be seen in individuals from any racial background. Patients with SSD or thalassemia are usually diagnosed through newborn screening or because all the clinically significant hemoglobinopathies produce some degree of anemia that comes to attention before any neurologic symptoms develop. It is rare for a neurologic complication to lead to the diagnosis of hemoglobinopathy.

Clinically the most important of these diseases are homozygous sickle cell disease (Hb SS or sickle cell anemia), sickle C (Hb SC) disease, and β-thalassemia (also called Cooley's anemia or thalassemia major), but many abnormal hemoglobin variants have been reported. More than one genetic abnormality may coexist in the same patient (e.g., sickle-thalassemia). Sickle β^0-thalassemia patients have a malignant course similar to Hb SS but sickle β^+-thalassemia shows a much milder course and is less likely to have neurologic complications. The bewildering array of molecular aberrations and abnormal hemoglobins, the complex and varying terminologies, and the coexistence of conditions makes it difficult for the neurologist to be confident that some of the less common hematologic abnormalities are related to the neurologic illness at hand. The amel
orat-

ing effect of fetal hemoglobin, which may be upregulated to levels much higher than normal in the presence of SCD, may partially negate the negative effect of Hb S. It is important to emphasize that whereas many case reports and small series exist in the literature only a few neurologic syndromes have been firmly associated with the hemoglobinopathies, most of these with homozygous Hb SS. The clinician is cautioned against assuming a causal relationship in such patients without first considering alternative and more common explanations for neurologic disease.

ACUTE MANIFESTATIONS

Bacterial meningitis and stroke are the most important acute CNS emergencies to consider in the Hb SS patient with acute brain dysfunction.

Meningitis

It is crucial to consider meningitis, for two reasons: (1) the association of meningitis with Hb SS is less well known than that of stroke, often leading to the erroneous assumption that all brain problems in Hb SS are due to stroke; and (2) treatment is effective if started early. Most cases are due to pneumococcus, and diagnosis and treatment with antibiotics and steroids should be undertaken as in any case with suspected or proven bacterial meningitis. This is primarily a problem in young children, many of whom now receive vaccine and prophylactic daily antibiotics. Chronic treatment with 250 mg of penicillin twice per day is common practice for children with Hb SS, which may complicate the interpretation of cerebrospinal fluid findings in cases of suspected meningitis. Hb SS patients are at risk of *Salmonella* osteomyelitis, and this agent may cause meningitis. Increased risk of *Haemophilus influenzae* and *Escherichia coli* infections has also been suggested. Bacterial meningitis is associated with at least a 15 percent incidence of long-term neurologic sequelae including seizures, sensorineural hearing loss, focal neurologic deficits, and hydrocephalus. Release of cytokines, believed to play a causative role in inflammatory injury to brain during the infection, can be reduced experimentally with steroids. Dexamethasone has been shown to improve outcome in childhood meningitis and should be used at a dose of 0.15 mg/kg intravenously every 6 hours for 4 days beginning at the start of antibiotic treatment. Cerebral ischemia and hearing loss resulting from bacterial meningitis do not seem to be more common in sickle cell disease even though these patients are already at higher risk for such problems due to their hemoglobinopathy. Susceptibility to infection is due to loss of splenic function and other abnormalities of the immune system. Adults with a history of frequent transfusions prior to 1985 must be considered at risk for human immunodeficiency virus infection. The initial manifestations, diagnostic tests, and management of the most important acute neurologic complications of Hb SS are shown in Table 190-1.

Stroke

Stroke is the most common neurologic complication of Hb SS. The prevalence of symptomatic cerebrovascular disease may reach 10 percent in the United States and as many as 15 to 20 percent of patients may have abnormal neuroimaging suggesting cerebrovascular disease. Unless otherwise specified, this discussion pertains only to symptomatic disease. In general,

TABLE 190-1. Neurologic Complications of Homozygous Sickle Cell Disease

Syndrome	Symptoms	Neurologic Examination Findings	Diagnosis	Iniital Treatment
Meningitis	Headache, lethargy, seizure, coma	Meningismus, stupor, coma	CSF abnormal; CT may show cerebral edema	Antibiotics; dexamethasone 0.15 mg/kg every hour for 4 days
Transient ischemia	Transient weakness numbness; alteration of behavior	Normal or focal, transient deficits	CT, EEG, and CSF exam normal; MRI or MRA with contrast may show abnormality	Transfusion; evaluate large vessels by angiography, TCD
Cerebral infarction	Hemiparesis, hemisensory loss, abnormal speech or vision	Hemiparesis, aphasia, or other cortical abnormalities	CT shows decreased attenuation; MRI shows decreased signal	Transfusion; hydration; repeat CT 3–4 days
Intraparenchymal hemorrhage	Headache, hemiparesis	Hemiparesis, may have lethargy or coma	CT shows intraparenchymal blood	Check for coagulopathy; treat cerebral edema as needed; angiography when stable
Subarachnoid or intraventricular hemorrhage	Sudden severe headache, vomiting, depression of consciousness	Stupor, coma, neck stiffness; may have normal exam	CT shows location of blood; MR may show aneurysm or moyamoya	Transfuse; close observation, nimodipine, 60 mg every 4 hours PO; intraventricular shunt for acute hydrocephalus; angiography when stable
Seizure	Tonic-clonic movements, impairment of consciousness	Postictal or normal; may have transient focal weakness	History, EEG, MRI with contrast may show cerebral infarct	Treat focal seizures as TIAs; generalized seizure treatment depends on etiology

Abbreviations: CSF, cerebrospinal fluid; CT, computed tomography; EEG, electroencephalogram; MRI, magnetic resonance imaging; MRA, magnetic resonance angiography; TCD, transcranial Doppler; TIA, transient ischemic attack.

cerebral infarction tends to occur in children and intracranial hemorrhage in adults, but many exceptions are seen, and all manifestations have been reported in all age groups.

Stroke may follow pain crisis, infection, and other systemic illness, but it is unclear whether such prodromes are characteristic or coincidental. Elevated blood levels of cytoadherance molecules may promote vaso-occlusion. Acute worsening of anemia was noted before 5 of 17 first-time strokes in one study, suggesting that sudden lowering of the oxygen-carrying capacity may cause ischemia in the presence of arterial stenosis. Other factors suggested to trigger symptoms include obstructive sleep apnea and transfusion after prolonged priapism. Most strokes, however, occur without a recognized prodrome.

Cerebral Infarction

Cerebral infarction typically presents with the sudden onset of symptoms of acute hemispheric dysfunction including hemiparesis, altered speech or aphasia, and hemisensory and visual deficits without alteration of consciousness. Seizures, often partial in onset, accompany about 20 percent of cases. Few are preceded by recognized transient ischemic attacks, although reporting of symptoms may be incomplete since infarction is especially common in young children with SSD. The initial cranial computed tomography (CT) often shows evidence of prior undetected brain lesions. Examination usually shows some degree of hemiparesis, which typically undergoes significant improvement in days to weeks after the ictus. Although motor symptoms improve, patients may show cognitive deficits. Posterior circulation syndromes and isolated cranial palsies due to central nervous system disease are rare and likely represent neuropathy rather than stroke.

Most patients with brain infarction who are studied with cerebral angiography show typical findings: (1) dilated vessels generally; (2) focal areas of stenosis or occlusion in the distal internal carotid artery and proximal middle and anterior cerebral arteries, (3) variable irregularities of more distal vessels; and (4) recruitment of willisian, leptomeningeal, and extracranial-intracranial collateral pathways. Although sickled cells do not pass well through the microcirculation, the simplistic notion that plugging is the cause of stroke is inadequate because both

the large arteries and microcirculation are involved. The most important lesions are those at the level of the circle of Willis. Although the cause is not known, the initiating event could be injury to endothelium followed by loss of the thromboresistant properties of the endothelium and either gradual formation of clot or acute blockage of vessels by thrombus. The anemia itself, which is associated with high blood flow rates, may also predispose to vessel wall damage.

Once initiated, the lesions are extended over time by endothelial hyperplasia, fibroblasts, fibrin thrombi, and even thrombus, with sickle red cells incorporated into the lesion. Acute thrombus formation causing total occlusion and hemodynamic failure may be the precipitating event, or stroke may be caused by artery-artery embolus. Hemodynamic failure is suggested by pathologic studies and neuroradiologic series showing a high incidence of so-called borderzone infarctions between major arterial territories and in subcortical areas. Moyamoya is present in up to 30 percent of patients who have been studied by angiography. The cervical carotid artery and the vertebrobasilar system show only dilation or narrowing believed to be secondary to intracranial disease.

The case shown in Figure 190-1 illustrates many of the typical features. This series is from a young girl who presented with left hemiparesis. Her initial scans showed old unrecognized infarcts, both deep and cortical lesions, and bilateral borderzone infarctions. Angiography showed severe bilateral distal internal carotid artery disease with moyamoya formation and evidence of circle of Willis, leptomeningeal, and extracranial-intracranial vessels providing collateral circulation.

Other potential causes of cerebral infarction in Hb SS are seldom noted in the literature, but these should be considered, especially in older patients and children without typical CT or angiographic findings. Patients with SSD often have cardiomyopathy, and cardiogenic embolus may be underdiagnosed. The danger is to assume that the stroke is caused by HB SS and fail to consider entities such as endocarditis, drug abuse coagulopathy, antiphospholipid antibodies, arterial dissection, paradoxical embolus, or venous disease.

Diagnosis is made from the clinical picture and either CT or magnetic resonance imaging (MRI) evidence of infarction. These techniques both allow the acute distinction between hem-

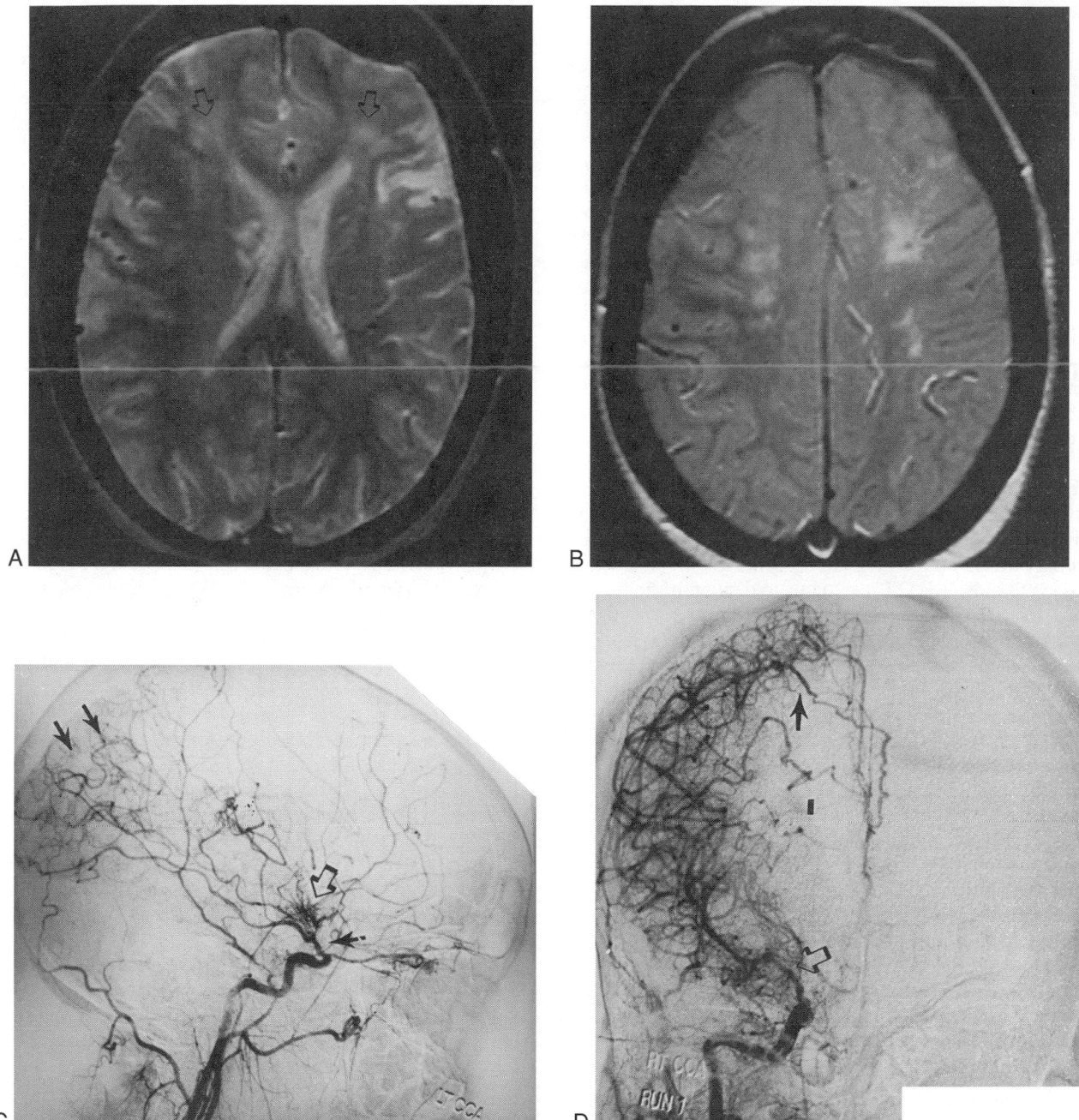

FIG. 190-1.   Series from a 12-year-old girl with sickle cell disease who presented with left hemiparesis. She had been under observation because a transcranial Doppler performed 9 months earlier had shown high velocities in the right internal carotid artery consistent with narrowing and an abnormally low left middle cerebral artery velocity, suggesting severe stenosis or occlusion. (**A**) Axial T2-weighted MRI showing deep and cortical high signal lesions consistent with infarction. The deep borderzone lesions (*arrows*) are particularly characteristic of sickle cell disease. Also typical is the presence of old hyposymptomatic lesions on MRI performed when these patients develop symptoms. (**B**) Axial proton-density MRI showing decreased signal in the right middle cerebral artery distribution and bilateral high signal areas in the centrum semiovale. (**C**) Lateral projection of a conventional angiogram during a left common carotid injection. A distal internal carotid artery occlusion and moyamoya (*open arrow*) are seen. The most distal patent segment of the internal carotid artery (*single black arrow*) is narrowed in the typical location just beyond the ophthalmic artery. This angiogram also demonstrates enlargement of the posterior communicator on the right with anterograde flow posteriorly. Typically the posterior cerebral artery, which is rarely involved in the sickle cell vasculopathy, will supply collateral flow to the anterior circulation through pericallosal collaterals or leptomeningeal collaterals (not shown) to the middle cerebral artery territory. Also depicted in this case are transdural collaterals from the external carotid circulation (*double arrows*). (**D**) Anteroposterior projection of the right common carotid artery injection showing distal internal carotid narrowing and apparent occlusion of the anterior cerebral artery (open arrow). Note that the middle cerebral branches are enlarged, another typical feature of sickle cell disease apparent on both angiography and MRI/ MRA, and there is evidence of leptomeningeal collateral flow from the middle to the anterior circulation on this side (*solid arrow*).

orrhage and infarction and provide evidence as to the vascular territories involved. Diagnostic testing addresses three questions: (1) what is the cause of the patient's symptoms? (2) if a stroke is the cause, are the symptoms due to cerebral infarction or hemorrhage? and (3) what is the likelihood of recurrence?

Management depends on prompt recognition of the cause of symptoms. The presenting symptoms and signs of four manifestations of cerebrovascular disease are described in Table 190-1, along with the results of diagnostic tests and initial management strategies. A patient presenting with a history of a transient focal neurologic deficit, especially hemiparesis, should be assumed to have had a transient ischemic attack or (less likely) a seizure with postictal weakness. Although cerebral ischemia (transient loss of brain blood flow) is the most likely, initial consideration should also be given to diseases other than stroke. If meningitis is suspected, treatment should be initiated with antibiotics at once and a CT scan performed followed by a lumbar puncture. The CT scan in the acute evaluation of a patient with neurologic symptoms is the best initial diagnostic test because it can be performed rapidly and requires little cooperation. It is not necessary to use intravenous contrast to rule out most emergency conditions, but diagnostic sensitivity is enhanced by its use for other conditions. Brain tumors may present with transient symptoms but more typically are associated with subacute or chronic symptoms. The CT also helps to distinguish these conditions.

Focal seizures should prompt evaluation for stroke risk. The electroencephalogram may help to localize the brain lesion, but imaging of the brain and assessment of the large vessels is necessary to evaluate cerebrovascular risk fully. The cause of generalized seizures, especially in adults, may be obvious from the history and an extensive workup may not be appropriate.

Cranial CT and/or MRI should be done in all patients with suspected stroke to eliminate other lesions and to identify hemorrhages. Cerebral angiography is clearly useful when the diagnosis of cerebrovascular disease is doubtful and chronic transfusion is being considered. This situation arises in young children with extremity symptoms that might represent stroke or painful crisis. In such cases the angiogram is used to decide on transfusion. Angiography is safe in Hb SS if the patient is prepared with hydration and reduction of Hb S to a low level, arbitrarily 30 percent or less. Transfusion is initiated if the angiogram shows extensive large-vessel disease and is withheld in the absence of impressive disease. Whether MR angiography or transcranial Doppler can substitute for angiography depends on local experience with these noninvasive techniques. Transcranial Doppler can identify children at risk for stroke before symptoms develop, but it is not clear that prophylactic transfusion is justified in asymptomatic patients on this basis alone.

If the CT is normal or shows new or old cerebral infarction, the standard treatment of children is hydration with transfusion. Acute treatment of a proved or suspected cerebral infarction consists of immediate partial or complete exchange transfusion and intravenous hydration with isotonic fluids. Although randomized study of the effects of this therapy on outcome have not been performed, the therapy seems reasonable on theoretical grounds and has become common practice. The optimal method of transfusion and target parameters have not been established. In theory, reduction of the Hb S level would be expected to improve blood viscosity and might improve cerebral blood flow in the region of an acute infarct. On this basis rapid rather than slow reduction is preferable because the therapeutic window for the brain is limited to a few hours after the onset of ischemia.

Simple transfusions are slower than exchange methods and risk increasing the hematocrit to levels that markedly increase blood viscosity, further impairing flow. On the other hand, the rate of exchange should not be so rapid as to risk cardiovascular instability, which could decrease brain perfusion. Given these considerations, partial exchange is recommended with the goal of reducing the Hb S to less than 30 percent as rapidly as can be safely accomplished. Therapeutic limits are 10 to 11 g/dl Hb and 30 to 33 percent hematocrit, being careful not to raise the hematocrit higher than 33 to 35 percent because doing so could impair cerebral blood flow due to elevated viscosity. Cautious hydration with colloid or normal saline and vigilance for seizures and increased intracranial pressure from cerebral edema are appropriate measures and may best be accomplished acutely in an intensive care setting.

The efficacy of transfusion has not been tested in the acute setting, but it seems to be a reasonable approach that might improve outcome by reducing blood viscosity. There is more support, although no randomized data, for the use of chronic transfusion on a long-term basis to prevent recurrent stroke, which occurs in most cases not treated with transfusion. For children with ischemic stroke the recommendation is for indefinite regular transfusions at least up to 18 to 20 years of age, frequent enough to maintain the level of Hb S to less than 30 percent of total hemoglobin. While on chronic transfusion patients may report transient episodes of worsening numbness or weakness, but recurrent infarction is rare.

The risk of stroke recurrence is not uniform and likely depends on the condition of the arterial system when symptoms first appear. Most patients who develop cerebrovascular symptoms have abnormal large arteries when studied with arteriography. It is reasonable to assume that risk is in part dependent on the degree of arterial stenosis, adequacy of collaterals, and number of vessels occluded. Other factors such as platelet or leukocyte count or viscosity probably modify risk. In patients with transient symptoms and no clear CT or MRI evidence for infarction, arteriography can identify patients with significant arterial stenoses. It is invasive and expensive but clearly demonstrates the status of the large arteries. Stroke has been reported as a complication of cerebral arteriography, but hydration and reduction of Hb to less than 30 percent has reduced the risk significantly. The risks of transfusion probably outweigh the benefits in patients with normal large arteries and should not be used indefinitely in such cases.

Prolonged transfusion is associated with cumulative hazards from iron overload, chelation therapy, and antibody formation. Iron accumulation can be attenuated by using chronic partial exchange rather than direct transfusion and treatment with chelation. Various surgical procedures to bypass the stenosis or occlusion associated with moyamoya disease have been tried and may be suitable for patients with sickle cell disease who have significant iron overload or problems with alloimmunization that make prolonged transfusion difficult or hazardous.

Enthusiasm is much lower for sustained transfusion in adults, and no consensus exists on the best means of secondary prevention in such patients. There is little experience with antiplatelet agents, but I recommend their use in adults who are not treated with transfusion. In theory, anticoagulants might be useful but could make the recognized problem of intracranial hemorrhage more likely in patients with extensive vascular disease and fragile moyamoya vessels.

Silent or hyposymptomatic brain infarction has been detected in 10 to 20 percent of SSD patients studied with MRI. These lesions may cause cognitive impairment or may predict future clinical stroke, or both, but proof of their significance at this point is inconclusive. They are not an indication for chronic transfusion.

Intracranial Hemorrhage

Intracranial hemorrhage usually presents with ominous symptoms and signs such as sudden, severe headache, vomiting, and alteration of consciousness with or without focal findings. The cranial CT is important not only in the diagnosis of intracranial bleeding but in the determination of blood location: subarachnoid, intraparenchymal, or intraventricular. Convulsions and coma suggest massive subarachnoid or intraventricular bleeding. Parenchymal bleeding is usually subcortical and presents with depressed alertness or stupor and focal findings. Arteriographic and pathologic investigation of SSD patients with intracranial hemorrhage identify several potential mechanisms including rupture of berry aneurysms or (less commonly) arteriovenous malformations, rupture of intraparenchymal or periventricular moyamoya-like small arteries, and no evident large artery disease (except for dilation), suggesting small vessel rupture as the presumed source. Aneurysms appear to be more common in Hb SS than in the general population, become manifest at a younger age, and may more often be multiple. Why aneurysms form is unclear, but hemodynamic stress due to elevated flow rates has been suggested. Deleterious effects on small vessels similar to what is seen in moyamoya disease probably account for intraparenchymal bleeding. Bleeding risk appears to be higher in patients who have experienced previous cerebral infarction, and it may not be reduced by the use of chronic transfusion.

If the CT scan shows hemorrhage the patient should be transfused and hydrated in preparation for cerebral angiography. The clinical condition may require urgent and intensive care to treat increased intracranial pressure or acute hydrocephalus, to manage seizures, or to treat vasospasm. Subarachnoid and intraventricular hemorrhage patients should receive nimodopine. Primarily intraventricular hemorrhage, often with third ventricular clot, is not uncommon in HB SS and is due to parenchymal hemorrhage in the deep subcortical areas with extension into the ventricular system. Such patients can undergo rapid deterioration after admission to hospital because of sudden blockage of the ventricular system (Fig. 190-2). Emergency ventriculostomy may be life saving and is associated with a good outcome if there has been relatively little parenchymal involvement in the hemorrhage.

The angiogram is important to determine the cause of the bleeding. Aneurysms should be repaired after preparation of the patient with reduction of Hb S. An intracranial bleed associated with extensive large-vessel intracranial occlusive disease should be followed by chronic transfusion, at least in younger patients. No data exist on the efficacy of chronic transfusion after aneurysm surgery, but continued transfusion indefinitely seems reasonable given the theories of aneurysm development in these patients.

Important alternative diagnoses to consider in cases of atypical hemorrhage, infarct, or brain injury are drug abuse-related strokes and child abuse. Drug intoxication may mimic stroke symptoms in young children.

Seizures

Seizures are more common in Hb SS because they occur in 15 to 30 percent of Hb SS patients with stroke and stroke is preva-

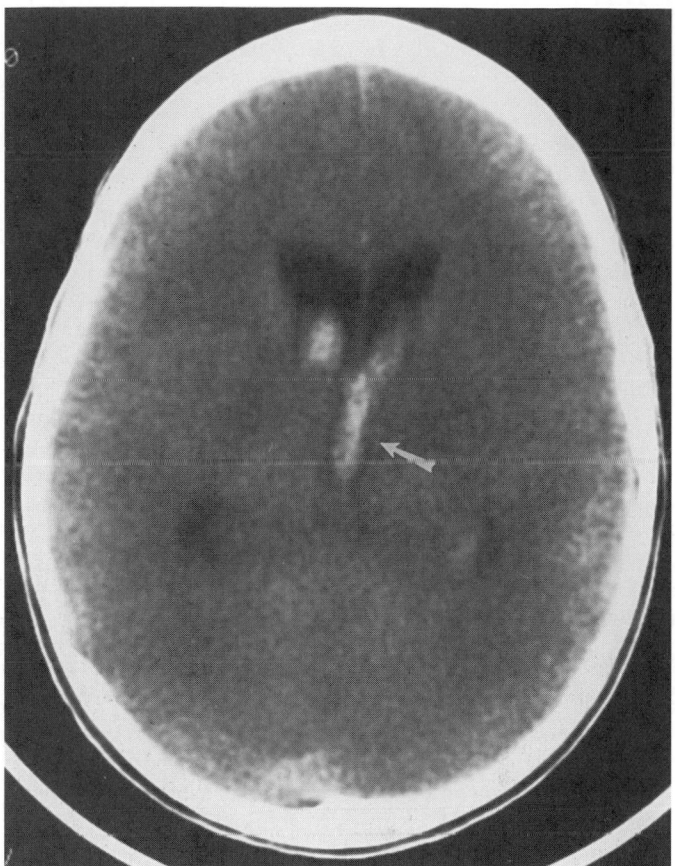

FIG. 190-2. Noncontrasted cranial CT taken shortly after this 7-year-old boy with sickle cell disease presented with severe headache, vomiting, and coma. Note the blood in the third *(arrow)* and lateral ventricles and early increase in ventricular size. The patient expired before reaching a neurosurgical center, where emergency ventriculostomy may have been life saving. Since his scan showed little parenchymal hemorrhage he is presumed to have died from acute ventricular obstruction. This patient had transcranial Doppler evidence of vasculopathy 2 years prior to his death. The presumed source of bleeding is rupture of moyamoya vessels.

lent in Hb SS. Two important points concerning seizures and Hb SS should be considered: (1) focal seizures in children may be the only symptom of unrecognized vascular disease; a workup for large vessel disease should be considered with an eye toward transfusion to prevent stroke if significant disease and cerebral infarction is present; and (2) in some settings patients with Hb SS receive demerol for management of pain; generalized seizures may be provoked by its metabolite nomeperidine and by toxic doses of other narcotic analgesics. Apart from these considerations the diagnostic and treatment approach to seizures is the same as in any other patient.

Comparative Risks

Despite an anemia that is more severe than that of Hb SS, little evidence shows that patients with β-thalassemia develop vascular disease or have increased risk of stroke. Intracranial hemorrhage with multiple blood transfusions has been reported, but this may have been due to coagulopathy. A syndrome of hypertension, convulsions, and cerebral hemorrhage was reported in thalassemia patients receiving blood transfusions but may have been a simple manifestation of malignant hypertension. Hb SC patients have a less severe anemia than those with

Hb SS and a less severe clinical course generally, including little if any increased risk of neurologic disease. They do get more retinopathy, however, presumably through a higher blood viscosity because they are less anemic.

Other Acute Manifestations

Other acute neurologic manifestations include sudden sensorineural hearing loss and vestibular dysfunction. These are usually caused by peripheral disease, but brainstem involvement is possible and MRI should be considered. Only a few cases of myelopathy from spinal cord infarction or compression from extramedullary hematatopoeisis have been reported. The differential diagnosis should first entertain more common causes such as transverse myelitis, demyelinating disease, or mass lesions (before Hb SS) when the spinal cord is involved. Central retinal artery occlusions have been reported. Visual disturbances may be part of a cerebrovascular syndrome or primarily retinal vascular, retinal (proliferative sickle retinopathy), or ocular from other sickle-related cases. Despite case reports, few data suggest that patients with sickle cell trait (Hb SA) are at increased risk for neurologic disease.

Consequences of Transfusion

It is important to mention that hemoglobinopathy patients treated with chronic transfusion are at increased risk of both acute and chronic consequences of this treatment. A partial list includes immediate transfusion reactions; delayed hemolytic transfusion reactions; hypertension and seizures after transfusion; iron overload with hepatic and cardiac hemosiderosis; chelation side effects including vision and hearing problems; infection with hepatitis B and C, human immunodeficiency virus, and possibly other agents.

CHRONIC MANIFESTATIONS

Frequent and bothersome headaches are reported in over 30 percent of patients. The headache pattern may suggest migraine but more commonly resembles tension-type headache. Unless it is part of a well-established migraine pattern, severe headache with vomiting should prompt an urgent CT scan because of the increased risk of intracranial hemorrhage. No evidence shows that chronic headache is more common in patients destined to have stroke. Treatment is approached as with any similar aged patient using episodic and prophylactic therapy as appropriate.

Children with Hb SS appear to have a but significant baseline small cognitive deficit when compared with sibling controls without the disease. This deficit becomes evident by early childhood and occurs outside the recognized cerebrovascular syndromes. The cause is unclear. A child with severe learning problems should be worked up for stroke with a CT or MRI. In the presence of extensive vessel and parenchymal disease and clear focal deficits transfusion should be considered. In most cases cerebral infarction is not found, however. Clinicians should be alert to the likelihood that children and adults with HB SS and perhaps other hemoglobinopathies may have special educational or training needs and should ensure that neuropsychological testing is conducted to assist in educational and vocational planning.

A few cases of peripheral neuropathy with Hb SS have been reported including mental neuropathy related to mandible infarctions.

SUGGESTED READINGS

Adams RJ: *Neurological complications* p. 599. Sickle Cell Disease: In Embury SH, Hebbel RP, Narla M, Steinberg MH (eds): Scientific Principles and Clinical Practice. Raven Press, New York, 1994

Adams RJ, Nichols FT: Sickle cell anemia, sickle cell trail and thalassemia. p. 503. In Vinken PJ, Bruyn GW, Klawans HL (eds): *Handbook of Clinical Neurology. Vascular Diseases III*. Vol. 11. Netherlands: Elsevier, Amsterdam, 1989

Adams RJ, McKie V, Nichols FT et al: *The use of transcranial ultrasonography to predict stroke in sickle cell disease*. N Engl J Med 326:605, 1992

Frempong KO: Stroke in sickle cell disease: demographic, clinical and therapeutic considerations. Semin Hematol 28:213, 1991

Hess DC, Adams RJ, Nichols: Sickle cell anemia and other hemoglobinopathies. Semin Neurol 11:314, 1991

Olopoinia L, Frederick W, Greaves W et al: Pneumococcal sepsis and meningitis in adults with sickle cell disease. South Med J 83:1002, 1990

Pavlakis SG: Neurologic complications of sickle cell disease. Adv Pediatr 36: 247, 1989

Powars ER, Wilson B, Imbus C et al: The natural history of stroke in sickle cell disease. Am J Med 65:461, 1978

Rothman SM, Fulling KH, Nelson JS et al: Sickle cell anemia and central nervous system infarction: a neuropathological study. Ann Neurol 20:684, 1986

Serjeant GR: The nervous system. In *Sickle Cell Disease*. 2nd Ed. Oxford University Press, New York, p. 292. 1992

SECTION 6. ENDOCRINOLOGY AND METABOLISM

191. NEUROLOGIC MANIFESTATIONS OF THE PORPHYRIAS

MELVIN GREER

The porphyrias are diseases caused by inherited or acquired deficiencies of enzymes in the heme biosynthetic pathway (Table 191-1). They manifest mainly as skin photosensitivity or neurologic abnormalities, or both. The enzyme deficiencies that underlie the eight porphyrias are each expressed predominantly in one of the two major sites of heme synthesis in the body: the liver and the erythropoietic system. This chapter presents four of the five hepatic porphyrias (which are associated with prominent neurologic effects): acute intermittent porphyria, variegate porphyria, hereditary coproporphyria, and δ-aminolevulinic acid (ALA) dehydratase deficiency porphyria. The erythropoietic porphyrias, by contrast, mainly cause skin photosensitivity, which may lead to mutilating skin lesions and hypertrichosis, and also may cause anemia and splenomegaly.

The rate-limiting step of the heme biosynthetic pathway is the first reaction, which is the synthesis of ALA from succinyl coenzyme A and glycine catalyzed by the enzyme ALA synthase (Fig. 191-1). Induction of this enzyme activates the pathway. Heme production is thought to exert feedback repression on the production of the enzyme, and various drugs and hormones can induce it. If a porphyria is present, the intermediates downstream from the deficient enzyme will tend to accumulate when the pathway is running at high volume, and derivatives of these intermediates will then be excreted in the urine or stool. Diagnosis of the porphyrias therefore depends on inducing the pathway and examining the urine and stool for enhanced excre-

tion of one or more of the relevant metabolites. The diagnosis can be confirmed by measuring the specific enzyme deficiency in erythrocytes, fibroblasts, or mitogen-stimulated lymphocytes.

Individuals with these enzyme deficiencies are clinically asymptomatic except when the pathway is strongly induced. The most common cause of disease attacks is administration of barbiturate drugs, although the hormone changes that occur during the menses may also precipitate an acute attack. The pathophysiology of the porphyrias represents not a deficiency in the manufacture of heme but rather the accumulation of heme synthesis intermediates.

ACUTE INTERMITTENT PORPHYRIA

Acute intermittent porphyria (AIP), also called Swedish porphyria and intermittent acute porphyria, is the most common of the hepatic porphyrias in the United States. It is caused by a defect in the gene for porphobilinogen deaminase (PGB deaminase), which is located on chromosome 11. The incidence of the defective gene is estimated to be about 5 to 10 in 100,000, but in the United States about 90 percent of the individuals who carry the genetic defect remain clinically unaffected. The incidence of clinical disease is much higher in Sweden (estimated at 1.5 in 100,000). Women are three times as likely as men to experience clinical disease.

PGB deaminase activity is about 50 percent of normal in ndividuals with the genetic defect. Clinical features emerge when such an individual is exposed to drugs that strongly induce ALA synthase, resulting in an overproduction of ALA and PBG. These drugs include steroids, barbiturates, and some other common lipid-soluble compounds. Chemicals that can induce P_{450} hemoproteins may also pose a risk. Severe dieting, infection, alcohol excess, surgery (including dental extraction), and severe stress have also been reported to cause clinical manifes-

TABLE 191-1. Porphyria Classification

	Enzyme Deficiency	Inheritance	Clinical Presentation	Increased Excretion	
				Urine	Stool
Hepatic porphyrias					
Acute intermittent porphyria (Swedish porphyria, intermittent acute porphyria)	3	AD	Neurologic	ALA, PBG	
Hereditary coproporphryia	6	AD	Neurologic Photosensitivity	ALA, PBG Coproporphyrin	Coproporphyrin
Variegate porphyria (South African porphyria)	7	AD	Neurologic Photosensitivity	ALA, PBG Coproporphyrin	Coproporphyrin Protoporphyrin
ALA dehydratase deficiency	2	AR	Neurologic	ALA	
Porphyria cutanea tarda	5	AD or acquired	Photosensitivity	Uroporphyrin	
Erythropoietic porphyrias					
Congenital erythropoietic protoporphyria	4	AR	Photosensitivity	Uroporphyrin Coproporphyrin	Coproporphyrin
Erythropoietic protoporphyria	8	AD	Photosensitivity		Protoporphyrin
Hepatoerythropoietic porphyria	5	AR	Photosensitivity	Uroporphrin	Isocoproporphyrin

Abbreviations: AD, autosomal dominant; AR, ausotomal recessive; ALA, δ-aminolevulinic acid; PBG, porphobilinogen.

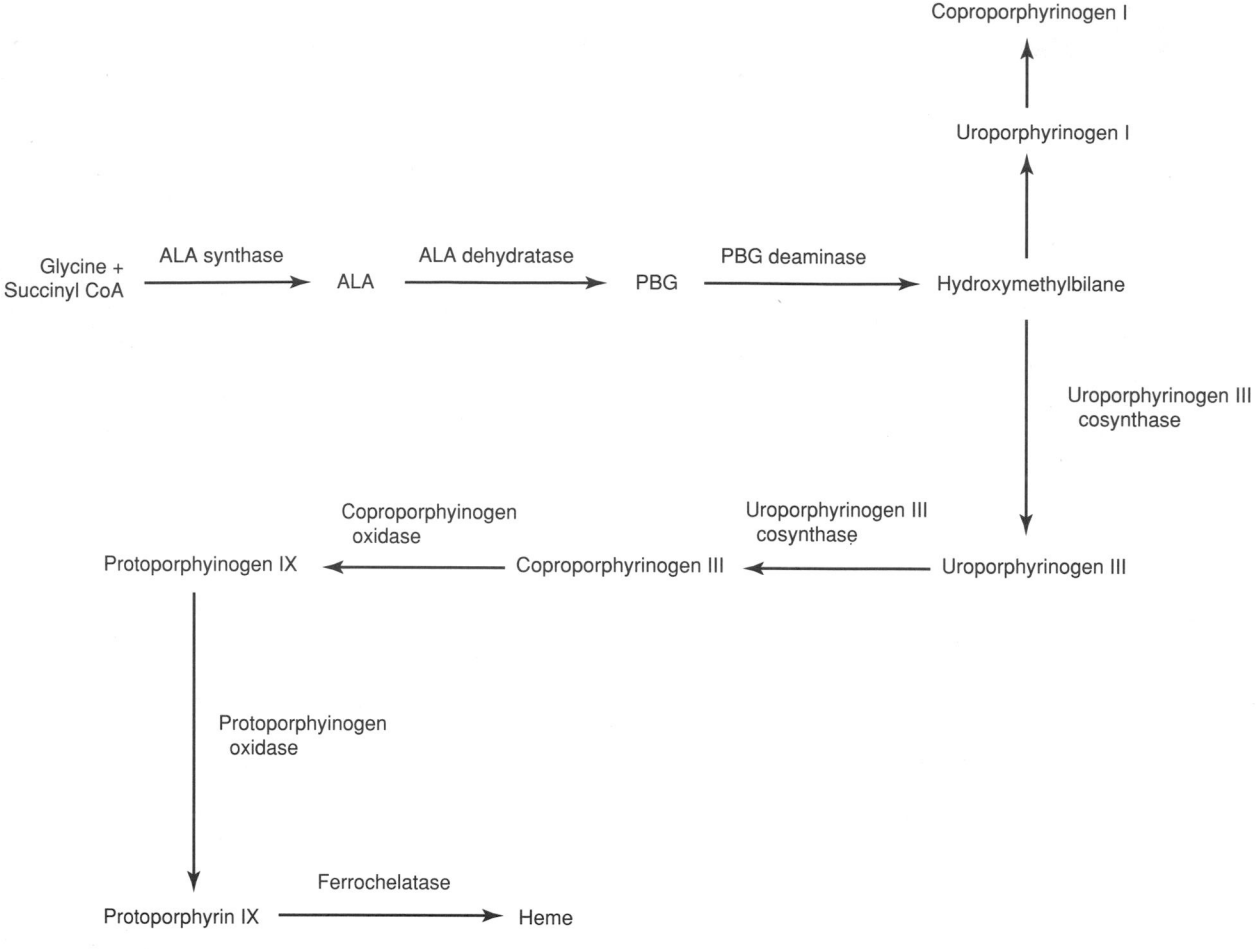

FIG. 191-1. The heme biosynethetic pathway. ALA, δ-aminolevulinic acid; PBG, porphobilinogen.

tations, and some women experience repeated attacks in relation to menstrual cycles. However, as these factors may not cause a clinical problem in a patient every time they occur, other, unknown circumstances evidently modify the response. In one study of 48 attacks in a series of patients, a specific inciting cause was found for 75 percent of the attacks, including barbiturate usage in 16 cases and the approach of menstruation in 6 patients.

In essence, the signs and symptoms reflect an acute problem of varying severity with abdominal pain usually the earliest manifestation (Table 191-2). This pain may be severe and colicky, localized or generalized, and may radiate to the back. In one series, abdominal pain occurred in 95 percent of patients and was the most common component of the acute attack; constipation, nausea, and vomiting were also described about half the time. Accompanying fever and leucocytosis often lead to laparotomy. Stasis and intestinal dilatation are observed by radiographic studies. These features are consistent with an abrupt change in splanchnic autonomic nervous system function.

Other features of the acute attack that imply a change in autonomic nervous system function include tachycardia (more than 100/bpm) (noted in 80 percent), hypertension (36 percent), postural hypotension (21 percent), bladder retention (12 percent), hyperhidrosis (12 percent), fever (9 percent), and fecal impaction (6 percent). In general, the presence and persistence of tachycardia is a useful indicator of the active process.

Extremity pain and paresthesias occurred in about 50 percent

of patients. In the more severely impaired patients, involvement of peripheral and cranial nerves was noted that, in one series progressed to flaccid quadriparesis in 11 of 35 patients. Weakness reflecting motor nerve dysfunction was proximal or distal, symmetrical or asymmetrical, and even focal. Patchy sensory impairment and dysesthesias were evident when motor deficits were pronounced. Selective truncal sensory deficits have been described. Tendon reflexes were depressed or absent, although they may be normal in the early phase of the neuropathy.

During the acute event, the emergence of hyponatremia secondary to gastrointestinal sodium loss, sodium-losing nephropathy, sodium-poor fluid administration, or the syndrome of inappropriate antidiuretic hormone excretion (SIADH) was noted in 40 percent of patients.

Behavioral changes that also may be witnessed in the acute attack include hallucinations, delirium, and altered consciousness. These changes in mentation, as well as seizures, are likely to be related to changes in fluid and electrolyte balance or to profound hypertension reflecting autonomic dysfunction. On the other hand, in one series, hyponatremia was considered the cause of hallucinations and mental confusion in only 3 of 16 patients. Other behavioral changes noted in the acute attack include such features as agitation, restlessness, anxiety, and depression. The relationship of these psychological responses to the accumulation of intermediates of porphyrin metabolism is uncertain. If they are not caused by hypertension or fluid and

TABLE 191-2. Signs and Symptoms in Acute Intermittent Porphyric Attack[a]

Sign or Symptom	% of Patients
Abdominal pain	85–95
Vomiting	43–88
Constipation	48–84
Diarrhea	5–12
Myalgia	50–52
Weakness	42–68
Sensory loss	9–38
Respiratory paralysis	9–14
Transient blindness	4–6
Mental changes	40–58
Convulsions	10–20
Hypertension	36–54
Tachycardia	28–80
Fever	9–37

[a] From a total of 417 patients described in Waldenstrom J: The porphyrias as inborn errors of metabolism. Am J Med, 22:758, 1957; Goldberg A: Acute intermittent porphyria: a study of 50 cases. Q J Med 28:183, 1959; and Stein JA, Tschudy DP: Acute intermittent porphyria. A clinical and biochemical study of 46 patients. Medicine 49:1, 1970.

electrolyte imbalance they may represent a reactive state based on premorbid psychological factors.

It is likewise uncertain whether the emergence of seizures can be accepted as a separate manifestation reflecting a toxic effect of the intermediates of porphyrin metabolism that accumulate in the body. In reports suggesting this phenomenon, the accompanying hypertension and hyponatremia are more likely to be causal.

The neurologic features reflect an acute progressive motor neuropathy that may mimic the Guillain-Barré syndrome, ascending from lower to upper extremities and leading to motor cranial nerve impairment. In certain circumstances a selective nerve impairment, usually the radial nerve, may be involved, leading to wrist drop, a feature similar to lead poisoning (in which a disturbance in porphyrin metabolism also occurs). In lead poisoning increased urinary ALA excretion but normal PBG excretion are noted.

Visual disturbances including transient blindness and subsequent optic atrophy have been noted, but here again the relationship to associated hypertension implies an effect on the basis of vascular insufficiency rather than a direct toxic process.

The duration of the neuropathy is variable. The patient's weakness may continue to progress even after the abdominal pain improves. The acute attack may last days or it may progress over a period of weeks to months. In women, an acute attack may occur with menses or during pregnancy. In this circumstance, the clinical features may be so severe that pregnancy may have to be terminated. On the other hand, most women with AIP tolerate gestation well. As a rule, the features of a porphyric attack are not seen before puberty or after menopause.

Variability in recurrent attacks is often seen in the same patient. Most patients experience an event that is time circumscribed followed by an asymptomatic state. Infrequently, however, the individual patient may exhibit a course of smoldering clinical abnormalities with episodes of exacerbation. The patient with severe motor neuropathy usually improves with supportive therapy; however, the duration of the deficit may be years, and incomplete recovery may be noted.

In one series of 3,867 subjects with chronic psychiatric disorders, 8 were found to have AIP by measurement of appropriate urine and blood tests. These patients, who had chronic problems such as schizoaffective disorders, agitated psychosis, and depression, did not exhibit other features of AIP such as episodic abdominal pain, autonomic dysfunction, or neuropathy.

Diagnostic Studies

The diagnosis is made on the basis of increased urinary excretion of ALA and PBG. The appearance of a port wine color of the urine on exposure to sunlight is due to porphobilin, an oxidation product of PBG, as well as to other degraded porphyrin compounds. The qualitative Watson-Schwartz or Hoesch tests are the most commonly performed screening diagnostic assays. A positive reaction only occurs when the concentration of PBG is three to five times the upper limit of normal. This is indicative of the acute attack. In the latent state the test results are often negative, although variably increased amounts may be excreted by carriers and by patients between attacks. Because of the incidence of false-positive reactions, certain quantitative confirmatory tests performed by column chromatography should be used to measure PBG and ALA. Periodic measurement of these excreted compounds provides a useful determinant of the activity of the porphyric attack; however, no strict correlation exists between the levels of urinary PBG and ALA and the severity of the attack. Measurement of elevated plasma levels of ALA and PBG will occur only in the acute attack. Increased urinary excretion of porphyrins is noted in lead poisoning and in hereditary tyrosinemia, as well as in other nonspecific infectious, toxic, or metabolic disorders. The selective increase of urinary ALA and PBG establishes the diagnosis of AIP. Confirmation of the diagnosis is based on the detection of a depressed level (about 50 percent) of reduced PBG deaminase in erythrocytes, fibroblasts, or mitogen-stimulated lymphocytes. This will identify the latent patient as well as the porphyric patient in the acute attack. Erythrocyte PBG deaminase is also decreased in uremia.

Stool porphyrin excretion is usually normal in AIP. Other biochemical changes that may be detected include hypercholesterolemia and hyper-β-lipoproteinemia. Abnormalities reflecting a disturbance of the pituitary-hypophyseal axis in the acute attack include SIADH, paradoxic glucose-stimulated growth hormone release, impaired corticotropin release, and increased prolactin release.

No cerebrospinal fluid abnormalities exist in the patient with porphyric polyneuropathy. Early in the course, the motor nerve conduction velocity tests and the F-wave responses are normal. Increase in the minimal-to-maximal latency difference of the nerve impulse is the earliest abnormality detected in the patient with porphyric neuropathy. Normal latency duration and amplitude of orthodromic sensory nerve action potentials are noted. Electromyography (EMG) is also normal early in the course; however, with maximal effort only a few motor unit potentials are recruited. With progressive weakness over time, nerve stimulation induces motor nerve conduction potentials with reduced amplitude. Orthodromic sensory nerve stimulation is likewise reduced in amplitude, but sensory conduction velocities and minimal latency are unchanged. Fibrillations and positive sharp waves are then noted by EMG. These findings are consistent with an axonal neuropathy: decreased amplitude of compound nerve and muscle action potentials and normal conduction velocity, fibrillation, and sharp waves.

Brain magnetic resonance imaging changes and EEG abnormalities have been described in patients having acute attacks in which changes in mentation and seizures exist. Concomitant hypertension as well as fluid and electrolyte abnormalities are likely interpretations for these changes. These abnormalities revert to normal after the attack subsides.

Pathology and Pathogenesis

Axonal changes are observed in the biopsied peripheral nerve as the primary area of change. Secondary features of peripheral nerve demyelination have also been described in patients whose neuropathic course was prolonged. In addition, at autopsy, anterior horn cell chromatolysis and vacuolation have been described. Splanchnic motor cells of the lateral horns, medullary nuclei, and dorsal vagal nuclei have also shown chromatolytic change. In the central nervous system, nonspecific neuronal changes, focal reactive glial changes, and perivascular demyelination have been described. With respect to the hormonal changes noted such as SIADH, the selective neuronal involvement of the supraoptic and paraventricular nuclei in the hypothalamus is of specific interest.

Although certain of the central nervous system changes may be attributable to the effects of acute hypertension and the often dramatic alteration in fluid balance, the selective hypothalamic change and the more common neuropathy imply a metabolic or toxic process. Nevertheless, no convincing evidence has indicated a causal relationship between a deficiency of heme or heme product or an excess of porphyrin intermediates.

Treatment

Preventive treatment for the porphyric patient is to emphasize the avoidance of inducing factors including drug ingestion and dietary indiscretion. The patient should be made aware of drugs considered safe (Table 191-3). Prompt treatment of infections and elimination of alcohol are also urged. In women who experience an acute attack perimenstrually, ovulatory suppressant

TABLE 191-3. Safe Drugs for Porphyria Patient[a]

Antibiotics
Penicillin
Streptromycin
Tetracycline
Nitrofurantoin (?)
Mandelamine
Chloramphenicol (?)
Analgesics/narcotics
Acetominophen
Aspirin
Narcotics
Anticonvulsants
Paraldehyde
Magnesium sulfate
Bromides
Diazepam (?)
Autonomic nervous system
Atropine
Propranolol
Guanethidine (?)
Epinephrine (?)
Labetalol (?)
Psychotropic drugs
Chloral hydrate
Phenothiazines
Amitriptylene
Others
Insulin
Adrenocorticosteroids
Succinylcholine
Ether

[a] ?, may be safe.

hormones may reduce the frequency and severity of the episode. On the other hand, caution is needed with respect to the use of steroid hormones, which may themselves induce an attack. Daily intranasal or subcutaneous luteinizing hormone treatment has been used with some success.

During the early phase of the attack, increased carbohydrate consumption may abort the event. If the signs and symptoms increase, intravenous 10 percent dextrose in water or other sugars that can be metabolized to glucose are indicated. A level as high as 500 g/d is recommended. Precautions are necessary in giving large fluid volumes intravenously: the risk of SIADH and hypertension may be enhanced.

Symptomatic treatment for pain with narcotics such as codeine and meperidine and the use of phenothiazines for agitation, hallucination, nausea, and vomiting are appropriate as well. Other drugs including chloral hydrate and diazepam may be offered for insomnia. Both the tachycardia and hypertension may be effectively treated with β-adrenergic blocking agents such as propranolol. The abdominal distress may also be benefited by this approach. If seizures occur, magnesium sulfate, paraldehyde, and diazepam are recommended. Hematin drugs such as heme arginase given intravenously at the dosage level of 3 to 4 mg/kg/24 h for 4 days appear to be effective in reducing the duration of the acute attack. The drug's beneficial effect is presumably related to a repression of ALA synthase activity. Its use is accompanied by a more rapid fall of urinary PBG. It needs to be given slowly over at least a 15-minute period, but a heightened risk of thrombophlebitis still exists. Other risks include coagulopathy and hemolysis.

Treatment for SIADH with fluid restriction is of primary concern for those patients with progressive evidence of encephalopathy and seizures. This need for fluid and electrolyte control should supersede treatment with other intravenous therapies in which large fluid volumes are necessary.

VARIEGATE PORPHYRIA (SOUTH AFRICAN PORPHYRIA, PROTOCOPROPORPHYRIA)

Both photosensitivity and features of neurologic involvement characterize variegate porphyria, heterozygous autosomal dominant hepatic porphyria. As in AIP, an overproduction of porphyrin metabolites exists after induction of ALA synthase. The enzyme deficiency is protoporphyrinogen oxidase. In the disease state excess urinary excretion of ALA, PBG, and coproporphyrin is found, as well as excess excretion of coproporphyrin and protoporphyrin in the stool.

This condition is most commonly observed in South Africa, where the incidence is 3 in 1,000. Elsewhere, it is less common than AIP. Moreover, the features of photosensitivity, not evident in AIP, often exist in the absence of neurovisceral symptoms. Skin lesions on exposed surfaces manifest as bullous eruptions and skin fragility. In time, hyperpigmented areas and hypertrichosis are observed as permanent residua.

Inducing factors including drugs, alcohol, and diets deficient in carbohydrates are known to cause the neurovisceral symptoms in a manner similar to AIP; however, the clinical features are usually not as severe. Rarely seen are patients in whom more than one enzyme deficiency exists. In other words, clusters of families exist in which variegate porphyria and AIP enzyme deficiency have been described in the same individual. Also, a homozygous form of variegate porphyria with onset in childhood has been identified. This is characterized by severe photosensitivity, growth restriction, and profound psychomotor retardation.

As with AIP, elevated urine porphyrin excretion may be measured; during an acute attack, however, in contrast to AIP, in which fecal excretion is not increased, in variegate porphyria marked fecal porphyrin excretion is noted.

The treatment approach, both prophylactically and for the acute attack, is similar to that recommended for AIP.

HEREDITARY COPROPORPHYRIA

Clinical features associated with hereditary coproporphyria are secondary to a heterozygous deficiency of coproporphyrinogen oxidase. This rare disorder is inherited in an autosomal dominant manner. The neurologic signs and symptoms are usually milder than those seen in AIP. Photosensitivity may be noted. In the very rare homozygous enzyme-deficient states, the clinical features are more severe. Abdominal pain, vomiting, and constipation are the hallmarks of the acute attack, which is induced particularly by drugs, as in other hepatic porphyrias; as in the other forms, recurrent attacks may also occur in menstruation. Neuropathy and psychiatric features may also be evident, although in such patients with hereditary coproporphyria neuropathy the signs and symptoms are usually not as severe as in AIP. In about 30 percent of patients skin photosensitivity exists and in some patients evidence of recurrent liver impairment has been noted with the attacks. This resolves after the attack subsides. In the rarer homozygous form that may be seen in childhood, hepatosplenomegaly, hemolytic anemia, and evidence of liver dysfunction are noted. Urine hyperexcretion of ALA, PBG, and coproporphyrin as well as increased fecal excretion of coproporphyrin are noted in the acute attack. The diagnosis is confirmed by measurement of the enzyme deficiency.

Treatment of the acute attack and prophylactic management are identical to that of AIP patients.

ALA DEHYDRATASE DEFICIENCY PORPHYRIA

ALA dehydratase deficiency porphyria, a very rare autosomal recessive disorder, is caused by a homozygous deficiency in ALA dehydratase. In an acute attack, neurologic signs and symptoms are similar to those described in the AIP patient, in whom abdominal pain, extremity pain, and a mixed motor and sensory polyneuropathy occur. Inducing factors such as drugs, alcohol ingestion, and decreased food intake are causal.

Increased urinary excretion of ALA but not PBG as well (as in AIP) is noted. The treatment approach for the acute attacks and the prophylactic management are similar to those used in AIP. Liver transplantation was performed in a child who had significant neurologic deficits from recurrent attacks of neuropathy. This did not affect the excess urinary excretion of porphyrin intermediates; however, fewer attacks occurred subsequent to the transplant.

SUGGESTED READINGS

Bourgeois F, Gu XF, Deybach JC et al: Denaturing gradient gel electrophoresis for rapid detection of latent carriers of a subtype of acute intermittent porphyria with normal erythrocyte porphobilinogen deaminase activity. Clin Chem 38:93, 1992

Goldberg A: Acute intermittent porphyria: a study of 50 cases. Q J Med 28: 183, 1959

Greer M: Porphyria. p. 429. In Vinken PJ, Bruyn GW (eds): Handbook of Clinical Neurology. Vol. 27. American Elsevier, New York, 1976

Greer M: Neuropathy of porphyria. p. 117. In de Jong JMBV (ed): Handbook of Clinical Neurology. Vol. 60. American Elsevier, New York, 1991

Herrick AL, Moore MR, McColl KEL et al: Controlled trial of haem arginate in acute hepatic porphyria. Lancet 1:1295, 1989

Kappas A, Sassa S, Galbraith RA et al: The porphyrias. p. 1305. In Scriver CR, Beaudet AL, Sly WS et al. (eds): The Metabolic Basis of Inherited Disease. Vol. I. McGraw-Hill, New York, 1989

King PH, Bragdon AC: MRI reveals multiple reversible cerebral lesions in an attack of acute intermittent porphyria. Neurology 41:1300, 1991

Stein JA, Tschudy DP: Acute intermittent porphyria. A clinical and biochemical study of 46 patients. Medicine 49:1, 1970

Thunell S, Henrichson A, Floderus YI: Liver transplantation in a boy with acute porphyria. Eur J Clin Chem Clin Biochem 30:599, 1992

Tishler PV, Woodward B, O'Connor J et al: High prevalence of intermittent acute porphyria in a psychiatric patient population. Am J Psychiatry 142: 1430, 1985

Waldenström J: The porphyrias as inborn errors of metabolism. Am J Med 22: 758, 1957

192. LYSOSOMAL STORAGE DISEASES

EDWIN H. KOLODNY

The lysosomal storage diseases are a clinically heterogeneous group of inherited diseases, more than 40 in all, with protean manifestations, including significant involvement of the central and peripheral nervous systems. They are a challenge to the physician because signs and symptoms of these disorders may lack specificity, and their clinical appearance may occur at almost any age. Prompt diagnosis greatly facilitates proper management, including, in certain instances, the initiation of treatments that may halt the progression of the disease. In the case of a young patient, early diagnosis also provides the child's family with the option for prenatal diagnosis of future pregnancies.

LYSOSOMAL METABOLISM

Lysosomes are sedimentable organelles present in the cytoplasm of all cells. They contain more than 50 hydrolytic enzymes capable of degrading both natural products of cellular metabolism and foreign materials ingested by the cell. They are vacuolar in appearance with a single limiting membrane that protects the cell from the potentially harmful effects of the degradative enzymes within it.

In 1955, C. DeDuve coined the term lysosome and first proposed its role in intracellular digestion. An endocytic vacuole containing either intracellular debris or foreign material of extracellular origin coalesces with a primary lysosome to form a secondary lysosome. The acidified environment of the secondary lysosome provides an optimal milieu for the degradative action of its hydrolytic enzymes. Any remaining undigested material is secreted from the cell in the form of a residual body to enter the urine, bile, or other excretory pathway.

Lysosomal enzymes are capable of catalyzing irreversibly the hydrolysis of lipids, carbohydrates, proteins, and nucleotides to their basic structural units. They are glycoproteins, which are first synthesized as preproteins on membrane-bound ribosomes attached to the rough endoplasmic reticulum (RER). To reach their final destination in lysosomes, they must undergo a series of post-translational modifications that involve protein and carbohydrate recognition signals. First, an amino-terminal signal peptide is attached to the nascent protein directing it into the lumen of the RER. A large preformed oligosaccharide is then transferred to the enzyme polypeptide by attachment to selected asparagine residues. The signal peptide is then cleaved and the asparagine-linked oligosaccharide partially degraded. The maturing lysosomal protein then enters the Golgi apparatus where it is acted upon by a phosphotransferase that transfers N-acetylglucosamine-1-phosphate from uridine diphosphate (UDP)-N-acetylglucosamine to mannose residues on the lysosomal enzyme. Subsequently, the N-acetylglucosamine residue is removed with the formation of mannose-6-phosphate (Man-6-P). This phosphomonoester serves as a recognition marker, directing the nascent enzyme to a prelysosomal endocytic compartment. The low pH within the endosome facilitates uncoupling of the Man-6-P receptor from its ligand and the receptor recycles back to the trans-Golgi apparatus. Further proteolytic modification and partial dephosphorylation of the enzyme proform occurs before the mature acid hydrolase enters the lysosome.

Not all the acid hydrolase proforms pass directly to lysosomes. Some are glycosylated with high mannose-type oligosaccharide, are further processed to complex type units containing galactose and sialic acid residues, and leave the trans-Golgi apparatus as secretory glycoproteins. Also, a fraction of the enzyme containing the Man-6-P recognition marker may leave the cell. These molecules are capable of subsequent recapture by binding to Man-6-P receptors on the cell surface. As a practical matter, the Man-6-P recognition system is of immense importance to the clinician, for it provides a rational basis for enzyme replacement therapy in the lysosomal storage diseases. There is evidence also for other mechanisms not involving Man-6-P receptors for delivery of acid hydrolases to the lysosome. Some of this comes from the study of I-cell disease fibroblasts which lack the ability to form the Man-6-P recognition marker.

One class of lysosomal membrane proteins contributes to the special properties of the lysosomal membrane, that is, maintenance of an acidic pH environment, sequestration of acid hydrolases, resistance to degradation by lysosomal enzymes, and the ability to fuse with other membrane organelles. Transport of these glycoproteins to the lysosome depends not on the attached N-glycans but on the character of the cytoplasmic tail in which a tyrosine residue is essential. Lysosomal acid phosphatase is one example of such Man-6-P independent targeting.

PATHOPHYSIOLOGY

The concept of an inborn disease of lysosomal enzyme metabolism was first proposed by Hers in 1965 based upon his studies of type II glycogen storage disease (Pompe disease). In this disorder, the deficiency of a specific lysosomal enzyme (acid α-glucosidase) results in the accumulation of its particular substrate (glycogen) within membrane-bound vesicles of lysosomal origin. As increasing amounts of the nonmetabolizable substrate accumulate within lysosomes, they hypertrophy, producing mechanical crowding within the cell, which in turn interferes with its normal functions and may eventually cause death of the cell.

The signs and symptoms of each inborn error of lysosomal metabolism vary according to the pattern of distribution of the nondegradable natural products and their usual rate of metabolic turnover in each tissue. In the classical infantile form of glycogenosis type II, glycogen is concentrated in heart and skeletal muscle, in the liver and in cortical and spinal cord neurons. Consequently, the affected child has extreme cardiomegaly, moderate hepatomegaly, and generalized hypotonia. Light microscopy of fresh frozen or ethanol-fixed paraffin-embedded sections of muscle demonstrate PAS-positive cytoplasmic granules, which disappear when the tissue is preincubated with diastase, an enzyme that digests glycogen. The concentration of certain types of macromolecules such as G_{M1}- and G_{M2}-gangliosides and the galactolipids, galactocerebroside, and sulfatide, is normally much higher in the central nervous system than in other tissues. Therefore, in diseases in which the hydrolysis of these compounds is defective, the signs and symptoms are almost exclusively confined to the nervous system, whereas in enzyme deficiencies affecting more widely distributed natural products such as glycoproteins and mucopolysaccharides, a variety of different organ systems, both neural and nonneural are affected. However, for nearly all lysosomal storage diseases there is a tendency for the nervous system to be preferentially affected. This is because the cells of visceral organ systems besieged by lysosomal hypertrophy are capable of replacing themselves, but neurons destroyed by lysosomal overcrowding are not replaceable. Thus, one might encounter a patient with marked hepatosplenomegaly with only minimal disturbance of hematologic parameters or of liver enzymes, yet even mild neuronal storage produces marked psychomotor delay and mental retardation.

Morphologic and histochemical studies alert the diagnostician not only to the presence of a lysosomal storage disease, but often to one particular class or form of lysosomal disease. Electron-microscopic analysis of readily available tissues such as white blood cells or skin may disclose the presence of increased numbers and size of intracytoplasmic vacuoles, alerting the clinician to the possibility of a lysosomal storage disease. The character of the inclusions may then permit further refinements in diagnosis. For example, alternating dark and light lines arranged in a circular lamellated pattern are a distinctive feature of the membranous cytoplasmic body (MCB), characteristic of the neuronal inclusions in Tay-Sachs disease (late-infantile G_{M2}-gangliosidosis). Such MCBs are also present within axons of dermal nerves not only in Tay-Sachs disease, but in later onset forms of G_{M2}-gangliosidosis as well. The presence of this same type of inclusion in cell types other than neurons or their axons is highly suggestive of mucolipidosis IV.

Parallel lamellar arrays in the form of zebra bodies is a distinguishing feature of the mucopolysaccharidoses. This type of inclusion may be found in several cell types, including muscle and connective tissues. Homogeneous dense bodies, membranovesicular and fingerprintlike inclusions are highly suggestive of the neuronal ceroid lipofuscinoses. Large empty vacuoles or vacuoles with a finely granular appearance are suggestive of a glycoprotein storage disorder such as fucosidosis, mannosidosis, or sialic acid storage disease. These may occasionally occur alongside other vacuoles containing laminated membrane structures and electron-dense bodies, suggesting the presence of different types of nondegradable compounds.

In certain forms of lysosomal storage disease with prominent involvement of the reticuloendothelial system, the bone marrow can be a source of distinctive cell types. Foam cells, enlarged histiocytes containing lipid droplets that impart a mulberry- or honeycomblike appearance to the cell, are found in Niemann-

Pick disease, G_{M1}-gangliosidosis, the Sandhoff variant of G_{M2}-gangliosidosis, sialidosis, mucolipidoses II and III, fucosidosis, α-mannosidosis, and Wolman's disease. Sea-blue histiocytes, revealing a blue or blue-green color with Giemsa and Wright stains are often an indication of Niemann-Pick disease type C. Another distinctive cell, the Gaucher cell, is similar in size to the foam cell, but contains rod-shaped inclusions imparting a wrinkled tissue paper or crumpled silk appearance to the cell. Bone marrow smears may also reveal Alder-Reilly bodies characteristic of Hurler's disease and multiple sulfatase deficiency.

GENETICS

Elucidation of the biochemical defect in many of the lysosomal storage diseases has followed a similar sequence. First, the nature of the accumulating material was discovered. As lysosomal enzymes are exohydrolases, that is, they cleave the terminally linked moiety from the nonreducing end of a complex lipid or carbohydrate, the chemical composition and structure of the stored substance provided a clue as to the nature of the defective enzyme. The enzyme was purified from normal tissues and subsequently shown to be deficient in activity in the tissues of affected individuals. The third step has been cloning of the gene coding for the enzyme or relevant enzyme subunit. In most cases, this was simplified by the availability of amino acid sequence for the protein product of the gene.

With the exception of Hunter's and Fabry's diseases, the inheritance of each lysosomal disease follows an autosomal recessive pattern. Equal numbers of males and females are affected, parental consanguinity is often present, and the recurrence risk in a family is 25 percent for each subsequent pregnancy. Except in the case of a gene occurring with high frequency in a population subgroup, as in the case of the Gaucher disease trait among Ashkenazi Jews, vertical transmission would be very rare. Therefore, it is unlikely for a lysosomal disease to occur in a family with a history of the disease in another branch of the family. The exceptions are Hunter's and Fabry's diseases, which are x-linked and therefore present as the full-blown disease in males only. Inheritance of these disorders would be through the carrier female, that is, the mother, and therefore a history of an affected maternal uncle might be expected.

The genes that are involved in the pathogenesis of most lysosomal diseases have been mapped and cloned and mutations in their genomic DNA structure identified. The chromosomal map position of these genes are shown in Table 192-1. The table also lists the substrate(s) in common use for the in vitro determination of the lysosomal enzyme activity known to be deficient in each disease. The fluorigenic 4-methylumbelliferyl derivatives are preferred by many biochemists. These artificial substrates contain the specific linkage targeted by the enzyme, although the lysosomal enzymes appear not to discriminate very critically with respect to the aglycan portion of the molecule. Before cleavage, the molecule is nonfluorigenic, but after its hydrolysis, free 4-methylumbelliferyl appears. This highly fluorigenic substance provides a high degree of sensitivity to the analysis of specific enzymes without the need to use radioactively labeled natural products as substrates. However, for certain enzyme determinations, the natural product is still required, and therefore such determinations can only be done in the few laboratories that have access to these compounds.

Carriers of the trait for a particular lysosomal disease will demonstrate reduced levels of activity of the relevant enzyme, but overlap with normal noncarrier values sometimes occurs so that enzyme determination is not an entirely dependable method for heterozygote identification. This problem can be circumvented when DNA from the affected family member is analyzed for the mutation(s) on both alleles. If these are known, then they can be sought in close relatives using DNA probes specific for the family mutation(s).

ONSET AND PROGRESSION

The lysosomal storage diseases are inborn errors of metabolism, so that the individual affected with one of these diseases will carry evidence of the disorder from the time of conception. Histologic signs of lipid accumulation have been found in spinal cord neurons of fetuses with G_{M1}- and G_{M2}-gangliosidoses as early as 20 weeks of gestation. Similarly, I am aware of Gaucher's disease detected in a fetus with hydrops in whom lipid-filled histiocytes were present in the lungs, liver, and other organs.

While histologic, biochemical, and molecular DNA evidence of a lysosomal storage disease can be found at birth or before, it is unusual for the disease to be manifest in the neonate. Dramatic exceptions are Pompe's disease, I-cell disease, G_{M1}-gangliosidosis, and infantile sialic acid storage disease. The infant with the Pompe type of glycogenosis presents as an alert youngster who is markedly hypotonic with flabby muscles and an enlarged heart and liver. Facial dysmorphism, hyperplastic gums, and restricted joint movements are characteristic of the neonate with I-cell disease. Some infants with G_{M1}-gangliosidosis can be spotted as neonates with frontal bossing, midfacial hypoplasia, macroglossia, broad hands, short stubby fingers, stiff joints, and edema of the extremities. The clinical appearance in the neonatal form of sialic acid storage disease is also very distinctive. Coarse facial features, ascites, hepatosplenomegaly, hypopigmented skin and hair, anemia, and renal failure are typical presenting features.

In the early neonatal period, Niemann-Pick disease type C, Gaucher's disease type 2, Farber's disease and Wolman's disease may be suspected. Neonatal jaundice and the appearance of a giant cell hepatitis on liver biopsy are early signs of type C Niemann-Pick disease. The infant with Farber's disease develops painful swollen joints, hoarseness, and feeding and respiratory difficulties. In the child with Wolman's disease, within the first few weeks of life there is the appearance of abdominal distention, forceful vomiting, diarrhea, hepatosplenomegaly, and anemia. The distinctive features of the neonate with type 2 Gaucher disease are a bilateral fixed strabismus, opisthotonic posturing, bulbar signs, limb rigidity, seizures, and severe hepatosplenomegaly.

Other lysosomal storage diseases will make their appearance later in the first year after a variable period of apparently normal development. These include Krabbe's disease, Niemann-Pick disease type A, the G_{M1}- and G_{M2}-gangliosidoses, the mucopolysaccharidoses, and the glycoproteinoses. Marked irritability and variability in muscle tone are characteristic of infants with Krabbe's disease. The Niemann-Pick type A child is beset with feeding problems, failure to thrive, and marked hepatosplenomegaly. Psychomotor retardation and cherry-red maculae are characteristic of the classical Tay-Sachs and Sandhoff variants of G_{M2}-gangliosidosis. An important feature distinguishing Krabbe's disease, Niemann-Pick disease type A, and the G_{M2}-gangliosidoses is that in these diseases the facial appearance remains normal, but in the mucopolysaccharidoses and glyco-

TABLE 192-1. Lysosomal Storage Diseases

Disorder	Stored Substance	Primary Deficiency	Enzyme Substrate[a]	Gene Location
Sphingolipidoses				
Fabry's disease	Ceramide trihexoside	α-Galactosidase A	4-MU-α-galactopyranoside + N-actylgalactosamine	Xq22
Farber's disease	Ceramide	Ceramidase	N-[1-^{14}C]lauroylsphingosine [^{14}C]cerebroside sulfate	
Gaucher's disease	Glucosylceramide, glycopeptides	Glucocerebrosidase	4-MU-β-glucopyranoside	1q21
G_{M1}-gangliosidosis	G_{M1}-ganglioside, galactosyl oligosaccharides, keratan sulfate	β-Galactosidase	4-MU-β-galactopyranoside	3p21-3pter
G_{M2}-gangliosidosis				
Tay-Sachs disease	G_{M2}-ganglioside	β-N-Acetylhexosaminidase α-subunit	4-MU-β-N-acetylglucosaminide, 4-MU-β-N-acetylglucosaminide sulfate	15q23-q24
Sandhoff's disease	G_{M2}-ganglioside, oligosaccharides, glycosaminoglycans	β-N-Acetylhexosaminidase β-subunit	4-MU-β-N-acetylglucosamimide	5q13
Activator deficiency	G_{M2}-ganglioside	G_{M2} activator	G_{M2}-ganglioside	5q32-q33
Krabbe's disease (globoid cell leukodystrophy)	Galactosylceramide Galactosylsphingosine	Galactocerebrosidase	Galactosylceramide	14q21-q31
Metachromatic leukodystrophy	Galactosylsulfatide Lactosylsulfatide	Arylsulfatase A (sulfatidase), sulfatide activator (saposin B)	p-Nitrocatechol sulfate, sulfatide	22q13 10 (activator)
Niemann-Pick disease				
Types A and B	Sphingomyelin, cholesterol	Sphingomyelinase	Sphingomyelin	11p15.1-p15.4
Type C	Unesterified cholesterol, bismonoacylglycerophosphate	Cholesterol esterification	Filipin staining LDL-cholesterol	18p
Schindler's disease	α-N-Acetylgalactosaminyl oligosaccharides and glycopeptides	α-N-Acetylgalactosaminidase (α-galactosidase B)	pNP-α-Gal NAC 4MU-α-Gal NAC	22q13
Neuronal Ceroid Lipofuscinoses				
Infantile form (Haltia-Santavuori)	Granular osmiophilic deposits	Acylthioyl palmityl	Electron microscopy	1p32
Late infantile form (Jansky-Bielschowsky)	Curvilinear bodies, subunit C of mitochondrial ATP synthase	Unknown	Electron microscopy	
Juvenile form (Spielmeyer-Sjögren)	Curvilinear and laminated (fingerprint) bodies, subunit C of mitochondrial ATP synthase	Unknown	Electron microscopy	16p12.1
Adult form (Kufs disease)	Mixed type, osmiophilic deposits and lamellar inclusions	Unknown	Electron microscopy	
Mucopolysaccharidoses				
Hurler's, Hurler-Scheie, Scheie's diseases (MPS-I)	Dermatan + heparan sulfate	α-Iduronidase	4-MU-α-L-iduronide	
Hunter's disease (MPS-II)	Dermatan + heparan sulfate	Iduronate sulfatase	L-O-(α-Iduronic acid-2-sulfate)-(1 → 4)-D-O-2.5-anhydro[1-^{3}H]mannitol-6-sulphate	
Sanfilippo's disease (MPS-III)				
Type A	Heparan sulfate	Heparan N-sulfamidase	[^{35}S]heparin	
Type B	Heparan sulfate	α-N-Acetylglucosaminidase	4-MU-α-N-acetyl-α-D-glucosaminide	
Type C	Heparan sulfate	AcetylCoA: α-glucosaminide acetyltransferase	4-MU-β-D-glucosaminide	
Type D	Heparan sulfate	N-Acetyl-α-glucosamine-6-sulfatase	4-MU-α-N-acetylglucosamine-6-sulphate	12q14
Morquio syndrome (MPS IV)				
Type A	Keratan sulfate Chondroitin-6-sulfate	Galactosamine-6-sulfatase		16q24
Type B	Keratin sulfate	β-Galactosidase	4-MU-β-galactopyranoside	
Maroteaux-Lamy syndrome (MPS-VI)	Dermatan sulfate	N-Acetylgalactosamine 4-sulfatase (arylsulfatase B)	p-Nitrocatechol sulfate	5q11-q13
Sly disease (MPS-VII)	Dermatan and heparan sulfate, chondroitin-4-6-sulfates	β-Glucuronidase	4-MU-β-glucuronide	7q21.11
Multiple sulfatase deficiency	Sulfated lipids, mucopolysaccharides	Arylsulfatases A, B, C, + other sulfatases	p-Nitrocatechol sulfate	
Glycoproteinoses				
Aspartylglucosaminuria	Aspartylgluosamine	Aspartylglucosaminidase	1-Aspartamido-β-N-acetylglucosamine	4q32-q33
Fucosidosis	Fucosyloligosaccharides	α-L-Fucosidase	4-MU-α-L-fucopyranoside	1p34
Galactosialidosis	Sialyloligosaccharides Galactosyloligosaccharides	Protective protein (β-galactosidase and α-neuraminidase)	4-MU-β-galactopyranoside 4-MU-α-D-N-acetylneuraminic acid	20q12-q13.1
α-Mannosidosis	α-Mannosyl-oligosaccharides	α-Mannosidase	4-MU-α-mannopyranoside	19p13.2-q12
β-Mannosidosis	β-Mannosyl-oligosaccharides	β-Mannosidase	4-MU-β-D-mannopyranoside	4

(continued)

TABLE 192-1. *(Continued)*

Disorder	Stored Substance	Primary Deficiency	Enzyme Substrate[a]	Gene Location
Mucolipidoses				
Sialidosis (mucolipidosis I)	Sialyloligosaccharides Sialylglycopeptides	α-Neuraminidase	4-MU-α-D-N-acetyl neuraminic acid	10pter-q23
Mucolipidosis II (I-Cell disease)	Sialyloligosaccharides, glycoproteins, glycolipids	UDP-N-Acetylglucosamine: lysosomal enzyme N-Acetylglucosamine-1-phosphotransferase	UDP-N-acetylglucosamine + α-methylmannose	4q21-q23
Mucolipidosis III (pseudo-Hurler polydystrophy)	Sialyloligosaccharides, glycoproteins, glycolipids	Same phosphotransferase as above	Same as above	4q21-q23
Mucolipoidosis IV	Gangliosides, phospholipids, mucopolysaccharides	Unknown	GM2-ganglioside turnover	
Other lysosomal diseases				
Acid lipase deficiency				
Wolman's disease	Cholesterol esters, triglycerides	Acid lipase	4-MU-oleate cholesteryl oleate	10q23.2-q23.3
Cholesterol ester storage disease	Cholesterol esters, triglycerides	Acid lipase	4-MU-oleate Cholesteryl oleate	10q23.2-q23.3
Glycogenosis type II (Pompe's disease)	Glycogen	α-Glucosidase (acid maltase)	4-MU-α-D-glucopyranoside	17q23
Sialic acid storage disease				
Infantile form	Free sialic acid	Sialic acid transport		
Salla's disease	Free sialic acid	Sialic acid transport		6q

[a] 4-MU, 4-methylumbelliferyl; pNP, p-nitrophenol.

proteinoses there is a slowly progressive infiltration of connective tissue with coarsening of the facial features, thickening of hair, skin, and ear cartilage, and skeletal dysmorphism. This may be plainly evident before the child is 1 year old, as in the severe form of Hurler's disease or may be more subtle and progress much more slowly as in Sanfilippo's disease or fucosidosis.

Within the second year, developmental delay or loss of motor milestones is usually the presenting feature. Multiple sulfatase deficiency, metachromatic leukodystrophy, and mucolipidosis IV may first become obvious during this period. However, it must be recognized that because of the slowly progressive nature of the lysosomal diseases, the child's developmental progress may continue, albeit more slowly than normal, for many months before a problem is recognized. This occurs less often in a family with older normal children who serve as a comparison than in the family with an only child. The tendency for delay in diagnosing a progressive degenerative disease may also exist when an acute illness or surgery intervenes. A febrile illness in a child with metachromatic leukodystrophy may cause prolonged weakness and apathy from which the child recovers only to become afflicted, several months later, with gait difficulty, loss of speech, and incoordination. Repeated ear infections in the youngster with a mucopolysaccharidosis may cause partial deafness and delay speech development. Following insertion of tubes into the tympanic membranes, hearing is improved, speech begins to develop, and the child's forward progress may obscure the underlying illness until further clinical signs appear.

In general, the earlier the onset, the more rapid the progression of the disease. Disorders with neuronal storage as the prime focus of their pathology progress more rapidly than disorders primarily affecting white matter. Cognition is most severely compromised in the gangliosidoses and in those mucopolysaccharidoses in which heparan sulfate is the principal accumulating substance, namely, the severe form of Hurler's disease and the various forms of Sanfilippo's disease. In the glycoproteinoses, that is, aspartylglucosaminuria, fucosidosis, mannosidosis, and juvenile-onset sialic acid storage disease, the impact of the biochemical lesion is most evident during the developmental period, so that in these patients there is little noticeable further cognitive decline after childhood.

LATER ONSET FORMS

The family members of patients who appear well for several years or even a decade or more before developing symptoms of a lysosomal storage disease frequently ask how a metabolic disease could be present for so many years without becoming manifest. If an infantile form of the disease is also known, then the question also arises as to what factor(s) exist in the later onset form to delay its appearance. Phenotype-genotype comparisons reveal that slightly more residual enzyme activity may be associated with the later onset forms and that the error in genomic DNA is also less severe. In a classical infantile form, the mutation may affect transcription, so that no enzyme protein is produced, resulting in a CRM⁻ situation, while the mutation in the late onset variant might result only in a single base substitution with the production of an enzyme protein differing in only one amino acid from the normal situation. Both residual enzyme analyses and molecular DNA studies are now regularly undertaken by laboratories with a special interest in one or another of the lysosomal diseases, but it is not yet possible in all cases to explain phenotypic differences within an inborn lysosomal disease. This presents a problem in genetic counseling, for one may encounter siblings with different degrees of expression of the same disease at the same age. I have noted this in families with later-onset Krabbe's disease, adult-onset glycogenosis type II, and chronic G_{M2}-gangliosidosis.

The onset of seizures, macular degeneration, and intellectual loss should alert the clinician to the possibility of a neuronal ceroid-lipofuscinosis. In the Jansky-Bielschowsky form, hyperactivity, ataxia, and seizures, typically between ages 2 and 4, precede the onset of visual failure and loss of intellect. The Spielmeyer-Sjögren form usually starts with retinitis pigmentosa and blindness at age 5 to 10. Seizures, an extrapyramidal movement disorder, cerebellar signs, and cognitive decline occur subsequently. Another cause for new onset seizures in the adolescent is the cherry-red spot myoclonus epilepsy syndrome (sialidosis type II). Grand mal attacks, especially on awakening in the morning, and intention myoclonus become very debilitating. Blindness eventually develops, but cognition may be retained for many years.

Niemann-Pick disease type C and Gaucher's disease type 3 have a wide range in age of onset. Vertical gaze paresis in the former and oculomotor apraxia in the latter are common eye signs. I have known of children age 3 to 5 years with Niemann-Pick disease type C who have massive hepatosplenomegaly and severe intellectual impairment progressing to death in the juvenile period, and others with the same disease, but only mild hepatosplenomegaly and adequate intellectual functioning into the third decade. Most patients with the type 3 subacute neuronopathic form of Gaucher disease are from the Norrbottnian region of northern Sweden and are homozygous for a base change at nucleotide 1448 of the gene for glucocerebrosidase.

Unlike classical Tay-Sachs disease, adolescents and young adults with late-onset G_{M2}-gangliosidosis are intellectually intact and seizure-free. However, proximal muscle weakness, first in the hips and later in the shoulders, tremor, dysarthria, and gait difficulties suggest a picture of Kugelberg-Welander disease or slowly progressive amyotrophic lateral sclerosis. Many patients also develop intermittent psychosis resembling the manic phase of bipolar disease or catatonia. Treatment of the psychiatric symptoms with major neuroleptics may cause worsening of the neurologic signs due to the lysosomotropic effect of these drugs. Carbamazepine, valproic acid, fluoxetine, and electrocortical shock therapy have been most helpful in managing the psychotic symptoms in this disease.

Fabry's disease, an x-linked disorder, presents in the preadolescent or adolescent male with bouts of a peculiar burning dysesthetic pain in the extremities. The pain is triggered by exercise, hot weather, or fever and may last minutes to hours. Abdominal complaints, including postprandial pain and diarrhea, are also common. Widespread vascular occlusive disease develops, leading to myocardial infarction, multiple small strokes, especially involving the brainstem, and kidney failure, usually requiring chronic renal dialysis. An early sign is the presence of purple angiokeratoma in the skin, especially at points of friction such as the umbilicus, over the elbows and knees, in the creases of the axillae and buttocks, and over the skin of the penis and scrotum. Affected patients and at least 90% of female carriers have feathery corneal opacities that are best seen in a slit lamp examination. Therapy of this progressive disabling neurovascular disease is directed against amelioration of pain using phenytoin, carbamazepine, acetaminophen, and increased use of fluids in hot weather and prevention of occlusive vascular disease with antiplatelet agents.

Glycogenosis type II can also present in the adult with proximal muscle weakness, especially of truncal musculature, leading to sudden unexpected respiratory failure. There is no cardiac involvement, and liver enlargement may be minimal. Assisted respiration at night during sleep may be required.

Variants of both metachromatic leukodystrophy and Krabbe's disease may also manifest in adults. Failing memory, behavioral changes, incontinence and ataxia suggest late-onset metachromatic leukodystrophy. The patient may preserve social chatter and some comprehension of his local environment, but, over many years, quadriparesis and dementia develop.

Club feet may, for years, be the only sign of incipient Krabbe's disease in the child or young adult. Patients with slow progression may have school difficulties, a suggestion of cortical blindness or a monoparesis. After months or years, weakness and spasticity spreads to involve the other limb on the same side of the body and then the limbs on the opposite side. Intellect in some cases observed by this author has been remarkably preserved. The oldest recorded patient developed limb weakness in her 40s and survived with intact sensorium into her 70s. Comparing the brain magnetic resonance imaging (MRI) findings of adult-onset metachromatic leukodystrophy with those of late-onset Krabbe's disease, one notices in the former a predilection for the loss of frontal white matter, including that of the genu of the corpus callosum, while in Krabbe's disease the white matter loss is primarily parieto-occipital with preferential involvement of the splenium of the corpus callosum.

Maroteaux-Lamy disease in the adult may not be recognized until signs of spinal cord compression supervene. Affected individuals are of normal intelligence, have short stature, and mildly dysmorphic facial features. Childbirth in affected women necessitates cesarean section due to cephalopelvic disproportion. Vertebral and lumbosacral radiculopathy develop as mucopolysaccharides infiltrate the dura and compress the spinal cord and adjacent nerve roots. This complication necessitates neurosurgical intervention with laminectomy and opening of the dural sheath to prevent further cord compression.

DIAGNOSIS

History

Suspicion of the possibility of a lysosomal storage disease should be raised on reviewing the history. Developmental delay alerts the pediatrician to scrutinize closely the prenatal history and birth history for any complication leading to a fixed encephalopathy, including, for example, cerebral dysgenesis from a chromosomal disorder, perinatal infection, and germinal matrix hemorrhage associated with prematurity. As the repertoire of a young infant is quite limited with respect to gross and fine motor control, language, and socialization, signs of early delays in development may not be appreciated, and consequently parents may insist that their child's early development was entirely normal until some event supervened such as a febrile illness, immunization, or injury requiring hospitalization. Therefore, it is important to try to document milestones in growth and neurologic development sequentially from birth and make comparisons with standard growth charts. This rigorous approach will help all concerned to appreciate the degree of developmental delay, to time its onset and to follow its trajectory. As a neurologist, I pay particular attention to the parents' assessment of their child's degree of alertness and responsiveness to stimuli, his ability to learn new skills and words, to understand what is being said to him, his motor milestones, and his play activity. Feeding behavior and sleep habits are also considered.

A family history is also taken to check on consanguinity and the occurrence in the family of a similar disorder, as well as other genetic diseases within the family. At this time, a pedigree is drawn up, which can be used subsequently for carrier testing and genetic counseling of other family members.

Physical Examination

Common physical signs associated with the lysosomal storage diseases are shown in Table 192-2. On inspection of the skin, only a diligent search may reveal angiokeratoma of Fabry's disease, whitish papules on the upper back of the 4-year-old with Hunter's disease, or thickening of the skin over the finger joints of the child with a mucopolysaccharidosis. Similarly, dysmorphism of facial features may be missed unless the child's

TABLE 192-2. Common Clinical Signs of Lysosomal Storage
Diseases

Skin
  Angiokeratoma: Fabry's disease, fucosidosis type 2, β-mannosidosis, Schindler's disease, type II
  White papules: Hunter's disease
  Peau de orange: mucopolysaccharidoses
  Fair complexion: infantile sialic acid storage disease
  Neonatal ascites (hydrops fetalis): Gaucher's disease, G_{M1}-gangliosidosis, infantile sialic acid storage disease, Sly's disease
  Neonatal jaundice: Niemann-Pick disease, type C
Eye
  Corneal clouding: Hurler's disease. Hurler-Scheie disease, Morquio's disease, Maroteaux-Lamy disease, Sly's disease, mucolipidosis II, mucolipidosis IV
  Lens opacities: Fabry's disease
  Macular degeneration: G_{M1}- and G_{M2}-gangliosidoses, neuronal ceroid lipofuscinoses
  Optic atrophy: metachromatic leukodystrophy, Krabbe's disease
  Ophthalmoparesis: Gaucher's disease, types 2 and 3, Niemann-Pick disease, type C
Coarse facies
  G_{M1}-gangliosidosis, glycoproteinoses, mucolipidoses II and III, mucopolysaccharidoses, multiple sulfatase deficiency, sialic acid storage disease
Skeletal abnormalities
  Gaucher's disease, G_{M1}-gangliosidosis, glycoproteinoses, mucolipidoses I-III, mucopolysaccharidoses, multiple sulfatase deficiency
Cardiomegaly
  Pompe's disease, Fabry's disease
Hepatosplenomegaly
  Cholesterol ester storage disease, Farber's disease, Gaucher's disease, glycoproteinoses, G_{M1}-gangliosidosis, mucopolysaccharidoses, Niemann-Pick disease, Wolman's disease

appearance is compared with that of his siblings and his parents. A broad forehead, flattening of the nasal bridge, fullness of the cheeks, and short underslung jaw may easily be missed on the first examination. Therefore I take full frontal and side view photographs of the face of every child I examine, using a Polaroid camera, so that I can study their features and make comparisons with their appearance on subsequent visits. I also measure the distance between the inner and outer canthi to determine whether there is hypo- or hypertelorism present. Other helpful measurements are head circumference, recumbent height, weight, length of the ears, distance between the root of the nose and upper lip, length of the hands and feet and upper body to lower body ratio.

Club feet may indicate long-standing hypertonicity in the legs as in late-onset Krabbe's disease. Contractures are appreciated if there is a systemic survey of all joints by passive range-of-motion testing. Claw hand will be found in Scheie's disease, Maroteaux-Lamy disease, and I-cell disease. A gibbus deformity provides a clue to an underlying deformity of the vertebral spine in I-cell disease and the mucopolysaccharidoses.

Abdominal swelling on the general physical examination leads to the suspicion of hepatosplenomegaly. The examiner should attempt to quantitate the size of the liver and spleen on repeated visits to gain a better idea as to the pace of the storage process. Marked hepatosplenomegaly as occurs in Gaucher's and Niemann-Pick diseases is associated with physical discomfort in the abdomen, digestive difficulties, stunting of growth, and emotional embarrassment to the child on account of his cosmetic appearance.

While the eye examination, especially in the child may require considerable patience and may need to be delayed until the end of the visit, it is often very revealing. Extraocular movements are abnormal in Gaucher's disease types 2 and 3, Niemann-Pick disease type C, and after blindness supervenes in the gangliosidoses, sialidosis, and leukodystrophies. Corneal clouding may be difficult to appreciate unless a penlight is directed obliquely at the cornea. The pupil should be dilated

with a mydriatic to carefully assess the retina for optic atrophy characteristic of the late-infantile leukodystrophies and the later stages of the gangliosidoses, for retinal pigmentation characteristic of the Spielmeyer-Sjögren form of neuronal ceroid-lipofuscinosis, and for macular degeneration as seen in the gangliosidoses, sialidosis type II, and the neuronal ceroid-lipofuscinoses.

As part of the neurologic examination, I look for macrocephaly indicative of communicating hydrocephalus in a child with a mucopolysaccharidosis or glycoproteinoses, or of megancephaly as in Tay-Sachs disease. Microcephaly or failure of the head to grow may suggest a leukodystrophy. Muscle tone is another important indicator. Tone is decreased in the early stages of many of the lysosomal diseases with central nervous system involvement, while in the late stages muscle hypertonicity is more common. In infantile Krabbe's disease, muscle tone is not consistent, varying from examination to examination. The presence of spinal cord compression as in Maroteaux-Lamy disease leads to spasticity in the extremities. Loss of knee and ankle deep tendon reflexes and sensory functions distally in the legs are consistent with the peripheral neuropathy of classical Krabbe's disease and late-infantile and juvenile metachromatic leukodystrophy.

Laboratory Workup

With a heightened awareness that your patient may have a lysosomal storage disease, how best should one proceed without doing a large battery of expensive tests? I favor a stepwise approach that targets in on one (presumably the correct) diagnosis as swiftly as possible. Several scenarios may be envisioned. A skin biopsy is the most direct way to screen for a lysosomal storage disease. Two specimens are taken, one for electron microscopy, (Figs. 192-1 to 192-6) and the second for fibroblast culture and subsequent biochemical studies as needed. A disposable 3-mm skin punch is used. The skin on the inner aspect of the upper arm adjacent to the axilla is preferred. This is an

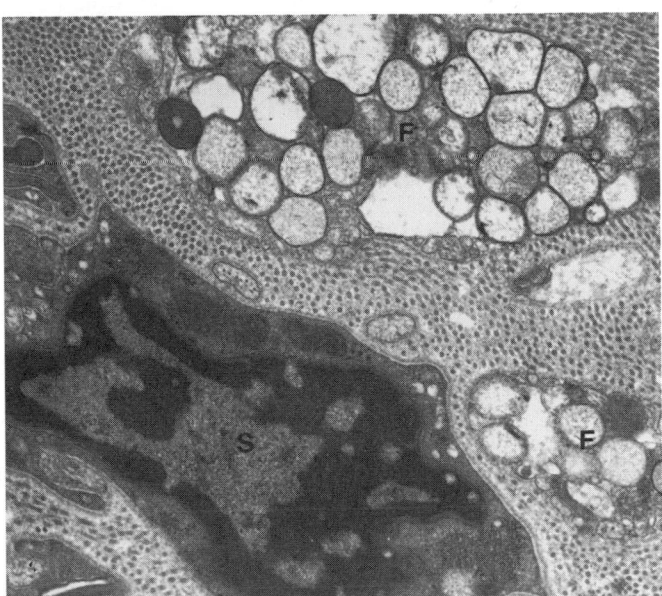

FIG. 192-1. Electron micrograph of a skin biopsy from a 5-year-old boy with mucopolysaccharidosis II illustrating Schwann cell *(S)* and two endoneural fibroblasts *(F)*. The fibroblasts are packed with secondary lysosomes filled with fine fibrillar material. (×14,200.)

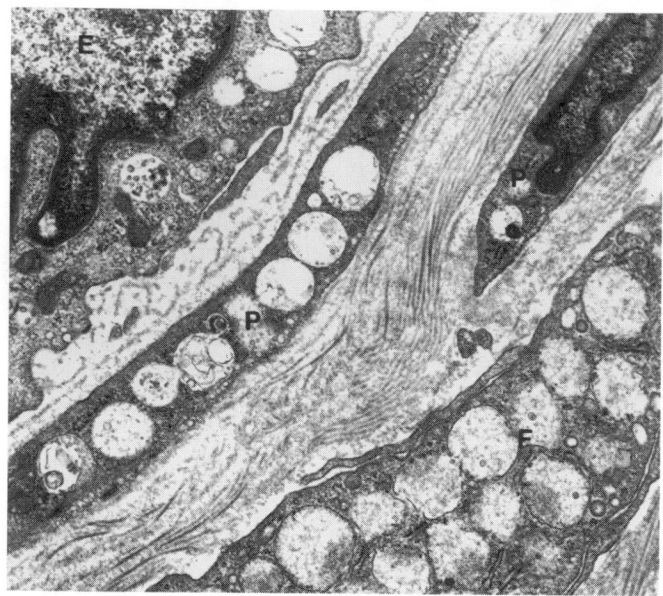

FIG. 192-2. Electron micrograph of a skin biopsy from a 9-year-old girl with hepatomegaly, retarded growth, and retarded mental development due to deficient activity of lysosomal α-fucosidase. The figure shows an endothelial cell *(E)*, two pericytes *(P)* and a fibroblast *(F)* containing numerous secondary lysosomes filled with fine fibrillar material and a few membrane fragments. ($\times$13,500.)

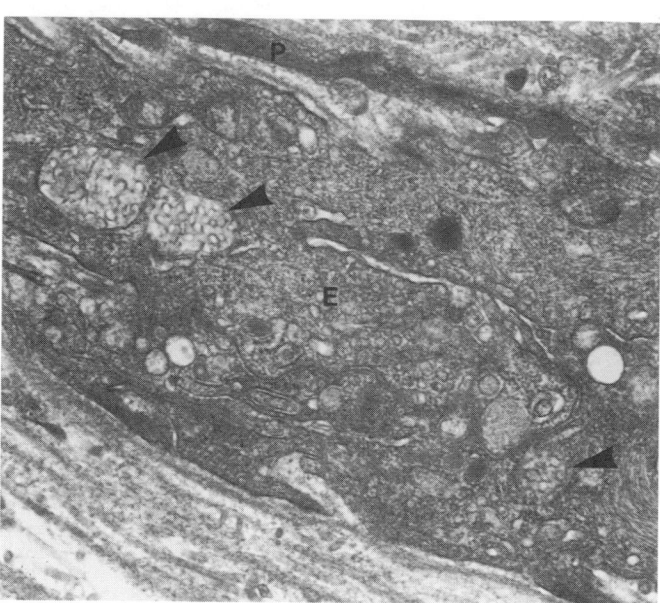

FIG. 192-4. Electron micrograph of a skin biopsy from a 20-year-old man who presented at the age of 5 with retinitis pigmentosa, intellectual decline, and progressively developing grand mal myoclonus and drop attacks. Demonstrated are vascular endothelium *(E)* and pericyte *(P)*. The endothelial cell has three secondary lysosomes filled with curvilinear bodies *(arrowheads)*. ($\times$21,700.)

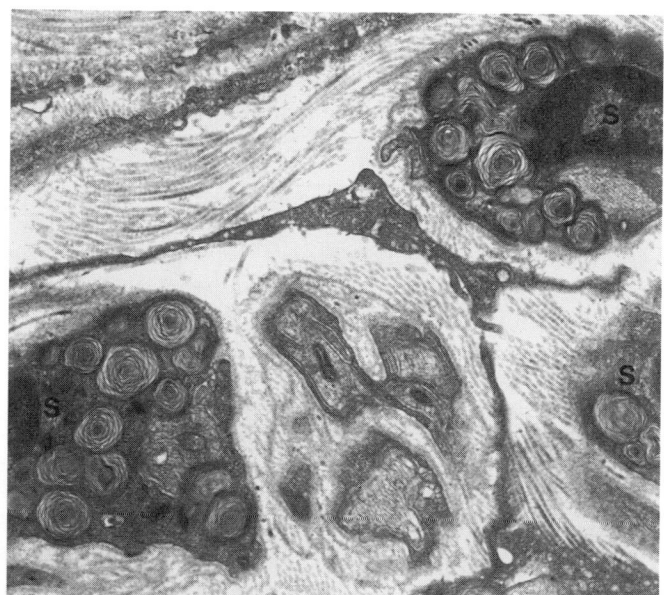

FIG. 192-3. Electron micrograph of a skin biopsy from a 22-month-old boy of Ashkenazi Jewish ancestry who presented at the age of 8 months with generalized hypotonia, microcephaly, and mild delays in motor and speech development. Visible are three Schwann cells *(S)* and unmyelinated axons. The Schwann cell contains numerous secondary lysosomes filled with fine lamellated membrane structures, which is consistent with ML IV. ($\times$13,500.)

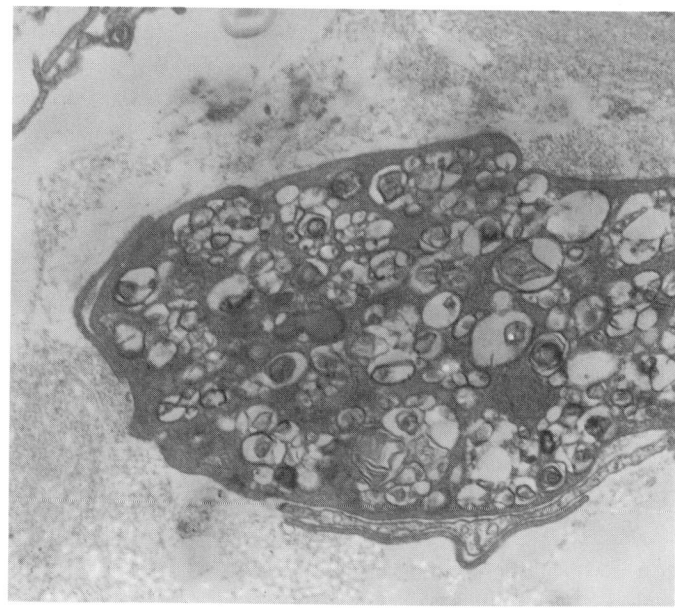

FIG. 192-5. Electron micrograph of a skin biopsy from a 34-year-old man who presented at age 28 with ruptured enlarged spleen that contained foamy macrophages. The figure shows a macrophage containing coarse lamellating membrane structures suggestive of Niemann-Pick type C. Cholesterol esterification assay that was performed following the biopsy confirmed the diagnosis. ($\times$13,500.)

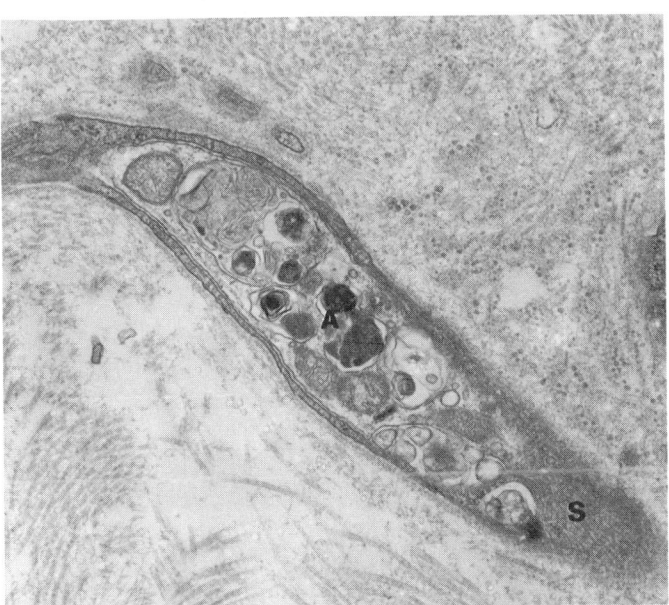

FIG. 192-6. Electron micrograph of a skin biopsy from a 50-year-old woman of Ashkenazi Jewish ancestry with adult form of G_{M2}-gangliosidosis. At age 28 she developed progressive neurologic signs, including oral dyskinesia, muscle weakness, and intermittent numbness. The figure shows a Schwann cell *(S)* and an axon *(A)*. The axon is enlarged and contains secondary lysosomes filled with lamellated membrane structures. ($\times 19,300$.)

area with a high density of dermal nerve endings, thus offering the opportunity to examine Schwann cells and nerve axons as well as sweat glands, vascular endothelia, and other cell types. The skin site is prepared with 70 percent alcohol. Skin preparations containing iodine should be avoided, since iodine may inhibit the growth of cells in tissue culture. A 1 to 2 percent solution of lidocaine is infiltrated within the skin surrounding the site to be biopsied. The specimen is placed in glutaraldehyde for electron microscopy and the other, in tissue culture media such as minimal essential media or Eagle's media. Both specimens should be delivered promptly to the respective laboratories but can be refrigerated overnight if there is to be a delay in delivery to the laboratory. They may also be forwarded by Express Mail without refrigeration.

Nonspecific Slowly Progressive Mental Retardation. Skin biopsy as a screening tool has allowed us to diagnose, for example, fucosidosis and juvenile sialic acid storage disease when there were few clues other than a clumsy child with little or no speech.

If a skin biopsy suggests the possibility of a lysosomal storage disease, then the ultrastructural features must be closely regarded for an indication as to the next steps. At this point, we generally favor analysis of urine for its content of mucopolysaccharides, oligosaccharides, sialyloligosaccharides, and free sialic acid. This will cover a large number of conditions, including the mucopolysaccharidoses, glycoproteinoses, sialidosis, Sandhoff's disease, G_{M1}-gangliosidosis, and sialic acid storage disease. The first morning void is preferred, as it is likely to be the most concentrated specimen of the day. A 24-hour collection is generally not needed, since most laboratories standardize their findings by comparing with the creatinine content of the specimen. For an infant or young child, the collection may be performed by affixing a specially designed plastic container

such as a Hollister U-bag adjacent to the perineum with the opening facing the urethra or penis. An adhesive edge around the opening maintains a closed system with the child's diaper placed over the bag to hold it in place. In the morning, the child is supported vertically while the bag and its contents are removed. The specimen should be kept frozen in a plastic container until it is delivered to the testing laboratory.

A spot test will reveal the presence of an excess of mucopolysaccharides, but quantitative tests for uronic acid and thin layer chromotography to separate the individual species, that is, dermatan sulfate, heparan sulfate, and other tests will help in further characterizing the type of mucopolysaccharidosis present. Similarly, thin layer chromatography is performed to separate the individual oligosaccharides and sialyloligosaccharides. The relative mobility of the individual compounds on the thin layer plate and their pattern may point to one particular form of glycoprotein storage disease.

Facial and Skeletal Dysmorphism. When developmental delay is associated with facial and skeletal dysmorphism, we will start by examining the urine for mucopolysaccharides, oligosaccharides, sialyloligosaccharides, and free sialic acid as described above. The diagnostic workup should also include an x-ray of the skull looking for thickening of the inner table and J-shaped sella, x-ray of the long bones and hands to check on cortical thickness and other evidence of dysplasia, and a lateral view of the spine for anterior beaking of the vertebrae and rounding of the edges of the vertebral bodies. Radiographic studies may also disclose pelvic bone dysplasia. If the urine and/or x-ray studies are suggestive, then blood and/or a skin biopsy are taken for lysosomal enzyme determinations.

Hepatosplenomegaly. Enlargement of the liver and/or spleen often signify a storage disease of the reticuloendothelial system. Examination of the peripheral blood smear can confirm the presence of storage vacuoles in lymphocytes and monocytes and Reilly-Alder bodies in granulocytes. Further investigations may include a bone marrow smear and biopsy for foam cells and Gaucher's cells, but eventually lysosomal enzyme studies on blood or cultured cells will be needed to make a definitive diagnosis.

Seizures. Seizures are a feature of the neuronal ceroid-lipofuscinoses, the gangliosidoses, sialidosis type 2, and Krabbe's disease. An electroencephalogram (EEG) is desirable to document epileptiform discharges as stimulus-provoked spasms can often be misinterpreted as seizures. A careful examination of the retina will also help to discern the presence of a cherry-red macula or other form of macular degeneration. Further evaluation will require a skin biopsy for ultrastructural analysis and enzyme analyses of cultured fibroblasts. In exceptional circumstances, one might elect to do a rectal biopsy or remove the appendix to search for neuronal storage in the cells of the myenteric plexuses.

Leukodystrophy. Brain white matter degeneration occurs primarily in Krabbe's disease, metachromatic leukodystrophy, and multiple sulfatase deficiency but also develops secondarily in the neuronal storage diseases as a consequence of nerve cell and axonal degeneration. A brain MRI examination, evoked potentials, and nerve conduction studies help to characterize the leukodystrophies. If metachromatic leukodystrophy or multiple sulfatase deficiency is being considered, collection of 100 ml of urine to quantitate sulfatide excretion greatly aids in differentiating pseudodeficiency of arylsulfatase A from true arylsulfatase A deficiency and also allows the detection of the activator deficiency form of metachromatic leukodystrophy in the presence of normal levels of arylsulfatase A activity. If clinical signs point to a leukodystrophy and tests for the lysosomal diseases are negative, other nonlysosomal leukodystrophies should be considered, including adrenoleukodystrophy, Alexander's disease, Canavan's disease, and Pelizaeus-Merzbacher disease. Biochemical and/or molecular tests for each of these diseases are available.

TREATMENT

The first obligation of the clinician when faced with the prospect of a lysosomal storage disease is to reach a definitive diagnosis as quickly as possible. This will save the family money and time that would otherwise be devoted to numerous fruitless diagnostic excursions. It will provide information that can be immediately utilized for the prenatal diagnosis of subsequent pregnancies and can provide therapists in early intervention programs with a more realistic view as to what types of progress they can expect for the child in the future. In certain of the mucopolysaccharidoses and leukodystrophies, if the diagnosis is made early enough, the child might be a candidate for enzyme replacement therapy through bone marrow transplantation.

For most lysosomal diseases, supportive care is all that can be offered with the expectation that the disease may continue to progress. Seizures can be treated with anticonvulsants, muscle spasms with diazepam and baclofen, and ankle contractures by orthoses placed in the shoe. A child who is not eating and losing weight may require a permanent gastrostomy. Heel cord lengthening and other types of tendon surgery may be required for severe contractures or clubfoot deformities. For Gaucher's disease types 1 and 3, specific enzyme therapy is available so that splenectomy is no longer done in this disease.

The neurologist should remain available to the patient with a lysosomal disease, offering to see the patient and his family at frequent intervals. In this way, each new complication can be recognized, its pathogenesis explained to the family, and strategies developed to minimize its effects. Also, frequent visits allow the physician the opportunity to update the patient and his family concerning new findings regarding the biochemistry and molecular genetics of the disease and what is happening locally, nationally, and internationally in research on the condition. Among present initiatives, gene therapy appears to offer the most promise to patients with lysosomal diseases, but considerable work with animal models is needed before human trials will become feasible.

ACKNOWLEDGMENT

I would like to thank Joseph Alroy, D.V.M., for preparing and providing the electron micrographs for Figures 192-1 to 192-6.

SUGGESTED READINGS

Adams RD, Lyon G, Kolodny EH: Neurology of Hereditary Metabolic Diseases of Children. 2nd Ed. McGraw-Hill, New York, 1995
Alroy J, Kolodny EH: Lysosomal metabolism and its relevance to skeletal muscle. pp. 708–738. In Engel AG, Franzini-Armstrong C (eds): *Myology*. 2nd Ed. McGraw-Hill, New York, 1994
Desnick RJ: Treatment of Genetic Diseases. Churchill Livingstone, New York, 1991
Kolodny EH, Tenembaum AL: Storage diseases of the reticuloendothelial system. pp. 1452–1491. In Nathan DG, Oski FA (eds): *Hematology of Infancy and Childhood*. 4th Ed. WB Saunders, Philadelphia, 1993
Scriver CR, Beaudet AL, Sly WS, Valle D: The Metabolic and Molecular Basis of Inherited Disease. Part 12. Lysosomal Enzymes. pp. 2427–2882. McGraw-Hill, New York; 1995
Suzuki K: Genetic disorders of lipid, glycoprotein, and mucopolysaccharide metabolism. pp. 793–812. In: *Basic Neurochemistry*. 5th Ed. Raven Press, New York, 1994

193. DIAGNOSIS AND MANAGEMENT OF MITOCHONDRIAL DISEASES

DONALD R. JOHNS

The mitochondrial encephalomyopathies are a diverse group of disorders that have in common functional, structural, or genetic abnormalities of mitochondria. A wide variety of neurologic symptoms occur in association with these disorders, (Table 193-1) affecting virtually the entire neuraxis. Cardinal neurologic manifestations include the following:

Chronic progressive external ophthalmoplegia (CPEO): ptosis and ophthalmoplegia
Mitochondrial encephalomyopathy, lactic acidosis, and strokelike episodes syndrome (MELAS): strokelike episodes
Myoclonic epilepsy with ragged red fibers (MERRF): myoclonus and seizures
Leber's hereditary optic neuropathy (LHON): optic neuropathy

Overlap neurologic manifestations include the following:

Myopathy
Fatiguability and exercise intolerance
Sensorineural hearing loss
Ataxia
Vascular headache
Dementia
Peripheral neuropathy
Seizures
Dystonia

In addition to these neurologic manifestations, a number of somatic organ systems may be prominently affected, and thus the internist may be in a pivotal position to recognize these patients and initiate a diagnostic evaluation. The main systemic manifestations are as follows:

Cardiac conduction defects
Cardiomyopathy
Diabetes mellitus
Short stature
Renal tubular dysfunction
Hepatopathy
Pigmentary retinopathy, cataracts
Sensorineural hearing loss
Episodic nausea/vomiting

Intestinal pseudo-obstruction
Hypoparathyroidism
"Horse-collar" lipomas

Recent advances in the molecular genetic analysis of these diseases have had a major impact on their diagnosis and management. Each of the mitochondrial diseases is a relatively rare entity, but the availability of specific molecular genetic assays for many of these diseases indicates that they have a higher prevalence than previously suspected on clinical grounds alone. Moreover, they represent some of the first molecularly proven examples of many cardinal types of neurologic disease: myopathy (CPEO), stroke (MELAS), seizures (MERRF), and optic neuropathy (LHON). Thus information gleaned from the detailed study of the pathophysiologic basis of these diseases may further our understanding of much more prevalent diseases such as stroke and epilepsy.

Mitochondria function to produce sufficient ATP to fuel the myriad energy-requiring cellular processes. Mitochondria contain their own mitochondrial DNA (mtDNA), which encodes essential components of oxidative phosphorylation. mtDNA has a number of properties that make it a unique genetic element, including exclusive maternal inheritance and a high mutation rate. The human mitochondrial diseases have been associated with a variety of pathogenetic mutations involving mtDNA-encoded genes.

Deletions of mtDNA, as opposed to point mutations, are not transmitted from one generation to the next. For this reason diseases caused by mtDNA deletions such as CPEO are usually sporadic, whereas diseases that result from point mutations of mtDNA such as MELAS, MERRF, and LHON may demonstrate a maternal pattern of inheritance. Unusual autosomal dominant families occur who have CPEO-plus on the basis of multiple mtDNA deletions. Not all persons who harbor a pathogenetic mtDNA point mutation will express the disease. Therefore, these mitochondrial diseases will often appear to occur sporadically despite the existence of the mutation in previous generations. The mitochondrial diseases exhibit variable penetrance and expressivity, as well as marked intrafamilial and interfamilial variation.

Consideration of the possibility of a mitochondrial disease depends on the recognition of characteristic clinical features or laboratory findings or a maternal pattern of inheritance. Many of the mitochondrial diseases have prominent neuro-ophthalmologic manifestations, and referral to an experienced neuro-ophthalmologist may be invaluable. The simplest tests for mitochondrial dysfunction are serum or cerebrospinal fluid lactate concentrations, which are often increased in patients with mitochondrial disease. Unfortunately, this increased concentration is rather insensitive and may be mild and present intermittently.

Skeletal muscle, a relatively accessible tissue, is clinically involved in many of these disorders and is the focus of most diagnostic procedures. Electromyography can document the presence of a myopathy even in the absence of clinically overt symptoms. In vivo phosphorus magnetic resonance spectroscopy of resting muscle is a powerful tool that may detect associated metabolic abnormalities, but it is not 100 percent specific and is not widely available.

Skeletal muscle biopsy, with appropriate histochemical stains, has remained the gold standard in the diagnosis of most mitochondrial diseases. Light microscopy may reveal ragged red fibers on Gomori trichrome stain or focal cytochrome oxidase-negative fibers. Ultrastructural analysis may reveal more direct evidence of abnormal, proliferating mitochondria. Skeletal muscle is suitable for biochemical analysis and provides appropriate material for the molecular genetic assays that have revolutionized the diagnostic workup of these diseases.

MAJOR CATEGORIES OF MITOCHONDRIAL DISEASE

The basic clinical features of each of the major mitochondrial encephalomyopathies are outlined here, with an emphasis on the molecular genetic testing now available for each of them and the evolving clinical conceptualizations of these diseases.

Chronic Progressive External Ophthalmoplegia

One of the cardinal manifestations of human mtDNA disorders is CPEO, which manifests as a slowly progressive disorder of extraocular muscle that is typically symmetric and unaccompanied by diplopia. The initial manifestation of this disorder is usually ptosis, but the ophthalmoparesis is progressive and eventually results in total ophthalmoplegia. CPEO may occur in isolation or may be accompanied by a number of other ophthalmologic, neurologic, and systemic features (termed *ophthalmoplegia-plus*). One subset of the ophthalmoplegia-plus disorders is the Kearns-Sayre syndrome, which is characterized by ophthalmoplegia, onset before 20 years of age, and pigmentary retinopathy plus at least one of the following: cardiac conduction defects, elevated cerebrospinal fluid protein concentration (more than 100 mg/dl), or cerebellar ataxia. Many of the neurologic and somatic findings in CPEO, other than ophthalmoplegia and ptosis, are also seen in other mtDNA diseases (see lists above).

Molecular genetic analysis of mtDNA from skeletal muscle will demonstrate large deletions in most patients with CPEO. The frequency of demonstrable mtDNA deletions depends on the presence of other features: 50 percent of patients with isolated CPEO harbor a deletion, whereas 80 percent of patients with CPEO and pigmentary retinopathy, and 90 percent of patients with the Kearns-Sayre syndrome, have deletions. At least some of the deletion-negative patients have pathogenetic mtDNA point mutations in transfer RNAs (tRNA), including the 3,243-mtDNA point mutation seen in most patients with MELAS syndrome. These deletions, which were the first proven examples of mtDNA abnormalities causing human disease, can be detected by several different molecular genetic methods. Size, location, and proportion of deleted mtDNA is poorly correlated with the phenotypic expression or associated biochemical abnormalities.

Mitochondrial Encephalomyopathy, Lactic Acidosis, and Strokelike Episodes Syndrome

The MELAS syndrome is a significant cause of stroke in the young. The strokelike episodes tend to occur in the setting of prolonged focal seizures or prolonged vascular headache. A number of molecularly confirmed MELAS patients were initially misdiagnosed as having herpes simplex encephalitis. Episodic nausea and vomiting are noted intercurrently and are particularly severe at the time of the strokelike events. The strokes do not follow vascular territories but have a definite posterior preponderance, so many patients develop cortical visual field defects. The strokes appear to be caused by an overwhelming defect in substrate utilization rather than the usual defect in substrate availability operative in occlusive vascular disease. The neurologic deficits may be reversible despite demonstrable signal abnormalities on magnetic resonance imaging (MRI) studies.

The availability of molecular genetic testing has broadened the clinical parameters of MELAS syndrome. The age of onset ranges from infancy to 45 years. Developmental delay and short stature may be noted in the early-onset cases, whereas dementia may predominate in older patients. Seizures are virtually always present and vascular headache occurs commonly. A host of other neurologic accompaniments common to many mitochondrial diseases are also found (see list above), and these may precede the development of strokelike episodes. Computed tomography (CT) may demonstrate basal ganglia calcification or evidence of tissue loss. MRI may reveal the signal abnormalities of new and old "infarcts" with a posterior predominance. The laboratory abnormalities found in all mitochondrial encephalopathies are as follows:

Myopathic potentials on electromyography
Ragged red fibers in skeletal muscle biopsy
Sensorineural hearing loss on audiogram
Cardiac conduction defects
Elevated serum and cerebrospinal fluid lactate concentration
Basal ganglia calcification or focal signal abnormalities on MRI
Axonal and demyelinating peripheral neuropathy on nerve conduction studies
Oxidative phosphorylation defects on biochemical studies
Molecular genetic demonstration of mtDNA mutation

MELAS syndrome has been linked to two-point mutations in the tRNA-leucine^{UUR} mtDNA gene. The mutation at position 3,243 accounts for 80 to 90 percent of patients with the MELAS phenotype and can be detected by molecular genetic analysis of polymerase chain reaction-amplified mtDNA. The mutation was originally described in DNA extracted from muscle, but DNA derived from noninvasive tissues such as blood and urine also contains a detectable proportion of the mutation.

Recognition of the MELAS syndrome in a young stroke patient may dramatically alter the extent and nature of the diagnostic workup and management. Since many of the strokelike episodes occur in the setting of prolonged seizures, we recommend aggressive treatment of the seizure disorder with vigilant attention to anticonvulsant levels. Genetic counseling must be individualized in each family and can be supplemented with molecular genetic testing of noninvasive tissues from maternal relatives. Most cases are sporadic, but mild oligosymptomatic manifestations may be seen in maternal relatives. One important goal of genetic counseling is to ensure an affected male proband that because of the strict maternal transmission of mtDNA he will not pass the disorder to his offspring. His maternal relatives are at risk for the disorder and the women may also act as carriers.

Myoclonic Epilepsy and Ragged Red Fibers

MERRF is the third major mitochondrial encephalomyopathy to have its molecular basis identified in recent years. The dominant clinical symptoms are myoclonus, seizures, and ataxia. A peculiar form of respiratory insufficiency is seen in the most severe cases. Some of the associated neurologic and somatic manifestations of mitochondrial encephalomyopathies (see above) are also seen. Most patients with MERRF have a point mutation in the tRNA-lysine gene at position 8,344 that can be detected by molecular genetic methods in skeletal muscle and blood. Characteristic "horse-collar" lipomas also occur in association with this mutation.

Leber's Hereditary Optic Neuropathy

LHON was the first human disease shown to be caused by a heritable defect in mtDNA. The core clinical phenotype is that of a painless optic neuropathy occurring in an otherwise healthy young person. Loss of central vision may occur rapidly or may progress slowly for several months. Visual symptoms often affect only one eye initially, but virtually always involve both eyes within 1 year. Most patients become symptomatic in the third or fourth decade of life, with a mean age at onset of 28 years (range, 6 to 80 years). Men are affected much more frequently than women (male/female ratio, 2 to 3:1). Since most patients with molecularly proven LHON have no documented family history of visual loss, the neurologist should not be dissuaded from the diagnosis of LHON in the absence of a suggestive family history.

The visual loss is severe, with a nadir of visual acuity ranging from 20/200 to hand motions and is accompanied by central or cecocentral scotomas. The funduscopic findings at the onset of visual loss are variable and may be entirely normal. Optic atrophy eventually supervenes in the chronic phase. Significant recovery of visual acuity is noted in some patients and is more commonly associated with certain LHON genotypes. Other neurologic accompaniments are infrequent and include peripheral neuropathy and demyelinating disease. The pathogenesis of acute visual loss in LHON appears to involve a complex interplay of genetic and epigenetic factors. Environmental factors that have been implicated include the use of tobacco and alcohol, diabetes mellitus, vitamin B$_{12}$ deficiency, head trauma, and occupational exposures.

Major diagnostic errors occur in a number of different situations of acute visual loss in patients who are eventually proven to have LHON on a molecular basis. LHON should be considered in any patient with an atypical optic neuritis (painless, bilateral, no recovery), a presumed toxic or nutritional optic neuropathy (especially alcohol/tobacco amblyopia), or anterior ischemic optic neuropathy. The most important dictum for the workup of suspected LHON is to have a high index of suspicion and to order appropriate molecular genetic testing.

The availability of reliable molecular genetic testing has revolutionized the diagnosis of LHON. Four primary pathogenetic mtDNA mutations have been described to date in LHON, and each can be readily detected with molecular genetic techniques. The first mutation at nucleotide position 11,778 in the ND-4 gene accounts for 50 to 55 percent of cases and can be detected with 100 percent sensitivity and specificity by molecular genetic analysis of polymerase chain reaction-amplified mtDNA extracted from a routine blood sample. The 11,778 mutation is a poor prognostic sign for significant recovery of visual acuity and in 5 percent of families is associated with demyelinating disease in maternal relatives.

Three other LHON-associated mtDNA mutations account for about 30 percent of cases and occur at nucleotide positions 3,460 (ND-1 gene), 15,257 (cytochrome b gene), and 14,484

(ND-6 gene) of mtDNA. The core clinical phenotype of painless visual loss is the same, but each mutation has some specific clinical features that distinguish it. The most notable distinctive feature is the prognosis for visual recovery, which varies nearly 10-fold among the various mutations: 4 percent (11,778 mutation); 22 percent (3,460 mutation); 28 percent (15,257 mutation); and 37 percent (14,484 mutation). The 15,257 mutation is associated with a higher prevalence of neurologic accompaniments, particularly spinal cord and peripheral nerve involvement, and with a pigmentary retinopathy.

Molecular genetic testing for each of the three primary mtDNA mutations is 100 percent specific but is only approximately 80 to 85 percent sensitive at present. This testing has proved useful in a number of different settings, including confirmation of the diagnosis in probable cases and establishment of the diagnosis in atypical or obscure cases of optic neuropathy. In addition to expediting the diagnostic workup of LHON, molecular genetic testing has implications for family counseling, risk factor intervention, prognosis for visual recovery, and therapy.

Coexistent systemic abnormalities that are occasionally associated with LHON such as cardiac conduction defects, migraine, and peripheral neuropathy should be recognized and treated appropriately. Referral for genetic counseling and low vision assessment are also important in the management of LHON patients.

Novel Mitochondrial Disease Phenotypes

The four disorders discussed above were for many years thought to have a mitochondrial etiology based on clinical, laboratory, or maternal inheritance characteristics. Recent advances in molecular genetics have established their precise etiologic basis. More recently a number of novel mitochondrial disease phenotypes have been identified on the basis of mtDNA defects. These include a family from England with a syndrome of peripheral neuropathy, ataxia, retinitis pigmentosa, seizures, developmental delay, and dementia (NARP) caused by an mtDNA mutation at nucleotide 8,993 in the ATPase 6 gene. This mutation was subsequently found in a subset of Leigh's disease patients who demonstrated maternal inheritance. We have identified a family with a syndrome of subacute optic neuropathy and myelopathy (Devic syndrome) that harbored mtDNA mutations in the cytochrome oxidase II gene and in the tRNA-aspartate gene. We predict that a wide array of neurologic and non-neurologic manifestations will be demonstrable in future novel mitochondrial disease phenotypes.

Movement disorders have only rarely been associated with mitochondrial diseases, but recently dystonia has emerged as a prominent manifestation in patients with several different mtDNA mutations. We have seen dystonia as the dominant clinical feature in patients with the 3,243 mtDNA mutation and with multiple mtDNA deletions who also had CPEO. Dystonia has also been prominent in exceptional maternal families with LHON-like visual loss and infantile bilateral striatal necrosis.

Mitochondrial dysfunction may also play a somewhat different role in some of the more prevalent neurodegenerative disorders, such as Parkinson's and Alzheimer's diseases. It is unclear at present if these mitochondrial abnormalities reflect a primary or secondary alteration in these diseases and a great deal of investigative interest is now focused on these issues. Perhaps most intriguing of all is the potential role of mtDNA mutations in aging (arguably the most prevalent condition in humans).

Molecular genetic analysis of mtDNA in human disease has had a rapid and profound impact on a number of different diseases that are of primary interest to the internist and neurologist. Although the diseases covered in this chapter are discussed as separate entities, many of the patients have clinical and laboratory features that overlap (see lists above). Internists and neurologists are in a pivotal position to recognize these patients and to guide their diagnosis and management. Many patients with mitochondrial diseases will present with partial or novel phenotypes and will require a high index of suspicion from an astute clinician. We anticipate that molecular genetic advances in the near future will allow us to diagnose more of these challenging patients definitively and will eventually guide their effective treatment.

TREATMENT

The treatment of mitochondrial diseases is similar to that of most other neurologic disorders in that no ''magic bullet'' is available and we must instead focus on broader therapeutic goals.

Detection and Correction of Co-Morbid Features

A number of signs and symptoms occur in the mitochondrial encephalomyopathies that contribute significantly to their morbidity and these could be rigorously pursued and corrected (see lists above). Seizures should be treated with carbamazepine or phenytoin if parenteral therapy is required; phenobarbital is avoided. Myoclonus may respond to clonazepam. Vascular headache in the proband or oligosymptomatic relatives should be treated with calcium channel-blockers (e.g., verapamil, sustained release 120 to 480 mg/d). Ptosis surgery should only be performed by an experienced oculoplastic surgeon who is aware of the need for undercorrection to avoid disabling exposure keratitis caused by concomitant facial weakness in patients with CPEO.

Sensorineural hearing loss is a correctable condition that contributes significantly to the disability caused by a number of different mitochondrial diseases and should be vigorously diagnosed and treated. Virtually every organ system can be affected in mitochondrial encephalomyopathy patients (see list above) and referral to the appropriate specialist is warranted. Cardiologic consultation can be particularly important since the cardiac manifestations may be life-threatening. Diabetes mellitus is very prevalent in the mitochondrial diseases and can be the dominant clinical feature in some families.

Avoidance of Inappropriate Therapy

In addition to having direct therapeutic implications, establishment of the correct diagnosis as a mitochondrial encephalomyopathy avoids inappropriate therapy for the wrong condition (e.g., treatment for myasthenia gravis in CPEO, anticoagulation in the MELAS syndrome, or high-dose steroids in LHON). Molecular genetic techniques may expedite the diagnostic workup and thereby avoid risks and complications of unnecessary procedures, such as angiography in the MELAS syndrome.

General Recommendations

Energy metabolism is compromised in patients with mitochondrial encephalomyopathies and thus overexertion to the point of fatigue and exhaustion should be avoided. Patients are advised to avoid prolonged fasting and to eat frequent light meals. Exposure to potential environmental cofactors, such as alcohol and tobacco use in LHON, should be eliminated. Fever is treated aggressively with acetaminophen and aspirin should be avoided. When antibiotic treatment is required, chloramphenicol and tetracycline should be avoided because of the toxicity to mitochondria.

Pharmacologic Therapy

Our knowledge of specific pharmacotherapy of the mitochondrial encephalomyopathies is limited by several factors, including their variable natural history (especially the MELAS syndrome) and their relatively low prevalence. A cohort of molecular genetically defined cases may provide an appropriate study population for future clinical trials. Our current knowledge is dominated by anecdotal experience and clinical trials with limited numbers of patients. Nevertheless, rational treatments have been formulated based on our knowledge of oxidative phosphorylation and intermediary metabolism.

Pharmacologic therapy is aimed at circumventing the biochemical deficit and preventing the secondary deleterious effects (e.g., the accumulation of reactive oxygen free radicals). One underlying principle is to avoid toxicity, and thus many agents are naturally occurring substances. Therapeutic monitoring can be accomplished by observation of the clinical response, changes in the levels of lactate and pyruvate at rest and with standardized exercise, and by phosphorous nuclear magnetic resonance spectroscopy.

Carnitine may become depleted from the muscle of mitochondrial encephalomyopathy patients, especially those with a significant lactic aciduria. Repletion with L-carnitine, 2 to 3 g/d, is advocated in patients with documented low levels in plasma or muscle. Coenzyme Q_{10} (ubiquinone) has been used in a number of mitochondrial encephalomyopathy patients at dosages ranging from 60 to 300 mg/d (average dose, 90 to 120 mg/d). The beneficial effects of coenzyme Q_{10} have been more prominent on skeletal muscle and cardiac muscle than on extraocular muscles. Coenzyme Q_{10} has been remarkably free of side effects, although some of our patients have complained of malodorous body secretions. Cofactors of oxidative phosphorylation have been given in pharmacologic dosages, including riboflavin (vitamin B_2, 100 mg/d) and thiamine (vitamin B_1 100 to 1,000 mg/d).

Free radical scavengers are used to allay the deleterious effects (e.g., lipid peroxidation) of excess free radicals that accumulate proximal to blocks in the electron transport chain. These include vitamin C (ascorbate, 2 to 4 g/d), vitamin E (tocopherol, 400 IU/d), and coenzyme Q_{10} (ubiquinone, 60 to 300 mg/d). Dichloroacetate, which stimulates pyruvate dehydrogenase, has been used to treat lactic acidosis of diverse etiologies, including mitochondrial encephalomyopathy cases. It is not available in the United States for routine use, however.

Corticosteroids are used in every neurologic condition for which definitive therapy is not available and the mitochondrial encephalomyopathies are no exception. Steroids have had anecdotal success in the treatment of MELAS syndrome patients, but they must be used with great caution in patients with mitochondrial diseases because of the frequent coexistence of impaired glucose tolerance.

Genetic Counseling and Therapy

The genetics of the mitochondrial encephalomyopathies are complicated, owing to the genetic composition of oxidative phosphorylation complexes by nuclear DNA and mtDNA-encoded proteins that must interact in a very precise manner. Most cases of CPEO-plus are sporadic and thus relatives are not at increased risk. Exceptional autosomal dominant CPEO cases have been noted that were caused by a defect in a nuclear-encoded factor involved in the maintenance of mtDNA fidelity. MERRF is maternally inherited, but a wide spectrum of clinical manifestations is found among maternal relatives. The MELAS syndrome is also maternally inherited, but only one or a few individuals tend to be overtly affected, and most relatives have a partial, oligosymptomatic presentation. LHON is strictly maternally inherited, but our extensive studies of molecularly confirmed cases reveal that only one or a few persons are affected in most families. One powerful genetic counseling principle for the maternally inherited disorders is the lack of paternal transmission, such that an affected male can be confidently assured he will not pass his condition to his offspring.

Our knowledge of the precise molecular basis of the mitochondrial encephalomyopathies is advancing rapidly and ultimately this information may guide effective genetic therapy.

SUGGESTED READINGS

Beal MF: Does impairment of energy metabolism result in excitotoxic neuronal death in neurodegenerative illness? Ann Neurol 31:119–30, 1992

Ciafaloni E, Ricci E, Shanske S et al: MELAS: clinical features, biochemistry, and molecular genetics. Ann Neurol 31:391–8, 1992

DiMauro S, Moraes CT: Mitochondrial encephalomyopathies. Arch Neurol 50: 1197–208, 1994

Holt IJ, Harding AE, Cooper JM, Morgan-Hughes JA: Mitochondrial myopathies: clinical and biochemical features of 30 patients with major deletions of mitochondrial DNA. Ann Neurol 26:699–708, 1989

Johns DR: Mitochondrial encephalomyopathy p. 329. In Johnson RT, Griffin JW (eds): Current Therapy in Neurologic Disease. Mosby-Year Book, St. Louis, 1993

Johns DR: Genotype-specific phenotypes in Leber's hereditary optic neuropathy. Clin Neurosci (in press)

Johns DR: Mitochondrial DNA mutations and eye disease. In Wiggs JL (ed): Molecular Genetics of Ocular Disorders. John Wiley & Sons, New York, 1994 (in press)

Johns DR, Stein AG, Wityk RJ: MELAS syndrome masquerading as herpes simplex encephalitis. Neurology 43:2471–3, 1993

Newman NJ: Leber's hereditary optic neuropathy: new genetic considerations. Arch Neurol 50:540–8, 1993

Zeviani M: Nucleus-driven mutations of human mitochondrial DNA. J Inherited Metab Dis 15:456–71, 1992

SECTION 7. TOXINS AND DRUG EFFECTS

194. NEUROLOGIC COMPLICATIONS OF ALCOHOLISM

MICHAEL E. CHARNESS

Alcohol ingestion and alcoholism are associated with protean changes in the nervous system. This chapter reviews the diagnosis and management of alcohol intoxication, alcohol withdrawal, and the nervous system complications of alcoholism. A review of the biochemical and physiologic effects of alcohol on the nervous system can be found in Charness (1992).

INTOXICATION, PHYSICAL DEPENDENCE, AND ALCOHOL WITHDRAWAL

Intoxication

Incoordination can be measured at blood ethanol concentrations of approximately 35 mg/dl. A blood ethanol concentration of 100 mg/dl legally defines intoxication in most states, although a few states have adopted a lower limit of 80 mg/dl. At these and higher concentrations, ethanol causes dysarthria, ataxia, encephalopathy, and sedation. In nonalcoholic individuals, blood ethanol concentration in excess of 450 mg/dl is frequently lethal, with death resulting from inhibition of medullary control of respiration.

Tolerance

Chronic consumption of ethanol produces significant tolerance to its intoxicating effects. In emergency rooms, literally hundreds of sober alcoholics are found to have blood ethanol concentrations well in excess of 100 mg/dl. The highest blood ethanol concentration ever reported, 1,510 mg/dl, was measured in an alcoholic described as "agitated and slightly confused but alert, responsive to questioning, and oriented to person and place (though unclear as to time)". The fact that some alcoholics show few signs of intoxication at blood ethanol concentrations that would prove lethal in nonalcoholic individuals attests to the remarkable capacity of the nervous system to adapt to ethanol. This adaptation begins during the first hours of drinking. During a single bout of drinking, naive subjects became sober at blood ethanol concentrations higher than those associated with initial intoxication. Animal studies confirm that tolerance to ethanol may occur after 30 minutes of ethanol administration.

Physical Dependence and the Withdrawal Syndrome

Physical dependence is a state in which ethanol is required to maintain normal central nervous system (CNS) function. Chronic ethanol ingestion provokes biochemical and physiologic adaptations that render CNS function normal in the pres-

ence of ethanol. These plastic CNS responses become maladaptive when ethanol intake is abruptly discontinued. There ensues a state of tremulousness, agitation, and autonomic hyperactivity, which is in many ways opposite to the clinical syndrome of acute intoxication. The alcohol withdrawal syndrome evolves gradually over hours to days after the cessation of drinking. Tremulousness appears after 8 to 12 hours followed in some instances by generalized tonic-clonic seizures. Delirium tremens, a state of autonomic hyperactivity, agitation, and hallucinations, typically begins 1 to 2 days after alcohol withdrawal and lasts for several days to a week or more. Delirium tremens may directly follow a series of alcohol withdrawal seizures, leading to a prolonged postictal alteration of sensorium.

Alcohol Withdrawal Seizures

Most alcohol withdrawal seizures occur between 12 and 48 hours after a sharp decline in blood alcohol concentrations. Some alcoholics will drink to control the tremulousness that sometimes precedes seizures; hence the smell of alcohol on the breath does not rule out the diagnosis of alcohol withdrawal seizures. Typically, alcohol withdrawal seizures are brief, may recur within a period of 6 to 12 hours and are self-limited. If the patient has recovered completely within this period of time, has a clear history of recent alcohol withdrawal, and a normal neurologic examination, then neuroimaging studies are unlikely to disclose a cerebral lesion. In contrast, prolonged or widely separated seizures, focal seizures, prolonged postictal state, or a focally abnormal neurologic examination should prompt a search for correctable structural lesions, metabolic abnormalities, or infection (Table 194-1). Nearly half of seizure admissions to a city hospital were attributable to alcohol withdrawal. Although only a small percentage of patients withdrawing from alcohol will develop status epilepticus, alcohol withdrawal may be a complicating factor in approximately one-fifth of all patients with status epilepticus. Likewise, alcohol withdrawal may precipitate seizures in patients with idiopathic or symptomatic epilepsy. The observation that some patients have ingested alco-

TABLE 194-1. Causes of Prolonged Postictal State After Alcohol Withdrawal Seizures

Trauma
Subdural hematoma
Traumatic subarachnoid hemorrhage
Intracerebral hemorrhage
Infection
Meningitis
Seizure
Nonconvulsive status epilepticus
Previous brain injury
Metabolic encephalopathy
Hypoglycemia
Wernicke's encephalopathy
Hyponatremia
Hepatic encephalopathy
Drug or toxin ingestion
Sepsis
Hypoxia

hol within an hour of a first seizure has led some investigators to postulate that ethanol intoxication can lower seizure threshold.

Treatment of alcohol withdrawal seizures is largely symptomatic. There is no evidence that the administration of anticonvulsants after an initial alcohol withdrawal seizure will prevent subsequent seizures during the same period of withdrawal. The long-term administration of anticonvulsants for uncomplicated ethanol-withdrawal seizures is unnecessary and possibly dangerous. Some alcoholics will abruptly withdraw from both alcohol and anticonvulsants, thereby increasing the risk of status epilepticus.

Management of the Alcohol Withdrawal Syndrome

Mild alcohol withdrawal syndromes can be managed effectively with oral benzodiazepines such as chlordiazepoxide, which may be titrated against agitation and tremulousness. Replacement of most vitamins and minerals can also be accomplished orally, although it is preferable to administer thiamine parenterally, since oral absorption of thiamine is unreliable in alcoholic and malnourished patients. Intravenous benzodiazepines, hydration, and replacement of magnesium and vitamins are the mainstays of therapy for severe alcohol withdrawal syndromes. The neuropharmacologic actions and therapeutic efficacies of most commonly used benzodiazepines are similar; hence the selection of a particular benzodiazepine is often based on pharmacokinetic considerations. Chlordiazepoxide, diazepam, and lorazepam are effective benzodiazepines that may be administered orally or parenterally. Oxazepam may be preferable in patients with liver disease because clearance of oxazepam is less dependent on hepatic metabolism than that of other benzodiazepines. Strikingly high doses of benzodiazepines may be required to control agitation due to alcohol withdrawal. Benzodiazepines produce sedation by potentiating the actions of γ-aminobutyric acid (GABA), the major inhibitory neurotransmitter in the CNS, and studies in animals suggest that chronic ethanol administration decreases the number and function of selective GABA receptor subunits. Clonidine has been reported to decrease the autonomic hyperactivity of alcohol withdrawal and β-adrenergic receptor blockers may be useful in suppressing tremulousness as well as autonomic hyperactivity.

Dehydration may develop rapidly during alcohol withdrawal because of agitation and diaphoresis. Vigorous intravenous hydration as well as sedation may be required to prevent hypotension. Venous access provides an opportunity to rapidly correct potential deficiencies of multiple vitamins and electrolytes. Symptomatic hyponatremia should be corrected slowly to prevent the occurence of central pontine myelinolysis, which occurs more frequently in alcoholics than in nondrinkers. It is important to administer multivitamins as well as additional supplements of thiamine (100 mg/day) because of the high incidence of unrecognized Wernicke's encephalopathy in alcoholics (see below). Magnesium deficiency is particularly common in alcoholics and may contribute to the alcohol withdrawal syndrome. Hypomagnesemia is associated with cardiac arrhythmias and complicates the correction of coexisting hypokalemia and hypocalcemia. Magnesium is also a cofactor for transketolase, one of the thiamine-dependent enzymes implicated in the pathogenesis of Wernicke's encephalopathy. Serum magnesium in alcoholics is frequently in the low-normal to low range despite the presence of significant magnesium deficiency. Metabolic studies have established magnesium deficits of approxi-

mately 2 mEq/kg in alcoholic patients; hence seemingly enormous quantities of magnesium must be administered to replete total body stores. One suggested regimen is to administer 6 g of magnesium (1 ampule of magnesium sulfate contains 1 g or 8.13 mEq of magnesium) over 3 hours in intravenous fluids followed by another 10 g of magnesium by continuous intravenous infusion over the next 24 hours and 6 g daily for an additional 3 days.

CENTRAL NERVOUS SYSTEM COMPLICATIONS OF ALCOHOLISM

Brain Lesions in Alcoholics

Alcoholism is complicated by a variety of neurologic disorders, most of which produce characteristic brain lesions. The most frequent causes of brain lesions in alcoholics are as follows:

Wernicke's encephalopathy
Alcoholic cerebellar degeneration
Hepatocerebral degeneration
Trauma
Central pontine myelinolysis
Fetal alcohol syndrome
Marchiafava-Bignami syndrome
Alcohol neurotoxicity
Pellagra

Malnutrition is common in alcoholics, who may derive most of their calories from ethanol (7 kcal/g). Thiamine deficiency is particularly frequent and leads to Wernicke's encephalopathy. Thiamine deficiency may also contribute to alcoholic cerebellar degeneration and alcoholic peripheral neuropathy. Pellagra is a disorder of dementia, dermatitis, and diarrhea resulting from a deficiency of nicotinic acid, which is now rare in the Western world. Alcoholics are subject to repeated episodes of head trauma. Alcoholic liver disease may cause hepatocerebral degeneration. Prenatal exposure to alcohol causes a variety of brain lesions associated with cognitive dysfunction. Finally, alcohol may directly damage the nervous system, although specific lesions of alcoholic neurotoxicity have not yet been described.

Cognitive Disorders in Alcoholics

Mild cognitive impairment can be demonstrated by neuropsychological testing in 50 to 70 percent of detoxified alcoholics, and several groups have reported that abstinence leads to an improvement in cognitive function, particularly in the first weeks after the cessation of drinking. Approximately 10 percent of alcoholics exhibit stable and severe cognitive dysfunction ranging from Korsakoff's amnestic syndrome, a selective anterograde and retrograde amnesia, to dementia. Both patterns of cognitive dysfunction have been documented in patients whose brains reveal only the lesions of nutritional deficiency.

Wernicke's Encephalopathy

Wernicke's encephalopathy is the neurologic manifestation of thiamine deficiency. The characteristic lesions occur symmetrically in structures surrounding the third ventricle, aqueduct and fourth ventricle. The mammillary bodies are involved in virtually all cases, and the dorsomedial thalamus, locus ceruleus, periaqueductal gray, ocular motor nuclei, and vestibular nuclei are commonly affected. Acute Wernicke lesions can be identified by endothelial prominence, microglial proliferation, and occasional petechial hemorrhages. In chronic lesions, there is demyelination, gliosis, and loss of neuropil with relative preservation of neurons. Atrophy of the mammillary bodies develops in up to 80 percent of cases after acute Wernicke's encephalopathy and occurs rarely in other disorders. In the Western world, Wernicke lesions are found most commonly in alcoholics.

In clinically based series, most patients with Wernicke's encephalopathy present with a classical triad of encephalopathy, oculomotor dysfunction, and gait ataxia. The encephalopathy is characterized by profound disorientation, indifference, and inattentiveness. Some patients exhibit an agitated delirium related to ethanol withdrawal. Ocular motor abnormalities include nystagmus, lateral rectus palsy, and conjugate gaze palsy. Gait ataxia is common, and is likely due to a combination of polyneuropathy, midline cerebellar involvement, and vestibular paresis. In contrast, ataxia of the arms and dysarthria or scanning speech are infrequent.

Computed tomography (CT) scanning may show symmetric, low-density abnormalities in the diencephalon and periventricular regions, which enhance after the injection of contrast. Gross hemorrhages are uncommon in acute Wernicke's encephalopathy, but have also been detected by CT. Symmetric areas of increased or decreased signal in the diencephalon, midbrain, and periventricular regions are relatively uncommon in other disorders, and when present in alcoholics, should strongly suggest the diagnosis of acute Wernicke's encephalopathy. However, the paucity of reports of such findings would suggest that CT is an insensitive method for their detection.

Magnetic resonance imaging (MRI) appears to be more sensitive than CT in detecting acute diencephalic and periventricular lesions. Patients with acute Wernicke's encephalopathy have exhibited areas of increased T2 signal surrounding the aqueduct and third ventricle and within the medial thalamus and mamillary bodies, consistent with the localization of the pathologic lesions (Fig. 194-1). Corresponding areas of decreased T1 signal have also been detected. The alterations in T1 and T2 signal have been shown to resolve over months, leaving an enlarged aqueduct and third ventricle. The sensitivity of MRI and CT in detecting Wernicke lesions has not been determined; hence a normal CT or MRI does not rule out acute Wernicke's encephalopathy.

Clinical recognition of Wernicke's encephalopathy is straightforward when alcoholics present with the classical triad of ataxia, oculomotor disorders, and encephalopathy. However, autopsy-based series suggest that many patients lack one or more elements of this triad, and in some, lethargy or coma is the predominant clinical feature. In these patients, the diagnosis of Wernicke's encephalopathy is frequently overlooked. Hence it is important to administer large doses of parenteral thiamine (100 mg/day for 5 days) to all patients with undiagnosed altered mental status, oculomotor disorders, or ataxia. Gastrointestinal absorption of thiamine is erratic in alcoholic and malnourished patients, making oral administration of thiamine an unreliable treatment for Wernicke's encephalopathy. With prompt administration of thiamine, ocular signs improve within hours to days, and ataxia and confusion within days to weeks. However, a majority of patients are left with horizontal nystagmus, ataxia, and Korsakoff amnestic syndrome.

Korsakoff Amnestic Syndrome

Many alcoholic patients recovering from classical Wernicke's encephalopathy exhibit the selective memory disturbance of Korsakoff amnestic syndrome. This striking neurologic disorder is characterized by marked deficits in anterograde and retrograde memory, apathy, an intact sensorium, and relative preservation of long-term memory and other cognitive skills. Confabulation is a feature of some cases. One alcoholic poet passed an hour with me reciting flawlessly the works of Wordsworth, but had no recollection of our meeting 1 minute after I stepped out of the room. Korsakoff amnestic syndrome may develop without an antecedent episode of Wernicke's encephalopathy. Some alcoholics with Wernicke lesions exhibit global abnormalities of higher cognitive function, leading to the mistaken diagnosis of Alzheimer's disease.

Mamillary body atrophy is a relatively specific abnormality in patients with chronic lesions of Wernicke's encephalopathy. A decrease in the volume of the mamillary bodies can be identified by MRI in approximately 80 percent of alcoholics with a history of classical Wernicke's encephalopathy and is not found in control subjects, patients with Alzheimer's disease, or alcoholics without a history of Wernicke's encephalopathy (Fig. 194-2). The finding of small mamillary bodies in a demented patient should raise the possibility that alcoholism and malnutrition have contributed to the dementia. Enlargement of the third ventricle, and by inference, shrinkage of the diencephalon, has been reported in patients with chronic Wernicke's encephalopathy. This finding is less specific than mamillary body atrophy in diagnosing chronic Wernicke's encephalopathy.

Ventricular Enlargement and Cognitive Dysfunction in Alcoholics

Imaging studies, neuropathologic observations, and animal experimentation suggest that ethanol neurotoxicity may contribute to chronic cognitive dysfunction in alcoholics. However, there is as yet no unequivocal evidence for a brain lesion in humans that is caused by chronic ethanol ingestion and is unrelated to coexisting nutritional deficiency, liver disease, or trauma. Reductions in brain weight in alcoholics are small and inconsistently reported. Brain volume, estimated by the volume of the pericerebral space—the cerebrospinal fluid (CSF)-filled region between the brain and skull—is reduced in alcoholics compared to controls, but this indirect measure of cerebral atrophy is most abnormal in alcoholics with liver disease or Wernicke's encephalopathy. Quantitative morphometry suggests that alcoholics, including those with liver disease and Wernicke's encephalopathy, lose a disproportionate amount of subcortical white matter as compared with cortical gray matter. This loss of cerebral white matter is also apparent when brains of nondemented alcoholics with liver disease are compared with those from patients with nonalcoholic liver disease; hence liver disease cannot be the sole cause of this selective loss of brain tissue. The loss of cerebral white matter is evident across a wide range of ages, is not accentuated in the frontal lobes, and is of sufficient magnitude (6 to 17 percent) to account for the associated ventricular enlargement.

CT and MRI show enlargement of the cerebral ventricles and sulci in a majority of alcoholics (Fig. 194-2); however, when corrected for the effects of aging, the radiographic indices do not correlate consistently with either the duration of drinking or the severity of cognitive impairment. The ventricles and sulci become significantly smaller within 1 month of abstinence, but brain water, estimated by MRI or chemical analysis, does not change consistently. Based on these findings, it has been hypothesized that changes in brain parenchyma, but not brain

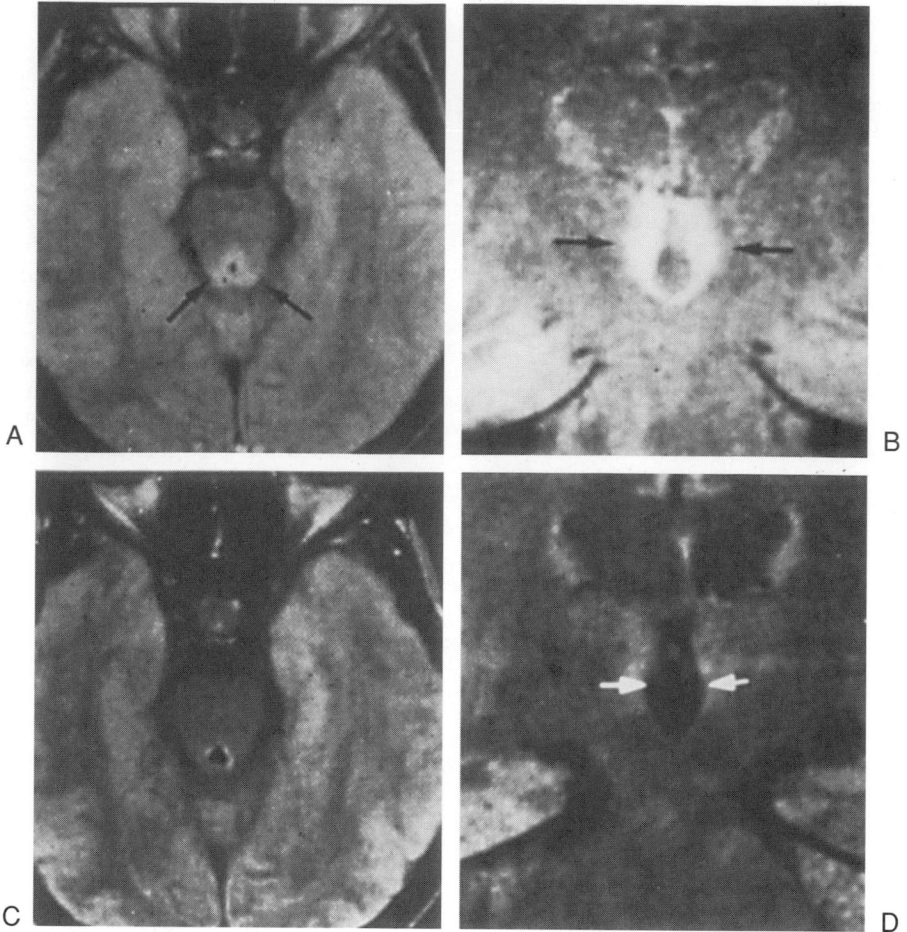

FIG. 194-1.   Resolution of areas of increased T2-weighted signal in acute Wernicke's encephalopathy. **(A)** Increased T2-weighted signal is seen surrounding the aqueduct (*arrows*) and **(B)** third ventricle (*arrows*). **(C)** A later study shows resolution of these abnormalities and enlargement of the aqueduct and **(D)** third ventricle (*white arrows*). (From Gallucci M, Bozzao A, Splendiani A et al: Wernicke encephalopathy: MR findings in five patients. AJR 155:1309, 1990, with permission.)

water, may account for the reversible radiographic and cognitive abnormalities of alcoholics. Reversible brain shrinkage, as determined by neuroimaging, is a nonspecific abnormality that has also been documented after treatment of anorexia nervosa and Cushing syndrome.

Alcoholic Cerebellar Degeneration

Some alcoholic patients develop a chronic cerebellar syndrome related to the degeneration of Purkinje cells in the cerebellar cortex. Midline cerebellar structures—especially the anterior and superior vermis—are predominantly affected, a pattern that resembles the distribution of cerebellar pathology in Wernicke's encephalopathy. Alcoholic cerebellar degeneration typically occurs only after 10 or more years of excessive ethanol use. It is usually a gradually progressive disorder that develops over weeks to months, but may also evolve over years or commence abruptly. Mild and apparently stable cases may become suddenly worse. As in Wernicke's encephalopathy, ataxia affects the gait most severely. Limb ataxia and dysarthria occur more often than in Wernicke's encephalopathy, whereas nystagmus is rare. The diagnosis of alcoholic cerebellar ataxia is based on the clinical history and neurologic examination. CT or MRI scans may show cerebellar vermian atrophy (Figs. 194-2 and 194-3), but one-half of alcoholic patients with this finding

are not ataxic on examination. It is unclear whether these represent subclinical cases in which symptoms will develop subsequently.

Marchiafava-Bignami Syndrome

Marchiafava-Bignami syndrome is a rare disorder of demyelination or necrosis of the corpus callosum and adjacent subcortical white matter, which occurs predominantly in malnourished alcoholics. In some cases there are associated lesions of Wernicke's encephalopathy or selective neuronal loss and gliosis in the third cortical layer. A few cases have been described in nonalcoholics, demonstrating that ethanol alone is not responsible for the lesion. The course may be acute, subacute, or chronic, and is marked by dementia, spasticity, dysarthria, and inability to walk. Patients may lapse into coma and die, survive for many years in a demented condition, or occasionally recover. An interhemispheric disconnection syndrome has been reported in survivors. The disorder was formerly diagnosed only at autopsy, but lesions can now be imaged using CT or MRI. CT may demonstrate hypodense areas in portions of the corpus callosum. MR typically shows cystic areas of decreased T1 signal (Fig. 194-3) or increased T2 signal (Fig. 194-4). The abnormalities may be restricted to one region of the corpus callosum or may be present diffusely throughout the corpus

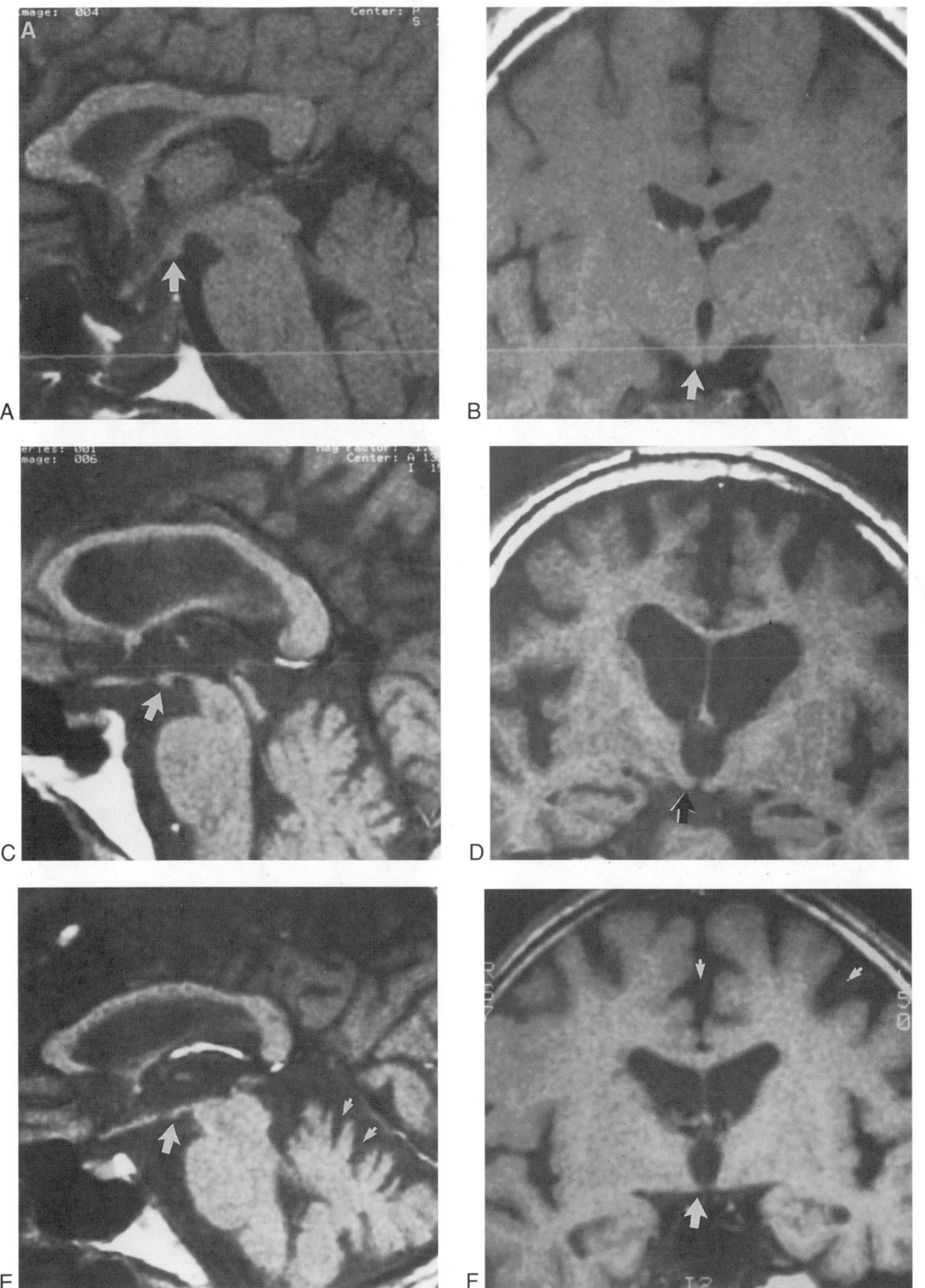

FIG. 194-2. MRI of chronic Wernicke's encephalopathy. **(A & B)** Normal control. **(C & D)** Alzheimer's disease. **(E & F)** Chronic Wernicke's encephalopathy. T1-weighted sagittal (Figs. A, C, E) and coronal (Figs. B, D, F) images in the plane of the mamillary bodies (*arrows*). The Wernicke patient shows atrophy of the mamillary bodies (arrows) and anterior superior cerebellar vermis (arrow heads) and enlargement of the third ventricle (black arrow heads), lateral ventricles, interhemispheric fissure (white arrow heads), and cerebral sulci (white arrow head). The Alzheimer patient exhibits greater cerebral atrophy and ventricular enlargement than the Wernicke patient, yet shows larger mamillary bodies. Images were acquired using TR 600, TE 25. (From Charness ME, De La Paz RL: Mamillary body atrophy in Wernicke's encephalopathy: centemortem identification using magnetic resonance imaging. Ann Neurol 22:595, 1987, with permission.)

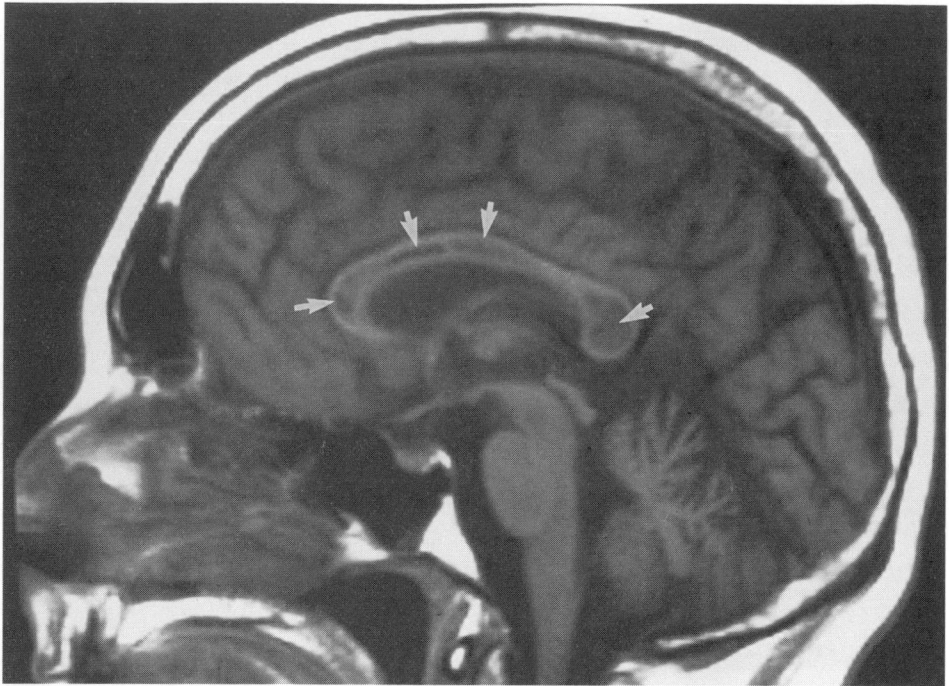

FIG. 194-3.   MRI of Marchiafava-Bignami Syndrome. T1-weighted image shows a cystic region of decreased signal throughout the corpus callosum (*arrows*). There is also atrophy of the mamillary bodies and anterior superior cerebellar vermis. (Courtesy of Professor Jaques Thiébot, Centre Hospitalier, Université de Rouen.)

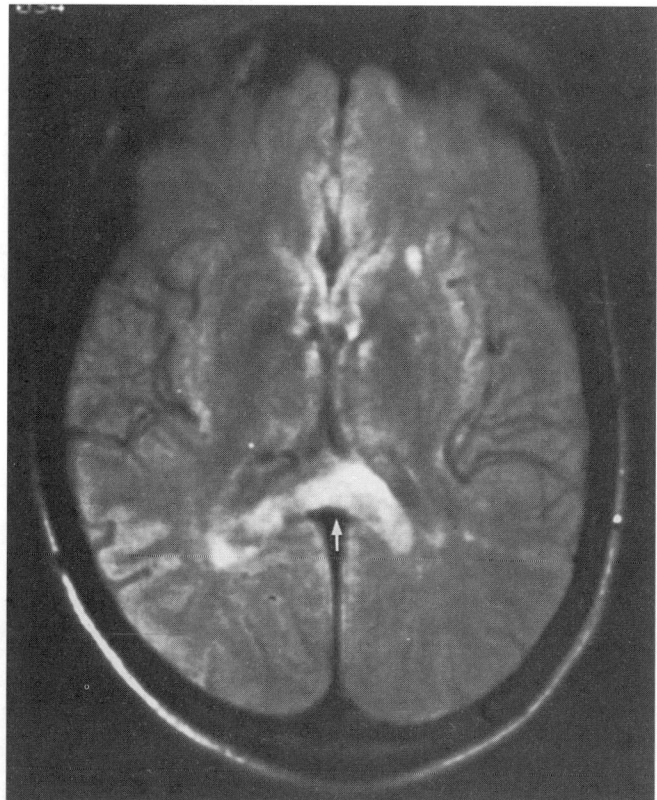

FIG. 194-4.   MRI of Marchiafava-Bignami syndrome. The splenium of the corpus callosum shows an area of increased T2-weighted signal (*arrow*). (TR 2000, TE 40). (From Charness ME: Brain lesions in alcoholics. Alcohol Clin Exp Res 17:2, 1993, with permission.)

callosum. The CT and MR findings may persist after the resolution of clinical signs.

Central Pontine Myelinolysis

Central pontine myelinolysis is a disorder of cerebral white matter that usually affects alcoholics, but also occurs in nonalcoholics with liver disease, including Wilson's disease, malnutrition, anorexia, burns, cancer, Addison's disease, and severe electrolyte disorders, such as thiazide-induced hyponatremia Central pontine myelinolysis is frequently associated with a rapid correction of hyponatremia; however, the majority of cases occur in alcoholics, suggesting that alcoholism may contribute to the genesis of central pontine myelinolysis in as yet undefined ways.

The most common macroscopic lesion is a triangular region of pallor in the base of the pons. Approximately 10 percent of cases also show symmetric extrapontine lesions, most frequently in the striatum, thalamus, cerebellum, and cerebral white matter. Microscopic examination reveals demyelinated axons with preserved cell bodies except in the center of lesions, which may reveal cavitation. Symptoms and signs of central pontine myelinolysis may be absent or obscured by associated conditions, such as ethanol withdrawal, Wernicke's encephalopathy, or hepatic encephalopathy. Treatment of these disorders may lead to an initial improvement in mental status, followed within days by confusion, lethargy, and coma due to central pontine myelinolysis. Involvement of the corticospinal tracts causes paraparesis or quadriparesis and demyelination of the corticobulbar tracts leads to dysarthria, dysphagia, and inability to protrude the tongue. The tendon reflexes may be increased, decreased, or normal, and Babinski signs may be present. Disorders of conjugate eye movement occur occasionally and may reflect extension of the lesion in the pons or associ-

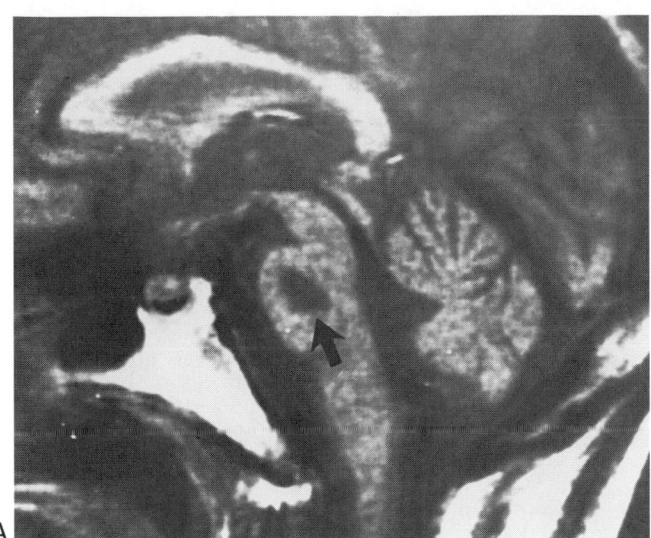
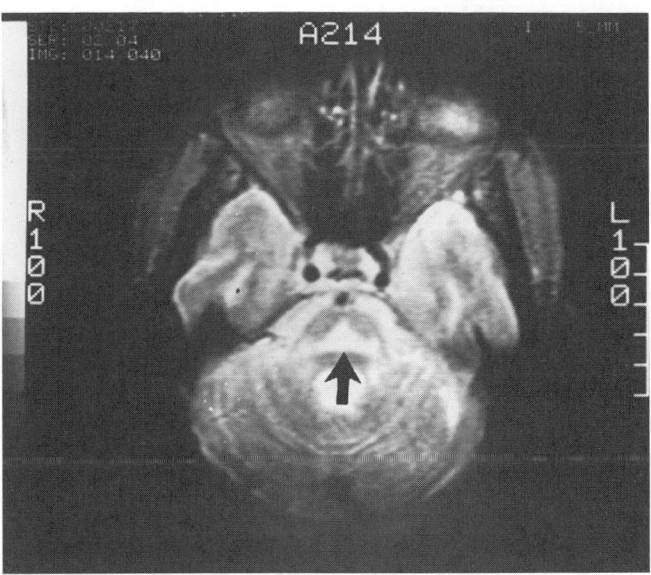

FIG. 194-5. MRI of central pontine myelinolysis in an alcoholic man. **(A)** T1-weighted sagittal image (TR 600, TE 25) reveals a sharply delineated zone of decreased signal in the midpons (*arrow*). **(B)** An axial image through the same region shows a triangular area of increased T2-weighted signal (TR 2000, TE 70) (*arrow*). (From Charness ME: Brain lesions in alcoholics: Alcohol Clin Exp Res 17:2, 1993, with permission.)

ated Wernicke lesions. Disproportionate involvement of motor function may produce the "locked-in" syndrome, with only limited ability to move the limbs or face despite a normal level of consciousness.

The lesions of central pontine myelinolysis can be visualized using CT scanning or MRI. MRI is more sensitive than CT in imaging the pontine lesions; however, even MRI may be unremarkable early in the course of central pontine myelinolysis. The most common MR finding is an area of decreased T1 signal or increased T2 signal within the basis pontis (Fig. 194-5). Symmetric extrapontine abnormalities have also been detected by CT and MRI in patients suspected of having central pontine myelinolysis. Other disorders, such as multiple sclerosis, multi-infarct dementia, and encephalitis, may produce areas of increased T2 signal in the pons that resemble those of central pontine myelinolysis, but also cause significant periventricular abnormalities and a distinctive clinical picture. Serial CT or MRI studies indicate that the radiographic lesions of central pontine myelinolysis may resolve in parallel with patient recovery; hence, the absence of lesions on MRI does not exclude a past episode of central pontine myelinolysis. Because small lesions of central pontine myelinolysis may be asymptomatic, typical MRI abnormalities can be an incidental finding in seriously ill patients.

Ethanol Neurotoxicity in the Developing Nervous System

Brain lesions in alcoholics may antedate birth. Alcoholism runs in families, and many alcoholics have been exposed to high concentrations of alcohol during critical stages of brain development. Fetal alcohol syndrome is characterized by pre- and postnatal growth retardation, microcephaly, neurologic abnormalities, facial dysmorphology, and other congenital anomalies. More often, heavy intrauterine exposure to ethanol is associated with a constellation of less severe "fetal alcohol effects," including mental retardation, intrauterine growth retardation, and minor, ungrouped congenital anomalies involving the cuta-

neous, genitourinary, musculoskeletal, and cardiac systems. Neuropathologic examination in fetal alcohol syndrome reveals microcephaly, cerebellar dysplasia, agenesis of the corpus callosum, and neuronal-glial heterotopias—lesions consistent with the decreased proliferation and disordered migration of neurons. MRI in a small number of children with fetal alcohol syndrome has identified agenesis or hypoplasia of the corpus callosum (Fig. 194-6) and selective reductions in the volume of the cerebrum, cerebellum, and basal ganglia. Agenesis of the corpus callosum occurs infrequently in the general population and its presence on MRI in the retarded offspring of an alcoholic mother should suggest the possibility of a neurodevelopmental abnormality related to gestational alcohol exposure.

PERIPHERAL NERVOUS SYSTEM COMPLICATIONS OF ALCOHOLISM

Neuropathy

Alcoholic patients have a high incidence of peripheral nerve disorders, including symmetric polyneuropathy and compression mononeuropathies. Alcoholic polyneuropathy is believed to result from inadequate nutrition, and particularly from deficiencies of thiamine and other B vitamins. A direct, neurotoxic effect of ethanol may also contribute to this disorder, because ethanol induces a disturbance of fast axonal transport that could promote alcoholic polyneuropathy.

Alcoholic polyneuropathy is a gradually progressive disorder of sensory, motor, and autonomic nerves. The clinical abnormalities are usually symmetric and predominantly distal. Symptoms include numbness, paresthesia, burning dysesthesia, pain, weakness, muscle cramps, and gait ataxia. The most common neurologic signs are loss of tendon reflexes, beginning with the ankle jerks, defective perception of touch and vibration sensation, and weakness. Autonomic disturbances are less common; when present, they may be associated with increased mortality.

"Saturday night palsies" occur when intoxicated patients fall asleep with their arms leaning against a firm surface,

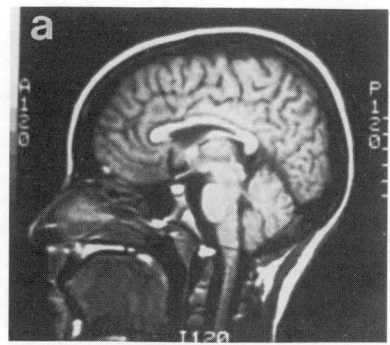
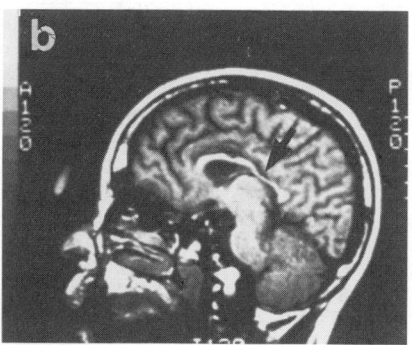
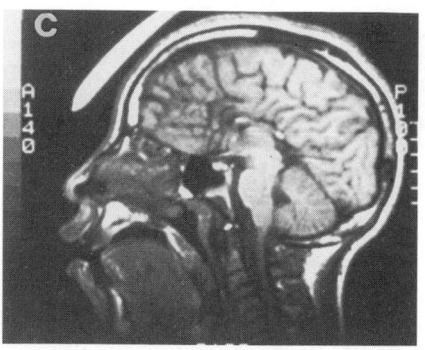

FIG. 194-6.   MRI showing agenesis of the corpus callosum after gestational exposure to alcohol. **(A)** Normal 13-year-old girl. **(B)** A 13-year-old boy with fetal alcohol syndrome and focal thinning (*arrow*) of the corpus callosum. **(C)** A 14-year-old boy with fetal alcohol syndrome and agenesis of the corpus callosum. (Courtesy of Edward P. Riley, M.D., San Diego State University San Diego, CA.)

thereby compressing the radial nerve against the spiral groove of the humerus. Alcoholic polyneuropathy also renders patients susceptible to compression of peripheral nerves at common sites of entrapment, including the median nerve at the carpal tunnel, the ulnar nerve at the elbow, and the peroneal nerve at the fibular head.

Because malnutrition may contribute to the development of alcoholic polyneuropathy, patients with this disorder should receive parenteral thiamine supplementation. Improved nutrition with cessation of drinking appears to be associated with a good prognosis for improvement. Low doses of tricyclic antidepressants are sometimes effective in controlling the burning dysesthesiae of alcoholic peripheral neuropathy.

Myopathy

Skeletal myopathy is an underrecognized complication of alcohol abuse. In recent studies, 46 percent of alcoholic patients visiting an ambulatory clinic and 60 percent of hospitalized alcoholics had biopsy evidence of myopathy. Skeletal muscle can be damaged by the administration of ethanol to well-nourished volunteers, and most patients with alcoholic myopathy are not demonstrably malnourished. Electrolyte abnormalities such as hypokalemia, which are often present in alcoholic patients, can also impair skeletal muscle function. However, studies of alcoholic patients and of ethanol-induced myopathy in rats show no correlation between hypokalemia and muscle damage. The biochemical basis for ethanol-induced muscle damage is unknown, although disturbances of sodium and potassium transport, mitochondrial function, calcium sequestration, and actin-myosin interaction have been proposed.

Alcoholic myopathy may present as either an acute, necrotizing disorder or as a more indolent process. The acute form develops over hours to days, often in relation to an alcoholic binge, and is characterized by weakness, pain, tenderness, and swelling of affected muscles. Animal studies suggest that fasting during a binge may precipitate muscle injury. The great majority of affected patients are men. Proximal muscles are often most severely involved, but the distribution of involvement may be asymmetric or focal. Dysphagia and congestive heart failure may occur. Laboratory findings include moderate to severe elevation of serum creatine kinase (CK), myoglobinuria, fibrillations and myopathic changes in the electromyogram, and muscle fiber necrosis on biopsy; type I muscle fibers defined by their low myosin adenosine triphosphatase activity

may be selectively vulnerable. Initial treatment is directed at correcting cardiac arrhythmias, renal failure due to rhabdomyolysis, and electrolyte disturbances such as hypophosphatemia or hypokalemia. Abstinence from ethanol is usually associated with gradual recovery.

Chronic alcoholic myopathy, which evolves over weeks to months, is a more common disorder. Pain is less prominent than in acute alcoholic myopathy, but muscle cramps may occur. On examination, the major findings are muscle weakness and atrophy, which affect predominantly the hip and shoulder girdles. Although a polyneuropathy coexists in many cases, the clinical and laboratory features of this disorder indicate a primary disturbance of muscle. Muscle biopsies show preferential atrophy of type II fibers defined by their high myosin adenosine triphosphatase activity. Serum CK is less elevated than in acute alcoholic myopathy and myoglobinuria does not occur. Cessation of drinking leads to improvement in most cases, while continued ethanol abuse may result in clinical deterioration.

ACKNOWLEDGMENTS

This work was supported by grants from NIAAA, the Alcoholic Beverage Medical Research Foundation, and the Medical Research Service, United States Department of Veterans Affairs.

SUGGESTED READINGS

Adams RD, Victor M, Mancall EL: Central pontine myelinolysis: a hitherto undescribed disease occurring in alcoholic and malnourished patients. Arch Neurol 81:154, 1959

Aminoff MJ, Simon RP: Status epilepticus: causes, clinical features and consequences in 98 patients. Am J Med 69:657, 1980

Brion S: Marchiafava-Bignami syndrome. p. 317. In Vinken PJ, Bruyn GW (eds): Metabolic and Deficiency Diseases of the Nervous System. Part 2. North-Holland Publishing, Amsterdam, 1976

Carlen PL, Wortzman G, Holgate RC et al: Reversible cerebral atrophy in recently abstinent chronic alcoholics measured by computed tomography scans. Science 200:1076, 1978

Charness ME: Brain lesions in alcoholics. Alcohol Clin Exp Res 17:2, 1993

Charness ME: Molecular mechanisms of ethanol intoxication, tolerance, and physical dependence. p. 155. In Mendelson JH, Mello NK (eds): Diagnosis and Treatment of Alcoholism. McGraw-Hill, New York, 1992

Charness ME, De La Paz RL: Mamillary body atrophy in Wernicke's encephalopathy: antemortem identification using magnetic resonance imaging. Ann Neurol 22:595, 1987

Charness ME, De La Paz RL: Periodic alternating nystagmus in an alcoholic with small mamillary bodies. Neurology 38(suppl):421, 1988

Charness ME, Simon RP, Greenberg DA: Ethanol and the nervous system. N Engl J Med 321:442, 1989 de la Monte SM: Disproportionate atrophy of cerebral white matter in chronic alcoholics. Arch Neurol 45:990, 1988

Earnest MP, Feldman H, Marx JA et al: Intracranial lesions shown by CT scans in 259 cases of first alcohol-related seizures. Neurology 38:1561, 1988

Earnest M, Yarnell PR: Seizure admissions to a city hospital: the role of alcohol. Epilepsia 17:387, 1976

Feussner JR, Linfors EW, Blessing CL, Starmer CF: Computed tomography brain scanning in alcohol withdrawal seizures: value of the neurologic examination. Ann Intern Med 94:519, 1981

Flink EB: Therapy of magnesium deficiency. Ann NY Acad Sci 162:901, 1969

Gallucci M, Bozzao A, Splendiani A et al: Wernicke encephalopathy: MR findings in five patients. AJR 155:1309, 1990

Harper CG, Giles M, Finlay-Jones R: Clinical signs in the Wernicke-Korsakoff complex: a retrospective analysis of 131 cases diagnosed at necropsy. J Neurol Neurosurg Psychiatry 49:341, 1986

Harper CG, Kril JJ: Brain atrophy in chronic alcoholic patients: a quantitative pathological study. J Neurol Neurosurg Psychiatry 48:211, 1985

Harper CG, Kril JJ, Holloway RL: Brain shrinkage in chronic alcoholics: a pathological study. Br Med J 290:501, 1985

Hillbom M, Muuronen A, Holm L, Hindmarsh T: The clinical versus radiological diagnosis of alcoholic cerebellar degeneration. J Neurol Sci 73:45, 1986

Johnson RA, Noll EC, Rodney WM: Survival after a serum ethanol concentration of 1 1/2% [Letter]. Lancet 2:1394, 1982

McLean RM: Magnesium and its therapeutic uses: a review. [Review]. Am J Med 96:63, 1994

Mirsky IR, Piker P, Rosenbaum M, Lederer H: 'Adaptation' of the central nervous system to varying concentrations of alcohol in the blood. Q J Stud Alcohol 2:35, 1941

Ng SKC, Hauser WA, Brust JCM, Susser M: Alcohol consumption and withdrawal in new-onset seizures. N Engl J Med 319:666, 1988

Streissguth AP, Landesman-Dwyer S, Martin JC, Smith DW: Teratogenic effects of alcohol in humans and laboratory animals. Science 209:353, 1980

Torvik A, Lindboe CF, Rodge S: Brain lesions in alcoholics: a neuropathological study with clinical correlation. J Neurol Sci 56:233, 1982

Urbano-Marquez A, Estruch R, Navarro-Lopez F et al: The effects of alcoholism on skeletal and cardiac muscle. N Engl J Med 320:409, 1989

Urso T, Gavaler JS, Van Thiel DH: Blood ethanol levels in sober alcohol users seen in an emergency room. Life Sci 28:1053, 1981

Victor M, Adams RD: The effect of alcohol on the nervous system. Res Publ Assoc Nerv Ment Dis 32:526, 1953

Victor M, Adams RA, Collins GH: The Wernicke-Korsakoff Syndrome and Related Disorders Due to Alcoholism and Malnutrition. FA Davis, Philadelphia, 1989

Victor M, Adams RD, Mancall EL: A restricted form of cerebellar cortical degeneration occurring in alcoholic patients. Arch Neurol 76:579, 1956

Victor M, Brausch C: The role of abstinence in the genesis of alcoholic epilepsy. Epilepsia 8:1, 1967

Warach SJ, Charness ME: Imaging the brain lesions of alcoholics. p. 503. In Greenberg JO (ed): Neuroimaging: a Companion to Adams and Victor's Principles of Neurology. McGraw-Hill, New York, 1995

195. DRUG DEPENDENCE

JOHN C. M. BRUST

This chapter addresses drugs of dependence other than ethanol and tobacco, with an emphasis on phenomena likely to be encountered in ambulatory patients. Although neurologists do not often treat drug intoxication, overdose, or withdrawal, it is worth remembering that the symptoms and signs associated with such conditions are often predominantly neurologic. Space limitations here dictate cursory attention to diverse agents and syndromes. Further information on any of the topics discussed can be found in Brust (1993).

DEFINITIONS

Psychic dependence is a psychic drive—a craving—to administer a drug periodically or continuously either to achieve pleasure or to avoid discomfort. *Physical dependence* is an adaptive state such that cessation of drug administration produces discomfort and objective physical signs. Depending on the drug and the setting, psychic and physical dependence can occur alone or together. *Addiction* refers to psychic dependence. *Tolerance* refers to the need for increasing doses of a substance in order to achieve the same desired effect or to avoid withdrawal symptoms. It may be the result of enhanced metabolism of the drug or of poorly understood adaptive responses in the brain. *Abuse* is a social judgment that may be based on a drug's perceived harmfulness or its legal status. (In the United States the harm a drug does—as in the case of ethanol and tobacco, for example—has little to do with its legality.)

TYPES OF DRUGS: INTOXICATION AND WITHDRAWAL

Opioids

Opioids include natural and synthetic agonists, antagonists, and mixed agonist-antagonists (Table 195-1). Acute effects of opioid agonists include euphoria or dysphoria, drowsiness, analgesia, nausea, vomiting, miosis, pruritus, dry mouth, sweating, suppression of the cough reflex, hypothermia, postural hypotension, respiratory depression, and constipation. Parenteral injection produces a "rush," a brief ecstatic feeling, followed by more lasting euphoria and either drowsy "nodding" or garrulous hyperactivity. Heroin, which is metabolized to morphine, must be taken more than once daily to avoid withdrawal symptoms, and the mental clouding it produces prevents normal social or occupational functioning. It is usually injected intravenously ("mainlining") or subcutaneously ("skinpopping"); fear of acquired immunodeficiency syndrome (AIDS) has made heroin sniffing and smoking increasingly popular. Methadone produces similar effects when taken parenterally; maintenance methadone therapy for heroin addiction is oral once daily and in most patients produces little if any cognitive disturbance.

Overdose from heroin or other antagonists produces the triad of coma, pinpoint (but reactive) pupils, and apnea. It is treated

TABLE 195-1. Major Opioids

Agonist
  Powdered opium
  Tincture of opium
  Camphorated tincture of opium (paregoric)
  Purified opium alkaloids
  Morphine
  Heroin
  Methadone
  Fentanyl
  Hydromorphone
  Codeine
  Oxycodone
  Meperidine
  Levorphanol
  Propoxyphene
Antagonist
  Naloxone
  Naltrexone
Mixed agonist-antagonist
  Pentazocine
  Butorphanol
  Nalbuphine
Partial agonist
  Buprenorphine

with respiratory support and titrated doses of the antagonist naloxone. Because the effects of naloxone are short-lived, hospitalization and close observation are necessary.

Withdrawal symptoms begin 4 to 6 hours after the last heroin dose and include irritability, lacrimation, rhinorrhea, sweating, yawning, myalgia, mydriasis, piloerection, nausea, vomiting, diarrhea, hot flashes, fever, tachypnea, tachycardia, muscle spasms, abdominal cramps, and orgasm. Craving is intense, but seizures, hallucinations, and delirium are not part of the syndrome, which in adults is rarely life-threatening. In neonates myoclonus and probably seizures do occur (they can be difficult to distinguish from jitteriness), and mortality is as high as 90 percent in untreated patients.

Treatment of withdrawal in adults is with methadone and in infants with paregoric.

Psychostimulants

Psychostimulants include amphetaminelike drugs and cocaine; the major drugs in this category are as follows:

Dextroamphetamine
Methamphetamine
Methylphenidate
Phenmetrazine
Diethylpropion
Fenfluramine
Phenylpropanolamine
Ephedrine
Pseudoephedrine
Cocaine

The major psychic effects are probably the result of dopamine agonism; in addition, cocaine has local anesthetic properties. Amphetaminelike drugs are taken orally or parenterally; methamphetamine can be smoked ("ice"). Cocaine hydrochloride is taken intranasally or parenterally; alkaloidal cocaine ("crack") is smoked. Acutely, psychostimulants produce euphoria and increased motor activity. Taken parenterally or smoked, they produce a "rush" that is subjectively different from an opioid rush. With repeated psychostimulant use stereotypic movements progress to bruxism and other dyskinesias, paranoia progresses to frank hallucinatory psychosis, and, especially with cocaine, there may be seizures. Overdose causes excitement, delirium, headache, chest pain, fever (sometimes severe), hypertensive crisis, tachycardia and atrial or ventricular arrhythmias, myoglobinuria, seizures, metabolic acidosis, coma, and death.

Treatment is complex and, depending on symptoms, includes benzodiazepines, oxygen, bicarbonate, anticonvulsants, antihypertensives, cardiorespiratory monitoring, and cooling.

Psychostimulant withdrawal produces few objective signs. There is exhaustion, hunger, and depression, which may be severe and require hospitalization. Craving can be intense.

Sedative Drugs

Sedative drugs include barbiturates, benzodiazepines, and miscellaneous agents (Table 195-2). Some recently developed sedative drugs, for example, buspirone and zolpidem, are believed free of dependence liability; sedative effects resemble ethanol intoxication; there is euphoria or dysphoria, impaired judgment, sleepiness, and ataxia. Overdose causes coma and respiratory depression (far less pronounced with benzodiazepines than with

TABLE 195-2. Major Sedatives/Hypnotics

Barbiturates
  Amobarbital
  Butalbital
  Pentobarbital
  Phenobarbital
  Secobarbital
Benzodiazepines
  Alprazolam
  Chlordiazepoxide
  Diazepam
  Lorazepam
  Oxazepam
  Flurazepam
  Triazolam
Nonbarbiturates/nonbenzodiazepines
  Bromides
  Chloral hydrate
  Ethchlorvynal
  Glutethimide
  Meprobamate
  Methaqualone
  Methylprylon
  Paraldehyde

barbiturates or ethanol). Withdrawal causes tremor, seizures, and, with barbiturates, potentially fatal delirium tremens.

Treatment of overdose or withdrawal often requires intensive care.

Cannabinoids

Marijuana is made from the tops and leaves of the hemp plant, *Cannabis sativa,* which contains numerous cannabinoid compounds, of which δ-9-tetrahydrocannabinol (δ-9-THC) is the principle psychoactive ingredient. Hashish, made from plant resin, has a high concentration of δ-9-THC. Acutely, marijuana causes relaxed dreamy euphoria ("stoned"), often with jocularity or silliness; there may be drowsiness, depersonalization, subjective time-slowing, conjunctival injection, tachycardia, and hypertension or postural hypotension. Higher doses impair judgment and coordination, and very high doses cause illusions or hallucinations and excitement or depression. Regular doses sometimes cause paranoia or panic, but fatal overdose has never been documented, and intoxication does not usually require treatment. Withdrawal can produce nervousness, headache, and craving, but objective signs are not evident.

Hallucinogens

For thousands of years hallucinogenic plants have been used ritualistically and recreationally. Today both natural and synthetic products are available in the United States, and during the early 1990s their popularity increased among American adolescents. The three major categories of hallucinogens are as follows:

Ergot-derived: *d*-lysergic acid diethylamide (LSD)
Indolalkylamines: psilocybin, psilocin
Phenylalkylamines: mescaline, dimethoxymethylamphetamine (DOM), dimethoxyethylamphetamine (DOET), methylenedioxyamphetamine (MDA), methylenedioxymethamphetamine (MDMA, "ecstasy")

Among these, methylenedioxymethamphetamine (MDMA; "ecstasy"), has both hallucinogenic and amphetaminelike effects. Drugs such as mescaline, psilocybin, and LSD produce illusions or hallucinations, often visual, formed, and elaborate, as well as depersonalization, elation, or paranoia, and, variably, tremor, ataxia, tachycardia, hypertension, and fever. Adverse reactions can lead to panic, accidents, or suicide, and some users have "flashbacks"—the spontaneous reappearance of symptoms days or weeks after use.

Treatment of overdose usually consists of calm reassurance; benzodiazepines can be given for severe agitation. There are no withdrawal symptoms.

Household Products Used as Recreational Inhalants

Among the variety of products recreationally inhaled are aerosols (e.g., refrigerants, hair sprays, antiseptics), spot removers, glues, lighter fluid, fingernail polish remover, bottled fuel gas, paints, thinners, gasoline, anesthetics, and "room odorizers" (amyl or butyl nitrite). Users are often children. Although the compounds inhaled are quite different (e.g., halogenated hydrocarbons, *n*-hexane, toluene, butane, nitrous oxide), their acute effects are similar and resemble ethanol intoxication. The need to inhale provides a check against overdose, but fatalities have resulted from accidents, cardiac arrhythmia, suffocation, or aspiration of vomitus.

Treatment of overdose is focused on cardiorespiratory monitoring. There does not appear to be a withdrawal syndrome, but psychic dependence is common.

Phencyclidine

Phencyclidine ("angel dust") was introduced as an anesthetic but withdrawn because it caused psychosis. It can be eaten, snorted, or injected, but is usually smoked, often with marijuana. Low doses produce euphoria or dysphoria, emotional lability, a sense of time-slowing, and a feeling of numbness. Higher doses cause sensory illusions, amnesia, agitation, "burst" nystagmus, sweating, hypersalivation, tachycardia, hypertension, and fever. With overdose there is psychosis with hallucinations or catatonia, dystonia, myoclonus, seizures, rhabdomyolysis, stupor (with a blank stare), and cardiorespiratory collapse.

Treatment includes a quiet environment—trying to "talk down" agitation only increases it—continuous gastric suctioning, activated charcoal, forced diuresis, cardiorespiratory monitoring, and, as needed, antihypertensives, anticonvulsants, benzodiazepines, or neuroleptics. (Neuroleptics, however, can aggravate seizures, hypotension, or myoglobinuria.) Symptoms can last days or even weeks. Although abstinence can produce craving, evidence of physical dependence is difficult to discern.

Anticholinergic Drugs

Around the world a number of plants are ingested recreationally for their anticholinergic properties. In the United States the most popular is the jimson weed, *Datura stramonium.* Users are often children. Other abused anticholinergic agents include antiparkinsonian drugs, antihistamines, and tricyclic antidepressants, especially amitriptyline. The desired effect is euphoria, but higher doses produce dry mouth, decreased sweating, tachycardia, mydriatic unreactive pupils, urinary retention, delirium, hallucinations, seizures, and coma.

The diagnosis is confirmed with physostigmine, which can then be continued in titrated doses as treatment. Other measures include gastric suctioning, activated charcoal, magnesium sulfate, cooling, bladder catheterization, fluids, cardiorespiratory monitoring, and anticonvulsants as needed. Phenothiazines are contraindicated. Symptoms can last days (especially mydriasis),

but fatalities are unusual. Few anticholinergic abusers use the drug on a daily basis, but some do develop withdrawal craving, tremor, nausea, and vomiting.

MEDICAL AND NEUROLOGIC COMPLICATIONS

Trauma

Violence among drug abusers has different causes. It may be secondary to altered behavior induced by the drug, to predatory activities required to procure it, or to the lifestyles and business methods of drug traffickers. In contrast to alcohol, which causes violence largely of the first type, violence and trauma associated with illicit drugs are overwhelmingly the consequence of activities related to their illegality. In 1986, for example, one-third of male homicides in Manhattan were drug-related, and in 1987 over 40 percent of New York City felony indictments were for drug law violations. Before the AIDS epidemic, the case fatality rate for New York City heroin addicts was 1 to 2 percent yearly, and approximately 40 percent of deaths were from violence.

Marijuana impairs judgment and coordination and contributes to automobile accidents. So do sedatives, including long-acting benzodiazepines taken the day before, which can interact synergistically with ethanol. Especially in the elderly, sedatives can produce paradoxical hyperactivity or agitation. Paranoia induced by psychostimulants and phencyclidine can make users a danger to others. Inhalant and hallucinogen users are prone to fatal accidents; some have committed self-mutilation and suicide.

Infection

Parenteral drug use of any kind causes infections that can affect the nervous system. Hepatitis predisposes to hepatic encephalopathy and hemorrhagic stroke. Endocarditis, bacterial or fungal, causes cerebral infarction or abscess, meningitis, and intracerebral or subarachnoid hemorrhage from ruptured septic ("mycotic") aneurysm. Vertebral osteomyelitis can cause radiculopathy or myelopathy, and cellulitis or local abscesses can damage peripheral nerves.

Tetanus, especially common in skin-poppers, tends to be severe in parenteral drug users, often requiring weeks of intensive care with neuromuscular blockade. Botulism can occur from local wound infection or, in intranasal cocaine users, from infected nasal sinuses. Malaria has occurred in epidemic form among needle sharers.

As of 1994, nonhomosexual drug abusers composed 23 percent of AIDS cases reported to the U.S. Centers for Disease Control, and an additional 7 percent were male homosexual or bisexual drug users. In New York City roughly two-thirds of subjects receiving methadone maintenance treatment are human immunodeficiency virus (HIV)-seropositive. Drug abusers with AIDS are subject to the same neurologic complications that affect other risk groups. Related to their often low socioeconomic status, they are at special risk of tuberculosis, including drug-resistant strains, and syphilis, which in such subjects, despite negative blood serology, can progress with unexpected rapidity to tertiary forms of neurosyphilis. Although, on the one hand, parenteral drug abusers are continually bombarding their immune systems with foreign material, and, on the other hand, a number of drugs (including ethanol) are themselves immunosuppressant, drug abuse per se does not appear to accelerate the emergence of AIDS in HIV-seropositive subjects.

Parenteral drug users are frequently seropositive for the retrovirus human T-cell lymphotropic virus type I (HTLV-I), and myelopathy has been reported in some.

Seizures

Seizures in drug abusers may be secondary to stroke, infection, recent or remote head injury, or concomitant use of ethanol. With some drugs, seizures are a feature of intoxication and with others, of withdrawal.

Although opioids lower seizure threshold, seizures are seldom encountered during heroin intoxication or overdose, and, except in neonates, they are not a feature of withdrawal. In either setting, therefore, additional disease—for example, other drugs, meningitis, or head injury—must be sought. For reasons that remain unclear, heroin use is a risk factor for new onset seizures not temporally related to use and independent of other risk factors, such as trauma or ethanol. Seizures have occurred during intoxication from parenterally administered pentazocine combined with the antihistamine tripelennamine (''T's and blues''), popular in the midwest during the 1980s.

Seizures are frequently encountered during psychostimulant intoxication. With amphetaminelike drugs overdose is usually obvious. Cocaine users, perhaps related to the drug's local anesthetic properties, appear to be more seizure-prone. Seizures often complicate overdose but can also occur without other signs of toxicity, sometimes emerging after extended use in a fashion suggestive of ''reverse tolerance'' or electrical ''kindling.'' Difficult-to-control status epilepticus is not unusual. Seizures have also occurred in users of the over-the-counter diet remedy and decongestant phenylpropanolamine.

Sedatives, including benzodiazepines, can cause seizures as a withdrawal phenomenon. Some sedatives, notably methaqualone (no longer available in the United States) and glutethimide, have reportedly caused seizures during intoxication.

A case-control study found marijuana to be protective against new-onset seizures. A possible explanation is the constituent cannabidiol, which is anticonvulsant.

Although in low dose it is anticonvulsant, phencyclidine overdose is often complicated by seizures or myoclonus. Seizures are also sometimes encountered during intoxication from hallucinogens, inhalants, or anticholinergics.

Stroke

That tobacco and heavy ethanol use are risk factors for stroke was established by epidemiologic case-control and cohort studies. By contrast, the relationship of illicit drug use to stroke is based on case reports and small series.

Parenteral drug users are at risk for stroke secondary to endocarditis, hepatitis, meningitis, or AIDS. Heroin nephropathy can cause hemorrhagic stroke. Occlusive and, less often, hemorrhagic strokes have also occurred in young heroin users without systemic disease or other risk factors. Cerebral angiography in some has suggested vasculitis. Hypotension accompanying heroin overdose can result in infarction of cerebral borderzones and endzones.

Intracranial hemorrhage, probably related to acute hypertension, has complicated amphetamine intoxication. Hemorrhagic and occlusive strokes without other obvious signs of overdose also occur in chronic users of amphetaminelike psychostimulants. In some, autopsy reveals systemic and cerebral vasculitis of medium-sized arteries, suggestive of polyarteritis nodosa. In others, changes more resemble small vessel hypersensitivity

TABLE 195-3. Cocaine-Related Stroke: Types and Numbers of Reported Cases

Type of Stroke	No. of Cases
Occlusive	181
TIA	11
Infarct	154
TIA or infarct	21
Occlusive and/or hemorrhagic	13
Hemorrhagic	163
ICH	66
SAH	62
ICH or SAH	29
Intraventricular hemorrhage	7
Hemorrhage and angiogram or autopsy done	125
Aneurysm	54
AVM	15
% with aneurysm or AVM	55%
Total stroke	347

Abbreviations: TIA, transient ischemic attack; ICH, intracerebral hemorrhage; SAH, subarachnoid hemorrhage; AVM, arteriovenous malformation.

angiitis. The diagnosis of vasculitis, however, has frequently been based on nonspecific angiographic signs, such as ''beading.''

By 1994 over 300 strokes, including stroke in neonates, had been reported in association with cocaine (Table 195-3). Roughly half were occlusive and half hemorrhage, and of those with intracranial hemorrhage who received angiography (or autopsy), roughly half had a saccular aneurysm or a vascular malformation. Occlusive strokes have included transient ischemic attacks and infarction of cerebrum, thalamus, brainstem, spinal cord, and retina. Possible mechanisms for stroke include cardioembolism in association with cocaine-induced myocardial infarction or cocaine cardiomyopathy, hypertensive surges during intoxication, and cerebral vasospasm. Cerebral vasculitis has been infrequently observed, and some autopsy cases have excluded it. For unclear reasons, cocaine hydrochloride is more often associated with hemorrhagic stroke, and alkaloidal cocaine is associated with occlusive and hemorrhagic stroke with roughly equal frequency. The rising prevalence of stroke since the ''crack'' epidemic began in the 1980s is probably related to plentiful supplies of an inexpensive drug taken in high doses, rather than to specific pharmacologic risk. Cocaine also influences platelet function and clotting factors.

LSD, a vasoconstrictor, has caused occlusive stroke in young users. Phencyclidine, also a vasoconstrictor, has caused both hemorrhagic stroke and hypertensive encephalopathy.

Altered Mentation

Whether abuse of drugs other than ethanol directly leads to lasting changes in cognition or behavior is a chicken versus egg question. Predrug psychometric baselines are seldom available, and, while there is no such thing as an ''addictive personality,'' many psychopathologic conditions are overrepresented among users of illicit agents. Additional confounders include concomitant ethanol use and many of the systemic and neurologic complications of drug use already discussed.

Heroin and other opioids appear to have little direct long-term adverse effects on cognition. Tolerant addicts tend to be depressed, apathetic, irritable, and socially withdrawn, but the great majority of patients receiving methadone maintenance therapy have normal social and occupational function.

Suggesting ''reverse tolerance,'' chronic amphetamine and cocaine users become progressively paranoid, sometimes to frank hallucinatory psychosis, but such symptoms clear with abstinence. Less certain is how long withdrawal depression can last. It has been speculated that chronic cocaine use causes lasting dopamine depletion in the limbic "reward circuit," producing a chronic anhedonic state. On the other hand, many psychostimulant abusers are unwittingly treating preexisting depression (or, in some instances, attention deficit disorder). Computed tomography (CT) scans in chronic cocaine users has revealed cerebral atrophy, with ventricular and sulcal enlargement, and positron-emission tomography (PET) and single-photon-emission computed tomography (SPECT) imaging have suggested patchy decreases in cerebral blood flow.

An alleged "antimotivational syndrome" in marijuana users consists of diminished drive, apathy, inattentiveness, decreased recent memory, and impaired visual-motor performance. Studies of such a relationship, conducted in many countries, have been conflicting, and, as with other drugs, even when such symptoms are found, it is difficult to distinguish cause from effect.

Although there is tolerance to the hypnotic effects of barbiturates, chronic users, with or without dosage escalation, often display lethargy, inattentiveness, and social deterioration. In small children barbiturates impair learning; whether such effects are permanent is unclear. In the elderly, barbiturates cause reversible dementia (as well as falls), and in both children and old people they can cause paradoxical hyperactivity or agitation.

In addition to drowsiness, benzodiazepines can cause amnesia lasting hours, including the day following their use as sleeping pills. Paradoxical agitation, confusion, and even hallucinations have been attributed to the benzodiazepine triazolam, although much of the "evidence" has been from the popular media rather than from the scientific literature. Long-term benzodiazepine use, with or without physical dependence, appears to be without lasting cognitive or behavioral consequence.

Bromides, long-associated with chronic cognitive impairment, are no longer present in over-the-counter sleeping pills.

Toluene sniffers have developed dementia with cerebral white matter changes, and gasoline sniffers have had lead encephalopathy.

The weight of evidence is against permanent mental change associated with hallucinogen use, but anxiety, depression, and insomnia have lasted weeks after use of "ecstasy," and LSD flashbacks have precipitated suicide.

Considerable attention has been paid to the psychopharmacology of phencyclidine, which, unlike amphetamine, reproduces both the "positive" (paranoia, delusions) and "negative" (loss of ego boundaries, apathy, loose associations) of schizophrenia. Psychotic symptoms can last days or weeks after single doses of phencyclidine, and chronic users often demonstrate persistent cognitive and behavioral abnormalities. As with other drugs, causality is difficult to establish.

Anticholinergic abuse does not appear to cause lasting mental impairment.

Fetal Effects

Similarly problematic are possible effects of illicit drugs on fetal development. Pregnant substance abusers often avoid prenatal care, abuse ethanol and tobacco, and following delivery are suboptimal mothers.

In utero exposure to opioids (including methadone) can cause a severe withdrawal syndrome, and such children are often small for gestational age and at risk for respiratory distress and sudden infant death. Hyperactivity, sleep disturbances, and cognitive impairment have been reported in later life. Others claim that such abnormalities tend to be outgrown.

In utero cocaine exposure has been associated with abruptio placentae, retarded fetal growth, microcephaly, and numerous congenital malformations, including the brain, spinal cord, and eye. Meta-analysis of a number of such reports, however, identified significant risk only for intrauterine death and genitourinary malformations. A prospective controlled study found a high incidence of hypertonus resembling cerebral palsy, which, however, tended to clear within the first two years of life. Clearly, media apprehension over an epidemic of "crack babies" paralyzing the American school system is premature.

Marijuana smoking during pregnancy is associated with decreased birth weight and length. Reports related to cognition and behavior have been inconsistent.

Detrimental cognitive effects of barbiturates on small children raises the fear that in utero exposure would be even more harmful, but evidence for such an association with either barbiturates or benzodiazepines is lacking.

Miscellaneous Effects

Heroin has been associated with peripheral neuropathy of Guillain-Barré type as well as with brachial and lumbosacral plexopathy, probably immune-mediated. (Brachial neuropathy has also occurred secondary to compression by a subclavian artery septic aneurysm; angiography should be considered in such patients.)

Severe sensorimotor peripheral neuropathy affects sniffers of glue containing *n*-hexane. Polyneuropathy has also affected gasoline sniffers. Rhabdomyolysis and renal failure can occur in users of heroin or cocaine with or without other signs of intoxication. Rhabdomyolysis in users of amphetamine or phencyclidine usually accompanies other obvious signs of overdose.

Myopathy affects gasoline and toluene sniffers.

Severe parkinsonism in California drug users was traced to a synthetic opioid contaminated with methylphenyltetrahydropyridine (MPTP). Symptoms responded dramatically to l-dopa but recurred when it was stopped. Positron emission tomography has shown reduced numbers of dopaminergic neurons in asymptomatic subjects exposed to MPTP, raising the fear that parkinsonism will emerge as they grow older.

A heroin user whose mixture contained large amounts of quinine became blind; vision improved when he switched to heroin lacking quinine.

Chronic cocaine use induces dystonia and other dyskinesias in a pattern suggestive of "reverse tolerance," and abnormal movements can persist for days or weeks despite abstinence. Cocaine has precipitated symptoms in otherwise well-controlled patients with Gilles de la Tourette syndrome.

Marijuana inhibits luteinizing hormone (LH) and follicle-stimulating hormone (FSH), causing impotence and sterility in men and menstrual irregularity in women. Symptoms are reversible with abstinence.

Cerebellar ataxia, with white matter changes, occurs in toluene sniffers.

European smokers of "heroin pyrolysate" ("chasing the dragon") have developed acute dementia, ataxia, quadriparesis, chorea, blindness, and death. Autopsies reveal cerebral white matter spongiform change. The responsible toxin has not been identified.

CONCLUSION

Regarding substance abuse, a practicing neurologist should keep several general points in mind:

1. Drug abusers are in no way stereotypic. Higher education, occupational success, and elevated socioeconomic standing do not exclude abuse of any substance.
2. Many drug abusers use more than one substance, including ethanol, leading to complex and confusing symptoms and signs. In fact, someone might be simultaneously intoxicated from one substance while withdrawing from another.
3. In known substance abusers, medical and neurologic complications as described above should be suspected or anticipated.
4. Conversely, in patients with trauma, seizures, infection, stroke, and cognitive or behavioral change, drug abuse should be considered.

SUGGESTED READINGS

Ballard PA, Tetrud JW, Langston JW: Permanent human parkinsonism due to 1-methyl-4-phenyl-1,2,3,6-tetrahydropyridine (MPTP): seven cases. Neurology 35:949, 1985

Barnes PF, Bloch AB, Davidson PT, Snider DE: Tuberculosis in patients with human immunodeficiency virus infection. N Engl J Med 324:1644, 1991

Bost RO: 3,4-Methylenedioxymethamphetamine (MDMA) and other amphetamine derivatives. J Forens Sci 33:576, 1988

Britton CB: HIV infection. Neurol Clin 11:605, 1993

Brown C, Osterlich J: Multiple severe complications from recreational ingestion of MDMA (''ecstasy''). JAMA 258:780, 1987

Brust JCM: Neurological Aspects of Substance Abuse. Butterworth-Heinemann, Stoneham, MA, 1993

Brust JCM, Dickinson PCT, Hughes JEO, Holtzman RHH: The diagnosis and treatment of cerebral mycotic aneurysms. Ann Neurol 27:238, 1990

Brust JCM, Richter RW: Quinine amblyopia related to heroin addiction. Ann Intern Med 74:84, 1971

Brust JCM, Richter RW: Stroke associated with addiction to heroin. J Neurol Neurosurg Psychiatry 39:194, 1976

Calne DB, Langston JW, Stoessl AJ et al: Positron emission tomography after MPTP: observations relating to the cause of Parkinson's disease. Nature 317:246, 1986

Caplan LR, Thomas C, Banks G: Central nervous system complications of addiction to ''T's and blues.'' Neurology 32:623, 1982

Chiriboga CA: Fetal effects. Neurol Clin 11:707, 1993

Chiriboga CA, Bateman DA, Brust JCM, Hauser WA: Neurological outcome of neonates exposed in-utero to cocaine. Pediatr Neurol 9:115, 1993

Citron BP, Halpern M, McCarron M et al: Necrotizing angiitis associated with drug abuse. N Engl J Med 283:1003, 1970

Delaney P: Intracranial hemorrhage associated with amphetamine use. Neurology 31:923, 1981

DesJarlais DC, Friedman SR, Novick DM et al: HIV-1 infection among intravenous drug users in Manhattan, New York City, from 1977 through 1987. JAMA 261:1008, 1989

Earnest MP: Seizures. Neurol Clin 11:563, 1993

Eastman JW, Cohen SN: Hypertensive crisis and death associated with phencyclidine poisoning. JAMA 231:1270, 1975

Fialip J, Aumaitre O, Eschalier A et al: Benzodiazepine withdrawal seizures: analysis of 48 case reports. Clin Neuropharmacol 10:538, 1987

Finnegan LP: The effects of narcotics and alcohol on pregnancy and the newborn. Ann NY Acad Sci 362:136, 1981

Fortenberry JD: Gasoline sniffing. Am J Med 79:740, 1985

Goldfrank LR, Bresnitz EA: Opioids. p. 433. In Goldfrank LR, Flomenbaum NE, Levin NA, et al (eds): Toxicologic Emergencies, 4th Ed. Appleton & Lange, Norwalk, CT, 1990

Goldfrank LR, Hoffman RS: The cardiovascular effects of cocaine. Ann Emerg Med 20:165, 1991

Hollister LE: Effects of hallucinogens in humans. p. 19. In Jacobs BL (ed): Hallucinogens: Neurochemical, Behavioral, and Clinical Perspectives. Raven Press, New York, 1984

Holman BL, Carvalho PA, Mendelson J et al: Brain perfusion is abnormal in cocaine-dependent polydrug users: a study using technetium-99M-HMPAO and ASPECT. J Nucl Med 32:1206, 1991

Hormes JT, Filley CM, Rosenberg NL: Neurologic sequelae of chronic vapor abuse. Neurology 36:698, 1986

Howrie DL, Wokfson JM: Phenylpropanolamine-induced seizure. J Pediatr 102:143, 1983

Jannsen RS, Kaplan JE, Khabbaz RF et al: HTLV-1 associated myelopathy/tropical spastic paraparesis in the United States. Neurology 41:1355, 1991

Kelly T: Prolonged cerebellar dysfunction associated with paint sniffing. Pediatrics 56:605, 1975

Kiokkinos J, Levine SR: Stroke. Neurol Clin 11:577, 1993

Kudrow DB, Henry DA, Haake DA et al: Botulism associated with *Clostridium botulinum* sinusitis after intranasal cocaine use. Ann Intern Med 109:984, 1988

Levine SR, Brust JCM, Futrell N et al: Cerebrovascular complications of the use of the ''crack'' form of alkaloidal cocaine. N Engl J Med 323:699, 1990

Levine SR, Brust JCM, Futrell N et al: A comparative study of the cerebrovascular complications of cocaine: alkaloidal versus hydrochloride: a review. Neurology 41:1173, 1991

Lolin Y: Chronic neurological toxicity associated with exposure to volatile substances. Hum Toxicol 8:293, 1989

Lutiger B, Graham K, Einarson TR, Koren G: Relationship between gestational cocaine use and pregnancy outcome: a meta-analysis. Teratology 44:405, 1991

McCarron MM, Schultze BW, Thompson GA et al: Acute phencyclidine intoxication: incidence of clinical findings in 1000 cases. Ann Emerg Med 10:237, 1981

Mikolich JR, Paulson GW, Cross CJ: Acute anticholinergic syndrome due to jimson seed ingestion. Ann intern Med 83:321, 1975

Morton HG: Occurrence and treatment of solvent abuse in children and adolescents. Pharmacol Ther 33:449, 1987

Musher DM, Hammill RJ, Baughn RE: The effect of human immunodeficiency virus infection on the course of syphilis and the response to treatment. Ann Intern Med 113:872, 1990

Ng SKC, Brust JCM, Hauser WA, Susser M: Illicit drug use and the risk of new onset seizures: contrasting effects of heroin, marijuana, and cocaine. Am J Epidemiol 40:1017, 1990

Pascual-Leone A, Anderson DC: Cerebral atrophy in habitual cocaine abusers: a planimetric CT study. Neurology 41:34, 1991

Pascual-Leone A, Dhuna A: Cocaine-associated multifocal tics. Neurology 40:999, 1990

Pascual-Leone A, Dhuna A, Altafallah I, Anderson DC: Cocaine-induced seizures. Neurology 40:404, 1990

Richter RW: Infections other than AIDS. Neurol Clin 11:591, 1993

Selwyn PA, Alcabes P, Hartel D et al: Clinical manifestations and predictors of disease progression in drug users with human immunodeficiency virus infection. N Engl J Med 327:1697, 1992

Shafer SQ: Disorders of spinal cord, nerve, and muscle. Neurol Clin 11:693, 1993

Sobel J, Espinas OE, Friedman SA: Carotid artery obstruction following LSD capsule ingestion. Arch Intern Med 127:290, 1971

Weinrieb RM, O'Brien CP: Persistent cognitive deficits attributed to substance abuse. Neurol Clin 11:663, 1993

Wolters ECH, Van Wijngaarden GK, Stan FC et al: Leukoencephalopathy after inhaling ''heroin pyrolysate.'' Lancet 2:1233, 1982

Zuckerman B, Frank DAD, Hingson R, et al: Effects of marijuana and cocaine use on fetal growth. N Engl J Med 320:762, 1989

196. NEUROLOGIC COMPLICATIONS OF COMMONLY PRESCRIBED DRUGS

JOHN C. M. BRUST

This chapter describes neurologic side effects of drugs taken by ambulatory patients and usually prescribed by nonneurologists. Neurologic complications of agents used to treat disorders such as seizures, migraine, multiple sclerosis, myasthenia gravis,

Parkinson's disease, Alzheimer's disease, and anxiety are addressed in other chapters. Drugs susceptible to abuse, for example, opioid analgesics, psychostimulants, and sedatives, are discussed in Chapter 196.

DRUGS TO TREAT INFECTION

Most drugs used to treat infection, whether bacterial, fungal, viral, or parasitic, are capable of causing neurologic complications (Tables 196-1 to 196-5). Nitrofurantoin polyneuropathy is usually seen with renal failure and with treatment of long duration. Penicillin G can cause altered mentation and seizures

TABLE 196-1. Drugs to Treat Bacterial Infection

Agent	Neurologic Complication
Sulfonamides	CNS-induced anorexia, nausea, vomiting Potentiate phenytoin
Trimethoprim- sulfamethoxazole	Headache, depression, hallucinations Aseptic meningitis Vertigo, ataxia Seizures Peripheral neuropathy
Quinolones (e.g., nalidixic acid, ciprofloxacin)	Headache, dizziness Potentiate methylxanthines (theophylline, caffeine)
Nitrofurantoin	Headache, vertigo, drowsiness, myalgia, nystagmus Peripheral neuropathy
Penicillins	Sciatic nerve injury after local injection Arachnoiditis, encephalopathy after intrathecal injection Lethargy, confusion, myoclonus, seizures with high dose or renal insufficiency Dizziness, tinnitus, headache, hallucinations, seizures with procaine penicillin G
Cephalosporins	Disulfiram-like ethanol reaction
Imipenem	Seizures with high dose or renal insufficiency
Aminoglycosides	Ototoxicity Neuromuscular blockade Optic neuropathy and peripheral neuropathy (streptomycin) Radiculopathy or myelopathy after intrathecal injection
Tetracyclines	Increased intracranial pressure
Chloramphenicol	Optic neuropathy Encephalopathy Peripheral neuropathy
Erythromycin	Transient hearing loss Potentiate carbamazepine
Clindamycin	Neuromuscular blockade
Spectinomycin	Dizziness, nausea, insomnia
Vancomycin	Ototoxicity

TABLE 196-2. Drugs to Treat Tuberculosis and Leprosy

Agent	Neurologic Complication
Isoniazid	Peripheral neuropathy Seizures Optic neuropathy Dizziness, ataxia, tinnitus Euphoria, impaired memory, psychosis, coma Hepatic encephalopathy Potentiation of phenytoin
Rifampin	Increased methadone metabolism, withdrawal symptoms
Ethambutol	Optic neuropathy Headache, dizziness, confusion, hallucinations Peripheral neuropathy
Pyrazinamide	Hepatic encephalopathy
Ethionamide	Postural hypotension, drowsiness, dizziness, tremor, headache, olfactory disturbance, diplopia, restlessness, depression, seizures, peripheral neuropathy
Sulfones (dapsone, etc.)	Peripheral neuropathy Headache, insomnia, anxiety, psychosis

TABLE 196-3. Antifungal Drugs

Agent	Neurologic Complication
Amphotericin B	Headache Uremic encephalopathy Hypokalemic myopathy
Flucytosine	Hepatic encephalopathy
Imidazoles (e.g., ketoconazole, fluconazole)	Hepatic encephalopathy Potentiate phenytoin
Griseofulvin	Headache Peripheral neuropathy Lethargy, confusion, Macular edema Hepatic encephalopathy Disulfiram-like ethanol reaction

TABLE 196-4. Antiviral Drugs

Agent	Neurologic Complication
Acyclovir, gancyclovir	Headache Encephalopathy
Vidarabine	Tremor, dizziness, ataxia Psychosis, hallucinations, seizures, coma
Amantadine	Insomnia, decreased concentration, confusion, hallucinations, seizures, coma
Ribavirin	Asthenia, seizures
Zidovudine	Headache, insomnia Seizures Wernicke's encephalopathy Myopathy
Didanosine	Peripheral neuropathy Retinal depigmentation
Dideoxycytidine	Peripheral neuropathy

TABLE 196-5. Antiparasitic Drugs

Agent	Neurologic Complication
Quinine	Tinnitus, deafness, vertigo Impaired color vision, constricted visual fields, blindness Headache, fever, vomiting, confusion, delirium, coma Tachypnea, respiratory depression Uremic encephalopathy
Chloroquine	Retinopathy Headache Myopathy Peripheral neuropathy Abnormal behavior
Metronidazole	Headache, dizziness, vertigo, ataxia, seizures Peripheral neuropathy Disulfiram-like ethanol reaction
Pentamidine	Headache, dizziness Hypoglycemia (tremor, altered behavior, seizures, coma)
Pyrimethamine	Headache, dizziness
Praziquantel	Headache, dizziness

when the concentration in cerebrospinal fluid (CSF) exceeds 10 μg/ml, and procaine in the preparation can contribute to symptoms. Streptomycin and gentamicin cause mainly vestibular toxicity; amikacin, kanamycin, and neomycin cause deafness; tobramycin causes both. Aminoglycoside-induced neuromuscular blockade, often in patients also receiving anesthetics, can precipitate myasthenic crisis. Tetracylcline-induced pseudotumor cerebri is most common in infants. Chloramphenicol-induced encephalopathy, seen in neonates and referred to as the "gray syndrome," includes vomiting, refusal to suck, irregular respiration, diarrhea, flaccidity, hypothermia, and metabolic acidosis.

Isoniazid-induced peripheral neuropathy occurs in about 2 percent of patients receiving usual doses of 5 mg/kg; polyneuropathy and CNS toxicity are prevented by giving pyridoxine.

Ethambutol-induced optic neuropathy causes reduced visual acuity as well as red-green color blindness.

Antifungal agents indirectly cause encephalopathy by damaging the liver or the kidneys. The antiviral agent acyclovir is directly encephalopathic but usually in association with renal failure and high blood concentrations. Wernicke's encephalopathy and myopathy can emerge after months of treatment with zidovudine. Peripheral neuropathy is less often encountered with dideoxycytidine than with didanosine.

Quinine retinopathy and ototoxicity are secondary to both ischemia and direct cellular injury. Chloroquine is directly retinotoxic. Metronidazole-induced peripheral neuropathy can be irreversible.

DRUGS TO TREAT PAIN, FEVER, INFLAMMATION, AND ARTHRITIS

Salicylism consists of ototoxicity and CNS stimulation, including hyperventilation and seizures, followed by depression (Table 196-6). Because of epidemiologic evidence linking aspirin with Reye syndrome, salicylates are contraindicated in children with varicella or influenza. Severe headache frequently develops in patients taking indomethacin for long periods. With the related drug sulindac drowsiness is common. Among so-called nonsteroidal anti-inflammatory drugs, ibuprofen has caused toxic amblyopia.

DRUGS TO REDUCE MUSCLE SPASM

Although their efficacy in reducing muscle spasm is questionable, a number of agents so promoted are widely prescribed (Table 196-7). Their use in the elderly is especially inappropriate.

TABLE 196-6. Drugs to Treat Pain, Fever, Inflammation, and Arthritis

Agent	Neurologic Complication
Salicylates	Headache, dizziness, tinnitus, high-tone deafness, hyperventilation, sweating, thirst, nausea, vomiting, drowsiness, confusion, progressing to seizures, delirium, hypoventilation, coma, cardiovascular collapse. Reye syndrome
Indomethacin, sulindac	Headache, lightheadedness, vertigo, drowsiness, confusion, psychosis, hallucinations. Hepatic encephalopathy
Propionic acid derivatives (ibuprofen, ketorolac, naproxen, etc.)	Headache, dizziness, tinnitus, anorexia, fatigue, confusion. Amblyopia. Aseptic meningitis
Piroxicam	Headache, dizziness, drowsiness
Diclofenac	Headache, dizziness
Acetaminophen	Hepatic encephalopathy. Uremic encephalopathy. Hypoglycemia (tremor, altered behavior, seizures, coma)
Phenylbutazone	Vertigo, insomnia, nervousness, euphoria, blurred vision
Gold	Encephalitis. Peripheral neuropathy. Hepatic encephalopathy. Uremic encephalopathy
Allopurinal	Headache, drowsiness
Probenecid	Headache, dizziness

TABLE 196-7. Drugs to Treat Acute Muscle Spasm

Agent	Neurologic Complication
Orphenadrine	Dizziness, syncope. Drowsiness, tremor. Anticholinergic effects (dry mouth, tachycardia, urinary hesitancy, blurred vision, agitation, hallucinations)
Carisoprodol	Drowsiness, nervousness, headache, dizziness, tremor, ataxia, syncope. Withdrawal: headache, nervousness, insomnia, muscle cramps
Methocarbamol	Headache, drowsiness, dizziness
Cyclobenzamine	Drowsiness, dizziness, dry mouth. Confusion, agitation. Taken with monoamine oxidase inhibitor: febrile crisis, seizures

TABLE 196-8. Cardiovascular Drugs

Agent	Neurologic Complication
Nitrates	Headache. Postural syncope
Digitalis	Headache, fatigue, drowsiness. Neuralgia, paresthesias. Confusion, aphasia, delirium, hallucinations. Blurred vision, chromatopsia, retrobulbar neuritis
Quinidine	Tinnitus, deafness, dizziness, headache, blurred vision, diplopia, altered color perception, confusion, delirium
Procainamide	Dizziness, psychosis, hallucinations
Tocainide, mexiletine	Dizziness, tremor
Amiodarone	Fatigue, tremor, abnormal movements, ataxia. Peripheral neuropathy. Hepatic encephalopathy. Hypo- and hyperthyroidism
Thiazide diuretics	Postural syncope. Hyponatremic encephalopathy. Hypokalemic myopathy. Exacerbation of hepatic encephalopathy
Ethacrynic acid, furosemide	Postural syncope. Hypokalemic myopathy. Deafness
Spironolactone, trimaterene	Hyperkalemic myopathy
Acetazolamide	Somnolence, paresthesias. Exacerbation of hepatic encephalopathy
Methyldopa, clonidine	Postural syncope. Somnolence, forgetfulness, dry mouth, headache, impotence, blurred vision, parkinsonism. Withdrawal headache, anxiety, tremor, sweating, tachycardia, abdominal pain
Guanethidine	Postural syncope. Delayed or retrograde ejaculation
Reserpine	Somnolence, decreased concentration, psychotic depression, parkinsonism
β-Adrenergic antagonists (propranolol, etc.)	Somnolence, insomnia, nightmares, depression, seizures. Paresthesias of hands
α-Adrenergic antagonists (prazosin, etc.)	Postural syncope. Headache, dizziness, drowsiness, nausea
Hydralazine, minoxidil	Postural syncope. Headache, dizziness, nausea. Anxiety, depression. Peripheral neuropathy
Angiotensin-converting enzyme inhibitors (captopril, enalapril, etc.)	Postural syncope. Loss of sense of taste
Calcium channel blockers (verapamil, diltiazem, nifedipine, etc.)	Postural syncope. Headache, nausea, dizziness, paresthesias of hands, somnolence

CARDIOVASCULAR DRUGS

Vasodilation is responsible for nitrate-induced headache and dizziness (Table 196-8). In digitalis toxicity, neuropathic, visual, and encephalopathic symptoms can be prominent. Both quinidine and procainamide directly cause psychosis and delirium; in procainamide-induced systemic lupus erythematosus the brain is spared. Amiodarone can cause neurologically symptomatic hypothyroidism or hyperthyroidism. Ethacrynic acid is more likely than furosemide to cause lasting deafness.

DRUGS FOR GASTROINTESTINAL DISORDERS

Among H$_2$ antihistamines (Table 196-9) cimetidine is most likely to cause mental change; it also, unlike ranitidine and other agents, prolongs the half-life of phenytoin, barbiturates, benzodiazepines, and tricyclic antidepressants. In patients with renal failure, aluminum-containing antacids have been implicated in the development of osteodystrophy, myopathy, and the dialysis dementia syndrome, which can progress to seizures and death. Metoclopromide is more likely than trimethobenzimide to cause extrapyramidal symptoms. Trimethobnzimide has been implicated in some cases of Reye syndrome, but the evidence is inconclusive.

DRUGS FOR NASAL CONGESTION AND ALLERGY

With the exception of the piperidines terfenadine and astemizole all H$_1$ antihistamines cause sedation, and overdose can cause seizures, delirium, and coma (Table 196-10). The serotonin antagonist cyprohepatidine also has H$_1$ antihistamine effects. Structurally similar to caffeine, theophylline causes CNS stimulation and is more likely than caffeine to cause seizures, sometimes without other signs of toxicity.

ANTINEOPLASTIC AND IMMUNOSUPPRESSANT DRUGS

Many antineoplastic drugs cause neurologic symptoms secondary to hepatic or renal injury (Table 196-11). They also cause nausea and vomiting and increase the risk of infection, including meningitis with such opportunists as cryptococcus and Listeria. Some, such as ifosfamide and methotrexate, are directly toxic to the brain. Acute cerebellar ataxia has followed fluoro-

TABLE 196-9. Drugs for Gastrointestinal Disorders

Agent	Neurologic Complication
H$_2$ antihistamines (cimetidine, ranitidine, etc.)	Sedation Headache, dizziness Confusion, agitation, psychosis, hallucinations
Omeprazole	Sedation Headache, dizziness
Aluminum-containing antacids (e.g., Maalox, Mylanta, Gelusil, sucralfate)	Myopathy Dialysis dementia, seizures
Bismuth compounds (e.g., Pepto-bismol)	Encephalopathy
Metoclopramide, trimethobenzamide	Extrapyramidal symptoms (acute dystonia, parkinsonism, akathisia, perioral tremor, tardive dyskinesia) Anxiety, depression Drowsiness Reye syndrome?
Laxatives	Electrolyte imbalance, especially hypokalemic myopathy

TABLE 196-10. Drugs for Nasal Congestion, Skin Allergy, or Asthma

Agent	Neurologic Complication
H$_1$ antihistamines (diphenhydramine, tripelennamine, hydroxyzine, meclizine, etc.)	Sedation Dizziness, tinnitus, blurred vision, tremor, nervousness, insomnia, euphoria Ataxia, athetosis, delirium, seizures, coma, mydriasis, apnea
Cyproheptadine	Sedation and other side effects of H$_1$ antihistamines
Theophylline	Nervousness, insomnia, tremor, delirium Seizures Nausea, vomiting
β$_2$-Adrenergic agonists (metaproterenol, terbutaline, albuterol, etc.)	Tremor Restlessness, anxiety, insomnia
Mixed α- and β-adrenergic agonists (pseudoephedrine, phenylpropanolamine, etc.)	Tremor Restlessness, anxiety, insomnia
Cromolyn	Headache (rare)

TABLE 196-11. Antineoplastic and Immunosuppressant Drugs

Agent	Neurologic Complication
Cyclophosphamide	Inappropriate secretion of antidiuretic hormone
Ifosfamide	Somnolence, dizziness, confusion, psychotic depression, hallucinations, cranial neuropathy, seizures
Chlorambucil	Tremor, agitation, ataxia, hallucinations, seizures
Carmustine, lomustine	Retinopathy Lethargy, confusion, ataxia, dysarthria
Methotrexate	Headache, sedation, blurred vision, seizures, coma
Fluorouracil, floxuridine	Headache Cerebellar ataxia Myelopathy
Cytarabine	Headache, dizziness, myalgia, sedation Altered behavior Peripheral neuropathy
Vincristine, vinblastine	Neuritic pain, peripheral neuropathy Constipation Seizures Optic neuropathy Inappropriate secretion of antidiuretic hormone
Taxol	Peripheral neuropathy Seizures (rare)
Etoposide	Peripheral neuropathy
Dactinomycin	Lethargy, myalgia
Mithramycin	Lethargy
L-Asparaginase	Lethargy, depression, agitation, hallucinations, coma Parkinsonism Nonketotic hyperosmolar hyperglycemia
Cisplatin, carboplatin	Tinnitus, deafness Peripheral neuropathy Tetany Myelopathy Loss of taste Seizures
Hydroxyurea	Headache, dizziness Confusion, hallucinations, seizures
Procarbazine	Sedation, nystagmus, ataxia Altered behavior, seizures, coma Peripheral neuropathy Disulfiram-like ethanol reaction
Tamoxifen	Headache, dizziness, depression Retinopathy
Cyclosporine	Tremor Seizures

TABLE 196-12. Drugs for Diabetes Mellitus

Agent	Neurologic Complication
Insulin	Hypoglycemia (tremor, sweating, hunger, blurred vision, weakness, altered behavior, confusion, seizures, coma, strokelike symptoms)
Sulfonylureas (tolbutamide, chlorpropamide, glyburide, glipizide)	Hypoglycemia Hyponatremic encephalopathy Disulfiramlike ethanol reaction Inappropriate secretion (or potentiation) of antidiuretic hormone Exacerbation of hepatic porphyria

uracil administration, and myelopathy has affected patients receiving the drug intrathecally. Neurotoxicity, especially peripheral neuropathy, is more often associated with vincristine than vinblastine. Mental change in patients receiving ɪ-asparaginase is often accompanied by elevated blood ammonia concentration. Ototoxicity, neurotoxicity, and nephrotoxicity are less often encountered with carboplatin than cisplatin.

DRUGS FOR DIABETES MELLITUS

The major complication of both insulin and oral sulfonylurea drugs is hypoglycemia, which causes symptoms either through epinephrine release (masked by beta-adrenergic blockers) or by direct CNS effects (Table 196-12). Focal signs can be present upon emerging from coma or a seizure; they can also occur in the absence of either, mimicking a stroke.

HORMONES AND ANTIHORMONES

Neurologic complications of adrenocortical steroids can be direct (altered mentation, myopathy), indirect (CNS infection, traumatic myelopathy, electrolyte abnormality), or the result of withdrawal (Table 196-13). Evidence for the association of occlusive and hemorrhagic stroke with oral contraceptive drugs, especially in smokers, is epidemiologic; the mechanism, poorly understood, is probably related to both the estrogen and progestin content of the preparations.[19]

ANTICOAGULANT AND ANTIPLATELET DRUGS

The major neurologic complication of anticoagulant and antiplatelet drugs is hemorrhage, centrally or into peripheral nerves

TABLE 196-13. Hormones and Antihormones

Agent	Neurologic Complication
Adrenocortical steroids	Altered behavior, psychotic depression Myopathy Vertebral compression fracture, myeloradiculopathy CNS infection Hypokalemia, weakness Withdrawal: addisonian crisis, pseudotumor cerebri
Estrogen	Nausea, anorexia
Progestins and oral contraceptives	Headache, fatigue Thromboembolic disease, occlusive and hemorrhagic stroke
Androgens	Increased muscle growth Virilization, feminization
Antithyroid thioureylenes (propylthiouracil, methimazole, etc.)	Headache, nausea, paresthesias, myalgia, loss of taste, drowsiness Hypoglycemia

TABLE 196-14. Anticoagulant and Antiviscosity Drugs

Agent	Neurologic Complication
Warfarin	Intracranial and intraspinal hemorrhage Nausea, anorexia
Aspirin and other nonsteroidal anti-inflammatory drugs	See Table 196-6
Dipyridamole	Headache, dizziness
Ticlopidine	Dizziness, anorexia
Pentoxifylline	Dizziness, nervousness

or roots (Table 196-14). Intraspinal hemorrhage can follow lumbar puncture in patients receiving warfarin.

LIPID-LOWERING DRUGS

Both clofibrate and hydroxymethylglutaryl (HMG)-CoA reductase inhibitors cause myopathy, which can range from asymptomatic creatine kinase elevation to acute rhabdomyolysis and renal shutdown (Table 196-15).

ANTIPSYCHOTIC AND ANTIDEPRESSANT DRUGS

Among neuroleptic agents, extrapyramidal side effects are especially common with fluphenazine, trifluoperazine, pimozide, and haloperidol, which in turn are less likely to cause sedation (Table 196-16). With chlorpromazine, mesoridazine, thioridazine, and chloroprothixene the opposite is true. Clozapine is far less likely to cause extrapyramidal signs but more likely to cause seizures. The potentially fatal neuroleptic malignant syndrome consists of severe akinetic parkinsonism, labile pulse and blood pressure, fever, elevated creatine kinase, and myoglobinuria. Among tricyclic antidepressants, anticholinergic side effects are especially prominent with amitriptyline and much less with desipramine. Priapism associated with trazadone is a medical emergency. Hemorrhagic stroke has occurred in patients taking monoamine oxidase inhibitors who ingested beer, wine, yeast, liver, pickled herring, chocolate, or other tyramine-containing foods. Neurologic side effects of lithium are usually associated with blood levels above 1.25 mEq/L.

VITAMINS

Hypervitaminosis A, including pseudotumor cerebri and visual loss, is most often seen in adolescents taking vitamin A in large doses for weeks or months (Table 196-17). Repeated ingestion of large doses of vitamin D causes hypercalcemia with a wide array of mental symptoms as well as life-threatening kidney damage. Although pyridoxine-induced sensory neuropathy is usually associated with "megadoses"—2 to 6 g daily for months—it has resulted from as little as 200 mg daily. Niacin overdose has caused retinal maculopathy, and lactic acidosis

TABLE 196-15. Drugs to Lower Blood Lipoprotein Concentrations

Agent	Neurologic Complication
Clofibrate	Headache, sedation, dizziness, blurred vision Elevated serum creatine kinase, polymyositis, rhabdomyolysis Potentiation of warfarin anticoagulation
Cholestyramine	Headache, dizziness, anxiety, sedation, myalgia
Lovastatin, pravastatin, etc.	Headache, dizziness Elevated serum creatinine kinase, polymyositis, rhabdomyolysis Altered taste

TABLE 196-16. Antipsychotic and Antidepressant Drugs

Agent	Neurologic Complication
Pheniothiazines, haloperidol	Sedation
	Extrapyramidal symptoms (acute dystonia, parkinsonism, akathisia, perioral tremor, tardive dyskinesia)
	Neuroleptic malignant syndrome
	Seizures
	Postural syncope
	Hyperprolactinemia, galactorrhea
	Anticholinergic effects (blurred vision, decreased sweating, dry mouth, constipation, urinary retention)
Clozapine	Sedation, dizziness, headache
	Restlessness, insomnia, confusion
	Tremor, akathisia, bradykinesia
	Seizures
	Blurred vision, increased sweating and salivation, dry mouth
	Neuroleptic malignant syndrome
	Postural syncope
Tricyclic antidepressants (imipramine, nortriptyline, amitriptyline, etc.)	Postural dizziness or syncope
	Anticholinergic effects
	Increased sweating
	Sedation, fatigue, weakness, tremor
	Manic excitement, delirium
	Seizures
	Inappropriate secretion of antidiuretic hormone
Trazodone	Postural dizziness or syncope
	Anticholinergic effects (very weak)
	Priapism
	Sedation, fatigue
Fluoxetine	Nervousness, insomnia, abnormal dreams, agitation
	Sedation, fatigue, dizziness
	Tremor
	Increased sweating
	Seizures
Bupropion	Anxiety, agitation, tremor, increased sweating
	Seizures
Monoamine oxidase inhibitors (phenylzine, tranylcypromine, isocarboxazid)	Tremor, nervousness, insomnia, agitation, confusion, hallucinations
	Increased sweating
	Seizures
	Hypertensive crisis, intracranial hemorrhage (when taken with sympathomimetic agents or tyramine-containing foods)
	Hyperthermic crisis (when taken with meperidine)
	Peripheral neuropathy (phenylzine and isocarboxazid)
Lithium salts	Sedation, tremor, dysarthria, ataxia, confusion, seizures, coma
	Polydipsia, polyuria
	Exacerbation of myasthenia gravis

TABLE 196-17. Vitamins

Agent	Neurologic Complication
Vitamin A (retinol, etc.)	Sedation, dizziness
	Increased intracranial pressure (headache, papilledema, diplopia)
Vitamin D (calciferol, cholecalciferol)	Weakness, fatigue, lassitude, disturbed sleep ("neurasthenia")
	Impaired memory, dementia, altered behavior, depression, paranoia, hallucinations, delirium, obtundation, coma
	Polydipsia, polyuria
Pyridoxine	Peripheral neuropathy
Folic acid	Correction of cobalamin deficiency anemia with progression of myeloneuropathy
Niacin	Retinopathy
	Lactic acidosis, delirium

with delirium has followed combined ingestion of niacin with ethanol.

SUGGESTED READINGS

Albin RL, Albers JW: Long-term follow-up of pyridoxine-induced acute sensory neuropathy—neuronopathy. Neurology 40:1319, 1990

Bateman DN, Dyson EH: Quinine toxicity. Adverse Drug React Acute Poisoning Rev 4:215, 1986

Bean B, Aeppli D: Adverse effects of high-dose intravenous acyclovir in ambulatory patients with acute herpes zoster. J Infect Dis 151:362, 1985

Bertino JS, Walker JW: Reassessment of theophylline toxicity. serum concentrations, clinical course, and treatment. Arch Intern Med 147:757, 1987

Brust JCM: Stroke and drugs. p. 517. In Toole JF (ed): Handbook of Clinical Neurology. Vol 11(55): Vascular Diseases, Part III. Elsevier Science, New York, 1989

Cedarbaum JM, Schleifer LS: Drugs for Parkinson's disease, spasticity, and acute muscle spasms. p. 463. In Gilman AG, Rall TW, Nies AS, Taylor P (eds): The Pharmacological Basis of Therapeutics. 8th Ed., Pergamon Press, New York, 1990

Coxon A, Pallis CA: Metronidazole neuropathy. J Neurol Neurosurg Psychiatry 39:403, 1979

Davtyan DG, Vinters HV: Wernicke's encephalopathy in AIDS patients treated with zidovudine. Lancet 1:919, 1987

Evans LS, Kleiman MB: Acidosis as a presenting features of chloramphenicol toxicity. J Pediatr 108:473, 1986

Lely AH, van Enter CHJ: Large-scale digitoxin intoxication. BMJ 3:737, 1970

Mach JR, Korchik WP, Mahowald MW: Dialysis dementia. Clin Geriatr Med 4:853, 1988

Malouf R, Brust JCM: Hypoglycemia: causes, neurological manifestations, and outcome. Ann Neurol 17:421, 1985

Millay RH, Klein ML, Illingworth DR: Niacin maculopathy. Ophthalmology 95:930, 1988

Moore RD, Smith CR, Lietman PS: Risk factors for the development of auditory toxicity in patients receiving aminoglycosides. J Infect Dis 149:23, 1984

Pinsky O, Hurwitz ES, Schonberger LB, Gunn WJ: Reye's syndrome and aspirin. Evidence for a dose-response effect. JAMA 260:657, 1988

Rybak LP: Pathophysiology of furosemide ototoxicity. J Otolaryngol 11:427, 1982

Saron BM, Gaind R: Lithium. Clin Toxicol 6:257, 1973

Schwab RA, Bachhuber BH: Delirium and lactic acidosis caused by ethanol and niacin ingestion. Am J Emerg Med 9.363, 1991

Sedman AJ: Cimetidine-drug interactions. Am J Med 76:109, 1984

Sokoll MD, Gergis SD: Antibiotics and neuromuscular function. Anesthesiology 55:148, 1981

Toole JF, Parrish ML: Nitrofurantoin polyneuropathy. Neurology 23:554, 1973

Walters BNJ, Gubbay SS: Tetracycline and benign intracranial hypertension: report of five cases. BMJ 282:19, 1981

Willcox M, Himmelstein DU, Woolhandler S: Inappropriate drug prescribing for the community dwelling elderly. JAMA 272:292, 1994

197. CLINICAL MANIFESTATIONS OF NEUROTOXIC EXPOSURE TO METALS

ROBERT G. FELDMAN

Metals are essential for certain metabolic processes, although their presence in living tissues at a level that interferes with normal functioning can produce serious and often fatal consequences. Early detection of the neurotoxicity of metals is important in clinical practice so that immediate removal from further exposure will prevent further intake, permit recovery of reversible effects, and minimize the risks of permanent damage. The mechanism of neurotoxicity of a metal may include interference with the actions of proteins in the enzyme systems, altering functions of the cell membranes, and affecting the oxidative processes of the organelles of the neurons. This chapter describes the neurologic manifestations of exposure to toxic levels of lead, arsenic, and mercury, three potential neurotoxicant metals most frequently considered in the differential diagnosis of neurologic disease in clinical practice. We begin with, a general review of an approach to detecting neurotoxic disease.

SYMPTOMATIC APPROACH TO DETECTING NEUROTOXIC DISEASE

Many cases of neurotoxic disease are overlooked or misdiagnosed because the individual is not questioned about possible exposures on the job or about working with hazardous substances in recreational activities or hobbies. The household, its water supply, and/or the soil where the individual may garden or play may be contaminated with neurotoxicants. A reasonable degree of suspicion and a systematic line of questioning will lead the examiner to an association between the presenting symptoms and a possible neurotoxic cause, if one exists. A medical history will provide the clinician with information about present and past discomforts and impairments of functions experienced by the patient. It should also reveal details about the patient's work history. Knowledge of the chemical substances used in various industrial processes and workplaces will alert the examiner to a potential risk for exposure (Table 197-1).

Neurologic signs and symptoms arise from alterations in the normal functioning of the various cellular elements and supportive structures of the central and peripheral nervous systems, regardless of the etiology. Thus, common symptoms such as headache, personality changes, disturbances of mood, cognitive functions (including language, memory, and problem-solving), weakness, tremor, ataxia, numbness, and tingling are found in cases of neurotoxic disease as well as in cases of nonneurotoxic disease. A detailed neurologic examination is necessary for the clinician to ascertain the physical signs of a lateralized intracranial lesion as opposed to a diffuse encephalopathic process more consistent with a toxic process, or the appearance of a focal peripheral nerve entrapment as contrasted with bilateral distal sensory losses and reflex changes usually associated with a mixed sensorimotor polyneuropathy.

Even after such discriminations, it is important to be able to confirm the fact that the patient has actually been exposed to a neurotoxicant by finding evidence of the suspected chemical or its metabolites in samples of blood, urine, hair, or nails. Proof of exposure can be obtained by careful sampling of the air, water, or soil sources to which the patient has been exposed. The contaminant is usually still present after the patient has left the site due to illness, but the blood and/or urine levels may have diminished or returned to normal because of excretion and no further exposure. Content of hair or nails may contain stored traces of the suspected neurotoxicant metal long after exposure has ended and urine and blood levels have returned to normal.

LEAD

Sources of Exposure

Lead has many commercial uses throughout the world. Lead ore is mined as a compound with other metals such as zinc, cadmium, and silver. The smelting process used to obtain pure lead releases particulate lead products into the atmosphere, exposing nearby populations. Urban lead air pollution is greatest where organic lead compounds are used as an antiknock agent in gasoline. Undue absorption of lead should be suspected to occur more in certain industries: ore mining and crushing, and smelting; battery manufacturing and battery recycling; radiator repair; paint and pigment manufacturing; soldering, welding, and cutting operations. Artists and craftspersons may use lead pigments in paint and pottery glazes, as well as in making lead glass objects. Recent ordinances have required lead removal from soils, housing, and other structures where it has been found. This has created a hazard among the laborers responsible for its removal, if they do not use proper protective measures. The ubiquitous nature of lead and lead products makes the risks of exposure a serious problem in modern society.

Absorption and Excretion

Particulate lead is inhaled and absorbed through the lungs. Larger size particles, however, do not reach the alveoli for absorption, but are brought to the oral pharynx. Ingested lead particles or lead compounds in food and other sources are absorbed through the gastrointestinal tract. Organic lead compounds are absorbed through the skin, although inorganic lead is not. Once in the bloodstream, lead, bound to the red blood cells, is carried throughout the body, where it is deposited in bone, teeth, liver, lung, kidney, brain, and spleen. Bone serves as a long-term storage site, and lead also crosses the blood-brain barrier and concentrates in neurons.

Lead is excreted mainly by the kidney, and unabsorbed lead may also be found in feces. During exposure, the rise in blood level and urine output reflect an increase in lead content of the body. Once distribution and storage of lead begins to take place, the blood level drops, and less lead may be found in the urine—an occurrence that can be misleading because the actual tissue content of lead may still be significant. For this reason, it is important to use the measures of heme synthesis defects rather than to use simply the blood lead concentration as a diagnostic test. When the blood level of zinc protoporphyrin is elevated (higher than 40 $\mu g/ml$), the concomitant disruption of heme synthesis, presumptively indicating the presence of stored lead as well as ongoing exposure to lead when the blood level of lead is no longer high, can be very helpful in early diagnosis.

Clinical Manifestations and Diagnosis

Symptoms of lead intoxication can be correlated with blood concentration. Toxic effects on the nervous system may not be

TABLE 197-1. Clinical Manifestations of Metal Neurotoxicity

Metal	Source of Exposure	Manifestation
Lead	Solder Lead shot Illicit whiskey Insecticides Auto body shop Storage battery manufacturing Foundries, smelters Lead-based paint Lead pipes	Acute: encephalopathy Chronic: encephalopathy and peripheral neuropathy
Arsenic	Pesticides Pigments Antifouling paint Electroplating industry Seafood Smelters Semiconductors	Acute: encephalopathy Chronic: peripheral neuropathy
Mercury	Scientific Instruments Electrical equipment Amalgams Electroplating industry Photography Felt making	Acute: headache, nausea, onset of tremor Chronic: ataxia, peripheral neuropathy, encephalopathy

the first symptoms recognized; early nonspecific complaints may include indigestion, constipation, or bloating. Fatigue, headache, myalgias, and weakness may be associated with anemia. At this point, the blood lead level may be 20 μg/dl or less. Developmental deficits in cognitive abilities and intellectual capacity have been reported in children exposed to very low levels of lead, showing blood lead concentrations as low as 10 μg./dl. Behavioral and cognitive impairments have been seen in adults at relatively low levels of lead (less than 70 μg/dl), as well. Headache, dizziness, and mood change occurs at higher concentrations (40 to 80 μg/dl); confusion, seizures, and coma associated with encephalopathy occur at higher levels. Death occurs after severe renal damage or when there has been extreme cerebral edema associated with the encephalopathy causing brainstem herniation and cardiorespiratory arrest.

Chronic low-level exposure results in symptoms and signs that become more serious and irreversible as the lead stores accumulate. A mixed sensory motor–peripheral neuropathy develops insidiously after several months. Distal weakness and mild sensory changes are found on neurologic examination. Electrophysiologic tests of nerve conduction velocity demonstrate slowing in motor fibers more than the sensory fibers. Carefully controlled studies of peripheral nerve conduction velocity in lead-exposed workers showed correlation between reduced velocity and amplitude, and blood levels above 70 μg/dl.

Treatment

Early diagnosis allows for time to eliminate and remove the patient from further exposure. If blood levels remain elevated (above 40 μg/dl) after the believed source of exposure has been eliminated, it may be necessary to suspect that there may be some other source of ongoing exposure. This may be due to an external contamination, or the continuing release of internal body stores of lead from muscle, liver, and spleen. Stored lead in bone is less mobilizable than it is from the soft tissues. If there is no continuing uptake of lead, then removal by chelation is necessary to prevent ongoing cellular damage and to eliminate symptoms.

A chelating agent combines with metalions in tissues and removes them. These compounds are then excreted in the urine. A baseline measure of lead in a 24-hour collection should be done before administering a chelating agent. The results can be compared with the output obtained after chelation. Total urinary output as well as urinary lead content are determined. Lead excretion is increased after the administration of several chelating agents. Calcium-sodium edathamil (ethylenediaminetetracetic acid; Ca-Na-EDTA) and penicillamine have been used for a long time with success, despite the risks of dose-related side effects, which include hypertension, rash, nausea, vomiting, headache, and numbness and tingling of extremities. Renal tubular necrosis and cardiac dysrhythmias are the most serious adverse effects, but they are reversible upon cessation of therapy. Dimercaprol, also known as British antilewisite (BAL), can be used in patients with known renal damage since it is excreted in the bile. However, the latter may produce side effects in as many as 50 percent of cases treated.

In the presence of severe encephalopathy and when blood levels exceed 100 μg/dl, treatment should begin with dimercaprol, 4 to 5 mg/kg given intramuscularly every 4 hours, followed by intravenous CaNa$_2$-EDTA, 2 mg/kg/day intravenously for 5 days. When the blood level is lower than 100 μg/dl, therapy can start with Ca-Na-EDTA omitting the dimercaprol. Intravenous Ca-Na-EDTA should be given slowly (maximum of 2 g/kg/be given over 24-hour infusion), while monitoring the electrocardiograph for dysrhythmias. Therapy is given for a period of 5 days and urinary levels are again tested after a rest period of several weeks. Another course of 5 days of chelation should be given if the blood and/or urine lead levels are still elevated. Ca-Na-EDTA is less effective given intramuscularly and not effective orally. Penicillamine is an oral chelating agent that can be given for mild cases, and over a prolonged period of time. A new agent, 2,33-dimercaptosuccinic acid (DSMA), has proven helpful and less noxious for treating lead poisoning in children and adults; it is an oral preparation related to dimercaprol.

ARSENIC

Sources of Exposure

Arsenic is found naturally in soil and water, especially in areas with high geothermal (i.e., volcanic) activity. Arsenic is mined from the earth as an ore usually mixed with other metals, such as copper, lead, and gold. Exposure to arsenic dust occurs among the workers who crush the ore and process it to separate the metals. Arsenic trioxide is released during the smelting process and can be a pollutant in the environment around smelting plants. Some of the many uses for arsenic are listed in Table 197-1. Contaminated ground water in areas where arsenic-containing insecticides are used can be a source for human consumption of arsenic. The most common source of arsenic intake by the general population is the ingestion of food and water containing the metal. Seafoods contain a high arsenic content. Accidental intake of arsenic occurs when the fumes of burning arsenic-treated wood are inhaled.

Absorption and Excretion

Arsenic enters the body by inhalation and ingestion. Dermal absorption is minimal. Airborne arsenic generally takes the form of arsenic trioxide. Arsine gas, the most toxic form of arsenic, enters by inhalation. Inorganic arsenic compounds are absorbed from the gastrointestinal tract most easily when they are in the pentavalent, water-soluble form. Trivalent forms are more lipid-soluble and are less readily absorbed by the gastrointestinal tract. Elemental arsenic has very low solubility and is not absorbed. In the bloodstream arsenic is localized in the erythrocyte, combining with the globin portion of hemoglobin. It also is found in leukocytes and bound to serum proteins. Arsenic clears from the bloodstream within 24 hours and becomes widely distributed in body tissues. If there is no further accumulation by continued exposure, clearance from these tissues takes at least 2 to 4 weeks.

Most arsenic is excreted in the urine. Other routes of elimination include desquamation of arsenic-containing skin and excretion through sweat, milk, and bile. Arsenic has a half-life of about 10 hours and 50 to 80 percent is excreted after 3 days. After a single meal of seafood known to contain large amounts of arsenic, a human subject eliminated 50 percent of the ''fish-arsenic'' after 20 hours. Methylation of arsenic in the liver is the process of detoxification. There is some interconversion between the more toxic pentavalent and the less toxic trivalent forms, but both forms are biomethylated. Organic arsenic compounds occur also in trivalent or pentavalent states. Organic trivalent compounds are more toxic than the organic pentavalent arsenic compounds, but both are less toxic than the inorganic trivalent form. Methylation efficiency increases with increasing arsenic dose in man. Subjects with poor nutrition have a lower capacity to methylate and, therefore, to detoxify inorganic arsenic. After low-level exposure to inorganic arsenic, most of the urinary arsenic is present as methylated metabolites (monomethylarsinic acid, dimethylarsinic acid, and trimethylarsinic acid). If the methylation capacity is exceeded, increased retention of arsenic in soft tissues occurs.

Clinical Manifestations and Diagnosis

The clinical manifestations of arsenic intoxication depend on the route, dose, and duration of exposure, the individual susceptibility of the exposed person, and the physiochemical characteristics of the arsenic taken in, such as the valence state, inorganic or organic compound, gas, solution, or powder. The mechanism of toxic effects of arsenic compounds, especially the trivalent forms, is related to the inhibition of sulfhydryl-containing enzymes in the body. Another possible mechanism, more likely to occur with pentavalent arsenic compounds, disrupts oxidative phosphorylation by replacing the stable phosphoryl with less stable arsenyl compounds, leading to rapid hydrolysis of the high-energy bonds in adenosone triphosphate (ATP) and disturbance of mitochondrial function.

Acute arsenic poisoning is accompanied by nausea, vomiting, colicky abdominal pain, and watery or bloody diarrhea. Serious fluid and electrolyte problems develop in extreme cases, often leading to cardiorespiratory failure and death. More commonly, the clinical picture of arsenic poisoning includes feelings of anxiety and mood change, headache, sleep disturbance, with an insidious emergence of behavioral and cognitive impairments as the exposure becomes more prolonged. With chronic exposure to arsenic the behavioral symptoms precede those of peripheral neuropathy. The typical symptoms of arsenical neuropathy are primarily sensory, consisting of numbness and tingling in the feet, then affecting the hands. These paresthesias often become very painful. Vibration sense is an early modality affected. Perception of pain and temperature is reduced as the neuropathy progresses. The lower extremities are more affected than are the upper ones. Electrical evidence of impaired conduction is seen in the sensory fibers more than in the motor fibers. Although sensory symptoms predominate, the secondary changes in myelin produce more motor signs, so that both sensory and motor neuropathies are seen in cases of arsenic intoxication.

Both short- and long-term exposure to arsenic result in encephalopathy. Chronic encephalopathy was considered to be more associated with exposure to organic arsenic in the past, but recently, with careful neuropsychological tests, subtle cognitive and affective disturbances are recognized in cases of exposure to inorganic arsenic compounds as well. Severe encephalopathy may be associated with memory disorders and seizures, as well as psychotic symptoms of hallucinations, delusions, paranoia, and delirium.

Diagnosis of arsenic poisoning is made by the usual careful and detailed history, and the ascertainment that the behavioral and peripheral nerve symptoms are not due to other medical conditions including alcoholism, diabetes, and/or nutritional problems. Confirmation of the etiology being arsenic in some form requires analysis of the urine content of arsenic. Baseline urine levels of arsenic in the general population not known to be exposed to arsenic range from zero to 130 μg/L, in those

with known dietary exposure the levels are 390 to 1,680 μg/L, and for those with known occupational intake of arsenic the level can be as much as 4 mg/L. Blood levels are useful only when there is ongoing exposure. After careful control to avoid measuring the external contamination, analysis of nails and hair shaft content of arsenic may reveal previous exposure at a time when the blood and urine levels are no longer elevated.

Treatment

Patients with suspected arsenic poisoning must immediately be removed from any source of continuing exposure and the body content of the arsenic must be reduced to safer levels. In cases of severe acute intoxication, stabilization of electrolytes and cardiorespiratory function in an intensive care unit may be needed. Gastric lavage must be used to remove any remaining ingested arsenic. Several remedies for reducing absorption and increasing excretion include administration of a mixture of 300 ml tincture of ferric chloride and 30 mg sodium carbonate in 120 ml water. Hemodialysis and plasma exchange may help clear the blood of any still-circulating arsenic.

Dimercaprol (BAL) is recommended for chelation in arsenic intoxication. The earlier it is given the greater the chance of recovery. Dimercaprol is given intramuscularly at an initial dose of 3 to 5 mg/kg of body weight every 4 to 5 hours for 2 days; it is given every 6 hours on the third day, then twice daily for 10 days. Urine output of arsenic should measured as a baseline every day during therapy and for several weeks thereafter to monitor the course of elimination as the symptoms are observed. Unless irreversible damage has already occurred, axonal regeneration and nerve fiber sprouting may be seen after several months. The degree of recovery depends upon the extent of initial axonal damage.

MERCURY

Sources of Exposure

Mercury is extracted from cinnabar ore, consisting of mercury sulfide. It is found in the environment in three forms: elemental, inorganic, and organic. Elemental mercury is known as quicksilver. Inorganic mercury, mercurous form, forms compounds that dissociate slowly in water or body fluids. Organic mercury compounds include long-chain alkyl and aryl compounds, and short-chain alkyl mercurial compounds. Elemental mercury and inorganic mercury are used in the manufacture of scientific instruments, in amalgams with copper, silver, or gold, in solder with lead, and in plating processes. It is found in industries that use photographic materials, paints and pigments, and dyes. Thermometers, batteries, vapor lamps, and taxidermy solutions contain elemental or inorganic mercury. Organic mercury compounds are used in certain embalming solutions, fungicides, insecticides, wood preservatives, and germicides.

The vaporization of elemental mercury at room temperature allows for inhalation of the metal fumes as they are exposed to the open air. Inorganic and organic mercury compounds can be ingested.

Absorption and Excretion

Mercury vapor is rapidly diffused through the alveolar membrane and is taken up to the brain by the red blood cells. Elemental mercury is highly lipophilic and can easily cross the blood-brain barrier. The concentration of mercury in the brain may remain elevated as long as 10 years after exposure. Inorganic mercurial compounds are highly corrosive and produce serious tissue necrosis of the mucosa of the mouth and of the gastrointestinal tract, usually preventing ingestion and thus absorption of large amounts of the material. Organic mercurial compounds are mainly taken in by ingestion of food, such as cereals that have been treated with mercury-containing fungicides, or accidental spills of organic mercury compounds in water ingested by fish, which in turn are eaten by man. Inorganic mercury in water sources may become methylated by the action of bacteria, forming organic compounds in the drinking water. Organic mercurial compounds are very lipid-soluble and are 90 percent absorbed through the gastrointestinal tract.

Widespread tissue distribution of mercurial compounds reaches the liver, kidney, blood, brain, hair, and epidermis. The amount of organic mercury in brain tissue, although less than in the liver and kidney, is greater than that found after inorganic mercury poisoning. Neurotoxic effects of mercury may be due to an alteration of cyclic adenosine monophosphate (cAMP) metabolism. Autopsy material from victims of a large outbreak of methylmercury poisoning in Japan showed severe cerebellar cell loss, atrophy of the calcarine, pre- and postcentral gyrus cortical neurons. There is a correlation between the exposure and the amount of mercury excreted in the urine and increased risk of neurotoxic effects. Deficits in finger-tapping and eye-hand coordination have been reported in mercury-exposed workers whose urine contained peak historical levels above 5 μg/dl.

Clinical Manifestations and Diagnosis

Clinical manifestations following exposure depend upon the chemical form of the mercury involved and the extent of the exposure. Acute ingestion of mercury salts or inhalation of vapors at toxic levels is followed immediately by gastrointestinal or respiratory effects; in those who do not die from renal shutdown, gastrointestinal bleeding, or pulmonary edema, neurologic manifestations appear within 24 hours. Ingestion of organic mercury leads to symptoms after a latency of weeks to months. These symptoms may increase in severity, even leading to death, if the exposure was sufficient and no treatment was received. Behavioral and cognitive disturbances are the earliest signs of chronic mercury poisoning, followed by movement disorders, including ataxia, tremor, and chorea, and peripheral neuropathy. A syndrome similar to motor neuron disease has been described after chronic mercury exposure.

The tremor of mercurialism, similar in nature to that seen in hyperthyroidism, is fine and rapid, it may worsen upon activity much like an essential tremor, and is faster than that seen in Parkinson's disease. It begins in the fingers and hands, then affects the eyelids, face, and eventually the head, neck, and torso. An electromyographic recording of the tremor and tests of eye-hand coordination, finger-tapping, and cerebellar functions may reveal the motor findings of mercury poisoning. For-

mal neuropsychological tests are helpful in documenting the cognitive impairments of mercurial encephalopathy. Nerve-conduction velocity studies demonstrate the slowing in the peripheral nerves if neuropathy has developed.

Laboratory diagnosis requires a 24-hour urine collection and analysis of the whole blood. Analysis of hair is not recommended because of the possibility of external contamination. Inorganic and elemental mercury are looked for in blood and urine samples. Organic mercury, which is concentrated in the red blood cells, is best found in blood samples. Blood levels normally contain less than 2 μg/dl, and should not exceed 5 μg/dl. Urine levels are normally less than 10 μg/L; exposed workers have been found to have urine levels between 50 and 100 μg/L. Paresthesias occur above 20 μg/L, and tremor is noticeable when urine contains over 50 μg/L.

Treatment

Persons at risk for increased intake of mercury should be monitored. A fourfold increase in urine mercury over baseline indicates a significant body burden, and action must be taken. Immediate removal from the source of exposure and serial urine analyses to ascertain that excretion is occurring satisfactorily must be accomplished. If symptoms have already been noted, then chelation therapy is necessary. Dimercaprol is used in cases of severe inorganic and elemental mercury poisoning. It is *contraindicated* in organic mercury poisoning because it has been shown to increase brain levels of the metal in mice.

Dimercaprol is given in doses of 3 to 5 mg/kg intramuscularly every 4 to 5 hours for 24 hours, every 12 hours for the second 24 hours, and then once a day for 3 days more. A 2-day rest is then followed by another 5-day course. This regimen is repeated until the urine level has come down to 50 μg/L or less. In less severely affected persons d-penicillamine (250 mg orally every 6 hours for 5 days, for adults; 100 mg/kg/day divided into four doses for children), is used. N-Acetyl-d,l,penicillamine (NAP), a water-soluble form of dimercaprol known as 2,3-dimercapto-propane-1-sulfonate (DMPS), and 2,33-dimercaptosuccinic acid (DMSA) have been used in treatment of all forms of mercury poisoning, including organic forms. DMSA is administered in dose of 10 mg/kg three times a day for 5 days, then twice daily for another 14 days. Two weeks of rest are taken between courses of therapy, as the urine is analyzed in this time for excreted mercury.

SUGGESTED READINGS

Bleeker ML: Occupational Neurology and Clinical Neurotoxicology. Williams & Wilkins, Baltimore, 1994

Feldman RG, Travers PH: Environmental and occupational neurology. pp. 191–213. In: Neurology: The Physician's Guide. Thieme, New York, 1984

Sullivan JB Jr, Krieger GR: Hazardous Materials Toxicology, Clinical Principles of Environmental Health. Williams & Wilkins, Baltimore, 1992

White RF, Feldman RG, Proctor SP: Neurobehavioral effects of toxic exposures. pp. 1–51. In White RF (ed): Clinical Syndromes in Adult Neurpsychology: The Practioner's Handbook. Elsevier, Amsterdam, 1992

SECTION 8.   ORGAN TRANSPLANTATION

198. NEUROLOGIC COMPLICATIONS OF ORGAN TRANSPLANTATION

ROY A. PATCHELL
MARTIN A. SAMUELS

Organ transplantation, begun in the midtwentieth century with renal transplantation, has burgeoned into one of the greatest advances in twentieth-century medicine. Considerable advances in immunology have allowed longer survival for transplant recipients, but this has resulted in the emergence of a number of neurologic problems in these patients, most of which will be presented to the primary care physician.

Three types of transplants exist: syngenic (identical twins), allogenic (different genetic origins), and autologous (patient's own tissue). When a new organ is implanted in place of an old one (e.g., liver transplantation), the transplant is said to be orthotopic. In most cases the transplants are allogenic and therefore the recipients require some form of lifelong immunosuppression to prevent rejection. Thus the neurologic complications of organ transplantation may be divided into two major categories: (1) those common to all allogenic transplants, due primarily to the effect of long-term immunosuppression and (2) those specific to particular transplants, due either to the underlying disease, which lead to the need for a transplant, or some phenomenon that is peculiar to the transplantation technique.

NEUROLOGIC COMPLICATIONS DUE TO THE LONG-TERM EFFECTS OF IMMUNOSUPPRESSIVE DRUGS

Cyclosporine

Cyclosporine, the most commonly used drug to prevent rejection, works by inhibiting lymphokine release. Its major toxicity is renal. The hypertension that nearly always complicates cyclosporine use is due in part to renal toxicity, but to a larger extent by the tendency of cyclosporine to stimulate the sympathetic nervous system by an unknown mechanism. Most, if not all, of its neurologic toxicity is due to its tendency to produce hypertension. The encephalopathy of cyclosporine toxicity is roughly correlated with blood levels (therapeutic level is 250 to 500 ng/ml of whole blood or 500 to 300 ng/ml of plasma), but is better correlated with the rate of change in blood pressure from the patient's baseline level. Cyclosporine neurotoxicity could be thought of as a forme fruste of hypertensive encephalopathy. It is characterized by tremor; abnormalities in mental states, ranging from mild inattention to coma; seizures; and various visual syndromes characteristic of dysautoregulation in distal arterial territories of the posterior circulation. These include visual hallucinations, visual field deficits, visual agnosias, Balint syndrome (i.e., the triad of simultanagnosia, abnormalities

in visually directed reaching, and difficulties with voluntary eye movements), and cortical blindness with denial of deficit (i.e., Anton syndrome).

Magnetic resonance imaging shows increased signal on T2-weighted images in the occipital white matter, a finding that may be quite evanescent and does not represent stroke. Flow studies such as single-photon-emission computed tomography demonstrate that this is due to increased flow with extravasation of water. These findings are identical to those found in patients with hypertensive encephalopathy, including the syndrome of toxemia of pregnancy. It should be emphasized that the patient's blood pressure need not be very high (i.e., in the range of malignant hypertension) for this syndrome to occur. The pathogenesis appears to be related to the rate of change of blood pressure combined with loss of cerebral autoregulation rather than the absolute level of blood pressure. Lowering of blood pressure by any means, including, but not exclusively, by lowering the blood level of cyclosporine will result in resolution of the clinical syndrome and the imaging abnormalities.

FK 506

FK 506 is an antirejection drug that works by a mechanism similar to cyclosporine. Although there is less experience with this drug, the range of side effects seems identical to cyclosporine, which is probably due to the same effects on blood pressure.

OK T3

OK T3 is a monoclonal antibody directed against T cells. Its major neurologic side effect is aseptic meningitis, which occurs in about 1 in 20 patients during the first 3 days of exposure to the drug. Cerebrospinal fluid analysis shows a lymphocytic pleocytosis with normal glucose and normal or slightly elevated protein. The syndrome is self-limited and benign, but one should be certain to perform a lumbar puncture and culture the spinal fluid, so as to exclude a bacterial or fungal meningitis before settling on the more benign diagnosis of OK T3-induced aseptic meningitis. The mechanism of the meningeal inflammation is probably allergic, similar to that seen in some patients placed on nonsteroidal anti-inflammatory drugs such as ibuprofen or in some patients treated with intravenous immunoglobulin (IV Ig). The ibuprofen syndrome appears to be more common in patients with rheumatic diseases such as lupus erythematosus. Whether this is also true for the IV Ig and OK T3-induced meningitis is, as yet, unknown. A more severe syndrome including variable degrees of mental status derangement, including seizures may occur even more rarely. It is associated with neuroimaging evidence of cerebral edema, but is also self-limited and benign, even if the OK T3 is continued. The long-term serious side effect of OK T3 use is the development of lymphoma, something which appears to be dose-related.

Antithymocyte and Antilymphoblast Globulins

Antithymocyte globulin and antilymphoblast globulin are antisera directed against thymocytes or lymphocytes. Rarely, patients develop an aseptic meningitis picture, similar to that seen with OK T3, which is also self-limited and benign in nature.

Corticosteroids

Corticosteroids are the oldest immunosuppressive drugs, and are less specific in their actions than the newer agents discussed above. Neurologic complications include psychosis and mania, a proximal myopathy, and, rarely, spinal cord compression due to epidural lipomatosis. Long-term use of steroids also predisposes to glucose intolerance, gastrointestinal bleeding, and osteoporosis, all of which have their own secondary neurologic effects. These are well known to most generalists and are covered in other sections of this text.

Neurologic Infections

Neurologic infections occur in about 10 percent of all transplant recipients, but are more important clinically than that number implies, since about half of the central nervous system (CNS) infections that occur in immunocompromised patients result in death. Nearly every conceivable organism has been reported to infect transplant recipients, but about 80 percent of the cases are due to infection with *Listeria monocytogenes, Cryptococcus neoformans,* and *Aspergillus fumigatus.* Central nervous system infections in immunocompromised hosts may be difficult to recognize because the usual signs of infection, such as fever and meningismus, may be minimally present or absent in such patients, since these signs depend on a vigorous immune response to the infection. Since the usual signs of central nervous system infection may be absent, and since nearly any organism—bacterium, fungus, parasite, or virus—can be responsible, the clinician should have a high suspicion index for infectious causes of neurologic deterioration in any transplant recipient. A few clues may be of help in determining the likely predominant organism.

An infection outside the nervous system should alert the clinician of a possible neurologic infection. Skin lesions may be found to harbor *cryptococcus,* and lung infection suggests *Aspergillus, Nocardia,* or *Cryptococcus.*

Acute meningitis is often due to *Listeria monocytogenes,* while chronic meningitis, often with cranial nerve palsies, suggest tuberculosis or fungal organisms. A progressive multifocal syndrome with hemiparesis visual symptoms, ataxia, dysarthria, and dementia should raise the specter of progressive multifocal leukoencephalopathy caused by the JC polyoma virus. A localized mass lesion (e.g., a brain abscess) is often due to multiple organisms, including anaerobes, but the predominant organism in the immunocompromised patient is usually *Aspergillus, Nocardia,* or *Toxoplasma.*

Another clue to the causative organism is the time period after transplantation. In the early period (up to 1 month after transplantation) infections are due to organisms common in the nonimmunocompromised patient. In the intermediate period (between 1 and 6 months after transplantation), the risk of neurologic infection peaks usually due to either virus (e.g., cytomegalovirus, Epstein-Barr virus) or opportunistic bacteria and fungi (e.g., *Listeria, Aspergillus,* and *Nocardia*). Late infections (more than 6 months after transplantation) are related to the chronic rise of potent antirejection medications such as steroids, monoclonal antibodies, and cyclosporine; the most common organisms at this time are *Cryptococcus, Listeria,* and *Nocardia.*

Lymphoproliferative syndromes occur after prolonged immunosuppression, ranging from apparently benign polyclonal lymphoid hyperplasia to monoclonal lymphoma. The nervous system is involved in about 20 percent of such patients. When the central nervous system is involved, it is the only apparent site of involvement 85 percent of the time. Post-transplant lymphoproliferative syndromes are strongly associated with Epstein-Barr virus infection, but primary central nervous system lymphomas in immunocompetent people are not associated with this virus. These B-cell lymphomas arise deep in the brain with a propensity for the perivascular spaces. Central nervous system lymphoma is distinguished from progressive multifocal leukoencephalopathy by the fact that the former produces mass effect and is enhanced with gadolinuim.

NEUROLOGIC COMPLICATIONS ASSOCIATED WITH SPECIFIC TRANSPLANT TYPES

Renal Transplantation

Renal Transplantation is most often performed in patients with glomerulonephritis (membranous or membranoproliferative) diabetes mellitus and hypertensive renal disease. Other underlying disease include polycystic kidney disease, lupus erythematosus, amyloidosis, analgesic nephropathy, and obstructive nephropathy.

Most of the neurologic complications of renal transplantation are due to the underlying disease for which the transplant was performed. For example, polycystic kidney disease may be associated with multiple cerebral berry aneurysms, hypertension with ischemic and hemorrhagic stroke, lupus erythematosus with antineuronal antibodies and mental states changes and uremic encephalopathy with hepatorenal syndrome. Rapid correction of hyponatremia may lead to central pontine myelinolysis, a syndrome that can range in severity from mild tetraparesis to deep coma or even death and can now be easily demonstrated in the pons or in extrapontine sites by magnetic resonance imaging.

The renal transplantation procedure itself is the oldest of all the organ transplants and now rarely causes any neurologic problems. Occasionally, peripheral nerve injuries (e.g., the lateral femoral cutaneous nerve of the thigh) may be caused by retractors or patient positioning during the surgical procedure, but these are usually reversible without specific treatment.

The most common postrenal transplantation neurologic complication is stroke related to underlying cerebrovascular and/or cardiac disease due to the risk factors of hypertension and diabetes, which are so often present in renal transplant recipients.

Bone Marrow Transplantation

Bone marrow transplants are performed for two major indications: (1) abnormal or absent marrow (e.g., aplastic anemia; genetic diseases such as lysosomal storage diseases or thalassemia major; acute leukemia, such as acute myelocytic, acute lymphoblastic, or chronic lymphocytic; or combined immunodeficiency disease); and (2) hazard to the marrow as the limiting factor in aggressive treatment of a disease (e.g., lymphoma, solid tumor autologous marrow programs, glioblastoma multiforme, breast cancer, or neuroblastoma).

Neurologic complications occur in about 70 percent of bone marrow transplant recipients and are the cause of death in 6 percent. The most common problem is metabolic encephalopathy caused by respiratory failure, hepatic failure, electrolyte disorders, or renal failure. The drugs used to prepare patients for the transplantation, including intrathecal methotrexate, busulfan, cyclophosphamide, and Adriamycin may also contribute to metabolic encephalopathy. Total body irradiation is often used (2,000 cGy or less), which can lead to long-term cognitive dysfunction, particularly in children.

Graft-versus-host disease (GVHD) occurs in about one-third of human leukocyte antigen (HLA)-matched and two-thirds of HLA-mismatched transplants. Acute GVHD, which occurs within 3 months of transplantation consists of rash, diarrhea, and hepatic dysfunction, but no neurologic complications have been reported. Chronic GVHD occurs in about a third of patients who survive more than 3 months after transplantation. It may have an autoimmune pathogenesis and has been associated with polymyositis, myasthenia gravis, and chronic inflammatory demyelinating polyneuropathy.

A leukoencephalopathy occurs in bone marrow transplant recipients who have been treated with methotrexate and whole-body irradiation. It appears that either high-dose intravenous or intrathecal methotrexate must be combined with radiation therapy to produce the leukoencephalopathy. Hemorrhages are usually related to severe thrombocytopenia (i.e., platelets fewer than 20,000/mm^3). Cerebral infarcts are largely caused by emboli from endocarditis, either infective or nonbacterial thrombotic endocarditis, which can occur as part of a generalized hypercoagulable state in bone marrow transplant recipients.

Cardiac Transplantation

Cardiac Transplantation is used to treat medically intractable dilated, hypertrophic, restrictive, and ischemic cardiomyopathies as well as some patients with rheumatic heart disease. Neurologic complications are very common, occurring in 50 to 60 percent of the patients. The cardiac transplantation procedure is associated with variable periods on extracorporeal circulation, which may result in diffuse hypoxic-ischemic injury or focal cerebral infarction related to thromboembolism or air embolism. Damage to the brachial plexus is also commonly seen, due to retraction of the chest wall, and the phrenic nerve may be damaged when the heart is packed in ice during the procedure.

Liver Transplantation

Liver transplantation is used to treat chronic advanced liver disease (e.g., cholestatic diseases, such as primary biliary cirrhosis and sclerosing cholangitis; hepatocellular diseases, such as alcohol or viral hepatitis; vascular diseases, such as the Budd-Chiari syndrome); hepatic malignancies (e.g., hepatoma, cholangiocarcinoma, and isolated hepatic metastasis as may be seen in carcinoid); fulminant hepatic failure (e.g., due to viral hepatitis or drug-induced liver damage with halothane or gold); and metabolic liver diseases (e.g., α_1-antitrypsin deficiency, Wilson's disease, glycogen storage diseases I and II, and protoporphyria).

Many neurologic complications are related to the underlying liver disease. Most patients have some degree of portosystemic

encephalopathy. In patients with Wilson's disease or acquired hepatocerebral degeneration, the neurologic syndrome is usually dramatic, consisting of dysarthria, movement disorder, dementia, and spasticity.

The transplantation procedure is particularly traumatic, often associated with a great deal of blood loss, requiring aggressive blood product and fluid replacement. Hypotension is common, often resulting in some degree of hypoxic-ischemic cerebral damage. Coagulation is frequently defective, leading to cerebral hemorrhages, and intraoperative cerebral infarctions may occur due to air or arterial embolism. Central pontine myelinolysis is particularly common in liver transplant patients, occurring in about 10 percent of autopsied cases. This is probably related to the fact that fluid and blood replacement often results in rapid rises in serum sodium concentrations, the presumed cause of central pontine myelinosis.

Pancreas Transplantation

Pancreas transplantation is used to treat patients with type I diabetes who have severe end-organ damage. Many times, it is done in conjunction with renal transplants, with the aim being to make the patient insulin-independent and reverse some of the end-organ damage. Neurologic complications are very common, occurring in perhaps as many as two-thirds of the patients. Much of the neurologic difficulty is related to the fact that all pancreas transplant recipients have retinopathy and neuropathy at the time of the transplant. In addition, nearly all patients have cerebrovascular disease related to the premature atherosclerosis associated with type I diabetes. The procedure involves either transplanting the whole pancreas into the abdomen or the transplantation of free islet cells. The former is thus far the most successful in correcting the diabetes and reversing or retarding damage to end organs. There are no unique neurologic complications caused by the procedure itself.

Lung Transplantation

Single and double lung transplantation as well as combined heart-lung transplantation is now being performed in specialized centers. No specific neurologic complications have been identified although the usual neurologic effects of metabolic encephalopathy are particularly common in patients undergoing these unusually complex procedures.

SUGGESTED READINGS

Adams HP, Dawson G, Coffman TJ, Corry MD: Stroke in renal transplant recipients. Arch Neurol 43:113–5, 1986

Estol CJ, Pessin MS, Martinez AJ: Cerebrovascular complications after orthotopic liver transplantation. Neurology 41:815–19, 1991

Hotson JR, Pedley T: The neurological complications of cardiac transplantation. Brain 99:673–94, 1976

Patchell RA: Neurological complications of organ transplantation. Ann Neurol 36:688–703, 1994

Patchell RA, White CL, Clark AW et al: Neurologic complications of bone marrow transplantation. Neurology 35:300–6, 1985

Textor SC, Canzanello VJ, Taler SJ et al: Cyclosporine-induced hypertension after transplantation. Mayo Clin Proc 69:1182–93, 1994

Vogt DP, Lederman RJ, Carey WD, Broughan TA: Neurologic complication of liver Transplantation. Transplantation 45:1057–61, 1988

SECTION 9. RHEUMATOLOGY

199. NEUROLOGIC MANIFESTATIONS OF RHEUMATIC DISEASES

PATRICIA M. MOORE

The rheumatic diseases comprise numerous conditions centering around inflammation of the joints, muscles, blood vessels, or connective tissue. The two largest categories, the connective tissue diseases and the vasculitides, typically manifest systemic inflammation and multiorgan injury. Diagnosis of these immunologically mediated diseases depends on clinical and histologic features. The pattern and extent of disease as well as specific serologic, histologic, and, occasionally, radiographic features render the individual diseases distinctive. Neurologic abnormalities, prominent in some disorders, occasionally herald disease. However, these diseases may be difficult to diagnose in their early stages.

The *connective tissue diseases* are multisystem diseases characterized by inflammation of joint, muscle, and skin, and the *vasculitides* are multiorgan or organ-specific diseases characterized by inflammation of blood vessels (Table 199-1). Ischemia is the common denominator of tissue injury caused by the vasculitides.

IMMUNOPATHOGENIC MECHANISMS

Lymphocytes and their products can mediate tissue damage. The complex interplay of lymphocyte subsets often makes it difficult to dissect components of an immune cascade. Genetic factors influence aspects of the immune system, particularly immunoregulatory mechanisms. The role of genetic factors explains the overlap in autoimmune diseases in patients and their relatives. Understanding mechanisms of immune-mediated diseases provides clues to appropriate diagnostic tests and will guide choices among the newer immunotherapies.

Autoantibodies and immune complexes predominate in some

TABLE 199-1. The Connective Tissue Diseases and Vasculitides

Connective tissue diseases
  Systemic lupus erythematosus
  Primary Sjögren's syndrome
  Mixed connective tissue disease
  Rheumatoid arthritis
  Systemic sclerosis
  Polymyositis/dermatositis
Vasculitides
  Polyarteritis nodosa
  Churg-Strauss angiitis
  Hypersensitivity vasculitis
  Wegener's granulomatosis
  Lymphomatoid granulomatosis
  Isolated angiitis of the CNS
  Temporal arteritis
  Takayasu's arteritis
  Behçet's disease
  Secondary vasculitis (caused by infections, neoplasia, toxins)

of these disorders. Transient autoantibody formation is a normal phenomenon in both humans and animals that likely performs a physiologic "housecleaning" function. Persistent autoantibodies occur and may be nonspecific manifestations of inflammation, as with antinuclear antibodies (ANA); markers for a specific disease, as with anti-Sm in systemic lupus erythematosus (SLE); or pathogenic. Autoantibody-mediated disease develops through several mechanisms. Antibodies binding to the cell surface may alter cell function or cause cell death. The antibodies to the acetylcholine receptor in myasthenia gravis and to a skin antigen in pemphigus are examples. Antibodies to intracellular autoantigens such as DNA and Sm produce renal and cutaneous damage largely by immune complex recruited inflammation. Deposition of circulating immune complexes or in situ immune complexes formation (with filtered or planted antigen) both occur. The immune complexes trapped along the basement membrane activate complement components. Complement-derived chemotactic factors (C3a, C5a, C567) cause accumulation of polymorphonuclear leukocytes.

The pathogenicity of other antibodies is uncertain. Antiphospholipid antibodies including anticardiolipin antibodies and lupus anticoagulant are strongly associated with recurrent fetal loss, venous thromboses, and some cases of stroke. Their role in stroke is uncertain. Another potentially pathogenic antibody is antineutrophilic cytoplasmic antibody (ANCA). Although the antigen is intracellular, there is a surface molecule on the neutrophils to which the antibodies bind. Binding of antibody to this surface molecule may induce a respiratory burst in neutrophils leading to degranulation with subsequent vessel wall injury.

Cell-mediated tissue damage is, increasingly, the focus of study in autoimmunity. These interactions occur over short distances (millimeters), and histology is central to understanding of cytotoxic mechanisms and diagnosis. Many of the vasculitic syndromes illustrate this. Endothelial cells are in an immunologically unique position: they direct traffic of lymphocytes by expression of cell surface adhesion molecules, they function as antigen presenting cells (APC), and they secrete cytokines. Cytokines, small proteins produced by lymphocytes, macrophages, and fibroblasts, affect gene expression in cells with cytokine receptors. Among other effects, cytokines amplify and perpetuate inflammation. Uncontrolled production of interleukin-1 (IL-1) and tumor necrosis factor (TNF) may result in tissue injury; the mechanisms appear to be intravascular coagulation, thrombosis, vasculitis, and tissue trauma. Interleukin 1 and other cytokines also induce thromboplastin, prostacyclin, and platelet activating factors from endothelial cells which result in altered vascular permeability and thrombosis. Other mediators released by the endothelium govern chemotaxis and adherence of leukocytes, changes in permeability of the vessel wall, and molecular and cellular transport across the endothelial barrier.

CONNECTIVE TISSUE DISEASES
Systemic Lupus Erythematosus

SLE is a multisystemic inflammatory disease that affects the skin, kidneys, blood, joints, muscles, heart, lungs, gastrointesti-

TABLE 199-2. Pathogenic Mechanisms in Neuro-SLE

Primary
  Immune-mediated
    Direct effects
      Immune complex
      Autoantibodies
    Indirect effects
      Vasculopathy
      Coagulopathy
      Cardiac emboli
Secondary
  Infectious
  Metabolic
  Toxic (including effects of medications)

nal tract, and nervous system. The course ranges from indolent to fulminant. Autoantibodies are a hallmark of SLE; patients and animals with this disease produce exaggerated responses to exogenous antigens and spontaneous production of autoantibodies, some to unique antigens. Autoantibodies to nuclear components, including nucleic acids, proteins, and nucleoprotein complexes are prominent. The particular pattern of autoantibody formation may be an important diagnostic feature. For example, anti-Sm antibodies rarely occur in any disease except SLE. Immune complex deposition with subsequent inflammation is the principal pathogenesis of the renal and cutaneous injury. Anemia, leukopenia, thrombocytopenia, and some coagulopathies likely result from direct antibody mediated effects.

Neurologic abnormalities (neuro-SLE) result from multiple pathogenic mechanisms (Table 199-2). Some clinical events develop from acute immunologic mechanisms and are treatable; others are the results of chronic injury, and therapy may produce more complications than benefit.

Primary manifestations (both acute and delayed) of the chronic hypergammaglobulinemia in SLE may result in neurologic abnormalities. Immune complex deposition occurs readily in the choroid plexus and perhaps some small cerebral vessels. Although these may provide the setting for later clinical effects or may alter the blood brain barrier, there is no direct correlation between the presence of immune complexes and clinical neurologic dysfunction as there is for renal disease. Direct antibody (antineuronal)-mediated effects are potentially important in many transient, diffuse neurologic abnormalities where alterations in cellular function occur without cytopathic effect. There is a correlation between certain neuron-reactive antibodies in the sera and cerebrospinal fluid (CSF) of patients with encephalopathies and psychiatric abnormalities but a specific pathogenic effect is not established. Vasculopathy-vasculitis occurs in visceral organs in SLE, but involvement of the neuraxis by frank arteritis is rare even in patients with recurrent vascular disease. Stroke in SLE more likely results from cardiac emboli, coagulopathies, and degenerative vasculopathies. The latter is histologically demonstrable, particularly in the small vessels. It is difficult to ascertain the pathogenesis because it develops slowly; chronically low levels of circulating immune complexes or cytokines may well be causative. The absence of inflammation is clinically important because there is minimal benefit to glucocorticoid or immunosuppressant therapy.

Secondary causes of neurologic abnormalities are frequently encountered, demand a high index of suspicion, and require different therapies from the primary manifestations. The most prominent of these are infections that remain a major cause of death in SLE patients. Bacterial infections are usually readily diagnosed; fungal infections may remain undetected antemor-

tem. Toxic (usually from medications, notably corticosteroids and antihypertensive agents) and metabolic (typically uremia) effects are consequential and treatable causes of encephalopathy.

Mixed Connective Tissue Disease

Mixed connective tissue disease was initially described on the basis of high titers of antibodies to ribonuclear protein (RNP). Clinically, it appears to be a mild variant of SLE. The clinical features of generalized systemic inflammation, scleroderma, and polymyositis associated with Raynaud's phenomenon suggest the disease. Titers of greater than 1:4000 anti-U1 RNP are typical. Neurologic manifestations occur in over half the patients and include aseptic meningitis, psychosis, febrile headaches, peripheral neuropathies, trigeminal neuropathy, and seizures.

Sjögren Syndrome

Sjögren syndrome is a chronic autoimmune inflammatory disease characterized by diminished lacrimal and salivary secretion resulting in keratoconjunctivits sicca and xerostomia. It is usually a relatively benign disease manifest primarily by exocrine gland impairment as a result of destructive mononuclear infiltrates. In a number of patients, however, visceral involvement occurs. A wide spectrum of extraglandular manifestations develops from lymphoid infiltration of lung, kidney, skin, thyroid gland, stomach, liver, and muscle. There exists a strong association between Sjogren and anti-Ro (SSA) antibodies, although anti-La antibodies also occur. The importance of these autoantibodies in the pathogenesis of the disease is not established. Diagnosis of Sjogren syndrome rests on clinical features, salivary or lacrimal gland biopsy showing lymphocyte infiltration, and, usually, circulating autoantibodies; also, attention to strict histologic criteria on the labial biopsy will be helpful in forming a more precise diagnosis.

Neurologic manifestations are more frequent in the peripheral than the central nervous system. The most distinctive neurologic abnormalities are the sensory and autonomic neuropathies. Cranial neuropathies particularly trigeminal neuropathy are also common and may occur in up to 40 percent of patients. Central nervous system abnormalities appear less often, although the exact incidence is not yet established. The two most likely pathogenic mechanisms for the neurologic abnormalities are direct mononuclear cell infiltration and vasculitis. Histologic studies are needed to better understand immunopathogenic mechanisms.

Rheumatoid Arthritis

Rheumatoid arthritis consists of progressive erosive inflammation of the joints. Activation of a cellular immune response in the genetically susceptible host generates the early stages; ensuing proliferation of polyclonal B cells results in proliferative synovitis; cytokines drive the proliferation of synovial cells, which invade and destroy articular cartilage. Because the damage to the joints is widespread, secondary injury to the nervous system occurs. Cervical spine abnormalities occur in up to 25 percent of patients. Potentially devastating is the dissolution of the transverse ligament allowing forward displacement of the skull and atlas. Physicians must be vigilant to prevent a high cervical myelopathy in these patients. Particularly in unconscious patients, neck manipulations should be performed carefully. Peripheral neuropathies develop from several mechanisms. Compression from swollen tissue and subcutaneous nodules typically result in the chronic, progressive neuropathies. Other pathogenic mechanisms of neuropathy include ischemia. Vascular occlusion, both from vasculitis and obliterative vasculopathy, causes neuropathies usually more acute in onset than the compressive neuropathies. Distal sensory neuropathies frequently occur. Central nervous system (CNS) abnormalities are less common and result from subcutaneous nodules or the systemic vasculitis that complicates a small percentage of patients with rheumatoid arthritis.

Progressive Systemic Sclerosis

Progressive systemic sclerosis (or scleroderma) involves the cardinal features of (1) proliferative intimal arterial lesions, (2) obliterative microvascular defects, and (3) atrophy and fibrosis of the involved organs. Largely a cell-mediated (T lymphocytes and mast cells) immune process, some distinctive autoantibodies may be markers of the disease. Neurologic abnormalities are unusual; in one large series they occurred in less than 1 percent of patients. When clinical neurologic disease does occur it is usually a consequence of accelerated hypertension, uremia, or pulmonary insufficiency. Rarely, a vasculitis complicates scleroderma, and this may involve the CNS. Because an inflammatory myopathy occurs occasionally, differentiation from mixed connective tissue disease may be required in the early stages of disease.

Other Connective Tissue Disorders

Patients may present with neurologic signs and serologic evidence of inflammation including autoantibodies yet defy clinical classification. Sometimes, this is an early manifestation of a specific syndrome. In other cases, the disease may remain undefined. After excluding infections, toxins and neoplasia as a cause of the abnormalities, I call many of these patients undifferentiated connective tissue disease.

VASCULITIS

Idiopathic Vasculitides

The vasculitides are a group of disorders characterized by inflammation and, usually, necrosis of the blood vessel wall. Ischemia is the common denominator of tissue injury. Classification of the vasculitic syndromes incorporates clinical, radiologic, and pathologic features. Sometimes the pattern of disease changes over time, and the diagnosis becomes clearer in retrospect. Identification of any underlying causes of vasculitis is central to the management as this guides treatment. Thus, clinically, primary vasculitides must be distinguished from the secondary vasculidites in patient evaluation.

Polyarteritis Nodosa

Classically a systemic necrotizing vasculitis, polyarteritis nodosa (PAN) targets small and medium-sized muscular arteries with a predilection for bifurcations and branchings. Clinically, the disease affects the kidneys, musculoskeletal system, nervous system, gastrointestinal tract, skin, heart, genitourinary system; hypertension is common. Laboratory features may reflect systemic inflammation but are not diagnostic. Although its role in the pathogenesis is not clear, about 20 to 30 percent of patients with polyarteritis nodosa have a hepatitis B antigenemia. Diagnosis of PAN depends on angiography and biopsy. Peripheral neuropathies, which may be the presenting manifestation of PAN, occur in 60 percent of patients. Six major patterns of neuropathy—mononeuropathy multiplex, extensive mononeuropathy multiplex, polyneuropathy, cutaneous neuropathy, brachial plexopathy, and radiculopathy—may appear. Central nervous system abnormalities develop in 40 percent of patients including encephalopathies, subarachnoid hemorrhage, seizures, strokes, cranial neuropathies. These usually occur later in the course of the disease then the peripheral neuropathies and are not typically a presenting manifestation of PAN.

Churg-Strauss Angiitis

Churg-Strauss angiitis affect small and medium-sized vessels with prominent involvement of pulmonary vessels, eosinophilic infiltrates, and granuloma. Neurologic abnormalities are similar to PAN, but encephalopathies occurring early in the course of the disease are more frequent. Peripheral neuropathies are common. Adult-onset asthma, particularly in association with eosinophilia, should suggest the diagnosis.

Hypersensitivity Vasculitis

Hypersensitivity vasculitis, the most frequently encountered of all the vasculitides, is a heterogeneous group of clinical syndromes characterized by inflammation of small vessels, mainly the venules. The skin is the predominantly affect organ. In many instances, the vessel inflammation can be identified as a response to a precipitating antigen such as a drug, foreign protein, or microbe. Several groups of hypersensitivity vasculitis including serum sickness, Henoch-Schonlein purpura and vasculitis with mixed cryoglobulinemia have distinctive clincopathologic characteristics. Involvement of the nervous system is variable. Neurologic abnormalities are frequent in serum sickness and include encephalopathy, seizures, stroke, brachial plexopathy, and peripheral neuropathies. In other subgroups of hypersensitivity vasculitis neurologic involvement is unusual, although reports of subarachnoid hemorrhage and peripheral neuropathies exist.

Wegener's Granulomatosis

Wegener's granulomatosis is a systemic necrotizing vasculitis with a characteristic organ specificity. The involvement of the upper and lower respiratory tracts with granulomatous vasculitis together with a necrotizing glomerluonephritis is quite distinctive. Histologically, granulomata are prominent in the vasculitic lesions. The diagnosis is often suggested by cough, hemopytis, or recurrent sinus abnormalities in a patient with evidence of systemic inflammation. Neurologic abnormalities, particularly cranial neuropathies may be among the presenting manifestations of disease. Two processes produce most of the neurologic abnormalities: contiguous extension of granulomas from primary sites in the nasopharynx (cranial neuropathies, cavernous sinus compression, diabetes insipitus), and vasculitis (peripheral neuropathies, encephalopathies, stroke). Ocular abnormalities, including proptosis and inflammation of the anterior structures of the eye occur just under half the patients. Wegener's is unusual among the vasculitides in the strong association between the disease and an autoantibody, antineutrophilic cytoplasmic antibody (cANCA). These autoantibodies are reactive with myeloperoxidase and proteinase 3. The pattern of binding within the cell varies. Classic ANCA (cANCA) is more strongly associated with Wegener's and microscopic polyarteritis while the peripheral (pANCA) is less specific in its associations. Controversy exists over whether these antibodies are serologic markers for disease activity, pathogenic, or neither.

Lymphomatoid Granulomatosis

Lymphomatoid granulomatosis a rare disease affecting the lungs, skin, and nervous system. Lung involvement is central and usually manifest as multiple nodular infiltrates, which tend to cavitate. Histologic lesions are characterized by infiltration of vessels with atypical lymphocytes, plasmacytes, and histiocytes in an angiocentric angiodestructive pattern. Granulomas are plentiful. Both central and peripheral nervous systems may be affected. CNS dysfunction is reported in 20 percent of patients and peripheral nervous system dysfunction in 15 percent. The spectrum of neurologic abnormalities is wide and includes visual loss, nystagmus, cranial neuropathies, ataxia, aphasia, encephalopathies, and upper motor neuron changes.

Giant Cell Arteritis

Two histologically similar but clinically distinct diseases are included under the term giant cell arteritis: temporal arteritis and Takayasu's arteritis.

Temporal Arteritis.   Temporal arteritis is a systemic panarteritis affecting mainly elderly patients. Despite the widespread nature of the vasculitis, symptoms below the neck are unusual. Neurologically, visual impairment and cranial neuropathies predominate. Because blindness is a frequently devastating complication of temporal arteritis, it is important for physicians remain vigilant for the disease. The disease should be considered in any patient over the age of 40 with new onset of headaches and/or visual changes. Jaw claudication, lingual ischemia, and occipital headache are alternate presenting manifestations. Immediate sedimentation rate and temporal artery biopsy guide diagnosis. The alkaline phosphatase is often elevated.

Takayasu's Arteritis.   Takayasu's arteritis a large-vessel arteritis affecting the aortic arch and its branches in young women. Often called the pulseless disease, absence of at least one arterial pulse is identified in 98 percent of patients. Bruits are often heard. The disease may be divided into an acute stage characterized by signs and symptoms of systemic inflammation, followed by a chronic phase marked by signs and symptoms of vascular occlusion. Typically the disease is recognized by ischemia secondary to the reduced blood flow to the extremities and other organs. Most of the neurologic abnormalities occur in the latter vaso-occlusive stage of the illness. Syncope is reported by over half the patients. Hypertension exacerbates the vascular disease. Neurologically, strokes, transient, ischemic attacks, and syncope are prominent.

Behçet's Disease

Behçet's disease, characterized by relapsing ocular lesions and recurrent oral and genital ulcers, is histologically a small-vessel vasculitis that mainly affects venules. A genetic role is suggested by the apparent increased incidence of the disease in patients from eastern Mediterranean countries. The disease is often benign, although the recurrent ulcers are symtomatically distressing. In some patients neurologic abnormalities are associated with a more serious course; 10 to 50 percent of patients have neurologic abnormalities including meningoencephalitis, brainstem abnormalities, and focal CNS changes.

Isolated Angiitis of the Central Nervous System

Isolated angiitis of the CNS is a recurrent, inflammatory disease of the small and medium-sized blood vessels of the brain and spinal cord. Initially included under the term granulomatous angiitis of the CNS, the name was changed because granulomas are a variable and often absent feature. The disease has been recognized with increasing frequency in the past decade, possibly because current treatment methods are so effective. The precise diagnosis may be difficult. Classically, appropriate clinical features, absence of evidence of systemic inflammation, angiographic and histologic data are necessary. In addition, because an occasional self-limited vasculopathy occurs, evidence of recurrent or persistent disease is necessary. Symptoms and signs are restricted to the nervous system and typically include headaches, encephalopathies, strokes, cranial neuropathies, and myelopathies. Notably symptoms and laboratory evidence of systemic inflammation are absent. Neurodiagnostic studies including computed tomography (CT) scan and magnetic resonance imaging (MRI) are often nonspecifically abnormal. Angiography is the most sensitive diagnostic study, although an occasional patient with only small vessel disease may have a normal angiogram. Of greater concern is the fact that the angiographic features are not specific for vasculitis; similar abnormalities may occur in noninflammatory vasculopathies as well as vasculitis secondary to infections, drugs, and neoplasia. Treatment is not recommended on the basis of angiogram alone. Clinical features that should suggest the diagnosis are headaches and encephalopathy particularly in association with multifocal signs. Angiography often shows single or multiple areas of beading along the course of a vessel, abrupt vessel terminations, hazy vessel margins, and neovascularization. The pathogenesis of the CNS vascular inflammation is not known. A cell-mediated process appears most likely.

Other Vasculitides

There are several reports and series of patients with neurologic abnormalities not readily classifiable in the above disease groups. Among these are a vasculitis restricted to the peripheral nervous system (although many of these patients later go on to develop systemic vasculitis) and a small vessel vasculitis restricted to the CNS, skin, and muscle. Another disorder of small vessel is more likely a microvasculopathy than a vasculitis, the retinocochlear encephalopathy, appears to be more prevalent in Europe. The syndrome consists of a subacute encephalopathy (often with early psychiatric features) sensorineural hearing loss, and retinal arteriolar occlusions. This hearing loss in association with vascular disease must be distinguished from Cogan syndrome (of nonsyphilitic interstitial keratitis and vestibuloauditory symptoms). Some patients with Cogan syndrome have a vasculitic component that is predominantly an aortitis.

Secondary Vasculitides

Central nervous system infections reveal the clearest association between a specific etiology and vasculitis. A wide range of infectious agents cause a vasculitis including: bacteria, fungi, viruses, treponemes, mycobacteria, rickettsia, and parasites. The infection may range in tempo and severity. At times, an infection is so indolent (such as aspergillosis) that only a rigorous search for the cause of a vasculitis reveals the pathogen. Multiple mechanisms can lead to vascular inflammation: direct infection of the vessel wall, immune complexes, or toxic products of the bacteria. Fungal infections may result in a vasculitis clinically indistinguishable from an idiopathic vasculitis. Herpes zoster ophthalmicus associated with contralateral hemiplegia is well described. Identifying an underlying infection in a patient is crucial. Corticosteroid or immunosuppressive therapy without appropriate antimicrobial agents could result in dissemination of disease.

The earliest reports of toxin associated vasculitis is probably sulfonamide-induced hypersensitivity vasculitides. Amphetamine abuse is associated with both a systemic necrotizing vasculitis and a vasculitis restricted to the CNS. More recently, cocaine is a frequently encountered cause of stroke; the underlying mechanism is usually a hemorrhagic vasculopathy, but occasionally a vasculitis occurs. Because drug use is currently prevalent in all socioeconomic sectors of society, a careful medication/drug history is important in all patients.

Neoplasia may cause a vasculitis by several mechanisms. Typically immune complex formation associated with a large tumor load causes nonspecific systemic inflammation. Hodgkin's disease, by an unknown mechanism, is associated with a vasculitis restricted to the central nervous system. A reported, although unusual, paraneoplastic complication of oat cell and ovarian carcinoma is a peripheral nerve vasculitis. Accurate diagnosis is important because the vasculitis resolves with treatment of the underlying disease.

DIAGNOSIS

The neurologist will encounter the rheumatic diseases primarily in two settings: (1) when a neurologic abnormality is the presenting complaint, and the physician must decide whether there is an underlying connective tissue disease or vasculitis, and (2) when a patient with an established diagnosis presents with a new neurologic event that may indicate either an undertreated disease, a complication of treatment, or a diagnosis that is inaccurate and must be revised. Tables 199-3 and 199-4 summarize some general points.

TABLE 199-3. General Points to Remember Regarding Rheumatic Diseases with Neurologic Manifestations

ANA, immune complexes, rheumatoid factor, and sedimentation rate are not tests for vasculitis; they neither confirm nor exclude a diagnosis.

Vasculitis has no pathognomonic radiographic features.

The erosive and destabilizing changes in the cervical spine in rheumatoid arthritis render the cord susceptible to compression and trauma.

The diagnosis of temporal arteritis rests on a high index of suspicion in any patient over 45 to 50 with new-onset headaches or visual changes. Extended treatment with corticosteroids (usually 1 year) is important to reduce the incidence of relapses.

Antiphospholipid antibodies occur in a variety of autoimmune diseases and are associated with strokes, but the pathogenesis of the antibodies is not yet established. Treatment directed at the antiphospholipid antibodies is usually reserved for patients who fulfill the criteria for the syndromes of recurrent fetal loss, recurrent thrombophlebitis, or stroke.

TABLE 199-4. Outline for the Evaluation and Treatment of Rheumatic Diseases with Neurologic Manifestations

Evaluation
  Delineate neurologic abnormalities (CNS/PNS; white/gray matter; mixed)
  Determine distribution of systemic disease (renal, cutaneous, cardiac, hepatic, ocular)
  Determine immunologic abnormalities (autoantibodies, immune complexes, cellular infiltrates)
  Discover any underlying conditions
Treatment
  Evaluate immunopathogenic mechanisms
  Remove any underlying causes
  Determine extent of tissue damage
  Determine the least toxic and most effective treatment
  Plan dose, duration, and goals of therapy

Features that would suggest a search for an underlying connective tissue disease or vasculitis include a young and/or female patient, evidence of multisystem disease, the presence of systemic inflammation, and previous unexplained neurologic or systemic abnormalities. The clinician relies on serologic and histologic studies for diagnosis, while realizing that in several of these diseases there may be no serologic markers of a progressive disease. Histology is central to the diagnosis is most of the vasculitides and is important in SLE and Sjögren's disease. Specific serologic studies (autoantibodies) may be diagnostic or at least narrow the diagnostic possibilities in cases with high titers of anti-DNA, anti-Sm, anti-Ro, anti-La, ENA, and ANCA. Angiography is useful in the medium- and large-vessel vasculitidies. Among the valuable information provided by angiography is the distribution of the disease and serial evaluations to show healing or progression.

The neurologist is also asked to evaluate patients with an identified connective tissue disease or vasculitis and new neurologic symptoms. In this situation the new features usually results from either inexorable disease progression, inadequate therapy, or a complication of the treatment regimen. Occasionally the initial diagnosis was incorrect and the clinicians must reevaluate the data for diagnosis.

Among the most important clinical concerns in this group are complications of therapy, largely avoidable or treatable. Because many of these patients are immunosuppressed, infections occur and contribute prominently to the morbidity and mortality. Diagnosis of infection may be overlooked because symptoms (malaise, fever, headache) and signs are attributed to the underlying disease. Specifically, the usually indolent CNS fungal infections are underdiagnosed. A high clinical index of suspicion, repeated CSF analyses and occasionally brain biopsy are important. Other complications of therapy include the side effects of medications. Corticosteroids are frequent causes of psychopathy, visual changes, myopathy. Antihypertensive medications may cause headaches and cognitive changes.

TREATMENT

The results of treatment vary from excellent to frustrating: Some regimens in individual diseases dramatically reduce morbidity and mortality, whereas in other disorders the optimal treatment remains empirical. The general guidelines to therapy are as follows:

1. Treat any precipitating causes such as infections or toxins in the secondary vasculitides.
2. Use the current, standard treatment in those primary vasculitides with known responsiveness to specific therapies (prednisone in temporal arteritis and prednisone/cyclophospha-

mide in Wegener's granulomatosis, PAN, and isolated angiitis of the CNS).

3. In the primary vasculitides with less well-defined treatments, such as lymphomatoid granulomatosus and Behçet's disease, compare the benefit/risk ratio for treatment in each patient and begin with the least toxic treatment.

4. Remember that in the later stages of vasculitic disease, ischemia may result from chronic scarring rather than acute inflammation; scarring is not responsive to immunosuppressive therapy, and the patient should be spared the side effects of ineffective medication.

Experience in the use of immunosuppressant medications is also important because of the wide range of potential and actual side effects. Side effects occur with any of these agents and the physician should be thoroughly acquainted with all potential side effects before initiating treatment. (Table 199-3).

Glucocorticoids

The efficacy of glucocorticoids, usually prednisone or methylprednisolone, varies. Undoubtedly it is the single most effective treatment in temporal arteritis. It must be remembered that the prednisone must be initiated in a dosage of 40 to 60 mg/day, although it can then usually be slowly tapered to a 20 to 30 mg/day and that treatment must be prolonged (more than 8 to 12 months) because shorter regimens have resulted in devastating relapses.

In some hypersensitivity vasculitides and in microangiopathic renal vasculitis, prednisone therapy alone may suffice. In other disorders, either the high dosage is unsustainable because of the considerable side effects or it is effective only as adjunct therapy. It is ineffective in well-established Wegener's granulomatosis. Patients with polyarteritis nodosa may develop new neurologic side effects while their disease is apparently quiescent on prednisone. Thus in these disorders experience with the underlying disease will enable the physician to determine when to use another agent such as cyclophosphamide.

In addition to the well described side effects of acute and chronic corticosteroid therapy, there are specific effects that impact vascular diseases particularly a potential to augment vasoconstriction and platelet aggregation. This may complicate treatment of vasculitis syndromes creating truly a "double-edged sword."

Cyclophosphamide

Cyclophosphamide dramatically reduces the mortality of Wegener's granulomatosus as well as isolated angiitis of the CNS and polyarteritis nodosa. In other diseases it is a useful adjunct either to reduce the dosage and side effects of prednisone or for corticosteroid failures. It is most often prescribed either in a daily oral dose or as an intermittent intravenous bolus. Oral cyclophosphamide usually prescribed at a dose of 1 to 2 mg/kg/day. Hydration is important to prevent hemorrhagic cystitis and potentially reduce incidence of bladder malignancies. Monitoring of white blood cell count for the limiting factor of neutropenia, less than 1,500, is essential in dosage management. Bolus intravenous cyclophosphamide, when effective, reduces the total dosage of medication used and, usually side effects.

Azathoprine

Azathoprine has less immunodepressive activity than other agents. It is used in the vasculitidies most often in patients

who cannot tolerate cyclophosphamide. A recent study reported azathioprine ameliorated the ocular manifestations of Behçet's disease.

Methotrexate

Methotrexate suppresses both cell-mediated and humoral immunity. Despite demonstrated efficacy in the therapy of rheumatoid arthritis, methotrexate is not established in the treatment of vasculitis. In several patients with isolated angiitis of the CNS, methotrexate did not control a relapse.

Cyclosporin

The efficacy of cyclosporin in various autoimmune diseases is under investigation. Cyclosporin administered along with an adrenergic blocking agent has minimized vessel permeability in rats with experimental retinal vasculitis. However, in the rabbit serum sickness model of vasculitis, cyclosporin pretreatment increased multifocal organ damage and hemorrhage ostensibly because of decreased endothelial cell prostacyclin production. The side effects of nephrotoxicity and hypertension limit its widespread use in human vasculitis, although therapeutic benefit is occasionally reportedly in patients who are refractory to traditional regimens.

Pheresis

Pheresis, the selective removal of plasma or cellular components from the blood, is effective in controlled studies of Goodpasture's syndrome, certain hyperviscosity states, thrombotic thrombocytopenic purpura, Guillan-Barré syndrome, and myasthenia gravis. Its efficacy in connective tissue and vasculitic diseases is unsubstantiated. Pheresis has been used in polyarteritis nodosa, particularly that associated with hepatitis B viremia. Plasma exchanges are able to remove immune complexes and to facilitate physiologic removal of complexes by the reticulendothelial system. Pheresis has been effective, albeit in a limited number of patients to date, in neurologic manifestations of SLE, especially those patients with presumed antineuronal antibody-mediated disease.

Monoclonal Antibodies

Monoclonal antibodies directed against surface markers on lymphocytes are potentially useful as selective therapeutic agents in a variety of immunologically mediated diseases. Current research utilizes antibodies that may block receptors for antigen, adhesion, or growth factors or may block effector cells (via complement activation or Fc binding). The more specific an antibody is the less likely there will be compromise of normal immune function. Anti-T cell monoclonal antibodies are an effective adjunct therapy in allograft rejection. Monoclonal antibodies to other molecules such as the interleukin-2 receptor might also modify recurrent inflammation. Monoclonal antibodies, anti-CD4, and campath-1H, have successfully induced a short-term remission in one patient with systemic vasculitis refractory to conventional immunosuppression.

Intravenous Immunoglobulin

Intravenous immunoglobulin, initially used about 10 years ago for the treatment of primary immunodeficiency disease effectively supplies anti-infectious agent antibodies by passive immunization. It was incidentally noted at the time to improve thrombocytopenia. Despite an occasional scattered report, its utility in the vasculitides is not established. Its use remains of concern in SLE and Sjögren syndrome, where dramatic autoantibody responses may occur.

Antiprostaglandins

Antiprostaglandins are a potentially useful adjunct in numerous vasculopathies. In the diseased blood vessel, endothelium dependent smooth muscle relaxation is impaired. Both vasoconstriction and secondary platelet aggregation accelerate. An endothelial peptide, endothelin, a smooth muscle contractor is increased in some diseases. Anti-inflammatory and antivasospastic effects of prostaglandin E_1 infusion are reported effective in several cases. The size of the vessel involved appears to be a restricting factor. There would be limited effects in peripheral neuropathy due to vasonervorum infarction and other small vessels too small to contain muscle cells. Side effects are unusual but noteworthy. The vasodilatory effect could result in hypotension (potentially serious in patients with ischemic bowel) and steal syndromes.

Antiplatelet Agents and Anticoagulation

Platelet activation, thrombus deposition, and vasoconstriction are prominent in most of the vasculitides. Low-dose aspirin during immunosuppressive therapy would appear to minimize many of these effects, although this has not been rigorously studied.

Anticoagulation with heparin or coumadin therapy, although theoretically useful, has practical limitations. Many of the vasculitides demonstrate histologic evidence of perivascular hemorrhage. The risk of intracranial hemorrhage is potentially high. In the vasculopathy associated with SLE, hemorrhage is a concern and anticoagulation should be used cautiously, if at all.

SUGGESTED READINGS

Alexander EL, Provost TT, Stevens MB et al: Neurologic complications of primary Sjögren's syndrome. Medicine 61:247–57, 1982

Alhalabi M, Moore PM: Serial angiography in isolated angiitis of the central nervous system. Neurology 44:1221–6, 1994

Boumpas DT, Yamada H, Patronas NJ et al: Pulse cyclophosphamide for severe neuropsychiatric lupus. Q J Med 81:975–84, 1991

Bourke BE: Central nervous system involvement in systemic lupus erythematosus are we any further forward? Br J Rheumatol 32:267–8, 1993

Calabrese LH, Gragg LA, Furlan AJ: Benign angiopathy: a distinct subset of angiographically defined primary angiitis of the central nervous system. J Rheumatol 20:2046–50, 1993

Calabrese LH, Mallek JA: Primary angiitis of the central nervous system. Report of 8 new cases, review of the literature, and proposal for diagnostic criteria. Medicine 67:20–39, 1988

Campion EW: Desperate diseases and plasmapheresis. N Engl J Med 326:1425–7, 1992

Citron BP, Halpern M, McCarron M et al: Necrotizing angiitis with drug abuse. N Engl J Med 283:1003–11, 1970

Conn DL, Tompkins RB, Nichols WL: Glucocorticoids in the management of vasculitis: a double edge sword? J Rheumatol 15:1181–83, 1988

Cupps TR, Moore PM, Fauci AS: Isolated angiitis of the central nervous system: prospective diagnostic and therapeutic experience. Am J Med 74:97–105, 1983

Delecocuillerie G, Poly P, Delara AC et al: Polymyalgia rheumatica and temporal arteritis: a retrospective analysis of prognostic features and different corticosteroid regiments. Ann Rheum Dis 47:733–9, 1988

Edwards KK, Lindsley HB, Lai C et al: Takayasu arteritis presenting as retinal and vertebrobasilar ischemia. J Rheumatol 16:1000–2, 1989

Greer JM, Longley S, Edwards NL et al: Vasculitis associated with malignancy. Experience with 13 patients and literature review. Medicine 67:220–30, 1988

Hall S, Barr W, Lie JT et al: Takayasu arteritis: a study of 32 north american patients. Medicine 64:89–99, 1985

Harris ED Jr: Rheumatoid arthritis. N Engl J Med 322:1277–89, 1990

Hart MN, Zsuzsanna F, Waldschmidt M et al: Lymphocyte interacting adhesion molecules on brain microvascular cells. Molec Immunol 27:1355–9, 1990

Herskovitz S, Lipton RB, Lautos G: Neuro-Behcet's disease: CT and clinical correlates. Neurology 36:260, 1986

Hickey WF: Migration of hematogenous cells through the blood-brain barrier and the initiation of CNS inflammation. Brain Pathol 1:97–105, 1991

Hoffman GS, Kerr GS, Leavitt RY et al: Wegener granulomatosis: an analysis of 158 patients. Ann Intern Med 116:488–98, 1992

Isenberg DA, Morrow WJW, Snaith ML: Methyl prednisolone pulse therapy in the treatment of systemic lupus erythematosus. Ann Rheum Dis 41:347–51, 1982

Jennette JC, Falk RJ, Andrassy K et al: Nomenclature of systemic vasculitides: proposal of an international consensus conference. Arthritis Rheum 37:187–92, 1994

Katzenstein AA, Carrington CD, Liebow AA. Lymphomatoid granulomatosis: a clinicopathologic study of 152 cases. Cancer 43:360–73, 1979

Krendel DA, Ditter SM, Frankel MR et al: Biopsy-proven cerebral vasculitis associated with cocaine abuse. Neurology 40:1092–4, 1990

Khamashta MA, Harris EN, Gharavi AE et al: Immune mediated mechanism for thrombosis: antiphospholipid antibody binding to platelet membranes. Ann Rheum Dis 47:849–54, 1988

Lanham JG, Elkon KB, Pusey CD et al: Systemic vasculitis with asthma and eosinophilia: a clinical approach to the Churg-Strauss syndrome. Medicine 63:65–81, 1984

Mader R, Keystone EC: Infections that cause vasculitis. Curr Opin Rheumatol 4:35–8, 1992

McCune WJ, Golbus J, Zeldes W et al: Clinical and immunologic effects of monthly administration of intravenous cyclophosphamide in severe systemic lupus erythematosus. N Engl J Med 318:1423–31, 1988

Mehler MF, Rainowich L: The clinical neuro-ophthalmologic spectrum of temporal arteritis. Am J Med 85:839–44, 1988

Moore PM: Diagnosis and management of isolated angiitis of the central nervous system. Neurology 39:167–73, 1989

Moore PM: Immune mechanisms in the primary and secondary vasculitides. J Neurol Sci 93:129–45, 1989

Moore PM, Cupps TR: Neurological complications of vasculitis. Ann Neurol 14:155–67, 1983

Moore PM, Fauci AS: Neurologic manifestations of systemic vasculitis: a retrospective and prospective study of the clinicopathologic features and responses to therapy in 25 patients. Am J Med Sci 71:517–24, 1981

Nakano KK, Schoene WC, Baker RA et al: The cervical myelopathy associated with rheumatoid arthritis: analysis of patients with 2 postmortem cases. Ann Neurol 3:144–51, 1978

Nishino H, Rubino FA, DeRemee RA et al: Neurological involvement in Wegener's granulomatosis: an analysis of 324 consecutive patients at the Mayo Clinic. Ann Neurol 33:4–9, 1993

Panegyres PK, Faull RJ, Russ GR et al: Endothelial cell activation in vasculitis of peripheral nerve and skeletal muscle. J Neurol, Neurosurg Psychiatry 55:4–7, 1992

Said G, Lacrois-Ciaudo C, Fujimura H: The peripheral neuropathy of necrotizing arteritis: a clinicopathologic study. Ann Neurol 23:461–5, 1988

Savage COS, Cooke SP: The role of the endothelium in systemic vasculitis. J Autoimmun 6:237–49, 1993

Schmidt BJ, Meagher-Villemure K, Carpio JD: Lymphomatoid granulomatosis with isolated involvement of the brain. Ann Neurol 15:478–81, 1984

Schneebaum AB, Singleton JD, Sterling G et al: Association of psychiatric manifestations with antibodies to ribosomal P proteins in systemic lupus erythematosus. Am J Med 90:54–62, 1991

Stern DM, Bank I, Nawroth PP et al: Self-regulation of procoagulant events on the endothelial cell surface. J Exp Med 162:1223–35, 1985

Tan EM, Cohen AS, Fries JF et al: The 1982 revised criteria for the classification of SLE. Arthritis Rheum 25:1271–7, 1982

Tervaert JWC, Woude FJ, Fauci AS et al: Association between active Wegner's granulomatosis and anticytoplasmic antibodies. Arch Intern Med 149:2461–5, 1989

Vanderzant C, Bromberg M, MacGuire A et al: Isolated small-vessel angiitis of the central nervous system. Arch Neurol 45:683–7, 1988

Walsh TJ, Hier DB, Caplan LR: Aspergillosis of the central nervous system: clinicopathological analysis of 17 patients. Ann Neurol 18:574–82, 1985

Wollheim FA: Acute and long-term complications of corticosteroid pulse therapy. Scand J Immunol 54:27–32, 1984

Yazici H, Pazarli H, Barnes CG et al: A controlled trial of azathioprine in Behcet's syndrome. N Engl J Med 322:281–5, 1990

HEADACHE AND PAIN

PART IX

SECTION 1. GENERAL ASPECTS OF HEADACHE

200. ANATOMY AND PHYSIOLOGY OF HEADACHE

EGILIUS L. H. SPIERINGS

The head hurts more often without harm having been done to it than any other part of the body. Pain in the head or headache affects 70 to 80 percent of the population, men and women alike. Fifty percent of the population has headache at least once a month, 15 percent at least once a week, and 5 percent, that is 1 of 20 people, suffers from headache daily.

Headaches are generally classified as mild, moderate, or severe. Mild headaches do not interfere with the ability to function, whereas moderate headaches do, and severe headaches disable the individual. Moderate and severe headaches affect women about twice as often as men; moderate headaches occur in 23 percent of women and 13 percent of men, and severe headaches occur in 12 percent of women and 6 percent of men. The prevalence of migraine is 16 percent for women and 9 percent for men.

Headaches are not only sex-dependent, but also age-dependent. The incidence of headache sharply increases during the first and second decades of life, then levels off until the age of 40. Thereafter the incidence gradually decreases.

In a recent epidemiologic study in Denmark, the lifetime prevalence of headache was 96 percent (93 percent for men and 99 percent for women) for a group ranging in age from 25 to 64 years. The headaches were diagnosed according to the classification criteria of the International Headache Society. The lifetime prevalence of migraine was found to be 16 percent (8 percent for men and 25 percent for women). The lifetime prevalence of tension-type headache was 78 percent (69 percent for men and 88 percent for women). Of those who ever had migraine, 87 percent also had tension-type headache at some time; 3 percent of the population had chronic tension-type headache with more than 180 days with headache per year.

EPIDEMIOLOGY OF MIGRAINE IN THE UNITED STATES

The prevalence of migraine was also a recent topic of study in the United States. All regions of the United States were included, and the segment of the population studied were those between 12 and 80 years of age. A self-administered questionnaire was sent to a stratified random sample of 15,000 households. A designated member of each household responded to the questionnaire by reporting the number of members in the household and the number who suffer from severe headaches. In addition, each household member with severe headaches was asked to complete the questionnaire.

Of the 15,000 households, 9,507 (63 percent) responded to the questionnaire for a total base population of 23,611 household members. The response rate was higher among whites (64 percent) than blacks (49 percent) and other race groups (38 percent). By age, it was highest among the elderly (76 percent) and lowest among adults between 18 and 29 years of age (52 percent). The response rate was also lower in the South Central United States (59 percent) than in other regions of the country. It did not differ by sex, urban versus rural residence, or household income.

Migraine was defined as at least one severe headache during the preceding 12 months which had one of the following features: (1) unilateral or pulsatile pain and either nausea or vomiting or photo- and phonophobia, or (2) visual or sensory aura preceding the headache. These criteria were derived from the definition of migraine by the International Headache Society (IHS).

A total of 6 percent of the men and 18 percent of the women in the base population of 23,611 household members was found to have migraine according to this definition. The prevalence of severe headaches per se was 14 percent in men and 27 percent in women, which are figures similar to what is reported above for the prevalence of moderate headaches. It is important to remember that ''severe'' in this study was self-defined and, therefore, not necessarily related to the impact of the headaches on the ability to function. Of those respondents diagnosed with migraine, 82 percent of the men and 86 percent of the women reported at least mild interference with the ability to function. No information is provided in the study with regard to the prevalence of severe disability, that is, headaches requiring bed rest, in those with severe headaches or migraine.

No differences in migraine prevalence were found for both men and women between urban and rural residence, or among the six regions of the United States studied. However, white men had a migraine prevalence twice that of black men (6 versus 3 percent). Also, for both men and women, the prevalence of migraine was the highest in the group with the lowest household income, less than $10,000 per year. There was also a clear age dependence in both men and women, with the highest prevalence between the ages of 25 and 45.

Of those identified, 29 percent of the men and 40 percent of the women had also been diagnosed with migraine by a physician. Of these individuals, 23 percent of the men and 15 percent of the women were not confirmed by the study as having migraine. When both sexes are taken together, this means that the physician and study diagnoses disagreed in 17 percent and agreed in 83 percent of cases. The IHS criteria were published in 1988 and the study was conducted in 1989, which means that the physician diagnosis was made mostly independent of the criteria but, nevertheless, agreed in the majority.

The proportion of respondents with a physician-diagnosis increased in the men from one-fifth to one-third and in the women from one-third to one-half with a rise in household income from less than $10,000 to more than $45,000 per year. There were no significant differences in physician-diagnosis of migraine between the races, urban versus rural residence and among the different regions of the United States, except in the North and South Central regions where it was lower in women. The headache features, which in both men and women were most strongly associated with a physician-diagnosis were vomiting, blurred vision, visual aura, and sensory aura. Physician-diagnosis was also found to be two times more frequently associated with severe disability, that is, headaches requiring bed rest (50 vs 25 percent).

With regard to medication use, 28 percent of the men and 40 percent of the women with migraine in the study population used prescription medications. This was almost twice as frequent as those in the study who reported severe headaches but who were not diagnosed with migraine. The use of prescription medications was more frequent among whites than blacks and was highest between the ages of 50 and 59. It did not depend to any great extent on household income or on rural versus urban residence. With regard to the different regions of the United States, it was highest in New England and in the Mountain region. In men, sensory aura (43 percent) and vomiting (38 percent) were associated with higher prescription-medication use, and in women, sensory aura (54 percent), vomiting (52 percent), and visual aura (48 percent). The use of prescription medications was also higher in both men and women with a migraine frequency of two to six attacks per week (40 and 48 percent, respectively). It was also higher in both men and women with a duration of migraine of 3 days or longer (56 and 49 percent, respectively).

Emergency-room services for headache were used by 13 percent of the men and 20 percent of the women with migraine. It was about three times higher in those who used prescription medications than those who used over-the-counter medications. Over-the-counter medications were used by 67 percent of the men and 57 percent of the women with migraine. Only 5 percent of the men and 3 percent of the women did not use any medications, but their use of emergency services was two to three times higher than those who used over-the-counter medications.

ANATOMY OF HEADACHE

In their location, headaches often not only involve the head proper but also the face and neck. Therefore, in this section on the anatomy of headache, also a description of the pain-sensitive structures of the face and neck will be included. The basic structures of the head, face, and neck—the bones—are insensitive to pain. However, they are enveloped in membranes—the periost—which are sensitive to pain. Most of what makes up the head—the brain—is also insensitive to pain. In this way the brain does not differ from other internal organs, which all derive their protection against nociceptive stimuli from the encapsulating membranes. The encapsulating membrane of the brain is the arachnoid, which is very sensitive to pain. It obtains its pain innervation from nerve fibers that travel along the blood vessels, both arteries and veins. As a result, the arachnoid is most sensitive to pain in areas adjacent to the blood vessels.

Like everywhere else in the body, the blood vessels of the brain—both arteries and veins—are sensitive to pain. However, in their course through the arachnoid, they give off their nerve fibers to innervate the arachnoid. As a result, the blood vessels gradually become less pain-sensitive as they travel toward the brain, to become insensitive to pain by the time they enter the brain itself. The pain fibers that travel along the (intracranial) carotid artery to the cerebral arteries come from the ophthalmic

branch of the trigeminal nerve. This so-called ophthalmic nerve gives off pain fibers to the carotid artery when it passes alongside it in the cavernous sinus. This is before it enters, with the ophthalmic artery, the orbit through the superior orbital fissure to innervate the contents of the orbit as well as the forehead and anterior vertex. The arteries innervated in this way by the ophthalmic nerve are the anterior, middle, and posterior cerebral arteries, as they are all branches of the carotid artery. Through nerve fibers that run along these arteries, the ophthalmic nerve provides pain innervation of the arteries and the arachnoid in the anterior and middle cranial fossae. In the central nervous system there is convergence of somatic and visceral pain information, resulting in referral of pain from stimulation of carotid and cerebral arteries and adjacent arachnoid to the ipsilateral eye and forehead.

The cerebral veins drain into the venous sinuses and derive their pain innervation from these structures. The venous sinuses lie embedded in the dura mater, which is essentially thickened periost of the inside of the skull. They are innervated by a branch of the ophthalmic nerve referred to as the tentorium nerve. This nerve originates from the ophthalmic nerve close to the ganglion and travels along the tentorium to the sagittal sinus in the falx in which the cerebral veins drain. Therefore, painful stimulation of the cerebral veins and sinuses refers pain to the area of somatic innervation of the ophthalmic nerve, the ipsilateral anterior vertex.

The dura mater is also innervated by nerve fibers which travel along the meningeal arteries. The main meningeal artery—the middle—is a branch of the maxillary artery. The middle meningeal artery divides into frontal and parietal branches, which vascularize most of the dura mater above the tentorium. Along with the meningeal arteries run branches of the mandibular nerve, which innervate the arteries and adjacent dura mater. The mandibular nerve also innervates, through the auriculotemporal nerve, the temple and anterior ear and, through the mental nerve, the anterior jaw. As a result, painful stimulation of the dura mater in the anterior or middle cranial fossa results in pain referred to the temple.

The pain-sensitive structures of the posterior fossa are innervated by the recurrent meningeal nerves of the first three cervical spinal nerves. These nerves originate from the anterior branches of the spinal nerves just distal to the ganglia and run back into the spinal canal through the intervertebral foramina. They innervate the dura mater and, through nerve fibers that run along the vertebral arteries, the basilar artery, its cerebellar branches and adjacent arachnoid. The first three cervical spinal nerves also innervate, through their posterior branches, the back of the head and upper neck. The medial side of the back of the head is innervated by the major occipital nerve (C2) and the lateral side by the minor occipital nerve (C3). Therefore, painful stimulation of structures in the posterior fossa causes pain referred to the back of the head and upper neck.

Apart from innervating the back of the head and neck, the posterior branches of the cervical spinal nerves also innervate the posterior neck muscles, the zygapophyseal joints and the interspinous ligaments. The anterior neck muscles and intervertebral disks are innervated by the anterior branches of the cervical spinal nerves, which, as mentioned above, through the recurrent meningeal nerves, also innervate the spinal dura mater and vertebral arteries.

The innervation of the face is through the three branches of the trigeminal nerve. The first branch, the ophthalmic nerve, innervates, through the supraorbital nerve, the forehead and anterior vertex. The second branch, the maxillary nerve, innervates, through the infraorbital nerve, the cheek. The third branch, the mandibular nerve, innervates, through the auriculotemporal nerve, the anterior ear and temple and, through the mental nerve, the anterior jaw. The posterior jaw is innervated by the auricular nerve, a branch of the C3 spinal nerve, which also innervates the inferior ear. The posterior ear is innervated by the minor occipital nerve, also a branch of the C3 spinal nerve, which also innervates the lateral side of the back of the head. The border between the innervation of the scalp by the trigeminal and cervical nerves is formed by an imaginary line that runs from ear to ear over the vertex.

Of the deeper structures of the face, in particular the nasal cavity and paranasal sinuses are important in relation to headache. As mentioned above, the bones making up these structures are insensitive to pain but their linings—the periost—and the linings of the cavities—the mucosal membranes—are sensitive to pain. The mucosal membranes are, in actual fact, very sensitive to pain where they cover the approaches to the paranasal sinuses. The turbinates in the lateral side of the nasal cavity are innervated by the nasal branches of the maxillary nerve. The maxillary nerve, through the infraorbital nerve, also innervates the maxillary sinus and, as mentioned above, the infraorbital nerve also innervates the cheek. As a result, painful stimulation of the nasal turbinates or maxillary sinus causes pain referred to the cheek. The upper part of the nasal septum and the ethmoid sinuses are, on the other hand, innervated, through the ethmoidal branches, by the ophthalmic nerve. The frontal sinus is also innervated by the ophthalmic nerve giving rise to pain referred to the forehead. The sphenoid sinus, although innervated by the maxilllary nerve, causes pain referred to the vertex.

In summary, the structures of the head, face, and neck that are sensitive to pain are the following:

Cerebral arteries, in particular those at the base of the brain
Dural venous sinuses and cerebral veins on the surface of the brain
Arachnoid adjacent to the pain-sensitive cerebral arteries and veins
Meningeal arteries
Dura mater adjacent to the meningeal arteries and dural venous sinuses
Mucosal membranes of the nasal cavity and paranasal sinuses, especially those covering the approaches to the sinuses
Temporomandibular and zygapophyseal joints
Vertebral arteries, intraspinous ligaments, and intervertebral disks
Extracranial arteries, veins, muscles, and skin

These structures are innervated predominantly by the trigeminal and cervical nerves with the border between the two innervation systems formed intracranially by the tentorium, separating the anterior and middle from the posterior cranial fossa, and extracranially by an imaginary line that runs from ear to ear over the vertex.

The nociceptive information from the trigeminal and cervical innervation systems of the head, face, and neck converges in the dorsal horn of the upper part of the cervical spinal cord, also known as cervicotrigeminal relay. The information from the trigeminal system reaches the cervicotrigeminal relay through the descending limb of the tract of the trigeminal nucleus, which runs from the port of entry of the trigeminal nerve—the pons—to the upper part of the cervical spinal cord. It is through the cervicotrigeminal relay that painful stinulation

of the face or head causes pain in the neck, and painful stimulation of the neck causes pain in the head or face. As mentioned above, in the central nervous system there is also convergence of somatic and visceral pain information resulting in referral of pain from stimulation of visceral structures to the corresponding somatic areas. In this way painful stimulation of structures within the anterior and middle cranial fossae causes pain referred mostly to the somatic areas innervated by the ophthalmic nerve, that is, the forehead and anterior vertex, and painful stimulation of structures in the posterior fossa to the somatic areas innervated by the upper three cervical nerves, that is, the back of the head and upper neck.

PHYSIOLOGY OF HEADACHE

The basic structures of the head, face, and neck—the bones—are insensitive to pain. Nevertheless, afflictions of the bones, such as inflammation (osteomyelitis) or neoplasm (metastasis), cause pain but they do so through chemical (inflammation) and/or mechanical stimulation (stretching) of the pain-sensitive membranes that envelop the bones—the periost. Most of what makes up the head—the brain—is also insensitive to pain, but afflictions of the brain do cause pain. However, in order to cause pain the afflictions have to involve pain-sensitive intracranial structures, either directly or indirectly. For example, a neoplasm of the brain, either primary or secondary, that is, metastatic, causes pain only when it causes a mass effect, either through its own size or through the induction of edema, to cause displacement and, thereby, stretching—mechanical stimulation—of major arteries and/or veins. It also causes pain, regardless of its mass effect, when it is in a strategic location, for example, to cause obstruction of cerebrospinal fluid flow or cause compression of a cranial nerve carrying sensory information, in particular the trigeminal nerve.

Obstruction of cerebrospinal fluid flow by a neoplasm due to its location is most likely to occur in the third ventricle (colloid cyst obstructing the interventricular foramina), the cerebral aqueduct in the mesencephalon (pinealioma) and the fourth ventricle (ependymoma). The obstruction of cerebrospinal fluid flow under these circumstances causes bi- or triventricular hydrocephalus with expansion of the ventricles, causing stretching of the major arteries and veins on the surface of the brain. Triventricular hydrocephalus can, of course, also be caused by a neoplasm or other lesion, such as an infarct or hematoma, in the cerebellum with enough mass effect to cause obstruction of the foramina in the roof of the fourth ventricle.

Similar to a neoplasm, an infarct, hematoma, or abscess of the brain causes pain when it has enough mass effect to cause displacement and, thereby, stretching of the major arteries and veins on the surface of the brain. A cerebral hematoma is usually caused by rupture of an intracerebral artery, which in itself is a painless event, as the intracerebral arteries are insensitive to pain, and the same is true for a cerebellar hematoma. The same is also true for a cerebral infarct when it is caused by obstruction of an intracerebral artery but not when it is caused by obstruction of a major artery due to thrombosis or embolism. In the latter case the obstruction of the major cerebral artery by thrombosis or embolism causes inflammation and distention of the blood vessel wall and, as a result, pain, and the same is true for a cerebellar infarct due to obstruction of a major cerebellar artery.

Displacement and, thereby, stretching of the major cerebral arteries and veins on the surface of the brain can also be caused by swelling of the brain, either locally as in encephalitis, for example, herpes encephalitis with swelling of a temporal lobe, or generally as in pseudotumor cerebri or benign intracranial hypertension. Inflammation of the brain—encephalitis—can be associated with inflammation of the membrane encapsulating the brain, the arachnoid, in meningoencephalitis with severe pain caused by the inflammation of the pain-sensitive meningeal membrane. The meningeal membrane can, of course, also be inflamed by itself, which is usually the case as in bacterial, viral, or fungal meningitis, subarachnoid hemorrhage or carcinomatous meningitis, conditions associated with severe generalized headache.

Subarachnoid hemorrhage is usually caused by rupture of an aneurysm and sometimes by rupture of an arteriovenous malformation or by a bleeding disorder. A cerebral aneurysm generally originates from a major artery at the base of the brain and would, therefore, be sensitive to pain. However, the pain caused by rupture of an aneurysm does not stand in any comparison to that caused by the subsequent subarachnoid hemorrhage. Pain from the aneurysm may be appreciated when the lesioning affecting it is not to the extent that it result in subarachnoid hemorrhage, such as in expansion of the aneurysm or bleeding in its wall. A cerebral arteriovenous malformation is a congenital abnormality that often also involves major, and therefore pain-sensitive, arteries and veins. It causes pain when subjected to inflammation, for example, due to thrombosis of blood vessels, in particular veins, involved in the malformation. A cerebral arteriovenous malformation can also affect the metabolism of the brain tissue with which it is in contact, resulting in seizures or migraine attacks.

Seizures are associated with increased metabolism of the brain, which, in turn, is associated with increased blood flow and dilation of the pain-sensitive major cerebral arteries causing generalized headache. Generalized dilation of the major cerebral arteries also occurs when cerebral metabolism is increased due to fever or when oxygen saturation is decreased, for example, due to high altitude, sleep apnea, carbon monoxide poisoning, or pulmonary insufficiency. Generalized cerebral vasodilation also occurs with hypercapnia, hypoglycemia (diabetes mellitus), and nitroglycerine, as well as when cerebral autoregulation is impaired, for example, after a concussion or carotid endarterectomy. The major cerebral arteries are distended in a generalized way when blood pressure rises abruptly, as in malignant hypertension, pheochromocytoma, toxemia of pregnancy, dysreflexia of the bladder or bowel in quadriplegics, and ingestion of a sympathomimetic agent in a patient treated with a monoamine oxidase inhibitor. Finally, apart from dilation and distention, inflammation can also affect the major cerebral arteries in a generalized way, such as in the arteritis seen in lupus erythematosus.

Inflammation of venous structures, such as major cerebral veins and dural venous sinuses, is generally associated with thrombosis and distention of the structures. The processes affecting the venous structures, that is, the inflammation and distention, cause pain, and pain can also be caused by swelling of the brain tissue drained by the affected structures, due to edema, infarction, and/or bleeding, with displacement and stretching of major arteries and veins on the surface of the brain. With regard to the venous structures, the inflammation can be primary, for example, of the saggital sinus due to scalp cellulitis, the sigmoid sinus due to otitis media, or the cavernous sinus due to a nasal carbuncle, or the thrombosis can be primary, such as during pregnancy or disseminated intravascular coagulation.

Displacement and concomitant stretching of the major veins on the surface of the brain also occurs with space-occupying lesions in the subdural space, that is, the space between the arachnoid and dura mater. Lesions that can occupy the subdural space are hematoma, acute or chronic, resulting from rupture of a cerebral vein due to trauma, or abscess. Stretching of the major cerebral veins can also occur due to traction by a downward displaced brain, such as is seen with low cerebrospinal fluid pressure, either following lumbar puncture or due to a (traumatic) fistula of the dural sac. Downward displacement of the brain can sometimes be associated with herniation of the cerebellar tonsils into the cervical spinal canal, which causes pain by stretching of the arachnoid.

Displacement and, thereby, stretching of the pain-sensitive meningeal arteries occurs with space-occupying lesions in the dura mater, such as a meningioma, hematoma, or abscess. A hematoma in the dura mater is referred to as an epidural hematoma and is caused by rupture of a middle meningeal artery due to trauma of the head; in persons over the age of 25 this trauma is always associated with a fracture of the skull crossing the artery.

The cranial nerves that carry sensory information, particularly the trigeminal nerve, causes pain when compressed by a neoplasm, for example, a neuroma or meningioma. They also cause pain when compressed chronically by a blood vessel, either artery or vein, such as is thought to be the case in trigeminal neuralgia or tic douloureux. Other processes that affect the sensory cranial nerves and cause pain are inflammation, for example, herpes zoster (zoster ophthalmicus), or demyelination, for example, multiple sclerosis (trigeminal neuropathy).

Extracranially in the head as well as in the face and in the neck, skeletal muscle makes up the largest component that causes pain by prolonged contraction, leading to accumulation of waste products and irritation of nerve fibers in the muscles. Prolonged contraction of the muscles can be caused by increased arousal due to psychosocial stress or excessive caffeine intake, muscle strain originating from the neck, eyes, or jaws, macrotrauma consisting of a stretch injury (whiplash), microtrauma resulting from a systemic viral infection, impaired relaxation due to fatigue, lack of sleep, exposure to cold (draft) or low thyroid function, or can be caused by reflex contraction of the muscles due to an irritative focus in the face (chronic sinusitis) or neck (arthrosis).

Second in line to the muscles in terms of causing headache are the extracranial arteries, which generally cause pain by a combination of dilation and inflammation. The dilation and inflammation create a vicious cycle in which the dilation causes stretching of the perivascular nerve fibers as a result of which the nerve fibers secrete inflammatory chemicals, such as substance P, calcitonin gene-related peptide, and neurokinin A, which further dilate the blood vessel, leading to further stretching of the nerve fibers, and so on. In giant cell or temporal arteritis, the initiating event is inflammation due to the presence of antibodies against the elastin in the wall of the arteries, but otherwise the initiating event tends to be dilation of the arteries, followed by inflammation, and so on. Dilation of the extracranial arteries can be caused by a great number of factors, such as prolonged contraction of the craniocervical muscles, overrelaxation, for example, poststress, oversleeping, or taking a nap, cardiovascular activation, for example, due to physical exertion, emotional excitement, or intercourse, estrogen introduction (postmenstruation) or estrogen withdrawal (premenstruation, ovulation), ingestion of a vasodilator agent, for example, alcohol, nitrites (cured meats), or histamine (red wine), withdrawal from a vasoconstrictor agent, for example, caffeine, tyramine (red wine), or phenylethylamine (dark chocolate), or a decrease in blood pressure, for example, as occurs nocturnally in hypertension or during renal dialysis.

The joints in the head and neck—the temporomandibular and zygapophyseal joints—cause pain due to arthrosis. The skin and the mucosal membranes of the nasal cavity and paranasal sinuses cause pain due to inflammation, referred to as cellulitis and rhinosinusitis, respectively. While cellulitis is bacterial, fungal, or parasitic in origin, rhinosinusitis can be viral or bacterial but can also be due to allergy or to mucosal contact, for example, a deviated nasal septum making contact with a turbinate, or can be due to vasomotor rhinitis.

In summary, the pain-sensitive structures of the head, face, and neck can be affected by a number of mechanisms, which in turn can be activated by a great variety of factors, conditions, and disorders. The resulting pain, that is, the headache, is in its location determined by the pain-sensitive structure(s) involved, the innervation of the structure(s), the extent of activation within the cervicotrigeminal relay, and the somatic projections of the neurons activated. Unilateral involvement of pain-sensitive structures causes pain limited to the ipsilateral side of the head, face, and/or neck with extension to the other side only when secondarily contralateral pain-sensitive structures get involved, most commonly consisting of contraction of craniocervical muscles secondary to the pain.

SUGGESTED READINGS

Celentano DD, Stewart WF, Lipton RB, Reed ML: Medication use and disability among migraineurs: a national probability sample survey. Headache 32:223–8, 1992

Dalessio DJ (ed): Wolff's Headache and Other Head Pain. 3rd Ed. Oxford University Press, New York, 1972

Goldstein M, Chen TC: The epidemiology of disabling headache. Adv Neurol 33:377–90, 1982

Lipton RB, Stewart WF, Celentano DD, Reed ML: Undiagnosed migraine headaches. Arch Intern Med 152:1273–8, 1992

Rasmussen BK, Jensen R, Schroll M, Olesen J: Epidemiology of headache in a general population: a prevalence study. J Clin Epidemiol 44:1147–57, 1991

Stewart WF, Lipton RB, Celentano DD, Reed ML: Prevalence of migraine headache in the United States. JAMA 267:64–9, 1992

201. APPROACH TO THE PATIENT WITH HEADACHE

FRED D. SHEFTELL

Pain is ultimately a personal and subjective experience. The patient is the expert in the report of his or her pain. First and foremost, patients are to be believed. The proper treatment must focus on the pain in the context of the entire patient. The Oslerian principle that it is more helpful to approach the person who has the disease than the disease the person has is well taken in regard to headache. One can take a logical approach to the diagnosis and treatment of headache and still miss the boat. All diagnosis and treatment takes place in the atmosphere of a relationship between the physician and patient. It is the quality of that atmosphere which often constitutes the difference between treatment success and failure. A nonbiased and nonjudgmental approach should be the template upon which diagnosis and treatment is built.

John R. Graham once wrote, "Any style will be effective providing it clearly demonstrates to the patient that the physician is interested in him and his life as a person, as well as in the details of the medical complaint." This quote catches the essence of the approach to the patient with headache. When Dr. Spierings asked me to write this chapter, I felt honored when he informed me that he would have offered it to Dr. Graham. I first met Dr. Graham in the 1970s when I became interested in headache. Of course, I was impressed by his abilities and contributions as a physician and researcher, but most of all I was impressed by his humanity, compassion, and warmth. He approached patients the same way as everyone else—with respect, interest, and a wonderful ability to truly make a person feel unique. A while ago a patient consulted me who had been a patient of Dr. Grahams many years ago. She suffered from chronic daily headache and was often debilitated by recurrent episodes of migraine. She had been an elementary school teacher for many years. At the end of her interview with Dr. Graham he commented "What a shame that your migraines have deprived your students of such a wonderful and dedicated teacher." In all her experiences with various physicians over the years, this comment above all else stood out in her memory.

In my own work with headache, the patient's scenario is often a familiar one. Patients who come to our center have often seen a variety of medical, dental, and other professionals. "The ear, nose, and throat doctor I saw told me my head pain was from sinus infections." "The allergist told me it was clearly allergic." "The nutritionist said it was hypoglycemia." "The dentist said I had problems with my temporomandibular joint." "The psychiatrist said I was overcontrolling, perfectionistic, and tense." I may add that one of our patients, while on vacation in the Virgin Islands, consulted a voodoo doctor who clearly identified the problem as being a curse and prescribed an appropriate remedy. So, who is right? One of them, none of them, all of them? While I do not pretend to have the ultimate answers, I will again stress that openness on the part of the physician during the history and examination is essential.

Before going into the essentials of the initial consultation, let me again remind you of the importance of getting to know the patient with the complaint of headache. You might ask yourself some of the following questions as you begin to explore the formal history: Who is this person? Why is he coming now? What are his expectations? What are his concerns, what are his fears? Is the fear of a tumor lurking somewhere in his mind? What has his experience with previous physicians been like? What were his dissatisfactions? What does he do for a living? What hobbies or interests does he have? How are things with his family and friends? I find it useful to ask a patient to describe a typical day from the time he gets up in the morning to the time he goes to sleep. One can get a very good idea about how he manages his time, to what extent is he overwhelmed, and how much time he leaves for himself. It is not unusual to see a patient who clearly has a lifestyle that is filled with demands and yet has no insight as to the extent of these demands and the effects on him. It is also important to understand what effect the patient's headaches have had on his life at work, home, and play. By the time you have completed the initial consultation you should have not only an idea in regard to diagnosis and initial treatment plan but also a good sense of who this person is. Finally, it is important to examine your own attitudes about headache complaints. Do you lean toward believing these patients are neurotics or do you prefer an exclusively neurobiologic and molecular explanation? While we have learned a great deal about the neurobiologic basis of headache, it is important to understand that whatever the pathophysiologic mechanisms are, they are occurring in the context of a human being. Pain is a multidimensional phenomenon influenced by neurologic, physiologic, psychological, social, ethnocultural, and cognitive factors. To tell a patient, ''The pain is all in your mind,'' is to invite treatment disaster and a major breach in the relationship with the patient. The patient should not be challenged about the reality, intensity, or debilitating quality of the pain.

STYLES OF PHYSICIAN/PATIENT INTERACTION

Roter and Hall's book, *Doctors Talking with Patients/Patients Talking with Doctors* explores the dynamics of the doctor/patient relationship and should be required reading for all medical students and residents as well as physicians in practice. The authors defined four typical types of doctor relationships: paternalism, consumerism, default, and mutuality. These relationships are based on relative degrees of physician and patient control. Where physician control is high and patient control is low, the relationship is paternalistic. The physician takes charge of decision-making, which is ultimately ''in the best interest'' of the patient; the patient's role is to cooperate and obey. Consumerism is characterized by high patient control and low physician control, where the physician accommodates the demands of the patient. Where both physician and patient control is low, the relationship is one of default, neither doctor nor patient taking responsibility for decisions and stagnation resulting. Finally, mutuality exists when patient and physician control is high and both take an active role in decision making. Another way of looking at this situation involves the concept of an internal versus external locus of control. Patients who have an external locus of control have a passive attitude and rely on the physician to make them better. They take no responsibility for their illness or its remediation. These patients will fit nicely with physicians who tend to be paternalistic. Studies have shown that patients who demonstrate an external locus of control have a poorer prognosis than patients with an internal locus of control. The latter take a more active attitude of, ''What can I do to help?'' These patients take more responsibility for their illness, are motivated to make changes in lifestyle, and comply better with regimens. The terms *alliance* or *partnership* can be used to describe what I believe is the best type of doctor/patient relationship.

THE INITIAL CONSULTATION

Now we can now move on to the initial consultation, which I divide into three phases: the history, the examination, and the ''close.''

The History

At our center, the initial consultation involves some 3 to 5 hours of history-taking, examinations, patient education, and treatment planning. This is done in the context of a multidisciplinary staff. Our center is a tertiary care center and, while

one may not need to spend this amount of time, I believe that exploration of the chief complaint of headache on the first visit should involve 1 or 2 hours. It would not be unusual for Dr. Graham to spend some 3 or 4 hours during this initial assessment.

We find it useful to have patients complete a questionnaire before their first visit. The questionnaire includes all previous pharmacologic (including nonprescription medications) and nonpharmacologic therapies, dosages, routes of administration, frequency of use, efficacy and side effects. We often see patients who have taken many headache medications without success secondary to either inappropriate dosing, timing of dosing, failure to use antiemetic therapy prior to ergotamine or dihydroergotamine, and, most importantly, many patients with chronic daily headache may have taken every known headache medication in the Physician's Desk Reference, but had never been taken off their daily use of prescription or nonprescription analgesics, ergotamine, etc., which decreases the effectiveness of all preventive pharmacologic and nonpharmacologic maneuvers. All previous examinations and tests for headaches are recorded, all potential triggers for headache are listed and explored. Medical and surgical history as well as pertinent family history is recorded. Nutritional status with attention paid to caffeine intake is important. These forms are used as a guideline for in-depth review at the time of the initial consultation.

We use a modified version of Dr. Lee Kudrow's format for the headache history. Since most headache patients present with more than one type of headache, we take the history by dividing headache intensity on a 1 to 3 scale. This information is recorded on the cover sheet shown in Figure 201-1. Severe or level 3 intensity includes only those episodes that render the patient totally incapacitated. The moderate or level 2, while annoying and clearly present, does not render the patient incapacitated, although it interferes with his ability to function. Finally, the dull or level 1 pain is mild, does not interfere with the patient's functioning and may not be noticed when the patient's attention is diverted. For each level of intensity we explore the following parameters:

1. Age of onset
2. Frequency
   (a) Previous
   (b) Current
3. Location: frontal, orbital, vertex, parietal, occipital, temporal, other.
4. Laterality: Is the pain on the right or left side? Is the pain bilateral? Does it alternate sides? In patients who have both right- and left-sided headache we determine whether or not one side predominates.
5. Description: Is the pain throbbing, pounding, pulsating, squeezing, pressing, aching, . . .? Most patients can accurately describe the quality of their pain, but for those who don't we will give them a list of pain descriptors.
6. Duration: We note the minimum and maximum duration of attacks as well as the average duration of untreated episodes.
7. Prodrome: This may be divided into nondescript prodrome prior to the onset of headache, such as changes in appetite, energy, mood, or sleep patterns, to more well-defined symptoms of aura, such as scintillating scotomata, field defects, or sensory/motor disturbances.
8. Associated symptoms: These include nausea, vomiting, appetite disturbances, diarrhea, dizziness, sensitivity to light

Name: _____   Date: _____   Ref.: _____

Age: _____   Sex: _____   Marital Status: S   M   W   D   D   D   SEP

Occupation: _____

Intensity	Severe	Moderate	Dull	Menstrual & Hormonal

Onset

┌─ Previous

Frequency   -   Habits (alcohol, tobacco, caffeine, sleep, drugs)

└─ Current

Location

RLBA   Medical   Surgical

Description   Trauma   LOC   S.D.

Duration   Min. Av. Max.

Prodrome

Association   NVAD
Stuffed/Running   dizzy
Red/Tearing   sono
Ptosis/Miosis   photo

Behavior

Diagnosis

Current Medication   Previous

Tests:

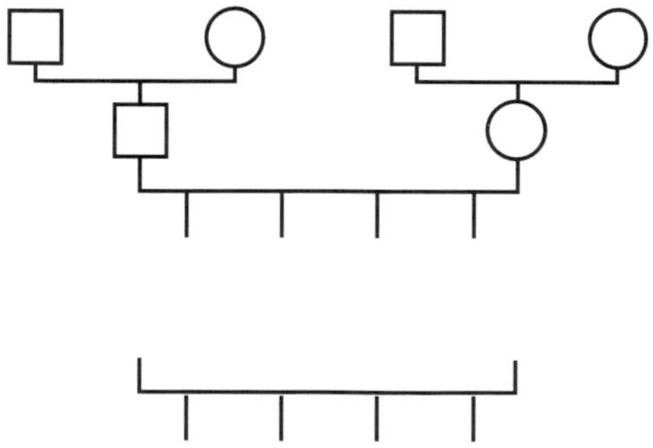

Fig. 201-1. Cover sheet of the headache history form used at the New England Center for Headache.

and sound, stuffed and running nostril, red and tearing eye, ptosis, miosis.

9. Behavior: We explore the patient's behavior during attacks. The migraine patient, of course, is more likely to retreat to a dark and quite room, while the cluster patient is restless, cannot sit or lie still and will pace, rock, etc.
10. Postdrome: Identify symptoms following the main attack, such as exhaustion, exhilaration, residual symptoms.
11. Diagnosis: We place the tentative diagnosis based on the above characteristics as well as incorporating other historical data related to family history, trigger factors, and the like.

Although this format was developed before the International Headache Society classification, we have found that it works very nicely. As a rule we find that migraine and cluster headache tend to fall primarily into the more severe categories with the dull category demonstrating tension-type headache. The moderate category may demonstrate any of the three primary headache disorders. As you will note in other chapters outlining the International Headache Society's criteria for primary headache disorders, one can clearly find these characteristics using this format of history-taking. While we certainly allow and encourage patients to describe their headaches in any manner that they see fit, many patients with chronic daily headache will state that they have headaches all the time which get worse from time to time. Using this intensity model one can tease out and separate the primary headache disorders and see how they relate to each other. We find that this model works well even for patients who have had both migraine and cluster headache in that the headaches are described differently, although both may fall into the severe category. One can also see how the headaches relate to each other. For example, patients may describe to us that their moderate headaches may escalate in intensity and move into the severe category with the characteristic associated symptoms of migraine or cluster headache, which may not be seen at the mild or moderate level.

You can see that the "face sheet" in Figure 201-1 summarizes pertinent identifying information. We then collate and review the overall history. All previous medications are listed and summarized as well as current medications. Again, be sure to include in your history nonprescription medications such as analgesics, sinus medications, allergy medications, and nasal sprays. Under habits we summarize alcohol intake, tobacco history, caffeine intake, sleep patterns, and recreational drugs. Under the menstrual and hormonal section we record the age of menarche and any possible association with the onset of headache. We record current or past use of oral contraceptives and possible association with headache. We record regularities or irregularities in the menstrual cycle. We record all pregnancies and live births. Where appropriate we record age of menopause and details of hormonal replacement therapy. We summarize medical and surgical histories with special attention to head trauma, loss of consciousness, and seizure disorder. We record all previous tests, examinations, and results, along with their dates. Notice the genogram in the lower right-hand corner. We find that this is very useful for outlining family history of headache, family medical history, age of siblings and parents, marital relationships, and offspring. A consideration of the major types of headache will show how their diagnostic criteria fit into this format. For example, age of onset is an important part of the history and may suggest a diagnosis. Cluster headache will generally tend to start in later life, while migraine is often

present by late adolescence or early 20s. It is important to note how the frequency and severity have changed over the years. Most patients with chronic daily headache start off with episodes of intermittent migraine which over a period of years transform to chronic daily headache and are often complicated by the overuse of analgesics and ergotamine. Cluster headache is almost entirely unilateral, migraine is often unilateral, and tension-type headaches are bilateral. The pain of migraine is often throbbing, while the pain of cluster is often boring, and the pain of tension-type headache is often dull, squeezing, or aching. The duration of cluster headache usually averages 45 minutes while migraine may go on for many hours and tension headache may last hours to days at a time. Migraine with aura is well defined, while no such aura or prodrome exists with tension-type headache. Migraine may be associated with nausea, vomiting, and sensitivity to light and sound while cluster and tension-type headache are not. Cluster headache, however, is usually associated with ipsilateral stuffed and running nostril, conjunctival injection, and lacrimation, as well as ptosis and miosis. Patients who have clear-cut episodes of migraine with aura will have a less "busy-looking" face sheet, while patients with more complex disorders and numerous symptoms and levels of intensity will require more information.

Danger signals to look for in the history include the following:

1. Sudden onset of new severe headache or the "first and worst headache"
2. Headaches that are worsening over time.
3. Headache onset associated with exertion, coughing, bending, sneezing, straining, or sexual activity (activity will always make migraine worse, but the concern here is that the headache comes on as a *result* of activity).
4. Changes in mentation and level of consciousness, such as drowsiness, confusion, or loss of memory (which may signal a structural lesion such as tumor or subarachnoid hemorrhage).
5. Chronic malaise, myalgias, and arthralgias in the older age group should alert you to the possibility of temporal arteritis.
6. The presence of fever should alert you to an infectious process such as meningitis or brain abscess—meningitis should be clearly suspect if neck pain or rigidity is present as well.
7. The presence of any neurologic symptom associated with headache should alert you to an organic basis for disease.
8. First headache occurring after the age of 50—while migraine and tension-type headache generally start earlier in life, the presence of headache in individuals over the age of 50 who have never experienced headache before should alert to the possibility of organic disease.

It is important not to neglect the psychosocial history and to be alert for psychological contributors and trigger factors. A variety of psychometric tests are extremely helpful in indicating the presence of disorders such as depression or anxiety, which tend to be comorbid with chronic daily headache. The Minnesota Multiphasic Personality Inventory (MMPI), the Hamilton Depression Scale, and the Beck Inventory are examples of these tools.

At the end of your history-taking please leave time to inquire as to whether there is anything you may have left out that the patient feels is important.

The Examination

A complete neurologic and physical examination should be done at the time of the initial consultation. Rather than review these examinations in their entirety, I will share with you the portion of the examinations that are useful in the diagnosis of headache disorders. Vital signs need to be taken, including blood pressure, pulse rate, respiration, and temperature.

Head and Neck.   One should observe the size and shape of the head. Look for signs of obvious deformity and unusual bumps. The size of the head should be measured, and this is especially important in children who may have headaches secondary to hydrocephalus. Note any obvious abnormalities related to the eyes such as ptosis, exopthalmus, asymmetric pupils, conjunctival injection, and strabismus.

Palpate the entire head and neck looking for signs of pericranial tenderness as well as excessive muscle contraction about the head and neck. Many patients with headaches may also complain of tightness of the neck, and some will have exquisitely tight neck musculature and not be aware of this. Palpate the trapezius and paracervical musculature as well as the cervical spine. Check the range of motion about the neck in flexion, extension, and rotation and ask if there is any pain on these movements. Some patients may demonstrate areas of explicit tenderness in the musculature that may or may not radiate. Pay attention to the occiput looking for tenderness of the greater and lesser occipital nerves and looking for referral of pain to other parts of the head. As stated, many patients are unaware of how tight they keep themselves. What I do is hold the patient's arm extended, holding the wrist with my hand. I tell him to make his muscles as loose as possible so when I let go at the count of three, his arm will drop by gravity into my other hand. It is not unusual to have a patient tell me that his muscles are relaxed and then to let go and find that there is no drop of the arm or that it is done voluntarily. Perception of muscle tension subjectively by the patient may be such that he is not aware of how tight his muscles are. Rigidity of the neck is a common symptom of meningitis and should be evaluated.

Gentle pressure may be applied to the orbits to check for increased pressure related to glaucoma or orbital tenderness related to meningitis. The temporomandibular joints should be checked by palpation and should be observed in regard to any pain when the jaw is opened and closed. Check for signs of deviation of the jaw on opening and check for any restriction of range of motion. The patient should be asked whether or not he experiences any pain in these joints when he is chewing. Auscultation may reveal evidence of clicks, pops, or crepitans. The internal pterygoids may be palpated as well for presumptive evidence of temporomandibular dysfunction.

Observe the temporal arteries for prominence and palpate them to determine presence or absence of palpation, tenderness, or rigidity.

The frontal and maxillary sinuses may be palpated for tenderness and swelling. One may also transilluminate the sinuses with the light from the otoscope to determine translucence, opacity, or the presence of an air fluid level.

Auscultation of the carotid arteries should be performed to rule out the presence of bruits. One may also auscultate the orbits with the bell of the stethoscope, which may reveal bruits secondary to arteriovenous malformation. The thyroid gland should be palpated. Look for adenopathy, which may reveal the presence of an infection such as sinusitis or an abscess.

Cranial Nerves.   A complete examination of the cranial nerves should be performed. This is necessary to rule out any organic factors. Fundoscopic examination is obviously key in

determining the presence of papilledema as evidence of increased intracranial pressure. This may be secondary to a structural lesion or secondary to idiopathic intracranial hypertension (pseudotumor cerebri). The latter may be found particularly in female patients with chronic daily headache and in fact there have been cases reported where no papilledema is found in spite of the existence of increased intracranial pressure. Look for hemorrhagic lesions in the retina, which may be secondary to a variety of disorders including hypertension and diabetes. Visual field defects such as hemianopsia or scotomata should be evaluated.

Look for lesions such as ptosis, asymmetric pupils, divergent strabismus, upward and outward deviation of the eye, and downward and inward deviation as well. Lesions of the fourth cranial nerve, though rare, may occur in meningitis and are characterized by an upward and inward turning of the affected eye. Patients may complain of double vision characterized by the image in the affected eye being lower than that of the normal eye (vertical diplopia). Lesions of the sixth nerve will cause an internal strabismus accompanied by double vision and are most often seen in meningitis, multiple sclerosis, and brain tumors. The trigeminal nerve, consisting of its three divisions, should be evaluated. The first or ophthalmic division is best evaluated through examination of the cornea reflex. The second or maxillary division as well as the third or mandibular division is evaluated by checking sensation to light touch and pin. Trigeminal neuralgia may be a differential diagnosis, particularly with cluster headache, and most commonly involves the second and third divisions of this nerve.

Lesions of the seventh or facial nerve may result in paralysis of the frontalis muscle and the orbicularis oris muscle. Patients should be asked to close their eyes as tightly as possible to evaluate any weakness. Lesions of the facial nerve as seen in Bell's palsy is characterized by absence of the nasolabial folds, drooping of the corner of the mouth, and inability to fully close the eye. Patients are not able to whistle or blow. Lesions of the facial nerve centrally will allow the patient to smile spontaneously which is not true of peripheral lesions.

The eighth nerve is best tested with a tuning fork using the Weber and Rinne testing.

Lesions of the ninth or glossopharyngeal nerve may be characterized by anesthesia of the upper parts of the pharynx and soft palate and difficulty in swallowing. Neuralgias may affect this nerve causing pain in the tonsillar area which may radiate to the ear.

Lesions of the tenth or vagus nerve and its various branches may effect swallowing and changes the character of the voice. The lesions of the cardiac branch may result in bradycardia and if paralysis is complete tachycardia.

The eleventh or spinal accessory nerve lesions are characterized by torticollis and may result from trauma to the neck, and large cervical lymph nodes or abscesses in the neck.

Finally, lesions of the twelfth or hypoglossal nerve will be demonstrated by deviation of the tongue pointing to the side of the lesion.

Sensory Functions.   Both light touch, pin prick, and vibratory sensations should be tested throughout. Many patients with migraine will demonstrate cold hands and feet secondary to excessive vasoconstriction of end arteries, which will be demonstrated by decreased sensation to cold stimuli. It is interesting to note that many of these patients will demonstrate subtle decreases in vibration sense when the tuning fork is applied to the toes. This does not necessarily reflect a neurologic lesion and is probably secondary to excessive vasoconstriction.

Motor System.   All muscle groups should be checked for tone and strength. Look for the presence of tremors, which may be evidence of a variety of disorders, including hyperthyroidism, Parkinson's disease, side effects secondary to drugs, multiple sclerosis, and anxiety. Check for symptoms such as ankle clonus or cogwheel phenomena.

Cerebellar System.   Evaluate the patient's gait and test for the integrity of coordination. Finger-to-nose testing, heel-to-shin, toe-walking, heel-walking, heel-to-toe should all be determined. A Romberg test should be performed as well.

Reflexes.   All reflexes should be tested including pupillary reflexes, corneal reflexes, as well as all deep tendon reflexes. Look for signs of pathologic reflexes such as the Babinski. Where meningitis is suspected look for Kernig's or Brudzinski's sign.

Mental Status.   Look for signs of depression and anxiety. These may include a blunted, restricted, sad, or labile affect. Look for signs of cognitive disturbance, including intrusive obsessional thoughts and inability to concentrate, check the patient's memory for both recent and remote events. Simple tests such as substraction of serial 7's, spelling five-letter words forward and backward, remembering phone numbers are all useful. Evaluations for the presence of depression or anxiety disorders such as panic anxiety are important, since these may be comorbid with many patients with chronic daily headache. The patients with posttraumatic headache may show deficits in concentration, memory, and ability to perform complex tasks.

Further Evaluations.   Further evaluations that are part of the general physical examinations should be performed as well. The heart and lungs should be auscultated. There is a higher incidence of mitral valve prolapse in patients with migraine, and if this is suspected an echocardiogram may be ordered to confirm the diagnosis. Comorbid medical disorders such as asthma, hypertension, coronary artery disease, peptic ulcer all need to be evaluated in terms of pharmacotherapy and potential side effects that may be detrimental to one or another of the comorbid conditions. For example, you would not want to prescribe nonsteroidal inflammatory agents to a patient with active peptic ulcer disease. You would not want to prescribe β-blockers to a patient with asthma. You would not want to prescribe vasoconstrictive agents such as ergotamine, dihydroergotamine or sumatriptan to a patient with active coronary artery disease and/or stroke. The physical and neurologic examination also provides an opportunity to evaluate the side effects of any medications that the patient may be on. These may include bradycardia or wheezing with patients on β-blockers, symptoms of ergot overuse such as decreased or absent pulsations, myalgias and nausea, and signs of ataxia, impaired concentration, and the like secondary to the overuse of butalbital, benzodiazepines, or narcotics. The latter may also produce symptoms of depression, impaired cognition, and impaired concentration. For patients who have been overusing narcotics, barbiturates, or benzodiazepines, one should be alert to the possible symptoms and signs of withdrawal if they have recently stopped these medications. This would be of most concern with withdrawal from barbiturates or benzodiazepines. Here one can look for symptoms and signs of irritability, tremors, hyperreflexia, dilated pupils, and piloerection.

The "Close"

The final consultation prior to completing the initial evaluation is as key as the initial history, physical, and neurologic examinations. All findings pertinent to the history and examination should be reviewed thoroughly with the patient in terms that are easily understandable. Your conclusions related to these findings and recommendations for further tests and treatment plan should be explained thoroughly. Let the patient ask questions and voice their concerns and feelings about your findings and suggestions. Here the role of patient education is of paramount importance and will go a long way toward maximizing compliance issues. One can follow precisely all the details of the history and examination and still wind up with an unhappy and dissatisfied patient if education is not included. A study by Dr. Russell Packard demonstrated that patients with headache come looking for an explanation of their disorder as well as relief of pain. With primary headache disorders in the absence of positive findings on the physical and neurologic examination, negative results from testing such as MRI, CT, and EEG, the patient is understandably concerned about the cause. There are a variety of materials that one can use to aid patient education. We have used a modification of the model suggested by Dr. John Graham demonstrated in Figure 201-2. Primary headache disorders may be described using this ''stick of dynamite'' model. Once it has been established that you are dealing with one of the primary headache disorders, this model is useful. If you believe that there may be an organic basis to the disorder, express your concerns based on your findings in the history and examination and be as reassuring as possible. If further testing is necessary, explain the reason for these tests and describe the procedure such as an MRI or electroencephalogram to the patient. For example, there are many patients who are claustrophobic and will not be able to tolerate the closed environment of the MRI. For these patients they may best be referred to an open magnet facility and if their anxiety level is determined to be high, it would not be inappropriate to prescribe a small dose of a benzodiazepine one hour before the test.

Again, once the headache is determined to be one of the primary headache disorders we explain that these headaches are definitely a valid biologic disorder. They are as valid as coronary artery disease, hypertension, ulcer, and the like. We explain that there are no biologic markers such as blood tests at this point that can determine or demonstrate the existence of the disorder. Our current thinking has demonstrated, for example, that migraine is a disorder of the brain involving changes in biochemistry or chemical messengers known as neurotransmitters. We explain that to the best of our knowledge migraine represents a cascade of complicated events, beginning in the brain and leading ultimately to changes in blood vessel activity. Once the biology or vulnerability is present there are a variety of factors that may *trigger* (not cause) the explosion. For example, these may involve hormones. We explain that the reason that migraine is more common in women is related to the cyclical nature of estrogens. Before puberty migraine is more common in boys than girls, but once menstruation occurs the ratio goes up to almost 3:1, male:female. Many women will have their headaches around the time of menstruation or ovulation, many will get worse on oral contraceptives, many will get better during the second 6 months of pregnancy, many will worsen

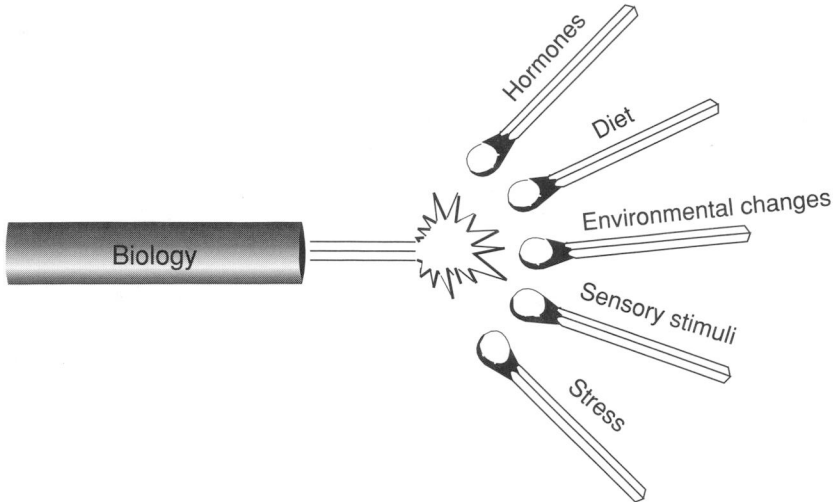

Fig. 201-2.   Diagrammatic representation of potential migraine triggers: a modified version of a model suggested by Graham.

around the time of menopause, and some will improve following menopause. We explain that it is not an abnormality of the hormones themselves but rather the way changes in estrogen levels effect the underlying biology of migraine.

We review the various dietary factors that may trigger migraine and cite alcohol as the most commonly identified food trigger. Providing a list of these foods is helpful and an entire overview of triggers if provided in Figure 201-3. These are used in conjunction with the headache calendars, which are described below. We suggest that these foods be eliminated for a period of approximately 1 month and we also provide the patients with a list of permissible foods. There are a number of lay books that can be helpful in (see the list of suggested readings at the end of this chapter).

We explain that migraine patients are very susceptible to changes in their environment both internal and external. Internal changes may be related to factors such as menstruation and sleep. External factors may be related to changes in seasons, weather, schedule changes, traveling, time zone changes, skipping meals, and the like. We make suggestions as to how patients may better regulate and respond to these environmental changes.

Migraine may be triggered by a variety of sensory stimuli including strong lights, flickering lights, and odors.

Last, but not least, we explain the role of stress. We state that if the biologic vulnerability were not present, than no matter what kind of stressors the patient is exposed to, no matter what kind of personality they have, and no matter what their ability to deal with stress, they will not get migraine. However, if the biology is present then a variety of factors not limited to, but not excluding stress, may provoke attacks. Behavioral patterns such as present in Type A individuals or maladaptive reactions to stress may indeed trigger migraine. We let patients know that migraine is more likely to occur during letdown periods than during times of active stress. Because of the nature of this biology, patients who tend to be intense, competitive, have high expectations of themselves and others, be rigid and perfectionistic, will find it to be useful to explore issues related to stress management, personality, and so on, and may be candidates for stress management and behavioral techniques such as biofeedback. If we find comorbid evidence of depression and anxiety, we review this thoroughly with the patient and suggest an ap-

propriate psychiatric or psychological referral. We do not do this in the context of communicating that we believe the patient's pain is ''all in their head'' or suggest that we are abandoning their treatment. Rather, we let him know that psychotherapy is an important adjunct to their treatment if applicable. We reassure him that we will continue to treat his headaches and are not abandoning him. We certainly will take the time to explore the patient's reaction to these kinds of suggestions.

We let the patient know that, although there are times that he can clearly identify a trigger for his attack, there are often times when he will not be able to identify a trigger for his attack as migraine attacks may occur spontaneously as a result of some innate periodicity. We do not want the patient to feel that he has somehow bought the attack on himself or say, ''What did I do now?''

We can also use the stick of dynamite model to review our treatment planning. Nonpharmacologic approaches include evaluating these trigger factors, nutritional changes, exercise, stress management techniques, adequate sleep, etc. The calendars provide very useful information about these factors. We next look at the frequency of attacks and where preventive medication is indicated, we let the patient know that the purpose of this medication is to reduce the frequency, intensity, and duration of the headaches. We review potential benefits and potential side effects and respond to patient's questions. We let him know that he will not necessarily be on medication for the rest of his life, but when the attack frequency is reduced sufficiently for a period of several months we can then begin to slowly titrate the preventive medication downward. Lastly, we explain that abortive medication will be used to treat the ''explosion'' when it occurs. Once again, we review a variety of options, benefits, and side effects. It is imperative that in prescribing abortive medications that strict limits be set on the frequency of use and again, the calendars are helpful in maintaining these limits. Limit setting on the use of abortive medication is key in preventing rebound phenomenon as described in other chapters.

For those patients who are overusing medication, such as analgesics, ergots, etc., we provide them with a structure and clear guidelines as to how to eliminate these medications and provide them with appropriate pharmacologic and nonpharmacologic tools. As a general guideline we educate patients thor-

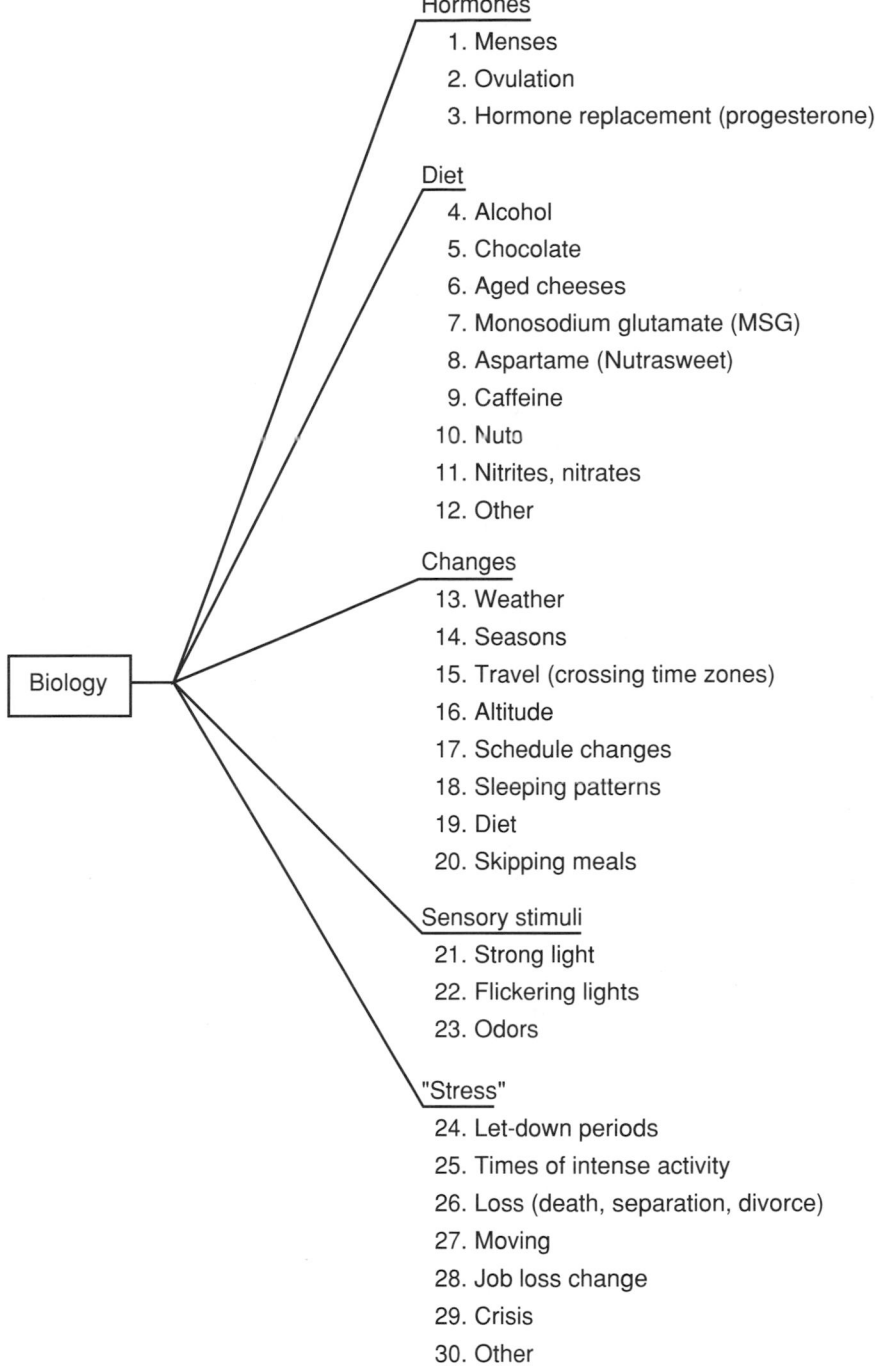

Fig. 201-3. Overview of possible headache triggers.

oughly as to the mechanism of rebound headache. They are told that as long these analgesics are maintained on a daily basis that their headaches are likely to remain chronic and unresponsive to a wide variety of pharmacologic and nonpharmacologic interventions. Initially, the patients are usually noted to be apprehensive about discontinuing the ongoing use of these medications because they are afraid of not being able to function. A variety of suggestions to treat analgesic or ergotamine rebound are found in the suggested readings and other chapters. For those patients who may require hospitalization the reasons and indications for hospitalization are explained as is length of

stay, description of hospital treatment, and goals of hospitalization. Here again, it is wise to stop and ask for questions and concerns.

USE OF HEADACHE CALENDARS

The use of a logging system or headache diary is absolutely key to successful treatment and to help minimize compliance issues. As stated earlier, the use of calendars and other behavioral tools are helpful in bringing patients around to an internal locus of control and having them truly take responsibility and be an active participant in their treatment plan. From the physician's point of view, the calendars provide detailed information as to frequency, intensity, and duration of the headaches. The calendar is demonstrated in Figure 201-4. Again, we use a three-point intensity scale, from 1 to 3, as explained earlier. The patients will note the levels of intensity, frequency, and duration using this numerical system on a daily basis with the day being divided up into three major areas. Underneath these data we place the medications that the patient is taking. The name of the medication and the dosages are clearly written along with specific guidelines for the use of both preventive and abortive medications. The times of menstruation and relationship, for example, of preventive medication to morning or evening or to mealtimes is clearly stated. Patients are given information sheets as to potential side effects. In regard to abortive medications, instructions for exact use and timing and routes of administration are given, as well as the limits on the frequency of administration. In regard to prescribing practices, we would recommend that until you get to know the patient that small amounts of as needed medications are prescribed that are nonrefillable. It is not useful as we have seen to prescribe butalbital compounds, #100 with five refills. Obviously, this is a gross exaggeration, but it has been seen in clinical practice. When dealing with the treatment of analgesic and ergotamine overuse,

tapering schedules and alternatives are given. We suggest that patients do not medicate with as needed medications for mild and if possible moderate headaches. We do make sure that they are given adequate abortive medication for their most severe episodes. Again, limits are set on the use of these abortive medications, and patients are instructed to call us if they are not able to stay within these limits.

We use a 0 to 3 relief code where zero means no relief and ''3'' is complete relief. We will also ask patients to include the names of other medications that other physicians are giving them so that interactions may be observed. Our patients find it useful to show these calendars to other physicians so that all prescribing persons are aware of the entire picture. Patients will also indicate their use, for example, of oral contraceptives or estrogen replacement to view possible trigger factors here as well.

Finally, on the front of the calendar women patients are asked to report the days of their periods by marking each appropriate box with an ''x''. The back of the calendar is demonstrated in Figure 201-3. These include a variety of potential trigger factors, and patients are asked to record these by number as appropriate.

These provide a reasonably objective picture of the headache story. Some patients are good historians, but even the best histo-

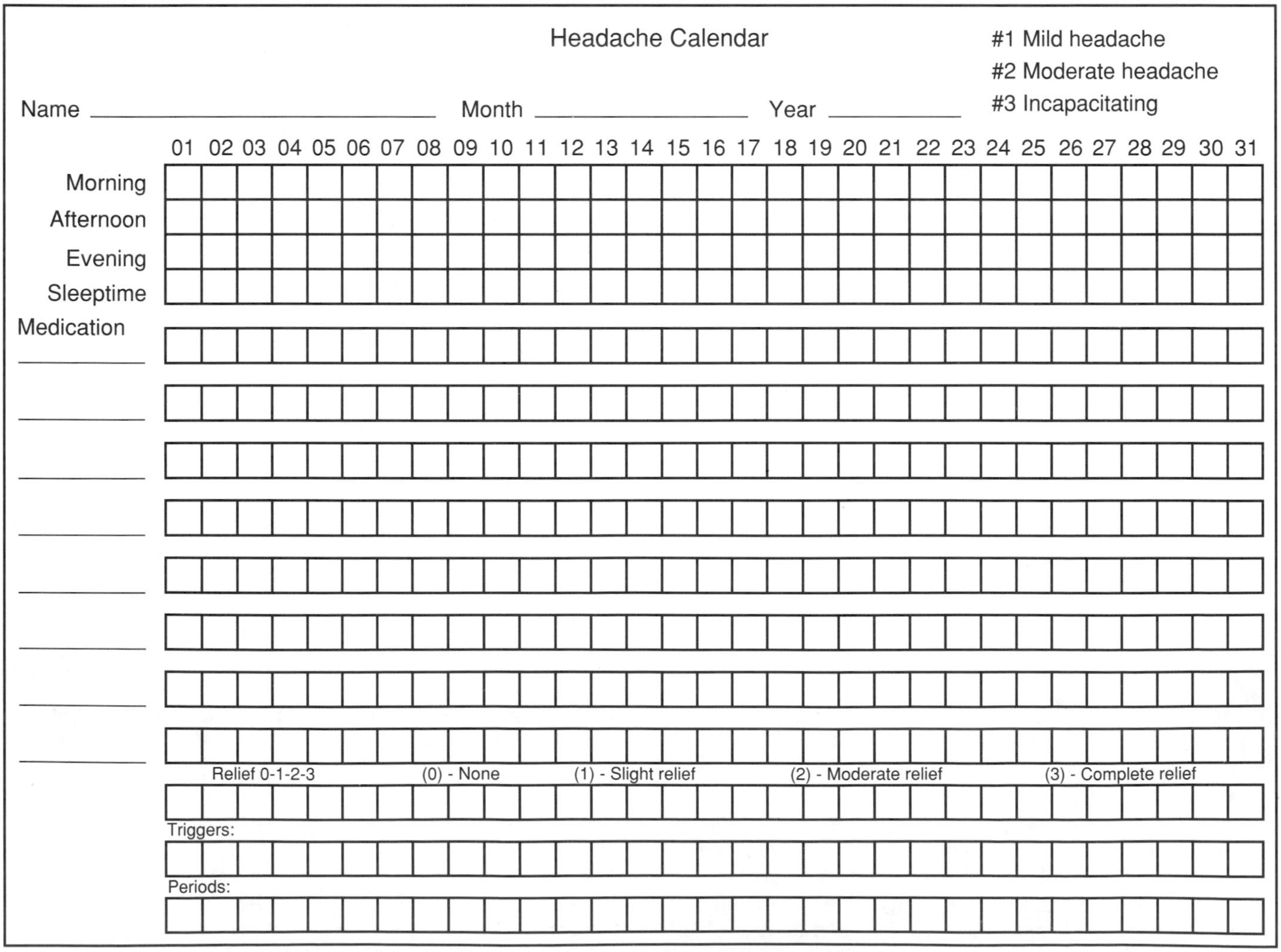

Fig. 201-4. Headache calendar given to patients at the New England Center for Headache.

rians, when asked to review their progress over several months, are not able to include the kinds of data and material that are necessary to make assessments. After the initial history is taken, we record baseline frequencies and intensities as a denominator. Let us take, for example, a patient with chronic daily headache. Where these headaches are occurring daily we may have the denominator "30" under the 1 or 2 intensities. The incapacitating or level 3 intensities are recorded separately and may show that a patient is having 4 attacks of incapacitating headache lasting an average of 36 hours. When the patient returns for follow-up visits we review their data on the calendars on a monthly basis and record current frequency, intensity, and duration as a denominator. This enables us to clearly evaluate the patient's progress and response to the preventive and abortive medications. I am reminded of one patient who returned for a follow-up visit and on initial questioning said that his headaches had remained unchanged. This was a patient with chronic daily headache who reported mild-to-moderate waxing and waning pain on a daily basis with three episodes of clear migrainous attacks lasting 24 hours. The patient had been placed on a β-blocker at the time of her initial evaluation. If we had gone on the verbal data alone, we would have likely increased the dosage of the medication if side effects were not a problem or changed to another medication. When her calendars were reviewed, though indeed she continued to have mild to moderate pain on a daily basis, she had experienced no incapacitating attacks of pain, had not missed work, and had not been confined to bed during that initial time period. It was clear that the β-blocker was successful in reducing the frequency and intensity of her migrainous episodes, but her daily background pain remained intact. This is but one example of the usefulness of headache calendars.

GUIDE TO SELF-ASSESSMENT

Roter and Hall review a number of questions and criteria for the patient to assess at the conclusion of his initial consultation. I will paraphrase this from the physician's point of view so that you may incorporate this into your thinking and assessment.

1. Have you informed the patient of your formulation of his problem and diagnosis?
2. Have you explained your concept of the cause of the problem in clearly understandable terms?
3. Have you discussed the prognosis, its potential seriousness, and how long you believe the problem will continue?
4. Have you explained thoroughly your treatment plan and have you explained why you believe this is the best and any alternatives that might exist?
5. If you have prescribed medication, does the patient know the name of the medication, how the medication works, when to take it, its side effects, including drowsiness or nausea? Are there interactions with any other medications including nonprescription medications or alcohol?
6. If you have ordered tests, have you explained the purpose of the tests, the nature of the tests, and how the results will be used?
7. Have you reviewed suggestions relating to lifestyle, such as nutrition, smoking, alcohol intake, exercise, or weight? If you have, have you explored with the patient any compliance issues? Did you tell the patient how much time it might take to notice a difference? Did you give the patient some directions as to how to go about making these changes?
8. Have you reviewed the patient's expectations of treatment?

For example, I believe it is important when talking about primary headache disorders to talk in terms of control and not cure. If the patient's expectations are total cure, this is obviously unrealistic, and the concept of decreased frequency, duration, and intensity of attacks needs to be explained. Although these headache disorders may remit on their own, they cannot at the present time be cured.

Again, the more education that you provide the patient and the more materials that are provided to the patient, the better compliance issues will be observed and the greater the likelihood of a spirit of partnership will be realized. It is important to communicate your expectations of the patient as well as listening to the patient's expectations of you.

FOLLOW-UP VISITS

The ongoing follow up visits are key, particularly in understanding that the great majority of headache patients present with a chronic disorder that is ongoing in nature. The frequency of follow-up visits obviously depends on the progress of the patient and the intensity of pharmacotherapy. We generally schedule a follow-up visit after the initial consultation within 2 to 4 weeks. The purpose of the follow-up visits is obviously to review progress via the patient's verbal reports, and a careful monitoring of the headache calendars. Treatment plans may be modified based on the patient's response to medication. Vital signs should be taken at each revisit and brief examinations as necessary may be performed. Review of efficacy and side effects will determine dosing regimens. As many patients may experience tachyphylaxis, changes of preventive regimens are necessary. Review of nonpharmacologic maneuvers related to diet, exercise, stress management, lifestyle, and so on, should also be reviewed. I find it useful to make small notes related to any upcoming important events in the patient's life or even a vacation that they are looking forward to. When I inquire about this in follow-up visits the patient can recognize interest and concern.

Phone calls between visits are important to note and record. While emergencies need to be responded to, major changes in preventive medications should not be made over the phone and should be reserved for discussion at follow-up visits. Ongoing follow-up via formal revisits and phone calls will begin to elucidate compliance issues such as failure to adhere to medical regimens, loss of prescriptions, receiving as needed medications from other physicians, missed visits, and the like. It is important to confront these issues directly and again, to review problems that the patient may have in adhering to these regimens. Pharmacists are often very helpful in alerting the physician to multiple prescribers. If we learn of these activities we will let patients know clearly that we can no longer go on prescribing or treating if they are getting medications from other sources without our knowledge. Patients with borderline personalities present some of the most difficult problems to the treating physician and clear limits, boundaries, and structure must be maintained. If patients cannot or will not adhere to these, then psychiatric referral must be considered. Only a very small percentage of headache patients comprise this population but can present with the highest frequency of phone contacts, missed visits, and misplaced or lost prescriptions.

Finally, please be aware of the changing headache. Primary headache disorders do not preclude or immunize a patient from developing organic disease such as tumor or aneurysm. It is important that you do not become complacent even after years of treating a chronic sufferer with primary headache. Be alert to changes in the characteristics and presentation of the patient's headache. When these are noted, proceed as if you are evaluating the patient for the first time and do what is necessary in regard to examination and tests.

IN CLOSING

Although patients with recurrent and chronic headache can present a challenge to the treating physician, they can also provide the physician with a great deal of satisfaction and gratification. To quote Dr. Marcia Angell, ''Few things a doctor does are more important than relieving pain . . . . pain is soul destroying . . . no patient should have to endure intense pain unnecessarily. The quality of mercy is essential to the practice of medicine.''

SUGGESTED READINGS

Adler CS, Morrisey SA, Packard RC: Psychiatric Aspects of Headache. Williams & Wilkins, Baltimore, 1987

American Council For Headache Education: Migraine: The Complete Guide. Dell Trade Paperbacks, New York, 1994

Angell M: The quality of mercy. N Engl J Med 306:98, 1982

Burks SL: Managing Your Migraine. Humane Press, Totowa, NJ, 1994

Headache: A Clinician's Guide to Diagnosis, Pathophysiology and Treatment Strategies. TMA Publishing, Cost de Mesa, CA, 1993

Packard RC: What does the headache patient want? Headache 19:370, 1979

Rapoport AM, Sheftell FD: Headache Relief. Fireside, New York, 1991

Rapoport AM, Sheftell FD: Headache associated with medication and substance withdrawal. p. 227. In Tollison CD, Kunkel RS (eds): Headache: Diagnosis and Treatment. 1st Ed. Williams & Wilkins, Baltimore, 1993

Rapoport AM, Sheftell FD: Conquering Headache. Empowering Press, Hamilton, Ontario, 1995

Roter DL, Hall JA: Doctor's Talking with Patients/Patients Talking with Doctors. Auburn Health, Westport, CT, 1992

Sheftell FD: Chronic daily headache. Neurology suppl. 2:32, 1992

Sheftell FD, Silberstein SD, Rapoport AM: Drug treatments for chronic headache. Drug Ther 22:47, 1992

Sheftell FD, Silberstein SD, Rapoport AM et al: Migraine in women: diagnosis, pathophysiology and treatment. J Women's Health 1:5, 1992

202. PSYCHOLOGICAL ASSESSMENT OF THE HEADACHE PATIENT

RANDALL E. WEEKS

Most clinicians agree that psychological factors are important considerations in the evaluation and treatment of headache patients. There is a lack of agreement as to exactly how psychological variables interact with underlying biochemical, biologic, and physiologic factors in the headache process, however. While psychological issues are primary causes of headache in a small number of patients, it is widely accepted that they more often coexist or are secondary to the pain process itself. Still, there remains a tendency for clinicians to attribute psychological causation to refractory headache patients more quickly than to patients with other medical diagnoses.

The purpose of this chapter is to provide a practical psychological assessment of headache patients, using a multimodal scheme that includes detailed discussion of (1) a clinical interview, (2) behavioral assessment, (3) self-report data, (4) interview with significant other(s), and (5) psychometric data. Such

an assessment will enable the clinician to make the proper headache diagnosis as well as highlight psychological factors that may be important treatment considerations. The final section lists primary psychiatric disorders from the Diagnostic and Statistical Manual of Mental Disorders, Third Edition, that may include headache as part of the symptom complex. Factors to consider at the initial consultation will be noted, but the diagnosis usually becomes apparent through the patient's reaction to the treatment course and their interactions with the health care professional.

CLINICAL INTERVIEW

The clinical interview includes a basic headache history as well as attention to psychological issues that may either contribute to head pain or be a result of head pain. It is important to assess the role medical factors, pharmacologic agents, and pain may play in the patient's psychological status. Care is taken to note the manner in which symptoms are described (dramatic, indifferent, obsessive, etc.) as well as whether the pain and/or associated symptoms are consistent with supposed underlying headache pathophysiology.

Intensity

Headaches are graded by intensity as either severe/incapacitating, moderate, or mild. Operationally, severe/incapacitating pain levels occur when a patient is no longer able to perform (e.g., has to leave work, hibernates in a dark, quiet room) or they attempt to continue functioning but with a greater than 50 percent reduction in performance. Moderate pain levels exist when pain is apparent and inhibits a patient's performance, but not in a severe way. Mild pain is described as slight pain that may not be apparent if the patient is distracted by work or other activities. It may only be noticeable when there is a ''break'' in their activity.

Care is taken to assess how many days out of the month the patient is, in fact, dysfunctional and the impact that severe pain has on current functioning (decreasing pleasurable events, causing greater social isolation, having enhanced feelings of guilt, etc.). Finally, it is noted whether there is a distinct pattern to changing levels of pain (e.g., in patients with chronic headache, those who are depressed may feel consistently worse in the morning but better as the day goes on).

Age of Onset

The age of headache onset is noted as well as any particular life circumstances or stressors that may have served as triggers. Attention is paid to periods of time when the frequency of head pain has increased as well as any contributing factor(s) the patient feels is relevant. The length of time that the frequency has been at its present rate is also noted.

Frequency

Each grade of headache intensity is reviewed with respect to how many days of the month a patient may have pain of that magnitude (e.g., 30 of 30 days would indicate daily headache). It is also important to note patterns of increased pain with respect to greater levels of stress versus letdown periods from stress, weather changes, dietary triggers, weekends versus regular routine, etc. Changes in a patient's headache pattern are noted if the patient is taking birth control pills or replacement hormone, and during and after pregnancy. An assessment is made of how menstrual patterns may relate to headache pain.

Location

The location for each kind of headache is described with close attention paid to the unilateral versus bilateral experience of pain. Changes in location (e.g., alternating sides with respect to pain) are also assessed.

Description of Pain

The patient is asked to describe the sensations of pain (throbbing, stabbing, pressure, etc.). Attention is paid to whether bending or physical exertion increases the pain and/or introduces a throbbing component. It is also important to note at what point in the pain process the patient will use abortive agents in an attempt to decrease pain. It is not unusual for some patients to medicate more to control their "fear of getting a bad headache" as opposed to responding to the intensity of the pain.

Duration

Duration is recorded for each headache and, if the patient has chronic daily headache, whether the pain waxes and wanes throughout the day. Patients using frequent abortive medications are asked the degree of relief and the "window" of reduced headache before the return of the headache. The impact of the pain on the patient's ability to perform regular work and to enjoy leisure activities is noted.

Prodrome

Prodromal activity is noted, with respect to changes in mood, "funny feelings," or formal aura before headaches. It is also important to make certain that the prodromal activity does, in fact, exist before the onset of pain and is not described as part of the pain process. How the patient handles the prodrome emotionally is also noted (e.g., feelings of helplessness and anxiety versus developing an effective "action plan" for treatment).

Associated Symptoms

Symptoms of cluster headache (stuffed and running nostril, red and tearing eye, ptosis, miosis, etc.) are noted, as well as migraine symptoms (nausea, vomiting, anorexia, diarrhea, dizziness, sonophobia, and photophobia). Care is taken to assess whether these symptoms are more pronounced when the pain is severe than during less intense or headache-free times and/or whether they may be a result of abortive medication.

Behavior During Headache

It is important to inquire about how the patient reacts to pain. Patients with cluster headache tend to have difficulty remaining still and often pace the floor and/or rock back and forth holding their head. Migraine patients prefer to hibernate in a dark, quiet room. Patients with tension-type headache may report a decrease in their pain with physical activity. The patient's thoughts and feelings during the headache are assessed for issues of helplessness and desperation ("I just wanted to die . . . I'm afraid the pain will never go away . . . It's getting harder to 'hide' the pain from other people . . . I feel guilty I can't be with my family . . .", etc.).

Medications

A complete medication history is recorded with respect to the various agents, doses, and the length of time the patient has been on that dose. This includes nonheadache medications and vitamins. Side effects are noted. Past medications are also listed, including the length of time they were taken and the efficacy of treatment. Side effects from those medications are also noted. Issues of analgesic or ergotamine rebound are assessed with respect to whether those agents may have compromised the effects of antidepressants and other prophylactic medications. Allergic reactions and any medication contraindications are noted.

It is also important to assess whether patients have been compliant in taking medications as prescribed. Medication compliance should never be taken for granted. There is a need to assess whether patients may be having prescriptions for headache medications written by more than one physician (corroboration by a close relative or friend of the patient is helpful in this).

From a psychological perspective, the chronic use and overuse of pain medication can lead to a depressed mood as well as a "mental dullness." Similarly, agents that contain caffeine may cause an alternation in mood of excitation and depression. Finally, a frequent side effect to the use of β-blockers is depression. In the psychological assessment of a headache patient it is important to assess what role, if any, adverse events from medications may be playing with respect to mood.

As mentioned previously, it is essential to note at what point patients medicate. Some patients will medicate to reduce their "fear of the headaches getting worse" as opposed to making it contingent on pain levels. Others may take abortive agents based on time factors and not pain ("I take two aspirin before I get out of bed each morning . . . I take two Fiorinal every four hours . . .", etc.) Patients will also tend to use (and overuse) medications in which they have little confidence in providing pain relief. It is important to assess expectancy of efficacy as this can contribute to medication effectiveness.

Medical History

A complete history is taken with respect to head or neck trauma, loss of consciousness, seizure disorder, or other neurologic events. Other systems are also reviewed (cardiac, gastrointestinal, pulmonary, endocrine, gynecologic (if appropriate), etc.). Patients are asked whether they have other types of pain (joint pain, back pain, neck and shoulder pain, etc.). Psychiatric history is reviewed with respect to any previous hospitalizations, psychotherapy experiences, or detoxification programs. Surgical history is also obtained.

Previous Testing

Patients are asked whether they have had a neurologic work up and formal neurologic testing (EEG, MRI, CT scan, etc.). In addition, they are asked the results of any blood studies they may have had previously (regarding Lyme disease, Epstein-Barr virus, thyroid function). There is an assessment of any previous psychological or neuropsychological testing.

Habit History

History regarding cigarette consumption, alcohol use or abuse, recreational drug use or abuse, and caffeine intake is noted. Issues of sleep difficulty and consistency of sleep are assessed.

Other triggers such as inconsistency in eating habits, sleep habits, and caffeine consumption are also assessed. Physiologic markers such as bruxism, neck and shoulder tightness, temporomandibular joint issues, cold extremities, and history of motion sickness are also noted.

Family History

The family history is assessed by the use of a genogram, which reviews the patient's position within the family unit. Areas of family conflict are identified as well as a description of the family's reaction to the patient's pain. Family history for headache, alcohol or substance use or abuse, psychiatric disturbance, and neurologic difficulties is also assessed. If family history of headache is positive, diagnostic and treatment information about other family members is gathered. Similarly, if family history is positive for psychiatric disturbance, information about diagnosis and treatment is also obtained.

Academic/Vocational History

The type of employment (or schooling) as well as the impact of headache on these systems is assessed. Absences from work or school due to headaches are noted as well as any particular pattern of increased headache during conflictual or demanding times within these systems. Evidence of secondary gain from pain is also assessed (e.g., school phobia).

Personal History

Assessment is made of pleasurable pursuits for the patient, amount of exercise and physical activity, as well as any history of biofeedback or relaxation training. In addition, other treatment modalities are noted (acupuncture, physical therapy, self-hypnosis, etc.).

Summary

The clinical interview provides data from which to make a headache diagnosis as well as to evaluate current psychological functioning. It explores the impact that a patient's head pain may have on his life and how it affects the other systems in his life. It generates questions that can be explored more fully in the rest of the assessment.

BEHAVIORAL CHECKLIST

The second part of the assessment gathers information as it pertains to symptomatic factors that are markers of underlying affective disturbance. Three factors should be kept in mind. First, many of these symptoms can be side effects from medication. Second, often patients develop psychological difficulties *as a result of pain,* and affective symptoms will markedly diminish as the patient's pain experience is ameliorated. Finally, affective disturbance secondary to other medical conditions needs to be ruled out (thyroid dysfunction, Lyme disease, etc.).

The patient (with corroboration by a significant other) is asked to identify which of the behavioral correlates in Table 202-1 currently exist; their intensity; and whether they are becoming increasingly disabling. Assessment is also made as to whether these symptoms existed before headaches became a serious problem.

As can be seen from Table 202-1, the clinician needs to carefully consider whether the behavioral correlates are, in fact

TABLE 202-1. Behavioral Markers of Depression

The DSM-IIIR lists the following behavioral correlates of depression:
 Poor appetite, significant weight loss (when not dieting)
 Increased appetite/significant weight gain
 Insomnia (initial, middle, or terminal)
 Hypersomnia
 Psychomotor agitation
 Psychomotor retardation (but not merely subjective feelings of restlessness or being slowed down)
 Loss of interest or pleasure in usual activities
 Decrease in sex drive
 Loss of energy/fatigue
 Feelings of worthlessness, self-reproach, or excessive or inappropriate guilt
 Difficulties with concentration/memory/ability to think
 Recurrent thoughts of death, suicidal ideation, wishes to be dead, or suicide attempt
 "Depressed mood" as perceived as distinctly different from the kind of feeling experienced following the death of a loved one
 "Depression" is regularly worse in the morning
 Excessive or inappropriate guilt
 Feelings of inadequacy
 Decreased effectiveness at work, school, or home
 Social withdrawal
 Less talkative than usual
 Pessimistic attitude toward the future or brooding about past events
 Tearfulness or crying

The following are behavioral correlates defined by the DSM-IIIR for symptoms of anxiety and panic disorders.
 Shortness of breath or smothering sensations
 Dizziness, unsteady feelings, or faintness
 Palpitations or accelerated heart rate
 Trembling or shaking
 Sweating
 Choking
 Nausea or abdominal distress
 Depersonalization or derealization
 Numbness or tingling sensations (paresthesias)
 Flushes (hot flashes or chills)
 Chest pain or discomfort
 Fear of dying
 Fear of going crazy or doing something uncontrolled
 Muscle tension, aches, or soreness
 Restlessness
 Sweaty or cold clammy hands
 Dry mouth
 Frequent urination
 Trouble swallowing or "lump in throat"
 Feeling keyed-up or on edge
 Exaggerated startle response
 Difficulty concentrating or "mind going blank" because of anxiety
 Irritability

independent of any underlying medical condition or medication side effect. It is usual for migraine patients to have coldness in the extremities and other autonomic signs that are also markers for anxiety. In addition, patients with frequent pain may develop "muscular tension" as part of a "bracing response," which is a reaction to pain and not an indication of affective disturbance. In sum, the purpose of the checklist is to provide an additional piece to the diagnostic puzzle with respect to entertaining hypotheses of affective disturbance in headache patients.

SELF-REPORT

An important part of the evaluation is to ask headache patients their impressions with respect to the following:

1. Why do they get headaches?
2. What factors contribute to their headaches (triggers, stress-related events, etc.)?
3. What impact do the headaches have on their life (low family tolerance for their having pain, guilt they feel when they have to important events, etc.)?
4. Do they feel depressed?
5. Do they feel anxious?
6. Do they think they are imagining or causing their headaches?

7. What do they think would help relieve or eliminate their headaches (pharmacologic and nonpharmacologic treatments)?
8. What treatments have been most effective in the past?
9. Do they think they will ever feel better?

Often, feelings of helplessness and frustration need to be managed through support and education. This information allows the clinician to better understand the patient's attitude about headache and treatment so as to more effectively engage the patient as an "active participant" in their own care.

INTERVIEW WITH SIGNIFICANT OTHER(S)

It is useful to have significant other(s) be part of the assessment to describe their perceptions of the patient's medical and psychological status. They provide additional data regarding the impact of the patient's pain experience on vocational, family, or academic functioning. Once again, issues of the family system's reaction to the headache patient are important with respect to whether they are supportive or punitive. Often, headache patients have to be "good actors" and attempt to suppress their pain because "other people do not understand it."

Significant others may also provide additional information with respect to the behavioral correlates of underlying affective factors as well as impressions about the psychological and cognitive functioning of the patient. Other dynamic factors may emerge, as the patient may be receiving empathy and nurturance from individuals around them because of their pain.

With children who have headache pain, it is important to explore family dynamics, peer relations, and reactions to the academic environment. Issues of school anxiety/school phobia need to be ruled out. In addition, there is often a great deal of family upheaval, which can lead to the experience of headache in children and/or occur as a result of the family struggling to deal with a child's headache problem.

PSYCHOMETRIC TESTING

A limitation in using traditional psychological tests with headache patients is that their performance on these tests may reflect headache symptomatology rather than psychopathology. Our group has raised this issue with respect to the Minnesota Multiphasic Personality Inventory (MMPI) and this notion has been extended to other tests by others as well.

Psychological tests provide important information with respect to the headache patient's present functioning but must be interpreted by an individual who is skilled in working with such patients as to not overestimate psychological issues. The following sections give a sample of traditional psychological test instruments used in assessment of headache patients.

Personality Assessment

Objective Tests. The MMPI is the most commonly employed personality inventory in the assessment of headache patients. It is a series of true/false questions yielding a personality profile across 3 validity scales and 10 clinical scales. There are a number of experimental and "special population" scales as well. Other personality inventories include the Spielberger State/Trait Personality Inventory and the Eysenck Personality Inventory.

Projective Tests. Projective tests are used less often as they are more complicated to administer and score, and their results are viewed as less "objective." The Thematic Apperception Test (adult and children's versions) is series of pictures from which the patient is to "make up a story" as to what is being observed. The pictures "pull for" information regarding interpersonal dynamics and reactions to classical human situations. This test can be useful in discovering more about family issues and attachment, relationship issues, mood variables, and body image. It can be especially useful in the evaluation of children. The Rorschach ink blots is another projective test.

Affective Inventories

The Beck Depression Inventory is a commonly used assessment instrument for headache patients. It contains 21 items reflecting different symptoms of depression. The patient is to indicate the magnitude of each symptom by giving it a score from 0 to 3. The score is the sum total of the 21 items indicating the degree of depression. Other inventories include the Zung Depression Inventory, the Spielberger State/Trait Anxiety Inventory, and the Beck Anxiety Inventory.

Locus of Control Scales

The Health Attribution Inventory was designed to assess issues regarding perceived cause of health and disease. It was based on theoretical premises, including locus of control and health attribution. It is a 22-item questionnaire that measures beliefs about causes and cures of illness. It yields scores on three scales regarding locus of control; these scores have been shown to predict behavioral reactions to illness and response to medical treatment. Other scales include Penzien's Headache Locus of Control Scales, Holroyd's Health Self-Efficacy Scale, and Rotter's Internal/External Locus of Control Scales.

Other Scales

There are a variety of other instruments used to provide additional personality data. Stress issues regarding life changes can be assessed by the Life Change Index Scale by Thomas Holmes. Daily hassles can be assessed by the Lazarus Hassles Scale. Issues of assertion can be measured by the Rathus Assertiveness Inventory and hopelessness through the Beck Hopelessness Scale. Finally, psychological factors and pain can be measured by the McGill Pain Questionnaire.

Summary

The foregoing list of psychological tests that have been used in the evaluation of headache patients is only a brief mention of traditional psychological instruments reported in the literature. Unfortunately, most of the tests were not standardized on headache populations (or, for that matter, medical patients in general). They tend, therefore, to overestimate psychopathology, as scores may be reflective of headache symptomatology and not purely psychological issues.

HEADACHE SECONDARY TO A PRIMARY PSYCHIATRIC DISORDER

In his review of psychiatric aspects of headaches, Bernard Shulman, offered the following eight questions to keep in mind looking for psychodynamic factors as causing headaches:

1. What role does the headache play in the person's life?
2. Is the invalid role useful to the patient?

3. What other person is most affected by the headaches?
4. Is the pain used to influence someone else's behavior?
5. What does the pain allow the patient to avoid?
6. What does the pain permit the patient to do (e.g., make demands on others)?
7. Is the patient angry? At whom?
8. Is the patient playing a martyr role?

By using these questions as a guideline, the clinician can begin to formulate more specific dynamic hypotheses regarding the individual patient. Primary psychiatric disorders are difficult to "tease out" in an initial consultation, but these points are useful for the clinician to consider as they get to know the patient more completely during the treatment course.

The DSM-III-R offers a listing of primary psychiatric disorders that may include headache as part of the symptom complex. The following sections discuss the most common psychiatric diagnoses that may exist as a primary cause of headache and "clues" the clinician should look for in the assessment.

A Factitious Disorder With Physical Symptoms

A factitious disorder with physical symptoms is defined as the intentional production or feigning of physical symptoms or the exacerbation/exaggeration of preexisting physical conditions. In such patients, there is a psychological need to assume a sick role with no apparent secondary gain. Medical history is often presented with a great dramatic flair, but individuals become more vague and inconsistent when questioned in detail.

Malingering

Malingering is the intentional production of false or grossly exaggerated physical or psychological symptoms with evidence of external incentives. Such patients rarely present symptoms in the context of emotional conflict, and secondary gain issues become more apparent as pain persists. Symptoms are not likely to be symbolically related to an underlying emotional need.

Somatoform Pain Disorders

A somatoform pain disorder should be suspected when a patient is extremely preoccupied with pain in the absence of adequate physical findings to account for the pain or its intensity. Often, the description of the pain symptom is inconsistent with the anatomic distribution of the nervous system or cannot adequately be accounted for by organic pathology. Other characteristics may include frequent physician's visits to obtain medical reassurance, excessive use of analgesics without any pain relief, requests for surgery, and the development of "sick role behavior" to the point of, potentially, becoming an invalid.

Conversion Disorders

Headache may also develop as part of a conversion disorder, where head pain occurs in addition to other purely psychological symptoms, such as paralysis or coordination disturbances. It is believed that these symptoms are produced unconsciously and may have a temporal relationship between symptom presentation and psychosocial stressors that represent an underlying psychological conflict or need.

Hypochondriasis

A diagnosis of hypochondriasis should be entertained when a patient has a preoccupation with a determined belief that headache is part of a serious disease process. Such a belief is based on the patient's interpretation of the physical symptoms and persists in spite of complete medical workup and reassurance to the contrary.

Delusional Disorders

A delusional (paranoid) disorder occurs when a predominant theme emerges that the person has some physical defect, disorder, or disease. This may occur as part of a psychotic process.

Major Depression

Headache may also exist as part of a major depression, where the affective state may serve as a trigger for underlying headache mechanisms. As mentioned previously, differential diagnosis is difficult, as symptoms of chronic daily headache or drug-induced headache have clinical correlates and behavioral markers that are consistent with depression.

Post-traumatic Stress Disorder

Reaction to head trauma may also involve a primary psychiatric diagnosis. One must rule out a post-traumatic stress disorder when an individual is involved in a psychological distressing event that is outside the range of human experience and has been experienced with intense fear, terror, and helplessness. Associated symptoms include reexperiencing the traumatic event, avoidance of stimuli associated with the event, and apparent increased arousal.

Adjustment Disorders

The adjustment disorders (with depression, anxiety, or mixed) are indicative of major life stressors, which tax coping skills and could lead to headache. These may include relatively common life situations that require adjustment, but can also include difficulties in the adjustment to the experience of pain itself.

Dependency and Withdrawal

Diagnoses of dependency and withdrawal are relevant as chronic headache patients may become dependent on pain medications, anxiolytics, or other agents that may require detoxification. Important issues center around the substances not being used in the absence of head pain and whether such patients resist withdrawal from these medications when the iatrogenic nature of their continued usage is explained to them.

Primary Addiction Disorder

Patients with a primary addiction disorder often present with a great deal of drug-seeking behavior. There may be a tendency to "lose" prescriptions for pain medications; to have difficulty sticking to detoxification limits; and to be found to be receiving pain medications from numerous sources. Such individuals require a great deal of limit setting and aggressive psychiatric rehabilitation and detoxification.

Summary

The above diagnoses are appropriate for individuals who either dramatically present with such symptoms or individuals in whom such symptoms manifest themselves throughout treatment. While a primary psychiatric diagnosis is indicated in only a small minority of patients, the clinician needs to consider these disorders as part of comprehensive treatment planning.

SUMMARY

This chapter presents a model for assessment of psychological factors in headache patients. Patients with frequent and severe head pain appear to have coexisting psychological factors that are related to (1) the biochemical aspects of the headache process itself (e.g., serotonin changes); (2) a reaction to the experience of frequent or chronic pain; or (3) a reaction to pharmacologic treatment. Psychological factors and affective disturbances are less apparent in patients with intermittent, less severe pain patterns. It is important to assess and treat psychological symptoms that are present but not to view their existence in a vacuum. The skilled clinician will appreciate the emotional trauma secondary to headaches and treat the patient accordingly.

Behavioral and dynamic considerations are put forth in this chapter to help the clinician more accurately assess psychological functioning in patients where headaches appear secondary to a primary psychiatric diagnosis. Identification of such psychological issues assists the practitioner in patient management and appropriate referral.

SUGGESTED READINGS

American Psychiatric Association Diagnostic and Statistical Manual of Mental Disorders. 3rd Ed. Washington, DC, 1981

Andrasik F: Psychologic and behavioral aspects of chronic headache. Neurol Clin Headache 8:961–76, 1990

Penzien DB, Rains JC, Holroyd KA: Psychological assessment of the recurrent headache sufferer. pp. 39–50. In Tollison CD, Kunkel RS (eds): Headache: Diagnosis and Treatment, Williams & Wilkins, Baltimore, 1993

Shulman BH: Psychiatric aspects of headache. Med Clin North Am 75:707–15, 1991

Weeks R, Baskin S, Rapoport A et al: A comparison of MMPI personality data and frontalis electromyographic readings in migraine with combination headache patients. Headache 23:75–82, 1983

203. CLASSIFICATION AND DIFFERENTIAL DIAGNOSIS OF HEADACHE

ROBERT S. KUNKEL

The diagnosis of headache is based on the history presented by the sufferer. The history will usually suggest whether or not the headache is due to some neurologic, pericranial, or systemic condition. Currently, the classification of headache is based on the symptoms and signs presented by the headache patient or elicited by the neurologic and physical examination.

Historically, headaches have been classified according to their presumed cause. Terms such as constipation headache, congestive headache, neuralgic headache, stress headache, allergy headache, emotional headache, and headache of monotony have been used in books written about headaches. Migraine has been called "sick headache" for years and this term is

still used by many today. Horton, who wrote the first detailed description of what is now known as cluster headache, called it histamine headache because he assumed that the pain was caused by the patients response to histamine.

Since the diagnosis of one of the three primary headache syndromes (migraine, tension-type, and cluster) is based on the history obtained from the patient, an accurate history is essential to making the correct diagnosis. Relatively few headaches are secondary to some underlying disease process or other condition; over 90 percent of patients complaining of head pain have either migraine, tension-type, or cluster headaches. However, it is essential to recognize the cases where headaches are caused by organic or structural conditions, as treatment of the underlying abnormality usually will lessen or bring an end to the headache. Specific symptomatology and causes of specific types of headache are discussed in detail in other chapters of this book.

Many classifications have been used over the years. In 1962 an ad hoc committee of the National Institutes of Health developed the first attempt at a comprehensive classification of headache (Table 203-1). This classification was used as a reference by nearly every author who wrote about headache in the subsequent years.

One of the most useful classifications of headache has been proposed by S. Diamond and D.J. Dalessio. Their classification is very helpful in clinical practice. Headaches are separated into those with vascular components (migraine and cluster), tension-type headache, or traction and inflammatory headaches. All headaches that are secondary to some underlying disease such as intracranial masses, hemorrhage, infection, or inflammation of the pericranial structures or due to some structural abnormality such as an Arnold-Chiari malformation or hydrocephalus are in this category. This simple scheme is both practical and adequate for most practitioners treating headache patients.

In 1988, after three years of deliberations, the International Headache Society (IHS) published a very detailed and complete headache classification, which was modeled after the DSM III (Diagnostic and Statistical Manual). (Table 203-2). This classification is now accepted throughout the world; the intention is that it will be revised after it has been used and tested in clinical practice. Diagnostic criteria are listed for the three primary headache syndromes and for nine categories of secondary headaches. This very detailed classification is not used extensively in the office practice of headache medicine. For reliable and comparable research however, it is essential that its diagnostic criteria be used.

This classification of the primary headache syndromes is based on symptoms, not on the pathophysiology or etiology of the headaches. Therefore, it is essential to get as much informa-

TABLE 203-1. Headache Classification—1962

1. Migrainous-vascular
    Classic
    Common
    Cluster
    Hemiplegic and ophthalmoplegic
    Lower-half
2. Muscle contraction
3. Combined: vascular and muscle contraction
4. Nasal vasomotor reaction
5. Delusional, conversion, or hypochondriacal
6. Nonmigrainous vascular
7. Traction
8. Overt cranial inflammation
9–13. Ocular, aural, nasal, sinus, dental, or other cranial or neck structure disorders
14. Cranial neuritides
15. Cranial neuralgias

TABLE 203-2. International Headache Society Classification—1988

1. Migraine
   1.1 Migraine without aura
   1.2 Migraine with aura
       1.2.1 Migraine with typical aura
       1.2.2 Migraine with prolonged aura
       1.2.3 Familial hemiplegic migraine
       1.2.4 Basilar migraine
       1.2.5 Migraine aura without headache
       1.2.6 Migraine with acute onset aura
   1.3 Ophthalmoplegic migraine
   1.4 Retinal migraine
   1.5 Childhood periodic syndromes that may be precursors to or associated with migraine
       1.5.1 Benign paroxysmal vertigo of childhood
       1.5.2 Alternating hemiplegia of childhood
   1.6 Complications of migraine
       1.6.1 Status migrainous
       1.6.2 Migrainous infarction
   1.7 Migrainous disorder not fulfilling above criteria

2. Tension-type headache
   2.1 Episodic tension-type headache
       2.1.1 Episodic tension-type headache associated with disorder of pericranial muscles
       2.1.2 Episodic tension-type headache unassociated with disorder of pericranial muscles
   2.2 Chronic tension-type headache
       2.2.1 Chronic tension-type headache associated with disorder of pericranial muscles
       2.2.2 Chronic tension-type headache unassociated wtih disorder of pericranial muscles
   2.3 Headache of the tension type not fulfilling above criteria

3. Cluster headache and chronic paroxysmal hemicrania
   3.1 Cluster headache
       3.1.1 Cluster headache periodicity undetermined
       3.1.2 Episodic cluster headache
       3.1.3 Chronic cluster headache
           3.1.3.1 Unremitting from onset
           3.1.3.2 Evolved from episodic
   3.2 Chronic paroxysmal hemicrania
   3.3 Cluster headachelike disorder not fulfilling above criteria

4. Miscellaneous headaches unassociated with structural lesion
   4.1 Idiopathic stabbing headache
   4.2 External compression headache
   4.3 Cold stimulus headache
       4.3.1 External application of a cold stimulus
       4.3.2 Ingestion of a cold stimulus
   4.4 Benign cough headache
   4.5 Benign exertional headache
   4.6 Headache associated with sexual activity
       4.6.1 Dull type
       4.6.2 Explosive type
       4.6.3 Postural type

5. Headache associated with head trauma
   5.1 Acute post-traumatic headache
       5.1.1 With significant head trauma and/or confirmatory signs
       5.1.2 With minor head trauma and no confirmatory signs
   5.2 Chronic post-traumatic headache
       5.2.1 With significant head trauma and/or confirmatory signs
       5.2.2 With minor head trauma and no confirmatory signs

6. Headache associated with vascular disorders
   6.1 Acute ischemic cerebrovascular disease
       6.1.1 Transient ischemic attack (TIA)
       6.1.2 Thromboembolic stroke
   6.2 Intracranial hematoma
       6.2.1 Intracerebral hematoma
       6.2.2 Subdural hematoma
       6.2.3 Epidural hematoma
   6.3 Subarachnoid hemorrhage
   6.4 Unruptured vascular malformation
       6.4.1 Arteriovenous malformation
       6.4.2 Saccular aneurysm
   6.5 Arteritis
       6.5.1 Giant cell arteritis
       6.5.2 Other systemic arteritides
       6.5.3 Primary intracranial arteritis
   6.6 Carotid or vertebral artery pain
       6.6.1 Carotid or vertebral dissection
       6.6.2 Carotidynia (idiopathic)
       6.6.3 Postendarterectomy headache

   6.7 Venous thrombosis
   6.8 Arterial hypertension
       6.8.1 Acute pressor response to exogenous agent
       6.8.2 Pheochromocytoma
       6.8.3 Malignant (accelerated) hypertension
       6.8.4 Preeclampsia and eclampsia
   6.9 Headache associated with other vascular disorder

7. Headache associated with nonvascular intracranial disorder
   7.1 High cerebrospinal fluid pressure
       7.1.1 Benign intracranial hypertension
       7.1.2 High pressure hydrocephalus
   7.2 Low cerebrospinal fluid pressure
       7.2.1 Post-lumbar puncture headache
       7.2.2 Cerebrospinal fluid fistula headache
   7.3 Intracranial infection
   7.4 Intracranial sarcoidosis and other noninfectious inflammatory diseases
   7.5 Headache related to intrathecal injections
       7.5.1 Direct effect
       7.5.2 Due to chemical meningitis
   7.6 Intracranial neoplasm
   7.7 Headache associated with other intracranial disorder

8. Headache associated with substances or their withdrawal
   8.1 Headache induced by acute substance use or exposure
       8.1.1 Nitrate/nitrite-induced headache
       8.1.2 Monosodium glutamate-induced headache
       8.1.3 Carbon monoxide-induced headache
       8.1.4 Alcohol-induced headache
       8.1.5 Other substances
   8.2 Headache induced by chronic substance use or exposure
       8.2.1 Ergotamine-induced headache
       8.2.2 Analgesics-abuse headache
       8.2.3 Other substances
   8.3 Headache from substance withdrawal (acute use)
       8.3.1 Alcohol withdrawal headache (hangover)
       8.3.2 Other substances
   8.4 Headache from substance withdrawal (chronic use)
       8.4.1 Ergotamine withdrawal headache
       8.4.2 Caffeine withdrawal headache
       8.4.3 Narcotics abstinence headache
       8.4.4 Other substances
   8.5 Headache associated with substances but with uncertain mechanism
       8.5.1 Birth control pills or estrogens
       8.5.2 Other substances

9. Headache associated with noncephalic infection
   9.1 Viral infection
       9.1.1 Focal noncephalic
       9.1.2 Systemic
   9.2 Bacterial infection
       9.2.1 Focal noncephalic
       9.2.2 Systemic (septicemia)
   9.3 Headache related to other infection

10. Headache associated with metabolic disorder
    10.1 Hypoxia
         10.1.1 High altitude headache
         10.1.2 Hypoxic headache
         10.1.3 Sleep apnea headache
    10.2 Hypercapnia
    10.3 Mixed hypoxia and hypercapnia
    10.4 Hypoglycemia
    10.5 Dialysis
    10.6 Headache related to other metabolic abnormality

11. Headache or facial pain associated with disorder of cranium, neck, eyes, ears, nose, sinuses, teeth, mouth, or other facial or cranial structures
    11.1 Cranial bone
    11.2 Neck
         11.2.1 Cervical spine
         11.2.2 Retropharyngeal tendinitis
    11.3 Eyes
         11.3.1 Acute glaucoma
         11.3.2 Refractive errors
         11.3.3 Heterophoria or heterotropia
    11.4 Ears
    11.5 Nose and sinuses
         11.5.1 Acute sinus headache
         11.5.2 Other diseases of nose and sinuses
    11.6 Teeth, jaws, and related structures
    11.7 Temporomanidular joint disease

TABLE 203-2. *(Continued)*

12. Cranial neuralgias, nerve trunk pain, and deafferentation pain
  12.1 Persistent (in contrast to ticlike) pain of cranial nerve origin
    12.1.1 Compression or distortion of cranial nerves and second or third cervical roots
    12.1.2 Demyelination of cranial nerves
      12.1.2.1 Optic neuritis (retrobulbar neuritis)
    12.1.3 Infarction of cranial nerves
      12.1.3.1 Diabetic neuritis
    12.1.4 Inflammation of cranial nerves
      12.1.4.1 Herpes zoster
      12.1.4.2 Chronic postherpetic neuralgia
    12.1.5 Tolosa-Hunt syndrome
    12.1.6 Neck-tongue syndrome
    12.1.7 Other causes of persistent pain of cranial nerve origin
  12.2 Trigeminal neuralgia
    12.2.1 Idiopathic trigeminal neuralgia

    12.2.2 Symptomatic trigeminal neuralgia
      12.2.2.1 Compression of trigeminal root or ganglion
      12.2.2.2 Central lesions
  12.3 Glossopharyngeal neuralgia
    12.3.1 Idiopathic glossopharyngeal neuralgia
    12.3.2 Symptomatic glossopharyngeal neuralgia
  12.4 Nervus intermedius neuralgia
  12.5 Superior laryngeal neuralgia
  12.6 Occipital neuralgia
  12.7 Central causes of head and facial pain other than tic douloureux
    12.7.1 Anesthesia dolorosa
    12.7.2 Thalamic pain
  12.8 Facial pain not fulfilling criteria in groups 11 or 12

13. Headache not classifiable

tion from the headache sufferer as possible in order to properly diagnose the type of headache present. As medication and possibly other treatments become more specific for the alleviation of various types of head pain, it is essential that an accurate diagnosis of headache be made.

In addition to the fact that the history may not be very accurate, many patients have more than one kind of headache. Perhaps the most significant ongoing controversy in the field of headache classification is related to this situation. The IHS classification does not contain the category of mixed headache or chronic daily headache, which are terms used repeatedly in the headache literature. Most headache clinics see many patients who have daily headache, which at times will fit the migraine criteria and at other times fit the chronic tension-type headache criteria. These headaches will often blend together, and it is impossible for the patient to separate them. The IHS classification states that each headache type should be diagnosed and listed separately. It is essential to remember that the IHS classification is a classification of headaches, not of patients.

Some new terms were introduced in the 1988 classification. Classic migraine is now known as migraine with aura and common migraine is migraine without aura. Migraine aura without headache is the new term for what has been known as migraine equivalents or acephalgic migraine. Tension-type headache is the term for what has been previously known as tension headache, psychogenic headache, muscle-contraction headache, ordinary headache, and many other terms.

The term tension-type headache was a compromise term. Most persons recognize this headache as being a pressure type of discomfort, which is nonlocalized and usually is not very intense. Most recently it had been known as muscle-contraction headache. Since studies have shown that the scalp muscles are not always in a state of increased contraction during the time of this headache, it was felt that muscle contraction was not an accurate term. For more details see Chapter 200.

One of the new categories in the IHS classification is headache due to substances or their withdrawal. There is increasing evidence that one of the most common causes of daily or near-daily headache is the persistent use or overuse of combination analgesics, narcotics, opiates, tranquilizers, caffeine, and ergotamine tartrate. Frequent use of these pharmacologic agents can cause a dependency with subsequent withdrawal or rebound headache when the use is not continued on a regular basis. Usually effective prophylactic drugs and other treatment modalities will not be beneficial as long as the other agents are used so frequently. It is therefore important that one gets a very accurate history of all drug use, including all of the over-the-counter preparations consumed. Many of these contain caffeine along with analgesic compounds.

Patients who are difficult to classify include those with a new onset of headache and those with many years of headache. The IHS classification requires that patients with tension-type headache, cluster, or migraine have several typical attacks before the diagnosis is made and the type of headache classified. Frequent drug ingestion may be an important factor in those with chronic headache. Patients who have had headache for many years may not remember some of the specific details about the symptoms that occurred when their headaches were beginning years previously. Hence symptoms that were suggestive of, and even diagnostic of, migraine when the headaches started years previously may have been forgotten. The patient may well have had migraine but now has a daily headache with very few migraine features. The primary headache may be migraine with the current headache being due to overusage of medications.

DIFFERENTIAL DIAGNOSIS OF HEADACHE

A reliable history from an observant patient should allow the clinician to come up with a reasonable differential diagnosis as to the cause of the headache present. The physical and neurologic examination will usually confirm the suspicion that the headache is due to an underlying disease. The overwhelming majority of patients have one of the primary headache syndromes, which are migraine, tension-type, and cluster. If it seems unlikely that the headache is one of these, then a search for neurologic, cranial, cervical, or systemic causes is indicated. There are systemic factors, such as hypertension, anemia, medication, and fever that may affect the frequency and intensity of migraine. If the pattern or frequency of migraine has changed, the reason for this should be pursued.

Typical attacks of migraine with aura and cluster headache rarely need any further investigation. Rarely, a lesion of the occipital lobe may cause visual symptoms that mimic the aura of migraine. It is often more difficult to be certain of the diagnosis of migraine without aura and tension-type headache.

CRANIAL AND CERVICAL CAUSES OF HEADACHE

Disease involving the head and upper neck can cause tension-type headache and, at times, headache indistinguishable from migraine without aura. Examination, however, will usually reveal disease or infection of the head or neck. Sinus and dental disease are the most common cephalgic problems causing headache. Sinus disease usually causes frontal or facial pains, but sphenoid sinusitis may cause pain in the vertex of the skull. Dental infection and periodontal disease may cause headaches. Dental abscesses or the cracked tooth syndrome are less common causes. Computed tomography scanning or magnetic resonance imaging (MRI) of the sinuses is very helpful in evaluating the extent of sinus disease.

Diseases of the eyes or ears are usually evident on examination. Refractive errors rarely cause headache. The headache caused by such diseases will occur during reading or close work with the eyes and will not be present upon awakening. Other diseases of the eye, such as glaucoma or inflammatory conditions, should be evident on examination and are usually of recent onset.

Tension-type headache that is secondary to some other problem is usually due to spasm in the muscles around the temporomandibular joint or the muscles of the cervical spine. Most pains that are related to the temporomandibular joint are secondary to clenching or grinding of the teeth. Rarely is there any significant disease in the joint or a symptomatic malalignment of the bite. Examination of the joint and inspection of the bite of the patient when opening and closing the mouth will usually demonstrate abnormalities. Radiographs and MRI of the temporomandibular joint will show disease of the joint if present. Degenerative changes in the cervical spine can be associated with neck and head pain, which is more often a muscular or tension type rather than a radicular or neuralgic type of pain. Associated spasm in the cervical and trapezius muscles with tender points that are often palpable on examination, and increased neck motion as well as sloping shoulders and a forward-positioned neck are often seen.

INTRACRANIAL DISEASE

Intracranial disease, if the cause of headache, is usually associated with neurologic symptoms and signs. It is most unusual to have headache as the only symptom of a central nervous system lesion or infection. A patient with a recent onset of headache should be investigated, as does one who has had a chronic headache but develops new neurologic symptoms or has a change in symptoms. The headache caused by a brain tumor will be of progressing intensity and will almost always be accompanied by neurologic symptoms and signs.

Aneurysms in the brain do not cause chronic headache unless they compress a cranial nerve, and neurologic signs should be evident. Ruptured aneurysms, of course, cause an acute severe headache and are often rapidly fatal. Subdural hematoma, Arnold-Chiari malformation, and hydrocephalus may cause headache of a subacute nature, but usually the headaches occurring with these conditions are not severe. Again, neurologic signs should be evident, and the headache is usually worsened by change of position or the Valsalva maneuver.

Intracranial infections may be the cause of acute pain and are usually accompanied by fever and neurologic abnormalities that are evident on examination. An abscess may not be associated with fever but usually will cause progressive symptoms as it expands. Meningitis and encephalitis, both of which are accompanied by headache, are usually also associated with alterations in mentation.

SYSTEMIC CAUSES OF HEADACHE

A vascular type of headache that is not episodic but persistent may be caused by fever, hypertension, anemia, or hypoxemia. This type of headache could be chronic or of recent onset depending on the underlying cause. Viral illnesses may cause a diffuse throbbing headache that is aggravated by Valsalva maneuvers such as bending, straining, coughing, and sneezing.

This type of headache is not at all uncommon and will tend to improve spontaneously, although it may take weeks or even months to subside. Often patients can remember that the headache started with an acute flulike illness; other systemic infections can cause headache, which may be caused by a "toxic effect" of the infection itself or secondary to fever.

Paroxysmal or episodic throbbing pain in the head, which is diffuse and nonlocalized, is a common symptom of acute hypertensive attacks of pheochromocytoma. Acute onset of exertional or orgasmic headache needs to be evaluated to exclude intercranial hemorrhage, intercranial obstruction, or conditions aggravated by exertion such as the Arnold-Chiari malformation. Studies that have been done in patients suffering acute orgasmic headache have demonstrated a vascular lesion on only very rare occasions. Benign orgasmic headache, although very frightening, is rarely due to any underlying disease.

Various endocrinopathies, such as thyroid dysfunction or hyperparathyroidism, can cause headache of a nonspecific type. Electrolyte abnormalities, hypoglycemia, and hypoxemia also are possible causes of headache, although quite rare. Anyone who awakens with a headache in the morning should raise suspicion of sleep apnea with subsequent hypoxemia. This usually is diagnosed by history from the spouse and confirmed by sleep studies.

Neuralgic pains involving the head usually occur in older persons. Tic douloureux or trigeminal neuralgia typically involves the second and third divisions of the fifth nerve. The characteristic of this headache is the triggering of sharp stabbing pains by touching the trigger zones about the face. Patients with tic douloureux will never rub or touch their face or head, but patients with almost all the other types of headaches will press, push, and rub their scalp in an effort to obtain relief. Occipital neuralgia is a headache involving the posterior part of the skull and can be associated with trauma or degenerative changes in the upper cervical spine. The location and type of pain is quite typical, and the diagnosis can be confirmed by local injection around the nerve, which causes an alleviation of the pain.

SUMMARY

The differential diagnosis of headache is extensive. The three primary headache syndromes,—migraine, tension-type headache, and cluster headache—are usually diagnosed by the history and lack of any demonstrable abnormalities on the neurologic and physical examination. Headaches, which by description do not fit one of the primary headache syndromes or are occurring with neurologic symptoms, need to be investigated for some specific underlying cause. The cause may be neurologic due to conditions of the central nervous system or may be due to problems in the cervical spine or systemic conditions. Any headache associated with signs on examination needs to be vigorously investigated in the hope that an underlying cause may be found and treated. It must be remembered, however, that some neurologic or systemic conditions will cause headache that may be indistinguishable, on history, from migraine or tension-type headache. It is unusual for the symptoms of cluster headache to be confused with any other condition.

SUGGESTED READINGS

Ad Hoc Committee on Classification of Headache, National Institute of Neurological Disease and Blindness: Classification of headache. JAMA 179: 717–18, 1962

Diamond S, Dalessio DJ: The Practicing Physician's Approach to Headache. 5th Ed. Williams & Wilkens, Baltimore, 1993

Headache Classification Committee of the International Headache Society: Classification and diagnostic criteria for headache disorders, cranial neuralgias and facial pain. Cephalalgia 8(suppl. 7), 1988

SECTION 2. HEADACHE SYNDROMES AND THEIR TREATMENT

204. MIGRAINE WITH AND WITHOUT AURA

RICHARD B. LIPTON
ALAN M. RAPOPORT

Migraine is a common headache disorder characterized by head pain and a combination of neurologic, gastrointestinal, and autonomic features. In a given year, 15 to 17 percent of women and about 6 percent of men have at least one migraine attack. Prevalence is highest from ages 25 to 55, so migraine affects people during their peak productive years. According to recent estimates, 23 million Americans currently suffer from migraine headaches and over 11 million experience significant levels of headache-related disability. The cost of migraine in the United States almost certainly exceeds 5 billion dollars per year. Yet, the majority of migraine sufferers are not diagnosed by doctors and are not treated with prescription drugs. Undiagnosed and untreated migraine is an important remedial public health problem. The overwhelming majority of migraine sufferers who seek care do so in the primary care setting. Therefore, primary care doctors have the best opportunity to improve the diagnosis of migraine and ultimately to improve the outcome of this potentially devastating disorder through effective treatment.

The diagnosis of migraine and other types of headache has been facilitated by the new formal criteria published in *Cephalalgia* in 1988 by the International Headache Society (IHS) (see Ch. 203). This classification system divides all headache disorders into two major groups: primary and secondary. In secondary disorders, the headache is symptomatic of some underlying condition such as a brain tumor, temporal arteritis, or medication rebound. In primary disorders, the headache is due to underlying biochemical, physiologic, and electrical dysfunction of the brain. The major categories of primary headaches are migraine, tension-type headache, and cluster headache. Based on international consensus, the criteria determine which headache features are required to establish or exclude the diagnosis of migraine.

The diagnosis of migraine is based largely on patient reports of headache characteristics and associated symptoms. There are no biologic markers or laboratory tests that can confirm the clinical diagnosis. The general medical and neurologic examinations, as well as laboratory studies, are usually normal save minor variations and serve to exclude secondary causes of headache. Therefore, the headache history is the key to accurate diagnosis (see Ch. 201).

In this chapter, we present an overview of the clinical characteristics of migraine, beginning with a description of the phases of the migraine attack. We then review the IHS diagnostic criteria for migraine and discuss their role in primary care. We close with an approach to the differential diagnosis of migraine.

DESCRIPTION OF THE MIGRAINE ATTACK

Blau has divided the migraine attack into five phases: (1) The prodrome is a change in mood or behavior that occurs hours or days before the headache. (2) The aura is a focal neurologic deficit often preceding the migraine headache. (3) The headache phase consists of pain and associated features. (4) In the termination phase, pain gradually subsides. (5) In the postdrome, residual symptoms persist after pain has remitted. Although most people with migraine experience more than one of these five phases, no single phase is obligatory for diagnosis. A description of the phases of the migraine attack provides a structured way to review the protean manifestation of migraine.

Prodrome

Prodromal features occur in about 60 percent of migraineurs, often hours to 1 or 2 days before headache onset. While prodromal features vary from person to person, for an individual sufferer, they may be quite stereotyped. Information about prodromal features is elicited by asking, ''Before the pain begins, do you know that a headache is coming? How do you know?'' Prodromes include changes in mood (depression, euphoria, irritability, restlessness), mental slowing, hyperactivity, sluggishness, fatigue, and drowsiness. Increased sensory sensitivity (photophobia and phonophobia), alterations in fluid balance (increased thirst, fluid retention, increased urination), changes in appetite (anorexia, food cravings), and alterations in gastrointestinal function (nausea, constipation, or diarrhea) may occur. Some people simply report a poorly characterized feeling that a migraine attack is coming. Prodromal features are believed to result from cerebral and brainstem dysfunction prior to pain onset, supporting the idea that migraine is primarily a disease of the brain, not of the blood vessels.

Aura

The migraine aura consists of focal neurologic symptoms that typically precede but may accompany the headache. About 20 percent of migraine sufferers experience auras. Therefore, if doctors require the presence of an aura to diagnose migraine, 80 percent of patients with migraine will not be diagnosed. Most aura symptoms develop slowly, over 5 to 20 minutes. They usually last 10 to 30 minutes, but almost always less than 60 minutes. The aura is characterized by visual, sensory, or motor features and may also involve language or brainstem disturbances. Headache usually occurs within 60 minutes of the end of the aura. Descriptions of auras can be improved through the use of diaries or by having patients draw pictures of their experience. Our knowledge of the phenomenology of auras is derived primarily from such patient accounts and drawings.

The most common type of migraine aura is the *visual aura*. The visual aura includes a range of positive visual phenomena such as scintillations (flickering lights), photopsias (flashes of light), and fortification spectra (jagged luminous zigzag lines, often in an overall crescentic shape). Scintillations may be so subtle that they are barely noticed or almost blinding in intensity. The visual aura often includes negative visual phenomena as well, in the form of a scotoma. Scotomas are areas of visual loss, which may take the form of a graying or blacking-out of vision. In the absence of positive visual features, scotomas may go unnoticed unless they are large, or unless patients walk or drive into objects in the involved visual field. Visual auras classically include a mix of positive and negative visual features, taking the form of a scintillating scotoma with flickering around the edges of a region of visual loss. Auras characteristically begin in the central vision, and expand laterally to encompass an enlarging segment of a homonymous visual field. Other patterns have been described. Scintillations less often begin laterally and travel medially across a visual field. Only the upper or lower half of a visual field may be involved. Occasionally, objects may change in size (micropsia or macropsia) or shape (metamorphopsia).

The *sensory aura* is the second most common type, occurring in about one-third of people who have migraine with aura. Like the visual aura, the sensory aura is also characterized by a mix of positive (tingling) and negative (numbness) features. Sensory aura frequently evolves in a cheiro-oral (hand-mouth) pattern, beginning in an isolated part of the hand (e.g., the thumb), expanding to involve the whole hand and then the perioral region. Involvement of half the tongue is common.

Motor aura occurs as a variable feature in up to 15 percent of patients who have migraine with aura. Although not well studied, it consists of paresis, usually developing in a focal region and gradually spreading to involve a larger area. Most patients with weakness also experience sensory symptoms. Motor phenomena are usually restricted to the hand and arm, although the face, arm, and leg may be involved in various combinations. Unilateral involvement is the rule; bilateral paresis is very rare, although a complaint of generalized weakness is common. A subgroup of patients with motor aura have an autosomal dominant disorder referred to as *familial hemiplegic migraine*. These individuals usually have episodes of hemiparesis and headache lasting from several hours to several days. Genetic linkage to chromosome 19 has been demonstrated in some but not all affected families.

There are a number of less common aura manifestations. *Basilar migraine* is characterized by various combinations of typical visual aura symptoms, vertigo, tinnitus, diplopia, ataxia, and a depressed level of awareness. This rare condition typically begins in childhood and adolescence. *Speech disturbances* may occur, usually with other symptoms indicating dominant hemisphere dysfunction, including right-sided motor or sensory disturbances. *Hemispatial neglect* as well as spatial disorientation have been described. A variety of deficits in higher integrative functions, including alexia (difficulty reading) or acalculia (difficulty calculating), and palinopsia (visual perseveration) have been reported.

The various types of migraine auras should not be regarded as discrete, mutually exclusive syndromes. More than one kind of aura may occur within a single attack; visual aura may be followed by sensory aura, for example. In addition, the type of aura may shift over time within individual sufferers. Someone with basilar migraine in childhood may develop typical visual aura in adolescence and migraine without aura in adult life. In families with several affected members, different patterns of aura may occur in different individuals, suggesting that aura characteristics are controlled by some nongenetic factors. Pa-

tients tend to have fewer attacks of migraine with aura as they get older, even if the frequency of migraine is unchanged or increasing.

Headache Phase

The frequency of various migraine symptoms are summarized in Table 204-1. The typical headache is unilateral, throbbing, moderate to in intensity, and aggravated by physical activity. Not all of these features are required for diagnosis. Pain may be bilateral at onset (in 40 percent of cases) or on one side and then become generalized. The headache of migraine can occur at any time of day or night, but occurs most frequently on arising in the morning. The onset is usually gradual; the pain typically increases over 0.5 to 2 hours, reaches a sustained plateau and then subsides slowly, lasting an average of 1 day with a range of 4 to 72 hours in adults and 2 to 48 hours in children.

The head pain varies greatly in intensity, although most people with migraine report severe or very severe pain. The pain is described as throbbing or pusatile in over 80 percent of cases. Throbbing pain is also often described in other types of headache. Pain is commonly aggravated by physical activity such as climbing stairs, bending over, simple head movement, coughing, or head rotation. The pain is hemicranial in 50 to 60 percent and tends to have a frontotemporal or retro-orbital location. Migraine sufferers will frequently experience momentary stabs and jabs of sharp, shooting pains at a variety of cephalic locations. These benign, idiopathic, stabbing pains tend to occur on the same side as migraine attacks and may frighten patients.

The pain of migraine is invariably accompanied by other "associated symptoms" (Table 204-1). Anorexia is common, although food craving can occur. Nausea occurs in 60 to 75 percent of patients, while vomiting occurs in about one-quarter of migraineurs. Reports of nausea, which begin only after the administration of medications (e.g., ergot alkaloids) should not be used to support the diagnosis. Many patients experience sensory hyperexcitability, as manifested by photophobia, phonophobia, and osmophobia. As many people are sensitive to light or sound at baseline, we ask about unusual or heightened sensory sensitivity. These reports are more convincing if they have a behavioral consequence such as going to a dark, quiet room to avoid light or sound. Some patients report lowering the window shades, turning off lights, or wearing sunglasses to limit light exposure. Patients may turn down the stereo, ask people to talk quietly, or wear ear plugs to avoid sound. During an attack, exposure to light or sound often exacerbates the pain; exposure to strong or noxious odors may exacerbate nausea.

Other systemic "associated symptoms" include blurred vision, nasal stuffiness, hunger, diarrhea, abdominal cramps, polyuria (sometimes followed by decreased urinary output after the attack), pallor (or, less commonly, redness) of the face, sensations of heat or cold, and sweating. There may be localized

TABLE 204-1. Proportion of Migraine Sufferers With Selected Symptoms

Symptom	Migraineurs Affected (%)	
	Females	Males
Throbbing pain	83	84
Unilateral pain	59	51
Nausea	72	60
Vomiting	28	21
Photophobia	72	66

edema of the scalp, the face, or under the eyes, tenderness of the scalp, unusual prominence of a vein or artery in the temple, stiffness of the neck, and tenderness of the cervical musculature. Difficulty with concentration is common; less often there is memory impairment. Depression, fatigue, anxiety, nervousness, and irritability may occur. There may be lightheadedness and a feeling of faintness. The distal extremities tend to be cold and moist. As discussed below, the IHS has selected particular associated symptoms as cardinal manifestations for diagnosis.

Termination and Postdrome

In the termination phase, the pain gradually decreases in intensity, usually over several hours. Migraine sufferers often find that sleep or vomiting will help end an attack. Following the headache, the patient often feels tired, washed out, irritable, and listless. Some report impaired concentration, scalp tenderness, or mood changes. Some people feel unusually refreshed or euphoric after an attack, while others note depression and malaise.

Exacerbating or Ameliorating Factors

Identifying factors that precipitate or aggravate migraine can help support the diagnosis. In addition, recognizing and avoiding these factors provides an opportunity to improve headache control. The most frequently reported trigger factors include menstruation (especially within a day of the onset of flow), stress or relaxation after stress, fatigue, changes in the sleep-wake cycle (excessive or insufficient sleep), or changes in weather conditions. Exposure to bright lights, loud noises, chemical fumes, and perfume may all trigger attacks.

Many migraine patients report dietary triggers. The most commonly reported precipitants include alcohol (especially red wine), followed by chocolate, aged cheese, aspartame, caffeine excess or withdrawal, and fermented foods. Individuals with diet-provoked migraine may have defects in the metabolism of particular dietary chemicals such as tyramine and phenolic compounds, increasing their vulnerability to these agents. It is unlikely that dietary triggers initiate attacks through true immunoglobulin E (IgE)-mediated allergic mechanisms.

Ameliorating factors vary from patient to patient, sometimes with the symptom profile of the migraine attack. For patients with photophobia and phonophobia, lying in a dark, quiet room can bring some relief. For people with movement sensitivity, lying motionless may decrease pain. Pressure on the extracranial arteries with hot or cold compresses often brings transient relief. Vomiting or sleep may terminate an attack. Effective medication is the major ameliorating factor for most patients. Migraine also often improves in the second two trimesters of pregnancy and after menopause, especially when replacement estrogens are avoided or used daily in low doses.

FORMAL DIAGNOSTIC CRITERIA OF THE INTERNATIONAL HEADACHE SOCIETY

To improve the classification of headache disorders both in clinical practice and in research, the IHS published diagnostic criteria for a broad range of headache disorders in 1988. These criteria, based on expert consensus, have had a major impact on clinical trials and on epidemiologic research, although they have not been widely employed in clinical practice, perhaps because of their complexity. The IHS system defines many

subtypes of migraine. For use in the primary care setting, we discuss two major types of migraine. Though the IHS criteria may be revised as empirical evidence and clinical experience accumulate, they provide the best currently available diagnostic "tool" for the clinician and investigator.

Migraine Without Aura (Common Migraine)

To establish a diagnosis of IHS *migraine without aura* (1.1), at least five attacks are required (Table 204-2). Each attack must last 4 to 72 hours and must have two of the following four pain characteristics: unilateral location, pulsating quality, moderate to severe intensity, and aggravation by routine physical activity. In addition, the attacks must have at least one of the following: nausea, vomiting, or photophobia and phonophobia. Using these criteria, no single characteristic is mandatory for diagnosing migraine. A patient who has moderate, nonthrobbing, bilateral pain aggravated by routine activity, with photophobia and phonophobia meets criteria, just like the more typical patient with unilateral, throbbing pain and nausea.

When a migraine attack lasts longer than 72 hours (3 days), the term *status migrainosus* is applied. The frequency of attacks is extremely variable, from a few per lifetime to several per week. The average migraineur experiences from one to three headaches per month. Migraine is, by definition, a recurrent phenomenon. The requirement for at least five attacks is imposed because headaches simulating migraine may be caused by organic disease, ranging from brain tumor to sinusitis to glaucoma. This is discussed in the section on differential diagnosis in Chapter 203. As the number of lifetime attacks increases, the probability of an ominous cause declines.

The IHS criteria also requires the exclusion of secondary headache disorders (Section E, Table 204-2) in one of several ways. Thus, migraine is both a diagnosis of inclusion, as specific combinations of symptoms are required, and a diagnosis of exclusion, as alternative causes of headache must be systematically eliminated.

Migraine with Aura (Classic Migraine)

The diagnosis of migraine with aura (1.2), requires at least two attacks with any three of the following four features: one or more fully reversible aura symptoms indicating brain dysfunction; aura developing over more than four minutes; aura lasting less than 60 minutes; and headache following aura with a free

TABLE 204-2. Migraine Without Aura: International Headache Society Criteria

Previously used terms: *common migraine, hemicrania simplex*
Diagnostic criteria:
A. At least 5 attacks fulfilling items B to D below.
B. Headache lasting 4 to 72 hours (untreated or unsuccessfully treated).
C. Headache with at least two of the following characteristics:
 1. Unilateral location.
 2. Pulsating quality.
 3. Moderate or severe intensity (inhibits or prohibits daily activities).
 4. Aggravation by walking stairs or similar routine physical activity.
D. During headache at least one of the following:
 1. Nausea and/or vomiting.
 2. Photophobia and phonophobia.
E. At least one of the following:
 1. History and physical and neurologic examinations do not suggest one of the disorders listed in groups 5–11 (organic disorders).
 2. History and/or physical and/or neurologic examinations suggest such disorder, but it is ruled out by appropriate investigations.
 3. Such disorder is present, but migraine attacks do not occur for the first time in close temporal relation to the disorder.

TABLE 204-3. Migraine With Aura: International Headache Society Criteria

Diagnostic criteria:
A. At least 2 attacks fulfilling item B below.
B. At least 3 of the following 4 characteristics:
  1. One or more fully reversible aura symptoms indicating brain dysfunction.
  2. At least one aura symptom develops gradually over more than 4 minutes or 2 or more symptoms occur in succession.
  3. No single aura symptom lasts more than 60 minutes.
  4. Headache follows aura with a free interval of less than 60 minutes (it may also begin before or simultaneously with the aura).
C. History, physical examination and, where appropriate, diagnostic tests exclude a secondary cause.

interval of less than 60 minutes (Table 204-3). If the first three criteria are met, migraine with aura can be diagnosed even in the absence of headache. Fewer attacks are required than for migraine without aura, based on the assumption that typical aura is highly specific for migraine. Other causes of this symptom complex must once again be excluded.

To utilize these criteria effectively, the clinician must make judgments about what features meet the criterion "one or more fully reversible aura symptoms indicating brain dysfunction." For example, if a patient sees spots of light for 10 seconds while climbing stairs during a headache, this "neurologic" event arguably meets criteria B1, B3, and B4 (Table 204-3). Recurrence on two occasions might qualify the patient for a diagnosis of migraine with aura. Similarly, 30 seconds of isolated tinnitus during a headache on two occasions may be judged to be migraine with aura. Most experienced clinicians would agree that these symptoms do not warrant a diagnosis of migraine with aura. More specific diagnostic criteria are therefore required. Methods for improving diagnostic criteria for headache disorders have been discussed elsewhere.

Migraine with aura is subdivided into migraine with typical aura (1.2.1) (homonymous visual disturbance, unilateral numbness or weakness, or aphasia); migraine with prolonged aura (1.2.2) (aura lasting more than 60 minutes); familial hemiplegic migraine (1.2.3); basilar migraine (1.2.4); migraine aura without headache (1.2.5); and migraine with acute-onset aura (1.2.6). Other varieties of migraine include ophthalmoplegic (1.3), retinal (1.4), and childhood periodic syndromes (1.5). The descriptive features of most of these syndromes are reviewed in the previous section.

Focal symptoms and signs of the aura may persist beyond the headache phase. Formerly termed *complicated migraine,* the IHS classification has introduced two more specific diagnostic categories. If the aura lasts for more than 1 hour but less than 1 week, the term *migraine with prolonged aura* is applied. If the signs persist for more than 1 week or a neuroimaging procedure demonstrates a stroke, a diagnosis of *migrainous infarction* is assigned. Particularly in middle or late life, the aura may occur without headache; it is then considered a *migraine equivalent* (migraine aura without headache [1.2.5]).

Atypical Migraine Without Aura

The IHS defines a group of people who fulfill all of the criteria for migraine but one (IHS 1.7). This group is sometimes termed "atypical migraine." Patients in this group may have fewer than five lifetime attacks, headache duration of less than 4 hours, typical pain features associated with photophobia or phonophobia (but not both), without nausea or vomiting. Features that are not part of the IHS criteria may help support the diagnosis. These features include the presence of a typical prodrome,

osmophobia, and an accurate family history of migraine in one or more first-degree relatives. Relief with sleep, exacerbation during menses, and the presence of dietary triggers (alcohol, tyramine-containing foods, chocolate) may also add diagnostic confidence in these atypical cases.

DIFFERENTIAL DIAGNOSIS

When evaluating a patient presenting with the complaint of headache, the primary care doctor must identify or exclude the myriad conditions that can cause secondary headache and then diagnose a specific primary headache disorder. In approaching this problem, the clinician looks for "alarms" or warning signals in the history, general medical, and neurologic examinations that suggest secondary headache. If those "alarms" are present, a directed workup is undertaken to determine whether or not an underlying condition is present. The patient's medical history provides a context for the evaluation of new headaches. The likely diagnoses in a previously well 30-year-old with new onset headache are quite different from those in a 30-year-old with AIDS or cancer.

Table 204-4 summarizes some important alarms, the diagnostic concerns they raise, and the initial diagnostic evaluations which should be considered. These issues are discussed in more detail in Chapter 203. If alarms are absent or the diagnostic evaluation is negative, the clinician then attempts to diagnose a specific primary headache disorder. If the patient has no alarms and meets criteria for a primary headache disorder, treatment is often initiated without additional diagnostic tests other than routine bloods and an electrocardiogram (ECG). Several recent studies suggest that in headache patients without alarms by history or examination, routine computed tomography (CT) and magnetic resonance imaging (MRI) have extraordinarily low yields.

If patients do not fit neatly into established diagnostic categories or if response to treatment is atypical, then the diagnosis should be revisited and neuroimaging should be considered. Some important causes of secondary headaches that simulate migraine are listed in Table 204-5.

Secondary Headaches

Headache is a common feature in transient ischemic attacks, thromboembolic stroke, and intracerebral hemorrhage. Like migraine with aura, these syndromes may be characterized by focal neurologic deficits associated with headache. In general, migraine begins in adolescence or early adult life, while stroke tends to occur with advancing years, simplifying the diagnostic problem. Most patients with stroke are not difficult to diagnose. For example, an elderly hypertensive man with a single episode of headache associated with the onset of a persistent neurologic deficit and an appropriate abnormality on a neuroimaging procedure has stroke and not migraine. On rare occasions, stroke may develop as a sequela of prolonged but otherwise typical migraine aura (migrainous infarction). In addition, the antiphospholipid (aPL) antibody syndromes (anticardiolipin antibody syndrome or lupus anticoagulant) with or without systemic lupus erythematosus (SLE) may predispose to both migrainelike headaches and cerebrovascular disease. Patients with atypical or prolonged aura should be evaluated for aPL antibody syndromes with a partial thromboplastin time and anticardiolipin antibody titers. Mitral valve prolapse and oral contraceptives may account for some strokes that occur in patients with migraine.

TABLE 204-4. Alarms in the Diagnosis of Headache Disorders

Headache Alarm	Selected Diagnostic Considerations	Possible Workup
Sudden onset headache	Subarachnoid hemorrhage Pituitary apoplexy Bleed into a mass or AVM Mass lesion (esp. posterior fossa)	Neuroimaging Lumbar puncture[a]
New onset headache after age 50	Temporal arteritis Mass lesion	Erythrocyte sedimentation rate Neuroimaging
Headache with fever, stiff neck, rash, systemic illness	Meningitis, encephalitis Lyme disease, systemic infection, collagen vascular disease	Neuroimaging Lumbar puncture[a] Blood tests
Accelerating pattern of headaches	Mass lesion Subdural hematoma Medication overuse	Neuroimaging
New-onset headache in a patient with cancer or HIV	Metastasis Meningitis (chronic or carcinomatous) Brain abscess (including toxoplasmosis)	Neuroimaging Lumbar puncture[a]
Focal neurologic symptoms or signs (other than typical aura)	Mass lesion AVM Stroke Collagen vascular disease (including aPL antibodies)	Neuroimaging Collagen vascular disease evaluation
Papilledema	Mass lesion Pseudotumor	Neuroimaging Lumbar puncture[a]

Abbreviations: AVM, arteriovenous malformation; HIV, human immunodeficiency virus; aPL, antiphospholipid.

[a] Lumbar puncture is performed for headache after the neuroimagery procedure, if the diagnosis remains in doubt. In suspected bacterial meningitis, in the absence of focal findings and papilledema, lumbar puncture should be performed immediately without delay.

Transient ischemic attacks (TIA), if accompanied by headache, and migraine with aura can be difficult to distinguish. Several features can facilitate differential diagnosis. TIAs are characterized primarily by negative features such as weakness, numbness, or visual loss. Migraine with aura is often characterized by a mix of positive and negative features. In TIA, symptoms evolve relatively quickly. In migraine, symptoms often spread slowly over a number of minutes before reaching their maximum distribution. In addition, the classical aura syndromes of migraine (e.g., the scintillating scotoma) are rarely due to TIA and classic TIA features (e.g., amaurosis fugax) are rarely due to migraine. Nonetheless, diagnostic evaluations to exclude cerebrovascular disease are often necessary.

TABLE 204-5. Selected Secondary Headaches in the Differential Diagnosis of Migraine

Cerebrovascular disease
  Thrombotic or embolic stroke
  Intracerebral hemorrhage
  Transient ischemic attack
  Subarachnoid hemorrhage
  Subdural hematoma
  Arteriovenous malformation
  Carotid or vertebral dissection
  Venous thrombosis
  Cranial vasculitis (i.e., giant cell arteritis, systemic lupus erythematosus)
Other neurologic disorders
  Primary or metastatic tumor
  Other mass lesions (i.e., brain abscess, granulomatous disease)
  Pseudotumor cerebri
  Epilepsy
  Chronic meningitis (i.e., Lyme)
  Parkinson's disease
  Post-traumatic headache
Toxic/metabolic systemic disorders
  Vasodilators: e.g., nitrates, nitrites, calcium channel blockers
  Respiratory disturbance: hypoxia or hypercarbia
  Hypoglycemia
  Fever and other systemic disease
  Other medications: tetracycline, caffeine, fluoxetine, trazodone, vitamin A, indomethacin
Disease of the cranium, neck, eyes, and skull
  Posterior fossa and cervical spine malformations
  Acute sinusitis
  Glaucoma
  Temporomandibular joint syndrome

Subarachnoid hemorrhage (SAH) enters the differential diagnosis of new or recent-onset migraine. Severe headache, neck stiffness, nausea, and vomiting are features of both conditions. The typical SAH patient, with the paroxysmal onset of a devastating headache and nuchal rigidity, usually receives the necessary diagnostic evaluation with CT and lumbar puncture. This is particularly true for patients with persistent neurologic deficits. But, patients with diagnosed SAH often report one or two headaches of sudden onset before diagnosis. These sentinel headaches most likely represent warning bleeds, which precede the major bleed. Often, patients with sentinel headache are sent out of emergency rooms and doctors' offices with the diagnosis of migraine. As early diagnosis and surgical clipping of an underlying aneurysm can save lives, these missed diagnostic opportunities are important.

Several features facilitate the differential diagnosis of SAH and migraine. While migraine pain typically intensifies over 30 minutes to 2 hours, SAH headache begins suddenly and is often maximal at onset. If patients are able to report exactly what they were doing at the precise moment the headache began, suspect SAH. In migraine, neck stiffness is common, but meningismus is rare. In SAH, there is often true meningismus, but it can take several hours to develop. Syncope or near syncope at onset, the worst headache ever, and persistent neurologic deficits (i.e., third nerve palsy) all suggest SAH. If the patient has had many similar attacks, SAH becomes much less likely.

The patient with a long history of migraine who develops the worst headache ever poses a serious diagnostic challenge. All migraineurs, sooner or later, have their "worst" headache. If that headache is of gradual onset and perfectly typical of their migraine, extensive diagnostic evaluation may be avoided. But if that headache is of sudden onset or atypical in its location and associated features, workup for SAH is advisable.

A number of vascular abnormalities can produce headaches that resemble migraine. *Arteriovenous malformations* (AVM) may mimic migraine. The headache tends to occur on the side of the vascular malformation. Dural AVMs may also produce migrainelike headaches. These conditions can sometimes be detected by auscultation of the skull, listening for a cranial bruit.

Carotid dissection causes pain that radiates to the eye or temple, often associated with an ipsilateral Horner syndrome and visual symptoms. A history of neck trauma is sometimes present. Workup of the suspected vessels by magnetic resonance angiography can usually spare the patient a gold standard assessment with cerebral angiography.

Arteritis produces headache with neurologic symptoms. The vasculitis that most seriously enters into the differential diagnosis of migraine is *systemic lupus erythematosus,* with the overlapping antiphospholipid antibody syndromes discussed above. The rare disorder, *primary vasculitis of the nervous system,* produces multifocal neurologic defects and headache, often in young adults. Diagnosis requires cerebral angiography and, at times, meningeal or cortical biopsy. Systemic tests for vasculitis are negative in this condition. *Giant cell arteritis* (GCA) rarely begins before age 55. When systemic features such as polymyalgia rheumatica, jaw claudication, tender temporal arteries with decreased pulses, anemia, and weight loss are present, diagnosis is usually not difficult. The headache in GCA has no characteristic pattern and can resemble migraine. It tends to be in one or both temples and associated with a tender temporal artery. When GCA is suspected, a high erythrocyte sedimentation rate warrants high-dose prednisone (60 mg daily) pending a temporal artery biopsy.

Headaches associated with *mass lesions* of all kinds may be unilateral (often on the side of the mass) with episodic exacerbations as well as nausea and vomiting. In this setting, headaches more often resemble tension-type headache than migraine. Episodic exacerbations of headache may be associated with transient elevations of intracranial pressure due to plateau waves or transient obstruction of the cerebrospinal fluid (CSF) pathways. In *pseudotumor cerebri,* there is an idiopathic elevation of intracranial pressure, often associated with papilledema.

The differential diagnosis of migraine and epilepsy can be challenging. Both conditions may produce episodic neurologic symptoms as well as headache. Migraine-like headaches and epilepsy occur together in the same person with much greater than chance frequency. Migraine aura can trigger seizures under certain circumstances. Seizures can activate the trigeminovascular system to produce ictal and postictal headache. Several features are helpful in differential diagnosis. Seizures typically produce positive symptoms such as tonic-clonic movements or tingling; migraine aura often produces a mix of positive and negative symptoms. In addition, the interictal electroencephalogram (EEG) is more likely to show spikes in patients with epilepsy than migraine. The ictal EEG shows characteristic sequences of spikes or sharp waves, which change in frequency and amplitude (electroencephalographic seizure pattern) during

seizures. These changes generally do not occur with migraine. Finally, both conditions can and do occur in the same individuals.

A number of drugs, both therapeutic and recreational, can trigger headaches. The key to diagnosis is to discover the association between drug use and the onset of the headache disorder. Nitrites, nitrates, certain calcium channel blockers, caffeine, tetracycline, monosodium glutamate, certain antihypertensives, and indomethacin can all cause headaches de novo. Many of these agents may also exacerbate an underlying headache disorder such as migraine. As discussed in the Chapter 205, the same agents used to treat headache may exacerbate headache through the mechanism of medication rebound. Cocaine intoxication and cocaine withdrawal can precipitate headache.

A number of metabolic derangements may also cause headache. Hypoxia, hypercarbia, hypoglycemia, fever, and a number of systemic diseases such as viremia may produce throbbing headache. Acute sinusitis, glaucoma, and post-traumatic headache all enter into the differential diagnosis of migraine.

Primary Headaches

A number of primary headache disorders should be considered in the differential diagnosis of migraine. For the major categories of primary headache, the keys to differential diagnosis are summarized in Table 204-6. *Cluster headaches* are of shorter duration and have a radically different temporal profile than migraine, with distinct associated autonomic features such as ipsilateral lacrimation, rhinorrhea, and ptosis. *Tension-type headache* is defined by features which distinguish it from migraine. In pure cases with bilateral nonpulsatile pain and no associated features, diagnosis is not difficult. Differential diagnosis can be challenging in patients with both disorders and in patients who have headaches with intermediate characteristics.

In *transformed migraine,* patients initially experience typical episodic migraine. Over a period of months to years, headaches gradually increase in frequency but decrease in intensity, leaving the patient with near-daily headaches of mild to moderate intensity, occasionally punctuated by attacks of more severe headache. The daily headaches often resemble tension-type headache. The more severe attacks, often meet criteria for migraine. The term transformed migraine is used for this clinical syndrome and encompasses both types of headache. In 80 percent of cases, the process of transformation is associated with medication overuse and the development of rebound headaches. This headache syndrome can occur in the absence of medication overuse, suggesting that it represents the natural history of a particularly pernicious part of the migraine spectrum. In pa-

TABLE 204-6. Primary Headache in the Differential Diagnosis of Migraine

Headache Type	Age of Onset (years)	Gender Ratio F:M	Location	Duration	Frequency/ Timing	Severity	Quality	Associated Features
Migraine	10–30	3:1	Hemicranial (60%)	Several hours to 3 days	Variable 1–3/mo	Moderate-severe	Throbbing (80%)	Nausea, vomiting, photo/phono/osmophobia scotomata, neurologic deficits
Tension-type	20–50	1:1	Bilateral (90%)	30 min to 7+ days	Variable	Mild, dull ache	Viselike, bandlike pressure, may wax/wane	Nausea or photo or phonophobia, no vomiting
Cluster headache	20–40	1:5	Unilateral/periorbital/retro-orbital (95%)	30–120 min nocturnal	1–3×/day	Excruciating	Boring, piercing	Ipsilateral conjunctival injection, lacrimation, nasal congestion, rhinorrhea, miosis, facial sweating

tients taking analgesics or ergot alkaloids on a daily basis, successful treatment requires breaking the pattern of daily medication use. If the patient emphasizes the daily headache disorder and the physician fails to inquire about the pattern of evolution, transformed migraine is often missed.

Occasionally, rare primary headache disorders are mistaken for migraine. In *hemicrania continua,* there is a constant unilateral pain that waxes and wanes in intensity. During exacerbations, pain is usually associated with autonomic features resembling those of cluster headache (Horner syndrome, lacrimation, rhinorrhea) but nausea and photophobia may occur. Patients may describe their exacerbations but not their background pain, giving the impression of an episodic disorder rather than a waxing and waning continuous disorder. The pain goes away completely in migraine but not in hemicrania continua or transformed migraine.

The syndromes of benign cough headache or benign exertional headache are occasionally confused with migraine. The headaches are of paroxysmal onset and relatively short duration (often minutes) brought on by coughing, sneezing, lifting, straining, or valsalva maneuvers of other kinds. Similar paroxysmal onset headaches are triggered by sexual activity. Although these headaches are usually benign, early in the course of subarachnoid hemorrhage, mass lesions, and other pathology (especially of the posterior fossa) must be considered in the differential diagnosis. A clear history of the temporal relationship to the provoking stimulus is the key to distinguishing these headaches from migraine.

SUGGESTED READINGS

Blau JN: Headache: history, examination, differential diagnosis and special investigations. pp. 43–58. In Vinken PJ, Bruyn GW, Klawans HL (eds): Handbook of Clinical Neurology. Vol. 48. Elsevier, New York, 1986

Campbell JK, Saki F: Diagnosis and differential diagnosis. pp. 227–81. In Olesen J, Tfelt-Hansen P (eds): The Headaches. Raven Press, New York 1993

Headache Classification Committee of the International Headache Society: Classification and diagnostic criteria for headache disorders, cranial neuralgias and facial pain. Cephalalgia 8(suppl 7):1–96, 1988

Rasmussen BK, Olesen J: Migraine with aura and migraine without aura: an epidemiological study. Cephalalgia 12:221–8, 1992

Selby G, Lance JW: Observations on 500 cases of migraine and allied vascular headache. J Neurol Neurosurg Psychiatry; 23:23–32, 1960

Silberstein S, Lipton RB: Overview of diagnosis and treatment of migraine. Neurology 44(suppl 7):6–16, 1944

205. PHARMACOLOGIC TREATMENT OF MIGRAINE

ALAN M. RAPOPORT
RICHARD B. LIPTON

The pharmacologic treatment of migraine begins after establishing a good doctor/patient relationship, diagnosing the patient's headache disorders, reviewing treatment options, including the nonpharmacologic ones, and reassuring the patient that on the basis of the history, examination, and appropriate testing, no other significant problems exist. Helping patients to identify and avoid headache triggers and to understand their condition is always an essential part of treatment.

In this chapter we focus on the pharmacotherapy of migraine. Pharmacotherapy is traditionally divided into acute and preventive medications. *Acute* treatment is intended to reverse attacks once they begin and to reduce the pain and associated symptoms. Some patients use only acute treatment and get fairly rapid and complete relief, especially if they use it early in the course of the headache.

Preventive (prophylactic) treatment is usually given to patients who have 3 or more days of headache-related disability per month and those who are not rapidly responsive to acute treatment. It is also given to patients who have very frequent headache of any intensity or to treat or avoid medication overuse and rebound headache. Patients who have one or two severe migraine attacks per month and a poor response or contraindications to acute treatment may also benefit from preventive medication. Even with effective preventive treatment, most patients require acute medications for breakthrough headaches.

PRINCIPLES OF PHARMACOLOGIC TREATMENT

Having made a specific diagnosis of migraine, the next task is to develop a treatment plan. That plan will almost certainly include suggestions for avoiding headache triggers and modifying lifestyle to decrease headache frequency. It will also include acute treatments to be taken at the time of the migraine attack. It may include preventive treatments if indicated.

Choosing from the myriad agents available for migraine can be difficult. In selecting from the agents of choice, the frequency and intensity of attacks, the patterns of associated features, the patient's other medical problems as well as the efficacy and side-effect profile of the drugs in question must all be considered. As the goals of migraine treatment are to relieve pain and restore normal function if possible, it is especially important to understand which features of the attack are most disturbing to the patient.

Preventing analgesic and ergotamine rebound headaches is one of the most important principals of pharmacotherapy in migraine (see Ch. 207). The overuse of acute medications may lead to rebound syndromes, especially analgesic or ergotamine rebound headaches. It can also lead to dependency on medications, especially narcotics, barbiturates, and benzodiazepines. A headache calendar will often help both patients and doctors accurately track patterns of headaches and medication use. Overuse of medications used to treat acute headaches not only worsens and perpetuates headaches, it often prevents prophylactic medications from working. We advise patients to limit analgesics to 3 days per week and ergotamine to 1 day per week.

All medications have possible side effects; patients should be advised of the most frequent ones and are told to contact their physician if they are not feeling well on medication. Women of childbearing age should be asked if they could be pregnant before treatment is initiated. They should be advised not to become pregnant on most headache medications.

All patients on preventive medications, especially those on β-blockers, should be warned not to abruptly discontinue their medication, but rather to taper it slowly as per the doctor's instructions. Patients should be told not to run out of their medication at night or on weekends because that is in effect abruptly stopping medication.

ACUTE MIGRAINE THERAPY

Principles of Acute Treatment

Most patients in the United States prefer taking oral medications, but during an acute migraine episode oral absorption may be limited. Accordingly, nasal sprays, sublingual preparations, transdermal patches, and self-administered injections are gaining wider use. Many patients initially do not like the idea of rectal suppositories or self-injection. But those who do not get adequate relief with oral drugs prefer these routes of administration to a severe long-lasting headache. There are no sublingual or inhalation preparations left at the present time to treat headache. Table 205-1 lists abortive medications used for migraine.

Simple Analgesics

Some patients can sucessfully treat migraine by taking simple analgesics, especially if treatment is taken early in the attack. Two regular aspirin tablets (650 mg) or two extra-strength acetaminophen tablets (1,000 mg) may be helpful. The use of the prokinetic drug, metoclopramide (Reglan), 5 or 10 mg given before oral analgesics, may improve absorption as well as the therapeutic response.

Nonsteroidal Anti-inflammatory Compounds

Various nonsteroidal anti-inflammatory drugs (NSAIDs) can be helpful in the acute treatment of migraine (Table 205-2). Lack of response to one agent does not preclude response to another; several NSAIDs should be tried before this approach is abandoned. Some patients do well with off-the-shelf brands such as ibuprofen (200 mg) or naproxen sodium (220 mg); the usual starting dose for migraine is two tablets at headache onset. Of the prescription NSAIDs, we favor naproxen (Naprosyn) 250 mg, two or three tablets immediately and repeat in 1 hour if needed; naproxen sodium (Anaprox) 275 mg, 2 tablets stat and repeat two tablets in 1 hour if needed; ketoprofen (Orudis) 75 mg, two tablets stat and repeat two tablets in 1 hour if needed;

TABLE 205-2. Selected Nonsteroidal Anti-inflammatory Drugs

Type	Available Size (mg)
Carboxylic acids	
Acetylated	
Aspirin	
Nonacetylated	
Choline magnesium trisalicylate (Trilisate)	500/750/100
Salsalate (Salflex, Disalcid)	500/750
Propionic acids	
Ibuprofen (Motrin, Advil)	200/400/600
Naproxen (Naprosyn)	250/375/500
Fenoprofen (Nalfon)	200/300/600
Naproxen sodium (Anaprox)	275/550
Ketoprofen (Orudis)	25/50/75
Aryl and heterocyclic acids	
Tolmetin (Tolectin)	200/400/600
Indomethacin (Indocin)	25/50/75
	50 rectal
Diclofenac (Voltaren)	25/50/75
Sulindac (Clinoril)	150/200
Fenamic acids	
Mefenamic acid (Ponstel)	250
Meclofenamate (Meclomen)	50/100
Enolic acids	
Phenylbutazone (Butazolidine)	100
Piroxicam (Feldene)	10/20
Pyrrolopyrrole	
Ketorolac (Toradol) (IM)	15/30/60
Ketorolac (Toradol) (PO)	10

(From Saper JR, Silberstein SD, Gordon CD, Hamel RL: Handbook of Headache Management. Williams & Wilkins, Baltimore, 1993, with permission.)

meclofenamate (Meclomen) 100 mg, two capsules stat and repeat two capsules in 1 hour if needed; and flurbiprofen (Ansaid) 100 mg, two tablets stat and repeat two tablets in 1 hour if needed. Ketorolac (Toradol) is an injectable NSAID; 60 mg IM relieves headache in 50 percent of migraineurs.

Combination Analgesics

Caffeine acts as an analgesic adjuvant in the treatment of headache and other pain disorders. Many patients treat themselves with simple analgesics and coffee. Others use off-the-shelf medications that contain caffeine such as Excedrin (250 mg aspirin, 250 mg acetaminophen, and 65 mg caffeine) and Ana-

TABLE 205-1. Abortive Medications[a]

Drug	Efficacy	Side Effects	Comorbid Condition Relative Contraindication[b]	Relative Indication
Aspirin	1+	1+	Kidney disease, peripheral vascular disease, Gastritis, (age <15)	CAD, TIA
Acetaminophen	1+	1+	Liver disease	Pregnancy
Caffeine adjuvant	2+	1+	Frequent headache	
Butalbital, caffeine, and analgesics	2+	2+	Use of other sedative; history of medication overuse	
Isomethepene	2+	1+	HTN (uncontrolled), CAD, PVD; use of MAOI	
NSAIDs	2+	1+	Ulcer, bleeding tendency	
Narcotics	3+	3+	Drug or substance abuse	Pregnancy; rescue medication
Ergotamine				
Tablets	2+	2+	Prominent nausea or vomiting; CAD, PVD, HTN	
Suppositories	3+	3+		
Sumatriptan				
SC injection	4+	1+	CAD, PVD; uncontrolled HTN	Vomiting, prominent nausea
Tablets	3+	1+	CAD, PVD; uncontrolled HTN	Vomiting, prominent nausea
Dihydroergotamine				
Injections (SC, IM, IV)	4+[c]	2+	CAD, PVD, HTN	
Intranasal	3+	1+	CAD, PVD, HTN	

Abbreviations: CAD, coronary artery disease; NSAIDs, nonsteroidal anti-inflammatory drugs; PVD, peripheral vascular disease; SC, subcutaneous; HTN, hypertension; MAOI, monoamine oxidase inhibitors.
[a] Ratings are on a scale from 1+ (lowest) to 4+ (highest)
[b] Caution is required in patients with frequent headaches
[c] Not well studied in double-blind placebo-controlled trials.

(Modified from Olesen J, Tfelt-Hansen P, Welch KMA: The Headaches. Raven Press, New York, 1993, with permission.)

TABLE 205-3. Major Ingredients in Off-the-Shelf Analgesics

Analgesic	Aspirin	Acetaminophen	Caffeine	Other
Advil				Ibuprofen 200
Anacin	400		32	
Anacin (maximum strength)	500		32	
Anacin II		325		
Anacin II (maximum strength)		500		
Aspirin	300–325			
Bayer Aspirin	325			
Bayer Aspirin (8-h time release)	625			
Bayer Aspirin (maximum)	500			
Bayer Aspirin (therapy)	325			
BC Powder	650		32	Salicylamide 195
Bufferin	325			Magnesium carbonate, calcium carbonate, magnesium oxide
Cope	421		32	Aluminum hydroxide 25 + Magnesium hydroxide 50
Datril		325		
Datril E.S.		500		
Ecotrin (enteric coated)	325			
Ecotrin (maximum strength)	500			
Empirin	325			
Excedrin (extra strength)	250	250	65	
Excedrin PM	500			Diphenhydramine citrate 38
Ibuprofen				Ibuprofen 200
Medipren				Ibuprofen 200
Midol	454		32.4	Cinnamedrine HCl 14.9
Motrin IB				Ibuprofen 200
Nuprin				Ibuprofen 200
Panadol		500		
Percogesic		325		Phenyltoloxamine citrate 30
Tylenol		325		
Tylenol (extra strength)		500		
Vanquish	227	194	33	Aluminum hydroxide 25 Magnesium hydroxide 50

[a] Table compiled by Robert W. Rosum, MS, RPH, Assistant Director of Pharmacy Services, Greenwich Hospital, Greenwich, Connecticut.
(From Rapoport AM, Sheftell FD: Headache Relief. Simon & Schuster, New York, 1990, with permission.)

cin (400 mg aspirin and 32 mg caffeine) (Table 205-3). These medications are helpful, but they can be overused by patients who have frequent headaches. At doses of 300 to 500 mg/day (3 to 4 cups of coffee), several days per week, caffeine can exacerbate the headache syndrome causing caffeine rebound and withdrawal headaches.

Butalbital-Containing Medications

When simple analgesics and caffeine-adjuvant compounds do not provide relief, the addition of butalbital may be very helpful. There are many butalbital-containing preparations, some of which also contain codeine. The most frequently used are Fiorinal (325 mg aspirin, 40 mg caffeine, and 50 mg butalbital), Fioricet or Esgic (325 mg acetaminophen, 40 mg caffeine, and 50 mg butalbital) and Phrenilin (325 mg acetaminophen and 50 mg butalbital, and no caffeine). Fiorinal and Fioricet are available in preparations which contain 30 mg of codeine. Codeine-containing preparations should be used only if other medications fail.

Butalbital may cause drowsiness or dependency, but many patients feel activated by the medication in small doses. Large doses may cause drowsiness, ataxia, difficulty with gait, and confusion. Other combination medications containing codeine are the aspirin/codeine and acetaminophen/codeine preparations. These and other opiates may be used if the more specific abortive medications are not advisable or the simpler analgesics and combination analgesics have not been effective.

An alternative combination analgesic contains isometheptene mucate 65 mg, acetaminophen 325 mg, and dichloralphenazone 100 mg (Midrin). Isometheptene mucate is a sympathomimetic amine which constricts blood vessels and may also work centrally. Dichloralphenazone is a mild tranquilizer. Midrin is often helpful in aborting a migraine attack and can also be used in tension-type headache. The adult dosage is two capsules immediately with additional doses every hour, if needed, for a total of four to five capsules per day, up to 3 days per week. Smaller doses can be helpful in children because it is effective and has few side effects. Although side effects are unusual, dizziness, drowsiness, and gastrointestinal (GI) symptoms may occur. This medication cannot be used when a patient is on a monoamine oxidase inhibitor (MAOI).

Opiates

Opiates should be used cautiously for migraine treatment. The specific migraine agents are preferable if they are effective. In addition to the codeine-containing products discussed above other oral opiates may be useful.

Percocet, Percodan, Darvon, Vicodin, Lortab, and Hydrocet may be used when absolutely necessary if no other medication is helpful. If a patient comes to a physician's office or an emergency room, intramuscular narcotics such as 75 mg meperidine (Demerol) combined with 50 mg promethazine are an option. Dihydroergotamine or sumatriptan usually provide more effective pain relief and better restoration of function.

Butorphanol is available as a nasal spray (Stadol), which is easy to use at home and is advantagious in patients who do not absorb oral medication during migraine attacks. Because it stimulates kappa rather than mu receptors, it may not be as addictive as other opiates and does not induce euphoria. It begins to work in 15 to 20 minutes. The dose is one spray in one nostril (1 mg) immediately, which may be repeated in 1 hour. If a third dose is necessary, 3 to 4 hours should elapse before it is taken. Although it is a good pain reliever for many patients, it may cause sedation and dizziness and patients should be warned to rest after taking it.

Ergot Alkaloids

Ergotamine tartrate has been available for over 50 years and has been used via oral, sublingual, injectable, inhaled, and rectal routes of administration. Ergotamine tartrate is erratically absorbed, and its bioavailability is less than 5 percent of the oral dose. Rectal dosing produces much better and more consistent absorption and more effective treatment of headache. The most commonly used ergotamine tartrate preparations are Cafergot or Wigraine tablets and suppositories. The tablets contain 1 mg ergotamine tartrate and 100 mg caffeine. The rectal suppositories contain 2 mg ergotamine tartrate and 100 mg caffeine. The starting dose is two tablets immediately followed by two more tablets in 1 hour if needed. Since the medication is better absorbed rectally, a smaller dose should be given. Start with only one-quarter of a Cafergot suppository, which can be repeated in 1 hour if needed. If this is not effective, then the treatment for the next headache should be one-half Cafergot suppository followed by one-half suppository in an hour if needed. The maximum dose is 4 mg/day and it should be used only 1 or 2 days/week.

As ergotamine tartrate often induces or exacerbates nausea or vomiting, pretreatment with an antinausea medication is often necessary. We prefer metoclopramide or promethazine. If a patient finds that nausea is not a problem, premedication may not be necessary.

Possible side effects of ergotamine preparations are an increase in nausea and vomiting, abdominal pain, distal paraesthesias, and muscle cramps. If used more than two times per week, even in low doses, ergotamine tartrate dependency and rebound headaches may develop. Ergotamine is contraindicated in pregnancy, uncontrolled hypertension, coronary artery disease, peripheral vascular disease, sepsis, and liver and kidney disease. It should not be given to a patient on erythromycin, which decreases its metabolism, and raises its blood level.

Dihydroergotamine. Dihydroergotamine (D.H.E. 45) is a hydrogenated ergot preparation available since the early 1940s. Although it is a weaker arterial constrictor and a stronger venoconstrictor than ergotamine tartrate, it is contraindicated in the same situations. It is approved for intravenous and intramuscular use in the United States. Subcutaneous use is approved else-

where. An intranasal preparation is available in some countries, and will soon be available in the United States.

The dose for intramuscular or subcutaneous administration is usually 0.5 mg to 1 mg at headache onset. The lower dose may be repeated in 1 hour if necessary. Pretreatment with an antinausea medication such as metoclopramide is usually not needed with intramuscular of subcutaneous administration.

Many intravenous protocols for the use of DHE have been published. The usual starting dose is 0.25 to 0.5 mg given by slow IV push over 5 to 10 minutes through a heparin lock. If the patient is in an office or emergency room and this dose is not effective in relieving the headache, another 0.5 mg can be given in 30 minutes if there are no side effects. If the patient is hospitalized for repetitive intravenous DHE, the usual dose is between 0.5 and 1 mg given slowly through a heparin lock every 8 hours over a period of 3 to 5 days. Intravenous administration is usually preceded by an antiemetic to prevent nausea.

DHE can be administered as a nasal spray giving 0.5 mg in each nostril for a total of 4 sprays, which equals a 2-mg dose. If this is not effective, a 3-mg dose can be given. Patients usually have fewer side effects with this route of administration, but will occasionally develop nasal stuffiness. The nasal spray is probably not quite as effective as intramuscular or intravenous administration, but is much easier to use. All forms of this medication have been found to be quite safe and effective in treating acute migraine. It is often helpful when taken well into the course of the migraine headache, but it should be taken as early as possible.

Sumatriptan

Sumatriptan (Imitrex) is a new, selective 5-HT$_1$ (serotonin) agonist for the acute treatment of migraine. It is available as a 6-mg subcutaneously self-injected preparation or 25- or 50-mg tablets. The injection works faster than the tablet, probably owing to more rapid absorption. Two large-scale randomized trials demonstrated that the injectable dose of 6 mg relieved pain in 70 percent of patients within 1 hour of administration. The drug also relieves nausea, photophobia, and phonophobia relative to placebo and rapidly restores normal functioning in 76 percent of subjects. A recent study from The New England Center for Headache showed that 84 percent of patients obtained effective relief in an average of 41 minutes.

Headache recurs in about one-third to one-half of subjects within 24 hours, but is usually relieved by a second dose of sumitriptan. Subcutaneous sumitriptan can be repeated 1 hour after the initial administration for a maximum of two doses in 24 hours. Retreatment should be for recurrence only; if the initial dose does not relieve pain, the second dose is unlikely to provide additional benefit.

The most common side effects are injection-site pain, distal paresthesias, flushing, heaviness, and non-cardiac chest pressure. The drug is contraindicated in Prinzmetal's angina, coronary artery disease, basilar and hemiplegic migraine, or uncontrolled hypertension. We obtain baseline electrocardiograms (EKGs) before giving this drug. In patients at risk for coronary artery disease the first dose should be given in a physician's office so that if chest symptoms occur, they can be evaluated by EKG.

Corticosteroids

Corticosteroids can be used as backup medication if the above treatments are contraindicated or ineffective. Our usual regimen

TABLE 205-4. Oral Antinausea Agents (Antiemetics)

Brand Name	Generic Name	Dose
Compazine	Prochlorperazine	5- or 10-mg tablet
Emetrol	Carbohydrate solution	1 or 2 tablespoonfuls
Phenergan	Promethazine	25- or 50-mg tablet
Reglan	Metoclopramide	10-mg tablet
Thorazine	Chlorpromazine	25- or 50-mg tablet
Tigan	Trimethobenzamide	250-mg capsule
Torecan	Thiethylperazine	10-mg tablet
Vistaril	Hydroxyzine	50-mg capsule
Zofran	Ondansetron	4-mg tablet

(From Rapoport AM, Sheftell FD: Conquering headache: an illustrated guide to understanding and control of headache. Empowering Press, Hamilton, Ontario, Canada, 1995, with permission.)

is oral dexamethasone 4 to 6 mg, which may be repeated in 3 hours if needed. This may work by decreasing neurogenic inflammation. An occasional dose rarely causes side effects. We permit patients to use it once or twice a month. The most common acute effects are reddening of the face, slight elevation of blood pressure, and insomnia. Long term frequent use should be avoided as it can produce avascular necrosis, osteoporosis, diabetes, hypertension, and other unwanted effects.

Treatment of Nausea

If nausea or vomiting are prominent, they should be treated (Table 205-4). We prefer promethazine (Phenergan), metoclopramide (Reglan), or prochlorperazine (Compazine). Promethazine is given at a dose of 25 or 50 mg by mouth, suppository, or injection. If the patient needs to remain alert, the prokinetic drug metoclopramide (Reglan) 10 mg by mouth or injection can prevent or treat nausea and improve absorption of other oral medications. Prochlorperazine (Compazine) 10 mg by mouth or intramuscularly, or 12.5 to 25 mg as a rectal suppository is often helpful in treating nausea. When given intravenously, 10 mg of this drug also effectively treats the pain of migraine. Trimethobenzamide (Tigan) 200 mg suppository or 250 mg capsule, and chlorpromazine (Thorazine) 25 or 50 mg by tablet or 50 or 100 mg by suppository can also be helpful. Hydroxyzine (Vistaril), a histamine receptor antagonist, can be helpful as an antinausea medication, pain reliever, or sedative. The usual dose is a 50 mg capsule immediately, which may be repeated in 2 hours. Side effects are drowsiness and dry mouth.

PREVENTIVE (PROPHYLACTIC) TREATMENT OF MIGRAINE

Principles of Preventive Treamtent

Preventive medications should be started at a low dose and gradually increased over a period of time if there are no side effects and if the drug has not yet been effective. Patients should be warned that preventive medications often take a minimum of 3 to 4 weeks to become effective and they should not discontinue the medication unless there are significant side effects.

The first-line agents for migraine prophylaxis include β-blockers, calcium channel blockers, antidepressants, and anticonvulsants (Table 205-5). We choose from among first-line drugs primarily based on their side effect profiles and the patient's comorbid conditions. For example, in the patient with asthma or Raynaud syndrome β-blockers are best avoided. But in the patient with migraine and hypertension, a β-blocker may

effectively treat both conditions. Though monotherapy is preferred, sometimes combinations of two or more medications at a low dose may be more effective with fewer side effects than a large dose of a single medication. Side effects can be numerous and significant and both patient and physician should be alert to them.

β-Adrenergic Blocking Drugs

β-Blockers are the most commonly used group of preventive medications for migraine. Propranolol (Inderal), the first β-blocker approved for migraine treatment, was accidentally found to prevent migraine when a patient being treated for angina pectoris noted that his long-standing migraine disappeared. The first controlled study established the value of propranolol in 1972. Both the lipophylic beta blockers that readily pass into the central nervous system (CNS) such as propranolol and metoprolol, and the hydrophilic atenolol and nadolol, which do not enter the CNS, are effective in treating migraine. Cardioselectivity also has no bearing on efficacy.

We prefer propranolol, nadolol, and atenolol, though timolol (Blocadren) and metoprolol (Lopressor) are also effective. Propranolol can be started at 10 to 20 mg bid and gradually increased. The usual effective dosage range is 80 to 160 mg daily. In patients with partial responses to lower doses, occasionally as much as 360 mg is given. Nadolol (Corgard) is started at 20 mg daily and raised to a usual range of 80 to 160 mg daily. Atenolol (Tenormin) is started at 25 mg daily and increased to a typical dose of 50 to 100 mg daily.

There are many possible adverse responses to the β-blockers, but they occur more commonly at higher doses. Patients may complain of fatigue, depression, impotence, reduced blood pressure and pulse rate, weight gain, GI side effects, reduced tolerance for physical activity, increased coldness in the extremities, dizziness on standing, and abnormal dreaming. These medications are contraindicated in certain cardiac disorders, asthma, chronic lung disease, diabetes, hypoglycemia, bradycardia, hypotension, Raynaud's disease, peripheral vascular disease, and severe depression. They should probably not be used in hemiplegic migraine. It is essential that patients be tapered off these drugs gradually, over a period of more than a week in many cases when they are stopped, as an abrupt cessation may produce rebound tachycardia, angina, or anxiety.

Calcium Channel Blocking Drugs (Calcium Antagonists)

The most widely used calcium channel antagonist for headache in the United States is verapamil (Calan, Isoptin). Flunarizine (Sibelium) is effective and commonly used in Europe. We often begin with verapamil 40 mg tid. The dose is increased after 1 or 2 weeks to 240 mg daily. The maximum recommended dose is 480 mg daily, although patients with partial responses at that level often benefit from further increases. Some patients tolerate as much as 720 mg daily. Our calcium channel blocker of second choice is diltiazem (Cardizem). The starting dose is 30 mg tid and we gradually raise it to 60 mg tid, but some patients have taken double that dose. Several newer calcium channel blockers such as isradipine (DynaCirc) and nicardipine (Cardene) may be effective. Nifedipine (Procardia) is occasionally helpful but at times actually worsens headache as it is a strong vasodilator.

The most common side effects are constipation and fluid

TABLE 205-5. Choices of Preventive Treatment in Migraine: Influence on Comorbid Conditions

Drug	Efficacy	Side Effects	Comorbid Condition	
			Relative Contraindication	Relative Indication
β Blockers	4+	2+	Asthma, depression, CHF, Raynaud syndrome, diabetes	Hypertension, angina
Antiserotonin				
Methysergide	4+	4+	Angina, PVD	Orthostatic hypotension
Calcium channel blockers				
Verapamil	2+	1+	Constipation; other antihypertensives	Migraine with aura, hypertension, angina, asthma
Antidepressants				
Amitriptyline	2+	3+	Urinary retention, heart block, MAOIs	Other pain disorders, depression, anxiety disorders, insomnia
Anticonvulsants				
Divalproex sodium	4+	3+	Liver disease, bleeding disorders	Mania, epilepsy, anxiety disorders
NSAIDs				
Naproxen	2+	2+	Ulcer disease, gastritis, bleeding disorders	Arthritis, other pain disorders

Abbreviations: NSAIDs, nonsteroidal anti-inflammatory drugs; CHF, congestive heart failure; PVD, peripheral vascular disease; MAOI, monoamine oxidase inhibitor. (Modified from Olesen J, Tfelt-Hansen P, Welch KMA: The Headaches. Raven Press, New York, 1993, with permission.)

retention. Less frequent but more significant side effects are cardiac dysfunction, hypotension, drowsiness, and dizziness. Calcium channel blockers are currently being investigated as male contraceptives. They should not be used in men who are actively trying to have children. These drugs are contraindicated in congestive heart failure, heart block, bradycardia, sick sinus syndrome, and other cardiac problems. If used concomitantly with a β-blocker, caution is required.

Antidepressants

There are three major categories of antidepressants: the tricyclic and tetracyclic antidepressants, the selective serotonin reuptake inhibitors, and the monoamine oxidase inhibitors. They are widely used for chronic tension-type headache and chronic daily headache, especially in patients with comorbid depression and sleep disorders. Only amitriptyline has demonstrated benefits in migraine clinical trials.

Tricyclics. Amitriptyline (Elavil) is the gold standard antidepressant for the treatment of headache and chronic pain. Although it has been used the longest and has been written about the most, it may cause prominent anticholinergic side effects. Nortriptyline (Pamelor) and doxepin (Sinequan) are often preferred because of their more favorable side-effect profiles. With all of these agents we start with 10 mg 30 to 60 minutes before bedtime and raise the dose in 10 mg increments every 3 to 7 nights as tolerated, to an average dose of 50 mg. Some patients require 100 mg or more if they have a significant sleep disorder, depression, or if they have only partial responses at lower doses. Most tricyclic antidepressants need to be given for 3 to 4 weeks before benefits develop.

Side effects include weight gain, drowsiness in the morning, dry mouth, constipation, blurred vision, and urinary retention. These drugs are contraindicated in cardiac arrhythmias, glaucoma, and urinary retention. Desipramine (Norpramin) in similar doses is somewhat more alerting. Nortriptyline has a therapeutic window for depression; we believe that underdosing or overdosing can attenuate the theraputic response. Blood levels should be monitored if the patient is not doing well.

Selective Serotonin Reuptake Inhibitors. The relatively new selective serotonin reuptake inhibitors may be helpful in the chronic headache syndromes, although their role in pure migraine in the absence of comorbid depression is controversial. As a class, these agents have fewer side effects than the tricyclic

antidepressants. Fluoxetine (Prozac) can be used in combination with the tricyclics to enhance therapeutic benefits. We often give a low dose of fluoxetine in the morning with a medium dose of a tricyclic at night. This will often promote better sleep at night and alertness in the morning. A typical starting dose is 10 mg fluoxetine at 7 am, which can be raised in approximately 2 weeks to 20 mg. A minimum of 3 to 6 weeks is necessary before full benefits develop.

Side effects include agitation (which often improves within 1 to 2 weeks), insomnia, tremor, anorgasmia, and other sexual dysfunction. A small percentage of patients have an increase in headaches. Patients should be warned to stop the drug if they have any alteration of mood or feel strange. Although most people are activated by the drug and have no change in their weight or possibly even weight loss, a minority of patients may become drowsy and may actually gain weight. Other potentially useful drugs in this category include sertraline (Zoloft) and paroxetine (Paxil).

Monoamine Oxidase Inhibitors. The third type of antidepressants are the monoamine oxidase inhibitors (MAOIs), which work well for frequent or daily headache and depression, as well as transformed migraine with daily milder headache and intermittent migraine. More than 80 percent of migraine sufferers report an improvement of at least 50 percent. Despite their efficacy MAOIs are not widely used in primary care because they require severe dietary limitations, and extreme caution regarding drug interactions. The most commonly used MAOI is phenelzine (Nardil), an MAO-A inhibitor.

Anticonvulsants

Anticonvulsants, especially divalproex sodium (Depakote), may be helpful in the preventive treatment of migraine as well as other conditions. Recently, there have been several randomized studies showing that divalproex sodium is effective in migraine prophylaxis. Divalproex sodium (Depakote) should be started at a low dose, 250 mg once daily, and increased slowly up to 250 mg in the morning and 550 mg in the evening. This dose usually produces a trough serum sodium valproate level below the therapeutic range of 50 to 100 $\mu g/ml$. If the patient is not doing well over a 3-week period, and there are no significant side effects, the dose can be gradually raised up to 2,000 mg. This will produce a higher blood level, in the 75 to 100 $\mu g/ml$ range, and a better theraputic response.

Side effects include weight gain, hair loss, tremor, GI problems, sedation, and cognitive changes. Children should be monitored closely for hepatotoxicity. If side effects occur, stopping the medication or reducing the dose usually resolves the problem, and it can then be restarted.

Sodium valproate is contraindicated in pregnancy because it produces neural tube defects and should also not be used in young children or patients with hepatic disease. It interacts with barbiturates and benzodiazepines; caution is required if these medications are combined. Butalbutal-containing analgesics must be given cautiously.

Serotonin (5-HT₂) Antagonists

The antihistamine cyproheptadine (Periactin) is a 5-HT$_2$ antagonist with calcium channel-blocking properties. It is rapidly absorbed and produces few side effects, other than dizziness, dry mouth, weight gain, and sedation, which can be beneficial in insomnia. The initial dose is 2 mg (half a tablet) 1 to 2 hours before bedtime, gradually increased over a period of 1 month up to 8 to 12 mg daily in divided doses. It is very effective in children and in some adults. It is contraindicated in closed-angle glaucoma and prostatic hypertrophy.

Methysergide. Methysergide (Sansert) is the oldest of the migraine preventive agents. The initial dose is 2 mg daily, gradually increased to 2 mg tid or qid. At full dose, the side effects include nausea, dizziness, muscle cramps, weight gain, abdominal pain, and psychiatric symptoms. The drug is contraindicated in coronary artery and peripheral vascular disease, pregnancy, peptic ulcer, phlebitis, lung, liver, and kidney disease.

The most significant side effect was first reported by John Graham and colleagues from Boston in 1967: retroperitoneal fibrosis. This process recedes when the drug is discontinued. Most of the patients with this side effect have used larger amounts of the drug for long periods, but some patients may develop this side effect idiosyncratically. The risk of developing this problem seems to be 1 in 1,500. It is common practice to give a patient a drug-free holiday every 6 months, but it is not clear if this will definitely prevent this complication.

Nonsteroidal Anti-inflammatory Drugs

NSAIDs, often used as acute treatment, can also prevent migraine. For menstrual migraine, these medications are used starting 4 days before the time of increased risk for headache and stopping when the time of increased risk is over. We favor naproxen sodium 275 mg tid with meals for this purpose, but several other medications are also effective. This treatment strategy requires headaches with relatively sterotyped timing in relation to menstrual flow. NSAIDs can also be used cautiously on a chronic basis. These medications should always be taken with food and consideration should be given to the use of histamine blockers to prevent peptic ulcer formation. Side effects may be gastric ulceration, dyspepsia, gastritis, diarrhea, and bleeding tendency. Contraindications include ulcers, liver and kidney disease, and anticoagulation.

Miscellaneous Drugs

Methylergonovine (Methergine) (0.2 mg tid) is used occasionally in migraine prophylaxis. It has the same contraindications as the other ergot alkaloids. It may cause muscle cramps.

Clonidine (Catapres), an α_2 adrenoceptor agonist, is used both to prevent migraine and sympathetic withdrawal symptoms in patients who are being detoxified from opiates. It may work best in women with increased migraine frequency in the perimenopausal period. It comes as a 0. 1 mg tablet and should be started at one-half tablet or 0.05 mg bid. The dose can be raised to 0.3 mg/day, cautiously. It is also available as a Catapres skin patch in doses of 0.1, 0.2, and 0.3 mg. Each patch can be worn for 1 week before changing and delivers the total dose evenly throughout the day. Major side effects are drowsiness and dizziness. It should not be used with beta blockers.

Patients with migraine and anxiety disorders may improve on a benzodiazepine such as *lorazepam (Ativan), alprazolam (Xanax), diazepam (Valium),* and *chlorazepate (Tranxene).* Sometimes the headache improves, but these medications are addictive, hard to control, and may even lead to worsening of headache. *Divalproex sodium (Depakote)* may be a more effective alternative in this setting. *Buspirone (Buspar)* is sometimes helpful. The major tranquilizers can be used with comorbid psychosis in treatment-refractory patients, but caution is advised.

Stimulant medication such as *dextroamphetamine (Dexedrine)* or *methylphenidate (Ritalin),* not usually used for headaches, can reduce the frequency and severity of migraine and related headaches. Some treatment-refractory patients do well on these medications. An initial dose is 5 mg of either Dexedrine or Ritalin in the morning, which can be raised to 20 mg slowly in divided doses, avoiding evening dose times. Side effects are few and tend to be those of sympathetic stimulation such as tachycardia, hyperalertness, insomnia, and anorexia.

Hormonal Therapy

Hormonal therapy is sometimes used in both the premenopausal and menopausal female. For women who have either pure menstrual migraine or marked worsening of their migraine perimenstrually, a burst of estrogen starting 4 days before menses and until the end of menses can be accomplished with the Estraderm skin patch or pure estradiol orally or sublingually in the form of Estrace.

Feverfew

Feverfew (*Tanacetum parthenium*) is an herb that is reported to decrease the frequency of migraine attacks when used on a daily basis. It seems to be more effective when patients chew fresh leaves, but also works as tablets. Studies show that it has an aspirinlike effect on platelets, but the exact mechanism of action is uncertain. Side effects seem to be limited to local effects on oral mucosa.

Papaverine

Papaverine works as a vasodilator, similar to the calcium channel blockers, to decrease the frequency of migraine. Its effectiveness is questionable and it has not become a frequently used medication. The usual dose is 300 to 600 mg/day and is well tolerated. The main side effect is nausea, but it may produce drowsiness or GI side effects as well.

Calcitonin

Calcitonin is a polypeptide secreted by the thyroid. It may work by increasing levels of β-endorphin, adrenocorticotropic hormone, and cortisol. The dose of salmon calcitonin is 100 IU/day, given either by injection or nasal spray, for 10 days. It is not a widely used preparation.

PERSISTENT MIGRAINE

When a patient develops persistent migraine, with frequent or daily headaches, often with analgesic overuse, depression, and sleep disturbance, most abortive and preventive migraine medications become ineffective. Part of the problem may be the intensity and chronicity of the headache syndrome, but much of the problem is often caused by analgesic and ergot rebound syndromes, which prevent usually effective daily medications from working. Although some of these patients can improve with outpatient analgesic withdrawal, appropriate behavioral treatments, and combinations of preventive medication, often they need hospitalization in an inpatient unit dedicated to the care of chronic and severe headache syndromes. The first step can be a referral to a neurologist or headache specialist for consultation.

The most important criteria for hospitalization are frequent and severe headaches with poor response to multiple outpatient treatment regimens; overuse of abortive headache medications producing rebound syndromes; comorbid medical and psychiatric illnessess that makes outpatient treatment ineffective or risky (such as coronary artery disease, hypertension, ulcer disease, severe depression, etc.); or status migrainosus of short or long duration of such intensity that the patient is unable to function at home and/or work.

Hospitalization usually begins with several medical evaluations, including, but not limited to, neurologic, psychological, social work, physical therapy, occupational therapy, and dietary. Patients are often started on repetitive, intravenous dihydroergotamine (D.H.E. 45) and sometimes steroids. They are put on a detoxification schedule of whatever medications that need to be stopped. Clonidine is sometimes used to prevent withdrawal symptoms if they are coming off opiates (narcotics). Phenobarbital is sometimes used to prevent withdrawal symptoms from butalbital-containing medication. Patients are usually started on 1 or 2 preventive medications and given a lot of behavioral therapy both in terms of relaxation therapy and relapse prevention training.

Long-term outcome studies of interdisciplinary inpatient headache unit patients indicate that 70 percent of them are markedly improved for as long as 6 to 12 months following discharge.

SUGGESTED READINGS

Callaham M, Raskin N: A controlled study of dihydroergotamine in the treatment of acute migraine headache, Headache 26:168–71, 1986

Delessio DJ, Silberstein SD (eds): Wolff's Headache and Other Head Pain. 6th Ed. New York, Oxford University Press, 1993

Edmeads J: Emergency room management of headache. Headache 28:675–9, 1988

Johnson ES, Ratcliffe DM, Wilkinson M: Naproxen sodium in the treatment of migraine. Cephalalgia 4:5–10, 1985

Kudrow L: Cluster Headache: Mechanisms and Management. 4th Ed. London, Oxford University Press, 1980

Lance JW, Curran DA, Anthony M: Investigations into the mechanism and treatment of chronic headache. Med J Aust 2:909–14, 1965

Lance JW: Mechanisms and Management of Headache, 5th Ed. Oxford, Butterworth-Heinemann, 1993

Rapoport AM, Sheftell FD: Headache Relief. New York, Simon & Schuster, 1990

Rapoport AM, Sheftell FD (eds): Headache: A Clinician's Guide to Diagnosis, Pathophysiology and Treatment Strategies. Costa Mesa, PMA Publishing, 1993

Rapoport A: Analgesic rebound headache: theoretical and practical implications. Cephalalgia 5(suppl 3):448–9, 1985

Raskin NH: Headache. 2nd Ed. New York, Churchill Livingstone, 1988

Saper JR: Headache Disorders: Current Concepts and Treatment Strategies. Boston, John Wright PSG, 1983

Saper JR, Silberstein SD, Gordon CD, Hamel RL: Handbook of Headache Management. Baltimore, Williams & Wilkins, 1993

Selby G, Lance JW: Observations on 500 cases of migraine and allied vascular headache. J Neurol Neurosurg Psychiatry 23:23–32, 1960

Subcutaneous Sumatriptan International Study Group: Treatment of migraine attacks with sumatriptan. N Engl J Med 325:316–321, 1991

206. CHRONIC TENSION-TYPE HEADACHE

GARY W. JAY

The diagnostic criteria for chronic tension-type headache (CTTH) are found in Table 206-1. It should be noted immediately that these criteria are not exact, nor do they encompass all clinical aspects of CTTH. The pathophysiology of acute or chronic tension-type headache is more illuminating, and is discussed below. The name *tension-type headache* is itself indicative of the uncertain etiology of this entity: physical, emotional, or a combination of both. It is more appropriate to determine the various aspects of the disorder by looking at the underlying central nervous system pathophysiology. The question of the possible transformation of episodic migraine into CTTH or chronic daily headache, felt by many clinicians to be nosologically similar, if not identical, will also be discussed.

SPECIFIC PATHOPHYSIOLOGY

Pathologic changes of the musculoskeletal system may initiate, modulate, or perpetuate CTTH. Chronic tension-type headache is, at least at first, a muscle-induced pain syndrome, and it is frequently found associated with the myofascial pain syndrome (MPS) as well as fibromyalgia.

The central nervous system controls muscle tone via systems including γ efferent neurons in the anterior horn cells of the spinal cord, which act on the α motor neurons supplying muscle spindles. Renshaw cells, probably via the inhibitory neurotransmitter, γ-aminobutyric acid (GABA), influence this synaptic system. There is also supraspinal control mediated by the cortical, subcortical, and limbic afferent and efferent systems. Physi-

TABLE 206-1. Diagnostic Criteria for Chronic Tension-Type Headache

A. Average headache frequency ≥15 days/month (180 days/year) for ≥6 months fulfilling criteria B to D:
B. At least 2 of the following pain characteristics:
  1. Pressing/tightening quality
  2. Mild or moderate severity (may inhibit, but does not prohibit activities)
  3. Bilateral location
  4. No aggravation by walking stairs or similar routine physical activity
C. Both of the following:
  1. No vomiting
  2. No more than one of the following: nausea, photophobia, or phonophobia
D. 1. History and physical and neurologic examinations do not suggest one of the disorders listed in groups 5–11 (of the IHS classification)
  2. History and/or physical and/or neurologic examinations do suggest such disorder, but it is ruled out by appropriate investigations
  3. Such disorder is present, but tension-type headache does not occur for the first time in close temporal relation to the disorder

ologic and emotional input interacts in the maintenance or flux in established muscle tone. Adverse influences from localized or regional myofascial nociception, with or without limbic (affective) stimulation may produce significant muscle spasm which, if prolonged, becomes tonic, with the additional aspects of an anxiety-increased or maintained muscle contraction–pain cycle.

Tonic or continued muscle contraction may induce hypoxia via compression of small blood vessels. Ischemia, the accumulation of pain-producing metabolites (bradykinin, lactic acid, serotonin, prostaglandins, etc.) may increase and potentiate muscle pain and reactive spasm. These nociceptive-enhancing chemicals may stimulate central mechanisms, which, through continued stimulation, may induce continued reactive muscle contraction and the maintenance of the myogenic nociceptive cycle.

Some researchers have confirmed a causal relationship between muscle spasm and headache, while others have felt that associated muscle spasm is an epiphenomenon, not the cause of headache, a reflexive response rather than an etiologic mechanism. Other authors indicated that muscle activity/spasm may be more pronounced in migraine than in tension-type/muscle contraction headaches.

A major problem with this research, in which information was obtained by electromyographic (EMG) studies, was that the authors evaluated different groups of muscles in different types of patients, many of which had poorly defined diagnoses. Other authors defined CTTH as an entity with or without associated pericranial muscle disorder. The concept of muscle fatigue was not taken into consideration.

In one study there was a positive correlation between pericranial muscle tenderness and headache intensity, and the former was felt to be the source of nociception. In another study it was found that pressure pain thresholds in patients with CTTH were highly dependent on myofascial factors. This study indicated that the generally lower pain thresholds in the CTTH patients suggested a dysmodulation of central nociception. A lower pain threshold in CTTH patients as compared to normal volunteers has also been reported.

Measurement of scalp muscle tenderness and sensitivity to pain in both migraine and tension-type headache patients, revealed that the pathophysiology of tension-type headache may involve a diffuse disruption of central pain modulating mechanisms.

Lower pain thresholds have also been found in patients diagnosed with myofascial pain syndromes, including lower back pain.

The CTTH patients frequently have a stereotypic posture, with their shoulders raised and their heads held in forward flexion. This tightly held posture, or muscular splinting, is effective in preventing unconscious head movement which may induce increased pain. The continued splinting, by maintaining tonic muscle contraction, also works to increase myogenic nociception.

The pericranial muscles are innervated by sensory fibers in nerves from the second or third cervical roots, and in the trigeminal nerve. The functions of these muscles contribute to the maintenance of posture and the stabilization of the head, as well as the withdrawal and protection of the head. These factors certainly contribute to their role in the myofascial aspects of CTTH.

Muscle fatigue, both metabolic and neurochemical in nature, which may follow prolonged or tonic muscle spasm, may also

be secondary to "sympatheticopenia," or the depletion of epinephrine and norepinephrine, the peripheral sympathetic transmitters. The muscle spindle is directly affected by the sympathetic nervous system via chemical products, particularly norepinephrine. Prolonged, sustained peripheral sympathetic activity may lead to depletion of norepinephrine at the synaptic receptors. Continued afferent sympathetic input from myogenic nociception, at least in part from buildup through ischemia of nociceptive metabolites, may result in sympatheticopenia.

Also correlated positively with pericranial muscle tenderness, is tenderness of the cervical, thoracic, and lumbar paravertebral muscles. It has been suggested that contraction of shoulder and cervical muscles, as well as emotional arousal, both contribute to tension-type headache.

Three mechanisms of muscle pain are thought to be relevant to CTTH, in that myogenic nociception may be induced by (1) low-grade inflammation associated with the release of algetic, or pain-inducing substances rather than signs of acute inflammation, (2) long-lasting relative ischemia, and (3) tearing of ligaments and tendons secondary to abnormal, sustained muscle tension.

MYOFASCIAL PAIN SYNDROME

The myofascial pain syndrome (MPS), clinically, involves a regional or localized pain complaint associated with tender trigger points located in taut bands of skeletal muscle. The trigger point may refer pain to the target area when it is palpated.

Trigger points may be active, with consistently reproducible pain on palpation, or latent, with no clinically associated complaints of pain, but with associated muscle dysfunction. Trigger points may shift between active and latent states. Clinically, continuous myogenic nociception from active trigger points appears to be a prime instigator of the central neurochemical nociceptive dysmodulation found in patients with CTTH.

Increased stiffness, weakness, fatigability, and a decreased range of motion may be found in muscles in which trigger points are found. These muscles may be shortened, with increased pain perceived on stretching. Patients may protect these muscles by adapting poor posture with sustained contraction (see above). The resulting muscular restrictions may perpetuate existing trigger points and aid in the development of others.

A large percentage of patients suffering from a MPS of the head and neck have been noted to have significant postural problems, with forward head tilt, rounded shoulders, as well as poor standing and sitting posture, all findings frequently seen in CTTH patients.

A MPS of the head and neck, via myofascial trigger point referred pain, may mimic other conditions, including migraine headache, tempromandibular joint disorders, sinusitis, and cervical neuralgias as well as various otologic problems including tinnitus, vertigo, ear pain, and dizziness.

Onset of an acute, single-muscle MPS may be associated with trauma, such as a slip and fall, or acceleration/deceleration injury. It may also come on insidiously, for example, in patients who work multiple hours typing or at the computer. The MPS, in many patients, may show a spontaneous regression to a latent status, with continued muscular dysfunction, but with significant diminution of the initial pain complaints. In other patients, the MPS may "metastasize" and involve associated musculature, becoming regional, or even involving multiple muscular regions.

OTHER CLINICAL ASPECTS

The exact role of emotional problems such as stress, anxiety, and depression is questionable: the literature is equivocal. Either way, most researchers agree that emotional/psychological factors may be important in the maintenance, if not the genesis of tension-type headaches. Depression has been linked to the initiation of tension-type headaches by some, while others are uncertain.

One difficulty in the literature is the fact that determinations of depression, anxiety, and stress occur in patients with CTTH. Without premorbid psychological analyses, it is obviously difficult to state with certainty whether these patients were depressed or anxious prior to the onset of their headache problems. It is therefore possible that the neurochemical changes associated with CTTH, such as a possible or probable central serotonergic dysfunction, initiated depression as a response of these pain-induced neurochemical changes.

Some authors noted the "conversion V" found in the hypochondriasis, depression, and hysteria scales of the Minnesota Multiphasic Personality Inventory (MMPI) was a marker for the tension-type headache patient, except that similar responses are found in chronic non-headache pain patients.

ASSOCIATED SLEEP DISORDERS

There appears to be an important relationship between sleep, headache, and the muscle-pain syndromes. Central biogenic amines, particularly serotonin and norepinephrine are important to sleep physiology as well as to the central pain modulating systems. Human and animal research indicates that central serotonin metabolism plays a role in pain modulation, affective states, and the regulation of non-REM sleep.

A high incidence of sleep disturbance has been noted in CTTH patients. Different sleep disorders may be associated with different headache entities. Migraine has been found to occur in association with REM sleep as well as excessive stage 3, 4, and REM sleep. CTTH has been found to be associated with frequent awakenings and decreased slow-wave sleep, an α-wave intrusion into stage 4 sleep. The latter sleep changes are similar to those seen in fibromyalgia.

A disturbance in stage 4 sleep has been reported as the first laboratory-based abnormality found in fibromyalgia. A similar non-α-wave REM pattern of α-wave intrusion in δ-wave sleep was induced in normal subjects by stage 4 sleep deprivation. The subjects subsequently developed musculoskeletal pain and affective changes comparable to those seen in fibromyalgia patients. Small doses of serotonergic tricyclic antidepressant medications, which reduced the α-wave intrusions into stage 4 sleep, were utilized to ameliorate the symptoms.

α-Wave intrusions into deep sleep have also been found in patients with other chronic pain syndromes, including rheumatoid arthritis. The α-wave non-REM disturbance has also been seen in asymptomatic people as well as in those who experience severe emotional stress, such as combat veterans. In the latter group, the veterans with this sleep disorder also complained of chronic headaches, diffuse pain, and emotional distress.

Sleep disturbance is associated with increased pain intensity. As noted above, chronic headache patients seem to have a higher incidence of sleep abnormalities than normal, pain-free subjects. Etiologic aspects of chronic headache may be linked to sleep abnormalities as an initiating element or as a result of the underlying pathologically dysmodulated neurochemical factors inducing a sleep disorder.

POSSIBLY ASSOCIATED FACTORS

There are two possible mechanical etiologies of CTTH. The first, cervical spondylosis, is defined as a degenerative disease affecting intervertebral discs and zygapophyseal joints of the cervical spine. While several authors note a possible correlation between cervical spondylosis and tension-type headache, others conclude to the contrary, suggesting that the basis of existing headache is secondary to muscle contraction.

The dental literature has been most active in reporting a possible correlation between temporomandibular joint dysfunction and tension-type headache. The relationship appears to depend mainly on tenderness of the masticatory muscles, which may have other etiologies and induce temporomandibular joint dysfunction, when it exists, on a secondary basis.

FIBROMYALGIA

Fibromyalgia is a systemic disorder clinically associated with a generalized increase in tenderness in susceptible areas over the entire body. These specific sites may induce a specific vulnerability to the central nociceptive pathways, much like myofascial trigger points. Patients with fibromyalgia are typically women between the ages of 30 and 50, with complaints of generalized pain with bilateral, symmetric tenderness for at least 3 months. On physical examination, at least 11 of 18 symmetric tender points must be found to confirm the diagnosis. The most common complaints found in these patients include morning stiffness, fatigue, chronic tension-type headaches, sleep disturbances, and the irritable bowel syndrome. Fibromyalgia and MPS may be two distinct entities, which may have the same underlying pathophysiology, as there are many similarities between the two syndromes, including trigger points found in fibromyalgia patients.

Similar to CTTH, EMG findings in fibromyalgia are typically negative or equivocal concerning the correlation of muscle tension with pain. No specific psychological findings are noted. The sleep disturbance is similar to that seen in CTTH, and may be linked to a deficiency of serotonin. Disturbances in oculomotor function are found in CTTH, to a lesser degree than in fibromyalgia patients. Sympathetic blockade has been found to diminish pain and decrease tender points, indicative of sympathetic hyperactivity and a related disturbance of microcirculation. The sympathetic aspects seen in the MPS and associated CTTH have already been mentioned.

Similar to CTTH, abnormalities of serotonin binding to platelets, a marker of central nervous system serotonergic efficacy, has also been found in fibromyalgia. Three groups of 20 patients with CTTH were analyzed with final diagnoses of CTTH, myofascial pain syndrome and fibromyalgia, on the basis of physical examination and published diagnostic criteria. A continuum of symptom intensity in the three groups was seen, including progressively increasing affective and physical problems as age, time in pain, and intensity increased. The findings were found to show a progression from CTTH, to the MPS group and finally to the fibromyalgia group. The signs and symptoms of CTTH were identified in the MPS and fibromyalgia groups. Localized trigger points were found in patients with simple tension-type headache.

PSYCHOPHYSIOLOGIC CHANGES

Less than half of tension-type headache patients complain of mild associated autonomic symptoms including lack of appetite, hyperirritability, dizziness, and increased light sensitivity. Notably, some of these symptoms may be secondary to the autonomic changes associated with active myofascial trigger points located in the head and neck.

While muscle contraction and tenderness may be interpreted as primary symptoms of tension-type headache, EMG activity and muscle tenderness increase more often during migraine than tension-type headache.

In research comparing tension-type headache (TTH) with common migraine patients exposed to auditory stimulation, TTH patients showed a lower heart rate reactivity than migraine patients. In another study it was shown that TTH patients exhibit the greatest cardiovascular arousal during headache. In yet another study, both migraine and TTH patients decreased pulse velocity in response to noise, while control subjects increased pulse velocity. In a psychophysiologic comparison of migraine and TTH, it was found that migraine patients are vasodilated and TTH patients are vasoconstricted both during and between headache attacks. During another study, administration of ergotamine tartrate, a vasoconstrictor, increased the pain of TTH, while amyl nitrate, a vasodilator, yielded only transient pain relief.

One study indicated greater sympathetic arousal during TTH as compared to controls. Another study reported both TTH and migraine patients to demonstrate cardiovascular sympathetic hypofunction, indicated by low basal levels of norepinephrine as well as orthostatic hypotension. It has also been suggested that TTH patients have phasic hypersympathetic activity, while migraineurs do not differ from controls during psychogalvanic response testing.

Evidence of pupillary sympathetic hypofunction and subtle anisocoria was found in both TTH and migraine patients. It was suggested that this may have reflected a central bioaminergic system dysfunction. Another study suggested a pupillary sympathetic system imbalance in CTTH patients, who showed asymmetric mydriasis after tyramine instillation and in the physiologic pupillary tests. Oculomotor dysfunction has also been noted in the amplitude and number of corrective saccads during testing of TTH patients.

Increased photophobia has been observed in TTH patients in comparison to controls. It has been hypothesized that changes in central modulation may induce increased sensitivity or hyperexcitability resulting in photophobia.

Episodic platelet abnormalities with associated serotonergic dysfunction has been well documented in migraine. Decreased platelet serotonin in CTTH patients has also been noted.

NEUROANATOMY AND NEUROCHEMISTRY

Central modulation of pain appears to originate in the brainstem, involving at least two systems. The inhibitory "descending" analgesia system, appears to regulate the spinal cord "gating" mechanisms. It includes the midbrain periaquaductal grey region, the medial medullary raphe nuclei and the adjacent reticular formation, and the dorsal horn neurons of the spinal cord. The "ascending" pain modulation system originates in the midbrain and projects to the thalamus. Both systems heavily utilize biogenic amines, opioid peptides and nonopioid peptides.

The ascending system appears to be more relevant to headache disorders. This system has a brainstem to medial thalamus projection, which includes both serotonergic and opiate receptors in large numbers. The midbrain dorsal raphe nucleus, a serotonergic nucleus, projects to the medial thalamus, and is associated with pain perception. The serotonergic projections to the forebrain have been implicated in sleep cycle regulation, mood changes, pain perception, and the hypothalamic regulation of hormone release.

In the central nervous system (CNS), the endogenous opiate system (EOS) may act as a nociceptive rheostat, setting pain modulation to a particular level. As this level changes, the individual's pain tolerance may also change. Fluctuations in the intensity of pain may be interpreted as being caused by fluctuations in the function of antinociceptive pathways. It has been suggested that patients with chronic neuropathic pain, who have been noted to have low β-endorphin levels, may be more prone to develop a pain syndrome not caused by excessive nociceptive stimulation, but by a deficiency in the EOS control mechanisms. Headache and other "nonorganic" central pain problems are thought to be the most common expression of impairment of the antinociceptive systems.

The endogenous opiates modulate the neurovegetative triad of pain, depression, and autonomic disturbances found in only two conditions, chronic headache and morphine abstinence. They are also implicated as primary protagonists in idiopathic headache. Reduced plasma concentrations of β-endorphin have been found in idiopathic headache patients, including CTTH. Increased levels of β-endorphin are found at the end of a headache attack, possibly associated with stress induced by the headache pain, suggested by the fact that ACTH and β-endorphin are located in the same hypothalamic neurons.

A primary relationship exists between the EOS and the biogenic amine systems. This relationship is intrinsic both to the pathophysiology of pain modulation, as well as to treatment. Clinical and pharmacologic information indicates that dysmodulated serotonergic neurotransmission probably generates chronic headache and head pain. It was also hypothesized that ordinary periodic headache may be the "noise" of serotonergic neurotransmission.

Serotonergic uptake mechanisms in the platelet are similar to those of neurons. Platelet serotonergic levels were found to be lower in patients with CTTH as compared to controls. Decreased levels of plasma serotonin were also found in CTTH patients. Decreased levels of serotonin in the platelets of TTH patients have been found, which was felt to indicate a central serotonergic disturbance, possibly an impairment of serotonergic metabolism in patients with CTTH.

Substance P, an excitatory neuropeptide, is found at all levels of the neuroaxis. Lower levels of substance P have been found in chronic neuropathic and idiopathic headache/pain patients than in normal volunteers.

Platelet GABA levels in CTTH patients are significantly increased compared to those seen in migraine patients and normal controls. Increased GABA levels may counterbalance neuronal hyperexcitability and may also be associated with depression.

Low levels of plasma norepinephrine are found in both migraine and CTTH patients in response to the cold pressor test, suggesting peripheral sympathetic hypofunction. Noradrenergic dysfunction may also participate in the etiology or maintenance of central opiod dysfunction.

Opioid receptor mechanisms are apparently very susceptible to desensitization, or the development of tolerance. In CTTH sufferers, opioid receptor hypersensitivity is marked, probably because of the chronically diminished secretion of neurotransmitters. This has been called the "empty neuron syndrome," indicating that it may involve both autonomic and nociceptive afferent systems, as well as be latent, subpathologic, or pathologic, with spontaneous manifestations.

The EOS modulates monoaminergic neurons. A chronic EOS deficiency would provoke transmitter leakage, both opioid and bioaminergic, leading to neuronal exhaustion and "emptying," as well as compensatory effector cell hypersensitivity. The most important phenomena of the hypoendorphin syndromes would appear to be the poor release of transmitter and cell/receptor hypersensitivity.

It has also been concluded that CTTH may result from a dysmodulation of nociceptive impulses, with sensitized receptors also being involved.

Chronic idiopathic headache may therefore be a "pain disease" linked to central dysmodulation of the nociceptive and antinociceptive systems, either latent or pathologic in nature. Research indicates that at least two arms of the main endogenous antinociceptive systems, the EOS and the serotonergic system, are involved in CTTH. This problem appears to be progressive, but it is uncertain whether the dysfunctions result from a genetic deficiency or neuronal exhaustion secondary to continuous activation of the systems.

PATHOPHYSIOLOGY OF CHRONIC TENSION-TYPE HEADACHE

Figure 206-1 summarizes the pathophysiological mechanisms of CTTH. Continuous peripheral stimulation from myofascial nociceptive input may effectively trigger a change in the central pain "rheostat" associated with nociceptive input, secondary to continuous need for pain modulating, antinociceptive neurotransmitters. The affective aspects of pain, secondary to

changes in neurotransmitters such as serotonin, which include depression, anxiety, and fear, can directly influence myofascial nociception, as well as further reinforce central neurochemical changes.

After 2 to 4 months (possibly sooner in some patients), changes in the central modulation of nociception can occur. Following continuous peripheral nociceptive stimulation, in association with affective changes, the central modulating mechanisms will assume a primary rather than a secondary or reactive role in pain perception, as well as antinociception, shifting pain perception initiation from the peripheral regions to the central nervous system.

This shift may make innocuous stimuli aggravating to the pain modulating systems. These already "dysmodulated" internal feedback mechanisms may react until central neurochemical mechanisms dominate, secondary to neurotransmitter exhaustion, receptor hypersensitivity, and abnormal biogenic amine metabolism/exhaustion occurs.

As previously discussed, the intrinsic neurochemical changes may induce and/or exacerbate a sleep disorder, which by itself may perpetuate the central neurochemical dysmodulation which is primarily responsible for CTTH.

Chronic post-traumatic tension-type headache, associated with a minor traumatic brain injury (MTBI) or not, has the same pathophysiologic mechanisms. In the presence of a MTBI there is the addition of (1) direct myofascial trauma, (2) diffuse axonal injury, which also affects the neurochemistry of the brain as neuronal degeneration and death occurs, (3) excitotoxic injury leading to cell death from overexuberant production of acetylcholine and glutamate. Affective changes typically follow, with

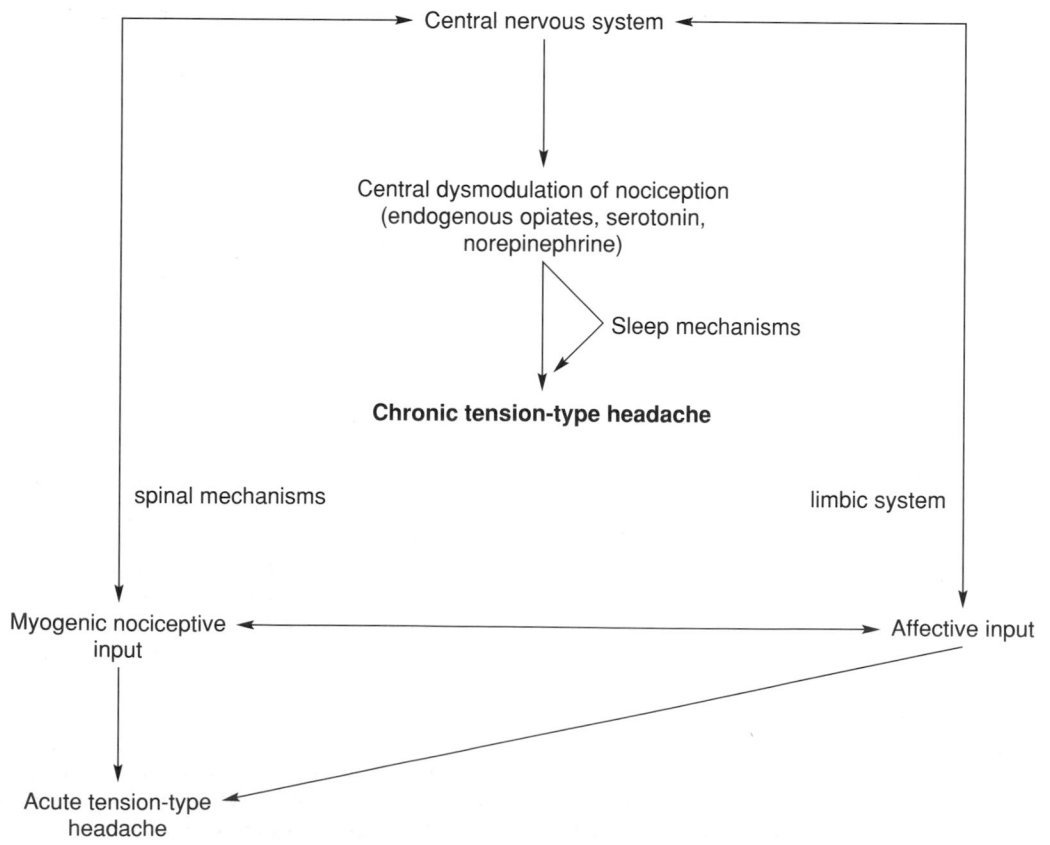

FIG. 206-1. Pathophysiology of acute and chronic tension-type headache.

the additional problem of possible cognitive changes occurring from a minor traumatic brain injury. The latter may make treatment more difficult, as treatment must involve patient education. Post traumatic tension-type headache is the most common sequelae of a minor traumatic brain injury. It may be associated with iatrogenic analgesic abuse. Before treatment of cognitive deficit is attempted, inappropriate medications must be stopped and the headache ameliorated.

TREATMENT

Treatment of CTTH is best accomplished via an interdisciplinary rehabilitation approach, the main purpose of which is *not* to "teach the patient to live with the headache," but to properly diagnose and effectively ameliorate or stop the headache.

Drug detoxification is the necessary first step, whether the patient is overutilizing simple, over-the-counter analgesics, or narcotics or barbiturates. Chronic daily analgesics appear to prevent appropriate functioning of the EOS (via negative neurochemical feedback loops) and other associated antinociceptive systems, inducing analgesic-rebound headaches, which are secondary problems from the medications that induce headache secondary to purely neurochemical/neurophysiologic changes. Vascular rebound headaches from overutilization of vasoconstrictors may also occur and must be stopped before other treatment is applied. Clinically, an effective way to detoxify CTTH patients is with the repetitive DHE-45 protocol. Concurrently, prophylactic medications should be started. The use of prophylactic medications, as well as physical therapy and other treatments given while a patient is enduring analgesic rebound headaches is an ineffectual waste of time and money.

After detoxification, an outpatient interdisciplinary headache rehabilitation program utilizing neuropharmacologic therapy (to restore neurochemical homeostasis), physical therapy, psychotherapy, and stress management (including biofeedback-enhanced neuromuscular re-education and muscle relaxation) is the most time and cost-effective treatment. Optimal psychotherapy or physical therapy regimens by themselves will not resolve myofascial difficulties or depression if the affective, sleep, and central nervous system neurochemical dysmodulation affecting them is not concurrently and appropriately treated. The interdisciplinary treatment paradigm also enables fine-tuning of diagnosis and possible determination of a secondary or "hidden" etiology for a patient's headaches.

Failure to treat the CTTH patient with an interdisciplinary, whole-person approach (Fig 206-1) is responsible for multiple treatment failures as well as monetary waste, as long-term response—headache remediation—is most often not achieved.

MIGRAINE AND TENSION-TYPE HEADACHE: TWO ENTITIES?

Much has been written about transformational headache, wherein episodic migraine may transform into CTTH, or migraine may transform from episodic TTH. There is no question that CTTH may evolve from episodic TTH, as the former is an extension and result of central changes induced over time by the latter.

It has been shown that CTTH is associated with systemic changes in serotonin metabolism as well as changes in the EOS and various other neurotransmitters and peptides. Migraine itself has associated serotonergic changes, possibly associated with EOS changes, which are not long lasting, and do not seem

to be secondary to a dysmodulation of the basic nociceptive/antinociceptive neurochemical substrates.

Rather than migraine and acute and CTTH being on two poles of a headache continuum, it appears more that both entities are different manifestations of the neurochemical/neurophysiologic dysmodulation of central pain-modulating systems. Migraine is episodic in nature, with seemingly specific, self-limited neurophysiologic and neurochemical changes. CTTH is associated with neurochemical changes which appear to be continuous, multifaceted, and similar in nature to those changes seen in other chronic pain syndromes, from pain arising from various places in the body. This appears to be true at least for those pain syndromes with myofascial/musculoskeletal etiologies, as differentiated from deafferentation induced neurochemical and neurophysiologic changes.

Perhaps, when looked at from this perspective, diagnosis, as well as treatment, can be more easily identified and routinely implemented.

SUGGESTED READINGS

Headache Classification Committee of the International Headache Society: Classification and diagnostic criteria for headache disorders, cranial neuralgias and facial pain. Cephalalgia 8(suppl 7), 1988

Jay GW: Chronic daily headache and myofascial pain syndromes: pathophysiology and treatment. pp. 211–33. In Cady RK, Fox AW (eds): Treating the Headache Patient. Marcel Dekker, New York, 1995

Jay GW: Pathophysiology of tension-type headache. p. 129. In Tollison CD, Kunkle RS (eds): Headache: Diagnosis and Treatment. Williams & Wilkins, Baltimore, 1993

Langemark M, Jensen K: Myofascial mechanisms of pain. p. 321. In Olesen J, Edvinsson L (eds): Basic Mechanisms of Headache. Elsevier Science Publishers, Amsterdam, 1988

Raskin NH: Headache. 2nd Ed. Churchill Livingstone, New York, 1988

Simons D: Muscular pain syndromes. p. 1. In Fricton JR, Awad E (eds): Advances in Pain Research and Therapy. Vol 17. Raven Press, New York, 1990

207. TRANSFORMED MIGRAINE

NINAN T. MATHEW

Traditionally, migraine and tension-type headache have been considered as distinct entities with defined cephalic vascular and myogenic mechanisms involved in their respective pathogeneses. A low-grade daily (or almost daily) chronic headache disorder without migrainous features that is clearly, but not necessarily, provoked by stress or other emotional factors has been referred to by clinicians as "tension headache." On the basis of this outdated concept, any historically nonspecific daily or near-daily headache was diagnosed as tension headache.

There is a trend for clinical opinion to view migraine and tension-type headache as physiologically related entities with a clinical expression that reflects a complex interaction of central (neurotransmitter centers of the brain), cephalic vascular and myogenic elements. The dichotomy of migraine and tension-type headache has been challenged by the observations of various authors. The primary headache disorders have also been described, as points on a "clinical continuum," with migraine

TABLE 207-1. Chronic Daily Headache (630 Cases)

Type	No.	Percentage	Male	Female	Age of Onset of Daily Headache
Chronic tension-type	84	13	36	48	28.5 ± 8.6
New daily persistent headache	57	9	18	39	32.4 ± 10.6
"Transformed" migraine	489	78	105	384	39.0 ± 11.2

with aura at one extreme and chronic tension-type headache at the other.

The classification and diagnostic criteria for headache disorders, cranial neuralgias, and facial pain, published by the Headache Classification Committee of the International Headache Society (IHS) primarily deals with individual headache attacks. The major drawback of this classification is that it ignores the fact that the same patient may suffer from different types of headache over time, or combinations of headache types. The IHS classification does not take into consideration the natural history of headache. For example, a person who suffers from migraine with aura, migraine without aura, chronic tension-type headache, and idiopathic stabbing headache will fall under four different diagnostic categories. Persons who initially manifest occasional migraines, but also suffer from interictal nondescript headaches, which eventually progress to a chronic daily or near-daily headache, are totally ignored in the classification.

CHRONIC DAILY HEADACHE

Chronic daily headache (CDH) is a widespread clinical problem, but limited data are available regarding its actual incidence and prevalence. It is a heterogeneous clinical entity with several subtypes occurring daily or near-daily over at least 6 months. Approximately 40 percent of patients seen in headache clinics suffer from CDH, a disorder given various other labels, including "chronic tension headache," "migraine with interparoxysmal headache," "transformed migraine," "evolutive migraine," "mixed headache syndrome," and "tension-vascular headache." The IHS classification does not consider chronic daily headache as a separate clinical entity. Chronic tension-type headache is the only variety of chronic daily or near-daily headache represented in the IHS classification. Most patients who present with daily or near-daily headache studied in our series, however, do not meet the IHS criteria for chronic tension-type headache. Of 630 cases of CDH (excluding those with post-traumatic headache), 489 were cases whose CDH evolved from previous migraine, 84 were cases of chronic tension-type; and 57 were cases of new daily persistent headache, unremitting from onset without previous history of headache (Table 207-1). An attempt was made to classify CDH to include the common varieties (Table 207-2). CDH, which evolved from previous migraine, is termed "transformed migraine" (TM). In practice, patients may present initially at different stages of evolution or transformation of their migraine. Earlier in this process of transformation, patients may present with distinct episodes of

TABLE 207-2. Clinical Types of Chronic Daily Headache[a]

Transformed migraine
  Drug-induced
  Non-drug-related
Chronic tension-type headache
New daily persistent headache
Post-traumatic headache

[a] Metabolic and structural causes are excluded.

migraine and frequent interictal tension-type headache. This is sometimes referred to as migraine with interparoxysmal headache.

CLINICAL FEATURES OF TRANSFORMED MIGRAINE

Traditionally, we have considered migraine as a purely episodic phenomenon, and daily headaches as muscle-contraction or tension headache. It has been reported that as many as 73 percent of patients with migraine have frequent low-grade headaches between attacks. It has been concluded that migraine is not just an episodic phenomenon, but a deviation from normal, because the biologic threshold for headache is lower in the migraine sufferer than in the general population. In another series of 750 migraine patients, 50 percent had interictal nondescript headaches. In his studies of the natural history of migraine, Graham observed that, in some individuals, headache attacks may show an increase in frequency until they become daily.

In 1982, reported a series of patients with a clear-cut past history of distinct attacks of migraine whose headaches evolved over the years into a daily or near-daily problem. Attacks of migraine, which are at first distinct in adolescence or the early twenties, over the years become more frequent, with the gradual development of nonspecific interictal headaches. By the age of 35 or 40, these patients suffer from daily or near-daily headaches, with mixed features of migraine and tension-type headache. Patients may suffer from migraine one day and tension-type headache the next day. The majority of the females in this group have menstruation related aggravation of the headaches. Transformed migraine is sometimes difficult to distinguish. Tension-type headache may progress to migraine after a few days. Migraine may gradually subside into a nagging, low-grade headache, often only to be followed by an even more severe attack with nausea, vomiting, and other migrainous features. It is important to take a detailed history of headaches from these patients; a clear-cut history of episodes of migraine will be obtained from most patients.

Table 207-3 deals with the transformed migraine group, and includes the age at first visit, the age of onset of distinct episodes of migraine, duration of migraine before the transformation occurred, age of transformation to chronic daily headache, and duration after the transformation to chronic daily headache. Between the age of 30 and 40, the incidence of chronic daily headache supersedes the incidence of distinct episodes of migraine in this group.

The diagnostic categorization of the types of migraine before CDH developed revealed that 45 (9.2 percent) patients suffered from migraine with aura and/or migraine with prolonged aura, and 444 (90.8 percent) patients had migraine without aura. Among the patients with aura 21 of 45 (4.2 percent of transformed migraine patients) had a clear history of transformation from migraine with aura to migraine without aura and then to CDH.

TRANSFORMATIONAL FACTORS

Table 207-4 lists the probable factors that influence transformation of episodic headaches to the chronic daily form. Analgesic

TABLE 207-3. Transformed Migraine

Age at First Visit	Mean Age of Onset of Episodic Migraine	Mean Duration of Episodic Migraine Before Transformation Occurred (years)	Mean Age of Transformation to Chronic Daily Headache	Mean Duration After Transformation
Mean 41 ± 12	Mean 22 ± 9.2	Mean 16 ± 11	Mean 39 ± 11.2	Mean 6 ± 5
Range 11–64	Range 3–53	Range 1–51	Range 12–65	

TABLE 207-4. Probable Factors in the Development of Chronic Daily Headache From Episodic Headache

	Mathew et al., 1982 N = 80 (%)	Manzoni et al., 1987 N = 250 (%)	Manzoni et al., 1991 N = 58 (%)	Solomon et al., 1992 N = 100 (%)
Analgesic/ergotamine overuse	52	59	67	50
Abnormal personality profile including depression	70.5	—	39.7	—
Stress	67	22	44	—
Traumatic life events	13	9	—	—
Hypertension	10	1.5	3.8	—
Nonheadache medications including sex hormones	—	1.5	3.8	—
Percentage with identifiable factors	—	78	—	—
Percentage without identifiable factors	—	22	—	—

or ergotamine overuse, comorbidity such as depression, anxiety, abnormal personality profile, and stress appear to top the list. Drug-induced and non-drug-induced are clearly identifiable. Analgesic or ergotamine overuse has been reported in 82 percent of patients who developed chronic migraine out of an episodic pattern. There may be a group of patients whose pain evolves spontaneously into a chronic daily headache, as a course in the natural history of the disease. It has been reported that in 22 percent of patients no apparent transformational factors could be found.

EVOLUTIONARY PATTERN

The evolutionary pattern of transformed migraine is shown in Table 207-5. Most patients maintained migraine attacks in addition to developing tension-type headache daily or nearly daily.

Others lost the temporal profile of migraine, but developed continuous headache with many migrainous features.

TRANSFORMED MIGRAINE VERSUS CHRONIC TENSION-TYPE HEADACHE

Table 207-6 compares the clinical characteristics of transformed migraine and chronic tension-type headache. In general, the transformed migraine group showed higher incidence of family history of headache, more neurologic and gastrointestinal symptoms, aggravation during menstruation, and relief during pregnancy, compared with other forms of chronic daily headaches, particularly CTH.

Patients with transformed migraine and chronic tension-type showed significantly elevated depression scales compared to patients with distinct episodes of migraine only. In addition,

TABLE 207-5. Natural History of Transformed Migraine

Manzoni et al. 1987 (N = 178)	118/178	Maintained migraine attacks and developed interparoxysmal tension-type headache Frequency of migraine was more than 1/week in only 35 patients
	60/178	Lost the distinct migraine attacks and developed either a "steady" (41 patients) or a "fluctuating" (19 patients) pattern
Manzoni et al. 1991 (N = 44)	28/44	Maintained migraine attacks and developed interparoxysmal tension-type headache Lost the distinct migraine attacks and developed a continuous headache that exhibited most of the features of migraine, except the temporal profile

TABLE 207-6. Comparison of Clinical Characteristics of Transformed Migraine and Chronic Tension Type

Transformed Migraine	Chronic Tension Type
Headache >15 days/month >180 days/year	Headache >15/month >180/year
Previous history of distinct migraine attacks	No history of distinct migraine attacks
Increased incidence of headache in the family	Positive family history less prominent
Retains migrainous characters to a significant degree, intermittently or continuously	Migrainous features absent or very insignificant
Increased neurologic and gastrointestinal symptoms	Neurologic and gastrointestinal symptoms minimal
Menstrual aggravation	No particular aggravation during menstruation
More relief during pregnancy	Less relief during pregnancy
Excessive intake of analgesics	Excessive intake of analgesics
Responds to antimigraine therapy	Response to antimigraine therapy occurs, but less striking
Behavioral and psychological factors prominent	Behavioral and psychological factors prominent

transformed migraine patients showed elevated type A behavioral pattern scores.

MMPI Scales

Based on the MMPI, an abnormal personality profile was found in 61 percent of patients with CDH, of which the majority were transformed migraine, compared to 12.2 percent of patients with distinct episodes of migraine group ($p < .01$). In this study, 56 percent of patients had elevations of scales I, II, and III, i.e., hyperchondriasis, depression, and hysteria, with the majority showing a typical V configuration. Thus, "neuroticism" was found to be significantly higher in CDHs. There was no statistical difference between the various types of CDHs; 21 percent also had various combinations of elevated scales of 6, 7, 8, and 9, often seen in the most persistent and intractable cases.

Our group showed that duration of the second exteroceptive silent period (ES_2) of the temporalis muscle was shorter and the degree of suppression lower in chronic daily headache of the transformed migraine type, even though not to the same degree as in CTH. The ES_2 abnormalities in our series of chronic headache patients support the concept of a continuum between migraine, transformed migraine, and CTH.

MIGRAINE-CHRONIC TENSION-TYPE HEADACHE COMPLEX EVOLVED FROM EPISODIC TENSION-TYPE HEADACHE (ETH)

A relatively small percentage of patients with CDH in the migraine-CTH headache complex, describe a history of evolution of the chronic headache from ETH; the percentages varied from 3 to 15 percent. The frequency of headaches with migrainous features is significantly less in this group compared with transformed migraine. Others also found a subset of patients who developed CDH from the onset, without a history of previous migraine or tension-type headache.

Subtypes of Transformed Migraine

The CDH patients in general overuse symptomatic medications: 73 percent of them used excessive amounts of analgesics, sedative/caffeine/analgesic combinations, or ergotamine on a daily basis. The use of daily symptomatic medication was more common in patients with transformed migraine than in patients with chronic tension-type or new daily persistent headache (transformed migraine, 87.2 percent; chronic tension-type, 67 percent and new daily persistent headache, 66 percent). When we analyzed our data, it was clear that there were two groups of patients in the transformed migraine type of CDH: one with clear-cut excessive use of symptomatic medications, the other where the chronic headache evolution was unrelated to medication. In the latter group, which was smaller, there appeared to be a natural transformation of episodic migraine to a chronic daily headache.

Withdrawal of daily symptomatic medications, institution of a low-tyramine, low-caffeine diet, initiation of prophylactic antimigraine therapy, biofeedback, and behavioral therapy resulted in 75 percent reduction in the headache index in 76 percent of CDH patients followed for a 6-month period. Based on these data and previous experience, we propose that transformed migraine, which comprises the majority of CDH, is a continuum of the migraine process, influenced and perpetuated by such factors as excessive use of symptomatic medications, abnormal personality profile, depression, stress, and traumatic life events. We further propose that the diagnosis of a separate entity of tension-type headache is not justified in these patients under such circumstances because the underlying biologic abnormality appears to be common to both entities.

Clinically relevant subtypes of transformed migraine are (1) transformed migraine related to excessive drug use, and (2) transformed migraine unrelated to excessive drug use.

Drug-Induced Transformed Migraine

Medications used for immediate relief of headache may perpetuate migraine if used frequently in excessive quantities. There are two main forms of such drug-induced headache. These are analgesic-rebound headache and ergotamine-rebound headache.

Table 207-7 gives the common daily symptomatic or immediate relief medications taken by a group of 200 patients with chronic daily headache. Table 207-8 gives the pattern of consumption of these medications; 22 percent of patients took more than three or more preparations concomitantly. The most common prescription medications that were overused for immediate relief were those containing butalbital, caffeine, and analgesic combinations with or without codeine. Many patients combined

TABLE 207-8. Pattern of Consumption of Symptomatic Medications

No. of Preparations of Symptomatic Medications Consumed Concurrently	No. of Patients (N = 200)	Patients (%)
1	70	35
2	86	43
3	44	22

(From Mathew NT, Kurman R, Perez F: Drug-induced refractory headache: clinical features and management. Headache 30:63, 1990, with permission.)

TABLE 207-7. Daily Symptomatic or Intermediate Relief Medications

Medications	Average No. of Tablets per Week	Range of No. of Tablets per Week	No. of Patients	Patients (%)
Butalbitol/aspirin Acetaminophen/caffeine with or without codeine	30	14–86	84	42
Natural or synthetic codeine-containing preparations	28	10–84	80	40
Aspirin or acetaminophen with caffeine	42	14–108	50	25
Ergotamine with or without phenobarbital	15 mg	6–42 mg	44	22
Acetaminophen	52	15–105	34	17
Propoxyphene	26	14–56	32	16
Nasal decongestants and antihistamines	14	6–30	24	12
Aspirin	28	10–64	8	4

(From Mathew NT, Kurman R, Perez F: Drug-induced refractory headache: clinical features and management. Headache 30:63, 1990, with permission.)

ergotamine with analgesics or analgesic/sedative/caffeine combinations.

Clinical Features of Analgesic-Related Transformed Migraine

The characteristic features of analgesic rebound headaches are a self-sustaining, rhythmic headache-medication cycle characterized by daily or near daily headache, and an irresistible and predictable use of pain medication as the only means of relieving headache attacks. The other characteristics are varying intensity, location, and type of headache. Headaches may be precipitated by minor physical or intellectual effort. Most of the time it is difficult to distinguish rebound headache from the primary headache disorders such as tension headache and migraine for which the medication is taken. The majority of those with a history of migraine exhibit features of migraine during some of the daily headache attacks, although rarely are the symptoms typical and distinct. Drug-induced headache can be throbbing. Accompanying symptoms are very striking in drug-induced headache and include asthenia, nausea, restlessness, irritability, memory problems, and difficulty in intellectual concentration and behavioral abnormalities such as depression.

Sleep Abnormalities. Difficulty in initiating and maintaining sleep and early morning awakening with severe headaches are very common in patients with analgesic-rebound headaches. This was observed in 71 percent of our patients. Predictable early morning (between 2 and 6 a.m.) headache occurred in 46 percent. There was usually a correlation between predictable early morning headache and high intake of butalbital, caffeine, or ergotamine. The majority of patients took analgesic or ergotamine tablets in the early morning hours upon awakening.

Tolerance. Tolerance to symptomatic medications may develop, resulting in a gradually increasing frequency of consumption and total quantity of medication. Analgesic medications may be taken in anticipation of headache or long before the actual headache attack occurs. Fear of an impending severe headache leads to consumption of symptomatic medications. This is mainly because there is no reliable way for a patient to predict which of the minor headaches will lead to a severe episode.

Withdrawal Headache and Related Symptoms. Abrupt cessation of analgesics may result in increased intensity of headache, accompanied by nausea, abdominal cramps, diarrhea, restlessness, sleeplessness, and mental anguish. These symptoms are especially common in patients who consume butalbital and caffeine/analgesic combinations. Seizures have been reported in certain instances. Increased headache intensity may start within 24 to 48 hours, and in most cases it may subside in 5 to 7 days.

Headache Improvement After Withdrawal of Analgesics. The most striking feature of analgesic-rebound headache is the continued decline in headache frequency and intensity, general well-being, and reduction in irritability, depression, and lethargy after the initial withdrawal period. In our series of 200 patients, mere discontinuation of symptomatic medications resulted in 52 percent improvement in the headache index. Addition of prophylactic medications, after discontinuation of daily analgesics resulted in a 78 percent improvement in a 12-week period.

Concomitant Prophylactic Agents. From our study, it is clear that daily excessive symptomatic medication nullifies the beneficial effects of prophylactic agents. Of our 200 patients, 58 were taking prophylactic antimigraine medications such as β-blockers, calcium channel blockers, methysergide, and tricyclic antidepressants in different combinations. Yet they continued to have daily headache. Withdrawal of daily symptomatic medication enhanced the effect of prophylactic medications in this series of patients.

Clinical Features of Ergotamine-Related Transformed Migraine

In the patients with ergotamine-rebound headache, a headache of migraine type occurs on an almost daily basis. As the effect of previous doses of ergotamine wanes, the headache gradually escalates until the next dose of ergotamine is taken. As time passes, psychological dependency on ergotamine intensifies, and patients take ergotamine in anticipation of headache. Sleep disturbance and depression also occur. The headache itself is strikingly sensitive to ergotamine but generally will not respond to alternate symptomatic or preventive medications that would otherwise be expected to have beneficial effect. Because migraine is characteristically a variable disorder, rarely occurring more than once or twice a week, a migrainelike headache occurring more than two to three times a week that is selectively responsive to ergotamine but refractory to other symptomatic or preventive medications should alert the physician to the possible presence of ergotamine-rebound headache. Anticipation of headache and resulting apprehension may lead to use of ergotamine even before a headache attack occurs.

All cases reported in the literature show an increasing pattern of usage of ergotamine. Weekly total dosage frequently exceeds safety limitations. In the majority of cases, weekly total dosage frequently exceeds safety limitations. In the majority of cases, weekly doses exceed 10 mg, with some patients taking as much as 10 to 15 mg/day. Surprisingly, peripheral ischemia or other signs of ergotism rarely occur in these patients. Therefore, ergotamine rebound should be distinguished from ergotamine toxicity.

Stopping ergotamine invariably causes predictable, protracted, and extremely debilitating headache accompanied by nausea, vomiting, at times diarrhea, and other physical and psychological complaints. Restlessness and sleeplessness are not uncommon. This withdrawal headache usually starts within 72 hours after stopping the drug and may last for another 72 or more hours once the headache begins. Spontaneous improvement after stopping of medication is common. Preventive medications previously without benefit become more effective when ergotamine is discontinued.

MANAGEMENT OF TRANSFORMED MIGRAINE

A multimodality approach is essential for satisfactory results. A combination of pharmacologic and behavioral intervention is necessary. Essential principles are as follows:

1. Discontinuation of the offending medications
2. Attempts to break the cycle of continuous headache by pharmacotherapeutic agents such as intravenous dihydroergotamine or subcutaneous sumatriptan
3. Initiation of prophylactic pharmacotherapy
4. Concomitant behavioral intervention, which includes bio-

feedback therapy, individual behavioral counseling, family therapy, physical exercise, and dietary instructions

5. Adequate instructions about ill effects of medications with special focus on analgesics
6. Continuity of care

The multimodality approach to treatment outlined above can be taken with either outpatients or inpatients. Indications for hospitalization would include the following:

1. Status migrainosus with nausea, vomiting, and dehydration associated with excessive narcotic/analgesic/ergotamine use
2. Chronic refractory headache with extreme narcotic or barbiturate habituation
3. Chronic refractory headache with severe psychiatric comorbidity such as depression and panic disorder
4. Refractory headache with associated medical problems such as uncontrolled hypertension or renal, gastric, or hepatic disease

Withdrawal of Analgesic/Narcotic/Ergotamine

In a hospitalized patient, offending medications can be discontinued abruptly, bearing in mind the possibility of withdrawal reactions. Usual withdrawal reactions are increased headache, restlessness, sleeplessness, excessive sweating, and diarrhea. These can be counteracted to a significant degree by use of a clonidine skin patch 0.2 mg. Serious withdrawal of reactions such as seizure can occur, specifically with abrupt withdrawal of butalbital-containing medications. In the hospital, such emergencies can be tackled effectively; it is unwise to ask a patient to stop butalbital abruptly as an outpatient.

Breaking the Cycle of Headache

Dihydroergotamine. In the hospital a heparin lock is used to administer intravenous fluids for rehydration and administration of antiemetics and dihydroergotamine (DHE). Unlike ergotamine, DHE does not appear to cause rebound headache and therefore can be substituted with repeated injections for 48 to 72 hours.

Side effects of intravenous DHE limit its use to some degree. Leg pain and cramps, nausea, and vomiting, despite using metoclopramide or phenothiazine, are drawbacks. There are instances of transient ischemic attacks and migrainous strokes developing in patients who were on DHE in the hospital. Angina can also occur. In general, DHE is contraindicated in (1) patients with migraine with prolonged aura (complicated migraine) or those with *frequent* migraine with aura, and (2) those who are heavy smokers or have other risk factors for stroke and vascular diseases such as severe diabetes, hyperlipidemia, hypertension, and positive anticardiolipin antibody. In spite of these limitations, DHE is useful in the majority of patients do break the cycles of headaches.

Sumatriptan. Sumatriptan administered subcutaneously has been used successful when withdrawing analgesics in patients with drug-induced headache. Sumatriptan can be given repeatedly without any major side effects. It is devoid of side effects such as nausea and vomiting, which are very frequent with DHE. In fact, sumatriptan by itself may ameliorate nausea and vomiting. It is conceivable that sumatriptan administered in repetitive doses will become the drug of choice in breaking the cycle of refractory migraine. As with DHE, the clinician has

to be careful in using sumatriptan in patients with high risk for stroke and vascular disease.

Prophylactic Pharmacotherapy

Simultaneously with analgesic/ergotamine withdrawal, adequate combinations of prophylactic pharmacotherapy can be started. Most of the patients in this category require copharmacy using one antimigraine agent and an antidepressant. Any of the agents used for prophylaxis of migraine can be used in chronic headache. Tricyclics are still the antidepressants of choice as they have an analgesic effect in addition to the antidepressant and sleep-enhancing properties, both of which are helpful to the chronic refractory headache patients. Fluoxetine (Prozac), which should theoretically be useful, as it is a specific 5-HT uptake inhibitor, has not yet been shown to have any antimigraine or analgesic effect. However, because of the lack of sedation, an anticholinergic side effect, many patients prefer fluoxetine to amitriptyline.

Valproate (Depakote) has been found to be particularly useful in the prophylactic management of chronic daily headache. Double-blind placebo-controlled studies have reported significant benefit with valproate as a prophylactic agent in patients with migraine. The usual dose is 500 to 1,000 mg/day to keep the blood level above 50 mg/ml; an occasional patient may require up to 2,000 mg/day.

Hepatic toxicity, which was a major concern when valproate was used in infants and young children for seizure control, is not a problem in adults in the headache age group. Certainly it should not be used in patients with active liver disease. Asthenia, tremor, weight gain, and hair loss occur in some patients. Valproate can be combined with antidepressants.

Behavioral Therapy

Behavioral therapy alone, using biofeedback, relaxation, or a combination of the two, gives only less than 50 percent improvement. The general experience is that when pharmacotherapy and behavioral therapy are combined, the improvement is greater than with one modality alone.

Behavioral therapy should include not only relaxation or biofeedback, but also short-term cognitive stress-management therapy and individual counseling. Family counseling may also be important, if a great deal of family stress is recognized.

SUGGESTED READINGS

Anderson PG: Ergotamine headache. Headache 15:118–21, 1975

Diener HC, Haab J, Peters C, Ried S et al: Subcutaneous sumatriptan in the treatment of headache during withdrawal from drug-induced headache. Headache 31:205–9, 1991

Isler H: Migraine treatment as a cause of chronic migraine. pp. 159–64. In Rose FC (ed): Advances in Migraine Research and Therapy. Raven Press, New York, 1982

Kudrow L: Paradoxical effects of frequent analgesic use. pp. 335–41. In Critchley M, Friedman A, Gorini S, Sicuteri F (eds): Advances in Neurology. Raven Press, New York, 1982

Mathew NT, Ali S: Valproate in the treatment of persistent chronic daily headache: an open label study. Headache 31:71–4, 1991

Mathew NT, Kurman R, Perez F: Drug induced refractory headache: clinical features and management. Headache 30:634–8, 1990

Mathew NT, Reuveni U, Perez F: Transformed or evolutive migraine. Headache 27:102–6, 1987

Mathew NT, Stubits E, Nigam MR: Transformation of episodic migraine into daily headache: analysis of factors. Headache 22:66–8, 1982

Raskin NH: Repetitive intravenous dihydroergotamine as therapy for intractable migraine. Neurology 36:995–7, 1986

Sands GH: A protocol for butalbital, aspirin, caffeine (BAC) detoxification in headache patients. Headache 30:491–6, 1990

Silverstein SD, Schulman EA, Hopkins MM: Repetitive intravenous DHE in the treatment of refractory headache. Headache 30:334–9, 1990

Solomon S, Lipton RB, Newman LC: Clinical features of chronic daily headache. Headache 32:325–9, 1992

Vanast WJ: New daily persistent headaches: definition of a benign syndrome. Headache 26:318, 1986

Ziegler DK, Hassanein RS, Couch JR: Headache syndrome suggested by statistical analysis of headache symptoms. Cephalalgia 2:125–34, 1982

208. CLUSTER HEADACHE AND PAROXYSMAL HEMICRANIA

LEE KUDROW

Of all primary headache disorders, cluster headache and paroxysmal hemicrania are most stereotypic in presentation and, in general, are the most amenable to medical management. Differences between the two disorders are so subtle as to present difficulties in their classification. As an example, both conditions share the same site of painful attacks, associated autonomic symptoms, and episodic and chronic states. While the frequency and duration of cluster headache attacks generally differ from those of the paroxysmal hemicranias, these features may overlap to make diagnosis difficult and to question the distinctiveness of these disorders. Yet there is one characteristic that distinguishes one disorder from the other; response to prophylactic medications. The diagnosis of paroxysmal hemicrania is assured when a complete response to indomethacin has occurred; with few exceptions, cluster headache will not respond to indomethacin prophylaxis. Conversely, cluster headache is quite responsive to prophylactic treatment with verapamil, lithium, or ergotamine, but paroxysmal hemicrania is completely refractory to these medications.

The currently accepted classification system holds that paroxysmal hemicrania represents a subcategory of cluster headache, as are other variants. Classification of these disorders, as recently established by The International Headache Society, is presented in Table 208-1. It should be noted that the current classification of headache disorders reflects only our current knowledge of this topic and is subject to change with improved understanding. Classification, therefore, is a dynamic process.

TABLE 208-1. Classification of Cluster Headache

Cluster headache	3.1
Periodicity undetermined	3.1.1
Episodic	3.1.2
Chronic	3.1.3
Primary chronic	3.1.3.1
Secondary chronic	3.1.3.2
Chronic paroxysmal hemicrania	3.2
Cluster headache-like syndrome	3.3

CLUSTER HEADACHE

Incidence, Age, and Sex

Cluster headache is believed to occur in approximately 0.4 percent of males and in one-fifth of that number for females. The ratio of males to females is approximately 5–6:1. The mean age of onset of this disorder is 30 years; the mean age of onset for women and chronic patients is older.

Familial History

Approximately 10 percent of cluster patients give a positive family history for one or more relatives; 3 percent of relatives of a cluster headache population are reported to have cluster headache. A recent study has shown that the family history of migraine among relatives of cluster patients was similar to that for relatives of migraine patients. These data suggested that inheritance of cluster headache may be dependent on a linkage to migraine genetics.

Clinical Presentation

The most frequently encountered cluster headache type is called episodic. Approximately 80 percent of all cluster sufferers are episodic types. This condition is defined by periods of attack susceptibility (cluster periods) followed by periods of nonattack susceptibility, called remissions. Cluster periods are most often found to recur cyclically, each lasting a mean of 2 months, followed by 1-year remissions. These periods may, however, range widely. The absence of a remission period of at least 1 year defines chronic cluster headache. A further distinction may be made for this chronic type: although it appears to be of little importance, chronic cluster is divided into two subtypes: primary (chronic from onset of the disorder) and secondary (converting to chronic from an episodic state).

The mean frequency of cluster attacks during active periods is 1 to 3 per day for episodic cluster headache and 2 to 4 per day in the chronic type. Attacks last an average of 45 minutes, ranging from 15 minutes to 3 hours. They most often occur when relaxing upon returning home from work, and almost as often, approximately 90 minutes after sleep onset. Cluster attacks least often occur during working hours. During cluster periods, and at no other time, attacks may be provoked by a small amount of ingested alcohol, sublingual nitroglycerin, intradermal histamine, or other vasodilating substances. Attack provocation under these conditions apply as well to chronic patients.

The pain of cluster headache attacks are reported to be of considerable intensity, known to cause some patients to drop to their knees, pounding their head on the ground or smash their fists into walls. (We have four patients who have fractured their hands after striking walls braced by two-by-fours). Celebrating this exquisite pain, patients commonly experience ipsilateral lacrimation, rhinorrhea and/or nasal stuffiness, conjuntival suffusion and less frequently, ipsilateral forehead sweating, miosis, and ptosis (partial Horner syndrome). Most significantly, patients tend to pace or rock forward and back in a chair during attacks, avoiding the supine position. Even when attempting to lie still the patient will writhe in a manner similar to one suffering from an attack of ureteral colic. These attack-related behavior patterns are pathognuemonic of cluster headaches. At the end of an attack the patient may be drained of all energy, yet feel euphoric. Between attacks, patients have no

TABLE 208-2. Differential Diagnosis of Cluster Headache

Disorders	Frequency	Duration	Intensity	Location	Quality	Other
Raeder syndrome	Constant	Persistent	Severe	Unilateral, supraocular	Burning, throb to nonthrob	Partial Horner syndrome
Pheochromocytoma	Daily to monthly	1 hour	Severe in supine position	Bilateral, occipital	Throbbing	Sweating, pallor, tachycardia, blood pressure elevation
Temporal arteritis	Constant	Persistent	Moderate	Unilateral, temporal	Burning, throb to nonthrob	Chewing claudication, Tender, torturous and pulseless temporal artery, elevated erythrocyte sedimentation rate, polymyalgia
Trigeminal neuralgia	Several/day	Seconds to minutes	Severe	Unilateral, 5th nerve distribution	Electric, lancinating	Facial trigger zones
Migraine	1–3/month	6–36 hours	Severe	Hemicranial 60%	Throbbing, 80%	Nausea, vomiting, photophobia, sonophobia
Paroxysmal hemicrania (chronic and episodic)	4–30/day	3–45 minutes	Severe	Unilateral, periorbital	Boring	1) See cluster headache 2) Response to indomethacin pathognomonic
Cluster headache	1–3/day	15–120 minutes	Severe	Unilateral, periorbital	Boring	Unilateral lacrimation, rhinorrhea, injection, partial Horner syndrome

pain but sense that they are still in a cluster period. This has been described as a warm cloud or feeling of warmth over the ipsilateral forehead and temple regions.

Differential Diagnosis

As mentioned earlier, the paroxysmal hemicranias most resemble cluster headache, and will be discussed in greater detail later. Other disorders to be differentiated from cluster headache include: Raeder's syndrome, pheochromocytoma, temporal arteritis, trigeminal neuralgia, and migraine (Table 208-2).

Raeder Syndrome. Raeders syndrome is similar to cluster headache sharing pain severity (early in its course), unilaterality, supraorbital distribution, and an associated partial Horner syndrome. Distinct from cluster headache, however, is the persistence of pain in Raeder syndrome. In the latter, there are no distinct attacks; pain is constant throughout.

Pheochromocytoma. Headache attacks of another rare disorder, pheochromocytoma, are similar to those of cluster headache in that they may recur daily, last less than an hour, and have associated symptoms of tachycardia, sweating, and blood pressure changes. Additionally, pain may be exacerbated in the supine position. The headache of pheochromocytoma, however, is most likely bilateral and occipital in location. It should be noted that in the rare case of cluster headache, bioccipital attacks have been documented.

Temporal Arteritis. The headache of temporal arteritis is generally unitemporal in laterality, and generally of dull to moderate intensity, but it may be severe. It is constant or waxing and waning, which distinguishes it from cluster headache. Other differentiating features include chewing claudication, a tender and pulseless temporal artery, and an elevated sedimentation rate. During some cluster attacks, however, the ipsilateral temporal artery may become distended, torturous, and tender, and, as in temporal arteritis, have a burning quality. The finding of giant cells on temporal artery biopsy is diagnostic of temporal arteritis.

Trigeminal Neuralgia. Trigeminal neuralgia is characterized by electric, lancinating paroxysms of only seconds duration,

often and solely triggered by a tactile stimulus on the face. None of these features resemble cluster headache. Also, trigeminal neuralgia is apt to occur initially at an older age. There is a condition, however, where trigeminal neuralgia seems to be part of cluster headache; symptoms and signs of both disorders may be present at the same or at different times. This is called cluster-tic syndrome.

Migraine Headaches. Finally, migraine headaches should be differentiated from cluster headache. For a majority of cases this presents little problem. Spontaneous migraine attacks are generally infrequent, occurring once or twice a month on average. Its duration is from 6 hours to 3 or 4 days. Migraines are bilateral in as many as 40 percent of cases, frequently associated with nausea and less often vomiting, and temporally related to hormonal-menstrual changes in as many as 80 percent of attacks in women. Except in rare cases migraine attacks are not associated with autonomic signs and symptoms, as characteristically found in cluster headache. It would seem from the foregoing that cluster headache could hardly be confused with migraine headaches. This is true until one sees a patient with a variant called *cluster-migraine*. Patients with this disorder may present two ways; migraine attacks having cluster headache periodicity or typical cluster attacks occurring monthly and having associated symptoms of both disorders.

It should be noted that cluster-tic syndrome and cluster-migraine headaches are classified under the term *cluster headache-like syndromes*. It is my opinion that these disorders will, in the near future, achieve recognition as true variants.

Pathophysiology

The etiology of cluster headache is unknown. The possible pathogenesis of this disorder, however, has been the subject of numerous reports. It is clear that its pathogenesis involves numerous systems, including central and peripheral neuronal and vascular systems involving cranial nerves, peptides, and neurohormones. It is the ordering of these systems into sequential events that has presented the greatest difficulty and challenge to researchers. Recently, this has been elucidated in a hypothesis, which holds that there are three clinicopathologic phases of cluster headache: the cluster period, attack onset or provocation, and attack signs and symptoms.

The Cluster Period. The cluster period appears to be the result of two major pathophysiologic changes. Evidence suggests that cyclic hypothalamic dysfunction may be associated with certain chronobiologic events, which cause an impaired sympathetic neuronal activity. These changes may be responsible for the altered physiologic state and attack susceptibility that characterizes the cluster period.

Attack Onset. While there may be disagreement, one hypothesis holds that hypoxemic events may induce cluster attacks. Studies have demonstrated that nitroglycerin-induced and spontaneous cluster attacks are preceded by mild but sustained oxygen desaturation. It was suggested that during the cluster period, chemoreceptor activity may become blunted as a result of impaired sympathetic function. A significant hypoxemic event may then hyperactivate chemoreceptors (denervation-hypersensitivity response). This model may also explain why oxygen inhalation rapidly aborts cluster attacks (blocks chemoreceptor activity). Others believe, however, that the beneficial affect of oxygen is mediated via its vasoconstrictive activity.

Attack Signs and Symptoms. The third phase of cluster headache is the attack itself. Most investigators would agree that pain and autonomic features, which comprise the "attack," probably result from the antidromal stimulation of the trigeminal nerve and release of neuropeptides, mediated via parasympathetic nerve activity and localizing to the region of the cavernous sinus. Thus the pain in cluster headache, as in migraine, may be due to dilatation and inflammation of extracerebral blood vessels mediated by peptides. That a similar pain mechanism is responsible for both disorders is supported by the similar beneficial response to sumatriptan, a 5-HT agonist.

Management

Successful treatment of cluster headache requires that patients are properly educated about this condition, that an appropriate prophylactic medication regimen is offered and that effective symptomatic treatment is provided.

Patient Education. During active cluster periods, patients should be advised to avoid using alcohol or vasodilating drugs, exposure to oil-based solvents, high altitude, or strenuous exercise, since such stimulants may induce cluster attacks. Patients should be encouraged by the recent advances in the treatment of this disorder and should be told of these advances. An appropriate prophylactic regimen should prevent 90 percent of attacks and breakthrough headaches may be rapidly aborted in most cases. Such "encouraging" news helps to diminish the anticipatory anxiety that accompanies this disorder

Prophylactic Medication. In episodic cluster headache the treatment of choice is verapamil, 80 mg four times a day, spread evenly over waking hours; and ergotamine tartrate, 1 mg an hour before bedtime. If contraindicated by medical conditions, intolerant, or allergic, one may substitute lithium carbonate, 300 mg, twice daily, for verapamil. Chronic cluster headache patients are more apt to be treatment-resistant than are episodic types (resistant cases are often found among those who have a history of drug abuse, neurosis, or a history of treatment resis-

tance). Thus, it may be preferable to initiate prophylactic lithium and ergotamine tartrate, in all cases of chronic cluster headache.

Failure to significantly reduce attack frequency may require "triple therapy," that is, the combination of verapamil, lithium, and ergotamine. Continued nonresponse may require an increased dosage schedule. Some patients respond quite dramatically to sodium valproate, 1,000 to 1,500 mg daily, in divided doses, alone or in combination with other prophylactic medications.

Symptomatic Treatment. The most effective symptomatic treatment of cluster headache is oxygen inhalation. Properly administered, oxygen inhalation should abort over 90 percent of attacks, in over 90 percent of patients. This compares to success rates of approximately 50 percent with 4.0 percent in tranasal lidocaine solution, 75 to 80 percent for sublingual or inhaled ergotamine tartrate, or injected dihydroergotamine or sumatriptan. Oxygen inhalation, however, has the distinction of being the most inconvenient.

Achieving maximal success rates with oxygen requires the proper equipment and technique. A portable or "E" tank, flow-rate regulator, and face mask without rebreathing apparatus may be rented from a medical supply store. Tanks may be refilled when needed.

At the onset of an attack, the patient should be seated, bent forward with elbows on the knees and face mask held loosely against the face. The flow rate should be preset at 7 L/min. The patient should breathe normally until the attack is aborted, but for no longer than 20 minutes. If unsuccessful, oxygen inhalation may be repeated after a 5-minute break. "Back-to-back" attacks, which may be experienced on occasion, may be similarly treated.

PAROXYSMAL HEMICRANIA

Of all primary headache disorders, paroxysmal hemicrania (PH) is the most clinically similar to cluster headache. There are two types; chronic paroxysmal hemicrania (CPH) and the more recently described episodic type, EPH. These differ from cluster headache in sex distribution, ratio of episodic to chronic, attack frequency and duration, and response to medication. CPH and EPH are indistinguishable from cluster headache in pain intensity, quality, and location. They also share associated signs and symptoms. (Table 208-2.)

The sex distribution of PH favors women, but to what extent, remains unknown. There also appears to be a greater occurrence of chronic over episodic types, but this may be due to earlier reports which suggested that PH existed solely in a chronic state; many EPH cases were dismissed as "prechronic" states. It is true, however, that as with secondary chronic cluster headache, EPH may convert to CPH.

The frequency of attacks of CPH has been reported to range from 4 to 38 per day, with a mean frequency of 14 attacks; that of cluster headache is 1 to 15 per day, with a mean of 1 to 2 per day. The difficulty of distinguishing cluster headache from PH occurs when attack frequencies are at the high end in the former or at the low end in the latter. This difficulty is also encountered when considering the duration of attacks. In PH, attack duration is usually quite short; the duration in CPH has been reported to range from 3 to 46 minutes, with a mean of 13 minutes. The duration of attacks of cluster headache may range from 15 minutes to 3 hours, with a mean of 45 minutes.

The major distinguishing feature of PH from cluster headache is response to indomethacin. While there is the occasional cluster patient found to be responsive to indomethacin, all patients with PH respond to it dramatically. Thus, the sole efficacious prophylactic medication for CPH or EPH is indomethacin, 75 to 100 mg/day, in divided doses. Attacks are generally arrested within 24 hours from onset of treatment. The dosage may be subsequently reduced to a maintenance level of 25 to 50 mg/day.

SUMMARY

Cluster headache and paroxysmal hemicrania are primary headache disorders that are characterized by their stereotypic presentations and consistent responses to specific treatment modalities. These features allow the clinician to recognize and effectively treat such cases. Our knowledge of the pathophysiology of cluster headache, has provided insight into the more recently described paroxysmal hemicranias. In neither case, however, has the etiology of these conditions been elucidated.

In this presentation cluster headache has been classified, described clinically, and its pathogenesis briefly reviewed. Differential diagnosis of this condition, with particular attention to paroxysmal hemicrania, was discussed. Finally, the most efficacious prophylactic and symptomatic treatment modalities were described.

SUGGESTED READINGS

Ekbom K: A clinical comparison of cluster headache and migraine. Acta Neurol Scand 46(suppl 41):1–48, 1970

Gabel IJ, Spierings ELH: Prophylactic treatment of cluster headache with verapamil. Headache 29:167–8, 1989

Headache Classification Committee of the International Headache Society: Classification and diagnostic criteria for headache disorders, cranial neuralgias and facial pain. Cephalalgia 8(suppl 7):9–96, 1988

Kudrow L: The pathogenesis of cluster headache. Curr Opin Neurol 7:278–82, 1994

Kudrow L: Cluster Headache: Mechanisms and Management. Oxford University Press, London, 1980

Kudrow L, Kudrow DB: Association of sustained oxyhemoglobin desaturation and onset of cluster headache attacks. Headache 30:474–80, 1990

Moskowitz MA: The neurobiology of vascular head pain. Ann Neurol 16: 157–68, 1984

Sjaastad O: Chronic paroxysmal hemicrania: clinical aspects and controversies. In Blau JN (ed): Migraine: Clinical, Therapeutic, Conceptual and Research Aspects. pp. 135–52. Chapman and Hall, London, 1987.

209. PSYCHOLOGICAL TREATMENT OF HEADACHE

STEVEN M. BASKIN

Psychobiologic models of headache posit that conditions that control chronic headache are multidimensional, involving cognitive/emotional factors as well as biologic processes. These models suggest that the underlying mechanisms present at the onset of the disorder may not be viable with chronicity and/or the same conditions that maintain the disorder. Many patients exhibit difficulty coping (both psychologically and biologically) with intermittent headache and gradually transform to chronic daily headache, where behavioral events become important maintenance factors. Psychobiologic processes are interactive, with biology affecting behavior and physiologic/neurochemical mechanisms routinely modified by environmental influences and learning. It is important to abandon the organic/psychogenic distinction and begin to ask how psychological and learning factors influence head pain; eventually examining underlying physiologic and neurochemical actions. Comprehensive interdiscipline treatment programs have emerged from this psychobiologic model to address various factors within migraine and tension-type headache.

This chapter describes an integrated psychological approach from a perspective of self-regulation and coping skills for the control of migraine and tension-type headache. The first phase of this approach includes a thorough assessment with multiple types of data collection, including clinical interview and psychophysiologic evaluation to set treatment goals. The second phase is interventional. The patient is encouraged to become an active treatment participant and learns various skills and techniques that target different aspects of the headache problem (physiologic, emotional, and behavioral). Patient education is a strong component of the program.

ASSESSMENT

Clinical Interview

A key aspect of the interview is educational, as patients often have many misconceptions about head pain. Many patients have a fear of significant brain pathology or are terrified that the clinician thinks that their problem is psychogenic. These patients may distort their history in relation to their own naive conceptualization of headache and may omit or distort certain key points. Patients often have consulted with many other professionals as well as family members and friends. Some are taking many medications, either self-prescribed or prescribed by a physician, that have paradoxical effects on their headache frequency and response to treatment. Often, these patients report "daily" migraine headaches that are in fact rebound headaches secondary to overuse of analgesics, ergotamines, and/or caffeine.

During psychological interviewing, it is important to assess whether the patient is having more than one type of headache. Patients often refer to only one type of headache without accurately differentiating other headache types. These patients typically have had intermittent migraine over the years complicated by a daily constant headache between migraine attacks; chronic, often excessive analgesic use; and psychobiologic mechanisms. With chronicity exist complicated maintenance patterns that may be relatively autonomous from "original" causative factors.

It is important to establish the ages and circumstances of onset for each of these headache types (e.g., menarche, head trauma, psychological stress). Psychological events and environmental factors may play a role in headache onset as well as headache maintenance, and careful questioning about the number and types of recent life changes as well as quality of life issues may be helpful. Some migraine patients notice that their headaches increase during a poststress "letdown," often on vacations or weekends. Levels of daily minor stress are positively correlated with headache activity, and headache patients sometimes engage in maladaptive coping behaviors in managing stress or headache. Clinical levels of psychopathology are seldom (less than 10 percent) observed in the headache population. Some researchers believe that measures that assess stress, cognitive and behavioral strategies for coping with stress, and beliefs about headache and headache related disability may be more useful than measures of psychopathology per se. Individuals with an internal locus of control (believing they have the skills to regulate headache, mood, and so on) are more likely to benefit from psychological interventions.

It is important to notice any prodromal symptoms for headache attacks even if they are vague. It has been my impression that close observation of migraine prodromes often improves outcome for both pharmacologic and nonpharmacologic therapies.

An extensive medication history should be taken. It is important to assess exact dosages of medication to see if patients have had an adequate trial and if they adhered to the drug regimen. It is important to assess analgesic, ergotamine, and benzodiazepine ''rebound'' phenomena. These will often paradoxically perpetuate their headache disorder and will interfere with standard, usually effective, preventative pharmacologic and behavioral therapies. It is also important to assess medication regimen adherence/compliance. Many patients have difficulty with active treatment participation, do not maintain an empiric attitude, and are often called ''poor historians.'' Poor adherence obviously limits the effectiveness of pharmacotherapy for many headache patients. Studies have shown that over 50 percent of headache patients fail to properly adhere to drug treatment regimens. Ergotamine often presents special problems for patients with headache because the effective use of this drug requires complex self-management skills. Studies have shown that approximately 50 to 70 percent of migraine sufferers fail to make optimum use of ergotamine tartrate. This often requires complex skills of accurately identifying migraine onset, knowing when to take the medicine and how to pretreat with an antiemetic, and adhering to limits to prevent overuse syndromes. One study showed that 18 percent of patients in an hospital outpatient clinic never filled their prescriptions upon leaving the clinic. Therefore, during the interview, it is important to assess patient compliance and understanding of particular drug regimens. This is a significant medical and psychological issue, as there are many consequences of nonadherence, including progressive disability and dysfunction, development of secondary complications including overuse of analgesics, increased emergency room visits, unnecessary prescriptions of ''more potent'' medications, treatment failures, and problematic interactions with other medications. There are numerous reasons for nonadherence to regimens, including lack of insight, receiving poor instructions, psychiatric problems, misconceptions about headache and the treatment strategies, inappropriate expectations, sociocultural reasons, strong belief systems (e.g., ''I don't need medicine''), helplessness and pessimism, anger and dissatisfaction with previous health-care providers, financial issues, complexity of the therapy regimen, the amount of behavior change required, and management of drug side effects. Finally, many patients have had poor continuity of care, with numerous medicine changes and a long waiting time between appointments, with resulting confusion.

It is important to take an in-depth habit history, in particular, assessing alcohol, nicotine, and ''recreational'' drug use. The amount of caffeine ingested daily should be noted, as many patients believe that because many abortive migraine medications contain caffeine, increased consumption of caffeine will

have an antimigraine effect. It must be explained to them that significant daily caffeine consumption increases the frequency of headache because of caffeine withdrawal and also has an anxiety-inducing effect. An exercise history is taken with the goal of getting patients gradually into an aerobic exercise program.

It is important to obtain a family history of headache, psychiatric disorder, and alcoholism/drug abuse. The clinician must thoroughly but subtly evaluate the symptoms of major depression as well as anxiety disorder. Often, it is helpful to ask about psychological problems as secondary to the headache problem. It is helpful to determine the psychological background as well as the general coping style of the patient. Careful questioning about family and marital functioning, occupational history, social/environmental stressors, abuse issues, disability, activity level, and general coping skills is helpful. It is also important to look at pain behaviors such as operant and respondent learning factors. In an operant model, the relationship of pain behavior to its consequences is important. It is important to see how family members attend to a patient's pain behavior and how the patient exhibits that behavior including any avoidance learning. Also, in the operant model, the reinforcing consequences of certain medications should be noted. In the respondent conditioning or classic conditioning model, biologic responses can be conditioned to all stimuli that are associated with painful stimulation. Therefore, some headache sufferers develop almost phobic reactions to the occurrence of intermittent severe headache.

Psychophysiologic Evaluation

Psychophysiologic evaluation is the second phase of the assessment after the clinical interview. This typically involves a physiologic stress profile, a diagnostic muscle scan, and sometimes a dynamic movement assessment to help identify certain physiologic/sensory targets for psychological intervention. A stress profile evaluates generalized arousal (some combination of electrodermal response, heart rate, and respiration dynamics), skeletal muscle responses (frontotemporal, masseter, trapezius), and smooth muscle/vascular changes (finger temperature, temporal pulse amplitude) in response to a variety of conditions. These include adaptation, baseline, mental and physical stressors, recovery, and relaxation. This profile is a clinical measure of autonomic reactivity.

A static muscle scan utilizes surface electrode electromyography (EMG) to assess different skeletal muscles in two positions, sitting and standing. Muscles assessed include frontalis, temporalis, masseter, sternocleidomastoid, cervical paraspinals, upper trapezius, and T1 paraspinals. These data are compared with normative data. This type of assessment is also helpful in identifying bracing and guarding behavior that may be problematic, although often secondary to headache. It is also helpful to assess muscular responses during dynamic movements, including mandibular range of motion, neck and shoulder movements, isometric contractions, and functional postural analysis. Many patients show diffuse hyperactivity and co-contraction of numerous muscles in the region.

There is much inconsistency and controversy in the literature concerning psychophysiologic profiling in headache. Although I endorse the primacy of neurogenic events in both migraine and tension-type headache, there appears to be a subgroup of patients with significant peripheral findings. In order to adequately look at EMG responses, one needs to look at baseline, peak contraction responses, recovery speed, symmetry, agonist/ antagonist, and synergist relationships. Therefore, there are so many data points that it is difficult to truly assess the role of muscle contraction in tension-type headache. Overall, there is a lack of consistent findings between measures of scalp and cervical surface EMG and headache levels in tension-type headache. However, I believe it is clinically useful for an individual patient to help identify certain sensory targets for intervention and any psychophysiologic stress-related aspects. Also, over the years, biofeedback therapies have incorporated some of the postural and movement evaluations that have come from physical medicine.

TREATMENT

Intervention proceeds from the detailed initial assessment. The program is built on a coping skills model, in which undifferentiated head pain is reduced to smaller and more manageable components that are susceptible to psychological intervention. This type of model helps self-regulation and increases a patient's sense of mastery and control. Even in strictly pharmacologic interventions, these coping skills can be important.

Psychological and pharmacologic treatments are ofen combined in order to provide a comprehensive multifaceted treatment program. The program is composed of (1) education about the causes, triggers, and treatment of headache in order to help the patient become an active participant and (2) coping skills that foster self-regulation, with a sensory and a reactive component. This coping skills model assumes that therapeutic gains are partially the result of changes in sensations, feelings, perceptions, and thought processes that accompany acute or chronic headache. The sensory component involves the patient's learning to control various physiologic responses. The reactive component is a combination of cognitive-behavioral interventions that examine and help change certain actions, thoughts, attitudes, expectations, and emotional states that may lead to problematic behavior, lowered pain threshold, and heightened levels of sympathetic arousal. Participation is encouraged, allowing the patient to assume partial responsibility for their treatment with individually tailored treatment strategies. This program exists in a series of appointments after the initial evaluation. The absolute number of sessions is determined by clinical considerations and is typically fewer than 15 appointments.

Education

A detailed educational program is undertaken, on the premise that headache is determined by a complicated interplay of biologic and psychological factors. These explanations may include headache predisposition, including genetic and familial aspects, biochemical factors, the physiology and psychology of the stress response, dietary factors, biologic rhythm factors, and relevant cognitive, emotional, and behavioral mechanisms. It is emphasized that the conditions that control chronic headache are multidimensional, and a rationale is given for psychological as well as pharmacologic management. Patients are taught that the conditions that lead to a disorder are often not the same as the conditions that maintain the disorder. Sensory and physiologic responses, biochemical events, and cognitive/emotional elements may be part of the maintenance process of chronic head pain.

Traditionally accepted myths regarding "perfectionistic" personality traits in headache are examined and exposed as untrue in the aggregate. It is important to educate the patient about the process of time-limited, goal-oriented psychological interventions. These treatments are very different from many patients' beliefs that psychological treatment involves long-term "reconstructive" psychotherapy.

Patients are taught to keep a headache calendar that is brought to each treatment session. The patient is taught how to self-monitor the frequency, intensity, and duration of each headache. Patients also monitor the type and amount of medications taken, both prescription and over-the-counter, as well as relief factors, environmental triggers (if known), and menstrual days. These calendars generate important data, help with outcome research, and are easy and efficient to use, given an adequate format. There is a relatively low correlation between self-report and objective calendar data; when pharmacologic treatment is based only on self-report, a practitioner can sometimes change medication orders without adequate information.

Skills Acquisition

A variety of factors may act as triggers for headache. These vary from person to person. Some individuals are affected by such factors as diet, sleep rhythm changes, acute stress, chronic stress, exertional factors, hormonal factors, or fasting and skipping meals, among others.

When appropriate, patients are put on an elimination diet to limit foods that have been shown to trigger headaches (Table 209-1). However, in line with a coping skills model, patients are encouraged to empirically validate this list for themselves, as dietary modification may be of limited benefit for many patients. Patients are taught that a variety of factors may act as headache triggers and they are given some general "hints" to help with headache control. They are encouraged to maintain consistent biologic rhythms, such as keeping to normal sleep–wake patterns, even on weekends. They are advised to eat nutritious meals at regular intervals without fasting for long periods, and to reduce their intake of caffeine and alcoholic

TABLE 209-1. Elimination Diet: Foods To Be Avoided[a]

Chocolate
Canned Figs
Nuts
Peanut butter
Onions
Pizza
Sour cream
Yogurt
Herring
Chicken livers
Avocado
Nutrasweet

Ripened cheeses (cheddar, Gruyère, Brie, Camembert, etc.); cheeses that are permissible are American, cottage, cream, and Velveeta
Vinegar; however, white vinegar is permissible
Anything that is fermented, pickled, or marinated
Hot, fresh breads; raised coffeecakes; doughnuts (due to activated yeast)
Pods of broad beans (lima, navy, and pea pods)
Monosodium glutamate—any foods containing large amounts (Chinese foods)
Citrus fruits (example: no more than 1 orange per day)
Bananas (no more than one-half a banana per day)
Pork—limit intake
Tea, coffee, cola beverages (excessive amounts)
Fermented sausage (bologna, salami, pepperoni, summer sausage, and hot dogs)
Alcoholic beverages: *to be avoided if possible;* of all possible food triggers for migraine, alcohol is most frequently cited

[a] It is recommended that the patient begin with a total elimination of the above for 1 month. If there occurs a decrease in frequency or severity of headache, foods may be slowly reintroduce *one* at a time and the effect observed. If headache increases, that food should be eliminated and the patient should continue to reintroduce foods one at a time.

beverages. Patients are helped to set behavioral goals, such as increasing pleasurable activities, decreasing "downtime," increasing aerobic exercise, and using time management. Aspects of the "type A" behavior pattern are assessed, including time urgency and hostility components, which often place excessive demands on the patient and those around them.

Brief educational interventions help better manage medication adherence and compliance. As stated previously, studies suggest that over 50 percent of chronic headache sufferers fail to adhere properly to drug regimens. Headache-abortive agents are often not optimally used, and noncompliance sometimes creates "rebound" phenomena, limiting the effectiveness of preventative interventions. Brief educational interventions, using a self-instruction model, will increase adherence to abortive medication regimens. These brief, time-limited meetings with health-care professionals — other than the prescribing physician — are helpful in teaching the complex self-management skills needed to maximize therapeutic gains. These interventions teach patients how to use a trial-and-error experimental approach in order to assess drug effectiveness. Patients are taught how to accurately identify migraine onset, to keep medication readily available, and to have clear written instructions as to dosage, repeating dosage, pretreatment with an antiemetic (if needed to limit nausea), and other necessary factors for adherence. Medication limits are set and patients are instructed to self-monitor with a headache calendar. It is important to take into account the patient's lifestyle in any drug regimen. Complex therapy regimens require complex behavioral repetoires in order to best manage side effects. Many patients on tricyclic antidepressants have a hard time with fatigue and soporific side effects and can often be managed relatively easily with modification in drug regimen (e.g., earlier dosing, slower titration). However, many of these patients are lost to follow-up when they stop taking a medication secondary to these side effects. Many patients need to be instructed about the "time lag" between beginning a medication and the onset of therapeutic gain. It is important to call a patient if an appointment is missed and to increase visits when headache control remains difficult. The involvement of spouses or significant others may enhance compliance with complex drug regimens. Thus, brief self-instruction training with the patient, including complete written instructions for headache-abortive drug regimens, specific drug titration schedules for prophylactic medications, and strategies for side effect management will increase drug therapy effectiveness.

In a coping-skills model to foster self-regulation of headache, patients learn to intervene on two components—sensory and reactive. The sensory component consists of the physical precursors to and the sensation of pain and teaches the patient to control various physiologic responses determined by both central and peripheral mechanisms. The reactive component is cognitive and affective and consists of thoughts and feelings that often precede or accompany headache attacks. Strategies that treat the reactive component of the "pain experience" help enhance pain tolerance and alter pain perception. In many of these chronic patients, the disorder has acquired a "life of its own." Environmental triggers become less important as the frequency of headache increases from intermittent to continuous. Some of the techniques discussed here were developed from the psychological literature on pain tolerance (Table 209-2).

The initial sessions of treatment are directed toward the sensory component, using relaxation exercises and biofeedback training to learn physiologic self-regulation. Later sessions focus on the thoughts and feelings that accompany headache—one's "internal dialogue"—and contribute to increased headache susceptibility. Biofeedback means biologic or physiologic feedback. Biofeedback facilitates self-regulation. The patient gains information about biologic processes that are normally out of his or her awareness, and learns to bring them more under voluntary control. This feedback may be visual and/or auditory and, via training, physiologic responses are "shaped" in the most adaptive directions (e.g., decreased muscle tension and increased finger temperature). Biofeedback also helps the patient to feel more in control of his or her internal environment. The type of training and sites used are based on the psychophysiologic evaluation. Biofeedback is a learning-based therapy, and thus cannot be applied where that process is impaired. Significant psychiatric problems, in which concentration and cognition are impaired or depression is severe, are relative contraindications until the disorders are adequately treated.

The biofeedback program is a step-by-step skill-building approach over a series of sessions (Table 209-3). Each step must be mastered before moving to the next one. EMG feedback is the most commonly used type of biofeedback in tension-type headache; it is done via the application of surface electrodes across various skeletal muscle groups. Thermal biofeedback, or hand temperature training, to increase peripheral blood flow is the most common type of biofeedback in migraine. EMG biofeedback therapy programs tend to move from general relaxation to more specific musculoskeletal training. For example, some programs teach EMG "functional" training of various muscle groups. For the upper trapezius muscle, they tend to teach various dynamic movements, including shoulder shrug and relaxation, shoulder abduction and relaxation, shoulder rotations and relaxation, and numerous postural changes all,

TABLE 209-2. Pain Tolerance

High Pain Tolerance	Low Pain Tolerance
Pain is perceived as a challenge that patient can control	Pain is perceived as an ordeal, with patient exhibiting much helplessness and "catastrophizing"
Patient orientation is task-specific, breaking down responses to manageable target behaviors	Patient is fatalistic
Patient exhibits action-oriented self-talk ("I have a plan of action") and sets realistic goals	Patient shows increased negative comments about self and ability to deal with pain; self-talk is often composed of "suffering" or "hope" without an action orientation

TABLE 209-3. Relaxation/Biofeedback Program

Step 1: Body awareness/diaphragmatic breathing

Step 2: Progressive muscle relaxation exercises and home practice with auditory tapes, electromyograms are monitored, as are respiration and finger temperature

Step 3: Passive relaxation using imagery and breathing as relaxation cues, with electromyography, respiration, and finger temperature monitor

Step 4: Scalp and facial relaxation/neck and shoulder relaxation, using electromyographic monitor

Step 5: Dynamic movement exercises of neck and shoulder with electromyographic monitor

Step 6: Smooth muscle relaxation, using autogenic phrases with thermal (hand-warming) biofeedback

Step 7: Generalization exercises

guided by EMG instrumentation. EMG functional training of facial and scalp muscles attempts to enhance the recovery of relaxation following a 10-second muscle contraction. Also, discrimination training can be helpful when patients are taught to attempt to discriminate differences between high, medium, and low levels of muscle contraction across different skeletal muscles. These programs tend to merge physical medicine approaches with general relaxation therapies, as they incorporate shoulder girdle and neck-stretching exercises with general muscle relaxation, all guided by EMG biofeedback instrumentation. Patients use generalization or "mini-exercises" throughout the day in order to heighten body awareness and increase muscle relaxation. A goal over time, other than a reduction of symptoms, is the eventual limitation of the need for biofeedback instruments via internal feedback mechanisms and the development of the ability to generalize the responses to the natural environment. Patients are taught to look for signs of tension throughout the day and to recognize when they are contracting muscles. Practicing these mini-exercises increases body awareness and leads to more "automatic" muscle relaxation.

In thermal biofeedback, a superficial thermistor is attached to a patient's index finger. Superficial skin temperature is largely determined by volume of blood flow to the area, as both blood flow and skin temperature usually change together. Some researchers believe that the mode of action of thermal biofeedback (hand warming) is a general decrease in sympathetic tone secondary to a retraining of the autonomic nervous system.

Since the mid-1980s, there have been several reviews of the biofeedback literature for both migraine and tension-type headache. Although many different biofeedback techniques are used, no single intervention has emerged as clearly more efficacious than any other. In biofeedback therapy, there has not been shown to be high correlations between the target physiologic response and headache outcome, especially in the EMG data. Outcome data is relatively good and, according to some studies, similar to that for single-pharmacologic interventions. The effects appear to be maintained over long-term follow-up, and positive changes in psychological state may also occur. My own view on EMG training in biofeedback parallels that of Jean Schoenen and his group (1991). Schoenen has shown that EMG levels of pericranial muscles are not significantly correlated with headache severity. Also, multiple EMG recording sites on pericranial, facial, and neck muscles are necessary in order to show that patients with chronic tension-type headache have increased EMG levels in relation to controls. However, EMG recordings of these muscles are of little diagnostic usefulness in headache patients. Also, as stated previously, there appears to be a weak correlation between improvement on headache calendar and maximal reduction of EMG level on various muscle groups. It is very likely that EMG biofeedback in chronic tension-type headache works less on peripheral mechanisms and more on the limbic input to the brainstem and its relays.

In the reactive component of treatment, patients learn to identify and modify maladaptive styles of thinking via cognitive therapy. Cognitive therapies emphasize the role of thoughts, belief systems, evaluations, and appraisals in influencing emotional states and behavior. Cognitive techniques are aimed at providing patients with a set of problem-solving and coping skills that can be used in a wide range of situations that trigger and maintain headache.

Distress-related cognitions and negative self-talk ("Why

me?"; "I can't believe I'm getting another migraine"; "It's no use") mediate poor outcome via a variety of mechanisms, including decreased mood, increased anxiety, and poor compliance, as in overuse of pain medications and tranquilizers. Patients are taught that this "reactive" component can be treated with coping strategies to help them actively "challenge" counterproductive automatic thinking processes. The clinician attempts to get the individual to increase a sense of control and to view pain as a challenge to be met rather than to become helpless.

Individuals with low pain tolerance make more negative comments about themselves and their ability to deal with pain. They tend to magnify the negative aspects of the entire situation, becoming fatalistic and appearing helpless. They focus on suffering and often look for the "magic pill" to take their pain away. These patients are taught self-statements to help develop alternative cognitive responses to the experience of recurrent severe pain or chronic, unremitting pain.

A form of cognitive therapy called self-instructional training involves approaching headache as a problem that can be solved and reducing global aspects into smaller, more manageable components. These self-instructions help the patient rehearse adaptive cognitive and behavioral responses to, for example, the development of a migraine. This involves a cognitive process in which the patient learns to appraise the nature of the problem and to develop task-relevant skills to manage the problem and reduce anxiety features that lead to symptom magnification. Self-instructions are broken down into (1) preparation for an attack, (2) managing initial symptoms, (3) handling critical moments, and (4) post-headache.

Migraine and tension-type headache can be significantly influenced by the patient's cognitive actions and reactions in dealing with the symptoms themselves. It is helpful to train patients to become keen observers and to be "prepared" to cope adaptively with the headache without being hypervigilant to pain sensations. Through classical conditioning, individuals associate numerous prodromal sensations with migraine, an intermittent, often unpredictable disorder, which often leads to fear responses. Therefore, many patients exhibit irrational ideation about loss of control or perceived threat of a future feared event and underestimate their coping skills. They frequently misinterpret bodily sensations and "catastrophize." One important aspect in cognitive treatment of these anxiety-related features is to help the patient accurately interpret and react to perceived danger signals with rational self-statements as per the forementioned self-instructional model. Patients use the following sequence of self-talk:

> What is it I have to do? What does the situation require? What strategies can I use? I will follow my plan, one step at a time. I can handle the attack, use many strategies, and take appropriate medicines at the appropriate amount and time. Just focus on what the situation requires, without worrying. I can use my relaxation skills and keep things under control without creating a catastrophe. Remember, I have many strategies to use if I stay focused. The last time, I did well, used my skills, and had only a small amount of time that I could not function. I am getting better at managing these attacks.

Patients with chronic daily headache who have completed our inpatient program do very well with this cognitive behavioral approach, as it appears to help in relapse prevention. As patients begin to have more clearheaded periods, these strategies help increase adherence to drug regimens and reduce headache-related distress at the time of an acute attack.

There are also some cognitive coping skills that increase pain tolerance via attention diversion. These are attention-based distraction exercises, frequently used in chronic pain programs that have been adapted for headache treatment. It is helpful to encourage patients to focus attention outside of themselves, away from the thought of pain, to—for example—music, photos, children, and so forth. Distraction can be helpful when patients focus on future plans (e.g., plan a vacation) and recall past enjoyable events from their personal history. Patients may also learn to make a mental movie of relaxing images incompatible with pain. Attentional strategies can also help a patient visualize success, in spite of the pain, as they overcome obstacles. High-pain–tolerance individuals view increased headache as a challenge to be met, that they will eventually exercise some degree of control. They believe they can alter the pain experiences by actively engaging in some type of coping strategy, including attention diversion. Data suggest that many of these coping strategies are more effective with episodic headache even when frequent, rather than with continuous pain.

Recent research has shown a comorbidity of migraine and depression. Some headache patients require cognitive therapy for depression. This involves modifying a patient's internal dialogue that predisposes the patient to helplessness and self-blame with an expectation of uncontrollability of future events. It is a time course-limited psychotherapeutic approach with proven efficacy, and it integrates well with pharmacologic therapies for depression. These cognitive behavioral therapies help the headache patient incorporate a variety of problem-solving skills to become an "active" collaborator with the health-care professional. These techniques are invaluable for patients with complex headache problems.

SUGGESTED READINGS

Andrasik F: Psychological and behavioral aspects of chronic headache. pp. 961–76. In Mathew NT (ed): Neurologic Clinics. WB Saunders, Philadelphia 1990

Bakal DA: The Psychobiology of Chronic Headache. Springer-Verlag, New York, 1982

Baskin SM, Weeks RE: The nonpharmacological treatment of migraine. pp. 107–13. In Tollison CD, Kunkel RS (eds): Headache. Williams & Wilkins, Baltimore, 1993

Blanchard EB: Psychological treatment of benign headache disorders. J Consult Clin Psychol 60:537–51, 1992

Cram JR: EMG muscle scanning and diagnostic manual for surface recordings. pp. 1–141. In Cram JR (ed): Clinical EMG for Surface Recordings. Vol. 2. Clinical Resources, Seattle, 1990

Flor H, Turk DC: Psychophysiology of chronic pain: do chronic pain patients exhibit symptom-specific psychophysiological responses? Psychol Bull 105:215–59, 1989

Holroyd KA, Cordingley GE, Pingel JD et al: Enhancing the effectiveness of abortive therapy: a controlled evaluation of self-management training. Headache 29:148–53, 1989

Holroyd KA, Nash JM, Pingel JD et al: A comparison of pharmacological (amitriptyline HCL) and nonpharmacological (cognitive-behavioral) therapies for chronic tension headaches. J Consult Clin Psychol 59:387–93, 1991

Meichenbaum D, Turk D: Facilitating Treatment Adherence: A Practitioner's Guidebook. Plenum, New York, 1987

Packard RC, O'Connel R: Medication compliance among headache patients. Headache 26:416–19, 1986

Schoenen J: Tension-type headache: pathophysiologic evidence for a disturbance of "limbic" pathways of the brain stem. Headache 20:314–5, 1990

Schoenen J, Gerard P, DePasqua V, Sianard-Gainko J: Multiple clinical and paraclinical analyses of chronic tension-type headache associated or unassociated with disorder of pericranial muscles. Cephalalgia 11:135–9, 1991

Taylor W: Dynamic EMG biofeedback in assessment and treatment using a neuromuscular re-education model. pp. 175–96. In Cram JR (ed): Clinical EMG for Surface Recordings: Vol. 2. Clinical Resources, Seattle, 1990

SECTION 3. SPECIAL HEADACHE PROBLEMS

210. POST-TRAUMATIC HEADACHE

WILLIAM G. SPEED

Ninety percent of cases of nervous system trauma are caused by injuries to the head, and in 30 percent of these cases, the trauma results in chronic headache and other post-traumatic symptoms. Unfortunately, the symptomatology of these impairments is often subtle and may not be recognized by the primary physician. The term *chronic post-traumatic headache* is used when the headache has persisted for more than 2 months after the injury. Many other chronic symptoms can also develop as a result of traumatic brain injury. The presence of such symptoms, with or without chronic headache, constitutes post-traumatic syndrome. The following is a partial list of symptoms that may be found in post-traumatic syndrome:

- Impaired short-term memory
- Impaired concentration
- Fatiguability
- Outbursts of anger ("short fuse")
- Depression and/or frustration
- Irritability
- Insomnia
- Lightheadedness and/or vertigo

PATHOGENESIS

Over the centuries, it has been recognized that closed-head injuries may produce headache and/or other symptomatology, but these symptoms were long attributed to psychological states rather than to structural and/or neurochemical impairment of the brain resulting from injury. Exactly how these structural or other findings relate to the symptoms produced as a result of head injury at the biochemical or cellular level remains to be

TABLE 210-1. Historical Summary of the Findings That Established the Organic Basis of Post-traumatic Headache and Syndrome

1941: In cats, it was shown that less force is needed to produce concussion when the head is free to move than when it is fixed.

1943: Using gelatin models of the brain, it was shown that acceleration of the brain was the force producing neurologic dysfunction, as opposed to impact itself.

1944: In guinea pigs, it was shown that there was structural alteration of the brain and loss of brain cells after closed-injury concussion.

1945: Guinea pigs with closed-injury concussion showed poor performance in maze-running tests.

1946: Observations using Lucite skulls in monkeys showed that there is significant brain movement on acceleration of the head.

1968: Widely scattered microglial clusters and axonal retraction balls (evidence of nerve damage) were found in humans following head injury.

1969: Nerve fiber degeneration in cerebral hemispheres and brainstem was found in humans in mild as well as severe head trauma.

1983: In cats, minor head injury produced extensive axonal injury, both anatomic and physiologic.

demonstrated. Table 210-1 gives a historical summary of the findings that led to the current concept of the organicity of the post-traumatic headache and syndrome.

DIAGNOSIS

Investigators of closed-head injury have found evidence of brain malfunction in some, but not all, closed-head-injured animals or humans consisting of (1) slowing of cerebral circulation lasting for months or years, (2) altered vasomotor regulation, (3) abnormal brain evoked potentials, and (4) altered neurotransmitter function. With the exception of brain evoked potentials, there are no other clinically practical tests in these areas. These combinations of structural and functional evidence of brain abnormalities lends strong supportive evidence to an organic brain damage concept of the post-traumatic syndrome, as opposed to a primary psychological disturbance. In addition, the symptoms experienced by these patients are so stereotyped from one patient to another that it highly suggests a common denominator—again, most likely of organic origin, resulting from the head injury.

Elicitation of an appropriate medical history is absolutely essential for physicians to understand patients with this problem. This history should include the following:

1. A complete description of the nature of the injury, consisting of how the patient felt immediately after the injury, and the status of the headache at that time, if that is part of the complaint when the patient is seen

2. Location of the headache (there may be various areas involved rather than one)

3. Variations in intensity of the headache

4. Duration of the headache (most of these will be constant, but when they are not, the variable duration rates should be noted)

5. Factors that aggravate or improve the headache

6. Characteristics of the pain (e.g., aching, throbbing, pounding, boring, pressure and so on)

7. Presence or absence of neurologic symptoms and their time relationship to the headache, if any

8. Presence or absence of symptoms associated with post-traumatic syndrome, as has been described above, and obtain the time factors after the injury when these were first noted by the patient.

A complete neurologic and musculoskeletal examination including the neck, as well as the presence or absence of tender-

ness over the occipital neurovascular bundle at the occipital ridge, is an important part of the evaluation. Blood counts, chemistries, and urinalysis are appropriate to obtain, but the results are usually found to be within normal limits. An electrocardiogram should be done because many of the medications used to treat these headaches may have an impact on the cardiovascular system. Imaging of the head, either by contrast-enhanced computed tomography scan or magnetic resonance imaging, should be undertaken if it has not been prior to your evaluation. Although results of imaging of the head will almost always prove to be normal, it is important to know that one is dealing with a clear playing field. Note that normal test results in these individuals in no way exclude the presence of underlying brain damage as a result of the injury. The fact is, with our relatively insensitive testing techniques, for most patients with symptomatic post-traumatic headache, there will not be positive test findings to support an organic basis for their complaints, but you will be relying on your skills as a clinician to support your diagnosis. The use of neuropsychological testing may or may not prove to be useful. Some of the symptoms are sufficiently obvious that no further help is needed to identify them, but in some patients with subtle symptomatology, resorting to such testing may be appropriate. Headache following closed-head injuries occurs, for the most part, immediately at the time of injury or within 24 hours thereof. Occasionally, there may appear to be a delay in the development of headache of up to 2 weeks following the injury, possibly because of significant memory deficit, impairment of concentration, and severe significant pain in other parts of the body, which in itself may prevent the patient's recognition of less severe pain in the head.

Chronic post-traumatic headache may mimic any of the chronic headache disorders. They are most likely to be constant, but at times they may be intermittent daily. They may involve any areas of the head (e.g., frontal, temporal, ocular, retroocular, parietal, vertex, occipital, and/or posterior cervical) singly, or in various combinations, or all of them together. Some of these headaches may be described as broad bands around the head, or as an ache deep inside the head, but more often they are described variously as aching, pressing, squeezing, burning, stabbing, expanding, and/or throbbing or pounding. They may be aggravated by jarring the head, bending over, coughing, sneezing, straining, exposure to lights, loud noises, physical exertion, alcohol, stress, or anxiety. These headaches are indistinguishable from those seen in the nontraumatic population of headaches, which include chronic tension-type, migraine, combinations of these, and, in rare instances, cluster headaches. The neck is frequently involved, producing what is called cervicogenic headache. It is common for the occipital neurovascular bundle to be tender to digital pressure where it goes over the occipital ridge.

MANAGEMENT

The management of post-traumatic headache is fundamentally the same regardless of the type of headache. Although there are no scientifically controlled double-blinded studies to determine the effectiveness of the low vasoactive–substance diet, the diet is certainly easy to implement and follow, and it appears, from long-term experience with these patients, to be effective. These vasoactive substances are tyramine, phenylethylamine, monosodium glutamate, sodium nitrate, or sodium nitrite. Foods containing one or more of these substances are chocolate, aged cheese, coffee, tea, citrus fruits and their juice (oranges, lemons, limes, and grapefruit), nuts, avocados, canned figs, chicken livers, onions, alcohol, bananas, pickled herring, yogurt, hot dogs, and fermented sausage (bologna, salami, and pepperoni).

There are many pharmacotherapeutic measures that are useful either singly or in various combinations:

1. Tricyclic compounds (amitriptyline, imipramine, doxepin, nortriptyline, asendin, ludiomil) and related compound (trazodone, fluoxetine, sertraline)
2. β-blockers (propranolol, metaprolol, nadalol, timolol, atenolol)
3. Monamine oxidase inhibitors (phenelzine sulfate [Nardil] and tranylcypramine [parnate])—it is essential that these compounds be employed only by physicians thoroughly familiar with their use; used properly, they are quite safe, but used improperly, they can cause death
4. Methysergide, cyproheptadine
5. Calcium channel-blockers (diltiazem, verapamil, nefedipine)
6. Dihydroergotamine (DHE45) and sumatriptan
7. Valproic acid
8. Ergonovine (not now available from pharmaceutical firms but can be mixed by a compounding pharmacist) or methylergonovine (which is available)

It is common, if there are no contraindications—such as the presence of asthma, the presence of significant neurologic manifestations of migraine, or a history of heart failure—to begin with a β-blocker combined with a tricyclic compound. Any one of the tricyclics or β-blockers may be used in combination, beginning with modest doses and gradually increasing, if needed, to the point of tolerance or maximum therapeutic allowance. I frequently begin with metoprolol 100 mg bid, and amitriptyline 25 mg qhs. If there is no response, the metoprolol may be increased gradually, perhaps at weekly intervals, to a relative maximum of 200 mg bid. Amitriptyline is increased by 25 mg every fourth night, to 75 mg qhs. Then after 2 or 3 weeks, at perhaps weekly intervals, this may be increased by 25 mg to a maximum of 150 mg qhs. Obviously, these suggestions are indicated only if there are no side effects such as—but not limited to—fatigue, sleepiness, or lightheadedness on standing (perhaps indicating a drop in blood pressure or a significant bradycardia). Some patients may not tolerate certain β-blockers or certain tricyclics (or related compounds). It is always worthwhile to explore other combinations within these groups of medications if good results are not obtained or poor tolerance is experienced.

If no beneficial results are obtained with these medications, one may wish, before leaving this group of medications, to add a monamine oxidase inhibitor, preferably beginning with phenelzine sulfate (Nardil). It may be used with any combination of the β-blockers and tricyclic compounds except for imipramine. Always add Nardil to this combination; do not do the reverse. Patients must be warned verbally and in writing that they must adhere to a low tyramine diet (the one described above is fine), and that they cannot use any sympathomimetic drugs, including over-the-counter nose drops, eye drops, and decongestant cold medications. They cannot use meperidine or morphine or related compounds, although codeine and hydrocodone are acceptable. To play it absolutely safe, I advise all my patients to call my office before using any over-the-counter medication on their own or before taking any medication prescribed by other physicians. Surprisingly, some physicians are

unaware of the potential serious interactions of some medications with Nardil. It is better overkill the safety factor than it is to have a regrettable error occur. A patient who understands and is forewarned will not have serious problems with this combination of medications. One can tell within 3 weeks whether this combination is going to be helpful; it may be discontinued in an appropriate manner if the headaches are not helped by then.

There are no solid guidelines concerning the order in which one may use the various medications. Calcium channel-blockers are also frequently helpful. They could be added to the β-blockers and tricyclic compounds or used alone. Only experience can give one a feel for how to make this determination. Either verapamil or diltiazem are equally effective, and sometimes one is tolerated better than the other. Long-acting forms make it easier for the patient to remember to take the medication, a problem that is not unusual in the post-traumatic headache patient. Long-acting drugs are more expensive but may still be more appropriate in that form. Remember that the headache response to the calcium channel-blockers is slow and may take up to 4 to 6 weeks to become manifest, so patients should be apprised of the need to have patience.

Methysergide (Sansert) is a useful and relatively safe medication to try. Although it may produce fibroproliferative effects, this phenomenon is not common and any significant problems related to this can usually be avoided by carefully monitoring the patient over time. Also avoid using it in patients who have cardiac murmurs or bruits, as the existence of these makes it difficult to assess changes in the cardiovascular system due to the medication. Sansert is a 2-mg tablet usually given three times a day. If no response is seen within 3 weeks, it is unlikely that further use will be effective. If good response does occur, then follow the manufacturer's guidelines for long-term use.

Sumatriptan (Imitrex) is not usually of benefit when post-traumatic headache is chronic. Even though it may relieve the headache, it will be only temporary, and another injection will soon be needed. This medication also has rebound properties and its use therefore should be limited to no more than 2 days a week. For this reason, it is not usually a satisfactory medication for this variety of headaches.

DHE45, on the other hand, may at times play a role in the management of this problem. The rebound phenomenon has never been seen with the use of this medication. For this reason, it is occasionally worth a try to give intramuscular DHE45 once or twice a day for a few days to assess its effectiveness. If good control is accomplished, then relatively long-term use may be justified, provided the patient is carefully followed. It is easy to teach patients the technique for self-administration.

Valproic acid should be started at a low dose, increasing the dose slowly in order to lessen possible gastrointestinal side effects. Begin with 125 mg bid for 1 week, and then increase to 125 mg tid, increase by 125-mg doses every third day if tolerated, to a maximum of 500 mg tid. It may take 1 month to 6 weeks to ascertain whether this medication is effective. Liver function should be determined before starting this medication and at occasional intervals thereafter.

Ergonovine or methylergonovine is used at 0.2 mg tid; if there is no response in a few days, the dose may be increased to 0.4 mg tid. It only takes 1 week or so to determine whether this is effective. If it is, then patients should be checked initially at 6-week to 2-month intervals, particularly for peripheral circulation. Ergot rebound has not been reported with these medications; if good response is obtained they may be continued for long periods.

Recently, physicians have begun to seriously look at the use of long-acting analgesics for those patients who continue to have chronic headache of sufficient degree to interfere with the ability to function with any appreciable degree or have a reasonable quality of life and who have shown no substantial improvement with the usual forms of management. This concept goes against the grain of everything that physicians have been taught regarding the proper use of narcotic medication in patients with nonterminal chronic pain syndromes. It appears, however, that this form of therapy in these special circumstances is safe, and seldom, if ever, results in addiction. As long as the dose is kept below that which causes sleepiness or sluggishness, and there is no evidence for the need to continue to increase the dose over time and the patient shows a significant improvement, there does not appear to be any logical reason, medical or otherwise, why a physician should not try this approach. Currently, however, it should be considered a last-ditch alternative to try to help these individuals whose quality of life has been destroyed by this devastating disorder. It should be used only in patients who are not taking any other form of analgesic medication. MS Contin or methadone may be used. MS Contin may be started at 15 mg bid and slowly increased to 15 mg tid or qid if required for relief. I am not happy with higher doses, but a few of our patients have been given up to 30 mg tid. This increase in dose given with the condition that there is no sleepiness, sluggishness, or other side effects. Methadone may also be used, starting with 2.5 mg bid and working up slowly, if needed, to 5 mg qid. Not enough experience with these medications in the chronic headache patient has been accumulated to be any more specific than this, but it does appear at this time that some patients treated in this way will be returned to a functional state. Further experience with these medications may ultimately alter the information given here. No analgesic rebound has yet been seen with this treatment.

Analgesic rebound, however, is an important part of many chronic headache syndromes, and this is certainly true of the chronic post-traumatic headache. It is well established that the frequent use of short-acting analgesics is likely to feed the headache mechanism in such a way as to perpetuate the headache itself, even though short-term temporary relief may occur, and also to interfere, probably totally, with any appropriate therapeutic management. Many physicians treating headache believe that taking analgesics more often than 2 days a week is likely to produce the analgesic rebound phenomenon. It does not seem to matter what the analgesic medication is or how low the dose may be; if the patient is taking something of this nature more than 2 days a week, be suspicious of this syndrome. It is likely that everything—from ibuprofin to aspirin to acetaminophen to meperidine to morphine, and so on—may produce this condition. It is imperative that all analgesics be discontinued if good response is to be seen with other forms of management. Since Fiorinal contains a short-acting barbiturate, sudden withdrawal, if a patient is taking more than 4 tablets a day, may precipitate a seizure. This can be avoided by allowing abrupt withdrawal and giving phenobarbital, 3 30-mg tablets qhs, decreasing by 1 tablet each week until the patient is off the medication. Most patients can accomplish abrupt analgesic withdrawal as outpatients. However, a few will find this impossible and will require a short period of hospitalization.

In addition to hospitalization for analgesic withdrawal, some patients with chronic post-traumatic headache will benefit from hospitalization to receive intravenous DHE 45. In general what is done is to withdraw all analgesics, ergots, and methysergide, if any of these are being used. Place a heparin lock in one arm and inject undiluted DHE45, using a syringe (initially, 0.5 mg), and if this is tolerated without side effects, the next dose should be 1 mg. The doses are given at 8-hour intervals for the length of the hospital stay. I also use intravenous hydrocortisone, which I believe benefits patients whose condition is severe enough to require hospitalization, but there are no double-blinded studies to prove this point. This is given as follows: 100 mg q6h for 24 hours, then 100 mg q8h for 24 hours, then 100 mg q12h for 24 hours, then no further dosages. The DHE45 is continued for a period of time, which must be individualized depending on the patient's response or lack thereof. The average length of hospital stay is 4 to 5 days, but under some circumstances, it could be as short as 3 days or as long as 6 or 7. About 80 percent of patients will have a significant response to this procedure. Also, during the time of hospitalization, various medications by mouth can be used and manipulated faster than can be done in an outpatient setting. DHE45 may need to be self-administered once or twice a day for 1 week or so after the patient is discharged from the hospital, but many patients do not need to do this.

Many patients with chronic post-traumatic headache will have tenderness to thumb pressure over the occipital neurovascular bundle, which resides about 1.5 inches lateral to the inion. If none of the former suggestions are bringing the headache under control, then an occipital nerve block at this site may prove beneficial. This is relatively easy to do by localizing the area of maximum specific tenderness with thumb pressure, but a Doppler device can be used to be certain that the area you are considering injecting is truly at the occipital artery. Since the artery, vein, and nerve run in a bundle at this site, if you have located the artery, you know that you are over the nerve. This area is then infiltrated with 8 ml of 1 percent xylocaine containing 4 mg of dexamethasone. This may be done unilaterally or bilaterally, as indicated by the headache locations. Remember that the descending root of the fifth nerve reaches down to the level of the nucleus of the second and third cervical nerves, so it is probable that this approximation has something to do with the fact that anterior head pain is often relieved by these posterior injections.

Biofeedback training is sometimes used in the treatment of this disorder. Its efficacy is somewhat reduced, however, by the memory and concentration impairment so often experienced by these patients.

When psychological factors appear to be playing a paramount role in the continuation of post-traumatic symptoms, consultation with psychologists, behavioral medicine specialists, or psychiatrists may be indicated. Are mood changes an understandable psychological reaction of the individual to a new and unpleasant cognitive or physical impairment or are they a direct consequence of the site of brain injury? There is considerable evidence to support the latter concept. It is clear that the symptoms generated by brain injury—chronic headache, impaired memory, impaired concentration, insomnia, easy fatiguability, irritability, anger outbursts, decreased libido, and depression—produce an enforced and distinctly unpleasant change in the patient's life routine. It is important for the physician to play a supporting role and to impart as much information as possible to aid comprehension not only in the patient but in the spouse and to lawyers as well, if they are involved. Psychological counseling may be very helpful in these patients.

PROGNOSIS

Predicting the outcome of headaches and other symptoms that follow trauma to the head and neck is based on literature reports and lengthy experience with these patients. It can predicted that after 2 months of symptoms, prolonged disability will ensue. Assuming that appropriate treatment has been tried and has failed, after 6 months, it is most likely that symptoms will not clear, although there is still a possibility (not a probability) that they might. The intensity of the injury, the presence or absence of compensation or litigation, or the presence pretraumatic headache appear to exert no influence on the ultimate prognosis of the post-traumatic symptoms.

SUGGESTED READINGS

Cartlidge NEF, Shaw DA: Head Injury. WB Saunders, Philadelphia,
Editorial: Financial compensation and head injury. Brain Inj 6:387–9, 1992
Goldstein J: Post-traumatic headache and the post-traumatic syndrome. Med Clin North Am 75:641–51, 1991
Mild head injury as a source of developmental disabilities. J Learn Disabil 24: 551–8, 1991
Nolte J: The Human Brain, an Introduction to Its Functional Anatomy. CV Mosby, St. Louis,
Packard H et al: Cognitive symptoms in patients with post-traumatic headache. Headache 33:365–8, 1993
Povlishock JT et al: Axonal change in minor head injury. J Neuropathol Exp Neurol 42:225–42, 1983
WG Speed: Psychiatric aspects of post-traumatic headaches. In Adler, Adler, Packard (eds): Psychiatric Aspects of Headache. Williams & Wilkins, Baltimore
Walker AE, Caveness WF: Head Injury Conference Proceedings. JB Lippincott, Philadelphia,
Wilson JTL et al: Intercorrelation of lesions detected by magnetic resonance imaging after closed head injury. Brain Inj 6:391–9, 1992
Wilson JTL, Wypert DJ: Neuroimaging and neuropsychological functioning following closed head injury: CT, MRI, and SPECT. Head Trauma Rehab 7:29–39, 1992

211. HEADACHE IN CEREBROVASCULAR DISEASE

THOMAS N. WARD

Headache may occur as a symptom of processes affecting the intra- or extracranial vasculature. The presence of headache in these situations may be a useful clue to the presence of underlying disease, and the nature of the headache may aid in localization and determination of pathogenesis. Evaluation of the patient with headache possibly symptomatic of an underlying condition requires elicitation of a detailed patient history—including risk factors for vascular disease, family history, medication history—and a carefully conducted physical examination.

OVERVIEW OF INNERVATION OF CEREBRAL STRUCTURES

Knowledge of the innervation of intra- and extracranial structures may allow the clinician to localize the source of headache.

The trigeminovascular system has been studied in great detail. The classic studies of Ray and Wolff have been confirmed and expanded upon. It is known that the parenchyma of the cerebral hemispheres and cerebellum and much of the intraparenchymal vessels are insensitive to stimulation of all forms. Pain-sensitive intracranial structures include the vessels of the circle of Willis, which are very sensitive in the proximal parts but become progressively less sensitive as they travel distally, the intracranial internal carotid artery, proximal 2 cm of the middle cerebral artery, and the anterior cerebral artery are also pain-sensitive structures, as are the vertebral arteries and basilar artery. Pain-sensitive structures above the tentorium are primarily innervated by branches of the trigeminal nerve, whereas pain-sensitive structures below the tentorium are largely innervated by branches of the upper cervical nerves as well as by the ninth and tenth cranial nerves and some branches from the trigeminal nerve. Disturbances involving these vessels may be indicated by pain referred to the appropriate nerve distribution. However, such information may be falsely localizing because of the phenomenon of convergence. The trigeminal system, as well as the upper cervical nerves, converge both anatomically and physiologically in the spinal nucleus of the trigeminal nerve. Therefore, pain from either system may be referred into the distribution of the other. The trigeminovascular system can antidromically release inflammatory neuropeptides (neurokinin A, calcitonin gene-related peptide, and substance P), thus effecting the blood vessels they innervate and causing painful neurogenic inflammation.

The presence of headache in the setting of an underlying disease is a useful clue, but it must be considered in the setting of associated symptoms and signs and knowing that the location of the headache may represent referred pain rather than local pain.

HYPERTENSION

The relationship of moderate elevations of blood pressure and headache has been controversial. It has been taught that patients with headaches related to hypertension suffer frontal or more often occipital headaches, which are most bothersome in the morning and tend to diminish as the day goes on. Most of the evidence suggests modest elevations of diastolic and systolic blood pressure are not associated with headache. With more dramatic elevations of blood pressure, however, especially in the setting of malignant hypertension or paroxysmal elevations of blood pressure, headache may well occur. Malignant hypertension, seen with elevated diastolic pressures often above 140 mmHg, is associated with severe diffuse headache, itself often associated with nausea and vomiting as well as papilledema, hypertensive retinal changes with visual loss, eventual renal failure, and death.

Dramatic changes in blood pressure, such as occur with pheochromocytoma or with the tyramine reaction seen in patients taking monoamine oxidase inhibitors, are frequently associated with headache. Symptoms of pheochromocytoma are episodic and include headaches that are often bilateral, pulsatile, and moderate to severe, but rather brief in duration. Most of the headaches last less than 1 hour and are often associated with palpitations, pallor, tremor, diaphoresis, and anxiety. The frequency of the headaches is variable but does appear to be related to sudden dramatic increase in blood pressure. Evaluation of the patient suspected of having pheochromocytoma includes 24-hour urine collection to assay for the chemical products of the tumor. In rare instances, the headache, which is typically bilateral and may be holocranial or bifrontal or bioccipital, is associated with generalized convulsions or stroke.

HEADACHE AND TRANSIENT ISCHEMIC ATTACK AND STROKE

Most reported series of headache and stroke find that only a minority of stroke patients complain of headache. Of those patients who do have headache associated with their stroke, approximately 60 percent will complain of headache prior to the onset of neurologic deficit, and 25 percent will complain of headache at the time of onset of the neurologic deficit. The headaches associated with transient ischemic attack (TIA) and stroke have variable features. Headaches are more frequently seen related to posterior circulation events rather than anterior circulation events, perhaps due to the more intense innervation of the posterior circulation meningeal vasculature. The headache may resemble prior headaches the patient has suffered, especially if the patient is younger but the intensity of the headache is unrelated to the size or location of the infarct. If the headache is lateralized to one side, it is usually to the side of the stroke. Perhaps 10 percent of patients with stroke will have had a sentinel headache (i.e., a headache occurring prior to the event). Headache is infrequent in lacunar strokes and most frequent in intracerebral hemorrhage, occurring perhaps 50 percent of the time. As a rule, when headache is related to a stroke in the carotid distribution, it is often located anteriorally, whereas vertebrobasilar territory events may produce headache that is posterior or anterior. Nausea and vomiting are more common with intracerebral hemorrhage than with ischemic stroke or lacunar events. It has been postulated that perhaps platelet aggregation with release of serotonin, prostaglandins, and other products causes vascular dilation and may be the cause of headache, at least in ischemic stroke.

In older patients, the differentiation of TIA from migraine aura can be difficult. TIA is usually abrupt in onset and often lasts less than 15 minutes. Migraine aura is usually more leisurely in evolution and may last somewhat longer, but generally less than 1 hour. The migraine aura need not be followed by headache. A prior history—even decades before—of migraine with aura is helpful; however, there are patients in whom no such history can be found. When there is doubt, a thorough evaluation for possible causes of stroke is mandatory.

Besides the more common varieties of stroke seen in older patients, headache may occur in the setting of stroke due to vasculitis and vascular involvement by diseases such as systemic lupus erythematosus and the antiphospholipid antibody syndrome. The headache of lupus commonly begins at the time of a stroke. The involved vessels may suffer occlusion by thrombus, involvement by vasculitis, dissection, or atherosclerosis. Cardiogenic embolism may also occur. Strokes may be recurrent in this situation. Headache occurring in patients with lupus who do not manifest neurologic signs or symptoms other than headache is not considered an indication of active central nervous system lupus.

The antiphospholipid antibody syndrome may present with migrainelike disturbances, transient or permanent visual loss, and stroke. Patients may appear to be afflicted with particularly severe migraine with aura. The pathogenesis is one of thrombotic occlusive vascular disease. Antiphospholipid antibodies clinically manifest as a thrombotic tendency and may occur in the absence of systemic lupus erythematosus. Patients with additional stroke risk factors beside antiphospholipid antibodies appear to be at even higher risk. These immunoglobins include the lupus anticoagulant, which may be detected by a false-positive VDRL, and increased partial, thromboplastin time or the anticardiolipin antibody. Beyond severe migraine, patients may suffer TIAs, cerebral venous thrombosis, seizures, or stroke. Treatment is controversial but may include aspirin, Coumadin (warfarin), or steroids.

Cerebral venous thrombosis may also present with headache. Headache is typically severe and may resemble migraine. It may be associated with photophobia, nausea, vomiting, and focal signs. The most notable form is superior sagittal sinus thrombosis. Venous thrombosis can be seen after trauma, in the setting of malignancy or malnutrition; postoperatively, with dehydration or sepsis; post-partum; and with parameningeal infection as well as other conditions such as Behçet's disease. Besides sudden headache, nausea, and vomiting, because medial parasagittal structures are involved, blurred vision, papilledema, and seizures (hemiplegia or bilateral crural paresis) may occur. Sixth nerve palsy may be seen, as may depressed level of consciousness and stiff neck. Sinus thrombosis may be imaged by magnetic resonance imaging (MRI) or conventional angiography. Treatment is directed against the underlying cause and is supportive. The use of anticoagulants and antifibrinolytic agents is controversial.

The condition known as mitochondrial myopathy, encephalopathy, lactic acidosis, and strokelike episodes (MELAS) is a condition with attacks often beginning prior to the age of 15 of frequent, severe, episodic sudden headache associated with vomiting and convulsions. Patients do manifest a myopathy, lactic acidosis, and suffer cumulative deficits from strokelike episodes.

SUBARACHNOID HEMORRHAGE AND HEADACHE

The clinical presentation of subarachnoid hemorrhage is often one of the most impressive in all of medicine. Perhaps 30 percent of patients will have had sentinel (warning) headaches prior to the aneurysmal rupture. The headache of aneurysmal rupture classically is bilateral and severe. Headache is present in nearly 100 percent of patients with subarachnoid hemorrhage. Initially, it may be ipsilateral to the aneurysm, but it rapidly becomes bilateral and will spread to involve the occipital region, neck, and eventually even the lumbar area. Its duration is usually longer than 24 hours. It should be noted, however, that misdiagnosis may occur when the headache presentation is not dramatic, or in patients who clinically may seem to be improving under observation or who have mild headaches. Besides sentinel headaches, prior to rupture of an aneurysm, patients may manifest a cranial neuropathy (often a third-nerve palsy), symptoms of ischemia in the circulation distal to the aneurysm, or headache due to mass effect. The headache may be due to aneurysmal thrombosis, expansion, meningeal inflammation, or may occur if the aneurysm causes TIAs or stroke. Approximately 5 to 7 percent of patients will have subhyaloid hemorrhages (hemorrhages in the preretinal layer on funduscopic examination), 5 percent will have a third-nerve palsy, 80 percent will have a stiff neck, and 15 percent may have seizures. Patients may also have depression of consciousness, electrocardiographic changes such as inverted T waves, or other signs of myocardial ischemia. Immediate performance of computed tomography (CT) scanning will reveal subarachnoid blood in approximately 85 percent of patients. In those patients in whom clinical suspicion is high, the remainder are typically diagnosed by immediate lumbar puncture. This is followed by four-vessel angiography, which is the gold standard for defining the location of the aneurysms; it must be remembered that perhaps 20 percent of aneurysms are multiple.

Clinical uncertainty can arise in the setting of so-called thunderclap headache. This has been reported as headache caused by expanding but unruptured aneurysms. CT scanning and lumbar puncture are negative. Day and Raskin reported a patient with just such a clinical scenario who had three severe thunderclap headaches and normal CT scan and lumbar puncture findings. Angiography, when performed, revealed diffuse vasospasm and a large right internal carotid artery aneurysm. Clinical confusion arises because some patients with migraine can present with a rather sudden onset of a severe headache. Further confusion is generated by the occurrence of so-called coital cephalgia. It is known that subarachnoid hemorrhage from either aneurysm or arteriovenous malformation is occasionally precipitated by sexual intercourse. Patients with benign coital cephalgia (similar to migraine) can manifest similar headache, which is severe and often occurs at the time of orgasm. However, in benign coital cephalgia, patients usually do not have nausea and vomiting, no alteration in the level of consciousness, no meningismus, and no focal deficits. The duration of headache is relatively brief. In patients in whom there are these findings, subarachnoid hemorrhage needs to be definitively ruled out and consideration ought to be given to performing angiography, especially if the patient has not been seen within 24 hours of the event.

The relationship between vascular malformations and headache remains controversial. Some authors believe that arteriovenous malformations may present as headaches, whereas others believe there is no relationship. Certainly, in a patient with headaches, an arteriovenous malformation might be suspected if the patient has had seizures, an intracranial bruit, neurologic deficit, or a subarachnoid hemorrhage. I have evaluated a number of patients who have had arteriovenous malformations resected only to find that their headaches persist. Others have been relieved of their headache problem by surgery (personal observations). The possibility exits that the arteriovenous malformation may by causing ischemia that then triggers migraine.

DISEASES OF THE CAROTID AND VERTEBRAL ARTERIES AND HEADACHE

Vascular dissection is due to hemorrhage into the wall of a blood vessel, leading to varying degrees of narrowing of the lumen. This dissection may be ''spontaneous'' (idiopathic) or secondary to a number of etiologies, including trauma. Dissection of the carotid and/or vertebral arteries may result in headache. The neural pathways for the sensation of pain from the carotid artery are not fully understood. They may involve the ninth, tenth, and fifth cranial nerves as well as branches from the second and third cranial nerves. Patients undergoing percutaneous angioplasty of the internal carotid artery have experienced neck pain; facial pain, especially in the gums and teeth; pain in the region of the eye; and also on the scalp and ear. Patients with internal carotid artery dissection experience headache as their most common initial symptom. The headache is typically ipsilateral and focal in and around the eye and often steady, although it may be throbbing or of a variable nature. It is usually severe. There may be pain and tenderness along the artery as well as a partial Horner syndrome (ptosis and miosis) and bruits. This pain typically lasts less than 3 months. Patients

with vascular dissection, of course, may have TIAs and stroke in the distribution of the vessel involved. More than one vessel may be involved, and patients presenting with these features, especially headache and neck pain referable to the carotid artery, should have evaluation, which may include ultrasound, MRI, or angiography. The vascular narrowing will manifest as a ''string sign.'' Treatment with anticoagulation may be life saving. It should also be noted that this problem can occur in young people, and early diagnosis is important to prevent permanent neurologic deficit.

Dissection of the vertebral arteries may also be spontaneous or secondary to other processes such as trauma. Dissection can be seen after a chiropractic manipulation. Most patients have neck pain and severe occipital pain that may radiate anteriorly to the forehead, periorbital region, or temple, or become generalized. The pain is usually sharp and severe but will gradually improve over 1 to 3 weeks. As with carotid artery dissection, TIA and/or stroke may occur either secondary to emboli or decreased perfusion distal to the stenotic segment. The interval from the onset of pain to neurologic deficit ranges from hours up to 3 weeks. Symptoms due to hypoperfusion in the vascular territory may include decrease in consciousness, vertigo, vomiting, paresthesias, motor deficits, diplopia, and hemianopia. Recognition of this condition and treatment of extracranial vertebral artery dissection with anticoagulation may be life saving. Diagnosis can be made either noninvasively by ultrasound or MRI, or by angiography.

Pain may either arise spontaneously from the carotid artery itself in a condition known as carotidynia, or headache may occur after procedures performed on the carotid artery such as carotid endarterectomy. Carotidynia is a condition seen more often in women than men. These patients often have a history of migraine, either personally or in their families. The artery is described as being tender and throbbing. Patients ranging in age from childhood to the elderly have been described. The pain is local, involving the carotid artery, but may radiate to the postauricular region. Treatment is the same as treatment for migraine and is generally effective. It has been noted that patients with migraine often have tender carotid arteries.

Patients who have undergone carotid endarterectomy may manifest postendarterectomy headaches. The original descriptions suggested a 36- to 72-hour headache-free interval followed by a self-limited headache lasting weeks to months, which could mimic migraine. Other studies, however, have suggested that headache may occur frequently, perhaps in even over one-half the patients undergoing endarterectomy. Most endarterectomy headaches typically occur within the first 5 days after the procedure, but headache may occur anywhere from minutes to 3 weeks after the procedure. It may be continuous or variable. It may mimic migraine or cluster headache or any other form of headache. It may be focal or diffuse. The etiology is unclear. Some forms of postendarterectomy headache may represent increased cerebral blood flow and disordered autoregulation. Some of these patients do have seizures and intercerebral hemorrhage in addition to their headaches. It has also been have suggested that these headaches may be due to inflammatory processes involving the carotid artery. It is difficult to explain the headache-free interval based simply on changes in cerebral blood flow. Postendarterectomy headache is diagnosed when postoperative vascular occlusion or dissection have been ruled out.

produced by mass lesions causes the pupil to dilate, then become unresponsive to light, followed by ptosis of the eyelid and by decreased vertical and medial eye movements. This pattern is especially seen with supratentorial tumors, mass effect of posterior communicating artery aneurysm, and with herniation of the medial temporal lobe through the tentorial notch. By contrast, the "metabolic" oculomotor palsy produced by ischemic neuropathy or diabetes typically produces pupil-sparing weakness of extraocular muscles, although it may also present with severe retro-orbital headache otherwise indistinguishable from a mass lesion or posterior communicating aneurysm.

Fever may be seen with headaches caused by masses in the region of the hypothalamus and diencephalon ("central fever"), causing disruption of temperature regulation. Brain and epidural abscess, meningitis, cerebritis, and encephalitis may all present with fever and a headache that is due to increased intracranial pressure and inflammation. Fever is a very nonspecific sign, for it may be seen in literally hundreds of diseases that present with headache.

Mass lesions also may produce other neurologic signs attributed to the anatomic localization of the mass and the surrounding edema. Focal muscular weakness, hyperreflexia, Babinski sign, and cerebellar and meningeal signs all may be found upon neurologic examination. Midline masses or progressive hydrocephalus may produce the typical triad of gait apraxia, spastic neurogenic bladder (with incontinence), and rapidly progressive dementia.

Comorbidity of cerebral masses and benign recurrent headaches is sometimes discovered. Structural causes of headache, although less common than benign causes such as migraine, may exactly mimic or even coexist with these more common forms. Migraine patients may have meningiomas or unruptured aneurysms that may not contribute to their headaches, but may be found during investigation.

Diagnosis

Mass lesions typically cause mild, intermittent, progressively worsening headaches that are milder than migraine and that begin in the recent past. The headache may have a variable pattern, being greatest in early morning, present on awakening, but improved by arising and activity. Nocturnal headache, awakening the patient from sleep, is also a common mode of presentation. These patterns are produced by changes in ICP in brain parenchyma around the mass. Recumbency decreases intracranial venous drainage and increases cerebral edema surrounding the tumor. Decreased venous drainage causes distention of venous sinuses and brain venules, increasing volume inside the hard box of the skull. This leads to increased ICP and headache.

Location of the pain may localize the mass. If it is above the tentorium, pain is referred to the forehead and temple, in the trigeminal nerve territory; below the tentorium, pain is referred to the nuchal and occipital areas in the territory of C2 and C3.

Mass lesions may produce stereotyped clinical syndromes, either nonspecific or indicative of focal anatomic localization. The nonspecific syndrome may present with brief headaches, blurred vision, syncope, transient focal weakness or paresthesias, somnolence, focal/generalized seizures, dysphasia, dementia, minor visual symptoms such as field defects, or gaze paresis. Symptoms and signs of progressive hydrocephalus may be seen, including a specific gait disturbance, apractic magnetic gait, in addition to gaze paresis, dementia, and urinary inconti-

TABLE 212-2. Cerebral Mass Lesions: Characteristic "Local Syndromes"

Regional Mass	Symptoms/Signs
Sellar and parasellar masses	Headache, bitemporal hemianopsia, galactorrhea, acromegaly, amenorrhea, diabetes insipidus, myxedema
Cerebellopontine angle tumors	Ipsilateral nerve deafness (VIII), then cranial nerve V, then peripheral nerve VII paresis; long-tract signs appear late
Sphenoid ridge tumors Medial Lateral	Syndrome of superior orbital foramen (III, IV, VI, V, late optic atrophy); minimal symptoms except headache until superior orbital fissure involved
Petrous apex (Gradenigo syndrome)	Temporal headache, progressive V with or without tic douloureux, late III, long tract signs
Subfrontal masses (Foster-Kennedy syndrome)	Ipsilateral anosmia, ipsilateral optic atrophy and blindness, contralateral papilledema
Foramen magnum tumors	Progressive clockwise development of weakness, occipito-nuchal headache
Midline tumors or obstructive hydrocephalus	Progressive gait apraxia, neurogenic bladder, incontinence, dementia

nence. Anatomically distinct masses may produce characteristic local syndromes (Table 212-2).

Mass lesions of the hemispheres may produce partial seizures, the pattern of which may have localizing value. Uncinate fits, indicating a lesion of the medial temporal lobe in the uncinate gyrus, have an olfactory aura followed by temporal lobe automatisms. Adversive seizures, from a lesion of the frontal hemisphere, produce rotation of head and eyes away from the involved hemisphere. Focal motor seizures, including typical Jacksonian march of progressive motor twitching, are seen with lesions of the motor strip, in the posterior frontal lobe.

Differentiation of headaches due to structural lesions from those due to benign recurring causes such as migraine can usually be accomplished by means of a complete neurologic history and review of systems, with attention to certain key questions (Table 212-3). The first five features listed in the table can usually help make the distinction between the two types of headache, but the remainder of questions may not differentiate the two. The most specific item is the presence of typical migrainous visual aura, with positive visual symptoms, such as teichopsia or photopsia, rather than loss of vision, such as amaurosis.

Complete neurologic examination is important even in patients suspected of having typical "benign" headaches, for cerebral masses may coexist with migraine or tension-type headaches.

Imaging studies are important for conclusively ruling out structural disease or for defining the extent of masses, edema, and degree of involvement. Cranial computed tomography (CT) imaging is gradually giving way to magnetic resonance imaging (MRI), because of its superior resolution, three-dimension spatial imaging, and lack of risk from x-rays and intravenous contrast material. MRI angiography has already reduced the use of conventional angiography, and this trend should continue.

Table 212-4 lists those conditions that should prompt reevaluation of the patient or the ordering of the appropriate imaging studies. Although some migraine patients have strictly hemicranial headaches, and many patients with chronic tension-type headache have chronic daily headaches, the new develop-

TABLE 212-3. Differentiating Structural Lesions from Benign Recurring Headaches

Historical Features	Benign Recurrent Headaches	Structural Lesions
Onset of headaches	Remote, usually childhood	Recent
Neurologic aura (before headache)	Frequent	Infrequent
Precipitants	Alcohol, odors, menses, foods, weather changes	Straining, coughing (increased intracranial pressure)
Prior headache history	Extensive	Rare
Family headache history	Extensive	Rare
Headache frequency	Intermittent to constant	Progressive increase
Pain quality	Pulsatile, neuritic, steady	Steady, wax and wane
Pain location	Global, hemicranial	Global, focal
Duration	Variable	Variable
Associated symptoms	Photophobia, muscle tension, nausea, vomiting, migrainous visual symptoms, transient focal central nervous system deficit	Focal central nervous system deficits without headache, nausea, vomiting, nonmigrainous visual symptoms, seizures

ment of either of these conditions should be cause for concern, as they may be associated with a more grave condition.

DECREASED DRAINAGE: VENOUS THROMBOSIS

General Principles: Approach to the Patient

Symptoms. Patients suffering from obstruction of the venous circulation of the brain, such as caused by thrombosis of the superior sagittal sinus or cortical vein thrombosis, may present with two main syndromes. These conditions produce damming back of blood into the draining cortical veins, producing bloody cortical infarcts that are quite irritative. Cortical irritation and inflammation produce focal headache and focal seizures, in addition to venous infarction produced in the cortex. This triad of focal headache, focal seizures, and focal neurologic signs should suggest the possibility of venous obstruction. If the lateral sinus or jugular system is occluded, collateral flow through the contralateral system may keep cerebral pressure near normal levels, without the development of focal cerebral infarction. These patients complain of focal headache, usually localized over the ipsilateral occipital area. The cortical form of venous thrombosis may be caused by pregnancy, hormonal treatments including oral contraceptives, coagulopathies such as thrombotic thrombocytopenic purpura or protein S deficiency, or circulating anticoagulant syndromes. Lateral sinus thrombosis may be produced by mastoiditis, petrous bone infections, or severe middle ear infections that extend intracranially.

Deep venous thrombosis, which usually begins with involvement of the great vein of Galen and the straight cerebral sinus, produces quite a different picture. Patients may complain of global headache, then gradually become somnolent, stuporous, and comatose, with very few focal or lateralizing signs until cerebral herniation is well under way. Bloody infarction of the deep structures of the brain, especially the diencephalon, basal

TABLE 212-4. Headache Danger Signals

New onset in headache-free individual
Headaches exclusively on one side
Chronic daily headaches
Fever, even if intermittent or low-grade
Change in pattern of stable headaches
Headaches awakening patient from sleep
Positional headaches, worse supine, with coughing/straining, relieved by sitting, standing
Neurologic signs or symptoms appearing with or without accompanying headache:
    Language or speech difficulties
    Visual loss or double vision
    Weakness in arm or leg
    Seizures, either focal or general, or loss of consciousness
    Motor clumsiness or tremor

ganglia, and thalami, creates an expanding midline deep mass that does not produce seizures, focal headache, or focal neurologic signs. Patients most at risk for the deep form of venous infarction are the elderly, especially if dehydrated or if cerebral venous return is compromised by factors that increase central venous pressure, such as congestive heart failure. Although the progressive development of headache, then rapid decline in mental status with few localizing neurologic findings (until late into the course) is fairly distinctive, few patients are diagnosed before death.

Signs. Many of the distinctive features discussed above for cerebral mass lesions may apply to patients with cerebral venous thrombosis. Focal headache is nearly universal in patients with the superficial forms of thrombosis. Focal neurologic findings may assist localization of the area of cortical infarction. The late stage of deep cerebral vein thrombosis produces the typical findings of progressive herniation, including pupillary changes, Cheyne-Stokes respiration, decorticate and decerebrate posturing, and Babinski signs.

Diagnosis and Treatment

The CT scan, without contrast, is quite sensitive for diagnosis of cerebral venous thrombosis, provided that hemorrhagic infarction has occurred. Early cases, or patients with occlusion of the lateral venous sinus or the jugular system, may need MRI scanning or magnetic resonance angiography to successfully image the lesions. Coronal sections, usually available only through MRI, are quite helpful in visualizing the volume of tissue infarcted. Electroencephalography is also important in patients with cortical venous thrombosis, even if seizures have not yet occurred. Laboratory testing to search for coagulopathies in such patients may be extremely involved, and may best be handled by consultation with specialists in coagulation disorders or hematology. Otolaryngology or neurosurgical consultation may be in order if imaging procedures reveal mastoiditis or petrous bone infection.

Therapy for patients with jugular or lateral sinus thrombosis focuses upon reducing intracerebral volume with steroids and/or with diuretics, such as furosemide or acetazolamide. In about 50 percent of such patients, the occluded segment may spontaneously recanalize, sometimes 1 year later. Cortical vein thrombosis is a more urgent matter, and usually requires admission to a hospital and treatment with anticonvulsants, heparin, and steroids to reduce ICP. Patients who are pregnant may require early cesarean delivery, whereas those found to have coagulation disorders may need heparin therapy for as long as 1 year. The long-term neurologic deficit of cerebral venous infarction seems to be much less than that of cerebral arterial infarction, owing to the superficial location of the infarcts. Persisting headaches following the acute illness may respond to drugs that increase central pain threshold, such as the tricyclics.

Therapy for patients with deep cerebral vein thrombosis is extremely difficult. Anticoagulation with heparin may only increase deep cerebral bleeding, whereas measures to reduce brain volume are usually ineffective.

BENIGN INTRACRANIAL HYPERTENSION (PSEUDOTUMOR CEREBRI)
General Principles: Approach to the Patient

Symptoms. Women who slowly develop daily persistent headaches may have chronically increased ICP, known as benign intracranial hypertension. This condition may mimic the symptoms of increased ICP produced by brain tumors, hence the name *pseudotumor*. Although typical patients described in the literature and textbooks are short, obese, hirsute, and have irregular menses, it is now recognized that this stereotype does not fit all patients. Pregnancy or hormonal therapy, including oral contraceptives, may initiate the syndrome. Some patients have recurrent attacks with each pregnancy. The headaches are dull, steady, and continuous; worsening with straining, coughing or sneezing, or taking a supine position; and improved by standing or sitting. As ICP rises, compression of the abducens nerve against the inner table may produce varying degrees of diplopia and abducens paresis. Further elevations in ICP produce optic nerve compression and centrocecal scotomas that may progress to blindness if untreated. Migrainous features of nausea, vomiting, photophobia, and sonophobia are absent, and the headaches are not exacerbated by the usual migraine trigger factors.

Other causes for benign intracranial hypertension are not restricted to women. Similar syndromes without the hormonal features may be caused by vitamin A poisoning (hypervitaminosis A), by tetracycline or its derivatives, during steroid withdrawal, or by chronic lead poisoning. The combination of isotretinoin (a vitamin A derivative, Accutane) and tetracycline or doxycycline for the treatment of acne has caused quite a few cases in otherwise healthy adolescents. Rare causes of benign intracranial hypertension include hypothyroidism or hypoparathyroidism, hyper- or hypoadrenalism, and treatment with phenothiazines or estrogens.

Signs. Papilledema with hemorrhages and exudates is seen in most patients, but some patients may show only absent/reduced venous pulsations on the optic discs, or even normal discs. Extraocular movements and visual testing may demonstrate abducens weakness, with diplopia on lateral gaze. Peripheral visual fields are usually normal, but testing central fields with a red-headed pin may detect enlargement of the physiologic blind spot surprisingly early. Later in the course, central blindness (a central scotoma) may develop, along with optic atrophy. Lumbar puncture reveals elevated CSF pressure, sometimes in the range of 400 to 500 mmCSF. Cerebral imaging is mandatory prior to lumbar puncture, to firmly exclude cerebral masses. It usually shows slitlike ventricles, and sometimes periventricular CT lucencies representing white-matter channels of CSF absorption. Empty sella syndrome may somehow deflect full CSF pressure from being manifested as papilledema, as it

has been reported in patients with benign intracranial hypertension with normal optic disks.

Pathophysiology. The cause of benign intracranial hypertension is open to speculation. Apparently, there is decreased resorption of CSF into the arachnoid granulations that line the superior sagittal sinus, so intracranial pressure rises. Accessory channels of CSF resorption are used, such as pinocytosis into cerebral venules and capillaries in the deep white matter. This may give a characteristic CT scan appearance. The cause of decreased CSF resorption is unknown. The contribution of obesity to the syndrome, although clinically observed, is totally obscure. Hormonal abnormalities are suspected in most patients because of menstrual irregularities and hirsutism, but clinical laboratory test results (including estrogen, progesterone, luteinizing hormone, follicle stimulating hormone) are usually normal. How such hormonal abnormalities could cause failure of CSF resorption is also unknown. Elevated levels of vasopressin have been found in the CSF of some patients. This peptide, in the goat, reduces CSF resorption and increases ICP.

Diagnosis and Treatment

Traditional recommendations for diagnosis of benign intracranial hypertension include CT scanning, then lumbar puncture to establish the diagnosis. Recurrent lumbar puncture may terminate the syndrome in as many as one-third of patients, with no need for further treatment. Drug therapy commences with prophylactic acetazolamide, a carbonic anhydrase inhibitor, which reduces the formation of CSF. Furosemide or thiazides may be needed in addition to acetazolamide. If visual field defects or retinal hemorrhages are present, a course of steroids may be necessary. The patient's papilledema, visual fields, and diplopia should be followed up concurrently by an ophthalmologist. Progressive deterioration of vision may necessitate ophthalmologic surgery (optic nerve sheath fenestration) to save vision. Lumbar peritoneal shunting of CSF may also be effective. Recommendations in the older literature to perform anterior temporal lobectomy for cranial decompression to save vision have been replaced by recommendations to perform the fenestration technique.

INTRACRANIAL HYPOTENSION

Headaches from lowered intracranial pressure may occur if there is obstruction to the generation of CSF, as with severe dehydration, arachnoiditis, or subarachnoid block from arachnoid tumors. Intracranial hypotension also occurs if there is a fistula that drains CSF faster than it can be manufactured, most frequently after lumbar puncture or dural puncture during the course of epidural anesthesia, but also following trauma or following spinal surgery. Idiopathic intracranial hypotension may also occur, with an occult cause.

POSTDURAL PUNCTURE HEADACHE
General Principles: Approach to the Patient

Symptoms. Headache usually starts within 24 hours of a dural puncture, but may be delayed up to 2 weeks if the patient is treated with bed rest. The natural course of the headache is gradual resolution over 4 hours to several weeks, although the average pain lasts 3 to 4 days. The longest recorded duration of headache is 19 months. The headache may be localized to the frontal area more than the occiput, or both regions or the entire head may be affected. Hemicranial, retro-orbital, or facial regions are not usually reported. The quality of the pain is usually a dull aching sensation, like a constricting band, sometimes with superimposed pulsations produced by changes in position or mild exercise. Typical descriptions include "a lead weight," a "heavy head," or a "vacuum in the head." The most typical feature of headache from intracranial hypotension is the rapid exacerbation of headache upon arising and the equally rapid relief with recumbency. Some authors suggest a correlation between the length of time spent upright and the length of time needed to improve headache when lying down again. Other exacerbating features may include shaking the head, jugular vein compression, coughing, or sneezing. Relief may also be obtained from a tight abdominal binder or other means of abdominal compression.

Symptoms that may be associated with postdural puncture headache include a mild degree of meningismus, nausea (but little vomiting), and low back pain, especially near the site of the dural puncture. Visual symptoms are infrequent, but nonspecific symptoms such as blurred vision, photophobia, photopsia, or scintillations occur in about 10 percent of patients. Vestibular and auditory symptoms occur with about the same frequency as visual symptoms, and include such vague feelings as intermittent vertigo, gait unsteadiness, tinnitus, decreased auditory acuity, and a sensation of ear obstruction or pressure.

Signs. No diagnostic signs are characteristic of intracranial hypotension. Neither objective meningismus nor Kernig sign is usually present. Ophthalmologic examination is usually unremarkable. Diplopia from abducens/lateral rectus palsy was seen in only 5 of 140 patients in one series.

Pathophysiology. The cause of headache from intracranial hypotension is the continued leakage of CSF through a hole made in the dura at the time of dural puncture. Because lumbar CSF pressure is higher than epidural pressure, especially in the upright position, CSF can be lost even faster than it is formed. The continued flow of CSF through the aperture serves to keep it open. As CSF volume is lost, the brain expands by dilating cerebral veins and expanding the vascular compartment. Stretching and traction of the dilated cerebral veins over the expanded brain hemispheres seems to produce a large part of the headache.

Many factors have been claimed to be important in determining who develops postdural puncture headache, but few have been substantiated by large reviews. It is more common in patients who have had prior bouts of postdural puncture headache, and there is a trend toward lower risk with smaller-caliber needles. In one series, there was a significant difference between 26-gauge needles (12 percent of patients had headache) and 22-gauge (36 percent had headache). Inadvertent dural puncture occurring during epidural anesthesia produces headache in 78 percent of patients, probably due to the very large caliber of the cannula used to insert the epidural catheter. The lower frequency of headache after spinal anesthesia (13 percent) than after diagnostic lumbar puncture (32 percent) may be a reflection of the different size needles used, and not the amount of fluid removed. Bevel direction is also important. Insertion of the needle with bevel perpendicular to the dural fibers raises the risk of headache twofold, compared to parallel insertion. These headaches are also less common in the elderly, for unclear reasons. It is speculated that channels for egress of CSF

from the epidural space are narrowed in the elderly by osteoarthritic thickening.

Factors that have failed to prove important in headache production include personality of the patient, position of the patient during the puncture (no difference between lying and sitting), total attempts or number of punctures made, and the amount of CSF removed. The duration of bed rest and degree of fluid intake after the spinal puncture likewise have no bearing on outcome.

Treatment

Treatment is often not necessary, as the natural course of most patients is resolution in 2 to 4 days. Most patients are headache-free as long as they lie supine, but this does not shorten the course. There is no evidence that forcing fluids or giving intravenous hydration can help. An abdominal binder can give symptomatic relief. Increased intra-abdominal pressure is transmitted to the epidural veins, where it then increases intraspinal pressure and relieves the headache.

Intravenous infusion of methylxanthines such as caffeine sodium benzoate (500 mg IV push over 2 to 3 minutes) has been shown effective in patients with headache after spinal anesthesia, with 75 percent gaining relief after one dose, and an additional 10 percent after two doses. Major cardiac arrhythmias may occur, so it is suggested that this treatment occur only in an intensive care or monitored environment. One small controlled study involving oral theophylline (300 mg tid) demonstrated decreased intensity and duration of headaches.

Infusion of epidural normal saline has been tested in headache after spinal anesthesia. Twenty ml saline gave 70 percent of patients permanent relief, and another 20 percent gained relief for 3 to 4 hours. Expected incidence of headache after inadvertent dural puncture in epidural anesthesia was reduced from 78 to 30 percent by continuous infusion of 1 to 1.5 L saline/h through the epidural catheter for 24 hours.

The most effective single treatment for postdural puncture headaches consists of an epidural blood patch, in which 20 ml autologous blood is injected carefully into the epidural space. The same interspace of the offending dural puncture may be used, or one level lower. The epidural blood produces immediate relief of headache by increasing epidural pressure, which is reflected back to the CSF to increase intraspinal pressure. Long-term relief is obtained by the formation of gelatinous clot, which tamponades the site of leakage, then by the formation of long-term fibrin to seal the dural laceration. Patients may be up and about after only a 30-minute rest, with up to 95 percent success after the first injection. Recurrent headache usually responds to a second blood patch, even if given several months later. The patch is usually successful when all other treatment has failed, even months after the original dural laceration. Follow-up studies as long as 2 years have shown no major complications, but included transient back pain in one-third of patients and radicular pain or paresthesias that usually resolved promptly. The patch does not obliterate the epidural space and does not produce arachnoiditis, so subsequent epidural injections or lumbar punctures can be carried out without difficulty.

SPONTANEOUS INTRACRANIAL HYPOTENSION

General Principles: Approach to the Patient

Symptoms. Headaches identical to those of postdural puncture headaches may develop suddenly in patients who have not had any form of lumbar puncture. The headache is worsened by the upright position and relieved by recumbency, usually has the same occipitofrontal location as postdural puncture headaches, and has other associated features of nausea, vomiting, dizziness, meningismus, and dizziness. The headache may develop after minor trauma, especially a fall upon the buttocks, but also after vigorous exercise, sexual intercourse, or violent coughing or sneezing. Occasionally, the syndrome develops gradually and precipitating factors cannot be identified.

Signs. The diagnosis is made by lumbar puncture, which usually demonstrates very low CSF pressure, less than 50 mm CSF. Occasionally, CSF must be aspirated by syringe because intraspinal pressure is too low to generate spontaneous flow. CSF protein is somewhat elevated, up to 100 mg/dl, in keeping with relative flow stasis. Small numbers of erythrocytes and lymphocytes may be found in the fluid, but culture results are negative. Subdural hematomas or hygromas are sometimes discovered on CT or MRI studies.

Pathophysiology. Prior speculation about impaired CSF production or increased absorption has now given way to the belief that spontaneous intracranial hypotension is produced by a dural tear with resulting chronic leakage of CSF. Most patients have an antecedent history of trauma or straining, and may have CSF leaks demonstrated by myelography, radioisotope cisternography, or MRI scanning. Falling upon the buttocks may produce deceleration injuries to the spinal dural root sleeves, resulting in CSF leakage. Subdural hematomas may arise from similar deceleration injuries when cerebral bridging veins are torn. CSF abnormalities such as erythrocytosis, leukocytosis, and elevated protein may result from these injuries or from meningeal inflammation at the site of a tear.

Treatment

The syndrome usually resolves spontaneously with the resolution of the underlying dural tear, but complete recovery may take several months. Conservative measures such as those discussed above for postdural puncture headaches may assist resolution, including rest in bed, analgesics, and an abdominal binder. Myelography, radioisotope cisternography, or MRI scanning (possibly with intrathecal contrast to image CSF flow) may be necessary to detect the site of leakage if pain is prolonged. Surgical intervention is sometimes called for, and usually can demonstrate the site of leakage and adjacent CSF soft-tissue accumulation. Epidural saline infusion and blood patches may offer relief even if the site of leakage has not been identified. Dural tears in the cervical or thoracic area may not respond to blood patching, however, as the site is above the level reached by the spreading epidural blood.

SUGGESTED READINGS

Bousser M-G, Chiras J, Bories J, Castaigne P: Cerebral venous thrombosis: a review of 38 cases. Stroke 16:199–213, 1985
Johnston I, Hawke S, Kalmagyi M, Antyeo C: The pseudotumor syndrome. Arch Neurol 48:740–7, 1991
Marcelis J, Silberstein SD: Idiopathic intracranial hypertension without papilledema. Arch Neurol 48:392–9, 1991
Marcelis J, Silberstein SD: Spontaneous low cerebrospinal fluid pressure headache. Headache 30:192–6, 1990
Rahman NU, al-Tahan AR: Computed tomographic evidence of an extensive thrombosis and infarction of the deep venous system. Stroke 24:744–6, 1993

Raskin NH: Lumbar puncture headache: a review. Headache 30:197–200, 1990
Sergott RC, Savino PJ, Bosley TM: Modified optic nerve sheath decompression provides long-term visual improvement for pseudotumor cerebri. Arch Ophthalmol 106:1384–90, 1988
Wall M: The headache profile of idiopathic intracranial hypertension. Cephalalgia 10:331–5, 1990

213. EXERTIONAL HEADACHE

C. DAVID GORDON

Exertional headache encompasses several headache syndromes, including effort migraine, cough headache, coital cephalgia, and benign exertional headache. In general, intracranial lesions and cerebrospinal fluid pathway obstruction must be ruled out before considering this condition benign. Approximately 90 percent of the time it is idiopathic and benign. Unfortunately, in the remaining 10 percent, it is due to a potentially more severe underlying pathology, such as Arnold-Chiari type I malformation, arteriovenous malformation, aneurysm, intracranial mass lesion, cerebral venous thrombosis, acute subdural hematoma, or even pheochromocytoma. In light of this differential diagnosis, exertional headache must be quickly evaluated clinically. It is recommended that magnetic resonance imaging be performed, as this visualizes the posterior fossa anatomy in far more detail than computed tomography, in addition to carotid noninvasive Doppler studies and urinary metanephrines. Table 213-1 lists treatment strategies for each type of exertional headache.

BENIGN EXERTIONAL HEADACHE

A 36-year-old previously healthy man presented to his family physician with the chief complaint of two bouts of excruciating headache that began 2 weeks after beginning an aggressive exercise program. He described the initial paroxysm of pain commencing after performing push-ups. It took the form of a left-sided throbbing pain accompanied by nausea, peaked to intolerable proportions almost immediately, lessening over several minutes, with a residual dull ache that persisted for another 2 hours. Leaning forward evidently relieved his discomfort significantly. Photosensitivity, emesis, and focal neurologic dis-

TABLE 213-1. The Pharmacologic Treatment of Exertional Headache Subtypes

Headache Subtype	Medication	Dosage
Effort migraine	Ergotamine (P)	0.5–1.0 mg PO before exercise
	Methysergide (P)	2 mg PO before exercise
	Acetylsalicylate	250–500 mg before exercise
	Indomethacin (P)	25–50 mg PO before exercise
Benign exertional	Indomethacin (P)	50 mg PO tid
	Methysergide (P)	1–2 mg PO PRN 30 minutes before exercise
Benign cough	Indomethacin (P)	50 mg PO tid
	Naproxen (P)	275–550 mg tid
	Ergonovine (P)	0.2–0.4 mg tid
	Phenelzine (P)	15–60 mg tid
Benign sex	Propranolol (P)	40–200 mg PO daily
	Diltiazem (P)	60 mg PO tid
	Indomethacin (P)	50 mg PO after dinner

turbance were decidedly absent. Weight-lifting brought on an identical headache several days later. Past medical history was negative, although his family history was significant for migraine on his mother's side, and his father was recently diagnosed with a ruptured saccular aneurysm. The patient took no medications and there were negative findings upon systems review. Initial assessment revealed a healthy middle-aged man in moderate pain, but the examination was otherwise unremarkable. On-site neuroimaging results were normal. The patient was diagnosed with benign effort migraine, recommended to refrain from aggressive exercise, and prescribed prophylactic oral indomethacin, 25 to 50 mg 1 hour before beginning his daily exercise routine. After 2 months, he had had no further headache activity.

Benign exertional headache is a sudden and severe condition brought on by any form of exercise, although weight-lifting, swimming, and short- or long-distance running are more typical precipitants. In contrast to benign cough headache, benign exertional headache occurs more commonly in younger patients, manifests as a typical migraine attack, and may thus be associated with nausea, vomiting, unilateral head pain, and both photo- and phonosensitivity. Treatment strategies typically include daily indomethacin, 50 mg tid, although 1 to 2 mg oral ergotamine tartrate or 1 to 2 mg oral methysergide given 30 minutes before exercise has been reported successful.

BENIGN COUGH HEADACHE

Benign cough headache typically presents as a paroxysmal unilateral or bilateral headache, brought on by bending over, lifting, coughing, sneezing, straining, laughing, stooping, or heavy running. The head pain often reaches peak intensity within seconds and may last minutes to several hours in duration. It is lateralized in approximately one-third of the cases, is usually unaccompanied by other traditional migraine symptoms, is sharp to throbbing in character, and almost always remits with indomethacin. Spontaneous improvement or total resolution occur in approximately one-third after 5 years, and in over two-thirds after 10 years.

Tinel first described this type of headache in the French literature in 1932, and Symonds (1956) attributed it to the distention of pain-sensitive posterior fossa structures. In 1968, Rooke considered this a variety of exertional headache, concluding a male to female ratio of occurrence of 4:1, often beginning following a respiratory infection with cough, with a 10 percent chance occurrence of Arnold-Chiari malformation, platybasia, subdural hematoma, and intracranial tumor. Between 1976 and 1980, Williams recorded cerebrospinal fluid pressures from the cisterna magna and lumbar region during coughing. He concluded that both intrathoracic and intra-abdominal pressure increased during coughing, transmitting a pressure wave via the epidural veins to the cerebrospinal fluid. Whenever cough headache occurs unilaterally, internal carotid artery stenosis should be considered.

The treatment of benign cough headache includes indomethacin, 50 mg tid, although intravenous dihydroertotamine has been used, in rare instances, for more refractory presentations. Raskin has found naproxen, ergonovine, and phenelzine also useful fallback measures should indomethacin prove ineffective.

COITAL CEPHALGIA

A 56-year-old healthy man presented acutely to his local emergency room complaining of "the worst headache of [his] life."

It reportedly began that night while making love with his wife, hitting him "like a bolt of lightning" at orgasm, at which point he developed severe nausea, emesis, and intolerable occipital pulsatile pain. On examination, he appeared to be in extreme pain, clutching his head, with obvious pallor and marked photosensitivity. He vomited twice. Apart from a blood pressure of 160/106 and a pulse of 96 beats/min, his examination results were otherwise unremarkable. Hematologic and cranial computed tomography study findings were normal. He was given parenteral meperidine and hydroxyzine and his condition improved. He was sent home with a diagnosis of thunderclap headache and told to take indomethacin, 50 mg orally, prior to sexual activity, and rectal phenergan, 50 mg, with Cafergot abortively if headache developed. However, at follow-up 2 weeks later, when he stated that headache activity continued, he was placed on nadolol, 40 mg bid, preventatively, with eventual cessation of all headache activity within 1 week.

Coital cephalgia, or "benign sex headache," occurs more often in men than women. It may present consistently with sexual activity, or it may remit for long periods despite continued sexual activity. It must be understood that although most headaches occurring during sexual activity are benign, on rare occasions, this type of physical exertion precipitates subarachnoid hemorrhage from aneurysmal rupture, or cerebral/brainstem infarction.

There are three types of coital headache: (1) the muscular tension-type headache, usually bilateral, associated with mounting sexual excitement, which may endure for up to 48 hours afterward; (2) orgasmic headache, which is throbbing, paroxysmal, and explosive, coming on at orgasm (so-called thunderclap headache) and thought to relate to increasing blood pressure; and (3) postural headache, suboccipitally localized, which presents on arising, much like the headache that develops after a lumbar puncture. This last type may in fact be due to a dural leak developing during aggressive sexual activity.

Evaluation of thunderclap headache should proceed as indicated above, although symptoms such as neck stiffness mandate spinal fluid examination. In addition, thunderclap headache presenting in the absence of sexual activity should be evaluated with computed tomography and spinal fluid examination. Raskin recommends lumbar puncture and angiography in the initial evaluation of coital headache to exclude the possibility of aneurysm.

The management of coital cephalgia may include avoidance of further sexual activity; however, indomethacin taken several hours earlier usually prevents the onset of headache altogether. In addition, prophylactic treatment with propranolol, 40 mg to 200 mg daily, may prevent these headaches by preventing elevation of blood pressure at orgasm.

EFFORT MIGRAINE

Effort migraine consists of migraine headache brought on as a result of aggressive exercise in the unconditioned individual. Attendant migrainous features, such as nausea, vomiting, and light and noise sensitivity, often ensue, though not as abruptly as the cephalgic component. This may be prevented by assuming a gradual exercise regimen, progressing as tolerated. It may be treated abortively by typical migraine medications, although it can often be pretreated if recognized, using anti-inflammatory (naproxyn sodium, indomethacin) or ergotamine-related drugs.

SUGGESTED READINGS

Lance JW: Mechanism and Management of Headache. 6th Ed. Butterworth Heineman, Oxford, 1993

Raskin NH: Headache. 2nd Ed. Churchill Livingstone, New York, 1988

214. ESTROGEN AND HEADACHE

SUSAN R. BELUK

Although migraine affects both men and women, estrogen physiology creates a significant gender bias. Four percent of prepubertal girls and boys are affected by migraines, but after menarche, girls outnumber boys. The gender ratio has been reported to fluctuate with age, increasing from menarche to age 42, with peak ratios from 2.5 to 3.8 : 1, and then declining. The ratio remains above 2.0 in the elderly. Migraine prevalence is highest between 25 and 55 years of age, ranging from 12.9 to 17.6 percent in women and from 3.4 to 6.1 percent in men. In a study of 1,955 headache sufferers, it was found that migrainous women link 60 percent of their headaches to menstruation, but true menstrual migraines occur only 14 percent of the time. The International Headache Society has not yet given menstrual migraine its own classification code but has specified that to be considered as menstrual migraine, 90 percent of headaches should occur within 48 hours prior to menses and up to the last day of flow. Many women show significant improvement in their migraine in the second and third trimester of pregnancy. A positive correlation between menstrual headache and absence of headache during pregnancy exists. Generally, migraine improves with age in the general population, yet headaches worsen in 47 percent of postmenopausal women.

MENSTRUAL PHYSIOLOGY

A review of the basic menstrual physiology is important to better understand the remainder of this chapter. Estrogen is a basic steroid hormone. Estradiol is the most potent naturally occurring estrogen. Estrogen is produced by two main sources: the ovaries and extraglandular tissue, primarily adipose cells. During the menstrual phase, the majority of estrogen produced by the ovaries is in the form of estradiol. The menstrual cycle can be divided into two phases: the follicular phase, during which time the follicles are developing, and the luteal phase, when the corpus luteum dominates.

During the first phase of the cycle, the hypothalamus produces gonadotropin releasing hormone in a pulsatile fashion, in turn stimulating the pituitary to release luteinizing hormone and follicle stimulating hormone. Follicle stimulating hormone stimulates the ovarian follicles, which produce estradiol. The estradiol has a negative feedback on the hypothalamus and on follicle stimulating hormone. A low level of estradiol has a negative effect on luteinizing hormone and high levels of circulating estradiol have a positive feedback effect on pituitary luteinizing hormone levels. Just prior to ovulation, estradiol levels reach a peak and then fall. In turn, luteinizing hormone surges and ovulation follows within 24 hours. The luteal phase is high-lighted by rises of both estrogen and progesterone, which will act to prime the uterine lining. This hormonal rise also has a negative feedback on gonadotropin release. Without fertilization and implantation, the corpus luteum begins to resolve. Circulating estrogen and progesterone levels drop. The endometrial lining prepares to slough, owing to intense vasospasm caused by locally produced prostaglandins.

ESTROGEN AND MIGRAINE

Fundamental work linking estrogen to migraine headaches was performed by Somerville in the early 1970s. A small group of women with known premenstrual or menstrual migraine were studied. Ten mg of estradiol valerate was injected during the premenstrual phase, resulting in a rapid rise, plateau, and gradual taper of estradiol levels. Treatment with the estradiol did not delay menstruation, but in all six patients, menstrual migraine was delayed 3 to 9 days, which corresponded to the decline of circulating estradiol. There was no clear threshold level below which migraine developed, but it was hypothesized that estradiol withdrawal triggered a sequence of events leading to the pathogenesis of menstrual migraine. During this study, progesterone withdrawal continued normally and was not associated with migraine. In later work, Somerville noted that patients required several days' exposure to high levels of estradiol to provoke a withdrawal headache. A study attempting to prevent menstrual migraine with estradiol implants failed, however. It is believed that the implant devices were likely to have been faulty, producing erratic estradiol levels and unpredictable headaches.

Somerville's data suggest that estrogen plays a role in menstrual migraine pathogenesis. Nerve cells not only respond to electrical stimulation but also respond more slowly and for a longer period of time to chemical messengers from within and outside of the brain. Steroid hormones are some of the most potent and specific chemical signals from outside the brain. The brain has receptors for all five classes of steroid hormones: estrogens, progestins, androgens, glucocorticords, and mineralcorticoids. Receptor sites occupy specific loci rather than being scattered diffusely. There is extensive occupation of estrogen receptors in the hypothalamus and limbic system.

The role of estrogen and central opioids in the production of migraine has been eloquently presented by Genazzani. Opiate receptors have many different subtypes and are diffusely distributed throughout the central nervous system. The μ receptor opioid subtype is primarily located in the arcurate nucleus of the hypothalamus, where opioids exert tonic inhibition of luteinizing hormone releasing hormone. Naloxone is a μ receptor antagonist that stimulates luteinizing hormone releasing hormone pulsatility and the resultant increase in luteinizing hormone. Both physiologic and surgical menopausal migraine sufferers were compared to controls. There was a lack of luteinizing hormone response to naloxone administered in the menopausal migraine subjects. Normal opioid tonus returned when the menopausal migraine patients were treated with estrogen and progesterone replacement. Progestins alone were not effective. Young women who underwent bilateral oopherectomy also lost the naloxone-induced luteinizing hormone rise. This suggests that central opioid tonus is modulated by ovarian steroid, namely estrogen, rather than being linked to a general aging process.

On the perivascular level, estrogens have been shown to selectively modulate serotonin receptors. In animal models, estrogen has been shown to block smooth muscle re-uptake of norepinephrine at the neurovascular junction and upregulate postsynaptic adrenergic subtype 1 receptor populations on vascular smooth muscle. In the vascular endothelium, estrogens also inhibit the enzymes catechol-o-methyltransferase and monoamine oxidase, which are responsible for the breakdown of norepinephrine, leading to increased levels circulating locally. Welch hypothesizes that the physiologic levels of estrogen may influence central aminergic and cerebrovascular function. In this model, when estrogen-"enhanced" receptors are sympathetically stimulated, they produce intense vasoconstriction. This oligemia is believed to correlate to the initial prodromal migraine phase, with ultimate vasodilation and headache secondary to local acidosis.

Estrogens both directly and indirectly stimulate prostaglandin (PG) biosynthesis via stimulation of prolactin secretion. Prostaglandins are directly implicated in the development of pain. Both intramuscular and subcutaneous injections of PGE_2 or $PGF_{2\alpha}$ cause intense local pain. PGE, when injected into humans, has been shown to trigger migrainous headaches. Prostaglandins also have the ability to sensitize pain receptors to chemical and mechanical stimulation. This prostaglandin hyperalgesia is probably caused by lowering the threshold of polymodal nociceptor C fibers. PGI_2 is one of the most important prostaglandins that protects against ischemia. Mean values of 6-keto-$PGF_{1\alpha}$, a stable metabolite of PGI_2, were measured at different phases of the menstrual cycle and during migraine crisis in patients known to have true menstrual migraine and in controls. 6-keto-$PGF_{1\alpha}$ levels were significantly decreased in the migraine patients throughout the hormone cycle as compared to controls. Baseline PGE_2 levels were slightly lower in the migraine patients than in the control patients. However, during a migraine crisis, levels significantly increased. Nattero's work suggests that the baseline deficit of PGI_2 in menstrual migraine individuals may be the contributing factor in vascular hypersensitivity to various ischemic events. Other models to support this mechanism in the pathogenesis of migraine are based on findings that PGI_2 levels are elevated during pregnancy, when migraine is less common, and that β-blockers, which increase 6-keto-$PGF_{1\alpha}$ levels, are effective in preventing migraine.

Although prostacycline appears to be the most potent vasodilating prostaglandin with hyperalgesic and inflammatory properties, it did not trigger migraine headaches when injected and is not likely to be a primary trigger in migraine pathogenesis.

Prolactin has been associated with migraine pathogenesis and the theory of central dysmodulation. The pituitary is stimulated to release prolactin by vasoactive intestinal peptide, angiotensin, and thryrotropin releasing hormone. Dopamine tonically inhibits prolactin release. Serotonin inhibits thyroid stimulating hormone indirectly via thyrotropin releasing hormone and directly at the pituitary level.

In a study of 11 females with migraine and 9 control subjects, exogenous injection of thyrotropin releasing hormone, luteinizing hormone releasing hormone, and insulin resulted in a significantly elevated prolactin level in the migrainous patients over controls. Thyroid stimulating hormone levels were also increased in controls versus migraine patients, but the increase was not statistically significant. In another study, the dopamine antagonists sulpride and domperidone, injected during the follicular phase, resulted in a significantly elevated luteinizing hormone release in both menstrual and nonmenstrual migraine patients compared to controls. If dopamine were the only focus

of dysmodulation, we should have seen marked elevation in the thyroid stimulating hormone in the previous study as well. Serotonin, however, triggers an increase in prolactin without elevation of thyroid stimulating hormone, suggesting serotonin hyperfunction in combination of dopaminergic hypofunction. Serotonin receptors in turn are modulated by estrogen. Other findings are consistent with the above theory, showing a marked prolactin response to thyrotropin releasing hormone during acute migraine attacks as compared to attack-free periods.

TREATMENT

Treatment of menstrual migraine is similar to that for other migraine conditions and is outlined elsewhere in Section 3, Part IX of this book. However, a brief review of a basic approach and some specific suggestions are highlighted here. Menstrual migraine is one of the most difficult headaches to manage, but we still begin with the basic principles when addressing this disorder: behavioral techniques, including regular exercise three times a week, which helps to increase β-endorphin levels; monitoring diet, specifically monosodium glutamate, nitrates, caffeine, and alcohol; and regular sleep and relaxation. For some lucky individuals, this may be the ticket to better control. If patients have only one headache a month associated with a predictable menstrual cycle, they may turn to "mini-prophylaxis" with β-blockers, nonsteroidal anti-inflammatory drugs, or ergotamine preparations, beginning 1 to 2 days before the typical headache begins and continuing through the length of the cycle. For individuals who have migraine headaches throughout the month and are already on prophylactic medicine yet who continue to have persistent breakthrough menstrual migraine, increasing the dose of medication premenstrually may be of some benefit. If this also is unsuccessful, this is an instance in which various prophylactic agents may have to be combined, with a second medicine added perimenstrually. Standard headache abortive agents are used for treating breakthrough headaches.

When a severe attack of menstrual migraine is recalcitrant to standard therapy, short-term high-dose corticosteroids, major tranquilizers, or intravenous dihydroergotamine can be used to break the cycle. If these treatments are relied on too heavily or fail to benefit, hormonal therapy should be tried. In 20 women with menstrual migraine and regular menstrual cycles, the prophylactic effect of 1.5 mg percutaneous estradiol was studied in a double-blind placebo-controlled crossover trial. Treatment was begun 2 days prior to expected migraine and was continued for 7 days each month. Migraine atttacks occured in 30.8 percent of the estradiol cycles, versus 96.3 percent of the placebo cycles. Migraine attacks were milder in nature and were of shorter duration than those under placebo treatment. In another study, 24 patients with refractory menstrual migraine were treated with subcutaneous estradiol implants for up to 5 years. Headaches in 23 patients improved with treatment. Twenty patients (83 percent) became almost headache-free. All these patients were able to stop previous therapies and believed that the implants had been the most effective migraine therapy. However, a follow-up placebo-controlled study on premenstrual syndrome was not as valuable. Now that estrogen implants are available in the United States, it is important to re-evaluate this treatment.

It has also been shown that danazol, an ethinytestosterone derivative, prevented hormonally mediated headache that had been unsuccessfully managed with standard therapies. Danazol prevents the rise in both estrogen and progesterone levels in the luteal phase of the menstrual cycle, maintaining a constant estrogen state. As mentioned earlier, migraine headaches were triggered by the late luteal drop in estrogens. In the initial study phase, 63 percent of patients reported relief of their hormonal migraine. Eighty-one women went onto continue the medication for a 6-month period, and 82 percent showed continued migraine prevention. Prophylaxis was maintained with 400 mg danazol taken 25 days each month in combination with a diuretic. Various side effects and significant drug interactions need to be addressed before prescribing this medication.

Tamoxifen has also been recommended for recalcitrant menstrual migraine. Tamoxifen is an antiestrogen (most known for its use in breast cancer). It binds to estrogen receptors and inhibits messenger RNA transcription. The drug is given for 7 to 14 days of the luteal cycle, with dosages ranging from 5 to 15 mg/day. Bromocriptine, in dosages of 2.5 to 5.0 mg/day given during the luteal phase, is also used to prevent premenstrual symptoms and headache.

Since migraine affects a significant number of women during their fertile years, physicians are often consulted regarding the appropriate use of oral contraceptive pills in these patients. The literature regarding this issue is very controversial; different works are difficult to compare, given the more current use of lower estrogen-progestin combinations. The safest pills contain the least amount of estrogen (35 μg or less) and the lowest possible progestin. In a study that parallels what we generally see in clinical practice, migrainous women who were placed on oral contraceptive pills, one-third had an increase in frequency of headaches, one-third had no change, and one-third experienced improvement. In a subset of women who begin oral contraceptive pills, new-onset migraine may develop within the first two cycles of therapy, but can also develop much later. Patients and clinicians may not recognize the association in the latter situation. Approximately 70 percent of individuals will show improvement after discontinuation; however, it may take several months or even years to return to baseline.

ORAL CONTRACEPTIVES AND THE MIGRAINE PATIENT

When should migraine patients be prescribed oral contraceptive pills? Headache specialists differ on the issue, with stances ranging from not recommending them at all to taking a somewhat less conservative approach. Oral contraceptive pill replacement may be appropriate for women with tension-type headache or migraine without aura who do not have other risk factors. If migraine patients develop increased headache frequency or intensity, or loss of manageability of the headaches, the pills should be discontinued. If neurologic symptoms develop, or aura or atypical aura occur, then oral contraceptives should be stopped immediately.

Stroke is the leading cause of acute neurologic impairment and the third highest cause of death in the United States. Data suggesting an increased risk of stroke among oral contraceptive pill users and migraine sufferers is often conflicting. Oral contraceptive pills are known to alter blood pressure, glucose metabolism, lipid metabolism, coagulation, and fibrinolyic synthesis, as well as to modify migraines. In a collaborative study of stroke in young women, it was confirmed that there is a definite increased relative risk of stroke in patients using oral contraceptive pills independent of other risk factors; the relative risk for thrombotic stroke and hemorragic stroke is approximately 4.2 and approximately 2.0, respectively. Unfortunately, the study could not correlate risk to dose strength. Twenty out of 24 patients who had thrombotic strokes were taking 100 μg of mestranol. The collaborative study also reported a twofold increased relative risk of thrombotic stroke in migraine sufferers on oral contraceptive agents. Several criticisms were addressed by the authors themselves, namely that arbitrary criteria were used to make migraine diagnoses. The results of this study are also difficult to interpret, given that current oral contraceptive pills have no more than 50 μg of synthetic estrogen.

A group of 310 patients with migraine and 30 patients with migrainous stroke were studied to see if predictive factors could be identified. A history of migraine with aura was significantly more common in the migrainous stroke group, (80 versus 46 percent of the migraine group), as was a history of previous stroke (30 versus 1.3 percent).

ESTROGEN AND CLIMACTERIC AND MENOPAUSE

This chapter would not be complete without addressing the role of estrogen and climacteric. *Climacteric* is defined as the transitional period from the reproductive to the nonreproductive years. Menopause, on the other hand, begins with the last menstrual period and generally occurs around age 51. Women who are 50 years old today can be expected to live into their late 80s. By the year 2000, women will be living one-third of their lives postmenopausally. In the general population, headaches tend to decrease with age. Headaches may flare up during climacteric, which may be partly due to fluctuating estrogen levels. Although many women obtain relief from their headaches after menopause, an unfortunate percentage of migraine patients show a worsening.

As the ovarian synthesis of estradiol comes to a halt, the adipose tissue becomes the primary site of estrogen aromatization into the form of estrone, which is the biologically weaker hormone. Interestingly, peripheral estrogen secretion may be enhanced in the obese perimenopausal individual. The lack of estrogen is felt throughout the female body. Thirty to 80 percent of postmenopausal women experience vasomotor instability. Although the pathogenesis of ''hot flashes'' is not certain, they have been correlated to the rapid decline of estrogen E_1 and E_2 levels. The hypothalamic pituitary axis remains intact into old age. It is believed that the estrogen influence on neurohormones has a parasympathomimetic stabilizing effect on the hypothalamus. Alterations of various neurohormones, catecholamines, prostaglandins, endorphins, and low estrogen levels may be responsible for the hypersympathomimetic attack associated with the vasomotor and mood changes seen with ''hot flashes.'' The instability of these factors may also be responsible for the erratic migraines often seen during this time.

Exogenous estrogens are commonly used in postmenopausal women to treat a variety of symptoms, ranging from osteoporosis to ''hot flashes.'' More than 30 percent of postmenopausal women have been given exogenous estrogen agents. The risk of stroke increases with age, and the decision to use estrogen replacement therapy needs to be weighed very carefully on an individual basis. Headache management becomes difficult when estrogen replacement therapy aggravates existing migraine. Although there is a limited body of literature addressing this topic, it has been shown that by decreasing estrogen dose and converting to continous therapy, there is a 60 percent improvement in headache control. There have been anecdotal reports that converting from oral estrogen to transdermal estrogen may also be better tolerated in the migrainous patient. Transdermal estradiol increases circulating estradiol and estrone, whereas oral conjugated estrogens primarily raise estrone. Fifty μg of transdermal estradiol is equivalent to .625 mg of oral estrogen. The transdermal estradiol was shown to elicit the favorable actions of estrogen while bypassing the hepatic metabolism. It is hoped that the heightened interest in the treatment of headaches will stimulate further research in this very important field.

SUGGESTED READINGS

Edelson R: Menstrual migraine and other hormonal aspects of migraine. Headache 25:376–9, 1985

Epstein MT, Hockaday TD: Migraine and reproductive hormones throughout the menstrual cycle. Lancet 543–8, 1975

Kudrow L: The relationship of headache frequency to hormone use in migraine. Headache, 15:36–49, 1975

Lignieres B, Vincens M, Mauvais-Jarvis P: Prevention of menstrual migraine by percutaneous oestradiol. Brit Med J 293:1540, 1986

Magos A, Zilkha K, Studd J: Treatment of menstrual migraine by oestradiol implants. J Neurol, Neurosurg, Psychiatry 46:1044–6, 1983

Rothrock J, North J, Madden K et al: Migraine and migrainous stroke: risk factors and prognosis. Neurology 43:2473–6, 1993

Ryan R: A controlled study of the effect of oral contraceptives on migraine. Headache 17:250–2, 1978

Silberstein S, Merriam G: Estrogens, progestins, and headache. Neurology 41:786–93, 1991

Somerville B: Estrogen-withdrawal migraine I: duration of exposure required and attempted prophylaxis by premenstrual estrogen administration. Neurology 25:239–44, 1975

Somerville B: Estrogen-withdrawal migraine II: attempted prophylaxis by continuous estradiol administration. Neurology 25:245–50 1975

Somerville B: The role of estradiol withdrawal in the etiology of menstrual migraine. Neurology 22:355–64, 1972

Welch K, Darnley D, Simkins R: The role of estrogen in migraine: a review and hypothesis. Cephalalgia 4:227–36, 1984

215. HEADACHES IN PREGNANCY

ELIZABETH LODER

The primary headache disorders of migraine and tension-type headache disproportionately affect women of childbearing age; consequently, the occurrence of headache in some form during pregnancy or the puerperium is common. Studies of the natural history and prevalence of headache during pregnancy and the puerperium show certain trends. In women with pre-existing benign headache disorders, tension-type headache is largely unaffected by pregnancy, with most women experiencing headaches of similar intensity and duration during and after pregnancy as before. The pathogenesis of tension-type headache is poorly understood, but hormonal factors are not generally thought to play a role in causing or aggravating these headaches. For that reason, the hormonal events of pregnancy presumably have little effect on the pre-existing headache pattern.

Well-conducted studies suggest that 67 percent of women whose headaches meet International Headache Society criteria for the diagnosis of migraine without aura prior to pregnancy will experience significant improvement in headaches during the second and third trimester of pregnancy. This improvement may be more likely to occur in women whose headaches have previously correlated with hormonal events, such as menarche, menstrual periods, or use of oral contraceptives. Headaches in these patients typically worsen again when menstrual cycles resume following delivery or cessation of breast-feeding. Women who suffer from migraine with aura prior to pregnancy are more likely to note no improvement in headache frequency or intensity—or even worsening—during pregnancy. Cluster headache and related conditions, such as paroxysmal hemicrania, are less common in women than men and therefore rarely complicate pregnancy. When they do, these headaches may be more resistant to treatment than those occurring in nonpregnant women. Women with pre-existing headache disorders may be more prone than other women to develop headache in response to epidural anesthesia during delivery.

In addition to changes in pre-existing headache conditions that can be provoked by pregnancy, headaches, particularly migraine with aura, frequently occur for the first time during pregnancy or following delivery. Thorough investigation or the passage of time generally reveal such headaches to be of benign origin. However, pregnancy and lactation do not confer immunity to such serious causes of headache as brain tumor, meningitis, or vasculitis. Therefore, evaluation of new or worsening headaches in the pregnant patient should be as thorough as that undertaken in nonpregnant patients. This may include imaging studies if clinically indicated. When a choice is possible between magnetic resonance imaging and computed tomography, the theoretic but undemonstrated risks of fetal exposure to the electromagnetic fields generated in magnetic resonance imaging are preferable to the known risks of exposure to ionizing radiation in computed tomography. In situations such as suspected intracranial hemorrhage, where computed tomography is clinically indicated and superior to magnetic resonance imaging, pregnancy should not deter its use.

The occurrence of some serious causes of headache, such as subarachnoid hemorrhage, is actually increased in pregnancy. It should also be borne in mind that new onset or worsening of pre-existing headache during pregnancy can be due to pregnancy-specific conditions. Most notable among these is pregnancy-induced hypertension, in which headache or other nonspecific neurologic complaints may precede objective signs of the disorder, such as hypertension or proteinuria. It has been theorized that pregnancy-induced hypertension is more common in migraine sufferers, but studies have produced conflicting data. Finally, a history of recurrent spontaneous abortions or thromboembolic disease in combination with migrainelike headaches should prompt a search for anticardiolipin antibodies.

Mild to moderate primary headache disorders occurring during pregnancy do not correlate with poor reproductive outcomes, and there is no evidence of an increased incidence of birth defects in the offspring of headache patients. Common sense and case reports in the medical literature suggest that pregnant patients whose headaches are severe enough to lead to intractable vomiting and poor weight gain, or who take frequent doses of headache medications, particularly those containing ergotamine, are at risk of pregnancy complications, including fetal malformation, intrauterine growth retardation, stillbirth, spontaneous abortion, and abruptio placentae.

Mention should be made of a situation common in clinical practice: a headache patient who has been in treatment for some time who discovers she is pregnant and has been taking various headache medications for much of her first trimester without realizing she is pregnant. This troublesome situation, which produces much anxiety for both patient and doctor, can be generally be avoided. It is helpful to remember that because women of childbearing potential are the majority of patients seeking headache evaluation and treatment, pregnancy, planned or unplanned, is likely to occur in many of them. It is therefore wise to include in the initial medical evaluation of any fertile woman a reminder to avoid any unnecessary medication if she plans to attempt pregnancy or has reason to think she might be pregnant. This recommendation should be documented in the medical record. Consideration should always be given to the fact that any female of childbearing age may already be pregnant, and a pregnancy test done if indicated. Patients seeking information on possible fetal harm from exposure to medication can be referred to one of several national telephone hotlines that provide available information about the teratogenic effects of many substances.

Whereas evaluation of headache in pregnancy is relatively straightforward, management of the disorder is not. Treatment of headache disorders in the pregnant patient, or the patient attempting pregnancy, is controversial and largely empiric. Because of concern about legal liability arising from potential harm to a fetus, women of childbearing potential have traditionally been excluded from drug studies. This has led to a serious lack of information about the effects of many drugs in pregnancy. Pregnant women with chronic illnesses of many kinds, including headache disorders, may be undertreated because of concern about theoretic adverse effects of medication on the fetus. In some instances, untreated headache or the complications of unprescribed or unsupervised medication use by a desperate headache patient may be far more dangerous to the mother or fetus than carefully prescribed and supervised medication regimens. Little is known about the extent of medication use among pregnant women with headache; clinical experience indicates that many pregnant patients with headache continue to use medications that are contraindicated in pregnancy, such as ergotamine-containing drugs, barbiturate-containing medications, and platelet-active agents such as aspirin or ibuprofen.

Ideally, headache patients who wish to become pregnant or who become pregnant while in treatment should be encouraged to discontinue all medications whenever possible. In most cases, both the pregnant patient and the physician will be eager to avoid the use of medication if at all possible. This resolve is generally aided by the previously mentioned improvement in headache that many patients experience. Most patients, with regular office visits to monitor their condition and offer psychosocial support, will be successful in tolerating headaches without the use of medication, or with the use of medication such as acetaminophen, which is generally accepted as safe for use in pregnancy.

Identification of headache trigger factors, although an important adjunct to treatment in any headache patient, is particularly important in the pregnant patient or the patient attempting pregnancy. Too often, such nonpharmacologic ''avoidance therapy'' is overlooked or underemphasized by physicians, who are more enthusiastic about pharmacologic approaches to headache. However, scrupulous avoidance of headache triggers can greatly reduce the need for medication in pregnant patients. Toward this end, dietary regimens should be carefully reviewed with patients who have migraine, and the avoidance of alcohol emphasized. Skipping meals should be discouraged. Caffeine intake should be avoided or minimized on a regular basis. Caffeine use in acute headache—for example, having a strong cup of coffee early in a headache episode—is very helpful for many patients and may obviate the need to use stronger medications later. Patients to whom this approach is suggested should be informed that a recent study has implicated caffeine in early spontaneous abortion; it may be wise to save this approach for the second and third trimesters, when the risk of spontaneous abortion is lower.

The importance of obtaining adequate rest cannot be overemphasized. The pregnant patient with job and family responsibilities may have great difficulty obtaining needed sleep. If headaches are intense enough that pharmacologic treatment is a possibility, serious consideration should be given to a reduction in work hours or a medical leave of absence from work. If effective, a temporary reduction in work responsibilities is clearly preferable to pharmacologic treatment of headache during pregnancy.

Psychosocial stressors during or after pregnancy may contribute to the burden of headache or render it intolerable; those patients may benefit from such interventions as counseling or relaxation training. Serious mood disturbances or emotional distress should prompt psychiatric referral. The incidence of postpartum depression in migraine patients has not been separately studied, but recent studies suggesting depression and anxiety are more common in migraine patients in general prompt concern that migraine patients may also be more vulnerable to postpartum depression as well; a high index of suspicion for the disorder should be maintained.

Biofeedback has been shown to reduce both frequency and intensity of migraine during pregnancy and should always be considered in place of or as an adjunct to medication in pregnant patients. Physical therapy interventions such as massage, postural training, and exercise can be helpful in nearly all headache patients, and should also be considered prior to a trial of medication. If clinically indicated, local anesthetic infiltration of trigger points in the head or neck region can be safely performed during pregnancy. With any nonpharmacologic treatment (as with any pharmacologic treatment), placebo response and patient expectation of benefit greatly influence the outcome of treatment, and should be exploited whenever possible.

The decision to use pharmacologic approaches to headache management in the pregnant patient should represent a consensus of the patient, her partner, and her obstetrician. Common sense dictates that the potential benefits of drug treatment should clearly outweigh the potential risks to the mother and fetus. The clinical situation will vary from patient to patient, and treatment must be individualized. Nonetheless, certain principles will apply in most cases:

1. Nonpharmacologic methods should be tried before medication is used, and even if suboptimally effective alone, should be continued with medication in most cases, as they may have a medication-sparing effect.
2. Whenever possible, pharmacologic treatment of headache should be delayed until the second and third trimesters, when organogenesis is complete.
3. The lowest effective dose of medication should be used for the shortest time possible.
4. Medications selected for use should be those that, on the basis of current knowledge, are least likely to pose a danger to mother or fetus.
5. Patients should be discouraged from using herbal or ''natural'' headache remedies about which little or no information

is available. A number of easily obtainable herbal preparations can be harmful to the pregnant woman or fetus.

For acute treatment of mild to moderate headache in pregnancy, acetaminophen is the drug of choice. If nausea or vomiting preclude oral use, it is available as a rectal suppository. Combined with rest, relaxation techniques, and perhaps caffeine, this reasonably safe approach will frequently be effective in the pregnant headache patient. Aspirin or nonsteroidal anti-inflammatory medications should be avoided in the pregnant patient. They interfere with platelet function and may increase the risk of hemorrhagic complications. They also interfere with prostaglandin synthesis. Late in pregnancy, this can theoretically produce early closure of the ductus arteriosus. Barbiturate-containing medications, though frequently used by nonpregnant patients for mild to moderate headache, should probably be avoided in pregnancy because of concern over possible neurobehavioral abnormalities and congenital malformations. Isometheptene-containing medications (Midrin) should be avoided, owing to vasoconstrictive properties and potential effects on uterine circulation. Ergotamine compounds (methylergonovine maleate, ergotamine tartrate, dihydroergotamine) are absolutely contraindicated during pregnancy because of concern over their stimulatory effects on uterine muscle. These drugs can be used for headache occurring after delivery, when they may be doubly useful in reducing the incidence of uterine atony.

For more severe headaches, narcotic medications may be appropriate, in combination with acetaminophen. Clear limits must be placed on frequency of use, to avoid habituation or dependence, and the drawback of sedation must be clearly explained. Nonetheless, narcotic medications, particularly meperidine and oxycodone, have been extensively used in pregnancy with no indication of major teratogenic effects. The one exception to this is codeine, which in several retrospective studies was associated with a number of congenital malformations. These results have not been verified by prospective studies, but it is probably wise to avoid codeine when possible, especially in the first trimester. Acetaminophen may be used in combination with narcotic medications to obtain synergistic pain relief.

Phenothiazines are sometimes used in severe headache to provide sedation and control of vomiting; these should be avoided in the pregnant patient if at all possible. Trimethobenzamide (Tigan) is believed to be a relatively safe alternative treatment for nausea and vomiting during pregnancy, and is therefore preferable if antiemetics are necessary. Parenteral ergotamine preparations, also used frequently for severe migraine, are absolutely contraindicated in the pregnant patient, owing to their effects on uterine muscle. Sumatriptan should likewise be avoided in pregnancy.

Among the commonly used prophylactic agents for headache, the anticonvulsants, lithium carbonate, and methysergide should not be used during pregnancy, because safer alternatives exist. The anticonvulsants and lithium have been convincingly linked to an increased incidence of fetal malformation, and methysergide may theoretically increase the risk of abortion or premature labor. If prophylaxis is thought to be necessary, it is probably wise to choose a β-blocker or a tricyclic antidepressant. There is accumulated and relatively reassuring experience with the use of these drugs in pregnant women with other chronic conditions. Calcium channel-blockers have been less extensively studied in pregnancy, but may also be an appropriate choice for prophylaxis. There is a theoretic possibility they can delay or lengthen labor, owing to tocolytic action on the uterine muscle. Fluoxetine, a serotonin re-uptake inhibitor, is useful in the prophylaxis of some headache disorders. A recent retrospective study found no increase in birth defects in infants born to women who used the drug during pregnancy.

The medical, legal, and ethical risks of pharmacologic management of headache disorders in pregnancy can be minimized by careful attention to all aspects of the doctor–patient relationship. It is important to review with the patient that the background risk of fetal malformation is 2 to 4 percent, and to inform her of the risks and benefits of any suggested approach to her headaches. Careful documentation of advice about avoiding medications should be entered in the chart; it is common for pregnant patients to say that they were never told not to use certain medications. If pharmacologic treatment is recommended, it may be wise to have the patient initial or sign a statement indicating that she has been informed of the potential risks and benefits of such treatment and of alternatives to treatment and that she consents to the proposed treatment.

It is remarkable how little formal attention has been paid to the problem of headache in pregnancy, given the frequency with which the two conditions occur together. Increased emphasis on research into disorders that primarily affect women and greater participation of women of childbearing age in clinical trials will eventually improve the treatment of pregnant women with headache disorders.

SUGGESTED READING

Berkowitz RL, Coustan DR, Mochizuki TK: Handbook for Prescribing Medications During Pregnancy. Little, Brown, Boston, 1986

Silberstein SD: Headaches and Women: Treatment of the pregnant and lactating migraineur. Headache 33:533–40, 1993

Welch KM: Migraine and pregnancy. Adv Neurol 64:77–81, 1994

SECTION 4. GENERAL ASPECTS OF PAIN

216. ANATOMY AND PHYSIOLOGY OF PAIN

ZAHID H. BAJWA
LANCE J. LEHMANN
SCOTT M. FISHMAN

Pain is the most common symptom reported to physicians. It has been a prominant concern of mankind since the beginning of recorded history. The word *pain* is originally derived from the Latin *poena*, meaning punishment. The International Association for the Study of Pain defines pain as ''an unpleasant sensory and emotional experience arising from the actual or potential tissue damage or described in terms of such damage.'' Over the past several years, the field of pain management has undergone a revolution marked by great advances in knowledge and therapeutic options. In order to better understand the anatomy and physiology of pain, this chapter subdivides pain into three major categories: neuropathic, nociceptive, and idiopathic pain. Before discussing specific neural pathways, it is useful to discuss some basic concepts and definitions.

BASIC CONCEPTS

Neuropathic pain is defined as pain due to dysfunction of the nervous system in the absence of ongoing tissue damage. Patients describe the pain as sharp, shooting, or burning. Pain sensation is usually felt in the area of sensory deficit and is worsened by mild stimuli that normally would not produce pain, such as light touch or cool air (allodynia). Many other labels are given to neuropathic pain, including nerve pain, neurogenic pain, deafferentation syndrome, and so on. Examples of neuropathic pain states include reflex sympathetic dystrophy, diabetic neuropathy, central pain syndromes, trigeminal and postherpetic neuralgia.

Nociceptive pain results from direct tissue damage and may occur with or without damage to the nervous system. Nociceptive pain results from the activation of nociceptors, intact peripheral afferent pain receptors. Arthritic, acute postoperative, and post-traumatic pain are in this category. Nociceptive pain is further subdivided into somatic and visceral pain, which can be distinguished by the quality of the pain and associated clinical features. Somatic pain is usually well localized and described as stabbing, aching, or throbbing. Visceral pain arises from the viscera and is characteristically dull, crampy, and poorly localized.

The term *idiopathic pain* has been used interchangeably with the term *psychogenic pain*. In our opinion, idiopathic pain is the more appropriate term because it implies a wider spectrum of poorly understood pain states. Myofascial pain syndrome and somatoform pain disorder are examples of idiopathic pain. In some patients, there is no evidence of an associated organic cause, whereas in others, pain and associated symptoms are grossly out of proportion to identifiable organic pathology. The recently revised *Diagnostic and Statistical Manual of Mental Disorders,* fourth edition (DSM-IV) avoids using the terms *psychogenic* or *idiopathic pain* altogether, instead using the broader term of *somatoform disorder* and distinguishing between ''pain disorder associated with psychologic factors (acute and chronic)'' and ''pain disorder associated with both psychologic factors and a general medical condition (acute and chronic).''

Finally, it is worth emphasizing that all pain has a psychological component. Psychological factors, which are often not obvious, as well as cultural and environmental factors, must be considered to fully evaluate pain patients. For example, emotional arousal can enhance nociception at the periphery. Heightened sympathetic activity with the release of norepinephrine at sympathetic terminals can sensitize or directly activate nociceptors. Similarly, reflex skeletal muscle spasm caused by anxiety can contribute to a positive feedback loop in which nociception fosters increased tone in muscle near the site of injury, eventually activating muscle nociceptors. Patients in clinical practice often exhibit more than one type of pain. One example are patients with cancer who may have pain of neuropathic, nociceptive, and myofascial origin.

Peripheral Pain Pathways

Nociception involves perception of pain and its subsequent response. An individual's perception of pain can be modified at any level from the periphery to the central nervous system (CNS). The peripheral sensory system becomes activated when nociceptors, which are free nerve endings of primary afferent neurons, are stimulated by mechanical, thermal, or chemical stimuli. With the exception of the CNS, all other tissues contain nociceptors, especially the skin, which is richly innervated. There are three major types of nociceptors: (1) A-δ high-threshold mechanoreceptors, which respond to noxious pressure; (2) A-δ mechanothermal receptors, which respond to both noxious mechanical and thermal stimuli; and (3) C-fiber polymodal nociceptors, which respond to noxious mechanical, thermal, and chemical stimuli. In addition, some A-δ fibers respond specifically to cold stimuli.

Nociceptive impulses, along with other sensory stimuli, are transmitted to the spinal cord and CNS via the dorsal roots (Fig. 216-1). Dorsal root ganglia are located outside of the spinal cord and contain cell bodies of sensory neurons. The summation theory states that any sensory stimulus if sufficiently intense can cause pain. Repetitive stimulation of a nocicepter can cause tissue damage, resulting in a decrease in the pain threshold. Clinical manifestations of this include enhanced pain (primary hyperalgesia), the ability of non-noxious stimuli to produce pain (allodynia), and an exaggerated response to noxious stimuli (hyperpathia). These nociceptors transduce the various forms of stimuli into electrical energy (via action potentials), which is transmitted to the CNS via peripheral nerves. Peripheral nerves consist of sensory, motor, and autonomic fibers, which are classified according to size, conduction velocity, and presence, absence, and thickness of the myelin sheath. To better illustrate

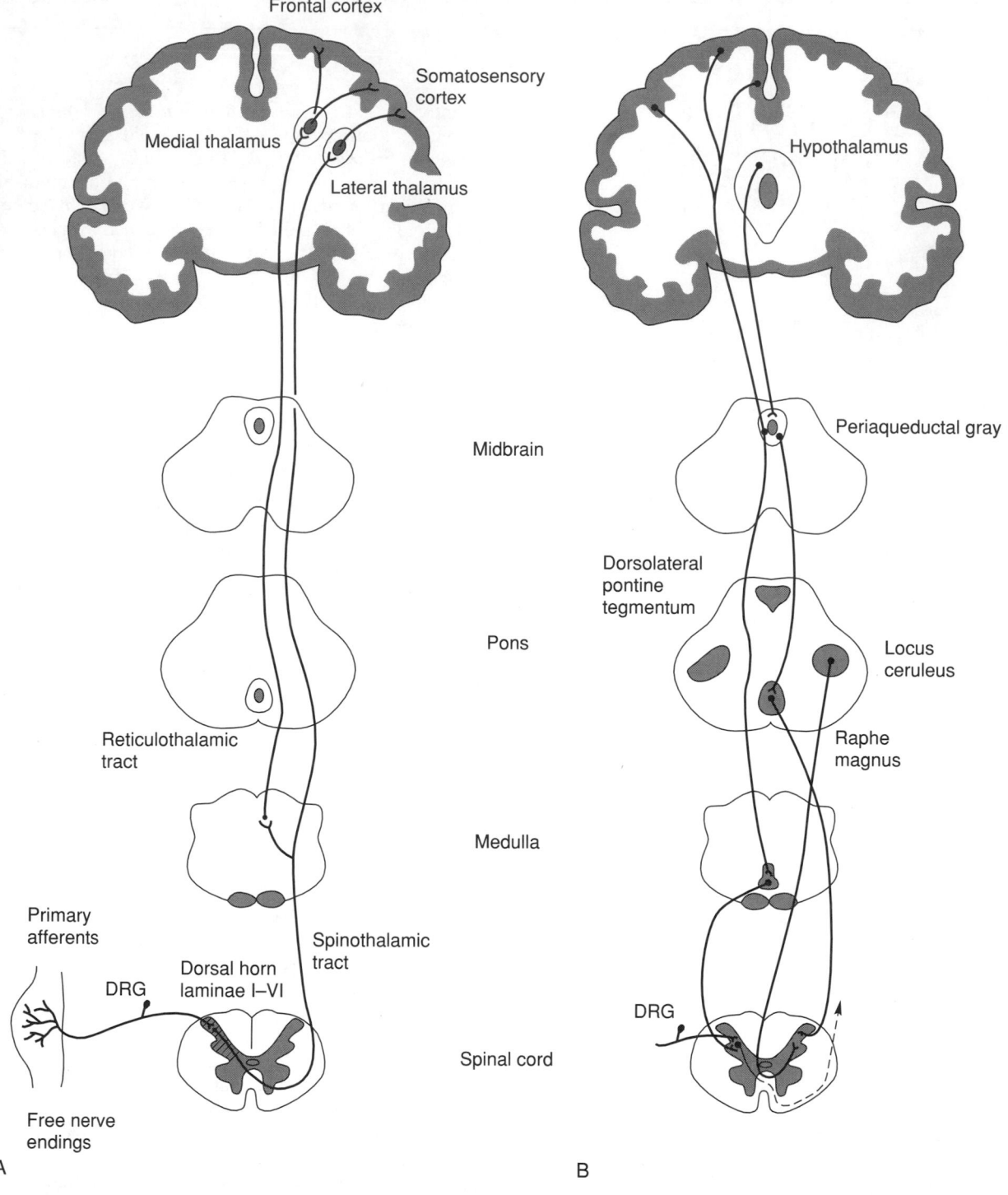

FIG. 216-1. A model of the ascending and descending systems that transmit and modulate pain. **(A)** The ascending transmission system starts with sensory afferents that synapse in the dorsal horn of the spinal cord and decussate to the enter the spinothalamic tract. At brainstem levels, some fibers leave the spinothalamic tract and ascend in the reticulothalamic tract. In the thalamus, spinothalamic projections terminate in both lateral and medial thalamic structures. The message is then relayed to both frontal and somatosensory cortex. **(B)** The descending modulation system involves direct projections to the dorsal horn of the spinal cord from cells in the pontine reticular formation, the locus ceruleus, and the nucleus raphe magnus. In addition, input from the somatosensory and frontal cortex and the hypothalamus activates cells in the midbrain, which control spinal pain transmission cells via cells in the rostroventral medulla.

the above concepts, let us consider visceral pain. Visceral pain tends to be diffuse and poorly localized, since the primary afferents of the viscera have large nociceptive fields. Viscera respond maximally to distention, torsion, and ischemia. The visceral afferents travel to the spinal cord with autonomic fibers, particularly the sympathetic fibers. Visceral pain can therefore be relieved by traditional sympathetic blockade.

DORSAL HORN

The dorsal horn is the first site within the CNS where incoming nociceptive information is processed and modulated. Modulation involves inhibition or augmentation of impulses along ascending and descending pathways via biochemical mediators. As was first described by Rexed in 1952, gray matter of the spinal cord is organized in laminae. There are 10 laminae, with laminae I through VI comprising the dorsal horn (very important in pain transmission and modulation) and laminae VII through X comprising the intermediate and ventral horns of the spinal cord (their role in pain transmission is less clear). There are two types of neurons in the dorsal horn that respond to incoming nociceptive stimuli: nociceptive-specific neurons, which respond to a specific type of stimulus, and wide dynamic range neurons, which respond to a wide variety of stimuli. Nociceptive-specific neurons have small receptive fields, are somatotopically organized, and are most abundant in lamina I. Wide dynamic range neurons have larger receptive fields and are the most prevalent cells in the dorsal horn.

Lissauer's tract is a superficial bundle made up of primary afferent fibers consisting of A-δ fibers, C-fibers, and propriospinal axons that run longitudinally between the surface of the spinal cord and the dorsal horn. Dorsal roots enter the spinal cord with fibers traversing through Lissauer's tract to enter the dorsal horn. A-δ fibers, upon entering Lissauer's tract, terminate in laminae I, II, V, and X. Likewise, C-fibers terminate in laminae I, II, and V. Lamina I is also called the marginal layer and it is the most superficial lamina. In addition to the nociceptive-specific and wide dynamic range neurons, the most abundant cell type in lamina I are projection cells. Some of these make up projection pathways, whereas others synapse with interneurons. Lamina II is called the substantia gelatinosa because of its gelatinous appearance. It also contains nociceptive-specific and wide dynamic range neurons. Lamina III through V are known as the nucleus proprius. Lamina III contains myelinated axons and dendrites from deeper laminae. The most common cell type in lamina IV are low-threshold mechanoreceptors, responding to tactile and thermal stimuli from the skin. Lamina V consists mainly of wide dynamic range neurons and axons that give rise to ascending systems. Lamina VI contains cells that provide information on movement.

The gate control theory of pain, as proposed by Wall and Melzack in 1965, states that the dorsal horn in the spinal cord acts as a gate upon which all nociceptive stimuli converge. Although this model does not explain all pain phenomena, the dorsal horn remains a pivotal landmark where excitation, inhibition, modulation, and integration of nociceptive impulses affect the expression of pain. More specifically, the substantia gelatinosa of the dorsal horn is an important area at which pain can be modulated. Specific "target" cells located in the dorsal horn are stimulated by both large mechanofibers and smaller pain-conducting fibers. These cells relay information to higher brain centers. The substantia gelatinosa acts primarily as an inhibitory structure. Small pain fibers inhibit the substantia gelatinosa,

reducing its inhibitory effect on fibers that stimulate target cells; thus, pain persists. The large fibers stimulate the substantia gelatinosa, enhancing its inhibitory effect; this tends to be self-limiting and would reduce painful stimuli from the same area. This pathway may explain the "counterirritation theory," which asserts that applying pressure or rubbing an area at the site of injury reduces pain perception by stimulation of large mechanofibers. Electrical stimulation of large afferent fibers has been shown to inhibit small primary afferents. This has been used to explain the therapeutic effectiveness of nervous system stimulation in reducing pain and may at least partially explain the mechanism of action of spinal cord stimulators and transcutaneous electrical nerve stimulators (TENS).

ASCENDING PATHWAYS

The ascending nociceptive pain pathways arise mainly from laminae I, II, and V. These include, but are not limited to, the following: spinothalamic tract, spinoreticular tract, dorsal columns, propriospinal system, and spinomesencephalic tract.

The spinothalamic tract is located in the anterolateral quadrant of the spinal cord and is involved with sensing mechanical or tactile stimuli as well as the transmission of nociceptive stimuli. Most of these axons cross in the ventral white commissure to ascend in the opposite anterolateral quadrant, whereas a smaller number of axons ascend ipsilaterally. The spinothalamic tract neurons separate into medial and lateral divisions as they approach the thalamus. Neurons projecting to the lateral thalamus arise from laminae I, II, and V and synapse with fibers that project to the somatosensory cortex. These neurons are thought to be involved with the sensory and discriminatory aspects of pain. Neurons projecting to the medial thalamus originate from the deeper laminae VI through IX, ultimately projecting to the reticular formation of the brainstem, periaqueductal gray matter, and hypothalamus. These fibers then synapse with neurons that project to the limbic system, somatosensory cortex, and other cortical centers.

Along with the spinothalamic tract, the spinoreticular tract and the spinomesencephalic tract are also located in the anterolateral quadrant. These tracts are similar in that each is involved with autonomic reflex responses and behavioral and motivational aspects of pain. Unlike the spinothalamic tract, the origin of spinoreticular tract neurons is not clear. They may predominantly arise from laminae VII and VIII and possibly also be from laminae I and V. Many of these cells are wide dynamic range neurons that transmit nociceptive stimuli, both ipsilaterally and contralaterally, to the reticular formation. The spinoreticular tract is most likely involved with the behavioral, autonomic, and motivational components of pain. The spinomesencephalic tract contains mostly nociceptive neurons that arise from laminae I and V. These neurons ascend contralaterally and terminate in a number of structures, including the periaqueductal gray matter, reticular formation, and limbic system.

The dorsal column system is thought to play an important role in proprioception and possibly inhibition of nociceptive transmission. In addition, it may provide information on the localization of pain. The cells in the dorsal column system are mainly large diameter myelinated primary afferents found in laminae III through IV. These fibers travel ipsilaterally in the nucleus gracilis and nucleus cuneatus, decussate in the brainstem, and terminate in the posterolateral thalamus.

The propriospinal system is composed of multisynaptic interneurons located in the spinal cord. This system may contribute to the transmission of nociception, possibly in a role of maintaining chronic pain states. The propriospinal system cell bodies are located in the deeper laminae, receiving input from visceral and deep structures; they then ascend within various laminae of the spinal cord, projecting to the medial thalamus and reticular formation.

The spinohypothalamic tract is a recently identified direct ascending pathway that has been and is currently the focus of intense research. Anatomically, it is as abundant as the spinothalamic tract and is hypothesized to play an important role role in affective and motivational aspects of pain.

SUPRASPINAL STRUCTURES

The supraspinal system comprises the reticular formation, thalamus, hypothalamus, limbic system, and cerebral cortex. Within this system are extensive communicating projections for ascending algesic and descending analgesic pathways.

The reticular formation extends through the entire length of the brainstem. The reticular formation receives input mainly from the spinoreticular tract as well as other structures in the supraspinal system. At the reticular formation level, receptive fields are usually extremely large, arising from both ipsilateral and contralateral parts of the body. The reticular formation controls the state of arousal and is important in autonomic reflex responses and in motivational and affective aspects of pain.

The thalamus consists of multiple nuclei and acts as the major relay station for incoming nociceptive stimuli. The thalamus is subdivided phylogenetically into either the paleothalamus, neothalamus, or by nuclei location. The paleothalamus is composed of medial and intralaminar nuclei. Input is mainly from the spinothalamic tract and the reticular formation. Its receptive fields are large and it is involved with motor reflexes and affective aspects of pain. The paleothalamus has extensive connections with the cerebral cortex. The neothalamus rests at the ventrobasal portion of the thalamus. The neothalamus, unlike the paleothalamus, is organized somatotopically and subdivided into the ventral posterolateral nucleus and the ventral posteromedial nucleus. The ventral posterolateral nucleus receives input mainly from the spinothalamic tract, but also from the dorsal column system and the somatosensory cortex. The ventral posteromedial nucleus receives input mainly from the trigeminothalmic tract, which carries sensory input from the head and face and projects to the somatosensory cortex, involved with craniofacial pain. Although most of the neothalamic neurons respond to mechanoreceptive input, some are nociceptive-specific and wide dynamic range neurons. The neothalamus appears to be involved with sensory and discriminative aspects of pain and, due to its somatotopic organization, the localization of pain. The posterior thalamus receives input from the spinothalamic tract, spinomesencephalic tract, and dorsal column system. It is characterized by large receptive fields and lack of somatotopic organization. It projects to the somatosensory cortex and appears to play a role in the sensory experience of pain.

The hypothalamus handles both noxious and non-noxious stimuli from the entire body, including deep tissues and the viscera. The neurons are not somatotopically organized and thus do not provide information about the discriminatory aspects or location of pain. Hypothalamic nuclei send projections to the pituitary gland via the hypophyseal stalk. These nuclei regulate the autonomic and neuroendocrine responses to stress and pain. The role of hypothalmus in pain perception and modulation is a fascinating and rapidly evolving area, but a detailed discussion of this area is beyond the scope of this chapter. The limbic system receives input from the thalamus, reticular formation, and perhaps many other areas of the CNS. It involves the frontal and temporal cortex and is important in the motivational and emotional aspects of pain, including mood and affect.

CEREBRAL CORTEX

The somatosensory cortex plays a major role in sensory and discriminative aspects of pain perception. It is located posterior to the central sulcus of the brain, and receives input from various nuclei of the thalamus, including the ventral posterolateral nucleus, ventral posteromedial nucleus, and posterior thalamus. The somatosensory cortex is cytoarchitecturally organized and therefore plays a role in the discriminatory aspect and localization of pain. Efferents from the it travel back to the thalamus and contribute to descending pathways. Information from the somatosensory cortex are transmitted to the limbic system. The frontal lobe receives input from the thalamus and limbic system with which it has an impact on behavioral and motivational aspects of pain.

Descending Modulation System

The first clear description of a descending pain modulation system was proposed by Melzack and Wall in their the gate-control theory of pain. Since then, tremendous efforts have been made to define the anatomy and physiology of this system. Despite recent advances, our knowledge of the descending modulatory system remains less than complete. This system modulates incoming information and is generally inhibitory in nature. The descending system can influence the transmission of nociceptive stimuli anywhere along its path from the brain to the periphery. Structures in the descending system include the (1) cortex, subcortical centers, and basal ganglia; (2) thalamus-hypothalamus system; (3) midbrain, pons, and medulla; and (4) the dorsal horn (Fig. 216-1).

Cortex, Subcortex, and Basal Ganglia.   Multiple areas of the cortex, subcortex and basal ganglia appear to play roles in pain modulation, but these pathways are incompletely understood. The role of the somatosensory cortex in pain modulation is somewhat better understood. Stimulation of the somatosensory cortex seems to have an inhibitory effect on wide dynamic range neurons of the spinothalamic tract and possibly other tracts involved in pain transmission. This inhibition may also be mediated by the corticospinal tract, which is primarily a motor system pathway that descends ipsilaterally, branching to the trigeminal system before crossing in the medulla to the opposite side, and partially terminating in the dorsal horn. Extrapyramidal pathways may also play a role in cortical inhibition of afferent transmission. Cortical structures in the limbic system, particularly insular cortex and amygdala, seem to exert modulatory effects via their input to the periaqueductal gray.

Thalamus-Hypothalamus System.   The thalamus-hypothalamus system seems to play an important role in pain transmission and modulation that is also not completely understood. Its descending analgesic properties are suggested by finding that electrical stimulation of specific hypothalamic regions produce analgesia. The paraventricular nucleus of the hypothalamus is thought to be involved in pain modulation, probably via its effects on the periaqueductal gray.

Midbrain, Pons, and Medulla. The midbrain, pons, and medulla contain not only reticular formation but also the periaqueductal gray, nucleus raphe magnus, locus ceruleus, dorsolateral pontomesencephalic tegmentum, and rostral ventromedial medulla, all participating in the descending analgesic system. These brainstem centers send projections via the dorsolateral funiculus to the dorsal horn of the spinal cord. Likewise, descending modulatory influences from the cortex, limbic system, hypothalamus and brainstem structures are also carried to the dorsal horn via the dorsolateral funiculus, which is located primarily in the spinal cord and represents the primary descending modulatory pathway. Thus, lesions of the dorsolateral funiculus block the inhibition by brainstem neurons of behavioral responses to noxious stimuli.

BIOCHEMICAL MEDIATORS

Neurotransmitters link one neuron to the next via chemical and receptor activity within the synaptic cleft between neurons. "Classic" neurotransmitters are small monoamines such as epinephrine, acetylcholine, or serotonin. Peptides are also recognized constituents of nerve cells and often coexist with "classic" neurotransmitters within the same nerve cell. Colocalization of transmitter molecules is well documented in endocrine cells. That a single neuron may produce, store, and release more than one messenger molecule significantly expands the complexity of possible interactions of pain signals.

Through varied mechanisms at the site of tissue damage, pain signals initiate and sustain an elaborate alarm of impending or ongoing damage. Nociception may be the first signal to activate local tissue reactions that promote defense, stimulate tissue repair, and enhance sensitivity to further physical or chemical insults. In response to noxious stimuli, nociceptors may release their algesic substances for purposes of afferent neurotransmission as well as modulation of local reactions such as inflammation and possibly tissue repair. Algesic substances trigger release of inflammatory mediators from mast cells, endothelial cells, and other surrounding neural and non-neural cells. Sensitization of nociceptors results in a reduced response threshold to noxious stimuli and enhanced activity once activated. Within the spinal cord, sensitization also takes place as the threshold for excitation of pain transmission decreases. The spontaneous firing rate and duration of nerve action ("windup") increases during repeated or ongoing nociceptive input. Sensitization underlies the experience of injured patients with hyperalgesia/hyperesthesia (exaggerated pain in response to noxious stimuli).

The large variety of mediators involved at the synaptic and circulatory levels allows for a multiplicity of pain-modulating signals. As described above, these may include positive and negative regulation of pain circuits and an elaborate system of fast or slow primary signals. The neurotransmitters involved in the processing of primary pain signals are not completely identified. The list of possible algesic and analgesic substances and neurotransmitters is rapidly expanding and presently includes substance P, calcitonin gene-related peptide, somatostatin, bradykinin, serotonin, histamine, acetylcholine, γ-aminobutyric acid, Leu- and Met-enkephalin, pancreatic polypeptide, neurotensin, vasoactive intestinal peptide, cholecystokinin, gastrin-releasing peptide, bombesin, angiotensin, adenosine, prostaglandins, leukotrienes, adenosine triphosphate, and the amino acids ʟ-glutamate and ʟ-aspartate (Table 216-1).

Endogenous opioids play a key role in the modulation of pain. Opiate receptors are found throughout many structures involved with pain, especially the dorsal horn. There are several types of opiate receptors: the μ receptor, found in the dorsal horn, limbic system, and brainstem; the κ-receptor, distributed in the dorsal horn, limbic system, brainstem and cerebral cortex, and the δ receptor, distributed throughout the spinal cord. The three classes of endogenous opioids each arise from specific precursors or prohormones: (1) enkephalin, which is derived from proenkephalin; (2) β-endorphin, derived from propiomelanocortin; and (3) dynorphin, derived from prodynorphin. These precursors are found in the highest concentrations in those structures thought to be involved with analgesia, including the dorsal horn, the raphe magnus, the periaqueductal gray, the hypothalamus, and the cingulate gyrus.

Noradrenergic receptors are found in the pons and dorsal horn. Activation of these neurons produces an inhibitory effect on nociception. Application of norepinephrine to the spinal cord has been shown to inhibit the transmission of nociceptive impulses. Tricyclic antidepressants provide analgesia in part by inhibiting the re-uptake of norepinephrine, and thus increasing its blood level. Clonidine, an α_2-agonist, can be given centrally or systematically to produce analgesia by inhibiting nociceptive impulses. Clonidine acts synergistically with opioids and can decrease the amount of opioids required for analgesia.

Serotonin is found, among other areas, in the medulla and spinal cord, especially laminae I and II. Like norepinephrine, stimulation of serotonin-containing neurons also inhibits nociceptive stimuli. Central application of serotonin induces analgesia. Tricyclic antidepressants can also inhibit the re-uptake of serotonin, producing an increase in its blood level. γ-Aminobutyric acid is an inhibitory amino acid found in high concentrations in laminae I and II. It principally acts at large primary afferents. The proposed mechanism of action of benzodiazepines is through alosteric binding and modulation of the γ-aminobutyric acid receptor, with resulting change of its chloride channels.

SUMMARY

Although pain has no molecular weight or DNA sequence, no other physiologic process has been more scrutinized. However,

TABLE 216-1. Key Neurotransmitters and Their Interaction With Common Analgesics

Excitatory Mediator	Drugs Affecting Excitatory Mediators	Inhibitory Mediator	Drugs Affecting Inhibitory Mediators
Glutamate and aspartate	NMDA antagonists (e.g., Memantine)		
Substance P	Capsaicin cream	Serotinin	Antidepressants
Bradykinin	Nonsteroidal anti-inflammatory drugs (e.g., aspirin)	Norepinephrine	Antidepressants
Histamine	Antihistamine drugs		
Prostaglandins	Nonsteroidal anti-inflammatory drugs	γ-Aminobutyric acid (GABA) Endogenous opioids (enkephalin, endorphin, dynorphin)	Baclofen and benzodiazepines Opioids

the central and peripheral mechanisms of pain remain incompletely understood. Although it may serve to maintain needed vigilance to protect tissues already damaged, the role of pain goes beyond a warning system and has significant impact on normal physiology. As such, there may be significant medical consequences to inadequate recognition or treatment of pain. Pain transmission is well integrated with other major physiologic processes such as immune, endocrine, cardiac, hemodynamic, gastrointestinal, and mental functions. A system of such complexity is a marvel of nature that may have devastating effects when malfunctioning. Continued advances in the understanding of the anatomy and physiology of pain will enhance health care for those in pain and offers hope for greater relief from suffering.

SUGGESTED READINGS

Bonica JJ: Anatomic and physiologic basis of nociception and pain. pp. 28–94. In: The Management of Pain. 2nd Ed. Lea & Febiger, Philadelphia, 1990
Bonica JJ: Biochemist and modulation of nociception and pain. pp. 95–121. In: The Management of Pain. 2nd Ed. Lea & Febiger, Philadelphia, 1990
Fields HL: Pain. pp. 1–78. McGraw-Hill, New York, 1987
Fields HL, Basbaum, AJ: Central nervous system mechanisms of pain modulation. pp. 243–56. In Wall PD, Melzack R (eds): Textbook of Pain. Churchill Livingstone, Edinburgh, 1994
Guilbaud G, Bernard JF, Besson JM: Brain areas involved in nociception and pain. pp. 113–128. In Wall PD, Melzack R (eds): Textbook of Pain. Churchill Livingstone, Edinburgh, 1994
Katz N, Ferrante FM: Nociception. pp. 17–67. In Ferrante FM, VadeBoncouer TR (eds): Postoperative Pain Management. Churchill Livingstone New York, 1993
Wilson PR, Lamer TJ: Pain mechanisms: anatomy and physiology. pp. 65–80. In Raj PP (ed): Practical Management of Pain. 2nd Ed. Mosby-Year Book, St. Louis, 1992
Woolf EJ: The dorsal horn: state-dependant sensory processing and the generation of pain. pp. 101–12. In Wall PD, Melzack R (eds): Textbook of Pain. Churchill Livingstone, Edinburgh, 1994

217. APPROACH TO THE PATIENT WITH CHRONIC PAIN

GERALD M. ARONOFF

Chronic pain is a major public health problem that inflicts not only tremendous personal suffering but also huge economic loss on individuals and on society as well. If the pain remains intractable, physicians and patients become increasingly uncertain as to the most appropriate course of treatment and both develop a sense of helplessness. As each becomes frustrated and disappointed in the other, their interaction becomes more strained and less direct.

Much more is known of the mechanisms and pathophysiology of acute pain and cancer pain than of chronic nonmalignant pain. Attempts to generalize from one to the other have resulted in dismal failures to control the pain, frequent iatrogenic complications, and inappropriate and excessive usage of medications. Current treatment approaches for chronic pain offer strategies for peripheral management of pain but increasingly emphasize central factors.

Pain is a subjective, unpleasant sensory and perceptual experience that may or may not be related to tissue damage. Try as we may to quantify, measure, and objectify it, we ultimately fall short. We attempt to incorporate the patient's subjective symptoms, objective signs, and the results of diagnostic testing with our own clinical interpretations (which include subjective biases). Yet finally, our response to a patient's complaint of pain depends heavily on the credibility of the patient.

Most physicians specializing in pain medicine believe that all pain is real, with the rare exception of malingering. Yet in my experience, it is still true, as it was decades ago, that we give more credence to the patient for whom there are well-documented, objective findings that support the complaint of pain than to the depressed, somatically preoccupied patient with a chronic pain syndrome not supported by objective findings. This is unfortunate and is often a disservice to the latter patient.

The United States has the most technologically advanced medical system in the world. However, in recent years, physician–patient relationships have deteriorated significantly. This is due both to medical bureaucracy and to the trend toward increased specialization and compartmentalization of patients' medical disorders. In the current traditional medical model, especially that practiced in most urban regions, it is now uncommon for one physician to be the primary caretaker for an individual and his or her family. Even within medical and surgical specialties, there are increasing subspecialties. The jogger who develops knee or ankle pain no longer contacts a general orthopaedist for care, but instead goes to a sports medicine clinic. The obese patient with chest pain is seen by an internist, often referred to a cardiologist, and then treated at a weight-loss clinic. Do health-care providers truly get to know the patients and their psychosocial dilemmas that, as studies indicate, often contribute to or cause the medical complaints, or is this lack of rapport an unavoidable consequence of the increasing depersonalization within the medical system? The now-antiquated model of the physician-healer who visited the patient's home has been replaced by the all-too-frequent scenario of the patient who takes a tranquilizer before going to the physician's office. Recognizing the impact of medical specialization has become crucial in the management of chronic pain, since studies indicate that of patients presenting to primary-care medical outpatient clinics with complaints of headaches, backaches, general myalgias, and other physical symptoms, for a large percentage, either there are no objective findings or the findings are inconsistent with the subjective complaints. Many receive treatment of their primary physical symptoms while the underlying problems continue.

Pain syndrome patients, in their desperate search for the elusive cure, often chase will-o'-the-wisps, convincing their physicians to perform myriad invasive tests and procedures. As a result of their pain behaviors, many experience iatrogenic complications, suffering, and disability. Those involved in their treatment must find improved ways to detect this highly susceptible population, establish a therapeutic alliance, and short-circuit their pain careers. Our health-care system cannot rely solely on the traditional methods of medical and surgical approaches so often used with this population.

Despite technologic advances in medicine, chronic pain syndromes remain among the most difficult problems to treat. Most treatment approaches have been based on a dichotomy between physiologic and psychological causes. This dualism greatly reduces the treatment available to the patient. It reinforces the tendency to isolate the symptoms from the individual experiencing the pain and to focus treatment on target organs. Although this dichotomy has not been universally rejected, medical science has made significant contributions to the theory of pain as a multidimensional phenomenon.

MEDICAL EVALUATION

Certainly, we should not ask people to live with pain if there is an acceptable way to alleviate it and if the potential benefits outweigh the potential risks and side effects. Therefore, I believe that all those involved in pain evaluations should begin with a comprehensive review of the patient's medical status as well as a detailed review of past medical evaluations and interventions. This should be performed by one experienced in the evaluation of chronic pain. Through the years, I have been distressed at the many clinical recommendations offered by inexperienced consultants. When seeing a chronic pain syndrome patient, they frequently order extensive diagnostic studies and invasive therapies, whereas more experienced consultants tend toward a more conservative course. As pain clinicians, our goal should be to develop and provide the most effective therapies for the various pains we treat. It is hoped that clinical research on the spectrum of pain disorders will help us delineate not only the treatments of choice but also the methods involved in their implementation.

One way to improve the cost-effectiveness of our system would involve the use of experienced consultants prior to surgery in populations thought to be at high risk of experiencing treatment failure. I suggest obtaining second opinions for all nonemergency surgeries for chronic pain patients in the following situations:

1. Those in which a patient has already undergone two or more pain-related surgeries without documented beneficial results.
2. Those in which a patient has undergone one or more pain-related surgeries with negative findings.
3. Those in which a patient is referred by attorneys and is actively involved in accident-related litigation.
4. Those involving a patient with known or highly suspected major psychopathology.
5. Those involving a patient with a past history indicative of excessive use of the health-care system without adequate justification.

In terms of choice of treatments, I believe that the same general rule that applies throughout all medical practice also holds true for chronic pain syndromes. That is, the least invasive treatment capable of bringing about the desired effect is not only the treatment of choice for the patient, but it is also the most cost-effective for society. All other factors being equal, a noninvasive therapy should be preferred over an invasive one.

The use of the term chronic pain syndrome is meant to be descriptive of an individual whose subjective pain complaints, resultant suffering, and pain behaviors are excessive and disproportionate to the actual pathophysiology. There is accompanying life disruption and maladaptive behavior. In an effort to expand the patient's choice of treatment modalities, the multidisciplinary pain center has emerged. In this setting the medical, psychological, and social contributions to chronic pain problems are addressed by staff from various disciplines. Physicians (most often anesthesiologists, neurologists, psychiatrists, internists, physiatrists, orthopaedists, neurosurgeons) participate in a coordinated treatment approach with nurses, psychologists, social workers, physical and occupational therapists, vocational counselors, and other health-care personnel. The multidisciplinary pain center team offers evaluation and treatment directed toward both modification of pain and drug-seeking behavior and interruption of the disability process.

Traditionally, individual physicians have been primarily responsible for pain management. Treatment options had generally included bed rest, physical therapy, analgesic medications, surgery, and nerve blocks. Unfortunately, these approaches often reinforce passive-dependent traits, which are common to many patients with chronic pain syndrome. Currently, bed rest is generally believed to be contraindicated for most chronic nonmalignant pain syndromes. Narcotics are used far more judiciously, and the indications for nerve blocks and surgery are being better defined and used more selectively. Characteristics common to this patient population include the following:

Preoccupation with pain
Strong and ambivalent dependency needs
Feelings of isolation and loneliness
Characterologic masochism (meeting others' needs at the expense of their own)
Inability to care for self-needs
Passivity
Lack of insight into self-defeating behavior patterns
Inability to deal appropriately with anger and hostility
Use of pain as a symbolic means of communication
Frequent secondary gain from pain
Feelings of being abused by the health-care system

Since the 1970s, research has demonstrated the importance of the multidisciplinary pain center team approach to chronic pain, particularly when the pain problem has eluded diagnosis and/or adequate treatment via conventional techniques. An assumption of virtually all multidisciplinary pain centers is that chronic pain syndromes always involve psychological, social, biologic, and medical factors. This assumption has been widely accepted throughout the community of pain clinicians. I have always emphasized the concept that any treatment program designed for chronic pain syndrome patients must be holistic in its orientation if it is to be effective. This assumption does not imply that psychosocial factors are merely sequelae to a more fundamentally medical disorder, nor that patients treated in a multidisciplinary pain center have primarily psychogenic pain. It does, suggest, however that regardless of our medical subspecialty, our treatment approach should be psychotherapeutic, assisting patients with the suffering component of the pain and encouraging them to discuss their fears, apprehensions, depressive feelings, and so on. If we do not feel equipped (or do not have the time) to personally treat the emotional components, these patients should be referred to an appropriate colleague. Emotional disorders associated with chronic pain syndromes include the following:

somatoform disorders
    somatization disorder
    conversion disorder
    pain disorder (formerly somatoform pain disorder)
    hypochondriasis
    atypical somatoform disorder
affective disorders
personality disorders
Psychological factors affecting physical conditions
malingering
schizophrenia

substance use disorders

Referral to a pain center is sometimes regarded as the treatment of last resort. Unfortunately, by the time most patients are referred for a pain management approach, their lives have become significantly disrupted by depression, disability, vocational difficulties, financial strain, difficulty in interpersonal relationships, and a general loss of productivity. It must be emphasized that early patient referrals may help eliminate needless or multiple surgeries, reduce health-care costs, and promote patients' return to productivity.

It is my belief that the majority of chronic pain syndrome patients (> 80 percent) can be effectively treated in an outpatient setting. This avoids costly hospitalization and more realistically simulates typical activities of daily living. Unfortunately, this has been one of the major problems with the hospital model since its inception. Many patients find that after being confined in a sheltered and artificial environment, they ultimately have a difficult transition back to the workplace or normal daily activities. Criteria for inpatient treatment include the following:

Unstable medical illness requiring around-the-clock medical/
  nursing supervision
Major substance dependence
Active suicidal ideation
Patients who are nonambulatory,
Failure of prior outpatient pain treatment

I have also found that having the inpatients participate with the outpatients is effective in shortening the inhospital portion of the treatment program.

Treatment is based on wellness model, recognizing that these patients, pain does not generally make them ''sick'' in the acute medical sense of the word, but that it interferes with optimal functioning in various areas of their lives. The main goal of treatment should be overcoming the disabling effects of chronic pain and return patients to productivity rather than continued dependency on the health-care system.

Staff in multidisciplinary pain centers generally view the chronic pain syndrome itself as the focal point of treatment, not merely as a symptom of an underlying pathophysiologic process. Thus, legitimate directions of treatment are to reduce pain behaviors, life disruption, medication dependence, secondary gain; to increase activity level (in spite of pain) and physical functioning; and to assist patients in returning to a more functional and productive lifestyle.

As other medical and surgical specialists are selective in choosing patients likely to benefit from a given treatment (e.g., blocks or surgery), so too must pain centers be selective in their admission process. As part of the pain center program, behavior modification to reinforce adaptive coping skills and extinguish self-defeating maladaptive behaviors requires use of the patient's capacity for insight and self-change. Some patients are incapable of this process and, if this is detected initially, they are recognized as being inappropriate candidates for inclusion in a pain center treatment program. Patients with major cognitive deficits from cerebrovascular accidents or dementing illnesses generally do not do well in this type of program. Individuals who have limited comprehension in the primary language used at the pain center also have difficulty in grasping the concepts of the program and interacting in a meaningful way with other patients or staff. Pain center personnel must be aware of the limitations that may place the treatment of many pain patients beyond their grasp.

PHARMACOLOGIC MANAGEMENT

It is beyond the scope of this chapter to discuss all aspects of pharmacologic management of chronic pain. However, several important areas are discussed, as their uses may not be well known to some primary-care physicians. These include the use of opioid analgesics, antidepressants, and benzodiazepines.

Opioid Analgesics

Although there is no doubt that opiates are often the drugs of choice for severe acute pain and chronic cancer pain, in my opinion, their use in chronic nonmalignant pain is extremely limited. However, there does appear to be a subgroup of patients with chronic nonmalignant pain whose pain can appropriately be managed for prolonged periods by opioids. Guidelines for maintenance opioid use are as follows:

1. There is a documented medical condition as the cause of pain.
2. Prior systemic therapeutic trials of alternative pain control regimens (analgesics, adjuvants, psychosocial interventions, appropriate medical treatments, and behavioral approaches) have been unsuccessful.
3. There is documentation that nonopioid treatments have resulted in inadequate analgesia impairing functional activities of daily living and continued suffering.
4. Prior to initiating opioid maintenance, nonalgologists should consult with an algologist or with a specialist in management of the specific problem being treated. The consultation report should document concurrence with opioid treatment.
5. Document detailed discussion of short- and long-term effects and risks of opioid maintenance. Signed informed consent is suggested.
6. One physician should be responsible for writing prescriptions (which should be on a time-contingent rather than pain-contingent basis) and monitoring clinical progress. The recommended initial frequency of appointments is at least monthly. Patients must be seen and records must show reason for continuing opioids.
7. Document whether maintenance opioids improve analgesia and function in activities of daily living and diminish suffering.
8. Use lowest clinically effective opioid dose. Peripherally acting nonopioids and adjuvants used concurrently may allow lower opioid usage.
9. A history of substance dependence and/or abuse is a relative contraindication.
10. Any evidence of drug-seeking behavior, obtaining opioids from multiple sources, or frequent requests for dose escalation without documentation of significant worsening of the clinical condition should be a cause for careful review and reconsideration of maintenance opioid use.

These individuals, who have a well-documented medical condition as the cause of their pain, have attempted alternative techniques of pain management and are being carefully monitored by a physician. In general, these are patients whose pain has responded neither to treatment with nonopioid analgesics or adjuvants, nor to alternative techniques of pain management (e.g., physical therapy, psychotherapy, relaxation training, and pain center therapy). In addition, it should be demonstrated that these patients remain functional while receiving opioid analgesics, but attempts to taper these result in diminished function, impairment in overall function in activities of daily living, and increased suffering. Patients with a history of substance abuse or dependence, significant psychopathology, or excessive environmental stressors contributing to their pain and suffering in general should not be maintained on opioids for nonmalignant pain. It needs to be emphasized that the majority of chronic pain syndrome patients can be effectively managed without the use of opioids. Yet in patients carefully selected for opioid maintenance, it should be noted that addiction is rarely a clinical problem.

Antidepressants

There is a complex interrelationship between pain and depression. Studies have found that a high percentage of psychiatric inpatients who presented with depression also experienced some form of pain; many psychiatric outpatients somatize; the majority of patients referred to pain centers have some degree of depression spectrum disorder, with most showing improvement in pain when treated with antidepressants. This depression is often masked by somatic symptoms rather than presenting as a mood disturbance.

There is growing evidence that depression lowers pain tolerance, increases analgesic requirements, and adds to the debilitating effects of pain. Patients in chronic pain often suffer from insomnia, with early onset latency, frequent awakenings, and early morning awakenings. These are also extremely common vegetative signs of depression. Although patients usually attribute insomnia to pain rather than depression, this may be because pain is the more socially acceptable malady. It is difficult to distinguish cause and effect with the pain-depression-insomnia cycle, but once established, the cycle becomes self-perpetuating and requires active intervention. Sedating tricyclic antidepressants may be useful in breaking this cycle. Although it has been suggested that the apparent analgesic effects of tricyclic antidepressants may be the result of changes in sleep, other studies suggest that these compounds are adjuvant analgesics independent of their action on sleep or on depression. There are many studies with clinical pain syndromes suggesting the efficacy of tricyclic antidepressants in migraine headaches, tension headaches, diabetic neuropathy, post-herpetic neuralgia, low-back pain, mixed arthritic and fibromyalgic disorders, atypical facial neuralgia, and others. The serotonergic-enhancing drugs have been the most studied including amitriptyline, doxepin, imipramine, and desipramine. Patient compliance is often a problem because of the high incidence of anticholinergic and antihistaminic side effects, with frequent complaints of weight gain, constipation, daytime somnolence, and dry mouth. Compliance is significantly higher with the more recently introduced selective serotonin re-uptake inhibitors (fluoxetine, sertraline, and paroxetine), since the incidence of adverse side effects is much reduced. Although further studies are needed to assess their efficacy as adjuvant analgesics, anecdotal reports and my initial trials with sertraline for chronic headaches and other pain disorders are encouraging. Serotonin re-uptake inhibitors often are used alone, or they may be used in combination with sedating tricyclics given in reduced doses in the evening in patients with insomnia. One must be aware that serotonin re-uptake inhibitors can increase serum tricyclic levels, and in patients already taking high doses of these agents, the serum tricyclic level should be monitored if these agents are used in combination. This effect on serum tricyclic level is more pronounced with coadministration of fluoxetine than it is with sertraline.

It should also be mentioned that pharmacologic agents will not treat underlying emotional conflicts, solve family problems, or resolve motivational issues. Therefore, in most cases, chronic pain coexisting with depression must be treated multidimensionally with agents such as antidepressants and a variety of other medical, psychotherapeutic, and social interventions.

Combinations of tricyclic antidepressants and phenothiazines have been used to treat a variety of pain syndromes. The only phenothiazine noted to have analgesic action is methotrimeprazine, but its clinical usefulness is limited by a high incidence of side effects. Because certain antihistamines, such as hydroxyzine, often seem to be as effective as phenothiazines when used for chronic pain patients, the long-term use of phenothiazines must be weighed against the potential risk of tardive dyskinesia.

Benzodiazepines

Many clinicians treating chronic pain syndromes are dismayed by the frequency with which the benzodiazepine drugs are prescribed for chronic pain patients with concurrent depression. Lipman has noted that benzodiazepines cause an increase in anger and hostility when given over a 9-week period. This can be an adverse response for this already difficult population of chronic pain sufferers. It has been suggested that one of the mechanisms by which the benzodiazepines and the barbiturates adversely affect pain is by actions on the neurotransmitters (depletion of α-aminobutyric acid). It is suggested that benzodiazepines deplete serotonin, often adding to depression, paradoxic rage, habituation, disrupted sleep, and hangovers due to alterations of stage 3 and 4 sleep and rapid-eye-movement sleep. It has also been suggested that the benzodiazepines inhibit serotonin release and may increase pain perception. These views, coupled with my 18-year experience at the Boston Pain Center, suggest that this class of medication should not be used for long-term treatment of chronic pain.

DISABILITY

Individuals with pain rarely are totally and permanently disabled from everything. If patients must live with pain, we do them a far greater service by helping them not be disabled and by teaching them how to cope with pain and resume a productive lifestyle than by promoting the sick role. Lack of productivity in our society almost always leads to lower self-esteem, passive-dependency, and depression. The importance of our authoritarian guidance as physicians should not be underestimated; it can take the form of supportive paternalism or maternalism. I believe that patients will either live up to our expectations that they need not be disabled or, conversely, become invalids unnecessarily through learned helplessness. It remains my conviction that the individual who must endure chronic pain suffers less when his or her life has purpose and meaning. Gainful employment frequently can serve as a distraction from pain.

Individuals with legitimate painful injuries should be appropriately compensated for pain and suffering. However, we need to have an alternative to the current reimbursement system that often rewards people more for remaining in a body jacket than for wearing a sports jacket. As physicians, we must rate impairment by objective criteria and not confuse our goal of being the patient's advocate with assigning him or her an unwarranted disability status. As clinicians, working together, we can continue to make the types of breakthroughs that will benefit our patients and contribute toward a more productive society. In doing so, we are living up to the meaning of the word *physician,* one skilled not only in the art of healing but also in helping to decrease suffering.

SUGGESTED READINGS

Aronoff GM: The role of pain clinics. pp. 481–92. In Warfield CA (ed.): Principles and Practice of Pain Management. McGraw-Hill, New York, 1993

Aronoff GM: Evaluation and Treatment of Chronic Pain. 2nd Ed. Williams & Wilkins, Baltimore, 1992

Aronoff GM: Chronic pain and the disability epidemic. Clin J Pain 7:330–8, 1991

Aronoff GM, Evans, WO: Evaluation and treatment of chronic pain at the Boston Pain Center. J Clin Psychiatry 43:4–8, 1982

Aronoff GM: Pain Centers: A Revolution in Health Care. Raven Press, New York, 1988

Aronoff GM, McAlary, PW: Multidisciplinary treatment of intractable pain syndromes. Adv Pain Ther 13:1990

Raj PP: Practical Management of Pain. 2nd Ed. Mosby-Year Book, St. Louis, 1992

Wall P, Melzack R: Textbook of Pain. 2nd ed. Churchill Livingstone, London, 1989

218. PSYCHOLOGICAL EVALUATION OF THE CHRONIC PAIN PATIENT

KENNETH KRAFT

The chronic pain patient presents the practitioner with a considerable challenge. The physician is accustomed to establishing linear causal associations in order to diagnose and treat medical illnesses. Acute pain can be treated in this fashion. With most acute pain, the physician can identify biologic causes and target them for treatment. However, although the patient with chronic pain may present with some objective findings, perhaps evidence of some soft or hard tissue damage, the degree of pain and the pervasiveness of symptoms often cannot be completely explained by this approach. The practitioner may continue to seek a biologic explanation for the problem and, finally exhausting all reasonable possibilities, may decide that the pain is "psychogenic" after all. This label is often applied after an exclusion of many diagnostic possibilities but without a true effort to explore the relevance of psychosocial factors, not as a total explanation of the problem but as part of a set of interactive causative factors.

A proper evaluation requires an identification of the biologic, psychological, and social factors and, most importantly, how they influence each other in shaping the course of the patient's illness. After such an evaluation, the clinician can select those treatments that are appropriate with a better understanding of the impact of each treatment on the complex web of biopsychosocial factors. Psychosocial issues can contribute to the generation, maintenance, or exacerbation of a chronic pain condition. In addition, nociceptive pain may over time have a crucial psychosocial impact that may itself cause increased pain, perpetuating and escalating the chronic pain cycle. Secondary biologic factors become important as heightened pain may lead to inactivity and physical deconditioning, once again intensifying the pain.

THE PSYCHOLOGICAL IMPACT OF PAIN

A critical aspect of the psychological assessment of chronic pain is an appreciation of the psychosocial impact on the individual. The degree of distress that the patient experiences is a function of how the pain is perceived. Here a distinction must be drawn between pain per se and suffering. *Pain* is the sensation understandable through the mediation of nociceptors, whereas *suffering* is the subjective interpretation or emotional response to the noxious or nociceptive stimulus. One may think that the greater the pain, the greater the suffering. However, this may not be so. For example, women in childbirth who are in severe pain may have such positive associations with the event that their suffering is considerably reduced. Patients are more likely to report suffering when the pain is experienced as out of control, is associated with a dire outcome, or appears to have no temporal end. Suffering is also correlated with how greatly the pain errodes the quality of life. Those individuals whose pain has severely affected their ability to function interpersonally, vocationally, or recreationally are under considerably more psychological strain than those who are less affected. The loss of the ability to function in ways that provide a basis for self-esteem can be devastating.

Patients who have greater difficulty mourning the losses suffered as a consequence of pain are more susceptible to depression. They have difficulty accepting the changes in their bodies, feeling a sense of hopelessness. At an impasse in the grieving process, they have a difficulty seeing new possibilities for themselves. Those individuals who make adjustments to the pain over a period of time may have a mild depressive or reaction that is associated with a depressed mood, tearfulness, nervousness, or negative cognitions. This reaction to pain is defined as an adjustment disorder, a maladaptive reaction to a recent stressor, according to the Diagnostic and Statistical Manual of Mental Disorders, fourth edition (DSM-IV). Such patients may have the resilience to refocus by getting satisfaction from other areas of their lives, making the pain less important. If so, the depression then will subside.

The pervasiveness and severity of depression can be evaluated by noting the extent of the depressed mood and associated pessimistic thoughts, which often have themes associated with guilt, self-deprecation, and worthlessness. In addition, nonverbal clues such as psychomotor agitation and retardation, slumped posture, sighing, and looking at the floor are important, particularly with patients who may be unwilling or unable to verbalize. Other symptoms associated with depression are appetite disturbances, sometimes causing significant weight loss or gain, daily insomnia or hypersomnia, lack of energy, poor concentration, anhedonia, and thoughts of death or suicide. The more seriously depressed patient must be evaluated for suicidal risk. According to DSM-IV, more severe depressions are categorized as major depressive disorders. In dysthymic disorder, the depression is chronic and not as profound or severe as in major depression. Depression is probably the most common psychological feature accompanying chronic pain. Within the larger group, there appear to be a subset of endogenously depressed pain patients who demonstrated vegetative or physical symptoms. They frequently have a premorbid and family history of depression, suggesting a possible genetic predisposition. These patients often respond well to antidepressant medications, which appears to help both the depression and the pain.

Sometimes the presentation of depressive symptomatology is not as straightforward as the above suggests. Certain patients deny the affective dimensions of depression and focus on somatic distress. *Alexithymia* refers to the lack of awareness or inability to articulate emotional experience. This syndrome may arise when parents are not attuned to the nuances of a child's emotional world, so that the ability to differentiate and label feelings is never developed. Alexithymic patients have considerable difficulty distinguishing between emotional and somatic sensations and often have an increased awareness of physical symptoms as their emotional distress heightens. They may not be able to tell the difference between anxiety and anger or depression and fatigue. Psychic suffering is disavowed.

Somatization tendencies refer to the characterologic use of physical explanations for emotional distress. The patient communicates via physical symptoms. The question of how to interpret the patient's pain—whether it is true somatic distress—is not always easy to answer. Those patients who have somatization tendencies tend to deny psychologic problems and often dramatically focus on their symptoms and disability. Another key indicator is that these patients have a history of biologic vulnerability, with clear bodily preoccupations, when stressed. Physical findings in such patients are mostly negative. Symptoms that are accompanied by objective findings are often greatly overstated. These patients tend to seek medical treatment, including unnecessary surgeries, as a way of keeping the focus on physical causes. DSM-IV classifies these somatizing patients under the category of somatoform disorders. Two important types of somatoform disorders are somatization disorder and pain disorder. Somatization disorder is characterized by physical complaints representing four categories: pain, gastrointestinal symptoms, sexual symptoms, and pseudoneurologic symptoms. Pain disorder refers to those patients for whom emotional factors specifically have a link to pain symptomatology.

Pain is perhaps the most common somatic pathway to convey emotional distress. Pain may therefore present a "depressive equivalent," or masked depression, suggesting an illness that the patient has no experience of. Typically these patients deny feeling depressed but generally show vegetative signs. They may have had a low-grade chronic dysthymic depression for years. Pain symptoms may increase during periods of stress. Pain, which may have a somatic origin but ordinarily would be mild enough not to interfere with a patient's life, is a vehicle for the expression of emotional distress for the somatizing patient.

The complicated relationship of pain and depression is central to the evaluative process. Often, depression is a sequela of pain, as the patient's physical suffering and disability impair the quality of life. On the other hand, pain may be an expression of emotional distress, an indicator of an underlying depression or "depressive equivalent," as mentioned above, or pain and depression may coincide secondary to some other psychiatric disorder. Pain and depression also affect each other in an interactive loop. If a patient in pain becomes depressed, the threshold for pain may be lowered, thus exacerbating suffering, leading to more depression, and so on.

Depression affects behavior, cognitions, and mood. As patients have more negative thoughts, they will convince themselves that they are unable to function; they will focus on the pain, which will increase in intensity. As this happens, they will become more dysfunctional and convinced of their incapacity. This slippery slope leads chronic pain patients toward what is often termed *chronic pain syndrome,* such that they learn a lifestyle of dysfunction. Pain becomes the focus of life; needs and experiences are interpreted through the prism of uncomfortable physical sensations. Patients become focused on "secondary gain" (i.e., getting attention and needs met by exaggerating and focusing on symptoms.) Secondary gain is a replacement for self-esteem needs that were previously met through more ordinary means of obtaining life's satisfaction, such as work, relationships, and recreation.

Illness behavior refers to those behaviors that patients demonstrate that perpetuate the chronic pain syndrome. Such patients may take on the identity of pain patients, viewing all of their experiences according to how they affect their body. Activities and relationships are focused around the pain. Pain becomes the central meaning of life. After a while, such patients may actually depend on the pain and would feel lost without it.

PREDISPOSING PSYCHOLOGICAL FACTORS

Pain, as indicated above, can produce psychological distress of varying levels of severity, with depression being the most prominent symptom. As has been suggested, the very emotional sequelae can actually increase the felt experience of pain and lead to a cascading downward spiral toward more dysfunction and illness behavior. In addition, various predisposing factors play an important role in chronic pain. The confluence of events both physical and psychosocial help to determine if pain will be acute, and resolve quickly, or be chronic and progressive. An understanding of developmental influences helps to illuminate the significance of predisposing factors.

Certain individuals are apparently vulnerable to a life of chronic pain by virtue of early childhood and familial experiences. Pain that is most clearly caused by psychological factors appears to be associated with pain-prone individuals. Although there may be some purely psychogenic pain, many of these patients do have some pain, for example from an injury, that ordinarily would not be troublesome. Yet with them, it becomes a significant problem. Often such patients easily feel guilt, pessimism, or depression. They may have an unconscious need to suffer to expiate their guilt. As stated by Engel (1959), the experience of felt pain may be a punishment for aggressive or sexual impulses that cannot be tolerated. There may be an identification with a punitive parent (particularly with a history of abuse), the pain representing punishment for having been "bad" in some way. That "badness" may be unacceptable dependency needs that are often awakened after an injury, when the patient feels the wish to be taken care of. Those who have a preinjury history of "workaholic" tendencies and an extreme drive toward self-sufficiency and repression of emotional needs are particularly vulnerable to this problem. When losing a significant person through death or separation, pain-prone individuals may identify part of the body with the lost person. The trauma of the loss is then represented by pain in that location, particularly when the patient has unacceptable aggressive feelings toward that individual.

Within a developmental context, children identify with family members who use somatization as a means to convey emotional distress. Intense affective states associated with emotional pain are too frightening and cannot be tolerated. These families are characterized by emotional denial and a particular inability to tolerate anger and provide nurturance. Often, patients will have parents (especially same-sex parents) and siblings who have a pain history, frequently the same pain complaints in the same location. There is often a family history of chronic depression and/or alcoholism.

A history of sexual or physical abuse is a significant influential factor, providing a predisposition for chronic pain. Trauma can have a devastating impact on personality development. Clinical experience indicates that a high percentage of chronic pain patients have suffered abuse, often by particularly cruel and sociopathic parents. Frequently, the chronic pain symptoms are at the same bodily location as the site of the original abuse. Often, pain patients fulfill the criteria for post-traumatic stress disorder, characterized by symptoms secondary to an extreme traumatic stressor, again commonly physical or sexual abuse. Patients may report intrusive re-experiencing or recollections of the trauma as well as extreme distress when exposed to anything associated with the trauma. They often have amnesia for aspects of the trauma and may feel a sense of emotional detachment and alienation from others. Other typical symptoms are insomnia, problems with anger, hypervigilance, and difficulty concentrating. Often, an injury such as a car accident has an intrusive, assaultive impact that causes a recrudescence of symptoms of post-traumatic stress in a patient who has a history of abuse. The pain that results from the injury often does not resolve until the underlying trauma is addressed in psychotherapy. It is not uncommon for patients who have an abuse history to present their pain complaints as their only outstanding problem. They may have no memory of the abuse or minimize its impact. The pain functions as a "traumatic equivalent" in these individuals.

Specific personality profiles may emerge with potential long-term impact on the development of chronic pain. Millon (1981) has clarified how the somatoform disorders mentioned earlier have particular configurations within the context of personality disorders. These patients tend to experience emotional conflicts somatically. Those with dependent personality disorders seek out attention and nurturance and utilize symptoms as a way of controlling others to get the caring and reassurances they want. Masochistic patients use illness as a form of punishment that they deserve and from which they derive pleasure. Histrionic patients also use physical symptoms as a way of receiving nurturance and warding off inner emptiness and loneliness. Thus, pain can evoke sympathy and serve as a center of meaning to fill the emptiness. Narcissistic patients may use pain to obtain "special treatment" or as an excuse to rationalize failure to achieve success. Sometimes after a narcissistic injury, such as abandonment by a loved one, they will experience pain as a way of deflecting from the intense disappointment. They may tyrannize others with their pain with constant demands for attention. Alternatively, narcissistically injured patients sometimes become preoccupied with their own pain as a way of turning inward because they find no trustworthy external sources of nurturances. This is their way of attempting to gain self-soothing. Schizoid and borderline patients may focus on pain as a way of experiencing themselves as "alive," the concrete feeling of reality it provides serving to ward off feelings of depersonalization. Borderline patients who have a fear of abandonment may use pain symptoms to secure their connection with others. Personality styles have a strong predisposing impact. Patients who do not have personality disorders may recover relatively quickly from pain resulting from injury. Those with personality disorders are more likely to use the pain in a maladaptive struggle with unresolved emotional issues.

THE ASSESSMENT PROCESS

The role of the physician or therapist is to collect the data in order to ascertain the relevant psychosocial factors, get a sense of their relative influence, and understand how they impact

TABLE 218-1. Evaluation of the Pain Patient

Current functioning:
    Description of pain complaint; patient provides description of pain including intensity, location, and variations over time in relation to current stressors; previous diagnoses and treatment, problems with addiction
    Psychological consequences of pain; impact on daily life, particularly occupational and interpersonal functioning since onset of pain; affective response to pain
    Mood or anxiety disorders; depressive equivalence, post-traumatic stress disorder, traumatic equivalence
    Evaluation of maintenance factors; maladaptive behaviors, cognitions, and coping style; motivation for change
Immediate precipitating factors
    Critical psychosocial event(s) and stresses around the beginning of pain complaint or with exacerbation of pain
Long-term predisposing factors
    Childhood emotional trauma; significant biopsychosocial events over the life cycle including important relationships, vocational and psychiatric history; relevant personality issues and somatoform disorders

upon each other. Although it is not wise to try to rigidly structure the assessment interviews, it is helpful to conceptualize the assessment into three steps as shown in Table 218-1. From this basis, one can develop an individualized treatment plan.

Most patients carry the conviction that they essentially have a physical problem. The more psychologically minded may have already hypothesized about the significance of psychosocial influences on their pain. Others will easily be prompted to draw such conclusions. However, most patients believe that their problem is entirely physical, and they may already have been given the message that their pain is "in their head," leading them to take a defensive stance.

The initial interview with the patient with chronic pain is an opportunity to broaden the area of inquiry. The patient is ordinarily focused on the experience of nociceptive pain. The physician or therapist is usually expected to treat that pain as a straightforward somatic phenomenon. He or she must first acknowledge to the patient that the pain is real, so that the patient's world view is accepted. This is not simply a device to ally oneself with the patient. A true biopsychosocial perspective accepts the credibility of the patient's experience and the likelihood of some somatic pain. However, this is viewed as an incomplete explanation. To reject the somatic explanation out of hand is so at variance with the patient's own experience that all opportunity for trust will break down.

The first area of inquiry, and that most acceptable to the patient, concerns the experience of the pain itself. What words are used to describe the pain? Some pain descriptors have biologic significance—for example, helping to distinguish neuropathic from myofascial pain. However, other pain descriptors suggest affective dimensions of pain: It is torturous, powerful, intrusive, frustrating, annoying. Descriptions of pain intensity and variations of that intensity are important (Table 218-1). Are there times when the pain is greater or lesser in intensity (e.g., evening or morning, weekday or weekend)? Consistent patterns of variation in pain intensity may correspond to exposure to various emotional stressors in the environment, such as work or interaction with particular individuals. Other patterns of variation may correspond to physical stressors, such as sitting or standing for long periods or activities requiring repetitive motion. Sometimes what appears to be the result of changes in physical activity is also associated with emotional stressors. It is helpful to ask what makes that pain better or worse to elicit any coping strategies. Those who are unable to discern a pattern of variation in their pain convey a sense of helplessness and loss of control.

In taking the pain history, it is important to note when the problem began, what the patient believes the cause to be, what health-care providers the patient has seen, what their diagnoses and treatments have been, and how successful the outcomes were. A careful exploration of the patient's assessment of past health-care providers may suggest useful information about prior obstacles to success, particularly how psychological factors may have determined success or failure. Such information is very useful in planning future treatment. Special attention must be paid to the use of medications, illicit drugs, or alcohol for pain control as a means of assessing potential for problems with addiction. Many chronic pain patients are addicts who need specific help for this problem as part of the overall treatment program.

The next area of exploration that is most acceptable to the patient is the range of psychological consequences of the pain. How is the patient affected by the pain? Does he or she feel stressed? depressed? anxious? panicked? What impact does the pain have on his or her daily life? relationships? sleeping? eating? work? recreation? household chores? children? These psychological issues are all too familiar to patients, and such questions are usually received as an expression of genuine interest in the complexity of the problem. As a patient becomes more comfortable with questions of a directly psychological nature, the examiner may venture to ask specific questions regarding the extent of depression and anxiety, seeking information about a possible underlying mood or anxiety disorder. Axis I disorders (DSM IV), such as major depression, adjustment disorder with depressed mood, panic disorder, and generalized anxiety disorder, and post-traumatic stress disorder, are typical of the diagnostic conclusions that might be drawn from these questions. The identification of such diagnoses will lead to appropriate referrals for psychotherapeutic and psychopharmacologic interventions.

The evaluation should continue with questions about some of the maintenance factors—that is, those psychological features that perpetuate the pain. How is the patient coping with the pain? Adaptively or maladaptively? What measures, if any, is the patient using to control the pain? What are the patient's cognitions like? Does he or she engage in catastrophic thinking? Is the patient using the pain to solicit attention or as a means of satisfying personal needs?

The term *pain behavior* refers to the observable repertory of behaviors that identify a person as in pain. Typical pain behaviors are overt communications of distress, such as moaning or sighing, or exaggerated gestures, such as rubbing or grimacing. Other significant pain behaviors are numerous medical consultations, reliance on pain medication, the use of devices such as cervical collars and canes, the self-imposed limitation of activity, and application for disability payments. Patients may describe pain symptoms that conform more to psychic organization of body image than anatomy—for example, whole leg pain or numbness. Pain that is described as unvarying in intensity with no periods of remission is characteristic. Often, such patients reports no benefit from any medical treatment, with some patients having an increase in pain and worsening of their condition with each additional intervention. During examination, patients may overreact with extreme responses such as collapsing, shaking, or appearing to be in agony.

Fordyce (1976) suggested that environmental factors, particularly interpersonal ones, may directly reward pain behaviors. Sometimes such reinforced pain behaviors are focused on receiving help from others. The patient limps, eliciting the spouse's concern. The behavior is now reinforced, prompting the patient to limp in order to get the spouse to respond. The

original nociceptive stimulus for the limp is replaced by a new psychosocial stimulus. Pain behaviors may be rewarded by the opportunity to avoid certain unpleasant tasks or responsibilities. Patients cannot go to work or school because they are in too much pain. The understanding employers or disability program representatives reward patients by allowing them to stay home without penalty. Ignoring or punishing well behaviors is as important as the reinforcement of pain behaviors. Fordyce indicated that when the patients' efforts to function despite the pain were ignored by those in their interpersonal environment, they were more likely to continue their pain behaviors. The evaluator must identify those pain behaviors or abnormal illness behaviors that are the outcome of environmental reinforcers. In addition, it is important to assess the interpersonal field of family, friends, employers, and health-care providers to better understand who may be reinforcing pain behaviors, to the detriment of the patient. A comprehensive treatment plan should include therapy that is behaviorally oriented in order to minimize these influences.

Pain behaviors cannot be completely understood without appreciating the cognitions that often correspond to a life of chronic pain. How do patients think about and cope with their pain? An individual's cognitive style is a critical factor in determining pain perception. Those who worry about their pain tend to have more negative thoughts, leading to anxiety, which may activate the autonomic nervous system and, hence, increase pain perception. They tend to feel ineffective about coping with pain associated with a perceived lack of control and, often, a fear of using their bodies. A cognitive approach to chronic pain suggests that the perception of the problem really is the problem. Catastrophic thinking—imaging the worst possible outcome—precipitates anxiety, keeping patients focused on their symptoms and enhancing and exacerbating their impact. This leads to more catastrophizing, and so on. Negativistic belief systems lead to self-doubt, perceived helplessness, and hopelessness, contributing to both anxiety and depression. Cognitive therapy has been found to be an effective treatment for dysfunctional thinking patterns.

Generalized anxiety disorder, which is associated with persistent worry that is difficult to control, is often accompanied by muscular tension, insomnia, irritability, fatigue, restlessness, or difficulty concentrating. Anxiety is also indicated by physiologic overreactivity, such as palpitations, shortness of breath, sweating, abdominal distress, and tingling sensations. If these sensations are severe and take place abruptly, the patient may be suffering from panic attacks. Intense fears about losing control, going crazy, fears of dying, or feelings of unreality can be associated with this disorder. Sometimes chronic pain patients have panic attacks precipitated by catastrophic thinking about their pain.

An associated factor that is relevant to cognitive style is coping or adaptation skill. Those who are subject to negativistic beliefs are likely to think that their pain will persist and will be more passive in their attempts to cope. *Coping* refers to the ability to contend with stress—the strain associated with marital or occupational roles and other demands in life. Pain patients learn to use coping strategies to deal with pain both as a somatic phenomenon and in relation to the major stresses at home and at work. Some useful coping strategies for pain are diverting attention, relaxation techniques, and using coping self-statements. Some maladaptive coping strategies are self-blaming, catastrophizing, and increasing pain behaviors. Hypnosis, biofeedback, and other relaxation approaches can be very useful at helping patients cope more effectively.

Finally, the most sensitive area of inquiry concerns the predisposing factors. The evaluator should first explore the immediate circumstances surrounding the beginning of the complaints of pain. The word *stress* is a sufficiently nonthreatening choice. What were the stresses in the person's life around the time of the initial pain compaint? Were there recent losses, changes in relationships, vocational stresses? It is helpful to create a picture of the patient's home and work life. Who is at home? Is there evidence of conflict or lack of support from other family members? It may be useful to interview them. Spouses may reveal or substantiate evidence of marital conflict, problems in parenting, or a tendency to reinforce the patient's pain behavior. The patient's pain may actually serve a defensive function for the couple by shifting the focus from underlying discord. Problems in the family system often indicate referral for marital or family therapy. Perhaps there is tension with other relatives or friends or feeling burdened by an aging parent. Younger patients may be struggling with separation from their parents. At work, there may be interpersonal conflicts with superiors or colleagues or a lack of enthusiasm or capacity to perform effectively. Financial pressures may be overwhelming.

Sometimes stressors are positive events. A new relationship, job, house, or baby may bring much joy to an individual but nonetheless be the source of considerable stress. Change, even positive change, will often produce stress. Some positive changes may be accompanied by emotional conflicts that can be quite painful. For example, a promotion may bring out feelings of inadequacy or fears of responsibility.

The physician or therapist attempts to establish the set of circumstances that might help to explain the onset or exacerbation of pain. These are the immediate precipitating factors. What changes took place in the patient's life just before or around the time of the onset of pain? There is often a critical psychosocial incident, frequently associated with a nociceptive trigger, which is the smoking gun that precipitates a cascading series of events leading to dysfunction and pain. The clinician must weigh the significance of organic findings within the context of psychosocial events to best grasp the entire picture.

Critical incidents may trigger one or more longer-term predisposing factors. A patient with an abuse history who has a car accident and interprets that experience as an assault may be more vulnerable to a chronic pain condition. A careful history of the family of origin should include parenting styles, sexual or physical abuse, and a family history of illness (particularly pain problems), drug abuse, depression, or other psychiatric disorder. Any significant traumatic events of childhood or adulthood, both physical and emotional, should be investigated. Have there been significant losses? Unresolved grief is a critical issue for many pain patients. The patient should provide information about any psychiatric disturbances and treatments. Is there a history of depression or drug use? Is there a tendency to somatize when emotionally stressed? A chronicle of significant relationships, marital status, and the evolving development of social support systems over time is important. Patients' vocational history should include responsibilities at work, job satisfaction, attitudes toward employers and coworkers, and degree of motivation and interest in work.

SUMMARY

The information sought in the comprehensive evaluation of patients with chronic pain is varied and complex and often must be developed slowly over time through skillful psychologically focused interviews. By integrating such information into a profile of the current level and manner of function and relevant immediate and long-term precipitating factors, it is possible to establish a broad-based psychological assessment to serve as a basis for constructive work with this difficult group of patients.

SUGGESTED READINGS

Blumer D, Heilbronni M: The pain prone patient: a clinical and psychological profile. Psychosomatics 22:395–402

Engel GL: Psychogenic pain and the pain-prone patient. Am J Med 26:899–918, 1959

Fields H: Pain. pp. 175–95. McGraw Hill, New York, 1987

First M: Diagnostic and Statistical Manual of Mental Disorders. 4th Ed. American Psychiatric Association, Washington, D.C., 1994

Fordyce W: Behavioral Methods for Chronic Pain and Illness. CV Mosby, St. Louis, 1976

Hanson R, Gerber K: Coping with Chronic Pain. Guilford Press, New York, 1990

Grezesiak R: Psychologic considerations in temporomandibular dysfunction. Dent Clin North Am 351:1, 209–226, 1991

Jamison R: Tutorial 3: Psychological assessment of chronic pain. Pain Digest 1:230–7, 1991

Miller T: Chronic Pain. International Universities Press, Madison, CT, 1990

Millon T: Disorders of Personality. John Wiley & Sons, New York, 1981

Rodin G, Craven J, Littlefield C: Depression in the Medically Ill. Brunner-Mazel, New York, 1991

Rome H, Harness D, Kaplan H: Psychologic and behavioral aspects of chronic facial pain in Jacobson AL Donlon W (eds): Headache and Facial Pain. Raven Press, New York, 1990

Rugh J: Psychological components of pain. Dent Clin North Am 31:4, 579–93, 1987

Waddell G, Turk D: Clinical assessment of low back pain. pp. 15–36. In Turk D, Melzack R (eds): Handbook of Pain Assessment. Guilford Press, New York, 1992

219. ADDICTION AND DETOXIFICATION IN CHRONIC PAIN

JOHN R. PETEET

Addiction presents two sets of challenges to clinicians treating pain: (1) the diagnosis and effective management of addiction in patients with chronic pain and (2) the assessment and adequate treatment of pain in patients with active or recovering addiction.

DIAGNOSIS OF ADDICTION

Growing acceptance of the use of opiates to treat chronic nonmalignant pain has engendered concerns that the treatment of pain will initiate or reactivate substance use disorders in susceptible patients. At the same time, clinicians' and patients' fears of addiction result in undermedication of patients with narcotics. This tension between these concerns about addiction and the practice of undermedication highlights the need for the development of clear and reliable guidelines for the diagnosis and management of addiction in patients with pain.

A lack of standard terminology has hampered this process. One recent review of 24 papers addressing the treatment of patients with chronic pain and drug and/or alcohol dependence or addiction concluded that only seven studies utilized acceptable diagnostic criteria and/or definitions for drug misuse diagnoses. Within these seven studies, the prevalence percentages for the diagnosis of drug misuse, drug dependence, and drug addiction in patients with chronic pain ranged between 3.2 and 18.9 percent. Standard psychiatric classification systems (e.g., *Diagnostic and Statistical Manual of Mental Disorders,* Revised Third and Fourth Editions) specify operational criteria for substance dependence and abuse but avoid the term addiction; as such, they do not adequately describe the problems of diagnosis in patients with pain treated with narcotics who may be physically dependent and preoccupied with receiving opiates but are not addicted in the usual sense. Accordingly, Portnoy recently proposed a definition of addiction in patients with pain that specifies: (1) an intense desire for the drug or an overwhelming concern about its continued availability (psychological dependence); (2) evidence for compulsive drug use (characterized, e.g., by unsanctioned dose escalation, continued dosing despite significant side effects, use of drug to treat symptoms not targeted by the therapy, or unapproved use during periods of no symptoms); and/or (3) evidence of one or more of a group of associated behaviors, including manipulation of the treating physician or medical system for the purpose of obtaining additional supplies of the drug (e.g., altering prescriptions), acquisition of drugs from other medical sources or from a non medical source, drug hoarding or sales, or unapproved use of other drugs (particularly alcohol or other sedative-hypnotics) during opioid therapy. In 1988, Rinaldi et al. also offered definitions that distinguish among drug addiction, drug abuse, physical dependence, psychological dependence, tolerance, and drug withdrawal syndromes.

The use of more precise definitions of addiction in the patient with pain has identified two major distinct addicted populations: street addicts and prescription drug abusers. Street addicts have a history of illicit polysubstance abuse, often dating from their teens and often including a history of intravenous drug abuse. Urine toxicology may identify the presence of other illicit drugs. Prescription drug abusers typically have initially obtained an opiate from a physician for a legitimate medical reason but have gradually increased the dose and frequency on their own. They resist reduction in medication claiming pain symptoms as a reason but actually fearing more the loss of its mood-altering effects. These patients may be difficult to distinguish without careful psychological assessment from a third category of patients with pain who are vulnerable to addiction, that is, those who can misuse medication to deal with anxiety or depression at times of stress, but who can use opiates appropriately at other times. Clear-cut distinctions among these categories of addicted or misusing patients may not always be possible, since a history of illicit polysubstance use is relatively common in the general population and anxiety, including anxiety over being adequately medicated, is also common in patients with pain.

A consensus exists that long-term opiate treatment for the management of chronic pain is at least relatively contraindicated for patients with a history of opiate addiction. Furthermore, efforts to predict which patients without an addiction history are likely to misuse narcotics prescribed for chronic pain has led clinicians to distinguish groups of patients with chronic pain on the basis of accumulated experience with their response to long-term opiate therapy. Most patients who misuse opiates have shown pain complaints and disability out of proportion to structural disease and have often used other medications such as benzodiazepines as well as opiates without sufficient relief. These patients are often resistant to trying nonopiate medications (e.g., tricyclic antidepressants or non steroidal anti-inflammatory agents) for pain management. Such patients are susceptible to a downhill spiral of pain and increasing opioid use often propelled by subtle withdrawal symptoms. By contrast, those patients who complain of mild to moderate pain appropriate to structural disease, with minimal disability and psychological difficulties, seem to respond better to long-term opiate treatment, particularly if they show evidence of adaptive coping. Further research and clinical experience is needed to determine the usefulness of such distinctions in predicting who will respond well to opioid treatment.

MANAGEMENT OF ADDICTION

Detoxification, or medically supervised withdrawal, the next step usually taken by the physician who has made a diagnosis of addiction, can be thought of as the short-term administration of an opiate or similarly acting substance that provides a steady reduction in dose on a schedule and rate that results in a tolerable level of discomfort and continued ability to function and that prevents the use of additional opiates or other drugs. The most appropriate setting for detoxification depends upon whether the patient is a street addict, a prescription drug abuser, or a patient undergoing methadone maintenance therapy.

Street addicts are best referred to a substance abuse treatment program, since detoxification is often difficult and relapse is common even following rehabilitation. Even if patients initially refuse referral for addiction treatment, collaboration among medical, pain, and substance abuse clinicians may be effective in engaging such patients in treatment over time.

Prescription drug abusers with pain can be detoxified more easily by medical clinicians using a schedule for tapering opiates to zero at a rate that minimizes withdrawal symptoms (e.g., over 7 to 10 days for inpatients and somewhat longer for outpatients), according to the duration and size of the patient's opiate requirement. More rapid detoxification may be possible, but slower tapering may be indicated if patients have been dependent on large doses for extended periods or if they are anxious about experiencing increased pain. Medically supervised withdrawal is made easier by converting the patient's medication to an equianalgesic dose of a longer acting opiate such as methadone or MS Contin to avoid peaks of euphoria and valleys of dysphoria. Patients who resist detoxification because of difficulty tolerating even mild withdrawal symptoms may also benefit from the adjunctive use of clonidine and from consultation with addiction medicine specialists.

Patients receiving methadone maintenance are best detoxified in conjunction with their methadone treatment providers, since a number of clinical considerations usually determine the methadone dose and the timing of detoxification. Two obstacles that interfere with complete withdrawal from opiates are psychosocial problems (such as hypochondriasis, depression, and disability) and pain masked by opiate dependency, which reemerges during attempts to decrease the opiate dose. Inpatient pain units are the most effective approach to the treatment of many patients with such problems since they are able to combine detoxification with the use of physical therapy, occupational and relaxation therapies, group meetings, and family therapy. A structured program in a controlled environment helps to achieve the goals of both freedom from drug dependence and improved overall functioning.

A further obstacle to the successful treatment of many addicted patients with chronic pain is the emotional responses they engender in caregivers. These may include frustration at patients' resistance to acknowledge addiction, anger at their manipulation, and guilt over the overly rigid or punitive interventions that these behaviors may provoke in clinicians. Collaboration with other members of the treatment team is important in maintaining the objectivity and perspective necessary to implement a consistent, comprehensive treatment approach. For example, it may be helpful to convene a ''summit'' meeting of the difficult patient's principal providers and to produce written recommendations for their treatment. Shared responsibility for such a treatment plan can markedly reduce the individual clinician's sense of helplessness and frustration and provide support during the treatment process.

ASSESSMENT OF PAIN

Not only is the problem of addiction difficult to recognize and treat in patients with chronic pain, but pain can be difficult to assess and treat effectively in patients with active addiction. Pain complaints almost always refer to the patient's real subjective experience. Emotions such as anxiety can influence this experience, and personality factors can influence its expression. Furthermore, cultural differences between addicts and clinicians and manipulative behavior of these patients can make pain in these patients more difficult to assess. The ability of clinicians to identify and address the issues of concern to addicted and recovering patients effectively can greatly reduce patients' anxiety and improve their management. While effective approaches to problematic behaviors of hospitalized drug-dependent patients such as drug-seeking behavior, poor compliance, and disruptive or violent behavior are beyond the scope of this chapter, several concerns of addicted patients are directly relevant to the adequate treatment of pain in these patients.

TREATMENT OF PAIN

A major concern for most addicted patients is that they will lose control of their habit of (self) medication. Many of these patients have become extremely attuned to managing or controlling physical and emotional distress by self-administering substances. Therefore, the prospect of relying on a physician to relieve their distress often increases, rather than diminishes, their anxiety. Mistrust that the physician is not taking their complaint seriously because of their addiction unnecessarily exacerbates this anxiety.

A related concern of addicted patients with pain admitted to the hospital is that they will be forced to experience withdrawal or untreated pain because narcotic medications will be withheld or inadequate. Unfortunately this concern may have a basis in reality since the principles of treating pain and withdrawal in hospitalized opiate addicts are not clearly understood by many medical practitioners. An example of these principles is that effective pain control in a patient stabilized or maintained on a stable dose of methadone (which may average 60 to 120 mg/day for patients in methadone treatment programs) requires the use of additional analgesics, as it would in any other patient. Another example is the unknowing use by physicians of agonist/antagonist drugs (e.g., pentazocine [Talwin]) in these patients, which may precipitate withdrawal. Finally, physicians may be reluctant to use methadone for the treatment of pain, although the Food and Drug Administration approved this use in 1947, because its use in the treatment of opiate addiction has been heavily regulated since 1973.

A third concern of addicted patients is that they will be reported to legal authorities, either because of the illegal nature of their procurement activities or because their substance use jeopardizes the health or welfare of others, such as their living or unborn children. Fear of discovery and efforts to hide addiction can contribute to under-reporting of illicit substance use, misdiagnosis, and in-hospital drug abuse. Resulting mistrust on the part of both patient and clinician in turn can increase anxiety and manipulation and can complicate the assessment and effective treatment of pain.

In addressing these concerns of addicts, early and frank discussion of the clinician's concerns and of the hospital's policies about substance abuse can help to prevent a destructive cycle of mistrust and anxiety. For example, clinicians do well to explain at the outset their expectation that patients agree to evaluation and recommended treatment by addiction consultants, and/or refrain from illicit substance use in order to continue to receive opiate medication. In some cases, urine screens can be a useful means of confirming or demonstrating compliance. The decision about whether to treat pain using opiates in addicts on an outpatient basis is best made in close consultation with an addiction treatment team, which can help monitor the appropriateness of drug use.

Although patients in methadone treatment may have concerns that their pain will not be adequately relieved because their maintenance methadone dose is assumed to be sufficient, other types of recovering addicts may have very different concerns. Many are reluctant to take opiates for pain for fear of reactivating their addiction or of compromising their record of ''clean time.'' Discussion of these concerns, reassurance that opiate prescription will be short-lived, clearly monitored, and different from the ones previously abused, as well as involvement of other supports from the patient's treatment or recovery community can help to avoid unnecessary suffering resulting from the patient's refusal of medication. This might include help from other members of the patient's recovery group in distinguishing ''medicine for pain'' from ''drugs for getting high.'' It might also include the use of a spouse, recovering friend, or sponsor in the management of pain medication (e.g., to hold the medication for them). Finally, the use of a specific medication schedule (e.g., every 4 to 6 hours) instead of an as-needed schedule may help patients structure appropriate use when they have had difficulty distinguishing the need for medication for pain from the craving of addiction.

For outpatients with chronic pain and recovering addiction, the risk of reactivated addiction needs to be carefully weighed against the relief of pain through the use of opiates. Other means of pain control such as behavioral approaches and the use of non-narcotic pain medications (e.g., nonsteroidal anti-inflammatory agents or tricyclic antidepressants) are particularly important to consider in this setting.

The concerns and emotional responses of clinicians can also have important effects on the assessment and treatment of pain in active or recovering addicts. These responses include fears of reactivating their addiction by administering opiates, anger at being manipulated, or a desire to rescue patients from overly punitive or rejecting behavior by other clinicians.

Given these concerns surrounding the use of opiates for pain in addicts, clinicians should clearly identify the goals of the treatment. Stabilization of the patient by preventing or minimizing withdrawal symptoms is an important initial goal. Respect for the patient's report of pain is also important in protecting the treatment relationship from mistrust and unnecessary struggles. Relief of the patient's pain within acceptable parameters of risk is a third important goal. Such risks include worsening of addiction and psychosocial functioning (difficult to evaluate in patients who deny their abuse or who are not engaged in addictions treatment), possible overdosage in the presence of unaccustomed drug use, and precipitation of withdrawal through the use of medications such as pentazocine, which contain opiate antagonists. An example of a novel attempt to minimize such risks is the report by Kennedy and Crowley in 1990 of a pilot study of methadone maintenance for patients with chronic non malignant pain and addiction who responded to a treatment program that included weekly routine urinalysis; weekly psychotherapy; and the use of quarterly self-report tests of mood, pain, and function to evaluate change. A fourth goal of treatment is to reduce patient anxieties that are contributing to the experience of pain. Effective means of doing this include the use of adequate doses of opiates (which are higher for those who have been dependent on opiates) and of measures to enhance control when possible, such as the use of patient-controlled analgesia pumps, regularly scheduled versus as-needed medications for persistent pain, and the avoidance of an excessive focus on the details of pain medication. Pain medication should never be used as a bargaining tool.

Both Portnoy and the California Medical Association recently proposed guidelines for the prescription of controlled substances for the treatment of chronic pain, emphasizing the need for adequate evaluation, diagnosis, documentation, informed consent, objectives, periodic review, and modification of treatment. Adaptation of such guidelines to the treatment of patients with both chronic pain and addiction requires careful attention to the multiple needs of these complex patients, awareness of the emotional responses they engender in their caretakers, and effective collaboration among all of the clinicians caring for them.

SUGGESTED READINGS

American Psychiatric Association: Diagnostic and Statistical Manual of Mental Disorders. 4th Ed. APA Press, Washington, DC, 1994
California Medical Association-Board of Medical Quality Assurance (CMA-BMQA): Guidelines for Prescribing Controlled Substances for Chronic Conditions: a Joint Statement by the BMQA and the CMA. Action report, BMQA. 1985
Fishbein DA, Rosomoff HL, Rosomoff RS: Drug abuse, dependence and addiction in chronic pain patients. Clin J Pain 8:77–85, 1992
Kennedy JA, Crowley TJ: Chronic pain and substance abuse: a pilot study of opioid maintenance. J Subst Abuse Treat 7:223–38, 1990
Portnoy RK: Chronic opioid therapy in non-malignant pain. J Pain Symptom Manage 5:546–62, 1990
Rinaldi RL, Steindler EM, Wilford BB, Goodwin D: Clarification and standardization of substance abuse terminology. JAMA 259:557–62, 1988
Savage SR: Addiction in the treatment of pain: significance, recognition, and management. J Pain Symptom Manage 8:265–78, 1993
Schofferman J: Long-term use of opioid analgesics for the treatment of chronic pain of non-malignant origin. J Pain Symptom Manage 8:279–88, 1993
Sees KL, Clark HW: Opioid use in the treatment of chronic pain: assessment of addiction. J Pain Symptom Manage 8:265–78, 1993
Washton AM, Resnick RB: Clonidine for opiate detoxification: outpatient clinical trials. Am J Psychiatry 137:1121–2, 1980

SECTION 5. GENERALIZED PAIN SYNDROMES

220. MYOFASCIAL PAIN SYNDROME

ZAHID H. BAJWA
JONATHAN P. ROZAN
CAROL A. WARFIELD

Chronic and disabling pains are commonly of musculoskeletal origin. These may arise from a pathologic process involving the joints, muscles and their ligamentous attachments, or both. When pain seems to be arising from one or more joints and can be confirmed by appropriate radiologic studies and objective signs of localized inflammation, the diagnosis of arthritis can be easily established. Another common form of musculoskeletal pain is persistent, deep aching pain that is not localized to the joints. It is commonly labeled as myofascial pain syndrome. As the name implies, this is a syndrome that encompasses a spectrum of symptoms, primarily involving muscles and their ligamentous attachments. It can be persistent, severe, and disabling and afflicts women about five times more commonly than men. Often it arises from mild trauma or muscular overuse and, if not properly treated, can persist for prolonged periods of time. Frequently, this syndrome is known by other names, including fibromyalgia, fibrositis, muscular rheumatism, nonarticular rheumatism, and idiopathic myalgia, among others. Traditionally, it is subdivided into localized and diffuse myofascial pain syndromes. The International Association for the Study of Pain defines it as "diffuse, aching musculoskeletal pain associated with discrete predictable tender points and stiffness." These tender areas are commonly known as trigger points. They are considered of vital importance in maintaining the pain syndrome and, by analogy, in treating it. Simple techniques directed at disarming trigger points are the mainstay of therapy. They are easy to perform in the office setting once the diagnosis of myofascial pain syndrome has been established.

CLINICAL FEATURES

A thorough history and physical examination are absolutely essential in diagnosing myofascial pain syndrome. Patients frequently describe diffuse muscular pain. Most often it is deep, continuous, dull, and aching in character. Rarely is it reported as throbbing or burning. Often no inciting event is remembered by the patient, but sometimes the pain begins abruptly, and an inciting event is precisely remembered. Mild trauma such as a whiplash injury from a motor vehicle accident may be noted. Simple increased physical activity, often found in "weekend athletes," can be the inciting event. Even increased office hours with resultant strain on back musculature from prolonged desk and computer work under the stress of approaching tests or deadlines can incite myofascial pain syndrome. Muscle spasm can be prominent, as can radiation of pain. Although most frequently located in the trunk and neck muscles, any muscle or group of muscles can be involved. The pain is frequently increased by stress; inadequate sleep; fatigue; and cold, humid weather. Continued use of the involved muscle group tends to aggravate the pain. Stiffness is an important feature, which is worse in the morning. Chronic exhaustion is a prominent symptom and may be associated with restless and unrefreshing sleep.

On physical examination, diffuse tenderness may be noted. Discrete areas of point tenderness overlying muscles and their ligaments are found. Although the patient is usually unaware of the presence and location of trigger points, they are exquisitely tender to palpation. Often they are approximately the size of the examiner's finger pad. A small lump of contracted muscle may be felt. These trigger points are usually located within taut bands of muscle, which can be rolled between the examiner's fingers. Usually, a "jump sign" will be elicited as the trigger point is palpated, and the patient may cry out and move away as the trigger point is located. A local muscle twitch is usually felt and occasionally seen during palpation of a trigger point. Reactive hyperemia to palpation may be seen, most commonly on the trunk. These trigger points are usually within the region of the patient's reported pain, but sometimes are not. Palpation of true trigger points, however, should reproduce the patient's typical pain. Well known patterns of radiation have been described. For example, trigger points over the neck and scapula tend to cause pain in the ipsilateral shoulder and arm. Those of the flank tend to cause pain in the ipsilateral buttock and those of the buttock, into the posterior thigh and calf. The radiation of pain should be regional and nondermatomal in nature. If the radiation pattern of peripheral nerve or root is observed, other causes such as herniated disc or nerve lesion should be sought out. It should be realized that the presence of trigger points is an essential feature of this syndrome but is not sufficient for the diagnosis of myofascial pain syndrome. Based on studies involving healthy and asymptomatic volunteers, up to 50 percent of the general population has been estimated to harbor latent trigger points, which are difficult to distinguish from true myofascial trigger points in patients suffering from myofascial pain. It is conceivable that a significant portion of the general population that harbors latent trigger points may be at increased risk for developing myofascial pain syndrome. These latent trigger points do not cause spontaneous pain at rest or with movement, as opposed to active trigger points. They are, however, painful to palpation, and they do cause radiation to typical reference areas. Latent trigger points may be activated by jerky movements or muscle overuse. They may persist for years after an episode of transient myofascial pain that resolves over time, leaving patients susceptible to painful relapse.

The appearance of the affected region tends to be normal but can occasionally show mild swelling and other signs of muscle spasm, particularly in the neck and shoulder region. There usually is no evidence of muscle wasting, although long-standing disuse of an extremity secondary to pain can be a cause of weakness, decreased range of motion, and atrophy. Heat and cold intolerance is not prominent. There should not be evidence of true allodynia (pain caused by a stimulus, e.g., light touch, which normally does not produce pain). If trophic changes and allodynia are present, a component of neuropathic and/or sympathetically maintained pain may be present, which may require further evaluation (see Ch. 222).

Myofascial pain syndrome is a common occurrence in pain clinic populations and is usually an easy and straightforward diagnosis, but many practicing physicians are not familiar with this syndrome. This is at least partly due to the absence of objective signs, normal radiologic studies, and lack of any diagnostic laboratory tests in myofascial pain syndrome. This is further complicated by the fact that it occurs in varying intensity, duration, and location and cannot be accurately diagnosed unless the affected muscles are properly examined. The following case studies from our own clinical experience illustrate some key points about myofascial pain syndrome. Readers are encouraged to consult references at the end of this chapter for a detailed review of this topic.

CASE STUDIES

Case Study 1

A 27-year-old woman was referred for evaluation with a 6-month history of severe, daily headaches involving the right side of her head after hitting her head against a window while at work. She had no immediate symptoms, and it was not considered an extraordinary incident. Gradually, over the next few days, she developed worsening headache, which did not respond satisfactorily to the Fiorinal (Sandoz, E. Hanover, NJ) prescribed by her primary care physician. The headaches continued and she was referred to a neurologist. After a neurologic evaluation and a normal computed tomographic scan of her brain, a diagnosis of "post-traumatic headache" was established. Daily amitriptyline in increasing doses was prescribed, and the patient was instructed to use acetaminophen or ibuprofen on an "as-needed" basis. At the time of her evaluation, she reported improved sleep with a single night-time dose of 125 mg of amitriptyline but continued to complain of daily headache during the day. She also reported worsening of pain on chewing and combing her hair.

Physical examination showed a healthy and fit-looking young woman complaining of right-sided headache. Her neurologic examination was completely normal but she had an exquisitely tender point in her right temporalis muscle (Fig. 220-1). Palpation of that "trigger point" reproduced her usual pain.

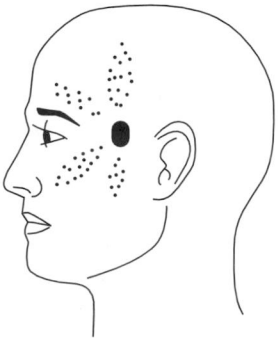

FIG. 220-1. The pattern of the myofascial pain syndrome in patient 1. The square represents the trigger point in the temporalis muscle, and the zones of stippling mark the areas of referred pain.

She initially declined to have an injection but could not tolerate occupational therapy manipulation. The tender spot was infiltrated with a 6-ml mixture of 1 percent lidocaine and 0.25 percent bupivacaine, which gave her lasting relief from headaches. Amitriptyline was slowly tapered.

Case Study 2

A manual laborer, aged 36, was referred for an evaluation. He had suffered for 8 months from low-back pain, radiating to his right hip and posterior thigh area. He could not recall a single precipitating event but remembered gradual worsening of his pain. He was referred to a local pain specialist who made a diagnosis of "lumbosacral radiculopathy" after a magnetic resonance imaging (MRI) scan of his spine showed disc bulges at L_4-L_5 and L_5-S_1 levels. The patient received two epidural steroid injections and bed rest over a 6-week period with partial and transient relief. His symptoms worsened, and he could not continue working. Physical examination showed a well-appearing and muscular man who walked with a slight limp. Neurologic examination was normal, but he had two tender spots in the quadratus lumborum muscle and one tender spot over the piriformis muscle (Fig. 220-2). Palpation over these trigger points reproduced his symptoms. The trigger points were infiltrated with a 20-ml mixture of 1 percent lidocaine, 0.25 percent bupivacaine, and 40 mg of triamcinolone, and he was referred for physical therapy. He was able to return to work in 2 months, during which he required repeat trigger point injections once and a course of physical therapy.

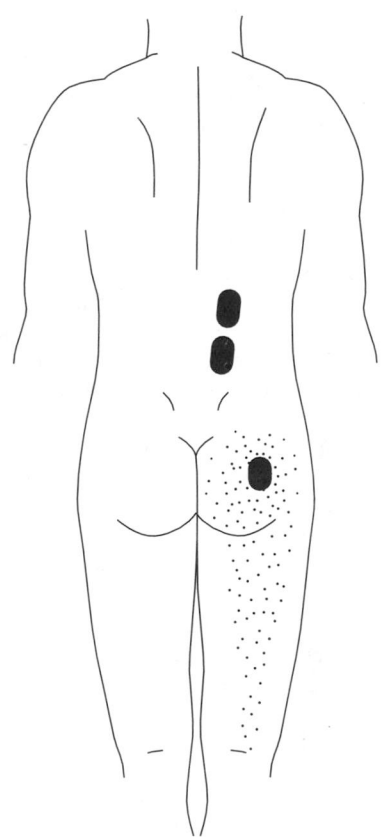

FIG. 220-2. The pattern of the myofascial pain syndrome in patient 2. The squares represent the trigger points in the quadratus lumborum and piriformis muscles, and the zones of stippling mark the areas of referred pain.

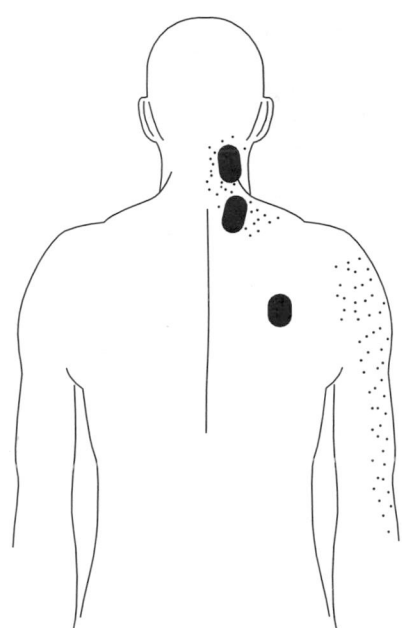

FIG. 220-3. The pattern of the myofascial pain syndrome in patient 3. The squares represent the trigger points in the levator scapulae and infraspinatus muscles, and the zones of stippling mark the areas of referred pain.

Case Study 3

A 29-year-old painter complained of progressive worsening of shoulder and neck pain, radiating to his right arm over a 3-month period. The pain was described as continuous, deep, and aching and was aggravated by any use of the right arm. He also complained of neck stiffness and had acute exacerbations of pain on any movement of his neck. He had well-defined trigger points in his right neck and scapular regions (Fig. 220-3). Palpation of these points produced referred pain in his neck, shoulder, and right arm. Over a 3-week period, he received multiple trigger point injections with local anesthetic and physical therapy three times per week. He reported significant pain relief for up to 3 to 4 hours after each session of trigger point injections followed by physical therapy. At this point, he was referred to our pain clinic. Physical examination showed a well-appearing muscular man, holding his head flexed to the right. All neck movements were greatly limited by pain. He did have two trigger points (Fig. 220-3). Palpation over these reproduced his typical referred pain but not numbness and the tingling sensation that was also felt in his hand and forearm on sudden movement of the neck. His neurologic examination was otherwise normal. We performed trigger point injections using long-acting local anesthetic and steroids in an attempt to provide him with long-lasting relief but also scheduled him to have an MRI scan of his cervical spine. This time, injections provided pain relief for 2 days. MRI scan showed a C6–C7 disc herniation impinging on the right neural foramen without other significant abnormalities. His pain finally responded to a combination of cervical traction, epidural steroid injections, and physical therapy.

PATHOPHYSIOLOGY

The exact mechanism of myofascial pain syndrome remains uncertain. Kellgren, who is credited for his pioneering work in this syndrome, demonstrated that injecting a particular muscle with an irritating solution consistently produces pain, which is felt over a much larger region than the muscle injected. He described classic cases of myofascial pain with trigger points that referred pain in the same pattern as in his earlier experiments. A contracted, hyperirritable spot in the muscle, known as a trigger point, is an integral part of this syndrome. How it is formed and maintained remains unclear. It is believed that overuse of deconditioned muscle and acute trauma contribute to formation and activation of trigger points. It has been speculated that trauma or muscle overload causes microscopic tissue injury involving sarcoplasmic reticulum. There is a resultant release of tissue humoral factors, which cause inflammation and pain. Local instability of calcium channels may occur. Increased levels of extracellular calcium may play a part in initiating and maintaining local muscle spasm. This produces a region of local vasoconstriction, ischemia, and uncontrolled metabolism within the muscles. Central and sympathetic nervous system reflexes may also be involved, leading to persistent inflammation, spasm, and pain. This process results in shortened muscle fibers in an area of increased metabolism and decreased circulation, which are palpable as a taut band in the muscle and give rise to the phenomena typically associated with palpation of trigger points.

After muscle injury, afferent impulses from damaged tissue bombard the central nervous system. Stress response systems intercede, leading to increased sympathetic activity in the affected muscle. Generalized fatigue and anxiety feed into this system. Local vasomotor changes occur. An area of increased metabolic demand secondary to continued spasm coupled with a decreased blood supply caused by sympathetic response develops. Local ischemia results in further release of humoral factors such as histamine, serotonin, kinins, and prostaglandins. A vicious cycle of local trigger point muscle spasm ensues, leading to vasomotor constriction with resultant continued pain and inflammation. This cycle can perpetuate itself long after the inciting event.

DIAGNOSIS

The diagnosis of myofascial pain syndrome is based on an extensive history and physical examination. Often a recent or remote episode of tissue trauma is elicited. A contralateral injury may be found to cause asymmetric body mechanics with resultant muscular stress of the painful muscle groups. Chronic muscle overload may be found. If a history of trauma is lacking and the pain has been gradual in onset, a thorough exploration into the patient's personal life is warranted. Significant emotional stressors should be elicited. Sleep patterns are important, as exhaustion can be a cause of myofascial pain syndrome in susceptible people. Depression is frequently found in these patients. Whether depression is a cause of this illness or rather a symptom is controversial. Certainly, any emotional derangement augments the pain cycle.

The pain may have been present for months to years and is frequently debilitating. Many patients are out of work secondary to pain. A complete list of previous medication trials and therapies should be sought. Radiation of pain is typical but should be regional and nondermatomal in character. History of paresthesia and numbness should be absent.

Trigger points are pathognomonic for myofascial pain syndrome. Their inactivation with resultant long-lasting relief of pain should therefore be considered diagnostic. Palpation for typical trigger points should be performed. These may be out-

side of the patient's described area of pain. Upon palpation, however, the typical referred pain will be elicited. Local tenderness is not considered a trigger point. Frequently a jump response is obtained. As mentioned, a taut band of muscle with a discrete trigger point within it may be felt as the muscle is rolled between the examiner's fingers. Reactive hyperemia may be found after trigger point palpation. Each trigger point should be labeled with a skin marker for later treatment. Deep tendon reflexes and sensory examination should be normal. Motor function may be diminished in patients with long-standing myofascial pain syndrome. Thermography of the skin overlying trigger points may show increased temperature secondary to the increased metabolism of a muscle in spasm, but that is a nonspecific finding and is not required to make this diagnosis. In fact, there are no radiographic or laboratory test abnormalities that are considered diagnostic of myofascial pain syndrome. Some cases of polymyalgia rheumatica, other inflammatory muscle diseases, and rheumatologic disorders may mimic myofascial pain syndrome. In those patients, erythrocyte sedimentation rate, muscle enzyme levels, antinuclear antibody, rheumatoid factor, and so forth become essential screening tools, and further management plans depend on the results of these tests. For all practical purposes, it is essentially a clinical diagnosis and sometimes a diagnosis of exclusion.

TREATMENT

The treatment of myofascial pain syndrome generally involves a multimodality approach. Inactivation of trigger points with local anesthetic injections, dry needling, and stretch and spray techniques form the mainstay of therapy. Physical therapy, transcutaneous electrical nerve stimulation, and massage therapy have also been used. Pharmacologic trials of anti-inflammatory medications are reported to help some patients in combination with other modalities. Biofeedback and relaxation therapy have also been used.

We most frequently use local anesthetic injections of trigger points with or without steroids. Steroids are generally most useful when hyperemia is present or there is history of prolonged pain after injection and should not be used frequently. Trigger points are located and marked during the physical examination. The skin overlying the trigger points is prepared with alcohol or povidone-iodine. A mixture of 20 to 40 mg of triamcinolone in 10 ml of 0.25 percent bupivacaine is generally used. The total volume of the solution depends on the size of the muscles involved and the number of trigger points to be injected. If a shorter duration of action is desired 1 to 1.5 percent lidocaine can be substituted for bupivacaine. A 1.5-inch 25-g needle on a 12-ml syringe is typically used. The trigger point is isolated between the physician's first and second fingers. The needle is introduced into the muscle after anesthetizing the skin overlying the trigger point. Often a local muscle twitch is felt and occasionally seen when the needle enters the trigger point, and the patient's typical referred pain may be reproduced. A total volume of 3 to 5 ml of local anesthetic is typically placed within the trigger point. Then the needle is withdrawn almost to the surface and redirected to the same depth, injecting other areas of the muscle surrounding the original injection site, thereby ensuring complete inactivation of the trigger point. Shortly after injection of each trigger point, the patient's pain should resolve or become markedly diminished, and muscle spasm should abate. Dry needling can be performed in a similar manner without the aid of local anesthetic, but we do not recommend dry needling because it is extremely painful and without any clear benefit over local anesthetic injections.

Stretch and spray can be performed when injection therapy is undesirable or contraindicated. The patient is placed in a comfortable position. The muscle to be treated is sprayed with a vapocoolant, such as ethyl chloride or chlorofluoromethane starting at the skin overlying the trigger point and continuing in the direction of the referred pain. The muscle is then very carefully stretched through its normal range of motion. This sequence of spray and stretch can be repeated a few times before rewarming. The involved muscle must reach its full stretch length in order to inactivate trigger points. This technique is particularly useful and preferred over trigger point injections in patients with diffuse myofascial pain.

Regardless of the technique chosen for trigger point inactivation, the patient should note prolonged pain relief. The relief should far outlast the duration of local anesthetic action. Frequently, patients may note prolonged pain relief after only one set of injections. Sometimes, however, a series of injections is performed as the effects of the last injections start to wane. Usually the interval between symptomatic recurrence will increase until the patient's myofascial pain syndrome has resolved. This may require a series of three to six sets of trigger point injections over a few weeks to months.

It is often useful to have patients treated with physical therapy after and between trigger point injections. Passive stretching and massage treatments can be instituted. Gradual increase in activity and gentle graduated exercise programs complement trigger point inactivation. Care must be used not to strain already compromised muscle groups. Especially vigorous physical therapy can aggravate the syndrome and often will alienate patients who either give up or go elsewhere for treatment. As patients improve, general exercise and body conditioning programs should be instituted. Transcutaneous electrical nerve stimulation may also be used during physical therapy. If patients respond, a portable unit may be taken home on a trial basis and later purchased or rented if effective.

Nonsteroidal anti-inflammatory medications are sometimes useful adjuncts in treating myofascial pain syndrome. They help reduce inflamation and are useful in treating the inherent soreness patients exhibit after the local anesthetic action of trigger point therapy abates. They are generally considered safe and offer the advantage of being nonaddicting. Other useful medications include tricyclic antidepressant medications. At relatively low doses, they certainly help with sleep and may, with time, help diminish pain. We would typically use amitriptyline or nortriptyline if anticholinergic side effects are especially undesirable. Ten- to 25-mg starting doses are generally well tolerated. This dose can then be titrated by the patient under strict guidelines every 4 to 7 days by the same starting increment. It must be remembered that nortriptyline is about twice as potent as amitriptyline and other tricyclic antidepressants commonly prescribed for chronic pain. Pain tends to improve within several days after reaching adequate dose of the medication with the maximum benefit found over weeks. Most patients respond to doses between 25 and 100 mg, although some may require much higher doses for effect. An adequate trial of these medications would require at least a few weeks of therapy at the highest dose tolerated. Biofeedback and relaxation techniques also afford significant pain relief in selected patients and should be considered as adjunct therapies.

PROGNOSIS

As with most pain syndromes, the prognosis is dependent on the chronicity of the pain. Patients with myofascial pain of short duration often respond to just a few trigger point injections. These patients tend still to be working and leading active, albeit dramatically modified lives. As the chronicity of the pain syndrome increases so, too, does the period of time needed to treat it and the modalities incorporated in its treatment. Frequently these patients are out of work and depressed. They might benefit from the antidepressant action of the tricyclic medications as much as from the pain relieving quality of it. Certainly physical therapy and psychological counseling with relaxation technique training is invaluable. With weeks to months of interdisciplinary therapy, these chronic pain sufferers tend to respond slowly.

SUGGESTED READINGS

Fischer AA: Pressure threshold measurements for diagnosis of myofascial pain and evaluation of treatment results. Clin J Pain 2:207, 1987

Frost FA, Jesson B, Siggaard-Anderson J: A control, double-blind comparison of mepivacaine injection versus saline injection for myofascial pain. Lancet 1:499, 1980

Gunn CC: Dry needling of muscle motor points for chronic low-back pain. Spine 5:279, 1980

Kellgren JH: A preliminary account of referred pains arising from muscle. BMJ 1:325–27, 1938

Reeves JL, Jaeger B, Graff-Radford SB: Reliability of the pressure algometer as a measure of myofascial trigger point sensitivity. Pain 24:313, 1986

Simons DG, Travell JG: Myofascial origins of low back pain. Postgrad Med 73:66–108, 1983

Sola AE: Treatment of myofascial pain syndromes. pp. 467–85. In Benedetti C et al (eds): Recent Advances in Pain Research and Therapy. Vol. 7. Raven Press, New York, 1984

Travell JG: Myofascial trigger points: clinical view. In Bonica JJ, Albe-Fessard D (eds): Advances in Pain Research and Therapy. Vol. 1. Raven Press, New York, 1976

Travell JG, Simons DG: Myofascial Pain and Dysfunction: The Trigger Point Manual. Vol. 1. Williams & Wilkins, Baltimore, 1983

Travell JG, Simons DG: Myofascial Pain and Dysfunction: The Trigger Point Manual. Vol. 2. Williams & Wilkins, Baltimore, 1991

221. ARTHRITIC PAIN

SIMON M. HELFGOTT

Arthritic pain is one of the most common subjective complaints encountered in clinical medicine. The term is often used synonymously with *musculoskeletal pain,* although, in fact, arthritic pain is only one of several types of pain related to the musculoskeletal system (Table 221-1). Arthritis pain must be distinguished from other causes of musculoskeletal pain to establish an accurate diagnosis and initiate appropriate treatment. Some clinicians use the term *arthritis pain* as a diagnostic label. As there are more than 100 disease states associated with arthritis, it is important to avoid this practice.

EVALUATION OF MUSCULOSKELETAL PAIN

Arthritis implies joint inflammation and the associated clinical features, including joint swelling, tenderness on palpation, limitation of motion, and warmth. Other types of musculoskeletal

TABLE 221-1. Types of Musculoskeletal Pain

	Associated Clinical Features
Arthritis	Joint swelling with limitation of motion, warmth, and occasional redness
Arthralgia	Joint achiness and tenderness without objective features such as swelling
Bursitis/tendonitis	Tenderness over involved area Limitation of joint motion (occasionally) Soft-tissue swelling, redness, and warmth are unusual
Myalgia	Achiness is nonarticular, felt to be muscular in origin Muscle tenderness on palpation may be noted
Myofascial pain	Diffuse achiness, poorly localized Associated with areas of trigger point tenderness Swelling, redness, and warmth are unusual
Neural entrapment	May be confused with other musculoskeletal pains Associated dysesthesias, vague distribution of symptoms No associated joint findings

pain include bursitis/tendonitis, neural entrapment syndromes, and soft tissue pain. Pain emanating from the bursae and tendons is typically described as a dull aching pain, which is rather diffuse in nature. Often the patient cannot describe the actual site of pain but points to a broad area surrounding the joint as being most painful. The pain is typically asymmetric; is present after, but not during, activities, and is often noted to be worse at night or when lying on the affected side. Commonly involved bursae and tendons include the rotator cuff; the radial tendons inserting into the wrists; the trochanteric and anserine bursae of the hip and knee joints, respectively, and the Achilles tendon (Table 221-2). Medial and lateral epicondylitides present with clinical syndromes very similar to those described for tendonitis syndromes elsewhere.

A nerve entrapment syndrome, such as carpal tunnel syndrome, can mimic arthritic pain. The symptoms intensify at night and are often seen in patients with associated arthritic disorders. The presence of dysesthesia and other neurologic symptoms and signs serves to distinguish the cause of this pain. The pain associated with soft-tissue disorders such as fibromyalgia is described elsewhere (see Ch. 22D). This pain can resem-

TABLE 221-2. Common Bursitis/Tendonitis Syndromes

Site Diagnosis	Clinical Features	Clinical Features
Shoulder	Supraspinatus tendonitis	Pain with forced abduction and external rotation Pain felt in deltoid muscle region
	Bicipital tendonitis	Pain over the insertion site of the long head of the biceps
Elbow	Epicondylitis Medial Lateral	Pain over relevant epicondyle (rarely simultaneous) Wrist squeeze exacerbates the pain
	Olecranon bursitis	Soft-tissue swelling over the olecranon Normal pronation and supination of the elbow exclude true elbow joint involvement
Wrist	de Quervain's tenosynovitis	Pain felt over radial tendons of the wrist Exacerbation by forced deviation of wrist to the ulnar side
Hip	Trochanteric bursitis	Maximal tenderness felt laterally over the greater trochanter
Knee	Anserine bursitis	Maximal tenderness over the inferomedial aspect of the knee joint
Ankle/foot	Achilles tendonitis	Pain and swelling over tendon
	Plantar fasciitis	Foot/heel pain May radiate upward into the shin

ble the tendonitis and bursitis syndromes, and in many patients there is some degree of overlap between these two entities.

CLINICAL EVALUATION OF ARTHRITIS

History

The site of the major area of pain, whether over the joint or distal to it, may serve to distinguish arthritis from other musculoskeletal pains. For example, arthritis pain in the small joints of the hands is usually described as being present over the affected joints. Similarly, arthritic knee pain is noted over the knee itself. Activity increases the pain, and rest generally alleviates it. Pain related to bursitis/tendonitis often develops after completion of the activity. It may increase during periods of rest or sleep and is the most common cause of night-time musculoskeletal pain, when laying on the affected area intensifies the discomfort.

Morning stiffness is often seen in association with inflammatory forms of arthritis such as rheumatoid arthritis and polymyalgia rheumatica. Stiffness associated with inflammatory disorders tends to be generalized and often involves both the upper and lower extremities. Patients have difficulty "getting going" after awakening. They describe a sense of stiffness as they try to dress themselves, and they have difficulty with grooming activities. Morning stiffness can be seen with mechanical joint disease such as osteoarthritis. However, the degree of stiffness tends to be shorter lasting (i.e., minutes rather than hours, as seen in inflammatory arthritis), and the area of involvement tends to be localized to the affected joint only.

The pattern of joint involvement can be diagnostically helpful. Rheumatoid arthritis is a symmetric polyarthritis, which almost always involves the hands. Arthritis associated with connective tissue diseases such as systemic lupus erythematosus (SLE) tends to be symmetric and polyarticular, as well, although the clinical findings of joint swelling and pain may be more subtle. Polymyalgia rheumatica is usually symmetric, with shoulder and sometimes hip girdle involvement. The seronegative spondyloarthropathies such as Reiter syndrome tend to be asymmetric, oligoarticular with a predilection for large joint involvement more often in the lower rather than the upper extremities. Osteoarthritis usually involves large joints such as the knees and hips. Hand involvement is restricted to the proximal interphalangeal, distal interphalangeal, and carpometacarpal joints of the hands. It is highly unusual to see involvement of the wrists, elbows, or shoulders in patients with primary osteoarthritis. Involvement of these joints or foot involvement is usually associated with a history of trauma to the joint. It may also suggest a secondary form of osteoarthritis caused by a metabolic disease such as hemachromatosis or hyperparathyroidism.

Crystal-induced arthritis (gout or pseudogout) usually involves the lower extremity joints, most commonly the first metatarsal phalangeal joints (podagra), the ankle, and the knee. Upper extremity involvement can be seen, particularly involving the wrist joint.

The arthritis associated with connective tissue disease and immune complex–mediated disease is generally symmetric, is polyarticular, and usually involves the hands. With some forms of immune complex–mediated arthritis, there is a history of exposure to an exogenous antigen such as ingestion of a drug (e.g., antibiotics) or exposure to viral antigens (e.g., hepatitis).

Bursitis/tendonitis syndromes (Table 221-2) are often related to history of extremity overuse. Patients with supraspinatus ten-

TABLE 221-3. Common Causes of Arthralgias

Viral syndromes	(e.g., Influenza, hepatitis, and parvovirus)
Immune complex mediated	(e.g., Cryoglobulins)
Drug induced	(lovastatin, zidovudine, intravenous immune globulin)
Post-transfusion	

TABLE 221-4. Causes of Night-Time Musculoskeletal Pain

	Areas of Involvement
Bursitis/tendonitis syndromes	(See text)
Polymyalgia rheumatica	Shoulder and hip girdle
Neural entrapment	Carpal and tarsal tunnel syndrome
End-stage joint disease	Any joint, confirm by radiography
Fibromyalgia syndrome	Diffuse achiness (see text)

donitis may recall excessive lifting activities or repetitive actions that require abduction and external rotation to the shoulder. Similarly, epicondylitis, either medial or lateral, is associated with excessive and repetitive hand functions that require squeezing maneuvers of the hand. Although commonly referred to as tennis elbow and golfer's elbow, respectively, lateral and medial epicondylitides are seen in a much wider range of the population. Excessive keyboard use is a common underlying factor.

PHYSICAL EXAMINATION

Rheumatoid Arthritis

The classic features of rheumatoid arthritis include joint swelling, pain on palpation, and increased warmth over the joint. Pain on range of motion is often seen. Joint swelling can easily be confirmed by physical examination of the wrists, small joints of the hands, and the knees. Joint swelling involving deeper joints such as the shoulders, elbows, and hips is difficult to ascertain by simple inspection of the joint and can only be inferred by noting a limitation of range of motion with associated pain. Radiographic imaging (magnetic resonance imaging and computed tomography) may be required to confirm the presence of a joint effusion. Although swelling around the ankles is often seen, it is not usually on the basis of true ankle joint arthritis. More common causes include fluid overload syndromes from congestive heart failure or renal disease. True ankle arthritis can be suspected by examining the patient's gait to assess for the degree of plantar and dorsi flexion of the foot.

Warmth over a particular joint is indicative of increased blood flow to the joint and possible underlying inflammation. Even with well-defined forms of inflammatory arthritis such as rheumatoid arthritis, its absence is not unusual. Increased warmth and redness over a joint suggests a crystal-induced or septic arthritis. Joint aspiration may be necessary to establish the diagnosis.

Pain on palpation of a joint or pain with range of motion of the joint needs to be interpreted in a broader context. Associated soft-tissue swelling helps to confirm a diagnosis of active arthritis in that joint. However, when pain is the only finding noted on physical examination, one must question whether the underlying process is indeed arthritis or simply arthralgia, that is, pain in a joint not necessarily accompanied by active inflammation. The distinction is crucial. Since many patients with a variety of nonarthritic disorders may complain of arthralgias, it is important to separate these diagnostic categories from those causing arthritis. Tables 221-3 lists several common causes of joint arthralgias.

The joint swelling seen in rheumatoid arthritis ranges from subtle to sizable. However, some degree of swelling must be evident to establish the diagnosis. Synovial thickening, a hallmark of chronic inflammatory synovitis, is felt by careful palpation of the joints, especially the wrists, metacarpophalangeal joints, and knees. A spongy sensation is felt. Other typical features of rheumatoid arthritis include symmetric joint involvement and involvement of the wrists and hands. Pain, stiffness,

and fatigue are common complaints. Night-time joint pain is unusual and suggests one of three possibilities, namely, bursitis/tendonitis, neural entrapment syndrome, or end-stage arthritic damage of a particular joint (Table 221-4).

Polymyalgia rheumatica is a syndrome consisting of proximal shoulder and hip girdle stiffness felt worst during the night and early morning hours. It develops in patients 50 years and older, rarely in nonwhites. Unlike rheumatoid arthritis, there is no distal joint (i.e., hand, wrist, knees or feet) involvement. An elevated erythrocyte sedimentation rate is usually seen. There is a reduction in the range of motion at the shoulders, particularly abduction and external rotation (hands behind the head). Hip rotation may also be limited. (Difficulty dressing and putting on shoes and socks.) Significant improvement, often dramatic, is noted following initiation of low-dose (10 to 15 mg/d of prednisone) corticosteroid therapy.

Osteoarthritis

Osteoarthritic joints typically are not swollen, but one can see and feel bony prominences surrounding the joint. These are known as Heberden's nodes when noted over the distal interphalangeal joints and Bouchard's nodes over the proximal interphalangeal joints. Osteoarthritis of the knee may be associated with structural changes such as a varus deformity. Arthritis pain can generally be recreated by active range of motion of the particular joint. With more progressive cartilage loss, crepitation may be felt with simple palpation. This generally indicates bone-on-bone apposition. End-stage changes caused by osteoarthritic damage may result in pain being felt even at rest.

Seronegative Spondyloarthropathies

These clinical entities share common features (Table 221-5). The association of the carriage of histocompatibility antigen HLA-B27 varies from 90 percent for ankylosing spondylitis to 20 to 30 percent for psoriatic arthritis. The variable specificity and sensitivity of HLA-B27 positivity coupled with its prevalence (5 to 12 percent) in the normal population makes the utility of HLA-B27 antigen testing questionable.

Sacroiliitis may be seen with any of the spondyloarthropathies. Low-back pain and stiffness, felt worse during the night and early morning, which improves with activity and hot show-

TABLE 221-5. HLA-B 27–Related Spondyloarthropathies

	Associated Features
Reiter syndrome	Conjunctivitis, uveitis, urethritis, balanitis, diarrhea
Ankylosing spondylitis	Loss of back flexibility, back pain and stiffness
Psoriatic arthritis	Skin, scalp, nail involvement
Inflammatory bowel disease	Ulcerative or granulomatous colitis
Reactive arthritis	Abdominal pain, diarrhea
Salmonella	
Shigella	
Yersinia	
Campylobacter	

ers, is characteristic. Direct examination of the sacroiliac joint is difficult. Tenderness on palpation may be seen with many types of back pain and is unreliable.

The Schober test, a measure of back flexibility, is abnormal in most symptomatic patients. A segment of lumbosacral spine 10 cm above and 5 cm below a line connecting the "dimples of Venus" is remeasured with the patient in full forward flexion. If the segment length does not enlarge by, at least, 4 to 5 cm, the test is considered abnormal and may be indicative of spondylitis.

The typical patient with a spondyloarthropathy is a young man. The arthritis is oligoarticular and asymmetric with a tendency toward lower extremity and foot involvement. Dactylitis with resultant sausage toe swelling can be disabling. Extraarticular features, when present, help to distinguish these arthritides from rheumatoid arthritis and connective tissue disorders (Table 221-5).

Crystal-Induced Disease

Crystal-induced synovitis is usually intensely painful (Table 221-6). The arthritis is monoarticular, although an asymmetric oligoarthritis may occur. Podagra, an acute arthritis of the first metatarsophalangeal joint, can be caused by any crystal, though it is usually due to gout. Whenever possible, joint aspiration and synovial fluid analysis should be performed to establish the diagnosis definitively. The presence of a red, swollen joint suggests a crystal-induced arthritis or sepsis, and it is essential that a joint aspiration be performed. Interestingly, one rarely sees coexisting sepsis and crystal-induced arthritis.

Connective Tissue Disease

The arthritis of the various connective tissue diseases ranges from arthralgias with objective joint findings to frank swelling, resembling rheumatoid arthritis. Symmetry and polyarticular involvement are the most commonly observed patterns of arthritis. Deformity is rarely observed, with the exception of the development of avascular necrosis of bone. This may be related to the underlying disease process (e.g., SLE) or to corticosteroid use. Commonly involved joints include the hips, knees, and shoulders. The onset of pain and gait disturbances may be fairly sudden. Diagnosis is confirmed by imaging studies.

Immune Complex Disease

The arthritis seen with circulating immune complex deposition (e.g., SLE and hepatitis B) or cryoglobulins (hepatitis C) presents with intense pain and discomfort. Again, there is a predilection for symmetry and hand involvement. Other clinical

TABLE 221-7. HIV-Associated Arthritides

Presentation	Pathogenesis
Arthralgias	?Immune complex Drug related (zidovudine)
Arthritis (monoarticular)	?Immune complex Septic joint
Arthritis (oligoarticular) (e.g., Reiter syndrome and psoriatic)	Reactive HLA-B27 related
Vasculitis (multisystem, including skin, joints, and muscle)	HIV or other viral antigen induced
Sjögren syndrome	Viral-mediated glandular destruction

Abbreviation: HIV, human immunodeficiency virus.

features such as jaundice, abdominal pain, or liver function test abnormalities develop concurrently or shortly afterward, helping to establish the correct diagnosis.

Human Immunodeficiency Virus

Human immunodeficiency virus-related arthropathies are outlined in Table 221-7. A CD8+ T-cell—mediated severe arthropathy resembling Reiter syndrome has been well described. Coexistent rheumatoid arthritis and acquired immunodeficiency syndrome have not been reported, probably because of the severe reductions in CD4+ T-cell populations, an integral cell in the pathogenesis of rheumatoid arthritis.

Bursitis/Supraspinatus Tendonitis

As noted earlier, there are a number of distinct bursitis/tendonitis syndromes (Table 221-2). The upper extremity shoulder pain related to supraspinatus tendonitis or an adhesive capsulitis may present in an identical fashion. Acutely, there is a history of increasing pain, usually felt over the upper portions of the humerus several centimeters distal to the shoulder joint itself. There is a significant limitation of abduction of the shoulder, and pain is also made worse with external rotation. A useful finding on physical examination is the accentuation of pain with forced abduction of the shoulder. Less common causes of shoulder pain include bicipital tendonitis. The pain is felt anteriorly over the upper portion of the humeral head at the site of insertion of the long head of the biceps tendon into the humerus. Unlike supraspinatus tendonitis, there is no restriction on the range of motion with abduction and/or external rotation. Acromioclavicular arthritis may mimic features of supraspinatus tendonitis. Pain is felt with abduction and external rotation. Unlike the former condition, there is tenderness felt over the acromioclavicular joint itself.

Pain around the elbows is most often due to an insertion syndrome, either medial or lateral epicondylitis. The most striking finding is pain on palpation of either epicondyle, which reproduces the characteristic discomfort. It can often be accentuated by having the patient clench the fist while palpating the epicondyle.

De Quervain's tenosynovitis results in pain extending into the distal forearm toward the base of the thumb. Finkelstein's maneuver (forced ulnar deviation of the hand) accentuates the pain.

In the lower extremities, the most common bursal pains include trochanteric and anserine bursitis. Trochanteric bursitis presents with lateral hip tenderness; the pain may radiate downward toward, but rarely beyond, the knee. Pain on palpation

TABLE 221-6. Crystal-Induced Arthritis

Condition	Crystal	Associated Clinical Clues
Gout	Sodium urate	Male, hyperuricemia Diuretic use Excessive ethanol intake Familial predisposition
Pseudogout	Calcium pyrophosphate	Older patient Chondrocalcinosis on radiograph Associated metabolic disorders (e.g., hemachromatosis, hyperparathyroidism, thyroid disease, Wilson's disease) occasionally seen
	Calcium hydroxyapatite	Calcific tendonitis Renal failure

TABLE 221-8. Therapies for Musculoskeletal Disorders

Drug therapies
   Nonsteroidal anti-inflammatory drugs
   Minor analgesics (e.g., acetaminophen)
   Tricyclic antidepressants (low dose)
   Corticosteroids
   Disease-modifying antirheumatic drugs (e.g., gold salts, hydroxychloroquine,
     methotrexate, and azathioprine)
   Intralesional corticosteroid (e.g., intra-articular, tendon sheath, or bursa)
Physical therapy
   Ultrasound
   Electrical stimulation
   Massage therapy
   Splinting

over the site of the bursa, the greater trochanter, confirms the diagnosis.

Anserine bursitis is associated with pain felt medial and inferior to the knee. Pain is felt maximally over the bursa, which is about 2 to 4 cm distal to the joint line on the medial side of the knee.

Foot pain caused by plantar fasciitis may present with heel discomfort and/or soreness in the medial part of the foot. Flattening of the medial arch is noted.

TREATMENT

First and foremost, the proper diagnosis must be established. Since there is considerable overlap among the diseases outlined, the presence or absence of systemic features, the degree of functional impairment, and the overall health of the individual are factors that must be considered. Table 221-8 outlines various treatment approaches fo the management of musculoskeletal pain.

SUGGESTED READINGS

Fauci AS, Haynes BF, Katz P: The spectrum of vasculitis: clinical, pathologic, immunologic and therapeutic considerations. Ann Intern Med 89:660, 1978

Harris ED: Rheumatoid arthritis: pathophysiology and implications for treatment. N Engl J Med 322:1277, 1990

Keat A: Reiter's syndrome and reactive arthritis in perspective. N Engl J Med 309:1606, 1983

Khan MA: An overview of the clinical spectrum and heterogeneity of spondyloarthropathies. Rheum Dis Clin North Am 18:1, 1992

Konttinen YT, Kemppinen, Segerberg M et al: Review: peripheral and spinal neural mechanisms in arthritis, with particular reference to treatment of inflammation and pain. Arthritis Rheum 37:965, 1994

Rheumatology Grand Rounds: Polyarthritis in a 78-year-old woman. Arthritis Rheum 37:1087, 1994

222. NEUROPATHIC PAIN

DAVID BORSOOK

A painful stimulus is conveyed to the central nervous system via *primary afferent fibers,* which have processes in the skin and tissue that synapse in the dorsal horn on *projection neurons* (e.g., spinothalamic and spinohypothalamic tract to the brainstem and basal forebrain structures, including the thalamus and limbic structures such as the hypothalamus and amygdala) and finally to the sensory cortex via *thalamocortical projections.* Under normal circumstances, the pain system detects and localizes painful stimuli and serves to protect the organism. However, with damage to the peripheral or central nervous system anywhere along the pain pathway, an unremitting painful syndrome may result. This damage anywhere along the peripheral nerve and spinothalamocortical pathway may produce a *neuropathic pain syndrome.* Although descending analgesic systems exist (e.g., periaqueductal gray-raphe magnus with descending pathways to the dorsal horn via the dorsolateral funiculus) there, it is unknown whether damage to these systems results in neuropathic pain. In some circumstances, damage to a peripheral nerve results in a particularly severe pain syndrome known as *sympathetically maintained pain* in which activity of the sympathetic nervous system seems to contribute to the maintenance of the pain. However, this occurs where there is damage to afferent nociceptive fibers.

CLINICAL FEATURES

Neuropathic pain may be defined as *a symptom resulting from neural injury, peripheral, central, or both, to a portion of the pain transmission system.* Such pain is often severe, delayed in the onset following injury, often burning or electrical in quality, and present in the absence of an ongoing source for the pain.

The history and physical examination of a patient with neuropathic pain should reveal the following symptoms: there may be clinical evidence of damage to peripheral nerve(s) or the central nervous system and the pain is most often in the area that has partial or complete sensory loss. Not always is there a history of obvious nerve damage. For example, seemingly trivial injuries such as a sprained ankle may result in swelling, burning pain, temperature changes, and motor dysfunction (i.e., the syndrome of sympathetically maintained pain). There may be *allodynia* (i.e., increased pain to a normally nonpainful stimulus, e.g., cold, wind, or vibration), *hyperalgesia* (i.e., increased sensitivity or decreased threshold to a usually painful stimulus), symptoms of burning, electrical sensations, or tingling. These symptoms may be spontaneous or triggered by a seemingly innocuous stimulus (e.g., the shooting pain in tic douloureux). Pain may increase with emotional stress. Often there is a significant component of suffering or depression. These topics are not dealt with here. The nature of the pain may be continuous or episodic. When continuous, it is usually burning or aching, and, when episodic, patients describe electric shocklike sensations. These pain sensations do not usually occur in a single form, but a burning pain may be associated with intermittent shocklike sensations. Pain may vary with activity and may have a circadian fluctuation, most often being more intense in the evening.

Physical signs of neuropathic pain include the loss of or altered sensation (pinprick and thermal) in the area of the pain. A classic example of this is the syndrome of pain in the area of sensory deficit following a thalamic stroke. In some neuropathic pain states, repetitive sharp stimuli in the area of the sensory deficit, as seen in patients with thalamic pain, may produce an increase in pain. Usually there is evidence of the underlying cause for the loss of sensation (e.g., peripheral trauma, stroke, and so forth). In cases of sympathetically maintained pain, the "classic signs" such as swelling or temperature changes are not always obvious or present. In fact, recent evidence indicates that clinical findings are not diagnostic of the condition and can only be correctly defined when the patient's pain is relieved by sympathetic blockade (see below).

The underlying cause of painful neuropathies may be varied. In many cases, it is not possible to determine the etiology for the painful symptom. Damage to a peripheral nerve may result from *infectious* (e.g., acquired immunodeficiency syndrome, Guillain-Barré syndrome, or herpes zoster), *endocrine* (e.g., diabetes), *toxic* (e.g., alcohol or arsenic), *inherited* (e.g., Fabry's disease or hereditary sensory neuropathy), or *entrapment causes* (e.g., carpal tunnel syndrome, herniated disc, or cancerous invasion of a plexus). Damage to the central nervous system may affect the *dorsal horn* (e.g., avulsion injuries), the *spinal cord* (e.g., trauma, tumors, syringomyelia, and demyelination), and the *thalamus* or *cortex* (e.g., stroke, demyelination, or tumor).

PATHOPHYSIOLOGY

The neurobiologic basis for neuropathic pain syndromes is not well understood. A number of models for neuropathic pain have been proposed, some of which have better experimental foundations than others. Nevertheless, these models allow us to formulate a working basis to understand better the reasons for painful syndromes, including the shooting pain or burning pain that may following nerve damage. Furthermore, these models have allowed for testing of new drug approaches in pain treatment. Below is a list of some of the abnormalities of neural function that are thought to take place in various neuropathic pain states.

1. *Ectopic impulses:* Under basal conditions, there is no electrical activity in pain fibers. Following nerve damage, abnormal spontaneous activity is present. The mechanisms for generating these spontaneous impulses are not well defined. Nevertheless, this process, which may take place in the central or peripheral nervous system, is probably the reason for the clinical phenomenon of shooting or dysesthetic pains
2. *Altered receptor numbers:* Following nerve damage, there is an increase in the number of adrenergic receptors on the sprouting terminals. These receptors are produced in the nerve body in the dorsal root ganglion and transported distally to the axon sprout. Neuromas, which are essentially a mangled bundle of neuronal sprouts emanating from the end-damaged nerve and represent attempted regrowth of the axons toward their normal targets, are usually very sensitive to norepinephrine and conditions of stress in which there is an endogenous release of epinephrine. Recent research has demonstrated that microneuromas form even after apparently minor trauma. Examples of this include after surgical skin incision or in postherpetic neuralgia.
3. *Altered neural connections in the dorsal horn:* Under normal conditions, A-δ and C-fibers synapse in the dorsal horn, predominantly in laminae I, II, and V. A-β fibers send collaterals to synapse in lamina IV. Under these conditions, light touch, which is conveyed by A-β fibers, does not produce pain. However, following nerve injury, the A-β fibers send new collaterals to lamina II and synapse on projecting spinothalamic neurons. In this manner, light touch sensation can be "misdirected" and activate pain pathways. It is not known whether there are altered connections in more central structures such as the thalamus following central nervous system damage.
4. *Ephaptic cross talk:* Under normal circumstances, activity in the nerve fiber remains confined to that fiber. Following

damage to the nerve, there may be the formation of abnormal electrical contacts called ephapses. This can result in activity from one fiber or group of fibers producing electrical activity in others. As a result, painful stimuli are not generated by normal sensory transduction.

5. *Altered levels of neurotransmitters and neuromodulators:* There are both excitatory and inhibitory neuromodulators in the dorsal horn. With nerve damage, there may be excessive release of excitatory transmitters or peptides (e.g., glutamate, calcitonin gene-related peptide, and substance P), which can produce excitotoxic damage to dorsal horn neurons. Inhibitory neurotransmitters and peptides may act as protectors of this damaging process. Providing opioids or local anesthetics prior to nerve damage, as in the case of surgical amputation of a limb, for example, may inhibit this process of excitatory neurotransmitter damage. This is called "pre-emptive analgesia."
6. *Coupling of sympathetic nerves and primary fibers in the dorsal root ganglion:* In animal models of neuropathic pain, noradrenergic axons form basket structures around large-diameter injured neurons. These may be the same large-fiber A-β neurons that send new collaterals into lamina II (see above). There may be other forms of coupling between the sympathetic nervous system and the primary nociceptive afferent fibers. It is hypothesized that these various forms of coupling are involved in sympathetically maintained pain, a pain syndrome that is rapidly relieved following blockade of the sympathetic nervous system.

DIAGNOSTIC APPROACH

As with any patient, a complete medical history and examination should be performed. However, there are two essential issues in the diagnostic approach to a patient with neuropathic pain: first, a specific history and physical examination, and, second, diagnostic tests for possible disease states. Figure 222-1 diagrams an approach to patients with possible neuropathic pain.

Specific History and Physical Examination

A neuropathic pain syndrome can be diagnosed on the basis of a history of nerve trauma combined with evidence for a sensory deficit in the painful area. Sometimes there is pain in a region of the body that has been removed, so-called deafferentation pain. A classic example is the pain seen in amputation stump pain and phantom limb pain. Examples of other phantom pains include phantom anal pain or phantom breast pain, which are seen in some patients following surgical removal of the anus or breast, respectively. It is unclear why some patients develop neuropathic pain and others do not. Animal studies point to a genetic component that is important in the development of neuropathic pain.

Special attention should be paid to factors that exacerbate or relieve the pain. Many patients with chronic pain do not sleep well, and this may contribute to the pain state. Although a careful history and examination may be performed, it is often difficult to define the type of neuropathic pain, particularly, the difference between pain that is sympathetically maintained and is completely abolished by sympathetic blockade and pain that is independent of sympathetic activity. In many cases, the clinical presentation may be very similar, and the previous notion

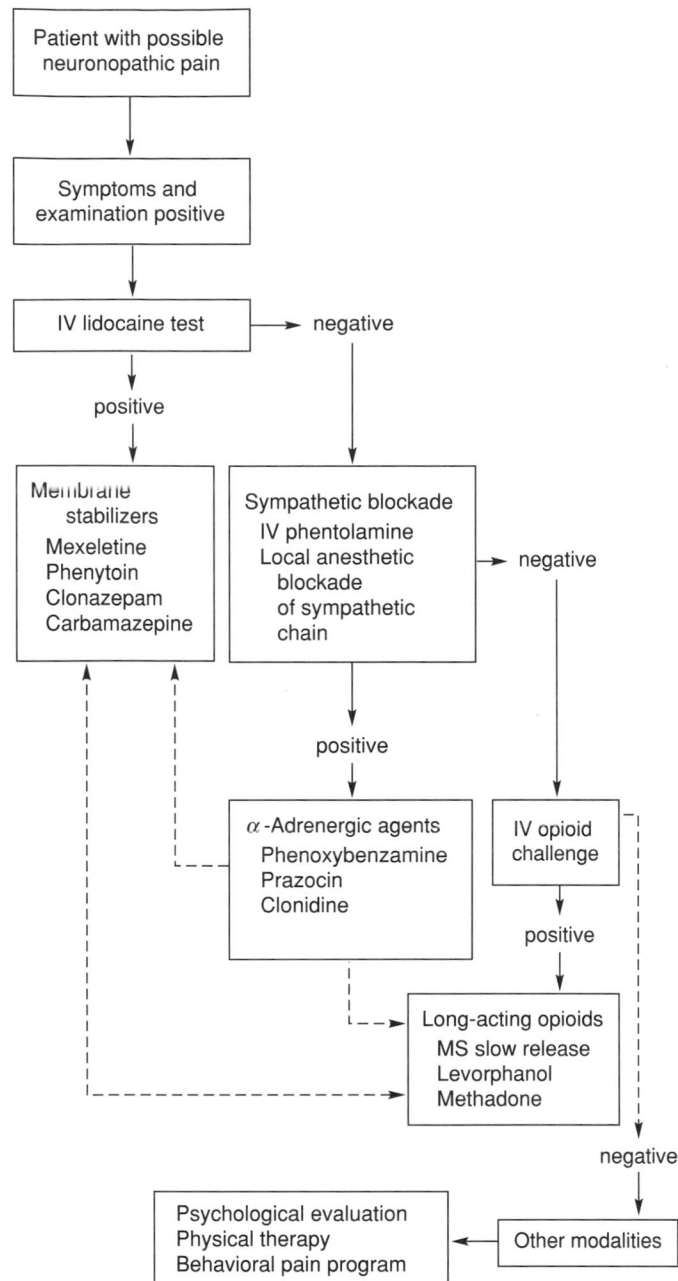

FIG. 222-1. Approach to patients with possible neuropathic pain.

TABLE 222-1 Anticonvulsants Used in the Treatment of Neuropathic Pain

Drug	Dose (mg)
Carbamazepine	200 tid
Clonazepam	0.5–2 tid
Phenytoin	300 qd

anesthetic blockade of the sympathetic ganglia (e.g., stellate or lumbar ganglia). If the pain is not affected by sympathetic blockade, it may be inhibited by the infusion of intravenous lidocaine? Lidocaine at 1 mg/kg has been shown to inhibit ectopic impulses in damaged nerves in animal models. In humans, analogues of lidocaine, tocainide, or mexiletine were initially used in the treatment of diabetic neuropathy. The infusion of the local anesthetic lidocaine, if it inhibits pain by 70 percent or more, may be a useful prerequisite to treating patients with oral analogues of the agent (see below). Finally, there is a subgroup of patients who do not respond to either of the above tests, and an infusion of an opioid may be a good approach to determine whether the neuropathic pain syndrome is responsive to opioids.

Diagnostic Tests

Specific blood tests for diabetes, hypothyroidism, or vitamin B_{12} deficiency should be routine when clinical evidence indicates the underlying cause. Such tests are used more in the diagnosis of generalized painful neuropathies. Unusual tests would be required when an unusual painful neuropathy such as Fabry's disease, porphyria, amyloidosis, or mitochondrial disease is suspected. In general, electromyography (EMG) is not particularly useful in the diagnosis of most pain syndromes since the clinical examination, if performed properly, will define the location, intensity, and etiology of the neuropathic pain states. In some cases, particularly entrapment neuropathies, EMG is very helpful. EMG may also be helpful in defining the progression of recovery, for example, in a patient with a traumatic peripheral nerve injury. Imaging studies are useful in the diagnosis of central lesions and cord or nerve root involvement. Thermography probably does not have a useful role in routine neurologic practice of the diagnosis and treatment of neuropathic pain. Thermal sensory testing is a useful diagnostic aid.

TREATMENT

Medical Treatment

For many patients, neuropathic pain syndromes may be very debilitating, that is, they cannot sleep or participate at work, during leisure, or at home because the pain is so severe and incapacitating. It is helpful to the patient for the physician to develop a treatment plan. The plan should address specific issues related to the pharmacologic treatment of neuropathic pain syndrome and more global issues such as the potential need for medications to promote sleep or the potential to increase activity at home and at work. With respect to these latter issues, referrals to physical therapy or psychology practitioners may be necessary. As noted above, the approach to neuropathic pain requires that all attempts are made to define the pathophysiology of the pain and the medication group (i.e., membrane stabilizers, sympathetic blockade, or opioids) to which the patient is most likely to respond. If the patient responds dramatically to one of these pharmacologic diagnostic approaches, it is useful

of the case of sympathetically maintained pain being obvious clinically is no longer tenable.

In order to define whether the pain arises from abnormal neural (ectopic) activity, one approach has been to administer intravenous lidocaine (1 mg/kg), either as a slow bolus or as a slow infusion. In patients, particularly those in which there is ongoing (e.g., diabetic neuropathy) or recent nerve damage (e.g., brachial plexus avulsion), intravenous lidocaine in most cases produces a decrease in the patient's pain by more than 50 percent. In these cases, patients are candidates for neuropathic pain medications (most of which stabilize membrane potentials). Thus, agents such as mexiletine, phenytoin, carbamazepine, clonazepam are the drugs of choice (Table 222-1).

Currently the two most common approaches to sympathetic blockade are the phentolamine test in which 0.5 to 1.0 mg/kg of phentolamine is given intravenously slowly or by local

TABLE 222-2. Antidepressant Medications Useful in the Treatment of Neuropathic Pain

| Drug | Uptake Blockade | | Ortho. Hypo. | Side Effects | | | Dose (mg/day) |
	NE	5HT		Sedation	Arrhythmia	Anticholinergic	
Amitriptyline	+ +	+ + + +	+ +	+ + + +	+	+ + + +	25–300
Desiprimine	+ + + +	+ +	+/−	+	+	+	50–300
Doxepin	+	+ +	+ +	+ + + +	+/−	+ +	75–400
Imipramine	+ +	+ + + +	+ + + +	+ +	+	+ +	75–400
Nortriptyline	+ +	+ + +	+/−	+ +	+	+ +	20–150

to start with medications that have the same effect. For, example, if intravenous lidocaine is beneficial, mexiletine, the oral analogue of lidocaine, is the drug of choice (see below).

Anticonvulsants. Anticonvulsants have been the mainstay of treatment for neuropathic pain and are particularly efficacious in patients with shooting pains. These drugs, which include phenytoin, carbamazepine, and clonazepam, are administered in the usual doses (Table 222-1), and the standard precautions are taken (e.g., complete blood count, liver function tests, and, when indicated, blood levels of the drug). These drugs can be used in combination with antiarrhythmics or opioids.

Antiarrhythmics. The antiarrhythmic tocainide was first used in the treatment of diabetic neuropathy. However, this agent produces bone marrow depression and is therefore not used. Mexiletine, another antiarrhythmic agent, can be used in patients who have a normal electrocardiogram. It seems to work well in patients with new-onset neuropathic pain and in patients with ongoing damage to peripheral nerves that produces pain such as in diabetic neuropathy or some of the neuropathies seen in acquired immunodeficiency syndrome. For dosing, 150 mg tid with meals is used as a starting dose, building up to a dose of 1,200 mg/d. Regular electrocardiograms should be obtained to monitor the drug's serious side effects.

Antidepressants. Antidepressants have been shown to have analgesic effects. The analgesic effect, unlike the antidepressant effect, is relatively rapid in onset (i.e., days versus weeks). Table 222-2 lists antidepressant medications that may be useful in the treatment of neuropathic pain. In elderly patients and in patients in whom the medication produces side effects (especially anticholinergic effects), low doses of these drugs or alternative drugs may still help. Furthermore, the antidepressants that produce more sedation (e.g., amitriptyline or doxepin) may be useful adjuncts in helping patients with sleep disorders.

Opioids. The use of opioids in neuropathic pain has been controversial. However, recent evidence and clinical experience indicates that opioids may be very useful in providing effective relief. It should be pointed out that concerns of addiction are, in general, unfounded since this is rare in patients who have no prior history of drug abuse or who are using opioids for the first time. The issue of tolerance is real since most, if not all,

patients will require increased doses owing to the development of tolerance. Nevertheless, opioids should be considered in all patients in whom other pharmacologic and nonpharmacologic options have not been proved to be beneficial. When this route is chosen, the risks (i.e., constipation, tolerance, or withdrawal if opioids are stopped suddenly) and benefits (i.e., pain relief) should be explained to the patient. Long-acting compounds such as sustained-release morphine, methadone, or levorphanol should be used (Table 222-3). The use of shorter acting compounds can be helpful in patients who have exacerbation with their pain during short intervals of regular activity. In these cases, a short-acting opioid may be given 20 minutes to 1 hour prior to the activity. It is very important to understand equivalent doses for various opioids since some patients, for reasons that are unclear, respond significantly better to one opioid over another.

Sympathetic Blockade

Sympathetically maintained pain may not only be diagnosed by sympathetic blockade (ganglion injections with local anesthetic) or with phentolamine, but, in some cases, a single injection, for example, may produce days to months of relief. Patients who respond well to sympathetic blockade should therefore receive repeated or continuous sympathetic blockade. These patients should be referred to anesthesia colleagues for repeated sympathetic chain injections or for continuous blockade via a catheter placed near the sympathetic chain, intrapleural (for upper limb pain) or epidural, which blocks the sympathetic afferents from the intermediolateral column of the spinal cord that egress via the ventral roots to the sympathetic ganglia.

Aggressive therapy, including medical and physical therapy, should be given to these patients. The mistake is often made not to treat aggressively in the early stages of the disease, and, in these patients, pain and other effects of the disease, including motor changes (tremor, dystonia, or weakness), may progress. Treatment of the pain in the late stages of the disease is very difficult. For reasons that remain poorly understood, physical therapy seems to be useful in this condition.

Medical therapy for patients with sympathetically mediated pain includes those agents that block sympathetic activity, that is, the release of norepinephrine at the terminal. Therefore agents that inhibit either α_1-adrenergic receptors (postsynaptic, e.g., phenoxybenzamine) or are α_2-adrenergic agonists (presy-

TABLE 222-3. Opioid Analgesic Starting Doses Used for Neuropathic Pain

Short-Acting Opioids	PO Dose (mg)	Long-Acting Opioids	PO Dose (mg)
Codeine	30–60 q3–4h	Morphine sustained release	15–30 bid, tid
Oxycodone	5–10 q3–6h	Levorphanol	2–4 q8h
		Methadone	5–20 q6–8h

TABLE 222-4. Drugs Used in the Treatment of Sympathetically Mediated Pain

Class	Drug	Dose (mg)
Oral sympatholytics	Clonidine	0.1 tid
	Prazosin	2 tid
	Phenoxybenzamine	30–120/day
Transdermal sympatholytics	Clonidine patch	0.1–0.4 q3–7 day
Opioids	Morphine (slow release)	15–60 bid
	Morphine elixir	5–20 q3h

naptic, e.g., clonidine) may be helpful. Other drug treatment approaches are given in Table 222-4. Agents such as the anticonvulsants or antidepressants may be tried with variable effect. Mexiletine and intravenous lidocaine are not helpful in these conditions. The phentolamine test (see above) is based on the idea that there is an upregulation of α_1-adrenergic receptors on the postsynaptic nerves (primary afferent nociceptive fibers), and blockade of the α_1-adrenergic receptors prevents abnormal or ectopic electrical activity in these afferent fibers.

Surgical Treatment

For nonmalignant pain, there is a very small role for surgical treatment. Removal of neuromas, sectioning or lesioning of somatic or sympathetic nerves, and surgery on the spinal cord or thalamus all have limited ability to provide long-term pain relief. Current understanding of the pain system and clinical experience has shown that, in most cases, pain returns in the original distribution and in the same intensity as that prior to the surgery. In some cases, for example, after sympathectomy, patients may experience new pain in regions different from their original pain at the level above or below the sympathectomy. One surgical procedure that may be useful in patients with brachial plexus avulsions is that of dorsal root entry zone surgery in which the afferent fibers together with laminae I to V are lesioned (recall that most nociceptive fibers terminate in laminae I, II, and V). Some institutions provide more aggressive surgical interventions such as thalamic surgery, implantation of spinal cord stimulators, or epidural or intrathecal subcutaneous pumps for administration of morphine. In selected patients, these may have a role, but large prospective clinical studies need to be performed.

Behavioral and Physical Treatment

Some patients with neuropathic pain syndromes may respond to physical therapy, behavioral therapy such as biofeedback, or psychiatric therapy. The mechanism by which these modalities work is not clear. The use of transcutaneous electrical nerve stimulation units is also controversial, although some patients seem to benefit from these.

Many patients with chronic pain are very difficult to treat, and psychological and/or psychiatric input is often necessary in the management of these patients. Since some pain syndromes have no cure, other psychosocial factors may contribute to the patient's pain. In these instances, appropriate referrals to centers that have multidisciplinary pain management teams may be helpful.

CONCLUSIONS

The treatment of neuropathic pain syndromes in benign and malignant pain can be difficult and challenging. Recent progress in the neurobiology of alterations in the nervous system that take place following peripheral or central damage to pain pathways has provided new insights into the mechanism of neuropathic pain. These developments will, no doubt, produce new pharmacologic agents that will help in the treatment of the pain that many patients suffer.

SUGGESTED READINGS

Awerbuch GI, Sandyk R: Mexiletine for thalamic pain syndrome. Int J Neurosci 55:129–33, 1990

Dejgard A, Petersen P, Kastrup J: Mexiletine for treatment of chronic painful diabetic neuropathy. Lancet 1:9–11, 1988

Fields HL, Liebeskind JC (eds): Pharmacological approaches to the treatment of chronic pain: new concepts and critical issues. Progress in Pain Research and Management. Vol. 1. IASP Press, Seattle, 1994

Gracely RH, Lynch SA, Bennett GJ: Painful neuropathy: altered central processing maintained dynamically by peripheral input published erratum appears in Pain 52:251–3. Pain 51:175–94, 1992

Jadad AR, Carroll D, Glynn CJ et al: Morphine responsiveness of chronic pain: double-blind randomized crossover study with patient-controlled analgesia. Lancet 339:1367–71, 1992

Leijon G, Bovie J, Johansson I: Central post stroke pain—neurological symptoms and characteristics. Pain 36:13–25, 1989

Max MB: Treatment of post-herpetic neuralgia: antidepressants. Ann Neurol 35:S50–3, 1994

Max MB, Lynch SA, Muri J et al: Effects of desipramine, amitriptyline and fluoxetine on pain in diabetic neuropathy. N Engl J Med 326:1250–6,

Portnoy RK, Foley KM, Inturrusi CE: The nature of opioid responsiveness and its implications for neuropathic pain: new hypotheses derived from studies of opioid infusions. Pain 43:273–86, 1990

Procacci P, Francini F, Zoppi M, Maresca M: Cutaneous pain threshold changes after sympathetic block in reflex dystrophies. Pain 1:167–75, 1975

Raja SN, Treede RD, Davis KD, Campbell JN: Systemic alpha-adrenergic blockade with phentolamine: a diagnostic test for sympathetically maintained pain. Anesthesiology 74:691–8, 1991

Rowbotham MC, Reisner-Keller LA, Fields HL: Both intravenous lidocaine and morphine reduce the pain of postherpetic neuralgia. Neurology 41:1024–8, 1991

Tanelian DL, Brose WG: Neuropathic pain can be relieved by drugs that are use-dependent sodium channel blockers: lidocaine, carbamazepine and mexiletine. Anesthesiology 74:949–51, 1991

Treede RD, Davis KD, Campbell JN, Raja SN: Plasticity of cutaneous hyperalgesia during sympathetic ganglion blockade in patients with neuropathic pain. Brain 115:607–21, 1992

223. CANCER PAIN

ALYSSA LEBEL

Cancer is a common and greatly feared diagnosis. More than 1 million new cases are identified in the United States each year, and the American Cancer Society predicts there will be more than 500,000 deaths caused by cancer this year. The World Health Organization estimates that cancer causes one of every 10 deaths worldwide and that, globally, more than 3.5 million people currently suffer from cancer pain.

The fear of cancer is due both to its high mortality rate and to the true perception that cancer is a painful disease. In the initial and intermediate stages of cancer, 30 to 45 percent of patients experience moderate to severe pain. In advanced disease, 70 to 80 percent of patients report pain, and 25 to 30 percent describe the pain as very severe. Fifty percent of patients report pain during cancer-related procedures, with an even higher percentage noted among pediatric patients. However, the reality of cancer pain is that most patients may be successfully treated with simple, inexpensive measures. Several studies show that pain may be controlled with oral morphine in 90 percent of patients, and an impressive array of alternative medications and techniques is available for resistant cases, including multiple opioids; adjuvant nonopiate medications; epidural, subarachnoid, and intraventricular routes of administration; neurolytic blockade; and ablative neurosurgery.

Paradoxically, cancer pain is undertreated. Several factors contribute to the undertreatment of pain and include fears of addiction by patients, physicians, and nurses; inadequate knowledge of the principles of cancer pain therapy; undue concerns about respiratory depression and other adverse effects of analgesics; and patient's reluctance to communicate pain, owing to concern about distracting the physician from the treatment of the primary disease, fear that pain means the disease is worse, and concern about not being a "good" patient. Barriers related to the health care system are the low priority given to cancer pain treatment, inadequate reimbursement, and restrictive regulation of controlled substances despite evidence that restriction decreases legitimate use with no effect on diversion. Efforts to eliminate these barriers to cancer pain management are a therapeutic and ethical imperative.

Effective cancer pain therapy depends on the clinician's understanding of the neuroanatomy and physiology of pain, ability to assess pain problems systematically and classify specific pain syndromes, and vigilant participation in comprehensive continuing care.

The physiology of pain is presented in detail in Chapter 216.

NEUROANATOMY/NEUROPHYSIOLOGY RELATED TO CANCER PAIN

An extensive plexus of receptors is found in the skin and viscera that responds to noxious stimuli. Mechanoreceptors and thermoreceptors are low-threshold nerve endings that respond to a wide range of noxious stimuli. If an actual or potential tissue-damaging event occurs, such as tumor infiltration, nociceptors are stimulated and transmit messages to the central nervous system. Tumor infiltration may also be associated with local tissue changes, such as vasodilation and edema, that outlast the initial stimulus and spread beyond its site of application. Inflammatory changes are generally accompanied by the release of algesic chemical mediators in the skin, bone, and viscera, which activate and sensitize nociceptors and which may promote spontaneous and continuous nociceptor activity, resulting in persistent pain. These diffusible substances may be released from damaged cells, such as potassium and bradykinin; be locally synthesized, such as prostaglandin E_2 and the leukotrienes; or be carried to the site by inflammatory cells, such as histamine by mast cells. Sensitization of nociceptors may also result in the release of substance P from primary nociceptive afferents, promoting further neural activation and inflammation and creating a vicious cycle of persistent pain. Chemical intermediaries of peripheral nociception include the following:

Histamine, mast cells, activates
Bradykinin, lymph, plasma, activates
Serotonin, platelets, activates
Norepinephrine, sympathetic efferents, activates
Prostaglandin E_1 and E_2 and leukotrienes, arachidonic acid metabolites, sensitizes
Substance P, primary afferents, activates

Also sensitization of peripheral afferents may be associated with an increase in expression of opioid receptors in the periphery, suggesting a peripheral role for exogenous and, possibly, endogenous opioids in areas of inflammation. Finally, efferent sympathetic activity may also sensitize myelinated (A-δ) nociceptors.

The algesic chemical mediators of inflammation are the targets of many pharmacologic agents, such as prostaglandin-synthesis inhibitors (nonsteroidal anti-inflammatory drugs [NSAIDs]), antihistamines (hydroxyzine), substance P antagonists (capsaicin), and sympatholytics (clonidine). For example, tumor metastasis to bone is a common cause of cancer-related pain, most frequently seen in cancers of the lung, breast, and prostate. Both myelinated and unmyelinated afferent fibers exist in bone and adjacent periarticular joints and soft tissue and are most prominent in the periosteum. Bony metastases result in osteolysis and osteoclasis, processes associated with prostaglandin synthesis and subsequent activation of local nociceptors. Therefore, corticosteroids and NSAIDs have an important role in the management of bony metastases.

Cutaneous and visceral nociceptive impulses are conducted in the central nervous system by A-δ afferents (thinly myelinated mechanoreceptors) and/or more slowly conducting C-afferent fibers (unmyelinated polynodal nociceptors). Classically, selective stimulation of A-δ fibers produces *first pain*, which is rapid in onset after injury, sharp, localized, and pricking. C-fiber stimulation produces *second pain*, which is slower in onset, prolonged, dull, aching, and poorly localized. Visceral afferents may be of A or C-caliber. Injury to afferent nerve fibers and the spinal cord by chemotherapy, radiation therapy, surgery, or tumor may activate the pain transmission system without stimulating nociceptors. The character of pain caused by this "deafferentation" is different from somatic or visceral pain from nociceptive activation of a normal nervous system and requires unique therapy.

Nociceptive afferent fibers enter the spinal cord through the dorsal root, travel in the dorsal root entry zone for one or two segments, and then enter the superficial layers of the cord where other interneurons may also synapse. Multiple incoming and descending stimuli combine to modulate the discharge patterns of dorsal horn cells, and multiple neurotransmitters are released. Again, this area of neural activity is the target of multiple analgesic pharmaceuticals. Under conditions of stimulation, such as produced by peripheral tissue injury, hypersensitivity of spinal nociceptive neurons occurs, a process that is exquisitely sensitive to treatment with opioid analgesics.

Nociceptive information is then relayed to the brain primarily via the spinothalamic tract, which consists of two subsystems: the neospinothalamic tract and the paleospinothalamic tract. The neospinothalamic tract ascends to the ventrolateral and posterior thalamus and the somatosensory cortex. This system is thought to transmit information about sharp, discriminative, well-localized pain. The paleospinothalamic tract branches widely in the brainstem to the reticular formation and, then, to the hypothalamus, medial and intrathalamic nuclei, and the limbic forebrain. It is thought to transmit information about poorly localized pain and generate affective and autonomic responses associated with painful stimuli. This extensive arborization of the ascending pain systems often limits the effectiveness of localized neuroablative surgical procedures and single pharmacologic agents for control of chronic pain.

In addition to ascending pathways, there is a descending analgesic system that terminates in the dorsal horn. Electrical stimulation of the midbrain periaqueductal gray region may activate cells in the nucleus raphe magnus, which then projects to the dorsal horn to produce analgesia. A pain-modulatory system also extends from the dorsolateral pons to the spinal cord. The pathway from the rostral medulla to the cord is partly serotonergic, and the pathway from the dorsolateral pons is partly noradrenergic. In addition to these biogenic amines, endogenous opioids are present in all regions implicated in pain modulation. The opioid-mediated analgesic system can be activated by electrical stimulation or by exogenous opioids, such as morphine. It can also be activated by stress, pain, and suggestion.

CLINICAL ASSESSMENT

Definition of pain is critical in the management of cancer pain. Specific factors to determine include

Temporal nature of the pain
Localization, that is, focal, generalized, or referred
Etiology, that is, specific pain syndromes
Pathophysiology, that is, somatic, visceral, or neuropathic
Concurrent problems, for example, physical, psychological, and social

Pain may be described as acute or chronic. Acute pain is first pain. It has a well-defined onset, is temporary, is provoked by injury and subsides with healing, is usually associated with autonomic signs, and is transmitted by normal sensory activity. Examples in patients with cancer include mucositis, pathologic fractures, ileus, and urinary retention.

Chronic pain occurs in the absence of a detectable tissue-damaging process or persists at least 1 month beyond healing, is not associated with autonomic signs, and may be associated with peripheral and central nervous system dysfunction (neuropathic pain). In the patient with cancer, both temporal categories usually exist simultaneously.

Localization of pain is straightforward if its origin is cutaneous and it corresponds to a dermatomal map. Visceral pain is frequently difficult to localize, is perceived in an area larger than the affected structure, and may be felt in a body region remote from the pathologic site.

Pain syndromes in patients with cancer are associated with direct tumor infiltration in approximately 75 percent of all cases, frequently presenting as bony (base of skull syndromes or vertebral body syndromes) or neuropathic (peripheral neuropathy, plexopathy, or leptomeningeal metastases) pain. Pain syndromes associated with cancer therapy (surgery, chemotherapy, and radiation) occur in approximately 20 percent of patients. Pain syndromes not associated with cancer or cancer therapy present in approximately 5 percent of cases and include such problems as osteoarthritis, diabetic neuropathy, aortic aneurysm, and herpes zoster infection, which is five times more common in patients with cancer than in the general population.

Pathophysiologic characterization of cancer pain most directly dictates appropriate therapy. *Somatic pain* occurs as a result of tissue injury, is aching or gnawing in quality, is generally well localized, and is initiated by nociceptive activation in cutaneous and deep tissues. It is usually manageable with anticancer therapy (radiation therapy) and common analgesics (morphine and NSAIDS). Examples include bone metastases, fractures, and postsurgical pain. *Visceral pain* is also associated with tissue injury, specifically infiltration, compression, distension, or stretching of thoracic and abdominal viscera. Surgical reaction of the viscera does not usually result in persistent pain. Visceral pain is aching, poorly localized, and often referred to distant cutaneous sites. *Neuropathic pain* results from injury to the peripheral and/or central nervous system by tumor, surgery, radiation, or chemotherapy. It is severe or dull pain, which is frequently associated with sensations of shooting or electrical pains superimposed on a background of burning and aching sensations. Pain is often felt in a region of sensory deficit, and mild stimuli may be perceived as painful (allodynia). Possible mechanisms of neuropathic pain include spontaneous hyperactivity of deafferented spinal pain transmission neurons, ectopic impulse generation in damaged nociceptive primary afferents, and central nervous system plasticity with the development or activation of aberrant inputs to deafferented central pain transmission neurons from spinal centers to the cerebral cortex.

The psychosocial assessment of the patient with cancer pain should address the following issues: the meaning of the pain to the patient and the family (i.e., severe pain implies a terminal state); the patient's typical coping response to stress and pain (i.e., would relaxation techniques, increased patient education individual or group support, or cognitive therapy be helpful?); the patient's concerns about using controlled substances such as opioids, anxiolytics, or stimulants; changes in mood such as depression and anxiety; and the economic effect of pain and its treatment.

The definition of pain is further enhanced by asking patients to assess the intensity of their present pain and pain at its least and worst. The most reliable and valid pain intensity scales are the simple descriptive scale, the 0 to 10 numeric scale, and the visual analog scale.

Clinical assessment naturally includes a thorough medical and neurologic examination and the use of appropriate diagnostic tools, within the framework of evaluation just described, to identify, ultimately, the source of pain or a specific cancer pain syndrome. However, unidentified cancer pain syndromes or prolonged diagnostic processes should not deter adequate pain treatment.

Some common pain syndromes defined by physical examination include bone metastases, spinal cord compression, plexopathies, and mucositis. Bone metastases commonly occur with cancer of lung, breast, and prostate and are found most frequently in the spine, pelvis, femur, and skull. The most common presenting symptom is pain, which is usually dull, aching, and aggravated by movement. Pain is typically somatic in character, well localized (but possibly in multiple sites), and occasionally accompanied by neuropathic pain from adjacent neural compression or invasion. Pathologic fractures and hypercalcemia may accompany the syndrome.

Spinal cord compression caused by epidural spinal metastases is a medical emergency. In general, patients who are ambulatory when they begin treatment remain so, about one-half of patients who have paraparesis pretreatment regain ambulation, and patients who are paraplegic rarely recover motor power. Symptomatic vertebral body metastases occur in 5 to 10 percent of all patients with cancer. In 8 percent of patients, symptomatic spinal metastases are the presenting symptom. In patients with epidural spinal cord compression, back pain is the presenting symptom in 90 percent of cases. Dull, aching, midline back pain is usually the first symptom of epidural metastases. It is often progressive and may be associated with sharp radicular pain, suggesting nerve root involvement. Generally, neurologic deficits develop 7 weeks after initial symptoms. Treatment includes high-dose steroids, radiation therapy, and, occasionally, surgical intervention. Cervical, brachial, and lumbosacral plexopathies may result from direct tumor infiltration or compression by fibrotic tissue from radiation therapy. In general, the pain of plexopathy caused by a tumor precedes neurologic deficits by weeks to months, whereas radiation plexopathy presents with a nonpainful loss of function. In brachial plexopathy, the lower plexus is most commonly involved, and the pain is described as a moderate to severe ache in the medial upper extremity, radiating to the fourth and fifth fingers.

Mucositis may be present in patients receiving cytotoxic chemotherapy or radiation therapy to the head and neck. Pain intensity is due to the extent of tissue damage and the degree of local inflammation. It is described as a burning sensation, and it is often associated with erythema. Management includes the aggressive use of potent analgesics (opioids) and appropriate antimicrobials.

The desired outcome of a comprehensive pain assessment is a practical treatment plan, which should consider the following factors: the treatment setting (inpatient or home), the therapeutic strategy (primary therapy of the cancer, medications, anesthetic blockade, or neurosurgical strategies), adjuvant therapies (social service, physical therapy, psychological support), a system for monitoring the pain and its side effects (patient diary, visual analog scale scores, and bedside vital sign sheets), and scheduled follow-up (primary physician emergency contacts, and pain clinic).

CANCER PAIN MANAGEMENT

The most effective therapy for cancer pain is primary treatment of the tumor with radiation therapy, surgery, and chemotherapy. However, medical therapy with the use of analgesics is a frequent adjuvant to primary therapy, especially during painful antitumor procedures, and is the treatment of choice for chronic cancer pain, such as pain as a sequela of antitumor therapy and secondary to metastases. Table 223-1 outlines a hierarchy of

TABLE 223-1. Cancer Pain Treatment Hierarchy

Medical therapy
  Opioids: morphine, hydromorphone, levorphanol, oxycodone
  Neuropathic pain medication: carbamazepine, clonazepam, lidocaine
  Antidepressants: amitriptyline, dextroamphetamine
  Anxiolytics: lorazepam, diazepam
  Anti-inflammatory medications: NSAIDs, steroids
  Radiotherapy
  Chemotherapy
Drug therapy and primary therapy

Spinal therapy, epidural/intrathecal catheters
  Epidural/intrathecal morphine
  Epidural fentanyl/bupivacaine mix
  Epidural clonidine

Neurosurgical therapy
  Pituitary ablation
  Intraventricular catheter
  Permanent epidural/intrathecal catheter
  Cordotomy
  Myelotomy

Abbreviation: NSAIDs, nonsteroidal anti-inflammatory drugs.

modalities that can be used in cancer pain treatment. Opioids are the mainstay of treatment for severe cancer pain. In 1982, the World Health Organization (WHO) declared that morphine was the drug of choice for cancer pain. This choice is based on several factors, including the frequent easy availability of this agent (with some exceptions in developing countries); a bioavailability of 35 to 75 percent; a half-life of 2 to 3 hours, which is equal to the duration of analgesia; linear pharmacokinetics with repeated dosing; and availability of multiple routes of administration.

The three major classes of analgesics are aspirin and NSAIDs, opioids, and adjuvant agents. The WHO has outlined the following guidelines in the use of these agents for cancer pain.

1. The three-step analgesic ladder is used, according to pain intensity. For mild to moderate pain, NSAIDs or other weak analgesics (acetaminophen) are chosen. For moderate to severe pain, weak narcotics, such as codeine and oxycodone, are added. For severe pain, potent opioids are used, such as morphine and hydromorphone. Adjuvant agents, which generally act centrally in specific pain states, may be added at each step for specific indications, such as the use of anticonvulsants for neuropathic pain and antidepressant agents for mood disturbance, insomnia, and neuropathic pain. Not all patients "climb" up all three ladder steps. For example, a patient presenting with severe pain caused by bony metastases is started on opioids (third step) as initial therapy, with or without NSAIDs and adjuvants. The guiding principle of care is individualization of therapy, frequently reassessment of the patient, and balancing of benefits and adverse effects.
2. Medications are administered orally whenever possible. Tolerance to opioids develops more slowly with this route, and painful intramuscular injections can be avoided.
3. Analgesics are administered "around the clock" rather than as needed.
4. Side effects are anticipated and vigorously treated.
5. Placebo treatment is never appropriate care.

Nonopioid Analgesics

The nonopioid analgesics (aspirin, acetaminophen, and the NSAIDs) are used for mild to moderate pain and are a heterogeneous group of substances with different chemical properties but some similar pharmacologic properties. They have antipyretic, antiplatelet, and anti-inflammatory effects, the latter owing to the inhibition of cyclo-oxygenase with subsequent blockage of prostaglandin synthesis. Prostaglandin E_2 and the leukotrienes are potent activators of peripheral and, possibly, central nociceptive neurons. The mechanism of acetaminophen remains obscure, but a central mechanism is likely, possibly involving central nervous system excitatory amino acid receptors. All nonopioids are not associated with tolerance, and all have a ceiling effect. Greater than 1,300 mg of aspirin will not provide increased efficacy, only toxicity. In general, the maximal recommended dose of these medications is 1.5 to 2.0 times the starting dose.

Side effects are common and dose dependent and include bleeding diathesis owing to platelet antiaggregation, gastroduodenopathy, and renal impairment. Less common side effects are confusion, dysphoria, and exacerbation of heart failure and hypertension. In patients with cancer and compromised blood clotting, the preferred agents are acetaminophen and choline magnesium trisalicylate (Trilisate). For all these agents, careful monitoring of blood count, fecal blood, and hepatic and renal function is suggested.

One useful effect of the nonopioids is their synergism with opioids, allowing one to use lower doses of each type of agent with minimal toxicity and maximal efficacy.

Opioid Analgesics

These agents are used to treat moderate to severe cancer pain. Morphine is the best-studied opioid and is usually the drug of choice. However, other opioids with different properties may be selected. The factors that influence this choice are analgesic potency, receptor binding affinity, medication half-life, route of administration, dosage, and drug toxicity.

Traditionally, opioids were classified as "weak" and "strong," a distinction based on customary use rather than significant pharmacologic differences. Weak opioids include codeine, oxycodone, hydrocodone, and propoxyphene. Of note, oxycodone and morphine have equal oral potency. However, oxycodone is usually commercially available in fixed-dose combinations with aspirin or acetaminophen, limiting the upward titration of the opioid component. Using oxycodone, 5-mg tablets, alone, when available, obviates this problem. Strong opioids are available in noncombination formulations with no ceiling effect and unlimited upward titration. For example, if a patient with cancer presents with mild pain, based on the WHO ladder approach, initial treatment with a NSAID, such as choline magnesium trisalicylate, is appropriate. The starting dose for this drug is usually 750 mg tid, increasing to a maximum of 2,000 mg bid if pain persists over several days. If the patient then complains of moderate pain, the next addition is a weak opioid, alone or as a combination drug. One could choose 5 mg of oxycodone and 325 mg of acetaminophen (Percocet), one to four tablets of 4 to 6 hours, being careful not to exceed the acetaminophen "ceiling" of 4,000 mg. If analgesia is still not achieved, one would add a strong opioid, such as 60 to 80 mg of oral morphine in divided doses, around the clock.

The choice of appropriate opioid is also influenced by its receptor-binding affinity. The pure agonist opioids, such as morphine, oxycodone, and hydromorphone, have high affinity to μ receptors and low affinity to κ (Table 223-2). Activation of μ receptors results in potent analgesia, and sedation, euphoria (with acute use), respiratory depression, bowel hypomotility, dependence, and tolerance. Of interest has been the characterization of two populations of μ receptors, μ_1 and μ_2, with the latter possibly being unassociated with the nonanalgesic effects of opioids. The agonist-antagonist opioids, such as pentazocine, butorphanol, and nalbuphine, produce analgesia predominantly by the activation of κ receptors, antagonizing the μ receptors and limiting adverse effects, such as respiratory depression. However, these agents have a ceiling effect and may not be given to patients receiving full opioid agonists, as mixed agents will likely produce opioid withdrawal and increased pain.

TABLE 223-2. Opioid Receptor Types and the Associated Activity of Selected Drugs

Receptor Type	Pharmacologic Effects
μ	Respiratory depression, euphoria, supraspinal analgesia, physical dependence
κ	Miosis, hypothermia (?), sedation
σ	Spinal analgesia
γ	Smooth msucle inhibition, ? spinal muscle analgesia

Therefore, these agents are rarely indicated for the treatment of cancer pain.

Opioids may also be selected according to the length of their half-lives. Morphine, hydromorphone, meperidine, oxycodone, and codeine have short half-lives, 3 to 4 hours. Levorphanol, methadone, and slow-release morphine (MS Contin, Oramorph SR) have half-lives of 8 to 12 hours. Of note, with the chronic use of methadone, the plasma half-life may increase to 24 to 48 hours, with the duration of analgesia remaining 8 to 12 hours. A similar discrepancy between analgesic duration and plasma half-life, with chronic use, is noted for levorphanol. Therefore, these medications are best considered second-line opioids and are most frequently used in patients with prior opioid exposure. Repetitive doses of opioids with long half-lives may lead to drug accumulation and adverse effects, necessitating careful drug titration, especially in the elderly population. If delirium and confusion occur, the use of an opioid with a short half-life is preferred.

Regarding meperidine, repetitive dosing may lead to the accumulation of its toxic metabolite, normeperidine, which has a half-life of 12 to 16 hours and which is associated with central nervous system stimulation, with subsequent tremor, delirium, and seizures. Normeperidine is two times more potent an anticonvulsant and 50 percent as potent an analgesic as meperidine. This toxic metabolite rapidly accumulates in patients with renal failure. In general, patients with cancer require both a long-acting opioid for constant, chronic pain and a short-acting agent for breakthrough pain.

The route of administration is also an important consideration in the choice of an opioid. Opioids are administered by the simplest, safest, and least invasive route that will provide adequate analgesia. The oral route is preferred during the early stages of cancer. In the terminal stages, two routes of administration are required in 60 percent of patients, and three routes are required in 25 percent. Most opioids are available in oral preparations, as tablets, or in liquid form. For chronic cancer pain, the general practice is to combine a opioid with a long half-life around the clock with an immediate-release form as needed for breakthrough pain. For example, sustained-release morphine, which provides 8 to 12 hours of analgesia, is combined with an immediate-release or short half-life opioid (morphine sulfate immediate-release tablets, morphine sulfate elixir, hydromorphone, or oxycodone).

Rectal opioid preparations are available for morphine, oxymorphone, and hydromorphone and are used in patients who are sedated or confused, have gastrointestinal obstruction, or are unable to tolerate parenteral medication. The dosage is equivalent to the parenteral dose of an opioid with a short half-life.

The intravenous route is the fastest way to achieve analgesia and is used in patients who have rapidly escalating or otherwise uncontrolled pain or who are unable to swallow (severe nausea or mucositis). The intramuscular route is contraindicated owing to pain with injection, a possible variable rate of absorption, and potential abscess formation or injection-site fibrosis. The onset of analgesia after intravenous bolus is within minutes. The duration is short, and prolonged analgesia requires continuous infusion. Patient-controlled analgesia offers, to the compliant patient, the possible combination of a basal, continuous infusion with rapid delivery, as needed of preselected bolus doses. This technique is most useful for patients with chronic and incident pain.

The subcutaneous route is applicable for either patient-controlled analgesia or continuous infusion and provides an alternative to the intravenous route in the home setting. The subcutaneous needle is changed every 3 days and generally is placed in the abdominal tissue. An external pump supplies a preselected dosage of medication. Dosing is equivalent to the intravenous route as are blood levels at steady state. Bolus doses have a delayed onset, lower peak effect, and longer duration of action compared with intravenous boluses.

The transdermal route is available for fentanyl with patches at constant doses of 25, 50, 75, and 100 μg/h. With initial application, plasma concentrations rise slowly, the peak effect occurs after approximately 15 hours, and the elimination half-life is more than 20 hours. Therefore, this route cannot be used to provide rapid analgesia or to titrate doses and is not the first choice for opioid-naive patients. The suggested equianalgesic dose of transdermal fentanyl 25 μg/h is 45 to 135 mg of oral morphine per day.

The intraspinal route (epidural and intrathecal) of opioid delivery is by intermittent injection through reservoir devices or by continuous infusion through implantable or external pumps. The advantage of spinal opioids is a long duration of analgesia (18 to 24 hours) with a small dose of opioid (5 to 10 mg of morphine sulfate) compared with parenteral doses. However, prolonged use of spinal administration results in increased plasma drug levels, systemic delivery to the central nervous system, and rostral cerebrospinal fluid redistribution of the drug, thus obviating the initial advantages. Side effects, such as nausea and vomiting, respiratory depression, sedation, and pruritus, may not be avoided with the spinal route. Also, tolerance may develop rapidly with this route. Finally, this technique is invasive and carries risks for patients with bleeding disorders and infection. However, in carefully selected cases, it may provide excellent analgesia with few difficulties. The principle of the use of spinal opioids is the binding of the injected agent to spinal opioid receptors.

Intraventricular morphine delivery has been used for patients with refractory head and neck pain and with advanced metastatic disease. The indications for this treatment have not been fully studied.

Additional, but as yet investigational, routes of opioid delivery are buccal, nasal, and sublingual. A nasal form of a mixed agonist-antagonist agent, butorphanol, is available, but, as previously mentioned, these medications are not recommended for patients with cancer pain.

Opioid Adverse Effects. Opioid side effects include constipation, nausea, vomiting, pruritus, sedation, confusion, and respiratory depression. Dry mouth, myoclonus, and urinary retention may also occur. These adverse effects are often readily treatable and should be anticipated in all patients who are receiving opioids.

Constipation is the most common adverse effect and does not diminish during the course of therapy. Morphine is known to increase sphincter tone, increase segmentation, increase electrolyte and water absorption, and impair the defecation reflex. Therefore, stool softeners and stimulating laxatives are concurrent treatments for patients receiving opioids. Rare patients with refractory constipation, with intact bowel mucosa, may undergo a brief trial of oral naloxone (i.e., 0.4 to 0.8 mg q4h) until a favorable effect occurs but not for greater than 24 to 48 hours. This oral antagonist putatively acts selectively on opioid receptors in the bowel.

Opioids may produce nausea and vomiting by central effects on the chemoreceptive trigger zone and vestibular system and by peripheral effects on the gastrointestinal tract. These effects most frequently occur with the initiation of opioid therapy, and tolerance often develops within weeks. Treatment includes antiemetics, such as neuroleptics, antihistamines, and benzodiazepines, and antivertiginous drugs, such as prochlorperazine or scopolamine.

Sedation is usually related to a marked increase in opioid dose. Tolerance to this effect develops rapidly. Persistent sedation may be treated with stimulants, such as dextroamphetamine or methylphenidate.

Confusion, hallucinations, and dysphoria may also occur with opioid therapy, especially in elderly patients. Opioids may be decreased initially by 75 percent without precipitating withdrawal and may then be converted into an agent with a short half-life to use as needed. Concurrent assessment for other potential contributory factors, such as a metabolic derangement, hypoxia, use of other medications, or cerebral metastases, is essential. Urinary retention may require opioid discontinuation or a change to an alternative opioid. Pruritus is treated with antihistamines and, for spinal opioids, with low-dose intravenous naloxone.

Respiratory depression is the most feared and least common adverse effect of opioid therapy, especially with chronic treatment. The risk of this problem is increased by rapid dose escalation; high titration of long-acting opioids, such as methadone and levorphanol; renal failure; and high-dose use in an opioid-naive patient. Pain is a potent respiratory stimulant. If the respiratory rate decreases to less than 6 to 8 breaths per minute, physical stimulation is often sufficient, and, rarely, diluted intravenous naloxone (0.1-mg increments) may be used cautiously.

Tolerance and physical dependence are normal pharmacologic responses to the chronic use of opioids. Tolerance is characterized by decreasing efficacy with repeated administration and is treated with an increased dosage. Physical dependence is characterized by withdrawal symptoms if treatment is stopped abruptly. Neither of these factors should limit appropriate opioid use. Addiction is psychological dependence, a behavioral pattern characterized by a craving for a drug and an overwhelming concern with obtaining it. Addiction is extremely rare in patients with cancer.

Adjuvant Analgesics Adjuvant drugs are a heterogeneous group of agents that either enhance the effectiveness of opioids and nonopioids or have independent analgesic effects in specific pain states, such as neuropathic pain. They may be indicated at each step in the WHO ladder. They include tricyclic antidepressants, anticonvulsants, stimulants (as already described), and corticosteroids.

Tricyclic antidepressants are considered to provide a direct analgesic effect by blocking the reuptake of serotonin and norepinephrine at central synapses and are used in patients with cancer and any neuropathic pain syndrome. Their analgesic effects are independent of their effects on mood. The most commonly used agent is amitriptyline, but imipramine, doxepin, nortriptyline, and desipramine are alternatives.

Anticonvulsants are particularly useful in treating chronic neuralgias or in any neuropathy characterized by paroxysmal, electrical pain. The putative mechanism of analgesia is sodium channel blockade in damaged axons. Carbamazepine and clonazepam are most commonly used; phenytoin or valproic acid may also be tried.

TABLE 223-3. Neuroinvasive Procedures

For generalized pain
  Hypophysectomy
  Bilateral cordotomy
For local pain
  Rhizotomy, chemical or surgical (head, neck, extremities, and pelvis/perineum)
  Chordotomy (extremities, chest, abdomen, and pelvis/perineum)
  Epidural or intrathecal morphine (chest, abdomen, pelvis/perineum)
  Celiac plexus block (epigastric/visceral)

Intravenous lidocaine and the oral lidocaine analogue (mexiletine) may also be useful in neuropathic pain via sodium channel blockade. They also have a poorly described spinal effect.

Baclofen may be adjuvant therapy for patients with facial pain, spasm, and neuropathic pain, putatively owing to its γ-aminobutyric acid agonist effects.

Corticosteroids are useful in relieving pain from bony metastases, nerve compression, spinal cord compression, and headache from raised intracranial pressure. They may also be used for mood enhancement and appetite stimulation.

Anesthetic Procedures

Anesthetic procedures may be either nondestructive or destructive. The former includes epidural and intrathecal use of opioids, with or without local anesthetics, and local anesthetic blockade of peripheral nerves and sympathetic ganglia. Destructive procedures include injections of lytic agents, such as phenol or alcohol near peripheral nerves and ganglia. The most commonly used destructive procedure is the celiac plexus lytic block. It has a greater than 80 percent efficacy in visceral pain, originating from both pancreatic and nonpancreatic intra-abdominal cancer. The duration of analgesia may last for months, and significant complications are rare.

Neurosurgical Procedures

Neurosurgical procedures for pain relief are indicated in a select minority of patients. These procedures only provide temporary pain relief and are associated with the risk of subsequent neurologic dysfunction and/or persistent deafferentation pain. These procedures include peripheral neurectomy, dorsal rhizotomy, anterolateral cordotomy, commissural myelotomy, and hypophysectomy (Table 223-3) (see Ch. 230). Unilateral cordotomy is indicated for persistent, contralateral somatic pain below spinal level C5. Bilateral cordotomies can be effective for bilateral somatic and visceral pain. Complications include respiratory failure (high cervical cordotomy), sexual and sphincter dysfunction, ataxia, and paresis below the cordotomy level. Hypophysectomy is indicated for refractory, widespread metastatic cancer pain. It is usually performed stereotactically via a transsphenoidal approach, putatively creating a deafferentation lesion of the hypothalamus and activating descending analgesic systems. Complications include diabetes insipidus, cerebrospinal fluid leakage, and optic or oculomotor nerve damage.

CONCLUSION

Pain control is but one part of a comprehensive approach to patients with cancer. Continuing care and assessment is essential to ensure the best quality of life. This goal necessitates a comprehensive medical evaluation and accurate diagnosis from initial therapy through the final stages of disease. Currently available treatments, especially analgesic medications, can relieve pain in the majority of patients. Patients with intractable and severe pain would benefit from referral to cancer pain and palliative care specialists.

SELECTED READINGS

American Pain Society: Principles of analgesic use in the treatment of acute pain and chronic cancer pain. In: A Concise Guide to Medical Practice. 3rd Ed. American Pain Society, Skokie 1992.

Bonica JJ, Buckley FP, Moricca G, Murphey TM: Neurolytic blockade and hypophysectomy. pp. 1980–2039. In Bonica JJ (ed): The management of pain. 2nd Ed. Vol. 2. Lea & Febiger, Philadelphia, 1990a

Cherney NI, Portenoy RK: Practical issues in the management of cancer pain. pp. 1437–67. In Wall PD, Melzack R (eds): Textbook of Pain. 3rd Ed. Churchill Livingstone, Edinburgh, 1994

Cleeland CS: Pain control: public and physician's attitudes. pp. 81–9. In Hill CS, Fields WS (eds): Drug Treatment of Cancer Pain in a Drug-Oriented Society. Advances in Pain Research and Therapy. Vol. 11. Raven Press, New York, 1989

Coyle N, Adelhardt J, Foley KM, Portenoy RK: Character of terminal illness in the advanced cancer patient: pain and other symptoms in the last four weeks of life. J Pain Symptom Manage 5:83–9, 1990

Jacox A, Carr DB, Payne R et al: Management of Cancer Pain. Clinical Practice Guideline no. 9. AHCPR publication no. 94-0592. Agency for Health Care Policy and Research, Department of Health and Human Services, Public Health Service, Rockville 1994

MacDonald N: The role of medical and surgical oncology in the management of cancer pain. pp. 27–39. In Foley KM, Bonica JJ, Ventafridda V (eds): Second International Congress on Cancer Pain. Advances in Pain Research and Therapy. Vol. 16. Raven Press, New York, 1990

Portenoy RK: Adjuvant analgesics pp. 187–203. In Doyle D, Hanks GW, MacDonald N (eds): Oxford Textbook of Palliative Medicine. Oxford University Press, Oxford, 1993

Walsh PR: Ablative neurosurgical procedures in pain related to malignancy. pp. 125–35. In Abram SE (ed): Cancer Pain. Kluwer Academic Publishers, Boston, 1988

World Health Organization: Cancer Pain Relief and Palliative Care. World Health Organization, Geneva, 1990

SECTION 6. REGIONAL PAIN SYNDROMES

224. FACE AND JAW PAIN

LARRY Z. LOCKERMAN

Facial pain has many unique characteristics owing to the innervation of the trigeminal nerve. The trigeminal nerve innervates many different structures in a region of the body that has a very strong psychological impact. In addition to that, serotonin receptor sites that are involved with migraine medications are in the trigeminal system. Research has also demonstrated that the trigeminal nerve travels in the cervical spinal cord and is influenced by cervical nerve input. All of this tends to cloud the issue of what is causing the facial pain and headache. By examining the patient, findings help in the decision of whether to manage the pain as mediated centrally, peripherally, or both. Physical medicine modalities should be considered when there is palpable pain, tenderness, and other observable signs. Centrally mediated pain is usually best managed with pharmacologic methods. With both types of pain, psychological involvement is always a factor.

Frequently patients are seen who appear to have a temporomandibular joint disorder but are actually suffering from another pain disorder. Since pain is a personal experience with complex psychological and physical overtones, it is very subjective. An examination and history must establish the generator for the pain. The diagnosis should locate the site of the pain, describe the pain, and determine if it is a primary or secondary pain problem.

ACUTE AND CHRONIC PAINS

There are two types of pain experienced: acute and chronic (4 to 6 months or more). Most medical and dental schools teach students to recognize acute pain. Often we are confronted with a patient who has a chronic pain that is being managed with acute pain modalities. Since chronic pain does not serve any biologic purpose, therapies that are effective for acute pain frequently are not effective and contraindicated with a chronic pain condition.

When pain has been present for a long period of time, it becomes centralized, and its clinical characteristics are intensified by psychological factors. For this reason, the pain can have overtones of several systems and might require several different specialists to help peel away the various systems involved. This is the reason why several different specialists can claim success when the pain is diminished.

PAIN CATEGORIES

Migraine headaches are considered a neurovascular event. Most facial pains can be clinically categorized as somatic, neurogenic, or vascular.

Somatic

Somatic pain can be primary or secondary. It is also divided into superficial and deep somatic pains. The most common pains are musculoskeletal pains, which are in the deep category. This type of pain has a dull, deep, depressing quality, which becomes more intense with movement of the affected structures. It can also refer pain to distant sites, which have the same dull steady pain description. When pain is referred, it can include autonomic effects such as local edema, skin flushing, and lacrimation.

Temporomandibular joint disorders are deep somatic pains. Patients describe a constant dull steady ache on the side(s) of the face. Usually as the level of pain increases, the pain spreads to the temple region and can be described as a muscle tension-type headache. Muscles in the neck can also refer pain to the temple region. If the temporomandibular joints are the primary cause of the pain, the headaches can be secondary and will not resolve until the temporomandibular joint disorder is diagnosed and managed.

Examination of the facial muscles and temporomandibular joint should include range of motion and palpation of the structures. Palpation of the temporomandibular joint is done by placing a finger at both joints with slight pressure and asking the patient to open and close. If there is inflammation at the joint, it will be painful, and any clicks and crepitus can be felt and noted. Records of the maximum opening are recorded by measuring the distance between the incisal edges of the anterior teeth. In most people, normal maximum opening is 35 mm or more, which is equivalent to the width of three of the patient's fingers. Asking the patient to protrude the jaw forward, to return to the normal bite position, and then to move the jaw to the left and right provides all excursive movements (usually 8 mm or more in each direction).

If the patient presents with limited opening of the mandible, the range-of-motion information enables the clinician to determine if the patient is unable to open owing to muscle spasm (limited opening about 20 mm or the width of two fingers or less) or if the joint has a displaced disc, which presents as limited opening and also limited lateral movement to the contralateral side and a deviated protrusive motion to the ipsilateral side.

Palpation of the muscles should include the masseter, temporalis, sternocleidomastoid, splenius capitis, and trapezius muscles. These muscles often are the primary or secondary pain generators for facial pains. The degree of tenderness should be noted. Limitation in the range of motion of the cervical spine should also be noted. In extremely tender muscles, the patient describes the pain as spreading to remote areas with palpation; this is a secondary pain. If an anesthetic is placed in the tender spot, the spreading or referred pain will stop.

Management of muscle spasm should include rest for the affected area. Physical therapy modalities can include ice, gradual stretching of the muscle, massage, and then moist heat. An oral retainer can be used for a bruxism habit and to relieve temporomandibular joint and associated muscle pain. The shape and bite position of a retainer is dependent on the type of pain and musculoskeletal dysfunction that is present. Medication can include nonsteroidal anti-inflammatory drugs and muscle relaxants. Narcotic medication for chronic pain is contraindicated; it only provides symptomatic relief and can cause psychological problems. If a patient is sleeping poorly and/or has muscle tenderness, a tricyclic antidepressant 10 to 75 mg at bedtime is the drug of choice. It takes approximately 1 to 2 weeks for the effect of the tricyclic antidepressant to be appreciated. The dose is titrated so that the patient does not feel very tired in the morning.

Many patients must have the three modalities mentioned occur simultaneously for best results: physical therapy, oral retainer management, and medication to relax the muscles (tricyclic antidepressant or other muscle relaxants). This helps the patient with both the centrally and peripherally mediated aspects of the pain.

Neurogenic

Intracranial pains are usually associated with additional neurologic signs and symptoms. Pain can occur from edema, hematoma, hemorrhage, aneurysm, or neoplasm. For pain to be present, pain sensitive structures must be involved, which can include the cranial nerves, meninges, and blood vessels. Pain referral to distant sites can occur when these structures experience pressure, distension, inflammation, and so forth. Any new headache or a change in the nature of chronic pain should be investigated.

Extracranial pains in the face should have various structures checked to rule out diseases that can often occur. The eyes, ears, nose, sinuses, throat, tongue, glands, and teeth must all be checked. Positive clinical and imaging signs should be obtained before any procedures are undertaken. Neuralgic pains are usually described as either burning, sharp, electric, or stabbing.

Trigeminal neuralgia (tic douloureux) is described as a unilateral brief electric shocktype pain limited to the distribution of any branch of the trigeminal nerve. Any movement or touching of the trigger site can evoke the pain, and it can also occur spontaneously. The pain is brief, lasting seconds or minutes. There is usually a latency period between attacks. Multiple sclerosis and tumors must be ruled out. Treatment can be pharmacologic (e.g., carbamazepine, baclofen, and so forth) and surgical. Surgical therapies can include alcohol blocks, neurectomy, glycerol or radiofrequency gangliolysis, microvascular decompression, and rhizotomy.

Glossopharyngeal neuralgia is uncommon in comparison with trigeminal neuralgia. It is characterized by paroxysms of pain in the pharyngeal area that radiates to the temporomandibular joint region and ear. It is often described as a burning, sharp, stabbing pain aggravated with swallowing, chewing, and talking. Topical anesthetic in the trigger area in the throat can temporarily stop the pain. Management involves the administration of medication that is used for other neuralgic conditions.

Sphenopalatine neuralgia is usually a deep pain located near the eye and nose. It can radiate pain to the maxilla, mandible, and ear. There can be nasal edema, rhinorrhea, and nasal obstruction. The diagnosis is made with topical or injection blockade. If repeated blockade does not resolve the pain, ganglionectomy can be considered.

Deafferentation pain refers to the total or partial loss of the sensory nerve supply. Injury or invasive procedures can damage the peripheral or central pathway. This type of pain can have a delayed onset and can have an area of diminished sensory sensations that cause pain. The pain can spread to other orofacial structures. Deafferentation pain is often maintained by the sympathetic nervous system, and highly emotional states can increase the pain levels.

Atypical odontalgia is considered a deafferentation pain that has been called "atypical facial pain." This pain has an aching, burning, or throbbing quality that can vary in intensity. Often dental procedures are done such as repeated endodontic (root canal) therapy and extractions, which may only temporally interrupt the pain pattern. Although peripheral activity can influence the pain, it is postulated that it is a centrally mediated mechanism.

Atypical odontalgia is not responsive to surgery, dental procedures, analgesics, or narcotics. It is responsive to serotonergic antidepressants. Amitriptyline 25 to 75mg has frequently been observed to give significant relief. The worst side effect is weight gain in the occasional patient.

Vascular

Carotidynia is considered a variant of migraine. There is a recurrent throbbing facial and neck pain lasting for several weeks. There is tenderness at the bifurcation of the carotid artery. It is a self-limiting syndrome and is managed with salicylates and steroids.

Temporal arteritis is a vascular inflammatory disease of autoimmune etiology. The patient presents with headache initially. Usually there can be fever, fatigue, prostration, and weight loss. In one-half of the patients, there can be painful mastication. Pain can also occur in the ear, mandible, scalp, and neck. Physical examination usually reveals a tortuous, very tender, enlarged temporal artery.

There is usually an elevated erythrocyte sedimentation rate, often greater than 100 mm/h. The most serious complication is blindness. Although a conformation of the diagnosis by biopsy is necessary, therapy should be initiated as soon as possible with prednisone 40 to 60 mg daily to alleviate the symptoms and prevent ocular complications.

SUMMARY

Successful diagnosis and management of facial pain is difficult. A team approach of practitioners of psychology, physical medicine, neurology, and dentistry is often necessary to provide comprehensive care.

SUGGESTED READINGS

Bell W: Temporomandibular Disorders: Classification, Diagnosis, Management, Year Book Medical Publishers, Chicago, 1990
Kaplan, Assael: Temporomandibular Disorders: Diagnosis and Treatment, WB Saunders, Philadelphia, 1991
Travell J, Simons D: Myofascial Pain and Dysfunction The Trigger Point Manual. Williams & Wilkins, Baltimore, 1983

225. NECK AND ARM PAIN

NATHANIEL KATZ

Pain in the neck and arm are among the most common complaints brought to the attention of the physician, particularly the primary physician, neurologist, or pain specialist. Among cases with legal or financial implications, the frequency appears to be even higher. The approach to these patients requires an awareness of the general principles of managing acute and chronic pain, as well as a detailed knowledge of the anatomy, neuroanatomy, and cardinal features of the painful disorders of this region of the body. Basic skills are required, including specific physical examination techniques, interviewing skills, and for some patients, injection skills. In the case of the chronic pain patient, a biopsychosocial approach is most useful, and multidisciplinary pain management may be indicated. Failure to recognize psychosocial contributions to the patient's distress may leave the physician perplexed at the failure of multiple treatment interventions. Even worse, such patients often report temporary success, inviting multiple repeated interventions with no long-term benefit and eventual complications.

This chapter assumes basic expertise in the multidimensional approach to the chronic pain patient and focuses on the medical diagnosis and treatment of conditions that present with neck and arm pain. The common disorders are presented, with emphasis on neurologic syndromes. For ease of discussion, disorders are presented sometimes by region (e.g., neck pain) and sometimes by system (e.g., neuropathies).

NECK PAIN

Cervical Anatomy

The cervical spine consists of seven vertebrae, C1 through C7, bounded rostrally by the occiput and caudally by the first thoracic vertebra (Fig. 225-1). The upper two vertebrae are unique in that the odontoid process projects rostrally from the body of C2, sitting within the ringlike body of C1. Each vertebra articulates with the one above and the one below by two paired facet (zygapophyseal) joints posteriorly, and for vertebrae

below C2, by discs anteriorly. The lateral aspects of the vertebral bodies are further interconnected by articulations called uncovertebral (Luschka's) joints. The spinal canal (Fig. 225-2) contains the spinal cord, surrounded by spinal fluid in the subarachnoid space, then the arachnoid, dura, epidural space, and finally the bony spinal canal. Eight cervical nerves (C1–C8) exit the cervical spine. All of the nerves exit above their respective vertebral level except C8, which exits below the C7 vertebral body (there is no C8 vertebral body). Upon exiting the neural foramena, the spinal nerves divide into anterior and posterior rami (Fig. 225-2). The anterior rami of C1–C4 combine to form the cervical plexus and the anterior rami of C4–T1, the brachial plexus (Fig. 225-3). The posterior ramus of C2 becomes the greater occipital nerve, of C3 the third occipital nerve, and of C4–C8 branches that innervate the facet joints, paraspinal muscles, and skin of the posterior midline.

The anatomy of the cervical spine permits rotation, mainly at C1–C2; flexion and extension, mainly at occiput-C1 and C2–C7; and lateral flexion, at multiple levels.

Approach to the Patient

The first priority in the approach to the patient with neck and arm pain is to exclude "diagnostic imperatives," illnesses that if overlooked will lead to dire consequences. Such diagnostic imperatives include the following:

Tumor: primary, metastatic
Infection: osteomyelitis, epidural abscess, discitis, meningitis, retropharyngeal abscess

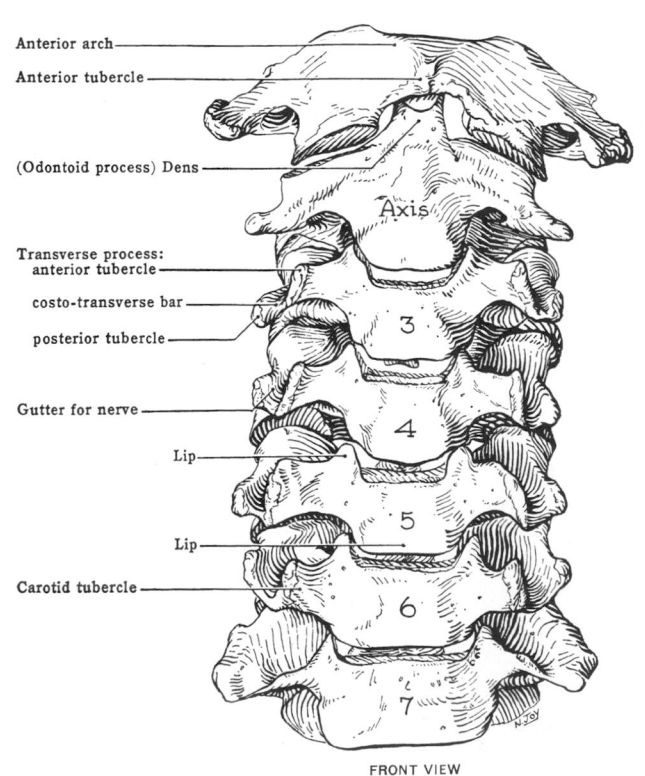

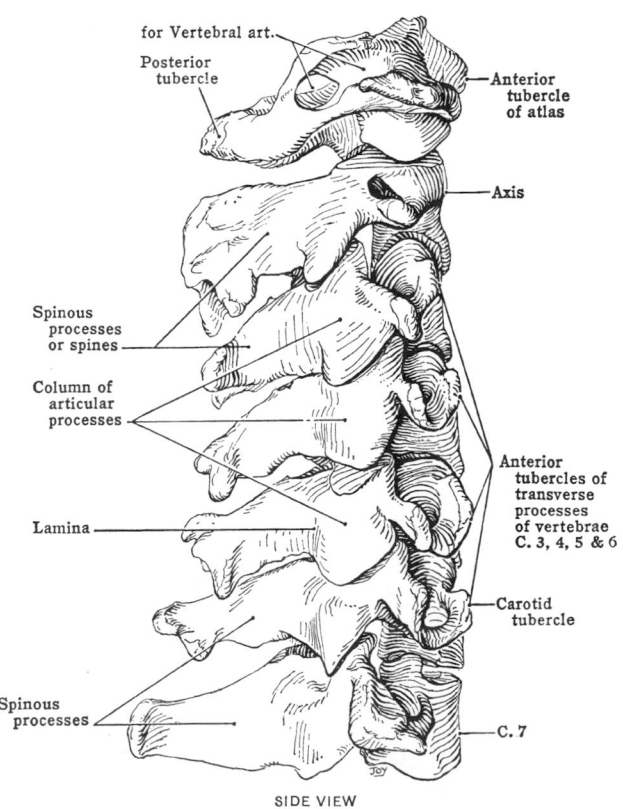

FIG. 225-1. **(A)** and **(B)** lateral views of the cervical spine. The facet (zygapophyseal) joints are best seen on the lateral view, forming the column of articular processes. The articulations of the uncovertebral joints (of Luschka) are labeled "lips." (From Anderson JE: Grant's Atlas of Anatomy. 7th Ed. Williams & Wilkins, Baltimore, 1978, with permission.)

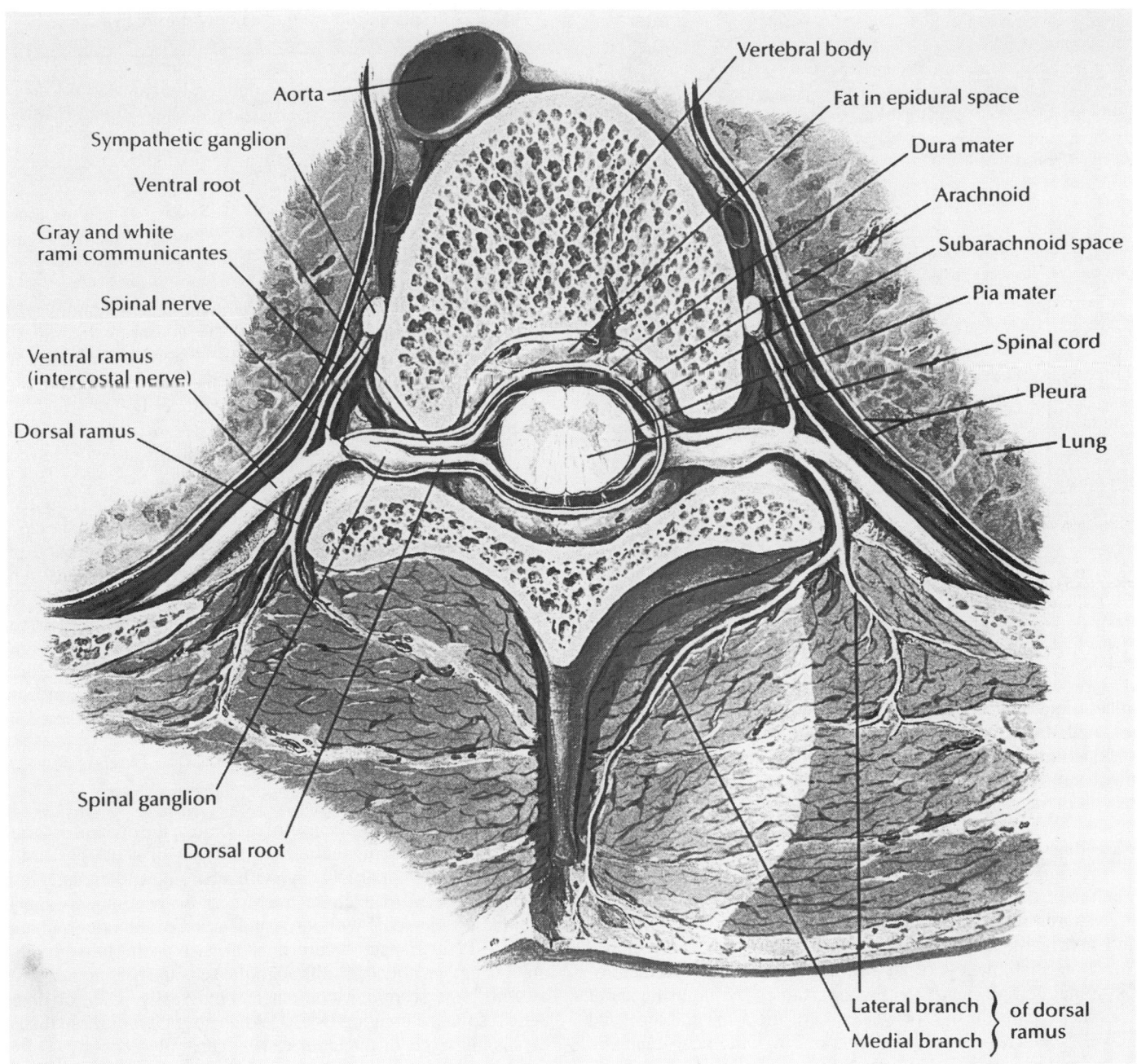

FIG. 225-2.   Cross section through a typical spinal cord segment, illustrating the layers surrounding the spinal cord. (From Netter FH. Atlas of Human Anatomy. Ciba-Geigy, Summit NJ, 1993, with permission.)

Spinal cord compression
Fracture/dislocation
Vertebral artery thrombosis/dissection

These disorders can generally be ruled out by thorough history and physical examination and plain x-rays, supplemented as needed by more sophisticated imaging studies and blood tests. Such patients do not often present in medical practice, and usually are the province of the emergency medicine physician, orthopaedist, or neurosurgeon.

A comprehensive diagnostic approach will usually lead to a treatable disorder, sparing patients the tragedy of chronic pain. In patients already suffering from the complete chronic pain syndrome, comprehensive assessment will most efficiently de-termine the most effective treatment approach, sparing partial approaches that do not address the patients' multidisciplinary needs.

For many patients, a precise diagnosis cannot be found, and they fall into the vague category of ''soft tissue pain.'' Many of these patients are told there is ''nothing wrong,'' and under-standably seek out alternative therapy, which is often helpful or even curative. The arrogance of confusing inability to make a diagnosis with absence of pain discredits the medical profes-sion and is best avoided, even in patients with prominent psy-chosocial factors contributing to the pain. Dismissing the pa-tient's concerns and problems benefits neither doctor nor patient. The balance between legitimization and reassur-

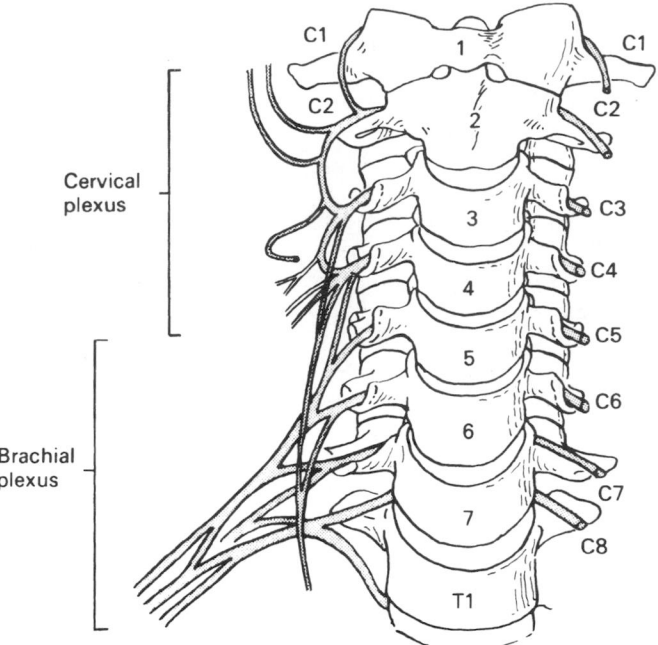

FIG. 225-3. Origin of the cervical plexus from the anterior rami of C1–C4, and the brachial plexus from the anterior rami of C4–T1. (From Bonica JJ (ed): The Management of Pain. 2nd Ed. JB Lippincott, Philadelphia, 1990, with permission.)

TABLE 225-1. Examination of the Major Nerves of the Upper Extremity

Nerve	Motor Test	Sensation Test
Radial	Wrist extension	Dorsal web space between thumb and index finger
Ulnar	Abduction of little finger	Distal ulnar aspect of little finger
Median	Thumb pinch; thumb opposition	Distal radial aspect of index finger
Axillary	Deltoid	Lateral arm at deltoid insertion
Musculocutaneous	Biceps	Lateral forearm

The *physical examination* starts with the general habitus, posture, and appearance of the patient. The key to examining the pain patient is to reproduce the pain, thereby determining its tissue of origin. Range of motion of the neck is checked, and may be reviewed segmentally to determine the abnormalities of the spine. Palpation is performed for myofascial trigger points. The spinous processes and facet joints are palpated for tenderness. The thyroid, hyoid, and styloids may be palpated for reproduction of pain. The neurologic examination (Fig. 225-4; Table 225-1) tests strength of the muscles of the shoulder girdle and arms, reflexes, and sensation over the occipital region, neck, and arms. In suspected nerve entrapment syndromes, the entire course of the nerve must be palpated for masses or a Tinel sign (elicitation of paresthesias in the distribution of the nerve when tapping the site of injury). The tone, strength, reflexes, and sensation of the legs may reveal signs of cord compression. The general physical examination may reveal important signs of systemic disease related to the etiology of the neck or arm pain.

Diagnostic Studies

Diagnostic studies may be useful to confirm the clinical diagnosis or exclude serious pathology. In cases of acute post-traumatic neck pain, particularly with neurologic deficits, plain films are useful to exclude fracture or dislocation. The neck cannot be "cleared" without visualization of the odontoid and the C7–T1 interspace. Plain films are also useful in excluding malignancy or infection, although the sensitivity is not as great as with bone scanning, computed tomography (CT), or magnetic resonance imaging (MRI). When suspicion of these disorders is high, one of the latter tests is generally necessary. MRI has become very useful in view of its high sensitivity to infection, neoplasm, and degenerative disease; its ability to visualize neural elements and demonstrate cord or root compression; and the ability to visualize the entire cervical spine in a single study. Its disadvantages are cost, lack of precise delineation of bony anatomy, and inability to perform dynamic studies. Electromyography (EMG) and nerve conduction studies are useful in documenting the presence or absence of a nerve lesion, and in delineating the anatomy of the lesion (e.g., distinguishing root from plexus lesion or localizing the site of a nerve entrapment).

It cannot be overemphasized that "objective" findings, such as those obtained by imaging studies and electrodiagnostic studies, often bear no relationship to the patient's symptoms. Imaging studies often disclose abnormalities that are common in the general population and of doubtful relevance in the individual patient. EMG and nerve conduction studies give no information about pain. A nerve lesion can be painful with negative EMG results. Documentation of a nerve lesion does not mean that it is the cause of the patient's pain or that it is painful at all (most

ance—that is, accepting the patient's complaints as legitimate and real, and conveying to the patient that complaints are taken seriously, but also reassuring the patient of hope for improvement and lack of life-threatening or potentially crippling illness—is the crux of the art of managing the pain patient.

History and Physical Examination

The medical history begins with eliciting symptoms and signs of systemic illness, such as weight loss, fatigue, fevers, chills, and involvement of multiple joints; the history may suggest infection, malignancy, or an arthritic disorder. Involvement of the spinal cord or nerve roots is ascertained by inquiring about numbness, paresthesias, or weakness of the arms and legs, and bowel, bladder, or sexual dysfunction. In acute post-traumatic pain, fracture or dislocation must be excluded, usually with x-rays. This approach serves to rule out the diagnostic imperatives. Next, the distribution of the pain is ascertained, and then the quality—somatic, neuralgic, or visceral. Learning about the provocative and palliative factors for the pain, such as which movements exacerbate the pain, gives insight into the tissue of origin.

Many patients present in the setting of accidents, work-related injuries, or psychosocial disturbances. Information about ongoing legal action, disability hearings, employment issues, use of controlled substances, psychological symptoms, and a personal or family history of substance abuse or mental issness must be elicited.

In patients with nerve injury, the distribution of pain often does not correlate precisely with the sensory distribution of the injured nerve. The distribution of paresthesias and, better yet, of neurologic signs is more reliable. Once the localization of the nerve injury is ascertained, its cause can be more easily determined.

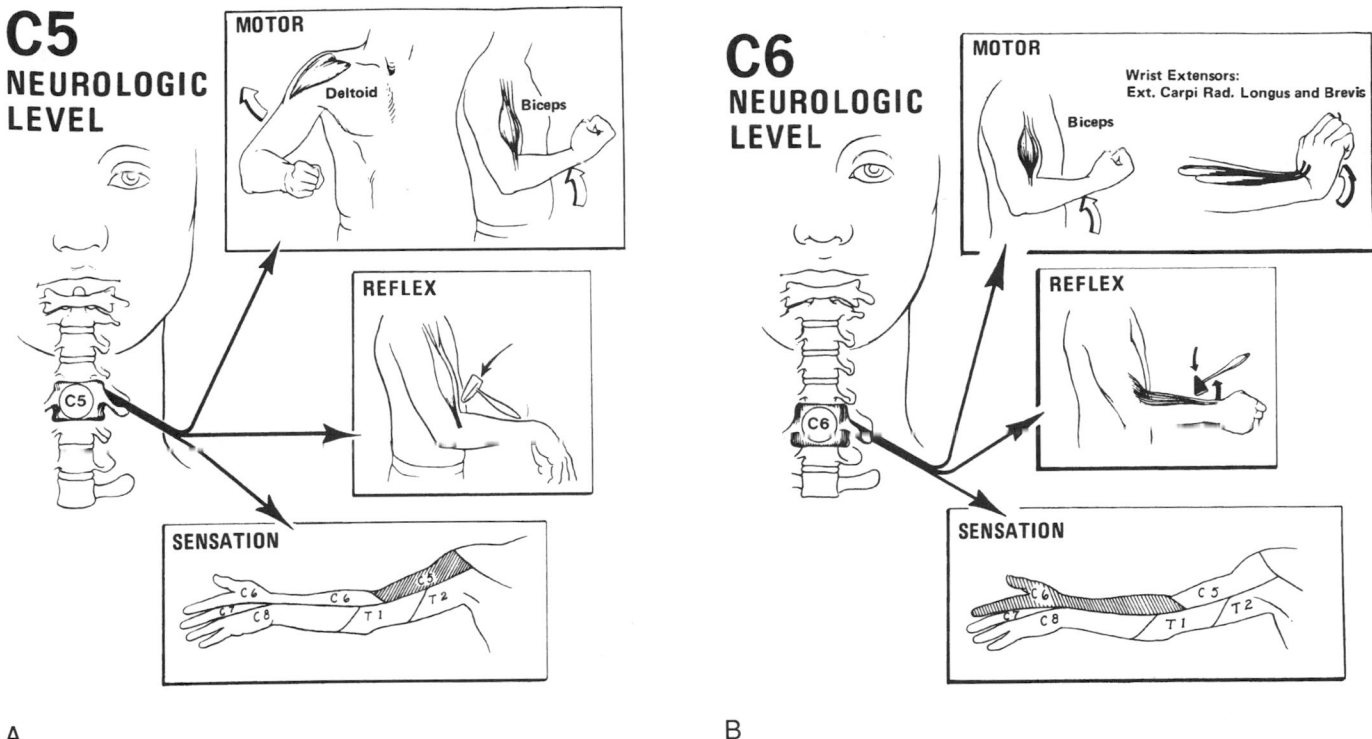

C5 NEUROLOGIC LEVEL

C6 NEUROLOGIC LEVEL

A   B

FIG. 225-4. **(A–F)** Major neurologic findings in cervical radiculopathy. (Figs. A–E from Hoppenfeld S: Physical Examination of the Spine and Extremities. Appleton-Century-Crofts, Norwalk, CT, 1976; Fig. F from Bonica JJ (cd): The Management of Pain. 2nd Ed. JB Lippincott, Philadelphia, 1990, with permission). (*Figure continues.*)

nerve lesions are not painful). The physician must keep the clinical syndrome foremost in mind, using studies to inform the clinical approach. The medicolegal system has encouraged the opposite approach, in which ''objective'' tests are given credence and the clinical impression is subject to debate and not worth much. This approach is destructive to the effective management of neck and arm pain.

Specific Disorders

Neuralgias. A *neuralgia* is defined as lancinating pain related to irritation of a nerve without evidence of damage to the nerve. (Pain in the presence of nerve damage is referred to as neuropathy.) The neuralgias are characterized by brief attacks of severe pain lasting seconds or less. Aside from possible trigger areas, physical examination results are by definition negative. The neck neuralgias are rare. *Glossopharyngeal neuralgia* presents with pain in the pharynx or base of the tongue, radiating to the ear or lateral neck. Some patients have bradycardia or syncope during attacks. Diagnosis can be confirmed by local anesthetic blockade of the nerve. Treatment is identical to that of trigeminal neuralgia: pharmacologic measures (Table 225-2) followed by decompressive surgery if necessary. *Superior laryngeal neuralgia* presents with pain the larynx, angle of the jaw, or other parts of the neck, and may be associated with hiccups, salivation, or coughing. Treatment is as for the other neuralgias.

Strictly speaking, *occipital neuralgia* refers to pain in the occipital region produced by entrapment of the occipital nerve. However, the term is usually used loosely to refer to any pain in the back of the head, and carries its own differential diagnosis (Table 225-3). Many patients have undergone inappropriate

section of the occipital nerve without adequate diagnostic approach. A history of neuralgic-type pain suggests true nerve entrapment, usually of the greater or lesser occipital nerves, or the C2 or C3 nerve roots. Pain that appears to arise from the neck or that is provoked by movement of the neck suggests cervical root pathology. A Tinel sign should be sought over the suspected nerves. The sensory examination may reveal hypesthesia in the distribution of the affected nerve (Fig. 225-4F). Aching or other non-neuralgic pain, while possibly neuropathic in origin, often indicates myofascial or joint pain. Myofascial pain is associated with palpable trigger points. Facet joint pain is provoked by neck extension or palpation of the joints. These syndromes are discussed in more detail below.

Cervical Disc Disease. Cervical disc disease is regarded as a common cause of acute and chronic neck pain. Precise estimates of the incidence of pain due to cervical disc disease vary, owing to the high incidence of disc ''abnormalities'' in asymptomatic patients, contributing to overdiagnosis of disc disease, with medicolegal implications. The normal disc consists of a small jellylike central *nucleus pulposus,* surrounded by a fibrous capsule, the *annulus fibrosus.* Over the years, the nucleus dehydrates, resulting in loss of disc height. Tears form in the annulus. If subjected to excess pressure, the nucleus may herniate into the annulus, perhaps causing it to bulge or extrude completely through the annulus. Which of these pathologic changes produces which, if any symptoms, is controversial. If the disc or annulus exerts pressure against the nerve roots or spinal cord, radiculopathy or myelopathy, respectively, results.

Patients with disc disease present with acute or chronic neck pain that may radiate into the periscapular region, occiput, thorax, or shoulder. Pain is worsened by maneuvers that in-

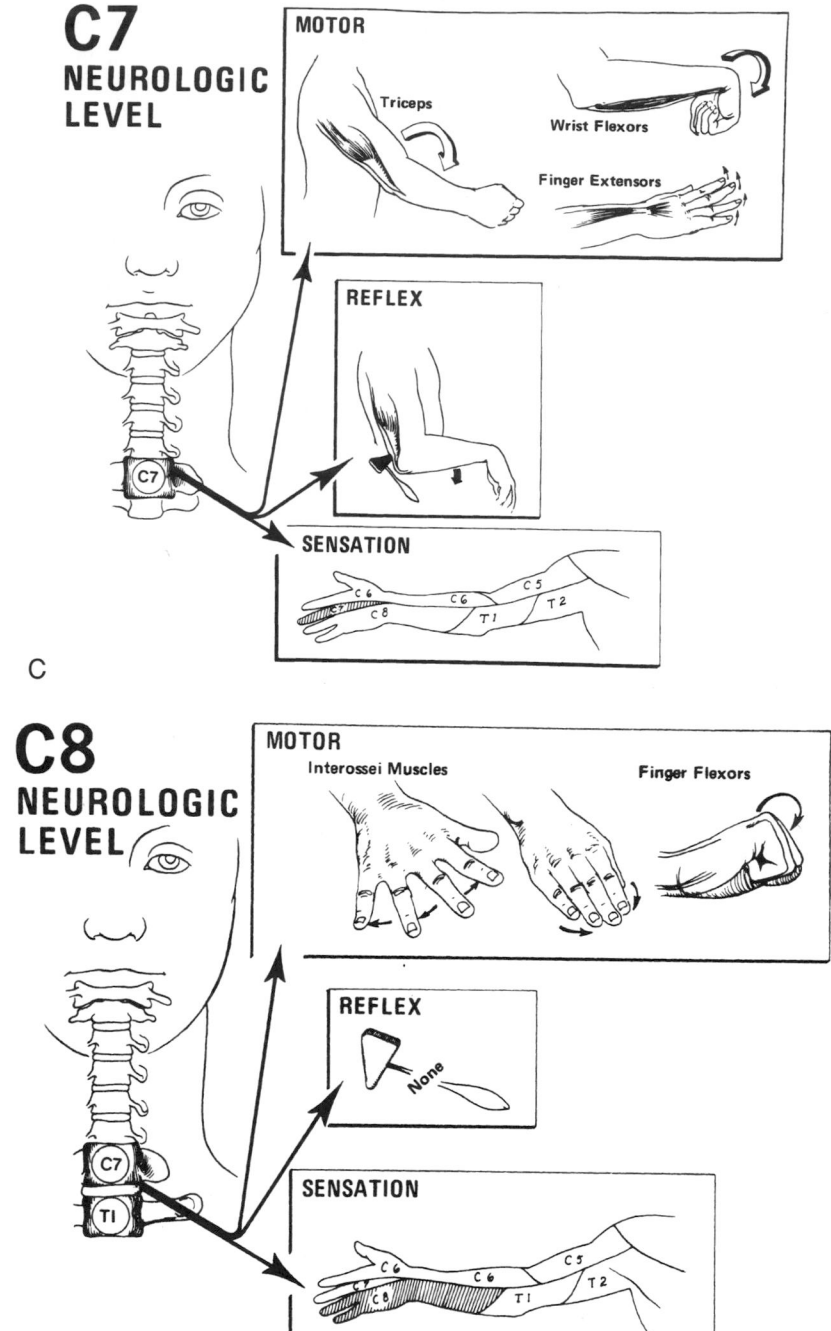

FIG. 225-4.   (*Continued*).

crease pressure in the epidural space: coughing, sneezing, Valsalva maneuver. The physical examination will demonstrate decreased range of motion (ROM), particularly flexion, and muscle spasm. Pressing downward on the head or neck flexion may reproduce pain. Lateral neck flexion with pressure on the head will reproduce neck or ipsilateral radicular pain (Spurling's test). If radiculopathy is present, patients will have pain and neurologic findings characteristic of the particular root. Pain may be decreased by manual distraction of the head. Cord compression will be manifested by weakness or sensory loss in the arms or legs, hyperreflexia and spasticity in the legs, Babinski and Hoffman signs, and bowel or bladder dysfunction. Patients with cervical cord compression may complain of aching in the thorax, low back, or legs.

The diagnosis of cervical disc disease may be confirmed by CT, MRI, or myelography. These tests are confounded by a high false-positive rate, and are appropriately used to confirm the clinical impression. The false-negative rate—that is, the percentage of patients with discogenic pain or radiculopathy with negative study results—is unknown, but false negatives cer-

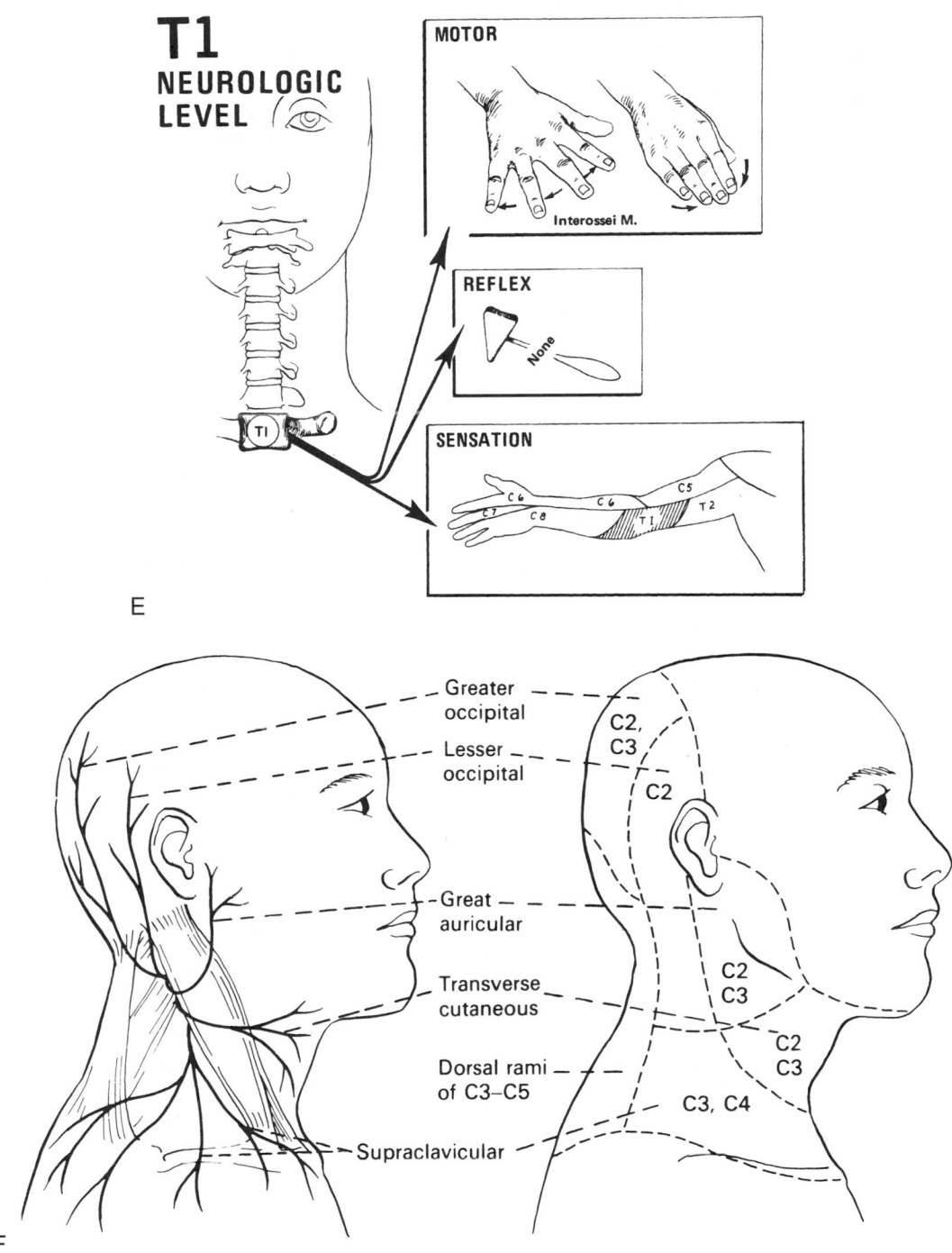

FIG. 225-4. (Continued).

tainly occur in daily practice. EMG/nerve conduction studies may be used to confirm the clinical impression of radiculopathy, but there are several limitations, as outlined above. These studies are probably not much more sensitive or specific than a thorough neurologic examination, have significant false positives and false negatives, and say nothing about pain. Discography involves the injection of dye into the disc and gives information on whether a disc is symptomatic by the radiographic appearance of the interior of the disc, as well as by reproduction of pain during the injection. Whether discography provides any useful information is controversial.

The natural history of pain due to disk herniation is favorable, with the vast majority of patients improving over time, although complete resolution may take years, and require lifestyle modifications during the healing process. The goals of treatment are to hasten resolution of symptoms, minimize psychological or vocational impact, and prevent relapses and chronicity.

Treatment consists of rest and immobilization with a cervical collar in the acute or flare-up phases, physical therapy, home use of modalities (e.g., ice or heat), traction, and analgesics. For subacute or chronic symptoms, treatment focuses on maximizing activity. Reliance on the collar is kept to a minimum.

TABLE 225-2. Approach to the Pharmacologic Management of Neuropathic Pain Syndromes[a]

Predominantly Lancinating Pain Syndromes	
Medication	Dose
Carbamazepine	Begin at 100 mg bid, titrate to effect
Baclofen	Begin at 5 mg tid, titrate to effect
Phenytoin	Begin at 100 mg tid, titrate to effect
Clonazepam	Begin at 0.5 mg tid, titrate to effect
Predominantly Constant Pain Syndromes	
Medication	Dose
Amitryptilene	Begin at 10 mg qhs, increase by 10 mg every 3–4 days to effect or side effects
Nortryptilene	As above
Desipramine	As above
Mexiletene	Begin at 150 mg bid, titrate to effect or side effects

[a] This table is intended to outline options. Prior to prescribing any of the above medications, one should consult a more detailed reference on the appropriate use and precautions.

Physical therapy may be employed with the goal of patient education about relapse prevention, and an independent exercise program. Care must be taken to avoid reliance on addicting medications; nonsteroidal anti-inflammatory drugs (NSAIDs) and tricyclic antidepressants are appropriate. Muscle relaxants have not been shown to specifically relax muscles, and whereas they are perhaps appropriate in the acute phase, their sedative properties and minimal efficacy make them undesirable for long-term use.

For patients whose pain is not relieved by conservative therapy, cervical epidural steroid injections are a safe alternative, most effective for radicular pain. Contraindications include local infection or tumor, bleeding diathesis, and major psychiatric contribution to the pain syndrome. Early surgical discectomy is appropriate for patients with symptomatic cord compression or progressive neurologic deficits. Surgery for pain alone is fraught with difficulty; the best candidates are patients with demonstrable radiculopathy, minimal psychological issues, and duration of symptoms less than approximately 6 months.

Cervical Spondylosis. The joints of the cervical spine are vulnerable to osteoarthritic degeneration, as are other joints. Cervical osteoarthritis can be part of primary generalized osteoarthritis, or can be a secondary ''wear and tear'' arthritis related to traumatic, metabolic, or congenital factors. The pathophysiology of secondary degeneration is controversial, but degeneration of the disc is thought to play a primary role, with loss of disc height, followed by abnormal apposition of the facet joints, leading to progressive degeneration of the functional unit. The results are the same: loss of disc height, disc bulge or protrusions, arthritis and hypertrophy of the facet and uncovertebral joint, hypertrophy of the intraspinal ligaments, and inflammatory changes of the periarticular tissues. Narrowing of the intervertebral foramina or spinal canal, with resultant radiculopathy or myelopathy may result.

TABLE 225-3. Differential Diagnosis of Occipital Neuralgia

Tumor, infection of the upper cervical spine
Upper cervical facet syndrome
    Osteoarthritis
    Rheumatoid arthritis
    Idiopathic
Myofascial pain
C2 or C3 root entrapment
True occipital nerve entrapment
Lesser occipital nerve entrapment

Patients present with symptoms related to (1) the joint pathology, (2) radiculopathy if present, and (3) myelopathy if present. In addition, osteophytic encroachment upon the vertebral artery or the esophagus may produce symptoms related to these structures. Osteoarthritis can present as acute, severe ipsilateral pain in the neck, usually resolving in 7 to 10 days. Different joints have characteristic (but overlapping) referral patterns: the upper cervical spine to the occiput or frontal region, the midcervical spine to the shoulder, and the lower cervical spine to the interscapular region. Torticollis may occur. Attacks may recur or may become longer, confluent, or constant. Stiffness and reduction of ROM supervene. Physical examination reveals decreased ROM, most notably extension, with fair preservation of flexion and rotation. The facet joints are tender.

If nerve root compression or irritation occurs, patients will complain of radiation of pain and paresthesias in characteristic distributions, discussed above under Cervical Disc Disease. Differences are (1) that in osteoarthritis, radiculopathy of the upper cervical nerve roots (C2–C4) may occur, (2) neck extension rather than flexion brings on radicular symptoms, and (3) the prognosis is less favorable. It is said that spondylitic radiculopathy is more likely to affect the sensory root, whereas discogenic radiculopathy is more likely to affect the motor root, owing to the posterior location of the motor root in the neural foramen. In patients with spondylitic myelopathy, L'hermitte sign (an electric sensation radiating down the spine upon neck flexion) may be noted. Signs of cord compression may be elicited. These signs include the following:

Leg weakness
Hyporeflexia (acute) or hyper-reflexia (chronic)
Sensory loss in the legs
Sensory level
Decreased sphincter tone
Babinski sign

These signs may accompany signs of radiculopathy in the arms. The combination of lower motor neuron signs in the arms and upper motor neuron signs in the legs may suggest amyotrophic lateral sclerosis.

Plain x-rays of the cervical spine are diagnostic of spondylosis, although the burden is on the physician to demonstrate the relevance of these findings in the individual patient. Radiologic findings include loss of disc height, sclerosis of bone and joints, osteophytes, irregular narrowing of joint spaces, and cyst formation. Oblique views demonstrate foraminal narrowing. CT shows details of bony anatomy best, and combined with myelography is the definitive study for the demonstration of bony impingement on neural structures. Many surgeons are becoming satisfied with MRI for surgical purposes, although it does not demonstrate bony detail as well.

The treatment of spondylitic pain consists of NSAIDs, short-term narcotics when needed, short-term use of the cervical collar and physical therapy, and exercise. Facet joint injections with local anesthesia and steroid are safe, easy to perform, and often helpful. For patients with chronic pain, radiofrequency denervation of the facet joints is safe in experienced hands, and provides 12 to 18 months of relief in 50 to 60 percent of patients. Cervical epidural steroid injections are helpful for radicular pain, although long-term benefit is uncertain.

For patients with myelopathy, treatment is similar, except with greater reliance on the collar, and less effort through exercise to improve ROM.

Surgical decompression is helpful for patients whose pain is clearly due to compression of specific neural structures, roots or cord. Poor prognostic factors for patients with myelopathy include advanced age, sphincter involvement, leg weakness out of proportion to spasticity, long-standing severe neurologic deficits, muscle atrophy, and severe concurrent medical problems.

Cervical Sprain. Probably the most common form of neck pain, sprain refers to acute injury without evidence of damage to neural or bony structures. The tissues affected are thought to include the ligaments, facet joint capsules, and muscles and tendons, which remain functional despite injury. The exact tissue traumatized in individual patients is difficult to ascertain. Symptoms include mild to moderate neck pain, headache, neck stiffness (which may develop days after the injury), dizziness, blurred vision, and gait imbalance. Physical examination reveals decreased ROM, tenderness of the spinous processes, muscle spasm, and sometimes referred tenderness in the shoulder and arm. Neurologic findings are absent. Radiographs are most important for what thay do not show (i.e., fracture, dislocation, or evidence of tumor or infection). Straightening of the cervical spine due to muscle spasm is characteristic.

Treatment consists of medication with NSAIDs, muscle relaxants, and short-term narcotics if necessary. Rest, gentle progressive exercise, heat and ice, and judicious use of a soft collar are the mainstays of therapy. Local anesthesia injections into tender areas may be helpful. Early mobilization and attention to psychosocial and vocational issues are important to avoid long-term disability.

Flexion–Extension (Whiplash) Injury. In our motor vehicle–based society, injuries to the cervical spine caused by acute hyperflexion followed by hyperextension, or vice versa, are common. When mild, the injury consists of stretching and microhemorrhage in the cervical muscles. When severe, the muscles suffer partial laceration, and stretching and tearing occurs in the ligaments, annulus, and facet joint capsules. Severe extension may cause chip fractures of the vertebrae and impaction of the facets, with potential contusion of nerve roots or spinal cord. The temporomandibular joint may be injured as the head suddenly extends back from the jaw.

Symptoms in mild cases are limited to neck pain, spasm, and reduced ROM beginning 1 to 2 days after the injury. In severe cases, symptoms begin right away. Headache, shoulder pain, and root or cord injury may be superimposed. Radiographs are used to exclude fracture or subluxation, and reveal straightening of the cervical lordosis.

The approach to the patient consists first of ensuring that bony injury requiring surgical treatment has been ruled out with plain films, and special views or CT if necessary. Injury to the brain, spinal cord, and nerve roots must then be addressed. From this point, treatment is conservative, as for cervical sprain, and with similar provisos to avoid chronicity. The term *whiplash* is best avoided owing to the suggestive legal implications. In cases of chronic pain after flexion–extension injury, psychosocial and legal issues must be dealt with when possible. Tricyclic antidepressants replace muscle relaxants and analgesics. Recent evidence supports radiofrequency facet denervation for prolonged pain relief.

Myofascial Pain. Myofascial pain refers to a regional disorder consisting of pain, muscle spasm, and decreased mobility related to tender nodules or bands of muscle spasm called *trigger points*. Patients complain of local and referred pain, subjec-

tive "numbness," fatigability, and stiffness. Symptoms are reproduced by palpating the trigger points. The syndrome may follow trauma to the muscle such as a cervical sprain, chronic strain related to poor posture or overuse, and psychological stress. Reactive muscle spasm also occurs in response to primary local pathology, such as osteoarthritis. The muscles most commonly giving rise to neck pain are the trapezius, levator scapulae, multifidi, erector spinae, and suboccipital group. These syndromes commonly produce referred pain to the head, eye, or arm. Spasm of the scalenes or pectoralis minor may constrict the brachial plexus, leading to a *myogenic thoracic outlet syndrome.*

The diagnosis depends on elicitation of an accurate history and a thoroughly conducted physical examination. Treatment consists of physical therapy and trigger-point injections. Physical therapy focuses on stretching and strengthening of the involved muscles; strengthening is critical but often overlooked. Patients are taught independent home programs. General conditioning, sleep, and proper dietary habits are encouraged. Trigger-point injections are highly effective, and often only a few treatments are needed.

Infectious, Inflammatory, and Neoplastic Disorders. *Infection* is an uncommon cause of neck pain in clinical practice. A number of types of infections may occur, including osteomyelitis, epidural abscess, and discitis. Whereas infection is rare, diagnosis is imperative, owing to the devastating consequences of dclayed treatment.

Symptoms can be mild and nonspecific. Neck pain radiating to the occiput or shoulders, decreased ROM, muscle spasm, and dysphagia occur. Physical examination results are also nonspecific and may disclose tenderness of the spinous processes, Spurling sign, and perhaps signs of radiculopathy or myelopathy. Diagnosis begins with plain films, which may have negative findings, especially early in the disease. Bone scanning and MRI are more sensitive and specific. An elevated white blood cell count, erythrocyte sedimentation rate, and anemia may occur, but their absence does not rule out infection. Biopsy may be needed for definitive diagnosis. Treatment consists of nonspecific measures, including immobilization and analgesics, antibiotics, and at times surgical intervention.

After osteoarthritis, the most common inflammatory disorders giving rise to neck pain are rheumatoid arthritis and ankylosing spondylitis. Rheumatoid arthritis is an inflammatory polyarthropathy that typically affects peripheral joints symmetrically. The cervical spine is commonly involved, particularly the upper portion. Symptoms include neck pain radiating to the occiput, temples, or retro-orbital regions. Upper cervical radiculopathy, with pain or numbness in the scalp, neck, or shoulder, may be present. Myelopathy or brainstem involvement may occur secondary to subluxation. Laboratory studies reveal anemia, elevated erythrocyte sedimentation rate, and positive rheumatoid factor in 80 percent of patients. X-rays show osteopenia, periarticular soft tissue swelling, and joint space erosions. Treatment of rheumatoid arthritis of the cervical spine, beyond standard medical treatment, includes gentle physical therapy to maintain mobility, judicious use of cervical collars, and surgical intervention for neurologic involvement or instability.

Ankylosing spondylitis is a polyarthropathy affecting mainly the joints of the axial skeletotn, including the facet, costovertebral, and sacroiliac joints. Ossification of the longitudinal ligaments and disc spaces may occur. Symptoms typically begin in the second to third decade, with low back pain radiating to the buttocks or legs, and morning stiffness. Decreased ROM, especially flexion, occurs, with loss of the lumbar lordosis. Sacroiliac joint x-rays are a useful early study, and show blurring of joint margins, then joint erosions, and finally joint fusion. Syndesmophytes and bone spurs are common. Ninety-five percent of patients have the HLA-B27 antigen. Treatment specific for cervical spine involvement includes physical therapy to maintain erect posture, sleeping prone or at least without a pillow when supine, and local steroid injections.

Tumors of the cervical spine are also an uncommon cause of neck pain. Most are metastatic, the most common from carcinoma of the lung, breast, or prostate. Primary tumors may be benign (giant cell tumor, bone cyst) or malignant (chondrosarcoma, osteosarcoma, Ewing's tumor). Symptoms are often nonspecific. Pain worse at rest or at night, torticollis, or constitutional symptoms arouse suspicion.

Metastasis to the odontoid complicated by fracture and subluxation presents with severe neck pain, with or without myelopathy. Plain films may need to be supplemented by CT for diagnosis. Involvement of the C7 and T1 vertebral bodies by either direct spread or hematogenous metastases, with or without radiculopathy, is another well-known syndrome. Plain x-rays do not rule out tumor; CT, MRI, and bone scanning are more useful.

Cervical Facet Syndrome. The term cervical facet syndrome refers to a group of patients with acute, subacute, or chronic pain with or without referral to the occiput, shoulder, arm, or periscapular region, accompanied by limitation of motion, particularly extension, and occasionally subjective neurologic symptoms in the arms, but neurologic examination findings are normal. Imaging studies correlate poorly with symptoms. Some patients have osteoarthritic changes of the facet joints, but most do not. The physical examination may show tenderness over the facet joints, decreased ROM, and reproduction of pain by neck extension or ipsilateral flexion. The physical therapist may report "hypomobility" or "locking" of the facet joints at segmentally specific levels. The origin of the pain of this syndrome has been hypothesized to be the cervical facet joints, and studies using local anesthetic blockade of the joint as a diagnostic tool have supported this claim. The syndrome is treated with physical therapy to restore mobility, analgesics, intra-articular steroid injections, and radiofrequency denervation of the facet joints. Patients whose pain does not respond to conservative measures are best referred to a pain management center with expertise in managing this syndrome.

Miscellaneous Disorders

Disorders of the Thyroid Gland. Neoplastic or inflammatory disorders of the thyroid can produce anterior neck pain, often with radiation to the ear, jaw, or occiput. *Thyroid malignancy* may be accompanied by signs of systemic illness. Physical examination will reveal enlargement, nodularity, and perhaps tenderness of the gland. Several types of thyroiditis can produce neck pain. *Pyogenic thyroiditis* is uncommon and usually results from hematogenous spread from a distant bacterial infection. *Riedel's thyroiditis* consists of intense fibrosis of the thyroid gland sometimes associated with retroperitoneal or mediastinal fibrosis. Subacute thyroiditis is a viral illness often occurring in the setting of an upper respiratory infection. Neck

pain and tenderness, often severe, may be accompanied by hyperthyroidism.

Diffuse Idiopathic Skeletal Hyperostosis. Diffuse idiopathic skeletal hyperostosis consists of idiopathic overproduction of bone, particularly of the spine, in men over the age of 50. Symptoms include pain, stiffness and tenderness to palpation. Cervical involvement is often accompanied by dysphagia. Plain radiographs are diagnostic and show dramatic osteophytosis and ossification of the anterior longitudinal ligament. Many cases are asymptomatic and are discovered during routine radiography. Treatment consists mainly of physical therapy and administration of NSAIDs.

Longus Colli Tendonitis. Tendonitis of the longus colli muscle can produce progressive anterior neck pain and dysphagia, worsened by head and neck movements. Physical examination is significant for reproduction of pain on palpation of the anterior cervical spine from C1 to C4.

Styloid (Eagle) Syndrome. An elongated styloid process is said to be responsible for this syndrome, often following tonsillectomy. Pain in the anterior neck radiating to the ear and persistent sore throat are the dominant symptoms. Diagnosis is supported by radiographic evidence of an elongated styloid process. Treatment is with local measures, analgesics, and surgical excision of the styloid if necessary.

Neuropathic Pain in the Upper Limb

Spinal Cord Disorders. Pathology of the cervical spinal cord may mimic disorders that produce cervical radiculopathy or radiculomyelopathy, particularly advanced cervical spondylosis. Furthermore, the radiographic changes and even clinical signs of cervical spondylosis are so common in the elderly that they often coexist with other disorders. *Spinal cord tumors* are rare and present with pain, sensory loss, reflex loss, and weakness in the arms. The presence of upper motor neuron signs in the legs, sphincter disturbance, involvement in the distribution of multiple cervical nerve roots, and dissociated sensory loss (loss of sensitivity to pinprick and temperature with preservation of sensitivity to position and vibration) suggest spinal cord involvement. *Syringomyelia* commonly affects the cervical cord, and may occur in relation to spinal cord neoplasm or after trauma. Clinical findings are similar to those of tumor. *Multiple sclerosis* with spinal cord involvement may produce a pseudoradiculopathy affecting the arm. MRI of the cervical spine is the diagnostic study of choice for these disorders, and may require supplementation with other studies, such cerebrospinal fluid analysis or biopsy.

Cervical Radiculopathy. The major causes of cervical radiculopathy are cervical spondylosis and disc herniation, discussed above. Other disorders discussed above, including the arthritides, trauma, tumor, and infection, may also produce cervical radiculopathy. Peripheral nerve tumors, including schwannomas and neurofibromas, present with a mass in the side of the neck, with the symptoms and signs of cervical radiculopathy. Noting the signs of von Recklinghausen's neurofibromatosis is relevant in such cases.

Herpes zoster may affect the cervical nerve roots, producing the characteristic vesicular rash, accompanied by severe pain, numbness, and weakness related to the affected roots. Treatment consists of antiviral therapy; topical applications to soothe, disinfect, and hasten healing of cutaneous lesions; and analgesics. Sympathetic blocks appear to decrease pain as well as to decrease the incidence of post-herpetic neuralgia.

The differential diagnosis of cervical radiculopathy begins with excluding non-neurologic disorders that produce referred pain in the neck and arm, such as tendinitis, bursitis, and arthritis of the shoulder, myocardial infarction, intrathoracic pathology, and cervical spine disorders. Central neurologic syndromes may cause confusion with cervical radiculopathy, such as thalamic infarction, which may present with surprisingly restricted pain and numbness in the arm; numbness in the ipsilateral face, trunk, or leg suggests a central disorder.

Cervical Plexopathy and Accessory Nerve Damage. The ventral rami of C1 to C4 anastomose to form the cervical plexus proper, which innervates the skin of the posterolateral scalp, neck, and epaulet region (Fig. 225-5). The dorsal rami innervate the midline skin over the neck, and as the occipital nerve, the posteromedial scalp. Muscular branches innervate the sternocleidomastoid, trapezius, and levator scapulae muscles, paraspinal muscles, and the diaphraghm.

Damage to the *superficial cervical plexus* is rare, and rarely symptomatic. Damage to the *occipital nerve* is discussed above. Damage to the greater auricular nerve occurs after surgical procedures, mainly facelift and carotid endarterectomy, from trauma, and from leprosy. Symptoms are sensory loss in the distribution of the nerve and neuropathic pain.

The *accessory nerve* arises from the cervical spinal cord, ascends within the spine through the foramen magnum into the skull, and exits the skull through the jugular foramen. It then descends deep to the sternocleidomastoid muscle, and penetrates it to cross the posterior triangle of the neck and end in the trapezius muscle. Damage to the nerve can be caused by intracranial lesions, in surgical procedures of the neck, from trauma, or may be idiopathic. Symptoms include shoulder pain,

paresthesias of the shoulder or arm, and weakness of shoulder elevation with winging of the scapula. Treatment may require surgical repair of the nerve or functional orthopaedic procedures.

Brachial Plexopathy. The brachial plexus (Fig. 225-6) arises from the C4–T1 nerve roots after they exit the cervical spine. The nerve roots exit the spine into the paravertebral space by passing between the anterior and middle scalene muscles, then combine to form the trunks of the plexus. The plexus then passes between the clavicle and first rib, then under the attachment of the pectoralis minor muscle to the coracoid process, to finally lie free in the axilla.

Several branches important in the evaluation of pain arise from the plexus: the long thoracic, suprascapular, axillary, and medial cutaneous nerves of the arm and forearm. In the axilla, the plexus gives rise to its major terminal branches, the median, ulnar, and radial nerves.

The brachial plexus can be damaged in a number of ways (Table 225-4). *Traumatic brachial plexopathy* occurs after motorcycle accidents, traction injuries, and penetrating wounds. Traumatic plexopathies are often combined with avulsion of roots from the spinal cord and injuries to individual nerve roots. Fracture or dislocation of the shoulder may cause acute injury to the brachial plexus; callus formation at the site of a clavicular fracture may cause chronic compression of the plexus. These lesions are often very painful. Management of the pain is similar to the management of neuropathic pain in general. Patients often fail conservative measures, and may derive tremendous benefit from spinal cord stimulation, spinal opioids, or neurosurgical procedures for pain control, particularly the dorsal root entry zone lesion.

Intraoperative injuries to the brachial plexus are common. Most are minimally symptomatic and resolve in the early postoperative period, although some can be associated with terrible neurologic deficits and devastating pain. The syndrome can be confused with postoperative ulnar neuropathy. The most common associated procedures are median sternotomy and thoracotomy. Management is as for traumatic plexopathy.

Acute brachial plexopathy, or Parsonage-Turner syndrome, presents with acute onset of pain in the shoulder radiating down the arm or into the neck, followed by weakness and numbness of the arm, which may resolve after a few weeks, or not for several years. The distribution of neurologic findings is variable. Worsening of pain by shoulder movements may lead to confusion with joint problems. A number of antecedent events have been described, including postimmunization, postinfectious, post-traumatic, and associated with autoimmune ill-

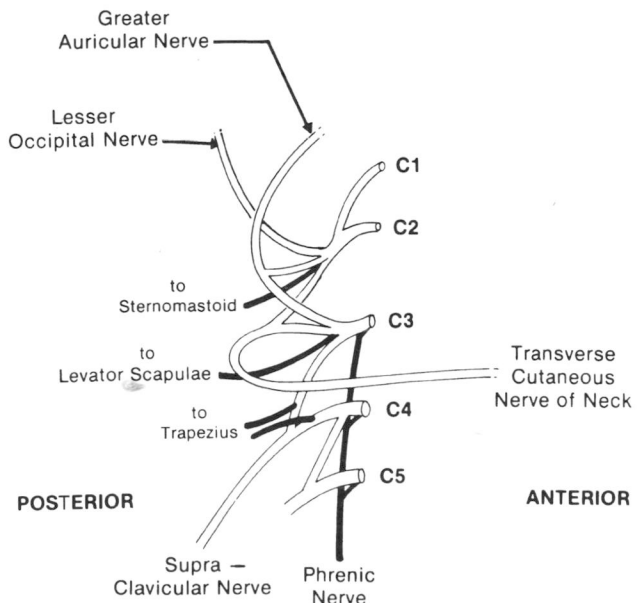

FIG. 225-5. The cervical plexus. (From Stewart JD: Focal Peripheral Neuropathies. Elsevier, New York, 1987, with permission.)

TABLE 225-4. Differential Diagnosis of Brachial Plexopathy

Trauma
Shoulder fracture-dislocation
Obstetric
Stingers and burners
Postoperative
Acute brachial plexus neuropathy
Hereditary
Malignancy
Radiation
Thoracic outlet syndrome
"Neurologic"
"Vascular"
Cervical rib
Scalenus anticus
Pectoralis minor
Costoclavicular

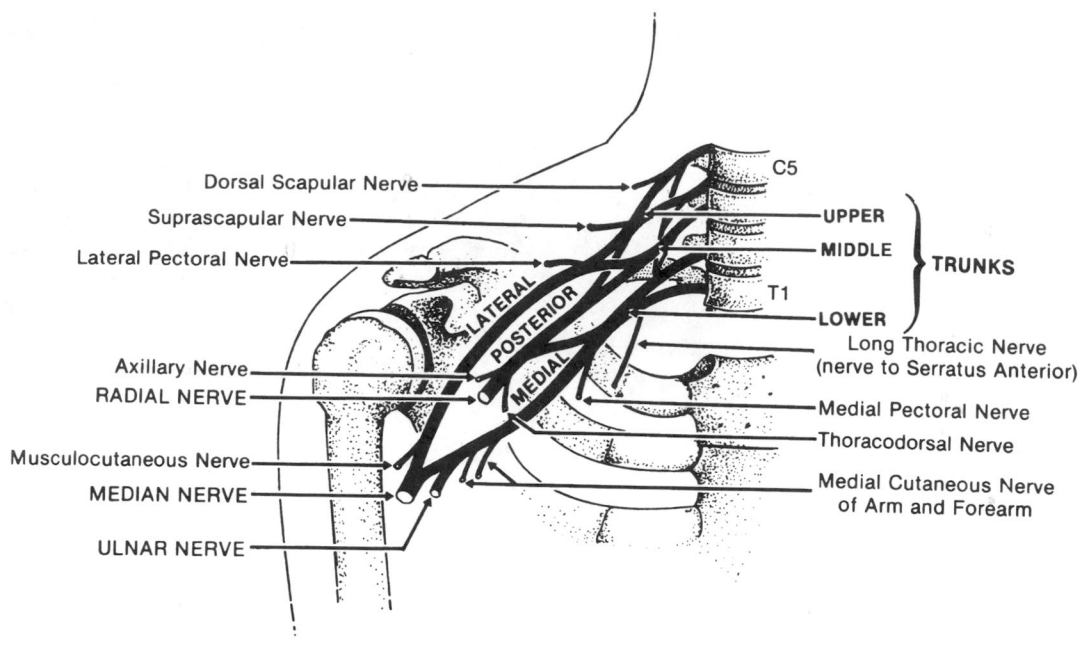

FIG. 225-6.   The brachial plexus. (From Stewart JD: Focal Peripheral Neuropathies. Elsevier, New York, 1987, with permission.)

nesses. An autoimmune etiology is hypothesized. Acute brachial plexus neuropathy may also occur in hereditary forms, in association with involvement of other nerves. Treatment options include systemic or locally injected steroids, physical therapy to prevent a frozen shoulder, and general treatment for neuropathic pain.

Malignant infiltration of the plexus presents with pain, followed by neurologic deficits, including a Horner syndrome. Most cases occur in patients with known metastatic disease, most commonly carcinoma of the breast; however, plexopathy can be the initial presentation of Pancoast tumor of the lung. Distinction from radiation plexopathy can be very difficult. The latter can begin months to years after radiotherapy and presents similarly. Several distinguishing features have been proposed: involvement of the lower trunk usually suggests tumor, whereas upper trunk involvement suggests radiation; tumor involvement presents with pain out of proportion to neurologic deficits, whereas radiation plexopathy presents with deficit greater than pain; and the EMG finding of myokymia suggests radiation plexopathy. Treatment for tumor plexopathy includes treatment of the primary tumor; radiation and steroids are particularly useful for palliation of pain. There is no specific treatment for radiation plexopathy, although revascularization procedures are gainng popularity. Aggressive pain control strategies, including neurolytic nerve blocks and neurosurgical procedures, are often necessary.

Thoracic Outlet Syndrome.   A variably accepted syndrome, thoracic outlet syndrome refers to compression of the brachial plexus or associated vasculature by a variety of structures, resulting in neck and arm symptoms. Patients present with pain in the neck, supraclavicular region, shoulder, or chest, radiating down the arm and often into the hand. Subjective paresthesias and weakness are common, but the neurologic examination and neurophysiologic test findings are negative. The physical examination may reveal tenderness, spasm, or reproduction of radiat-

ing pain by palpation of the scalene muscles or pectoralis minor. Various maneuvers have been suggested as helpful in diagnosing thoracic outlet syndrome, but none have been demonstrated to be accurate. Psychological or work-related issues commonly appear. Imaging studies may reveal an elongated transverse process of C7 (''cervical rib''), but this is also seen in asymptomatic patients. Treatment focuses on improving strength, flexibility, and posture related to the neck and upper extremities, and is best carried out by a physical therapist experienced with the syndrome. Attention should be paid to mental health and work-related issues. Diagnoses that are uncertain should be used sparingly in view of the legal implications. Surgery is probably overdone and should be left as a last resort in psychologically stable patients with a well-defined syndrome. Surgical options include resection of a cervical rib and first rib resection.

Injuries to individual branches of the brachial plexus may give rise to pain and neurologic dysfunction. Injury to the long thoracic nerve may result from trauma, surgery, general anesthesia, or as part of an acute brachial plexus neuropathy. Patients present with difficulty using the shoulder and aching of the shoulder and chest wall; physical examination shows winging of the scapula and weakness of the serratus anterior muscle.

The *suprascapular nerve* may be injured by trauma, especially scapular fracture, ligamentous or bony compression in the suprascapular notch, or as part of an acute brachial plexus neuropathy. Patients present with shoulder pain and weakness of shoulder abduction. The main differential diagnosis is rotator cuff injury. The diagnosis can be confirmed by electrodiagnostic studies. Treatment consists of local injections; surgical decompression may be necessary.

The *axillary nerve* can be damaged by trauma, usually shoulder dislocation or humerus fracture, compression, or injections. Deltoid weakness is the most prominent symptom and sensory loss may be detectable over the area of the deltoid insertion. Pain is not a prominent feature. The *musculocutaneous nerve*

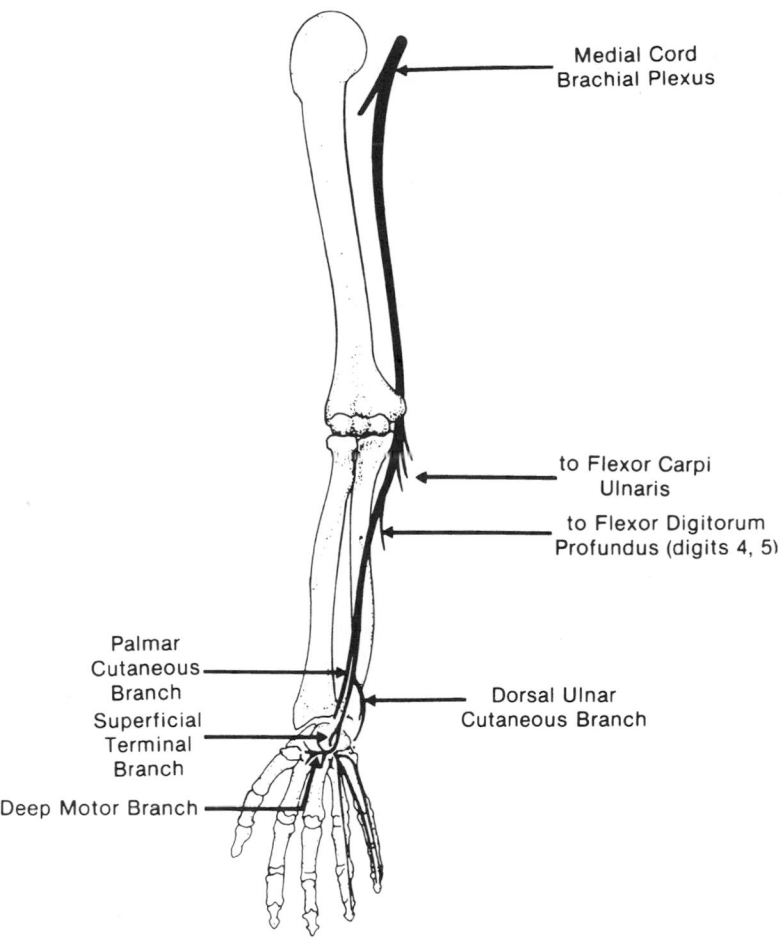

Medial Cord
Brachial Plexus

to Flexor Carpi
Ulnaris

to Flexor Digitorum
Profundus (digits 4, 5)

Palmar
Cutaneous
Branch

Superficial
Terminal
Branch

Deep Motor Branch

Dorsal Ulnar
Cutaneous Branch

FIG. 225-7. The course of the ulnar nerve. (From Stewart JD: Focal Peripheral Neuropathies. Elsevier, New York, 1987, with permission.)

may also be damaged by a variety of causes. Weakness of the biceps and sensory loss over the lateral forearm are the prominent features, with pain less significant.

Ulnar Neuropathy. The ulnar nerve (Fig. 225-7) derives from the C8 and T1 roots via the lower trunk and medial cord of the brachial plexus, and passes down the medial aspect of the upper arm. It then passes through the ulnar groove of the elbow, then under the aponeurosis of the flexor carpi ulnaris muscle to lie in the so-called *cubital tunnel.* At the wrist, the nerve passes through Guyon's canal, finally splitting into superficial and deep terminal branches. The nerve may be injured at any of these sites. In the axilla, the nerve is most commonly injured by deep sleep or coma with prolonged pressure on the nerve, or misplaced crutches. At the elbow, the most common site of damage, injury may result from old fractures or other bony deformities, trauma, scar tissue, tumors and masses, external pressure such as during anesthesia, supracondylar spurs, prolapse of the nerve, and leprosy. The nerve may also be damaged in the cubital tunnel by the aponeurosis of the flexor carpi ulnaris muscle, particularly after repetitive or prolonged flexion.

Damage to the nerve at the wrist is uncommon and may occur in several locations, related to lacerations, fractures, ganglia, disorders of the ulnar artery, bony disorders and abnormal muscle or connective tissue bands.

The approach to the patient begins with careful elicitation of a medical history and a thorough physical examination. Neurophysiologic studies are usually necessary, and imaging studies of the potential sites of entrapments may reveal local pathology. The exact site of injury can be quite difficult to determine even with sophisticated neurophysiologic testing. Even with surgical exploration, findings indicative of nerve pathology are difficult to distinguish from findings in asymptomatic patients.

The pain of ulnar neuropathy is often in the distribution of the sensory branches of the nerve, and may concentrate around the elbow. However, the pain may also be quite spread out through the arm and provide no localizing value. Other clinical features include sensory loss, weakness, and wasting of muscles, depending on the site of injury. Treatment depends upon accurate diagnosis and treatment of the underlying disorder. For patients with focal nerve injury, local injections at the site of injury may relieve symptoms. In patients with neuropathy at the elbow, avoiding leaning on the nerve and use of elbow padding to prevent flexion may be very helpful. Surgical exploration with decompression or transposition of the nerve may afford relief.

Median Neuropathy. The median nerve (Fig. 225-8) derives from contributions from C5–T1 cervical nerve roots, via union of parts of the lateral and medial cords of the brachial plexus.

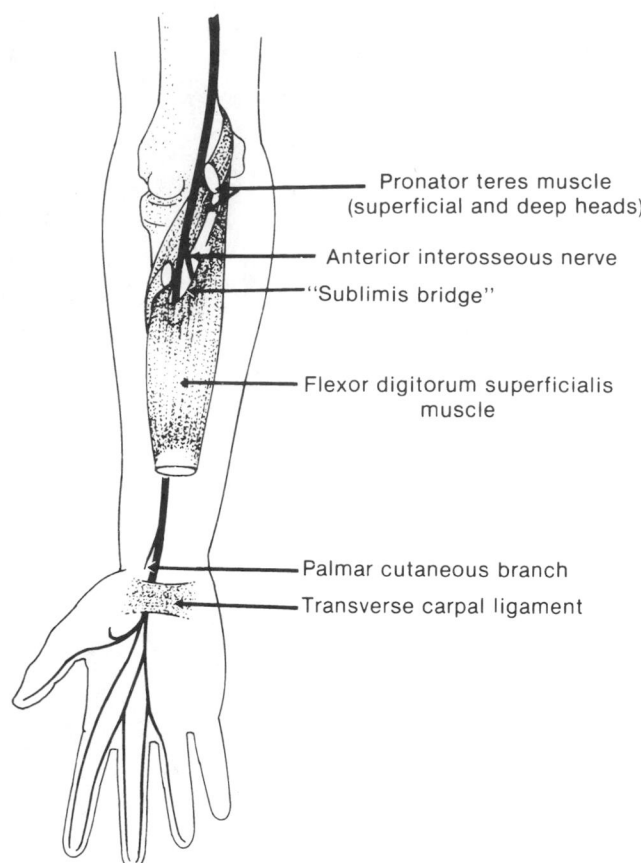

FIG. 225-8.   The median nerve (From Stewart JD: Focal Peripheral Neuropathies. Elsevier, New York, 1987, with permission.)

The nerve courses in the medial arm to cross the antecubital fossa in proximity to the brachial artery and biceps tendon. The nerve then passes beneath the bicipital aponeuross, and between the heads of the pronator teres muscle, after which it gives rise to the anterior interosseus nerve. The median nerve then passes under a tendinous structure called the sublimis bridge, and courses down the forearm to enter the carpal tunnel. Beyond the carpal tunnel, the nerve divides into a number of branches that innervate intrinsic hand muscles.

The median nerve may be damaged in several locations. Compression in the axilla is unusual and may be caused by crutches, sharp trauma, sleep palsies, aneurysms from dialysis shunts, and axillary arteriography. Damage at the elbow is more common and may be due to supracondylar spurs or anomalous ligaments, fractures or dislocations, injections, or compression by the bicipital aponeurosis or by bands within the pronator teres muscle.

By far the most common cause of compression of the median nerve is the *carpal tunnel syndrome.* Most cases are idiopathic, and relate to excessive hand activity as in manual laborers. Specific causes relate to anatomic compression in the carpal tunnel due to tenosynovitis, osteophytes, ganglia, or other lesions; increased susceptibility of nerves to compression, such as diabetes; and miscellaneous conditions including pregnancy and hypothyroidism.

Clinical features of the median neuropathies include neuropathic pain, usually in the region of the compression and in

the distribution of the nerve, but pain and paresthesias may be widespread. For example, in carpal tunnel syndrome most patients have wrist pain radiating into the first three fingers of the hand, but pain and paresthesias may radiate into all five fingers, or proximally even to the neck, creating diagnostic confusion with cervical radiculopathy. In addition to pain, weakness and sensory loss in the distribution of the nerve may be discernable.

Diagnosis and treatment parallels that of the other focal peripheral neuropathies. The history and physical examination focus on identifying compressive lesions and predisposing factors. Electrodiagnostic studies and imaging of the putative region of compression may be diagnostic. Splinting to avoid nerve irritation, local injections, and as a last resort surgical decompression are effective.

Radial Neuropathy.   The radial nerve (Fig. 225-9) consists of contributions from C5–T1 cervical nerve roots, and is the continuation of the posterior cord of the brachial plexus. The nerve winds around the humerus in the spiral groove, descends into the forearm between the biceps and brachioradialis muscles, and divides at the elbow into a motor (the posterior interosseus) and sensory (superficial radial) branches. The radial nerve may be injured in the upper arm by external compression, fractures, blunt trauma, injections, and tourniquets. Posterior interosseus neuropathies may be painful, and present similarly to tennis elbow, often accompanied by weakness of the wrist and finger extensors. Causes include the types of trauma and injuries described for the other neuropathies, as well as compression by abnormal fibrous bands around the elbow. The superficial radial nerve may be injured by injections, tight handcuffs or watch bands, or trauma. Patients present with a distinct syndrome of neuropathic pain in the distribution of the nerve.

Diagnosis and treatment of these syndromes is analogous to that described above.

Reflex Sympathetic Dystrophy.   Reflex sympathetic dystrophy is a poorly understood disorder consisting of the following triad: spontaneous burning pain, allodynia (extreme pain during stimulation with a normally nonpainful stimulus), and autonomic or trophic changes in the limb (e.g., atrophy, pitting of nails, loss of hair, changes in color, temperature, or sweating). Symptoms usually follow minor trauma, and involve the distal aspect of the limb, not respecting peripheral nerve territories, and occurring in the absence of injury to a nerve. Similar symptoms following nerve injury are termed *causalgia.* Many patients improve after blockade of the sympathetic nervous system. The syndrome is recognized to be nonspecific, and the pathophysiology is not understood. The basis of treatment consists of sympathetic blocks and active physical therapy. These patients are best managed in a multidisciplinary pain management center with experience in treating the disorder.

REGIONAL MUSCULOSKELETAL SYNDROMES

A number of syndromes of musculoskeletal dysfunction may cause pain in the upper extremity. The pain of these syndromes is typically regional, concentrated in the area of the pathology, although referred pain may be prominent, and may even overshadow the origin of the pain. The pain is typically described as sharp, aching, and constant, increased by physical activity

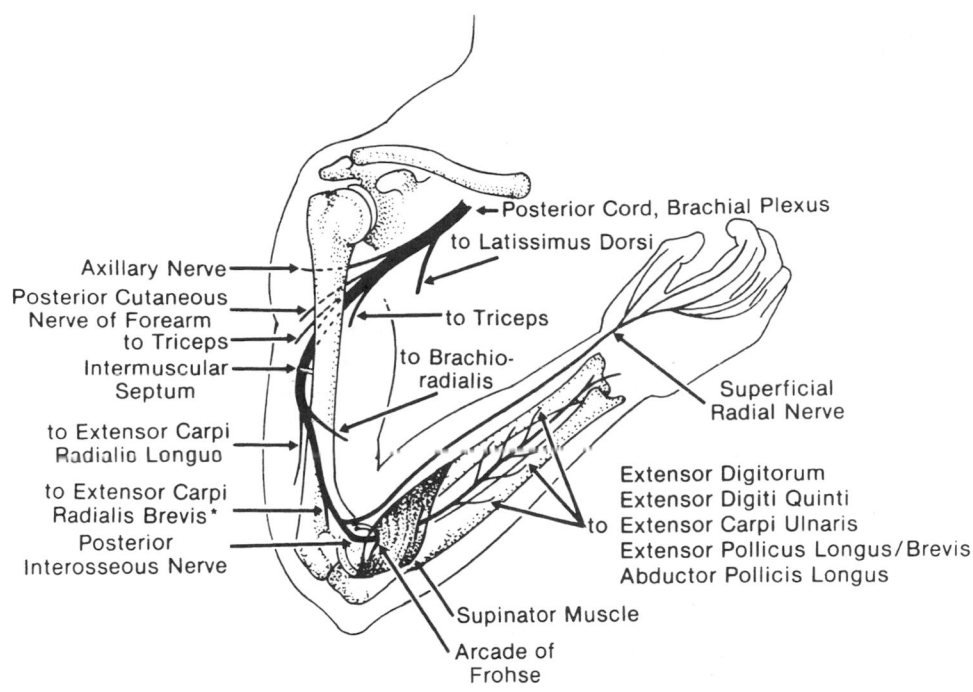

FIG. 225-9.   The radial nerve. (From Stewart JD: Focal Peripheral Neuropathies. Elsevier, New York, 1987, with permission.)

of the affected parts. Although patients may complain of subjective "heaviness," "weakness," or "numbness" of the limb, neurologic findings are absent.

General principles apply to the diagnosis and treatment of these syndromes. Patients with acute injury must be evaluated for intactness of neurologic and vascular function. Even when symptoms arise acutely, underlying disease must be kept in mind, such as infection or neoplasm. Most acute injuries can be treated with ice, compression, immobilization, and analgesics titrated to effect, with appropriate follow-up the most important next step. Follow-up care typically involves gradual remobilization, exercises to restore strength, flexibility, and function, tapering off of analgesics as appropriate, and ensuring that psychosocial complications do not ensue, with particular emphasis on the injured worker.

In the patient with chronic symptoms, accurate diagnosis is the first step in rational care. This may require subspecialty or physical therapy consultation, and evaluation should incorporate the full components of a chronic pain assessment. The first question is whether a specific syndrome can be diagnosed; if so, specific treatment can be instituted. If not, general measures will be indicated. Physical therapy with the goal of restoring function may be pivotal. Injections of cortisone and local anesthesia into an area of localized pain and tenderness may be surprisingly effective even in the absence of a definitive diagnosis (with the usual precautions). Nonspecific measures for the treatment of chronic pain—analgesics, antidepressants, psychological techniques, pain programs—may be the only indicated approaches, and may make a tremendous difference in pain, function, and quality of life.

The discussion below focuses on the most common regional musculoskeletal pain syndromes. Although not strictly "neurologic" they often present in the context of the neurologic evaluation of the patient with upper extremity pain.

Shoulder and Upper Arm

Rotator Cuff Tendinitis and Subacromial Bursitis.   The pain may be diffuse or located on the lateral aspect of the shoulder. Arm abduction is painful, and other motions may be as well. Flexion and elevation of the shoulder may be painful, the so-called impingement sign. Tenderness may be present in the subacromial region. If inflammation extends from the rotator cuff to the adjacent subacromial bursa, bursitis may result. The finding of true weakness on examination suggests rotator cuff tear; true limitation of ROM suggests the development of adhesive capsulitis or a "frozen shoulder."

Acute symptoms are treated by the general measures described above. Subacute or chronic symptoms are treated with ice or heat, active exercises to restore mobility and prevent frozen shoulder, and local steroid injections. Lack of response to conservative therapy or suggestion of a tear requires orthopaedic referral.

Biceps Tendinitis.   Shoulder pain with tenderness over the biceps tendon suggests this diagnosis. The biceps tendon is palpated by externally rotating the shoulder and palpating anteriorly. Resisted forearm flexion or supination also is painful. Treatment is analogous to that for rotator cuff tendinitis.

Acromioclavicular Joint Arthritis.   Pain is diffuse, exacerbated by arm elevation, with associated tenderness of the acromioclavicular joint. Treatment is as above.

Adhesive Capsulitis (Frozen Shoulder).   Frozen shoulder is a common end stage for any painful shoulder pathology, as well as for neurologic conditions that diminish active shoulder movement. Patients present with progressive diffuse shoulder pain and decreased active and passive range of motion. Physical examination reveals diffuse tenderness and painful limitation of ROM; signs of the inciting injury may be evident. Treatment depends on restoration of mobility with exercise; therefore, adequate analgesia with medications or injections is imperative.

Osteoarthritis of the Glenohumeral Joint. Patients present with chronic pain increased with activity, in the setting of advanced age or trauma. X-rays are confirmatory. Treatment consists of exercise, analgesia, injections, and as a last resort, surgery for shoulder replacement.

Elbow and Forearm

Lateral Epicondylitis. Patients present with diffuse elbow pain concentrated around the lateral epicondyle, increased with resisted wrist or finger extension. Predisposing factors include repetitive wrist extension, thus the term *tennis elbow*. Treatment or persistent cases includes a wrist splint or tennis elbow band, exercises, injections, and as a last resort, one of several surgical options.

Medial Epicondylitis. Otherwise known as golfer's elbow, medial epicondylitis occurs as a consequence of repetitive wrist flexion and pronation. Treatment is analogous to that of lateral epicondylitis.

Arthritis of the Elbow. As in shoulder arthritis, patients present with diffuse pain increased with activity, generally in older patients or after trauma. Treatment is analogous to shoulder arthritis.

Olecranon Bursitis. The olecranon bursa sits between the olecranon process and the triceps tendon, and may become inflamed owing to repetitive motion or leaning on the elbow. Differential diagnoses include joint infection and gout, or other arthritides, and tapping the joint may be necessary for diagnosis. Treatment, in addition to the general measures described above, includes aspiration of the bursa and instillation of steroid; surgical removal of the bursa is a last resort.

Wrist

DeQuervain's Tenosynovitis. A fairly common syndrome, DeQuervain's tenosynovitis consists of pain and tenderness over the radial aspect of the wrist. Physical examination shows a positive Finklestein test—that is, increased pain on ulnar flexion of the wrist with the patient holding the thumb in the closed fist. Predisposing factors include repetitive wrist movements, including knitting or using a wrench. Treatment, in addition to the general measures, includes temporary casting, steroids, injection, or surgery.

Wrist Tendonitis. Tendonitis can occur at any of the wrist tendons, and presents with pain and tenderness that may be localized or diffuse, particularly in the setting of excessive use of the wrist, as in typists. As a component of the so-called *repetitive strain* or *overuse syndrome* there are frequent psychosocial or work-related issues. Signs of infection suggest infectious tenosynovitis, mandating immediate orthopaedic referral. Treatment is as for the other tendinitis syndromes.

Arthritis of the First Carpometacarpal Joint. Arthritis in the first carpometacarpal joint occurs in patients with chronic use of the joint, such as mail carriers. Diagnostic features include tenderness of the joint and positive radiologic findings. Treatment options include splinting and joint injection.

Ganglia. Cystic masses overlying the wrist may arise from outpouchings of the synovium of the wrist joint or adjacent tendon sheaths. They may or may not be painful. If the mass is pulsatile or noncystic, further evaluation is necessary. Treatment options include splinting, aspiration, and surgical removal.

Miscellaneous Disorders

Polymyalgia Rheumatica. The syndrome of polymyalgia rheumatica consists of severe aching pain and stiffness in the proximal arms and legs, occurring in older patients. Elevation of the erythrocyte sedimentation rate is characteristic. Constitutional symptoms may occur. Some cases are associated with temporal arteritis. Signs of muscle inflammation are absent. Response to steroids is dramatic, with nearly complete elimination of symptoms with low doses.

Vascular Disease. A number of vascular diseases can present with upper extremity pain. The syndromes of *acute and chronic arterial ischemia* related to thrombotic or embolic disease are well known. Patients present with pain, pallor, paresthesias, and in the end, paralysis. Symptoms may be mild from small peripheral emboli, or devastating from acute large vessel occlusion. Upper extremity compartment syndrome may result, and cause further pain and neurologic injury. *Thromboangiitis obliterans* presents in young smokers, predominantly in the legs, but often with pain or claudication in the arms as well.

The vasospastic disorders include *Raynaud's, acrocyanosis, and livedo reticularis.* Raynaud's disease consists of idiopathic spasm of the microcirculation, resulting in blanching of the fingers, followed by cyanosis, then hyperemia, often in response to cold. Attacks may be severe enough to be disabling. *Raynaud's phenomenon* refers to the syndrome in the setting of an underlying disease (e.g. rheumatoid arthritis). Therapy consists of administration of systemic vasodilators, and in severe cases, sympathectomy. *Acrocyanosis* is is a syndrome of unknown etiology consisting of constant coldness, cyanosis, and sometimes edema and hyperhidrosis. Trophic changes and gangrene, unlike in Raynaud's phenomenon, do not occur. Treatment is the same as for Raynaud's. *Livedo reticularis* is a bluish mottling of the skin of the extremities that may occur in the setting of underlying disease. The disorder is painful in some patients, and may result in recurrent ulcerations. Treatment is again as for Raynaud's.

The most important of the vasodilating disorders is *erythromelalgia,* a condition of hot, red, and painful extremities that is usually idiopathic, but may occur in the setting of myeloproliferative and other disorders. The pathophysiology is uncertain but may relate to abnormal sensitization of receptors for warm and cold. Treatment consists of avoiding heat, application of cold, treatment of any underlying disorder, and administration of aspirin; several other agents have been suggested as well.

SUGGESTED READINGS

Adams RD, Victor M: Principles of Neurology. 4th Ed. McGraw Hill, New York, 1989

Birnbaum JS: The Musculoskeletal Manual. 2nd Ed. WB Saunders, Philadelphia, 1990

Bland JH: Disorders of the Cervical Spine: Diagnosis and Medical Management. WB Saunders, Philadelphia, 1987

Bonica JJ, Cailliet R: General considerations of pain in the neck and upper limb. Ch. 46. In Bonica JJ (ed): The Management of Pain. 2nd Ed. JB Lippincott, Philadelphia, 1990

Cailliet R: Neck and Arm Pain. FA Davis, Philadelphia, 1992

Stewart JD: Focal Peripheral Neuropathies. Elsevier, New York, 1987

226. LOW BACK PAIN

STEVEN FESKE

Those complaining of back pain represent a significant percentage of the patients in any general neurologist's practice. Epidemiologic information is problematic, because it is often based on data acquired from self-reporting of pain or from the interaction of back pain with working life as measures of time lost from work or compensation claims; however, a few statistics give a sense of the magnitude of the problem. An estimated 50 to 80 percent of adults will have low back pain during their lifetimes (Loeser 1991). Although most of this number represents benign, self-limited pain, a significant percentage of those affected will seek medical attention. Back pain is the single greatest cause of lost work days in the United States. Data from the U.S. Census Bureau estimate that from 1984 to 1985, 14 percent of workers missed 1 or more workdays owing to back pain during this period. About 2 percent of workers submit claims for compensation for back pain each year (Loeser 1991). By such parameters, the incidence of back pain has been rising since the 1960s, although it is likely that this increase represents more a change of the interaction of back pain and societal trends than a true change in the nature and frequency of back pain itself.

This chapter discusses the evaluation and management of acute and chronic back pain. We begin with a brief review of some of the relevant anatomy. The next section mentions some of the important and most serious diseases to consider in the diagnosis. This discussion of the causes of back pain is then expanded by a more detailed discussion of the most common causes, the various skeletal, muscular, and neurologic syndromes. There follows a discussion of the approach to patients with acute and chronic back pain. Other chapters in Part IX of this book discuss more fully the many issues of chronic pain in general.

ANATOMY OF THE LUMBOSACRAL SPINE

Figures 226-1 to 226-3 show the relationships of the bones, intervertebral discs, and ligaments of the lumbosacral spine. The ligaments, the periosteum, and the outer ligamentous portions of the intervertebral discs are all innervated by nociceptive afferents from the spinal nerves. The periosteum is also innervated for pain perception. Figure 226-4 shows the relationships of the lower spinal cord and roots to the bony spine. Pain can arise from involvement of the meninges, which are innervated by nociceptive fibers or by disease of the roots, commonly compressive, or of pain-mediating networks within the spinal cord.

ETIOLOGY

A multitude of illnesses can cause back pain. Although it is true that the great majority of patients who present with acute back pain will have minor musculoskeletal disorders and the majority with chronic back pain will have degenerative disorders, it is a major part of the initial task of assessment to properly diagnose those who do have other diseases. To do so efficiently, it is helpful to have access to a broad list of differential diagnoses. It is not feasible try to list them all; however, an extended list is offered in Table 226-1. It is also helpful to have access to a detailed description of the differential diagnosis of the various musculoskeletal disorders, since their proper management depends on accurate diagnosis.

Common Skeletal and Muscular Causes

Lumbosacral Strain and Sprain. Lumbosacral strain and sprain is the most common diagnosis made in cases of acute low back pain and implies stress to the musculoskeletal tissues without a precise anatomic localization or pathologic definition.

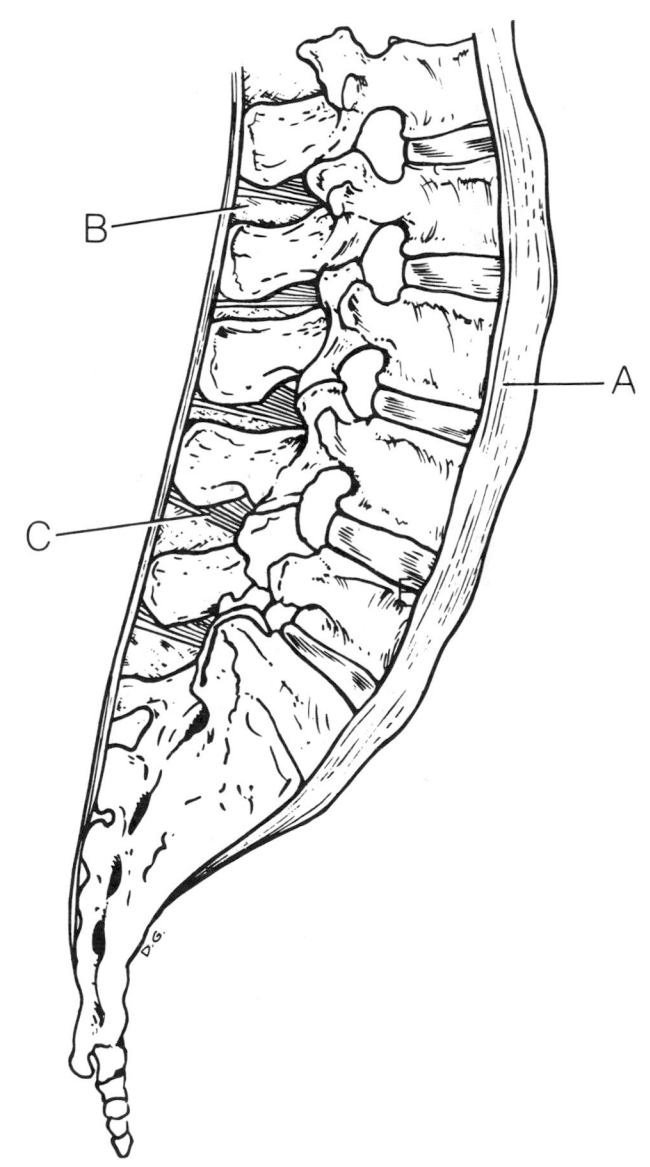

FIG. 226-1. Lumbosacral spine viewed from the side. *(A)* Anterior longitudinal ligament; *(B)* supraspinous ligament; *(C)* interspinous ligament. (From Dupuis PR: The anatomy of the lumbosacral spine. p. 15. In Kirkaldy-Willis WH, Burton CV (eds): Managing Low Back Pain. 3rd Ed. Churchill Livingstone, New York, 1992, with permission.)

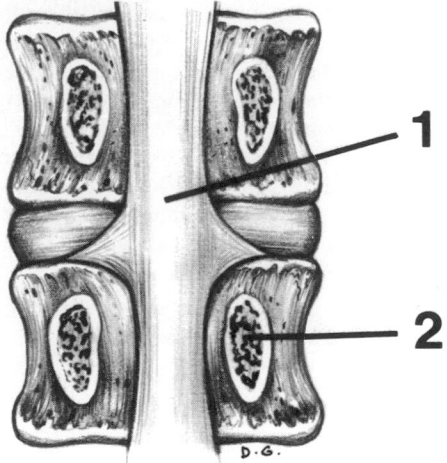

FIG. 226-2. Posterior longitudinal ligament. The spine is viewed from the back with posterior elements removed. *1,* posterior longitudinal ligament with lateral expansions; *2,* pedicle. (From Dupuis PR: The anatomy of the lumbosacral spine. p. 15. In Kirkaldy-Willis WH, Burton CV (eds): Managing Low Back Pain. 3rd Ed. Churchill Livingstone, New York, 1992, with permission.)

The medical history is usually that of acute onset of low back pain after a minor injury, such as those due to lifting or twisting. Sometimes onset is spontaneous or the pain is present upon waking. The pain is usually in the lumbosacral area at the midline or slightly to one side. It often radiates into the buttocks and posterolateral thighs, occasionally below the knee. The pain is typically exacerbated by movement and partially relieved by

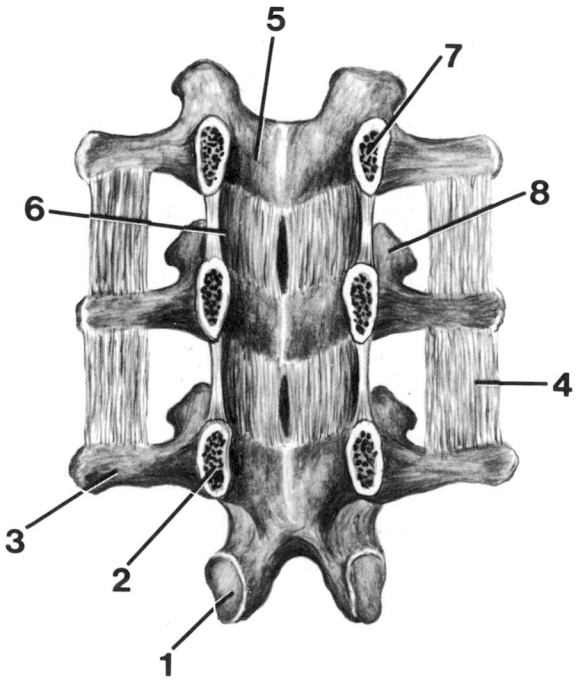

FIG. 226-3. View of the posterior lumbar spine from the front, with vertebral body excised. *1,* inferior articular facet; *2,* pedicle; *3,* transverse process; *4,* intertransverse process; *5,* lamina; *6,* ligamentum flavum; *7,* pedicle; *8,* superior articular facet. (From Dupuis PR, Kirkaldy-Willis WH: The spine: integrated function and pathophysiology. In Cruess RL, Rennie WRJ (eds): Adult Orthopaedics. Churchill Livingstone, New York, 1984, with permission.)

rest, although significant resting pain is often present. Physical examination shows a decreased range of motion and marked sensitivity to movement in many cases. There is often mild to moderate tenderness in the low back along the spine and in the paraspinal muscle mass. Palpable muscle spasm may be present but is difficult to distinguish from voluntary contraction or guarding. Straight-leg raising may be limited by pain in the back and tightness in the hamstrings, but it does not cause shocklike radiaton in a dermatomal distribution. If there are no features to suggest more serious disease (see section on Management) and there is no serious trauma to the area, and the patient is less than 50 years old, no further testing is necessary in most cases.

The mainstays of treatment have been rest, non-narcotic analgesics, physical therapy, including exercises, and patient education to reduce the risk of future injury. Weisel and colleagues (1980) compared bed rest and ambulatory controls in military recruits and found that bed rest speeded recovery. Deyo and colleagues (1986) found 2 days of bed rest no different from 7 for recovery, but found that the 2 days lead to briefer periods of missed work. Malmivaara and colleagues (1995) compared 2 days of bed rest, light exercises, and a control group undertaking normal activity limited by symptoms only. The control group recovered most quickly with the least pain. The patients restricted to bed rest fared the worst. If we equate ambulatory status in the military with a significant level of exercise, these data suggest that bed rest is not helpful and that ordinary light levels of activity may promote the most rapid recovery from acute nonspecific low back pain. If rest is recommended, it should be brief to avoid deconditioning and reinforcement of the sick role.

Various physical therapies have traditionally been recommended for acute low back pain: heat or cold application, exercises, traction, ultrasound, and diathermy. Data concerning the benefits of exercise are conflicting. As noted above, Malmivaara recently found ordinary activity better than extension and lateral bending exercises. Prior studies had also failed to show a benefit of exercise over usual care with information and analgesics (Faas et al., 1993). Other studies have found a benefit of back extension exercises compared to education only (Stankovic and Johnell, 1990). Flexibility training and strengthening and conditioning exercises still have their advocates and likely do provide benefit to some patients, especially those with inactive lifestyles. Contrary to the conflicting data on acute low back pain, when pain of this type becomes chronic, there is much evidence in favor of exercise. The application of heat and cold may provide some relief of symptoms and is safe if done properly. There is little support in the literature for its use or for the use of other modalities, such as ultrasound, diathermy, or traction. Manipulation is a controversial topic. In his review, Frymoyer (1988) states that the data support some short-term benefit from manipulation in the amelioration of pain and improvement of function but that there is no evidence for long-term benefit.

Nonsteroidal analgesics and strictly time-limited dosages of muscle relaxants and, in case of severe pain, narcotics may be used for acute pain. Nonsteroidal agents and antidepressants may be used for chronic pain. Pharmacologic treatment of acute and chronic pain is discussed in more detail below under Management.

Acute Disc Herniation.   Acute lumbosacral disc herniation may cause isolated pain of a nonspecific sort, radicular pain

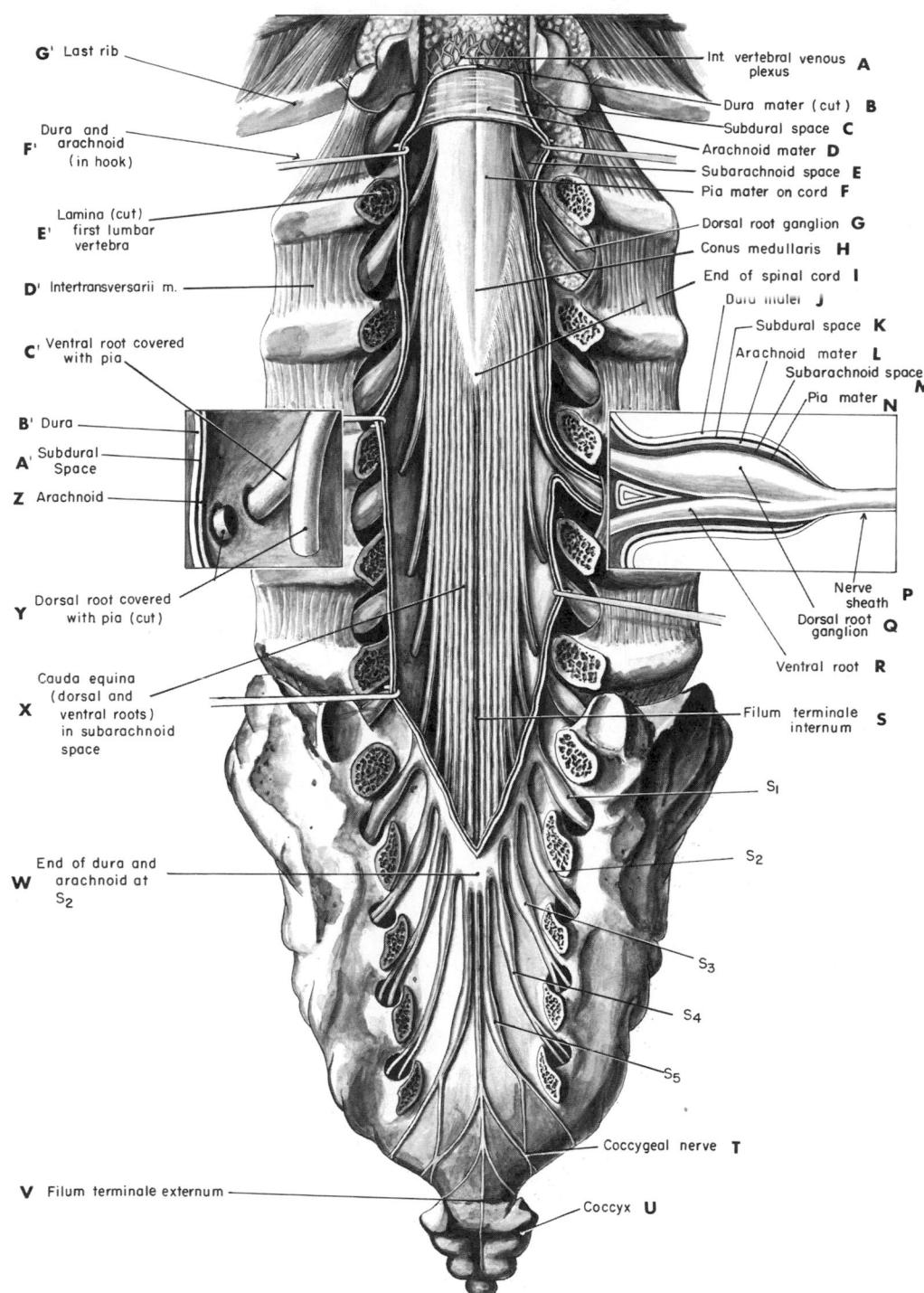

G' Last rib

Int. vertebral venous plexus **A**

Dura and arachnoid (in hook) **F'**

Dura mater (cut) **B**
Subdural space **C**
Arachnoid mater **D**
Subarachnoid space **E**
Pia mater on cord **F**

Lamina (cut) first lumbar vertebra **E'**

Dorsal root ganglion **G**
Conus medullaris **H**
End of spinal cord **I**
Dura mater **J**

Intertransversarii m. **D'**

Subdural space **K**
Arachnoid mater **L**
Subarachnoid space **M**

Ventral root covered with pia **C'**

Pia mater **N**

Dura **B'**
Subdural Space **A'**
Arachnoid **Z**

Dorsal root covered with pia (cut) **Y**

Nerve sheath **P**
Dorsal root ganglion **Q**
Ventral root **R**

Cauda equina (dorsal and ventral roots) in subarachnoid space **X**

Filum terminale internum **S**

S₁
S₂
S₃
S₄
S₅

End of dura and arachnoid at S₂ **W**

Coccygeal nerve **T**

Filum terminale externum **V**

Coccyx **U**

FIG. 226-4. Distribution of nerves in the lumbosacral region, showing the dorsal and ventral roots (cauda equina, X) with their coverings of pia streaming inferiorly to emerge from the proper intervertebral foramen. The enlargement on the left side shows a dorsal (Y) and ventral (C') root emerging through the arachnoid and dura via separate openings. The enlargement on the right has been turned, showing the distribution of the dorsal and ventral roots and how they blend to form the nerve sheath. (From Crafts RC: A Textbook of Human Anatomy. 3rd Ed. p. 101. John Wiley & Sons, New York, 1985, with permission.)

TABLE 226-1. Major Causes of Back Pain

Musculoskeletal disorders
  Trauma
    Fracture
    Contusion
    Hematoma
  Degenerative disease
    Disc herniation
      Ligamentous
      Radicular
      Myelopathic
      Conus or cauda equina syndrome
      Postoperative
      "Failed back"
      Litigous/compensation-seeking
    Arthritis
      Facet arthritis
      Osteophyte impingement of neural foramina or central canal (spinal stenosis)
        with radicular syndrome
      Spondylolisthesis
      Spondylolysis
      Anklyosing spondylitis
  Ligamentous strain
  Muscle strain and spasm

Congenital disorders
  Scoliosis and spinal anomalies
  Tethered cord
  Meningocele
  Spina bifida
  Lipoma, teratoma, and other congenital tumors

Infectious diseases
  Abscess
    Discitis
    Osteomyelitis
    Epidural abscess
  Meningitis
  Urologic infection
  Herpes zoster reactivation

Parainfectious disorders and autoimmune disorders
  Transverse myelitis
  Guillain-Barré syndrome
  Multiple sclerosis (Lhermitte sign)
  Inflammatory arthritides
    Ankylosing spondylitis
    Reiter's syndrome and other spondyloarthropathies

Neoplasm
  Multiple myeloma
  Metastatic cancer
    Lung
    Breast
    Prostate
    Melanoma
    Renal cell carcinoma
    Others
  Lymphoma
  Primary tumors affecting the spinal cord or roots
    Astrocytoma
    Ependymoma
    Schwannoma
    Meningioma
    Others
  Tumors in the retroperitoneum
    Pancreatic carcinoma
    Retroperitoneal sarcoma
    Renal cell carcinoma
    Others
  Tumors infiltrating the pelvis and lumbosacral plexus

Vascular disorders
  Epidural hematoma
  Spinal dural arteriovenous fistula (subacute necrosis of the spinal cord)
  Aortic dissection
  Aortic aneurysm
  Splenic and renal infarction and other renal causes

Metabolic disorders
  Paget's disease
  Osteoporosis, compression fractures
  Retroperitoneal fibrosis

due to protrusion into the lateral recess and neural foramen, or cauda equina syndrome due to massive central herniation. The onset of the pain is often sudden with severe radicular symptoms. This is commonly precipitated by a lifting or twisting injury. The symptoms are classically exacerbated by coughing and straining. The L5–S1 disc is the most often involved with posterolateral herniation such that it entraps the S1 root as it descends to emerge below S1. Sciatica with S1 dermatomal (posterolateral leg, lateral heel and sole) pain, paresthesias, and sensory loss are most common (Table 226-2). The pain and paresthesias can be elicited by straight-leg raising, often with radiation to the sole of the foot. The smaller the angle of elevation necessary to elicit the pain, the greater the predictive value of the test for disc herniation (Troup 1981). A positive test with elevation of the contralateral leg is even stronger evidence of root compression (Scham 1971). The ankle jerk is diminished, and there may be weakness in the S1 myotome (gastrocnemius and hamstrings). A more lateral protrusion of the L5–S1 disc may entrap the L5 root exiting at that level, causing sciatica with L5 dermatomal (anterolateral lower leg and dorsum of foot) and myotomal (tibialis anterior group, extensor hallicus longus, peroneii [foot eversion], and tibialis posterior [foot inversion]) deficits. Again, straight-leg raising is positive, eliciting dermatomal signs. In both cases, the sciatic nerve may be tender to palpation through the gluteus muscle mass at the sciatic notch in the buttocks and below. Less commonly, L4–L5 disc herniation occurs. Herniations at other levels are much less common and may cause correspondingly higher radicular symptoms and signs. The massive central herniation of a lumbosacral disc may cause acute compression of multiple lower roots, leading to the cauda equina syndrome. In this syndrome, one finds radicular pain, paresthesias, and sensory loss at multiple and bilateral, though often asymmetric, sites, bilateral leg weakness, and loss of lower extremity reflexes. There may be varying degrees of bowel and bladder dysfunction. When severe, there is perianal sensory loss, loss of anal tone and reflexes (reflex sphincter constriction to skin stimulation [wink], bulbocavernosus reflex), and fecal and urinary retention and incontinence. When more subtle, there may be no bowel or bladder

TABLE 226-2. Some Causes of Sciatica[a]

Herniated nucleus pulposus
Congenital abnormality of the spine (trefoil canal)
  Congenital spinal stenosis
  Anomalous roots (e.g., conjoined root)
Degenerative disease of the lumbosacral spine
  Osteophyte impingement
  Spondylolisthesis/spondylolysis
  Spinal stenosis
  Synovial cysts
Spinal osteochondrosis (Sheuermann's disease)
Neoplasms
  Schwannoma, meningioma, and other primary tumors
  Osseous tumors
  Metastatic tumor
  Lymphoma
Epidural hematoma
Infections
  Epidural abscess
  Herpes zoster
Retroperitoneal and intrapelvic tumors outside of the spine
Local compression
  Wallets
  Toilet seats, etc.
Piriformis syndrome

[a] See also Table 226-1.

(From Frymoyer JW: Back pain and sciatica. N Engl J Med 315:1090, 1988, with permission.)

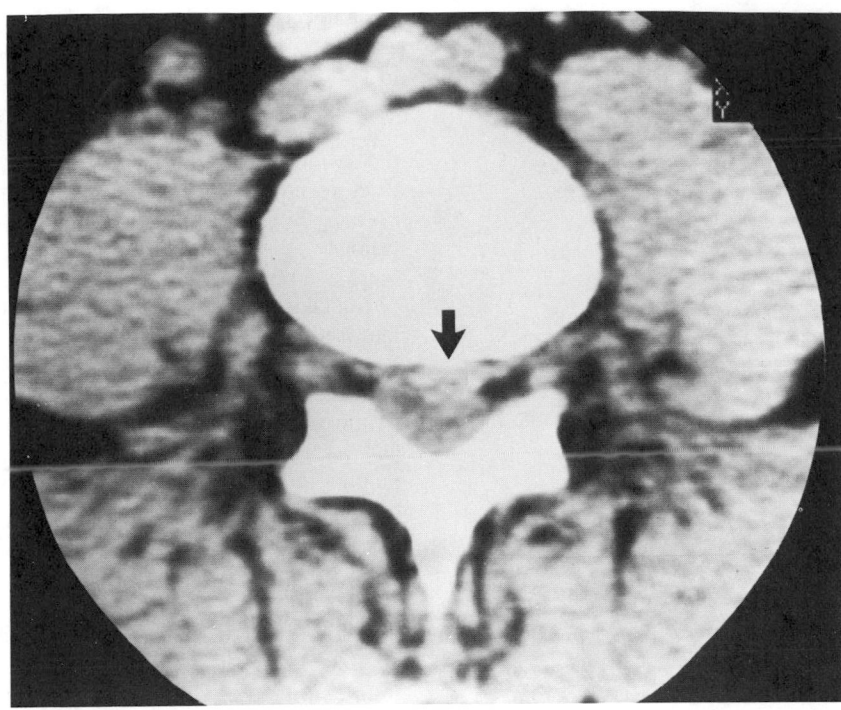

FIG. 226-5. Axial computed tomography scan through and L4–L5 intervertebral disc level demonstrating a posterolateral left-sided disc herniation (*arrow*), resulting in impingement of the traversing left L5 nerve root. (From Gundry CR, Heithoff KB: Lumbar spine imaging. p. 176. In Kirkaldy-Willis WH, Burton CV (eds): Managing Low Back Pain. 3rd Ed. Churchill Livingstone, New York, 1992, with permission.)

symptoms, but there may be a large retained postvoid residual volume noted upon catheterization.

Further evaluation will depend on the level of suspicion for disease other than benign disc disease, such as cancer or abscess (see Section on Management) and on the severity of the symptoms and neurologic deficit. When the bowel or bladder are acutely involved, patients should receive immediate intravenous dexamethasone and undergo imaging to define the lesion. In most cases, magnetic resonance imaging (MRI) is preferred, although computed tomography (CT) may better define bony pathology (Fig. 226-5), and CT or myelography with CT may substitute for or complement MRI. This situation demands immediate neurosurgical consultation and surgery to optimize functional recovery. In patients in whom there are major radicular findings, early imaging is indicated. In those with significant motor deficits, early surgery for demonstrated disc herniation corresponding to the clinical deficit is indicated for patients who desire it. This may optimize early recovery; however, long-term functional recovery is probably not compromised by a delay of many weeks. Those with a significant motor deficit should go to surgery within 12 weeks to achieve the best long-term outcome. (Weber 1978, Thomas 1983). It is crucial to correlate symptoms and signs with the lesions found on imaging, because the rates of abnormalities of CT scans (Rothman 1984, Wiesel 1984), myelograms (Hitselberger 1968) and MRI scans (Boden 1990, Jensen 1994) are high in asymptomatic patients.

For the more common patients, in whom there are mild to moderate radicular findings or none at all, one-half will recover in 6 weeks. All patients with radicular findings should probably have at least pain x-rays to look for unexpected lesions. If the clinical diagnosis of disc herniation and mild radiculopathy is made and conservative treatment is planned, then no further immediate imaging is needed. When diagnosis is in doubt or when guidance is needed for later therapy (e.g., epidural sterioid injection or surgery), imaging may be needed. Electromyography (EMG) can help in questionable cases to define a radiculopathy. Initially, the EMG will typically be normal. If axonal loss develops, the amplitude of the compound muscle action potential will be reduced, and the EMG will begin to show changes of acute denervation in the myotome in question after 1 to 2 weeks (see Ch. 20).

In these milder cases, conservative treatment consists of rest and analgesics and sometimes short-term corticosteroids (e.g., prednisone 30 to 60 mg daily for 7 to 10 days) for anti-inflammatory effect in acutely painful discs. During the recuperative phase, patients may benefit from physical therapy and education about prevention of back injury. Manipulation should be avoided. Patients whose pain fails to improve over 6 weeks of follow-up and who have neurologic deficits or intractable pain are candidates for surgical therapy for decompression. When pain is the indication for more aggressive therapy, epidural injection of corticosteroids at the site of the herniation may promote symptomatic relief. The large majority of patients with disc herniation can be managed successfully without surgery, although this approach will probably result in more short-term disability in many patients.

Spondylolisthesis and Spondylolysis. Spondylolisthesis is a slippage of one lumbar vertebra on another or of the L5 vertebra on the sacrum. In degenerative disease, this usually occurs at L4–L5 and does not include fracture of the vertebral arch (Fig. 226-6). Spondylolysis is a fracture of the pars interarticularis of the arch that often accompanies such slippage. A simple classification of spondylolisthesis based on the degree of displacement facilitates communication and guides decision mak-

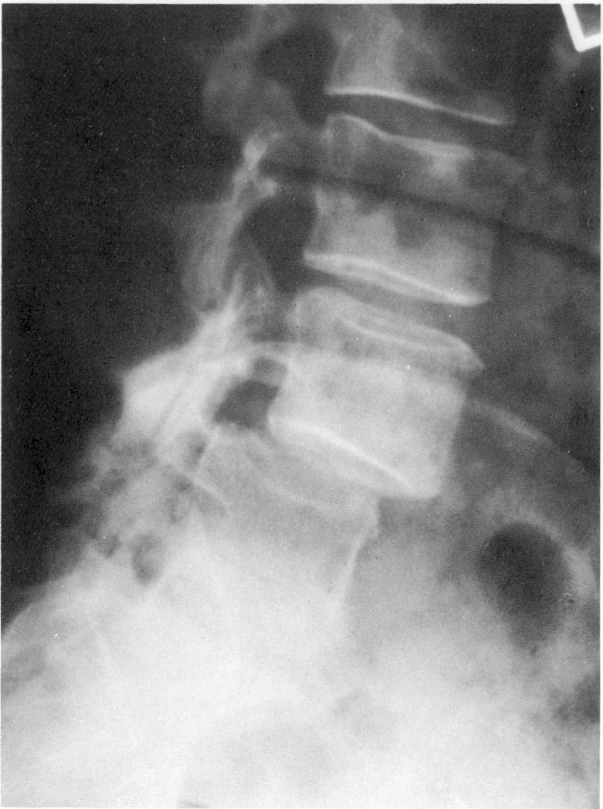

FIG. 226-6. Degenerative spondylolisthosis of the fourth to the fifth lumbar vertebra. (From Kirkaldy-Willis WH, Burton CV, Cassidy JD: The site and nature of the lesion. p. 114. In Kirkaldy-Willis WH, Burton CV (eds): Managing Low Back Pain. 3rd Ed. Churchill Livingstone, New York, 1992, with permission.)

ing: grade 1; less than 25 percent; grade 2, 25 to 50 percent; grade 3, 50 to 75 percent; and grade 4, greater than 75 percent. The abnormality is due to abnormal development, trauma, or degenerative or other structural disease. An etiologic classification has also been proposed, as detailed in Table 226-3.

Spondylolisthesis is common, occurring in about 5 percent of the general population. Isthmic spondylolysis with spondylolisthesis is thought to be due to stress fracture of the pars interarticularis. Participation in demanding athletic pursuits, such as football and gymnastics, greatly increases the risk of developing this lesion.

Although it may occur acutely after trauma, this lesion is usually asymptomatic or may present with persistent low back pain. The pain is probably due to (1) abnormalities of the pain-sensitive ligaments and joints, (2) root compression, or (3) lumbar spinal stenosis and, correspondingly, may be nonspecific

TABLE 226-3. Etiologic Classification of Spondylolisthesis

1. Dysplastic
2. Isthmic
   a. Lytic—fatigue fracture of the pars
   b. Elongated, intact pars
   c. Acute fracture of the pars
3. Degenerative
4. Traumatic (fracture elsewhere than the pars)
5. Pathologic

(From Wiltse LL, Newman PH, MacNab I: Classification of spondylolisthesis and spondylolysis. Clin Orthop 117:23, 1976, with permission.)

in character or have radicular features or symptoms typical of spinal stenosis. It is usually aggravated by activity and relieved in part by rest.

When low back pain is persistent, spinal x-rays should be obtained to look for this lesion. Oblique views may demonstrate the spondylolytic fracture. Sclerosis of the borders of such a fracture indicate a chronic lesion, and healing cannot be expected. Bone scanning may help to differentiate acute active lesions with potential to heal from chronic sclerotic ones when there is doubt. Flexion and extension x-rays allow quantitation of translational and angular movements large enough to correlate with instability of the spinal segment. MRI and CT can demonstrate associated root compression and spinal stenosis.

In the more common degenerative and isthmic lytic varieties, treatment is usually conservative—rest for acute pain, and non-narcotic analgesics and external supportive devices. Surgery may be indicated in some cases for decompression of root entrapment and spinal stenosis. For acute lytic fractures with healing potential, external bracing may promote healing. The detailed evaluation and management of spondylolisthesis and spondylolysis is complex, and patients with acute lesions or chronic lesions with persistent symptoms are best referred to an orthopaedic surgeon for expert care.

Lumbar Spinal Stenosis. Spinal stenosis may result from degenerative changes of the bony spine and ligaments or from a congenital anomaly of the spine, usually a shortening of the pedicles. Degenerative disease leads to posterior bulging of intervertebral discs, osteophyte formation, hypertrophy of the ligamentum flavum and other ligaments within the spinal canal, hypertrophy of the facet joints, spondylolisthesis without spondylolysis, and abnormal angulation of the spine. All of these features may compromise the space available to neural structures. The characteristic symptom is neural claudication. This is low back pain, often radiating to the buttocks and anterior thighs, that is brought on by extension and relieved by flexion of the spine. A typical history might be the onset of aching pain while walking with relief by seated rest but not by rest while standing (in contradistinction to vascular claudication). Walking downhill exacerbates the pain by demanding spinal extension. When pain is severe, patients may have difficulty standing upright and hence may bend forward when walking. Many patients will have only mechanical symptoms and signs. Others will have, in addition, radicular symptoms and signs from stenosis involving the lateral recess or degenerative compromise of the neural foramina. Evaluation includes imaging by CT or MRI. MRI simultaneously visualizes bony and neural tissues. This can demonstrate the stenotic bony canal and the effacement of the surrounding cerebrospinal fluid on T2-weighted images (Fig 226-7). CT is good for evaluation of lateral recess stenosis, whereas MRI may underestimate the degree of bony overgrowth. A transverse interfacet dimension of less than 16 mm is low, and less than 10 mm represents severe stenosis. An anteroposterior dimension of less than 12 mm suggests stenosis but is insensitive. A lateral recess of 3 mm or less is likely stenotic. When lateral stenosis is significant, compression of the root can be seen within the recess. Although these dimensions are guidelines, again, clinical correlation of symptoms and anatomy is crucial to selection of patients for successful surgery. Symptomatic therapy is as for other causes of chronic low back pain. Surgical therapy to decompress the stenotic canal is an option when disability and pain are significant.

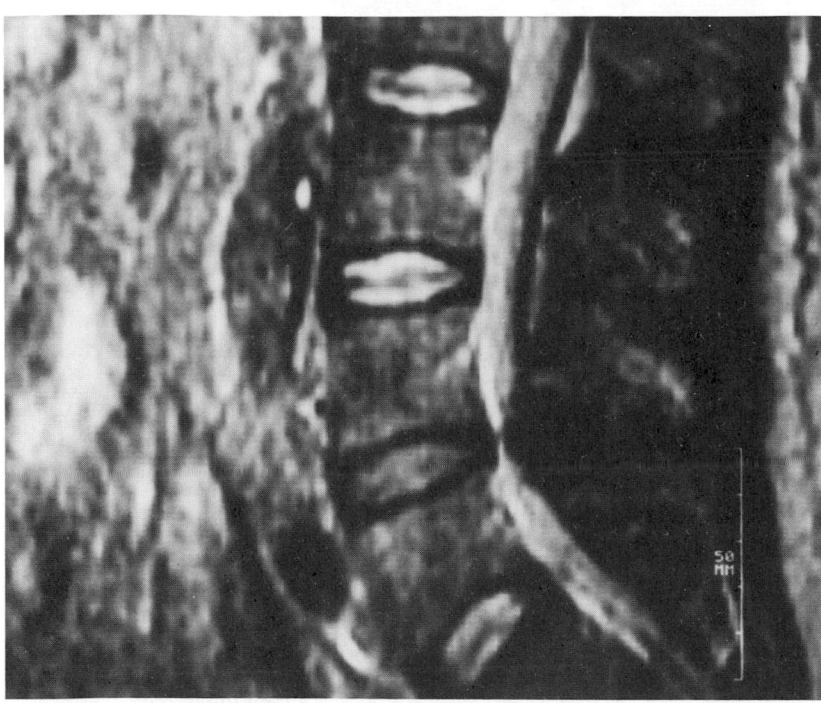

FIG. 226-7. Sagittal magnetic resonance image of a patient with neurogenic claudications. The image shows central spinal stenosis caused by hypertrophy of the ligamentum flavum and posterior protrusion of the annulus fibrosus. (From Bernard TN, Kirkaldy-Willis WH: Making a specific diagnosis. p. 210. In Kirkaldy-Willis WH, Burton CV (eds): Managing Low Back Pain. 3rd Ed. Churchill Livingstone, New York, 1992, with permission.)

Facet Syndrome. This diagnosis remains controversial. It has been argued that radicular chronic low back pain exacerbated by hyperextension and twisting and tenderness over a facet joint in hyperextesion in the context of facet degenerative arthritis on imaging studies suggest the diagnosis of the facet syndrome as a primary source of chronic low back pain. However, there are no more objective criteria of diagnosis. Some practitioners advocate direct or fluoroscopy- or CT-guided injections of depocorticosteroid and local anesthetics into the presumed affected facet joint or around the joint capsule for more definitive diagnosis and specific control of symptoms. However, the joint injection is itself considered the best diagnostic test, and there is no reliable way to predict responders. Otherwise, treatment is as for other forms of chronic low back pain.

Disc-Disruption Syndrome. The annulus fibrosus can tear circumferentially between adjacent fibrous layers without a complete disruption of the structure containing the nucleus pulposus, or it can rupture radially with a disruption of the disc but without prolapse of nuclear material. There may be a history of a twisting or lifting injury, often in a young patient, followed by severe and persistent back pain with radiation to the hip and leg. The examination findings are unremarkable or may show nonspecific, nonradicular signs. Imaging studies may show a small lesion indenting the dural sac but do not show prolapse or root compression. In the past, diagnosis was made by contrast discography, which can demonstrate the annulus tear and reproduce the characteristic pain. MRI may be as accurate, but clearly, it is difficult to correlate MRI abnormalities and the nonspecific symptoms of this syndrome. Conservative management is as for other types of chronic low back pain. Occasionally, such patients will come to surgery for disc removal and interbody fusion.

Piriformis Syndrome. There is controversy about the existence of this syndrome of sciatic entrapment by the tendinous origin of the piriformis muscle. Normally, the sciatic nerve passes just beneath the piriformis muscle as it exits the pelvis through the sciatic notch. In about 6 percent of cadavers, the sciatic nerve passes between the two parts of the tendinous origin of this muscle. Internal rotation of the thigh presses the sciatic nerve against the origin of the muscle. The nerves to the gluteus medius, gluteus minimus, and tensor fascia lata branch off of the sciatic trunk before this crossing. Nerves to all other structures innervated by the sciatic nerve branch after it. Rare cases of symptomatic proximal sciatic compression, presumably due to compression by an inflamed or shortened muscle and tendon, have been reported (Table 226-2). The typical history is of a runner who develops local pain in the gluteus area with radiation into the posterior thigh and lower leg. There might be mild weakness of knee flexion and movements below the knee. Images of the lumbosacral spine reveal no cause. Nerve conduction is normal; however, EMG shows normal lumbar paraspinals, gluteus medius, gluteus minimus, and tensor fascia lata with signs of denervation in the gluteus maximus and all muscles of the leg innervated by the sciatic nerve. This must be distinguished from other causes of proximal sciatic compression. Conservative treatment with anti-inflammatory agents and analgesics should be tried. Operative decompression, removing one of the heads of the muscle, has reportedly been successful (Nakano, 1987; Dawson, 1990).

Postoperative Back Pain. Back pain after spinal surgery, sometimes called the failed back syndrome, can have many causes. Causes amenable to correction by a second operation include (1) those causing root compression, (2) those causing spinal instability, and (3) those due to any prior yet unrecognized surgically responsive lesion. Compression of a spinal root after surgery may be due to retained disc material, especially a lateral disc herniation, recurrent disc herniation, or postoperative scar acting as a mass. Spinal instability may be caused by spondylolisthesis, surgical disruption of joints, or degenerative disease with incompetent ligaments. With careful selection, a small number of patients may benefit from reoperation to address such diagnoses. Nonsurgical causes of postoperative pain include adhesive epidural scar (probably), intraneural scar, arachnoiditis, and, on rare occasions, pseudomeningocele or disc space infection. Unfortunately, the majority of patients with chronic postoperative pain will fall into the category of patients with degenerative disease and chronic low back pain without a discrete medical explanation.

Arachnoiditis. Arachnoiditis refers to adhesive fibrosis of the lumbosacral roots. This usually occurs after some prior inflammatory incitement. Causes include the following:

Meningitis
Trauma
Chemical radiculitis (after subarachnoid injections of contrast, steroids, or other agents)
Postoperative (after hemorrhage, trauma, infection, or the use of hemostatic agents such as Gelfoam)

Modern water-soluble contrast agents are much less likely to cause arachnoiditis than the older oil-based agents. Symptoms usually emerge long after the inciting event. These include low back pain radiating to the buttocks and legs and later weakness and wasting. Examination reveals positive findings from the straight-leg raising test and weakness, atrophy, and diminished deep tendon reflexes in the legs, implicating multiple roots. MRI and CT or myelogram can demonstrate thickening and clumping of the roots of the cauda equina and adherence to the dura. There is no effective treatment. Therefore, efforts should be made to prevent it by using water-soluble contrast agents for myelogram and by careful neurosurgical technique (Jayson 1987).

APPROACH TO THE PATIENT

History

The patient history should include a description of the manner of onset of the pain, whether it can be associated with a particular event such as an injury or whether the onset was gradual and insidious. A description of the character and location of the pain will help to establish whether it is radicular or mechanical. Establishing its time course, whether it is acute, subacute, or chronic or recurrent, and whether it is associated primarily with movement like mechanical back pain, with axial loading and increased intra-abdominal pressure like disc herniation, with extension and walking like that in spinal stenosis, or, perhaps, with quiet rest at night like the pain of malignancy or spinal infection, will all supply clues to its cause. A history of risk factors for low back pain may suggest both a cause and steps in management. Obtaining an occupational history is important to explore risk factors. The major risk factor is occupational lifting. Others are exposure to vibrations caused by machinery or vehicles and cigarette smoking. A psychological profile may establish a context for the problem of chronic low back pain. Such patients are often depressed, anxious, or hypochondriacal and may have Minnesota Multiphasic Personality Inventory profiles suggesting hysteria. Other problems of living, such as alcoholism or divorce, and other medical problems, such as

ulcer disease, may accompany chronic low back pain at a rate greater than otherwise expected. All patients should be questioned about bowel and bladder symptoms since the presence of retention or incontinence will suggest possible disease of the spinal cord, conus, or cauda equina and, if acute, demand prompt evaluation.

This history is relevant to the most common types of back pain. One of the major priorities in the initial evaluation of patients with back and leg pain is to identify those with less common, and especially treatable, causes of pain. Much of this work can be done during history taking by use of a battery of screening questions designed to elicit suspicion for those diseases and disorders listed in Table 226-1. Is there a history of cancer? Metastatic breast cancer, melanoma, and renal cell carcinoma may present years after the original tumor, in which case the patient may not volunteer the old diagnosis without a specific question. Back pain may be a major clue to the initial diagnosis of multiple myeloma. Constitutional symptoms—weight loss, fever, sweats—and local symptoms—cough, urinary and rectal blood—all call for an aggressive search for the cause of the back pain itself and further evaluation into the possibility of cancer. A history of fever, intravenous drug abuse, surgical procedures, and impaired immunity, including diabetes mellitus, should prompt a search for an abscess. Regional infections may also occasionally predispose to epidural abscess formation, as in the diabetic patient with urinary tract infection. Herpes zoster reactivation may cause a persistent back and leg pain before the telltale rash appears. Patients with inflammatory disorders will usually carry the diagnosis of a rheumatic disease or have other characteristic features of the disease in question, such as conjunctivitis and urethritis in Reiter syndrome. Back pain, though present, is rarely the only or primary complaint in those with multiple sclerosis, transverse myelitis, or Guillain-Barré syndrome. Patients should be questioned concerning any congenital or developmental spinal problems. Achondroplasia predisposes to shortened pedicles and congenital spinal stenosis. Scoliosis and other less common congenital spinal disorders may underlie the pain. Patients writhing in pain should raise the suspicion of an intra-abdominal disorder or vascular lesion. A patient with coagulopathy or on anticoagulant therapy should raise suspicion for a possible epidural hematoma. Although the differential diagnosis list is long, the screening history can quickly eliminate most of the diagnoses in most cases and allow a selection of particular features to focus on during the physical examination.

Patient Examination

The examiner goal is finding evidence of a localizing neurologic deficit and of features associated with particular diseases noted above and in Table 226-1. Inspection of the spine for deformities, such as scoliosis, or clues of congenital anomalies, such as tufts of hair and dimples in the sacral region, or features of achondroplasia should take place early in the examination. It is informative to observe the patients walk into the room and to note how they stand. Patients with lumbar and sacral root compression may avoid full weightbearing on the heel of the affected side. Posture should be noted. Flexed posture, for example, is seen in severe lumbar spinal stenosis. Spinal mobility is tested by observing range of motion during extension, flexion, lateral flexion, and rotation. Direct palpation of the spine can identify local areas of concern. In cases of tumor and abscess, tapping each vertebral spine with a reflex hammer may localize the lesion at the tender site. Palpation of the sciatic nerve through the gluteus maximus at the sciatic notch and distally may demonstrate sensitivity in cases of compression. With the patient in the supine position, straight-leg raising is performed with each leg, noting the angle of elevation at which pain and paresthesias arise and their character and location. Lowering the leg to an angle just less than that causing pain and then dorsiflexing the elevated foot may reproduce the pain and help to confirm that it is from sciatic stretch. In acute musculoskeletal pain, any movement may elicit back pain. With root compression, consistent localizing radicular symptoms may emerge with elevation of either leg. Pain on passive extension of the hip and leg with the patient prone is said to suggest benign disease of posterior spinal elements, as opposed to tumor-related pain, which almost always includes the vertebral bodies; however, this sign is not reliable for differentiation. The examiner should inspect muscles for signs of denervation (atrophy, fasciculations). Muscle power testing is done to identify weakness and localize it to a root or to multiple roots as in cauda equina syndrome, to the conus or spinal cord, or to a peripheral nerve, as in femoral or peroneal palsies (see Ch. 102). With root lesions, the tone will be normal or reduced. Spastic tone suggests a lesion at the level of the thoracic bony spine or above. Sensory testing is done to look for dermatomal patterns of loss or signs of isolated neuropathies. Patients with cauda equina syndrome and conus compression may have hyin the perianal area and perineum in addition to the legs. Especially in conus lesions, the saddle hypesthesia tends to occur early. A sensory level is sought on the torso by applying light touch, pinprick, and warm or cold stimuli. If reporting is a problem, an autonomic level can be demonstrated by scratching a line down the torso, looking for an abrupt termination of a normal flare response below the level of a deficit. The ankle jerk (S1) may be lost in L5–S1 herniation. In some patients, a posterior tibial reflex (L5) can be elicited by tapping just posteroinferiorly to the medial malleolus. Asymmetries may occasionally help to localize an L5 lesion. Involvement of the L2–L4 roots may dampen the knee jerk. Hyperreflexia and bilateral signs and extensor plantar responses support a myelopathy. A screening general physical examination should be conducted to seek evidence of such associated disorders as those in Table 226-1.

Further Evaluation and Treatment of Acute Back Pain Without Neurologic Signs or Suspicion of Serious Disease

The great majority of patients without neurologic signs or in whom there is no suspicion of serious disease have a minor, self-limited disorder that will improve without specific treatment. When these patients are young and healthy, no further tests may be necessary. If the patient is older or if there has been significant trauma, plain x-ray should screen for major abnormalities. Many patients are satisfied to receive confident reassurance that there is no major problem and that they should quickly return to full health. Short-term amelioration with non-narcotic analgesic agents, light activity, and physical measures, such as heat or cold application, may be recommended. If rest is recommended, it should be brief, usually no more than 2 days. The management of these patients is discussed in greater detail under the section Lumbosacral Strain and Sprain, above.

Further Evaluation and Treatment of Acute Back Pain With Neurologic Signs or Suspicion of Serious Disease

Minor radicular signs in patients at low risk of other disease may be screened with plain x-ray and managed as described above under the section Acute Disc Herniation. In those with major neurologic deficits, sufficient study should be done promptly to establish a diagnosis. This will allow treatment to be directed to specific remediable lesions. When the history or examination raises the possibility of associated illness—patients with cancer or symptoms raising the question of a new diagnosis of cancer, those with fever, those with coagulation disorders or on anticoagulants—one should pursue an evaluation adequate to uncover potential serious causes of the pain. Tests will be individualized, but at times it will be appropriate to pursue MRI scanning in the absence of neurologic deficits. When cancer is present or suspected, plain x-ray is not sensitive enough to eliminate the diagnosis of bony metastases. Bone scanning or MRI with contrast are both sensitive for such lesions. The issues of spinal metastases are discussed in Chapter 167.

Further Evaluation and Treatment of Chronic Back Pain

The assessment and management of chronic low back pain is complex. All patients should have plain x-rays to look for major bony abnormalities. When instability is suspected, flexion and extension views should be included to look for displacement. If further study is needed, MRI is preferred, since it most easily visualizes both bony and soft tissue structures. This should include gadolinium contrast for those with a history of spinal surgery, those for whom there is a suspicion of tumor or infection, and to better characterize certain lesions seen on prior noncontrast scans. CT scanning substitutes for MRI in those with contraindications or prohibitive claustrophobia—although most patients tolerate MRI if they can be safely sedated. CT may surpass MRI in visualizing bony lesions due to trauma or other bony abnormalities. As noted above, asymptomatic patients have many abnormalities on imaging studies of all kinds; therefore, care must be taken to correlate images with symptoms and signs. EMG may help to clarify questionable findings on the neurologic examination.

When surgically correctable causes are identified, treatment may be relatively straightforward. Orthopaedic or neurosurgical consultation should also be obtained when there is doubt about the need for surgery, further work-up, or the indications for and proper use of further therapies, such as bracing. For the large majority of patients without surgical lesions, a constructive, multidisciplinary approach should emphasize functional recovery using non-narcotic analgesics and pain-modulating medications (e.g., tricyclic agents), exercise, nutrition, smoking cessation, education ("back school"), psychological support, and vocational rehabilitation. The services of physical therapists, psychologists, and physicians skilled in the management of chronic pain are invaluable. Several authors have reported significant rates of successful rehabilitation with aggressive programs of exercise and a multidisciplinary attack.

When beginning pharmacologic therapy, it should be made clear that the goal of therapy is functional rehabilitation and that drugs are only a limited part of the therapy program. It should also be emphasized that the drugs are not expected to rid the patient of all pain but to limit it and to aid physical therapy and functional recovery. Available medications include acetaminophen, aspirin, and other nonsteroidal anti-inflammatory analgesics, several medications with unclear mechanisms but commonly referred to as "muscle relaxants," and tricycle antidepressants. Although they may be effective for short-term use in acute back pain and for occasional flares of chronic pain, most authors agree that narcotics have little role in the treatment of chronic low back pain. Nonsteroidal agents may be given as needed or on a time schedule. In general, patients with persistent pain tend to take less medication when a time schedule is established. Acetaminophen use should be limited, owing to its renal and hepatic toxicity. Aspirin and other nonsteroidal agents are limited by their gastrointestinal side effects and, less commonly, by renal side effects. When one agent does not work, it is worthwhile to try another, since patients may respond differently to particular members of this loose class of drugs. The ''muscle relaxants'' include diazepam and other benzodiazepines. These do, in fact, suppress the spinal reflex arc and may truly relieve spasm. However, it may take high and sustained doses to achieve this effect. Since their abuse potential is high, this use is problematic, and their use for back pain and muscle spasm should be strictly short term. Other so-called muscle relaxants are methocarbamol, carisoprodol, and cyclobenzaprine. These all have no establish effect on the spinal reflex arc and do have central sedative effects. These effects may account for any positive responses and certainly cause most of the common side effects. These agents also have abuse potential, and their use should also be short term. Tricyclic agents have antidepressant properties and pain-modulating effects independent of this antidepressant effect. These drugs may be helpful as long-term adjuvant therapy. Many patients will challenge these simple recommendations, and ultimately the therapy of chronic low back pain will require the range of skills needed to treat all chronic pain.

General issues of chronic pain evaluation and management relevant to the care of those with chronic back pain are discussed in detail in Chapters 217 through 219 and 227 through 230.

SUGGESTED READINGS

Boden SD, Davis DO, Dina TS et al: Abnormal magnetic-resonance scans of the lumbar spine in asymptomatic subjects. J Bone Joint Surg [Am] 72: 403, 1990

Dawson DM, Hallet M, Millender LH: Entrapment Neuropathies. pp. 270–4. 2nd Ed. Little, Brown, Boston, 1990

Deyo RA, Diehl AK, Rosenthal M: How many days of bed rest for acute low back pain? A randomized clinical trial. N Engl J Med 315:1064, 1986

Faas A, Chavannes AW, van Eijk JThM, Gubbels JW: A randomized, placebo-controlled trial of exercise therapy in patients with acute low back pain. Spine 18:1388, 1993

Fredrickson BE, Baker D, McHolick WJ et al: The natural history of spondylolysis and spondylolisthesis. J Bone Joint Surg 66A:699, 1984

Frymoyer JW, Rosen JC, Clements J, Pope MH: Psychologic factors in low-back-pain disability. Clin Orthop 195:178, 1985

Frymoyer JW: Back Pain and sciatica. N Engl J Med 318:291, 1988

Hadler MN: Regional back pain. N Engl J Med 315:1090 1986

Hitselberger WE, Witten RM: Abnormal myelograms in asymptomatic patients. J Neurosurg 28:204, 1968

Long DM: Failed back syndrome. Neurosurg Clin 2:899, 1991

Mayer TG, Gatchel RJ, Kishino N et al: Objective assessment of spine function following industrial injury: a prospective study with comparison group and one-year follow-up. Spine 10:482, 1985

Mooney V: Facet joint syndrome. In Jayson MIV (ed): The Lumbar Spine and Back Pain. 3rd Ed. Churchill Livingstone, Edinburgh, 1987

Jensen MC, Brant-Zawadzki MN, Obuchowski N et al: Magnetic resonance imaging of the lumbar spine in people without back pain. N Engl J Med 331:69, 1994

Kirkwood RJ: Essentials of Neuroimaging. pp. 393–5. Churchill Livingstone, New York, 1990

Loeser JD, Volinn E: Epidemiology of low back pain. Neurosurg Clin 2:713, 1991

Malmivaara A, Häkkinen U, Aro T et al: The treatment of acute low back pain—bed rest, exercises, or ordinary activity? N Engl J Med 332:351, 1995

Meyerding: Spondylolisthesis. Surg Gynae Obst 54:371, 1932

Mooney V, Robertson J: The facet syndrome. Clin Orthop 115:149, 1976

Nachemson AL: Instability of the lumbar spine: pathology, treatment, and clinical evaluation. Neurosurg Clin 2:785, 1991

Nakano KK: Sciatic nerve entrapment: the piriformis syndrome. J Musculoskeletal Med 4:33, 1987

Pyhtinen J, Lähde S, Tanska E-L, Laitinen J: Computed tomography after lumbar myelography in lower back and extremity syndromes. Diagn Imag 52:19, 1983

Rothman RH: A study of computer-assisted tomography: Introduction. Spine 9:548, 1984

Scham SM, Taylor TKF: Tension signs in lumbar disc prolapse. Clin Orthop 75:195, 1971

Stankovic R, Johnell O: Conservative treatment of acute low-back pain: a prospective randomized trial: McKenzie method of treatment versus patient education in ''mini back school.'' Spine 15:120, 1990

Thomas M, Grant N, Marshall J, Stevens J: Surgical treatment of low backache and sciatica. Lancet 2:1437, 1983

Troup JDG: Straight-leg raising (SLR) and the qualifying tests for increased root tension: their predictive value after back and sciatic pain. Spine 6: 526, 1981

Waddell G: Low back disability: a syndrome of western civilization. Neurosurg Clin 2:719, 1991

Waddell G, McCulloch JA, Kummel E, Wenner RM: Nonorganic physical signs in low-back-pain. Spine. 5:117, 1980

Weber H: Lumbar disc herniation: a controlled prospective study with ten years of observation. Spine 8:131, 1983

Weber H: Lumbar disc herniation: a prospective study of prognostic factors including a controlled trial. Part I. J Oslo City Hosp 28:33, 1978

Wiesel SW, Cuckler JM, Deluca F et al: Acute low-back pain: an objective analysis of conservative therapy. Spine 5:324, 1980

Wiesel SW, Tsourmas N, Feffer HI et al: A study of computer-assisted tomography. I. The incidence of positive CAT scans in an asymptomatic group of patients. Spine 9:549, 1984

Wiltse LL, Newman PH, Macnab I: Classification of spondylolisthesis and spondylolysis. Clin Orthop 117:23, 1976

SECTION 7. TREATMENT OF PAIN

227. PHARMACOLOGIC (ANALGESIC) TREATMENT OF PAIN

GILBERT J. FANCIULLO

Analgesic therapy includes pharmacologic prescription of opioids; nonsteroidal anti-inflammatory drugs (NSAIDs); and neuropsychiatric, adjunctive, and other analgesic drugs. The use of these drugs results in greater benefit if the psychosocial and behavioral components of pain are addressed. The emphasis on pharmacologic therapy is based on the familiar model of diagnosis and treatment of acute disease and relies on drug prescription as a major strategy. When painful conditions are treated, drugs are important but psychological and environmental factors are equally consequential. These factors can amplify pain and influence response to therapy and, if ignored, contribute to many failures in treatment that would have been successes had they been considered.

OPIOIDS

Opioids remain the benchmark for effective therapy for moderate and severe pain. The word opium derives from the Greek word for juice. Opium, the juice of the poppy, *Papaver somniferum,* is seldom used today, but its alkaloid extracts and synthetic derivatives are commonly utilized and represent our modern-day opioids. Opiate is a term that describes drugs directly derived from opium. The expression, narcotic, derives from the Greek word for stupor and typically describes agents that are morphinelike and have the capability to produce physical or psychological dependence or addiction. The word opioid refers to any substance produced outside the body that binds specifically to one or more of the subpopulations of receptors that, when occupied, produce at least some morphinelike effects.

Societal and individual prejudices and fear of causing addiction in patients have greatly limited the use of these agents except for acute pain and pain from cancer. The use of opioids for chronic nonmalignant pain remains controversial. The efficacy of long-term opioid use has never been demonstrated. The risk of addiction in patients without a history of alcoholism or drug addiction has been demonstrated to be very slight, in the range of 1 in 3,000 patients. Prescribing these agents can be problematic, and colleagues, pharmacists, nurses, family members, and the patients themselves question their use. Strict limit setting with patients can reduce the number of issues that can develop in patients receiving chronic opioid therapy. A controlled-substance agreement (Fig. 227-1) can be helpful in management and assist physicians and patients who may be benefiting only marginally or not at all from opioid therapy. Pain and activity levels should be well documented both before and during opioid use to determine efficacy.

Opioids act as agonists at stereospecific receptor sites in the brain, spinal cord, and other tissue localities. Opioids mimic the action of endogenous morphinelike substances (endorphins), activating pain-modulating pathways. It appears that opioid side effects result from binding to receptors different from those that produce analgesia. It is likely that opioids will be developed that are specific for analgesia, and many of the side effects will become of historical interest only. Opioid agonists bind to μ receptors, which results in supraspinal and intense analgesia. Agonist-antagonists are agonists at κ receptors, which produce analgesia to a ceiling, at which point increased doses do not produce greater analgesia. They are antagonists at μ receptors and can precipitate withdrawal in patients dependent on opioid agonists. Activation of κ receptors results in little or no respiratory depression. The δ receptors modulate μ receptors. The σ receptor activation results in psychotomimetic side effects such as dysphoria and hallucinations. Agonist-antagonist agents are potent σ agonists.

Naloxone is a pure opioid antagonist. It is most potent as a μ receptor antagonist but also has effects at κ and σ sites. It does not reverse the psychotomimetic σ-mediated effects. Its elimination half-life is 60 to 90 minutes, much shorter than that of morphine. If used to treat an opioid overdose, a naloxone drip is often necessary. It is usually possible to titrate the reversal of the respiratory depression effect while still maintaining analgesia.

Opioid Agonists

Opioid agonists (Table 227-1) include morphine, meperidine, hydromorphone, oxycodone, hydrocodone, methadone, fentanyl, codeine, and propoxyphene. Agonists that are not discussed in this chapter include alfentanil and sufentanil. Opioid agonists particularly suitable for chronic pain because of their longer duration of action include methadone, fentanyl transdermal, and continuous-release morphine preparations. Because of more sustained serum levels, around-the-clock dosing schedules are almost always more advantageous than as needed dosing

Morphine. Morphine was isolated from opium and named after the god of dreams, Morpheus, in 1803. It is the prototypic opioid agonist against which all others are compared. Morphine produces analgesia, sedation, and euphoria. It can also produce nausea, vomiting, pruritus (often around the nose), constipation, lightheadedness, dysphoria, respiratory depression, and feelings of warmth of the body and heaviness of the extremities. Morphine is well absorbed after intramuscular injection with onset of action in 15 minutes and a peak effect in 45 to 90 minutes. Intravenous administration results in peak activity in approximately 20 minutes. The intravenous route is always preferred over the intramuscular route, both for patient comfort and pharmacokinetic reasons. The peak effect of intramuscular morphine often occurs when no one is nearby to observe the patient.

Morphine is metabolized in the liver and kidneys, and metabolites are eliminated in the urine. Principal metabolites include morphine-6-glucuronide (M-6-G) and morphine-3-glucuron-

Pain Management Center
Patient Controlled Substance Agreement
Informed Consent Form

The following agreement relates to my use of controlled substances for chronic pain prescribed by a physician at the Pain Management Center at Holy Name Hospital. I recognize that there are policies regarding the use of controlled substances which are followed by the staff at the Pain Management Center. I will be provided controlled substances while actively participating in this program only if I adhere to the following regulations:

1. I will use the substances only within the parameters given by the medical physician.

2. I will not receive replacement medications for "lost" or "stolen" medications.

3. I will receive controlled substances only from the Holy Name Hospital pain staff. Information that I have been receiving other controlled substances not prescribed by other than at the Pain Management Center may lead to a discontinuation of treatment.

4. I will not expect to receive additional medication prior to the time of my next scheduled refill, even if my prescription runs out.

5. I will not request that "brand name medically necessary" be written on my prescription, nor will I request split prescriptions.

6. If it appears that there are no demonstrable benefits to my daily function or quality of life from the controlled substance, I will gradually taper my medication as prescribed by the physician. I will not hold any member of the Pain Management Center liable for problems caused by discontinuance of controlled substances, provided that I receive 30 days notice of termination.

7. I agree to submit to urine and blood screens to detect the use of non-prescribed medications at any time.

8. I recognized that my chronic pain represents a complex problem which may benefit from physical therapy, psychotherapy and behavioral medicine strategies. I also recognize that my active participation in the management of my pain is extremely important. I agree to actively participate in all aspects in the Pain Management Program to secure increased functioning and improve coping with my conditon.

_____

Patient Signature   Date

_____

Physician Signature   Date

_____

Family Member or Significant Other Signature   Date

FIG. 227-1.   An example of a patient's controlled-substance agreement.

ide, which is pharmacologically inactive. M-6-G produces analgesia, respiratory depression, and sedation. In patients with normal renal function, the ratio of M-6-G to morphine may be as high as 10:1 within 90 minutes. In patients with impaired renal function, this ratio rises to 45:1. Elimination of morphine glucuronides, is delayed in patients with impaired renal function, and unexpected sedation and respiratory depression may result from low doses. Unexplained sedation and respiratory depression in patients with deteriorating renal function who are receiving stable doses of morphine may also be attributable to accumulation of morphine metabolites. Morphine is a poor choice for analgesia in patients with impaired renal function. Despite the complicated pharmacokinetics, morphine is well tolerated in patients with impaired hepatic function.

The elimination half-time is 114 minutes. Elderly patients have higher plasma concentrations of morphine owing to delayed metabolism and excretion. Elderly patients have also been shown to be more sensitive to morphine than younger patients. There is at least a fivefold variation in requirement for morphine in any age group, and this variation is not readily predictable

TABLE 227-1. Opioid Analgesic in Opioid-Naive Patients Weighing Greater Than 50 kg and Less Than 60 Years of Age

Drug (Brand Name Examples)	Equianalgesic Dose		Starting Dose for Moderate to Severe Pain	
	Oral	Parenteral	Oral	Parenteral
Opioid agonists				
Morphine	30 mg q3–4h	10 mg q3–4h	15–30 mg q3–4h	10 mg q3–4h
Morphine, controlled release (MS Contin, Oramorph)	90–120 mg q12h	N/A	30–120 mg q12h	N/A
Hydromorphone (Dilaudid)	7.5 mg q3–4h	1.5 mg q3–4h	2–6 mg q3–4h	1.5 mg q3–4h
Levorphanol (Levo-Dromoran)	4 mg q6–8h	2 mg q6–8h	4 mg q6–8h	2 mg q6–8h
Meperidine (Demerol)	300 mg q2–3h	100 mg q3–4h	N/R	100 mg q3–4h
Methadone (Dolophine)	20 mg q6–8h	10 mg q6–8h	20 mg q6–8h	10 mg q6–8h
Oxymorphone (Numorphan)	N/A	1 mg q3–4h	N/A	1 mg q3–4h
Opioid-NSAID combinations				
Codeine (with aspirin or acetaminophen)	180–200 mg q3–4h	130 mg q3–4h	60 mg q3–4h	60 mg q2h (IM or SC)
Hydrocodone (in Lorcet, Lortab, Vicodin)	30 mg q3–4h	N/A	10 mg q3–4h	N/A
Oxycodone (Percocet, Percodan, Tylox, Roxicodone)	30 mg q3–4h	N/A	10 mg q3–4h	N/A

Abbreviation: N/A, not applicable.

based on weight or other factors. Dosages of morphine and other opioids should be individualized.

Side effects described for morphine also apply to other opioid agonists, although there may be differences in incidence or magnitude. These differences are pointed out in reference to individual drugs.

All opioid agonists produce dose-dependent depression of ventilation. Respiratory depression is via depression of medullary and pontine centers that regulate the responsiveness to carbon dioxide and centers that regulate the rhythm of breathing. This can result in a shift of the carbon dioxide response curve to the right with an elevation in resting partial arterial carbon dioxide pressure and prolonged pauses between breaths or periodic breathing. It can also result in increased respiratory rate and a decrease in tidal volume with an overall decrease in minute ventilation. High doses of opioids result in apnea. Patients often remain conscious and will breath if asked to do so. Pain stimulates patients to breath, and patients who are complaining of pain are unlikely to have significant respiratory depression. Death from opioids is a result of respiratory depression.

Morphine can cause the release of histamine and result in hypotension owing to histamine-induced vasodilation. Administration of 1 mg/kg of intravenous morphine over 10 minutes results in a significant decrease in systemic vascular resistance and blood pressure. Supine, euvolemic patients who receive analgesic doses of morphine are at low risk for development of hypotension. Morphine does not increase the incidence of arrhythmias as long as normocarbia and oxygen saturation are maintained. Analgesic doses of opioids do not cause myocardial depression or bradycardia.

Morphine should be used with caution in patients with head injury because of miosis and the decrease in wakefulness associated with its use and the risk of respiratory depression with subsequent rise in CO_2 levels.

Opioids increase intrabiliary pressure and can cause biliary colic. The pain of opioid-induced biliary colic is reversible with naloxone, glucagon, or nitroglycerin. The pain of angina pectoris is reversible only with nitroglycerin and not glucagon or naloxone. Meperidine may increase intrabiliary pressure to a lesser extent than morphine, but all opioid agonists increase intrabiliary pressure.

Opioids impair peristalsis and increase sphincter pressure in the gastrointestinal tract, causing constipation. Tolerence to constipation does not occur. Senna compound (Senokot) is a colon-specific agent that stimulates Auerbach's plexus, increasing peristalsis. It directly antagonizes the constipating effects

of opioids and, used on a regular basis, prevents opioid-induced constipation.

Morphine can cause nausea and vomiting that is often dose related and eliminated by decreasing doses. This effect seems to be drug specific and can be eliminated by changing to another opioid agonist. Morphine can cause urinary retention by increasing the tone of the vesicle sphincter, particularly in older men or men with prostatic hypertrophy. Opioids are not teratogenic, but hypercarbia is. Pregnant patients should be watched carefully when receiving opioids, particularly during organogenesis. The respiratory depressant effect of morphine and other opioids can be augmented by combination with benzodiazepines, phenothiazines, and antidepressants.

Morphine is available for parenteral administration and as an elixir, a suppository, an immediate-release form, and a sustained-release form.

Meperidine. Meperidine is one-tenth as potent as morphine. It was developed as an atropinic agent and has many properties more similar to atropine than to opioids. It is the only opioid to cause mydriasis. It increases the heart rate at increased doses rather than decreases it, as other opioids do. Meperidine can lower the seizure threshold in and of itself. Accumulation of normeperidine in patients with impaired renal function has resulted in death in some cases. Meperidine interacts with monoamine oxidase inhibitors and can cause hyperpyrexia, hypertension, and death. Meperidine has an extensive first-pass hepatic effect and is a very poor drug for oral administration. Because of the myriad side effects associated with the use of meperidine, it should be considered an opioid of last resort and used only when other opioid agonists are not tolerated or unavailable. Meperidine is available for parenteral and oral administration.

Hydromorphone. Hydromorphone is eight times as potent as morphine and has a duration of action of only 3 hours. Indications are the same as for morphine. It is available in a parenteral form, as a liquid, and as a suppository.

Oxycodone. Oxycodone is available alone or in many combination preparations with acetaminophen or aspirin. It is equally potent with morphine and is available as a tablet or a solution.

Hydrocodone. There are 41 formulations available in the United States that include hydrocodone. It is a semisynthetic analgesic and antitussive with efficacy similar to that of codeine. It is available in many combination tablet forms and as a syrup.

Methadone. Methadone has an elimination half-life of 35 hours but an analgesic duration of action of only 8 hours by the oral route. This long analgesic duration of action combined with its low cost and efficacy similar to morphine make it an attractive drug for the treatment of chronic pain. Methadone is metabolized in the liver to inactive end products and excreted in the urine and bile. Methadone is available for parenteral administration and as tablets, in a liquid form, and as diskets, which are tablets with insoluble excipients to prevent intravenous use of the tablets.

Fentanyl. Fentanyl is approximately 100 times as potent as morphine and is available in an intravenous form and as a transdermal system. Fentanyl has no metabolically active end products and is excreted in the urine only minimally unchanged. It produces no histamine release even at very high doses. It has a duration of action when administered intravenously in usual doses of only 30 minutes. The transdermal patches are useful in patients who are unable to take tablets and must be changed every 48 to 72 hours.

Codeine. Codeine is a commonly used analgesic and antitussive opioid agonist. There appears to be a ceiling effect on its analgesic properties, thus limiting its usefulness to mild or moderate pain. Maximum analgesia is produced with a dose of 60 mg and is equivalent to 650 mg of aspirin.

Propoxyphene. Propoxyphene is another commonly used opioid with potency similar to aspirin. It is indicated only for mild or moderate pain.

Opioid Agonist-Antagonists

Commonly used opioid agonist-antagonists include pentazocine, butorphanol, nalbuphine, and buprenorphine. Because of their ceiling effect on analgesia and the high incidence of psychotomimetic side effects, these drugs are rarely indicated. They were initially popularized by the belief that they were not addictive. This has been repeatedly disproved. Intranasal butorphanol may be useful because of its unique route of administration.

NONSTEROIDAL ANTI-INFLAMMATORY DRUGS

NSAIDs have been used for hundreds of years (Table 227-2). The bark of the willow tree was described as a treatment for rheumatism as long ago as 1763 and is still available in health food stores. NSAIDs produce analgesia, antipyrexia, and anti-inflammatory effects by the inhibition of cyclo-oxygenase and a decrease in the production of prostaglandins. There is interpatient variability in efficacy of NSAIDs. Treatment failure with one agent does not eliminate the entire group of drugs as potentially beneficial. Failure with a trial of three agents should eliminate NSAIDs as an efficacious class of drugs. Most patients who use opioids can benefit from concomitant use of a NSAID, and this in fact is recommended by many authorities. There are 24 available NSAIDs in the United States, and they should be selected based on their unique properties and side effect profiles.

NSAIDs represent the most commonly prescribed drugs in the United States. They are the most common cause of gastric mucosal abnormalities. NSAIDs decrease the production of gastric mucus, which is prostaglandin dependent. The mucosa is thus more sensitive to gastric acid; this can result in a very characteristic pattern of gastric erosion. H_2 blockers do not prevent gastric erosion because the problem is not with gastric acid but with loss of the protective mucosal layer. Misoprostol is a prostaglandin analogue that maintains the mucous layer and may provide prophylaxis against NSAID-induced ulceration and erosion. Nabumetone, compared with aspirin and naproxen, has been shown to have a lower incidence of gastropathy. Choline magnesium trisalicylate may also have a reduced incidence of gastric erosion.

NSAIDs prolong bleeding time and should be used with caution in patients at increased risk of bleeding. Aspirin irreversibly inhibits platelet aggregation and can prolong bleeding time for up to 11 days, the life of the platelet. Nonaspirin NSAIDs reversibly inhibit platelet aggregation. Ibuprofen, for example, prolongs bleeding time for approximately five half-lives. The half-life of ibuprofen is approximately 5 hours. Platelet aggregation is inhibited 25 hours after stopping ibuprofen. Choline magnesium trisalicylate may have less of an effect on inhibition of platelet aggregation than other NSAIDs and may be a logical choice when bleeding is a risk but an NSAID is indicated.

Choline magnesium trisalicylate is available as an oral suspension, as is ibuprofen, indomethacin, and naproxen. Indomethacin is the only NSAID available as a suppository. Only indomethacin and ketorolac are available in a parenteral formulation. Intravenous indomethacin is associated with a high incidence of gastropathy and nephropathy in infants and is not used often as an analgesic. Indomethacin is predominantly an anti-inflammatory agent with less activity as an analgesic. It may be useful to use a low dose (25 mg) of indomethacin at bedtime to prevent early morning stiffness and pain.

Ketorolac has a side effect profile similar to other NSAIDs and is the only NSAID indicated for moderate to severe pain. Parenteral ketorolac when used for more than 5 days is associated with an increased incidence of gastropathy. Duration of therapy greater than 14 days with the oral form is also associated with an increased incidence of gastropathy. One-half the usual dose of parenteral ketorolac should be used in persons over the age of 65 years, less then 50 kg in weight, or with impaired renal function.

NSAIDs cause elevation of hepatic transaminases in 15 percent of patients. The risk associated with "idiopathic transaminasemia" is unknown, but, when noted, the drug should be stopped. Another agent can be instituted. Some authorities recommend routine testing of transaminases at 8 and 24 weeks after starting a NSAID. Acute hepatic necrosis has been reported rarely with the use of NSAIDs.

NSAIDs can cause nephrotoxicity by a variety of mechanisms. Papillary necrosis, interstitial nephritis, and the nephrotic syndrome have all been reported. Renal damage is usually reversible if detected in time and the drug is discontinued. Urinalysis to detect protein is the best single screening test for NSAID-induced nephropathy. Sulindac may be associated with a decreased risk of nephropathy, although this is controversial.

Allergy to NSAIDs is rare, but manifestations can be severe. Patients with the triad of asthma, nasal polyposis, and aspirin hypersensitivity are at high risk of manifesting anaphylactoid reactions to other NSAIDs. Patients who are allergic to aspirin may cross react to all other NSAIDs.

Phenylbutazone is a potent anti-inflammatory agent that is

TABLE 227-2. Oral Doses of Nonsteroidal Anti-Inflammatory Drugs

Generic Name	Trade Name	Dosing Schedule	Recommended Starting Dose (mg/d)	Recommended Maximum Dose (mg/d)
Acetaminophen	Tylenol, Datril, Panadol	q4–6h	2,600	6,000
Aspirin	Bayer	q4–6h	2,600	6,000
Choline magnesium trisalicylate	Trilisate	q8–12h	1,500	4,000
Diclofenac	Voltaren	q6–12h	75	200
Diflunisal	Dolobid, Dolobis	q12h	1,000	15,000
Etodolac	Lodine	q6–8h	800	1,200
Fenoprofen	Nalfon	q6h	800	3,200
Flurbiprofen	Ansaid	q8–12h	100	300
Ibuprofen	Motrin, Advil, Nuprin	q4–8h	1,200	4,200
Indomethacin	Indocin	q8–12h	75	200
Ketoprofen	Orudis	q6–8h	150	300
Ketorolac	Toradol	q6h	40	40
Meclofenamate	Meclomen	q6–8h	150	400
Mefenamic acid	Ponstel	q6–8h	400	1,000
Nabumetone	Relafen	q24h	1,000	2,000
Naproxen	Aleve, Naprosyn	q12h	500	1,000
Oxaprozin	Daypro	q24h	1,200	1,800
Phenylbutazone	Butazolidin	q6–8h	300	400
Piroxicam	Feldene	q24h	20	40
Salsalate	Disalcid	q8–12h	1,500	4,000
Sulindac	Clinoril	q12h	300	400
Tolmetin	Tolectin	q6–8h	600	2,000

useful in the treatment of acute gout and rheumatoid arthritis. Because of the frequent occurrence of anemia and agranulocytosis, phenylbutazone use should be limited to 7 days.

Phenacetin and its active metabolite acetaminophen may have some anti-inflammatory activity and may be classified as NSAIDs. They do have antipyretic and analgesic properties. They do not produce gastric irritation, platelet inhibition, or bleeding abnormalities. Phenacetin may cause hemolytic anemia and methemoglobinemia in patients with glucose-6-phosphate deficiency.

Piroxicam is a frequently used drug owing largely to its long duration of action, enabling once-a-day administration. Other once-a-day agents include nabumetone and oxaprozin. Diclofenac is unique in that it accumulates in bone and synovial fluid to an extent that may be greater than that of other NSAIDs. It is a potent analgesic and is used three times a day. An association between diclofenac and acute hepatic necrosis has limited its use. There is probably no greater risk of hepatic necrosis with diclofenac than with any other NSAID; however, transaminase levels should be checked periodically when using this drug.

The properties of all 24 NSAIDs cannot be enumerated or compared in this short chapter. Clinicians treating pain should familiarize themselves with half a dozen or so of these agents, know them well, and be able to use them interchangeably.

NEUROPSYCHIATRIC DRUGS

Antiepileptics

Antiepileptic drugs are discussed only briefly in this chapter. The effective analgesic doses are not known, and therefore these drugs should be dosed as if epilepsy were being treated. These drugs are most useful in the treatment of neuropathic pain, particularly if there is a shooting, electrical, or lancinating component. They may also add efficacy when combined with antidepressants to treat the burning or dysesthetic components of

neuropathic pain. Most investigation has been with carbamazepine, but there is work also with phenytoin and valproic acid. Clonazepam is becoming more widely used because of its advantageous side effect profile. The use of these agents in the treatment of specific diseases such as trigeminal neuralgia is discussed elsewhere in this text.

Tricyclic Antidepressants and Related Drugs

Antidepressants are the treatment of first choice for burning pain (Table 227-3). There are data to suggest analgesic onset within hours of administration to healthy volunteers in a model of acute pain and also data that suggest a delay of analgesic efficacy for as long as 2 weeks in patients with diabetic neuropathy. Nortriptyline is the demethylated derivative of amitriptyline, and desipramine is the principal metabolite of imipramine. Trazodone, fluoxetine, sertraline, and paroxetine are structurally unrelated to the tricyclics and tetracyclics. The analgesically useful mechanism of action of these agents is the same as

TABLE 227-3. Trade Name and Dose Range of Antidepressant Medications Possibly Useful in Neuropathic Pain[a]

Generic Name	Trade Name	Dose Range
Amitriptyline	Elavil, Endep	10–300
Desipramine	Norpramine	20–300
Imipramine	Tufranil	75–300
Nortriptyline	Pamelor	50–100
Trazodone	Desyrel	50–600
Fluoxetine	Prozac	20–40
Paroxetine	Paxil	20–50
Sertraline	Zoloft	50–150

[a] Values listed reflect the range between the minimum and maximum recommended doses for the treatment of depression. When used to treat pain, the usual effective dose is in the lower end of the spectrum, with initial doses often being the lowest possible dose.

TABLE 227-4. Side Effect[a] Profiles of Antidepressant Medications

Drug	Anticholinergic	Sedation	Orthostatic Hypotension	Cardiac Arrhythmia	Weight Gain
Amitriptyline	4	4	4	3	4
Desipramine	1	1	2	2	1
Imipramine	3	3	4	3	3
Nortriptyline	1	1	2	2	1
Trazodone	0	4	1	1	1
Fluoxetine	0	0	0	0	0
Paroxetine	0	0	0	0	0
Sertraline	0	0	0	0	0

[a] 0, absent; 2, moderate; 4, common.

for the tricyclics and is the potentiation of the biogenic amines norepinephrine and serotonin. These amines are neurotransmitters in pain-modulating pathways.

Side effects with these agents are frequent and are manifested as either anticholinergic, cardiovascular, or sedating (Table 227-4). Salutary effects of these drugs include not only analgesia but also a restoration of disrupted sleeping patterns. Increase in appetite is usual with amitriptyline, nortriptyline, desipramine, and imipramine. Decrease in appetite is characteristic of fluoxetine, sertraline, and paroxetine. Bupropion is not considered an analgesic because of its nonserotonergic and non-noradrenergic mechanism of action.

Anticholinergic side effects are manifested as dry mouth, blurred vision, tachycardia, constipation, memory impairment, urinary retention, and delayed gastric emptying. Fluoxetine, sertraline, and paroxetine have only very slight if any anticholinergic effects and are usually alerting as opposed to sedating. These agents have half-lives ranging from 21 to 72 hours and can be given once a day. Trazodone is extremely sedating but has a very low anticholinergic profile. It has no effect on norepinephrine, and there is some question of whether trazodone has analgesic properties at all. Of amitriptyline, nortriptyline, desipramine, and imipramine, the agent with the stongest anticholinergic profile is amitriptyline, and the weakest is desipramine. Amitriptyline is the most sedating of these drugs, and imipramine and desipramine are less sedating. Tolerance to the anticholinergic and sedating side effects of these drugs frequently occurs.

Orthostatic hypotension and tachycardia are the most common cardiovascular side effects of these drugs. Prolongations of the Q-T or P-R intervals have unknown significance in the absence of overdose. Amitriptyline, nortriptyline, desipramine, and imipramine should be used with caution in patients with prolonged conduction times or heart block and with great caution in patients receiving type 1 antiarrhythmics such as quinidine. Fluoxetine, sertraline, and paroxetine are not associated with postural hypotension, conduction system abnormalities, or anticholinergic effects. There are no clinically significant changes in the electrocardiogram in patients treated with these agents.

ADJUNCTIVE AND OTHER ANALGESICS

Dextroamphetamine and methylphenidate are useful agents to decrease sedation associated with high doses of opioids (Table

TABLE 227-5. Miscellaneous Analgesic Drugs

Generic Name	Trade Name	Dose Range
Mexiletine	Mexitil	600–900 mg/day
Dextroamphetamine	Dexedrine	5–20 mg q6–12h
Methylphenidate	Ritalin	5–20 mg bid

227-5). They are structurally related to central nervous system stimulants. They may enhance the analgesia produced by concomitantly administered opioids. Methylphenidate has been shown to eliminate the cognitive dysfunction associated with fluctuating doses of opioids in patients with cancer pain. Dosing is typically at 7 AM and 2 PM, thus enabling the patient to sleep during the night.

Mexiletine is a class 1B antidysrhthmic, which is a lidocaine analogue and may be useful in the treatment of neuropathic pain.

Capsaicin cream is an extract of the seeds and membranes of certain species of plants of the nightshade family. Capsaicin stimulates and then blocks nociceptive sensory afferents from the skin and mucous membranes that contain substance P, somatostatin, and calcitonin gene-related peptide. These fibers have been implicated in mediating cutaneous pain and pathologic itch. The basis of capsaicin's action is its ability to enhance the release of substance P and prevent its reaccumulation in these fibers. Several studies have demonstrated success in relieving postherpetic neuralgia and pain associated with peripheral neuropathy.

EMLA cream is an eutectic mixture of local anesthetics, lidocaine and prilocaine, with a boiling point less than either drug individually. This accounts for its ability to be absorbed and provide analgesia also for peripheral neuropathic pain or postherpetic neuralgia.

CONCLUSIONS

Successful treatment of both acute and chronic pain requires a commitment to understanding the nature of the patient's pain and the psychosocial and environmental history. Selection of an agent within a group is often possible, but trial-and-error approaches are often necessary. The patient should be warned that it may take months to develop an optimum regimen and that only rarely will pain be eradicated completely.

SUGGESTED READINGS

Bonica JJ: The Management of Pain. 2nd Ed. Lea & Febiger, Philadelphia, 1990

Carr DB, Jacox AK: Acute Pain Management Clinical Practice Guidelines. Publication no. 92-0032. Agency for Health Care Policy and Research, Department of Health and Human Services, Rockville, 1992

Casey KL: Pain and Central Nervous System Disease. Raven Press, New York, 1991

Fields HL: Pain Syndromes in Neurology. Butterworths, London, 1990

Jacox AK, Carr DB: Management of Cancer Pain: Clinical Practice Guidelines. Publication no. 94-0592. Agency for Health Care Policy and Research, Department of Health and Human Services, Rockville, 1994

Mann RD: The History of the Management of Pain. Parthenon Publishing, Carnforth, 1988.

Patt RB: Cancer Pain. JB Lippincott, Philadelphia, 1993

Turk DC, Melzack R: Handbook of Pain Assessment. Guilford Press, New York, 1992

Wall PD, Melzack R: Textbook of Pain. 3rd Ed. Churchill Livingstone, Edinburgh, 1994

228. PHYSICAL THERAPY AND TRANSCUTANEOUS NERVE STIMULATION

NATHANIEL KATZ
SUSAN LAVIOLETTE

In the first author's experience, the most useful consultant in the management of chronic pain is the physical therapist (PT) (with the psychologist a close second). Once diagnostic imperatives have been excluded, most patients are diagnosed with musculoskeletal pain syndromes, the conservative treatment of which may be most effectively carried out by the PT. The PT provides an array of services:

1. Diagnostic assessment of the patient's condition and function
2. Treatment of specific conditions
3. Symptomatic reduction of pain
4. Patient education
5. Restoration of function

Occupational therapists (OTs) also carry out these functions, and distinguishing between PT and OT services can be confusing. Generally, OTs train patients to carry out their activities of daily living, including their jobs and therefore focus on the upper extremities. In practice, differences between PTs and OTs depend to a great extent on individual interest, referral patterns, and the community setting. For the purposes of this chapter, the term *PT* is understood to include the activities of the OT, recognizing the potential disservice of this oversimplification.

For specific presenting complaints, the PT can provide a diagnostic opinion and treat with the goal of cure. Treatments offered include passive modalities, (treatments performed by the therapist on a passive patient) and active treatments performed by the patient under the therapist's guidance, such as exercise and relaxation techniques. For patients whose disease process may not be curable, such as those patients with fibromyalgia, the therapist provides patient education in self-management techniques, including home pain-control strategies, pacing, proper body mechanics and posture, general or regional conditioning, and the use of aids or special techniques to maximize function. Methods for symptomatic reduction of pain are offered. In patients with specific functional goals, such as achievements in work or athletics, the PT may perform a functional capacity assessment, in order to provide rational recommendations for return to activity, for modifications of activity, or for a tailored functional restoration program designed to achieve specific realistic goals.

The following sections elaborate on the above points with the goal of helping the physician maximize the effectiveness of a relationship with the PT.

DIAGNOSTIC ASSESSMENT

The PT is trained to perform in-depth musculoskeletal assessment. Sprains, myofascial pain, tendonitis, bursitis, facet joint syndromes, and other such entities can pose diagnostic dilemmas to the neurologist or medical physician that the PT can often clarify. These syndromes often have underlying causes, such as poor posture, a suboptimal work station, repetitive strain, or inadequate strength of a group of muscles to meet their demand. These predisposing biomechanical factors are often overlooked by the physician, resulting in recurrence of symptoms after "successful" treatment. For example, trochanteric bursitis may result from tightness of the tensor fascia lata muscle; injection of the bursa will temporarily correct the problem, only to be followed inevitably by recurrence until the underlying muscle problem is addressed.

Along with many others, the senior author (N.K.) has acknowledged for some time the existence of a group of musculoskeletal disorders, recognized and treated by osteopaths, chiropractors, and manually trained PTs, for which there is scant language or acceptance in the orthodox medical community. Examples include misalignment of the joints of the spine, "subluxations," and a variety of soft-tissue syndromes. Such syndromes may be classified under the rubric of "manual medicine." Whereas orthodox physicians may dispute the existence of these syndromes and the hypotheses offered to explain symptoms, the manually trained PT can help recognize such syndromes and discuss them in a language acceptable to physicians.

In addition to diagnosing the patient's condition, the PT is enormously useful in diagnosing the patient's function. Functional assessment, although addressed in some way by all PTs, has evolved into a full subspecialty. The PT can compare the patient's present functional abilities to those required by his or her employment, sport, or demands at home, set reasonable goals, and guide the patient through a functional restoration program, designed to achieve those goals. Such assessments and programs are particularly useful in the patient with a work-related injury or disability. Formal functional capacity assessment documents the patient's abilities at the time of the assessment. The physician can use this information to make rational and consistent recommendations regarding return to work or other activities, which among other advantages reduces the liability of returning an injured worker to the job.

In summary, referral to the PT for diagnostic assessment is most useful when the patient suffers from a musculoskeletal disorder the exact nature of which is unclear, when underlying biomechanical predisposing factors may exist, and when functional assessment and goal setting are important, such as in the injured worker.

PASSIVE TREATMENT MODALITIES

Modalities are defined as passive treatments performed by the PT on the patient. In general the PT applies treatment modalities to aid in the recovery from acute injury, to reduce pain during the initiation phase of an active exercise program and to prevent or reduce exacerbations produced by individual exercise sessions. Modalities alone are frowned upon in the chronic pain setting, as they do not contribute to resolution of the painful disorder, do not resolve deconditioning, do not restore function, are not logically time-limited, and promote further dependence of the patient on the health-care provider. We have been frustrated numerous times by the patient who has exhausted insurance physical therapy benefits on a useless course of passive modalities, only to be denied potentially effective therapy when properly evaluated. The common passive modalities are described below.

Ice

Little scientific data exist to determine whether ice or heat is preferable. Ice is preferred in acute injuries because it decreases inflammation, swelling, and muscle spasm; heat worsens inflammatory injury. Ice is also helpful in chronic pain, especially after activity or during flare-ups. The analgesic effect of ice appears to last longer than that of heat. The benefits of ice are thought to derive from vasoconstriction, decreased nerve conduction velocity, a counterirritant effect, decreased vascular permeability and leukocyte activity, and decreased muscle spindle activity leading to reduced muscle spasm. Ice may be applied via a variety of commercially available cold packs, immersion in ice water, or application of an ice stick. Perhaps the major advantage of ice is that patients can be taught to apply it at home with minimal expense or difficulty. Relative contraindications include vascular insufficiency, anesthetic skin, vasospastic disorders, and poorly healing wounds.

Heat

Heat application is one of the oldest treatments for pain. Benefits include improved tissue circulation, relief of muscle spasm, analgesia, and increased flexibility of muscle and connective tissue. Heat is generally used prior to exercise to increase flexibility of tight muscles and stiff joints and for flare-ups of pain. Relative contraindications include acute injury (to avoid increased swelling), cardiorespiratory failure (due to the increased cardiac output when much of the body is warmed), circulatory compromise, sensory impairment or obtundation, and multiple sclerosis. Numerous methods for applying heat have been developed. Hot packs are simple, effective, and least expensive. The heat remains superficial; thus, the mechanism of relief of muscle spasm is not clear. Hydrocollator packs contain a silicone gel that retains heat for approximately 30 minutes and have similar effects to the heating pad. Electric heating pads are more expensive and must be used with caution, especially if they do not automatically shut off. An extremity can be dipped in a hot paraffin bath, which coats the limb with hot paraffin wax and heats the limb as the wax solidifies and cools. Whirlpools can be used to immerse a limb or the whole body, and to go one step further, exercise can be performed in a heated pool. These treatments are used for patients with widespread joint or muscular involvement, as in rheumatoid arthritis or fibromyalgia. Infrared radiation is used to apply heat, but it heats superficially and probably has no advantage over a hot pack.

Heating of deeper tissues requires one of the following methods. In short-wave diathermy, the patient is placed in an electromagnetic field. The impedance of the patient completes the circuit, causing tissue heating. Muscles may be directly heated using this method. Although in common use and theoretically attractive, the clinical advantages of this method are unclear. In microwave diathermy, the patient is placed in a microwave field, producing deep heating mainly of muscle and subcutaneous tissue. Ultrasound is a popular method that produces deep, localized heat, particularly at the soft tissue–bone interface. It has been found to be particularly useful in bursitis, periarthritic conditions, joint contractures, scar syndromes, and myofascial pain.

Electrotherapy

Electricity has been used since antiquity to treat a variety of ailments. Today electricity may be applied in several different forms. Direct current or galvanic stimulation is used to stimulate muscle contraction to prevent atrophy and speed muscular rehabilitation. Its use for pain is less well documented. Interferential therapy utilizes alternating current. Two pairs of electrodes are situated on the skin and aligned so that the two electric fields intersect at the site of pain. This allows the operator to selectively stimulate and heat deep-tissue structures. Transcutaneous electrical nerve stimulation (TENS) is described below.

Massage

Massage has a long and venerable history in the treatment of pain and as a general health tonic. We have yet to meet anyone who would deny the beneficial and invigorating effects of a massage on mind and body. Massage enhances the flexibility of muscle and connective tissue, improves peripheral circulation, helps restore lymph flow, and can loosen scar or tight connective tissue. Massage can help prepare tissues for active exercise. Long-term regular massage therapy, while pleasurable and temporarily analgesic for many musculoskeletal conditions, like the other passive modalities can lead to a dependence on the part of the patient, and in chronic pain patients, usually does not contribute to enduring symptom resolution. Therefore, massage as sole treatment is generally not appropriate in the management of chronic pain.

Traction

Traction refers to the application of a tonic force to a part of the body to distract soft tissues and joints. Benefits include pain relief, rest, immobilization, restoration of proper alignment, and preparation of tissues for active exercise or manipulation. Sufficient weight and proper angle of pull are important. For cervical traction, weight begins at about 25 lb., applied at an angle of 20 degrees of flexion. Pelvic traction for lumbar pain begins at about 80 lb., at an angle of about 20 degrees of flexion. Studies have demonstrated minimal if any benefit of traction for lumbar pain, but significant benefit for cervical disorders. Home traction units are available. Contraindications include tumor, cord compression, infection, and severe arthritis or osteoporosis.

Immobilization

Rest or splinting of an injured part is probably the oldest treatment for acute injuries, is the first step toward healing of an injured part, and remains a mainstay in the treatment of acute pain. Even in chronic pain, rest and immobilization are useful for acute flare-ups or as part of a pacing regimen when activity increases pain. Immobilization can be achieved by simple rest or by use of supportive devices. For example, judicious use of a cervical collar in patients with chronic neck pain can allow patients to increase their function or to manage activity-induced flare-ups. In the patient with low-back pain, rest after a period of activity constitutes healthy pacing. Supportive devices can be used to allow continued work that would otherwise be impossible, such as the wrist splint for the typist with carpal tunnel syndrome.

Long-term immobilization, however, has caused much misery and disability. Consequences include weakness and atrophy of muscles, deconditioning, joint contractures, and osteoporosis. Prolonged immobilization probably causes a number of chronic pain syndromes, including reflex sympathetic dystrophy and some myofascial pain. For low-back pain, about 2 days of bedrest are probably optimal; more does not help and probably hurts. Therefore rest and immobilization must be prescribed judiciously, usually combined with an active exercise program.

Supportive Devices

The PT can be very helpful in the prescription of supportive devices to reduce pain, improve function, or increase activities of daily living. Examples include canes to improve balance and increase ambulation, back braces to reduce back pain and allow increased activity, and gripping devices to aid in removing bottle tops or manipulating clothing. The cautions mentioned above for immobilization apply.

Manipulation

Manipulation refers to the movement by the therapist of joints or periarticular tissues to restore normal alignment or range of motion. Although strictly a passive modality, manipulation is somewhat different in that resolution of the underlying disorder is the goal. Several types of manipulation are performed, classified according to whether the structure is moved within its normal range, to the end point of its range, or beyond the physiologic range, and, according to the velocity of motion. Different schools train practitioners in different techniques: chiropractic incorporates high-velocity thrusts often accompanied by a snapping sound, osteopathy uses somewhat gentler techniques, and PTs may be trained in a variety of manipulative techniques. Debate on the relative merits of these techniques is imbued with heated argument over philosophical, historical, and economic issues, with little scientific evidence to rely upon. Little can be stated regarding manipulation that would not be disputed by one or another camp. The senior author has found the advice of a PT experienced in manipulation indispensable.

Most authorities and experienced clinicians agree on the following principles. If no improvement is noted after a few (3 to 10) manipulative treatments, treatment should be stopped and reassessed. High-velocity manipulation of the neck is probably dangerous and is best shunned (vertebral artery stroke has resulted). Manipulation without exercises to maintain proper alignment and function is often a sign of an inadequate practitioner. Manipulation is contraindicated in the presence of infection, tumor, fracture, severe osteoporosis, and neural compression.

ACTIVE TREATMENT

Therapeutic exercise is one of the cornerstones of chronic pain management and is indispensable to the restoration of function after acute injuries. During the healing phase of an acute injury, passive range of motion is often prescribed to prevent stiffness and contractures that may impede the rehabilitative process.

During therapy sessions exercise is often preceded and followed by the use of passive modalities. In patients with chronic pain, the goals of exercise are increased range of motion and flexibility, increased strength and endurance, decreased muscle spasm, and improved general conditioning and function. A balance must be maintained between "giving in" to the pain and not exercising sufficiently and overexercising to the point of relapse. Specific exercises to restore particular functions constitute the final phase of rehabilitation prior to return to previous activities. Educating patients to properly pace their exercise programs is one of the major contributions of the PT to the management and rehabilitation of chronic pain. Aerobic fitness seems to decrease pain perception and is often taught, owing to its beneficial effects on the sense of well-being, general health, and psychological health.

The specific exercise regimen prescribed depends upon precise diagnosis and the judgment of the therapist. Whereas much energy has been expended debating the relative merits of different exercise regimens for various conditions, literature demonstrating important differences is scant. Several principles are accepted. Diagnosis must be accurate and should be re-evaluated if the patient does not respond as expected to therapy. Passive modalities alone are not useful. A program will often begin with passive modalities followed by gentle exercises to restore mobility. Such exercises include range of motion, stretching, and isometric strengthening, which are not very painful. However, these exercises do little to restore normal functioning and should be advanced to more natural activities, such as biking, swimming, and walking.

TREATMENT OF SPECIFIC CONDITIONS

Little systematic study has addressed whether these treatments are better than natural history, which treatments are best, what is the most effective or cost-effective manner of applying them or how effectiveness compares with that of other forms of treatment (e.g., medications, injections, and operations). Designing the treatment program is thus left to the judgment of the individual PT, according to principles as outlined above. Treatment programs can be so variable that to state that a patient has already had "physical therapy" without specifying exactly what therapy was performed is equivalent to stating that a patient has already had "medication" for an ailment without specifying which medication.

In general, physical therapy for pain is a short-term proposition. Acute injuries generally resolve rapidly, and the role of the PT is to aid resolution, prevent complications, and educate the patient in a home exercise program, preventive measures, and the use of passive modalities to prevent or treat recurrence. For chronic pain, the goals are to train patients to treat themselves with home modalities, exercises to enhance general conditioning, and exercises to improve the underlying disorder or at least to improve function even if the pain cannot be reduced. In the chronic pain patient, reducing fear of reinjury and enabling the patient to enjoy normal movement is another explicit goal. Many PTs experienced in the treatment of chronic pain also teach relaxation techniques, biofeedback, and other specific treatments.

Arthritis

For acute flare-ups of arthritis pain, short-term immobilization and analgesics are indicated. For subacute or chronic symptoms, a number of modalities are used to provide symptomatic relief and to permit therapeutic exercise. Paraffin, whirlpool, short-wave diathermy, microwave, or ultrasound may be used to heat the tissues. For widespread arthritis, a heated pool is a godsend. Exercises including stretching, strengthening, and general mobilization, and conditioning may be performed during the period of relative comfort following the use of modalities.

Myofascial Pain

The principles of treating myofascial pain are restoring the strength and flexibility of the involved muscles, using passive modalities initially to facilitate exercise, and eliminating underlying factors such as emotional tension or poor posture. Whereas any of the modalities can be used initially, patients graduate to home use of ice or heat. Exercises begin with gentle stretching and general conditioning and progress to include strengthening and aerobic activities. Education to empower the patient to eliminate predisposing factors, including stress, complete the therapy.

Bursitis, Tendonitis

The acute phase of bursitis or tendinitis is treated with ice, immobilization and analgesics. Later, passive modalities, usually ice or heat, are applied, followed by passive and active range-of-motion exercise. Strengthening exercises follow when tolerated, with instruction on proper body mechanics to avoid recurrence of pain.

Back and Neck Pain

Aerobic conditioning, "back school," and stretching and strengthening exercises are the only treatments, other than surgical discectomy, supported by controlled studies on the treatment of low-back pain. The vast majority of cases of acute back or neck pain resolve without medical intervention. Bed rest is appropriate for a few days, followed by remobilization. Passive modalities are useful in this stage for pain relief and to allow mobilization. The patient can be quickly advanced to a supervised home program consisting of ice or heat application, followed by strengthening and flexibility exercises and aerobic conditioning. In certain patients, manual therapy to restore normal alignment and mobility of the spine at segmental levels may be needed; not all PTs are trained in these techniques.

In patients with chronic pain, the general rules listed above apply. Functional restoration, reduction of fear of reinjury, muscle relaxation techniques, and general conditioning are the pillars of treatment. Manual therapy may be helpful. Return-to-work issues may dominate the picture, and the PT may be helpful in assessing functional capacity, setting functional goals, and advising on the appropriateness of particular jobs. A work conditioning program, designed to recondition the patient in a general way to meet the physical demands of the work environment, or a work hardening program, designed to restore the function needed to perform a specific occupational task, may be required. These programs are usually directed by a PT or physiatrist.

Scar Pain

Pain in the region of a surgical scar is a common chronic pain syndrome, worth recognizing in view of its good response to treatment. A variety of physical therapy techniques are employed; two of the most useful are friction massage and cortisone phonophoresis.

TRANSCUTANEOUS ELECTRICAL NERVE STIMULATION

Ancient Egyptians and Greeks were the first to use electricity to treat painful disorders by applying electric fish to the affected areas of desperate patients. Electrical therapy did not become practical until the nineteenth century, when devices to store and deliver electrical energy became readily available. These devices lost popularity in the early twentieth century, but after publication of the gate control theory of pain in 1965, interest was renewed. The theory implied that stimulation of large myelinated afferent fibers in the peripheral nerve would have an inhibitory effect on pain. Efforts began to implant electrostimulating devices to stimulate the peripheral nerves and spinal cord. TENS was developed as a method to screen patients who might benefit from spinal cord stimulation but became a therapy in its own right as its effectiveness became known.

Technical Considerations

The TENS unit consists of one or more pairs of electrodes attached by cables to a hand-held electrical stimulator. Stimulation is generally delivered in either conventional mode, which elicits paresthesias, or acupuncture-like mode, which produces muscle contractions. The wave form refers to the contour of each electrical pulse and may be monophasic or biphasic. The frequency of stimulation determines whether paresthesias or muscle contractions are felt. Conventional TENS uses 20 to 100 Hz; acupuncture-like TENS uses 1 to 2 Hz. The pulse width and amplitude are adjusted to produce as strong a paresthesia in the painful area as is comfortable to the patient. Although many recommendations specifying the best electrical parameters and electrode placements have been given, there are no adequate scientific studies comparing the different parameters to each other.

Technique

Clinical experience suggests beginning with the conventional mode and placing electrodes to achieve paresthesias in the painful area. Placing electrodes over the area itself or over the nerve innervating the area can be effective. A second pair of electrodes can be placed paraspinally at the level of the pain. If conventional TENS fails, acupuncture-like TENS can be tried.

Indications

TENS has been best studied in the relief of acute postoperative pain. Controlled studies have demonstrated benefit after thoracotomy, upper abdominal surgery, and knee surgery, with improvement in pain and function and decreased opioid requirements. Controlled studies have also demonstrated good results in labor pain with no adverse effects on the fetus.

In chronic pain, well-controlled studies are scant. Evidence does suggest that pain related to peripheral nerve injury responds well. Musculoskeletal pain may respond as well, although one controlled study for patients with chronic low-back pain showed no benefit. Visceral and psychogenic pains do not respond well.

Contraindications

The major adverse effect of TENS is skin irritation from the electrodes or tape. Placing the stimulator on anesthetic areas of skin can result in burns. Patients with demand pacemakers should not use TENS.

Effectiveness

TENS is a useful form of therapy, particularly in certain postoperative pain states, neuropathic pain, and regional musculoskeletal pains. Its lack of serious side effects makes it attractive. Effectiveness requires an experienced provider. The unit should be prescribed for long-term use only after a successful trial.

SUGGESTED READINGS

Birnbaum JS: The Musculoskeletal Manual. 2nd Ed. WB Saunders, Philadelphia, 1986
Cotter DJ: Overview of transcutaneous electrical nerve stimulation for treatment of acute postoperative pain. Med Instrum 17:289, 1983
Kottke FJ, Stillwell GK, Lehmann JF et al: Krusen's Handbook of Physical Medicine and Rehabilitation. 3rd Ed. WB Saunders, Philadelphia, 1982
Lee MHM, Itoh M, Yang GF, Eason A: Physical therapy and rehabilitation medicine. pp. 1769–88. In Bonica JJ (ed): The Management of Pain. 2nd Ed. Lea & Febiger, Philadelphia, 1990
Lehmann JF: Therapeutic Heat and Cold. 3rd Ed. Williams & Wilkins, Baltimore, 1982
Melzack R, Wall P: Pain mechanisms: a new theory. Science, 150:971, 1965

229. PSYCHOLOGICAL AND BEHAVIORAL TREATMENT

ROBERT N. JAMISON

Chronic nonmalignant pain is a costly syndrome that influences every aspect of a person's functioning. Profound changes in quality of life are associated with intractable chronic pain. Significant interference with sleep, employment, social functioning, and daily activities is common. Patients with chronic pain frequently complain of depression, anxiety, irritability, sexual dysfunction, and decreased energy. Family roles are altered, and worries about financial limitations and future consequences of a restricted lifestyle are prevalent. Patients with chronic pain generally present with a history of multiple medical procedures and minimal physical findings. The treatments for acute pain are often insufficient or inappropriate in managing chronic pain.

In this chapter, an overview of psychological and behavioral interventions for chronic nonmalignant pain is presented within the context of a multidisciplinary pain management program. A description of a group-based interdisciplinary pain program is presented, which is similar to one found in many clinics. Included is a rationale for a group-based program along with roles of a team, program goals, patient selection criterion, components of the program, and information on program evaluation.

ISSUES OF CHRONIC PAIN ASSESSMENT

The process of initially assessing the patient with chronic pain is much like piecing together parts of a puzzle and then using the collected information to determine a prognosis and the best course of treatment. Important components that must be evaluated in this process include pain intensity, functional capacity, mood and personality, coping and pain beliefs, and medication usage. In addition, a behavioral analysis should be conducted, and information on psychosocial history, adverse effects of treatment, and health care utilization should be obtained.

Attempts to distinguish reliably between organic and psychogenic pain have been largely unsuccessful. Many practitioners incorrectly believe that chronic pain represents either organic pathology or psychogenic pain. If there are inadequate physical findings to account for a report of chronic pain, then pain is perceived to be a largely psychological phenomenon. Whether an individual presents with organic pathology or not may be independent of whether there is significant psychopathology. An individual may have a major psychiatric illness and clinical migraine or low-back pain. It is generally unwarranted to assume that psychological factors are the cause of pain.

TRADITIONAL TREATMENT APPROACHES

There are many therapeutic modalities for treating chronic pain. Some of these include medications, manipulation, injections, acupuncture, ultrasound treatments, hot packs, transcutaneous electrical nerve stimulation, psychotherapy, and surgery. Traditionally, these modalities would be tried one at a time, in the hope that the pain would eventually subside. Although the majority of patients with acute pain benefit from this regimen, the pain and suffering of many patients with chronic pain continue; in some patients, a pattern of failure and disability develops.

When a unimodal treatment for chronic pain fails to take away the patient's pain, the patient would then be seen by another health care professional who might institute some other therapy. The cycle of being treated by many clinicians with many individual therapies results in multiple evaluations, medications, and often hospitalizations and leads to increased depression, dependence, and deconditioning.

An alternative strategy for those patients with persistent chronic pain would be to offer a structured, goal-oriented program in which persons from different disciplines work together to manage the pain. In addition, emphasis is placed on active participation of the patient in the treatment plan.

BENEFITS OF A PAIN MANAGEMENT PROGRAM

Interdisciplinary pain management programs have been shown to be more effective than unimodal approaches. In a meta-analysis of outcome data from 65 studies, it was found that (1) combined treatments are superior to single treatments or no treatments for chronic nonmalignant pain; (2) participation in an interdisciplinary pain program increases return-to-work percentage (average 43 percent) and decreases health care utilization; (3) the benefits of an interdisciplinary pain program are maintained over time; and (4) there are no differences in age, pain duration, worker's compensation status, or treatment duration between patients who benefit from treatment and those who do not.

Pain programs are cost effective. Patients who complete a multidisciplinary pain program return to work or vocational rehabilitation more often than similar patients who do not enter a pain program. Multidisciplinary pain programs also produce marked subjective and functional improvements in patients with chronic pain, that is, pain ratings decrease from admission to discharge, reliance on medication decreases, and physical functioning increases. These positive treatment outcomes have been shown to be maintained 2 to 3 years after discharge.

Roles of a Multidisciplinary Team

Chronic pain involves a complex interaction of physiologic and psychosocial factors, and successful intervention requires the coordinated effort of a treatment team with expertise in a variety of therapeutic disciplines. Although some pain centers offer a unimodal treatment approach, most programs use a blend of medical, psychological, vocational, and educational techniques. Treatment modalities for chronic pain generally include medical assessment, medication management, pain-reduction treatments, didactic instruction, relaxation training, biofeedback, physical therapy, psychotherapy, and vocational counseling.

Most interdisciplinary pain treatment programs have as their core staff one or more physicians, a clinical psychologist, and a physical therapist. Other health professionals who may play important roles include clinical nurse specialists, occupational therapists, vocational rehabilitation counselors, and exercise physiologists. Physicians from specialty areas (e.g., rheumatology, orthopaedic surgery, physical medicine, and internal medicine) are often available for consultation. The physician's primary responsibility is to oversee the medical aspects of treatment and to offer medication and procedures when needed. The psychologist, psychiatrist, or social worker addresses the mental health and behavioral aspects of the patient's program. This team member facilitates the pain management classes and group therapy sessions and offers biofeedback and instruction in relaxation strategies. The physical therapist and exercise physiologist coordinate daily group exercises and assist the patients in setting up and following individual exercise programs. An interdisciplinary staff coordinates efforts to rehabilitate the patient with pain and provides a comprehensive discharge and follow-up plan designed to meet the patient's short-term and long-term needs. The patient's active participation is strongly encouraged. Among the predictors of success in a multidisciplinary pain program are the patient's motivation to cope with pain and the external support provided.

Program Structure

A multidisciplinary pain program is highly structured, time limited, and organized along a specific treatment schedule. The patient goals include an increase in physical, social, and emotional functioning and a decrease in pain and reliance on health care services. The patient is expected to attend clinic sessions and to participate actively in all aspects of the program. These expectations are made clear. To this end, patients sign a treatment contract that spells out the general program requirements and their individual treatment goals. In addition to helping patients understand exactly what is expected of them, such a contract is a means of identifying those patients who, prior to treatment, lack motivation or may have difficulty conforming to the structure of the program. Patients are asked to keep a daily written record of their pain intensity, medication use, and activity levels. Noncompliance is grounds for discharge from the program.

Goals of the Program

At the start of a program, each patient identifies specific goals, which may include the following:

1. *Reduction of pain intensity.* Although they rarely, if ever, report that pain is eliminated, patients often report a reduction in the amount of pain by the conclusion of the program. A persistent pain problem is the reason most patients enter a pain management program. Patients are taught, however, not to set pain reduction as their primary goal. Instead they are encouraged to focus on other more attainable goals.

2. *Increased physical functioning.* Group-based pain programs support regular exercise, including stretching, cardiovascular reconditioning, and weight training. Patients are encouraged to exercise regularly and to increase their activity at a progressive rate while under supervision. The goal is to increase function gradually without exceeding predetermined limits of pain and discomfort. Patients have been known to increase their physical strength and endurance from 50 to 100 percent over a 3-month period.

3. *Proper use of medication.* Through education and daily monitoring, most patients are able to gain control in using prescription pain medication responsibly. Participants are requested to monitor their medication for 1 week before entering a program and to record their daily medication at the end of a structured program.

4. *Improvement of sleep, mood, and interaction with others.* Most patients admit to being depressed and to having problems relating to others. At the conclusion of a group-based pain program, patients show evidence of decreased emotional distress and increased self-esteem.

5. *Return to work or to normal daily activities.* Patients who set as their goal eventual return to work often are successful. Follow-up helpfulness ratings indicate that patients who have a positive pain program experience tend to return to work and/or maintain an active productive lifestyle.

Patient Screening

Not all patients with chronic pain need a structured pain program. Patients who are in crisis and require ongoing supportive therapy may not benefit from a group experience. Some patients are unwilling to accept a rehabilitation model in managing pain. They may expect that a suitable medical treatment will eventually be offered to resolve the pain. As a result, they may lack the motivation to participate fully in a pain management program.

Patients who demonstrate limited intelligence or who have an inability to grasp basic concepts of rehabilitation are at a distinct disadvantage. Also, patients with a severe physical handicap that makes ambulation and/or sitting for up to 1 hour extremely difficult are not good candidates. Finally, patients with a history of alcohol or medication abuse may be at risk for drop out from a structured pain program. Patients should be carefully screened and may be excluded if they are found to have an ongoing addiction. Patients coerced to attend a pain program rarely succeed. Rather, patients who attend of their own free will are the most successful.

Program Components

Education.   Most people with chronic pain have an inadequate understanding of the nature of their painful condition. It is important for them to be knowledgeable about their pain and the treatments designed for them. Information is given through video presentations, handouts, or individual sessions. An optimal way to educate patients is through didactic groups. Topics for these group sessions include physiology of pain, medication for chronic pain, exercise and pain, stress management, sleep disturbance, assertiveness training, posture and body mechanics, problem solving, weight management and nutrition, vocational rehabilitation, sexual issues, positive thinking, and relapse prevention. In general, patients who understand their condition and who have been exposed to relevant management techniques maintain a perception of control over their pain and show higher rates of success in meeting their goals.

Emphasis is placed on active learning techniques. Active involvement includes periodic completion of surveys, checklists, or questionnaires and solicitation of ideas from group members.

Some recurrent themes are highlighted throughout a structured program as follows: (1) you will most likely not be "cured" (2) you need to expect "ups" and "downs" (3) rarely does pain intensity remain exactly the same over time; (4) you need to have a "fall back" plan for those times when you have a flare up of pain; (5) what you do about your pain may be as beneficial as anything that is done to you; and (6) you need to work toward gaining control over your condition with the help of medical treatments and psychological pain management strategies. Acceptance of these themes is crucial to a pain management approach. These themes are repeated throughout the class sessions to ensure that the patients leave with an understanding of these important principles.

Relaxation Training.   Patients with chronic pain tend to experience substantial residual muscle tension as a function of the bracing, posturing, and emotional arousal often associated with pain. Such responses, maintained over a long period, can exacerbate pain in injured areas of the body and increase muscular discomfort. For example, it is common for patients with low-back pain or limb injuries to develop neck stiffness and tension-type headaches. Relaxation training leads to pain reduction through the relaxation of tense muscle groups, the reduction of symptoms of anxiety, the use of distraction, and the enhancement of self-efficacy. In addition, this training increases the patient's sense of control over physiologic responses. In a pain management program, patients are taught and encouraged to practice a variety of relaxation strategies, including diaphragmatic breathing, progressive muscle relaxation, autogenic relaxation, self-hypnosis, and cue-controlled relaxation techniques. Biofeedback training is also commonly used. All participants are encouraged to practice each of the techniques during the group relaxation sessions and at home. Cassette tapes are made or purchased for practice purposes.

Group Therapy.   Patients with pain frequently show signs of emotional distress, with evidence of depression, anxiety, and irritability. Group therapy with a cognitive/behavioral orientation is designed to help patients gain control of the emotional reactions associated with chronic pain. Specific problem-solving strategies are offered during group therapy sessions, including (1) identifying maladaptive and negative thoughts, (2) disputing "irrational" thinking, (3) constructing and repeating positive self-statements, (4) learning distraction techniques, (5) working to prevent future "catastrophizing," and (6) examining ways to increase social support. In addition, group therapy presents an opportunity to discuss concerns or problems that patients have in common. Unlike psychotherapists in traditional group sessions, group therapists in a pain management program are active facilitators. They redirect the discussion so that every member has an opportunity to speak and no one individual monopolizes the session. Participants are also offered individual therapy sessions in which to deal with personal relationship issues.

Certain group members may initially be reluctant to discuss personal problems related to their pain. The group therapist's role is to prevent other group members from being overly judgmental and negative. Group members are told that they are there to learn from each other and to support each other in gaining control over their condition. Individuals who display overt negative pain behaviors (e.g., resting on a table or floor, grimacing throughout the session, arriving late, or leaving early without explanation) are asked to meet with their case manager to determine whether this behavior can be changed. In order to maintain a positive group atmosphere, certain participants who show excessive negative behavior are asked to leave.

Cognitive/Behavioral Therapy.   There are a number of objectives of cognitive/behavioral therapy. The first is to help patients change their view of their problem from overwhelming to manageable. Patients who are prone to catastrophize benefit from examining the way they view their situation. What could be perceived as a hopeless condition can be reframed as a difficult yet manageable condition over which they can exercise some control.

The second objective of cognitive/behavioral therapy is to help convince patients that the treatment is relevant to their problem and that they need to be actively involved in their treatment and rehabilitation. They need to understand how relaxation training, cognitive restructuring, adaptive coping skills, and pacing behaviors can help decrease their pain. They also need to reorient their view away from that of passive victim to that of proactive, competent problem-solver. When individuals are successful in managing difficult painful episodes, their views change. Patients eventually begin to believe themselves capable of overcoming any acute flare-up of pain.

The third objective is to teach patients to monitor maladaptive thoughts and substitute positive thoughts. Persons with chronic pain are plagued, either consciously or unconsciously, by negative thoughts related to their condition. These negative thoughts have a way of perpetuating pain behaviors and feelings of hopelessness. Demonstrating how and when to attack these negative thoughts and when to substitute positive thoughts and adaptive management techniques for chronic pain is an important component of cognitive restructuring. Patients are encouraged to attribute success to their own efforts; they are taught to feel that they are responsible for the gains they make. Finally, anticipation of problems and lapses are discussed so that the patient will have a "game plan" to manage short-term setbacks.

Family Therapy.   Chronic pain has a significant impact on all members of a family. Family members are educated about the goals of therapy and are given an opportunity to share their concerns. Moreover, active involvement of family members helps ensure the patient's long-term success. Therefore, both patients and members of their families are invited to attend family therapy sessions. At these sessions, the facilitator encourages family members to ask questions about the pain management program, to discuss their concerns and expectations, and to express their feelings. Besides enhanced communication, important outcomes of these sessions are that family members learn how to help the person in pain achieve and maintain goals and that they come to understand that they are not alone in their dealings with the person in pain.

Physical Activity and Exercise.   Most patients are physically deconditioned because of their reluctance to exercise and because of a perceived need to protect themselves. Some patients have been medically advised to restrict activity when pain increases. Patients with chronic pain learn that exercise is important. Some stretching, cardiovascular activity, and weight training is encouraged. Patients are asked to keep track of their activity in an exercise record. An exercise quota is set so that the patient will work to meet a weekly goal. The exercise plan is initially determined by the patient and reviewed and supervised by a physical therapist or exercise physiologist. Offering a time for group members to stretch and exercise together improves compliance and encourages those who are anxious about worsening their condition. Patients are instructed to stretch before and after each exercise session.

The cardiovascular component of the exercise program is designed to increase endurance and self-confidence and is individualized for each patient. Patients are encouraged to begin cautiously by doing only a little during the first week of the program. This may include a 10-minute walk, 5 minutes on a treadmill, or 5 minutes on a stationary bike once or twice a day. Some patients have a tendency to push themselves too far, which may negatively affect their belief that exercise is beneficial. Prevention of overexertion is emphasized. A common scenario is for patients to feel good about their first day of exercise and then report a significant increase in pain and discomfort on the following day. Patients are encouraged to exercise in a creative way in order to find out which exercise is best for them and to minimize any exacerbation of their pain.

Attempts at an exercise program of patients with chronic pain often produce disappointment and perceived failure. Patients often make excellent gains only to experience a flare-up of their condition. These setbacks are anticipated so that the patient does not become excessively disappointed. Behavioral research suggests that compliance with exercise is best achieved in a structured setting where patients are monitored and given encouragement for their accomplishments. Unfortunately, persons with chronic pain tend not to continue with a regular exercise regimen 6 months after a treatment program is concluded. Ways to improve compliance such as organizing an exercise period with others, joining a health club, or combining exercise with another everyday activity are explored.

Vocational Counseling.   The goal of vocational rehabilitation is the return to work of the patient with chronic pain. After an extended period out of work, patients become both physically and psychologically deconditioned to the demands and stresses of the workplace. Together, a vocational rehabilitation counselor and the patient develop a plan that incorporates both long-range employment goals and short-term objectives based on medical, psychological, social, and vocational information. Vocational rehabilitation counselors are specialists in the assessment of aptitudes and interests, transferable skills, physical capacity, modifications in the workplace, skills training, and job readiness.

Many patients with chronic pain receive workers' compensation benefits or social security disability income. Patients frequently fear that their benefits will be jeopardized if they return to work. A vocational rehabilitation counselor helps a patient negotiate with an employer a return-to-work trial that will not

jeopardize the patient's income. Through counseling strategies and assessment tools, a patient's suitability for returning to work or retraining is determined. Patients are exposed to the Americans with Disabilities Act in order to know their rights regarding discrimination owing to a pain-related disability.

Relapse Prevention.   Most patients with chronic pain need support after completing a pain treatment program in order to maintain the gains they have achieved. Patients are encouraged to identify and anticipate situations that place them at risk for returning to previous maladaptive behavior patterns. They are also encouraged to rehearse problem-solving techniques and behavioral responses that will enable them to avoid a relapse. The goals of relapse prevention are to help the patient (1) maintain a steady level of activity, emotional stability, and appropriate medication use; (2) anticipate and deal with situations that cause setbacks; and (3) acquire skills that will decrease reliance on the health care system.

Follow-up has been shown to be vital in helping to prevent relapse. A specific written follow-up plan is made for each patient before the end of a pain program. The participant is offered structured follow-up services such as participation in a monthly support group session. Individual sessions may also be needed. Individuals who are unable to complete a structured program may to invited to repeat the program at another time.

Pain Treatment Program Outcome

An important component of any group-based pain program is its ability to measure its own effectiveness. A number of recommendations for effective program evaluation have been put forward by the Commission on the Accreditation of Rehabilitation Facilities. A system is in place for obtaining follow-up information from patients on the use of medications, use of health care services, return to gainful employment, functional activities, ability to manage pain, and subjective pain intensity. Provisions are made for periodic contact after discharge. A data-based system is developed from which information on patients who have completed a program can be obtained on a regular basis. This type of system not only helps determine how a program meets the needs of individual patients but also offers substantive information on overall efficacy. Program evaluation encompasses goals and objectives that are achievable and end results that are measurable. A program evaluation report includes primary objectives, measures, time of measurement, source of information, expectancies, and outcome. Finally, program evaluation helps identify which types of services are most effective in the treatment of patients with chronic pain.

SUGGESTED READINGS

Caudill M, Schnable R, Zuttermeister P et al: Decreased clinic use by chronic pain patients: response to behavioral medicine intervention. Clin J Pain 7:305–10, 1991

Cinciripini PM, Floreen A: An evaluation of a behavioral program for chronic pain. J Behav Med 5:375, 1982

Commission on the Accreditation of Rehabilitation Facilities: Standards Manual for Organizations Serving People with Disabilities, Commission on the Accreditation of Rehabilitation Facilities, Tucson, 1994

Deardoff WW, Rubin HS, Scott DW: Comprehensive multidisciplinary treatment of chronic pain: a follow-up study of treated and untreated groups. Pain 45:35, 1991

Flor H, Fydrich, Turk DC: Efficacy of multidisciplinary pain treatment centers: a meta-analytic review. Pain 49:221–30, 1992

Jamison RN: Mastering Chronic Pain: A Manual for Persons with Chronic Pain. Professional Resource Press, Sarasota, 1995 (in press)

Rains JC, Penzien DB, Jamison RN: A structured approach to the management of chronic pain. pp. 521–39. In VandeCreek L, Knapp S, Jackson TJ (eds): Innovations In Clinical Practice: A Source Book. Vol 11. Professional Resource Press, Sarasota, 1992

Turk DC, Meichenbaum D, Genest M: Pain and Behavioral Medicine: A Cognitive-Behavioral Perspective. The Guilford Press, New York, 1983

Wilson PH (ed): Principles and Practice of Relapse Prevention. The Guilford Press, New York, 1992

Wright G: Total Rehabilitation. Little, Brown, Boston, 1980

230. NEUROSURGICAL TREATMENT AND IMPLANTABLE DEVICES

THORKILD VAD NORREGAARD

Individuals suffering from chronic pain often seek a surgical solution to their problem. This is indeed a logical approach and significant time is often required explaining physiologic and pharmacologic aspects of pain transmission for the patient to understand why this approach may or may not be a viable solution to their problem. Anatomic and physiologic studies have been very helpful in elucidating pathways transmitting acute pain. The exact mechanisms underlying chronic pain are, however, much less well known. Since appropriate chronic animal pain models are scarce, neurosurgical intervention has often been based on knowledge derived from acute pain.

Neurosurgical interventions in chronic pain management are often, and appropriately, reserved for conditions intractable to other less invasive measures. A chronic pain condition can be either initially largely insensitive to pharmacologic manipulation or can develop a tolerance to the same. Interruption of peripheral and central pain pathways may initially be effective but subsequently lose its effectiveness after the emergence of either a similar or slightly different pain. This might be thought of as a "tolerance" to destructive lesions in the nervous system and serve as an example of pain being a very essential protective mechanism for the individual and evolution having provided strong mechanisms for its upkeep.

Neurosurgical pain management should be seen in a multidisciplinary setting. The overall treatment of an individual in chronic pain should follow an algorithm in which treatment attempts follow a logical ladder from least invasive to more invasive and from few side effects to more potential side effects. The treating team has to be sure that the pain is not amenable to direct attack. The team must generate a background of sympathetic understanding of the patient's personality and general medical problems. Also, they must clearly understand the limitations inherent to the use of drugs, nerve blocks, central administration of drugs into the ventricular system or subarachnoid space, electrical stimulation of the central and peripheral nervous system, and classic ablative neurosurgery.

INTRATHECAL OR EPIDURAL ADMINISTRATION OF PHARMACOLOGIC AGENTS

Discovery of morphine receptors in the spinal cord and subsequent experimental studies showing the analgesic effect of intrathecal administration of opiates prompted extensive use of this modality for the treatment of pain in human beings. Morphine sulfate is by far the most common agent used in this context. Morphine sulfate is highly hydrophilic and diffuses throughout the intrathecal space. The exact position of the catheter tip in the intrathecal space is therefore less important. This is in contrast to lipophilic substances such as fentanyl, which binds rapidly and locally and therefore is dependent on the exact site of administration for its efficacy. When using a mixture of morphine sulfate and, for instance, bupivacaine, one is again faced with the importance of catheter tip location.

Spinal administration of narcotics is extremely potent. Ten and 1 percent of an intravenous dose administered in the epidural space or subarachnoid space, respectively, produce an equianalgesic effect. It should be kept in mind that a patient whose pain is not responding well to narcotics will not have a better response when the drug is given by an intraspinal route. The best candidate for intraspinal administration of narcotics is the individual who has good analgesic effect from systemic narcotics but intolerable side effects such as constipation or sedation. Pain of a nociceptive nature such as from cancer or from certain degenerative conditions is usually a good candidate for this approach. The combination of narcotics and local anesthetics offer certain clear-cut advantages. Local anesthetics such as bupivacaine can be given in a dose up to 20 mg per 24 hours in the subarachnoid space without causing motor disturbances. There can, however, periodically be slight tingling in lower extremities.

Subarachnoid administration is preferable to epidural administration since there is a tendency for scarring around the catheter tip and decreased diffusion, necessitating an increase in doses with systemic side effects as a consequence.

A candidate for spinal narcotics first undergoes a test trial. During the test, a percutaneously inserted catheter is hooked up to a minipump that delivers the drug on a continuous basis. This allows for titration and assessment of the effect. During this phase, the patient is fully ambulatory but initially needs to be observed for respiratory depression, which rarely occurs. If the projected survival time, for example, in a patient with cancer, is 1 or 2 months, one can continue with percutaneous administration using this concept. For patients with longer survival times and certainly for those with benign pain conditions responding to this treatment, a subcutaneous reservoir could be implanted. This reservoir can be filled via a percutaneous needle stick, and the delivery rate can be electronically altered. More complex infusion rates, including automatic bolus, can also be programmed into the pump.

Infection around the implanted system is usually the most serious complication, which would necessitate explantation of the system. In addition to the above-mentioned possibility of respiratory depression, there can be urinary retention; nausea and vomiting, which usually is transient; and tolerance.

For certain pain syndromes related to the face and pain related to cancer of head and neck, intraventricular administration of morphine should be considered.

ELECTRICAL STIMULATION OF PERIPHERAL NERVES AND CENTRAL NERVOUS SYSTEM

Melzack and Wall's gate control theory presented in 1965 predicted a possible effect on pain transmission from stimulation of different parts of the nervous system. This indeed has also turned out to be a powerful tool for the control of pain. The following years have seen a significant development and improvement of implantable stimulating devices. Completely implantable devices, including implantable stimulating units and complex electrode configurations, are now available for implantation.

Patient selection is still difficult, thereby also necessitating a test trial. Pain of a neuropathic nature seems to respond better than pain of a nociceptive nature. Luckily the latter is often more amenable to pharmacologic control than neuropathic pain. It is still not completely understood how electrical stimulation causes pain relief. The gate control theory, implying a modulatory effect from stimulation of large fibers, can explain certain aspects but, for instance, not explain why often, after turning the stimulator off, there is pain relief lasting minutes to hours. Measurement of transmitters in spinal fluid during stimulation has indicated an involvement of certain neurotransmitters such as substance P. From a practical point of view, it is important to notice the need for stimulation-induced paresthesia to cover the geographic area of pain in order to obtain pain relief. When dealing with causalgia or other pain syndromes clearly referable to a single peripheral nerve, it is natural to consider stimulation of the actual nerve in question. This involves the surgical implantation of test electrodes, allowing the patient to stimulate the nerve until a clear-cut answer can be given as to its effect.

Pain covering more than a single peripheral nerve territory is common. Chronic sciatica and failed low-back syndrome, including cases of multiple back surgeries and/or arachnoiditis, typically fall into this category. Phantom pain, postherpetic neuralgia, and sympathetically mediated pain such as reflex sympathetic dystrophy also fall into this category. After careful medical trials and evaluation by a multidisciplinary pain group, including psychological assessment, it may be reasonable to proceed with a trial of spinal cord stimulation.

Most spinal cord stimulators are inserted using a percutaneous technique in which a Tuohy needle is positioned in the epidural space and a spinal cord test stimulator lead is inserted into the epidural space under fluoroscopic guidance. If large areas are to be covered, it is often beneficial to insert more than one electrode with multiple stimulation sites on each electrode. The leads are then exteriorized through a separate stab incision, and the patient is typically discharged wearing an external stimulator unit. The individual will then go through a careful trial period in which pain intensity during stimulation is charted and compared with pain during stimulation-free periods. If the patient experiences at least 50 percent pain relief and considers this a valuable asset, then permanent implantation takes place. Depending on the electrode configuration used, a stimulating unit is either implanted subcutaneously or a subcutaneous receiver is implanted and this receiver is then stimulated using an external stimulator taped to the skin.

When applying strict selection criteria, success rates can be as high as 80 to 85 percent, with the long-term success rate being in the 60 to 65 percent range. Good results usually indicate more than 50 percent pain relief. Some individuals have a spectacular 100 percent pain relief; other individuals fall short of this desirable level of relief.

Deep brain stimulation focuses on two areas. As a rule, somatic nociceptive pain responds better to periventricular gray and periaqueductal gray stimulation; neurogenic pain seems to respond better to stimulation of the ventral posteromedial and ventral posterolateral areas of the thalamus. The technique involves stereotactic implantation of electrodes, and the final electrode site is reached during test stimulation. Deep brain stimulation seems overall to have a 50 to 60 percent or more pain reduction in 50 to 60 percent of implants.

Electrical stimulation on the peripheral and central nervous system is overall a safe modality. Infections can occur, which necessitate explantation of the system. Injury to peripheral nerves or the central nervous system rarely occurs. Why there is an overall reduction in efficacy over time is not entirely known. Local mechanical factors such as electrode migration can obviously play a role, but it seems apparent that neural physiologic aspects also play a role.

Together with intrathecal administration of drugs, the concept of stimulating the peripheral and central nervous system is minimally invasive and testable, and patients do not run the risk of worse outcome from trying these modalities, which otherwise can be the case in, for instance, repeated spinal surgery.

NEUROABLATIVE PROCEDURES

All of the following procedures have in common an irreversible destruction of nociceptive pathways in the peripheral or central nervous system. They are associated with variable degrees of neurologic deficits, which usually are well tolerated. There is a risk from a few percent to 10 to 15 percent of anesthesia or analgesia dolorosa (i.e., a painful or unpleasant sensation in the anesthetic or analgesic area). Excellent pain relief over time can decrease, and the original pain can recur.

Peripheral Neurectomies

Morton's metatarsalgia and trigeminal neuralgia are well known cases in which resection of a peripheral postganglionic nerve branch can result in pain relief. If it is possible clearly to locate the nerve with the tip of a needle, a percutaneous destructive lesion can also be performed, either using a neurolytic agent such as alcohol or phenol or by applying radiofrequency heat. The latter application has been well established for the treatment of trigeminal neuralgia. Through this procedure, a needle with an uninsulated tip is inserted percutaneously, under fluoroscopic guidance, through the oval foramen into the trigeminal ganglion. Gentle stimulation in the awake patient verifies the needle's position with reference to the three different divisions. The advantage of this technique is the possibility of applying gradually increasing heat and at the same time performing a sensory examination. The goal is a moderate hypalgesia with otherwise preserved sensation. This procedure is associated with 95 to 100 percent initial pain relief and a recurrence rate below 25 to 30 percent. The procedure can be repeated with an equally good up-front response. Other invasive procedures for trigeminal neuralgia include glycerol injection into Meckel's cave; percutaneous insertion of inflatable balloons, causing compression of the trigeminal ganglion; and posterior fossa microvascular decompression of the trigeminal root. The latter procedure is based on the remarkable observation that, when explored, up to 80 to 90 percent of patients with trigeminal neuralgia have compression by a vessel loop against the trigeminal root. Pain relief is accomplished when this vessel is dissected and gently repositioned in a noncompressing manner or when a piece of Teflon, for instance, is interpositioned between the nerve root and the vessel loop. A successful microvascular decompression is associated with pain relief and no sensory deficits. In the absence of a major vascular compression, a partial rhizotomy can be performed. A percutaneous radiofrequency lesion of the trigeminal nerve is usually the treatment of choice when medical treatment fails in the elderly individual and is well tolerated by people in their 70s and 80s. Careful blood pressure control during the procedure is necessary since hypertension often occurs during the lesion. Intravenous and intra-arterial access is therefore mandatory.

Cluster headache or its more chronic variant, chronic migrainous neuralgia, when medical treatment fails, can be treated along the guidelines of radiofrequency ablation of the gasserian ganglion. This should, in general, be preceded by a diagnostic lidocaine block of the gasserian ganglion under induced attack. In the absence of effect of a radiofrequency lesion in this condition, lesions at the cervicomedullary junction should be entertained. The cephalic pain pathways loop down into the upper cervical cord with a fairly predictable relationship to surrounding structures before synapsing on second-order neurons in the nucleus caudalis. Fibers from not only cranial nerve V but also VII, IX, and X are associated with this, the so-called descending nociceptive tract. A carefully placed lesion of the tract around the level of the obex can render the entire ipsilateral face, oral cavity, and pharynx analgesic with preserved sensation to touch. This procedure has been utilized in the treatment of chronic migrainous neuralgia with success. In a variant of the same procedure using a radiofrequency technique, the entire nucleus caudalis is destroyed, resulting in successful treatment of the pain of postherpetic neuralgia and anesthesia or analgesia dolorosa of the face.

The much less common vagoglossopharyngeal neuralgia can be treated according to similar guidelines using percutaneous rhizotomy or open exploration with microvascular decompression or rhizotomy of ninth and parts of the tenth cranial nerve.

These procedures are primarily aimed toward benign cephalic pain conditions. When used in a setting of head and neck cancer not responding to narcotics, nucleus caudalis nucleotomy is usually indicated, including dorsal root entry zone lesions of the upper cervical dorsal root zones.

Procedures Directed Toward Dorsal Roots and Dorsal Root Entry Zones

Dorsal rootlets can be sectioned through an open intradural procedure. The dorsal root ganglion can also be resected, and this procedure often has more merit since some sensory fibers travel through the ventral rootlets. Removing the entire ganglion should therefore also result in degeneration of fibers in the ventral root. These procedures have been used in chronic benign pain such as chronic radiculopathies and in cancer pain. Particularly patients with Pancoast tumors have benefited from these procedures. Since these two described procedures result in complete analgesia and anesthesia of the involved areas, other less invasive procedures should be tested first. There is also a not insignificant risk of postlesion dysesthesia and recurrence of pain owing to the plasticity of the central nervous system. These considerations spurred interest in the dorsal root entry zone where open radiofrequency lesions in Rexed's laminae have been proposed and successfully applied, particularly in brachial plexus avulsion injuries. These so-called dorsal root entry zone lesions can again be associated with denervation paresthesias and, not infrequently, transient motor weakness. An open superficial surgical lesion of the dorsolateral aspect of the nerve root entry zone is an anatomically more pleasing

procedure aimed at interrupting the small-diameter pain fibers. Collectively, these procedures should be reserved for otherwise intractable cases in which spinal cord stimulation or intrathecal drug administration has failed.

Lesions in the Spinal Cord

Interruption of the spinothalamic tract in the anterior cord can be an extremely successful procedure for pain in the extremities and trunk when the pain is clearly off the midline. This procedure can be offered in malignant pain conditions and more benign pain conditions, particularly pain in an amputation stump. This so-called anterolateral cordotomy can be performed either through an open procedure or through a percutaneous procedure using a radiofrequency technique. The procedure can be performed either in the high thoracic or high cervical region. When performed bilaterally, there is not infrequently an often transient bladder paralysis. Bilateral high cervical anterolateral cordotomy can be associated with respiratory failure owing to lesion of the descending respiratory pathways controlling involuntary breathing.

Pain located in the midline of the body, such as, for instance, pelvic pain, is more difficult to control surgically. These pain conditions can be associated with pelvic or rectal cancer. A procedure for this often-debilitating pain condition is commissural myelotomy. This procedure takes into account the fact that pain fibers, after ascending one or two cord segments, cross to the contralateral hemicord. Since pain fibers are the only crossing fibers, it is feasible to eliminate pain, for instance, from pelvic structures by dividing the spinal cord over several segments in a vertical anteroposterior plane. A peculiar phenomenon of this procedure is that the resulting sensory deficits can be rather moderate in spite of the successful pain relief.

Cerebral Lesions for Pain Control

Lesions in the diencephalon are thalamotomy and hypothalamotomy. Both of these procedures, and, in particular, the latter, should be reserved for otherwise completely intractable conditions. Thalamotomy, as other procedures, can be associated with dysesthesia and only transient effect. Additional research based on lesion experiments and stimulation of these nuclei may result in a better understanding and possibly better results in the future.

Pituitary ablation can be, for reasons that are not completely known, an effective procedure for the control of severe cancer pain refractory to other therapeutic attempts.

Cingulotomy is a bilateral lesion of the cingulate gyrus. This procedure can be done with remarkable effect, again, in highly selected cases. There is remarkable absence of side effects from this procedure when utilized in pain treatment and for obsessive-compulsive disorders.

Sympathectomy for Pain Control

The sympathetic nervous system clearly plays a role in a number of pain conditions. More modern nomenclature collectively refers to these pain conditions as sympathetically mediated pain. These conditions include causalgia and post-traumatic reflex sympathetic dystrophy. Any pain condition considered to belong to this category should initially be treated with local anesthetic blocks of the relevant portions of the sympathetic nervous system. Since a number of neurolytic drugs are available and stereotactic placement of needles is also available, it is often possible to execute a chemical interruption of the relevant sympathetic pathways. Open surgical sympathetectomy is therefore called on less and less frequently. There is, unfortunately, a tendency to not insignificant recurrence of pain after an initial successful period lasting a few months.

CONCLUSION

Neurosurgical intervention can be extremely helpful and effective in the treatment of chronic pain. This modality should, however, clearly be seen in the context of a multidisciplinary approach in which an appropriate algorithm is supplied, striving for optimal effect utilizing the simplest means possible. This should also take into consideration a conscious effort toward minimizing potential side effects and long-term complications.

SUGGESTED READINGS

Burchiel KJ, Steege TD, Howe JF, Loeser JD: Comparison of a subcutaneous radiofrequency gangliolysis and microvascular decompression for the surgical management of tic douloreux. Neurosurgery 9:111, 1981

De LaPort C, Siegfried J: Lumbosacral fibrosis (spinal arachnoiditis): its diagnosis and treatment by spinal cord stimulation. Spine 8:593, 1983

Gybelis JM, Sweet WH: Neurosurgical Treatment of Persistent Pain. Karger, Basel, 1989

North RB, Ewend MG, Lawton MT et al: Failed back surgery syndrome: 5-year follow-up after spinal cord stimulator implantation. Neurosurgery 28: 692, 1991

Onofrio BM, Yaksh TL: Long term pain relief produced by intrathecal morphine infusion in 53 patients. J Neurosurg 72:200, 1990

Sampson JH, Nashold BS, Jr: Facial pain due to vascular lesions in the brain stem relieved by dorsal root entry zone lesions in the nucleus caudalis. J Neurosurg 77:473, 1992

Tasker RR, DeCarvalho GTC, Dolan EJ: Intractable pain of spinal cord origin: clinical features and implications for surgery. J Neurosurg 77:373, 1992

INDEX

Page numbers followed by f *indicate figures; those followed by* t *indicate tables.*